SECTION NINE
Problems of Ingestion, Digestion, Absorption, and Elimination

SECTION TEN
Problems of Urinary Function

SECTION ELEVEN
Problems Related to Regulatory and Reproductive Mechanisms

SECTION TWELVE
Problems Related to Movement and Coordination

SECTION THIRTEEN
Care in Specialized Settings

APPENDIXES

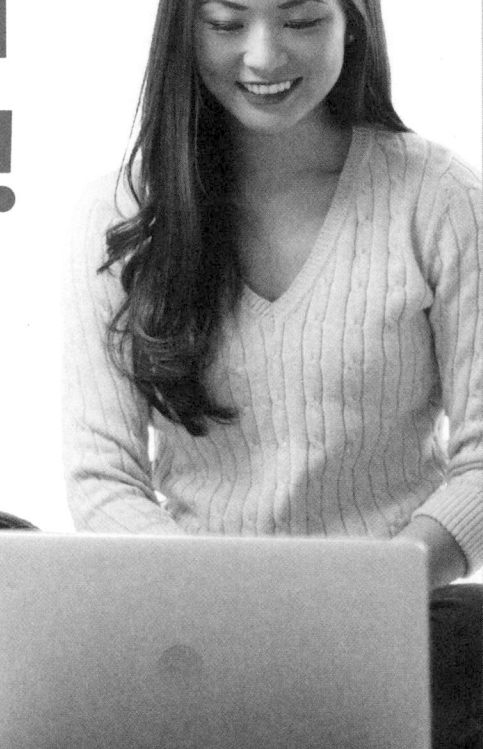
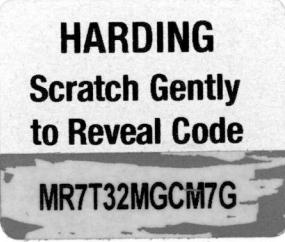
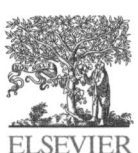

Lewis's
Medical-Surgical Nursing

Assessment and Management of Clinical Problems   Eleventh Edition

Mariann M. Harding, RN, PhD, FAADN, CNE
Professor of Nursing
Kent State University at Tuscarawas
New Philadelphia, Ohio

Section Editors

Jeffrey Kwong, RN, DNP, MPH, ANP-BC, FAAN, FAANP
Professor
Division of Advanced Nursing Practice
School of Nursing
Rutgers University
Newark, New Jersey

Dottie Roberts, RN, EdD, MSN, MACI, OCNS-C, CMSRN, CNE
Executive Director
Orthopaedic Nurses Certification Board
Chicago, Illinois

Debra Hagler, RN, PhD, ACNS-BC, CNE, CHSE, ANEF, FAAN
Clinical Professor
Edson College of Nursing and Health Innovation
Arizona State University
Phoenix, Arizona

Courtney Reinisch, RN, DNP, FNP-BC
Undergraduate Program Director
Associate Professor
School of Nursing
Montclair State University
Montclair, New Jersey

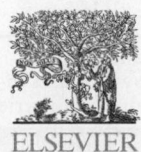

ELSEVIER

Elsevier
3251 Riverport Lane
St. Louis, Missouri 63043

Senior Content Strategist: Jamie Blum
Senior Content Development Specialist: Rebecca Leenhouts
Publishing Services Manager: Julie Eddy
Book Production Specialist: Clay S. Broeker
Design Direction: Amy Buxton

Printed in Canada

Last digit is the print number: 9 8 7 6 5 4 3 2 1

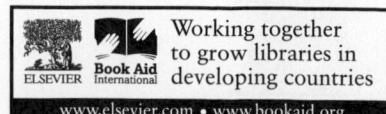

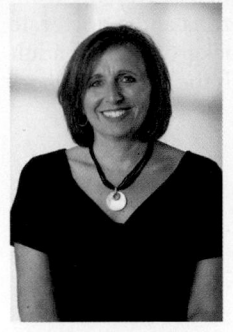

MARIANN M. HARDING, RN, PHD, FAADN, CNE

Mariann Harding is a Professor of Nursing at Kent State University Tuscarawas, New Philadelphia, Ohio, where she has been on the faculty since 2005. She received her diploma in nursing from Mt. Carmel School of Nursing in Columbus, Ohio; her Bachelor of Science in nursing from Ohio University in Athens, Ohio; her Master of Science in Nursing as an adult nurse practitioner from the Catholic University of America in Washington, DC; and her doctorate in nursing from West Virginia University in Morgantown, West Virginia. Her 29 years of nursing experience have primarily been in critical care nursing and teaching in licensed practical, associate, and baccalaureate nursing programs. She currently teaches medical-surgical nursing, health care policy, and evidence-based practice. Her research has focused on promoting student success and health promotion among individuals with gout and facing cancer.

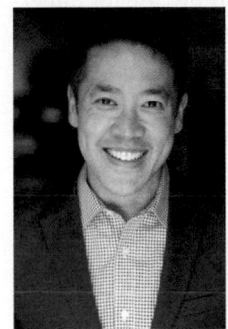

JEFFREY KWONG, RN, DNP, MPH, ANP-BC, FAAN, FAANP

Jeffrey Kwong is a Professor at the School of Nursing at Rutgers, the State University of New Jersey. He has worked for over 20 years in the area of adult primary care with a special focus on HIV. He received his undergraduate degree from the University of California—Berkeley, his nurse practitioner degree from the University of California—San Francisco, and completed his doctoral training at the University of Colorado—Denver. He also has a Master of Science Degree in public health with a focus on health education and behavioral sciences from the University of California—Los Angeles, and he was appointed a Hartford Geriatric Interprofessional Scholar while completing his gerontology education at New York University. In addition to teaching, Dr. Kwong maintains a clinical practice at Gotham Medical Group in New York City. He is a Fellow in the American Association of Nurse Practitioners.

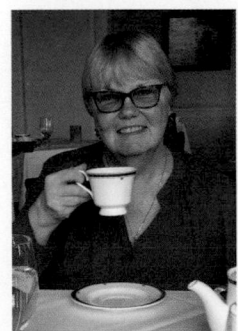

DOTTIE ROBERTS, RN, EdD, MSN, MACI, CMSRN, OCNS-C, CNE

Dottie Roberts received her Bachelor of Science in nursing from Beth-El College of Nursing, Colorado Springs, Colorado; her Master of Science in adult health nursing from Beth-El College of Nursing and Health Sciences; her Master of Arts in curriculum and instruction from Colorado Christian University, Colorado Springs, Colorado; and her EdD in healthcare education from Nova Southeastern University, Ft. Lauderdale, Florida. She has over 25 years of experience in medical-surgical and orthopaedic nursing and holds certifications in both specialties. She has also taught in two baccalaureate programs in the Southeast and is certified as a nurse educator. She currently serves as contributing faculty for the RN-BSN program at Walden University. For her dissertation, Dottie completed a phenomenological study on facilitation of critical-thinking skills by clinical faculty in a baccalaureate nursing program. She has been Executive Director of the Orthopaedic Nurses Certification Board since 2005 and editor of *MEDSURG Nursing,* official journal of the Academy of Medical-Surgical Nurses, since 2003. Her free time is spent traveling, reading, and cross-stitching.

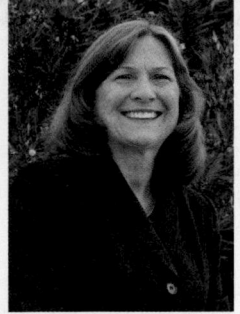

DEBRA HAGLER, RN, PhD, ACNS-BC, CNE, CHSE, ANEF, FAAN

Debbie Hagler is a Clinical Professor in the Edson College of Nursing and Health Innovation at Arizona State University in Phoenix. She is Deputy Editor of *The Journal of Continuing Education in Nursing*. She received her Practical Certificate in Nursing, Associate Degree in Nursing, and Bachelor of Science in Nursing from New Mexico State University. She earned a Master of Science from the University of Arizona and a doctorate in Learning and Instructional Technology from Arizona State University. Her clinical background is in adult health and critical care nursing. Her current role focuses on supporting students through the Barrett Honors program and helping faculty members develop their scholarly writing for publication.

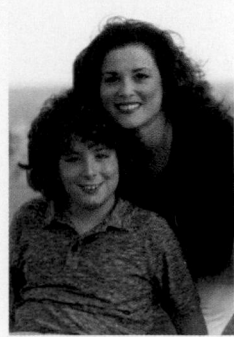

COURTNEY REINISCH, RN, DNP, FNP-BC

Courtney Reinisch is the Undergraduate Program Director and Associate Professor for the School of Nursing at Montclair State University. She earned her Bachelor of Arts in biology and psychology from Immaculata University. She received her Bachelor of Science in nursing and Masters of Science in family practice nurse practitioner degree from the University of Delaware. She completed her Doctor of Nursing Practice degree at Columbia University School of Nursing. Courtney's nursing career has focused on providing care for under-served populations in primary care and emergency settings. She has taught in undergraduate and graduate nursing programs in New York and New Jersey. Courtney enjoys playing tennis, snowboarding, reading, and spending time with her family and dogs. She is the biggest fan for her nieces and nephews at their soccer games, cross-country events, and track meets. She is an active volunteer in the Parents Association of her son's school and advocates for the needs of students with learning differences and the LGBTQ community.

Vera Barton-Maxwell, PhD, APRN, FNP-BC, CHFN
Assistant Professor
Advanced Nursing Practice, Family Nurse
    Practitioner Program
Georgetown University
Washington, District of Columbia
    Nurse Practitioner
Center for Advanced Heart Failure
West Virginia University Heart and Vascular
    Institute
Morgantown, West Virginia

Cecilia Bidigare, MSN, RN
Professor
Nursing Department
Sinclair Community College
Dayton, Ohio

Megan Ann Brissie, DNP, RN, ACNP-BC, CEN
Acute Care Nurse Practitioner
Neurosurgery
Duke Health
Durham, North Carolina
Adjunct Instructor
College of Nursing
University of Cincinnati
Cincinnati, Ohio

Diana Taibi Buchanan, PhD, RN
Associate Professor
Biobehavioral Nursing and Health Systems
University of Washington
Seattle, Washington

Michelle Bussard, PhD, RN
RN to BSN Online eCampus Program Director
College of Health and Human Services
Bowling Green State University
Bowling Green, Ohio

Kim K. Choma, DNP, APRN, WHNP-BC
Women's Health Nurse Practitioner
Independent Consultant and Clinical
    Trainer
Kim Choma, DNP, LLC
Scotch Plains, New Jersey

Marisa Cortese, PhD, RN, FNP-BC
Research Nurse Practitioner
Hematology/Oncology
White Plains Hospital
White Plains, New York

Ann Crawford, RN, PhD, CNS, CEN
Professor
Department of Nursing
University of Mary Hardin-Baylor
Belton, Texas

Kimberly Day, DNP, RN
Clinical Assistant Professor
Edson College of Nursing and Health Innovation
Arizona State University
Phoenix, Arizona

Deena Damsky Dell, MSN, RN, APRN, AOCN(R), LNC
Oncology Advanced Practice Registered
    Nurse
Sarasota Memorial Hospital
Sarasota, Florida

Hazel Dennison, DNP, RN, APNc, CPHQ, CNE
Director of Continuing Nursing Education
College of Health Sciences, School of Nursing
Walden University
Minneapolis, Minnesota
Nurse Practitioner
Urgent Care
Virtua Health System
Medford, New Jersey

Jane K. Dickinson, PhD, RN, CDE
Program Director/Lecturer
Diabetes Education and Management
Teachers College Columbia University
New York, New York

Cathy Edson, MSN, RN
Nurse Practitioner
Emergency Department
Team Health—Virtua Memorial
Mt. Holly, New Jersey

Jonel L. Gomez, DNP, ARNP, CPCO, COE
Nurse Practitioner
Ophthalmic Facial Plastic Surgery
    Specialists
Stephen Laquis, MD
Fort Myers, Florida

Sherry A. Greenberg, PhD, RN, GNP-BC, FGSA
Courtesy-Appointed Associate Professor
Nursing
Rory Meyers College of Nursing
New York University
New York, New York

Diana Rabbani Hagler, MSN-Ed, RN, CCRN
Staff Nurse
Intensive Care Unit
Banner Health
Gilbert, Arizona

Julia A. Hitch, MS, APRN, FNPCDE
Nurse Practitioner
Internal Medicine—Endocrinology
Ohio State University Physicians
Columbus, Ohio

Haley Hoy, PhD, APRN
Associate Professor
College of Nursing
University of Alabama in Huntsville
Huntsville, Alabama
Nurse Practitioner
Vanderbilt Lung Transplantation
Vanderbilt Medical Center
Nashville, Tennessee

Melissa Hutchinson, MN, BA, RN
Clinical Nurse Specialist
MICU/CCU
VA Puget Sound Health Care System
Seattle, Washington

Mark Karasin, DNP, APRN, AGACNP-BC, CNOR
Advanced Practice Nurse
Cardiothoracic Surgery
Robert Wood Johnson University Hospital
New Brunswick, New Jersey
Adjunct Faculty
Center for Professional Development
School of Nursing
Rutgers University
Newark, New Jersey

Patricia Keegan, DNP, NP-C, AACC
Director Strategic and Programmatic
    Initiatives
Heart and Vascular Center
Emory University
Atlanta, Georgia

Kristen Keller, DNP, ACNP-BC, PMHNP-BC
Nurse Practitioner
Trauma and Acute Care Surgery
Banner Thunderbird Medical Center
Glendale, Arizona

Anthony Lutz, MSN, NP-C, CUNP
Nurse Practitioner
Department of Urology
Columbia University Irving Medical Center
New York, New York

Denise M. McEnroe-Petitte, PhD, RN
Associate Professor
Nursing Department
Kent State University Tuscarawas
New Philadelphia, Ohio

**Amy Meredith, MSN, RN, EM Cert/
Residency**
APN-C Lead and APN Emergency
    Department
Emergency Department
Southern Ocean Medical Center
Manahawkin, New Jersey

Helen Miley, RN, PhD, AG-ACNP
Specialty Director of Adult Gerontology
Acute Care Nurse Practitioner Program
School of Nursing
Rutgers University
Newark, New Jersey

Debra Miller-Saultz, DNP, FNP-BC
Assistant Professor of Nursing
School of Nursing
Columbia University
New York, New York

Eugene Mondor, MN, RN, CNCC(C)
Clinical Nurse Educator
Adult Critical Care
Royal Alexandra Hospital
Edmonton, Alberta
Canada

Brenda C. Morris, EdD, RN, CNE
Clinical Professor
Edson College of Nursing and
    Health Innovation
Arizona State University
Phoenix, Arizona

Janice A. Neil, PhD, RN, CNE
Associate Professor
College of Nursing, Department of
    Baccalaureate Education
East Carolina University
Greenville, North Carolina

**Yeow Chye Ng, PhD, CRNP, CPC,
AAHIVE**
Associate Professor
College of Nursing
University of Alabama in Huntsville
Huntsville, Alabama

Mary C. Olson, DNP, APRN
Nurse Practitioner
Medicine, Division of Gastroenterology and
    Hepatology
New York University Langone Health
New York, New York

**Madona D. Plueger, MSN, RN, ACNS-BC
CNRN**
Adult Health Clinical Nurse Specialist
Barrow Neurological Institute
Dignity Health
St. Joseph's Hospital and Medical Center
Phoenix, Arizona

Matthew C. Price, MS, CNP, ONP-C, RNFA
Orthopedic Nurse Practitioner
Orthopedic One
Columbus, Ohio
Director
Orthopedic Nurses Certification Board
Chicago, Illinois

Margaret R. Rateau, PhD, RN, CNE
Assistant Professor
School of Nursing, Education, and Human
    Studies
Robert Morris University
Moon Township, Pennsylvania

Catherine R. Ratliff, RN, PhD
Clinical Associate Professor and Nurse
    Practitioner
School of Nursing/Vascular Surgery
University of Virginia Health System
Charlottesville, Virginia

Sandra Irene Rome, MN, RN, AOCN
Clinical Nurse Specialist
Blood and Marrow Transplant Program
Cedars–Sinai Medical Center
Los Angeles, California
Assistant Clinical Professor
University of California Los Angeles School
    of Nursing
Los Angeles, California

Diane M. Rudolphi, MSN, RN
Senior Instructor of Nursing
College of Health Sciences
University of Delaware, Newark
Newark, Delaware

**Diane Ryzner, MSN, APRN, CNS-BC,
OCNS-C**
Clinical Nursing Transformation Leader
Orthopedics
Northwest Community Healthcare
Arlington Heights, Illinois

Andrew Scanlon, DNP, RN
Associate Professor
School of Nursing
Montclair State University
Montclair, New Jersey

**Rose Shaffer, MSN, RN, ACNP-BC,
CCRN**
Cardiology Nurse Practitioner
Thomas Jefferson University Hospital
Philadelphia, Pennsylvania

Tara Shaw, MSN, RN
Assistant Professor
Goldfarb School of Nursing
Barnes-Jewish College
St. Louis, Missouri

**Cynthia Ann Smith, DNP, APRN,
CNN-NP, FNP-BC**
Nurse Practitioner
Renal Consultants, PLLC
South Charleston, West Virginia

Janice Smolowitz, PhD, DNP, EdD
Dean and Professor
School of Nursing
Montclair State University
Montclair, New Jersey

Cindy Sullivan, MN, ANP-C, CNRN
Nurse Practitioner
Department of Neurosurgery
Barrow Neurological Institute
Phoenix, Arizona

Teresa Turnbull, DNP, RN
Assistant Professor
School of Nursing
Oregon Health and Science University
Portland, Oregon

Kara Ann Ventura, DNP, PNP, FNP
Director
Liver Transplant Program
Yale New Haven
New Haven, Connecticut

**Colleen Walsh, DNP, RN, ONC, ONP-C,
CNS, ACNP-BC**
Contract Assistant Professor of Nursing
College of Nursing and Health Professions
University of Southern Indiana
Evansville, Indiana

Pamela Wilkerson, MN, RN
Nurse Manager
Primary Care and Urgent Care
Department of Veterans Affairs
Veterans Administration, Puget Sound
Tacoma, Washington

Daniel P. Worrall, MSN, ANP-BC
Nurse Practitioner
Sexual Health Clinic
Nurse Practitioner
General and Gastrointestinal Surgery
Massachusetts General Hospital
Boston, Massachusetts
Clinical Operations Manager
The Ragon Institute of MGH, MIT, and
    Harvard
Cambridge, Massachusetts

AUTHORS OF TEACHING AND LEARNING RESOURCES

TEST BANK

Debra Hagler, RN, PhD, ACNS-BC, CNE, CHSE, ANEF, FAAN
Clinical Professor
Edson College of Nursing and Health Innovation
Arizona State University
Phoenix, Arizona

CASE STUDIES
Interactive and Managing Care of Multiple Patients Case Studies

Mariann M. Harding, RN, PhD, FAADN, CNE
Professor of Nursing
Kent State University at Tuscarawas
New Philadelphia, Ohio

Brenda C. Morris, EdD, RN, CNE
Clinical Professor
Edson College of Nursing and Health Innovation
Arizona State University
Phoenix, Arizona

POWERPOINT PRESENTATIONS

Bonnie Heintzelman, RN, MS, CMSRN
Assistant Professor of Nursing
Pennsylvania College of Technology
Williamsport, Pennsylvania

Michelle A. Walczak, RN, MSN
Associate Professor of Nursing
Pennsylvania College of Technology
Williamsport, Pennsylvania

TEACH FOR NURSES

Margaret R. Rateau, RN, PhD, CNE
Assistant Professor
School of Nursing, Education, and Human Studies
Robert Morris University
Moon Township, Pennsylvania

Janice Sarasnick, RN, PhD, CHSE
Associate Professor of Nursing
Robert Morris University
Moon Township, Pennsylvania

NCLEX EXAMINATION REVIEW QUESTIONS

Mistey D. Bailey, RN, MSN
Lecturer, Nursing
Kent State University Tuscarawas
New Philadelphia, Ohio

Shelly Stefka, RN, MSN
Lecturer, Nursing
Kent State University Tuscarawas
New Philadelphia, Ohio

STUDY GUIDE

Collin Bowman-Woodall, RN, MS
Assistant Professor
Samuel Merritt University
San Francisco Peninsula Campus
San Mateo, California

CLINICAL COMPANION

Debra Hagler, RN, PhD, ACNS-BC, CNE, CHSE, ANEF, FAAN
Clinical Professor
Edson College of Nursing and Health Innovation
Arizona State University
Phoenix, Arizona

EVIDENCE-BASED PRACTICE BOXES

Linda Bucher, RN, PhD, CEN, CNE
Emerita Professor
University of Delaware
Newark, Delaware

NURSING CARE PLANS

Collin Bowman-Woodall, RN, MS
Assistant Professor
Samuel Merritt University
San Francisco Peninsula Campus
San Mateo, California

REVIEWERS

Kristen Ryan Barry-Rodgers, RN, BSN, CEN
Emergency Department Charge and Staff Nurse
Virtua Memorial Hospital
Mt. Holly, New Jersey

Michelle Bussard, PhD, RN
RN to BSN Online eCampus
    Program Director
College of Health and Human Services
Bowling Green State University
Bowling Green, Ohio

Margaret A. Chesnutt, MSN, FNP, BC, CORLN
Nurse Practitioner
Primary Care
Veterans Administration Medical Center
Decatur, Georgia

Ann Crawford, RN, PhD, CNS, CEN
Professor
Department of Nursing
University of Mary Hardin-Baylor
Belton, Texas

Jonel L. Gomez, DNP, ARNP, CPCO, COE
Nurse Practitioner
Ophthalmic Facial Plastic Surgery Specialists
Stephen Laquis, MD
Fort Myers, Florida

Jennifer Hebert, MSN, RN-BC, NE-BC
Manager, Patient Care Services
Nursing Administration
Sentara Princess Anne Hospital
Virginia Beach, Virginia

Haley Hoy, PhD, APRN
Associate Professor
College of Nursing
University of Alabama in Huntsville
Huntsville, Alabama
Nurse Practitioner
Vanderbilt Lung Transplantation
Vanderbilt Medical Center
Nashville, Tennessee

**Coretta M. Jenerette, PhD, RN,
CNE, AOCN**
Associate Professor
School of Nursing
University of North Carolina at
    Chapel Hill
Chapel Hill, North Carolina

Beth Karasin, MSN, APN, AGACNP-BC, RNFA, CNOR
Advanced Practice Nurse
Neurosurgery
Atlantic Neurosurgical Specialists
Morristown, New Jersey

Mark Karasin, DNP, APRN, AGACNP-BC, CNOR
Advanced Practice Nurse
Cardiothoracic Surgery
Robert Wood Johnson University Hospital
New Brunswick, New Jersey
Adjunct Faculty
Center for Professional Development
School of Nursing
Rutgers University
Newark, New Jersey

Kristen Keller, DNP, ACNP-BC, PMHNP-BC
Nurse Practitioner
Trauma and Acute Care Surgery
Banner Thunderbird Medical Center
Glendale, Arizona

Suzanne M. Mahon, DNSc, RN, AOCN(R), AGN-BC
Professor
Division of Hematology/Oncology
Department of Internal Medicine
Adult Nursing, School of Nursing
Saint Louis University
St. Louis, Missouri

Helen Miley, RN, PhD, AG-ACNP
Specialty Director of Adult Gerontology
Acute Care Nurse Practitioner Program
School of Nursing
Rutgers University
Newark, New Jersey

Linda L. Morris, PhD, APN, CCNS, FCCM
Clinical Nurse Educator
Associate Professor of Physical Medicine and Rehabilitation
    and Anesthesiology
Academy Department
Shirley Ryan Ability Lab
Northwestern University Feinberg School of Medicine
Chicago, Illinois

Louise O'Keefe, PhD, CRNP
Assistant Professor and Director
Faculty and Staff Clinic
College of Nursing
University of Alabama in Huntsville
Huntsville, Alabama

Catherine R. Ratliff, RN, PhD
Clinical Associate Professor and Nurse Practitioner
School of Nursing/Vascular Surgery
University of Virginia Health System
Charlottesville, Virginia

Lori M. Rhudy, RN, PhD, CNRN, ACNS-BC
Clinical Associate Professor
School of Nursing
University of Minnesota
Minneapolis, Minnesota
Nurse Scientist
Division of Nursing Research
Mayo Clinic
Rochester, Minnesota

Cynthia Ann Smith, DNP, APRN, CNN-NP, FNP-BC
Nurse Practitioner
Renal Consultants, PLLC
South Charleston, West Virginia

Janice Smolowitz, PhD, DNP, EdD
Dean and Professor
School of Nursing
Montclair State University
Montclair, New Jersey

Charity L. Tan, MSN, ACNP-BC
Acute Care Nurse Practitioner
Neurological Surgery
University of California Davis Health
Sacramento, California

Kara Ann Ventura, DNP, PNP, FNP
Director
Liver Transplant Program
Yale New Haven
New Haven, Connecticut

Robert M. Welch, MSN, FNP, CRNO
Nurse Practitioner
Ophthalmology—Retina
Neveda Retina Associates
Reno, Nevada

Mary Zellinger, APRN-CCNS, MN, ANP-BC, CCRN-CSC, FCCM
Clinical Nurse Specialist
Cardiovascular Critical Care
Nursing Department
Emory University Hospital
Atlanta, Georgia

To the Profession of Nursing and to the Important People in Our Lives

Mariann

*My husband Jeff, our daughters
Kate and Sarah,
and my parents, Mick and Mary.*

Jeff

*My parents, Raymond and Virginia,
thank you for believing in me and
providing me the opportunity to become a nurse.*

Dottie

*My husband Steve and my children Megan, E.J., Jessica, and Matthew, who have
supported me through four college degrees and countless writing projects; and to
my son-in-law Al, our grandsons Oscar and Stephen, and my new daughter-in-law
Melissa.*

Debbie

*My husband James, our children Matthew,
Andrew, Amanda, and Diana, and our granddaughter Emma.*

Courtney

To future nurses and the advancement of health care globally.

The eleventh edition of *Lewis's Medical-Surgical Nursing: Assessment and Management of Clinical Problems* incorporates the most current medical-surgical nursing information in an easy-to-use format. This textbook is a comprehensive resource containing the essential information that students need to prepare for class, examinations, clinical assignments, and safe and comprehensive patient care. The text and accompanying resources include many features to help students learn key medical-surgical nursing content, including patient and caregiver teaching, gerontology, interprofessional care, cultural and ethnic considerations, patient safety, genetics, nutrition and drug therapy, evidence-based practice, and much more.

To address the rapidly changing practice environment, all efforts were directed toward building on the strengths of the previous editions while delivering this more effective new edition. To help students and faculty members focus on the most important concepts in patient care, most chapters open with a conceptual focus that introduces students to the common concepts shared by patients experiencing the main exemplars discussed in the chapter. This edition features more body maps and has many new illustrations. Lengthy diagnostic tables in the assessment chapters have been separated into specific categories, including radiologic studies and serology studies. The previously combined visual and auditory content is now in separate chapters focusing on the assessment and management of vision and hearing disorders. New Promoting Population Health boxes address strategies to improve health outcomes.

For a text to be effective, it must be understandable. In this edition, great effort has been put into improving the readability and lowering the reading level. Students will find more clear and easier-to-read language, with an engaging conversational style. The narrative addresses the reader, helping make the text more personal and an active learning tool. The language is more positive. For example, particular side effects and complications are referred to as *common,* as opposed to *not uncommon.*

International Classification for Nursing Practice (ICNP) nursing diagnoses, one of the terminologies recognized by the American Nurses Association, are used throughout the text and ancillary materials. The language is similar to that of NANDA-I. ICNP nursing diagnoses are used in many facilities worldwide to document nursing care in electronic health records. By introducing students to the ICNP nursing diagnoses, students will learn a more shared vocabulary. This should translate into the more accurate use of diagnostic language in clinical practice across healthcare settings.

Contributors were selected for their expertise in specific content areas; one or more specialists in a given subject area have thoroughly reviewed each chapter to increase accuracy. The editors have undertaken final rewriting and editing to achieve internal consistency. The comprehensive and timely content, special features, attractive layout, full-color illustrations, and student-friendly writing style combine to make this the textbook used in more nursing schools than any other medical-surgical nursing textbook.

ORGANIZATION

Content is organized into 2 major divisions. The first division, Sections 1 through 3 (Chapters 1 through 16), discusses general concepts related to the care of adult patients. The second division, Sections 4 through 13 (Chapters 17 through 68), presents nursing assessment and nursing management of medical-surgical problems. At the beginning of each chapter, the Conceptual Focus helps students focus on the key concepts and integrate concepts with exemplars affecting different body systems. Learning Outcomes and Key Terms assist students in identifying the key content for that chapter.

The various body systems are grouped to reflect their interrelated functions. Each section is organized around 2 central themes: assessment and management. Chapters dealing with assessment of a body system include a discussion of the following:

1. A brief review of anatomy and physiology, focusing on information that will promote understanding of nursing care
2. Health history and noninvasive physical assessment skills to expand the knowledge base on which treatment decisions are made
3. Common diagnostic studies, expected results, and related nursing responsibilities to provide easily accessible information

Management chapters focus on the pathophysiology, clinical manifestations, diagnostic studies, interprofessional care, and nursing management of various diseases and disorders. The nursing management sections are presented in a consistent format, organized into assessment, nursing diagnoses, planning, implementation, and evaluation. To emphasize the importance of patient care in and across various clinical settings, nursing implementation of all major health problems is organized by the following levels of care:

1. Health Promotion
2. Acute Care
3. Ambulatory Care

SPECIAL FEATURES

The 6 competencies for registered nursing practice identified by QSEN serve as the foundation of the text and are highlighted in the core content, case studies, and nursing care plans.

- *New!* **Nursing Management** tables and boxes focus on the actions nurses need to take to deliver safe, quality, effective patient care.
- *New!* **Diagnostic Studies** tables focus on the specific type of study, such as interventional, serologic, or radiologic, with more detailed information on interpreting results and associated nursing care.
- **Cultural and ethnic health disparities** content and boxes in the text highlight risk factors and important issues related to the nursing care of various ethnic groups. A special Culturally Competent Care heading denotes cultural and ethnic content related to diseases and disorders. Chapter 2 (Health Equity and Culturally Competent Care) discusses health status differences among groups of people related to access to care, economic aspects of health care, gender and cultural issues, and the nurse's role in promoting health equity.
- **Interprofessional care** is highlighted in special Interprofessional Care sections in all management chapters and Interprofessional Care tables throughout the text.

- **Focused Assessment boxes** in all assessment chapters provide brief checklists that help students do a more practical "assessment on the run" or bedside approach to assessment. They can be used to evaluate the status of previously identified health problems and monitor for signs of new problems.
- **Safety Alert boxes** highlight important patient safety issues and focus on the National Patient Safety Goals.
- **Pathophysiology Maps** outline complex concepts related to diseases in a flowchart format, making them easier to understand.
- **Patient and caregiver teaching** is an ongoing theme throughout the text. Chapter 4 (Patient and Caregiver Teaching) emphasizes the increasing importance and prevalence of patient management of chronic illnesses and conditions and the role of the caregiver in patient care.
- *New!* **Conceptual Focus** at the beginning of each chapter helps students focus on the key concepts and integrate concepts with exemplars affecting different body systems.
- **Gerontology and chronic illness** are discussed in Chapter 5 (Chronic Illness and Older Adults) and included throughout the text under Gerontologic Considerations headings and in Gerontologic Differences in Assessment tables.
- **Nutrition** is highlighted throughout the textbook. Nutritional Therapy tables summarize nutritional interventions and promote healthy lifestyles in patients with various health problems.
- *New!* **Promoting Population Health boxes** present health care goals and interventions as they relate to specific disorders, such as diabetes and cancer, and to health promotion, such as preserving hearing and maintaining a healthy weight.
- **Extensive drug therapy** content includes Drug Therapy tables and concise Drug Alerts highlighting important safety considerations for key drugs.
- **Genetics content** includes:
  - Genetics in Clinical Practice boxes that summarize the genetic basis, genetic testing, and clinical implications for genetic disorders that affect adults
  - A genetics chapter that focuses on practical application of nursing care as it relates to this important topic
  - Genetic Risk Alerts in the assessment chapters, which call attention to important genetic risks
  - Genetic Link headings in the management chapters, which highlight the specific genetic bases of many disorders
- **Gender Differences** boxes discuss how women and men are affected differently by conditions such as pain and hypertension.
- **Check Your Practice boxes** challenge students to think critically, analyze patient assessment data, and implement the appropriate intervention. Scenarios and discussion questions are provided to promote active learning.
- **Complementary & Alternative Therapies boxes** expand on this information and summarize what nurses need to know about therapies such as herbal remedies, acupuncture, and yoga.
- **Ethical/Legal Dilemmas boxes** promote critical thinking for timely and sensitive issues that nursing students may deal with in clinical practice—topics such as informed consent, advance directives, and confidentiality.
- **Emergency Management tables** outline the emergency treatment of health problems most likely to require emergency intervention.

- **Nursing care plans** on the Evolve website focus on common disorders or exemplars. These care plans incorporate ICNP nursing diagnoses, Nursing Interventions Classification (NIC), and Nursing Outcomes Classification (NOC) in a way that clearly shows the linkages among NIC, NOC, and nursing diagnoses and applies them to nursing practice.
- Coverage on delegation and prioritization includes:
  - Specific topics and skills related to delegation and the nurse's role in working with members of the interprofessional team, which are detailed in Nursing Management tables.
  - Delegation and prioritization questions in case studies and Bridge to NCLEX Examination Questions.
  - Nursing interventions throughout the text, listed in order of priority.
  - Nursing diagnoses in the nursing care plans, listed in order of priority.
- **Assessment Abnormalities tables** in assessment chapters alert the nurse to commonly encountered abnormalities and their possible etiologies.
- **Nursing Assessment tables** summarize the key subjective and objective data related to common diseases. Subjective data are organized by functional health patterns.
- **Health History tables** in assessment chapters present key questions to ask patients related to a specific disease or disorder.
- **Evidence-based practice** is covered in Applying the Evidence boxes and evidence-based practice-focused questions in the case studies. Applying the Evidence boxes use a case study approach to help students learn to use evidence in making patient care decisions.
- **Informatics boxes and content** in Chapter 4 (Patient and Caregiver Teaching) reflect the current use and importance of technology as it relates to patient self-management.
- **Bridge to NCLEX® Examination Questions** at the end of each chapter are matched to the Learning Outcomes and help students learn the important points in the chapter. Answers are provided just below the questions for immediate feedback, and rationales are provided on the Evolve website.
- **Case Studies** with photos bring patients to life. Management chapters have case studies at the end of the chapters. These cases help students learn how to prioritize care and manage patients in the clinical setting. Unfolding case studies are included in each assessment chapter, and case studies that focus on managing care of multiple patients are included at the end of each section. Discussion questions with a focus on prioritization, delegation, and evidence-based practice are included in all case studies. Answer guidelines are provided on the Evolve website.

LEARNING SUPPLEMENTS FOR STUDENTS

- The handy **Clinical Companion** presents approximately 200 common medical-surgical conditions and procedures in a concise, alphabetical format for quick clinical reference. Designed for portability, this popular reference includes the essential, need-to-know information for treatments and procedures in which nurses play a major role. An attractive and functional four-color design highlights key information for quick, easy reference.
- An exceptionally thorough **Study Guide** contains over 500 pages of review material that reflect the content found in

the textbook. It features a wide variety of clinically relevant exercises and activities, including NCLEX-format multiple choice and alternate format questions, case studies, anatomy review, critical thinking activities, and much more. It features an attractive four-color design and many alternate-item format questions to better prepare students for the NCLEX examination. An answer key is included to provide students with immediate feedback as they study.

- The **Evolve Student Resources** are available online at *http://evolve.elsevier.com/Lewis/medsurg* and include the following valuable learning aids organized by chapter:
  - Printable **Key Points** summaries for each chapter.
  - 1000 NCLEX examination **Review Questions.**
  - **Answer Guidelines** to the case studies in the textbook.
  - **Rationales for the Bridge to NCLEX® Examination Questions** in the textbook.
  - 55 **Interactive Case Studies** with state-of-the-art animations and a variety of learning activities, which provide students with immediate feedback. Ten of the case studies are enhanced with photos and narration of the clinical scenarios.
  - Customizable **Nursing Care Plans** for over 60 common disorder or exemplars.
  - **Conceptual Care Map Creator.**
  - **Audio glossary** of key terms, available as comprehensive alphabetical glossary and organized by chapter.
  - **Fluids and Electrolytes Tutorial.**
  - **Content Updates.**
- More than just words on a screen, **Elsevier eBooks** come with a wealth of built-in study tools and interactive functionality to help students better connect with the course material and their instructors. In addition, with the ability to fit an entire library on one portable device, students have the ability to study when, where, and how they want.

TEACHING SUPPLEMENTS FOR INSTRUCTORS

- The **Evolve Instructor Resources** (available online at *http://evolve.elsevier.com/Lewis/medsurg*) remain the most comprehensive set of instructor's materials available, containing the following:
  - **TEACH for Nurses Lesson Plans** with electronic resources organized by chapter to help instructors develop and manage the course curriculum. This exciting resource includes:
    - Objectives
    - Pre-class activities
    - Nursing curriculum standards
    - Student and instructor chapter resource listings
    - Teaching strategies, with learning activities and assessment methods tied to learning outcomes
    - **Case studies** with answer guidelines
  - The **Test Bank** features over 2000 NCLEX examination test questions with text page references and answers coded for NCLEX Client Needs category, nursing process, and cognitive level. The test bank includes hundreds

of prioritization, delegation, and multiple patient questions. All alternate-item format questions are included. The ExamView software allows instructors to create new tests; edit, add, and delete test questions; sort questions by NCLEX category, cognitive level, nursing process step, and question type; and administer and grade online tests.
- The **Image Collection** contains more than 800 full-color images from the text for use in lectures.
- An extensive collection of **PowerPoint Presentations** includes over 125 different presentations focused on the most common diseases and disorders. The presentations have been thoroughly revised to include helpful instructor notes/teaching tips, unfolding case studies, illustrations and photos not found in the book, new animations, and updated audience response questions for use with iClicker and other audience response systems.
- Course management system.
- Access to all student resources listed above.
- The **Simulation Learning System (SLS)** is an online toolkit that helps instructors and facilitators effectively incorporate medium- to high-fidelity simulation into their nursing curriculum. Detailed patient scenarios promote and enhance the clinical decision-making skills of students at all levels. The SLS provides detailed instructions for preparation and implementation of the simulation experience, debriefing questions that encourage critical thinking, and learning resources to reinforce student comprehension. Each scenario in the SLS complements the textbook content and helps bridge the gap between lecture and clinical. The SLS provides the perfect environment for students to practice what they are learning in the text for a true-to-life, hands-on learning experience.

ACKNOWLEDGMENTS

The editors are especially grateful to many people at Elsevier who assisted with this revision effort. In particular, we wish to thank the team of Jamie Blum, Rebecca Leenhouts, Denise Roslonski, Clay Broeker, and Julie Eddy. In addition, we want to thank Kristin Oyirifi in marketing. We also wish to thank our contributors and reviewers for their assistance with the revision process.

We are particularly indebted to the faculty, nurses, and student nurses who have put their faith in our textbook to assist them on their path to excellence. The increasing use of this book throughout the United States, Canada, Australia, and other parts of the world has been gratifying. We appreciate the many users who have shared their comments and suggestions on the previous editions.

We sincerely hope that this book will assist both students and clinicians in practicing truly professional nursing.

Mariann M. Harding
Jeffrey Kwong
Dottie Roberts
Debra Hagler
Courtney Reinisch

CONTENTS

CONCEPTS EXEMPLARS

Acid–Base Balance
Chronic Kidney Disease
Diarrhea
Metabolic Acidosis
Metabolic Alkalosis
Respiratory Acidosis
Respiratory Alkalosis

Cellular Regulation
Anemia
Breast Cancer
Cervical Cancer
Colon Cancer
Endometrial Cancer
Head and Neck Cancer
Leukemia
Lung Cancer
Lymphoma
Melanoma
Prostate Cancer

Clotting
Disseminated Intravascular
 Coagulopathy
Pulmonary Embolism
Thrombocytopenia
Venous Thromboembolism

Cognition
Alzheimer's Disease
Delirium

Elimination
Benign Prostatic Hypertrophy
Chronic Kidney Disease
Constipation
Diarrhea
Intestinal Obstruction
Pyelonephritis
Prostatitis
Renal Calculi

Fluids and Electrolytes
Burns
Hyperkalemia
Hypernatremia
Hypokalemia
Hyponatremia

Gas Exchange
Acute Respiratory Failure
Acute Respiratory Distress Syndrome
Asthma

Chronic Obstructive Pulmonary Disease
Cystic Fibrosis
Lung Cancer
Pulmonary Embolism

Glucose Regulation
Cushing's Syndrome
Diabetes Mellitus

Hormonal Regulation
Addison's Disease
Hyperthyroidism
Hypothyroidism

Immunity
Allergic Rhinitis
Anaphylaxis
HIV Infection
Organ Transplantation
Peptic Ulcer Disease

Infection
Antimicrobial Resistant Infections
Health Care–Associated Infections
Hepatitis
Pneumonia
Tuberculosis
Urinary Tract Infection

Inflammation
Appendicitis
Cholecystitis
Glomerulonephritis
Pancreatitis
Pelvic Inflammatory Disease
Peritonitis
Rheumatoid Arthritis

Intracranial Regulation
Brain Tumor
Head Injury
Meningitis
Seizure Disorder
Stroke

Mobility
Fractures
Low Back Pain
Multiple Sclerosis
Osteoarthritis
Parkinson's Disease
Spinal Cord Injury

Nutrition
Gastroesophageal Reflux Disease
Inflammatory Bowel Disease
Metabolic Syndrome
Malnutrition
Obesity

Perfusion
Acute Coronary Syndrome
Atrial Fibrillation
Cardiogenic Shock
Endocarditis
Heart Failure
Hyperlipidemia
Hypertension
Hypovolemic Shock
Mitral Valve Prolapse
Peripheral Artery Disease
Septic Shock
Sickle Cell Disease

Reproduction
Early Pregnancy Loss
Ectopic Pregnancy
Infertility

Sleep
Insomnia
Sleep Apnea

Sensory Perception
Cataracts
Glaucoma
Hearing Loss
Macular Degeneration
Otitis Media

Sexuality
Erectile Dysfunction
Leiomyomas
Menopause
Sexually Transmitted Infection

Thermoregulation
Frostbite
Heat Stroke
Hyperthyroidism

Tissue Integrity
Burns
Pressure Injuries
Wound Healing

DIAGNOSTIC STUDIES TABLES

DRUG THERAPY TABLES

EMERGENCY MANAGEMENT TABLES

ETHICAL/LEGAL DILEMMAS BOXES

EVIDENCE-BASED PRACTICE BOXES

FOCUSED ASSESSMENT BOXES

GENDER DIFFERENCES BOXES

NURSING ASSESSMENT TABLES

NURSING MANAGEMENT BOXES

NUTRITIONAL THERAPY TABLES

PATIENT & CAREGIVER TEACHING TABLES

PROMOTING HEALTH EQUITY

PROMOTING POPULATION HEALTH BOXES

Professional Nursing

Mariann M. Harding

Caring is the essence of nursing.

Jean Watson

ⓔ http://evolve.elsevier.com/Lewis/medsurg/

CONCEPTUAL FOCUS

Care Competencies
Leadership

Professional Identity

LEARNING OUTCOMES

1. Describe professional nursing practice in terms of domain, definitions, and recipients of care.
2. Compare the different scopes of practice available to professional nurses.
3. Describe the role of critical thinking skills and using the nursing process to provide patient-centered care.
4. Apply the SBAR procedure and effective communication techniques in the clinical setting.
5. Explore the role of the professional nurse in delegating care to licensed practical/vocational nurses and unlicensed assistive personnel.
6. Discuss the role of integrating safety and quality improvement processes into nursing practice.
7. Evaluate the role of informatics and technology in nursing practice.
8. Apply concepts of evidence-based practice to nursing practice.

KEY TERMS

advanced practice registered nurse (APRN), p. 2
case management, p. 7
clinical pathways, p. 9
clinical reasoning, p. 8
critical thinking, p. 8

delegation, p. 9
electronic health records (EHRs), p. 13
evidence-based practice (EBP), p. 13
interprofessional team, p. 8
nursing, p. 2

nursing process, p. 4
SBAR (Situation-Background-Assessment-Recommendation), p. 9
serious reportable event (SRE), p. 10
telehealth, p. 8

This chapter presents an overview of professional nursing practice, discussing the wide variety of roles and responsibilities that nurses fulfill to meet society's health care needs. This overview includes several key concepts that are part of competent nursing practice. These include safety, quality, informatics, and collaboration.

PROFESSIONAL NURSING PRACTICE

Domain of Nursing Practice

Nursing practice today consists of a wide variety of roles and responsibilities necessary to meet society's health care needs. As a nurse, you are the frontline professional of health care (Fig. 1.1). You can practice in virtually all health care settings and communities. You have never been more important to health care than you are today. As a nurse, you (1) offer skilled care to those recuperating from illness or injury, (2) advocate for patients' rights, (3) teach patients to manage their health, (4) support patients and their caregivers at critical times, and (5) help them navigate the complex health care system. Although many nurses work in acute care facilities, nurses also practice in long-term care, home care, community health, public health centers, schools, and ambulatory or outpatient clinics. Wherever you practice, recipients of your care include individuals, families, groups, or communities.

The American Nurses Association (ANA) states that the authority for nursing practice is based on a contract with society that acknowledges professional rights and responsibilities, as well as mechanisms for public accountability.[1] The knowledge and skills that make up nursing practice are based on

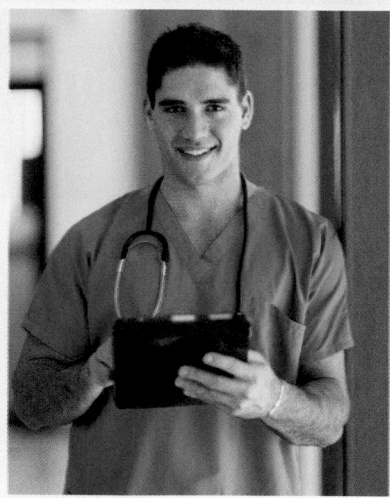

FIG. 1.1 Nurses are frontline professionals of health care. (© Michael Jung/iStock/Thinkstock.)

society's expectations and needs. Nursing practice continues to evolve according to society's health care needs and as knowledge and technology expand. This chapter introduces concepts and factors that affect professional nursing practice.

Definitions of Nursing

Well-known definitions of nursing show that the basic themes of health, illness, and caring have existed since Florence Nightingale described nursing. Following are 2 such examples:

- Nursing is putting the patient in the best condition for nature to act (Nightingale).[2]
- The nurse's unique function is to aid patients, sick or well, in performing those activities contributing to health or its recovery (or to peaceful death) that they would perform unaided if they had the necessary strength, will, or knowledge—and to do this in such a way as to help them gain independence as rapidly as possible (Henderson).[3]

In 1980 the ANA defined **nursing** as "the diagnosis and treatment of human responses to actual and potential health problems."[1] In this context, your care of a person with a fractured hip would focus on the patient's response to impaired mobility, pain, and loss of independence. The 2010 edition of the ANA's *Nursing: A Social Policy Statement* provided a new definition of nursing that reflects the continuing evolution of nursing practice:

> ***Nursing*** *is the protection, promotion, and optimization of health and abilities, prevention of illness and injury, alleviation of suffering through the diagnosis and treatment of human response, and advocacy in the care of individuals, families, communities, and populations.[1]*

Nursing's View of Humanity

A person has physiologic (or biophysical), psychologic (or emotional), sociocultural (or interpersonal), spiritual, and environmental components or dimensions. In this book, we consider a person to be in constant interaction with a changing environment. A person is composed of interrelated dimensions and not separate entities. Thus a problem in 1 dimension may affect 1 or more of the other dimensions. A person's behavior is meaningful and oriented toward fulfilling needs, coping with stress, and developing one's self. However, at times a person needs help to meet these needs, cope successfully, or develop his or her unique potential.

Scope of Nursing Practice

The essential core of nursing practice is to deliver holistic, patient-centered care. It includes assessment and evaluation, giving a variety of interventions, patient and family teaching, and being a member of the interprofessional health care team.

The extent that nurses engage in their scope of practice depends on their educational preparation, experience, role, and state law. To enter practice, a nurse must complete an accredited program and pass an examination verifying that the nurse has the knowledge necessary to provide safe care. Entry-level nurses with associate or baccalaureate degrees are prepared to function as generalists. At this level, nurses provide direct health care and focus on ensuring coordinated and comprehensive care to patients in a variety of settings. Nurses work collaboratively with other health care providers to manage the needs of persons and groups.

With experience and continued study, nurses may specialize in a specific practice area. Certification is a formal way for nurses to obtain professional recognition for having expertise in a specialty area. A variety of nursing organizations offer certification in nursing specialties.[4] Certification usually requires a certain amount of clinical experience and successful completion of an examination. Recertification usually requires ongoing clinical experience and continuing education. Common nursing specialties include critical care, women's health, geriatric, medical-surgical, perinatal, emergency, psychiatric/mental health, and community health nursing.

Additional formal education and experience can prepare nurses for advanced practice. An **advanced practice registered nurse (APRN)** is a nurse educated at the master's or doctoral level, with advanced education in pathophysiology, pharmacology, and health assessment and expertise in a specialized area of practice. APRNs include clinical nurse specialists, nurse practitioners, nurse midwives, and nurse anesthetists. APRNs play a vital role in the health care delivery system. In addition to managing and delivering direct patient care, APRNs have roles in leadership, quality improvement, evidence-based practice, and informatics.

The doctor of nursing practice (DNP) degree is a practice-focused terminal nursing degree. With raising the educational preparation for APRNs to the doctoral level, nursing is at the same level as other health professions that offer practice doctorates (e.g., pharmacy [PharmD], physical therapy [DPT]). Nurses with a research-focused doctorate (PhD) typically are used in health care settings as nurse faculty, clinical experts, researchers, and health care system executives.

Standards of Professional Nursing Practice

To guide nurses in how to perform professionally, the ANA defined Standards of Professional Nursing Practice. There are 2 parts, Standards of Practice and Standards of Professional Performance.[5] The Standards of Practice describe a competent level of nursing care, based on the nursing process. The Standards of Professional Performance describe behavioral competencies expected of a nurse. You are following the performance standards when you practice ethically and use evidence-based practice. Communicating effectively and staying competent in practice are important. You must be able to work in collaboration with other interprofessional team members, patients, and caregivers.

INFLUENCES ON PROFESSIONAL NURSING PRACTICE

Expanding Knowledge and Technology

Ever-changing technology and rapidly expanding clinical knowledge add to the complexity of health care. The increased treatment, diagnostic, and care options available are changing care delivery and extending patients' lives. Discoveries in genetics are changing the way we think about diseases such as cancer and heart disease. For example, genetic information guides breast cancer screening. If a woman has cancer, this information allows for treatment and drug therapy based on her genetic makeup. Ethical dilemmas and controversies arise about the use of new scientific knowledge and the disparities that exist in patients' access to technologically advanced health care. Throughout this book, genetics, informatics, and ethical/legal boxes highlight expanding knowledge and technology's impact on nursing practice.

Diverse Populations

Patient populations are more diverse than ever. Americans are living longer, with the number of people with chronic illnesses and multiple co-morbidities increasing. Unlike those who receive acute, episodic care, patients with chronic illnesses have complex needs. They see different health care providers in various settings over an extended period. With care shifting from hospitals and nursing homes to managed care in the community, you need to be able to manage and coordinate care when patients are transitioning among different settings.

At the same time, you will be caring for a more culturally and ethnically diverse population. When delivering care, you must consider the patient's and caregiver's cultural beliefs and values. Immigrants, particularly undocumented immigrants, often lack the resources necessary to access health care. Inability to pay for health care is related to a tendency to delay seeking care, resulting in illnesses that are more serious at the time of diagnosis. Boxes throughout this book emphasize the influence of such factors as gender, culture, and ethnicity on nursing practice.

Consumerism

Health care is a consumer-focused business, and patients today are more involved in their health care. They want more control over their health care and expect high-quality, coordinated, and financially reasonable care. Health information is readily available. Many patients are very knowledgeable about their health and seek information about health problems and health care from media and Internet sources. They gather information so that they can have a voice in making decisions about their health care. As a nurse, you must be able to help patients access, interpret, and use safe health care information (Fig. 1.2).

Health Care Financing

High health care costs are a growing problem. There are many reasons for the continued increase in costs. These include the rising use of prescription medications, administrative costs, and new medical innovations and treatments.[6] Many changes in health care systems that influence nursing care delivery are

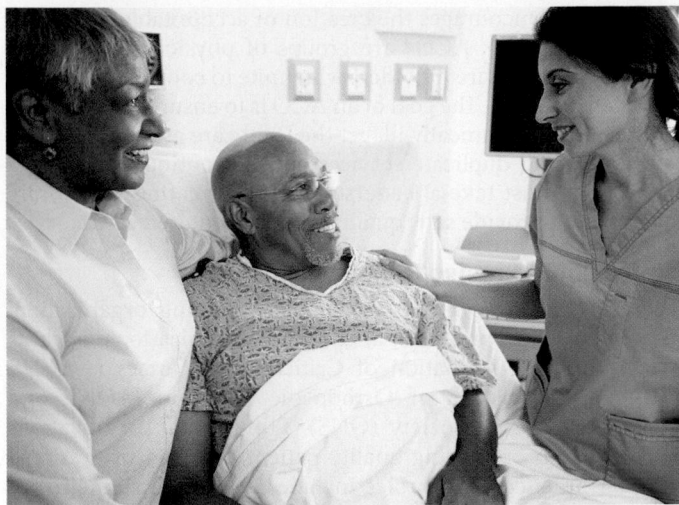

FIG. 1.2 The patient, family, and nurse collaborate as part of coordinating high-quality care. (© monkeybusinessimages/iStock/Thinkstock.)

started by the government, employers, insurance companies, and regulating agencies. They are usually in effort to contain spending and provide more cost-effective health care. Historically, the most notable event related to reimbursement was the establishment of prospective payment systems in the Medicare program. With this system, payment for hospital services for Medicare patients are based on flat fees determined by the diseases and problems treated during the admission. For example, if a patient had a total knee replacement, the hospital receives a set sum of money, such as $45,000, for the patient's care.

Other health care systems followed by introducing managed care systems that use prospective payment as a means of offering cost-effective health care delivery. In health maintenance organizations (HMOs) and preferred provider organizations (PPOs), charges are negotiated before the delivery of care using fixed reimbursement rates or capitation fees for medical care, hospitalization, and other health care services.

Now, quality and performance initiatives are driving further changes in health care financing. Value-based purchasing programs base reimbursement to health care providers on their performance on certain quality measures. These quality measures include clinical outcomes, patient safety, patient satisfaction, and the provider's adherence to evidence-based practice. Those who provide quality care at a lower cost may receive more payment.

As part of value-based purchasing, payment for care can be withheld if a patient experiences events such as developing a pressure injury during a hospital stay or having something happen that is considered preventable (e.g., a fall-related injury, having wrong-site surgery).[7] This type of event is considered a *serious reportable event (SRE)*. SREs are discussed later in this chapter on p. 10.

Health Policy

Legislation has serious implications for health care delivery and nursing practice. The 2010 Patient Protection and Affordable Care Act (ACA) was the most important health care legislation since the creation of Medicare in 1965. The ACA triggered changes throughout the health care system. The ACA's main goal was to increase access to health care. The ACA created new health care delivery and payment models that emphasized teamwork, care coordination, and quality care.

The ACA encourages the creation of accountable care organizations (ACOs). ACOs are groups of physicians, hospitals, and other health care providers who unite to coordinate care for Medicare patients. The goal of an ACO is to ensure that patients, especially the chronically ill, get the right care at the right time, while avoiding duplicate services and preventing errors. As a nurse, you must take a leadership role in creating health care systems that provide safe, quality, patient-centered care.

Professional Nursing Organizations

The ANA is the primary professional nursing organization. There are many professional specialty organizations, such as the American Association of Critical-Care Nurses (AACN), National Association of Orthopedic Nurses (NAON), and Oncology Nursing Society (ONS). Professional organizations play a role in promoting quality patient care and professional nursing practice. These roles include developing standards of practice and codes of ethics, supporting research, and lobbying for legislation and regulations. Major nursing organizations promote research into the causes of errors, develop strategies to prevent future errors, and address nursing issues that affect the nurse's ability to deliver patient care safely. Nurses join a professional organization to keep current in their practice and network with others who are interested in a specific practice area.

A program that supports nurses is the American Nurses Credentialing Center's Magnet Recognition Program. The Magnet program "recognizes health care organizations for quality patient care, nursing excellence and innovations in professional nursing practice."[8] Magnet designation shows a high quality of nursing care and achievement of a positive practice environment for nurses. Nurses who work in Magnet facilities have low turnover and burnout rates and more opportunities for professional and personal growth. This leads to better patient outcomes and greater career satisfaction.

Nursing Core Competencies

Several high-profile reports over the past 20 years have highlighted problems with the quality of health care. One of these reports, *The Future of Nursing: Leading Change, Advancing Health,* acknowledged the link between professional nursing practice and health care delivery. The report discussed how health care providers, including nurses, were not being adequately prepared to provide the highest quality care possible. It recommended making changes so that nurses will have the skills to advance health care and play leadership roles in the health care system[9] (Table 1.1).

To address nursing's role in solving these problems, the Robert Wood Johnson Foundation funded the *Quality and Safety Education*

TABLE 1.1 Key Messages for the Future of Nursing

- Nurses should practice to the full extent of their education and training.
- Nurses should achieve high education and training through an improved education system that promotes seamless academic progression.
- Nurses should be full partners with physicians and other health professionals in redesigning health care.
- Effective workforce planning and policy making require better data collection and information infrastructure.

Source: IOM (now HMD) recommendations. Retrieved from *www.thefutureofnursing.org/recommendations.*

---

for Nurses (QSEN) Institute. QSEN has made a major contribution to nursing by defining specific competencies that nurses need to have to practice safely and effectively in today's complex health care system. The rest of this chapter describes each of the 6 QSEN nursing core competencies and the knowledge, skills, and attitudes (KSAs) necessary in each area: (1) patient-centered care, (2) teamwork and collaboration, (3) safety, (4) quality improvement, (5) informatics, and (6) evidence-based practice[10] (Table 1.2). When you are licensed as a registered nurse, you accept responsibility to base your practice on these core competencies.

PATIENT-CENTERED CARE

Nurses have long shown that they deliver patient-centered care based on each patient's unique needs and understanding of the patient's preferences, values, and beliefs. Patient-centered care is interrelated with quality and safety. In a patient-centered care model, patients and caregivers seek and receive care from competent and knowledgeable health care professionals. In addition, patients and caregivers are involved in making decisions and coordinating care.

Nursing Process

Nurses provide patient-centered care using an organizing framework called the *nursing process.* The nursing process is a problem-solving approach to the identification and treatment of patient problems that is the foundation of nursing practice. The nursing process framework provides a structure for delivering nursing care and the knowledge, judgments, and actions that nurses use to achieve best patient outcomes. Once started, the nursing process is continuous and cyclic.

The nursing process consists of 5 phases: assessment, diagnosis, planning, implementation, and evaluation (Fig. 1.3). There is a basic order to the nursing process, beginning with assessment. *Assessment* is the collection of subjective and objective patient information on which you will base your plan of care. *Diagnosing* is the act of analyzing the assessment data and making a judgment about the nature of the data. It includes your identifying nursing diagnoses or problems and collaborative problems. During *planning,* you use nursing diagnoses and problems to develop patient outcomes or goals and identify nursing interventions to accomplish the outcomes. *Implementation* is the activation of the plan with the use of nursing interventions. *Evaluation* is a continual activity. During evaluation you decide whether the patient outcomes have been met because of the nursing interventions. If the outcomes were not met, a review of the steps of the process is necessary to figure out why not. You may need to revise the assessment (data collection), nursing diagnoses, planning (determining patient outcomes), or implementation (nursing interventions).

Standard Nursing Terminologies

The demands of the health care system challenge nursing to define its contribution to health care. The nursing profession can describe its unique role by answering questions such as: What do nurses do? How do they do it? How does it make a measurable difference in the health of those for whom they care? How are nursing's contributions different from those of medicine?

In response to these questions, nursing uses standard terminologies (also called *classification systems* or *taxonomies*) to define and evaluate nursing care. This promotes continuity of patient care and gives data showing nursing's impact on patient outcomes. Instead of using a variety of words to describe the

TABLE 1.2 QSEN Competencies

Competency	Knowledge, Skills, and Attitudes
Patient-Centered Care Recognize the patient and caregiver as full partners in providing compassionate and coordinated care based on respect for patient's preferences, values, and needs	• Provide care with sensitivity and respect, taking into consideration the patient's perspectives, beliefs, and cultural background • Assess level of comfort and treat appropriately • Engage the patient in an active partnership that promotes health, well-being, and self-care management • Facilitate patient's informed consent for care
Teamwork and Collaboration Function effectively within nursing and interprofessional teams	• Value the expertise of each interprofessional member • Initiate appropriate referrals • Follow communication practices that minimize risks associated with hand-offs and transitions in care • Take part in interprofessional rounds
Safety Minimize risk of harm to patients and providers	• Follow recommendations from national safety campaigns • Appropriately communicate concerns related to hazards and errors • Contribute to designing systems to improve safety
Quality Improvement Use data to monitor the outcomes of care and to improve the quality and safety of health care systems	• Use quality measures to understand performance • Identify gaps between local and best practices • Take part in investigating the circumstances surrounding a sentinel event (never event) or serious reportable event (SRE)
Informatics Use information and technology to communicate, manage knowledge, reduce errors, and support decision making	• Protect confidentiality of patient's protected health information • Document appropriately in electronic health records • Use communication technologies to coordinate patient care • Respond correctly to clinical decision-making alerts
Evidence-Based Practice Integrate best current evidence with clinical expertise and the patient/family preferences and values for delivery of optimal health care	• Read research, clinical practice guidelines, and evidence reports related to area of practice • Base patient care plan on patient's values, clinical expertise, and evidence • Continuously improve clinical practice based on new knowledge

Source: QSEN competencies. Retrieved from *www.qsen.org/competencies*.

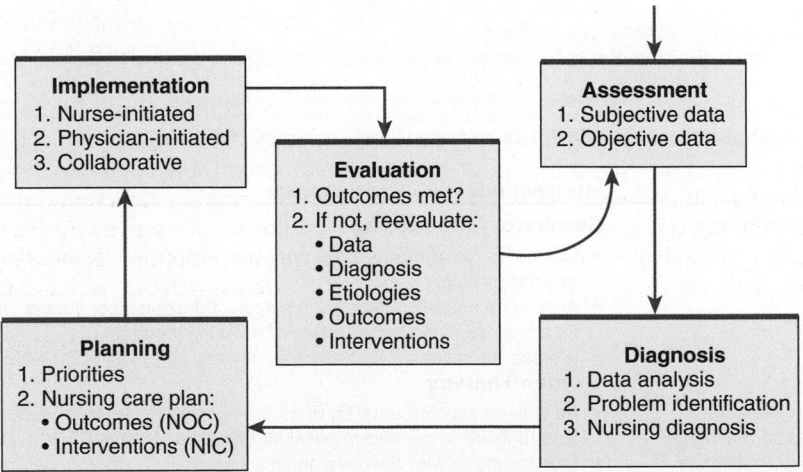

FIG. 1.3 *Nursing process.*

same patient problems and nursing interventions, nurses use a common language to improve communication.

Standard languages are essential in exchanging information between different electronic records systems. The need for quality care makes it necessary to be able to share information in a meaningful way across care settings. Using the same language reduces ambiguity and confusion. For example, do the patient problems of pressure injury and skin breakdown mean the same thing? Does turning the patient every 2 hours mean the same

thing as repositioning the patient every 2 hours? If you turn or reposition the patient every 2 hours, what is the result? Does placing the patient on a pressure-relieving mattress or a standard mattress change the results? When you use a standard language, each nurse reading and documenting in the electronic record understands the diagnosis, can provide the interventions, and can measure the outcome.

The ANA recognizes several nursing and multidisciplinary languages. Three nursing languages focus on specific phases of the nursing process: (1) NANDA International (NANDA-I): Nursing Diagnoses, Definitions, and Classification; (2) the Nursing Outcomes Classification (NOC); and (3) the Nursing Interventions Classification (NIC). Two other nursing languages, each with their own nursing diagnoses, outcomes, and interventions, include the International Classification of Nursing Practice (ICNP) and the Clinical Care Classification (CCC).

Nursing Diagnoses. The ANA defines a nursing diagnosis as the nurse's clinical judgment about the patient's response to actual or potential health conditions or needs.[11] You determine nursing diagnoses based on your analysis of the assessment data. Delivering care based on accurately identified nursing diagnoses results in more effective and safer patient care. They are the basis for selecting nursing interventions to achieve patient outcomes for which nursing is accountable. This book uses the ICNP nursing diagnosis terminology (see Appendix B).

Outcome Identification. The next step is to create the framework for delivering care by identifying outcomes and goal indicators. After choosing an outcome, you need to identify short- and/or long-term measurable goals and then list the behaviors or observations you will use to determine if the goal was attained. By identifying the right outcomes and goals, you can measure and evaluate the impact of the interventions you provide as part of your nursing practice. They also guide the interprofessional team so that we are all working to achieve the same outcomes. The outcomes achieved by patients are the most important indicator of quality in health care.[12]

Nursing Interventions. An intervention is "a single nursing action, treatment, procedure, activity, or service designed to achieve an outcome of a nursing or medical diagnosis for which the nurse is accountable."[13] This includes treatments that you perform in all settings and includes direct and indirect care. The ICNP includes more than 1100 interventions. That many interventions may seem overwhelming. You will discover the interventions you will use most often with your patient population. When planning care for a patient, choose specific interventions for the patient based on the nursing diagnosis and desired patient outcomes. You make the crucial decision of when and which interventions to use for a specific patient and situation based on your knowledge of the patient and the patient's condition.

Nursing Care Plans

In any clinical setting, you are responsible for providing a custom plan of care that includes nursing diagnoses, outcomes, and interventions. In clinical practice, electronic care plans often follow a standard format that has been adapted for that specific setting. These plans are guides for routine nursing care. You customize each to your patient's unique needs and problems.

In nursing education, the nursing process is often documented differently from clinical practice. The nursing process is often recorded in nursing care plans similar to those found on the website for this book (http://evolve.elsevier.com/Lewis/medsurg). These nursing care plans are teaching and learning tools. You practice and learn the nursing process by collecting assessment data, identifying nursing diagnoses, and selecting patient outcomes and nursing interventions. You usually should give rationales for the selected interventions.

◉ NURSING CARE PLAN 1.1

*Patient With Heart Failure**

Nursing Diagnosis†*

Impaired Gas Exchange

Etiology: Increased preload, alveolar-capillary membrane changes
Supporting data: Abnormal O_2 saturation, hypoxemia, dyspnea, tachypnea, tachycardia, restlessness, patient's statement, "I am so short of breath"

Patient Goal

Maintains adequate O_2/CO_2 exchange at the alveolar-capillary membrane to meet O_2 needs of the body

Outcomes (NOC)	Interventions (NIC) and Rationales
Respiratory Status: Gas Exchange	**Respiratory Monitoring**
• O_2 saturation ___	• Monitor pulse oximetry, respiratory rate, rhythm, depth, and effort of respirations *to detect changes in respiratory status.*
• Arterial pH ___	• Auscultate breath sounds, noting areas of decreased or absent ventilation and presence of adventitious sounds *to detect presence of pulmonary edema.*
• PaO_2 ___	• Monitor for increased restlessness, anxiety, and work of breathing *to detect increasing hypoxemia.*
• $PaCO_2$ ___	**Oxygen Therapy**
• Chest x-ray findings ___	• Administer supplemental O_2 or other noninvasive ventilator support (e.g., bilevel positive airway pressure [BiPAP]) as needed *to maintain adequate O_2 levels.*
Measurement Scale	• Monitor the O_2 liter flow rate and placement of O_2 delivery device *to ensure O_2 is adequately delivered.*
1 = Severe deviation from normal range	• Change O_2 delivery device from mask to nasal prongs during meals as tolerated *to sustain O_2 levels while eating.*
2 = Substantial deviation from normal range	• Monitor the effectiveness of O_2 therapy *to identify hypoxemia and establish range of O_2 saturation.*
3 = Moderate deviation from normal range	**Positioning**
4 = Mild deviation from normal range	• Position patient to alleviate dyspnea (e.g., semi-Fowler's position), as appropriate, to improve ventilation by decreasing venous return to the heart and increasing thoracic capacity.
5 = No deviation from normal range	
• Dyspnea with exertion ___	
• Dyspnea at rest ___	
• Restlessness ___	
• Impaired cognition ___	
Measurement Scale	
1 = Severe	
2 = Substantial	
3 = Moderate	
4 = Mild	
5 = None	

*This example presents 1 nursing diagnosis for heart failure. The complete nursing care plan for heart failure is available on *http://evolve.elsevier.com/Lewis/medsurg*.
†Nursing diagnoses are listed in order of priority.

The nursing care plans associated with this book list nursing diagnoses, in order of priority, based on the ICNP, along with outcomes and interventions (NCP 1.1). When you use these care plans, you will need to customize the plan for your specific patient. You must use critical thinking to continually evaluate the situation and revise the nursing diagnoses, outcomes, and interventions to fit each patient's unique care needs.

Collaborative problems are certain physiologic complications that nurses must monitor to detect the onset of or changes in patient status.[14] Nurses manage collaborative problems using physician and nurse prescribed interventions to prevent morbidity and mortality. You identify these risks during the diagnosis phase of the nursing process. Identifying collaborative problems requires knowledge of pathophysiology and possible complications of medical treatment. Collaborative problem statements are usually written as "potential complication: _____" or "PC: _____" without a *related to* statement. An example is "PC: pulmonary embolism."

A *concept map* is another method of recording a nursing care plan. A concept map records the nursing process in a visual diagram. The map displays patient problems and interventions and shows relationships among clinical data. Nurse educators use concept mapping to teach nursing process and care planning. There are various formats for concept maps.

Conceptual care maps blend a concept map and a nursing care plan. On a conceptual care map, assessment data used to identify the patient's primary health concern are centrally positioned. Diagnostic test data, treatments, and medications surround the assessment data. Positioned below are nursing diagnoses or problems that represent the patient's responses to the health state. Listed with those are the supporting assessment data, outcomes, nursing interventions with rationales, and evaluation. After completing the map, you draw connections between identified relationships and concepts. A conceptual care map creator is available online on the website for this book. Concept maps for select case studies at the end of management chapters are available on the website at *http://evolve.elsevier.com/Lewis/medsurg.*

Continuum of Patient Care

Nursing is part of health care at all points along the patient care continuum. Depending on their health status, patients often move among a multitude of different health care settings. For example, a young man is in a trauma unit of an acute care hospital following a motor vehicle crash. After he is stable, he is transferred to a general medical-surgical unit and then to an acute rehabilitation facility. After rehabilitation is complete, he is discharged home to continue with outpatient rehabilitation, with follow-up by home health care nurses and care in an ambulatory clinic.

Decisions about the best setting for obtaining health care often depend on the cost of care and the patient's health care insurance plan and personal finances. Although the hospital is the mainstay for acute care interventions, community-based settings offer patients the opportunity to live or recover in settings that maximize their independence and preserve human dignity.

Community-based health care settings include ambulatory care, transitional care, and long-term care. *Transitional care* settings provide care in between the acute care and the home or long-term care setting. Patients may receive transitional care at an acute rehabilitation facility after head trauma or a spinal cord injury.

Long-term care refers to the care of patients for a period longer than 30 days. It may be needed for those who are severely developmentally disabled, who are mentally impaired, or who have physical deficits requiring continuous medical and nursing care (e.g., patients who are ventilator dependent or have Alzheimer's disease). Long-term care facilities include skilled nursing facilities, assisted living facilities, and residential care facilities.

There is a new emphasis on care coordination when patients transition between care settings. *Transitions of care* refer to patients moving among health care practitioners, settings, and home as their condition and care needs change.[15] As a nurse, you are an essential part of care coordination by stressing actions that meet patients' needs and facilitate safe, quality care. Collaborating with other members of the interprofessional team is critical. A lack of communication can result in an ineffective care transition, leading to drug errors and higher hospital readmission rates. For example, you are a nurse in acute care admitting a long-term care patient who has been receiving propranolol 20 mg/5 mL twice a day. The admitting orders read "propranolol 20 mg/mL, give 5 mL twice a day." You avert a potential drug error by using communication techniques to reconcile the difference.

Delivery of Nursing Care

Nurses deliver patient-centered care in collaboration with the interprofessional health care team and within the framework of a care delivery model. A care delivery model outlines how responsibilities and authority are structured to carry out patient care.[16] More positive care outcomes occur when the number and type of care providers match patient needs and there is a designated care coordinator.

In acute care settings, 2 basic models are used: team care and total patient care. *Team care* models involve a group of providers who work together to deliver care. A professional nurse is usually the team leader. As team leader, you manage and coordinate care with others, such as licensed practical/vocational nurses (LPN/VNs) and unlicensed assistive personnel (UAP). You have accountability for the quality of care delivered by team members during a work period. In total patient care models, you are responsible for planning and providing all care.

Other care models include case management and telehealth. Case management is "a collaborative process of assessment, planning, facilitation, care coordination, evaluation, and advocacy for options and services to meet an individual's and family's comprehensive health needs through communication and available resources to promote quality, cost-effective outcomes."[17] Although health care agencies implement case management in various ways, it involves managing the patient's care with other interprofessional team members across multiple care settings and levels of care.

A professional nurse often serves as the case manager. In this role, the nurse assesses the needs of patients and/or caregivers, coordinates services for them, makes appropriate referrals, and evaluates the progress toward meeting care goals. For example, a nurse case manager in an outpatient clinic has been working for 3 months with an older male patient who has multiple co-morbidities, including severe coronary artery disease, diabetes, and osteoarthritis. After he is scheduled for a coronary artery bypass, the nurse manager coordinates his care with other members of the interprofessional team. She arranges his preoperative appointments and informs the other team members so that all health care providers understand the patient's unique needs. After the patient has surgery, he develops a deep venous thrombosis in his leg. The case manager then works with the interprofessional team to evaluate the patient's discharge needs and decide whether rehabilitation or home health care is necessary for the patient. With the patient and caregiver, the team decides to discharge the patient to a rehabilitation facility. The case manager helps with the transition, again coordinating care so that the providers at the rehabilitation facility are aware of the patient's needs.

Telehealth nursing is the delivery of health care and information through telecommunication technologies, including high-speed Internet, wireless, satellite, and video communications.[18] Among the many uses of telehealth are triaging patients, monitoring patients with chronic or critical conditions, helping patients manage symptoms, providing patient and caregiver education and emotional support, and providing follow-up care. Telehealth can increase access to care. The nurse engaged in telehealth can assess the patient's health status, deliver interventions, and evaluate the outcomes of nursing care while separated geographically from the patient (Fig. 1.4).

Critical Thinking

Complex health care environments require that you use critical thinking and clinical reasoning skills to make decisions that lead to the best patient outcomes. **Critical thinking**, your ability to focus your thinking to get the results you need in various situations, has been described as knowing how to learn, be creative, generate ideas, make decisions, and solve problems.[19]

Critical thinking is not memorizing a list of facts or the steps of a procedure. Instead, it is the ability to make judgments and solve problems by making sense of information. Learning and using critical thinking is a continual process that occurs inside and outside of the clinical setting.

Clinical reasoning is using critical thinking to examine and analyze patient care issues.[19] It involves understanding the medical and nursing implications of a patient's situation when making decisions about patient care. You use clinical reasoning when you identify a change in a patient's status, consider the context and concerns of the patient and caregiver, and decide what to do about it.

Given the complexity of patient care today, nurses need to learn and implement critical thinking and clinical reasoning skills before they gain those skills through experience in professional practice. Various experiences in nursing school offer opportunities for you to learn and make decisions about patient care. Various education activities, including interactive case studies and simulation exercises, promote practice in critical thinking and clinical reasoning. Throughout this book, select boxes, case studies, and review questions promote your use of critical thinking and clinical reasoning skills.

TEAMWORK AND COLLABORATION

Interprofessional Team

To deliver high-quality care, you need to have effective working relationships with members of the health care team. The **interprofessional team** is made up of providers from various disciplines, working together and sharing their expertise to provide customized care. It may consist of physicians, nurses, pharmacists, occupational and physical therapists, and others (Table 1.3). To be competent in interprofessional practice, you must collaborate in many ways by exchanging knowledge, sharing responsibility for problem solving, and making patient care decisions. You may be responsible for coordinating care among the team members, taking part in interprofessional

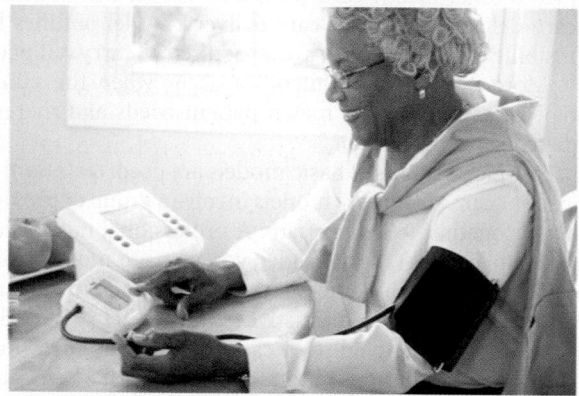

FIG. 1.4 An older adult performing remote blood pressure monitoring. (From Cooper K, Gosnell K: *Foundations of nursing,* St Louis, 2015, Elsevier.)

TABLE 1.3 Interprofessional Team Members	
Team Member	**Description of Services Provided**
Dentist	Provides preventive and restorative treatments for problems affecting the teeth and mouth
Dietitian	Provides general nutrition services, including dietary consultation about health promotion or specialized diets
Occupational therapist (OT)	May help patient with fine motor coordination, performing activities of daily living, cognitive-perceptual skills, sensory testing, and the construction or use of assistive or adaptive equipment
Pastoral care	Offers spiritual support and guidance to patients and caregivers
Pharmacist	Prepares medications and infusion products
Physical therapist (PT)	Works with patients on improving strength and endurance, gait training, transfer training, and developing a patient education program
Physician (medical doctor [MD])	Practices medicine and treats illness and injury by prescribing medication, performing diagnostic tests and evaluations, performing surgery, and providing other medical services and advice
Physician assistant	Conducts physical exams, diagnoses and treats illnesses, and counsels on preventive health care in collaboration with a physician
Respiratory therapist	May provide oxygen therapy in the home, give specialized respiratory treatments, and teach the patient or caregiver about the proper use of respiratory equipment
Social worker	Assists patients with developing coping skills, meeting caregiver concerns, securing adequate financial resources or housing, or making referrals to social service or volunteer agencies
Speech pathologist	Focuses on treatment of speech defects and disorders, especially by using physical exercises to strengthen muscles used in speech, speech drills, and audiovisual aids that develop new speech habits

TABLE 1.4 Guidelines for Communicating Using SBAR

Purpose: SBAR is a model for effective transfer of information by providing a standard structure for concise factual communications from nurse-to-nurse, nurse-to-physician, or nurse-to–other health professionals.

Steps to Use: Before speaking with a physician or other health care professional about a patient problem, assess the patient yourself, read the most recent physician progress and nursing notes, and have the patient's chart available.

S **Situation**	• What is the situation you want to discuss? What is happening right now? • Identify self, unit. State: I am calling about: *patient, room number.* • Briefly state the problem: what it is, when it happened or started, and how severe it is. State: I have just assessed the patient and am concerned about: *describe why you are concerned.*
B **Background**	• What is the background or circumstances leading up to the situation? State pertinent background information related to the situation that may include: • Admitting diagnosis and date of admission • List of current medications, allergies, IV fluids • Most recent vital signs • Date and time of any laboratory testing and results of previous tests for comparison • Synopsis of treatment to date • Code status
A **Assessment**	• What do you think the problem is? What is your assessment of the situation? State what you think the problem is: • Changes from prior assessments • Patient condition unstable or worsening
R **Recommendation/Request**	• What should we do to correct the problem? What is your recommendation or request? State your request. • Specific treatments • Tests needed • Patient needs to be seen now

Source: Institute for Health Care Improvement: SBAR technique for communication: A situational briefing model. Retrieved from *www.ihi.org/resources/Pages/Tools/SBAR-TechniqueforCommunicationASituationalBriefingModel.aspx.*

team meetings or rounds, and making referrals when you need expertise in specialized areas to help the patient. To do so, you must be aware of the knowledge and skills of other team members and be able to communicate effectively with them.

To help you develop the competencies necessary to practice within an interprofessional clinical environment, you may take part in education activities with students from other disciplines. Throughout this book, case studies and review questions discuss the roles others have in managing patient care.

Coordinating Care

Communication. Effective communication is key to fostering teamwork and coordinating care. To provide safe, effective care, everyone involved in a patient's care should understand the patient's condition and needs. Unfortunately, many issues result from a breakdown in communication. Miscommunication often occurs during transitions of care. One structured model used to improve communication is the SBAR (Situation-Background-Assessment-Recommendation) technique (Table 1.4). This technique offers a way to talk about a patient's condition among members of the health care team in a predictable, structured

manner. Other ways to enhance communication during transitions include using bedside rounds, having standard processes for patient hand-offs, and conducting interprofessional rounds to identify risks and develop a plan for delivering care.

Clinical Pathways. Clinical pathways, also known as care maps, are interprofessional care plans that outline the care and desired outcomes for a specific time period for patients with a specific diagnosis. Think of a clinical pathway as a road map the patient and health care team should follow. As the patient progresses along the road, the patient should receive specific care and accomplish specific goals. If a patient's progress differs from the planned path, a variance has occurred. A negative variance occurs when specific goals are not met. The nurse usually identifies when a negative variance is present and works with the interprofessional team to create a plan to address the issue.[16]

The exact content and format of clinical pathways vary among agencies and settings. Each agency usually develops its own pathways based on evidence-based practice guidelines. Common components include assessment guidelines, laboratory and diagnostic testing, medications, activity, diet, and teaching. In acute care, clinical pathways often describe which patient care components are needed at specific times (Fig. 1.5). The case types selected for this type of pathway are usually those that are high volume or high risk and predictable, such as myocardial infarction and surgical procedures (e.g., endoscopy, cholecystectomy, cataract surgery).

Delegation and Assignment. As a registered nurse (RN), you will delegate nursing care and supervise those who are qualified to deliver care. Delegation allows a care provider to perform a specific nursing activity, skill, or procedure that is beyond their usual role.[20] Delegating and assigning nursing activities is a process that, when used appropriately, results in safe, effective, and efficient patient care. Delegating can allow you more time to focus on complex patient care needs. Delegating care and supervising others will be one of your essential roles as a professional nurse.

Delegation usually involves tasks and procedures that licensed practical/vocational nurses (LPN/VNs) and unlicensed assistive personnel (UAP) perform. Nursing interventions that require independent nursing knowledge, skill, or judgment (e.g., initial assessment, patient teaching, evaluating care) are your responsibility and cannot be delegated. State nurse practice acts and agency policies identify activities that you can delegate to LPN/VNs and UAP. You will use professional judgment to select which activities to delegate. Your decision will be based on the patient's needs, the LPN/VN's and UAP's education and training, and the amount of supervision needed. The most common delegated nursing actions occur during the implementation phase of the nursing process. For example, you can delegate measuring oral intake and urine output to UAP, but you use your nursing judgment to decide if the intake and output are adequate.

The general guideline for LPN/VN practice is that they can function independently in a stable, routine situation. However, they must work under the direct supervision of a professional nurse in acute, unstable situations in which a patient's condition can rapidly change. In most states, LPN/VNs may give medications, perform sterile procedures, and perform a wide variety of interventions planned by the RN. The procedure itself is not the issue when an RN is determining what to delegate. Rather, the stability of the patient determines whether it is appropriate for an RN to delegate a procedure to an LPN/VN. For example, the LPN/VN can change a dressing on an abdominal surgical wound, but the RN should do the first dressing change and wound assessment.

Patient Name _____   Date _____

DRG# _____   Expected LOS ___<23 hours___

	Preprocedure	Preoperative	Intraoperative	Postoperative Phase I PACU	Postoperative PHASE II PACU	Discharge	Postoperative PHASE II PACU
Medication	Review medical history	Start IV	Administer meperidine, propofol, midazolam	Administer naloxone, flumazenil pm	Pain med prn	Start on Rx omeprazole	Continue medications
Diagnostic tests	H-&-P chest x-ray, ECG, blood work	Review tests	Endoscopy procedure	None, unless complications	None	None	None
Diet	Regular	NPO	NPO	NPO	Clear liquids & progress	Regular	Regular
Activity	Not restricted	Ambulate	None	Turn, cough, and deep breathe	Increase activity to ambulation	Normal ambulation	Not restricted
Nursing action	Assessment	Vital signs	Vital signs, O₂ saturation	Vital signs, level of consciousness, O₂ saturation	Monitor as before	Prepare for discharge	Follow-up evaluation via phone
Teaching/ discharge planning	Phone call	Patient education about procedure	Transport to PACU	Discharge when Aldrete criteria I met	Discharge when Aldrete criteria II met	Instructions reviewed	Phone call for follow-up

FIG. 1.5 Clinical pathway for endoscopy. (From Arnold EC, Boggs KU: *Interpersonal relationships,* ed 6, St Louis, 2011, Mosby.)

UAP hold many titles, including nurse aides, certified medication aides, nursing assistants, patient care assistants, or technicians. The activities UAP perform typically include obtaining routine vital signs on stable patients, feeding and helping patients at mealtimes, ambulating stable patients, and helping patients with bathing and hygiene.

Delegation can occur among professional nurses. For example, if 1 RN has accountability for an outcome and asks another RN to perform a specific intervention related to that outcome, that is delegation. This type of delegation typically occurs when 1 RN leaves the unit/work area for a meal break.

Assignment is different from delegation. The term *assign* is used when you direct an LPN/VN or UAP to do an activity or procedure that is part of their everyday job.[20] An assignment must be within the authorized scope of practice of the LPN/VN or part of the routine function of the UAP. For example, you can assign an LPN/VN to give medications to a patient, because this is within the LPN/VN's scope of practice. You cannot assign an LPN/VN to a patient who needs an admission assessment because an RN must perform the initial patient assessment.

Whether you delegate or are working with staff to whom you assign tasks, you are responsible for the patient's total care during your work period. You need to decide what patient care tasks must be carried out during the given period, identify who will do them, and prioritize the order in which the tasks must be completed. You are responsible for supervising UAP or LPN/VNs. Clearly communicate the tasks that must be done and give

necessary guidance. Because you are accountable for ensuring that delegated tasks are completed in a competent manner, evaluate the care given, follow up as needed, and make sure no care was missed.

Delegation is a skill that is learned, and you must practice to be proficient in managing patient care. You need to use critical thinking and professional judgment to ensure that you follow the 5 Rights of Delegation (Table 1.5). To help you, information on delegation is presented in the nursing management tables and case study questions at the end of the management chapters.

SAFETY

It is estimated that about 250,000 patients each year die because of preventable medical errors.[21] Several groups are addressing this issue by outlining safety goals for health care organizations and identifying safety competencies for health professionals. By implementing various procedures and systems that improve patient safety, health care systems are working to attain a culture that minimizes the risk of harm to the patient. Because of your closeness to patients, you are in a unique position to promote patient safety.

Serious Reportable Events

The National Quality Forum (NQF) uses the term serious reportable event (SRE), also called a *never event,* to describe

TABLE 1.5 5 Rights of Delegation

The 5 Rights of Delegation

The registered nurse uses critical thinking and professional judgment to be sure that the delegation or assignment is:

1. The right task
2. Under the right circumstances
3. To the right person
4. With the right directions and communication
5. Under the right supervision and evaluation

Rights of Delegation	Description	Questions to Ask
Right Task	One that can be delegated for a specific patient	Is it appropriate to delegate based on legal and agency factors? Has the person been trained and evaluated in performing the task? Is the person able and willing to do this specific task?
Right Circumstances	Appropriate patient setting, available resources, and considering relevant factors, including patient stability	What are the patient's needs right now? Is staffing such that the circumstances support delegation strategies?
Right Person	Right person is delegating the right task to the right person to be performed on the right person	Is the prospective delegatee a willing and able employee? Are the patient needs a "fit" with the delegatee?
Right Directions and Communication	Clear, concise description of task, including its objective, limits, and expectations	Have you given clear communication about the task? With directions, limits, and expected outcomes? Does the delegatee know what and when to report? Does the delegatee understand what needs to be done?
Right Supervision and Evaluation	Appropriate monitoring, evaluation, intervention, and feedback	Do you know how and when you will interact about patient care with the delegatee? How often do you need to directly observe? Will you be able to give feedback to the staff member if needed?

Source: National Guidelines for Nursing Delegation. Retrieved from *www.ncsbn.org/1625.htm.*

serious, largely preventable, and harmful clinical events.[22] The current list of SREs consists of 29 events. These events include such things as a patient acquiring a stage III or greater pressure injury while hospitalized and death or disability from a fall or hypoglycemia.

To reduce the occurrence of SREs, the NQF has a list of effective *Safe Practices* that health care settings should use to provide safe patient care *(www.qualityforum.org)*. You are implementing NQF practices when you perform a time-out before a surgical procedure, reconcile medication records, and implement interventions to prevent hospital-acquired infections, pressure injuries and falls.

National Patient Safety Goals

The Joint Commission (TJC), the accrediting agency for health care organizations, gathers and reports data on serious errors they call sentinel events. A *sentinel event* is a patient safety event not related to the patient's illness or underlying condition that reaches a patient and results in death, permanent harm, or severe temporary harm.[23] Events are "sentinel" because they signal the need for immediate investigation and response. Many sentinel events are also serious reportable events. If the patient undergoes a wrong-site or wrong-procedure surgery, experiences an assault in the health care setting, or receives an incompatible blood product, the occurrence is both a sentinel event, reportable to TJC, and a serious reportable event, reportable to NQF.

To address specific patient safety concerns, TJC issues National Patient Safety Goals (NPSGs).[24] NPSGs promote patient safety by offering evidence-based solutions to common safety problems. The 2017 NPSGs are listed in Table 1.6.

The latest safety goal, focusing on improving the safety of clinical alarm systems, greatly affects nursing. Patient monitoring systems provide vital information. Alarms that work well improve patient safety and care by telling you when a patient needs your attention. However, so many alarms can go off that *alarm fatigue* occurs, and nurses can become desensitized to the sounds. By better managing alarms, we reduce alarm fatigue and improve patient safety.

Because you have the greatest amount of interaction with patients, you play a key role in promoting safety. Many describe nurses as the patient's last line of defense. Every nurse has the responsibility to ensure the patient receives care in a manner that prevents errors and promotes patient safety. Throughout this book, safety alerts highlighting patient care issues and NPSGs will help you in learning to apply safety principles.

QUALITY IMPROVEMENT

Quality care and safety are related: the higher the culture of safety, the better the quality of care. Health care systems focused on quality outcomes use practice standards and protocols based on best evidence while considering the patient's unique preferences and needs. Your role is to coordinate the complex aspects of patient care, including the care delivered by others, and identify and correct issues associated with poor quality and unsafe care.

Quality improvement (QI) programs involve systematic actions that monitor, assess, and improve health care quality. QI is an interprofessional team effort that is required by accrediting agencies. As part of professional nursing practice, you need to be able to collect data using QI tools, implement interventions to improve quality of care, and monitor patient outcomes. Several public and private groups focusing on improving health care quality have developed standard QI measures. These performance measures assess how well the health care team cares

TABLE 1.6 National Patient Safety Goals

Safety Goal	Examples
Identify patients correctly	• Use at least 2 ways to identify patients (e.g., have them state full name and date of birth). • Give the correct patient the correct blood with every blood transfusion.
Improve communication among the health care team	• Get critical test results to the right person on time.
Use medicines safely	• Before a procedure, label all medicines. Discard any found unlabeled. • Use proper precautions with patients who take anticoagulants. • Find out what medicines each patient is taking. Make certain that it is safe for the patient to take any new medicines with his or her current ones. • Give a medication list to the patient and the caregiver before discharge. Explain the list.
Use alarm systems safely	• Respond to alarms promptly. • Do not turn alarms off.
Prevent health care–associated infections	• Use soap, water, and hand sanitizer before and after every patient contact. • Use evidence-based practices to prevent infections related to central lines, indwelling urinary catheters, and multidrug-resistant organisms
Identify patient safety risks	• Assess patients at risk for suicide. • Assess any risks, such as fires, for patients who are getting home oxygen therapy.
Prevent mistakes in surgery	• Conduct a time-out before the start of any surgery. • Confirm correct patient, procedure, and site.

Adapted from The Joint Commission (TJC): *2016 National patient safety goals,* Oakbrook Terrace, IL. Retrieved from *www.jointcommission.org/assets/1/6/2017_NPSG_HAP_ER.pdf.*

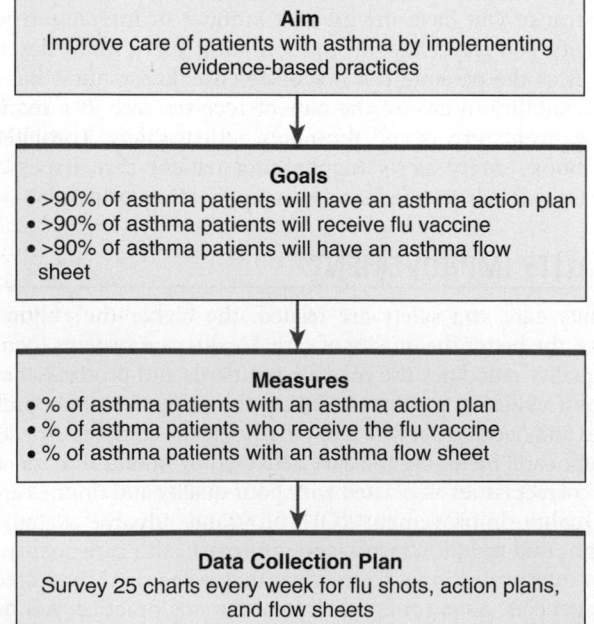

Aim
Improve care of patients with asthma by implementing evidence-based practices

↓

Goals
• >90% of asthma patients will have an asthma action plan
• >90% of asthma patients will receive flu vaccine
• >90% of asthma patients will have an asthma flow sheet

↓

Measures
• % of asthma patients with an asthma action plan
• % of asthma patients who receive the flu vaccine
• % of asthma patients with an asthma flow sheet

↓

Data Collection Plan
Survey 25 charts every week for flu shots, action plans, and flow sheets

FIG. 1.6 Quality improvement system. (Adapted from Courtlandt CD, Noonan L, Leonard GF: Model for improvement—Part 1: A framework for health care quality, *Pediatr Clin North Am* 56:757, 2009.)

for a patient with a certain condition or receives a specific treatment. They describe what data the team must collect and monitor. Fig 1.6 shows an example of a QI system for adult patients with asthma. In this example, you would review patient medical records to decide if the rate of flu vaccine administration exceeds 90%. You would share the results with the team and, if the identified standard was not met, work as a team to implement measures to correct the deficiency.

National Database of Nursing Quality Indicators

The National Database of Nursing Quality Indicators (NDNQI) provides data on nursing-sensitive measures to evaluate the impact of nursing care on patient outcomes. Patient outcomes are nursing sensitive if they improve with a greater quantity or quality of nursing care. NDNQI outcomes are unique because they identify how nursing workforce factors, including nurse staffing and skill mix, directly influence patient outcomes. NDNQI data show the incidence of falls and health care–associated pressure injuries and infections decreases with adequate staffing and increased nurse education and satisfaction with the work environment. Table 1.7 lists the current NDNQI.

INFORMATICS

Nursing is an information-intense profession. Advances in informatics and technology have changed the way nurses plan, deliver, document, and evaluate care. All nurses, regardless of their setting or role, use informatics and technology every day in practice. Informatics has changed how you obtain and review diagnostic information, make clinical decisions, communicate with patients and health care team members, document, and provide care.

Technology advances have increased the efficiency of nursing care, improving the work environment and the care nurses provide. Computers and mobile devices allow you to document at the time you deliver care and give you quick and easy access to information, including clinical decision-making tools, patient education materials, and references. Texting, video chat, and e-mail enhance communication among health care team members and help you deliver the right message to the right person at the right time.

Technology plays a key role in providing safe, quality patient care. Medication administration applications improve patient

TABLE 1.7 National Database of Nursing Quality Indicators

• Structure indicators
  • RN turnover rate
  • Nursing hours per patient day
  • RN education and certification
  • Staff mix: RNs, LPN/VNs, UAP, agency staff
• Process and outcome indicators
  • Patient falls and falls with injury
  • Pressure injury rate
  • RN surveys on job satisfaction and practice environment scale
• Outcome indicators
  • Physical/sexual assault rate
  • Restraint use
• Health care–associated infections (HAI) rate

Source: National Database of Nursing Quality Indicators. Retrieved from *www.nursingquality.org.*

safety by flagging potential errors, such as look-alike and sound-alike medications and adverse drug interactions, before they can occur. Computerized provider order entry (CPOE) systems can reduce errors caused by misreading or misinterpreting handwritten orders. Sensor technology can decrease the number of falls in high-risk patients. Care reminder systems give cues that decrease the amount of missed nursing care.

Being able to use technology skills to communicate and access information is now an essential part of your professional nursing practice. You must be able to use word processing software, communicate by e-mail and book messaging, access information, and follow security and confidentiality rules. You need to have the ability to safely use patient care technologies and navigate electronic documentation systems.

Protected health information (PHI) is highly sensitive. *The Health Insurance Portability and Accountability Act (HIPAA)* is part of federal legislation that addresses actions for how PHI is used and disclosed. With the increased use of informatics and

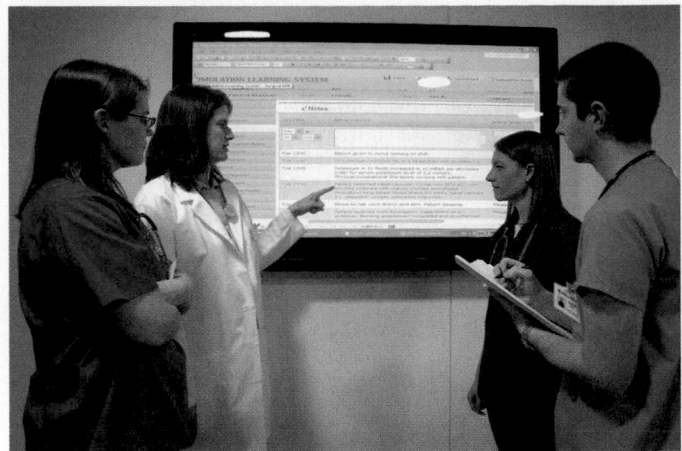

FIG. 1.7 Members of the interprofessional team review a patient's electronic health record. (From Arnold EC, Boggs KU: *Interpersonal relationships*, ed 6, St Louis, 2011, Mosby.)

technology come new concerns on how to comply with HIPAA regulations and maintain a patient's privacy. Wireless technologies, increased use of e-mail and computer networking, and the ongoing threat of computer viruses increase the need for properly protecting a patient's privacy. We must assure patients of their privacy and that only those with a right to know are accessing protected information.

As a nurse, you have an obligation to ensure the privacy of your patient's health information. To do so, you need to understand your agency's policies about the use of technology. You need to know the rules about accessing patient records and releasing PHI, what to do if information is accidentally or intentionally released, and how to protect any passwords you use. If you are using social networking, you must be careful not to place any individually identifiable PHI online. Throughout this book, Informatics in Practice boxes offer suggestions on how to use informatics in your practice.

Electronic Health Records

The largest use of informatics is **electronic health records (EHRs)**, also called *electronic medical records*. An EHR is a computerized record of patient information. It is shared among all health care team members involved in a patient's care and moves with the patient—to other providers and across care settings. The ideal EHR provides a single place for team members to review and update a patient's health record, document care given, and enter patient care orders, including medications, procedures, diets, and diagnostic and laboratory tests (Fig. 1.7).

Several obstacles are still in the way of fully implementing EHRs. Systems are technologically complex, requiring many resources and training to implement and maintain. Communication is still lacking among computer systems and software applications. Finally, perceived challenges in the use of EHRs, including increased workload and the need for work-arounds, affect implementation.

EVIDENCE-BASED PRACTICE

Evidence-based practice (EBP) is a problem-solving approach to clinical decision making. Using the best available evidence (e.g., research findings, QI data), combined with your expertise

---

ETHICAL/LEGAL DILEMMAS

Social Networking: HIPAA Violation

Situation

You log into a closed group on a social networking site and read a posting from a fellow nursing student. The posting describes in detail the complex care the student gave to an older patient in a local hospital the previous day. The student comments on how stressful the day was and asks for advice on how to deal with similar patients in the future.

Ethical/Legal Points for Consideration

- Protecting and maintaining patient privacy and confidentiality are basic obligations defined in the Code of Ethics for Nurses, which nurses and nursing students should uphold.[1]
- As outlined in the Health Insurance Portability and Accountability Act (HIPAA), a patient's private health information is any information that relates to the person's past, present, or future physical or mental health. This includes not only specific details such as a patient's name or picture but also information that gives enough details that someone may be able to identify that person.
- You may unintentionally breach privacy or confidentiality by posting patient information (diagnosis, condition, situation) on a social networking site. Using privacy settings or being in a closed group does not guarantee the secrecy of posted information. Others can copy and share any post without your knowledge.
- Potential consequences for improperly using social networking vary based on the situation. These may include (1) disciplinary action by the state board of nursing; (2) being disciplined, suspended, or fired by an employer; (3) dismissal from a nursing program; and (4) civil and/or criminal charges.
- A student nurse who experienced a stressful day and is looking for advice and support from peers (e.g., "Today my patient died. I wanted to cry.") could share the experience by clearly limiting the posts to the student's personal perspective and not sharing any identifying information. This is 1 area in which it is safest to err on the side of caution to avoid the appearance of impropriety.

Discussion Questions

1. How would you deal with the situation involving the fellow nursing student?
2. How would you handle a situation in which you saw a staff member who violated HIPAA?

Reference

1. Code of Ethics for Nurses. Retrieved from *www.nursingworld.org/ DocumentVault/Ethics-1/Code-of-Ethics-for-Nurses.html*.

TABLE 1.8 Steps of Evidence-Based Practice (EBP) Process

1. Ask the clinical question using the **PICOT** format:
   Patients/population
   Intervention
   Comparison or comparison group
   Outcome(s)
   Time (as applicable)
2. Search for the best evidence based on the clinical question.
3. Critically appraise and synthesize the evidence.
4. Implement the evidence in practice.
5. Evaluate the practice decision or change.
6. Share the outcomes of the decision or change.

and the patient's unique circumstances and preferences, leads to better clinical decisions and improved patient outcomes. EBP closes the gap between research and practice, providing more reliable and predictable care than that based on tradition, opinion, and trial and error.

EBP does not mean that you conduct a research study. Instead, EBP depends on you to take an active role in using the best available evidence when delivering care. You need to have an ongoing curiosity about what are the best nursing practices and routinely ask questions about your patient's care. Recognize when you need more information. When you base your practice on valid evidence, you are solving problems and supporting best patient outcomes.

Steps of EBP Process

The EBP process has 6 steps (Table 1.8).

Step 1. Step 1 is asking a clinical question in the PICOT format. Developing the clinical question is the key step in the EBP process.[25] A good clinical question sets the context for integrating evidence, clinical judgment, and patient preferences. In addition, the question guides the literature search for the best evidence to influence practice.

An example of a clinical question in PICOT format is, "In adult abdominal surgery patients (**P** = patients/population) is splinting with an elasticized abdominal binder (**I** = intervention) or a pillow (**C** = comparison) more effective in reducing pain associated with ambulation (**O** = outcome) on the first postoperative day (**T** = time period)?" A clinical question may not have all components of PICOT. Some only include 4 components. The (T) timing or (C) comparison components are not appropriate for every question. The (C) component of PICOT may include a comparison with a specific intervention, the usual standard of care, or no intervention at all.

Step 2. Step 2 is searching for the best evidence that applies to the clinical question. Technology provides you with ready access to data. You can easily search several online resources and collect large amounts of clinical information and evidence. It is important to evaluate all data sources for their credibility and reliability. Not all evidence is equal. Fig. 1.8 presents the hierarchy of evidence. As you go down the pyramid, the strength of the evidence becomes weaker. Systematic reviews and evidence-based clinical practice guidelines save time and effort in the EBP process. However, they are available for only a limited number of clinical topics and may not suit all types of clinical questions. When insufficient research exists to guide practice, recommendations from expert panels and authority figures may be the best evidence available.

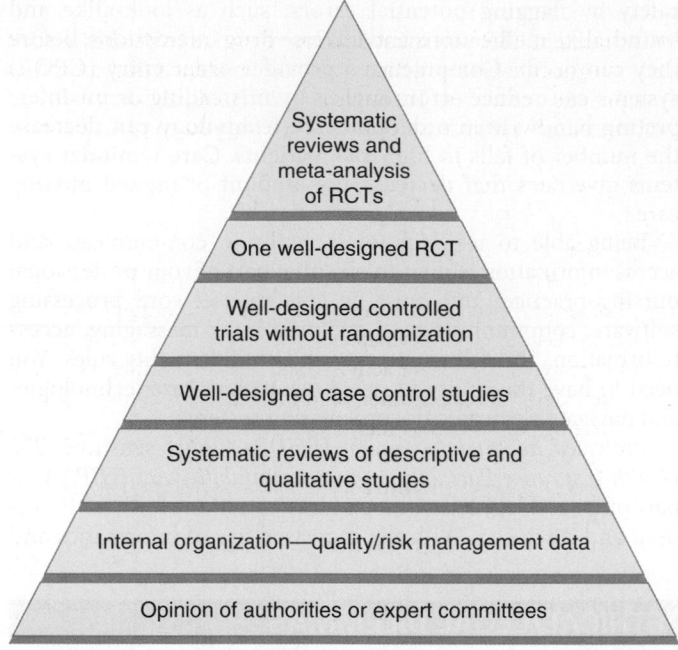

FIG. 1.8 Hierarchy of evidence. (Modified from Melnyk BM, Fineout-Overholt E: *Evidence-based practice in nursing and healthcare: A guide to best practice,* ed 3, Philadelphia, 2014, Lippincott Williams & Wilkins.)

Step 3. Step 3 is to critically appraise the evidence you found. A successful critical appraisal process focuses on 3 essential questions: (1) What are the results? (2) Are the results reliable and valid? and (3) Will the results help me in caring for my patients? You decide the strength of the evidence and synthesize the findings related to the clinical question to conclude what is the best practice. For example, you find strong evidence supporting effectiveness of elasticized binders and pillows in reducing pain associated with ambulation. However, the binder appears to be more effective if the patient is obese or has had prior abdominal surgery.

Step 4. Step 4 involves implementing the evidence in practice. The decision to implement change is made by combining the evidence, clinical judgment, and preferences and values of patients and caregivers. You may be part of an interprofessional team charged with implementing a practice change or applying evidence in a specific patient care situation. This may include developing clinical practice guidelines, policies and procedures, or new assessment, teaching, or documentation tools. For example, you may be part of a team implementing a new postoperative protocol focused on using elasticized abdominal binders with patients who are obese or had prior abdominal surgery.

Step 5. Step 5 is evaluating the outcome of the practice change. After implementing the change for a specific period, you should monitor outcomes to determine whether the change has improved patient outcomes. Accrediting bodies require documentation of outcome measures to show that the organization is using evidence to improve patient care.

Step 6. Step 6 is sharing the results of the EBP change. If you do not share the outcomes of EBP, then other health care providers and patients cannot benefit from what you learned from your experience. You can share information locally using unit- or hospital-based newsletters and posters and regionally and nationally through journal publications and presentations at conferences.

Implementing EBP

To implement EBP, you must develop the skills to be able to seek and incorporate into practice scientific evidence that supports best patient outcomes. Throughout this book, Evidence-Based Practice boxes provide an opportunity for you to practice your critical thinking skills in applying EBP to patient scenarios. To help you identify the use of evidence in this book, an asterisk (*) in the reference list at the end of each chapter indicates evidence-based information for clinical practice.

■ BRIDGE TO NCLEX EXAMINATION

The number of the question corresponds to the same-numbered outcome at the beginning of the chapter.

1. An example of a nursing activity that best reflects the American Nurses Association's definition of nursing is
   a. treating dysrhythmias that occur in a patient in the coronary care unit.
   b. diagnosing a patient with a feeding tube as being at risk for aspiration.
   c. setting up protocols for treating patients in the emergency department.
   d. offering antianxiety drugs to a patient with a disturbed sleep pattern.

2. A nurse working on the medical-surgical unit at an urban hospital would like to become certified in medical-surgical nursing. The nurse knows that this process would most likely require
   a. a bachelor's degree in nursing.
   b. formal education in advanced nursing practice.
   c. experience for a specific period in medical-surgical nursing.
   d. membership in a medical-surgical nursing specialty organization.

3. The nurse is assigned to care for a newly admitted patient. Number in order the steps for using the nursing process to prioritize care. (Number 1 is the first step, and number 5 is the last step.)
   ___ Evaluate whether the plan was effective.
   ___ Identify any health problems.
   ___ Collect patient information.
   ___ Carry out the plan.
   ___ Decide a plan of action.

4. Using the SBAR format, number in order the steps for how the nurse would communicate information with the provider. (Number 1 is the first step, and number 4 is the last step.)
   ___ "I would like you to order an IV medication and come evaluate the patient as soon as possible."
   ___ "This is Nurse M.H. I am calling from the unit because your patient, D.R., has a new onset of atrial fibrillation."
   ___ "The atrial fibrillation started about 10 minutes ago. The heart rate is 124; BP 90/60. The patient is experiencing dizziness."
   ___ "D.R., who is 2 days postoperative for a bowel resection for diverticulitis, has a history of mitral valve disease."

5. The nurse is caring for a diabetic patient in the ambulatory surgical unit who has undergone wound debridement. Which task is appropriate for the nurse to delegate to unlicensed assistive personnel (UAP)?
   a. Check the patient's vital signs.
   b. Assess the patient's pain level.
   c. Palpate the patient's pedal pulses.
   d. Monitor the patient's IV catheter site.

6. The nurse's role in addressing the National Patient Safety Goals established by The Joint Commission includes (select all that apply)
   a. answering all patient monitoring alarms promptly.
   b. memorizing all the rules published by The Joint Commission.
   c. obtaining a correct list of the patient's medications on admission.
   d. encouraging patients to be actively involved in their own health care.
   e. using side rails and alarm systems as necessary to prevent patient falls.

7. Advantages of using informatics in health care delivery are (select all that apply)
   a. reduced need for nurses in acute care.
   b. increased patient anonymity and confidentiality.
   c. the ability to achieve and maintain high standards of care.
   d. access to standard plans of care for many health problems.
   e. improved communication of the patient's health status to the health care team.

8. When using evidence-based practice, the nurse
   a. must use clinical practice guidelines developed by national health agencies.
   b. should use findings from randomized controlled trials to plan care for all patient problems.
   c. uses clinical decision making and judgment to decide what evidence is appropriate for a specific clinical situation.
   d. analyzes the relationship of nursing interventions to patient outcomes to discover evidence for patient interventions.

1. b, 2. c, 3. 5, 2, 1, 4, 3, 4. 4, 1, 3, 2, 5. a, 6. a, c, e, 7. c, d, e, 8. c.

For rationales to these answers and even more NCLEX review questions, visit *http://evolve.elsevier.com/Lewis/medsurg.*

ⓔ EVOLVE WEBSITE/RESOURCES LIST

http://evolve.elsevier.com/Lewis/medsurg
Review Questions (Online Only)
Key Points
Answer Key for Questions
• Rationales for Bridge to NCLEX Examination Questions
Conceptual Care Map Creator
Audio Glossary
Content Updates

REFERENCES

1. American Nurses Association: *Nursing: A social policy statement,* 3rd ed, Washington, DC, 2010, The Association. (Classic)
2. Nightingale F: *Notes on nursing: What it is and what it is not* (facsimile edition), Philadelphia, 1946, Lippincott. (Classic)
3. Henderson V: *The nature of nursing,* New York, 1966, Macmillan. (Classic)
4. American Nurses Credentialing Center. Certification. Retrieved from *www.nursingworld.org/ancc/.*

5. American Nurses Association. *Nursing: Scope and standards of practice,* Washington, DC, 2010, The Association. (Classic)

6. Thorpe KE The rise in health care spending and what to do about it, *Health Affairs* 24:1436, 2017.

7. Robert Wood Johnson Foundation. Achieving the potential of health care performance measures. Retrieved from *www.rwjf.org.*

8. ANCC Magnet Recognition Program. Retrieved from *www.nursingworld. org/organizational-programs/magnet/.*

9. Committee on the Robert Wood Johnson Foundation Initiative on the Future of Nursing at the Institute of Medicine. *The future of nursing: Leading change, advancing health,* Washington, DC, 2011, National Academies Press. (Classic)

10. QSEN Institute. Retrieved from *http://qsen.org.*

11. American Nurses Association: The nursing process. Retrieved from *www. nursingworld.org/practice-policy/workforce/what-is-nursing/the-nursing-process/.*

12. Rabelo-Silva ER, Dantas Cavalcanti AC, Ramos MC, et al: Advanced nursing process quality: Comparing the ICNP with the NANDA-International and Nursing Interventions Classification, *J Clinical Nurs* 26:379, 2017.

13. Clinical Care Classification. Nursing interventions. Retrieved from *www. sabacare.com/framework/nursing-interventions/.*

14. Carpenito LJ: *Handbook of nursing diagnoses.* 17th ed, Philadelphia, 2017, Lippincott Williams & Wilkins.

15. The Joint Commission: Transitions of care portal. Retrieved from *www. jointcommission.org/toc.aspx.*

16. Motacki K, Burke K. *Nursing delegation and management of patient care.* 2nd ed, St Louis, 2016, Elsevier.

17. What is a case manager? Retrieved from *www.cmsa.org.*

18. Zerwekh J, Garneau AZ. *Nursing today: Transitions and trends,* 9th ed, St Louis, 2017, Elsevier.

19. Alfaro-LeFevre R. *Critical thinking, clinical reasoning, and clinical judgment,* 6th ed, St Louis, 2017, Saunders.

20. Delegation. Retrieved from *www.ncsbn.org/1625.htm.*

*21. Makary MA, Daniel M: Medical error—The third leading cause of death in the US, *BMJ* 3:353, 2016.

22. Safe practices for better healthcare. Retrieved from *www.qualityforum. org/Topics/Patient_Safety.aspx.*

23. Sentinel events policy and procedures. Retrieved from *www.jointcommission. org/sentinel_event_policy_and_procedures/.*

24. National patient safety goals. Retrieved from *www.jointcommission.org/ standards_information/npsgs.aspx.*

25. Melnyk BM, Gallagher-Ford L, Fineout-Overholt E: *Implementing the evidence-based practice competencies in healthcare: A practical guide for improving quality, safety, and outcomes,* Indianapolis, 2016, Sigma Theta Tau.

*Evidence-based information for clinical practice.

Health Equity and Culturally Competent Care

Andrew Scanlon

We may have different religions, different languages, different colored skin, but we all belong to one human race. We all share the same basic values.

Kofi Annan

http://evolve.elsevier.com/Lewis/medsurg/

CONCEPTUAL FOCUS

Culture

Health Disparities

LEARNING OUTCOMES

1. Identify the key determinants of health and equity.
2. Describe the factors that contribute to health disparities and health equity.
3. Define the terms *culture, values, acculturation, ethnicity, race, stereotyping, ethnocentrism, cultural imposition, cultural competency,* and *culture-bound syndrome.*
4. Explain how culture and ethnicity may affect a person's physical and psychologic health.
5. Apply strategies for incorporating cultural information in the nursing process with all patients.
6. Describe the role of nursing in promoting health equity.
7. Examine ways that your own cultural background may influence nursing care.
8. Describe strategies for successfully communicating with a person who speaks a language that you do not understand.

KEY TERMS

acculturation, p. 21
cultural competence, p. 22
culture, p. 20
culture-bound syndromes, p. 27
determinants of health, p. 17
ethnicity, p. 18
ethnocentrism, p. 21

folk healers, p. 23
health disparities, p. 18
health equity, p. 18
health status, p. 17
lesbian, gay, bisexual, transgender, and queer or questioning (LGBTQ), p. 20
place, p. 19

race, p. 18
sexuality, p. 20
stereotyping, p. 21
transcultural nursing, p. 22
values, p. 20

This chapter discusses health disparities and culture. Health is a cultural concept because culture frames and shapes our experiences. Cultural beliefs influence health promotion practices and attitudes about seeking health care. Cultural differences can lead to problems that decrease the chance of receiving equitable health care. Nurses play a key role in recognizing and reducing health disparities. Understanding the concept of culture is important in your ability to provide patient-centered care.

DETERMINANTS OF HEALTH

Why are there differences in people's health status? How do these differences occur? The determinants of health are factors that (1) influence the health of individuals and groups and (2) help explain why some people experience poorer health than others.[1] Where people are born, grow up, live, work, and age helps determine their health status, behaviors, and care.

Health status is a holistic concept that is more than the presence or absence of disease. It encompasses life expectancy as well as self-assessment of health. As such, many measures make up the concept of health status. For individuals, this means the sum of their current health problems plus their coping resources (e.g., family, financial resources). For a community, health status is the combination of health measures for all people living in the community. Community health measures include birth and death rates, life expectancy, access to care, and morbidity and mortality rates related to disease and injury.

Factors in a person's social and physical environment, including personal relationships, workplace, housing, transportation, and neighborhood violence, contribute to health status.[1] For example, the risk of youth homicide is much higher in neighborhoods with gang activity and high crime rates. The physical environment in which one lives, works, and plays may expose a person to such risks as environmental hazards (workplace injuries), toxic agents (chemical spills, industrial pollution), unsafe traffic patterns (lack of sidewalks), or absence of fresh and healthy food choices.

A person's behavior is influenced by his or her environment, education, and economic status. Behaviors such as tobacco and illicit drug use are strongly linked to many health conditions (e.g., lung cancer, liver disease). A person's biologic makeup, such as genetics and family history of disease (e.g., heart disease), can increase the risk for specific diseases.

The availability of health care also contributes to a person's health. Though government initiatives are striving to reduce the number of uninsured Americans, millions remain uninsured and have limited access to care. This affects both individual and community health.

HEALTH DISPARITIES AND HEALTH EQUITY

Health disparities are differences in the incidence, prevalence, mortality rate, and burden of diseases that exist among specific population groups. In the United States this is because of social, economic, or environmental disadvantages. Health disparities can affect population groups based on gender, age, ethnicity, socioeconomic status, education, location, sexual orientation, or disability status.[2] Health equity is achieved when every person has the opportunity to attain his or her health potential, and no one is disadvantaged.

ETHICAL/LEGAL DILEMMAS
Health Disparities

Situation

E.M., a 47-yr-old Mexican American woman living with type 2 diabetes mellitus, comes to the clinic to have her blood glucose measured. It has been 12 months since her last visit. At that time, the nurse asked that she bring along her glucometer and strips to show how she checks her blood glucose because her glucose values were high at her previous visits.

When you check E.M.'s equipment and glucose strips, you find that the strips are for a different machine and they expired more than 2 years ago. When you inquire about the situation, E.M. explains that she cannot afford to come to the clinic or to buy new equipment and supplies to check her blood glucose level. During the day, E.M. cares for her 3 grandchildren so her daughter can work. E.M. spends most of her income on food for her family, so she has little money left for her health care.

Ethical/Legal Points for Consideration

- Ethnic minorities and other vulnerable or disadvantaged groups experience certain chronic illnesses at higher rates. Limited access to high-quality, accessible, and affordable health care services is associated with an increased incidence of illness and complications, as well as a reduced life span.
- People with certain health problems such as diabetes may have difficulty obtaining health care insurance. Consider these issues in the broader context of social justice.
- In many states, the legal definition of the role of the professional nurse includes patient advocacy. Advocacy includes the obligation to provide adequate follow-up care for all patients, especially those who are experiencing health care disparities.
- A nurse who observes disparities must consider the possibility of discrimination and abuse. Professional nurses are legally and ethically responsible for patient advocacy. The nurse may incur legal liability if failure to fulfill this obligation results in patient harm.

Discussion Questions

1. How would you work with E.M. to help her obtain the necessary resources and knowledge to care for her diabetes?
2. What can you do to begin working on the problems of health disparities in your community?

Factors and Conditions Leading to Health Disparities

Many factors and conditions can lead to the development of health disparities (Table 2.1). Awareness of these factors will help you provide optimal care for your patients.

Ethnicity and Race. The terms ethnicity and race are subjective and based on self-report. These terms are used interchangeably in conversation and are not defined by genetic markers. Social context and lived experiences influence people's decision about the ethnic and race category to which they identify or are assigned. For example, ethnic and race categories may differ on a person's birth certificate and death certificate.

People often identify their own ethnicity and race for health data collection (e.g., health plans, birth certificates). Collection of health data based on self-reported ethnic and race categories is important for research, to inform policy, and to understand and eliminate disparities. People identify their race using 1 or more categories. Law requires federal agencies to list a minimum of 5 race categories: white, black, American Indian or Alaska Native, Asian, and Native Hawaiian or other Pacific Islander. Federal agencies must also list a minimum of 2 ethnicities for people who self-identify as either *Hispanic or Latino* and *Not Hispanic or Latino*. A Hispanic or Latino is typically a person of Cuban, Mexican, Puerto Rican, South or Central American, or other Spanish descent, regardless of race. In this book, we use the terms *ethnicity* and *race* interchangeably or together.

Although dramatic improvements in treatments have prolonged life and improved quality of life for many, racial and ethnic minorities have benefited far less from these advances. Disparities are generally determined by comparing population groups. In the United States, minority groups include Hispanics/Latinos (17.8% of the U.S. population), blacks (13.3%), Asian Americans (5.7%), Native Hawaiians and other Pacific Islanders (0.2%), Native Americans and Native Alaskans (1.3%), and 2 or more races (2.6%) population.[3] The number for most of these groups is expected to increase in the coming decades.

Obesity and chronic illness rates for diabetes, hypertension, chronic obstructive pulmonary diseases, cancer, and stroke are higher among minority people. Racial, ethnic, and cultural differences exist in health services, treatments provided, and access to health care providers (HCPs). Race and ethnicity also influence disease risk and outcomes. For example, after myocardial infarction, minority patients are at greater risk of rehospitalization and death but are less likely than nonminority patients to receive potentially beneficial treatments.[4] Native Americans have a higher incidence of several types of cancers and are often diagnosed at later stages of disease, resulting in a poorer prognosis.[5] Numerous strategies are being developed to promote health equity and reduce disparities.

TABLE 2.1 Factors and Conditions Leading to Health Disparities

- Age	- Income status
- Disability status	- Lack of health care services access
- Education	
- Ethnicity and race	- Language barrier
- Gender	- Occupation or unemployment
- Health care provider attitudes/biases	- Place
- Health literacy	- Sexual orientation

PROMOTING HEALTH EQUITY

Promoting Health Equity Boxes Throughout Book

Place. Place refers to the geographic and environmental location where a person is born, grows, lives, works, and ages. Place affects the use of health services, health status, and health behaviors.

About 20% of Americans live in nonurban or rural areas.[6] Differences in access to health care services between rural and urban settings can create geographic health disparities. For example, rural populations and Native Americans living on reservations may need to travel long distances to receive health care. This can result in inadequate or less-frequent access to health care services. Some parts of the rural United States are "medically underserved" because of decreased numbers of HCPs per population.

People living in rural areas have higher rates of cancer, heart disease, diabetes, depression, and injury-related deaths than people living in urban areas. For example, in rural Appalachia the rates of lung, colon, cervical, and colorectal cancer are higher than the national average. Rural populations tend to be older than urban populations. Many rural areas have higher rates of obesity and chronic disease. The impact of social and physical environment on health choices can be illustrated by the problem of intimate partner violence in rural communities.[7] The decision to seek help is affected by geographic isolation, traditional gender roles, patriarchal attitudes, fear of lack of confidentiality, and economic factors that exist in some small rural communities.

Living in urban centers may also predispose a person to health disparities. Concerns about personal safety (e.g., clinics located in high-crime neighborhoods) can make patients reluctant to visit HCPs. High rates of chronic health problems and premature deaths occur in neighborhoods with social inequalities, including high poverty rates and residential segregation.

Among the most obvious health behaviors affected by place are physical activity and nutrition. Safe, walkable neighborhoods with playgrounds and sources of healthy foods promote physical activity and healthy eating. Social support positively affects coping with illness. Social networks are more likely to be found in communities where neighbors interact and rely on one another.

Income, Education, and Occupation. People of lower income, education, or occupational status experience worse health. In addition, they die at a younger age than those who are more affluent. Adults without a high school diploma or equivalent are 3 times more likely to die before age 65 than those with a college degree. Health care costs are 1 of the key factors that contribute to health disparities. People who have no insurance, are underinsured, or lack financial resources to pay for treatment of diseases may forgo health care visits, screenings, and treatments. Patients who lack the knowledge and/or access to apply for government assistance programs (e.g., Medicaid) are also at risk. Hazardous work environments and high-risk occupations of laborers increase health risk and contribute to higher rates of illness, injury, and death.

Health Literacy. *Health literacy* is defined as the degree to which a person has the capacity to obtain, process, and understand basic health information and services needed to make appropriate health decisions. This includes the ability to (1) read, understand, and analyze information; (2) understand instructions; (3) weigh risks and benefits; and (4) make decisions and take action. Low health literacy is associated with more hospitalizations, greater use of emergency department care, decreased use of cancer screening and influenza vaccine, decreased ability to use medications correctly, and higher mortality rates among older adults.

On a daily basis, patients need to self-manage conditions such as diabetes and asthma. For example, patients with diabetes may not be able to maintain adequate blood glucose levels if they cannot read or understand the numbers on the home glucose monitoring system. The inability to read and understand medication labels can result in taking medications at the wrong time or in the wrong dose. See Chapter 4 for more about health literacy.

Gender. Health disparities exist between men and women. Adult women use health care services more than men. Women may not receive the same quality of care (Fig. 2.1). For example, women are less likely than men to receive procedures (e.g., coronary angiography) for cardiovascular disease.[8] When gender is combined with racial and ethnic differences, the disparities are

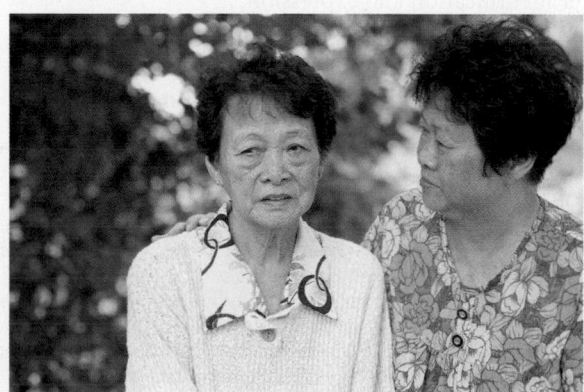

FIG. 2.1 Older Asian women are especially at risk for health disparities. (© szefei/iStock/Thinkstock.)

even greater. Gender Differences boxes throughout this book highlight gender differences in disease risk, manifestations, and treatment.

Age. Older adults are at risk for experiencing health disparities in the number of diagnostic tests done and aggressiveness of treatments used. Biases toward older adults that affect their care, or ageism, are discussed in Chapter 5. Older people of low socioeconomic status experience greater disability, more limitations in activities of daily living, and more frequent and rapid cognitive decline. Black and Latino older adults, in particular, are disproportionately affected by chronic illnesses, disability, depression, and substandard quality of life.[9]

Sexual Orientation. *Sexuality* is defined as a person's romantic, emotional, or sexual attraction to another person.

Lesbian, Gay, Bisexual, Transgender, and Queer or Questioning. Lesbian, gay, bisexual, transgender, and queer or questioning (LGBTQ) is a term that refers to the sexual orientation of these groups of people. LGBTQ persons encompass all races and ethnicities, religions, and social classes. Being LGBTQ places a person at risk for health disparities resulting from social, economic, or environmental disadvantages. Personal, family, and social acceptance of sexual orientation and gender identity affects the mental health and personal safety of LGBTQ persons. Discrimination against LGBTQ people has been associated with high rates of psychiatric disorders, substance abuse, and suicide.

LGBTQ people are more likely to be obese when compared with their heterosexual counterparts. Lesbian and bisexual women have higher rates of breast cancer and increased risk factors for cardiovascular disease. Gay and bisexual men have higher rates of human immunodeficiency virus and hepatitis infections than other groups.[10] Older LGBTQ persons may face added barriers to health because of isolation and a lack of social services and culturally competent providers.[9]

Understanding the cause of disparities among LGBTQ persons is essential to providing safe and high-quality care. One of the barriers to accessing high-quality health care by LGBTQ adults is the current lack of HCPs who are knowledgeable about their health needs. LGBTQ people may also experience fear of discrimination in health care settings.

Some health care settings are addressing the negative stereotypes that health care professionals may have, but of which they may not be aware. The Joint Commission (TJC) requires that patients be allowed the presence of a support person of their choice. In addition, hospitals must adopt policies that bar discrimination based on factors such as sexual orientation and gender identification and expression.

♥ **PROMOTING POPULATION HEALTH**

Improving the Health and Well-Being of LGBTQ Persons

- Provide supportive social services to reduce suicide among young LGBTQ persons.
- Inquire about and be supportive of a patient's sexual orientation to enhance the patient-provider interaction and patient's regular use of care.
- Implement antibullying policies in schools.
- Provide health care professionals with knowledge of the health needs of the LGBTQ community and training on LGBT mental health issues.
- Continue efforts to expand domestic partner health insurance coverage.
- Establish community advisory boards and LGBTQ health centers.
- Disseminate effective HIV and sexually transmitted infections interventions.

Health Care Provider Attitudes. Certain behaviors and biases of the HCP can contribute to health disparities. Factors such as bias and prejudice can affect health care-seeking behavior in minority populations. The health care system may also contribute to the problem of health disparities. For example, a clinic located in an area with a large population of Vietnamese immigrants that does not provide interpreters or educational materials and financial forms in Vietnamese may limit these families' ability to understand how to access health care.

Discrimination and *bias* based on a patient's race, ethnicity, gender, age, body size, sexual orientation, or ability to pay are likely to result in less aggressive or negative treatment practices. Discrimination can result in the delay of a proper diagnosis due to assumptions made about the patient. Sometimes discrimination is hard to recognize, especially when it occurs at the institutional level.

Because an HCP's overt discriminatory behavior may not be clear to the patient or yourself, it may be difficult to confront. Even well-intentioned providers who try to eliminate bias in their care can show their prior beliefs or prejudices through nonverbal communication. Many policies are in place to eliminate discrimination, but it still exists.

CULTURE

Culture is a way of life for a group of people. It includes the behaviors, beliefs, values, traditions, and symbols that the group accepts, generally without thinking about them. This way of life is passed along by communication and imitation from 1 generation to the next. You can also think of culture as cultivated behavior that one acquires through social learning. It is the totality of a person's learned, accumulated experience that is socially transmitted. The 4 classic characteristics of culture are described in Table 2.2.

Values are the sets of rules by which persons, families, groups, and communities live. They are the principles and standards that serve as the basis for beliefs, attitudes, and behaviors. Although all cultures have values, the types and expressions of those values differ from 1 culture to another. These cultural values develop over time, guide decision making and actions, and may affect a person's self-esteem. Cultural values often unconsciously develop early in life as a child learns about acceptable and unacceptable behaviors. The extent to which a person's cultural values are internalized influences that person's tendency toward judging other cultures, while usually using his or her own culture as the accepted standard. Table 2.3 provides some examples of cultural characteristics of different ethnic groups in the United States.

Although persons within a cultural group may have many similarities through their shared values, beliefs, and practices, there is also diversity within groups (Fig. 2.2). Each person is culturally unique. Such diversity may result from different perspectives and interpretations of situations. These differences may be based on age, gender, marital status, family structure, income, education level, religious views, and life experiences. Within any cultural group, there are smaller groups that may not hold all the values of the dominant culture. These smaller cultural groups have experiences that differ from those of the dominant group. These differences may be related to ethnic background, residence, religion, occupation, health, age, gender, education, or other factors that unite the group. Members

TABLE 2.2 Basic Characteristics of Culture

- *Dynamic* and ever-changing
- *Not always shared* by all members of a cultural group
- *Adapted* to specific conditions such as environmental factors
- *Learned* through oral and written histories, as well as socialization

TABLE 2.3 Cultural Characteristics of Different Ethnic Groups

Asian American
- Cultural foods
- Family loyalty
- Folk healing
- Harmonious relationships
- Harmony and balance within body vital for preservation of life energy
- Respect for elders
- Respect for one's parents and ancestors

Black
- Cultural foods
- Family networks
- Folk healing
- Importance of religion
- Interdependence within ethnic group
- Music and physical activities valued

European American
- Equal rights of genders
- Independence and freedom
- Individualistic and competitive
- Materialistic
- Self-reliance valued
- Youth and beauty valued

Hispanic/Latino
- Cultural foods
- Folk healing

- Extended family valued
- Interdependence and collectivism
- Involvement of family in social activities
- Religion and spirituality highly valued
- Respect for elders and authority

Native American
- Doing the honorable thing
- Folk healing
- Living in harmony with people and nature
- Respect for tribal elders and children
- Respect for all things living
- Return what is taken from nature
- Spiritual guidance

Pacific Islander American
- Collective concern and involvement
- Kinship alliance among nuclear and extended family
- Knowledge is collective; belongs to group, not a person
- Natural order and balanced relationships

Adapted from Andrews MM, Boyle JS: *Transcultural concepts in nursing care,* ed 7, Philadelphia, 2016, Lippincott Williams & Wilkins; and Giger JN, Davidhizar RE: *Transcultural nursing: Assessment and intervention,* ed 7, St Louis, 2016, Mosby.

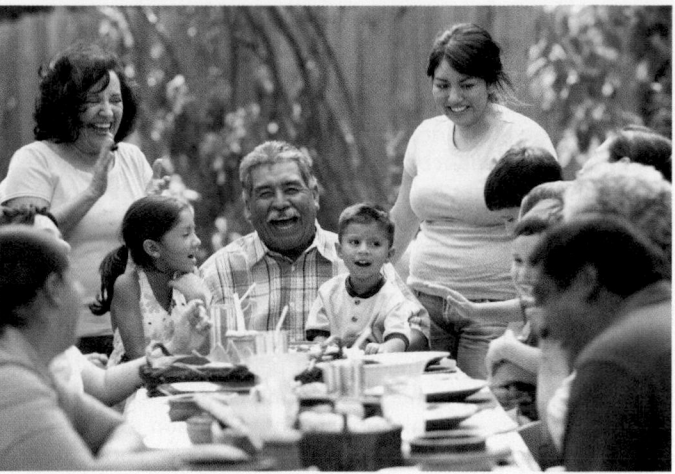

FIG. 2.2 Members of this family share a common heritage. (© Jack Hollingsworth/Photodisc/Thinkstock.)

Acculturation is the lifelong process of incorporating cultural aspects of the contexts in which a person grows, lives, works, and ages.[11] Acculturation is often bidirectional. In other words, the context changes as a person's culture influences it. Change may be in attitudes, behaviors, and values. For example, a sedentary person who loves to cook may change his or her attitude toward exercise when living with athletic roommates, who in turn also change as they begin to appreciate cooking. Behaviors change when an immigrant child learns the local language while influencing the conduct of classmates. A deeply held value such as self-sufficiency may change for a person exposed to a culture in which reliance on others dominates.

Newcomers may adopt both the strengths and limitations of the dominant culture. This is relevant when considering health behaviors and the quality of health care delivered by professionals. For example, an immigrant may be negatively influenced by a dominant cultural context in which unhealthy eating habits prevail.[12]

The result of acculturation may be new cultural variations in attitudes, behaviors, and values. All people take part in this process over their lives. People who move to a new cultural context are more aware of the acculturation experience than people who are not exposed to new experiences. Exposure to new cultural contexts increases a nurse's cultural competency.

Stereotyping refers to an overgeneralized viewpoint that members of a specific culture, race, or ethnic group are alike and share the same values and beliefs. This oversimplified approach does not consider the individual differences that exist within a culture. Being a member of a particular cultural, ethnic, or racial group does not make the person an expert on other members of that same group. Such stereotyping can lead to false assumptions and affect a patient's care. For example, it would be inappropriate for you to assume that just because a nurse is Mexican American, he would know how a Mexican American patient's beliefs may affect that patient's health care practices. As another example, a young Mexican American nurse born and raised in a large city has experienced a different culture than the older patient who was born and raised in a rural area of Mexico.

Ethnocentrism refers to the belief that one's own culture and worldview are superior to those of others from different cultural, ethnic, or racial backgrounds.[11] Comparing others' ways to your own can lead to seeing others as different or inferior. HCP's ethnocentrism can result in poor communication,

of a subculture share certain aspects of culture that are different from those of the overall cultural group. For example, among Hispanics some seek professional health care right away when symptoms appear. Other Hispanics rely first on folk healers. Others first seek the opinion of family and friends before seeking formal health care.

Cultural beliefs about symptom tolerance and health care–seeking behavior can contribute to health disparities. Some cultures consider pain something to be endured or ignored, and as a result, the patient does not seek help. Some cultures may view diseases or problems fatalistically; that is, people see no reason to seek treatment because they believe it is unlikely to have any benefit. Some cultures view the signs and symptoms of an illness as "God's will" or as a punishment for some prior behavior. In some cultures, it may not be acceptable to see an HCP who is not of the same gender or ethnic group. Such beliefs can result in delays in seeking health care or inadequate treatment.

patient alienation, and potentially inadequate treatment. To avoid ethnocentrism, you need to remain open to a variety of perspectives and maintain a nonjudgmental view of the values, beliefs, and practices of others. Failure to do this can result in ethnic stereotyping or cultural imposition.

Cultural imposition occurs when we impose our own cultural beliefs and practices on another person or group of people. In health care, it can result in disregarding or trivializing a patient's health care beliefs or practices. Cultural imposition may happen when an HCP is unaware of the patient's cultural beliefs and plans and implements care without taking them into account.

Cultural safety describes care and advocacy for a person of another culture determined by that person or family. Care that is culturally safe prevents cultural imposition. Culturally safe practice requires cultural competency and action to ensure that cultural histories, experiences, and traditions of patients, their families, and communities are valued and shape health care approaches and policies.[13]

Madeleine Leininger coined the term **transcultural nursing** in the 1950s. Transcultural nursing is a specialty that focuses on the comparative study and analysis of cultures and subcultures. The goal of transcultural nursing is the discovery of culturally relevant facts that can guide the nurse in providing culturally appropriate care.[11]

CULTURAL COMPETENCE

Cultural competence is the ability to understand, appreciate, and work with people from cultures other than your own. It involves an awareness and acceptance of cultural differences, self-awareness, knowledge of the patient's culture, and adaptation of skills to meet the patient's needs. The 4 components of cultural competence are (1) cultural awareness, (2) cultural knowledge, (3) cultural skill, and (4) cultural encounter (Table 2.4).

We present specific information throughout this book to help you develop an awareness of cultural differences and learning assessment skills for different cultural groups. Table 2.8 (later in this chapter) presents a cultural assessment guide. It may be helpful to review general cultural characteristics associated with a cultural group when preparing to interview a patient. However, recognize that the patient may not identify with the assumed cultural group and the provider's own biases and stereotypes may affect the patient and result in more patient-provider barriers.

Providing culturally competent care may increase patient satisfaction, promote health equity, increase patient safety, and prevent misunderstandings between you and your patients.[14] It also involves integrating cultural practices into Western medicine. For example, before some diagnostic procedures and interventions, it is typical to have patients remove personal objects they are wearing on the body. Ask patients whether they wear personal objects and the significance of their removal, since they may have cultural or spiritual significance. You should know whether wearing these objects will compromise patient safety, test results, or outcomes of the intervention.

CULTURAL DIVERSITY IN THE HEALTH CARE WORKPLACE

Poorer health outcomes for minorities are linked to the shortage of culturally and ethnically diverse HCPs, who have historically

TABLE 2.4 **How to Develop Cultural Competence**

Description	Role of Nurse
Cultural Awareness	
• Ability to understand patients' unique cultural needs	• Understand your own cultural background, values, and beliefs, especially as related to health and health care.
	• Examine your own cultural biases toward people whose cultures differ from your own culture.
Cultural Knowledge	
• Process of learning key aspects of a group's culture, especially as it relates to health and health care practices	• Learn basic general information about predominant cultural groups in your geographic area. Cultural pocket guides can be a good resource.
• Patients are best source of information about their culture	• Assess patients for presence or absence of cultural traits based on an understanding of generalizations about a cultural group.
	• Do not make assumptions based on cultural background because the degree of acculturation varies among persons.
	• Read research studies that describe cultural differences.
	• Read ethnic newspaper articles and books.
	• View documentaries about cultural groups.
Cultural Skill	
• Ability to collect relevant cultural data	• Be alert for unexpected responses with patients, especially as related to cultural issues.
• Performance of a cultural assessment	• Become aware of cultural differences in predominant ethnic groups.
	• Develop assessment skills to do a competent cultural assessment for any patient (see Table 2.8).
	• Learn assessment skills for different cultural groups, including cultural beliefs and practices.
Cultural Encounter	
• Direct cross-cultural interactions between people from culturally diverse backgrounds	• Create opportunities to interact with predominant cultural groups.
• Extended contact with a cultural group to enhance understanding of its values and beliefs	• Attend cultural events, such as religious ceremonies, significant life passage rituals, social events, and demonstrations of cultural practices.
	• Visit markets and restaurants in ethnic neighborhoods.
	• Explore ethnic neighborhoods, listen to different types of ethnic music, and learn games of various ethnic groups.
	• Visit or volunteer at health fairs in local ethnic neighborhoods.
	• Learn about prominent cultural beliefs and practices and incorporate this knowledge into planning nursing care.

been underrepresented in the health professions. A diversity gap exists between the ethnic composition of the interprofessional health care team and the overall population in the United States (Fig. 2.3). For example, the diversity of nurses in the United States is increasing but still lags that of the overall population. Blacks, Hispanic/Latino Americans, and Native Americans make up more than 35% of the population but only

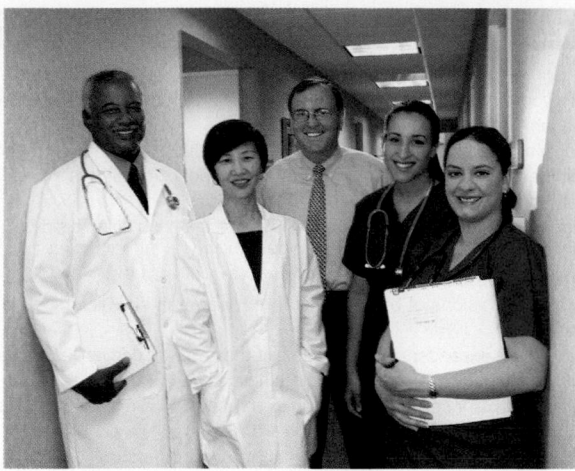

FIG. 2.3 Interprofessional team working together in a multicultural health care environment. (© Thinkstock/Stockbyte/Thinkstock.)

24% of the nation's nurses.[3,15] Biased behaviors against nurses of diverse cultural and ethnic backgrounds by patients and health care professionals may contribute to their underrepresentation.

Cultural differences exist in how well patients think they can communicate with their HCP. In the United States, minority patients are more likely to have difficulty communicating with their HCP.[16] Communication issues include not understanding the HCP, feeling that they are not listened to, and having questions but not asking them. As more internationally educated nurses join the workforce, sufficient training and transitional support must be in place to ensure communication and quality of care.

When HCPs from different cultures work together as members of the health care team, opportunities for miscommunication and conflict can occur. This is termed *cultural conflict*. The cultural origins of miscommunication and conflict in the workplace are often interconnected with cultural beliefs, values, and etiquette. Seeking clarification about misperceptions and misunderstandings is a communication strategy to foster effective teamwork among a multicultural health care team. To ensure the recruitment and retention of nurses from minority populations, all members of the health care team and leadership must create an environment that promotes effective cross-cultural communication and reduces bias and discrimination.

CULTURAL FACTORS AFFECTING HEALTH AND HEALTH CARE

Many cultural factors affect the patient's health and health care. Several potential factors are outlined in Table 2.5.

Folk Healers and Traditions

Many cultures have folk healers, who are also known as *traditional healers*. Most folk healers speak the person's native language and cost less than conventional HCPs. Among the many folk healers found worldwide, Hispanics, particularly from regions in Mexico and Central and South America, may choose to use a *curandero* (or *curandera*); blacks may visit a *hougan*; Native Americans may seek help from a medicine man or *shaman*; and Asian Americans may use folk healers such as a Chinese herbal therapist. In addition to folk healers, some cultures involve lay midwives (e.g., *parteras* for Hispanic women) in the care of pregnant women.

TABLE 2.5 Cultural Factors Affecting Health and Health Care

Beliefs and Practices
- Care provided in established health care programs may not be perceived as culturally relevant.
- Religious reasons, beliefs, or practices may affect a person's decision to seek (or not seek) health care.
- Patients may delay seeking health care because of fear or dependence on folk medicine and herbal remedies.
- Patients may stop treatment or visits for health care because the symptoms are no longer present and they think that further care is not needed.
- Some patients associate hospitals and extended care facilities with death.
- The patient may have had a previous negative experience with culturally incompetent HCPs or discriminatory practices.
- Some people mistrust the majority population and institutions dominated by them.
- Some patients may feel apprehensive about unfamiliar diagnostic procedures and treatment options.

Communication and Language
- Patients may not speak English and may not be able to communicate with the HCP.
- It may be hard to communicate, even with interpreters.

Economic Factors
- Patients may not get health care because they cannot pay for it or because of the costs associated with travel for health care.
- Refugee or undocumented immigrant status may deter some patients from using the health care system.
- Immigrant women who are heads of households or single mothers may not seek health care for themselves because of child care costs.
- Patients may lack health insurance.

Health Care System
- Patients may not make or keep appointments because of the time lag between the onset of an illness and an available appointment.
- Hours of operation of health care facilities may not accommodate patients' need to work or use public transportation.
- Requirements to access some types of care may discourage some patients from taking the steps to qualify for health care or health care payment assistance.
- Some patients have a general distrust of HCPs and health care systems.
- Lack of ethnic-specific health care programs may deter some people from seeking health care.
- Transportation may be a problem for patients who must travel long distances for health care.
- Adequate interpreter services may be unavailable.
- Patients may not have a primary HCP and may use emergency departments or urgent care centers for health care.
- Shortages of HCPs from specific ethnic groups may deter some people from seeking health care.
- Patients may lack knowledge about the availability of existing health care resources.
- Facility policies may not be culturally competent (e.g., hospital policy may limit the number of visitors, which is problematic for cultures that value having many family members present).

Time Orientation
- For some cultures, it is more important to attend to a social role than to arrive on time for an appointment with an HCP.
- Some cultures are future oriented; others are past or present oriented.

TABLE 2.6 Health-Related Beliefs and Practices of Selected Religious Groups

Amish
- Prohibit drinking alcoholic beverages
- Prohibit abortion, artificial insemination, and stem cell use
- Seldom buy commercial health insurance
- Prohibit drugs unless prescribed by HCPs

Buddhism
- Prohibit drinking alcoholic beverages and using illicit drugs
- Practice moderation in diet and avoidance of extremes
- Central tenets are maintaining right views, intentions, speech, actions, livelihood, effort, mindfulness, and concentration

Catholicism
- Fast and abstain from meat and meat products on Ash Wednesday and the Fridays of Lent
- Prohibit artificial contraception and direct abortion
- Indirect abortion (e.g., treatment of uterine cancer in a pregnant woman) may be morally justified
- Sacrament of the Sick includes anointing of sick with oil, blessing by a priest, and communion (unleavened wafer made of flour and water)

Church of Jesus Christ of Latter-Day Saints (Mormons)
- Strict dietary code called Word of Wisdom prohibits all alcoholic beverages, hot drinks (nonherbal teas and coffee), tobacco, and recreational drugs
- Fast for a 24-hour period each month on "Fast Sunday"
- During hospitalization or serious illness, an elder anoints the ill person with oil while a second elder seals the anointing with a prayer and blessing (laying on of hands)
- Prohibit abortion except when the mother's life is in danger

Hinduism
- Prohibit eating meat because it involves harming a living creature
- Cremation is the usual form of body disposal, but fetuses or newborns are sometimes buried

Islam
- Fasting during daytime hours occurs during a month-long period called Ramadan
- Perform a ritual cleansing with water before eating and before prayer
- Prohibit eating pork or taking medicines with pork derivatives
- Prohibit drinking alcoholic beverages
- Artificial insemination is permissible only if from the husband to his own wife

Jehovah's Witness
- Prohibit transfusions of blood in any form or agents in which blood is an ingredient
- Blood volume expanders are acceptable if they are not derivatives of blood
- Prohibit transplants that involve bodily mutilation
- Prohibit artificial insemination and therapeutic and on-demand abortions

Judaism
- Prohibit eating pork, shellfish, or predatory fowl or mixing milk dishes and meat dishes when preparing foods
- Certain foods and drinks are designated as kosher, which means "proper." All animals must be ritually slaughtered
- On the eighth day after birth, boys are circumcised in a ritual called Brit Milah. Girls are given a dedication ceremony involving prayers and blessings
- Prohibit abortion except when the mother's life is in danger
- Organized support system for the sick includes a visit from the rabbi. The rabbi may pray with the sick person alone or in a minyan, a group of 10 adults over age 13
- If an autopsy is done, all body parts must be returned for burial

Seventh-Day Adventism
- Encourage a vegetarian diet
- Nonvegetarian members do not eat foods derived from any animal having a cloven hoof that chews its cud (e.g., pigs, goats).
- Prohibit eating shellfish; eating fish with fins and scales is acceptable
- Prohibit drinking alcoholic beverages
- Healthy church members practice voluntary fasting

Data from Andrews MM, Boyle JS: *Transcultural concepts in nursing care,* ed 7, Philadelphia, 2016, Lippincott Williams & Wilkins.

Folk medicine and traditions are culturally based forms of prevention and treatment. They traditionally rely on oral transmission of healing techniques from 1 generation to the next. The patient may not use the term *folk medicine* but thinks of these as cultural home remedies or treatment practices. A patient can be practicing folk medicine at home without using a folk healer. It is important to assess whether the patient is practicing traditional or folk healing.

Some traditions that are practiced as a rite of passage in some cultures are considered harmful in the dominant culture in the United States. For example, female genital cutting is a tradition that is illegal in most countries yet still practiced in many countries in Africa and the Middle East. It results in physical and emotional trauma and may affect childbirth. Nurses can advocate for immigrant women who have experienced this trauma and to prevent return of young girls to their country of origin for the procedure.

Spirituality and Religion

Spirituality and religion are aspects of culture that may affect a person's beliefs about health, illness, and end-of-life care. They may also play a role in nutrition and decisions related to health, wellness, and how to respond to or treat an illness.

Spirituality refers to a person's effort to find purpose and meaning in life. It is influenced by a person's unique life experiences and reflects one's personal understanding of life's mysteries. Spirituality relates to the soul or spirit more than to the body, and it may provide hope and strength for a person during an illness.

Religion is a more formal and organized system of beliefs, including belief in or worship of God or gods. Religious beliefs include the cause, nature, and purpose of the universe and involve prayer and rituals. Religion is based on beliefs about life, death, good, and evil. You can use several interventions to meet a patient's religious and spiritual needs, including prayer, scripture reading, listening, and referral to a chaplain, rabbi, or priest.

Many patients find that rituals help them during times of illness. Rituals help a person make sense of life experiences and may take the form of prayer, meditation, or other rituals that the patient may create. You should include spiritual questions in your patient assessment and plan care accordingly. Table 9.5 has a spiritual assessment guide that may be used with patients. Table 2.6 summarizes health-related beliefs and practices of selected religious groups.

Cross-Cultural Communication

Communication refers to an organized, patterned system of behavior that may be verbal or nonverbal (Fig. 2.4). *Verbal communication* includes not only one's language or dialect, but also voice tone, volume, timing, and ability to share thoughts and feelings. More than 45 million people in the United States speak a language other than English in their home, with Spanish being

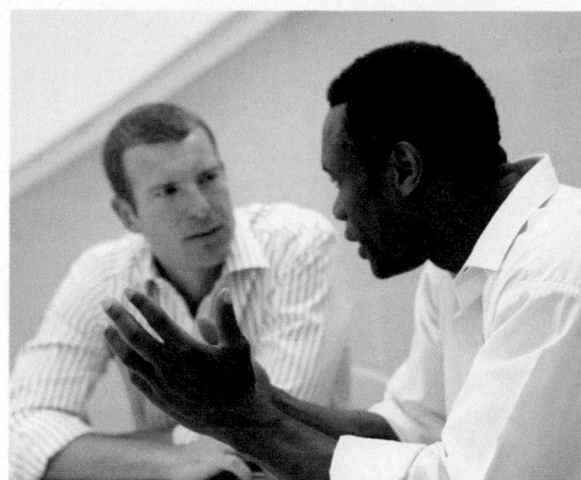

FIG. 2.4 Co-workers from different cultures communicate with verbal and nonverbal cues. (© BananaStock/Thinkstock.)

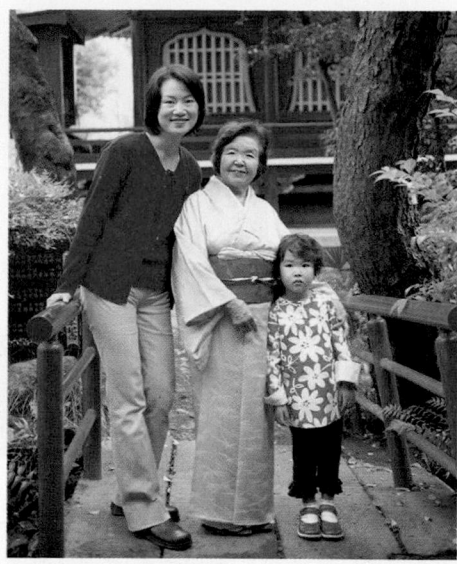

FIG. 2.5 Family roles and relationships differ from 1 culture to another. (© Jupiterimages/Photos.com/Thinkstock.)

the most common. Hispanic people who do not speak English at home are less likely to receive a variety of health care services even if they are comfortable speaking English.

Nonverbal communication may take the form of writing, gestures, body movements, posture, facial expressions, and personal dress in some cultures. It also includes eye contact, use of touch, body language, style of greeting, and spatial distancing. Eye contact varies greatly among cultural groups. Patients who are Asian, Arab, or Native American may avoid direct eye contact and consider it disrespectful or aggressive. Hispanic patients may expect you to look directly at them but may not return that direct gaze. Other variables to consider include the role of gender, age, acculturation, status, or appropriate eye contact. For example, Muslim-Arab women exhibit modesty when avoiding eye contact with men other than their husbands and when in public situations.

Silence has many meanings. It is important to understand the meaning of silence for different cultural groups. Some people are comfortable with silence. Others become uncomfortable and may speak to decrease the amount of silent time. It is important to clarify what silence means in an interaction with a patient. Patients sometimes nod their head or say "yes" as if agreeing with you or to show they understand. Actually, they may be doing this because it is a culturally acceptable manner of showing respect, not because they understand or agree.

Many Native Americans are comfortable with silence and interpret silence as essential for thinking and carefully considering a response. In these interactions, silence shows respect for the other person and shows the importance of the remarks. In traditional Japanese and Chinese cultures, the speaker may stop talking and leave a period of silence for the listener to think about what was said before continuing. Silence may show respect for the speaker's privacy. In some cultures (e.g., French, Spanish, and Russian) the person may interpret silence as meaning agreement. Asian Americans may use silence to show respect for elders. Blacks may use silence as a response to what they perceive to be an inappropriate question.

Racism and microaggression affect communication. *Racism* is a belief that differences among the various racial/ethnic groups determine cultural or individual achievement. It usually involves the idea that one's own race/ethnicity is superior and

has the right to dominate others or that a particular racial/ethnic group is inferior to the others.

Microaggression is social exchanges in which a person says or does something that can either intentionally or unintentionally belittle or alienate a person, especially someone of a different racial/ethnic group. It is imperative that nurses seek to understand racism and microaggression through education, self-awareness, and open dialogue with peers.[17]

Family Roles and Relationships

Family roles differ from 1 culture to another (Fig. 2.5). It is important for you to determine who should be involved in communication and decision making related to health care. Some cultural groups emphasize interdependence rather than independence. In the United States, many in the mainstream culture have strong beliefs related to autonomy. We expect a patient to sign consent forms when receiving health care. In some cultural groups, the patient may expect a family member to make health care decisions. When you encounter a patient who values interdependence over independence, the health care system may have difficulty with how the patient makes decisions. We may have to delay treatment while the patient waits for family members to arrive before giving consent for a procedure or treatment. In other instances, the patient may make a decision that is best for the family despite adverse outcomes for the patient. Being aware of such values will better prepare you to advocate for the patient.

Some cultural differences relate to expectations of family members in providing care. In some cultures, family members expect to provide care for the patient even in the hospital. The patient may expect that the family, along with the HCPs, will provide all care. This view is the opposite of the predominant Western expectation that the patient will assume self-care as quickly as possible.

Ask about culturally relevant gender relationships. For example, in some cultures, such as many Arab groups, it is not appropriate for a man to be alone with a woman other than his wife. Nor is it appropriate for a woman other than a man's wife

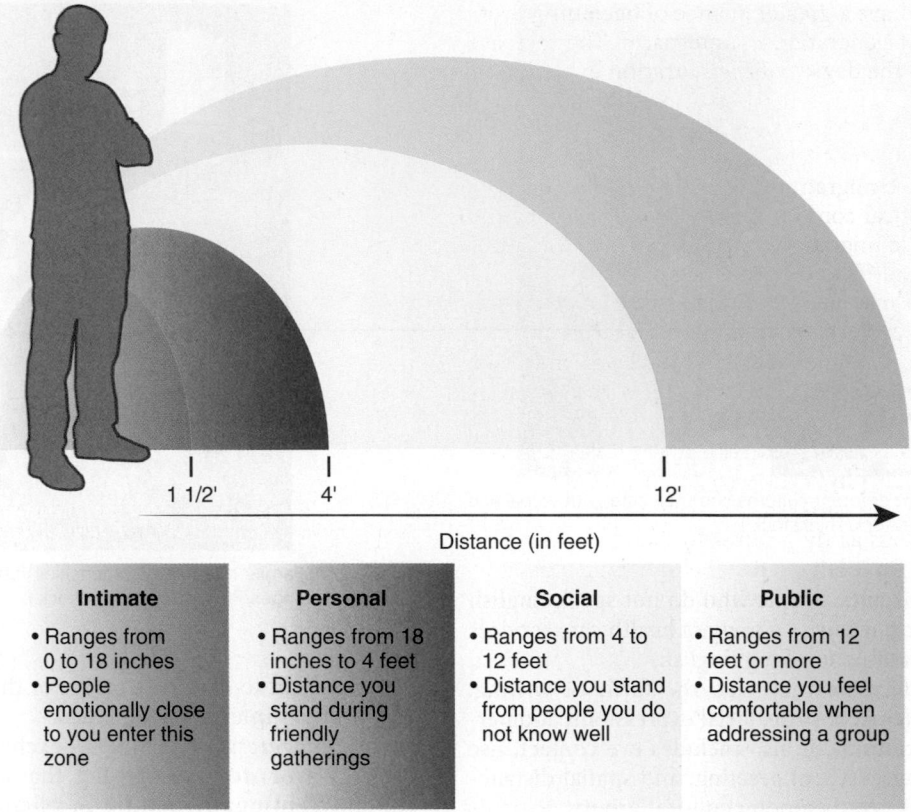

FIG 2.6 Personal space zones.

Intimate	Personal	Social	Public
• Ranges from 0 to 18 inches • People emotionally close to you enter this zone	• Ranges from 18 inches to 4 feet • Distance you stand during friendly gatherings	• Ranges from 4 to 12 feet • Distance you stand from people you do not know well	• Ranges from 12 feet or more • Distance you feel comfortable when addressing a group

to provide physical care for him. The clinical implication of this cultural belief is that for many patients from Arab cultures, nurses cannot provide direct physical care for patients of the opposite gender. In some instances, patients may only receive procedures or treatments from providers of the opposite gender if a third party is present.

Personal Space

Personal space zones are the variable and subjective distance at which 1 person feels comfortable talking to another. A representative example of personal space zones for European Americans is shown in Fig. 2.6. Personal space distances vary from culture to culture, as well as within a culture. As a nurse, you often interact with patients in the intimate or personal distance, which may be uncomfortable for the patient.

Cultural groups have wide variations in their perception of appropriate distances. An American nurse of European descent may be comfortable with a certain distance. A person from a Hispanic or Middle Eastern background may believe that the distance is too far and will move closer, perhaps causing you to feel uncomfortable. If you then move away to a more comfortable distance, this may cause the other person to think that you are unfriendly or the person may be offended.

Touch

Physical contact with patients conveys various meanings depending on the culture. Performing a comprehensive assessment requires touching a patient. Many people of Asian and Hispanic heritage believe that touching a person's head is a sign of disrespect because the head is the source of one's

strength and/or soul. Many people in the world believe in the evil eye, or *mal ojo*. In this culture-bound syndrome, the illness—usually in a child or a woman—resulted from excessive admiration by another person. In some cultures, the proper way to ward off the evil eye is to touch the area of admiration. For example, if the person admires the hair, the top of the head may be touched. It is important for you to ask permission before touching anyone, particularly if it is necessary to touch the person's head.

Nutrition

An important part of cultural practices is food, including both the foods that are eaten and rituals and practices associated with food. Muslims fast during the daytime during the Islamic month of Ramadan. Such practices may affect when and how patients take medications. Patients may need to make major changes in their diets because of health problems. A person may use food to cope with life changes such as homesickness. Specific foods may be considered essential to good health during pregnancy or other life stages. The HCP should consider food-related cultural beliefs, practices, and habits when discussing nutrition with patients and planning their diets.

When people immigrate to an area that is very different from their country of origin, they may experience unfamiliar foods, food-storage systems, and food-buying habits. They may come from countries that have limited food supplies because of poverty, wars, and poor sanitation. They may arrive with conditions such as malnutrition, diarrhea, and dental caries. Other problems may develop after the person arrives in the new country. For example, second-generation

Hispanic immigrants have a greater chance of becoming overweight than their first-generation counterparts. The increase in weight is related to the degree of acculturation experienced by the immigrant.

Immigrants and Immigration

Several conditions drive migration, such as overcrowding, natural disasters, geopolitical conflict, persecution, and economic forces. Because of these migrations, a rich diversity of cultures exists in many communities and countries today (Fig. 2.7).

Recent immigrants may be at risk for physical and mental health problems for many reasons. Conditions in their countries of origin (e.g., malnutrition, poor sanitation, civil war) may have resulted in chronic health problems. In addition, recent immigrants are at increased risk for health problems after arriving in a new area. Relocation is associated with many losses and can cause economic hardship, physical stress, and mental distress.

As new immigrants go through the acculturation process, many have cultural stress as they adjust to their new environment, especially if they have left relatives behind or are unable to return to their home country. Older immigrants are especially affected by changes in role and social position. This may result in depression. Immigrants who have survived wars and violence may have posttraumatic stress disorder. Immigrants may face barriers to social acceptance, such as prejudice or discrimination, and experience a lack of ethnic and cultural resources. For some, it may mean loss of the social status that they experienced in their countries of origin.

Another potential problem is tuberculosis (TB). Two-thirds of the TB cases in the United States occur in people born outside the country.[18] Those who have recently immigrated from areas that have a high endemic rate of TB are more likely to have TB. Foreign-born Hispanics and Asians combined account for 48% of the nation's TB cases. The top 5 countries of the origin of foreign-born people with TB are Mexico, Philippines, Vietnam, India, and China. The *Refugee Health Guidelines* from the Centers for Disease Control and Prevention supports early identification and treatment.[19]

During the past 45 years, the migration pattern of North America has shifted. Once most immigrants came from Europe. Now, most originate from Asia, Latin America, and Africa. Additionally, an increased number of first- and second-generation immigrants enter the United States after visiting friends and relatives. They have a higher risk for malaria, typhoid fever, cholera, and hepatitis A than people born in the United States. Many immigrants lack health insurance and may primarily obtain their health care in emergency departments and urgent care clinics. Therefore nurses in all settings need to be aware of refugee health screening, treatment recommendations, and resources for access to health care and social services.

Drugs

Genetic differences among people from diverse ethnic or racial groups may explain differences in drug choice, dosage, or administration. For example, some drugs are more effective in certain ethnic groups than others. Side effects may vary among persons from diverse backgrounds.

Genetic variations can affect how the body processes a drug and the overall effect of selected drugs on the body. Although race and ethnicity are imprecise indicators of genetic differences, they can be helpful in predicting variations in the

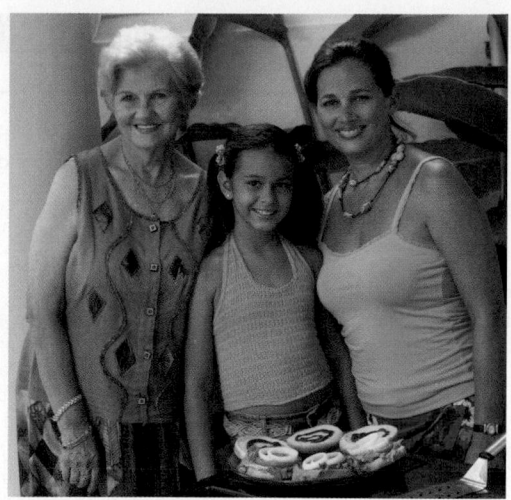

FIG. 2.7 Recently arrived immigrants join a neighbor for a barbecue, a common American tradition. (© Jack Hollingsworth/Photodisc/Thinkstock.)

response to drugs. For example, European Americans respond better to angiotensin-converting enzyme (ACE) inhibitors and β-blockers than blacks. Genetics and drug metabolism are discussed in Chapter 12.

Regardless of their cultural origins, many people use cultural remedies and prescription drugs to treat illness. Problems can result from interactions of these substances. For example, some Mexican Americans may treat gastrointestinal problems with preparations that contain lead. Some people may self-treat their depression with St. John's wort, which can result in adverse effects if taken with prescription antidepressants.

Patients may avoid standard Western medicine until herbs and other remedies become ineffective or the illness becomes acute. The challenge for you is to try to accommodate the patient's desire for traditional aspects of care while using evidence-based approaches that are appropriate and acceptable to the patient. Evaluate the safety and appropriateness of the patient's traditional cultural healing therapies.

Develop a collaborative, trusting relationship with patients and encourage them to discuss their traditional approaches to healing. Seek out information on potential drug and herbal product interaction from the pharmacist. Honor the patient's choices, if safe and effective, since this will enhance collaboration and may have a positive impact on health outcomes.

Psychologic Factors

Symptoms are interpreted through a person's cultural norms and may vary from the recognized interpretations of Western medicine. All symptoms have meaning, and the meanings may vary from 1 culture to another. For example, the degree of depression following a cardiac diagnosis is mediated by cultural views. It is important to ask patients what their illness means to them, what they believe is the cause, and what they think is the best treatment.

Culture-bound syndromes are illnesses or afflictions that are recognized only within a cultural group (Table 2.7). The symptoms, course of the illness, and people's reactions to the illness are limited to specific cultures. Culture-bound syndromes are expressed through psychologic or physical symptoms.

TABLE 2.7 Culture-Bound Syndromes

Syndrome	Description
Blacks	
Brain Fag	Term describing brain "fatigue" caused by the challenges of school. Symptoms include difficulties concentrating, remembering, and thinking.
Thin Blood	Affects older adults, women, and children. Weakens a person and increases susceptibility to illness.
Cambodians	
Koucharang or Kit Chroeun	Translates as "thinking too much," brought about by having seen or experienced a horrific trauma. Characterized by physical and emotional exhaustion, immobilization, and constant preoccupation with past suffering and loss.
Caribbean and Southern United States	
Falling Out	Characterized by a sudden collapse, which may sometimes be preceded by dizziness or "swimming" in the head. The person can hear but is unable to move.
Chinese	
Shenjing Shuairuo	Characterized by physical and mental fatigue, headaches and other pains, dizziness, sleep disturbances, and concentration difficulties.
Hispanics/Latinos	
Bilis or Colera	Caused by strong anger or rage. Anger results in excess bile that gets into the systemic circulation. Symptoms include acute nervous tension, headache, trembling, screaming, stomach disturbances, and, in severe cases, loss of consciousness.
Ataque de Nervios	Brought on by a stressful family event (e.g., death, divorce). Symptoms may include uncontrollable shouting, crying, trembling, and verbal or physical aggression.
Empacho	The perception that an undigested food bolus is "stuck" somewhere in the gastrointestinal tract, causing nausea, pain, and diarrhea.
Susto	Sometimes referred to as "fright sickness" or "soul loss." A traumatic anxiety-depressive state that may result from a frightening experience, such as a loud sound or some threat. Can cause anxiety, insomnia, listlessness, loss of appetite, and social withdrawal. One treatment is to have the affected person lie on the floor. The healer then sweeps indigenous herbs over the person's body while praying to release the evil wind.
Koreans	
Hwa-Byung	Ailment characterized by resentment that is brought about by bitterness and discontent.
Native Americans	
Ghost Sickness	Condition sometimes associated with witchcraft and a preoccupation with death. Symptoms include general weakness, loss of appetite, a feeling of suffocation, recurring nightmares, and a pervasive feeling of terror

❖ NURSING MANAGEMENT: PROMOTING HEALTH EQUITY AND INCREASING CULTURAL COMPETENCY

Nurse's Self-Assessment

The first step in promoting health equity and providing culturally competent care is for you to assess your own cultural background, values, and beliefs, especially those that are related to health and health care. Many tools are available to help you with this process (http://nccc.georgetown.edu).

Table 2.4 suggests ways for you to improve your cultural competence. This information can help you better understand patients and provide culturally competent care. It is important to understand that cultures evolve and change over time. Culturally competent care requires continual learning and self-reflection. Many other important aspects of culture related to health care are included in the Culturally Competent Care sections throughout this book.

In today's increasingly multicultural environment, you will meet patients, families, significant others, and members of the health care team from many different cultures. You will find yourself in patient care situations that require an understanding of the patient's cultural beliefs and practices. Even when you provide care for patients from your own cultural background, you may be from a different subculture than the patient. For example, there are more than 550 federally recognized Native American tribes in the United States. It would be inappropriate for you to assume that a Native American nurse can give culturally appropriate care to a Native American patient when the nurse may be from a different tribe. A white nurse from an urban upbringing may find cultural differences with a white patient from a rural community. Cultural competence is a lifelong process that involves self-reflection and continual learning.[20]

Patient Assessment

HCPs play a key role in promoting health equity. However, the causes of health disparities are not always easy to identify. Assess patients for their risk for reduced health care services because of limited access, inadequate resources, age, or low health literacy.

A cultural assessment should be included in the nursing process.[21] Table 2.8 lists important components of the assessment. Determine the patient's (1) health beliefs and health care practices and (2) perspective of the meaning, cause, and preferred treatment of illness. Ask questions that you are comfortable with based on your own culture.

How can you be aware of the differences among ethnic groups? Using guides for cultural assessment will facilitate the nursing process when working with patients, families, or other groups who are from different cultures. Although guides can help in this process, you need to be careful not to stereotype or assume that common cultural characteristics pertain to each patient. Use guides to explore the degree to which patients share commonalities with the traits attributed to their cultural group. You need to know about traditional characteristics of cultural groups while recognizing that culture is constantly evolving and unique for each person.

Nursing Implementation

Although the issues associated with health disparities can seem overwhelming, several strategies are available to reduce and eliminate health disparities. Table 2.9 presents nursing interventions to promote health equity.

Advocacy. The solutions to reduce health disparities often rest with the policymakers. Economic issues often determine health care delivery. Access and public policy decisions determine who is eligible for federal and state health insurance coverage. You, along with the social worker, can help by identifying key resources in the community, including transportation services,

TABLE 2.8 Cultural Assessment

A cultural assessment should include the following:
- Brief history of the cultural group with which person identifies
- Communication
- Cultural sanctions and restrictions
- Educational background
- Health-related beliefs and practices
- Nutrition
- Organizations providing cultural support
- Religious affiliation
- Socioeconomic considerations
- Spiritual considerations
- Values orientation

Adapted from Jarvis C: *Physical examination and health assessment,* ed 7, Philadelphia, 2016, Saunders.

TABLE 2.9 Nursing Management

Interventions to Promote Health Equity
- Treat all patients equally.
- Be aware of your own biases or prejudices and work toward eliminating them.
- Learn about services and programs that focus on specific cultural/ethnic groups.
- Inform patients about health care services available for their specific cultural/ethnic group.
- Make sure the same standards of care are followed for all patients regardless of culture or ethnicity.
- Recognize health care practices and cultural practices that are important to cultural and ethnic identity.
- Take part in research focused on understanding and improving care to culturally and ethnically diverse populations.
- Identify stereotypic attitudes toward a culture/ethnic group that may interfere with getting appropriate health care.
- Support patients who are fearful about traveling outside the accepted neighborhood for health care services.
- Advocate for patients of specific cultural/ethnic groups to receive health care services that pay special attention to English-language limitations and cultural health practices.
- Learn advocacy and interpersonal strategies from leaders of specific cultural/ethnic groups. For example, blacks may respond to themes such as "do it for your loved ones." Asian Americans may respond to fear of dependency themes.
- Ensure availability of culturally appropriate patient educational resources.

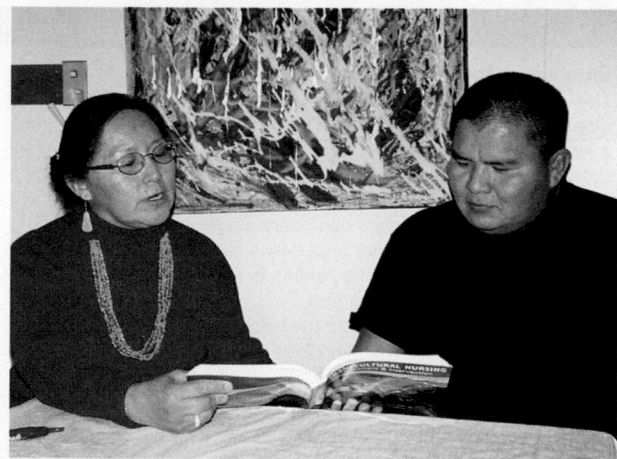

FIG. 2.8 A Navajo nurse teaching a Navajo patient. (From Giger JN: *Transcultural nursing,* ed 7, St Louis, 2016, Mosby.)

The National Standards for Culturally and Linguistically Appropriate Services in Health Care (CLAS standards) are guidelines that improve the quality of health care.[22] The CLAS standards provide practical guidance for care of people with limited English proficiency and of diverse cultural backgrounds.

Communication. Improving interpersonal skills is an important first step in providing culturally competent care. To show respect for the patient, consider the patient's usual communication style. For instance, conduct a health history in an unhurried manner and in a way that is appropriate for the culture. In some cultures, it is best to start with general rather than direct questions. For some cultures, it is most effective to engage in "small talk," with the discussion including answers that may seem to be unrelated to the questions. If you appear to be "too busy," communication may be impaired.

When meeting patients or family members, introduce yourself and indicate how you would like them to address you—whether they should use first names; Mr., Ms., or Mrs.; or a title, such as Nurse. Ask the patient how he or she prefers to be addressed. This shows respect and will help you begin the relationship in a culturally appropriate manner.

If you need to gather personal information, it is important to understand the most effective approach to use. For instance, when talking with people from some cultural groups, it is imperative that you take time to establish trust and listen to the patient's responses to questions. There may be long silences as the person thinks about the question, showing respect by giving the question proper consideration before answering. Take time to listen and help establish trust.

Consider how the patient's age may affect his or her views and communication. For example, black older adults with mental health concerns may struggle with shame, uncertainty, and lack of trust in the system.

Do not try to serve as an interpreter if your patient does not understand English, because this could lead to misunderstandings. Get the help of a person who is qualified to do medical interpretation when you cannot speak the patient's primary language (Table 2.10). Interpreters are available by phone anywhere in the United States through a fee-based service. Use them rather than a family member. Table 2.11 offers guidelines for communicating when no interpreter is available.

reduced-fee screening programs, and appropriate federal and state offices for Medicaid and Medicare.

You can be an advocate in your health care setting by helping to create a community advisory group. Such a group can be very helpful when setting up health programs within a community. This can increase the distribution of culturally sensitive information. Another powerful strategy is to increase the number of underrepresented populations in the health care professions (Fig. 2.8).

Standardized Guidelines. The use of standardized, evidence-based care guidelines can reduce disparities in diagnosis and treatments. For example, the management of hypertension should be based on guidelines and the patient's BP, symptoms, history, and laboratory values rather than other characteristics such as gender, age, or culture. Following the guidelines reduces racial or cultural differences in outcomes. In addition, recommendations related to cultural competency will guide you in your learning and practice.

TABLE 2.10 Using a Medical Interpreter

Choosing an Interpreter

- Use an agency interpreter if possible.
- Use a trained medical interpreter who knows how to interpret, has a health care background, understands patients' rights, and can help with advice about the cultural relevance or appropriateness of the health care plan and instructions.
- Use a family member only if necessary. Be aware of limitations if the family member does not understand medical terms, is younger or a different gender from the patient, or is not aware of the health care procedures or medical ethics.
- Interpreter should be able to do the following:
  - Interpret the patient's nonverbal as well as verbal communication.
  - Translate the message into understandable terms.
  - Act as a patient advocate to represent the patient's needs to the health care team.
  - Be culturally competent and understand how to give teaching instructions.

Strategies for Working With an Interpreter

- If possible, have the interpreter meet with the patient ahead of time to establish rapport before the interpreting begins.
- Speak slowly.
- Maintain eye contact with the patient.
- Talk to the patient, not the interpreter.
- Use simple language with as few medical terms as possible.
- Speak 1 or 2 sentences at a time to allow for easier interpretation.
- Avoid raising your voice during the interaction.
- Obtain feedback to be certain the patient understands.
- Plan to take twice as long to complete the interaction.

INFORMATICS IN PRACTICE

Use of Translation Applications

- Communication barriers can negatively affect the type of care received by non–English-speaking patients.
- Use a language translation app to help you translate 1 language into another language.
- Some apps allow you to speak critical phrases and the translation is immediately spoken back to you or the patient in a natural human voice with the proper accent.
- Check the policy of the health care institution on the use of medical interpreters or translators, including the use of translation apps.

A dictionary that translates from both your language and the patient's language (e.g., Spanish-English/English-Spanish dictionary) is useful. Patients may find it helpful if you have a list of questions and potential answers in several languages prepared by using these types of dictionaries. Many websites and applications translate words and documents from 1 language into another (see Informatics in Practice box). It is helpful to have resources for persons from cultural groups who often use the health care facility. This is especially beneficial when a qualified medical interpreter is not readily available, and you need to learn important phrases in another language.

TABLE 2.11 Overcoming Language Barriers

1. Be polite and formal.
2. Pronounce name correctly. If unsure, ask about the correct pronunciation of the name. Use proper titles of respect, such as "Mr.," "Mrs.," "Ms.," "Dr." Greet the person using the last or complete name.
3. Gesture to yourself and say your name.
4. Offer a handshake or nod. Smile.
5. Proceed in an unhurried manner. Pay attention to any effort by the patient or family to communicate.
6. Speak in a low, moderate voice and avoid excess hand gestures. Remember that there is a tendency to raise the volume and pitch of your voice when the listener appears not to understand. The listener may perceive that you are shouting or angry.
7. Use any words that you might know in the person's language. This shows that you are aware of and respect his or her culture.
8. Use simple words such as "pain" instead of "discomfort." Avoid medical jargon, idioms, and slang. Avoid using contractions (e.g., don't, can't, won't). Use nouns repeatedly instead of pronouns. *Example:*
   Do not say: "He has been taking his medicine, hasn't he?"
   Do say: "Does Juan take medicine?"
9. Pantomime words and simple actions while you say them.
10. Give instructions in the proper sequence. *Example:*
   Do not say: "Before you rinse the bottle, sterilize it."
   Do say: "First, wash the bottle. Second, rinse the bottle."
11. Discuss 1 topic at a time. Avoid using conjunctions. *Example:*
   Do not say: "Are you cold and in pain?"
   Do say: "Are you cold [while pantomiming]? Are you in pain?"
12. Validate whether the person understands by having him or her repeat instructions, demonstrate the procedure, or act out the meaning.
13. Write out several short sentences in English and determine the person's ability to read them.
14. Try a third language. Many Indochinese people speak French. Europeans often know 2 or more languages. Try Latin words or phrases. Use English words that have Latin roots (e.g., use precipitation instead of rain).
15. Ask the person's family and friends who could serve as an interpreter.
16. Use websites that translate words from 1 language to another. Some of them also have audio to help you know how to say the word correctly.
17. Obtain phrase books from a library or bookstore, make or purchase flash cards, contact hospitals for a list of interpreters, and use both a formal and an informal network to find a suitable interpreter.

Source: Jarvis C: *Physical examination and health assessment*, ed 7, Philadelphia, 2016, Saunders.

CASE STUDY

Health Disparities

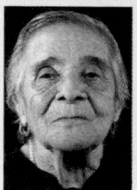

(© Luevanos/ iStock/ Thinkstock.)

Patient Profile

M.S. is an 81-yr-old woman who came to the United States from India 4 years ago with her son and daughter-in-law and their 4 children. She has several health problems, including coronary artery disease, hypertension, osteoarthritis in her right hip, and diabetes. Her daughter-in-law is the primary caregiver and often brings her to the urban community health clinic for a variety of health-related problems. Recently, M.S. has been having memory problems.

The entire family comes to the health clinic with M.S. Because English is a second language (Hindustani is their first language) for all the adult family members, the staff relies on the oldest granddaughter to interpret.

At this clinic visit, M.S. is presenting with shortness of breath. Through her granddaughter's interpretation, she tells the nurse that she is having trouble walking up the stairs in the apartment building. The nurse does the history and assessment, checks her blood glucose (which is within normal limits), and tells her that she should get more exercise. Given M.S.'s memory problems and limited English, the nurse does not complete a 24-hour dietary recall or teach her or the family about diabetes management. M.S. is scheduled for an appointment with the cardiologist for an evaluation of her hypertension and heart disease. Two weeks later, when she sees the cardiologist, her shortness of breath is much worse, and she is having chest pain. She is hospitalized immediately.

Meanwhile, the clinic supervisor is completing a chart audit for the clinic's quality review program. She is reviewing M.S.'s chart and notices that, although she has been a patient in the clinic for 3 years, she has never received instructions on blood glucose monitoring or general diabetes management. The clinic has a nurse diabetes educator who teaches individual patients and groups of patients with diabetes. The clinic manager reviews these findings with the nurse and asks why she has not recommended that M.S. see the diabetes educator. The nurse states that with M.S.'s memory problems and the language barrier, she assumed that M.S. and her family would not benefit from the consultation.

Discussion Questions

1. What type of health disparity has M.S. experienced?
2. What factors led to her not receiving the standard of care?
3. What other assessment should have been done at the initial visit?
4. *Patient-Centered Care:* What strategies may have worked to enhance patient education?
5. *Patient-Centered Care:* How would you assess M.S.'s religious and spiritual needs?
6. *Quality Improvement:* If you were the clinic manager, how would you recommend that the nurse improve her practice?

Answers available at *http://evolve.elsevier.com/Lewis/medsurg.*

■ BRIDGE TO NCLEX EXAMINATION

The number of the question corresponds to the same-numbered outcome at the beginning of the chapter.

1. What are the *leading* determinants of a patient's health *(select all that apply)?*
   a. Genetics
   b. Health behaviors
   c. Family history of disease
   d. Social and physical environment
   e. Type and quality of medical care received

2. In identifying patients at the *greatest* risk for health disparities, the nurse would note that
   a. patients who live in urban areas have readily available access to health care services.
   b. cultural differences exist in patients' ability to communicate with their health care provider.
   c. a patient receiving care from a health care provider of a different culture will have decreased quality of care.
   d. men are more likely than women to have their cardiovascular disease symptoms ignored by a health care provider.

3. Forcing one's own cultural beliefs and practices on another person is an example of
   a. stereotyping.
   b. ethnocentrism.
   c. cultural relativity.
   d. cultural imposition.

4. Which statement *most* accurately describes cultural factors that may affect health?
   a. Diabetes and cancer rates differ by cultural/ethnic groups.
   b. There are limited ethnic variations in physiologic responses to drugs.
   c. Most patients find that religious rituals help them during times of illness.
   d. Silence during a nurse-patient interaction means the patient understands the instructions.

5. As part of the nursing process, cultural assessment is *best* accomplished by
   a. judging the patient's cultural values based on observations.
   b. using a cultural assessment guide as part of the nursing process.
   c. seeking guidance from a nurse from the patient's cultural background.
   d. relying on the nurse's previous experience with patients from that cultural group.

6. Nurses play a key role in promoting health equity. An important mechanism to do this is to
   a. discourage use of evidence-based practice guidelines.
   b. insist that patients adhere to established clinical guidelines.
   c. teach patients to use the Internet to find resources related to their health.
   d. engage in active listening and establish relationships with patients and families.

7. What is the *first* step in developing cultural competence?
   a. Create opportunities to interact with a variety of cultural groups.
   b. Examine the nurse's own cultural background, values, and beliefs about health and health care.
   c. Learn about a multitude of folk medicines and herbal substances that different cultures use for self-care.
   d. Learn assessment skills for different cultural groups, including cultural beliefs and practices and physical assessments.

8. When communicating with a patient who speaks a language that the nurse does not understand, it is important to *first* attempt to
   a. have a family member interpret.
   b. use a trained medical interpreter.
   c. use specific medical terminology so there will be no mistakes.
   d. focus on the translation rather than nonverbal communication.

1. a, b, d. 2. b. 3. d. 4. a. 5. b. 6. d. 7. b. 8. b.

For rationales to these answers and even more NCLEX review questions, visit *http://evolve.elsevier.com/Lewis/medsurg.*

ⓔ EVOLVE WEBSITE/RESOURCES LIST

http://evolve.elsevier.com/Lewis/medsurg
Review Questions (Online Only)
Key Points
Answer Keys for Questions
- Rationales for Bridge to NCLEX Examination Questions
- Answer Guidelines for Case Study on p. 31

Conceptual Care Map Creator
Audio Glossary
Content Updates

REFERENCES

1. World Health Organization: Health impact assessment. Retrieved from *www.who.int.hia.en.*
2. Kaiser Family Foundation: Disparities in health and health care. Retrieved from *www.kff.org/disparities-policy/issue-brief/disparities-in-health-and-health-care-five-key-questions-and-answers/.*
3. U.S. Census Bureau : Population estimates. Retrieved from *www.census.gov/programs-surveys/popest.html.*
*4. Hess CN, Kaltenbach LA, Doll JA, et al Race and sex differences in post-myocardial infarction angina frequency and risk of 1-year unplanned rehospitalization, *Circulation* 135:532, 2017.
*5. Willman CL: Cancer health disparities in American Indian and Alaskan Native populations, *Cancer* 77:13, 2017.
6. U.S. Census Bureau: Measuring America, our changing landscape. Retrieved from *www.census.gov/library/visualizations/2016/comm/acs-rural-urban.html.*
*7. DeKeseredy WS, Hall-Sanchez A, Dragiewicz M, et al Intimate violence against women in rural communities. In Donnermeyer JF, editor: *The Routledge international handbook of rural criminology,* London, 2016, Routledge.
*8. Shaw LJ, Pepine CJ, Xie J, et al Quality and equitable health care gaps for women: Attributions to sex differences in cardiovascular medicine, *J Am Coll Cardiol* 70:373, 2017.
9. Correa-de-Araujo R: *Health disparities: Access and utilization,* New York, 2017, Springer.
10. Cigna: LGBT and health disparities. Retrieved from *www.cigna.com/healthwellness/lgbt/lgbt-disparities.*
11. Giger JN: *Transcultural nursing: Assessment and intervention,* ed 7, St Louis. 2016, Mosby.
12. Schwartz SJ, Unger J. *The Oxford handbook of acculturation and health,* New York, 2017, University Press.
*13. Darroch F, Giles A, Sanderson P, et al The United States does CAIR about cultural safety, *J Transcult Nurs* 28:269, 2017.
*14. Betancourt JR, Green AR, Carrillo JE, et al Defining cultural competence: A practical framework for addressing racial/ethnic disparities in health and health care, *Public Health Rep* 118:293, 2016.
15. Minority Nurse: *Nursing statistics.* Retrieved from *http://minoritynurse.com/nursing-statistics/.*
*16. Han W, Lee S: Racial/ethnic variation in health care satisfaction: The role of acculturation, *Soc Work Health Care* 55:694, 2016.
*17. Hall JM, Carlson K: Marginalization, *Adv Nurs Sci* 39:200, 2016.
*18. Schmit KM: Tuberculosis—United States 2016, *MMWR* 66:289, 2017.
19. Centers for Disease Control and Prevention: Refugee health guidelines. Retrieved from *www.cdc.gov/immigrantrefugeehealth/guidelines/refugee-guidelines.html.*
20. American Association of Colleges in Nursing: Cultural competency in baccalaureate nursing education. Retrieved from *www.aacnnursing.org/Education-Resources/Tool-Kits/Cultural-Competency-in-Nursing-Education.*
21. Jarvis C: *Physical examination and health assessment,* ed 7, Philadelphia, 2016, Saunders.
22. U.S. Department of Health and Human Services: Think cultural health. Retrieved from *www.ThinkCulturalHealth.hhs.gov.*

*Evidence-based information for clinical practice.

3

Health History and Physical Examination

Courtney Reinisch

We make a living by what we get, but we make a life by what we give.

Winston Churchill

ℯ http://evolve.elsevier.com/Lewis/medsurg/

CONCEPTUAL FOCUS

Clinical Judgment
Collaboration

Communication

LEARNING OUTCOMES

1. Explain the purpose, components, and techniques of a patient's health history and physical examination.
2. Obtain a nursing history using a functional health pattern format.

3. Select appropriate techniques of inspection, palpation, percussion, and auscultation for physical examination of a patient.
4. Distinguish among emergency, comprehensive, and focused types of assessment in terms of indications, purposes, and components.

KEY TERMS

auscultation, p. 38
database, p. 33
functional health patterns, p. 35

inspection, p. 38
nursing history, p. 34
objective data, p. 34

palpation, p. 38
percussion, p. 38
subjective data, p. 34

During the assessment phase of the nursing process, you will obtain a patient's health history and perform a physical examination. This serves as part of the interprofessional team evaluation. The interprofessional team, also known as an interdisciplinary, transdisciplinary, or multidisciplinary team, is made up of a number of health care professionals who provide care to a patient. The findings of your nursing assessment (1) contribute to a database that identifies the patient's current and past health status and (2) provide a baseline against which future changes can be evaluated. The purpose of the nursing assessment is to enable you to make clinical judgments about your patient's health status.[1] Assessment is the first step of the nursing process. It is performed continually throughout the nursing process to validate nursing diagnoses, evaluate nursing interventions, and determine whether patient outcomes and goals have been met.

The language of assessment is complex, with many overlapping and confusing terms. In this text, *assessment* describes a hands-on data collection process and a *database* identifies a specific list of information (data) to collect.

DATA COLLECTION

The **database** is all the health information about a patient. It includes (1) nursing history and physical examination, (2) the medical history and physical examination, and (3) laboratory and diagnostic test results. A nurse and health care provider (HCP) perform a patient history and a physical examination using formats and data based on each discipline's focus.

Medical Focus

A *medical history* is designed to collect data to be used primarily by the HCP to determine risk for disease and diagnose medical conditions. The medical history is usually collected by a member of the health care team (e.g., physician, advanced practice nurse [APN], resident, physician's assistant, medical student). The HCP's physical examination and diagnostic tests aid in establishing medical diagnoses and implementing and monitoring the medical treatment plan. The information collected and reported by the HCP is used by nurses and other health care team members (e.g., pharmacist, physical therapist, dietitian, social worker) based on the focus of their care. For example, the abnormal results of a neurologic examination by an APN may aid in diagnosing a stroke. You may use the same results to identify a priority nursing diagnosis of fall risk. A physical therapist may use this information to plan therapy involving range-of-motion exercises.

Nursing Focus

The focus of nursing care is the diagnosis and treatment of human responses to actual or potential health problems or life processes. The information obtained from the **nursing history** and physical examination is used to determine the patient's strengths and responses to a health problem. For example, a patient with a diagnosis of diabetes may respond with anxiety or a lack of knowledge about self-managing the condition. This patient may experience the physical response of fluid volume deficit because of the abnormal fluid loss caused by hyperglycemia. These human responses to the condition of diabetes are diagnosed and treated by nurses. During the nursing history interview and physical examination, you will obtain and record the data to support the identification of nursing diagnoses (Fig. 3.1).

Types of Data

The database includes subjective and objective data. **Subjective data**, also known as *symptoms*, are collected by interviewing the patient and/or caregiver during the nursing history. This type of data includes information that can be described or verified only by the patient or caregiver. It is what the person tells you either spontaneously or in response to a direct question.

Objective data, also known as *signs*, are data that can be observed or measured. You obtain this type of data using inspection, palpation, percussion, and auscultation during the physical examination. Objective data are also acquired by diagnostic testing. Patients often provide subjective data while you are performing the physical examination. You will observe objective signs while interviewing the patient. All the findings related to a specific problem, whether subjective or objective, are known as *clinical manifestations* of that problem.

Interview Considerations

The purpose of the patient interview is to obtain a health history (i.e., subjective data) about the patient's past and present health state. Effective communication is needed in the interview process. Creating a climate of trust and respect is critical to establishing a therapeutic relationship.[2] You need to communicate acceptance of the patient as a person by using an open, responsive, nonjudgmental approach. You communicate through spoken language, as well as in your manner of dress, gestures, and body language. Culture influences the words, gestures, and postures one uses and the information that is shared with others (see Chapter 2).

In addition to understanding the principles of effective communication, you will develop a personal style of relating to patients. One style of communication does not fit all. The wording of questions can increase the likelihood of obtaining the needed information. The ease of asking questions, particularly those related to sensitive areas such as sexual functioning, comes with training and experience.

The amount of time you need to complete a nursing history varies with the format used and your experience. The nursing history may be completed in 1 or several sessions, depending on the setting and patient. For example, an older adult patient with a low energy level may need a few brief interviews to allow time for the patient to give the needed information. You must make a judgment about the amount of information to collect on initial contact with the patient. In interviews with patients with chronic disease, patients in pain, and patients in emergency situations, ask only those questions that are pertinent to a specific problem. You can complete the health history interview at a more appropriate time.

Judge the reliability of the patient as a historian. An older adult may give a false impression about his or her mental status because of a prolonged response time or visual and hearing impairments. The complexity and long duration of health problems may make it hard for an older adult or a chronically ill younger patient to be an accurate historian.

It is important for you to determine the patient's priority concerns and expectations, since your priorities may be different from the patient's. For example, your priority may be to complete the health history, while the patient is interested only in relief from symptoms. Until the patient's priority need is met, you will probably be unsuccessful in obtaining complete and accurate data.

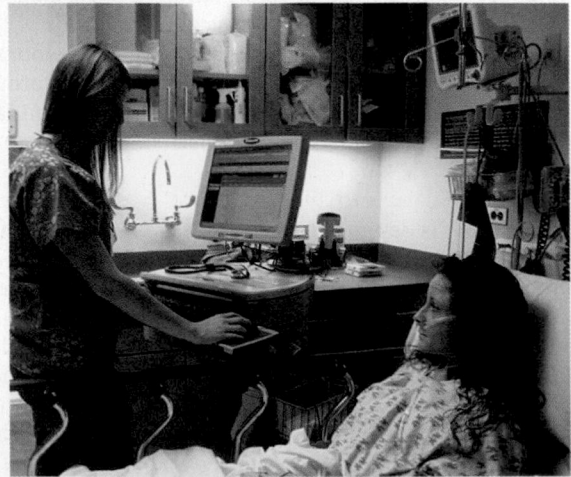

FIG. 3.1 Conducting a nursing focused interview. (Courtesy Linda Bucher, RN, PhD, CEN, CNE, Staff Nurse, Virtua Memorial Hospital, Mt. Holly, N.J.)

⬛ NURSING MANAGEMENT
Assessment and Data Collection

In acute care, a registered nurse (RN) must complete the initial (admission) nursing assessment within the timeframe determined by the agency. Ongoing data collection is expected of all members of the health care team.

- On admission, complete a comprehensive assessment (Table 3.4).
- Obtain patient's health history by interviewing patient and/or caregiver.
- Perform physical examination using inspection, palpation, percussion, and auscultation as appropriate.
- Document findings from the health history and physical examination in the patient's record.
- Organize patient data into functional health patterns (Table 3.2).
- Develop and prioritize nursing and collaborative problems for the patient.
- Throughout hospitalization, perform focused assessments based on patient's history or clinical manifestations (Table 3.7).
- Oversee aspects of data collection by UAP.
  - Vital signs, including oxygen saturation
  - Height and weight, oral intake, and output
  - Per agency policy, point-of-care testing (e.g., glucose)

Symptom Investigation

At any time during the assessment the patient may report a symptom such as pain, fatigue, or weakness. Because we do not observe symptoms patients experience, the symptoms must be explored. Table 3.1 shows a mnemonic (PQRST) to help you remember the areas to explore when a symptom is reported. The information you receive may help determine the cause of the symptom. A common symptom that you will assess is pain (see Chapter 8). For example, if a patient states that he has "pain in his leg," you would assess and record the data using PQRST.

Has right midcalf pain that usually occurs at work when climbing stairs after lunch (P). Pain is alleviated by stopping and resting for 2 to 3 minutes. Patient states he has been "eating a banana every day for extra potassium" but "it hasn't helped" (P). Pain is described as "stabbing" and is non-radiating (Q, R). Pain is so severe (rating 9 on 0-10 scale) that patient cannot continue activity (S). Onset is abrupt, occurring once or twice daily. It last occurred yesterday while cutting the lawn (T).

Data Organization

You must systematically obtain and organize assessment data so you can readily analyze and make judgments about the patient's health status and any health problems. Some assessment forms are organized using body systems. Although helpful, these types of forms may be incomplete because they may omit areas such as health promotion behaviors, sleep, coping, and values.

Functional health patterns, developed by Gordon,[3] provide the framework used throughout this book for obtaining a nursing history. This format includes an initial collection of important health information followed by assessment of 11 areas of health status or function (Table 3.2). Data organized in this format allow for the identification of areas of wellness (or positive function) and health problems.[2]

Culturally Competent Care: Assessment

The process of obtaining a health history and performing a physical examination is an intimate experience for you and the patient. Culture influences patterns of communication and the information one shares with others. During the interview and physical examination, be sensitive to issues of eye contact, space, modesty, and touching, as discussed in Chapter 2. Knowing the cultural norms related to male-female relationships is especially important during the physical examination. To avoid violating any culturally based practices, ask the patient about cultural values. Determine if the patient would like to have someone present during the history or physical examination or someone of the same gender to perform the history and physical examination.[1]

NURSING HISTORY: SUBJECTIVE DATA

Important Health Information

Important health information offers an overview of past and present medical conditions and treatments. Past health history, medications, allergies, and surgery or other treatments are included in this part of the history.

Past Health History. The past health history provides information about the patient's prior state of health. Ask the patient about major childhood and adult illnesses, injuries, hospitalizations, and surgeries. Specific questions are more effective than simply asking whether the patient has had any illness or health problems in the past. For example, asking "Do you have a history of diabetes?" elicits better information than asking "Do you have any chronic health problems?"

Medications. Ask the patient for specific details related to past and current medications, including prescription and illicit drugs, over-the-counter (OTC) drugs, vitamins, herbs, and dietary supplements. Patients often do not consider herbs and dietary supplements as drugs. It is important to specifically ask about their use because they can interact adversely with existing or newly prescribed medications (see the Complementary & Alternative Therapies box).

COMPLEMENTARY & ALTERNATIVE THERAPIES

Assessment of Use of Herbs and Dietary Supplements

Why Assessment Is Important

- Herbs and dietary supplements may have side effects or may interact adversely with prescription or OTC drugs.
- Patients at high risk for drug-herb interactions include those taking anticoagulant, antihypertensive, antidepressant, or immune-regulating therapy and patients undergoing anesthesia. Most herbs must be stopped 2 to 3 weeks before surgery.
- Many patients do not tell HCPs that they are using herbs and dietary supplements. They may fear HCPs will disapprove of their use.
- Many herbal preparations have a variety of ingredients. Ask the patient or caregiver to bring labeled containers to the health care site to determine product composition.

Nurse's Role

- Patients typically share information about the use of herbs and dietary supplements with you if you ask them.
- Create an accepting and nonjudgmental attitude when assessing use or interest in herbs or dietary supplements.
- Use open-ended questions such as, "What types of herbs, vitamins, or supplements do you take?" and "What effects have you noticed from using them?"
- Document the use of any herb(s) or dietary supplements in the patient record, including the name, amount, frequency of use, and any side effects.
- Inform patients of the following:
  - Risks and benefits associated with herbal use, including drug-herb interactions
  - Health food store employees are not licensed HCPs
  - Importance of carefully reading the labels of herbal therapies and dietary supplements and taking only the recommended amount
  - Moisture, sunlight, and heat may change the components of herbs
  - Many herbal therapies have side effects. Report these to the HCP at once.

Question older adult and chronically ill patients about medication routines. Look for issues related to medication cost and polypharmacy. Changes in absorption, metabolism, and elimination of drugs can pose serious potential problems for these patients.[4]

Allergies. Explore the patient's history of allergies to drugs, latex, contrast media, food, and the environment (e.g., pollen). Include a detailed description of any allergic reaction(s) reported by the patient.

Surgery or Other Treatments. Record all surgeries, along with the date, reason for the surgery, and outcome. The outcome includes whether the problem was resolved or has residual effects. Ask about and record any blood products the patient has received.

TABLE 3.1   Investigation of Patient-Reported Symptom

	Factor	Questions for Patient and Caregiver	Record
P	Precipitating and Palliative	Were there any events that came before the symptom? What makes it better? Worse? What have you done for the symptom? Did this help?	Influence of physical and emotional activities. Patient's attempts to alleviate (or treat) the symptom
Q	Quality	Tell me what the symptom feels like (e.g., aching, dull, pressure, burning, stabbing).	Patient's own words (e.g., "Like a pinch or stabbing feeling")
R	Radiation	Where do you feel the symptom? Does it move to other areas?	Region of body. Local or radiating, superficial or deep
S	Severity	On a scale of 0–10, with 0 meaning no pain and 10 being the worst pain you could imagine, what number would you give your symptom?	Pain rating number (e.g., 5/10)
T	Timing	When did the symptom start? Was it sudden or gradual? Any particular time of day, week, month, or year? Has the symptom changed over time? Has the symptom happened before? What are you doing when the symptom occurs?	Time of onset, duration, periodicity, and frequency. Course of symptoms. Where patient is and what patient is doing when the symptom occurs

Functional Health Patterns

Assess the patient's functional health patterns to identify effective, dysfunctional, and potential dysfunctional health patterns. *Dysfunctional health patterns* occur with disease. *Potential dysfunctional patterns* identify risk conditions for problems. You may identify patients with effective health function who want a higher level of wellness. Table 3.2 gives examples of possible questions to ask the patient related to functional health patterns.

Health Perception–Health Management Pattern. This pattern focuses on the patient's perceived level of health and well-being and on personal practices for maintaining health. Ask the patient to describe his or her personal health and any concerns about it. Explore the patient's feelings of effectiveness at staying healthy by asking what helps and what hinders his or her well-being. Ask the patient to rate his or her health as excellent, good, fair, or poor. When possible, record this information in the patient's own words.

Next, ask about the type of HCP the patient uses. For example, if the patient is Native American, a medicine man may be considered the primary HCP. If the patient is of Hispanic origin, a *curandero,* a Hispanic healer who uses folk medicine and herbs to treat patients, may be the primary HCP (see Chapter 2).

Other questions seek to identify risk factors by obtaining a thorough family history (e.g., heart disease, cancer, genetic disorders), history of personal health habits (e.g., tobacco, alcohol, drug use), and history of exposure to environmental hazards (e.g., asbestos). If the patient is hospitalized, ask about the expectations for this experience. Have the patient describe his or her understanding of the current health problem, including its onset, course, and treatment. These questions obtain information about a patient's knowledge of the health problem and ability to use appropriate resources to manage the problem.

Nutritional-Metabolic Pattern. This pattern assesses the processes of ingestion, digestion, absorption, and metabolism. Obtain a 24-hour diet recall from the patient to evaluate the quantity and quality of foods and fluids consumed. If a problem is found, ask the patient to keep a 3-day food diary for a more careful analysis of dietary intake. Assess the impact of psychologic factors such as depression, anxiety, stress, and self-concept on nutrition. Evaluate socioeconomic and cultural factors such as food budget, who prepares the meals, and food preferences. Determine whether the patient's present condition has interfered with eating and appetite by exploring any symptoms of nausea, intestinal gas, or pain. Food allergies should be distinguished from food intolerances, such as lactose or gluten intolerance.

Elimination Pattern. This pattern involves bowel, bladder, and skin function. Ask the patient about the frequency of bowel and bladder activity. Ask about urgency, incontinence, and diuretic use. Inquire about stool consistency, color, and laxative use. Assess the skin in the elimination pattern in terms of its excretory function.

Activity-Exercise Pattern. Assessing this pattern looks at the patient's usual pattern of exercise, work activity, leisure, and recreation. Question the patient about his or her ability to perform activities of daily living (ADLs) and note any specific problems. Table 3.2 includes a scale for rating the functional levels of common activities.

Sleep-Rest Pattern. This pattern describes the patient's perception of his or her pattern of sleep, rest, and relaxation in a 24-hour period. Elicit this information by asking, "Do you feel rested when you wake up?"

Cognitive-Perceptual Pattern. Assessing this pattern involves a description of all the senses and cognitive functions. Assess pain as a sensory perception (see pain assessment in Chapter 8). Ask the patient about any sensory deficits that affect the ability to perform ADLs. Record ways in which the patient compensates for any sensory-perceptual problems. Ask the patient how he or she learns best and in what language. Ask what he or she understands about the illness and treatment plan. Plan patient teaching according to identified needs and preferences (see Chapter 4 for details on patient teaching).

Self-Perception–Self-Concept Pattern. This pattern describes the patient's self-concept, which is critical in determining the way the person interacts with others. Included are attitudes about self, perception of personal abilities, body image, and general sense of worth. Ask the patient for a self-description and about how his or her health condition affects self-concept. Patients' expressions of hopelessness or loss of control often reflect an inability to care for one's self.

TABLE 3.2 Health History

Functional Health Pattern Format

Demographic Data
Name, address, age, occupation, gender
Race, ethnicity, culture, spirituality

Important Health Information
Past health history
Medications, supplements
Allergies
Surgery or other treatments

Health Perception–Health Management Pattern
1. Reason for visit?
2. General state of health?
3. Most important things done to keep healthy? Testicular self-examination? Colorectal cancer, hypertension, and heart disease risk screening? Papanicolaou (Pap) test? Immunizations such as tetanus, pneumonia, hepatitis, and flu vaccines?
4. Who is your primary health care provider?
5. Health adherence problems?
6. Cause of illness? Action taken? Results?
7. Things important to you while here?
8. Family health history (e.g., cardiovascular disease, hypertension, cancer, diabetes, psychiatric illness, genetic disorders)?
9. Illness and injury risk factors (e.g., sexual abuse, intimate partner abuse, violence, use of tobacco or alcohol, substance abuse)?

Nutritional-Metabolic Pattern
1. Typical daily food intake (describe)? Supplements?
2. Typical daily fluid intake (describe)?
3. Weight loss or gain (amount, time span, intentional)?
4. Desired weight?
5. Appetite?
6. Food or eating: Discomfort? Diet restrictions?
7. Change in appetite with anxiety?
8. Heal well or poorly?
9. Skin problems: Lesions? Dryness?
10. Dentition: Dental problems? Well-fitting dentures?
11. Food preferences?
12. Food allergies?

Elimination Pattern
1. Bowel elimination pattern (describe): Frequency? Character? Discomfort? Laxatives? Enemas?
2. Urinary elimination pattern (describe): Frequency? Problem in control? Diuretics?
3. Any external devices?
4. Excess perspiration? Odor problems? Itching?

Activity-Exercise Pattern
1. Sufficient energy for desired or required activities?
2. Exercise pattern? Type? Regularity?
3. Spare time (leisure) activities?
4. Dyspnea? Chest pain? Palpitations? Stiffness? Aching? At rest? With activity?
5. Perceived ability for (rate Functional Level 0–III for each):
   Eating __ Cooking __ Grooming __
   Transfer (e.g., bed to chair) __ Toileting __
   Bathing __ Dressing __ Shopping __ General mobility __

   Functional Levels
   Level 0: Full self-care
   Level I: Requires use of equipment or device
   Level II: Needs help or supervision from another person
   Level III: Is dependent and does not participate

Sleep-Rest Pattern
1. Generally rested and ready for daily activities after sleep?
2. Sleep onset problems? Aids (e.g., drugs, CPAP)? Dreams (nightmares)? Early awakening?
3. Usual sleep rituals?
4. Usual sleep pattern?

Cognitive-Perceptual Pattern
1. Hearing impairment? Hearing aids?
2. Vision? Wear glasses? Wear contact lens? Last checked?
3. Any change in taste? Any change in smell?
4. Any recent change in memory?
5. Easiest way to learn things?
6. Any discomfort? Pain (rating on scale of 0–10)? How managed?
7. Ability to communicate (e.g., primary language)?
8. Understanding of illness?
9. Understanding of treatments?

Self-Perception–Self-Concept Pattern
1. Self-description? Self-perception?
2. Effect of illness on self-image?

Role-Relationship Pattern
1. Live alone? Family/caregiver? Family structure?
2. Family problems?
3. Family problem solving?
4. Family dependence on you for things? How managing?
5. Family's and others' feelings about illness or hospitalization?*
6. Problems with children? Hard to handle?*
7. Belong to social groups? Have close friends? Feel lonely (frequency)?
8. Work (school) satisfaction? Income sufficient for needs?*
9. Feel part of or isolated from neighborhood where living?

Sexuality-Reproductive Pattern
1. Any changes or problems in sexual relations?*
2. Effect of illness?
3. Use of contraceptives? Problems?
4. When menstruation started? Last menstrual period? Menstrual problems? Gravida? Para?†
5. Effect of present condition or treatment on sexuality?
6. Sexually transmitted infections?

Coping–Stress Tolerance Pattern
1. Tense a lot of the time? What helps? Use any drugs, alcohol?
2. Have someone to confide in? Available to you now?
3. Recent life changes?
4. Problem-solving techniques? Effective?

Value-Belief Pattern
1. Satisfied with life?
2. Religion important in your life?
3. Conflict between treatment and beliefs?

Modified from Gordon M: *Manual of nursing diagnosis*, ed 13, Boston, 2014, Jones & Bartlett.
CPAP, Continuous positive airway pressure.
*If appropriate.
†For women.

Role-Relationship Pattern. This pattern reveals the patient's roles and relationships, including major responsibilities. Ask the patient to describe family, social, and work roles and relationships and to rate his or her performance of the expected behaviors related to these. Determine whether patterns in these roles and relationships are satisfactory or whether strain is evident. Note the patient's feelings about how the present condition affects his or her roles and relationships.

Sexuality-Reproductive Pattern. This pattern describes satisfaction or dissatisfaction with personal sexuality and describes reproductive issues. Assessing this pattern is important because many illnesses, surgical procedures, and drugs affect sexual function. A patient's sexual and reproductive concerns may be expressed. Teaching needs may be identified through information obtained in this pattern.

You may feel uncomfortable obtaining information related to sexuality. However, it is important to take a health history and screen for sexual function and dysfunction in a nonjudgmental way. Provide appropriate information or refer the patient to a more experienced HCP.

Coping–Stress Tolerance Pattern. This pattern describes the patient's general coping and the effectiveness of the coping mechanisms. Assessing this pattern involves analyzing the specific stressors or problems that confront the patient, the patient's perception of the stressors, and the patient's response to the stressors. Document any major losses or stressors experienced by the patient in the previous year. Note strategies used by the patient to deal with stressors and relieve tension. Ask about persons and groups that make up the patient's social support networks.

Value-Belief Pattern. This pattern describes the values, goals, and beliefs (including spiritual) that guide health-related choices. Document the patient's ethnic background and effects of culture and beliefs on health practices. Note and respect the patient's wishes about continuation of religious or spiritual practices and the use of religious articles.

PHYSICAL EXAMINATION: OBJECTIVE DATA

General Survey

After the nursing history, make a *general survey statement*. This is your general impression of a patient, including behavioral observations. The initial survey begins with your first encounter with the patient and continues during the health history interview.

The major areas included in the general survey statement are (1) body features, (2) mental state, (3) speech, (4) body movements, (5) obvious physical signs, (6) nutritional status, and (7) behavior. Vital signs and body mass index (BMI) (calculated from height and weight [kg/m²]) may be included. The following is a sample of a general survey statement:

> A.H. is a 34-yr-old Hispanic woman, BP 130/84, P 88, R 18. No distinguishing body features. Alert but anxious. Speech rapid with trailing thoughts. Wringing hands and shuffling feet during interview. Skin flushed, hands clammy. Overweight relative to height (BMI = 28.3 kg/m²). Sits with eyes downcast, shoulders slumped, and avoids eye contact.

Physical Examination

The *physical examination* is the systematic assessment of a patient's physical status. Explore any positive findings using the same criteria used when investigating a symptom in the nursing history (Table 3.1). A *positive finding* shows that the patient has

or has had the particular problem or sign under discussion (e.g., if the patient with jaundice has an enlarged liver, it is a positive finding). Relevant information about this problem should then be gathered.

Negative findings may be significant. A pertinent *negative finding* is the absence of a sign or symptom usually associated with a problem. For example, peripheral edema is common with advanced liver disease. If edema is not present in a patient with advanced liver disease, specifically note this as "no peripheral edema."

Techniques. Four major techniques are used in performing the physical examination: inspection, palpation, percussion, and auscultation. The techniques are usually performed in this sequence: inspection, palpation, percussion, and auscultation. The abdominal examination is an exception. Inspection is first, followed by auscultation, percussion, and palpation. Performing percussion and palpation before auscultation can alter bowel sounds and produce false findings. Not every assessment area requires the use of all 4 assessment techniques (e.g., musculoskeletal system requires only inspection and palpation).

Inspection. Inspection is the visual examination of a part or region of the body to assess normal conditions or deviations. Inspection is more than just looking. This technique is deliberate, systematic, and focused. Compare what is seen with the known, generally visible characteristics of the body part that you are inspecting. For example, most 30-yr-old men have hair on their legs. Absence of hair may indicate a vascular problem and the need for further investigation, or it may be normal for a patient of a particular ethnicity (e.g., Filipino men have little body hair). Always compare 1 side of the patient's body to the other to assess bilaterally for any abnormal findings.

Palpation. Palpation is the examination of the body using touch. Using light and deep palpation can yield information related to masses, pulsations, organ enlargement, tenderness or pain, swelling, muscular spasm or rigidity, elasticity, vibration of voice sounds, crepitus, moisture, and texture. Different parts of the hand are more sensitive for specific assessments. For example, use the palmar surface (base of fingers) to feel vibrations, the dorsa (backs) of your hands and fingers to assess skin temperature, and tips of your fingers to palpate the abdomen[1] (Fig. 3.2).

Percussion. Percussion is a technique that produces a sound and vibration to obtain information about the underlying area (Fig. 3.3). The sounds and vibrations are relative to the underlying structures. A change from an expected sound may indicate a problem. For example, dullness in the right lower quadrant instead of the normal sound of tympany should be explored. Specific percussion sounds of various body parts and regions are discussed in the appropriate assessment chapters.

Auscultation. Auscultation involves listening to sounds produced by the body with a stethoscope to assess normal and abnormal conditions. This technique is useful in evaluating sounds from the heart, lungs, abdomen, and vascular system. The bell of the stethoscope is more sensitive to low-pitched sounds (e.g., heart murmurs). The diaphragm of the stethoscope is more sensitive to high-pitched sounds (e.g., bowel sounds). Some stethoscopes have only a diaphragm, designed to transmit low- and high-pitched sounds. To listen for low-pitched sounds, hold the diaphragm lightly on the skin. For high-pitched sounds, press the diaphragm firmly

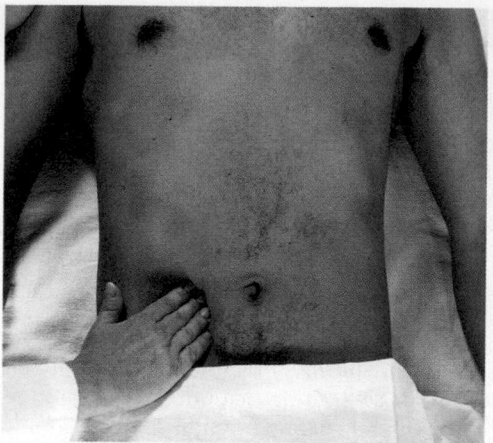

FIG. 3.2 Palpation is the examination of the body using touch. (From Jarvis C: *Physical examination and health assessment*, ed 7, St Louis, 2015, Saunders.)

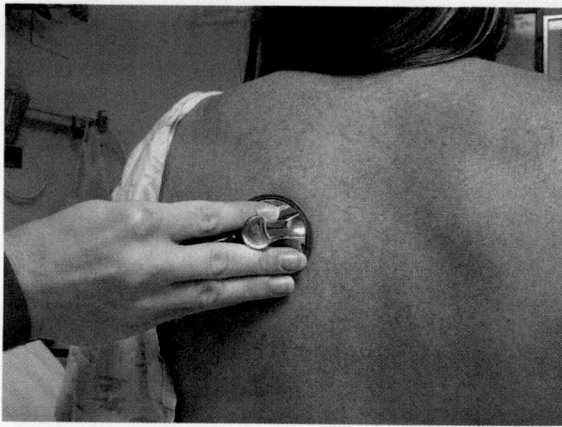

FIG. 3.4 Auscultation is listening to sounds produced by the body to assess normal conditions and deviations from normal. (Courtesy Linda Bucher, RN, PhD, CEN, CNE, Staff Nurse, Virtua Memorial Hospital, Mt. Holly, N.J.)

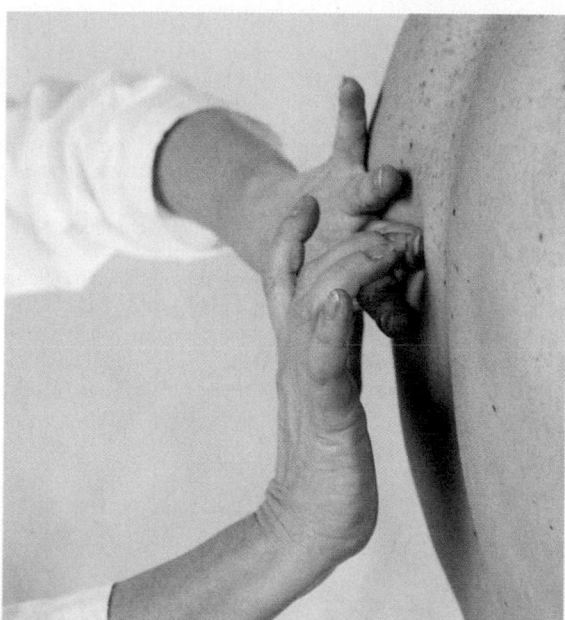

FIG. 3.3 Percussion is tapping of the patient's skin with the middle finger or striking finger of the dominant hand. Hyperextend the middle finger of the nondominant hand and place its distal joint and tip firmly on the patient's skin. Normal percussion sounds: *resonant*—lung tissue; *tympany*—air-filled viscus (e.g., intestines); *dull*—dense organs (e.g., liver); *flat*—no air present (e.g., bone, muscle). (Adapted from Jarvis C: *Physical examination and health assessment*, ed 7, St Louis, 2015, Saunders.)

TABLE 3.3 **Common Physical Examination Equipment**
• Alcohol swabs
• Blood pressure cuff
• Cotton balls
• Examining table or bed
• Eye chart (e.g., Snellen eye chart)
• Paper cup with water
• Patient gown
• Pocket flashlight
• Reflex hammer
• Stethoscope (with bell and diaphragm or a dual-purpose diaphragm; tubing 15–18 inches [38–46 cm])
• Tongue blades
• Watch (with second hand or digital)

on the skin (Fig. 3.4).[1] Specific sounds and auscultation techniques are discussed in the appropriate assessment chapters.

Equipment. Collect the equipment needed for the physical examination before you begin (Table 3.3). This saves time and energy for you and the patient. It promotes trust by showing a level of professionalism. The use of specific equipment is discussed in the appropriate assessment chapters.

Organization of Examination. Perform the physical examination systematically and efficiently. Give explanations to the patient as the examination proceeds and consider the patient's comfort, safety, and privacy. Follow the same sequence every time to avoid omitting a procedure, a step in the sequence, or a part of the body. Table 3.4 presents a comprehensive, organized physical examination outline.

Adapting the physical examination is often useful for the older adult patient, who may have age-related problems such as decreased mobility, limited energy, and perceptual changes.[5] An outline listing some useful adaptations is found in Table 3.5.

A nurse with appropriate education can perform advanced techniques. A retinal reflex examination would be done with an eye examination. Speculum and bimanual examination of women and the prostate gland examination of men would be performed after inspecting the genitalia.

Recording Physical Examination. At the end of the examination, record the normal and abnormal findings in the patient's health record. See Table 3.6 for an example of how to record findings of a normal physical examination of a healthy adult. See Table 5.5 to find age-related assessment findings in the book.

TYPES OF ASSESSMENT

Different types of assessment are used to obtain information about a patient. These approaches are divided into 3 types: emergency, comprehensive, and focused (Table 3.7). Decide what type of assessment to perform based on the clinical situation. Sometimes the health care agency provides guidelines, and other times it is a nursing judgment.

Emergency Assessment

An *emergency assessment* may be done in an emergency or life-threatening situation. This involves a rapid history and examination of a patient while supporting vital functions.

TABLE 3.4 Physical Examination Outline

1. General Survey
Observe general state of health (patient is seated).
- Body features
- Mental state and level of orientation
- Speech
- Body movements
- Physical appearance
- Nutritional status
- Behavior

2. Vital Signs
Record vital signs.
- Blood pressure—both arms for comparison
- Apical/radial pulse
- Respiration
- Temperature
- Oxygen saturation

Record height and weight; calculate body mass index (BMI).

3. Integument
Inspect and palpate skin for the following:
- Color
- Integrity (e.g., lacerations, lesions, breakdown)
- Scars, tattoos, piercings
- Bruises, rash
- Edema
- Moisture
- Texture
- Temperature
- Turgor
- Vascularity

Inspect and palpate nails for the following:
- Color
- Lesions
- Size
- Shape
- Angle
- Capillary refill time

4. Head and Neck
Inspect and palpate head for the following:
- Shape and symmetry of skull
- Masses
- Tenderness
- Condition of hair and scalp
- Temporal arteries
- Temporomandibular joint
- Sensory (CN V, light touch, pain)
- Motor (CN VII, shows teeth, purses lips, raises eyebrows)
- Looks up, wrinkles forehead (CN VII)
- Raises shoulders against resistance (CN XI)

Inspect and palpate (occasionally auscultate) neck for the following:
- Skin (vascularity and visible pulsations)
- Symmetry
- Range of motion
- Pulses and bruits (carotid)
- Midline structure (trachea, thyroid gland, cartilage)
- Lymph nodes (preauricular, postauricular, occipital, mandibular, tonsillar, submental, anterior and posterior cervical, infraclavicular, supraclavicular)

Test visual acuity.
Inspect and lightly palpate eyes/eyebrows for the following:
- Position and movement of eyelids (CN VII)
- Visual fields (CN II)
- Extraocular movements (CN III, IV, VI)
- Cornea, sclera, conjunctiva
- Pupillary response (CN III)
- Red reflex

Inspect and palpate nose and sinuses for the following:
- External nose: Shape, blockage
- Internal nose: Patency of nasal passages, shape, turbinates or polyps, discharge
- Frontal and maxillary sinuses

Inspect and palpate ears for the following:
- Placement
- Pinna
- Auditory acuity (whispered voice, ticking watch) (CN VIII)
- Mastoid process
- Auditory canal
- Tympanic membrane

Inspect and palpate mouth for the following:
- Lips (symmetry, lesions, color)
- Buccal mucosa (Stensen's and Wharton's ducts)
- Teeth (absence, state of repair, color)
- Gums (color, receding from teeth)
- Tongue for strength (asymmetry, ability to stick out tongue, side to side, fasciculations) (CN XII)
- Palates
- Tonsils and pillars
- Uvular elevation (CN IX)
- Posterior pharynx
- Gag reflex (CN IX and X)
- Jaw strength (CN V)
- Moisture
- Color
- Floor of mouth

5. Extremities
Observe size and shape, symmetry and deformity, involuntary movements. Inspect and palpate arms, fingers, wrists, elbows, shoulders for the following:
- Strength
- Range of motion
- Joint pain
- Swelling
- Pulses (radial, brachial)
- Sensation (light touch, pain, temperature)
- Test reflexes: Triceps, biceps, brachioradialis

Inspect and palpate legs for the following:
- Strength
- Range of motion
- Joint pain
- Swelling, edema
- Hair distribution
- Sensation (light touch, pain, temperature)
- Pulses (dorsalis pedis, posterior tibialis)
- Test reflexes: Patellar, Achilles, plantar

6. Posterior Thorax
Inspect for muscular development, scoliosis, respiratory movement, approximation of AP diameter.
- Palpate for symmetry of respiratory movement, tenderness of CVA, spinous processes, tumors or swelling, tactile fremitus
- Percuss for pulmonary resonance
- Auscultate for breath sounds
- Auscultate for egophony, bronchophony, whispered pectoriloquy

7. Anterior Thorax
- Assess breasts for configuration, symmetry, dimpling of skin
- Assess nipples for rash, direction, inversion, retraction
- Inspect for apical impulse, other precordial pulsations
- Palpate the apical impulse and the precordium for thrills, lifts, heaves, tenderness
- Inspect neck for venous distention, pulsations, waves
- Palpate lymph nodes in the subclavian, axillary, brachial areas
- Palpate breasts
- Auscultate for rate and rhythm; character of S_1 and S_2 in the aortic, pulmonic, Erb's point, tricuspid, mitral areas; bruits at carotid, epigastrium

TABLE 3.4 Physical Examination Outline—cont'd

8. Abdomen
- Inspect for scars, shape, symmetry, bulging, muscular position and condition of umbilicus, movements (respiratory, pulsations, presence of peristaltic waves)
- Auscultate for peristalsis (i.e., bowel sounds), bruits
- Percuss then palpate to confirm positive findings; check liver (size, tenderness), spleen, kidney (size, tenderness), urinary bladder (distention)
- Palpate femoral pulses, inguinofemoral nodes, abdominal aorta

9. Neurologic

Observe motor status:
- Gait
- Toe walk
- Heel walk
- Drift

Observe coordination:
- Finger to nose
- Romberg sign
- Heel to opposite shin

Observe the following:
- Proprioception (position sense of great toe)

10. Genitalia

Male External Genitalia
- Inspect penis, noting hair distribution, prepuce, glans, urethral meatus, scars, ulcers, eruptions, structural changes, discharge
- Inspect epidermis of perineum, rectum
- Inspect skin of scrotum; palpate for descended testes, masses, pain

Female External Genitalia
- Inspect hair distribution; mons pubis, labia (minora and majora); urethral meatus; Bartholin's, urethral, Skene's glands (may be palpated, if indicated); introitus; any discharge
- Assess for presence of cystocele, prolapse
- Inspect perineum, rectum

AP, Anteroposterior; *CN,* cranial nerve; *CVA,* costovertebral angle.

 ## TABLE 3.5 Gerontologic Assessment Differences

Adaptations in Physical Assessment Techniques

General Approach
Keep patient warm and comfortable because loss of subcutaneous fat decreases ability to stay warm. Adapt positioning to physical limitations. Avoid unnecessary changes in position. Perform as many activities as possible in the position of comfort for the patient.

Skin
Handle with care because of fragility and loss of subcutaneous fat.

Head and Neck
Provide a quiet environment free from distraction because of possible sensory impairments (e.g., decreased vision, hearing).

Extremities
Use gentle movements and reinforcement techniques. Avoid having patient hop on 1 foot or perform deep knee bends if patient has limited range of motion of the extremities, decreased reflexes, or diminished sense of balance.

Thorax
Adapt examination for changes related to decreased force of expiration, weakened cough reflex, and shortness of breath.

Abdomen
Use caution in palpating patient's liver because it is readily accessible because of a thinner, softer abdominal wall. The older adult patient may have diminished pain perception in the abdominal wall.

Comprehensive Assessment

A *comprehensive assessment* includes a detailed health history and physical examination of all body systems. This is typically done on admission to the hospital or onset of care in a primary care setting.

Focused Assessment

A *focused assessment* is an abbreviated health history and examination. It is used to evaluate the status of previously identified problems and monitor for signs and symptoms of new problems. It can be done when a specific problem (e.g., pneumonia) is identified. The patient's clinical manifestations guide a focused assessment. For example, abdominal pain signals the need for a focused assessment of the abdomen. Some problems need a focused assessment of more than 1 body system. A patient with a headache may need musculoskeletal, neurologic, and head and neck examinations. Examples of focused assessments for the various body systems are found in each assessment chapter of this book.

Using Assessment Approaches

Assessment in an inpatient, acute care hospital setting is different from assessment in other settings. Focused assessment of the hospitalized patient is frequent and performed by many different HCPs. A team approach demands a high degree of consistency among HCPs from a variety of disciplines.

As you gain experience, you will be able to form a mental image of a patient's status from a few basic details, such as "85-yr-old Hispanic woman admitted for COPD exacerbation." Details from a complete verbal report, including length of stay, laboratory results, physical findings, and vital signs will help you make a clearer picture. Next, perform your own assessment using a focused approach. During your assessment, you will confirm or revise the findings that you read in the medical record and what you heard from other HCPs.

Remember, the process does not end once you have done your first assessment on a patient during rounds. Continue to gather information about all your patients throughout your shift. Everything you learned previously about each patient is considered in light of new information. For example, when you are doing a respiratory assessment on your patient with COPD, you hear crackles in her lungs. This finding should lead you to

TABLE 3.6 Findings From a Physical Examination of a Healthy Adult

Example

General Status

Well-nourished, well-hydrated, well-developed white (woman) or (man) in NAD, appears stated age, speech clear and evenly paced; is alert and oriented ×3; cooperative, calm; BMI 23.8

Skin

Clear s̄ lesions, warm and dry, trunk warmer than extremities, normal skin turgor, no ↑ vascularity, no varicose veins

Nails

Well-groomed, round 160-degree angle s̄ lesions, nail beds pink, capillary refill <2 sec

Hair

Thick, brown, shiny, normal (male, female) distribution

Head

Normocephalic, nontender

Eyes

Visual fields intact on gross confrontation

Visual acuity: Right eye   20/20
          Left eye   20/20
          Both eyes   20/20
          s̄ glasses

EOM: Intact on all gazes s̄ ptosis, nystagmus
Pupils: PERRLA, negative cover and uncover tests

Ears

Pinna intact, in proper alignment; external canal patent; small amount of cerumen present bilaterally; TMs intact; pearly gray LM, LR visible, not bulging; whisper heard at 3 ft bilaterally

Nose

Patent bilaterally; turbinates pink, no swelling
Sinuses nontender

Mouth

Moist and pink, soft and hard palates intact, uvula rises midline on "ahh," 24 teeth present and in good repair

Throat

Tonsils surgically removed, no redness

Tongue

Moist, pink, size appropriate for mouth, no lesions

Neck

Supple, s̄ masses, s̄ bruits, lymph nodes nonpalpable and nontender
Thyroid: Palpable, smooth, not enlarged
ROM: Full, intact strong
Trachea: Midline, nontender

Breasts

Soft, nonpendulous, s̄ venous pattern, s̄ dimpling, puckering
Nipples: s̄ inversion, point in same direction, areola dark and symmetric, no discharge, no masses, nontender

Axilla

Hair present, no lesions, no palpable lymph nodes

Thorax and Lungs

Respiratory rate 18, regular rhythm, oxygen saturation 98% on room air; AP < transverse diameter, no ↑ in tactile fremitus, no tenderness, lungs resonant throughout, diaphragmatic excursion 4 cm bilaterally, chest expansion symmetric, lung fields clear throughout

Heart

Rate 82, regular rate and rhythm; blood pressure: RA: 122/76, LA: 120/78; no lifts, heaves
Apical impulse: 5th ICS at MCL; no palpable thrills; S_1, S_2 louder, softer in appropriate locations; no S_3, S_4; no murmurs, rubs, clicks
Carotid, femoral, pedal, and radial pulses present; equal, 2+ bilaterally

Abdomen

No pulsations visible, rounded, positive bowel sounds in 4 quadrants, no bruits or CVA tenderness, no palpable masses

Liver

Lower border percussed at costal margin, smooth, nontender; approx. 9-cm span

Spleen

Nonpalpable, nontender

Neurologic System

Cranial nerves I–XII intact
Motor (drift, toe stand) intact
Coordination (FN, Romberg) intact
Reflexes: See diagram

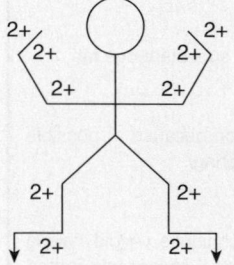

Grading Scale

0 No response
1+ Diminished
2+ Normal
3+ Increased
4+ Hyperactive
Sensation (touch, vibration, proprioception) normal bilaterally, upper and lower extremities

Musculoskeletal System

Well developed, no muscle wasting; s̄ crepitus, nodules, swelling; no scoliosis
ROM: Full and equal bilaterally, upper and lower extremities
Strength: Equal, strong 5/5 bilaterally, upper and lower extremities
Gait: Walks erect 2-foot steps, arms swinging at side s̄ staggering

TABLE 3.6 Findings From a Physical Examination of a Healthy Adult—cont'd

Female Genitalia*

External genitalia: No swelling, redness, tenderness in BUS; normal hair distribution, no cysts

Vagina: No lesions, discharge; bulging, pink

Cervix: Os closed; pink, no lesions, erosions, nontender

Uterus: Small, firm, nontender

Adnexa: No enlargement; nontender

Rectovaginal: Sphincter intact; confirms above findings

Male Genitalia*

Normal male hair distribution, negative inguinal hernia

Penis: Urethral opening patent; no redness, swelling, discharge; no lesions, structural changes

Scrotum: Testes descended; no redness, masses, tenderness

Rectal: No lesions, redness; sphincter intact; prostate small, nontender

AP, Anterior-posterior; *BMI*, body mass index; *BUS*, Bartholin's gland, urethral meatus, Skene's duct; *CVA*, costovertebral angle; *EOM*, extraocular movements; *FN*, finger to nose; *ICS*, intercostal space; *LA*, left arm; *LM*, landmarks; *LR*, light reflex; *MCL*, midclavicular line; *NAD*, no acute distress; *PERRLA*, pupils equal, round, reactive to light and accommodation; *RA*, right arm; *ROM*, range of motion; $\overline{s}$, without; S_1, S_2, S_3, and S_4, heart sounds; *TM*, tympanic membrane.

*Some data would be obtained only if the nurse has the appropriate education.

TABLE 3.7 Types of Assessment

The following describes types of assessment that you may use in various situations.

Description	When and Where Performed	Where to Find in Book
Emergency		
• Limited to assessing life-threatening conditions (e.g., inhalation injuries, anaphylaxis, myocardial infarction, shock, stroke) • Conducted to ensure survival. Focuses on elements in primary survey (e.g., airway, breathing, circulation, disability) • After life-saving interventions are started, perform brief systematic assessment to identify other injuries or problems	• Performed in any setting when signs or symptoms of a life-threatening condition appear (e.g., emergency department, critical care unit, surgical setting)	• Chapter 68, Table 68.3 and Table 68.5 • Emergency management tables throughout the book and listed in Table 68.1
Comprehensive		
• Detailed assessment of all body systems (head-to-toe assessment)	• Onset of care in primary or ambulatory care setting • On admission to hospital, rehabilitation, or long-term care setting • On initial home care visit	• Assessment chapters for each body system • Physical examination outline (Table 3.4) • Findings from physical examination of a healthy adult (Table 3.6)
Focused		
• Abbreviated assessment that focuses on 1 or more body systems that are the focus of care • Includes an assessment related to a specific problem (e.g., pneumonia, specific abnormal laboratory findings) • Monitors for signs and symptoms of new problems	• Throughout hospital admission—at beginning of a shift and as needed throughout shift • Revisit in ambulatory care setting or home care setting	• Focused assessment boxes in each assessment chapter • Tables on nursing assessment of specific diseases throughout book

do a cardiovascular assessment because heart problems (e.g., heart failure) can also cause crackles. As you gain experience, the importance of new findings will be more obvious to you. Assessment case studies integrated into all the assessment chapters will help you develop your assessment skills and knowledge.

Table 3.8 shows how you perform different types of assessments based on a patient's progress through a given hospitalization. When a patient arrives at the emergency department with a life-threatening condition, you will perform an emergency assessment based on the elements of a primary survey (e.g., airway, breathing, circulation, disability) (see Table 68.3).

Once the patient is stable, you can begin a focused assessment of related body systems. After the patient is admitted, a comprehensive assessment of all body systems is completed.

PROBLEM IDENTIFICATION

After completing the history and physical examination, analyze the data to develop a list of nursing and collaborative problems. See Chapter 1 for a description of the nursing process, including the identification of nursing and collaborative problems.

TABLE 3.8 Clinical Applications for Types of Assessment

The following is an example of how different types of assessment would be used as a patient progresses from the emergency department to a clinical unit of a hospital.

Timeline	Type of Assessment
Emergency Department Patient arrives in acute respiratory distress. Problem is found, and critical interventions are performed. Patient stabilizes.	• Perform emergency assessment (see Table 68.3). • Conduct a focused assessment of the respiratory and related body systems (e.g., cardiovascular). • May begin comprehensive assessment of all body systems.
Clinical Unit Patient is admitted to a monitored clinical unit. Beginning of each shift: Reassess per orders and more frequently as determined by the nurse.	• Complete comprehensive assessment of all body systems within proper timeframe. • Perform focused assessment of respiratory system and other related body systems per agency protocol. • Perform focused assessment of appropriate body system(s) if new symptoms are reported.

■ BRIDGE TO NCLEX EXAMINATION

The number of the question corresponds to the same-numbered outcome at the beginning of the chapter.

1. The patient health history and physical examination provide the nurse with information primarily to
   a. diagnose a medical problem.
   b. investigate a patient's signs and symptoms.
   c. classify subjective and objective patient data.
   d. identify nursing diagnoses and collaborative problems.
2. The nurse would place information about the patient's concern that his illness is threatening his job security in which functional health pattern?
   a. Role-relationship
   b. Cognitive-perceptual
   c. Coping–stress tolerance
   d. Health perception–health management

3. The nurse is preparing to examine a patient's abdomen. Place in order the proper steps for an abdominal assessment, using the numbers 1–4, with 1 = the first technique and 4 = the last technique:
   ___ Inspection
   ___ Palpation
   ___ Percussion
   ___ Auscultation
4. Which situation would require the nurse to obtain a focused assessment *(select all that apply)*?
   a. A patient denies a current health problem.
   b. A patient reports a new symptom during rounds.
   c. A previously identified problem needs reassessment.
   d. A baseline health maintenance examination is needed.
   e. A patient with an emergent problem needs immediate care.

1. d, 2. a, 3. 1, 4, 3, 2, 4. b, c.

For rationales to these answers and even more NCLEX review questions, visit *http://evolve.elsevier.com/Lewis/medsurg.*

ⓔ EVOLVE WEBSITE/RESOURCES LIST

http://evolve.elsevier.com/Lewis/medsurg
Review Questions (Online Only)
Key Points
Answer Key for Questions
• Rationales for Bridge to NCLEX Examination Questions
Conceptual Care Map Creator
Audio Glossary
Content Updates

REFERENCES

1. Jarvis C: *Physical examination and health assessment*, ed 7, St Louis, 2015, Saunders.
2. Wilson S: Giddens J. *Health assessment for nursing practice*, ed 6, St Louis, 2016, Mosby.
3. Gordon M: *Manual of nursing diagnosis*, ed 13, Boston, 2014, Jones & Bartlett.
4. Lehne R: *Pharmacology for nursing care*, ed 9, St Louis, 2016, Saunders.
5. Touhy T, Jett J: *Ebersole and Hess' gerontological nursing and healthy aging*, ed 5, St Louis, 2017, Mosby.

Patient and Caregiver Teaching

Brenda C. Morris

True compassion lies in what you can do for someone else.

Billy Graham

ⓔ http://evolve.elsevier.com/Lewis/medsurg/

CONCEPTUAL FOCUS

Adherence

Communication

Health Promotion

Patient Education

Self-Management

LEARNING OUTCOMES

1. Apply the teaching-learning process to diverse patient populations.
2. Apply strategies to support patient learning.
3. Evaluate the role of the caregiver in patient teaching.
4. Relate the physical, psychologic, and sociocultural characteristics of the patient and caregiver to the teaching-learning process.
5. Prioritize patient teaching goals for patients and caregivers.
6. Choose appropriate teaching strategies for patients and their caregivers.
7. Choose appropriate methods to evaluate patient and caregiver teaching.

KEY TERMS

caregivers, p. 48

health literacy, p. 50

learning, p. 46

learning needs, p. 51

motivational interviewing, p. 46

positive reinforcement, p. 51

self-efficacy, p. 47

teaching, p. 46

teaching plan, p. 45

teaching process, p. 49

This chapter describes the process of patient and caregiver teaching and strategies that contribute to successful teaching and learning experiences. The concept of patient and caregiver (family member or significant other) teaching is central to delivering quality patient care. It is a dynamic, interactive process that involves a change in a patient's knowledge, behavior, and/or attitude to maintain or improve health. You will find that teaching is 1 of your most challenging and rewarding roles. Teaching patients and caregivers is a key nursing intervention that makes a difference in their lives.

ROLE OF PATIENT AND CAREGIVER TEACHING

The general goals of patient teaching include health promotion, disease prevention, management of illness, and appropriate choice and use of treatment options. In patients with acute and chronic health problems, teaching can prevent complications and promote recovery, self-care, and independence. Chronic diseases are responsible for 7 of 10 deaths each year in the United States.[1] Whether patients adequately manage their health problems and maintain quality of life depends on what they learn about their conditions and what they do with this knowledge. Patients who have the knowledge, skills, and desire to take responsibility for managing their health are less likely to visit the emergency department or be readmitted.[2]

Teaching may occur wherever you work. Although agencies may employ advanced practice nurses and patient educators to establish and oversee patient teaching programs, you are always responsible for patient and caregiver teaching.[3] It is a responsibility that cannot be delegated to unlicensed assistive personnel (UAP).

Every interaction with a patient and a caregiver is a potential *teachable moment*. On any given day, more informal opportunities to teach occur than formal opportunities. Take advantage of and document all these moments. For example, when you teach a patient with asthma how to use a peak flow meter, you do not need a formal teaching plan. However, when your patient has a specific learning need about health promotion or management of a health problem, you should develop a teaching plan. A **teaching plan** includes (1) assessment of the patient's ability and readiness to learn, (2) identification of teaching needs, (3) development of learning goals with the patient, (4) implementation of the teaching, and (5) evaluation of the patient's learning.

TEACHING-LEARNING PROCESS

Teaching is "a complex process intended to facilitate learning" (p. 75).[4] When a nurse is teaching a patient about health, the nurse becomes the teacher and the patient becomes the learner. Nurses often teach patients using various methods such as direct instruction, coaching, counseling, and behavior modification. Teaching may be formal, such as giving a planned presentation to a group of patients and their caregivers, or informal such as teaching a patient about medications prior to giving them.

Learning is the act of a person acquiring knowledge, skills, or attitudes that may result in a permanent change.[4] Observation of this change is an indication that learning has occurred. However, learning may not result in any observable change. A patient who understands the instruction and is fully informed may choose not to change behavior.

Although learning may occur without teaching, a teacher helps to organize information and skills to make learning more efficient. In patient teaching, the teaching-learning process involves the patient, the patient's caregiver(s), and you.

Adult Learner

Adult Learning Principles. Understanding how and why adults learn is important for you to effectively teach patients and their caregivers. Many theories of adult learning have evolved from the work of Malcolm Knowles. He identified 6 principles of *andragogy* (adult learning) that are important for you to consider when teaching adults (Table 4.1).[5]

Models to Promote Health. Patients and their caregivers may progress through a series of steps before they are willing or able to accept a change in health behaviors. Prochaska and Velicer proposed 6 stages of change in their *Transtheoretical Model of Health Behavior Change* (Table 4.2).[6] This model is often used for planning to help patients stop smoking, manage diabetes, and lose weight.

Motivational interviewing uses nonconfrontational interpersonal communication techniques to motivate patients to change behavior.[7] This strategy includes interventions that enhance the patient's motivation for change (Table 4.3). The techniques used in motivational interviewing are linked to the stages of change identified by Prochaska and Velicer.

During the process of change, relapse and recycling through the stages are expected. Sometimes patients do not change behaviors, or they return to previous behaviors after a period of change. This may mean that the interventions used did not consider the patient's stage of change. Identify the patient's current stage of readiness for change and the stage to which the patient is moving. Patients who are in the early stages of change need and use different kinds of motivational support than patients at later stages of change.

For example, a hospitalized patient who smokes cigarettes may be in the *precontemplation* or *contemplation* stage of change. In the precontemplation stage, patients are not concerned about

TABLE 4.1	**Adult Learning Principles Applied to Patient and Caregiver Teaching**	
Principles	**Teaching Implications for Nurse**	**Examples**
Need to know	• Patients need to know why they should learn something, what they need to learn, and how it will help them. • Ask the patient questions such as, "What do you think you need to learn about this topic?"	Your patient and his caregiver ask what they need to know about exercise guidelines after a heart attack.
Readiness to learn	• Readiness and motivation to learn are high when facing new tasks. • Health crises provide opportunities for patients to learn and change behavior. • Stress and anxiety may interfere with learning, thus requiring frequent reinforcement of content.	While recovering from a transient ischemic attack, your patient tells you that she is ready to learn about the changes she needs to take to reduce her risk for stroke.
Prior experiences	• Motivation is increased when one already knows something about the subject from past experiences. • Identification of past knowledge and experiences can help find familiar ground to increase patients' confidence.	Your patient needs to begin injections of enoxaparin. She tells you that she gives her father insulin injections and is ready to learn how to give this medication.
Motivation to learn	• Patients prefer to apply learning at once. • Long-term goals may have less appeal than short-term goals. • Focus teaching on information that the patient views as needed right now.	Your patient is scheduled for discharge in the morning. Both she and her caregiver have received instruction on wound care and have watched the procedure. The caregiver tells you that he wants to perform the wound care today.
Orientation to learning	• Patients seek out various resources for specific learning and prefer choices. • When the patient does not recognize the relevancy of the teaching, offer explanations of the value of the learning. • Teaching should target the specific problem or circumstance.	Your patient, who is newly diagnosed with diabetes mellitus, tells you that he is worried about the diet changes he will need to make. Share several options with him to learn about diet changes (e.g., cooking classes, Web-based tutorials, mobile applications, individual sessions with the dietitian, brochures).
Self-concept	• Patients need control and self-direction (sense of autonomy) to maintain their sense of self-worth. • Patients do not learn when we treat them like children and tell them what they must do.	Your patient has a temporary colostomy. She says she is not ready to look at the stoma. Work out a schedule with her for learning colostomy care that meets her need for control and prepares her for self-care.

TABLE 4.2	Stages of Change in Transtheoretical Model	
Stage	**Patient Behavior**	**Nursing Implications**
1. Precontemplation	Is not considering a change. Is not ready to learn	Provide support, increase awareness of condition. Describe benefits of change and risks of not changing
2. Contemplation	Thinks about a change. May state recognition of need to change. Says "I know I should," but identifies barriers	Introduce what is involved in changing the behavior. Reinforce the stated need to change
3. Preparation	Starts planning the change, gathers information, sets a date to start change, shares decision to change with others	Reinforce the positive outcomes of change, give information and encouragement, develop a plan, help set priorities, and identify sources of support
4. Action	Begins to change behavior through practice. Tentative and may experience relapses	Reinforce behavior with reward, encourage self-reward, discuss choices to help minimize relapses and regain focus. Help patient plan to deal with potential relapses
5. Maintenance	Practices the behavior regularly. Able to sustain the change	Continue to reinforce behavior. Provide more teaching on the need to maintain change.
6. Termination	Change has become part of lifestyle. Behavior no longer considered a change	Evaluate effectiveness of the new behavior. No further intervention needed.

Adapted from Prochaska J, Velicer W: The transtheoretical model of health behavior change, *Am J Health Promot* 12:38, 1997. (Classic).

TABLE 4.3 Key Aspects of Motivational Interviewing
• Listen rather than tell.
• Adjust to, rather than oppose, patient resistance.
• Express empathy through reflective listening.
• Focus on the positive. Do not criticize the patient.
• Gently persuade with the understanding that change is up to the patient.
• Focus on the patient's strengths to support the hope needed to make changes.
• Avoid argument and direct confrontation, which can cause defensiveness and a power struggle.
• Help the patient recognize the "gap" between where he or she is and where he or she hopes to be.

their cigarette smoking and are not considering changing their behavior. During this stage, it is important to help the patient increase awareness of risks and problems related to smoking and create doubt about using cigarettes. Ask the patient what he or she thinks could happen if the behavior is continued. Give evidence of the problem (e.g., x-ray changes), and share facts about the risks of smoking. Although patients may not be ready to change behavior while experiencing an acute health problem, the seeds of doubt are sown. In other cases, such as when a patient has a life-threatening condition (e.g., heart attack), there may be an immediate awareness of the problem and motivation to change.

A patient in the *contemplation* stage of change often is ambivalent. The patient understands that the behavior is a problem and that change is necessary. However, he or she believes that change is too hard or that the pleasures of the behavior are worth the risks. This is seen in the patient who says, "I know that I have to stop smoking. This heart attack really scared me. I know I need to lose weight and start exercising, but I can't change everything all at once. Smoking helps me control my eating; I can't stop until I lose some weight." During this stage of change, help the patient consider the positive and negative aspects of his or her behavior (e.g., tobacco use), gently trying to tip the balance in favor of positive behavior. Helping the

patient discover internal motivators in addition to those external motivators (e.g., second heart attack, lung disease) that push the patient toward change can move the patient from contemplating change to preparation and action. Throughout this process, emphasize the patient's personal choices and responsibilities for change.

As the patient moves from contemplation to *preparation,* we can help strengthen the commitment to change by helping the patient develop self-efficacy. This is the belief that one can succeed in a given situation. In this case, it is the patient's belief that they can change tobacco-use behaviors. Support even the smallest effort to change. Movement through action and maintenance stages of change requires continued support to increase the patient's involvement and participation in treatment. You can find a comprehensive discussion of motivational interviewing in the Treatment Improvement Protocols available at *www.ncbi.nlm.nih.gov/books/NBK14856.*

The resolution of acute health problems or discharge from the hospital often occurs before the patient moves to the preparation and action stages of change. As the patient develops readiness in the contemplative stage of change, continue to support him or her with referral to appropriate community and outpatient resources.

Nurse as Teacher
Required Competencies
Knowledge of Subject Matter. Although it is impossible to be an expert in all subject areas, develop confidence as a teacher by becoming knowledgeable about the topic. For example, if you are teaching patients about managing hypertension, you must be able to explain what hypertension is and why treating it is important. Teach patients what they need to know about exercise, diet, medication side effects, monitoring BP, and situations that must be reported to the health care provider (HCP). Last, provide the patient with resources such as credible websites, brochures, and information about support organizations (e.g., American Heart Association).

Sometimes you will not be able to answer patients' or caregivers' questions. Clarify the questions to be sure of what they are asking. When you do not know the answer, tell this to the patient and caregiver. Seek help from co-workers, patient educators, and other reliable sources to answer the question.

Communication Skills. Patient teaching depends on effective communication between you and the patient or caregiver. Medical jargon can be intimidating and frightening. Introduce medical words and define their meanings. Limit the use of acronyms (e.g., CABG for coronary artery bypass graft) and abbreviations (e.g., IV) when talking with patients. Have the patient and caregiver clarify their understandings of the disease process. Ask them to explain what they know in their own words. For example, if we tell a patient he has leukopenia, define this term in words that mean something to him. Explain that *leuko-* refers to a leukocyte, a white blood cell that fights infections, and that *penia* refers to a shortage. To enhance learning, use a brief explanation such as, "You have a shortage of white blood cells, the cells that fight infection."

Nonverbal communication is critical when teaching. Cultural practices often guide nonverbal communication. For example, in Western culture, sitting in an open, relaxed position facing the patient with eyes at the same level delivers a positive nonverbal message (Fig. 4.1). Raise the patient's bed or sit in a chair at the bedside. Open body gestures communicate interest and a willingness to share. Patients from Eastern cultures may prefer that you avoid direct eye contact and give health information to a family spokesperson rather than directly to the patient.

Develop the art of *active listening* by paying attention to what the patient says, observing the patient's nonverbal cues, and not interrupting. Nod in response to the patient's statements and restate what the patient is saying to help clarify communication.

Empathy is the courage to enter the world of another in a manner that does not judge or correct but tries to understand. Empathy means putting aside your own self and stepping into the patient's shoes. Active listening, combined with empathy, is a powerful way to communicate caring and prepare the patient to learn.

Challenges to Nurse-Teacher Effectiveness. Teaching patients and caregivers has many challenges, including (1) lack of time, (2) your own feelings as a teacher, (3) nurse-patient differences in learning goals, and (4) rapid or early discharge from the health care system.

Lack of time can be a barrier to effective teaching. For example, the patient's physical needs may compete for time that you could use for teaching. To make the most of limited time, it is critical to set learning priorities with the patient. Tell the patient at the beginning of the interaction how much time you can devote to the session. Deliver or reinforce teaching during every contact with the patient or caregiver. For example, when giving medications, explain the purpose and side effects of each. Reinforcing small pieces of information over time is an effective teaching strategy, especially if information is new or complex.

Other barriers are your *own feelings as a teacher* and insecurity about your own knowledge and skill. Teaching is a skill that will take time to master. Become familiar with the resources for patient teaching available at your agency. Consult with nurse educators or experienced co-workers for further help with developing your teaching skills.

Sometimes disagreements arise among the patient, the caregiver, and you about the expectations or outcomes of teaching. Having realistic discussions about discharge plans, timelines,

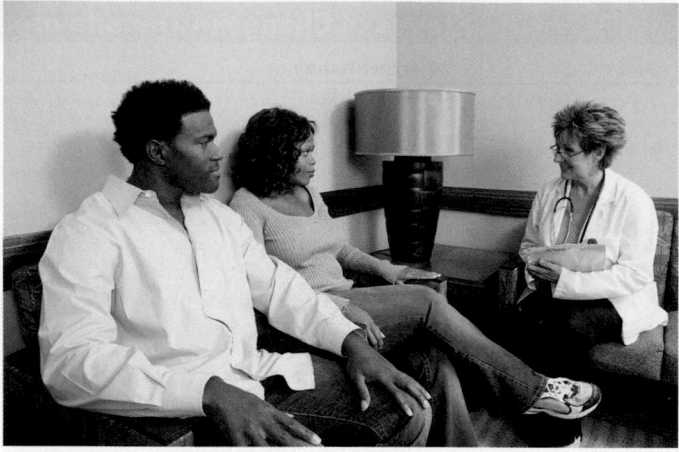

FIG. 4.1 Open, relaxed positioning of patient, spouse, and nurse at eye level promotes communication in teaching and learning. (© Jupiterimages/Photos.com/Thinkstock.)

and home care options can emphasize the need for learning. For example, after a diagnosis of heart failure due to aortic valve insufficiency and subsequent emergent valve surgery, the patient and caregiver may reject teaching efforts until they realize and accept the seriousness of the patient's health problem.

Another important challenge to patient teaching relates to patients having early and quick discharges from the health care system. Shortened lengths of hospital stays have resulted in patients having only basic teaching plans implemented; thus it is important to begin teaching patients soon after admission to the health care system.

Caregiver Support in the Teaching-Learning Process

The teaching and learning process applies to the caregiver as well as the patient. Caregivers are people who care for those who cannot care for themselves. Most caregivers are family members or significant others who (1) give or help with direct patient care; (2) provide emotional, social, spiritual, and possibly financial support for the patient; and (3) manage and coordinate health care services.

About 1 in 4 American adults serves as a caregiver to a person with a long-term disability or illness.[8] We often categorize caregivers by their relationship to the patient. The most common caregivers are spouses, adult children, parents, grandparents, and life partners. Identify the key caregiver(s) and assess their roles and relationships to the patient. Because the patient's health problem affects family roles and functions, it is important to identify the needs of caregivers. If the caregiver's needs are unmet, this may interfere with the ability to assist the patient (Table 4.4).

Consider cultural differences when assessing the caregiver. In some cultures, a male family member may be the designated spokesperson to receive and communicate information among family members and the patient. In this type of situation, the caregivers who will actually provide care for the patient and the family spokesperson should be included in discharge planning (see Chapter 2 for more information on culturally competent care).

When possible, teach the caregiver along with the patient. Explain the goals of the teaching plan. Caregivers may need

TABLE 4.4 Assessment of Caregiver Needs
Ask caregivers the following questions: 1. How are you coping with your caregiver role?   2. Do you have any problems performing your caregiver responsibilities?   3. How much support do you get from outside sources (e.g., other family members, friends)?   4. Are you aware of and do you use community resources (e.g., disease-specific professional organizations [such as Alzheimer's Association, American Heart Association], adult day care centers, church, synagogue)?   5. Do you know about resources that are available for respite (someone caring for your loved one while you have time to yourself)?   6. What kind of help or services do you need now and in the near future?   7. How can I or other health care providers help you in your caregiving role?

TABLE 4.5 The Joint Commission's Speak Up Initiative
Speak up if you have questions or concerns. If you still do not understand, ask again. It is your body and you have a right to know.   **P**ay attention to the care you get. Always make sure you are getting the right treatments and medicines by the right health care professionals. Do not assume anything.   **E**ducate yourself about your illness. Learn about the medical tests you get and your treatment plan.   **A**sk a trusted family member or friend to be your advocate (advisor or supporter).   **K**now what medicines you take and why you take them. Medicine errors are the most common health care mistakes.   **U**se a hospital, clinic, surgery center, or other type of health care organization that has been carefully checked out.   **P**articipate in all decisions about your treatment. You are the center of the health care team.

Source: The Joint Commission: To prevent health care errors, patients are urged to Speak Up (poster). Retrieved from *www.jointcommission.org/assets/1/18/SpeakUp_Poster.pdf.*

help to learn the physical and technical requirements of care, find resources for home care, find equipment and supplies, and rearrange the home to accommodate the patient. Sources of support for the transition from hospital to home include community-based agencies, Medicare and Medicaid offices, and case managers at the hospital and insurance companies.

Patients and caregivers may have different teaching needs. For example, the priority of an older patient with a diabetic leg ulcer may be to learn how to transfer from a bed to a chair in the least painful manner. On the other hand, the caregiver may be most concerned about learning the technique for dressing changes. Both the patient's and caregiver's learning needs are important. The patient and caregiver may also have differing or conflicting views of the illness and treatment options. Developing a successful teaching plan requires you to view the patient's needs within the context of the caregiver's needs. For instance, you may teach a patient with right-sided *paresis* (weakness) self-feeding techniques with special tools, but at a home visit you find the caregiver feeding the patient. On questioning, the caregiver reveals that it is too hard to watch the patient struggle with feeding, it takes too long, and it is messy. As a result, the caregiver decided that it is easier to feed the patient. This is an example of a situation in which the patient and caregiver need more teaching about goals for self-care.

Discuss the potential that support groups, family and friends, and community resources have for providing ongoing resources. Support groups help by people sharing experiences and information, offering understanding and acceptance, and suggesting solutions to common problems and concerns.

Regulatory Mandates for Patient Teaching

Several important agencies have specific mandates related to teaching hospitalized patients. The Joint Commission's (TJC's) accreditation standards, National Patient Safety Goals,[9] and the American Hospital Association's Patient Care Partnership[10] state that patients have a fundamental right to receive information about their care. This information includes their diagnosis, treatment, and prognosis in terms that they can understand. For example, this means that written materials must be at the patient's reading level. One program started by TJC, Speak Up, was developed to encourage patients to become more involved and informed about their plan of care (Table 4.5).[11] Another program implemented by the Institute for Healthcare Improvement's National Patient

Safety Foundation is Ask Me 3.[12] Both programs encourage patients to ask specific questions about their care.

PROCESS OF PATIENT TEACHING

We use many different approaches in the process of patient teaching. However, the approach used most often by nurses parallels the nursing process. The teaching process and the nursing process involve the development of a plan that includes assessment, goal setting, implementation, and evaluation. The teaching process, like the nursing process, may not always flow in linear order, but the steps serve as checkpoints.

Assessment

During the general nursing assessment, gather data to determine if the patient has learning needs. For example, what does the patient know about the health problem? How does he or she perceive the problem? If you identify a learning need, you need a more detailed assessment, and address that problem with the teaching plan. Include caregivers in the assessment as you determine their role and ability to care for the patient at home. Key questions to use in the assessment are outlined in Table 4.6.

Physical Factors. The patient's age is a factor to consider in the teaching plan. Age affects the patient's experiences and rate of learning. Some effects of increased age on learning may be obvious, but the inexperience of younger people can also affect learning. For example, a man in his twenties who has never thought about his own mortality may be unable to accept the long-term health implications of diabetes mellitus.

Sensory impairments (e.g., hearing or vision loss) decrease sensory input and can alter learning. Cognition may be affected by disorders of the nervous system (e.g., stroke, head trauma) and by other diseases (e.g., liver impairment, heart failure). Patients with altered cognition may have a hard time learning and need more caregiver involvement in the teaching process. You need manual dexterity to perform skills such as giving injections or BP monitoring.

Pain, fatigue, and certain drugs influence the patient's ability to learn. No one can learn effectively when in pain.

TABLE 4.6 Assessment of Factors Affecting Patient Teaching

Key Factors and Questions

Physical
- What is the patient's age?
- Is the patient acutely ill?
- Is the patient fatigued or in pain?
- What is the primary diagnosis?
- Are there other medical problems?
- What is the patient's current mental status?
- What is the patient's hearing ability? Visual ability? Motor ability?
- What drugs does the patient take that may affect learning?

Psychologic
- Does the patient appear anxious, afraid, depressed, defensive?
- Is the patient in a state of denial?
- What is the patient's level of motivation? Self-efficacy?

Sociocultural
- What are the patient's beliefs about his or her illness or treatment?
- Is the proposed teaching consistent with the patient's cultural values?
- What is the patient's educational experience, reading ability, primary language?
- What is the patient's present or past occupation?
- How does the patient describe his or her financial status?
- What is the patient's living arrangement?
- Does the patient have family or close friends?

Learner
- What does the patient already know about his or her health problem?
- What does the patient think is most important to learn?
- What prior learning experiences could act as a frame of reference for current learning needs?
- Is the patient ready to learn? Change behavior?
- How does the patient learn best (e.g., reading, listening, looking at pictures, doing, playing games)?
- In what kind of environment does the patient learn best? Formal classroom? Computer/Web-based setting? Informal setting, such as home? Alone or in a group?
- In what way should the caregiver(s) be involved in patient teaching?

Provide teaching after the patient's pain is controlled. A tired, weak patient cannot learn effectively because of the inability to concentrate. Sleep disruption is common during hospitalization, and patients are often sleep deprived at the time of discharge. Drugs that cause central nervous system depression, such as opioids and sedatives, decrease mental alertness and can affect the patient's ability to learn new information. Adjust the teaching plan by setting high-priority goals based on need-to-know information and realistic expectations. Patients often need a referral for follow-up so that teaching continues and learning is confirmed after discharge.

Psychologic Factors. Psychologic factors have a major influence on the patient's ability to learn. Anxiety and depression are common reactions to illness. Although mild anxiety increases the learner's perceptual and learning abilities, moderate or severe anxiety limits learning. Anxiety and depression can negatively affect the patient's motivation and readiness to learn. For instance, the patient newly diagnosed with diabetes who is depressed about the diagnosis may not listen or respond to instructions about glucose testing. Discussions with the patient about these concerns or referrals to an appropriate support group may help the patient to learn that management of diabetes is possible.

Patients respond to the stress of illness with a variety of defense mechanisms, such as denial, rationalization, or even humor. A patient who denies having cancer will not be receptive to information related to treatment options. Similarly, a caregiver may have a hard time accepting a terminal diagnosis. A patient using rationalization will imagine any number of reasons for avoiding change or for rejecting teaching. For example, a patient with heart disease who does not want to change dietary habits will relate stories of people who have eaten bacon and eggs every day and lived to be 100. Some patients use humor to filter reality or decrease anxiety. They may use laughter to escape from the experience of facing threatening situations. Humor in the teaching process is important and useful but notice when humor is used excessively or inappropriately to avoid reality.

One important factor in successful adoption of new behaviors is the patient's sense of self-efficacy. There is a strong relationship between self-efficacy and outcomes of illness management. Self-efficacy increases when a person gains new skills in managing a threatening situation. It decreases if the person has repeated failure, especially early in the course of events. Plan easily achievable goals early in the teaching sessions. Proceed from simple to more complex content to support a feeling of success.

Sociocultural Factors

Health Literacy. Literacy is the ability to use printed and written information to function in society. **Health literacy** is the degree to which a person can obtain and understand basic health information needed to make appropriate health decisions.[13] As many as 50% of U.S. adults have limited literacy skills, and almost 90% have limited health literacy skills.[14]

Improving health literacy will advance population health. Currently, only 64% of adults report receiving easy-to-understand instructions from their HCPs and only 24% report that a HCP asked them to describe how they will follow the instructions provided.[15] Patients with low levels of health literacy have trouble understanding and acting on health information, placing them at greater risk for hospital readmissions.[16] Even patients with high levels of health literacy may have a hard time understanding complex health information if they are sick or stressed. Health illiteracy results in poor patient outcomes, not following treatment plans, limited self-management skills, and increased health disparities.[16]

It is challenging to assess health literacy, because patients may be embarrassed to admit that they are having trouble understanding health information. Health professionals often over-estimate the health literacy of patients, so it is important to routinely assess health literacy level. Easy-to-use assessment tools are available. The Single-Item Literacy Screener (SILS) uses 1 question to identify adults who need help with reading.[17] The question is, "How often do you need to have someone help you when you read instructions, pamphlets, or other written material from your doctor or pharmacy?"

Another approach is to implement health literacy universal precautions. These are the steps to take when we assume that all patients may have difficulty understanding important health

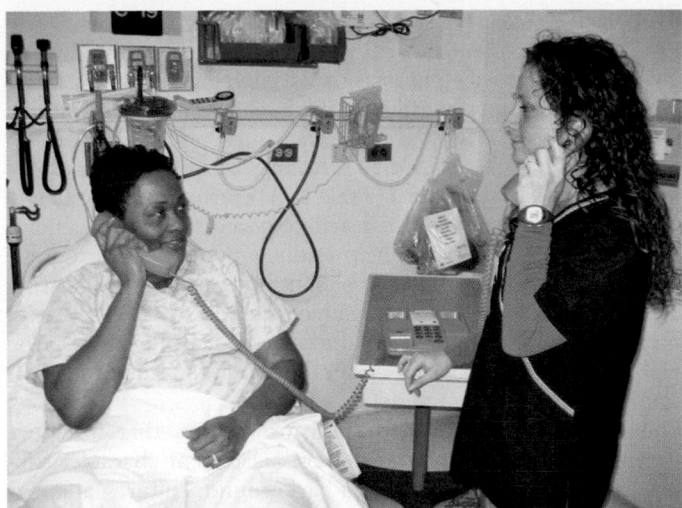

FIG. 4.2 Nurse communicating with a non–English-speaking patient using a translation phone service. (Courtesy Linda Bucher, RN, PhD, CEN, CNE, Staff Nurse, Virtua Memorial Hospital, Mt. Holly, N.J.)

information and accessing health services. These include using simple communications about health information and verifying patient understanding.[14]

TJC states that we must tailor patient teaching to the patient's literacy needs. For example, teach patients and give them written materials in their primary language. Teaching materials are available in multiple languages. It is preferable to use medical interpreters instead of family members or friends, to protect patient privacy (Fig. 4.2). Medical interpreters are discussed in Chapter 2 in Table 2.10. Choose patient teaching materials written at the fifth-grade or lower reading level. Other interventions to help patients with low levels of health literacy include using the teach-back method, highlighting key text, and teaching content in small increments.

Cultural Considerations. The wider culture to which a patient belongs influences learning. Cultural traditions influence our health practices, beliefs, and behavior. These traditions, which can affect patient teaching, can be identified in a cultural assessment (see Table 2.3). TJC requires that patient teaching be tailored to the patient's cultural needs.[18] Ask patients to describe their beliefs about health and illness.

One cultural element that specifically affects the teaching-learning process is a conflict between the patient's cultural beliefs and values and the behaviors promoted by the health care team. For example, you can teach a patient who values a trim figure to use diet and exercise to keep that figure while at the same time improving BP control. However, being heavier may be valued in another patient's culture. This patient may have more difficulty accepting the need for diet and exercise in BP control.

Assess the patient's use of cultural remedies and healing practices (see the Complementary & Alternative Therapies Box: Assessment of Use of Herbs and Dietary Supplements in Chapter 3, p. 35). Consider the cultural remedies that may interfere with or are contraindicated by the treatment plan.

Last, it is important to know who has authority in the patient's culture. The patient may defer to the authority, such as an elder or a spiritual leader, for decisions. In this case, identify and work with the patient and the decision makers in the

patient's cultural group. See Chapter 2 for more information on cultural competence.

Socioeconomic Considerations. Consider a variety of socioeconomic factors when preparing to teach patients. Knowing the patient's present or past occupation may help you determine the vocabulary to use during teaching. For example, an auto mechanic may understand the volume overload associated with heart failure as flooding an engine. An engineer may understand the principles of physics associated with gravity and pressures when discussing vascular problems.

Ask the patient about living arrangements. Whether the patient lives alone, with friends, or with family influences who you include in the teaching process. You may need to change the teaching plan if the patient does not have access to electricity or phones. If the patient has unmet learning needs by the time of discharge, arrange for ongoing teaching after discharge.

Learner Factors. Last, assess learner factors, including the patient's learning needs, readiness to learn, and learning style.

Learning Needs. Learning needs are the new knowledge and skills that a person must have to meet a goal. The assessment of learning needs determines what the patient already knows and any past experiences with health problems. Patients with long-standing health problems may have different learning needs from those patients with newly diagnosed health problems.

What patients should learn about managing an illness or what behaviors promote health may seem obvious to you. However, what you think is important may be different from what patients want to know. Remember, adults learn best when the teaching gives information that they view as being needed at once (Table 4.1). Ask patients to prioritize what they see as the most critical information. Start by giving the patient a list of the recommended topics and then ask the patient to identify other topics not on the list. Having patients prioritize their own learning needs lets you begin with the patient's most important needs. Explain why critical information is "need to know."

Readiness to Learn. Readiness to learn and motivation depend on multiple factors, such as perceived need, attitudes, and beliefs. When teaching adults, identify what information the person values. Readiness to learn is increased if the patient perceives a need for information, has a belief that a behavior change has value, or perceives the learning activities as new and stimulating.[5]

Before implementing the teaching plan, determine where the patient is in the stages of change (Table 4.2). If the patient is in the precontemplation stage, provide support and increase the patient's awareness of the problem until the patient is ready to consider a change in behavior. Nurses in outpatient settings and home health care can continue to assess the patient's readiness to learn and implement the teaching plan as the patient moves through the stages of change. Reinforcement throughout the change process is a strong motivational factor for achieving a desired behavior. Positive reinforcement involves rewarding the target behavior with positive feedback or other rewards to maintain the behavior.[6]

Learning Style. Each person has a distinct style of learning. The 3 general learning styles are (1) *visual* (reading, pictures), (2) *auditory* (listening), and (3) *physical* (doing things). People often use more than 1 learning style to gain new knowledge or skills. To assess a patient's preferred learning style, ask how the patient likes to learn and has learned effectively in the past.

When assessing the patient's learning style, identify the patient who does not read or who has low health literacy. For example, the patient may tell you that he or she does not read much but likes to learn from television. In addition, assess the patient's *ehealth literacy*. This refers to the degree that patients use digital information (e.g., webinars, online health management tools) and communication technologies (e.g., online communication with HCP, online support groups) to improve their health (Fig. 4.3).[19] When possible, use the patient's or caregiver's preferred learning style.

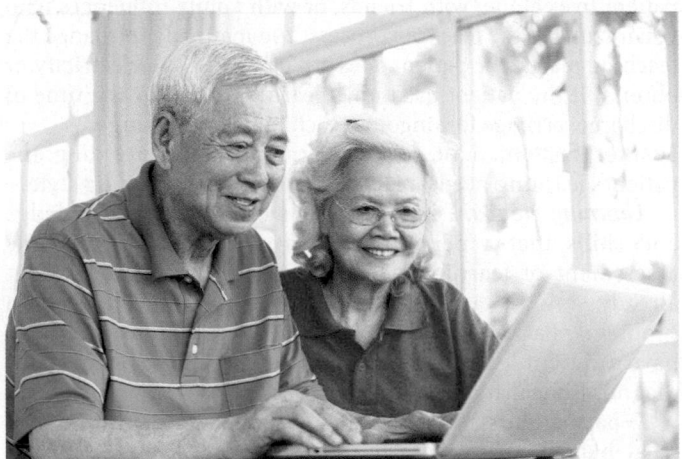

FIG. 4.3 Older couple accessing the Web for health information. (© monkeybusinessimages/iStock/Thinkstock.)

Planning

Prioritize the patient's learning needs and agree on learning goals. If the patient's physical or psychologic condition interferes with participation, involve the patient's caregiver(s) in the planning phase.

Setting Goals. It is important to have clear and measurable learning goals or outcomes (Table 4.7). Learning goals relate to the intended outcome of the learning process, guide the choice of teaching strategies, and help evaluate the patient's progress. Learning goals are parallel to patient outcomes in the nursing care plan (NCP). Most settings have standardized NCPs with preset goals and interventions for specific learning needs. You will modify these NCPs based on the patient's unique sociocultural and learner characteristics.

Choosing Teaching Strategies. Three factors that influence the choice of teaching strategies are (1) patient characteristics (e.g., learning style, educational background, culture, language skills), (2) subject matter, and (3) available resources. Table 4.8 summarizes learner characteristics and recommends teaching approaches based on the generation of the patient or caregiver.

Consider various strategies (Table 4.9) in the teaching plan. We often use multiple teaching strategies to improve learning (Fig. 4.4). Discussion is the most common type of interaction used in teaching patients and caregivers. A type of group teaching involves *peer teaching*, as occurs in support groups. Patients dealing with common problems such as cancer, alcoholism, and eating disorders can receive help from peer teaching.

Adapt your teaching methods when teaching patients with a disability how to care for themselves or how to take part in

---

TABLE 4.7 Writing Learning Goals

Elements of Learning Goals

Learning goals (also called outcomes or objectives) are written statements that define exactly how patients demonstrate their knowledge of the content. Goals address the following 4 questions:

1. Who Will Perform the Activity or Acquire the Desired Behavior?
Examples:
I (the patient) will
I (the caregiver) will
We (patient's family/caregivers) will

2. What Is the Actual Behavior That the Learner Will Exhibit to Show Mastery of the Goal?
Examples:
List the symptoms.
Self-administer an insulin injection.
Choose from a hospital menu.

3. What Are the Conditions Under Which the Behavior Is to Be Demonstrated?
Examples:
In front of the nurse
From a random list
Using sterile technique

4. What Are the Specific Criteria That Will Be Used to Measure the Patient's Success, Such as Time and Degree of Accuracy?
Examples:
With 100% accuracy
Over the next week
Before discharge

Verbs in Learning Goals

Avoid vague, ambiguous verbs that are hard to measure:	*Use verbs that have precise descriptions with few interpretations:*
• Appreciate	• Identify
• Learn	• List
• Understand	• Describe
• Enjoy	• Demonstrate
• Feel	• Perform
• Value	• Choose

Poorly and Well-Written Learning Goals

Example of Poorly Written Learning Goal	**Examples of Well-Written Learning Goals**
• The patient will understand the importance of managing his own colostomy. *Analysis:* It is not clear how the patient will show that he "understands" the importance of managing his colostomy, when and to whom he will demonstrate this behavior, or what criteria will be used to determine whether the goal has been met.	• The patient will describe to the nurse the basic steps for changing the colostomy pouch and skin barrier by 2/14/21. • Using correct technique, the patient will empty his colostomy pouch when one-third full. • The patient's caregiver will perform colostomy care, including changing the pouch and skin barrier. • Given a list of signs and symptoms related to complications of a colostomy, the patient and caregiver will identify signs and symptoms to report to a health care provider before discharge. *Analysis:* When learning goals are clear and specific and documented in the patient's record, all members of the health care team can work together to achieve the same outcomes.

TABLE 4.8 Learner Characteristics and Teaching Strategies by Generation

Birth Year	Learner Characteristics	Recommended Teaching Strategies
Millennials (Generation Y, Yers, Nexters, Digital Natives)		
1981–2000	• Multitaskers • Prefer interactive and virtual environments • Technologically focused • Need flexibility • Short attention span • Team players • Prefer more structured learning compared to Xers • Accustomed to learning whatever, wherever, whenever	• Integrate technology and media in teaching • Discuss reliable health-related mobile apps and websites • Download health information to smart phones, tablets, or similar devices • Consider group teaching • Consider active learning approaches
Generation X (Xers, Digital Natives)		
1965–1980	• Self-directed or self-paced learning • Self-reliant • Consumers of education • Short attention span	• Integrate technology and media in teaching • Discuss reliable websites • Consider health-related mobile applications • Give Web-based education materials • Provide education materials that are brief and easy to read • Encourage questions
Baby Boomers (Digital Immigrants)		
1946–1964	• Emphasis on self-knowledge • Solve problems by action • Acquisition of knowledge from authoritative sources • Receptive to feedback • Prefer text over graphics • Process (step-by-step) oriented	• Assess ehealth literacy and consider strategies as appropriate • Consider lecture or lecture-discussion (e.g., PowerPoint presentation) • Use patient education TV channels • Provide printed materials
Veterans (Traditionalists, Digital Immigrants)		
Born before 1946	• Emphasis on rote learning • Memorization of knowledge • Follow rules	• Assess ehealth literacy and consider strategies as appropriate • Consider lecture or lecture-discussion • Use pictures and printed materials such as books

Compiled from Bradshaw M, Lowenstein A: *Innovative teaching strategies in nursing*, ed 7, Burlington, Mass, 2017, Jones & Bartlett Learning; and Hart S: Today's learners and educators: bridging the generational gaps, *Teach Learn Nurs* 12:253, 2017.

their own care. It is essential to know how to modify teaching methods to meet the needs of patients with cognitive impairment, hearing loss, limited manual dexterity, or vision loss. Magnifying glasses, bright lighting, and materials printed in a large font may help the patient with impaired vision read teaching materials. More visual stimuli can help people with hearing loss. Using adaptive equipment may help those with problems performing manual skills. Table 4.10 presents strategies for teaching patients with disabilities.

Learning Materials. Use learning materials in multiple formats. Learn what resources are available in your agency and from support services and professional groups. The use of CDs/DVDs and online videos is helpful, particularly when teaching visual content such as the steps of a procedure (e.g., suctioning a tracheostomy). The health care agency's television system may show high-quality, professionally produced patient teaching programs on demand or on a rotating schedule (Fig. 4.4).

Printed materials are useful for teaching patients and caregivers, especially for those whose preferred learning style is reading. Some health-related organizations, such as the American Cancer Society and the American Heart Association provide quality patient education materials free of charge. Some governmental organizations, such as the National Institutes of Health and the Centers for Disease Control and Prevention, have learning materials for patients and caregivers. These materials can be used in combination with other teaching strategies. For instance, after a discussion on the effects of smoking on health, you may use material from the American Cancer Society to reinforce the information.

When writing teaching materials, use several techniques to keep the reading level at a fifth-grade level. These include (1) organize the content logically; (2) highlight or place key information in bold or italics; (3) use short, common words of 1 or 2 syllables; (4) define medical words in simple language; (5) keep sentences short, between 10 and 15 words; (6) use pictures or drawings; and (7) use active voice in the same manner in which you would normally speak.[20] Whenever possible, appraise written materials for readability level using word processing (e.g., Microsoft Word) or Web-based (e.g., *www.wordscount.info*) programs.

Using Technology. Patients may use the Internet and other digital technology (e.g., smart phones) to obtain information and manage their health. Patients can quickly do a Web search or open a software application for access to information about diseases, drugs, treatments, and surgeries. Your job is to help patients sift through the information and determine if it is valid, reliable, and usable. Encourage patients to use websites established by the government, universities, or reputable health-related organizations (e.g., American Diabetes Association, American Heart Association, National Institutes of Health, U.S. Food and Drug Administration). Understanding the principles of Web searching for health information and teaching patients how to find valid information are critical skills. The presence of Internet connections in many patient rooms provides an opportunity for you to teach patients about their illness and how to use the Web to find related information.

Overall, the digital health divide for older adults has narrowed. However, adults older than 75 years of age, those with less than a high school education, and those with very low income are less likely to access the Internet for health-related Internet use.[21] Organizations dedicated to improving the quality of life for older adults promote the development of user-friendly websites (e.g., *www.nlm.nih.gov/pubs/checklist.pdf*) and publish guides to help evaluate Web-based health information (e.g., *www.mlanet.org/resources/userguide.html*).

The quantity and complexity of digital health care technology available to you and your patients will continue to increase. *Telehealth,* a broad term that refers to the delivery of

TABLE 4.9   Comparison of Teaching Strategies

Description	Advantages	Limitations
Discussion ("Teach Back")		
• Purpose is to exchange points of view about a topic or to arrive at a decision or conclusion • Can be done with patient, with patient and caregiver, or with group • *Example:* Weight loss	• Allows for an active exchange of information and previous experiences among participants • Good choice when patients have previous experience with subject and have information to share • Nonthreatening format • Can use peers (patients with common problems) to teach	• May need more time depending on topic and number of participants
Lecture-Discussion		
• Useful when group of patients and caregivers can benefit from basic information • Lecture portion is short (i.e., 15–20 min) • Discussion ("teach back") follows lecture • *Example:* Basic principles of cardiac rehabilitation (e.g., exercise, nutrition)	• Combines short lecture to present basic information with time for discussion • Provision of printed material related to lecture content is useful and recommended	• Need to limit number of lecture topics to 3 to 5 • May need more time depending on topic and number of participants
Demonstration/Return Demonstration ("Show Back")		
• Purpose is to teach patient and caregiver to perform a skill • Return demonstration ("show back") can show patient's ability to perform skill (see Fig. 4.5) • *Examples:* Dressing change, injection	• Provides for learning and practice of physical skills • Dividing skill into series of smaller steps helps mastery and provides reinforcement	• May need more time for practice needed to master skill • Patients with limited manual dexterity may have difficulty
Use of Teaching Resources		
• Audiovisual aids to supplement teaching • Printed materials (e.g., brochures) • CDs/DVDs • Hospital-based TV (see Fig. 4.4) • Digital and communication technologies (e.g., mobile applications, Web-based patient education programs, game-based education, online support groups) • Telehealth	• Enhances the presentation through visual and/or auditory stimulation • Best used in combination with other teaching strategies • Use of digital and communication technologies for health information is the preferred choice for many • Web access in patient rooms is standard in most health care agencies • Health information can be given and reinforced to patients remotely	• Review materials for accuracy, reading level, completeness, etc., before using • Evaluate websites, games, applications, programs, etc., for validity of information • May not be appropriate for all learners (e.g., lack of interest, decreased mental capacity) • Finances (e.g., equipment purchase, Internet service) may be a limiting factor to using digital technology

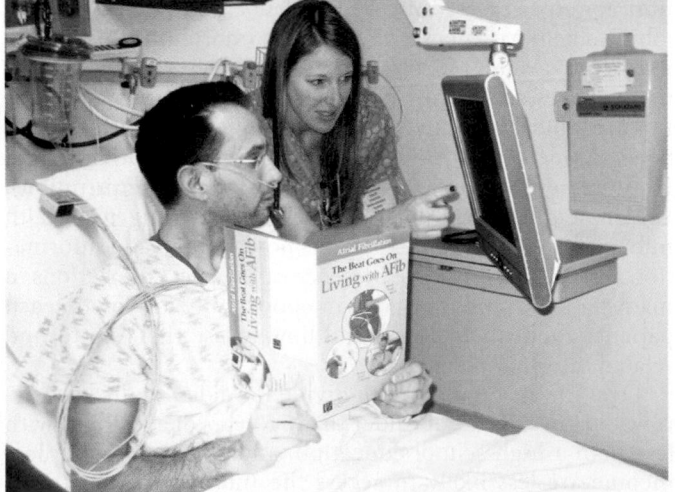

FIG. 4.4 Effective teaching using a variety of strategies (written materials, computer-based patient education programs). (Courtesy Linda Bucher, RN, PhD, CEN, CNE, Staff Nurse, Virtua Memorial Hospital, Mt. Holly, N.J.)

health-related services and information via telecommunications technologies, allows for (1) remote HCP-patient consultations *(telemedicine)*; (2) monitoring of vital signs, weight, heart rhythm, blood glucose, etc.; and (3) ongoing patient teaching.

Learn about these technologies and determine how useful they may be when teaching patients.

Implementation

During the implementation phase, use the planned strategies to present information and teach new skills (Table 4.10). Incorporate verbal and nonverbal communication skills, active listening, and empathy into the process. Based on the assessment of the patient's physical, psychologic, sociocultural, and learner characteristics, determine how much the patient can participate. Whenever possible and appropriate, involve the patient's caregiver(s) in the teaching-learning process.

Remember the principles and characteristics of the adult learner. Although reinforcement and reward are important, phrases such as, "Aren't you doing well!" in a tone one would use with a child can be condescending to adult learners.

Evaluation

Evaluation, the last step in the learning process, is a measure of the degree to which the patient has achieved the learning goals. You can use various evaluation techniques (Table 4.11). Use techniques such as "teach back" to determine the knowledge and skill levels of the patient and/or caregiver throughout the teaching and learning process (Fig. 4.5). If goals are not reached, reassess the patient and revise the teaching plan as needed.

TABLE 4.10 Teaching Patients With Disabilities

Hearing Loss[22]
- Sit in front of the patient at eye level with the light shining on your face
- Use assistive listening devices to amplify sound
- Speak slowly and clearly, using short, simple sentences
- Create a quiet environment that eliminates or minimizes background noises
- Assess patient's preferred communication method (sign language or lip reading)
- If patient prefers to use sign language:
  - Leave as much freedom as possible for their dominant hand to allow for signing
  - Use a sign language interpreter to preserve patient privacy and confidentiality
  - If using a sign language interpreter, speak to the patient, not the interpreter
- If the patient prefers lip-reading:
  - Make sure the patient can see your lips
  - Face the patient and maintain eye contact
  - Ensure there is good lighting on your lips
  - Speak in a normal rhythm and tone
  - Use facial expressions to help convey meaning

Limited Manual Dexterity
- Provide assistive (ease of use) devices to help the patient perform necessary tasks to perform a skill

Mild Cognitive Impairment[23]
- Explain what you will be doing
- Use simple wording
- Present 1 instruction at a time
- Ask yes/no questions
- Avoid open-ended questions
- Be patient
- Answer repeated questions as if it were the first time the question was asked
- Reinforce instructions often
- Create a quiet environment and minimize distractions

Vision Loss[24,25]
- Use low-vision aids, such as magnifiers, high-power reading glasses, or handheld or mounted telescopes
- Use technology, such as screen readers that read text on the computer screen using a speech synthesizer or convert text to braille
- Use electronic tablets or smart phones with adjustable text size
- Use large print publications
- Ensure that there is good lighting in the environment
- Minimize distractions and eliminate background noise
- Give educational materials available in braille
- Provide verbal or tactile instruction instead of written instruction

TABLE 4.11 Evaluating Patient and Caregiver Learning

Technique	Strategy and Examples
Observe patient or caregiver directly	• Ask person to show you how to change the dressing • Return demonstration ("show back") determines whether: • Skill has been mastered • Further instruction is needed • Patient and caregiver are ready for new or more content
Observe verbal and nonverbal cues	• Teaching may have to be delayed, more teaching needed, or different strategy used if patient or caregiver: • Asks you to repeat instructions • Loses eye contact • Begins to doze in chair or bed • Becomes restless or fidgety • Does not speak English
Ask open-ended questions ("teach back")	• Open-ended questions provide more information about understanding than closed-ended questions, which need only a "yes" or "no" • Ask questions such as: • "How often do you need to change the dressing?" • "What will you do if you develop chest pain at home?"
Talk with caregiver ("teach back")	• Involve caregiver in the evaluation process • Ask questions such as: • "What medications is she taking?" • "When does he use his oxygen?"
Seek the patient's self-evaluation of progress	• Ask patient's opinion about his or her progress • Assess what evidence the patient has that the goals are being met • Assess if the patient is ready to learn new material

Documentation is an essential part in the teaching-learning process. Record everything from the assessment through plans for evaluation and follow-up. Because members of the health care team use these records in different settings and for various reasons, the teaching goals, strategies, and evaluation results need to be clear, complete, and available to the team members.

The patient may not have been giving himself enough insulin for some time. The patient's vision had declined, and he now needs special equipment to correctly draw up the insulin. The lesson here is that assumptions about a patient's knowledge and skills are dangerous. Confirm prior knowledge even as you are teaching new skills.

Long-term evaluation of learning goals often requires follow-up after discharge. Provide a written schedule of visits and other appropriate referrals before the patient leaves the hospital or clinic. It is important to share this information with the patient's caregiver(s) so that everyone involved in the patient's long-term progress has the same information.

⚉ CHECK YOUR PRACTICE

Your patient is a 53-yr-old man with type 1 diabetes who entered the hospital with a blood glucose level of 550 mg/dL (30.53 mmol/L). He is now stable and soon will be discharged.

You prepare his insulin and plan to give him the syringe to let him do his own injection. Before you go to his room, your preceptor suggests that you observe his technique of preparing the insulin as well as the injection. This comment puzzles you because he has had diabetes for 32 years and should know how to do it.

When you go to his room, you ask him to prepare the insulin injection ("show back"). You notice that he filled the syringe with 30 units of insulin and 10 units of air, instead of 40 units of insulin. After correcting the dose and questioning the patient more fully ("teach back"), you wonder what happened.

What are possible reasons that he did not draw up the correct amount of insulin?

CASE STUDY
Patient and Caregiver Teaching

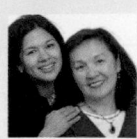

Patient Profile

M.L., a 60-yr-old Asian woman, is admitted to the hospital with a diagnosis of exacerbation of chronic obstructive pulmonary disease (COPD).

(© Thomas M Perkins/
Shutterstock.)

Subjective Data

- History of COPD for 10 years. Admitted twice in the past 8 months for exacerbations of COPD. Reports a chronic cough but denies any recent change in sputum color. States: "I stopped smoking last year, but my son-in-law smokes in the house."
- Past medical history: Gastroesophageal reflux disease; macular degeneration in right eye.
- Social history: Widowed 5 years ago. Lives with daughter and son-in-law, who work full time. Cares for 2 young grandchildren after school. English is M.L.'s second language.

Objective Data

Physical Examination

- Alert, cognitively intact, anxious, thin woman with dyspnea on minimal exertion. Speaks in short phrases. States: "I have no energy."
- Oxygen via nasal cannula at 2 L/min
- Weight 100 lb, height 5 ft 2 in

Diagnostic Studies

- Chest x-ray negative for acute infection
- Arterial blood gases on room air: pH 7.35, $PaCO_2$ 47 mm Hg, PaO_2 75 mm Hg, HCO_3^- 30 mEq/L
- O_2 saturation (via pulse oximetry) during 6-minute walk test on room air = 83%
- Forced expiratory volume in 1 second of expiration (FEV_1) = 60% of predicted

Interprofessional Care

- Medications: bronchodilator therapy (inpatient nebulizer therapy, inhalers at home), oral corticosteroids
- Continuous home O_2 therapy 2 L/min via nasal cannula
- Pulmonary rehabilitation: inpatient and outpatient

Discussion Questions

1. ***Priority Decision:*** What are M.L.'s priority learning needs?
2. ***Patient-Centered Care:*** What factors (e.g., sociocultural, physical, psychologic) noted in the assessment may influence M.L.'s response to teaching?
3. ***Patient-Centered Care:*** What potential challenges might you expect when planning to teach M.L.? How would you manage them?
4. ***Priority Decision:*** Choose 2 of M.L.'s priority learning needs. Develop a teaching plan for M.L. for each of these needs.

Answers available at *http://evolve.elsevier.com/Lewis/medsurg.*

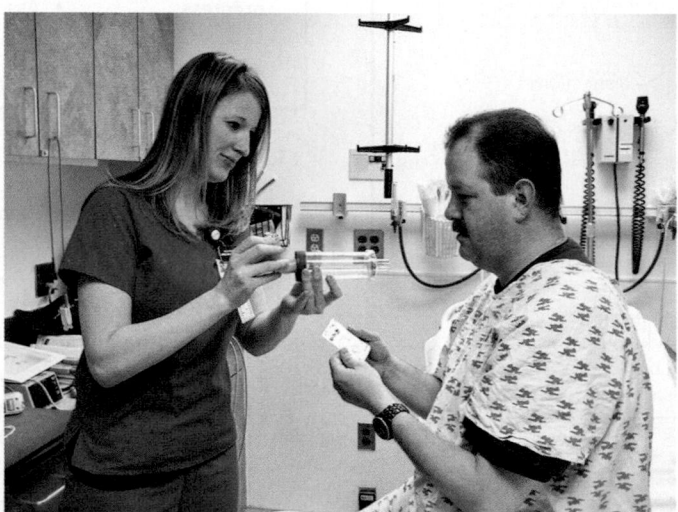

FIG. 4.5 Teaching using discussion ("teach back") and demonstration/return demonstration ("show back") increases successful learning by the patient. (Courtesy Linda Bucher, RN, PhD, CEN, CNE, Staff Nurse, Virtua Memorial Hospital, Mt. Holly, NJ.)

BRIDGE TO NCLEX EXAMINATION

The number of the question corresponds to the same-numbered outcome at the beginning of the chapter.

1. Which technique is *most* appropriate when using motivational interviewing with a patient who tells you that he is ready to start a weight-loss program?
   a. Confirm that the patient is serious about losing weight.
   b. Insist that the patient consider an organized group weight-loss program.
   c. Focus on the patient's strengths to support his optimism that he can successfully lose weight.
   d. Ask a prescribed set of questions to increase the patient's awareness of his dietary behaviors.

2. Which is the *priority* patient teaching strategy when limited time is available?
   a. Setting realistic goals that have high priority for the patient
   b. Referring the patient to a nurse educator in private practice
   c. Observing more experienced nurse-teachers to learn how to teach faster and more efficiently
   d. Providing reading materials for the patient instead of discussing information the patient needs to learn

3. The nurse needs to include caregivers in patient teaching primarily because *(select all that apply)*
   a. caregivers provide all the care for patients after discharge.
   b. they might feel rejected if they are not included in the teaching.
   c. patients have better outcomes when their caregivers are involved.
   d. the patient may be too ill or too stressed to fully understand the teaching.
   e. caregivers are responsible for the overall management of the patient's care.

4. Which patient characteristic enhances the teaching-learning process?
   a. Moderate anxiety
   b. High self-efficacy
   c. Being in the precontemplative stage of change
   d. Being able to laugh about the current health problem

5. What would be the *priority* teaching goal for a middle-aged Hispanic woman about methods to relieve symptoms of menopause?
   a. Prevent the development of future disease.
   b. Maintain the patient's current state of health.
   c. Provide information on possible treatment options.
   d. Change the patient's beliefs about herbal supplements.

6. A patient tells the nurse that she enjoys talking with others and sharing experiences but often falls asleep when reading. Which teaching strategy would be *most* effective with this patient?
   a. Formal lecture
   b. Journal writing
   c. Web-based program
   d. Small group discussion

7. The nurse has taught a family caregiver how to administer insulin. Evaluation of the caregiver's learning would include
   a. monitoring the patient's glucose readings.
   b. arranging for follow-up with a home care nurse.
   c. asking the caregiver to "show back" the ability to administer insulin.
   d. asking the caregiver what was helpful about the teaching experience.

1. c, 2. a, 3. c,d, 4. b, 5. c, 6. d, 7. c.

For rationales to these answers and even more NCLEX review questions, visit *http://evolve.elsevier.com/Lewis/medsurg.*

EVOLVE WEBSITE/RESOURCES LIST

http://evolve.elsevier.com/Lewis/medsurg
Review Questions (Online Only)
Key Points
Answer Keys for Questions
- Rationales for Bridge to NCLEX Examination Questions
- Answer Guidelines for Case Study on p. 56
Conceptual Care Map Creator
Audio Glossary
Content Updates

REFERENCES

1. Centers for Disease Control and Prevention: Chronic disease prevention and health promotion. Retrieved from *www.cdc.gov/chronicdisease/index.htm.*
*2. Jenq GY, Doyle MM, Belton BM, Herrin J, Horwitz LI, et al: Quasi-experimental evaluation of the effectiveness of a large-scale readmission reduction program, *JAMA Intern Med* 176:681, 2016.
3. American Nurses Association: *Nursing scope and standards of practice,* ed 3, Washington, DC, 2015, The Association. (Classic)
4. Oermann M, Shellenbarger T, Gaberson K: *Clinical teaching strategies in nursing,* ed 5, New York, 2018, Springer.
5. Knowles MS, Holton EF, Swanson RA: *The adult learner: the definitive classic in adult education and human resource development,* ed 7, St Louis, 2011, Mosby. (Classic)
*6. Prochaska J, Velicer W. The transtheoretical model of health behavior change. *Am J Health Promotion* 12:38, 1997. (Classic)
7. Rollnick S, Miller WR, Yahne CE: *Motivational interviewing in health care: Helping patients change behavior,* New York, 2008, Guilford Press. (Classic)
8. Centers for Disease Control and Prevention: Healthy aging, Caregiving. Retrieved from *www.cdc.gov/aging/caregiving/index.htm.*
9. The Joint Commission: National patient safety goals. Retrieved from *www.jointcommission.org/standards_information/npsgs.aspx.*
10. American Hospital Association: The patient care partnership. Retrieved from *www.aha.org/advocacy-issues/communicatingpts/pt-care-partnership.shtml.*
11. The Joint Commission: Speak Up initiatives, 2016. Retrieved from *www.jointcommission.org/facts_about_speak_up/.*
12. Institute for Healthcare Improvement, National Patient Safety Foundation: Ask Me 3. Retrieved from *http://www.npsf.org/?page=askme3.*
13. National Institutes of Health: Health literacy. Retrieved from *www.nih.gov/institutes-nih/nih-office-director/office-communications-public-liaison/clear-communication/health-literacy.*
14. Agency for Healthcare Research and Quality: Health literacy universal precautions toolkit. Retrieved from *www.ahrq.gov/professionals/quality-patient-safety/quality-resources/tools/literacy-toolkit/index.html.*
15. Office of Disease Prevention and Health Promotion: Health communication and health information technology. Retrieved from *www.healthypeople.gov/2020/topics-objectives/topic/health-communication-and-health-information-technology.*
*16. Sand-Jecklin K, Daniels CS, Lucke-Wold N: Incorporating health literacy screening into patients' health assessment, *Clinical Nurs Res* 26:176, 2017.
*17. Morris NS, MacLean CD, Chew LD, et al: The single item literacy screener: Evaluation of a brief instrument to identify limited reading ability, *BMC Fam Pract* 7:21, 2006. (Classic)
18. The Joint Commission: Health equity. Retrieved from *www.jointcommission.org/assets/1/6/HLCOneSizeFinal.pdf.*

19. Oh H, Rizo C, Enkin M, et al What is e-health: A systematic review of published definitions, *J Med Internet Res* 7:1, 2005. (Classic)

20. Medline Plus: How to write easy-to-read health materials. Retrieved from *www.nlm.nih.gov/medlineplus/etr.html.*

*21. Hong YA, Cho J: Has the digital health divide widened? Trends of health-related internet use among older adults from 2003 to 2011. *J Gerontol* 72:856, 2017.

22. National Institutes of Health, National Institute on Deafness and Other Communication Disorders: Hearing loss and older adults. Retrieved from *www.nidcd.nih.gov/health/hearing-loss-older-adults.*

23. National Institute on Aging: Communicating with a confused patient. Retrieved from *www.nia.nih.gov/health/communicating-confused-patient.*

24. U.S. National Library of Medicine, Medline Plus: Living with vision loss. Retrieved from *www.medlineplus.gov/ency/patientinstructions/000526. htm.*

25. American Foundation for the Blind: Technology resources for people with vision loss. Retrieved from *www.afb.org/info/living-with-vision-loss/ using-technology/12.*

*Evidence-based information for clinical practice.

5

Chronic Illness and Older Adults

Sherry A. Greenberg

Helping one person might not change the whole world,
but it could change the world for the one person.

Unknown

e http://evolve.elsevier.com/Lewis/medsurg/

CONCEPTUAL FOCUS

Cognition

Family Dynamics

Functional Ability

Mobility

Nutrition

Sensory Perception

LEARNING OUTCOMES

1. Describe the prevention and major causes of chronic illness.
2. Explain the characteristics of a chronic illness.
3. Describe the demographics of aging.
4. Explain the needs of special populations of older adults.
5. Describe nursing interventions to assist older adults with chronic illnesses.
6. Describe common problems of older adults related to hospitalization and acute illness and the nurse's role in assisting them.
7. Differentiate among care alternatives to meet needs of older adults.
8. Describe the nurse's role in health promotion and managing the special needs of older adults.

KEY TERMS

ageism, p. 63

elder mistreatment (EM), p. 65

ethnogeriatric, p. 65

frail older adult, p. 62

gerontologic nursing, p. 68

Medicaid, p. 67

Medicare, p. 67

old-old adult, p. 62

young-old adult, p. 62

This chapter discusses issues related to chronic illness and aging. The population of older adults is growing rapidly. You need to consider their multiple, complex health care conditions and needs when planning and providing comprehensive nursing care. Functional ability in those with chronic illness and older adults is interrelated with several concepts, including mobility, perfusion, nutrition, cognition, and sensory perception. Family dynamics and caregiving shape the care provided to those who need help to meet their needs.

CHRONIC ILLNESS

Illness can be categorized as either acute or chronic (Table 5.1). The U.S. health care system faces a growing burden of chronic illness as the population ages. Chronic illnesses account for 70% of all deaths in the United States. Chronic illness results in limitations in physical functioning, work productivity, and quality of life for nearly 1 out of 10 Americans. Many older adults live with more than 1 chronic illness, some live with 6 or more. A sizable portion of U.S. health care dollars goes toward treating chronic illnesses.[1] Managing a chronic illness greatly affects the lives of the older adult, family, and caregiver. Table 5.2 presents the impact of some chronic illnesses.

In addition to people living longer, other societal changes have contributed to the increase in chronic illnesses. These include insufficient physical activity, lack of access to fresh fruits and vegetables, and tobacco and alcohol use.[1]

Trajectory of Chronic Illness

The person with a chronic illness can move from a level of optimum functioning, with the illness well controlled, to a period of physical instability. Corbin and Strauss proposed a view of chronic illness as a trajectory (Fig. 5.1) with overlapping phases[2] (Table 5.3). This trajectory characterizes the common course of most chronic conditions. In addition, Corbin and Strauss identified the 7 tasks of those who are chronically ill (Table 5.4). These tasks are discussed in the following sections.

Preventing and Managing a Crisis. Most chronic illnesses have the potential for an acute exacerbation of symptoms, which may result in further disability or death. Examples include the patient with heart disease who has another myocardial infarction or the patient with asthma who has a severe attack. A major task for the patient and caregiver is to learn to prevent or manage the crisis. First, the patient and caregiver need to understand the potential for the crisis to occur. Second, they need to know ways to prevent or modify the threat. This often involves adhering to a prescribed medical plan. Patients

need to know the signs and symptoms of the onset of a crisis or exacerbation. Depending on the chronic illness, signs and symptoms may occur suddenly (e.g., bleeding in a patient with inflammatory bowel disease) or slowly (e.g., heart failure in a person with untreated hypertension). It is important for the patient and caregiver to develop a plan to manage a crisis that is likely to occur.

Carrying Out Prescribed Treatment Plan. Treatment plans vary in degree of difficulty and the impact they have on the person's lifestyle. Treatment plans may be challenging or time consuming, such as changing a dressing multiple times a day or following a toileting program. However, they generally save time and prevent complications.

Controlling Symptoms. An important task for those with chronic illnesses is to learn to control symptoms so that they can continue desired activities. Some redesign their lifestyle by learning to plan ahead. People with heart failure adjust the time they take diuretics when going out for the day to avoid needing to rush to a bathroom. Encourage independence in decision making and collaborating with the health care provider (HCP) about treatment plans to avoid an exacerbation of the illness. Others may redesign their living space. Patients and their families and/or caregivers need to learn about the pattern of symptoms, such as typical onset, duration, and severity, so that lifestyle may be changed accordingly, while maintaining safety.

Reordering Time. People with chronic illness often report having too much or too little time. Treatment plans that require large amounts of time for the person, as well as caregivers, may require changing schedules or eliminating other activities. For example, the patient with a new ileostomy needs to plan for increased time in the bathroom to change the drainage bag.

TABLE 5.1 Characteristics of Acute and Chronic Illness

Description	Characteristics
Acute Illness	
Diseases that have a rapid onset and short duration *Examples:* colds, influenza, acute gastroenteritis	• Usually self-limiting • Responds readily to treatment • Complications infrequent • After illness, return to previous level of functioning
Chronic Illness	
Diseases that are prolonged, do not resolve spontaneously, and are rarely cured completely *Examples:* Table 5.2	• Permanent impairments or deviations from normal • Irreversible pathologic changes • Residual disability • Special rehabilitation needed • Need for long-term medical and/or nursing management

TABLE 5.2 Impact of Chronic Illnesses

Chronic Illness	Impact	CONTENT IN BOOK	
		Chapter	Page
Alzheimer's disease	• Affects 5.5 million people • Sixth leading cause of death among all adults; fifth leading cause of death among those age 65 and above	59	1386
Arthritis	• Affects 1 in 5 people • One of most common chronic illnesses • Leading cause of disability	64	1499
Cancer	• Second leading cause of death • Risk increases with age	15	232
Cardiovascular disease, including heart disease and stroke	• Affects about 17 million adults • Account for 31% of U.S. deaths annually • Heart disease is leading cause of death in United States • Heart failure is a common cause of hospitalization and rehospitalization • Stroke is fifth leading cause of death • Stroke is a common cause of serious disability	33	698
Chronic obstructive pulmonary disease (COPD)	• Affects many older adults • Third leading cause of death	28	560
Diabetes	• Affects >29 million Americans • 25% of adults in United States do not know they have diabetes • Seventh leading cause of death	48	1108
Human immunodeficiency virus (HIV)	• 45% of those living with HIV in the United States are over 50 years old • Older adults more likely to receive diagnosis of HIV infection later in course of disease	14	216
Obesity	• Affects about 1 in 3 adults • Major contributor to other health problems and chronic diseases	40	869

Data from Centers for Disease Control and Prevention: CDC's chronic disease press releases. Retrieved from *www.cdc.gov/chronicdisease/resources/publications/aag.htm* and *www.cdc.gov/hiv/group/age/olderamericans/index.html.*

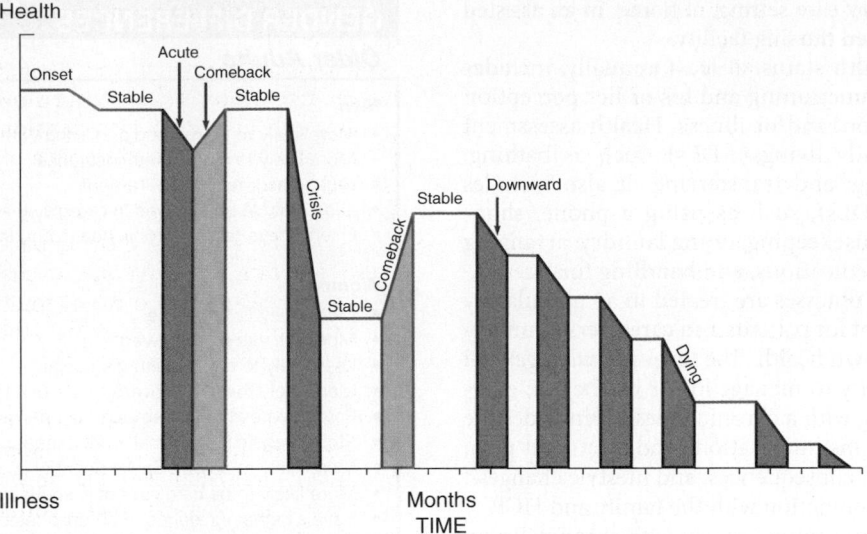

FIG. 5.1 The Chronic Illness Trajectory is a theoretical model of chronic illness. The trajectory model of chronic illness recognizes that chronic illness will have many phases (Table 5.3). (From Woog P: *The chronic illness trajectory framework: The Corbin and Strauss nursing model*, New York, 1992, Springer.)

TABLE 5.3 Chronic Illness Trajectory

Phases	Description
Onset	• Signs and symptoms are present • Disease diagnosed
Stable	• Illness course and symptoms controlled by treatment plan • Person maintains everyday activities
Acute	• Active illness with severe and unrelieved symptoms or complications • Hospitalization may be needed for management
Comeback	• Gradual return to an acceptable way of life
Crisis	• Life-threatening situation occurs • Emergency services are necessary
Unstable	• Unable to keep symptoms or disease course under control • Life becomes disrupted while patient works to regain stability • Hospitalization not required
Downward	• Gradual and progressive deterioration in physical or mental status • Accompanied by increasing disability and symptoms • Continuous changes in everyday life activities
Dying	• Patient has to relinquish everyday life interests and activities, let go, and die peacefully • Immediate weeks, days, hours preceding death

Source: Woog P: *The chronic illness trajectory framework: The Corbin and Strauss nursing model*, New York, 1992, Springer.

TABLE 5.4 7 Tasks of People With Chronic Illness

1. Prevent and manage a crisis
2. Carry out prescribed treatment plan
3. Control symptoms
4. Reorder time
5. Adjust to changes in course of disease
6. Prevent social isolation
7. Attempt to normalize interactions with others

Source: Corbin JM, Strauss A: A nursing model for chronic illness management based upon the trajectory framework, *Sch Inq Nurs Pract* 5:155, 1991.

Adjusting to Changes in the Course of Disease. Some diseases, such as multiple sclerosis, have unpredictable courses that make planning activities difficult. Part of the person's task is to develop a personal identity that includes the chronic illness and to adjust to the necessary lifestyle changes. For example, a person taking warfarin due to a mechanical heart valve may need to avoid extreme physical sports that have a high potential for injury.

Preventing Social Isolation. Social isolation may occur with chronic illness. The person may choose to withdraw from social activities or others withdraw from the chronically ill person. For example, a woman who has aphasia secondary to a stroke may not want to go out in public because of embarrassment related to communication issues.

Attempting to Normalize Interactions With Others. Most persons with chronic illness try to manage symptoms so that they can hide their disabilities or disfigurement. This may involve wearing a prosthesis or showing that they can function the same as a person without a disability or chronic illness. An example of this is the woman with heart failure who stops walking to catch her breath but appears to be inspecting a plant or looking in a store window.

Prevention of Chronic Illness

Chronic illnesses are often preventable. *Primary prevention* refers to measures such as eating a healthy diet, getting proper exercise, and receiving immunizations that prevent a specific disease. Appropriate immunizations for older adults include influenza, pneumococcal, herpes zoster, tetanus/diphtheria/pertussis (Td/Tdap), and hepatitis A and B. *Secondary prevention* refers to actions aimed at health screening and early detection of disease. This can lead to interventions to prevent disease progression, such as colon cancer screening or breast cancer screening. *Tertiary prevention* refers to activities that limit disease progression such as rehabilitation.

❖NURSING MANAGEMENT: CHRONIC ILLNESS

Diagnosis and treatment of the acute phase or acute exacerbations of a chronic illness sometimes take place in a hospital. Other phases of a chronic illness are regularly assessed and managed in an ambulatory care setting, at home, in an assisted living facility, or in a skilled nursing facility.

An assessment of health status, at least annually, includes a person's level of daily functioning and his or her perception of relative health, function, and/or illness. Health assessment includes activities of daily living (ADLs), such as bathing, dressing, eating, toileting, and transferring. It also includes instrumental ADLs (IADLs), such as using a phone, shopping, preparing food, housekeeping, doing laundry, arranging transportation, taking medications, and handling finances.[3]

Because most chronic illnesses are treated in an ambulatory care setting, it is important for patients and caregivers to understand and manage their own health. The term *self-management* refers to the person's ability to manage his or her health, especially in response to living with a chronic illness. It includes the ability to manage symptoms, medications and treatment plan, physical and psychosocial consequences, and lifestyle changes.[4] Self-management is in conjunction with the family and HCP.

You play a key role in managing patients with chronic illness. This includes conducting a comprehensive history and physical assessment, teaching the patient and caregiver about the treatment plan, implementing strategies for symptom management, and evaluating patient outcomes.

Family caregivers (e.g., spouses, partners, adult children) often have important roles in the life of the chronically ill person. The ideal situation is 1 in which family caregivers work together with the patient to manage the chronic condition(s). This collaboration begins under the direction of the health care team at the time of diagnosis. When the caregiver is a spouse or partner who is also older, he or she may have a chronic illness or multiple chronic conditions as well. This may add a level of complexity to the coordination of care.[5]

OLDER ADULTS

DEMOGRAPHICS OF AGING

The older adult population (those 65 years of age and older) continues to outpace the rest of the population. Nearly 1 in 7 U.S. residents, more than 47.8 million people, or 14.9% of the population, were age 65 or older in 2016.[6] This is projected to more than double to 98 million in 2060. The U.S. Census Bureau predicts life expectancy to continue to increase for both men and women. Those reaching 65 years have an average life expectancy of an added 19.4 years, specifically 20.6 years for females and 18 years for males.[6] Whether this gender difference is due to differences in health behaviors (e.g., smoking, alcohol use) or occupation is not known.

The fastest-growing segment of older Americans is people ages 85 or older. The 85 and older population is projected to increase from 6.3 million in 2015 to 14.6 million in 2040.[6] The increase in life span is due to declining infant mortality, new drug therapies, mechanical devices, and improved surgical interventions. A greater emphasis on health promotion, disease prevention, and earlier detection as well as better care management has led to more Americans living past 85 years.

In 2016, 22% of the U.S. population age 65 years or older were of racial or ethnic minority populations, including 9% black; 4% Asian or Pacific Islanders; and 0.5% Native American. People of Hispanic ethnicity (who may be of any race) represented 8% of the older population.[6] The number of older adults of racial or ethnicity populations in the United States is projected to increase from 10.6 million in 2015 (22% of older adults) to 21.1 million in 2030 (28% of older adults).[6]

GENDER DIFFERENCES
Older Adults

Men
- More likely to be married and living with spouse or partner
- More likely to have health insurance
- Higher income after retirement
- Less likely to be involved in caregiving activities
- Overall have fewer chronic health conditions

Women
- More likely to live alone
- More likely to be widowed
- Less likely to have health insurance
- More likely to live in poverty
- Poverty rates highest among minority women
- More likely to lack formal work experience, leading to lower income
- More likely to rely on Social Security as major source of income
- More likely to be caregiver of ill spouse or partner
- Have a higher incidence of chronic health conditions such as arthritis, hypertension, stroke, and diabetes

Upcoming cohorts of older adults will likely have increased access to higher education, employment, technology, and resources than previous cohorts. Between 1970 and 2015, the percent of older adults who had completed high school rose from 28% to 85%.[6] In 2016, about 28% of the population 65 and older have earned a bachelor's degree or higher.[6]

The terms **young-old adult** (65–74 years of age) and **old-old adult** (85 years of age and older) describe 2 groups of older adults with distinct characteristics, needs, and living arrangements. The number of older adults age 65 living in nursing homes increases with age; 1% of those age 65 to 74, 3% of those age 75 to 84, and 9% of those 85 and older live in nursing homes. The old-old adult is often a widowed, divorced, or single woman dependent on family for support or care. Many old-old adults have outlived children, spouses or partners, and siblings.

The **frail older adult** is usually over age 75 with multiple physical, cognitive, and/or mental conditions. These often interfere with self-management and the ability to perform daily activities independently. Frail older adults are discussed later in this chapter on page 64.

ATTITUDES TOWARD AGING

Who is old? The answer to this question often depends on the respondent's age and attitude. Your "real" age is set by a date in time. Many factors influence how "old" you feel. These include emotional and physical health, developmental stage, socioeconomic status, culture, and ethnicity. We all age. As we do, we are exposed to new and different life experiences. The accumulation of these differences makes older adults more diverse than any other age-group.

As you assess older adults, consider and value their diversity and life history. Assess their feelings of what it means to be an older adult. Most older adults report having good-to-excellent health despite having a chronic condition. However, those with poor health often report a higher perceived age and lower sense of well-being when compared with healthy older adults. Age is important, but it may not be the most relevant factor in determining the appropriate care of an individual older adult.

Myths and stereotypes about aging are often supported by media reports of older adults who are "problematic." These misconceptions may lead to omissions or errors in assessment and unnecessary limitations or interventions. For example, if you think that all older people are rigid in their thinking, you may not present new ideas to a patient.[7]

Ageism is a negative attitude based on age. Ageism leads to discrimination and disparities in the care given to older adults. If you have negative attitudes, it may be because you fear your own aging process. Or, you are not knowledgeable about aging and the health care needs of the older adult.

BIOLOGIC AGING

From a biologic view, *aging* reflects the changes that occur over time. Biologic aging is a multifactorial process involving genetics, diet, and environment.[8] In part, we view biologic aging as a balance of positive and negative factors (Fig. 5.2). Research is directed at increasing the average life span, functional status, and quality of life of older adults. The hope is that we can develop new antiaging therapies to slow down or reverse age-related changes that result in chronic illness and disability.

AGE-RELATED PHYSIOLOGIC CHANGES

Age-related changes affect every body system. These changes are normal and occur as people age. However, the age at which specific changes occur differs from person to person and within the same person. For instance, a person who has gray hair at age 45 may have relatively unwrinkled skin at age 80. As a nurse, you will assess for age-related changes. Table 5.5 shows where you can find tables outlining specific age-related assessment findings throughout the book.

SPECIAL OLDER ADULT POPULATIONS

Chronically Ill Older Adults

Daily living with chronic illness is a reality for many older adults. The incidence of chronic illness triples after age 45. Most people 65 years of age and older have at least 1 chronic condition, and many have multiple conditions.[1] The most common chronic conditions in older adults are hypertension, heart failure, coronary artery disease, chronic obstructive pulmonary disease (COPD), cancer, diabetes, and osteoarthritis. Other common chronic conditions include Alzheimer's disease, vision and hearing deficits, osteoporosis, stroke, Parkinson's disease, and depression.

Cognitively Impaired Older Adults

Most healthy older adults have no noticeable decline in cognitive abilities (Table 5.6). Older adults may have a mild decline in memory and may need more time to recall events or new information. This differs from cognitive impairment. New learning may be slower. Refer older adults with memory loss to their HCP for an evaluation. Teach them to use memory aids, attempt recall in a calm and quiet environment, and actively engage in enhancing memory. Memory aids include clocks, calendars, notes, marked pillboxes, safety alarms on stoves, and identification necklaces or bracelets. Memory techniques include word association, mental imaging, and mnemonics.

Dementia, delirium, and depression can occur and may coexist in older adults. Declining physical health and acute illness are important factors that may influence cognition. For example, an older adult who undergoes surgery may have an acute change in mental status known as *delirium*.[9] Delirium superimposed on dementia may signify an acute or emergent condition such as heart failure. Hence, it is important to distinguish signs

TABLE 5.5 Gerontologic Assessment Differences

Summary of Tables

Body System	Table Number	Page
Visual	20-1	352
Auditory	21-1	378
Integumentary	22-1	398
Respiratory	25-2	460
Hematologic	29-3	591
Cardiovascular	31-1	661
Gastrointestinal	38-5	835
Urinary	44-2	1012
Endocrine	47-3	1095
Reproductive	50-3	1178
Nervous	55-2	1287
Musculoskeletal	61-1	1434

TABLE 5.6 Gerontologic Assessment Differences

Cognitive Function

Effect of Aging	Cognitive Function
Improves with aging	• Vocabulary and verbal reasoning • Crystallized intelligence (ability to use skills, knowledge, and experience)
Declines during middle age	• Mental performance speed • Synthesis of new information • Fluid intelligence (ability to think logically and solve problems in new situations)
Declines during old age	• Short-term recall memory
Constant (no changes with aging)	• Long-term recall memory

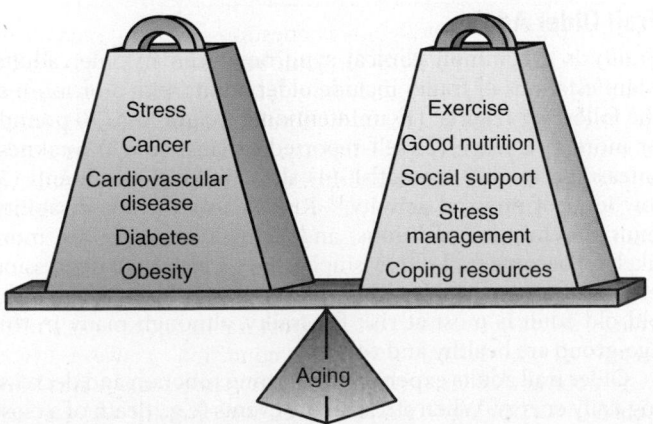

FIG. 5.2 The aging process can be viewed as a balance between negative and positive factors.

(Left weight: Stress, Cancer, Cardiovascular disease, Diabetes, Obesity. Right weight: Exercise, Good nutrition, Social support, Stress management, Coping resources. Fulcrum: Aging)

and symptoms of each. Cognitive impairment, delirium, and dementia are discussed in Chapter 59.

Rural Older Adults

Key barriers to health care access for rural older adults are transportation, limited supply of health care workers and facilities, lack of quality health care, social isolation, and financial limitations. Particularly vulnerable are older adults of racial or ethnic minority living in rural areas, who have even less access to HCPs. Older adults who live in rural areas may be less likely to engage in health-promoting activities.

When you work with older adults in rural areas, recognize lifestyle values and practices of rural life (Fig. 5.3). In planning care, be aware that transportation is the number 1 barrier to health care for rural older adults. Alternative service approaches such as computer-based Internet sources, DVDs, radio, community centers, and church social events may be used to promote healthy practices or to conduct health screening (Fig. 5.4).

The use of telehealth devices for monitoring patients in their home environments has enhanced the ability to provide care, including to those more isolated.[10] We must continue to develop innovative models of nursing practice to help the rural older adult. Older adults are increasingly using technology in their daily lives. Most older adults use the Internet and own a cell phone.[10]

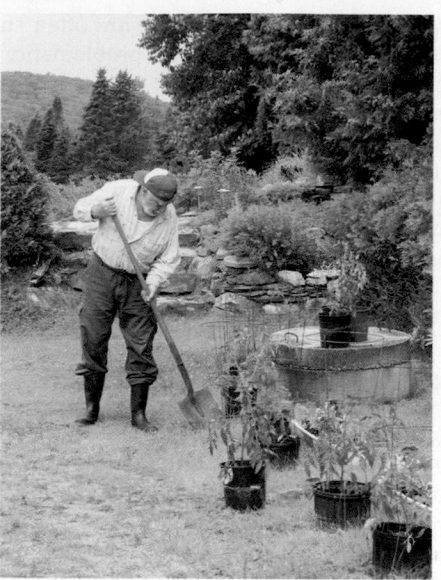

FIG. 5.3 Older adults living in rural areas often enjoy outside activities, such as gardening. (© iStockphoto/Thinkstock.)

INFORMATICS IN PRACTICE

Older Adults and Internet Use

- Sixty-seven percent of older adults use the Internet, as of 2016.
- Older adults may use the Internet to look for health information.
- Many track their weight, diet, and exercise using apps.
- Older adults are more likely to accept as true what they read on the Internet.
- Teach those who use the Internet as a source of information how to assess the credibility of a website.
- Suggest the use of websites and apps that include senior-friendly design elements.

Source: *www.pewinternet.org/2017/05/17/technology-use-among-seniors/.*

Homeless Older Adults

The number of older adults who are homeless is increasing. Key factors associated with homelessness include (1) having a low income, (2) having reduced cognitive capacity, (3) living alone, and (4) living in a community that lacks affordable housing. Homeless older adults may be chronically homeless or recently homeless because of a crisis in either health, economic, or social status.

Mortality rates for homeless older adults are higher than for older adults who have housing. Older homeless adults are at higher risk for more health problems because many aging network services are not designed to reach out to homeless people. They are less likely to use shelters or meal site services than younger homeless people. This may be due to fear of institutionalization. Care for homeless older adults requires an interprofessional approach (including nurses, physicians, social workers, clerical workers, and transporters) that links shelters with outreach, primary care clinics, Medicare and Medicaid offices, pharmacies, senior centers, and Area Agencies on Aging. Long-term care placement is often an alternative to homelessness, especially when the person is cognitively impaired.

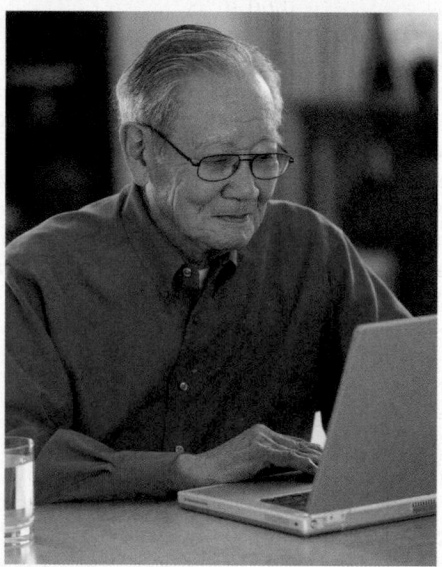

FIG. 5.4 Older adults are using computers more often and accessing health care information on the Internet. (© iStockphoto/Thinkstock.)

Frail Older Adults

Frailty is a common clinical syndrome seen in older adults. Manifestations of frailty include older adults with 3 or more of the following criteria: (1) unintentional weight loss (10 pounds or more in a year); (2) self-reported exhaustion; (3) weakness (measured by grip strength); (4) slow walking speed; and (5) low level of physical activity.[11] Risk factors include disability, multiple chronic conditions, and dementia. People are more likely to become frail if they smoke, have a history of depression or long-term medical health problems, or are underweight. The old-old adult is most at risk for frailty, although many in this age-group are healthy and robust.

Older frail adults experience declining function and decreasing daily energy. When stressful life events (e.g., death of a close friend) and daily strain (e.g., caring for an ill spouse) occur, frail older adults often have ineffective coping mechanisms and, as a result, may become ill. Common health problems of frail older

TABLE 5.7 SCALES: Nutritional Assessment of Older Adults

The acronym SCALES can remind you to assess important nutritional indicators:

Sadness, or mood change
Cholesterol, high
Albumin, low
Loss or gain of weight
Eating problems (e.g., mechanical problems, such as impaired swallowing, poor dentition)
Shopping and food preparation problems

adults include mobility limitations, sensory impairment, cognitive decline, and falls.

Frail older adults may tire easily, have little physical reserve, and are at risk for physical dependence and institutionalization. They are especially at risk for malnutrition and dehydration. These are related to factors such as living alone, depression, and low socioeconomic status. Other factors, such as dementia, inadequate dental care, sensory deficits, fatigue, and limited mobility increase the risk for malnutrition and dehydration. Monitor frail older adults for adequate calorie, protein, iron, calcium, vitamin D, and fluid intake. Use the *SCALES* tool to assess the risk factors for poor nutritional status in older adults (Table 5.7). Once you identify an older adult's nutritional needs, common interventions include home-delivered meals, dietary supplements, Supplemental Nutrition Assistance Program (SNAP), dental referrals, and vitamin supplements.[12] Because medications may affect appetite or interact with nutrients, perform a thorough medication review, including prescription drugs, over-the-counter (OTC) drugs, vitamins, minerals, supplements, herbs, and cultural remedies. Nutrition is discussed in Chapter 39.

Culturally Competent Care: Older Adults

The term **ethnogeriatric** describes the specialty area of providing culturally competent care to older adults.[13] As American society changes, ethnic institutions and neighborhoods may also change. For the older adult with strong ethnic and cultural roots, there may be a loss of friends who speak the native language, a loss of the religious institution that supports social ethnic activities, and a loss of stores that carry desired ethnic foods. This sense of loss is increased when children and others deny or ignore ethnic and cultural practices. Support for older adults of racial or ethnic minority is most often found in the family, religious practices, and isolated geographic or community ethnic clusters.

Ethnic populations of older adults face unique situations. Older adults may live in neighborhoods where physical security and personal safety related to crime may be a concern. Those who identify with particular ethnic groups often have disproportionately lower incomes and may not be able to afford Medicare deductibles or drugs needed to treat chronic illnesses. Older adults from minority populations such as Hispanics use health care services less often when compared to nonminority groups.[13]

Assess each older adult's ethnic and cultural background. Assume that ethnicity and culture are important and of value to older adults and their families unless they tell you otherwise during an assessment. For you to be effective with the ethnic older adult, a sense of respect and clear communication are critical. Nursing interventions to help meet the needs of ethnic populations are described in Table 2.9.[14] Culturally competent care is discussed in Chapter 2.

SOCIAL SUPPORT FOR OLDER ADULTS

Social support for older adults occurs at 3 levels. First, family members are the primary and preferred providers of social support. Second, semiformal support is found in clubs, religious (faith-based) organizations, neighborhoods, adult day care, and senior centers. Third, older adults may be linked to formal systems of social welfare agencies, health facilities, and government support. Generally, you, as a nurse, are part of the formal support system.

Family Caregivers

Many older adults need caregiving by family members. This includes those with multiple chronic conditions, those needing help with ADLs and IADLs, and older adults with dementia. The most common caregivers are spouses, adult children, parents, grandparents, and life partners. Older adult women, age 65 or older, are the most common family caregivers.[15] Other examples include husbands who care for wives with Alzheimer's disease, adult children who care for a parent with a stroke, grandparents who care for a grandchild with a developmental disorder, and parents who care for an adult child with a spinal cord injury. Many family caregivers are caring for themselves, their aging parents, and their children and grandchildren.

The caregiver usually takes on responsibilities gradually. For example, a caregiver may initially need only to adjust work schedules to accommodate a patient's health care appointments. Later, as the patient's needs become greater, the caregiver may have to reduce work hours and provide more help with ADLs.

Caregiving is an experience for which most people are not prepared. It is common for caregivers to become physically, emotionally, and economically overwhelmed by the responsibilities and demands of caring for a loved one. The stress of caregiving may lead to emotional problems such as depression, anger, and resentment. Signs of caregiver stress include irritability, inability to concentrate, fatigue, and sleeplessness. The caregiver often experiences decreased social interactions and may be at risk for social isolation. Multiple commitments, fatigue, and, at times, the patient's socially inappropriate behaviors contribute to the caregiver's social isolation. Stress can progress to burnout and result in negligence and abuse of the patient by the caregiver. Consider collaborating with a social worker if caregiver stress or strain is present and caregivers need respite.

Encourage caregivers to take care of themselves. Suggest journaling or joining a support group to help them share feelings that may be hard to express. Remind caregivers that getting regular exercise and sleep and eating balanced meals will enhance their well-being. Encourage contact with others to give emotional support. Finally, humor is important. Sometimes its use by caregivers can provide distraction and relieve stress-filled situations.

Elder Mistreatment

Elder mistreatment (EM) describes intentional acts of omission or commission by a caregiver or "trusted other" that cause harm or serious risk for harm to a vulnerable older adult. EM may occur in community (home or assisted living facility) or long-term care (institutional) settings.

Between 2 and 10% of community-dwelling older adults in the United States are abused, neglected, or exploited by trusted others.[16] The prevalence of EM in institutional settings is unknown, but it is thought to be widespread. Although EM rates are similar in women and men, most victims are women because of the predominance of women in older age cohorts. Victims of EM have a mortality risk that is 3 times higher than that of nonmistreated peers. The higher mortality risk is not due to the abuse or neglect itself but may be due to stress-related illnesses associated with prolonged mistreatment.[16]

EM is a hidden problem. For every reported case in the community setting, more than 5 cases go unreported. Underreporting may be higher based on immigration status, ethnic background, or sexual orientation. Victims are unlikely to report mistreatment by "trusted others" because of isolation; impaired cognitive or physical function; feelings of shame, guilt, or self-blame; fear of reprisal; pressure from family members; fear of long-term care; or cultural norms. HCPs also underreport EM, possibly from a failure to suspect or recognize EM, perceived inability to successfully intervene, desire to avoid responsibility for further action, or ageism.

Family members are responsible for up to 90% of domestic EM.[16] Adult children who abuse, neglect, or exploit their parents are usually dependent on their parent(s) for housing and financial support, have a history of violence, are unemployed, and/or are disabled from substance use or mental illness. Abusive spouses or partners may either begin intimate partner violence in older age or continue a lifelong pattern of abuse.

Many factors put community-dwelling older adults at risk for domestic EM. These include (1) physical or cognitive dysfunction that leads to an inability to perform ADLs (and therefore produces dependence on others for care), (2) any psychiatric diagnoses, including dementia and depression, (3) alcohol misuse and abuse, (4) decreased social support; (5) living with a large number of household members other than a spouse and (6) low income.[17] In long-term care settings the same factors that lead to institutionalization are risk factors for mistreatment by staff, visitors, and others. These include dependence on others for care because of physical or cognitive limitations.

Types of EM, characteristics, and manifestations are shown in Table 5.8. In institutional settings, EM includes the types described in Table 5.8 as well as failure to follow the plan of care, unauthorized use of physical or chemical restraints, overuse or underuse of medication, or isolation as punishment.

Follow your organization's protocols for EM screening and interventions. Perform a thorough history and physical examination that includes screening for mistreatment. It is important that you interview people alone. If mistreatment is occurring, they may not disclose it in the presence of the person who is with them, especially if that person is the abuser. Be especially attentive to explanations about injuries that are not consistent with what you observe, contradictory explanations between the patient and the caregiver, or behavioral clues that suggest the patient is being threatened or intimidated. Other nursing assessments and interventions are listed in Table 5.9. In most states, health care workers are among those mandated to report suspected or actual EM to Adult Protective Services (APS) and/or law enforcement. Know your legal responsibilities by checking the laws in your state.

Self-Neglect

Most referrals made to APS are for self-neglect. Older adults who self-neglect are often unable to meet their basic needs and refuse help; have multiple, untreated medical or psychiatric conditions; and live alone and often in squalor. Older community-dwelling adults who self-neglect face a higher risk for mortality than peers who do not self-neglect.[18] Nursing interventions include assessment for possible self-neglect, referrals for long-term interprofessional case management, and referral to APS.

TABLE 5.8   Types of Elder Mistreatment

Characteristics	Manifestations
Abandonment	
Desertion of an older person by a person who has assumed responsibility for providing care or by a person with physical custody.	Older adult's reports of being abandoned; deserting an older adult at a hospital or skilled nursing facility, shopping center, or other public place.
Financial Abuse	
Denying access to personal resources, stealing money or possessions. Coercing to sign contracts or durable power of attorney. Making changes in will or trust.	Living situation below level of personal resources. Sudden change in personal finances, sudden transfer of assets.
Neglect	
Failure or refusal to provide basic life needs, including food, water, medications, clothing, hygiene. Failure to provide physical aids such as dentures, eyeglasses, hearing aid. Failure to ensure safety.	Older adult's report of being neglected. Untreated or infected pressure injuries on sacral area, heels. Weight loss, malnutrition. Laboratory values showing dehydration. Poor personal hygiene. Lack of adherence with medical treatment.
Failure to provide social stimulation. Leaving alone for long periods. Failure to provide companionship.	Depression, withdrawn behavior, agitation. Ambivalent attitude toward caregiver or family member.
Physical Abuse	
Slapping, striking, restraining, incorrect positioning. Oversedation with medications.	Bruises, bilateral injuries (upper arms, ankles, wrists), repeated injuries in various stages of healing, burn marks, oversedation. Use of several emergency departments.
Psychologic Abuse	
Berating verbally, harassment, intimidation, threats of punishment, or deprivation. Childlike treatment, isolation.	Depression, withdrawn behavior, agitation. Ambivalent attitude toward caregiver or family member.
Sexual Abuse	
Nonconsensual sexual contact, including touching inappropriately. Forced sexual contact.	Older adult's report of sexual abuse. Unexplained vaginal or anal bleeding, bruised breasts, unexplained sexually transmitted or genital infections.
Violation of Personal Rights	
Denying right to privacy or right to make decisions about health care or living environment. Forcible eviction.	Sudden inexplicable changes in living situation, confusion.

SOCIAL SERVICES FOR OLDER ADULTS

A network of services supports older adults in the community and health care facilities. In the United States, most older adults are the beneficiaries of at least 1 social or governmental service. To understand the older adult's situation, learn about government structures that fund and regulate programs for older adults. The

TABLE 5.9 Nursing Management

Elder Mistreatment

When elder mistreatment is suspected, it is important to do the following:
- Screen for possible elder mistreatment, including domestic violence.
- Conduct a thorough history and head-to-toe physical assessment. Document your findings, including any statements made by the older adult or accompanying adult.
- If the older adult appears to be in immediate danger, develop and implement a safety plan in collaboration with the interprofessional team involved in the person's care.
- Identify, collect, and preserve physical evidence (e.g., dirty or bloody clothing dressing sheets).
- After obtaining consent, take photographs to document physical findings of suspected abuse or neglect. If possible and appropriate, do this before treating or bathing the alleged victim.
- If you suspect that mistreatment is occurring, report your findings to the state agency and/or law enforcement as mandated by the laws in your state.
- Initiate appropriate consultations with social work, forensic nursing, and adult protective services.

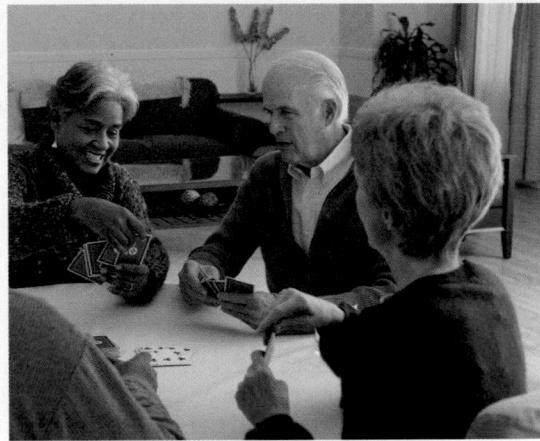

FIG. 5.5 Senior centers offer places for older adults who live independently to meet and gather with friends. (© Jupiterimages/Comstock/Thinkstock.)

Administration on Aging (AoA), which is part of the Department of Health and Human Services, is the federal agency responsible for many older adult programs. Funding from the AoA is given to state and local Area Agencies on Aging (AAAs).

MEDICARE AND MEDICAID

Medicare is a federally funded health insurance program for people ages 65 years or older. It also covers people under age 65 with certain disabilities and people of any age with end-stage renal disease (ESRD) requiring dialysis or a kidney transplant.

Medicare has 4 options for coverage: A, B, C, and D. Part A covers inpatient hospital care and partially covers skilled nursing facility care, hospice, and home health care. Part A coverage is "free" because workers support Medicare through payroll taxes. Medicare Part B partially covers outpatient care, physicians' or primary care providers' services, and home health care. It also covers some preventive services, such as mammograms. Medicare Part B is voluntary and has a monthly premium and an annual deductible before payment begins. Medicare Advantage Plans, sometimes called "Part C" or "MA Plans," are offered by private companies approved by Medicare to provide Part A and Part B benefits. Part D is available to Medicare enrollees and provides a prescription drug benefit. Members pay a yearly deductible, monthly premium, and copayment. People with lower incomes and limited assets may qualify for extra help to pay for prescriptions.

Medicare does not cover long-term care, custodial ADLs or IADLs care, dental care or dentures, hearing aids, or eyeglasses. (More information is available at *www.medicare.gov.*) Out-of-pocket expenditures for people on Medicare continue to rise. The costs increase with age, functional disabilities, number of chronic conditions, and number of hospitalizations.[19]

Medicaid is a state-administered, needs-based program to help eligible low-income people, including Medicare beneficiaries, with certain medical expenses. Those who qualify for both Medicare and Medicaid are referred to as *dual-eligible*. Eligibility and coverage vary by state. For qualified Medicare beneficiaries, Medicaid pays Medicare premiums, deductibles, and co-insurance, as well as long-term care and home health expenses. In the United States most long-term care is paid for by Medicaid or private pay. (More information is available at *www.medicaid.gov.*)

CARE ALTERNATIVES FOR OLDER ADULTS

Older adults with special care needs include people who are homeless, in need of help with ADLs, cognitively impaired, homebound, or no longer able to live at home. Older adults may be served by adult day care, adult day health care, home health care, and long-term care. Continuing care retirement communities, congregate housing, and assisted living facilities are housing options for older adults.

Adult Day Care and Adult Day Health Care

Adult day care centers provide social, recreational, and health-related services to people in a safe, community-based environment (Fig. 5.5). This includes daily supervision, social activities, opportunities for social interaction, and ADLs help for 2 groups of adults: (1) those who are cognitively impaired and (2) those who have problems independently performing ADLs. Adult day care programs provide individualized services based on need. Programs designed for adults who are cognitively impaired offer therapeutic recreation, support for family, family counseling, and social involvement.

Adult day health care centers are like adult day care but provide care to meet the needs of older adults and people with disabilities who need a higher level of care. This might include health monitoring, therapeutic activities, 1-on-1 ADLs training, and personal services.

Adult day care centers and adult day health care centers may offer respite to allow continued employment for the caregiver and delay institutionalization of older adults. States set standards and regulate centers. Medicare does not cover costs. Adult day health care is tax deductible as dependent care. Appropriate placement in adult care programs that match participants' needs is important. You can help by knowing the available centers in your area and assessing the needs of older adults and their families. You will then be able to help them make good decisions about their care.

Home Health Care

Home health care (HHC) can be a cost-effective care alternative for older adults who are homebound, have health needs that are intermittent or acute, and have supportive caregiver involvement. HHC is not an alternative for adults in need of 24-hour help with ADLs or continuous safety supervision. Private duty care may be an alternative in these situations. HHC services require physician orders and skilled nursing care for Medicare reimbursement. Unless one meets these requirements, Medicare will not pay for home health aides for ADLs management or a homemaker for IADLs management.

In addition to HHC, caregivers often seek homemaker services and respite and personal care through organizations that provide nonmedical assistance. These services help older adults stay at home.

Long-Term Care Facilities

Three factors appear to precipitate placement in a long-term care facility: (1) rapid patient deterioration, (2) caregiver inability to continue care because of stress and burnout, and (3) a change in or loss of the family support system. Progressive dementia, urinary incontinence, or a major health event (e.g., stroke) can hasten long-term care placement.

The conflicts and fears faced by older adults and their families make placement a difficult transition. Common caregiver concerns include: (1) Will the older adult resist the admission process? (2) Will the level of care given by staff be insufficient? (3) Will the resident be lonely? and (4) Will nursing care be affordable?

The physical relocation of the older adult may lead to adverse health effects. *Relocation stress syndrome* is associated with the disruption, confusion, and challenges that older adults face when moving to a new environment. Older adults may have anxiety, depression, and disorientation. Appropriate interventions can reduce the effects of relocation. Whenever possible, involve older adults in the decision to move and fully inform them about the location. Caregivers can share information, pictures, or a video recording of the new location. Staff members at the institution can send a welcome message. On arrival, they can greet new residents and provide orientation. To bridge the relocation, new residents can be "buddied" with seasoned residents (Fig. 5.6).

Programs for All-Inclusive Care for the Elderly (PACE)

Programs for All-Inclusive Care for the Elderly (PACE) provide care for adults age 55 and older. PACE services include primary care including prescription medications and wound care; physical, occupational, recreational, and speech therapy; adult day care; dental; podiatry; social services; and home health care.

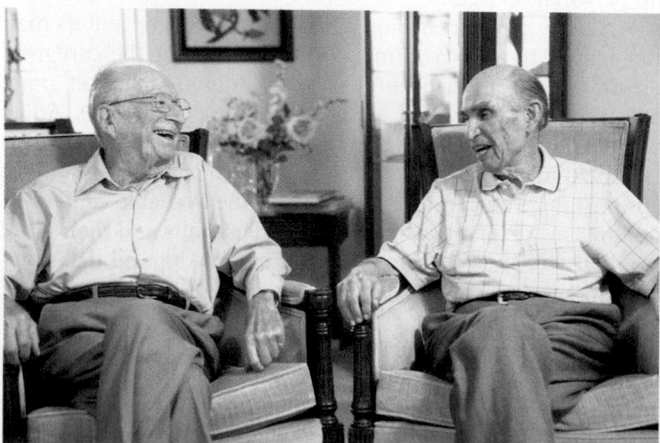

FIG. 5.6 Social interaction and acceptance are important for older adults. (©Hemera/Thinkstock.)

Respite care, hospitalization, short-term rehabilitation, and long-term care are provided as needed.[20]

A person who has Medicaid will not have to pay a monthly premium for the long-term portion of the PACE benefit. A person who does not qualify for Medicaid but has Medicare must pay a monthly premium to cover the long-term care portion.

LEGAL AND ETHICAL ISSUES

Legal guidance and assistance is needed by many older adults. Legal issues include advance directives, estate planning, taxation issues, appeals for denied services (e.g., disability), financial decisions, or exploitation by strangers or "trusted others."

Advance directives are written statements of a person's wishes about medical care. A health care proxy may be appointed to make medical decisions if a person is unable to make his or her own medical decisions. These documents allow people to direct their own care at end of life. Advance directives are discussed in detail in Chapter 9 and Table 9.6.

When working with older adults, you may find several ethical issues that influence practice, such as the assessment of older adults' ability to make decisions. Other ethical issues related to end-of-life care include decisions about resuscitation, treatment of infections, nutrition and hydration, and transfer to more intensive treatment units and the hospital. These situations are often complex, especially during emotionally difficult times. You can assist the older adult, family, and other health care workers by (1) keeping current on the ethical issues, (2) acknowledging when an ethical dilemma is present, and (3) advocating for an institutional ethics committee to help provide guidance in the decision-making process and assist when differences of opinion occur.

❖ NURSING MANAGEMENT: OLDER ADULTS

Gerontologic nursing is the care of older adults based on the specialty body of knowledge of gerontology and nursing. These specialty nurses provide care for older adults using a whole-person (physical, psychologic, functional, developmental, socioeconomic, cultural) perspective. Care of older adults is complex and presents challenges that require skilled assessment and creative nursing interventions tailored to this population.

Diseases and conditions in older adults may be hard to accurately assess and diagnose. Older adults may underreport symptoms and try to manage these symptoms by changing their functional status. For example, a woman having loss of feeling in her feet because of neuropathy may start using a walker to get around, while not reporting the symptom to her HCP. The older adult may attribute a new symptom to "aging" and ignore it. The older adult may eat less, sleep more, or "wait it out."

In older adults, disease symptoms are often atypical. For example, confusion may be a sign of an infection. A patient being treated for a urinary tract infection may be diagnosed with asymptomatic heart disease. Pathologic conditions with similar symptoms can be confused. For example, depression may be misdiagnosed and treated as dementia. The most common atypical illness presentations are "delirium" or "acute change in mental status" and change in functional status. A caregiver may say that a relative "is acting differently," "doesn't appear as him/herself," or is no longer taking part in usual activities or self-care.

In older adults a *cascade disease pattern* may occur. For example, a person who has insomnia treats the condition with a sleeping medication becomes lethargic and delirious and falls, sustaining a hip fracture. This decreases activity and mobility, leading to pneumonia and/or pressure injuries. Nurses play a vital role in preventing this downward trajectory.

For older adults, the stress of an illness may lead to fear and anxiety. They may view health care personnel as helpful but perceive institutions as negative and potentially harmful places. Communicate a sense of concern and care by use of direct and simple statements, appropriate eye contact, direct touch, and gentle humor. These actions help the older adult relax in this stressful situation.

◆ Nursing Assessment

Prior to assessment, attend to the person's primary needs. For example, ensure that older adults are comfortable and ask if they need to use the bathroom. If older adults normally use eyeglasses and hearing aids, ask them to use these during the assessment. Place all assistive devices, such as walkers, within reach. Assess your patient's level of fatigue and pause the interview if necessary. Allow adequate time to offer information and time for the person to respond to questions. Interview both the older adult and his or her family or caregivers. You can do this separately, unless the patient is cognitively impaired or specifically requests the caregiver's presence. Although the health history may be lengthy, it is important to obtain. Review medical records and determine what information is most relevant or needs more detail.

The focus of a comprehensive geriatric assessment is to determine appropriate interventions to support and enhance the health, quality of life, function, and independence of older adults. At a minimum, it includes the medical history, functional assessment, medication review, cognitive and mood evaluation, social resources, and physical examination followed by recommended diagnostic tests. Comprehensive geriatric assessment is often conducted by an interprofessional geriatric assessment team. This team minimally includes a staff nurse, an HCP such as a physician or adult-geriatric nurse practitioner, and a social worker. It may also include a physical and/or occupational therapist, dietitian, podiatrist, ophthalmologist, dentist, and pastoral care representative. After the assessment is complete, the interprofessional team meets with the patient and family to present the team's findings and recommendations.

Specific elements in a comprehensive nursing assessment include a thorough history, mood assessment, functional assessment including ADLs and IADLs, mental status evaluation, social-environmental assessment, and physical assessment. Evaluation of mental status is particularly important for older adults because these results often determine the potential for independent living. *SPICES,* an effective tool for obtaining assessment data in older adults, may be used as an initial nursing assessment in any setting (Fig. 5.7). Multiple evidence-based geriatric assessment tools and best practice approaches to nursing care for older adults are available from the *Try This* Series at the Hartford Institute for Geriatric Nursing (available at *www. consultgeri.org/tools*).

A comprehensive geriatric assessment includes fall risk, fear of falling, cause(s) of past falls, and post-fall assessment. Those at increased risk for falls have a history of falls or a fear of falling. Many factors increase the risk for falls, including prescription and nonprescription medications; infection; orthostatic hypotension; dehydration; electrolyte imbalance or other laboratory abnormalities; arthritis; changes in gait, balance, and mobility; neurologic impairment (e.g., stroke, Parkinson's disease); decreased muscle strength; and decreased visual acuity. Assess for symptoms of dizziness or lightheadedness upon standing. Other risk factors include environmental hazards, feet abnormalities, poor footwear, clutter, throw rugs, incorrect use of an assistive device such as a walker or cane, shiny or waxy floors, slippery floors, poor lighting, bed in an incorrect position such as too high, and uneven pavement.

Evaluation of the results of a comprehensive nursing assessment helps determine the service and potential long-term placement needs of older adults. Collect data about community resources that will help older adults and their caregivers in supporting maximal function. The goal is to plan and implement actions that help older adults stay as functionally independent as possible and to promote their quality of life.

◆ Planning

When setting goals with older adults, identify their strengths and abilities. Include caregivers in planning. Priority goals may include gaining a sense of control, feeling safe, and reducing stress.

◆ Nursing Implementation

When carrying out a plan of action for older adults, adjust your approach and actions based on their physical, functional, and mental status. The small body size common in frail older adults may require the use of pediatric equipment (e.g., BP cuff). Safety is a primary concern when caring for an older adult. Those with bone and joint changes often need transfer assistance, altered positioning, and use of gait belts and lift devices. Older adults with declining energy reserves may need extra time to complete tasks. A slower approach and the use of other adaptive equipment may be needed. Cognitive impairment, if present, requires that you offer careful explanations and a calm approach to avoid producing anxiety and resistance. Depression can result in apathy and poor cooperation with the treatment plan.

◆ Health Promotion.
Health promotion and prevention of health problems for older adults focus on 3 areas: (1) increased participation in health promotion and disease prevention activities (Fig. 5.8), (2) reduction in diseases and health-related issues, and (3) increased use of services that reduce health hazards. Programs exist for screening for chronic health conditions, tobacco cessation, geriatric foot care, vision and hearing screening, stress reduction, exercise

Patient name:		Date:	
SPICES		**EVIDENCE**	
		Yes	No
Sleep disorders			
Problems with eating or feeding			
Incontinence			
Confusion			
Evidence of falls			
Skin breakdown			

FIG. 5.7 SPICES. (Adapted from Fulmer T: The geriatric nurse specialist role: a new model. *Nurs Manag* 22:91, 1991. © Lippincott Williams & Wilkins, *www.lww.com.*)

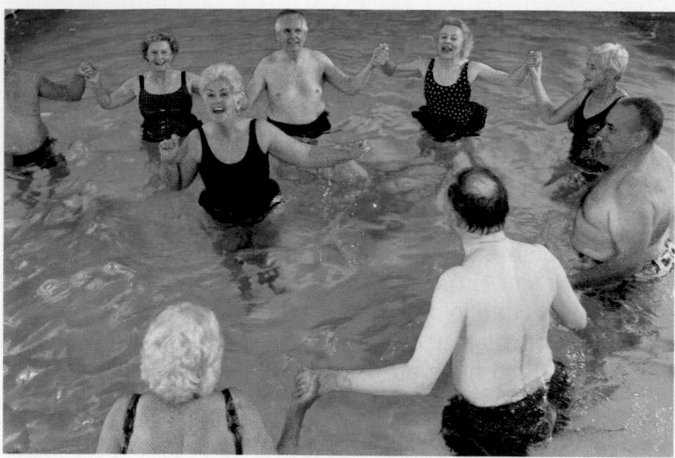

FIG. 5.8 Water aerobics is an example of a health promotion activity for older adults. (© Purestock/Thinkstock.)

programs, fall prevention programs, drug usage, crime prevention, elder mistreatment, and home safety assessment.[3] Teach older adults about the need for specific preventive services and available programs.

♥ PROMOTING POPULATION HEALTH
Promoting Health in Older Adults

- Get influenza, pneumococcal, shingles, and tetanus vaccines as needed.
- Create a living environment free of hazards to reduce the risk for falling.
- Drink plenty of liquids. Limit drinks with lots of added sugar or salt.
- Be physically active 3 to 5 days each week.
- Maintain an appropriate weight based on a nutrient-rich diet.
- Use medications, herbs, and supplements according to your HCP's direction.

Include health promotion and disease prevention in nursing interventions and plans at any setting or level of care in which nurses and older adults interact. You can use health promotion activities to increase personal responsibility for health and independent functioning. Teaching and reinforcement are important tools for you to use to enhance self-care practices by older adults. Patient teaching is discussed in Chapter 4.

◆ **Acute and Ambulatory Care.** The hospital may be the first point of contact for older adults with the health care system. Conditions that often result in hospitalization include falls, dysrhythmias, heart failure, stroke, fluid and electrolyte imbalances (e.g., hyponatremia, dehydration), pneumonia, urosepsis, and hip fractures. Hospitalized older adults often have multiple problems.

When older adults are being cared for in the acute care setting, both patients and caregivers need help with a variety of functions (Table 5.10). The outcome of hospitalization for older adults varies. Of special concern are patients undergoing high-risk surgical procedures (e.g., hip replacement) and those who have delirium while hospitalized.

Care Transitions. The time of a care transition to another setting (e.g., acute care hospital to rehabilitation) is challenging for many older adults. While in the hospital, patients and caregivers are counseled on how to prepare for posthospital care. Those with multiple health conditions have a particularly high risk for rehospitalization.

Medicare regulations require a registered nurse, social worker, or qualified person to develop a care transition plan for patient discharge. Safe and effective care transitions are most

▓ TABLE 5.10 Nursing Management
Care of the Hospitalized Older Adult

Give special consideration to the following nursing interventions when caring for hospitalized older adult:
- Identify older adults at risk for consequences of medical and/or surgical treatments).
- Consider discharge and postacute needs early in the hospital stay, especially assistance with activities of daily living and medications.
- Encourage the development and use of interprofessional teams, special care units, and providers who focus on the special needs of older patients.
- Implement standard protocols to screen for at-risk conditions common in the hospitalized older adult, such as urinary tract infection and delirium.
- Implement mobility and exercise programs to prevent functional decline.
- Monitor for and prevent skin integrity changes.
- Implement measures focused on safety (e.g., fall prevention).
- Refer patients to the appropriate community-based services.

likely to occur when interprofessional team members work together with the patient and family to coordinate care.

The Transitional Care Model (TCM) is an evidence-based, innovative approach to care coordination and management of the complex needs of older adults.[21] In this model a transitional care nurse delivers and coordinates care by nurses and other team members throughout potential and acute episodes of illness. Those most likely to benefit from transitional care nursing include those of older age and those with functional deficits, behavioral or psychiatric issues, multiple chronic conditions, polypharmacy, a recent hospitalization, lack of a support system, low health literacy, and history of non-adherence to treatment.[21]

Rehabilitation. The goal of rehabilitation is to help older adults adapt to or recover from disability or an acute functional decline. Rehabilitation may occur in acute inpatient rehabilitation, subacute rehabilitation, or long-term care settings. With proper training, assistive equipment, and attendant personal care, people with functional deficits may live independently. Older adults, primarily through Medicare reimbursement, can receive rehabilitative assistance through acute inpatient rehabilitation (limited days) and home health care programs (Fig. 5.9).

Older adults with chronic conditions, such as arthritis, have increased risk for functional decline. Decreased function or disabilities lead to increased self-care deficits, increased rates of institutionalization, decreased quality of life, and higher mortality rates.

Several factors influence the rehabilitation of older adults. First, preexisting conditions associated with decreased reaction time, visual acuity, fine motor ability, physical strength, and cognitive function affect the short- and long-term rehabilitation potential. Older adults may have anxiety, fear, or concern about falling. Poor nutrition and financial issues may limit the rehabilitation process. Encouragement, support, and acceptance from the interdisciplinary team members as well as their caregivers can help older adults remain motivated for potentially physically challenging rehabilitation.

Second, older adults often lose function because of inactivity and immobility. This deconditioning can occur because of unstable acute medical conditions, lack of assistive devices, and a lack of motivation to stay fit. The effect of inactivity leads to "use it or lose it" consequences. Older adults can improve flexibility, strength, and aerobic capacity even into very old

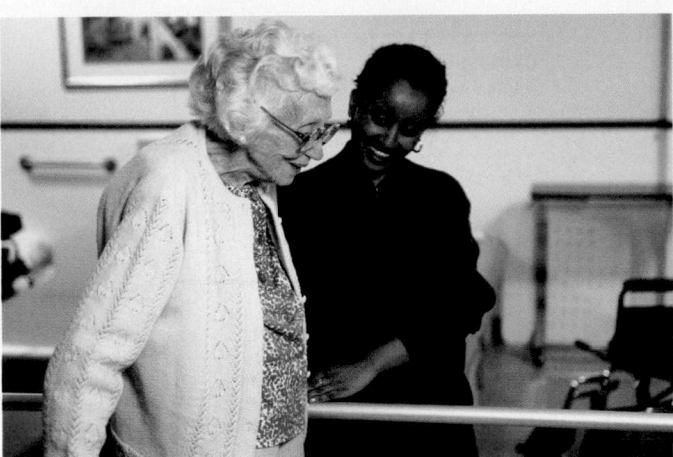

FIG. 5.9 The nurse assists a patient in a geriatric rehabilitation facility. (© KeithBrofsky/Photodisc/Thinkstock.)

age. Passive and active range-of-motion exercises are used with all older adults to preserve muscle tone and strength and prevent deconditioning and subsequent functional decline.

Last, the goal of rehabilitation is to strive for maximal function and physical capabilities considering the person's current health and functional status. For example, on admission to an acute or long-term care facility and home health services, assess for fall risk as well as the person's fear of falling. Initiate appropriate fall prevention interventions and assess for ongoing risk. Conduct comprehensive foot and peripheral vascular assessments for all older adults, especially those with diabetes, and arrange appropriate follow-up care.

Assistive Devices. Consider the use of assistive devices as interventions for older adults. Using appropriate assistive devices such as dentures, glasses, hearing aids, walkers, wheelchairs, adaptive utensils, elevated toilet seats, and skin protective devices can increase function. Include these tools and devices in the older adult's care plan when needed and teach the proper use of the devices. For example, using a cane correctly may decrease fall risk.

Technology can help with rehabilitation and living with functional impairments. For example, we can use electronic monitoring equipment to monitor heart rhythm and BP. Monitoring can locate a person with dementia who has wandered away from home or a long-term care facility. Computerized assistive devices may help patients with speech difficulties after a stroke. Small electronic devices can serve as memory aids.

Safety. Safety is crucial in the health maintenance of older adults. When compared to younger adults, older adults are at higher risk for accidents due to normal sensory changes, slowed reaction time, decreased thermal and pain sensitivity, changes in gait and balance, and medication effects. Most accidents occur in or around the home. Falls, motor vehicle accidents, and fires are common causes of accidental death in older adults. Declining thermoregulation impairs the older person's ability to adapt to extremes in environmental temperatures. The bodies of older adults can neither conserve nor dissipate heat as efficiently as those of younger adults. Therefore both hypothermia and hyperthermia occur more readily. The older adult age-group accounts for most deaths during severe cold spells and heat waves.

You can review environmental changes that can improve safety for older adults. Measures such as colored step strips, tub

and toilet grab bars, and stairway handrails can be effective in "safety-proofing" the living spaces of older adults. Uncluttered floor space (e.g., removal of throw rugs), railings, and increased lighting and night-lights are some of the easiest and most practical adaptations. Social workers may help older adults implement these environmental changes. You can advocate for home fire and security alarms.

Other interventions to decrease the risk for falling include exercise, physical therapy, and management of foot and footwear issues. Encourage the patient's use of glasses and hearing aids as ordered. Fear of falling can affect the older adults' decisions about the activities that they engage in and how active they remain.

Older adults who are new to inpatient or long-term care settings need a thorough orientation to the environment. Reassure the older adult that he or she is safe. Answer all questions and refer to interprofessional team members and specialists as needed. Foster orientation by displaying large-print clocks, keeping wall designs simple, clearly designating doors and exits, and using simple bed and nurse or family-call controls. Provide diffuse lighting while avoiding glare.

Medication Use. Medication use in older adults requires thorough and regular assessment, care planning, and evaluation. Nonadherence to medication plans by older adults is common. Many older adults are unable to read prescription drug labels and understand the health information that we provide them.

Age-related changes alter the pharmacodynamics and pharmacokinetics of drugs. Drug-drug, drug-nutrient, and drug-disease interactions influence the absorption, distribution, metabolism, and excretion of drugs. The most dramatic changes with aging are related to drug metabolism (Fig. 5.10). Hepatic blood flow and the enzymes responsible for drug metabolism decrease markedly with aging. These increase drug half-life in older adults and lead to greater risk for drug toxicity and adverse drug events. Overall, by age 75 to 80, there is a 50% decline in the renal clearance of drugs. Older adults with altered renal function may need a lower dose and/or decreased frequency of administration of a drug excreted by the kidney. When drug level monitoring is available (e.g., digoxin), identify toxic levels by serum monitoring at regular intervals, especially when there is a change of dose and/or frequency of administration.

Older adults may have difficulty managing medication due to cognitive impairment, altered sensory perception, and limited hand mobility or dexterity. Table 5.11 lists common reasons for drug errors made by older adults.

Polypharmacy (the use of multiple medications by a person who has more than 1 health problem), overdose, and addiction to prescription drugs are major causes of illness in older adults.[22] Potential medication errors include the (1) taking both brand and generic medications, (2) refilling medications too soon or too late (resulting in taking the medication incorrectly), and (3) drug-drug interactions. These errors can be prevented by having a pharmacist review medications regularly. Suggest the use of 1 pharmacy for filling all prescription medications.

The effects of medications in older adults with multiple health problems are particularly challenging to assess and manage. As 1 disease is treated, another may be affected. For example, the use of a drug such as oxybutynin, which is given to treat overactive bladder, may cause confusion. To accurately assess medication knowledge and use, ask older adults to bring all medications (OTC drugs, prescription drugs, vitamins and supplements, laxatives, sleep aids, and herbal remedies) that they take regularly or

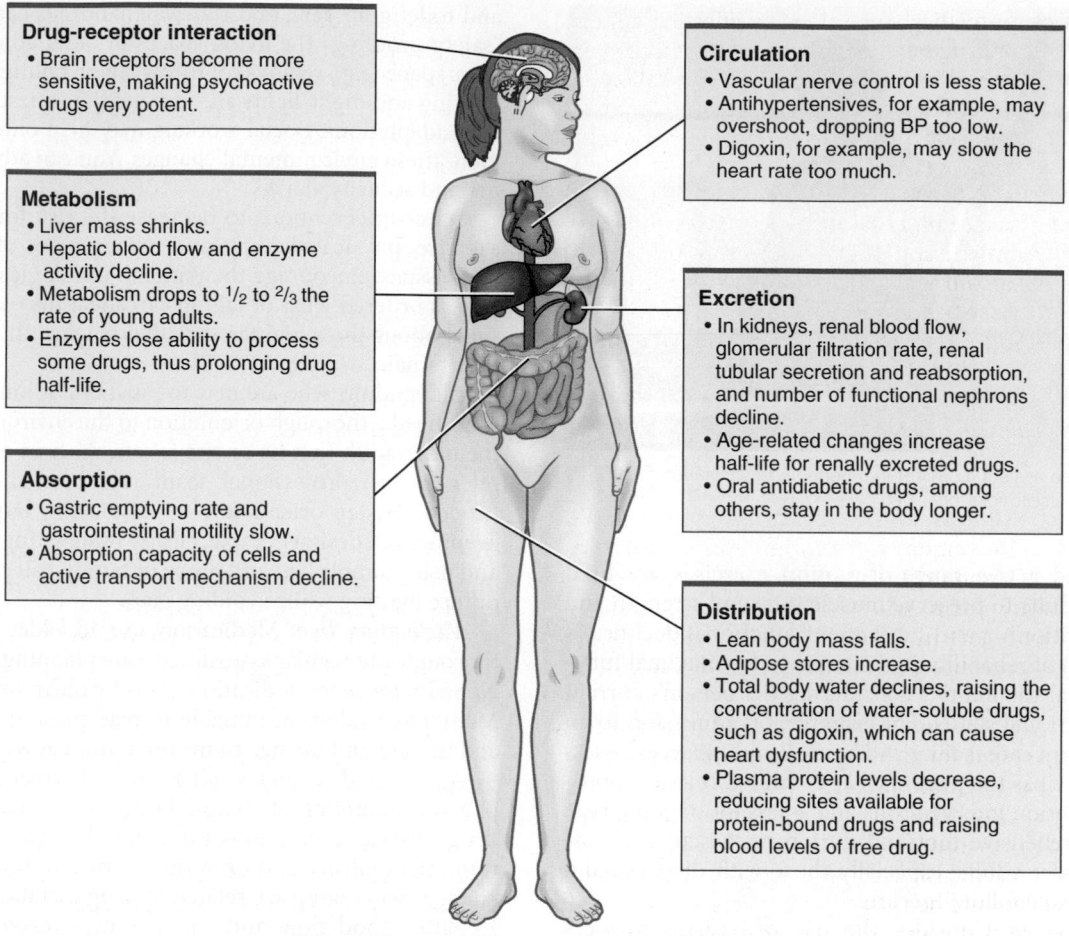

Drug-receptor interaction
- Brain receptors become more sensitive, making psychoactive drugs very potent.

Metabolism
- Liver mass shrinks.
- Hepatic blood flow and enzyme activity decline.
- Metabolism drops to $\frac{1}{2}$ to $\frac{2}{3}$ the rate of young adults.
- Enzymes lose ability to process some drugs, thus prolonging drug half-life.

Absorption
- Gastric emptying rate and gastrointestinal motility slow.
- Absorption capacity of cells and active transport mechanism decline.

Circulation
- Vascular nerve control is less stable.
- Antihypertensives, for example, may overshoot, dropping BP too low.
- Digoxin, for example, may slow the heart rate too much.

Excretion
- In kidneys, renal blood flow, glomerular filtration rate, renal tubular secretion and reabsorption, and number of functional nephrons decline.
- Age-related changes increase half-life for renally excreted drugs.
- Oral antidiabetic drugs, among others, stay in the body longer.

Distribution
- Lean body mass falls.
- Adipose stores increase.
- Total body water declines, raising the concentration of water-soluble drugs, such as digoxin, which can cause heart dysfunction.
- Plasma protein levels decrease, reducing sites available for protein-bound drugs and raising blood levels of free drug.

FIG. 5.10 The effects of aging on drug metabolism.

TABLE 5.11 Drug Therapy
Causes of Medication Errors by Older Adults

- Decreased vision
- Forgetting to take drugs
- Use of nonprescription over-the-counter drugs
- Use of medications prescribed for someone else
- Lack of financial resources to obtain prescribed medication
- Refusal to take medication because of undesirable side effects
- Failure to understand instructions or importance of drug treatment

TABLE 5.12 Drug Therapy
Safe Medication Use by Older Adults

When older adults are using medications, it is important to take the following measures to prevent medication errors:
- Assess cognitive function and monitor for changes.
- Try to reduce medication use that is not essential by consulting the HCP and pharmacist.
- Assess ability to self-administer medication and overall medication use, including prescription drugs; OTC drugs; pain treatments; antihistamines; cough syrups; vitamins, minerals, and supplements; sleep remedies; and herbal remedies.
- Assess alcohol and illicit drug use.
- Encourage the use of written or electronic medication-reminder systems.
- Encourage the use of 1 pharmacy.
- Work with HCPs and pharmacists to set up routine drug profiles on all older adult patients.
- Advocate for low-income prescription support services.

---

occasionally to their health care appointment. You will then be able to accurately assess all medications that the patient is taking, including drugs that the person may have omitted or thought unimportant. The American Geriatrics Society (AGS) Beers Criteria are designed to reduce problems with medications in older adults.[22] Table 5.12 describes other nursing interventions to help older adults follow a safe medication routine.

Depression. Depression is not a normal part of aging. However, it is often an underrecognized problem in older adults. Around 15% of older adults living in their homes have manifestations of depression. Rates of depressive symptoms in older adults in institutional settings are higher. The second highest rate of suicide occurs in those over 75.

Depression is associated with female gender, being divorced or separated, low socioeconomic status, poor social support, and a recent adverse and unexpected event. Depression in older adults tends to arise from a loss of self-esteem and may be related to life situations, such as retirement or loss of a spouse or partner. Problems such as pain, insomnia, lethargy, agitation, weight loss, and dementia are associated with depression.

Late-life depression often occurs together with medical conditions, such as heart disease, stroke, diabetes, and cancer.

Depression can worsen medical conditions by affecting adherence to diet, exercise, or drug regimens. It is important that your assessment include physical examination and interpretation of laboratory results for physical disorders that may have symptoms similar to those of depression (e.g., thyroid disorders, vitamin deficiencies).

Encourage older adults who have depressive symptoms to seek treatment. Because older adults with depression may feel unworthy, withdrawn, and isolated, the support of the family or others in encouraging older adults to seek treatment is important. Assist older adult caregivers who have depressive symptoms to seek medical attention, and help them in secure respite services and support for their caregiving role.

Restraint Use. *Physical restraints* are devices, materials, and equipment that physically prevent persons from moving freely, such as walking, standing, lying, transferring, or sitting. *Chemical restraints* are drugs used to restrict a patient's freedom of movement or in some cases to sedate a patient. The current standard is to provide safe care without using restraints of any form, whether physical or chemical. Restraints are a last resort in the care of older adults. Only use restraints to ensure the person's safety or the safety of others.

Before considering the use of any restraint, completely assess the perceived need for the restraint and document the assessment. Behavioral symptoms, such as crying and shouting, may arise from co-morbidities, pain, medication effects, unmet needs, and/or environmental factors. When behavioral manifestations are present, ask the following questions to better understand the patient's behavior: Is the person able to say what she or he needs and wants? People with dementia may respond by speaking, gesturing, nodding, or making eye contact. Questions that use "yes" or "no" answers are better than open-ended questions for gathering assessment information. Ask family, friends, or staff members from previous care settings about the patient's (1) history; (2) usual communication style and cues to indicate pain, fatigue, hunger, or a need to urinate or defecate; (3) abilities in ADLs; and (4) daily routines (e.g., "Is he often awake at night or an early riser?" "Does she prefer breakfast before dressing? Take an afternoon nap? Have a routine for dressing?").

Evaluate whether disruptive behaviors signal unmet physiologic or psychosocial needs. For example, a patient who tries to get out of bed without help may be trying to reach the toilet.

A toileting schedule will help to curtail such attempts and prevent incontinence.

Long-term care regulations and The Joint Commission set standards for restraint use. These include time limit, observation and care, mandating use of least restrictive measures (e.g., mittens), and alternatives to restraint use. Restraint alternatives include low beds, body props, and electronic devices (such as bed and chair alarm signaling). Such approaches support the development of a "restraint-free," safe environment. Alternatives to restraints require vigilant, creative, and sensitive nursing care.

All restraints require an order from an HCP. Carefully document restraint use and the reason for use. It is not appropriate to use restraints to prevent falls, avoid interference with medical devices, or reduce irritating behaviors, such as calling out. Frequent scheduled reviews of the ongoing need for the restraint are done with consideration of when to discontinue the restraint.

Sleep. Adequacy of sleep is often a concern for older adults because of altered sleep patterns. Older people have a marked decrease in deep sleep and are easily aroused. Many older adults report difficulty going to sleep and staying sleep. They may feel "unrefreshed" after sleep. See Chapter 7 for more about the sleep problems of older adults.

◆ Evaluation

The evaluation phase of the nursing process is similar for all patients. The results of evaluation direct you to continue the plan of care or revise as needed. When evaluating nursing care with older adults, focus on functional improvement and quality of life. Useful questions to consider when evaluating the plan of care for older adults are outlined in Table 5.13.

TABLE 5.13 **Evaluating Nursing Care for Older Adults**
Use the following questions to evaluate the effectiveness of care for older adults:
• Is there an identifiable change in function, mental status, or signs and symptoms of exacerbation of chronic condition(s)?
• Does the person consider his or her health state to be improved?
• Does the person think the plan is helpful?
• Do the person and caregiver think the care is worth the time and cost?
• Can you document positive changes that support the interventions?

CASE STUDY
Older Adults

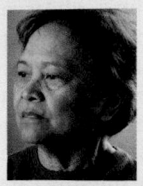

Patient Profile

C.L., a 73-yr-old Taiwanese woman, was admitted through the emergency department with shortness of breath. She was diagnosed with community-acquired pneumonia. Her medical history includes COPD, hypertension, diabetes, mild cognitive impairment, depression, macular degeneration, and significant hearing loss.

(© azndc/iStock/Thinkstock.)

Subjective Data

- A stroke 5 years ago and has right-sided weakness
- A 100 pack-year history of tobacco use but quit smoking after her stroke
- Not seen primary care physician in 1 year
- In past year has had an unplanned weight loss of 15 pounds
- Spends her days either in bed or in a recliner watching television
- Shortness of breath for past 5 days

Psychosocial Data

- Came to the United States 15 years ago from Taiwan
- Speaks Mandarin Chinese with limited English proficiency
- Lives with her unemployed adult son who provides help with ADLs and IADLs
- Has 3 daughters who live within a 2-hour drive
- Limited financial resources but has Medicare and Medicaid benefits
- Daughters raise concerns about their mother's care and safety at home, given their brother's history of anger issues and a gambling addiction
- When daughters ask their brother about how he is caring for his mother, he says, "I'm doing the best I can. She refuses help. She refuses to go to the doctor. What do you want me to do? She's old. She's crazy. She's going to die anyway!"
- Daughters state their mother does not want to go to a nursing home

Objective Data

Physical Examination

- Unwashed, matted hair, poor oral hygiene, overgrown toenails
- 2 Stage 3 sacral pressure injuries

- Unstageable right heel pressure injury
- Multiple small bruises on her forearms and shins
- 5- × 10-cm bruise in the middle of her back

Diagnostic Tests

- Serum albumin 2.4 g/dL
- X-ray reveals consolidation in lower left and right lung lobes

Discussion Questions

1. What other information do you need to assess C.L.'s condition? How should you address questions about potential elder mistreatment?
2. Define ageism, and explain how it may be manifested in this case.
3. Identify the stage of Corbin and Strauss chronic illness trajectory that describe C.L.'s current status. Which stage is the goal of your nursing care?
4. *Patient-Centered Care:* What is your assessment of C.L.'s ability to manage her chronic illnesses? What will you include in your care planning to optimize her self-care ability?
5. *Priority Decision:* Based on your assessment of C.L., what are the priority nursing diagnoses?
6. *Safety:* To ensure C.L.'s safety, what nursing interventions are necessary during her hospitalization?
7. *Collaboration:* How would you use unlicensed assistive personnel (UAP) on the hospital unit to carry out the priorities that you identified in question 4?
8. What risk factors does C.L. have for developing frailty? Which factors are modifiable?
9. Based on your knowledge of care alternatives for older adults, what setting would be most appropriate for C.L. upon hospital discharge?
10. *Collaboration:* Because she has an expressed desire to return home, what referrals would be indicated if this were the plan?
11. What risk factors does C.L. have for becoming a victim of elder mistreatment? List and provide the rationale for nursing interventions and legal and ethical responsibilities in this case.

Answers available at *http://evolve.elsevier.com/Lewis/medsurg.*

▌ BRIDGE TO NCLEX EXAMINATION

The number of the question corresponds to the same-numbered outcome at the beginning of the chapter.

1. Examples of primary prevention strategies include
   a. colonoscopy at age 50.
   b. avoidance of tobacco products.
   c. teaching the importance of exercise to a patient with hypertension.
   d. intake of a diet low in saturated fat in a patient with high cholesterol.
2. A characteristic of a chronic illness is that it *(select all that apply)*
   a. has reversible pathologic changes.
   b. has a consistent, predictable clinical course.
   c. results in permanent deviation from normal.
   d. is associated with many stable and unstable phases.
   e. always starts with an acute illness and then progresses slowly.
3. Among older Americans in the United States
   a. more than 30% live in nursing homes.
   b. women are less likely to live in poverty.
   c. the number of those who completed college is lower than in previous decades.
   d. those 85 years or older account for the fastest growing segment of the population.

4. An ethnic older adult may feel a loss of self-worth when the nurse *(select all that apply)*
   a. prohibits visits from a faith healer.
   b. informs the patient about ethnic support services.
   c. allows a patient to rely on ethnic health beliefs and practices.
   d. emphasizes that a therapeutic diet does not allow ethnic foods.
   e. uses a medical interpreter to provide explanations and teaching.
5. An important nursing action to help a chronically ill older adult is to
   a. avoid discussing future lifestyle changes.
   b. ensure the patient that the condition is stable.
   c. treat the patient as a competent manager of the disease.
   d. encourage the patient to "fight" the disease as long as possible.
6. Older adults who become ill are more likely than younger adults to
   a. report symptoms to their health care providers.
   b. refuse to carry out lifestyle changes to promote recovery.
   c. seek medical attention because of limitations on their lifestyle.
   d. alter their daily living activities to accommodate new symptoms.

7. An appropriate care choice for an older adult who lives with an employed daughter but needs help with activities of daily living is
   a. adult day care.
   b. long-term care.
   c. a retirement center.
   d. an assisted living facility.

8. Nursing interventions directed at health promotion in the older adult are primarily focused on
   a. disease management.
   b. controlling symptoms of illness.
   c. teaching positive health behaviors.
   d. teaching about nutrition to enhance longevity.

1. b, 2. c, d, 3. d, 4. a, d, 5. c, 6. d, 7. a, 8. c.

For rationales to these answers and even more NCLEX review questions, visit *http://evolve.elsevier.com/Lewis/medsurg*.

ⓔ EVOLVE WEBSITE/RESOURCES LIST

http://evolve.elsevier.com/Lewis/medsurg
Review Questions (Online Only)
Key Points
Answer Keys for Questions
- Rationales for Bridge to NCLEX Examination Questions
- Answer Guidelines for Case Study on p. 74
Conceptual Care Map Creator
Audio Glossary
Content Updates

REFERENCES

1. Centers for Disease Control and Prevention: Chronic diseases and health promotion. Retrieved from *www.cdc.gov/chronicdisease*.
2. Corbin JM, Strauss A: A nursing model for chronic illness management based upon the Trajectory Framework, *Sch Inq Nurs Pract* 5:155, 1991. (Classic)
3. Hartford Institute for Geriatric Nursing: Try This: Series. Retrieved from *www.consultgeri.org/tools/try-this-series*.
4. Department of Health and Human Services: Self-management for health in chronic conditions. Retrieved from *www.grants.nih.gov/grants/guide/pa-files/PA-14-344.html*.
5. Schulz R, Beach SR, Friedman EM, et al: Changing structures and processes to support family caregivers of seriously ill patients. *J Palliat Med*. 2018;21:S36.
6. Administration on Aging: A profile of older Americans: 2016. Retrieved from *www.acl.gov/sites/default/files/Aging%20and%20Disability%20in%20America/2016-Profile.pdf*.
*7. Wilson DM, Nam MA, Murphy J, et al: A critical review of published research literature reviews on nursing and healthcare ageism, *J Clin Nurs* 26:23, 2017.
*8. Cellerino A, Terzibasi ET: Biology of aging: New models, new methods, *Semin Cell Dev Biol* 70:98, 2017.
9. Denny DL, Lindseth G: Preoperative risk factors for subsyndromal delirium in older adults who undergo joint replacement surgery, *Ortho Nurs* 36:402, 2017.
10. Czaja S: The potential role of technology in supporting older adults, *Public Policy & Aging Report*, 27:44, 2017.
11. Li G, Thabane L, Papaioannou A, et al: An overview of osteoporosis and frailty in the elderly, *BMC Musculoskelet Disord*, 18:46, 2017.
12. U.S. Department of Agriculture Food and Nutrition Service: Supplemental Nutrition Assistance Program. Retrieved from *www.fns.usda.gov/snap/snap-special-rules-elderly-or-disabled*.
13. Manuel JI: Racial/ethnic and gender disparities in health care use and access, *Health Serv Res* 53:1407, 2018.
14. Stanford Medicine Geriatric Education Center: A national resource center in ethnogeriatrics. Retrieved from *http://sgec.stanford.edu/*.
15. Administration on Aging Family Caregiver Alliance: Selected caregiver statistics. Retrieved from *https://www.caregiver.org/caregiver-statistics-demographics*.
16. National Center for Elder Abuse: What we do. Retrieved from *https://ncea.acl.gov/*.
17. National Center for Elder Abuse: Preventing elder abuse and neglect in older adults: Tools and tips. Retrieved from *https://ncea.acl.gov/resources/publications.html*.
*18. Dong X: Elder self-neglect: Research and practice, *Clin Interv Aging* 12:949, 2017.
19. Kaiser Family Foundation: How much is enough? Out-of-pocket spending among Medicare beneficiaries. Retrieved from *www.kff.org/medicare/report/how-much-is-enough-out-of-pocket-spending-among-medicare-beneficiaries-a-chartbook/*.
20. National PACE Association: Eligibility requirements. Retrieved from *www.npaonline.org/*.
21. Penn Nursing Science: Transitional care model. Retrieved from *www.nursing.upenn.edu/ncth/transitional-care-model/*.
*22. Levy HB: Polypharmacy reduction strategies, *Clin Geriatr Med* 33:241, 2017.

*Evidence-based information for clinical practice.

6

Stress Management

Margaret R. Rateau

You may not be able to change the stressors in your life, but you can change your reaction or response to them.

Florence Nightingale

ℰ http://evolve.elsevier.com/Lewis/medsurg/

CONCEPTUAL FOCUS

Coping   Stress

LEARNING OUTCOMES

1. Distinguish between the terms *stressor* and *stress*.
2. Describe the role of the nervous and endocrine systems in the stress process.
3. Describe the effects of stress on the immune system.
4. Discuss the effects of stress on health.

5. Explain the role of coping in managing stress.
6. Select coping and relaxation strategies that you, a patient, or a caregiver experiencing stress can use.
7. Describe the nursing assessment and management of a patient experiencing stress.

KEY TERMS

biofeedback, p. 83
coping, p. 81
emotion-focused coping, p. 81
imagery, p. 83

massage, p. 84
meditation, p. 83
mind-body-spirit connection, p. 80
problem-focused coping, p. 81

psychoneuroimmunology (PNI), p. 79
relaxation breathing, p. 82
stress, p. 76
stressors, p. 77

All people experience stress. Stress has a powerful effect on the mind and therefore a significant effect on one's health and well-being. The concept of stress directly relates to multiple other concepts. Chronic stress is a major factor in causing and worsening chronic health conditions. This in turn is a major driver of escalating health care costs.

High levels of stress are common among patients and caregivers. How they deal with their stress is critical to their well-being. As a nurse, you play a key role in helping them recognize stress and manage stressful events. This chapter focuses on how stress can affect the mind, body, and spirit and how a person can effectively cope with stress.

WHAT IS STRESS?

Stress is the inability to cope with perceived (real or imagined) demands or threats to one's mental, emotional, or spiritual well-being.[1] What 1 person perceives as stressful may not be perceived as stressful to someone else. Responses to the same stressor vary greatly. Stress might be more prevalent in women than men, although it may be that women are more willing to admit they are experiencing stress.[2] *Perception* of the potential stressor influences the way a person responds to that stressor. This is shown in the following examples:

- B.J., a 43-yr-old woman, becomes depressed after a laparoscopic hysterectomy for fibroids. She is unwilling to take part in normal self-care activities. You are surprised by her response. You think she had a simple surgery and should get on with her life. After further assessment, you discover that removing her uterus is a great psychologic stressor because she perceives it as a loss of her womanhood and femininity.
- K.R., a 52-yr-old woman, has just been told by her health care provider (HCP) of her new diagnosis of type 2 diabetes. After the HCP's visit with her, you are prepared to provide emotional

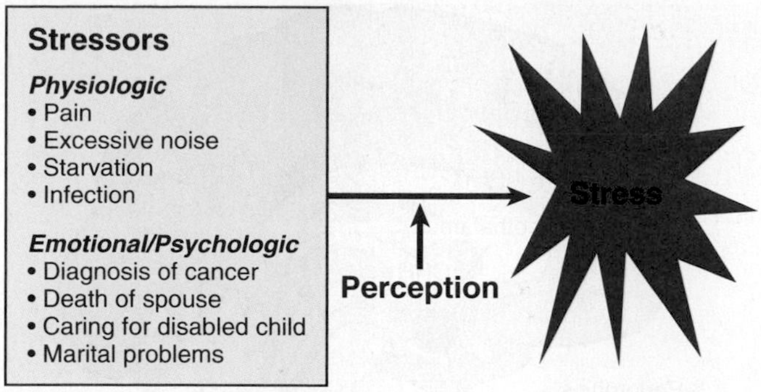

Stressors

Physiologic
- Pain
- Excessive noise
- Starvation
- Infection

Emotional/Psychologic
- Diagnosis of cancer
- Death of spouse
- Caring for disabled child
- Marital problems

Perception → Stress

FIG. 6.1 Stressors can be physiologic or emotional/psychologic. Your perception of these stressors will determine whether they cause stress. Events or circumstances become stressful when you perceive them to be.

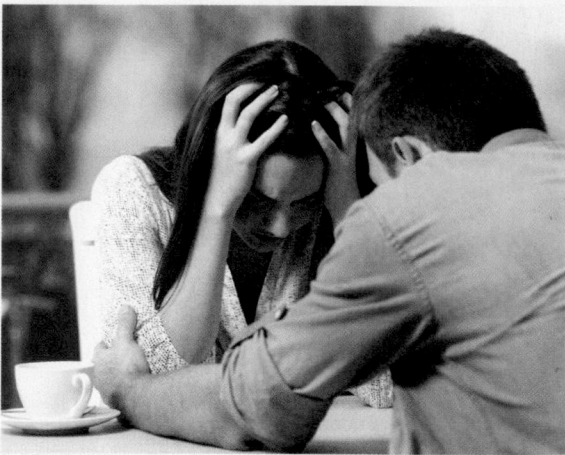

FIG. 6.2 During stressful situations, the demands seem to exceed the resources. (© iStock.com/AntonioGuillem.)

support. However, you are puzzled when she is smiling and feeling relieved. You think that this diagnosis should be stressful. However, K.R. tells you that she is so relieved because for weeks she was worried that her symptoms were caused by cancer.

Many different events or factors can be **stressors**. They can be physiologic or emotional/psychologic (Fig. 6.1). The emotional/psychologic stressors can be positive or negative. For example, the birth of a baby is usually a positive stressor. Marital discord is a negative stressor.

Is Stress Bad or Good?

We tend to think of stress as bad or a threat. Actually, any event or situation that is out of the ordinary can be a stressor. This includes events that we normally consider happy or enjoyable (e.g., getting married, going on a vacation).

Stress can be helpful. A little stress can motivate you. Stress can actually inspire you to achieve a goal and become more confident or stronger physically.

The body does not distinguish between bad stress and good stress or real or imaginary stress. It responds to the stressor with the same stress response. This stress response is the way our bodies react both physically and emotionally to any change, be it good, bad, real, or imagined.

For you as a nursing student, a test can be a stressful situation. A little bit of stress related to the upcoming test makes you study and become better prepared. If you feel mildly stressed during the test, it may help your test performance as a little stress heightens your awareness and increases your mental acuity. However, if you are overly stressed, it causes mental blocks, lack of concentration, and inability to remember things.

Stress is a key for survival, but too much stress can be detrimental. That is why it is important for you and your patients to learn to cope more effectively with the stressors in life.

Factors Affecting Response to Stress

Why do people respond so differently to stress? Why do some people cope better with stress than others? Interestingly, some people experience significant adverse life events but do not succumb to the effects of stress.

Differences in the responses to a stressor can be based on the duration of a stressor (acute or chronic) and intensity of a stressor (mild, moderate, or severe). For example, a person dealing with the chronic stress of caring for a loved one may be exposed to many acute stressors (e.g., car accident, influenza). The type, duration, and intensity of a stressor are important variables that can influence a person's response (Fig. 6.2).

TABLE 6.1 Factors Affecting Response to Stress

Internal
- Age
- Attitude
- Genetic background
- Hardiness
- Health status
- Nutritional status
- Optimistic outlook
- Personality characteristics
- Previous experience with stressors
- Resilience
- Sleep status

External
- Cultural and ethnic influences
- Number of stressors already experiencing
- Religious or spiritual influences
- Socioeconomic status
- Social support
- Timing of stressors

Factors that affect a person's response to stress include internal and external influences (Table 6.1). These factors show the importance of using a holistic approach when assessing the impact of stress on a person. Key personal characteristics that buffer the effects of stress are attitude, hardiness, being optimistic, and resilience.

Resilience is being resourceful and flexible and having good problem-solving skills. People who have a high degree of resilience are not as likely to perceive an event as stressful.

Hardiness is a combination of 3 characteristics: commitment, control, and openness to change. Together they give the courage and motivation needed to turn stressful circumstances from potential calamities into opportunities for personal growth.[3]

Attitude can influence the effect of stress on a person. People with positive attitudes view situations differently from those with negative attitudes. A person's attitude also influences how he or she manages stress. To some extent, positive emotional attitudes can prevent disease and prolong life.[4]

PATHOPHYSIOLOGY MAP

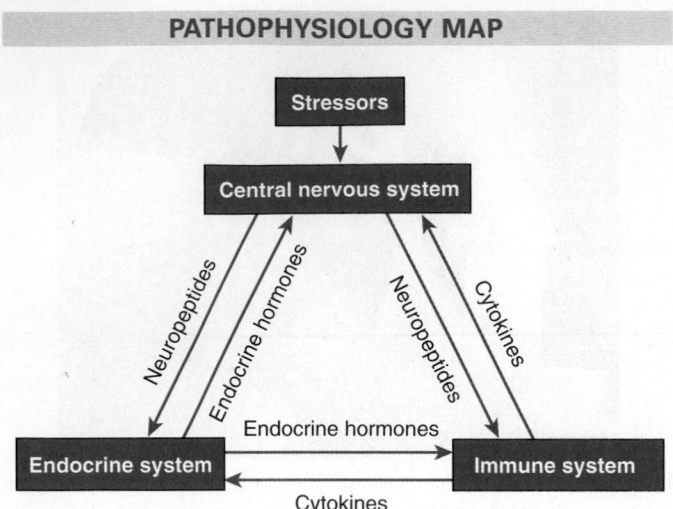

FIG. 6.3 Neurochemical links among the nervous, endocrine, and immune systems. The communication among the systems is bidirectional.

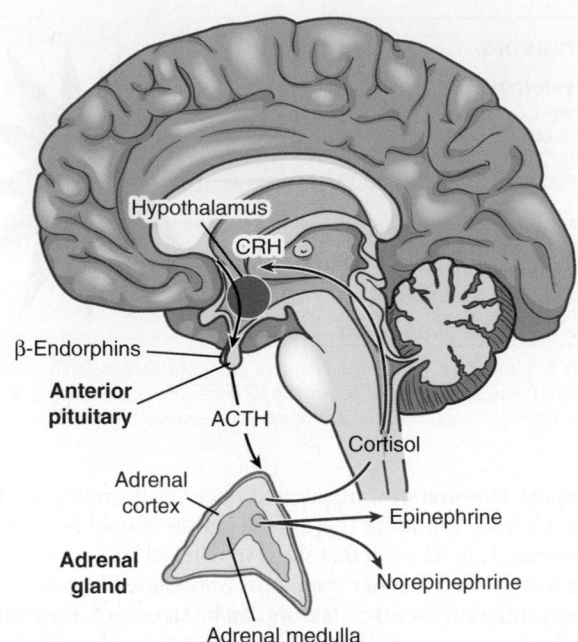

FIG. 6.4 Hypothalamic-pituitary-adrenal axis. *ACTH,* Adrenocorticotropic hormone; *CRH,* corticotropin-releasing hormone.

Being optimistic can help you cope more effectively with stress. Optimism also reduces a person's chances of developing stress-related illnesses. When optimistic people do become ill, they tend to recover more quickly. Pessimists are likely to deny the problem, distance themselves from the stressful event, focus on stressful feelings, or allow the stressor to interfere with achieving a goal. People with a more pessimistic attitude tend to report poorer health than people with optimistic attitudes.[4]

In addition to personal characteristics, external factors play a vital role in one's ability to cope with stress. Being surrounded by a strong social support system and receiving positive support from friends and family have a large impact on a person's ability to cope with stressors.

PHYSIOLOGIC RESPONSE TO STRESS

The nervous, endocrine, and immune systems are primarily involved in the stress response. These systems are interrelated, and that interrelationship is reflected in a person's physiologic response to stress (Fig. 6.3). Further, stress activation of these systems affects other body systems, such as the cardiovascular, respiratory, gastrointestinal, renal, and reproductive systems. A person's response to a stressor (real or imagined and physiologic or emotional/psychologic) determines the impact that stress will have on the body.

Nervous System
Cerebral Cortex. The areas of the cerebral cortex, or cerebrum, involved in the control of cognition, affect, and movement influence how we perceive stressors. We evaluate the stressor in light of past experiences and future consequences. This gives us some control over our response to stress. The motor areas also send signals to the adrenal medulla that directly relate to how stressors are managed.[5]

Limbic System. The *limbic system* lies in the inner midportion of the brain near the base of the brain. The limbic system is an important mediator of emotions and behavior. When the limbic system is stimulated, emotions, feelings, and behaviors can occur that ensure survival and self-preservation.

Reticular Formation. The *reticular formation* is located between the lower end of the brainstem and thalamus. It contains the *reticular activating system* (RAS), which sends impulses contributing to alertness to the limbic system and cerebral cortex. When the RAS is stimulated, it increases its output of impulses, leading to wakefulness. Stress usually increases the degree of wakefulness and can lead to sleep disturbances.

Hypothalamus. The hypothalamus, which lies at the base of the brain just above the pituitary gland, has many functions that aid in adaptation to stress. Stress activates the limbic system, which in turn stimulates the hypothalamus. Because the hypothalamus secretes neuropeptides that regulate the release of hormones by the anterior pituitary, it is central to the connection between the nervous and endocrine systems in responding to stress (Fig. 6.4).

The hypothalamus plays a primary role in the stress response by regulating the function of both the sympathetic and parasympathetic branches of the autonomic nervous system. When a person perceives a stressor, the hypothalamus sends signals that initiate both the nervous and endocrine responses to the stressor. It does this primarily by sending signals via nerve fibers to stimulate the sympathetic nervous system (SNS) and by releasing corticotropin-releasing hormone (CRH), which stimulates the pituitary to release adrenocorticotropic hormone (ACTH) (see Chapter 47).

Endocrine System
Once the hypothalamus is activated in response to stress, the endocrine system becomes involved. The SNS stimulates the adrenal medulla to release epinephrine and norepinephrine (catecholamines). The effect of catecholamines and the activation of the SNS, including the response of the adrenal medulla, is referred to as the *sympathoadrenal response.* Epinephrine and norepinephrine prepare the body for the *fight-or-flight response* (Fig. 6.5).

Stress activates the hypothalamic-pituitary-adrenal (HPA) axis. In response to stress, the hypothalamus releases CRH, which stimulates the anterior pituitary to release proopiomelanocortin (POMC). Both ACTH (a hormone) and β-endorphin (a neuropeptide) are derived from POMC.

PATHOPHYSIOLOGY MAP

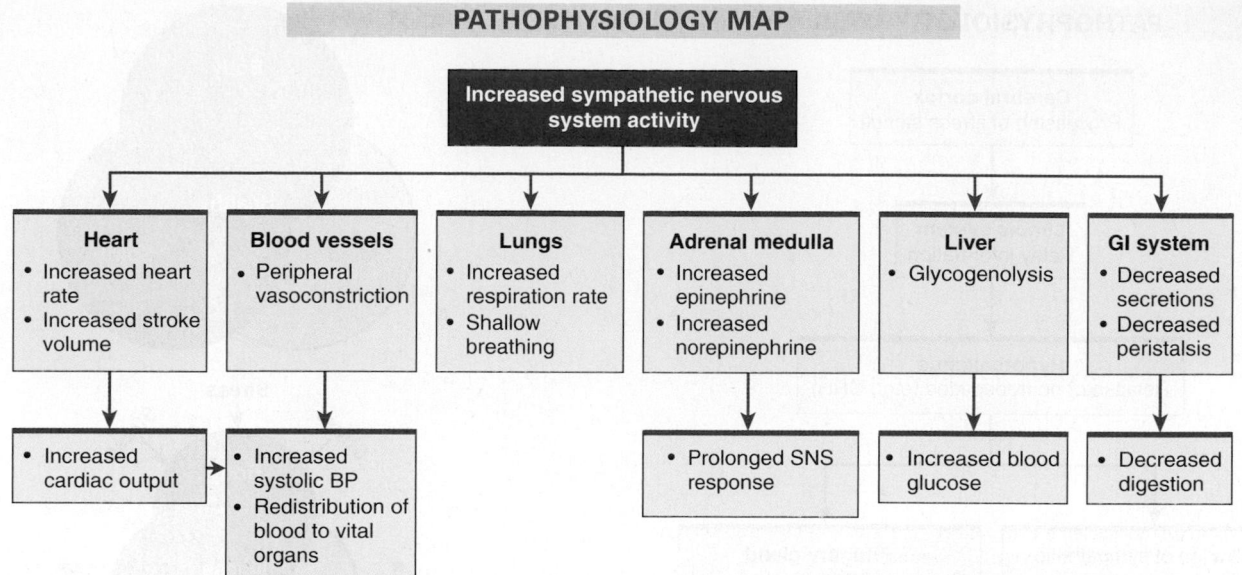

FIG. 6.5 "Fight-or-flight" reaction. Alarm reaction responses resulting from increased sympathetic nervous system *(SNS)* activity.

Endorphins have analgesic-like effects and blunt pain perception during stress situations involving pain stimuli. ACTH in turn stimulates the adrenal cortex to synthesize and secrete corticosteroids (e.g., cortisol) and, to a lesser degree, aldosterone.

Corticosteroids are essential for the stress response. Cortisol produces several physiologic effects, such as increasing blood glucose levels, intensifying the action of catecholamines on blood vessels, and inhibiting the inflammatory response. Corticosteroids play an important role in "turning off" or blunting the stress response, which, if uncontrolled, can become self-destructive. This is shown by their ability to suppress the release of proinflammatory mediators, such as the cytokines tumor necrosis factor (TNF) and interleukin-1 (IL-1). The persistent release of such mediators is believed to initiate organ dysfunction in conditions such as sepsis or autoimmune disease. Thus corticosteroids act not only to support the body's adaptive response to a stressor but also to suppress an overzealous and potentially self-destructive response.

The stress response involves increases in (1) cardiac output (resulting from the increased heart rate and increased stroke volume), (2) blood glucose levels, (3) oxygen consumption, and (4) metabolic rate (Fig. 6.5). In addition, dilation of skeletal muscle blood vessels increases blood supply to the large muscles and supports quick movement. Increased cerebral blood flow increases mental alertness. For example, in the case of stressful situations (e.g., blood loss from trauma), the increased blood volume (from increased extracellular fluid and the shunting of blood away from the gastrointestinal system) helps to maintain adequate circulation to vital organs.

Summary of Stress Response

In summary, the fight-or-flight response is an important and necessary adaptive mechanism of the body to acute stress. We activate this response to stressors whether they are physiologic

(e.g., acute pain) or emotional/psychologic (e.g., death of a child, loss of a home through fire, fear).

Acute stress leads to physiologic changes that are important to a person's survival. This is your "alarm system." It puts you on high alert. The acute stress response is a state of physiologic and psychologic arousal characterized by increased SNS activity that leads to increased heart and respiratory rate, increased BP, increased muscle tension, increased brain activity, and decreased skin temperature.

Immune System

Stress has an impact on the immune system. **Psychoneuro-immunology (PNI)** is an interdisciplinary science that studies the interactions among psychologic, neurologic, and immune responses. Because neuroanatomic and neuroendocrine pathways connect the brain to the immune system, stressors have the potential to lead to changes in immune function (Fig. 6.6).

Nerve fibers extend from the nervous system and synapse on cells and tissues of the immune system (i.e., spleen, lymph nodes). In turn, the cells of the immune system have receptors for many neuropeptides and hormones. This allows them to respond to nervous and neuroendocrine signals. As a result, the mediation of stress by the central nervous system leads to corresponding changes in immune cell activity.

Both acute and chronic stress can cause immunosuppression. Stress affects immune function by (1) decreasing the number and function of natural killer cells; (2) decreasing lymphocyte proliferation; (3) altering production of *cytokines* (soluble factors secreted by white blood cells and other cells, e.g., interferon, interleukins); and (4) decreasing phagocytosis by neutrophils and monocytes. This stress-induced immunosuppression may worsen or increase the risk for progression of immune-related diseases such as multiple sclerosis, asthma, rheumatoid arthritis, and cancer.[6] Natural killer cells, lymphocytes, and cytokines are discussed in Chapter 13.

PATHOPHYSIOLOGY MAP

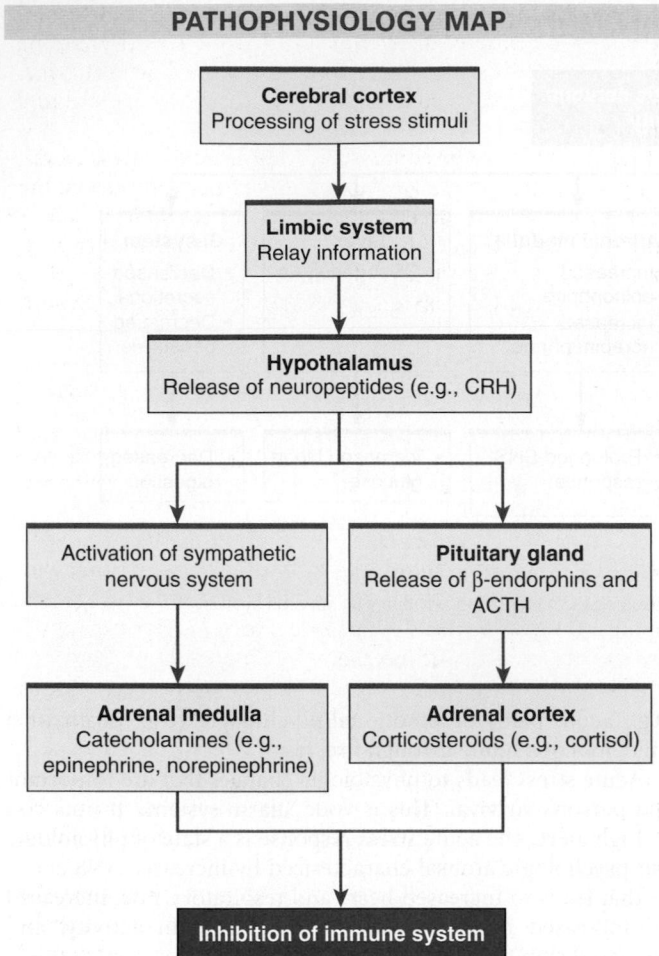

FIG. 6.6 The cerebral cortex processes stressful stimuli and relays the information via the limbic system to the hypothalamus. Corticotropin-releasing hormone *(CRH)* stimulates the release of adrenocorticotropic hormone *(ACTH)* from the pituitary gland. ACTH stimulates the adrenal cortex to release corticosteroids. Sympathetic nervous system stimulation results in the release of epinephrine and norepinephrine from the adrenal medulla. The result is the inhibition of the immune system.

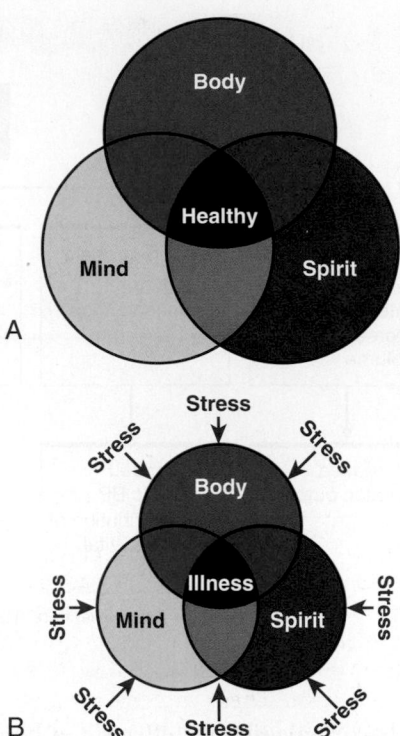

FIG. 6.7 The connections among the mind, body, and spirit can lead to a person being healthy (A) or the effects of stress on the mind, body, and spirit connections can lead to illness (B).

Importantly, the network that links the brain and immune system is bidirectional (Fig. 6.3). Signals from these systems travel back and forth, allowing for communication among these systems. Consequently, not only do emotions influence the immune response, but products of immune cells send signals back to the brain and alter its activity. Many of the communication signals sent from the immune system to the brain are mediated by cytokines, which are central to the coordination of the immune response. For example, IL-1 (a cytokine made by monocytes) acts on the temperature regulatory center of the hypothalamus and initiates the febrile response to infectious pathogens (see Fig. 11.4).

Many questions about stress and the immune response are unanswered. For example, it is not known how much stress (intensity or chronicity) is needed to cause changes or how much of a change in the immune system is necessary before disease susceptibility occurs.

MIND-BODY-SPIRIT CONNECTION

The **mind-body-spirit connection** shows the relationship and interconnectedness among the parts that make up a person:

mind, body, and spirit (Fig. 6.7). All 3 parts are important in your life and in determining who you are. What goes on in your mind influences every part of the body. Your mind is 1 of the most powerful weapons you have to deal with and conquer stress. You have a choice in how you respond to a crisis or a difficult time. Even if the outcome of the situation is not what a person desired, one can emerge with a winning attitude.

How you deal with difficult situations or stressful times greatly influences your overall well-being: your mind, body, and spirit. When your mind is healthy, your body can resist illness better. When your body is healthy, your feelings are more positive. Your spirit is renewed and energized.

As a nurse, stress can have a significant effect on you. A primary source of stress for a nurse can be the work environment, which includes extreme physical demands and the potential for violence.[7] The mind-body-spirit connection also influences your ability to provide nursing care. Your ability to maintain the mind-body-spirit balance is important in providing proper care to your patients and in maintaining a healthy and meaningful life for yourself.

EFFECTS OF STRESS ON HEALTH

As previously mentioned, the acute stress response is your alarm system and puts you on alert. However, your body was not meant to be on high alert all the time. If stress is excessive or prolonged, these same "helpful" physiologic responses can lead to harm and disease. When a person sustains chronic, unrelieved stress, the body's defenses can no longer keep up with the demands. Therefore stress plays a role in the development and/or progression of diseases of adaptation, or stress-related illnesses (Table 6.2).

TABLE 6.2 Common Disorders With a Stress Component

- Depression
- Dyspepsia
- Eating disorders
- Erectile dysfunction
- Fatigue
- Fibromyalgia
- Headaches
- Hypertension
- Insomnia
- Irritable bowel syndrome
- Low back pain
- Menstrual irregularities
- Peptic ulcer disease
- Sexual dysfunction

Stress is linked to leading causes of death, including cancer, accidents, and suicides. Stress can have effects on cognitive function, including poor concentration, memory problems, distressing dreams, sleep disturbances, and impaired decision making. It can also cause a wide variety of changes in behavior. These include people withdrawing from others, becoming quiet or unusually talkative, changing eating habits, drinking alcohol excessively, or becoming irritable.[8] Long-term exposure to catecholamines resulting from excessive SNS activation may increase the risk for cardiovascular diseases such as atherosclerosis and hypertension.[9] Other conditions that are precipitated or worsened by stress include migraine headaches, irritable bowel syndrome, and peptic ulcers.[10] Stress affects the control of metabolic conditions, such as diabetes mellitus. Behavioral interventions aimed at stress reduction and relaxation have helped manage these diseases in conjunction with standard medical therapy.[11]

Stressful life events can make a person more susceptible to infection. For example, psychologic stress may increase one's risk for developing the common cold. In a landmark study, researchers intranasally inoculated healthy people with low doses of upper respiratory tract viruses. The people underwent psychologic testing to measure the occurrence of stressful events in their lives and their reactions to such stresses. The results showed that the rates of both viral infection and clinical colds increased with the degree of psychologic stress. In this study, social support buffered the harmful effects of stress.[12]

At the cellular level, stress may promote earlier onset of age-related diseases. There is a link between stress and telomere length. Telomeres are the protective end caps on chromosomes. Their diminishing size is a sign of age. Telomeres are highly susceptible to stress and depression. Telomeres are shorter in people who are stressed and depressed than in healthy people. Thus chronic stress can have a long-term effect on our overall health by changing our DNA and accelerating the rate at which our cells age.[13]

COPING STRATEGIES

Coping is a person's efforts to manage stressors.[14] *Coping strategies* are what you do (your behaviors and actions) to help deal with stress. Coping can be either positive or negative. Positive coping includes activities such as exercise and spending time with friends and family. Healthy coping helps you handle your stressors so that they do not overwhelm you. Negative coping may include substance use and denial.

Unfortunately, some coping strategies make the stress worse. Sometimes coping strategies temporarily relieve the stress, but in the long run they increase the stress. For example, you may really enjoy watching a favorite TV show as a form of coping. However, if you become fixated on several reality shows, then TV becomes an addiction and an escape from dealing with your real stressors.

> You cannot always choose your destiny in life, but you can choose how you cope with it.
>
> **Norman Vincent Peale**

We can use a number of coping strategies to cope with stress. Table 6.3 has examples of coping strategies that you can use in your life and teach to your patients and caregivers. Coping strategies can be divided into 2 broad categories: emotion-focused coping and problem-focused coping. **Emotion-focused coping** involves managing the emotions that a person feels when a stressful event occurs. When a situation is unchangeable or uncontrollable, emotion-focused coping may predominate. The primary purpose of emotion-focused coping is to help decrease negative emotions and create a feeling of well-being. Examples include discussing feelings with a friend or taking a hot bath.

Problem-focused coping involves attempts to resolve the problems causing the stress. If you can change or control a problem, this strategy is the most helpful. Problem-focused coping strategies allow a person to look at a challenge objectively, act to address the problem, and thereby reduce the stress. Setting priorities, collecting information, and seeking advice are examples of problem-focused coping.

We often use a combination of strategies to cope with the same stressor. Table 6.4 gives examples of emotion- and problem-focused coping when applied to the same stressful situation.

RELAXATION STRATEGIES

The *relaxation response* is a state of physiologic and psychologic rest. It is opposite of the stress response. The relaxation response is characterized by decreased SNS activity, which leads to decreased heart and respiratory rate, decreased BP, decreased muscle tension, decreased brain activity, and increased skin temperature.

We can use a variety of relaxation strategies to elicit the relaxation response (Table 6.5). Regular elicitation of the relaxation response is an effective treatment for a wide range of stress-related disorders, including chronic pain, insomnia, and hypertension. People who regularly engage in relaxation strategies better cope with their stressors, increase their sense of control over stressors, and reduce their tension.[15]

Relaxation Breathing

The way one breathes affects every aspect of one's life. When a person is stressed, muscles tense and breathing becomes shallow

TABLE 6.3 Coping Strategies

Strategy	Description	How to Implement	Strategy	Description	How to Implement
Aromatherapy	• Use of essential oils (fragrant molecules from plants) for inhalation or topical application • Variety of essential oils, including lavender, peppermint, rosemary, eucalyptus, sandalwood, etc.	• Place 5–8 drops in a full bath and agitate water before bathing. • Place a few drops on a tissue or in diffuser or vaporizer.	Humor	• Can take the form of laughter, cartoons, funny movies, videos, riddles, comic books, and joke books	• Keep a "tickler" scrapbook with funny photos, cartoons, etc. • Humor carts can be set up in many clinical settings for patient and family use.
Art therapy	• Allows a person to nonverbally express and communicate feelings, emotions, and thoughts • Can reduce stress, promote relaxation, and help process experiences • Based on the belief that the creative process is healing and life enhancing	• Close your eyes and draw a line on a piece of paper. Open your eyes. Continue to build on that line and draw whatever comes to mind. • Get a piece of paper and doodle. Do not edit. • Get a coloring book and crayons and just start coloring.	Journaling	• Allows a person to express self in writing • Enhances personal development and awareness through self-reflection	• Use a journaling notebook or computer to write down thoughts, feelings, memories, and perceptions.
Exercise	• Any form of movement, especially aerobic movement • Can be viewed as meditation in motion	• Walk, swim, garden, bicycle, dance, climb stairs, take part in group exercises.	Pet therapy (animal-assisted therapy) (Fig. 6.8) Social support	• Use of animals as a form of treatment • Improves a patient's social, emotional, or cognitive functioning • Relationships with family and friends • Self-help groups and professional help	• Pet therapist or family member or friend brings a pet with which patient can socialize. • Get together with family and friends on a regular basis. • Join a support group that specifically helps to meet needs (e.g., grief support group).

🌿 COMPLEMENTARY & ALTERNATIVE THERAPIES

Yoga

Yoga is an ancient system of relaxation, exercise, and healing with origins in Indian philosophy. The goal of yoga is physical and mental well-being achieved using stretching, postures, breathing practices, and meditation.

Scientific Evidence

Yoga can be used to treat hypertension and reduce stress and anxiety in cancer patients.[16]

Nursing Implications

• Deep abdominal relaxation breathing is a main component of all types of yoga. It helps one to focus on the inner self and promote the relaxation response.
• Yoga is used to promote relaxation, decrease stress, improve flexibility, and enhance overall health.
• Yoga is considered safe. Patients with certain medical conditions or illnesses should avoid some postures.

TABLE 6.4 Problem- and Emotion-Focused Coping

Stressor	Problem-Focused Coping	Emotion-Focused Coping
Failing an examination	Obtaining a tutor	Going for a run
Being diagnosed with diabetes	Attending education classes about diabetes	Getting a massage
Receiving questionable mammogram results	Scheduling follow-up testing for ultrasound	Expressing feelings of anxiety to friends and nurse

TABLE 6.5 Common Relaxation Strategies

• Biofeedback
• Imagery
• Massage
• Meditation
• Muscle relaxation
• Music
• Qigong
• Relaxing breathing
• Tai Chi
• Yoga

and rapid. Therefore 1 of the simplest and most effective ways to stop the stress response is to breathe deeply and slowly. It is hard to stay tense when breathing in a slow, deep, and relaxed pattern. **Relaxation breathing** forms the basis for most relaxation strategies. It is especially useful during a stressful or anxious situation to reduce stress. You can do relaxation breathing while sitting, standing, or lying down. It is natural for newborns and sleeping adults.

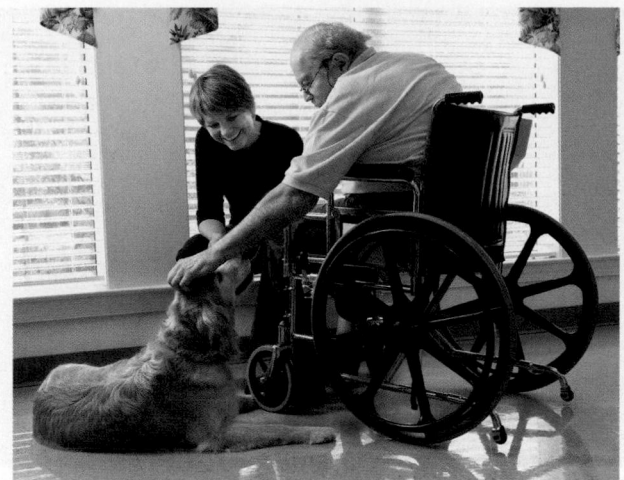

FIG. 6.8 Pet therapy can be used in a variety of settings including rehabilitation. (© RonChappleStudios/Hemera/Thinkstock.)

Before practicing relaxation breathing, it is important to assess one's normal breathing pattern (Table 6.6). Chest breathing, which involves the upper chest and shoulders, is inefficient. We often use it during times of anxiety and distress.

Relaxation breathing is a more efficient type of breathing. It involves the primary use of the diaphragm and less use of the upper chest and shoulders to help in each breath. In this type of breathing, the abdomen gently moves in and out during exhalation and inhalation. The breaths should be slow, steady, and deep.

One basic technique for relaxation breathing is as follows: (1) Inhale slowly and deeply, pushing the abdomen out. Think about breathing in peace. (2) Exhale slowly, letting the abdomen come in and all the muscles relax. Think about breathing out tension. (3) Repeat these deep breaths 10 times without interruption. As with any breathing exercise, if a light-headed feeling arises, stop for 30 seconds, and then start again.

Other methods used to teach relaxation breathing are the 4 × 4 technique and relaxation sigh. Breathing techniques are discussed in the Stress-Busting Kit for Nursing Students available on the website for this book.

Initially, relaxation breathing may feel unusual. With practice it becomes easier, and its relaxing benefits are soon obvious. You should personally learn to use relaxation breathing before teaching it to patients and their caregivers. Once learned, you can easily teach relaxation breathing to patients in a variety of settings, particularly when they are undergoing stressful and painful procedures.

Biofeedback

Biofeedback helps a person become more aware of involuntary body responses such as breathing, heart rate, and muscle activity. Electrodes attached to the skin or, in some cases, hand-held sensors measure these processes and display them on a monitor. This feedback allows the person to learn to control their responses. This gives a person the power to use thoughts to control the body, often to improve a health condition or physical performance.[15]

TABLE 6.6 Relaxation Breathing Techniques
Breathing Assessment
1. Begin by placing 1 hand gently on your abdomen below your waistline.
2. Place the other hand on the center of your chest on the sternum.
3. Without changing the normal breathing pattern, take several breaths. During inhalation notice which hand rises the most.
4. When relaxation breathing is done properly, the hand on the abdomen should rise more than the hand on the chest.
4 × 4 Technique
1. Sit up straight with your back flush to the support of the chair and your feet flat on the floor.
2. Rest your arms on your lap, thighs, or arms of the chair.
3. Take in a deep breath through your nose to a count of 4 (1 … 2 … 3 … 4).
4. Hold your breath to a count of 4 (1 … 2 … 3 … 4).
5. Release your breath through your mouth to a count of 4 (1 … 2 … 3 … 4).
6. Rest for a count of 4 (1 … 2 … 3 … 4).
7. Repeat the cycle 4 times.
Relaxing Sigh
1. Sit up straight with your back against the support of the chair and your feet flat on floor.
2. Inhale a natural breath and then sigh deeply. Let out a sound of relief as the air rushes out of your lungs.
3. Do not think about inhaling at the end of the sigh; just let the air come in naturally as you breathe deeply.
4. Repeat this sigh about 4 to 6 times very slowly.
5. You can repeat this exercise whenever you need it.

Meditation

Meditation is a practice of concentrated focus on a sound, object, visualization, the breath, or movement. The purpose of meditation is to increase awareness, reduce stress, promote relaxation, and enhance personal and spiritual growth.

It is best to practice meditation in a quiet place, free of distractions. Table 6.7 gives some basic guidelines on how to meditate. Meditation is often practiced while seated, and it is important to maintain a comfortable posture. Meditation can be done while walking and focusing on a single action such as the movement of the feet. In the beginning, you typically start with just 5 to 10 minutes of meditation at a time. Increase the time as the practice becomes more comfortable. Meditation exercises are available in the Stress-Busting Kit for Nursing Students on the website for this book.

Imagery

Imagery is the use of one's mind to generate images that have a calming effect on the body. It involves focusing the mind and incorporates all the senses to create physiologic and emotional changes. It is a simple relaxation technique that needs no equipment other than an active imagination. *Guided imagery* is a variation of imagery in which another person (either live or through technology) suggests the images to you.

You can use imagery in your own life or use guided imagery with your patients. One of the uses of imagery is to create a special place for a mental retreat. Table 6.8 describes the steps involved in creating a special place. More imagery exercises are available in the Stress-Busting Kit for Nursing Students on the website for this book.

TABLE 6.7 **Guide to Meditation**

You can teach yourself the basics of meditation by following a few simple steps:

1. Find a quiet place.
2. Make sure there are no distractions.
3. Sit in a comfortable position.
4. Close your eyes.
5. Shut out the world so that your brain can stop processing information coming from your senses.
6. Pick a focus word, short phrase, song verse (melody), or prayer that is firmly rooted in your belief system, such as *one, peace, The Lord is my shepherd, Hail Mary full of grace,* or *shalom.*
7. Breathe slowly and practice relaxation breathing. Say your focus word, short phrase, song verse, or prayer silently to yourself as you exhale.
8. Say the word or phrase again and again.
9. Try saying the word or phrase silently to yourself with every exhalation. The monotony will help you focus.
10. Relax your muscles, progressing from your feet to your calves, thighs, abdomen, shoulders, head, and neck.
11. Do not be concerned when other thoughts come to mind. Just acknowledge them and return calmly to your word or phrase.
12. Continue for 10 to 20 minutes, but even 5 minutes can leave you feeling calm and refreshed. Rise slowly.
13. Practice once or twice daily.

TABLE 6.8 **Imagery**

Creating Your Special Place

1. Begin by closing your eyes and taking several slow, deep breaths.
2. Imagine a place where you feel completely comfortable and peaceful. It may be a real place or 1 you imagine: 1 from your past or a place you have always wanted to go.
3. Allow this special place to take form, slowly. As it takes form, look around to your left, to your right. Enjoy the scenery: the colors, the texture, the shapes.
4. Listen carefully to the sounds of your place. What do you hear?
5. Is there a gentle breeze or sunshine warming your face? Pick up or touch some favorite objects from your special place.
6. Take in a deep breath through your nose and notice the rich smells around you. Perhaps your favorite flower is in bloom, or you smell the scents of the ocean.
7. Take another deep breath and relax. Enjoy the peace, comfort, and safety of your special place.
8. This is your special place. You relax and feel thankful that you are here, in your special place.
9. You can return to this place any time that you wish.

It is best to perform imagery in a comfortable position. Take slow, deep breaths. Focus should involve all senses (sight, hearing, touch, smell). For example, you can use an image, such as Fig. 6.9, engaging all the senses as you focus on the image.

Imagery can be used in many clinical settings for stress reduction and pain relief. Benefits of imagery include anxiety reduction, decreased muscle tension, improved comfort during medical procedures, enhanced immune function, decreased recovery time after surgery, and reduction in sleeping problems. It can specifically target a disease, problem, or stressor. Table 6.9 describes some suggestions for using imagery in specific diseases or disorders.

A person can use imagery to enhance performance or process stressful or difficult tasks. For example, an athlete or musician can use imagery to achieve greater success. Imagery allows one to mentally rehearse the difficult or challenging situation.

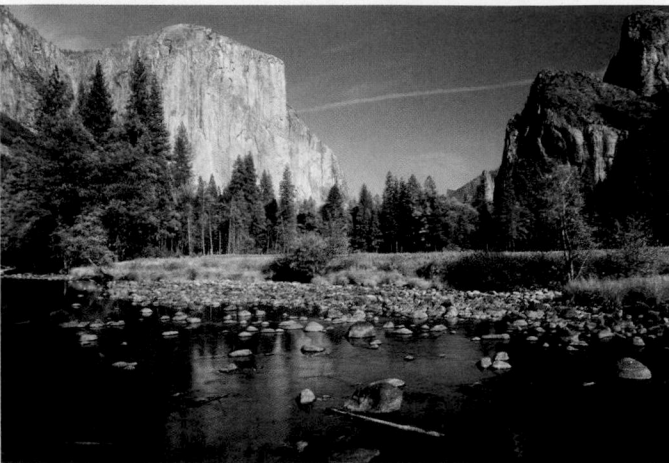

FIG. 6.9 In imagery, special places are created involving all the senses, such as a place where one can hear rustling water, smell flowers, feel the wind, and see a colorful landscape. (© iStockphoto/Thinkstock.)

TABLE 6.9 **Examples of Imagery**

Imagery can be used to relieve stress and promote health and healing in conjunction with regular medical care. Special images can be created to ease symptoms or treat diseases or disorders. The image should be strong and vivid for the person, using many senses to create the image. Below are some examples that some people have found useful.

Disease or Disorder	Images
Asthma	• Tiny elastic rubber bands that constrict the airways pop open
Cancer	• Shark gobbles up cancer cells • Radiation or chemotherapy treatments enter the body like healing rays of light; they destroy cancer cells
Coronary artery disease	• Water flows freely through a wide, open river
Depression	• Attach troubles and feelings of sadness to big colorful helium balloons that float off into a clear blue sky
Infection	• White blood cells with flashing red sirens arrest and imprison harmful germs
Pain	• Wash away pain by a cool calm river flowing through the entire body
Weakened immune system	• White blood cells rapidly multiply like millions of seeds bursting from a ripe seed pod

Adapted from Sobel DS, Ornstein R: *Healthy mind, healthy body*, New York, 1996, Patient Education Materials, Time Life.

Imagery can help a fearful nurse start an IV line or perform a difficult procedure. It can be used with a patient who is afraid to have a stressful or painful procedure (e.g., bone marrow biopsy).

Massage

Massage includes a range of techniques that manipulate the soft tissues and joints of the body. Involving touch and movement, massage is typically delivered with the hands. It reduces muscle tension and positively affects mental and emotional states.

Massage is an important form of touch. It is a form of caring, communication, and comfort. Your role related to massage differs from that of the registered massage therapist. A massage therapist can provide more comprehensive massage therapies. As a nurse, you can use specific massage techniques as part of nursing care. For example, you can give a back massage to help promote sleep. For a bedridden patient, gentle massage can stimulate circulation and help prevent skin breakdown. A simple hand massage can have a calming and relaxing effect, especially for patients who are anxious or agitated. During end-of-life care, hospice nurses may include massage into their nursing care as the massaging touch can lessen pain and restlessness.

When you identify that massage may be useful, first assess the patient's preference about touch and massage. Consider cultural and social beliefs and discuss potential benefits with the patient. You can teach family members to massage their loved one, giving a way for family members to take part in patient care. This can be therapeutic for the patient and family, even when the loved one is cognitively impaired or unresponsive.

Music

Music can help achieve relaxation and bring about healthy changes in emotional or physical states. Listening to relaxing music can divert one's focus from a stressful situation.

Music can be used in many clinical settings. It is noninvasive, safe, inexpensive, and easy to use. Music decreases anxiety and elicits the relaxation response. Music helps people with insomnia go to sleep. It can decrease muscle tension, pain sensation, and emotional stress.[17]

Each person considers different types of music to be relaxing. Music that has 60 to 80 beats/min is considered soothing. Many find low-pitched tones and music without words best for relaxation. Mozart's music is popular for relaxation. On the other hand, fast-tempo music can stimulate and uplift a person. Assess each patient's interest and preference in music, and find music that best matches the person's needs and circumstance. Create a listening environment by helping the patient find a comfortable position and minimizing interruptions. Evaluate patients' responses to the music, asking them how it sounds and how it makes them feel.

Prayer

Prayer can be a form of meditation. It is a spiritual communion with God or an object of worship. Many people find deep comfort in their faith. Religious services, conversations with clergy, and personal worship and prayer may help to ease a person's stress and give 1 greater perspective, strength, and inspiration.

❖ NURSING MANAGEMENT: STRESS

◆ Nursing Assessment

Patients and caregivers face many potential stressors that can have health consequences. As a nurse, you are in a key position to (1) assess stress in patients and their caregivers, (2) help them identify high-risk periods for stress, and (3) implement stress management strategies that can prevent the negative consequences of stress on their health (Fig. 6.10).

The first step in managing stress is to become aware of its presence. This includes identifying what the stressors are and the person's response to them. Be aware of situations that are likely to result in stress. Assess the number of stressors, duration of these stressors, and prior experience with similar demands.

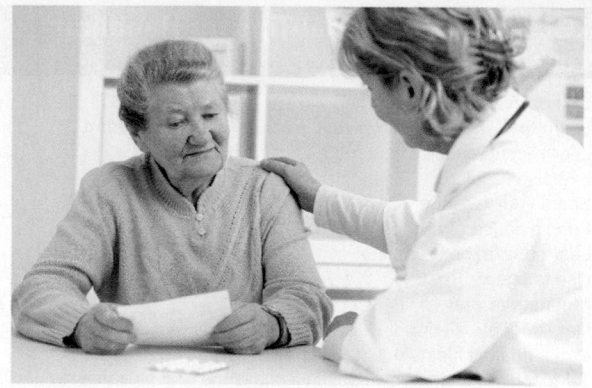

FIG. 6.10 As a nurse, you have a key role in helping patients deal with stress. (© AlexRaths/iStock/Thinkstock.)

Assess the personal meaning attached to the stressful situation to provide useful insight for planning stress management strategies with the patient.

Be specific with your questions: Have you experienced this stressor before? How did you handle it? What worked well and what did not? Although the manifestations of stress may vary from person to person, assess the patient for the signs and symptoms of the stress response, including an increased heart rate and BP, hyperventilation, sweating, headache, musculoskeletal pain, gastrointestinal upset, loss of appetite, insomnia, and fatigue. In addition, the patient may show stress-related illness (Table 6.2).

Behavioral manifestations of stress may include an inability to concentrate, accident proneness, impaired speech, anxiety, crying, frustration, and irritability. Work-related responses to stress may include absenteeism or tardiness at work, decreased productivity, and job dissatisfaction. Cognitive responses include self-reports about the inability to make decisions and forgetfulness. Some of these responses may be apparent to significant others.

Consider the caregivers' responses to the stressors. A patient's illness often causes stress for the caregiver and other family members. Assess what aspects of the illness are the most stressful for the patient and caregiver. These may include the patient's physical health, job responsibilities, finances, and children. This information is valuable because it helps you to understand the patient's perspective of the stressors. Knowledge of stressors, the feelings these stressors evoke, and the psychologic effects they can produce will help you recognize potential and actual sources of stress and their effect on the patient.

Nursing Implementation

Your role is to facilitate and enhance the patient's coping and adaptation. Nursing interventions depend on the severity of the stress experience. For example, a patient with multiple trauma expends energy to physically survive. As a nurse, you direct efforts toward life-supporting interventions and approaches aimed at reducing added stressors for the patient. The patient is much less likely to adapt or recover if faced with more stressors, such as sleep deprivation or an infection. You can assume a primary role in implementing stress management strategies. Some personal tips for handling stress are shown in Table 6.10. These tips will help you personally and enhance your own level of health and wellness. It is essential that you first care for yourself before you can help the patients who need your care.

TABLE 6.10 Personal Tips for Handling Stress

- Do not try to be superhuman.
- Learn to "let go" of things that are outside of your control.
- Learn acceptance of yourself.
- Exercise regularly.
- Share your feelings.
- Keep a sense of humor; laugh often.
- Learn relaxation breathing.
- Use imagery.
- Meditate or pray.
- Get adequate sleep.
- Live a healthy lifestyle.
- Try to look at change as a positive challenge, not as a threat.
- Solve the little problems, since this can help you gain a feeling of control.
- Work to resolve conflicts with other people.
- If needed, get professional counseling.

TABLE 6.11 How to Implement Stress Management in Practice

1. Learn relaxation breathing. It is the easiest method of relaxation to use.
2. Practice teaching relaxation breathing with peers, then patients.
3. Pick coping strategies (Table 6.4) and relaxation strategies that are appropriate for your clinical area.
4. Practice using the strategy yourself. It becomes easier with time.
5. Take advantage of opportunities to teach coping and relaxation strategies to patients.
6. If you have setbacks, think about what went wrong. Do NOT quit!
7. Attend seminars and workshops on stress management to learn more.

Many professional organizations, such as the American Nurses Association, offer resources to help you manage stress (*www.nursingworld.org*). Once you included these strategies into your life, you can share them with patients and caregivers.

Ideas for how to include stress management strategies into nursing practice are described in Table 6.11. Although some require additional training, many stress management strategies are within the scope of nursing practice. These include relaxation breathing, imagery, music, exercise, massage, meditation, art therapy, and journaling. More resources are in the Stress-Busting Kit for Nursing Students on the website for this book.

Coping strategies used should be helpful and not a source of added stress for the patient. You can teach most coping and relaxation strategies to patients in 10 to 15 minutes. Choose a coping or relaxation strategy to best suit the patient and situation. Effective stress management provides a sense of control of the stressful situation. As stress management practices become part of daily activities, the person can increase his or her confidence and self-reliance and limit the emotional response to the stressful circumstances. Having a sense of control can prevent the harmful effects of a stress response.

As a nurse, you are in an ideal situation to integrate stress management in clinical practice. You are well equipped to develop and test the effectiveness of new ways to manage stress and promote positive health outcomes. However, it is very important to recognize when you need to refer the patient or caregiver to a professional with advanced training in counseling.

CASE STUDY
Stress-Induced Illness

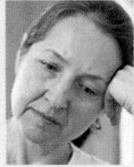

(© JackF/ iStock/ Thinkstock.)

Patient Profile

K.F., a 48-yr-old woman, recently moved to the United States from Romania with her 2 teenage children. She has no family in the country and was recently divorced. She has taken a job as a waitress in a hectic restaurant and works as a seamstress out of her home in the evenings.

She has developed some unusual symptoms and comes to see the nurse practitioner at a community clinic. Although she says that she was in good health when she left Romania, she now presents with fatigue, inability to sleep, and aches all over her body. Even when she gets some extra sleep, she still feels exhausted. Her co-worker told her she has fibromyalgia.

Discussion Questions

1. Consider K.F.'s situation and describe the stressors with which she is dealing. Describe the possible effects of these stressors on her health.
2. *Priority Decision:* What are the priority coping strategies that you should include in K.F.'s plan of care?
3. What limitations should you consider when discussing specific coping strategies?
4. *Patient-Centered Care:* What cultural considerations should you include in the plan of care?

Answers available at *http://evolve.elsevier.com/Lewis/medsurg.*

▐ BRIDGE TO NCLEX EXAMINATION

The number of the question corresponds to the same-numbered outcome at the beginning of the chapter.

1. Determination of whether an event is a stressor is based on a person's
   a. tolerance.
   b. perception.
   c. adaptation.
   d. stubbornness.

2. The nurse would expect which finding in a patient because of the physiologic effect of stress on the reticular formation?
   a. An episode of diarrhea while awaiting painful dressing changes
   b. Refusal to communicate with nurses while awaiting a cardiac catheterization
   c. Inability to sleep the night before beginning to self-administer insulin injections
   d. Increased blood pressure, decreased urine output, and hyperglycemia after a car accident

3. The nurse uses knowledge of the effects of stress on the immune system by encouraging patients to
   a. sleep for 10 to 12 hours per day.
   b. avoid exposure to upper respiratory tract infections.
   c. receive regular immunizations when they are stressed.
   d. use emotion-focused rather than problem-focused coping strategies.

4. The nurse recognizes that a person who has chronic stress could be at higher risk for (select all that apply)
   a. osteoporosis.
   b. fibromyalgia.
   c. colds and flu.
   d. high blood pressure.
   e. high serum cholesterol.

5. The nurse recognizes that a patient with newly diagnosed breast cancer is using an emotion-focused coping process when she
   a. joins a support group for women with breast cancer.
   b. considers the pros and cons of the various treatment options.
   c. delays treatment until her family can take a weekend trip together.
   d. tells the nurse that she has a good prognosis because the tumor is small.

6. During a stressful circumstance that is unchangeable, which type of coping strategy is the *most* effective?
   a. Avoidance
   b. Coping flexibility
   c. Emotion-focused coping
   d. Problem-focused coping

7. An appropriate nursing intervention for a hospitalized patient who says she cannot cope with her illness is
   a. controlling the environment to prevent sensory overload and promote sleep.
   b. encouraging the patient's family to offer emotional support by frequent visiting.
   c. arranging for the patient to phone family and friends to maintain emotional bonds.
   d. asking the patient to describe previous stressful situations and how she managed to resolve them.

1. b, 2. c, 3. b, 4. b, c, d, 5. a, 6. c, 7. d.

For rationales to these answers and even more NCLEX review questions, visit *http://evolve.elsevier.com/Lewis/medsurg.*

ⓔ EVOLVE WEBSITE/RESOURCES LIST

http://evolve.elsevier.com/Lewis/medsurg
Review Questions (Online Only)
Key Points
Answer Keys for Questions
  • Rationales for Bridge to NCLEX Examination Questions
Answer Guidelines for Case Study on p. 86
Conceptual Care Map Creator
Stress-Busting Kit for Nursing Students
Audio Glossary
Content Updates

REFERENCES

1. Seward BL: *Managing stress: Principles and strategies for health and well-being,* 9th ed, Burlington, MA, 2017, Jones & Bartlett.
2. The Physiological Society: Stress in modern Britain: Making sense of stress, our 2017 theme. Retrieved from *www.physoc.org/sites/default/files/press-release/4042-stress-modern-britain.pdf.*
*3. Maddi SR: Hardiness: The courage to grow from stresses, J Pos Psych, 1:160, 2006. (Classic)
4. Mayo Clinic: Positive thinking. Retrieved from *www.mayoclinic.org/healthy-living/stress-management/in-depth/positive-thinking/art-20043950.*
*5. Dum RP, Levinthal DJ, Strick PL: Motor, cognitive, and affective areas of the cerebral cortex influence the adrenal medulla, *PNAS* 113:9922, 2016.
6. American Institute of Stress: Effects of stress. Retrieved from *www.stress.org.*
7. Yoder L: Nursing: The balance of mind, body, and spirit, *MEDSURG Nursing* 26:75, 2017.
8. Bergland C: Chronic stress can damage brain structure and connectivity. Retrieved from *www.psychologytoday.com/blog/the-athletes-way/201402/chronic-stress-can-damage-brain-structure-and-connectivity.*
9. American Heart Association: Stress and heart health. Retrieved from *www.heart.org/HEARTORG/Conditions/More/MyHeartandStrokeNews/Stress-and-Heart-Health_UCM_437370_Article.jsp.*
10. U.S. Department of Health and Human Services: Stress and migraines. Retrieved from *www.womenshealth.gov/publications/our-publications/fact-sheet/migraine.html.*
11. National Institutes of Health: Feeling stressed? Stress relief might help your health. Retrieved from *http://newsinhealth.nih.gov/issue/Dec2014/Feature1.*
*12. Cohen S, Tyrrell DA, Smith AP: Psychological stress and susceptibility to the common cold, *N Engl J Med* 325:606, 1991. (Classic)
13. American Psychological Association: Stress in America: Our health at risk. Retrieved from *www.apa.org/news/press/releases/stress.*
14. Lazarus R, Folkman S: Stress, appraisal, and coping, New York, 1984, Springer. (Classic)
15. National Center for Complementary and Integrative Health: Relaxation techniques for health. Retrieved from *https://nccih.nih.gov/health/stress/relaxation.htm.*
16. Mayo Clinic: Alternative cancer treatments. Retrieved from *www.mayoclinic.org/diseases-conditions/cancer/in-depth/cancer-treatment/art-20047246.*
*17. Collingwood J: The power of music to reduce stress. Retrieved from *http://psychcentral.com/lib/the-power-of-music-to-reduce-stress/000930.*

*Evidence-based information for clinical practice.

7

Sleep and Sleep Disorders

Diana Taibi Buchanan

I slept and dreamt that life was joy. I awoke and saw that life was service. I acted and behold, service was joy.

Rabindranath Tagore

ⓔ http://evolve.elsevier.com/Lewis/medsurg/

CONCEPTUAL FOCUS

Functional Ability

Mood and Affect

Sleep

LEARNING OUTCOMES

1. Define sleep.
2. Describe the stages of sleep.
3. Explain the relationship of various diseases/disorders and sleep disorders.
4. Describe the etiology, clinical manifestations, and interprofessional and nursing management of insomnia.

5. Describe the etiology, clinical manifestations, and interprofessional and nursing management of obstructive sleep apnea.
6. Describe clinical manifestations and interprofessional management of narcolepsy, parasomnias, and circadian rhythm disorders.
7. Select strategies for managing sleep problems associated with shift work sleep disorder.

KEY TERMS

circadian rhythms, p. 89
continuous positive airway pressure (CPAP), p. 96
insomnia, p. 91
jet lag disorder, p. 97
narcolepsy, p. 98

obstructive sleep apnea (OSA), p. 95
parasomnias, p. 98
periodic limb movement disorder (PLMD), p. 97
shift work sleep disorder, p. 99
sleep, p. 88

sleep-disordered breathing (SDB), p. 95
sleep disorders, p. 88
sleep disturbance, p. 88
sleep hygiene, p. 92
wake behavior, p. 89

SLEEP

Sleep is a state in which a person lacks conscious awareness of environmental surroundings but can be easily aroused. Sleep is distinct from unconscious states such as coma, in which the person cannot be aroused. Sleep is a basic, dynamic, highly organized, and complex behavior that is essential for healthy functioning and survival. Over a life span of 80 years, a person who sleeps 7 hours each night will spend around 24 years sleeping. Sleep influences mood, behavior, and physical functioning. Some physical functions affected by sleep are memory, mood, hormone secretion, glucose metabolism, immune function, and body temperature.

Most adults need 7 to 8 hours of sleep within a 24-hour period.[1] Adequate sleep is defined as the amount of sleep one needs to be fully awake and alert the next day. *Insufficient sleep* means getting less than the recommended amount of sleep. *Fragmented sleep* means a person wakes up or almost wakes (called an arousal), interrupting continuous sleep. *Nonrestorative sleep* means that a person sleeps the recommended amount but does not feel refreshed and alert the next day.

Sleep disturbance is a broad term that refers to poor sleep quality from various causes. Sleep disturbance may be related to environmental factors such as noise or light. It can be caused by health-related factors such as pain or by **sleep disorders**, which are problems unique to sleep. Sleep disorders discussed in this chapter include insomnia, obstructive sleep apnea syndrome, periodic limb movement disorder, circadian sleep disorders, narcolepsy, and parasomnias.

Sleep disturbances and sleep disorders can result in insufficient sleep. Many people get insufficient sleep because they simply are not in bed long enough to allow for an adequate amount of sleep. About 35% of Americans get less than the recommended 7 hours of sleep per night. An estimated 50 to 70 million people in the United States have a sleep disorder.[2] Many are unaware that they have a problem (Fig. 7.1). People with chronic illnesses have the greatest risk for sleep disturbances.

Untreated sleep disorders cause considerable health, safety, and economic consequences. Daytime sleepiness can be so severe that it interferes with work and social functioning. Driving while drowsy is related to 100,000 accidents

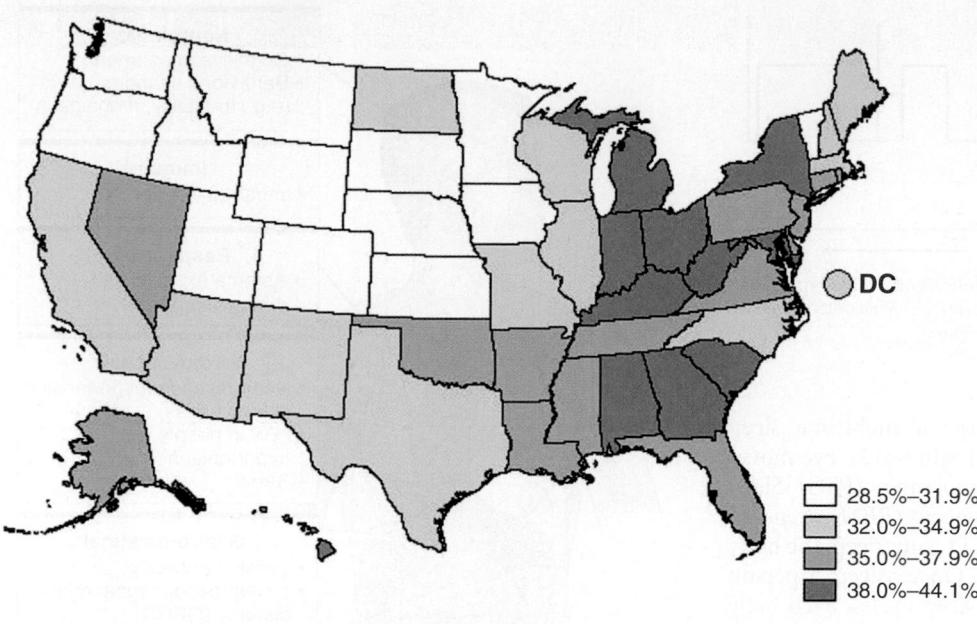

FIG. 7.1 Prevalence among U.S. adults of obtaining less than 7 hours of sleep each night. (Modified from *www.cdc.gov/sleep/data_statistics.html*.)

Legend:
- 28.5%–31.9%
- 32.0%–34.9%
- 35.0%–37.9%
- 38.0%–44.1%

and 1500 traffic fatalities per year.[3] Sleep disorders, sleep loss, and excessive daytime sleepiness cost the United States billions of dollars each year from the cost of health care, work-related accidents, and lost productivity.[4] Opportunities to address sleep problems are often missed because health care providers (HCPs) do not ask and patients do not readily talk about them.

PHYSIOLOGIC SLEEP MECHANISMS

Sleep-Wake Cycle

The brain controls the cyclic changes between sleep and waking. Complex networks in the areas of the forebrain (cerebral cortex, hypothalamus, thalamus) and brainstem interact to regulate the sleep-wake cycle.

Wake Behavior. Wake behavior is maintained by an integrated network of arousal systems from the brainstem and forebrain. A cluster of neuron structures in the brainstem, called the *ascending reticular activating system (ARAS),* promote general activation of the cerebral cortex, which is responsible for higher brain functions. This activation gives rise to typical wake behaviors such as alertness and attention. Various neurotransmitters (glutamate, acetylcholine, norepinephrine, dopamine, histamine, serotonin) promote wake behavior.[5]

People with Alzheimer's disease lose cholinergic neurons in the forebrain, which results in sleep disturbances. In Parkinson's disease, dopamine neurons in the ARAS degenerate, which causes excessive daytime sleepiness. Histamine neurons in the hypothalamus stimulate cortical activation and wake behavior.[6] The sedating properties of many over-the-counter (OTC) medications (e.g., diphenhydramine) result from inhibiting histamine-related arousal systems.[7]

Orexin (also called hypocretin) is a neuropeptide found in the hypothalamus. Orexin is involved in regulating the sleep-wake cycle. It plays an important role in keeping people awake. Decreased levels of orexin or its receptors lead to difficulties staying awake, which is a syndrome called *narcolepsy.*[8] Narcolepsy is discussed later in this chapter on p. 98.

Sleep Behavior. An area in the hypothalamus just above the optic chiasm contains many sleep-promoting neurons. These neurons inhibit the ARAS and promote sleep.[5] Sleep is stimulated by a variety of sleep-promoting neurotransmitters and peptides, including γ-aminobutyric acid (GABA), galanin, melatonin, adenosine, somatostatin, growth hormone–releasing hormone (GHRH), delta-sleep–inducing peptide, prostaglandins, and proinflammatory cytokines. When a person has an infection, proinflammatory cytokines (interleukin-1, tumor necrosis factor, interleukin-6) contribute to sleepiness and lethargy. Peptides released by the gastrointestinal tract after food ingestion (e.g., cholecystokinin) may mediate sleepiness after eating (called *postprandial sleepiness*).

Melatonin is a hormone made by the pineal gland in the brain. Melatonin secretion is linked to the environmental light-dark cycle. Release of the hormone signals the time for sleep by "turning off" the mechanisms that promote wakefulness. Under normal day-night conditions, we release melatonin in the evening as it gets dark. Light exposure at night can suppress melatonin secretion.[7]

Circadian Rhythms. Many biologic rhythms of behavior and physiology fluctuate within a 24-hour period. These 24-hour patterns are called circadian (*circadian,* about a day) rhythms. The suprachiasmatic nucleus (SCN) in the hypothalamus is the master clock of the body. The SCN synchronizes the genetic clocks within individual cells and regulates the 24-hour sleep-wake cycle. Circadian rhythm timing is synchronized to the environmental light and dark periods through specific light detectors in the retina. Pathways from the retina reach the SCN, and pathways from the SCN innervate brain regions controlling wake and sleep behavior.[7]

Light is the strongest time cue for the sleep-wake rhythm. Thus we can use light as a therapy to shift the timing of the sleep-wake rhythm. For example, bright light used early in the morning will cause the sleep-wake rhythm to move to an earlier time; bright light used in the evening will cause the sleep-wake rhythm to move to a later time. For some people, being outside in daylight (without sunglasses) may be helpful. Others need light therapy, which is given through a device that makes very bright light.

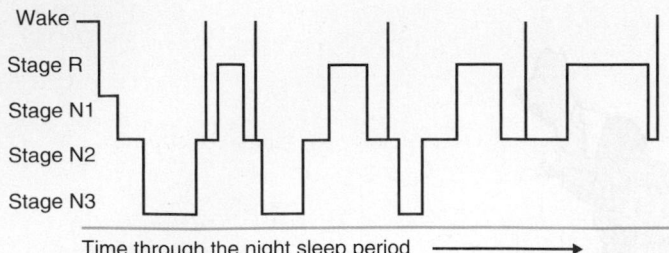

FIG. 7.2 Sleep stages graphed across a complete sleep cycle. (From Goldman L, Schafer AI: *Goldman's Cecil medicine*, ed 25, Philadelphia, 2016, Saunders.)

Sleep Architecture

Sleep architecture refers to the pattern of nighttime sleep recorded from physiologic measures of brain waves, eye movements, and muscle tone called *polysomnography* (PSG). Sleep consists of 2 basic states: *rapid eye movement (REM) sleep* and *non–rapid eye movement (NREM) sleep*. During sleep, the body cycles between NREM and REM sleep. Once asleep, a person goes through 4 to 6 NREM and REM sleep cycles, each cycle lasting 60 to 110 minutes (Fig. 7.2).

NREM Sleep. Healthy adults spend about 75% to 80% of sleep time in NREM sleep. NREM sleep is subdivided into 3 stages.[9] However, you may see the older version of sleep staging that used 4 stages. The newer, 3-stage approach combines the old stages 3 and 4 into N3.

N1 is the stage that occurs at the beginning of sleep. It is characterized by slow eye movements and is a transition phase from wakefulness to sleep. During this period the person can be easily awakened.

N2 is the stage that takes up most of the night's sleep. The heart rate slows down and body temperature drops. N2 is associated with specific brain wave forms measured by electroencephalograph (EEG) that represent sleep-maintaining neural activity.

N3 is the deepest stage of sleep. It is called slow-wave sleep (SWS) because large, low-frequency EEG waves are characteristic. N3 is associated with large EEG waveforms, called delta waves. They are a measure of sleep intensity. SWS declines as people age. Most adults over 60 years of age have little NREM stage 3 sleep.

REM Sleep. REM sleep accounts for 20% to 25% of sleep. REM sleep follows NREM sleep in a sleep cycle. In this stage, brain waves resemble wakefulness and postural muscles are inhibited, leading to greatly reduced skeletal muscle tone. During REM sleep a person cannot initiate muscle movement (e.g., cannot stand up). REM sleep is the period when the most vivid dreaming occurs.

INSUFFICIENT SLEEP AND SLEEP DISTURBANCES

Insufficient sleep is associated with changes in body function (Fig. 7.3) and health problems (Table 7.1). Impaired cognitive function and impaired performance on simple behavioral tasks occur within 24 hours of sleep loss. The effects of sleep loss are cumulative.[10] Those who report less than 6 hours of sleep a night are more likely to be obese. The risk for developing glucose intolerance and diabetes is higher in those with a history of insufficient sleep. Chronic loss of sleep places people at risk for depression, impaired daytime functioning, social isolation, and overall reduction in quality of life.[11]

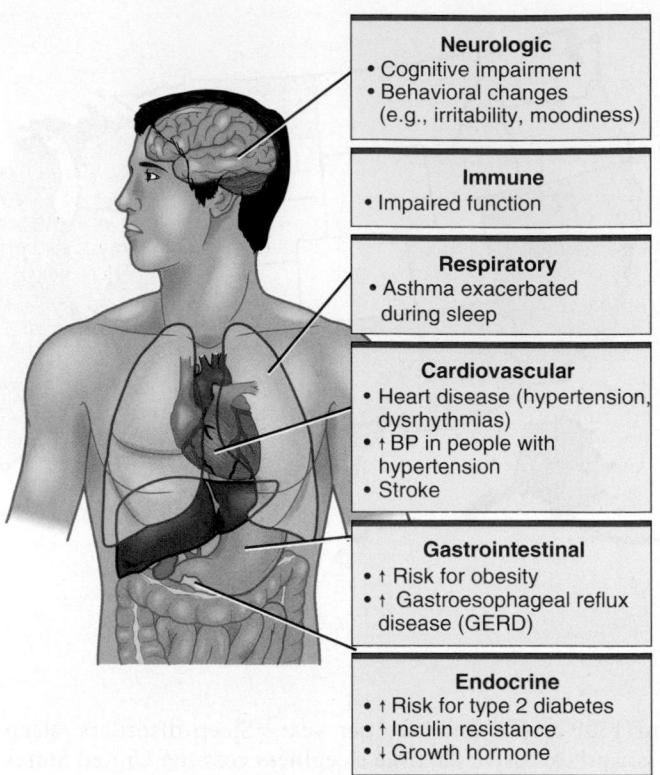

FIG. 7.3 Effects of sleep deprivation and sleep disorders on the body.

SLEEP DISTURBANCES IN THE HOSPITAL

Hospitalized patients, especially in the intensive care unit (ICU), may have decreased total sleep time, disrupted normal sleep stages, and disrupted circadian rhythms.[12] In the hospital, environmental sleep-disruptive factors, psychoactive medications, and acute and critical illness contribute to poor sleep. Contributing environmental factors include around-the-clock noise, light, and patient care activities. Hospital and ICU noise often persists both day and night from sources such as staff paging system, ventilator alarms, bedside monitors, infusion alarms, and staff conversations near patients (e.g., in hallways). Bright lights during the night disrupt sleep and reduce melatonin levels. Patient care activities including dressing changes, blood draws, vital sign monitoring, and medication administration often disrupt patients' ability to get sound, continuous sleep. This includes when we provide care to a patient's roommate in a shared room. Inactivity, boredom, and napping during the day and evening that can affect nighttime sleep. Patient symptoms, including pain, dyspnea, and nausea, can contribute to sleep loss in the acutely ill patient. Commonly used medications can further contribute to sleep loss. Preexisting sleep disorders may be worsened or triggered in those who are hospitalized.

Decreased sleep duration and sleep loss cause patients to be more sensitive to pain and less able to tolerate pain.[13] Adequate pain management may improve total sleep time, but many medications used to relieve pain, especially opioids, alter sleep quality and place a person at risk for sleep-disordered breathing.

You play a key role in creating an environment conducive to sleep. This includes the scheduling of medications and procedures, including those performed by unlicensed assistive personnel (UAP). Reducing light and noise levels can promote opportunities for sleep. Hypnotic sleep-aid medications are often available on an as-needed basis or can be discussed with the HCP.

TABLE 7.1 Relationship of Sleep Disturbances to Diseases and Disorders

Disease or Disorder	Sleep Disturbance
Cardiovascular (CV)	
Coronary artery disease	• People with sleep apnea or sleep disorders are at increased risk for CV disorders, including hypertension, dysrhythmias, and coronary artery disease
Heart failure (HF)	• Sleep problems (insomnia, PLMD, SDB) are common • Cheyne-Stokes breathing and central apnea are signs of HF exacerbation related to fluid overload
Hypertension	• Inadequate sleep in people with hypertension can lead to further elevations in BP
Endocrine	
Diabetes	• Insufficient sleep linked to increased risk for type 2 diabetes • Sleep deprivation in healthy people increases insulin resistance
Gastrointestinal	
Obesity	• Short sleep duration may result in metabolic changes that are linked to obesity • Higher body mass index (BMI) in those who sleep <6 hours compared with those who sleep >8 hours • Risk factor for SDB
Gastroesophageal reflux disease (GERD)	• Reflux of gastric contents into the esophagus occurs during sleep because of incompetent lower esophageal sphincter • Swallowing is depressed during sleep
Liver disease	• Associated with excessive sleepiness, nocturnal arousal, and RLS
Immune Disorders	
Human immunodeficiency virus (HIV)	• Sleep problems and fatigue highly prevalent and associated with increased morbidity and mortality
Musculoskeletal	
Arthritis	• Increased rates of RLS and SDB • Disease activity linked to sleep complaints
Fibromyalgia	• Co-morbid insomnia, especially complaint of nonrestorative sleep • Increased rates of PLMD and RLS • Lower levels of sleep-dependent hormones (growth hormone, prolactin)
Systemic exertion intolerance disease (chronic fatigue syndrome)	• Co-morbid insomnia • Increased rates of SDB
Neurologic	
Alzheimer's disease	• Many have SDB (frequently sleep apnea) • Circadian rhythm changes with nocturnal wandering, daytime sleepiness, and sleep disruption and awakening
Cancer	• Higher rates of insomnia • Chemotherapy for cancer treatment associated with fragmented sleep and fatigue
Pain (acute and chronic)	• Decreases quantity and quality of sleep • Poor sleep can intensify pain
Parkinson's disease	• Associated with difficulty initiating or maintaining sleep, parasomnias, and excessive daytime sleepiness
Renal	
End-stage renal disease (ESRD)	• Disrupted nocturnal sleep with excessive daytime sleepiness • Patients on dialysis have a high incidence of SDB and RLS, which are both significant predictors of mortality
Respiratory	
Asthma	• Worse during sleep
Chronic obstructive pulmonary disease (COPD)	• Associated with poor sleep quality, nocturnal oxygen desaturation, and coexisting sleep apnea
Obstructive sleep apnea (OSA)	• Linked with heart disease (hypertension, stroke, heart failure, coronary artery disease, dysrhythmias) • Results in impaired glucose control like that which occurs in type 2 diabetes

Source: National Center on Sleep Disorders and National Heart, Lung, and Blood Institute: National Sleep Disorders Research Plan: Section 4: Sleep and health. Retrieved from *www.cdc.gov/sleep/about_sleep/chronic_disease.html.*
PLMD, Periodic limb movement disorder; *RLS*, restless legs syndrome; *SDB*, sleep-disordered breathing.

SLEEP DISORDERS

INSOMNIA

The most common sleep disorder is insomnia. It affects 1 in 3 adults. Insomnia is characterized by difficulty falling asleep, difficulty staying asleep, waking up too early, or waking up feeling unrefreshed. The main problem people with insomnia report is overall dissatisfaction with sleep quality and quantity.

Acute insomnia refers to difficulties falling or remaining asleep at least 3 nights per week for less than a month. *Chronic insomnia* is defined by the same symptoms and a daytime problem related to poor sleep (e.g., fatigue, poor concentration, interference with social or family activities) that persist for 3 months or longer. Chronic insomnia occurs in 10% to 15% of Americans. It is more common in women than men. Insomnia is more common in people who are divorced, widowed, and separated than in those who are married. It is more prevalent in people with low socioeconomic status and less education.[14]

Etiology and Pathophysiology

Behaviors, lifestyle, diet, physical and mental conditions, and medications may contribute to insomnia. Insomnia is worsened or perpetuated by behaviors such as keeping irregular sleep-wake schedules (varying one's bedtime and rise time), taking long naps in the afternoon, spending time awake in bed trying to sleep, sleeping late in the morning, and exercising near bedtime. Lifestyle factors can contribute to insomnia. Although the sedative effects of alcohol help people fall asleep, it suppresses REM sleep and causes restlessness and awakenings later in the night. Use of various stimulants, including nicotine in tobacco products, caffeine, or methamphetamine, can cause restlessness and sleep disruption, worsening insomnia. Insomnia is a common side effect of many medications (e.g., antidepressants, antihypertensives, corticosteroids, psychostimulants, analgesics).

The physiologic and psychologic causes of chronic insomnia may be related to varied factors. Often people report that the onset occurred after a stressful life event, such as losing a job or the death of a loved one. In other cases, psychiatric illnesses, medical conditions, medications, or substance use may precipitate insomnia. Patients with psychiatric or medical conditions are more likely to have insomnia than those without these conditions. Once insomnia becomes chronic, symptoms are likely to persist over time.

Clinical Manifestations

Manifestations of insomnia include 1 or more of the following symptoms: (1) difficulty falling asleep *(long sleep latency)*, (2) frequent awakenings *(fragmented sleep)*, (3) prolonged nighttime awakenings or awakening too early and not being able to fall back to sleep *(difficulty maintaining sleep)*, and (4) awakening feeling unrefreshed *(nonrestorative sleep)*.[14] Daytime or functional consequences of insomnia include fatigue, having trouble concentrating at work or school, and having an altered mood. Behavioral manifestations of poor sleep include irritability, sleepiness during the day, forgetfulness, and attention and concentration problems.

Diagnostic Studies

Self-Report. The diagnosis of insomnia is made based on subjective complaints and an evaluation of a 1- or 2-week sleep diary completed by the patient. A diary or log usually includes the number and times of naps, times of going to bed, awakening, and getting up, number of awakenings, and overall sleep quality ratings.

In ambulatory care settings, the evaluation of insomnia requires a comprehensive sleep history. This establishes the type of insomnia and screens for possible psychiatric, medical, or other sleep disorders that would require specific treatment. Questionnaires, such as Pittsburgh Quality Sleep Index, Insomnia Severity Index, and Epworth Daytime Sleepiness, are often used to assess sleep quality and negative daytime symptoms related to insomnia.

Actigraphy. *Actigraphy* is a relatively noninvasive method of monitoring rest and activity cycles. An actigraph is a device that measures overall motor activity. It is worn on the wrist like commercially available activity monitors. Actigraphs used for sleep medicine and research are more accurate and sensitive than consumer-based devices. The unit continuously records the patient's movements, producing data that are downloaded to a computer and analyzed. Activity

TABLE 7.2	Interprofessional Care
Insomnia	

Diagnostic Assessment **History**	**Drug Therapy (Table 7.4)**
• Self-report sleep log or diary	• Benzodiazepines
• Sleep assessment (Table 7.5)	• Benzodiazepine-receptor–like agents
• Pittsburgh Sleep Quality Index	• Orexin-receptor antagonist
• Insomnia Severity Index	• Melatonin-receptor agonist
• Epworth Sleepiness Scale	• Antidepressants
Management **Nondrug Therapy**	**Complementary and Alternative Therapy**
• Sleep hygiene (Table 7.3)	• Melatonin
• Cognitive-behavioral therapies for insomnia (CBT-I)	

corresponds to time spent awake, and continuous inactivity corresponds to time spent asleep. Actigraphy is not necessary for diagnosing insomnia, but it is useful for confirming patient's sleep self-reports and monitoring the effects of treatments.

Polysomnography. A polysomnography (PSG) study is not recommended to diagnose insomnia. A PSG study is done only if there are symptoms or signs of another sleep disorder, such as sleep-disordered breathing (discussed later in the chapter). In a PSG study, electrodes simultaneously record physiologic measures that define the main stages of sleep and wakefulness. These measures include (1) muscle tone recorded using an electromyogram (EMG), (2) eye movements recorded with an electrooculogram (EOG), and (3) brain activity recorded through EEG. To determine additional characteristics of specific sleep disorders, other measures made during PSG include airflow at the nose and mouth, respiratory effort around the chest and abdomen, heart rate, noninvasive oxygen saturation, and EMG of the anterior tibialis muscles (used to detect periodic leg movements). Finally, cameras and microphones continuously monitor a patient's gross body movements.

Interprofessional Care

Insomnia treatments are directed toward changing behaviors that perpetuate insomnia and managing symptoms (Table 7.2). The goal is to (1) prevent acute insomnia from becoming chronic and (2) treat chronic insomnia. An important first step is to provide teaching about sleep along with behavioral strategies. **Sleep hygiene** is a variety of different practices that are important to have normal, quality nighttime sleep and daytime alertness (Table 7.3). Patients often have some familiarity with sleep hygiene principles, but they may still benefit from coaching on how to use these principles effectively.

Cognitive-Behavioral Therapy for Insomnia. Although teaching about sleep hygiene practices is useful, those with chronic insomnia need more in-depth *cognitive-behavioral therapy for insomnia (CBT-I)*.[14] CBT-I is based on structured treatment plans that include cognitive and behavioral components. The cognitive part of CBT-I may include stress management techniques (e.g., relaxation breathing, imagery) or cognitive strategies to address misconceptions about sleep. The specific approach used varies based on the patient's need. The behavioral

TABLE 7.3   Patient Teaching

Sleep Hygiene

Include the following instructions when teaching a patient who has a sleep disturbance or disorder.

- Do not go to bed unless you are sleepy.
- If you are not asleep after 20 minutes, get out of bed and do a non-stimulating activity. Return to bed only when you are sleepy.
- Adopt a regular pattern in terms of bedtime and awakening.
- Begin rituals (e.g., warm bath, light snack, reading) that help you relax each night before bed.
- Get a full night's sleep on a regular basis.
- Make your bedroom quiet, dark, and a little bit cool.
- Do not read, write, eat, watch TV, talk on the phone, or use technologies such as smart phones and tablet computers in bed.
- Avoid caffeine, nicotine, and alcohol at least 4–6 hours before bedtime.
- Do not go to bed hungry, but do not eat a big meal near bedtime either.
- Avoid strenuous exercise within 6 hours of your bedtime.
- Avoid sleeping pills, or use them cautiously.
- Practice relaxation techniques (e.g., relaxation breathing) to help you cope with stress.

Adapted from American Academy of Sleep Medicine: Healthy sleep habits, 2017. Retrieved from *www.sleepeducation.org/treatment-therapy/healthy-sleep-habits/*.

TABLE 7.4   Drug Therapy

Insomnia

Benzodiazepines
- Temazepam (Restoril)
- Triazolam (Halcion)

Benzodiazepine-Receptor–Like Agents
- Eszopiclone (Lunesta)
- Zaleplon (Sonata)
- Zolpidem (Ambien, Ambien CR, Edluar, Intermezzo, Zolpi-Mist)

Orexin-Receptor Antagonist
- Suvorexant (Belsomra)

Melatonin-Receptor Agonist
- Ramelteon (Rozerem)

Antidepressants
- Amitriptyline
- Doxepin

Source: U.S. Food and Drug Administration: Sleep disorder (sedative-hypnotic) drug information, 2017. Retrieved from *www.fda.gov/Drugs/DrugSafety/PostmarketDrugSafetyInformationforPatientsandProviders/ucm101557.htm*.

part of CBT-I includes instructions to (1) limit the amount of time a person can stay in bed, (2) set a scheduled time to get up in the morning, (3) go to bed only when feeling sleepy, and (4) get out of bed when unable to sleep. CBT-I includes focused teaching and coaching on how to effectively use sleep hygiene practices (Table 7.3). CBT-I requires people to change behavior, which can be hard.

Although full CBT-I treatment should be delivered by trained HCPs, you can apply many of the principles to help patients. Teach the person with insomnia to avoid naps. Older adults may have difficulty fully avoiding naps. You can teach them that naps are less likely to affect nighttime sleep if they are limited to 15 to 20 minutes, once per day, and scheduled no later than 7 to 9 hours after waking in the morning. Regular exercise may enhance sleep quality but should not be done within several hours of bedtime.

Drug Therapy. Most medications for insomnia work by producing sleepiness to promote the onset or maintenance of sleep. Based on the characteristics (onset, half-life, and mechanism of action), certain medications may be recommended for specific patterns of insomnia but not for others. They can treat problems falling asleep (sleep onset), waking during the night and having trouble falling back asleep (sleep maintenance), or both. Medications that treat insomnia can cause next-day drowsiness and impair driving and other activities that require alertness. People can be impaired even when they feel fully awake. Many people become used to taking OTC or prescription medications to treat insomnia and risk becoming dependent on them, psychologically and physically. *Rebound insomnia* is worsening of sleep that may occur when one abruptly stops certain sleep medications.

Medications are generally recommended for short-term treatment of insomnia. There is little evidence to support the use of medications for chronic insomnia. In 2017 the American Academy of Sleep Medicine (AASM) published new guidelines for pharmacologic treatment of chronic insomnia.[15] Drug classes used to treat insomnia include benzodiazepines, benzodiazepine-receptor agonists, orexin-receptor antagonist, melatonin-receptor agonist, antidepressants, and antihistamines (Table 7.4).[16] Use of hypnotic medications in older adults is controversial due to side effects and safety concerns, such as fall risk.[17]

Benzodiazepine Hypnotics. Benzodiazepines activate GABA receptors to promote sleep. These agents are no longer recommended as first-line therapy for insomnia. Only 2 benzodiazepines are included in the 2017 AASM guidelines: triazolam (Halcion) is recommended for sleep onset insomnia, and temazepam (Restoril) is recommended for both sleep onset and sleep maintenance insomnia.[15] Some benzodiazepines are recommended for treating anxiety but not insomnia (e.g., diazepam, alprazolam). However, you may still encounter patients who are prescribed these medications for insomnia. Other benzodiazepines (estazolam, flurazepam, oxazepam) lack enough research to support clinical recommendations. The prolonged half-life of some of these drugs can result in daytime sleepiness, amnesia, dizziness, and rebound insomnia. Tolerance develops, and there is a risk for dependence and the potential for misuse. They should be used for only 2 to 3 weeks. In addition, they interact with alcohol and other central nervous system (CNS) depressants.

Non-Benzodiazepine Hypnotics. Non-benzodiazepine hypnotics act at GABA receptors but have more selective action than benzodiazepines, resulting in better safety.[16] These agents are considered first-line for pharmacologic treatment of insomnia. The 2017 AASM guidelines recommend zaleplon (Sonata) for sleep onset insomnia and zolpidem (Ambien) and eszopiclone (Lunesta) for sleep onset and sleep maintenance insomnia.[15] These drugs are effective and safe for use from 3 months to a year.[16] Food has the potential to delay onset of action and should not be taken with these agents. These agents have short half-lives, making their duration of action short and reducing the risk for daytime sedation. Newer formulations have improved specific therapeutic uses. A controlled-release formulation of zolpidem (Ambien CR) lengthens the action of the medication, improving its use for sleep maintenance insomnia. Zolpidem (Intermezzo) is available in a quick-acting sublingual tablet that may be taken for middle-of-the-night awakenings. A dissolvable tablet form of zolpidem (Edluar) and an oral spray formulation (ZolpiMist) may be used with those who have difficulty swallowing pills or are on restricted oral fluid intake.

Orexin-Receptor Antagonist. Suvorexant (Belsomra) is the first approved orexin-receptor antagonist. It promotes sleep by blocking the effects of orexin. Suvorexant should be taken no more than once per night, within 30 minutes of going to bed, with at least 7 hours remaining before the planned time of waking. It is recommended only for sleep maintenance insomnia.[15] The most common side effect is drowsiness.

Melatonin-Receptor Agonist. Ramelteon (Rozerem) is a melatonin-receptor agonist. It has a rapid onset that is effective for sleep onset. Ramelteon does not cause tolerance, but it is not always effective in improving sleep quality. Ramelteon is recommended for insomnia with sleep onset difficulty, not for sleep maintenance problems.[15]

Antidepressants. Certain tricyclic antidepressants (e.g., doxepin, amitriptyline) are used as sleep aids due to their side effects of sedation. The insomnia dose is much lower than the antidepressant dose. The AASM recommends doxepin for sleep maintenance insomnia.[15] Doxepin improves sleep without next-day drowsiness in older and middle-aged adults with chronic primary insomnia.

Trazodone, an atypical antidepressant, is 1 of the most common agents prescribed to treat insomnia, especially in older adults. Giving this drug to older adults is controversial. Daytime sleepiness is a common side effect. Tolerance can develop within a few weeks. The AASM recommends against using trazodone because there is not enough research to determine if the benefit outweighs risks for side effects.[15]

Antihistamines. Many people self-medicate with OTC sleep aids. These include doxylamine (Unisom) and several agents that contain diphenhydramine. Diphenhydramine is in many "nighttime" pain medicines. The AASM guidelines do not recommend diphenhydramine for insomnia because research does not show that it effectively improves sleep. It should not be used by older adults. Antihistamines have anticholinergic side effects, including daytime sleepiness, impaired cognitive function, blurred vision, urinary retention, constipation, and risk for increased intraocular pressure. The AASM guidelines do not mention doxylamine.[15]

Complementary and Alternative Therapy. Many types of complementary and alternative therapies are used as sleep aids (see Complementary & Alternative Therapies: Melatonin box). Melatonin is not recommended for treatment of insomnia,[15] but it may be effective for improving sleep disturbance associated with jet lag.[18] It also helps night shift workers sleep during the daytime. Valerian is an herb that has been used for many years as a sleep aid and to relieve anxiety. Although valerian is safe, it is not effective in treating insomnia. Other sleep aids include white noise devices or relaxation strategies.

🌿 COMPLEMENTARY & ALTERNATIVE THERAPIES
Melatonin

Scientific Evidence
Overall, the scientific evidence suggests melatonin may help people who take it for jet lag. It may also decrease the time it takes to fall asleep (sleep latency).

Nursing Implications
- Regarded as safe in recommended doses for short-term use.
- Avoid in patients using warfarin (Coumadin).
- Avoid in patients using central nervous system depressants.
- Common side effects are headache, nausea, dizziness, and drowsiness.

Source: Based on a systematic review of scientific literature. Retrieved from *www.naturalmedicines.therapeuticresearch.com.*

TABLE 7.5 Nursing Assessment
Sleep

Use the following questions to do an initial sleep assessment.
1. What time do you normally go to bed at night? What time do you normally wake up in the morning?
2. Do you often have trouble falling asleep at night?
3. About how many times do you wake up at night?
4. If you do wake up during the night, do you usually have trouble falling back asleep?
5. Does your bed partner say or are you aware that you frequently snore, gasp for air, or stop breathing?
6. Does your bed partner say or are you aware that you kick or thrash about while asleep?
7. Are you aware that you ever walk, eat, punch, kick, or scream during sleep?
8. Are you sleepy or tired during much of the day?
9. Do you usually take 1 or more naps during the day?
10. Do you usually doze off without planning to during the day?
11. How much sleep do you need to feel alert and function well?
12. Are you currently taking any type of medication or other preparation to help you sleep?

❖ NURSING MANAGEMENT: INSOMNIA

◆ Nursing Assessment

As a nurse, you are in a key position to assess sleep problems in patients and their caregivers. Sleep assessment is important in helping patients identify personal habits and environmental factors that contribute to poor sleep. Family caregivers may have sleep disruptions from the need to provide care to patients in the home. These sleep disruptions can increase the burden of caregiving.

Self-report and objective data are used to assess sleep duration and quality. Many patients do not tell their HCP about their sleep problems. Make sure to ask patients about their sleep and problems with sleep. A sleep history includes characteristics of sleep such as sleep duration, the pattern of sleep, and daytime alertness (Table 7.5). Healthy adults should have 7 to 8 hours of sleep a night. Occasional difficulty getting to sleep or awakening during the night is not unusual. However, sleep disturbances longer than 1 month are problematic. Assess the diet and caffeine intake.

Ask the patient about sleep aids. This includes OTC and prescription medications. Note the drug dose, frequency of use, and any side effects (e.g., daytime drowsiness, dry mouth). Ask about alcohol consumption and whether it is used as a sleep aid. Many people consume herbal or dietary supplements that they believe will improve sleep. Common supplements include valerian, melatonin, hops, passion flower, kava, and skullcap. Tell the patient that many of these products are sold as dietary supplements and do not have U.S. Food and Drug Administration (FDA) approval or regulatory oversight. The exact components and concentrations of herbs and supplements often are unknown. Patients may have adverse effects or herb-drug interactions. Certain agents such as kava are associated with liver toxicity.

Encourage the patient to keep a sleep diary for 1 to 2 weeks. A free sleep diary is available from the National Sleep Foundation (*www.sleepfoundation.org/sites/default/files/SleepDiaryv6.pdf*). You can help the patient choose 1 of the many sleep diary smartphone applications that track information about sleep. Commercially available activity monitors can track sleep, but these vary in accuracy. Encourage people with sleep problems to share this information with their HCP to help identify sleep patterns.

The patient's medical history can provide important information about factors that contribute to poor sleep. For example, a man with benign prostatic hyperplasia may report frequent awakenings during the night for voiding. Psychiatric problems (e.g., depression, anxiety, posttraumatic stress disorder [PTSD], drug use) are associated with sleep disturbances. Some patients being seen for sleep problems may complete short questionnaires to screen for mood disturbances. Sleep disturbances often develop as a result or complication of a chronic or terminal condition (e.g., heart disease, dementia, cancer). Painful conditions such as arthritis may contribute to nighttime awakenings.

Ask about work schedules and cross-country and international travel. Shift work contributes to reduced or poor-quality sleep. Work-related behaviors resulting from poor sleep may include poor performance, decreased productivity, and job absenteeism.

◆ Nursing Diagnoses

Nursing diagnoses related to sleep include sleep deprivation and impaired sleep pattern.

◆ Nursing Implementation

Nursing care depends on the severity and duration of the sleep problem. Although teaching about sleep hygiene practices (Table 7.3) is beneficial, patients with chronic insomnia need more in-depth intervention using CBT-I strategies. An important part of sleep hygiene is reducing dietary intake of caffeine-containing substances (Table 7.6). Caffeine has a half-life of about 6 hours and possibly as long as 9 hours in older adults. Patients should avoid consuming caffeinated beverages after 12 noon.

Suggest and implement changes in home and institutional environments to enhance sleep. Reducing light and noise levels enhances sleep. Awareness of time passing and watching the clock adds to anxiety about not falling asleep or returning to sleep. Keeping the bedroom dark and cool is conducive to good sleep.

Teach patients about sleeping medications. With the benzodiazepines, non-benzodiazepine hypnotics, and melatonin-receptor agonists, teach the patient to take the drug right before bedtime and be prepared to get a full night's sleep of at least 6 to 8 hours. Tell patients not to plan activities the next morning that require highly skilled psychomotor coordination. Advise patients not to take these medications with high-fat food (delays absorption), alcohol, or other CNS depressants. Patient follow-up about medications is important. Ask about daytime sleepiness, nightmares, and any difficulties in activities of daily living.

OBSTRUCTIVE SLEEP APNEA

The term **sleep-disordered breathing (SDB)** describes abnormal respiratory patterns associated with sleep. These include snoring, apnea (temporary cessation of respiration), and hypopnea (temporary restriction of respiration without full cessation) with increased respiratory effort leading to frequent arousals. SDB results in frequent sleep disruptions and changes in sleep stages. Obstructive sleep apnea is the most commonly diagnosed SDB problem.

Obstructive sleep apnea (OSA), also called *obstructive sleep apnea–hypopnea syndrome* (OSAHS), is characterized by partial or complete upper airway obstruction during sleep. *Apnea* is the cessation of respiratory airflow (90% or greater

TABLE 7.6 Caffeine Content of Select Beverages

Food or Beverage	Caffeine (mg)
Coffee, brewed (8 oz)	95–165
Coffee, instant (8 oz)	7.63
Coffee, espresso (1 oz)	47.64
Coffee, decaffeinated	2–5
Cola (8 oz)	24–46
Energy drink (8 oz)	27.164
Energy shot (1 oz)	40–100
Hot chocolate (8 oz)	5
Root beer, most brands (8 oz)	0
Sprite, 7up (12 oz)	0
Tea, black (8 oz)	25–48
Tea, green (8 oz)	25–297

Source: Mayo Clinic: Caffeine content for coffee, tea, soda and more, 2017. Retrieved from *www.mayoclinic.org/healthy-lifestyle/nutrition-and-healthy-eating/in-depth/caffeine/art-20049372.*

reduction) lasting longer than 10 seconds. *Hypopnea* is a condition characterized by shallow respirations (30%–90% reduction in airflow).[9] Airflow obstruction in OSA occurs because of (1) narrowing of the air passages with relaxation of muscle tone during sleep and/or (2) the tongue and soft palate falling backward to partially or completely obstruct the pharynx (Fig. 7.4). Each obstruction may last from 10 to 90 seconds. During the apneic period the patient can have *hypoxemia* (decreased PaO_2 or SpO_2) and *hypercapnia* (increased $PaCO_2$). These changes are ventilatory stimulants and cause brief arousals, but the patient may not fully awaken.

The patient has a generalized startle response, snorts, and gasps, which cause the tongue and soft palate to move forward and the airway to open. Apnea and arousal cycles occur repeatedly throughout the night. Apneic episodes occur most often during REM sleep, when airway muscle tone is lowest.

There is no single cause for OSA. The condition is related to multiple factors that influence airway patency and the tone of airway musculature. Risk factors include obesity (body mass index [BMI] greater than 30 kg/m²), age older than 65 years, neck circumference greater than 17 inches, craniofacial abnormalities that affect the upper airway, and acromegaly (acromegaly is discussed in Chapter 49). Smokers are more likely to have OSA. OSA is more common in men than in women until after menopause, when the prevalence of the disorder is equal.[19] Women with OSA have higher mortality rates than men with OSA. OSA patients with excessive daytime sleepiness have increased mortality.

Clinical Manifestations

Clinical manifestations of sleep apnea include frequent arousals during sleep, insomnia, excessive daytime sleepiness, and witnessed apneic episodes. The patient's bed partner may complain about the patient's loud snoring. Other symptoms include morning headaches (from hypercapnia or increased BP that causes vasodilation of cerebral blood vessels), personality changes, and irritability.

A major risk of OSA is cardiovascular complications. Apnea during sleep causes hypoxia, nocturnal arousals, and increased pressure in the thoracic cavity. These events can lead to negative physiologic consequences, including overactivation of the sympathetic nervous system, increased

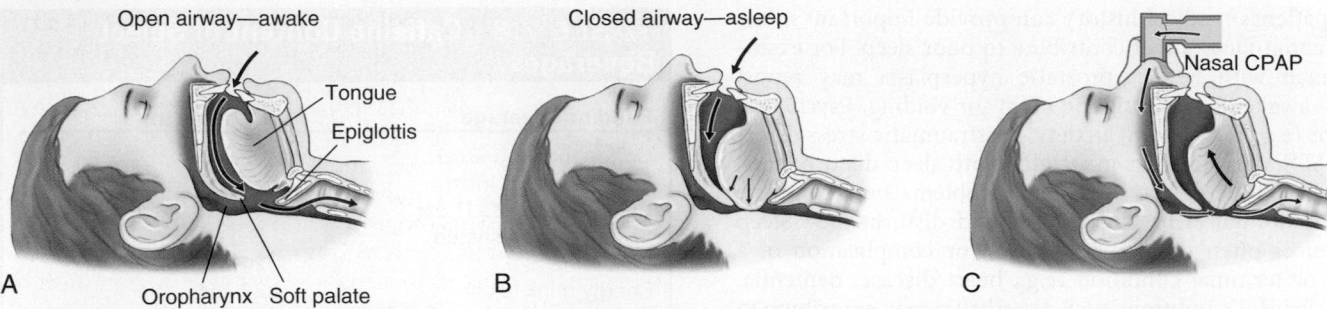

FIG. 7.4 How sleep apnea occurs. A, The patient predisposed to obstructive sleep apnea (OSA) has a small pharyngeal airway. B, During sleep, the pharyngeal muscles relax, allowing the airway to close. Lack of airflow results in repeated apneic episodes. C, Continuous positive airway pressure *(CPAP)* splints the airway open, preventing airflow obstruction. (Modified from LaFleur Brooks M: *Exploring medical language: A student-directed approach,* ed 8, St Louis, 2012, Mosby.)

vascular resistance, and reduced oxygenation of the heart muscle. Long-term effects include hypertension, cardiac dysrhythmias, arteriosclerosis, heart failure, and cardiovascular-related mortality.[20]

Chronic sleep loss predisposes the person to diminished ability to concentrate, impaired memory, failure to complete daily tasks, and interpersonal difficulties. Men may have impotence. Hypercapnia and arousals contribute to daytime sleepiness in people with OSA. Driving accidents may occur due to excessive daytime sleepiness. Family life and the patient's ability to maintain employment are often compromised. As a result, the patient may become depressed. Cessation of breathing reported by the bed partner is usually a source of great anxiety because of the fear that breathing may not resume.

Diagnostic Studies

Assessment of the patient with OSA includes a thorough sleep and medical history. Tools used to screen for OSA are the Berlin questionnaire and the STOP-BANG questionnaire, which assesses for clinical manifestations highly suspicious of OSA.[19]

Typically, OSA is diagnosed by PSG done in a clinical sleep laboratory. The patient's chest and abdominal movement, oral and nasal airflow, SpO_2, eye movement, and heart rate and rhythm are monitored. In some instances, portable sleep studies are done in the home setting. Overnight pulse oximetry assessment may be done to determine whether nocturnal oxygen supplementation is needed.

A diagnosis of sleep apnea requires documentation of apneic events or hypopneas of at least 10 seconds' duration. OSA is defined as more than 5 apnea/hypopnea events per hour with a 3% to 4% decrease in oxygen saturation. Severe apnea can be associated with apneic events of more than 30 to 50 per hour of sleep.[9]

INFORMATICS IN PRACTICE

Sleep Apnea Diagnosis and Monitoring

- Home respiratory monitoring is a cost-effective alternative to diagnose and manage SDB that allows patients the convenience of sleeping in their own home.
- It is used as part of a comprehensive sleep evaluation and in patients likely to have moderate to severe OSA but without heart failure, obstructive lung disease, or neuromuscular disease.
- Home respiratory monitoring is used to monitor the effectiveness of non-CPAP therapies for patients with sleep-related breathing disorders.
- Wireless monitors can detect changes in vital signs and pulse oximetry, raising an alarm if values fall outside of set parameters.

❖ NURSING AND INTERPROFESSIONAL MANAGEMENT: SLEEP APNEA

◆ Conservative Treatment

Mild sleep apnea (5–10 apnea/hypopnea events per hour) may respond to simple measures. Conservative treatment at home begins with sleeping on one's side rather than on the back (called *positional therapy*), which reduces the effects of gravity on the airway. Elevating the head of the bed may eliminate OSA in some patients.

Medications that relax airway muscle tone often make OSA worse. Teach the patient to avoid taking sedatives or consuming alcoholic beverages for 3 to 4 hours before sleep. Sleep medications often make OSA worse. Excess weight worsens sleep apnea as the pressure of adipose tissue in the neck and on the chest restricts ventilation. Referral to a weight loss program may be needed. Bariatric surgery may also reduce OSA.[19] Teach the patient the dangers of driving or using heavy equipment due to the profound sleepiness that is common in people with OSA. Insomnia is common in people with OSA. They may need specific treatment for the insomnia (such as CBT-I).

Symptoms may resolve in up to half of patients with OSA who use a special mouth guard, also called an oral appliance, during sleep to prevent airflow obstruction. Oral appliances bring the mandible and tongue forward to enlarge the airway space, thereby preventing airway occlusion.[19] Some find a support group helpful, because they can express concerns and feelings and discuss strategies for resolving problems.

In patients with more severe symptoms (>15 apnea/hypopnea events/hour), continuous positive airway pressure (CPAP) by mask is the treatment of choice. With CPAP, the patient applies a nasal mask that is attached to a high-flow blower (Fig. 7.5). The blower is adjusted to maintain enough positive pressure (5–25 cm H_2O) in the airway during inspiration and expiration to prevent airway collapse.

Some patients cannot adjust to wearing a mask over the nose or mouth or to exhaling against the high pressure. A technologically more sophisticated therapy, bilevel positive airway pressure (BiPAP), can deliver a higher inspiration pressure and a lower pressure during expiration. With BiPAP, the apnea can be relieved with a lower mean pressure and may be better tolerated.

CPAP reduces apnea episodes, daytime sleepiness, and fatigue. It improves quality of life ratings and returns cognitive functioning to normal. Benefits of CPAP are dose-dependent

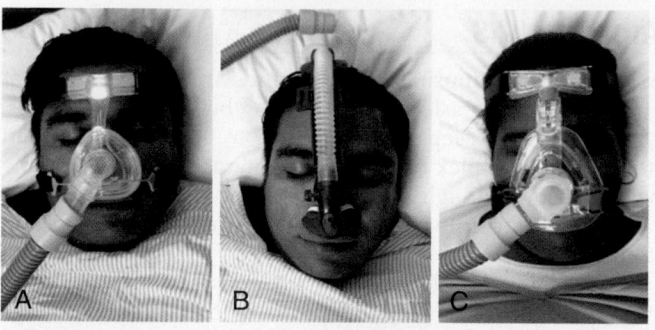

FIG. 7.5 Examples of positive airway pressure devices for sleep apnea. **A,** Patient wearing a nasal mask and headgear (positive pressure only through nose). **B,** Patient wearing nasal pillows (positive pressure only through nose). **C,** Patient wearing a full face mask (positive pressure to nose and mouth). (From Goldman L, Schafer AI: *Goldman's Cecil medicine*, ed 24, Philadelphia, 2012, Saunders.)

based on how long the device is used during the night. It must be used a minimum of 4 hours each night to reduce/reverse the negative cardiovascular effects of OSA.[20] Although CPAP is a highly effective treatment, patients have problems with using it every day. About two-thirds of those using CPAP report side effects such as nasal stuffiness.

First, assess the patient's knowledge about OSA and CPAP. Involve the bed partner in teaching. Assess the patient for nasal resistance. To ensure successful adherence to CPAP treatment, patients need to be involved in choosing the mask and device before the start of therapy. Patient-centered care may improve patient outcomes given that OSA treatment requires behavioral and lifestyle changes. You can facilitate goal-setting discussions between patients and HCPs to arrive at treatment plans that are feasible and mutually agreed upon.

When patients with a history of OSA are hospitalized, be aware that giving opioid analgesics and sedating medications (benzodiazepines, hypnotics) may worsen OSA symptoms by depressing respirations. Check with the HCP in charge of the patient's care to determine if a patient who uses home CPAP or BiPAP should continue this therapy in the hospital. If so, it is important for these patients to wear the device when resting or sleeping. Many patients can use their own equipment but check hospital policy to be certain it can be used.

◆ Surgical Treatment

If other measures fail, OSA can be managed surgically. The goal of OSA surgery is to reduce collapsibility and increase patency of the upper airway, including oral, nasal, and pharyngeal passages. The most common procedures are uvulopalatopharyngoplasty (UPPP or UP3) and genioglossal advancement and hyoid myotomy (GAHM). UPPP involves excision of the tonsillar pillars, uvula, and posterior soft palate to remove the obstructing tissue. GAHM involves advancing the attachment of the muscular part of the tongue on the mandible. When GAHM is performed, UPPP is generally done as well. Depending on the site of the obstruction, symptoms are relieved in up to 80% of patients.

Radiofrequency ablation (RFA) of obstructive tissues alone or in combination with other surgical techniques is also used. RFA is the least invasive surgical intervention. New treatments involve surgically implanted neurostimulators. One type

stimulates the hypoglossal nerve to increase the tone of airway muscles. This treatment for OSA is still being tested for effectiveness and safety.[19]

After surgery, complications of airway obstruction or hemorrhage occur most often in the immediate postoperative period. Patients are usually discharged home within 1 day after the procedure. Before going home, teach the patient what to expect during the postoperative recovery period. Tell patients that their throat will be sore. They may have a foul breath odor that may be reduced by rinsing with diluted mouthwash and then salt water for several days. Snoring may persist until the inflammation has subsided. Follow-up after surgery is important. A repeat PSG is done 3 to 4 months after surgery.

PERIODIC LIMB MOVEMENT DISORDER

Periodic limb movement disorder (PLMD) is characterized by *periodic limb movements in sleep* (PLMS): involuntary, repetitive movement of the limbs that affects people only during sleep.[21] PLMD usually involves the legs and rarely involves the arms. Sometimes abdominal, oral, and nasal movement accompanies PLMD. Movements typically occur for 0.5 to 10 seconds, in intervals separated by 5 to 90 seconds. PLMD causes poor-quality sleep and excessive daytime sleepiness. The causes of PLMD are not fully understood. Iron deficiency and dopamine dysfunction in the CNS have been implicated.[21]

PLMS can occur with medical disorders (e.g., sleep apnea, narcolepsy) and certain medications. For a diagnosis of PLMD, the occurrence of PLMS must not be due to another disorder. PLMS affects many people with restless legs syndrome (RLS). RLS is discussed in Chapter 58.

PLMD is diagnosed using a detailed history from the patient and/or bed partner and doing PSG. PLMD is treated by medications aimed at reducing or eliminating the limb movements or the arousals. Clonazepam, a benzodiazepine, is used to treat PLMD. It likely helps patients by improving sleep quality rather than reducing limb movements. Other medications shown to be effective are valproic acid, an antiseizure drug that reduces muscle activity, and selegiline, a dopaminergic agent. Dopamine agonists (pramipexole, ropinirole) are used to treat RLS, but there is little research on their efficacy for PLMD. However, it is common practice for HCPs to prescribe these drugs treat PLMD.

CIRCADIAN RHYTHM DISORDERS

Circadian rhythm disorders can occur when the circadian time-keeping system loses synchrony with the environment. Lack of synchrony between the circadian time-keeping system and environment disrupts the sleep-wake cycle and affects the patient's ability to have quality sleep. The common symptoms are insomnia and excessive sleepiness. Jet lag disorder and shift work sleep disorder (see Special Sleep Needs of Nurses section on p. 99) are the most common types of circadian rhythm disorders.

Jet lag disorder occurs when a person travels across multiple time zones. The result is your body's time is not synchronized with environmental time. Most persons crossing at least 3 time zones get jet lag. The number of time zones crossed affects the severity of symptoms and the time it takes to recover. Resynchronization of the body's clock occurs at a rate of about

1 hr/day when traveling eastward and 1.5 hr/day when traveling westward. Melatonin and exposure to daylight help to synchronize the body's rhythm.

Several strategies may help to reduce the risk for developing jet lag. Before travel the person can start to get in harmony with the time schedule of the destination. When time at destination is brief (i.e., 2 days or less), keeping home-based sleep hours rather than adopting destination sleep hours may reduce sleepiness and jet lag symptoms.

NARCOLEPSY

Narcolepsy is a chronic neurologic disorder caused by the brain's inability to regulate sleep-wake cycles normally. At various times throughout the day, people with narcolepsy have uncontrollable urges to sleep. Patients with narcolepsy often go directly into REM sleep from wakefulness.[21] This does not occur in normal sleep and is a unique feature of narcolepsy. Patients with narcolepsy also have fragmented and disturbed nighttime sleep. There are 2 types of narcolepsy: with cataplexy (type 1) and without cataplexy (type 2).[21] Cataplexy is a brief and sudden loss of skeletal muscle tone. It can manifest as a brief episode of muscle weakness or complete postural collapse and falling. Laughter, anger, or surprise often triggers episodes.

The onset of narcolepsy typically occurs in adolescence or early in the third decade. Head trauma, a sudden change in sleep-wake habits, and infection may trigger the onset of narcolepsy symptoms. The cause of narcolepsy is unknown. It is associated with destruction of neurons that make orexin. The resulting deficiency of orexin causes instability of wake and transitions from wake to sleep that occur unpredictably. The loss of neurons may be due to an autoimmune process.[22]

Narcolepsy is diagnosed based on a history of sleepiness, PSG, and daytime *multiple sleep latency tests* (MSLTs).[21] For the MSLT, patients undergo an overnight PSG evaluation followed by 4 or 5 naps scheduled every 2 hours during the next day. Short sleep latencies and onset of REM sleep in more than 2 MSLTs are diagnostic signs of narcolepsy.

Narcolepsy cannot be cured. Management is focused management of common symptoms: excessive daytime sleepiness, nighttime sleep disturbance, and cataplexy (Table 7.3). Provide teaching about sleep and sleep hygiene. Advise the patient to take 3 or more short (15-minute) naps throughout the day and to avoid large or heavy meals and alcohol.[22] You can play a key role in ensuring patient safety by teaching safety behaviors and encouraging adherence to the prescribed medication regimen. Safety precautions, especially when driving, are critically important for patients with narcolepsy. The behavioral therapies for insomnia are also used to address the sleep disturbances. Stimulants are used to counter daytime sleepiness.

Modafinil (Provigil) and armodafinil (Nuvigil) are nonamphetamine wake-promotion drugs that are considered a first-line drug therapy. Sodium oxybate (Xyrem), a metabolite of GABA, is another wake-promoting medication that is effective for treating both daytime sleepiness and cataplexy. Antidepressants are used to treat cataplexy. Tricyclic antidepressants used to be commonly used, but selective serotonin reuptake inhibitors (SSRIs) (e.g., fluoxetine [Prozac], venlafaxine) are becoming favored for the management of cataplexy.[22]

PARASOMNIAS

Parasomnias are unusual and often undesirable behaviors that occur while falling asleep, transitioning between sleep stages, or arousing from sleep.[21] They are due to CNS activation and often involve complex behaviors. The parasomnia is generally goal directed, although the person is not aware or conscious of the act. Parasomnias may result in fragmented sleep and fatigue.

Sleepwalking and sleep terrors are arousal parasomnias that occur during NREM sleep. *Sleepwalking* behaviors can range from sitting up in bed, moving objects, and walking around the room to driving a car. During a sleepwalking event the person may not speak and may have limited or no awareness of the event. On awakening, the person does not remember the event. In the ICU, a parasomnia may be misinterpreted as ICU psychosis. Sedated ICU patients can have manifestations of a parasomnia.

Sleep terrors (night terrors) are characterized by a sudden awakening from sleep along with a loud cry and signs of panic. The person has marked increases in heart rate and respiration and diaphoresis. Factors in the ICU such as sleep disruption and deprivation, fever, stress, and exposure to noise and light can contribute to sleep terrors.

Nightmares are a parasomnia characterized by recurrent awakening with recall of a frightful or disturbing dream. These normally occur during REM sleep during the final third of sleep. In critically ill patients, nightmares are common and likely due to medications. Drug classes most likely to cause nightmares are sedative-hypnotics, β-adrenergic antagonists, dopamine agonists, and amphetamines.

Gerontologic Considerations: Sleep

Older age is associated with overall shorter total sleep time, decreased sleep efficiency, and more awakenings (Fig. 7.6). A common misconception is that older people need less sleep than younger people. In fact, the amount of sleep needed as a person ages stays relatively constant. Other sleep disorders (e.g., sleep-disordered breathing) increase with age and may manifest with symptoms of insomnia. Some older adults have a shift in their circadian sleep timing so that they get sleepy earlier in the evening and awaken early in the morning.[23]

Multiple factors impair older adults' ability to obtain quality sleep. Insomnia symptoms in older adults often occur with depression, cardiovascular disease, pain, and cognitive problems. Chronic conditions that are common in older adults (chronic obstructive pulmonary disease [COPD], diabetes, dementia, chronic pain, cancer) can affect sleep quality. Medications used to treat these conditions can contribute to sleep problems. OTC medications can lead to sleep problems. Stimulating OTC medications include cough and cold medications, especially those containing pseudoephedrine; caffeine-containing drugs; and drugs containing nicotine (e.g., nicotine gum, transdermal patches).

Awakening and getting out of bed during the night (e.g., to use the bathroom) increase the risk for falls. Older adults may use OTC medications or alcohol as a sleep aid. This practice can further increase the risk for falls at night. Chronic disturbed sleep in older adults can result in disorientation, delirium, impaired intellect, disturbed cognition, and increased risk for accidents and injury.

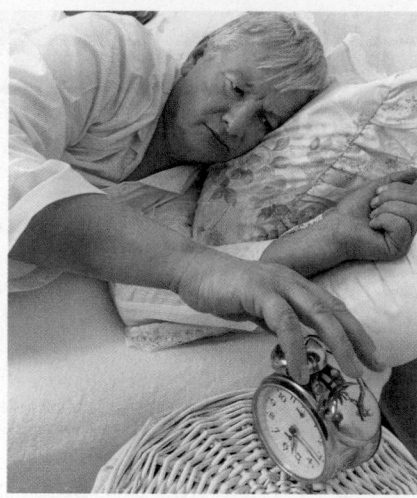

FIG. 7.6 Many older people have sleep problems. (© Studio-Annika/iStock/Thinkstock.)

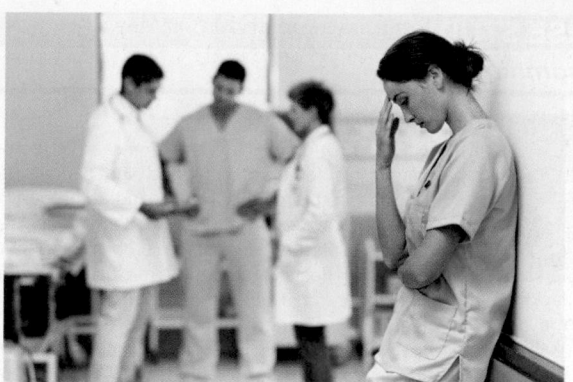

FIG. 7.7 Sleep disturbances are common among nurses. (© iStock.com/kupicoo.)

Because older adults may attribute their disturbed sleep to normal aging, they may fail to report symptoms of sleep disorders to their HCPs. Use a sleeping assessment (Table 7.5) to detect sleep disturbances in older adults.

Sleep medications should be used with great caution in older adults. Diphenhydramine, alone or in combination with other drugs, is sedating with anticholinergic effects. Any OTC medication labeled "PM" probably has diphenhydramine and should be used cautiously by older adults. Metabolism of most hypnotic drugs decreases with aging. Older adults have increased sensitivity to hypnotic and sedative medications. Thus drug therapies for sleep disturbances are started at lower doses and monitored carefully.[17] Whenever possible, long-acting benzodiazepines should be avoided. Older adults receiving benzodiazepines are at increased risk of daytime sedation, falls, and cognitive and psychomotor impairment.

❖ SPECIAL SLEEP NEEDS OF NURSES

Nursing is 1 of several professions that needs night shift and rotating shift schedules. In many settings, nurses work a variety of day and night shifts, often alternating and rotating them. Unfortunately, nurses who do shift work often report less job satisfaction and more job-related stress.[24]

Nurses on permanent night or rapidly rotating shifts are at increased risk for experiencing shift work sleep disorder. It is characterized by insomnia, sleepiness, and fatigue. Nurses on rotating shifts get the least amount of sleep. With repeated periods of inadequate sleep, the sleep debt grows. Chronic fatigue

in nurses doing shift work poses challenges for the individual nurse's health and for patient safety (Fig. 7.7).[24]

Shift work alters the synchrony between circadian rhythms and the environment, leading to sleep disruption. Nurses working the night shift are often too sleepy to be fully alert at work and too alert to sleep soundly the next day. Sustained changes in circadian rhythms such as those imposed by rotating shift work are linked to increased morbidity and mortality risks associated with cardiovascular problems. Mood disorders such as anxiety are higher in nurses who work rotating shifts.

From a safety perspective, disturbed sleep and subsequent fatigue can result in errors and accidents for nurses as well as for their patients. Fatigue diminishes or distorts perceptual skills, judgment, and decision-making capabilities. Lack of sleep reduces the ability to cope and handle stress and may result in physical, mental, and emotional exhaustion.

The problem of sleep disruption is critically important to nursing. Several strategies may help reduce the distress associated with rotating shift work. These include brief periods of on-site napping. Maintaining a consistent sleep-wake schedule even on days off is best but somewhat unrealistic. For night shift work, scheduling the sleep period just before going to work increases alertness and vigilance, improves reaction times, and decreases accidents during night shift work. Nurses who have control over their work schedules appear to have less sleep disruption than those whose schedule is imposed. As a nurse, you need to manage the impact of sleep disruption by using sleep hygiene practices.

CASE STUDY

Insomnia

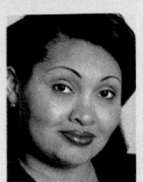

(© JackF/ iStock/ Thinkstock.)

Patient Profile

G.P., a 49-yr-old black woman, is seen in the primary care clinic for chronic fatigue and disturbed sleep. She is postmenopausal based on self-report. In the past year, since the end of her periods, she has had daily hot flashes and sleep problems. She denies any other health problems. On a usual workday she drinks 2 cups of hot tea in the morning and a can of diet cola in the late afternoon. Currently she is taking OTC diphenhydramine for sleep. Her partner, who has accompanied her to the clinic, states that her snoring has gotten worse, and it is interfering with his sleep.

Subjective Data

- Reports hot flashes and nighttime sweating
- Reports daytime tiredness and fatigue
- States she has trouble getting to sleep and staying asleep

Objective Data

Physical Examination

- Laboratory evaluations within normal limits
- Height 5'6"
- Weight 190 lb

Diagnostic Studies

- Nighttime PSG study reveals episodes of obstructive sleep apnea

Interprofessional Care

- CPAP nightly
- Referred for weight reduction counseling
- Education about sleep hygiene

Discussion Questions

1. What are G.P.'s risk factors for sleep apnea?
2. What are the major health risks for G.P. from sleep apnea?
3. *Priority Decision:* Based on the assessment data provided, what are the priority nursing diagnoses?
4. How does CPAP work?
5. *Priority Decision:* Based on your assessment of G.P., what are the priority nursing interventions for her?
6. *Collaboration:* For the interventions that you identified in the previous question, which can you delegate to unlicensed assistive personnel (UAP)?
7. *Patient-Centered Care:* What specific sleep hygiene practices could G.P. use to improve the quality of her sleep?
8. *Collaboration:* What referrals may be indicated for G.P.?

Answers available at *http://evolve.elsevier.com/Lewis/medsurg.*

BRIDGE TO NCLEX EXAMINATION

The number of the question corresponds to the same-numbered outcome at the beginning of the chapter.

1. Sleep is *best* described as a
   a. loosely organized state similar to coma.
   b. quiet state in which there is little brain activity.
   c. state in which a person has reduced sensitivity to pain.
   d. state in which a person lacks conscious awareness of the environment.

2. Which statements are true about rapid eye movement (REM) sleep (*select all that apply*)?
   a. The EEG pattern is quiescent.
   b. Muscle tone is greatly reduced.
   c. It occurs only once in the night.
   d. It is physiologically similar to NREM sleep.
   e. The most vivid dreaming occurs during this phase.

3. Insufficient sleep is associated with (*select all that apply*)
   a. increased body mass index.
   b. increased insulin resistance.
   c. impaired cognitive functioning.
   d. improved immune responsiveness.
   e. increased daytime body temperature.

4. When teaching the patient with primary insomnia about sleep hygiene, the nurse should emphasize
   a. the importance of daytime naps.
   b. the need for long-term use of hypnotics.
   c. the need to exercise about 1 hour before bedtime.
   d. the importance of avoiding caffeine 6 to 9 hours before bedtime.

5. An overweight patient with sleep apnea would like to avoid using a nasal CPAP device. To help him reach this goal, the nurse suggests that the patient
   a. lose excess weight.
   b. take a nap during the day.
   c. eat a high-protein snack at bedtime.
   d. use mild sedatives or alcohol at bedtime.

6. While caring for a patient with a history of narcolepsy with cataplexy, the nurse can delegate which activity to the unlicensed assistive personnel (UAP)?
   a. Teaching about the timing of medications
   b. Walking the patient to and from the bathroom
   c. Developing a plan of care with a family member
   d. Planning an appropriate diet that avoids caffeine-containing foods

7. Strategies to reduce sleepiness during nighttime working include
   a. exercising before work.
   b. taking melatonin before working the night shift.
   c. sleeping for at least 2 hours immediately before work time.
   d. walking for 10 minutes every 4 hours during the night shift.

1. d, 2. b, e, 3. a, b, c, 4. d, 5. a, 6. b, 7. c

For rationales to these answers and even more NCLEX review questions, visit *http://evolve.elsevier.com/Lewis/medsurg.*

(e) EVOLVE WEBSITE/RESOURCES LIST

http://evolve.elsevier.com/Lewis/medsurg
Review Questions (Online Only)
Key Points
Answer Keys for Questions
- Rationales for Bridge to NCLEX Examination Questions
- Answer Guidelines for Case Study on p. 100

Conceptual Care Map Creator
Audio Glossary
Content Updates

REFERENCES

1. National Heart, Lung, and Blood Institute: How much sleep is enough? Retrieved from *www.nhlbi.nih.gov/health-topics/sleep-deprivation-and-deficiency*.
2. Centers for Disease Control and Prevention: Short sleep duration among U.S. adults. Retrieved from *www.cdc.gov/sleep/data_statistics.html*.
3. National Sleep Foundation: Facts and stats. Retrieved from *www.drowsy-driving.org/about/facts-and-stats/*.
4. Centers for Disease Control and Prevention: Insufficient sleep is a public health problem. Retrieved from *www.cdc.gov/features/dssleep/*.
*5. Saper CB, Fuller PM: Wake-sleep circuitry: An overview, *Curr Opin Neurobiol* 44:186, 2017.
6. Bhat S, Chokroverty S: Hypersomnia in neurodegenerative diseases, *Sleep Med Clin* 12:443, 2017.
7. Equihua-Benitez AC, Guzman-Vasquez K, Drucker-Colin R: Understanding sleep-wake mechanisms and drug discovery, *Expert Opin Drug Discov* 12:643, 2017.
8. Chow M, Cao M: The hypocretin/orexin system in sleep disorders: Preclinical insights and clinical progress, *Nat Sci Sleep* 8:81, 2016.
9. Berry RB, Brooks R, Gamaldo C, et al: *The American Academy of Sleep Medicine: The AASM manual for the scoring of sleep and associated events*, Westchester, IL, 2017, American Academy of Sleep Medicine.
*10. Lowe CJ, Safati A, Hall PA: The neurocognitive consequences of sleep restriction: A meta-analytic review, *Neurosci Biobehav Rev* 80:58, 2017.
*11. Hossin MZ: From habitual sleep hours to morbidity and mortality: Existing evidence, potential mechanisms, and future agenda, *Sleep Health* 2:146, 2016.
*12. Boyko Y, Jennum P, Nikolic M, et al: Sleep in intensive care unit: The role of environment, *J Crit Care* 37:99, 2017.
*13. Simpson NS, Scott-Sutherland J, Gautam S, et al : Chronic exposure to insufficient sleep alters processes of pain habituation and sensitization. *Pain* 159:33, 2018.
*14. Sorscher AJ: Insomnia: Getting to the cause, facilitating relief, *J Fam Pract* 66:216, 2017.
*15. Sateia MJ, Buysse DJ, Krystal AD, et al: Clinical practice guideline for the pharmacologic treatment of chronic insomnia in adults: An AASM clinical practice guideline, *J Clin Sleep Med* 13:307, 2017.
*16. Asnis GM, Thomas M, Henderson MA: Pharmacotherapy treatment options for insomnia: A primer for clinicians, *Int J Mol Sci* 17:50, 2016.
*17. Markota M, Rummans TA, Bostwick JM, et al: Benzodiazepine use in older adults: Dangers, management, and alternative therapies, *Mayo Clin Proc* 91:1632, 2016.
*18. Noyek S, Yaremchuk K, Rotenberg B: Does melatonin have a meaningful role as a sleep aid for jet lag recovery? *Laryngoscope* 126:1719, 2016.
*19. Semelka M, Wilson J, Floyd R. Diagnosis and treatment of obstructive sleep apnea in adults. *Am Fam Physician.* 2016; 94:355.
*20. Abuzaid AS, Al Ashry HS, Elbadawi A, et al: Meta-analysis of cardiovascular outcomes with continuous positive airway pressure therapy in patients with obstructive sleep apnea, *Am J Cardiol* 120:693, 2017.
21. American Academy of Sleep Medicine: *International classification of sleep disorders*, Darien, IL, 2014, American Academy of Sleep Medicine. (Classic)
*22. Bhattarai J, Sumerall S: Current and future treatment options for narcolepsy: A review, *Sleep Sci* 10:19, 2017.
23. National Sleep Foundation: Aging and sleep. Retrieved from *www.sleepfoundation.org/sleep-topics/aging-and-sleep*.
*24. Tahghighi M, Rees CS, Brown JA, et al: What is the impact of shift work on the psychological functioning and resilience of nurses? An integrative review, *J Adv Nurs* 73:2065, 2017.

*Evidence-based information for clinical practice.

8

Pain

Debra Miller-Saultz

One word frees us of all the weight and pain of life. That word is love.

Sophocles

ⓔ http://evolve.elsevier.com/Lewis/medsurg/

CONCEPTUAL FOCUS

Coping

Functional Ability

Pain

LEARNING OUTCOMES

1. Define pain.
2. Describe the neural mechanisms of pain and pain modulation.
3. Distinguish between nociceptive and neuropathic types of pain.
4. Explain the physical and psychologic effects of unrelieved pain.
5. Interpret the subjective and objective data that are obtained from a comprehensive pain assessment.

6. Describe effective interprofessional pain management techniques.
7. Describe drug and nondrug methods of pain relief.
8. Explain your role and responsibility in pain management.
9. Discuss ethical and legal issues related to pain and pain management.
10. Evaluate the influence of one's own knowledge, beliefs, and attitudes about pain assessment and management.

KEY TERMS

analgesic ceiling, p. 111
breakthrough pain (BTP), p. 108
central sensitization, p. 105
complex regional pain syndrome (CRPS), p. 107
equianalgesic dose, p. 117
modulation, p. 106

multimodal analgesia, p. 110
neuropathic pain, p. 106
nociception, p. 103
nociceptive pain, p. 106
pain, p. 102
patient-controlled analgesia (PCA), p. 119

patient-controlled epidural analgesia (PCEA), p. 119
peripheral sensitization, p. 104
transduction, p. 104
transmission, p. 104
trigger point, p. 120

Pain is a complex, multidimensional experience that can cause suffering and decreased quality of life. Pain is 1 of the major reasons that people seek health care. To effectively assess and manage patients with pain, you need to understand the physiologic and psychosocial dimensions of pain. Pain is interrelated with many concepts. Culture and spirituality influence the expression of pain. Acute pain adversely affects mobility and sleep, leading to fatigue. Having pain is a stressor that can lead to depression. Those with severe or chronic pain are more likely to describe their health as poor and have increased mortality. This chapter presents evidence-based information to help you assess and safely manage pain in collaboration with other interprofessional team members.

MAGNITUDE OF PAIN PROBLEM

Millions of people suffer from pain. Each year in the United States, at least 25 million people have acute pain because of injury or surgery. Common chronic pain conditions, such as arthritis, migraine headache, and back pain, affect more than 1 million American adults.[1] Of the 1.7 million people diagnosed with cancer each year, about 60% have pain during treatment.[2] Despite the high prevalence and costs of acute and chronic pain, inadequate pain management occurs. Consequences of unrelieved acute pain are shown in Table 8.1.

DEFINITIONS AND DIMENSIONS OF PAIN

In 1968 Margo McCaffery, a nurse and pioneer in pain management, defined **pain** as "whatever the person experiencing the pain says it is, existing whenever the person says it does."[3] The International Association for the Study of Pain (IASP) defines *pain* as "an unpleasant sensory and emotional experience associated with actual or potential tissue damage, or described in terms of such damage."[1]

TABLE 8.1 Negative Consequences of Unrelieved Acute Pain

Response	Possible Consequences
Cardiovascular	
↑ Heart rate	Hypertension
↑ Cardiac output	Unstable angina
↑ Peripheral vascular resistance	Myocardial infarction
↑ Myocardial oxygen consumption	Deep vein thrombosis
↑ Coagulation	
Endocrine and Metabolic	
↑ Adrenocorticotropic hormone (ACTH)	Weight loss (from ↑ catabolism)
↑ Cortisol	↑ Respiratory rate
↑ Antidiuretic hormone (ADH)	↑ Heart rate
↑ Epinephrine and norepinephrine	Shock
↑ Renin, ↑ aldosterone	Glucose intolerance
↓ Insulin	Hyperglycemia
Gluconeogenesis	Fluid overload
Glycogenolysis	Hypertension
Muscle protein catabolism	Urinary retention, ↓ urine output
Gastrointestinal	
↓ Gastric and intestinal motility	Constipation
	Anorexia
	Paralytic ileus
Immunologic	
↓ Immune response	Infection
Musculoskeletal	
Muscle spasm	Immobility
Impaired muscle function	Weakness and fatigue
Neurologic	
Impaired cognitive function	Confusion
	Impaired ability to think, reason, and make decisions
Renal and Urologic	
↓ Urine output	Fluid imbalance
Urinary retention	Electrolyte disturbance
Respiratory	
↓ Tidal volume	Atelectasis
Hypoxemia	Pneumonia
↓ Cough, sputum retention	

TABLE 8.2 Dimensions of Pain

Dimension	Description
Affective	• Emotional responses to pain include anger, fear, depression, and anxiety • Negative emotions impair patient's quality of life
Behavioral	• Observable actions (e.g., grimacing, irritability, coping skills) are used to express or control pain • People unable to communicate may have behavioral changes (e.g., agitation, combativeness)
Cognitive	• Beliefs, attitudes, memories, and meaning attributed to pain influence the ways in which a person responds to pain
Physiologic	• Genetic, anatomic, and physical determinants of pain influence how painful stimuli are processed, recognized, and described
Sociocultural	• Age and gender influence nociceptive processes and responses to opioids • Families and caregivers influence patient's response to pain through their beliefs, behaviors, and support • Culture affects pain expression, medication use, pain-related beliefs, and coping methods

GENDER DIFFERENCES
Pain

Men
- Are less likely to report pain than women
- Report more control over pain
- Are less likely to use alternative treatments for pain

Women
- More often have migraine headache, back pain, arthritis, fibromyalgia, irritable bowel syndrome, neuropathic pain, abdominal pain, and foot ache
- Are more likely to be diagnosed with a nonspecific, somatic disorder
- Are less likely to receive analgesics for symptoms of chest and abdominal pain

These definitions emphasize the subjective nature of pain, in which the patient's self-report is the most valid means of assessment. Although understanding the patient's experience and relying on his or her self-report is essential, this view is problematic for many patients. For example, patients who are comatose or who have dementia, patients who are mentally disabled or challenged, and patients with expressive aphasia have varying abilities to report pain. In these instances, you must include nonverbal information, such as observed behaviors, into your pain assessment.

The emotional distress of pain can cause *suffering*, which is the state of distress associated with loss. Suffering can result in a sense of insecurity, lack of control, and spiritual distress. It is important to assess the ways in which a person's spirituality influences and is influenced by pain.[4]

The meaning of the pain to the person is important. For example, a woman in labor may have severe pain but can manage it without analgesics because for her it is associated with a joyful event. Moreover, she may feel control over her pain because of the training she received in prenatal classes and the knowledge that the pain is time-limited. In contrast, a woman with chronic, undefined musculoskeletal pain may be stressed by thoughts that her pain is "not real," is uncontrollable, or is caused by her own actions. Perceptions influence the ways in which a person responds to pain and must be included in a comprehensive treatment plan.

Some people cope with pain by distracting themselves. Others convince themselves that the pain is permanent, untreatable, and overwhelming. People who believe their pain is uncontrollable and overwhelming are more likely to have poor outcomes.[5] The biopsychosocial model of pain includes the physiologic, affective, cognitive, behavioral, and sociocultural dimensions of pain (Table 8.2).

Families and caregivers influence the patient's response to pain through their beliefs and behaviors. For example, families may discourage the patient from taking opioids because they have preconceived notions and fears that the patient may become addicted. Understanding these beliefs helps you address them through patient and family teaching.

Pain Mechanisms

Nociception is the physiologic process by which information about tissue damage is communicated to the central nervous system (CNS). It involves 4 processes: (1) transduction, (2) transmission, (3) perception, and (4) modulation (Fig. 8.1).

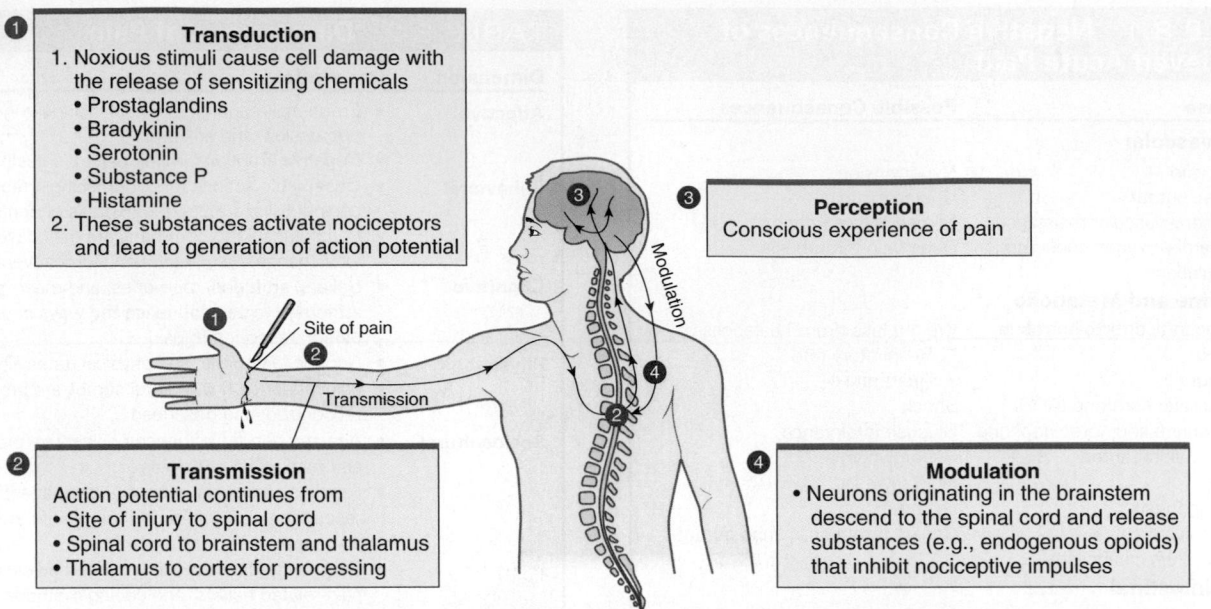

FIG. 8.1 Nociceptive pain originates when the tissue is injured. 1, Transduction occurs when there is release of chemical mediators. 2, Transmission involves the conduct of the action potential from the periphery (injury site) to the spinal cord and then to the brainstem, thalamus, and cerebral cortex. 3, Perception is the conscious awareness of pain. 4, Modulation involves signals from the brain going back down the spinal cord to modify incoming impulses. (Developed by McCaffery M, Pasero C, Paice JA. Modified from McCaffery M, Pasero C: *Pain: Clinical manual*, ed 2, St Louis, 1999, Mosby.)

Transduction. Transduction involves the conversion of a noxious mechanical, thermal, or chemical stimulus into an electrical signal called an action potential. Noxious (tissue-damaging) stimuli, including thermal (e.g., sunburn), mechanical (e.g., surgical incision), or chemical (e.g., toxic substances) stimuli, cause the release of chemicals, such as substance P and adenosine triphosphate (ATP), into the damaged tissues. Other chemicals are released from mast cells (e.g., serotonin, histamine, prostaglandins) and macrophages (e.g., cytokines). These chemicals activate nociceptors, which are specialized receptors, or free nerve endings, which respond to painful stimuli. Activation of nociceptors results in an action potential that is carried from the nociceptors to the spinal cord primarily by small, rapidly conducting, myelinated A-delta fibers and slowly conducting unmyelinated C fibers.

In addition to stimulating nociceptors, inflammation and the subsequent release of chemical mediators lower nociceptor thresholds. As a result, nociceptors may fire in response to stimuli that previously were insufficient to elicit a response. They may also fire in response to non-noxious stimuli, such as light touch. We call this increased susceptibility to nociceptor activation peripheral sensitization. Leukotrienes, prostaglandins, cytokines, and substance P are involved in peripheral sensitization. Cyclooxygenase (COX), produced in the inflammatory response, also plays a key role in peripheral sensitization. A clinical example of this process is sunburn. This thermal injury causes inflammation that results in a sensation of pain when the affected skin is lightly touched. Peripheral sensitization amplifies signal transmission, which in turn contributes to central sensitization (discussed under Dorsal Horn Processing). The pain from activation of peripheral nociceptors is called nociceptive pain (described later in the chapter on p. 106).

Therapies that change either the local environment or sensitivity of the peripheral nociceptors can prevent transduction and initiation of an action potential. Decreasing the effects of chemicals released at the periphery is the basis of several drug approaches to pain relief. For example, nonsteroidal antiinflammatory drugs (NSAIDs), such as ibuprofen (Advil), exert their analgesic effects by blocking the action of COX (see Fig. 11.4).

Transmission. Transmission is the process by which pain signals are relayed from the periphery to the spinal cord and then to the brain. Nerves that carry pain impulses from the periphery to the spinal cord are called *primary afferent fibers*. These include A-delta and C fibers. Each is responsible for a different pain sensation. A-delta fibers conduct pain rapidly and are responsible for the initial, sharp pain that accompanies tissue injury. C fibers transmit painful stimuli more slowly and produce pain that is typically aching or throbbing. Primary afferent fibers end in the dorsal horn of the spinal cord. Activity in the dorsal horn integrates and modulates pain inputs from the periphery.

The movement of pain impulses from the site of transduction to the brain is shown in Fig. 8.1. Three segments are involved in nociceptive signal transmission: (1) transmission along the peripheral nerve fibers to the spinal cord, (2) dorsal horn processing, and (3) transmission to the thalamus and cerebral cortex.

Drugs that stabilize the neuronal membrane act on peripheral sodium channels to inhibit movement of nerve impulses. These medications include local anesthetics (e.g., injectable or topical lidocaine, bupivacaine [Sensorcaine]) and antiseizure drugs (e.g., gabapentin [Neurontin]).

Transmission to Spinal Cord. The *first-order neuron* extends the entire distance from the periphery to the dorsal horn with no synapses. For example, an afferent fiber from the great toe travels from the toe through the fifth lumbar nerve root into

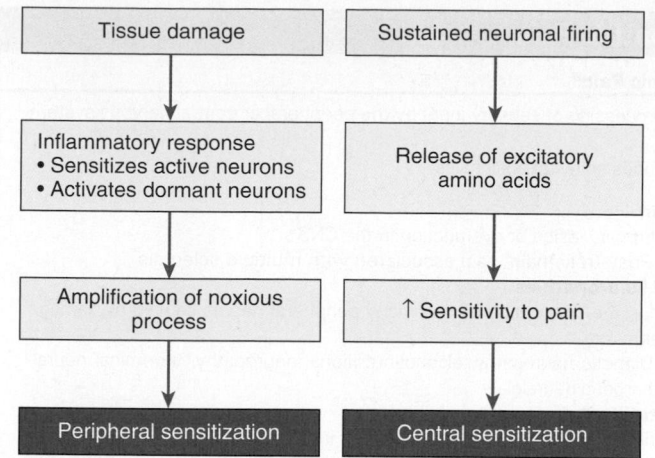

FIG. 8.2 Sequence of mechanisms leading to peripheral and central sensitization. Increased susceptibility to nociceptor activation is called *peripheral sensitization.* Increased sensitivity and hyperexcitability of neurons in the CNS is called *central sensitization.*

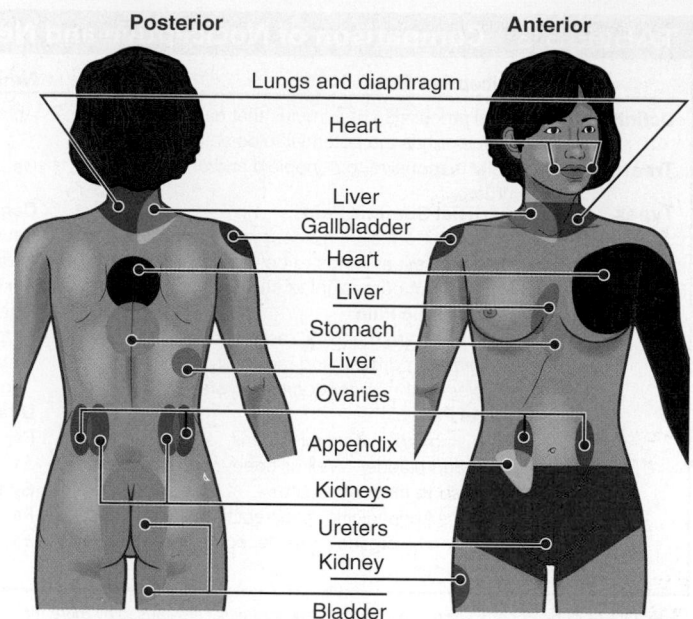

FIG. 8.3 Typical areas of referred pain.

the spinal cord; it is 1 cell. Once generated, an action potential travels all the way to the spinal cord unless it is blocked by a sodium channel inhibitor (e.g., local anesthetic) or disrupted by a lesion, such as a dorsal root entry zone lesion.

The way nerve fibers enter the spinal cord is central to the notion of spinal dermatomes. *Dermatomes* are areas on the skin that are innervated primarily by a single spinal cord segment. The distinct pattern of the rash caused by herpes zoster (shingles) across the back and trunk is determined by dermatomes (see Fig. 23.7). Different dermatomes and their innervations are shown in Fig. 55.7.

Dorsal Horn Processing. Once a nociceptive signal arrives in the spinal cord, it is processed within the dorsal horn. Neurotransmitters released from the afferent fiber bind to receptors on nearby cells. Some of these neurotransmitters (e.g., glutamate, substance P) produce activation. Others (e.g., γ-aminobutyric acid [GABA], serotonin) inhibit activation of nearby cells. In this area, exogenous and endogenous opioids (e.g., encephalin, β-endorphin) play a vital role by binding to opioid receptors and blocking the release of neurotransmitters, especially substance P. They produce analgesic effects similar to those of exogenous opioids, such as morphine. The neurons that project to the thalamus are called *second-order neurons.*

Increased sensitivity and hyperexcitability of neurons in the CNS is called **central sensitization**. With central sensitization, the central processing circuits are altered. Peripheral tissue damage or nerve injury can cause central sensitization. Continued nociceptive input from the periphery maintains it (Fig. 8.2). In some cases, central sensitization can be long-lasting due to multiple changes that occur in the periphery and CNS.[6]

Because of the increased excitability of CNS neurons, normal sensory inputs cause abnormal sensing and responses to painful and other stimuli. This explains why some people have significant pain from touch or tactile stimulation in and around the areas of tissue or nerve injury. We call this *allodynia,* pain from a stimulus that is not typically painful. It also explains why some people have *hyperalgesia,* an exaggerated or increased pain response to noxious stimuli.

With ongoing stimulation of slowly conducting unmyelinated C-fiber nociceptors, firing of specialized dorsal horn neurons gradually increases. These inputs can lead to the sprouting of wide dynamic range (WDR) neuron dendrites and

the induction of glutamate-dependent *N*-methyl-D-aspartate (NMDA) receptors. This results in an increased capacity to transmit a broader range of stimuli-producing signals, which are then passed up the spinal cord and to the brain. This process is known as *wind-up.*[7] Activation of NMDA receptors also plays a role in wind-up. NMDA receptor antagonists, such as ketamine (Ketalar), potentially interrupt or block mechanisms that lead to or sustain central sensitization. Wind-up is like central sensitization and hyperalgesia in that it occurs in response to C-fiber inputs. Wind-up is different, however, in that it can be short-lasting, while central sensitization and hyperalgesia persist over time.

It is important for you to understand that acute, unrelieved pain leads to chronic pain through central sensitization. Even brief intervals of acute pain can induce long-term neuronal remodeling and sensitization *(plasticity),* chronic pain, and lasting psychologic distress.

Neuroplasticity refers to processes that allow neurons in the brain to compensate for injury and adjust their responses to new situations or changes in their environment.[8] Neuroplasticity contributes to adaptive mechanisms for reducing pain but can result in maladaptive mechanisms that enhance pain sensitivity.

Genetic variability may play a key role in changes that occur in the CNS and the response to different analgesic therapies to treat pain. Understanding this phenomenon helps explain individual differences in response to pain and why some patients develop chronic pain conditions and others do not.[9] *Referred pain* must be considered when interpreting the location of pain reported by the person with an injury or a disease involving visceral organs. The location of a stimulus may be distant from the pain location reported by the patient (Fig. 8.3). For example, pain from liver disease often occurs in the right upper abdominal quadrant. It also can be referred to the anterior and posterior neck region, shoulder area, and posterior flank area. If we do not consider referred pain when evaluating a pain location report, diagnostic tests and therapy could be misdirected.

TABLE 8.3 Comparison of Nociceptive and Neuropathic Pain

	Nociceptive Pain	Neuropathic Pain*
Definition	Normal processing of stimulus that damages normal tissue or has the potential to do so if prolonged	Abnormal processing of sensory input by the peripheral or central nervous system
Treatment	Usually responsive to nonopioid and/or opioid drugs	Usually includes adjuvant analgesics
Types	**Superficial Somatic Pain**	**Central Pain**
	Pain arising from skin, mucous membranes, subcutaneous tissue. Tends to be well localized	Caused by primary lesion or dysfunction in the CNS
	Examples: Sunburn, skin contusions	*Examples:* Poststroke pain, pain associated with multiple sclerosis
	Deep Somatic Pain	**Peripheral Neuropathies**
	Pain arising from muscles, fasciae, bones, tendons. Localized or diffuse and radiating	Pain felt along the distribution of 1 or many peripheral nerves caused by damage to the nerve
	Examples: Arthritis, tendonitis, myofascial pain	*Examples:* Diabetic neuropathy, alcohol-nutritional neuropathy, trigeminal neuralgia, postherpetic neuralgia
	Visceral Pain	**Deafferentation Pain**
	Pain arising from visceral organs, such as the GI tract and bladder. Well or poorly localized. Often referred to cutaneous sites	Pain resulting from a loss of or altered afferent input
		Examples: Phantom limb pain, postmastectomy pain, spinal cord injury pain
	Examples: Appendicitis, pancreatitis, cancer affecting internal organs, irritable bowel and bladder syndromes	**Sympathetically Maintained Pain**
		Pain that persists secondary to autonomic nervous system dysfunction
		Examples: Phantom limb pain, complex regional pain syndrome

*Some types of neuropathic pain (e.g., postherpetic neuralgia) are caused by more than 1 neuropathologic mechanism.

Transmission to Thalamus and Cortex. From the dorsal horn, nociceptive stimuli are communicated to the *third-order neuron,* primarily in the thalamus. Fibers of dorsal horn projection cells enter the brain through several pathways, including the spinothalamic tract and spinoreticular tract. Distinct thalamic nuclei receive nociceptive input from the spinal cord and have projections to several regions in the cerebral cortex, where the perception of pain is presumed to occur.

Therapeutic approaches that target pain transmission include opioid analgesics that bind to opioid receptors on primary afferent and dorsal horn neurons. These agents mimic the inhibitory effects of endogenous opioids. Another medication, baclofen (Lioresal), inhibits pain transmission by binding to GABA receptors, thus mimicking the inhibitory effects of GABA.

Perception. *Perception* occurs when pain is recognized, defined, and assigned meaning by the person experiencing the pain. In the brain, nociceptive input is perceived as pain. There is no single, precise location where pain perception occurs. Instead, pain perception involves several brain structures. For example, it is thought that the reticular activating system is responsible for warning the person to attend to the pain stimulus; the somatosensory system is responsible for localization and characterization of pain; and the limbic system is responsible for the emotional and behavioral responses to pain.

Cortical structures are crucial to constructing the meaning of the pain. Therefore behavioral strategies, such as distraction and relaxation, are effective pain-reducing therapies for many people. Meditation and imagery can affect pain perception. By directing attention away from the pain sensation, patients can reduce the sensory and affective components of pain.

Modulation. Modulation involves the activation of descending pathways that exert inhibitory or facilitatory effects on the transmission of pain (Fig. 8.1). Depending on the type and degree of modulation, nociceptive stimuli may or may not be perceived as pain. Modulation of pain signals can occur at the level of the periphery, spinal cord, brainstem, and cerebral cortex. Descending modulatory fibers release chemicals, such as serotonin, norepinephrine, GABA, and endogenous opioids, which can inhibit pain transmission.

Several antidepressants exert their effects through the modulatory systems. For example, tricyclic antidepressants (e.g., amitriptyline) and serotonin norepinephrine reuptake inhibitors (SNRIs) (e.g., venlafaxine) are used to manage chronic noncancer and cancer pain. These agents interfere with the reuptake of serotonin and norepinephrine, thereby increasing their availability to inhibit noxious stimuli.

CLASSIFICATION OF PAIN

We categorize pain in several ways. Most often, pain is categorized as nociceptive or neuropathic based on underlying pathology (Table 8.3). Another useful scheme is to classify pain as acute or chronic (Table 8.4).

Nociceptive Pain

Nociceptive pain is caused by damage to somatic or visceral tissue. *Somatic pain* often is further categorized as superficial or deep. *Superficial pain* arises from skin, mucous membranes, and subcutaneous tissues. It is often described as sharp, burning, or prickly. *Deep pain* is often described as aching or throbbing. It originates in bone, joint, muscle, skin, or connective tissue.

Visceral pain comes from the activation of nociceptors in the internal organs and lining of the body cavities, such as the thoracic and abdominal cavities. Visceral nociceptors respond to inflammation, stretching, and ischemia. Stretching of hollow viscera in the intestines and bladder that occurs from tumor involvement or obstruction can produce intense cramping pain. Examples of visceral nociceptive pain include pain from a surgical incision, pancreatitis, and inflammatory bowel disease.

Neuropathic Pain

Neuropathic pain is caused by damage to peripheral nerves or structures in the CNS. Although neuropathic pain is often associated with diabetic neuropathy and other neuropathic pain syndromes, around 8% of the general population has pain with neuropathic characteristics.[9] Typically described as numbing, hot, burning, shooting, stabbing, sharp, or electric shock–like,

TABLE 8.4 Differences Between Acute and Chronic Pain

	Acute Pain	Chronic Pain
Onset	Sudden	Gradual or sudden
Duration	<3 mo or as long as it takes for normal healing to occur	>3 mo. May start as acute injury or event but continues past the normal time for recovery
Severity	Mild to severe	Mild to severe
Cause of pain	Usually can identify a precipitating event (e.g., illness, surgery)	May not be known. Original cause of pain may differ from mechanisms that maintain the pain.
Course of pain	Decreases over time and goes away as recovery occurs	Typically pain does not go away Characterized by periods of increasing and decreasing pain
Typical physical and behavioral manifestations	Manifestations vary but can reflect sympathetic nervous system activation: • ↑ Heart rate, respiratory rate, BP • Diaphoresis, pallor • Anxiety, agitation, confusion • Urine retention	Common behavioral manifestations: • Flat affect • ↓ Physical activity • Fatigue • Withdrawal from social interaction
Usual goals of treatment	Pain control with ability to take part in recovery activities Minimize side effects of treatment	Pain control to the extent possible Focus on enhancing function and quality of life

neuropathic pain can be sudden, intense, short lived, or lingering. Paroxysmal firing of injured nerves is responsible for shooting and electric shock-like sensations. Common causes of neuropathic pain include trauma, inflammation, metabolic diseases (e.g., diabetes), alcoholism, nervous system infections (e.g., herpes zoster, human immunodeficiency virus), tumors, toxins, and neurologic diseases (e.g., multiple sclerosis). Examples of neuropathic pain conditions include phantom limb sensation, diabetic neuropathy, and trigeminal neuralgia. No single sign or symptom is diagnostic for neuropathic pain.

CNS lesions or dysfunction cause *central pain*. *Deafferentation pain* results from loss of or altered afferent input secondary to either peripheral nerve injury (e.g., amputation) or CNS damage, including a spinal cord injury. Painful peripheral polyneuropathies (pain felt along the distribution of multiple peripheral nerves) and painful mononeuropathies (pain felt along the distribution of a damaged nerve) arise from damage to peripheral nerves. They generate pain that people may describe as burning, paroxysmal, or shock-like. The patient may have positive or negative motor and sensory signs, including numbness, allodynia, or change in reflexes and motor strength.

Sympathetically maintained pain is associated with a group of conditions that have a degree of changes in autonomic nervous system. One particularly debilitating type is **complex regional pain syndrome (CRPS)**. Typical features include dramatic changes in the color and temperature of the skin over the affected limb or body part, accompanied by intense burning pain, skin sensitivity,

sweating, and swelling. CRPS type I is often triggered by tissue injury, surgery, or a vascular event, such as stroke.[10] CRPS type II includes all these features and a peripheral nerve lesion.

Neuropathic pain is often not well controlled by opioid analgesics alone. Treatment often requires a multimodal approach combining various adjuvant analgesics from different drug classes. These include tricyclic antidepressants (e.g., amitriptyline), SNRIs (e.g., bupropion [Wellbutrin, Zyban]), antiseizure drugs (e.g., pregabalin [Lyrica]), transdermal lidocaine, and α_2-adrenergic agonists (e.g., clonidine). NMDA receptor antagonists, such as ketamine, have shown promise in alleviating neuropathic pain refractory to other drugs.

Acute and Chronic Pain

Acute pain and chronic pain differ in their cause, course, manifestations, and treatment (Table 8.4). Examples of *acute pain* include postoperative pain, labor pain, pain from trauma (e.g., lacerations, fractures, sprains), pain from infection (e.g., dysuria from cystitis), and pain from acute ischemia. For acute pain, treatment includes analgesics for symptom control and treatment of the underlying cause (e.g., splinting for a fracture, antibiotic therapy for an infection). Normally, acute pain decreases over time as healing occurs. However, acute pain that persists can lead to disabling chronic pain states. For example, pain associated with herpes zoster subsides as the acute infection resolves, usually within a month. However, sometimes the pain persists and develops into a chronic pain state called *postherpetic neuralgia*. Because of the connection between inadequately treated acute pain and chronic pain, it is important to treat acute pain aggressively.

Chronic pain, or *persistent pain*, lasts for longer periods, often defined as longer than 3 months or past the time when an expected acute pain or acute injury should subside. The severity and functional impact of chronic pain often are disproportionate to objective findings because of changes in the nervous system not detectable with standard tests. Although acute pain functions as a signal, warning the person of potential or actual tissue damage, chronic pain does not appear to have an adaptive role. Chronic pain can be disabling and often is accompanied by anxiety and depression.

PAIN ASSESSMENT

Assessment is an essential, although often overlooked, step in pain management. Regularly screen all patients for pain and, when present, perform a more thorough pain assessment. The key to accurate and effective pain assessment is to consider the principles of pain assessment (Table 8.5).

The goals of a nursing pain assessment are to (1) describe the patient's pain experience to identify and implement appropriate pain management techniques and (2) identify the patient's goal for therapy and resources for self-management.

Elements of a Pain Assessment

Most components of a pain assessment involve direct interview or observation of the patient. Diagnostic studies and physical examination findings complete the initial assessment. Although the assessment differs according to the clinical setting, patient population, and point of care (i.e., whether the assessment is part of an initial workup or a reassessment of pain following therapy), the evaluation of pain should always be multidimensional (Table 8.6).

Before beginning any assessment, recognize that patients may use words other than "pain." For example, older adults may deny that they have pain but respond positively when asked

TABLE 8.5   Principles of Pain Assessment

Principles	Nursing Implications
1. Patients have the right to appropriate assessment and management of pain.	• Assess pain in *all* patients.
2. Pain is always subjective.	• Patient's self-report of pain is the single most reliable indicator of pain. • Accept and respect this self-report unless there are clear reasons for doubt.
3. Physiologic and behavioral signs of pain (e.g., tachycardia, grimacing) are not reliable or specific for pain.	• Do not rely primarily on observations and objective signs of pain unless the patient is unable to self-report pain.
4. Pain is an unpleasant sensory and emotional experience.	• Address physical and psychologic aspects of pain when assessing pain.
5. Assessment approaches, including tools, must be appropriate for the patient population.	• Special considerations are needed for assessing pain in patients with difficulty communicating. • Include family members in the assessment process (when appropriate).
6. Pain can exist even when no physical cause can be found.	• Do not attribute pain that does not have an identifiable cause to psychologic causes.
7. Different patients have different levels of pain in response to comparable stimuli.	• A uniform pain threshold does not exist.
8. Patients with chronic pain may be more sensitive to pain and other stimuli.	• Pain tolerance varies among and within persons depending on several factors (e.g., genetics, energy level, coping skills, prior experience with pain).
9. Unrelieved pain has adverse consequences. Acute pain that is not adequately controlled can result in physiologic changes that increase the chance of developing persistent pain.	• Encourage patients to report pain, especially patients who are reluctant to discuss pain, deny pain when it is probably present, or fail to follow through on prescribed treatments.

if they have soreness or aching. Document the specific words that the patient uses to describe pain. Then consistently ask the patient about pain using those words.

Pain Pattern. Assessing pain *onset* involves determining when the pain started. Patients with acute pain resulting from injury, acute illness, or treatment (e.g., surgery) typically know exactly when their pain began. Those with chronic pain may be less able to relate when the pain started. Establish the *duration* of the pain (how long it has lasted). This information helps to determine whether the pain is acute or chronic and helps identify the cause of the pain. For example, a patient with advanced cancer who has chronic low back pain from spinal stenosis reports a sudden, severe pain in the back that began 2 days ago. Knowing the onset and duration can lead to a diagnostic workup that may reveal new metastatic disease in the spine.

The pain pattern gives clues about the cause of the pain and directs its treatment. Many types of chronic pain (e.g., arthritis pain) can increase and decrease over time. A patient may have pain all the time (around-the-clock pain), as well as discrete periods of intermittent pain.

Breakthrough pain (BTP) is transient, moderate to severe pain that occurs in patients whose baseline persistent pain is otherwise mild to moderate and fairly well controlled. The average peak of BTP can be 3 to 5 minutes and can last up to 30 minutes or even longer. BTP can be either predictable or unpredictable. Patients can have 1 to many episodes per day. Several transmucosal fentanyl products are used specifically to treat BTP.

End-of-dose failure is pain that occurs before the expected duration of a specific analgesic. It should not be confused with BTP. Pain that occurs at the end of the duration of an analgesic often leads to a prolonged increase in the baseline persistent pain. For example, in a patient on transdermal fentanyl (Duragesic patches) the typical duration of action is 72 hours. An increase in pain after 48 hours on the drug would be an end-of-dose failure. End-of-dose failure signals the need for changes in the dose or scheduling of the analgesic. Episodic, procedural, or *incident pain* is a transient increase in pain that is caused by a specific activity or event that precipitates pain. Examples include dressing changes, movement, position changes, and procedures, such as catheterization.

TABLE 8.6   Nursing Assessment

Pain

Subjective Data

Important Health Information

Health history: Pain history includes onset, location, intensity, quality, patterns, aggravating and alleviating factors, and expression of pain. Coping strategies. Past treatments and their effectiveness. Review health care use related to the pain problem (e.g., emergency department visits, treatment at pain clinics, visits to primary HCPs and specialists)

Medications: Use of any prescription or over-the-counter, illicit, or herbal products for pain relief. Alcohol use

Nondrug measures: Use of therapies, such as massage, heat or ice, Reiki, aromatherapy, acupuncture, hypnosis, yoga, or meditation

Functional Health Patterns

Health perception–health management: Social and work history, mental health history, smoking history. Effects of pain on emotions, relationships, sleep, and activities. Interviews with family members. Records from psychologic/psychiatric treatment related to the pain

Elimination: Constipation related to opioid drug use, other medication use, or pain related to elimination

Activity-exercise: Fatigue, limitations in ability to perform activities of daily living (ADLs), instrumental activities of daily living (IADLs), and pain related to use of muscles

Sexuality-reproductive: Decreased libido

Coping–stress tolerance: Psychologic evaluation using standardized measures to examine coping style, depression, anxiety

Objective Data

Physical examination, including evaluation of functional limitations
Psychosocial evaluation, including mood

Location. Determining the *location* of pain helps us identify possible causes and treatment. Some patients may be able to specify the precise location(s) of their pain. Others may describe general areas or comment that they "hurt all over." The location of the pain may be referred from its origin to another site (Fig. 8.3). For example, myocardial infarction can result in pain in the left shoulder. Pain can radiate from its origin to another site. For example, angina pectoris can radiate from the chest to the jaw or down the left arm. We refer to this as radiating pain. *Sciatica* is pain that follows the course of the sciatic nerve. It may originate

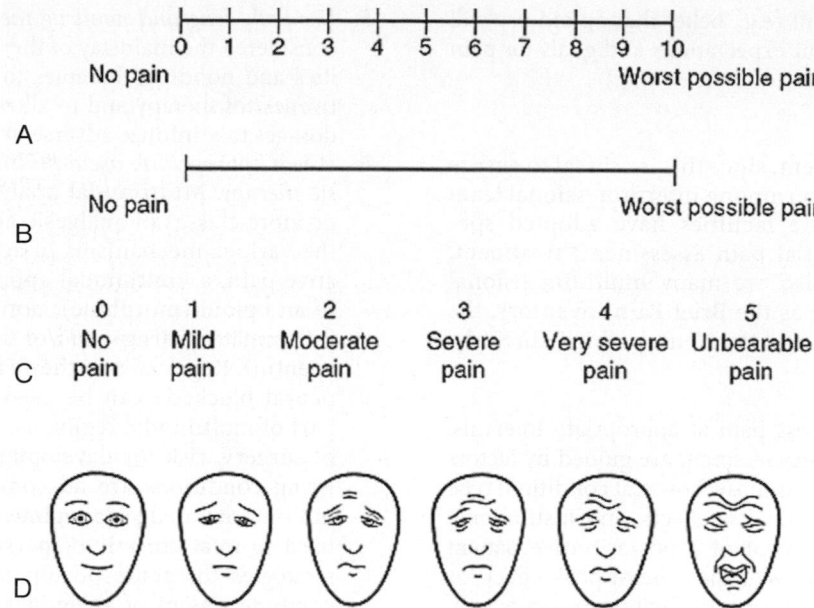

FIG. 8.4 Pain intensity scales. **A,** 0 to 10 numeric scale. **B,** Visual analog scale. **C,** Descriptive scale. **D,** Faces Pain Scale. (Modified from Baird M: *Manual of critical care nursing: Nursing interventions and collaborative management,* ed 2, St Louis, 2015, Elsevier.)

from joints or muscles around the back or from compression or damage to the sciatic nerve. The pain is projected along the course of the peripheral nerve, causing painful shooting sensations down the back of the thigh and inside of the leg to the foot.

Obtain information about the location of pain by asking the patient to (1) describe the site(s) of pain, (2) point to painful areas on the body, or (3) mark painful areas on a pain map. Because many patients have more than 1 site of pain, make certain that the patient describes every location.

Intensity. Assessing the severity, or *intensity,* of pain provides a reliable measure to determine the type of treatment and its effectiveness. Pain scales help the patient communicate pain intensity. Base your choice of a scale on the patient's developmental needs and cognitive status (Fig. 8.4). Most adults can rate the intensity of their pain using a numeric rating scale (e.g., 0 = no pain, 10 = the worst pain). Patients who wish to have word choices to quantify pain may prefer a verbal descriptor scale (e.g., none, mild, moderate, severe). For those oriented to vertical representations, the Pain Thermometer Scale is an option. Other visual pain measures, such as the Wong-Baker FACES pain tool, are useful for patients with cognitive or language barriers to describe their pain.[11] Pain assessment measures for cognitively impaired adults and nonverbal adults are addressed later in this chapter.

Although intensity is an important factor in determining analgesic approaches, do not dose patients with opioids solely based on reported pain scores.[12] Opioid "dosing by numbers" without considering a patient's sedation level and respiratory status can lead to unsafe practices and serious adverse events. Safer analgesic administration can be achieved by balancing an amount of pain relief with analgesic side effects and using a multimodal approach. (Multimodal approach is described later in this chapter.) Adjustments in therapy can be made to promote better pain control and minimize adverse outcomes.

Quality. The pain *quality* refers to the nature or characteristics of the pain. For example, patients often describe neuropathic pain as burning, numbing, shooting, stabbing, electric shock–like, or itchy. Nociceptive pain may be described as sharp, aching, throbbing, dull, and cramping. Since the quality of pain relates

to a degree to the classification of pain (e.g., neuropathic, nociceptive), these descriptors can help to guide treatment options that best address the specific mechanism of pain.

Associated Symptoms. *Associated symptoms,* such as anxiety, fatigue, and depression, may worsen or be worsened by pain. Patients with pain often report poor sleep and subsequent daytime sleepiness. Poor sleep can further increase pain perception. Ask about aggravating factors that increase pain as well as activities and situations that alleviate pain. For example, musculoskeletal pain may be increased or decreased with movement and ambulation. Resting or immobilizing a painful body part can decrease pain. Knowing what makes pain better or worse can help characterize the type of pain and be helpful in selecting treatments.

Management Strategies. As people experience and live with pain, they may cope differently and be more or less willing to try different strategies to manage it. Some strategies are successful, while others are not. To maximize the effectiveness of the pain treatment plan, ask patients what they are using now to control pain, what they have used in the past, and the outcomes of these methods. Strategies include prescription and nonprescription drugs and nondrug therapies, such as hot and cold applications, complementary and alternative therapies (e.g., acupuncture), and relaxation strategies (e.g., imagery). It is important to document both those that work and those that are ineffective.

Impact of Pain. Pain can have a profound influence on a patient's quality of life and functioning. Assess the effect of the pain on the patient's ability to sleep, enjoy life, interact with others, perform work and household duties, and engage in physical and social activities. Assess the impact of pain on the patient's mood.

In an acute care setting, time limitations may dictate a shortened assessment. At a minimum, assess the effects of the pain on the patient's sleep and daily activities, relationships with others, physical activity, and emotional well-being. Include the ways in which the patient describes the pain and strategies used to cope with and control the pain.

Patient's Beliefs, Expectations, and Goals. Patient and family beliefs, attitudes, and expectations influence responses to pain and pain treatment. Assess for attitudes and beliefs that may hinder effective treatment (e.g., belief that opioid use will result in addiction). Ask about expectations and goals for pain management.

Documentation

Document the pain assessment, since this is critical to ensure safe, effective communication among interprofessional team members. Many health care facilities have adopted specific tools to record an initial pain assessment, treatment, and reassessment. There also are many multidimensional pain assessment tools, such as the Brief Pain Inventory, the McGill Pain Questionnaire, and the Neuropathic Pain Scale.

Reassessment

It is critical for you to reassess pain at appropriate intervals. The frequency and scope of reassessment are guided by factors such as pain severity, physical and psychosocial condition, type of intervention and risks for adverse effects, and institutional policy. For example, reassessment of a postoperative patient may be done frequently, such as at the time of peak effect for each analgesic dose. In a long-term care facility, residents with chronic pain are reassessed at least quarterly or with a change in condition or functional status.

PAIN TREATMENT

Basic Principles

All pain treatment plans are based on the following 10 principles and practice standards:

1. *Follow the principles of pain assessment* (Table 8.5). Remember that pain is a subjective experience. The patient is not only the best judge of his or her own pain but also the expert on the effectiveness of each pain treatment.
2. *Use a holistic approach to pain management.* The pain experience affects all aspects of a person's life. Thus a holistic approach to assessment, treatment, and evaluation is required.
3. *Every patient deserves adequate pain management.* Many patient populations, including ethnic minorities, cognitively impaired adults, and people with past or current substance abuse, are at risk for inadequate pain management. Be aware of your own biases and ensure that all patients are treated respectfully.
4. *Base the treatment plan on the patient's goals.* Discuss with the patient realistic goals for pain relief during the initial pain assessment. Although goals can be described in terms of pain intensity (e.g., the desire for average pain to decrease from "8/10" to "3/10"), with chronic pain conditions, encourage functional goal setting (e.g., a goal of performing certain daily activities, such as socializing and recreational activities). Encourage functional activities for the patient with acute pain as well. For example, the pain must be at a level that allows the patient to use the incentive spirometer, get out of bed, and ambulate. Over time, reassess these goals and progress made toward meeting them. The patient, in collaboration with the interprofessional team, determines new goals. If the patient has unrealistic goals for therapy, such as wanting to be completely rid of all chronic arthritis pain or be completely pain free after a major surgery, work with the patient to establish a more realistic goal.

5. *Use both drug and nondrug therapies.* Although drugs are considered the mainstay of therapy, include self-care activities and nondrug therapies to increase the overall effectiveness of therapy and to allow for the reduction of drug dosages to minimize adverse drug effects.
6. *When appropriate, use a multimodal approach to analgesic therapy.* **Multimodal analgesia** employs the use of 2 or more classes of analgesic agents to take advantage of the various mechanisms of action. For acute, postoperative pain, a multimodal approach may include the use of an opioid (morphine), nonopioid (nonsteroidal antiinflammatory drug), and/or antiseizure drug (e.g., gabapentin). Regional anesthesia and continuous peripheral neural blockade can be used with local anesthetics as part of multimodal regimens.[13] Factors such as age, type of surgery, risk for developing chronic pain, and coexisting conditions are all considered when designing a multimodal analgesic regimen. Multimodal analgesia is used to treat chronic or persistent pain. Similar to the strategies for acute postoperative pain, the goal is to combine classes of analgesics for the maximum benefit of relieving pain with minimum doses to achieve relief and reduce adverse events from analgesics. Multimodal regimens achieve superior pain relief, enhance patient satisfaction, and decrease adverse effects of individual drugs.[14]
7. *Address pain using an interprofessional approach.* The expertise and perspectives of an interprofessional team are often necessary to provide effective assessment and therapies for patients with both acute and chronic pain. For hospitalized patients or those with complex acute or chronic pain issues, anesthesiology-based pain services may be available to manage patients with technology-supported pain care (e.g., patient-controlled analgesia or regional analgesia). Team members for these services can include pain management nurses, nurse practitioners, clinical nurse specialists, anesthesiologists, and clinical pharmacists. These teams help to establish realistic goals with patients and families to facilitate recovery and discharge. Many outpatient pain management centers or clinics are available. Some provide comprehensive pain care and employ multiple providers, including anesthesiologists, rehabilitation physicians, nurses, psychologists, physical and occupational therapists, and social workers. Services may focus on medication management, pain interventional therapies, psychologic counseling, cognitive and behavioral therapies, rehabilitative therapies (physical and occupational therapy), and social services. Specialized pain treatment centers may also offer more holistic therapies, such as massage, music and art therapy, and acupuncture. Advise patients seeking specialized pain care from outpatient treatment centers to check about services that are provided.
8. *Evaluate the effectiveness of all therapies to ensure that they are meeting the patient's goals.* Achievement of an effective treatment plan often requires trial and error. Adjustments in drug, dosage, or route are common to achieve maximal benefits while minimizing adverse effects. This trial-and-error process can become frustrating for the patient and caregivers. Reassure them that pain relief, if not pain cessation, is possible and that the interprofessional team will continue to work with them to achieve adequate pain relief.

TABLE 8.7 Drug Therapy
Managing Side Effects of Pain Medications

Side effects can be managed by 1 or more of the following methods:
- Decreasing the dose of analgesic by 10% to 15%
- Changing to a different medication in the same class
- Adding a drug to counteract the adverse effect of the analgesic (e.g., using a stool softener for patients experiencing opioid-induced constipation)
- Using an administration route that minimizes drug concentrations (e.g., intraspinal administration of opioids used to minimize high drug levels that produce sedation, nausea, and vomiting)

9. *Prevent and/or manage medication side effects.* Side effects or adverse events are a major reason for treatment failure and nonadherence. Side effects are managed in 1 of several ways, as described in Table 8.7. You play a key role in monitoring for and treating side effects and in teaching patients and caregivers how to minimize these effects.

10. *Include patient and caregiver teaching throughout assessment and treatment.* Content should include information about the causes of the pain, pain assessment methods, treatment goals and options, expectations of pain management, proper use of drugs, side effect management, and nondrug and self-help pain relief measures. Document the teaching and include evaluation of patient and caregiver comprehension.

Drug Therapy for Pain

Pain medications generally are divided into 3 categories: non-opioids, opioids, and adjuvant drugs. Patient-centered treatment regimens may include medications from 1 or more of these groups. Mild pain often can be relieved using nonopioids alone. Moderate to severe pain usually requires an opioid. Certain types of pain, such as neuropathic pain, typically require adjuvant drug therapy alone or in combination with an opioid or another class of analgesics. Pain caused by cancer may be treated with chemotherapy or radiation therapy, as well as pain medications.

Nonopioids. Nonopioid analgesics include acetaminophen, aspirin and other salicylates, and NSAIDs (Table 8.8). These agents are characterized by (1) their analgesic properties have an **analgesic ceiling**; that is, increasing the dose beyond an upper limit provides no greater analgesia; (2) they do not produce tolerance or physical dependence; and (3) many are available without a prescription. To provide safe care, monitor over-the-counter (OTC) analgesic use to avoid serious problems related to drug interactions, side effects, and overdose.

Nonopioids are effective for mild to moderate pain. They are often used in conjunction with opioids because they allow for effective pain relief using lower opioid doses (thereby causing fewer opioid side effects). This phenomenon is called the *opioid-sparing effect.*

Aspirin is effective for mild pain, but its use is limited by its common side effects, including increased risk for bleeding, especially gastrointestinal (GI) bleeding. Other salicylates, such as choline magnesium trisalicylate (Trilisate), cause fewer GI problems and bleeding abnormalities. Similar to aspirin, acetaminophen (Tylenol) has analgesic and antipyretic effects. Unlike aspirin, it has no antiplatelet or antiinflammatory effects. Acetaminophen is well tolerated. It is metabolized by the liver.

TABLE 8.8 Drug Therapy
Selected Nonopioid Analgesics

Drug	Nursing Considerations
Nonsalicylate acetaminophen (Tylenol)	• Chronic overdose: Liver toxicity • Sustained release, rectal suppository, and injectable forms (OFIRMEV) available • Maximum daily dose of 3 g • Oral doses of >3 g may cause hepatotoxicity • Acute overdose: Acute liver failure • Chronic overdose: Liver toxicity • Maximum daily IV dose should not exceed 4 g/day for adults ≥50 kg
Nonsteroidal Antiinflammatory Drugs (NSAIDs)	
celecoxib (Celebrex)	• Causes fewer GI side effects (e.g., bleeding) than other NSAIDs, but risk still present • More costly than other NSAIDs • May increase risk for serious cardiovascular thrombotic events, myocardial infarction, and stroke • Risks may increase with duration of use, preexisting cardiovascular disease, or risk factors for cardiovascular disease
diclofenac K	• Use lowest effective dose for shortest possible duration • Available in oral, ophthalmic, topical preparations
ibuprofen (Advil)	• Use lowest effective dose for shortest possible duration • Increased risk for serious GI adverse events (bleeding, ulceration, perforation), especially in older adults • May increase risk for serious cardiovascular thrombotic events, myocardial infarction, and stroke • May increase risk for hypertension and renal insufficiency
ketorolac	• Limit treatment to 5 days • May precipitate renal failure in dehydrated patients
naproxen (Naprosyn, Aleve)	• Use lowest effective dose for shortest possible duration • Increased risk for serious GI adverse events (bleeding, ulceration, perforation), especially in older adults • Contraindicated for the treatment of perioperative pain in setting of coronary artery bypass graft (CABG) surgery
Salicylates	
aspirin	• Rectal suppository and sustained-release preparations available • Chance of upper GI bleeding • Used more often in low doses as a cardioprotective measure than for its analgesic properties
choline magnesium trisalicylate (Trilisate)	• Unlike aspirin and NSAIDs, does not increase bleeding time

Hepatotoxicity may result from chronic dosing of more than 3 g/day, acute overdose, or use by patients with severe preexisting liver disease.[15] Adding acetaminophen to opioid therapy produces an opioid-sparing effect, lower pain scores, and fewer side effects. This is the reason for opioid-acetaminophen combinations.

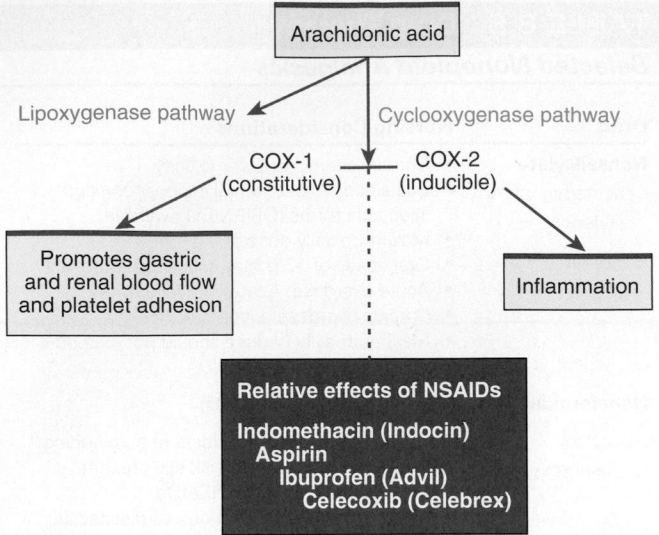

FIG. 8.5 Arachidonic acid is oxidized by 2 different pathways: lipoxygenase and cyclooxygenase. The cyclooxygenase pathway leads to 2 forms of the enzyme cyclooxygenase: COX-1 and COX-2. COX-1 is known as *constitutive* (always present), and COX-2 is known as *inducible* (its expression varies markedly depending on the stimulus). Nonsteroidal antiinflammatory drugs (NSAIDs) differ in their actions, with some having more effects on COX-1 and others more on COX-2. Indomethacin acts primarily on COX-1. Ibuprofen is equipotent on COX-1 and COX-2. Celecoxib primarily inhibits COX-2.

IV acetaminophen (Ofirmev) is used alone for the treatment of acute mild to moderate pain and as an adjunct to opioid analgesics or part of a multimodal analgesic regimen for moderate to severe pain. It must be given over 15 minutes and has a short duration of action. The daily dose should not exceed 4 g/day.

NSAIDs represent a broad class of drugs with varying efficacy and side effects. All NSAIDs inhibit COX, the enzyme that converts arachidonic acid into prostaglandins and related compounds. The enzyme has 2 forms: COX-1 and COX-2. COX-1 is found in almost all tissues. It is responsible for several protective physiologic functions. In contrast, COX-2 is made mainly at the sites of tissue injury, where it mediates inflammation (Fig. 8.5). Inhibition of COX-1 causes many of the untoward effects of NSAIDs, such as impairment of renal function, bleeding tendencies, GI irritation, and ulceration. COX-2 inhibition is associated with the therapeutic, antiinflammatory effects of NSAIDs. (Celecoxib [Celebrex] is a COX-2 inhibitor.) Older NSAIDs, such as ibuprofen, inhibit both forms of COX. We refer to them as nonselective NSAIDs.

Patients vary greatly in their responses to a specific NSAID. So, when 1 NSAID does not provide relief, another should be tried. NSAIDs are associated with many side effects, including GI problems ranging from dyspepsia to life-threatening ulceration and hemorrhage. NSAIDs can cause cognitive impairment and hypersensitivity reactions with asthma-like symptoms.

Patients at risk for NSAID-associated GI toxicity include those who have a recent history of peptic ulcer disease, patients who are older than 65, and those concurrently using corticosteroids or anticoagulants. If NSAIDs are used in patients at risk for GI bleeding, they should have concomitant therapy with misoprostol (Cytotec) or a proton pump inhibitor, such as omeprazole. NSAIDs should not be given concurrently with aspirin since this increases the risk for GI bleeding.

> **💊 DRUG ALERT   Nonsteroidal Antiinflammatory Drugs (NSAIDs)**
> - NSAIDs, except aspirin, have been linked to a higher risk for cardiovascular events, such as myocardial infarction, stroke, and heart failure.
> - Patients who have just had heart surgery should not take NSAIDs.

Opioids. Opioids (Table 8.9) produce their effects by binding to receptors in the CNS. This results in (1) inhibition of the transmission of nociceptive input from the periphery to the spinal cord, (2) altered limbic system activity, and (3) activation of the descending inhibitory pathways that modulate transmission in the spinal cord. Thus opioids act on several nociceptive processes.

Types of Opioids. Opioids are categorized according to their physiologic action (i.e., agonist, antagonist) and binding at specific opioid receptors (e.g., mu, kappa, delta). The most commonly given subclass of opioids is the pure opioid agonists, or morphine-like opioids, which bind to mu receptors.

Opioid agonists are used for acute and chronic pain. Although nociceptive pain seems to be more responsive to opioids than neuropathic pain, opioids may be used to treat both types of pain. In the treatment of neuropathic pain, antineuropathic pain drugs, such as antidepressants and antiseizure drugs, are recommended as first-line agents. Pure opioid agonists include morphine, oxycodone (OxyContin), hydrocodone, codeine, methadone, hydromorphone (Dilaudid), and levorphanol (Table 8.9). These drugs are effective for moderate to severe pain because they are potent, theoretically have no analgesic ceiling, and can be given by several routes. When opioids are prescribed for moderate pain, they are usually combined with a nonopioid analgesic, such as acetaminophen with codeine or hydrocodone plus acetaminophen or ibuprofen. Adding acetaminophen limits the total daily dose that we can give.

> **💊 DRUG ALERT   Morphine**
> - Morphine may cause respiratory depression.
> - If respirations are 12 or fewer breaths per minute, withhold medication and contact the health care provider (HCP).

Methadone has a unique mechanism of action as an NMDA receptor antagonist and mu opioid receptor agonist. It is used primarily in the treatment of chronic pain but can be used for acute pain. It produces analgesic effects independent of its action as an opioid.[16]

> **💊 DRUG ALERT   Methadone (Dolophine)**
> - Methadone may cause respiratory depression.
> - Methadone can cause cardiac toxicity, specifically QT prolongation.

Mixed agonist-antagonists (e.g., pentazocine [Talwin], butorphanol) bind as agonists on kappa receptors and as weak antagonists or partial agonists on mu receptors. Because of this difference in binding, mixed agonist-antagonists produce less respiratory depression than drugs that act only at mu receptors. These drugs cause more dysphoria and agitation. In addition, opioid agonist-antagonists have an analgesic ceiling and can precipitate withdrawal if used by a patient who is physically dependent on mu agonist drugs. Partial opioid agonists (e.g.,

TABLE 8.9   Drug Therapy

Opioid Analgesics

Drug	Routes of Administration	Nursing Considerations
Mu Agonists		
codeine oral (with acetaminophen [Tylenol #3]), codeine injectable	PO, subcutaneous	• Associated with higher incidence of nausea and constipation than other mu agonists • Many codeine preparations are combined with acetaminophen • 5%–10% of European Americans lack the enzyme to metabolize codeine to morphine
fentanyl (Sublimaze [IV]), Duragesic [transdermal], Actiq [transmucosal], Fentora [buccal tablet], Abstral [sublingual], Lazanda [nasal spray]	IV, epidural, intrathecal, transmucosal, transdermal	• Immediate onset after IV route, 7–8 min after IM route, 5–15 min after transmucosal route, up to 6 hr after transdermal route • For procedures, IV fentanyl often combined with benzodiazepines for analgesia and sedation • Very potent; dosage is in micrograms (mcg) • Transdermal fentanyl used only for chronic pain and should not be given to opioid-naive patients
hydrocodone with acetaminophen (Norco), hydrocodone with bitartrate (Hysingla, Zohydro ER), hydrocodone with ibuprofen (Reprexain)	PO (short-acting and long-acting)	• Used for moderate or moderately severe pain • For short-term management of acute pain (e.g., trauma, musculoskeletal)
hydromorphone (Dilaudid)	PO (short-acting and long-acting forms), rectal, IV, subcutaneous, epidural, intrathecal	• Slightly shorter duration than morphine • For moderate to severe pain • Tablets for sustained-release preparations are to be swallowed whole and must not be broken, chewed, dissolved, or crushed • Preparations for neuraxial administration must be preservative free
levorphanol	PO, IV, IM, subcutaneous	• Accumulates with repeated dosing
methadone (Dolophine)	PO, IV, IM	• High oral and rectal bioavailability • Accumulates with repeated dosing • Use with caution in older adults • Risk for QT interval prolongation
morphine (MS Contin, Kadian, Duramorph, Embeda)	PO (short-acting and sustained-release forms), rectal, IV, subcutaneous, epidural, intrathecal, sublingual, intranasal	• Standard of comparison for opioid analgesics (Table 8.12) • For moderate to severe pain • Can stimulate histamine release, leading to pruritus, with systemic administration • Tablets for sustained-release preparations are to be swallowed whole and must not be broken, chewed, dissolved, or crushed • Preparations for neuraxial administration must be preservative free
oxycodone (Roxicodone) oxycodone extended-release (OxyContin) oxycodone plus acetaminophen (Percocet) oxycodone plus aspirin (Percodan)	PO (short-acting and extended-release forms)	• Available as single entity and in combination with a nonopioid • Used similarly to oral morphine for moderate to severe pain • Often combined with a nonopioid for acute, moderate pain • Extended-release indicated for chronic pain
tapentadol (Nucynta)	PO (short-acting and extended release)	• Dual mechanism of action: Mu opioid agonist and blocks reuptake of norepinephrine and serotonin
tramadol (Ultram)	PO (short-acting and extended release)	• Dual mechanism of action: Mu opioid agonist and blocks reuptake of norepinephrine and serotonin • Used for moderate pain
Mu Mixed Agonist-Antagonists		
butorphanol	Nasal spray, injectable form Not available orally	• Psychotomimetic effects lower than with pentazocine • May precipitate withdrawal in opioid-dependent patients • Injectable used for acute pain • Nasal spray given for migraine headaches
pentazocine (Talwin)	IM, IV, subcutaneous	• May cause psychotomimetic effects (e.g., hallucinations) and may precipitate withdrawal in opioid-dependent patients • Not recommended for treatment of chronic pain and rarely for acute pain
Partial Agonists		
buprenorphine buprenorphine plus naloxone sublingual (Suboxone)	Sublingual, injectable, implant	• Sublingual form should not be chewed or swallowed • Lower abuse potential than morphine • Does not produce psychotomimetic effects • May precipitate withdrawal in opioid-dependent patients. Not readily reversed by naloxone • Buprenorphine plus naloxone used as a sublingual preparation to treat opioid dependence for easier withdrawal when necessary to taper from opioids

buprenorphine [Buprenex]) can produce some pain relief but bind tightly to mu receptors and can block the effect of other drugs. Agonist-antagonists and partial agonists currently have limited clinical application in pain management.

Dual-Mechanism Agents. Some analgesics have 2 distinct actions, or dual mechanisms. Tramadol (Ultram) is a weak mu agonist and inhibits the reuptake of norepinephrine and serotonin. It is effective in low back pain, osteoarthritis, fibromyalgia, diabetic peripheral neuropathic pain, polyneuropathy, and postherpetic neuralgia. The most common side effects are like those of other opioids, including nausea, constipation, dizziness, and sedation. As with other medications that increase serotonin and norepinephrine, avoid this drug in patients with a history of seizures because it lowers seizure threshold.

Tapentadol (Nucynta) is a centrally acting analgesic that works at mu receptors and inhibits norepinephrine reuptake. It is approved for management of moderate to severe acute pain. For chronic moderate to severe pain, an extended-release formula is available. The side effects are like those of conventional opioids, except that this drug is associated with less nausea and constipation.

Opioids to Avoid. Some opioids should be avoided for pain relief because of limited efficacy and/or toxicities. Meperidine (Demerol), or pethidine, is associated with neurotoxicity (e.g., seizures) caused by accumulation of its metabolite, normeperidine. Its use is limited for very short-term (i.e., less than 48 hours) treatment of acute pain when other opioid agonists are contraindicated.

 DRUG ALERT   Meperidine (Demerol)

> The American Pain Society does not recommend the use of meperidine as an analgesic.

Side Effects of Opioids. Common side effects of opioids include constipation, nausea and vomiting, sedation, respiratory depression, and pruritus. With continued use, many side effects diminish; the exception is constipation. Less common side effects include urinary retention, myoclonus, dizziness, confusion, and hallucinations. *Constipation* is the most common side effect of opioids. Left untreated, it may increase the person's pain and can lead to fecal impaction and paralytic ileus.

Because tolerance to opioid-induced constipation does not develop, a bowel regimen should be started at the beginning of opioid therapy and continued for as long as the person takes opioids. Although dietary fiber, fluids, and exercise should be encouraged, these measures alone may not be enough. Most patients should use a gentle stimulant laxative (e.g., senna) plus a stool softener (e.g., docusate sodium [Colace]). Other agents (e.g., Milk of Magnesia, bisacodyl, polyethylene glycol, lactulose) can be added if needed. Methylnaltrexone (Relistor), naldemedine (Symproic), and naloxegol (Movantik) are peripheral opioid receptor antagonists used for opioid-induced constipation when the response to traditional laxative and stool softener therapy is insufficient.

Nausea is often a problem in opioid-naive patients. The use of an antiemetic, such as ondansetron (Zofran), metoclopramide (Reglan), transdermal scopolamine, or hydroxyzine (Vistaril), can prevent or minimize nausea and vomiting until tolerance develops, usually within 1 week. Opioids delay gastric emptying (patient relates gastric fullness). Metoclopramide can reduce this effect. If nausea and vomiting are severe and persistent, changing to a different opioid may be needed.

Sedation is usually seen in opioid-naive patients being treated for acute pain. Regularly monitor patients receiving opioid analgesics for acute pain, especially in the first few days (e.g., after surgery). Be aware that the risk for unintended sedation in postoperative patients is greatest within 4 hours after leaving the postanesthesia care unit. Opioid-induced sedation resolves with the development of tolerance. Persistent sedation with chronic opioid use can be effectively treated with psychostimulants, such as caffeine, dextroamphetamine (Dexedrine), methylphenidate (Ritalin), or the anticataleptic drug modafinil (Provigil).

The risk for *respiratory depression* is higher in opioid-naive, hospitalized patients who are treated for acute pain. Clinically significant respiratory depression is rare in opioid-tolerant patients and when opioids are titrated to analgesic effect. Patients most at risk for respiratory depression include those who are age 65 or older, have a history of snoring or witnessed apneic episodes, report excessive daytime sleepiness, have underlying heart or lung disease, are obese (body mass index greater than 30 kg/m^2), have a history of smoking (more than 20 pack-years), or are receiving other CNS depressants (e.g., sedatives, benzodiazepines, antihistamines). For postoperative patients the greatest risk for opioid-related respiratory adverse events is within the first 24 hours after surgery. Clinically significant respiratory depression cannot occur in patients who are fully awake.

❓ CHECK YOUR PRACTICE

A 74-yr-old male patient returned to the clinical unit after surgery for a hip replacement. You are having difficulty arousing him with either verbal or physical stimulation. His wife tells you to just let him sleep. His respiratory rate ranges from 8 to 10 breaths/min.
• What should you do?

Frequently monitor both the sedation level and respiratory rate in patients receiving opioid analgesics.[17] A sedation scale can be used for monitoring and providing appropriate interventions based on the level of sedation (Table 8.10).

⚠ SAFETY ALERT   Sedation and Respiratory Depression

• If the patient's respiratory rate falls below 8 or 10 breaths/min and the sedation level is 3 or greater, you should vigorously stimulate the patient and try to keep the patient awake.
• If the patient becomes oversedated, apply oxygen.
• In this situation, the opioid dose should be reduced.

For patients who are excessively sedated or unresponsive, we can give naloxone, an opioid antagonist that rapidly reverses the effects of opioids. Naloxone can be given IV, subcutaneously, or intranasally. Evzio (hand-held autoinjector containing naloxone) can be used by a caregiver or family member to treat a person known or suspected to have had an opioid overdose.

If the patient has been taking opioids regularly for more than a few days, use naloxone carefully because it can precipitate severe, agonizing pain; profound withdrawal symptoms; hypertension; and pulmonary edema. Because naloxone's half-life is shorter than that of most opioids, frequently monitor the patient.

Pruritus (itching) is another common side effect of opioids. It occurs most often when opioids are given by neuraxial (i.e., epidural, intrathecal) routes. Managing opioid-induced pruritus in noncancer patients may include low-dose infusions of naloxone.

TABLE 8.10 Pasero Opioid-Induced Sedation Scale (POSS) With Interventions

Level of Sedation	Nursing Intervention
S = Sleep, easy to arouse	• Acceptable • No action necessary • May increase opioid dose if needed
1. Awake and alert	• Acceptable • No action necessary • May increase opioid dose if needed
2. Slightly drowsy, easily aroused	• Acceptable • No action necessary • May increase opioid dose if needed
3. Frequently drowsy, arousable, drifts off to sleep during conversation	• Unacceptable • Monitor respiratory status and sedation level closely until sedation level is stable at <3 and respiratory status is satisfactory • Decrease opioid dose 25%–50% or notify HCP or anesthesiologist for orders • Consider giving a nonsedating, opioid-sparing nonopioid, such as acetaminophen or an NSAID, if not contraindicated
4. Somnolent, minimal or no response to verbal or physical stimulation	• Unacceptable • Stop opioid • Consider giving naloxone • Notify HCP or anesthesiologist • Monitor respiratory status and sedation level closely until sedation level is stable at <3 and respiratory status is satisfactory

Adapted from Pasero C: Assessment of sedation during opioid administration for pain management, *J PeriAnesthesia Nurs* 24:186, 2009.

A rare but concerning problem with long-term and even short-term use of high-dose opioids is *opioid-induced hyperalgesia* (OIH). OIH is a state of nociceptive sensitization caused by exposure to opioids. It is characterized by a paradoxical response in which patients become more sensitive to certain painful stimuli and report increased pain with opioid use. The exact mechanism is not clearly understood, but it may be due to neuroplasticity changes. This may explain why opioids tend to lose their effectiveness in certain patients over time.

Adjuvant Analgesic Therapy. Analgesic adjuvants are drugs that can be used alone or in conjunction with opioid and nonopioid analgesics (Table 8.11). Generally, these agents were developed for other purposes (e.g., antiseizure drugs, antidepressants) and found to be effective for treating pain.

α_2-Adrenergic Agonists. We think clonidine and tizanidine (Zanaflex), the most widely used α_2-adrenergic agonists, work on the central inhibitory α-adrenergic receptors. These agents may also decrease norepinephrine release peripherally. They are given for chronic headache and neuropathic pain.

Antidepressants. Tricyclic antidepressants (TCAs) enhance the descending inhibitory system by preventing the cellular reuptake of serotonin and norepinephrine. Higher levels of serotonin and norepinephrine in the synapse inhibit the transmission of nociceptive signals in the CNS. Other potential beneficial actions of TCAs include sodium channel modulation, α_1-adrenergic antagonist effects, and a weak NMDA receptor modulation. They are effective for a variety of pain syndromes, especially neuropathic pain syndromes. However, side effects, such as sedation, dry mouth, blurred vision, and weight gain,

limit their usefulness. Antidepressants that selectively inhibit reuptake of serotonin and norepinephrine (SNRIs) are effective for many neuropathic pain syndromes and have fewer side effects than the TCAs. These agents include venlafaxine, desvenlafaxine (Pristiq), milnacipran (Savella), and bupropion.

Antiseizure Drugs. Antiseizure drugs affect peripheral nerves and the CNS in several ways, including sodium channel modulation, central calcium channel modulation, and changes in excitatory amino acids and other receptors. Agents such as gabapentin, lamotrigine, and pregabalin are valuable adjuvant agents in chronic pain therapy and are being used more in the treatment of acute pain.

GABA-Receptor Agonist. Baclofen, an agonist at GABA receptors, can interfere with the transmission of nociceptive impulses. It is used for muscle spasms and neuropathic pain. It crosses the blood-brain barrier poorly and is much more effective for spasticity when delivered intrathecally.

Corticosteroids. Corticosteroids include dexamethasone, prednisone, and methylprednisolone (Medrol). They are used for managing acute and chronic cancer pain, pain secondary to spinal cord compression, and inflammatory joint pain syndromes. Mechanisms of action may be related to the ability of corticosteroids to decrease edema and inflammation.

Corticosteroids have many side effects, especially when given chronically in high doses. These include hyperglycemia, fluid retention, dyspepsia and GI bleeding, impaired healing, muscle wasting, osteoporosis, adrenal suppression, and susceptibility to infection. Because they act through the same final pathway as NSAIDs, do not give corticosteroids at the same time as NSAIDs.

Local Anesthetics. For acute pain from surgery or trauma, local anesthetics, such as bupivacaine and ropivacaine, can be given epidurally by continuous infusion or by intermittent or continuous infusion with regional nerve blocks. Systemic lidocaine given in an IV infusion is sometimes used for neuropathic and postoperative visceral pain. Topical applications are used to interrupt transmission of pain signals to the brain. For example, 5% lidocaine patch (Lidoderm) is a first-line agent for the treatment of several types of neuropathic pain. In the treatment of chronic severe neuropathic pain that is refractory to other analgesics, oral therapy with mexiletine (Mexitil) may be tried.

Cannabinoids. Cannabinoid-derived medications show promise in the treatment of neuropathic pain, certain pain syndromes, and some symptoms. However, these preparations have sparked considerable controversy and confusion, mostly because cannabinoids are related to the cannabis plant, also known as marijuana. Synthetic cannabinoids (e.g., dronabinol [Marinol]) have been approved for medical use. Smoking marijuana or cannabis rapidly increases plasma levels of tetrahydrocannabinol (THC). The increase depends on composition of the marijuana cigarette and inhalation technique. As a result, this form of use is associated with variable pain relief. With commercially available oral preparations, the absorption and bioavailability are more reliable and predictable.

Cannabinoids exert their analgesic effects primarily through the cannabinoid-1 (CB1) and CB2 receptors. Activation of cannabinoid receptors modulates neurotransmission in the serotoninergic, dopaminergic, and glutamatergic systems, as well as other systems. Cannabinoids also enhance the endogenous opioid system. Other beneficial effects include alleviating nausea and increased appetite. They may have opioid-sparing effects, possibly reducing opioid tolerance and symptoms of opioid withdrawal.[18]

TABLE 8.11 Drug Therapy

Adjuvant Drugs Used for Pain

Drug	Specific Indication	Nursing Considerations
α₂-Adrenergic Agonists		
clonidine (Duraclon) tizanidine (Zanaflex)	Particularly useful for neuropathic pain when given intrathecally	• Side effects include sedation, orthostatic hypotension, dry mouth • Often combined with anesthetics (e.g., bupivacaine)
Anesthetics: Local		
capsaicin (active compound of chili peppers)	Pain associated with arthritis, postherpetic neuralgia, diabetic neuropathy	• Apply very sparingly onto affected area. • Use gloves or wash hands with soap and water after application • Monitor for side effects: Skin irritation (burning, stinging) at application site and cough when inhaled
lidocaine (L-M-X)	Topical local anesthetic cream applied to intact skin before venipuncture or lumbar puncture. May be effective for postherpetic neuralgia	• Apply bubble layer to intact skin and wait at least 20–30 min before wiping and performing painful procedure • Duration is around 60 min after wiped from skin • Available without prescription
lidocaine 2.5% + prilocaine 2.5% (topical eutectic mixture of local anesthetics [EMLA])	Longer time to take effect than L-M-X	• Apply under an occlusive dressing (e.g., Tegaderm, Duo-Derm) or on an anesthetic disk • Side effects include mild erythema, edema, skin blanching
Anesthetics: Oral or Systemic		
5% lidocaine-impregnated transdermal patch (Lidoderm patch)	Postherpetic neuralgia	• Local skin reactions (e.g., change in color, colored spots, irritation, itching, rash, burning) occur at the site of application; typically mild
mexiletine	Diabetic neuropathy Neuropathic pain	• Monitor for side effects: High incidence of nausea, dizziness, perioral numbness, paresthesias, tremor, seizures (at high doses), dysrhythmias, and myocardial depression • Avoid in patients with preexisting heart disease
Antidepressants *Tricyclic Antidepressants*		
amitriptyline desipramine (Norpramin) doxepin imipramine (Tofranil) nortriptyline (Pamelor)	Neuropathic pain	• Side-effect profile differs for each agent and is often dose-dependent • Common side effects include anticholinergic effects (e.g., dry mouth) and sedation • Monitor for anticholinergic side effects • Titrate slowly over days to weeks to reach optimal therapeutic doses
Serotonin Norepinephrine Reuptake Inhibitor (SNRI) Antidepressants		
duloxetine (Cymbalta) milnacipran (Savella) venlafaxine (Effexor)	Neuropathic pain Multimodal therapy for acute pain (venlafaxine) Fibromyalgia (duloxetine, milnacipran)	• Side effects vary with each agent • Decreased arousal and desire for sex
Other Antidepressants		
bupropion (Wellbutrin)	Neuropathic pain Headaches	• Low risk for sexual problems and sedation • Distinguished from TCAs and SNRIs as an inhibitor of norepinephrine and dopamine uptake
Antiseizure Drugs		
First generation: carbamazepine (Tegretol) phenytoin (Dilantin) Second generation: gabapentin (Neurontin) lamotrigine (Lamictal) pregabalin (Lyrica)	Neuropathic pain Multimodal therapy for acute pain (gabapentin, pregabalin) Fibromyalgia (pregabalin)	• Start with low doses, increase slowly • Side effects vary with each agent
Cannabinoids		
dronabinol (Marinol)	Neuropathic pain Certain pain syndromes	• May relieve nausea and increase appetite • May have opioid-sparing effects, possibly reducing opioid tolerance and symptoms of opioid withdrawal
Corticosteroids		
dexamethasone (Decadron)	Inflammation	• Avoid high doses for long-term use
GABA-Receptor Agonist		
baclofen (Lioresal)	Neuropathic pain Muscle spasms	• Monitor for weakness, urinary dysfunction • Avoid abrupt discontinuation because of CNS irritability

Adapted from Pasero C, Polomano RC, McCaffery M, etal: Adjuvant analgesics. In Pasero C, McCaffery M, editors: *Pain: Assessment and pharmacological management*, New York, 2011, Mosby.

Administration

Scheduling. Appropriate analgesic scheduling focuses on preventing or controlling pain, rather than providing analgesics only after the patient's pain has become severe. Premedicate a patient before procedures and activities that will likely produce pain. Similarly, a patient with constant pain should receive analgesics around the clock rather than on an "as needed" (PRN) basis. These strategies control pain before it starts and usually result in lower analgesic requirements. Use fast-acting drugs for incident or breakthrough pain, while long-acting analgesics are more effective for constant pain. Examples of fast-acting and sustained-release analgesics are described later in this section.

Titration. Analgesic titration is dose adjustment based on assessment of the adequacy of analgesic effect versus the side effects produced. The amount of analgesic needed to manage pain varies widely, and titration is an important strategy in addressing this variability. An analgesic can be titrated upward or downward, depending on the situation. For example, in a postoperative patient the dose of analgesic decreases over time as the acute pain resolves. On the other hand, opioids for chronic, severe cancer pain may be titrated upward many times over the course of therapy to maintain adequate pain control. The goal of titration is to use the smallest dose of analgesic that provides effective pain control with the fewest side effects.

Equianalgesic Dosing. The term equianalgesic dose refers to a dose of 1 analgesic that is equivalent in pain-relieving effects to a given dose of another analgesic (Table 8.12). This equivalence helps guide opioid dosing when changing routes or opioids when a specific drug is ineffective or causes intolerable side effects. Equianalgesic charts and conversion programs are widely available in clinical guidelines, in health care facility pain protocols, and on the Internet. They are useful tools, but you need to understand their limitations since these doses are estimates. To ensure safety, all changes in opioid therapy must be carefully monitored and adjusted for the individual patient.

Administration Routes. We can deliver opioids and other analgesic agents by many routes. This flexibility allows the HCP to (1) target a particular anatomic source of the pain, (2) achieve therapeutic blood levels rapidly when necessary, (3) avoid certain side effects through localized administration, and (4) provide analgesia when patients are unable to swallow. The following discussion highlights the uses and nursing considerations for analgesic agents delivered through a variety of routes.

Oral. Generally, oral administration is the route of choice for the person with a functioning GI system. Most pain medications are available in oral preparations, such as liquid and tablet. For opioids, larger oral doses are needed to achieve the equivalent analgesia of doses given IM or IV (Table 8.12). For example, 10 mg of parenteral morphine is equivalent to around 30 mg of oral morphine. The reason larger doses are needed is related to the *first-pass effect* of hepatic metabolism. This means that oral opioids are absorbed from the GI tract into the portal circulation and shunted to the liver. Partial metabolism in the liver occurs before the drug enters the systemic circulation and becomes available to peripheral receptors or can cross the blood-brain barrier and access CNS opioid receptors, which is needed to produce analgesia. Oral opioids are as effective as parenteral opioids if the dose is large enough to compensate for the first-pass metabolism.

Many opioids are available in short-acting (immediate-release) and long-acting (sustained-release or extended-release) oral preparations. Immediate-release products are effective in providing rapid, short-term pain relief. Sustained-release or extended-release preparations generally are given every 8 to 12 hours, although some preparations (e.g., Kadian, Exalgo) may be dosed every 24 hours.

> **⚠ SAFETY ALERT** Sustained-Release or Extended-Release Preparations
> - These should not be crushed, broken, dissolved, or chewed. These drugs are to be swallowed whole.
> - If all the medicine is released into a person at once, serious side effects can occur, including death from overdose.

Transmucosal and buccal routes. Although morphine has historically been given sublingually to people with cancer pain who have difficulty swallowing, little of the drug is absorbed from the sublingual tissue. Instead, most of the drug dissolves in saliva and is swallowed, making its absorption similar to that of oral morphine.

Several transmucosal fentanyl products are used for the treatment of breakthrough pain. These include (1) oral transmucosal fentanyl citrate (OTFC) (Actiq), with the fentanyl embedded in a flavored lozenge on a stick that is absorbed by the buccal mucosa after being rubbed actively over it when given as the lozenge (not sucked as a lollipop); (2) fentanyl buccal tablet (FBT) (Fentora) in the form of a buccal tablet that disintegrates; and (3) fentanyl sublingual (Abstral). Transmucosal absorption allows the drug to enter the bloodstream and travel directly to the CNS. Pain relief typically occurs 5 to 7 minutes after administration. These formulations should be used only for patients who are already receiving and are tolerant to opioid therapy.[19]

Intranasal route. Intranasal administration allows delivery of medication to highly vascular mucosa and avoids the first-pass effect. Butorphanol is given for acute headache and other intense, recurrent types of pain. A transmucosal fentanyl nasal spray (Lazanda) is available for the treatment of breakthrough pain.

Rectal. The rectal route is often overlooked but is particularly useful when the patient cannot take an analgesic by mouth, such as with severe nausea and vomiting. Analgesics that are available as rectal suppositories include hydromorphone, oxymorphone, morphine, and acetaminophen. If rectal preparations are not available, many oral formulations can be given rectally if the patient is unable to take medications by mouth.

TABLE 8.12	Opioid Equianalgesic Doses*	
Drug	**DOSE EQUAL TO PARENTERAL MORPHINE 10 mg**	
	Oral (mg)	**Parenteral (IM, IV, Subcutaneous) (mg)**
Codeine	200	120–130
Fentanyl	NA	0.1 (100 mcg)
Hydrocodone	30	NA
Hydromorphone	7.5	1.5
Levorphanol	4	2
Meperidine	300	75
Morphine	30	10
Oxycodone	15–30	NA

*All equivalencies are approximations. These amounts can be affected by many factors, including interpatient variability, type of pain, and tolerance. Monitor patients for effectiveness and adverse reactions and adjust the dose accordingly.

Transdermal route. Transdermal patches are designed for systemic drug delivery (e.g., Duragesic) or for topical or local delivery (e.g., Lidoderm). Fentanyl (Duragesic) is useful for the patient who cannot tolerate oral analgesic drugs. Absorption from the patch is slow. It takes 12 to 17 hours to reach full effect with the first application. Therefore transdermal fentanyl is not suitable for rapid dose titration but can be effective if the patient's pain is stable and the dose needed to control it is known. Patches may have to be changed every 48 hours rather than the recommended 72 hours based on individual patient responses. Patches are applied to intact, nonhairy skin. Rashes caused by the patch's adhesive may be reduced by preparing the skin 1 hour before placement with a weak corticosteroid cream. Biocclusive dressings are available if the patch keeps falling off because of sweating. A transdermal patient-controlled analgesia (PCA) system (iontophoretic transdermal system [ITS]) is available.

> 💊 **DRUG ALERT**   **Fentanyl Patches**
> - Fentanyl patches (Duragesic) may cause death from overdose.
> - Signs of overdose include trouble breathing or shallow respirations; tiredness, extreme sleepiness, or sedation; inability to think, talk, or walk normally; and faintness, dizziness, or confusion.

A 5% lidocaine-impregnated transdermal patch (Lidoderm patch) is used for postherpetic neuralgia. The patch is placed directly on the intact, nonhairy skin in the area of postherpetic pain and left in place for up to 12 hours. There are few systemic side effects, even with chronic use.

Creams and lotions containing 10% trolamine salicylate (Aspercreme, Myoflex Creme) are available for joint and muscle pain. This aspirin-like substance is absorbed locally. This route avoids GI irritation but not the other side effects of high-dose salicylates. Topical diclofenac solution and a diclofenac patch (Flector) are effective for osteoarthritic pain of the knee.

Other topical analgesic agents, such as capsaicin (e.g., Zostrix) and lidocaine (L-M-X cream), also provide analgesia. Derived from red chili pepper, capsaicin acts on C-fiber heat receptors. If used 3 or 4 times a day for 4 to 6 weeks, it will cause the C nociceptor fibers to become inactive. The result is neuronal resistance to painful stimuli. Capsaicin may control pain associated with diabetic neuropathy, arthritis, and postherpetic neuralgia. L-M-X cream is useful for control of pain associated with venipunctures. Cover the targeted area of intact skin with a layer of L-M-X for at least 20 to 30 minutes, then wipe it off prior to beginning a painful procedure.

Parenteral routes. The parenteral routes include IV and subcutaneous administration. Single, repeated, or continuous dosing (IV or subcutaneous) is possible with parenteral routes. IV administration is the best route when immediate analgesia and rapid titration are needed. Continuous IV infusions provide excellent steady-state analgesia through stable blood levels.

Onset of analgesia after subcutaneous administration is slow, and thus the subcutaneous route is rarely used for acute pain management. However, continuous subcutaneous infusions are effective for pain management at the end of life. This route is especially helpful for people with abnormal GI function and limited venous access.

The IM route is not recommended because injections cause significant pain and result in unreliable absorption. With chronic use, IM injections can result in abscesses and fibrosis.

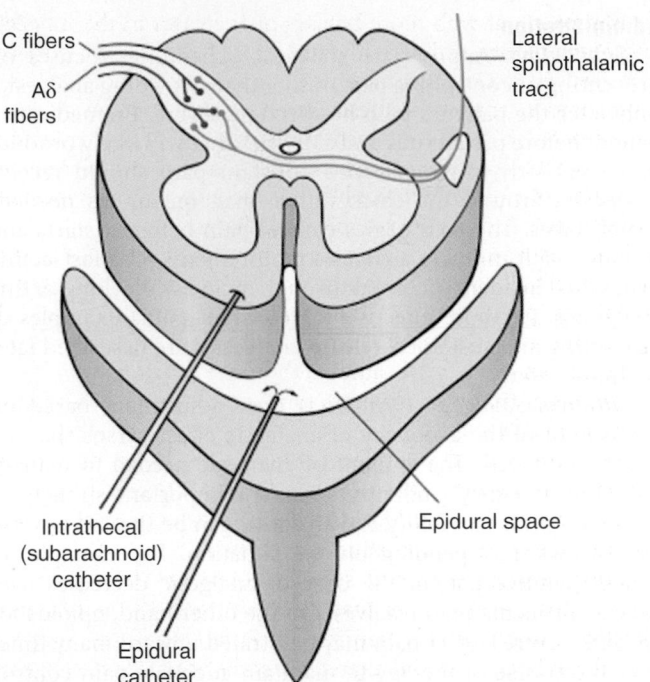

FIG. 8.6 Cross section of spinal cord with placement of catheters into the subarachnoid space (intrathecal delivery) and the epidural space (epidural delivery). (From Urden LD, Stacy KM, Lough ME: *Critical care nursing: Diagnosis and management,* ed 8, St Louis, 2018, Elsevier.)

Intraspinal delivery. Intraspinal or neuraxial opioid therapy involves inserting a catheter into the subarachnoid space *(intrathecal delivery)* or the epidural space *(epidural delivery)* (Fig. 8.6). Analgesics are injected either by intermittent bolus doses or continuous infusion.

Percutaneously placed temporary catheters are used for short-term therapy (2 to 4 days), and surgically implanted catheters are used for long-term therapy. Although the lumbar region is the most common site of placement, epidural catheters may be placed at any point along the spinal column (cervical, thoracic, lumbar, or caudal). The tip of the epidural catheter is placed as close to the nerve supplying the painful dermatome as possible. For example, a thoracic catheter is placed for upper abdominal surgery, and a high lumbar catheter is used for lower abdominal surgery. Fluoroscopy ensures correct placement of the catheter.

Intraspinal analgesics are highly potent because they are delivered close to the receptors in the spinal cord dorsal horn. Smaller doses of analgesics are needed than with other routes, including IV. For example, 1 mg of intrathecal morphine equals 10 mg of epidural morphine, 100 mg of IV morphine, and 300 mg of oral morphine. Drugs delivered intraspinally include morphine, fentanyl, sufentanil (Sufenta), alfentanil (Alfenta), hydromorphone, clonidine, and ziconotide, a calcium channel receptor modulator for use in neuropathic pain syndromes. Nausea, itching, and urinary retention are common side effects of intraspinal opioids.

Complications of intraspinal analgesia include catheter displacement and migration, accidental infusions of neurotoxic agents, epidural hematomas, and infection. Clinical manifestations of catheter displacement or migration depend on catheter location and the drug being infused. A catheter that migrates out of the intrathecal or epidural space causes a decrease in pain relief with no improvement with more boluses or increases in the infusion rate. If an epidural catheter migrates into the subarachnoid space, increased side effects become quickly apparent. Somnolence, confusion, and increased anesthesia (if the infusate contains an anesthetic) occur. Check with institutional policy before aspirating cerebrospinal fluid to determine intrathecal catheter placement. Migration of a catheter into a blood vessel may cause an increase in side effects because of systemic drug distribution.

Many drugs and chemicals are highly neurotoxic when given intraspinally. These include antibiotics, chemotherapy agents, potassium, parenteral nutrition, and many preservatives, such as alcohol and phenol. To avoid inadvertent injection of IV drugs into an intraspinal catheter, the catheter should be clearly marked as an intraspinal access device. Only preservative-free drugs should be used.

Infection is a rare but serious complication of intraspinal analgesia. Assess the skin around the exit site for inflammation, drainage, or pain. Manifestations of an intraspinal infection include diffuse back pain, pain or paresthesia during bolus injection, and unexplained sensory or motor deficits in the lower limbs. Fever may or may not be present. Acute bacterial infection (meningitis) is manifested by photophobia, neck stiffness, fever, headache, and altered mental status. Regular, meticulous wound care and using sterile technique when caring for the catheter and injecting drugs reduces infection risk.

Long-term epidural catheters may be placed for terminal cancer patients or patients with certain pain syndromes that are unresponsive to other treatments. If a long-term indwelling epidural catheter is used, bacterial filters are recommended.

Implantable pumps. Intraspinal catheters can be surgically implanted for long-term pain relief. The surgical placement of an intrathecal catheter to a subcutaneously placed pump and reservoir allows for the delivery of drugs directly into the intrathecal space. The pump, which is normally placed in a pocket made in the subcutaneous tissue of the abdomen, may be programmable or fixed.

We make changes reprogramming the pump, changing the mixture, or concentration of drug in the reservoir. The pump is refilled every 30 to 90 days depending on flow rate, mixture, and reservoir size.

Patient-controlled analgesia. Patient-controlled analgesia (PCA) (demand analgesia) is a method that allows the patient to self-administer preset doses of an analgesic within a prescribed time period by activating an infusion pump. Routes of administration include oral, IV, epidural, inhaled, nasal, and transcutaneous. In acute care, PCA often refers to an electronically controlled infusion pump that delivers the medication by an IV or epidural route (patient-controlled epidural analgesia [PCEA]). PCEA often combines an opioid and local anesthetic. PCA also can be adapted for oral administration. With PCA/PCEA, a dose of opioid is delivered when the patient decides a dose is needed. PCA/PCEA uses an infusion system in which the patient pushes a button to receive a bolus infusion of an analgesic. PCA/PCEA is used widely for the management of acute pain, including postoperative pain and cancer pain.

Opioids, such as morphine and hydromorphone, are often given via PCA therapy for acute and chronic pain. Sometimes IV PCA is given with a continuous or background infusion called a *basal rate,* depending on the patient's opioid requirement. Adding a basal rate in opioid-naive patients and those at risk for adverse respiratory outcomes (e.g., older age, obstructive sleep apnea, lung disease) may lead to serious respiratory events. Basal rates are often used with epidural catheter pain management. Because the medication is delivered directly into the epidural space, the amount of opioid is 10 times less than is needed by IV route. This lessens the risk for respiratory depression but does not eliminate it.

Patient teaching is very important with the use of PCA/PCEA. Help the patient understand the mechanics of getting a drug dose and how to titrate the drug to achieve good pain relief. Teach the patient to self-administer the analgesic before pain is severe. Assure the patient that he or she cannot "overdose" because the pump is programmed to deliver a maximum number of doses per hour. The patient will not receive more analgesic once the maximum dose has been reached. If the maximum dose is inadequate to relieve pain, the pump can be reprogrammed to increase the amount or frequency of dosing. In addition, you can give bolus doses if they are part of the HCP's orders. To make a smooth transition from infusion PCA to oral drugs, the patient should receive increasing doses of oral drug as the PCA analgesic is tapered.

Patient-controlled delivery systems are intended for use by the patient. An *authorized agent controlled analgesia (AACA)* is a method of delivery performed by a consistently available and competent person for patients who are unable to independently activate PCA devices.[20] This authorized agent must be carefully selected, taught the principles of PCA, and capable of recognizing pain and the appropriate times to give medication via the PCA device. Understand your institution's policies about PCA and AACA.

Interventional Therapy

Therapeutic Nerve Blocks. Nerve blocks involve 1-time or continuous infusion of local anesthetics into a particular area to produce pain relief. These techniques are also called *regional anesthesia.* Nerve blocks interrupt all afferent and efferent transmission to the area and thus are not specific to nociceptive pathways. They include local infiltration of anesthetics into a surgical area (e.g., chest incisions, inguinal hernia) and injection of anesthetic into a specific nerve (e.g., occipital, pudendal nerve) or nerve plexus (e.g., brachial, celiac plexus). Nerve blocks can be used during and after surgery to manage pain. For longer term relief of chronic pain syndromes, local anesthetics can be given by a continuous infusion.

Adverse effects of nerve blocks are similar to those for local anesthetics delivered by other systemic routes. Effects include systemic toxicity resulting in dysrhythmias, confusion, nausea and vomiting, blurred vision, tinnitus, and metallic taste. Temporary nerve blocks affect motor function and sensation and typically last 2 to 24 hours, depending on the agent and the site of injection. Motor ability generally returns before sensation.

Neuroablative Techniques. Neuroablative interventions are done for severe pain that is unresponsive to all other therapies. They involve destroying nerves, thereby interrupting pain transmission. Destruction is by surgical resection or thermocoagulation, including radiofrequency coagulation. Neuroablative interventions that destroy the sensory division of a peripheral or spinal nerve are classified as *neurectomies, rhizotomies,* and *sympathectomies.* Neurosurgical procedures that ablate the lateral spinothalamic tract are classified as *cordotomies* if the tract is interrupted in the spinal cord or *tractotomies* if the interruption is in the medulla or midbrain of the brainstem (Fig. 8.7). Cordotomy and tractotomy can

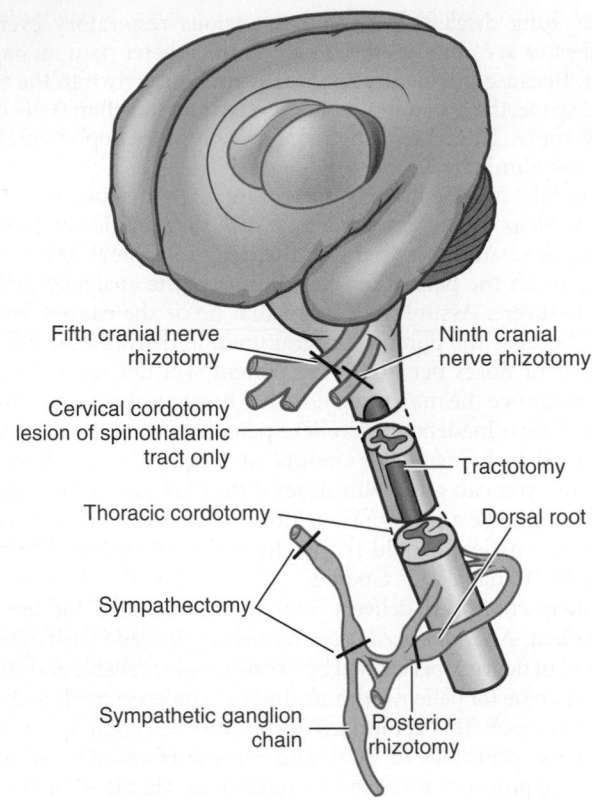

FIG. 8.7 Sites of neurosurgical procedures for pain relief.

- Fifth cranial nerve rhizotomy
- Ninth cranial nerve rhizotomy
- Cervical cordotomy lesion of spinothalamic tract only
- Tractotomy
- Thoracic cordotomy
- Dorsal root
- Sympathectomy
- Sympathetic ganglion chain
- Posterior rhizotomy

TABLE 8.13   Nondrug Therapies for Pain
Physical Therapies
• Acupuncture
• Application of heat and cold (Table 8.14)
• Exercise
• Massage
• Transcutaneous electrical nerve stimulation (TENS)
Cognitive Therapies
• Distraction
• Hypnosis
• Imagery
• Relaxation strategies (see Chapter 6)
• Art therapy
• Imagery
• Meditation
• Music therapy
• Relaxation breathing

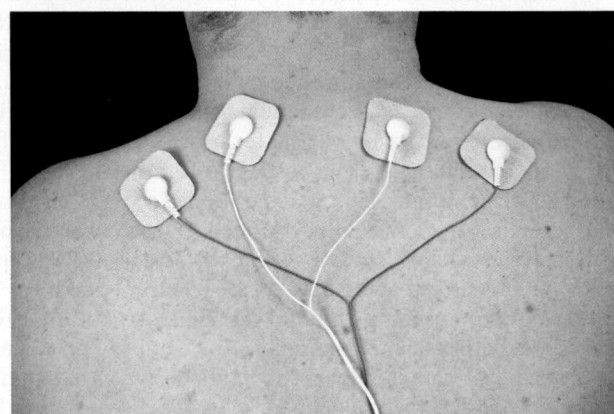

FIG. 8.8 Treatment of pain with transcutaneous electrical nerve stimulation (TENS) treatment after shoulder surgery. (© Noel Moore/Hemera/Thinkstock.)

be done with the aid of local anesthesia by a percutaneous technique under fluoroscopy.

Neuroaugmentation. *Neuroaugmentation* involves electrical stimulation of the brain and spinal cord. Spinal cord stimulation (SCS) is done much more often than brain stimulation. The most common use of SCS is for chronic back pain secondary to nerve damage that is unresponsive to other therapies. Other uses include CRPS, spinal cord injury pain, and interstitial cystitis. Potential complications include those related to the surgery (bleeding and infection), migration of the generator (which usually is implanted in the subcutaneous tissues of the upper gluteal or pectoralis area), and nerve damage.

Nondrug Therapies for Pain

Nondrug strategies play an important role in pain management (Table 8.13). They can reduce the dose of an analgesic needed to relieve pain and thereby minimize side effects of drug therapy. Moreover, they increase the patient's sense of personal control about managing pain and increase coping skills. Some strategies are thought to alter ascending nociceptive input or stimulate descending pain modulation mechanisms. These nondrug therapies are useful for both acute and chronic pain.

Physical Pain Relief Strategies

Massage. Massage is useful for acute and chronic pain. Many different massage techniques exist, including moving the hands or fingers over the skin slowly or briskly with long strokes or in circles (superficial massage) or applying firm pressure to the skin to maintain contact while massaging the underlying tissues (deep massage). Another type is trigger point massage. A **trigger point** is a circumscribed hypersensitive area within a tight band of muscle. It is caused by acute or chronic muscle strain. It feels like a tight knot under the skin. Trigger point massage is done

by applying strong, sustained digital pressure; deep massage; or gentler massage with ice followed by muscle heating. Massage is discussed in Chapter 6.

Exercise. Exercise is an essential part of the treatment plan for patients with chronic pain, particularly those with musculoskeletal pain. Many patients become physically deconditioned from their pain, which in turn leads to more pain. Exercise acts via many mechanisms to relieve pain. It enhances circulation and cardiovascular fitness, reduces edema, increases muscle strength and flexibility, and enhances physical and psychosocial functioning. Tailor an exercise program to the patient's physical needs and lifestyle. It may include aerobic exercise, stretching, and strengthening exercises. Trained personnel (e.g., physical therapist) should supervise the program.

Transcutaneous Electrical Nerve Stimulation. *Transcutaneous electrical nerve stimulation* (TENS) involves the delivery of an electric current through electrodes applied to the skin surface over the painful region, at trigger points, or over a peripheral nerve. A TENS system consists of 2 or more electrodes connected by lead wires to a small, battery-operated stimulator (Fig. 8.8). Usually a physical therapist is responsible for delivering TENS therapy, although nurses can be trained in the technique.

TENS may be used for acute pain, including postoperative pain and pain associated with physical trauma. The effects of TENS on chronic pain are less clear, but it may be effective in these cases.[21]

TABLE 8.14 Patient & Caregiver Teaching

Heat and Cold Therapy

Include the following instructions when teaching the patient and caregiver about superficial heat or cold techniques:

Heat Therapy

- Do not use heat on an area that is being treated with radiation therapy, is bleeding, has decreased sensation, or has been injured in the past 24 hours.
- Do not use any menthol-containing products (e.g., Ben-Gay, Vicks, Icy Hot) with heat applications because this may cause burns.
- Cover the heat source with a towel or cloth before applying to the skin to prevent burns.

Cold Therapy

- Cover the cold source with a cloth or towel before applying to the skin to prevent tissue damage.
- Do not apply cold to areas that are being treated with radiation therapy, have open wounds, or have poor circulation.
- If it is not possible to apply the cold directly to the painful site, try applying it right above or below the painful site or on the opposite side of the body on the corresponding site (e.g., left elbow if the right elbow hurts).

Acupuncture. Acupuncture is a technique of Traditional Chinese Medicine in which very thin needles are inserted into the body at designated points. Acupuncture is used for many kinds of pain. Acupuncture is described in Chapter 6.

Heat Therapy. Heat therapy is the application of either moist or dry heat to the skin. Heat therapy can be either superficial or deep. We can apply superficial heat using an electric heating pad (dry or moist), a hot pack, hot moist compresses, warm wax (paraffin), or a hot water bottle. To expose large areas of the body, patients can immerse themselves in a hot bath, shower, or whirlpool. Physical therapy departments provide deep-heat therapy through techniques such as short-wave diathermy, microwave diathermy, and ultrasound therapy. Patient and caregiver teaching about heat therapy is described in Table 8.14.

Cold Therapy. Cold therapy involves the application of either moist or dry cold to the skin. Dry cold can be applied by using an ice bag, moist cold by using towels soaked in ice water, cold hydrocollator packs, or immersion in a bath or under running cold water. Icing with ice cubes or blocks of ice made to resemble Popsicles is another technique used for pain relief. Cold therapy is thought to be more effective than heat for a variety of painful conditions, including acute pain from trauma or surgery, acute flare-ups of arthritis, muscle spasms, and headache. Patient and caregiver teaching about cold therapy is described in Table 8.14.

Cognitive Therapies. Techniques to alter the affective, cognitive, and behavioral components of pain include a variety of cognitive strategies and behavioral approaches. For example, patients can identify and challenge negative pain-related thoughts and replace them with more positive coping thoughts. Some techniques need little training and often are adopted independently by the patient. For others, a trained therapist is needed.

Distraction. Distraction involves redirection of attention away from the pain and onto something else. It is a simple but powerful strategy to relieve pain. Distraction involves engaging the patient in any activity that can hold his or her attention (e.g., watching TV or a movie, conversing, listening to music). It is

important to match the activity with the patient's energy level and ability to concentrate.

Hypnosis. Hypnotherapy is a structured technique that enables a patient to achieve a state of heightened awareness and focused concentration that can be used to alter the patient's pain perception. Hypnosis should be delivered and monitored only by specially trained clinicians.

Relaxation Strategies. Relaxation strategies reduce stress, decrease acute anxiety, distract from pain, ease muscle tension, combat fatigue, promote sleep, and enhance the effectiveness of other pain relief measures.[22] Relaxation strategies include relaxation breathing, music, imagery, meditation, muscle relaxation, and art (see Chapter 6).

❖ NURSING AND INTERPROFESSIONAL MANAGEMENT: PAIN

You are an important member of the interprofessional pain management team. You provide input into the assessment and reassessment of pain. You help in planning and implementing treatments, including teaching, advocacy, and support of the patient, caregiver, and family. Because patients in any care setting can have pain, you must be knowledgeable about current therapies and flexible in trying new approaches to pain management.

Together with the patient, develop a written agreement or treatment plan that describes the pain management. The plan should ensure that pain will be treated based on the patient's perception and report of pain. When appropriate, the plan outlines the gradual tapering of the analgesic dose, with eventual substitution of parenteral analgesics with long-acting oral preparations and possibly cessation of opioids.

Many nursing roles are described earlier in this chapter, including assessing pain, giving treatment, monitoring for side effects, and teaching patients and caregivers. However, the success of these actions depends on your ability to establish a trusting relationship with the patient and caregiver and to address their concerns about pain and its treatment.

◆ Effective Communication

Because pain is a subjective experience, patients need to feel confident that their reporting of pain will be believed and will not be perceived as "complaining." The patient and caregiver need to know that you consider the pain significant and understand that pain may profoundly disrupt a person's life. Communicate concern and commit to helping the patient obtain pain relief and cope with any unrelieved pain. Support the patient and caregiver through the period of trial and error that may be necessary to implement an effective therapeutic plan. It is important to clarify responsibilities in pain relief. Help the patient understand the role of the interprofessional team members, as well as the patient's roles and expectations.

In addition to addressing specific aspects of pain assessment and treatment, evaluate the impact that the pain has on the lives of the patient and caregiver. Table 8.15 addresses teaching needs of patients and caregivers related to pain management.

◆ Challenges to Effective Pain Management

Common challenges to effective pain management include misunderstandings about tolerance, physical dependence, and addiction. It is important for you to understand and be able to explain these concepts. Table 8.16 lists barriers to pain management and strategies to address them.

NURSING MANAGEMENT

Pain Management

- Assess pain characteristics (pattern and onset, area or location, intensity, quality, associated symptoms, and management strategies).
- Develop treatment plan for patient's pain (including drug and nondrug therapies).
- Give ordered pain medications.
- Evaluate whether current treatment plan is effective.
- Teach patient and caregiver about treatment plan.
- Implement discharge teaching about pain management.
- Provide effective supervision of UAP:
  - Help with screening for pain and notify RN if patient expresses pain.
  - Take and report vital signs before and after pain medications are given.
  - Note and report if patient is refusing to take part in ordered activities, such as ambulation (since this may indicate inadequate pain management).

TABLE 8.15   Patient & Caregiver Teaching

Pain Management

Include the following information in the teaching plan for the patient with pain and caregiver:
- Self-management techniques
- Realistic goals for pain control
- Negative consequences of unrelieved pain
- Need to maintain a record of pain level and effectiveness of treatment
- Treat pain with drugs and/or nondrug therapies before it becomes severe
- Medication may stop working after it is taken for a period of time, and dosages may have to be adjusted
- Potential side effects and complications associated with pain therapies can include nausea and vomiting, constipation, sedation and drowsiness, itching, urinary retention, and sweating.
- Need to report when pain is not relieved to tolerable levels

---

◆ **Tolerance.** *Tolerance* occurs with chronic exposure to a variety of drugs. In the case of opioids, tolerance to analgesia is characterized by the need for an increased opioid dose to maintain the same degree of analgesia. Although the development of tolerance to side effects (except constipation) is more predictable, the incidence of clinically significant analgesic opioid tolerance in chronic pain patients is unknown, since dosage needs may increase as the disease (e.g., cancer) progresses. It is essential to assess for increased analgesic needs in patients on long-term therapy. The interprofessional team must evaluate and rule out other causes of increased analgesic needs, such as disease progression or infection.

If significant tolerance to opioids develops and the opioid is losing its effectiveness, or intolerable side effects are associated with escalation of doses, the practice of *opioid rotation* may be considered. This involves switching from 1 opioid to another, assuming that the new opioid will be more effective at lower equianalgesic doses. However, very high opioid doses can result in OIH rather than pain relief. This means that increases in the dose can lead to higher pain levels. (OIH is discussed on p. 115.)

◆ **Physical Dependence.** Like tolerance, physical dependence is a normal physiologic response to ongoing exposure to drugs. It is manifested by a withdrawal syndrome when the drug is abruptly decreased. Manifestations of opioid withdrawal are listed in Table 8.17. When opioids are no longer needed to provide pain relief, a tapering schedule should be used in conjunction with careful monitoring. A typical tapering schedule may involve reducing the dose by 20% to 50% per day. The goal is to reduce the amount of medication and at the same time minimize adverse and withdrawal effects.

◆ **Pseudoaddiction.** Inadequate treatment of pain can lead to a phenomenon called *pseudoaddiction*. This occurs when patients show behaviors associated with addiction (e.g., frequent requests for analgesic refills or higher dosages), but the behaviors resolve with adequate treatment of the patient's pain. These patients are often labeled as drug seeking, which can result in mistrust between the patient and HCP. This problem can be avoided by effective communication strategies and optimal pain management.

◆ **Addiction.** *Addiction* is a complex neurobiologic condition characterized by aberrant behaviors arising from a drive to obtain and take substances for reasons other than the prescribed therapeutic value (see Chapter 10). Tolerance and physical dependence are not indicators of addiction. Rather, they are normal physiologic responses to chronic exposure to certain drugs, including opioids. Addiction rarely occurs in patients who receive opioids for pain control. If addiction is suspected, it must be investigated and appropriately diagnosed. It should not be implied without evidence because this interferes with pain management. The hallmarks of addiction include (1) compulsive use, (2) loss of control of use, and (3) continued use despite risk of harm.

◆ **Risk Monitoring.** Several opioid risk assessments are available to help clinicians assess patients for abuse, misuse, and addiction. A controlled substance agreement for those at risk for addiction may be used. Addiction risk assessment tools, such as the Opioid Risk Tool *(www.drugabuse.gov/sites/default/files/files/OpioidRiskTool.pdf)* and the Screener and Opioid Assessment for Patient Pain *(www.nhms.org/sites/default/files/Pdfs/SOAPP-14.pdf)* are available. Patient monitoring with urine drug screens and access to state prescription monitoring programs to track prescriptions are effective in detecting misuse of drugs. The risk for addiction should not prevent HCPs from using opioids to effectively treat moderate to severe acute and chronic pain.

INSTITUTIONALIZING PAIN EDUCATION AND MANAGEMENT

Besides patient and caregiver barriers, other barriers to effective and safe pain management include inadequate HCP education and lack of institutional support. Traditionally, medical and nursing school curricula have spent little time teaching future physicians and nurses about pain and symptom management. The lack of emphasis on pain has contributed to inadequate training of HCPs.

We have made progress overcoming these barriers. Medical and nursing schools devote more time to addressing pain. Numerous professional organizations have published evidence-based guidelines for assessing and managing pain in many patient populations and clinical settings.

Institutional commitment and practices are changing clinical practice. One major step in institutionalizing pain management is the development and adoption of The Joint Commission (TJC) guideline on pain.[23] TJC is the accrediting body for most health care facilities (hospitals, nursing homes, and health care clinics). Under these standards, health care facilities are required to (1) recognize the patient's right to appropriate assessment and management of pain; (2) identify pain in patients during their initial assessment and as needed, during ongoing, periodic reassessments; (3) teach HCPs about pain assessment and management and ensure competency; and (4) teach patients and their families about pain management.

TABLE 8.16 Patient & Caregiver Teaching

Reducing Barriers to Pain Management

When teaching the patient and caregiver about pain management discuss the following barriers:

Barrier	Nursing Considerations
Fear of addiction	• Explain that addiction is uncommon in patients taking opioids as directed by the HCP for pain.
Fear of tolerance	• Teach that tolerance is a normal physiologic response to chronic opioid therapy. If tolerance does develop, the drug may have to be changed (e.g., morphine in place of oxycodone).
	• Teach that there is no absolute upper limit to pure opioid agonists (e.g., morphine). Dosages can be increased, and patient should not save drugs for when the pain is worse.
	• Teach that tolerance develops more slowly to analgesic effects of opioids than to side effects (e.g., sedation, respiratory depression). Tolerance does not develop to constipation; thus a regular bowel program should be started early.
Concern about side effects	• Teach methods to prevent and to treat common side effects.
	• Stress that side effects, such as sedation and nausea, decrease with time.
	• Explain that different drugs have unique side effects, and other pain drugs can be tried to reduce the specific side effect.
Fear of injections	• Explain that oral medicines are preferred.
	• Stress that even if oral route becomes unusable, transdermal or indwelling parenteral routes can be used rather than injections.
Desire to be "good" patient	• Discuss that patients are partners in their care and that partnership requires open communication by both patient and nurse.
	• Stress to patients that they have a responsibility to keep you informed about their pain.
Desire to be stoic	• Explain that although stoicism is a valued behavior in many cultures, failure to report pain can result in undertreatment and severe, unrelieved pain.
Forgetting to take analgesic	• Provide and teach use of pill containers.
	• Provide methods of record keeping for drug use.
	• Recruit caregivers to help with the analgesic regimen.
Concern that pain indicates disease progression	• Explain that increased pain or the need for analgesics may reflect tolerance.
	• Stress that new pain may come from a non–life-threatening source (e.g., muscle spasm, urinary tract infection).
	• Use drug and nondrug strategies to reduce anxiety.
	• Ensure that patient and caregivers have current, accurate, comprehensive information about the disease and prognosis.
	• Provide psychologic support.
Sense of fatalism	• Explain that pain can be managed in most patients.
	• Explain that most therapies require a period of trial and error.
	• Stress that side effects can be managed.
Ineffective medication	• Teach that there are multiple options within each category of medication (e.g., opioids, NSAIDs), and another medication from the same category may provide better relief.
	• Discuss that finding the best treatment regimen may require trial and error.
	• Include nondrug approaches in treatment plan.

TABLE 8.17 Manifestations of Opioid Withdrawal Syndrome

	Early Response (6–12 hr)	Late Response (48–72 hr)
Psychosocial Secretions	• Anxiety • Lacrimation • Rhinorrhea • Diaphoresis	• Excitation • Diarrhea
Other	• Yawning • Piloerection • Shaking, chills • Dilated pupils • Anorexia • Tremor	• Restlessness • Fever • Nausea and vomiting • Abdominal cramping pain • Hypertension • Tachycardia • Insomnia

ETHICAL ISSUES IN PAIN MANAGEMENT

Fear of Hastening Death by Giving Analgesics

A common concern of health care professionals and caregivers is that giving a sufficient amount of drug to relieve pain will hasten or precipitate death of a terminally ill person. However, there is no scientific evidence that opioids can hasten death, even among patients at the very end of life. Moreover, you have a moral obligation to provide comfort and pain relief at the end of life. Even if there is a concern about the possibility of hastening death, the rule of double effect provides ethical justification. This rule states that if an unwanted consequence (i.e., hastened death) occurs because of an action taken to achieve a moral good (i.e., pain relief), the action is justified if the nurse's intent is to relieve pain and not to hasten death.

Requests for Assisted Suicide

Unrelieved pain is 1 of the reasons that patients make requests for assisted suicide. Aggressive and adequate pain management may decrease the number of such requests. Assisted suicide is a complex issue that extends beyond pain and pain management. Physician-assisted suicide is legal in some states (e.g., Oregon, Washington). To address the legal and ethical issues about this situation, the International Association for Hospice and Palliative Care prepared a position paper on this topic.[24]

Use of Placebos in Pain Assessment and Treatment

Placebos are still sometimes used to assess and treat pain. Using a placebo involves deceiving patients by making them think they are receiving an analgesic when they are receiving an inert substance, such as saline. Many professional organizations condemn the use of placebos to assess or treat pain.

Gerontologic Considerations: Pain

Persistent pain is a common problem in older adults and is often associated with physical disability and psychosocial problems.

The prevalence of chronic pain among community-dwelling older adults exceeds 50% and among older nursing home patients is around 80%. The most common painful conditions among older adults are musculoskeletal conditions, such as osteoarthritis and low back pain. Chronic pain often results in depression, sleep problems, decreased mobility, increased health care use, and physical and social role dysfunction. Despite its high prevalence, pain in older adults is often inadequately assessed and treated.

Several barriers to pain assessment in the older patient exist. Older adults and their HCPs often believe that pain is a normal, inevitable part of aging and that nothing can be done to relieve the pain. Older adults may not report pain for fear of being a "burden" or a "complainer." They may fear taking opioids. In addition, older patients are more likely to use words such as "aching," "soreness," or "discomfort" rather than "pain." Be persistent in asking older adults about pain. Carry out the assessment in an unhurried, supportive manner.

Another barrier is the increased prevalence of cognitive, sensory-perceptual, and motor problems that interfere with a person's ability to process information and communicate. Examples include dementia and delirium, poststroke aphasia, and other communication barriers. Hearing and vision deficits may complicate assessment. Therefore pain assessment tools may have to be adapted for older adults. For example, you many need to use a large-print pain intensity scale. Most older adults, even those with mild to moderate cognitive impairment, can use quantitative scales accurately and reliably.

In older patients with chronic pain, perform a thorough physical examination and history to identify causes of pain, possible therapies, and potential problems. Assess for depression and functional impairments, because they are also common among older adults with pain.

Treatment of pain in older adults is complicated by several factors. First, older adults metabolize drugs more slowly than younger people and thus are at greater risk for higher blood levels and adverse effects. The adage "start low and go slow" must be applied to analgesic therapy in this age group. Second, the use of NSAIDs in older adults is associated with a high frequency of GI bleeding. Third, older adults often are taking many drugs for 1 or more chronic conditions. The addition of analgesics can result in dangerous drug interactions and increased side effects. Fourth, cognitive impairment and ataxia can be worsened by analgesics, such as opioids, antidepressants, and antiseizure drugs. This requires that HCPs titrate drugs slowly and monitor carefully for side effects.

Treatment regimens for older adults must include nondrug modalities. Exercise and patient teaching are important nondrug interventions for older adults with chronic pain. Include family and caregivers in the treatment plan (Tables 8.15 and 8.16).

MANAGING PAIN IN SPECIAL POPULATIONS

Patients Unable to Self-Report Pain

Although the patient's self-report is the gold standard of pain assessment, many illnesses and conditions affect a patient's ability to report pain. These diagnoses and conditions include dementia and delirium. For these people, behavioral and physiologic changes may be the only indicators of pain. You must be astute at recognizing behavioral symptoms of pain.

TABLE 8.18   **Assessing Pain in Nonverbal Patients**
The following assessment techniques are recommended: • Obtain a self-report when possible. • Never assume a nonverbal person is unable to communicate pain; blinking, writing, hand gestures, or nodding can be ways to express pain or the absence of pain. • Investigate potential causes of pain. • Observe patient behaviors that indicate pain (e.g., grimacing, frowning, rubbing a painful area, groaning, restlessness). • Obtain surrogate reports of pain from professional and family caregivers. • Try to use analgesics and reassess the patient to observe for a decrease in pain-related behaviors.

Modified from Herr K, Coyne PJ, McCaffery M, et al: Position statement from the American Society for Pain Management Nursing (ASPMN): Pain assessment in the patient unable to self-report—Position statement with clinical practice recommendations, *Pain Manag Nurs* 12:230, 2011.

A guide for assessing pain in nonverbal patients is outlined in Table 8.18. Several scales are available to assess pain-related behaviors in nonverbal patients, particularly those with advanced dementia and the critically ill. Links to several pain assessment tools are available at the City of Hope Pain and Palliative Care Resource Center website (*http://prc.coh.org*).

Patients With Substance Use Problems

HCPs are often reluctant to give opioids to patients at risk for addiction or those with substance-abuse disorders for fear of promoting or worsening addictions. However, there is no evidence that providing opioid analgesia to these patients in any way worsens their addictive disease. In fact, the stress of unrelieved pain may contribute to relapse in the recovering patient or increased drug use in the patient who is actively abusing drugs.

❓ **CHECK YOUR PRACTICE**
A 36-yr-old male patient is recovering from abdominal surgery to remove his spleen after an automobile accident. He is a known drug user. You are taking care of him, and he is very irritable because he is not getting enough pain medication. You are reluctant to give him his PRN morphine for fear that you will contribute to his addiction problem. • What should you do?

Guidelines for pain management in patients with addictive disease have been established by the American Society for Pain Management Nursing (ASPMN). These guidelines reflect your role in a team approach in which patients with addictive disease and pain have the right to be treated with dignity, respect, and the same quality of pain assessment and management as all other patients.

If the patient acknowledges substance use, determine the types and amounts of drugs used. Avoid exposing the patient to the misused drug. Effective equianalgesic doses of other opioids may be determined if daily drug doses are known. If a history of drug use is unknown or if the patient does not acknowledge substance use, be suspect when normal doses of analgesics do not relieve the patient's pain.

Aggressive behavior patterns and signs of withdrawal may occur. Withdrawal symptoms can worsen pain and lead to drug-seeking behavior or illicit drug use. Toxicology screens may be helpful in determining recently used drugs. Discussing these findings with the patient may help gain the patient's cooperation in pain control.

Severe pain should be treated with opioids and at much higher doses than those used with drug-naive patients. The use of a single opioid is preferred. Avoid using a mixed opioid agonist-antagonist (e.g., butorphanol) or a partial agonist (e.g., buprenorphine) because these drugs may precipitate withdrawal symptoms. Nonopioid and adjuvant analgesics and nondrug pain relief measures may be used as needed. To maintain opioid blood levels and prevent withdrawal symptoms, provide analgesics around the clock. Use supplemental doses to treat breakthrough pain. IV or PCA infusions may be considered for acute pain management.

Pain management for people with addiction is challenging and needs an interprofessional team approach. When possible, the team includes pain management and addiction specialists. Team members need to be aware of their own attitudes about people with substance use problems, which may result in undertreatment of pain.

CASE STUDY

Pain

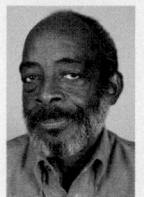

(© iStock.com/XiXinXing.)

Patient Profile

K.C. is a 280-lb (127-kg) 68-yr-old black man with diabetes, peripheral neuropathy, hypertension, and gout, who was admitted for an incision and drainage of a right abdominal abscess. He is being discharged on his second postoperative day. His daughter will perform dressing changes at home.

Subjective Data

- Lives alone
- Desires 0 pain but will accept 1 or 2 on a scale of 0 to 10
- Reports incision area pain as a 2 or 3 between dressing changes and as a 6 during dressing changes
- States sharp pain persists 1 to 2 hours after dressing change
- Reports pain between dressing changes controlled by 2 oxycodone tablets
- Has history of peripheral neuropathy and describes chronic pain in his feet

Objective Data

- Needs dressing changes 4 times per day after discharge
- For discharge, oxycodone (2 tablets q4hr for pain PRN) is prescribed.

Discussion Questions

1. Describe the assessment data that are important for determining whether K.C. has adequate pain management.
2. *Priority Decision:* Based on the data presented, what are the priority nursing diagnoses? Are there any collaborative problems?
3. *Priority Decision:* What are the priority nursing interventions for K.C.?
4. How long should the daughter wait after the oxycodone is given to begin the dressing change?
5. *Patient-Centered Care:* What other pain therapies might you plan to help K.C. through the dressing change?
6. *Safety:* What side effects might he have because of his pain medication? How can these be safely managed?
7. *Collaboration:* To whom can you delegate teaching K.C. and his daughter the plan of care at home?
8. *Evidence-Based Practice:* K.C.'s daughter asks you if any other strategies could be used to help decrease her father's incisional pain and his peripheral neuropathy pain.

Answers available at *www.evolve.elsevier.com/Lewis/medsurg.*

BRIDGE TO NCLEX EXAMINATION

The number of the question corresponds to the same-numbered outcome at the beginning of the chapter.

1. Pain is *best* described as
   a. a creation of a person's imagination.
   b. an unpleasant, subjective experience.
   c. a maladaptive response to a stimulus.
   d. a neurologic event resulting from activation of nociceptors.

2. A patient is receiving a PCA infusion after surgery to repair a hip fracture. She is sleeping soundly but awakens when the nurse speaks to her in a normal tone of voice. Her respirations are 8 breaths/min. The *most* appropriate nursing action in this situation is to
   a. stop the PCA infusion.
   b. obtain an oxygen saturation level.
   c. continue to closely monitor the patient.
   d. administer naloxone and contact the provider.

3. Which words are *most* likely to be used to describe neuropathic pain (*select all that apply*)?
   a. Dull
   b. Itching
   c. Burning
   d. Shooting
   e. Shock-like

4. Unrelieved pain is
   a. not expected after major surgery.
   b. expected in a person with cancer.
   c. dangerous and can lead to many physical and psychologic complications.
   d. an annoying sensation, but it is not as important as other physical care needs.

5. A cancer patient who reports ongoing, constant moderate pain with short periods of severe pain during dressing changes is
   a. probably exaggerating his pain.
   b. in need of a referral for surgical treatment of his pain.
   c. best treated by receiving a long-acting and a short-acting opioid.
   d. best treated by regularly scheduled short-acting opioids plus acetaminophen.

6. An example of distraction to provide pain relief is
   a. TENS.
   b. music.
   c. exercise.
   d. biofeedback.

7. Appropriate nonopioid analgesics for mild pain include *(select all that apply)*
   a. oxycodone.
   b. ibuprofen (Advil).
   c. lorazepam (Ativan).
   d. acetaminophen (Tylenol).
   e. codeine with acetaminophen (Tylenol #3).

8. An *important* nursing responsibility related to pain is to
   a. leave the patient alone to rest.
   b. help the patient appear to not be in pain.
   c. believe what the patient says about the pain.
   d. assume responsibility for eliminating the patient's pain.

9. Giving opioids to an actively dying patient who has moderate to severe pain
   a. may cause addiction.
   b. will likely be ineffective.
   c. is an appropriate nursing action.
   d. will likely hasten the person's death.

10. A nurse believes that patients with the same type of tissue injury should have the same amount of pain. This statement reflects
    a. a belief that will contribute to appropriate pain management.
    b. an accurate statement about pain mechanisms and expected goals of pain therapy.
    c. a belief that will not have any effect on the type of care provided to people in pain.
    d. a lack of knowledge about pain mechanisms, which is likely to contribute to poor pain management.

1. b, 2. c, 3. b, c, d, e, 4. c, 5. c, 6. b, 7. b, d, 8. c, 9. c, 10. d.

For rationales to these answers and even more NCLEX review questions, visit *http://evolve.elsevier.com/Lewis/medsurg.*

ⓔ EVOLVE WEBSITE/RESOURCES LIST

http://evolve.elsevier.com/Lewis/medsurg
Review Questions (Online Only)
Key Points
Answer Keys for Questions
- Rationales for Bridge to NCLEX Examination Questions
- Answer Guidelines for Case Study on p. 125
Student Case Study
- Patient With Pain
Conceptual Care Map Creator
Audio Glossary
Content Updates

REFERENCES

1. Centers for Disease Control and Prevention. Guideline for prescribing opioids for chronic pain. Retrieved from *www.cdc.gov/drugoverdose/prescribing/guideline.html.*
*2. Van den Beuken-Van Everdingen MH, Hochstenbach LM, Joosten EA, et al: Update on prevalence of pain in patients with cancer: Systematic review and meta-analysis, *J Pain Symptom Manage* 51:6, 2016.
3. McCaffery M. *Nursing practice theories related to cognition, bodily pain and man-environmental interactions*, Los Angeles, 1968, UCLA Students Store. (Classic)
*4. Goncalves JPB, Lucchetti G, Menezes PR, et al: Complimentary religious and spiritual interventions in physical health and quality of life: A systematic review of randomized controlled clinical trials, *PLoS One* 12:10, 2017.
5. Jensen MP, Tomé-Pires C, de la Vega C, et al: What determines whether a pain is rated as mild, moderate, or severe? *Clin J Pain* 33:414, 2017.
6. Nix WA: *Muscles, nerves, and pain.* Berlin, 2017, Springer.
*7. Tesarz J, Eich W, Treede RD, et al: Altered pressure pain thresholds and increased wind-up in adult patients with chronic back pain with a history of childhood maltreatment: A quantitative sensory testing study, *Pain* 157:1799, 2016.
*8. Parker RS, Lewis, GN, Rice DA, et al: Is motor cortical excitability altered in people with chronic pain? A systematic review and meta-analysis, *Brain Stimul* 9:4, 2016.
*9. Blyth FM: The global burden of neuropathic pain, *Pain* 159:614, 2018.

*10. Kuttikat A, Maliha S, Oomatia A, et al: Novel signs and their clinical utility in diagnosing complex regional pain syndrome: A prospective observational cohort study, *Clin J Pain* 33:496, 2017.
11. Hale D, Marshall K. Assessing and treating pain in the cognitively impaired geriatric home care patient, *Home Health Now* 25:116, 2017.
*12. Gordon DB, Dahl J, Phillips P, et al: The use of "as-needed" range orders for opioid analgesic in the management of acute pain: A consensus statement of the American Society of Pain Management Nurses and the American Pain Society, *Pain Manag Nurs* 5:53, 2004. (Classic)
*13. Kumar K, Kirksey MA, Duong S, et al: A review of opioid-sparing modalities in perioperative pain management: methods to decrease opioid use postoperatively, *Anesth Analg* 125:1749, 2017.
14. Tawfic Q, Kumar K, Pirani Z, et al: Prevention of chronic post-surgical pain: The importance of early identification of risk factors, *J Anesth* 31:424, 2017.
15. Yoon E, Barbar A, Choudhary M, et al: Acetaminophen-induced hepatotoxicity: A comprehensive update, *J Clin Transl Hepatol* 4:131, 2016.
16. Kharasch ED: Current concepts in methadone metabolism and transport, *Clin Pharmacol Drug Dev* 6:125, 2017.
*17. Gupta K, Prasad A, Nagappa M, et al: Risk factors for opioid-induced respiratory depression and failure to rescue, *Curr Opin Anaesthesiol* 31:110, 2018.
*18. Mu A, Weinberg E, Moulin DE, et al: Pharmacologic management of chronic neuropathic pain: Review of the Canadian Pain Society consensus statement, *Can Fam Physician* 63:844, 2017.
19. Janknegt R, van den Beuken M, Schiere S, et al: Rapid acting fentanyl formulations in breakthrough pain in cancer: Drug selection by means of the System of Objectified Judgement Analysis. *Eur J Hosp Pharm Sci Pract*, 25:e2, 2018.
20. Webb RJ, Shelton CP: The benefits of authorized agent controlled analgesia (AACA) to control pain and other symptoms at the end of life, *J Pain Symptom Manage* 50:371, 2015.
21. Coutaux A. Non-pharmacological treatments for pain relief: TENS and acupuncture, *Joint Bone Spine* 84:657, 2017.
*22. Felix MM, Ferreira MB, da Cruz LF, et al: Relaxation therapy with guided imagery for postoperative pain management: An integrative review, *Pain Manag Nurs* 35:342, 2017.
23. The Joint Commission: Revised standard on pain assessment and management, 2018. Retrieved from *www.jointcommission.org.*
24. De Lima L, Woodruff R, Pettus K, et al: International Association for Hospice and Palliative Care position statement: Euthanasia and physician-assisted suicide, *J Palliat Med* 20:8, 2017.

*Evidence-based information for clinical practice.

9

Palliative and End-of-Life Care

Denise M. McEnroe-Petitte

> *Those who have the strength and the love to sit with a dying patient in the silence that goes beyond words will know that this moment is neither frightening nor painful, but a peaceful cessation.*
>
> ***Elisabeth Kübler-Ross***

ℯ http://evolve.elsevier.com/Lewis/medsurg/

CONCEPTUAL FOCUS

Coping

Ethics

Family Dynamics

Health Care Organizations

Palliation

Spirituality

LEARNING OUTCOMES

1. Distinguish the purpose of palliative care at the end of life and hospice care.
2. Describe the physical and psychologic manifestations at the end of life.
3. Explain the process of grief and bereavement at the end of life.
4. Examine the cultural and spiritual issues related to end-of-life care.
5. Discuss ethical and legal issues in end-of-life care.
6. Describe the nursing management of the dying patient.
7. Explore the special needs of family caregivers in end-of-life care.
8. Discuss the special needs of the nurse who cares for dying patients and their families.

KEY TERMS

advance directives, p. 133
bereavement, p. 131
brain death, p. 129
Cheyne-Stokes respiration, p. 130

death, p. 129
death rattle, p. 130
end of life, p. 129
grief, p. 131

hospice, p. 128
palliative care, p. 127
spirituality, p. 132

PALLIATIVE CARE

Palliative care is any form of care or treatment that focuses on reducing the severity of disease symptoms. The overall goals of palliative care are to (1) prevent and relieve suffering and (2) improve quality of life for patients with serious life-limiting illnesses[1] (Fig. 9.1). Specific goals of palliative care are listed in Table 9.1.

Ideally, all patients receiving curative or restorative health care should receive palliative care at the same time. Palliative care extends into the period of end-of-life (EOL) care and offers patient and family support while planning for EOL needs.[2] Bereavement care follows the patient's death (Fig. 9.2).

Palliative care originated as EOL care in the 1960s. Initially, this care focused on providing symptom relief and emotional support to the patient, family, and significant others during the terminal phases of a serious life-limiting disease. We now call that phase of palliative care *palliative care at the end of life*, which is the focus of this chapter.

The role of palliative care at the EOL is increasing in our current health care environment. Demographic changes are increasing the demand for palliative care. A growing number of Baby Boomers are turning 65. Improvements in health care technology have led to longer life expectancies and an increased number of older adults. The growing number of people with conditions such as diabetes and heart disease contribute to the increased use of palliative care.[2]

Older adults often have multiple chronic illnesses resulting in increased health care use.[3] Palliative care has been shown to (1) improve quality of life for those with chronic illness, (2) decrease the associated economic costs for their health care, and (3) ease caregiver burden for those with chronic and terminal illnesses.

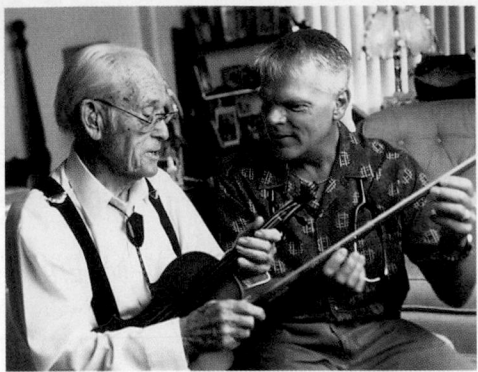

FIG. 9.1 One goal of palliative care is to improve the quality of the patient's remaining life. (Courtesy Kathleen A. Pollard, RN, MSN, CHPN, Phoenix, AZ.)

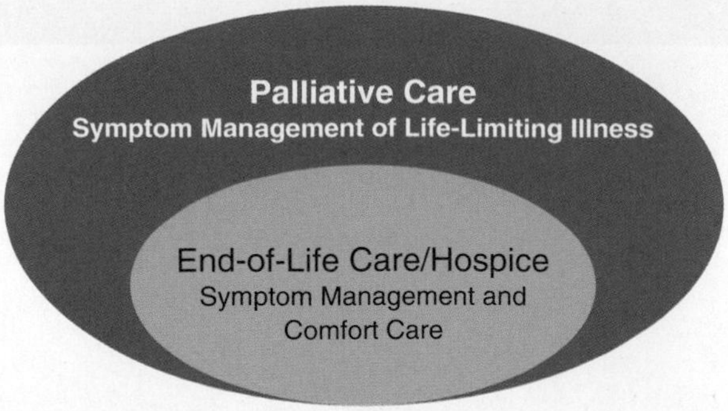

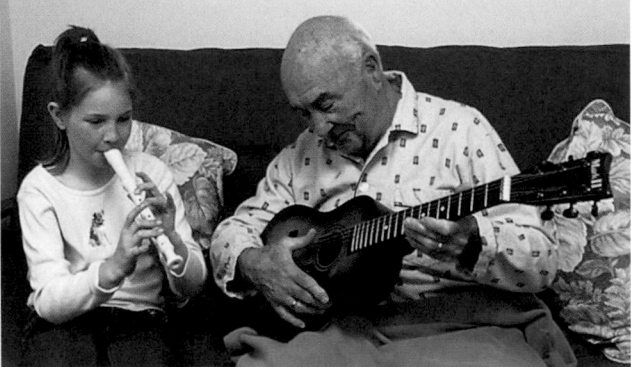

FIG. 9.3 Relationship of palliative care and end-of-life care/hospice. (From Rosenberg M, Lamba S, Misra S: Palliative medicine and geriatric emergency care: Challenges, opportunities, and basic principles, *Clin Geriatr Med* 29:1, 2013.)

TABLE 9.1 **Goals of Palliative Care**
• Regard dying as a normal process
• Provide relief from symptoms, including pain
• Affirm life and neither hasten nor postpone death
• Support holistic patient care and enhance quality of life
• Offer support to patients to live as actively as possible until death
• Offer support to the family during the patient's illness and in their own bereavement

Adapted from World Health Organization: WHO definition of palliative care. Retrieved from *www.who.int/cancer/palliative/definition/en.*

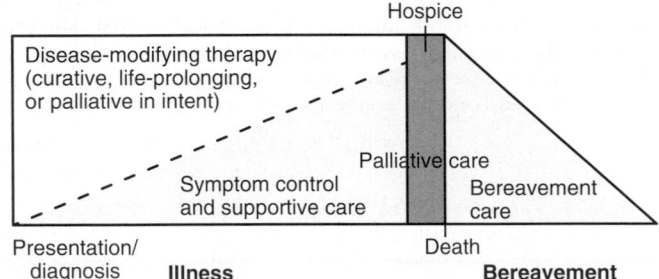

FIG. 9.2 Continuum-of-care model showing integration of curative care, palliative and end-of-life/hospice care, and bereavement care. (Redrawn from Robert Wood Johnson Foundation: *The EPEC Project: Elements and models of end-of-life care,* 1999.)

FIG. 9.4 Hospice care is designed to provide compassion, concern, and support for the dying. (From Rick Brady, Riva, MD.)

concern, and support for persons in the last phases of a terminal disease (Fig. 9.4). The main goals of hospice care are to assist the patient to live as fully and comfortably as possible while dying with dignity. Hospice programs provide care with an emphasis on symptom management, advance care planning, spiritual care, and family support.

The major difference between palliative care and hospice care is that palliative care allows a person to simultaneously receive curative and palliative treatments. Hospice care is an option when the physician determines a person has 6 months or less to live and that person or health care proxy decides to forgo curative treatments. Hospice is often underused, as many assume the person must be actively dying before hospice is necessary. On the contrary, it is important that the person be referred to hospice as soon as possible to ease the physical, emotional, and spiritual distress so common at the EOL.

Almost half of the patients who die in the United States are under the care of a hospice program.[4] More than three-quarters of persons in hospice programs are over the age of 65 years, and the majority are white. Most patients have cancer, dementia, stroke, or heart or respiratory conditions.[4]

Hospice programs are organized under a variety of models. Some are hospital-based programs, others are part of existing home health care agencies, and others are freestanding or community-based programs.

Like palliative care, hospice care is provided in a variety of locations, including the home, inpatient settings, acute and long-term care facilities, and rehabilitation centers. Hospice services are available 24 hours a day, 7 days a week to help

To optimize the benefits of palliative care, it should be started after a person receives a diagnosis of a life-limiting illness, such as cancer, heart failure, chronic obstructive pulmonary disease, dementia, or end-stage kidney disease. The palliative care team is an interprofessional collaboration involving physicians, nurses, social workers, pharmacists, chaplains, and other health care professionals. Communication among the patient, family, and interprofessional palliative team is important to provide optimal care.

Patients may receive palliative care services in multiple settings, including the home, long-term and acute care, mental health facilities, rehabilitation centers, and prisons. Many institutions have established interprofessional palliative and hospice care teams.[1]

HOSPICE CARE

Palliative care often includes hospice care before or at the EOL (Fig. 9.3). **Hospice** is a concept of care that provides compassion,

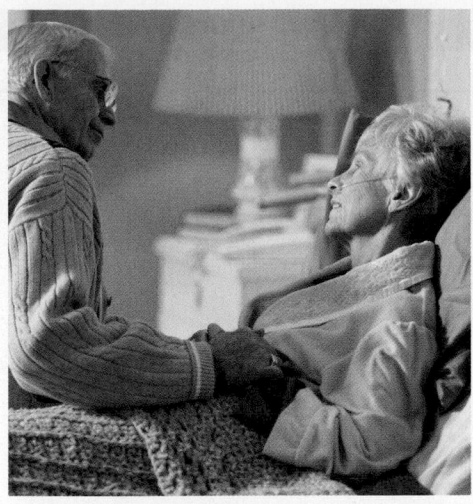

FIG. 9.5 Inpatient hospice settings are designed to make the atmosphere as relaxed and homelike as possible. (© Photodisc/Thinkstock.)

patients and families in their homes. Inpatient hospice settings often have a relaxed and homelike atmosphere (Fig. 9.5). Staff and volunteers are available for the patient and family.

A medically supervised interprofessional team and volunteers provide holistic hospice services. The hospice nurse plays a pivotal role in coordination of the hospice team.[5] Hospice nurses work with other interprofessional team members to provide care and support to the patient and family. Hospice nurses focus on pain control and symptom management, spiritual assessment, and assessment and management of family needs. To meet patient and family needs, the hospice nurse needs excellent teaching skills, compassion, flexibility, cultural competence, and adaptability.

The decision to begin hospice care is hard for several reasons. Many patients, families, physicians, and other health care providers (HCPs) lack information about hospice care. Some cultural/ethnic groups may not use hospice because of a lack of awareness of hospice services, a desire to continue with potentially curative therapies, and concerns about lack of minority hospice workers. Physicians may be reluctant to give referrals because they sometimes view a patient's decline as their personal failure. Some patients or family members see hospice care as "giving up" or receiving second-rate care.

It is important to consider potential barriers to hospice care in vulnerable populations. These may include veterans, homeless, immigrants, impoverished, disabled, or institutionalized persons. In these populations, besides the hospice team, you may need to collaborate with community partners to facilitate support services to meet the needs of the patient and family.[5]

Medicare, Medicaid, and many private insurance agencies cover hospice services. Admission to a hospice program has 2 criteria. The first criterion is that the patient must want the services and agree in writing to use only hospice care, not curative care, to treat the terminal illness. The second criterion is that the patient must be medically eligible for hospice. Medicare, Medicaid, and other insurers require that 2 physicians certify that the patient's prognosis is terminal, with less than 6 months to live. After this initial certification, only 1 physician (e.g., the hospice medical director) is needed to recertify the patient. It is important to realize that the physician who certified that a hospice patient is terminal does not "guarantee" death within

6 months. If a patient in hospice survives beyond 6 months, Medicare and other reimbursement organizations will continue to reimburse for an extended period if the patient still meets enrolment criteria.

Hospice patients can receive care for other health problems that are not related to the terminal illness. However, the hospice, Medicare, Medicaid, or patient's insurance company may not cover those services.[6] They can voluntarily withdraw from the program at any time. Occasionally, a patient's condition stabilizes, and the patient may be discharged from hospice care. This decision is made after review of the current treatment plan and input from members of the interprofessional hospice team.

DEATH

Death occurs when all vital organs and body systems cease to function. It is the irreversible cessation of cardiovascular, respiratory, and brain function.

Brain death is an irreversible loss of all brain functions, including those of the brainstem. Brain death is a clinical diagnosis. It occurs when the cerebral cortex stops functioning or is irreversibly destroyed.

With the growing use of technology that assists in supporting life, controversies have arisen over the exact definition of death. Questions and discussions have focused on whether brain death occurs when the whole brain (cortex and brainstem) ceases activity or when function of the cortex alone stops. The American Academy of Neurology developed the diagnostic criteria guidelines for clinical diagnosis of brain death. The criteria include coma or unresponsiveness, absence of brainstem reflexes, and apnea. Physicians must perform specific assessments to confirm each of the criteria.[7]

Currently, legal and medical standards require that all brain function must cease to be able to pronounce brain death and disconnect life support. Diagnosing brain death is of special importance when organ donation is an option. In some states and under specific circumstances, a registered nurse is legally allowed to pronounce death. Policies and procedures may vary from state to state and among health care institutions.

END-OF-LIFE CARE

End of life generally refers to the final phase of a patient's illness when death is imminent. The time from diagnosis of a terminal illness to death varies depending on the patient's diagnosis and extent of disease.

The National Academy of Medicine defines *end of life* as the period during which a person copes with declining health from a terminal illness or from the frailties associated with advanced age, even if death is not clearly imminent.[8] In some cases it is obvious to HCPs that the patient is at the EOL. In other cases, they may be uncertain if the EOL is near. This uncertainty adds to the challenge of answering the common question asked by the patient and family, "How much time is left?"

End-of-life care (EOL care) is the term used for issues and services related to death and dying. EOL care focuses on physical and psychosocial needs for the patient and family. The goals for EOL care are to (1) provide comfort and supportive care during the dying process, (2) improve the quality of the patient's remaining life, (3) help ensure a dignified death, and (4) provide emotional support to the family.

TABLE 9.2 Physical Manifestations at End of Life

System	Manifestations
Cardiovascular system	• Increased heart rate; later slowing and weakening of pulse • Irregular rhythm • Decreased BP • Delayed absorption of drugs given IM or subcutaneously
Gastrointestinal system	• Slowing or cessation of GI function (may be enhanced by pain-relieving drugs) • Gas accumulation • Distention and nausea • Loss of sphincter control, producing incontinence • Bowel movement before imminent death or at time of death
Integumentary system	• Mottling on hands, feet, arms, and legs • Cold, clammy skin • Cyanosis of nose, nail beds, knees • "Waxlike" skin when very near death
Musculoskeletal system	• Gradual loss of ability to move • Sagging of jaw resulting from loss of facial muscle tone • Difficulty speaking • Swallowing becoming more difficult • Difficulty maintaining body posture and alignment • Loss of gag reflex • Jerking seen in patients on high doses of opioids
Respiratory system	• Increased respiratory rate • Cheyne-Stokes respiration • Inability to cough or clear secretions resulting in grunting, gurgling, or noisy congested breathing (death rattle or terminal secretions) • Irregular breathing, gradually slowing down to terminal gasps (may be described as guppy breathing)
Sensory system Hearing Sight Taste and smell Touch	 • Usually last sense to disappear • Blurring of vision • Sinking and glazing of eyes • Blink reflex absent • Eyelids stay half-open • Decreased with disease progression • Decreased sensation • Decreased sense of pain and touch
Urinary system	• Gradual decrease in urine output • Incontinence of urine • Inability to urinate

Physical Manifestations at End of Life

As death approaches, metabolism reduces and the body gradually slows down until all functions end. Respiratory changes are common. Respirations may be rapid or slow, shallow, and irregular. Breath sounds may become wet and noisy, both audibly and on auscultation. Mouth breathing and accumulation of mucus in the airways cause noisy, wet-sounding respirations, termed the **death rattle** or terminal secretions. **Cheyne-Stokes respiration** is a pattern of breathing characterized by alternating periods of apnea and deep, rapid breathing. When respirations cease, the heart stops beating within a few minutes. The physical manifestations of approaching death are listed in Table 9.2.

Psychosocial Manifestations at End of Life

A variety of feelings and emotions can affect the dying patient and family at the EOL (Table 9.3). Most patients and families struggle with a terminal diagnosis and the realization that there is no cure. The patient and family may feel overwhelmed, fearful, powerless, and fatigued. The family's response depends in part on the type and length of the illness and their relationship with the person.

The patient's needs and wishes must be respected. Patients need time to think and express their feelings. Response time

TABLE 9.3 Psychosocial Manifestations at End of Life

- Altered decision making
- Anxiety about unfinished business
- Decreased socialization
- Fear of loneliness
- Fear of meaninglessness of one's life
- Fear of pain
- Helplessness
- Life review
- Peacefulness
- Restlessness
- Saying goodbyes
- Unusual communication
- Vision-like experiences
- Withdrawal

to questions may be sluggish because of fatigue, weakness, and confusion.

Bereavement and Grief

Although we often use the terms interchangeably, *bereavement* refers to the state of loss and *grief* refers to the reaction to loss.

TABLE 9.4   Kübler-Ross Model of Grief

Stage	What Person May Say	Characteristics
Denial	No, not me. It cannot be true.	Denies the loss has taken place and may withdraw. This response may last minutes to months
Anger	Why me?	May be angry at the person who inflicted the hurt (even after death) or at the world for letting it happen. May be angry with self for letting an event (e.g., car accident) take place, even if nothing could have stopped it
Bargaining	Yes me, but . . .	May make bargains with God, asking, "If I do this, will you take away the loss?"
Depression	Yes me, and I am sad.	Feels numb, although anger and sadness may remain underneath
Acceptance	Yes me, but it is okay.	Anger, sadness, and mourning have tapered off. Accepts the reality of the loss

Adapted from Kübler-Ross E: *On death and dying,* New York, 1969, Macmillan. (Classic)

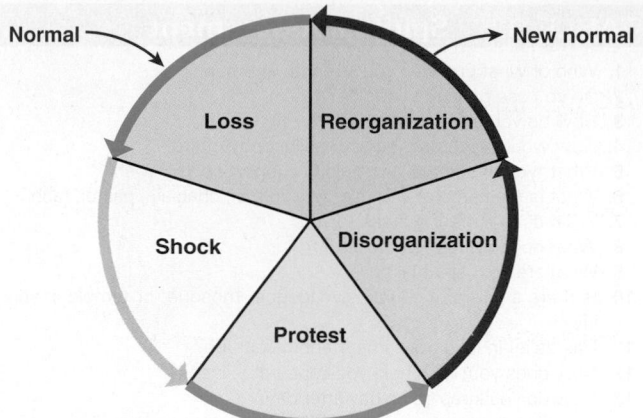

FIG. 9.6 The grief wheel model begins with the normal state at the bottom. After a person goes through the grief process, eventually the grief will resolve. However, because of the loss, the normal state is different from before. The challenge is to accept the "new normal."

Bereavement is the period after the death of a loved one during which we experience grief and mourning occurs. The time spent in bereavement depends on several factors, including how attached one was to the person who died and how much time one spent expecting the loss.

Grief is a normal reaction to loss. Grief occurs in response to the real loss of a loved one and the loss of what might have been. Grief is dynamic and includes both psychologic and physiologic responses after a loss. Psychologic responses include anger, guilt, anxiety, sadness, depression, and despair. Physiologic reactions include sleeping problems, changes in appetite, physical problems, and illness.

Grief is a powerful emotional state that affects all aspects of a person's life. It is a complex and intense emotional experience. In the Kübler-Ross model of grief, there are 5 stages[9] (Table 9.4). Not every person experiences all the stages of grieving, and they are not always progressive. It is common to reach a stage and then go backward. For example, a person may have reached the stage of bargaining and then revert to the denial or anger stage.

Another model of grief is the grief wheel (Fig. 9.6). After a person has a loss, he or she feels *shock* (numbness, denial, inability to think straight). Next is the *protest* stage, in which a person may have anger, guilt, sadness, fear, and searching. Then comes the *disorganization* stage, in which a person feels despair, apathy, anxiety, and confusion. The next stage is *reorganization,* in which a person gradually returns to normal functioning, but he or she feels different. The last stage is the *new normal.* Eventually the destabilization experienced in grief resolves and a normal state can begin. However, because of the loss, the normal state is different from before. The challenge is to accept the new normal. Trying to go back to the "old" normal (which is not there anymore) is what causes a great deal of anxiety and stress.

The way a person grieves depends on factors such as the relationship with the person who has died (e.g., spouse, parent), physical and emotional coping resources, concurrent life stresses, cultural beliefs, and personality. Other factors that affect the grief response include mental and physical health, economic resources, religious influences or spiritual beliefs, family relationships, social support, and time spent preparing for the death. Issues that occurred before the death (e.g., marital problems) may affect the grief response.[10]

The grief experience for the caregiver of the patient with a chronic illness often begins long before the actual death event. This is called *anticipatory grief.* Patients at the EOL also can have anticipatory grief.

Working in a positive way through the grief process helps to adapt to the loss. Grief that helps the person accept the reality of death is called *adaptive grief.* It is a healthy response. It may be associated with grieving before death occurs or when the inevitability of the death is known. Indicators of adaptive grief include the ability to see some good resulting from the death and positive memories of the deceased person.

Dysfunctional reactions to loss can occur, and the physical and psychologic impact of the loved one's death may persist for years. *Prolonged grief disorder,* formerly called *complicated grief,* is a term used to describe prolonged and intense mourning. Prolonged grief disorder can include symptoms such as recurrent and severe distressing emotions and intrusive thoughts related to the loss of a loved one, self-neglect, and denial of the loss for longer than 6 months. About 1 in 5 bereaved persons has prolonged grief disorder. Those with prolonged grief disorder have a higher risk for illness and may have work and social impairments.

Bereavement and grief counseling are core parts of patient- and family-centered palliative care. The goal of a bereavement program is to provide support and to help survivors in the transition to a life without the deceased person. Incorporate grief support into the plan of care for the family and significant others during the patient's illness and after the death.

TABLE 9.5	Spiritual Assessment

1. Who or what provides you strength and hope?
2. Do you use prayer in your life?
3. How do you express spirituality?
4. How would you describe your philosophy of life?
5. What type of spiritual or religious support do you wish?
6. What is the name of your clergy, minister, chaplain, pastor, rabbi?
7. What does suffering mean to you?
8. What does dying mean to you?
9. What are your spiritual goals?
10. Is there a role of a church, synagogue, mosque, or temple in your life?
11. Has belief in God been important in your life?
12. How does your faith help you cope with illness?
13. How do you keep going day after day?
14. What helps you get through this health care experience?
15. How has illness affected you and your family?

© The Joint Commission. Adapted with permission.

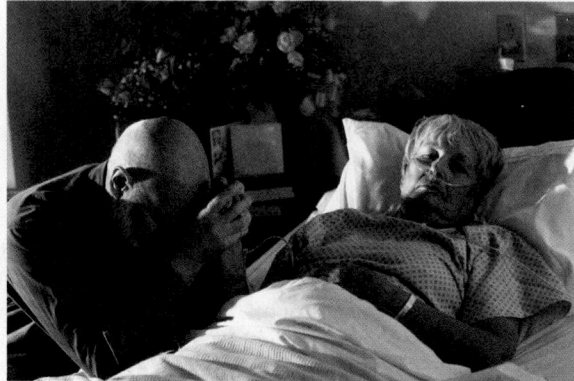

FIG. 9.7 Spiritual needs are an important consideration in end-of-life care. (© Photodisc/Thinkstock.)

Priority interventions for grief focus on providing an environment that allows the patient and family to express their feelings, such as anger, fear, and guilt. Discussing feelings helps the patient and family work toward resolution of the grief process. Respect for the patient's privacy and need or desire to talk (or not to talk) is important. Honesty in answering questions and giving information is essential.

Spiritual Needs

Assessment of spiritual needs in EOL care is a key consideration (Table 9.5). **Spirituality** is a broad concept that encompasses beliefs, values, and purpose that relate to the search for existential meaning and purpose.[11] Some define spirituality as a relationship with a supreme being that directs beliefs and practices. Spiritual needs do not necessarily equate to religion or belief in a higher power. A person may not be part of a particular religion but have a deep spirituality. Assess the patient's and family's preferences related to spiritual guidance or pastoral care services and make appropriate referrals.

Deep-seated spiritual beliefs may surface for some patients when they deal with their terminal diagnosis and related issues. Patients may question their beliefs about a higher power, their journey through life, religion, and an afterlife (Fig. 9.7). Spiritual distress may occur.[11] Characteristics of spiritual distress include anger toward God or a higher being, change in behavior and mood, desire for spiritual assistance, or displaced anger toward clergy.

Spirituality has been associated with decreased despair in patients at EOL. Some dying patients are secure in their faith about the future. It is common to see patients relinquish material possessions of life and focus on values that they believe will lead them on to another place. Many turn to religion because it gives order to the world even in the presence of physical decline, social losses, suffering, and impending death. Religion may offer an existential meaning that offers a sense of peace and recognition of one's place in the broader cosmic context.[11]

Culturally Competent Care: End of Life

Culture and ethnicity are important considerations for patients who are receiving palliative and EOL care and their families. Cultural beliefs affect a person's understanding of and reaction to death or loss. In some cultural/ethnic groups, death and dying are private matters shared only with significant others. Often feelings are repressed or internalized. People who believe in "toughing it out" or "being strong" may not express themselves when they are experiencing a loss. Some cultural groups, such as blacks and Hispanic/Latinos, may easily express their feelings and emotions. Kinship tends to be strong in the Hispanic culture, and immediate and extended family provide support for one another. Expressing feelings of loss is encouraged and accepted easily.

Culture and ethnicity affect decision making about life support, withholding and withdrawing treatments, and using palliative or hospice care.[12] In some cultures, such as the Filipino American culture, it may be appropriate to first discuss a terminal diagnosis with the family before informing the patient. For Hispanics, often spouses and daughters are involved in decisions about palliative care and hospice. Blacks and Asian Americans use hospice care less often, with blacks being more likely to prefer aggressive treatment.

Rituals associated with dying are part of all cultures. In certain cultures, the family may want to keep constant vigil in the room of a dying patient or in the waiting area. For example, some Jewish Americans believe that the spirit should not be alone when it leaves the body at the time of death. Therefore someone who is terminally ill should never be alone. The Jewish culture believes all body tissues must be buried with the person. Once a death has occurred, some cultures, such as the Puerto Rican American culture, may want to kiss and touch the body to say goodbye. In the Islamic cultures, the traditional rites of washing, shrouding, funeral prayers, and burial are done as soon as possible.

Cultural variations exist in symptom expression (e.g., pain expression) and use of health care services. Providing culturally competent care requires assessment of nonverbal cues, such as grimaces, body position, and decreased or guarded movements. See Chapter 8 for issues related to pain assessment and management.

Many differences exist among cultural beliefs and values in relation to death and dying. Assess beliefs and preferences on an individual basis to avoid stereotyping patients with different cultural belief systems. Assess and document the patient's cultural background, concerns, health practices, and attitudes about suffering. Ask the patient and family to describe their desires for care before death and care of the body after death. Use this assessment to guide the patient's plan of care and evaluation. You can suggest or plan grief and bereavement counseling for the family.

Make accommodations related to the patient's language, diet, and cultural beliefs and practices. Families with non–English-speaking members are at risk for receiving less information about their family member's critical illness and prognosis.[13] When appropriate, access medical interpreter services so that the patient's wishes are known. Culturally competent care is discussed in Chapter 2.

LEGAL AND ETHICAL ISSUES AFFECTING END-OF-LIFE CARE

Patients and families struggle with many decisions during the terminal illness and dying experience. Many people decide that the outcomes related to their care should be based on their own wishes and values. It is important to provide information to help patients with these decisions. The decisions may involve the choice for (1) organ and tissue donations, (2) advance directives (e.g., medical power of attorney, living wills), (3) resuscitation, (4) mechanical ventilation, and (5) feeding tube placement.

Decisional capacity refers to the ability to consent to or refuse care. It means that the person has an understanding and appreciation of the information received and has the capacity to engage in the reasoning process.

Organ and Tissue Donation

Persons who are legally competent may choose organ donation. You can donate any body part or the entire body. The decision to donate organs or to provide anatomic gifts may be made by a person before death or by immediate family after death. Family permission must be obtained at the time of donation.[14]

Some people carry donor cards. Some states mark organ donation wishes on drivers' licenses. The names of agencies that handle organ donation vary by state and community. Common names for such an agency may be the organ bank, organ-sharing network, and organ-sharing alliance. Organ and tissue donations follow specific legal guidelines. Follow those requirements and facility policies for organ or tissue donation. Notify the proper personnel at once when organ donation is intended, because some tissues must be used within hours after death.

Advance Care Planning and Advance Directives

Advance care planning is a process that involves having patients (1) think through their values and goals for treatment, (2) talk about their values and goals with others, and (3) document them. Advance directives are the written documents that provide information about the patient's wishes and his or her designated spokesperson (Table 9.6).

The first advance directive was known by laypersons as a *living will*. Most states have replaced the idea of living wills with *natural death acts,* which may include *directive to physicians* (DTPs), *durable power of attorney for health care* (DPAHC), *medical power of attorney* (MPOA), and *power of attorney for health care* (POAH). Under the natural death acts, a person can tell the HCP exactly what treatment is or is not desired. Each state has its own unique requirements. Patients often change their minds about desired treatments as their disease state progresses. It is important to reassess a patient's advance directives. For cognitively impaired older adults, consider the person's values and manner of life to make health care decisions consistent with decisions they made when they were cognitively intact.

People can get copies of state-specific forms from local medical associations and on the Internet. However, a person may write his or her wishes without special forms. Verbal directives can be given to the attending physician in the presence of 2 witnesses. The physician may use a Physician Order for Life-Sustaining Treatment (POLST) or Medical Order for Life-Sustaining Treatment (MOLST) to outline current treatment options that honor the person's desire for treatment (Table 9.6).

The person should keep a copy of the order to use in case of an emergency in which the primary physician is not available for consultation. Attorneys and notaries may not be needed to develop these directives. If the person is not capable of communicating his or her wishes, the surrogate decision maker (most often family or significant other) decides the measures that will or will not be taken. In this case, the physician and nurse can discuss the available options with the family. Then it is important to document the family's decision. This is important because often nurses and other medical professionals do not know who can legally make EOL decisions for patients when they no longer have decisional capacity.

Resuscitation

Cardiopulmonary resuscitation (CPR) is common practice in health care. Patients who have respiratory or cardiac arrest receive CPR unless the physician gives a *do-not-resuscitate (DNR) order*. A DNR order is a written medical order that documents a patient's wishes about resuscitation and, more important, the patient's desire to avoid CPR.[15]

There are several types of CPR decisions. Complete and total heroic measures, which may include CPR, drugs, and mechanical ventilation, can be referred to as a *full code.* Some people choose variations of the full code. A *chemical code* involves the use of drugs for resuscitation without the use of CPR. A "no code," or a DNR order, allows the person to die with comfort measures only and without the interference of technology. Some states have implemented a form called *out-of-hospital DNR* for use by terminally ill patients who wish to have no heroic measures used to prolong life after they leave an acute care facility.

Allow natural death (AND) is a term being used to replace "no code" or DNR. This term more accurately conveys our actions. It is sometimes referred to as *"comfort measures only"* status. The patient receives all comfort measures associated with pain control and symptom management, but the natural physiologic progression to death is not delayed or interrupted. The use of this type of language means that we do not withhold care, but care is supportive while allowing nature to take its course. It is meant to promote comfort and dignity at the EOL.

An advance directive includes whether to withhold or withdraw certain treatments. The directive must clearly state what is to be done and what is not to be done. The American Nurses Association (ANA) states that the decision to withhold artificial nutrition and hydration should be made by the patient or surrogate together with the interprofessional team. It is important we continue to provide expert nursing care for patients who are no longer receiving artificial nutrition and hydration.

You need to be aware of legal issues and have a primary role in supporting the patient's wishes. Advance directives and organ donor information should be in the medical record and identified on the patient's record and/or the nursing care plan. All caregivers responsible for the patient need to know the patient's wishes. Additionally, you need to be familiar with state, local, and agency procedures in EOL care documentation.

TABLE 9.6   Common Documents Used in End-of-Life Care

Document	Description	Special Considerations
Advance directive	General term used to describe documents that give instructions about future medical care and treatments and who should make the decisions in the event the person is unable to communicate	• Should adhere to guidelines established by state of residence
Allow natural death (AND)	Written order acknowledging that comfort measures only are being provided to patient. Used in many palliative care and hospice settings to indicate that patient wants to die naturally with dignity and comfort	• In many settings, may be used in conjunction with DNR terminology to ensure patient/family wishes for advance directives are followed (DNR/AND)
Directive to physicians (DTP)	Written document specifying the patient's wish to be allowed to die without heroic or extraordinary measures	• Indicates specific measures to be used or withheld
Do not resuscitate (DNR)	Written physician's order instructing HCPs not to attempt CPR. DNR order often requested by family	• Must indicate any specific measures to be used or withheld • Must be signed by a physician to be valid
Living will	Lay term used to describe any documents that give instructions about future medical care and treatments or the wish to be allowed to die without heroic or extraordinary measures should the patient be unable to communicate for self	• Must identify specific treatments that a person wants or does not want at end of life
Medical power of attorney (MPOA)	Term used by some states to describe a document used for listing the person(s) to make health care decisions should a patient become unable to make informed decisions for self	• May be the same as durable power of attorney for health care, health care proxy, or appointment of a health care agent or surrogate • Specifies measures to be used or withheld • Person appointed may be called a health care agent, surrogate, attorney-in-fact, or proxy
Physician Order for Life-Sustaining Treatment (POLST) or Medical Order for Life-Sustaining Treatment (MOLST)	A standardized physician order guided by the patient's medical condition and based upon personal preferences stated by patient or expressed in advance directive	• Only for those whose illness may limit life to <12 mo • Guides current treatments. Differs from advance directive, which guides future treatments • Physician completes form based on discussion with patient or authorized representative, or in review of advance directive • Signed by physician, patient, or patient representative • Printed on bright pink paper
Power of attorney for health care (POAH)	Term used by some states to describe a document used for listing the person(s) to make health care decisions should a patient become unable to make informed decisions for self	• May be the same as medical power of attorney • Indicates specific measures to be used or withheld

Euthanasia is the deliberate act of hastening death. The ANA statement on active euthanasia states that the nurse should not take part in active euthanasia, because such an act is in direct violation of the Code for Nurses, ethical traditions and goals of the profession, and its covenant with society.

Physician-assisted suicide is legal in some states. In this case, the physician provides the means and/or information about how the patient can commit suicide. As a nurse, you have an obligation to provide prompt, humane, comprehensive, and compassionate EOL care. Some confuse euthanasia with *palliative sedation,* which is the use of medications to intentionally produce sedation to relieve intractable symptoms and distress in a patient who is imminently dying. The intent of palliative sedation is to relieve pain and suffering and not to shorten life or to hasten death, as is the case with euthanasia.

The use of opioids for symptom management at the EOL is often misunderstood and feared by patients, families, and HCPs. For this reason, many patients refuse to take opioids, which leads to physical and emotional suffering due to uncontrolled pain and symptoms. Your ethical obligation is to relieve suffering. This includes giving medications that have the potential of producing harm, such as with opioids. The *principle of double effect* refers to a principle that regards it morally permissible to give a medication that has the potential for harm if it is given with the intent of relieving pain and suffering and not intended to hasten death.

As a nurse, your role is to teach the patient and family about addiction and tolerance to and dependence on medications. The person with terminal illness should not be concerned with addiction when the goal of treatment is comfort. Pain management is discussed in Chapter 8.

ETHICAL/LEGAL DILEMMAS
End-of-Life Care

Situation

A.P. is a terminally ill 50-yr-old woman with metastatic breast cancer who is hospitalized with severe bone pain. She moans at rest and shows severe pain with any movement to reposition her. The present dose of IV morphine is not controlling her pain. At the team conference, the nurses discuss the need for more effective pain control but are concerned that more pain medicine could hasten her death.

Ethical/Legal Points for Consideration

- Adequate pain relief is an important outcome for all patients, especially patients who are terminally ill.
- The *Code of Ethics for Nurses* addresses the responsibility of the nurse to relieve suffering and have conversations with patients and families about pain and symptom management.[1]
- The *principle of beneficence* means that we provide care to benefit patients. The goal of adequate pain control in the terminally ill to ease suffering is based on the *principle of nonmaleficence* (preventing or reducing harm to the patient). The secondary effect of hastening the patient's death is ethically justified and known as the *double effect*.
- Legally, the *standard of care* is used to define the nursing acts that are required for safe and competent nursing practice. When the actual nursing care falls below the standard of care, it is considered negligent and unsafe, and the nurse is at risk for being found incompetent.
- In a court of law, the standard of care in nursing is determined by nursing experts and evidence-based practices. The increasing use of technology to access the latest scientific findings is changing the standard of nursing care to a national, if not global, standard defined by research findings and nationally recognized expert testimony. Standards for providing expert nursing care and counseling at EOL are available.[1]
- In A.P.'s situation the standard of care is that the patient will have pain relief. Failure of the nurse to act assertively to achieve pain relief for the patient and failure to effectively use resources to obtain that pain relief will be considered below the standard of care and unsafe and incompetent practice.

Discussion Questions

1. What types of discussions need to occur among the health care team, patient, and family as the terminally ill patient approaches this phase of care?
2. Distinguish between promotion of comfort and relief of pain in dying patients and between assisted suicide and euthanasia.

Reference

1. ANA: Code of ethics for nursing. Retrieved from *www.nursingworld. org/DocumentVault/Ethics-1/Code-of-Ethics-for-Nurses.html.*

❖ NURSING MANAGEMENT: END OF LIFE

Nurses spend more time with patients near the EOL than any other health care professionals. Nursing care of terminally ill and dying patients is holistic and encompasses all psychosocial and physical needs. Respect, dignity, and comfort are important for the patient and family. Although there is no cure for the person's disease, the treatment plan still consists of assessment, planning, implementation, and evaluation. The main difference is that the focus of care is on the management of the symptoms of the disease, not necessarily the disease itself. Nurses who care for the dying need to recognize their own needs when dealing with grief and dying.

◆ Nursing Assessment

Assessment of the terminally ill or dying patient varies with the patient's condition. Be sensitive and do not impose repeated, unnecessary assessments on the dying patient. When possible, use health history data that are available in the medical record rather than tiring the patient with an interview.

Document the specific event or change that brought the patient into the health care setting. Record the patient's medical diagnoses, medication profile, and allergies.

If the patient is alert, do a brief review of the body systems. Assess for discomfort, pain, nausea, and dyspnea so that you can implement interventions using evidence-based tools for symptom assessment. These include numeric scales or visual analog scales for pain rating. Evaluate and manage co-morbidities or acute episodes of problems, such as diabetes mellitus or headache. Elicit information about the patient's abilities, food and fluid intake, patterns of sleep and rest, and response to the stress of terminal illness. Assess the patient's ability to cope with the diagnosis and prognosis of the illness. Determine the family's ability to manage the needed care and to cope with the illness and its consequences.

The physical assessment is abbreviated and focuses on changes that accompany terminal illness and the specific disease process. Pay attention to patients who are nonverbal for subtle changes in their condition.[16] The frequency of assessment depends on the patient's stability. Assessment is done at least every 8 hours in the institutional setting. For patients cared for in their homes by hospice programs, assessment may occur weekly. As changes occur, you may have to complete assessment and documentation more often. If the patient is in the final hours of life, we may limit the physical assessment to essential data.

Key elements of a social assessment include determining the relationships and patterns of communication among the family. If multiple family members are present, listen to concerns from different members. Differences in expectations and interpersonal conflict can produce disruptions during the dying process and after the death of the loved one. Social assessment also includes evaluating the goals of the patient and family.

As death approaches, monitor the patient for multiple systems that often are failing during the EOL period. This requires vigilance and attention to often subtle physical changes. Neurologic assessment is especially important and includes level of consciousness, presence of reflexes, and pupil responses. Evaluation of vital signs, skin color, and temperature shows changes in circulation. Monitor and describe respiratory status, character and pattern of respirations, and characteristics of breath sounds. Assess nutritional and fluid intake, urine output, and bowel function, since this gives data about renal and gastrointestinal functioning. Assess skin condition on an ongoing basis, because skin becomes fragile and may easily break down.

In the last hours of life, limit assessments to only those that you need to determine patient comfort. Assessment of pain and respiratory status may be the most important during this time. It may be more peaceful and comforting to the patient and family to refrain from overstimulation that may occur from certain types of assessments, such as measuring BP or checking for pupillary response. As death approaches, your efforts may be better spent providing emotional support to the patient and family rather than performing tasks that will have no impact on the patient's physical care.

◆ Planning

The patient and family need to be involved in planning and coordinating EOL care. In some cases, a family conference may be helpful to develop a coordinated plan of care.

Develop a comprehensive plan to support, teach, and evaluate patients and families. Nursing care goals during the last stages of life involve comfort and safety measures and care of the patient's emotional and physical needs. These goals may include determining where the patient would like to die and whether this is possible. For example, the patient may want to die at home, but the family may object. Many factors contribute to the patient and family's decision. Interprofessional EOL care that includes the physician, social worker, chaplain, and other members of the palliative and/or hospice care team is important. Advocate for the patient so that their wishes are met as much as possible.

The last hours or days of the patient experiencing brain death (e.g., from trauma) are often spent in the ICU. Planning for EOL care may be particularly challenging in the ICU environment. At this time, some families are approached about organ donation. Consultation from palliative care specialists may help the family plan and cope with EOL issues.

◆ Nursing Implementation

Psychosocial care and physical care are interrelated for both the dying patient and family. Teaching them is an important part of EOL care. Families need ongoing information on the disease, the dying process, and any care you will be providing. They need information on how to cope with the many issues during this period of their lives. Denial and grieving may be barriers to learning and understanding at the EOL for both the patient and family.

◆ **Psychosocial Care.** As death approaches, respond appropriately to the patient's psychosocial manifestations at the EOL (Table 9.7).

Anxiety and Depression. Patients often show signs of anxiety and depression during the EOL period. Causes of anxiety and depression may include uncontrolled pain and dyspnea, psychosocial factors related to the disease process or impending death, altered physiologic states, and drugs used in high dosages. Anxiety is often related to fear. Encouragement, support, and teaching decrease some of the anxiety and depression. Management of anxiety and depression may include both medications and nonpharmacologic interventions. Relaxation strategies, such as relaxation breathing, muscle relaxation, music, and imagery, may be useful (see Chapter 6).

Anger. Anger is a common and normal response to grief. A grieving person cannot be forced to accept the loss. The surviving family members may be angry with the dying loved one who is leaving them. Encourage the expression of feelings, but at the same time realize how hard it is to come to terms with loss. As a nurse, you may be the target of the anger. You need to understand what is happening and not react on a personal level.

Hopelessness and Powerlessness. Feelings of hopelessness and powerlessness are common during the EOL period. Encourage realistic hope within the limits of the situation. Allow the patient and family to deal with what is within their control and help them recognize what is beyond their control. When possible, support the patient's involvement in decision making about care to foster a sense of control and autonomy.

TABLE 9.7   Nursing Management

Psychosocial Care at End of Life

Manifestations	Nursing Management
Saying Goodbyes	
It is important for the patient and family to acknowledge their sadness, mutually forgive one another, and say goodbye.	Encourage the dying person and family to share their feelings of sadness, loss, forgiveness and to touch, hug, cry. Allow the patient and family privacy to express their feelings and comfort one another.
Spiritual Needs	
Patient or family may request spiritual support, such as the presence of a chaplain.	Assess spiritual needs. Allow patient to express his or her spiritual needs. Encourage visit by appropriate spiritual care service provider, chaplain, or family member.
Unusual Communication	
This may indicate that an unresolved issue is preventing the dying person from letting go. Patient may become restless and agitated or perform repetitive tasks (may also indicate terminal delirium).	Encourage the family to talk with and reassure the dying person.
Vision-Like Experiences	
Patient may talk to persons who are not there or see places and objects not visible. Vision-like experiences help the dying person in coming to terms with meaning in life and transition from it.	Affirm the dying person's experience as a part of transition from this life.
Withdrawal	
Patient near death may seem withdrawn from the physical environment, maintaining the ability to hear but unable to respond	Converse as though the patient were alert, using a soft voice and gentle touch.

Fear. Fear is a typical feeling associated with dying. Specific fears associated with dying are fear of pain, fear of shortness of breath, fear of loneliness and abandonment, and fear of meaninglessness.

Fear of pain. Many people assume that pain always accompanies death. Physiologically, there is no absolute indication that death is always painful. Psychologically, pain may occur based on the anxieties and separations related to dying. Patients can take part in their own pain relief by discussing pain relief measures and their effects. Most patients want their pain relieved without the side effects of grogginess or sleepiness. Pain relief measures do not have to deprive the patient of the ability to interact with others.

Patients with physical pain should have pain-relieving drugs available. Assure the patient and family that drugs will be given promptly when needed and that side effects of drugs can and will be managed. As many EOL patients are unable to swallow, other routes, such as patches, sublingual, and rectal routes, may be used.[17] Consider alternative methods like massage, music, aromatherapy, and mindfulness.

Fear of shortness of breath. Respiratory distress and dyspnea are common near the EOL. The sensation of air hunger results in anxiety for the patient and family. Current therapies

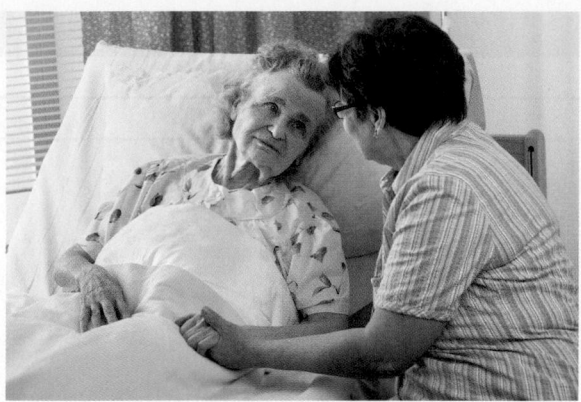

FIG. 9.8 Dying patients typically want someone whom they know and trust to stay with them. (© iStockphoto/Thinkstock.)

include opioids, bronchodilators, and oxygen, depending on the cause of the dyspnea. Anxiety-reducing agents (e.g., anxiolytics) may help produce relaxation.

Fear of loneliness and abandonment. Most terminally ill and dying people fear loneliness and do not want to be alone. Many dying patients are afraid that loved ones who are unable to cope with the patient's imminent death will abandon them. Simply being present offers support and comfort (Fig. 9.8). Holding hands, touching, and listening are important nursing interventions. Providing companionship allows the dying person a sense of security.

Fear of meaninglessness. Fear of meaninglessness leads people to review their lives. They review their intentions during life, examining actions and expressing regrets about what might have been. *Life review* helps patients recognize the value of their lives. Assist patients and their families to identify the positive qualities of the patient's life. Practical ways of helping may include looking at photo albums or collections of important mementos. Sharing thoughts and feelings may enhance spirituality and provide comfort. Respect and accept the practices and rituals associated with the patient's life review while staying nonjudgmental.

Communication. Communication among the interprofessional team, patient, and family is essential at the EOL. Empathy and active listening are essential parts of communication in care. *Empathy* is the identification with and understanding of another's situation, feelings, or motives. *Active listening* is paying attention to what is said, observing the patient's nonverbal cues, and not interrupting.

There may be silence. Often silence is related to the overwhelming feelings experienced at the EOL. Silence can also allow time to gather thoughts. Listening to the silence sends a message of acceptance and comfort. Communication must be respectful of the patient's ethnic, cultural, and religious backgrounds.

Patients and family members may have difficulties expressing themselves emotionally. Allow time for them to express their feelings and thoughts. Make time to listen and interact in a sensitive way to enhance the relationship among you, the patient, and the family. A family conference is 1 way to create a good environment for communication.

Prepare family members for changes in emotional and cognitive function that occur as death nears. Unusual communication by the patient may take place. The patient's speech may become confused, disoriented, or garbled. Patients may speak to or about family members or others who have predeceased them

or give instructions to those who will survive them. Active, careful listening allows for the identification of specific patterns in the dying person's communication and decreases the risk for inappropriate labeling of behaviors.

◆ **Physical Care.** Nursing management related to physical care at the EOL focuses on symptom management and comfort rather than treatment for curing a disease or disorder (Table 9.8). The priority is meeting the patient's physiologic and safety needs. Physical care focuses on the needs for oxygen, nutrition, pain relief, mobility, elimination, and skin care. People who are dying deserve and require the same physical care as people who are expected to recover. If possible, it is important to discuss with the patient and family the goals of care before treatment begins. An advance directive should be completed so that the patient and family wishes are followed.

Postmortem Care. After the patient is pronounced dead, prepare or delegate preparing the patient's body for immediate viewing by the family with consideration for cultural customs and in accord with state law and agency policies and procedures (Table 9.9). In some cultures and in some types of death, it may be important to allow the family to prepare or help in caring for the patient's body. When the death is unexpected, preparing the patient's body for viewing or release to a funeral home depends on state law and agency policies and procedures.

Care of and discussion related to the person should continue to be respectful even after death. Allow the family privacy and as much time as they need with the deceased person. Never refer to the deceased person as "the body."

SPECIAL NEEDS OF CAREGIVERS AND NURSES IN END-OF-LIFE CARE

Special Needs of Family Caregivers

Family caregivers are important in meeting the patient's physical and psychosocial needs. Their role includes working and communicating with the patient and other family members, supporting the patient's concerns, and helping the patient resolve any unfinished business. Families often face emotional, physical, and economic consequences from caring for a family member who is dying. The caregiver's responsibilities do not end when the patient is admitted to an acute care, inpatient hospice, or long-term care facility.[18]

An understanding of the grieving process as it affects both the patient and family is important. Being present during a family member's dying process can be highly stressful. Recognize signs and behaviors among family members who may be at risk for abnormal grief reactions and be prepared to intervene if needed. Warning signs may include dependency and negative feelings about the dying person, inability to express feelings, sleep disturbances, a history of depression, difficult reactions to previous losses, perceived lack of social or family support, low self-esteem, multiple previous bereavements, alcoholism, or substance abuse. Caregivers with concurrent life crises (e.g., divorce) are especially at risk.

Family caregivers and other family members need encouragement to continue their usual activities as much as possible. They need to discuss their activities and maintain some control over their lives. Inform caregivers about resources for support, including respite care. Community counseling and local support may help some people in working through their grief.

Encourage caregivers to build a support system of extended family, friends, faith community, and clergy. The caregivers

TABLE 9.8   **Nursing Management**

Physical Care at End of Life

Manifestation	Nursing Management
Anorexia, Nausea, and Vomiting • May be caused by complications of disease process • Drugs contribute to nausea • Constipation, impaction, and bowel obstruction can cause anorexia, nausea, and vomiting	• Assess the patient for nausea or vomiting • Assess possible contributing causes of nausea or vomiting • Provide antiemetics before meals if ordered • Offer and provide frequent meals with small portions of favorite foods • Offer culturally appropriate foods • Provide frequent mouth care, especially after vomiting • Ensure uninterrupted mealtimes • If ordered, give drugs (e.g., megestrol, corticosteroids) to increase appetite • Teach family that appetite naturally decreases at end of life and hunger is rare • Do not force the patient to eat
Bowel Patterns • Immobility, opioid medication use, depression, lack of fiber in the diet, and dehydration can cause constipation • Diarrhea may occur as muscles relax or from a fecal impaction related to the use of opioids and immobility	• Assess bowel function • Assess for and remove fecal impactions • Encourage movement and physical activities as tolerated • Encourage fiber in the diet if appropriate • Encourage fluids if appropriate • Use suppositories, stool softeners, laxatives, or enemas if ordered • Assess for confusion, agitation, restlessness, and pain, which may be signs of constipation
Candidiasis • White, cottage cheese–like oral plaques • Fungal overgrowth in the mouth due to chemotherapy and/or immunosuppression	• If ordered, give oral antifungal nystatin • Clean dentures and other dental appliances to prevent reinfection • Provide oral hygiene and use soft toothbrush
Dehydration • May occur during the last days of life • Hunger and thirst are rare in the last days of life • As the end of life approaches, patients tend to take in less food and fluid	• Assess mucous membranes often for dryness, which can lead to discomfort • Maintain complete, regular oral care to provide for comfort and hydration of mucous membranes • Encourage consumption of ice chips and sips of fluids or use moist cloths to provide moisture to the mouth • Use moist cloths and swabs for unconscious patients to avoid aspiration • Apply lubricant to the lips and oral mucous membranes as needed • Do not force the patient to drink • Teach family that thirst is rare in the last days of life • Reassure family that cessation of food and fluid intake is a natural part of the process of dying
Delirium • A state characterized by confusion, disorientation, restlessness, clouding of consciousness, incoherence, fear, anxiety, excitement, and often hallucinations • May be misidentified as depression, psychosis, anger, or anxiety • May be caused by using opioids or corticosteroids • Underlying disease process may contribute to delirium • Considered a reversible process	• Perform a thorough assessment for reversible causes of delirium, including pain, constipation, and urinary retention • Provide a room that is quiet, well lit, and familiar to reduce the effects of delirium • Reorient the dying person to person, place, and time with each encounter • Give ordered benzodiazepines and sedatives as needed • Stay physically close to frightened patient Reassure in a calm, soft voice with touch and slow strokes of the skin • Provide family with emotional support and encouragement in their efforts to cope with the behaviors associated with delirium
Dysphagia • May occur because of extreme weakness and changes in level of consciousness • Difficulty swallowing • Aspiration of liquids and/or solids • Drooling/inability to swallow secretions	• Identify the least invasive alternative routes of administering drugs needed for symptom management • Suction orally as needed • Modify diet as tolerated/desired • Hand feed small meals • Elevate the head for meals and at least 30 minutes after • If necessary, use alternative (rectal, buccal, transdermal) medication routes • Discontinue nonessential medications • Discuss risk for aspiration
Dyspnea • Subjective symptom • Accompanied by fear of suffocation and anxiety • Underlying disease process can worsen dyspnea • Coughing and expectorating secretions become difficult	• Assess respiratory status regularly • Elevate the head and/or position patient on side to improve chest expansion • Use a fan or air conditioner to help movement of cool air • Teach and encourage the use of pursed-lip breathing • Give supplemental oxygen as ordered • Suction PRN to remove accumulation of mucus from the airways. Suction cautiously in the terminal phase • Give an expectorant as ordered

TABLE 9.8   Nursing Management—cont'd

Physical Care at End of Life

Manifestation	Nursing Management
Myoclonus • Mild to severe jerking or twitching sometimes associated with use of high dose of opioids • Patient may have involuntary twitching of extremities	• Assess for initial onset, duration, and any discomfort or distress • If myoclonus is distressing or becoming more severe, discuss possible drug therapy modifications with the HCP • Changes in opioid medication may decrease myoclonus
Pain • May be a major symptom associated with terminal illness and the 1 most feared • Can be acute or chronic • Bone pain can be caused by metastases, fractures, arthritis, immobility • Physical and emotional stressors can worsen pain	• Assess pain thoroughly and regularly to determine the quality, intensity, location, and contributing and alleviating factors • Minimize irritants, such as skin irritations from wetness, heat or cold, pressure • Give medications around the clock, in a timely manner, and on a regular basis to provide constant relief rather than waiting until the pain is unbearable and then trying to relieve it • Provide complementary and alternative therapies, such as guided imagery, massage, and relaxation techniques as needed (see Chapter 6) • Evaluate effectiveness of pain relief measures frequently to ensure that the patient is on a correct, adequate drug regimen • Do not delay or deny pain relief measures to a terminally ill patient
Restlessness • May occur as death approaches and cerebral metabolism slows • May occur with tachypnea, dyspnea, sweating	• Assess for previous anxiety disorder • Assess for spiritual distress and/or concerns related to death as causes of restlessness and agitation • Assess for urinary retention and stool impaction • Do not restrain • Use soothing music and slow, soft touch and voice • Limit the number of persons at the bedside
Skin Breakdown • Skin integrity is hard to maintain at the end of life • Immobility, urinary and bowel incontinence, dry skin, nutritional deficits, anemia, friction, and shearing forces lead to a high risk for skin breakdown • Disease and other processes may impair skin integrity • As death approaches, circulation to the extremities decreases and they become cool, mottled, and cyanotic	• Assess skin for signs of breakdown • Implement protocols to prevent skin breakdown by controlling drainage and odor and keeping the skin and any wound areas clean • Perform wound assessments as needed • Follow appropriate nursing management protocol for dressing wounds • Follow appropriate nursing management protocol for a patient who is immobile, but consider realistic outcomes of skin integrity vs. maintenance of comfort • Follow appropriate nursing management to prevent skin irritations and breakdown from urinary and bowel incontinence • Use blankets to cover for warmth. Never apply heat
Urinary Incontinence • May result from disease progression or changes in the level of consciousness • As death becomes imminent, the perineal muscles relax	• Assess urinary function • Use absorbent pads for urinary incontinence • Follow appropriate nursing protocol for the consideration and use of indwelling or external catheters • Follow appropriate nursing management to prevent skin irritations and breakdown from urinary incontinence
Weakness and Fatigue • Expected at the end of life • Metabolic demands related to disease process contribute to weakness and fatigue	• Assess the patient's tolerance for activities • Time nursing interventions to conserve energy • Help the patient identify and complete valued or desired activities • Provide support as needed to maintain positions in bed or chair • Give frequent rest periods

TABLE 9.9   Nursing Management

Postmortem Care

- Close the patient's eyes and jaw.
- Replace dentures; remove jewelry and eyeglasses.
- Wash the body as needed then apply a clean gown and bed linen.
- Place a waterproof pad or incontinence brief to absorb urine and feces.
- Comb and arrange the hair neatly.
- Remove tubes and dressings (if appropriate).
- Straighten the body, placing the arms at their sides or across the abdomen with palms down.
- Place a pillow under the head.

should have people to call on at any time to express any feelings they are experiencing.

Special Needs of Nurses

Many nurses who care for dying patients do so because they are passionate about providing high-quality EOL care. Caring for patients and their families at the EOL is challenging and rewarding but also intense and emotionally charged. A bond or connection may develop between you and the patient or family. Be aware of how grief personally affects you. When you provide care for terminally ill or dying patients, you are not immune to feelings of loss. It is common to feel helpless and powerless when dealing with death. Express feelings of sorrow, guilt, and frustration. It is important to recognize your own values, attitudes, and feelings about death. Common ethical concerns include lack of adequate communication, lack of effective decision making, when to stop life-prolonging interventions, and concerns with symptom treatment, especially with use of opioids.

Interventions are available that may help ease your physical and emotional stress. Be aware of what you can and cannot control. Recognizing personal feelings allows openness in exchanging feelings with the patient and family. Realizing that it is okay to cry with the patient or family during the EOL may be important for your well-being.

To meet your personal needs, focus on interventions that will help decrease your stress. Get involved in hobbies or other interests, schedule time for yourself, ensure time for sleep, maintain a peer support system, and develop a support system beyond the workplace. Many hospice agencies offer support groups and discussion sessions that can help you cope.

CASE STUDY

Spiritual Distress at End of Life

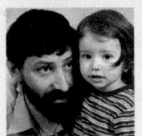

(© Mocker_bat/iStock/Thinkstock.)

Patient Profile

G.M. is a 42-yr-old Orthodox Jewish man. He is being seen by the hospice nurse for increasing abdominal pain, nausea, vomiting, lack of appetite, and constipation. He was diagnosed 6 months ago with pancreatic cancer that has metastasized to the liver and lungs. He quit work 1 month later. Two weeks ago, he ended the drug trial he was on for 5 months and enrolled in hospice. Currently, he is taking oral opioids for pain, ondansetron for nausea and vomiting, sertraline for depression, and megestrol for appetite. His wife is worried that he will become addicted to the pain medication.

Subjective Data

- States that he is angry at God for giving him this illness
- Reports fatigue and lack of appetite
- Reports pain at 7 (0–10 point scale) not relieved by medication
- States he is worried about the loss of his health benefits and what will happen to his young family, including a son age 3, when he is gone

Objective Data

Physical Examination

- Underweight (20% less than ideal body weight for height)
- Skin is jaundiced
- Yellow sclera

Interprofessional Care

- Review pain medications for dosage adjustment.
- Hospice social worker to review medical benefits and disability application
- Ensure that advance directives are in place.

Discussion Questions

1. What are G.M.'s risk factors for spiritual distress?
2. Based on the data given, what are the major health problems for G.M.?
3. **Patient-Centered Care:** What specific palliative care needs does G.M. have?
4. **Priority Decision:** Based on your assessment of G.M., what are the priority nursing interventions for him?
5. **Collaboration:** For the interventions that you identified in the previous question, which personnel could be responsible for implementing them: RN, LPN/VN, unlicensed assistive personnel (UAP)?
6. **Collaboration:** What referrals may be indicated?

Answers available at *http://evolve.elsevier.com/Lewis/medsurg.*

▌BRIDGE TO NCLEX EXAMINATION

The number of the question corresponds to the same-numbered outcome at the beginning of the chapter.

1. An 80-yr-old female patient is receiving palliative care for heart failure. The *primary* purpose(s) of her receiving palliative care is (are) to (*select all that apply*)
   a. improve her quality of life.
   b. assess her coping ability with disease.
   c. have time to teach patient and family about disease.
   d. focus on reducing the severity of disease symptoms.
   e. provide care that the family is unwilling or unable to give.

2. A 67-yr-old woman was recently diagnosed with inoperable pancreatic cancer. Before the diagnosis, she was very active in her neighborhood association. Her husband is concerned because his wife is staying at home and missing her usual community activities. Which common EOL psychologic manifestation is she *most* likely demonstrating?
   a. Peacefulness
   b. Decreased socialization
   c. Decreased decision making
   d. Anxiety about unfinished business

3. For the past 5 years, Tom has repeatedly asked his mother to donate his deceased father's belongings to charity, but his mother has refused. She sits in the bedroom closet, crying and talking to her long-dead husband. What type of grief is Tom's mother experiencing?
   a. Adaptive grief
   b. Disruptive grief
   c. Anticipatory grief
   d. Prolonged grief disorder

4. While caring for his dying wife, the husband states that his wife is a devout Roman Catholic, but he is a Baptist. Who is considered the *most* reliable source for spiritual preferences concerning EOL care for the dying wife?
   a. A priest
   b. Dying wife
   c. Hospice staff
   d. Husband of dying wife

5. The family attorney informed a patient's adult children and wife that the patient did not have an advance directive after he suffered a serious stroke. Who is responsible for making the decision about EOL measures when the patient cannot communicate his or her specific wishes?
   a. Notary and attorney
   b. Physician and family
   c. Wife and adult children
   d. Physician and nursing staff

6. The home health nurse visits a 40-yr-old patient with metastatic breast cancer who is receiving palliative care. The patient has pain at a level of 7 (0–10 point scale). In prioritizing activities for the visit, what should the nurse do *first*?
   a. Auscultate for breath sounds.
   b. Give as needed pain medication.
   c. Check pressure points for skin breakdown.
   d. Ask family about patient's food and fluid intake.

7. The children caregivers of an older patient whose death is imminent have not left the bedside for the past 36 hours. In the nurse's assessment of the family, what findings indicate the potential for an abnormal grief reaction to occur (*select all that apply*)?
   a. Family cannot express their feelings to one another.
   b. Dying patient is becoming more restless and agitated.
   c. A family member is going through a difficult divorce.
   d. Family talks with and reassures the patient at frequent intervals.
   e. Siblings who were estranged from each other have now reunited.

8. A nurse has been working full-time with terminally ill patients for 3 years. He has been experiencing irritability and mixed emotions when expressing sadness since 4 of his patients died on the same day. To optimize the quality of his nursing care, he should examine his own
   a. full-time work schedule.
   b. past feelings toward death.
   c. patterns for dealing with grief.
   d. demands for involvement in patient care.

1. a, 2. b, 3. d, 4. b, 5. c, 6. b, 7. a, c, 8. c.

For rationales to these answers and even more NCLEX review questions, visit *http://evolve.elsevier.com/Lewis/medsurg.*

ⓔ EVOLVE WEBSITE/RESOURCES LIST

http://evolve.elsevier.com/Lewis/medsurg
Review Questions (Online Only)
Key Points
Answer Keys for Questions
- Rationales for Bridge to NCLEX Examination Questions
- Answer Guidelines for Case Study on p. 140
Student Case Study
- Patient With Chronic Myelogenous Leukemia Including End-of-Life Care
Conceptual Care Map Creator
Audio Glossary
Content Updates

REFERENCES

1. National Coalition for Hospice and Palliative Care: Clinical practice guidelines for quality palliative care. Retrieved from *www.nationalcoalitionhpc.org/ncp/.*
*2. Cleary A: Integrating palliative care into primary care for patients with chronic, life-limiting conditions, *TNP* 41:42, 2016.
3. Centers for Disease Control and Prevention: *Healthy aging.* Retrieved from *www.cdc.gov/aging.*
4. National Hospice and Palliative Care Organization: Facts on hospice and palliative care. Retrieved from *www.nhpco.org/hospice-statistics-research-press-room/facts-hospice-and-palliative-care.*
5. Hospice and Palliative Nurses Association: *HPNA position statements.* Retrieved from *https://advancingexpertcare.org/HPNA/Leadership/Position_Statements/HPNA/Leadership_Advocacy/Position_Statements.aspx?hkey=a794c17f-c88f-42d9-a09f-caf413e42aa3.*
6. National Hospice and Palliative Care Organization: Palliative care costs and benefits. Retrieved from *www.caringinfo.org/i4a/pages/index.cfm?pageid=3297.*
7. Lungu M, Lupu MN, Voinescu CD: The neurologist's responsibilities in declaring the time of brain death and organ donation, *Acta Medica* 22:15, 2017.
8. Field M, Cassel C: *Approaching death: Improving care at the end of life,* Washington, DC, 1997, National Academy Press. (Classic)
9. Kübler-Ross E: *On death and dying,* New York, 1969, Macmillan. (Classic).
10. National Cancer Institute: PDQ: Grief, bereavement, and coping with loss. Retrieved from *www.cancer.gov/cancertopics/pdq/supportivecare/bereavement/HealthProfessional.*
11. O'Brien ME: *Spirituality in nursing,* 3rd ed, Burlington, MA, 2017, Jones & Bartlett Learning.
*12. LoPresti MA, Dement F, Gold HT: End-of-life care for people from ethnic minority groups: A systematic review, *Am J Hosp Palliat Care* 33:291, 2016.
*13. Hagerty TA, Velázquez Á, Schmidt JM, et al: Assessment of satisfaction with care and decision-making among English and Spanish-speaking family members of neuroscience ICU patients, *App Nurs Res.* 29:262, 2016.
14. U.S. Department of Health and Human Services: U.S. government information on organ donation and transplantation. Retrieved from *www.organdonor.gov/index.html.*
*15. Robinson EM, Cadge W, Zollfrank AA, et al: After the DNR: Surrogates who persist in requesting cardiopulmonary resuscitation, *Hastings Center Report* 47:10, 2017.
*16. Davies P: Pharmacologic pain management at the end of life, *TNP* 41:26, 2016.
*17. Paez K, Gregg M, Massion C, et al: A new intervention for rapid end-of-life symptom control in the home setting, *JHPN* 18:498, 2016.
18. Marrelli T: Caregivers and caregiving: An important part of the healthcare team, *Home Healthcare Now* 35:427, 2017.

*Evidence-based information for clinical practice.

10

Substance Use Disorders

Mariann M. Harding

You can accomplish with kindness what you cannot by force.

Publilius Syrus

ⓔ http://evolve.elsevier.com/Lewis/medsurg/

LEARNING OUTCOMES

1. Relate the effects of substance use to its resulting major health complications.
2. Distinguish among the effects of the use of stimulants, depressants, and cannabis.
3. Explain your role in promoting the cessation of smoking and tobacco use.
4. Summarize the nursing and interprofessional management of patients who experience toxicity or withdrawal from stimulants and depressants.
5. Apply the Screening, Brief Intervention, and Referral to Treatment approach in clinical situations.
6. Describe the incidence and effects of substance use in the older adult.

Substance use is a serious problem affecting society and the health care system. Substance-related disorders involve several types of substances, ranging from widely used and accepted tobacco and alcohol to illegal, brain-altering drugs such as heroin and cocaine. The *Diagnostic and Statistical Manual of Mental Disorders V (DSM-V)* outlines criteria used to identify the presence of substance use disorder (SUD)[1] (Table 10.1).

Whether SUD is mild, moderate, or severe depends on the person's pattern of use and the functional impact of use on the person's daily life. Knowing the severity of substance use allows the health care team to tailor treatment according to a patient's needs. For example, a person who binge drinks may not have alcohol SUD but is at increased risk for it. On the other hand, a person who uses heroin or cocaine is likely to have severe SUD because these substances are highly addictive.

Many patients with substance use problems receive acute care for problems associated with substance use. SUD does not exist in isolation. There are many interrelated concepts depending on the patient situation. Every drug associated with SUD harms some tissue or organ. Substance use causes specific health problems, such as liver damage related to alcohol use or lung cancer related to smoking. Other problems result from injuries associated with substance use, such as falls or motor vehicle accidents. Common health problems related to substance use are outlined in Table 10.2.

This chapter focuses on the role of the medical-surgical nurse in identifying and managing the patient with SUD in the acute care setting. A hospitalized patient who uses substances can develop withdrawal when substance use abruptly stops. You need to be able to recognize substance use and its effects on health problems and manage withdrawal. The health care setting offers an opportunity for screening and providing teaching about substance use. It is your responsibility to motivate the patient to change behavior and refer the patient to programs that offer treatment.

DRUGS ASSOCIATED WITH SUBSTANCE USE DISORDER

NICOTINE

You are most likely to encounter people with **tobacco use disorder (TUD)**. People with TUD are dependent on the drug nicotine due to using tobacco products. Several products contain

TABLE 10.1 Criteria for Substance Use Disorder

The following criteria (clustered in 4 groups) can be used to identify substance use disorder (SUD). The severity of SUD can be classified as mild (2-3 criteria), moderate (4-5 criteria), or severe (6 or more criteria).

Impaired Control
- Taking more or for longer than intended
- Not quitting use despite multiple times of trying to do so
- Spending a great deal of time obtaining, using, or recovering from use
- Craving the substance

Social Impairment
- Missing school, work, or other responsibilities due to use
- Continuing use despite problems caused or worsened by use
- Giving up or reducing important activities because of use

Risky Use
- Recurrent use in hazardous situations
- Continued use despite causing or worsening problems

Pharmacologic Dependence
- Physical tolerance to effects of the substance
- Presence of withdrawal symptoms when not using or using less

Source: American Psychiatric Association: *The diagnostic and statistical manual of mental disorders*, ed 5, Arlington, VA, 2013, The Association.

TABLE 10.2 Health Problems Related to Substance Use

Substance	Health Problems*
Amphetamines	• Cardiac dysrhythmias, myocardial ischemia and infarction • Liver, lung, kidney damage • Mood disturbances, violent behavior, psychoses
Cannabis	• Bronchitis, chronic cough • Depression, anxiety, schizophrenia • Memory impairment
Cocaine	• Cardiac dysrhythmias, myocardial ischemia and infarction • Seizures, stroke • Psychosis
Inhalants	• Cognitive and motor impairment • Acute and chronic kidney injury
Opioids	• Sexual dysfunction • Gastric ulcers • Glomerulonephritis
Sedative-hypnotics	• Memory impairment • Personality changes, depression
Behaviors	
Injecting drugs	• Blood clots, phlebitis, skin infections • Hepatitis B and C • HIV/AIDS • Other infections: endocarditis, tuberculosis, pneumonia, meningitis, tetanus, bone and joint infections, lung abscesses
Personal neglect	• Malnutrition, impaired immunity • Accidental injuries
Risky sexual behavior	• HIV/AIDS • Hepatitis B and C • Sexually transmitted infections
Snorting drugs	• Nasal sores, septal necrosis or perforation • Chronic sinusitis

Adapted from National Institute on Drug Abuse: Medical consequence of drug abuse. Retrieved from *www.drugabuse.gov/related-topics/medical-consequences-drug-abuse*.

*Health problems related to SUD are discussed in the appropriate chapters throughout the text where they are identified as risk factors for these problems.

nicotine, including smoked tobacco (cigarettes, cigars, pipes), smokeless tobacco (chew, snuff, dip), and some electronic cigarettes. Cigarette smoking is the main form of tobacco use in the United States.

Effects of Use and Complications

Nicotine is a central nervous system stimulant. Within seconds of entering the body, nicotine reaches the brain, causing the release of adrenaline and creating feelings of a "high" or a "buzz." The effects last about 1 to 2 hours before withdrawal symptoms occur, leaving the person feeling tired, irritable, and anxious. The need to have the "high" or "buzz" feelings again makes the person crave more nicotine, leading to addiction.

Smoked tobacco is the most harmful method of nicotine use. Smoking harms nearly every organ in the body and reduces the general health of smokers. More than 14 million persons in the United States have a smoking related disease.[2] Smoking causes lung disease, cardiovascular disease, and lung and other cancers and is a major factor in many other conditions (Fig. 10.1).

Although those who use smokeless tobacco have less risk for lung disease, use can cause serious health problems. Holding tobacco in the mouth is associated with periodontal disease and cancer of the mouth, cheek, tongue, throat, and esophagus. Smokeless tobacco users experience the systemic effects of nicotine on the cardiovascular system, increasing the risk for heart attack and stroke.[3]

The use of electronic cigarettes, or e-cigs, continues to increase. E-cigs have a similar look and feel of traditional cigarettes. These battery-operated devices turn nicotine and other chemicals, including propylene glycol and flavorings, into an aerosol. Emerging information shows e-cigs can be harmful. E-cigs may affect the respiratory and immune systems. Those containing nicotine may increase the risk for cardiovascular problems and influence brain development in adolescents and pregnant users.[4] Other problems, such as poisonings and facial burns from device explosions, have occurred. Although some believe using an e-cig may aid in smoking cessation, no e-cigs are FDA approved. Do not recommend them as a smoking cessation aid.

❖ NURSING AND INTERPROFESSIONAL MANAGEMENT: TOBACCO USE DISORDER

◆ Tobacco Cessation

As a nurse, you have a professional responsibility to help people stop smoking or using tobacco. The Joint Commission mandates that every health professional must identify tobacco users and provide them with information on ways to stop using tobacco. Patients who receive even brief advice and intervention from you are more likely to quit than those who receive no intervention.

With each patient encounter, encourage the patient to quit and offer specific smoking cessation interventions. The Agency for Healthcare Research and Quality has issued clinical practice guidelines for clinicians, including nurses, to use to motivate users to quit[5] (Tables 10.3 and 10.4). Use these brief clinical interventions, called the "5 *As*," with each patient encounter. These interventions will help you identify tobacco users, encourage

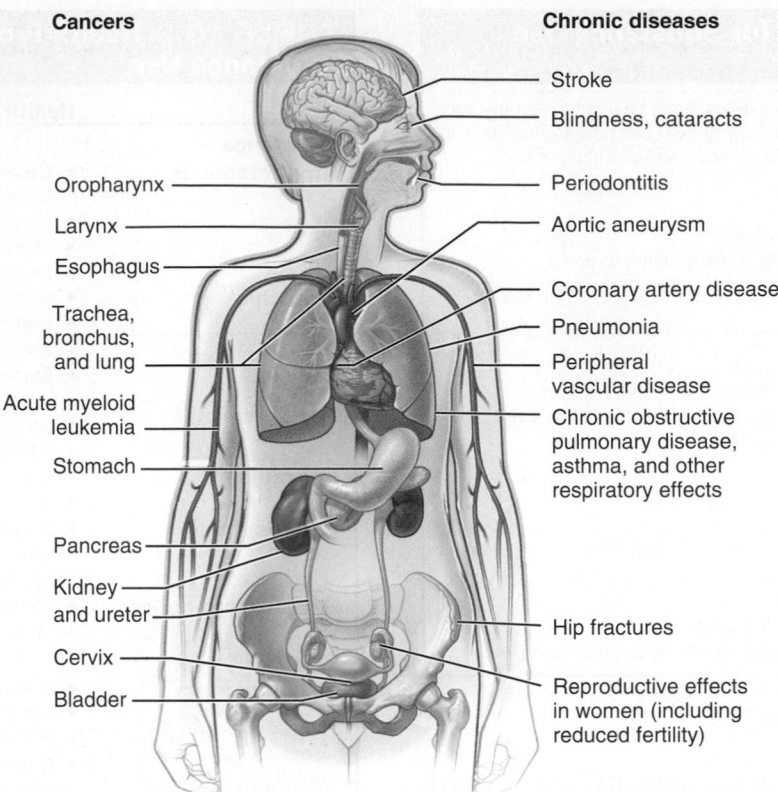

FIG 10.1 Health effects of smoking. (From Samet JM: Tobacco smoking, *Thorac Surg Clin* 23[2]:103, 2013.)

TABLE 10.3 Clinical Practice Guideline

Treating Tobacco Use Disorder

The 5 *A*s for Users Who Want to Quit	The 5 *R*s for Users Unwilling to Quit
1. **Ask:** Identify all tobacco users at every contact.	1. **Relevance:** Ask the patient to say why quitting is personally relevant (e.g., health).
2. **Advise:** Strongly urge all tobacco users to quit.	2. **Risks:** Ask the patient to identify his or her potential risks/consequences of tobacco use.
3. **Assess:** Determine willingness to make a quit attempt.	3. **Rewards:** Ask the patient to relate potential benefits of stopping tobacco use.
4. **Assist:** Develop a plan with the patient to help the patient quit (e.g., counseling, medication).	4. **Roadblocks:** Ask patient to identify barriers or impediments to quitting.
5. **Arrange:** Schedule follow-up contact.	5. **Repetition:** Repeat process every clinic visit.

Source: Agency for Healthcare Research and Quality: *AHCPR supported clinical practice guideline: Treating tobacco use and dependence—2008 update,* Washington, DC, 2008, U.S. Public Health Service.

TABLE 10.4 Inpatient Tobacco Cessation Interventions

Take the following steps for every hospitalized patient:
- Ask each patient on admission if he or she uses tobacco and document tobacco use status.
- For current tobacco users, list tobacco use status on the admission problem list and as a discharge diagnosis.
- Use counseling and medication to help all tobacco users stay abstinent and to treat withdrawal symptoms.
- Give advice and assistance on how to quit during hospitalization and stay abstinent after discharge.
- Arrange for follow-up about smoking status. Provide supportive contact for at least a month after discharge.

Source: Agency for Healthcare Research and Quality: *AHCPR supported clinical practice guideline: Treating tobacco use and dependence: 2008 update,* Washington, DC, 2008, U.S. Public Health Service.

them to quit, determine their willingness to quit, assist them in quitting, and arrange for follow-up. A patient teaching guide (Table 10.5) expands on the fourth strategy, *Assist,* to help you aid the user willing to quit. If a tobacco user is unwilling to quit, using the "5 *R*s" may motivate the user to quit in the future.

A variety of smoking cessation products are available to help support users in quitting. These include prescription medicines as well as over-the-counter (OTC) products such as skin patches, lozenges, and gum. Nicotine replacement products are 1 type of smoking cessation product. These products reduce the craving and withdrawal symptoms associated with cessation by supplying the body with smaller amounts of nicotine (Table 10.6).

Because most health care facilities are tobacco-free environments, admitted patients who are addicted to nicotine may experience withdrawal symptoms since they are unable to smoke. These symptoms are the same as for the person who stops using tobacco "cold turkey." Offering nicotine replacement therapy to every patient who wants to quit will help control withdrawal symptoms during hospitalization and promote continued cessation after discharge.

Non-nicotine products also play a role in helping users quit. Varenicline (Chantix) is a drug used to aid smoking cessation. Varenicline is unique in that it has both agonist and antagonist

TABLE 10.5 **Patient Teaching**

Smoking and Tobacco Use Cessation

The following interventions are methods that work for quitting tobacco use. Tobacco users have the best chance of quitting if they use more than 1 method.

Develop a Quit Plan
- Set a quit date, ideally within 2 weeks.
- Talk to your HCP about getting help to quit.
- Tell family, friends, and co-workers about quitting and request understanding and support.
- Expect withdrawal symptoms and challenges when quitting.
- Before quitting, avoid smoking in places where you spend a lot of time (work, car, home).
- Throw away all tobacco products from your home, car, and work.
- Have support options in place by your quit date.

Use Approved Nicotine Replacement Systems
- Use a nicotine replacement agent unless you are a pregnant or nursing woman (Table 10.6).
- Do not use other forms of tobacco when using nicotine replacement systems.

Support and Encouragement
- Joining a quit-tobacco support group will increase your chances of stopping permanently.
- If you get the urge for tobacco, call someone to help talk you out of it—preferably an ex-user.
- Be proud every time you reach a quit milestone and reward yourself.
- Do not be afraid to talk about how you feel while quitting, especially fears of not being able to quit for good. Ask your spouse or partner, friends, and co-workers to support you. Self-help materials, mobile phone applications, and hot lines are available:
  - American Lung Association: 800-586-4872; *www.lung.org*
  - American Cancer Society: 800-227-2345; *www.cancer.org*
  - National Cancer Institute: LiveHelp; *www.smokefree.gov*

Dealing With Urges to Use Tobacco
- Identify situations that may cause you to want to smoke or use other tobacco, such as being around other smokers, being under time pressure, feeling sad or frustrated, and drinking alcohol.
- Avoid difficult situations while you are trying to quit. Try to lower your stress level.

- Exercise can help, such as walking, jogging, or bicycling.
- Distract yourself from thoughts of smoking and the urge to use tobacco by talking to someone, going to a movie, getting busy with a task, or having a game night with friends.
- Drink a lot of water.
- Keep your hands busy with a pen or toothpick.

Avoiding Relapse
Most relapses occur within the first 3 months after quitting. Do not be discouraged if you start using tobacco again. Remember, most people try several times before they finally quit. Explore different ways to break habits. You may have to deal with some of the following triggers that cause relapse.
- *Change your environment.* Get rid of cigarettes, tobacco (in any form), and ashtrays in your home, car, and place of work. Get rid of the smell of cigarettes in your car and home.
- *Alcohol.* Consider limiting or stopping alcohol use while you are quitting tobacco.
- *Other smokers at home.* Encourage housemates to quit with you. Work out a plan to cope with others who smoke and avoid being around them.
- *Weight gain.* Tackle 1 problem at a time. Work on quitting tobacco first. You will not necessarily gain weight, and increased appetite is often temporary. Eat healthy and exercise.
- *Negative mood or depression.* If these symptoms persist, talk to your HCP. You may need treatment for depression.
- *Withdrawal symptoms.* Your body will go through many changes when you quit tobacco. You may have a dry mouth, cough, or scratchy throat, and you may feel irritable. The nicotine patch or gum may help with cravings (Table 10.6).
- *Focus on the benefits of quitting:*
  - Your BP and heart rate will lower almost at once.
  - Your risk for a heart attack declines within 24 hours. The blood will become less likely to clot, making dangerous blood clots less likely.
  - Within a few weeks, you will be less short of breath, cough less, and have more energy. Your ability to smell and taste should improve.
  - Your immune system will be stronger, so you will be less likely to be sick.
  - Quitting will improve your night vision and help preserve your overall vision.

Adapted from National Cancer Institute: 18 ways smoking affects your health. Retrieved from *www.smokefree.gov/health-effects.*

actions. Its agonist activity at 1 subtype of nicotinic receptors provides some nicotine effects to ease withdrawal symptoms. If the person does resume smoking, its antagonist action blocks the effects of nicotine at another subtype of nicotinic receptor, making smoking less enjoyable. Bupropion (Zyban), an antidepressant drug, reduces the urge to smoke, reduces some symptoms of withdrawal, and helps prevent weight gain associated with smoking cessation.

> **💊 DRUG ALERT**   Varenicline (Chantix) and Bupropion (Zyban)
> - Serious neuropsychiatric symptoms such as changes in behavior, hostility, agitation, depressed mood, suicidal thoughts and behavior, and attempted suicide can occur.
> - Tell patients to stop taking these drugs and contact the HCP at once if they have any of these manifestations.

Along with using a smoking cessation product, users who wish to quit are more likely to succeed if they take part in a tobacco cessation program. You should be aware of available community resources. Cessation programs may involve hypnosis, acupuncture, behavioral interventions, aversion therapy, group support programs, individual therapy, and self-help options. Many of these programs teach users to avoid high-risk situations for smoking relapse (e.g., those that promote cue-induced craving) and help them develop coping skills, such as cigarette refusal skills, assertiveness, alternative activities, and peer support systems.

ALCOHOL

Of Americans ages 18 and older, 70% consume alcohol. Most people use alcohol in moderation.[6] *Risky drinking* is consuming more alcohol than the amounts in guidelines established by the National Institute on Alcohol Abuse and Alcoholism (Fig. 10.2). Risky drinking can have negative physical, emotional, and social consequences. **Alcohol use disorder (AUD)**, or alcoholism, affects about 6.2% of U.S. adults.[6] A higher percent engages in periodic excess alcohol use. **Binge drinking** is consuming 5 or more alcoholic drinks for males or 4 or more alcoholic drinks for females on the same occasion at least once per month.

TABLE 10.6 Drug Therapy

Smoking Cessation*

Agents	Common Side Effects	Considerations
Nicotine Replacement Agents		
Nicotine Gum (OTC) Nicorette 2 mg, 4 mg • Use up to 12 wk • Use 1 piece q1–2hr for 6 wk then q2–4hr for 3 wk • Maximum dose: 24 pieces/day	Hiccups, mouth/jaw pain, mouth ulcers, indigestion, throat irritation, nausea	Specific 30-min chewing regimen with periods of holding the gum between cheek and teeth. Take only water 15 min before and during use. Hard to use with dentures.
Nicotine Lozenge (OTC) Commit 2 mg, 4 mg • Use 8–12 wk • Use 1 lozenge q1–2hr tapering to 1 lozenge q4–8hr in 12 wk	Insomnia, nausea, sore throat, hiccups, cough, heartburn, headache	Dissolves in mouth in 20–30 min. Do not chew or swallow. Avoid food and drink during use. Occasionally rotate around the mouth.
Nicotine Patch (OTC) NicoDerm CQ, Habitrol, Nicotine transdermal system • 18- or 24-hr doses • Use ≥8 wk	Local skin irritation, insomnia, nausea, headache	Provides steady level of nicotine and is easy to use. Cannot be used by those with adhesive allergies. Rotate site to diminish skin irritation.
Nicotine Nasal Spray Nicotrol NS • 1–2 doses (2 sprays)/hr • Use ≥6 mo	Nose and throat irritation, sneezing, rhinitis, headache, cough	Requires a prescription. Provides fastest nicotine delivery. Do not sniff or inhale while dosing. Tilt head back slightly for best results.
Nicotine Inhaler Nicotrol nicotine inhalation system • Use 1 cartridge q1–2hr • Use 3–6 mo	Cough, mouth and throat irritation, headache, nausea, hiccups	Requires a prescription. Simulates smoking with mouthpiece and nicotine cartridge. May not be advisable for those with asthma or pulmonary disease
Non-Nicotine Agents		
bupropion (Zyban) • 150 mg/day for 3 days, then 150 mg bid • Use 12 wk; can use up to 6 mo	Insomnia, dry mouth, irritability, rash, tremors, anorexia	Contraindicated with history of seizures or eating disorders. Promotes weight loss. First choice for smokers with depression
varenicline (Chantix)† • 0.5 mg/day for 3 days, 0.5 mg bid for 4 days, then 1 mg bid • Use 12 wk; additional 12 wk may be used in select patients	Nausea, sleep disturbances, constipation, flatulence, vomiting, headache	If taken concurrently with nicotine replacement therapy, incidence of nausea, headache, vomiting, dizziness, dyspepsia, and fatigue is increased, but nicotine pharmacokinetics not affected.

*OTC nicotine replacement agents are also available in generic forms. More information and patient instructions are available from the American Lung Association at *www.lungusa.org*.
†See the Drug Alert for varenicline on p. 145.

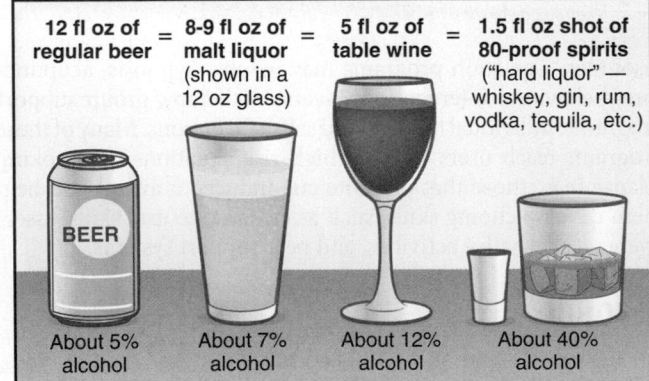

About 5% alcohol — About 7% alcohol — About 12% alcohol — About 40% alcohol

The percent of "pure" alcohol, expressed here as alcohol by volume (alc/vol), varies by beverage.

FIG 10.2 U.S. standard drink equivalents. The National Institute on Alcohol Abuse and Alcoholism (NIAAA) guidelines for alcohol use state that healthy men younger than 65 should consume no more than 14 standard drinks per week or 4 drinks per drinking occasion. Healthy, nonpregnant women and adults older than 65 should consume no more than 7 standard drinks per week or 3 drinks per drinking occasion. (From NIAAA: *What's a standard drink?* Retrieved from *www.niaaa.nih.gov*.)

Effects of Use and Complications

Alcohol affects almost all cells of the body. It changes levels of neurotransmitters in the central nervous system (CNS), affecting all areas and functions of the CNS. These include centers that control our impulses, mood, and behavior; coordinate motor activity; and promote respiratory and cardiac function. The immediate effects of alcohol depend on a person's susceptibility to alcohol and the blood alcohol concentration (BAC).

For the person who is not dependent on alcohol, the BAC generally predicts alcohol's effects. The relationship between BAC and behavior is different in a person who has developed tolerance to alcohol and its effects. The *tolerant person* is usually able to drink large amounts without obvious impairment and perform complex tasks without problems at BAC levels much higher than levels that would produce obvious impairment in the *nontolerant drinker*. Women have higher blood alcohol levels than men do after the same amount of alcohol intake.

Alcohol use is linked to many health problems (Table 10.7), which are often the reason that people seek health care. Long-term alcohol use can lead to hypertension, heart disease, stroke, liver disease, and digestive problems. Short-term, excess alcohol

TABLE 10.7 Effects of Chronic Alcohol Use

BODY SYSTEM	EFFECTS
Cardiac	Hypertension, atrial fibrillation, cardiomyopathy, stroke, coronary artery disease, sudden cardiac death
Gastrointestinal	Gastritis, gastroesophageal reflux disease (GERD), peptic ulcer, esophagitis, esophageal varices, gastrointestinal bleeding, pancreatitis, oropharyngeal cancer, colorectal cancer
Hematologic	Bone marrow depression, anemia, leukopenia, thrombocytopenia, blood clotting abnormalities
Hepatic	Alcoholic hepatitis, cirrhosis, liver cancer
Integumentary	Palmar erythema, spider angiomas, rosacea, rhinophyma
Musculoskeletal	Myopathy, osteoporosis, gout
Neurologic	Alcoholic dementia, Wernicke-Korsakoff syndrome, impaired cognitive function, psychomotor skills, abstract thinking, and memory. Depression, anxiety, attention deficit, labile moods, seizures, insomnia, peripheral neuropathy, chronic headache
Nutrition	Diabetes, anorexia, malnutrition, vitamin deficiencies (especially thiamine)
Reproductive	Breast cancer, testicular atrophy, decreased beard growth, decreased libido, decreased sperm count, gynecomastia
Urinary	Diuretic effect from inhibition of antidiuretic hormone

use increases the risk for injury from motor vehicle crashes, falls, firearms, assault, drowning, and burns. Patients with AUD undergoing surgery have increased in-hospital death rates and longer lengths of stay.

Complications may arise from the interaction of alcohol with commonly prescribed or OTC medications. Those that interact with alcohol in an additive manner include antihypertensives, antihistamines, and antianginals. Alcohol taken with aspirin may cause or worsen GI bleeding. Alcohol taken with acetaminophen may increase the risk for liver damage. Taking a CNS depressant with alcohol can increase, or potentiate, the effect of both. An alcohol-dependent person may have cross-tolerance, needing higher doses of CNS depressants to achieve the desired effect.

❖ NURSING AND INTERPROFESSIONAL MANAGEMENT: ALCOHOL USE DISORDER

◆ Alcohol Toxicity

Acute alcohol toxicity occurs when a person has a high level of alcohol in the blood, generally after ingesting a large amount of alcohol. This leads to behavior changes and alcohol-induced CNS depression, resulting in respiratory and circulatory

failure. Unconsciousness, coma, and death can occur. Other common effects include hypokalemia, hypomagnesemia, and hypoglycemia.

Obtain as accurate a health history as possible and assess for injuries, diseases, and hypoglycemia. No antidote for alcohol is available. Implement supportive care measures to maintain airway, breathing, and circulation (the ABCs) until the alcohol metabolizes. Frequently monitor vital signs and level of consciousness. Treat alcohol-induced hypotension with IV fluids.

Patients with hypoglycemia may receive glucose-containing IV solutions. IV thiamine may be given before or with IV glucose solutions to prevent *Wernicke-Korsakoff syndrome*, which can cause seizures and brain damage.[7] Many patients have low serum magnesium levels and other signs of malnutrition, so HCPs often add multivitamins and magnesium to the IV fluids.

Agitation and anxiety are common. Stay with the patient as much as possible, orienting as necessary. Assess the patient for increasing belligerence and a potential for violence. Since the patient is at risk for injury because of lack of coordination and impaired judgment, use protective measures.

◆ Alcohol Withdrawal Syndrome

Alcohol withdrawal syndrome (AWS) can develop in a hospitalized patient when the use of alcohol abruptly stops. The onset of AWS is variable depending on the quantity, frequency, pattern, and duration of alcohol use. The early signs usually develop within a few hours after the last drink. They peak after 24 to 48 hours and then disappear unless the withdrawal progresses to alcohol withdrawal delirium.

Alcohol withdrawal delirium is a serious complication that can occur from 2 to 3 days after the last drink and last 2 to 3 days. The greater the patient's dependence on alcohol, the greater the risk for alcohol withdrawal delirium. Death may result from multiorgan dysfunction, dysrhythmias, or peripheral vascular collapse.[8]

Management begins with identifying at-risk persons. Use a symptom assessment tool, such as the Clinical Institute Withdrawal Assessment of Alcohol Scale, Revised (CIWA-Ar), to determine treatment[7] (Table 10.8). Table 10.9 presents the clinical manifestations and suggested treatment for AWS. A nursing care plan (eNursing Care Plan 10.1) for a patient with AWS is available on the website at *http://evolve.elsevier.com/Lewis/medsurg*.

? CHECK YOUR PRACTICE

A 34-yr-old male patient was admitted for multiple trauma following a car accident. His girlfriend tells you that he always drinks too much and she knew he would get in trouble someday.
- What signs and symptoms would alert you to the presence of AWS?
- What measures would you use to protect his safety?
- How would you involve members of the interprofessional team in planning patient care?

■ USE OF OTHER SUBSTANCES

STIMULANTS

Amphetamine-related stimulants are highly addictive substances. While the use of crack cocaine and methamphetamine is illegal, amphetamines have a role in treating narcolepsy, obesity, and attention deficit disorder. Though most people responsibly use

TABLE 10.8 Clinical Institute Withdrawal Assessment of Alcohol Scale, Revised (CIWA-Ar)

CIWA-AR CATEGORIES	SCORE RANGE IN EACH CATEGORY
Agitation	0–7
Anxiety	0–7
Auditory disturbances	0–7
Headache	0–7
Clouding of sensorium	0–4
Paroxysmal sweats	0–7
Tactile disturbances	0–7
Tremor	0–7
Visual disturbances	0–7

Source: University of Maryland School of Medicine. Available at *www.umem.org/files/uploads/1104212257_CIWA-Ar.pdf.*

TABLE 10.9 Manifestations and Treatment of Alcohol Withdrawal

Manifestations	Interprofessional Care
Alcohol Withdrawal Syndrome	
• Agitation • Anxiety • ↑ Heart rate • ↑ BP • Sweating • Nausea • Tremors • Insomnia • Hyperactivity	• Benzodiazepines (e.g., lorazepam, diazepam) to prevent seizures and delirium • Thiamine to prevent Wernicke-Korsakoff syndrome • Multivitamins (e.g., folic acid, B vitamins) • Magnesium sulfate to treat low serum magnesium • IV glucose solution to treat hypoglycemia • β-Blockers (e.g., atenolol) or α₂-agonists (e.g., clonidine) to stabilize vital signs • Respiratory support
Alcohol Withdrawal Delirium	
• Disorientation • Visual, tactile, or auditory hallucinations • Seizures	• Continued use of benzodiazepines • Valproic acid or gabapentin to treat seizures • Antipsychotic agents (haloperidol [Haldol]) • Chlordiazepoxide if psychosis persists after benzodiazepine administration

prescribed stimulants, prescription stimulants are often misused. All stimulants increase cardiac activity and excite the CNS by increasing levels of norepinephrine, serotonin, and dopamine. People use these drugs to produce feelings of euphoria, increase alertness, and boost their energy. Health problems associated with using stimulants are outlined in Table 10.2.

❖ NURSING AND INTERPROFESSIONAL MANAGEMENT: STIMULANT USE

◆ Toxicity

Patients with stimulant toxicity present with *sympathetic overdrive* (increased stimulation of the sympathetic nervous system). The patient has restlessness, agitation, delirium, impaired judgment, and paranoia with psychotic symptoms. Physical effects include hypertension, tachycardia, fever, pupil dilation,

TABLE 10.10 Emergency Management
Stimulant Toxicity

ASSESSMENT FINDINGS	INTERVENTIONS
Cardiovascular • Palpitations • Tachycardia • ↑ BP • Dysrhythmias • Myocardial ischemia • Chest pain **Central Nervous System** • Agitation • Euphoria • Insomnia • Combativeness • Seizures • Hallucinations • Confusion • Paranoia • Fever	• Ensure patent airway. • Establish IV access and start appropriate fluid replacement. • Obtain a 12-lead ECG and start ECG monitoring. • Treat ventricular dysrhythmias as needed. • Treat hypertension and chest pain with nitrates or calcium channel blockers. • Aspirin may be given to lower the risk for myocardial infarction. • Give IV diazepam or lorazepam for seizures. • Give IV antipsychotic drugs for psychosis and hallucinations. • Monitor vital signs and level of consciousness. • Begin cooling measures for hyperthermia. • Treat insomnia with trazodone, hydroxyzine, or diphenhydramine at bedtime. • Start gastric lavage in cases of recent ingestion.

seizures, confusion, and diaphoresis. Death may occur from stroke, dysrhythmias, or myocardial infarction.[1]

The emergency management depends on the clinical manifestations at the time of treatment (Table 10.10). A specific antidote for stimulant toxicity is not available. Treatment focuses on supportive care measures.

◆ Withdrawal

Stimulant withdrawal is usually not an emergency. Abrupt cessation can lead to a "crash." The patient may be depressed and experience fatigue, disturbed sleep, vivid dreams, general aching, irritability, increased appetite, and mood swings.[9] Craving for the drug is intense during the first hours to days of drug cessation and may continue for weeks. Supportive care includes providing a safe, quiet environment and allowing the patient to sleep and eat as desired. If a patient has severe depression, initiate suicide precautions and refer for further treatment.

DEPRESSANTS

Commonly used depressants include sedative-hypnotics and opioids. Depressants have a rapid development of tolerance and dependence. Their use is associated with many medical emergencies involving toxicity and withdrawal. The majority of drug overdose deaths involve an opioid, either alone or in combination with another depressant (e.g., opioid and benzodiazepine).[10] Common health problems resulting from depressant use are outlined in Table 10.2.

Sedative-Hypnotics

Common sedative-hypnotic agents include barbiturates, benzodiazepines, and barbiturate-like drugs. Sedative-hypnotic drugs depress the CNS, causing sedation at low doses and sleep at high doses. Their use produces a euphoria and intoxication that resembles that of alcohol. Tolerance develops rapidly to the effects of these drugs, requiring higher doses to achieve euphoria. However, tolerance may not develop to the brainstem-depressant effects. As a result, an increased dose may trigger hypotension and respiratory depression, resulting in death.

Opioids

Opioids include substances directly derived from the opium poppy (e.g., morphine), semisynthetics (e.g., heroin, hydromorphone), and synthetic compounds (e.g., fentanyl). Persons dependent on opioids include those who use illegal drugs sold on the street and those who misuse prescription opioids. Opioids act on opiate receptors and neurotransmitter systems in the CNS, causing sedation and analgesia. The person taking an opioid experiences euphoria, mood changes, mental clouding, drowsiness, and pain reduction. While this makes prescription opioids useful in treating a number of medical conditions, their pleasurable effects promote misuse. Misusing oxycodone or fentanyl can result in the same harmful consequences as abusing heroin.

❖ NURSING AND INTERPROFESSIONAL MANAGEMENT: DEPRESSANT USE

◆ Toxicity

Overdoses can occur when a person purposefully misuses a depressant or takes 1 prescribed for someone else. Unintentional overdose often occurs, especially when depressants are used with alcohol or other drugs. Depressant toxicity can cause death from respiratory and CNS depression. The priority of care is always the patient's ABCs. Supporting respiratory and cardiovascular function and continuous monitoring of neurologic status is critical until the patient is stable. The emergency management depends on the substance used and the clinical manifestations (Table 10.11).

TABLE 10.11 Emergency Management
Depressant Toxicity

Assessment Findings	Interventions
• Aggressive behavior	• Ensure patent airway.
• Agitation	• Expect intubation if respiratory
• Confusion	distress present.
• Lethargy	• Establish IV access.
• Stupor	• Obtain temperature.
• Hallucinations	• Obtain 12-lead ECG and start
• Depression	continuous ECG monitoring.
• Slurred speech	• Obtain information about sub-
• Pinpoint pupils	stance (name, route, when taken,
• Nystagmus	amount).
• Seizures	• Obtain specific drug levels or
• Cold, clammy skin	comprehensive toxicology screen.
• Rapid, weak pulse	• Obtain a health history, including
• Slow or rapid shallow	drug use and allergies.
respirations	• Give the right antidotes.
• Decreased O₂ saturation	• Perform gastric lavage if
• Hypotension	necessary.
• Dysrhythmias	• Give activated charcoal and
• ECG changes	cathartics as needed.
• Cardiac or respiratory	• Monitor vital signs, level of
arrest	consciousness, and O₂ saturation.

◆ **Sedative-Hypnotics.** On occasion, a patient with a benzodiazepine overdose may receive flumazenil, a specific benzodiazepine antagonist. Because flumazenil may have a shorter duration of action than some benzodiazepines, repeated doses may be needed until the benzodiazepine is metabolized. Place the patient on safety precautions as flumazenil can cause seizures.

There are no antagonists for barbiturates or other sedative-hypnotic drugs. The patient receives supportive care, including passive rewarming, hydration, and vasopressors, along with treatments to promote drug elimination. If the airway can be maintained, activated charcoal is an option. Dialysis can be used in certain situations.

◆ **Opioids.** Overdose in the inpatient setting may occur when a patient inadvertently receives an incorrect dose, or when opioids are aggressively dosed, given to patients with new kidney or liver impairment, or given with drugs that potentiate respiratory depression.[11] Treatment includes supporting respiratory function and giving the opioid antagonist naloxone. Naloxone reverses respiratory depression and other manifestations of toxicity. Monitor the patient closely because naloxone has a shorter duration of action than most opioids. Repeated doses or IV infusion of naloxone may be needed until the opioid is metabolized.

Overdose in the community setting can occur when a person deliberately misuses an illegal or prescription opioid, takes an opioid in combination with other depressants, or takes an opioid prescribed for someone else. In many areas, naloxone is publicly available. This allows police, first responders, family members, and friends to give someone naloxone in emergencies, thus reversing the effects of an overdose sooner. As a result, you may see more patients requiring postreversal care.

◆ Withdrawal

◆ **Sedative-Hypnotics.** Withdrawal from sedative-hypnotics can be life threatening. The manifestations and treatment are similar to those of AWS. Early, the patient may have tremors, anxiety, insomnia, fever, orthostatic hypotension, and disorientation. Since the patient may experience delirium, seizures, and respiratory and cardiac arrest within 24 hours after the last dose, closely monitor the patient. Treatment consists of giving a long-acting benzodiazepine in a tapered dose. IV diazepam is an option for severe manifestations. Supportive care includes implementing patient safety and comfort measures, frequently assessing neurologic status and vital signs, and providing reassurance and orientation.

◆ **Opioids.** Opioid withdrawal symptoms depend on the opioid used, route of administration, and duration of use. It is usually not life threatening but can be extremely uncomfortable. Manifestations include intense drug craving, diaphoresis, gastrointestinal distress, restlessness, fever, insomnia, watery eyes, tremors, muscle aches, runny nose, and anxiety.[1] With shorter acting drugs, withdrawal may begin 4 to 6 hours after the last dose, peak in 36 to 72 hours, and last 7 to 10 days. With longer acting drugs, manifestations may begin 24 to 48 hours after last dose and peak in 3 to 4 days.[11]

Treatment focuses on relieving symptoms and often requires drug therapy. Substituting a long-acting opioid (e.g., methadone, buprenorphine) at low doses or α₂-adrenergic agonists (e.g., clonidine) decreases withdrawal symptoms. Other therapies include medications for GI distress (e.g., loperamide, ondansetron), acetaminophen or nonsteroidal antiinflammatory agents for muscle aches and fever, and antihistamines for acute anxiety and sleep disturbances.

INHALANTS

Persons with inhalant use disorder inhale hydrocarbon-based fumes, such as those found in glues or paints, to change their mental state.[1] Inhalants are rapidly absorbed and reach the CNS quickly. Most are depressants with effects like those of alcohol. They cause a brief period of euphoria, followed by drowsiness and lightheadedness. Long-term use can result in neurologic problems, including damage to parts of the brain that control cognition, movement, vision, and hearing (Table 10.2).

The patient with inhalant toxicity may have lethargy, dizziness, slurred speech, blurry vision, tremors, and impaired coordination.[1] The effects usually resolve within minutes to a few hours. Inhalant toxicity is managed with supportive care. However, in some cases, users need emergency treatment for dysrhythmias, heart failure, or CNS hyperactivity (e.g., seizures). Using some inhalants (e.g., toluene) can result in nephrotoxicity; so, you must monitor renal function. Withdrawal is rare as most inhaled substances have a very short duration. Any manifestations that may occur require supportive care.

CANNABIS

The use of cannabis, also called marijuana or weed, continues to increase in the United States. Cannabis is available in forms that can be smoked, vaporized, or ingested. The main ingredient is tetrahydrocannabinol (THC). At low to moderate doses, THC produces euphoria, reduced anxiety, and improved appetite. Adverse effects include impaired memory, impaired motor coordination, altered judgment, and, in high doses, paranoia and psychosis. Long-term use is associated with a wide range of effects, particularly on cardiopulmonary and mental health (Table 10.2).

Legalizing cannabis for recreational and medical use is controversial. Sales for recreational use continue to grow. More than half of the states have legalized its use for specific medical reasons. If an HCP in 1 of those states determines a patient has a disorder that qualifies for medical cannabis use, the HCP can give the patient an *authorization for use*. This form allows the patient to buy cannabis at special dispensaries or have a limited number of cannabis plants. THC-based medications, dronabinol (Marinol) and nabilone (Cesamet), are available to control nausea and vomiting from cancer chemotherapy. Dronabinol is also used to stimulate appetite in patients with acquired immunodeficiency syndrome (AIDS). Illegal synthetic cannabinoid drugs (e.g., K2, Spice) have some of the same properties as THC. They contain varying amounts of different ingredients. The result is that these products have unpredictable effects and are more toxic. Sometimes, death has occurred with 1 use.

Patients with *acute marijuana toxicity* can present with acute psychotic episodes, especially if the patient used a synthetic derivative. Cannabis can induce tachycardia and hypertension, triggering dysrhythmias and myocardial infarction. Support the patient's ABCs. Panic and flashbacks are managed by maintaining a quiet environment and reassuring the patient. Benzodiazepines give symptom relief.[12]

Withdrawal can occur in a hospitalized patient who uses cannabis. The patient may have irritability, insomnia, anorexia, cramping, mild agitation, and nausea.[13] This peaks about 48 hours after cessation and may be more severe in women. There

is no specific drug therapy for treating withdrawal. Supportive care includes measures to promote sleep, safety, and patient comfort, including analgesics and hydration.

CAFFEINE

Caffeine is the most widely used psychoactive substance in the world. It is very weak when compared with the other stimulants. Most people use it to promote wakefulness. Other uses include promoting motor activity and treating headaches. Its use is safe in most people. Problems from high doses of caffeine have occurred in association with specialized drinks. A large caffeine intake can cause cardiac dysrhythmias, hypertension, disturbed sleep, seizures, and anxiety. Treatment consists of seizure control with benzodiazepines and supportive care until the effects wear off. In a hospitalized patient, caffeine withdrawal can result in muscle pain or stiffness, drowsiness, irritability, and headaches after general anesthesia or during restrictions on usual caffeine intake.[1]

❖ NURSING MANAGEMENT: SUBSTANCE USE

◆ Nursing Assessment

You need to be able to determine if patients use substances in a way that places them at risk or if SUD is present. Screening is a simple, effective way to identify patients who need further assessment. Use the Screening, Brief Intervention, and Referral to Treatment (SBIRT) approach (Fig. 10.3). SBIRT consists of 3 parts: (1) screening to quickly identify and assess the severity of any substance use problems, (2) providing a brief intervention or teaching patients about the consequences of substance use, and (3) referring those who screen positive for further treatment.[14]

Screening is the first part of SBIRT. Use screening tools to identify those who may have problems with substance use. As a baseline, ask every patient about the use of all substances, including prescribed medications, OTC medications, caffeine, tobacco, and recreational drugs. Use simple 1 or 2 question screening tests to detect alcohol, tobacco, and/or other substance use problems (Table 10.12). If a patient has a positive screen, follow up with a detailed assessment to identify specific problems. A screening tool for AUD, the Alcohol Use Disorders

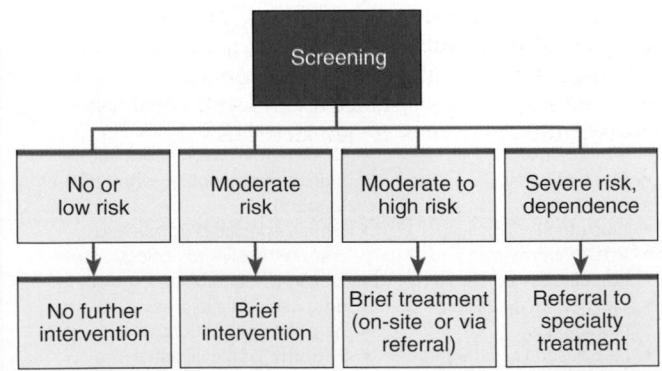

FIG 10.3 Screening, Brief Intervention, and Referral to Treatment approach. (From Substance Abuse and Mental Health Services Administration [SAMHSA]: Systems-level implementation of screening, brief intervention, and referral to treatment, Technical Assistance Publication [TAP] Series 33. HHS Publication No. 13-4741, Rockville, MD, 2013, SAMHSA. Retrieved from *www.integration.samhsa.gov/SBIRT/tap33.pdf*.)

TABLE 10.12 Brief Screening Tools for Substance Use

Single Question Tests
Use 1 of the following questions to screen for the presence of alcohol, drug, or tobacco use.
- How often in the past year have you had 5 (men) or 4 (women) or more drinks in a day?
- How many times in the past year have you used illegal drugs or prescription medications for nonmedical reasons?
- In the past year, how often have you used tobacco products?

2-Question Tests
Use the following 2 questions to screen for alcohol or drug use.
- In the past year, have you ever drunk or used drugs more than you meant to?
- Have you felt you wanted or needed to cut down on your drinking or drug use in the past year?

Adapted from Strobbe S: Prevention and screening, brief intervention, and referral to treatment for substance use in primary care, *Prim Care Clin Office Pract* 41:185, 2014.

TABLE 10.13 Alcohol Use Disorders Identification Test (AUDIT)

Please answer each question by checking 1 of the circles in the second column.

		Score
1. How often do you have a drink containing alcohol?	• Never	(0)
	• Monthly or less	(1)
	• 2 to 4 times per month	(2)
	• 2 to 4 times per week	(3)
	• 4+ times per week	(4)
2. How many drinks containing alcohol do you have on a typical day when you are drinking?	• 1 or 2	(0)
	• 3 or 4	(1)
	• 5 or 6	(2)
	• 7 to 9	(3)
	• 10 or more	(4)
3. How often do you have 6 or more drinks on 1 occasion?	• Never	(0)
	• Less than monthly	(1)
	• Monthly	(2)
	• Weekly	(3)
	• Daily or almost daily	(4)
4. How often during the last year have you found that you were not able to stop drinking once you had started?	• Never	(0)
	• Less than monthly	(1)
	• Monthly	(2)
	• Weekly	(3)
	• Daily or almost daily	(4)
5. How often in the last year have you failed to do what was normally expected of you because you were drinking?	• Never	(0)
	• Less than monthly	(1)
	• Monthly	(2)
	• Weekly	(3)
	• Daily or almost daily	(4)
6. How often during the last year have you needed a first drink in the morning to get yourself going after a heavy drinking session?	• Never	(0)
	• Less than monthly	(1)
	• Monthly	(2)
	• Weekly	(3)
	• Daily or almost daily	(4)
7. How often during the last year have you had a feeling of guilt or remorse about drinking?	• Never	(0)
	• Less than monthly	(1)
	• Monthly	(2)
	• Weekly	(3)
	• Daily or almost daily	(4)
8. How often during the last year have you been unable to remember what happened the night before because you had been drinking?	• Never	(0)
	• Less than monthly	(1)
	• Monthly	(2)
	• Weekly	(3)
	• Daily or almost daily	(4)
9. Have you or someone else been injured as a result of your drinking?	• No	(0)
	• Yes, but not in the last year	(2)
	• Yes, during the last year	(4)
10. Has a relative, friend, or other health worker been concerned about your drinking or suggested that you cut down?	• No	(0)
	• Yes, but not in the last year	(2)
	• Yes, during the last year	(4)

Scoring for AUDIT: Questions 1 through 8 are scored 0, 1, 2, 3, or 4. Questions 9 and 10 are scored 0, 2, or 4 only. The minimum score (nondrinkers) is 0 and the maximum possible score is 40. A score of 9 or more indicates hazardous or harmful alcohol consumption.
Source: Babor TF, Higgins-Biddle JC, Saunders JB, Monteiro M: *The alcohol use disorders identification test*, ed 2, Geneva, Switzerland, 2001, WHO Press.

Identification Test, is shown in Table 10.13. A score of 8 points or more in men or 7 or more in women is concerning. Another useful tool is the Drug Abuse Screening Test (DAST-10), shown in Table 10.14.

If there is any sign of substance use, figure out when the patient last used the substance. Knowing this information will let you know when to expect the onset of withdrawal and help you anticipate drug interactions. Assess for factors that influence the onset of withdrawal, including the substance used, dose taken, method of intake, and length of time the patient has used the substance. You may discover that the patient is dealing with *polysubstance use,* or the use of more than 1 substance. Alert the HCP as these patients need care tailored to the combination of substances used.

You may find problems associated with substance use during your physical assessment. Assess the patient's general appearance and nutritional status. Examine the abdomen, skin, and cardiovascular, respiratory, and neurologic systems. The presence of a mental health disorder, such as anxiety, bipolar disorder, or depression, increases the risk for SUD. Serum and urine drug screens can identify the type and amounts of drugs present in the body. A complete blood count, serum electrolytes, blood urea nitrogen, creatinine, and liver function tests evaluate for electrolyte imbalances and cardiac, kidney, or liver dysfunction.

During your assessment, look for patient behaviors such as denial, avoidance, underreporting or minimizing substance use, or giving inaccurate information. Behaviors and physical manifestations suggesting substance use are outlined in Table 10.15. However, these behaviors are not all inclusive.

◆ Nursing Diagnoses

Nursing diagnoses for the patient with substance use disorder include:
- Substance abuse, drug, alcohol and/or tobacco
- Risk for injury
- Acute confusion
- Altered perception

◆ Planning

Nursing care focuses on the priority problems of reducing the risk for injury and managing acute confusion. The overall goals are that the patient with a substance use problem will (1) have normal physiologic functioning, (2) acknowledge a substance use problem, (3) explain the psychologic and physiologic effects of substance use, (4) abstain from substance use, and (5) cooperate with a proposed treatment plan.

TABLE 10.14 Drug Abuse Screening Test (DAST-10)

In the last 12 months:

		No	Yes
1.	Have you used drugs other than those required for medical reasons?	No	Yes
2.	Do you abuse more than 1 drug at a time?	No	Yes
3.	Are you always able to stop using drugs when you want to?	No	Yes
4.	Have you had "blackouts" or "flashbacks" as a result of drug use?	No	Yes
5.	Do you ever feel bad or guilty about your drug use?	No	Yes
6.	Does your spouse (or parents) ever complain about your involvement with drugs?	No	Yes
7.	Have you neglected your family because of your use of drugs?	No	Yes
8.	Have you engaged in illicit activities in order to obtain drugs?	No	Yes
9.	Have you ever experienced withdrawal symptoms or felt sick when you stopped taking drugs?	No	Yes
10.	Have you had medical problems as a result of your drug use?	No	Yes

© 1982 by Harvey A. Skinner, PhD, and the Centre for Addiction and Mental Health, Toronto, Canada. You may reproduce this instrument for noncommercial use (clinical, research, training purposes) as long as you credit the author, Dr. Harvey A. Skinner, Dean, Faculty of Health, York University, Toronto, Canada.

TABLE 10.15 Findings Suggesting Substance Use

Physiologic
- Fatigue
- Insomnia
- Headaches
- Seizure disorder
- Changes in mood
- Anorexia, weight loss
- Vague physical complaints
- Appearing older than stated age, unkempt appearance
- Sexual dysfunction, decreased libido, erectile dysfunction
- Failure of standard doses of sedatives to have a therapeutic effect

Behavioral
- Overuse of mouthwash or toiletries
- Citations for driving while intoxicated or impaired
- Leisure activities that involve alcohol and/or other drugs
- Trauma secondary to falls, auto accidents, fights, or burns
- Financial problems, including those related to spending for substances
- Defensive or evasive answers to questions about substance use and its importance in the person's life
- Problems in areas of life function (e.g., frequent job changes; marital conflict, separation, or divorce; work-related accidents, tardiness, absenteeism; legal problems; social isolation, estranged from friends or family)

◆ Nursing Implementation

Health Promotion. Your role in health promotion includes prevention and early detection of substance use. Prevention measures include abstaining from harmful substances and limiting alcohol use. These measures decrease the risk for substance-related injury or illness. You can help prevent substance use problems by (1) teaching about the effects and negative outcomes of substance use and (2) providing support. Through screening, you have an opportunity to prevent patients from becoming dependent on alcohol and drugs. You can do this by using brief interventional techniques and helping patients access appropriate care through referral to treatment if they show risky behaviors or are already dependent.

Acute Intervention. The immediate result of overconsumption is acute toxicity or overdose. The patient may also present with trauma or injuries. The priority of care is supporting the patient's ABCs, especially respiratory status. In addition to treating injuries, provide supportive care until detoxification can occur. Nursing care includes frequently assessing neurologic status and vital signs, giving IV fluids to prevent dehydration, orienting to time and place, and implementing patient safety measures.

Sometimes, uncertainty exists as to what substances are involved. If the patient used multiple substances, a complex clinical picture can result. For example, a patient presents with toxicity and the health care team does not know what substances are involved. Although blood and urine tests will help identify the substances, treatment is started while waiting for the test results. The patient in this situation would usually receive naloxone. If the substance used is a barbiturate or another CNS depressant, naloxone will not help the patient, but it will not hurt the patient either. If the patient does not respond to a total dose of 10 mg of naloxone, it is unlikely opioids are involved.

Once acute health issues are resolved, provide a brief intervention to teach patients about the consequences of substance use and support behavioral change. When patients have a substance use problem, it is critical to motivate the patient to engage in long-term treatment. You are in a unique position to facilitate behavior change. When a patient seeks care for health problems related to substance use or when hospitalization interferes with the usual pattern of use, the patient's awareness of any substance use problem increases. Intervention at this time can promote behavior change. Take an active role in performing motivational interviewing and providing counseling aimed at cessation. (Motivational interviewing is discussed in Chapter 4.) Discuss the risks associated with substance use and provide feedback and advice. If the patient agrees, assist with referral to counseling or behavioral therapy.

Gerontologic Considerations: Substance Use

Substance use in older adults is a fast-growing and often hard to recognize problem. Older adults do not fit the image of users. For example, older users are less likely to binge drink and use different substances than younger users. The effects of alcohol and drugs can be mistaken for medical conditions common among older adults (e.g., hypertension, dementia). So, we may attribute substance use problems to another cause and not offer treatment. Some use alcohol or drugs to cope with grief and loss issues, such as the death of a spouse.[15]

Because of the higher rate of coexisting medical problems, older adults are at greater risk for medical problems associated with substance use. Common problems include liver damage and cardiovascular, GI, and endocrine problems. Substance use may cause confusion, delirium, memory loss, and neuromuscular impairment. Physiologic changes may lead to toxicity at levels that may not have been a problem at a younger age. Withdrawal symptoms may be more severe than in younger persons.

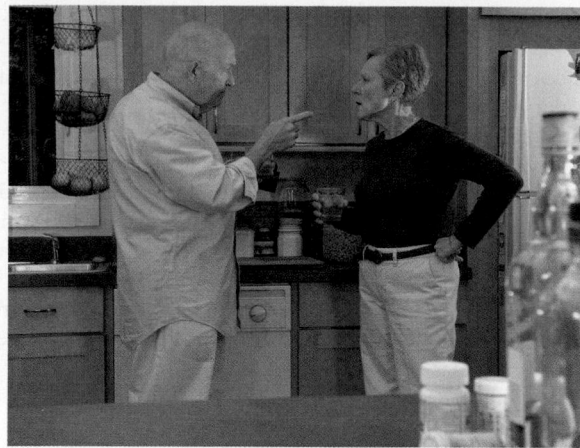

FIG 10.4 Older adults are often unaware of their substance use problems. (© Ned White/iStock/Thinkstock.)

It is important to screen older adults for substance use. Family members are important sources of information (Fig. 10.4). Other potential sources include friends, home health aides, meal delivery personnel, and staff members at senior citizen centers and long-term care facilities. It is important for you to discuss drug and alcohol use with older adult patients, including OTC and herbal drug use. Assess the patient's knowledge of currently used drugs. Common screening questionnaires may not identify an older adult with a substance use problem. The Short Michigan Alcoholism Screening Test–Geriatric version (SMAST-G) is a short-form alcoholism screening instrument for older adults (*www.consultgerirn.org*) that can identify older adults with potential AUD.

Smoking and other tobacco use is another issue. Those who have smoked for decades may feel unable to stop or believe there is no benefit to stopping at an advanced age. However, smoking contributes to and worsens many chronic illnesses found in the older adult population. Smoking cessation at any age is beneficial. The information about smoking cessation discussed earlier is appropriate for helping older adults with smoking cessation (Tables 10.3 to 10.6).

Patient teaching for the older adult includes teaching about the desired effects, possible side effects, and proper use of prescribed and OTC drugs. When you suspect alcohol or substance use, refer the patient for treatment. It is a mistaken belief that older people have little to gain from alcohol and drug dependence treatment. The rewards of treatment can lead to greater quality and quantity of life for older adults.

CASE STUDY

Substance Use Disorder

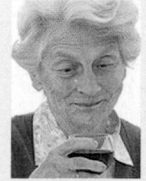

(©JPC-PROD/ iStock/Think-stock.)

Patient Profile

C.M., a 78-yr-old woman, is admitted to the emergency department after falling and injuring her right hip. She has been widowed for 4 years and lives alone. Recently her best friend died. Her only family is a daughter who lives out of town. When contacted by phone, the daughter tells the nurse that her mother has appeared more disoriented and confused over the past few months when she has talked to her on the phone.

Subjective Data

- Describing severe pain in her right hip
- Admits she had some wine in the late afternoon to stimulate her appetite
- Has experienced several falls in the past 2 months
- Reports that she fell after taking a prescribed sleeping pill because she does not sleep well
- Speech is hesitant and slurred
- Says she smokes about a half pack of cigarettes a day

Objective Data

Physical Examination

- Oriented to person and place, but not time
- BP 162/94, pulse 92, respirations 24
- Severe pain and tenderness in the right hip region
- Bilateral hand tremors

Diagnostic Tests

- X-ray reveals a subtrochanteric fracture of the right femur requiring surgical repair
- Blood alcohol concentration (BAC) 120 mg/dL (0.12%)
- Complete blood count: Hemoglobin 10.6 g/dL, hematocrit 33%

Discussion Questions

1. What other information is needed to assess C.M.'s condition?
2. How should you address questions about these areas?
3. What factors may contribute to C.M.'s substance use?
4. *Priority Decision:* Based on the assessment data given, what are the priority nursing diagnoses? Are there any collaborative problems?
5. *Priority Decision:* What are the priority nursing interventions during C.M.'s preoperative period?
6. What possible complications and injury risks may occur during C.M.'s postoperative recovery?
7. *Safety:* To ensure C.M.'s safety, what nursing interventions are necessary after surgery?
8. *Delegation Decision:* How would you use the unlicensed assistive personnel (UAP) on the postoperative unit to carry out the interventions that you identified in question 5?
9. *Collaboration:* What referrals are indicated?

Answers available at *http://evolve.elsevier.com/Lewis/medsurg.*

BRIDGE TO NCLEX EXAMINATION

The number of the question corresponds to the same-numbered outcome at the beginning of the chapter.

1. When admitting a patient, the nurse must assess the patient for substance use based on the knowledge that long-term use of addictive substances leads to
   a. the development of coexisting psychiatric illnesses.
   b. a higher risk for complications from underlying health problems.
   c. potentiation of effects of similar drugs taken when the person is drug free.
   d. increased availability of dopamine, resulting in decreased sleep requirements.

2. The nurse would suspect cocaine toxicity in the patient who is experiencing
   a. agitation, dysrhythmias, and seizures.
   b. blurred vision, restlessness, and irritability.
   c. diarrhea, nausea and vomiting, and confusion.
   d. slow, shallow respirations; bradycardia; and hypotension.

3. The *most* appropriate nursing intervention for a patient who is being treated for an acute exacerbation of chronic obstructive pulmonary disease who is not interested in quitting smoking is to
   a. accept the patient's decision and not intervene until the patient expresses a desire to quit.
   b. ask the patient to identify the risks and benefits of quitting and what barriers to quitting are present.
   c. realize that some smokers never quit, and trying to assist them increases the patient's frustration.
   d. motivate the patient to quit by describing how continued smoking will worsen the breathing problems.

4. While caring for a patient who is experiencing alcohol withdrawal, the nurse should *(select all that apply)*
   a. monitor neurologic status on a routine basis.
   b. provide a quiet, nonstimulating, dimly lit environment.
   c. pad the side rails and place suction equipment at the bedside.
   d. orient the patient to environment and person with each contact.
   e. give antiseizure drugs and sedatives to relieve withdrawal symptoms.

5. A patient admitted for scheduled surgery has a positive brief screening test result for an alcohol use disorder. Which initial action is *most* appropriate?
   a. Notify the health care provider.
   b. Complete a detailed alcohol use assessment.
   c. Initiate a referral to a specialty treatment center.
   d. Provide patient teaching on postoperative health risks.

6. Substance use problems in older adults are usually related to
   a. use of drugs and alcohol as a social activity.
   b. continuing the use of illegal drugs started during middle age.
   c. misuse of prescribed and over-the-counter medications and alcohol.
   d. a pattern of binge drinking for weeks or months with periods of sobriety.

1. b, 2. a, 3. b, 4. a, c, d, e, 5. b, 6. c

For rationales to these answers and even more NCLEX review questions, visit *http://evolve.elsevier.com/Lewis/medsurg*.

ⓔ EVOLVE WEBSITE/RESOURCES LIST

http://evolve.elsevier.com/Lewis/medsurg
Review Questions (Online Only)
Key Points
Answer Keys for Questions
- Rationales for Bridge to NCLEX Examination Questions
- Answer Guidelines for Case Study on p. 153
- Answer Guidelines for Managing Care of Multiple Patients Case Study (Section 2) on p. 155
Nursing Care Plan
- eNursing Care Plan 10.1: Patient in Alcohol Withdrawal
Conceptual Care Map Creator
Audio Glossary
Content Updates

REFERENCES

1. American Psychiatric Association: *The diagnostic and statistical manual of mental disorders*, 5th ed, Arlington, VA, 2013, The Association. (Classic)
2. Centers for Disease Control and Prevention: Adult cigarette smoking in the U.S. Retrieved from *www.cdc.gov/tobacco/data_statistics/fact_sheets/adult_data/cig_smoking*.
3. Centers for Disease Control and Prevention: Health effects of cigarette smoking. Retrieved from *www.cdc.gov/tobacco/data_statistics/fact_sheets/health_effects/effects_cig_smoking/#overview*.
*4. Breland A, Soule E, Lopez A, et al: Electronic cigarettes: What are they and what do they do? *Ann NY Acad Sci* 1394:5, 2017.
5. Agency for Healthcare Research and Quality: Treating tobacco use and dependence: 2008 update. Retrieved from *www.ahrq.gov/professionals/clinicians-providers/guidelines-recommendations/tobacco/index.html*.
6. Alcohol facts and statistics. Retrieved from *www.niaaa.nih.gov/alcohol-health/overview-alcohol-consumption/alcohol-facts-and-statistics*.
*7. Gortney JS, Raub JN, Patel P, et al: Alcohol withdrawal syndrome in medical patients, *Cleve Clin J Med* 83:67, 2016.
*8. Sutton LJ, Jutel A: Alcohol withdrawal syndrome in critically ill patients: Identification, assessment, and management, *Crit Care Nurse* 36:28, 2016.
*9. Rasimas JJ, Sinclair CM: Assessment and management of toxidromes in the critical care unit, *Crit Care Clin* 33:521, 2017.
10. Centers for Disease Control and Prevention: Understanding the epidemic. Retrieved from *www.cdc.gov/drugoverdose/epidemic/index.html*.
*11. Donroe JH, Holt SR, Tetrault JM: Caring for patients with opioid use disorder in the hospital, *CMAJ* 188:17, 2016.
*12. Phillips J, Lim F, Hsu R: Synthetic cannabinoid poisoning: A growing health concern, *Nursing* 46:34, 2016.
*13. Bonnet U, Preuss UW: Cannabis withdrawal syndrome: Current insights, *Subst Abuse Rehabil* 8:9, 2017.
14. SAMSA-HRSA Center for Integrated Health Solutions: SBIRT. Retrieved from *www.samhsa.gov/sbirt*.
*15. Masferrer L, Garre-Olmo J, Caparrós B: Is complicated grief a risk factor for substance use? *Addict Research Theory* 9:1, 2017.

*Evidence-based information for clinical practice.

CASE STUDY
Managing Care of Multiple Patients

You are assigned to care for the following 5 patients on a medical-surgical unit. Your team consists of yourself, a new LPN still on orientation, and a UAP.

Patients

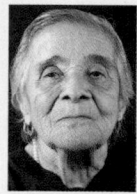

M.S. is an 81-yr-old woman who came to the United States from India 4 years ago with her daughter, son-in-law, and their 4 children. She speaks minimal English, relying on her oldest granddaughter to translate. M.S., who has a history of diabetes, was admitted to the hospital yesterday with a diagnosis of heart failure.

(© Luevanos/ iStock/Thinkstock.)

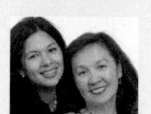

M.L. is a 60-yr-old Asian woman who was admitted to the hospital with a diagnosis of exacerbation of chronic obstructive pulmonary disease (COPD). She is receiving O_2 at 2 L/min via nasal cannula. Her condition is currently stable.

(© Thomas M Perkins/ Shutterstock.)

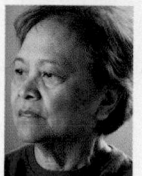

C.L. is a 73-yr-old Taiwanese woman who was brought to the ED by her son. Her chief complaint is shortness of breath. She has a history of COPD, hypertension, and diabetes. She was diagnosed with community-acquired pneumonia, which is being treated with IV antibiotics.

(© azndc/iStock/ Thinkstock.)

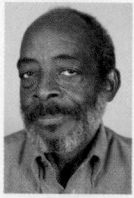

K.C. is a 280-lb (127-kg) 68-yr-old black man with diabetes who was admitted for incision and drainage of a right abdominal abscess. He is being discharged on his second postoperative day. His daughter will assist with dressing changes at home.

(© azndc/iStock/ Thinkstock.)

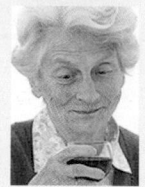

C.M. is a 78-yr-old woman who was admitted from the ED after falling and fracturing her right hip. She is in Buck's traction and is scheduled to undergo surgical repair later this morning. She has a history of substance use, and her blood alcohol content (BAC) was 120 mg/dL (0.12 %) on admission. The night nurse reports that she has been confused and restless overnight.

(© JPC-PROD/ iStock/Thinkstock.)

Discussion Questions

1. ***Priority Decision:*** After receiving report, which patient should you see first? Provide rationale.
2. ***Collaboration:*** Which morning task(s) could you delegate to the LPN (*select all that apply*)?
   a. Obtain a capillary blood glucose reading on K.C.
   b. Assess C.L.'s IV site for signs of phlebitis or infiltration.
   c. Access the hospital's available translation services for M.S.
   d. Provide discharge teaching on wound care for K.C. and her daughter.
   e. Titrate M.L.'s O_2 to obtain a pulse oximetry reading of 95% (as ordered by the HCP).
3. ***Priority and Collaboration:*** When you and the LPN enter M.S.'s room, you find her sitting up in bed with labored respirations. Although you cannot

understand what she is saying, you note that she is unable to say more than a few words without stopping for a breath. Which initial action would be the most appropriate?
   a. Give M.S.'s cardiac and respiratory medications and reassess her in 30 minutes.
   b. Ask the LPN to stay with M.S. while you go to the nurse's station to call the HCP.
   c. Have the LPN find M.S.'s granddaughter so that she can translate what M.S. is trying to tell you.
   d. Ask the LPN to obtain an O_2 saturation and vital signs while you perform a respiratory assessment.

Case Study Progression

M.S.'s assessment reveals bibasilar crackles, 2+ dependent pitting edema, BP 175/84, pulse 116, RR 32, temp 36.8°C, and pulse oximetry 88% on room air. You apply O_2 at 4 L/min via nasal cannula and obtain an order from M.S.'s HCP for furosemide 40 mg IV stat. After giving the diuretic, M.S.'s granddaughter arrives and you discuss her grandmother's condition. She tells you that her grandmother asked her to bring in potato chips and soda yesterday. She did not think her grandmother should be eating salt, but M.S. insisted that the dietitian said that she could eat them.

4. On further investigation, the dietitian tells you that an interpreter (translator) was not available when she saw M.S. yesterday. Because the dietitian did not understand what the patient was saying, she could not respond to her questions. She planned to visit M.S. today when the granddaughter is present. Being a culturally competent nurse, you realize that M.S. most likely interpreted the dietitian's silence as
   a. agreement with what A.Z. was asking.
   b. demonstrating a lack of respect for A.Z.'s wishes.
   c. a lack of understanding by the dietitian as to what she was asking.
   d. a need for the dietitian to get more information before answering her questions.
5. Which assessment findings may suggest elder mistreatment by C.L.'s son with whom she lives (*select all that apply*)?
   a. 2 sacral ulcers
   b. Asking when her son is coming to visit
   c. Multiple small bruises on her forearms and shins
   d. Matted hair, poor oral hygiene, overgrown toenails
   e. C.L. becomes totally silent when her son comes to visit
6. Knowing that C.M.'s confusion and restlessness overnight may indicate acute alcohol withdrawal, you perform a more thorough assessment. Your assessment reveals a score of 11 on the Clinical Institute Withdrawal Assessment for Alcohol Scale. To prevent alcohol delirium, you plan to give which medication per the HCP's order?
   a. morphine
   b. naloxone
   c. lorazepam
   d. IV thiamine
7. ***Priority Decision:*** You assess C.M. and find her trying to pull out the IV line and remove the Buck's traction. What action should you do *first*?
   a. Have the UAP stay with C.M.
   b. Ask C.M.'s daughter to stay with her.
   c. Obtain a restraint order from the HCP.
   d. Move C.M. to a room closer to the nurse's station.
8. ***Management Decision:*** The UAP informs you that the LPN is not following C.L.'s fall risk protocol. What is your most appropriate action?
   a. Notify the unit manager as soon as possible.
   b. Ask the UAP to explain hospital protocol to the LPN.
   c. Write up the LPN's actions so they will be included in her evaluation.
   d. Talk to the LPN about the importance of following protocol to prevent C.L. from sustaining a fall-related injury.

Answers available at *http://evolve.elsevier.com/Lewis/medsurg*.

11

Inflammation and Healing

Catherine R. Ratliff

A kind gesture can reach a wound only compassion can heal.

Steve Maraboli

http://evolve.elsevier.com/Lewis/medsurg/

CONCEPTUAL FOCUS

Health Promotion	Pain	Tissue Integrity
Inflammation	Perfusion	
Nutrition	Sensory Perception	

LEARNING OUTCOMES

1. Describe the inflammatory response, including vascular and cellular responses and exudate formation.
2. Explain local and systemic manifestations of inflammation and their physiologic bases.
3. Describe the drug therapy, nutrition therapy, and nursing management of inflammation.
4. Distinguish among healing by primary, secondary, and tertiary intention.
5. Describe the factors that delay wound healing and common complications of wound healing.
6. Describe the nursing and interprofessional management of wound healing.
7. Explain the etiology and clinical manifestations of pressure injuries.
8. Apply a patient risk assessment for pressure injuries to measures used to prevent the development of pressure injuries.
9. Discuss nursing and interprofessional management of a patient with pressure injuries.

KEY TERMS

adhesions, Table 11.7, p. 163
dehiscence, Table 11.7, p. 163
evisceration, Table 11.7, p. 163
fibroblasts, p. 162

hypertrophic scars, Table 11.7, p. 163
inflammatory response, p. 156
pressure injury, p. 168
regeneration, p. 161

repair, p. 161
shear, p. 168

This chapter focuses on inflammation, wound healing, and pressure injury prevention and management. Maintaining skin and tissue integrity is a key nursing role. Multiple concepts are closely related to tissue integrity. Adequate nutrition and perfusion are essential so that the body has the necessary factors to promote healing when injury occurs. Impaired mobility and sensory perception increase the risk for injury. When injury does occur, pain and problems regulating temperature and fluid and electrolyte balance are common.

INFLAMMATORY RESPONSE

The **inflammatory response** is a sequential reaction to cell injury. It neutralizes and dilutes the inflammatory agent,

removes necrotic materials, and establishes an environment suitable for healing and repair. The term *inflammation* is often incorrectly used as a synonym for *infection*. Inflammation is always present with infection, but infection is not always present with inflammation. However, a person who is neutropenic may not be able to mount an inflammatory response. An infection involves invasion of tissues or cells by microorganisms, such as bacteria, fungi, and viruses. In contrast, heat, radiation, trauma, chemicals, allergens, and an autoimmune reaction also can cause inflammation.

The mechanism of inflammation is basically the same regardless of the injuring agent. The intensity of the response depends on the extent and severity of injury and on the injured person's reactive capacity. The inflammatory response can be

PATHOPHYSIOLOGY MAP

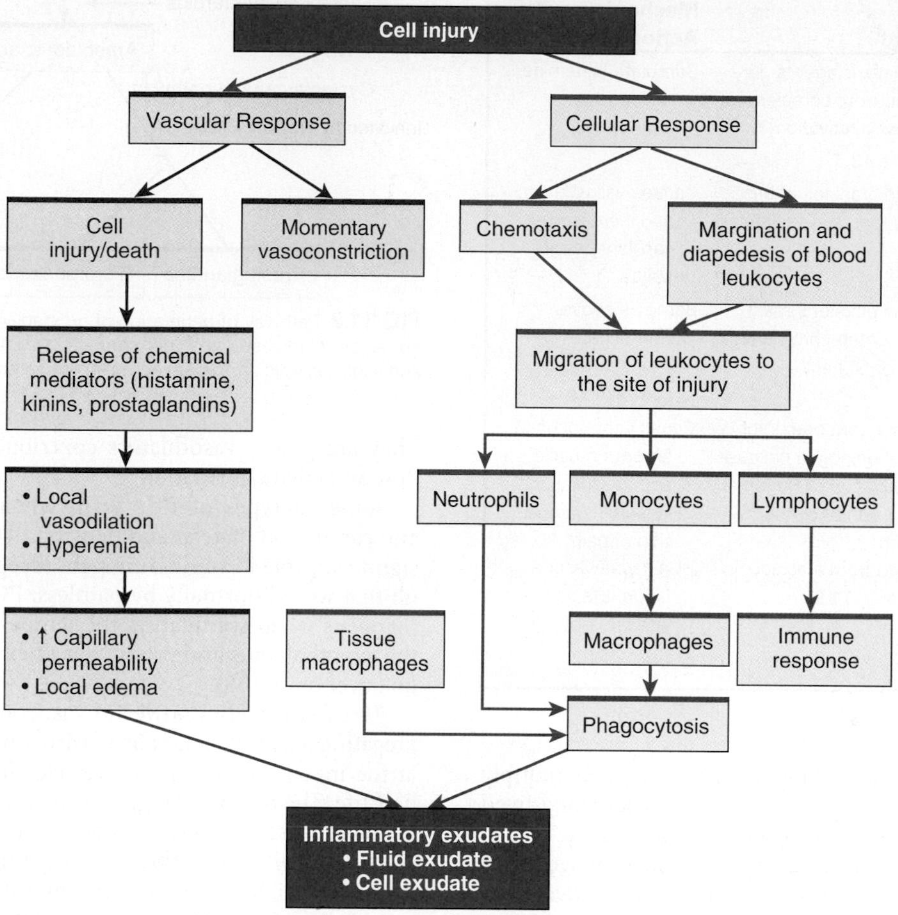

FIG 11.1 Vascular and cellular responses to tissue injury.

divided into a vascular response, cellular response, formation of exudate, and healing. Fig. 11.1 shows the vascular and cellular response to injury.

Vascular Response

After cell injury, local arterioles briefly undergo transient vasoconstriction. After release of histamine and other chemicals by the injured cells, the vessels dilate. Chemical mediators cause increased capillary permeability and facilitate fluid movement from capillaries into tissue spaces. At first this inflammatory exudate is made up of serous fluid. Later, it contains plasma proteins, primarily albumin. These proteins exert oncotic pressure that further draws fluid from blood vessels. Both vasodilation and increased capillary permeability are responsible for redness, heat, and swelling at the site of injury and the surrounding area.

As the plasma protein fibrinogen leaves the blood, it is activated to fibrin by the products of the injured cells. Fibrin strengthens a blood clot formed by platelets. In tissues, the clot functions to trap bacteria, prevent their spread, and serve as a framework for the healing process. Platelets release growth factors that start the healing process.

Cellular Response

Neutrophils and monocytes move from circulation to the site of injury (Fig. 11.1). *Chemotaxis* is the directional migration of white blood cells (WBCs) to the site of injury, resulting in an accumulation of neutrophils and monocytes at the site.

Neutrophils. Neutrophils are the first WBCs to arrive at the injury site (usually within 6 to 12 hours). They phagocytize (engulf) bacteria, other foreign material, and damaged cells. With their short life span (24 to 48 hours), dead neutrophils soon accumulate. In time, a mixture of dead neutrophils, digested bacteria, and other cell debris accumulates as a creamy substance called *pus*.

To keep up with the demand for neutrophils, the bone marrow releases more neutrophils into circulation. This results in a high WBC count, especially the neutrophil count. Mature neutrophils are called *segmented neutrophils*. Sometimes the demand for neutrophils increases to the extent that the bone marrow releases immature forms of neutrophils *(bands)* into circulation. We call an increased number of band neutrophils in circulation a *shift to the left*. It is common in patients with acute bacterial infections. (See Chapter 29 for a discussion of neutrophils.)

Monocytes. Monocytes are the second type of phagocytic cells that migrate from circulating blood. They usually arrive at the site within 3 to 7 days after the onset of inflammation. On entering the tissue spaces, monocytes transform into macrophages. Together with the tissue macrophages, these newly arrived macrophages help in phagocytosis of the inflammatory debris. The macrophage role is important in cleaning the area before healing

TABLE 11.1	Mediators of Inflammation	
Mediator	**Source**	**Mechanisms of Action**
Complement components (C3a, C4a, C5a)	Anaphylatoxic agents generated from complement pathway activation	Stimulate histamine release and chemotaxis
Cytokines	See Table 13.3	
Histamine	Stored in granules of basophils, mast cells, platelets	Causes vasodilation and increased capillary permeability
Serotonin	Stored in platelets, mast cells, enterochromaffin cells of GI tract	Same as above. Stimulates smooth muscle contraction
Kinins (e.g., bradykinin)	Produced from precursor factor kininogen because of activation of Hageman factor (XII) of clotting system	Cause contraction of smooth muscle and vasodilation. Result in stimulation of pain
Prostaglandins (PGs) **and leukotrienes** (LTs)	Produced from arachidonic acid (Fig. 11.2)	PGs cause vasodilation. LTs stimulate chemotaxis

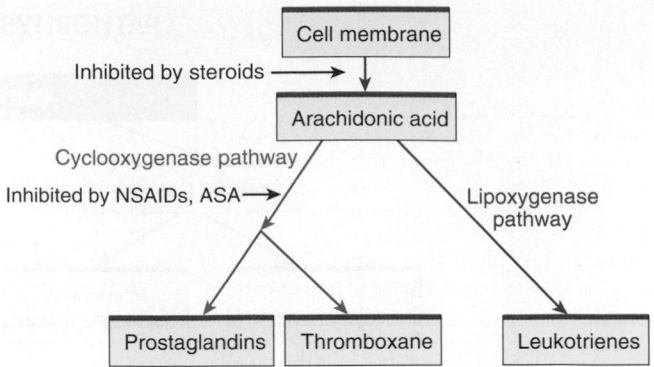

FIG 11.2 Pathway of generation of prostaglandins, thromboxane, and leukotrienes. Corticosteroids, nonsteroidal antiinflammatory drugs *(NSAIDs)*, and acetylsalicylic acid *(ASA)* act to inhibit various steps in this pathway.

can occur. Macrophages have a long life span. They can multiply and may stay in the damaged tissues for weeks. These long-lived cells are important in orchestrating the healing process.

When particles are too large for a single macrophage, macrophages accumulate and fuse to form a *multinucleated giant cell.* Collagen encapsulates this giant cell, leading to the formation of a granuloma. A classic example of this process occurs in tuberculosis of the lung. While the *Mycobacterium* bacillus is walled off, a chronic state of inflammation exists. The granuloma formed is a cavity of necrotic tissue.

Lymphocytes. Lymphocytes arrive later at the site of injury. Their primary role is related to humoral and cell-mediated immunity (see Chapter 13).

Chemical Mediators

Mediators of the inflammatory response are outlined in Table 11.1.

Complement System. The complement system is an enzyme cascade (C1 to C9) consisting of pathways to mediate inflammation and destroy invading pathogens. Major functions of the complement system are enhanced phagocytosis, increased vascular permeability, chemotaxis, and cellular lysis. All these activities are important mediators of the inflammatory response and healing.

Cell lysis occurs when the final components create holes in the cell membranes and cause targeted cell death by membrane rupture. In autoimmune disorders, complement activation and the resulting inflammatory response can damage healthy tissue. Examples of this include rheumatoid arthritis and systemic lupus erythematosus.

Prostaglandins and Leukotrienes. When cells are activated by injury, the arachidonic acid in the cell membrane is rapidly converted to produce prostaglandins (PGs), thromboxane, and leukotrienes (Fig. 11.2). PGs are considered proinflammatory.

They are potent vasodilators contributing to increased blood flow and edema formation.

Some subtypes of PGs form when platelets are activated and can inhibit platelet and neutrophil aggregation. PGs have a significant role in sensitizing pain receptors to arousal by stimuli that would normally be painless. PGs have a pivotal role as pyrogens when stimulating the temperature-regulating area of the hypothalamus and producing a febrile response (see section on Fever on p. 158).

Thromboxane is a powerful vasoconstrictor and platelet-aggregating agent. It causes brief vasoconstriction and skin pallor at the injury site and promotes clot formation. It has a short half-life. The pallor soon gives way to vasodilation and redness, which is caused by PGs and histamine.

Leukotrienes form the slow-reacting substance of anaphylaxis (SRS-A). SRS-A constricts smooth muscles of the bronchi, causing narrowing of the airway, and increases capillary permeability, leading to airway edema.

Exudate Formation

Exudate consists of fluid and WBCs that move from the circulation to the site of injury. The nature and quantity of exudate depend on the type and severity of the injury and tissues involved (Table 11.2).

Clinical Manifestations

The *local* manifestations of inflammation include redness, heat, pain, swelling, and loss of function (Table 11.3 and Fig. 11.3). *Systemic* manifestations include an increased WBC count with a shift to the left, malaise, nausea and anorexia, increased pulse and respiratory rate, and fever.

Leukocytosis results from the increased release of WBCs from the bone marrow. The causes of other systemic manifestations may be related to complement activation and the release of *cytokines* (soluble factors secreted by WBCs and other types of cells that act as intercellular and intracellular messengers). Some cytokines (e.g., interleukins [ILs], tumor necrosis factor [TNF]) are important in causing fever and other systemic manifestations of inflammation. An increase in pulse and respiration follows the rise in metabolism because of an increase in body temperature. (Cytokines are discussed in Chapter 13.)

Fever. The release of cytokines triggers the onset of fever. Cytokines cause fever by initiating metabolic changes in the temperature-regulating center in the hypothalamus (Fig. 11.4). The synthesis of PGs is the most critical metabolic change. PGs

TABLE 11.2 Types of Inflammatory Exudate

Type	Description	Examples
Catarrhal	Found in tissues where cells produce mucus Inflammatory response accelerates mucus production	Runny nose associated with upper respiratory tract infection
Fibrinous	Occurs with increasing vascular permeability and fibrinogen leakage into interstitial spaces Excessive amounts of fibrin that coats tissue surfaces may cause them to adhere	Adhesions, gelatinous ribbons seen in surgical drain tubing Frequently covers fluid-exuding wounds, such as venous injuries
Hemorrhagic	Results from rupture or necrosis of blood vessel walls	Hematoma, bleeding after surgery or tissue trauma
Purulent (pus)	Consists of WBCs, microorganisms (dead and alive), liquefied dead cells, and other debris	Furuncle (boil), abscess, cellulitis (diffuse inflammation in connective tissue)
Serosanguinous	Found during the midpoint in healing after surgery or tissue injury Composed of RBCs and serous fluid, which is semiclear pink and may have red streaks	Surgical drain fluid
Serous	Results from outpouring of fluid. Seen in early stages of inflammation or when injury is mild	Skin blisters, pleural effusion

TABLE 11.3 Local Manifestations of Inflammation

Manifestations	Cause
Heat	Increased metabolism at inflammatory site
Loss of function	Swelling and pain
Pain	Change in pH. Nerve stimulation by chemicals (e.g., histamine, prostaglandins). Pressure from fluid exudate
Redness	Hyperemia from vasodilation
Swelling	Fluid shift to interstitial spaces. Fluid exudate accumulation

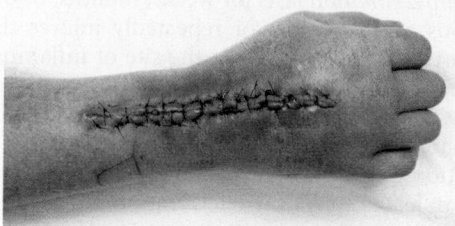

FIG 11.3 Inflammation secondary to postoperative deep wound infection after wrist surgery. (From Hayden RJ, Jebson PJL: Wrist arthrodesis, *Hand Clin* 21[4]:631, 2005.)

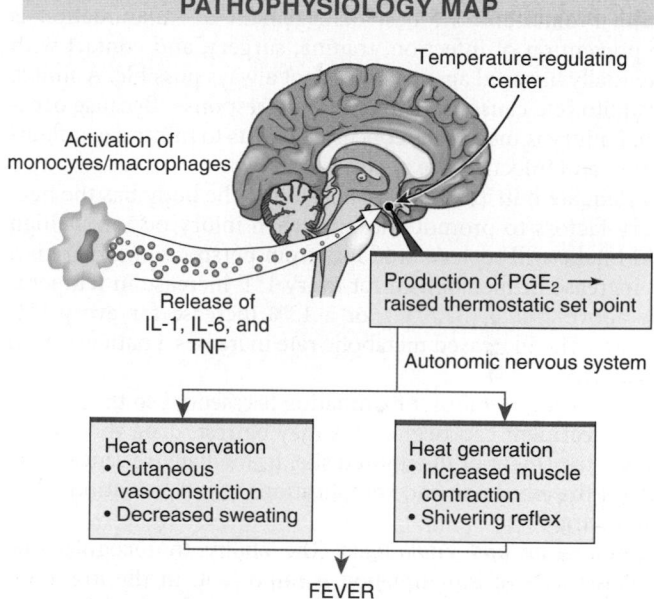

FIG 11.4 Production of fever. When monocytes/macrophages are activated, they secrete cytokines such as interleukin-1 *(IL-1)*, interleukin-6 *(IL-6)*, and tumor necrosis factor *(TNF)*, which reach the hypothalamic temperature-regulating center. These cytokines promote the synthesis and secretion of prostaglandin E_2 *(PGE_2)* in the anterior hypothalamus. PGE_2 increases the thermostatic set point, and the autonomic nervous system is stimulated, resulting in shivering, muscle contraction, and peripheral vasoconstriction.

act directly to increase the thermostatic set point. The hypothalamus then activates the autonomic nervous system to stimulate increased muscle tone and shivering and decreased perspiration and blood flow to the periphery. Epinephrine released from the adrenal medulla increases the metabolic rate. The net result is fever.

With the physiologic thermostat raised to a higher-than-normal temperature, the body increases heat production and conservation until the temperature reaches that new set point. At this point, the person feels chilled and shivers. The shivering response is the body's method of raising the body's temperature to the new set point.[1] This seeming paradox is dramatic: the body is hot, yet the person piles on blankets and may go to bed to get warm. When the body temperature reaches the set point, the chills and warmth-seeking behavior cease.

The released cytokines and the fever that they trigger activate the body's defense mechanisms. Beneficial aspects of fever include increased killing of microorganisms, increased phagocytosis by neutrophils, and increased proliferation of T cells. Higher body temperatures may enhance the activity of interferon, the body's natural virus-fighting substance (see Chapter 13).

Types of Inflammation

The basic types of inflammation are acute, subacute, and chronic. In *acute inflammation*, the healing occurs in 2 to 3 weeks and usually leaves no residual damage. Neutrophils are the predominant cell type at the site of inflammation. A *subacute inflammation* has the features of the acute process but lasts longer. For example, infective endocarditis is a smoldering infection with acute inflammation, but it lasts for weeks or months (see Chapter 36).

Chronic inflammation lasts for weeks, months, or even years. The injurious agent persists or repeatedly injures tissue. The predominant cell types present at the site of inflammation are lymphocytes and macrophages. Examples of chronic inflammation include rheumatoid arthritis and osteomyelitis. The prolongation and chronicity of any inflammation may be the result of an alteration in the immune response (e.g., autoimmune disease) and can lead to physical deterioration.

❖ NURSING AND INTERPROFESSIONAL MANAGEMENT: INFLAMMATION

◆ Nursing Implementation

◆ **Health Promotion.** The best management of inflammation is the prevention of infection, trauma, surgery, and contact with potentially harmful agents. This is not always possible. A simple mosquito bite causes an inflammatory response. Because occasional injury is inevitable, concerted efforts to minimize inflammation and infection are needed.

Adequate nutrition is essential so that the body has the necessary factors to promote healing when injury occurs. A high fluid intake will replace fluid loss from perspiration. There is a 7% increase in metabolism for every 1°F increase in temperature above 100°F (37.8°C), or a 13% increase for every 1°C increase. The increased metabolic rate increases a patient's need for calories.

Early recognition of inflammation is essential so that appropriate treatment can begin. This may be rest, drug therapy, or specific treatment of the injured site. Immediate treatment may prevent the extension and complications of inflammation.

◆ Acute Care

Observation and Vital Signs. The ability to recognize the manifestations of inflammation is important. In the immunosuppressed person (e.g., taking corticosteroids, receiving chemotherapy), the classic manifestations of inflammation may be masked. The early symptoms of inflammation may be malaise or "just not feeling well."

Vital signs are important to note with any inflammation, especially when an infectious process is present. With infection, the temperature may rise, and pulse and respiration rates may increase.

Fever. An important aspect of fever management is determining its cause. Although many regard fever as harmful, an increase in body temperature is an important host defense mechanism. In the seventeenth century, Thomas Sydenham noted that "fever is a mighty engine which nature brings into the world for the conquest of her enemies."[2]

Steps are often taken to lower body temperature to relieve anxiety of the patient and health care professionals. Because mild to moderate fever usually does little harm, imposes no great discomfort, and may help host defense mechanisms, antipyretic drugs are rarely essential to patient welfare. Moderate fevers (up to 103°F [39.4°C]) usually produce few problems in most patients. However, if the patient is very young or very old, is extremely uncomfortable, or has a significant medical problem (e.g., severe heart or lung disease, brain injury), antipyretic use should be considered. Fever in the immunosuppressed patient should be treated immediately with antibiotic therapy because infections can rapidly progress to septicemia. (Neutropenia is discussed in Chapter 30 on pp. 631.)

Fever, especially if greater than 104°F (40°C), can damage body cells, and delirium and seizures can occur. At temperatures

TABLE 11.4 Drug Therapy
Inflammation and Healing

Drug	Mechanism of Action
Antipyretic Drugs	
Acetaminophen (Tylenol)	Inhibits synthesis of prostaglandins (PGs). Lowers temperature by action on heat-regulating center in hypothalamus
NSAIDs (e.g., ibuprofen [Advil])	Inhibit synthesis of PGs
Salicylates (aspirin)	Inhibit synthesis of PGs (Fig. 11.2). Lower temperature by action on heat-regulating center in hypothalamus, resulting in peripheral vasodilation and heat loss
Antiinflammatory Drugs	
Corticosteroids (e.g., prednisone)	Interfere with tissue granulation, induce immunosuppressive effects (decreased lymphocyte synthesis), prevent liberation of lysosomes
NSAIDs (e.g., ibuprofen, piroxicam [Feldene])	Inhibit synthesis of PGs
Salicylates (aspirin)	Inhibit synthesis of PGs, reduce capillary permeability
Vitamins	
Vitamin A	Accelerates epithelialization
Vitamin B complex	Acts as coenzymes
Vitamin C	Aids in synthesis of collagen and new capillaries
Vitamin D	Facilitates calcium absorption

greater than 105.8°F (41°C), the hypothalamic temperature control center becomes impaired. Damage can occur to many cells, including those in the brain.

Older adults have a blunted febrile response to infection. The body temperature may not rise to the level expected for a younger adult, or there may be a delay in the onset of the rise. The blunted response can delay diagnosis and treatment. By the time fever (as defined for younger adults) is present, the illness may be more severe. Patients who are taking nonsteroidal antiinflammatory drugs (NSAIDs) on a regular basis (e.g., for rheumatoid arthritis) may have a blunted febrile response.

Although sponge baths increase evaporative heat loss, they may not decrease the body temperature unless the person received antipyretic drugs to lower the set point. Otherwise, the body will initiate compensatory mechanisms (e.g., shivering) to restore body heat. The same principle applies to the use of cooling blankets. They are most effective in lowering body temperature after the set point has been lowered.

A nursing care plan for the patient with a fever (eNursing Care Plan 11.1) is available on the website for this chapter at *http://evolve.elsevier.com/Lewis/medsurg.*

Drug Therapy. Drugs can decrease the inflammatory response and lower the body temperature (Table 11.4). Aspirin blocks PG synthesis in the hypothalamus and elsewhere in the body. Acetaminophen acts on the heat-regulating center in the hypothalamus. Some NSAIDs (e.g., ibuprofen [Motrin, Advil]) have antipyretic effects. Corticosteroids are antipyretic through the dual actions of preventing cytokine production and PG synthesis. This results in dilation of superficial blood vessels, increased skin temperature, and sweating.

CHECK YOUR PRACTICE

A 76-yr-old female patient has acute osteomyelitis after a fractured femur. You are checking her temperature every 2 hours and giving acetaminophen when it is higher than 102°F. However, you notice that her temperature is fluctuating from 96° to 103°F.
• What should you do?

Antipyretics cause a sharp decrease in temperature. They should be given around the clock to prevent acute swings in temperature. Giving them intermittently can induce or perpetuate chills. When the antipyretic wears off, the body may initiate a compensatory involuntary muscular contraction (i.e., chill) to raise the body temperature back up to its previous level. We can prevent this unpleasant side effect by giving them regularly at 2- to 4-hour intervals.

Antihistamine drugs may be used to inhibit the action of histamine. Antihistamines are discussed in Chapters 13 and 26.

RICE. Rest, ice, compression, and elevation (RICE) is a key concept in treating soft tissue injuries and related inflammation.

Rest. Rest helps the body use its nutrients and O_2 for the healing process. The repair process is facilitated by allowing fibrin and collagen to form across the wound edges with little disruption.

Cold and heat. Cold application is usually appropriate at the time of the initial trauma. Use promotes vasoconstriction and decreases swelling, pain, and congestion from increased metabolism in the area of inflammation. Heat may be used later (e.g., after 24 to 48 hours) to promote healing by increasing the circulation to the inflamed site and subsequent removal of debris. Heat is used to localize the inflammatory agents. Warm, moist heat may help debride the wound site if necrotic material is present.

Compression and immobilization. Compression counters the vasodilation effects and development of edema. Compression by direct pressure over a laceration occludes blood vessels and stops bleeding. Compression bandages support injured joints when tendons and muscles are unable to provide support on their own. Assess distal pulses and capillary refill before and after application of compression to evaluate whether compression has compromised circulation (e.g., pale color of skin, loss of feeling).

Immobilization of the inflamed or injured area promotes healing by decreasing the tissues' metabolic needs. Immobilization with a cast or splint supports fractured bones and prevents further tissue injury from sharp bone fragments that could sever nerves or blood vessels, causing hemorrhage. As with compression, evaluate the patient's circulation after application and at regular intervals. Swelling can occur within the closed space of a cast and compromise circulation.

Elevation. Elevating the injured extremity above the level of the heart reduces the edema at the inflammatory site by increasing venous and lymphatic return. Elevation helps reduce pain associated with blood engorgement at the injury site. Elevation may be contraindicated in patients with significantly reduced arterial circulation.

TABLE 11.5 Regenerative Ability of Different Types of Tissues

Tissues	Cell Type	Description
Skin, lymphoid organs, bone marrow, and mucous membranes	Labile cells	Cells divide constantly. Injury to these organs is followed by rapid regeneration.
Liver, pancreas, kidney, and bone cells	Stable cells	Retain their ability to regenerate but do so only if the organ is injured. Regeneration is slow.
Neurons of the central nervous system (CNS) and skeletal and cardiac muscle cells	Permanent cells	Do not divide. Damage to CNS neurons or skeletal or heart muscle can lead to permanent loss. Healing of skeletal and cardiac muscle will occur by repair with scar tissue. If neurons in the CNS are destroyed, the tissue is generally replaced by glial cells. Neurogenesis may occur from stem cells (see Chapter 55).

HEALING PROCESS

The last phase of the inflammatory response is healing. Healing includes 2 major components: regeneration and repair.

Regeneration

Regeneration is the replacement of lost cells and tissues with cells of the same type. The ability of cells to regenerate depends on the cell type (Table 11.5).

Repair

Repair is healing, with connective tissue replacing lost cells. Repair is the more common type of healing and usually results in scar formation. Repair is a more complex process than regeneration. Most injuries heal by connective tissue repair. Repair healing occurs by primary, secondary, or tertiary intention (Fig. 11.5).

Primary Intention. Primary intention healing takes place when wound margins are neatly approximated, as in a surgical incision or a paper cut. A continuum of processes is associated with primary healing (Table 11.6). These processes include 3 phases.

Initial Phase. In the *initial* (inflammatory) phase, the edges of the incision are aligned and sutured (or stapled) in place. The incision area fills with blood from the cut blood vessels, blood clots form, and platelets release growth factors to begin the healing process. This forms a matrix for WBC migration. An acute inflammatory reaction occurs.

The area of injury is composed of fibrin clots, erythrocytes, neutrophils (dead and dying), and other debris. Macrophages ingest and digest cellular debris, fibrin fragments, and red blood cells (RBCs). Extracellular enzymes derived from macrophages and neutrophils help digest fibrin. As the wound debris is removed, the fibrin clot serves as a meshwork for future capillary growth and migration of epithelial cells.

Granulation Phase. The *granulation* phase is the second step. The components of granulation tissue include proliferating

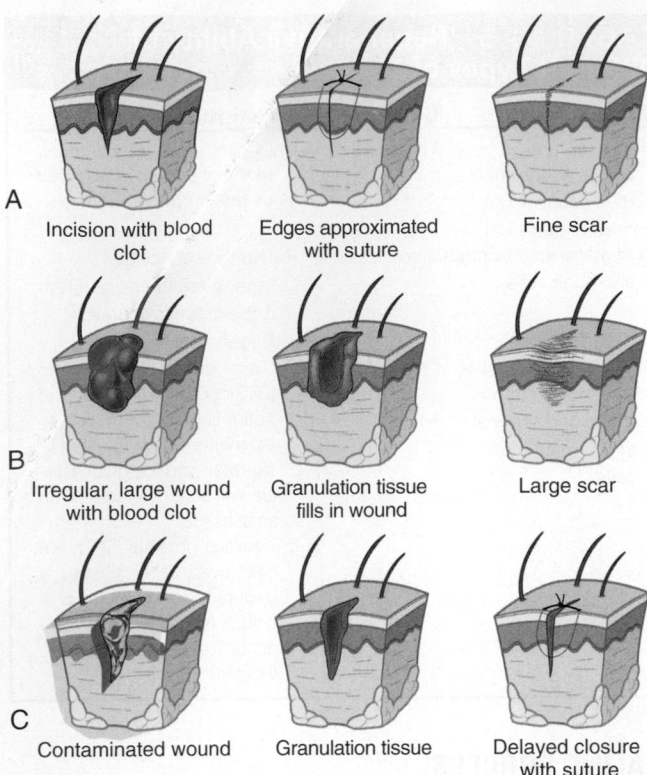

FIG 11.5 Types of wound healing. **A,** Primary intention. **B,** Secondary intention. **C,** Tertiary intention.

TABLE 11.6	**Phases in Primary Intention Healing**	
Phase	**Duration**	**Description**
Initial	3 to 5 days	Approximation of incision edges. Migration of epithelial cells. Clot serving as meshwork for starting capillary growth
Granulation	5 days to 4 weeks	Migration of fibroblasts. Secretion of collagen. Abundance of capillary buds. Wound fragile
Maturation and scar contraction	7 days to several months	Remodeling of collagen. Strengthening of scar

fibroblasts; proliferating capillary sprouts *(angioblasts);* various WBCs; exudate; and loose, semifluid, ground substance.

Fibroblasts are immature connective tissue cells that migrate into the healing site and secrete collagen. In time, the collagen is organized and restructured to strengthen the healing site. At this stage, it is called *fibrous* or *scar tissue.*

During the granulation phase, the wound is pink and vascular. Numerous red granules (young budding capillaries) are present. At this point, the wound is friable, at risk for dehiscence (Fig. 11.6), and resistant to infection.

Surface epithelium at the wound edges begins to regenerate. In a few days, a thin layer of epithelium migrates across the wound surface in a 1-cell-thick layer until it contacts cells spreading from

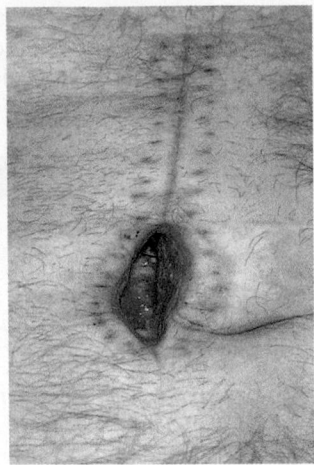

FIG 11.6 Dehiscence after a cholecystectomy. (From Bale S, Jones V: *Wound care nursing: A patient-centered approach,* ed 2, St Louis, 2006, Mosby.)

the opposite direction. The epithelium thickens and begins to mature, and the wound now closely resembles the adjacent skin. In a superficial wound, re-epithelialization may take 3 to 5 days.

Maturation Phase and Scar Contraction. The *maturation* phase, during which scar contraction occurs, overlaps with the granulation phase. It may begin 7 days after the injury and continue for several months or years. This is the reason abdominal surgery discharge instructions limit lifting for up to 6 weeks.

Collagen fibers are further organized, and the remodeling process occurs. Fibroblasts disappear as the wound becomes stronger. The active movement of the myofibroblasts causes contraction of the healing area, helping to close the defect and bring the skin edges closer together. A mature scar is then formed. In contrast to granulation tissue, a mature scar is virtually avascular and pale. The scar may be more painful at this phase than in the granulation phase.

Secondary Intention. Wounds that occur from trauma, injury, and infection have large amounts of exudate and wide, irregular wound margins with extensive tissue loss. These wounds may have edges that cannot be *approximated* (brought together). The inflammatory reaction may be greater than in primary healing. This results in more debris, cells, and exudate. We may have to clear the debris away *(debride)* before healing can take place.

The process of healing by secondary intention is essentially the same as healing by primary intention. The major differences are the greater defect and the gaping wound edges. Healing and granulation take place from the edges inward and from the bottom of the wound upward until the wound is filled. There is more granulation tissue, and the result is a much larger scar.

Tertiary Intention. *Tertiary intention* (delayed primary intention) healing occurs with delayed suturing of a wound in which 2 layers of granulation tissue are sutured together. This occurs when a contaminated wound is left open and sutured closed after the infection is controlled. It also occurs when a primary wound becomes infected, is opened, allowed to granulate, and then sutured. Tertiary intention usually results in a larger and deeper scar than primary or secondary intention.

Wound Classification

A *wound* is a break or opening into the skin. Wounds often occur because of accidents or injuries. Types of wounds can range from minor scrapes to deep wounds involving bones, blood vessels, and nerves.

Identifying the cause of a wound is essential to classifying the wound properly. Wounds can be classified by their cause (surgical or nonsurgical; acute or chronic) or the depth of tissue affected (superficial, partial thickness, or full thickness). A *superficial wound* involves only the epidermis. *Partial-thickness* wounds extend into the dermis. *Full-thickness* wounds have the deepest layer of tissue destruction. They involve the subcutaneous tissue and sometimes extend into the fascia and underlying structures, including muscle, tendon, or bone.

A *skin tear* is a wound caused by shear, friction, and/or blunt force resulting in separation of skin layers. A skin tear can be partial thickness or full thickness. This type of wound is common, especially in older adults and critically or chronically ill adults.[3]

Complications of Healing

Certain factors can interfere with wound healing and lead to complications (Table 11.7).

TABLE 11.7 Complications of Wound Healing

Adhesions
- Bands of scar tissue that form between or around organs
- May occur in the abdominal cavity or between the lungs and the pleura
- Those in the abdomen may cause an intestinal obstruction.

Contractions
- Wound contraction is a normal part of healing.
- Complications occur when excessive contraction results in deformity.
- Shortening of muscle or scar tissue, especially over joints, results from excessive fibrous tissue formation.

Dehiscence
- Separation and disruption of previously joined wound edges (Fig. 11.6)
- Usually occurs when a primary healing site bursts open
- May be caused by:
  - Infection causing an inflammatory process
  - Granulation tissue not strong enough to withstand forces imposed on wound
  - Obesity, because adipose tissue has less blood supply and may slow healing
  - Pocket of fluid (seroma, hematoma) developing between tissue layers and preventing the edges of the wound from coming together

Evisceration
- Occurs when wound edges separate to the extent that intestines protrude through wound
- Usually needs immediate surgical treatment

Excess Granulation Tissue ("Proud Flesh")
- Excess granulation tissue may protrude above surface of healing wound.

- If the tissue is cauterized or cut off, healing continues in normal manner.

Fistula Formation
- An abnormal passage between organs or a hollow organ and skin (abdominal or perianal fistula)

Infection (Fig. 11.3)
- ↑ Risk for infection when wound contains necrotic tissue or blood supply is ↓, patient's immune function is ↓ (e.g., from immunosuppressive drugs), undernutrition, multiple stressors, and hyperglycemia in diabetes.

Hemorrhage
- Abnormal internal or external blood loss may be caused by suture failure, clotting abnormalities, dislodged clot, infection, or erosion of a blood vessel by a foreign object (tubing, drains) or infection process.

Hypertrophic Scars
- Inappropriately large, raised red and hard scars (Fig. 11.7)

- Occur when an overabundance of collagen is made during healing

Keloid Formation
- Great protrusion of scar tissue that extends beyond wound edges and may form tumor-like masses of scar tissue (Fig. 11.8)

- Permanent without any tendency to subside
- Patients often have tenderness, pain, and hyperparesthesia, especially in early stages.
- Thought to be a hereditary condition occurring most often in dark-skinned people.

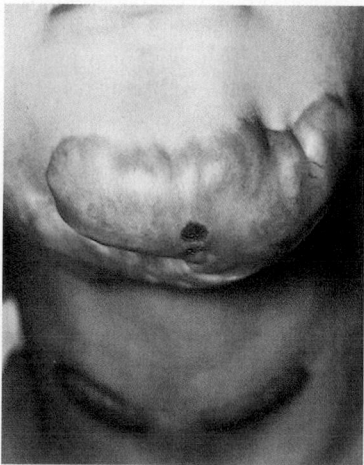

FIG 11.7 Hypertrophic scarring. (Reproduced with kind permission from Dr. C. Lawrence, Wound Healing Research Unit, Cardiff. In Bale S, Jones V, eds: *Wound care nursing: A patient-centered approach,* ed 2, St Louis, 2006, Mosby.)

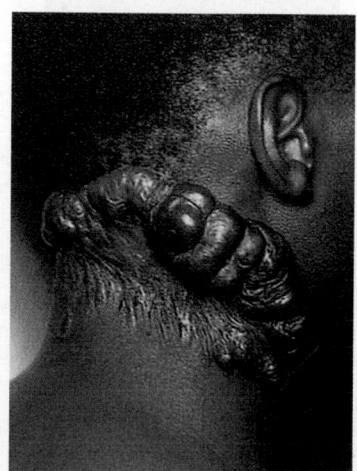

FIG 11.8 Keloid scarring. (Reproduced with kind permission from Dr. C. Lawrence, Wound Healing Research Unit, Cardiff. In Bale S, Jones V, editors: *Wound care nursing: A patient-centered approach,* ed 2, St Louis, 2006, Mosby.)

❖ NURSING AND INTERPROFESSIONAL MANAGEMENT: WOUND HEALING

◆ Nursing Assessment

The first step in wound care is to carefully assess and document the characteristics of the wound and surrounding area. This includes the location, size (longest length and widest width), depth, undermining and tunneling, wound margin (e.g., normal, macerated, erythema), and wound base (e.g., eschar, slough, exudate). There are several ways to measure a wound. One way is shown in Fig. 11.9. Record the consistency, color, and odor of any drainage and report if abnormal for the situation. *Staphylococcus* and *Pseudomonas* are common organisms that cause purulent, draining wounds.

Thoroughly assess the wound on admission, or first clinic visit, and on a regular basis thereafter. In healthy people, wounds heal at a normal, predictable rate. Assess for factors that may delay wound healing and contribute to chronic nonhealing wounds (Table 11.8). If deterioration in the wound occurs, you need to assess and document changes more often.[4]

Chronic wounds are those that do not heal within the normal time (around 3 months). If a wound does not heal as expected, assess and identify factors that may delay healing. Refer the patient to an HCP specializing in wound management. Time does not heal all wounds. While caring for patients during the healing process, you need to continually assess for complications (e.g., infection) associated with healing (Table 11.7).

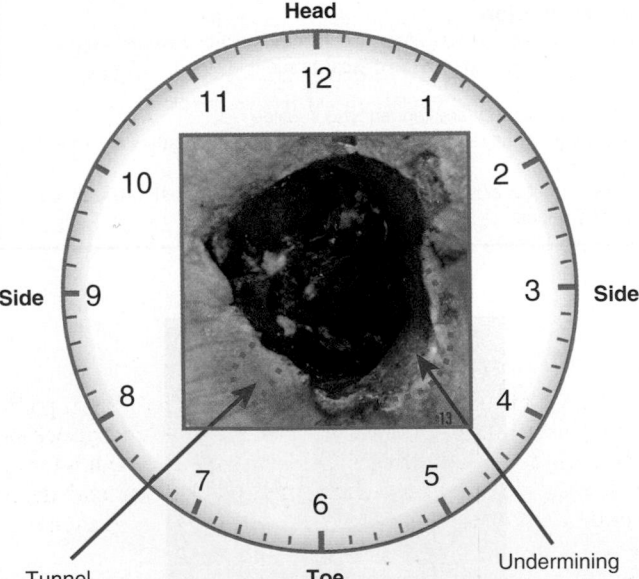

FIG 11.9 Wound measurements are made in centimeters. The first measurement is oriented from head to toe, the second is from side to side, and the third is the depth (if any). If there is any tunneling (when cotton-tipped applicator is placed in wound, there is movement) or undermining (when cotton-tipped applicator is placed in wound, there is a "lip" around the wound), this is charted in respect to a clock, with 12 o'clock being toward the patient's head. This wound would be charted as a full-thickness, red wound, 7 × 5 × 3 cm, with a 3-cm tunnel at 7 o'clock and 2 cm undermining from 3 o'clock to 5 o'clock. (Courtesy Robert B. Babiak, RN, BSN, CWOCN, San Antonio, TX.)

◆ Nursing Implementation

The type of wound management and dressings needed depend on the type, extent, and characteristics of the wound and the phase of healing. The purposes of wound management include (1) protecting a clean wound from trauma so that it can heal normally, (2) cleaning a wound to remove any dirt and debris from the wound bed, and (3) treating infection to prepare the wound for healing.

Clean Wounds. Superficial skin injuries may only need cleansing. Material used to close wounds include adhesive strips (e.g., Steri-Strips, butterflies), sutures (stitches), staples, and tissue adhesives (fibrin sealants). We use adhesive strips instead of *sutures* for some injuries because they decrease scarring and it is easier to care for them. Sutures are used to close wounds because suture material provides the mechanical support needed to sustain closure. A wide variety of suturing materials are available. Tissue adhesives are a biologic adhesive that can be applied alone or with sutures or tape.

A dressing material that keeps the wound surface clean and slightly moist is best to promote epithelialization. For wounds that heal by primary intention, it is common to cover the wound or incision with a dry, sterile dressing. It is removed as soon as

TABLE 11.8	Factors Delaying Wound Healing
Factor	**Effect on Wound Healing**
Advanced age	Slows collagen synthesis by fibroblasts, impairs circulation, needs longer time for epithelialization of skin, alters phagocytic and immune responses
Anemia	Supplies less O_2 at tissue level
Corticosteroid drugs	Impair phagocytosis by WBCs, inhibit fibroblast proliferation and function, depress formation of granulation tissue, inhibit wound contraction
Diabetes	Decreases collagen synthesis, delays capillary growth, impairs phagocytosis (result of hyperglycemia), reduces supply of O_2 and nutrients secondary to vascular disease
Inadequate blood supply	Decreases supply of nutrients to injured area, decreases removal of exudative debris, inhibits inflammatory response
Infection	Increases inflammatory response and tissue destruction
Mechanical friction on wound	Destroys granulation tissue, prevents apposition of wound edges
Nutritional deficiencies	
Vitamin C	Delays formation of collagen fibers and capillary development
Protein	Decreases supply of amino acids for tissue repair
Zinc	Impairs epithelialization
Obesity	Decreases blood supply in fatty tissue
Poor general health	Causes generalized absence of factors necessary to promote wound healing
Smoking	Nicotine, a potent vasoconstrictor, impedes blood flow to healing areas

TABLE 11.9 Types of Wound Dressings

Type of Dressing	Description	Uses	Examples
Alginates	Derived from processed seaweed or kelp. Form a nonstick gel on contact with draining wound. Highly absorbent. Easy to use over irregular-shaped wounds. Require a secondary dressing	Wounds with moderate to heavy exudates (e.g., pressure injuries, infected wounds)	Algisite, CalciCare, Kalginate, Melgisorb
Antimicrobials	Alter the wound bed bioburden. Often contain silver, iodine, chlorhexidine, honey, or polyhexamethylene biguanide (PHMB). Available as sponges, impregnated woven gauzes, film dressings, absorptive products, nylon fabric, nonadherent barriers, or a combination of materials		Aquacel, Acticoat, Curity AMD, Iodoflex, Medihoney, SilverSorb, Silvercel
Foams	Film-coated gel or polyurethane. Absorption of minimal to heavy exudate, nonadherent. May need to be affixed with a secondary dressing	Primary dressing for absorption, secondary dressing for wounds with packing. Used for prevention of sacral pressure injuries	Allevyn, Cutimed, Hydro-cell, Lyofoam, Mepilex, PolyMem
Gauze	Made of woven or nonwoven material. Absorb exudates. Most often combined with another kind of dressing	Can be used on almost any kind of wound. Cleansing, packing, and covering a variety of wounds	Numerous products available (e.g., Curity, Kerlix)
Hydrocolloids	Gelatin, pectin, or carboxymethylcellulose bonded to a film or sheet. Produce a flat occlusive dressing that forms a gel on wound surface. Occlusion does not interfere with wound healing. Support autolytic debridement and prevent secondary infections	Wounds with light to moderate drainage	Bursamed, Comfeel, Duo-Derm, Primacol
Hydrogels	Available in gels, gel-covered gauze, or sheets. Give moisture to a dry wound and maintain a moist environment. Can rehydrate wound tissue. Debridement (autolytic) because of moisturizing effects. Require a secondary dressing	Dry wounds. Wounds with minimal drainage. Necrotic wounds. May have a cooling effect to help decrease pain	Aquasite, Curasol, IntraSite, Purilon, Solosite
Nonadherent	Woven or nonwoven dressings. May be impregnated with saline, petrolatum, or antimicrobials. Minimally absorbent	Minor wounds or as a second dressing	Adaptic, Vaseline gauze, Xeroform
Transparent films	Generally composed of polyurethane. Transparency allows visualization of the wound. Minimally absorbent. Use with caution over superficial wounds. Can result in further tissue loss in fragile wounds (e.g., skin tears). In other wounds, can draw in moisture, increasing risk for infection	Dry, uninfected wounds or wounds with minimal drainage	Bioclusive, OpSite, Suresite, Tegaderm, Transeal

For more information, see *www.woundsource.com/product-category/dressings.*

the drainage stops or in 2 to 3 days. Medicated sprays that form a transparent film on the skin may be used for dressings on a clean incision or injury. Transparent film or adhesive semipermeable dressings (e.g., OpSite, Tegaderm) are occlusive dressings that are permeable to oxygen. The wound is then usually covered with a sterile dressing. Sometimes an HCP will leave a surgical wound uncovered or remove the dressing within 48 hours after surgery.[5] Examples of types of wound dressings are described in Table 11.9.

Clean wounds that are granulating and re-epithelializing should be kept slightly moist and protected from further trauma until they heal naturally.[6] Do not let a wound that has the potential to heal dry out. Dryness is an enemy of wound healing. "Airing out" a wound is a great mistake. Wounds need a moist environment to heal. Unnecessary manipulation during dressing changes may destroy new granulation tissue and break down fibrin formation.

Topical antimicrobials and antibactericidals (e.g., povidone-iodine [Betadine], Dakin's solution [sodium hypochlorite]), should be used with caution in wound care because they can damage the new epithelium of healing tissue and delay healing. They should never be used in a clean granulating wound.

Sometimes drains are inserted into the wound to help remove fluid. The Jackson-Pratt drain is a suction drainage device consisting of a flexible plastic bulb connected to an internal plastic drainage tube (Fig. 11.10).

Contaminated Wounds. If the wound is contaminated, it must be converted into a clean wound before healing can occur normally. Debridement of a wound that has debris or dead tissue may be needed. Another option is absorptive dressings. They can be used to absorb exudate and clean the wound surface. These dressings work by drawing excess drainage from the wound surface. The amount of wound secretions determines the number of dressing changes.

In hydrocolloid dressings, such as DuoDerm, the inner part of the dressing interacts with the exudate, forming a hydrated gel over the wound. When the dressing is removed, the gel separates and stays over the wound. The wound must be cleansed gently to prevent damage to newly formed tissue. We can leave these dressings in place for up to 7 days or until leakage occurs around the dressing.

Debridement is done to remove dead tissue.[7] The debridement method used depends on the amount of debris and the condition of the wound tissue (Table 11.10).

◆ **Negative-Pressure Wound Therapy.** Negative-pressure wound therapy (NPWT) is used to treat acute and chronic wounds. A vacuum source creates continuous or intermittent negative pressure inside the wound to remove fluid, exudates, and infectious materials to prepare the wound for healing and closure. We do not know exactly how NPWT promotes healing. It is thought that NPWT pulls excess fluid from the wound, reduces bacterial load, and encourages blood flow into the wound base.

NPWT systems consist of a vacuum pump, drainage tubing, a foam or gauze wound dressing, and an adhesive film dressing

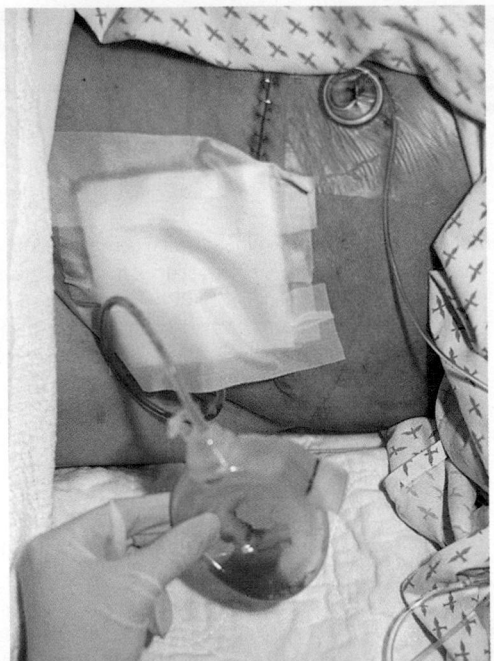

FIG 11.10 Jackson-Pratt drainage device. (From Perry AG, Potter PA, Elkin MK: *Nursing interventions and clinical skills,* ed 5, St Louis, 2012, Mosby.)

NURSING MANAGEMENT
Wound Care

In general, the registered nurse (RN) manages wound care for complex or nonhealing wounds. Wound, ostomy, and continence (WOC) nurses may treat and manage pressure injuries, traumatic and draining wounds, surgical incisions, and tubes and fistulas. State nurse practice acts vary in the wound care actions allowed by licensed practical/vocational nurses (LPNs/VNs). In general, the role of the RN includes:

- Assess all patients at risk for pressure injury at time of first hospital and/or home visit or whenever the patient's condition changes. Thereafter, assess at regular intervals based on care setting (every 24 hours for acute care or every visit in home care).
- Assess patients for factors that may delay wound healing and develop a plan of care to address these factors.
- Assess and document initial wound appearance, including wound size, depth, color, and drainage.
- Develop a plan of care to prevent the development of pressure injuries.
- Plan nursing actions to aid with wound healing, including wound care, positioning, and nutritional interventions.
- Choose dressings and therapies for wound treatment (in conjunction with the HCP and/or wound care specialist).
- Implement wound care for complex or new wounds, including negative-pressure wound therapy and hyperbaric O₂ therapy.
- Evaluate whether wound care is effective in promoting wound healing.
- Provide teaching to patient and caregivers about home wound care and pressure injury prevention.
- Oversee LPN/VN:
  - Perform sterile dressing changes on acute and chronic wounds.
  - Apply ordered topical antimicrobials and antibactericidals to wounds.
  - Apply prescribed dressings or medications for wound debridement.
  - Collect and record data about wound appearance.
- Collaborate with dietitian to:
  - Assess and monitor patient's nutritional status.
  - Outline diet to support proper wound healing.

TABLE 11.10 Types of Debridement

Type	Description
Autolytic debridement	• Moisture-retentive semiocclusive or occlusive dressings (e.g., hydrocolloids, transparent films, hydrogels) (Table 11.9) that soften dry eschar by autolysis • Must assess area around wound for maceration
Biologic debridement (larval therapy)	• Application of sterile fly larvae to dead tissue
Conservative sharp	• Use of scalpels, curettes, scissors to remove nonviable tissue • Ensure adequate vascular blood supply
Enzymatic debridement	• Drug applied topically to dissolve necrotic tissue and then covered with moist dressing (e.g., saline-moistened gauze) • Process can be slow, and thick eschar may have to be scored with scalpel

Mechanical debridement	• Methods:
	  • *Wet-to-dry dressings,* in which open-mesh gauze is moistened with normal saline, lightly packed into wound surface, and outer layer allowed to dry. Wound debris adheres to dressing and then dressing is removed
	  • *Wound irrigation.* Make certain bacteria are not accidentally driven into wound with high irrigation pressure
	• Noncontact low-frequency ultrasound and ultrasonic mist

Surgical/sharp debridement	• Quick method of debridement to prevent, control, or remove infection • Used when large amounts of nonviable tissue are present • Prepares wound bed for healing, skin grafting, or flaps

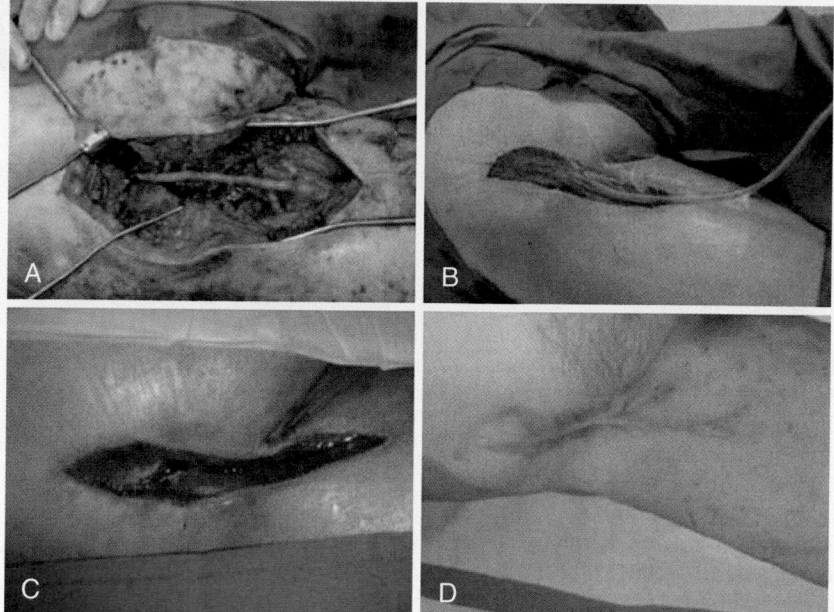

FIG 11.11 Negative-pressure wound therapy in woman with history of IV drug abuse. **A,** The completely destroyed femoral artery was reconstructed with a homograft. **B,** A black open-pore polyurethane foam was directly applied to the vascular reconstruction and negative pressure applied to wound. **C,** Wound site 16 days after surgery. **D,** Healed wound at 28 months without reinfection. (Reprinted from Mayer D, Hasse B, Koelliker J, et al: Long-term results of vascular graft and artery preserving treatment with negative pressure wound therapy in Szilagyi grade III infections justify a paradigm shift, *Ann Surg* 254:754, 2011. © Southeastern Surgical Congress.)

that covers and seals the wound.[8] In NPWT, the wound is cleansed and a gauze or foam dressing is cut to the dimensions of the wound. A large occlusive dressing is applied, with a small hole made over the gauze or foam dressing where the tubing is attached (Fig. 11.11). The tubing is connected to a pump, which creates a negative pressure in the wound bed.

Monitor the patient's serum protein levels and fluid and electrolyte balance because of losses from the wound. Also, monitor the patient's coagulation studies (platelet count, prothrombin time [PT], partial thromboplastin time [PTT]).

◆ **Hyperbaric Oxygen Therapy.** Hyperbaric O_2 therapy (HBOT) is the delivery of O_2 at increased atmospheric pressures. It can be given topically by creating a chamber around the injured limb. It also can be given systemically with the patient in an enclosed chamber, receiving 100% O_2 at 1.5 to 3 times the normal atmospheric pressure.

HBOT allows O_2 to diffuse into the serum, rather than RBCs, and be transported to the tissues. By increasing the O_2 content in the serum, HBOT moves the O_2 past narrowed arteries and capillaries where RBCs cannot go.

In addition, high O_2 levels stimulate *angiogenesis* (production of new blood vessels), kill anaerobic bacteria, and increase the killing power of WBCs and certain antibiotics (e.g., fluoroquinolones, aminoglycosides). HBOT accelerates granulation tissue formation and wound healing.

Most systemic treatments last from 90 to 120 minutes. The number of treatments is highly variable (from 10 to 60), depending on the condition being treated.

◆ **Drug Therapy.** Platelet-derived growth factor is released from the platelets and stimulates cell proliferation and migration. Becaplermin (Regranex), a recombinant human platelet–derived growth factor gel, actively stimulates wound healing. It is used to treat foot injuries in patients with diabetes (see Chapter 48). Becaplermin should be used only when the wound

is free of dead tissue and infection. It should not be used if cancer is suspected in the wound.

◆ **Nutritional Therapy.** Special nutritional measures promote wound healing. A high fluid intake is needed to replace fluid loss from perspiration and exudate formation. An increased metabolic rate intensifies water loss. Persons at risk for wound healing problems are those with malabsorption problems (e.g., Crohn's disease, GI surgery, liver disease), deficient intake or high energy demands (e.g., cancer, major trauma or surgery, sepsis, fever), and diabetes.

Undernutrition puts a person at risk for poor healing. A diet high in protein, carbohydrate, and vitamins with moderate fat intake is necessary to promote healing. Protein is needed to correct the negative nitrogen balance resulting from the increased metabolic rate. It is also needed for the synthesis of immune factors, WBCs, fibroblasts, and collagen, which are the building blocks for healing. Carbohydrates are needed to meet the increased metabolic energy required for healing. If there is a carbohydrate deficit, the body will break down protein for the needed energy. Fats help in the synthesis of fatty acids and triglycerides, which are part of the cellular membrane.[9]

Vitamin C is needed for capillary synthesis and collagen production by fibroblasts. The B-complex vitamins are necessary as coenzymes for many metabolic reactions. If a vitamin B deficiency develops, a disruption of protein, fat, and carbohydrate metabolism will occur. Vitamin A aids in epithelialization. It increases collagen synthesis and tensile strength of the healing wound.

If the patient is unable to eat, enteral feedings and supplements should be the first choice if the GI tract is functional. Parenteral nutrition is indicated when enteral feedings are contraindicated or not tolerated. (Enteral and parenteral nutrition are discussed in Chapter 39.)

◆ **Infection Prevention and Control.** You and the patient must scrupulously follow aseptic procedures, including hand washing, for keeping the wound free from infection. Do not allow the patient to touch a recently injured area. The patient's environment should be as free as possible from contamination from items introduced by roommates and visitors. Some patients may receive prophylactic antibiotics.

If an infection develops, a culture and sensitivity test is done to determine the organism and the most effective antibiotic for that specific organism. Obtain the culture before the first dose of antibiotic is given. We can obtain cultures by needle aspiration, tissue culture, or swab technique. HCPs perform needle and tissue punch biopsies.

As a nurse, you can obtain cultures using the swab technique. This is done using Levine's technique, which involves rotating a culture swab over a cleansed 1-cm^2 area near the center of the wound. Use enough pressure to extract wound fluid from deep tissue layers. Take a culture of the clean tissue because exudate and necrotic tissue will not provide an accurate sample.[10] The sample must be sent to the laboratory within 1 hour.

◆ **Psychologic Implications.** The patient may be distressed at the thought or sight of an incision or wound because of fear of scarring or disfigurement. Drainage and odor from a wound often cause alarm. The patient needs to understand the healing process and normal changes that occur as the wound heals.

When changing a dressing, avoid inappropriate facial expressions that may alert the patient to problems with the wound or raise doubts about your ability to care for it. Wrinkling your nose may convey disgust to the patient. Be careful not to focus on the wound to the extent that you are not treating the patient as a total person.

◆ **Patient Teaching.** Because patients are being discharged earlier after surgery and many have surgery as outpatients, it is important that the patient and caregiver know how to care for the wound and perform dressing changes. Wound healing may not be complete for 4 to 6 weeks or longer. Emphasize the importance of adequate rest and good nutrition throughout this time. Physical and emotional stress should be minimal. Observing the wound for complications, such as contractures, adhesions, and secondary infection, is important. Teach the patient and caregiver the signs and symptoms of infection. Have them note changes in the wound color and amount of drainage. Teach the patient to notify the HCP of any signs of abnormal wound healing.

Drugs may be given for a time after recovery from the acute infection. Review drug-specific side effects and adverse effects with the patient and caregiver, as well as methods to prevent side effects (e.g., taking with food). Teach the patient to contact the HCP if any of these effects occur. Discuss the need to complete the entire course of therapy. For example, a patient who needed to take an antibiotic for 10 days decides to stop taking the drug after 5 days because of absent symptoms. However, the organism was not entirely eliminated. It becomes resistant to the antibiotic, and the patient develops a more severe infection.

PRESSURE INJURIES

Etiology and Pathophysiology

A **pressure injury** is localized damage to the skin and/or underlying soft tissue. It usually occurs over a bony prominence or is related to a medical or other device. The injury occurs because of intense and/or prolonged pressure or pressure in combination with shear. The most common site for pressure injuries is the sacrum, with heels being second.

TABLE 11.11   **Risk Factors for Pressure Injuries**
• Advanced age
• Anemia
• Contractures
• Critically ill, cared for in critical care setting
• Diabetes
• Fever
• Friction (rubbing of surfaces together)
• Hip fracture
• Immobility
• Incontinence
• Long and/or extensive surgical procedure
• Low diastolic blood pressure (<60 mm Hg)
• Major trauma
• Mental deterioration
• Neurologic disorders
• Pain
• Peripheral vascular disease
• Spinal cord injury

Factors that influence the development of pressure injuries include the amount of pressure (intensity), length of time the pressure is exerted on the skin (duration), and ability of the patient's tissue to tolerate the externally applied pressure. Other factors that contribute to pressure injury formation include shear (pressure exerted on the skin when it adheres to the bed and the skin layers slide in the direction of body movement [e.g., when pulling the patient up in bed]) and *excessive moisture* (increases risk for skin breakdown). The tolerance of soft tissue for pressure and shear are affected by microclimate, nutrition, perfusion, co-morbidities, and condition of the soft tissue.[11]

Factors that put a patient at risk for developing a pressure injury are outlined in Table 11.11. Patients at risk include those who are older, incontinent, unable to reposition or unaware of the need to reposition (e.g., spinal cord injury), and bed- or wheelchair-bound.

Clinical Manifestations

The manifestations of pressure injuries depend on the extent of the tissue involved. The injury can present as intact skin or an open injury and may be painful. We stage pressure injuries based on the visible or palpable tissue in the injury bed. Table 11.12 shows the pressure injury stages based on the National Pressure Injury Advisory Panel (NPUAP).[11]

If the pressure injury becomes infected, the patient may have signs of infection (e.g., leukocytosis, fever). The pressure injury may increase in size, odor, and drainage; have necrotic tissue; and be indurated, warm, and painful. Untreated pressure injuries may lead to *cellulitis* (spreading of inflammation to subcutaneous or connective tissue), chronic infection, sepsis, and possibly death. The most common complication of a pressure injury is recurrence. Therefore it is important to note the location of previously healed pressure injuries on a patient's admission assessment.

◆ NURSING AND INTERPROFESSIONAL MANAGEMENT: PRESSURE INJURIES

In 1859, Florence Nightingale wrote, "If he has a bedsore, it is generally not the fault of the disease, but of the nursing."[12] Her comment emphasizes the critical role that nurses have in prevention and treatment of pressure injuries.

TABLE 11.12   Pressure Injuries

Pressure Injuries

Stage 1 Pressure Injury: Non-Blanchable Erythema of Intact Skin

Intact skin with a localized area of non-blanchable erythema, which may appear differently in dark skin. Blanchable erythema or changes in sensation, temperature, or firmness may precede visual changes.

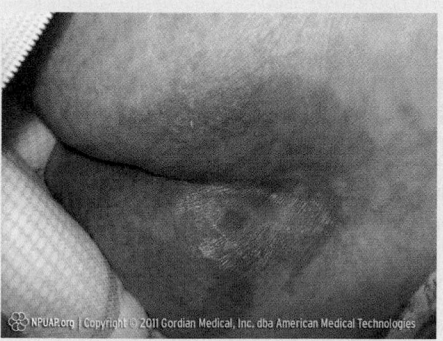

Stage 2 Pressure Injury: Partial-Thickness Skin Loss With Exposed Dermis

Partial-thickness loss of skin with exposed dermis. The wound bed is viable, pink or red, and moist. May present as an intact or ruptured serum-filled blister. Adipose and deeper tissues are not visible. Often result from adverse microclimate and shear in the skin over the pelvis and shear in the heel.

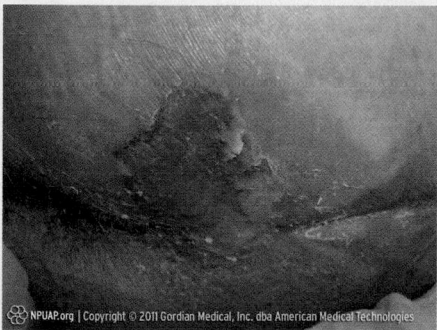

Stage 3 Pressure Injury: Full-Thickness Skin Loss

Full-thickness loss of skin, in which adipose is visible in the injury. Granulation tissue and epibole (rolled wound edges) are often present. Slough and/or eschar (types of dead tissue) may be visible. The depth of tissue damage varies by anatomical location; areas of significant adiposity can develop deep wounds. Undermining and tunneling may occur.

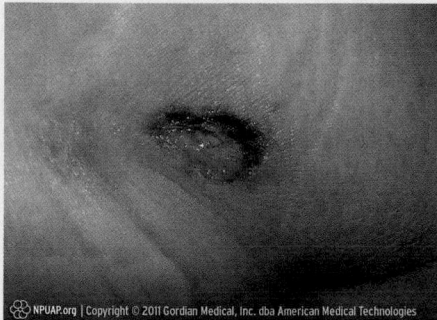

Stage 4 Pressure Injury: Full-Thickness Skin and Tissue Loss

Full-thickness skin and tissue loss with exposed or directly palpable fascia, muscle, tendon, ligament, cartilage, or bone in the injury. Slough and/or eschar may be visible. Epibole, undermining, and/or tunneling often occur. Depth varies by anatomical location.

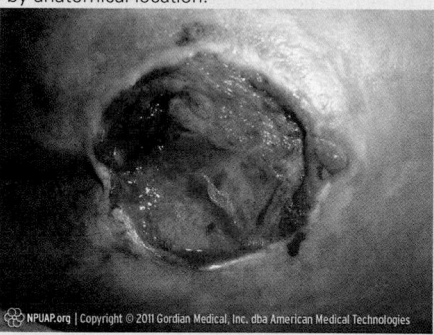

Unstageable Pressure Injury: Obscured Full-Thickness Skin and Tissue Loss

Full-thickness skin and tissue loss in which the extent of tissue damage within the injury cannot be confirmed because it is obscured by slough or eschar. A Stage 3 or Stage 4 pressure injury is present after removing slough or eschar. Stable eschar (i.e., dry, adherent, intact without erythema or fluctuance) on the heel or ischemic limb should not be softened or removed.

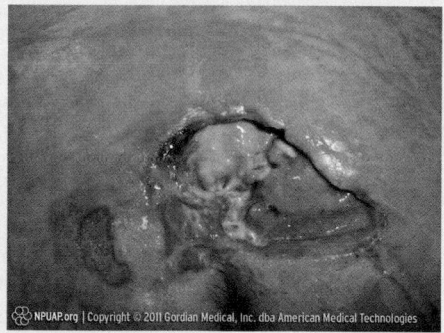

Deep Tissue Pressure Injury (DTPI): Persistent Non-Blanchable Deep Red, Maroon, or Purple Discoloration

Intact or non-intact skin with localized area of persistent non-blanchable deep red, maroon, purple discoloration, or epidermal separation revealing a dark wound bed or blood-filled blister. Pain and temperature change often precede skin color changes. Discoloration may appear differently in dark skin. Results from intense and/or prolonged pressure and shear forces at the bone-muscle interface. May evolve rapidly to reveal the actual extent of tissue injury or may resolve without tissue loss. Visible necrotic tissue, subcutaneous tissue, granulation tissue, fascia, muscle, or other underlying structures indicates a full-thickness pressure injury (Unstageable, Stage 3 or Stage 4). Do not use DTPI to describe vascular, traumatic, neuropathic, or dermatologic conditions.

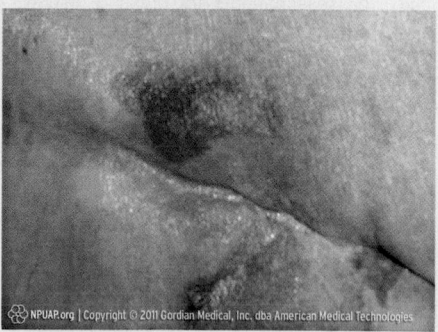

TABLE 11.12 **Pressure Injuries—cont'd**

Pressure Injuries

Medical Device–Related Pressure Injury
Results from the use of devices designed and applied for diagnostic or therapeutic purposes. The resultant injury generally conforms to the pattern or shape of the device. Stage the injury using the staging system.

Mucosal Membrane Pressure Injury
Found on mucous membranes with a history of a medical device in use at the site of the injury. These injuries cannot be staged due to the anatomic location.

Photos used with permission of the National Pressure Injury Advisory Panel. Retrieved from *www.npuap.org/resources/educational-and-clinical-resources/ pressure-injury-staging-illustrations/*.

TABLE 11.13 **Assessing Patients With Dark Skin**

- Look for changes in skin color, such as skin that is darker (purplish, brownish, bluish) than surrounding skin.
- Use natural or halogen light source to accurately assess the skin color. Fluorescent light casts blue color, which can make skin assessment difficult.
- Assess the area for the skin temperature using your hand. The area may feel initially warm, then cooler.
- Touch the skin to feel its consistency. Boggy or edematous feel may indicate a Stage 1 pressure injury.
- Ask the patient if he or she has any pain or itchy sensation.

⚠ **SAFETY ALERT** **Pressure Injuries**

- Stage 3 or 4 (full skin–thickness injury) pressure injury acquired after admission to a health care setting is considered a serious reportable event (SRE) (never event).[13] (SREs are discussed in Chapter 1.)

Nursing and interprofessional management are discussed together because the activities are interrelated. In addition to the nurse, other members of the health team, such as the wound care specialist, plastic surgeon, dietitian, physical therapist, and occupational therapist, can provide valuable input into the complex treatment necessary to prevent and treat pressure injuries.

◆ **Nursing Assessment**

Assess patients for pressure injury risk initially on admission and at periodic intervals based on the patient's condition. Conduct a thorough head-to-toe assessment on admission to identify and document any pressure injuries. After admission, conduct periodic reassessments of the skin and wounds.

⚠ **SAFETY ALERT** **Assessing for Pressure Injuries**

- In acute care, reassess patients for pressure injuries every 24 hours.
- In long-term care, reassess residents weekly for the first 4 weeks after admission and then at least monthly or quarterly.
- In home care, reassess patients at every nurse visit.

To do a risk assessment, use a validated assessment tool, such as the Braden Scale (available at www.bradenscale.com). Knowing the level of risk can help determine how aggressive preventive measures should be.

Identification of skin changes may be hard in patients with dark skin. Table 11.13 presents techniques to help assess darker skin.

TABLE 11.14 **Nursing Assessment**

Pressure Injuries

Subjective Data
Important Health Information
Past health history: Stroke, spinal cord injury; prolonged bed rest or immobility; circulatory impairment; poor nutrition; altered level of consciousness; prior history of pressure injury; immunologic abnormalities; advanced age; diabetes; anemia; trauma
Medications: Use of opioids, hypnotics, systemic corticosteroids
Surgery or other treatments: Recent surgery

Functional Health Patterns
Nutritional-metabolic: Obesity, emaciation; decreased fluid, calorie, or protein intake; vitamin or mineral deficiencies; clinically significant malnutrition as shown by low serum albumin, decreased total lymphocyte count, and decreased body weight (15% less than ideal body weight)
Elimination: Incontinence of urine, feces, or both
Activity-exercise: Weakness, debilitation, inability to turn and position body; contractures
Cognitive-perceptual: Pain or altered cutaneous sensation in pressure injury area; decreased awareness of pressure on body areas; capacity to follow treatment plan

Objective Data
General
Fever

Integumentary
Diaphoresis, edema, and discoloration, especially over bony areas, such as sacrum, hips, elbows, heels, knees, ankles, shoulders, and ear rims, progressing to increased tissue damage characteristic of injury stages

Possible Diagnostic Findings
Leukocytosis, positive cultures for microorganisms from pressure injury

Subjective and objective data that should be obtained from a person with or at risk for a pressure injury are outlined in Table 11.14.

◆ **Nursing Diagnoses**

Nursing diagnoses for the patient with a pressure injury may include:
- Impaired tissue integrity
- Risk for infection

◆ **Planning**

The overall goals are that the patient with a pressure injury will (1) have no deterioration of the wound, (2) not develop an infection in the pressure injury, (3) have healing of pressure injuries, and (4) have no recurrence.

◆ **Nursing Implementation**

◆ **Health Promotion.** The primary nursing responsibilities are (1) identifying patients at risk for developing pressure injuries (Tables 11.11 and 11.14) and (2) implementing pressure injury prevention strategies for those who are at risk. Prevention is the best treatment for pressure injuries. Implementing evidence-based pressure injury prevention programs can reduce the occurrence of health care–acquired pressure injuries.[14,15]

EVIDENCE-BASED PRACTICE

Repositioning and Pressure Injuries

You are doing discharge planning with L.H., an obese 76-yr-old woman with a history of diabetes, hypertension, and macular degeneration. L.H. has spent most of her time while hospitalized in a bed or wheelchair and now has a stage 1 pressure injury on her sacrum. You explain the importance of skin care with her son, who is her primary caregiver.

Making Clinical Decisions

Best Available Evidence. Repositioning is the primary method of reducing the risk for pressure injury. Pressure relief schedules should be developed. Pressure-reducing devices (e.g., foam mattress, padded commode, wheelchair seats) may be used but are not be a substitute for repositioning. In addition, develop a nutrition care plan based on the patient's nutritional and hydration needs, feeding route, and care goals.

Clinician Expertise. You know patients with pressure injury should be repositioned at least every 2 hours while in bed and every hour when in a chair.

Caregiver Preferences and Values. L.H.'s caregiver states he will reposition his mother during the day and have the home health care aide reposition her more often at night.

Implications for Nursing Practice

1. In addition to repositioning, what information is important to discuss with L.H.'s son to prevent further skin injury?
2. What are the risk factors for L.H. to develop worsening pressure injury?
3. What is important for the home health care nurse to monitor on her visits to L.H. related to pressure injuries and healing?

References for Evidence

Edsberg LE, Black JM, Goldberg M, et al: Revised National Pressure Advisory Panel Pressure Injury Staging System, *J Wound Ostomy Continence Nurs* 43(585), 2016. National Pressure Injury Advisory Panel. Retrieved from *www.npuap.org/wp-content/uploads/2014/08/Updated-10-16-14-Quick-Reference-Guide-DIGITAL-NPUAP-EPUAP-PPPIA-16Oct2014.pdf.*

⚠ SAFETY ALERT   Preventing Pressure Injuries

- Use devices to reduce pressure and shear (e.g., low-air-loss mattresses, foam mattresses, wheelchair cushions, padded commode seats, boots [foam, air], lift sheets) as appropriate. These devices do not replace the need for frequent repositioning.
- Reposition patients often to prevent pressure injuries.

In the past, the "standard" was to turn and reposition patients every 2 hours. However, this "policy" is not evidence-based. Individualize time schedules and frequency based on risk factors, patient's overall condition, and type of mattress and support surface. For example, some high-risk patients may need to be turned and repositioned every hour, while others at lower risk may need to be turned and repositioned only every 3 to 4 hours.[11,14]

◆ **Acute Care.** Care of a patient with a pressure injury requires wound care and support measures of the whole person, including adequate nutrition, pain management, control of other medical conditions, and redistributing pressure. Both conservative and surgical strategies are used in the treatment of pressure injuries, depending on the stage and condition of the injury.

Once a pressure injury has developed, initiate interventions based on the injury characteristics (e.g., stage, size, location, amount of exudate, type of wound, presence of infection or pain) and the patient's general status (e.g., nutritional state, age, cardiovascular status, level of mobility). Carefully document the size of the pressure injury. A wound-measuring card or tape can be used to note the injury's maximum length and width in centimeters. To find the depth of the injury, take a sterile cotton-tipped applicator and soak it with saline. Gently place it into the deepest part of the injury, and then measure the length of the part of the applicator that probed the injury. Documentation of the healing wound can be done using several available pressure injury healing tools, such as the NPUAP Pressure Injury Scale for Healing (PUSH) tool (available at *www.npuap.org/wp-content/uploads/2012/03/push3.pdf*).

Some agencies require that pictures of the pressure injury be taken initially and at regular intervals during treatment. The Informatics box has suggestions for digital imaging.

INFORMATICS IN PRACTICE

Digital Images

To monitor wound progress, use digital photography. For the best images:

- Include a ruler with date, length, width, and depth of the wound in each photo.
- Position the patient the same way for each photo.
- Take the photo from the same angle each time. Pointing perpendicularly at the wound is best.
- Use natural light, without flash, whenever possible.
- Show the wound on a solid background, avoiding shiny underpads.
- Avoid patient identifiers, such as jewelry, tattoos, or visible family members.

Pressure injuries generally fall under the category of healing by secondary intention. Care may involve debridement, wound cleaning, application of a dressing, and offloading pressure. It is important to choose the right pressure-redistributing techniques (e.g., mattress replacement, mattress overlay, integrated bed system, seat cushion, seat cushion overlay) to move pressure off areas of pressure injury. Whenever possible, do not turn the patient onto a body surface that has blanchable erythema. Massage is contraindicated in the presence of acute inflammation and where there is the possibility of damaged blood vessels or fragile skin.

Sliding down in bed causes shear. Encourage patients to reposition themselves by lifting rather than sliding and to use a trapeze if needed. Use lift sheets to move patients up in bed or to transfer them.

A pressure injury that has necrotic tissue or eschar (except for dry, stable necrotic feet or heels) should have the tissue removed by surgical, mechanical, enzymatic, or autolytic debridement methods. Once the pressure injury has been successfully debrided and has a clean granulating base, the goal is to provide a wound environment that supports moist wound healing and prevents disruption of the newly formed granulation tissue. Reconstruction of the pressure injury site by surgical repair, including skin grafting, skin flaps, musculocutaneous flaps, or free flaps, may be necessary.

Clean pressure injuries with noncytotoxic solutions (e.g., normal saline) that do not kill or damage cells, especially fibroblasts. Cytotoxicity is a concern when applying a topical agent to a pressure injury. However, if there is a delay in healing due to infection, then antimicrobial use (e.g., sodium hypochlorite [Dakin's solution], povidone-iodine, cadexomer iodine) overrides the toxicity concern. Hydrogen peroxide is cytotoxic and should not be used. It is important to use enough irrigation pressure (4 to 15 psi) to adequately clean the pressure injury without causing trauma or damage to the wound. You can achieve this pressure using a 30-mL syringe and a 19-gauge needle.

After the pressure injury has been cleansed, cover it with an appropriate dressing. Keep a pressure injury slightly moist, rather than dry, to enhance re-epithelialization. Some factors to consider when choosing a dressing are maintaining a moist environment, preventing the wound from drying out, ability to absorb the wound drainage, location of the wound, amount of caregiver time required to change the dressing, cost of the dressing, presence of infection, clean versus sterile dressings, and care delivery setting. Dressings are described in Table 11.9.

Stages 2 through 4 pressure injuries are considered contaminated or colonized with bacteria. Remember that in people who have chronic wounds or are immunocompromised, the signs and symptoms of infection (purulent exudate, odor, erythema, warmth, tenderness, edema, pain, fever, high WBC count) may not be present even when the pressure injury is infected.

Maintaining adequate nutrition is an important nursing responsibility for the patient with a pressure injury. Often the patient is debilitated and has a poor appetite secondary to inactivity. Oral feedings must be adequate to meet the patient's nutritional requirements. The caloric intake needed to correct and maintain nutritional balance may be 30 to 35 calories/kg/day and 1.25 to 1.50 g of protein/kg/day.

Enteral feedings can supplement oral feedings. When oral and enteral feedings are inadequate, parenteral nutrition consisting of amino acid and glucose solutions is used. Parenteral and enteral nutrition are discussed in Chapter 39.

◆ **Ambulatory Care.** Pressure injuries affect the quality of life of patients and their caregivers. Because pressure injuries often recur, teaching prevention techniques to the patient and caregiver is extremely important (Table 11.15). A sixth-grade level

TABLE 11.15   Patient & Caregiver Teaching

Pressure Injury

When teaching the patient and caregiver to prevent and care for pressure injuries, do the following:

1. Identify and explain risk factors and cause of pressure injuries.
2. Teach the caregiver techniques for incontinence. If incontinence occurs, cleanse skin at time of soiling and use absorbent pads or briefs.
3. Demonstrate correct positioning to decrease risk for skin breakdown. NEVER position the patient directly on the pressure injury if possible.
4. Teach caregiver to reposition a bed-bound patient at least every 2 hours and a chair-bound patient every hour.
5. Review the available resources (i.e., caregiver's availability and skill, finances, equipment) of patients who need pressure injury care at home.
6. Teach patient and/or caregiver to place clean dressings over sterile dressings using "no touch" technique when changing dressings. Review the disposal of contaminated dressings.
7. Teach patient and caregiver to inspect skin daily. Tell them to report any significant changes to the HCP.
8. Teach patient and caregiver the importance of good nutrition to enhance injury healing.
9. Evaluate program effectiveness.

version of the patient guide to pressure injury prevention is available for use in patient teaching at *www.npuap.org/wp-content/uploads/2016/04/Pressure-Injury-Prevention-Points-2016.pdf.*

The caregiver needs to know the cause of pressure injuries, prevention techniques, early signs, nutritional support, and care techniques for actual pressure injuries. Because the patient with a pressure injury often needs extensive care for other health problems, it is important that the nurse support the caregiver with the added responsibility for pressure injury treatment. eNursing Care Plan 11.2 (available on the website for this chapter at *http://evolve.elsevier.com/Lewis/medsurg*) outlines the care for the patient with a pressure injury.

◆ **Evaluation**

The expected outcomes are that the patient with a pressure injury will have
• Healing of pressure injury(s)
• Intact skin with no further breakdown

CASE STUDY

Inflammation and Infection

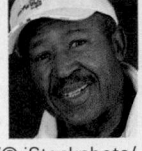
(© iStockphoto/Thinkstock.)

Patient Profile

G.N., a 65-yr-old black man, was admitted to the hospital emergency department with partial-thickness burns that involved his face, neck, and upper trunk. He also had a lacerated right leg. His injuries occurred about 36 hours earlier when he fell out of a tree onto his lit gas grill while trimming tree branches.

Subjective Data

• Reports a slightly hoarse voice and irritated throat
• States that he tried to treat himself because he does not have health insurance
• Has been coughing up sooty sputum
• Describes severe pain in left hip

Objective Data

Physical Examination

• Leg wound is gaping and has drainage: temperature 101.1°F (38.4°C)
• X-rays reveal a fractured right tibia and fractured left hip

Laboratory Studies

• WBC count 26,400/μL (26.4 × 10⁹/L) with 80% neutrophils (10% bands)

Interprofessional Care

• Surgery was done to repair the left hip.

Continued

CASE STUDY—cont'd

Inflammation and Infection

Discussion Questions

1. What manifestations of inflammation did G.N. exhibit, and what are their pathophysiologic mechanisms?
2. What type of exudate formation did he develop?
3. What is the basis for the development of the temperature?
4. What is the significance of his WBC count and differential?
5. Because his wound was gaping, primary tissue healing was not possible. How would you expect healing to take place? What complications could he develop?
6. What risk factors does G.N. have to develop a pressure injury?
7. **Priority Decision:** Based on the assessment data provided, what are the priority nursing diagnoses? Are there any collaborative problems?
8. **Collaboration:** What nursing activities related to wound care can be delegated to unlicensed assistive personnel (UAP)?
9. **Quality Improvement:** What outcomes would indicate that interprofessional care was effective?

Answers available at *http://evolve.elsevier.com/Lewis/medsurg.*

▌ BRIDGE TO NCLEX EXAMINATION

The number of the question corresponds to the same-numbered outcome at the beginning of the chapter.

1. A patient 1 day postoperative after abdominal surgery has incisional pain, 99.5°F temperature, slight erythema at the incision margins, and 30 mL serosanguinous drainage in the Jackson-Pratt drain. Based on this assessment, what conclusion would the nurse make?
   a. The patient has a normal inflammatory response.
   b. The abdominal incision shows signs of an infection.
   c. The abdominal incision shows signs of impending dehiscence.
   d. The patient's health care provider must be notified about her condition.

2. The nurse assessing a patient with a chronic leg wound finds local signs of erythema, and the patient reports pain at the wound site. What would the nurse expect to be ordered to assess the patient's systemic response?
   a. Serum protein analysis
   b. WBC count and differential
   c. Punch biopsy of center of wound
   d. Culture and sensitivity of the wound

3. A patient in the unit has a 103.7°F temperature. Which intervention would be *most* effective in restoring normal body temperature?
   a. Using a cooling blanket while the patient is febrile
   b. Giving antipyretics on an around-the-clock schedule
   c. Providing increased fluids and have the UAP give sponge baths
   d. Giving prescribed antibiotics and placing warm blankets for comfort

4. A nurse is caring for a patient who has a pressure injury that is treated with debridement, irrigations, and moist gauze dressings. How would the nurse expect healing to occur?
   a. Cell regeneration
   b. Tertiary intention
   c. Secondary intention
   d. Remodeling of tissues

5. Which patient has the *greatest* risk for experiencing delayed wound healing?
   a. A 65-yr-old woman with stress incontinence
   b. A 52-yr-old obese woman with type 2 diabetes
   c. A 78-yr-old man who has a history of hypertension
   d. A 30-yr-old man who drinks 2 alcoholic beverages per day

6. Which order should a nurse question in the plan of care for an older adult, immobile stroke patient with a pink, clean stage 3 pressure injury?
   a. Pack the wound with foam dressing.
   b. Turn and position the patient every hour.
   c. Clean the wound every shift with Dakin's solution.
   d. Assess for pain and medicate before dressing change.

7. An 85-yr-old patient has a score of 16 on the Braden Scale. What should the nurse include in the plan of care?
   a. Implementing a 1-hour turning schedule with skin assessment.
   b. Elevating the head of bed to 90 degrees when the patient is supine.
   c. Continuing with weekly skin assessments with no special precautions.
   d. Placing a silicone foam dressing on the patient's sacrum to prevent breakdown.

8. Which patients are at *most* risk for pressure injuries? *Select all that apply.*
   a. A patient with right sided-paralysis and fecal incontinence
   b. An older adult who is alert and needs assistance to ambulate
   c. A young adult patient with paraplegia after a gunshot wound
   d. A morbidly obese patient who has an open abdominal wound
   e. An ambulatory patient who has occasional stress incontinence
   f. A young adult with a tibial fracture from a motor vehicle accident

9. An 82year-old man is being cared for at home by his family. A pressure injury on his right buttock measures 1 × 2 × 0.8 cm in depth, and pink subcutaneous tissue is completely visible on the wound bed. Which stage would the nurse document on the wound assessment form?
   a. Stage 1
   b. Stage 2
   c. Stage 3
   d. Stage 4

1. a, 2. b, 3. b, 4. c, 5. b, 6. c, 7. a, 8. a, c, d, 9. c

For rationales to these answers and even more NCLEX review questions, visit *http://evolve.elsevier.com/Lewis/medsurg.*

ⓔ EVOLVE WEBSITE/RESOURCES LIST

http://evolve.elsevier.com/Lewis/medsurg

Review Questions (Online Only)

Key Points

Answer Keys for Questions
- Rationales for Bridge to NCLEX Examination Questions
- Answer Guidelines for Case Study on p. 172

Student Case Study
- Patient With Pressure Injury

Nursing Care Plans
- eNursing Care Plan 11.1: Patient With a Fever
- eNursing Care Plan 11.2: Patient With a Pressure Injury

Conceptual Care Map Creator

Audio Glossary

Content Updates

REFERENCES

*1. Schieber AM, Ayres JS: Thermoregulation as a disease tolerance defense strategy, *Pathogens and Disease* 1:74, 2016.

2. Atkins E: Fever: Its history, cause, and function, *Yale J Biol Med* 55:283, 1982. (Classic)

*3. LeBlanc K, Baranoski S, Christensen D, et al: The art of dressing selection: A consensus statement on skin tears and best practice, *Adv Skin Wound Care* 29:32, 2016.

4. Nix DP: *Acute and chronic wounds: Current management concepts,* 5th ed, St Louis, 2016, Mosby.

5. Whitney JD: Surgical wounds and incision care. In *Acute and chronic wounds: Current management concepts,* 5th ed, St Louis, 2016, Mosby.

*6. Sibbald RG, Elliott JA, Verma L, et al: Topical antimicrobial agents for chronic wounds, *Adv Skin Wound Care* 30:438, 2017.

*7. International Wound Infection Institute: Wound infection in clinical practice. Retrieved from *www.woundinfection-institute.com/wp-content/uploads/2017/07/IWII-Consensus_Final-2017.pdf.*

*8. Driver VR, Eckert KA, Carter MJ, et al: Cost-effectiveness of negative pressure wound therapy in patients with many comorbidities and severe wounds of various etiology, *Wound Repair Regen* 24:1041, 2016.

*9. Molnar JA, Vlad LG, Gumus T, et al: Nutrition and chronic wounds: Improving clinical outcomes, *Plast Reconstr Surg* 138:71S, 2016.

*10. Stallard Y: When and how to perform cultures on chronic wounds? *J Wound Ostomy Continence Nurs* 45:179, 2018.

*11. National Pressure Injury Advisory Panel: Prevention and treatment of pressure ulcers. Retrieved from *www.npuap.org/resources/educational-and-clinical-resources/.*

12. Nightingale F: Notes on nursing, Philadelphia, 1859, Lippincott. (Classic)

*13. Elsabrout K, Orbacz E, McMahon LA, et al: Large-scale hospital mattress switch-out leads to reduction hospital-acquired pressure injuries: Operationalization of a multidisciplinary task force, *Worldviews Evid Based Nurs* 15:161, 2018.

*14. Jocelyn CH, Thiara E, Lopez V, et al: Turning frequency in adult bedridden patients to prevent hospital-acquired pressure injury: A scoping review, *Int Wound J* 15:225, 2018.

*15. Pickham D, Berte N, Pihulic M, et al: Effect of a wearable patient sensor on care delivery for preventing pressure injuries in acutely ill adults: A pragmatic randomized clinical trial, *Int J Nurs Stud* 80:12, 2018.

*Evidence-based information for clinical practice.

12

Genetics

Janice Smolowitz

The things you do for yourself are gone when you are gone, but the things you do for others remain as your legacy.

Kalu Ndukwe Kalu

http://evolve.elsevier.com/Lewis/medsurg/

CONCEPTUAL FOCUS

Cellular Regulation

Ethics

LEARNING OUTCOMES

1. Describe common terms related to genetics and genetic disorders: autosomal, carrier, heterozygous, homozygous, mutation, recessive, and X-linked gene.
2. Distinguish between the 2 common causes of genetic mutations.
3. Compare and contrast the 3 most common inheritance patterns of genetic disorders.
4. Describe the most common classifications of genetic disorders.

5. Explore the complex ethical and social implications of genetic testing.
6. Analyze the role of pharmacogenomics and pharmacogenetics in developing personalized drug therapy.
7. Discuss your role in assisting the patient and family in dealing with genetic and genomic issues.

KEY TERMS

epigenetics, p. 180
genes, p. 175
genetics, p. 175
genome, p. 175

genomics, p. 175
hereditary, Table 12.1, p. 176
heterozygous, Table 12.1, p. 176
homozygous, Table 12.1, p. 176

mutation, p. 178
pharmacogenetics, p. 183
pharmacogenomics, p. 183

GENETICS AND GENOMICS

Genes are the basic units of heredity. They are composed of sequences of DNA found along a person's chromosomes. Genes are passed from 1 generation to the next. The **genome** is the complete set of DNA. It includes all the organism's genes. An organism's genome has all the information it needs to build and maintain itself.[1]

Genetics is the study of genes and their role in inheritance. Genetics determines the way that certain traits or conditions are passed down through genes. A person's genes can have a profound impact on health and disease. More than 4000 diseases are thought to be related to altered genes.

Genomics is the study of all a person's genes (the *genome*), including interactions of these genes with each other and with the person's environment. Genomics includes the study of complex diseases, such as heart disease, diabetes, and cancer, because these diseases are typically caused by a combination of genetic and environmental factors rather than by a single gene.

Genomics may help us understand why some people who eat healthy diets and exercise regularly die at a young age of cancer, and some people eat unhealthy diets and never exercise and yet live to an old age. Common terms used in genetics and genomics are defined in Table 12.1.

Important advances in genetic and genomic research and technology have affected the delivery of health care services.[2] In response to these scientific developments, nursing organizations have established practice standards that provide a framework for applying the nursing process to the care of persons with genetic and genomic concerns. Other standards outline competencies and education in relation to professional practice and genetics.

The identification of a genetic basis for many diseases has the potential to strongly influence the care of patients at risk for or diagnosed with a disease that has a genetic link. You need to know the basic principles of genetics, be familiar with the impact that genetics and genomics have on health and disease and be prepared to aid the patient and family with genetic issues.

TABLE 12.1 Glossary of Genetic and Genomic Terms

Term	Definition
Allele	One of a series of alternative forms (genotypes) at a specific region (locus) of a chromosome
Autosome	A chromosome other than X or Y. The human genome has 44 autosomes (22 pairs of autosomes)
Carrier	A person who is heterozygous for a gene variant that causes autosomal recessive or X-linked recessive disease. Used to describe heterozygotes for risk alleles of complex traits with variable penetrance, regardless of inheritance type
Carrier rate	Frequency of carriers in a population
Carrier testing	Clinical method used to identify at-risk family members of populations, who are usually asymptomatic but may have a pathogenic variant for an autosomal recessive or X-linked disorder
Chromosome	Microscopic structures in the cell nucleus composed of chromatin, which contain genetic information. Each cell normally has 46 chromosomes in 23 pairs (22 autosome pairs and 2 sex chromosomes)
Codominance	Expression of each pair of alleles when present in the heterozygous state (e.g., AB blood type)
Congenital	Present at birth
Consanguineous	Reproduction between 2 persons from the same bloodline, such as first or second cousins. Consanguineous parentage increases the probability of a rare recessive disease
Dominant allele	Gene that is expressed in the phenotype of a heterozygous person
Familial disorder	A trait that appears with higher frequency among close relatives than in the general population
Gene	Functional unit of heredity. A gene is a unit of DNA sequence that encodes for a specific functional product, such as RNA
Genetic risk	Probability that a trait will occur or recur in a family, based on knowledge of its genetic pattern of transmission
Genetics	Study of genes and their role in inheritance
Genome	All the DNA contained in a person. A person's genetic constitution
Genome-wide association study (GWAS)	A type of genetic mapping study design that involves scanning complete sets of DNA (genomes) of many people to find genetic variations associated with a particular disease
Genomics	Study of how genes interact and influence people's biologic and physical characteristics
Genotype	Genetic identity of a person, comprised of the entire complex of genes inherited from both parents
Haploid	Cells or organisms that have 1 copy of each autosomal chromosome and 1 copy of each sex chromosome. Ova and sperm are haploid. Fertilization results in an embryo with 1 set of chromosomes from each parent (diploid embryo)
Hereditary	Transmission of a disease, condition, or trait from parent to children
Heterozygous	Having 2 different alleles for 1 given gene, 1 inherited from each parent
Homozygous	Having 2 identical alleles for 1 given gene, 1 inherited from each parent
Locus	Position of a gene on a chromosome
Mutation	A change in a gene that affects function. Types include nonsense, missense silent, and frameshift. A mutation associated with a disease is called a *pathogenic variant*. Sometimes mutations are passed from parent to children.
Oncogene	Gene that contributes to the conversion of normal cells to cancer cells. Usually dominant
Pedigree	A graphic representation that shows family relationships, gender, age, and presence of diseases for each family member
Pharmacogenetics	Study of variability of drug metabolism related to variations in single genes
Pharmacogenomics	Study of variability of drug metabolism in relation to variations in and interactions of multiple genes or the person's genome
Phenotype	Observable characteristics of a person. Can be measured categorically or quantitatively
Protooncogene	Genes that can be turned into oncogenes by a dominant activating mutation. Oncogenes synthesize structurally altered proteins that result in cancer
Recessive allele	Allele that has no noticeable effect on the phenotype in a heterozygous person
Trait	Physical characteristic that one inherits, such as hair or eye color
X-linked gene	Gene found on the X chromosome rather than an autosome. In general, sex-linked disorders are seen in males

Basic Principles of Genetics

Genes. We think there are around 30,000 genes in each person's genome. Genes carry the instructions (encode) for making proteins that direct the activities of cells. Genes control how a cell functions, including how quickly it grows, how often it divides, and how long it lives. To control these functions, genes make proteins that perform specific tasks and act as messengers for the cell. It is essential that each gene have the correct instructions, or "code," for making its protein so that the protein can perform the proper function for the cell.

Genes are arranged in a specific linear formation along a chromosome (Fig. 12.1). Each gene has a specific location on a chromosome, termed a *locus*. An *allele* is 1 of 2 or more alternative forms of a gene that occupy corresponding loci on *homologous chromosomes* (a pair of chromosomes having corresponding deoxyribonucleic acid [DNA] sequences, with 1 coming from the mother and the other from the father). Each allele codes for a specific inherited characteristic.

When there are 2 different alleles, the allele that is fully expressed is the *dominant allele*. The other allele that lacks the ability to express itself in the presence of a dominant allele is the *recessive allele*. The actual genetic makeup of the person is called the *genotype*. Physical traits expressed by a person are called the *phenotype*.

Chromosomes. *Chromosomes* are found in the cell nucleus. They occur in pairs. Humans have 23 pairs of chromosomes. Twenty-two of the 23 pairs of chromosomes are *homologous* and are termed *autosomes*. Autosomes are the same in both

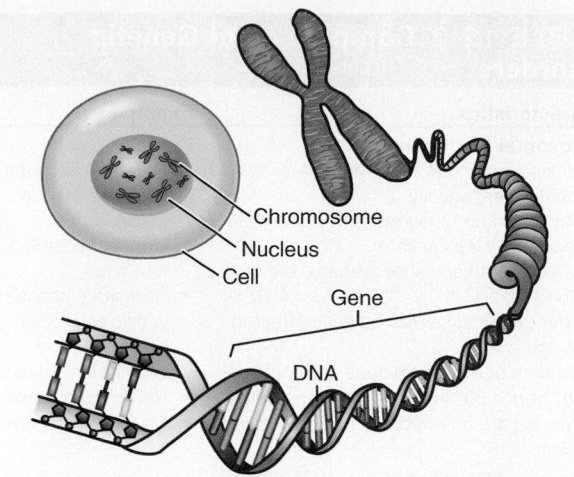

FIG. 12.1 The long, stringy DNA that makes up genes is spooled within chromosomes inside the nucleus of a cell. (Note that a gene would be a much longer stretch of DNA than what is shown here.) (Adapted from *The new genetics*, Bethesda, MD, 2010, National Institute of General Medical Science, National Institutes of Health, U.S. Department of Health and Human Services.)

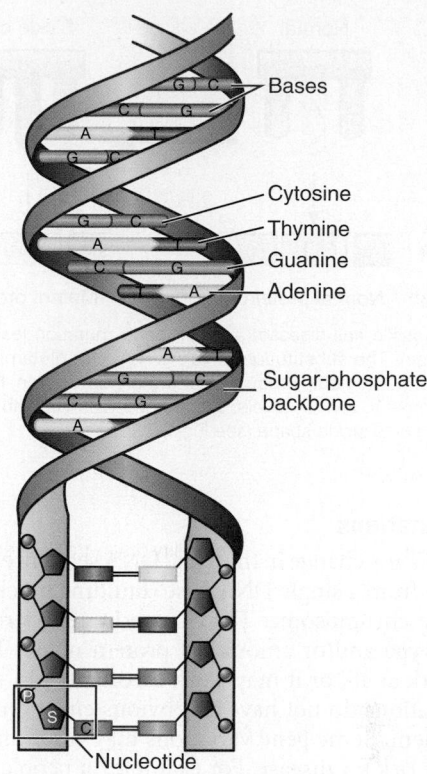

FIG. 12.2 DNA consists of 2 long, twisted chains made up of nucleotides. Each nucleotide contains a base, a phosphate molecule *(P)*, and the sugar molecule deoxyribose *(S)*. The bases in DNA nucleotides are adenine *(A)*, thymine *(T)*, cytosine *(C)*, and guanine *(G)*. (Adapted from *The new genetics*, Bethesda, MD, 2010, National Institute of General Medical Science, National Institutes of Health, U.S. Department of Health and Human Services.)

males and females. The sex chromosomes make up the twenty-third pair of chromosomes. A female has 2 X chromosomes, and a male has 1 X and 1 Y chromosome. One chromosome of each pair is inherited from the mother and one from the father. Half of each child's chromosomes (and therefore the genetic makeup) comes from his or her father and half from his or her mother.

DNA. Genes are made up of a nucleic acid called *deoxyribonucleic acid* (DNA). DNA stores genetic information and encodes the instructions for synthesizing specific proteins needed to maintain life. DNA also dictates the rate at which proteins are made. Every somatic cell in a person's body has the same DNA.

The information in DNA is stored as a code made up of 4 nitrogenous bases: adenine (A), guanine (G), cytosine (C), and thymine (T). Human DNA consists of about 3 billion bases, and more than 99% of those bases are the same in all people. The order, or sequence, of these bases determines the information for building and maintaining an organism. This is similar to the way we use letters of the alphabet to create words and sentences.

DNA bases pair up with each other, A with T and C with G, to form units called *base pairs*. Each base is attached to a sugar molecule and a phosphate molecule (Fig. 12.2). Together, a base, sugar, and phosphate are called a *nucleotide*. Nucleotides are arranged in 2 long strands that form a spiral called a *double helix*. The structure of the double helix is like a ladder, with the base pairs forming the ladder's rungs and the sugar and phosphate molecules forming the ladder's vertical sidepieces.

DNA can *replicate* or make copies of itself. Each strand of DNA in the double helix can serve as a pattern for duplicating the sequence of bases. When cells divide, each new cell must have an exact copy of the DNA that was in the parent (original) cell.

If you uncoiled the chromosomes in a cell and placed it end to end, the DNA would be about 6 feet long. If all the DNA in your body were connected, it would stretch about 67 billion miles.[2]

RNA. *Ribonucleic acid* (RNA) is similar to DNA but with some significant differences. RNA contains the nitrogenous bases adenine, guanine, and cytosine, but it contains uracil instead of thymine. RNA is single, not double, stranded. It contains ribose instead of deoxyribose sugar. RNA transfers the genetic information obtained from DNA to the proper location for protein synthesis.

Protein Synthesis. Protein synthesis, or the making of proteins, occurs in 2 steps: *transcription* and *translation*. Transcription is the process by which messenger RNA (mRNA) is made from single-stranded DNA. The mRNA becomes attached to a ribosome, where translation occurs. At this point another specialized type of RNA, transfer RNA (tRNA), arranges the amino acids in the correct sequence to assemble the protein. Once the protein is complete, it is released from the ribosome and able to perform its specific function in the cell.

Mitosis. *Mitosis* is a type of cell division that results in the formation of genetically identical daughter cells. Before cell division, the chromosomes duplicate, and each new cell (called *daughter cells*) receives an exact replica of the chromosomes from the original cell (called the *parent cell*).

Meiosis. Meiosis occurs only in germline, or sexual reproductive, cells. Two consecutive nuclear divisions, meiosis I and meiosis II, occur without chromosomes replicating in between. This results in the production of 4 haploid sex cells. Each has a single copy of each chromosome.

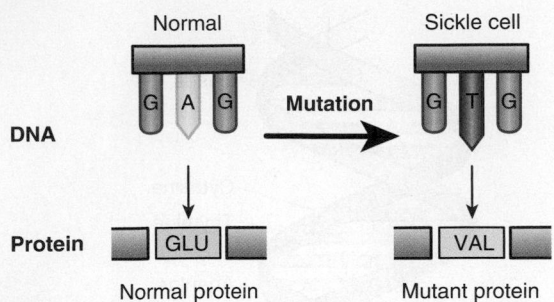

FIG. 12.3 In sickle cell disease, a single gene mutation leads to mutant (incorrect) protein. The substitution of valine *(VAL)* for glutamic acid on the β-globin chain of hemoglobin produces abnormal hemoglobin, hemoglobin S *(Hb S)*. In response to low O_2 levels, the erythrocytes with Hb S stiffen and elongate, taking on a sickle shape (see Fig. 30.3).

Genetic Mutations

A **mutation** is any change in the usual DNA sequence. Mutations range in size from a single DNA base (building block) to a large segment of a chromosome. The change in gene structure may change the type and/or amount of protein made. The protein may not work at all, or it may work incorrectly. In some cases, genetic mutations do not have an obvious effect on the people who have them. Some gene variations may result in disease or an increased risk for disease. For example, in people with sickle cell disease, a substitution of a single base (adenine is replaced by thymine) in a single gene (β-globin gene) causes the disease (Fig. 12.3).

Types of Mutations. Genetic mutations occur in 2 ways. They can be inherited from a parent (germline mutation) or acquired (somatic mutation) during a person's lifetime.

Germline mutations are passed from parent to child. These mutations are present in the oocyte and sperm cells. This type of mutation is present throughout a person's life in virtually every cell in the body.

Acquired (somatic) mutations occur in the DNA of a cell at some time during a person's life. An acquired mutation is passed on to all cells that develop from that single cell. These mutations in somatic cells cannot be passed on to the next generation. Acquired mutations can occur if (1) a mistake is made as DNA replicates during cell division or (2) environmental factors alter the DNA.

Mutations can occur when a cell is dividing. During replication, occasionally mistakes, such as deletions, insertions, or duplication of DNA material, can occur. Although DNA repair enzymes can correct replication errors, mistakes can go uncorrected.

DNA damage can also occur from environmental factors. For example, ultraviolet (UV) radiation can cause DNA damage, leading to skin cancer. Toxins in cigarettes can lead to lung cancer. Many chemotherapy drugs used to treat cancer target the DNA of cancer cells and healthy cells. In the process, these drugs increase a person's risk for developing secondary cancers (see Chapter 15).

Cells have built-in mechanisms that catch and repair most of the changes that occur during DNA replication or from environmental damage. However, as we age, our DNA repair does not work as effectively and we accumulate changes in our DNA.

Inheritance Patterns

Genetic conditions can be inherited in several ways, including autosomal dominant, autosomal recessive, X-linked, and

TABLE 12.2 Comparison of Genetic Disorders

Characteristics	Examples
Autosomal Dominant	
• Males and females are affected, or have the disease, equally • More common than recessive disorders and usually less severe • Affected persons show variable expression • Affected persons may have an affected parent • Children of a heterozygous (affected) parent have a 50% chance of being affected • Persons are affected in successive generations	• Breast and ovarian cancer related to *BRCA* genes • Familial hypercholes-terolemia • Hereditary nonpolyposis colorectal cancer • Huntington's disease • Neurofibromatosis • Marfan's syndrome
Autosomal Recessive	
• Males and females are affected equally • Heterozygotes are carriers and usually asymptomatic • Affected persons may have unaffected parents who are heterozygous for trait • Children of 2 heterozygous parents have a 25% chance of being affected and a 50% chance of being carriers (Fig. 12.9) • Often no family history of disease	• Cystic fibrosis • Phenylketonuria • Sickle cell disease • Tay-Sachs disease • Thalassemia
X-Linked Recessive	
• Most affected persons have unaffected parents • Affected persons are usually male • Daughters of affected males are carriers • Sons of affected males are unaffected (unless mother is a carrier)	• Duchenne muscular dystrophy • Hemophilia • Wiskott-Aldrich syndrome

Y-linked disorders. If the mutant gene is found on an autosome, the genetic disorder is called *autosomal.* If the mutant gene is on the X chromosome, the genetic disorder is called *X-linked.* These patterns are considered mendelian patterns of inheritance. They occur less often than multifactorial or complex traits and disorders. Table 12.2 compares characteristics of autosomal dominant, autosomal recessive, and X-linked recessive conditions. Family pedigrees for autosomal recessive and dominant disorders and X-linked recessive disorders are shown in Figs. 12.4 and 12.5. These diagrams will be discussed later in this chapter in the context of documenting a pedigree and family history.

Autosomal dominant disorders are caused by a mutation of a single gene pair (heterozygous) on a chromosome. A dominant allele prevails over a normal allele. *Penetrance* describes the chance that a carrier of a dominant mutation will show signs of the disorder. *Incomplete penetrance* occurs when a person with a genetic mutation does not have signs of the disorder. It explains why a parent who has a genetic disorder may not have signs of the disorder, but the child does. Autosomal dominant disorders show variable expressivity. *Expressivity* describes the way the phenotype manifests. This accounts for how symptoms of a disorder vary from person to person, even though they have the same mutated gene. Symptoms are also influenced by other, usually unknown, genetic factors, gene-environment interactions, and chance events.

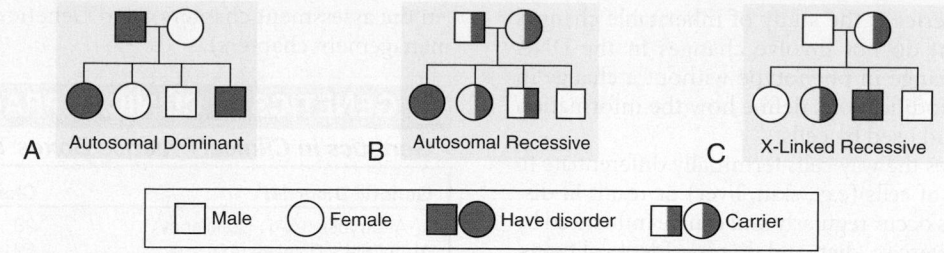

FIG. 12.4 Examples of family pedigrees showing inheritance of (A) autosomal dominant, (B) autosomal recessive, and (C) X-linked recessive disorders.

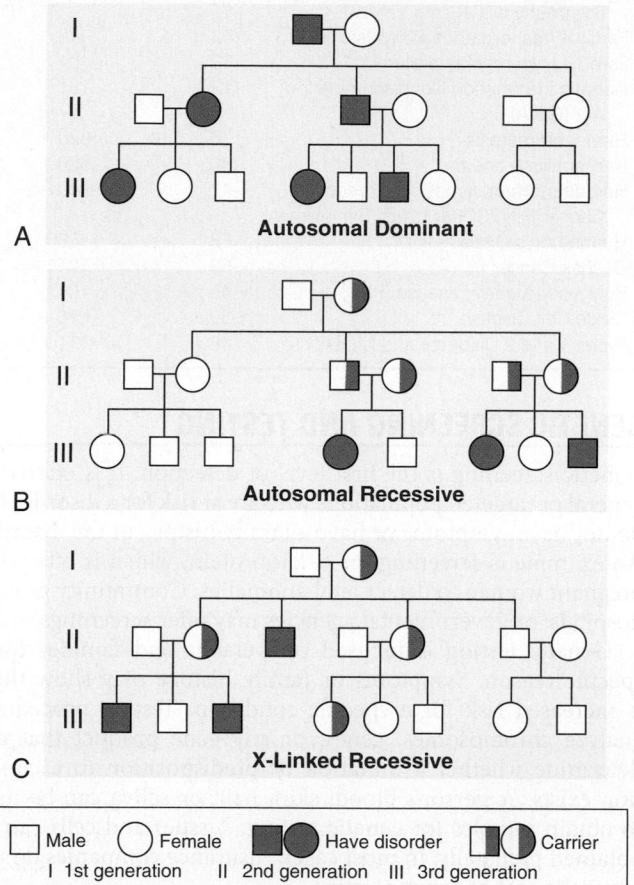

FIG. 12.5 Family pedigrees showing 3 generations. A, Family pedigree suggestive of an autosomal dominant disorder. B, Family pedigree suggestive of an autosomal recessive disorder. C, Family pedigree suggestive of an X-linked recessive disorder.

Autosomal recessive disorders are caused by mutations of 2 gene pairs (homozygous) on a chromosome. A person who inherits 1 copy of the recessive allele does not develop the disease because the normal allele predominates.[3] However, this person is a *carrier*. Several children of 1 couple may be affected. Males and females are affected with equal frequency and severity. These disorders occur in 1 generation and more often among children of parents who are blood relatives, such as first cousins.

X-linked recessive disorders are caused by a mutation on the X chromosome. Men can be severely affected because they have only 1 X chromosome. Women who carry the mutated gene on 1 X chromosome have another X chromosome to compensate

for the mutation. Women who carry the mutated gene can transmit it to their offspring.

Y chromosomal inheritance occurs for genes that are only on the Y chromosome. An affected father transmits the disorder to all his sons. Only men are affected.

Human Genome Project

The Human Genome Project (HGP), which was completed in 2003, mapped the entire human genome.[4] Analysis of the data will continue for many years. The knowledge gained through the HGP will (1) help improve the diagnosis of diseases, (2) allow for earlier detection of genetic predisposition to diseases, and (3) play a critical role in determining risk assessment for genetic-related diseases. In addition, the results of the HGP help match organ donors with transplant recipients.

GENETIC DISORDERS

A *genetic disorder* is caused in whole or in part by a change in the DNA sequence. They can be inherited (person born with altered genetic code) or they can be acquired (e.g., replication errors, damage to DNA from toxins).[3] Genetic disorders can be caused by (1) a mutation in 1 gene (single gene disorder); (2) mutations in multiple genes (multifactorial inheritance disorder), which are often related to environmental factors; or (3) damage to chromosomes (changes in the number or structure of chromosomes).

Classification of Genetic Disorders

Single Gene Disorders. Some genetic disorders result from a single gene mutation (Fig. 12.6, *A*). Examples include cystic fibrosis, sickle cell disease, and polycystic kidney disease. The pattern of inheritance for single gene disorders can be autosomal dominant, autosomal recessive, or X-linked. Single gene disorders are relatively rare compared with more commonly occurring multifactorial genetic disorders.

Multifactorial Inherited Conditions. *Multifactorial inherited conditions* are complex diseases that result from inherited variations in genes acting together with environmental factors (Fig. 12.6, *B*). These disorders run in families but do not show the same inherited characteristics as the single gene mutation conditions. Heart disease, diabetes, and most cancers are examples of such disorders.[5]

Many diseases can also be caused by rare hereditary mutations in a single gene. In these cases, genetic mutations that cause or strongly predispose a person to these diseases run in a family. These mutations can significantly increase each family member's risk for developing the disease. One example is breast cancer, in which inheritance of a mutated *BRCA1* or *BRCA2* gene confers significant risk for developing the disease.

Epigenetics. Epigenetics is the study of inheritable changes in gene expression that do not involve changes in the DNA sequence. There is a change in phenotype without a change in genotype. Epigenetic modifications define how the information in genes is expressed and used by cells.

Epigenetics influences the way cells terminally differentiate to become different types of cells (e.g., skin, liver) or result in disease. Epigenetic changes occur regularly and can be influenced by age, the environment, exercise, diet, and disease. Identical twins, who have the same genetic makeup, do not always develop the same diseases or at the same rate. Twins share the same genes, but their environments become different as they age. This unique aspect of twins makes them an excellent model for understanding how genes and the environment contribute to certain traits, especially complex behaviors and diseases.[6]

Chromosome Disorders. *Chromosome disorders* are caused by structural changes within chromosomes or by an excess or deficiency of the genes that are found on chromosomes. For example, an extra copy of chromosome 21 causes Down syndrome (called *trisomy 21*), so there are 3 copies of this chromosome instead of 2. In Down syndrome, there is no individual abnormal gene on the chromosome.

Chronic myelocytic leukemia can be caused by a chromosomal translocation, in which portions of 2 chromosomes (chromosomes 9 and 22) are exchanged. This translocation is called the *Philadelphia chromosome.*

Throughout the book, genetic disorders are highlighted in Genetics in Clinical Practice boxes, Genetic Risk Alert boxes

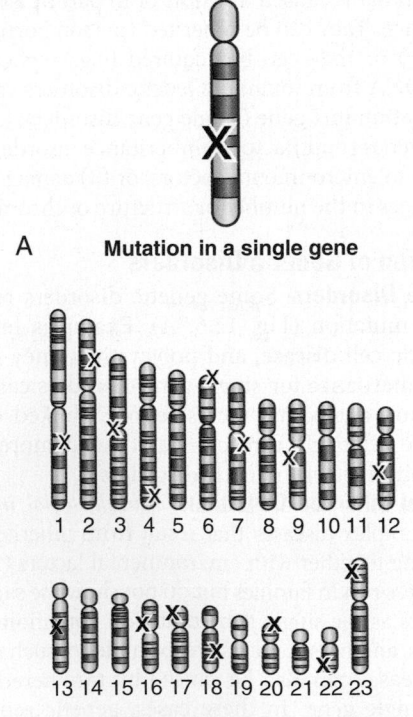

A   **Mutation in a single gene**

1 2 3 4 5 6 7 8 9 10 11 12

13 14 15 16 17 18 19 20 21 22 23

B   **Mutations in multiple genes**

FIG. 12.6 A, Genetic disorders can be caused by a mutation in a single gene (e.g., sickle cell disease, cystic fibrosis, hemophilia). **B,** Most genetic disorders are multifactorial genetic disorders caused by a combination of mutations in multiple genes, often interacting with environmental factors. Examples include cancer, diabetes, obesity, and hypertension.

(in the assessment chapters), and Genetic Links content (in the management chapters).

GENETICS IN CLINICAL PRACTICE

Genetics in Clinical Practice Boxes Throughout Book

Genetic Disorder	Chapter	Page
α_1-Antitrypsin (AAT) Deficiency	28	561
Alzheimer's Disease (AD)	59	1387
Ankylosing Spondylitis	64	1517
Breast Cancer	51	1195
Cystic Fibrosis (CF)	28	577
Duchenne and Becker Muscular Dystrophy (MD)	63	1484
Familial Adenomatous Polyposis (FAP)	42	948
Familial Hypercholesterolemia	33	701
Genetic Information Nondiscrimination Act (GINA)	12	181
Hemochromatosis	30	620
Hemophilia A and B	30	626
Hereditary Nonpolyposis Colorectal Cancer (HNPCC) or Lynch Syndrome	42	949
Huntington's Disease (HD)	58	1380
Ovarian Cancer	53	1244
Polycystic Kidney Disease (PKD)	45	1042
Sickle Cell Disease	30	616
Types 1 and 2 Diabetes and MODY	48	1110

GENETIC SCREENING AND TESTING

Genetic screening is the first level of detection. It is offered to general or targeted populations who are at risk for a disorder but do not have symptoms or have a family history of the disorder. An example is screening for α-fetoprotein, which is offered to pregnant women to detect fetal anomalies. Community groups, hospitals, or governmental agencies may offer screenings.

Genetic testing is focused on persons and families for a specific reason. Symptoms or family history may show there is increased risk for a specific condition. Testing procedures analyze chromosomes, genes, or any gene product that can determine whether a mutation or predisposition to a condition exists. A person's blood, skin, hair, or saliva can be used to obtain samples for genetic testing. Tissues and cells can be obtained prenatally. In most cases, insurance companies do not cover the cost of genetic testing.

Genetic testing has been very useful in health care (Table 12.3). Genetic tests have been developed for more than 2000 diseases. Most tests assess single genes and are used to diagnose genetic disorders, such as cystic fibrosis or Duchenne muscular dystrophy.[7] Some genetic tests look at rare inherited mutations of otherwise protective genes, such as *BRCA1* and *BRCA2*, which are responsible for some types of hereditary breast and ovarian cancers.[8]

Test results are used to assess risk or diagnose a disorder, an important step in providing ongoing care for the person and family. It is important to identify people at high risk for conditions that may be preventable. For example, persons who have inherited a gene for familial adenomatous polyposis (FAP) need ongoing monitoring.[8] FAP is discussed in Chapter 42 on p. 948.

Genetic testing may raise ethical questions. People considering genetic testing should receive counseling about the various issues. They should be aware that test results in their medical records might not be private and there is the potential for discrimination by employers and insurance companies. To protect people from discrimination by employers and health insurance companies, the federal government passed the Genetic Information Nondiscrimination Act (GINA) in 2008.

GENETICS IN CLINICAL PRACTICE

Genetic Information Nondiscrimination Act (GINA)

The Genetic Information Nondiscrimination Act (GINA) is a federal law that prohibits discrimination in health care coverage and employment based on genetic information. Genetic information is any data about a person's genetic tests, family members' genetic tests, and family history of a genetic disease or disorder.

- Addresses concerns about discrimination that might prevent people from seeking genetic tests
- Enables people to take part in research studies without fear that their DNA information may be used against them in the workplace or prevent them from getting health insurance
- Prevents health insurers from denying health insurance coverage and discriminating against a person based solely on genetic or family history information
- Prevents health insurers from asking that a person have a genetic test
- Prohibits most employers from using genetic information for hiring, firing, or promotion decisions and for any decisions about terms of employment
- Protection does not extend to life insurance, disability insurance, and long-term care insurance

For more information see:

- www.genome.gov/Pages/PolicyEthics/GeneticDiscrimination/GINAInfoDoc.pdf.
- Frequently Asked Questions about GINA at *www.dol.gov/sites/default/files/ebsa/about-ebsa/our-activities/resource-center/faqs/gina.pdf*.

If a person has genetic testing, it may uncover information that may affect a family member who was not tested. These persons may not have taken part in the decision-making process to undergo testing. Similarly, if a whole family is tested, the results may show that a biologic relationship is not what the family believed it to be. For more information about genetic testing, see www.cdc.gov/genomics/gtesting/index.htm.

Interpreting Genetic Test Results

The results of genetic tests are not always straightforward, which often makes them challenging to interpret and explain. When interpreting test results, HCPs need to consider the reason the test was done, pretest counseling provided, the person's medical history, the family history, and the type of genetic test.[8]

A *positive test* result means that the laboratory found a change in a particular gene, chromosome, or protein that was being tested. Depending on the purpose of the test, this result may confirm a diagnosis (e.g., Huntington's disease), show that a person is a carrier of a particular genetic mutation (e.g., cystic fibrosis), identify an increased risk for developing a disease (e.g., breast cancer), or suggest a need for further testing. A positive result of a predictive or presymptomatic genetic test usually cannot establish the absolute risk for developing a disorder. A positive test also cannot predict the course or severity of a condition.

In some situations, it is difficult to interpret a positive result because some people who have the genetic mutation never develop the disease. For example, having the *apolipoprotein E-4 (Apo E-4)* allele increases the risk for developing Alzheimer's disease. However, many people who test positive for *Apo E-4* never develop Alzheimer's disease (see Chapter 59).

A *negative test* result means that the laboratory did not find an altered form of the gene, chromosome, or protein under consideration. This result generally means a person is not affected by a particular disorder, is not a carrier of a specific genetic mutation, or does not have increased risk for developing a certain disease. It is possible that the test missed a disease-causing genetic alteration. Many tests cannot detect all the genetic changes that cause a particular disorder. Further testing may be needed to confirm a negative result.

Direct-to-Consumer Genetic Tests

Direct-to-consumer genetic tests are marketed directly to people (consumers) via television, print advertisements, or the Internet. The test kit is mailed to the person instead of being ordered through an HCP's office. The test typically involves collecting a DNA sample at home, often by swabbing the inside of the cheek, and mailing the sample back to the laboratory. In some cases, the person must visit a health clinic to have blood drawn. People are notified of their results by mail, over the telephone, or online. In some cases, a genetics counselor or other HCP is available to explain the results and answer questions.

ETHICAL/LEGAL DILEMMAS

Genetic Testing

Situation

A 30-yr-old woman informs you that she is 3 months pregnant. She has 2 children with her current husband. This pregnancy was unplanned, and her youngest child has cystic fibrosis (CF). She expresses concern about the chance of having another child with CF. She mentions that she would like to have genetic testing on her fetus. Her husband asks you what the chance is of having another child with CF.

Ethical/Legal Points for Consideration

- With genetic testing, the patient and her family can find out whether their child will have CF. The woman and her husband can then make an informed decision.
- Genetic counseling is recommended before and after genetic testing because of the complexity of the information and the emotional issues involved with implications and options.
- Knowing that CF is an autosomal recessive condition, you can use Punnett squares (Fig. 12.9) or a family pedigree (Figs. 12.4 and 12.5) to show the woman and her husband the probability of having another child with CF.
- Be mindful of the privacy and confidentiality of genetic information and the potential conflict between 1 person's right to privacy and another person's right to information.

Discussion Questions

1. What information would you give the patient and her husband about genetic testing for them to make an informed decision?
2. What options are available for this couple?
3. How would you help this couple as they are considering ending the pregnancy if the results of the genetic testing reveal that the fetus will have CF?

TABLE 12.3 Use of Genetic Tests

Type of Test	Description	Examples
Carrier screening	• Can be used to identify unaffected persons who carry 1 copy of a gene • Offered to persons who have a family history of a genetic disorder and to those in ethnic groups with an increased risk for specific genetic conditions • If both parents are tested, the test can provide information about a couple's risk for having a child with a genetic condition	• Cystic fibrosis • Sickle cell disease • Hemophilia
Diagnostic testing	• Used to diagnose, rule out, or confirm a specific genetic or chromosomal condition • Used to confirm findings when patient's signs and symptoms suggest a genetic disorder • Can be done at any time during a person's life but is not available for all genes or all genetic conditions	• Cystic fibrosis • Sickle cell disease • Polycystic kidney disease • Hemophilia • Familial hypercholesterolemia
Forensic testing	• Done to identify a person for legal purposes	• Identify crime or victims in catastrophic situations • Rule out or implicate a crime suspect
Newborn screening	• Most widespread use of genetic testing • Early intervention to treat these disorders can eliminate or reduce symptoms that may otherwise cause a lifetime of disability	• Phenylketonuria • Congenital hypothyroidism • Cystic fibrosis
Parental testing	• Establish biologic relationships between people	• Paternity testing
Pharmacogenomic testing	• Identifies genetic variations that influence a person's response to drugs • Results provide information to help choose drug therapy that is best for the person	• Warfarin (Coumadin) dose
Predictive testing	• Can identify mutations that increase a person's risk for developing disorders • If results are positive, person can have prophylactic measures (e.g., mastectomy, oophorectomy) to prevent development of cancer	• Breast cancer • Ovarian cancer
Preimplantation genetic diagnosis (PGD)	• Fertilized embryos tested before implantation and pregnancy • Allows embryos free of particular disorders to be placed into the uterus • Embryos that test positive for genetic disorders can be destroyed	• For persons known to have or be a carrier for a genetic mutation (e.g., Huntington's disease)
Prenatal diagnostic testing	• Fluid obtained from amniocentesis or tissue from chorionic villus used to obtain fetal cells. Can obtain fetal samples from mother's blood • Used to detect changes in genes or chromosomes of fetus before birth • Type of testing offered to a couple with an increased risk for having a baby with a genetic or chromosomal disorder • Can decrease a couple's uncertainty or help them decide whether to end a pregnancy	• Down syndrome • Other genetic alterations in fetuses
Presymptomatic testing	• Used to detect genetic mutations associated with disorders that appear later in life • Can be helpful to people who have a family member with a genetic disorder but who have no features of the disorder themselves at the time of testing • Results can provide information about a person's risk for developing a specific disorder and help with making decisions about treatment	• Huntington's disease • Adult polycystic kidney disease • Hemochromatosis • Familial adenomatous polyposis • Hereditary nonpolyposis colorectal cancer syndrome

Direct-to-consumer genetic tests have significant risks and limitations. People may want their genetic information, but they may not understand what it means. They are vulnerable to being misled by the results of unproven or invalid tests. Without guidance from an HCP, they may make important decisions about disease treatment or prevention based on inaccurate, incomplete, or misunderstood information about their health. People may experience an invasion of genetic privacy if testing companies use their genetic information in an unauthorized way. When people are considering using these kinds of genetic tests, nurses should provide education and suggest they discuss the issue with their HCP or a genetics counselor. Teaching related to genetic testing is outlined in Table 12.4.

Genetic Technology

DNA Fingerprinting. DNA (genetic) fingerprinting begins by extracting DNA from the cells in a sample of blood, saliva, semen, or other appropriate fluid or tissue. *Polymerase chain reaction (PCR)* is a quick, easy method to provide unlimited copies of a DNA or RNA sequence using only a small amount of sample. PCR involves the artificial replication of a DNA or RNA sequence. The DNA or RNA strands can be separated to form new templates that are used for replication.

PCR is a key element in *genetic fingerprinting*. It is an essential technique to finding mutations in genes. It is used in forensic medicine to identify the DNA of criminal suspects by using samples from blood, hair, saliva, and semen. It has been used to free persons who are wrongly incarcerated. PCR is used in paternity testing and as a confirmatory test in human immunodeficiency virus (HIV) testing. This is especially important when an infant of a mother who is HIV-antibody positive tests HIV positive. In this situation, PCR will determine if the baby is infected with HIV or if the antibodies are from the mother.

DNA Microarray (DNA Chip). Although all a person's somatic cells have identical genetic material, the same genes are not active in every cell. Studying which genes are active and which

TABLE 12.4 Patient & Family Teaching
Genetic Testing

Genetic Counselors

- People who are considering genetic testing should meet with a genetics counselor who is specially trained in medical genetics and counseling.
- Counseling is advised to help you understand the purpose of genetic testing, considerations before testing, and the emotional and medical impact of the test results.
- Genetics counseling can help you understand the pros and cons of genetic testing before making a decision to undergo a genetic test.

General Information

The following includes some important general information about genetic testing:

- Genetic testing can be expensive and may not be included in your medical insurance policy.
- Genetic testing may determine whether you are predisposed to developing an inherited disease.
- A particular genetic test will only tell you whether there is a specific genetic variant or mutation. Positive tests do not mean you will develop that disease or disorder. Neither can the results tell you when you will develop the disease.
- If a genetic test shows a genetic predisposition to an inherited disorder, the news can be depressing.
- Knowledge of a genetic predisposition to a disease may give you the motivation to take preventive measures (e.g., taking drugs for familial hypercholesterolemia) or make lifestyle changes to lower the risk for a disease (e.g., exercising to decrease the risk for type 2 diabetes).
- If a genetic test reveals you are at risk for a specific genetic disorder, there is the chance that other family members may be at risk.
- If a genetic test reveals you are at risk for developing an inherited disease, whether you decide to share that information with family members is a personal and an ethical decision that you will have to make.
- Genetic testing may provide important information that you can use when making decisions about having children.

are inactive in different cell types helps to understand (1) how these cells function normally and (2) how they are affected when various genes do not perform properly.

Gene expression profiling uses a technology called *DNA microarrays* (DNA chips). DNA chips can identify changes in gene sequences or if certain genes are turned off in cells and tissues. It can serve as a diagnostic test or determine if certain medications might have a better therapeutic effect for certain people. The chip is a small glass plate enclosed in plastic. The surface of each chip has thousands of short, synthetic, single-stranded DNA sequences. Together they represent the normal gene, as well as known variations of the gene.

To determine if a mutation is present for a specific disease, a sample of DNA from the blood of the person with suspected disease and a control sample, which does not have a mutation in the gene, are obtained. The DNA in the samples is separated into single-stranded molecules and then cut into small fragments. The fragments are labeled using fluorescent dye. Different colors are used to identify the control and test samples. Both sets are inserted into the chip, where they bind to the synthetic DNA on the chip. If the person does not have a mutation for the gene, both samples will bind to the normal sequences on the chip. If a mutation is present, the person's DNA will bind to the sequence on the chip that represents the mutated DNA.

Genome-Wide Association Study (GWAS)

Genome-wide association study (GWAS) is an approach that involves rapidly scanning complete sets of DNA, or genomes, of many people to find genetic variations associated with the development or progression of a particular disease.

Until recently, researchers looked at single genes and the proteins that they encoded. With GWAS, researchers study large numbers of genes and proteins, including how they act and interact. This gives a more complete picture of what goes on in a person. After the genetic associations are found, researchers may be able to learn how to stop or jump-start genes on demand, change the course of a disease, or prevent it from ever happening. GWAS is particularly useful in finding genetic variations that contribute to multifactorial inherited disorders, such as cancer and heart disease.

To carry out a GWAS, researchers use 2 groups of people: those with the disease and similar people without the disease. Each person's complete set of DNA, or genome, is purified from the blood or cells, placed on tiny chips, and scanned on automated laboratory machines. The machines quickly survey each person's genome for strategically selected markers of genetic variation.

If certain genetic variations are significantly more common in people with the disease compared to people without the disease, the variations are said to be "associated" with the disease. The associated genetic variations can serve as powerful pointers to the region of the human genome where the disease-causing problem exists.

The potential impact of GWAS is substantial, since it lays the groundwork for personalized medicine. This changes the "1-size-fits-all" approach to health care. It provides a mechanism for providing more individualized plans of care. The information will help the HCP tailor prevention programs.

PHARMACOGENOMICS AND PHARMACOGENETICS

Patients vary widely in their response to drugs. Although the reasons for this are complex, genetic factors may account for a large percentage of individual variability. **Pharmacogenomics** looks at how drugs affect and interact with the genome and output expression. Pharmacogenomics allows for the identification of variations in multiple genes that affect drug response. **Pharmacogenetics** is the study of variable drug responses, including adverse events from differences in inheritable genes. These terms are often used interchangeably when describing the relationship between pharmacology and genetic variability in determining a person's response to drugs. Pharmacogenetics has a narrower focus than pharmacogenomics.[9]

Pharmacogenetic and pharmacogenomic studies could lead to the development of drugs that can be tailor-made or adapted to each person's particular genetic makeup. This will make it possible to have personalized medicine by choosing the right drug and the right dose for the right person.[8] HCPs are starting to use pharmacogenomic information to prescribe drugs. Examples are shown in Table 12.5.

One important area of study has focused on the hepatic cytochrome P450 (CYP450) enzyme system, which is responsible for oxidizing many drugs and chemicals.[8] The enzymes in this system share certain amino acid sequences. Each is coded by a separate gene. People with a less active form of the enzyme (who metabolize the drug slowly) may get too much of the drug. People with a more active form of the enzyme (who metabolize

TABLE 12.5 Examples of Pharmacogenetics

Drug	Role of Pharmacogenetics
abacavir (Ziagen)	• Some people are at greater risk for serious allergic reactions when first starting treatment with this drug. • Genetic testing for *HLA-B*5701* before taking the drug can identify those who carry a genetic marker that is associated with life-threatening hypersensitivity reactions.
clopidogrel (Plavix)	• For clopidogrel to work, cytochrome P450 enzymes in the liver (particularly CYP2C19) must convert the drug to its active form. • About 2% to 14% of the population are poor metabolizers of the drug. These patients may not receive the full benefits of the drug. • Genetic tests are available to identify genetic differences in CYP2C19 function.
crizotinib (Xalkori)	• Used to treat patients with late-stage, non–small cell lung cancers (NSCLCs) who express the abnormal anaplastic lymphoma kinase *(ALK)* gene. • *ALK* gene abnormality causes cancer development and growth. • Blocks certain proteins called *kinases,* including the protein made by the abnormal *ALK* gene. • Drug was approved for use with a companion genetic diagnostic test that determines whether a patient with NSCLC has the abnormal *ALK* gene.
trastuzumab (Herceptin)	• In breast cancer, drug works only for women whose tumors have genes that lead to the overproduction of a protein called HER-2. • Drug is a monoclonal antibody to HER-2. After the antibody attaches to the antigen, it kills the cells. • Genetic testing provides information on which women are good candidates for treatment with drug. • Drug does not work for women whose tumor genes do not express HER-2.
vemurafenib (Zelboraf)	• Approved for patients with late-stage (metastatic) or unresectable melanoma. • Indicated for the treatment of patients with melanoma whose tumors express a gene mutation called *BRAF V600E.* • To be considered for treatment, patients must first have genetic testing to determine whether melanoma cells have the *BRAF V600E* mutation.
warfarin (Coumadin) (see Fig. 12.7)	• Genetic variants in the genes *VKORC1* and cytochrome P450 2C9 *(CYP2C9)* have a significant impact on people's sensitivity to warfarin (Fig. 12.7). • Persons with particular variations in these genes need a lower warfarin dose to maintain therapeutic levels of anticoagulation. • Persons with other variations need higher doses. • Together, these genetic variations explain about 50% of the required dose difference between persons. • Testing for *CYP2C9* and *VKORC1* genotype information can assist in choosing the starting dose.

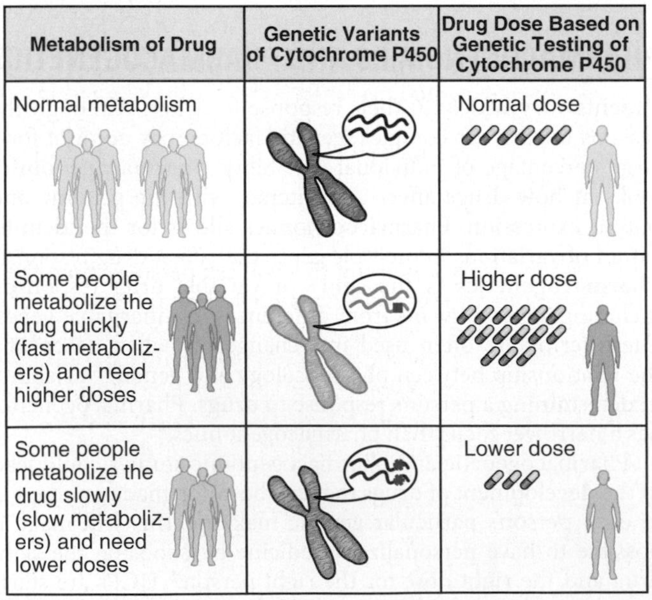

Metabolism of Drug	Genetic Variants of Cytochrome P450	Drug Dose Based on Genetic Testing of Cytochrome P450
Normal metabolism		Normal dose
Some people metabolize the drug quickly (fast metabolizers) and need higher doses		Higher dose
Some people metabolize the drug slowly (slow metabolizers) and need lower doses		Lower dose

FIG. 12.7 People respond differently to the drug warfarin (Coumadin). The diversity of responses is partially due to genetic variants in 1 of the cytochrome *P450* genes.

the drug quickly) may get too little of the drug. It may appear that the medication is not effective. These persons may need more frequent dosing. So, pharmacogenomic testing can help HCPs in prescribing the right dose of medicine based on a patient's particular genetic makeup (Fig. 12.7).

GENE THERAPY

Gene therapy is an investigational technique used to treat the underlying cause of a disease. Gene therapy may be used to supply a missing gene, avoid the missing gene's role, or enhance treatment of a disease. The goal is to provide a normally functioning gene to a person with a pathogenic gene variant. A carrier molecule called a *vector* must be used to deliver the therapeutic gene to the person's target cells.[10] Currently, the most common vector is a virus that has been genetically altered to carry normal human DNA.[11] The vector can be injected or given intravenously directly into specific tissue. The vector unloads its genetic material containing the therapeutic human gene into the target cell. If the treatment is successful, the new gene will make a functional protein and restore the target cell to a normal state. A diagram of gene therapy is shown in Fig. 12.8.

Although gene therapy is a promising treatment for a number of diseases (including inherited disorders, some types of cancer, certain viral infections), the technique is still under study. In 2017 the FDA approved the first 2 gene therapies. Tisagenlecleucel (Kymriah) is used to treat certain pediatric and young adult patients with a form of acute lymphoblastic leukemia. The other gene therapy treats vision loss from a congenital retinal degenerative disorder. The cost of that 1-time gene therapy is currently $850,000.[12]

STEM CELL THERAPY

Stem cells are the subject of much discussion because they may offer treatment for many diseases.[8] The use of stem cells may

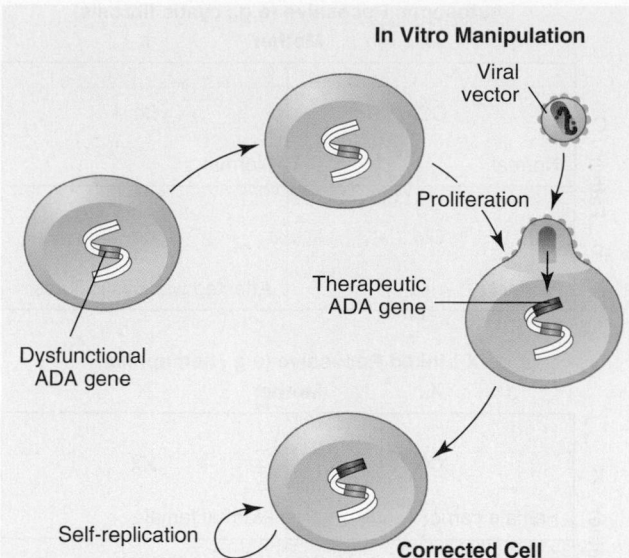

In Vitro Manipulation

Viral vector

Proliferation

Therapeutic ADA gene

Dysfunctional ADA gene

Self-replication

Corrected Cell

FIG. 12.8 Gene therapy for adenosine deaminase *(ADA)* deficiency tries to correct this immunodeficiency state. The viral vector containing the therapeutic ADA gene is inserted into the patient's lymphocytes. These cells can then make the ADA enzyme.

allow for the regeneration of lost tissue and restoration of function in various diseases.

Stem cells are unspecialized cells in the body that have the ability to (1) remain in their unspecialized state and divide or (2) differentiate and develop into specialized cells. Stem cells can be derived from human embryos or adult somatic tissues. Stem cells can be totipotent, pluripotent, multipotent, or unipotent. Totipotent cells can produce all the cell types of the developing organism. Pluripotent cells can make any body cell because they make all cells of the embryo. Multipotent cells only make cells within a specific germ layer. Unipotent cells make a single cell type.

Adult stem cells are undifferentiated cells that are found in small numbers in many organs and tissues, including brain, bone marrow, peripheral blood, blood vessels, skeletal muscle, skin, teeth, heart, GI tract, liver, ovarian epithelium, and testes. The primary roles of adult stem cells are to maintain and repair the tissues in which they are found. They are usually thought of as multipotent cells, giving rise to a closely related family of cells within the tissue. For example, skin stem cells produce new skin cells. Hematopoietic stem cells found within the bone marrow can form all the various blood cells. These cells are prolific by design.

Stems cells are used to treat persons with many different disorders, including severe burns and orthopedic conditions that require bone grafting. For the past 20 years, hematopoietic stem cell transplantation has been a standard for treatment for hematologic cancers and bone marrow failure (see Chapter 15). Medical researchers are investigating the use of stem cells to repair or replace damaged body tissues, similar to whole organ transplants.

❖ NURSING MANAGEMENT: GENETICS AND GENOMICS

You need to understand genetics and genomics to assist persons and families seeking information and making decisions related to genetic issues.[13] By understanding the profound influence that genetics has on health and illness, you can aid the patient and family in making critical decisions related to genetic issues, such as genetic testing. You can facilitate access to resources and provide education in response to questions.

You will collaborate with other health care team members, including genetics nurses and genetics counselors. A genetics nurse is a licensed professional nurse with specialized education and training in genetics. Nurses with *GCN* after their names are baccalaureate-prepared licensed registered nurses who have received specialty credentialing as a Genetic Clinical Nurse (GCN). Nurses with *APNG* after their names are registered nurses with a master's degree who have received specialty credentialing as an Advanced Practice Nurse in Genetics (APNG).

The specialized knowledge and counseling skills of a genetics nurse or genetics counselor are often important when genetic testing is considered. Genetic testing may raise many emotional issues. Knowledge of carrier status of a genetic disorder may influence a person's career, marriage, and childbearing decisions. It may also affect family members, as they contemplate potentially serious life and health care issues.

For example, how should a wife deal with a husband who has tested positive for Huntington's disease and shows early signs of cognitive impairment? Should their children be tested for the disease? Consider the situation of a woman who has a family history of breast cancer and is now diagnosed with breast cancer. She asks whether she and her teenage daughters should have *BRCA* testing. What do you tell her?

Genetic testing raises ethical questions. Who should know the results of a genetic test? Who should protect the privacy of test results and prevent persons from discrimination? People may be reluctant to share or disclose information about family history or genetic test results. They fear they are vulnerable to discrimination based on their DNA. As a nurse, you need to understand how different health care policies relate to genetic testing. Discuss how the Genetic Information Nondiscrimination Act (GINA) protects persons from discrimination by employers and health care insurance companies (see Genetics in Clinical Practice Box on p. 181).[14]

◆ Nursing Assessment: Family History

As a nurse, it is very important that you ask persons about their family history and identify and assess inheritance patterns by constructing a family pedigree (Figs. 12.4 and 12.5). The family health history is a written or graphic record of the diseases and health conditions present in one's family (see Chapter 3). A pedigree is a graphic representation of the family history. The family history and pedigree should include a minimum of 3 generations.

To help people record information about their family history, the Centers for Disease Control and Prevention (CDC) has collaborated with the U.S. Surgeon General and other federal agencies to develop a Web-based tool called My Family Health Portrait (*https://phgkb.cdc.gov/FHH/html/index.html*). Other Web-based programs are available to help create pedigree diagrams based on the information entered. Or, you can draw a pedigree by hand.

When constructing the pedigree, start with the proband, or person being interviewed. Identify that person with an arrow. For each family member, document date of birth, any medical illnesses or health conditions and the age when diagnosed, and age and cause of death, if the person is deceased. Comment on ancestors' racial and ethnic information, information that is unknown, and presence of consanguinity. After recording the family history or pedigree, review the information to identify key features that may increase a person's risk for genetic-related diseases. These include:

- Disease in more than 1 close relative
- Disease that does not usually affect a certain gender (e.g., breast cancer in a male)
- Disease that occurs at an earlier age than expected (e.g., myocardial infarction before age 35)
- Certain combinations of diseases within a family (e.g., breast and ovarian cancer, heart disease, and diabetes)

If 1 or more of these features are identified, the family history may hold important clues about a person's risk for a genetic disease. These persons may benefit from further clinical investigation, screening, and diagnostic testing. As a nurse, you may refer these persons to a specialist for information about the benefits and risks of genetic screening and testing.

Genetic Risk Alert boxes in the assessment chapters of this book highlight persons' risks related to genetic diseases and disorders. You can use the information in these boxes to assess the family history.

As a nurse, you can support the person and family by providing education and reinforcing the information they receive throughout the process. You can use the family history, pedigree, and Punnett squares (Fig. 12.9) to explain the risk for inheritable disease. When a diagnosis is confirmed, you can discuss health promotion activities. People with multifactorial disorders may benefit from lifestyle modification that addresses unhealthy behaviors (e.g., smoking, poor eating habits). You can help the person and family understand how evidence-based guidelines are used for monitoring, screening, and ongoing follow-up. For example, it is important to monitor cholesterol levels in a person with a family history of familial hypercholesterolemia. Throughout this process, maintain the person's confidentiality and respect his or her values and beliefs.

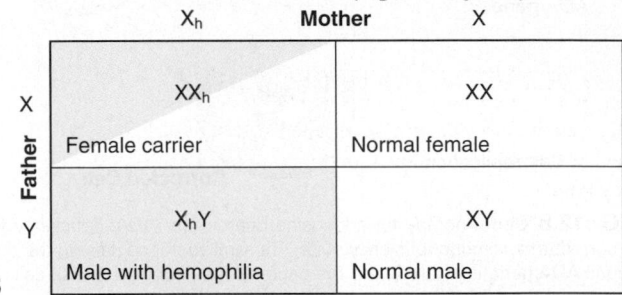

FIG. 12.9 Punnett squares illustrate inheritance possibilities. **A,** If the mother and father are both carriers for cystic fibrosis, there is a 25% chance that offspring will have cystic fibrosis. **B,** If the mother is a carrier for the hemophilia gene and the father has a normal genotype, there is a 50% chance that any male offspring will have hemophilia. There is a 50% chance that any female offspring will be a carrier. **C,** If the mother has a normal genotype and the father has Huntington's disease, there is a 50% chance that offspring will have the disease.

BRIDGE TO NCLEX EXAMINATION

The number of the question corresponds to the same-numbered outcome at the beginning of the chapter.

1. If a person is heterozygous for a given gene, it means that the person
   a. is a carrier for a genetic disorder.
   b. is affected by the genetic disorder.
   c. has 2 identical alleles for the gene.
   d. has 2 different alleles for the gene.

2. Common causes of genetic mutations include (select all that apply)
   a. DNA damage from toxins.
   b. DNA damage from UV radiation.
   c. inheritance of altered genes from father.
   d. inheritance of altered genes from mother.
   e. inheritance of somatic mutations from either parent.

3. A father who has an X-linked recessive disorder and a wife with a normal genotype will
   a. pass the carrier state to all his children.
   b. pass the carrier state to his male children.
   c. pass the carrier state to his female children.
   d. not pass on the genetic mutation to any of his children.

4. What characterizes multifactorial genetic disorders?
   a. Often caused by single gene alterations
   b. Genetic testing available for most disorders
   c. Many family members report having the disorder
   d. Caused by complex interactions of genetic and environmental factors

5. If a person tests positive for a genetic mutation, it means *(select all that apply)*
   a. the laboratory found an alteration in a gene.
   b. the person is predisposed to develop a genetic disease.
   c. there is the chance other family members may be at risk.
   d. the person will develop the disease at some point in time.
   e. the person should not have any children or any more children.

6. What role does pharmacogenomics have in health care?
   a. It can assess individual variability to many drugs.
   b. It can be used to assess the effectiveness of a drug.
   c. It provides important assessment data for gene therapy.
   d. It can assess the variability of drug responses due to single genes.

7. A couple who recently had a son with hemophilia A is consulting with a nurse. They want to know if their next child will have hemophilia A. The nurse can tell the parents that if their child is a
   a. boy, he will have hemophilia A.
   b. boy, he will be a carrier of hemophilia A.
   c. girl, she will be a carrier of hemophilia A.
   d. girl, there is a 50% chance she will be a carrier of hemophilia A.

1. d, 2. a, b, c, d, 3. c, 4. d, 5. a, c, 6. d, 7. d

For rationales to these answers and even more NCLEX review questions, visit *http://evolve.elsevier.com/Lewis/medsurg.*

ⓔ EVOLVE WEBSITE/RESOURCES LIST

http://evolve.elsevier.com/Lewis/medsurg
Review Questions (Online Only)
Key Points
Answer Key for Questions
  • Rationales for Bridge to NCLEX Examination Questions
Conceptual Care Map Creator
Audio Glossary
Content Updates

REFERENCES

1. National Human Genome Research Institute: Your guide to understanding genetic conditions. Retrieved from *www.ghr.nlm.nih.gov/primer/hgp/genome.*
2. National Human Genome Research Institute: An animation of the interactive timeline found on genome. Retrieved from *www.unlockinglifescode.org/timeline?tid=4.*
3. U.S. National Library of Medicine: Different ways genetic conditions can be inherited. Retrieved from *www.ghr.nlm.nih.gov/primer/inheritance/inheritancepatterns.*
4. U.S. Department of Energy: Human Genome Project information. Retrieved from *www.ornl.gov.*
5. National Center for Biotechnology Information: Genes and diseases. Retrieved from *www.ncbi.nlm.nih.gov/books/NBK22183.*
6. Schwab TL, Hogenson TL: Effect of epigenetic differences in identical twins, *Handbook of Nutrition, Diet, and Epigenetics,* 1, 2017.
7. National Center for Biotechnology Information: Gene tests. Retrieved from *www.ncbi.nlm.nih.gov/sites/GeneTests.*
8. Kasper CE, Schneidereith TA, Lashley FR: *Lashley's essentials of clinical genetics in nursing practice,* ed 2, New York, 2017, Springer.
9. Singh DB: Pharmacogenomics: Clinical perspective, strategies, and challenges. In *Translational bioinformatics and its application,* Dordrecht, 2017, Springer.
10. U.S. National Library of Medicine: Gene therapy. Retrieved from *www.ghr.nlm.nih.gov/handbook/therapy/genetherapy.*
*11. Lee CS, Bishop ES, Zhang R, et al: Adenovirus-mediated gene delivery: Potential applications for gene and cell-based therapies in the new era of personalized medicine, *Genes Dis* 4:43, 2017.
12. Food and Drug Administration News Release (2017). FDA approves novel gene therapy to treat patients with a rare form of inherited vision loss. Retrieved from *www.fda.gov/NewsEvents/Newsroom/PressAnnouncements/UCM589467.htm?utm_campaign=12192017_PR_FDA%20approves%20first%20gene%20therapy%20treatment&utm_medium=email&utm_source=Eloqua.*
*13. Montgomery S, Brouwer WA, Everett PC, et al Genetics in the clinical setting, *American Nurse Today* 12:10, 2017.
14. International Society of Nurses in Genetics: Position statements: Privacy and confidentiality of genetic information. Retrieved from *www.isong.org/resources/Documents/PS_Privacy_Confidentiality.pdf.*

*Evidence-based information for clinical practice.

Immune Responses and Transplantation

Haley Hoy and Yeow Chye Ng

Compassion is the ultimate expression of your highest self.

Russell Simmons

ℯ http://evolve.elsevier.com/Lewis/medsurg/

CONCEPTUAL FOCUS

Functional Ability

Immunity

Infection

Inflammation

Tissue Integrity

LEARNING OUTCOMES

1. Describe the components and functions of the immune system.
2. Characterize the 5 types of immunoglobulins.
3. Distinguish among the 4 types of hypersensitivity reactions in terms of immunologic mechanisms and resulting alterations.
4. Outline the clinical manifestations and emergency management of a systemic anaphylactic reaction.
5. Describe the assessment and interprofessional care of a patient with chronic allergies.

6. Describe the etiologic factors, clinical manifestations, and treatment modalities of autoimmune diseases.
7. Describe the etiologic factors and categories of immunodeficiency disorders.
8. Explain the relationship between the human leukocyte antigen system and certain diseases.
9. Distinguish among the types of rejections after transplantation.
10. Identify the types and side effects of immunosuppressive therapy.

KEY TERMS

anergy, p. 193
antigen, p. 189
autoimmunity, p. 202
cell-mediated immunity, p. 193

cytokines, p. 191
human leukocyte antigen (HLA), p. 204
humoral immunity, p. 193
hypersensitivity reactions, p. 194

immunocompetence, p. 193
immunodeficiency, p. 203
immunosuppressive therapy, p. 206

Our bodies have several defense mechanisms for protecting ourselves. One of the most complex is the immune response. Immune processes must be functioning properly for the body to defend itself against the presence of foreign substances. This response is critical to maintaining health. Thus many problems occur when the immune response is altered. These problems are closely related to the concepts of inflammation, infection, and tissue integrity. You will find that the care of patients with immune disorders discussed in this chapter will be similar to the care of patients with inflammation (Chapter 11), neutropenia (Chapter 30), and general infection (Chapter 14).

NORMAL IMMUNE RESPONSE

Immunity is the body's ability to resist disease. Immune responses serve the following 3 functions:

1. *Defense:* The body protects against invasions by microorganisms and prevents the development of infection by attacking foreign antigens and pathogens.
2. *Homeostasis:* Damaged cellular substances are digested and removed. Through this mechanism, the body's different cell types stay uniform and unchanged.
3. *Surveillance:* Mutations continually arise but are recognized as foreign cells and destroyed.

TABLE 13.1 Types of Acquired Specific Immunity

Type	Natural	Artificial
Active	Natural contact with antigen through actual infection (e.g., chicken-pox, measles, mumps)	Immunization with antigen (e.g., vaccines for chicken-pox, measles, mumps)
Passive	Transplacental and colostrum transfer from mother to child (e.g., maternal immunoglobulins passed to baby)	Injection of serum with antibodies from 1 person (e.g., injection of hepatitis B immune globulin) to another person who does not have antibodies

Antigens

An antigen is a substance that elicits an immune response. Most antigens are composed of protein. However, other substances such as large polysaccharides, lipoproteins, and nucleic acids can act as antigens. All the body's cells have antigens on their surface that are unique to that person and enable the body to recognize itself. The immune system normally becomes "tolerant" to the body's own molecules. Therefore it is nonresponsive to "self" antigens.

Types of Immunity

We classify immunity as innate or acquired.

Innate Immunity. *Innate immunity* is present at birth. Its primary role is first-line defense against pathogens. This type of immunity involves a nonspecific response, and neutrophils and monocytes are the primary white blood cells (WBCs) involved. Innate immunity is not antigen specific. So, it can respond within minutes to an invading microorganism without prior exposure to that organism.

Acquired Immunity. *Acquired immunity* is the development of immunity, either actively or passively (Table 13.1).

Active Acquired Immunity. *Active acquired immunity* results from the invasion of the body by foreign substances such as microorganisms and the subsequent development of antibodies and sensitized lymphocytes. With each reinvasion of the microorganisms, the body responds more rapidly and vigorously to fight off the invader. Active acquired immunity may result naturally from a disease or artificially through immunization. Because the body makes antibodies, immunity takes time to develop but is long lasting.

Passive Acquired Immunity. In *passive acquired immunity,* the host receives antibodies to an antigen rather than making them. This may take place naturally through the transfer of immunoglobulins across the placental membrane from mother to fetus. Artificial passive acquired immunity occurs through injection with gamma globulin (serum antibodies). The benefit of this immunity is its immediate effect. Unfortunately, passive immunity is short lived because the person does not make the antibodies and memory cells for the antigen.

Lymphoid Organs

The lymphoid system is composed of central (or primary) and peripheral lymphoid organs. The *central lymphoid organs* are the thymus gland and bone marrow. The *peripheral lymphoid organs* are the lymph nodes; tonsils; spleen; and gut-, genital-, bronchial-, and skin-associated lymphoid tissues (Fig. 13.1).

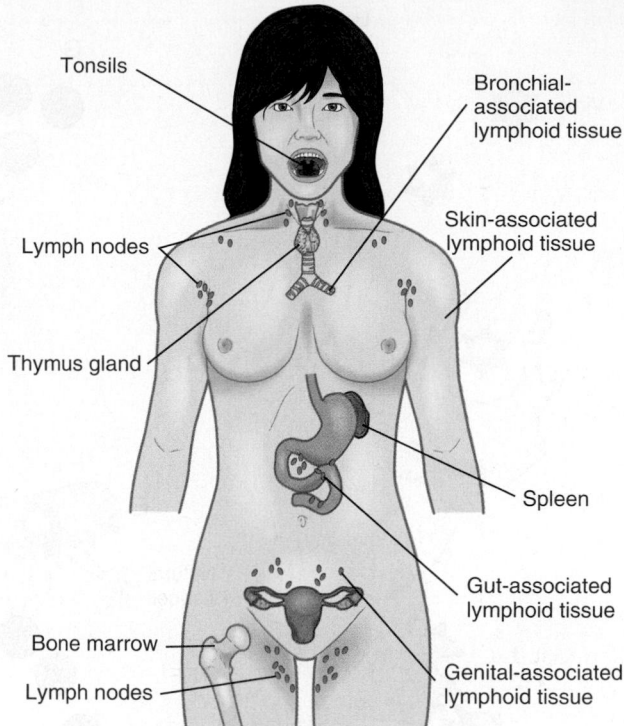

FIG. 13.1 Organs of the immune system.

Lymphocytes are made in the bone marrow. They eventually migrate to the peripheral organs. The thymus is involved in the differentiation and maturation of T lymphocytes and is therefore essential for a cell-mediated immune response. The thymus is its largest during childhood. After puberty, the thymus starts to slowly shrink and become replaced by fat. By age 75, the thymus is little more than fatty tissue and produces few T lymphocytes.

When antigens enter the body, they may be carried by the bloodstream or lymph channels to regional lymph nodes. The antigens interact with B and T lymphocytes and macrophages in the lymph nodes. The 2 major functions of lymph nodes are (1) filtration of foreign material brought to the site and (2) circulation of lymphocytes.

The tonsils are an example of lymphoid tissue. The spleen, a peripheral lymph organ, is important as the primary site for filtering foreign antigens from the blood. Lymphoid tissue is found in the submucosa of the GI (gut-associated), genitourinary (genital-associated), and respiratory (bronchial-associated) tracts. This tissue protects the body from external microorganisms.

The skin-associated lymph tissue consists primarily of lymphocytes and Langerhans' cells (type of dendritic cell) found in the epidermis of skin. When Langerhans' cells are depleted, the skin cannot initiate an immune response. Therefore a delayed hypersensitivity reaction (as determined by skin testing with injected antigens) does not occur.

Cells Involved in Immune Response

Mononuclear Phagocytes. The *mononuclear phagocyte system* includes monocytes in the blood and macrophages found throughout the body. Mononuclear phagocytes have a critical role in the immune system. They are responsible for capturing, processing, and presenting the antigen to the

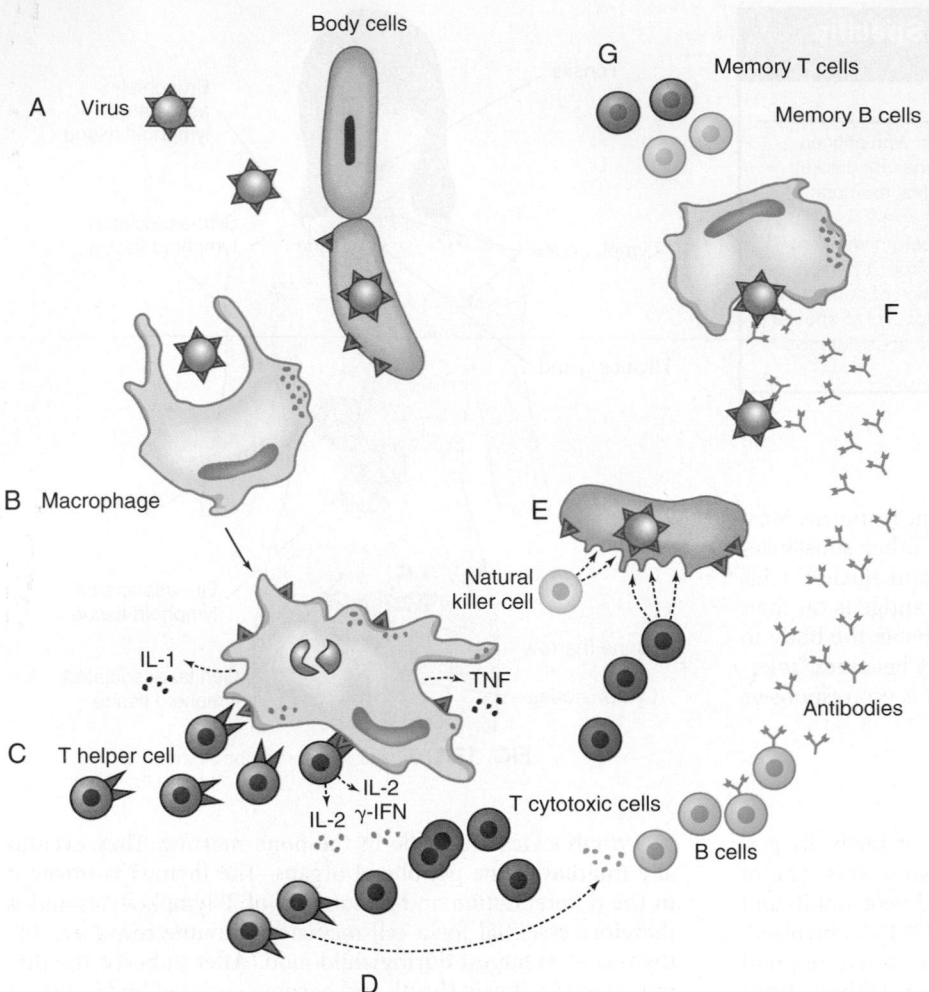

FIG. 13.2 The immune response to a virus. **A,** A virus invades the body through a break in the skin or another portal of entry. The virus must make its way inside a cell to replicate itself. **B,** A macrophage recognizes the antigens on the surface of the virus. The macrophage digests the virus and displays pieces of the virus (antigens) on its surface. **C,** T helper cell recognizes the antigen displayed and binds to the macrophage. This binding stimulates the production of cytokines (interleukin-1 *[IL-1]* and tumor necrosis factor *[TNF]*) by the macrophage and interleukin-2 *(IL-2)* and γ-interferon *(γ-IFN)* by the T cell. These cytokines are intracellular messengers that provide communication among the cells. **D,** IL-2 instructs other T helper cells and T cytotoxic cells to proliferate (multiply). T helper cells release cytokines, causing B cells to multiply and make antibodies. **E,** T cytotoxic cells and natural killer cells destroy infected body cells. **F,** The antibodies bind to the virus and mark it for macrophage destruction. **G,** Memory B and T cells stay behind to respond quickly if the same virus attacks again.

lymphocytes. This stimulates a humoral or cell-mediated immune response. Capturing is accomplished through phagocytosis. The macrophage-bound antigen, which is highly immunogenic, is presented to circulating T or B lymphocytes and thus triggers an immune response (Fig. 13.2).

Lymphocytes. Lymphocytes are made in the bone marrow (Fig. 13.3). They then differentiate into B and T lymphocytes.

B Lymphocytes. In the early research on *B lymphocytes* (bursa-equivalent lymphocytes) in birds, we discovered that they mature under the influence of the bursa of Fabricius, hence the name *B cells.* However, this lymphoid organ does not exist in humans. The bursa-equivalent tissue in humans is the bone marrow. B cells differentiate into *plasma cells* when activated. Plasma cells make antibodies (immunoglobulins) (Table 13.2).

T Lymphocytes. Cells that migrate from the bone marrow to the thymus differentiate into *T lymphocytes* (thymus-dependent cells). The thymus secretes hormones, including thymosin, that stimulate the maturation and differentiation of T lymphocytes. T cells make up 70% to 80% of the circulating lymphocytes. They are primarily responsible for immunity to intracellular viruses, tumor cells, and fungi. T cells can live from a few months to the life span of a person. They account for long-term immunity.

T lymphocytes can be categorized into T cytotoxic and T helper cells. Antigenic characteristics of WBCs can be classified using monoclonal antibodies. These antigens are classified as

clusters of differentiation, or *CD antigens.* We refer to many types of WBCs, especially lymphocytes, by their CD designations. All mature T cells have the CD3 antigen.

T cytotoxic cells. T cytotoxic (CD8) cells are involved in attacking antigens on the cell membrane of foreign pathogens and releasing cytolytic substances that destroy the pathogen. These cells have antigen specificity and are sensitized by exposure to the antigen. Much like B cells, some sensitized T cells do not attack the antigen but remain as memory T cells. As in the humoral immune response, a second exposure to the antigen results in a more intense and rapid cell-mediated immune response.

T helper cells. T helper (CD4) cells are involved in the regulation of cell-mediated immunity and the humoral antibody response. T helper cells differentiate into subsets of cells that make distinct types of cytokines (discussed in a later section). These subsets are called T_H1 cells and T_H2 cells. T_H1 cells stimulate phagocyte-mediated ingestion and killing of microbes, the key component of cell-mediated immunity. T_H2 cells stimulate eosinophil-mediated immunity, which is effective against parasites and is involved in allergic responses.

Natural Killer Cells. Natural killer (NK) cells are involved in cell-mediated immunity. These cells are not T or B cells but are large lymphocytes with many granules in the cytoplasm. NK cells do not need prior sensitization for their generation. These cells are involved in recognition and killing of virus-infected

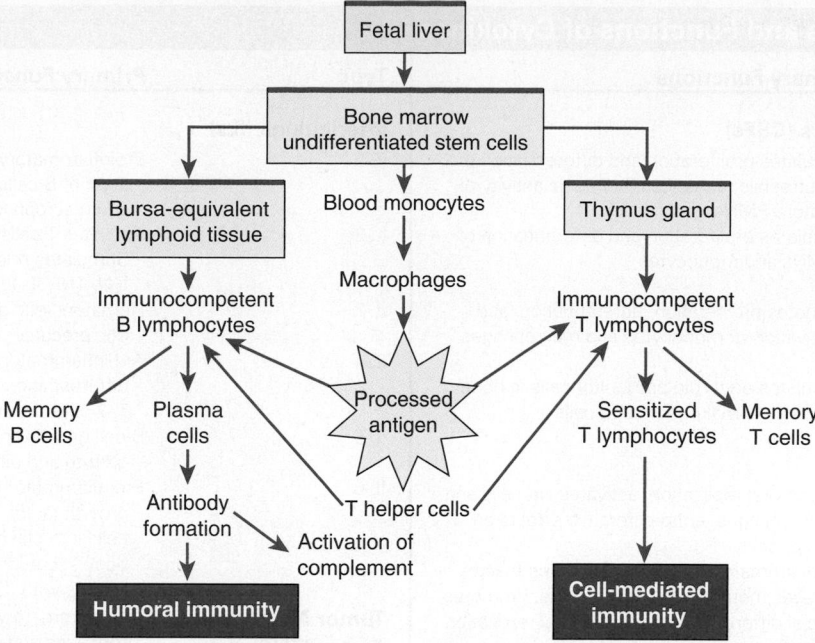

FIG. 13.3 Relationships and functions of macrophages, B lymphocytes, and T lymphocytes in an immune response.

TABLE 13.2	Characteristics of Immunoglobulins		
Class	**Serum Concentration (%)**	**Location**	**Characteristics**
IgG	76	Plasma, interstitial fluid	Only immunoglobulin that crosses placenta Responsible for secondary immune response
IgA	15	Body secretions, including tears, saliva, breast milk, colostrum	Lines mucous membranes and protects body surfaces
IgM	8	Plasma	Responsible for primary immune response Forms antibodies to ABO blood antigens
IgD	1	Plasma	Present on lymphocyte surface Aids in the differentiation of B lymphocytes
IgE	0.002	Plasma, interstitial fluids	Causes symptoms of allergic reactions Fixes to mast cells and basophils Aids in defense against parasitic infections

cells, tumor cells, and transplanted grafts. NK cells have a vital role in immune surveillance for malignant cell changes. We do not fully understand the mechanism of recognition.

T Dendritic Cells. *Dendritic cells* make up a system of cells that is important to the immune system, especially the cell-mediated immune response. They have an atypical shape with extensive dendritic processes that form and retract. They are found in many places in the body, including the skin (where they are called *Langerhans' cells*) and the lining of the nose, lungs, stomach, and intestine. There are many immature dendritic cells in the blood.[1]

Dendritic cells function primarily to capture antigens at sites of contact with the external environment (e.g., skin, mucous membranes) and then transport the antigen until it meets a T cell with specificity for that antigen. In this role, they have an important function in activating the immune response.

Cytokines

The immune response involves complex interactions of T cells, B cells, monocytes, and neutrophils. These interactions depend on **cytokines** (soluble factors secreted by WBCs and a variety of other cells in the body) that act as messengers among the cell types. Cytokines instruct cells to alter their proliferation, differentiation, secretion, or activity.

Currently, we know of more than 100 different cytokines. They can be classified into distinct categories. Some of these cytokines are listed in Table 13.3. In general, the interleukins (ILs) act as immunomodulatory factors. Colony-stimulating factors act as growth-regulating factors for hematopoietic cells. Interferons are antiviral and immunomodulatory.

The net effect of an inflammatory response is determined by a balance between proinflammatory and antiinflammatory mediators. We can sometimes classify cytokines as proinflammatory or antiinflammatory. However, it is not that clear-cut, since many other factors (e.g., target cells, environment) influence the inflammatory response to a given injury or insult.

Cytokines have a beneficial role in hematopoiesis and immune function. They can have detrimental effects such as those seen in chronic inflammation, autoimmune diseases, and sepsis. Cytokines such as colony-stimulating factors, interferons, and IL-2 have clinical uses (Table 13.4).

Interferon helps the body's natural defenses attack tumors and viruses. We know of 3 types of interferon (Table 13.3). Interferon is not directly antiviral but produces an antiviral

TABLE 13.3   Types and Functions of Cytokines

Type	Primary Functions	Type	Primary Functions
Colony-Stimulating Factors (CSFs)		**Interleukins (ILs)**	
Granulocyte colony-stimulating factor (G-CSF)	Stimulates proliferation and differentiation of neutrophils, enhances functional activity of mature PMNs	IL-1	Proinflammatory mediator. Promotes proliferation of B cells. Activates T cells, NK cells, and macrophages
Granulocyte-macrophage colony-stimulating factor (GM-CSF)	Stimulates proliferation and differentiation of PMNs and monocytes	IL-2	Activates T cells, NK cells, and macrophages. Stimulates release of other cytokines (α-IFN, TNF, IL-1, IL-6)
Macrophage colony-stimulating factor (M-CSF)	Promotes proliferation, differentiation, and activation of monocytes and macrophages	IL-3	Hematopoietic growth factor for hematopoietic precursor cells
Erythropoietin	Stimulates erythroid progenitor cells in bone marrow to make red blood cells	IL-4	Antiinflammatory mediator. B cell growth and differentiation. Induces differentiation into T_H2 cells. Stimulates growth of mast cells
		IL-5	B-cell growth and differentiation. Promotes growth and differentiation of eosinophils
Interferons (IFNs)		IL-6	Proinflammatory mediator. T- and B-cell growth factor, promotes differentiation of B cells into plasma cells and stimulates antibody secretion. Induces fever. Synergistic effects with IL-1 and TNF
α-IFN β-IFN	Inhibits viral replication, activates NK cells and macrophages, antiproliferative effects on tumor cells		
γ-IFN	Proinflammatory mediator. Activates macrophages, neutrophils, and NK cells. Promotes B cell differentiation. Inhibits viral replication	**Tumor Necrosis Factor (TNF)**	Proinflammatory mediator. Activates macrophages and granulocytes. Promotes immune and inflammatory responses. Kills tumor cells. Responsible for weight loss associated with chronic inflammation and cancer

NK, Natural killer; *PMNs,* polymorphonuclear neutrophils.

TABLE 13.4   Clinical Uses of Cytokines

Cytokine	Clinical Uses
Colony-Stimulating Factors	
G-CSF filgrastim (Neupogen) pegfilgrastim (Neulasta)	Chemotherapy-induced neutropenia
GM-CSF sargramostim (Leukine)	Neutropenia, myeloid recovery after bone marrow transplantation
Erythropoietin epoetin alfa (Epogen, Procrit), darbepoetin alfa (Aranesp)	Anemia related to chronic kidney disease, cancer, and chemotherapy
IL-1 Receptor Antagonist anakinra (Kineret)	Rheumatoid arthritis
Interferons	
α-Interferon (Roferon-A, Intron A)	Hairy cell leukemia, chronic myelogenous leukemia, malignant melanoma, renal cell cancer, ovarian cancer, multiple myeloma, Kaposi sarcoma, hepatitis B and C
β-Interferon (Betaseron, Avonex, Rebif)	Multiple sclerosis
Interleukins	
Interleukin-2 aldesleukin (Proleukin)	Metastatic renal cell cancer, metastatic melanoma
Interleukin 11 (platelet growth factor) oprelvekin (Neumega)	Thrombocytopenia related to chemotherapy
Soluble TNF Receptor etanercept (Enbrel)	Rheumatoid arthritis

G-CSF, Granulocyte colony-stimulating factor; *GM-CSF,* granulocyte-macrophage colony-stimulating factor; *TNF,* tumor necrosis factor.

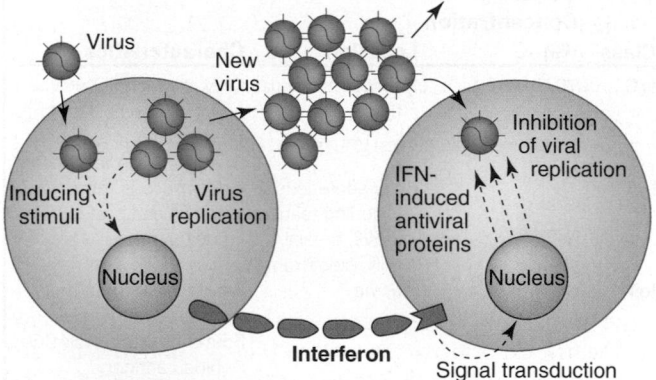

FIG. 13.4 Mechanism of action of interferon *(IFN).* When a virus attacks a cell, the cell begins to make viral DNA and IFN. IFN serves as an intercellular messenger and induces the production of antiviral proteins. Then the virus is not able to replicate in the cell.

effect in cells by reacting with them and inducing the formation of a second protein termed *antiviral protein* (Fig. 13.4). This protein mediates the antiviral action of interferon by changing the cell's protein synthesis and preventing new viruses from becoming assembled.

Comparison of Humoral and Cell-Mediated Immunity

Humans need both humoral and cell-mediated immunity to remain healthy. Each type of immunity has unique properties, different methods of action, and reactions against particular antigens. Table 13.5 compares humoral and cell-mediated immunity.

TABLE 13.5 Comparison of Humoral and Cell-Mediated Immunity

Characteristics	Humoral Immunity	Cell-Mediated Immunity
Cells involved	B lymphocytes	T lymphocytes, macrophages
Products	Antibodies	Sensitized T cells, cytokines
Memory cells	Present	Present
Protection	Bacteria	Fungus
	Viruses (extracellular)	Viruses (intracellular)
	Respiratory and GI pathogens	Chronic infectious agents
		Tumor cells
Examples	Anaphylactic shock	Tuberculosis
	Atopic diseases	Fungal infections
	Transfusion reaction	Contact dermatitis
	Bacterial infections	Graft rejection
		Destruction of cancer cells

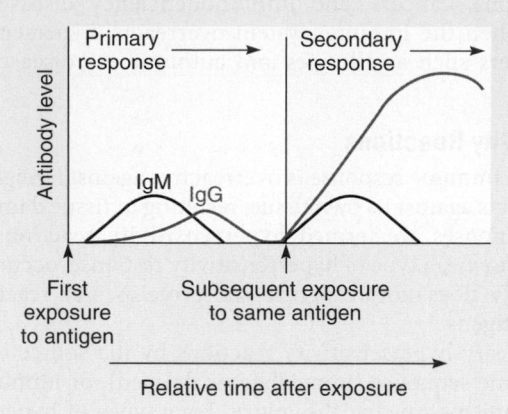

FIG. 13.5 Primary and secondary immune responses. The introduction of antigen induces a response dominated by 2 classes of immunoglobulins, IgM and IgG. IgM predominates in the primary response, with some IgG appearing later. After the host's immune system is primed, another challenge with the same antigen induces the secondary response, in which some IgM and large amounts of IgG are made.

Humoral Immunity. Humoral immunity consists of antibody-mediated immunity. The term *humoral* comes from the Greek word *humor*, which means body fluid. Since antibodies are made by plasma cells (differentiated B cells) and found in plasma, the term *humoral immunity* is used. Antibody production is an essential part of the humoral immune response. Each of the 5 classes of immunoglobulins (Igs) (IgG, IgA, IgM, IgD, IgE) has specific characteristics (Table 13.2).

When a pathogen (especially bacteria) enters the body, it may encounter a B cell that is specific for antigens found on that bacterial cell wall. In addition, a monocyte or macrophage may phagocytize the bacteria and present its antigens to a B cell. The B cell recognizes the antigen because it has receptors on its cell surface specific for that antigen. When the antigen comes in contact with the cell surface receptor, the B cell becomes activated, and most B cells differentiate into plasma cells (Fig. 13.3). The mature plasma cell secretes immunoglobulins. Some stimulated B cells remain as memory cells.

The primary immune response becomes evident 4 to 8 days after the first exposure to the antigen (Fig. 13.5). IgM is the first type of antibody formed. Because of the large size of the IgM molecule, IgM is confined to the intravascular space. As the immune response progresses, we make IgG. IgG can move from intravascular to extravascular spaces.

When a person is exposed to the antigen the second time, a secondary antibody response occurs. This response occurs faster (1 to 3 days), is stronger, and lasts for a longer time than a primary response. Memory cells account for the memory of the first exposure to the antigen and the more rapid production of antibodies. IgG is the primary antibody found in a secondary immune response.

IgG crosses the placental membrane. It provides the newborn with passive acquired immunity for at least 3 months. Infants may get some passive immunity from IgA in breast milk and colostrum.

Cell-Mediated Immunity. Immune responses that are initiated through specific antigen recognition by T cells are termed cell-mediated immunity. Several cell types and factors are involved in cell-mediated immunity. These include T cells, macrophages, and NK cells. Cell-mediated immunity is of primary importance in (1) immunity against pathogens that survive inside of cells, including viruses and some bacteria (e.g., mycobacteria); (2) fungal infections; (3) rejection of transplanted tissues; (4) contact hypersensitivity reactions; and (5) tumor immunity.

Gerontologic Considerations: Effects of Aging on the Immune System

With advancing age, there is a decline in the function of the immune response (Table 13.6). The main evidence of *immunosenescence* is the high incidence of cancer in older adults. Older people are also more susceptible to infections (e.g., influenza, pneumonia) from pathogens that they were more immunocompetent against earlier in life. Bacterial pneumonia is the leading cause of death from infections in older adults. The antibody response to immunizations (e.g., flu vaccine) in older adults is considerably lower than in younger adults.[1]

The bone marrow is unaffected by increasing age. Immunoglobulin levels decrease with age, leading to a suppressed humoral immune response in older adults. The thymus shrinks with age, along with decreased numbers of T cells. These changes in the thymus gland are a primary cause of immunosenescence. Both T and B cells show deficiencies in activation, transit time through the cell cycle, and subsequent differentiation. However, the most significant changes involve T cells. As thymic output of T cells diminishes, the differentiation of T cells increases. Consequently, there is an accumulation of memory cells rather than new precursor cells responsive to previously unencountered antigens.

The delayed hypersensitivity reaction, as determined by skin testing with injected antigens, is often decreased or absent in older adults. This altered response reflects anergy (an immunodeficient condition characterized by lack of or diminished reaction to an antigen or a group of antigens).

ALTERED IMMUNE RESPONSE

Immunocompetence exists when the body's immune system can identify and inactivate or destroy foreign substances. When the immune system is incompetent or underresponsive, severe infections, cancers, and immunodeficiency diseases may occur. When the immune system overreacts, hypersensitivity disorders such as allergies and autoimmune diseases may develop.

Hypersensitivity Reactions

Sometimes the immune response is overreactive against foreign antigens or reacts against its own tissue, resulting in tissue damage. These responses are termed hypersensitivity reactions. *Autoimmune disease,* a type of hypersensitivity response, occurs when the body does not recognize self-proteins and reacts against self-antigens.

We can classify hypersensitivity reactions by the source of the antigen, time sequence (immediate or delayed), or immunologic mechanisms causing the injury. Four types of hypersensitivity reactions exist (Table 13.7). Types I, II, and III are immediate and are examples of humoral immunity. Type IV is a delayed hypersensitivity reaction and is related to cell-mediated immunity.

TABLE 13.6 Gerontologic Assessment Differences

Effects of Aging on the Immune System

- Thymic shrinkage
- ↓ Cell-mediated immunity
- ↓ Delayed hypersensitivity reaction
- ↓ IL-1 and IL-2 synthesis
- ↓ Expression of IL-2 receptors
- ↓ Proliferative response of T and B cells
- ↓ Primary and secondary antibody responses
- ↑ Autoantibodies

IL, Interleukin.

Type I: IgE-Mediated Reactions. *Anaphylactic reactions* are type I reactions that occur only in susceptible people who are highly sensitized to specific allergens. IgE antibodies, made in response to the allergen, have a characteristic property of attaching to mast cells and basophils (Fig. 13.6; see Fig. 28.2). Within these cells are granules containing potent chemical mediators (histamine, serotonin, leukotrienes, eosinophil chemotactic factor of anaphylaxis [ECF-A], kinins, and bradykinin). Chemical mediators of inflammation are discussed in Chapter 11 and Table 11.1.

On the first exposure to the allergen, IgE antibodies are made and bind to mast cells and basophils. On any subsequent exposures, the allergen links with the IgE bound to mast cells or basophils and triggers degranulation of the cells and the release of chemical mediators from the granules. In this process, the mediators that are released attack target tissues, causing clinical symptoms of an allergic response. These effects include smooth muscle contraction, increased vascular permeability, vasodilation, hypotension, increased secretion of mucus, and itching. Fortunately, the mediators are short acting and their effects are reversible. The mediators are listed in Table 13.8.

A genetic predisposition to the development of allergic diseases exists. The capacity to become sensitized to an allergen, rather than the specific allergic disorder, appears to be the inherited trait. For example, a father with asthma may have a son who has allergic rhinitis.

The manifestations of an anaphylactic reaction depend on whether the mediators remain localized or become systemic or whether they affect specific organs. When the mediators are localized, a cutaneous response termed the *wheal-and-flare reaction* occurs. This reaction is characterized by a pale wheal containing edematous fluid surrounded by a red flare from the hyperemia. The reaction occurs in minutes or hours and is usually not dangerous. A classic example of a wheal-and-flare reaction is the mosquito bite. The wheal-and-flare reaction serves a

TABLE 13.7   Types of Hypersensitivity Reactions

Type I: IgE-Mediated	Type II: Cytotoxic	Type III: Immune-Complex	Type IV: Delayed Hypersensitivity
Antigen			
Pollen, food, drugs, dust	Cell surface of RBCs Cell basement membrane	Extracellular fungal, viral, bacterial	Intracellular or extracellular
Rate of Development			
Immediate	Minutes to hours	Hours to days	Several days
Complement Involved			
No	Yes	Yes	No
Mediators of Injury			
Histamine	Complement lysis	Neutrophils	Cytokines
Mast cells	Macrophages in tissues	Complement lysis	T cytotoxic cells
Leukotrienes		Monocytes, macrophages	
Prostaglandins		Lysosomal enzymes	
Examples			
Allergic rhinitis	Transfusion reaction	SLE	Contact dermatitis (e.g., to poison ivy)
Asthma	Goodpasture syndrome	Rheumatoid arthritis	
Atopic dermatitis	Immune thrombocytopenic purpura	Acute glomerulonephritis	
Urticaria	Graves' disease		
Angioedema			
Skin Test			
Wheal and flare	None	Erythema and edema in 3–8 hr	Erythema and edema in 24–48 hr (e.g., TB test)

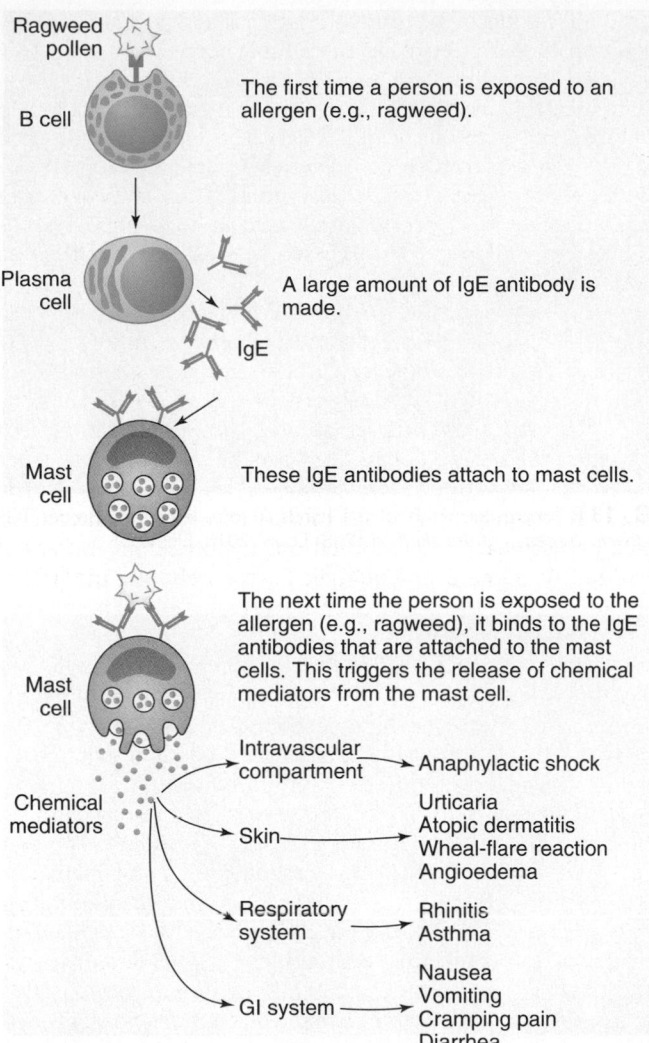

FIG. 13.6 Steps in a type I allergic reaction.

TABLE 13.8	Mediators of Allergic Response

- Anaphylatoxins (C3a, C4a, C5a from complement activation)
- Histamine
- Kinins
- Leukotrienes
- Platelet-activating factor
- Prostaglandins
- Serotonin

diagnostic purpose as a means of showing allergic reactions to specific allergens during skin tests.

Common allergic reactions include anaphylaxis and atopic reactions.

Anaphylaxis. *Anaphylaxis* can occur when mediators are released systemically (e.g., after injection of a drug, after an insect sting). The reaction occurs within minutes and can be life-threatening because of bronchial constriction and subsequent airway obstruction and vascular collapse. The target organs affected are shown in Fig. 13.7. Initial symptoms include edema and itching at the site of exposure to the allergen. Shock can occur rapidly and is manifested by rapid, weak pulse;

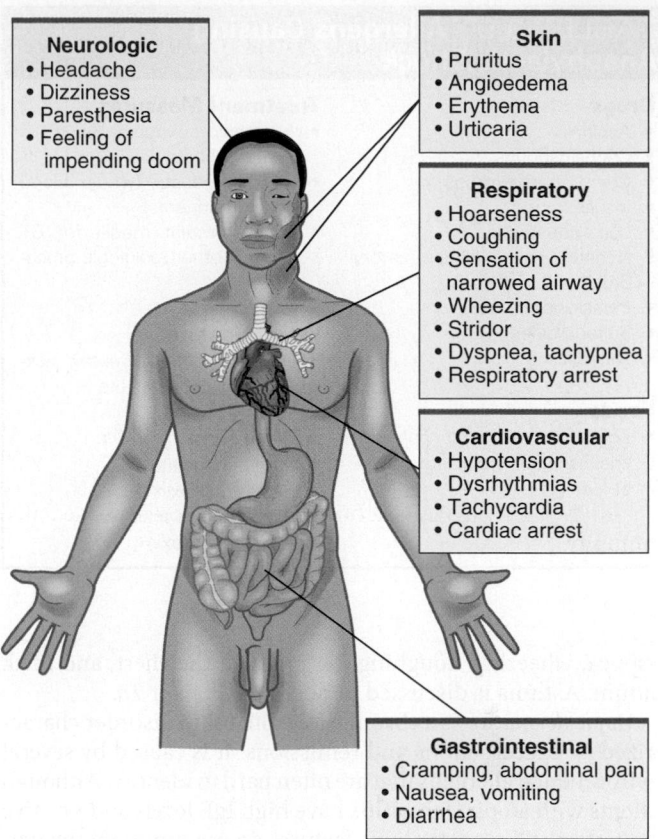

FIG. 13.7 Manifestations of a systemic anaphylactic reaction.

hypotension; dilated pupils; dyspnea; and possibly cyanosis. Bronchial edema and angioedema can compound shock. Death will occur without emergency treatment. Some of the important allergens that can cause anaphylactic shock in hypersensitive people are listed in Table 13.9. Drugs are the leading cause of anaphylaxis-related deaths.[2]

Atopic Reactions. Around 20% of the population is *atopic,* having an inherited tendency to become sensitive to environmental allergens. The atopic diseases that can result are allergic rhinitis, asthma, atopic dermatitis, urticaria, and angioedema.

Allergic rhinitis, or hay fever, is the most common type I hypersensitivity reaction. It may occur year-round (perennial allergic rhinitis), or it may be seasonal (seasonal allergic rhinitis). Airborne substances such as pollens, dust, and molds are the primary causes of allergic rhinitis. Dust, molds, and animal dander often cause perennial allergic rhinitis. Seasonal allergic rhinitis is often caused by pollens from trees, weeds, or grasses. The target areas affected are the conjunctiva of the eyes and the mucosa of the upper respiratory tract. Symptoms include nasal discharge; sneezing; tearing; mucosal swelling with airway obstruction; and pruritus around the eyes, nose, throat, and mouth. Treatment of allergic rhinitis is discussed in Chapter 26 on p. 480.

Many patients with *asthma* have an allergic component to their disease. These patients often have a history of atopic disorders (e.g., infantile eczema, allergic rhinitis, food intolerances). Inflammatory mediators produce bronchial smooth muscle constriction, excess secretion of thick mucus, edema of the mucous membranes of the bronchi, and decreased lung compliance. Because of these physiologic changes, patients have

TABLE 13.9 Allergens Causing Anaphylactic Shock

Drugs
- Aspirin
- Cephalosporins
- Chemotherapy drugs
- Insulins
- Local anesthetics
- Nonsteroidal antiinflammatory drugs
- Penicillins
- Sulfonamides
- Tetracycline

Foods
- Eggs, milk, nuts, peanuts, shellfish, fish, chocolate, strawberries

Treatment Measures
- Allergenic extracts used in immunotherapy
- Blood products (whole blood and components)
- Iodine-contrast media for CT scan or other radiologic procedures

Insect Venoms
- Wasps, hornets, yellow jackets, bumblebees, ants

Animal Sera
- Diphtheria antitoxin
- Rabies antitoxin
- Snake venom antitoxin
- Tetanus antitoxin

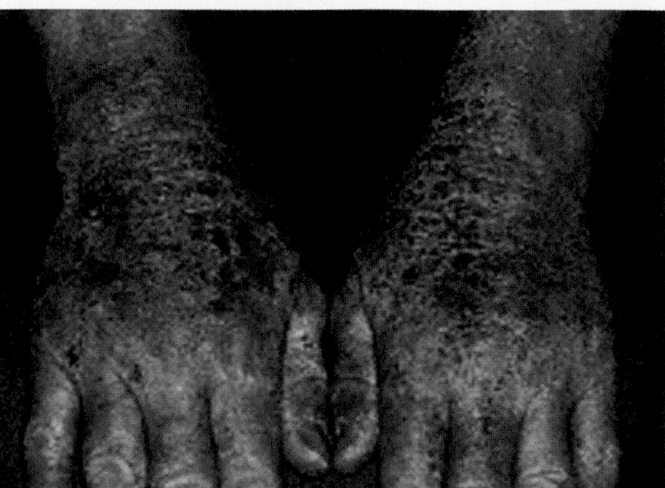

FIG. 13.8 Atopic dermatitis of the hands. (From James W, Berger TG: *Andrews' diseases of the skin,* ed 12, St Louis, 2016, Elsevier.)

dyspnea, wheezing, coughing, tightness in the chest, and thick sputum. Asthma is discussed in depth in Chapter 28.

Atopic dermatitis is a chronic, inherited skin disorder characterized by exacerbations and remissions. It is caused by several environmental allergens that are often hard to identify. Although patients with atopic dermatitis have high IgE levels and positive skin tests, the histopathologic features do not represent the typical, localized wheal-and-flare type I reactions. The skin lesions are more generalized and involve vasodilation of blood vessels, resulting in interstitial edema with vesicle formation (Fig. 13.8). Dermatitis is discussed in Chapter 23.

Urticaria (hives) is a cutaneous reaction against systemic allergens occurring in atopic people. It is characterized by transient wheals (pink, raised, edematous, pruritic areas) that vary in size and shape and may occur all over the body. Urticaria develops rapidly after exposure to an allergen and may last minutes or hours. Histamine causes localized vasodilation (erythema), transudation of fluid (wheal), and flaring. Flaring is due to dilated blood vessels on the edge of the wheal. Histamine is responsible for the pruritus associated with the lesions. Urticaria is discussed in Chapter 23.

Angioedema is a localized cutaneous lesion similar to urticaria but involving deeper layers of the skin and submucosa. The principal areas of involvement include the eyelids, lips, tongue, larynx, hands, feet, GI tract, and genitalia (Fig. 13.9). Swelling usually begins in the face and then progresses to the airways and other parts of the body. Dilation and engorgement of the capillaries secondary to the release of histamine cause the diffuse swelling. Welts are not present as in urticaria. The outer skin appears normal or has a reddish hue. The lesions may burn, sting, or itch and can cause acute abdominal pain if in the GI tract. The swelling may occur suddenly or over several hours and usually lasts for 24 hours.

Type II: Cytotoxic and Cytolytic Reactions. Cytotoxic and cytolytic reactions are type II hypersensitivity reactions involving the direct binding of IgG or IgM antibodies to an antigen on the cell surface. Antigen-antibody complexes activate the complement system, which mediates the reaction. Cellular tissue is destroyed by either (1) activation of the complement system resulting in cytolysis or (2) enhanced phagocytosis.

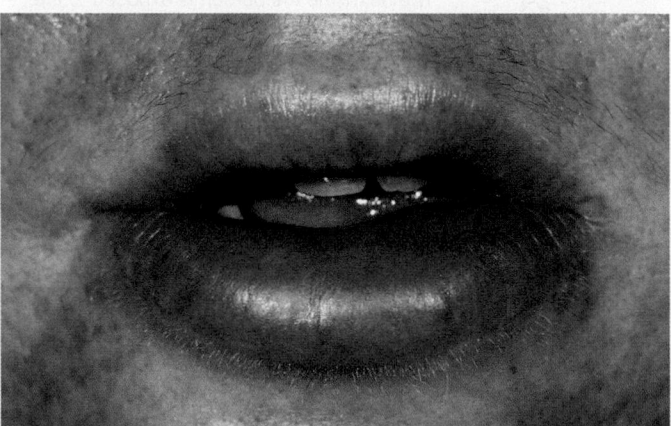

FIG. 13.9 Allergic reaction with angioedema of the lip. (From Habif TP: *Clinical dermatology,* ed 6, Philadelphia, 2016, Saunders.)

Target cells often destroyed in type II reactions are erythrocytes, platelets, and leukocytes. The tissue damage usually occurs rapidly. Some of the antigens involved are the ABO blood group, Rh factor, and drugs. Pathophysiologic disorders characteristic of type II reactions include ABO incompatibility transfusion reaction, Rh incompatibility transfusion reaction, autoimmune and drug-related hemolytic anemias, leukopenias, thrombocytopenias, erythroblastosis fetalis (hemolytic disease of the newborn), and Goodpasture syndrome.

Hemolytic Transfusion Reactions. A classic type II reaction occurs when a recipient receives ABO-incompatible blood from a donor. Naturally acquired antibodies to antigens of the ABO blood group are in the recipient's serum but are not present on the erythrocyte membranes (see Table 29.9). For example, a person with type A blood has anti-B antibodies, a person with type B blood has anti-A antibodies, a person with type AB blood has no antibodies, and a person with type O blood has anti-A and anti-B antibodies.

If the recipient is transfused with incompatible blood, antibodies immediately coat the foreign erythrocytes, causing *agglutination* (clumping). The clumping of cells blocks small blood vessels in the body, uses existing clotting factors, and depletes them, leading to bleeding. Within hours, neutrophils and macrophages phagocytize the agglutinated cells. The complement system is activated. Cell lysis occurs, which causes the release of hemoglobin into the urine and plasma. Acute kidney injury can result from the hemoglobinuria. Blood transfusions are discussed in Chapter 30.

Goodpasture Syndrome. *Goodpasture syndrome* is a disorder involving the lungs and kidneys. An antibody-mediated autoimmune reaction occurs involving the glomerular and alveolar basement membranes. The circulating antibodies combine with tissue antigen to activate the complement system, which causes deposits of IgG to form along the cell basement membranes of the lungs or kidneys. This reaction may result in pulmonary hemorrhage and glomerulonephritis. Goodpasture syndrome is discussed in Chapter 45.

Type III: Immune-Complex Reactions. Tissue damage in immune-complex reactions, which are type III reactions, occurs secondary to antigen-antibody complexes. Soluble antigens combine with IgG and IgM to form complexes that are too small to be effectively removed by the mononuclear phagocyte system. Therefore the complexes deposit in tissue or small blood vessels. They cause activation of the complement system and release of chemotactic factors that lead to inflammation and destruction of the involved tissue.

Type III reactions may be local or systemic and immediate or delayed. The manifestations depend on the number of complexes and the location in the body. Common sites for deposit are the kidneys, skin, joints, blood vessels, and lungs. Severe type III reactions are associated with autoimmune disorders such as systemic lupus erythematosus (SLE), acute glomerulonephritis, and rheumatoid arthritis. SLE and rheumatoid arthritis are discussed in Chapter 64. Acute glomerulonephritis is discussed in Chapter 45.

Type IV: Delayed Hypersensitivity Reactions. A *delayed hypersensitivity reaction*—a type IV reaction—is a *cell-mediated immune response*. Although cell-mediated responses are usually protective mechanisms, tissue damage occurs in delayed hypersensitivity reactions.

The tissue damage in a type IV reaction does not occur in the presence of antibodies or complement. Rather, sensitized T cells attack antigens or release cytokines. Some of these cytokines attract macrophages into the area. The macrophages and enzymes released by them are responsible for most of the tissue destruction. In the delayed hypersensitivity reaction, it takes 24 to 48 hours for a response to occur.

Examples of delayed hypersensitivity reactions include contact dermatitis (Fig. 13.10); hypersensitivity reactions to bacterial, fungal, and viral infections; and transplant rejections. Some drug sensitivity reactions also fit this category.

Contact Dermatitis. *Allergic contact dermatitis* is an example of a delayed hypersensitivity reaction involving the skin. The reaction occurs when the skin is exposed to substances that easily penetrate the skin to combine with epidermal proteins. The substance then becomes antigenic. Over a period of 7 to 14 days, memory cells form to the antigen. On subsequent exposure to the substance, a sensitized person develops eczematous skin lesions within 48 hours. The most common antigenic substances are metal compounds (e.g., those containing nickel or mercury); rubber compounds; poison ivy, poison oak, and poison sumac; cosmetics; and some dyes.

In acute contact dermatitis, the skin lesions appear erythematous and edematous and are covered with papules, vesicles, and bullae. The involved area is pruritic but may burn or sting. When

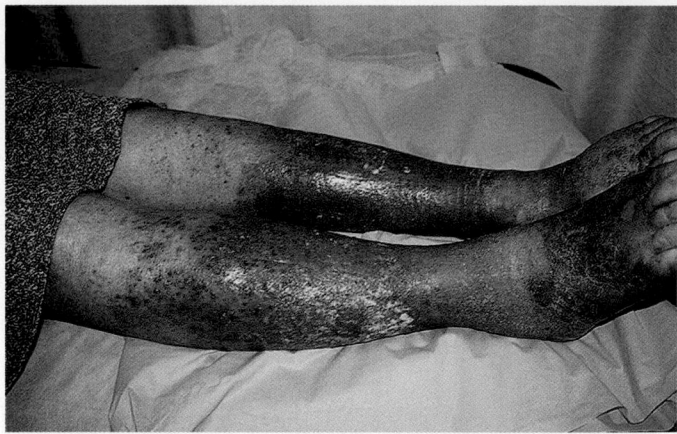

FIG. 13.10 Contact dermatitis to rubber. (From Morison MJ: *Nursing management of chronic wounds,* Edinburgh, 2001, Mosby.)

contact dermatitis becomes chronic, the lesions resemble atopic dermatitis because they are thickened, scaly, and lichenified. The main difference between contact dermatitis and atopic dermatitis is that contact dermatitis is localized and restricted to the area exposed to the allergens. Atopic dermatitis is usually widespread.

Microbial Hypersensitivity Reactions. The classic example of a microbial cell-mediated immune reaction is the body's defense against the tubercle bacillus. Tuberculosis results from invasion of lung tissue by the highly resistant tubercle bacillus. The organism itself does not directly damage the lung tissue. However, antigenic material released from the tubercle bacilli reacts with T cells, initiating a cell-mediated immune response. The resulting response causes extensive caseous necrosis of the lung.

After the first cell-mediated reaction, memory cells persist, so subsequent contact with the tubercle bacillus or an extract of purified protein from the organism causes a delayed hypersensitivity reaction. This is the basis for the purified protein derivative (PPD) tuberculosis skin test, which we read 48 to 72 hours after injecting the PPD intradermally. Tuberculosis is discussed in Chapter 27.

ALLERGIC DISORDERS

Assessment

For a thorough assessment of a patient with allergies, obtain a complete history and perform a comprehensive physical examination, diagnostic workup, and skin testing for allergens. Obtain information from the patient about family allergies, past and present allergies, and social and environmental factors.

Family history, including information about atopic reactions in relatives, is especially important in identifying at-risk patients. Note past and present allergies. Obtain information about the manifestations and course of allergic reaction. The time of year when an allergic reaction occurs can be a clue to a seasonal allergen. Ask about any over-the-counter or prescription medications used to treat the allergies.

Social and environmental factors, especially the physical environment, are important. Ask about pets, trees and plants on the property, pollutants in the air, floor coverings, houseplants, and cooling and heating systems in the home and workplace. Note any reactions to medication. A daily or weekly food diary with a description of any untoward reactions may be useful.[3] Ask about the patient's lifestyle and stress level in connection with the allergic symptoms.

TABLE 13.10 Nursing Assessment

Allergies

Subjective Data

Important Health Information

Past health history: Recurrent respiratory problems, seasonal exacerbations. Unusual reactions to insect bites or stings; past and present allergies

Medications: Unusual reactions to any medications; use of over-the-counter drugs or medications for allergies

Functional Health Patterns

Health perception–health management: Family history of allergies; malaise

Nutritional-metabolic: Food intolerances, vomiting

Elimination: Abdominal cramps, diarrhea

Activity-exercise: Fatigue; hoarseness, cough, dyspnea

Cognitive-perceptual: Itching, burning, stinging of eyes, nose, throat, or skin; chest tightness

Role-relationship: Altered home and work environment, presence of pets

Objective Data

Integumentary

Rashes, including urticaria, wheal and flare, papules, vesicles, bullae; dryness, scaliness, scratches, irritation

Eyes, Ears, Nose, and Throat

Eyes: Conjunctivitis, lacrimation, rubbing or excessive blinking, dark circles under the eyes ("allergic shiner")

Ears: Diminished hearing, immobile or scarred tympanic membranes, recurrent ear infections

Nose: Nasal polyps, nasal voice, nose twitching, itchy nose, rhinitis; pale, boggy mucous membranes; sniffling, repeated sneezing; swollen nasal passages; recurrent, unexplained nosebleeds; crease across the bridge of nose ("allergic salute")

Throat: Continual throat clearing, swollen lips or tongue, red throat, palpable neck lymph nodes

Respiratory

Wheezing, stridor; thick sputum

Possible Diagnostic Findings

Eosinophilia of serum, sputum, or nasal and bronchial secretions; increased serum IgE levels; positive skin tests; abnormal chest and sinus x-rays

---

Table 13.10 outlines subjective and objective data to obtain. During the physical examination, focus attention on the site of the allergic manifestations.

Diagnostic Studies

Various immunologic techniques are used to detect abnormalities of lymphocytes, eosinophils, and immunoglobulins. A complete blood count (CBC) with WBC differential is done, with an absolute lymphocyte count and eosinophil count. Immunodeficiency is diagnosed if the lymphocyte count is below 1200/μL (1.2×10^9/L). T cell and B cell quantification is used to diagnose specific immunodeficiency syndromes. The eosinophil count is high in type I hypersensitivity reactions involving IgE. The serum IgE level is also generally high in type I hypersensitivity reactions and serves as a diagnostic indicator of atopic diseases.

We can test sputum and nasal and bronchial secretions for the presence of eosinophils. Pulmonary function tests, especially for forced expiratory volume, are helpful for patients with asthma.

Skin testing for allergens is the preferred method. Sometimes skin testing is contraindicated and blood allergy testing is used. Allergy blood testing is recommended if a person (1) is using a drug that interferes with skin test results (e.g., antihistamines, corticosteroids) and cannot stop taking it for a few days, (2) cannot tolerate the many needle scratches needed for skin testing, or (3) has a skin disorder (e.g., severe eczema, dermatitis, psoriasis).

Skin Tests. Skin testing is used to identify the specific allergens that are causing the allergy symptoms. With the use of empiric allergy medications as the treatment of choice for most allergic rhinitis, it has become common practice to omit skin testing for specific allergens in these patients. However, diagnosing an allergy to a specific antigen allows the patient to avoid an allergen and makes him or her a candidate for immunotherapy. Unfortunately, we cannot do skin testing on patients who cannot stop taking drugs that suppress the histamine response or patients with food allergies.

Procedure. We can do skin testing by 3 different methods: (1) a scratch or prick test, (2) an intradermal test, or (3) a patch test. The areas of the body usually used in skin testing are the arms and back. Allergen extracts are applied to the skin in rows with a corresponding control site opposite the test site. Saline or another diluent is applied to the control site. In the *scratch test* a drop of allergen is placed on the skin, and then a pricking device is used so that the allergen can enter the skin. In the *intradermal test* the allergen extract is injected under the skin, similar to a PPD test for TB. In the *patch test* an allergen is applied to a patch that is placed on the skin.

Results. In the scratch and intradermal tests, the reaction occurs in 5 to 10 minutes. In the patch test the patches must be worn for 48 to 72 hours. If the person is hypersensitive to the allergen, a positive reaction will occur within minutes after insertion in the skin and may last for 8 to 12 hours. We will see a local wheal-and-flare response with a positive reaction.

The size of the positive reaction does not always correlate with the severity of allergy symptoms. False-positive and false-negative results may occur. Negative results from skin testing do not always mean the person does not have an allergic disorder. Positive results do not always mean that the allergen was causing the manifestations. Positive results imply that the person is sensitized to that allergen. Therefore correlating skin test results with the patient's history is important.

Precautions. A highly sensitive person is always at risk for developing an anaphylactic reaction to skin tests. Therefore never leave a patient during the testing period. If a severe reaction does occur with a skin test, the extract is immediately removed and antiinflammatory topical cream is applied to the site. For intradermal testing, the arm is best so that a tourniquet can be applied during a severe reaction. A subcutaneous injection of epinephrine may be needed.

Interprofessional and Nursing Management

After an allergic disorder is diagnosed, treatment is aimed at reducing exposure to the offending allergen, treating the symptoms, and, if needed, desensitizing the person through immunotherapy.

✚ TABLE 13.11 Emergency Management

Anaphylactic Shock

Etiology
- Injection of, inhalation of, ingestion of, or topical exposure to substance that produces profound allergic response (Table 13.9)

Assessment Findings
- See Fig. 13.7

Interventions

Initial
- Ensure patent airway. Intubation if evidence of impending obstruction
- Remove insect stinger if present
- Establish IV access
- Epinephrine (1 mg/mL preparation): Give 0.3–0.5 mg IM preferably in the mid-outer thigh. Can repeat every 5–15 min.
- Give high-flow O_2 (8–10 L/min) via face mask. Can give up to 100% as needed
- Nebulized albuterol for bronchospasm resistant to epinephrine
- Diphenhydramine IV for urticaria and itching
- Corticosteroids: Methylprednisolone IV

Hypotension
- Place recumbent and elevate legs
- IV normal saline rapid bolus of 1–2 L
- Maintain BP with fluids, volume expanders, vasopressors (e.g., dopamine)

Ongoing Monitoring
- Monitor vital signs, respiratory effort, O_2 saturation, level of consciousness, cardiac rhythm, and urine output
- Anticipate intubation with severe respiratory distress
- Anticipate cricothyrotomy or tracheostomy with severe laryngeal edema

Anaphylaxis. Anaphylactic reactions occur suddenly in hypersensitive patients after exposure to the offending allergen. They may occur after parenteral injection of drugs (especially antibiotics) or blood products and after insect stings. The cardinal principle in management is speed in (1) recognizing signs and symptoms of an anaphylactic reaction, (2) maintaining a patent airway, (3) giving drugs, and (4) treating for shock. Table 13.11 outlines the emergency treatment of anaphylactic shock.

Epinephrine is the drug of choice to treat an anaphylactic reaction. It must be given parenterally (IM, IV). Patients receiving β-blockers may be resistant to treatment with epinephrine and can develop refractory hypotension and bradycardia. Glucagon should be given to these patients because it has inotropic and chronotropic effects that are not mediated through β-receptors. Severe cases of anaphylaxis may result in hypovolemic shock because of the loss of intravascular fluid into interstitial spaces that occurs due to increased capillary permeability.[4] Peripheral vasoconstriction and stimulation of the sympathetic nervous system occur to compensate for the fluid shift. However, unless shock is treated early, the body will no longer be able to compensate and irreversible tissue damage will occur, leading to death. (Hypovolemic shock is discussed in Chapter 66.)

❓ CHECK YOUR PRACTICE

You are caring for a patient who has been receiving IV antibiotic therapy for 2 days. Several minutes after starting the latest infusion, the patient states that his chest feels tight and begins coughing. You take his BP and it is 100/64 and his pulse is 124.
- What should you do?

All health care workers must be prepared for the rare but life-threatening anaphylactic reaction, which requires immediate medical and nursing interventions. It is extremely important to list all the patient's allergies on the chart, nursing care plan, and medication record.

Chronic Allergies. Most allergic reactions are chronic. They are characterized by remissions and exacerbations of symptoms. Treatment focuses on identification and control of allergens, relief of symptoms through drug therapy, and hyposensitization of a patient to an offending allergen.

Allergen Recognition and Control. You play a key role in helping the patient make lifestyle adjustments so that there is minimal exposure to offending allergens. Reinforce that, even with drug therapy and immunotherapy, the patient will never be totally desensitized or completely symptom free. Help the patient use various preventive measures to control the allergic symptoms.

Of primary importance is the need to identify the offending allergen. Sometimes this is done through skin testing. In the case of food allergies an elimination diet is sometimes valuable. If an allergic reaction occurs, all foods eaten shortly before the reaction should be eliminated and gradually reintroduced 1 at a time until the offending food is detected.

Many allergic reactions, especially asthma and urticaria, may be worsened by fatigue and emotional stress. Help the patient plan a stress management program. Have the patient practice relaxation techniques when coming in for frequent immunotherapy treatments.

Sometimes control of allergic symptoms requires environmental control, including changing an occupation, moving to a different climate, or giving up a favorite pet. In the case of airborne allergens, sleeping in an air-conditioned room, damp dusting daily, covering mattresses and pillows with hypoallergenic covers, and wearing a mask outdoors may be helpful.

If the allergen is a drug, have the patient avoid the drug. The patient has the responsibility to make any drug allergies known to all health care team members. The patient should wear a Medic Alert bracelet listing the drug allergy and have the drug allergy listed on all medical and dental records.

For a patient allergic to insect stings, commercial kits containing automatic injectable epinephrine are available. Teach the patient and family how to use the injector and have them practice assembling and using the non–drug containing training device (Table 13.12). This patient should wear a Medic Alert bracelet and carry an insect-sting kit whenever going outdoors.

Drug Therapy. The major categories of drugs used for symptomatic relief of chronic allergic disorders include antihistamines, sympathomimetic/decongestant drugs, corticosteroids, antipruritic drugs, and mast cell–stabilizing drugs. Many of these drugs can be bought OTC and are often misused by patients.

TABLE 13.12 Patient and Caregiver Teaching

Automatic Epinephrine Injectors

Include the following information when teaching the patient and caregiver how to use an automatic epinephrine injector.

1. Fill the prescription at once and keep at least 2 doses available.
2. Always keep at least 1 autoinjector with you.
3. Keep an autoinjector in a place where others can easily find it in case of an emergency. Tell family and friends where it is stored.
4. Keep the autoinjector in the original case, at room temperature, away from extremes of cold and heat.
5. Mark on your calendar when the autoinjector expires, although an expired autoinjector may be used if there is no alternative. Replace solutions that are discolored or contain particles.
6. Use the device if you have any sign of anaphylaxis, such as trouble breathing or feeling tightness in the throat or lightheaded.
7. When needed:
   - Inject the drug into the top of the thigh, slightly to the outside, at a 90-degree angle. Hold in place for at least 2 to 3 seconds.
   - You can inject the drug through clothes. Avoid pockets and seams where the fabric is thick.
   - After use, call 911 and get to the nearest hospital for monitoring. Take the autoinjector with you.

Antihistamines. Antihistamines are the best drugs for treatment of allergic rhinitis and urticaria (see Chapter 26, Table 26.2). They are less effective for severe allergic reactions. They act by competing with histamine for H_1-receptor sites, thus blocking the effect of histamine. Results are best if they are taken as soon as allergy symptoms appear. Antihistamines can be used effectively to treat edema and pruritus. They are ineffective in preventing bronchoconstriction. With seasonal rhinitis, antihistamines should be taken during peak pollen seasons.

Sympathomimetic/Decongestant Drugs. The major sympathomimetic drug is epinephrine (Adrenalin). Epinephrine is made by the adrenal medulla and stimulates α- and β-adrenergic receptors. Stimulation of the α-adrenergic receptors causes vasoconstriction of peripheral blood vessels. β-Receptor stimulation relaxes bronchial smooth muscles. Epinephrine also acts directly on mast cells to stabilize them against further degranulation. The action of epinephrine lasts only a few minutes.

Minor sympathomimetic drugs differ from epinephrine because they are taken orally or nasally and last for several hours. Included in this category are drugs containing phenylephrine and pseudoephedrine. The minor sympathomimetic drugs are used mainly to treat allergic rhinitis (see Chapter 26 and Table 26.2).

Corticosteroids. Nasal corticosteroid sprays are effective in relieving the symptoms of allergic rhinitis (see Chapter 26 and Table 26.2). Occasionally patients have such severe manifestations of allergies that they are truly incapacitated. In these situations, a brief course of oral corticosteroids can be used.

Antipruritic Drugs. Topically applied antipruritic drugs are most effective when the skin is intact. These drugs protect the skin and provide relief from itching. Common OTC drugs include calamine lotion, coal tar solutions, and camphor. Menthol and phenol may be added to other lotions to produce an antipruritic effect.

Mast Cell–Stabilizing Drugs. Cromolyn is a mast cell–stabilizing agent that inhibits the release of histamines, leukotrienes, and other agents from the mast cell after antigen-IgE interaction. It is available as an inhalant nebulizer solution or a nasal spray. Cromolyn is used in the management of allergic rhinitis (see Chapter 26).

Leukotriene Receptor Antagonists. Leukotriene receptor antagonists (LTRAs) block leukotriene, 1 of the major mediators of the allergic inflammatory process (see Table 26.2). These medications can be taken orally. They are used to treat allergic rhinitis and asthma.

Immunotherapy. Immunotherapy is the recommended treatment for control of allergic symptoms when the allergen cannot be avoided and drug therapy is not effective. Few patients with allergies have symptoms so intolerable that they need allergy immunotherapy. Immunotherapy is definitively indicated for those with anaphylactic reactions to insect venom.

Immunotherapy involves giving small titers of an allergen extract in increasing strengths until hyposensitivity to the specific allergen is achieved. For best results, teach the patient to avoid the offending allergen whenever possible because complete desensitization is impossible. Unfortunately, not all allergy-related conditions respond to immunotherapy. Food allergies cannot be safely treated with this therapy. Eczema may worsen with immunotherapy.

Mechanism of Action. The IgE level is high in atopic people. When IgE combines with an allergen in a hypersensitive person, a reaction occurs, releasing histamine in various body tissues. Allergens more readily combine with IgG than with other immunoglobulins. Therefore immunotherapy involves injecting allergen extracts that will stimulate increased IgG levels. The goal of long-term immunotherapy is to keep "blocking" IgG levels high. By increasing IgG levels, IgE is blocked from binding to the allergen. This prevents mast cell degranulation. In addition, allergen-specific T suppressor cells develop in those receiving immunotherapy.

Method of Administration. The allergens included in immunotherapy are chosen based on the results of skin testing with a panel of allergens. Results are best when immunotherapy is given throughout the year.

Subcutaneous immunotherapy. *Subcutaneous immunotherapy (SCIT)* involves the subcutaneous injection of titrated amounts of allergen extracts biweekly or weekly. The dose is small at first and then increased slowly until a maintenance dosage is reached. Generally, it takes 1 to 2 years of immunotherapy to reach the maximal therapeutic effect. Therapy may continue for about 5 years. After that, some patients may stop therapy. Many have a sustained decrease in symptoms after the treatment is stopped. Those with severe allergies or sensitivity to insect stings may continue maintenance therapy indefinitely.

Sublingual immunotherapy. *Sublingual immunotherapy (SLIT)* involves allergen extracts taken under the tongue. SLIT has been used in Europe for decades. Recently the first sublingual products have become available in the United States. These include a 5-grass pollen tablet (Oralair), a single grass pollen tablet (Grastek), and a ragweed pollen tablet (Ragwitek).[5]

Patients usually take SLIT once daily at home. The first dose is usually given under medical supervision. Some patients have local application site reactions (e.g., oral pruritus, throat irritation, tongue swelling). Local reactions subside in many patients within a few days to a week. Systemic allergic reactions are markedly fewer than with SCIT.

SLIT has the advantage of being a convenient, self-administered oral therapy. Its primary disadvantage is that the patient must consistently adhere to the therapy.[6]

❖ NURSING MANAGEMENT: IMMUNOTHERAPY

You will often be the person responsible for giving SCIT. Immunotherapy always carries the risk for a severe anaphylactic reaction. Therefore an HCP, emergency equipment, and essential drugs should be available whenever injections are given. Always anticipate adverse reactions, especially when using a new dose strength, after a previous reaction, or after a missed dose. Early manifestations of a systemic reaction include pruritus, urticaria, sneezing, laryngeal edema, and hypotension. If these occur, initiate emergency measures for anaphylactic shock at once.

Describe any local reaction according to the degree of redness and swelling at the injection site. If the area is greater than the size of a quarter in an adult, report the reaction to the HCP so that the allergen dosage may be decreased.

Record keeping must be accurate and can help prevent an adverse reaction to the allergen extract. Before giving an injection, check the patient's name against the name on the vial. Next, determine the vial strength, amount of last dose, date of last dose, and any reaction information.

Always give the allergen extract in an extremity away from a joint so that a tourniquet can be applied for a severe reaction. Rotate the site for each injection. After giving the injection, carefully observe the patient for 20 to 30 minutes, since systemic reactions are most likely to occur immediately. However, warn the patient that a delayed reaction can occur as long as 24 hours later.

Latex Allergies

Allergies to latex products have become an increasing problem, affecting patients and health care workers. The increase in allergic reactions has coincided with the sharp increase in glove use. The more frequent and prolonged the exposure to latex, the greater the risk for developing a latex allergy.[7]

Besides gloves, we use many other latex-containing products in health care. These include BP cuffs, stethoscopes, tourniquets, IV tubing, syringes, electrode pads, O_2 masks, tracheal tubes, colostomy and ileostomy pouches, urinary catheters, anesthetic masks, and adhesive tape. Latex proteins can become aerosolized through powder on gloves and can result in serious reactions when inhaled by sensitized persons. All health care facilities should use powder-free gloves to avoid respiratory exposure to latex proteins.[8]

Types of Latex Allergies. Two types of latex allergies can occur: type IV allergic contact dermatitis and type I allergic reactions. *Type IV contact dermatitis* is caused by the chemicals used in the manufacturing process of latex gloves. It is a delayed reaction that occurs within 6 to 48 hours. Typically, the person first has dryness, pruritus, fissuring, and cracking of the skin, followed by redness, swelling, and crusting at 24 to 48 hours. Chronic exposure can lead to lichenification, scaling, and hyperpigmentation. The dermatitis may extend beyond the area of physical contact with the allergen.

A *type I allergic reaction* is a response to the natural rubber latex proteins and occurs within minutes of contact with the proteins. The manifestations of type I reactions can vary from skin redness, urticaria, rhinitis, conjunctivitis, or asthma to full-blown anaphylactic shock. Systemic reactions to latex may result from exposure to latex protein via various routes, including the skin, mucous membranes, inhalation, and blood.

Latex-Food Syndrome. Because some proteins in rubber are similar to food proteins, some foods may cause an allergic reaction in people who are allergic to latex. This is called *latex-food syndrome.* The most common of these foods are banana, avocado, chestnut, kiwi, tomato, water chestnut, guava, hazelnut, potato, peach, grape, and apricot. Most people with latex allergy have a positive allergy test to at least 1 related food.

TABLE 13.13 Guidelines for Preventing Allergic Latex Reactions
• Use nonlatex gloves for activities that are not likely to involve contact with infectious materials (e.g., food preparation, housekeeping).
• Use appropriate barrier protection when handling infectious materials.
• If you choose latex gloves, use powder-free gloves with reduced protein content.
• Do not use oil-based hand creams or lotions when wearing latex gloves.
• Frequently clean work areas that are contaminated with latex-containing dust (e.g., carpets, ventilation ducts).
• Learn to recognize the symptoms of latex allergy: Skin rash; hives; flushing; itching; nasal, eye, or sinus symptoms; asthma; and shock.
• If symptoms of latex allergy develop, avoid direct contact with latex gloves and products.
• Wear a Medic Alert bracelet and carry an epinephrine pen (e.g., EpiPen, Symjepi).

Source: National Institute for Occupational Safety and Health (NIOSH). Retrieved from *www.cdc.gov/niosh.*

❖ NURSING AND INTERPROFESSIONAL MANAGEMENT: LATEX ALLERGIES

Identifying patients and health care workers sensitive to latex is crucial to prevent adverse reactions. Obtain a thorough health history and history of any allergies, especially for patients with any history of latex contact symptoms. We cannot identify all latex-sensitive people, even with a careful and thorough history. The greatest risk factor is long-term multiple exposures to latex products (e.g., health care personnel, those who have had multiple surgeries, rubber industry workers). Other risk factors include a patient history of allergic rhinitis, asthma, and allergies to certain foods (listed earlier).

Use latex precaution protocols for those patients with a positive latex allergy test or a history of signs and symptoms related to latex exposure. Many health care facilities have created latex-free product carts to use with patients with latex allergies. The National Institute for Occupational Safety and Health (NIOSH) has published recommendations for preventing allergic reactions to latex in the workplace (Table 13.13).

Because of the potential for severe symptoms of food allergy, teach patients to avoid those foods. Other recommendations for people with latex and food allergies include wearing a Medic Alert bracelet or necklace and carrying an injectable epinephrine pen.

Multiple Chemical Sensitivity

Multiple chemical sensitivity (MCS) is a subjective illness marked by recurrent, vague, nonspecific symptoms attributed to low levels of chemical, biologic, or physical agents.

Commonly accused substances include smoke, pesticides, plastics, synthetic fabrics, scented products, petroleum products, and paint fumes. Women between the ages of 30 and 50 are more likely to develop the symptoms. MCS is a controversial diagnosis. It is not recognized as an illness by the American Medical Association or other authorities.[9]

The symptoms that people report are wide-ranging and not specific. They include headache, fatigue, dizziness, nausea, congestion, itching, sneezing, sore throat, chest pain, breathing problems, muscle pain or stiffness, skin rash, diarrhea, bloating, gas, confusion, difficulty concentrating, memory problems, and mood changes. These symptoms are usually subjective, with no evidence of a pathologic condition or physiologic dysfunction.

Diagnosis is usually made based on a patient's health history. There is no established test to diagnose MCS. The most effective treatment for MCS is to avoid the chemicals that may trigger the symptoms and create a chemical-free and odor-free home and workplace.

Psychotherapy is the recommended treatment. In patients who are unwilling to undergo psychotherapy but willing to accept medications, antidepressants, including selective serotonin reuptake inhibitors (SSRIs) (e.g., citalopram [Celexa]), are options. Drugs for anxiety and sleep also have been used.

AUTOIMMUNITY

Autoimmunity is an immune response against self in which the immune system no longer differentiates self from nonself. For some unknown reason, immune cells that are normally unresponsive (tolerant to self-antigens) are activated. In autoimmunity, autoantibodies and autosensitized T cells cause pathophysiologic tissue damage.

The cause of autoimmune diseases is still unknown. Age may play some role because the number of circulating autoantibodies increases in people over age 50. However, the principal factors in the development of autoimmunity are (1) the inheritance of susceptibility genes, which may contribute to the failure of self-tolerance, and (2) initiation of autoreactivity by triggers, such as infections, which may activate self-reactive lymphocytes.

Autoimmune diseases tend to cluster. A given person may have more than 1 autoimmune disease (e.g., rheumatoid arthritis, Addison's disease), or the same or related autoimmune diseases may be found in other members of the same family. This observation has led to the concept of genetic predisposition to autoimmune disease. Most of the genetic research in this area correlates certain human leukocyte antigen (HLA) types with an autoimmune condition. (HLAs and disease association are discussed later in this chapter on p. 204.)

Even in a genetically predisposed person, some trigger is needed to initiate autoreactivity. This may include infectious agents such as a virus. Viral infections can change cells or tissues that are not normally antigenic. The virally induced changes make the cells or tissues antigenic. Viruses may be involved in the development of diseases such as type 1 diabetes. Rheumatic fever and rheumatic heart disease are autoimmune responses triggered by streptococcal infection and mediated by antibodies against group A β-hemolytic streptococci that cross-react with heart muscles and valves and synovial membranes.

Drugs can be precipitating factors in autoimmune disease. Hemolytic anemia can result from methyldopa administration. Procainamide can induce the formation of antinuclear antibodies and cause a lupus-like syndrome.

Gender and hormones have a role in autoimmune disease. More women than men have autoimmune disease. During pregnancy, many autoimmune diseases get better. After delivery, the woman with an autoimmune disease often has an exacerbation.

Autoimmune Diseases

Generally, autoimmune diseases are grouped according to organ-specific and systemic diseases (Table 13.14). SLE is a classic

---

TABLE 13.14   Examples of Autoimmune Diseases

Systemic Diseases
- Rheumatoid arthritis
- Scleroderma (systemic sclerosis)
- Systemic lupus erythematosus

Organ-Specific Diseases
Blood
- Autoimmune hemolytic anemia
- Hemochromatosis
- Immune thrombocytopenic purpura (ITP)

Central Nervous System
- Guillain-Barré syndrome
- Multiple sclerosis

Endocrine System
- Addison's disease
- Graves' disease
- Hypothyroidism
- Thyroiditis
- Type 1 diabetes

Eye
- Uveitis

Gastrointestinal System
- Celiac disease
- Inflammatory bowel disease
- Pernicious anemia

Heart
- Rheumatic fever

Kidney
- Glomerulonephritis
- Goodpasture syndrome

Liver
- Autoimmune hepatitis
- Primary biliary cirrhosis

Muscle
- Myasthenia gravis

---

example of a systemic autoimmune disease characterized by damage to multiple organs. The cause is unknown, but there appears to be a loss of self-tolerance for the body's own DNA antigens.

In SLE, tissue injury appears to be the result of the formation of antinuclear antibodies. For some reason (possibly a viral infection), the cell membrane is damaged and DNA is released into the systemic circulation, where it is viewed as nonself. This DNA is normally sequestered inside the nucleus of cells. On release into the circulation, the DNA antigen reacts with an antibody. Some antibodies are involved in immune complex formation, and others may cause damage directly. Once the complexes are deposited, the complement system is activated and further damages the tissue, especially the renal glomerulus. SLE is discussed in Chapter 64.

Apheresis

Apheresis is a procedure to separate components of the blood followed by the removal of 1 or more of these components. It is an effective treatment for several autoimmune diseases and other diseases and disorders. Compound words are often used to describe a specific apheresis procedure, depending on the blood components being collected. *Plateletpheresis* is the removal of platelets, usually for collection from normal persons to infuse into patients with low platelet counts (e.g., patients taking chemotherapy who develop thrombocytopenia). *Leukocytapheresis* is a general term indicating the removal of WBCs. It is used in chronic myelogenous leukemia to remove high numbers of leukemic cells.

Apheresis is used in hematopoietic stem cell transplantation to collect stem cells from peripheral blood. These stem cells can then be used to repopulate a person's bone marrow after high-dose chemotherapy (see Chapter 15 for more on hematopoietic stem cell transplants).

Plasmapheresis. *Plasmapheresis* is the removal of plasma containing components causing or thought to cause disease. It can be used to get plasma from healthy donors to give to patients as replacement therapy.

Plasmapheresis involves the removal of whole blood through an IV device, and then the blood circulates through the apheresis machine. Inside the machine the blood is divided into plasma and its cellular components by centrifugation or membrane filtration. The plasma is generally replaced with normal saline, lactated Ringer's solution, fresh-frozen plasma, plasma protein fractions, or albumin. When we manually remove blood, we can only take 500 mL at 1 time. However, with the use of apheresis procedures, more than 4 L of plasma can be pheresed in 2 to 3 hours.

Plasmapheresis has been used to treat autoimmune diseases such as SLE, glomerulonephritis, Goodpasture syndrome, myasthenia gravis, rheumatoid arthritis, and Guillain-Barré syndrome. Many of these disorders have circulating autoantibodies (usually of the IgG class) and antigen-antibody complexes. The reason for performing therapeutic plasmapheresis in autoimmune disorders is to remove pathologic substances present in plasma. Immunosuppressive therapy has been used to prevent recovery of IgG production, and plasmapheresis to prevent antibody rebound.

Plasmapheresis may remove inflammatory mediators (e.g., complement) that are responsible for tissue damage. In the treatment of SLE, plasmapheresis is usually reserved for the patient having an acute attack who is unresponsive to conventional therapy.

You need to be aware of side effects associated with plasmapheresis. The most common complications are hypotension and citrate toxicity. Hypotension is usually the result of a vasovagal reaction or transient volume changes. Citrate, used as an anticoagulant, may cause hypocalcemia, which may cause headache, paresthesias, and dizziness.

IMMUNODEFICIENCY DISORDERS

When the immune system does not adequately protect the body, immunodeficiency exists. Immunodeficiency disorders involve an impairment of 1 or more immune mechanisms, which include (1) phagocytosis, (2) humoral response, (3) cell-mediated response, (4) complement, and (5) a combined humoral and cell-mediated deficiency. Immunodeficiency disorders are *primary* if the immune cells are improperly developed or absent and *secondary* if an illness or treatment causes the deficiency. Primary immunodeficiency disorders are rare and often serious. Secondary disorders are more common and less severe.

Primary Immunodeficiency Disorders

The basic categories of primary immunodeficiency disorders are (1) phagocytic defects, (2) B-cell deficiency, (3) T-cell deficiency, and (4) a combined B-cell and T-cell deficiency (Table 13.15).

Secondary Immunodeficiency Disorders

Key factors that may cause secondary immunodeficiency disorders are listed in Table 13.16. Drug-induced immunosuppression is the most common. Immunosuppressive therapy is prescribed for patients to treat autoimmune disorders and to prevent transplant rejection. Immunosuppression is a serious side effect of drugs used in cancer chemotherapy. Generalized leukopenia often results, leading to a decreased humoral and cell-mediated response. Therefore secondary infections are common in immunosuppressed patients.

Malnutrition alters cell-mediated immune responses. When protein is deficient over a prolonged period, the thymus gland atrophies and lymphoid tissue decreases. In addition, an increased susceptibility to infections always exists.

TABLE 13.15   Primary Immunodeficiency Disorders

Disorder	Affected Cells	Genetic Basis
Ataxia-telangiectasia	B, T	Autosomal recessive
Bruton's X-linked agammaglobulinemia	B	X-linked
Chronic granulomatous disease	PMNs, monocytes	X-linked
Common variable hypogammaglobulinemia	B	—
DiGeorge syndrome (thymic hypoplasia)	T	—
Graft-versus-host disease	B, T	—
Job syndrome	PMNs, monocytes	—
Severe combined immunodeficiency disease	Stem, B, T	X-linked or autosomal recessive
Selective IgA, IgM, or IgG deficiency	B	Some X-linked
Wiskott-Aldrich syndrome	B, T	X-linked

Ig, Immunoglobulin; *PMNs,* Polymorphonuclear neutrophils.

TABLE 13.16   Causes of Secondary Immunodeficiency

Age
- Infants
- Older adults

Diseases or Disorders
- Acquired immunodeficiency syndrome (AIDS)
- Burns
- Cancers
- Chronic kidney disease
- Cirrhosis
- Diabetes
- Hodgkin's lymphoma
- Severe infection
- Systemic lupus erythematosus
- Trauma

Drug-Induced Immunodeficiency
- Chemotherapy drugs
- Corticosteroids

Malnutrition
- Cachexia
- Dietary deficiency

Stress
- Chronic stress
- Trauma (physical or emotional)

Therapies
- Anesthesia
- Radiation
- Surgery

Hodgkin's lymphoma impairs the cell-mediated immune response, and patients may die from severe viral or fungal infections (see Chapter 30). Viruses, especially rubella, may cause immunodeficiency by direct cytotoxic damage to lymphoid cells. Systemic infections can place such a demand on the immune system that resistance to a secondary or another infection is impaired.

Radiation can destroy lymphocytes either directly or through depletion of stem cells. As the radiation dose is increased, more bone marrow atrophies, leading to severe pancytopenia and suppression of immune function. Splenectomy in children is especially dangerous. They may develop sepsis from a simple respiratory tract infection.

Stress may alter the immune response. This response involves interrelationships among the nervous, endocrine, and immune systems (see Chapter 6).

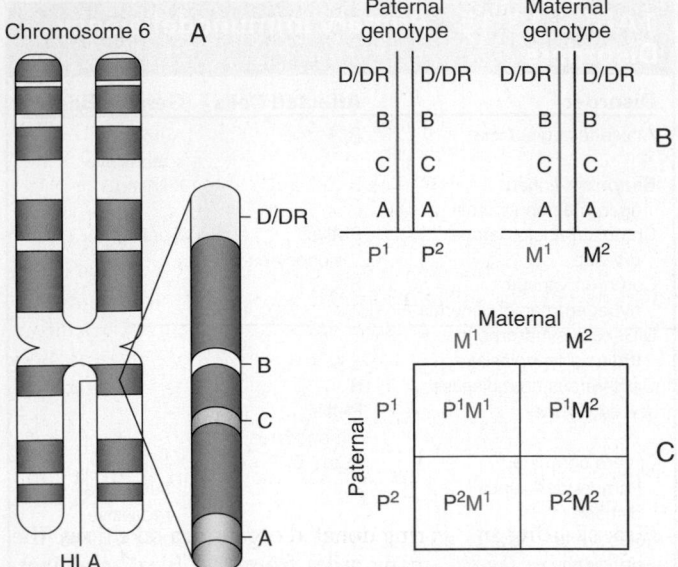

FIG. 13.11 Patterns of human leukocyte antigen (HLA) inheritance. **A,** HLA genes are found on chromosome 6. **B,** The 2 haplotypes of the father are labeled P^1 and P^2, and the haplotypes of the mother are labeled M^1 and M^2. Each child inherits 2 haplotypes, one from each parent. **C,** Therefore only 4 combinations—P^1M^1, P^1M^2, P^2M^1, and P^2M^2—are possible, and 25% of the offspring will have identical HLA haplotypes.

HUMAN LEUKOCYTE ANTIGEN SYSTEM

The antigens responsible for rejection of genetically unlike tissues are called the *major histocompatibility antigens*. These antigens are products of histocompatibility genes. In humans, they are called the **human leukocyte antigen (HLA)** system. The genes for the HLA antigens are linked and occur together on the sixth chromosome. HLAs are present on all nucleated cells and platelets. We primarily use the HLA system in matching organs and tissues for transplantation.

An important characteristic of HLA genes is that they are highly *polymorphic* (variable). Each HLA locus can have many different possible alleles, and thus many combinations exist. Each person has 2 alleles for each locus, 1 inherited from each parent. Both alleles of a locus are expressed independently (i.e., they are codominant). The proteins encoded by certain genes are known as *antigens*.

The entire set of A, B, C, D, and DR genes (the HLA genes) on 1 chromosome is termed a *haplotype*. A complete set is inherited as a unit (haplotype). One haplotype is inherited from each parent (Fig. 13.11). This means that a person has HLA genes that are half identical to those of each parent. The HLA genes of 1 person have a 25% chance of being identical to the HLA genes of a sibling.

In organ transplantation A, B, and DR are primarily used for compatibility matching. The specific allele at each locus is identified by a number. For example, a person could have an HLA of A2, A6, B7, B27, DR4, and DR7. Currently more than 8000 HLA alleles have been identified for the various HLA genes.

Human Leukocyte Antigen and Disease Associations

The early interest in HLAs was stimulated by the role of HLAs in matching donors and recipients of organ transplants. Since that time, the interest in the association between HLAs and disease

has grown. Several diseases show significant associations with specific HLA alleles. People who have these alleles are much more likely to develop the associated disease than those who do not have the alleles. However, having a particular HLA allele does not mean that the person will necessarily develop the associated disease—only that the relative risk is greater than in the general population.

Most of the HLA-associated diseases are classified as autoimmune disorders. Examples of HLA types and disease associations include (1) HLA-B27 and ankylosing spondylitis; (2) HLA-DR2, HLA-DR3, and SLE; (3) HLA-DR3, HLA-DR4, and diabetes; and (4) HLA-DR2 and narcolepsy.

The discovery of HLA associations with certain diseases was a major breakthrough in understanding the genetic bases of these diseases. It is now known that at least part of the genetic bases of HLA-associated diseases lies in the HLA region, but the actual mechanisms involved in these associations are still unknown. However, most people who inherit a specific HLA type (e.g., HLA-DR3) that is associated with a disease will never develop that disease.

Currently the association between HLAs and certain diseases is of minimal practical clinical importance. Nevertheless, there is promise for the development of clinical applications in the future. For example, with certain autoimmune diseases, it may be possible to identify members of a family at greatest risk for developing the same or a related autoimmune disease. These people would need close medical supervision, implementation of preventive measures (if possible), and early diagnosis and treatment to prevent chronic complications.

ORGAN TRANSPLANTATION

Transplantation success has improved with advances in surgical technique, advances in histocompatibility testing, and more effective immunosuppressant drugs. Common tissue transplants include corneas, skin, bone marrow, heart valves, bone, and connective tissues (Fig. 13.12). Cornea transplants can prevent or correct blindness. Skin grafts are used in managing burn patients. Donated bone marrow can help patients with leukemias and other cancers.

Transplanted organs currently come from many different body systems. These organs include the heart, lung, liver, kidney, pancreas, and intestine. Multiple organs can be transplanted together, such as kidney and pancreas, kidney and liver, kidney and heart, or the complete intestinal tract. For example, some patients with diabetes who receive a pancreas transplant also receive a kidney transplant because the diabetes has not only impaired the pancreas but also led to renal failure.

Some organs can be transplanted in parts or segments instead of transplanting an entire organ. Liver and lung lobes (rather than the whole organ) may be transplanted, or an intestine may be used in segments, thus allowing for 1 person's organ donation to help many recipients. This technique enables living donors to donate part of an organ or 1 of their organs, in the case of kidneys.

Organ donations come from either deceased (cadaver) or living donors. Most organs and tissues currently come from deceased donors. However, because of the shortage of organs from deceased donors, the use of related and living unrelated donor organs is increasing.

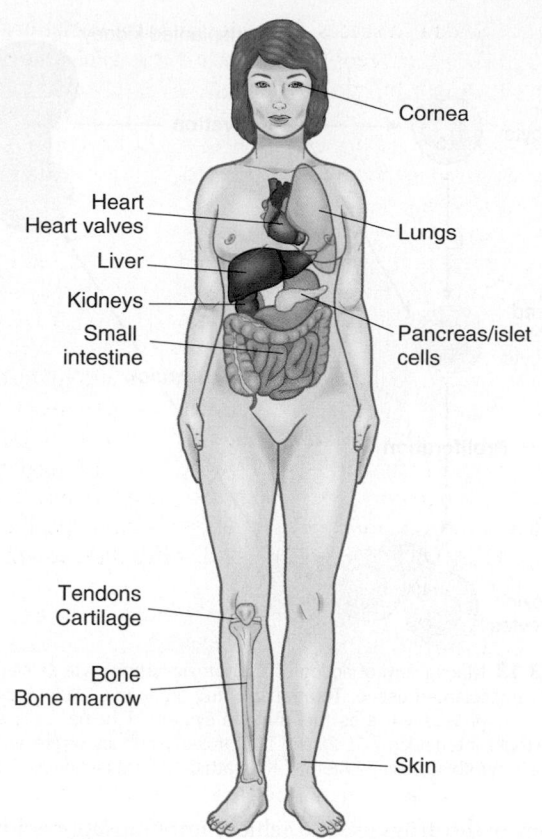

Cornea

Heart
Heart valves

Lungs

Liver

Kidneys

Small
intestine

Pancreas/islet
cells

Tendons
Cartilage

Bone
Bone marrow

Skin

FIG. 13.12 Tissues and organs that can be transplanted.

People can indicate their wish to become a donor when they sign a donor card or driver's license or join a donor registry (depending on the state). However, on their death or imminent death, the person's legal next of kin may need to consent to the donation. Legal requirements and the facility's policy for a donor's legal next of kin to consent regardless of whether the donor's wishes varies from state to state and from facility to facility.

Currently more than 116,000 people are on the organ procurement and transplantation network's national waiting list. This list is maintained by the United Network for Organ Sharing (UNOS). However, fewer than 35,000 people receive transplants annually. The organs in highest demand are kidneys, hearts, and livers. These are also the most often transplanted organs.[10] The Uniform Anatomical Gift Act regulates organ and tissue donations to allow for fair and consistent transplantation laws among all states.[11] Patients are matched to available donors based on a number of factors: ABO blood and HLA typing, medical urgency, time on the waiting list, and geographic location.

Tissue Typing

The recipient usually receives a transplant from an ABO blood group–compatible donor (see Table 29.9). The donor and recipient do not need to share the same Rh factor.

HLA Typing. HLA typing is done on potential donors and recipients. Currently we think only the A, B, and DR antigens are clinically significant for transplantation. Because each locus has 2 alleles that encode for antigens, a total of 6 antigens is identified. In transplantation we try to match as many antigens as possible between the HLA-A, HLA-B, and HLA-DR loci. Antigen matches of 5 and 6 antigens and some 4-antigen matches have

better clinical outcomes (i.e., the patient is less likely to reject the transplanted organ), especially in kidney and bone marrow transplants.

The degree of HLA matching needed or suitable for successful solid organ transplantation depends on the type of organ and degree of acceptable risk. Certain organ and tissue transplants need a closer histocompatibility match than other organs. For example, a cornea transplant can be accepted by nearly anyone because corneas are avascular and therefore no antibodies reach the cornea to cause rejection. In kidney and bone marrow transplantation, HLA matching is very important, since these transplants are at high risk for graft rejection. On the other hand, for liver transplants, HLA mismatches have little impact on graft survival. Heart and lung transplants fall somewhere in between but minimizing HLA mismatches significantly improves survival. For liver, lung, and heart transplants, few donors are available and it is hard to get good HLA matches.

Transporting and storing donated organs can take time. The "best" match may live many miles from the "ideal" recipient. The need to have the "best" matches must be balanced against the time it takes to procure and transport a donated organ and then transplant it.

Panel of Reactive Antibodies. A *panel of reactive antibodies (PRA)* shows the recipient's sensitivity to various HLAs before receiving a transplant. To detect preformed antibodies to HLA, the recipient's serum is mixed with a randomly selected panel of donor lymphocytes to determine reactivity. The potential recipient may have been exposed to HLA antigens by previous blood transfusions, pregnancy, or a previous organ transplant.

PRA allows for the determination of whether a recipient is of high or low reactivity to potential donors. The results for the PRA are calculated in percentages. A high PRA indicates that the person has a large number of cytotoxic antibodies and is highly sensitized, which means there is a poor chance of finding a crossmatch-negative donor. In patients awaiting transplantation, a PRA panel is usually done on a regular basis. In highly sensitized patients (high PRA), plasmapheresis and IV immunoglobulin (IVIG) can be used to lower the number of antibodies.

Crossmatch. A crossmatch is done to determine the existence of antibodies against the potential donor. A crossmatch uses serum from the recipient mixed with donor lymphocytes to test for any preformed anti-HLA antibodies to the potential donor organ. The crossmatch can be used as a screening test when possible living donors are being considered or once a cadaver donor is chosen.

A negative crossmatch means that no preformed antibodies are present, and it is safe to go ahead with transplantation. A positive crossmatch means that the recipient has cytotoxic antibodies to the donor, which is an absolute contraindication in living donor transplants. Live donor transplants may be done for patients with a positive crossmatch if no other live donors (with a negative crossmatch) exist. In this situation, plasmapheresis or IVIG can be done to remove antibodies.

It is not always possible to complete a crossmatch prior to transplantation. If a retrospective crossmatch is done, the results will have implications for immunosuppression protocols after the transplant. A prospective crossmatch is especially important for kidney transplants. It may not be done for lung, liver, and heart transplants.

Transplant Rejection

Rejection is 1 of the major problems after organ transplantation. Organ rejection occurs as a normal immune response to foreign tissue. The risk for rejection is reduced by using immunosuppression therapy, performing ABO and HLA matching, and ensuring that the crossmatch is negative. Unfortunately, many different HLAs exist. A perfect match is nearly impossible unless the tissue is from one's self, an identical twin, or in some cases a sibling. Rejection can be hyperacute, acute, or chronic. Prevention, early diagnosis, and treatment of rejection are essential for long-term graft function.

Hyperacute Rejection. *Hyperacute rejection* occurs within 24 hours after transplantation because the blood vessels are rapidly destroyed. It occurs because the person had preexisting antibodies against the transplanted tissue or organ. There is no treatment for hyperacute rejection, and we must remove the transplanted organ. Fortunately, hyperacute rejection is a rare event because of improved immunosuppression medications and because the final testing prior to transplantation usually determines whether the recipient is sensitized to any of the donor HLAs.

Acute Rejection. *Acute rejection* most often occurs in the first 6 months after transplantation. This type of rejection is usually a cell-mediated immune response by the recipient's lymphocytes, which have been activated against the donated (foreign) tissue or organ (Fig. 13.13). In addition to cell-mediated rejection, another type of acute rejection occurs when the recipient develops antibodies to the transplanted organ (humoral rejection).

It is common to have at least 1 rejection episode, especially with organs from deceased donors. These episodes are usually reversible with additional immunosuppressive therapy. This may include increased corticosteroid doses or polyclonal or monoclonal antibodies. Unfortunately, immunosuppressants increase the risk for infection. To combat acute rejection, all patients with transplants need long-term use of immunosuppressants, putting them at a high risk for infection, especially in the first few months after transplant when the immunosuppressive doses are highest.

Chronic Rejection. *Chronic rejection* is a process that occurs over months or years and is irreversible. Chronic rejection can occur for unknown reasons or from repeated episodes of acute rejection. Large numbers of T and B cells infiltrate the transplanted organ, indicating ongoing, low-grade, immune-mediated injury. Chronic rejection results in fibrosis and scarring. In heart transplants it manifests as accelerated coronary artery disease. In lung transplants it manifests as bronchiolitis obliterans. In liver transplants, we see a loss of bile ducts. In kidney transplants it manifests as fibrosis and glomerulopathy.

There is no definitive therapy for this type of rejection. Treatment is primarily supportive. This type of rejection is hard to manage and is not associated with the optimistic prognosis of acute rejection.

Immunosuppressive Therapy

Immunosuppressive therapy requires a lifelong balance between rejection and infection. On 1 hand, the immune response must be suppressed to prevent rejection of the transplanted organ. On the other hand, an adequate immune response must be maintained to prevent overwhelming infection and the development of cancers.[12]

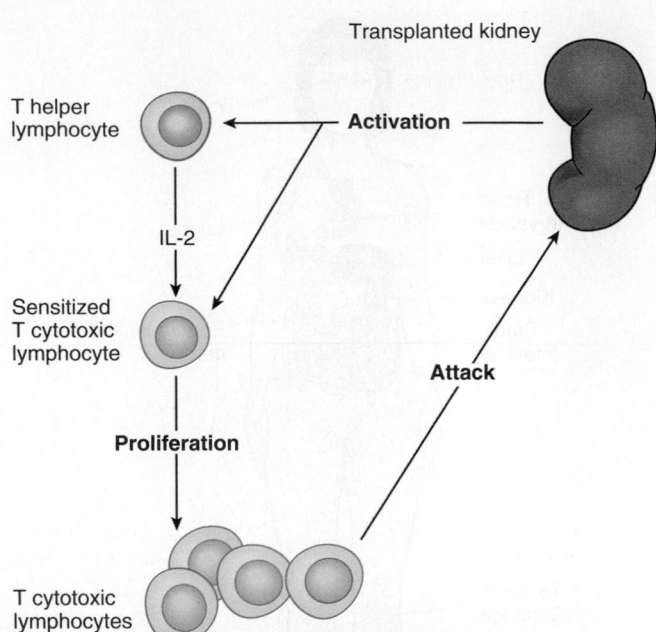

FIG. 13.13 Mechanism of action of T cytotoxic lymphocyte activation and attack of transplanted tissue. The transplanted organ (e.g., kidney) is recognized as foreign and activates the immune system. T helper cells are activated to make interleukin-2 *(IL-2)*, and T cytotoxic lymphocytes are sensitized. After the T cytotoxic cells proliferate, they attack the transplanted organ.

Many of the drugs used to achieve immunosuppression have significant side effects. Because transplant recipients must take immunosuppressants for life, the risk for toxicity continues for the rest of their lives.

Immunosuppressant drugs are listed in Table 13.17. With the use of a combination of agents that work during different phases of the immune response (Fig. 13.13), we can give lower doses of each drug to produce effective immunosuppression while minimizing side effects.

The major immunosuppressive agents are (1) calcineurin inhibitors; (2) corticosteroids (prednisone, methylprednisolone); (3) purine synthesis antagonists, including mycophenolate mofetil (CellCept, Myfortic) and azathioprine (Imuran); and (4) sirolimus. Muromonab-CD3 (Orthoclone OKT3) and either horse antithymocyte globulin (Atgam) or rabbit antithymocyte globulin (ATG) are IV medications used for short periods to prevent early rejection or reverse acute rejection.

Immunosuppression protocols are highly variable among transplant centers, with different combinations of medications being used. Most patients are initially on triple therapy. The standard triple therapy usually includes a calcineurin inhibitor, a corticosteroid, and mycophenolate mofetil.

The doses of immunosuppressant drugs are reduced over time after the transplant. The trend in many transplant centers is to follow an immunosuppression protocol that uses minimal corticosteroids because of their many side effects. Patients taking corticosteroids may be weaned off after a few years.

Calcineurin Inhibitors. This group of drugs, including tacrolimus (Prograf) and cyclosporine (Sandimmune), is the foundation of most immunosuppression regimens. As the most effective immunosuppressants, these drugs prevent a cell-mediated attack against the transplanted organ (Fig. 13.14). They are generally used in combination with corticosteroids, mycophenolate mofetil, and sirolimus. Tacrolimus is the most widely used calcineurin inhibitor. Cyclosporine is being used less often.

TABLE 13.17 **Drug Therapy**

Immunosuppressive Therapy

Agent	Route	Mechanism of Action	Side Effects
Calcineurin Inhibitors			
cyclosporine (Sandimmune, Neoral, Gengraf)	PO, IV	Acts on T helper cells to prevent production and release of IL-2 Inhibits proliferation of T and B cells	Nephrotoxicity, ↑ risk for infection, neurotoxicity (tremors, seizures), hepatotoxicity, lymphoma, hypertension, tremors, hirsutism, leukopenia, gingival hyperplasia
tacrolimus (Prograf)	PO, IV	Same as cyclosporine but more effective	Same as cyclosporine
Corticosteroids			
prednisone, methylprednisolone	PO, IV	Suppress inflammatory response Inhibit cytokine production (IL-1, IL-6, TNF) and T-cell activation and proliferation	Peptic ulcers, hypertension, osteoporosis, Na$^+$ and H$_2$O retention, muscle weakness, easy bruising, delayed healing, hyperglycemia, ↑ risk for infection
Cytotoxic (Antiproliferative) Drugs			
azathioprine (Imuran)	PO, IV	Inhibits purine synthesis Suppresses proliferation of T and B cells	Bone marrow suppression (neutropenia, anemia, thrombocytopenia)
cyclophosphamide	PO, IV	Cross-links DNA, leading to cell injury and death. Results in decrease in number and activity of T and B cells	Neutropenia, hemorrhagic cystitis
everolimus (Zortress)	PO	Binds to mechanistic target of rapamycin (mTOR), thereby suppressing T-cell activation and proliferation	Peripheral edema, constipation, hypertension, nausea, anemia, urinary tract infection, hyperlipidemia
mycophenolate mofetil (CellCept, Myfortic)	PO, IV	Inhibits purine synthesis Suppresses proliferation of T and B cells	Diarrhea, nausea and vomiting, neutropenia, thrombocytopenia, ↑ risk for infection, ↑ incidence of cancer
sirolimus (Rapamune)	PO	Same as everolimus	↑ Risk for infection, leukopenia, anemia, thrombocytopenia, hyperlipidemia, hypercholesterolemia, arthralgias, diarrhea. ↑ incidence of cancer
Monoclonal Antibodies			
alemtuzumab (Campath)	IV	Monoclonal antibody that targets the CD52 antigen on T and B cells, monocytes, and macrophages Causes prolonged T cell depletion	Fever, chills, dyspnea, chest pain, nausea, vomiting. Neutropenia, anemia, thrombocytopenia Increased risk for opportunistic infections
basiliximab (Simulect)	IV	Monoclonal antibody that targets IL-2 receptor and inhibits T cell activation and proliferation	Can cause acute hypersensitivity reaction, including anaphylaxis
daclizumab (Zenapax)	IV	Same as basiliximab	Same as basiliximab
muromonab-CD3 (Orthoclone OKT3)	IV push	Monoclonal antibody that binds to CD3 receptors on T cells, causing cell lysis. Inhibits function of T cells	Fever, chills, dyspnea, chest pain, nausea, vomiting Anaphylactic reactions include pulmonary edema, cardiac or respiratory arrest
Other			
belatacept (Nulojix)	IV	Prevents the activation of T cells	Anemia, diarrhea, constipation, urinary tract infection, peripheral edema
Polyclonal Antibodies			
Horse antithymocyte globulin (Atgam) Rabbit antithymocyte globulin (Thymoglobulin, ATG)	IV	Prepared by immunizing horse or rabbit with human thymocyctes or T cells. Polyclonal antibodies directed against T cells, thus depleting them	Fever, chills, dyspnea, myalgia, chest pain, nausea and vomiting, anaphylaxis, leukopenia, thrombocytopenia, rash, ↑ risk for infection

They do not cause bone marrow suppression or change the normal inflammatory response. Many of the side effects are dose related. These drugs are potentially nephrotoxic. We monitor drug levels closely to prevent toxicity.

 DRUG ALERT Tacrolimus and Cyclosporine

• A substance in grapefruit and grapefruit juice prevents metabolism of these drugs.
• Consuming grapefruit or grapefruit juice while using these drugs can increase their toxicity.

Mycophenolate Mofetil. Mycophenolate mofetil inhibits purine synthesis with suppressive effects on T and B cells. The major limitation of this drug is GI toxicity, including nausea, vomiting, and diarrhea. In many cases the side effects can be lessened by lowering the dose or giving smaller doses more often.

 DRUG ALERT Mycophenolate Mofetil

• When given IV, it can only be reconstituted in D$_5$W.
• Do not give as IV bolus. Give over 2 or more hours.

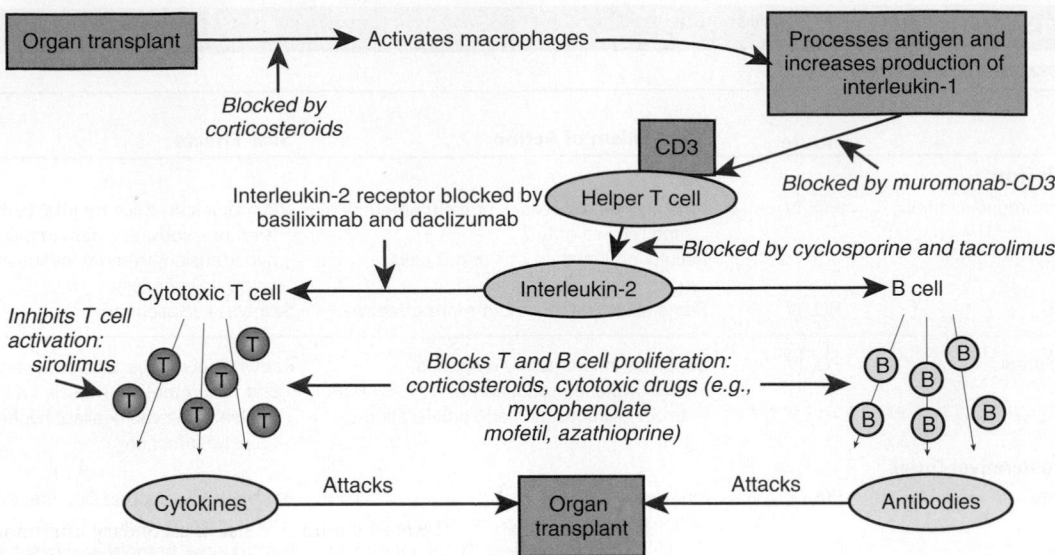

FIG. 13.14 Sites of action for immunosuppressive agents. (Adapted from McKenry L, Tessier E, Hogan M: *Mosby's pharmacology in nursing,* St Louis, 2006, Mosby.)

Sirolimus. Sirolimus (Rapamune) suppresses T-cell activation and proliferation. It is used in combination with corticosteroids, cyclosporine, and/or tacrolimus.

Monoclonal Antibodies. Monoclonal antibodies are used to prevent and treat acute rejection episodes. Muromonab-CD3 was the first of these monoclonal antibodies to be used in clinical transplantation. It is a mouse monoclonal antibody that binds with the CD3 antigen found on the surface of human thymocytes and mature T cells. It interferes with the function of T cells, the pivotal cells involved in rejection. All T cells are affected, rather than just the subset active in graft rejection. It is given by IV bolus. Within minutes after the first infusion of muromonab-CD3, the number of circulating T cells decreases significantly.

A flu-like syndrome occurs during the first few days of treatment because of cytokine release. Side effects include fever, rigors, headache, myalgias, and various GI disturbances. To reduce the expected side effects of muromonab-CD3, give patients acetaminophen, diphenhydramine, and IV methylprednisolone beforehand.

Newer generation monoclonal antibodies are a hybrid of mouse and human antibodies and have fewer side effects than muromonab-CD3 because they have been "humanized." These include daclizumab (Zenapax) and basiliximab (Simulect), which target the IL-2 receptor and impair lymphocyte proliferation. Another monoclonal antibody is alemtuzumab (Campath), which targets the CD52 antigen found on T and B cells, monocytes, and macrophages. It can cause prolonged T-cell depletion.

Polyclonal Antibodies. Polyclonal antibodies to T cells include horse antithymocyte globulin (Atgam) and rabbit antithymocyte globulin (thymoglobulin, ATG). These agents are derived by injecting animals (rabbit or horse) with human lymphoid cells, then procuring and purifying the resultant antibody. They are often used for induction immunosuppression and treatment of acute rejection.

Allergic reactions to the foreign proteins from the host animal, manifested by fever, arthralgias, and tachycardia, are common but usually not severe enough to prevent use. These side effects can be decreased by giving the preparation slowly, over 4 to 6 hours, and premedicating patients with acetaminophen, diphenhydramine, and methylprednisolone. The main toxicities of polyclonal antibodies are leukopenia and thrombocytopenia. They are caused by antibody contaminants that are not completely removed during preparation of the antibodies.

GRAFT-VERSUS-HOST DISEASE

Graft-versus-host disease (GVHD) occurs when an immunoincompetent (immunodeficient) patient receives immunocompetent cells. A GVHD response is most common in hematopoietic stem cell transplants. In most transplantation situations, the biggest concern is the patient's (host's) rejection of the organ or transplant. However, in GVHD disease, the graft (donated tissue) rejects the host (recipient) tissue.[12]

The GVHD response may begin 7 to 30 days after transplantation. Once the reaction is started, little can be done to change its course. The exact mechanism involved in this reaction is not completely understood. However, it involves donor T cells attacking and destroying vulnerable host (recipient) cells.

The target organs for the GVHD phenomenon are the skin, liver, and GI tract. The skin disease may be a maculopapular rash, which may be pruritic or painful. It initially involves the palms and soles of the feet but can progress to a generalized erythema with bullous formation and desquamation (shedding of the outer layer of skin). The liver disease may range from mild jaundice with high liver enzymes to hepatic coma. GI manifestations may include mild to severe diarrhea, severe abdominal pain, GI bleeding, and malabsorption.

The biggest problem with GVHD is infection, with different types of infections seen in different periods. Bacterial and fungal infections predominate right after transplantation when granulocytopenia exists. The development of interstitial pneumonitis is the primary concern later.

There is no adequate treatment of GVHD once it is established. Although corticosteroids are often used, they enhance the susceptibility to infection. The use of immunosuppressive agents (e.g., methotrexate, cyclosporine) has been most effective as a preventive rather than a treatment measure. Radiating blood products before they are given is another way to prevent T-cell replication. Ibrutinib (Imbruvica), a kinase inhibitor that is used to treat several forms of leukemia and lymphoma, is an option for some patients with chronic GVHD.[13]

BRIDGE TO NCLEX EXAMINATION

The number of the question corresponds to the same-numbered outcome at the beginning of the chapter.

1. The function of monocytes in immunity is related to their ability to
   a. stimulate the production of T and B lymphocytes.
   b. make antibodies after exposure to foreign substances.
   c. bind antigens and stimulate natural killer cell activation.
   d. capture antigens by phagocytosis and present them to lymphocytes.

2. The reason newborns are protected for the first 3 months of life from bacterial infections is because of the maternal transmission of
   a. IgA.
   b. IgE.
   c. IgG.
   d. IgM.

3. In a type I hypersensitivity reaction the primary immunologic disorder appears to be
   a. binding of IgG to an antigen on a cell surface.
   b. deposit of antigen-antibody complexes in small vessels.
   c. release of cytokines used to interact with specific antigens.
   d. release of chemical mediators from IgE-bound mast cells and basophils.

4. The nurse is alerted to possible anaphylactic shock immediately after a patient has received IM penicillin by the development of
   a. edema and itching at the injection site.
   b. sneezing and itching of the nose and eyes.
   c. a wheal-and-flare reaction at the injection site.
   d. chest tightness and production of thick sputum.

5. The nurse tells a friend who asks him to administer his allergy shots that
   a. it is illegal for nurses to administer injections outside of a medical setting.
   b. he is qualified to do it if the friend has epinephrine in an injectable syringe provided with his extract.
   c. avoiding the allergens is a more effective way of controlling allergies, and allergy shots are not usually effective.
   d. immunotherapy should only be administered in a setting where emergency equipment and drugs are available.

6. A patient is undergoing plasmapheresis for treatment of systemic lupus erythematosus. The nurse explains that plasmapheresis is used in treatment to
   a. remove T lymphocytes in her blood that are producing antinuclear antibodies.
   b. remove normal particles in her blood that are being damaged by autoantibodies.
   c. exchange her plasma that contains antinuclear antibodies with a substitute fluid.
   d. replace viral-damaged cellular components of her blood with replacement whole blood.

7. The *most* common cause of secondary immunodeficiencies is
   a. drugs.
   b. stress.
   c. malnutrition.
   d. human immunodeficiency virus.

8. Association between HLA antigens and diseases is *most* commonly found in what disease conditions?
   a. Cancers
   b. Infectious diseases
   c. Neurologic diseases
   d. Autoimmune disorders

9. What accurately describes rejection after transplantation?
   a. Hyperacute rejection can be treated with OKT3.
   b. Acute rejection can be treated with sirolimus or tacrolimus.
   c. Chronic rejection can be treated with tacrolimus or cyclosporine.
   d. Hyperacute reaction can be avoided if crossmatching is done before transplantation.

10. In a person having an acute rejection of a transplanted kidney, what would help the nurse understand the course of events (*select all that apply*)?
    a. A new transplant should be considered.
    b. Acute rejection can be treated with OKT3.
    c. Repeated episodes of acute rejection can lead to chronic rejection.
    d. Corticosteroids are the most successful drugs used to treat acute rejection.
    e. Acute rejection is common after a transplant and can be treated with drug therapy.

1. d, 2. c, 3. d, 4. a, 5. d, 6. c, 7. a, 8. d, 9. d, 10. b, c, e

For rationales to these answers and even more NCLEX review questions, visit *http://evolve.elsevier.com/Lewis/medsurg*.

ⓔ EVOLVE WEBSITE/RESOURCES LIST

http://evolve.elsevier.com/Lewis/medsurg
Review Questions (Online Only)
Key Points
Answer Key for Questions
- Rationales for Bridge to NCLEX Examination Questions
Conceptual Care Map Creator
Audio Glossary
Supporting Media
- Animations
- Antibodies and Antigens
- Vaccination
Content Updates

REFERENCES

1. Banasik, Jacquelyn L: *Pathophysiology*, 6th ed, St. Louis, 2018, Elsevier.
*2. Lee SE: Management of anaphylaxis, *Otolaryng Clin N Amer* 50:1175, 2017.
3. American Academy of Allergy, Asthma & Immunology: Food allergy. Retrieved from *www.aaaai.org/conditions-and-treatments/allergies/food-allergies*.
4. American Academy of Allergy, Asthma & Immunology: Anaphylaxis. Retrieved from *www.aaaai.org/conditions-and-treatments/allergies/anaphylaxis*.
5. American Academy of Allergy, Asthma & Immunology: SLIT treatment for allergic rhinitis. Retrieved from *www.aaaai.org/conditions-and-treatments/library/allergy-library/sublingual-immunotherapy-for-allergic-rhinitis*.
6. American Academy of Allergy, Asthma & Immunology: Practice parameters and other guidelines. Retrieved from *www.aaaai.org/practice-resources/statements-and-practice-parameters/practice-parameter-guidelines*.
7. Asthma and Allergy Foundation of America: Allergies. Retrieved from *www.aafa.org/page/latex-allergy.aspx*.
8. Centers for Disease Control and Prevention: Preventing allergic reactions to natural rubber latex in the workplace. Retrieved from *www.cdc.gov/niosh/docs/97-135/pdfs/97-135.pdf*.
9. U.S. Department of Labor: Multiple chemical sensitivities. Retrieved from *www.osha.gov/SLTC/multiplechemicalsensitivities/*.
10. United Network of Organ Sharing (UNOS). Retrieved from *www.unos.org*.
11. U.S. Department Health and Human Services: Organ procurement and transplantation network. Retrieved from *https://optn.transplant.hrsa.gov/*.
12. Cupples SA, Lerret S, McCalmont V, et al: *Core curriculum for transplant nurses*, 2nd ed, Philadelphia, 2017, Wolters Kluwer.
13. Voelker R: Relief for graft-vs-host disease, *JAMA* 318:996, 2017.

14

Infection

Jeffrey Kwong

Always be kind, for everyone you meet is fighting a harder battle.

Plato

ⓔ http://evolve.elsevier.com/Lewis/medsurg/

CONCEPTUAL FOCUS

Adherence	Functional Ability	Inflammation
Coping	Immunity	Nutrition
Fatigue	Infection	

LEARNING OUTCOMES

1. Evaluate the impact of emerging and reemerging infections on health care.
2. Identify interventions to reduce health care–associated infections.
3. Explain the transmission of human immunodeficiency virus (HIV) and factors that affect transmission.
4. Describe the pathophysiology of HIV infection.
5. Apply the diagnostic criteria for acquired immunodeficiency syndrome (AIDS).
6. Describe methods used to test for HIV infection.
7. Discuss the role of HIV antiretroviral therapy.
8. Summarize the characteristics of opportunistic diseases associated with AIDS.
9. Describe the potential complications associated with long-term treatment of HIV infection.
10. Compare and contrast HIV prevention methods.
11. Describe the nursing management of HIV-infected patients and HIV-at-risk patients.

KEY TERMS

acquired immunodeficiency syndrome (AIDS), p. 219
antiretroviral therapy (ART), p. 217
emerging infection, p. 213
health care–associated infections (HAIs), p. 214

human immunodeficiency virus (HIV), p. 216
opportunistic diseases, p. 218
postexposure prophylaxis (PEP), p. 225
preexposure prophylaxis (PrEP) p. 222
standard precautions, p. 216

transmission-based precautions, p. 216
viral load, p. 218
window period, p. 219

This chapter presents a brief overview of the concept of emerging and health care–associated infections (HAIs). This includes identifying persons most at risk, recognizing signs and symptoms of infection, and understanding ways to treat or manage infection. Infection, immunity, and inflammation are closely related. Infection stimulates an inflammatory response and affects thermoregulation. The patient may have fatigue and pain. Maintaining adequate nutrition and rest is important to combating infection and supporting immune function. The chapter closes with a comprehensive discussion of human immunodeficiency virus (HIV) infection, focusing on transmission, pathophysiology, and interprofessional and nursing management.

INFECTIONS

Infections, such as lower respiratory tract infections, malaria, HIV, and tuberculosis (TB), are responsible for a significant number of deaths worldwide. Infection occurs when a *pathogen* (a microorganism that causes disease) invades the body, multiplies, and produces disease, usually causing harm to the host. The signs and symptoms of infection are a result of specific pathogen activity, which triggers inflammation and other immune responses.

We categorize infections as localized, disseminated, or systemic. A *localized* infection is limited to a small area. A *disseminated* infection has spread to areas of the body beyond the initial site of infection. *Systemic* infections have spread extensively throughout the body, often via the blood.

TYPES OF PATHOGENS

The many kinds of pathogens are classified into several groups, including bacteria, viruses, fungi, protozoa, and prions. *Bacteria* are one-celled organisms that are common throughout nature.

Many bacteria are normal flora. They live harmoniously in or on the human body without causing disease under normal circumstances. Normal flora protect the human body by preventing the overgrowth of other microorganisms. For example, *Escherichia coli* is part of the normal flora in the large intestine.

Bacteria cause disease in 2 ways: by entering the body and growing inside human cells (e.g., TB) or by secreting toxins that damage cells (e.g., *Staphylococcus aureus*). Bacteria are classified based on the shape of their cells. *Cocci*, such as streptococci and staphylococci, are round. *Bacilli* are rod shaped and include tetanus and TB. *Curved rods* include *Vibrio* bacteria, one of which causes cholera. *Spirochetes* are spiral shaped. They include the organisms that cause leprosy and syphilis. Table 14.1 lists common bacteria that cause disease.

Viruses, unlike bacteria, do not have a cellular structure. They are simple infectious particles that consist of a small amount of genetic material (either ribonucleic acid [RNA] or deoxyribonucleic acid [DNA]) and a protein envelope. Viruses can reproduce only after releasing their genetic material into the cell of another living organism. Examples of diseases caused by viruses are shown in Table 14.2.

Fungi are organisms similar to plants, but they lack chlorophyll. *Mycosis* is any disease caused by a fungus. Pathogenic fungi cause infections that are usually localized but can become disseminated in an immunocompromised person. Tinea pedis (athlete's foot) and tinea corporis (ringworm) are common mycotic infections. Some fungi are normal flora in the body, but when overgrowth occurs, disease can result. Overgrowth of *Candida albicans*, for example, can cause candidiasis in the mouth (thrush), esophagus, intestines, and vagina. Table 14.3 lists other fungi and their respective mycotic infections.

Protozoa are single-cell, animal-like microorganisms. Protozoa normally live in soil and bodies of water. When

TABLE 14.1 Disease-Causing Bacteria

Bacteria	Diseases Caused
Chlamydia trachomatis	Chlamydia, lymphogranuloma venereum
Clostridia	
• Clostridium botulinum	Food poisoning with progressive muscle paralysis
• Clostridium tetani	Tetanus (lockjaw)
Corynebacterium diphtheriae	Diphtheria
Escherichia coli	UTIs, peritonitis, hemolytic-uremic syndrome
Haemophilus	
• Haemophilus influenzae	Nasopharyngitis, meningitis, pneumonia
• Haemophilus pertussis	Pertussis (whooping cough)
Helicobacter pylori	Peptic ulcers, gastritis
Klebsiella-Enterobacter organisms	UTIs, peritonitis, pneumonia
Legionella pneumophila	Pneumonia (Legionnaires' disease)
Mycobacteria	
• Mycobacterium leprae	Hansen's disease (leprosy)
• Mycobacterium tuberculosis	Tuberculosis
Neisseriae	
• Neisseria gonorrhoeae	Gonorrhea, pelvic inflammatory disease, proctitis
• Neisseria meningitidis	Meningococcemia, meningitis
Proteus species	UTIs, peritonitis
Pseudomonas aeruginosa	UTIs, meningitis
Salmonella	
• Salmonella typhi	Typhoid fever
• Other Salmonella organisms	Food poisoning, gastroenteritis
Shigella	Shigellosis; diarrhea, abdominal pain, and fever (dysentery)
Staphylococcus aureus	Skin infections, pneumonia, UTIs, acute osteomyelitis, toxic shock syndrome
Streptococci	
• Streptococcus faecalis	Genitourinary infection, infection of surgical wounds
• Streptococcus pneumoniae	Pneumococcal pneumonia
• Streptococcus pyogenes (group A β-hemolytic streptococci)	Pharyngitis, scarlet fever, rheumatic fever, acute glomerulonephritis, erysipelas, pneumonia
• S. pyogenes (group B β-hemolytic streptococci)	UTIs
• Streptococcus viridans	Bacterial endocarditis
Treponema pallidum	Syphilis

TABLE 14.2 Disease-Causing Viruses

Virus	Diseases Caused
Adenoviruses	Upper respiratory tract infection, pneumonia
Arbovirus	Syndrome of fever, malaise, headache, myalgia; aseptic meningitis; encephalitis
Coronavirus	Upper respiratory tract infection
Coxsackieviruses A and B	Upper respiratory tract infection, gastroenteritis, acute myocarditis, aseptic meningitis
Ebola	Hemorrhagic fever
Echoviruses	Upper respiratory tract infection, gastroenteritis, aseptic meningitis
Hepatitis A, B, C	Viral hepatitis
Herpesviruses	
• Cytomegalovirus CMV)	Gastroenteritis; pneumonia and retinal damage in immunosuppressed persons, infectious mononucleosis-like syndrome
• Epstein-Barr	Mononucleosis, Burkitt's lymphoma (possibly)
• Herpes simplex type 1	Herpes labialis ("fever blisters"), genital herpes infection
• Herpes simplex type 2	Genital herpes infection
• Varicella-zoster	Chickenpox, shingles
Human immunodeficiency virus (HIV)	HIV infection, AIDS
Influenza A and B	Upper respiratory tract infection, H1N1 (swine) flu, H5N1 avian (bird) flu
Mumps	Parotitis, orchitis in postpubertal males
Papillomavirus	Genital warts, cervical and anal cancer
Parainfluenza 1-4	Upper respiratory tract infection
Parvovirus	Gastroenteritis
Poliovirus	Poliomyelitis
Pox viruses	Smallpox, Molluscum contagiosum
Reoviruses 1, 2, 3	Upper respiratory tract infection
Respiratory syncytial virus	Gastroenteritis, respiratory tract infection
Rhabdovirus	Rabies
Rhinovirus	Upper respiratory tract infection, pneumonia
Rotaviruses	Gastroenteritis
Rubella	German measles
Rubeola	Measles
West Nile virus	Flu-like symptoms, meningitis, encephalitis
Zika virus	Flu-like symptoms, fetal microcephaly

TABLE 14.3 Disease-Causing Fungi

Fungi	Diseases Caused	Organs Affected
Aspergillus fumigatus	Aspergillosis	Lungs*
	Otomycosis	Ears
Blastomyces derma-titidis	Blastomycosis	Lungs,* various organs
Candida albicans	Candidiasis	Intestines
	Vaginitis	Vagina
	Thrush	Skin,† mouth
Coccidioides immitis	Coccidioidomycosis	Lungs*
Epidermophyton	Tinea corporis	Skin†
Microsporum	Tinea capitis	Skin†
Pneumocystis jiroveci	Pneumocystis pneumonia (PCP)	Lungs*
Sporothrix schenckii	Sporotrichosis	Skin, lymph vessels
Trichophyton	Tinea pedis	Skin†

*See Table 27.14: Fungal Infections of the Lung.
†See Table 23.8, Common Fungal Infections of the Skin.

TABLE 14.4 Emerging Infections

Microorganism	Related Disease
Bacteria	
Borrelia burgdorferi	Lyme disease
Campylobacter jejuni	Diarrhea
Escherichia coli O157:H7	Hemorrhagic colitis, hemolytic-uremic syndrome
Helicobacter pylori	Peptic ulcer disease
Legionella pneumophila	Pneumonia (Legionnaires' disease)
Vibrio cholerae 0139	New strain associated with epidemic cholera
Virus	
Chikungunya	Fever, muscle aches, rash
Ebola virus	Ebola hemorrhagic fever
H1N1	H1N1 (swine) flu
Hantavirus	Hemorrhagic fever associated with severe pulmonary syndrome
Hepatitis C virus	Parenterally transmitted hepatitis
Hepatitis E virus	Enterically transmitted hepatitis
Human immunodeficiency virus (HIV)	HIV infection and AIDS
Human herpesvirus 6 (HHV-6)	Roseola subitum
Human herpesvirus 8 (HHV-8)	Associated with Kaposi sarcoma in immunosuppressed patients, including people with HIV infection
West Nile virus	West Nile fever
Zika virus	Fever, rash, muscle aches; microcephaly in children born to infected mothers
Parasite	
Cryptosporidium parvum	Acute and chronic diarrhea

introduced into the human body, they can cause infection. Protozoal parasites cause amoebic dysentery and giardiasis. A sporozoan called *Plasmodium malariae* causes malaria.

Prions are infectious particles that have abnormally shaped proteins. Not all prions cause disease. Those that do typically affect the nervous system. They can cause a group of illnesses called *transmissible spongiform encephalopathies (TSEs)*. Examples of TSEs are Creutzfeldt-Jakob disease and bovine spongiform encephalopathy in cattle (also known as mad cow disease).

EMERGING INFECTIONS

An **emerging infection** is an infectious disease that has recently increased in incidence or that threatens to increase in the immediate future.[1] Table 14.4 lists examples of emerging infections. Emerging infectious diseases can originate from unknown sources or from contact with animals, changes in known diseases, or biologic warfare. For example, severe acute respiratory syndrome (SARS) and the Ebola virus come from animal sources. Others emerged when a previously treatable organism developed resistance to antibiotics.

The battle against infection is not new, but modern technologies have changed the rules of the game. Global travel, population density, encroachment into new environments, misuse of antibiotics, and bioterrorism have increased the risk for widespread distribution of emerging infections.

Additionally, some diseases thought to be under control, such as TB, measles, and pertussis, have reemerged. Newer infections include Middle Eastern respiratory syndrome (MERS), severe acute respiratory syndrome (SARS), Zika virus, and zoonotic influenza viruses (e.g., H1N1, H5N1).

Studies in *zoonosis* (science of transmission of diseases from animals to humans) have shown that many known infectious diseases come from animal and insect vectors. The SARS outbreak in China in 2003, for instance, was linked to the civet cat, a small carnivorous mammal found throughout much of Asia and Africa. SARS is discussed in Chapter 67.

West Nile virus is carried and transmitted by mosquitoes. Mosquitoes acquire the virus as they draw blood from infected animals and humans. The virus does not cause illness in the mosquito. The mosquito transfers the virus to uninfected animals and humans when it feeds. Bird deaths are an early warning sign of a West Nile virus outbreak, which can spread quickly if action is not taken promptly. West Nile virus is discussed in Chapter 56.

Influenza viruses are examples of how disease can spread between animals and humans. Variants of influenza A viruses are responsible for many influenza epidemics. We traced the 2009 influenza A (H1N1) outbreak back to pigs, hence the name *swine flu*. In 1997 and 2003, outbreaks of the influenza A (H5N1) strain of avian flu resulted from transmission of influenza virus from chickens to humans.

Ebola virus has been an ongoing public health challenge since it was first seen in 1976. In 2014, rates of Ebola increased significantly in East Africa and the first cases of Ebola occurred in the United States. These initial cases were primarily from travelers or medical aid workers who were working in Africa. Ebola virus can cause severe hemorrhagic fever and is usually lethal. Therapeutic and preventive measures are limited. The natural reservoir and path of transmission are unknown, which makes it impossible to effectively combat Ebola virus and the disease it causes.

Reemerging Infections

Advances in the development of medications and vaccines has led to the near eradication of some infections (e.g., smallpox, polio), but infective agents can reemerge under the right conditions. Table 14.5 presents some diseases that have shown resurgence in recent decades. For example, infections such as measles and pertussis have had sporadic resurgences.[2] This is in part due to people not receiving recommended vaccines.

TABLE 14.5 Reemerging Infections

Microorganism	Infection	Description
Bacteria		
Corynebacterium diphtheriae	Diphtheria	Localized infection of mucous membranes or skin
Bordetella pertussis	Pertussis	Acute, highly contagious respiratory disease characterized by loud whooping inspiration. Also known as whooping cough
Mycobacterium tuberculosis	Tuberculosis	Chronic infection transmitted by inhalation of infected droplets (see Chapter 27)
Virus		
Dengue viruses (flaviviruses)	Dengue fever	Acute infection transmitted by mosquitoes. Occurs mainly in tropical and subtropical regions
Rubeola	Measles	Fever, malaise, cough, and maculopapular rash
Parasite		
Giardia	Giardiasis	Diarrheal illness that usually originates in water contaminated with fecal matter. Also known as traveler's diarrhea

TABLE 14.6 Common Antibiotic-Resistant Organisms and Treatment

Bacteria	Resistant to	Preferred Treatment
Enterococcus faecalis	vancomycin streptomycin gentamicin	daptomycin (Cubicin) linezolid (Zyvox) oritavancin (Orbactiv) tigecycline (Tygacil)
Enterococcus faecium	vancomycin streptomycin gentamicin	daptomycin (Cubicin) linezolid (Zyvox) tigecycline (Tygacil)
Klebsiella pneumoniae	carbapenems (e.g., imipenem, meropenem)	ceftazidime and avibactam (Avycaz)
Staphylococcus aureus	methicillin*	vancomycin
Staphylococcus epidermidis	methicillin*	vancomycin
Streptococcus pneumoniae	penicillin G	ceftriaxone cefotaxime

*This drug is no longer available in the United States.

International travel has created a new obstacle for the local eradication of diseases. For example, measles is no longer endemic in the United States but is still a leading cause of death in developing countries. Domestic outbreaks have typically occurred in areas with low vaccination rates. Some cases occurred in people who have recently traveled to measles-endemic areas outside the United States.[3]

Antimicrobial-Resistant Organisms

Resistance occurs when pathogenic organisms change in ways that decrease the ability of a drug (or a family of drugs) to treat disease.[4] Microorganisms can become resistant to classic treatments (e.g., penicillin) as well as to newer antibiotics and antiviral agents. Microorganisms are highly adaptable. They have evolved genetic and biochemical mechanisms to defend against antimicrobials. Genetic mechanisms include mutation and acquisition of new DNA or RNA. Biochemically, bacteria can resist antibiotics by producing enzymes that destroy or inactivate the drugs. Drug target sites are then altered so that the antibiotic cannot bind to or enter the bacteria. If the drug cannot enter the cell, it cannot kill the bacteria. Table 14.6 describes common antibiotic-resistant bacteria.

Methicillin-resistant *S. aureus* (MRSA), vancomycin-resistant enterococci (VRE), vancomycin-resistant *S. aureus* (VRSA), carbapenem-resistant Enterobacteriaceae (CRE), and penicillin-resistant *Streptococcus pneumoniae* are examples of emerging strains of antibiotic-resistant organisms. These drug-resistant bacteria were first seen in health care settings but are becoming more prevalent in the community. For example, we initially considered MRSA, a form of *S. aureus* that does not respond to methicillin- or penicillin-based therapies, a health care–associated infection (HA-MRSA). However, a variant strain of MRSA that is primarily acquired in the community (community-acquired MRSA [CA-MRSA]) has emerged.[5] This strain of MRSA is more *virulent* (able to cause disease or infection) compared with HA-MRSA. CA-MRSA can cause rapidly forming skin infections and systemic diseases, including pneumonia and sepsis. VRE infection is another concern for patients and health care workers. VRE are more virulent than MRSA and can survive on environmental surfaces for weeks. Although antibiotic-resistant bacteria can infect anyone, hospitalized patients and those with a suppressed immune system are more likely to be exposed to these bacteria and to develop infection.

HCPs have contributed to the development of drug-resistant microorganisms by (1) giving antibiotics for viral infections, (2) succumbing to patient pressure to prescribe unnecessary antibiotic therapy, (3) using inadequate drug regimens to treat infections, or (4) using broad-spectrum or combination agents for infections that should be treated with first-line medications.

Patients can contribute to resistance development by (1) skipping doses, (2) not taking antibiotics for the full duration of prescribed therapy, or (3) saving unused antibiotics "in case I need them later." In addition, limited resources and access to medications make it hard for some patients to get adequate treatment for infections. Teaching patients and their families the proper use of antibiotics (Table 14.7) is crucial to treatment success and prevention of drug-resistant pathogens. The Centers for Disease Control and Prevention (CDC), the Infectious Diseases Society of America (IDSA), and many health care organizations campaign for greater vigilance in minimizing the misuse of antibiotics in reaction to this growing concern.

Although antibiotics are a class of drugs that we typically think of when discussing drug-resistant organisms, any organism (virus, fungi, parasite) can develop drug resistance to agents typically used to treat them. Hence, we now use the term *antimicrobial resistance* to describe the phenomena of resistance across different classes of organisms.

HEALTH CARE–ASSOCIATED INFECTIONS

Health care–associated infections (HAIs) are infections that are acquired because of exposure to microorganisms in a health care setting.[6] About 722,000 HAIs occur annually, and nearly 1 in every 25 hospitalized patients has at least 1 HAI.

TABLE 14.7 Patient & Caregiver Teaching

Decrease Risk for Antibiotic-Resistant Infection

Include the following instructions when teaching patients or their caregivers how to decrease the risk for antibiotic-resistant infection.

1. Only Take Antibiotics Prescribed for You
- This decreases your risk for developing resistant infection.
- You may need antibiotics before certain surgeries and dental work or in the presence of immune dysfunction.

2. Wash Your Hands Frequently
- Hand washing is the single most important thing you can do to prevent infection.

3. Follow Directions When Taking Antibiotics
- Not taking your antibiotic as prescribed or skipping doses can allow antibiotic-resistant bacteria to develop.

4. Do Not Request an Antibiotic for Flu or Colds
- If your HCP says that you do not need an antibiotic, chances are you do not.
- Antibiotics are effective against bacterial infections but not viruses, which cause colds and flu.

5. Finish Your Antibiotic
- Do not stop taking your antibiotic when you feel better.
- If you stop taking your antibiotic early, the hardiest bacteria survive and multiply.
- Eventually you could develop an infection resistant to any antibiotics. You should never have leftover antibiotics.

6. Do Not Take Leftover Antibiotics
- Do not save unfinished antibiotics for later use or borrow leftover drugs from family or friends.
- This is dangerous because (1) the leftover antibiotic may not be appropriate for you, (2) your illness may not be a bacterial infection, (3) old antibiotics can lose their effectiveness and, in some cases, can be fatal, and (4) there will not be enough doses in a leftover bottle to provide full treatment.

TABLE 14.8 OSHA Requirements for Personal Protective Equipment

The following equipment minimizes exposure to blood-borne pathogens.

Equipment	Indications for Use
Gloves	• Must be used when the employee can reasonably expect having contact with blood or other potentially infectious materials, when performing vascular access procedures, and when handling or touching contaminated items or surfaces. • Gloves must be replaced if torn, punctured, or contaminated or their ability to function as a barrier is compromised.
Clothing (gowns, aprons, caps, boots)	• Must be used when occupational exposure is expected. • The type and characteristics depend on the task and degree of exposure expected.
Face protection (mask and glasses with solid side shields or a chin-length face shield)	• Must be used when splashes, sprays, spatters, or droplets of blood or other potentially infectious materials pose a hazard to the eyes, nose, or mouth.

Source: Occupational Safety and Health Administration (OSHA): Bloodborne pathogens and needlestick prevention. Retrieved from *www.osha.gov/ SLTC/bloodbornepathogens.*

Improvements in infection control have resulted in fewer infections in recent years.[7] We have seen decreases in several of the major types of HAIs, including central line–associated bloodstream infections, surgical site infections, *Clostridium difficile* infections, and methicillin-resistant *S. aureus* bacteremia. Any organism can cause HAIs, but certain bacteria, including *E. coli, S. aureus, Enterobacter aerogenes,* and various types of streptococci, are the more common culprits. Some bacteria that do not normally cause disease can cause infections in high-risk patients because of illness or treatment of illness. Surgical and immunocompromised patients are at highest risk.

Around one-third of HAIs are preventable. HCPs often transmit HAIs from patient to patient through direct contact. First lines of defense to prevent the spread of HAIs include hand washing (or using an alcohol-based hand sanitizer) before and after patient contact or procedures, appropriate use of personal protective equipment such as gloves, and decontamination of equipment used for patient care.[8] Isolated infections also can be caused when bacteria that normally stay in one area of the body are introduced into another area. Therefore you must take care to change gloves and wash hands when moving from one task to another, even when working with the same patient. Most facilities have developed and implemented guidelines on reducing and controlling the spread of disease in health care settings, especially of antimicrobial-resistant organisms (Table 14.8).[9] Nurses and all HCPs have the responsibility of using appropriate measures, including transmission-based precautions, to help protect patients from HAIs.

 Gerontologic Considerations: Infections in Older Adults

For older adults, the rate of HAIs is 2 to 3 times higher compared to younger patients. Persons in long-term care facilities are at higher risk for HAI. Age-related changes (e.g., impaired immune function) and co-morbidities, such as diabetes and physical disabilities, contribute to higher infection rates in older adults.[10]

Infections common in older adults include pneumonia, urinary tract infections (UTIs), skin infections, and TB. UTIs are more common in those who live in long-term care facilities. Patients with indwelling catheters are at particular risk.

? CHECK YOUR PRACTICE

You are working in a long-term care facility. One of your residents, a 76-yr-old man who is recovering from a stroke, seems very confused today. You discuss your concerns with the unlicensed assistive personnel (UAP). You explain that he seemed so alert yesterday and wonder if he may have an infection, such as pneumonia or a UTI. The UAP says, "I just took his temperature and it is normal. I don't think he has an infection."
- How should you follow up with the resident and the UAP?

Infections in older adults often have atypical manifestations, such as cognitive and behavioral changes, before the emergence of fever, pain, or changes in laboratory values. Do not rely on the presence of fever to indicate infection in older adults because many have lower core body temperatures and decreased immune responses. Suspicion of disease should typically begin if a patient shows changes in the ability to perform daily activities or in cognitive function. In addition, underlying diseases, increased frequency of drug reactions, and institutionalization can complicate the management of an older adult with infection.

INFECTION PREVENTION AND CONTROL

Occupational Safety and Health Administration (OSHA) Guidelines

OSHA is a federal agency that protects workers from injury and illness in places of employment and supports activities that minimize or eliminate exposure to infectious materials in the workplace. OSHA mandates that any employer whose employees could be exposed to potentially infectious materials implement standard policies and procedures to protect those employees. Employees must be provided with appropriate personal protective equipment (PPE) and safety equipment at no cost to the employee.[11] These include gloves, gowns, facial protection, and disposal systems for sharps (Table 14.8). PPE also must be provided in the right sizes. Hypoallergenic gloves or similar alternatives must be made available to those who have an allergic sensitivity to gloves. Appropriate PPE varies depending on the situation. You need to use sound judgment when deciding when and how to use protective equipment.

Infection Precautions

The CDC has established guidelines with 2 levels of precautions: (1) standard precautions, designed for the care of all patients in hospitals and health care facilities and (2) transmission-based precautions, designed for specific diseases.[12] The purpose of these precautions is to prevent the transmission of organisms from patients to HCPs, from HCPs to patients, from patients to other patients, and from health care personnel and patients to people outside of the hospital (Table 14.9).

The *standard precautions* system applies to (1) blood; (2) all body fluids, secretions, and excretions; (3) non-intact skin; and (4) mucous membranes. Standard precautions are designed to reduce the risk for transmission of microorganisms in hospitals. Standard precautions should be applied to *all* patients regardless of diagnosis or presumed infection status. The CDC's standard precautions incorporate all the OSHA blood-borne pathogens standard requirements.

Transmission-based precautions are used for patients known to be or suspected of being infected with highly transmissible or epidemiologically important pathogens that require additional precautions to interrupt transmission and prevent infection. Transmission-based precautions include airborne precautions, droplet precautions, and contact precautions. *Airborne precautions* are used if the organism can cause infection over long distances when suspended in the air (e.g., TB, rubeola). *Droplet precautions* minimize contact with pathogens that spread through the air at close contact and that affect the respiratory system or mucous membranes (e.g., influenza, pertussis). *Contact precautions* minimize the spread of pathogens that are acquired from direct or indirect contact, especially multidrug-resistant organisms (e.g., MRSA, VRE, CRE). Transmission-based precautions may be combined for diseases that have multiple routes of transmission. Whether used alone or in combination, transmission-based precautions should always be used in conjunction with standard precautions.

HUMAN IMMUNODEFICIENCY VIRUS INFECTION

Human immunodeficiency virus (HIV) is a retrovirus that causes immunosuppression. Persons with HIV are more susceptible to infections that people normally control through immune responses. The terms *HIV disease* and *HIV infection* are used interchangeably. With advances in treatment, we view HIV as a chronic disease since people with the disease are living longer.

More than 1 million people are currently living with HIV in the United States, with about 37,600 new infections occurring each year.[13] With the availability of effective HIV treatment, there has been a dramatic drop in the number of deaths attributable to HIV. In North America HIV is most prevalent among men who have sex with men (MSM).

Transmission of HIV

HIV can be transmitted through contact with infected blood, semen, vaginal secretions, or breast milk.[14] HIV transmission occurs through sexual intercourse with an infected partner; exposure to HIV-infected blood or blood products; and perinatal transmission during pregnancy, at delivery, or through breastfeeding. HIV is not spread casually. The virus cannot be transmitted through hugging, dry kissing, shaking hands, sharing eating utensils, using toilet seats, or casual encounters in any setting. It is not spread by tears, saliva, urine, emesis, sputum, feces, sweat, respiratory droplets, or enteric routes. Health care personnel have a low risk for acquiring HIV at work, even after a needle-stick injury.[15]

Sexual Transmission. The most common mode of HIV transmission is unprotected sexual contact with an HIV-infected partner. Sexual activity involves contact with semen, vaginal secretions, and/or blood, all of which have lymphocytes that may contain HIV. During any form of sexual intercourse (anal, vaginal, oral), the risk for infection is greater for the partner who receives the semen. This is because the receiver has prolonged contact with infected fluids. It helps explain why it is easier to infect women than men during heterosexual intercourse. Sexual activities that cause trauma to local tissues can increase

TABLE 14.9 Types of Isolation Precautions Used in Health Care Settings

Type	Examples
Standard Precautions	
• Used for care of all patients, regardless of their diagnosis or presumed infection status	Includes the use of hand washing and appropriate personal protective equipment
Transmission-Based Precautions	
• Recommended to provide additional precautions beyond standard precautions to prevent transmission of pathogens	**Airborne precautions:** Used for infections spread in small particles in the air, such as chickenpox (varicella), measles, and TB
• Can be used for patients known or suspected to be infected or colonized with pathogens that can be transmitted by airborne or droplet transmission, or by contact with dry skin or contaminated surfaces	**Droplet precautions:** Used for infections spread in large droplets by coughing, talking, or sneezing, such as influenza and bacterial meningitis
• These precautions should be used in addition to standard precautions	**Contact precautions:** Used for infections spread by skin-to-skin contact or contact with other surfaces, such as *C. difficile*, MRSA, and VRE

the risk for transmission. In addition, genital lesions from other sexually transmitted infections (e.g., herpes, syphilis) significantly increase the chance of transmission.

Contact With Blood and Blood Products. HIV can be transmitted from exposure to blood when sharing drug-using paraphernalia. Needles, syringes, straws, and other equipment may be contaminated with HIV or other blood-borne organisms. Sharing this equipment can result in disease transmission.

Routine screening of blood donors to identify at-risk persons and testing donated blood for the presence of HIV have

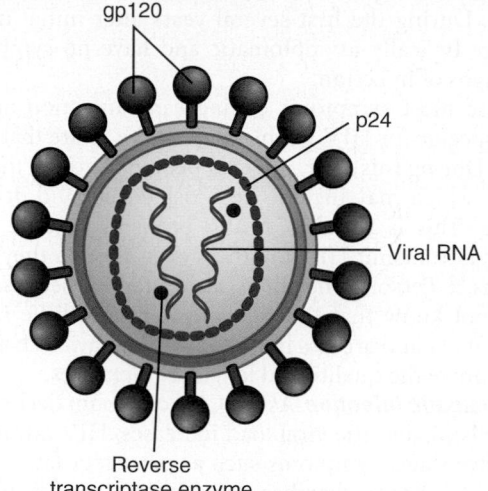

FIG. 14.1 HIV is surrounded by an envelope made up of proteins (including gp120) and a core of viral RNA and proteins.

improved the safety of the blood supply. In countries that routinely test donated blood, HIV infection because of blood transfusions or hemophilia clotting factors is unlikely.

Puncture wounds are the most common means of work-related HIV transmission. The risk for infection after a needlestick exposure to HIV-infected blood is 0.3% to 0.4% (or 3 or 4 out of 1000).[15] The risk is higher if the exposure involves blood from a patient with a high level of circulating HIV, a deep puncture wound, a needle with a hollow bore and visible blood, or a device used for venous or arterial access. Splash exposures of blood on skin with an open lesion present some risk, but it is much lower than from a puncture wound.

Perinatal Transmission. Perinatal transmission from an HIV-infected mother to her infant can occur during pregnancy, delivery, or breastfeeding. On average, 25% of infants born to women with untreated HIV infection are born with HIV. Fortunately, the risk for transmission is less than 2% in settings in which pregnant women are routinely tested for HIV infection and, if found to be infected, treated with **antiretroviral therapy (ART)**, a combination of medications used to control and suppress HIV replication.[16]

Pathophysiology

HIV is an RNA virus. RNA viruses are called *retroviruses* because they replicate in a "backward" manner (going from RNA to DNA). Like all viruses, HIV cannot replicate unless it is inside a living cell.[17] The *CD4+ T cell (CD4 cell)*, a type of lymphocyte, is the target cell for HIV. HIV enters the CD4 cell by binding to protein receptors on the outside of the cell (Fig. 14.1). This process is known as *fusion* (Fig. 14.2).

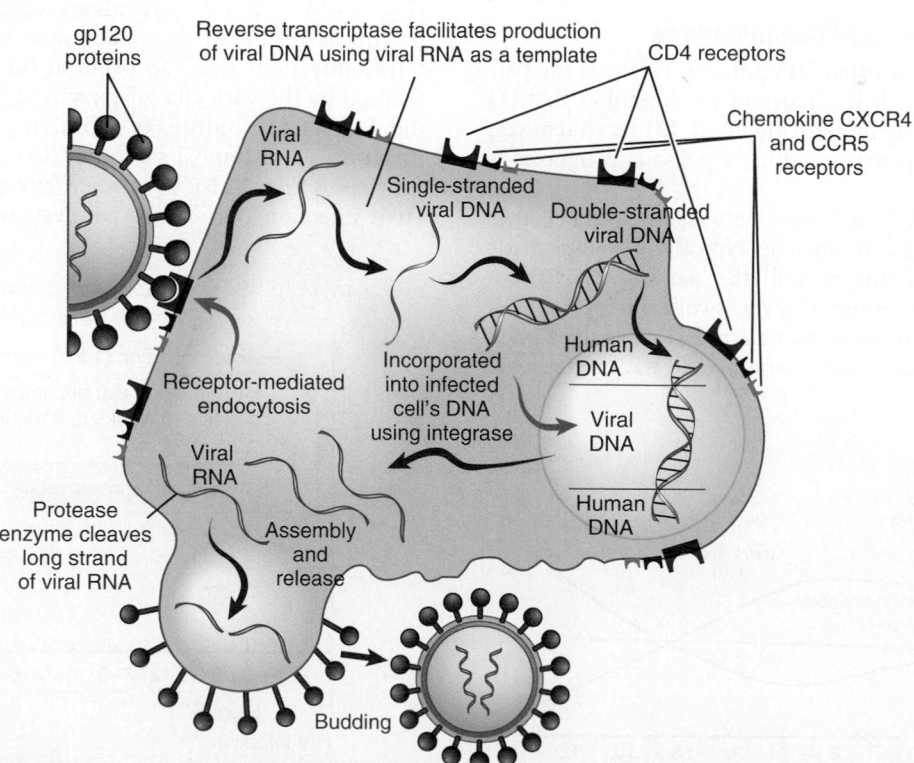

FIG. 14.2 HIV has gp120 glycoproteins that attach to CD4 and chemokine CXCR4 and CCR5 receptors on the surface of CD4 cells. Viral RNA then enters the cell, produces viral DNA in the presence of reverse transcriptase, and incorporates itself into the cellular genome in the presence of integrase, causing permanent cellular infection and the production of new virions. New viral RNA develops initially in long strands that are cut in the presence of protease and leave the cell through a budding process that contributes to cellular destruction.

Once HIV is attached and fused with the CD4 cell, HIV RNA enters the CD4 cell. This triggers the release of *reverse transcriptase,* an enzyme that transforms HIV RNA into a single strand of DNA. This strand copies itself, becoming double-stranded viral DNA. Another enzyme, called *integrase,* allows the newly formed double-stranded DNA to integrate itself into the host' genetic structure. This action has 2 consequences: (1) because all genetic material is replicated during cell division, all daughter cells are infected and (2) viral DNA in the genome directs the cell to make new HIV.

Protease, another enzyme involved in the replication process, cleaves the newly formed strands of HIV genetic material into smaller pieces. New HIV virions are then formed and released. The CD4 cell is then destroyed after the HIV virions are released.[17]

HIV destroys about 1 billion CD4 cells every day. For many years, the body can make new CD4 cells to replace the destroyed cells. However, over time the ability of HIV to destroy CD4 cells exceeds the body's ability to replace the cells. The decline in the CD4 cell count impairs immune function. Generally, the immune system remains healthy with more than 500 CD4 cells/μL. Immune problems begin to occur when the count drops below 500 CD4 cells/μL. Severe problems develop with fewer than 200 CD4 cells/μL.

With HIV, a point is eventually reached at which so many CD4 cells have been destroyed that not enough are left to regulate immune responses (Fig. 14.3). This allows **opportunistic diseases** (infections and cancers that occur in immunosuppressed patients) to develop. Opportunistic diseases are the main cause of disease, disability, and death in patients with HIV infection.

Clinical Manifestations and Complications

The typical course of untreated HIV infection follows the pattern shown in Fig. 14.4. It is important to remember that (1) disease progression is highly individualized, (2) treatment can significantly alter this pattern, and (3) a person's prognosis is unpredictable.

Acute Infection. About 2 to 4 weeks after someone becomes newly infected with HIV, the person typically develops *acute HIV infection.* During this period, the person can have a mononucleosis-like syndrome of fever, swollen lymph nodes, sore throat, headache, malaise, nausea, muscle and joint pain, diarrhea, and/or a diffuse rash. Some people have neurologic

complications, such as aseptic meningitis, peripheral neuropathy, facial palsy, or Guillain-Barré syndrome.[18] During this time, there is a high **viral load,** the amount of HIV circulating in the blood. CD4 cell counts fall temporarily but quickly return to baseline or near-baseline levels (Fig. 14.3). Many people, including HCPs, mistake acute HIV symptoms for a bad case of the flu. People are most infectious during the acute infection stage because of the high amounts of circulating HIV.

Chronic HIV Infection

Asymptomatic Infection. The time between initial HIV infection and a diagnosis of AIDS is about 10 years in untreated infection. During the first several years after initial infection, people are typically asymptomatic and have no symptoms or limited signs of infection.

Because most symptoms during early infection are vague and nonspecific for HIV, people may not be aware that they are infected. During this time, infected people continue their usual activities, which may include high-risk sexual and drug-using behaviors. This is a public health problem because infected persons can transmit HIV to others even though they have no symptoms.[19] Personal health is also affected because people who do not know that they are infected have little reason to seek treatment and are less likely to make behavior changes that could improve the quality and length of their lives.

Symptomatic Infection. As the CD4 cell count declines closer to 200 cells/μL and the viral load increases, HIV advances to a more active stage. Symptoms such as persistent fever, frequent night sweats, chronic diarrhea, recurrent headaches, and severe fatigue may develop.

One of the more common infections associated with this phase of HIV infection is oropharyngeal candidiasis (thrush) (Fig. 14.5). *Candida* organisms rarely cause problems in healthy adults but are more common in HIV-infected people. Other infections that can occur at this time include shingles (caused by the varicella-zoster virus); persistent vaginal candidal infections; outbreaks of oral or genital herpes; bacterial infections; and Kaposi sarcoma (KS), caused by human herpesvirus 8 (Fig. 14.6). *Oral hairy leukoplakia,* an Epstein-Barr virus infection that causes painless, white, raised lesions on

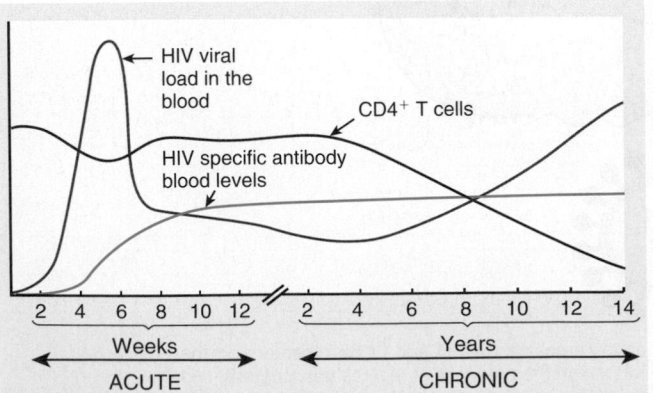

FIG. 14.3 Viral load in the blood in relationship to number of CD4 cells over the spectrum of untreated HIV infection.

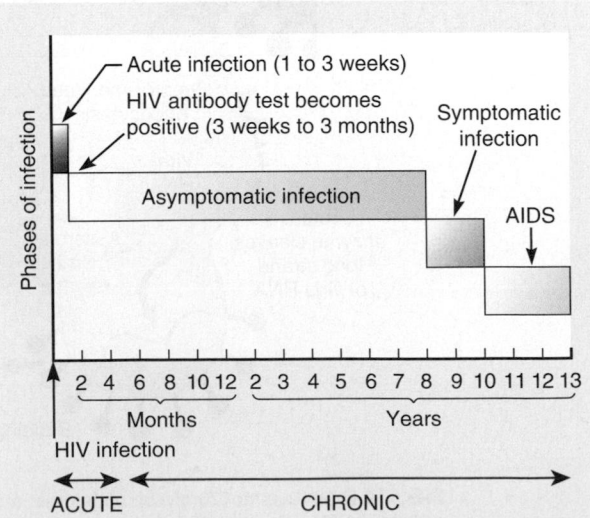

FIG. 14.4 Timeline for the spectrum of untreated HIV infection. The timeline represents the course of untreated illness from the time of infection to clinical manifestations of disease.

the lateral aspect of the tongue (Fig. 14.7), is another sign of disease progression.

AIDS. A diagnosis of **acquired immunodeficiency syndrome (AIDS)** is made when an HIV-infected patient meets criteria established by the CDC.[20] This occurs when the immune system becomes severely compromised (Table 14.10). Opportunistic diseases generally do not occur in the presence of a functioning immune system. Many infections, a variety of cancers, wasting, and HIV-related cognitive changes can occur in patients with immune impairment (Table 14.11). Organisms that do not cause severe disease in people with functioning immune systems can cause debilitating, life-threatening infections during this stage. Several opportunistic diseases may occur at the same time, increasing the difficulties of diagnosis and treatment. Advances in HIV treatment have decreased the occurrence of opportunistic diseases.

Diagnostic Studies

Diagnosis of HIV Infection. Diagnosis of HIV infection is made by testing for HIV antibodies and/or antigens.[21] HIV screening tests can be done using blood or saliva. Typically it takes several weeks after infection before a screening test can detect evidence of HIV (Fig. 14.3). This delay is known as the **window period**. The typical window period for most tests to detect HIV infection is about 3 weeks (Table 14.12). If a newly infected person is tested during the window period, the test may not be able to detect infection and they will have a false negative result.

Laboratory Studies in HIV Infection. Two laboratory tests are used for monitoring HIV progression: CD4 cell count and viral load. The CD4 cell count is a marker of immune function. As the disease progresses, the number of CD4 cells usually decreases (Fig. 14.3). The normal range for CD4 cells is 800 to 1200 cells/μL. Laboratory tests that measure viral levels provide an assessment of disease progression. The lower the viral load, the less active the disease. In HIV, viral loads are reported as

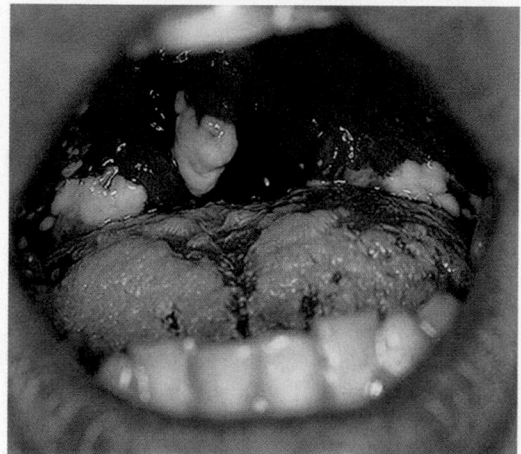

FIG. 14.5 Oral thrush involving hard and soft palate. (From Emond R, Welsby P, Rowland H: *Colour atlas of infectious diseases,* ed 4, Edinburgh, 2003, Mosby.)

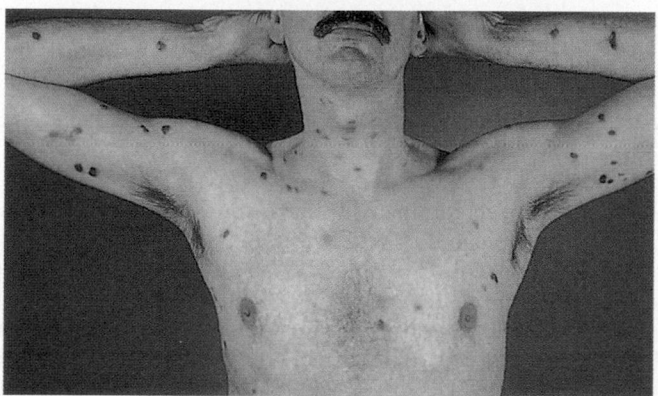

FIG. 14.6 Kaposi sarcoma (KS). KS lesions can appear anywhere on the skin surface or on internal organs. Lesions vary in size from pinpoint to large and may appear in a variety of shades. (From Friedman-Kien AE: Color atlas of AIDS, Philadelphia, 1989, Saunders.)

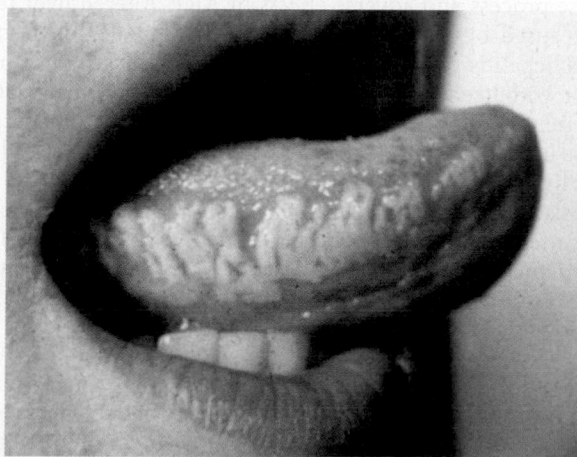

FIG. 14.7 Oral hairy leukoplakia on the lateral aspect of the tongue. (Set of slides published in 1992 by Jon Fuller, MD, and Howard Libman, MD, at Boston University School of Medicine, Boston, MA.)

TABLE 14.10 Diagnostic Criteria for AIDS

AIDS is diagnosed when a person with HIV develops at least one of the following conditions:

1. CD4+ T cell count drops below 200 cells/μL.
2. One of the following opportunistic infections (OIs):
   - *Bacterial:* *Mycobacterium tuberculosis* (any site); any disseminated or extrapulmonary mycobacteria, including *Mycobacterium avium* complex (MAC) or *Mycobacterium kansasii;* recurrent pneumonia; recurrent *Salmonella* septicemia
   - *Fungal:* Candidiasis of bronchi, trachea, lungs, or esophagus; *Pneumocystis jiroveci* pneumonia (PCP); disseminated or extrapulmonary coccidioidomycosis; disseminated or extrapulmonary histoplasmosis
   - *Protozoal:* Toxoplasmosis of the brain, chronic intestinal isosporiasis, chronic intestinal cryptosporidiosis
   - *Viral:* Cytomegalovirus (CMV) disease other than liver, spleen, or nodes; CMV retinitis (with loss of vision); herpes simplex with chronic ulcer(s) or bronchitis, pneumonitis, or esophagitis; progressive multifocal leukoencephalopathy (PML); extrapulmonary cryptococcosis
3. One of the following opportunistic cancers:
   - Burkitt's lymphoma
   - Immunoblastic lymphoma
   - Invasive cervical cancer
   - Kaposi sarcoma (KS)
   - Primary lymphoma of the brain
4. Wasting syndrome. *Wasting* is defined as a loss of 10% or more of ideal body mass.

Modified from Centers for Disease Control and Prevention: 1993 Revised classification system for HIV infection and expanded surveillance case definition for AIDS among adolescents and adults, 1993. Retrieved from *www.cdc.gov/mmwr/preview/mmwrhtml/rr5710a1.htm?s_cid=rr5710a1_e.*

TABLE 14.11 Common Opportunistic Diseases Associated With HIV Infection

Organism or Disease	Clinical Manifestations
Candida albicans	Thrush (Fig. 14.5), esophagitis, vaginitis. Whitish yellow patches in mouth, esophagus, GI tract, vagina
Coccidioides immitis	Pneumonia and fever, weight loss, cough
CNS lymphoma	Cognitive dysfunction, motor impairment, aphasia, seizures, personality changes, headache
Cryptococcus neoformans	Meningitis, cognitive impairment, motor dysfunction, fever, seizures, headache
Cryptosporidium muris	Gastroenteritis, watery diarrhea, abdominal pain, weight loss
Cytomegalovirus (CMV)	*Retinitis:* retinal lesions, blurred vision, loss of vision
	Esophagitis, stomatitis: difficulty swallowing, colitis or gastritis: bloody diarrhea, pain, weight loss
	Pneumonitis: respiratory symptoms
	Neurologic disease: central nervous system (CNS) manifestations
Hepatitis B virus (HBV)	Jaundice, fatigue, abdominal pain, loss of appetite, nausea, vomiting, joint pain. Some have no signs or symptoms
Hepatitis C virus (HCV)	Jaundice, fatigue, abdominal pain, loss of appetite, nausea, vomiting, dark urine. Many have no signs or symptoms
Herpes simplex virus (HSV)	*HSV-1 (type 1):* orolabial and mucocutaneous vesicular and ulcerative lesions. Keratitis, visual changes, encephalitis, CNS manifestations
	HSV-2 (type 2): genital and perianal vesicular and ulcerative lesions
Histoplasma capsulatum	*Pneumonia:* fever, cough, weight loss
	Meningitis: CNS manifestations, disseminated disease
JC papovavirus	Progressive multifocal leukoencephalopathy (PML), CNS manifestations, mental and motor declines
Kaposi sarcoma (KS) caused by human herpesvirus 8 (HHV-8)	Vascular lesions on the skin (Fig. 14.6), mucous membranes, and viscera with wide range of presentation: firm, flat, raised, or nodular; pinpoint to several cm in size; hyperpigmented, multicentric. Can cause lymphedema and disfigurement. Usually not serious unless occurring in the respiratory or GI system
Mycobacterium avium complex (MAC)	Gastroenteritis, watery diarrhea, weight loss
Mycobacterium tuberculosis (MTB, TB)	Respiratory and disseminated disease. Productive cough, fever, night sweats, weight loss
Pneumocystis jiroveci pneumonia (PCP)	Pneumonia, nonproductive cough, hypoxemia, progressive shortness of breath, fever, night sweats, fatigue
Toxoplasma gondii	Encephalitis, cognitive dysfunction, motor impairment, fever, altered mental status, headache, seizures, sensory abnormalities
Varicella-zoster virus (VZV)	*Shingles:* erythematous maculopapular rash along dermatomal planes, pain, pruritus
	Ocular: progressive outer retinal necrosis (PORN)

TABLE 14.12 HIV Testing

HIV-Antibody/Antigen Testing

A highly sensitive test detects antibodies and antigens associated with HIV. Blood samples that are negative for HIV infection are reported as negative. The antigen/antibody testing algorithm includes confirmation with HIV viral load testing for any indeterminate results.
- If the patient has a negative HIV antibody/antigen test, but reports recent risky behaviors, encourage retesting in 4 to 6 weeks. Persons at ongoing risk should be assessed or counseled for risk reduction interventions, including preexposure prophylaxis (PrEP).
- If the results are positive and consistent with HIV infection, assist the patient in getting appropriate counseling, support, and follow-up HIV primary care.

Rapid HIV-Antibody Testing

1. The Centers for Disease Control and Prevention strongly recommends rapid testing. Results are highly accurate. It can be done in a variety of settings (mobile health units, HCP offices, privacy of a person's home). Results are typically available within 20 minutes.
2. In-home HIV test kits are available. Testing is done on saliva.
3. Follow a negative rapid test with a risk assessment to determine the need for repeat tests.
4. Positive rapid tests can be disclosed to the patient but must be confirmed with a standard HIV assay. This step necessitates a blood draw and a return appointment to get results.

the virus has been eliminated from the body or that the person can no longer transmit HIV to others. Rather, it refers to the fact that the amount of circulating HIV in the blood is below the level of detection of the test.

Abnormal blood test results are common in HIV infection. They may be caused by HIV, opportunistic diseases, or complications of therapy. Decreased white blood cell (WBC) counts, especially below-normal numbers of lymphocytes (lymphopenia) and neutrophils (neutropenia), often occur. HIV, antiplatelet antibodies, or drug therapy can cause low platelet counts (thrombocytopenia). Anemia is associated with the chronic disease process and adverse effects of ART. Altered liver function, caused by HIV infection, drug therapy, or co-infection with a hepatitis virus, is common. Early identification of co-infection with hepatitis B virus (HBV) or hepatitis C virus (HCV) is extremely important. These infections have a more serious course in patients with HIV, may limit options for ART, and can cause liver-related morbidity and mortality.[22]

Resistance tests can determine if a patient's HIV is resistant to drugs used for ART. *Genotype* and *phenotype* assays help HCPs know which medications can best control a patient's infection. These tests are similar to culture and sensitivity testing used for antibiotic selection.

Interprofessional Care

Interprofessional care of the HIV-infected patient focuses on (1) monitoring HIV disease progression and immune function, (2) initiating and monitoring ART, (3) preventing the development of opportunistic diseases, (4) detecting and

real numbers (e.g., 1260 copies/µL). The goal of treatment is to suppress the viral load to the lowest level possible, which is below the level of detection on a commercial assay. This is often referred to as "undetectable." "Undetectable" does *not* mean that

TABLE 14.13 Drug Therapy

HIV Infection

Drug Classification	Mechanism of Action	Drug Names
Attachment Inhibitors Entry Inhibitors	Interrupts the ability of HIV to attach to the CD4 cell. Prevent binding of HIV to cells, thus preventing entry of HIV into cells where replication would occur	ibalizumab-uiyk (Trogarzo) enfuvirtide (Fuzeon) maraviroc (Selzentry)
Integrase Inhibitors	Bind with integrase enzyme and prevent HIV from incorporating its genetic material into the host cell	bictegravir* dolutegravir (Tivicay) elvitegravir* raltegravir (Isentress)
Protease Inhibitors (PIs)	Prevent the protease enzyme from cutting HIV proteins into the proper lengths needed to allow viable virions to assemble and bud out from the cell membrane	atazanavir (Reyataz) darunavir (Prezista) fosamprenavir (Lexiva) indinavir (Crixivan) lopinavir + ritonavir (Kaletra) nelfinavir (Viracept) ritonavir (Norvir)† saquinavir (Fortovase, Invirase) tipranavir (Aptivus)
Reverse Transcriptase Inhibitors		
Nonnucleoside Reverse Transcriptase Inhibitors (NNRTIs)	Inhibit the action of reverse transcriptase	efavirenz (Sustiva) etravirine (Intelence) delavirdine (Rescriptor) nevirapine (Viramune XR) rilpivirine (Edurant)
Nucleoside Reverse Transcriptase Inhibitors (NRTIs)	Insert a piece of DNA into the developing HIV DNA chain, blocking further development of the chain and leaving the production of the new strand of HIV DNA incomplete	abacavir (Ziagen) didanosine (Videx, Videx-EC) doravarine (Pifeltro) emtricitabine (Emtriva) lamivudine (Epivir) stavudine (Zerit) zidovudine (Retrovir)
Nucleotide Reverse Transcriptase Inhibitor (NtRTI)	Combines with reverse transcriptase enzyme to block the process needed to convert HIV RNA into HIV DNA	tenofovir (Viread)

*Elvitegravir and bictegravir are integrase inhibitors that are available only in fixed-dose combinations with tenofovir AF and emtricitabine (Table 14.14).
†Most often used in low doses with other PIs to boost effect.

treating opportunistic diseases, (5) managing symptoms, (6) preventing or decreasing complications of treatment, and (7) preventing further transmission of HIV. To achieve these goals, ongoing assessment, clinician-patient interactions, and patient teaching and support are needed.

The first patient visit provides an opportunity to gather baseline data and start establishing rapport. A complete history and physical examination, including an immunization history and psychosocial and dietary evaluations, should be done. Findings from the history, assessment, and laboratory tests help determine patient needs. This is a good time to complete the case reports required by the state health department. Initiate patient teaching about the spectrum of HIV disease, treatment, prevention of transmission to others, improvements in health, and family planning at this meeting. Use patient input to develop a plan of care and determine the need for referrals. Remember that a newly diagnosed patient may not be able to retain or understand information. Be prepared to repeat and clarify information over the course of several months.

Drug Therapy for HIV Infection. The goals of drug therapy in HIV infection are to (1) decrease the viral load, (2) maintain or increase CD4 cell counts, (3) prevent HIV-related symptoms and opportunistic diseases, (4) delay disease progression, and

(5) prevent HIV transmission. HIV cannot be cured, but ART can delay disease progression by decreasing viral replication.[23] When taken consistently and correctly, ART can reduce viral loads by 90% to 99%. This makes adherence to treatment regimens extremely important.

Drugs used to treat HIV work at various points in the HIV replication cycle (Tables 14.13 and 14.14). The major advantage of using drugs from different classes is that combination therapy can inhibit viral replication in different ways. This makes it more difficult for the virus to recover and decreases the chance of drug resistance. A major problem with most drugs used in ART is that resistance develops rapidly when they are used alone *(monotherapy)* or taken in inadequate doses. This is why patients receive combinations of 3 or more drugs.

⚠ SAFETY ALERT Interaction of ART With Other Drugs

- Significant interactions with ARTs occur with over-the-counter (OTC) drugs, including antacids, proton pump inhibitors, and certain supplements.
- Many ARTs have interactions with other commonly used drugs and herbal therapies (e.g., St. John's wort).
- Be sure to ask patients about prescribed and OTC drugs as well as herbal products and supplements.

TABLE 14.14 Fixed-Dose Drug Combination Products

HIV Infection

Mechanism of Action	Evotaz (atazanavir + cobicistat[†])
More than one drug combined into a single tablet. Drugs may be from the same or different classes.	Genvoya (tenofovir AF + emtricitabine + elvitegravir + cobicistat[†])
	Juluca (dolutegravir + rilpivirine)
	Odefsey (tenofovir AF + emtricitabine + rilpivirine)
Examples	Prezcobix (darunavir + cobicistat[†])
Atripla (tenofovir DF + emtricitabine + efavirenz)	Temixys (tenofovir DF + lamivudine)
	Triumeq (abacavir + lamivudine + dolutegravir)
Biktarvy (tenofovir AF + emtricitabine + bictegravir)	Trizivir (abacavir + lamivudine + zidovudine)
Combivir (lamivudine + zidovudine)	
Complera (tenofovir DF + emtricitabine + rilpivirine)	Truvada (tenofovir DF + emtricitabine)
Delstrigo (tenofovir DF + lamivudine + doravarine)	Stribild (tenofovir DF + emtricitabine + elvitegravir + cobicistat[†])
Descovy (tenofovir AF + emtricitabine)	Symtuza (tenofovir AF + emtricitabine + darunavir + cobicistat[†])
Epzicom (abacavir + lamivudine)	

[†]Cobicistat is a pharmacologic booster that enhances the potency of some HIV antiretrovirals. It has no direct effects against HIV.
AF, Alafenamide. *DF,* disoproxil fumarate.

Drug Therapy for Opportunistic Diseases. Management of HIV is complicated by the many opportunistic diseases that can develop as the immune system deteriorates (Table 14.11). Prevention is the preferred approach to opportunistic diseases. Several opportunistic diseases associated with HIV can be delayed or prevented with adequate ART, vaccines (including hepatitis B, influenza, pneumococcal), and disease-specific prevention measures.[24] Although it is usually not possible to eradicate opportunistic diseases once they occur, prophylactic medications can significantly decrease morbidity and mortality rates. Advances in the prevention, diagnosis, and treatment of opportunistic diseases have contributed significantly to increased life expectancy.

Preventing Transmission of HIV. Preexposure prophylaxis (PrEP) is a comprehensive HIV prevention strategy to reduce the risk for sexually acquired HIV infection in adults at high risk.[25] PrEP should be used in conjunction with other proven prevention interventions such as condoms, risk reduction counseling, and regular HIV testing.

Currently, certain antiretrovirals are approved for both treatment of HIV in persons living with HIV, as well as prevention of HIV infection in persons without HIV infection. Various formulations have been studied for PrEP. The first medications approved for PrEP were tenofovir disoproxil fumarate (Tenofovir DF) in combination with emtricitabine. Other medications, including injectable options, will soon be available. As PrEP, these medications reduce the risk for HIV infection in uninfected people who are at significant risk for acquiring HIV. Tenofovir and emtricitabine are also used in combination with other antiretroviral agents for the treatment of HIV-infected people.

❖ NURSING MANAGEMENT: HIV INFECTION

◆ Nursing Assessment

Nursing assessment of people not known to have HIV infection should focus on behaviors that put the person at risk for HIV and other sexually transmitted and blood-borne infections. Assess patients for risky behaviors on a regular basis. Do not assume that someone is without risk because he or she is too old, too young, heterosexual, or married.

Assess risk by asking some basic questions: (1) Have you ever had a blood transfusion or used clotting factors? If so, was it before 1985? (2) Have you ever shared drug-using equipment with another person? (3) Have you ever had a sexual experience in which your penis, vagina, rectum, or mouth came into contact with another person's penis, vagina, rectum, or mouth? (4) Have you ever had a sexually transmitted infection? (5) Have you ever had sexual contact with someone known to have HIV? These questions provide the minimum information needed to initiate a risk assessment. Follow up a positive response to any of these questions with an in-depth exploration of issues related to the identified risk.

A person who has HIV infection needs specific, ongoing assessment. Subjective and objective data are outlined in Table 14.15. Repeated nursing assessments over time are essential because people's circumstances change. Early recognition and treatment can slow the progression of HIV infection and prevent new infections. A complete history and thorough systems review can help identify and address problems in a timely manner.

◆ Nursing Diagnoses

Nursing diagnoses for the patient with HIV disease may include:

- Risk for infection
- Lack of knowledge
- Difficulty coping
- Impaired nutritional status

◆ Planning

Nursing interventions can help the patient (1) adhere to drug regimens; (2) adopt a healthy lifestyle that includes avoiding exposure to other sexually transmitted infections and blood-borne diseases; (3) protect others from HIV; (4) maintain or develop healthy and supportive relationships; (5) maintain activities and productivity; (6) explore spiritual issues; (7) come to terms with issues related to disease, disability, and death; and (8) cope with symptoms caused by HIV and its treatments.

❖ Nursing Implementation

The complexity of HIV disease is related to its chronic nature. As with most chronic and infectious diseases, primary prevention and health promotion are the most effective health care strategies. When prevention fails, disease results. Table 14.15 shows a summary of nursing goals, assessments, and interventions throughout the course of HIV infection.

◆ Health Promotion. Even with recent successes in HIV treatment, prevention is key in controlling the epidemic. In addition, health promotion encourages early detection of the disease so that, if primary prevention has failed, early intervention can be initiated.

TABLE 14.15 Nursing Assessment

HIV-Infected Patient

Subjective Data

Important Health Information

Past health history: Route of infection. Hepatitis, other sexually transmitted infections, tuberculosis. Frequent viral, fungal, and/or bacterial infections
Medications: Use of immunosuppressive drugs

Functional Health Patterns

Health perception–health management: Perception of illness. Alcohol and drug use. Malaise
Nutritional-metabolic: Weight loss, anorexia, nausea, vomiting. Lesions, bleeding, or ulcerations of lips, mouth, gums, tongue, or throat. Sensitivity to acidic, salty, or spicy foods. Difficulty swallowing, abdominal cramping. Skin rashes, lesions, or color changes
Elimination: Persistent diarrhea, change in character of stools. Painful urination, low back pain
Activity-exercise: Chronic fatigue, muscle weakness, difficulty walking. Cough, shortness of breath
Sleep-rest: Insomnia, night sweats, fatigue
Cognitive-perceptual: Headaches, stiff neck, chest pain, rectal pain, retrosternal pain. Blurred vision, photophobia, diplopia, loss of vision. Hearing impairment. Confusion, forgetfulness, attention deficit, changes in mental status, memory loss, personality changes. Paresthesias, hypersensitivity in feet, pruritus
Role-relationship: Support system(s), career or job, financial resources
Sexuality-reproductive: Lesions on genitalia or anus (internal or external), pruritus or burning in vagina, penis, or anus. Painful sexual intercourse, rectal pain or bleeding, changes in menstruation, vaginal or penile discharge. Use of birth control measures, pregnancies, desire for future children
Coping–stress tolerance: Stress levels, previous losses, coping patterns, self-concept; social withdrawal

Objective Data

General

Lethargy, persistent fever, lymphadenopathy, peripheral wasting, fat deposits in truncal areas and upper back

Eyes

Presence of exudates, retinal lesions or hemorrhage, papilledema

Integumentary

Decreased skin turgor, dry skin, diaphoresis. Pallor, cyanosis. Lesions, eruptions, discolorations, bruises of skin or mucous membranes. Vaginal or perianal excoriation. Alopecia. Delayed wound healing

Respiratory

Tachypnea, dyspnea, intercostal retractions. Crackles, wheezing, productive or nonproductive cough

Cardiovascular

Pericardial friction rub, murmur, bradycardia, tachycardia

Gastrointestinal

Mouth lesions, including blisters (HSV), white-gray patches (*Candida* infection), painless white lesions on the side of the tongue (hairy leukoplakia), discolorations (Kaposi sarcoma). Gingivitis, tooth decay or loosening. Redness or white patchy lesions of throat. Vomiting, diarrhea, incontinence, rectal lesions, hyperactive bowel sounds, abdominal masses, hepatosplenomegaly

Musculoskeletal

Muscle wasting, weakness

Neurologic

Ataxia, tremors, lack of coordination. Sensory loss, slurred speech, aphasia. Memory loss, peripheral neuropathy, apathy, agitation, depression, inappropriate behavior. Decreasing levels of consciousness, seizures, paralysis, coma

Reproductive

Genital lesions or discharge, abdominal tenderness secondary to pelvic inflammatory disease (PID)

Possible Diagnostic Findings

Positive HIV antibody/antigen assay. Detectable viral load. ↓ CD4 cell count, ↓ WBC count, lymphopenia, anemia, thrombocytopenia. Electrolyte imbalances, abnormal liver function tests. ↑ cholesterol, triglycerides, and blood glucose

---

ETHICAL/LEGAL DILEMMAS

Individual vs. Public Health Protection

Situation

A nurse in a community clinic is having a follow-up visit with V.T., a 38-yr-old woman who was diagnosed with HIV infection during her annual examination 2 weeks ago. During the visit, V.T. discloses that her partner verbally and physically abuses her. V.T. says she had not yet told her partner about the HIV diagnosis because she is afraid that he will hurt her. She has not used any protection during sex with him since she learned of her test results because she suspects he infected her.

Ethical/Legal Points for Consideration

- You face a conflict between preventing further harm to V.T. (possible increase in intimate partner violence), providing care to her partner (his need for an HIV test, diagnosis, and treatment), and protecting the public health (potential spread of HIV infection to her partner or from her partner to others in the community). Patient teaching and support are essential because your primary obligation is to the patient.
- Because relevant law varies from state to state, your first step is to be familiar with your state law concerning mandated reporting for domestic partner abuse and infectious diseases.
- Federal laws about protection of privacy in HIV testing apply everywhere.
- In many states, reporting domestic abuse is mandatory only when the reporter actually witnesses the abuse or when the immediate effects of the abuse (e.g., wounds, contusions, broken bones) are witnessed.[1]

- You should be familiar with crisis counseling services for V.T. and offer her the following advice: Collect and stash a set of car keys or taxi money in a safe place, keep a bag packed and hidden or even stored in a locker somewhere accessible, develop a code phrase to use with a friend or family member to call for help, keep a cell phone charged, and have money hidden in a safe place.

Discussion Questions

1. Within the parameters of your state's requirements for reportable conditions, how can you protect the patient's confidentiality to prevent further intimate partner violence?
2. What services does your state offer to notify a partner without disclosing the source patient's name? How would V.T. access those services in your state?
3. How can you protect the partner from possible infection while also protecting V.T. from further violence?
4. How can you best address the issue of intimate partner violence? What resources would V.T. have in your community?
5. Discuss the benefits of universal, voluntary testing in light of V.T.'s case.

Reference

National Coalition Against Domestic Violence. Retrieved from *www.ncadv.com.*

Prevention of HIV Infection. HIV infection is preventable. Avoiding or modifying risky behaviors is the most effective prevention tool. Nursing interventions to prevent disease transmission are based on an assessment of the person's risk behaviors. Provide culturally sensitive, language-appropriate, and age-specific teaching and behavior change counseling. Nurses who are comfortable with and know how to talk about sensitive topics such as sexuality and drug use are best prepared to provide prevention education.

❤ PROMOTING POPULATION HEALTH

Prevention and Early Detection of HIV

- Increase safer sexual practices, including condom use
- Decrease equipment sharing among IV drug users
- Increase clinician skills to assess for risk factors for HIV infection, recommend HIV testing, and provide counseling for behavior change
- Make voluntary HIV testing a routine part of health care
- Increase access to new HIV testing technologies, especially rapid testing
- Increase access to HIV testing facilities in traditional health care settings and alternative sites, such as drug and alcohol treatment facilities and community-based organizations
- Increase risk assessment and individualized behavior change messages to people with HIV to prevent new infections
- Decrease perinatal HIV infection by offering voluntary HIV testing as a part of routine prenatal care
- Provide counseling and appropriate HIV therapy to those who are infected

A wide variety of activities can reduce the risk for HIV infection.[26] Help people choose the methods that best fit their needs and circumstances. Prevention techniques are divided into *safe sexual activities* (those that eliminate risk) and *risk-reducing sexual activities* (those that decrease, but do not eliminate, risk).

The goal is to develop safer, healthier, and less risky behaviors. The more consistently and correctly one uses prevention methods, the more effective they are in preventing HIV infection. It is a good idea to use a combination of prevention methods (e.g., using condoms, decreasing the number of sex partners) to increase the prevention effect.

Decreasing risks related to sexual intercourse. *Safe sexual activities* eliminate the risk for exposure to HIV in semen and vaginal secretions. Abstaining from all sexual activity is an effective way to achieve this goal, but there are safe options for those who cannot or do not wish to abstain. Limiting sexual behavior to activities in which the mouth, penis, vagina, or rectum does not come into contact with a partner's mouth, penis, vagina, or rectum eliminates contact with blood, semen, or vaginal secretions. Safe activities include masturbation, mutual masturbation ("hand job"), and other activities that meet the "no contact" requirements. *Insertive sex* between partners who are not infected with HIV and not at risk of becoming infected with HIV is considered safe.

Risk-reducing sexual activities decrease the risk of contact with HIV through the use of barriers. Barriers should be used when engaging in insertive sexual activity (oral, vaginal, anal) with a partner who has HIV or whose HIV status is not known. The most commonly used barrier is the male condom. Male condoms offer protection during anal, vaginal, and oral intercourse. Female condoms are an alternative to male condoms. Squares of latex (known as dental dams) can be used as a barrier during oral sexual activity.

Decreasing risks related to drug use. Drug use, including alcohol and tobacco, can cause immunosuppression, poor nutrition, and a host of psychosocial problems. However, drug use does not cause HIV infection. The major risk for HIV related to using drugs involves sharing equipment or having unsafe sexual experiences while under the influence of drugs. Basic risk reduction rules are (1) do not use drugs; (2) if you use drugs, do not share equipment; and (3) do not have sexual intercourse when under the influence of any drug, including alcohol, that impairs decision making.[27]

The safest method is to abstain from drugs, but this may not be a practical option for users who are not prepared to quit or have no access to drug treatment services. The risk for HIV infection for these persons is eliminated if they do not share equipment. Injecting equipment ("works") includes needles, syringes, cookers (spoons or bottle caps used to mix the drug), cotton, and rinse water. Blood can contaminate equipment used to snort (straws) or smoke (pipes) drugs and should not be shared.

Access to sterile equipment is an important risk elimination tactic. Some communities have needle and syringe exchange programs (NSEPs) that provide sterile equipment in exchange for used equipment. Opposition to these programs is related to the fear that access to injecting supplies will increase drug use. However, studies have shown that in communities with NSEPs, drug use does not increase, rates of HIV and other blood-borne

EVIDENCE-BASED PRACTICE

Condom Use and HIV

As a nurse in an HIV clinic, you are counseling M.J., a 27-yr-old gay man and his partner. M.J. is on antiretroviral therapy (ART). His viral load is very low, and his CD4 cell count is normal. He tells you that since the drugs are working, he and his partner (who is HIV-negative) are considering not using condoms in the future.

Making Clinical Decisions

Best Available Evidence. One of the best ways to prevent HIV transmission from an infected person to an uninfected person continues to be the consistent and correct use of latex condoms. Those with HIV who take ART and get and keep an undetectable viral load (<200 copies/mL) have effectively no risk for transmitting HIV to their HIV-negative sexual partners. Behavior change programs provided by HCPs, peers, and others can significantly reduce risk behaviors among those with HIV and the transmission of the virus to others.

Clinician Expertise. You know that risk-reducing sexual activities in this situation include the continued use of condoms. However, you also know that although an undetectable viral load decreases the risk for HIV transmission, the risk may not be completely eliminated.

Patient Preferences and Values. M.J. tells you that he and his partner are in a committed relationship, have no other partners, and do not like using condoms.

Implications for Practice

1. What information would you discuss with M.J. related to HIV transmission, ART and viral load, and the risks of unprotected sexual activity?
2. What measures besides condom use would you discuss with M.J. to reduce the risk for HIV transmission?

References for Evidence

Centers for Diseases Control and Prevention. Evidence of HIV treatment and viral suppression in preventing the sexual transmission of HIV. Retrieved from *www.cdc.gov/hiv/pdf/risk/art/cdc-hiv-art-viral-suppression.pdf.*
Centers for Diseases Control and Prevention. Proven HIV prevention methods. Retrieved from *www.cdc.gov/nchhstp/newsroom/docs/factsheets/hiv-proven-prevention-methods-508.pdf.*

infections are controlled, and an overall cost benefit results.[28] Appropriately cleaning equipment before use can reduce risk by decreasing the chance of blood contact.

Providing support for patients with substance use and referring them to professionals who can assist with managing the psychologic aspects of substance use is important. Other self-help programs (e.g., Narcotics Anonymous, Alcoholics Anonymous) may be helpful.

Decreasing risks of perinatal transmission. The best way to prevent HIV infection in infants is to prevent HIV infection in women. Women infected with HIV should be asked about their reproductive desires. Those who choose not to have children need to have family planning methods discussed in detail. Should they become pregnant, we need to discuss their options, including the possibility of maintaining the pregnancy and using ART to decrease the risk for transmission or having an abortion.

If HIV-infected pregnant women are appropriately treated during pregnancy, the rate of perinatal transmission decreases from 25% to less than 2%. ART has significantly decreased the risk for infants born to HIV-infected women, and more of these women are now becoming mothers. The current standard of care is for all women who are pregnant or contemplating pregnancy to receive HIV counseling, be offered access to voluntary HIV-antibody testing, and, if infected, offered optimal ART.[29]

Decreasing risks at work. The risk for infection from occupational exposure to HIV is small but real. OSHA requires employers to protect workers from exposure to blood and other potentially infectious materials (Table 14.8). Precautions and safety devices decrease the risk for direct contact with blood and body fluids. Should exposure to HIV-infected fluids occur, postexposure prophylaxis (PEP) with combination ART can significantly decrease the risk for infection.[15] The need for timely treatment and counseling makes it critical for nurses to report all blood exposures.

HIV Testing. An estimated 14% of people living with HIV in the United States are not aware that they are infected. People who do not know they are infected are more likely to transmit the infection to others. Current guidelines recommend universal, voluntary testing as part of routine medical care.[30,31] The goal is to normalize the test, decrease the stigma related to HIV testing, find hidden cases, get infected persons into care, and prevent new cases of infection.

◆ **Acute Care**

Early Intervention. Early intervention after detection of HIV infection can promote health and limit disability. The nursing assessment in HIV disease should focus on early detection of symptoms, opportunistic diseases, and psychosocial problems (Table 14.16).

Initial response to diagnosis of HIV. Reactions to an HIV diagnosis are similar to the reactions of people who are diagnosed with any life-threatening, debilitating, or chronic illness. These reactions include anxiety, panic, fear, depression, denial, hopelessness, anger, and guilt.[32] Unfortunately, all these emotions are overlaid with the stigma and discrimination that continue to infuse societal reactions to HIV. The patient's family members, friends, and caregivers experience many of the same reactions. As time passes, patients and their loved ones will be confronted with complex treatment decisions; feelings of loss, anger, powerlessness, depression, and grief; social isolation; the possibility of death; and/or thoughts of suicide.

Antiretroviral therapy. ART can significantly slow the progression of HIV. However, treatment regimens can be complex, the drugs have side effects, ART does not work for everyone, and it is expensive. These factors can contribute to problems with adherence to treatment, a dangerous situation because of the high risk for developing drug resistance.

❓ CHECK YOUR PRACTICE

You are working in an outpatient HIV clinic, and one of the patients, a 34-yr-old single parent with HIV infection, tells you, "I've been feeling well lately. I've been so busy taking care of my kids and working, I have not been taking my HIV meds."

• How would you respond to this patient?

Interventions include teaching about (1) advantages and disadvantages of new treatments, (2) dangers of poor adherence to therapeutic regimens, (3) how and when to take each drug, (4) drug interactions to avoid, and (5) side effects to report to the HCP. Table 14.17 outlines patient and caregiver teaching on HIV treatment and initial follow-up.

Clinical guidelines provide information on initial drug regimens.[23] However, one of the most important considerations for initiating therapy is patient readiness for treatment. Adherence to ART is a critical part of successful drug therapy for people with HIV infection. Nurses are uniquely prepared to provide assistance with adherence to the drug regimen (Table 14.18). Taking drugs as prescribed (right dose and time) is important for all drug therapy, but with HIV infection, missing even a few doses can lead to drug resistance. We can help patients adhere to difficult treatment regimens with electronic reminders, beepers, timers on pillboxes, and calendars. Group support and individual counseling can help. The best approach is to learn about the patient's life and assist with problem solving related to taking medications within the confines of that life.

INFORMATICS IN PRACTICE

Use of Internet and Mobile Devices to Manage HIV

• The Internet offers resources and support for patients that can help them cope with their illness and teach them about signs and symptoms of serious illness.
• By monitoring their health and quickly spotting warning signs of serious illnesses, patients are able to alert their HCPs and receive earlier treatment.
• These systems can help the patient manage antiretroviral therapy by sending medication reminders by text or e-mail.

Delaying disease progression. Promoting a healthy immune system, whether the patient chooses to take ART or not, may delay the progression of HIV disease. Useful interventions for HIV-infected patients include (1) getting nutritional support to maintain lean body mass and ensure appropriate levels of vitamins and micronutrients; (2) moderating or eliminating alcohol, tobacco, and drug use; (3) keeping up to date with recommended vaccines; (4) getting adequate rest and exercise; (5) reducing stress; (6) avoiding exposure to new infectious agents; (7) accessing counseling; (8) getting involved in support groups and community activities; and (9) developing a consistent relationship with HCPs, including attending regular appointments.

TABLE 14.16 **Nursing Management**

HIV Infection

Nursing Care and Goals	Assessment	Interventions
Health Promotion **Prevent HIV infection**	*Risk factors:* What behaviors or social, physical, emotional, pathogenic, or immune factors place the patient at risk?	• Education, including knowledge, attitudes, and behaviors, with emphasis on risk reduction to the following: • *General population:* Cover general information • *Pregnant women:* General information and information specific to HIV infection and pregnancy • *Individual patient:* Specific to assessed need • Empower patients to take control of prevention measures.
Detect HIV infection early	Does the patient need to be tested for HIV?	• Provide HIV antibody/antigen testing with appropriate counseling.
Acute Care **Promote health and limit disability**	*Physical health:* Is the patient experiencing problems? *Mental health:* How is the patient coping? *Resources:* Does the patient have family or social support? Is the patient accessing community services? Is money or insurance a problem? Does the patient have access to spiritual support as desired?	• Provide case management or refer to interprofessional team, including social work. • Teach about HIV, the spectrum of infection, options for care, signs and symptoms to report, treatment options, immune enhancement, risk reduction, and ways to adhere to treatment regimens. • Establish long-term, trusting relationship with patient, family, and significant others. • Provide emotional and spiritual support. • Develop resources for legal needs: discrimination prevention, wills and advance directives, child care wishes. • Empower the patient to identify needs, direct care, and seek services.
Manage problems caused by HIV infection	*Physical health:* Has the patient had an acute exacerbation of problems related to immunodeficiency, opportunistic disease, or risk factors (e.g., substance use)? *Mental health status:* Has the patient's ability to cope with psychosocial issues deteriorated?	• Provide care during acute exacerbations: recognition of life-threatening developments, life support, rapid intervention with treatments and drugs, comfort, and hygiene needs. • Support patient and family during crisis. • Assist the patient with mental health issues and provide referral to mental health specialist as needed.
Ambulatory Care **Maximize quality of life**	*Physical health:* Are new symptoms developing? Is the patient experiencing drug side effects or interactions?	• Continue case management. • Teach about changing treatment options and continued adherence. • Empower patient to continue to direct care and to make desires known to family members and significant others.
Resolve life and death issues	*Mental health:* How is the patient coping? What adjustments have been made? *Finances:* Can the patient maintain health care and basic standards of living? *Family, social, and community support:* Are these available? Is the patient using support in an effective manner? Do family or significant others need teaching, encouragement, or stress relief? *Spirituality issues:* Does the patient desire support from a religious organization or spiritual counselor? What assistance does the patient desire?	• Continue physical care for chronic disease process: treatments, drugs, comfort, and hygiene needs. • Encourage health promotion measures (as above). • Refer the patient to resources to support finances. • Support patient and family or significant others in a trusting relationship. • Assist with end-of-life issues: resuscitation orders, comfort measures, funeral plans, estate planning, child care, etc. • Assess desires and refer to resources that will help in meeting spiritual needs.

Teach patients to recognize symptoms that may indicate disease progression and/or drug side effects so that prompt medical care can be initiated. Table 14.19 gives an overview of symptoms that patients should report.

Acute Exacerbations. Acute exacerbations of recurring problems characterize chronic disease. This is especially true in HIV disease in which infections, cancers, debility, and psychosocial or economic issues may interact to overwhelm the patient's ability to cope. Nursing care becomes more complex as the patient's immune system declines and new problems arise to compound existing difficulties. When opportunistic diseases or difficult treatment side effects develop, the patient needs symptom management, teaching, and emotional support.

Nursing care can help prevent the many opportunistic diseases associated with HIV infection. The best way to prevent opportunistic disease is to ensure that the patient is adhering to an effective ART regimen and, if appropriate, taking prophylactic medications for opportunistic infections. Should an opportunistic disease occur, nursing care is an essential part of helping the patient adhere to medications and providing supportive care specific to the opportunistic disease. For example, if the patient has *Pneumocystis jiroveci* pneumonia (PCP) (Fig. 14.8), nursing interventions can ensure adequate oxygenation. If the patient has cryptococcal meningitis, an important nursing concern is maintaining a safe environment for a confused patient.

TABLE 14.17 Patient & Caregiver Teaching
Antiretroviral Drugs

Resistance to antiretroviral drugs is a major problem in treating HIV infection. Include the following instructions when teaching the patient and/or caregiver to decrease the risk for developing resistance.

1. Discuss options with your HCP to find the best regimen for you.
2. Know the drugs you are taking and how to take them (some have to be taken with food, some must be taken on an empty stomach, some cannot be taken together). If you do not understand, ask. Have your nurse write the instructions for you.
3. Take the full dose prescribed and take it on schedule. If you cannot take the drug because of side effects or other problems, report it to your HCP immediately.
4. Take all your medications as prescribed. Do not quit taking one drug while continuing the others. If you cannot tolerate even one of your drugs, talk to your HCP, who will recommend a way to deal with the side effects or a new set of drugs.
5. Many antiretroviral drugs interact with other drugs, including many common drugs you can buy without a prescription. Be sure your HCP and pharmacist know all the drugs that you are taking. Do not take any new drugs without checking for possible interactions.
6. The goals of antiretroviral therapy are to decrease the amount of virus in your blood (your viral load) and to keep your CD4 cell count high. The best results reduce your viral load below detectable levels and keep your CD4 cell count high. Most HCPs do routine laboratory work every 3 to 6 months whether you are taking antiretroviral drugs or not.
7. At 2 to 4 weeks after you start on drug therapy or change your therapy, your HCP will test your viral load to find out how the drugs are working.
   - Your viral load is reported in absolute numbers. All you need to know is that you want to see the viral load drop.
   - Your CD4 cell count is reported in absolute numbers or percentages. It is best for your CD4 cell count to be above 500 cells/µL. If reported in percentages, you would like your CD4 cell value to be above 14%.
8. An undetectable viral load means that the amount of virus is extremely low, and HIV cannot be found in the blood using current testing technology. It does not mean that the virus is gone because the virus can be in lymph nodes and organs that blood tests cannot detect. It also does not mean that you are no longer able to transmit HIV to others. You will need to continue protecting all your sexual and drug-using partners from HIV.

TABLE 14.18 Patient & Caregiver Teaching
Improving Adherence to Antiretroviral Therapy

The following are strategies that you can use to improve a patient's adherence to using antiretroviral therapy:

1. Determine whether the patient understands the importance of adherence and is ready to start therapy.
2. Provide teaching on medication dosing.
3. Review potential side effects of drugs.
4. Assure the patient that side effects can be treated. If not, medication regimens can be changed.
5. Use teaching and memory aids, including pictures, pillboxes, and calendars.
6. Engage family and friends in the teaching process. Solicit their support to help the patient take treatment.
7. Simplify regimens, dosing, and food requirements as much as possible.
8. Use a team of nurses, HCPs, pharmacists, case managers, and mental health and peer counselors to support the patient.
9. Help the patient integrate the medication regimen into his or her typical life activities and work schedules.

Modified from Centers for Disease Control and Prevention: Guidelines for the use of antiretroviral agents in HIV-1-infected adults and adolescents, 2015. Retrieved from *www.aidsinfo.nih.gov.*

TABLE 14.19 Patient & Caregiver Teaching
Signs and Symptoms HIV-Infected Patients Need to Report

Teach the patient with HIV infection and the caregiver to report the following signs and symptoms.

Report Immediately
- Any change in level of consciousness: lethargic, hard to arouse, unable to be aroused, unresponsive, unconscious
- Headache accompanied by nausea and vomiting, changes in vision, changes in ability to perform coordinated activities, or after any head trauma
- Vision changes: blurry or black areas in vision field, new floaters, double vision
- Persistent shortness of breath related to activity and not relieved by a short rest period
- Nausea and vomiting accompanied by abdominal pain
- Vomiting blood
- Dehydration: unable to eat or drink because of nausea or mouth lesions; severe diarrhea or vomiting; dizziness when standing
- Yellow discoloration of the skin
- Any bleeding from the rectum that is not related to hemorrhoids or trauma (e.g., from anal sexual intercourse)
- Pain in the flank with fever and inability to urinate for more than 6 hours
- Blood in the urine
- New onset of weakness in any part of the body, new onset of numbness that is not obviously related to pressure, new onset of difficulty speaking
- Chest pain not obviously related to cough
- Seizures
- New rash accompanied by fever
- New oral lesions accompanied by fever
- Severe depression, anxiety, hallucinations, delusions, or thoughts of causing danger to self or others

Report the Following Signs and Symptoms Within 24 Hours
- New or different headache; constant headache not relieved by over-the-counter medication
- Headache accompanied by fever, nasal congestion, or cough
- Burning, itching, or discharge from the eyes
- New or productive cough
- Vomiting 2 or 3 times a day
- Vomiting accompanied by fever
- New, significant, or watery diarrhea (more than 6 times a day)
- Painful urination, bloody urine, urethral discharge
- Significant new rash (widespread; painful; or following a path down the leg or arm, around the chest, or on the face)
- Difficulty eating or drinking because of mouth lesions
- Vaginal discharge, pain, or itching

◆ **Ambulatory Care.** HIV infection has no cure, continues for life, causes physical disability, and contributes to impaired health. In many cases it can lead to death. HIV infection affects the entire range of a person's life from physical health to social, emotional, economic, and spiritual well-being. As a nurse, you are often the person who works most closely with patients who are trying to cope with living with HIV.

Stigma of HIV. HIV-infected patients share problems experienced by all those with chronic diseases, but these problems are worsened by negative social attitudes and beliefs surrounding HIV. HIV-infected people may be thought to lack control over urges to have sex or use IV drugs. Some people conclude that people with HIV brought the disease

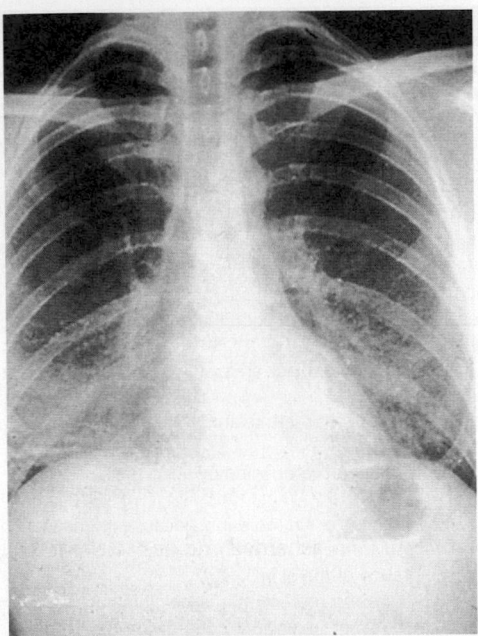

FIG. **14.8** Chest x-ray showing interstitial infiltrates as the result of *Pneumocystis jiroveci* pneumonia. (From the Centers for Disease Control and Prevention. Courtesy Jonathan W. M. Gold, MD, New York, NY.)

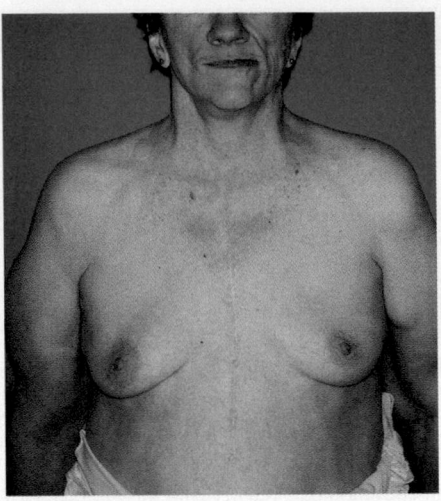

FIG. **14.9** Lipodystrophy manifestations. (From James WD, Berger T, Elston D: *Andrews' diseases of the skin: Clinical dermatology,* ed 11, St Louis, 2011, Saunders.)

on themselves and deserve to be sick. Some view behaviors associated with HIV infection as immoral (e.g., homosexuality, promiscuity). Other behaviors are sometimes illegal (e.g., using drugs, sex work). The fact that infected people can transmit HIV to others creates fear, which leads to stigma and discrimination in all areas of life.[33]

In the United States, HIV-infected people have lost jobs, homes, and insurance, although the Americans with Disabilities Act (ADA) prohibits these forms of discrimination. HIV-related stigma is a global problem that is often more severe for women. Discrimination can lead to social isolation, dependence, frustration, low self-image, loss of control, and economic pressures.

Disease and Drug Side Effects. Physical problems related to HIV or its treatment can interfere with the patient's ability to maintain a desired lifestyle. HIV-infected patients often have anxiety, fear, depression, diarrhea, peripheral neuropathy, pain, nausea, vomiting, and fatigue. Nursing interventions for these symptoms are similar to what they would be for the patient who does not have HIV infection. For example, nursing management of diarrhea includes helping patients collect specimens, recommending diet changes, encouraging fluid and electrolyte replacement, teaching the patient about skin care, and managing skin breakdown around the perianal area. Nursing approaches for fatigue in HIV include teaching patients to assess fatigue patterns; determine contributing factors; set activity priorities; conserve energy; schedule rest periods; exercise regularly; and avoid substances such as caffeine, nicotine, alcohol, and other drugs that may disturb sleep.

Some HIV-infected patients, especially those who have been infected and on ART for a long time, may develop a set of metabolic disorders. These include (1) lipodystrophy (changes in body shape caused by a redistribution of fat in the abdomen, upper back, and breasts along with fat loss in the arms, legs, and face) (Fig. 14.9); (2) hyperlipidemia (high triglycerides, high low-density lipoproteins, and decreased high-density lipoproteins); (3) insulin resistance; (4) hyperglycemia; (5) bone disease (osteoporosis, osteopenia, avascular necrosis); (6) lactic acidosis; (7) renal disease; and (8) cardiovascular disease.[34]

It is still not clear why these disorders develop, but it is likely a combination of factors such as long-term infection with HIV, side effects of ART, genetic predisposition, and chronic stress. Management of metabolic disorders focuses on detecting problems early, dealing with symptoms, and helping the patient cope with emerging problems and changes to treatment regimens. It is important to recognize and treat these problems early, especially because cardiovascular disease and lactic acidosis are potentially fatal complications.

A frequent first intervention is to change ART medications because some drugs are more often associated with these disorders. Lipid abnormalities are generally treated with lipid-lowering drugs (see Table 33.6), diet changes, and exercise. Insulin resistance is treated with hypoglycemic drugs and weight loss. Exercise, diet changes, and calcium and vitamin D supplements may improve bone disease.

End-of-Life Care. Despite new developments in the treatment of HIV infection, many patients eventually have disease progression, disability, and death. Sometimes these occur because treatments do not work for the patient. Sometimes the patient's HIV becomes resistant to all available drug therapies. In addition, ART is now allowing people living with HIV to live longer and to develop diseases of aging, such as cardiovascular and endocrine problems that lead to death.

Nursing care during the terminal phase of any disease should focus on keeping the patient comfortable, facilitating emotional and spiritual acceptance of the finite nature of life, helping the patient's significant others deal with grief and loss, and maintaining a safe environment.[35] As a nurse, you are the pivotal care provider during this phase of illness, whether at home, through hospice, or in a health care facility. End-of-life care is discussed in Chapter 9.

◆ **Evaluation**

The expected outcomes are that the patient at risk for HIV infection will:

- Develop and implement a personal plan to decrease personal risk factors
- Have testing for HIV

The expected outcomes are that the patient with HIV infection will:

- Adhere to treatment for HIV disease
- Work with the health care team to achieve optimal health
- Prevent transmission of HIV to others

 Gerontologic Considerations: HIV Infection

The number of older adults who have HIV disease is increasing because (1) HIV treatment has been effective in reducing the number of deaths from HIV-related opportunistic infections and (2) people 60 and older are being infected at increasing rates. The number of people over the age of 60 living with HIV is expected to grow.

Remember that older people living with HIV are susceptible to the same diseases as non–HIV-infected older people. These include heart disease, cancer, diabetes, bone disease, arthritis, hypertension, kidney disease, and cognitive impairment. However, people with HIV infection may develop these diseases at an earlier age (compared with non–HIV-infected people) and be at higher risk for co-morbidities related to ART.[36] For example, some HIV medications are associated with increased lipids and altered insulin metabolism. Focusing nursing care on early identification of these complications, and helping patients reduce their risk for heart disease, diabetes, or other chronic disease, are critical aspects of caring for the older HIV patient.

 CHECK YOUR PRACTICE

You are receiving report on a patient newly admitted to the rehabilitation unit. He is a 68-yr-old male patient who had a hip replacement 3 days ago. The nurse giving the report casually mentions, "Oh, by the way, he has AIDS. Can you believe that an old man like that has HIV?"
- How would you respond?

The impact of polypharmacy is another consideration with the aging HIV population. In general, older adults take multiple medications to manage various chronic diseases. Some medications may interact with or be potentiated by HIV medications. Therefore careful monitoring and assessment of possible drug interactions is important when providing care to this population.

Older adults may be ashamed and hesitate to tell anyone that they have an HIV infection. This may make it hard for them to get the appropriate health care and support. As a nurse, you need to recognize that HIV will affect an increasing number of older adults and be prepared to help the older person who is living with HIV infection.

CASE STUDY

HIV Infection

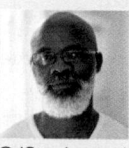

(© iStock.com/ Cecilie_Arcurs.)

Patient Profile

J.N., a 69-yr-old black male with HIV, chronic hepatitis B, and hypertension, was admitted 2 days ago with *Pneumocystis jiroveci* pneumonia (PCP).

Subjective Data

- Diagnosed with HIV infection at age 56 after his male partner was diagnosed with Kaposi's sarcoma
- Has had issues taking ART consistently, "Too many side effects"
- Has fatigue and frequent oral candidiasis outbreaks
- Expresses concern about his future, "I don't know who will take care of me. I don't have any family around"

Objective Data

Physical Examination

- 5 ft 10 in tall, 150 lb, temperature 100.4° F (38° C), O_2 saturation 92% on 3 L of O_2 via nasal cannula

Laboratory Studies

- CD4 cell count 185 cells/µL
- Viral load 155,328 copies/µL

Interprofessional Care

- Trimethoprim/sulfamethoxazole
- Combination antiretroviral therapy: tenofovir alafenamide and emtricitabine (Descovy), with dolutegravir (Tivicay)

Discussion Questions

1. Why was trimethoprim/sulfamethoxazole ordered, and what are its common side effects?
2. **Priority Decision:** What priority teaching needs should be covered before J.N. is discharged from the hospital to return home?
3. How can J.N. be helped to adhere to his medication schedule?
4. **Priority Decision:** What are the priority nursing interventions? What nursing care will he need after discharge?
5. **Collaboration:** Older lesbian, gay, bisexual, transgender (LGBT) adults often lack familial social support as they age. What barriers could this cause for J.N.'s treatment? How could the interprofessional team assist in addressing these issues? What referrals may be made?
6. **Safety:** The nurse needs to start an IV for fluid replacement on J.N. Before inserting the IV what type of personal protective equipment is recommended for this situation?

Answers available at *http://evolve.elsevier.com/Lewis/medsurg*.

BRIDGE TO NCLEX EXAMINATION

The number of the question corresponds to the same-numbered outcome at the beginning of the chapter.

1. Emerging and reemerging infections affect health care by *(select all that apply)*
   a. reevaluating vaccine practices.
   b. revealing antimicrobial resistance.
   c. limiting antibiotics to those with life-threatening infection.
   d. challenging researchers to discover new antimicrobial therapies.

2. Interventions to prevent health care–associated infections include *(select all that apply)*
   a. following hand-washing protocols.
   b. limiting visitors to persons over age 18.
   c. placing high-risk patients in private rooms.
   d. decontaminating equipment used for patient care.
   e. appropriately using personal protective equipment.

3. Transmission of HIV from an infected person to another most often occurs because of
   a. unprotected anal or vaginal sexual intercourse.
   b. low levels of virus in the blood and high levels of CD4+ T cells.
   c. transmission from mother to infant during labor and delivery and breastfeeding.
   d. sharing eating utensils, dry kissing, hugging, using toilet seats, or shaking hands.

4. During HIV infection
   a. reverse transcriptase helps HIV fuse with the CD4+ T cell.
   b. HIV RNA uses the CD4+ T cell's mitochondria to replicate.
   c. the immune system is impaired predominantly by the eventual widespread destruction of CD4+ T cells.
   d. a long period of dormancy develops during which HIV cannot be found in the blood and there is little viral replication.

5. A diagnosis of AIDS is made when an HIV-infected patient has
   a. a CD4+ T cell count below 200/μL.
   b. a high level of HIV in the blood and saliva.
   c. lipodystrophy with metabolic abnormalities.
   d. oral hairy leukoplakia, an infection caused by Epstein-Barr virus.

6. Screening for HIV infection generally involves
   a. detecting CD8+ cytotoxic T cells in saliva.
   b. laboratory analysis of saliva to detect CD4+ T cells.
   c. analysis of lymph tissues for the presence of HIV RNA.
   d. laboratory analysis of blood to detect HIV antigen and/or antibody.

7. HIV antiretroviral drugs are used to
   a. cure acute HIV infection.
   b. decrease viral RNA levels.
   c. treat opportunistic diseases.
   d. decrease symptoms in terminal disease.

8. Opportunistic diseases in HIV infection
   a. are usually benign.
   b. are generally slow to develop and progress.
   c. occur in the presence of immunosuppression.
   d. are curable with appropriate drug interventions.

9. Which statements about metabolic side effects of ART are true *(select all that apply)*?
   a. These are annoying symptoms that are ultimately harmless.
   b. ART-related body changes include fat redistribution and peripheral wasting.
   c. Lipid problems include increases in triglycerides and decreases in high-density cholesterol.
   d. Insulin resistance and hyperlipidemia can be treated with drugs to control glucose and cholesterol.
   e. Compared to uninfected people, insulin resistance and hyperlipidemia are harder to treat in HIV-infected patients.

10. Which strategy can the nurse teach the patient to eliminate the risk for HIV transmission?
    a. Using sterile equipment to inject drugs
    b. Cleaning equipment used to inject drugs
    c. Taking lamivudine (Epivir) during pregnancy
    d. Using latex or polyurethane barriers to cover genitalia during sexual contact

11. What is the *most* appropriate nursing intervention to help an HIV-infected patient adhere to a treatment regimen?
    a. Set up a drug pillbox for the patient every week.
    b. Give the patient a video and a brochure to view and read at home.
    c. Tell the patient that side effects of ART are bad but that they go away.
    d. Assess the patient's routines and find adherence cues that fit into the patient's life circumstances.

1. a, b, d, 2. a, d, e, 3. a, 4. c, 5. a, 6. d, 7. b, 8. c, 9. b, c, d, 10. a, 11. d

For rationales to these answers and even more NCLEX review questions, visit *http://evolve.elsevier.com/Lewis/medsurg.*

ⓔ EVOLVE WEBSITE/RESOURCES LIST

http://evolve.elsevier.com/Lewis/medsurg
Review Questions (Online Only)
Key Points
Answer Keys for Questions
- Rationales for Bridge to NCLEX Examination Questions
- Answer Guidelines for Case Study on p. 229.

Student Case Study
- Patient With Human Immunodeficiency Virus (HIV) Infection and Acquired Immunodeficiency Syndrome (AIDS)

Conceptual Care Map Creator
Audio Glossary
Content Updates

REFERENCES

1. Centers for Disease Control and Prevention: National Center for Emerging and Zoonotic Infectious Diseases (NCEZID). Retrieved from *www.cdc.gov/ncezid.*
2. Hall V, Banerjee E, Kenyon C, et al: Measles outbreak—Minnesota April–May 2017, *MMWR* 66:713, 2017.
3. Grobusch MP, Rodriguez-Morales AJ, Wilson ME: Measles on the move, *Travel Med Infect Dis* 18:1, 2017.
4. Infectious Disease Society of America: Antimicrobial resistance. Retrieved from *www.idsociety.org/topic_antimicrobial_resistance.*
*5. Ray SM: Preventing methicillin-resistant *Staphylococcus aureus* (MRSA) disease in urban US hospitals-now for the hard part: More evidence pointing to the community as the source of MRSA acquisition, *JID* 215:1631, 2017.

6. Centers for Disease Control and Prevention: Healthcare-associated infections. Retrieved from *www.cdc.gov/HAI.*

7. Centers for Disease Control and Prevention: Healthcare-associated infections (HAI) progress report. Retrieved from *www.cdc.gov/hai/surveillance/progress-report/index.html.*

*8. Dunne CP, Kingston L, Slevin B, et al: Hand hygiene and compliance behaviors are the under-appreciated human factors pivotal to reducing hospital-acquired infections, *J Hosp Infect* 98:4, 2018.

9. Office of Disease Prevention and Health Promotion: Health care-associated infections. Retrieved from *www.health.gov/hcq/prevent-hai.asp.*

10. Katz MJ, Roghmann MC: Healthcare-associated infections in the elders: What's new, *Curr Opin Infect Dis* 29:388, 2016.

11. U.S. Food and Drug Administration: Personal protective equipment for infection control. Retrieved from *www.fda.gov/MedicalDevices/ProductsandMedicalProcedures/GeneralHospitalDevicesandSupplies/PersonalProtectiveEquipment/default.htm.*

*12. Centers for Disease Control and Prevention: Transmission-based precautions. Retrieved from *www.cdc.gov/infectioncontrol/basics/transmission-based-precautions.html.*

13. Centers for Disease Control and Prevention: HIV in the United States: At a glance. Retrieved from *www.cdc.gov/hiv/statistics/overview/ataglance.html.*

14. Centers for Disease Control and Prevention: HIV transmission. Retrieved from *www.cdc.gov/hiv/basics/transmission.html.*

15. Centers for Disease Control and Prevention: Occupational HIV transmission and prevention among health care workers. Retrieved from *www.cdc.gov/hiv/workplace/healthcareworkers.html.*

*16. Beste S, Essajee S, Siberry G, et al: Optimal antiretroviral prophylaxis in infants at high risk of acquiring HIV: A systematic review, *Pediatr Infect Dis J* 37:169, 2018.

17. US Department of Health and Human Services: The HIV life cycle. Retrieved from *www.aidsinfo.nih.gov/understanding-hiv-aids/fact-sheets/19/73/the-hiv-life-cycle.*

*18. Hoenigl M, Green N, Camacho M, et al: Signs or symptoms of acute HIV infection in a cohort undergoing community-based screening, *Emerg Infect Dis* 22:532, 2016.

*19. Rutstein SE, Ananworanich J, Fidler S, et al: Clinical and public health implications of acute and early HIV detection and treatment: A scoping review, *J Int AIDS Soc* 20:21579, 2017.

20. US Department of Health and Human Services: AIDS case definition. Retrieved from *www.aidsinfo.nih.gov/understanding-hiv-aids/glossary/2925/aids-case-definition.*

21. Centers for Disease Control and Prevention: 2018 Quick reference guide: Recommended laboratory HIV testing algorithm for serum or plasma specimens. Retrieved from *https://stacks.cdc.gov/view/cdc/50872.*

22. Centers for Disease Control and Prevention: HIV/AIDS and viral hepatitis. Retrieved from *www.cdc.gov/hepatitis/populations/hiv.htm.*

*23. Panel on Antiretroviral Guidelines for Adults and Adolescents: Guidelines for the use of antiretroviral agents in adults and adolescents living with HIV. Retrieved from *www.aidsinfo.nih.gov/guidelines/html/1/adult-and-adolescent-treatment-guidelines/0.*

*24. Panel on Opportunistic Infections in HIV-Infected Adults and Adolescents: Guidelines for the prevention and treatment of opportunistic infections in HIV-infected adults and adolescents. Retrieved from *www.aidsinfo.nih.gov/guidelines/html/4/adult-and-adolescent-opportunistic-infection/0.*

*25. Smith DK, Koenig LJ, Martin M, et al: Preexposure prophylaxis for the prevention of HIV infection: A clinical practice guideline. Retrieved from *www./stacks.cdc.gov/view/cdc/23109.*

26. Corey L, Gray GE: Preventing acquisition of HIV is the only path to an AIDS-free generation, *Proc Natl Acad Sci USA* 114:3798, 2017.

27. US Department of Health and Human Services: Alcohol and drug use and HIV risk. Retrieved from *www.hiv.gov/hiv-basics/hiv-prevention/reducing-risk-from-alcohol-and-drug-use/alcohol-and-drug-use-and-hiv-risk.*

*28. Mackesy-Amiti ME, Boodram B, Spiller MW, et al: Injection-related risk behavior and engagement in outreach, intervention and prevention services across 20 US cities, *J Acquir Immune Defic Syndr* S3:S316, 2017.

*29. Panel on Treatment of Pregnant Women with HIV Infection and Prevention of Perinatal Transmission: Recommendations for use of antiretroviral drugs in transmission in the United States. Retrieved from *www.aidsinfo.nih.gov/guidelines/html/3/perinatal/0.*

30. Centers for Disease Control and Prevention: Revised guidelines for HIV testing of adults, adolescents, and pregnant women in health-care settings. Retrieved from *www.cdc.gov/mmwr/preview/mmwrhtml/rr5514a1.htm.*

31. US Preventive Services Task Force: Human immunodeficiency virus (HIV) infection: Screening. Retrieved from *www.uspreventiveservicestaskforce.org/Page/Document/UpdateSummaryFinal/human-immunodeficiency-virus-hiv-infection-screening.*

32. University of California San Francisco HIV InSite: Coping with HIV/AIDS: Mental health. Retrieved from *http://hivinsite.ucsf.edu/insite?page=pb-daily-mental.*

*33. Davtyan M, Olshansky EF, Lakon C: Addressing HIV stigma in health care, *Am J Nurs* 118:11, 2018.

34. Mirza FS, Luthra P, Chirch : Endocrinological aspects of HIV infection, *J Endocrinol Invest* 41:881-899, 2018.

35. Goodkin K, Kompella S, Kendell SF: End-of-life care and bereavement issues in human immunodeficiency virus–AIDS, *Nurs Clin North Am* 53:123, 2018.

*36. The HIV and Aging Consensus Project: Clinical recommendations. Retrieved from *www.hiv-age.org/clinical-recommendations/.*

*Evidence-based information for clinical practice.

15

Cancer

Marisa Cortese

So long as you can sweeten another's pain, life is not in vain.

Helen Keller

e http://evolve.elsevier.com/Lewis/medsurg/

CONCEPTUAL FOCUS

Cellular Regulation
Coping

Health Promotion

LEARNING OUTCOMES

1. Describe the incidence, survival, and mortality rates of cancer in the United States.
2. Describe the processes involved in the biology of cancer.
3. Outline the stages of cancer development.
4. Describe the role of the immune system related to cancer.
5. Discuss the role of the nurse in the prevention, detection, and diagnosis of cancer.
6. Explain the use of surgery, chemotherapy, radiation therapy, immunotherapy, targeted therapy, and hormone therapy in the treatment of cancer.
7. Identify the classifications of chemotherapy agents and methods of administration.

8. Distinguish between external beam radiation and brachytherapy.
9. Describe the effects of radiation therapy and chemotherapy on normal tissues.
10. Identify the types and effects of immunotherapy and targeted therapy.
11. Describe the nursing management of patients receiving chemotherapy, radiation therapy, immunotherapy, and targeted therapy.
12. Describe nutritional therapy for patients with cancer.
13. Identify complications associated with advanced cancer.
14. Describe support interventions for cancer patients, cancer survivors, and their caregivers.

KEY TERMS

brachytherapy, p. 247
cancer, p. 232
carcinogens, p. 235
carcinoma in situ (CIS), p. 239
chemotherapy, p. 243
external beam radiation, p. 247
hematopoietic stem cell transplantation (HSCT), p. 258
histologic grading, p. 238

immunologic surveillance, p. 237
immunotherapy, p. 255
malignant neoplasms, p. 238
metastasis, p. 235
oncogenes, p. 234
peripheral stem cell transplantation (PSCT), p. 258
protooncogenes, p. 234
staging, p. 238

targeted therapy, p. 255
tumor angiogenesis, p. 236
vesicants, p. 245

Cancer is a group of diseases characterized by uncontrolled and unregulated growth of cells. The resulting problems may be directly related to the cancer, a consequence of treating the cancer, or a combination of both. The combined physiologic, psychologic, and social impact of cancer on patients and their caregivers is considerable. Despite advances in treatment and care, a great deal of anxiety and fear continue to be associated with a diagnosis of cancer.

Educating health care professionals and the public is essential to promote realistic attitudes about cancer and cancer treatment. You are in a strategic position to lead efforts for changing attitudes about cancer. You can (1) help people decrease their risk for cancer development, (2) increase rates of cancer screening, (3) help patients adhere to cancer management plans, and

(4) support patients and caregivers as they cope with the effects of cancer and related treatment. You need to be knowledgeable about specific types of cancer, treatment options, management of side effects of therapy, and supportive therapies for cancer.

Cancer is often considered a disease of aging, with most cases diagnosed in those over age 55 years. However, it occurs in people of all ages. An estimated 1.7 million people in the United States are diagnosed annually with invasive cancer (excluding basal and squamous cell skin cancers).[1]

Overall both the incidence and mortality rates of cancer have been declining.[2] The incidence of many cancers, such as colorectal, lung, breast, and oropharyngeal cancers, have declined largely because of preventive efforts. However, the incidence of other types of cancers, such as kidney, thyroid, pancreas, liver, uterus, skin melanoma, multiple myeloma, and non-Hodgkin's lymphoma, is increasing.[3]

Overall cancer incidence is higher in men than women. Gender differences in incidence and death rates for specific cancers are shown in the Gender Differences box and Tables 15.1 and 15.2.

GENDER DIFFERENCES

Cancer

Men

- More men than women die from cancer-related deaths each year.
- Mortality rate from lung cancer is higher in men.
- Cancer with the highest incidence among men is prostate cancer.
- Men are more likely to develop liver cancer.
- Head and neck cancers occur more often in men.

Women

- Cancer with the highest death rate among women is lung cancer.
- Cancer with the highest incidence among women is breast cancer.
- Thyroid cancer is more prevalent in women.
- Women are less likely to have colon cancer screenings.

TABLE 15.1 Cancer Incidence by Site and Gender*

MALE		FEMALE	
Type	%	Type	%
Prostate	19	Breast	30
Lung	14	Lung	13
Colon/rectum	9	Colon/rectum	7
Urinary bladder	7	Uterus	7
Melanoma of the skin	5	Thyroid	5
Kidney and renal pelvis	5	Melanoma of the skin	4
Non-Hodgkin's lymphoma	5	Non-Hodgkin's lymphoma	4
Oral cavity and pharynx	4	Pancreas	3
Leukemia	4	Leukemia	3
Liver and intrahepatic bile duct	4	Kidney and renal pelvis	3

Source: American Cancer Society: *Cancer facts & figures 2018*, Atlanta, 2018, American Cancer Society.

*Numbers are estimates and exclude basal and squamous cell skin cancers and carcinoma in situ.

TABLE 15.2 Cancer Deaths by Site and Gender

MALE		FEMALE	
Type	%	Type	%
Lung and bronchus	26	Lung and bronchus	25
Prostate	9	Breast	14
Colon/rectum	8	Colon/rectum	8
Pancreas	7	Pancreas	7
Liver and intrahepatic bile ducts	6	Ovary	5
Leukemia	4	Leukemia	4
Esophagus	4	Uterus	4
Urinary bladder	4	Non-Hodgkin's lymphoma	3
Non-Hodgkin's lymphoma	4	Liver and intrahepatic bile ducts	3
Kidney and renal pelvis	3	Brain and other nervous system	3

Source: American Cancer Society: *Cancer facts & figures 2018*, Atlanta, 2018, American Cancer Society.

Although mortality rates from all cancers combined are on the decline, it is still the second most common cause of death in the United States. Cancer is the leading cause of death of people 40 to 79 years of age. Each year about 609,640 Americans are expected to die because of cancer, which is more than 1600 people per day.[1,2]

Considerable progress has been made in controlling cancer for long periods. More than 15.5 million Americans are alive today who have a history of cancer. This includes those who have cancer and are undergoing treatment, are disease free, or are in remission.[2] Cancer survivors are discussed later on pp. 264-265.

BIOLOGY OF CANCER

Two major dysfunctions present in the process of cancer development are defective cell proliferation (growth) and defective cell differentiation.

Defect in Cell Proliferation

Normally, most tissues have a population of undifferentiated cells known as stem cells. These stem cells ultimately differentiate and become mature, functioning cells of a specific tissue.

Cell proliferation starts in the stem cell and begins when the stem cell enters the cell cycle (Fig. 15.1). The time from when a cell enters the cell cycle to when the cell divides into 2 identical cells is called the *generation time* of the cell. A mature cell continues to function until it degenerates and dies.

All the body's cells are controlled by an intracellular mechanism that determines when cell proliferation is necessary. Under normal conditions, there is a state of dynamic equilibrium. This means cell proliferation equals cell degeneration or death. Normally, the process of cell division and proliferation is activated only in the presence of cell degeneration or death *(apoptosis)*. Cell proliferation also occurs if the body has a physiologic need for more cells. For example, a normal increase in white blood cell (WBC) count occurs with infection.

Another means of proliferation control in normal cells is *contact inhibition*. Normal cells respect the boundaries and territory of the cells surrounding them. They will not invade a territory that is not their own. We think the neighboring cells inhibit cell growth through the physical contact of the surrounding cell membranes. Cancer cells grown in tissue culture have a loss of contact inhibition. They have no regard for cell boundaries and grow on top of one another and on top of or between normal cells.

The rate of normal cell proliferation (from the time of cell birth to the time of cell death) differs in each body tissue. In some tissues, such as bone marrow, hair follicles, and epithelial lining of the gastrointestinal (GI) tract, the rate of cell proliferation is rapid. In other tissues, such as myocardium and cartilage, cell proliferation does not occur or is slow.

Cancer cells proliferate at the same rate as the normal cells of the tissue from which they arise. However, cancer cells respond differently from normal cells to the intracellular signals that regulate cell proliferation and death. The result is that the proliferation of the cancer cells is indiscriminate and continuous. Sometimes they produce more than 2 cells at the time of mitosis. In this way, there is continuous growth of a tumor mass: $1 \times 2 \times 4 \times 8 \times 16$ and so on. This is termed the *pyramid effect*. The time needed for a tumor mass to double in size is known as its *doubling time*.

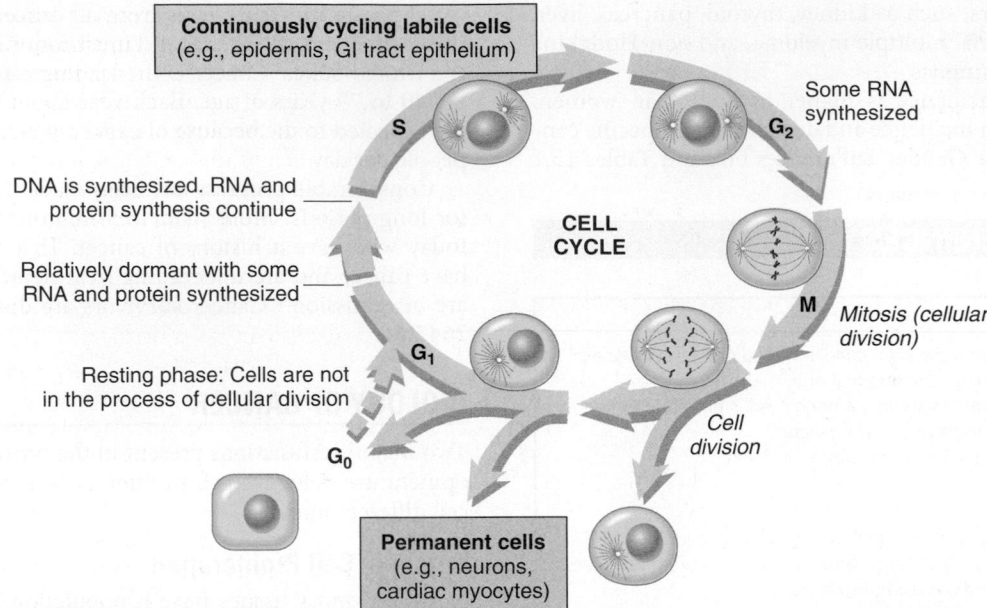

FIG. 15.1 Cell life cycle and metabolic activity. Generation time is the period from *M* phase to *M* phase. Cells not in the cycle but capable of division are in the resting phase *(G₀)*. (Adapted from Kumar V, Abbas AK, Fausto N, et al: *Robbins and Cotran pathologic basis of disease*, ed 8, Philadelphia, 2010, Saunders.)

Defect in Cell Differentiation

Cell differentiation is normally an orderly process that progresses from a state of immaturity to a state of maturity. Because all body cells are derived from the fertilized ova, all cells have the potential to perform all body functions. As cells differentiate, this potential is repressed, and the mature cell can perform only specific functions. With cell differentiation, there is a stable and orderly phasing out of cell potential. Under normal conditions, the differentiated cell is stable and will not *dedifferentiate*, or return to its previous undifferentiated state.

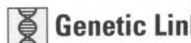 ## Genetic Link

Cancer involves the malfunction of genes that control differentiation and proliferation. Two types of normal genes that can be affected by mutation are *protooncogenes* and *tumor suppressor genes*. **Protooncogenes** are normal cell genes that are important regulators of normal cell processes. Protooncogenes promote growth. Tumor suppressor genes suppress growth. Mutations that change the expression of protooncogenes can cause them to function as **oncogenes** (tumor-inducing genes).

The protooncogene has been described as the genetic lock that keeps the cell in its mature functioning state. When this lock is "unlocked," as may occur through exposure to *carcinogens* (agents that cause cancer) or oncogenic viruses, genetic alterations and mutations occur. The abilities and properties that the cell had in fetal development are again expressed. Oncogenes can change a normal cell to a malignant one. This cell regains a fetal appearance and function. For example, some cancer cells make new proteins characteristic of the embryonic and fetal periods of life. These proteins, found on the cell membrane, include carcinoembryonic antigen (CEA) and α-fetoprotein (AFP). They can be found in the blood by laboratory studies. Other cancer cells, such as small cell cancer of the lung, make hormones that are usually made by cells arising from the same embryonic cells as the tumor cells. See Complications of Cancer later in this chapter on pp. 260-263.

Tumor suppressor genes regulate cell growth. They prevent cells from going through the cell cycle. Mutations can change tumor suppressor genes and make them inactive. This results in a loss of their tumor-suppressing action. Examples of tumor suppressor genes are *BRCA1* and *BRCA2*. Alterations in these genes increase a person's risk for breast and ovarian cancer. Another tumor suppressor gene is the *APC* gene. Mutations in this gene increase a person's risk for familial adenomatous polyposis, a precursor for colorectal cancer (see Chapter 42). Mutations in the *p53* tumor suppressor gene have been found in many cancers, including bladder, breast, colorectal, esophageal, liver, lung, and ovarian cancers.

Development of Cancer

The following is a theoretical model of cancer development. The cause and development of each type of cancer are likely to be multifactorial. A common misbelief is that cancer development is a rapid, haphazard event. However, cancer is usually an orderly process that occurs over time. It has 3 stages: initiation, promotion, and progression (Fig. 15.2).

Initiation. Cancer cells arise from normal cells because of changes in genes. The first stage, *initiation*, involves a mutation in the cell's genetic structure. A *mutation* is any change in the usual DNA sequence.

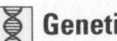 ## Genetic Link

Gene mutations can occur in 2 ways: *inherited* from a parent (passed from one generation to the next) or *acquired* during a person's lifetime. (Mutations are discussed in Chapter 12.)

The genetic predisposition to cancer is thought to play a role in about 5 to 10% of all cancers. These genetic alterations lead to a high risk for developing a specific type of cancer. However, most cancers do not result from inherited genes. They are acquired from damage to genes occurring during one's lifetime. An acquired mutation is passed on to all cells that develop from that single cell. The damaged cell may die or repair itself. However, if cell death or repair does not occur before cell

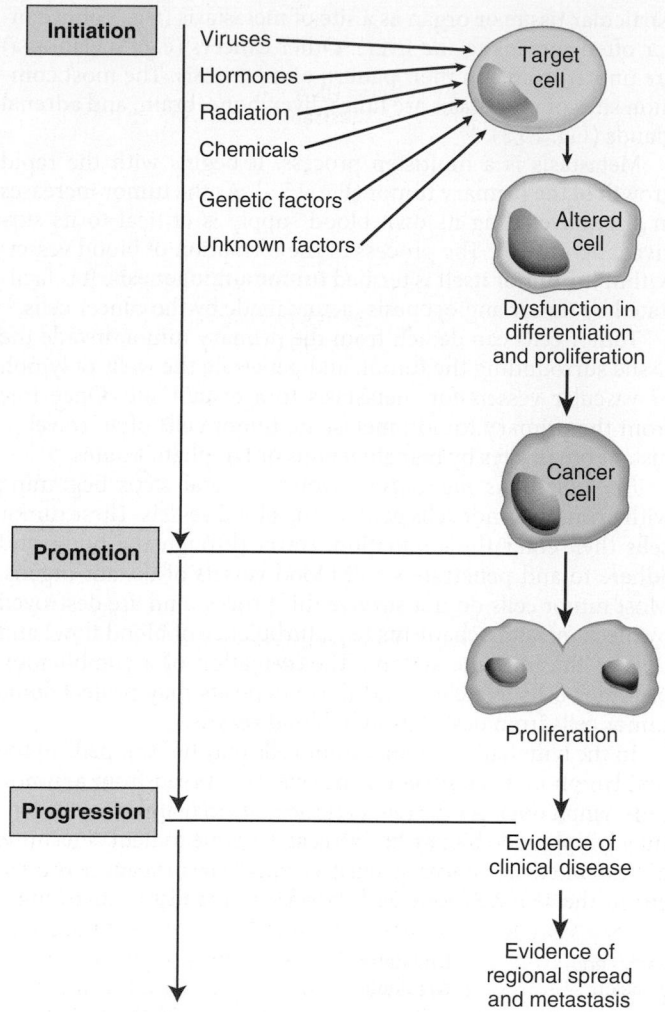

FIG. 15.2 Process of cancer development.

division, the cell will replicate into daughter cells, each with the same genetic alteration.

Carcinogens. Many carcinogens (cancer-causing agents capable of producing cell alterations) are detoxified by protective enzymes and harmlessly excreted. If this protective mechanism fails, carcinogens can enter the cell's nucleus and alter deoxyribonucleic acid (DNA). Carcinogens may be chemical, radiation, or viral.

Chemical carcinogens. Chemicals were identified as cancer-causing agents in the latter part of the 18th century. Percival Pott noted that chimney sweeps had a higher incidence of cancer of the scrotum associated with exposure to soot residue in chimneys. As the years passed, we have found many chemicals that are carcinogens (e.g., benzene, arsenic, formaldehyde). People exposed to these chemicals over time have a greater incidence of certain cancers than others. The long latency period from the time of exposure to the development of cancer makes it hard to identify cancer-causing chemicals.

Radiation. Radiation can cause cancer in almost any body tissue. When cells are exposed to a source of radiation, damage occurs to DNA. Certain cancers are correlated with radiation as a carcinogenic agent:

• The incidence of leukemia, lymphoma, and thyroid cancer increased in the general population of Hiroshima and Nagasaki after the atomic bomb explosions.

• A higher incidence of bone cancer occurs in people exposed to radiation in certain occupations, such as radiologists, radiation chemists, and uranium miners.

Ultraviolet (UV) radiation has long been associated with melanoma and squamous and basal cell skin cancers. Skin cancer is the most common type of cancer among whites in the United States. Sunlight exposure is the main source of UV exposure, giving off UVA and UVB rays. UV radiation from tanning beds also causes skin cancer.[4]

Viral carcinogens. Certain DNA and ribonucleic acid (RNA) viruses, termed *oncogenic,* can alter the cells they infect and induce malignant transformation. These viruses have been identified as causative agents of cancer in animals and humans. Burkitt's lymphoma is associated with Epstein-Barr virus (EBV).[5] People with acquired immunodeficiency syndrome (AIDS), which is caused by human immunodeficiency virus (HIV), have a high incidence of Kaposi sarcoma (see Chapter 14). Other viruses linked to cancer development include hepatitis B virus, which is associated with hepatocellular cancer, and human papillomavirus (HPV). HPV is thought to cause lesions that progress to squamous cell cancers, such as cervical, anal, and head and neck cancers.

Promotion. A single alteration of the genetic structure of the cell is not enough to cause cancer. However, the odds of cancer development are increased with the presence of promoting agents. *Promotion,* the second stage in cancer development, is characterized by the reversible proliferation of the altered cells. An increase in the altered cell population further increases the likelihood of more mutations.

An important distinction between initiation and promotion is that the activity of promoters is reversible. This is a key concept in cancer prevention. Promoting factors include agents such as dietary fat, obesity, cigarette smoking, and alcohol use. Changing a person's lifestyle to modify these risk factors can reduce the chance of cancer development. Around one third of cancer-related deaths in the United States are related to tobacco use, unhealthy diet, physical inactivity, and obesity.[1]

Several promoting agents have activity against specific types of body tissues. So, these agents tend to promote specific kinds of cancer. For example, cigarette smoke is a promoting agent in lung cancer. In conjunction with alcohol use, it promotes esophageal and bladder cancers.

Some carcinogens, termed *complete carcinogens,* are capable of both initiating and promoting cancer development. Cigarette smoke is an example of a complete carcinogen.

A period of time elapses between the first genetic alteration and the actual clinical evidence of cancer. This period, called the *latent* period, includes both the initiation and promotion stages in the natural history of cancer. The variation in the length of time that elapses before the cancer becomes clinically evident is related to the mitotic rate of the tissue of origin and environmental factors. In most cancers, this process is years or even decades in length.

For the disease process to become clinically evident, the cells must reach a critical mass. A tumor that is 1.0 cm (0.4 inch) (the size usually detectable by palpation) has 1 billion cancer cells. A 0.5-cm tumor is the smallest that can be detected by current diagnostic measures, such as MRI.

Progression. *Progression* is the last stage in the natural history of a cancer. This stage is characterized by increased growth rate of the tumor, increased invasiveness, and metastasis (spread of the cancer to a distant site). Certain cancers have an affinity for a

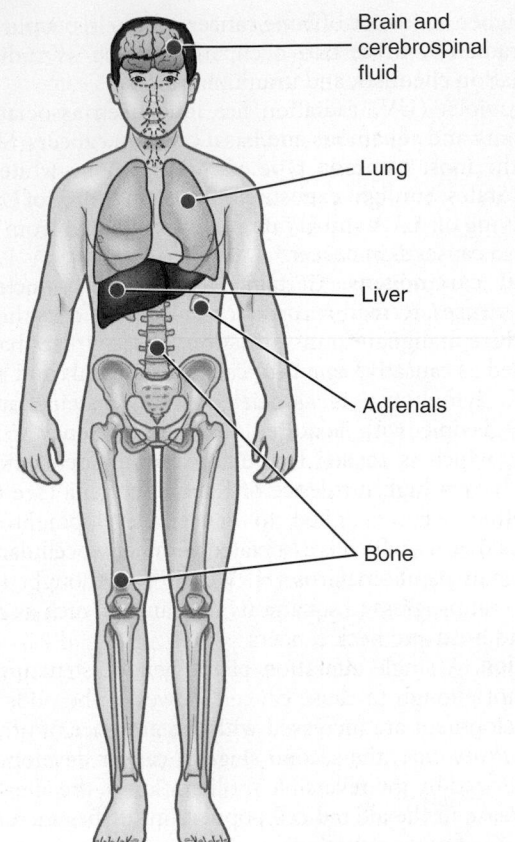

Brain and
cerebrospinal
fluid

Lung

Liver

Adrenals

Bone

FIG. 15.3 Main sites of metastasis. (Adapted from Stevens A, Lowe J: *Pathology: An illustrated review in colour*, ed 2, London, 2000, Mosby.)

particular tissue or organ as a site of metastasis (e.g., colon cancer often spreads to the liver). Other cancers (e.g., melanoma) are unpredictable in their pattern of metastasis. The most common sites of metastasis are lungs, liver, bone, brain, and adrenal glands (Fig. 15.3).

Metastasis is a multistep process. It begins with the rapid growth of the primary tumor (Fig. 15.4). As the tumor increases in size, developing its own blood supply is critical to its survival and growth. The process of the formation of blood vessels within the tumor itself is termed **tumor angiogenesis**. It is facilitated by tumor angiogenesis factors made by the cancer cells.

Tumor cells can detach from the primary tumor, invade the tissue surrounding the tumor, and penetrate the walls of lymph or vascular vessels for metastasis to a distant site. Once free from the primary tumor, metastatic tumor cells often travel to distant organ sites by hematogenous or lymphatic routes.

Hematogenous metastasis involves several steps beginning with primary tumor cells penetrating blood vessels. These tumor cells then enter the circulation, travel through the body, and adhere to and penetrate small blood vessels of distant organs. Most tumor cells do not survive this process and are destroyed by mechanical mechanisms (e.g., turbulence of blood flow) and cells of the immune system. The formation of a combination of tumor cells, platelets, and fibrin deposits may protect some tumor cells from destruction in blood vessels.

In the lymphatic system, tumor cells may be "trapped" in the first lymph node confronted and likely to spread from a tumor. This lymph node is referred to as the *sentinel lymph node*. A sentinel lymph node biopsy (SLNB) can be done to help determine the extent of the cancer. A positive SLNB means cancer is present in the sentinel node and may have spread to other lymph

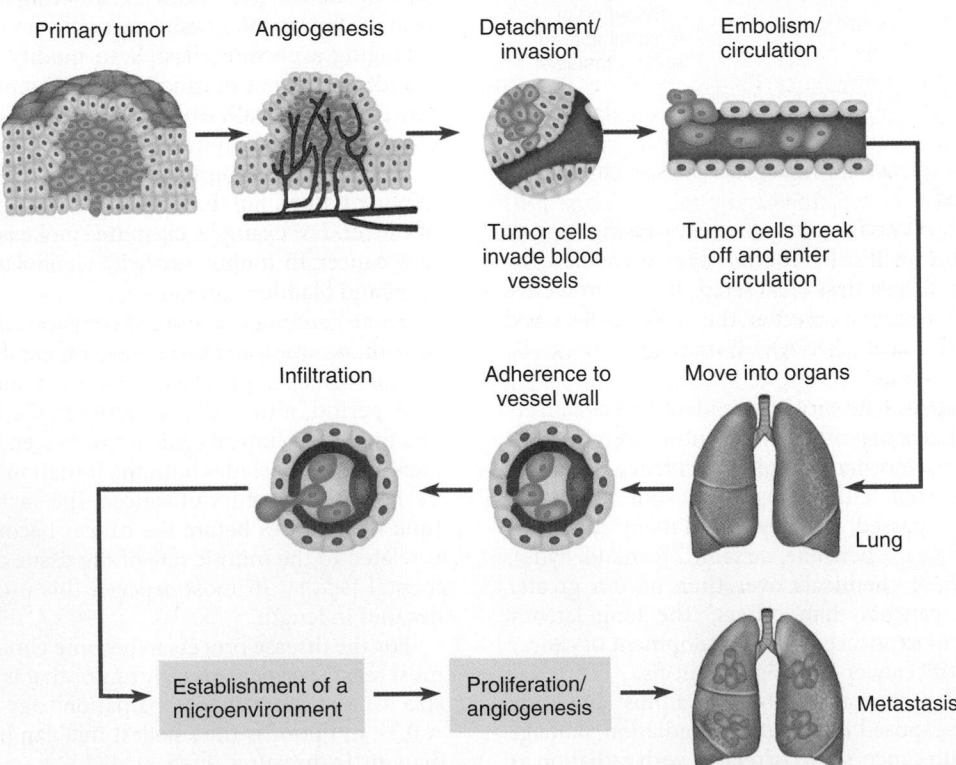

Primary tumor

Angiogenesis

Detachment/
invasion

Embolism/
circulation

Tumor cells
invade blood
vessels

Tumor cells break
off and enter
circulation

Infiltration

Adherence to
vessel wall

Move into organs

Lung

Establishment of a
microenvironment

Proliferation/
angiogenesis

Metastasis

FIG. 15.4 The pathogenesis of cancer metastasis. To produce metastases, tumor cells must detach from the primary tumor and enter the circulation, survive in the circulation to rest in the capillary bed, adhere to capillary basement membrane, gain entrance into the organ parenchyma, respond to growth factors, proliferate, induce angiogenesis, and evade host defenses. (Adapted from Fidler IT: The pathogenesis of cancer metastasis: The "seed and soil" hypothesis revisited, *Nat Rev Cancer* 3:453, 2003.)

nodes and organs. Sometimes, the tumor cells may bypass local lymph nodes and travel to distant lymph nodes, a phenomenon termed *skip metastasis.*

Tumor cells that survive the process of metastasis must create an environment in the distant organ site that promotes their growth and development. Growth and development are facilitated by the tumor cells' ability to evade cells of the immune system and produce a vascular supply within the metastatic site like that of the primary tumor site. Vascularization is critical to the supply of nutrients to the metastatic tumor and the removal of waste products.

Role of the Immune System

This section is limited to a discussion of the role of the immune system in the recognition and destruction of tumor cells. For a detailed discussion of immune system function, see Chapter 13.

The immune system has the potential to tell normal (self) cells from abnormal (nonself) cells. For example, cells of transplanted organs can be recognized by the immune system as *nonself* and thus elicit an immune response. This response can result in organ rejection. Similarly, cancer cells can be perceived as nonself. This can elicit an immune response, resulting in their rejection and destruction. However, unlike transplanted cells, cancer cells arise from normal human cells and, although they are mutated and thus different, the immune response that is mounted against cancer cells may be inadequate to effectively kill them.

Cancer cells may have altered cell-surface antigens because of malignant transformation. These antigens are termed *tumor-associated antigens (TAAs)* (Fig. 15.5). We think that the immune system responds to TAAs through a process termed **immunologic surveillance**. In this process, lymphocytes continuously check cell-surface antigens. They detect and destroy cells with abnormal or altered antigenic determinants. Under most circumstances, immune surveillance prevents transformed cells from developing into clinically detectable tumors.

Immune response to cancer cells involves cytotoxic T cells, natural killer (NK) cells, macrophages, and B cells. *Cytotoxic T cells* play a dominant role in resisting tumor growth. These cells can kill tumor cells. T cells are important in the production of cytokines (e.g., interleukin-2 [IL-2], γ-interferon), which stimulate T cells, NK cells, B cells, and macrophages.

Natural killer (NK) cells can directly lyse tumor cells spontaneously without any prior sensitization. γ-Interferon (made by T cells) and IL-2 (released from T cells) stimulate NK cells, resulting in increased cytotoxic activity.

Monocytes and *macrophages* have several important roles in tumor immunity. γ-Interferon can activate macrophages

to become nonspecifically lytic for tumor cells. Macrophages secrete cytokines, including IL-1, tumor necrosis factor (TNF), and colony-stimulating factors (CSFs). The release of IL-1, coupled with the presentation of the processed antigen, stimulates T-cell activation and production. α-Interferon augments the killing ability of NK cells. TNF causes hemorrhagic necrosis of tumors and exerts cytocidal or cytostatic actions against tumor cells. CSFs regulate the production of various blood cells in the bone marrow and stimulate the function of various WBCs.

B cells can make specific antibodies that bind to tumor cells. These antibodies are often detectable in the patient's serum and saliva.

Escape Mechanisms From Immunologic Surveillance. The process by which cancer cells evade the immune system is termed *immunologic escape.* Possible mechanisms by which cancer cells escape immunologic surveillance include (1) suppression of factors that stimulate T cells to react to cancer cells; (2) weak surface antigens allowing cancer cells to "sneak through" immunologic surveillance; (3) development of tolerance of the immune system to some tumor antigens; (4) suppression of the immune response by products secreted by cancer cells; (5) induction of suppressor T cells by the tumor; and (6) blocking antibodies that bind TAAs, thus preventing their recognition by T cells (Fig. 15.6).

Oncofetal Antigens and Tumor Markers. *Oncofetal antigens* are a type of tumor antigen. They are found on the surfaces and the inside of cancer cells and fetal cells. These antigens are an expression of the shift of cancerous cells to a more immature metabolic pathway. This expression is usually associated with embryonic or fetal periods of life. The reappearance of fetal antigens in cancer is not well understood. We think it is the result of the cell regaining its embryonic capability to differentiate into many different cell types.

Examples of oncofetal antigens are CEA and AFP. CEA is found on the surfaces of cancer cells from the GI tract and normal cells from the fetal gut, liver, and pancreas. Normally, CEA disappears during the last 3 months of fetal life. CEA was originally isolated from colorectal cancer cells. However, high CEA levels can be found in nonmalignant conditions (e.g., cirrhosis of the liver, ulcerative colitis, heavy smoking).

Oncofetal antigens can be used as *tumor markers* that may be clinically useful to monitor the effect of therapy and indicate tumor recurrence. However, they are not 100% specific for tumor recurrence. Tumor markers are affected by various factors that

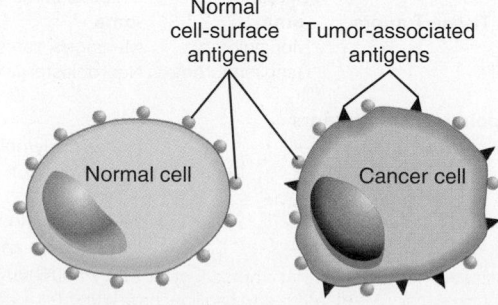

FIG. 15.5 Tumor-associated antigens appear on the cell surface of cancer cells.

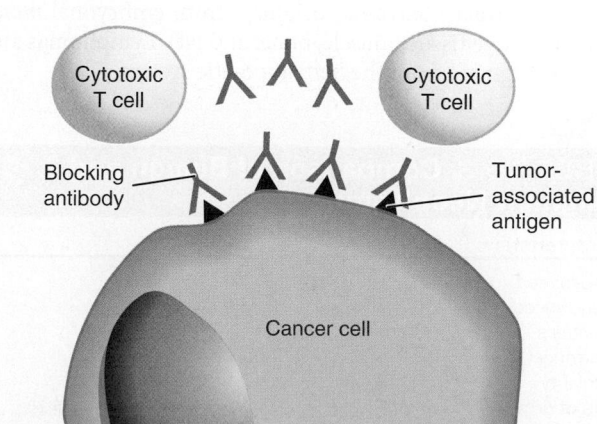

FIG. 15.6 Blocking antibodies prevent T cells from interacting with tumor-associated antigens and from destroying the cancer cell.

must be accounted for when reviewing these results. For example, the persistence of high preoperative CEA titers after surgery means that the tumor is not completely removed. A rise in CEA levels after chemotherapy may mean recurrence or spread of the cancer. Or, it may be due to chronic lung disease and smoking.

AFP is made by malignant liver cells and fetal liver cells. AFP has diagnostic value in primary liver cancer (hepatocellular cancer). It is also made when metastatic liver growth occurs. This makes AFP valuable in tumor detection and determination of tumor progression. AFP levels are also high in some cases of testicular cancer and viral hepatitis.

Other examples of oncofetal antigens are CA-125 (ovarian cancer), CA-19-9 (pancreatic and gallbladder cancer), prostate-specific antigen (PSA) (prostate cancer), and CA-15.3 and CA-27-29 (breast cancer). Molecular markers for specific tumors include kRAS (expression of oncogene in colon cancer), epidermal growth factor receptor (EGFR) often overexpressed in lung cancer, and human epidermal growth factor receptor-2 (HER-2) expression in breast cancer.

BENIGN VERSUS MALIGNANT NEOPLASMS

Tumors can be classified as benign or malignant. In general, *benign neoplasms* are well differentiated. Malignant neoplasms range from well differentiated to undifferentiated. The ability of malignant tumor cells to invade and metastasize is the major difference between benign and malignant neoplasms. Other differences are outlined in Table 15.3.

CLASSIFICATION OF CANCER

Tumors can be classified according to anatomic site, histology (grading), and extent of disease (staging). Tumor classification systems provide a standardized way to (1) communicate the status of the cancer to all members of the interprofessional care team, (2) assist in determining the most effective treatment plan, (3) evaluate the treatment plan, (4) predict prognosis, and (5) compare groups for statistical purposes.

Anatomic Site Classification

In the *anatomic classification* of tumors, the tumor is identified by the tissue of origin, anatomic site, and behavior of the tumor (e.g., benign or malignant) (Table 15.4). *Carcinomas* originate from embryonal *ectoderm* (skin and glands) and *endoderm* (mucous membrane linings of the respiratory tract, GI tract, and genitourinary [GU] tract). *Sarcomas* originate from embryonal *mesoderm* (connective tissue, muscle, bone, and fat). Lymphomas and leukemias originate from the hematopoietic system.

Histologic Classification

In histologic grading of tumors, the appearance of cells and degree of differentiation are evaluated pathologically. For many tumor types, 4 grades are used to evaluate abnormal cells based on the degree to which the cells resemble the tissue of origin. Tumors that are poorly differentiated (undifferentiated) have a poorer prognosis than those that are closer in appearance to the normal tissue of origin (well differentiated):

Grade I: Cells differ slightly from normal cells (mild dysplasia) and are well differentiated (low grade).

Grade II: Cells are more abnormal (moderate dysplasia) and moderately differentiated (intermediate grade).

Grade III: Cells are very abnormal (severe dysplasia) and poorly differentiated (high grade).

Grade IV: Cells are immature, primitive *(anaplasia),* and undifferentiated; cell of origin is hard to determine (high grade).

Grade X: Grade cannot be assessed.

Extent of Disease Classification

Classifying the extent and spread of disease is termed staging. Staging is based on the anatomic extent of disease. Although there are similarities in the staging of various cancers, there are many differences for specific types of cancer.

Clinical Staging. The clinical staging classification system determines the anatomic extent of the malignant disease process by stages:

Stage 0: Cancer in situ

Stage I: Tumor limited to the tissue of origin; localized tumor growth

Stage II: Limited local spread

Stage III: Extensive local and regional spread

Stage IV: Metastasis

Clinical staging has been used as a basis for staging a variety of tumor types, including colorectal cancer (see Fig. 42.7) and Hodgkin's lymphoma (see Fig. 30.15). Other cancers (e.g., leukemia) do not use this staging approach.

TABLE 15.3 Comparison of Benign and Malignant Neoplasms

Characteristic	Benign	Malignant
Encapsulated	Usually	Rarely
Differentiated	Normally	Poorly
Metastasis	Absent	Capable
Recurrence	Rare	Possible
Vascularity	Slight	Moderate to marked
Mode of growth	Expansive	Infiltrative and expansive
Cell characteristics	Fairly normal, like parent cells	Cells abnormal, become more unlike parent cells

---

TABLE 15.4 Anatomic Classification of Tumors

Site	Benign	Malignant
Epithelial Tissue Tumors*	**-oma**	**-carcinoma**
Surface epithelium	Papilloma	Carcinoma
Glandular epithelium	Adenoma	Adenocarcinoma
Connective Tissue Tumors†	**-oma**	**-sarcoma**
Fibrous tissue	Fibroma	Fibrosarcoma
Cartilage	Chondroma	Chondrosarcoma
Striated muscle	Rhabdomyoma	Rhabdomyosarcoma
Bone	Osteoma	Osteosarcoma
Nervous Tissue Tumors	**-oma**	**-oma**
Meninges	Meningioma	Meningeal sarcoma
Nerve cells	Ganglioneuroma	Neuroblastoma
Hematopoietic Tissue Tumors		
Lymphoid tissue	—	Hodgkin's lymphoma, non-Hodgkin's lymphoma
Plasma cells	—	Multiple myeloma
Bone marrow	—	Lymphocytic and myelogenous leukemia

*Body surfaces, lining of body cavities, and glandular structures.
†Supporting tissue, fibrotic tissue, and blood vessels.

TNM Classification System. The *TNM classification system* (Table 15.5) is used to determine the anatomic extent of the disease involvement according to 3 parameters: tumor size and invasiveness (T), presence or absence of regional spread to the lymph nodes (N), and metastasis to distant organ sites (M). Examples of the TNM classification system can be found in Tables 27.17 and 51.6. TNM staging cannot be applied to all cancers. For example, leukemias are not solid tumors and cannot be staged using these guidelines.

The latest cancer staging guidelines for some cancers add nonanatomic factors when making the final determination of stage. Staging is still based on the TNM classification, but it now adds grade and hormone receptor expression. When appropriate, it also includes genomic profile results (e.g., Oncotype DX, Mammaprint). This information should allow a more accurate determination of prognosis and better guide therapy.

Carcinoma in situ (CIS) refers to a cancer whose cells are localized and show no tendency to invade or metastasize to other tissues. CIS has its own designation in the system (T_{is}) because it has all the histologic characteristics of cancer except invasion—a key feature of the TNM staging system.

Staging of the disease can be done initially and at several points. Clinical staging is done at the completion of the diagnostic workup to guide treatment selection. Examples of diagnostic studies that may be done to assess for extent of disease include bone and liver scans, ultrasonography, and CT, MRI, and positron emission tomography (PET) scans.

Surgical staging refers to the extent of the disease as determined by surgical excision, exploration, and/or lymph node sampling. For example, a laparotomy and splenectomy may be done to stage Hodgkin's lymphoma. During a staging laparotomy, lymph node biopsies may be done, and margins of any masses may be marked with metal clips for use during radiation therapy. Exploratory surgical staging is being used less often as noninvasive diagnostic technology becomes more sophisticated.

After the extent of the disease is determined, the stage classification is set. The original description of the extent of the tumor stays part of the record. If more treatment is needed, or if treatment fails, retreatment staging is done to determine the extent of the disease before retreatment. "Restaging" classification (rTNM) is differentiated from the stage at diagnosis, since the clinical significance may be different. Staging can never

decrease, but the stage can increase. For example, a patient may initially be a stage 3. After treatment failure, the tumor metastasizes, and now the patient is a stage 4.

In addition to tumor classification systems, other rating scales can be used to describe and document the status of patients with cancer at the time of diagnosis, treatment, and retreatment and at each follow-up examination. For example, the Karnofsky Performance Scale and Katz Index of Independence in Activities of Daily Living describe patient's functional performance.

PREVENTION AND EARLY DETECTION OF CANCER

We can reduce the incidence of cancer through a stronger emphasis on prevention through promoting healthy lifestyles. As a nurse, you have an essential role in the prevention and early detection of cancer. Reducing risk factors reduces the incidence of cancer. For example, rates of smoking-related cancers (e.g., lung and head and neck cancers) have declined with a reduction in smoking rates.[1]

Early detection and prompt treatment are responsible for increased survival rates in patients with cancer. Colonoscopy is important in reducing colon cancer mortality both by early detection of colon cancers and prevention (e.g., excision of adenomatous polyps).

The goals of public education are to (1) motivate people to recognize and change behaviors that may negatively affect health and (2) encourage awareness of and participation in health-promoting behaviors. When you teach about cancer, try to minimize the fear that surrounds the diagnosis.

Teach people to be familiar with their bodies. Review how to perform self-examinations and the 7 warning signs of cancer (Table 15.6). Encourage them to seek immediate medical care if they notice a change in what is normal for them or if cancer is suspected. Following recommended cancer screening guidelines for breast, colon, cervical, and prostate cancer from the American Cancer Society (ACS) is important.[6]

TABLE 15.5 TNM Classification System

Primary Tumor (T)

T_0	No evidence of primary tumor
T_{is}	Carcinoma in situ
T_{1-4}	Ascending degrees of increase in tumor size and involvement
T_x	Tumor cannot be measured or found

Regional Lymph Nodes (N)

N_0	No evidence of disease in lymph nodes
N_{1-4}	Ascending degrees of nodal involvement
N_x	Regional lymph nodes unable to be assessed clinically

Distant Metastases (M)

M_0	No evidence of distant metastases
M_{1-4}	Ascending degrees of metastatic involvement, including distant nodes
M_x	Cannot be determined

♥ PROMOTING POPULATION HEALTH
Prevention and Early Detection of Cancer

Teach patients and the public about cancer prevention and early detection, including:

- Limit alcohol use.
- Get regular physical activity (e.g., 30 minutes or more of moderate physical activity 5 times weekly).
- Maintain a normal body weight.
- Have regular physical examinations.
- Obtain regular colorectal screenings.
- Avoid cigarette smoking and other tobacco use.
- Get regular mammography screening and Pap tests.
- Be familiar with your own family history and risk factors for cancer.
- Obtain adequate, consistent periods of rest (at least 6 to 8 hours per night).
- Use sunscreen with a sun protection factor of 15 or higher. Avoid the use of tanning beds.
- Eliminate, reduce, or change the perception of stressors and enhance the ability to effectively cope with stress (see Chapter 6).
- Eat a balanced diet that includes vegetables and fresh fruits, whole grains, and adequate amounts of fiber. Reduce dietary fat and preservatives, including smoked and salt-cured meats with high nitrite concentrations.

Diagnosis of Cancer

When a patient has a possible diagnosis of cancer, it is a stressful time for the patient and caregivers. Patients may undergo several days to weeks of diagnostic studies. During this time, fear of the unknown may be more stressful than the actual diagnosis of cancer. Patients may be overwhelmed or confused by the need for multiple diagnostic studies and consultations. Help coordinate care between multiple specialists. Explain the purpose of required tests and any special preparation needed for them.

Some facilities have comprehensive oncology teams and services that are all housed in the same building to help coordinate care among the cancer specialists. These centers combine appointments to make the experience convenient and comfortable for patients and their caregivers.

While patients are waiting for the results of diagnostic studies, be available to actively listen to their concerns. Their anxiety may arise from myths and misconceptions about cancer (e.g., cancer is a "death sentence," cancer treatment is worse than the illness). Correcting those misconceptions can help to minimize their anxiety.

Learn to recognize your own discomfort during difficult conversations. Avoid communication patterns that may hinder exploration of feelings and meaning. These include providing false reassurances (e.g., "It's probably nothing"), redirecting the discussion (e.g., "Let's discuss that later"), generalizing (e.g., "Everyone feels this way"), and using overly technical language. These self-protective strategies deny patients the opportunity to share the meaning of their experience. They can jeopardize your ability to build a trusting relationship with your patients.

During this time of high anxiety, the patient may need repeated explanations of the diagnostic workup. Include as much information as needed by the patient and caregivers. Give clear, understandable explanations and reinforce them as needed. Written information is helpful to reinforce verbal information.

A diagnostic plan for the person suspected of having cancer includes the health history (including a history of present illness), identifying risk factors, the physical examination, and specific diagnostic studies. For many people, cancer is diagnosed after the findings of an abnormal screening test (e.g., mass on mammogram). For others, they are alerted to the presence of cancer by a presenting symptom or cluster of symptoms (e.g., cough and hemoptysis, anorexia and weight loss).

Concentrate on risk factors for cancer. Obtain information about any family and personal history of cancer and any exposure to or use of known carcinogens (e.g., cigarette smoking, occupational pollutants or chemicals, radiation exposure). Review the medical history for diseases characterized by chronic inflammation or immunosuppression (e.g., ulcerative colitis) and treatments (e.g., hormone therapy, previous anticancer therapies). Assess factors that may call for additional supportive care during therapy, including alcohol or drug use, living situation, social support, and coping strategies for perceived stressors.

Diagnostic studies depend on the suspected primary or metastatic site(s) of the cancer. (Specific procedures as they relate to each body system are discussed in the respective assessment chapters.) Examples of diagnostic studies include:

- Cytology studies (e.g., Pap test, bronchial washings)
- Tissue biopsy
- Chest x-ray
- Complete blood count (CBC), chemistry profile
- Liver function studies (e.g., aspartate aminotransferase [AST])
- Endoscopic examination: upper GI, sigmoidoscopy, or colonoscopy (including guaiac test for occult blood)
- Radiographic studies (e.g., mammography, ultrasound, CT scan, MRI)
- Radioisotope scans (e.g., bone, lung, liver, brain)
- PET scan (Fig. 15.7)
- Tumor markers (e.g., CEA, AFP, PSA, CA-125)
- Genetic markers (e.g., *BRCA1, BRCA2*)
- Molecular receptor status (e.g., estrogen and progesterone receptors)
- Bone marrow examination (if a hematolymphoid malignancy is suspected or to document metastatic disease)

Biopsy. A *biopsy* is the removal of a tissue sample for pathologic analysis. Various methods are used to obtain a biopsy depending on the location and size of the suspected tumor. *Percutaneous biopsy* is often done for tissue that can be safely reached through the skin. *Endoscopic biopsy* may be used for lung or other intraluminal lesions (esophageal, colon, bladder).

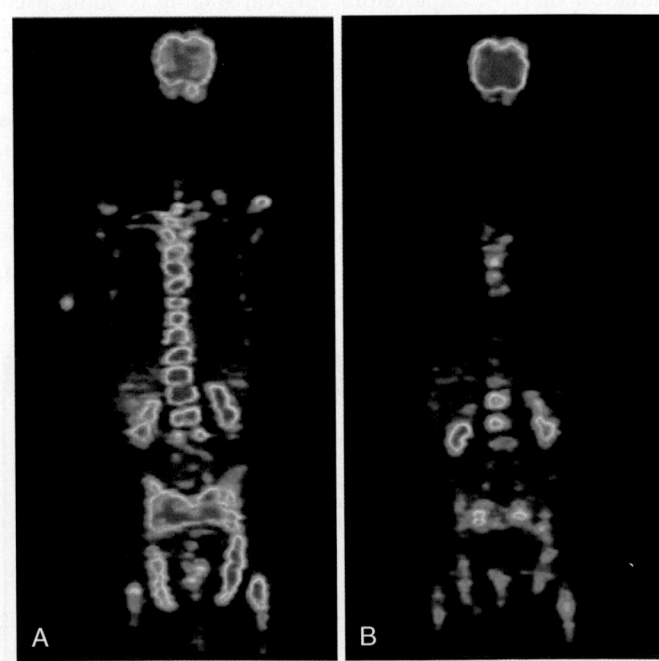

FIG. 15.7 PET scan before treatment (A) showing metastasis throughout the body. PET scan after treatment (B) shows the effects of therapy. More radioactive material accumulates in areas that have higher levels of activity. This often corresponds to areas of disease and shows up as brighter spots on the PET scan. (From Shimizu N, Masuda H, Yamanaka H, et al: Fluorodeoxyglucose PET scan of prostate cancer bone metastases with flare reaction after endocrine therapy, *J Urol* 151:609, 1999.)

TABLE 15.6 **7 Warning Signs of Cancer**
Change in bowel or bladder habits
A sore that does not heal
Unusual bleeding or discharge from any body orifice
Thickening or a lump in the breast or elsewhere
Indigestion or difficulty in swallowing
Obvious change in a wart or mole
Nagging cough or hoarseness

When a tumor is not easily accessible, a *surgical procedure* (laparotomy, thoracotomy, craniotomy) is often needed to obtain a piece of the tumor tissue. Many radiographic techniques may be used in conjunction with the biopsy procedure (e.g., CT, MRI, ultrasound-guided biopsy, stereotactic biopsy) to improve tissue localization.

Various types and sizes of biopsy needles are available and chosen according to the type of tissue to be sampled. *Fine-needle aspiration* (FNA) may be done with a small-gauge aspiration needle that provides cells from the mass for cytologic examination. *Large-core biopsy* cutting needles deliver an actual piece of tissue (core) that can be analyzed. An advantage is that it preserves the histologic architecture of the tissue specimen. *Excisional biopsy* involves the surgical removal of the entire lesion, lymph node, nodule, or mass. So, it is therapeutic as well as diagnostic. If an excisional biopsy is not feasible, an *incisional biopsy* (partial excision) may be done with a scalpel or dermal punch.

Pathologic evaluation of a tissue sample is the only definitive way to diagnose cancer. The pathologist examines the tissue to determine (1) whether it is benign or malignant, (2) the anatomic tissue from which the tumor arises *(histology)*, and (3) the degree of cell differentiation *(histologic grade)*. Other information that can be obtained includes the extent of malignant involvement (size of tumor and depth), evidence of invasiveness (extracapsular, lymphatic), adequacy of surgical excision (positive or negative surgical margin status), and nuclear grade (mitotic rate). Special staining techniques may give insight into responsiveness of the tumor to treatment or disease behavior (receptor status, tumor markers).

INTERPROFESSIONAL CARE

TREATMENT GOALS

The goals of cancer treatment are cure, control, and palliation (Fig. 15.8). When caring for the patient with cancer, knowing the treatment goals will help you appropriately communicate with, teach, and support the patient. The main factors that determine what therapy is used are the tumor histology and staging outcomes. Other crucial factors are the patient's physiologic status (e.g., presence of co-morbid illnesses), psychologic status, and personal desires (e.g., active treatment versus palliation).

These factors influence (1) the modalities chosen for treatment (e.g., surgery, radiation therapy, chemotherapy, immunotherapy, targeted therapy, hormone therapy), (2) how therapies are sequenced, and (3) the length of time the treatment is prescribed. Each type of therapy can be used alone or in any combination during initial treatment, as maintenance therapy, and in retreatment if the disease does not respond or recurs after remission.

For many cancers, 2 or more of the treatment modalities (known as *multimodality therapy* or *combined modality therapy*) are used to achieve the goal of cure or control for a long time. Multimodality therapy has the benefit of being more effective (because it takes advantage of more than one mechanism of action), but often at the expense of greater toxicity.

Cure

When *cure* is the goal, treatment is expected to have the greatest chance of eradicating the cancer. Curative cancer therapy

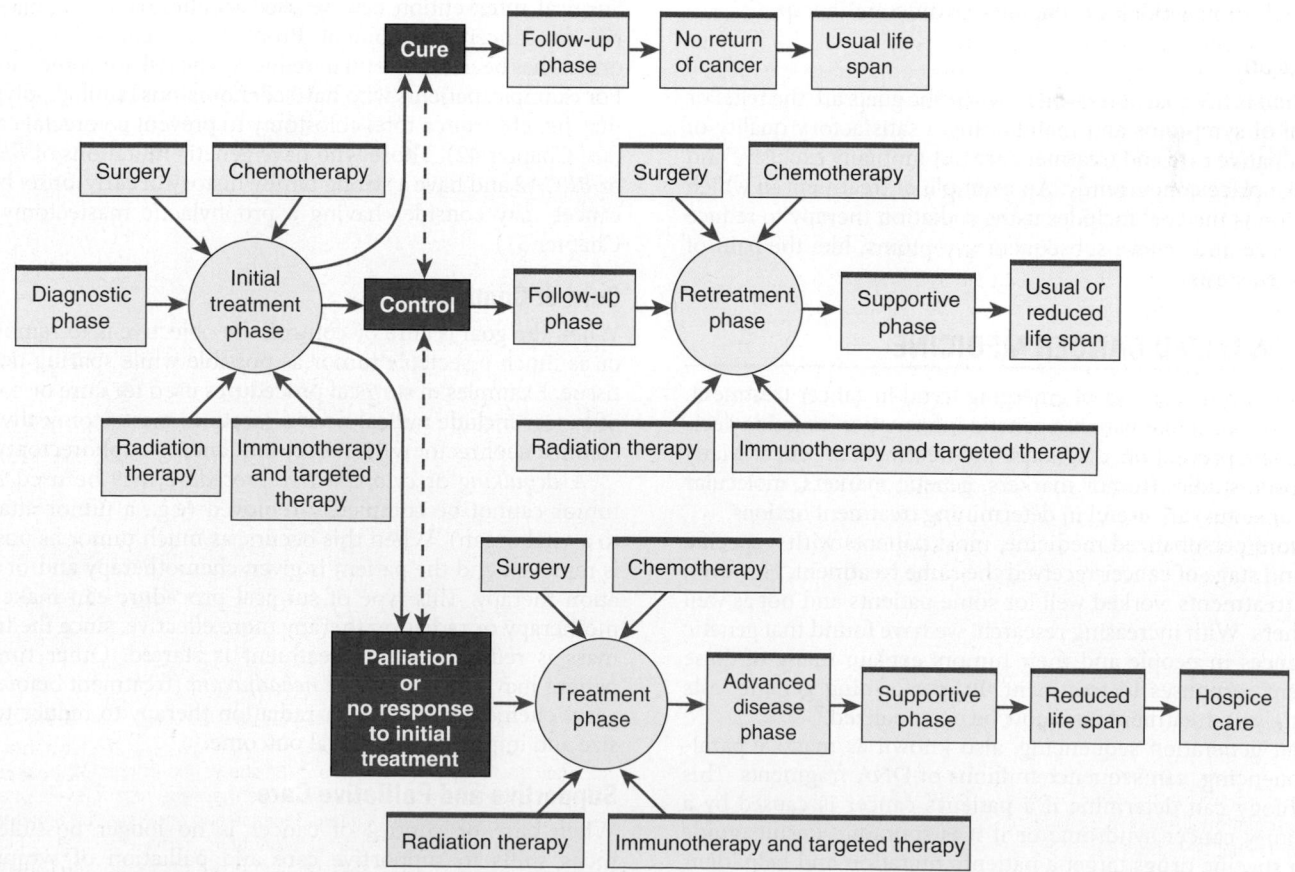

FIG. 15.8 Goals of cancer treatment.

differs according to the cancer being treated. It may involve local therapies (e.g., surgery or radiation) alone or in combination, with or without periods of adjunctive systemic therapy (e.g., chemotherapy).

For example, basal cell skin cancer is usually cured by surgical removal of the lesion and several weeks of radiation therapy. In the treatment plan for acute promyelocytic leukemia (which has curative potential), several chemotherapy drugs are given on a scheduled basis over many months to several years. Testicular cancer can be cured with a combination of surgery, chemotherapy, and radiation.

There is no benchmark that ensures "cure" for most cancers. In general, the risk for recurrent disease is highest after treatment completion. It gradually decreases the longer the patient is disease free after treatment. Cancers with a higher mitotic rate (e.g., testicular cancer) are more likely to recur than cancers with slower mitotic rates (e.g., postmenopausal breast cancer). So, the timeframe to consider a person "cured" may differ according to the tumor and its characteristics.

Control

Control is the goal of treatment for cancers that cannot be completely eradicated but are responsive to anticancer therapies. As with other chronic illnesses (e.g., diabetes, heart failure), cancer can be controlled for long periods with therapy. Examples include multiple myeloma and chronic lymphocytic leukemia (see Chapter 30). Patients may undergo an initial course of treatment followed by maintenance therapy for as long as the disease is responding. Patients are monitored closely for early signs and symptoms of disease recurrence or progression and the cumulative effects of therapy. Evidence of tumor resistance (e.g., disease progression) may call for changing to a different therapy.

Palliation

Palliation is the goal of treatment when the goals are the relief or control of symptoms and maintaining a satisfactory quality of life. Palliative care and treatment are not mutually exclusive and can take place concurrently. An example of treatment in which palliation is the goal includes using radiation therapy to reduce tumor size and relieve subsequent symptoms, like the pain of bone metastasis.

PERSONALIZED CANCER MEDICINE

Personalized medicine is an emerging trend in cancer treatment. It involves using the patient's genetic information to guide decisions about prevention, diagnosis, and treatment of cancer. Many diagnostic studies (tumor markers, genetic markers, molecular receptor status) are useful in determining treatment options.

Before personalized medicine, most patients with a specific type and stage of cancer received the same treatment. However, some treatments worked well for some patients and not as well for others. With increasing research, we have found that genetic differences in people and their tumors explain many of these different responses to treatment. By performing genetic tests and analysis, treatments can now be personalized.[7]

Next-generation sequencing, also known as massive parallel sequencing, can sequence millions of DNA fragments. This technology can determine if a patient's cancer is caused by a hereditary cancer syndrome or if it is sporadic. Results guide which specific drugs target a patient's mutation and help identify clinical trials specific to the genetic mutation.[8]

Targeted therapy (Table 15.13) targets a cancer's specific genes or proteins that contribute to cancer growth and survival. Treatment with a targeted therapy depends on assessing whether the tumor has the specific target. This is usually done by testing a sample of the tumor obtained through a biopsy.

Pharmacogenomics and *pharmacogenetics* is the study of genomic variation associated with drug responses.[9] Examples of how the results of genetic testing can be applied to the use of cancer drugs are shown in Table 12.5. For example, vemurafenib (Zelboraf) is used to treat patients with metastatic melanoma. However, it is indicated only for the treatment of patients with melanoma whose tumors express a gene mutation called *BRAF V600E*.

Despite the promises of personalized cancer treatments, not all types of cancer have personalized treatment options. Genetic testing may be costly and time consuming. Many insurance plans do not cover the costs of these tests. Some personalized treatments, such as targeted treatments, can be expensive.[7]

SURGICAL THERAPY

Surgery is the oldest form of cancer treatment. The treatment of choice for many years was to remove the cancer and as much of the surrounding normal tissue as possible. What this approach did not fully consider was the ability of cancer cells to travel from the original tumor site to other locations, making surgical cure possible only when the tumor was localized and relatively small. Today surgery is used to meet a variety of goals (Fig. 15.9). The trend is toward less radical surgeries.

Prevention

Surgical intervention can be used to eliminate or reduce the risk for cancer development. Prophylactic removal of nonvital organs has been successful in reducing the risk for some cancers. For example, patients who have adenomatous familial polyposis may benefit from a total colostomy to prevent colorectal cancer (see Chapter 42). Those who have genetic mutations of *BRCA1* or *BRCA2* and have a strong family history of early-onset breast cancer may consider having a prophylactic mastectomy (see Chapter 51).

Cure or Control

When the goal is cure or control, the objective is to remove all or as much resectable tumor as possible while sparing normal tissue. Examples of surgical procedures used for cure or control of cancer include radical neck dissection, mastectomy, thyroidectomy, nephrectomy, hysterectomy, and/or oophorectomy.

A *debulking* or *cytoreductive procedure* may be used if the tumor cannot be completely removed (e.g., a tumor attached to a vital organ). When this occurs, as much tumor as possible is removed and the patient is given chemotherapy and/or radiation therapy. This type of surgical procedure can make chemotherapy or radiation therapy more effective, since the tumor mass is reduced before treatment is started. Other times, a patient may need to receive *neoadjuvant* (treatment before surgery) chemotherapy and/or radiation therapy to reduce tumor size and improve the surgical outcome.

Supportive and Palliative Care

When cure or control of cancer is no longer possible, the focus shifts to supportive care and palliation of symptoms. Surgical procedures may be used to provide supportive care

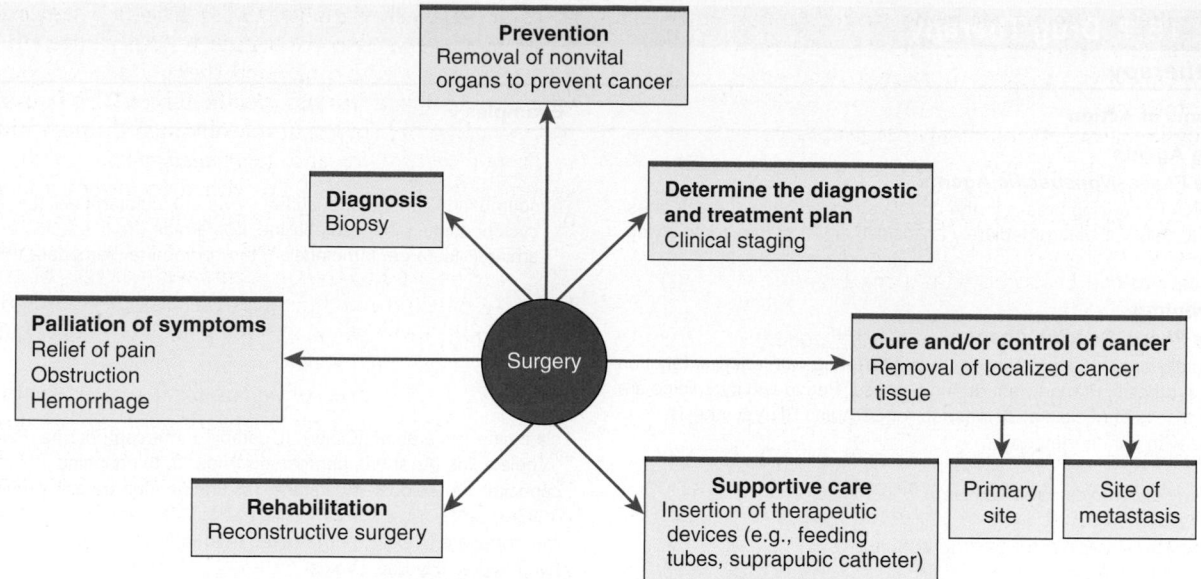

FIG. 15.9 Role of surgery in the treatment of cancer.

that maximizes bodily function or facilitates cancer treatment. Examples of supportive surgical procedures include:

- Insertion of a feeding tube to maintain nutrition during head and neck cancer treatment
- Placement of a central venous access device to deliver chemotherapy agents
- Prophylactic surgical fixation of bones at risk for pathologic fracture

Effects of treatment or symptoms from metastatic cancer may require surgical intervention for palliation. Examples include (1) tumor debulking to relieve pain or pressure, (2) colostomy for the relief of a bowel obstruction (see Chapter 42), and (3) laminectomy for the relief of a spinal cord compression (see Chapter 60).

CHEMOTHERAPY

Chemotherapy (antineoplastic therapy) is the use of chemicals as a systemic therapy for cancer. In the 1970s, chemotherapy was proven an effective treatment for cancer. Chemotherapy is now a mainstay of cancer treatment for most solid tumors and hematologic cancers (e.g., leukemias, lymphomas). Chemotherapy can offer cure for some cancers, control other cancers for long periods, and in some cases, offer palliative relief of symptoms when cure or control is no longer possible (Fig. 15.10).

Effect on Cells

The goal of chemotherapy is to eliminate or reduce the number of cancer cells in the primary and metastatic tumor site(s). All cells (cancer cells and normal cells) enter the cell cycle for replication and proliferation (Fig. 15.1). The effects of the chemotherapy drugs are described in relation to the cell cycle.

The 2 major categories of chemotherapy drugs are cell cycle phase–nonspecific and cell cycle phase–specific drugs. *Cell cycle phase–nonspecific chemotherapy drugs* have their effect on the cells during all phases of the cell cycle. This includes the process of cell replication and proliferation and the resting phase (G_0). *Cell cycle phase–specific chemotherapy drugs* have their greatest effects during specific phases of the cell cycle (e.g., when cells

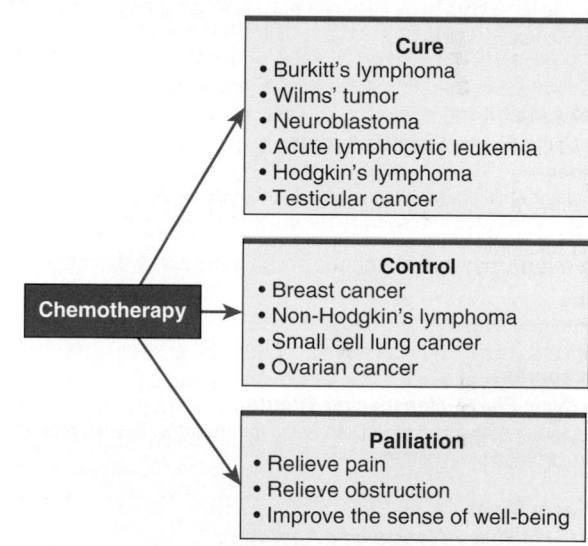

FIG. 15.10 Goals of chemotherapy.

are in the process of replication or proliferation during G_1, S, G_2, or M). Cell cycle phase–specific and cell cycle phase–nonspecific agents are often given together to maximize effectiveness by using agents that function in different ways and throughout the cell cycle.

When cancer first begins to develop, most of the cells are actively dividing. As the tumor increases in size, more cells become inactive and convert to a resting state (G_0). Because most chemotherapy agents are effective against dividing cells, cells can escape death by staying in the G_0 phase. A major challenge is to overcome the effect of resistant resting and noncycling cells.

Classification of Chemotherapy Drugs

Chemotherapy drugs are classified in general groups according to their molecular structure and mechanisms of action (Table 15.7). Each drug in a particular class has many similarities. However, there are major differences in how the drugs work and the unique side effects associated with drugs in each class.

TABLE 15.7 Drug Therapy

Chemotherapy

Mechanisms of Action	Examples
Alkylating Agents	
Cell Cycle Phase–Nonspecific Agents	
Damage DNA by causing breaks in the double-stranded helix. If repair does not occur, cells will die immediately (cytocidal) or when they try to divide (cytostatic).	bendamustine (Treanda), busulfan (Myleran), chlorambucil (Leukeran), cyclophosphamide, dacarbazine, ifosfamide (Ifex), mechloreth-amine (Mustargen), melphalan, temozolomide (Temodar), thiotepa
Antimetabolites	
Cell Cycle Phase–Specific Agents	
Mimic naturally occurring substances, thus interfering with enzyme function or DNA synthesis. Primarily act during S phase. Purine and pyrimidine are building blocks of nucleic acids needed for DNA and RNA synthesis.	
• Interfere with purine metabolism	cladribine, clofarabine (Clolar), fludarabine, mercaptopurine (Purixan), nelarabine (Arranon), pentostatin (Nipent), thioguanine
• Interfere with pyrimidine metabolism	capecitabine (Xeloda); cytarabine, floxuridine, fluorouracil, gemcitabine (Gemzar)
• Interfere with folic acid metabolism	methotrexate (Trexall), pemetrexed (Alimta)
• Interfere with DNA synthesis	hydroxyurea (Hydrea, Droxia)
Antitumor Antibiotics	
Cell Cycle Phase–Nonspecific Agents	
Bind directly to DNA, thus inhibiting the synthesis of DNA and interfering with transcription of RNA.	bleomycin, dactinomycin (Cosmegen), daunorubicin, doxorubicin (Doxil), epirubicin (Ellence), idarubicin, mitomycin, mitoxantrone, valrubicin (Valstar)
Mitotic Inhibitors	
Cell Cycle Phase–Specific Agents	
Taxanes	albumin-bound paclitaxel (Abraxane), docetaxel (Taxotere), paclitaxel (Taxol)
Antimicrotubule agents that interfere with mitosis. Act during the late G_2 phase and mitosis to stabilize microtubules, thus inhibiting cell division.	
Vinca Alkaloids	vinblastine, vincristine, vinorelbine (Navelbine)
Act in M phase to inhibit mitosis.	
Others	estramustine (Emcyt), ixabepilone (Ixempra), eribulin (Halaven)
Microtubular inhibitors.	
Nitrosoureas	
Cell Cycle Phase–Nonspecific Agents	
Like alkylating agents, break DNA helix, interfering with DNA replication. Cross blood-brain barrier.	carmustine (BiCNU, Gliadel), lomustine (Gleostine), streptozocin (Zanosar)
Platinum Drugs	
Cell Cycle Phase–Nonspecific Agents	
Bind to DNA and RNA, miscoding information and/or inhibiting DNA replica-tion, and cells die.	carboplatin, cisplatin, oxaliplatin
Topoisomerase Inhibitors	
Cell Cycle Phase–Specific Agents	
Inhibit topoisomerases (normal enzymes) that function to make reversible breaks and repairs in DNA that allow for flexibility of DNA in replication.	etoposide, irinotecan (Camptosar), topotecan (Hycamtin)

Preparation of Chemotherapy

Only persons specifically trained in chemotherapy handling techniques should be involved with the preparation and admin-istration of cancer drugs.[10] They may pose an occupational hazard to health care professionals who do not follow safe handling guidelines. A person preparing, transporting, or giv-ing chemotherapy may absorb the drug through inhalation of particles when reconstituting a powder or through skin contact from exposure to droplets or powder. There may be some risk in handling the body fluids and excretions of people during the first 48 hours after they receive chemotherapy. Guidelines for the safe handling of chemotherapy agents have been developed by the National Institute for Occupational Safety and Health (OSHA) and the Oncology Nursing Society (ONS).[11]

Methods of Administration

Chemotherapy can be given by multiple routes (Table 15.8). With advances in drug formulation techniques, more oral che-motherapy agents are available. With oral agents, the patient will need to be taught about storage and side effects.

The IV route is the most common method of giving che-motherapy. Major concerns associated with IV chemotherapy administration include venous access problems, device- or cath-eter-related infection, and *extravasation*.[10] It is the infiltration of

TABLE 15.8 Drug Therapy Methods of Chemotherapy Administration

Method	Examples
Oral	cyclophosphamide, capecitabine (Xeloda), temozolomide (Temodar)
Intramuscular	bleomycin
Intravenous	doxorubicin, vincristine, cisplatin, fluorouracil, paclitaxel (Taxol)
Intraarterial	dacarbazine, fluorouracil, methotrexate
Intracavitary (pleural, peritoneal)	Radioisotopes, alkylating agents, methotrexate
Intrathecal	methotrexate (preservative free), cytarabine
Perfusion	Alkylating agents
Subcutaneous	cytarabine, bortezomib
Topical	fluorouracil

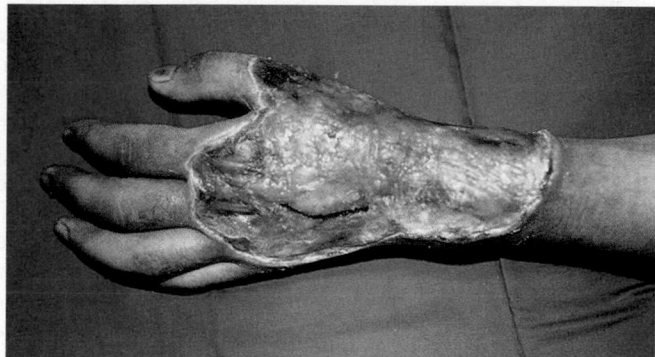

FIG. 15.11 Extravasation injury from infiltration of chemotherapy drug. (From Weinzweig N, Weinzweig J: *The mutilated hand*, Philadelphia, 2005, Mosby.)

drugs into tissues surrounding the infusion site, causing local tissue damage (Fig. 15.11).

Many chemotherapy drugs are either irritants or vesicants. *Irritants* will damage the intima of the vein, causing phlebitis and sclerosis and limiting future peripheral venous access. They will not cause tissue damage if infiltrated. However, vesicants, if inadvertently infiltrated into the skin, may cause severe local tissue breakdown and necrosis. It is extremely important to monitor for and promptly take action if extravasation of a vesicant occurs. To minimize discomfort, emotional distress, and risks of infection and infiltration, IV chemotherapy can be given through a *central venous access device* (CVAD). CVADs are placed in large blood vessels and allow frequent, continuous, or intermittent administration of chemotherapy, immunotherapy, and targeted therapy, and other products, thus avoiding multiple venipunctures for vascular access. (CVADs are discussed in Chapter 16.)

Regional Chemotherapy Administration

Regional treatment with chemotherapy involves delivery of the drug directly to the tumor site. The advantage of this method is that higher concentrations of the drug can be delivered to the tumor with less systemic toxicity. Several regional delivery methods have been developed. These include intraarterial, intraperitoneal, intrathecal, intraventricular, and intravesical bladder chemotherapy.

Intraarterial Chemotherapy. Intraarterial chemotherapy delivers the drug to the tumor through the arteries supplying the

tumor. This method has been used for the treatment of osteogenic sarcoma; cancers of the head and neck, bladder, and cervix; melanoma; primary liver cancer; and metastatic liver disease. One method of intraarterial drug delivery involves the surgical placement of a catheter that is connected to an external or implanted infusion pump for infusion of the chemotherapy agent.

Intraperitoneal Chemotherapy. Intraperitoneal chemotherapy involves the delivery of chemotherapy to the peritoneal cavity. It is a treatment for peritoneal metastases from primary colorectal and ovarian cancers and malignant ascites. Temporary Silastic catheters (Tenckhoff, Hickman, Groshong) are percutaneously or surgically placed into the peritoneal cavity for short-term administration of chemotherapy. An implanted port also can be used to give chemotherapy intraperitoneally. Chemotherapy is generally infused into the peritoneum in 1 to 2 L of fluid and allowed to *dwell* in the peritoneum for 1 to 4 hours. After the *dwell time*, the fluid is drained from the peritoneum.

Intrathecal or Intraventricular Chemotherapy. Cancers that metastasize to the central nervous system (CNS) are hard to treat because the blood-brain barrier often prevents distribution of chemotherapy to this area. One method used to treat metastasis to the CNS is intrathecal chemotherapy. This method involves a lumbar puncture and injection of chemotherapy into the subarachnoid space. To reduce the need for repeated lumbar punctures, patients may have an Ommaya reservoir inserted. An Ommaya reservoir is a Silastic, dome-shaped disk with an extension catheter that is surgically implanted through the cranium into a lateral ventricle.

Intravesical Bladder Chemotherapy. *Intravesical bladder chemotherapy* involves instilling chemotherapy into the bladder. This is done through a urinary catheter. The solution is retained for 1 to 3 hours.

Effects of Chemotherapy on Normal Tissues

Chemotherapy agents cannot selectively distinguish between normal cells and cancer cells. Chemotherapy-induced side effects are the result of the destruction of normal cells, especially those that are rapidly proliferating. These include those in the bone marrow, lining of the GI system, and integument (skin, hair, nails) (Table 15.9). The general and drug-specific adverse effects of these drugs are classified as acute, delayed, or chronic.

Acute toxicity occurs during and right after drug administration. It includes anaphylactic and hypersensitivity reactions, extravasation or a flare reaction, anticipatory nausea and vomiting, and dysrhythmias.

Delayed effects are numerous. They include delayed nausea and vomiting, mucositis, alopecia, skin rashes, bone marrow suppression, altered bowel function (diarrhea, constipation), and a variety of cumulative neurotoxicities.

Chronic toxicities involve damage to organs, such as the heart, liver, kidneys, and lungs. Chronic toxicities can be either long-term effects that develop during or right after treatment and persist or late effects that are absent during treatment and manifest later.

Some side effects fall into more than 1 category. For example, nausea and vomiting can be both acute and delayed.

Treatment Plan

Although single-drug chemotherapy is sometimes prescribed, the most common modality is combining agents in multidrug regimens. Multidrug treatment targets more than one signaling

TABLE 15.9 Cells With Rapid Rate of Proliferation

Cells	Generation Time	Effect of Cell Destruction
Bone marrow stem cell	6–24 hr	Myelosuppression (infection, bleeding, anemia)
Epithelial cells lining the GI tract	12–24 hr	Anorexia, mucositis (including stomatitis, esophagitis), nausea, vomiting, diarrhea
Hair follicle cells	24 hr	Alopecia
Neutrophils	12 hr	Leukopenia, infection
Ova or testes	24–36 hr	Reproductive problems

pathway and is more effective in managing most cancers. The regimens involve drugs with different mechanisms of action and varying toxicity profiles. However, when chemotherapy agents are used in combination, patients can have an increase in toxicities.

Drug regimens are chosen based on evidence supporting their use in specific cancers. Sometimes they are customized to meet the needs of an individual patient. Chemotherapy is most effective when the tumor burden is low, therapy is not interrupted, and the patient receives the intended dose. The dose of each drug is based on the person's body weight and height using the body surface area calculation.

Mutation of cancer cells within the tumor can result in cells that are resistant to chemotherapy. With multiple drugs working at different places in the cell cycle, cancer cells can be more effectively killed. Thus mutation and resistance of cancer cells can be decreased.

INFORMATICS IN PRACTICE
Managing Cancer Patients' Symptoms

- Patients arriving at some clinics are handed a tablet computer. While in the waiting room or chemotherapy infusion unit, with the touch of a finger they select the symptoms that they are having.
- Health care team members can review the information and provide care aimed at managing the patient's specific symptoms.
- After the visit, the notes are stored in the patient's electronic health record. This system can help determine if standards of care were followed.

RADIATION THERAPY

Along with surgery, radiation therapy is one of the oldest methods of cancer treatment. It was first used to treat a woman with breast cancer in 1896. Although the patient responded locally, she died later of metastatic disease. It was not until the 1960s that advances in equipment and treatment planning facilitated the delivery of adequate radiation doses to tumors and tolerable doses to normal tissues. Today many cancer patients receive radiation therapy at some point in their treatment.

Effects of Radiation

Radiation is energy that is emitted from a source and travels through space or some material. Delivery of high-energy beams, when absorbed into tissue, produces ionization of atomic particles. The energy in ionizing radiation acts to break the chemical bonds in DNA. The DNA is damaged, causing cell death.

Different types of ionizing radiation are used to treat cancer, including *electromagnetic radiation* (e.g., x-rays, gamma rays) and *particulate radiation* (e.g., alpha particles, electrons, neutrons, protons). High-energy x-rays (photons) are generated by an electric machine, such as a linear accelerator.

Technologic advances have expanded and refined the sources and methods of delivering radiation therapy. This allows for more accurate and less invasive treatment options. Most radiation centers in the United States use megavoltage linear accelerator technology. Larger facilities may offer a combination of machines that give patients more options at that site.

Principles of Radiobiology

As the radiation beam passes through the treatment field, energy is deposited. *Low-energy beams* (e.g., electrons) expend energy quickly on impact with matter, so they penetrate only a short distance. They are clinically useful in treating superficial skin lesions. *High-energy beams* (e.g., photons) have greater depth of penetration, not reaching full intensity until they reach a certain depth. This makes them suitable for delivering optimal doses to internal targets while sparing the skin.

Technically, all cancer cells could be killed with radiation given in high enough doses. However, to avoid serious toxicity and long-term complications of treatment, radiation to surrounding healthy tissue must be limited to the *maximal tolerated dose* for that specific tissue. Advances in planning and in delivery technology (e.g., *intensity-modulated radiation therapy [IMRT]* and *image-guided radiation therapy [IGRT]*) have greatly improved the ability to deliver maximal doses while sparing critical structures (e.g., spinal cord, carotid arteries, optic chiasm) as much as possible.

Historically, the radiation dose was expressed in units called *rads* (radiation absorbed doses). Now we use *gray* (Gy) or *centigray* (cGy). A *centigray* is equal to 1 rad; 100 centigray equals 1 gray. Once the total dose to be delivered is determined, that dose is divided into daily *fractions*. Doses between 180 and 200 cGy/day are considered *standard fractionation*. They are typically delivered once a day Monday through Friday for a period of 2 to 8 weeks, depending on the desired total dose.

Certain cancers are more responsive to the effects of radiation than others (Table 15.10). Radiosensitivity is the relative responsiveness of cells and tissues to the effects of radiation. In highly responsive tumors (such as lymphomas), even a large tumor is affected by radiation therapy. In less responsive tumors, there may be a slower or incomplete response. Localized prostate cancer responds very slowly to radiation (several months after treatment is completed).

Simulation and Treatment Planning

Simulation is a process by which the radiation treatment fields are defined, filmed, and marked out on the skin. The radiation oncologist specifies the dose and volume of area to be treated. Treatment volumes include the (1) *gross target volume* (GTV), which is the gross extent of the tumor identified by examination or imaging; (2) the *clinical target* volume (CTV), which is the GTV plus additional margin to encompass any potential microscopic or subclinical disease; and (3) the *planning target* volume (PTV), which is the GTV/CTV plus additional margin to allow for organ motion or variance in daily set-up position.

During the simulation, the patient is positioned on a simulator. It is a diagnostic x-ray machine that re-creates the actions of the linear accelerator. The radiation fields are marked on the

TABLE 15.10 Tumor Radiosensitivity

High Radiosensitivity
- Hodgkin's lymphoma
- Neuroblastoma
- Non-Hodgkin's lymphoma
- Ovarian dysgerminoma
- Testicular seminoma
- Wilms' tumor

Moderate Radiosensitivity
- Bladder carcinoma
- Breast adenocarcinoma
- Esophageal carcinoma
- Oropharyngeal carcinoma
- Prostate carcinoma
- Uterine and cervical carcinoma

Mild Radiosensitivity
- Colon adenocarcinoma
- Gastric adenocarcinoma
- Renal adenocarcinoma
- Soft tissue sarcomas (e.g., chondrosarcoma)

Poor Radiosensitivity
- Osteosarcoma
- Malignant glioma
- Melanoma
- Testicular nonseminoma

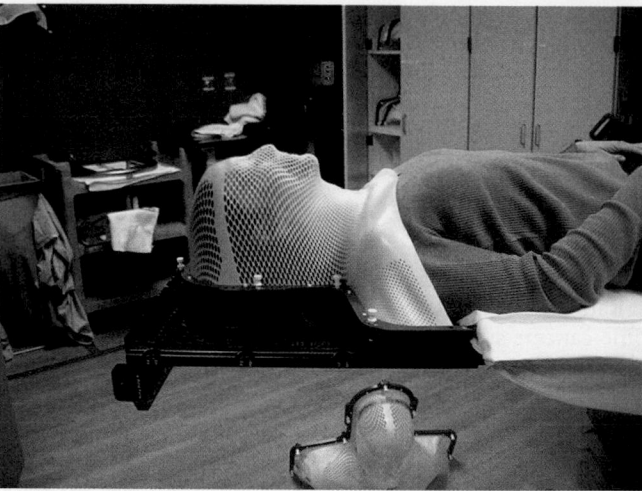

FIG. 15.12 Immobilization device. A head holder and an immobilization mask may be used to ensure accurate positioning for daily treatment of head and neck cancer. (Courtesy Jormain Cady, Virginia Mason Medical Center, Seattle, WA.)

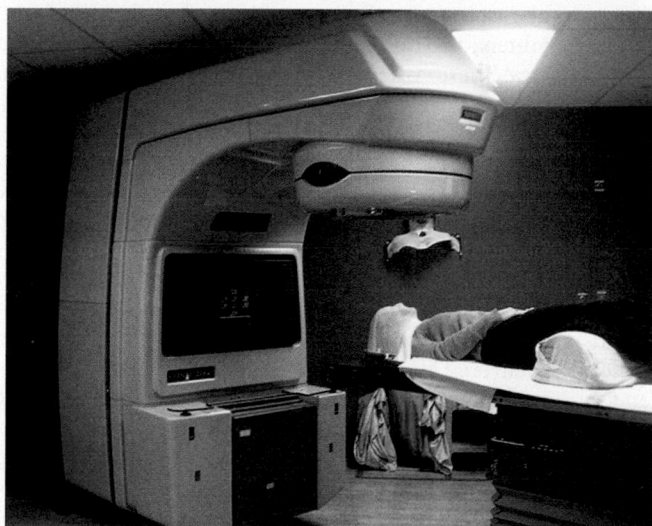

FIG. 15.13 Linear accelerator. Varian Clinac EX linear accelerator with multiple photon and electron energies available for use according to the treatment plan. Patient is positioned on radiation treatment table for treatment of head and neck cancer. (Courtesy Jormain Cady, Virginia Mason Medical Center, Seattle, WA.)

patient's skin. Immobilization devices (e.g., casts, bite blocks, thermoplastic face masks) are typically used to help the patient keep a stable position (Fig. 15.12).

The target is defined using a variety of imaging techniques (e.g., x-rays; CT, MRI, PET scans), physical examination, and surgical reports. Small tattoos may be placed to ensure the patient position is precisely reproduced each treatment.

Treatment

Radiation is used to treat a carefully defined area of the body. Since radiation affects only tissues within the treatment field, it is not appropriate as the main treatment for systemic disease. However, radiation may be used by itself, in combination with chemotherapy or surgery to treat primary tumors, or for palliation of metastatic lesions.

External Radiation. Radiation can be delivered externally *(external beam radiation therapy)* or internally *(brachytherapy).* **External beam radiation** is the most common form of radiation treatment delivery. With this technique, the patient is exposed to radiation from a megavoltage treatment machine. The beam passes through the external tissues to reach the internal target. A linear accelerator, which generates ionizing radiation from electricity and can have multiple energies, is the most commonly used machine for delivering external beam radiation (Fig. 15.13). *Gamma knife technology* (used to deliver highly accurate stereotactic treatment to a localized treatment volume) uses a cobalt source.

Internal Radiation. Radiation can be delivered as **brachytherapy**, which means "close" or internal radiation treatment. It consists of the implantation or insertion of radioactive materials directly into the tumor (interstitial) or near the tumor (intracavitary or intraluminal). This allows for direct delivery of radiation to the target with minimal exposure to surrounding healthy tissues. It is often used in combination with external radiation as a supplemental "boost" treatment. It may be a primary or adjuvant therapy.

Sources of radiation for brachytherapy include temporary sealed sources (e.g., iridium-192, cesium-137) and permanent sealed sources (e.g., iodine-125, gold-198, palladium-103). These are supplied in the form of seeds or ribbons. With a temporary implant, the source may be placed into a special catheter or metal tube that has been inserted into the tumor area. It is left in place until the prescribed dose of radiation has been reached in the calculated number of hours.

Brachytherapy may be delivered as high-dose-rate (HDR) treatment (e.g., several doses given at varying intervals over a few minutes each time) or low-dose-rate (LDR) treatment (e.g., continuous treatment over several hours or days). A remote "afterloading" technique (e.g., the source is inserted after the applicator is in place) is designed to enhance HCP and patient safety. It is used for HDR brachytherapy with iridium-192. These methods are often used for head and neck, lung, breast, and gynecologic cancers.

Permanent implants, such as for prostate brachytherapy, involve the insertion of radioactive seeds directly into the tumor tissue, where they stay permanently. As interstitial seeds used for treatment emit low energies with limited tissue penetration, patients are not considered radioactive. However, some initial radiation precautions may be recommended because of a small risk of seed dislodgement. Over time, the isotopes that are used decay and are no longer radioactive. The timeframe for side effects induced by treatment can be predicted based on the rate of decay for the specific isotope used.

Radioactive drugs, or radiopharmaceuticals, are used to treat some cancers systemically. They may be given orally as a capsule or drink (e.g., iodine-131 for thyroid cancer), or IV as with yttrium-90 given for resistant lymphomas or samarium-153 used to treat bone metastases. The drug is sometimes bound to monoclonal antibodies. The antibodies attach to the cancer cell, directly delivering the radiation. This may minimize the effects of the radiation on healthy cells.

Caring for the person undergoing brachytherapy or receiving radioactive drugs requires that you be aware when the patient is emitting radioactivity. Patients with temporary implants are radioactive only while the source is in place. In those with permanent implants, because the sources have short half-lives and are weak emitters, the radioactive exposure to the outside and to others is low. These patients may be discharged with minimal precautions.

The principles of *ALARA (as low as reasonably achievable)* and *time, distance,* and *shielding* are vital to our safety when caring for the person with a source of internal radiation. Organize care to limit the time spent in direct contact with the patient. To minimize anxiety and confusion, tell the patient the reason for time and distance limitations before the procedure.

The radiation safety officer will say how much time at a specific distance can be spent with the patient. This is determined by the dose delivered by the implant. Because the source is nonpenetrating, small differences in distance are critical. Only care that must be delivered near the source, such as checking placement of the implant, is done in close proximity. Use shielding, if available. Do not deliver care without wearing a film badge (dosimeter) showing cumulative radiation exposure. Do not share the film badge. Do not wear it anywhere but at work and return it according to the agency's protocol.

❖ NURSING MANAGEMENT: CHEMOTHERAPY AND RADIATION THERAPY

You play a key role in helping patients deal with the side effects of chemotherapy and radiation therapy. Before starting teaching, assess the patient's ability to process information. Customize teaching to meet the patient's and caregiver's learning needs.

Common side effects of chemotherapy and radiation are outlined in Table 15.11. Bone marrow suppression, fatigue, GI disturbances, skin and mucosal reactions, and pulmonary and reproductive effects are discussed in this section.

◆ Nursing Implementation
◆ **Bone Marrow Suppression.** Myelosuppression is one of the most common effects of chemotherapy. To a lesser extent, it can occur with radiation. Treatment-induced myelosuppression can result in life-threatening and distressing effects. These include infection, hemorrhage, and overwhelming fatigue. The major

difference in manifestations between radiation therapy and chemotherapy is that radiation (a local therapy) only affects bone marrow within the treatment field. Chemotherapy (a systemic therapy) affects bone marrow function throughout the body. When the therapies are combined, the risk for myelosuppression greatly increases.

In general, the onset of bone marrow suppression is related to the life span of the type of blood cell. WBCs (especially neutrophils) are affected first (within 1 to 2 weeks), platelets in 2 to 3 weeks, and red blood cells (RBCs), with a longer life span of 120 days, later. The severity of myelosuppression depends on the chemotherapy drugs used, drug dosages, and the radiation treatment field. Radiation to large marrow-containing regions of the body produces the most clinically significant myelosuppression. In the adult, most of the active marrow is in the pelvis and thoracic and lumbar vertebrae.

Monitor the CBC, especially the neutrophil, platelet, and RBC counts, in patients receiving chemotherapy or radiation. Patients often have the lowest blood cell counts (called the *nadir*) between 7 and 10 days after starting therapy. However, the exact onset depends on the drug regimen.

Neutropenia is more common in patients receiving chemotherapy than radiation therapy. It is a serious risk factor for life-threatening infection and sepsis. Significant neutropenia will prompt treatment delay or adjustments (e.g., lower dosages). Take every measure to prevent infections in these patients. Hand hygiene is the mainstay of patient protection. Patients and their contacts, including health care team members, should follow hand-washing guidelines.

Monitor temperature routinely. Any sign of infection should be treated promptly, since fever in the presence of neutropenia is a medical emergency. WBC growth factors (e.g., filgrastim [Neupogen], pegfilgrastim [Neulasta]) are routinely used to reduce the duration of chemotherapy-induced neutropenia. They are used as a prophylactic measure to prevent neutropenia when highly myelosuppressive chemotherapy drugs are used.[12] (Neutropenia is discussed in Chapter 30. See the patient teaching guide in Table 30.23 and eNursing Care Plan 30.3 on the website for that chapter.)

Thrombocytopenia can result in spontaneous bleeding or major hemorrhage. Avoid invasive procedures. Teach patients to avoid activities that place them at risk for injury or bleeding (including excessive straining). Risk for serious bleeding is generally not present until the platelet count falls below 50,000/μL. Platelet transfusions may be necessary and are usually given when platelet counts fall below 20,000/μL. (Thrombocytopenia is discussed in Chapter 30. See the patient teaching guide in Table 30.15 and eNursing Care Plan 30.2 on the website for that chapter.)

Anemia is common in patients undergoing either radiation therapy or chemotherapy. It generally has a later onset (about 3 to 4 months after starting treatment). For patients with low hemoglobin levels, RBC growth factors (e.g., darbepoetin [Aranesp], epoetin [Procrit]) may be given according to clinical guidelines. In extreme circumstances (e.g., symptomatic anemia), RBC transfusions may be needed. However, in general, RBC transfusions are avoided. (Hematopoietic growth factors are discussed later in this chapter and in Table 15.15.)

◆ **Fatigue.** *Fatigue* is the persistent subjective sense of tiredness that interferes with usual day-to-day functioning. Fatigue is a nearly universal symptom affecting most patients with cancer. It is often reported by patients as the most distressful of

TABLE 15.11 Nursing Management

Problems Caused by Chemotherapy and Radiation Therapy

Etiology	Nursing Management
Biochemical	
Hyperuricemia	
Increased uric acid levels due to chemotherapy-induced cell destruction. Can cause secondary gout and obstructive uropathy.	• Monitor uric acid levels. • Allopurinol may be given as a prophylactic measure. • Maintain increased fluid intake.
Cardiovascular	
Cardiotoxicity	
Some chemotherapy drugs (e.g., anthracyclines, taxanes) can cause ECG changes and rapidly progressive heart failure.	• Monitor heart with ECG and cardiac ejection fractions. • Drug therapy may need to be changed for symptoms or deteriorating cardiac function studies. • Administer antidysrhythmic drugs as ordered.
Pericarditis and Myocarditis	
Inflammation from radiation injury. Complication from chest wall radiation. May occur up to 1 year after treatment. Side effect of some chemotherapy drugs.	• Monitor for manifestations of these disorders (e.g., dyspnea).
Comfort	
Fatigue	
Anabolic processes result in accumulation of metabolites from cell breakdown.	• Assess for reversible causes of fatigue and address them as indicated. • Reassure patient that fatigue is a common side effect of therapy. • Encourage patient to rest when fatigued, to maintain usual lifestyle patterns, as much as possible, and to pace activities in accordance with energy level. • Encourage moderate exercise as tolerated.
Gastrointestinal System	
Anorexia	
Release of TNF and IL-1 from macrophages has appetite-suppressant effect. Therapy-induced GI effects (mucositis, nausea, vomiting, bowel problems) and anxiety reduce appetite.	• Monitor weight. • Encourage patient to eat small, frequent meals of high-protein, high-calorie foods. • Gently encourage patient to eat, but do not nag. • Recommend keeping a food diary to track daily calories and fluids. • Serve food in pleasant environment.
Constipation	
Autonomic nervous system dysfunction decreases intestinal motility. Caused by neurotoxic effects of plant alkaloids (vincristine, vinblastine).	• Teach patients to take stool softeners as needed, eat high-fiber foods, and increase fluid intake. • Teach patients to increase activity (e.g., walking) if tolerated.
Diarrhea	
From denuding of epithelial lining of intestines. Side effect of chemotherapy. Follows radiation to abdomen, pelvis, lumbosacral areas.	• Give antidiarrheal drugs as needed. • Encourage low-fiber, low-residue diet. • Encourage fluid intake of at least 3 L/day.
Hepatotoxicity	
Toxic effects from chemotherapy drugs (usually transient and resolve when drug is stopped).	• Monitor liver function tests.
Nausea and Vomiting	
Release of intracellular breakdown products stimulates vomiting center in brain. Drugs stimulate vomiting center in brain (see Fig. 41.1). Radiation and chemotherapy destroy lining of GI tract.	• Encourage patient to eat and drink when not nauseated. • Give prophylactic antiemetics before chemotherapy and on as-needed basis. • Teach patients to take antiemetics on a scheduled basis for 2–3 days after highly emetogenic chemotherapy. • Use diversional activities (if appropriate).

Continued

TABLE 15.11 Nursing Management—cont'd

Problems Caused by Chemotherapy and Radiation Therapy

Etiology	Nursing Management
Stomatitis, Mucositis, and Esophagitis	
Epithelial cells are destroyed by chemotherapy or radiation treatment when located in field (e.g., head and neck, stomach, esophagus). Rapid cell destruction causes inflammation and ulceration.	• Assess oral mucosa daily and teach patient to do this. • Encourage nutritional supplements (e.g., Ensure, Carnation Instant Breakfast) if intake is decreasing. • Be aware that eating, swallowing, and talking may be difficult and patient may need analgesics. • Teach avoidance of irritating spicy or acidic foods or too hot or too cold food (extremes in temperature). • Teach how to choose moist, bland, and softer foods. • Encourage patient to keep oral cavity clean and moist by frequent oral rinses with saline or salt and soda solution. • Encourage patient to use artificial saliva to manage dryness (radiation). • Discourage use of irritants, such as tobacco and alcohol. • Apply topical anesthetics (e.g., viscous lidocaine, oxethazaine).
Genitourinary Tract **Hemorrhagic Cystitis**	
Chemotherapy (e.g., cyclophosphamide, ifosfamide) destroys cells lining the bladder Side effect of radiation when in the treatment field.	• Encourage increased fluid intake 24–72 hr after treatment as tolerated. • Monitor for urgency, frequency, and hematuria. • Give cytoprotectant agent (mesna [Mesnex]) and hydration. • Give supportive care agents to manage symptoms (e.g., flavoxate).
Nephrotoxicity	
Exposure to nephrotoxic agents (cisplatin and high-dose methotrexate) directly damages renal cells. Precipitation of metabolites of cell breakdown (tumor lysis syndrome [TLS]).	• Monitor BUN and serum creatinine levels. • Avoid potentiating drugs. • Alkalinize the urine by adding sodium bicarbonate to IV infusion • Give allopurinol or rasburicase for TLS prevention.
Reproductive Problems	
Therapy damages cells of testes or ova.	• Discuss possibility with patients before treatment initiation. • Offer opportunity for sperm and ova banking before treatment for patients of childbearing age.
Hematologic System **Anemia**	
Therapy causes bone marrow depression. Malignant infiltration of bone marrow by cancer.	• Monitor hemoglobin and hematocrit levels. • Give iron supplements and erythropoietin. • Encourage intake of foods that promote RBC production (see Table 30.5).
Leukopenia	
Chemotherapy or radiation therapy causes bone marrow depression. Infection most frequent cause of morbidity and death in cancer patients. Respiratory and genitourinary system are usual sites of infection.	• Monitor WBC count, especially neutrophils. • Tell patient to report temperature elevation and any other manifestations of infection. • Teach patient to avoid large crowds and people with infections. • Give WBC growth factors (Table 15.15). • For patient teaching, see Table 30.23.
Thrombocytopenia	
Chemotherapy causes bone marrow depression. Malignant infiltration of bone marrow crowds out normal marrow. Spontaneous bleeding can occur with platelet counts ≤20,000/μL.	• Observe for signs of bleeding (e.g., petechiae, ecchymosis). • Monitor platelet counts. • For patient teaching, see Table 30.15.
Integumentary System **Alopecia**	
Chemotherapy or radiation to scalp destroys hair follicles. Hair loss usually is temporary with chemotherapy, but usually permanent in response to radiation.	• Suggest ways to cope with hair loss (e.g., hair pieces, scarves, wigs). • Cut long hair before therapy. • Avoid excessive shampooing, brushing, and combing of hair. • Avoid use of electric hair dryers, curlers, and curling rods. • Discuss impact of hair loss on self-image.

TABLE 15.11 Nursing Management—cont'd

Problems Caused by Chemotherapy and Radiation Therapy

Etiology	Nursing Management
Chemotherapy-Induced Skin Changes Acneiform eruptions. Acral erythema. Hyperpigmentation. Photosensitivity. Telangiectasia.	• Alert patient to potential skin changes. • Encourage patient to avoid sun exposure. • Implement symptomatic management as needed depending on specific skin effect (e.g., application of lotions, corticosteroid creams).
Radiation Skin Changes (dry to moist desquamation) Radiation damages skin.	• See Table 15.12 for patient management details.
Nervous System **Cognitive Changes ("chemo brain")** Occur during and after treatment (especially with chemotherapy). Problems with concentration, memory lapses, trouble remembering details, taking longer to finish tasks. May happen quickly and last a short time. Some people have mild long-term effects.	• Teach patients to: • Use detailed daily planner. • Get enough sleep and rest. • Exercise brain (learn something new, do word puzzles). • Focus on one thing (no multitasking).
Intracranial Pressure May result from radiation edema in central nervous system.	• Monitor neurologic status. • May be controlled with corticosteroids.
Peripheral Neuropathy Paresthesias, areflexia, skeletal muscle weakness, and smooth muscle dysfunction can occur as a side effect of plant alkaloids, taxanes, and cisplatin.	• Monitor for manifestations in patients on these drugs. • Consider temporary chemotherapy dose interruption or reduction until symptoms improve. • Antiseizure drugs (e.g., gabapentin [Neurontin]) may be considered.
Respiratory System **Pneumonitis** Radiation pneumonitis develops 2–3 mo after start of treatment. After 6–12 mo, fibrosis occurs and is evident on x-ray. Side effect of some chemotherapy and immunotherapy drugs.	• Monitor for dry, hacking cough; fever; and dyspnea with exertion. • Encourage activity and respiratory exercises.

treatment-related side effects. Fatigue may persist long after treatment has ended.

Anemia is one cause of fatigue. Other causes may be related to the (1) accumulation of toxic substances that are left in the body after cells are killed by cancer treatment, (2) need for extra energy to repair and heal body tissue damaged by treatment, and (3) lack of sleep caused by some chemotherapy drugs. Assess for reversible causes of fatigue, such as anemia, hypothyroidism, depression, anxiety, insomnia, dehydration, or infection.

Help patients recognize that fatigue is a common side effect of therapy. Teach them energy conservation strategies. Help patients identify days or times during the day when they typically feel better. Encourage them to be more active during that period.

Resting before activity and having others help with work or home tasks may be necessary. Ignoring the fatigue or overstressing the body when fatigue is tolerable may lead to an increase in symptoms. Maintaining exercise and activity within tolerable limits is often helpful in managing fatigue. Walking programs are a way for most patients to keep active without overtaxing themselves. Staying active helps improve mood and avoid the debilitating cycle of fatigue-depression-fatigue that can occur in patients with cancer. Guidelines for the evaluation and management of cancer-related fatigue are available.[13]

? CHECK YOUR PRACTICE

Your 56-yr-old female patient with breast cancer has just completed 4 cycles of a chemotherapy regimen of CAF (cyclophosphamide, doxorubicin, fluorouracil). At her clinic visit today, she reports being so tired that she "can barely get out of bed." She then becomes tearful, sharing "who knows what my future holds, and now I am missing so many things with my grandchildren."
• How would you respond?

◆ **Gastrointestinal Effects.** The cells of the mucosal lining of the GI tract are highly proliferative. The epithelial cells are replaced every 2 to 6 days. The intestinal mucosa is one of the most sensitive tissues to radiation and chemotherapy. The cause of GI reactions is related to a variety of mechanisms. These include (1) the release of serotonin from the GI tract, which then stimulates the chemoreceptor trigger zone (CTZ) and the vomiting center in the brain and (2) cell death and resulting damage to GI mucosa. Radiation to treatment fields that contain GI structures (e.g., abdominopelvic, lumbosacral, lower thoracic areas) and selected chemotherapy agents cause direct injury to GI epithelial cells. These injuries cause a variety of GI effects, including nausea and vomiting, diarrhea, mucositis, and anorexia. These problems can significantly affect the patient's hydration and nutritional status and sense of well-being.

Nausea and Vomiting. Nausea and vomiting are common effects of chemotherapy and sometimes radiation therapy. Chemotherapy-induced nausea and vomiting (CINV) may occur within 1 hour of chemotherapy administration. Vomiting may start a few hours after radiation therapy to the chest or abdomen. It may persist for 24 hours or more. Several antiemetic drugs are available (see Table 41.1).

Serotonin (5-HT_3) receptor antagonists (ondansetron [Zofran], granisetron, palonosetron [Aloxi]) and neurokinin-1 receptor antagonists (NK_1RA), (e.g., aprepitant [Emend], netupitant, rolapitant [Varubi]) can reduce CINV. Dexamethasone is given with other antiemetics to manage acute and delayed CINV. Akynzeo is a fixed combination of palonosetron (a 5-HT_3 receptor antagonist) and netupitant (a NK_1RA antagonist).

Anticipatory nausea and vomiting can develop if a patient has poorly controlled nausea and vomiting after chemotherapy administration. In this phenomenon, encountering the cues even without receiving treatment may precipitate nausea and vomiting. Aggressive emesis control, including giving prophylactic antiemetic and antianxiety medication 1 hour before treatment, is recommended. The patient may find that eating a light meal of nonirritating food before treatment is helpful.

Delayed nausea and vomiting can develop 24 hours to a week after treatment. Assess patients who have nausea and vomiting for signs and symptoms of dehydration and metabolic alkalosis. Nausea and vomiting can be successfully managed with antiemetic drugs, diet adjustments, and other nondrug interventions (e.g., relaxation breathing).

Diarrhea. Diarrhea is a reaction of the bowel mucosa to radiation and some chemotherapy drugs. It is characterized by an increase in frequency and liquidity of stool. The small bowel is extremely sensitive and does not tolerate significant radiation doses. With pelvic radiation, patients may be treated with a full bladder. This moves the small bowel out of the treatment field. Both radiation- and chemotherapy-induced diarrhea are best managed with diet adjustments, antidiarrheals, antimotility agents, and antispasmodics (see Table 42.2).

Recommend a diet low in fiber and residue before chemotherapy known to cause diarrhea. This includes limiting foods high in roughage (e.g., fresh fruits, vegetables, seeds, nuts). To prevent diarrhea, other foods to avoid include fried, fatty, or highly seasoned foods and foods that are gas producing. Bowel mucosal injury from radiation may cause temporary lactose intolerance. So, avoiding milk products is helpful for some patients during and right after treatment.

Depending on the severity of the diarrhea, hydration and electrolyte supplementation are recommended. Lukewarm sitz baths may ease discomfort and cleanse the rectal area if significant rectal irritation has developed. The rectal area must be kept clean and dry to maintain skin integrity. Inspect the perianal area for evidence of skin breakdown. Systemic analgesia may be used for painful skin irritations. Note the number, volume, consistency, and character of stools per day. Have patients keep a diary or log to record episodes and aggravating and alleviating factors.

Mucositis. Mucositis is irritation, inflammation, and/or ulceration of the mucosa. Chemotherapy or radiation therapy can cause mucositis. Patients diagnosed with head and neck cancer who receive radiation are at high risk. Like the bowel mucosa, the mucosal linings of the oral cavity, oropharynx, and esophagus are extremely sensitive to the effects of radiation and chemotherapy.

Certain factors can compound the problem. For example, patients undergoing head and neck radiation may face the added challenge of radiation-induced parotid gland dysfunction. This may result in decreased salivary flow, causing acute or chronic *xerostomia* (dry mouth). Dryness or thick saliva compromises the protective salivary functions of assisting with cleansing teeth, moistening food, and swallowing. Meticulous oral care during and for a long time after treatment reduces the risk for cavities, which may occur due to decreased saliva. Teach patients to continue regular dental follow-up every 6 months. They should use fluoride supplements as recommended by their dentist. Saliva substitutes may be offered to patients with xerostomia. Many patients find that drinking small amounts of water frequently has a similar effect.

Dysgeusia (taste loss) may develop during therapy. By the end of treatment, patients often report that all food has lost its flavor. Ultimately, nutritional status may be compromised. *Dysphagia* (difficulty swallowing), which marks pharyngeal and/or esophageal involvement, further impedes eating. Patients may report feeling that they have a "lump" as they swallow and that "foods get stuck." The patient with *odynophagia* (painful swallowing) caused by oropharyngeal or esophageal irritation and ulceration may need analgesics before meals.

Oral assessment and meticulous intervention to keep the oral cavity moist, clean, and free of debris are essential to prevent infection and promote nutritional intake. Implementing standard oral care protocols that address prevention and management of mucositis promotes routine assessment, patient and caregiver teaching, and intervention.

Routinely assess the oral cavity, mucous membranes, characteristics of saliva, and ability to swallow. Having a dentist perform all necessary dental work before starting treatment is recommended. Teach the patient to self-examine the oral cavity and how to perform oral care. Oral care should be done at least before and after each meal, at bedtime, and as needed through the day. A saline solution of 1 tsp of salt in 1 L of water is an effective cleansing agent; 1 tsp of sodium bicarbonate may be added to the oral care solution to decrease odor, ease pain, and dissolve mucin. Have the patient use a soft bristled toothbrush.

Mucositis or pain in the throat can be eased by systemic and/or topical analgesics and antibiotics if infection is present. Monitor and get prompt treatment for oral candidiasis (which often occurs with mucositis). Frequent cleansing with saline and water and topical application of anesthetic gels directly to the lesions are standard care.

Anorexia. Anorexia (loss of appetite) is a common occurrence in patients with cancer. It is a side effect of the cancer as well as of cancer treatment. Anorexia may be related to an inflamed mouth or esophagus, which creates difficulty chewing or swallowing, or to emotions, such as anxiety or depression. It is important to have a dietitian involved in patient care before cancer treatment starts.

Patients with nausea and vomiting, bowel problems, mucositis, and taste changes typically have little desire to eat. Anorexia seems to peak at about 4 weeks of treatment. It resolves more quickly than fatigue when treatment ends.

Monitor patients with anorexia during and after treatment to ensure that weight loss does not become excessive. Observe for dehydration. Small, frequent meals of high-protein, high-calorie foods are better tolerated than large meals. Nutritional supplements can be helpful, too. Enteral or parenteral nutrition may be needed if the patient is severely malnourished, if symptoms are expected to interfere with nutrition for a time, or if the bowel is being rested. Monitor for and manage other symptoms that may interfere with appetite (e.g., nausea, vomiting, pain, depression).

◆ Skin Reactions

Radiation Skin Changes. With radiation therapy, skin effects are local, occurring only in the treatment field. Radiation-induced skin changes can be acute or chronic depending on the area irradiated, dosage, and technique. The skin-sparing ability of modern radiation equipment limits the severity of these reactions.

Erythema may develop 1 to 24 hours after a single treatment. It generally occurs progressively as the treatment dose accumulates. It is an acute response followed by dry desquamation (Fig. 15.14). If the rate of cell sloughing is faster than the ability of the new epidermal cells to replace dead cells, a wet desquamation occurs with exposure of the dermis and weeping of serous fluid (Fig. 15.15). Skin reactions are especially evident in areas of skinfolds or where skin is subjected to pressure. This includes behind the ear; in gluteal folds; on the perineum, breast, or collar line; and bony prominences.

Although skin care protocols vary, basic skin care principles apply. The goal is to prevent infection and promote wound healing. Protect radiated skin from temperature extremes. Do not use heating pads, ice packs, and hot water bottles in the treatment field. Avoid constricting garments, rubbing, harsh chemicals, and deodorants, since they may traumatize the skin. Dry reactions are uncomfortable and result in pruritus. Lubricate

dry skin with a nonirritating lotion emollient that contains no metal, alcohol, perfume, or additives. These can be irritating. Calendula ointment and topical hyaluronic acid cream are effective for managing radiation dermatitis. Aloe vera gel is useful for preventing skin problems.

Wet desquamation of tissues generally causes pain, drainage, and increased risk for infection. Skin care to manage moist desquamation includes keeping tissues clean with normal saline compresses or modified Burow's solution soaks. Protect the skin from further damage with moisture vapor–permeable dressings or Vaseline petrolatum gauze. Because protocols vary widely, you should verify the guidelines in Table 15.12 with your agency' s radiation oncology department.

Chemotherapy Skin Changes. Chemotherapy causes a wide range of skin toxicities. These can range from mild erythema and hyperpigmentation to more distressing effects, such as acral erythema and *erythrodysesthesia syndrome* (also called palmar-plantar erythrodysesthesia or hand-foot syndrome).

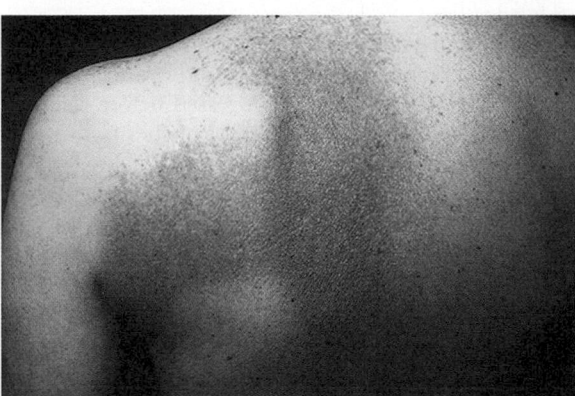

FIG. 15.14 Dry desquamation.

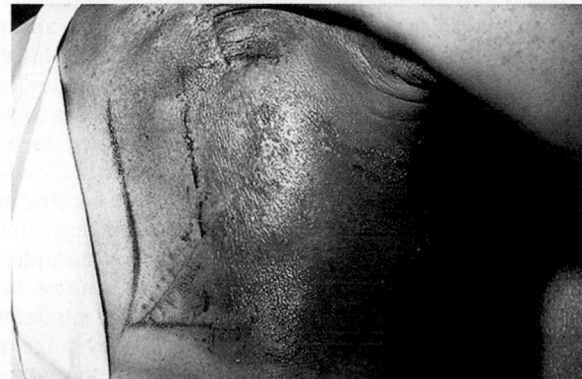

FIG. 15.15 Wet desquamation.

TABLE 15.12 Patient & Caregiver Teaching

Radiation Skin Reactions

Include the following instructions when teaching the patient and caregiver to clean and protect the skin in a radiation treatment area:

1. Gently cleanse the skin in the treatment field using a mild soap (Ivory, Dove), tepid water, a soft cloth, and a gentle patting motion. Rinse thoroughly and pat dry.
2. Apply nonmedicated, nonperfumed, moisturizing lotion or cream, such as calendula ointment, aloe gel, Aquaphor, or Biafine cream, to alleviate dry skin. Some substances must be gently cleansed from the treatment field before each treatment and reapplied. Over-the-counter hydrocortisone cream 1% may reduce itching.
3. Rinse the area with saline solution. Expose the area to air as often as possible. If copious drainage is present, use astringent compresses (such as Domeboro solution) and nonadhesive absorbent dressings. Change dressings as soon as they become wet.
4. Observe the area daily for signs of infection.
5. Avoid wearing tight-fitting clothing, including brassieres and belts, over the treatment field.
6. Avoid wearing harsh fabrics, such as wool and corduroy. A lightweight cotton garment is best. If possible, expose the treatment field to air.
7. Use gentle detergents (e.g., Dreft, Ivory Snow) to wash clothing that will come in contact with the treatment field.
8. Avoid direct exposure to the sun. If the treatment field is in an area that is exposed to the sun, wear protective clothing, such as a wide-brimmed hat, when out in the sun and apply sunscreen lotion.
9. Avoid all sources of excessive heat (hot water bottles, heating pads, sunlamps) on the treatment field.
10. Avoid exposing the treatment field to cold temperatures (ice bags or cold weather).
11. Avoid swimming in saltwater or in chlorinated pools during the time of treatment.
12. Avoid the use of potential irritants (e.g., perfumes, powders, or cosmetics) on the skin in the treatment field. Review the use of other topical medications or lotions with your HCP during treatment. Avoid tape, dressings, and adhesive bandages unless allowed by the radiation therapist.
12. Continue to protect sensitive skin after the treatment is completed. Do the following:
    - Avoid direct exposure to the sun. A sunscreen agent and protective clothing must be worn if the potential of exposure to the sun is present.
    - Use an electric razor if shaving is needed in the treatment field.

Erythrodysesthesia syndrome can cause mild symptoms of redness and tingling of the palms of the hands and soles of the feet. It may also cause severe symptoms of painful moist desquamation, ulceration, blistering, and pain.

Alopecia is an easily recognizable effect of cancer treatment. Hair loss associated with radiation is local. Chemotherapy affects hair throughout the body. The degree and duration of hair loss depends on the type and dose of the chemotherapy agent. Scalp cooling during chemotherapy may reduce alopecia. Cold caps are placed on the head before, during, and after chemotherapy treatment. Common side effects are headache and cold sensation.[14]

Alopecia caused by chemotherapy agents is usually reversible. Usually the hair does not grow back until 3 to 4 weeks after the end of therapy. Often the new hair is a different color and texture than the hair that was lost.

Patients have a range of emotions at the prospect of losing their hair and when hair loss occurs. These may include anger, grief, embarrassment, or fear. Hair loss is a visible reminder of their cancer and the challenges of treatment. For some people, the hair loss is one of the most stressful events experienced during treatment. The ACS's "Look Good, Feel Better" program is an excellent support and resource for people with hair loss and body image changes.

◆ **Pulmonary Effects.** Both chemotherapy and radiation have the potential to cause irreversible and progressive lung damage. Distinguishing between the complications of treatment and those related to disease is challenging. The effects of radiation on the lung include both acute and late reactions. Acute effects can be alarming to patients because they may mimic symptoms (e.g., cough, dyspnea) that precipitated the cancer diagnosis.

Pneumonitis is a delayed acute inflammatory reaction that may occur within 1 to 3 months after completing thoracic radiation. This reaction is often asymptomatic, although an increase in cough, fever, and night sweats may occur. Some patients may develop pulmonary fibrosis (with or without prior pneumonitis), which is a late effect of therapy.

The most common toxicities associated with chemotherapy include pulmonary edema (noncardiogenic) related to capillary leak syndrome or fluid retention, hypersensitivity pneumonitis, interstitial fibrosis, and pneumonitis due to an inflammatory reaction or destruction of alveolar-capillary endothelium.

◆ **Cardiovascular Effects.** Radiation to the thorax can damage the pericardium, myocardium, valves, and coronary blood vessels. The pericardium is most often involved. Pericardial effusion and pericarditis are key problems. Patients with preexisting coronary artery disease are especially at risk.

Anthracyclines (e.g., doxorubicin, daunorubicin) cause cardiotoxicity. Acute cardiotoxicities may cause electrocardiographic (ECG) changes. Late effects cause left ventricular dysfunction and heart failure. Baseline and periodic echocardiograms to monitor left ventricular function during treatment are usually done.

◆ **Cognitive Effects.** Cognitive effects can happen at any time during cancer, especially after treatment. This change in mental function, often described by patients as mental cloudiness or fog, is commonly called *chemo brain*.[15] Patients can have thinking and memory problems. Although the brain will usually recover over time, the effects can last a short time or for years. The effects can be so severe that patients may be unable to be involved in any activities that need mental effort, including school, work, or social activities.

◆ **Reproductive Effects.** Reproductive problems from radiation and chemotherapy vary according to the radiation treatment field and dosage, the chemotherapy agent and dosage, and host factors (e.g., age). Treatment can cause temporary or permanent gonadal failure. Reproductive problems occur most often when reproductive organs are included in the radiation treatment field and when alkylating agents are used.

The testes are highly sensitive to radiation. They should be protected with a testicular shield whenever possible. Pretreatment status may be a significant factor. A low sperm count and loss of motility are seen in those with testicular cancer and Hodgkin's lymphoma before any therapy is begun. Combined modality treatment or prior chemotherapy with alkylating agents enhances and prolongs the effects of radiation on the testes. When radiation is used alone with conventional doses and appropriate shielding, testicular recovery often occurs. Men may have erectile dysfunction after pelvic radiation.

The radiation dose that induces ovarian failure changes with age. Unlike the testes, there is no way to repair ovarian function. When radiation therapy is given, the ovaries are shielded whenever possible. Other factors that influence reproductive or sexual functioning in women include reactions in the cervix and endometrium. These tissues withstand a high radiation dose with minimal sequelae. This accounts for the ability to treat endometrial and cervical cancer with high external and brachytherapy doses. Acute reactions, such as tenderness, irritation, and loss of lubrication, compromise sexual activity. Late effects of combined internal and external radiation therapy include vaginal shortening related to fibrosis and loss of elasticity and lubrication.

The patient and partner need information about the expected effects of treatment related to reproductive and sexual issues. Fertility preservation should be addressed before starting cancer treatment. Pretreatment harvesting of sperm, ova, or ovarian tissue may be considered.[16]

Potential infertility can be a significant consequence, and counseling may be needed. However, in no case should the patient think that conception is not possible during treatment. Specific suggestions that have an impact on sexual function include using a water-soluble vaginal lubricant and a vaginal dilator after pelvic irradiation. Encourage discussion of issues related to reproduction and sexuality, offer specific suggestions, and make referrals for ongoing counseling when needed.

LATE EFFECTS OF RADIATION AND CHEMOTHERAPY

Cancer survivors are achieving long-term remission and survival with advancements in treatment modalities. However, therapy (especially radiation therapy and chemotherapy) may cause long-term effects *(late effects)* that occur months to years after therapy.[17] Every body system can be affected to some extent by radiation therapy or chemotherapy.

Acute radiation effects generally manifest as transient inflammatory changes in highly proliferative cells (e.g., epithelial tissues). In contrast, late radiation effects occur most often in post-mitotic cells (e.g., liver, kidney, lung, heart, muscle, bone, connective tissues). Once they occur, the late effects may be progressive and generally are permanent. Examples range from skin telangiectasias to strictures, fistulas, or radiation necrosis.

Alteration of the lymphatic channels (e.g., axillary lymph node dissection) may contribute to lymphedema.

Long-term effects of chemotherapy include cardiac toxicity, cataracts, arthralgia, endocrine problems, renal insufficiency, hepatitis, osteoporosis, neurocognitive problems, or other effects depending on the agents. The additive effects of multiagent chemotherapy before, during, or after a course of radiation therapy can significantly increase the resulting late effects.

The cancer survivor may be at risk for secondary cancers, including leukemia, angiosarcoma, and skin cancer. Patients treated with alkylating agents and those treated with high-dose radiation have an increased risk. The potential risk for developing a secondary cancer does not contraindicate the use of cancer treatment.

IMMUNOTHERAPY AND TARGETED THERAPY

Immunotherapy uses the immune system, the body's main defense against infection and disease, to fight cancer. Some types of immunotherapy are called *biologic therapy*. Immunotherapy can (1) boost or manipulate the immune system and create an environment that is not conducive for cancer cells to grow or (2) attack cancer cells directly. Types of immunotherapy include cytokines, vaccines, and monoclonal antibodies (Table 15.13). Antibodies are proteins made by the immune system that bind to a target antigen on the cell surface. Monoclonal antibodies (drugs ending in -mab) are the most successful immunotherapy. Because each antibody is specific to an antigen, that mechanism is used to develop specific drugs to treat cancer. Many of the monoclonal antibodies are targeted therapies.

Targeted therapy interferes with cancer growth by targeting specific cell receptors and pathways that are important in tumor growth.[18,19] Targeted therapies work at sites that are on the cell surface, at the intracellular level, or in the extracellular domain (Fig. 15.16 and Table 15.13). Targeted therapies are more selective for specific molecular targets than chemotherapy drugs. Thus they act on specific targets that are associated with cancer. A major advantage of targeted therapy is that it does less damage to normal cells.

As we identify more oncogene targets, agents are being developed that target those specific oncogenes. Targeted therapies provide personalized treatment based on the biology of the tumor. Examples of some targeted therapies are discussed in the next few paragraphs.

A major class of targeted therapy is tyrosine kinase inhibitors (Table 15.13). Tyrosine kinases are enzymes responsible for activating many proteins by signal transduction cascades. EGFR is a transmembrane molecule that works by activating intracellular tyrosine kinase (TK). Overexpression of EGFR is associated with unregulated cell growth and a poor prognosis. Drugs that inhibit EGFR suppress cell proliferation and promote *apoptosis* (programmed cell death).

EGFRs belong to the same receptor family as human epidermal growth factor receptor-2 (HER-2). It is the target for trastuzumab (Herceptin), a drug mainly used to treat breast cancer. HER-2 is overexpressed in certain cancers (especially breast cancers). It is associated with more aggressive disease and decreased survival. Trastuzumab is a monoclonal antibody (MoAb) that binds to HER-2. It is given IV to inhibit the growth of breast cancer cells that overexpress the HER-2 protein. Lapatinib (Tykerb) is an oral agent used for breast cancer that overexpresses HER-2.

Chronic myeloid leukemia (CML) cells make an abnormal active enzyme called BCR-ABL tyrosine kinase. Drugs, such as imatinib (Gleevec), that inhibit this enzyme suppress proliferation of CML cells and promote cell death.

Angiogenesis inhibitors work by preventing the mechanisms and pathways necessary for vascularization of tumors. Bevacizumab (Avastin), a recombinant human MoAb, binds with vascular endothelial growth factor (VEGF), a compound that stimulates blood vessel growth. When bevacizumab binds with VEGF, it prevents VEGF from binding with its receptors on vascular endothelial cells and promoting new vessel formation. As a result, further tumor growth is inhibited.

Proteasomes are intracellular multienzyme complexes that degrade proteins. In cancer cells, proteasome inhibitors (e.g., bortezomib [Velcade]) promote accumulation of proteins that leads to cell death.

Cancer cells can become resistant to targeted therapies. This can occur because the (1) target changes through mutation and the therapy no longer interacts with it and (2) the tumor finds a new growth pathway and no longer depends on the target. Because of the possibility of resistance, targeted therapies work best in combination or in combination with a chemotherapy drug.

Side Effects of Immunotherapy and Targeted Therapy

The administration of one type of immunotherapy usually induces the endogenous release of other agents. The release and action of these agents result in systemic immune and inflammatory responses. The toxicities and side effects are related to dose and schedule.

Common side effects include flu-like symptoms, including headache, fever, chills, myalgias, fatigue, malaise, weakness, photosensitivity, anorexia, and nausea. Those receiving interferon therapy almost always have flu-like symptoms. Their severity generally decreases over time. Acetaminophen given every 4 hours, as prescribed, and large amounts of fluids often reduce the severity of the flu-like syndrome. The patient is often premedicated with acetaminophen to try to prevent or decrease the intensity of these symptoms.

Tachycardia and orthostatic hypotension are common. IL-2 and MoAbs can cause *capillary leak syndrome,* which can result in pulmonary edema. Other toxic and side effects may involve the CNS, renal and hepatic systems, and cardiovascular system. These effects are found with interferons and IL-2.

A wide range of neurologic problems can occur with interferon and IL-2 therapy. The nature and extent of these problems are not yet completely understood. They are frightening to the patient and caregivers. Teach them to observe for neurologic problems (e.g., confusion, memory loss, difficulty making decisions, insomnia), report their occurrence, and institute safety and support measures.

MoAbs are given by infusion. Patients may have infusion-related symptoms, including fever, chills, urticaria, mucosal congestion, nausea, diarrhea, and myalgias.

Skin rashes are common in patients receiving EGFR inhibitors. They manifest generally as erythema and acneiform-like rash that can cover a large part of the upper body. Angiogenesis inhibitors can cause arterial thrombi, hemorrhage, hypertension, impaired wound healing, and proteinuria. Other toxicities of MoAbs include hepatotoxicity, bone marrow depression, and CNS effects.

TABLE 15.13 Drug Therapy

Select Immunotherapies and Targeted Therapies

Mechanism of Action	Examples
Angiogenesis Inhibitors	
Bind vascular endothelial growth factor (VEGF), thereby inhibiting angiogenesis.	bevacizumab (Avastin)
	pazopanib (Votrient)
	ramucirumab (Cyramza)
CD20 Monoclonal Antibodies	
Bind CD20 antigen, causing cytotoxicity and radiation injury.	ibritumomab tiuxetan/yttrium-90 (Zevalin)
Bind CD20 antigen, causing cytotoxicity.	ofatumumab (Arzerra)
	rituximab (Rituxan)
CD52 Monoclonal Antibody	
Bind CD52 antigen (found on T and B cells, monocytes, natural killer [NK] cells, neutrophils).	alemtuzumab (Campath)
Cytokines (see Table 13.4)	
Inhibit DNA and protein synthesis. Suppress cell proliferation. Increase cytotoxic effects of NK cells.	α-interferon (Intron A)
Stimulate proliferation of T and B cells.	interleukin-2 (aldesleukin [Proleukin])
Activate NK cells.	
Human Epidermal Growth Factor Receptor-2 (HER-2)	
Monoclonal antibody to HER-2 that attaches to the antigen. It is taken into the cells and eventually kills them.	pertuzumab (Perjeta)
	trastuzumab (Herceptin)
Trastuzumab connected to a chemotherapy drug called DM1.	ado-trastuzumab emtansine (Kadcyla)
Immunomodulatory Drugs (IMiDs)	
Inhibit production of TNF, IL-6, and VEGF (which leads to its antiangiogenic effects). Stimulate T and NK cells and increase γ-interferon and IL-2 production.	apremilast (Otezla)
	lenalidomide (Revlimid)
	pomalidomide (Pomalyst)
	thalidomide (Thalomid)
Kinase Inhibitors	
Anaplastic Lymphoma Kinase (ALK) Inhibitors	
Inhibit anaplastic lymphoma kinase (ALK).	ceritinib (Zykadia)
	crizotinib (Xalkori)
BCR-ABL Tyrosine Kinase Inhibitors	
Inhibit BCR-ABL TK. Primarily used in chronic myeloid leukemia.	bosutinib (Bosulif)
	dasatinib (Sprycel)
	imatinib (Gleevec)
	nilotinib (Tasigna)
BRAF and MEK Kinase Inhibitors	
Inhibit BRAF and MEK enzymes.	dabrafenib (Tafinlar)
	trametinib (Mekinist)
	vemurafenib (Zelboraf)
	cobimetinib (Cotellic)
EGFR Tyrosine Kinase (TK) Inhibitors	
Inhibit epidermal growth factor receptor (EGFR) TK.	cetuximab (Erbitux)
	erlotinib (Tarceva)
	gefitinib (Iressa)
	panitumumab (Vectibix)
Inhibit EGFR-TK and binds HER-2.	lapatinib (Tykerb)
Multi-Tyrosine Kinase Inhibitors	
Inhibit multiple TKs.	axitinib (Inlyta)
	cabozantinib (Cometriq)
	pazopanib (Votrient)
	regorafenib (Stivarga)
	sorafenib (Nexavar)
	sunitinib (Sutent)
	vandetanib (Caprelsa)
mTOR Kinase Inhibitors	
Inhibit a specific protein known as the mechanistic target of rapamycin (mTOR).	everolimus (Afinitor)
	temsirolimus (Torisel)

TABLE 15.13 Drug Therapy—cont'd

Select Immunotherapies and Targeted Therapies

Mechanism of Action	Examples
Programmed Death Receptor (PD)-1 Blockers	
Block PD-1, a protein on T cells that normally helps keep these cells from attacking other cells. This boosts immune response against cancer cells.	nivolumab (Opdivo) pembrolizumab (Keytruda)
Proteasome Inhibitors	
Inhibit proteasome activity, which functions to regulate cell growth.	bortezomib (Velcade) carfilzomib (Kyprolis)
Vaccines	
Live attenuated strain of *Mycobacterium bovis* induces immune response. Used intravesically to treat bladder cancer (see Chapter 45).	BCG vaccine
Vaccine against prostate cancer that stimulates the immune system against the cancer (see Chapter 54).	sipuleucel-T (Provenge)

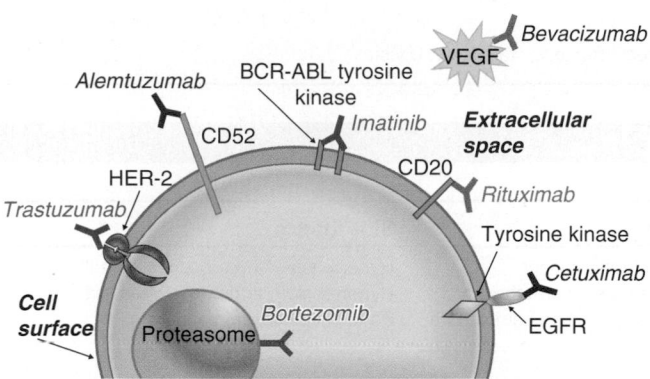

FIG. 15.16 Sites of action of targeted therapy. Examples of targeted therapy drugs that work at the specific site of action are shown in colored, italicized font. *EGFR*, Epidermal growth factor receptor; *HER-2*, human epidermal growth factor receptor-2; *VEGF*, vascular endothelial growth factor.

❖ NURSING MANAGEMENT: IMMUNOTHERAPY AND TARGETED THERAPY

Some problems experienced by the patient receiving immunotherapy and targeted therapy are different from those seen with more traditional forms of cancer treatment. These effects occur more acutely and are dose limited (e.g., effects resolve when therapy is over). Patients may be hesitant to inform the HCP of intolerable side effects. Some may be afraid to discuss side effects because they may think that the drug will be stopped. Or, they decide to stop the drug because of side effects. Assess and evaluate the patient's side effects and tolerance. Appropriate proactive nursing care can prevent these problems because you are able to intervene.

Capillary leak syndrome and pulmonary edema are problems that require critical care nursing. Bone marrow depression is generally more transient and less severe than that seen with chemotherapy. Fatigue associated with immunotherapy and targeted therapy can be so severe that it is a dose-limiting toxicity. When these agents are combined with chemotherapy, the spectrum of therapy-related effects expands.

Nursing interventions for flu-like syndrome include giving acetaminophen before treatment and every 4 hours after treatment. IV meperidine (Demerol) has been used to control the severe chills or rigors associated with some agents. Other nursing measures include monitoring vital signs and temperature, planning for periods of rest for the patient, assisting with activities of daily living (ADLs), and monitoring for adequate oral intake.

HORMONE THERAPY

Hormones are substances that are made in endocrine glands and function as chemical messengers in the body. The hormones estrogen and progesterone can enhance the growth of some breast cancers. Androgen (testosterone) can enhance the growth of some prostate cancers. When given as a cancer treatment, drugs (hormone therapy) can block the effects of the hormone and stop the growth of cancer cells (Table 15.14).

Corticosteroids are used in combination with many drug regimens for cancer. They are antiinflammatory agents that reduce swelling and inflammation, which may be contributing to cancer pain. They may be used with other drugs, such as ondansetron and aprepitant, to control and prevent nausea and vomiting caused by chemotherapy.

In addition to drug manipulation of hormones, surgical interventions (oophorectomy, castration) can be used to remove the effects of the hormone on cancer growth.

HEMATOPOIETIC GROWTH FACTORS

Hematopoietic growth factors are used to support patients through their cancer treatment (Table 15.15). Colony-stimulating factors (CSFs) are a family of glycoproteins made by various cells. CSFs stimulate production, maturation, regulation, and activation of cells of the hematologic system. The name of the CSF is based on the specific cell line it affects.

Erythropoiesis-stimulating agents (ESAs) should be used only when treating anemia specifically caused by chemotherapy. ESA use is avoided in patients receiving chemotherapy with the intent to cure the disease. Their use has raised safety concerns. They can cause potential harm (thromboembolic events, shorter survival) and increase the risk for death and serious cardiovascular events when given to achieve a target hemoglobin of greater than 12 g/dL. Thus the lowest dose should be used that will gradually increase hemoglobin to the lowest level sufficient to avoid the need for blood transfusion. Monitor the hemoglobin level regularly.

TABLE 15.14 Drug Therapy

Hormone Therapy

Androgen Receptor Blockers Selectively attach to androgen receptors, blocking androgen from binding. Inhibits tumor growth.	flutamide, bicalutamide (Casodex), enzalutamide (Xtandi)
Aromatase Inhibitors Inhibit aromatase, thus preventing the production of estrogen.	anastrozole (Arimidex), exemestane (Aromasin), letrozole (Femara)
Corticosteroids Disrupt the cell membrane and inhibit synthesis of protein. Decrease circulating lymphocytes, inhibit mitosis, depress immune system, increase sense of well-being.	cortisone, dexamethasone, hydrocortisone, methylprednisolone, prednisone
Estrogens Interfere with the effect of testosterone.	estradiol, estramustine (Emcyt), estrogen (Menest)
Estrogen Receptor Blockers Selectively attach to estrogen receptors, blocking estrogen from binding. Inhibits tumor growth.	fulvestrant (Faslodex), tamoxifen, toremifene (Fareston)
Estrogen Receptor Modulator Has both estrogen-agonistic effects on bone and estrogen-antagonistic effects on breast tissue.	raloxifene (Evista)

TABLE 15.15 Drug Therapy

Hematopoietic Growth Factors Used in Cancer Treatment

Growth Factor	Drug Name	Indications	Side Effects
Erythropoietin	epoetin alfa (Epogen, Procrit) darbepoetin alfa (Aranesp)	Anemia of chronic cancer Anemia related to chemotherapy	Hypertension, thrombosis, headache Hypertension, thrombosis, headache
Granulocyte colony-stimulating factor (G-CSF)	filgrastim (Neupogen) filgrastim-sndz (Zarxio) pegfilgrastim (Neulasta) tbo-filgrastim (Granix)	Chemotherapy-induced neutropenia	Bone pain, nausea, vomiting
Granulocyte-macrophage colony-stimulating factor (GM-CSF)	sargramostim (Leukine)	Myeloid cell recovery after bone marrow transplantation	Nausea, vomiting, diarrhea, fever, chills, myalgia, headache, fatigue
Interleukin-11 (platelet growth factor)	oprelvekin (Neumega)	Thrombocytopenia related to chemotherapy	Fluid retention, peripheral edema, dyspnea, tachycardia, nausea, mouth sores

HEMATOPOIETIC STEM CELL TRANSPLANTATION

Hematopoietic stem cell transplantation (HSCT) and **peripheral stem cell transplantation (PSCT)** are effective, lifesaving procedures for the treatment of several malignant and nonmalignant diseases (Table 15.16). Both allow for the safe use of very high doses of chemotherapy agents and/or radiation therapy in patients whose tumors have developed resistance (refractory) or did not respond to standard doses of chemotherapy and radiation. Although these procedures are lifesaving, patients may have long-term or delayed complications that can affect their quality of life.

This therapeutic approach was referred to as bone marrow transplant because the bone marrow was the original source of stem cells when the procedure was first developed. However, advances in harvesting and cryopreservation technologies have opened new pathways to the collection of stem cells from the peripheral blood.[20] Consequently, the terminology has changed. Overall cure rates are steadily increasing. Even when cure is not achieved, transplantation can result in a period of remission.

The approach in HSCT is to eradicate diseased tumor cells and/or clear the bone marrow of its components to make way for engraftment of the transplanted, healthy stem cells. This is done by giving higher than usual dosages of chemotherapy with or without radiation therapy. Life-threatening consequences

TABLE 15.16 Indications for Hematopoietic Stem Cell Transplantation

Malignant Diseases
- Acute and chronic lymphocytic leukemia
- Acute and chronic myelogenous leukemia
- Hodgkin's lymphoma
- Multiple myeloma
- Myelodysplastic syndrome
- Non-Hodgkin's lymphoma

Nonmalignant Diseases
- Aplastic anemia
- Chronic granulomatous disease
- Fanconi's anemia
- Hematologic diseases
- Immunodeficiency diseases
- Severe combined immunodeficiency disease (SCID)
- Sickle cell disease (severe)
- Thalassemia
- Wiskott-Aldrich syndrome

associated with pancytopenia and other adverse effects can result from this procedure. After chemotherapy and radiation therapy are over, healthy stem cells are infused. These healthy stem cells "rescue" the damaged bone marrow through subsequent proliferation and differentiation of the donated stem cells in the recipient.

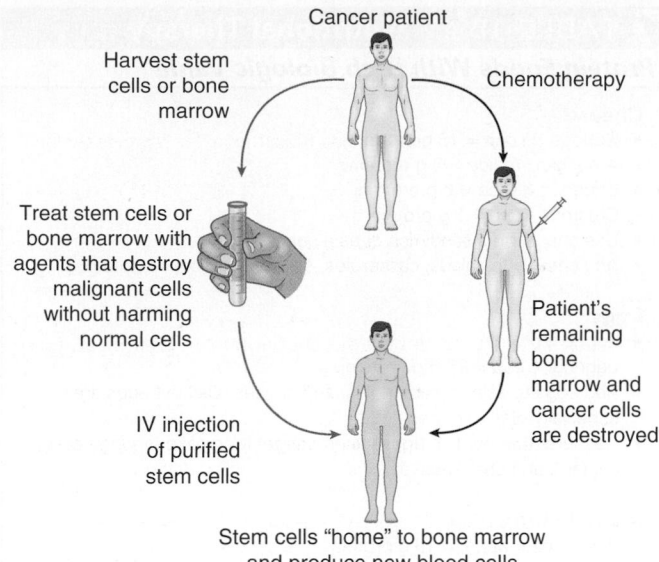

Cancer patient

Harvest stem cells or bone marrow

Chemotherapy

Treat stem cells or bone marrow with agents that destroy malignant cells without harming normal cells

Patient's remaining bone marrow and cancer cells are destroyed

IV injection of purified stem cells

Stem cells "home" to bone marrow and produce new blood cells

FIG. 15.17 Autologous stem cell transplant.

HSCT is an intensive procedure with many risks. Some patients die from treatment-related complications or from recurrence of the original disease. Because it is a highly toxic therapy, the patient must weigh the significant risks for treatment-related death or treatment failure (relapse) against the hope of cure.

Types of Hematopoietic Stem Cell Transplants

HSCTs are categorized as allogeneic, syngeneic, or autologous. The sources of stem cells include the bone marrow, peripheral circulating blood, and umbilical cord blood. In *allogeneic transplantation,* stem cells are acquired from a donor (graft) who, through human leukocyte antigen (HLA) tissue typing, has been determined to be HLA matched to the recipient (host). HLA typing involves testing WBCs to identify genetically inherited antigens common to both donor and recipient that are important in compatibility of transplanted tissue. (HLA tissue typing is discussed in Chapter 13.) The donor is often a family member. It may be an unrelated donor found through a national or international bone marrow registry (e.g., National Marrow Donor Program). These are known as matched unrelated donor (MUD) transplants. Increased risks and toxicities may be associated with a MUD. Common indications for allogeneic transplant are certain leukemias, multiple myeloma, and lymphoma.

Syngeneic transplantation is a type of allogeneic transplant that involves obtaining stem cells from one identical twin and infusing them into the other. Identical twins have identical HLA types and are a perfect match

In *autologous transplantation,* patients receive their own stem cells back after *myeloablative* (destroying bone marrow) chemotherapy (Fig. 15.17). The aim of this approach is purely "rescue." It allows patients to receive intensive chemotherapy and/or radiation by supporting them with their previously harvested stem cells until their marrow generates blood cells again on its own. Restoration usually takes about 4 to 6 weeks.

The newer, nonmyeloablative or reduced intensity transplant uses lower doses of radiation or chemotherapy that result in less toxicity and myelosuppression. HSCT continues to be investigated in managing some solid tumors resistant to treatment.

Procedures

Harvest Procedures. Hematopoietic stem cells are *harvested* from a donor (for allogeneic transplantation) or from the recipient (for autologous transplantation) via 2 methods. The procedure used for harvesting stem cells from bone marrow is done in the operating room using general or spinal anesthesia. Multiple bone marrow aspirations (usually from the iliac crest, but sometimes from the sternum) are carried out to obtain stem cells. The harvested marrow is processed to strain out bone fragments. The entire bone marrow harvest procedure takes about 1 to 2 hours. The patient can be discharged after recovery. Postharvest, the donor may have pain at the collection site that lasts up to 7 days. It can be treated with mild analgesics. The donor's body will replenish the removed bone marrow in a few weeks.

In the other procedure, peripheral stem cell transplants are obtained from the peripheral blood in an outpatient procedure. It is done using cell separator equipment that automatically separates the stem cells from the blood circulating through the machine and returns the remaining blood components to the donor. The process averages about 2 to 4 hours. Sometimes it takes longer depending on donor factors and the quality of the venous access. Often it takes more than one procedure to obtain enough stem cells. Because the blood has fewer stem cells than the bone marrow, "mobilization" of stem cells from the bone marrow into the peripheral blood can be achieved with chemotherapy and/or hematopoietic growth factors.

To increase stem cell production for collection, common growth factors that are used are granulocyte-macrophage colony-stimulating factor (GM-CSF) and granulocyte colony-stimulating factor (G-CSF) (see Table 15.15). When patients are given growth factors for mobilization, stem cells are harvested 4 or 5 days after growth factor injections.

After collection, the marrow or peripheral stem cells are used immediately or bagged with preservative for cryopreservation and storage until they are needed. Since they come from the patient, autologous stem cells are sometimes treated (purged) to remove undetected cancer cells. Many different pharmacologic, immunologic, physical, and chemical agents are used for this purpose.

Umbilical cord blood is rich in hematopoietic stem cells. Successful allogeneic transplants have been done using this source. Cord blood can be HLA-typed and cryopreserved. A disadvantage of cord blood is the possibility of insufficient numbers of stem cells to allow transplant to adults. Considerable research is currently ongoing to define the optimal use of this technology.

Preparative Regimens and Stem Cell Infusions. Patients receive myeloablative dosages of chemotherapy with or without adjunctive radiation to treat the underlying disease. Total-body irradiation (TBI) can be used for immunosuppression or to treat the disease. These preparative therapies are known as the *conditioning regimen.*

Stem cell infusions are given IV. They can be injected via the slow bolus method or infused much like a blood transfusion (using tubing without a filter). The infused stem cells reconstitute the bone marrow elements, "rescuing" the recipient's hematopoietic system. It usually takes 2 to 4 weeks for the transplanted marrow to start making hematopoietic blood cells. During this period the patient has pancytopenia. The patient must be protected from exposure to infectious agents and supported with electrolyte supplements, nutrition, and blood component transfusions (as needed) to maintain adequate levels of circulating RBCs and platelets.

Complications. Bacterial, viral, and fungal infections are common after HSCT. Prophylactic therapies are used to reduce their incidence. A potentially serious complication of allogeneic transplant is graft-versus-host disease. This occurs when the T cells from the donated marrow (graft) recognize the recipient (host) as foreign and begin to attack certain organs, such as the skin, liver, and GI tract. (Graft-versus-host disease is discussed in Chapter 13.)

The occurrence and severity of posttransplant complications depend on the drugs used (some are more toxic than others) and the stem cell source. Because stem cells in the peripheral blood are more mature than those harvested from the marrow, the hematologic recovery period in PSCT is shorter, and fewer, less severe complications are seen.

GENE THERAPY

Gene therapy is an experimental therapy that involves introducing genetic material into a person's cells to fight disease. At this time, the use of gene therapy is investigational. (Gene therapy is discussed in Chapter 12.)

COMPLICATIONS OF CANCER

The patient may develop complications related to the continual growth of the cancer into normal tissue or to the side effects of treatment.

NUTRITIONAL PROBLEMS

Malnutrition

The patient with cancer may have protein and calorie malnutrition characterized by fat and muscle depletion. The assessment of malnutrition is discussed in Chapter 39.

Soft, nonirritating high-protein and high-calorie foods should be eaten throughout the day. Foods suggested for increasing the protein intake are shown in Table 15.17. High-calorie foods that provide energy and minimize weight loss are shown in Table 15.18. Foods in a high-calorie, high-protein diet are outlined in Table 39.10.

Teach the patient to avoid extremes of temperature, tobacco, alcohol, spicy or rough foods, and other irritants. Encourage nutritional supplements (e.g., Ensure) as an adjunct to meals and fluid intake. Weigh the patient at least twice each week to monitor for weight loss.

Suggest a referral for nutritional counseling to the patient or HCP as soon as a 5% weight loss is noted or if the patient has the potential for protein and calorie malnutrition. Monitor albumin and prealbumin levels. Once a 10-lb (4.5-kg) weight loss occurs, it may be hard to maintain the patient's nutritional status.

Teach the patient to use nutritional supplements in place of milk when cooking or baking. Foods to which nutritional supplements can be easily added include scrambled eggs, pudding, custard, mashed potatoes, cereal, and cream sauces. Packages of instant breakfast can be used as indicated or sprinkled on cereals, desserts, and casseroles.

Caregivers are an integral part of the health care team. As symptom severity increases, the caregiver's role in helping the patient eat becomes increasingly critical.

If the malnutrition cannot be treated with dietary intake, it may be necessary to use enteral or parenteral nutrition. (Enteral and parenteral nutrition are discussed in Chapter 39.)

TABLE 15.17 Nutritional Therapy

Protein Foods With High Biologic Value

Cheese
- Cottage: ½ cup = 15 g protein.
- American: 1 slice = 3 g protein.
- Cheddar: 1 slice = 6 g protein.
- Cream: 1 Tbsp = 1 g protein.
- Use cheese in a sandwich or as a snack.
- Add cheese to salads, casseroles, sauces, and baked potatoes.

Eggs
- Egg: 6 g protein.
- Eggnog: 1 cup = 15.5 g protein.
- Add eggs to salads, casseroles, and sauces. Deviled eggs are especially well tolerated.
- Desserts that contain eggs include angel food cake, sponge cake, custard, and cheesecake.

Meat, Poultry, Fish
- Pork: 3 oz = approx. 19 g protein.
- Chicken: ½ breast = approx. 26 g protein.
- Fish: 3 oz = approx. 30 g protein.
- Tuna fish: 6½ oz = approx. 44.5 g protein.
- Add meat, poultry, and fish to salads, casseroles, and sandwiches.
- Add strained and junior baby meats to soups and casseroles.

Milk
- Whole milk: 1 cup = 9 g protein.
- Double-strength milk (1 quart of whole milk plus 1 cup of dried skim milk blended and chilled): 1 cup = 14 g protein.
- Milk shake (1 cup of ice cream plus 1 cup of milk): 15 g protein, 415 cal.
- Use evaporated milk, double-strength milk, or half-and-half to make casseroles, hot cereals, sauces, gravies, puddings, milk shakes, and soups.
- Yogurt (regular and frozen): Select brands with high protein content: 1 cup = 10 g protein

TABLE 15.18 Nutritional Therapy

High-Calorie Foods

Mayonnaise	1 Tbsp	=	101 cal
Butter or margarine	1 tsp	=	35 cal
Sour cream	1 Tbsp	=	72 cal
Peanut butter	1 Tbsp	=	94 cal
Whipped cream	1 Tbsp	=	53 cal
Corn oil	1 Tbsp	=	119 cal
Jelly	1 Tbsp	=	49 cal
Ice cream	1 cup	=	256 cal
Honey	1 Tbsp	=	64 cal

Altered Taste Sensation (Dysgeusia)

Cancer cells may release substances that stimulate the bitter taste buds. The patient may have changes in the sweet, sour, and salty taste sensations. Meat may taste bitter or bland. We do not know the cause of these taste changes.

Teach patients with altered taste problems to avoid foods that they dislike. Often, the patient may feel compelled to eat certain foods that are believed to be beneficial. Tell the patient to try different ways to mask the taste changes. Some find stronger seasonings and spices effective. Others find it better to avoid strong flavors and eat more bland foods. Avoiding strong smells, drinking more water with food, oral care before eating, eating smaller amounts more often, and using plastic utensils may help.[21]

Cancer Cachexia

Cancer cachexia (wasting syndrome) is a complex, multifactorial syndrome characterized by anorexia and/or unintended loss of weight and appetite. It is accompanied by generalized tissue wasting, skeletal muscle atrophy, immune dysfunction, and metabolic problems. The weight loss cannot be reversed nutritionally. Patients with upper GI and pancreatic cancers are prone to cachexia. As cancer progresses, cachexia can affect many cancer patients. It is associated with increased morbidity.[22]

The best management of cancer cachexia is to effectively treat the cancer. Unfortunately, this is not a realistic goal for patients with advanced cancer. A second option is to increase nutritional intake, but this does not completely reverse the wasting associated with cachexia. A third option is to use megestrol acetate (Megace). It is a synthetic form of the hormone progesterone, which stimulates appetite in patients with cachexia.

INFECTION

Infection is a leading cause of death in the patient with cancer. The usual sites of infection include the lungs, GU system, mouth, rectum, peritoneal cavity, and blood (septicemia). Infection occurs because of the ulceration and necrosis caused by the tumor, the tumor compressing vital organs, and neutropenia from the cancer or cancer treatment.

Teach patients at risk for neutropenia to call their HCP if they have a temperature of 100.4° F (38° C) or greater. Assessment often includes signs and symptoms of fever, determination of possible cause (e.g., sinuses, mucous membranes, respiratory, GI, urinary, sites of any tubes or lines), and CBC.

Many patients are neutropenic when an infection develops. In these persons, infection may cause significant morbidity. It may be rapidly fatal if not treated promptly. The classic manifestations of infection are often subtle or absent in a patient with neutropenia and a depressed immune system. (Neutropenia was discussed earlier in this chapter on p. 248. It is also discussed in Chapter 30.)

ONCOLOGIC EMERGENCIES

Oncologic emergencies are life-threatening emergencies that can occur because of cancer or cancer treatment. These emergencies can be obstructive, metabolic, or infiltrative (Table 15.19).

Obstructive Emergencies

Obstructive emergencies are mainly caused by tumor obstruction of an organ or blood vessel. They include superior vena cava syndrome (Fig. 15.18), spinal cord compression syndrome, third space syndrome, and intestinal obstruction.

Metabolic Emergencies

Metabolic emergencies are caused by the production of ectopic hormones directly from the tumor or from metabolic problems caused by the cancer or cancer treatment. Ectopic hormones arise from tissues that do not normally make these hormones. Cancer cells return to a more embryonic form, thus allowing the cells' stored potential to become evident.

Metabolic emergencies include syndrome of inappropriate antidiuretic hormone secretion (Chapter 49), hypercalcemia (Chapter 16), tumor lysis syndrome, septic shock (Chapter 66), and disseminated intravascular coagulation (Chapter 30).

Infiltrative Emergencies

Infiltrative emergencies occur when cancer infiltrates major organs or from cancer treatment. The most common infiltrative emergencies are cardiac tamponade and carotid artery rupture.

CANCER PAIN

Moderate to severe pain occurs in around 50% of patients who are receiving active treatment for their cancer and in 80% to 90% of patients with advanced cancer.[23] What is concerning is that these statistics have not changed in the past 30 years. Undertreatment of cancer pain is common. It causes needless suffering, decreases quality of life, and increases the burden on caregivers.

Pain Assessment

Inadequate pain assessment is the single greatest barrier to effective pain management. Data, such as vital signs and patient behaviors, are not reliable indicators of pain, especially long-standing, chronic pain. It is important to know if pain is persistent or episodic, positional, or breakthrough pain. It is essential that a comprehensive pain assessment include a detailed history to elicit the characteristics of pain. This includes the quality, location, intensity, duration, and precipitating and alleviating factors. Distinguishing between types of pain (e.g., visceral, bone, neuropathic) is important in developing an effective pain management plan.

Assess pain on an ongoing basis to determine the effectiveness of the treatment plan. Obtain data and document at regular intervals the location and intensity of the pain, what it feels like, and how it is relieved. Assess change in pain (e.g., a change in the intensity, character, worsening, or location of pain) to determine the cause (e.g., progression of disease).

Always believe the patient's report and accept it as the primary source of assessment data. Table 15.20 presents assessment questions that may facilitate data collection. Have patients keep a pain management diary.[23]

Pain Management

Pain management for the cancer patient must address both persistent and breakthrough components of pain if they are present. Adjuvant therapies need to be delivered specific to the type or nature of the pain.

Drug therapy, including NSAIDs (e.g., ibuprofen), opioids (e.g., morphine), and adjuvant pain medications, should be used and selected based on the character and/or cause of the pain. Opioids normally are prescribed for the treatment of moderate to severe cancer pain. Drug dosages are adjusted to control pain with the fewest side effects. Analgesic medications (e.g., morphine, fentanyl) should be given on a regular schedule (around the clock) with more doses available as needed for breakthrough pain. In general, oral administration is preferred. Other routes (e.g., transdermal, transmucosal) are options.

Treatment plans should be developed that balance analgesia and side effects to maintain optimal functional status. It is important for you to pay attention to common side effects of pain medications (e.g., constipation) to ensure the patient's well-being and adherence with the pain management program. NSAIDs often serve as helpful adjuncts to opioid therapy, especially for bone pain. Antidepressant and antiseizure drugs may be helpful in managing neuropathic pain, which is often resistant to opioids.

TABLE 15.19 Oncologic Emergencies

Description	Manifestations	Management
Obstructive Emergencies		
Spinal Cord Compression		
• Neurologic emergency caused by cancer in epidural space of spinal cord. • Common causes are breast, lung, prostate, GI, renal cancers, melanoma. • Lymphomas can invade epidural space.	• Intense, localized, and persistent back pain with vertebral tenderness. • Motor weakness, sensory paresthesia and loss. • Autonomic dysfunction (e.g., change in bowel or bladder function).	• Radiation therapy, corticosteroids. • Surgical decompressive laminectomy. • Activity limitations and pain management.
Superior Vena Cava Syndrome (SVCS)		
• Results from obstruction of superior vena cava by tumor or thrombosis. • Common causes are lung cancer, non-Hodgkin's lymphoma, metastatic breast cancer. • Presence of central venous catheter and previous mediastinal radiation increase risk.	• Facial edema, periorbital edema. • Distention of veins of head, neck, and chest (Fig. 15.18). • Headache, seizures. • Mediastinal mass on chest x-ray.	• Considered a serious medical problem. • Radiation therapy to site of obstruction. • Chemotherapy for tumors more sensitive to this therapy.
Third Space Syndrome		
• Shifting of fluid from vascular space to interstitial space. • Occurs due to extensive surgical procedures, immunotherapy, septic shock.	• Signs of hypovolemia: hypotension, tachycardia, low central venous pressure, decreased urine output.	• Fluid, electrolyte, plasma protein replacement. • During recovery hypervolemia can occur, causing hypertension, increased central venous pressure, weight gain, shortness of breath.
Metabolic Emergencies		
Hypercalcemia		
• Occurs in metastatic disease of bone or multiple myeloma, or when a parathyroid hormone–like substance is secreted by cancer cells. • Immobility and dehydration can contribute to or worsen hypercalcemia.	• Serum calcium higher than 12 mg/dL (3 mmol/L) often produces symptoms. • Apathy, depression, fatigue, muscle weakness, ECG changes, polyuria and nocturia, anorexia, nausea, vomiting. • High calcium elevations can be life threatening. • Chronic hypercalcemia can result in nephrocalcinosis and irreversible renal failure.	• Treat primary disease. • Hydration (3 L/day) and bisphosphonate therapy. • Diuretics (especially loop diuretics) used to prevent heart failure or edema. • Infusion of bisphosphonate zoledronate (Zometa) or pamidronate (Aredia).
Syndrome of Inappropriate Antidiuretic Hormone (SIADH)		
• Tumor cells can produce abnormal or sustained production of antidiuretic hormone (ADH). • Many chemotherapy agents may contribute to ectopic ADH production or potentiate ADH effects.	• Water retention and hyponatremia (hypotonic hyponatremia) (see Chapter 49). • Weight gain without edema, weakness, anorexia, nausea, vomiting, personality changes, seizures, oliguria, decrease in reflexes, coma.	• Treat underlying cancer. • Take measures to correct sodium-water imbalance, including fluid restriction, oral salt tablets or isotonic (0.9%) saline administration, and IV 3% sodium chloride solution (severe cases). • Furosemide (Lasix) used in early phases. • Monitor sodium level. Correcting SIADH quickly may cause seizures or death.
Tumor Lysis Syndrome (TLS)		
• Metabolic complication characterized by rapid release of intracellular components in response to chemotherapy and radiation therapy (less often). • Massive cell destruction releases intracellular components (potassium, phosphate, DNA, RNA) that are metabolized to uric acid by liver.	• *Hallmark signs*: hyperuricemia, hyperphosphatemia, hyperkalemia, hypocalcemia. • Weakness, muscle cramps, diarrhea, nausea, vomiting. • Occurs within 24–48 hr after starting chemotherapy. • May last 5–7 days. • Metabolic abnormalities and concentrated uric acid (which crystallizes in distal tubules of kidneys) can lead to acute kidney injury.	• Identify patients at risk. • Increase urine production using hydration therapy. • Decrease uric acid concentrations using allopurinol. • Use IV sodium bicarbonate to counter effects of acidic properties that are released.
Infiltrative Emergencies		
Cardiac Tamponade		
• Fluid accumulation in pericardium. • Caused by constriction of pericardium by tumor or pericarditis from radiation therapy to the chest.	• Heavy feeling over chest, shortness of breath, tachycardia, cough, dysphagia, hiccups, hoarseness. • Nausea, vomiting, excessive perspiration. • Decreased level of consciousness, distant or muted heart sounds. • Extreme anxiety.	• Decrease fluid around heart using (1) surgery to create a pericardial window or an (2) indwelling pericardial catheter. • Administer O_2 therapy, IV hydration, and vasopressor therapy.
Carotid Artery Rupture		
• Invasion of arterial wall by tumor or erosion following surgery or radiation therapy. • Occurs most often in patients with head and neck cancer.	• Bleeding: ranges from minor oozing to spurting of blood in the case of a "blowout" of artery.	• Give IV fluids and blood products. • Surgery: ligation of carotid artery above and below rupture site and reduction of local tumor.

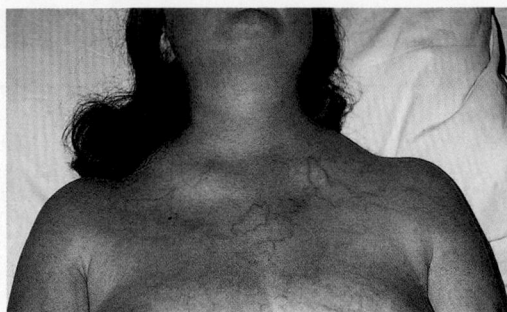

FIG. 15.18 Superior vena caval obstruction in bronchial cancer. Note the swelling of the face and neck and the development of collateral circulation in the veins. (From Forbes CD, Jackson WF: *Colour atlas and text of clinical medicine,* ed 3, London, 2003, Mosby.)

TABLE 15.20 Pain Assessment in Cancer Patients

Characteristic	Questions to Ask
Location	• Where is the pain? • Is the pain in more than one place? Is the pain in a new location? • Does location of pain correlate with known diagnosis?
Intensity	• How bad is the pain? • Rate the pain on a scale of 0 to 10. (See Chapter 8 for rating scales.)
Quality	• What does the pain feel like—sharp, dull, burning, shooting, aching, or other? (See Chapter 8 for descriptors.)
Pattern	• Has the pain changed? • Is the pain getting better, worse, or unchanged? • What makes the pain better or worse?
Relief measures	• What do you do to control your pain? • Do you use medications? • Do the relief measures help much? How much?

TABLE 15.21 Factors Affecting How Patients Cope With Cancer

Factor	Description
Ability to cope with stressful events in the past	How patients coped with previous stressful events (e.g., loss of job, major disappointment, significant traumatic event) affects how they cope with diagnosis of cancer.
Ability to express feelings and concerns	Patients who express feelings and needs and ask for help cope better than those who internalize feelings and needs.
Age at the time of diagnosis	Age determines coping strategies to a great degree. For example, a young mother with cancer may have different concerns than a 70-yr-old woman with cancer.
Attitude associated with the cancer	Patients who feel in control and have a positive attitude about cancer and cancer treatment cope better with the diagnosis and treatment of cancer than those who feel hopeless, helpless, and out of control.
Availability of significant others	Patients who have effective support systems cope better than those who do not.
Disruption of body image	Disruption of the body image (e.g., radical neck dissection, alopecia, mastectomy) may intensify the psychologic impact of cancer.
Extent of disease	Cure or control of the disease process is usually easier to cope with than the reality of terminal illness.
Past experience with cancer	Negative experiences with cancer (personal or in others) influence perceptions about the current situation.
Symptoms	Symptoms such as fatigue, nausea, diarrhea, and pain may intensify the psychologic impact of cancer.

Radioactive drugs (e.g., samarium-153) may help patients with diffuse bone pain, especially if no further chemotherapy is planned. Patients may have an initial pain *flare* after administration. Nerve blocks or epidural or intrathecal analgesia may be used to treat patients with unrelieved pain or to minimize the use of opioids.

Discuss the goals of analgesic therapy with patients, especially those needing large or chronic doses of opioids. You need to assess the patient for risk factors for opioid misuse. Patient teaching should clarify myths and misconceptions and reassure patients and caregivers that cancer pain can be effectively relieved. Fear of addiction is not warranted. However, it must be addressed as part of patient teaching. It is a significant barrier for patients and nurses in appropriate pain management. Stress that addiction and tolerance are not problems associated with effective cancer pain management. Nondrug interventions, including relaxation therapy and imagery, can be effectively used to manage pain (see Chapter 6). Other strategies to relieve pain are discussed in Chapter 8.

COPING WITH CANCER AND TREATMENT

You have a key role in assisting patients in coping with the psychosocial issues associated with cancer and cancer treatment. The patient may have a variety of concerns, including fears of dependency, loss of control, family and relationship stress, financial burden, and fear of death. Anxiety and fear may occur throughout the cancer continuum, including at diagnosis, during or after treatment, and in association with long-term follow-up.

Repetitive office visits or hospitalizations, continuing medications, and frequent laboratory testing force the patient to confront the cancer on a daily basis. Treatment-related uncertainties and fears are often most evident at the beginning of therapy. However, anxiety and fear may be present throughout treatment and when therapy is completed (e.g., fear of recurrence, less available support).

Adaptation and coping with a cancer diagnosis may be influenced by a variety of patient factors. These include demographics, prior coping skills and strategies, social support, and religious and spiritual beliefs (Table 15.21). You are in a key position to assess the patient's and caregiver's responses and support positive coping strategies. To promote effective coping and to support them during the various stages of cancer, you should:

- Be available and continue to be available, especially during difficult times.
- Exhibit a caring attitude.
- Listen actively to fears and concerns.
- Help provide relief from distressing symptoms.
- Provide accurate, essential information about cancer and cancer care.

- Help establish realistic expectations about what the patient will experience.
- Maintain a relationship based on trust and confidence. Be open, honest, and caring in the approach.
- Use touch to show caring. A squeeze of the hand or a hug may at times be more effective than words.
- Help the patient in setting realistic, reachable short-term and long-term goals.
- Help the patient maintain usual lifestyle patterns.
- Maintain hope, which is the key to effective cancer care.

Hope varies, depending on the patient's status—hope that the symptoms are not serious, hope that the treatment is curative, hope for independence, hope for relief of pain, hope for a longer life, hope to achieve meaningful goals, or hope for a peaceful death. Hope provides control over what is occurring and is the basis of a positive attitude toward cancer and cancer care.

Tell patients that they will be followed, and reassure them that support is ongoing. Give information and support to help minimize the negative impact of cancer treatment on quality of life. Patient teaching and symptom management help patients to self-manage their illness (e.g., adjusting treatment schedules to allow patients to work when possible, making referrals to support groups). Work with the oncology nurse navigators, who serve as the liaison between the patient and members of the interprofessional care team.

Arrange for patients to meet with people who have successfully completed therapy. This can increase their hopefulness and confidence. Make regular supportive telephone contacts between office visits. Assist with planning for transportation, nutrition, and emotional support.

Do not forget the caregivers. They need education and support throughout the trajectory of diagnosis, treatment, and follow-up. Patients and caregivers may benefit from a variety of psychosocial interventions. These include supportive listening, stress management techniques, individual or group counseling, and cognitive-behavioral therapy. Assess the psychosocial concerns and emotional responses of patients, caregivers, and families so you can connect them with appropriate supportive care resources. Use the available resources in the community, such as the ACS, Cancer Lifeline, churches, and other community resources.

Gerontologic Considerations: Cancer

Cancer is usually a disease of aging, with 78% of cancers occurring in people 55 years or older.[1] Cancer mortality rates are exceedingly high in older adults. Of all deaths due to cancer, 70% occur in those over age 65. This is especially important since the normal life span is increasing and the proportion of the population who are older than 65 years is increasing.

Manifestations of cancer in older adults may be mistakenly attributed to age-related changes and ignored by the person.[24] Older adults are especially at risk for complications of both cancer and cancer treatment. This is due to their decline in physiologic functioning, social and emotional resources, and cognitive function.

The older adult's functional status should be taken into consideration when developing a treatment plan. Age alone is not a good predictor of tolerance or response to treatment. Advances in cancer treatment are making cancer therapies beneficial to more older adults, including those with suboptimal health.

ETHICAL/LEGAL DILEMMAS
Medical Futility

Situation

D.M., a 65-yr-old Asian woman, has breast cancer with metastasis to the liver and bone. The family asks you why their mother is not receiving chemotherapy. They want to make sure that she will be resuscitated should her heart stop. They are aware of her diagnosis and that she only has a few months to live. In morning rounds, you were told that D.M. does not want any more treatment that would prolong her life.

Ethical/Legal Points for Consideration

- Although court decisions have varied, legally there is substantial consensus about the right to privacy (a constitutional right), right to informed consent and refusal of treatment, and rights about end-of-life decision making. The *Code of Ethics for Nurses* addresses the key components in the informed consent process that nurses must address.[1]
- A patient who is an adult and is competent (defined as capable of understanding and interpreting information, making choices, and communicating those choices) solely retains the right to make personal health care decisions.
- The Patient Self-Determination Act requires that the patient be asked on admission whether they have an advance directive. If available, it is placed in the medical record. If the patient does not have an advance directive, it must be documented.
- The National POLST Paradigm is an approach to end-of-life planning that emphasizes patients' wishes about the care they receive. The POLST Paradigm is an approach to end-of-life planning emphasizing the medical orders and includes coverage regardless of location (e.g., hospital, home, assisted living).[2]
- Often families have difficulty accepting the finality of a terminal diagnosis.
- Sometimes family members have conflicting interests (e.g., finances, property, inheritance rights) that influence their decision-making abilities.

Discussion Questions

1. How can you help D.M. communicate her wishes to her family?
2. How can you and the interprofessional team help the family in planning end-of-life care that incorporates their mother's wishes?
3. What are the cultural issues in D.M.'s case?

References

1. Code of Ethics for Nurses. Retrieved from. *www.nursingworld.org/practice-policy/nursing-excellence/ethics/code-of-ethics-for-nurses/*.
2. Physician Orders for Life Sustaining Treatment (POLST) Paradigm. Retrieved from. *www.polst.org*.

Assess the patient at the time of diagnosis to identify important issues that may affect decisions about treatment options. Issues to assess include projected life expectancy, estimate of morbidity from cancer, co-morbidities that would affect treatment, and patient decision-making capacity and wishes.

Some important questions to consider when an older adult is diagnosed with cancer include: Will the treatment provide more benefits than harm? Will they be able to tolerate the treatment safely? Is there a need to treat co-morbidities or nutritional or functional status before starting treatment? What are the patient's preferences and wishes?

CANCER SURVIVORSHIP

As the overall death rate from cancer decreases, the number of cancer survivors continues to increase. It is estimated that there are currently more than 14.5 million cancer survivors in the

TABLE 15.22 Patient Teaching

Cancer Survivors

You can help cancer survivors by doing the following:

1. Provide all cancer patients with a treatment summary and care plan outlining treatment exposures, risk for late effects, preventive care recommendations, and follow-up surveillance plan after completion of treatment.
   - Care plans should clearly identify all members of the interprofessional team and their responsibilities for follow-up care.
   - Include referrals to appropriate supportive care and community resources that would help the patient in recovery or ongoing care.
2. Coordinate care among the oncology team, primary HCP, and other specialists.
3. Teach HCPs about the needs of cancer survivors, including long-term effects of cancer and cancer treatments.
4. Teach cancer survivors to look for and report any ongoing symptoms resulting from treatment, including late effects of radiation therapy and chemotherapy.
5. Teach cancer survivors healthy behaviors:
   - *Prevention:* good nutrition, exercise, smoking avoidance, maintaining proper weight, cardiac risk reduction, bone health.
   - *Early detection:* routine health screenings (e.g., breast, colon), cholesterol, diabetes, osteoporosis screening as recommended.
6. Encourage cancer survivors to have regular follow-up examinations with their HCP.
7. Assess for psychologic, financial, health insurance, or vocational problems related to cancer. Assist patients in getting appropriate help if necessary.

TABLE 15.23 Resources for Cancer Survivors

Organization	Purpose
ACS Cancer Survivors Network	Provides survivorship information and resources and online forum for connecting with others affected by cancer. (*https://csn.cancer.org/*)
CancerCare	Provides a variety of free support services delivered by professional oncology social workers for patients and anyone else affected by cancer. (*www.cancer-care.org*)
Cancer.Net	American Society of Clinical Oncology (ASCO) patient support site that includes extensive information and resources for cancer survivors. (*www.cancer.net*)
National Cancer Institute Office of Cancer Survivorship	Supports research into the short- and long-term physical, social, emotional, and economic effects of cancer survivorship. Offers educational and support resources for cancer survivors, caregivers, and advocates. (*www.cancercontrol.cancer.gov/ocs/*)
National Coalition for Cancer Survivorship	Advocates for quality cancer care. Seeks to teach patients and advocates about issues that affect the quality of life of cancer survivors. (*www.canceradvocacy.org*)

United States. Some of these persons are cancer free. Others still have evidence of cancer and may be receiving treatment. The increase in survivorship is attributed to the aging and growth of the population and improvements in early detection and treatment. Survival statistics vary by the type and stage of cancer.[1,25]

The rapid increase in cancer survivors has been accompanied by a greater awareness of the long-term health and quality-of-life issues that a cancer diagnosis imposes. Cancer survivors have a variety of long-term and late effects after treatment. You need to be aware of the effects of the various treatments so that you can teach patients and their caregivers.

The impact of cancer and its treatment confers greater risk for non–cancer-related death and co-morbidities (e.g., heart disease, diabetes, metabolic syndrome, endocrine dysfunction, osteoporosis) among cancer survivors. Cancer survivors may continue to have symptoms or functional impairment related to treatment for years after treatment.

The impact of a cancer diagnosis can affect many aspects of a patient's life. Cancer survivors often report financial, vocational, marital, and spiritual concerns long after treatment is over. Psychosocial and emotional issues can play a profound role in a patient's life after cancer. Many find living in uncertainty challenging.

Some patients may wish to return to their normal lives as soon as possible. They may not go to scheduled follow-up appointments. Others become cancer advocates or active members of a cancer support group. Still others allow their lives to revolve around the cancer and may even resist giving up the illness role.

Tips to help cancer survivors are described in Table 15.22. Connecting cancer survivors to online support and resources is a strategy to enhance positive health outcomes (Table 15.23).

 Culturally Competent Care: Cancer

Cancer incidence and death rates are disproportionately higher in blacks than in whites and other minority groups. Although overall racial disparities in cancer death rates have been declining, death rates continue to be higher among blacks than whites. Blacks are more likely to have later stage disease at the time of diagnosis than whites.[1]

PROMOTING HEALTH EQUITY

Cancer

- Cancer incidence and death rates for men are highest among blacks, followed by whites, Hispanics, and Asians/Pacific Islanders.
- Cancer incidence rates for women are highest among whites, followed by blacks, Hispanics, and Asians/Pacific Islanders.
- Cancer death rates for women are highest among blacks, followed by whites, Hispanics, and Asians/Pacific Islanders.

Differences in survival rates from cancer are attributed to a combination of factors. These include poverty, difficult access to and poorer quality of health care, more co-morbid conditions, and differences in tumor biology. Disparities in cancer care exist throughout the continuum from cancer prevention and screening to end-of-life care and survivorship. The disparity in prevention and screening results in cancer being in advanced stages at the time of diagnosis.[1,2]

Culturally competent care in oncology is needed to meet the needs of diverse groups. It involves awareness of personal background, how culture affects care delivery, and how to adapt to meet cultural needs. Nurses need to actively seek to understand cultural differences to meet the patient's needs. Culture is discussed in Chapter 2. Culturally competent care related to specific cancers is in the chapters in which the cancer is discussed.

BRIDGE TO NCLEX EXAMINATION

The number of the question corresponds to the same-numbered outcome at the beginning of the chapter.

1. Trends in the incidence and death rates of cancer include the fact that
   a. a higher percent of women than men have lung cancer.
   b. lung cancer is the most common type of cancer in men.
   c. blacks have a higher death rate from cancer than whites.
   d. breast cancer is the leading cause of cancer deaths in women.

2. What features of cancer cells distinguish them from normal cells *(select all that apply)*?
   a. Cells lack contact inhibition.
   b. Cells undergo rapid proliferation.
   c. Cells return to a previous undifferentiated state.
   d. Proliferation occurs when there is a need for more cells.
   e. New proteins characteristic of embryonic stage emerge on cell membrane.

3. A characteristic of the stage of progression in cancer development is
   a. oncogenic viral transformation of target cells.
   b. a reversible steady growth facilitated by carcinogens.
   c. a period of latency before clinical detection of cancer.
   d. proliferation of cancer cells despite host control mechanisms.

4. The primary protective role of the immune system related to malignant cells is
   a. surveillance for cells with tumor-associated antigens.
   b. binding with free antigens released by all cancer cells.
   c. producing blocking factors that immobilize cancer cells.
   d. reacting to a new set of antigenic determinants on cancer cells.

5. The nurse is caring for a 59-year-old woman who had surgery 1 day ago to remove an ovarian cancer mass. The patient is awaiting the pathology report. She is tearful and says that she is scared to die. The *most* effective nursing intervention at this point is to use this opportunity to
   a. motivate change in an unhealthy lifestyle.
   b. teach her about the 7 warning signs of cancer.
   c. discuss healthy stress relief and coping practices.
   d. let her communicate about the meaning of this experience.

6. The goals of cancer treatment are based on the principle that
   a. surgery is the single most effective treatment for cancer.
   b. initial treatment is always directed toward cure of the cancer.
   c. a combination of treatment modalities is effective for controlling many cancers.
   d. although cancer cure is rare, quality of life can be increased with treatment modalities.

7. The *most* effective method of administering a chemotherapy agent that is a vesicant is to
   a. give it orally.
   b. give it intraarterially.
   c. use an Ommaya reservoir.
   d. use a central venous access device.

8. The nurse explains to a patient undergoing brachytherapy of the cervix that she
   a. must undergo simulation to locate the treatment area.
   b. requires the use of radioactive precautions during nursing care.
   c. may have desquamation of the skin on the abdomen and upper legs.
   d. requires shielding of the ovaries during treatment to prevent ovarian damage.

9. A patient on chemotherapy and radiation for head and neck cancer has a WBC count of $1.9 \times 10^3/\mu L$, hemoglobin of 10.8 g/dL, and a platelet count of $99 \times 10^3/\mu L$. Based on the CBC results, what is the *most* serious clinical finding?
   a. Cough, rhinitis, and sore throat
   b. Fatigue, nausea, and skin redness at site of radiation
   c. Temperature of 101.9° F, fatigue, and shortness of breath
   d. Skin redness at site of radiation, headache, and constipation

10. To prevent fever and shivering during an infusion of rituximab (Rituxan), the nurse should premedicate the patient with
    a. aspirin.
    b. acetaminophen.
    c. sodium bicarbonate.
    d. meperidine (Demerol).

11. The nurse counsels the patient receiving radiation therapy or chemotherapy that
    a. effective birth control methods should be used for the rest of the patient's life.
    b. after successful treatment, patients can expect a return to their previous level of function.
    c. the cycle of fatigue-depression-fatigue that may occur during treatment may be reduced by restricting activity.
    d. nausea and vomiting can usually be managed with antiemetic drugs, diet modification, and other interventions.

12. A patient on chemotherapy for 10 weeks started at a weight of 121 lb. She now weighs 118 lb and has no sense of taste. Which nursing intervention would be a *priority*?
    a. Discuss with the provider the need for parenteral nutrition.
    b. Teach the patient to eat foods that are fatty, fried, or high in calories.
    c. Tell the patient to drink a nutritional supplement beverage three times a day.
    d. Have the patient try various spices and seasonings to enhance the flavor of food.

13. A 70-year-old male patient has multiple myeloma. His wife calls to report that he sleeps most of the day, is confused when awake, and reports nausea and constipation. Which complication of cancer is this *most* likely caused by?
    a. Hypercalcemia
    b. Tumor lysis syndrome
    c. Spinal cord compression
    d. Superior vena cava syndrome

14. A patient has recently been diagnosed with early stages of breast cancer. What is *most* appropriate for the nurse to focus on?
    a. Maintaining the patient's hope
    b. Preparing a will and advance directives
    c. Discussing replacement child care for the patient's children
    d. Discussing the patient's past experiences with her grandmother's cancer

1. c, 2. a, c, e, 3. d, 4. a, 5. d, 6. c, 7. d, 8. b, 9. c, 10. b, 11. d, 12. d, 13. a, 14. a

For rationales to these answers and even more NCLEX review questions, visit *http://evolve.elsevier.com/Lewis/medsurg*.

ⓔ EVOLVE WEBSITE/RESOURCES LIST

http://evolve.elsevier.com/Lewis/medsurg
Review Questions (Online Only)
Key Points
Answer Keys for Questions
- Rationales for Bridge to NCLEX Examination Questions
Conceptual Care Map Creator
Supporting Media
- Animations
  - Chemotherapy
  - Radiation Therapy
Audio Glossary
Content Updates

REFERENCES

1. American Cancer Society: Cancer facts & figures 2018. Retrieved from *www.cancer.org/research/cancer-facts-statistics/all-cancer-facts-figures/cancer-facts-figures-2018.html.*

*2. Siegel RL, Miller KD, Jemal A: Cancer statistics 2018, *CA Cancer J Clin* 68:7, 2018.

3. National Cancer Institute: Cancer trends progress report. Retrieved from *www.progressreport.cancer.gov.*

4. Centers for Disease Control and Prevention: Skin cancer. Retrieved from *www.cdc.gov/cancer/skin/.*

5. Kanabar AH, Sacher RA, Besa EC: Burkitt lymphoma and Burkitt-like lymphoma. Retrieved from *https://emedicine.medscape.com/article/1447602-overview.*

*6. American Cancer Society: Cancer screening guidelines. Retrieved from *www.cancer.org/healthy/find-cancer-early/cancer-screening-guidelines.html.*

7. American Society of Clinical Oncology: What is personalized cancer medicine? Retrieved from *www.cancer.net/navigating-cancer-care/how-cancer-treated/personalized-and-targeted-therapies/what-personalized-cancer-medicine.*

*8. Kamps R, Brandao RD, van den Bosch BJ, et al: Next-generation sequencing in oncology: genetic diagnosis, risk prediction and cancer classification, *Int J Mol Sci* 18:1, 2017.

9. Patel JN: Cancer pharmacogenomics, challenges in implementation and patient focused perspectives. Retrieved from *www.ncbi.nlm.nih.gov/pmc/articles/PMC4948716/.*

10. Polovich M, Olsen M, LeFebvre K: *Chemotherapy and biotherapy guidelines and recommendations for practice,* ed 4, Pittsburgh, 2014, Oncology Nursing Society.

11. National Institute for Occupational Safety and Health: Safe handling of chemotherapy agents. Retrieved from *www.cdc.gov/niosh/topics/antineoplastic.*

*12. Mhaskar R, Clark OA, Lyman G, et al: Colony-stimulating factors for chemotherapy-induced febrile neutropenia, *Cochrane Database Syst Rev* 10:CD003039, 2014. (Classic)

13. National Cancer Institute: Fatigue (PDQ^R)—Health professional version. Retrieved from *www.cancer.gov/about-cancer/treatment/side-effects/fatigue/fatigue-hp-pdq.*

*14. Rugo HS, Voight J: Scalp hypothermia for preventing alopecia during chemotherapy: a systematic review and meta-analysis of randomized controlled trials, *Clin Breast Cancer* 18:19, 2018.

*15. Loh KP, Janelsins MC, Mohile SG, et al: Chemotherapy-related cognitive impairment, *J Geriatr Oncol* 7:270, 2016.

*16. Oktay K, Harvey BE, Partridge AH, et al: Fertility preservation in patients with cancer: ASCO clinical practice guideline update, *J Clin Oncol* 36:1994, 2018.

*17. Langer T, Grabow D, Steinmann D, et al: Late effects and long-term follow-up after cancer in childhood, *Oncol Res Treatment* 40:746, 2017.

18. American Cancer Society (ACS): What is targeted cancer therapy? Retrieved from *www.cancer.org/treatment/treatments-and-side-effects/treatment-types/targeted-therapy/what-is.html.*

19. National Cancer Institute: Targeted cancer therapies. Retrieved from *www.cancer.gov/about-cancer/treatment/types/targeted-therapies/targeted-therapies-fact-sheet.*

20. Gratwohl A: Global perspectives on hematopoietic stem cell transplants. In *Establishing a hematopoietic stem cell transplantation unit,* New York, 2018, Springer.

*21. Munankarmi D: Management of dysgeusia related to cancer, *JLMC* 5:3, 2017.

*22. Arends J, Baracos V, Bertz H, et al: ESPEN expert group recommendations for action against cancer-related malnutrition, *Clin Nutr* 36:1187, 2017.

23. National Comprehensive Cancer Network: *National clinical practice guidelines in oncology: Adult cancer pain,* version 1, 2018. Retrieved from www.nccn.org/.

24. National Institute on Aging: Global health and aging. Retrieved from *www.nia.nih.gov/sites/default/files/2017-06/global_health_aging.pdf.*

*25. Miller KD, Siegel RL, Lin CC, et al: Cancer treatment and survivorship statistics, 2016, *CA Cancer J Clin* 66:271, 2016.

*Evidence-based information for clinical practice.

16

Fluid, Electrolyte, and Acid-Base Imbalances

Margaret R. Rateau

Even the smallest act of caring for another person is like a drop of water. It will make ripples throughout the entire pond.

Jessy Mateo

http://evolve.elsevier.com/Lewis/medsurg/

CONCEPTUAL FOCUS

Acid-Base Balance   Nutrition
Fluids and Electrolytes

LEARNING OUTCOMES

1. Describe the composition of the major body fluid compartments.
2. Define processes involved in regulating the movement of water and electrolytes between the body fluid compartments.
3. Describe the etiology, laboratory diagnostic findings, clinical manifestations, and nursing and interprofessional management of the following disorders:
   a. Extracellular fluid volume imbalances: fluid volume deficit and fluid volume excess
   b. Sodium imbalances: hypernatremia and hyponatremia
   c. Potassium imbalances: hyperkalemia and hypokalemia
   d. Magnesium imbalances: hypermagnesemia and hypomagnesemia
   e. Calcium imbalances: hypercalcemia and hypocalcemia
   f. Phosphate imbalances: hyperphosphatemia and hypophosphatemia
4. Identify the processes involved in maintaining acid-base balance.
5. Discuss the etiology, diagnostic findings, clinical manifestations, and nursing and interprofessional management of the following acid-base imbalances: metabolic acidosis, metabolic alkalosis, respiratory acidosis, and respiratory alkalosis.
6. Describe the composition of and indications for common IV fluid solutions.
7. Discuss the types and nursing management of commonly used central venous access devices.

KEY TERMS

acidosis, p. 285
alkalosis, p. 285
anions, p. 269
buffers, p. 285
cations, p. 269
central venous access devices (CVADs), p. 292

electrolytes, p. 269
fluid spacing, p. 272
hydrostatic pressure, p. 271
hypernatremia, p. 276
hypertonic, p. 271
hyponatremia, p. 278

hypotonic, p. 271
isotonic, p. 271
oncotic pressure, p. 271
osmolality, p. 271
osmotic pressure, p. 270

HOMEOSTASIS

Body fluids and electrolytes play an important role in maintaining *homeostasis,* the body's stable internal environment. Body fluids are in constant motion transporting nutrients, electrolytes, and oxygen to cells and carrying waste products away from cells. The body uses many adaptive responses to keep the composition and volume of fluids and electrolytes within narrow limits to maintain homeostasis and promote health.

Many diseases and their treatments affect fluid and electrolyte balance. Conceptually, these imbalances are often reflected by changes in perfusion, gas exchange, mobility, and cognition. For example, a patient with metastatic colon cancer may develop hypercalcemia because of bone destruction from tumor invasion and have severe muscle weakness and confusion. Chemotherapy used to treat the cancer may result in nausea and vomiting, which causes dehydration and acid-base imbalances.

When correcting dehydration with IV fluids, the patient needs close monitoring to prevent fluid overload.

It is important to anticipate the potential for fluid and electrolyte imbalances associated with certain disorders and medical therapies, recognize the signs and symptoms of imbalances, and intervene with the appropriate action. This chapter describes the (1) normal control of fluids, electrolytes, and acid-base balance; (2) conditions that disrupt homeostasis and resulting manifestations; and (3) actions that the health care provider and you can take to manage fluid, electrolyte, and acid-base imbalances and restore homeostasis.

WATER CONTENT OF THE BODY

The body is composed primarily of water. It accounts for about 50% to 60% of body weight in the adult. Water content varies with body mass, gender, and age (Fig. 16.1). Lean body mass has

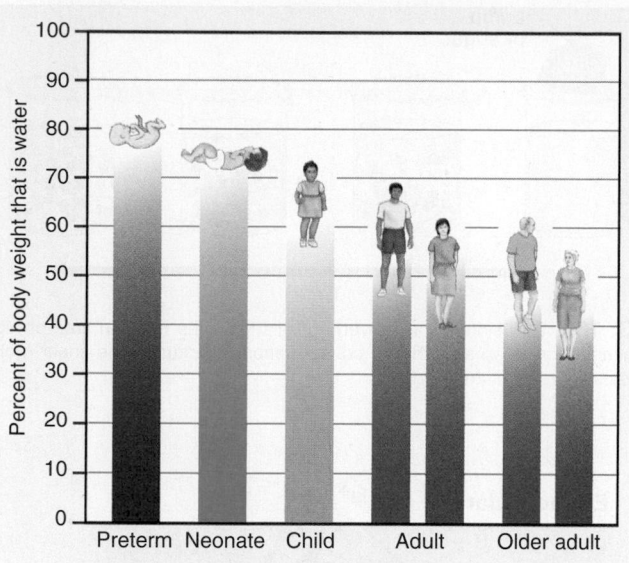

FIG. 16.1 Body water over the life span.

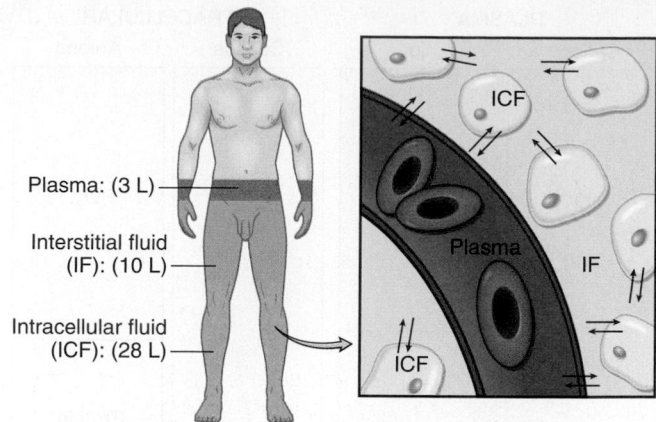

FIG. 16.2 Relative volumes of 3 body fluids. Values represent fluid distribution in a young male adult.

a higher percentage of water, while adipose tissue has a lesser percentage of water. So, the more fat present in the body, the less the total water content. Women generally have a lower percentage of body water because they tend to have less lean body mass than men. Older adults also tend to have less lean body mass, resulting in a lower percentage of body water when compared to younger adults. In older adults, body water content averages 45% to 50% of body weight. This places them at a higher risk for fluid-related problems than young adults.

Body Fluid Compartments

The 2 fluid compartments in the body are the *intracellular space* (inside the cells) and the *extracellular space* (outside the cells) (Fig. 16.2). About two thirds of body water is found within cells and is termed *intracellular fluid* (ICF). ICF makes up about 40% of body weight of an adult. This means a 70-kg young man would have about 42 L of water, with about 28 L of that water within his cells.

The fluid in the extracellular space is *extracellular fluid* (ECF). The 2 main compartments containing ECF are the *interstitial fluid*, or the fluid in the spaces between cells, and the *intravascular fluid* or *plasma*, the liquid part of blood. Other ECF compartments include lymph and *transcellular fluids*. Transcellular fluids include cerebrospinal fluid; fluid in the gastrointestinal (GI) tract and joint spaces; and pleural, peritoneal, intraocular, and pericardial fluid. ECF makes up about one third of the body water; this amounts to about 14 L in a 70-kg man. About one third of ECF is in the intravascular space as plasma (3 L in a 70-kg man), and two thirds is in the interstitial space (10 L in a 70-kg man). The fluid in the transcellular spaces totals about 1 L at any given time.

Calculation of Fluid Gain or Loss

One liter of water weighs 2.2 lb. (1 kg). Body weight change, especially sudden change, is an excellent indicator of overall fluid volume loss or gain. For example, if a patient drinks 240 mL (8 oz) of fluid, weight gain will be 0.5 lb (0.23 kg). A patient receiving diuretic therapy who loses 4.4 lb (2 kg) in 24 hours has a fluid loss of about 2 L. An adult patient who is fasting may lose 1 to 2 lb/day. A weight loss exceeding this is likely due to loss of body fluid.

ELECTROLYTES

Electrolytes are substances whose molecules dissociate, or split, into ions when placed in water. *Ions* are electrically charged particles. Cations are positively charged ions. Examples include sodium (Na^+), potassium (K^+), calcium (Ca^{2+}), and magnesium (Mg^{2+}) ions. Anions are negatively charged ions. Examples include bicarbonate (HCO_3^-), chloride (Cl^-), and phosphate (PO_4^{3-}) ions. Most proteins bear a negative charge and thus are anions.

Measurement of Electrolytes

The concentration of electrolytes in body fluids is expressed in milliequivalents (mEq) per liter. Since electrolytes are active chemicals, it is useful to express their concentration according to their chemical activity, or the number of electrolytes able to combine chemically. Ions combine milliequivalent for milliequivalent. For example, 1 mEq (1 mmol) of sodium combines with 1 mEq (1 mmol) of chloride.

Electrolyte Composition of Fluid Compartments

Electrolyte composition varies between ECF and ICF. The overall concentration of electrolytes is nearly the same in the ECF and ICF. However, concentrations of specific ions differ greatly (Fig. 16.3). In ECF the main cation is sodium, with small amounts of potassium, calcium, and magnesium. The primary ECF anion is chloride, with small amounts of bicarbonate, sulfate, and phosphate anions.

In ICF the prevalent cation is potassium, with small amounts of magnesium and sodium. The prevalent ICF anion is phosphate, with some protein and a small amount of bicarbonate. Table 16.1 lists normal serum electrolyte values.

MECHANISMS CONTROLLING FLUID AND ELECTROLYTE MOVEMENT

The movement of electrolytes and water between ICF and ECF to maintain homeostasis involves many different processes, including simple diffusion, facilitated diffusion, and active transport. Water moves as driven by 2 forces: hydrostatic pressure and osmotic pressure.

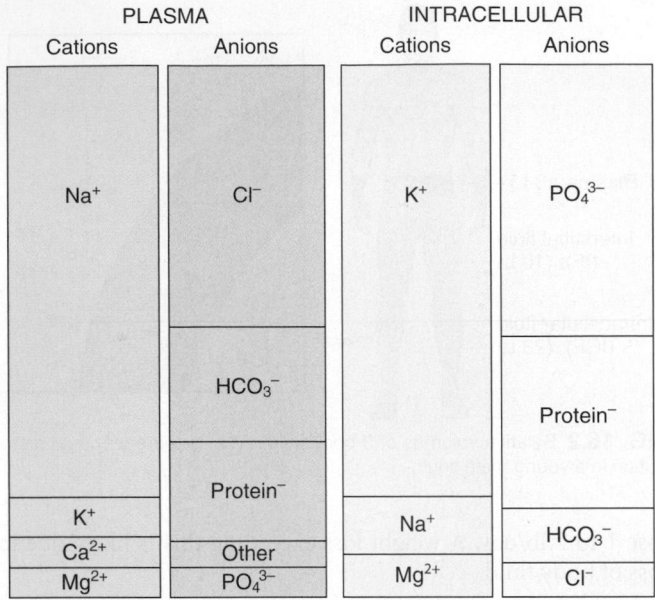

FIG. 16.3 The relative concentrations of the major cations and anions in the intracellular space and the plasma.

TABLE 16.1 Normal Serum Electrolyte Values	
Electrolyte	**Reference Interval**
Anions	
Bicarbonate (HCO₃⁻)	22–26 mEq/L (22–26 mmol/L)
Chloride (Cl⁻)	98–106 mEq/L (98–106 mmol/L)
Phosphate (PO₄³⁻)	3.0–4.5 mg/dL (0.97–1.45 mmol/L)
Cations	
Calcium (Ca²⁺) (total)	9.0–10.5 mg/dL (2.25–2.62 mmol/L)
Calcium (ionized)	4.5–5.6 mg/dL (1.05–1.3 mmol/L)
Magnesium (Mg²⁺)	1.3–2.1 mEq/L (0.65–1.05 mmol/L)
Potassium (K⁺)	3.5–5.0 mEq/L (3.5–5.0 mmol/L)
Sodium (Na⁺)	136–145 mEq/L (136–145 mmol/L)

Diffusion

Diffusion is the movement of molecules from an area of high concentration to low concentration (Fig. 16.4). Net movement of molecules stops when the concentrations are equal in both areas. It occurs in liquids, gases, and solids. Simple diffusion requires no external energy.

Facilitated Diffusion

Facilitated diffusion involves the use of a protein carrier in the cell membrane. The protein carrier combines with a molecule, especially one too large to pass easily through the cell membrane, and helps move the molecule across the membrane from an area of high to low concentration. Like simple diffusion, facilitated diffusion is passive and requires no energy. An example of facilitated diffusion is glucose transport into the cell. The large glucose molecule must combine with a carrier molecule to be able to cross the cell membrane and enter most cells.

Active Transport

Active transport is a process in which molecules move against the concentration gradient. External energy is needed for this

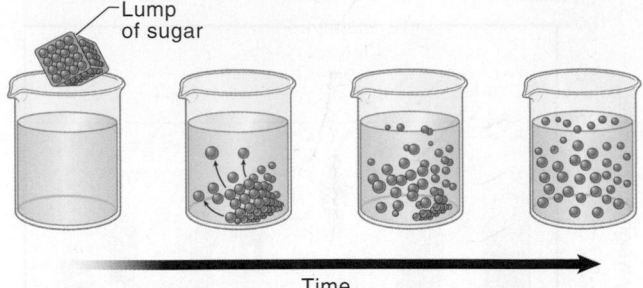

FIG. 16.4 Diffusion is the movement of molecules from an area of high concentration to an area of low concentration. Eventually, the sugar molecules are evenly distributed.

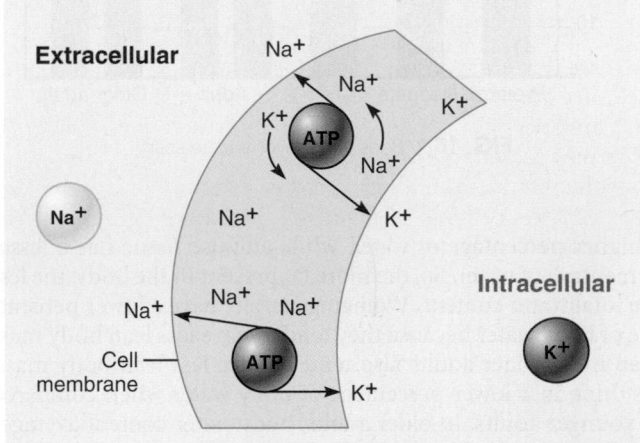

FIG. 16.5 Sodium-potassium pump. As sodium *(Na⁺)* diffuses into the cell and potassium *(K⁺)* diffuses out of the cell, an active transport system supplied with energy delivers Na⁺ back to the extracellular compartment and K⁺ to the intracellular compartment. *ATP,* Adenosine triphosphate.

process. An example is the sodium-potassium pump. The concentrations of sodium and potassium differ greatly intracellularly and extracellularly (Fig. 16.3). To maintain this concentration difference, the cell uses active transport to move sodium out of the cell and potassium into the cell (Fig. 16.5). The energy source for this movement is adenosine triphosphate (ATP), which is made in the cell mitochondria.

Osmosis

Osmosis is the movement of water "down" a concentration gradient, that is, from a region of low solute concentration to one of high solute concentration, across a semipermeable membrane. Osmosis requires no outside energy sources. It stops when the concentration differences disappear or when hydrostatic pressure builds and opposes any further movement of water. Imagine a chamber with 2 compartments separated by a semipermeable membrane, one that allows only the movement of water (Fig. 16.6). If you add albumin to one side, water will move from the less concentrated side (has more water) to the more concentrated side of the chamber (has less water) until the concentrations are equal.

Whenever dissolved substances are contained in a space with a semipermeable membrane, they can pull water into the space by osmosis. The concentration of the solution determines the strength of the osmotic pull. The higher the concentration, the greater a solution's pull, or **osmotic pressure**. Osmotic pressure is measured in milliosmoles (mOsm). It may be expressed as

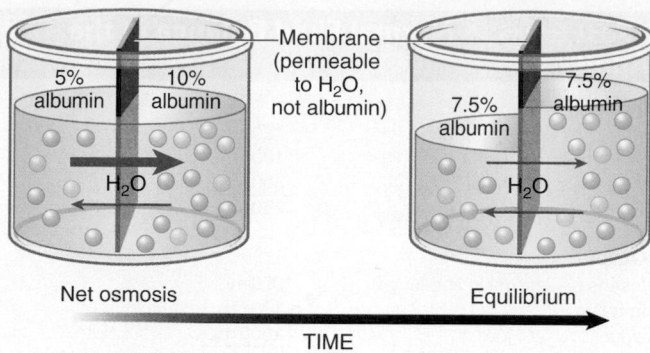

FIG. 16.6 Osmosis is the process of water movement through a semipermeable membrane from an area of low solute concentration to an area of high solute concentration.

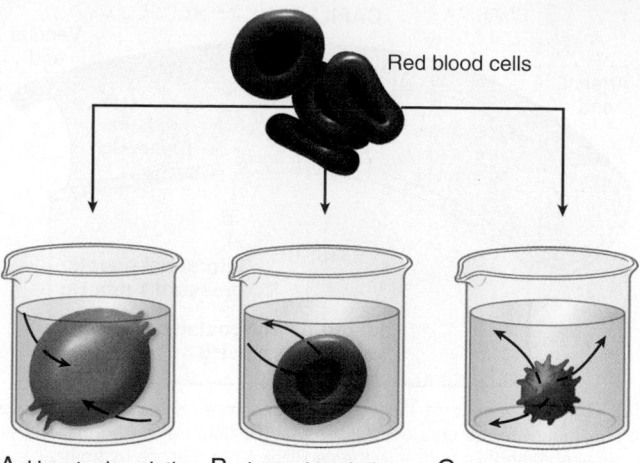

A Hypotonic solution **B** Isotonic solution **C** Hypertonic solution

FIG. 16.7 Effects of water status on red blood cells. **A,** Hypotonic solution (H_2O excess) results in cellular swelling. **B,** Isotonic solution (normal H_2O balance) results in no change. **C,** Hypertonic solution (H_2O deficit) results in cellular shrinking.

either fluid osmolarity or fluid osmolality. Although you will often see the terms *osmolarity* and *osmolality* used interchangeably, they are different measurements. *Osmolarity* measures the total milliosmoles per liter of solution, or the concentration of molecules per volume of solution (mOsm/L). **Osmolality** measures the number of milliosmoles per kilogram of water, or the concentration of molecules per weight of water. Osmolality is the preferred measure to evaluate the concentration of plasma, urine, and other body fluids, as changes in the ECF osmolality can significantly influence changes in the ICF osmolality. These changes can affect normal cell function.[1]

Measurement of Osmolality. Osmolality is nearly the same in the various body fluid spaces. Therefore measuring or estimating plasma osmolality is a useful way to assess the state of the body's water balance. Calculate the plasma osmolality using the following formula.[2]

$$\text{Plasma osmolality} = (2 \times \text{Na}) + (\text{BUN}/2.8) + (\text{Glucose}/18)$$

Normal plasma osmolality is between 280 and 295 mOsm/kg. A value greater than 295 mOsm/kg indicates that the concentration of solute is too great, or the water content is too little. This condition is termed *water deficit.* A value less than 275 mOsm/kg indicates too little solute for the amount of water or too much water for the amount of solute. This condition is termed *water excess.* Both conditions are clinically significant.

Urine osmolality can range from 100 to 1300 mOsm/kg. It depends on fluid intake, the amount of antidiuretic hormone (ADH) in circulation, and the renal response to ADH.

Osmotic Movement of Fluids. The osmolality of the fluid surrounding cells affects them. Fluids with the same osmolality as the cell interior are **isotonic.** Normally, ECF and ICF are isotonic to one another, so no net movement of water occurs.

Changes in the osmolality of ECF change the volume of cells. Solutions in which the solutes are less concentrated than in the cells are **hypotonic** (hypoosmolar). If a cell is surrounded by hypotonic fluid, water moves into the cell, causing it to swell and possibly burst. Fluids with solutes more concentrated than in cells, or an increased osmolality, are **hypertonic** (hyperosmolar). If hypertonic fluid surrounds a cell, water leaves the cell to dilute ECF. The cell shrinks and may eventually die (Fig. 16.7).

Hydrostatic Pressure

Hydrostatic pressure is the force of fluid in a compartment pushing against a cell membrane or vessel wall. In the blood vessels, hydrostatic pressure is the BP generated by the heart's contraction. Hydrostatic pressure in the vascular system

gradually decreases as the blood moves through the arteries until it is about 30 mm Hg in the capillary bed. At the capillary level, hydrostatic pressure is the major force that pushes water out of the vascular system and into the interstitial space.

Oncotic Pressure

Oncotic pressure (colloidal osmotic pressure) is the osmotic pressure caused by plasma colloids (large molecules) in solution. The major colloids in the vascular system contributing to osmotic pressure are proteins, such as albumin. Plasma has large amounts of protein, while the interstitial space has very little. Plasma protein molecules attract water, pulling fluid from the tissue space to the vascular space. Under normal conditions, plasma oncotic pressure is about 25 mm Hg. The small amount of protein found in the interstitial space exerts an oncotic pressure of about 1 mm Hg.

FLUID MOVEMENT IN CAPILLARIES

As plasma flows through the capillary bed, 4 factors determine if fluid moves out of the capillary and into the interstitial space or if fluid moves back into the capillary from the interstitial space. The amount and direction of movement are determined by the interaction of (1) capillary hydrostatic pressure, (2) plasma oncotic pressure, (3) interstitial hydrostatic pressure, and (4) interstitial oncotic pressure.

Capillary hydrostatic pressure and interstitial oncotic pressure move water out of the capillaries. Plasma oncotic pressure and interstitial hydrostatic pressure move fluid into the capillaries. At the arterial end of the capillary, capillary hydrostatic pressure exceeds plasma oncotic pressure, and fluid moves into the interstitial space. At the venous end of the capillary, the capillary hydrostatic pressure is lower than plasma oncotic pressure, drawing fluid back into the capillary by the oncotic pressure created by plasma proteins (Fig. 16.8).

Fluid Shifts

If capillary or interstitial pressures change, fluid may abnormally shift from one compartment to another, resulting in edema or dehydration.

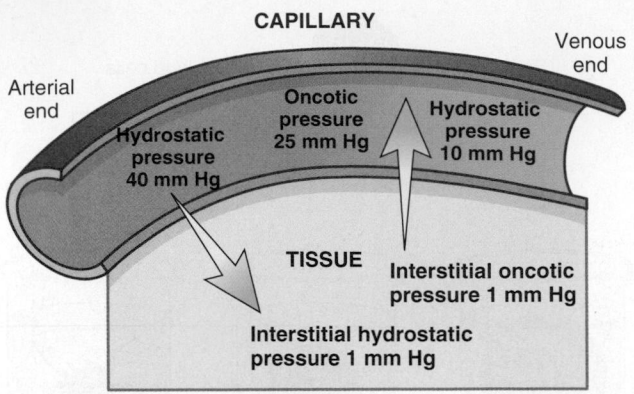

CAPILLARY

FIG. 16.8 Dynamics of fluid exchange between a capillary and tissue. An equilibrium exists between forces filtering fluid out of the capillary and forces absorbing fluid back into the capillary. Note that the hydrostatic pressure is greater at the arterial end of the capillary than at the venous end. The net effect of pressures at the arterial end of the capillary causes a movement of fluid into the tissue. At the venous end of the capillary, there is net movement of fluid back into the capillary.

TABLE 16.2 Normal Fluid Balance in the Adult

Intake	
Fluids	1200 mL
Solid food	1000 mL
Water from oxidation	300 mL
Total	2500 mL
Output	
Insensible loss (skin and lungs)	900 mL
In feces	100 mL
Urine	1500 mL
Total	2500 mL

Shifts of Plasma to Interstitial Fluid. *Edema,* an accumulation of fluid in the interstitial space, occurs if venous hydrostatic pressure rises, plasma oncotic pressure decreases, or interstitial oncotic pressure rises. Edema may also develop if an obstruction of lymphatic outflow causes a decrease in the removal of interstitial fluid.

Elevation of Venous Hydrostatic Pressure. Increasing the pressure at the venous end of the capillary inhibits fluid movement back into the capillary, which results in edema. Causes of increased venous pressure include fluid overload, heart failure, liver failure, obstruction of venous return to the heart (e.g., tourniquets, restrictive clothing, venous thrombosis), and venous insufficiency (e.g., varicose veins).

Decrease in Plasma Oncotic Pressure. Fluid stays in the interstitial space if the plasma oncotic pressure is too low to draw fluid back into the capillary. Low plasma protein content decreases oncotic pressure. This can result from excess protein loss (renal disorders), deficient protein synthesis (liver disease), and deficient protein intake (malnutrition).

Elevation of Interstitial Oncotic Pressure. Trauma, burns, and inflammation can damage capillary walls and allow plasma proteins to accumulate in the interstitial space. This increases interstitial oncotic pressure, draws fluid into the interstitial space, and holds it there.

Shifts of Interstitial Fluid to Plasma. An increase in the plasma osmotic or oncotic pressure draws fluid into the plasma from the interstitial space. This could happen when we give colloids, dextran, mannitol, or hypertonic solutions. Increasing the tissue hydrostatic pressure is another way of causing a shift of fluid into plasma. Wearing elastic compression gradient stockings or hose to decrease peripheral edema is a therapeutic application of this effect.

FLUID SPACING

Fluid spacing is a term used to describe the distribution of body water. *First spacing* describes the normal distribution of fluid in ICF and ECF compartments. *Second spacing* refers to an abnormal accumulation of interstitial fluid (i.e., edema). *Third spacing* occurs when excess fluid collects in the nonfunctional area between cells. This fluid is trapped where it is difficult or impossible for it to move back into the cells or blood vessels. Third spacing occurs with ascites; fluid leaking into the abdominal cavity with peritonitis or pancreatitis; and edema associated with burns, trauma, or sepsis.

REGULATION OF WATER BALANCE

Many factors are involved in maintaining the finely tuned balance among water intake, use, and excretion. For proper fluid balance, an average healthy adult needs a daily water intake between 2000 and 3000 mL (Table 16.2). This amount replaces what the body loses in urinary output and insensible losses. Oral fluid intake accounts for most of the water intake. Water intake also includes water from food metabolism and water present in solid foods.

Insensible water loss, which is invisible vaporization from the lungs and skin, helps regulate body temperature. Accelerated body metabolism, which occurs with increased body temperature and exercise, increases the amount of water lost and may result in the need for additional water replacement.

Do not confuse water loss through the skin with the vaporization of water excreted by sweat glands. Insensible perspiration causes only water loss. Excess sweating *(sensible perspiration)* caused by exercise, fever, or high environmental temperatures may lead to large losses of water and electrolytes.

Hypothalamic-Pituitary Regulation

Water ingestion equals water loss in the person who has free access to water, intact thirst and ADH mechanism, and normally functioning kidneys. A body fluid deficit or increase in plasma osmolality activates osmoreceptors in the hypothalamus. This stimulates thirst and the release of ADH from the posterior pituitary gland. ADH acts on the distal tubules and collecting ducts in the kidney by making them more permeable to water. The result is increased water reabsorption from the tubular filtrate into the blood and decreased excretion in the urine. Because ADH is only able to regulate how much water the body holds onto, an intact thirst mechanism is our main protection against developing dehydration or hyperosmolality. Thirst causes us to increase the amount of water we drink. Together these result in increased free water in the body, decreasing plasma osmolality and restoring fluid volume.

Many factors influence ADH secretion and thirst. Decreased BP, nausea, pain, hypoglycemia, and hypoxemia stimulate ADH release. In the postoperative patient, the stress response to surgery and receiving analgesics and anesthesia cause ADH release and decreased osmolality. The unconscious or cognitively

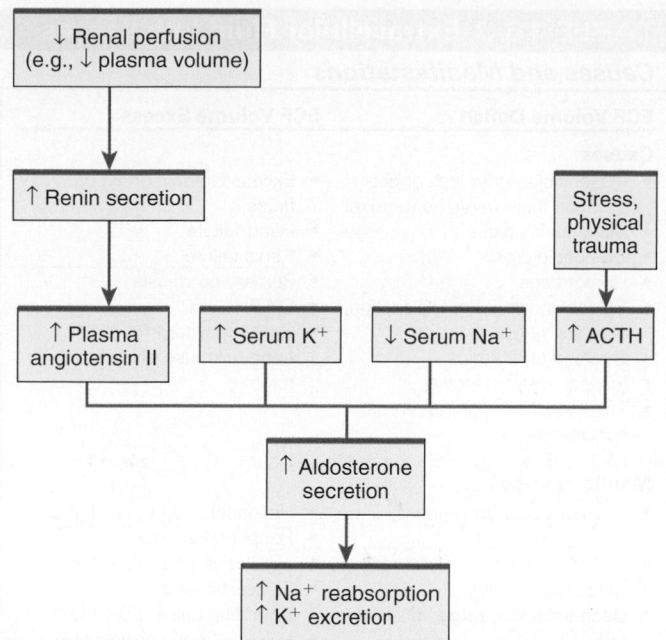

FIG. 16.9 Factors affecting aldosterone secretion. *ACTH,* Adrenocorticotropic hormone.

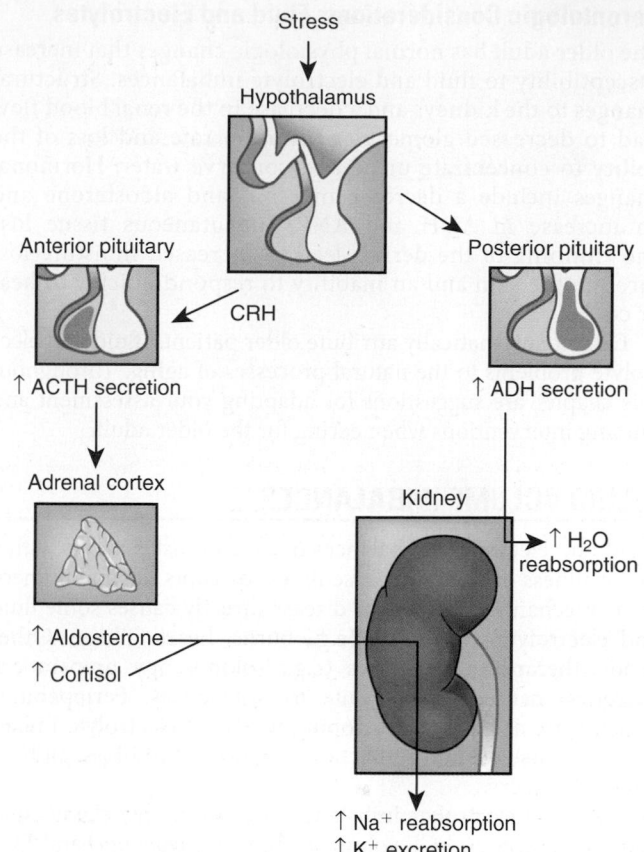

FIG. 16.10 Effects of stress on fluid and electrolyte balance. *ACTH,* Adrenocorticotropic hormone; *ADH,* antidiuretic hormone; *CRH,* corticotropin-releasing hormone.

impaired patient is at increased risk for fluid deficit and hyperosmolality because of an inability to express thirst and act on it. A dry mouth will cause a person to drink, even when there is no body water deficit.

Renal Regulation

The primary function of the kidneys is to regulate fluid and electrolyte balance by adjusting urine volume and the excretion of most electrolytes (see Chapter 44). The kidneys filter the total plasma volume many times each day. In the average adult, the kidneys reabsorb 99% of this filtrate, producing around 1.5 L of urine per day. Under the influence of ADH, aldosterone, and other hormones, selective reabsorption and secretion of water and electrolytes in the renal tubules result in urine that is different in composition and concentration from plasma. This process helps maintain normal plasma osmolality, electrolyte balance, blood volume, and acid-base balance.

With severely impaired renal function, the kidneys cannot maintain fluid and electrolyte balance. This condition results in edema, potassium and phosphate retention, acidosis, and other electrolyte imbalances (see Chapter 46).

Adrenal Cortical Regulation

Glucocorticoids and mineralocorticoids secreted by the adrenal cortex help regulate water and electrolyte balance. The glucocorticoids (e.g., cortisol) primarily have an antiinflammatory effect and increase serum glucose levels. The mineralocorticoids (e.g., aldosterone) enhance sodium retention and potassium excretion (Fig. 16.9). When sodium is reabsorbed, water follows because of osmotic changes.

Aldosterone is a mineralocorticoid with strong sodium-retaining and potassium-excreting capabilities. Decreased renal perfusion or decreased sodium in the distal part of the renal tubule activates the renin-angiotensin-aldosterone system (RAAS), resulting in aldosterone secretion. In addition to the RAAS, increased serum potassium, decreased serum sodium, and adrenocorticotropic hormone (ACTH) stimulate

aldosterone secretion. Aldosterone increases sodium and water reabsorption in the renal distal tubules, decreasing plasma osmolality and restoring fluid volume.

Cortisol is the most abundant glucocorticoid. In large doses, cortisol has both glucocorticoid (glucose-elevating and antiinflammatory) and mineralocorticoid (sodium-retention) effects. Normally cortisol secretion is in a diurnal or circadian pattern. Increased cortisol secretion occurs in response to physical and psychologic stress. This affects many body functions, including fluid and electrolyte balance (Fig. 16.10).

Cardiac Regulation

Natriuretic peptides, including atrial natriuretic peptide (ANP) and b-type natriuretic peptide (BNP), are hormones made by cardiomyocytes. They are made in response to increased atrial pressure (increased volume, such as occurs in heart failure) and high serum sodium levels. They are natural antagonists to the RAAS and suppress secretion of aldosterone, renin, and ADH, and the action of angiotensin II. In the renal tubules, peptides promote excretion of sodium and water, decreasing blood volume and BP.

Gastrointestinal Regulation

In addition to oral intake, the GI tract normally secretes around 8000 mL of digestive fluids each day. The GI tract normally reabsorbs most of this fluid, with only a small amount eliminated in feces. This is why diarrhea and vomiting, which prevent GI reabsorption of secreted fluid, can lead to significant fluid and electrolyte loss.

Gerontologic Considerations: Fluid and Electrolytes

The older adult has normal physiologic changes that increase susceptibility to fluid and electrolyte imbalances. Structural changes to the kidneys and a decrease in the renal blood flow lead to decreased glomerular filtration rate and loss of the ability to concentrate urine and conserve water. Hormonal changes include a decrease in renin and aldosterone and an increase in ADH and ANP. Subcutaneous tissue loss and thinning of the dermis lead to increased moisture lost through the skin and an inability to respond quickly to heat or cold.

Do not automatically attribute older patients' fluid and electrolyte problems to the natural processes of aging. Throughout this chapter are suggestions for adapting your assessment and nursing interventions when caring for the older adult.

FLUID VOLUME IMBALANCES

Fluid and electrolyte imbalances occur in most patients with a major illness or injury because illness disrupts normal homeostatic mechanisms. Illness or disease directly causes some fluid and electrolyte imbalances (e.g., burns, heart failure). Other times, therapeutic measures (e.g., colonoscopy preparation, diuretics) cause or contribute to imbalances. Perioperative patients are at risk for developing fluid and electrolyte imbalances because of fluid restrictions, blood or fluid loss, and the stress of surgery.

Fluid and electrolyte imbalances are commonly classified as *deficits* or *excesses*. ECF volume deficit *(hypovolemia)* and ECF volume excess *(hypervolemia)* are common clinical conditions. ECF volume imbalances are usually accompanied by one or more electrolyte imbalances, particularly changes in the serum sodium level.

Although each imbalance is discussed separately in this chapter, it is common for more than one imbalance to occur in the same patient. For example, a patient with prolonged nasogastric (NG) suction will lose sodium, potassium, hydrogen, and chloride ions. This may result in sodium and potassium deficiencies, a fluid volume deficit, and metabolic alkalosis caused by the loss of HCl acid.

FLUID VOLUME DEFICIT

Fluid volume deficit can occur with abnormal loss of body fluids (e.g., diarrhea, vomiting, hemorrhage, polyuria), inadequate fluid intake, or a shift from plasma to interstitial fluid. Though often used interchangeably, *fluid volume deficit* and *dehydration* are not the same. *Dehydration* refers to loss of pure water alone without a corresponding loss of sodium. Table 16.3 lists causes and manifestations of fluid volume deficit.

Interprofessional Care

Managing fluid volume deficit involves correcting the underlying cause and replacing both water and any needed electrolytes. Replacement therapy depends on the severity and type of volume loss. In mild losses, we can use oral rehydration. If the deficit is more severe, we replace volume with blood products or balanced IV solutions, such as isotonic (0.9%) sodium chloride or lactated Ringer's solution. The choice of fluid depends on the cause and patient's electrolyte status. For rapid volume replacement, 0.9% sodium chloride is preferred. Blood is given when volume loss is due to blood loss.

TABLE 16.3 Extracellular Fluid Imbalances

Causes and Manifestations

ECF Volume Deficit	ECF Volume Excess
Causes	
• ↑ Insensible water loss or perspiration (high fever, heatstroke)	• Excess isotonic or hypotonic IV fluids
• Diabetes insipidus	• Heart failure
• Osmotic diuresis	• Renal failure
• Hemorrhage	• Primary polydipsia
• GI losses: vomiting, NG suction, diarrhea, fistula drainage	• SIADH
• Overuse of diuretics	• Cushing syndrome
• Inadequate fluid intake	• Long-term use of corticosteroids
• Third-space fluid shifts: burns, pancreatitis	
Manifestations	
• Restlessness, drowsiness, lethargy, confusion	• Headache, confusion, lethargy
• Thirst, dry mucous membranes	• Peripheral edema
• Cold clammy skin	• Jugular venous distention
• Decreased skin turgor, ↓ capillary refill	• S_3 heart sound
• Postural hypotension, ↑ pulse, ↓ CVP	• Bounding pulse, ↑ BP, ↑ CVP
• ↓ Urine output, concentrated urine	• Polyuria (with normal renal function)
• ↑ Respiratory rate	• Dyspnea, crackles, pulmonary edema
• Weakness, dizziness	• Muscle spasms
• Weight loss	• Weight gain
• Seizures, coma	• Seizures, coma

FLUID VOLUME EXCESS

Fluid volume excess may result from excess intake of fluids, abnormal retention of fluids (e.g., heart failure, renal failure), or a shift of fluid from interstitial fluid into plasma fluid. Weight gain is the most consistent manifestation of fluid volume excess. Table 16.3 lists causes and manifestations of fluid volume excess.

Interprofessional Care

Managing fluid volume excess involves treating the underlying cause and removing fluid without producing abnormal changes in the electrolyte composition or osmolality of ECF. Diuretics and fluid restriction are the primary forms of therapy. Some patients also need sodium restrictions. If the fluid excess leads to ascites or pleural effusion, an abdominal paracentesis or thoracentesis may be needed.

❖ NURSING MANAGEMENT: FLUID VOLUME IMBALANCES

◆ Nursing Diagnoses

Nursing diagnoses and collaborative problems for the patient with a fluid imbalance include:
ECF volume deficit:
- Fluid imbalance
- Impaired cardiac output
- Acute confusion
- Potential complication: hypovolemic shock
ECF volume excess:
- Fluid imbalance
- Impaired gas exchange

- Impaired tissue integrity
- Activity intolerance
- Disturbed body image
- Potential complications: pulmonary edema, ascites

◆ Nursing Implementation

◆ **Daily Weights.** Daily weights are the most accurate measure of volume status. An increase of 1 kg (2.2 lb) is equal to 1000 mL (1 L) of fluid retention, provided the person has maintained usual dietary intake or has not been on NPO status. Obtain the weight under standardized conditions. Weigh the patient at the same time every day, wearing the same clothes and on the same carefully calibrated scale. Remove excess bedding and empty all drainage bags before the weighing. If items are present that are not there every day, such as bulky dressings or tubes, note this along with the weight.

◆ **Intake and Output.** Intake and output records give valuable information about fluid and electrolyte problems. An accurately recorded intake and output will identify sources of excess intake or fluid losses. Intake should include oral and IV fluids, tube feedings, and retained irrigation solutions. Output includes urine, excess perspiration, wound or tube drainage, vomitus, and diarrhea. Estimate fluid loss from wounds and perspiration. Note the amount and color of the urine and measure the urine specific gravity. Readings greater than 1.025 mean urine is concentrated, while readings less than 1.010 mean urine is dilute.

◆ **Laboratory Findings.** Monitor laboratory results when available and calculate the serum osmolality. The patient with a fluid volume deficit often has increased blood urea nitrogen (BUN), sodium, and hematocrit levels with increased plasma and urine osmolality. With fluid volume excess, the patient will have decreased BUN, sodium, and hematocrit levels, with decreased plasma and urine osmolality.

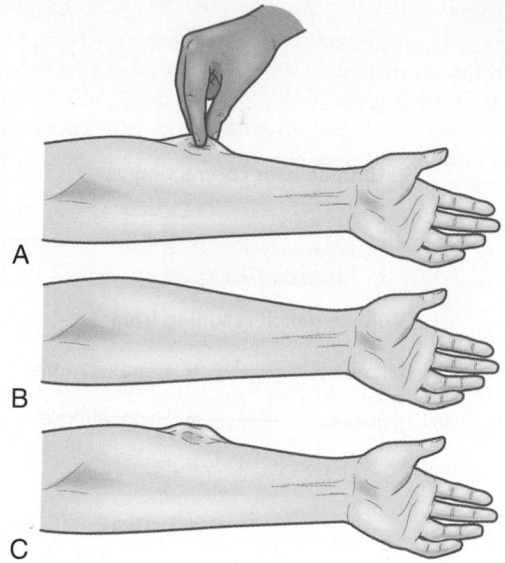

FIG. 16.11 Assessment of skin turgor. **A** and **B,** When normal skin is pinched, it resumes shape in seconds. **C,** If the skin stays wrinkled for 20 to 30 seconds, the patient has poor skin turgor.

▓ NURSING MANAGEMENT

Fluid Volume Changes

- Assess patient for manifestations of fluid imbalances.
- Give IV fluids and medications as ordered.
- Give O₂ therapy as ordered.
- Implement fall precautions.
- Monitor patient for effectiveness of therapy.
- Oversee UAP:
  - Obtain daily weights and vital signs.
  - Offer frequent oral care.
  - Record accurate intake and output.
  - Perform skin care and frequent position changes.
  - Elevate edematous extremities.
  - Encourage oral fluids as appropriate.

◆ **Cardiovascular Care.** Monitor vital signs and perform a thorough cardiovascular assessment as needed. Changes in BP, central venous pressure, pulse force, and jugular venous distention reflect ECF volume imbalances. In fluid volume excess, the pulse is full, bounding, and not easily obliterated. Increased volume causes distended neck veins (jugular venous distention), increased central venous pressure, and high BP. Auscultate heart sounds, being alert for the presence of an S₃.

In mild to moderate fluid volume deficit, sympathetic nervous system compensation increases the heart rate and results in peripheral vasoconstriction to try to keep BP within normal limits. Pulses may be weak and thready. Assess for orthostatic changes. A change in position from lying to sitting or standing may decrease BP or further increase the heart rate (orthostatic hypotension). In more severe deficits, hypotension may be present.

Respiratory Care. Monitor pulse oximetry and auscultate lung sounds as needed. ECF excess can cause pulmonary congestion and pulmonary edema, as increased hydrostatic pressure in the pulmonary vessels forces fluid into the alveoli. The patient will have shortness of breath and moist crackles on auscultation. The patient with ECF deficit will have an increased respiratory rate because of decreased tissue perfusion and resultant hypoxia. Give O₂ as ordered.

Patient Safety. The patient with fluid volume deficit is at risk for falls because of orthostatic hypotension, muscle weakness, and changes in level of consciousness. Assess level of consciousness, gait, and muscle strength. Implement fall precautions. If orthostatic hypotension is present, teach the patient to change positions slowly when rising from a bed or chair. Place alarm monitors on patients who are confused and try to get out of bed without help.

Skin Care. Assess the skin for turgor and mobility. Normally, a fold of skin, when pinched, will readily move and, on release, rapidly return to its former position. In ECF volume deficit, there is diminished skin turgor with tenting, or a lag in the pinched skinfold's return to its original state. Skin areas over the sternum, abdomen, and anterior forearm are the usual sites we use to assess turgor (Fig. 16.11). In older people, decreased skin turgor is less predictive of fluid deficit because of the loss of tissue elasticity.

In mild fluid deficits, the skin may appear warm, dry, and wrinkled. These signs may be hard to assess in the older adult because the person's skin may be normally dry, wrinkled, and non-elastic. In more severe deficits, the skin may be cool and moist if there is vasoconstriction to compensate for the decreased fluid volume. Oral mucous membranes will be dry, the tongue may be furrowed, and the person often is thirsty. Routine oral care is critical for the comfort of a patient who is dehydrated or on a fluid restriction.

Edematous skin may feel cool because of fluid accumulation and a decrease in blood flow secondary to the pressure of the

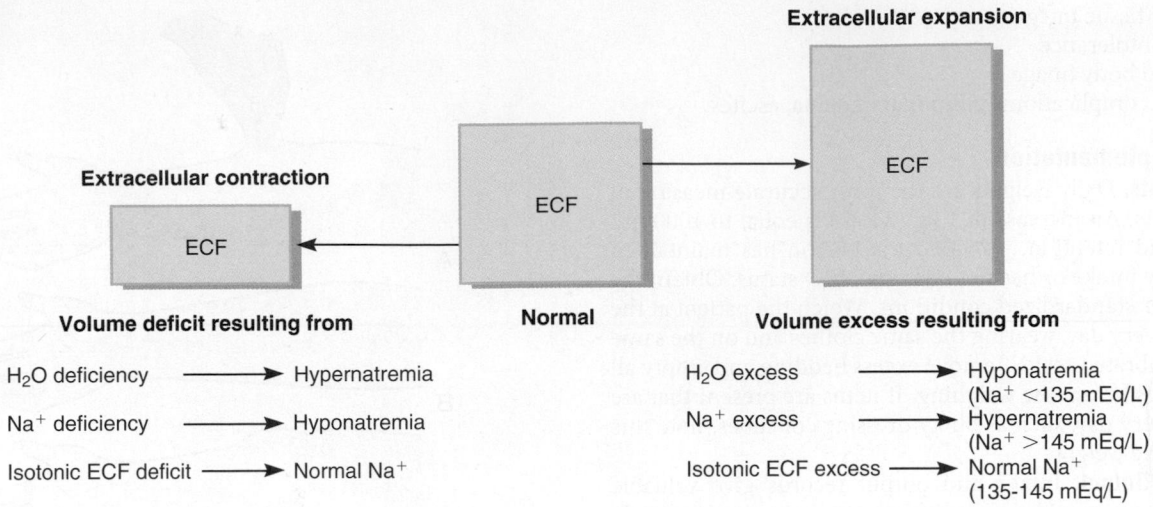

FIG. 16.12 Differential assessment of extracellular fluid (ECF) volume.

fluid. The fluid can stretch the skin, causing it to feel taut and hard. Assess edema by pressing with a thumb or forefinger over the edematous area. Use a grading scale to standardize the description if an indentation (ranging from 1+ [slight edema; 2-mm indentation] to 4+ [pitting edema; 8-mm indentation]) remains when pressure is released. Assess for edema in areas where soft tissues overlie a bone, particularly the tibia, fibula, and sacrum.

Good skin care is important. Protect tissues from extremes of heat and cold, prolonged pressure, and trauma. Frequent skin care and changes in position will prevent skin breakdown. Elevate edematous extremities to promote venous return and fluid reabsorption. Dehydrated skin needs frequent care without the use of soap. Applying moisturizing creams or oils increases moisture retention and stimulates circulation.

◆ **Fluid Therapy.** Give IV fluids as ordered. Carefully monitor the rates of infusion of IV fluid solutions, especially when you are giving large volumes of fluid. This is especially true in patients with heart, renal, or neurologic problems.

In the presence of fluid volume deficit, you can use several interventions to maintain adequate oral intake. Assess the patient's ability to obtain adequate fluids independently, express thirst, and swallow effectively. Fluids should be easily accessible. Provide a variety of fluids that the patient likes.[3] Serve fluids at a temperature preferred by the patient. Offer fluids every 1 to 2 hours and at select times, such as when giving medications. Remind the patient to finish all drinks.

If the patient is choosing to limit intake to decrease nocturia or incontinence, make it easier for the patient to reach the toilet when needed.[3] Help those with physical limitations, such as arthritis, to open and hold containers. Involve the dietitian, speech therapist, or occupational therapist for help with patients with dysphagia or physical limitations.

SODIUM IMBALANCES

Sodium, the main cation of ECF, plays a major role in maintaining the concentration and volume of ECF and influencing water distribution between ECF and ICF. Sodium is important in generating and transmitting nerve impulses, muscle contractility, and regulating acid-base balance.

The serum sodium level reflects the ratio of sodium to water, not necessarily the amount of sodium in the body. Changes in the serum sodium level can reflect a primary water imbalance, primary sodium imbalance, or combination of the two. Sodium imbalances are typically associated with imbalances in ECF volume (Figs. 16.12 and 16.13). Because sodium is the primary determinant of ECF osmolality, sodium imbalances are typically associated with parallel changes in osmolality.

The GI tract absorbs sodium from foods. Typically, daily intake of sodium far exceeds the body's daily requirements. Sodium leaves the body through urine, sweat, and feces. The kidneys primarily regulate sodium balance. The kidneys control ECF sodium concentration by excreting or retaining water under the influence of ADH. Aldosterone plays a smaller role in sodium regulation by promoting sodium reabsorption from the renal tubules.

HYPERNATREMIA

Hypernatremia (high serum sodium) may occur with inadequate water intake, excess water loss, or, rarely, sodium gain. Because sodium is the major determinant of ECF osmolality, hypernatremia causes hyperosmolality. ECF hyperosmolality causes water to move out of the cells to restore equilibrium, leading to cellular dehydration. As discussed earlier, the primary protection against the development of hyperosmolality is thirst. Hypernatremia is not a problem in an alert person who has access to water, can sense thirst, and is able to swallow. Hypernatremia from water deficiency is often the result of an impaired level of consciousness or inability to obtain fluids.

Several clinical states can produce hypernatremia from water loss (Table 16.4). A deficiency in the synthesis or release of ADH from the posterior pituitary gland (central diabetes insipidus) or a decrease in kidney responsiveness to ADH (nephrogenic diabetes insipidus) can result in profound diuresis, producing a water deficit and hypernatremia. Hyperosmolality with osmotic diuresis can result from hyperglycemia associated with uncontrolled diabetes or giving concentrated hyperosmolar tube feedings.

Excess sodium intake with inadequate water intake can also lead to hypernatremia. Examples of sodium gain include IV administration of hypertonic saline or sodium bicarbonate, use of sodium-containing drugs, excess oral intake of sodium (e.g., ingesting seawater), and *primary aldosteronism* (excess aldosterone secretion) caused by a tumor of the adrenal glands.

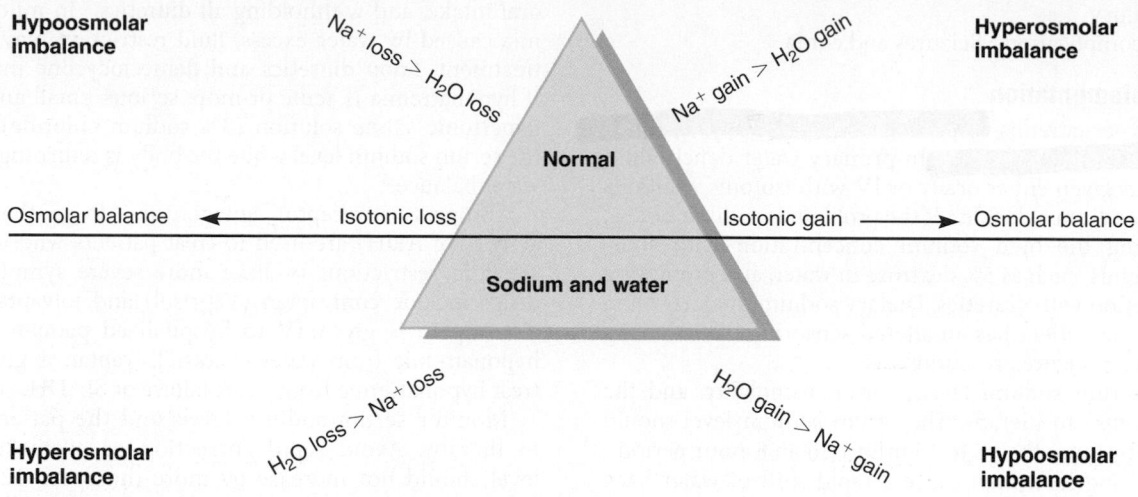

FIG. 16.13 Isotonic gains and losses affect mainly the extracellular fluid (ECF) compartment, with little or no water movement into the cells. Hypertonic imbalances cause water to move from inside the cell into the ECF to dilute the concentrated sodium, causing cell shrinkage. Hypotonic imbalances cause water to move into the cell, causing cell swelling.

TABLE 16.4 Sodium Imbalances

Causes and Manifestations

Hypernatremia (Na⁺ >145 mEq/L [mmol/L])	Hyponatremia (Na⁺ <136 mEq/L [mmol/L])
Causes	**Causes**
Excess Sodium Intake	**Excess Sodium Loss**
• IV fluids: hypertonic NaCl, excess isotonic NaCl, IV sodium bicarbonate	• *GI losses:* diarrhea, vomiting, fistulas, NG suction
• Hypertonic tube feedings without water supplements	• *Renal losses:* diuretics, adrenal insufficiency, Na⁺ wasting renal disease
• Near-drowning in salt water	• *Skin losses:* burns, wound drainage
Inadequate Water Intake	**Inadequate Sodium Intake**
• Unconscious or cognitively impaired persons	• Fasting diets
Excess Water Loss (↑ sodium concentration)	**Excess Water Gain (↓ sodium dilution)**
• ↑ Insensible water loss (high fever, heatstroke, prolonged hyperventilation)	• Excess hypotonic IV fluids
• Osmotic diuretic therapy	• Primary polydipsia
• Diarrhea	
Diseases	**Diseases**
• Diabetes insipidus	• SIADH
• Primary hyperaldosteronism	• Heart failure
• Cushing syndrome	• Primary hypoaldosteronism
• Uncontrolled diabetes	• Cirrhosis
Manifestations	
With Decreased ECF Volume	**With Decreased ECF Volume**
• Restlessness, agitation, lethargy, seizures, coma	• Irritability, apprehension, confusion, dizziness, personality changes, tremors, seizures, coma
• Intense thirst, dry swollen tongue, sticky mucous membranes	• Dry mucous membranes
• Postural hypotension, ↓ CVP, weight loss, ↑ pulse	• Postural hypotension, ↓ CVP, ↓ jugular venous filling, ↑ pulse, thready pulse
• Weakness, muscle cramps	• Cold and clammy skin
With Normal or Increased ECF Volume	**With Normal or Increased ECF Volume**
• Restlessness, agitation, twitching, seizures, coma	• Headache, apathy, confusion, muscle spasms, seizures, coma
• Intense thirst, flushed skin	• Nausea, vomiting, diarrhea, abdominal cramps
• Weight gain, peripheral and pulmonary edema, ↑ BP, ↑ CVP	• Weight gain, ↑ BP, ↑ CVP

Clinical Manifestations

The manifestations of hypernatremia are primarily the result of water shifting out of cells into ECF with resultant dehydration and shrinkage of cells (Table 16.4). Dehydration of brain cells results in changes in mental status, ranging from drowsiness, restlessness, confusion, and lethargy to seizures and coma.[4] If there is an accompanying ECF volume deficit, manifestations such as postural hypotension, tachycardia, and weakness occur.

❖ NURSING AND INTERPROFESSIONAL MANAGEMENT: HYPERNATREMIA

◆ Nursing Diagnoses

Nursing diagnoses and collaborative problems for the patient with hypernatremia include:

• Electrolyte imbalance
• Fluid imbalance

- Risk for injury
- Potential complications: Seizures and coma

◆ Nursing Implementation

Managing hypernatremia depends on the underlying cause and the patient's volume status. In primary water deficit, fluid replacement is given either orally or IV with isotonic solutions such as 0.9% sodium chloride.[2] If the problem is sodium excess, expect diluting the high sodium concentration with sodium-free IV fluids, such as 5% dextrose in water, and promoting sodium excretion with diuretics. Dietary sodium intake is often restricted. If the patient has an altered sensorium or is having seizures, initiate seizure precautions.

Monitor serum sodium levels, serum osmolality, and the patient's response to therapy. The serum sodium level should not decrease by more than 8 to 15 mEq/L in an 8-hour period.[2] Quickly reducing levels can cause a rapid shift of water back into the cells, causing cerebral edema and neurologic complications. This risk is greatest in the patient who developed hypernatremia over several days or longer.

HYPONATREMIA

Hyponatremia (low serum sodium) may result from a loss of sodium-containing fluids, water excess in relation to the amount of sodium (dilutional hyponatremia), or a combination of both (Table 16.4). Hyponatremia is usually associated with ECF hypoosmolality from the excess water. To restore balance, fluid shifts out of the ECF and into the cells, leading to cellular edema.

Common causes of hyponatremia from loss of sodium-rich body fluids include draining wounds, diarrhea, vomiting, and primary adrenal insufficiency. Inappropriate use of sodium-free or hypotonic IV fluids causes hyponatremia from water excess. This may occur in patients after surgery or major trauma, or if we give fluids to patients with renal failure. Patients with psychiatric disorders may have an excess water intake. Syndrome of inappropriate antidiuretic hormone secretion (SIADH) results in dilutional hyponatremia caused by abnormal retention of water (see Chapter 49).

Clinical Manifestations

The manifestations are due to cellular swelling and first appear in the central nervous system (CNS). Mild hyponatremia has minor, nonspecific neurologic symptoms, including headache, irritability, and difficulty concentrating. More severe hyponatremia can cause confusion, vomiting, seizures, and even coma. If hyponatremia is severe and develops rapidly, irreversible neurologic damage or death from brain herniation can occur.

❖ NURSING AND INTERPROFESSIONAL MANAGEMENT: HYPONATREMIA

◆ Nursing Diagnoses

Nursing diagnoses and collaborative problems for the patient with hyponatremia include:

- Electrolyte imbalance
- Risk for injury
- Acute confusion
- Potential complication: seizures and coma

◆ Nursing Implementation

Managing hyponatremia from fluid loss includes replacing fluid using isotonic sodium-containing solutions, encouraging oral intake, and withholding all diuretics.[2] In mild hyponatremia caused by water excess, fluid restriction may be the only treatment. Loop diuretics and demeclocycline may be given. If hyponatremia is acute or more serious, small amounts of IV hypertonic saline solution (3% sodium chloride) can restore the serum sodium level while the body is returning to a normal water balance.[5]

Vasopressor receptor antagonists (drugs that block the activity of ADH) are used to treat patients who cannot tolerate fluid restrictions or have more severe symptoms.[6] These drugs include conivaptan (Vaprisol) and tolvaptan (Samsca). Conivaptan is given IV to hospitalized patients with severe hyponatremia from water excess. Tolvaptan is given orally to treat hyponatremia from heart failure or SIADH.

Monitor serum sodium levels and the patient's response to therapy. Avoid rapid correction or overcorrection. The level should not increase by more than 6 to 12 mEq/L per hour in the first 24 hours and 18 mEq/L or less per hour within 48 hours.[6] Quickly increasing sodium levels can cause osmotic demyelination syndrome with permanent damage to nerve cells in the brain. An accurate urine output record is essential. The patient may need a urinary catheter placed if unable to help with monitoring output. If the patient has an altered sensorium or is having seizures, initiate seizure precautions.

POTASSIUM IMBALANCES

Potassium is the major ICF cation, with 98% of the body potassium being in cells. For example, potassium concentration within muscle cells is around 140 mEq/L; potassium concentration in ECF is 3.5 to 5.0 mEq/L. The sodium-potassium pump in cell membranes maintains this concentration difference by pumping potassium into the cell and sodium out. Insulin helps by stimulating the sodium-potassium pump.

Because the ratio of ECF potassium to ICF potassium is the major factor in the resting membrane potential of nerve and muscle cells, potassium imbalances often affect neuromuscular and cardiac function. Potassium is involved with regulating intracellular osmolality and promoting cellular growth. It is required for glycogen to be deposited in muscle and liver cells. It also plays a role in acid-base balance (discussed in the section on Acid-Base Regulation later in this chapter).

Diet is the main source for potassium. The typical Western diet contains roughly 50 to 100 mEq of potassium daily, mainly from protein-rich foods and various fruits and vegetables. Many salt substitutes used in low-sodium diets have substantial potassium. Patients may receive potassium from parenteral sources, including IV fluids; transfusions of stored, hemolyzed blood; and certain medications (e.g., potassium penicillin).

The kidneys are the primary route for potassium loss, eliminating about 90% of the daily potassium intake. Potassium excretion depends on the serum potassium level, urine output, and renal function. When serum potassium is high, urine potassium excretion increases, and when serum levels are low, excretion decreases. Large urine output can cause excess potassium loss. Impaired kidney function can cause potassium retention. There is an inverse relationship between sodium and potassium reabsorption in the kidneys. Factors that cause sodium retention (e.g., low blood volume, hyponatremia, aldosterone secretion) cause potassium excretion.

HYPERKALEMIA

Hyperkalemia (high serum potassium) may result from impaired renal excretion, a shift of potassium from ICF to ECF, a massive intake of potassium, or a combination of these factors (Table 16.5). The most common cause of hyperkalemia is renal failure. Adrenal insufficiency with subsequent aldosterone deficiency leads to potassium retention. Factors that cause potassium to move from ICF to ECF include acidosis, massive cell destruction (as in burn or crush injury, tumor lysis, severe infections), and intense exercise. In metabolic acidosis, potassium ions shift from ICF to ECF in exchange for hydrogen ions moving into the cell.

Digoxin-like drugs and β-adrenergic blockers (e.g., propranolol) can impair entry of potassium into cells, resulting in higher ECF potassium concentrations. Several drugs, such as NSAIDs, potassium-sparing diuretics, angiotensin II receptor blockers (e.g., losartan), and angiotensin-converting enzyme (ACE) inhibitors (e.g., lisinopril), can contribute to hyperkalemia by reducing the kidney's ability to excrete potassium.[7]

Clinical Manifestations

The increased potassium concentration outside the cell changes the normal ECF and ICF ratio. This results in increased cell excitability and changes in impulse transmission to the nerves and muscles. The most clinically significant problems are the changes in cardiac conduction. The initial finding is tall, peaked T waves. As potassium increases, cardiac depolarization decreases, leading to loss of P waves, a prolonged PR interval, ST segment depression, and widening QRS complex (Fig. 16.14). Heart block, ventricular fibrillation, or cardiac standstill may occur.[7]

The patient may have fatigue, confusion, tetany, muscle cramps, paresthesias, and weakness. As potassium increases, loss of muscle tone and weakness or paralysis of other skeletal muscles, including the respiratory muscles, can occur, leading to respiratory arrest. Abdominal cramping, vomiting, and diarrhea occur from hyperactivity of GI smooth muscles.

❖ NURSING AND INTERPROFESSIONAL MANAGEMENT: HYPERKALEMIA

◆ Nursing Diagnoses

Nursing diagnoses and collaborative problems for the patient with hyperkalemia include:

- Electrolyte imbalance
- Activity intolerance
- Impaired cardiac output
- Potential complication: dysrhythmias

TABLE 16.5 Potassium Imbalances

Causes and Manifestations

Hyperkalemia (K⁺ >5.0 mEq/L [mmol/L])	Hypokalemia (K⁺ <3.5 mEq/L [mmol/L])
Causes	
Excess Potassium Intake	***Potassium Loss***
• Excess or rapid parenteral administration	• *GI losses:* diarrhea, vomiting, fistulas, NG suction, ileostomy drainage
• Potassium-containing drugs (e.g., potassium penicillin)	• *Renal losses:* diuretics, hyperaldosteronism, magnesium depletion
• Potassium-containing salt substitute	• *Skin losses:* diaphoresis
	• Dialysis
Shift of Potassium Out of Cells	***Shift of Potassium Into Cells***
• Acidosis	• Increased insulin release (e.g., IV dextrose load)
• Tissue catabolism (e.g., fever, crush injury, sepsis, burns)	• Insulin therapy (e.g., with diabetic ketoacidosis)
• Intense exercise	• Alkalosis
• Tumor lysis syndrome	• ↑ Epinephrine (e.g., stress)
Failure to Eliminate Potassium	***Lack of Potassium Intake***
• Renal disease	• Starvation
• Adrenal insufficiency	• Diet low in potassium
• *Medications:* Angiotensin II receptor blockers, ACE inhibitors, heparin, potassium-sparing diuretics, NSAIDs	• Failure to include potassium in parenteral fluids if NPO
Clinical Manifestations	
• Fatigue, irritability	
• Muscle weakness, cramps	• Fatigue
• Loss of muscle tone	• Muscle weakness, leg cramps
• Paresthesias, decreased reflexes	• Soft, flabby muscles
• Abdominal cramping, diarrhea, vomiting	• Paresthesias, decreased reflexes
• Confusion	• Constipation, nausea, paralytic ileus
• Irregular pulse	• Shallow respirations
• Tetany	• Weak, irregular pulse
	• Hyperglycemia
ECG Changes	**ECG Changes**
• Tall, peaked T wave	• Flattened T wave
• Prolonged PR interval	• Presence of U wave
• ST segment depression	• ST segment depression
• Widening QRS	• Prolonged QRS
• Loss of P wave	• Peaked P wave
• Ventricular fibrillation	• Ventricular dysrhythmias
• Ventricular standstill	• First- and second-degree heart block

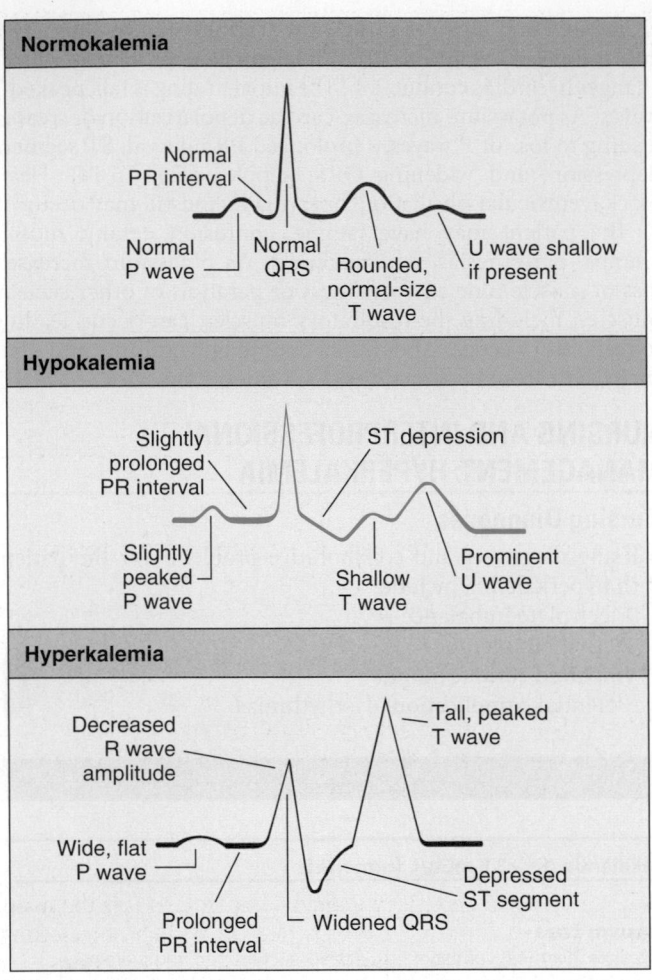

Normokalemia

Normal PR interval

Normal P wave

Normal QRS

Rounded, normal-size T wave

U wave shallow if present

Hypokalemia

Slightly prolonged PR interval

ST depression

Slightly peaked P wave

Shallow T wave

Prominent U wave

Hyperkalemia

Decreased R wave amplitude

Tall, peaked T wave

Wide, flat P wave

Prolonged PR interval

Widened QRS

Depressed ST segment

FIG. 16.14 ECG changes associated with changes in potassium levels.

◆ Nursing Implementation

Management of hyperkalemia consists of the following:
1. Stop oral and parenteral potassium intake (Table 16.6).
2. Increase potassium excretion. This may be done with loop or thiazide diuretics, dialysis, patiromer (Veltassa), and/ or sodium polystyrene sulfonate (Kayexalate). Kayexalate, given orally or rectally, is used acutely to bind potassium in the bowel. Each gram of the drug removes roughly 1 mEq of potassium. Patients with renal failure need hemodialysis.[7] Patiromer, given orally, also binds potassium in the GI tract. It takes several hours to days to work and is best for patients with chronic hyperkalemia. Patiromer binds with many other oral drugs and reduces their effectiveness. You should not give it within 6 hours of other drugs.
3. Force potassium from ECF to ICF. A combination of IV regular insulin with dextrose and a β-adrenergic agonist stimulates the sodium-potassium pump, shifting potassium into cells. Using these drugs together is more effective than using either alone. Both metered-dose inhalers and nebulized β-adrenergic agonists (e.g., nebulized albuterol) are equally effective. IV sodium bicarbonate is an option if the patient is acidotic.[7]
4. Stabilize cardiac membranes. IV calcium chloride or calcium gluconate does not lower the potassium but serves as an antagonist to reverse the toxic effects on the cardiac cell membrane. This protects the patient from life-threatening dysrhythmias.[7]

TABLE 16.6 Nutritional Therapy

High-Potassium Foods

Fruits	Vegetables	Other Foods
• Apricot, raw (medium)	• Baked beans	• Bran or bran products
• Avocado (¼ whole)	• Butternut squash	• Chocolate (1.5–2 oz)
• Banana (¼ whole)	• Refried beans	• Granola
• Cantaloupe	• Black beans	• Milk, all types (1 cup)
• Dried fruits	• Broccoli, cooked	• Nutritional supplements (use only under the direction of physician or dietitian)
• Grapefruit juice	• Carrots, raw	
• Honeydew	• Greens, except kale	
• Orange (medium)	• Mushrooms, canned	• Nuts and seeds (1 oz)
• Orange juice	• Potatoes, white and sweet	• Peanut butter (2 Tbsp)
• Prunes	• Spinach, cooked	• Salt substitutes, Lite Salt
• Raisins	• Tomatoes or tomato products	• Salt-free broth
	• Vegetable juices	• Yogurt

When the potassium elevation is mild and the kidneys are functioning, it may be enough to (1) withhold potassium from the diet and IV sources and (2) increase renal potassium excretion by giving fluids and loop or thiazide diuretics. Patients with severe hyperkalemia or symptomatic patients should receive treatment to force potassium into cells.

Use continuous ECG monitoring for all patients with clinically significant hyperkalemia to detect dysrhythmias and monitor the effects of therapy. The patient with dangerous dysrhythmias should receive IV calcium immediately. Monitor BP because giving calcium rapidly can cause hypotension. When giving insulin, monitor for hypoglycemia and give glucose as needed. Monitor serum potassium levels as appropriate.

HYPOKALEMIA

Hypokalemia (low serum potassium) can result from an increased loss of potassium, an increased shift of potassium from ECF to ICF, or, rarely, from deficient dietary potassium intake. The most common causes are abnormal losses from either the kidneys or GI tract. GI tract losses are associated with diarrhea, laxative misuse, vomiting, and ileostomy drainage. Renal losses occur when a patient is diuresing or has a low magnesium level. Low magnesium levels stimulate renin and aldosterone release, resulting in potassium excretion.

Among the factors causing potassium to move from ECF to ICF are insulin therapy, especially in conjunction with diabetic ketoacidosis, and β-adrenergic stimulation (catecholamine release in stress, coronary ischemia). Alkalosis can cause a shift of potassium into cells in exchange for hydrogen, lowering potassium in ECF and causing symptomatic hypokalemia.

Clinical Manifestations

Hypokalemia alters the resting membrane potential, resulting in hyperpolarization (an increased negative charge within the cell) and impaired muscle contraction. Therefore the manifestations of hypokalemia involve changes in cardiac and muscle function (Table 16.5).

The most serious clinical problems are cardiac changes, including impaired repolarization, resulting in a flattened T wave, depressed ST segment, and the presence of a U wave. The P waves peak and the QRS complex is prolonged (Fig. 16.14). There is an increased incidence of heart block and potentially lethal ventricular dysrhythmias.

As with hyperkalemia, skeletal muscle weakness and paresthesias may occur. Severe hypokalemia can cause paralysis. This usually involves the extremities but can involve the respiratory muscles, leading to shallow respirations and respiratory arrest. Changes in smooth muscle function may lead to decreased GI motility (e.g., constipation, paralytic ileus). Finally, hypokalemia impairs insulin secretion, leading to glucose intolerance and hyperglycemia.

❖ NURSING AND INTERPROFESSIONAL MANAGEMENT: HYPOKALEMIA

◆ Nursing Diagnoses

Nursing diagnoses and collaborative problems for the patient with hypokalemia include:

- Electrolyte imbalance
- Activity intolerance
- Impaired cardiac output
- Potential complication: dysrhythmias

Nursing Implementation

Managing hypokalemia consists of oral or IV potassium chloride (KCl) supplements and increased dietary intake of potassium. Consuming potassium-rich foods can usually correct mild hypokalemia. See Table 16.6 for foods that are high in potassium. Clinically significant hypokalemia requires giving oral or IV KCl.

> ⚠ **SAFETY ALERT IV KCl**
> - Always dilute IV KCl and do not give in concentrated amounts.
> - Never give KCl via IV push or as a bolus.
> - Invert IV bags containing KCl several times to ensure even distribution in the bag.
> - Do not add KCl to a hanging IV bag to prevent giving a bolus dose.

IV KCl infusion rates should not exceed 10 mEq/hr unless the patient is in a critical care setting with continuous ECG monitoring and central line access for administration.[5] IV KCl must be given by infusion pump to ensure correct administration rate. Because KCl is irritating to the vein, assess IV sites at least hourly for phlebitis and infiltration. Infiltration can cause necrosis and sloughing of the surrounding tissue.

Patients who are critically ill and those at risk for hypokalemia should have continuous ECG monitoring to detect cardiac changes. Monitor serum potassium levels and urine output as appropriate.

> 🔎 **CHECK YOUR PRACTICE**
>
> You are taking care of a 78-yr-old female patient with heart failure. She is taking furosemide (Lasix) and digitalis.
> - What should you be alert for in a patient who takes both drugs?

KCl is usually given only if the urine output is at least 0.5 mL/kg of body weight per hour. Because patients on digoxin therapy have an increased risk for toxicity if their serum potassium

TABLE 16.7 Patient & Caregiver Teaching
Prevention of Hypokalemia
Include the following instructions when teaching at-risk patients how to prevent hypokalemia: 1. For all patients at risk: • Report the signs and symptoms of hypokalemia (Table 16.5) to the HCP. • Have serum potassium levels checked regularly. • Regularly include foods high in potassium in your diet (Table 16.6). • Consume alcohol in moderation only. • Avoid consuming large amounts of licorice. 2. For patients taking oral potassium supplements: • Take the medication as prescribed to prevent overdosing. • Take the supplement with a full glass of water. Do not crush or chew tablets.

level is low, monitor the patient for digitalis toxicity. Patients who have confusion, lethargy, or GI problems, including nausea/vomiting or poor appetite, may have digitalis toxicity. Visual problems, including blurred vision and changes in color vision, may be seen in digitalis toxicity.[8]

Teach patients ways to prevent hypokalemia (Table 16.7). Patients at risk should have regular monitoring of serum potassium levels. Teach the patient taking digitalis to report signs and symptoms of digoxin toxicity at once to the HCP.

CALCIUM IMBALANCES

Calcium has a role in many metabolic processes. It is the major cation in bones and teeth. Calcium plays a role in blood clotting, transmission of nerve impulses, myocardial contractions, and muscle contractions. The major source for calcium is dietary intake. Calcium absorption requires the active form of vitamin D. Vitamin D is obtained from foods or made in the skin by the action of sunlight on cholesterol.

The total body content of calcium is about 1200 g. The bones contain 99% of the body' calcium; the rest is in plasma and body cells. Of the calcium in plasma, 50% is bound to plasma proteins, primarily albumin; 40% is in a free or ionized form, and the rest is found bound with phosphate, citrate, or carbonate. The ionized or free calcium is biologically active. The serum pH influences how much calcium is ionized or bound to albumin. A decreased plasma pH (acidosis) decreases calcium binding to albumin, leading to more ionized calcium. An increased plasma pH (alkalosis) increases calcium binding, leading to decreased ionized calcium.

Serum calcium levels reflect the total level of all forms of plasma calcium. Serum albumin levels affect the interpretation of total calcium levels. Total calcium values increase or decrease directly with serum albumin levels. Ionized calcium levels are measured using special laboratory techniques or calculated using a formula. Albumin levels do not affect ionized calcium levels.

Parathyroid hormone (PTH) and calcitonin regulate calcium levels. Since the bones serve as a readily available store of calcium, the body can usually keep calcium levels normal by regulating the movement of calcium into or out of the bone. Low serum calcium levels stimulate the parathyroid glands to make and release PTH. PTH increases bone resorption (movement of calcium out of bones), increases GI absorption of calcium, and increases renal

TABLE 16.8 Calcium Imbalances
Causes and Manifestations

Hypercalcemia (Ca²⁺ >10.5 mg/dL [2.62 mmol/L])	Hypocalcemia (Ca²⁺ <9.0 mg/dL [2.25 mmol/L])
Causes	
Increased Total Calcium	***Decreased Total Calcium***
• Hyperparathyroidism	• Primary hypoparathyroidism
• Hematologic cancer	• Renal insufficiency
• Cancers with bone metastasis	• Acute pancreatitis
• Prolonged immobilization	• High phosphate level
• Vitamin A or D overdose	• Vitamin D deficiency, malnutrition
• Paget's disease	• Low magnesium level
• Adrenal insufficiency	• Bisphosphonates
• Thyrotoxicosis	• Tumor lysis syndrome
• Thiazide diuretics	• Loop diuretics
• Excess dairy intake	• Chronic alcohol use
• Calcium-containing antacids	• Diarrhea
• *Mycobacterium* infection	• ↓ Serum albumin
Increased Ionized Calcium	***Decreased Ionized Calcium***
• Acidosis	• Alkalosis
	• Receiving excess citrated blood
Manifestations	
• Lethargy, weakness, fatigue	• Weakness, fatigue
• Decreased memory	• Depression, irritability, confusion
• Depressed reflexes	• Hyperreflexia, muscle cramps
• ↑ BP	• ↓ BP
• Confusion, psychosis	• Numbness and tingling in extremities and region around mouth
• Anorexia, nausea, vomiting	• Chvostek's sign
• Bone pain, fractures	• Trousseau's sign
• Polyuria, dehydration	• Laryngeal and bronchial spasms
• Nephrolithiasis	• Tetany, seizures
• Seizures, coma	
ECG Changes	***ECG Changes***
• Shortened ST segment	• Elongation of ST segment
• Shortened QT interval	• Prolonged QT interval
• Ventricular dysrhythmias	• Ventricular tachycardia
• Increased digitalis effect	

tubule reabsorption of calcium. High serum calcium levels stimulate the release of calcitonin from the thyroid gland. Calcitonin has the opposite effect of PTH. It lowers the serum calcium level by increasing calcium deposition into bone, increasing renal calcium excretion, and decreasing GI absorption.

HYPERCALCEMIA

Hypercalcemia (high serum calcium) is caused by hyperparathyroidism in about two thirds of persons. Cancers, especially hematologic, breast, and lung cancers, cause the remaining third. Cancers lead to hypercalcemia through tumor-producing factors that prompt osteoclastic activity and bone resorption.[9] More rare causes include thiazide diuretic use, prolonged immobilization, and increased calcium intake (e.g., use of calcium-containing antacids).

Excess calcium acts like a sedative, leading to reduced excitability of muscles and nerves. Neurologic manifestations begin with fatigue, lethargy, weakness, and confusion and progress to hallucinations, seizures, and coma. Changes in cardiac conduction can lead to dysrhythmias, including heart block and ventricular tachycardia. Table 16.8 lists the causes and manifestations of hypercalcemia.

❖ NURSING AND INTERPROFESSIONAL MANAGEMENT: HYPERCALCEMIA

◆ Nursing Diagnoses

Nursing diagnoses and collaborative problems for the patient with hypercalcemia include:
• Electrolyte imbalance
• Acute confusion
• Impaired physical mobility
• Potential complication: dysrhythmias

◆ Nursing Implementation

Management depends on the degree of hypercalcemia, patient's condition, and underlying cause. Patients with mild hypercalcemia should stop any medications related to hypercalcemia, start a diet low in calcium, increase weight-bearing activity, and maintain adequate hydration. The patient must drink 3000 to 4000 mL of fluid daily to promote the renal excretion of calcium and decrease the chance of kidney stone formation. Fluids that promote urine acidity (cranberry or prune juice) will help to prevent formation of stones.

Managing severe hypercalcemia includes giving IV isotonic saline, a bisphosphonate, and calcitonin. IV saline therapy requires careful monitoring. Fluid overload can occur in patients who cannot excrete the excess sodium because of impaired renal function. Bisphosphonates (e.g., pamidronate, zoledronic acid) are the gold standard in treating hypercalcemia, particularly when caused by cancer. They interfere with the activity of osteoclasts, cells that break down bone. Because it takes 2 to 4 days for them to achieve maximum effect, patients receive calcitonin injections for an immediate effect. Calcitonin rapidly increases renal calcium excretion. However, therapy is effective for only a few days and may cause tachycardia. For patients who do not respond to bisphosphonates or have renal impairment, denosumab (Prolia) may be used as an alternative treatment.[9] Dialysis is an option in life-threatening situations.

HYPOCALCEMIA

Hypocalcemia (low serum calcium) can result from any condition associated with PTH deficiency. This may occur with surgical removal of part of, or injury to, the parathyroid glands during thyroid or neck surgery or with neck radiation. The patient who receives multiple blood transfusions can develop hypocalcemia because citrate, used as an anticoagulant in blood bags, binds with calcium, decreasing ionized calcium levels. Sudden alkalosis may result in symptomatic hypocalcemia despite a normal total serum calcium level. The high pH increases calcium binding to protein, decreasing the amount of ionized calcium. Table 16.8 lists causes and manifestations of hypocalcemia.

Low ionized calcium levels decrease the threshold for activating the sodium channels that cause cell membrane depolarization. This results in increased nerve excitability and sustained muscle contraction, or *tetany*. Clinical signs of tetany include Chvostek's sign and Trousseau's sign. *Chvostek's sign* is contraction of facial muscles in response to a tap over the facial nerve in front of the ear (Fig. 16.15, *A*). *Trousseau's sign* refers to carpal spasms induced by inflating a BP cuff on the arm (Fig. 16.15, *B* and *C*). When you inflate the cuff above the systolic pressure, carpal spasms occur within 3 minutes if hypocalcemia is

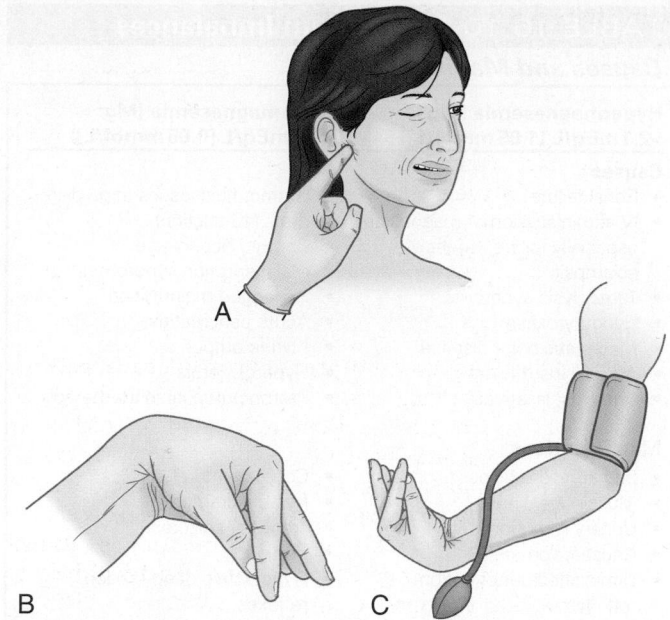

FIG. 16.15 Tests for hypocalcemia. **A,** Chvostek's sign is contraction of facial muscles in response to a light tap over the facial nerve in front of the ear. **B,** Trousseau's sign is a carpal spasm induced by **(C)** inflating a BP cuff above the systolic pressure for a few minutes.

present. Other manifestations of tetany are laryngeal stridor, dysphagia, paresthesia, and numbness and tingling around the mouth or in the extremities. Cardiac effects include decreased cardiac contractility and ECG changes. A prolonged QT interval may develop into ventricular tachycardia.

❖ NURSING AND INTERPROFESSIONAL MANAGEMENT: HYPOCALCEMIA

◆ Nursing Diagnoses

Nursing diagnoses and collaborative problems for the patient with hypocalcemia include:

- Electrolyte imbalance
- Impaired breathing
- Activity intolerance
- Potential complications: fracture, respiratory arrest

◆ Nursing Implementation

Managing hypocalcemia depends on the underlying cause and the presence of symptoms. Treating mild or asymptomatic hypocalcemia involves a diet high in calcium-rich foods and calcium and vitamin D supplementation. Symptomatic hypocalcemia is treated with IV calcium gluconate.[10] Measures to promote CO_2 retention, such as breathing into a paper bag or sedating the patient, can control muscle spasm and other symptoms of tetany until the calcium level is corrected. Patients taking loop diuretics may need to change to thiazide diuretics to decrease urinary calcium excretion. Closely assess any patient who had thyroid or neck surgery in the immediate postoperative period for manifestations of hypocalcemia because of the proximity of the surgery to the parathyroid glands. Adequately treat pain and anxiety because hyperventilation-induced respiratory alkalosis can precipitate hypocalcemic symptoms.

PHOSPHATE IMBALANCES

Phosphorus is the primary anion in ICF and the second most abundant element in the body after calcium. Most phosphorus is in bones and teeth as calcium phosphate. The remaining phosphorus is metabolically active in the form of phosphate salts. Thus, we use the terms *phosphorus* and *phosphate* interchangeably in this text. Phosphate is essential to the function of muscle, red blood cells, and the nervous system. It is involved in the acid-base buffering system; the mitochondrial formation of ATP; cellular uptake and use of glucose; and carbohydrate, protein, and fat metabolism.

PTH maintains serum phosphate levels and balance. Proper phosphate balance requires adequate renal functioning because the kidneys are the major route of phosphate excretion. When the phosphate level in the glomerular filtrate falls below normal or PTH levels are low, the kidneys reabsorb more phosphate. A reciprocal relationship exists between phosphate and calcium. This means a low serum calcium level will result in a high phosphate level and vice-versa.[10]

HYPERPHOSPHATEMIA

Hyperphosphatemia (high serum phosphate) is common in patients with acute kidney injury or chronic kidney disease, which alter the kidney's ability to excrete phosphate. Other causes include excess phosphate intake from the use of phosphate-containing laxatives or enemas or a shift of phosphate from ICF to ECF. This may occur in patients with tumor lysis syndrome or rhabdomyolysis. Hypoparathyroidism and vitamin D intoxication cause increased kidney phosphate reabsorption. Table 16.9 describes causes and manifestations of hyperphosphatemia.

Hyperphosphatemia can be asymptomatic unless calcium binds with phosphate, leading to manifestations of hypocalcemia. These include tetany, muscle cramps, paresthesias, hypotension, dysrhythmias, and seizures.[10] Long-term, increased phosphate levels result in the development of calcified deposits outside of the bones. These calcium deposits can be found in soft tissues, such as joints, arteries, skin, corneas, and kidneys, and cause organ dysfunction, notably renal failure.

Managing hyperphosphatemia involves identifying and treating the underlying cause. Restrict the intake of foods and fluids high in phosphorus (e.g., dairy products). Oral phosphate-binding agents (e.g., calcium carbonate) limit intestinal phosphate absorption and increase phosphate secretion in the intestine. With severe hyperphosphatemia, hemodialysis may be used to rapidly decrease levels. Volume expansion and forced diuresis with a loop diuretic may increase phosphate excretion. If hypocalcemia is present, institute measures to correct calcium levels. See Chapter 46 for more information about treating hyperphosphatemia associated with kidney disease.

HYPOPHOSPHATEMIA

Hypophosphatemia (low serum phosphate) can result from decreased intestinal absorption, increased urinary excretion, or ECF to ICF shifts. Malabsorption, diarrhea, and phosphate-binding antacids lead to decreased absorption. Phosphate shifts occur in respiratory alkalosis, treatment of diabetic ketoacidosis, and refeeding syndrome (reinstitution of nutrition to patients who are severely malnourished). Hypophosphatemia

TABLE 16.9 Phosphate Imbalances

Causes and Manifestations

Hyperphosphatemia (PO$_4^{3-}$ >4.5 mg/dL [1.45 mmol/L])	Hypophosphatemia (PO$_4^{3-}$ <3.0 mg/dL [0.97 mmol/L])
Causes	
• Renal failure	• Malabsorption syndromes
• Phosphate enemas (e.g., Fleet Enema)	• Chronic diarrhea
• Excess ingestion (e.g., phosphate-containing laxatives)	• Malnutrition, vitamin D deficiency
• Rhabdomyolysis	• Parenteral nutrition
• Tumor lysis syndrome	• Chronic alcohol use
• Thyrotoxicosis	• Phosphate-binding antacids
• Hypoparathyroidism	• Diabetic ketoacidosis
• Sickle cell anemia, hemolytic anemia	• Hyperparathyroidism
• Hyperthermia	• Refeeding syndrome
	• Respiratory alkalosis
Manifestations	
• Hypocalcemia	• CNS depression (confusion, coma)
• Numbness and tingling in extremities and region around mouth	• Muscle weakness, including respiratory muscle weakness
• Hyperreflexia, muscle cramps	• Polyneuropathy, seizures
• Tetany, seizures	• Heart problems (dysrhythmias, heart failure)
• Calcium-phosphate precipitates in skin, soft tissue, cornea, viscera, blood vessels	• Osteomalacia, rickets
	• Rhabdomyolysis

TABLE 16.10 Magnesium Imbalances

Causes and Manifestations

Hypermagnesemia (Mg$^+$ >2.1 mEq/L [1.05 mmol/L])	Hypomagnesemia (Mg$^+$ <1.3 mEq/L [0.65 mmol/L])
Causes	
• Renal failure	• GI tract fluid losses (e.g., diarrhea, NG suction)
• IV administration of magnesium, especially for treatment of eclampsia	• Chronic alcohol use
• Tumor lysis syndrome	• Malabsorption syndromes
• Hypothyroidism	• Prolonged malnutrition
• Metastatic bone disease	• Acute pancreatitis
• Adrenal insufficiency	• ↑ Urine output
• Antacids, laxatives	• Hyperglycemia
	• Proton pump inhibitor therapy
Manifestations	
• Lethargy, drowsiness	• Confusion
• Muscle weakness	• Muscle cramps
• Urinary retention	• Tremors, seizures
• Nausea, vomiting	• Vertigo
• Diminished deep tendon reflexes	• Hyperactive deep tendon reflexes
• Flushed, warm skin, especially facial	• Chvostek's and Trousseau's signs
• ↓ Pulse, ↓ BP	• ↑ Pulse, ↑ BP, dysrhythmias

may occur in those who are malnourished or receive parenteral nutrition with inadequate phosphorus replacement. Table 16.9 lists causes and manifestations of hypophosphatemia.

Most of the manifestations of hypophosphatemia result from impaired cellular energy and O$_2$ delivery due to low levels of cellular ATP and 2,3-diphosphoglycerate (2,3-DPG), an enzyme in RBCs that facilitates O$_2$ delivery to the tissues. Mild to moderate hypophosphatemia is often asymptomatic. Severe hypophosphatemia may be fatal because of decreased cellular function. Acute manifestations include CNS depression, muscle weakness and pain, respiratory failure, and heart failure. Chronic hypophosphatemia alters bone metabolism, resulting in rickets and osteomalacia.

Managing mild phosphate deficiency involves increasing oral intake with dairy products or phosphate supplements. Dairy products are better tolerated because phosphate supplements are often associated with adverse GI effects, including diarrhea and bloating.[11] Symptomatic hypophosphatemia can be fatal and usually requires IV administration of sodium phosphate or potassium phosphate. During IV replacement, monitor serum calcium and phosphate levels every 6 to 12 hours.[11] Perform frequent assessment during IV therapy, as complications include hypocalcemia, hyperkalemia, hypotension, and dysrhythmias.

MAGNESIUM IMBALANCES

Magnesium, the second most abundant intracellular cation, plays a key role in essential cellular processes. It is a cofactor in many enzyme systems, including those responsible for carbohydrate metabolism, DNA and protein synthesis, blood glucose control, and BP regulation. Magnesium is needed for the production and use of ATP, the energy source for the sodium-potassium pump. Muscle contraction and relaxation, normal neurologic function, and neurotransmitter release depend on magnesium.

About 50% to 60% of the body's magnesium is stored in muscle and bone; 30% is in cells, with only 1% in ECF. The kidneys and GI system regulate serum magnesium by controlling the amount of magnesium reabsorbed in the ascending loop of Henle and distal tubules and absorption in the small intestine. GI absorption and renal reabsorption increase when magnesium levels are low.

HYPERMAGNESEMIA

Hypermagnesemia (high serum magnesium level) usually occurs only with increased magnesium intake accompanied by renal insufficiency or failure. A patient with chronic kidney disease who ingests products containing magnesium (e.g., Maalox, Milk of Magnesia) will have a problem with excess magnesium. Magnesium excess could develop in a pregnant woman receiving magnesium sulfate for the treatment of eclampsia or in patients taking laxatives and antacids that contain magnesium. Table 16.10 lists the causes and manifestations of hypermagnesemia.

Excess magnesium inhibits acetylcholine release at the myoneural junction and calcium movement into cells, impairing nerve and muscle function. Initial manifestations include hypotension, facial flushing, lethargy, urinary retention, nausea, and vomiting. As the serum magnesium level increases, deep tendon reflexes are lost, followed by muscle paralysis and coma. Respiratory and cardiac arrest can occur.

Management begins with avoiding magnesium-containing drugs and limiting dietary intake of magnesium-containing foods (e.g., green vegetables, nuts, bananas, oranges, peanut butter, chocolate). If renal function is adequate, increased fluids and diuretics promote urinary excretion of magnesium. The patient with impaired renal function may need dialysis. If hypermagnesemia is symptomatic, giving IV calcium gluconate will oppose the effects of the excess magnesium on cardiac muscle.[12]

HYPOMAGNESEMIA

Hypomagnesemia (low serum magnesium level) occurs in patients with limited magnesium intake or increased GI or renal losses. Causes of hypomagnesemia from insufficient food intake include prolonged fasting or starvation and chronic alcohol use. Another potential cause is prolonged parenteral nutrition without magnesium supplementation. Fluid loss from the GI tract, acute pancreatitis, and poorly controlled diabetes may contribute to hypomagnesemia. Diuretics, proton-pump inhibitors, and certain antibiotics may lead to magnesium loss.[12] Table 16.10 lists the causes and manifestations of hypomagnesemia.

Clinically, hypomagnesemia resembles hypocalcemia. Neuromuscular manifestations are common, such as muscle cramps, tremors, hyperactive deep tendon reflexes, Chvostek's sign, and Trousseau's sign. Neurologic manifestations include confusion, vertigo, and seizures. Dysrhythmias, such as torsades de pointes and ventricular fibrillation, can occur.

Management depends on the underlying cause and the patient's symptoms. Mild magnesium deficiency involves oral supplements and increased dietary intake of foods high in magnesium. If the deficiency is severe or if hypocalcemia is present, IV magnesium (e.g., magnesium sulfate) is given. Monitor vital signs and use an infusion pump, since rapid administration can lead to hypotension and cardiac or respiratory arrest.

ACID-BASE IMBALANCES

The body normally maintains a steady balance between the acids continually produced during normal metabolism and the bases that neutralize and promote the excretion of the acids. Because these acids alter the body's internal environment, their regulation is necessary to maintain homeostasis and acid-base balance. Many health problems may lead to acid-base imbalances. Patients with diabetes, chronic obstructive pulmonary disease (COPD), and kidney disease often develop acid-base imbalances.

Remember that an acid-base imbalance is not a disease but a symptom of an underlying health problem. Always consider the possibility of acid-base imbalance in patients with serious illnesses.

pH AND HYDROGEN ION CONCENTRATION

The acidity or alkalinity of a solution depends on its hydrogen ion (H^+) concentration. An increase in H^+ concentration leads to acidity; a decrease leads to alkalinity. H^+ concentration is usually expressed as a negative logarithm (symbolized as *pH*). The use of the negative logarithm means that the lower the pH, the higher is the H^+ concentration.

The pH of a chemical solution may range from 1 to 14. A solution with a pH of 7 is considered neutral. An acid solution has a pH less than 7, and an alkaline solution has a pH greater than 7. Blood is slightly alkaline and has a normal arterial pH of 7.35 to 7.45. Medically, if the pH drops below 7.35, a person has acidosis. If the blood pH is greater than 7.45, the person has alkalosis (Fig. 16.16).

ACID-BASE REGULATION

The body uses 3 mechanisms to regulate acid-base balance and keep the pH between 7.35 and 7.45. These are the buffer systems, respiratory system, and renal system. Each mechanism reacts at different speeds. Buffers are the fastest, reacting immediately.

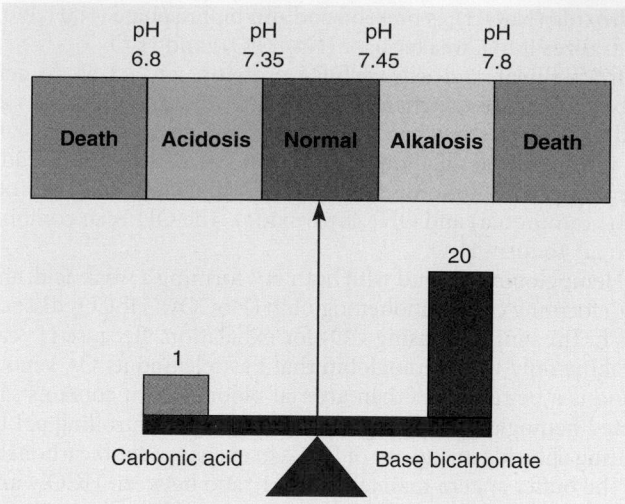

FIG. 16.16 The normal range of plasma pH is 7.35 to 7.45. A normal pH is maintained by a ratio of 1 part carbonic acid to 20 parts bicarbonate.

The respiratory system responds in minutes and reaches maximum effectiveness in hours. The renal response occurs hours to days after a change in pH. The kidneys can maintain balance indefinitely in patients with chronic imbalances. But, if the person has impaired kidney function, the kidneys will not be effective in maintaining acid-base balance.

Buffer System

Buffering is the primary regulator of acid-base balance. **Buffers** act chemically to change strong acids into weaker ones or bind acids to neutralize them. This minimizes the effect of acids on blood pH until they can be excreted from the body. Buffers can maintain pH only if the respiratory and renal systems function adequately.

All body fluids contain buffers. The major buffer in ECF is the carbonic acid–bicarbonate system (H_2CO_3/HCO_3^-). Other buffer systems include phosphate, protein, and hemoglobin. The cell can act as a buffer by shifting H^+ in and out of the cell. When ECF levels of H^+ are increased, H^+ enters the cell in exchange for potassium. This may result in hyperkalemia as potassium moves into the ECF. Conversely, with decreased H^+ levels, H^+ enters plasma in exchange for potassium. This is why a patient with alkalosis can develop hypokalemia.

A buffer consists of a weak acid, which releases H^+ when fluid is too alkaline, or a base and its salt, which takes up H^+ when fluid is too acidic. The carbonic acid–bicarbonate buffer system neutralizes hydrochloric acid (HCl), a strong acid, by combining it with a strong base. This prevents the acid from making a large decrease in pH.

$$\underset{\text{Strong Acid}}{HCL} + \underset{\text{Strong Base}}{Na_2CO_3} \rightarrow \underset{\text{Salt}}{NaCl} + \underset{\text{Weak Acid}}{H_2CO_3}$$

The carbonic acid is broken down into H_2O and CO_2. The lungs excrete CO_2, either combined with insensible H_2O as carbonic acid or alone as CO_2.

The phosphate, protein, and hemoglobin buffer systems act in the same way as the bicarbonate system. The main components of the phosphate system are monohydrogen phosphate (HPO_4^{2-}) and dihydrogen phosphate ($H_2PO_4^-$). A phosphate, combined with sodium, can neutralize a strong acid, such as HCl, by forming sodium chloride (NaCl) and sodium biphosphate (NaH_2PO_4), a weak acid. If a strong base, such as sodium hydroxide (NaOH), is present, sodium biphosphate (NaH_2PO_4) neutralizes it to a weaker base (Na_2HPO_4) and H_2O.

Intracellular and extracellular proteins can act as an acid or base. Because the chemical structure of amino acids has an acid and a base, they can accept H^+ if pH decreases or release H^+ if fluid is too alkaline. Some amino acids have basic radicals (NH_3OH [ammonium hydroxide]) that can dissociate into NH_3^+ (ammonia) and OH^- (hydroxide). The OH^- can combine with H^+ to form H_2O.

Hemoglobin can bind with both H^+, forming a weak acid, and CO_2, forming carbaminohemoglobin ($HbCO_2$). $HbCO_2$ dissociates in the lungs, releasing CO_2 for exhalation. Because H^+ can combine only with hemoglobin that has released its O_2, venous blood is a better buffer than arterial blood, which contains saturated hemoglobin. Hemoglobin also aids in controlling pH by shifting chloride in and out of RBCs in exchange for bicarbonate.

The buffer system maintains a 20:1 ratio between HCO_3^- and carbonic acid in ECF. The body's ability to keep this ratio is important in controlling pH. For example, excess carbonic acid increases the ratio and decreases pH, resulting in acidosis. In response, the body can increase HCO_3^- levels to keep the ratio 20:1 and keep the pH near normal, a state called *compensation*. For example, a ratio of 40:2 is present in compensated acid-base balance.

Respiratory System

The lungs help maintain a normal pH by excreting CO_2 and water, which are by-products of cellular metabolism. When released into the circulation, CO_2 enters RBCs and combines with H_2O to form H_2CO_3. Carbonic acid dissociates into H^+ and HCO_3^-. Hemoglobin buffers the free H^+, and the HCO_3^- diffuses into the plasma. This process is reversed in the pulmonary capillaries, forming CO_2 that is excreted by the lungs.

The amount of CO_2 in the blood directly relates to carbonic acid and H^+ concentration. With increased respirations, more CO_2 is expelled and less stays in the blood. This leads to less carbonic acid and less H^+. With decreased respirations, more CO_2 stays in the blood. This leads to increased carbonic acid and more H^+.

The respiratory center in the medulla controls the rate of excretion of CO_2. If increased amounts of CO_2 or H^+ are present, the respiratory center stimulates an increased rate and depth of breathing to "blow off" CO_2 through hyperventilation. If the center senses low H^+ or CO_2 levels, respirations are reduced and CO_2 retained. The older adult has an impaired compensatory ability due to decreased respiratory function.

Renal System

Under normal conditions, the body depends on the kidneys to reabsorb and conserve all the HCO_3^- they filter and excrete some of the acid produced by cellular metabolism. The 3 mechanisms of acid excretion include (1) secreting small amounts of free hydrogen into the renal tubule, (2) combining H^+ with ammonia (NH_3) to form ammonium (NH_4^+), and (3) excreting weak acids.

The kidneys normally excrete acidic urine (average pH is 6). As a compensatory mechanism, the pH of the urine can decrease to 4 or increase to 8. To compensate for acidosis, the kidneys can reabsorb more HCO_3^- and excrete excess H^+. This increases the blood pH and decreases the urine pH. In the older adult, the kidneys are less able to compensate for acid load.

ALTERATIONS IN ACID-BASE BALANCE

An acid-base imbalance results when there is a change in the ratio of 20:1 between base and acid content. This occurs when a

disease or process alters one side of the ratio (e.g., CO_2 retention in pulmonary disease) and the compensatory processes that maintain the other side of the ratio (e.g., increased renal HCO_3^- reabsorption) either fail or are inadequate. The compensatory process may be inadequate because either the pathophysiologic activity is overwhelming or there is not enough time for the compensatory process to work.

Acid-base imbalances are classified as respiratory or metabolic. *Respiratory imbalances* result from changes in carbonic acid concentration. *Metabolic imbalances* affect the base HCO_3^-. Acidosis occurs with an increase in carbonic acid (respiratory acidosis) or decrease in HCO_3^- (metabolic acidosis). Alkalosis occurs with a decrease in carbonic acid (respiratory alkalosis) or increase in HCO_3^- (metabolic alkalosis). Imbalances are further classified as acute or chronic. Chronic imbalances allow greater time for compensatory changes.

Respiratory Acidosis

Respiratory acidosis (carbonic acid excess) occurs when a person has hypoventilation (Table 16.11). Hypoventilation leads to a buildup of CO_2, resulting in an accumulation of carbonic acid in the blood. Carbonic acid dissociates, releasing H^+ and decreasing pH. If CO_2 is not eliminated from the blood, acidosis results from the accumulation of carbonic acid (Fig. 16.17, *A*).

During acute respiratory acidosis, the renal compensatory mechanisms begin to work within 24 hours. The kidneys conserve HCO_3^- and secrete increased H^+ into the urine. Until the renal mechanisms have an effect, the serum HCO_3^- level will usually be normal and then increase.

Respiratory Alkalosis

Respiratory alkalosis (carbonic acid deficit) occurs with hyperventilation, or an increase in respiratory rate or volume (Table 16.11). The primary cause of respiratory alkalosis is hypoxemia from acute pulmonary disorders (e.g., pneumonia, pulmonary embolus). Hyperventilation can occur as a physiologic response to metabolic acidosis and increased metabolic demands (e.g., fever). Pain, anxiety, and some CNS disorders can increase respirations without a physiologic need. The decrease in the arterial CO_2 level leads to decreased carbonic acid concentration in the blood and an increased pH (Fig. 16.17, *A*).

Compensated respiratory alkalosis is rare. In acute respiratory alkalosis, aggressive treatment of the cause of hypoxemia is essential and usually does not allow time for compensation to occur. If the respiratory alkalosis is caused by significant pain, anxiety, or panic, breathing into a closed system to rebreathe eliminated CO_2 can aid in the compensatory process. Some buffering may occur with shifting of HCO_3^- into cells in exchange for chloride ions (Cl^-). In chronic respiratory alkalosis that occurs with pulmonary fibrosis or CNS disorders, compensation may include renal excretion of HCO_3^-.

Metabolic Acidosis

Metabolic acidosis (base bicarbonate deficit) occurs when an acid other than carbonic acid accumulates in the body or when bicarbonate is lost in body fluids (Table 16.11 and Fig. 16.17, *B*). Ketoacid accumulation in diabetic ketoacidosis and lactic acid accumulation with shock are examples of acid accumulation. Severe diarrhea resulting in loss of HCO_3^- is an example of a base deficit. In renal disease, the kidneys lose their ability to reabsorb HCO_3^- and secrete H^+. To compensate for metabolic acidosis, the kidneys try to excrete extra acid and the lungs

TABLE 16.11 Acid-Base Imbalances

Causes	Pathophysiology	Laboratory Findings

Respiratory Acidosis
• Chronic respiratory disease (e.g., COPD)
• Barbiturate or sedative overdose
• Chest wall abnormality
• Severe pneumonia
• Atelectasis
• Respiratory muscle weakness
• Mechanical hypoventilation
• Pulmonary edema
	• ↑ CO_2 retention from hypoventilation
	• Compensatory response is ↑ HCO_3^- retention by kidney
		↓ Plasma pH
		↑ $PaCO_2$
		HCO_3^- normal (uncompensated)
		↑ HCO_3^- (compensated)
		Sample ABG
		Uncompensated:
		  pH 7.31
		  $PaCO_2$ 54 mm Hg
		  HCO_3^- 25 mEq/L

Respiratory Alkalosis
• Hyperventilation (e.g., hypoxia, anxiety, fear, pain, exercise, fever)
• Stimulated respiratory center (e.g., septicemia, stroke, meningitis, encephalitis, brain injury, salicylate poisoning)
• Liver failure
• Mechanical hyperventilation
	↑ CO_2 excretion from hyperventilation
	Compensatory response is ↑ HCO_3^- excretion by kidney
		↑ Plasma pH
		↓ $PaCO_2$
		HCO_3^- normal (uncompensated)
		↓ HCO_3^- (compensated)
		Sample ABG
		Uncompensated:
		  pH 7.52
		  $PaCO_2$ 27 mm Hg
		  HCO_3^- 24 mEq/L

Metabolic Acidosis
• Diabetic ketoacidosis
• Lactic acidosis
• Starvation
• Diarrhea
• Renal tubular acidosis
• Renal failure
• GI fistulas
• Shock
	• Gain of fixed acid, inability to excrete acid or loss of base
	• Compensatory response is ↑ CO_2 excretion by lungs
		↓ Plasma pH
		$PaCO_2$ normal (uncompensated)
		↓ $PaCO_2$ (compensated)
		↓ HCO_3^-
		Sample ABG
		Uncompensated:
		  pH 7.29
		  $PaCO_2$ 38 mm Hg
		  HCO_3^- 18 mEq/L

Metabolic Alkalosis
• Vomiting
• NG suctioning
• Diuretic therapy
• Hypokalemia
• Excess $NaHCO_3$ intake
• Mineralocorticoid use
	• Loss of strong acid or gain of base
	• Compensatory response is ↑ CO_2 retention by lungs
		↑ Plasma pH
		$PaCO_2$ normal (uncompensated)
		↑ $PaCO_2$ (compensated)
		↑ HCO_3^-
		Sample ABG
		Uncompensated:
		  pH 7.50
		  $PaCO_2$ 40 mm Hg
		  HCO_3^- 34 mEq/L

increase CO_2 excretion. The patient often develops *Kussmaul respirations* (deep, rapid breathing) when trying to compensate for metabolic acidosis.

If metabolic acidosis is present, calculating the anion gap helps determine the source of the acidosis. The *anion gap* is the difference between the measured serum cations and anions in ECF.

$$Anion\ gap = Na^+ - (HCO_3^- + Cl^-)$$

A normal anion gap is 8 to 12 mmol/L. The anion gap increases in metabolic acidosis associated with acid gain (e.g., lactic acidosis, diabetic ketoacidosis) but is normal in metabolic acidosis caused by bicarbonate loss (e.g., diarrhea).

Metabolic Alkalosis

Metabolic alkalosis (base bicarbonate excess) occurs when a loss of acid (e.g., from prolonged vomiting or gastric suction) or a gain in HCO_3^- (e.g., from ingestion of baking soda) occurs (Table 16.11 and Fig. 16.17, *B*). Renal excretion of HCO_3^- occurs in response to metabolic alkalosis. The lung's compensatory response is limited. The respiratory rate decreases to retain plasma CO_2. However, once hypoxemia occurs or plasma

CO_2 reaches a certain level, stimulation of chemoreceptors will increase respirations.

Mixed Acid-Base Disorders

A mixed acid-base disorder occurs when 2 or more disorders are present at the same time. The pH depends on the type, severity, and acuity of each disorder involved and any compensatory mechanisms at work. Respiratory acidosis combined with metabolic alkalosis (e.g., a patient with atelectasis and NG suction) may result in a near-normal pH. Respiratory acidosis combined with metabolic acidosis causes a greater decrease in pH than either disorder alone. An example of a mixed acidosis is a patient in severe shock with poor perfusion and hypoventilation. Mixed alkalosis can occur in a patient hyperventilating because of postoperative pain who is losing acid from NG suctioning.

CLINICAL MANIFESTATIONS OF ACID-BASE IMBALANCES

The manifestations of acidosis and alkalosis are outlined in Tables 16.12 and 16.13. In both respiratory and metabolic acidosis, the

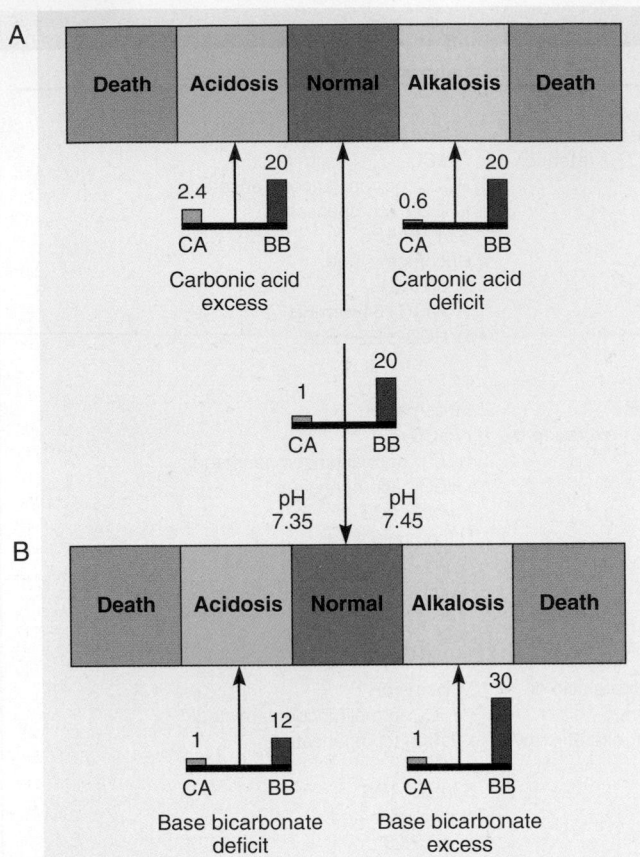

FIG. 16.17 Kinds of acid-base imbalances. **A,** Respiratory imbalances caused by carbonic acid *(CA)* excess and carbonic acid deficit. **B,** Metabolic imbalances caused by base bicarbonate *(BB)* deficit and base bicarbonate excess.

TABLE 16.12 Manifestations of Acidosis

Respiratory ($\uparrow$ PaCO$_2$)	Metabolic ($\downarrow$ HCO$_3^-$)
Neurologic	
Lethargy	Lethargy
Confusion	Confusion
Dizziness	Dizziness
Headache	Headache
Coma	Coma
Cardiovascular	
$\downarrow$ BP	$\downarrow$ BP
Ventricular fibrillation (related to hyperkalemia from compensation)	Dysrhythmias (related to hyperkalemia from compensation)
Warm, flushed skin	Cold, clammy skin
Gastrointestinal	
No significant findings	Nausea, vomiting, diarrhea, abdominal pain
Neuromuscular	
Seizures	Muscle weakness
Respiratory	
Hypoventilation with hypoxia	Deep, rapid respirations

CNS is depressed. Headache, lethargy, weakness, and confusion develop, leading eventually to coma and death. Compensatory mechanisms also produce specific manifestations. For example, the deep, rapid (Kussmaul) respirations of a patient with metabolic acidosis occur with respiratory compensation.

TABLE 16.13 Manifestations of Alkalosis

Respiratory ($\downarrow$ PaCO$_2$)	Metabolic ($\uparrow$ HCO$_3^-$)
Neurologic	
Dizziness	Irritability
Light-headedness	Lethargy
Confusion	Confusion
Headache	Headache
Cardiovascular	
Tachycardia	Tachycardia
Dysrhythmias (related to hypokalemia from compensation)	Dysrhythmias (related to hypokalemia from compensation)
Gastrointestinal	
Nausea, vomiting, diarrhea	Nausea, vomiting
Epigastric pain	Anorexia
Neuromuscular	
Tetany	Tetany
Numbness	Tremors
Tingling of extremities	Tingling of fingers and toes
Hyperreflexia	Muscle cramps, hypertonic muscles
Seizures	Seizures
Respiratory	
Hyperventilation (lungs are unable to compensate if there is a respiratory problem)	Hypoventilation (compensatory action by lungs)

TABLE 16.14 Normal Arterial Blood Gas Values

Parameter	Reference Interval
pH	7.35–7.45
PaCO$_2$	35–45 mm Hg
Bicarbonate (HCO$_3^-$)	22–26 mEq/L (mmol/L)
PaO$_2$*	80–100 mm Hg
SaO$_2$	>95%
Base excess	$\pm$2.0 mEq/L

*Decreases above sea level and with increasing age.

In both types of alkalosis, symptoms usually result from an accompanying electrolyte abnormality rather than the alkalosis. Hypocalcemia occurs due to increased calcium binding with albumin, lowering the amount of ionized, active calcium. Therefore muscle cramping and symptoms of CNS excitability, including tingling and numbness of the fingers and tetany, occur. If left untreated, respiratory alkalosis can be life-threatening.[13]

Blood Gas Values

Arterial blood gas (ABG) values give objective information about a patient's acid-base status, the underlying cause of an imbalance, and the body's ability to regulate pH. Knowing the patient's clinical situation and the extent of renal and respiratory compensation allows you to identify acid-base disorders and the patient's ability to compensate. Blood gas analysis also shows the partial pressure of arterial O$_2$ (PaO$_2$) and O$_2$ saturation. Table 16.14 lists normal blood gas values. These values help you evaluate the patient's overall oxygenation status and identify hypoxemia. Table 16.15 shows *ROME*, a quick memory device for understanding acid-base imbalances.

TABLE 16.15 ROME
Memory Device for Acid-Base Imbalances

For acid-base imbalances, use this quick memory device (mnemonic).
In **Respiratory** conditions, the pH and the $PaCO_2$ go in **Opposite** directions.
- In respiratory alkalosis, the pH is ↑ and the $PaCO_2$ is ↓.
- In respiratory acidosis, the pH is ↓ and the $PaCO_2$ is ↑.

In **Metabolic** conditions, the pH and the HCO_3^- go in the same direction **(Equal)**. The $PaCO_2$ may also go in the same direction.
- In metabolic alkalosis, pH and HCO_3^- are ↑ and the $PaCO_2$ is ↑ or normal.
- In metabolic acidosis, pH and HCO_3^- are ↓ and the $PaCO_2$ is ↓ or normal.

To interpret the results of an ABG, perform the following 5 steps:

1. Look at each of the values. If the pH is between 7.35 and 7.45, and the CO_2, HCO_3^-, and PaO_2 are within normal limits, the ABGs are normal. If any value is out of normal, then continue.
2. Look at the pH first. Values less than 7.35 indicate acidosis and values greater than 7.45 indicate alkalosis. A normal pH means there is normal acid-base status, compensation is occurring, or a mixed disorder is present.
3. Use ROME (Table 16.15) to figure out if the origin is respiratory or metabolic. Remember respiratory opposite and metabolic equal.
4. Once the metabolic or respiratory origin is determined, look at the remaining value, either the CO_2 or HCO_3^-, to figure the level of compensation. If the value is moving in the opposite direction, the body is trying to compensate. If the remaining value moving to compensate is abnormal and the pH is higher or lower than normal, *partial compensation* has occurred. If the pH is within normal limits, *full compensation* has occurred.
5. Assess the PaO_2 and O_2 saturation. If these values are abnormal, hypoxemia is present.

Table 16.16 explains how to analyze ABG results. The laboratory findings section of Table 16.11 shows ABG findings of the 4 major acid-base imbalances. See Chapter 25 for further discussion of ABGs.

ASSESSMENT OF FLUID, ELECTROLYTE, AND ACID-BASE IMBALANCES

Assessing patients for fluid, electrolyte, and acid-base imbalances is an important part of your nursing practice. In addition to assessing for the manifestations discussed earlier in this chapter, obtain subjective and objective data from any patient with suspected fluid, electrolyte, or acid-base imbalances.

Subjective Data
Important Health Information

Past Health History. Question the patient about any history of problems involving the kidneys, heart, GI system, or lungs that could affect the present fluid, electrolyte, and acid-base balance. Ask about specific diseases such as diabetes, diabetes insipidus, COPD, renal failure, ulcerative colitis, and Crohn's disease. Assess for any prior fluid, electrolyte, or acid-base disorders.

Medications. Assess the patient's current and past use of medications. The ingredients in many drugs, especially over-the-counter drugs, are often hidden sources of sodium, potassium,

TABLE 16.16 Applying Arterial Blood Gas (ABG) Analysis

Sample ABG Values	Analysis
pH 7.32 $PaCO_2$ 30 HCO_3^- 16 PaO_2 95	1. Look at each of the values. If the pH is between 7.35 and 7.45, and the CO_2, HCO_3^-, and PaO_2 are within normal limits, the ABGs are normal. If any value is out of normal, then continue. *The pH, CO_2, HCO_3^- are all abnormally low. Continue with analysis.* 2. Look at the pH first. Values less than 7.35 indicate acidosis and values greater than 7.45. *The pH is below 7.35, indicating acidosis.* 3. Use ROME to figure out if the origin is respiratory or metabolic. Remember respiratory opposite and metabolic equal. *Using ROME, the pH and CO_2 are not going in the opposite direction (the disorder is not respiratory in origin). The pH and HCO_3^- are moving in the same or equal direction, so the disorder is metabolic in origin.* 4. Once the metabolic or respiratory origin is determined, look at the remaining laboratory value (either CO_2 or HCO_3^-) to figure the level of compensation. *Since the disorder is metabolic in origin, review the remaining laboratory value (in this case the CO_2) The CO_2 is low, meaning the lungs are trying to compensate by lowering acid levels.* 5. Assess the PaO_2 and O_2 saturation. If these values are abnormal, hypoxemia is present. *The PaO_2 is normal and does not indicate hypoxemia.*

Interpretation
This ABG is interpreted as metabolic acidosis with partial compensation. Partial compensation is occurring because the pH remains abnormal. Full compensation would occur after the pH returns within normal limits.

calcium, magnesium, and other electrolytes. Many prescription drugs, including diuretics, corticosteroids, and electrolyte supplements, can cause fluid and electrolyte imbalances.

Surgery or Other Treatments. Ask the patient about past or present renal dialysis, kidney surgery, or bowel surgery resulting in a temporary or permanent external collecting system, such as an ileostomy.

Functional Health Patterns

Health Perception–Health Management Pattern. If the patient currently has a problem related to fluid, electrolyte, and acid-base balance, obtain a careful description of the illness, including onset, course, and treatment. Ask the patient about any recent changes in body weight.

Nutritional-Metabolic Pattern. Ask the patient about diet and any special dietary practices. Weight reduction diets, fad diets, or any eating disorders, such as anorexia or bulimia, can lead to fluid and electrolyte problems. If the patient is on a special diet, such as low sodium or high potassium, assess the ability to adhere to the dietary prescription.

Elimination Pattern. Make note of the patient's usual bowel and bladder habits. Carefully document any deviations from the expected elimination pattern, such as diarrhea, oliguria, polyuria, or incontinence.

Activity-Exercise Pattern. Ask about the patient's exercise pattern and any excess perspiration. Determine if the patient is exposed to extremely high temperatures during leisure or work activity. Ask the patient what he or she does to replace fluid and electrolytes lost through excess perspiration. Assess the patient's activity level to determine any functional problems that could lead to lack of ability to obtain food or fluids.

Cognitive-Perceptual Pattern. Ask about any changes in sensations, such as numbness, tingling, or muscle weakness, which could indicate a fluid and electrolyte problem. Ask the patient and caregiver if there have been any changes in mentation or alertness, such as confusion, memory impairment, or lethargy.

Objective Data

Physical Examination. Perform a complete physical examination because fluid, electrolyte, and acid-base balance affects all body systems. As you assess each system, check for manifestations that you would expect with an imbalance. Common abnormal assessment findings of major body systems offer clues to possible imbalances (Table 16.17).

TABLE 16.17 Assessment Abnormalities

Fluid and Electrolyte Imbalances

Finding	Possible Cause
Blood Pressure	
Hypotension	Fluid volume deficit, low Ca^{2+}, high Mg^{2+}
Hypertension	Fluid volume excess, high Ca^{2+}, low Mg^{2+}
Muscular	
Chvostek's sign	Low Ca^{2+}, high PO_4^{3-}, low Mg^{2+}
Muscle cramping	High K^+, low Ca^{2+}, high PO_4^{3-}, low Mg^{2+}
Muscle weakness	High or low K^+, high Ca^{2+}, low PO_4^{3-}, high Mg^{2+}
Trousseau's sign	Low Ca^{2+}, high PO_4^{3-}, low Mg^{2+}
Neurologic	
Confusion	Fluid volume excess, high or low Na^+, high or low K^+, low Ca^{2+}, high or low Mg^{2+}, low PO_4^{3-}
Decreased level of consciousness	Fluid volume deficit or excess, high or low Na^+, low PO_4^{3-}
Fatigue	Fluid volume deficit, low K^+, high Ca^{2+}
Irritability	Low Na^+, high K^+, low Ca^{2+}, high PO_4^{3-}
Tremors, seizures	High Na^+, low K^+, low Ca^{2+}, high PO_4^{3-}, low Mg^{2+}
Respirations	
Crackles	Fluid volume excess
Dyspnea	Fluid volume excess
Rapid respirations	Fluid volume deficit
Restricted airway	Low Ca^{2+}, high PO_4^{3-}
Pulse	
Bounding pulse	Fluid volume excess
Rapid, weak, thready pulse	Fluid volume deficit
Weak, irregular, rapid pulse	Severe low K^+, low Mg^{2+}
Weak, irregular, slow pulse	Severe high K^+, high Mg^{2+}
Skin	
Cold, clammy skin	Fluid volume deficit, low Na^+
Flushed, dry skin	High Na^+, High Mg^{2+}
Pitting edema	Fluid volume excess
Poor skin turgor	Fluid volume deficit

Laboratory Values. Assessing serum electrolyte values is a good starting point for evaluating fluid and electrolyte balance (Table 16.1). Serum electrolytes can also provide important information about a patient's acid-base balance. Changes in the serum HCO_3^- (often reported as total CO_2 or CO_2 content on an electrolyte panel) indicate metabolic acidosis (low HCO_3^- level) or alkalosis (high HCO_3^- level).

> ⚠ **SAFETY ALERT** **Managing Critical Test Results**
> • Promptly report critical laboratory values to the HCP.
> • Assess the patient and take appropriate actions (e.g., ECG monitoring).

Remember that serum electrolyte values often provide limited information. They reflect the concentration of that electrolyte in ECF but not necessarily in ICF. For example, most potassium is found in the cells. Changes in serum potassium values may be the result of a true deficit or excess of potassium or reflect the movement of potassium into or out of the cell during acid-base imbalances. An abnormal serum sodium level may reflect a sodium problem or, more likely, a water problem.

Other useful laboratory tests include serum and urine osmolality, serum glucose, blood urea nitrogen, serum creatinine, venous blood gas sampling, urine specific gravity, and urine electrolytes.

ORAL FLUID AND ELECTROLYTE REPLACEMENT

In all cases of fluid, electrolyte, and acid-base imbalances, the primary treatment involves correcting the underlying cause. Oral rehydration solutions containing water, potassium, sodium, and glucose may be used to correct mild fluid and electrolyte deficits. Glucose not only provides calories but also promotes sodium and water absorption in the small intestine. Commercial oral rehydration solutions are now available for home use. Avoid cola drinks because they do not contain adequate electrolyte replacement, and the sugar content may lead to osmotic diuresis.

IV. FLUID AND ELECTROLYTE REPLACEMENT

IV fluid and electrolyte therapy are necessary to treat many different fluid and electrolyte imbalances. Many patients need maintenance IV fluid therapy when they cannot take oral fluids (e.g., during and after surgery). Other patients need corrective or replacement therapy for losses that are ongoing or have already occurred. The amount and type of solution is determined by the normal daily maintenance requirements and by imbalances identified by laboratory results. We classify IV replacement solutions by their concentration or tonicity (Table 16.18). Tonicity is a key factor in determining the appropriate solution to correct imbalances.

Solutions

Hypotonic. A hypotonic solution has a lower osmolality when compared to plasma.[14] Infusing a hypotonic solution dilutes ECF, lowering serum osmolality. Osmosis then produces a movement of water from ECF to interstitial spaces and cells, causing cells to swell. After achieving equilibrium, ICF and ECF have the same osmolality. Hypotonic solutions (e.g., 0.45% NaCl) are useful in treating patients with hypernatremia. They are a good maintenance fluid because normal daily losses are hypotonic. They are not good for replacement because they can deplete ECF and lower BP. Because hypotonic solutions have the potential to cause cellular swelling, monitor patients for changes in mentation that may indicate cerebral edema.

Although 5% dextrose in water is technically an isotonic solution, the dextrose quickly metabolizes. The net result is the administration of hypotonic free water with equal expansion of ECF and ICF. One liter of a 5% dextrose solution provides 50 g of dextrose, or 170 calories. While this amount of dextrose is not enough to meet caloric requirements, it helps prevent ketosis associated with starvation.

Isotonic. An isotonic solution has an osmolality similar to plasma.[14] Because of this similarity, giving an isotonic solution expands only ECF and the fluid does not move into cells. This makes isotonic solutions the ideal fluid replacement for patients with ECF volume deficits. Examples of isotonic solutions include 0.9% NaCl and lactated Ringer's solution.

Isotonic saline (0.9% NaCl), or *normal saline*, has a sodium concentration (154 mEq/L) slightly higher than that of plasma (135 to 145 mEq/L) and a chloride concentration (154 mEq/L) significantly higher than the plasma chloride level (96 to 106 mEq/L). Therefore giving too much isotonic saline has the potential to increase sodium and chloride levels. Isotonic saline is used when a patient has had both fluid and sodium losses (e.g., diarrhea, vomiting).

Lactated Ringer's solution contains sodium, potassium, chloride, calcium, and lactate (the precursor of bicarbonate) in about the same concentrations as ECF. This makes it the ideal fluid in certain situations, such as surgery, burns, or GI fluid losses. Patients with liver dysfunction, hyperkalemia, and severe hypovolemia should not receive lactated Ringer's because they have a decreased ability to convert the lactate to bicarbonate.

Hypertonic. A hypertonic solution has a higher osmolality than plasma.[14] The higher osmotic pressure draws water out of the cells into ECF. It is useful in the treatment of hyponatremia and trauma patients with head injury. Those receiving hypertonic

TABLE 16.18 Common Crystalloid Solutions

Solution	Tonicity	mOsm/kg	Contents	Indications and Considerations
Dextrose in Water				
5%	Isotonic, but physiologically hypotonic	278	50 g/L dextrose	• Contains free water only, no electrolytes • Provides 170 cal/L • Used to replace water losses and treat hypernatremia
10%	Hypertonic	556	100 g/L dextrose	• Contains free water only, no electrolytes • Provides 340 cal/L • Used with parenteral nutrition
Saline				
0.45%	Hypotonic	154	77 mEq/L Na+ 77 mEq/L Cl-	• Contains free water, Na+, and Cl-, no calories • Used to treat hypernatremia and uncontrolled hyperglycemia • Used as a maintenance solution
0.9%	Isotonic	308	154 mEq/L Na+ 154 mEq/L Cl-	• Contains Na+ and Cl- in excess of plasma levels • Does not contain free water or calories • Used to expand intravascular volume and replace extracellular fluid losses • Only solution given with blood products • May cause volume overload in patients with heart or kidney disease
3.0%	Hypertonic	1026	513 mEq/L Na+ 513 mEq/L Cl-	• Contains Na+ and Cl- in excess of plasma levels • Used to treat symptomatic hyponatremia and trauma patients with head injury • Give slowly because it may cause volume overload and pulmonary edema
Dextrose in Saline				
5% in 0.25%	Isotonic	355	50 g/L dextrose 34 mEq/L Na+ 34 mEq/L Cl-	• Provides Na+, Cl-, and free water • Used to replace hypotonic losses and treat hypernatremia • Provides 170 cal/L
5% in 0.45%	Hypertonic	432	50 g/L dextrose 77 mEq/L Na+ 77 mEq/L Cl-	• Provides Na+, Cl-, and free water • Used as a maintenance solution
5% in 0.9%	Hypertonic	586	50 g/L dextrose 154 mEq/L Na+ 154 mEq/L Cl-	• Contains Na+ and Cl- in excess of plasma levels • Used to treat metabolic alkalosis and volume deficits in patients with hyponatremia
Multiple Electrolyte Solutions				
Ringer's solution	Isotonic	309	147 mEq/L Na+ 156 mEq/L Cl- 4 mEq/L K+ 4 mEq/L Ca2+	• Similar in composition to plasma except that it has excess Cl-, no Mg2+, no HCO3- • Does not provide free water or calories • Used to expand the intravascular volume and replace extracellular fluid losses
Lactated Ringer's (Hartmann's) solution	Isotonic	273	130 mEq/L Na+ 109 mEq/L Cl- 4 mEq/L K+ 3 mEq/L Ca2+ 28 mmol/L lactate	• Similar in composition to normal plasma except does not contain Mg2+ • Does not provide free water or calories • Used to treat hypovolemia, burns, and GI fluid losses • Cannot be used in patients with alkalosis or lactic acidosis

solutions need frequent monitoring of BP, lung sounds, and serum sodium levels because of the risk for intravascular fluid volume excess.

Although concentrated dextrose and water solutions (10% dextrose or greater) are hypertonic solutions, once the dextrose is metabolized, the net result is the administration of water. This free water ultimately expands ECF and ICF. The primary use of these solutions is providing calories as part of parenteral nutrition (see Chapter 39). You may give solutions containing 10% dextrose or less through a peripheral line. You must use a central line to give solutions with dextrose concentrations greater than 10%.

IV Additives. Additives in basic IV solutions replace specific losses. KCl, CaCl$_2$, MgSO$_4$, and HCO$_3^-$ are common additives. The use of each was described earlier in the discussion of the specific electrolyte deficiencies. Many premixed IV solutions containing specific additives are available. Using these solutions reduces error as the solution contains the correct amount of the electrolyte in the proper volume and type of IV solution.

Colloids. Colloid solutions contain large molecules that increase oncotic pressure and pull fluid into the blood vessels. Because this action restores blood volume, colloids are also called *volume expanders* or *plasma expanders*. Colloids include human plasma products (albumin, fresh frozen plasma, blood) and semisynthetic solutions (dextran, starches).

Albumin is available in 5% and 25% solutions. The 5% solution has an albumin concentration similar to that of plasma and results in plasma volume expansion equal to the volume infused. This makes it ideal for treating hypovolemic patients. In contrast, 25% albumin solution is hypertonic and draws fluid from the interstitial space. This makes it useful in treating patients with burns, hepatic failure, and ascites.

Dextran solutions are synthetic complex sugar solutions. There are 2 types: low-molecular-weight dextran (dextran 40) and high-molecular-weight dextran (dextran 70). Because dextran metabolizes slowly, it stays in the vascular system for a prolonged period. It pulls fluid into the intravascular space, expanding it by more volume than what is infused. Hydroxyethyl starches (e.g., Hespan) are synthetic colloids that work similarly to dextran to expand plasma volume.

Colloids can lead to circulatory overload because they pull fluid into ECF. Monitor vital signs and urine output frequently and assess for signs and symptoms of fluid volume excess. All colloids affect blood coagulation, with dextran and starches having the strongest anticoagulation effect.[14] Monitor coagulation times and implement any necessary precautions. Fatal anaphylactic reactions have occurred with Hespan and dextran. Monitor the patient closely for a hypersensitivity reaction and stop an infusion at once if a reaction occurs.

If the patient has lost blood, whole blood or packed RBCs are given. Packed RBCs have the advantage of giving the patient primarily RBCs rather than RBCs and fluid volume. Although packed RBCs have a decreased plasma volume, they increase the oncotic pressure and pull fluid into the intravascular space. The use of whole blood, with its added fluid volume, may cause circulatory overload, particularly in patients who are susceptible to complications from excess circulating volume (e.g., heart failure). To prevent fluid volume excess, loop diuretics may be given with blood and colloids. See Chapter 30 for more information on giving blood and blood products.

NURSING MANAGEMENT

IV Therapy

- Assess patient for manifestations of fluid and electrolyte imbalances.
- Determine if ordered IV therapies are appropriate.
- Choose and insert appropriate IV catheters and infusion devices.
- Give IV fluids and medications.
- Monitor for adverse reactions to IV fluids or medications.
- Assess for manifestations of fluid overload or hypovolemia and initiate appropriate changes in IV fluids.
- Evaluate if IV therapies are addressing patient's fluid and electrolyte needs.
- Collaborate with the pharmacist to:
  - Determine appropriateness of IV therapies and need for dose adjustments.
  - Prepare IV infusions and medications.
  - Screen for potential problems, such as compatibility issues.
  - Monitor response to therapy.

CENTRAL VENOUS ACCESS DEVICES

Central venous access devices (CVADs) are catheters placed in large blood vessels (e.g., subclavian vein, jugular vein) of people who need frequent or special access to the vascular system. There are 3 main types of CVADs: centrally inserted catheters, peripherally inserted central catheters (PICCs), and implanted ports.

Advantages of CVADs include immediate access to the central venous system, a reduced need for multiple venipunctures, and decreased risk for extravasation injury. CVADs permit frequent, continuous, rapid, or intermittent administration of fluids and medications. They allow for the administration of drugs that are potential *vesicants* (agents that can cause tissue damage), blood and blood products, and parenteral nutrition. CVADs can provide a means to perform hemodynamic monitoring and obtain venous blood samples. They are useful with patients who have limited peripheral vascular access or who have a projected need for long-term vascular access. CVADs also can be used to inject radiopaque contrast media. Table 16.19 gives examples of when CVADs are used.

The major disadvantages of CVADs are an increased risk for systemic infection and the invasiveness of the procedure. Extravasation (leakage of fluid) can still occur if there is displacement of or damage to the device.

Centrally Inserted Catheters

The tip of centrally inserted catheters (also called central venous catheters [CVCs]) rests in the distal end of the superior vena cava near its junction with the right atrium (Fig. 16.18). The other end of the catheter exits through a separate incision on the chest or abdominal wall. *Nontunneled catheters* are usually placed in the subclavian or internal jugular vein, more rarely in the femoral vein. They are best for patients with short-term needs in an acute care setting. *Surgically placed tunneled catheters* (e.g., Hickman, Broviac, Groshong) are suitable for long-term needs. Tunneling of the catheter through subcutaneous tissue and the synthetic cuff used to anchor the catheter provide stability and decrease infection risk. After the site heals, the catheter does not need a dressing, making it easier for the patient to maintain the site at home.

CVCs are available with single-, double-, or triple-lumens. Multilumen catheters are useful in the critically ill patient

TABLE 16.19 Common Indications for Central Venous Access Devices (CVADs)

Condition	Indications for Use
Autoimmune disorders	Perform plasmapheresis
Blood sampling	Multiple blood draws for diagnostic tests over time
Blood transfusions	Infusion of blood or blood products
Heart failure	Perform ultrafiltration
Hemodynamic monitoring	Used to measure central venous pressure to assess fluid balance
Medication administration	
• Cancer	Chemotherapy, infusion of irritating or vesicant medications
• Contrast media	Inject radiopaque contrast media for diagnostic testing
• Infection	Long-term administration of antibiotics
• Pain	Long-term administration of pain medication
• Drugs at risk for causing phlebitis	Epoprostenol (Flolan) Calcium chloride Potassium chloride Amiodarone
Nutritional replacement	Infusion of parenteral nutrition Infusion of high percentage dextrose solutions
Renal failure	Perform hemodialysis (especially on an acute basis) or continuous renal replacement therapy
Shock, burns	Infusion of high volumes of fluid and electrolyte replacement

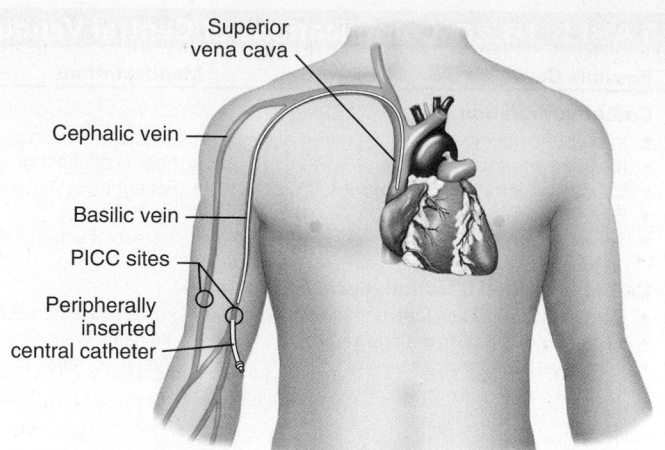

FIG. 16.19 Peripherally inserted central catheter (PICC) can be inserted using the basilic or cephalic vein.

need vascular access for 1 week to 6 months, but they can be in place for longer periods.

Advantages of a PICC over a CVC are lower infection rate, fewer insertion-related complications, decreased cost, and ability to insert at the bedside or in an outpatient area. PICCs, however, are associated with an increased risk for deep vein thrombosis and phlebitis (Table 16.20). If phlebitis occurs, it usually happens within 7 to 10 days after insertion. Do not use the arm with the PICC to take a BP reading or draw blood. When the BP cuff is inflated, the PICC can touch the vein wall, increasing the risk for vein damage and thrombosis.

Implanted Infusion Ports

An implanted infusion port consists of a surgically implanted CVC connected to a reservoir or port (Fig. 16.20, A). The catheter tip lies in the desired vein. The port lies in a surgically created subcutaneous pocket on the upper chest or arm. It consists of a titanium or plastic reservoir covered with a self-sealing silicone septum. You access the port by using a special noncoring needle with a deflected tip. This prevents damage to the septum that could make the port useless (Fig. 16.20, B).

Drugs are placed in the reservoir either by a direct injection or through injection into an established IV line. The reservoir then slowly releases the medicine into the bloodstream. Implanted ports are good for long-term therapy and have a low risk for infection. The hidden port offers the patient cosmetic advantages and overall has less maintenance than other types of CVADs. Monitor accessed ports for infiltration that can occur if the needle is not in place or dislodges.

Midline Catheters

Midline catheters technically are peripheral catheters because they do not enter a central vein. However, their use and care are similar to a PICC. A specially trained nurse can insert a midline catheter. A catheter can be from 3 to 8 inches long and have single or double lumens. They are inserted in the antecubital area through either the basilic or cephalic vein, often under ultrasound guidance. The basilic vein is best since it has a larger diameter. The tip rests right below the axilla, staying below the shoulder joint to reduce the risk for vein irritation from moving the shoulder. These lines can stay in place for up to 4 weeks.

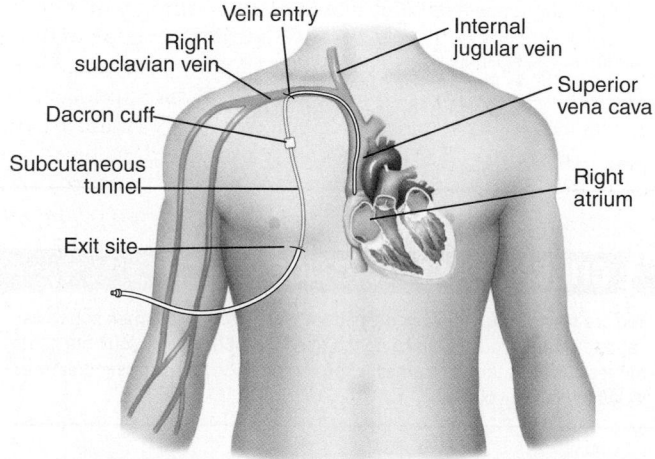

FIG. 16.18 Tunneled central venous catheter. Note tip of the catheter in the superior vena cava.

because each lumen can be used simultaneously to provide a different therapy. For example, incompatible drugs infuse in separate lumens without mixing while a third lumen gives access for blood sampling.

Peripherally Inserted Central Catheters

Peripherally inserted central catheters (PICCs) are CVCs inserted into a vein in the arm. The basilic vein is best because of its large diameter (Fig. 16.19). The cephalic, median cubital, or brachial veins are other options. Single-, double-, or triple-lumens are available. Double lumens are preferred because they allow for simultaneous uses. PICCs are used with patients who

TABLE 16.20 Complications of Central Venous Access Devices (CVADs)

Possible Cause	Manifestations	Management
Catheter Migration • Improper suturing • Insertion site trauma • Changes in intrathoracic pressure • Forceful catheter flushing • Spontaneous	• Sluggish infusion or aspiration • Edema of chest or neck during infusion • Patient reports gurgling sound in ear • Dysrhythmias • Increased external catheter length	• Prepare for fluoroscopy to verify position • Assist with removal and new CVAD placement
Catheter-Related Infection (Local or Systemic) • Contamination during insertion or use • Migration of organisms along catheter • Immunosuppressed patient	• *Local:* redness, tenderness, purulent drainage, warmth, edema • *Systemic:* fever, chills, malaise	Local • Culture drainage from site • Apply warm, moist compresses • Remove catheter if needed Systemic • Take blood cultures • Give antibiotic therapy • Give antipyretic therapy • Remove catheter if needed
Catheter Occlusion • Clamped or kinked catheter • Tip against wall of vessel • Thrombosis • Precipitate buildup in lumen	• Sluggish infusion or aspiration • Inability to infuse and/or aspirate	• Have patient change position, raise arm, and cough • Assess and alleviate any clamping or kinking • Flush with normal saline using a 10-mL syringe. Do not force flush • Instill anticoagulant or thrombolytic agent
Embolism • Catheter breaking • Dislodgment of thrombus • Entry of air into circulation	• Chest pain • Respiratory distress (dyspnea, tachypnea, hypoxia, cyanosis) • Hypotension • Tachycardia	• Apply O_2 • Clamp catheter • Place patient on left side with head down (air emboli) • Notify provider
Pneumothorax • Perforation of visceral pleura during insertion	• Decreased or absent breath sounds • Respiratory distress (cyanosis, dyspnea, tachypnea) • Chest pain • Distended unilateral chest	• Apply O_2 • Place in semi-Fowler's position • Prepare for chest tube insertion

Complications

CVADs always have a potential for complications. Careful monitoring and assessment will help you to identify potential complications early. Table 16.19 lists common complications, potential causes, manifestations, and interventions.

❖ NURSING MANAGEMENT: CENTRAL VENOUS ACCESS DEVICES

Nursing management of CVADs includes assessment, dressing changes and cleansing, injection cap changes, and maintenance of catheter patency. The exact frequency and procedures for these requirements vary by type of CVAD and facility, so it is important to follow your facility's policies and procedures. The following section discusses some general guidelines.

Catheter and insertion site assessment includes inspecting the site for redness, edema, warmth, drainage, tenderness, or pain. Observing the catheter for misplacement or slippage is important. Perform a comprehensive pain assessment, particularly noting any reports of chest or neck discomfort, arm pain, or pain at the insertion site. Do not use a newly placed CVAD until the tip position is verified with a chest x-ray.

❓ CHECK YOUR PRACTICE

You are taking care of a 74-yr-old patient with a left triple-lumen subclavian catheter. When you are changing the transparent dressing, you note some redness at the site with a small amount of yellow, foul-smelling drainage.
• What should you do?

Before manipulating a catheter for any reason, perform hand hygiene. Perform dressing changes and cleanse the catheter insertion site using strict sterile technique. Typical dressings include transparent semipermeable dressings or gauze and tape. If the site is bleeding, a gauze dressing may be preferable. Otherwise, transparent dressings are best. They allow observation of the site without having to remove the dressing. Transparent dressings may be left in place for up to 1 week. Change any dressing at once if it becomes damp, loose, or soiled.

Cleanse the skin around the catheter insertion site according to facility policy. A chlorhexidine-based preparation is the cleansing agent of choice. Its effects last longer than either povidone-iodine or alcohol, offering improved killing of bacteria.[15] When using chlorhexidine, cleansing the skin with friction is critical to preventing infection. When applying a new dressing, allow the area to air dry completely. Secure the lumen ports to

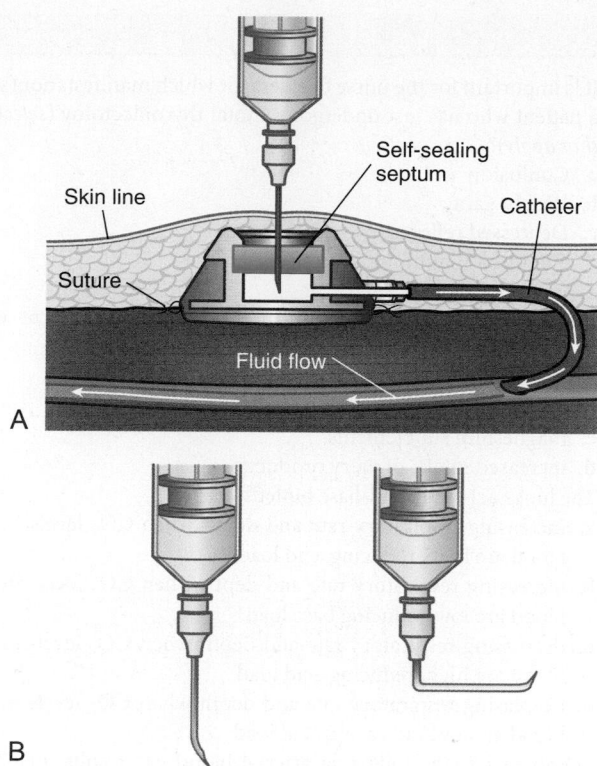

FIG. 16.20 A, Cross section of implantable port displaying access of the port with the Huber-point needle. Note the deflected point of the Huber-point needle, which prevents coring of the port's septum. **B,** 2 Huber-point needles used to enter the implanted port. The 90-degree needle is used for top-entry ports for continuous infusion.

the skin above the dressing site. Document the date and time of the dressing change and initial the dressing.

Disinfect catheter hubs, needleless connectors, and injection ports before accessing the catheter. Use an alcoholic chlorhexidine preparation, 70% alcohol, or povidone-iodine. Change injection caps at regular intervals according to facility policy, or if they have damage from excess punctures. Use strict sterile technique.

Teach the patient to turn the head to the opposite side of the insertion site during cap change. If you cannot clamp the catheter, have the patient lie flat in bed and perform the Valsalva maneuver whenever the catheter is open to air to prevent an air embolism.

Flushing is one of the most effective ways to maintain catheter patency. It also keeps incompatible drugs or fluids from mixing. Use a normal saline solution in a syringe that has a barrel capacity of 10 mL or more to avoid excess pressure on the catheter. If you feel resistance, do not apply force. This could result in a ruptured catheter or create an embolism if a thrombus is present. Because of the risk for contamination and infection, use solution from prefilled syringes or single-dose vials rather than multiple-dose vials when flushing catheters. If you are not using a positive-pressure valve cap, clamp any unused lines after flushing.

Use the push-pause technique when flushing all catheters. Push-pause creates turbulence within the catheter lumen, promoting the removal of debris that adheres to the catheter lumen and decreasing the chance of occlusion. This technique involves injecting saline with a rapid alternating push-pause motion, instilling 1 to 2 mL with each push on the syringe plunger. If you are using a negative-pressure cap or neutral pressure cap, clamp the catheter while maintaining positive pressure while instilling the last 1 mL of saline. This prevents reflux of blood back into the catheter. If a positive-pressure valve cap is present, it works to prevent the reflux of blood and resultant catheter lumen occlusion. Remove the syringe before clamping the catheter to allow the positive pressure valve to work correctly.

CVAD Removal

Removing a CVAD is done according to agency policy and the nurse's scope of practice. In many agencies, nurses with demonstrated competency can remove PICCs and nontunneled central venous catheters. The procedure involves removing any sutures and then gently withdrawing the catheter. Have the patient perform the Valsalva maneuver as the last 5 to 10 cm of the catheter is withdrawn. Immediately apply pressure to the site with sterile gauze to prevent air from entering and to control bleeding. Inspect the catheter tip to determine that it is intact. After bleeding has stopped, apply an antiseptic ointment and sterile dressing to the site.

CASE STUDY

Fluid and Electrolyte Imbalance

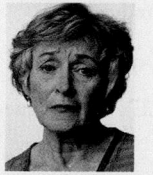

(© Kevin Peterson/ Photodisc/Think-stock.)

Patient Profile

S.S., a 63-yr-old white woman with acute lymphocytic leukemia, has been receiving chemotherapy on an outpatient basis. She completed her third treatment 5 days ago and has had nausea and vomiting for 2 days despite using ondansetron (Zofran). S.S.'s daughter brings her to the hospital, where she is admitted to the medical unit. As the admitting nurse, you perform a thorough assessment.

Subjective Data

- Reports lethargy, weakness, dizziness, and dry mouth
- States she has been too nauseated to eat or drink anything for 2 days

Objective Data

- Heart rate 110 beats/min, pulse thready
- BP 100/65
- Weight loss of 5 lb since she received her chemotherapy treatment 5 days ago
- Dry oral mucous membranes

Discussion Questions

1. Based on her manifestations, what fluid imbalance does S.S. have?
2. What additional assessment data should you obtain?
3. What are her risk factors for fluid and electrolyte imbalances?
4. You draw blood for a serum chemistry evaluation. What electrolyte imbalances are likely and why?
5. S.S. is at risk for which acid-base imbalance? Describe the changes that would occur in S.S.'s ABGs with this acid-base imbalance. How would the body compensate?
6. *Priority Decision:* What are the priority nursing interventions for S.S.?
7. *Collaboration:* Who should be the primary members of the interprofessional team in caring for S.S.? What is the interprofessional team's priority at this time for S.S.?
8. The provider orders dextrose 5% in 0.45% saline to infuse at 100 mL/hr. What type of solution is this, and how will it help S.S.'s fluid imbalance?
9. *Evidence-Based Practice:* S.S. has a double-lumen PICC in her left arm. One lumen is connected to the IV infusion; the other is unused. What is the recommended practice for maintaining the patency of the unused lumen?
10. *Quality Improvement:* What outcomes will indicate that interprofessional care was effective?

Answers available at *http://evolve.elsevier.com/Lewis/medsurg.*

BRIDGE TO NCLEX EXAMINATION

The number of the question corresponds to the same-numbered outcome at the beginning of the chapter.

1. During the postoperative care of a 76-year-old patient, the nurse monitors the patient's intake and output carefully, knowing that the patient is at risk for fluid and electrolyte imbalances primarily because
   a. older adults have an impaired thirst mechanism and need reminding to drink fluids.
   b. water accounts for a greater percentage of body weight in the older adult than in younger adults.
   c. older adults are more likely than younger adults to lose extracellular fluid during surgical procedures.
   d. small losses of fluid are significant because body fluids account for 45% to 50% of body weight in older adults.

2. During administration of a hypertonic IV solution, the mechanism involved in equalizing the fluid concentration between ECF and the cells is
   a. osmosis.
   b. diffusion.
   c. active transport.
   d. facilitated diffusion.

3a. An older woman is admitted to the medical unit with GI bleeding. Assessment findings that indicate fluid volume deficit include (*select all that apply*)
   a. weight loss.
   b. dry oral mucosa.
   c. full bounding pulse.
   d. engorged neck veins.
   e. decreased central venous pressure.

3b. The nursing care for a patient with hyponatremia and fluid volume excess includes
   a. fluid restriction.
   b. administration of hypotonic IV fluids.
   c. administration of a cation-exchange resin.
   d. placement of an indwelling urinary catheter.

3c. The nurse should be alert for which manifestations in a patient receiving a loop diuretic?
   a. Restlessness and agitation
   b. Paresthesias and irritability
   c. Weak, irregular pulse and poor muscle tone
   d. Increased blood pressure and muscle spasms

3d. Which patient is at *greatest* risk for developing hypermagnesemia?
   a. 83-year-old man with lung cancer and hypertension
   b. 65-year-old woman with hypertension taking β-adrenergic blockers
   c. 42-year-old woman with systemic lupus erythematosus and renal failure
   d. 50-year-old man with benign prostatic hyperplasia and a urinary tract infection

3e. It is important for the nurse to assess for which manifestation(s) in a patient who has just undergone a total thyroidectomy (*select all that apply*)?
   a. Confusion
   b. Weight gain
   c. Depressed reflexes
   d. Circumoral numbness
   e. Positive Chvostek's sign

3f. The nurse expects the long-term treatment of a patient with hyperphosphatemia from renal failure will include
   a. fluid restriction.
   b. calcium supplements.
   c. magnesium supplements.
   d. increased intake of dairy products.

4. The lungs act as an acid-base buffer by
   a. increasing respiratory rate and depth when CO_2 levels in the blood are high, reducing acid load.
   b. increasing respiratory rate and depth when CO_2 levels in the blood are low, reducing base load.
   c. decreasing respiratory rate and depth when CO_2 levels in the blood are high, reducing acid load.
   d. decreasing respiratory rate and depth when CO_2 levels in the blood are low, increasing acid load.

5. A patient has the following arterial blood gas results: pH 7.52, $PaCO_2$ 30 mm Hg, HCO_3^- 24 mEq/L. The nurse determines that these results indicate
   a. metabolic acidosis.
   b. metabolic alkalosis.
   c. respiratory acidosis.
   d. respiratory alkalosis.

6. The typical fluid replacement for the patient with a fluid volume deficit is
   a. dextran.
   b. 0.45% saline.
   c. lactated Ringer's solution.
   d. 5% dextrose in 0.45% saline.

7. The nurse is unable to flush a central venous access device and suspects occlusion. The *best* nursing intervention would be to
   a. apply warm moist compresses to the insertion site.
   b. try to force 10 mL of normal saline into the device.
   c. place the patient on the left side with the head down.
   d. have the patient change positions, raise arm, and cough.

1. d, 2. a, 3a. a, b, e, 3b. a, 3c. c, 3d. c, 3e. a, d, e, 3f. b, 4. a, 5. d, 6. c, 7. d

For rationales to these answers and even more NCLEX review questions, visit *http://evolve.elsevier.com/Lewis/medsurg*.

ⓔ EVOLVE WEBSITE/RESOURCES LIST

http://evolve.elsevier.com/Lewis/medsurg
Review Questions (Online Only)
Key Points
Answer Keys for Questions
- Answer Guidelines for Case Study on p. 295
- Rationales for Bridge to NCLEX Examination Questions
- Answer Guidelines for Managing Care of Multiple Patients Case Study (Section 3) on p. 298

Student Case Study
- Patient With Hyponatremia/Fluid Volume Imbalance
Conceptual Care Map Creator
Audio Glossary
Fluids and Electrolytes Tutorial
Content Updates

REFERENCES

1. Henderson R: Osmolality, osmolarity, and fluid homeostasis. Retrieved from *www.patient.info/doctor/osmolality-osmolarity-and-fluid-homeostasis*.

2. Reddi AS: *Fluid, electrolyte and acid-base disorders*, ed 2, New York, 2018, Springer.

*3. Oates LL, Price CI: Clinical assessments and care interventions to promote oral hydration amongst older patients: A narrative systematic review, *BMC Nurs* 16:4, 2017.

4. Hew-Butler T, Weisz K: Focus the secret stories of sodium: hypernatremia, *Clin Lab Sci* 29:3, 2016.

*5. Hoorn EJ, Zietse R: Diagnosis and treatment of hyponatremia: compilation of the guidelines, *J Am Soc Nephrol* 28:1340, 2017.

6. Rafiq MF: Hyponatremia still remains largely undiagnosed and untreated, *Anaesth Pain Intensive Care* 21:1, 2017.

*7. Douglas M, Rizzolo D, Kruger D: Hyperkalemia in adults: Review of a common electrolyte imbalance, *Clin Rev* 3:40, 2017.

8. Pincus M: Management of digoxin toxicity, *Austr Prescr* 39:1, 2016.

9. Body JJ, Niepel D, Tonini G: Hypercalcemia and hypocalcemia: Finding the balance, *Support Care Cancer* 25:5, 2017.

10. Walker M: Fluid and electrolyte imbalance: interpretation and assessment, *J Infusion Nurs* 39:6, 2016.

11. Boyle SM, Goldfarb S: *Phosphate deficiency and the phosphate-depletion syndrome: Pathophysiology, diagnosis, and treatment*, New York, 2017, Springer.

12. Hiner A: Electrolyte series: magnesium, *Nursing2018 Crit Care* 13:15, 2018.

13. Perkins A: Alkalosis in brief, *Nursing Made Incredibly Easy* 14:13, 2016.

14. Naisbitt C, Buckley H, Kishen R: Crystalloids, colloids, blood products, and blood substitutes, *Anaesth Intensive Care* 17:308, 2016.

*15. Septimus EJ, Moody J: Prevention of device-related healthcare-associated infections, *F1000Res* 14:5, 2016.

*Evidence-based information for clinical practice.

CASE STUDY

Managing Care of Multiple Patients

You and another RN are assigned to care for the following 3 patients in the intensive care unit. There is also an unlicensed assistive personnel (UAP) on duty.

Patients

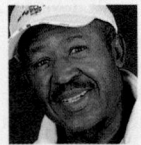

(© Stockphoto/Thinkstock.)

G.N., a 65-yr-old black man, was admitted to the ICU after falling into a lit gas grill. He has partial-thickness burns on his face, neck, and upper trunk. He has undergone surgical repair of right tibia and left hip fractures and debridement of a severely lacerated right leg. His voice is slightly hoarse, and he is coughing up sooty sputum. He is receiving O_2 at 4 L/min via nasal cannula, and his O_2 saturation is 93%. His WBC count is 26,400/μL (26.4 × 10^9/L) with 80% neutrophils (10% bands).

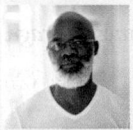

(© iStock.com/Cecilie_Arcurs.)

J.N., a 65-yr-old black man, was transferred to the ICU from the clinical unit last evening with acute respiratory failure. He was diagnosed 2 days ago with AIDS and *Pneumocystis jiroveci* pneumonia (PCP). Prior to this hospital admission he was started on oral trimethoprim/sulfamethoxazole (Bactrim) and combination antiretroviral therapy. However, his respiratory distress worsened, and he was transferred to the ICU for intubation and mechanical ventilation. He is now receiving IV Bactrim.

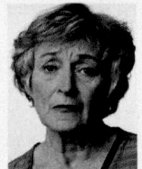

(© Kevin Peterson/Photodisc/Thinkstock.)

S.S., a 63-yr-old white woman with acute lymphocytic leukemia, has been receiving chemotherapy on an outpatient basis. She completed her third treatment 5 days ago and has been experiencing nausea and vomiting for 2 days despite using ondansetron (Zofran). She was initially admitted to the clinical unit but was transferred to the ICU for close monitoring after becoming severely hypotensive overnight. Her most recent blood pressure was 98/50, HR 82 and regular, O_2 saturation 95% on 2 L via nasal cannula, RR 22 and regular.

Discussion Questions

1. **Priority Decision:** After receiving report, which patient should you see first? Provide your rationale.
2. **Collaboration:** Which morning tasks should you delegate to the UAP (select all that apply)?
   a. Take BP readings on S.S.
   b. Perform respiratory assessment on G.N.
   c. Document strict intake and output on S.S.
   d. Provide oral care around the endotracheal tube for J.N.
   e. Titrate S.S.'s IV infusion rate based on her BP reading.
3. **Priority Decision and Collaboration:** When you enter J.N.'s room, the ventilator alarms are going off. The UAP had just finished providing oral care, and she tells you that J.N. has become increasingly agitated within the last 5 minutes. Which *initial* action would be *most* appropriate?
   a. Suction J.N.'s endotracheal tube.
   b. Have the UAP stay with J.N. while you obtain IV sedation for him.
   c. Ask the UAP to describe exactly what she did when she was providing oral care.
   d. Assess the ventilator to identify what alarm is going off and to make sure all connections are secure.

Case Study Progression

J.N.'s ventilator tubing became disconnected. You quickly reconnect his tubing, and as he settles down his oxygenation improves. You ask the UAP to obtain vital signs on your other patients while you begin a more thorough assessment of J.N.

4. During your assessment of J.N., you note gray-white patches on the inside of his mouth. You recognize these as *most* likely caused by
   a. *Candida albicans.*
   b. poor oral hygiene.
   c. *Coccidioides immitis.*
   d. irritation from recent mouth care.
5. G.N.'s family asks you why surgery was performed on his leg wound. Your response is based on the knowledge that debridement *(select all that apply)*
   a. is used to remove infected tissue.
   b. is used to remove nonviable tissue.
   c. prepares the wound bed for healing.
   d. can be accomplished only in surgery.
   e. is necessary in any burn wound involving the skin.
6. S.S.'s morning laboratory results reveal a serum potassium level of 2.8 mEq/L. You notify the health care provider and obtain an order for IV potassium. During infusion of the potassium replacement, you prioritize assessment of S.S.'s
   a. bowel function.
   b. cardiac rhythm.
   c. muscle strength.
   d. level of consciousness.
7. **Priority Decision:** As the day continues, you find that you are getting busy. Which nursing task should be your priority?
   a. Changing the sterile dressings on G.N.'s leg wounds
   b. Performing routine suctioning of J.N.'s endotracheal tube
   c. Starting a 500-mL fluid bolus to S.S., whose most recent BP is 76/42
   d. Calling the hospital chaplain to speak with S.S., who is upset over her condition
8. **Priority Decision:** Which medication should you administer first?
   a. Daily subcutaneous enoxaparin to G.N.
   b. IV Bactrim, ordered twice daily, to J.N.
   c. IV proton pump inhibitor, ordered twice daily, to S.S.
   d. As needed IV morphine to G.N., who reports pain at a level 9 (1 to 10 scale)
9. **Management Decision:** While sitting at the computer charting your patients' morning assessments, you overhear the UAP telling a nursing student that J.N. deserves what he got because HIV is God's way of punishing those who sin. Your *most* appropriate response would be to
   a. report the UAP's actions to the supervisor.
   b. ask the UAP to keep her opinions to herself.
   c. ignore the conversation because it does not affect patient care.
   d. talk to the UAP and student about keeping personal feelings separate from patient care.

Answers available at *http://evolve.elsevier.com/Lewis/medsurg.*

17

Preoperative Care

Janice A. Neil

From caring comes courage.

Lao Tzu

ⓔ http://evolve.elsevier.com/Lewis/medsurg/

CONCEPTUAL FOCUS

Anxiety

Patient Education

Safety

LEARNING OUTCOMES

1. Distinguish the common purposes and settings of surgery.
2. Apply knowledge of the purpose and components of a preoperative nursing assessment.
3. Interpret the significance of data related to the preoperative patient's health status and operative risk.
4. Analyze the components and purpose of the patient's informed consent for surgery.

5. Examine the nursing role in the physical, psychological, and educational preparation of the surgical patient.
6. Prioritize the nursing responsibilities related to day-of-surgery preparation for the surgical patient.
7. Discern the purposes and types of common preoperative medications.
8. Apply knowledge of the special considerations of preoperative preparation for the older adult surgical patient.

KEY TERMS

ambulatory surgery, p. 300

elective surgery, p. 300

emergency surgery, p. 300

informed consent, p. 307

same-day admission, p. 300

surgery, p. 299

Surgery is the art and science of treating diseases, injuries, and deformities by operation and instrumentation. The total surgical episode is called the *perioperative period*. This period includes the time before surgery (preoperative period), the time spent during the actual surgical procedure (intraoperative period), and the period after the surgery is over (postoperative period).

The surgical experience involves an interprofessional team, including the patient, surgeon, anesthesia care provider (ACP), nurse, and other health care team members. Preparing patients for surgery is an important nursing role. This chapter discusses preoperative care that applies to all surgical patients. Preparation measures for specific surgical procedures (e.g., abdominal, thoracic, or orthopedic surgery) are discussed in the appropriate chapters of this book.

Surgery is performed for many reasons. These include:

- *Diagnosis:* Determine the presence and extent of a pathologic condition (e.g., lymph node biopsy, bronchoscopy).

- *Cure:* Eliminate or repair a pathologic condition (e.g., removal of ruptured appendix or benign ovarian cyst).
- *Palliation:* Alleviate symptoms without cure (e.g., cutting a nerve root [rhizotomy] to reduce pain, creating a colostomy to bypass an inoperable bowel obstruction).
- *Prevention:* Reduce risk of developing a condition (e.g., removal of a mole before it becomes malignant, removal of the colon in a patient with familial polyposis to prevent cancer).
- *Cosmetic improvement:* Alter physical appearance (e.g., repairing a burn scar, breast reconstruction after a mastectomy).
- *Exploration:* Determine the nature or extent of a disease (e.g., laparotomy). With the use of advanced diagnostic tests, exploration is less common because we can identify many problems noninvasively.

Surgical procedures are usually described by combining specific suffixes with a body part or organ (Table 17.1).

TABLE 17.1 Suffixes Describing Surgical Procedures

Suffix	Meaning	Example
-ectomy	Excision or removal of	Appendectomy
-lysis	Destruction of	Electrolysis
-orrhaphy	Repair or suture of	Herniorrhaphy
-oscopy	Looking into	Endoscopy
-ostomy	Creation of opening into	Colostomy
-otomy	Cutting into or incision of	Tracheotomy
-plasty	Repair or reconstruction of	Mammoplasty

SURGICAL SETTINGS

Surgery may be a carefully planned event (elective surgery) or may arise with unexpected urgency (emergency surgery). Both elective and emergency surgeries are done in a variety of settings. The type of surgery, potential complications, and the patient's health status influence the setting where a patient can safely undergo a surgical procedure

For inpatient surgery, patients who are going to be admitted to the hospital are usually admitted on the day of surgery (same-day admission). Patients who are in the hospital before surgery are usually there because of acute or chronic medical conditions.

Most surgical procedures are performed as ambulatory surgery (also called *same-day* or *outpatient surgery*). Many of these surgeries use minimally invasive techniques (e.g., laparoscopic techniques). Ambulatory surgery often occurs in endoscopy clinics, physicians' offices, freestanding surgical clinics, and outpatient surgery units in hospitals. These procedures can involve the use of general, regional, or local anesthetic. Patients require less than a 24-hour stay after surgery. Many go home with a caregiver within hours of surgery.

Patients and HCPs often prefer ambulatory surgery. Generally, it requires fewer laboratory tests and medications and reduces the patient's risk for health care–associated infections. Patients like the convenience of recovering at home. HCPs prefer the flexibility in scheduling. The costs are usually less for the patient and the insurer.

You play an essential role in preparing the patient for surgery, caring for the patient during surgery, and aiding the patient's recovery after surgery. To perform these functions effectively, first know the reason the patient is undergoing surgery and any co-morbidities. Second, identify the individual patient's response to the stress of surgery. Third, know the results of preoperative diagnostic tests. Last, identify potential risks and complications associated with the surgical procedure and any special considerations that should be addressed in the plan of care. The nurse caring for the patient before surgery is likely to be different from the nurse in the operating room (OR), postanesthesia care unit (PACU), surgical intensive care unit (SICU), or surgical unit. Communication and documentation of important preoperative assessment findings are essential for quality care.

PATIENT INTERVIEW

One of the most important nursing actions is the preoperative interview. The nurse who works in the physician's office, ambulatory surgery center, or hospital may do the interview.

The preoperative interview can occur in advance or on the day of surgery. The primary purposes of the patient interview are to (1) obtain the patient's health information, including drug and food allergies; (2) provide and clarify information about the planned surgery, including anesthesia; and (3) assess the patient's emotional state and readiness for surgery, including his or her expectations about the surgical outcomes. The interview gives the patient and caregiver an opportunity to ask questions about the surgery, anesthesia, and postoperative care. Often patients ask about taking their routine drugs, such as insulin, anticoagulants, or heart medications, and if they will have pain. By being aware of the patient's and caregiver's needs, you can provide the information and support needed during the perioperative period.

NURSING ASSESSMENT OF PREOPERATIVE PATIENT

The overall goal of the preoperative assessment is to identify risk factors and plan care to ensure patient safety throughout the surgical experience. To achieve this, you will need to do the following:

- Establish baseline data for comparison in the intraoperative and postoperative period.
- Determine the patient's psychologic status to reinforce the use of coping strategies during the surgical experience.
- Determine physiologic factors directly or indirectly related to the surgical procedure that may contribute to operative risk factors.
- Participate in the identification and documentation of the surgical site according to agency protocol.
- Identify prescription drugs, over-the-counter (OTC) drugs, and herbs taken by the patient that may result in drug interactions affecting the surgical outcome.
- Review the results of all preoperative diagnostic studies in the patient's record and share this information with the appropriate HCPs.
- Identify cultural and ethnic factors that may affect the surgical experience.
- Determine if the patient received adequate information from the surgeon to make an informed decision to have surgery and that the consent form is signed and witnessed.

Subjective Data

Psychosocial Assessment. Surgery is a stressful event, even when the procedure is minor. The psychologic and physiologic reactions to surgery may elicit the stress response (e.g., elevated BP and heart rate). The stress response enables the body to meet the demands in the perioperative period. If stressors or the responses to the stressors are excessive, the stress response can be magnified and may affect recovery. Many factors influence the patient's reaction to stress, including age, past experiences with illness and pain, current health, and socioeconomic status.

The use of common language and avoidance of medical jargon are essential. Use words and language that are familiar to the patient to help the patient understand the surgery. Familiar language also helps reduce anxiety.

Your role in psychologically preparing the patient for surgery is to assess the patient for potential or actual stressors that could negatively affect surgery (Table 17.2). Communicate all concerns to the appropriate surgical team member, especially if the concern requires intervention later in the surgical experience.

TABLE 17.2 Psychosocial Assessment of Preoperative Patient

Situational Changes
- Define current degree of personal control, decision making, and independence
- Determine the presence of hope and anticipation of positive results
- Consider the impact of surgery and hospitalization and possible effects on lifestyle
- Identify support systems, including family, other caregivers, and religious and spiritual groups

Concerns With the Unknown
- Identify degree of anxiety and fears related to the surgery (e.g., pain)
- Identify expectations of surgery, changes in current health status, effects on daily living, and sexual activity (if appropriate)

Concerns With Body Image
- Identify current roles or relationships and view of self
- Determine perceived or potential changes in roles or relationships and their impact on body image

Past Experiences
- Review previous surgical experiences, hospitalizations, and treatments
- Determine responses to those experiences (positive and/or negative)
- Identify current perceptions of surgical procedure in relation to the above and information from others (e.g., a friend's view of a personal surgical experience)

Lack of Knowledge
- Determine the amount and type of information the patient wants
- Assess understanding of surgical procedure, including preparation, care, interventions, preoperative activities, restrictions, and expected outcomes
- Review the accuracy of information the patient has received from others, including health care team, family, friends, and media

EVIDENCE-BASED PRACTICE
Music and Preoperative Anxiety

You are taking care of D.G., a 67-yr-old woman scheduled for a renal mass biopsy to rule out metastatic disease. She was admitted early this morning to the preoperative unit. Unfortunately, an emergency surgery has resulted in at least a 4-hour delay of her procedure. You note that she has a high level of anxiety.

Making Clinical Decisions

Best Available Evidence. Complementary and alternative therapies include a variety of interventions, such as mental imagery, aromatherapy, acupuncture, and music. Music intervention in the preoperative period, including listening to pre-recorded music or individually tailored music given by a trained therapist, can help reduce anxiety. While sedatives and antianxiety drugs are often given before surgery, these drugs can have negative side effects, especially in the older adult.

Clinician Expertise. Anxiety can increase BP and pulse rate and may lengthen postoperative recovery. Excessive anxiety can even result in surgery being canceled.

Patient Preference and Values. D.G. tells you that she cannot relax and would like "a strong pill" to help her calm down. D.G.'s family mentioned to you earlier that she enjoys listening to classical music at home.

Implications for Practice

1. What information would you share with D.G. related to the use of drugs to reduce her anxiety?
2. How would you respond to D.G. when she asks how music could possibly help in reducing her anxiety?

Reference for Evidence

Bradt J, Dileo C, Shim M: Music interventions for preoperative anxiety, *Cochrane Database Syst Rev* 6:CD006908, 2013. (Classic)

Because many patients are admitted directly into the preoperative area from their homes, you must be skilled in assessing important psychologic factors in a short time. The most common psychologic factors are anxiety, fear, and hope.

Anxiety. Most people are anxious when facing surgery because of the unknown. This is normal and is an inborn survival mechanism. However, a high anxiety level can impair cognition, decision making, and coping abilities.

Anxiety can arise from lack of knowledge. This can range from not knowing what to expect to uncertainty about the outcome and may result from past experiences or stories heard through friends or the media. You can decrease some anxiety for the patient by giving information about what to expect. This is often done through classes or Web-based or audiovisual teaching materials before surgery. Inform the surgeon if the patient needs more information or has excessive anxiety.

Patients may have anxiety when surgery conflicts with their religious or cultural beliefs. Identify, record, and communicate patient decisions about the possibility of blood transfusions. For example, Jehovah's Witnesses may choose to refuse blood or blood products.[1]

Common Fears. Patients fear surgery for many reasons. The most common fear is the risk for death or permanent disability resulting from surgery. Sometimes the fear comes after hearing or reading about the risks during the informed consent process. Other fears are related to pain, change in body image, or results of diagnostic procedures.

Fear of death can be extremely harmful. Notify the HCP if the patient has a strong fear of death. A patient's strong fear of impending death may prompt the HCP to delay the surgery because the emotional state influences the stress response and thus the surgical outcome.

Fear of pain and discomfort during and after surgery is common. If the fear is extreme, notify the ACP or the surgeon. Reassure the patient that drugs are available for anesthesia and analgesia during surgery. For pain after surgery, tell patients to ask for pain medication before pain becomes severe. Teach the patient how to use a pain intensity scale (e.g., 0 to 10, FACES). See Chapter 8 for more on pain scales.

The patient may receive drugs that provide an amnesic effect so that the patient will not remember what occurs during surgery. Tell the patient that helps decrease anxiety after surgery.

Fear of mutilation or an *altered body image* can occur whether the surgery is radical, such as amputation, or minor, such as a breast biopsy. Even a small scar on the body can upset some, and others fear keloid development (overgrowth of a scar). Listen to and assess the patient's concern about this fear with an accepting attitude.

Fear of anesthesia may arise from the unknown, personal experience, or tales of others' bad experiences. These concerns can also result from information about the risks of anesthesia (e.g., brain damage, paralysis). Many patients fear losing control while under anesthesia. If you identify any of these fears, inform the ACP at once so that he or she can talk further with the patient.

Fear of disruption of life functioning may be present in varying degrees. It can range from fear of permanent disability to concern about not being able to engage in activities of daily living for a few weeks. You may find concerns about loss of role function, separation from family, and how the family will manage. Financial concerns include dealing with an expected loss of income and the costs of surgery.

If you find any of these fears, a consult with the patient's caregiver, a social worker, a spiritual advisor, or a psychologist may be appropriate. Financial advisors at the hospital may be able to give information about financial support.

> ### ❓ CHECK YOUR PRACTICE
>
> Your 19-yr-old male patient is in the holding area. He is scheduled for an orchiectomy for testicular cancer. He is visibly sweating and agitated. When you ask him how he is doing, he responds, "I am scared. Wouldn't you be?"
> * What can you do to reduce his fear?

Hope. Although many psychologic factors related to surgery seem to be negative, hope is a positive attribute. Hope may be the patient's strongest method of coping. To deny or minimize hope may negate the positive mental attitude necessary for a quick and full recovery. Some patients hopefully anticipate surgery. These can be the surgeries that repair (e.g., plastic surgery for burn scars), rebuild (e.g., total joint replacement to reduce pain and improve function), or save and extend life (e.g., repair of aneurysm, organ transplant). Assess and support the presence of hope and the patient's anticipation of positive results.

Past Health History. Ask the patient about any previous health problems and surgeries. Determine if the patient understands the need for surgery. For example, the patient scheduled for a total knee replacement may say that increasing pain and immobility are the reasons for the surgery.

Record the reason for any past hospitalizations, including previous surgeries and the dates. Identify any problems with previous surgeries. For example, the patient may have had a wound infection or a reaction to a drug.

Ask women about their menstrual and obstetric history. This includes the date of their last menstrual period, the number of pregnancies, and any history of cesarean section.

When obtaining a family health history, ask the patient and caregiver about any inherited traits, since they may contribute to the surgical outcome. Record any family history of heart and endocrine diseases. For example, if a patient reports a parent with hypertension, sudden cardiac death, or myocardial infarction, this should alert you to the possibility that the patient may have a similar predisposition or condition. Obtain information about the patient's family history of adverse reactions to or problems with anesthesia. For example, malignant hyperthermia has a genetic predisposition. If present, measures will be taken to decrease complications associated with this condition (see Chapter 18).

Medications. Document all current medication use, including OTC drugs and herbs. Many surgery centers ask patients to bring their medications with them when reporting for surgery.

This helps to accurately assess and document the name and dosage of medications.

The interaction of the patient's current drugs and anesthetics can increase or decrease the desired physiologic effect of anesthetics. Consider the effects of opioids and prescribed drugs for chronic health conditions (e.g., heart disease, hypertension, depression, seizure disorder, diabetes). For example, certain antidepressants can potentiate the effect of opioid agents used for anesthesia or pain control. Antihypertensive drugs may predispose the patient to shock from the combined effect of the drug and the vasodilator effect of some anesthetic agents. Insulin or oral hypoglycemic drugs may need adjustments during the perioperative period because of increased body metabolism, decreased oral intake, stress, and anesthesia. Antiplatelet drugs (e.g., aspirin, clopidogrel [Plavix]) and nonsteroidal antiinflammatory drugs (NSAIDs) inhibit platelet aggregation and may contribute to postoperative bleeding.

HCPs may have patients withhold medications before surgery. Specific timeframes for withholding medications depend on the medication and the patient. Patients on long-term anticoagulation therapy (e.g., warfarin [Coumadin], rivaroxaban [Xarelto], dabigatran [Pradaxa], apixaban [Eliquis]) present a unique challenge. The options for these patients include (1) continuing therapy, (2) withholding therapy for a time before and after surgery, or (3) withholding the therapy and starting subcutaneous or IV heparin therapy during the perioperative period. The management strategy selected is based on the patient history and the nature of the surgery.[2]

Ask about the use of herbs and dietary supplements because their use is so common. Many patients do not think to include supplements in their list of medications. They believe that herbal and dietary supplements are "natural" and do not pose a surgical risk.[3] Excess use of vitamins and herbs can cause harmful effects in patients undergoing surgery. In those taking anticoagulants or antiplatelets, herbal supplements can produce excess postoperative bleeding that may require a return to the OR.[3] The Complementary & Alternative Therapies box lists the effects of specific herbs that are of concern during the perioperative period.

> ### 🌿 COMPLEMENTARY & ALTERNATIVE THERAPIES
> #### *Herbal Products and Surgery*
>
> Use the following as a guide for patient teaching:
> * Notify your HCP of all vitamins, herbs, and dietary supplements that you are taking.
> * Avoid astragalus and ginseng, since they can increase BP before and during surgery.
> * Avoid garlic, vitamin E, ginkgo, and fish oils because they can increase bleeding.
> * Avoid kava and valerian because they can cause excessive sedation.
> * In general, stop taking all herbs 2 to 3 weeks before any surgical procedure. Consult your HCP for specific instructions.
> * Take multivitamins until the day before surgery. Taking them on the day of surgery on an empty stomach may contribute to nausea and vomiting after surgery.

Ask the patient about any substance use. The most likely used substances include tobacco, alcohol, opioids, marijuana, cocaine, and amphetamines. Ask questions about use in a frank manner. Stress that substance use may affect the type and amount of anesthesia the patient will need. When patients become aware of the potential interactions of these substances with anesthetics, most patients respond honestly about using them.

Chronic alcohol use can place the patient at risk because of lung, GI, or liver damage. Decreased liver function prolongs the metabolism of anesthetic agents, alters nutritional status, and increases the potential for postoperative complications. Alcohol withdrawal can occur during lengthy surgery or in the postoperative period. Proper planning and management are needed to avoid this life-threatening event (see Chapter 10).

Record and share all findings of the drug history with the perioperative health care team. The ACP will decide the best schedule and dose of the patient's routine drugs before and after surgery. Ensure that you identify all the patient's drugs, implement any changes in the medication plan, and monitor the patient for potential interactions and complications.

Allergies. Ask the patient about drug intolerances and drug allergies. Drug intolerance usually results in side effects that are unpleasant for the patient but are not life threatening. These effects can include nausea, constipation, diarrhea, or *idiosyncratic* (opposite than expected) reactions. A true drug allergy produces hives and/or an anaphylactic reaction, causing cardiopulmonary compromise (e.g., hypotension, tachycardia, bronchospasm). Being aware of drug intolerances and drug allergies helps the health care team maintain patient comfort and safety.

Record all drug intolerances and allergies and, if needed, place an allergy identification band on the patient on the day of surgery.

> **! SAFETY ALERT Allergies**
> • Some local anesthetic agents contain bisulfite preservatives.
> • Notify the ACP if the patient reports an allergy to sulfur-containing drugs.

Ask about nondrug allergies, specifically food and environmental (e.g., latex, pollen, animals) allergies. The patient with a history of any allergic reactions has a greater potential for hypersensitivity reactions to drugs given during anesthesia. Screen all patients for latex allergies by gathering data about:

- Risk factors
- Contact dermatitis
- Contact urticaria (e.g., hives)
- Aerosol reactions
- History of reactions that suggest an allergy to latex

Risk factors for latex allergy include long-term, multiple exposures to latex products, such as those experienced by health care and rubber industry workers. Other risk factors include a history of hay fever, asthma, and allergies to certain foods (e.g., eggs, avocados, bananas, chestnuts, potatoes, peaches).[4] Latex allergies are discussed in Chapter 13.

Review of Systems. The last part of the patient history is the body systems review. Ask specific questions to confirm the presence or absence of any diseases. Current health problems can alert you to areas that you will need to examine in the preoperative physical examination. The combined review of systems and patient history provide essential data to determine the specific preoperative tests that the patient needs.

Cardiovascular System. Evaluate cardiovascular (CV) function to determine preexisting disease or problems (e.g., coronary artery disease, prosthetic heart valve). In reviewing the CV system, you may find a history of hypertension, angina, dysrhythmias, heart failure, or myocardial infarction (MI). Ask about the patient's current treatment for any CV condition (e.g., drugs) and the level of functioning. A cardiology consult is often needed before surgery if the patient has a significant CV history (e.g., recent MI, valvular heart disease, implantable cardioverter-defibrillator).

If indicated, the patient should have a 12-lead electrocardiogram (ECG) and coagulation studies and the results should be on the chart before surgery. The CV assessment provides data on what other measures the patient needs. For example, the patient who is on diuretic therapy needs to have a serum potassium level drawn before surgery. If the patient has hypertension, the ACP may give vasoactive drugs to maintain adequate BP during surgery. The patient with a prosthetic heart valve may receive antibiotic prophylaxis before surgery to decrease the risk for infective endocarditis (see Chapter 36).

Venous thromboembolism (VTE), a condition that includes deep vein thrombosis and pulmonary embolism, is a concern for any surgical patient. Patients at high risk for VTE include those with a history of previous thrombosis, blood-clotting disorders, cancer, varicosities, obesity, tobacco use, heart failure, or chronic obstructive pulmonary disease (COPD).[5] People are also at risk for developing a VTE because of immobility and positioning during the operative procedure. Intermittent pneumatic compression devices (IPCs) may be applied in the preoperative holding area.

Respiratory System. Ask the patient about any recent or chronic respiratory disease or infections. Elective surgery may be postponed if the person has an upper respiratory tract infection. Upper airway infections may increase the risk for bronchospasm, laryngospasm, decreased O_2 saturation, and problems with respiratory secretions. Report a patient's history of dyspnea at rest or with exertion, coughing (dry or productive), or hemoptysis (coughing blood) to the ACP and surgeon.

If a patient has a history of asthma, ask about the use of inhaled or oral corticosteroids and bronchodilators, as well as the frequency and triggers of asthma attacks. The patient with a history of COPD is at high risk for pulmonary complications, including hypoxemia and atelectasis.

Gather information about the patient's tobacco use. The HCP and you should encourage the patient to stop smoking at least 6 weeks before surgery. Smoking increases the risk for pulmonary complications during and after surgery. Report conditions likely to affect respiratory function such as sleep apnea, obesity, and spinal, chest, and airway deformities. For example, patients are often asked to bring their sleep apnea devices with them to the hospital or surgical center. Depending on the patient's history and physical examination, baseline pulmonary function tests and arterial blood gases may be done before surgery.

Neurologic System. Evaluation of neurologic functioning includes assessing the patient's ability to respond to questions, follow commands, and maintain orderly thought patterns. Changes in the patient's hearing and vision may affect responses and the ability to follow directions throughout the perioperative assessment and evaluation. Record the patient's ability to pay attention, concentrate, and respond appropriately to establish a baseline for postoperative comparison.

If you note deficits in cognitive function, determine the extent of the problems and whether they can be corrected before surgery. If the problems cannot be corrected, it is important to involve a legal guardian or person with durable power of attorney for health care to aid the patient and provide informed consent for surgery.

Preoperative assessment of the older person's baseline cognitive function is especially crucial for comparison during and after surgery. The older adult may have intact mental abilities before surgery but is more prone to adverse outcomes during and after surgery than the younger adult. This is due to the added stressors of the surgical procedure, dehydration, hypothermia, and anesthesia and adjunctive drugs. These factors may contribute to the development of *emergence delirium,* a condition that may be falsely labeled as senility or dementia.

In the review of the neurologic system, obtain about any history of strokes, transient ischemic attacks, or spinal cord injury. Ask about neurologic diseases, such as myasthenia gravis, Parkinson's disease, and multiple sclerosis, and any treatments used.

Genitourinary System. Assess for a history of renal or urinary tract diseases, such as chronic kidney disease or repeated urinary tract infections. Record the present disease state and current treatment. Renal dysfunction is associated with several problems, including fluid and electrolyte imbalances, coagulopathies, increased risk for infection, and impaired wound healing. Because the kidneys metabolize and excrete many drugs, a decrease in renal function can lead to an altered response to drugs and unpredictable drug elimination. Renal function tests (e.g., serum creatinine, blood urea nitrogen [BUN]) are often done before surgery.

Record and share with the perioperative team if the patient has problems voiding (e.g., incontinence, hesitancy). Older male patients may have an enlarged prostate that can interfere with the insertion of a bladder catheter or impair voiding after surgery.

For a woman of childbearing age, determine if she is pregnant or thinks she could be pregnant. Most agencies perform a pregnancy test for all women of childbearing age before surgery.[6] Immediately tell the surgeon if the patient states that she may be pregnant. Maternal and fetal exposure to anesthetics should be avoided during the first trimester.

Hepatic System. The liver is involved in glucose homeostasis, fat metabolism, protein synthesis, drug and hormone metabolism, and bilirubin formation and excretion. The liver detoxifies many anesthetics and adjunctive drugs. The patient with hepatic dysfunction may have an increased perioperative risk for clotting abnormalities and adverse responses to drugs. Consider the presence of liver disease if there is a history of jaundice, hepatitis, alcohol abuse, or obesity.

Integumentary System. Ask about a history of skin problems. Assess the current condition of the skin, especially at the incision site, for rashes, breakdown, or other skin conditions. A patient with a history of pressure injuries may need extra padding during surgery. Skin problems can affect wound healing.

Body art such as tattoos and piercings are increasingly common. When possible, select pigment-free areas for injections, IV sites, and laboratory draws.

Musculoskeletal System. Note any musculoskeletal and mobility problems, especially in the older adult. If the patient has arthritis, identify all affected joints. Mobility restrictions may influence intraoperative and postoperative positioning and ambulation. Spinal anesthesia may be difficult if the patient cannot flex the lumbar spine enough to allow easy needle insertion. If the neck is affected, intubation and airway management may be difficult. Any mobility aids (e.g., cane, walker) should be with the patient on the day of surgery.

Endocrine System. The patient with diabetes is especially at risk for adverse effects of anesthesia and surgery. Hypoglycemia, hyperglycemia, delayed wound healing, and infection are common complications of diabetes during the perioperative period. Clarify with the surgeon or ACP whether the patient should take the usual dose of insulin or oral hypoglycemic agents on the day of surgery. ACPs may vary the usual insulin dose based on the patient's status and history of glucose control. Measure serum or capillary glucose levels the morning of surgery to establish baseline levels. Assess the patient's glucose levels regularly and, if necessary, manage according to agency protocol.

Determine if the patient has a history of thyroid dysfunction. Hyperthyroidism or hypothyroidism can place the patient at surgical risk because of changes in metabolic rate. If the patient takes a thyroid replacement drug, check with the ACP about administering the drug on the day of surgery. If the patient has a history of thyroid dysfunction, laboratory tests may be done to determine current levels of thyroid function.

The patient with Addison's disease needs special consideration during surgery. Addisonian crisis or shock can occur if a patient abruptly stops taking replacement corticosteroids. The patient may need additional IV corticosteroid therapy from the stress of surgery[7] (see Chapter 49).

Immune System. Note if the patient has a history of a compromised immune system or takes immunosuppressive drugs. Corticosteroids used in immunosuppressive doses may be tapered before surgery. Impairment of the immune system can lead to delayed wound healing and increased risk for infections.[8] Elective surgery may be cancelled if the patient has an acute infection (e.g., sinusitis, influenza). Patients with active chronic infections such as hepatitis B or C, acquired immunodeficiency syndrome, or tuberculosis may have surgery if needed. However, when preparing the patient for surgery, remember to take infection control precautions for the protection of the patient and staff. Infection control guidelines are discussed in Chapter 14.

Fluid and Electrolyte Status. Ask the patient about any recent conditions that increase the risk for fluid and electrolyte imbalances, such as vomiting, diarrhea, or completing a bowel prep. Identify drugs that change fluid and electrolyte status, such as diuretics. Serum electrolyte levels are often assessed before surgery. Many patients may have restricted fluids for a specific period of time before surgery. They could develop dehydration if surgery is delayed. A patient with or at risk for dehydration may need more fluids and electrolytes before or during surgery.

Complete a preoperative fluid balance history for all patients. This is especially critical for older adults. Their reduced adaptive capacity leaves a narrow margin of safety between overhydration and underhydration.

Nutritional Status. Nutritional problems include overnutrition and undernutrition, both of which need considerable time to correct. However, knowing that a patient has a nutritional problem can help the health care team provide more customized care. For example, if the patient is thin, place more padding than usual on the OR table. Notify the team if a patient is severely obese (body mass index [BMI] greater than 40 kg/m^2) to allow time to obtain special equipment needed for the patient's care (e.g., longer instruments for abdominal surgery).

Obesity stresses the heart and lung systems and makes access to the surgical site and anesthesia administration more difficult.[9] It predisposes the patient to wound dehiscence, wound infection, and incisional herniation after surgery. Adipose tissue is less vascular than other types of tissue. The patient may be slower to recover from anesthesia because adipose tissue absorbs and stores inhalation agents, so they leave the body more slowly. See Chapter 40 for the special needs of obese patients undergoing surgery.

Nutritional problems impair the ability to recover from surgery. Remember that the obese patient or the very thin patient can be protein and vitamin deficient. If the problem is severe, surgery may be postponed. Protein and vitamins A, C, and B complex deficiencies are particularly important because these substances are essential for wound healing.[10] Patients who are malnourished may receive supplemental nutrition during the perioperative period. The older adult is often at risk for malnutrition and fluid volume deficits.

Identify patients who consume large quantities of coffee or caffeinated soft drinks. In many cases, withholding caffeinated beverages before surgery or for some time after surgery can lead to severe withdrawal headaches.[11] These headaches can be confused with spinal headaches if the preoperative data are not recorded. Giving caffeinated beverages after surgery, when possible, may prevent these headaches.

Objective Data

Physical Examination. The Joint Commission requires that all patients admitted to the OR have a documented history and physical examination (H&P) in their chart.[12] This may be done in advance of surgery or on the day of surgery. Any qualified HCP, including advanced practice nurses, physicians, physician assistants, or ACPs, may perform the H&P. Findings from the H&P enable the ACP to assign the patient a physical status rating for anesthesia administration (Table 17.3). This rating is an indicator of the patient's perioperative risk and may influence perioperative decisions. It uses a scale of P1 to P6. A rating of P6 is reserved for a brain-dead patient undergoing organ procurement. Patients undergoing surgery in ambulatory or outpatient settings generally have ratings of P1, P2, or P3. Other designations can be added to the ASA status (e.g., "E" to designate an "emergent" procedure).

Complete a physical examination of the patient before surgery (Table 17.4). Review the documentation already present in the patient's chart, including the H&P, to better proceed with

TABLE 17.3 American Society of Anesthesiologists' (ASA) Physical Classification System

Rating	Definition
P1 (ASA I)	Normal healthy person
P2 (ASA II)	Patient with mild systemic disease
P3 (ASA III)	Patient with severe systemic disease
P4 (ASA IV)	Patient with severe systemic disease that is a constant threat to life
P5 (ASA V)	Moribund patient who is not expected to survive without surgery
P6 (ASA VI)	Declared brain-dead patient whose organs are being removed for donor purposes

Source: American Society of Anesthesiologists: ASA physical status classification system, 2014. Retrieved from *www.asahq.org/resources/clinical-information/asa-physical-status-classification-system*.

TABLE 17.4 Health Assessment and Physical Examination of Preoperative Patient*

Cardiovascular System
- Identify acute or chronic problems. Note presence of angina, hypertension, heart failure, recent myocardial infarction.
- Identify any drugs (e.g., aspirin) or herbs (e.g., ginkgo) that may affect coagulation.
- Identify patients with prosthetic heart valves, pacemakers, or implantable cardioverter-defibrillators.
- Assess for edema (including dependent areas), noting location and severity.
- Inspect neck veins for distention.
- Obtain bilateral baseline BPs.
- Assess capillary refill and pulses for rate, rhythm, and quality: apical, radial, and pedal.

Gastrointestinal System
- Determine patterns of food and fluid intake and any recent changes in weight.
- Review usual pattern of bowel movements, including date of last bowel movement.
- Assess for presence of dentures and bridges (loose dentures or teeth may be dislodged during intubation).
- Weigh patient.
- Auscultate abdomen for presence of bowel sounds.

Genitourinary System
- Identify any infection or preexisting disease.
- Determine ability to void.
- Note color, amount, and characteristics of urine.
- Determine pregnancy status (if appropriate).

Hepatic System
- Review any substance use, especially alcohol and IV drug use.
- Inspect skin color and sclera of eyes for any signs of jaundice.

Immune System
- Note any immunodeficiency or autoimmune disorders.
- Assess for use of corticosteroids or other immunosuppressant drugs.

Integumentary System
- Determine skin status. Note any current or previous skin problems (e.g., pressure injuries, eczema, bruising).
- Inspect skin for rashes, boils, or infection, especially around the planned surgical site.
- Inspect mucous membranes and skin turgor for signs of dehydration.
- Assess skin moisture and temperature.

Musculoskeletal System
- Examine skin around bone pressure points.
- Assess for limitations in joint range of motion and muscle strength.
- Assess for joint or muscle pain.
- Assess mobility, gait, and balance.

Neurologic System
- Determine orientation to person, place, and time.
- Assess baseline mental status. Note any confusion, disorderly thinking, or inability to follow commands.
- Identify any history of strokes, transient ischemic attacks, or neurologic diseases (e.g., Parkinson's disease, multiple sclerosis).

Respiratory System
- Identify acute or chronic problems. Note presence of infection, chronic obstructive pulmonary disease, or asthma.
- Note use of continuous positive airway pressure (CPAP) machine.
- Assess tobacco history, including date/time of last cigarette and number of pack-years.
- Determine baseline O_2 saturation and respiratory rate and rhythm.
- Observe for cough, dyspnea, and use of accessory muscles of respiration.
- Auscultate lungs for normal and adventitious breath sounds.

*See specific body system chapters for more detailed assessments and related laboratory studies.

TABLE 17.5 Common Preoperative Diagnostic Studies

Test	Assessment
ABGs, pulse oximetry	Respiratory and metabolic function, oxygenation status
Blood glucose	Metabolic status, diabetes
Blood urea nitrogen, creatinine	Renal function
Chest x-ray	Lung disorders, cardiac enlargement, heart failure
CBC: RBCs, Hgb, Hct, WBCs	Anemia, immune status, infection
Electrocardiogram	Heart disease, dysrhythmias
Electrolytes	Metabolic status, renal function, diuretic side effects
hCG	Pregnancy status
Liver function tests	Liver status
PT, PTT, INR, platelet count	Coagulation status
Pulmonary function studies	Pulmonary status
Serum albumin	Nutritional status
Type and crossmatch	Blood available for replacement (elective surgery patients may have own blood available)
Urinalysis	Renal status, hydration, urinary tract infection

CBC, Complete blood count; *hCG,* human chorionic gonadotropin; *Hct,* hematocrit; *Hgb,* hemoglobin; *INR,* international normalized ratio; *PT,* prothrombin time; *PTT,* partial thromboplastin time.

your examination. Record all findings and share any relevant findings at once with the surgeon or ACP.

Diagnostic Studies. Obtain and assess the results of diagnostic studies ordered before surgery (Table 17.5). For example, a patient taking an antiplatelet drug (e.g., aspirin) may have a coagulation profile done or a patient on diuretic therapy may have a potassium level checked. A woman of childbearing age may receive a pregnancy test. An ECG is done for many who take drugs for dysrhythmias or have high blood pressure. Patients with diabetes undergo blood glucose monitoring. In many settings, patients are tested for methicillin-resistant *Staphylococcus aureus.* Those with positive results are prescribed antibiotics for several days before surgery.[13]

Ideally, preoperative tests are ordered based on the patient's H&P. However, many agencies and insurers have protocols for preoperative tests, which may not include all those in Table 17.5. In addition, some tests may be done days before surgery. Ensure that all laboratory and diagnostic reports are in the patient's chart. Missing reports may result in a delay or cancellation of the surgery.

❖ NURSING MANAGEMENT: PREOPERATIVE PATIENT

Base the preoperative nursing interventions on the nursing assessment, depending on the patient's specific needs. The pending surgery and routines of the surgery setting guide the patient's physical preparation. Preoperative teaching may be minimal or extensive. The Association of periOperative Registered Nurses (AORN) provides standards and recommended practices to guide nursing interventions in all perioperative settings.[5]

◆ Preoperative Teaching

The patient has a right to know what to expect and how to take part effectively during the surgical experience. Preoperative teaching increases patient satisfaction and can reduce postoperative fear, anxiety, and stress.[14] Teaching may decrease the

development of complications, length of hospitalization, and recovery time after discharge.

In most surgical settings, patients often arrive only a short time before their surgery. Preoperative teaching for these patients generally occurs in the surgeon's office or a preadmission surgical clinic and is reinforced on the day of surgery. After ambulatory surgery, the patient usually goes home several hours after recovery, depending on the patient's progress and procedure-specific needs. Teaching must include information that focuses on the patient's safety. Give written materials for patients and caregivers to use for review and reinforcement at home. Discharge teaching is required for all patients (see Chapter 19).

When delivering teaching, find a balance between explaining so much that the patient is overwhelmed and telling so little that the patient is unprepared. If you observe and listen carefully to the patient, you can usually figure out how much information is enough. Remember that anxiety and fear may limit learning ability. Assess what the patient wants to know and give priority to those concerns.

Generally, preoperative teaching includes 3 types of information: sensory, process, and procedural. Different patients, with varying cultures, backgrounds, and experience, may want different types of information. See Table 4.6 for factors affecting patient teaching.

With *sensory information,* patients find out what they will see, hear, smell, and feel during the surgery. For example, you may tell them that the OR will be cold, but they can ask for a warm blanket; the lights in the OR are bright; or many unfamiliar sounds and specific smells will be present.

Patients wanting *process information* may not want specific details but just the general flow of what is going to happen. This information would include the patient's transfer to the holding area, visits by the nurse and the ACP before transfer to the OR, and waking up in the PACU.

With *procedural information,* patients desire details that are more specific. For example, this information would include saying an IV line will be started while the patient is in the holding area and the surgeon will mark the operative area with an indelible marker to verify the surgical site.[5]

Share the preoperative teaching given to the patient with the nurses providing postoperative care to evaluate learning and avoid duplication of teaching. Because there is limited time for teaching, a team approach is often used. For example, teaching may start in the outpatient setting. Your responsibility is to assess the patient's understanding of this teaching and fill in the gaps at this point in the surgical process.

Record all teaching in the patient's chart. A guide for preoperative patient and caregiver teaching is outlined in Table 17.6. See Chapter 4 for more on patient and caregiver teaching.

◆ General Surgery Information. Unless it is contraindicated (e.g., after craniotomy, tonsillectomy), all patients should receive instruction about deep breathing, coughing, and early ambulation postoperatively. This is essential because patients may not want to do these activities after surgery unless they know the reason for them and practice them before surgery. Tell patients and caregivers if tubes, drains, monitoring devices, or special equipment will be used after surgery. Explain that these devices help you to safely care for the patient. Examples of specific teaching may include how to use incentive spirometers or patient-controlled analgesia pumps. Patients should have a clear understanding of how to rate their pain and how their pain will be managed[10] (see Chapter 8).

TABLE 17.6 Patient & Caregiver Teaching

Preoperative Preparation

Include the following information in the preoperative teaching plan for the patient and caregiver.

Sensory Information
- Preoperative holding area may be noisy
- Drugs and cleaning solutions may be odorous
- Operating room (OR) can be cold. Forced air warming devices may be used. Warm blankets are available
- Talking may be heard but may be distorted because of masks. Ask questions if something is not understood
- OR bed will be narrow. A safety strap will be applied over the thighs
- Lights in the OR may be bright
- Monitoring machines may be heard (e.g., beeping noises) when awake

Procedural Information
- What to bring and what type of clothing to wear to the surgery center
- Any changes in time of surgery
- Fluid and food restrictions
- Physical preparation needed (e.g., shower, bowel, or skin preparation)
- Purpose of frequent vital signs assessment
- Pain control and other comfort measures
- Why turning, deep breathing, and coughing after surgery are important. Do practice sessions
- Insertion of IV lines
- Procedure for anesthesia administration
- Surgical site may be marked with indelible ink or marker

Process Information
Information About General Flow of Surgery
- Admission area
- Preoperative holding area, OR, and postanesthesia care unit (PACU)
- Caregivers can usually stay in preoperative holding area until surgery
- Caregivers will be able to see patient after discharge from the PACU or possibly in PACU once the patient is awake
- Identification of any technology that may be present on awakening, such as monitors, central lines, intermittent pneumatic compression devices

Where Caregivers Can Wait During Surgery
- Encourage caregivers to ask questions and express any concerns
- OR staff will update caregivers during surgery and when surgery is over
- Surgeon will usually talk with caregivers after surgery

TABLE 17.7 Preoperative Fasting Recommendations

Liquid and Food Intake	Minimum Fasting Period (hr)
Clear liquids (e.g., water, clear tea, black coffee, carbonated beverages, fruit juice without pulp)	2
Breast milk	4
Nonhuman milk, including infant formula	6
Light meal (e.g., toast and clear liquids)	6
Regular meal (may include fried or fatty food, meat)	8 or more

Source: Practice guidelines for preoperative fasting and the use of pharmacologic agents to reduce the risk of pulmonary aspiration: Application to healthy patients undergoing elective procedures, *Anesthesiology* 126:376, 2017.

before surgery. Evidence-based guidelines for healthy patients of all ages undergoing elective surgery (except women in labor) from the American Society of Anesthesiologists are less strict[15] (Table 17.7). Restricting fluids and food is designed to reduce the risk for pulmonary aspiration and nausea and vomiting. Protocols may vary for patients having local anesthesia or surgery scheduled late in the day. Follow the NPO protocol of each surgical setting. The patient who has not followed the NPO instructions may have surgery delayed or cancelled. It is critical that the patient understands the reason for and follows all restrictions.

◆ **Legal Preparation for Surgery**

Legal preparation for surgery consists of checking that all required forms have been correctly signed and are present in the patient's chart and that the patient and caregiver clearly understand what is going to happen. Standard consent forms include those for the surgical procedure and blood transfusions. Other forms may include advance directives and durable power of attorney for health care (see Chapter 9).

◆ **Consent for Surgery.** Before nonemergency surgery can be legally performed, the patient must voluntarily sign an informed consent form in the presence of a witness. Informed consent is an active, shared decision-making process between the HCP and recipient of care. Three conditions must be met for consent to be valid. First, there must be *adequate disclosure* of the (1) diagnosis; (2) nature and purpose of the proposed treatment; (3) risks and consequences of the proposed treatment; (4) probability of a successful outcome; (5) availability, benefits, and risks of alternative treatments; and (6) prognosis if treatment is not instituted. Second, the patient must show a clear *understanding* of the information before receiving sedating preoperative drugs. If a patient is sedated prior to signing the consent, surgery may be cancelled or delayed. Third, the recipient of care must *give consent voluntarily.* The patient must not be persuaded or coerced in any way by anyone to undergo the procedure.

The surgeon is ultimately responsible for obtaining the patient's consent for surgical treatment. You may be asked to witness the patient's signature on the consent form. At this time, you must be a patient advocate, verifying that the patient understands the information in the consent and the implications of consent, and that consent for surgery is truly voluntary. If the patient is unclear about the surgical plans, contact the surgeon about the patient's need for more information. The patient

The patient should also receive surgery-specific information. For example, a patient having a total joint replacement may have an immobilizer after surgery. Tell a patient having open heart surgery about waking up in the intensive care unit.

◆ **Ambulatory Surgery Information.** The ambulatory surgery patient or the patient admitted to the hospital the day of surgery needs to receive information before admission. Some ambulatory surgical centers telephone patients several days before the procedure to obtain health information, give instructions, and answer questions. Each center has policies and procedures for communicating this information.

In addition to specifics on the procedure, patients need information on day-of-surgery events such as arrival time, registration, parking, what to wear, what to bring, and the need to have a responsible adult present for transportation home after surgery.

Traditionally, we tell patients having elective surgery to have nothing by mouth (NPO) starting at midnight on the night

should be aware that consent, even when signed, can be withdrawn at any time.

If the patient is a minor, unconscious, or mentally incompetent to sign the permit, a legally appointed representative or responsible family member may give written permission. An *emancipated minor* is one who is younger than the legal age of consent but is recognized as having the legal capacity to provide consent.[10] Procedures for obtaining consent vary among states and agencies. Follow your state's nurse practice act and agency policies that apply to a specific situation.

ETHICAL/LEGAL DILEMMAS
Informed Consent

Situation
J.S., a 72-yr-old woman, is waiting in the preoperative holding area. You are discussing her impending surgery when you realize that this competent adult does not fully understand her surgery and was not informed of the alternatives to this surgery. Although she has previously signed a consent form, your assessment is that she was not fully informed about her treatment options or does not recall them.

Ethical/Legal Points for Consideration
• Informed consent requires that patients have complete information about the proposed treatment, as well as alternative treatments, risks and benefits of each treatment option, and possible consequences of the surgical procedure. The person (usually the surgeon) performing the procedure usually has this responsibility.
• An opportunity to have questions answered about the various treatment options and their possible outcomes is a crucial element of informed consent.
• A patient can revoke the consent at any time, even at the very last minute. It is essential that you report any circumstance that suggests that the patient does not understand the information or is revoking the informed consent to the person who obtained the consent.
• In most states, the registered nurse's legal role is to witness the signing of the document. This means that as a nurse, you attest to the fact that the patient's signature was valid.

Discussion Questions
1. What do you think you should do next?
2. What is your role as a patient advocate in the informed consent process?
3. What should you do if the patient states that she does not want to know about the surgical procedure or alternatives to surgery?

A true medical emergency may override the need to obtain consent.[10] The next of kin may give consent when immediate medical treatment is necessary to preserve life or prevent serious impairment to life or limb and the patient is incapable of giving consent. If reaching the next of kin is not possible, the HCP may begin treatment without written consent. A note in the chart must document the medical necessity of the procedure. In the case of an emergency in which consent cannot be obtained, you will usually need to complete an event report because it is an occurrence that is inconsistent with routine agency practices.

◆ Day-of-Surgery Preparation
◆ **Nursing Role.** Day-of-surgery preparation varies a great deal depending on whether the patient is an inpatient or an ambulatory surgical patient. Your responsibilities immediately before surgery include final preoperative teaching, assessment, and communication of pertinent findings. In addition, ensure that all preoperative orders are done and that the chart is complete

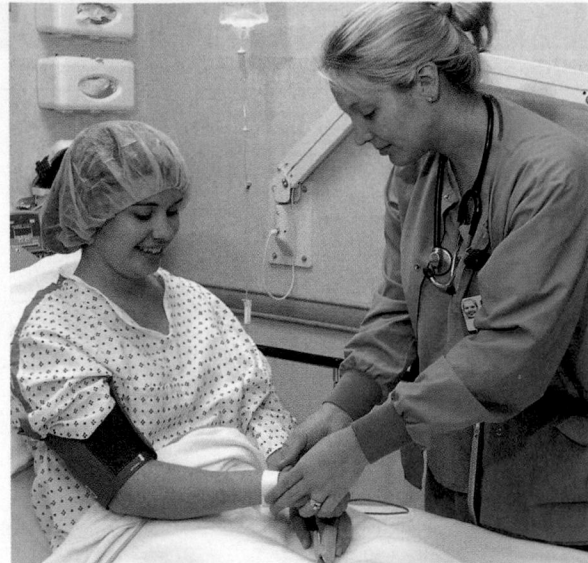

FIG. 17.1 The nurse performs a safety check by verifying that the patient has an identification band (wristband) as part of the preoperative preparations before she goes to surgery. (Courtesy Susan R. Volk, RN, MSN, CCRN, CPAN, Staff Development Specialist, Christiana Care Health System, Newark, DE.)

and goes with the patient to the OR. It is especially important to verify the presence of a signed informed consent form, results of laboratory and diagnostic studies, an H&P, a record of any consultations, baseline vital signs, proper skin preparation, and completed nursing notes. The surgical site is identified and marked with an indelible marker by the surgeon and documented to show that the patient agrees.[5]

Hospitals often require that a patient wear a hospital gown with no underclothes. Surgical centers may allow the patient to wear underwear, depending on the procedure. The patient should remove any cosmetics, since observation of skin color is important. Remove nail polish and artificial nails so you can assess capillary refill and pulse oximetry. Place an identification band on the patient and, if applicable, an allergy band (Fig. 17.1). Return all patient valuables to a caregiver or secure according to agency policy. All prostheses, including dentures, contact lenses, and glasses, are generally removed to prevent loss or damage. If electrocautery devices will be used during surgery, jewelry in piercings must be removed as a safety measure. Leave hearing aids in place to allow the patient to better follow instructions. Return glasses to the patient as soon as possible after surgery.

Encourage the patient to void before you give preoperative drugs and before transfer to the OR. An empty bladder prevents involuntary elimination under anesthesia and reduces the risk for urinary retention during the early postoperative recovery.

Many preoperative drugs interfere with balance and increase the risk for a fall during ambulation. Carefully assess each patient for responses to drugs given and adjust the plan of care as needed.

? CHECK YOUR PRACTICE
You are caring for an older female patient who received a dose of alprazolam (Xanax) for preoperative anxiety. One hour later, she requests to use the bathroom. You ask her if she can walk and she replies "yes." When helping her to stand, she becomes dizzy and almost falls. You return her to bed.
• Instead of trying to help this patient ambulate to the bathroom, what should have you done?

TABLE 17.8 Drug Therapy

Commonly Used Preoperative Medications

Class	Drug	Purpose
Antibiotics	cefazolin	Prevent postoperative infection
Anticholinergics	atropine glycopyrrolate	↓ Oral and respiratory secretions
	scopolamine (Transderm Scop)	Prevent nausea and vomiting
		Provide sedation
Antidiabetics	insulin (Humulin R)	Stabilize blood glucose
Antiemetics	metoclopramide (Reglan)	↑ Gastric emptying
	ondansetron (Zofran)	Prevent nausea and vomiting
Benzodiazepines	diazepam (Valium)	↓ Anxiety, induce sedation, amnesic effects
	lorazepam (Ativan)	
	midazolam	
β-Blockers	labetalol	Manage hypertension
Histamine (H$_2$)-receptor antagonists	famotidine	↓ HCl acid secretion, ↑ pH, ↓ gastric volume
	ranitidine	
Opioids	fentanyl	Relieve pain during preoperative procedures
	morphine	

◆ **Preoperative Medications** . Preoperative medications are used for a variety of reasons (Table 17.8). A patient may receive a single drug or a combination of drugs. Benzodiazepines are used for their sedative and amnesic properties. Anticholinergics are sometimes given to reduce secretions. Opioids may be given to decrease pain and anesthetic requirements during surgery. Antiemetics can decrease nausea and vomiting.

Other drugs that may be given before surgery include antibiotics, eyedrops, and routine prescription drugs. Antibiotics may be given throughout the perioperative period for patients with a history of prosthetic heart valve to prevent infective endocarditis and for patients with previous joint replacement. They also may be given when wound contamination is a potential risk (e.g., GI surgery). Antibiotics are most often given IV. We often give a single or first dose within 30 to 60 minutes of the surgical incision.

INFORMATICS IN PRACTICE

Computer-Based Timing for Antibiotic Administration

- A patient who receives the appropriate preoperative antibiotic has a decreased risk for a health care–associated infection.
- Using a computer to time antibiotic administration can decrease the incidence of wound infections.
- Computer-based timing systems aid with quality of care by tracking patient outcomes.
- You can look at the time patients received antibiotics and compare the rate of wound infections for those who did and did not receive timely treatment.

People with known hypertension or coronary artery disease may receive β-adrenergic blockers (β-blockers) to control BP or reduce the chances of MI and cardiac arrest.[16] Those with diabetes are carefully monitored and may receive insulin in the preoperative period.[10] Eyedrops are often given prior for the patient undergoing cataract and other eye surgery. Many times, the patient will need multiple sets of eyedrops given at 5-minute intervals. It is important to give these drugs as ordered and on time to adequately prepare the eye for surgery.

Patients may or may not receive drugs they routinely take on the day of surgery. To aid patient teaching and remove confusion about which drugs patients are taking, carefully check written preoperative orders and clarify the orders with the surgeon and/or ACP if there is any question.

Preoperative drugs may be given by mouth (PO), IV, or subcutaneously. Provide PO drugs with a small sip of water 60 to 90 minutes before the patient goes to the OR unless otherwise ordered. Subcutaneous injections (e.g., insulin) and IV drugs are usually given to the patient after arrival in the preoperative holding area. Teach the patient about the expected effects of the drugs (e.g., drowsiness).

! **SAFETY ALERT Preoperative Checklist**
- Use a preoperative checklist (Table 17.9) to make sure you have completed all required preparations.
- This is especially important to do before the patient receives any sedating drugs.

◆ Transportation to the Operating Room

For inpatients, transport staff move the patient by stretcher to the OR. Help the patient in moving from the bed to the stretcher and raise the side rails. Ensure that the completed chart and any needed equipment goes with the patient. In many agencies, the caregiver may go with the patient to the holding area.

In an ambulatory surgical center, the patient may go to the OR by stretcher or wheelchair. If no sedatives have been given, the patient may even walk with someone to the OR. In all cases, it is important to ensure patient safety during transport. Record the method of transportation and the person who transports the patient to the OR. Provide the hand-off communication to the nurse receiving the patient. This allows each of you to ensure you have shared all pertinent information about the patient. To avoid adverse events related to miscommunication, AORN recommends the use of the Situation-Background-Assessment-Recommendation (SBAR) model for the hand-off process in this setting[5] (see Table 1.4).

Show the caregiver where to wait for the patient during surgery. Many hospitals have a surgical waiting room where OR staff communicate the patient's status to the caregiver(s) and let them know when the surgery is complete. The surgeon can find the caregiver in this room after surgery to discuss the outcome. Some hospitals give pagers to caregivers so that they may eat or do errands during the surgery.

TABLE 17.9 Preoperative Checklist

Preoperative Data	Initials	Day of Surgery	Initials
Height _____ Weight _____		Surgical site marked Y or NA	
Isolation Y or N Type _____		ID band on patient Y or N	
Allergies noted on chart Y or N		Allergy band on patient Y or NA	
Vital signs (baseline) T _____ P _____ R _____ BP _____ Pulse Ox _____		Vital signs Time _____ T _____ P _____ R _____ BP _____ Pulse Ox _____	
Chart Review		**Procedures**	
H&P on chart		NPO since _____	
H&P within 30 days? Y or N		Capillary blood glucose Time _____ Result: _____ NA	
Signed and witnessed informed consent form on chart Y or N		Voided/catheter Time _____	
Signed consent for blood administration Y or NA		Preoperative drugs given Time _____ NA	
Blood type and crossmatch Y or NA		Preoperative antibiotics given Time _____ NA	
Diagnostic Results		Preoperative skin prep Y or NA Shower____ Scrub____ Clip____	
Hgb/Hct _____ /_____ NA		Makeup, nail polish, false fingernails, and false eyelashes removed Y or NA	
PT/INR/PTT _____ /_____ /_____ NA		Hospital gown applied Y or NA	
CXR _____ NA		**Valuables**	
ECG _____ NA hCG _____ Negative _____ Positive _____ NA		Dentures Y or N	
Other labs:		Wig or hairpiece Y or N	
Final Chart Review		Eyeglasses Y or N	
Additional forms attached:		Contact lenses Y or N	
		Hearing aid Y or N	
		Prosthesis Y or N	
		Jewelry Y or N Piercings with jewelry Y or N	
		Clothing Y or N	
		Disposition of valuables: Hearing aid in place Y or NA	

Time to OR _____ Date _____
Transported to OR by _____
Final check by _____ RN _____

Culturally Competent Care: Preoperative Patient

Include cultural considerations when assessing and implementing care for the patient's preoperative needs. For example, culture often determines one's expression of pain, family expectations, and ability to verbally express needs. One's culture may require that the family be included in any decision making. For example, many older Hispanic women may defer to their family for the decision whether to have surgery. Respect these decisions. If the patient or caregiver does not speak English, you must use a qualified interpreter (translates orally) or translator (interprets written text) communication system.[17] See more on culturally competent care in Chapter 2.

Gerontologic Considerations: Preoperative Patient

Many patients older than 65 years of age undergo surgery. Surgery on older adults requires careful evaluation. Frequently performed procedures in older adults include cataract extraction, coronary and vascular procedures, prostate surgery, cholecystectomy, and joint repair or replacement. Communication is important. The patient's primary HCP is usually not the surgeon. Often several HCPs are involved in the patient's care.

Be particularly alert when assessing and caring for the older adult surgical patient. An event that has little effect on a younger adult may be overwhelming to the older patient. Hospitalization may represent a physical decline and loss of health, mobility, and independence. The older adult may view the hospital as a place to die or as a stepping-stone to a nursing home. Help to decrease anxieties and fears while maintaining the self-esteem of the older adult during the surgical experience.

The risks associated with anesthesia and surgery increase in the older patient. In general, the older the patient, the greater are the risks for complications after surgery. In planning care, consider the patient's physiologic status, not only the chronologic age. The surgical risk in the older adult relates to normal physiologic aging and changes that compromise organ function, reduce reserve capacity, and limit the body's ability to adapt to stress. This decreased ability to cope with stress, often compounded by the burden of one or more chronic illnesses, and the surgery itself increase the risk for complications.

Confirm and document the patient's goals and treatment preferences. In those with advance directives, discuss any new risks associated with the surgical procedure. Make sure the approach for treating any potential problems is consistent with the patient's preferences.[18]

Older adults may have some sensory deficits. Bright lights may bother those with eye problems. They can have reduced vision and hearing. Thought processes and cognitive abilities may be slowed or impaired. Assess and record baseline sensory and cognitive function. Physical reactions are often slowed because of mobility and balance problems. Because of these changes, the older adult may need more time to complete preoperative testing and understand preoperative instructions.

These changes also require you to pay more attention to promote patient safety and prevent injury.

When older adults live in a long-term care or assisted living facility, you may need to coordinate transportation from these facilities so that timely arrival allows for surgery preparation. A legal representative of the patient must be present to provide consent for surgery if the patient cannot sign for himself or herself.

Finally, determine the presence of or need for caregiver support for the older adult undergoing surgery. With the increase in outpatient surgical procedures and shorter length of stays after surgery, caregiver support is critical in the continuity of care for this population.

CASE STUDY

Preoperative Patient

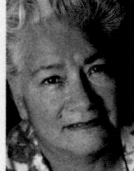

(© Ryan McVay/
Photodisc/
Thinkstock.)

Patient Profile

F.D., a 72-yr-old Hispanic retired librarian, is admitted to the hospital with compromised circulation of the right lower leg and a necrotic right foot. She has diabetes and takes insulin to maintain appropriate blood glucose levels. She has been NPO since midnight. It is now 10 AM on the morning of the surgery.

Subjective Data

- History of type 2 diabetes for 30 years; states, "My blood sugar is hard to control" and "I just started taking insulin"
- History of hypertension and peripheral vascular disease
- History of stage 2 chronic kidney disease
- History of macular degeneration in right eye; reports poor vision
- Surgical history: cesarean section at age 30, cholecystectomy at age 65; reports poor wound healing after last surgery
- States her Social Security checks barely cover her living expenses
- States she often runs out of her drugs and cannot always afford to refill them right away
- Reports chronic burning pain in both legs and has trouble sleeping at night
- Lives alone but has family who want her to move in with them after surgery
- Uses herbs to control blood glucose levels and often skips her insulin

Objective Data

Physical Examination

- Alert, cognitively intact, anxious, older woman with numbness and lack of feeling in right leg
- Weight 190 lb, height 5 ft 3 in
- BP 180/94, pulse 84 and slightly irregular
- Wears glasses for close work and reading

Diagnostic Studies

- Admission serum blood glucose level 272 mg/dL (15.2 mmol/L), glycosylated hemoglobin (Hb A1C) 14%
- Morning capillary blood glucose level 198 mg/dL (11 mmol/L)
- Doppler pulses for right lower leg weak, absent in right foot
- Doppler pulses in left lower leg present, weak in left foot
- Serum creatinine 2.0 mg/dL (176 mmol/L)

Interprofessional Care

- Scheduled for a below-the-knee amputation of the right leg at 1 PM today

Discussion Questions

1. What factors may influence F.D.'s response to hospitalization and surgery?
2. **Priority Decision:** Given F.D.'s history, what priority preoperative nursing assessments would you want to complete and why?
3. What potential perioperative complications may you expect for F.D.?
4. **Priority Decision:** What priority topics would you include in F.D.'s preoperative teaching plan?
5. **Priority Decision:** Based on the assessment data presented, identify the priority nursing diagnoses and related interventions. Are there any collaborative problems?
6. **Collaboration:** Identify appropriate interventions that could be delegated to unlicensed assistive personnel (UAP).
7. **Safety:** To ensure F.D.'s safety, what preoperative nursing interventions are essential?
8. **Evidence-Based Practice:** F.D. asks you why she received insulin this morning when she has not eaten anything since midnight. How would you respond to her?

Answers available at *http://evolve.elsevier.com/Lewis/medsurg.*

▮ BRIDGE TO NCLEX EXAMINATION

The number of the question corresponds to the same-numbered outcome at the beginning of the chapter.

1. An overweight patient (BMI 28.1 kg/m²) is scheduled for a laparoscopic cholecystectomy at an outpatient surgery setting. The nurse knows that
   a. surgery will involve multiple small incisions.
   b. this setting is not appropriate for this procedure.
   c. surgery will involve removing a part of the liver.
   d. the patient will need special preparation because of obesity.

2. The patient tells the nurse in the preoperative setting that she has noticed she has a reaction when wearing rubber gloves. What is the *most* appropriate action?
   a. Notify the surgeon so that the surgery can be cancelled.
   b. Ask additional questions to assess for a possible latex allergy.
   c. Notify the OR staff at once so they can use latex-free supplies.
   d. No action is needed because the patient's rubber sensitivity has no bearing on surgery.

3. A 59-yr-old man scheduled for a herniorrhaphy in 2 days reports that he takes ginkgo daily. What is the *priority* intervention?
   a. Inform the surgeon, since the procedure may have to be rescheduled.
   b. Notify the anesthesia care provider, since this herb interferes with anesthetics.
   c. Ask the patient if he has noticed any side effects from taking this herbal supplement.
   d. Tell the patient to continue to take the herbal supplement up to the day before surgery.

4. A 17-yr-old patient with a leg fracture who is scheduled for surgery is an emancipated minor. She has a statement from the court for verification. Which intervention is *most* appropriate?
   a. Witness the permit after the surgeon obtains consent.
   b. Call a parent or legal guardian to sign the permit since the patient is under 18.
   c. Notify the hospital attorney that an emancipated minor is consenting for surgery.
   d. Obtain verbal consent since written consent is not necessary for emancipated minors.

5. A *priority* nursing intervention to aid a preoperative patient in coping with fear of postoperative pain would be to
   a. inform the patient that pain medication will be available.
   b. teach the patient to use guided imagery to help manage pain.
   c. describe the type of pain expected with the patient's particular surgery.
   d. explain the pain management plan, including the use of a pain rating scale.

6. A patient is scheduled for surgery requiring general anesthesia at an ambulatory surgical center. The nurse asks him when he ate last. He replies that he had a light breakfast a couple of hours before coming to the surgery center. What should the nurse do *first*?
   a. Tell the patient to come back tomorrow, since he ate a meal.
   b. Have the patient void before giving any preoperative medications.
   c. Proceed with the preoperative checklist, including site identification.
   d. Notify the anesthesia care provider of when and what the patient last ate.

7. A patient who normally takes 40 units of glargine insulin (long acting) at bedtime asks the nurse what to do about her dose the night before surgery. The *best* response would be to have her
   a. skip her insulin altogether the night before surgery.
   b. get instructions from her surgeon or HCP on any insulin adjustments.
   c. take her usual dose at bedtime and eat a light breakfast in the morning.
   d. eat a moderate meal before bedtime and then take half her usual insulin dose.

8. Preoperative considerations for older adults include *(select all that apply)*
   a. using only large-print educational materials.
   b. speaking louder for patients with hearing aids.
   c. recognizing that sensory deficits may be present.
   d. providing warm blankets to prevent hypothermia.
   e. teaching important information early in the morning.

1. a, 2. b, 3. a, 4. a, 5. d, 6. d, 7. b, 8. c, d

For rationales to these answers and even more NCLEX review questions, visit *http://evolve.elsevier.com/Lewis/medsurg*.

⊚ EVOLVE WEBSITE/RESOURCES LIST

http://evolve.elsevier.com/Lewis/medsurg
- Review Questions (Online Only)
- Key Points
- Answer Keys for Review Questions
  - Rationales for Bridge to NCLEX Examination Questions
  - Answer Guidelines for Case Study on p. 311
- Conceptual Care Map Creator
- Audio Glossary
- Content Updates

REFERENCES

1. Jehovah's Witnesses: Why don't Jehovah's Witnesses accept blood transfusions? Retrieved from *www.jw.org/en/jehovahs-witnesses/faq/jehovahs-witnesses-why-no-blood-transfusions/*.
*2. Ebner M, Birschmann I, Peter A, et al: Point-of-care testing for emergency assessment of coagulation in patients treated with direct oral anticoagulants, *Critical Care* 21:32, 2017.
3. Society of Gastroenterology Nurses and Associates: Patient safety issues with use of herbal supplements. Retrieved from *www.sgna.org/Practice/GI-Nurse-Sedation/Patient-Care-Safety*.
4. American College of Allergy, Asthma, and Immunology: Latex allergy. Retrieved from *https://acaai.org/allergies/types/latex-allergy*.
5. Association of periOperative Registered Nurses: *Guidelines for perioperative practice*. Denver, 2017, AORN.
*6. Bock M, Fritsch G, Hepner D: Preoperative laboratory testing, *Anesthesiol Clin* 34:43, 2016.
*7. Troy HK, Stikkelbroeck NM, Smans LC, et al: Adrenal crisis: Still a deadly event in the 21st century, *AJM* 129:339, 2016.
8. Wound Care Centers: How diabetes affects wound healing. Retrieved from *www.woundcarecenters.org/article/living-with-wounds/how-diabetes-affects-wound-healing*.
*9. Prabhaker A, Helander E, Chopra N, et al: Preoperative assessment for ambulatory surgery, *Curr Pain Headache Rep* 21:43, 2017.
10. Rotruck JC: *Alexander's care of the patient in surgery*, ed 16, St Louis, 2018, Elsevier.
*11. Martin VT, Vij B: Diet and headache, *Headache* 56:1543, 2016.
12. The Joint Commission: History and physical content. Retrieved from *www.jointcommission.org/standards_information/jcfaqdetails.aspx?StandardsFaqId=1851&ProgramId=46*.
*13. Torres EG, Lindmair JM, Langan JW, et al: Is preoperative nasal povidone-iodine as efficient and cost-effective as standard MRSA screening protocol in total joint arthroplasty? *J Arthroplasty* 31:215, 2016.
*14. Wilson RA, Watt-Watson J, Hodnett E, et al: A randomized controlled trial of an individualized preoperative education intervention for symptom management after total knee arthroplasty, *Orthopaedic Nursing* 35:20, 2016.
*15. Practice guidelines for preoperative fasting and the use of pharmacologic agents to reduce the risk of pulmonary aspiration: Application to healthy patients undergoing elective procedures, *Anesthesiology* 126:376, 2017.
16. Smeltz A, Kumar P: Angiotensin axis blocking drugs in the perioperative period, *Anesthesiol News*, 2016. Retrieved from *www.anesthesiologynews.com/Review-Articles/Article/02-16/Angiotensin-Axis-Blocking-Drugs-In-the-Perioperative-Period/35357/ses=ogst*.
17. The Joint Commission: Standard FAQ details. Retrieved from *www.jointcommission.org/standards_information/jcfaqdetails.aspx?StandardsFaqId=1490&ProgramId=46*.
*18. Mohanty S, Rosenthal RA, Russell MM, et al: Optimal perioperative management of the geriatric patient: A best practices guideline from the American College of Surgeons NSQIP and the American Geriatrics Society, *JACS* 222:930, 2016.

*Evidence-based information for clinical practice.

18

Intraoperative Care

Mark Karasin

*Unless someone like you cares a whole awful lot,
nothing is going to get better, it's not.*

Dr. Seuss

ⓔ http://evolve.elsevier.com/Lewis/medsurg/

CONCEPTUAL FOCUS

Gas Exchange	Perfusion	Tissue Integrity
Pain	Safety	

LEARNING OUTCOMES

1. Distinguish various areas of perioperative department and appropriate attire.
2. Outline the roles and responsibilities of interprofessional surgical team members.
3. Prioritize needs of patients undergoing surgery.
4. Analyze role of a perioperative nurse in the management of patients undergoing surgery.
5. Apply basic principles of infection prevention and aseptic technique in the operating room.
6. Recognize operating room safety measures related to patients, equipment, and anesthesia.
7. Distinguish various anesthesia techniques and common anesthesia drugs.

KEY TERMS

anesthesia care provider (ACP), p. 315
anesthesiology, p. 315
epidural block, p. 325

general anesthesia, p. 320
local anesthesia, p. 324
malignant hyperthermia (MH), p. 325

nurse anesthetist, p. 315
regional anesthesia, p. 324
spinal anesthesia, p. 324

Historically, surgery took place in the traditional environment of the hospital operating room (OR). Now, many surgical procedures are done as ambulatory surgery (outpatient surgery). In addition, the use of *minimally invasive surgery* (MIS) is rapidly increasing. More procedures use endoscopes, robotics, and other advanced technologies that lead to decreased blood loss, incision size, pain, recovery time, and hospital length of stay. Hybrid ORs, which allow for MIS, such as endovascular procedures, and the traditional open incision approach within the same room, are becoming more common. This chapter discusses the basics of intraoperative care that apply to all surgical patients regardless of where or how the surgery is done.

PHYSICAL ENVIRONMENT OF THE OPERATING ROOM

Department Layout

The surgery department is a controlled environment designed to minimize the spread of pathogens and allow a smooth flow of patients, staff, and equipment needed to give safe surgical patient care. The department is divided into 3 distinct zones: (1) unrestricted, (2) semirestricted, and (3) restricted (Fig. 18.1). The *unrestricted zone* is where people in street clothes interact with those in scrub attire. These areas typically include the points of entry for patients (e.g., holding area), staff (e.g., locker rooms), and information (e.g., nursing station or control desk). The *semirestricted zone* includes the surrounding support areas and corridors. Only authorized staff are allowed access to semirestricted areas. All staff in the semirestricted area should wear clean surgical attire. This includes scrub attire that was laundered in an accredited laundry facility, long-sleeved jacket, shoes dedicated for surgery use or shoe covers, surgical head cover and mask that covers all head and facial hair, and any appropriate personal protective equipment (e.g., face shield). The *restricted zone* is found within the semirestricted area. It includes the surgical suite (OR) where the invasive procedure takes place and the sterile core (Fig. 18.2). Masks should be worn and traffic minimized whenever sterile supplies are open in the restricted area.[1]

The physical layout is designed to reduce cross-contamination. The flow of clean and sterile supplies and equipment is separate from contaminated supplies, equipment, and waste by space, time, and traffic patterns. Staff members move supplies from clean areas, such as the sterile core, through the OR for surgery, and on to the instrument decontamination and sterilization area (e.g., central processing department [CPD]).

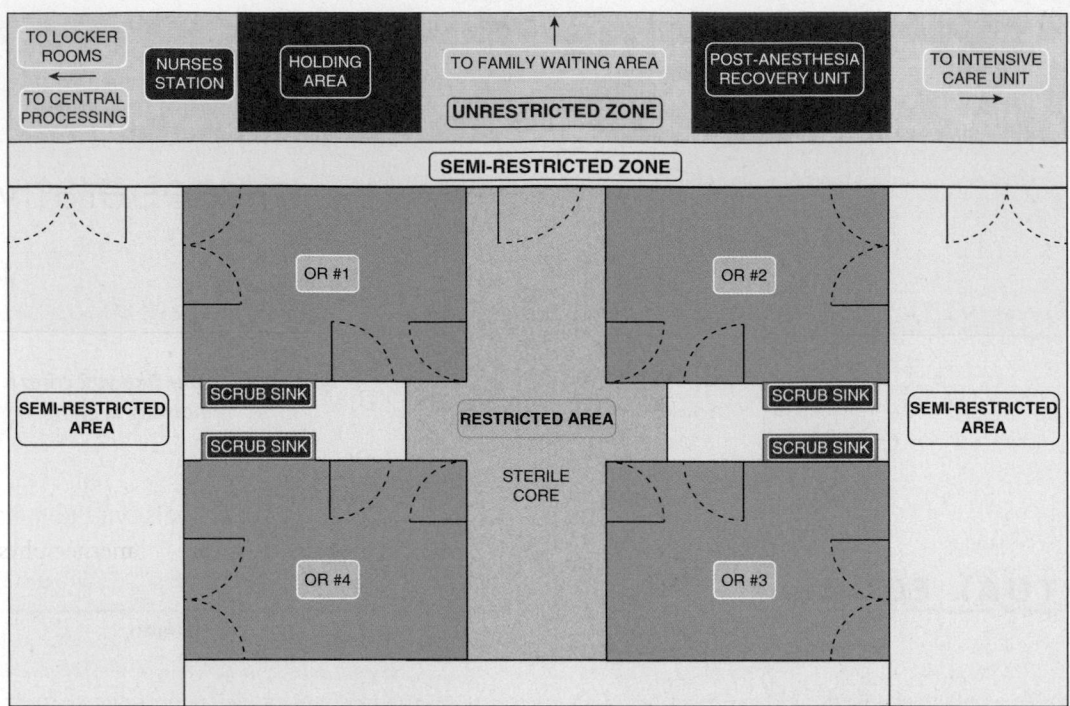

FIG. 18.1 Perioperative department layout.

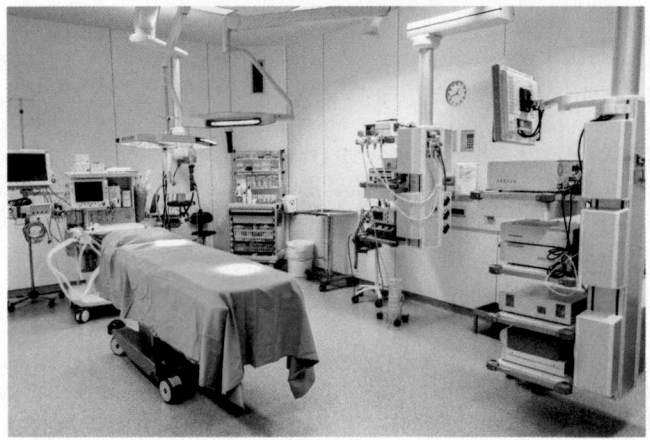

FIG. 18.2 Typical OR. (© iStock.com/windslegend.)

Holding Area

The *holding area,* often called the *preoperative holding area,* is an unrestricted zone where patient identification and assessment take place. The size can range from a large centralize area that handles many patients to a small designated area right outside of the OR.

In some settings, the holding area is called the *admission, observation, and discharge* (AOD) unit. An AOD unit is designed to allow early morning admission for outpatient surgery, same-day admission, and inpatient holding before surgery. The patient is identified and assessed before and after surgery, before being discharged home or transferred to an inpatient room. The AOD unit is important in outpatient surgery and prevents unnecessary overnight stays in the inpatient setting.

Operating Room

The traditional OR is a unique setting separate from other clinical units. This restricted zone is controlled geographically, environmentally, and aseptically (Fig. 18.1). It is best to have the OR next to the postanesthesia care unit (PACU) and the surgical intensive care unit. This allows for quick transport of the patient after surgery and close proximity to anesthesia staff if complications occur.

We use several methods to prevent the transmission of infection in the OR. Filters and controlled airflow in the ventilating systems provide dust control. Positive air pressure in the rooms prevents air from entering the OR from the halls and corridors. ORs are kept within a narrow range of temperature and humidity to prevent bacteria growth. ORs follow strict protocols for cleaning between cases and terminal cleaning at the end of the day. The use of ultraviolet lighting reduces the number of microorganisms in the air.[2]

Using OR furniture that is adjustable, easy to clean, and easy to move promotes safety and comfort. All equipment is checked frequently to ensure proper functioning and electrical safety. The lighting is designed to give a low- to high-intensity range for a precise view of the surgical site. A communication system offers a way to deliver routine and emergency messages.[3]

SURGICAL TEAM

Registered Nurse

The *perioperative nurse* is a registered nurse (RN) who collaborates with the rest of the surgical team and implements the patient's plan of care during perioperative period. Depending on the size of the OR department, this role may include three domains: (1) preoperative RN, (2) OR RN, and (3) PACU RN. As an OR RN, you are the patient's advocate during surgery. This includes (1) maintaining the patient's safety, dignity, and confidentiality; (2) communicating with the patient, the surgical team, and other departments (e.g., CPD, PACU, laboratory); and (3) providing nursing care discussed in the Nursing Management section of this chapter.

TABLE 18.1 Intraoperative Nursing Activities

Circulating, Nonsterile Activities
- Helps prepare room, ensuring that supplies and equipment are available, in working order, and sterile
- Maintains aseptic technique in all required activities
- Monitors practices of aseptic technique in self and others
- Checks mechanical and electrical equipment and environmental factors
- Conducts a preprocedure verification process
- Assesses patient's physical and emotional status
- Confirms and implements facility protocols and safety measures
- Plans and coordinates intraoperative nursing care
- Checks chart and relates pertinent data to team members
- Helps with applying monitoring devices and insertion of invasive lines and other devices
- Assists with and ensures patient safety in transferring and positioning patient
- Aids with anesthesia induction
- Monitors draping
- Takes part in surgical time-out
- Records intraoperative care
- Prepares, records, labels, and sends blood, pathology, and any anatomic specimens to proper locations
- Measures blood, urine output, and other fluid loss
- Confirms, dispenses, and records drugs used, including local anesthetics
- Coordinates all intraoperative activities with team members and other staff and departments
- Works with scrubbed personnel to keep correct count of sponges, needles, instruments, and medical devices
- Facilitates patient transfer to PACU
- Gives hand-off report to PACU nurse with information relevant to care of patient

Scrubbed, Sterile Activities
- Helps prepare the OR
- Completes surgical hand antisepsis and gowns and gloves self and other members of surgical team
- Prepares instrument table and arranges sterile equipment for functional use
- Assists with draping
- Takes part in surgical time-out procedure
- Passes instruments to surgeon and assistants by anticipating their needs
- Keeps correct count of sponges, needles, instruments, and medical devices that could be retained in the patient
- Monitors practices of aseptic technique in self and others
- Keeps track of irrigation solutions used for calculation of blood loss
- Accepts, verifies, and reports drugs used by surgeon and/or ACP, including local anesthetics

During surgery, the OR RN assumes functions that involve either sterile or unsterile activities (Table 18.1). The *scrub nurse* (sterile) follows the designated surgical hand antisepsis and glove and gown sterile attire and prepares and manages the sterile field and instrumentation. The *circulating nurse* stays in the unsterile field, facilitates the progress of the procedure, and keeps documentation.[4] Examples of nursing activities that occur during each phase of the surgical experience are outlined in Table 18.2.

After meeting specific criteria (e.g., 2 years of experience), perioperative RNs can obtain OR certification (CNOR). CNOR certification is an objective measure (written test) that validates a nurse has essential knowledge and skills in perioperative nursing.[5]

Licensed Practical/Vocational Nurse and Surgical Technologist

Depending on the state's nurse practice act, an LPN/VN or a surgical technologist may fill the role of the circulating or scrub nurse. Surgical technologists attend an associate degree program or a vocational, hospital, or military training program. The Association of Surgical Technologists sets the standards for education, provides continuing education opportunities, and offers certification for surgical technologists.[6]

If the circulating nurse is not an RN, the LPN/VN or surgical technologist must always have access to an RN. As an OR RN, you take on responsibility for supervising an LPN/VN or surgical technologist performing delegated nursing tasks.[7]

Surgeon and Assistant

The *surgeon* is the physician who does the surgical procedure. The surgeon is primarily responsible for:
- Preoperative medical history and physical assessment, directing preoperative testing, and postoperative management Obtaining informed consent
- Leading the surgical team and directing the course of a procedure

The *surgeon's assistant* can be another physician, registered nurse first assistant (RNFA), physician's assistant, surgical resident or fellow, medical student, or a certified surgical first assistant. The assistant usually holds retractors to expose surgical areas and helps with hemostasis and suturing. In some agencies, especially in educational settings, the assistant may perform some portions of the surgery under the surgeon's direct supervision.

Registered Nurse First Assistant

The *registered nurse first assistant* (RNFA) works with the surgeon to achieve an optimal surgical outcome for the patient. The Association of periOperative Registered Nurses (AORN) states that you must have formal education for this role and work collaboratively with the surgeon, patient, and surgical team.[8] CNOR nurses or nurse practitioners can complete RNFA program to assume this expanded role. RNFAs can obtain certification (C-RNFA).

Anesthesia Care Provider

Anesthesiology is a medical specialty that focuses on clinical management of the patient in the perioperative period, pain management, critical care, trauma, airway management, and cardiopulmonary resuscitation. The anesthesia care provider (ACP) is the person responsible for administering anesthetic agents and managing vital life functions (e.g., breathing, BP) during the perioperative period.[9] This can be an anesthesiologist, nurse anesthetist, or anesthesiologist assistant (AA).

A nurse anesthetist is a master's or a doctorate prepared RN who has graduated from an accredited nurse anesthesia program and completed a national certification examination to become a certified registered nurse anesthetist (CRNA).

The CRNA's scope of practice includes:[10]
- Performing and documenting a preanesthetic assessment and evaluation
- Developing and implementing a plan for delivering anesthesia
- Choosing, obtaining, and administering anesthesia, adjuvant drugs, and fluids
- Choosing, applying, and inserting appropriate monitoring devices
- Managing a patient's airway and pulmonary status
- Managing emergence and recovery from anesthesia
- Releasing or discharging patients from a PACU
- Ordering, starting, or modifying pain relief therapy
- Responding to emergency situations by providing airway management

TABLE 18.2 Common Perioperative Nursing Activities

Before Surgery	During Surgery	After Surgery
Home, Clinic, Holding Area	**Safety Maintenance**	**Postanesthesia, Discharge Area**
• Starts preoperative assessment	• Ensures integrity of sterile field	• Determines patient's response to surgical intervention
• Plans teaching appropriate to patient's needs	• Ensures that sponge, needle, instrument, and medical device counts are correct	• Monitors ABCs, vital signs, level of consciousness
• Involves caregiver	• Positions patient to ensure correct alignment, exposure of surgical site, and prevention of injury	• Safely gives ordered drugs
Surgical Unit	• Prevents chemical injury from prepping solutions, drugs, etc.	**Clinical Unit**
• Completes preoperative assessment	• Ensures safe use of electrical equipment	• Evaluates effectiveness of nursing care in OR using patient outcome criteria
• Coordinates patient teaching with staff	• Safely gives ordered drugs	• Determines patient's level of satisfaction with care given
• Develops a plan of care that reflects patient's level of function and ability		• Assesses patient's psychologic status
• Safely gives ordered drugs	**Monitoring Physical Status**	• Helps with discharge planning
	• Monitors and reports changes in patient's vital signs	
Surgical Suite	• Monitors blood loss and urine output	**Home, Clinic**
• Conducts preprocedure verification		• Seeks patient's perception of surgery in terms of effects of anesthetic agents, impact on body image, immobilization
• Assesses patient's level of consciousness, skin integrity, mobility, emotional status, and functional limitations	**Monitoring Psychologic Status**	• Determines caregiver's perceptions of surgery
• Reviews chart	• Gives emotional support to patient	
• Ensures all supplies and equipment needed are available, functioning, and sterile, if appropriate	• Ensures patient's right to privacy	
	• Communicates patient' emotional status to health care team	

An AA is a master's-prepared health professional who serves under the direction of an anesthesiologist. AAs have completed an accredited program and passed a national certification examination. They take part in all types of anesthesia. This includes giving drugs, obtaining vascular access, applying and interpreting monitors, maintaining airways, and helping with preoperative assessment.

❖ NURSING MANAGEMENT: PATIENT BEFORE SURGERY

The preoperative assessment of the surgical patient provides baseline data for intraoperative and postoperative care and is used to plan intraoperative care. Preoperative care of the patient is discussed in Chapter 17.

Provide physical and emotional comfort for the patient and caregivers along with teaching about the upcoming surgery. This is particularly important in the same-day surgery settings, where caregivers must assume greater responsibility for postoperative care.

◆ Psychosocial Assessment

Knowing about the activities that occur when a patient moves into the OR allows you to provide teaching and comfort, especially to the anxious patient. You can usually answer general questions about surgery and anesthesia, such as, "When will I go to sleep?" "Who will be in the room?" "When will my surgeon arrive?" "How much of my body will be exposed?" "Will I be cold?" "When will I wake up?" Refer specific questions about the details of the surgery and anesthesia to the surgeon or ACP. For patients who do not speak English, use a qualified interpreter (see Table 2.10).

Separation from caregivers just before surgery can produce anxiety for the patient. Allowing the caregiver to wait with the patient in the holding area until we transfer the patient to the OR can reduce anxiety.

◆ Physical Assessment

Perform a thorough physical assessment during the preoperative preparation of the patient (see Chapter 17).

◆ Chart Review

Required chart data vary with agencies, patient conditions, and surgical procedures. Tables 17.2 and 17.4 provide examples of data we obtain during the preoperative assessment. This information gives an understanding of past and present medical history and an opportunity to anticipate and prepare for potential needs during surgery, such as obtaining equipment or drugs. You can discuss any abnormal findings or concerns for infection and other complications with the surgeon or ACP.

? CHECK YOUR PRACTICE

Your patient has arrived in the holding area. As you review the chart, you realize the patient has not signed the consent for blood. You see the patient has Alzheimer's disease and is not mentally competent to give consent.
• How would you proceed?

◆ Admitting the Patient

Agency policy guides the protocol you follow when admitting the patient to the holding area and OR. A general routine includes initial greeting, proper identification, and offer of human contact and warmth.

The admitting process continues with reassessment of the patient and time for last-minute questions. Determine if any other tasks need to be done. Complete the chart review for the previously mentioned data and note any problems or changes. Ask the patient about valuables, prostheses, and last intake of food and fluid. Confirm that any ordered preoperative drugs were given. Provide a pillow or adjust the patient's position if requested. Most agencies require the patient's hair to be covered just before transfer to the OR suite to reduce potential shedding.

You may offer complementary and alternative therapies, such as aromatherapy, music therapy, guided imagery, and distraction (see the Complementary & Alternative Therapies box).

These therapies may decrease anxiety, promote relaxation, and reduce pain.[11] Some agencies start these therapies before the patient is admitted to the OR. In others, such as ambulatory settings, they may start after the patient arrives in the holding area.

COMPLEMENTARY & ALTERNATIVE THERAPIES

Music Therapy

Music is an ancient healing tool recognized in the writings of Plato.

Scientific Evidence

Strong evidence supports using music therapy to reduce stress and anxiety and enhance mood.

Nursing Implications

- To be effective, the music used must be appropriate for the situation. Music can have many different physiologic effects.
- Listening to calming music can result in slower, deeper breathing and a decrease in heart rate and BP. Both indicate relaxation.
- Music with a faster pace can energize a person and promote mental alertness.
- Music therapy is safe in combination with other treatment approaches.

Source: Daniel E: Music used as anti-anxiety intervention for patients during outpatient procedures: a review of the literature, *Complement Ther Clin Pract* 22:21, 2016.

❖ NURSING MANAGEMENT: PATIENT DURING SURGERY

Patient care in the surgical setting is dynamic and depends on the knowledge, skills, and judgment of the RN.[4] The circulating nurse is responsible for implementing the intraoperative plan of care and serving as the patient's advocate. The circulating nurse focuses on the whole patient. This involves ongoing assessment, reassessment, and adjusting the care plan to promote the best surgical outcomes.

◆ Room Preparation

Before transferring the patient into the OR, prepare the room to ensure privacy, prevention of infection, and safety. Individualized preparation is essential to achieve the expected patient outcomes.

When a patient is severely obese, extra staff and special equipment may be needed to safely position and transfer the patient to and from the OR bed. During surgery, special equipment (e.g., extra-long instrumentation, bariatric OR bed) may be used.

CHECK YOUR PRACTICE

You are assigned to observe in the OR. A severely obese patient is admitted to the holding area. The circulating nurse tells you that the team will address the unique needs of the patient for a safe surgical experience.
- What special considerations are needed for this patient?

All people entering the OR wear surgical attire (Fig. 18.3). All electrical and mechanical equipment is checked for proper functioning. Each surgical item is opened and placed on the instrument table using aseptic technique. Sponges, needles, instruments, and small medical devices (e.g., surgical clip

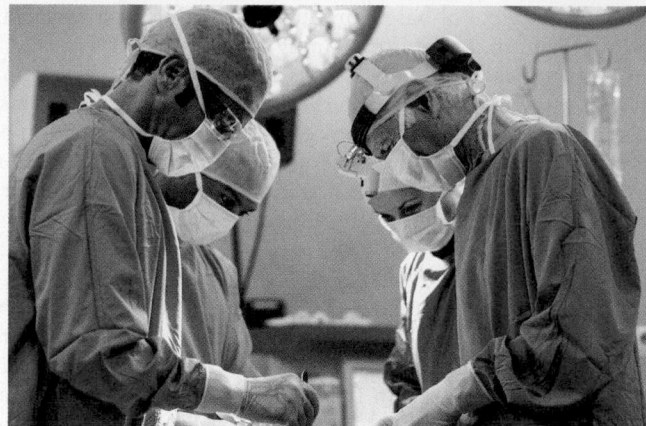

FIG. 18.3 All surgical personnel wear surgical attire. (© iStock.com/Ridofranz.)

cartridges, universal adapters) are counted according to strict processes to ensure accurate retrieval at the end of the procedure. Any retained surgical supplies, devices, or instruments are sentinel events (never events) or serious reportable events (SREs) that can result in negative outcomes for the patient.[1,4] (Sentinel events and SREs are discussed in Chapter 1.)

During room preparation and the surgical procedure, the scrub person does surgical hand antisepsis, dons sterile gown and gloves, and touches only items in the sterile field. The circulating nurse stays in the unsterile field and does those activities that involve contact with all unsterile items and the patient. This coordinated effort allows for smooth functioning throughout the procedure.

◆ Transferring Patient

The patient is moved into the OR after the preoperative assessment is complete and the surgical suite is ready. Always maintain privacy during transfers through public areas by covering the patient with a gown and/or blanket. Each time a patient is transferred between beds, the wheels of each must be locked. Enough staff members using ergonomic tools for safe patient handling and movement should be available to lift, guide, and prevent accidental falling or injury to staff and the patient. Once the patient is on the OR bed, ensure that there is always someone on both sides of the patient until a safety strap is secured to prevent falls. The monitor leads (e.g., ECG leads), BP cuff, and pulse oximeter are usually applied after the patient is safe on the OR bed.

◆ Scrubbing, Gowning, and Gloving

Surgical hand antisepsis is required of all sterile members of the surgical team (scrub nurse, surgeon, assistant). When wet scrubbing is the chosen method for surgical hand antisepsis, your finger nails are cleaned first, followed by scrubbing each plane of individual fingers, palms, and forearms in the distal to proximal fashion. The hands should always be held away from surgical attire and higher than the elbows. This prevents contamination from clothing or detergent suds and water from draining from the unclean area above the elbows to the clean and previously scrubbed areas of the hands and fingers.

Waterless, alcohol-based agents are replacing soap and water in many agencies. When using an alcohol-based surgical hand-scrub product, prewash hands and forearms with soap and dry completely before applying the alcohol-based product. After applying the alcohol-based product, rub hands and forearms thoroughly until dry before donning sterile attire.[1,4]

Once surgical hand antisepsis is completed, the team members enter the OR to put on sterile gowns and 2 pairs of gloves. This protects patients and themselves from the transmission of microorganisms.[1,4] Because the gowns and gloves are sterile, those who have scrubbed can manipulate and organize all sterile items for use during the procedure.

◆ Basic Aseptic Technique

Aseptic technique is practiced in the OR to prevent infection. This is done through the creation and maintenance of a sterile field. The center of the sterile field is the site of the surgical incision. Items used in the sterile field, including surgical instruments and equipment, have been sterilized by appropriate sterilization methods.

Team members must understand specific principles to practice aseptic technique (Table 18.3). If these principles are not followed, the patient's safety is compromised and the risk for infection is increased.[1,4]

The surgical team is also responsible for following the guidelines established by the U.S. Occupational Safety and Health Administration (OSHA) and the AORN to protect the patient and the team from exposure to blood-borne pathogens.[12] These guidelines emphasize (1) standard and transmission-based precautions, (2) engineering and work practice controls, and (3) the use of personal protective equipment, such as gloves, gowns, caps, face shields, masks, and protective eyewear. This is especially important in the OR because of the high potential for exposure to blood-borne pathogens.

◆ Assisting Anesthesia Care Provider

While you check the OR to complete the final preparations, the ACP prepares the patient for receiving anesthesia. You need to understand the effects of the anesthetic agents and know the location of all emergency drugs and equipment.

If you are the circulating nurse, you may be involved in placing monitoring devices used during the procedure (e.g., ECG leads). If the patient is having general anesthesia, stay at the patient's side to ensure safety and aid the ACP. These responsibilities may include measuring BP and helping maintain the patient's airway. During the procedure, you are a vital communication link for the ACP to other departments, such as the laboratory or blood bank.

◆ Positioning Patient

The surgical team carefully plans the patient's positioning and monitors the patient throughout the procedure. Positioning is a critical part of every procedure and usually follows induction of anesthesia. The ACP says when to begin positioning. The patient's position should allow for accessibility to the operative site, administering and monitoring of anesthetic agents, and maintaining the patient's airway. We use a variety of surgical positions, including supine, prone, lateral, lithotomy, or sitting. The supine is the most common position. It allows operating on most body systems, including the abdomen, heart, chest, or head. The prone position is often used in spine surgery (e.g., laminectomy). The lithotomy position is used for various gynecological, genitourinary, and colon procedures.

With any position, take great care to prevent injury to the patient. Take care to (1) provide correct musculoskeletal alignment; (2) prevent undue pressure on nerves, skin over bony prominences, earlobes, and eyes; (3) provide for adequate thoracic excursion; (4) prevent occlusion of arteries and veins; (5) provide modesty in exposure; and (6) recognize and respect individual needs, such as previously assessed pains or deformities. It is your responsibility to secure the extremities, provide adequate padding and support, and have physical or mechanical help to avoid unnecessary straining of the staff and patient.

Because anesthesia blocks the sensory nerve impulses, the patient will not feel pain, discomfort, or stress placed on nerves, muscles, bones, and skin. General anesthesia causes peripheral vessels to dilate. Position changes affect where the pooling of blood occurs. If the head of the OR bed is raised, the lower torso will have increased blood volume and the upper torso may become compromised. Hypovolemia and cardiovascular disease can further compromise the patient's status. Improper positioning can potentially result in muscle strain, joint damage, pressure injuries, nerve damage, and other untoward effects.

◆ Electrosurgery and Smoke

Care must be taken to correctly place the grounding pad and all electrosurgical equipment to prevent injury from burns or fire. When an electrosurgical unit is in use, the patient must be properly grounded to prevent unintended injury (Fig. 18.4). Excess hair, adipose tissue, bony prominences, fluid (edema), adhesive failure, and scar tissue can compromise safety. Fire in the OR can have devastating consequences for the patient. Fortunately, we can prevent surgical fires with awareness of the hazards and emphasis on safe practices.[13]

◆ Preparing Surgical Site

The purpose of skin preparation, or "prepping," is to reduce the number of microorganisms available to migrate to the surgical wound. The circulating nurse, surgeon, or surgical assistant completes the task of prepping before surgery.

TABLE 18.3 Principles of Aseptic Technique in Operating Room

- All materials that enter the sterile field must be sterile.
- If a sterile item comes in contact with an unsterile item, it is contaminated.
- Contaminated items are removed at once from the sterile field. If the unsterile item is small (e.g., unopened suture), once it is removed, the area is marked off (i.e., covered with a sterile drape). If the entire field is contaminated, it should be set up again with all new materials.
- The surgical team working in the operative field must wear sterile gowns and gloves. Once dressed for procedure, they must recognize that the only parts of the gown considered sterile are the front from chest to table level and sleeves to 2 inches above elbow.
- A wide margin of safety is maintained between sterile and unsterile fields.
- Tables are sterile only at tabletop level. Items extending beneath this level are contaminated.
- The edges of a sterile package are contaminated once the package has been opened. If a sterile package (e.g., package of sutures) is placed on the sterile field, that entire package stays sterile even when opened.
- Microorganisms travel on airborne particles and will enter the sterile field with excessive air movements and currents.
- Microorganisms travel by capillary action through moist fabrics, resulting in contamination.
- Microorganisms on the patient's and team members' hair, skin, and respiratory tracts must be confined by proper attire.

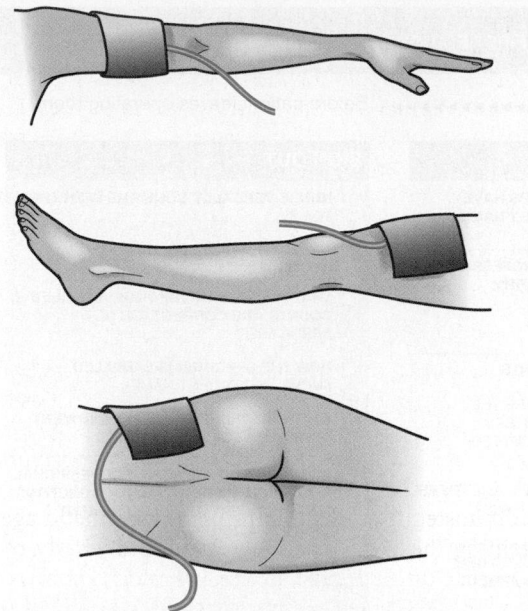

FIG. 18.4 A well-vascularized muscle mass is the best site for grounding. (Courtesy Covidien, Mansfield, MA.)

The skin is prepared by mechanically scrubbing or cleansing the surgical site with an antimicrobial agent specific to the procedure. Follow manufacturer's instructions for proper application of the prepping agent. The principle of scrubbing from the clean area (site of the incision) to the dirty area (distal to the incision) is always followed.

Antiseptic agents used for skin preparation may contain alcohol and therefore are flammable. Skin injury can occur if these agents pool under the patient. Care must be taken to ensure that these agents are properly confined and allowed to fully dry. After the skin is prepped and the fumes are allowed to dispel to reduce the risk for fire, the sterile members of the surgical team drape the area. Only the site to be incised is left exposed.

◆ Safety Considerations

All surgical procedures put the patient at risk for injury. These injuries include infections, physical trauma from positioning or equipment used, or physiologic effects of surgery itself. Although technical skills, such as operating equipment or proper instrument handling, are a critical part of OR RN competency, there is strong research supporting that nontechnical skills (NTS) also have a high impact on outcomes. These include proper and clear communication, teamwork, situational awareness (e.g., anticipatory cognitive skills), and stress and fatigue management.[14] Considering the importance of NTS skills, especially in crisis events, some agencies use special training programs to develop these skills. There are standard approaches, such as a variety of communication tools, that promote safe patient care and minimize the potential negative effects of human factors.

◆ Communication.
Many team members care for patients as they move through the perioperative continuum. Chances for error arise whenever team members share information. The Joint Commission requires that all health care providers use a standardized approach to hand-off communication. As a RN, use SBAR (see Table 1.4) to ensure that a complete and accurate hand-off is done every time patient care is transferred to

another provider (e.g. change of shift, surgeon to nurse, OR RN to PACU RN).

◆ Surgical Care Improvement Project.
The *Surgical Care Improvement Project* (SCIP) is a national quality partnership of organizations focused on improving surgical care by significantly reducing the number of complications from surgery.[2] Specific SCIP measures include (1) a prophylactic antibiotic started within 30 to 60 minutes before the surgical incision to decrease risk for infection, (2) applying a warming blanket to prevent unintended hypothermia, and (3) applying intermittent pneumatic compression devices (IPCs) to minimize the risk for VTE.

◆ Time Out and Surgical Checklist.
The National Patient Safety Goals (NPSGs) require a preprocedure verification process. This includes verification of relevant documentation (e.g., history and physical examination, signed consent forms, nursing and preanesthetic assessment) and the results of any diagnostic studies (e.g., x-rays, biopsy reports). Any needed blood products, implants, devices, and special equipment must be available.

The *Universal Protocol,* one of the NPSGs, is followed to prevent wrong site, wrong procedure, and wrong surgery. Wrong surgical procedure and surgery on the wrong body part or wrong patient are *sentinel events (never events)* or *SREs* (described in Chapter 1). The AORN has a position statement about correct site surgery and guidelines for implementing the Universal Protocol.[15] The surgeon marks the procedure site. If possible, the marking is done with the patient's involvement.[3]

A patient safety checklist for ORs is the cornerstone of a major focus to make surgery safer. Using the World Health Organization (WHO) Surgical Safety Checklist has improved compliance with standards and decreased complications from surgery (Fig. 18.5). In addition, OR staff complete a fire risk assessment to identify and reduce the potential for a fire.

> **! SAFETY ALERT** Surgical Time-Out
> - Before anesthesia induction, ask the patient to confirm name, birthdate, procedure and site, and consent.
> - All members of the surgical team stop what they are doing just before the procedure starts to verify patient identification, procedure, and surgical site.

❖ NURSING MANAGEMENT: PATIENT AFTER SURGERY

Through constant observation of the surgical process, the ACP anticipates the end of the procedure. The ACP gives proper types and doses of anesthetic agents so that their effects will be minimal at the end of the surgery. This allows greater physiologic control of the patient during the transfer to the PACU.

The ACP and you or another member of the surgical team go with the patient to the PACU. The hand-off, including the patient's status and the procedure done, is communicated to the nurse receiving the patient in the PACU to promote safe, ongoing care.

❚ ANESTHESIA

The American Society of Anesthesiologists (ASA) defines anesthesia according to the effect that it has on the patient's sensorium and pain perception. These definitions include minimal

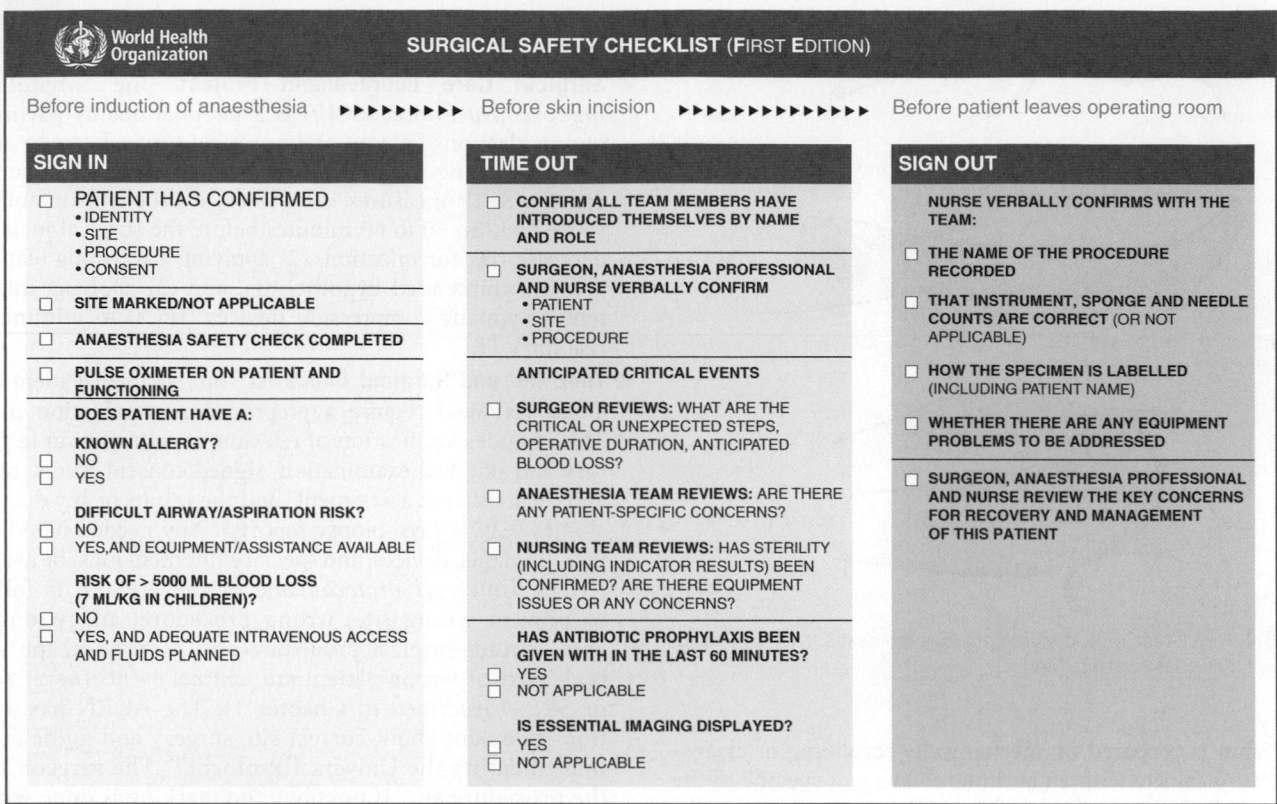

FIG. 18.5 WHO Surgical Safety Checklist.

sedation (e.g., anxiolysis), moderate sedation/analgesia, deep sedation/analgesia, and general anesthesia. The science of providing anesthesia continues to evolve. For example, noninvasive electroencephalogram-based technology allows ACPs to track the level of patient awareness (i.e., *awareness monitoring*) during surgery and adjust anesthesia as needed.

The anesthetic technique and agents are chosen by the ACP in collaboration with the surgeon and patient. The ACP has ultimate responsibility for the choice of anesthesia. Contributing factors include the patient's current physical and mental status, age, allergies, pain history, expertise of the ACP, and factors related to the procedure (e.g., length, site, discharge plans). An absolute contraindication to any anesthetic technique or agent is patient refusal.

The ACP obtains anesthesia consent, writes orders for preoperative and postoperative drugs, and assigns the patient an anesthesia classification. The ASA physical status classification system is based on the patient's physiologic status. It uses a scale of P1 to P6 (see Table 17.3). An intraoperative complication is more likely to develop with a higher classification number.

ANESTHESIA TECHNIQUES

Types of anesthesia techniques include moderate to deep sedation, monitored anesthesia care (MAC), general anesthesia, and local and regional anesthesia (Table 18.4).

Moderate to Deep Sedation

Moderate to deep sedation is used for procedures done outside of the OR (e.g., reduction of dislocated joints in the emergency department). The presence of an ACP is not needed. Trained RNs who are allowed by agency protocols and state nurse practice acts can provide this type of anesthesia.[16] It is given by the nurse under the direct supervision of a physician.

Monitored Anesthesia Care

Monitored anesthesia care (MAC) is used for diagnostic or therapeutic procedures done in or outside of the OR (e.g., endoscopy clinic). It includes varying levels of sedation, analgesia, and anxiolysis. A critical part of MAC is the assessment and management of any physiologic problems that may develop. The provider of MAC must be an ACP since it may be necessary to change to general anesthesia during the procedure.

General Anesthesia

The goals of anesthesiology include the (1) control of excessive biologic responses induced by a variety of stressors and (2) protection of patients from stress-induced complications. To this end, *total intravenous anesthesia (TIVA)* and newer inhalation agents have a fast onset, fast elimination, and fewer undesirable side effects than earlier agents. These factors promote early discharge from the PACU and ambulatory surgery centers.

General anesthesia is the technique of choice for patients who are having surgical procedures that are of significant duration, need skeletal muscle relaxation, require uncomfortable operative positions because of the location of the incision site, or require control of ventilation. Other reasons include patient refusal of local or regional techniques, contraindications to other techniques, and uncooperative patients. Patients may be uncooperative due to intoxication, emotional lability, head injury, impaired cognition, or inability to remain immobile for any length of time. Phases of general anesthesia are outlined in Table 18.5.

TABLE 18.4 Anesthesia Techniques and Effects

Technique	Patient Effects
General anesthesia	• Loss of sensation with loss of consciousness • Combination of hypnosis, analgesia, and amnesia • Usually involves use of inhalation agents • Skeletal muscle relaxation • Elimination of coughing, gagging, vomiting, and sympathetic nervous system responsiveness • Requires advanced airway management
Local anesthesia	• Loss of sensation without loss of consciousness • Induced topically or via infiltration, intracutaneously, or subcutaneously • Topical applications may be aerosolized or nebulized
Moderate sedation/analgesia (formerly called *conscious sedation*)	• Sedative, anxiolytic, and/or analgesic drugs used • Does not include use of inhalation agents • Patient responsive and breathes without assistance • Not expected to induce level of sedation that would impair patients' ability to protect their airway • Most often used for minor therapeutic procedures (e.g., fracture realignment in the emergency department)
Monitored anesthesia care (MAC)	• Sedative, anxiolytic, and/or analgesic drugs used • Does not usually involve inhalation agents • Patient less responsive and may need airway management • Gives greatest flexibility to match sedation level to patient needs and procedural requirements • Often used in conjunction with regional or local anesthesia • Often used for minor therapeutic and diagnostic procedures (e.g., eye surgery, colonoscopy)
Regional anesthesia	• Loss of sensation to a region of body without loss of consciousness • Involves blocking a specific nerve or group of nerves by administering a local anesthetic • Includes spinal, caudal, and epidural anesthesia and IV and peripheral nerve blocks (e.g., interscalene, axillary, infra-/supra-clavicular, popliteal, femoral, sciatic)

Source: American Society of Anesthesiologists: *Distinguishing monitored anesthesia care ("MAC") from moderate sedation/analgesia (conscious sedation)*, Schaumburg, Ill, 2013, The Society.

TABLE 18.5 Phases of General Anesthesia

Preinduction	Induction	Maintenance	Emergence
Description			
• Period starting with initiation of IV or arterial access, application of monitors (e.g., ECG), administration of preoperative drugs	• Initiation of drugs that make patient unconscious • Airway secured with airway assist devices	• Period during which procedure is done • Patient stays in an unconscious state with measures to ensure airway safety	• Period when procedure is completed • Patient is prepared for return to consciousness and removal of airway assist devices
Role of Anesthesia Care Provider			
• Determine anesthetic care plan • Insert and monitor IV or arterial access • Confirm antibiotic prophylaxis • Give drugs for anxiety, aspiration prophylaxis	• Give appropriate drugs • Secure airway • Position patient appropriately for procedure	• Monitor patient's physiologic status • Give drugs and titrate fluids as appropriate	• Reverse residual neuromuscular blocking agents • Assess for return of all protective reflexes • Remove airway assist devices • Assess pain
Role of Perioperative Nurse			
• Complete preoperative assessment • Check and confirm signed informed consent • Complete surgical time-out	• Help with application of monitors (noninvasive and invasive) • Assist with airway management	• Adjust patient position as needed • Monitor patient safety	• Help place dressing • Protect patient during return of reflexes • Prepare patient to move to PACU
Classes of Drugs Used (Tables 17.8, 18.6, and 18.7)			

• Benzodiazepines
• Opioids
• Antibiotics
• Aspiration prophylaxis:
  • H_2 receptor blockers (e.g., ranitidine)
  • Gastric motility agents (e.g., metoclopramide)
  • Anticholinergics (e.g., scopolamine)
	• Benzodiazepines
	• Opioids
	• Barbiturates
	• Hypnotics
	• Volatile gases
		• Benzodiazepines
		• Opioids
		• Barbiturates
		• Hypnotics
		• Volatile gases
		• Neuromuscular blocking agents
			• Reversal agents (PRN):
			  • Anticholinesterases (e.g., neostigmine)
			  • Opioid antagonists (e.g., naloxone)
			  • Benzodiazepine antagonists (e.g., flumazenil)
			  • Neuromuscular block reversal of rocuronium [Zemuron] and vecuronium [Norcuron] (e.g., sugammadex [Bridion])
			• Supplemental opioids (PRN)
			• Antiemetics (PRN)

General anesthesia may be induced by IV or inhalation and maintained by either or a combination of the two (Table 18.6). A *balanced technique,* using adjunctive drugs to complement the induction, is the most common approach used for general anesthesia.

IV Agents. All routine general anesthetics begin with an IV induction agent, whether it is a hypnotic, an anxiolytic, or a dissociative agent. When used during the initial period of anesthesia, these agents induce sleep with a rapid onset of action. A single dose lasts only a few minutes. This is long enough for placement of a laryngeal mask airway (LMA) or an endotracheal (ET) tube. Once this is done, the ACP gives the inhalation and IV agent(s).

Recent advances in IV hypnotics (e.g., dexmedetomidine [Precedex]) and opioids (e.g., remifentanil [Ultiva]) have led to the more frequent use of TIVA. However, the patient may still need advanced airway management (e.g., LMA, ET tube) to receive oxygen/air mixtures.

Inhalation Agents. Inhalation agents are the cornerstone of general anesthesia. They may be volatile liquids or gases. Volatile liquids are given through a specially designed vaporizer after being mixed with oxygen as a carrier gas. This gas mixture is then delivered to the patient through the anesthesia circuit. Waste gases are removed using negative evacuation pressure venting to the outside of the agency.

TABLE 18.6 **Drug Therapy**

General Anesthesia

Drugs	Advantages	Adverse Effects	Nursing Interventions
IV Agents			
Barbiturates			
methohexital (Brevital)	Rapid induction, duration of action <5 min.	Cardiac effects (e.g., myocardial depression), hypotension, respiratory depression, excitation, involuntary movement.	Usually have minimal effects after surgery because of short duration of action. Increased incidence of nausea in patients with barbiturate sensitivity, histamine-triggered nausea, vomiting.
Nonbarbiturate Hypnotics			
etomidate (Amidate)	Has little effect on cardiovascular function. Useful for hemodynamically unstable patients. Only minor respiratory depression. No histamine release.	Myoclonia, nausea and vomiting, hiccups, adrenocortical inhibition.	Observe for myoclonia, nausea and vomiting, hiccups, hypotension, hypoglycemia.
propofol (Diprivan)	Ideal for short outpatient procedures because of rapid onset of action, metabolic clearance. May be used for induction and maintenance of anesthesia.	Bradycardia and other dysrhythmias, hypotension, apnea, transient phlebitis, nausea and vomiting, hiccups. May cause hypertriglyceridemia.	Monitor for hypotension, bradycardia. Monitor serum triglycerides q24hr when sedated >24 hr.
Inhalation Agents			
Gaseous Agents			
nitrous oxide	Potentiates volatile agents, thus speeding induction and reducing total dosage and side effects. Weak anesthetic, rarely used alone. Good analgesic potency.	Little or no toxicity at therapeutic concentrations.	Avoid in patients with bone marrow depression. Must be given with O₂ to prevent hypoxemia. Avoid in patients with strong history of nausea and vomiting.
Volatile Liquids			
desflurane (Suprane) isoflurane (Forane) sevoflurane (Ultane)	All cause skeletal muscle relaxation. *desflurane:* Fastest onset and emergence, widely used in ambulatory settings. Least postoperative cognitive dysfunction. Potential airway irritant. *isoflurane:* No increase in ventricular irritability. Does not cause liver or renal toxicity. Resistant to metabolic breakdown. *sevoflurane:* Predictable effects on cardiovascular and respiratory systems, rapid acting. Preferred for inhalation induction as nonirritating to respiratory tract.	All cause respiratory depression, hypotension, myocardial depression. *desflurane and isoflurane:* May be unsuitable for patients with coronary artery disease. *sevoflurane:* May be associated with emergence delirium (see Chapter 19) and atypical seizure-like activity.	Assess and treat pain during early anesthesia recovery. Assess for adverse reactions such as cardiopulmonary depression with hypotension and prolonged respiratory depression. Monitor for nausea and vomiting.
Dissociative Anesthetic			
ketamine (Ketalar)	Given IV or IM. Potent analgesic and amnesic.	May cause hallucinations and nightmares, ↑ intracranial and intraocular pressure, ↑ heart rate, ↑ BP.	Anticipate use of a benzodiazepine if agitation and hallucinations occur. Calm, quiet environment is essential in postoperative care.

Inhalation agents enter the body through the alveoli in the lungs. Ease of administration and rapid excretion by ventilation make them desirable agents. One undesirable trait is the irritating effect some inhalation agents (e.g., desflurane [Suprane]) have on the respiratory tract. Complications include coughing, laryngospasm, and increased secretions.

Once the patient has been induced with an IV agent, the choice for delivering inhalation agents is usually through an ET tube or LMA. The ET tube allows control of ventilation and protects the airway from aspiration. LMAs are currently an important option for patients with difficult airways, but they do not provide access to the trachea or airway protection with the same certainty as ETs. Complications of ET tube or LMA use are primarily related to insertion and removal. These include failure to intubate, damage to teeth and lips, laryngospasm, laryngeal edema, sore throat, and hoarseness caused by injury or irritation of the vocal cords or surrounding tissues.

Adjuncts to General Anesthesia. General anesthesia is rarely limited to a single agent. Drugs added to an inhalation anesthetic (other than an IV induction drug) are termed *adjuncts*. Adjuncts are added to the anesthetic regimen to achieve unconsciousness, analgesia, amnesia, muscle relaxation, or autonomic nervous system control. They include opioids, benzodiazepines, neuromuscular blocking agents (muscle relaxants), and antiemetics (Table 18.7). It is important to know that we often give these drugs in combination and they may have synergistic or

TABLE 18.7 Drug Therapy

Adjuncts to General Anesthesia

Agents	Intended Effect	Adverse Effects	Nursing Interventions
Antiemetics (See Table 41.1) aprepitant (Emend) granisetronmetoclopramide (Reglan) ondansetron (Zofran) palonosetron prochlorperazine promethazine rolapitant (Varubi)	Counteract emetic effects of inhalation agents and opioids. Prophylactic prevention of nausea and vomiting related to histamine release, vagal stimulation, vestibular disturbance, procedure (e.g., abdominal laparoscopy).	Headache, dizziness, IV irritation, dysrhythmias, dysphoria, dystonia, dry mouth, central nervous system sedation.	• Monitor heart rhythm, cardiopulmonary status, level of central nervous system excitation or sedation, ability to move limbs, presence of nausea or vomiting.
Benzodiazepines diazepam (Valium) lorazepam (Ativan) midazolam (Versed)	Reduce anxiety, induce and maintain anesthesia, induce amnesia, treat emergence delirium. Supplement sedation in local and regional anesthesia and MAC.	Synergistic effect with opioids, increasing potential for respiratory depression. Hypotension and tachycardia. Prolonged sedation or confusion.	• Monitor level of consciousness. Assess for respiratory depression, hypotension, and tachycardia. • Reverse severe benzodiazepine-induced respiratory depression with flumazenil (Romazicon).
Neuromuscular Blocking Agents *Depolarizing agent:* succinylcholine (Anectine) *Nondepolarizing agents:* • atracurium • cisatracurium (Nimbex) • pancuronium • rocuronium	Promote endotracheal intubation, promote skeletal muscle relaxation (paralysis) to enhance access to surgical sites. Effects of nondepolarizing agents are usually reversed toward end of surgery by giving anticholinesterase agents (e.g., neostigmine).	Apnea related to paralysis of respiratory muscles. Duration of action of nondepolarizing agents may be longer than surgery. Reversal agents may not completely eliminate effects. Confusion and nausea. Recurrence of muscle weakness with correction of hypothermia.	• If intubated, monitor return of muscle strength, level of consciousness, and ventilation. • Maintain patent airway. Monitor respiratory rate and rhythm until patient able to cough and return to previous levels of muscle strength. Ensure availability of nondepolarizing reversal agents (e.g., neostigmine) and emergency respiratory support equipment. • Monitor temperature and levels of muscle strength with temperature changes.
Opioids alfentanil (Alfenta) fentanyl (Sublimaze) hydromorphone (Dilaudid) morphine sulfate remifentanil (Ultiva) sufentanil (Sufenta)	Induce and maintain anesthesia, reduce stimuli from sensory nerve endings, provide analgesia during surgery and recovery in PACU.	Respiratory depression, vomiting, bradycardia, peripheral vasodilation (when combined with anesthetics). High risk for pruritus with both regional and IV administration.	• Assess respiratory rate and rhythm, monitor pulse oximetry, protect airway in anticipation of vomiting. • Use standing orders for antipruritics and antiemetics. • Reverse opioid-induced respiratory depression with naloxone. If used, reversal of analgesic effects also occurs.
Other Agents dexmedetomidine (Precedex)	Induces and maintains sedation in nonintubated patients prior to and/or during surgery.	Hypotension, bradycardia, sinus arrest, transient hypertension during administration of loading dose.	• Monitor heart rate and rhythm, and BP for side effects.

antagonistic effects. You may see deeper levels of sedation or more drug-related side effects beyond those seen with inhalation anesthetics alone. If needed, drugs are available to reverse the effects of some of these adjuncts.

Dissociative Anesthesia. *Dissociative anesthesia* interrupts associative brain pathways while blocking sensory pathways. The patient may appear catatonic, is amnesic, and has profound analgesia that lasts into the postoperative period. Ketamine (Ketalar) (given IV or IM) is a common dissociative anesthetic. It is a potent analgesic and amnesic. Ketamine is given to asthmatic patients because it promotes bronchodilation. In trauma patients, it increases heart rate and helps maintain cardiac output. Because ketamine is a phenyl cyclohexyl piperidine (PCP) derivative, the drug may cause hallucinations and nightmares, limiting its usefulness. Concurrent use of midazolam (Versed) can reduce or eliminate the hallucinations. Providing a quiet, unhurried environment in the PACU is especially important for all patients receiving dissociative anesthesia.

Local and Regional Anesthesia

Local anesthesia interrupts the generation of nerve impulses by changing the flow of sodium into nerve cells. The result is autonomic nervous system blockade, anesthesia, and skeletal muscle flaccidity or paralysis. Local anesthetics are topical, ophthalmic, nebulized, or injected. A local anesthetic is applied to a specific area of the body by the surgeon or ACP. It does not involve sedation or loss of consciousness.

Regional anesthesia (or block) using a local anesthetic is always injected. It involves a central nerve (e.g., spinal) or group of nerves (e.g., plexus) that innervate a site remote to the point of injection. Administration of a local or regional anesthetic may involve concurrent use of MAC or moderate to deep sedation (Table 18.4), either preinjection or intraoperatively. Regional blocks are used as preoperative analgesia, during surgery to manage surgical pain, and after surgery to control pain. Indwelling catheters that deliver local anesthetic to the surgical site through a pump implanted during surgery can give continuous pain relief up to 72 hours after surgery.

Advantages of local and regional anesthesia include rapid recovery and discharge with continued postoperative analgesia without any accompanying cognitive dysfunction. They can be safely used in patients who have co-morbidities that prevent the use of general anesthesia.

Disadvantages include the potential for technical problems, discomfort at the injection site, and the inability to precisely match the agent's duration of action to the duration of the procedure. Another disadvantage is the risk for inadvertent vascular injection leading to local anesthetic systemic toxicity (LAST). LAST first presents as confusion, metallic taste, oral numbness, and dizziness.[17] Without treatment, seizures, coma, and dysrhythmias may occur.

The topical applications of creams, ointments, aerosols, and liquids are standard methods to administer local anesthesia. The drug is applied directly to the skin, mucous membranes, or open surface. Eutectic mixture of local anesthetics (EMLA cream, a combination of prilocaine and lidocaine) is an example. It is applied to the site 30 to 60 minutes before a procedure. The success of injected local anesthetics may be limited by prolonged duration of procedure or infection at the injection site that interferes with drug absorption.

In ambulatory or outpatient procedures, you may aid the ACP in administering a peripheral or regional block. You must be familiar with the drugs, including the methods of

administration and adverse and toxic effects. Initial assessment of the patient should include the patient's history with the use of local anesthetics and any adverse events associated with their use by the patient or blood relatives.

Many patients report "allergies" to local anesthetics. Although true allergies to local anesthetics occur, they are rare. Allergies are likely to be a result of additives or preservatives in the preparation. Some local anesthetics are combined with epinephrine to provide localized vasoconstriction. This decreases absorption and extends the action of the agent. However, if the local anesthetic is absorbed in the tissues or inadvertently injected IV and enters the general circulation, the patient may have tachycardia, hypertension, and a general feeling of panic.

Examples of common regional nerve blocks include brachial plexus block; IV regional anesthesia (IVRA) or Bier block anesthesia; and femoral, axillary, cervical, sciatic, ankle, and retrobulbar blocks. For IVRA or Bier block, the patient has a double-cuff tourniquet applied as a safety measure.

You can promote the success of regional anesthesia by properly positioning the patient, monitoring vital signs during block delivery, applying oxygen therapy, and using supporting devices (at the direction of the ACP) that contribute to the anesthesia (e.g., ultrasound imaging, nerve stimulator, tourniquets). When a patient is receiving regional anesthesia, airway equipment, emergency drugs, and a cardiac monitor/defibrillator should be available to provide advanced airway and cardiopulmonary support if needed.

Spinal and Epidural Anesthesia. Spinal anesthesia and epidural anesthesia are also types of regional anesthesia. **Spinal anesthesia** involves the injection of a local anesthetic into the cerebrospinal fluid in the subarachnoid space, usually below the level of L2 (Fig. 18.6, A). The local anesthetic mixes with cerebrospinal fluid. Depending on the extent of its spread, various levels of anesthesia are achieved. Because the local anesthetic is given directly into the cerebrospinal fluid, a spinal anesthetic produces an autonomic, sensory, and motor blockade. Patients develop vasodilation and may become hypotensive from the autonomic block. They feel no pain because of the sensory block. They cannot move because of the motor block. The duration of action of the spinal anesthetic depends on the drug used and the dose

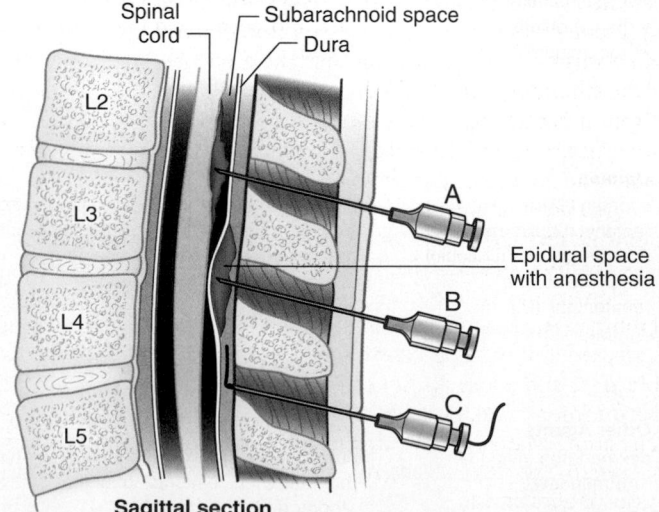

Sagittal section

FIG. 18.6 Location of needle point and injected anesthetic relative to dura and spinal cord. A, Spinal anesthesia. B, Single-injection epidural. C, Epidural catheter. (Interspaces most often used are L2-3, L4-5, L3-4.)

given. A spinal anesthetic may be used for procedures involving the extremities (e.g., joint replacements) and lower gastrointestinal, prostate, and gynecologic surgeries.

An epidural block involves injection of a local anesthetic into the epidural space via a thoracic or lumbar approach (Fig. 18.6, *B*). The anesthetic agent does not enter the cerebrospinal fluid but binds to nerve roots as they enter and exit the spinal cord. With the use of a low concentration of local anesthetic, sensory pathways are blocked but motor fibers are still intact. In higher doses, sensory and motor fibers are blocked. Epidural anesthesia may be the sole anesthetic for a surgical procedure. In addition, a catheter may be placed to allow for intraoperative use and continued analgesia in the postoperative period (Fig. 18.6, *C*). For postoperative analgesia, lower doses of epidural local anesthetic, usually in combination with an opioid, are used. Epidural anesthesia is often used for analgesia or in combination with MAC or general anesthesia, in obstetrics, vascular procedures involving the lower extremities, lung resections, and renal and midabdominal surgeries. The desirable effects of vasodilation and analgesia contribute to better surgical outcomes.

With spinal or epidural anesthesia, the patient can stay fully conscious, receive MAC, or choose general anesthesia. The onset of spinal anesthesia is more rapid than that of epidural anesthesia. Both may be extended in duration using indwelling catheters, thus allowing for more doses of anesthetic.

With either anesthesia, closely observe the patient for manifestations of autonomic nervous system blockade. These include hypotension, bradycardia, nausea, and vomiting. There is less autonomic nervous system blockade with epidural anesthesia than with spinal anesthesia. Should "too high" a block be present, the patient may have tingling in the arms and hands or inadequate breathing and apnea. Other complications include postdural puncture headache, back pain, isolated nerve injury, and meningitis.

🧍 Gerontologic Considerations: Patient During Surgery

Although anesthetic agents have become safer and more predictable, the aging process affects the absorption, distribution, and metabolism of drugs. This results in changes in their onset, peak, and duration independent of the route of administration. Because of this, anesthetic drugs need to be carefully titrated when given to older adults. Physiologic changes in aging may also change the patient's response to blood and fluid loss and replacement, hypothermia, pain, and tolerance of the procedure and positioning. Carefully monitor the older adult's response to all anesthetic agents. Postoperative delirium is a common complication in this population and associated with adverse surgical outcomes.[18] Assess the postoperative recovery from anesthesia before the patient is transferred out of the PACU.

Some older adults may have a hard time communicating and following directions because of problems with hearing or vision. These factors increase the need for clear and concise communication in the OR, especially when preoperative sedation is combined with already existing sensory deficits. Because of decreased ability to perceive discomfort or pressure on vulnerable areas and a loss of skin elasticity, the older adult's skin is at risk for injury from tape, electrodes, warming and cooling blankets, and certain types of dressings. Pooling of solutions used to prepare the skin in dependent areas can quickly create skin burns or abrasions.

Care and vigilance are needed in preparing and positioning the older patient. The older adult often has osteoporosis and/or osteoarthritis. Misalignment, pressure, or other insults to arthritic joints desensitized from an anesthetic may create long-term injury and disability. Older adults are at a greater risk for perioperative hypothermia. Consider using warming devices and carefully monitor them when used.

PERIOPERATIVE CRISIS EVENTS

Although the incidence of crisis events has significantly decreased with scientific advancements, there is an inherent risk with surgery for an adverse outcome, which may be of critical nature. Some events may be expected (e.g., cardiac arrest in an unstable patient, massive blood loss during trauma surgery). Others may occur without warning (e.g., air embolism, hypoxia), demanding immediate intervention by all members of the OR team. More rare events include anaphylactic reactions and malignant hyperthermia.

Anaphylactic Reactions

Anaphylaxis is the most severe form of an allergic reaction, manifesting with life-threatening pulmonary and circulatory complications. ACPs give patients a variety of drugs, including anesthetics, antibiotics, and blood products. Anesthetic agents, antibiotics, and latex cause many allergic reactions. Vigilance and rapid intervention are essential. Anesthesia may mask the initial manifestations of anaphylaxis. An anaphylactic reaction causes hypotension, tachycardia, bronchospasm, and pulmonary edema. Anaphylaxis is discussed in Chapter 13.

Latex allergy has become a concern in the surgical setting. Gloves, catheters, and many devices contain natural rubber latex. Latex allergy protocols should be set up in each agency to provide a latex-safe environment for susceptible patients.[19] Latex allergies are discussed in Chapter 13.

Malignant Hyperthermia

Malignant hyperthermia (MH) is a rare disorder characterized by hyperthermia with skeletal muscle rigidity. It can result in death. MH occurs in susceptible people when they are exposed to certain anesthetic agents. Succinylcholine (Anectine), especially when given with volatile inhalation agents, is the primary trigger of MH. Other factors include stress, trauma, and heat. When MH does occur, it is usually during general anesthesia. It may occur in the recovery period, too.[20]

MH is an autosomal dominant trait. It is variable in its genetic manifestation, so predictions based on family history are important but not reliable. The fundamental defect is hypermetabolism of skeletal muscle resulting from altered control of intracellular calcium. This leads to muscle contracture, hyperthermia, hypoxemia, lactic acidosis, and hemodynamic and cardiac problems. Tachycardia, tachypnea, hypercarbia, and ventricular dysrhythmias may occur but are nonspecific to MH.

MH is diagnosed after ruling out other causes of the hypermetabolism. The rise in body temperature is not an early sign of MH. Unless promptly detected and treated, MH can result in cardiac arrest and death. The definitive treatment of MH is prompt administration of dantrolene (Dantrium, Ryanodex).[20] Dantrolene slows metabolism, reduces muscle contraction, and mediates the catabolic processes associated with MH.

To prevent MH, take a careful family history and be alert to the development of MH perioperatively. The patient known or suspected to be at risk for this disorder can receive anesthesia with minimal risks if proper precautions are taken. Patients with MH need to be aware of the condition so that family members may be genetically tested.

CASE STUDY

Intraoperative Patient

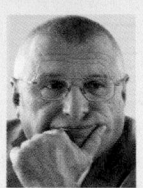

(© shironosov/ iStock/Thinkstock.)

Patient Profile

G.S., a 63-yr-old retired accountant, was admitted to the hospital for severe pain from acute cholecystitis. G.S.'s medical history includes hypertension and type 2 diabetes. His pain has been managed with hydromorphone (Dilaudid) using patient-controlled analgesia. Intractable nausea and vomiting required the placement of a NG tube. He is scheduled for a laparoscopic cholecystectomy. The surgery will be done under general anesthesia.

Subjective Data

- G.S. is awake and able to identify himself, his birth date, procedure, and surgical site
- Rates pain as a 4 on a 0- to 10 scale on arrival to the holding area

Objective Data

- Admitted to the holding area with an NG tube in place and one peripheral IV catheter
- Capillary blood glucose 1 hour ago was 125 mg/dL
- Oxygen saturation 96% on room air

Interprofessional Care

- Vital signs per holding area routine
- 0.9 normal saline solution at 100 mL/hr
- Titrate O_2 therapy to keep O_2 saturation >90%
- NG tube connected to low, intermittent suction

Discussion Questions

1. What are the potential intraoperative problems that you may expect with G.S.?
2. **Priority Decision:** What priority nursing interventions would be appropriate to prevent these complications from occurring?
3. **Collaboration:** What are the interprofessional team's priorities for G.S.?
4. **Evidence-Based Practice:** G.S. tells you that he is cold despite a blanket in place. Why is it important that G.S. stays warm?
5. **Safety:** Identify 2 areas of risk for injury to G.S. What actions can be taken to ensure patient safety?

Answers available at *http://evolve.elsevier.com/Lewis/medsurg.*

■ BRIDGE TO NCLEX EXAMINATION

The number of the question corresponds to the same-numbered outcome at the beginning of the chapter.

1. Proper attire for the semirestricted area of the surgery department is
   a. street clothing.
   b. surgical attire and head cover.
   c. scrub attire, head cover, shoe covers.
   d. street clothing with the addition of shoe covers.
2. Activities that the nurse might perform in the role of a scrub nurse during surgery include *(select all that apply)*
   a. checking electrical equipment.
   b. preparing the instrument table.
   c. assisting with draping the patient.
   d. passing instruments to the surgeon and assistants.
   e. documenting activities occurring in the operating room.
3. The nurse is caring for a patient undergoing surgery for a knee replacement. What is critical to the patient's safety during the procedure *(select all that apply)*?
   a. Universal protocol is followed.
   b. The ACP is an anesthesiologist.
   c. The patient has adequate health insurance.
   d. The patient's family is in the surgery waiting area.
   e. The patient's allergies are conveyed to the surgical team.
4. The nurse's *primary* responsibility for the care of the patient undergoing surgery is
   a. developing an individualized plan of nursing care for the patient.
   b. carrying out specific tasks related to surgical policies and procedures.
   c. ensuring that the patient has been assessed for safe administration of anesthesia.
   d. performing a preoperative history and physical assessment to identify patient needs.

5. When scrubbing at the scrub sink, the nurse should
   a. scrub from elbows to hands.
   b. scrub without mechanical friction.
   c. scrub for a minimum of 10 minutes.
   d. hold the hands higher than the elbows.
6. When positioning a patient in preparation for surgery, the nurse understands that injury to the patient can occur because of *(select all that apply)*
   a. loss of pain perception.
   b. incorrect musculoskeletal alignment.
   c. vasoconstriction of the peripheral vessels.
   d. hypovolemia contributing to decreased perfusion.
   e. inability to sense pressure over bony prominences.
7. IV induction for general anesthesia is the method of choice for *most* patients because
   a. the patient is not intubated.
   b. the agents are nonexplosive.
   c. induction is rapid and controlled.
   d. emergence is longer but with fewer complications.

1. c, 2. b, c, d, 3. a, e, 4. a, 5. d, 6. a, b, d, e, 7. c

For rationales to these answers and even more NCLEX review questions, visit *http://evolve.elsevier.com/Lewis/medsurg.*

ⓔ EVOLVE WEBSITE/RESOURCES LIST

http://evolve.elsevier.com/Lewis/medsurg
Review Questions (Online Only)
Key Points
Answer Keys for Questions
- Rationales for Bridge to NCLEX Examination Questions
- Answer Guidelines for Case Study on p. 326

Conceptual Care Map Creator
Audio Glossary
Content Updates

REFERENCES

*1. Association of periOperative Registered Nurses: *2018 Guidelines for perioperative practice.* Denver, 2018, AORN.

2. The Joint Commission: Surgical care improvement project core measure set. Retrieved from *www.jointcommission.org/assets/1/6/Surgical%20 Care%20Improvement%20Project.pdf.*

3. The Joint Commission: National patient safety goals. Retrieved from *www.jointcommission.org/standards_information/npsgs.aspx.*

4. Rothrock JC: *Alexander's care of the patient in surgery,* ed 16, St Louis, 2018, Mosby.

5. Competency and Credentialing Institute: CNOR certification. Retrieved from *www.cc-institute.org/cnor/about.*

6. Association of Surgical Technologists: About the profession. Retrieved from *www.ast.org/AboutUs/About_AST.*

*7. Association of periOperative Registered Nurses: AORN position statement on allied health care providers and support personnel in the perioperative practice setting. Retrieved from *www.aorn.org/-/media/aorn/guidelines/ position-statements/posstat-personnel-allied-health-care.pdf.*

*8. Association of periOperative Registered Nurses: AORN position statement on RN first assistants. Retrieved from *www.aorn.org/-/media/aorn/ guidelines/position-statements/posstat-rnfa.pdf.*

9. American Society of Anesthesiologists: Types of careers in anesthesia. Retrieved from *https://www.asahq.org/education-and-career/career-resources/anesthesia-as-a-career/types-of-careers-in-anesthesia.*

10. American Association of Nurse Anesthetists. *Scope of nurse anesthesia practice.* Retrieved from *www.aana.com/docs/default-source/practice-aana-com-web-documents-(all)/scope-of-nurse-anesthesia-practice. pdf?sfvrsn=250049b1_2.*

*11. Hudson BF, Ogden J: Exploring the impact of intraoperative interventions for pain and anxiety management during local anesthetic surgery: A systematic review and meta-analysis, *J PeriAnesthesia Nurs* 31:118, 2016.

12. Occupational Safety and Health Administration: Occupational safety and health standards, toxic and hazardous substances: Bloodborne pathogens. Retrieved from *www.osha.gov/pls/oshaweb/owadisp.show_document?p_ id=10051&p_table=STANDARDS.*

13. Spruce L: Back to basics: Surgical fire prevention, *AORN J* 104:217, 2017.

14. Sanchez JA, Barach P, Johnson J: *Surgical patient care: Improving safety, quality and value,* New York, 2017, Springer.

*15. Association of periOperative Registered Nurses: Prevention of sentinel events. Retrieved from *www.aorn.org/education/staff-development/ prevention-of-sentinel-events .*

16. American Association of Nurse Anesthetists: *Non anesthesia provider procedural sedation and analgesia.* Retrieved from *www.aana.com/docs/ default-source/practice-aana-com-web-documents-(all)/non-anesthesia-provider-procedural-sedation-and-analgesia.pdf?sfvrsn=670049b1_2.*

17. Wadlund DL: Local anesthetic systemic toxicity, *AORN J* 106:367, 2017.

*18. Mohanty S, Rosenthal R, Russell M, et al: Optimal perioperative management of the geriatric patient: A best practices guideline from the American College of Surgeons NSQIP and the American Geriatrics Society, *JACS* 222:930, 2016.

19. Seifert P: Crisis management of anaphylaxis in the OR, *AORN J* 105:219, 2017.

20. Malignant Hyperthermia Association of the United States: Emergency treatment for an acute MH event. Retrieved from *www.mhaus.org/ healthcare-professionals/managing-a-crisis.*

*Evidence-based information for clinical practice.

Postoperative Care

Diane M. Rudolphi

Three things in human life are important. The first is to be kind. The second is to be kind. And the third is to be kind.

Henry James

e http://evolve.elsevier.com/Lewis/medsurg/

CONCEPTUAL FOCUS

Gas Exchange	Pain	Tissue Integrity
Fluids and Electrolytes	Perfusion	
Infection	Safety	

LEARNING OUTCOMES

1. Prioritize nursing responsibilities related to managing patients in the postanesthesia care unit (PACU).
2. Prioritize nursing responsibilities to maintain patient safety and prevent postoperative complications in the PACU and clinical unit.
3. Apply data from the initial nursing assessment to the management of the patient after transfer from the PACU to the clinical unit.
4. Select nursing interventions to manage potential problems during the postoperative period.
5. Distinguish discharge criteria from Phase I and Phase II postanesthesia care.

KEY TERMS

airway obstruction, p. 332	delayed emergence, p. 337	patient-controlled analgesia (PCA), p. 338
atelectasis, p. 332	emergence delirium, p. 337	postoperative ileus (POI), p. 340

The postoperative period begins immediately after surgery and continues until the patient is discharged from medical care. This chapter focuses on the multiple concepts central to postoperative nursing. Nursing plays a vital role in supporting ventilation and perfusion, maintaining fluid and electrolyte balance, promoting comfort, reducing infection, and promoting safety. Specific surgical procedures and related postoperative care are discussed in the appropriate chapters of this text.

POSTOPERATIVE CARE OF SURGICAL PATIENT

The patient's immediate recovery period is managed in a *postanesthesia care unit (PACU)*. It is usually next to the operating room (OR). This location limits transportation of the patient right after surgery and gives ready access to anesthesia and OR staff. The goals of PACU care are to maintain patient safety during recovery from anesthesia and identify actual and potential patient problems that may occur because of anesthesia and surgery and intervene appropriately.

Postanesthesia Care Unit Admission

The patient's admission to the PACU is a joint effort among the anesthesia care provider (ACP), OR nurse, and PACU nurse. This collaboration fosters a smooth transfer of care to the PACU and helps determine which phase we assign the patient.

PACU Progression. There are 3 phases of postanesthesia care. During each phase, we provide different levels of care depending on the patient's needs[1] (Table 19.1). How patients move through the phases of care is determined by their condition and the type of anesthesia they received. If a patient assigned to Phase I care on admission to the PACU is stable and recovering well, the patient may rapidly progress through Phase I to either Phase II care or an inpatient unit. This accelerated progress is called rapid postanesthesia care unit progression (RPP). Another accelerated system of care is fast-tracking, which involves admitting ambulatory surgery patients directly to Phase II care. Although RPP and fast-tracking can result in time and cost savings, the patient's safety is the primary factor determining where and at what level we provide postoperative care.

TABLE 19.1 Phases of Postanesthesia Care

Phase I
- Care during the immediate postanesthesia period
- ECG and more intense monitoring (e.g., arterial BP monitoring, mechanical ventilation)

Goal: Prepare patient for transfer to Phase II level of care, an inpatient unit, or intensive care setting

Phase II
- Ambulatory surgery patients
- Fast-tracking (i.e., patients who have bypassed Phase I level of care)

Goal: Prepare patient for transfer to extended observation, home, or extended care facility

Extended Observation
- Extended care or observation after transfer/discharge from Phase I or Phase II levels of care

Goal: Prepare patient for self-care

Blended Levels of Care
- Various levels of care offered in the same environment

Source: American Society of PeriAnesthesia Nurses: *2015-2017 Perianesthesia nursing standards, practice recommendations and interpretive statements,* Cherry Hill, NJ, 2015, The Society.

TABLE 19.2 PACU Hand-Off Report

General Information
- Patient name and age
- Surgeon and anesthesia care provider
- Surgical procedure
- Presence of tubes, drains, catheters, and IV lines
- Type of anesthesia (e.g., general, regional, monitored anesthesia care)
- Use of any reversal agents
- Airway status (artificial airway and/or interventions to maintain adequate oxygenation)
- Pain management interventions
- NPO status and postoperative orders that need started

Patient History
- Indication for surgery
- Medical history, medications, allergies
- Preoperative or baseline vital signs, laboratory and diagnostic findings
- Level of consciousness, orientation
- Specific patient characteristics (e.g., hearing loss, vision impairment, mobility limitations)
- Patient preferences (e.g., cultural, personal beliefs/restrictions)
- Patient emotional status on arrival to OR

Intraoperative Management
- Anesthetic agents
- Other drugs received preoperatively or intraoperatively
- Last dose of opioid administration/pain management plan
- Total fluid replacements, including blood transfusions
- Total fluid losses (e.g., blood, nasogastric drainage)
- Urine output

Intraoperative Course
- Unexpected anesthetic events or reactions
- Unexpected surgical events
- Most recent vital signs and monitoring trends
- Results of laboratory tests and x-rays

Phase I Initial Assessment. On admission of the patient to the PACU, the ACP gives you a postanesthesia hand-off report (Table 19.2). Hand-off reports should be standardized and interactive, allowing you to ask questions and clarify information.[2] The ACP should stay in the PACU until you accept responsibility for the care of the patient. Potential problems in the postoperative period are shown in Fig. 19.1. Table 19.3 describes key parts of a PACU assessment.

Begin your initial assessment by evaluating the patient's airway, breathing, and circulation (ABC) status. Residual neuromuscular blockade, opioid use, and patient characteristics such as sleep-disordered breathing (e.g., obstructive sleep apnea [OSA], abnormal airway anatomy) affect oxygenation and ventilation. Be alert for signs of inadequate oxygenation and ventilation (Table 19.4). Any sign of respiratory distress needs prompt intervention.

Pulse oximetry monitoring is a noninvasive means of assessing oxygenation and can provide an early warning of hypoxemia. *Transcutaneous carbon dioxide ($PtcCO_2$) and end-tidal CO_2 ($PetCO_2$) (capnography) monitoring* are used to detect respiratory depression in high-risk patients.[3] Volumetric capnography and acoustic respiratory rate monitoring can help you detect respiratory distress early.[4] Pulse oximetry, capnography, $PtcCO_2$, and $PetCO_2$ are discussed in Chapter 25.

Note and assess changes in ECG findings from the preoperative baseline. Measure the BP and compare it with baseline readings. Invasive monitoring (e.g., arterial BP) may be needed. Assess body temperature, peripheral pulses, capillary refill, and skin condition (e.g., color, moisture). Any signs of inadequate tissue perfusion need prompt intervention.

Focus the initial neurologic assessment on level of consciousness; orientation; sensory and motor status; and size, equality, and reactivity of the pupils. The patient may be awake, drowsy but arousable, or asleep. Because hearing is the first sense to return in the unconscious patient, explain all activities to the patient from the time of admission to the PACU. If the patient received a regional anesthetic (e.g., spinal, epidural), sensory and motor blockade may still be present and you should assess dermatome levels (Fig. 19.2). During recovery from regional anesthesia, sensory and motor function first returns distal to the site where the anesthetic was given. This means the areas near the site of injections are the last to recover.

> **⚠ SAFETY ALERT Regional Anesthesia**
> - Monitor for complications of regional anesthesia.
> - Be alert for respiratory distress, hypotension, dysrhythmias, changes in heart rate, bleeding or hematoma at site, headache, neurologic deficit or prolonged block, urinary retention, nausea, and pruritis.
> - Implement treatment protocols and notify the health care provider (HCP) as needed.

Assess the urinary system by measuring intake and output and determining fluid balance. Intraoperative fluid totals are part of the ACP report. Note the presence of all IV lines; all irrigation solutions and infusions; and all output devices, including catheters and wound drains. Assess the surgical site. Note the condition of any dressings and the type and amount of any drainage. Implement orders related to incision care.

The rest of this chapter discusses the nursing management of select problems. You can apply this information to patients in both the PACU and clinical unit.

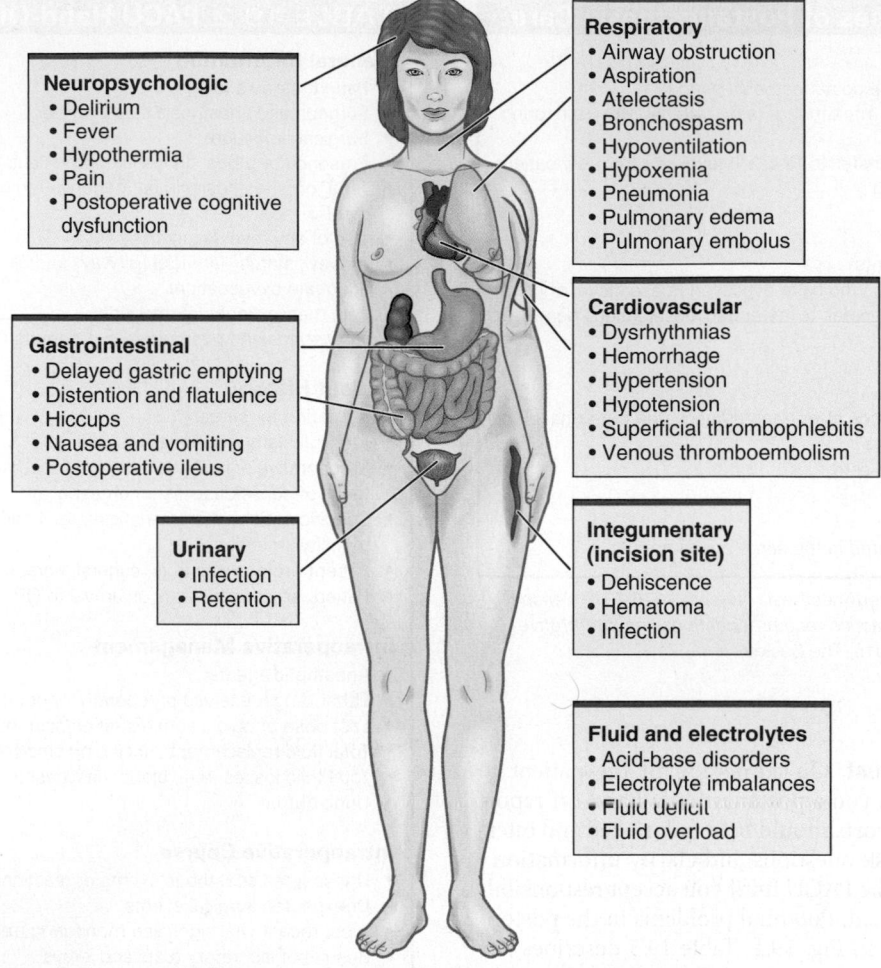

Neuropsychologic
- Delirium
- Fever
- Hypothermia
- Pain
- Postoperative cognitive dysfunction

Respiratory
- Airway obstruction
- Aspiration
- Atelectasis
- Bronchospasm
- Hypoventilation
- Hypoxemia
- Pneumonia
- Pulmonary edema
- Pulmonary embolus

Gastrointestinal
- Delayed gastric emptying
- Distention and flatulence
- Hiccups
- Nausea and vomiting
- Postoperative ileus

Cardiovascular
- Dysrhythmias
- Hemorrhage
- Hypertension
- Hypotension
- Superficial thrombophlebitis
- Venous thromboembolism

Urinary
- Infection
- Retention

Integumentary (incision site)
- Dehiscence
- Hematoma
- Infection

Fluid and electrolytes
- Acid-base disorders
- Electrolyte imbalances
- Fluid deficit
- Fluid overload

FIG. 19.1 Potential problems in the postoperative period.

TABLE 19.3 Initial PACU Assessment

Airway
- Patency
- Oral or nasal airway
- Laryngeal mask airway
- Endotracheal tube with ventilator settings

Breathing
- Respiratory rate and quality
- Auscultated breath sounds
- Pulse oximetry
- Capnography or other technology-supported monitoring if indicated
- Supplemental O_2

Circulation
- ECG monitoring: rate and rhythm
- BP: noninvasive or arterial line
- Hemodynamic pressure readings (if applicable)
- Temperature
- Capillary refill
- Color, temperature, moisture of skin
- Apical and peripheral pulses

Neurologic
- Level of consciousness
- Orientation
- Sensory and motor status
- Pupil size and reaction

Surgical Site
- Dressings and visible incisions
- Drains: type, patency, and drainage
- IV assessment: location and condition of sites, solutions infusing

Genitourinary
- Urine output

Gastrointestinal
- Nausea, vomiting
- Intake (fluids, irrigations)
- Output (vomitus)
- Bowel sounds

Pain
- Incision
- Other

Patient Safety Needs
- Patient position
- Fall risk assessment

TABLE 19.4 Signs of Inadequate Oxygenation

Cardiovascular System
- Hypertension
- Hypotension
- Tachycardia
- Bradycardia
- Dysrhythmias
- Delayed capillary refill
- Weak peripheral pulses
- Decreased O_2 saturation

Central Nervous System
- Restlessness
- Agitation
- Confusion
- Muscle twitching
- Seizures
- Coma

Integumentary System
- Flushed, cool, or moist skin
- Cyanosis

Renal System
- Urine output <0.5 mL/kg/hr

Respiratory System
- Increased to absent respiratory effort
- Use of accessory muscles
- Abnormal breath sounds
- Abnormal arterial blood gas values

NURSING MANAGEMENT

Caring for the Postoperative Patient

In the PACU, patients need frequent assessment and intervention by RNs. On the clinical units, the RN is responsible for assessment, developing an individualized plan of care, implementing and evaluating the plan of care, and discharge teaching. The RN can delegate much of the care to LPNs/VNs and UAP. Respiratory and physical therapy may have a role in the patient's care, depending on the type of surgery and the patient's past medical history.

PACU

- Assess patient's initial airway, breathing, and circulation status.
- Evaluate for the return to consciousness, ability to maintain airway and breathing.
- Perform ongoing assessments for postoperative problems (e.g., airway obstruction, hypoventilation, hypotension or hypertension, dysrhythmias, emergence delirium).
- Administer and titrate O_2 based on agency protocols.
- Give analgesics and IV fluids.
- Evaluate patient's readiness for transfer to clinical unit or discharge from ambulatory surgery.
- Give hand-off report to RN about patient status when transferring patient to clinical unit.
- Provide discharge teaching for patient and caregiver after ambulatory surgery.
- Oversee UAP:
  - Assist with positioning of patients in the lateral recovery position.
  - Obtain vital signs, pulse oximetry and capillary blood glucose levels (per agency policy). Report abnormal levels to RN.
  - Aid patient with elimination needs.

Clinical Unit

- Assess patient on initial admission to the unit.
- Assess for complications (e.g., atelectasis, hemodynamic instability, cognitive dysfunction, pain, fluid and electrolyte imbalance, fever or hypothermia, nausea and vomiting, urinary retention, wound infection).
- Develop and implement an individualized plan of care based on identification of patient risk factors and potential complications.
- Titrate O_2 administration according to prescribed parameters.
- Monitor pain level and give prescribed analgesics.
- Give medications.
- Provide wound care, including dressing changes.
- Insert urinary catheter as prescribed for urinary retention.
- Develop and implement individualized patient and caregiver education, including discharge teaching.
- Oversee UAP:
  - Record oral intake and output.
  - Obtain vital signs, pulse oximetry and capillary blood glucose levels (per agency policy). Report abnormal levels to RN.
  - Aid patient with nutrition, elimination, and hygienic needs.
  - Reposition and ambulate patient as instructed.
  - Help patient with deep breathing and coughing exercises.

Collaborate With Interprofessional Team

Respiratory Therapist

- Provide respiratory care modalities that support patient recovery from anesthesia (e.g., O_2 therapy, nebulizer treatments, pulmonary drainage procedures, mechanical ventilation, and airway support).
- Institute extubation protocols.
- Monitor pulse oximetry, capnography, or other technology-assisted means of assessing hypoxemia or hypoventilation.
- Assist with O_2 and/or ventilation management during patient transport.
- Perform arterial blood gas sampling in the absence of an arterial line.

- Institute rapid intubation protocols if needed in the absence of ACP.
- Provide respiratory care modalities (e.g., O_2 therapy, nebulizer treatments, pulmonary drainage procedures).
- Assist with O_2 and/or ventilation support during patient transport.
- Monitor pulse oximetry and capnography and titrate O_2 as needed.
- Perform arterial blood gas sampling as needed.

Physical Therapist

- Perform initial assessment to determine normal functioning level if surgery was emergent.
- Support patient motion and joint mobility.

- Support patient motion and joint mobility.
- Support patient return to baseline functional mobility following surgery.
- Support nursing staff on best measures for joint positioning, transferring from bed to chair, and/or ambulation.

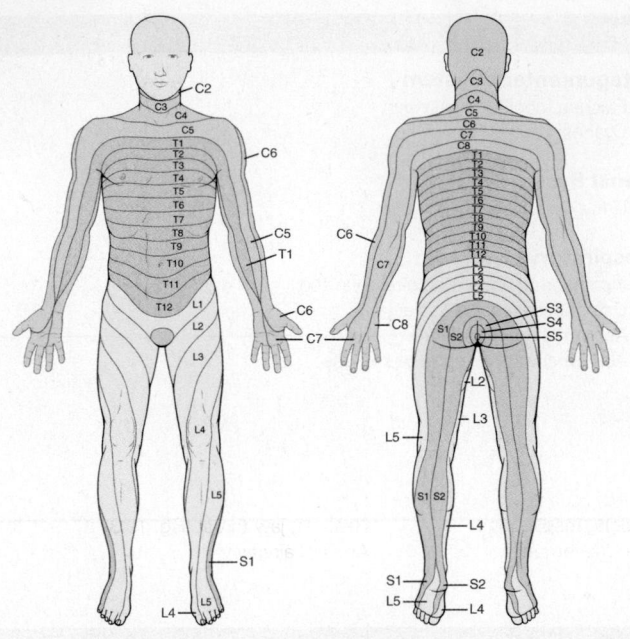

Sensory level anesthesia necessary for surgical procedures

Sensory level	Type of surgery
S2-S5	Hemorrhoidectomy
L2-L3 (knee)	Foot surgery
L1-L3 (inguinal ligament)	Lower extremity surgery
T10 (umbilicus)	Hip surgery Transurethral resection of the prostate Vaginal delivery
T6-T7 (xiphoid process)	Lower abdominal surgery Appendectomy
T4 (nipple)	Upper abdominal surgery Cesarean section

FIG. 19.2 Sensory innervation by spinal nerves and sensory level required for various surgical procedures. (From Pardo M, Miller R: *Basics of anesthesia*, ed 7, St Louis, 2018, Elsevier.)

RESPIRATORY PROBLEMS

Etiology

PACU. In the immediate postanesthesia period the most common causes of airway compromise include obstruction, hypoxemia, and hypoventilation (Table 19.5). Patients at high risk include those who (1) have had general anesthesia; (2) are older than 55 years of age; (3) have a history of tobacco use; (4) have preexisting lung disease and/or sleep-disordered breathing; (5) are obese; (6) have co-morbidities (e.g., renal disease, diabetes, hypertension); or (7) have undergone airway, thoracic, or abdominal surgery. Pulmonary complications pose the greatest risk to patients in the postanesthesia period and in the immediate postoperative period. High-risk patients should be monitored in a critical care or postanesthesia care unit.[5]

Airway obstruction is often caused by the patient's tongue blocking the airway (Fig. 19.3). The base of the tongue falls backward against the soft palate and occludes the pharynx. It is most pronounced in the supine position and in the patient who is extremely sleepy after surgery.

Hypoxemia, a partial pressure of arterial oxygen (PaO_2) less than 60 mm Hg, is characterized by a variety of nonspecific clinical signs and symptoms, ranging from agitation to somnolence, hypertension to hypotension, and tachycardia to bradycardia. Pulse oximetry will show low O_2 saturation (less than 92%).

The most common cause of hypoxemia after surgery is atelectasis. Atelectasis (alveolar collapse) may be the result of bronchial obstruction caused by retained secretions, decreased respiratory excursion, or general anesthesia. Atelectasis occurs when mucus blocks bronchioles or there is not enough alveolar surfactant (substance that holds the alveoli open) (Fig. 19.4). As air becomes trapped beyond the plug and is absorbed, the alveoli collapse. Atelectasis may affect a part of or an entire lobe of the lung.

Other causes of hypoxemia include pulmonary edema, pulmonary embolism (PE), aspiration, and bronchospasm. An accumulation of fluid in the alveoli can cause *pulmonary edema.* It may be the result of fluid overload, heart failure, prolonged airway obstruction, sepsis, or aspiration.

After surgery patients are at risk for *aspiration* of gastric contents into the lungs. This can occur because anesthesia depresses the respiratory protective airway reflexes. Gastric aspiration is a potentially serious emergency. It may result in laryngospasm, pneumonia, and pulmonary edema. Because of the grave consequences of aspiration of gastric fluids, prevention is the goal.

Bronchospasm is the result of an increase in bronchial smooth muscle tone with resulting closure of small airways. Airway edema develops, causing secretions to build up in the airway. The patient will have wheezing, dyspnea, use of accessory muscles, hypoxemia, and tachypnea. Bronchospasm may be due to aspiration, endotracheal intubation, pharyngeal suctioning, or an allergic response. (Allergic responses are discussed in Chapter 13.) Bronchospasm may occur in any patient. It occurs more often in patients with a history of smoking, asthma, and chronic obstructive pulmonary disease (COPD).

Hypoventilation, a common complication in the PACU, is characterized by a decreased respiratory rate or effort, hypoxemia, and increasing hypercapnia (increasing $PaCO_2$). It may result from depression of the central respiratory drive (from anesthesia or use of opioids), poor respiratory muscle tone (from neuromuscular blockade or disease), or a combination of both.

> **! SAFETY ALERT Hypoventilation**
> - Always assess for respiratory depression when giving opioids.
> - Use a sedation assessment scale (e.g., Richmond Agitation and Sedation Scale, available at *www.icudelirium.org/docs/RASS.pdf*) to assess for levels of sedation and promote patient safety when giving opioids in the PACU.
> - Begin emergency management protocols if hypoventilation is present.

Clinical Unit. Common causes of respiratory problems are atelectasis and pneumonia, especially in patients with co-morbidities (e.g., OSA, COPD, heart failure) and after abdominal and thoracic surgery.[6,7] The development of mucous plugs and decreased surfactant production is directly related to hypoventilation, immobility and bed rest, ineffective coughing, and history of tobacco use. Increased bronchial secretions occur when the respiratory passages have been irritated by heavy smoking, COPD, pulmonary infection, or dry mucous membranes that occurs with intubation, inhalation anesthesia, and dehydration. Without intervention, atelectasis can progress to pneumonia.

TABLE 19.5 Postoperative Respiratory Complications

Complications	Mechanisms	Manifestations	Interventions
Airway Obstruction			
Laryngeal edema	Allergic drug reaction Mechanical irritation from intubation Fluid overload	Similar to laryngospasm	O_2 therapy Antihistamines Corticosteroids Sedatives Possible intubation
Laryngospasm	Irritation from endotracheal tube, anesthetic gases, or gastric aspiration Most likely to occur after removal of endotracheal tube	Inspiratory stridor (crowing respirations) Sternal retraction Acute respiratory distress	O_2 therapy Positive pressure ventilation IV muscle relaxant Lidocaine Corticosteroids
Retained thick secretions	Secretion stimulation by anesthetic agents Dehydration of secretions	Noisy respirations Coarse crackles	Suctioning Deep breathing and coughing IV hydration Chest PT
Tongue falling back	Muscular flaccidity associated with ↓ consciousness and muscle relaxants	Use of accessory muscles Snoring respirations ↓ Air movement	Patient stimulation Head tilt, jaw thrust (Fig. 19.3) Artificial airway
Hypoxemia			
Aspiration	Inhalation of gastric contents into lungs	Unexplained tachypnea Bronchospasm ↓ O_2 saturation Atelectasis Interstitial edema Alveolar hemorrhage Respiratory failure	O_2 therapy Cardiopulmonary support Antibiotics
Atelectasis	Bronchial obstruction caused by retained secretions or ↓ lung volumes	↓ Breath sounds ↓ O_2 saturation	Humidified O_2 therapy Deep breathing Incentive spirometry Early mobilization
Bronchospasm	↑ Smooth muscle tone with closure of small airways	Wheezing Dyspnea Tachypnea ↓ O_2 saturation	O_2 therapy Bronchodilators
Pulmonary edema	Fluid overload ↑ Hydrostatic pressure ↓ Interstitial pressure ↑ Capillary permeability	↓ O_2 saturation Crackles Infiltrates on chest x-ray	O_2 therapy Diuretics Fluid restriction
Pulmonary embolism	Thrombus dislodged from peripheral venous system and lodged in pulmonary arterial system	Acute tachypnea Dyspnea Tachycardia Hypotension ↓ O_2 saturationBronchospasm	O_2 therapy Cardiopulmonary support Anticoagulant therapy
Hypoventilation			
Depressed central respiratory drive	Medullary depression from anesthetics, opioids, sedatives	Shallow respirations ↓ Respiratory rate, apnea ↓ PaO_2 ↑ $PaCO_2$	Start capnography or other technology-supported respiratory monitoring Stimulation Reversal of opioids or benzodiazepines Mechanical ventilation
Mechanical restriction	Tight casts, dressings, abdominal binders Positioning and obesity preventing lung expansion	As above	Elevate head of bed Repositioning Loosen dressings
Pain	Shallow breathing to prevent incisional pain	↑ Respiratory rate Hypotension Hypertension ↓ $PaCO_2$ ↓ PaO_2 Reports of pain Guarding behavior	Opioid analgesic drug therapy Nonsteroidal antiinflammatory drug therapy Complementary and alternative therapies (e.g., music, imagery)
Poor respiratory muscle tone	Neuromuscular blockade Neuromuscular disease	As above	Reversal of paralysis Mechanical ventilation

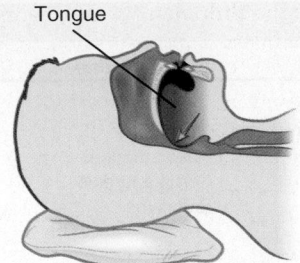

Tongue occluding airway

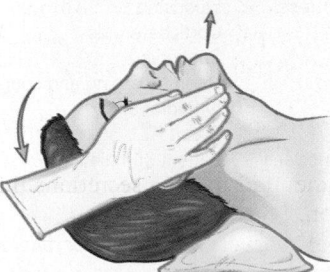

Manually elevate the jaw while tilting the head back

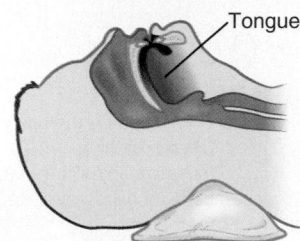

Airway cleared

FIG. 19.3 Etiology and relief of airway obstruction.

❖ NURSING MANAGEMENT: RESPIRATORY PROBLEMS

◆ Nursing Assessment

Respiratory assessment requires evaluation of airway patency; chest symmetry; and depth, rate, and character of respirations. Impaired ventilation may first be seen as slowed breathing or reduced chest and abdominal movement during breathing. Abdominal or accessory muscle use may occur with respiratory distress. Auscultating breath sounds will alert you to decreased or absent breath sounds. These findings may mean airflow is diminished or obstructed. Arouse patients with poor respiratory effort, noisy respirations, or other signs of respiratory distress at once and have them take deep breaths.

Regular monitoring of vital signs, including pulse oximetry, capnography, or other technology-supported monitoring (e.g., acoustic monitoring), and a thorough respiratory assessment allow you to recognize early signs of respiratory problems. Manifestations of hypoxemia include tachypnea, gasping, anxiety, restlessness, confusion, and a rapid or thready pulse.

Note and record the characteristics of sputum or mucus. Mucus from the trachea and throat is normally colorless and thin in consistency. Sputum from the lungs and bronchi is normally thick with a pale, yellow tinge. Changes in sputum (e.g., color) may indicate a respiratory infection.

◆ Nursing Diagnoses

Nursing diagnoses and collaborative problems related to respiratory problems include:

- Impaired airway clearance
- Impaired breathing
- Impaired gas exchange
- Risk for aspiration
- Potential complications: pneumonia, atelectasis

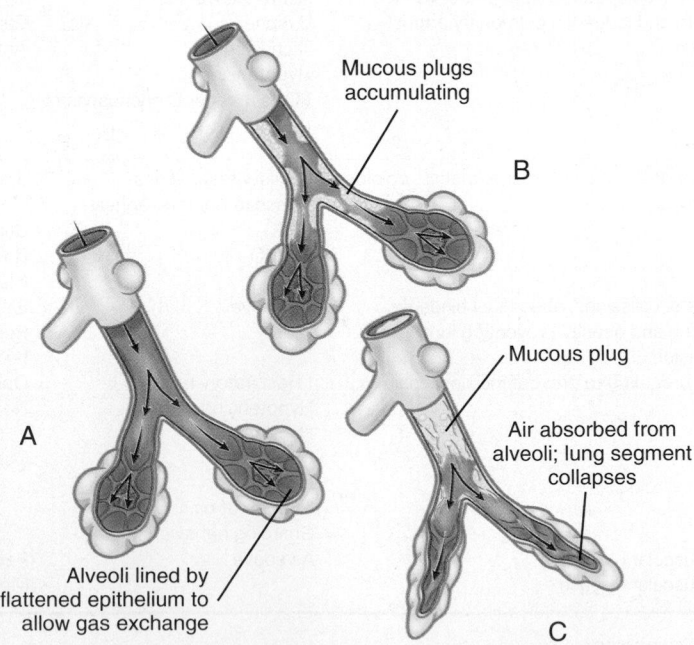

FIG. 19.4 Postoperative atelectasis. **A,** Normal bronchiole and alveoli. **B,** Mucous plug in bronchiole. **C,** Collapse of alveoli resulting from atelectasis after absorption of air.

◆ Nursing Implementation

In the PACU, nursing interventions are aimed at preventing and treating respiratory problems. Proper positioning of the patient aids breathing and protects the airway.

> ⚠ **SAFETY ALERT Postoperative Patient Positioning**
> • Position the unconscious patient in a lateral "recovery" position (Fig. 19.5).
> • This position keeps the airway open and reduces the risk for aspiration if vomiting occurs.

Once conscious, place the patient in a supine position with the head of the bed elevated. This position maximizes expansion of the thorax by decreasing the pressure of the abdominal contents on the diaphragm.

Start O_2 therapy via nasal cannula or face mask if ordered. O_2 helps to eliminate anesthetic gases and meet the increased demand for O_2 resulting from decreased blood volume or increased metabolism.

All postoperative patients are at risk for atelectasis. Encourage deep breathing to aid gas exchange and promote the return to consciousness. Once the patient is more awake, deep breathing, coughing, and use of an incentive spirometer help prevent alveolar collapse and move respiratory secretions to larger airway passages for expectoration. One technique, known as *sustained maximal inspiration,* requires the patient to inhale as deeply as possible and, at the peak of inspiration, hold the breath for a few seconds, and then exhale. This is followed by another deep breath and cough.

The use of an incentive spirometer helps by giving visual feedback of respiratory effort (Fig. 19.6). Diaphragmatic or abdominal breathing involves inhaling slowly and deeply through the nose, holding the breath for a few seconds, and then exhaling slowly and completely through the mouth. Place the patient's hands lightly over the lower ribs and upper abdomen so that the patient can feel the abdomen rise during inspiration and fall during expiration. Unless contraindicated, have the patient perform these maneuvers 10 times every hour while awake.

Effective coughing is essential in mobilizing secretions. If secretions are in the respiratory tract, deep breathing often moves them up and stimulates the cough reflex. Splinting an abdominal incision with a pillow or a rolled blanket supports the incision and aids in coughing and expectorating secretions (Fig. 19.7).

Change the patient's position every 1 to 2 hours to allow full chest expansion and increase perfusion of both lungs. Help the patient sit in a chair and ambulate as soon as ordered. Provide adequate and regular pain medication. Incisional pain often is the greatest barrier to patient participation in effective breathing exercises and ambulation. Reassure the patient that these activities will not cause the incision to open. Adequate hydration, either parenteral or oral, is essential to maintain the integrity of mucous membranes and to keep secretions thin and loose for easy expectoration.

Other nursing interventions for specific respiratory problems are detailed in Table 19.5. A nursing care plan for the postoperative patient (eNursing Care Plan 19.1) is available on the website for this chapter.

INFORMATICS IN PRACTICE
Respiratory Monitoring

- Continuous monitoring of respiratory rate is important for those receiving patient-controlled analgesia (PCA) for pain management, as opioids can cause respiratory depression and place patients at risk for serious injury or death.
- Acoustic respiration rate (RRa) is a new measurement that allows for the noninvasive and continuous assessment of patients' breathing. RRa uses a sensor with an acoustic transducer that is placed on the patient's neck.
- The respiratory signal is displayed as a continuous respiration rate.

CARDIOVASCULAR PROBLEMS

Etiology

PACU. In the immediate postanesthesia period the most common cardiovascular problems include hypotension, hypertension, and dysrhythmias. Patients at greatest risk for altered

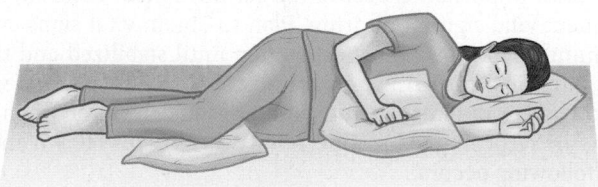

FIG. 19.5 Position of patient during recovery from general anesthesia.

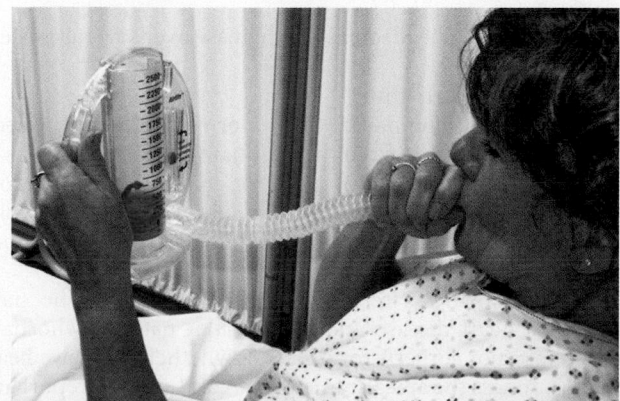

FIG. 19.6 Proper use of an incentive spirometer. (Courtesy Christine R. Hoch, MSN, RN, ACNS-BC, Nursing Instructor, University of Delaware, Newark, DE.)

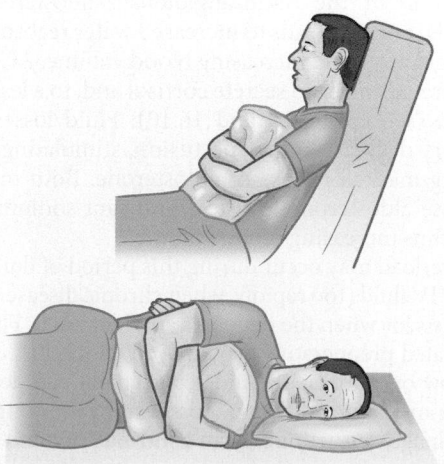

FIG. 19.7 Techniques for splinting incision when coughing.

cardiovascular function include those with altered respiratory function, those with a history of cardiovascular disease, older adults, the debilitated, and the critically ill.

Hypotension can cause hypoperfusion to the vital organs, especially the brain, heart, and kidneys. Clinical signs of disorientation, loss of consciousness, chest pain, and oliguria reflect hypoperfusion, hypoxemia, and the loss of physiologic compensation. Intervention must be prompt to prevent the devastating complications of cardiac ischemia or infarction, cerebral ischemia, renal ischemia, and bowel infarction.

The most common cause of hypotension in the PACU is fluid and blood loss, which may lead to hypovolemic shock. Hemorrhage is always a risk of surgery. Marked blood loss is possible when cauterization or sutures fail. Hemorrhage most often occurs internally. Assess for changes in level of consciousness and vital signs. If detected, treatment is aimed toward restoring circulating volume. If there is no response to fluid administration, heart dysfunction may be the cause of hypotension.

Primary heart dysfunction, which may occur in myocardial infarction, cardiac tamponade, or PE, results in an acute drop in cardiac output. Secondary heart dysfunction occurs because of the negative *chronotropic* (rate of heart contraction) and negative *inotropic* (force of heart contraction) effects of drugs, such as β-adrenergic blockers, digoxin, or opioids. Other causes of hypotension include decreased systemic vascular resistance and dysrhythmias.

Hypertension most often occurs from sympathetic nervous system stimulation. This may be the result of pain, anxiety, bladder distention, or respiratory distress. Hypertension may be related to hypothermia and preexisting hypertension.

Many problems can cause dysrhythmias. These include hypoxemia, hypercapnia, electrolyte and acid-base imbalances, circulatory instability, preexisting heart disease, hypothermia, pain, surgical stress, and many anesthetic agents.

Clinical Unit. On the clinical unit, postoperative fluid and electrolyte imbalances are contributing factors to heart problems. Such imbalances may result from a combination of the body's normal response to the stress of surgery, excessive fluid losses, and IV fluid replacement. The body's fluid status directly affects cardiac output.

Fluid retention during postoperative days 1 to 3 can result from the stress response, which maintains both blood volume and BP. Fluid retention results from the release of antidiuretic hormone (ADH) and adrenocorticotropic hormone (ACTH) and activation of the renin-angiotensin-aldosterone system (RAAS). ADH release leads to increased water reabsorption and decreased urine output, increasing blood volume. ACTH stimulates the adrenal cortex to secrete cortisol and, to a lesser degree, aldosterone (see Figs. 16.9 and 16.10). Fluid losses resulting from surgery decrease kidney perfusion, stimulating the RAAS and causing marked release of aldosterone. Both mechanisms that increase aldosterone lead to significant sodium and fluid retention, thus increasing blood volume.

Fluid overload may occur during this period of fluid retention if we infuse IV fluids too rapidly, when chronic disease (e.g., heart, kidney) exists, or when the patient is an older adult. Fluid deficits from untreated preoperative dehydration, blood loss during surgery, or slow or inadequate fluid replacement can decrease cardiac output and tissue perfusion. Losses from vomiting, bleeding, wound drainage, or suctioning can contribute to fluid deficits.

Hypokalemia can result from urinary and gastrointestinal (GI) tract losses. Low serum potassium levels directly affect the heart's contractility and may contribute to decreases in cardiac output and tissue perfusion. The patient can receive potassium replacement, usually 40 mEq/day, if renal function is adequate. A urine output of at least 0.5 mL/kg/hr and a normal serum creatinine are considered indicative of adequate renal function.

The state of tissue perfusion or blood flow affects cardiovascular status. The stress response contributes to an increase in clotting tendencies by increasing platelet production. A *venous thromboembolism (VTE)* may form in leg veins because of venous stasis, vein injury, or a hypercoagulable state. VTE is especially common in older adults, obese persons, immobilized patients, and patients with a history of PE or predisposition to clotting. It is a potentially life-threatening complication because it may lead to PE and infarction. Suspect PE in any patient with tachypnea, chest pain, hypotension, agitation, tachycardia, and dyspnea, especially when the patient is already receiving O_2 therapy. Superficial thrombophlebitis is an uncomfortable but less serious complication. It may develop in a leg vein because of venous stasis or in the arm veins because of irritation from IV catheters or solutions. (PE and VTE are discussed in Chapters 27 and 37, respectively.)

Syncope (fainting) may result from decreased cardiac output, fluid deficits, or defects in cerebral perfusion. Syncope often occurs because of postural hypotension when the patient ambulates. It is more common in the older adult or in the patient who has been immobile for long periods. Normally when the patient stands up quickly, the arterial baroreceptors respond to the accompanying fall in BP with sympathetic nervous system stimulation. This produces vasoconstriction and maintains BP. These sympathetic and vasomotor functions may be diminished in the older adult, immobile, or postanesthesia patient.

❖ NURSING MANAGEMENT: CARDIOVASCULAR PROBLEMS

◆ Nursing Assessment

The most important aspect of the cardiovascular assessment is frequent vital sign monitoring. Plan to obtain vital signs every 15 minutes in Phase I, or more often until stabilized and then less often in Phase II. Compare postoperative vital signs with preoperative and intraoperative findings to determine when the signs are returning to baseline. Notify the ACP or HCP if any of the following occurs:

- Systolic BP <90 mm Hg or >160 mm Hg
- Pulse rate <60 beats/min or >120 beats/min
- Pulse pressure (difference between systolic and diastolic BP) narrows
- BP trends gradually decrease or increase over several consecutive readings
- Change in heart rhythm

Hypotension accompanied by a normal pulse and warm, dry, pink skin is usually from the residual vasodilating effects of anesthesia and suggests only a need for continued observation. Hypotension accompanied by a rapid or weak pulse and cold, clammy, pale skin may indicate impending hypovolemic shock and needs immediate treatment.

ECG monitoring is recommended for patients who have a history of heart disease and for all older patients who have undergone major surgery, regardless of whether they have heart problems. Assess the apical-radial pulse carefully and report any deficits or irregularities. Assess peripheral pulses and skin color, temperature, and moisture for valuable information about tissue perfusion.

◆ Nursing Diagnoses

Nursing diagnoses and collaborative problems related to cardiovascular problems include:

- Altered blood pressure
- Impaired cardiac output
- Risk for bleeding
- Potential complications: hypovolemic shock, VTE

◆ Nursing Implementation

◆ **PACU.** Begin treatment of hypotension with O_2 therapy to promote oxygenation of hypoperfused organs. Because the most common cause of hypotension is fluid loss, give IV fluid boluses to normalize BP. Inspect the surgical incision to determine if excess bleeding is the cause of volume loss. Primary heart dysfunction may require drug intervention. Peripheral vasodilation and hypotension may require vasoconstrictive drugs to increase systemic vascular resistance.

Treatment of hypertension centers on removing the cause of sympathetic nervous system stimulation. This may include giving analgesics, assisting with voiding, and correcting respiratory problems. Rewarming corrects hypothermia-induced hypertension. The patient with preexisting hypertension or who has undergone heart or vascular surgery usually needs drug therapy to reduce BP.

Since most dysrhythmias seen in the PACU have identifiable causes, treatment is directed toward removing the cause. Correcting the cause usually corrects the dysrhythmias. With life-threatening dysrhythmias (e.g., ventricular tachycardia), follow your agency's protocol for advanced cardiac life support.

◆ **Clinical Unit.** Continue to monitor vital signs. Keep an accurate intake and output record, monitor laboratory findings (e.g., electrolytes, hematocrit), and manage IV therapy after surgery.

Early ambulation is the most significant general nursing measure to prevent complications. The exercise associated with walking (1) increases muscle tone; (2) stimulates circulation, which prevents venous stasis and VTE, and speeds wound healing; and (3) increases vital capacity and supports normal respiratory function. Begin progression to ambulation by first raising the head of the patient's bed for 1 to 2 minutes. Then help the patient to sit, with legs dangling, while monitoring the pulse rate. If you do not note changes or problems, start ambulation with ongoing monitoring of the pulse. If you note changes in the pulse or dizziness occurs, sit the patient in a nearby chair. The patient should stay in this location until the BP and pulse are stable. Then help the patient back to the bed. If dizziness occurs, it is often frightening for the patient. Injury can result from a fall, so take measures to ensure patient and staff safety.

❓ CHECK YOUR PRACTICE

You are caring for an older, obese male patient who is 1 day post colon resection with activity orders for moving out of the bed to a chair. While he is in bed, you help him to a sitting position with his legs dangling. He tells you that he feels dizzy. You take his BP and it is 108/64 and his pulse is 124.

- What should you do?

NEUROLOGIC AND PSYCHOLOGIC PROBLEMS

Etiology

PACU. Postoperatively, emergence delirium is a short-term neurologic change manifested by behaviors such as restlessness, agitation, disorientation, thrashing, and shouting. If delirium occurs, first suspect hypoxia. Other causes include anesthetic agents, bladder distention, pain, long duration of preoperative fasting, residual neuromuscular blockade, or the presence of an endotracheal tube.

Delayed emergence can be a problem after surgery. Patients with delayed emergence spend longer periods in the PACU and have prolonged hospital courses. Identifying the causative factors is critical for determining appropriate interventions.[8] The most common cause of delayed emergence after anesthesia is drug-related. This includes anesthetic agents as well as drugs used during the perioperative period. Contributory nonpharmacologic causes include metabolic disorders, electrolyte imbalances, hypertension, liver disease, uremia, central anticholinergic syndrome, and hypothyroidism. Other causes can include hypoxia, hypercapnia, hemorrhage, and embolism.

Clinical Unit. Two types of cognitive impairments seen in surgical patients are *postoperative cognitive dysfunction (POCD)* and *delirium.* POCD is a decline in the patient's cognitive function (e.g., memory, ability to concentrate) for weeks or months after surgery. POCD occurs primarily in the older surgical patient. Preexisting cognitive impairment, duration of anesthesia, complications during surgery, and infection contribute to the development of POCD. Quickly and thoroughly investigate any changes in mental status as the causes may be life threatening.

Postoperative delirium is more common in the older patient, but it can occur in patients of any age. Delirium may be the result of severe pain, fluid and electrolyte imbalances, hypoxemia, drug effects, sleep deprivation, and sensory deprivation or overload. Signs include cognitive dysfunction, varying levels of consciousness, altered psychomotor activity, and a disturbed sleep/wake cycle. See Chapter 59 for more about delirium.

Anxiety and depression may occur and correlate with an increased likelihood for complications.[9] These responses may be part of grieving for lost body parts or altered body function or for loss of independence during recovery and rehabilitation.

Alcohol withdrawal delirium results from the patient undergoing alcohol withdrawal. It is characterized by restlessness, insomnia, nightmares, irritability, and auditory or visual hallucinations. Chapter 10 discusses the identification and management of alcohol withdrawal delirium.

❖ NURSING MANAGEMENT: NEUROLOGIC AND PSYCHOLOGIC PROBLEMS

◆ Nursing Assessment

Assess the patient's level of consciousness, orientation, memory, and ability to follow commands. Determine the size, reactivity, and equality of the pupils. Assess the patient's sleep/wake cycle and sensory and motor status. Determine the possible cause if the patient has an altered neurologic status. If the patient was mentally alert before surgery and becomes cognitively impaired after surgery, you need to do further assessment to rule out hypoxia, delirium, or POCD.

◆ Nursing Diagnoses

Nursing diagnoses related to neurologic and psychologic problems include:

- Confusion
- Disturbed body image
- Sleep deprivation

◆ **Nursing Implementation**

◆ **PACU.** The most common cause of agitation in the PACU is hypoxemia. So, you need to focus attention on evaluating respiratory function. Once you have ruled out hypoxemia or other known causes of postoperative delirium, sedation may be beneficial in controlling agitation. Because the most common cause of delayed emergence is prolonged drug action, delays in awakening usually spontaneously resolve with time. If necessary, antagonists can reverse the effects of benzodiazepines and opioids.

Interventions to prevent perioperative delirium, other than reducing the depth of anesthesia, have not significantly reduced the incidence of emergence delirium [10] Until the patient is awake and able to communicate effectively, you are responsible for patient safety. This includes monitoring physiologic status, having the side rails up and the call bell available, securing equipment (e.g., IV lines, artificial airways), using 2 patient identifiers before giving drugs or completing treatments, and verifying allergies.

◆ **Clinical Unit.** To prevent or manage postoperative delirium or POCD, address any potential contributing factors. Maintain normal physiologic function by achieving fluid and electrolyte balance, adequate nutrition and sleep, pain management, proper bowel and bladder function, and early mobilization. To help orient the patient, use specific aids, such as clocks, calendars, and photos.

To prevent or limit psychologic problems, provide adequate support for the patient. This includes listening to and talking with the patient, offering explanations and reassurance, and encouraging the presence and aid of the patient's caregiver(s). Evaluate the patient's behavior to distinguish a normal reaction to a stressful situation from one that is becoming abnormal or excessive. Recognizing alcohol withdrawal delirium can be a challenge. Record and report any unusual or disturbed behavior so that a diagnosis can be made and treatment started.

PAIN AND DISCOMFORT

Etiology

Despite the availability of pain-relieving drugs and techniques, pain is a common problem and a significant fear for patients. Pain is caused by the interaction of several physiologic and psychologic factors. The incision and retraction during surgery traumatize the skin and underlying tissues. In addition, there may be reflex muscle spasms around the incision. Anxiety and fear, sometimes related to the anticipation of pain, create tension and further increase muscle tone and spasm. Positioning during surgery and the use of internal devices such as an endotracheal tube or catheters may also cause discomfort. The effort and movement associated with deep breathing, coughing, and ambulating may worsen pain by creating tension on the incision area. Other sources of discomfort include nausea and vomiting, environmental noises, noxious odors, and shivering.

The patient does not feel pain when the internal viscera are cut. Pain, does, however, come from pressure in the internal viscera. This means deep visceral pain may signal a complication such as intestinal distention, bleeding, or abscess formation. Pain increases the risk for atelectasis and impaired respiratory function.

❖ NURSING MANAGEMENT: PAIN

◆ **Nursing Assessment**

Assess the patient on arrival to the PACU and at frequent intervals. The patient's self-report is the single most reliable indicator of pain. Use a pain scale, such as a numeric or FACES pain scale, to assess the severity or intensity of pain. (Pain scales are discussed in Chapter 8.) Assess pain levels at rest and during activities. Since verbalization of pain is not always possible in the PACU, assess the patient for other indications of pain (e.g., restlessness, grimacing, changes in vital signs). You need to identify the location of the pain. Expect that patients will have incisional pain, especially with movement, and with certain procedures (e.g., removal of drains). Other causes of pain, such as a full bladder, may be present.

Always involve patients in the assessment and management of their pain. Assessing patients from different cultures or who do not speak English may be challenging. Take extra time to explore the pain experience with these patients. Adapt care as needed to meet the patient's unique needs and expectations for pain control.

◆ **Nursing Implementation**

Begin before surgery to develop a plan for pain control that includes behavioral modalities and control of anxiety. Evaluate any adjustments to or continuation of drugs used to treat any chronic pain during the preoperative phase. During this time, teach patients to report pain and how it will be managed after surgery. Share pain management plans during the hand-off report.

The acute pain of surgery almost always requires the use of analgesics. Organizational approaches can reduce pain intensity with fewer side effects associated with the analgesic use. These approaches include using procedure-specific pain management guidelines with titration of analgesia based on specific patient needs.[11]

Pain control techniques include the use of single modalities (e.g., opioid drugs, PCA, regional analgesic [local anesthetic infiltration]), or multimodal analgesia. *Multimodal analgesia,* or the use of 2 or more analgesics with different mechanisms of action (e.g., an opioid and a nonsteroidal antiinflammatory drug [NSAID]), is recommended. Multimodal analgesia reduces pain, opioid use, and opioid-related adverse effects. It also enhances recovery and increases patient satisfaction.[12] These drugs may be given via the same or different routes. The choice of modalities should be procedure and patient specific.

The HCP often writes orders for pain medication and other comfort measures on an as-needed (PRN) basis. Time giving analgesics to ensure that they are in effect during activities that may be painful, such as walking. Although opioid analgesics are often essential for the patient's comfort, there are undesirable side effects. The most common include constipation, nausea and vomiting, respiratory and cough depression, and hypotension.

Before giving any analgesic, first assess the patient's pain, including location, quality, and intensity; vital signs; and level of consciousness. Treat incisional pain as ordered. If the patient reports chest or leg pain, analgesics may mask a complication (e.g., VTE). If it is gas pain, opioids can worsen it. If the analgesic either does not relieve the pain or makes the patient lethargic or somnolent, notify the HCP and request a change in the order.

Patient-controlled analgesia (PCA) allows the self-administration of predetermined doses of analgesia by the patient. The goals of PCA are to provide immediate analgesia and maintain an acceptable level of pain control. Continuous infusions allow for a steady blood level of analgesia with additional patient doses used prior to painful events (e.g., walking, deep breathing, and coughing) or for breakthrough pain. Opioid-tolerant patients may need patient-administered boluses. The route of delivery may be IV, oral, epidural, or transdermal. The transdermal route is for short-term pain management and may offer advantages over the IV route (e.g., needleless, low infection risk, decreased drug errors associated with pump malfunction or inaccurate programming). Some advantages of PCA are early ambulation, better pain management than with as-needed analgesia, and greater patient satisfaction. (PCA is discussed in Chapter 8.)

> **! SAFETY ALERT Patient-Controlled Analgesia (PCA)**
> - Carefully check the HCP's order and properly program the pump for IV or epidural PCA to deliver the ordered dose of analgesic (e.g., continuous rate, bolus dose, maximum dose).
> - A patient's death or serious injury associated with a drug error (e.g., wrong drug, wrong dose, wrong patient, wrong rate) is a serious reportable event (never event).

Epidural analgesia is the infusion of opioid analgesics through a catheter placed into the epidural space surrounding the spinal cord. The goal of epidural analgesia is delivery of the drug directly to opiate receptors in the spinal cord. Administration methods include intermittent bolus dosing, continuous infusion, and epidural PCA. This technique results in a constant circulating level and a reduced total dose of medication. The use of epidural analgesia for managing pain after surgery is increasing.

Perineural local anesthesia, the infiltration of a nonopioid drug into the surgical site, is another way to manage postoperative pain. A disposable or mechanical infusion pump delivers the local anesthetic via a catheter directly to the surgical incision site. A single dose of bupivacaine liposome injectable suspension (Exparel) provides pain relief with reduced opioid needs for up to 72 hours.

Complementary and alternative therapies such as music therapy, guided imagery, relaxation exercises, and aromatherapy are effective adjuncts in pain management. Nondrug approaches such as repositioning, massage, and distraction can enhance pain management.

> **? CHECK YOUR PRACTICE**
>
> Although PCA is infusing as ordered, your postoperative patient reports ongoing pain that is rated 8 on a 0 to 10 scale.
> - What steps would you take next to manage this patient's pain more effectively?

TEMPERATURE CHANGES

Etiology

Knowing the patient's temperature in the postoperative period is valuable (Table 19.6). We are giving increased attention to the importance of maintaining a normal body temperature.

Perioperative temperature management is a quality measure by the Surgical Care Improvement Project (SCIP), a national partnership of organizations whose goal is to reduce surgical site infections (SSIs).[13]

Hypothermia. Perioperative *hypothermia* is a core body temperature less than 96.8°F (36°C). Hypothermia occurs when heat loss exceeds heat production. Heat loss may occur due to skin exposure, use of cold irrigants, skin preparations, and unwarmed inhaled gases. Although all patients are at risk for postoperative hypothermia, patients with low preoperative core body temperatures, those with systolic BP less than 140 mm Hg, older patients, female patients, and patients who receive epidural or spinal anesthesia are at a higher risk.[1] Long surgical procedures, open cavity procedures (e.g., abdominal or thoracic) and prolonged anesthetic administration lead to redistribution of body heat from the core to the periphery. This places the patient at an increased risk for hypothermia and complications.[14]

Complications associated with hypothermia can include vasoconstriction with resulting hypertension, compromised immune function, bleeding, untoward cardiac events, SSIs, altered drug metabolism, increased pain, and shivering. Shivering can increase resting energy expenditure and O_2 consumption up to 500%, which can lead to hypoxemia and myocardial ischemia (angina). Shivering can also increase carbon dioxide production; increase heart rate, BP, and intracranial pressure; and significantly affect the patient's comfort level.[1]

Fever. Fever may occur at any time after surgery (Table 19.6). SSI, particularly from aerobic organisms, is often accompanied by a fever that spikes in the afternoon or evening and returns to near-normal levels in the morning. The respiratory tract may be infected from stasis of secretions in areas of atelectasis. Urinary tract infections (UTIs) may occur from catheterization. Superficial thrombophlebitis may occur at the IV site. VTE in the leg veins may raise temperature.

Surgical patients who receive antibiotic therapy are at risk for *Clostridium difficile* infections. Manifestations of *C. difficile* may include fever, diarrhea, and abdominal pain.

Intermittent high fever accompanied by shaking chills and diaphoresis suggests septicemia. This may occur at any time after surgery. It can result from microorganisms being introduced into the bloodstream during surgery, especially in GI or genitourinary (GU) procedures. Septicemia may occur later from a wound or UTI.

Malignant hyperthermia (MH) is a muscle metabolism disorder that is triggered by general anesthetic agents. Although often a late sign, it is characterized by a rapid rise in core body temperature and severe muscle rigidity. Other signs of MH include tachycardia, hypercarbia, metabolic and respiratory acidosis, myoglobinuria, and elevated creatine kinase levels. MH is a life-threatening complication. While most cases of MH occur during general anesthesia, the 1-hour period right after surgery (e.g., in the PACU) is a critical time.[1]

TABLE 19.6 Postoperative Temperature Changes

Time After Surgery	Temperature	Possible Causes
Up to 12 hr	Hypothermia: ≤96.8°F (36°C)	Effects of anesthesia, body heat loss during surgical procedure
First 48 hr (postoperative days 1 and 2)	Mild elevation: ≤100.4°F (38°C)	Inflammatory response to surgical stress
	Moderate elevation: >100.4°F (38°C)	Lung congestion, dehydration
After first 48 hr (postoperative day 3 and later)	Elevation >100°F (37.8°C)	Infection (e.g., wound, urinary, respiratory)

❖ NURSING MANAGEMENT: TEMPERATURE CHANGES

◆ Nursing Assessment

Take the patient's temperature on arrival to the PACU and every hour if the patient stays normothermic. If the patient is hypothermic, take the temperature every 15 minutes until normothermia is reached. Use the same route of measuring temperature during the patient's stay in the PACU.

Assess the color and temperature of the skin. Communicate risk factors for hypothermia or MH to all members of the perioperative team. Observe the patient for early signs of inflammation and infection that may precede a fever so that any complications can be treated promptly.

◆ Nursing Diagnoses

Nursing diagnoses related to altered temperature include:
- Hypothermia
- Hyperthermia

◆ Nursing Implementation

Passive warming measures include the use of warmed cotton blankets, socks, and reflective blankets and limiting skin exposure. *Active warming measures* involve the application of external warming devices, including forced air warmers; heated water mattresses; radiant warmers; heated, humidified O_2; and warmed IV fluids. When using any external warming device, record body temperature and the patient's comfort level at 15-minute intervals. In addition, take care to prevent skin injuries.

Apply O_2 therapy via nasal cannula or mask to treat the increased demand for O_2 caused by shivering. Shivering can be treated with opioids (e.g., meperidine). Keep the supplies readily available to manage MH. Treatment for MH includes the administration of dantrolene (Dantrium), measures to cool the patient (e.g., ice packs), and correcting acid-base imbalances.

Use meticulous asepsis with wound and IV site care. Encourage airway clearance with deep breathing, coughing, and use of the incentive spirometer. If fever develops, chest x-rays may be taken, and antipyretic drugs given. Depending on the suspected cause of the fever, obtain cultures of the wound, sputum, urine, or blood. If a bacterial infection is the source of the fever, start antibiotics as soon as you obtain cultures. If the fever rises above 103°F (39.4°C), you may use body-cooling measures.

GASTROINTESTINAL PROBLEMS

Etiology

Postoperative nausea and vomiting (PONV) are the most common complications affecting as many as 80% of high-risk patients. Risk factors include younger age (under 50 years of age), gender (female), history of motion sickness or previous PONV, nonsmoking status, action of anesthetics or opioids, and duration and type of surgery.[2] Delayed gastric emptying and slowed peristalsis that result from handling of the bowel during abdominal surgery contribute to PONV, as does starting oral intake too soon after surgery.

Constipation may occur after surgery. It can be due to anesthetics used during surgery that may paralyze the intestine; immobility; changes in diet and fluid intake; and the use of opioids for pain relief. Opioids contribute to constipation by decreasing peristalsis and slowing fecal transport through the intestinal tract. They may also decrease a patient's urge to defecate.

Postoperative ileus (POI) is the temporary impairment of gastric and bowel motility after surgery. It results from the handling or reconstruction of the intestine during surgery and limited dietary intake before and after surgery. POI is normal after abdominal surgery and may occur after nonabdominal surgery. After abdominal surgery, motility in the large intestine may be reduced for 2 to 7 days. Motility in the small intestine resumes within several hours after surgery.

Risk factors for POI include the use of opioids, immobility, older age, prior abdominal surgery, and early postoperative feeding. Use of opioid analgesia may prolong the duration of POI. Abdominal cramps, increasing abdominal distention, constipation, nausea, vomiting, and dehydration often accompany POI.[15]

Hiccups (singultus) are intermittent spasms of the diaphragm caused by irritation of the phrenic nerve, which innervates the diaphragm. The phrenic nerve may be irritated after surgery by gastric distention, intestinal obstruction, intraabdominal bleeding, or a subphrenic abscess. Indirect irritation of the phrenic nerve may occur with acid-base and electrolyte imbalances. Reflex irritation may come from drinking hot or cold liquids or from the presence of a nasogastric (NG) tube. Hiccups usually last a short time and stop spontaneously.

❖ NURSING MANAGEMENT: GASTROINTESTINAL PROBLEMS

◆ Nursing Assessment

Ask the patient about feelings of nausea. If nausea is present, assess the severity using a verbal descriptor or numeric scale. If vomiting occurs, determine the quantity, characteristics, and color of the vomitus. Assess the abdomen for distention and presence of bowel sounds. Because bowel sounds are often absent or diminished right after surgery, auscultate all 4 quadrants to determine the presence, frequency, and characteristics of the sounds. The return of normal bowel motility is usually accompanied by passing gas or stool and the ability to tolerate oral intake without nausea or vomiting.

◆ Nursing Diagnoses

Nursing diagnoses and collaborative problems related to GI problems include:
- Nausea and vomiting
- Electrolyte imbalance
- Fluid imbalance
- Potential complications: POI, hiccups

◆ Nursing Implementation

When the patient is NPO, give IV fluids to maintain fluid and electrolyte balance. Begin oral fluids as ordered and tolerated. Depending on the type of the surgery, the patient may begin oral intake as soon as the gag reflex returns. When starting oral intake, offer clear liquids first and continue the IV fluids, usually at a reduced rate. If the patient tolerates oral intake, the IV fluids are stopped.

Be alert to prevent aspiration if the patient vomits while still sleepy from anesthesia. Position the patient in the lateral recovery position and have suction equipment available. Interventions for PONV include monitoring fluid status and giving antiemetic drugs (see Table 41.1). Consider prophylactic antiemetic drugs for patients at high risk for PONV.[16] Complementary and alternative therapy interventions for PONV (e.g., imagery, music, aromatherapy, acupressure) may help.

Constipation may be prevented using bowel protocols that include the use of a stool softener and laxative. Assess the patient regularly to detect the return of peristalsis. Encourage the patient to expel gas. Gas pains tend to become pronounced on the second or third postoperative day. Ambulation and frequent repositioning may provide relief. Positioning the patient on the right side permits gas to rise along the transverse colon and aids its release. Bisacodyl (Dulcolax) suppositories may be given to stimulate colonic peristalsis and expulsion of gas and stool. Resuming a normal diet after bowel sounds have returned also aids the return of normal peristalsis.

The goal of treatment for POI is the relief of associated symptoms and return of normal GI function. Management includes bowel rest or the withholding of solid foods with a gradual reintroduction of food starting with clear liquids. Advance the diet to solid food with an ongoing assessment of tolerance to oral intake.

An NG tube may be needed to decompress the stomach to prevent nausea, vomiting, and abdominal distention. Oral care is critical for comfort and stimulation of salivary glands when the patient is NPO or has an NG tube.

URINARY PROBLEMS

Etiology

Low urine output (800 to 1500 mL) in the first 24 hours after surgery may be expected regardless of fluid intake. Causes include increased aldosterone and ADH secretion resulting from the stress of surgery; fluid restriction before surgery; and fluid loss through surgery, drainage, and diaphoresis. By the second or third day, after fluid has been mobilized and the immediate stress reaction subsides, the patient will begin to have increasing urine output.

Acute urinary retention can occur for a variety of reasons. Anesthesia depresses the nervous system, including the micturition reflex arc and the higher centers that influence it. This allows the bladder to fill more completely than normal before the patient feels the urge to void. Anesthesia also impedes voluntary micturition. Anticholinergic and opioid drugs interfere with the ability to start voiding or to empty the bladder completely.

Urinary retention is more likely to occur after lower abdominal or pelvic surgery because spasms or guarding of the abdominal and pelvic muscles interferes with their normal function in micturition. Pain may alter perception and interfere with the patient's awareness of bladder filling. Immobility and bed rest impair voiding ability. The supine position reduces the ability to relax the perineal muscles and external sphincter.

Oliguria (diminished output of urine) can be a sign of renal failure and is a less common, although more serious, problem after surgery. It may result from renal ischemia caused by inadequate renal perfusion.

❖ NURSING MANAGEMENT: URINARY PROBLEMS

◆ Nursing Assessment

Examine the urine for both quantity and quality. Note the color, amount, and odor of the urine. Assess indwelling catheters for patency. Urine output should be at least 0.5 mL/kg/hr. To

decrease the risk for catheter-associated urinary tract infection (CAUTI), remove the catheter as soon as possible or within 24 hours, unless there is a reason to continue its use. Most patients void within 6 to 8 hours after surgery. If no voiding occurs, scan or percuss the suprapubic area for signs of bladder fullness or distention.

◆ Nursing Diagnoses

Nursing diagnoses and collaborative problems related to urinary problems include:
- Urinary retention
- Potential complication: CAUTI, acute kidney injury

◆ Nursing Implementation

Reassure the patient about the ability to void. You can promote voiding by helping the patient into a normal position. Other helpful techniques include providing privacy, running water, offering water for the patient to drink, or pouring warm water over the perineum. Walking, preferably to the bathroom, and the use of a bedside commode are other measures to help with voiding.

The HCP often leaves an order to catheterize the patient in 6 to 8 hours if voiding has not occurred. Because of the risk for CAUTI, first confirm that the bladder is full. Consider fluid intake during and after surgery and determine bladder fullness (e.g., discomfort with bladder palpation). Scan the bladder with a portable ultrasound to assess volume of urine in the bladder and avoid unnecessary catheterization. If catheterization is needed, a straight catheterization, as compared to an indwelling catheter, is preferred to limit the risk for CAUTI.

INTEGUMENTARY PROBLEMS

Etiology

Surgery generally involves an incision through the skin and underlying tissues, disrupting the protective skin barrier. Wound healing is a major concern after surgery. One of the greatest risks during the perioperative period is SSI. SSIs account for 14% to 16% of hospital-acquired infections and are associated with prolonged hospitalizations, increased costs, and poor patient outcomes.[17] Many are preventable with using evidence-based strategies (e.g., hand hygiene; selection, timing, and duration of prophylactic antibiotics; surgical site skin preparation; maintaining perioperative normothermia).[18] Adhering to these strategies can reduce the incidence of SSIs, a major goal of the SCIP initiative.[14]

SSIs may result from wound contamination from 3 major sources: (1) exogenous flora present in the environment and on the skin, (2) oral flora, and (3) intestinal flora. The incidence of SSI is higher in patients who are malnourished, immunosuppressed, or older, or who have had a long hospital stay or a lengthy surgical procedure (more than 3 hours). Patients post bowel surgery, particularly after a traumatic injury, are at high risk. SSI may involve the entire incision and may extend downward through deeper tissues. An abscess may form locally, or it may spread throughout entire body cavities, as in peritonitis.

Evidence of SSI usually does not become clear before the third to fifth postoperative day. Local manifestations include redness, swelling, and increasing pain and tenderness at the site. Systemic manifestations are fever and leukocytosis.

An accumulation of fluid in a wound may create pressure, impair circulation and wound healing, and predispose the patient to infection. To allow for drainage, the HCP may place a drain in the incision or make a stab wound next to the incision. Drains may be of soft rubber and drain into a dressing, or firm catheters attached to a Hemovac or other source of gentle suction.

Adequate nutrition is essential for wound healing. The patient who is well nourished before surgery can tolerate the lack of nutritional intake for several days. However, the patient with preexisting nutritional deficits that occur with chronic diseases (e.g., diabetes, ulcerative colitis, alcoholism) is more prone to problems of wound healing. The patient who cannot meet nutritional needs may need enteral or parenteral nutrition to promote healing.

❖ NURSING MANAGEMENT: SURGICAL WOUNDS

◆ Nursing Assessment

Assessment of the wound and dressing requires knowledge of the type of wound, the drains inserted, and expected drainage related to the specific type of surgery. Immediately after surgery, check the wound every 15 to 30 minutes or as ordered. When drainage appears on the dressing, record the type, amount, color, and odor of drainage. Assess the effect of position changes on drainage. A small amount of serous drainage is common from any type of wound. If a drain is in place, assess the amount of drainage and compare to what is expected. Expected drainage from tubes is outlined in Table 19.7. An abdominal incision with an accompanying drain will likely

have a moderate amount of serosanguineous drainage in the first 24 hours. In contrast, an inguinal herniorrhaphy should have only minimal serous drainage.

In general, expect the drainage to change from sanguineous (red) to serosanguineous (pink) to serous (clear yellow). Purulent drainage may occur with an SSI. The drainage should decrease over hours or days, depending on the type of surgery. *Wound dehiscence* (separation and disruption of previously joined wound edges) may be preceded by a sudden discharge of brown, pink, or clear drainage. (Wound dehiscence is discussed in Chapter 11.) Notify the HCP of any excess or abnormal drainage or significant changes in vital signs.

◆ Nursing Diagnoses

Nursing diagnoses related to surgical wounds include:
- Surgical wound
- Risk for infection

◆ Nursing Implementation

The incision may be covered with a dressing right after surgery. Many HCPs prefer to change the first postoperative dressing. If the initial operative dressing is saturated, follow agency policy as to whether you should change or simply reinforce the dressing. Skin graft dressings may stay in place for 3 to 5 days to avoid disturbing the graft site and promote graft acceptance. Specially trained nurses may change these dressings. (Skin grafts are discussed in Chapter 23.)

TABLE 19.7 Output From Tubes, Drains, and Catheters

Substance	Daily Amount	Color	Odor	Consistency
Indwelling Catheter				
Urine	800–1500 mL for first 24 hr Minimum expected output: 0.5 mL/kg/hr	Clear, yellow	Ammonia	Watery
Nasogastric Tube or Gastrostomy Tube				
Gastric contents	<1500 mL/day	Pale, yellow-green Bloody after GI surgery	Sour	Watery
Open Drains (e.g., Penrose)				
Wound drainage	Varies with procedure May decrease over hours or days	Varies with procedure Initially may be sanguineous or sero- sanguineous, changing to serous	Same as wound dress- ing Foul odor may indicate infection	Thin, watery
Closed Suction Drains (e.g., Hemovac, Jackson-Pratt)				
Wound drainage	Varies with procedure May decrease over hours or days	Varies with procedure Initially may be sanguineous or sero- sanguineous, changing to serous	Little to no odor Foul odor may indicate infection	Thin, watery
T-Tube				
Bile	500 mL	Bright yellow to dark green	Acid	Thick
Mediastinal Chest Tube				
Wound drainage post car- diothoracic surgery	Varies with procedure Should decrease over several hours after surgery	Sanguineous or serosanguineous	N/A	Thin
Pleural Chest Tube				
Fluid that has collected in the pleural space	Varies with procedure Decreases over hours or days>100 mL/hr is considered excessive	Varies with indication for insertion and fluid collected in the pleural spaces	N/A	Varies with indication for insertion

When you change a dressing, note the number and type of drains present and avoid dislodging the drains. Inspect the incision site carefully. The area around the sutures may be slightly reddened and swollen, which is an expected inflammatory response. However, the skin around the incision should be of normal color and temperature. If the wound is healing by primary intention, has little or no drainage, or has no drains in place, a single-layer dressing or no dressing is sufficient. Use a multilayer dressing when drains are in place, moderate to heavy drainage is occurring, or healing occurs other than by primary intention. (Wound healing and care are discussed in Chapter 11.)

DISCHARGE FROM THE PACU

The choice of discharge site is based on patient acuity, access to follow-up care, and the potential for complications. The decision to discharge the patient from the PACU is based on written discharge criteria approved by the agency's anesthesiology and medical staff[1] (Table 19.8). Standardized scoring systems (e.g., *Modified Aldrete Scoring System*) are often used to determine the patient's general condition and readiness for discharge from the PACU.

Discharge to Clinical Unit

Before discharging the patient from the PACU to the clinical unit, give a hand-off report about the patient to the receiving nurse. The report summarizes the operative and postanesthesia period. It should include information as to where the patient's caregivers are waiting. Nurse-to-nurse communication must be accurate and allow for questions. The use of a standardized communication tool, such as SBAR (*Situation-Background-Assessment-Recommendation*), provides a complete report and enhances a safe transfer of the patient from PACU to the clinical unit (Table 19.9).

When you receive the patient on the clinical unit, assist the PACU transport staff to safely move the patient from the stretcher to the bed. Take care to protect IV lines, drains, and traction devices. Obtain vital signs and compare the patient status with the report provided by the PACU nurse. After this, perform a more focused assessment and initiate postoperative orders and nursing care (Table 19.10).

TABLE 19.8 Surgery Discharge Criteria

PACU Discharge Criteria (Phase I)
- Patient awake, easily arousable (or baseline)
- Vital signs at baseline or stable
- No excess bleeding or drainage
- No respiratory depression
- O_2 saturation >90%
- Pain controlled or acceptable
- Nausea and vomiting controlled
- Report given

Ambulatory Surgery Discharge Criteria (Phase II or Extended Observation)
- All PACU discharge criteria (Phase I) met
- No IV opioid drugs for last 30 minutes
- Voided if appropriate to surgical procedure or orders
- Able to ambulate if not contraindicated
- Responsible adult present to accompany and drive patient home
- Written discharge instructions given and patient and caregiver understanding confirmed

---

TABLE 19.9 Postoperative SBAR Hand-Off Communication

Situation
Patient _____ Date of birth _____
Transferring to Room # _____ Surgeon _____
ACP _____ Type of Anesthesia _____
Procedure _____
Surgical site(s) _____
Past medical history _____
Code status _____ Isolation precautions _____

Background
Allergies _____
Medications received in PACU _____
IV site/fluids _____
Dressings and/or drains _____
Significant OR events _____

Assessment
PACU vital signs T _____ P _____ RR _____ BP _____ O_2 Sat _____
O_2 source _____ FIO_2 _____
Pain rating at discharge _____
Method of pain management _____
Last dose of pain medication _____
Mental status _____
Nausea/vomiting at discharge _____
Intake _____ Output _____
Laboratory tests _____
Recovery comments _____

Recommendations
Equipment needed _____
Orders to be completed _____
Family _____
Other notes _____
Transferring RN _____ Phone # for questions _____
Receiving RN _____

TABLE 19.10 Nursing Assessment

Care of Patient on Admission to Clinical Unit
1. Record time of patient's return to unit and assess airway, breathing, and circulation.
2. Obtain baseline vital signs, including O_2 saturation.
3. Assess neurologic status, including level of consciousness and movement of extremities.
4. Assess level of pain:
   - Last dose and type of pain control
   - Current pain rating
5. Assess wound, dressing, and drainage tubes:
   - Type and amount of drainage
   - Tubing connected to gravity or suction drainage (per orders)
6. Assess color, temperature, and appearance of skin.
7. Position for airway maintenance, comfort, and safety (bed in low position, side rails up).
8. Check IV infusion:
   - Type of solution
   - Amount of fluid remaining
   - Patency and flow rate
   - Condition of insertion site and size of catheter
9. Assess urinary status:
   - Time of voiding
   - Presence of catheter, patency, and total output
   - Bladder distention or urge to void
10. Assess for any nausea or vomiting.
    - Availability of emesis basin and tissues
11. Position call bell within reach, and orient patient to use of call bell.
12. Determine emotional state and provide support as needed.
13. Check for presence of caregiver.
    - Patient and caregiver oriented to immediate environment
14. Check and carry out postoperative orders.

AMBULATORY SURGERY

Phase II and Extended Observation

Advances in minimally invasive and noninvasive procedures, anesthesia, and analgesia have resulted in an increase in ambulatory surgical procedures. Ambulatory surgery patients include those patients receiving Phase II and extended observation postoperative care (Table 19.1). PONV and pain are common problems after ambulatory surgery. These can lead to delirium, prolonged PACU stay, delayed discharge, readmission, delayed resumption of usual activities, and decreased patient satisfaction.

Ambulatory Surgery Discharge

The patient leaving an ambulatory surgery setting must be hemodynamically stable, mobile, alert, and able to provide a degree of self-care when discharged to home (Table 19.8). PONV and pain must be under control. Overall, the patient must be stable and near the level of preoperative functioning for discharge from the unit. The patient may not drive and must be accompanied by an adult at the time of discharge. Carefully assess the patient's readiness for discharge and home care needs. Determine availability of caregivers (e.g., family, friends) and access to (1) a pharmacy for prescriptions, (2) a phone in the case of an emergency, and (3) follow-up care.

INFORMATICS IN PRACTICE

Discharge Teaching

- When discharging a patient who needs a complex dressing change and the written instructions are not adequate, consider using a video. This may be available on the hospital's television system or the Internet (e.g., YouTube).
- If using a video from the Internet, check to ensure that the procedure is properly performed.
- The patient and caregiver can view the video or pictures at home as a reference when performing the procedure.
- Have the patient and/or caregiver provide teach back information and/or demonstration.

Planning for Discharge and Follow-up Care

Preparation for the patient's discharge is an ongoing process that begins before surgery. Include the patient and caregiver in discharge planning and provide them with the information and support to make informed decisions about ongoing care. The informed patient is prepared as events unfold and gradually assumes more responsibility for self-care during the postoperative period.

As discharge approaches, be sure that the patient and caregiver(s) have the following information:

- Symptoms to report (e.g., fever, increased incisional drainage, unrelieved incisional pain, discomfort in other parts of the body)
- When and how to take prescribed drugs and possible side effects
- Care of incision and any dressings, including bathing recommendations
- Activities allowed and prohibited, when various activities can be resumed safely (e.g., driving, return to work, sexual intercourse, leisure activities)
- Dietary restrictions or modifications

- Where and when to return for follow-up appointment
- Answers to any questions or concerns

Common reasons patients seek help after discharge include unrelieved pain, need for advice about drugs, and wound issues (e.g., drainage). Attention to complete discharge instructions may prevent needless distress for the patient and caregiver. Standardized, preprinted discharge instructions that are surgery specific and easy to read ensure that information is complete.

Record the discharge teaching in the chart. For the patient, the postoperative phase of care continues and extends into the recuperative period. Assessment and evaluation of the patient after discharge may be done with a follow-up call or by a visit from a home health nurse, who can address any specific questions and concerns.

Increasingly, patients are discharged from the hospital with many care needs. They may be transferred to transitional care facilities, to long-term care facilities, or directly to their homes. When discharged directly to home, the patient is expected to continue self-care, with help from caregivers or home health care personnel (e.g., nurses, physical therapists). The care may include dressing changes, wound care, catheter or drain care, home antibiotics, or continued physical therapy. Working together with the discharge planner or case manager, ensure the patient's safe transition from hospital-based care to community- or home-based care.

Gerontologic Considerations: Postoperative Patient

The older surgical patient deserves special consideration. The older adult has decreased respiratory function, including decreased ability to cough and decreased thoracic compliance. These changes lead to an increase in the work of breathing and a decreased ability to eliminate drugs. Carefully monitor reactions to anesthetic drugs. Pneumonia is a common complication in older adults.

Altered vascular function in the older adult is due to atherosclerosis and decreased elasticity in the blood vessels. Cardiac function is often compromised with limited compensatory responses to changes in BP and volume. Circulating blood volume decreases. Hypertension is common. Cardiovascular status needs to be monitored closely throughout surgery and the postoperative period.

Drug toxicity is a potential problem in the older adult. Renal perfusion normally decreases, along with a reduced ability to remove drugs that the kidneys excrete. Decreased liver function leads to reduced drug metabolism and increased drug activity. Carefully assess renal and liver function to prevent drug overdose and toxicity.

Observing for changes in mental status is an important part of postoperative care in older adults. Factors such as age, history of alcohol abuse, poor baseline cognition, hypoxia, metabolic imbalances, hypotension, and polypharmacy can contribute to postoperative delirium. Anesthetics, especially anticholinergic and benzodiazepine drugs, increase the risk for delirium.

Pain control in the older patient is challenging because of possible preexisting cognitive deficits, impaired communication, and physiologic changes that affect drug metabolism. Patients may hesitate to ask for pain medication because they believe pain is inevitable with surgery. Some older patients may fear addiction or be nervous about using PCA machines. Thoroughly assess pain in a surgical patient who does not report any pain. Encourage the use of analgesics. Explain to the patient and caregiver that untreated pain has a negative effect on recovery.

CASE STUDY
Postoperative Patient

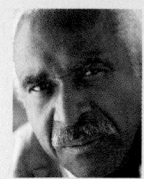

(© BananaStock/
BananaStock/
Thinkstock.)

Patient Profile

E.G., a 74-yr-old retired college professor, has just undergone surgery for a fractured hip. He fell off a ladder while painting his house. E.G.'s medical history includes type 2 diabetes and COPD. The surgery, done while he was under general anesthesia, lasted 3 hours.

Subjective Data

- Active walker in his home community
- Smokes 1 pack of cigarettes per day × 58 years
- Always had problems sleeping
- Difficulty hearing, wears hearing aid
- Upset with injury and its impact on life
- Is a widower and has no relatives nearby or friends to assist with care
- Reports pain is 8 on a 0 to 10 scale on arrival to PACU

Objective Data

- Admitted to PACU with abduction pillow between his legs, one peripheral IV catheter, a self-suction drain from the hip dressing, an indwelling urinary catheter
- O_2 saturation 91% on 40% O_2 face mask

Interprofessional Care
Postoperative Orders

- Vital signs per PACU routine
- Capillary blood glucose level on arrival and every 4 hours. Call for blood glucose level <70 mg/dL or >250 mg/dL. Follow agency guidelines for management of hypoglycemia.
- 0.45 normal saline at 100 mL/hr
- Morphine via patient-controlled analgesia 1 mg q10min (20 mg max in 4 hr) for pain
- Advance diet as tolerated
- Incentive spirometry q1hr × 10 while awake
- O_2 therapy to keep O_2 saturation >90%

- Respiratory: albuterol 2.5 mg via nebulizer every 4 hours PRN for wheezing
- Neurovascular checks q1hr × 4 hr
- Empty and measure self-suction drain every shift
- Strict intake and output

Discussion Questions

1. What are the potential postanesthesia problems you may expect with E.G.?
2. **Priority Decision:** What priority nursing interventions would be appropriate to prevent these problems from occurring?
3. **Collaboration:** Which interventions could you delegate to unlicensed assistive personnel (UAP)?
4. What factors predispose E.G. to the following problems: atelectasis, SSI, and VTE?
5. How would you determine E.G. is sufficiently recovered from general anesthesia to be discharged to the clinical unit?
6. What potential postoperative problems on the clinical unit might you expect?
7. What are risk factors for his developing postoperative delirium? What are the signs and symptoms of delirium?
8. Why is drug toxicity a potential problem for E.G.?
9. **Priority Decision:** Based on the assessment data, identify 3 priority nursing diagnoses. Are there any collaborative problems?
10. **Evidence-Based Practice:** E.G. tells you he does not want the "catheter" out because he does not want anyone to help him to the bathroom. How would you respond to this request?
11. **Patient-Centered Care:** What teaching will you provide so that E.G. can successfully self-manage his care?
12. **Collaboration:** What referrals may be indicated based on E.G.'s medical history?
13. **Safety:** Identify 2 areas of risk for injury to E.G. What actions can you take to ensure patient safety?
14. **Quality Improvement:** What outcomes would indicate that interprofessional care with respiratory therapy was effective?

Answers available at *http://evolve.elsevier.com/Lewis/medsurg.*

BRIDGE TO NCLEX EXAMINATION

The number of the question corresponds to the same-numbered outcome at the beginning of the chapter.

1. What are the *priority* interventions the nurse performs when admitting a patient to the PACU?
   a. Assess the surgical site, noting presence and character of drainage.
   b. Assess the amount of urine output and the presence of bladder distention.
   c. Assess for airway patency and quality of respirations and obtain vital signs.
   d. Review results of intraoperative laboratory values and medications received.

2. A patient is admitted to the PACU after major abdominal surgery. During the initial assessment the patient tells the nurse he thinks he is going to "throw up." A *priority* nursing intervention is to
   a. increase the rate of the IV fluids.
   b. give antiemetic medication as ordered.
   c. obtain vital signs, including O_2 saturation.
   d. position patient in lateral recovery position.

3. After admitting a postoperative patient to the clinical unit, which assessment data require the *most* immediate attention?
   a. O_2 saturation of 85%
   b. Respiratory rate of 13/min
   c. Temperature of 100.4° F (38° C)
   d. Blood pressure of 90/60 mm Hg

4. A 70-kg postoperative patient has an average urine output of 25 mL/hr during the first 8 hours. The *priority* nursing intervention(s) given this assessment would be to
   a. notify the surgeon and expect obtaining blood work to evaluate renal function.
   b. perform a straight catheterization to measure the amount of urine in the bladder.
   c. continue to monitor the patient because this is a normal finding during this time period.
   d. evaluate the patient's fluid volume status since surgery and obtain a bladder ultrasound.

5. Discharge criteria for the Phase II patient include (*select all that apply*)
   a. no nausea or vomiting.
   b. ability to drive self home.
   c. no respiratory depression.
   d. written discharge instructions understood.
   e. opioid pain medication given 45 minutes ago.

1. c, 2. d, 3. a, 4. d, 5. c, d, e

For rationales to these answers and even more NCLEX review questions, visit *http://evolve.elsevier.com/Lewis/medsurg.*

EVOLVE WEBSITE/RESOURCES LIST

REFERENCES

1. Schick L, Windle P: *Perianesthesia nursing core curriculum: Preprocedure, phase i and phase II PACU nursing*, ed 3, St Louis, 2016, Elsevier.

2. Odom-Forren J: *Drain's perianesthesia nursing: A critical care approach*, ed 7, St Louis, 2018, Elsevier.

*3. Smallwood CD, Walsh BK: Noninvasive monitoring of oxygen and ventilation, *Respir Care* 62:6, 2017.

*4. Patino M, Kalin M, Griffin A, et al: Comparison of postoperative respiratory monitoring by acoustic and transthoracic impedance technologies in pediatric patients at risk of respiratory depression, *Anesthes Analg* 124:6, 2017.

*5. Gillies M, Sander M, Shaw A, et al: Current research priorities in perioperative intensive care medicine, *Intensive Care Med* 43:9, 2017.

*6. Auffret V, Becerra Munoz V, Loirat A, et al: Transcatheter aortic valve implantation versus surgical aortic valve replacement in lower surgical risk patients with chronic obstructive pulmonary disease, *Am J Cardiol* 120:10, 2017.

*7. Feng B, Lin J, Jin J et al: Thirty–day postoperative complications following primary total knee replacement arthroplasty: A retrospective study of incidence and risk factors at a single center in China, *Chin Med J* 130:21, 2017.

*8. Misal U, Joshi S, Shaikh M: Delayed recovery from anesthesia: A postgraduate educational review, *Anesth Essays Res* 10:2, 2016.

*9. Takagi H, Ando T, Umemoto T: Perioperative depression or anxiety and postoperative mortality in cardiac surgery: A systematic review and meta-analysis, *Heart Vessels* 32:12, 2017.

*10. Oh E, Fong, T, Hsheih T, et al: Delirium in older persons advances in diagnosis and treatment, *JAMA* 318:12, 2017.

*11. Singh K, Bohl D, Ahn J, et al: Multimodal analgesia versus intravenous patient-controlled analgesia for minimally invasive transforaminal lumbar interbody fusion procedures, *Spine* 42:15, 2017.

12. Polomano R, Fillman M, Giordano N et al: Multimodal analgesia for acute postoperative and trauma-related pain, *AJN* 117:3, 2017.

13. The Joint Commission: Specifications manual for national hospital inpatient quality measures. Retrieved from *www.jointcommission.org/specifications_manual_for_national_hospital_inpatient_quality_measures.aspx*.

*14. Ziolkowski N, Rogers A, Xiong W, et al: The impact of operative time and hypothermia in acute burn surgery, *Burns* 43:1673, 2017.

*15. Venara A, Neunlist M, Slim K et al: Postoperative ileus: Pathophysiology, incidence, and prevention, *J Visc Surg* 153:6, 2016.

*16. Cao X, White, P, Ma, H: An update on the management of postoperative nausea and vomiting, *J Anesthes* 31:617, 2017.

17. Rothrock J: *Alexander's care of the patient in surgery*, ed 15, 2015, St Louis.

18. Berrios-Torres S, Umscheid C, Bratzler D, et al: Centers for Disease Control and Prevention guidelines for the prevention of surgical site infection, *JAMA Surg* 152:784, 2017.

*Evidence-based information for clinical practice.

CASE STUDY
Managing Care of Multiple Patients

You have been called into work at 10:00 AM to cover patients for a nurse who had a family emergency. You take over care for the following 3 patients on a surgical unit. You have 1 UAP available who is assigned to help you. Two other RNs are on the unit.

Patients

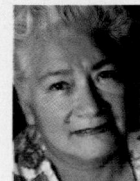

(© Ryan McVay/Photodisc/Thinkstock.)

F.D., a 72-yr-old woman, was admitted to the hospital with compromised circulation of the right lower leg and a necrotic right foot as a complication of her diabetes. She is scheduled for a below-the-knee amputation of the right leg at 1:00 PM today. She has been NPO since midnight. Her morning capillary blood glucose level was 198 mg/dL. She received 4 units of regular insulin at 8 AM. She has an IV of normal saline infusing at 125 mL/hr.

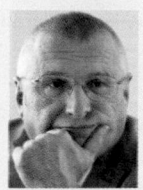

(© shironosov/iStock/Thinkstock.)

G.S., a 63-yr-old man, was admitted to the hospital for severe pain and intractable vomiting from acute cholecystitis. G.S.'s medical history includes hypertension and type 2 diabetes. He had a laparoscopic cholecystectomy yesterday afternoon. His capillary blood glucose 1 hour ago was 135 mg/dL.

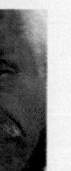

(© BananaStock/BananaStock/Thinkstock.)

E.G., a 74-yr-old man, had surgery for a fractured hip yesterday. He is currently receiving dextrose 5% in 0.45 normal saline at 100 mL/hr, morphine via patient-controlled analgesia at 1 mg q10min (20 mg max in 4 hr) for pain, heparin 5000 units subcutaneously every 12 hours, and O_2 to keep O_2 saturation >93%. He has a self-suction drain in place at the surgical site. He has good respiratory effort when using his incentive spirometer.

Discussion Questions

1. **Priority Decision:** After receiving report, which patient should you see first? Provide a rationale for your decision.
2. **Collaboration:** Which tasks should you delegate to the UAP? *(select all that apply)*
   a. Explain discharge instructions to G.S.
   b. Obtain noon vital signs on E.G. and F.D.
   c. Measure capillary blood glucose levels on F.D. and G.S.
   d. Confirm E.G.'s understanding of how to use the PCA pump.
   e. Remind E.G. and G.S. to use their incentive spirometers every hour.
3. **Priority Decision and Collaboration:** When you enter F.D.'s room, you find her somewhat withdrawn and lethargic. Her face is cool and slightly clammy. What initial action would be most appropriate?
   a. Give 1 ampule of D_{50} IV stat.
   b. Increase F.D.'s IV rate to 150 mL/hr.
   c. Obtain a stat capillary blood glucose level.
   d. Ask the UAP to give F.D. a glass of orange juice.

Answers available at *http://evolve.elsevier.com/Lewis/medsurg*.

Case Study Progression

F.D.'s capillary blood glucose reading was 52 mg/dL. You notify her HCP and give 1 ampule of D_{50} IV dextrose as ordered. You then change her IV infusion to D_5 ½NS. You check her capillary blood glucose within 15 minutes and then monitor her blood glucose levels each hour.

4. A preoperative checklist for F.D. is used to ensure completion of *(select all that apply)*
   a. removal of nail polish and jewelry.
   b. signed and witnessed informed consent.
   c. patient understanding of sensory information.
   d. identification of surgical site with surgical skin marker.
   e. notification of family of where to wait during the surgery.
5. F.D. tells you that she is afraid they may amputate the wrong leg. She tells you she has read stories of that happening at other hospitals. Your *best* response to F.D. would be to
   a. ask her if she would like a sedative to calm her fears.
   b. reassure her that it has never happened in this hospital.
   c. explain the "time-out" procedure for preventing such errors.
   d. offer to go to the operating room with her to ensure the correct leg is amputated.
6. **Priority Decision:** The laboratory calls to report that E.G.'s aPTT (activated partial thromboplastin time) is 84 seconds. You assess him and find that the hip dressing is saturated with serosanguinous drainage. The next dose of heparin is due at 2100 this evening; the last dose was at 0900 this morning. His blood pressure is 92/54 with a heart rate of 110 bpm. Respiratory rate is 30 breaths/min, and O_2 saturation is 98% on 2 L of O_2. The nursing *priority* for this patient would be to
   a. notify physical therapy that his session today will have to be postponed until evening.
   b. notify the previous RN that a medication error occurred with the patient's heparin dose at 0900.
   c. send an order to the laboratory for stat CBC and type and screen for 4 units of packed red blood cells.
   d. notify the provider of the aPTT result and anticipate orders for reversal agent, such as protamine.
7. **Collaboration:** Which instructions should you give to the UAP who will be helping E.G. with ADLs? *(Select all that apply.)*
   a. Use a soft toothbrush for oral care.
   b. Provide an emery board for nail care.
   c. Avoid overinflating blood pressure cuffs.
   d. Use an electric razor to shave the patient.
   e. Offer mouthwash with alcohol for rinsing.
8. **Management Decision:** When providing discharge instructions to G.S., he tells you that the UAP told him that he could do whatever activity he was comfortable doing—to let pain guide his progress. Your *initial* reaction to this statement should be to
   a. ask the UAP to clarify what was said to G.S.
   b. report the UAP's actions to the nurse manager.
   c. teach G.S. about the reason for activity restrictions.
   d. clarify the discharge instructions with the health care provider.

20

Assessment and Management: Visual Problems

Jonel L. Gomez

Be the beacon of light in someone's darkness.

Randi Fine

ⓔ http://evolve.elsevier.com/Lewis/medsurg/

CONCEPTUAL FOCUS

Coping

Functional Ability

Infection

Sensory Perception

LEARNING OUTCOMES

1. Describe the structures and functions of the visual system.
2. Explain the physiologic processes involved in normal vision.
3. Obtain significant subjective and objective assessment data related to the visual system.
4. Perform a physical assessment of the visual system using the appropriate techniques.
5. Distinguish normal from common abnormal findings of a physical assessment of the visual system.
6. Link the age-related changes in the visual system to differences in assessment findings.

7. Describe the purpose, significance of results, and nursing responsibilities related to diagnostic studies of the visual system.
8. Compare and contrast the types of refractive errors and appropriate corrections.
9. Describe the common causes and assistive measures for severe visual impairment.
10. Discuss nursing measures that promote eye health.
11. Explain the pathophysiology, clinical manifestations, and interprofessional and nursing management of the patient with ocular disorders.
12. Discuss the general preoperative and postoperative care of patients undergoing surgery of the eye.

KEY TERMS

VISUAL SYSTEM

For people to be as independent as possible and take part in fulfilling activities, it is important that the visual system is as functional as possible. The impact of poor vision or blindness can be devastating to activities of daily living (ADLs) and independence. The psychosocial consequences can include decreased quality of life, social isolation, depression, and loss of self-esteem. Vision loss also takes a huge toll on caregivers. This makes our being involved in vision-loss prevention, detection, and treatment strategies important.

STRUCTURES AND FUNCTIONS OF VISUAL SYSTEM

The visual system is part of the central nervous system (CNS). It consists of 2 main parts, the eyes, which contain the image receptors, and the brain. The brain functions to process and interpret the information transmitted from the receptors into images. Anatomically, the visual system is made up of the orbit, the ocular adnexa (external tissues and structures surrounding the eye), the eye, and the visual pathway (optic nerve, optic chiasm, lateral geniculate nucleus, and visual cortex). The entire visual system is important for visual function.

Periocular Structures

Orbit. The orbits, or eye sockets, are the bony structures that house the eyeballs. Seven bones form the orbit: frontal, zygoma, maxilla, ethmoid, sphenoid, lacrimal, and palatine (Fig. 20.1). The average orbit is 35 mm high and 40 mm wide. In addition to the eye, the orbits contain the associated muscles, nerves, blood vessels, and fat.[1]

Within the orbit are 3 main orbital openings, or *fissures,* the optic canal, the superior orbital fissure, and the inferior orbital fissure. They are all important conduits for arteries, veins, and nerves. The optic canal is located at the top of the socket. It provides an entry point for the optic nerve (CN II). The superior orbital fissure is a small slit in the posterior orbit. It is the main entry point for several other cranial nerves to enter the orbit from the brain. These include the oculomotor nerve (CN III),

trochlear nerve (CN IV), trigeminal nerve (CN V), and abducens nerve (CN VI). The inferior orbital fissure is in the floor of the orbit. It holds the zygomatic branch of the maxillary nerve.

There are 6 extraocular muscles: (1) superior and inferior rectus muscles, (2) medial and lateral rectus muscles, and (3) superior and inferior oblique muscles. They emerge from the apex of the orbit and attach to the eye to stabilize and move it (Fig. 20.2). Neuromuscular coordination produces simultaneous movement of the eyes in the same direction.

Ocular Adnexa. The ocular adnexa include the eyebrows, eyelids, eyelashes, and lacrimal system. Eyebrows, eyelids, and eyelashes are vital in protecting the eye. They are a physical barrier to dust and foreign particles. Blinking protects the eye from injury, distributes tears over the anterior surface of the eyeball, and supplies necessary nourishment to surface cells.

The upper and lower eyelids join at the medial and lateral canthi. Eyelid skin is the thinnest skin in the human body, measuring less than 1 mm thick. The upper eyelids contain the levator palpebrae superioris muscle, innervated by the superior division of CN III. This muscle elevates and retracts the upper eyelid. The eyelids close through the action of the orbicularis muscle, which is innervated by CN VII.

Lacrimal System. The lacrimal system includes the structures needed for tear production and drainage. The main lacrimal gland and accessory lacrimal glands make tears. The lacrimal glands, in the superotemporal orbit, are exocrine glands. They make and secrete the aqueous layer of tear film and are responsible for reflex tear production. The tear film moistens the eye and supplies oxygen to the cornea. The accessory lacrimal glands, the *glands of Wolfring* and *glands of Krause,* are found within the conjunctiva of the upper eyelid. They are responsible for baseline tear production. Tears pass over the surface of the eye and then enter the nasolacrimal system. The nasolacrimal drainage system includes the puncta, canaliculi, lacrimal sac, and nasolacrimal duct (Fig. 20.3).

Eyeball. The eyeball, or globe, is composed of 3 layers (Fig 20.4). The tough outer layer is composed of the cornea, conjunctiva, and sclera. The middle layer consists of the uveal tract (iris, choroid

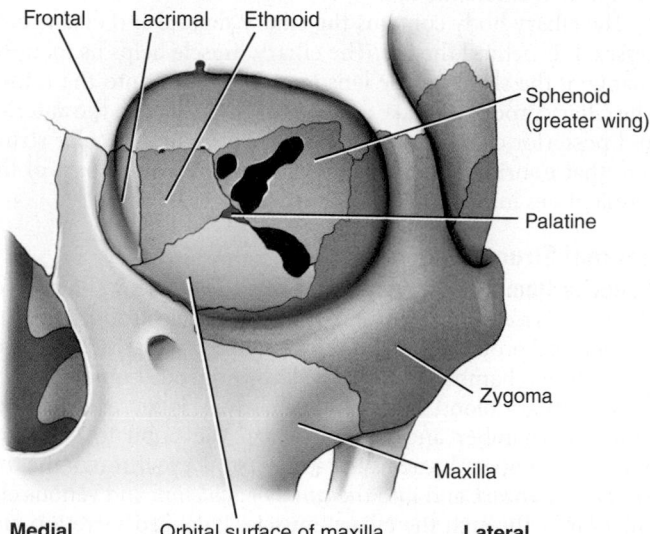

FIG. 20.1 Bones that form the orbit, or eye socket. (From Lampignano J, Kendrick L: *Bontrager's textbook of radiographic positioning and related anatomy,* ed 9, St Louis, 2018, Mosby.)

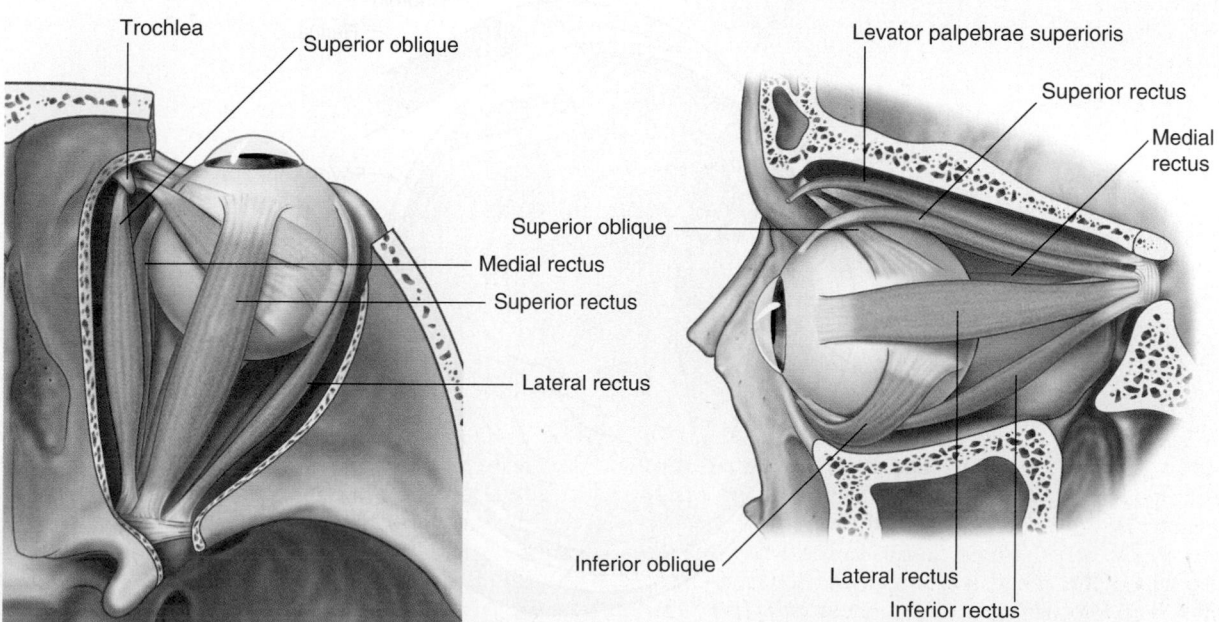

FIG. 20.2 The 6 extraocular muscles. (From Drake R, Vogl AW, Mitchell AWM: *Gray's anatomy for students,* ed 3, Philadelphia, 2015, Churchill Livingstone.)

and ciliary body), and the innermost layer, the retina. The *anterior cavity* is divided into the anterior and posterior chambers. The anterior chamber lies between the iris and posterior surface of the cornea. The posterior chamber lies between the anterior surface of the lens and posterior surface of the iris. The *posterior cavity* lies in the large space behind the lens and in front of the retina.

External Ocular Structures

The conjunctiva is a transparent mucous membrane that covers the inner surfaces of the eyelids and extends over the sclera. Glands in the conjunctiva secrete mucus and tears. Tenon's capsule, also called the fascia bulbi, is a thin layer of fascia that encases the eyeball behind the conjunctiva. The capsule extends posteriorly, ultimately fusing with the optic nerve.

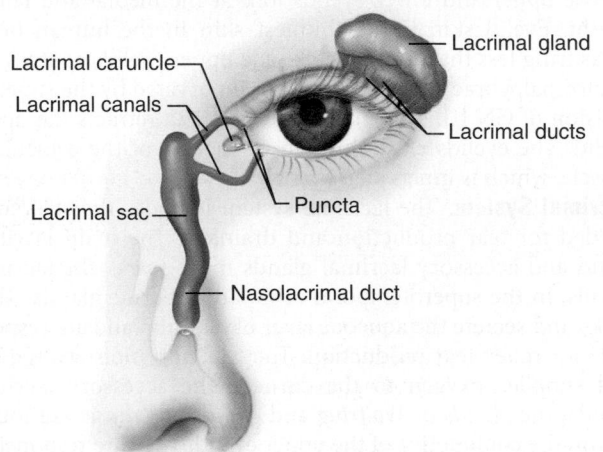

FIG. 20.3 External eye and lacrimal apparatus. Tears made in the lacrimal gland pass over the surface of the eye and enter the lacrimal canal. From there the tears are carried through the nasolacrimal duct to the nasal cavity. (Modified from Patton KT, Thibodeau GA: *Anatomy and physiology,* ed 8, St Louis, 2013, Mosby.)

The cornea allows light to enter the eye. It is transparent and avascular. Its curved shape refracts or bends incoming light rays to help focus them on the retina. The cornea has 6 layers: epithelium, Bowman's layer, stroma, Descemet's membrane, Dua's layer, and endothelium.

The sclera, the white part of the eye, is a fibrous connective tissue layer that protects the eye and helps the eye maintain its shape and structure. The sclera extends from the cornea to the optic nerve. We call the junction of the sclera and cornea the limbus.

Middle Ocular Structures

The iris gives the eye its color. It has a small round opening in the center, the *pupil,* which allows light to enter the eye. The pupil constricts by action of the iris sphincter muscle (under parasympathetic control) and dilates by action of the iris dilator muscle (under sympathetic control). This controls the amount of light that enters the eye.

The ciliary body contains the ciliary muscle and ciliary processes. It is behind the iris. The ciliary muscle helps us focus by changing the shape of the lens to refract light onto the retina. The ciliary processes make aqueous humor for both the anterior and posterior chamber. The choroid is a highly vascular structure that nourishes the ciliary body, iris, and outer part of the retina. It lies inside and parallel to the sclera.

Internal Structures

Aqueous Humor. Aqueous humor fills the anterior chamber of the eye. It is a clear watery fluid composed of electrolytes, growth factors, and proteins. It nourishes the nonvascular structures of the anterior chamber, such as the lens. Aqueous humor is made from capillary blood in the ciliary body. It is secreted into the posterior chamber and flows through the pupil to enter the anterior chamber. Aqueous humor exits the eye through the *trabecular meshwork* and into the *canal of Schlemm* and venous circulation or through the ciliary muscle. Balanced secretion and excretion of aqueous humor is important. Excess production or

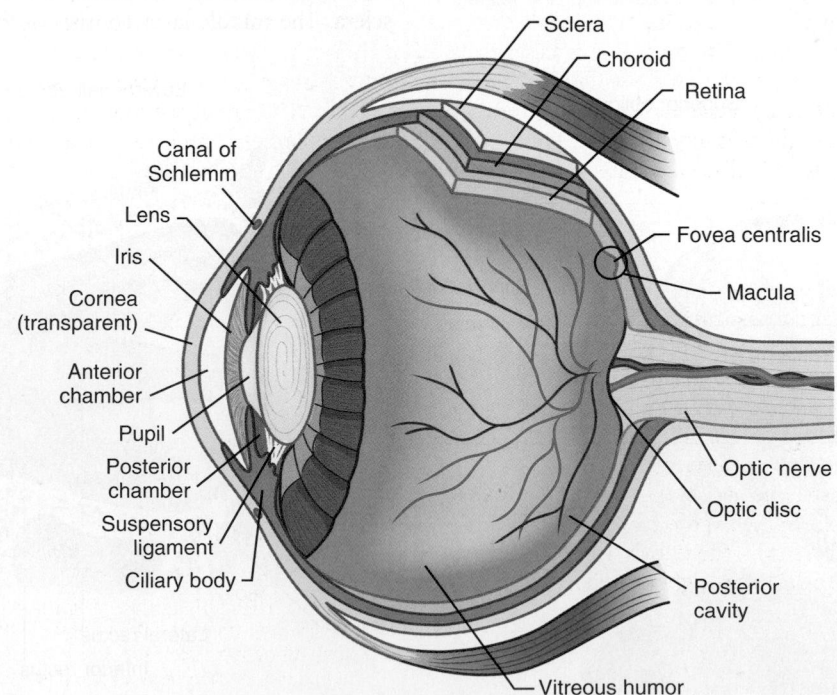

FIG. 20.4 The human eye. (Modified from Patton KT, Thibodeau GA: *Anatomy and physiology,* ed 8, St Louis, 2013, Mosby.)

decreased outflow can increase intraocular pressure (IOP) above the normal 10 to 21 mm Hg, a condition termed *glaucoma*.

Lens. The lens is a biconvex structure behind the iris. It is kept in place by small fibers collectively called the suspensory ligament, or the zonule. The ligament is a series of microscopic wire-like threads that connect the lens to the ciliary body. The primary function of the lens is to change shape to alter the focal distance of the eye. It works with the cornea to refract, or bend light. The lens shape is changed by action of the ciliary body as part of accommodation, a process that allows a person to focus. An example of accommodation is the ability to focus on near objects, such as when reading.

Vitreous Humor. The retina lines the back of the eye, extending from the area of the optic nerve to the ciliary body (Fig. 20.4). Neurons make up most of the retina. Therefore retinal cells are unable to regenerate if destroyed. The retina converts images into a form that the brain can understand and process as vision.

The retina has 2 main parts, the peripheral retina and central retina. The central retina contains the macula and fovea. The macula is about 6 mm in diameter. It is responsible for the central visual field. The fovea is at the center of the macula. This area provides the sharpest visual acuity, which we need for activities in which detail is important, like reading and driving.

The retina contains light-sensitive structures called photoreceptor cells. There are 2 types of photoreceptors, rods and cones. Rods and cones convert light to neural signals, which the nervous system translates into vision. Rods are mostly found in the peripheral retina. They are responsible for most of our peripheral vision and night vision. Rods only perceive light and dark and do not contribute to color vision. Cones are in the central retina, condensed mostly in the fovea. They are responsible for central vision and color vision. There are 3 types of cone cells, red, green, and blue. They all work together to create the full color spectrum.

The retina receives oxygen and nutrients from the choroid and the retinal vasculature. The central retinal artery carries blood and nutrients into the retina. The central retinal vein carries blood away from the retina.

Optic Nerve. The optic nerve, or CN II, transmits visual information from the retina to the brain. The optic nerve begins at the optic disc, which is the region of the retina where the optic nerve and vessels leave the retina. Because there are no photoreceptor cells over the optic disc, there is an anatomic blind spot in this area. In the center of the optic disc is a white, cup-shaped area called the optic cup.

VISUAL PATHWAY

For light to reach the retina, it must pass through many structures: the cornea, aqueous humor, lens, and vitreous humor. These structures must be clear for light to reach the retina and stimulate the photoreceptor cells. Once the image travels through the refractive media, it is focused on the retina (Fig. 20.5). From the retina, the impulses travel through the optic nerve to the optic chiasm, where the nasal fibers of each eye cross over to the other side. Fibers from the left field of both eyes form the left optic tract and travel to the left occipital cortex. The fibers from the right field of both eyes form the right optic tract and travel to the right occipital cortex.

Gerontologic Considerations: Effects of Aging on the Visual System

Every structure of the visual system is subject to changes as a person ages. While many of these changes are relatively benign,

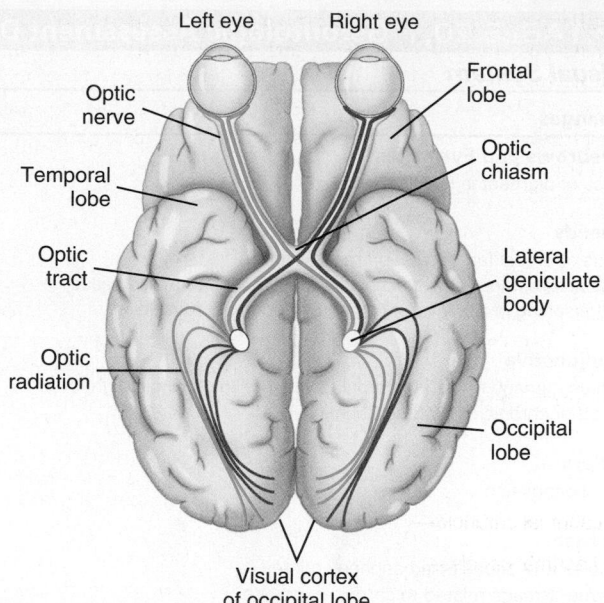

FIG. 20.5 The visual pathway. Fibers from the nasal portion of each retina cross over to the opposite side of the optic chiasma, ending in the lateral geniculate body of the opposite side. Location of a lesion in the visual pathway determines the resulting visual defect.

others may result in severely compromised visual acuity in the older adult. Age-related changes in the visual system and differences in assessment findings are shown in Table 20.1.

ASSESSMENT OF VISUAL SYSTEM

Assessment of the visual system may be as simple as determining a patient's visual acuity or as complex as collecting complete subjective and objective data pertinent to the visual system. The patient in a clinic or office setting is often seeking routine eye care or a change in the prescription of eyewear. However, the patient may have some underlying concerns that he or she does not mention or even recognize. To perform an appropriate visual evaluation, assess what is necessary for the specific patient. While many of these assessments are within your scope of practice, some require special training.

CASE STUDY
Patient Introduction

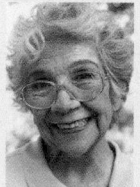

F.M. is an 81-yr-old Hispanic woman who comes to the emergency department with visual changes. F.M. states that her vision "looks like everything is covered with a spider web." She reports seeing periodic light flashes and small white spots "floating" in the air.

(© Jack Hollingsworth/Photodisc/Thinkstock.)

Discussion Questions

1. What are the possible causes of F.M.'s vision problems?
2. What type of assessment would be most appropriate for F.M.: comprehensive, focused, or emergency?
3. What assessment questions will you ask her?

You will learn more about F.M. and her condition as you read through this assessment chapter.

(See p. 354 for more information on F.M.)

Answers available at *http://evolve.elsevier.com/Lewis/medsurg.*

TABLE 20.1 Gerontologic Assessment Differences

Visual System

Changes	Differences in Assessment Findings
Eyebrows and Eyelashes	
Loss of pigment in hair	Graying of eyebrows, eyelashes
Eyelids	
Loss of orbital fat, decreased muscle tone	Entropion, ectropion
Tissue atrophy and stretching, prolapse of fat into eyelid tissue, loosening of the levator palpebrae superioris muscle	Dermatochalasis (excess upper lid skin), ptosis
Conjunctiva	
Tissue damage related to chronic exposure to ultraviolet light or to other chronic environmental exposure	Pinguecula (small yellowish spot usually on medial aspect of conjunctiva)
Sclera	
Lipid deposition	Scleral color yellowish as opposed to bluish
Cornea	
Cholesterol deposits in peripheral cornea	Arcus senilis (milky white-gray ring encircling periphery of cornea) (Fig. 20.6)
Tissue damage related to chronic exposure	Pterygium (thickened, triangular bit of pale tissue that extends from inner canthus of eye to nasal border of cornea)
Decrease in water content, atrophy of nerve fibers	Decreased corneal sensitivity and corneal reflex
Epithelial changes	Loss of corneal luster
Accumulation of lipid deposits	Blurring of vision
Lacrimal Apparatus	
Decreased tear secretion	Dryness
Malposition of eyelid and punctal eversion resulting in tears overflowing lid margins instead of draining through puncta	Tearing, irritated eyes
Iris	
Increased rigidity of iris	Decreased pupil size
Dilator muscle atrophy or weakness	Slower recovery of pupil size after light stimulation
Loss of pigment	Change of iris color
Ciliary muscle becoming smaller, stiffer	Decrease in near vision and accommodation
Lens	
Biochemical changes in lens proteins, oxidative damage, chronic exposure to ultraviolet light	Cataracts
Increased rigidity of lens	Presbyopia
Opacities in lens (also may be related to opacities in cornea and vitreous)	Reports of glare, night vision impaired
Accumulation of yellow substances	Yellow color of lens
Retina	
Retinal vascular changes related to atherosclerosis and hypertension	Narrowed, pale, straighter arterioles. Acute branching
Decrease in number of cones	Changes in color perception, especially blue and violet
Loss of photoreceptor cells, retinal pigment, epithelial cells, and melanin	Decreased visual acuity
Age-related macular degeneration because of vascular changes	Loss of central vision, presence of yellow deposits, atrophy of macular retinal pigment
Vitreous	
Liquefaction and detachment of vitreous	Increased "floaters"

Subjective Data

Important Health Information

Past Health History. Take information about the patient's past health history, including the ocular and nonocular history. The patient's nonocular history can be significant in assessing and treating an eye condition. Ask the patient about systemic diseases that may have ocular manifestations. These include diabetes, hypertension, cancer, rheumatoid arthritis, syphilis and other sexually transmitted infections (STIs), acquired immunodeficiency syndrome (AIDS), muscular dystrophy, myasthenia gravis, multiple sclerosis, inflammatory bowel disease, and hypothyroidism or hyperthyroidism. Include any history of stroke or neurologic problems as these have the potential to result in visual field defects.

Obtain a history of tests for visual acuity, including the date of the last examination and change in glasses or contact lenses. Ask the patient about a history of strabismus, amblyopia, cataracts, retinal detachment, refractive surgery, or glaucoma. Note any trauma to the eye, its treatment, and sequelae.

Obtain information about allergies. Allergies often cause eye symptoms, such as itching, burning, watering, drainage, and blurred vision.

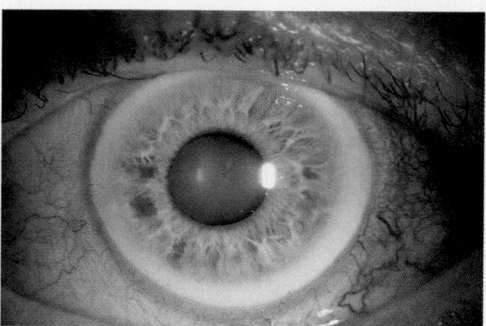

FIG. 20.6 Arcus senilis, or age-related degeneration of the cornea. (From Kanski JJ: *Clinical ophthalmology: A synopsis*, ed 2, New York, 2009, Butterworth-Heinemann.)

Medications. Obtain a complete medication history, including dosage and frequency of over-the-counter (OTC) medicines, eyedrops, herbal therapies, and dietary supplements. Many of these drugs have ocular effects. For example, many cold preparations contain a form of epinephrine (e.g., pseudoephedrine) that can dilate the pupil. Note the use of any antihistamine or decongestant, since these drugs can cause ocular dryness. Ask whether the patient uses any prescription drugs, such as corticosteroids, thyroid medications, or oral hypoglycemics and insulin. Long-term use of corticosteroid preparations can contribute to the development of glaucoma or cataracts.[2] Note whether the patient is taking any β-blockers, since β-blockers used to treat glaucoma can potentiate their effects. Hydroxychloroquine, which is used to treat rheumatoid arthritis and other autoimmune diseases, has the potential to result in retinal toxicity. It is important that these patients have annual comprehensive eye examinations.

Surgery or Other Treatments. Obtain a comprehensive history of both ocular and nonocular surgeries. Include laser-based surgery and invasive treatments, such as retinal injections.

Functional Health Patterns. The focus of the functional health pattern assessment depends on the presence or absence of vision loss and whether the loss is permanent or temporary. Table 20.2 lists suggested health history questions related to the functional health patterns.

Health Perception–Health Management Pattern. Patient characteristics, such as gender, ethnicity, and age, are important in assessing eye problems. Men are more likely than women to have color blindness. The leading cause of blindness among blacks is glaucoma.[3]

The patient's visual health can affect activities at home or at work. It is important to know how the patient perceives the current health problem. As outlined in Table 20.2, guide the patient in describing the current problem. Assess the patient's ability to perform self-care, especially any eye care related to the patient's eye problem.

The patient may not recognize the importance of eye-safety practices, like wearing protective eyewear during potentially hazardous activities or avoiding noxious fumes and other eye irritants. Ask about the use of sunglasses in bright light. Prolonged exposure to ultraviolet (UV) light can affect the retina. Ask about night driving habits and any problems encountered. Today, millions of people wear contact lenses, but many do not care for them properly. The type of contact lenses used and the patient's wearing and care habits may provide an opportunity for teaching.

Hereditary systemic diseases (e.g., sickle cell anemia) can significantly affect eye health. In addition, many refractive

errors and other eye problems are hereditary. Ask whether the patient has a family history of arteriosclerosis, diabetes, thyroid disease, hypertension, arthritis, or cancer. Determine whether the patient has a family history of eye problems, including cataracts, tumors, glaucoma, refractive errors (especially myopia, hyperopia), and retinal degenerative conditions (e.g., macular degeneration, retinal detachment).

📋 TABLE 20.2 Health History

Visual System

Health Perception–Health Management
- Describe the change in your vision. Describe how this affects your daily life.
- Do you wear protective eyewear (sunglasses, safety goggles, hats)?*
- Do you wear contact lenses? If so, how do you take care of them?
- If you use eyedrops, how do you instill them?
- Do you have any allergies that cause eye symptoms?*
- Do you have a family history of cataracts, glaucoma, or macular degeneration?*

Nutritional-Metabolic
- Do you take any nutritional supplements?*
- Does your visual problem affect your ability to obtain and prepare food?*

Elimination
- Do you have to strain to void or defecate?*

Activity-Exercise
- Are your activities limited in any way by your eye problem?*
- Do you take part in any leisure activities that have the potential for eye injury?*

Sleep-Rest
- Is your vision affected by the amount of sleep you get?*
- Does your eye problem affect your sleeping patterns?*

Cognitive-Perceptual
- Does your eye problem affect your ability to read?*
- Do you have any eye pain?*
- Do you have any eye itching, burning, or foreign body sensation?*

Self-Perception–Self-Concept
- How does your eye problem make you feel about yourself?

Role-Relationship
- Do you have any problems at work or home because of your eyes?*
- Have you made any changes in your social activities because of your eyes?*

Sexuality-Reproductive
- Has your eye problem caused a change in your sex life?*
- For women: Are you pregnant? Do you use birth control pills?*
- For men: Do you use any erectile dysfunction drugs? Any vision problems with their use?*

Coping–Stress Tolerance
- Do you feel able to cope with your eye problem?*
- How do you feel that your eye problem has affected your life, and how do you cope with these changes?*

Value-Belief
- Do you have any conflicts about the treatment of your eye problem?*

* If yes, describe.

Nutritional-Metabolic Pattern. High doses of vitamins containing antioxidant, carotenoids, and omega-3 fatty acids (vitamins C and E, beta-carotene, zinc) may be important to ocular health. Some patients with age-related macular degeneration (AMD) may benefit from supplements of these vitamins.

Elimination Pattern. Straining to defecate (Valsalva maneuver) can raise IOP. After patients have eye surgery, many HCPs do not want them to strain. Assess the patient's usual pattern of elimination and determine whether there is the potential for constipation in the patient who has had eye surgery.

Activity-Exercise Pattern. The patient's usual level of activity or exercise may be affected by reduced vision, symptoms accompanying an eye problem, or activity restrictions after surgery. Ask about leisure activities during which the patient may incur an eye injury. For example, gardening, woodworking, and other craft activities can result in corneal or conjunctival foreign bodies or even penetrating injuries of the globe. Sports activities, such as racquetball, baseball, and tennis, carry risks for blunt trauma to the eyes. People should wear protection goggles for these sports.

Sleep-Rest Pattern. In the otherwise healthy person, lack of sleep may cause ocular irritation, especially if the patient wears contact lenses. Painful eye problems, such as corneal abrasions, may disrupt normal sleep patterns.

Cognitive-Perceptual Pattern. Assess for other cognitive or perceptual problems. For example, the functional ability of a patient with a visual deficit will be further compromised if the patient also has hearing problems. The patient who cannot see to read may find it harder to follow discharge instructions if he or she also has trouble hearing or remembering verbal instructions. Eye pain is always an important symptom to assess. If eye pain is present, ask the patient about treatment and response.

Self-Perception–Self-Concept Pattern. The loss of independence that can follow a partial or complete loss of vision, even if the condition is temporary, can have devastating effects on the patient's self-concept. Evaluate the potential effect of vision loss on the patient's self-image. For instance, disabling glare from a cataract may prevent nighttime driving. In today's highly mobile society, losing the ability to drive can represent a significant loss of independence and self-esteem.

Role-Relationship Pattern. Eye problems can negatively affect the patient's ability to take part in roles and responsibilities in the home, work, and social environments. For example, with decreased visual acuity, the patient may no longer adequately function at work. Many occupations place workers in conditions in which eye injury may occur. For example, factory workers may be at risk from flying metal debris. Eye-safety practices, such as the use of goggles or safety glasses, are now a legal requirement in some workplaces. The patient with diabetes may not be able to see well enough to self-administer insulin. This patient may resent dependence on a caregiver who takes over this function. Sensitively ask if the problem has affected the patient's preferred roles and responsibilities.

Sexuality-Reproductive Pattern. The patient with severe vision loss may develop such a poor self-image that the ability to be sexually intimate is lost. Assure the patient that low vision or blindness does not affect a person's ability to be sexually expressive. Often touch is more important than vision.

Coping–Stress Tolerance Pattern. The patient with temporary or permanent visual problems may have emotional stress. Assess the patient's coping strategies and availability of support systems.

Value-Belief Pattern. Be sensitive to each patient's individual values and spiritual beliefs as these may guide decisions about eye care. It can be hard to understand why a patient refuses treatment that has potential benefit or wants treatment that may have limited potential benefit.

CASE STUDY
Subjective Data

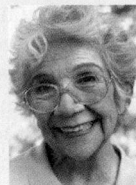

(© Jack Hollingsworth/ Photodisc/ Thinkstock.)

A focused subjective assessment of F.M. revealed the following information:
- **PMH:** Extraocular extraction of cataract on right eye (OD) with implantation of intraocular lens 2 mo ago. Type 2 diabetes, hypothyroidism, and hypertension.
- **Medications:** Glucophage 500 mg twice daily, levothyroxine 100 mcg daily, metoprolol 50 mg daily.
- **Health Perception–Health Management:** States she used antibiotic and corticosteroid eyedrops after surgery as directed and followed-up with surgeon. Recovery was uneventful. Eyedrops were stopped 2 wk ago. Does not have allergies. Had excellent eyesight until today.
- **Elimination:** Has had problems moving bowels with increased straining. Trying prune juice to help.
- **Activity-Exercise:** Walks in the mall at least ½ mile 3 times a week. No resistance or isotonic exercises.
- **Cognitive-Perceptual:** Denies eye pain, itching, or tearing. Having difficulty reading.
- **Coping–Stress Tolerance:** Afraid she is having a stroke.

Discussion Questions
1. Which subjective assessment findings are of most concern to you?
2. What should be included in the physical assessment? For what would you be looking?
3. How will you individualize the assessment based on her age, ethnic/cultural background, and condition?
   You will learn more about the physical assessment of the visual system in the next section.
   (See p. 358 for more information on F.M.)

Answers available at *http://evolve.elsevier.com/Lewis/medsurg.*

Objective Data
Physical Examination. Physical examination of the visual system includes inspecting the ocular structures and determining the status of their respective functions. Physiologic functional assessment includes (1) assessing the patient's visual acuity, ability to judge closeness and distance, and extraocular muscle function; (2) evaluating visual fields; (3) checking pupil function; and (4) measuring IOP. Assessment of ocular structures should include examining the ocular adnexa, external eye, and internal structures. Some structures, such as the retina, blood vessels, and optic disc, must be assessed with an ophthalmoscope.

TABLE 20.3 Normal Physical Assessment of Visual System

- Visual acuity 20/20 OU. No diplopia
- External eye structures symmetric and without lesions or deformities
- Lacrimal apparatus nontender and without drainage
- Conjunctiva clear. Sclera white
- PERRLA (pupils equal, round, reactive to light and accommodation)
- Lens clear
- EOMs intact (extraocular movements intact)
- Optic disc margins sharp
- Retinal vessels without hemorrhages or spots

FOCUSED ASSESSMENT

Visual System

Use this checklist to make sure the key assessment steps have been done.

Subjective

Ask the patient about any of the following and note responses.

Changes in vision (e.g., acuity, blurred)	Y	N
Eye redness, itching, discomfort	Y	N
Drainage from eyes	Y	N

Objective: Physical Examination
Inspect

Eyes for any discoloration or drainage	✓
Conjunctiva and sclera for color and vascularity	✓
Lens for clarity	✓
Eyelid for ptosis	✓

Assess

Vision based on patient looking at nurse or Snellen chart	✓
Extraocular movements (EOMs)	✓
Peripheral vision	✓
PERRLA	✓

PERRLA, Pupils equal, round, reactive to light and accommodation.

TABLE 20.4 Nursing Assessment

Assessment Techniques: Visual System

Description	Purpose
Color Vision Testing In the Ishihara test, a patient identifies numbers or paths formed by pattern of dots in series of color plates.	Determines ability to distinguish colors
Confrontation Visual Field Test Patient faces examiner, covers one eye, fixates on examiner's face, and counts number of fingers that examiner brings into patient's field of vision.	Determines if patient has a full field of vision, without obvious blind spots or vision loss
Intraocular Pressure Testing: Tonometry Covered end of probe is gently touched several times to anesthetized corneal surface. Examiner records several readings to obtain a mean IOP.	Measures IOP. Normal pressure is 10–21 mm Hg
Keratometry Examiner aligns projection and notes readings of corneal curvature. Often done before fitting contact lenses, before refractive surgery, or after corneal transplantation.	Measures corneal curvature
Ophthalmoscopy Examiner holds ophthalmoscope close to patient's eye, shining light into back of eye and looking through aperture on ophthalmoscope. Examiner adjusts dial to choose the ophthalmoscope lens that produces desired amount of magnification to inspect retina.	Provides magnified view of retina and optic nerve (Fig. 20.7)
Pupil Function Testing Examiner shines light into patient's pupil and checks pupillary response. Each pupil is examined independently. Examiner also checks for consensual and accommodative response.	Determines if patient has normal pupillary response
Visual Acuity Testing Patient reads from Snellen chart at 20 ft (distance vision test) or Jaeger chart at 14 in (near vision test). Examiner notes smallest print patient can read on each chart.	Determines distance and near visual acuity

Normal physical assessment of the visual system is outlined in Table 20.3. Assessment techniques related to vision are described in Table 20.4. Table 20.5 shows select assessment abnormalities.

A *focused assessment* is used to evaluate the status of previously identified visual problems and to monitor for signs of new problems. A focused assessment of the visual system is shown in the box above.

Initial Observation. Your initial observation of the patient can provide information that will help focus the assessment. A patient dressed in clothing with unusual color combinations may have a color-vision deficit. Note an unusual head position. The patient with diplopia may hold the head in a skewed position to try to see a single image. The patient with a corneal abrasion or photophobia will cover the eyes with the hands to try to block out room light. Make a crude estimate of depth perception by extending a hand for the patient to shake.

During the initial observation, observe the patient's overall facial and eye appearance. The eyes should be symmetric and normally placed on the face. The globes should not have a bulging or sunken appearance.

Assessing Functional Status

Visual acuity. Always record the patient's visual acuity for medical and legal reasons. When doing a physical examination of the eyes, assess the right eye first and then the left eye. Use the abbreviations right eye "OD," left eye "OS," and both eyes "OU." Record the patient's visual acuity before the patient receives any eye care.

To assess visual acuity, position the person on a mark exactly 20 ft (6 m) from the Snellen eye chart. If the person wears glasses or contacts, leave them on. Using an occlude, cover one eye at a time during the test. Ask the person to read down the lines of the chart to the smallest line of letters and numbers possible. Record the result using the numeric fraction at the end of the last successful line read. Indicate whether any letters

TABLE 20.5 Assessment Abnormalities

Visual System

Finding	Description	Possible Etiology and Significance
Subjective Data		
Blurred vision	Gradual or sudden inability to see clearly	Refractive errors, corneal opacities, cataracts, migraine aura, retinal changes (detachment, macular degeneration)
Diplopia	Double vision	Abnormal extraocular muscle action related to muscle or cranial nerve pathologic condition
Dryness	Discomfort, sandy, gritty, irritation, or burning	Decreased tear formation or changes in tear composition because of aging or various systemic diseases
Pain	Foreign body sensation	Superficial corneal erosion or abrasion. Can result from contact lens wear or trauma. Conjunctival or corneal foreign body
	Severe, deep, throbbing	Anterior uveitis, acute glaucoma, infection. Acute glaucoma also associated with nausea, vomiting
Photophobia	Persistent abnormal intolerance to light	Inflammation or infection of cornea or anterior uveal tract (iris and ciliary body)
Spots, floaters	Patient describes seeing spots, "spider webs," "curtain," or floaters within the field of vision	Most common cause is vitreous liquefaction (benign phenomenon). Other causes include hemorrhage into the vitreous humor, retinal holes or tears
Objective Data		
Eyelids		
Allergic reactions	Redness, excessive tearing, and itching of lid margins	Many possible allergens. Associated eye trauma can occur from rubbing itchy eyelids
Blepharitis	Redness, swelling, and crusting along lid margins	Bacterial invasion of lid margins. Often chronic
Dermatochalasis	Excess eyelid skin	May eventually obstruct superior and peripheral vision
Ectropion	Outward turning of lower lid margin	Age-related tissue changes, posttraumatic changes, facial paralysis
Entropion	Inward turning of upper or lower lid margin, unilateral or bilateral	Age-related tissue changes, posttraumatic changes, facial paralysis
Hordeolum (sty) (Fig. 20.8)	Small, superficial white nodule along lid margin	Infection of meibomian gland of eyelid. Causative organism is usually bacterial (most often *Staphylococcus aureus*)
Ptosis	Drooping of upper eyelid, unilateral or bilateral	Myasthenia gravis, congenital, or mechanical causes from eyelid tumors or excess skin
Conjunctiva		
Conjunctivitis	Redness, swelling of conjunctiva. May be itchy	Bacterial or viral infection. May be allergic response or inflammatory response to chemical exposure
Subconjunctival hemorrhage	Appearance of blood spot on sclera. May be small or can affect entire sclera	Conjunctival blood vessels rupture, leaking blood into the subconjunctival space.
Cornea		
Corneal abrasion	Localized painful disruption of the epithelial layer of cornea. Can be seen with fluorescein dye	Trauma. Overwear or improper fit of contact lenses
Globe		
Exophthalmos (Fig. 20.9)	Protrusion of globe beyond its normal position within bony orbit. Sclera often visible above iris when eyelids are open	Intraocular or periorbital tumors Hyperthyroidism
Pupil		
Abnormal response to light or accommodation	Pupils respond asymmetrically or abnormally to light stimulus or accommodation	CNS disorders, general anesthesia
Anisocoria	Pupils unequal (constricted)	CNS disorders. Slight difference in pupil size is normal in some people
Extraocular Muscles		
Strabismus	Deviation of eye position in one or more directions	Overaction or underaction of one or more extraocular muscles
Lens		
Cataract	Opacification of lens. Pupil can appear cloudy or white when opacity is visible behind pupil opening.	Aging, trauma, diabetes, long-term systemic corticosteroid therapy
Visual Field Defect		
Central	Loss of central vision	Macular disease
Peripheral	Partial or complete loss of peripheral vision	Glaucoma. Interruption of visual pathway (e.g., tumor). Migraine headache

were missed and if corrective lenses were worn (e.g., "Right eye, 20/30-2, with contacts"). Next ask the patient to cover the other eye and repeat the process. Normal visual acuity is 20/20. The first number indicates the distance the person is standing or sitting from the chart. The second number gives the distance at which a normal eye can read the particular line. *Legal blindness* is defined as the best-corrected vision in the better eye of 20/200 or less.

If the patient reports near vision difficulty or is 40 years of age or older, use a hand-held vision screener with varying print sizes (e.g., a Jaeger chart). Hold the card at 14 in (35 cm) from the eye in good light to assess near vision. Examine each eye separately, with glasses on if worn. A normal result is "14/14" in each eye, read without hesitancy and without the patient moving the card. If you must assess near visual acuity without access to a Jaeger eye chart, you can still make an accurate assessment using newsprint or the label on a container. Record the acuity as "reads newspaper headline at X inches." If the patient is unable to read any of the lines on both the near and distant visual acuity charts, the next step is to assess whether they can see hand motion and light perception.

Extraocular muscle functions. Assess the corneal light reflex to evaluate for weakness or imbalance of the extraocular muscles. In a darkened room, ask the patient to look straight ahead while shining a penlight directly on the cornea. The light reflection should be in the center of both corneas as the patient faces the light source.

To assess eye movement, hold a finger or an object within 10 to 12 inches of the patient's nose. Ask the patient to follow with eyes only the movement of the object or finger in the 6 cardinal positions of gaze. This test can indicate weakness or paralysis in the extraocular muscles and cranial nerves (CN III, CN IV, and CN VI).

Pupil function and intraocular pressure. Pupil function is determined by inspecting the pupils and their reactions to light. The normal finding is often abbreviated as PERRL (pupils are equal [in size], round, and reactive to light). The pupils should react to light directly (pupil constricts when a light shines into the eye) and consensually (pupil constricts when a light shines into the opposite eye). In a small number of people, the pupils are normally unequal in size (*anisocoria*).

To test for accommodation, ask the person to focus on a distant object. This process dilates the eyes. Then have the person shift the focus to a near object (e.g., your finger held about 3 inches from the person's nose). A normal response is constriction of the eyes and convergence (inward movement of both eyes toward each other). When accommodation is assessed with the pupillary light reflex, a normal response is *PERRLA* (pupils are equal, round, and reactive to light and accommodation).

IOP (Table 20.4) is measured by a variety of methods, including tonometry. Normal IOP ranges from 10 to 21 mm Hg.

Assessing Structures. We assess the visual system structures primarily by inspection. The visual system is unique because we can inspect not only the external structures but also many of the internal structures. The iris, lens, vitreous, retina, and optic nerve can be seen directly through the clear cornea and pupil opening.

This direct inspection requires special observation equipment, such as the slit lamp microscope or ophthalmoscope. These permit examination of the conjunctiva, sclera, cornea, anterior chamber, iris, lens, vitreous, and retina under magnification. The *ophthalmoscope* is a hand-held instrument with a light source and magnifying lenses that is held close to the patient's eye to visualize the posterior part of the eye. Little pain or discomfort is associated with these examinations.

Eyebrows, eyelashes, and eyelids. All structures should be present and symmetric, without deformities, redness, or swelling. Eyelashes extend outward from the lid margins. In normal closing, the upper and lower eyelid margins just touch. The lacrimal puncta should be open and positioned properly against the globe.

Conjunctiva and sclera. The conjunctiva and sclera are easily examined at the same time. Assess the color, smoothness, and presence of lesions or foreign bodies. The conjunctiva covering the sclera is normally clear, with fine blood vessels visible. These blood vessels are more common in the periphery.

The sclera is normally white. A slight yellow cast may be found in some dark-skinned people, such as blacks and Native Americans, or in the older adult from lipid deposition. A pale blue cast caused by scleral thinning can be normal in older adults.

Cornea. The cornea should be clear, transparent, and shiny. The iris should appear flat and not bulge toward the cornea. The area between the cornea and iris should be clear, with no blood or purulent material visible in the anterior chamber.

Iris. Both irises should be of similar color and shape. However, a color difference between the irises occurs normally in a small number of people.

Retina and optic nerve. We can get vital information about the vascular system and CNS through direct visualization with an ophthalmoscope. It is used to magnify the retina and optic nerves and bring them into crisp focus (Fig. 20.7). Skilled use of this instrument takes practice.

Examine the optic nerve or disc for size, color, and abnormalities. The optic disc is creamy yellow with distinct margins. A central depression in the disc, called the *physiologic cup*, may be seen. This area is the exit site for the optic nerve. The cup should be less than half the diameter of the disc. Normally, no hemorrhages or exudates are present in the fundus (retinal background). Careful inspection of the fundus can reveal retinal holes, tears, detachments, or lesions. Small hemorrhages can be associated with diabetes or hypertension and can appear in various shapes, such as dots or flames. Finally, examine the macula for shape and appearance. This area is normally devoid of any blood vessels.

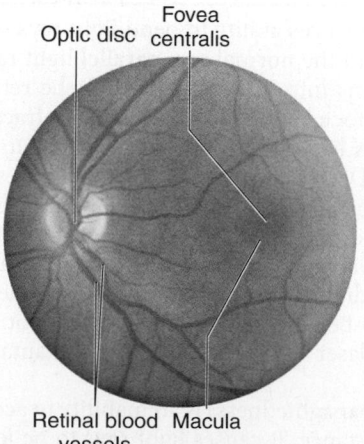

FIG. 20.7 Magnified view of retina through the ophthalmoscope. (From Newell FW: *Ophthalmology: Principles and concepts,* ed 7, St Louis, 1992, Mosby.)

Special Assessment Techniques

Color Vision. Testing the patient's ability to distinguish colors is an important part of the overall assessment. Some occupations require accurate color discrimination. The Ishihara color test determines the patient's ability to distinguish a pattern of color in a series of color plates.

Stereopsis. Stereoscopic vision allows a patient to see objects in 3 dimensions. An event that causes a patient to have monocular vision (e.g., enucleation, patching) results in the loss of stereoscopic vision. Without stereopsis, the person's ability to judge distances or the height of a step is impaired. This can have profound consequences if the person trips over a step when walking or follows too closely behind another vehicle when driving.

CASE STUDY

Objective Data: Physical Examination and Diagnostic Studies

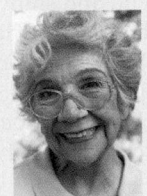

(© Jack Hollingsworth/ Photodisc/ Thinkstock.)

Physical examination findings of F.M. were as follows:
- PERRL. No abnormalities noted on visual examination of external eye structures. EOMs intact and symmetric.

The HCP performs an ophthalmoscopic examination and finds a partial retinal detachment. Ultrasonography confirms the diagnosis.

Discussion Questions
1. Are these the diagnostic studies that you expected to be ordered?
2. Which diagnostic study results are of most concern to you?

Answers available at *http://evolve.elsevier.com/Lewis/medsurg*.

DIAGNOSTIC STUDIES OF VISUAL SYSTEM

Diagnostic studies of the visual system provide vital information in monitoring the patient's condition and planning appropriate interventions. These studies are considered objective data. Table 20.6 presents common diagnostic studies of the visual system.

VISUAL PROBLEMS

REFRACTIVE ERRORS

Refraction is the eye's ability to bend light rays so that they fall on the retina. In the normal eye, parallel light rays are focused through the lens into a sharp image on the retina. When the light does not focus properly, it is called a refractive error. This defect prevents light rays from converging into a single focus on the retina. Defects are a result of irregularities of the corneal curvature, focusing power of the lens, or length of the eye.

Refractive errors are the most common visual problem. Blurred vision is the major symptom. In some cases, the patient may have eye discomfort, eyestrain, or headaches. Most refractive errors can be corrected using eyeglasses or contact lenses, refractive eye laser surgery, or surgical implantation of an artificial lens.

Myopia (nearsightedness) is an inability to accommodate for objects at a distance. It causes light rays to be focused in front of the retina. This means the person can see near objects but objects in the distance are blurry. Myopia may occur because of excessive light refraction by the cornea or lens or because of

---

TABLE 20.6 Diagnostic Studies

Visual System

Study	Description, Purpose, and Nursing Responsibility
Amsler Grid test	Self-administered test using a hand-held card printed with a grid of lines (like graph paper) (Fig. 20.15). Using one eye at a time, patient fixates on center dot and records any abnormalities of grid lines, such as wavy, missing, or distorted areas. Used to monitor macular problems.
Fluorescein angiography	Fluorescein injected IV into peripheral vein followed by serial photographs (over 10-min period) of retina through dilated pupils Provides diagnostic information about flow of blood through retinal vessels. If extravasation occurs, fluorescein is toxic to tissue. Tell patient that dye can sometimes cause transient nausea or vomiting. Yellow-orange discoloration of urine and skin may occur.
Perimetry (visual field) testing	Can detect changes in central and peripheral vision, which may be caused by various conditions, including glaucoma, stroke, brain tumors, or other neurologic deficits. Person sits and looks inside a bowl-shaped instrument called a *perimeter*. While staring at the center of bowl, a light flashes, and the person presses a button each time flash is seen. A computer records the results, and a printout shows if there are areas where flashes of light are not seen.
Refractometry	Measure of refractive error. Patient sits looking through apertures at Snellen acuity chart and lenses are changed. Patient chooses lenses that make acuity sharpest. Dilation of eyes may help visualize retina and optic nerves. Procedure is painless. Pupil dilation, which may last 3–4 hr, makes it difficult to focus on near objects.
Ultrasonography	*A-scan* determines the right power of a lens implant before cataract surgery. *B-scan* used to diagnose ocular pathologic conditions, including intraocular foreign bodies or tumors, vitreous opacities, retinal detachments.

---

an abnormally long eye. Myopia is the most common refractive error. About 30% of Americans have this disorder.[4] There is strong evidence that many people inherit myopia, or at least the tendency to develop myopia.[4]

Hyperopia (farsightedness) is an inability to accommodate for near objects. It causes the light rays to focus behind the retina and requires the person to use accommodation to focus the light rays on the retina for near objects. The person with hyperopia can see distant objects clearly. This type of error occurs when the cornea or lens does not have adequate focusing power or when the eyeball is too short.

Presbyopia is the loss of accommodation associated with age. One usually begins to notice this condition in the early to mid-40s. As the eye ages, the lens becomes larger, firmer, and less elastic. These changes, which progress with aging, result in an inability to focus on near objects.

Astigmatism is an uneven or irregular curvature of the cornea. The irregularity causes the incoming light rays to be bent unequally. Thus, the light rays do not come to a single point of focus on the retina, which results in visual distortion. Astigmatism can occur in conjunction with any of the other refractive errors.

Aphakia is the absence of the lens. Rarely, the lens may be absent congenitally, or it may be removed during cataract surgery. A lens that is traumatically injured is removed and replaced with an intraocular lens (IOL) implant. The absence of the lens results in a significant refractive error. Without the focusing ability of the lens, images are projected behind the retina.

Nonsurgical Corrections
Corrective Glasses. The right corrective lenses can enhance vision in those with myopia, hyperopia, presbyopia, and astigmatism. Glasses for presbyopia are often called "reading glasses" because they are usually worn only for close work. Presbyopic correction may be combined with a correction for another refractive error, such as myopia or astigmatism. In these combined glasses, the presbyopic correction is in the lower part of the spectacle lens. A traditional bifocal or trifocal has visible lines. However, most lenses today that correct vision at various distances do not have visible lines. The prescription varies throughout the lens, allowing distance focusing in the top two thirds and near focus in the bottom one third of the lens.

Contact Lenses. Contact lenses are another way to correct refractive errors. Contact lenses are made from various plastic and silicone substances. They are highly permeable to oxygen and have a high water content. These features allow for increased wearing time with greater comfort. If the oxygen supply to the cornea is decreased, it becomes swollen, visual acuity decreases, and the patient has severe discomfort.

In general, you need to know whether the patient wears contact lenses, the pattern of wear (daily versus extended), and care practices. Shining a light obliquely on the eyeball can help visualize a contact lens. Contact lenses are associated with microbial keratitis, a severe sight-threatening complication. Risk factors for keratitis include poor hand cleaning, poor lens case hygiene, and inadequate lens cleaning. Teach the patient the importance of following recommended cleaning practices and reporting redness, sensitivity, vision problems, and pain to the eye care provider. Teach the patient to remove contact lenses at once if any of these problems occur.

Surgical Therapy
Surgery can eliminate or reduce the need for eyeglasses or contact lenses and correct refractive errors by changing the focus of the eye. Surgical management for refractive errors includes laser surgery and IOL implantation.

Laser. *Laser-assisted in situ keratomileusis* (LASIK) may be considered for patients with low to moderately high amounts of myopia or hyperopia, with or without astigmatism. The procedure first involves using a laser or surgical blade to create a flap in the cornea. The flap is folded back, exposing the middle section (stroma) of the cornea. Pulses from a computer-controlled laser vaporize a part of the stroma. The flap is then repositioned, adhering on its own without sutures in a few minutes.[5]

Photorefractive keratectomy (PRK) is indicated for low to moderate amounts of myopia or hyperopia, with or without astigmatism. It is a good option for a patient with insufficient corneal thickness for a LASIK flap. In PRK, the epithelium is removed and the laser sculpts the cornea to correct the refractive error. *Laser-assisted subepithelial keratomileusis* (LASEK) is similar to PRK, except that the epithelium is replaced after surgery.

Implant. *Refractive intraocular lens* (refractive IOL) implantation is an option for patients with a high degree of myopia or hyperopia. Like cataract surgery, it involves removing the patient's natural lens and implanting an IOL. The IOL implant used is a special lens designed to correct the patient's refractive error. Refractive IOLs can correct both myopia and presbyopia.

Phakic intraocular lenses (phakic IOLs) are sometimes called *implantable contact lenses*. They are implanted into the eye without removing the eye's natural lens. They are used for patients with high degrees of myopia or hyperopia. Unlike refractive IOLs, the phakic IOL is placed in front of the eye's natural lens. Leaving the natural lens preserves the eye's ability to focus for reading vision.

🌐 PROMOTING HEALTH EQUITY
Visual Problems

- Glaucoma has an increased incidence and severity among blacks compared with whites.
- Hispanic Americans have an increased incidence of diabetic retinopathy.
- Whites have a higher incidence of macular degeneration than Hispanics, blacks, and Asian Americans.

VISUAL IMPAIRMENT

Visual impairment describes vision that cannot be fully corrected by corrective lenses, medical treatment, or surgery. The term *visual impairment* includes conditions ranging from low vision to the absence of all vision (total blindness). Many terms are used when people refer to visual impairment, including:

- *Low vision* refers to impaired vision that cannot be improved by conventional eyeglasses, contact lenses, medications, or surgery in which some good usable vision remains.
- *Severe visual impairment* describes visual impairment in people who are unable to read ordinary newsprint even with correction. People with a severe visual impairment may or may not be legally blind.
- *Legal blindness* refers to central visual acuity of 20/200 or less in the better eye with correction or a peripheral visual field of 20 degrees or less.[6]

Most blindness in the United States is the result of common eye diseases, including cataracts, glaucoma, age-related macular degeneration, and diabetic retinopathy.

❖ NURSING MANAGEMENT: VISUAL IMPAIRMENT
◆ Nursing Assessment

It is important to assess how long the patient has had a visual impairment. Recent loss of vision has different implications for nursing care. Determine how the patient's visual impairment affects normal functioning. Ask the patient about the level of difficulty involved in doing certain tasks. For example, how hard is it for the patient to read, write a check, move from one room to the next, or view the television? Other questions can help determine the personal meaning that the patient attaches to the visual impairment. Ask how the vision loss has affected specific aspects of the patient's life, whether the patient has lost a job, or what activities the patient does not engage in because of the visual impairment.

Determine the patient's emotional reactions, coping strategies, and support systems. The patient may attach many negative meanings to the impairment because of societal views of blindness. For example, the patient may view the impairment as punishment or view themselves as useless and burdensome.

◆ Planning

The overall goals are that the patient with impaired vision will (1) make a successful adjustment to the impairment, (2) discuss feelings related to the loss, (3) identify personal strengths and support systems, and (4) use appropriate coping strategies. If the patient has been functioning at an appropriate or acceptable level, the goal is to maintain the current level of function.

◆ Nursing Implementation

◆ **Health Promotion.** Encourage the patient with preventable causes of further visual impairment to seek appropriate health care. For example, the patient with vision loss from glaucoma may be able to prevent further visual loss by with prescribed therapies and eye examinations.

◆ **Acute Care.** Provide emotional support and direct care to the patient with recent visual impairment. Allow the patient to express fear, anger, and grief. Help the patient identify positive coping strategies. Caregivers are intimately involved in the experiences that occur with vision loss. With the patient's knowledge and permission, include caregivers in discussions and encourage them to express their concerns.

Many people are uncomfortable around a person with visual impairment because they are not sure what behaviors are appropriate. Being sensitive to the patient's feelings without being overly worried or smothering the patient's independence is vital in creating a therapeutic nursing presence. Always communicate in a normal conversational tone and manner with the patient and address the patient, not the caregiver. Common courtesy dictates introducing yourself and any other people who approach the patient. It is important to say good-bye when leaving the patient's presence. Making eye contact with the patient achieves several goals. It ensures that you are speaking while facing the patient so that the patient has no difficulty hearing. Your head position confirms that you are attentive to the patient. In addition, establishing eye contact ensures that you can observe the patient's facial expressions and reactions.

Help the patient using a *sighted-guide technique*. Stand slightly in front and to one side of the patient and offer an elbow for the patient to hold. Serve as the sighted guide, walking slightly ahead of the patient with the patient holding the back of your arm. As you walk, describe the environment to help orient the patient. For example, "We're going through an open doorway and approaching 2 steps down." Help the patient sit by placing one of his or her hands on the seat of the chair.

◆ **Ambulatory Care.** In working with the patient who is visually impaired, remember that a person classified as legally blind may have some useful vision. Rehabilitation after partial or total loss of vision can foster independence, self-esteem, and productivity. Know what services and devices are available and make appropriate referrals. For the legally blind patient the primary resource for services is the state agency for rehabilitation of the blind. Legally blind persons are often eligible for federal and state assistance and income tax benefits. A list of agencies that serve the partially sighted or blind patient is available from the American Foundation for the Blind (*www.afb.org*).

Braille or audio books for reading and a cane or guide dog for ambulation are examples of vision substitution techniques. These are usually best for the patient with no functional vision. For most patients who have some remaining vision, vision enhancement techniques can help in learning to ambulate, read printed material, and perform ADLs.

Optical Devices for Vision Enhancement. A wide range of newer technologies are available to help people with low vision. These devices include desktop video magnification/closed circuit units, electronic hand-held magnifiers, text-to-speech scanners (material read aloud to you), E-readers, and computer tablets (material read aloud, magnification, image zooming, brighter screen, voice recognition). Many of these devices require some training by an assistive technology professional. Encourage patients to practice with the technologic device to ensure they can use it successfully.

Nonoptical Methods for Vision Enhancement. Approach magnification is a simple way to enhance the patient's residual vision. Recommend that the patient sit closer to the television or hold books closer to the eyes. Contrast enhancement techniques include watching television in black and white, using a black felt-tip marker, and using contrasting colors (e.g., a red stripe at the edge of steps or curbs). Increased lighting can be provided by halogen lamps, direct sunlight, or gooseneck lamps that are aimed directly at the reading material or other near objects. Large type is often helpful, especially when used with other vision enhancements.

Non–24-Hour Sleep/Wake Disorder. A common problem that can occur in blind people, especially those who are totally blind, is *non–24-hour sleep/wake disorder (Non-24)*. It is a circadian rhythm sleep disorder in which a person's biologic clock does not synchronize to a 24-hour day.[7] It is caused by lack of light input to the circadian clock.

People with Non-24 have problems falling asleep or staying asleep at night. During the day, they may have an uncontrollable urge to sleep. This can result in severe sleep issues, including insomnia, excessive sleepiness, changing patterns of when a person sleeps, and social and work consequences.

Taking melatonin can shift the circadian clock earlier (an advance) or later (a delay). Tasimelteon (Hetlioz), a melatonin receptor agonist, also can be used for treatment. It works by targeting receptors in the brain that control the timing of the sleep/wake cycle.

◆ Evaluation

The overall expected outcomes are that the patient with visual impairment will:

• Follow treatment plan to prevent further loss of vision
• Be able to use adaptive coping strategies
• Maintain self-esteem and take part in social interactions
• Function safely within her or his own environment

♥ PROMOTING POPULATION HEALTH
Responsible Eye Care

• Regular hand washing prevents the spread of disease from one eye to the other.
• Seeking appropriate health care can lead to early detection of disease and prevent further loss of vision in patients with certain types of partial vision loss.
• Wearing sunglasses and practicing proper nutrition may help prevent cataract development and age-related macular degeneration.
• Wearing eye protection during potentially hazardous work, hobby, and sport activities reduces the risk for eye injuries.

Gerontologic Considerations: Visual Impairment

The older adult is at an increased risk for vision loss caused by eye disease. They may have other deficits, such as cognitive impairment or limited mobility, that further affect the ability to function in usual ways. Societal devaluation of older adults may compound the self-esteem or isolation issues associated with visual impairment. Financial resources may be inadequate to secure vision services or assistive devices.

The older patient may become increasingly confused or disoriented when visually compromised. The combination of decreased vision and confusion increases the risk for falls, which can have serious consequences. Decreased vision may compromise the older patient's ability to function, resulting in concerns about independence and a diminished self-image. Decreased manual dexterity may make instilling prescribed eyedrops hard. Those with low vision are more likely to make medication errors that are potentially dangerous, such as taking too much insulin or mistaking one drug for another.

EYE TRAUMA

Although the eyes are well protected by the bony orbit and fat pads, everyday activities can result in eye trauma. The most common eye injuries in the United States are due to falls and fights. Injuries at home may be caused by cleaning, gardening, power tool use, and home repair work. Sport- and work-related injuries are other causes of eye trauma.[8]

CHECK YOUR PRACTICE

You are working in your garden when your neighbor comes running into your yard. She is screaming and waving her arms. Her husband was using a chain saw to cut down a tree when a piece of wood chip flew into his eye. When you go to your neighbor's yard, the husband is on the ground crying in pain and you assess that the wood chip is embedded in his eye.
• What should you do next?

Table 20.7 outlines the emergency management of the patient with an eye injury. Chemical burns can be devastating to the eye and need immediate attention. Alkaline chemicals with a pH greater than 7 are the most harmful. They can penetrate the eye and damage the inner components. Acidic chemicals with a pH of less than 7 are unable to penetrate the eye but can damage the cornea. Both types of injury have the potential to result in blindness.

A *Morgan lens* may be used to provide continuous irrigation of an injured eye. It consists of a sterile plastic device resembling a contact lens that floats over the eye (never physically touches it) and allows copious irrigation of the eye. The device is connected to tubing that delivers irrigating solution. The Morgan lens provides relief for chemical or thermal burns and removes nonembedded foreign materials in the eye.

Trauma is often a preventable cause of visual impairment. Many eye injuries could be prevented by wearing protective eyewear. Your role in individual and community education is extremely important in reducing the incidence of eye trauma.

EXTRAOCULAR DISORDERS

INFLAMMATION AND INFECTION

One of the most common eye conditions is inflammation or infection of the external eye. Many external irritants or microorganisms can affect the eye, conjunctiva, and avascular cornea.

An external hordeolum (or a *sty*) is an infection of the meibomian glands in the lid margin (Fig. 20.8). The most common bacterial infective agent is *Staphylococcus aureus*. A red, swollen, circumscribed, and acutely tender area develops rapidly. Have the patient apply warm, moist compresses at least 4 times a day until it improves. This may be the only treatment needed. If it tends to recur, teach the patient to do lid scrubs daily. On occasion, antibiotic ointments or drops may be needed.

A *chalazion* is a chronic inflammatory granuloma of the meibomian glands in the lid. It may evolve from a hordeolum or

TABLE 20.7 Emergency Management

Eye Injury

Etiology	Assessment Findings	Interventions
Chemical Burn • Acid • Alkaline **Foreign Bodies** • Ceramics • Glass • Metal • Plastic • Wood **Thermal Burn** • Direct burn from hot surface • Indirect burn from UV light (e.g., welding torch, looking directly at sun) **Trauma** • Blunt (e.g., fist) • Penetrating (e.g., glass, metal, or wood fragments; knife, stick, other object)	• Pain • Photophobia • Redness—diffuse or localized • Swelling • Bruising • Tearing • Blood in the anterior chamber • Absent eye movements • Fluid drainage from eye (e.g., blood, aqueous humor) • Abnormal or decreased vision • Visible foreign body • Prolapsed globe • Abnormal IOP • Visual field defect	**Initial** • Determine mechanism of injury. • Ensure airway, breathing, and circulation. • Assess for other injuries. • Assess for chemical exposure. • Begin ocular irrigation *immediately* in case of chemical exposure. Do not stop until emergency personnel arrive to continue irrigation. Use sterile saline or water if sterile saline is unavailable. • Assess visual acuity. • Do not put pressure on the eye. • Tell patient not to blow nose. • Do not try to treat the injury (except as noted above for chemical exposure). • Stabilize foreign objects. • Cover the eye(s) with dry, sterile patches and a protective shield. • Do not give the patient food or fluids. • Elevate head of bed 45 degrees. • Give proper analgesia. **Ongoing Monitoring** • Reassure the patient. • Monitor pain. • Anticipate surgical repair for penetrating injury, globe rupture, or globe avulsion.

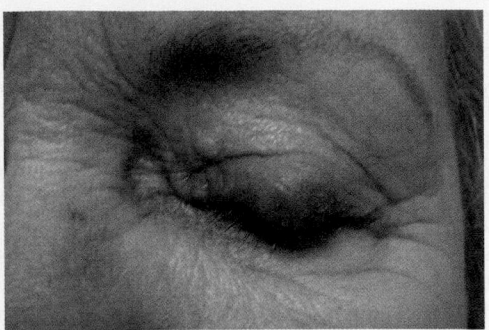

FIG. 20.8 Hordeolum (sty) on the upper eyelid caused by staphylococcal infection. (Courtesy Stephen J. Laquis, MD, FACS Ophthalmic Facial Plastic Surgery Specialists, Fort Myers, FL.)

occur in response to the material released into the lid when a blocked gland ruptures. The chalazion usually appears on the upper lid as a swollen, tender, reddened area that may be painful. Initial treatment is like that for a hordeolum. If warm, moist compresses are ineffective in promoting spontaneous drainage, the HCP may drain the lesion or inject it with corticosteroids.

Blepharitis is a common chronic bilateral inflammation of the lid margins. The lids are red rimmed with many scales or crusts on the lid margins and lashes. The patient mainly has itching but may also have burning, irritation, and photophobia.

If a staphylococcal infection caused blepharitis, an eye antibiotic ointment must be used. Often blepharitis is caused by both staphylococcal and seborrheal microorganisms. The treatment must be more vigorous to avoid hordeolum, *keratitis* (inflammation of the cornea), and other eye infections. Emphasize thorough cleaning practices of the skin and scalp. Gentle cleansing of the lid margins with baby shampoo or lid scrubs can effectively soften and remove crusting.

Conjunctivitis

Conjunctivitis is an infection or inflammation of the conjunctiva. Infections may be bacterial or viral. Conjunctival inflammation may result from exposure to allergens or chemical irritants. Careful hand washing and use of individual or disposable towels help prevent spreading the condition.

Bacterial Infections. Acute bacterial conjunctivitis *(pinkeye)* is a common infection. Although it occurs in every age group, epidemics are common among children. *S. aureus* is the most common cause. The patient with bacterial conjunctivitis may have discomfort, pruritus, redness, and a mucopurulent drainage. Although it typically occurs initially in one eye, it generally spreads to the unaffected eye. It is usually self-limiting, but treatment with antibiotic drops shortens the course of the disorder. Teach patients the importance of hand washing and avoiding contact with an infected person.

Viral Infections. Many different viruses cause conjunctival infections. The patient with viral conjunctivitis may have tearing, foreign body sensation, redness, and mild photophobia. This condition is usually mild and self-limiting. However, it can be severe, with increased discomfort and subconjunctival hemorrhaging. Adenovirus conjunctivitis may be contracted in contaminated swimming pools and through direct contact with an infected patient.

Epidemic keratoconjunctivitis (EKC) is the most serious ocular adenoviral disease. EKC is spread by direct contact. In the medical setting, contaminated hands and instruments can be

the source of spread. The patient may have tearing, redness, photophobia, and foreign body sensation. In most patients, the disease involves only one eye. Treatment is primarily palliative and includes ice packs and dark glasses. Therapy for severe cases can include mild topical corticosteroids to temporarily relieve symptoms and topical antibiotic ointment. Teach the patient the importance of good hygiene practices to avoid spreading the disease.

Chlamydial Infections. *Trachoma* is a chronic conjunctivitis caused by *Chlamydia trachomatis* (serotypes A through C). It is a major cause of blindness worldwide. Trachoma is most often seen in underdeveloped countries. It is transmitted mainly by the hands and by flies. Adult inclusion conjunctivitis (AIC) is caused by *C. trachomatis* (serotypes D through K). AIC is becoming more prevalent in the United States because of the increase in sexually transmitted chlamydial infection.[9]

Manifestations of both trachoma and AIC are mucopurulent eye discharge, irritation, redness, and lid swelling. For unknown reasons, AIC does not carry the long-term consequences of trachoma. Antibiotic therapy is usually effective for trachoma and AIC. Patients with AIC have a high risk for concurrent chlamydial genital infection and STIs that may need treatment.

Allergic Conjunctivitis. Conjunctivitis caused by exposure to an allergen can be mild and transitory, or it can be severe enough to cause significant swelling. The defining symptom of allergic conjunctivitis is itching. The patient may have burning, redness, and tearing. The patient may develop allergic conjunctivitis in response to pollens, animal dander, ocular solutions, and medications. Teach the patient to avoid known allergens if possible. Artificial tears can be effective in diluting the allergen and washing it from the eye. Topical medications include antihistamines and corticosteroids.

Keratitis

Keratitis is an inflammation or infection of the cornea. It is caused by a variety of microorganisms or by other factors. The condition may involve the conjunctiva and/or the cornea. When it involves both, the disorder is termed *keratoconjunctivitis*.

Bacterial Infections. The cornea can become infected by a variety of bacteria. Risk factors include mechanical or chemical corneal epithelial damage, contact lens wear, nutritional deficiencies, immunosuppressed states, and contaminated products (e.g., lens care solutions and cases, topical medications, cosmetics). Treatment includes topical antibiotics. In some cases, the patient may need subconjunctival antibiotic injection or, in severe cases, IV antibiotics.

Viral Infections. Herpes simplex virus (HSV) keratitis is the most common infectious cause of corneal blindness in the Western hemisphere. It is a growing problem, especially with immunosuppressed patients. The corneal ulcer has a characteristic dendritic (tree-branching) appearance. Pain and photophobia are common.

Current treatment for HSK includes acyclovir, ganciclovir, trifluorothymidine, penciclovir, and valacyclovir.[10] Therapy may also involve corneal debridement. Topical corticosteroids are usually contraindicated because they contribute to a longer course and possible deeper ulceration of the cornea.

The varicella-zoster virus (VZV) causes both chickenpox and herpes zoster ophthalmicus (HZO). HZO may occur by reactivation of an endogenous infection that has persisted in a latent form after an earlier attack of varicella or by contact with a patient with chickenpox or herpes zoster. It occurs most often in the older adult and immunosuppressed patient. Care of the patient with acute HZO may include analgesics for pain, topical corticosteroids to reduce inflammation, antiviral agents to reduce viral replication, mydriatic agents to dilate the pupil and relieve pain, and topical antibiotics to combat secondary infection. The patient may apply warm compresses and povidone-iodine gel to the affected skin.

Other Causes of Keratitis. Keratitis may be caused by fungi, such as *Aspergillus, Candida,* and *Fusarium* species. This is especially true in the case of eye trauma in an outdoor setting where fungi are prevalent in the soil and moist organic matter.

Acanthamoeba keratitis is caused by a parasite that is associated with contact lens wear, usually from contaminated lens care solutions or cases. Homemade saline solution is particularly susceptible to *Acanthamoeba* contamination. Teach the patient who wears contact lenses about good lens care practices. The treatment of *Acanthamoeba* keratitis is difficult since the organism is resistant to most drugs. Antifungal agents (e.g., ketoconazole) may be given. If antimicrobial therapy fails, the patient may need a corneal transplant.

Exposure keratitis occurs when the eyelids cannot adequately close. The patient with *exophthalmos* (protruding eyeball) from thyroid eye disease or masses posterior to the globe is susceptible to exposure keratitis (Fig. 20.9).

Corneal Ulcer. Tissue loss caused by a corneal infection produces a *corneal ulcer* (infectious keratitis) (Fig. 20.10). The infection can be due to bacteria, viruses, or fungi. Corneal ulcers are often painful. The patient may feel as if there is a foreign body in the eye. Other symptoms can include tearing, purulent or watery

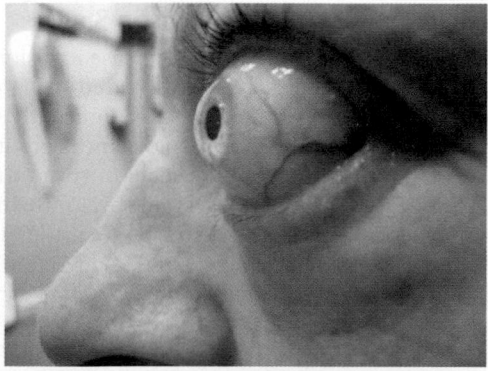

FIG. 20.9 Exophthalmos. (Courtesy Stephen J. Laquis, MD, FACS Ophthalmic Facial Plastic Surgery Specialists, Fort Myers, FL.)

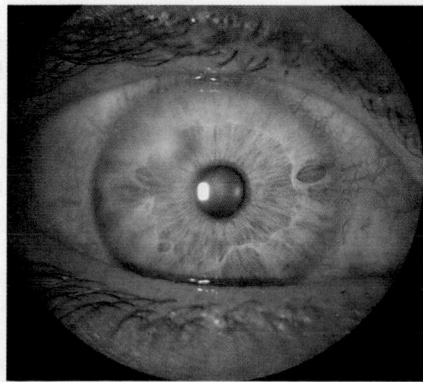

FIG. 20.10 Corneal ulcer. Infection associated with poor contact lens care. (Courtesy Cory J. Bosanko, OD, FAAO, Eye Centers of Tennessee, Crossville, TN.)

discharge, redness, and photophobia. Treatment is aggressive to avoid permanent vision loss. Antibiotic, antiviral, or antifungal eyedrops may be given as often as every hour for the first 24 hours. An untreated corneal ulcer can result in corneal scarring and perforation, or hole in the cornea. A corneal transplant may be needed.

❖ NURSING MANAGEMENT: INFLAMMATION AND INFECTION

Assess ocular changes, such as edema, redness, decreased visual acuity, feelings that a foreign body is present, or discomfort. Record the findings in the patient's record. Consider the psychosocial aspects of the patient's condition, especially when vision is impaired.

The patient's primary need is for information about prescribed care and how to perform that care. Careful asepsis and frequent, thorough hand washing are essential to prevent spreading organisms from one eye to the other, to other patients, to caregivers, and to health care team members. Teach the patient and caregivers how to avoid sources of ocular irritation or infection and to respond appropriately if an eye problem occurs. The patient with infective disorders that may have a sexual mode of transmission needs specific information about those disorders.

Apply warm or cool compresses as needed. Darkening the room and giving an analgesic are other comfort measures. If the patient's visual acuity is decreased, modify the environment and activities for safety. Suggest alternative ways to perform daily activities and self-care.

The patient may need eyedrops as often as every hour. If the patient receives 2 or more different drops, stagger the eye drops to promote maximum absorption. For example, if 2 different eyedrops are ordered hourly, give 1 drop on the hour and 1 drop on the half hour (unless otherwise prescribed). The patient who needs to instill eyedrops frequently may have sleep deprivation. Review the proper technique for eye drop instillation.

Review the use and care of lenses and lens care products. Teach the patient who wears contact lenses and develops infections to discard all opened or used lens care products and cosmetics. This will decrease the risk for reinfection from contaminated products.

DRY EYE DISORDERS

Keratoconjunctivitis sicca (dry eyes) is a common problem, especially in older adults and people with certain systemic autoimmune diseases, such as scleroderma, systemic lupus erythematosus, and Sjögren's. It is caused by a decrease in the quality or quantity of the tear film. Patients with dry eyes report irritation or "sand in my eye." The sensation typically worsens through the day.

Treatment is aimed at the underlying cause. With decreased tear secretion, the patient may use artificial tears or ointments. Cyclosporine ophthalmic emulsion (Restasis) helps to increase the eyes' natural ability to make tears. In severe cases, closure of the lacrimal puncta may be done.

STRABISMUS

Strabismus is a condition in which a person cannot consistently focus both eyes simultaneously on the same object. One eye may deviate in (*esotropia*), out (*exotropia*), up (*hypertropia*), or down *(hypotropia).* Strabismus in an adult may be caused by thyroid disease, neuromuscular problems of the eye muscles, retinal detachment repair, or cerebral lesions. The primary problem is double vision.

CORNEAL DISORDERS

Corneal Scars

Any wound (e.g., trauma, infection) to the cornea can cause it to become scarred and opacified, thus decreasing the normal transparency. The treatment is a corneal transplant.

Keratoconus

Keratoconus is a noninflammatory, usually bilateral disease with a familial tendency. Keratoconus usually appears during adolescence and slowly progresses between ages 20 and 60 years. The anterior cornea thins and protrudes forward, taking on a cone shape. The only symptom is blurred vision. The astigmatism may be corrected with glasses or rigid contact lenses.

Intacs inserts are generally used to delay the need for a corneal transplant when contact lenses or glasses no longer help a patient achieve adequate vision. They are clear plastic lenses surgically inserted on the cornea perimeter to reduce astigmatism and myopia.

Sometimes, the cornea can perforate as central corneal thinning progresses. In these cases, a corneal transplant is done before the cornea can perforate.

Corneal Transplant. Around 46,000 corneal transplants are done in the United States each year. The surgery is one of the fastest and safest of all tissue or organ transplant surgeries.[11] Indications for corneal transplants (keratoplasty) are corneal scarring and keratoconus. Types include penetrating (full thickness) corneal transplant and lamellar corneal transplant.

Penetrating (full thickness) cornea transplant involves transplanting all the layers of the cornea using a donor cornea. In this procedure, the HCP removes the full thickness of the patient's cornea and replaces it with a donor cornea that is sutured into place (Fig. 20.11). Vision may not be restored for up to 12 months.

During a *lamellar cornea transplant,* only some layers of the cornea are replaced with the transplant. This can include the deepest layer, called the *endothelium* (posterior lamellar cornea transplant). Versions of this procedure include Descemet's stripping endothelial keratoplasty (DSEK) or Descemet's membrane endothelial keratoplasty (DMEK). Lamellar transplants may be better than full penetrating transplants when the disease process is limited to only part of the cornea.

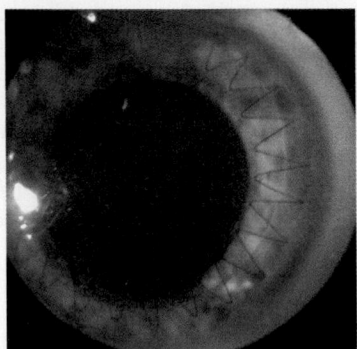

FIG. 20.11 Sutures on a donated cornea after penetrating keratoplasty (corneal transplant). (Courtesy Cory J. Bosanko, OD, FAAO, Eye Centers of Tennessee, Crossville, TN.)

The time between the donor's death and the removal of the tissue should be as short as possible. Eye banks test donors for human immunodeficiency virus (HIV) and hepatitis B and C. The tissue is preserved in a special nutritive solution. Improved methods of tissue procurement and preservation, postoperative topical corticosteroids, and careful follow-up have decreased graft rejection. Matching the blood type of the donor and recipient improves the success rate.

INTRAOCULAR DISORDERS

CATARACT

A cataract is an opacity within the lens. The patient may have a cataract in one or both eyes. If cataracts are present in both eyes, one may affect the patient's vision more than the other. Cataract removal is the most common surgery in the United States.[12]

Etiology and Pathophysiology

Although most cataracts are age related *(senile cataracts),* they can be associated with other factors. These include blunt or penetrating trauma, smoking, alcohol use, radiation or UV light exposure, certain drugs (e.g., steroids), and ocular inflammation. The rate of cataract development varies from patient to patient. The patient with diabetes tends to develop cataracts at a younger age.[13]

In senile cataract formation, altered metabolic processes within the lens cause an accumulation of water and changes in the lens fiber structure. These changes affect lens transparency, causing vision changes.

Clinical Manifestations and Diagnostic Studies

The patient with cataracts may have a decrease in vision, abnormal color perception, and glare. Glare is due to light scatter caused by the lens opacities. It may be significantly worse at night when the pupil dilates. The visual decline is gradual.

Diagnosis is based on decreased visual acuity or other visual problem. The opacity is directly observable by ophthalmoscopic or slit lamp microscopic examination. A totally opaque lens creates the appearance of a white pupil. Table 20.6 lists other diagnostic studies that may be helpful in evaluating a cataract.

Interprofessional Care

The presence of a cataract does not necessarily indicate a need for surgery. For many patients the diagnosis is made long before they decide to have surgery. Interprofessional care for cataracts is outlined in Table 20.8.

Nonsurgical Therapy. Currently, no treatment is available to "cure" cataracts other than surgical removal. Often changing the patient's eyewear prescription can improve visual acuity, at least temporarily. Other visual aids, such as strong reading glasses or magnifiers, may help the patient with near vision. Increasing the amount of light to read or do other near-vision tasks is useful. The patient may be willing to adjust his or her lifestyle to adjust to visual decline. For example, if glare makes it hard to drive at night, a patient may choose to drive only during daylight hours or to have a someone else drive at night. Sometimes, informing and reassuring the patient about the disease process makes the patient comfortable about choosing nonsurgical measures, at least temporarily.

Surgical Therapy. When palliative measures no longer provide an acceptable level of visual function, the patient is a

TABLE 20.8 Interprofessional Care

Cataract

Diagnostic Assessment

- History and physical examination
- Visual acuity measurement
- Ophthalmoscopy (direct and indirect)
- Slit lamp microscopy
- Glare testing, potential acuity testing in selected patients
- Keratometry and A-scan ultrasound (if surgery is planned)
- Other tests (e.g., visual field perimetry) to determine cause of visual loss

Management
Nonsurgical

- Change in glasses prescription
- Strong reading glasses or magnifiers
- Increased lighting
- Lifestyle adjustment

Acute Care: Surgical Therapy
Preoperative

- Mydriatic, cycloplegic agents
- Nonsteroidal antiinflammatory drugs
- Topical antibiotics
- Antianxiety medications

Surgery

- Removal of lens
- Phacoemulsification
- Extracapsular extraction
- Correction of surgical aphakia
- Intraocular lens implantation (most frequent type of correction)
- Contact lenses

Postoperative

- Topical antibiotic
- Topical corticosteroid or other antiinflammatory agent
- Mild analgesia, if necessary
- Eye patch or shield and activity as prescribed

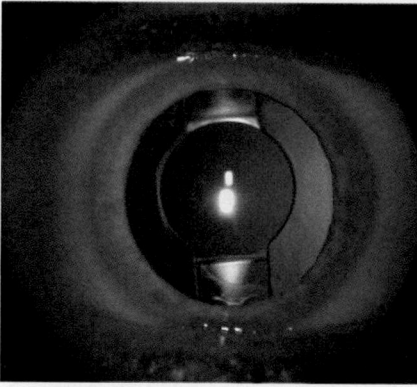

FIG. 20.12 Intraocular lens implant after cataract surgery. (Courtesy Cory J. Bosanko, OD, FAAO, Eye Centers of Tennessee, Crossville, TN.)

muscle. Another type of drug is a *cycloplegic*, such as tropicamide (Mydriacyl), which are anticholinergic agents. They block the effects of acetylcholine on the ciliary body muscles. This produces paralysis of accommodation (cycloplegia), and on the iris sphincter muscle, pupillary dilation (mydriasis). The patient may receive antianxiety medication before surgery.

 DRUG ALERT Cycloplegics and Mydriatics

- Teach the patient to wear dark glasses to minimize photophobia.
- Monitor for signs of systemic toxicity (e.g., tachycardia, CNS effects).

Intraoperative Phase. The most common form of cataract surgery is *phacoemulsification*. In this procedure, a very small incision is made in the surface of the eye in or near the cornea. A thin ultrasound probe is inserted into the eye and ultrasonic vibrations are used to dissolve the clouded lens into fragments. These pieces are then suctioned out through the same ultrasound probe. The small incisions are self-sealing and usually do not need sutures.

An *extracapsular cataract extraction procedure* is used for very advanced cataracts where the lens is too dense to dissolve into fragments. This technique requires a larger incision so that the cataract can be removed in one piece without being fragmented inside the eye. Sutures are needed to close the larger wound, and visual recovery is often slower.

Most patients have an IOL implanted at the time of cataract extraction surgery (Fig. 20.12). The lens of choice is a posterior chamber lens that is placed in the capsular bag behind the iris. At the end of the procedure, other drugs, such as antibiotics and corticosteroids, may be given.

Postoperative Phase. Unless complications occur, the patient is usually ready to go home as soon as the effects of sedative agents have worn off. Postoperative medications usually include antibiotic drops to prevent infection and corticosteroid drops to decrease the inflammatory response. The eyedrops are gradually reduced in frequency and then stopped when the eye has healed.

Recommendations for activity restrictions and nighttime eye shielding vary based on the HCP's preference. Many prefer that the patient avoid activities that increase the IOP, such as bending or stooping, coughing, or lifting.

During each postoperative examination, the HCP measures the patient's visual acuity, checks anterior chamber depth, assesses corneal clarity, and measures IOP. Even on the operative

candidate for surgery. The patient's occupational needs and lifestyle changes are also factors affecting the decision to have surgery. In some instances, factors other than the patient's visual needs may influence the need for surgery. Lens-induced problems, such as increased IOP, may require lens removal. Opacities may prevent the HCP from getting a clear view of the retina in the patient with diabetic retinopathy or other sight-threatening pathologic conditions. In those cases, the cataract is removed to allow visualization of the retina and adequate management of the problem.

Preoperative Phase. Before surgery, obtain an appropriate history and physical examination. Because most patients have local anesthesia, they do not need extensive preoperative physical assessment. However, most patients with cataracts are older adults who may have several medical problems that should be evaluated and controlled before surgery. Most patients are admitted on an outpatient basis. The patient normally presents several hours before surgery to allow time for preoperative procedures.

The patient receives a nonsteroidal antiinflammatory eyedrop to reduce inflammation and dilating drops. One type of drug used for dilation is a *mydriatic*, an α-adrenergic agonist that produces pupillary dilation by contracting the iris dilator

day, the patient's uncorrected visual acuity in the operative eye may be good. However, it is not unusual if the patient's visual acuity is reduced right after surgery. Multifocal IOL can correct for both near and far vision. Some patients may still need glasses or contact lenses to achieve their best visual acuity.

❖ NURSING MANAGEMENT: CATARACTS

◆ Nursing Assessment

Assess the patient's distance and near visual acuity. If the patient is going to have surgery, especially note the visual acuity in the patient's unoperated eye. Use this information to determine how visually compromised the patient may be while the operative eye is healing. Assess the psychosocial impact of the visual disability and the level of knowledge about the disease process and therapeutic options. After surgery, assess the patient's level of comfort and ability to follow the discharge plan.

◆ Planning

Preoperatively, the overall goals are that the patient with a cataract will (1) make informed decisions about therapeutic options and (2) have minimal anxiety. Postoperatively, the overall goals are that the patient with a cataract will (1) understand and follow discharge instructions, (2) maintain an acceptable level of physical and emotional comfort, and (3) remain free of infection and other complications.

◆ Nursing Implementation

◆ Health Promotion. There are no proven measures to prevent cataract development. However, it is wise to suggest that the patient wear sunglasses, avoid unnecessary radiation, and maintain appropriate intake of antioxidant vitamins (e.g., vitamins C, E) and good nutrition. Provide information about vision enhancement techniques for the patient who chooses not to have surgery.

◆ Acute Care. Before surgery, the patient with cataracts needs accurate information about the disease process and treatment options, since cataract surgery is considered an elective procedure. Be available to the patient and caregiver to help them make an informed decision about treatment. For the patient having surgery, provide information, support, and reassurance about the surgical and postoperative experience to reduce anxiety.

Photophobia is common when receiving pupil dilation medications. Therefore decreasing the room lighting is helpful. These medications produce transient stinging and burning.

After cataract surgery the patient usually has little or no pain but may have some scratchiness or blurriness in the operative eye. Mild analgesics are usually enough to relieve any pain. If the pain is intense, the patient should notify the HCP because this may indicate hemorrhage, infection, or increased IOP. A nursing care plan for the patient after eye surgery (eNursing Care Plan 20.1) is available on the website for this chapter.

◆ Ambulatory Care. Patients with cataracts who have surgery remain in the surgical facility for only a few hours. The patient and caregiver are responsible for almost all postoperative care. Give them written and verbal instructions before discharge. Include the caregiver in the instructions because some patients may have difficulty with self-care activities, especially if the vision in the unoperated eye is poor. Table 20.9 outlines patient and caregiver teaching after eye surgery.

Most patients have little visual impairment after surgery. IOL implants provide immediate visual improvement. Many

---

TABLE 20.9 Patient & Caregiver Teaching

After Eye Surgery

Include the following information in the teaching plan for the patient and caregiver after eye surgery:

- Proper hygiene and eye care techniques to ensure that medications, dressings, and/or surgical wound is not contaminated during eye care
- Signs and symptoms of infection (e.g., increased or purulent drainage, increased redness, any decrease in visual acuity) and when and how to report these to allow for early recognition and treatment of possible infection
- Importance of following restrictions on head positioning, bending, coughing, and Valsalva maneuver to optimize visual outcomes and prevent increased IOP
- How to instill eye medications using aseptic techniques and adherence with prescribed eye medication routine to prevent infection
- How to take pain medication and report pain not relieved by medication
- Importance of continued follow-up as recommended to maximize potential visual outcomes

---

patients achieve a usable level of visual acuity within a few days after surgery.

A few patients may have significant visual impairment after surgery. These include patients who do not have an IOL implanted at the time of surgery, those who need several weeks to achieve a usable level of visual acuity after surgery, or those with poor vision in their unoperated eye. For those patients, the time between surgery and receiving glasses or contacts can be a period of significant visual disability. Suggest ways the patient and caregiver can modify activities and the environment to maintain an adequate level of safe functioning. Suggestions may include getting help with steps, removing area rugs and other potential obstacles, preparing meals for freezing before surgery, or obtaining audio books for diversion until visual acuity improves.

If a patch is used, tell patients that they will not have depth perception until the patch is removed. This makes special measures to avoid falls or other injuries necessary. The patient with significant visual impairment in the unoperated eye needs more help while the operative eye is patched. Some patients may need 1 or 2 weeks for the visual acuity in the operated eye to reach an adequate level for most visual needs. These patients need special assistance until the vision improves.

◆ Evaluation

The overall expected outcomes are that the patient after cataract surgery will:
- Have improved vision
- Be better able to take care of self
- Have minimal to no pain
- Be optimistic about expected outcomes

👤 Gerontologic Considerations: Cataracts

Most patients with cataracts are older. When the older patient is visually impaired, even temporarily, the patient may have a loss of independence, lack of control over her or his life, and a significant change in self-perception. Societal devaluation of the older adult complicates these experiences. The older patient often needs emotional support and encouragement, as well as specific suggestions to allow a maximum level of independent function. Assure the older patient that cataract surgery can be done safely and comfortably with minimal sedation.

RETINOPATHY

Retinopathy is a process of microvascular damage to the retina. It can develop slowly or rapidly and lead to blurred vision and progressive vision loss. Retinopathy occurs most often in adults with diabetes or hypertension.

Diabetic retinopathy is a common complication of diabetes, especially in patients with long-standing uncontrolled disease.[13] *Nonproliferative retinopathy* is the most common form of diabetic retinopathy. It is characterized by capillary microaneurysms, retinal swelling, and hard exudates. Macular edema represents a worsening of the retinopathy as plasma leaks from macular blood vessels. As capillary walls weaken, they can rupture, leading to intraretinal "dot or blot" hemorrhaging (Fig. 20.13). A severe loss in central vision can result. As the disease advances, *proliferative retinopathy* may occur. New blood vessels grow, but they are abnormal, fragile, and predisposed to leak, thus causing severe vision loss. (Diagnosis and treatment of diabetic retinopathy are discussed in Chapter 48.)

Hypertensive retinopathy is caused by blockages in retinal blood vessels from hypertension. (Hypertension is discussed in Chapter 32.) These changes may not initially affect a person's vision. On a routine eye examination, retinal hemorrhages, anoxic cotton-wool spots, and macular swelling can be seen. Sustained, severe hypertension can cause sudden visual loss from swelling of the optic disc and nerve *(papilledema)*. Treatment, which may be an emergency, focuses on lowering the BP. Normal vision is usually restored by treating hypertension.

RETINAL DETACHMENT

A retinal detachment is a separation of the sensory retina and the underlying pigment epithelium, with fluid accumulation between the 2 layers. In the patient with no other risk factors who has had a retinal detachment in one eye, the risk for detachment in the second eye is as high as 25%.[14] Most patients with an untreated, symptomatic retinal detachment become blind in the involved eye.

Etiology and Pathophysiology

Retinal detachment has many causes. The most common is a retinal break. *Retinal breaks* are an interruption in the full thickness of the retinal tissue. They can be classified as tears or holes. *Retinal holes* are atrophic retinal breaks that occur spontaneously. *Retinal tears* can occur as the vitreous humor shrinks during aging and pulls on the retina. The retina tears when the traction force exceeds the strength of the retina. Once the retina has a break, liquid vitreous can enter the subretinal space between the sensory layer and the retinal pigment epithelium layer, causing a *rhegmatogenous* retinal detachment. Risk factors for retinal detachment are listed in Table 20.10.

Clinical Manifestations and Diagnostic Studies

Patients with a detaching retina describe symptoms that include *photopsia* (light flashes), floaters, and a "cobweb," "hairnet," or ring in the field of vision. Once the retina has detached, the patient describes a painless loss of peripheral or central vision, "like a curtain" coming across the field of vision.

The area of visual loss corresponds inversely to the area of detachment. For example, if the retinal detachment involves the superior retina, the defect is seen in the inferior visual field. If the detachment is small or develops slowly, the patient may not be aware of a visual problem.

Visual acuity measurements should be the first diagnostic procedure with any report of vision loss (Table 20.11). The HCP

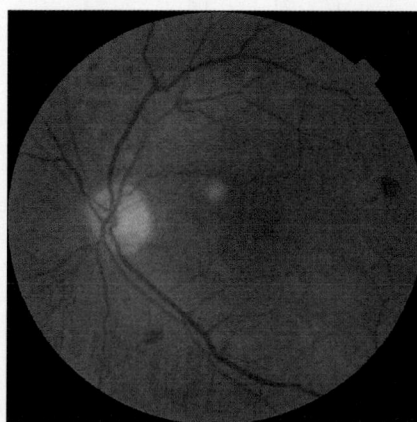

FIG. 20.13 Diabetic retinopathy. Intraretinal dot or blot hemorrhages. (Courtesy Cory J. Bosanko, OD, FAAO, Eye Centers of Tennessee, Crossville, TN.)

TABLE 20.10 Risk Factors for Retinal Detachment

- Age
- Cataract surgery
- Eye trauma
- Family or personal history of retinal detachment
- Severe myopia

Source: National Eye Institute, National Institutes of Health: Retinal detachment. Retrieved from *www.nei.nih.gov/health/retinaldetach.*

TABLE 20.11 Interprofessional Care

Retinal Detachment

Diagnostic Assessment

- History and physical examination
- Visual acuity measurement
- Ophthalmoscopy (direct and indirect)
- Slit lamp microscopy
- Ultrasound if cornea, lens, or vitreous is hazy or opaque

Management

Preoperative

- Mydriatic, cycloplegic agents
- Photocoagulation of retinal break that has not progressed to detachment

Surgery

- Laser photocoagulation
- Cryopexy
- Scleral buckling procedure
- Vitrectomy
- Intravitreal bubble

Postoperative

- Topical antibiotic
- Topical corticosteroid
- Analgesia
- Mydriatics
- Positioning and activity as prescribed

can see a retinal detachment using direct and indirect ophthalmoscopy or slit lamp microscopy in conjunction with a special lens to view the far periphery of the retina. Ultrasound may be useful in finding a retinal detachment if the retina cannot be directly visualized (e.g., when the cornea, lens, or vitreous is hazy or opaque).

Interprofessional Care

Some retinal breaks are not likely to progress to detachment. In these situations, the HCP simply monitors the patient and teaches the patient to seek immediate evaluation if warning signs and symptoms of impending detachment occur. The goals of treatment are to re-attach the retina and seal any retinal breaks. Several techniques are used to meet these goals.

Surgical Therapy

Laser Photocoagulation and Cryopexy. These techniques seal retinal breaks by creating an inflammatory reaction that causes a chorioretinal adhesion or scar. *Laser photocoagulation* involves using an intense, precisely focused light beam to create an inflammatory reaction. The light is directed at the area of the retinal break. *Cryopexy* involves freezing (cryotherapy) the retinal break by placing a probe on the ocular surface at the location of the break. The probe is activated with compressed nitrous oxide gas that temporarily freezes the break. The freeze thaw reaction creates scarring in the area that will seal the break.

For retinal breaks accompanied by significant detachment, photocoagulation or cryopexy may be used intraoperatively in conjunction with scleral buckling. Tears or holes without accompanying retinal detachment may be treated prophylactically with laser photocoagulation or cryopexy if there is a high risk for progression to a retinal detachment. When used alone, laser photocoagulation and cryopexy therapy are outpatient procedures. They usually require topical anesthesia. The patient may have minimal adverse symptoms during or after the procedure.

Scleral Buckling. *Scleral buckling* is an extraocular surgical procedure that involves placing a band around the globe to move the pigment epithelium, choroid, and sclera toward the detached retina. A silicone implant is sutured against the sclera, causing the sclera to buckle inward. An encircling band may be placed over the implant if there are multiple retinal breaks, if suspected breaks cannot be found, or if there is widespread inward traction on the retina (Fig. 20.14). If present, subretinal fluid may be drained using a small-gauge needle. This promotes contact between the retina and buckled sclera. Scleral buckling is usually done as an outpatient procedure.

Intraocular Procedures. Intraocular procedures are used on occasion. *Pneumatic retinopexy* is the intravitreal injection of a gas to form a temporary bubble in the vitreous that closes retinal breaks and provides apposition of the separated retinal layers. Because the intravitreal bubble is temporary, this technique is combined with laser photocoagulation or cryopexy. The patient with an intravitreal bubble must position the head so that the bubble is in contact with the retinal break. The patient may need to maintain this position as much as possible for up to several weeks.

Vitrectomy (surgical removal of the vitreous) may relieve traction on the retina, especially when the traction results from proliferative diabetic retinopathy. Vitrectomy may be combined with scleral buckling to provide a dual effect in relieving traction.

Postoperative Considerations. Visual prognosis varies, depending on the extent, length, and area of detachment. After surgery, the patient may be on bed rest and need special positioning to maintain proper position of an intravitreal bubble. The level of activity restriction after retinal detachment surgery varies. Verify the prescribed level of activity with the HCP and help the patient plan for any help needed related to activity restrictions.

The patient may need multiple topical medications, including antibiotics, antiinflammatory agents, or dilating agents. Give prescribed pain medications and teach the patient to take the medication as prescribed after discharge.

In most cases, retinal detachment is an urgent situation, and the patient is suddenly confronted with the need for surgery. The patient needs emotional support, especially during the immediate preoperative period when preparations for surgery can lead to more anxiety.

The patient may go home within a few hours of surgery or may remain in the hospital for several days, depending on the surgeon and type of repair. Discharge planning and teaching are important and should begin early. Patient and caregiver teaching after eye surgery is discussed in Table 20.11. Because the patient is at increased risk for retinal detachment in the other eye, teach the patient the signs and symptoms of retinal detachment. Promote the use of proper protective eyewear to help avoid damage related to trauma.

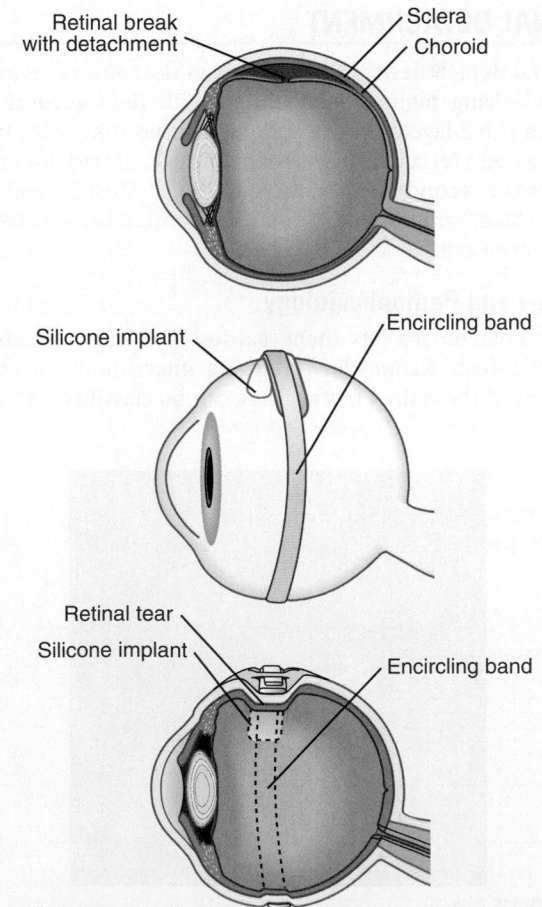

FIG. 20.14 Retinal break with detachment and surgical repair by scleral buckling technique.

AGE-RELATED MACULAR DEGENERATION

Age-related macular degeneration (AMD) is the most common cause of irreversible central vision loss in people over age 60 in the United States. AMD is classified as dry (nonexudative) or wet (exudative). *Dry AMD* is the more common form, accounting for 90% of all cases. Those with dry AMD often notice that close vision tasks become harder. In dry AMD, the macular cells start to atrophy. This leads to a slowly progressive and painless vision loss.

Wet AMD is the more severe form. It accounts for most cases of AMD-related blindness. Wet AMD has a more rapid onset of vision loss. With wet AMD there is the development of abnormal blood vessels in or near the macula. Many patients with wet AMD have dry AMD first.

Etiology and Pathophysiology

AMD is related to retinal aging. Genetic factors also play a major role, and family history is a major risk factor for AMD.[15] Other risk factors include light-colored irises, high C-reactive protein levels, smoking, and hypertension.

Dry AMD starts with the abnormal accumulation of yellowish extracellular deposits called *drusen* in the retinal pigment epithelium. Over time atrophy and degeneration of macular cells occur. In wet AMD, vascular endothelial growth factor (VEGF) promotes the growth of new blood vessels in an abnormal location in the retinal epithelium. As the new blood vessels grow, they leak fluid and can bleed, causing scar tissue to gradually form.

Clinical Manifestations and Diagnostic Studies

Acute vision loss may occur from either the dry or wet forms of AMD. The patient may have blurred and darkened vision, *scotomas* (blind spots in the visual field), and *metamorphopsia* (distortion of vision). If only one eye is affected, the patient may not notice early changes in vision.

In addition to visual acuity measurement, the primary diagnostic procedure is ophthalmoscopy. The HCP looks for drusen and other fundus changes associated with AMD. The Amsler grid test may help define the involved area. It provides a baseline for future comparison (Fig. 20.15). Fundus photography and IV angiography with fluorescein and/or indocyanine green dyes may help to further determine the extent and type of AMD. Retinal anatomy can be analyzed using optical coherence tomography (OCT) or scanning laser ophthalmoscopy.

Interprofessional Care

Visual prognosis varies greatly. Limited treatment options for patients with wet AMD include medications that are injected

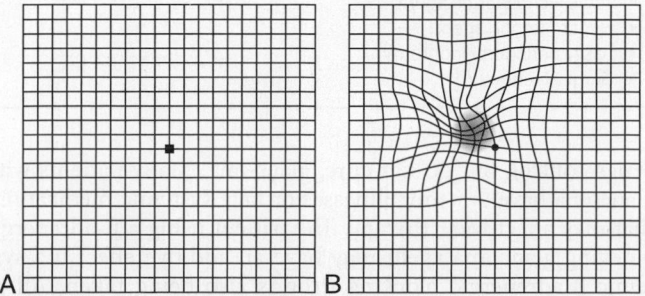

FIG. 20.15 Amsler grid. A, Normal grid. B, Abnormal grid as seen by person with macular degeneration.

directly into the vitreous cavity. Ranibizumab (Lucentis), bevacizumab (Avastin), aflibercept (Eylea), and pegaptanib (Macugen) inhibit VEGF. This helps slow vision loss by stopping new vessels from forming.[15] Side effects can include blurred vision, eye irritation, eye pain, and photosensitivity. Injections are given at 4- to 6-week intervals, depending on treatment response. Disease stability is determined by OCT, which looks at pathology in the macula. The findings determine the need for continued intravitreal injections.

Photodynamic therapy (PDT) uses verteporfin (Visudyne) IV and a "cold" laser to excite the dye. The PDT procedure is used in wet AMD to damage the abnormal blood vessels. Verteporfin is a photosensitizing drug that becomes active when exposed to the low-level laser light wave. Until the drug is completely excreted by the body, it can be activated by exposure to sunlight or other high-intensity light, such as halogen. Have patients avoid direct exposure to sunlight and other intense forms of light for 5 days after treatment. Exposure of the skin to sunlight could activate the drug in that area, causing a chemical burn.

Nutritional factors may play a role in the progression of AMD. Dietary supplements of vitamin C, vitamin E, beta-carotene, and zinc decrease the progression of AMD. Lutein/zeaxanthin supplements may help some patients. Teach the patient to eat dark green, leafy vegetables containing lutein (e.g., kale and spinach) and fatty fish at least twice a week.[16] Smoking cessation may help in halting the progression of dry AMD to a more advanced stage.

The management of the patient with visual impairment discussed on p. 359 is appropriate for the patient with AMD. Many patients with low-vision assistive devices can continue reading and keep a license to drive during the daytime and at lowered speeds. The permanent loss of central vision has significant psychosocial implications for nursing care. Avoid giving the impression that "nothing can be done" about the problem when caring for the patient with AMD. Although therapy may not recover lost vision, much can be done to augment the remaining vision.

GLAUCOMA

Glaucoma is a group of disorders characterized by increased IOP and its' consequences, optic nerve atrophy, and peripheral visual field loss. Glaucoma is the second leading cause of permanent blindness in the United States and the leading cause of blindness among blacks.[3,17] Many people with glaucoma are unaware of their condition. The incidence of glaucoma increases with age. Blindness from glaucoma is largely preventable with early detection and proper treatment. Genetic factors play a role in some types of glaucoma.[17]

Etiology and Pathophysiology

A proper balance between the rate of aqueous production (*inflow*) and the rate of aqueous reabsorption (*outflow*) is essential to maintain the IOP within normal limits. We call the place where the outflow occurs the *angle* because it is the angle where the iris meets the cornea. When the rate of inflow is greater than the rate of outflow, IOP can increase above the normal limits. If IOP stays increased, permanent vision loss may occur.

Primary open-angle glaucoma (POAG) is the most common type of glaucoma. In POAG the outflow of aqueous humor is decreased in the trabecular meshwork. The drainage channels become clogged, like a clogged kitchen sink. Damage to the optic nerve can then result.

Angle-closure glaucoma (ACG) is due to a reduction in the outflow of aqueous humor that results from angle closure. Usually, this is caused by the lens bulging forward because of the aging process. Angle closure may also occur because of pupil dilation in the patient with anatomically narrow angles. Acute angle-closure glaucoma (AACG) may be precipitated by situations in which the pupil stays partially dilated long enough to cause an acute and significant rise in the IOP. This may occur because of drug-induced mydriasis, emotional excitement, or darkness. Drug-induced mydriasis may occur from topical eye preparations or many systemic medications (both prescription and OTC). Check medication records before giving medications to the patient with ACG. Teach the patient not to take any mydriatic medications.

Clinical Manifestations

POAG develops slowly and without symptoms of pain or pressure. The patient usually does not notice the gradual visual field loss until peripheral vision has been severely compromised. Eventually, the patient with untreated glaucoma has "tunnel vision," with only a small center visual field. All peripheral vision is absent.

AACG causes definite symptoms, including sudden, severe pain in or around the eye. The patient often has nausea and vomiting. Visual symptoms include seeing colored halos around lights, blurred vision, and ocular redness.

Manifestations of subacute or chronic ACG appear more gradually. The patient who had a previous, unrecognized episode of subacute ACG may report blurred vision, seeing colored halos around lights, ocular redness, or eye or brow pain.

Diagnostic Studies

IOP is usually increased in glaucoma (normal is 10 to 21 mm Hg). In the patient with increased pressures, the measurements are repeated over time to verify the elevation. In POAG, IOP is usually between 22- and 32-mm Hg. In AACG, IOP may be more than 50 mm Hg.

In POAG, slit lamp microscopy reveals a normal angle. In ACG, there may be a markedly narrow or flat anterior chamber angle, an edematous cornea, a fixed and moderately dilated pupil, and ciliary injection (hyperemia of the ciliary blood vessels produces a red color).

Measures of peripheral and central vision provide more diagnostic information. While central acuity may remain 20/20 even in the presence of severe peripheral visual field loss, visual field perimetry may reveal subtle changes in the peripheral vision early in the disease process, long before actual scotomas develop. In ACG, central visual acuity is reduced if the patient has corneal edema, and the visual fields may be markedly decreased. As glaucoma progresses, *optic disc cupping* may be one of the first signs of chronic POAG. The optic disc becomes wider, deeper, and paler (light gray or white), which is visible with direct or indirect ophthalmoscopy (Fig. 20.16).

Interprofessional Care

The primary focus of glaucoma therapy is to keep the IOP low enough to prevent the patient from developing optic nerve damage. Therapy varies with the type of glaucoma. The diagnostic and interprofessional care of glaucoma is outlined in Table 20.12. **Chronic Open-Angle Glaucoma.** Drug therapy is the initial treatment in POAG (Table 20.13). The patient must understand that continued treatment and supervision are needed because the

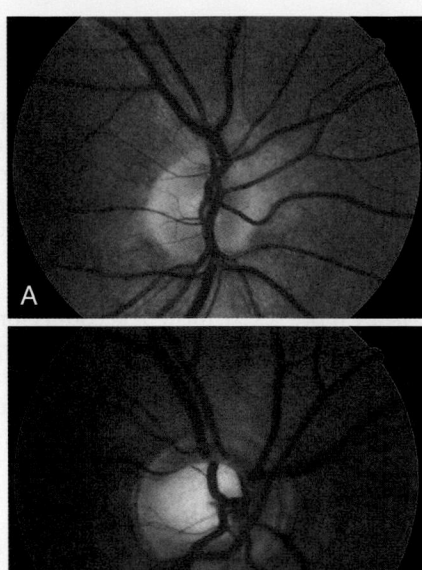

FIG. 20.16 A, In the normal eye the optic cup is pink with little cupping. B, In glaucoma the optic cup is bleached and optic cupping is present. (Note the appearance of the retinal vessels, which travel over the edge of the optic cup and appear to dip into it.)

TABLE 20.12 **Interprofessional Care**
Glaucoma

Diagnostic Assessment
- History and physical examination
- Visual acuity measurement
- Tonometry
- Ophthalmoscopy (direct and indirect)
- Slit lamp microscopy
- Gonioscopy
- Visual field perimetry

Management
Chronic Open-Angle Glaucoma
Drug Therapy (Table 20.13)
- β-Adrenergic blockers
- α-Adrenergic agonists
- Cholinergic agents (miotics)
- Carbonic anhydrase inhibitors

Surgical Therapy
- Argon laser trabeculoplasty (ALT)
- Trabeculectomy with or without filtering implant

Acute Angle-Closure Glaucoma
- Topical cholinergic agent
- Hyperosmotic agent
- Laser peripheral iridotomy
- Surgical iridectomy

drugs control, but do not cure, glaucoma. Many patients with glaucoma have systemic illnesses or take systemic medications that may affect their therapy. The patient using a β-adrenergic blocking glaucoma agent may have an additive effect if a systemic β-adrenergic blocking drug is also being taken. All β-adrenergic blocking glaucoma agents are contraindicated in the patient with bradycardia, heart block greater than first-degree

TABLE 20.13 Drug Therapy

Acute and Chronic Glaucoma

Drug	Action	Side Effects	Nursing Considerations
α-Adrenergic Agonists			
apraclonidine (Iopidine), brimonidine (Alphagan)	↓ Aqueous humor production	Ocular redness, irregular heart rate	Topical drops Used to control or prevent acute postlaser IOP rise (used before and immediately after ALT and iridotomy, Nd:YAG laser capsulotomy) Teach patient at risk for systemic reactions to occlude puncta
α- and β-Adrenergic Agonists			
dipivefrin (Propine)	Converted to epinephrine inside the eye aqueous humor production, enhances outflow facility	Ocular discomfort and redness, tachycardia, hypertension	Topical drops Contraindicated in patient with narrow-angle glaucoma Teach punctal occlusion if patient at risk for systemic reactions
epinephrine	Same as dipivefrin	Same as dipivefrin, but can be more pronounced	Topical drops Same as dipivefrin
β-Adrenergic Blockers			
betaxolol (Betoptic)	β₁ cardioselective ↓ IOP, ↓ aqueous humor production	Transient discomfort Systemic reactions rarely reported but include bradycardia, heart block, pulmonary distress, headache, depression	Topical drugs Contraindicated in patient with bradycardia, cardiogenic shock, or heart failure Systemic absorption can have additive effect with systemic β₁-blocking agents
levobunolol (Betagan) timolol maleate (Timoptic, Istalol)	β₁ and β₂ noncardioselective blockers ↓ IOP, ↓ aqueous humor production	Transient ocular discomfort, blurred vision, photophobia, bradycardia, decreased BP, bronchospasm, headache, depression	Topical drops Same as betaxolol Contraindicated in patients with asthma or COPD
Carbonic Anhydrase Inhibitors			
Systemic			
acetazolamide (Diamox) dichlorphenamide (Daranide) methazolamide	↓ Aqueous humor production	Paresthesias, especially "tingling" in extremities, hearing problems or tinnitus, loss of appetite, taste changes, GI problems, drowsiness, confusion	Oral nonbacteriostatic sulfonamides Anaphylaxis and other sulfa-type allergic reactions may occur in patient allergic to sulfa Diuretic effect can ↓ electrolyte levels Do not give to patient on high-dose aspirin therapy
Topical			
brinzolamide (Azopt) dorzolamide (Trusopt)	↓ Aqueous humor production	Transient stinging, blurred vision, redness	Anaphylaxis and other sulfa-type allergic reactions may occur in patient allergic to sulfa
Cholinergic Agents (Miotics)			
carbachol (Miostat, Isopto Carbachol)	Parasympathomimetic Stimulates iris sphincter contraction, causing miosis and opening of trabecular meshwork, facilitating aqueous outflow Partially inhibits cholinesterase	Transient ocular discomfort, headache, blurred vision, decreased adaptation to the dark, syncope, salivation, dysrhythmias, vomiting, diarrhea, hypotension	Topical drops Caution patient about ↓ visual acuity caused by miosis, particularly in dim light
pilocarpine (Isopto Carpine, Pilocar)	Parasympathomimetic Stimulates iris sphincter contraction, causing miosis and opening of trabecular meshwork, facilitating aqueous humor outflow	Same as carbachol	Topical drops Same as carbachol
Prostaglandin Agonists			
bimatoprost (Lumigan) latanoprost (Xalatan) tafluprost (Zioptan) travoprost	↓ Outflow of aqueous humor between the uvea and sclera and the usual exit through the trabecular meshwork	Increased brown iris pigmentation, ocular discomfort and redness, dryness, itching, and foreign body sensation	Topical drops Teach patient to only administer 1 drop per day Have patient remove contact lens 15 min before instilling

ALT, Argon laser trabeculoplasty; *Nd:YAG,* neodymium-doped yttrium aluminum garnet (laser).

heart block, cardiogenic shock, and heart failure. The noncardioselective β-adrenergic blocking glaucoma agents are contraindicated in the patient with chronic obstructive pulmonary disease (COPD) or asthma. The hyperosmolar agents may precipitate heart failure or pulmonary edema in the susceptible patient. The patient on high-dose aspirin therapy should not take carbonic anhydrase inhibitors. The α-adrenergic agonists can cause tachycardia or hypertension. This may have profound consequences in the older patient.

Argon laser trabeculoplasty (ALT) is a noninvasive way to lower IOP when medications are not successful or when the patient either cannot or will not use the drug therapy as recommended. ALT is an outpatient procedure that uses topical anesthetic. The laser stimulates scarring and contraction of the trabecular meshwork, which opens the outflow channels. ALT reduces IOP most of the time. The patient uses topical corticosteroids for 3 to 5 days after the procedure. The most common complication is an acute rise in IOP. The HCP examines the patient at 1 week and again at 4 to 6 weeks after surgery.

Filtration surgery, also called a *trabeculectomy,* may be used if medical management and laser therapy are not successful.

Acute Angle-Closure Glaucoma. AACG is an ocular emergency that needs immediate intervention. Miotics (Table 20.13) and oral or IV hyperosmotic agents, including glycerin liquid (Ophthalgan), isosorbide solution (Ismotic), and mannitol solution (Osmitrol), are usually successful in immediately lowering IOP. A laser peripheral iridotomy or surgical iridectomy is necessary for long-term treatment and prevention of more episodes. These procedures allow the aqueous humor to flow through a newly created opening in the iris and into normal outflow channels. A procedure may be done on the other eye as a precaution because many patients often have an acute attack in the other eye.

 DRUG ALERT Miotics

- Warn patients about decreased visual acuity, especially in dim light.

❖ NURSING MANAGEMENT: GLAUCOMA

◆ Nursing Assessment

Because glaucoma is a chronic condition requiring long-term management, assess the patient's ability to understand and adhere to the therapy plan. Assess the patient's psychologic reaction to the diagnosis of a potentially sight-threatening chronic disorder. Include the patient's caregiver in the assessment process because the chronic nature of this disorder affects them too. For example, caregivers may become the eyedrop administrator if the patient is unwilling or unable.

◆ Nursing Diagnoses

Nursing diagnoses for the patient with glaucoma include:
- Risk for injury
- Acute pain

◆ Planning

The overall goals are that the patient with glaucoma will (1) have no progression of visual impairment, (2) follow the treatment plan, and (3) have no complications.

◆ Nursing Implementation

◆ **Health Promotion.** Loss of vision because of glaucoma is a preventable problem. Teach the patient and caregiver about the risk

for glaucoma and that it increases with age. Stress the importance of early detection and treatment in preventing visual impairment. A comprehensive eye examination is important in identifying people with glaucoma or those at risk for developing glaucoma. The current recommendation is for an eye examination every 2 to 4 years for people between ages 40 and 64 years, and every 1 to 2 years for people age 65 years or older. Blacks in every age category should have one more often because of the increased incidence and more aggressive course of glaucoma.[17]

◆ **Acute Care.** Acute nursing interventions are directed primarily toward the patient with AACG and the surgical patient. The patient with AACG needs medication immediately to lower the IOP. Most surgeries for glaucoma are outpatient procedures. Provide care to relieve any discomfort related to the procedure. Patient and caregiver teaching after eye surgery is discussed in Table 20.9.

◆ **Ambulatory Care.** Because of the chronic nature of glaucoma, teach the patient to follow the therapy plan and follow-up recommendations prescribed by the HCP. Provide accurate information about the disease process and treatment options, including the reason for each option. In addition, the patient needs information about the purpose, frequency, and technique for administering antiglaucoma drugs. Encourage adherence by helping the patient set up a medication administration schedule and advocating a change in therapy if the patient reports unacceptable side effects.

◆ Evaluation

The overall expected outcomes are that the patient with glaucoma will:
- Have no further loss of vision
- Adhere to the recommended therapy
- Safely function within own environment
- Have relief from pain associated with the disease and surgery

INTRAOCULAR INFLAMMATION AND INFECTION

The term *uveitis* is used to describe inflammation of the uveal tract, retina, vitreous body, or optic nerve. Inflammation may be caused by bacteria, viruses, fungi, or parasites. *Cytomegalovirus retinitis* (CMV retinitis) is an opportunistic infection that occurs in patients with acquired immunodeficiency syndrome (AIDS) and in other immunosuppressed patients. The cause of sterile intraocular inflammation includes autoimmune disorders, AIDS, cancer, or disorders associated with systemic diseases, such as inflammatory bowel disease. Pain and photophobia are common symptoms.

Endophthalmitis is an extensive intraocular inflammation of the vitreous cavity. Bacteria, viruses, fungi, or parasites can induce this serious inflammatory response. The mechanism of infection may be endogenous, in which the infecting agent arrives at the eye through the bloodstream, or exogenous, in which the infecting agent is introduced through a surgical wound or a penetrating injury. Although rare, endophthalmitis is a devastating complication of intraocular surgery or penetrating ocular injury. It can lead to irreversible blindness within hours or days. Manifestations include ocular pain, photophobia, decreased visual acuity, headaches, reddened and swollen conjunctiva, and corneal edema.

Treatment depends on the underlying cause. Intraocular infections require antimicrobial agents. They may be delivered topically, subconjunctivally, intravitreally, systemically, or in some combination. Inflammatory responses require antiinflammatory medications (e.g., corticosteroids). The patient with intraocular inflammation is usually uncomfortable and may be noticeably anxious and frightened. Provide accurate information and emotional support to the patient and caregiver. In severe cases, enucleation may be needed. When the patient has lost visual function or even the entire eye, the patient will grieve the loss. Your role includes helping the patient through the grieving process.

OCULAR TUMORS

Benign and cancerous tumors can occur in many areas of the eye, including the conjunctiva, retina, and orbit.[18] Eyelid cancers include basal cell and squamous cell cancers (see Chapter 23).

Uveal melanoma is a cancer of the iris, choroid, or ciliary body. It more often occurs in light-skinned people with light eye color, who are over age 60, and have chronic UV exposure.[19] Uveal melanoma can arise from preexisting nevi in the eye. Tumors may be asymptomatic or associated with vision loss. This depends on their size and location and presence of hemorrhage and retinal detachment. As with other cancers, cancer stage and cell type are important variables in the prognosis. Diagnostic testing may include ultrasound, MRI, and fine-needle aspiration biopsy. Uveal melanoma often appears as a dome-shaped, well-circumscribed, solid brown to golden pigment in the iris, choroid, or ciliary body (Fig. 20.17).

Depending on the status of the involved eye, treatment options can include enucleation, radiation therapy (brachytherapy), external beam radiation, transpupillary photocoagulation, eye wall resection, and eye removal. Many patients do not lose their eye. Some may have good vision after treatment in the affected eye.

ENUCLEATION

Enucleation is the removal of the eye. The primary reason for enucleation is a blind, painful eye. This may result from glaucoma, infection, or trauma. Enucleation may be used to treat ocular cancer. The surgical procedure includes severing the extraocular muscles close to their insertion on the globe, inserting an implant to maintain the intraorbital anatomy, and suturing the ends of the muscles over the implant. The conjunctiva covers the joined muscles, and a clear conformer is placed over the conjunctiva until the permanent prosthesis is fitted. A pressure dressing helps prevent bleeding.

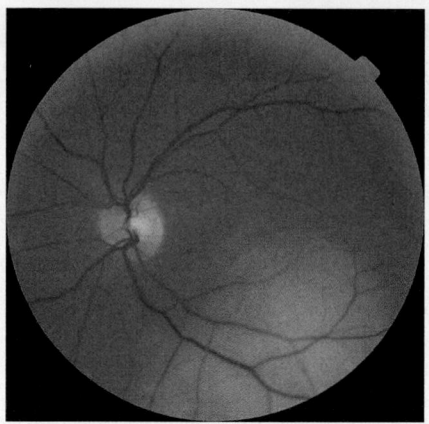

FIG. 20.17 Uveal melanoma. A large tumor in the choroid, the most common location in the eye for melanoma. (Courtesy Cory J. Bosanko, OD, FAAO, Eye Centers of Tennessee, Crossville, TN.)

After surgery, observe the patient for signs of complications, including excess bleeding or swelling, increased pain, displacement of the implant, and fever. Patient teaching should include the instillation of topical ointments or drops and wound cleansing. Teach the patient how to insert the conformer into the socket in case it falls out. The loss of an eye is often devastating, even when enucleation occurs after a lengthy period of painful blindness. Recognize the patient's emotional response and provide support to the patient and caregivers.

About 6 weeks after surgery, the wound is sufficiently healed for the permanent prosthesis. An ocularist fits the prosthesis and designs it to match the remaining eye. Teach the patient how to remove, cleanse, and insert the prosthesis. Special polishing is needed periodically to remove dried protein secretions.

OCULAR MANIFESTATIONS OF SYSTEMIC DISEASES

Many systemic diseases have significant ocular manifestations. Ocular signs and symptoms may be the first finding or complaint in the patient with a systemic disease. One example is the patient with undiagnosed diabetes who seeks eye care for blurred vision. A careful history and examination can reveal that the underlying cause of the blurred vision is lens swelling from hyperglycemia. Another example is the patient who seeks care for a conjunctival lesion. AIDS may be diagnosed based on the presence of a conjunctival Kaposi sarcoma (KS).

CASE STUDY

Glaucoma and Diabetic Retinopathy

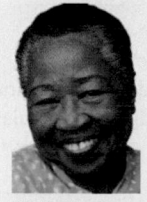

(© Kevin Peterson/Stockbyte/ Thinkstock.)

Patient Profile

J.K. is a 68-yr-old black woman with a history of osteoarthritis and type 2 diabetes for the past 15 years. She now has diabetic retinopathy. She returns to the eye clinic with her daughter for continued care of primary open-angle glaucoma (POAG) and reexamination for changes in diabetic retinopathy. Her current drug therapy for POAG includes topical timolol maleate 0.5% extended (Timoptic-XE) once daily in both eyes (OU) and latanoprost (Xalatan) 0.005% OU daily at bedtime. At her last examination, she had microaneurysms and hard exudates of the retina.

Subjective Data

- She can no longer read the newspaper and reports that medication labels are difficult to read.
- States she is not always successful in getting the eyedrops instilled because her hands are gnarled and painful from osteoarthritis.

Objective Data

- Distant and near visual acuity are stable at 20/60 (OD) and 20/50 (OS). This is a reduction from 20/40 (OU) at her last visit.
- Intraocular pressure (IOP) stable at 20 mm Hg (OU).
- There is a new scotoma on visual field testing in the OS.
- Fluorescein angiography reveals diabetic macular edema OU.

Continued

CASE STUDY

Glaucoma and Diabetic Retinopathy—cont'd

Interprofessional Care

- Brimonidine 0.15% (OS) 15 min before and immediately after argon laser trabeculoplasty (ALT)
- Argon laser (OU) to seal leaking microaneurysms from macular edema
- Check IOP 1 hr after ALT
- Continue previous glaucoma drop regimen
- Follow-up examination for in 2 wk for possible ALT of OD

Discussion Questions

1. Explain the cause of the new scotoma.
2. Why is ALT an appropriate therapy for J.K.?

3. What is the purpose of the eyedrops before and immediately after ALT?
4. What is the cause of the vision loss from diabetic retinopathy?
5. Priority Decision: Based on the assessment data, what are the priority nursing diagnoses? Are there any collaborative problems?
6. ***Priority Decision:*** What are the priority nursing interventions for J.K.?
7. ***Patient-Centered Care:*** What are the priority topics that should be discussed in discharge teaching with J.K.?
8. ***Evidence-Based Practice:*** J.K. wants to know if her glaucoma is related to her diabetes. How would you respond to her question?

Answers available at *http://evolve.elsevier.com/Lewis/medsurg.*

BRIDGE TO NCLEX EXAMINATION

The number of the question corresponds to the same-numbered outcome at the beginning of the chapter.

1. In a patient who has a hemorrhage in the posterior cavity of the eye, the nurse knows that blood is accumulating
   a. in the aqueous humor.
   b. between the lens and retina.
   c. between the cornea and lens.
   d. in the space between the iris and lens.

2. Increased intraocular pressure may occur because of
   a. edema of the corneal stroma.
   b. dilation of the retinal arterioles.
   c. blockage of the lacrimal canals and ducts.
   d. increased aqueous humor production by the ciliary process.

3. Ask patients using eyedrops to treat their glaucoma about
   a. use of corrective lenses.
   b. their usual sleep pattern.
   c. a history of heart or lung disease.
   d. sensitivity to opioids or depressants.

4. Always assess the patient with an eye problem for
   a. visual acuity.
   b. pupillary reactions.
   c. intraocular pressure.
   d. confrontation visual fields.

5. When examining the patient's eyes, which finding would be of *most* concern to the nurse?
   a. Intraocular pressure of 16 mm/Hg
   b. Slightly yellowish cast of the sclera
   c. Outward turning of the lower lid margin
   d. Small, white nodule on the upper lid margin

6. Presbyopia occurs in older people because
   a. the eyeball elongates.
   b. the lens becomes inflexible.
   c. the corneal curvature becomes irregular.
   d. light rays are focusing in front of the retina.

7. Before injecting fluorescein for angiography, it is important for the nurse to *(select all that apply)*
   a. obtain an emesis basin.
   b. ask if the patient is fatigued.
   c. administer a topical anesthetic.
   d. inform patient that skin may turn yellow.
   e. assess for allergies to iodine-based contrast media.

8. A patient says she was diagnosed with astigmatism. When she asks what that is, what is the best explanation the nurse can give to the patient?
   a. "It happens because the lens of the eye is absent."
   b. "People with astigmatism have abnormally long eyeballs."
   c. "The cornea of the eye is uneven or irregular with astigmatism."
   d. "Astigmatism occurs because the eye muscles weaken with age."

9. Which intervention would be part of the plan of care for a patient who has new vision loss?
   a. Allow the patient to express feelings of grief and anger.
   b. Have the UAP perform all self-care activities for the patient.
   c. Address any family present first when discussing care concerns.
   d. Speak loudly and clearly, addressing the patient with each contact.

10. Which patient behaviors would the nurse promote for healthy eyes *(select all that apply)*?
    a. Protective sunglasses when bicycling
    b. Taking part in a smoking cessation program
    c. Supplementing diet intake of vitamin C and beta-carotene
    d. Washing hands thoroughly before putting in or taking out contact lenses
    e. A woman avoiding pregnancy for 4 weeks after receiving MMR immunization

11. The *most* important intervention for the patient with epidemic keratoconjunctivitis is
    a. cleansing the affected area with baby shampoo.
    b. monitoring spread of infection to the opposing eye.
    c. regular instillation of artificial tears to the affected eye.
    d. teaching the patient and caregivers good hygiene techniques.

12. What should be included in the discharge teaching for the patient who had cataract surgery *(select all that apply)*?
    a. Eye discomfort is often relieved with mild analgesics.
    b. A decline in visual acuity is common for the first week.
    c. Stay on bed rest and limit activity for the first few days.
    d. Notify the provider if an increase in redness or drainage occurs.
    e. Following activity restrictions is essential to reduce intraocular pressure.

1. b, 2. d, 3. c, 4. a, 5. d, 6. b, 7. a, d, 8. c, 9. a, 10. a, b, c, d, 11. d, 12. a, d, e

For rationales to these answers and even more NCLEX review questions, visit *http://evolve.elsevier.com/Lewis/medsurg.*

e EVOLVE WEBSITE/RESOURCES LIST

http://evolve.elsevier.com/Lewis/medsurg
Review Questions (Online Only)
Key Points
Answer Keys for Questions
- Rationales for Bridge to NCLEX Examination Questions
- Answer Guidelines for Case Study on pp. 351, 354, 358, and 373

Student Case Study
- Patient Undergoing Cataract Surgery

eNursing Care Plan
- eNursing Care Plan 20.1: Patient After Eye Surgery

Conceptual Care Map Creator
Audio Glossary
Supporting Media
- Animations
- Cataract Removal
- LASIK
- Myringotomy
- Scleral Buckling

Content Updates

REFERENCES

1. Lampignano J, Kendrick L: *Bontrager's textbook of radiographic positioning and related anatomy*, ed 9, St Louis, 2018, Elsevier.
*2. Martin E, Patrianakos T, Giovingo M: Medication induced glaucoma, *Disease-a-Month* 63:54, 2017.
3. National Eye Institute: Statistics and data. Retrieved from *www.nei.nih.gov/eyedata*.
4. American Optometric Association: Myopia. Retrieved from *www.aoa.org/patients-and-public/eye-and-vision-problems/glossary-of-eye-and-vision-conditions/myopia?sso=y*.
5. US Food and Drug Administration: LASIK. Retrieved from *www.fda.gov/medicaldevices/productsandmedicalprocedures/surgeryandlifesupport/lasik/default.htm*.
6. American Optometric Association: Low vision. Retrieved from *www.aoa.org/patients-and-public/caring-for-your-vision/low-vision*.
*7. Salva MA, Hartley S, Léger D, et al : Non-24-hour sleep–wake rhythm disorder in the totally blind: Diagnosis and management., *Front Neurol* 8:686, 2017.
8. American Academy of Ophthalmology: Preventing eye injuries. Retrieved from *www.aao.org/eye-health/diseases/preventing-injuries*.
*9. Satpathy G, Behera HS, Ahmed NH: Chlamydial eye infections: Current perspectives, *Indian J Ophthalmol* 65:97, 2017.
*10. Azher TN, Yin XT, Tajfirouz D, et al: Herpes simplex keratitis: Challenges in diagnosis and clinical management, *Clin Ophthalmol* 11:185, 2017.
11. Saving Sight: Important information about saving sight. Retrieved from *www.saving-sight.org/cornea-donation-facts*.
12. Date RC, Al-Mohtaseb ZN: Advances in preoperative testing for cataract surgery, *Internat Ophthalmol Clin* 57:99, 2017.
13. American Diabetes Association: Standards of medical care in diabetes—2018, *Diabetes Care* 1:S105, 2018.
14. Schachat AP, Sadda SR, Hinton DR, et al: *Ryan's retina: Principles and practice*, ed 6, St Louis, 2018, Elsevier.
15. American Macular Degeneration Foundation: About macular degeneration. Retrieved from *www.macular.org/about-macular-degeneration*.
*16. Carneiro Â, Andrade JP: Nutritional and lifestyle interventions for age-related macular degeneration: A review, *Oxid Med Cell Longev*, 2017.
17. Glaucoma Research Foundation: Glaucoma. Retrieved from *www.glaucoma.org/glaucoma/*.
18. International Society of Ocular Oncology: Eye tumors. Retrieved from *www.isoo.org/tumors*.
*19. Pandiani C, Béranger GE, Leclerc J, et al : Focus on cutaneous and uveal melanoma specificities, *Genes Dev* 31:724, 2017.

*Evidence-based information for clinical practice.

21

Assessment and Management: Auditory Problems

Mariann M. Harding

Kindness is a language which the deaf can hear and the blind can see.

Mark Twain

http://evolve.elsevier.com/Lewis/medsurg/

CONCEPTUAL FOCUS

Coping
Functional Ability

Infection
Sensory Perception

LEARNING OUTCOMES

1. Describe the structures and functions of the auditory system.
2. Obtain significant subjective and objective assessment data related to the auditory system from a patient.
3. Perform a physical assessment of the auditory system using the appropriate techniques.
4. Distinguish normal from common abnormal findings of a physical assessment of the auditory system.
5. Link the age-related changes in the auditory system to differences in assessment findings.
6. Describe the purpose, significance of results, and nursing responsibilities related to diagnostic studies of the auditory system.

7. Explain the pathophysiology, clinical manifestations, and nursing and interprofessional management of common ear problems.
8. Compare the common causes, management, and rehabilitative potential of conductive and sensorineural hearing loss.
9. Explain the use, care, and patient teaching related to assistive devices for ear problems.
10. Describe measures used to assist the patient in adapting to decreased hearing.

KEY TERMS

acoustic neuroma, p. 387
benign paroxysmal positional vertigo (BPPV),
  p. 387
external otitis, p. 383

Ménière's disease, p. 386
nystagmus, p. 378
otosclerosis, p. 385
presbycusis, p. 378

tinnitus, p. 378
vertigo, p. 378

AUDITORY SYSTEM

Hearing is a complex process that allows us to interact with the environment. It is the basis for social interaction and communication. Having a hearing impairment can lead to major challenges that can negatively affect well-being. In the adult, difficulties with related concepts, including functional ability and cognition, may be present with hearing loss. This chapter presents an overview of auditory function and discusses care when problems occur.

STRUCTURES AND FUNCTIONS OF AUDITORY SYSTEM

The auditory system is composed of the peripheral auditory system and central auditory system. The peripheral auditory system includes the structures of the ear itself: external, middle, and inner ear (Fig. 21.1). This system is involved with the reception and perception of sound. The inner ear functions in hearing and balance.

The central auditory system integrates and assigns meaning to what one hears. This system includes the vestibulocochlear nerve (cranial nerve [CN] VIII) and auditory cortex of the brain. The brain and its pathways transmit and process sound and sensations that maintain a person's equilibrium.

The role of the external and middle part of the ear is to conduct and amplify sound waves from the environment. This part of sound conduction is termed *air conduction.* Problems in these two parts of the ear may cause *conductive hearing loss,* resulting in a decrease in sound intensity and/or a distortion in sound.[1]

Disturbances in equilibrium can impair coordination, balance, and orientation. Damage to or an abnormality of the inner ear or along the nerve pathways results in *sensorineural hearing loss.* In addition to causing distortion or faintness of sound, sensorineural hearing loss may affect the ability to understand speech or cause complete hearing loss. Impairment within the auditory pathways of the brain causes *central hearing loss.* This type of hearing loss causes difficulty in understanding the meaning of words the person heard. Types of hearing loss are discussed later in this chapter on pp. 387-389.

External Ear

The external ear consists of the *auricle* (pinna), external auditory canal, and *tympanic membrane (TM).* The auricle is composed of cartilage and connective tissue covered with epithelium, which also lines the external auditory canal (Fig. 21.1). The external auditory canal is a slightly S-shaped tube about 1 inch (2.5 cm) in length in the adult. The lining of the proximal one third of the canal contains fine hairs (cilia), sebaceous (oil) glands, and ceruminous (wax) glands. The oil and wax lubricate the ear canal, keep it free from debris, and kill bacteria. Thin epithelium lines the distal two thirds of the canal. It is over bone and very sensitive.

The function of the external ear and canal is to collect and transmit sound waves to the TM, or eardrum. The TM is a shiny, translucent, pearl-gray membrane. It is made up of epithelial cells, connective tissue, and mucous membrane. It serves as a partition and transmits sounds between the external auditory canal and middle ear.

Middle Ear

The middle ear cavity is an air space in the temporal bone. Mucous membrane lines the middle ear and is continuous from the nasal pharynx via the eustachian (auditory) tube. The eustachian tube equalizes atmospheric air pressure between the middle ear and throat. This allows the TM to move freely. It is normally closed, opening only with yawning, swallowing, and chewing. Blockage of the tube can occur with allergies, nasopharyngeal infections, or enlarged adenoids. A tube that stays open is called *patulous.* When this occurs, *autophony,* or hearing your own voice, may be present.

The middle ear contains the *ossicles,* the 3 smallest bones in the body: *malleus, incus,* and *stapes.* Vibrations of the TM cause the ossicles to move and transmit sound waves to the oval window. The superior part of the middle ear is the *epitympanum,* or the attic. It also communicates with air cells within the mastoid bone. The mastoid is the posterior part of the temporal bone. The facial nerve (CN VII) traverses above the oval window of the middle ear. The thin, bony covering of the facial nerve can become damaged by chronic ear infection, skull fracture, or trauma during ear surgery. Problems may occur related to voluntary facial movements, eyelid closure, and taste discrimination. Permanent damage to the facial nerve can result.

Inner Ear

The inner ear consists of 3 spaces in the temporal bone, assembled in a system called the bony labyrinth. The space is filled with watery fluid called perilymph. Within the perilymph is the membranous labyrinth. It follows the shape of the bony labyrinth and holds a thicker fluid called *endolymph.*

The inner ear holds the functional organs for hearing and balance. The receptor organ for hearing is the *cochlea,* a coiled structure that contains the *organ of Corti.* Its tiny hair cells respond to stimulation of select portions of the basilar membrane according to pitch. This stimulus is converted into an electrochemical impulse. It is transmitted by the acoustic part

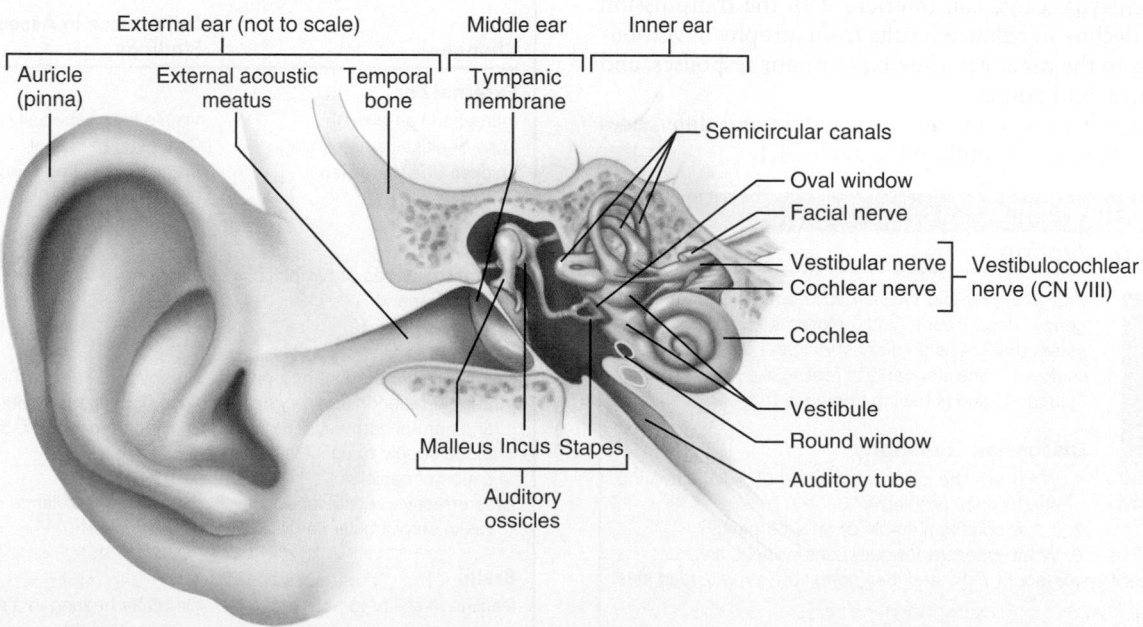

FIG. 21.1 External, middle, and inner ear. (Modified from Patton KT, Thibodeau GA: *Anatomy and physiology,* ed 8, St Louis, 2013, Mosby.)

of the vestibulocochlear nerve (CN VIII) to the temporal lobe of the brain to process and interpret the sound.

Three *semicircular canals* and the *vestibule* make up the organ of balance. The semicircular canals sit at right angles to each other. Structures in each canal and the vestibule generate nerve impulses in response to our movements. The vestibule is beside the oval window between the semicircular canals and the cochlea. Nerves from receptors in the vestibule join those from the semicircular canals to form the vestibular nerve, which joins with the cochlear nerve to form the *vestibulocochlear nerve,* or CN VIII.

Transmission of Sound

Sound waves travel by air (air conduction) and are picked up by the auricles and auditory canal. Sound waves strike the TM, causing it to vibrate. The central part of the TM is connected to the malleus, which then starts to vibrate. The malleus transmits the vibration to the incus and then the stapes. As the stapes moves back and forth, it pushes the membrane of the oval window in and out. Movement of the oval window makes waves in the perilymph.

Once sound waves are transmitted to the liquid medium of the inner ear, the vibration is picked up by the tiny sensory hair cells of the cochlea, which initiate nerve impulses. These impulses are carried by nerve fibers to the main branch of the acoustic portion of CN VIII and then to the brain. The bones of the skull can also transmit sound directly to the inner ear (bone conduction).

Gerontologic Considerations: Effects of Aging on Auditory System

Presbycusis, or hearing loss due to aging, is the third most common health issue in older adults, after arthritis and heart disease.[2] Sound transmission is diminished by calcification of the ossicles. Tinnitus, or ringing in the ears, may accompany the hearing loss that results from the aging process. Cerumen glands atrophy, causing cerumen (earwax) to be much drier. The hair in the ear becomes thicker and coarser, entrapping the hard, dry cerumen in the canal. Accumulation of dry cerumen in the external canal can interfere with the transmission of sound. A decline in balance results from atrophy of vestibular structures in the inner ear, slowing of motor responses, and musculoskeletal limitations.

Age-related changes in the auditory system and differences in assessment findings are outlined in Table 21.1.

CASE STUDY

Patient Introduction

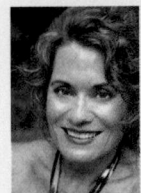
(© iStock.com/ EyeMark.)

R.S. is a 57-yr-old woman who comes to the emergency department with extreme dizziness. R.S. states that she is so dizzy she "can't do anything but lie down." She also reports feeling like her right ear is "plugged" and is having ringing in that ear.

Discussion Questions

1. What are the possible causes of R.M.'s hearing and balance problems?
2. Is her condition stable or an emergency?
3. What assessment questions will you ask her?

You will learn more about R.S. and her condition as you read this chapter.

(See p. 380 for more information on R.S.)

Answers available at *http://evolve.elsevier.com/Lewis/medsurg.*

ASSESSMENT OF AUDITORY SYSTEM

Assessment of the auditory system should include assessment of hearing and equilibrium because the auditory and *vestibular* (balance) systems are closely related. It is often hard to separate symptoms related to these two systems. Help the patient describe symptoms and problems to determine the source of the problems. Health history questions to ask a patient with an auditory problem are listed in Table 21.2.

Problems with balance may manifest as vertigo or nystagmus. Vertigo is a sense that the person or objects around the person are moving or spinning. It is usually stimulated by head movement. *Dizziness* is a sensation of being off-balance that occurs when standing or walking. Nystagmus is an abnormal eye movement that may be seen as a twitching of the eyeball or described by the patient as a blurring of vision with head or eye movement.

At first, try to determine symptoms that are related to balance and separate them from those related to hearing loss or tinnitus. The symptoms can be combined later in the assessment to help make a diagnosis and care plan for the patient.

Subjective Data
Important Health Information

Past Health History. Many ear problems result from childhood illnesses or problems of adjacent organs. This makes a careful assessment of past health problems is important.

Ask the patient about previous ear problems, especially during childhood. Record the (1) frequency of acute middle ear infections (otitis media); (2) surgical procedures (e.g., myringotomy); (3) perforations of the eardrum; (4) drainage; and (5) history of mumps, measles, or scarlet fever. Assess for systemic

TABLE 21.1 Gerontologic Assessment Differences

Auditory System

Changes	Differences in Assessment Findings
External Ear	
Increased hair growth	Visible hair, especially in men
Loss of elasticity in cartilage	Collapsed ear canal
Thicker, drier cerumen	Impacted cerumen, potential hearing loss
Middle Ear	
Atrophic changes of tympanic membrane	Conductive hearing loss
Inner Ear	
Hair cell degeneration, neuron degeneration in auditory nerve and central pathways, reduced blood supply to cochlea, calcification of ossicles	Presbycusis, diminished sensitivity to high-pitched sounds, impaired speech reception, tinnitus
Less effective vestibular apparatus in semicircular canals	Alterations in balance and body orientation
Brain	
Decline in ability to filter out unwanted and unnecessary sound	Difficulty hearing in a noisy environment, heightened sensitivity to loud sounds

conditions, including hypertension, rheumatoid arthritis, and inflammatory bowel disease, that are associated with hearing loss.[3] Document head injury because it may result in hearing loss. Information about food and environmental allergies is important because they can cause the eustachian tube to become edematous and prevent aeration of the middle ear.

Record symptoms such as vertigo, tinnitus, and hearing loss in the patient's words. Ask for specific details of the sensations and situations that may cause them or make them worse. Information about family members with hearing loss and type of hearing loss is important. Some congenital hearing loss is hereditary. The age of onset of presbycusis also follows a familial pattern.

Medications. Obtain information about present or past use of ototoxic drugs (cause damage to CN VIII). These include aspirin, some antibiotics (aminoglycosides, erythromycin, vancomycin), loop diuretics, nonsteroidal antiinflammatory drugs (NSAIDs), antimalarial agents, and certain chemotherapy drugs (e.g., bleomycin, cyclophosphamide, cisplatin). Ask about hearing and balance problems, such as hearing loss, tinnitus, and vertigo, in patients receiving these drugs. For many, the hearing loss may be reversible if treatment is stopped. Chemicals used in industry (e.g., toluene, carbon disulfide, mercury) may damage the inner ear.

Surgery or Other Treatments. Document previous hospitalizations for ear surgery, including myringotomy (ventilation holes placed in the TM with or without tubes), tympanoplasty (surgical repair of TM), tonsillectomy, and adenoidectomy. Record the use of and satisfaction with a hearing aid. Note any problems with impacted cerumen.

Functional Health Patterns. Hearing and balance problems can affect all aspects of a person's life. To assess the impact of hearing loss, ask health history questions based on a functional health patterns approach (Table 21.2).

Health Perception–Health Management Pattern. Note the onset of hearing loss, whether sudden or gradual, and who noted the onset (e.g., patient, family, significant others). Gradual hearing losses are often noted by those who communicate with the patient. Sudden losses and those worsened by other condition are often reported by the patient.

Assess the patient for personal measures used to preserve hearing. The use of protective ear covers or earplugs is good practice for people in high-noise environments. Document if the patient is a swimmer and the frequency and duration of swimming and use of ear protection. Note the type of water (pool, lake, ocean) in which the swimming takes place to help identify contact with contaminated water. Assess for the placement of any item in the ear, including hearing aids, which can cause trauma to the canal and TM.

Nutritional-Metabolic Pattern. Alcohol, sodium, and dietary supplements affect the amount of endolymph in the inner ear system. Patients with Ménière's disease may notice some

---

TABLE 21.2 Health History

Auditory System

Health Perception–Health Management	Activity-Exercise
Hearing	• Do you need help with certain activities (e.g., lifting, bending, climbing stairs, driving, speaking) because of symptoms?*
• Have you had a change in your hearing?* If yes, how does this change affect your daily life?	
• Do you use any devices to improve your hearing (e.g., hearing aid, special volume control, headphones for television or stereo)?*	**Sleep-Rest**
• How do you protect your hearing?	• Is your sleep disturbed by noises or ringing in the ears or by a sensation of spinning?*
• Do you have any allergies that result in ear problems?*	
	Cognitive-Perceptual
Equilibrium	• Do you experience ear pain?* What relieves the pain? What makes it worse? Does the pain affect your hearing or balance?
• When did the dizziness or spinning sensation first occur?	• Have you noticed any problem with communicating or understanding what people are saying?*
• Does this sensation occur when you first stand up, when you are lying down, or both?	
• Have you ever fallen because of the dizziness?*	**Self-Perception–Self-Concept**
• Can you drive or walk alone? If no, elaborate.	• Have changes in your hearing affected how you feel about yourself or your feeling of independence?*
• Are there any times of the day when your symptoms are worse?*	
	Role-Relationship
Tinnitus	• What effect has your ear problem had on your work, family, or social life?
• How long have you experienced ringing in your ears? Has it changed?* Describe the ringing (e.g., buzzing, ringing, roaring). Do you also have a feeling of fullness or pressure?*	• Are you able to recognize the effects of your ear problems on your life?*
• When does it bother you the most?	
• What things have you tried that help or have not helped?	**Sexuality-Reproductive**
• What medications are you taking?	• Has your ear problem caused a change in your sex life?*
Nutritional-Metabolic	**Coping–Stress Tolerance**
• Do you notice any differences in symptoms with changes in diet?*	• Do you consider your ear problem a source of stress?*
• Does your ear problem cause nausea that interferes with your food intake?*	• How do you cope when you are experiencing symptoms?
• Does chewing or swallowing cause you any ear discomfort?*	
	Value-Belief
Elimination	• Do you have a conflict between what your health care provider would like you to do and what you believe you should do?
• Does straining during a bowel movement cause ear pain?*	

* If yes, describe.

improvement in their symptoms with alcohol restriction and a low-sodium diet. Note changes in symptoms with food intake. Ask the patient about any ear pain (otalgia) or discomfort associated with chewing or swallowing. These symptoms are often associated with middle ear problems.

Assessment of clenching or grinding of the teeth helps distinguish problems of the ear from referred pain of the temporomandibular joint (TMJ). Ask about dental problems and dentures.

Elimination Pattern. Elimination patterns are of interest in the patient with perilymph fistula and after surgical procedures. Frequent constipation or straining with bowel or bladder elimination may interfere with healing or repair of a perilymph fistula. After middle ear surgery (stapedectomy) the patient needs to prevent increased intracranial (and consequent inner ear) pressure associated with straining during bowel movements. Stool softeners may be needed after surgery for the patient who reports chronic problems with constipation.

Activity-Exercise Pattern. A review of the patient's activity-exercise pattern is essential when assessing for balance problems. Ask the patient about the onset, duration, and frequency of symptoms. Identify activities that relieve or worsen symptoms and how they relate to the time of the day. For example, patients with Ménière's disease are less able to compensate for environmental input as the day progresses.

Sleep-Rest Pattern. Ask the patient with chronic tinnitus about sleep problems. Find out if the patient has tried anything to minimize the tinnitus (e.g., having fan on, using white noise devices). Assess for snoring. It can be caused by swelling or hypertrophy of tissue in the nasopharynx. This excess tissue can impair eustachian tube function and cause the sensation of ear fullness or pain.

Cognitive-Perceptual Pattern. Pain is associated with some ear problems, particularly those involving the middle ear and auditory canal. If pain is present, ask the patient to describe the pain, presence of drainage (*otorrhea*), history of teeth grinding, and treatments used for relief. Note the effect on the pain level when you move the auricle or palpate the tragus.

Note the patient's ability to pay attention and follow directions. Problems with these tasks may be an early indicator of hearing loss. The patient may not recognize a gradual hearing loss. Ask caregivers if they have noted any change in the patient's hearing.

Self-Perception–Self-Concept Pattern. Ask the patient to describe how the ear problem has affected his or her personal life and feelings about himself or herself. Hearing loss and chronic vertigo are particularly distressing for the patient. Hearing loss can result in embarrassing social situations that affect the patient's self-concept. People may think a patient with chronic vertigo is intoxicated. Sensitively question the patient about such situations. Clarify the symptom history with the patient and consider an evaluation with a hearing specialist.

Role-Relationship Pattern. Ask the patient about the effect that an ear problem or vertigo has had on family life, work responsibilities, and social relationships. Hearing loss can result in strained relationships and misunderstandings.

Ask about employment or contact with environments that have excessive noise levels, such as work with jet engines and machinery and electronically amplified music. Document the use of preventive devices worn in noisy environments. Many jobs rely on the ability to hear accurately and respond appropriately. If a hearing loss is present, gather detailed information on the effect this has on the patient's job. The unpredictability of vertigo attacks can have devastating effects on all aspects of life. Ordinary activities, such as driving, cooking, and work, that require balance all have an element of danger.

Sexuality-Reproductive Pattern. Determine whether hearing loss or vertigo has interfered with having a satisfactory sex life. Although intimacy does not depend on the ability to hear, hearing loss can interfere with establishing or maintaining a relationship.

Coping–Stress Tolerance Pattern. Ask the patient about his or her usual coping style, stress management strategies, and available support. If the patient seems unable to manage the situation, outside intervention may be needed. Denial is a common response to a hearing problem and should be assessed.

Value-Belief Pattern. Ask the patient about any conflicts produced by the problem or treatment related to values or beliefs. Make every effort to resolve the problem so that the patient does not have added stress. Ask about the use of home remedies such as hot oil in the ear.

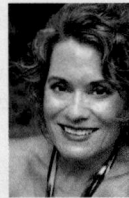
Objective Data

Physical Examination. During the interview to obtain a health history, obtain objective data about the patient's ability to hear. Look for cues that a patient cannot hear (Table 21.3). Record these observations. This is important because the patient is often unaware of hearing loss or does not admit to changes in hearing until moderate losses have occurred.

A normal assessment of the auditory system is shown in Table 21.4. Age-related changes of the auditory system and differences in assessment findings are found in Table 21.1.

TABLE 21.3 Indicators of Possible Hearing Loss

- Does not respond to or understand oral communication
- Has excessively loud or soft speech
- Answers questions inappropriately
- Tilts head, leans forward when listening
- Constantly needs to clarify conversation
- States other people mumble all the time
- Increases the volume of radio or TV
- Difficulty hearing over the phone

TABLE 21.4 Normal Physical Assessment of Auditory System

- Ears symmetric in location and shape
- Auricles and tragus nontender, without lesions
- Canal clear, tympanic membrane intact, landmarks and light reflex intact
- Able to hear low whisper at 30 cm. Weber test results, no lateralization. Rinne test results AC > BC

AC, Air conduction; *BC,* bone conduction.

A *focused assessment* is used to evaluate the status of previously identified auditory problems and monitor for signs of new problems. A focused assessment of the auditory system is presented in the box below.

FOCUSED ASSESSMENT
Auditory System

Use this checklist to make sure the key assessment steps have been done.

Subjective
Ask the patient about any of the following and note responses.

Changes in hearing	Y	N
Ear pain	Y	N
Ear drainage	Y	N
Tinnitus	Y	N

Objective: Physical Examination
Inspect

Alignment and position of ears on head	✓
Size, shape, symmetry, color, and skin intactness	✓
External auditory meatus for discharge or lesions	✓

Assess

Hearing based on ability to respond to conversation, respond to a whisper, or hear a ticking watch	✓

External Ear. Inspect and palpate the external ear before examining the external canal and tympanum. Observe the auricle, preauricular area, and mastoid area for symmetry, color of skin, swelling, redness, and lesions. Then palpate the auricle and mastoid areas for tenderness and nodules. Grasping the auricle or pressing on the tragus may cause pain, especially if the external ear or canal is inflamed.

External Auditory Canal and Tympanum. Before inserting an otoscope, inspect the canal opening for patency, palpate the tragus, and gently move the auricle to check for discomfort. Select

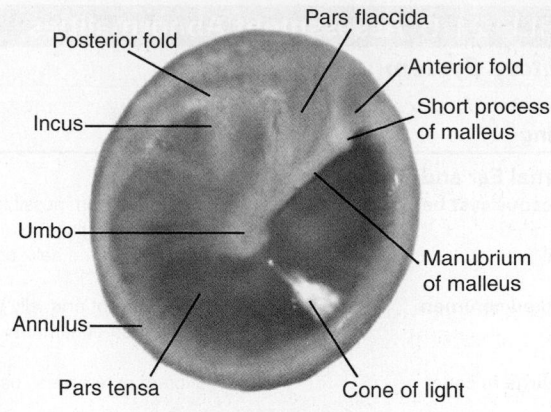

FIG. 21.2 Normal tympanic membrane. (From Jarvis C: *Physical examination and health assessment,* ed 7, St Louis, 2015, Elsevier.)

a speculum slightly smaller than the size of the ear canal. Tip the patient's head to the opposite shoulder. Grasp the top of the auricle and gently pull up and backward to straighten the canal. Hold the otoscope while stabilizing it with your fingers on the patient's cheek, and then insert it slowly. A pneumatic otoscope creates negative pressure to pull at the TM and is helpful in confirming TM retraction or fluid behind the membrane. A tight seal of the speculum is essential during this step of the examination. Observe the canal for size and shape and the color, amount, and type of cerumen. Be careful when clearing the canal of cerumen. Damage can occur to the middle ear if the TM is perforated.

Inspect the TM for color, fluid behind the membrane, landmarks, contour, and intactness (Fig. 21.2). The TM is normally pearl gray, white, or pink; shiny; and translucent. The handle (manubrium) of the malleus and its short process (umbo) should be visible through the membrane. The position and dome (concave) shape of the TM cause the light from the otoscope to reflect in a cone shape with crisp edges. If the TM is bulging or retracted, the edges of the light reflex will be fuzzy (diffuse) and may spread over the TM. The middle and inner ear cannot be examined with the otoscope.

Table 21.5 summarizes assessment abnormalities of the auditory system.

CASE STUDY
Objective Data: Physical Examination

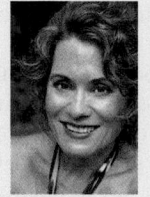
(© iStock.com/ EyeMark.)

Physical examination findings of R.S. were as follows:
- Neurologic and otoscopic examinations normal
- Unable to hear whisper on the right at 30 cm
- Vision normal. PERRLA without nystagmus
- Gait unsteady. No motor weakness
- Skin pale, warm, and dry
- Heart rate 84 beats/min, temperature 97.4° F (36.3° C)

Discussion Questions
1. What physical assessment findings concern you most?
2. What diagnostic studies might you expect to be ordered?

As you continue to read this chapter, consider diagnostic studies that you would expect being performed for R.S.

(See p. 382 for more information on R.S.)

TABLE 21.5 Assessment Abnormalities

Auditory System

Finding	Description	Possible Etiology and Significance
External Ear and Canal		
Sebaceous cyst behind ear	Usually within skin, possible presence of black dot (opening to sebaceous gland)	Removal or incision and drainage if painful
Tophi	Hard nodules in the helix or antihelix consisting of uric acid crystals	Associated with gout, metabolic disorder. Further diagnosis needed
Impacted cerumen	Wax that has not normally been excreted from the ear. No visualization of eardrum	Decreased hearing possible, pain, sensation of fullness in auditory canal, removal necessary before otoscopic examination
Discharge in canal	Infection of external ear, usually painful	Swimmer's ear, infection of external ear. Possibly caused by ruptured eardrum and otitis media
Swelling of pinna, pain	Infection of glands of skin, hematoma caused by trauma	Aspiration (for hematoma)
Scaling or lesions	Change in usual appearance of skin	Seborrheic dermatitis, actinic keratosis, basal or squamous cell carcinoma
Exostosis	Bony growth extending into canal causing narrowing of canal	Possible interference with visualizing tympanum. Usually asymptomatic
Tympanum		
Retracted eardrum	Appearance of shorter, more horizontal malleus. Absent or bent cone of light	Vacuum in middle ear, blockage of eustachian tube, negative pressure in middle ear
Hairline fluid level, yellow-amber bubbles above fluid level	Caused by transudate of blood and serum, meniscus of fluid producing hairline appearance	Serous otitis media
Bulging red or blue eardrum, lack of landmarks	Fluid-filled middle ear, pus, blood	Acute otitis media, perforation possible
Perforation of eardrum (Fig. 21.3)	Previous perforations of the eardrum that have failed to heal. Thin, transparent layer of epithelium surrounding eardrum	Chronic otitis media, mastoiditis, drainage
Recruitment	Perception that sounds are getting too loud too fast	Sensorineural hearing loss. Hearing aid hard to use

DIAGNOSTIC STUDIES OF AUDITORY SYSTEM

Table 21.6 describes common diagnostic studies used to assess the auditory system.

Audiometry

Audiometry is beneficial as a screening test for hearing acuity and as a diagnostic test to determine the degree and type of hearing loss. The most common test performed by the audiologist is pure-tone audiometry. The audiometer produces pure tones at varying intensities to which the patient can respond. Sound is characterized by the number of vibrations or cycles that occur each second. Hertz (Hz) is the unit of measurement used to classify the frequency of a tone. The higher the frequency is, the higher the pitch.

Hearing loss can affect certain sound frequencies. The specific pattern produced on the audiogram by these losses can help in diagnosing the type of hearing loss. The intensity or strength of a sound wave is expressed in terms of decibels (dB), ranging from 0 to 110 dB. The intensity of a sound needed to make any frequency barely audible to the average normal ear is 0 dB. Threshold refers to the signal level at which pure tones are detected (pure-tone thresholds) or the signal level at which the patient correctly hears 50% of the signals (speech detection thresholds).

Normal speech is around 40 to 65 dB; a soft whisper is 20 dB. Normally, a child and a young adult can hear frequencies from about 16 to 20,000 Hz, but hearing is most sensitive between 500 and 4000 Hz. This is similar to normal speech frequencies.

A 40- to 45-dB loss in these frequencies causes moderate difficulty in hearing normal speech. A hearing aid may be helpful because it makes sound information louder but not clearer. A hearing aid may not be helpful to the patient who has problems with discrimination of sounds or sound information because the consonants are still not heard well enough to make speech understandable.

Specialized Tests

More sophisticated tests are available to determine the cause of certain hearing losses (Table 21.6). CT scan and MRI can detect lesions such as a tumor of the auditory nerve.

CASE STUDY
Objective Data: Diagnostic Studies

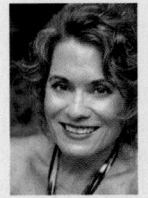

The Weber's test shows lateralization to the left. An audiogram confirms low-frequency, sensorineural hearing loss with normal speech discrimination. An MRI of the head is normal.

Discussion Questions

1. Are these the diagnostic studies that you expected to be ordered?
2. Which diagnostic study results are of most concern to you?

(© iStock.com/ EyeMark.)

(See p. 393 for more information on R.S.)

TABLE 21.6 Diagnostic Studies

Auditory System

Study	Description, Purpose, and Nursing Responsibility
Auditory	
Audiometry	*Pure-tone audiometry* quantifies hearing loss. Sounds are presented through earphones in soundproof room. Patient responds when sound is heard. Response is recorded on an audiogram. Purpose is to determine patient's hearing range in terms of decibels (dB) and Hertz (Hz) for diagnosing hearing loss. Tinnitus can cause inconsistent results. *Speech audiometry* includes speech reception threshold (measure of intensity at which speech is recognized) and word recognition score (ability to discriminate among various speech sounds).
Auditory brainstem response (ABR)	Study measures electrical peaks along auditory pathway of inner ear to brain and provides diagnostic information related to acoustic neuromas, brainstem problems, and stroke.
Auditory evoked potential (AEP)	Procedure is like an electroencephalogram (see Chapter 55 and Table 55.10). Electrodes are placed typically at vertex, mastoid process, and forehead. A computer is used to isolate auditory from other electrical activity of brain. Patient should avoid loud noises for 24 hours before the test.
Electrocochleography	Test records electrical activity in cochlea and auditory nerve. Electrode placed on or through the eardrum. Used to assess and monitor patients with dizziness.
Tympanometry	Used to check middle ear and mobility of eardrum. A probe is placed snugly into external ear canal, and positive and negative pressures are applied. Measurements are made of movement of eardrum.
Tuning Fork Tests	
Rinne test	Compares hearing by bone conduction (BC) and air conduction (AC). Stem of vibrating tuning fork held against mastoid bone (for BC of sound) and time noted. When the sound is no longer perceived behind the ear (BC of sound), time is noted once again and the still-vibrating fork is moved close to the pinna (AC of sound). Have the patient report when the sound next to the ear canal (AC) is no longer heard and note time. Normally, sound is heard twice as long in front of the ear as it is on the bone. With conductive hearing loss, the relationship is reversed; BC is longer than AC. With sensorineural hearing loss, both AC and BC are reduced, but AC remains longer.
Weber test	Stem of vibrating tuning fork is placed on midline of skull or forehead. Patient asked to indicate where the sound is heard best. In normal auditory function, the patient perceives a midline tone and the sound is heard equally in both ears. If a patient has conductive hearing loss in one ear, the sound will be heard louder (lateralizes) in that ear. If sensorineural loss is present, the sound is louder (lateralizes) in the normal (unaffected) ear.
Vestibular Tests	
Electronystagmography (ENG)	Used to diagnose diseases of vestibular system such as dizziness and balance disorders. Electrodes are placed near patient's eyes, and eye movement (nystagmus) is recorded on graph during specific eye movements and when ear is irrigated. Caloric test may be part of testing to measure responses to warm and cold water circulated into the ear canal. Have patient eat a light meal before test to avoid nausea. Observe patient for vomiting. Ensure patient safety.
Posturography	Balance test that can isolate one semicircular canal from others to determine site of lesion. Test is done in a boxlike device in which floor moves in response to a correction in balance by patient. Tell patient that test may be uncomfortable. Test can be stopped at any time at patient's request.
Rotary chair testing	Evaluates peripheral vestibular system. Patient is seated in a chair driven by a motor under computer control. Test is usually done in the dark. Tell patient to eat light meal before test to avoid nausea. Observe patient for vomiting. Ensure patient safety.

AUDITORY PROBLEMS: EXTERNAL EAR AND CANAL

EXTERNAL OTITIS

The skin of the external ear and canal is subject to the same problems as skin anywhere on the body. External otitis involves inflammation or infection of the epithelium of the auricle and ear canal. Swimming may change the flora of the external canal because of chemicals and contaminated water. This can result in an infection often referred to as "swimmer's ear." Trauma from picking the ear or using sharp objects (e.g., hairpins) often causes the initial break in the skin. Piercing of cartilage in the upper part of the auricle also places the patient at higher risk for infection.

Infections and skin conditions may cause external otitis. Bacteria or fungi may be the cause. *Pseudomonas aeruginosa* is the most common bacterial cause. Fungi, especially *Candida albicans* and *Aspergillus*, thrive in warm, moist climates. The warm, dark environment of the ear canal provides a good growth medium for microorganisms.

Malignant external otitis is a serious infection caused by *P. aeruginosa*. It occurs mainly in older patients with diabetes. The infection, which can spread from the external ear to the parotid gland and temporal bone (osteomyelitis), is usually treated with antibiotics.

Ear pain *(otalgia)* is one of the first signs of external otitis. Even in mild cases, the patient may have significant discomfort with chewing, moving the auricle, or pressing on the tragus. Swelling of the ear canal can muffle hearing. There may be serosanguineous (blood-tinged fluid) or purulent (white to green thick fluid) drainage. Fever occurs when the infection spreads to surrounding tissue.

❖ NURSING AND INTERPROFESSIONAL MANAGEMENT: EXTERNAL OTITIS

External otitis is diagnosed by otoscopic examination of the ear canal. Take care to avoid pain when pulling on the pinna to straighten out the canal or when inserting the otoscope speculum. The eardrum may be hard to see due to swelling in the

TABLE 21.7 Patient & Caregiver Teaching

Prevention of External Otitis

Include the following instructions when teaching the patient and caregiver:

1. Do not put anything in your ear canal unless requested by your health care provider.
2. Report itching if it becomes a problem.
3. Earwax is normal.
   * It lubricates and protects the canal.
   * Report chronic excess cerumen if it impairs your hearing.
4. Keep your ears as dry as possible.
   * Use earplugs if you are prone to swimmer's ear.
   * Turn your head to each side for 30 seconds at a time to help water run out of the ears.
   * Do not dry with cotton-tipped applicators.
   * A hair dryer set to low and held at least 6 inches from the ear can speed water evaporation.

canal. Culture and sensitivity studies of the drainage may be done. Moist heat, mild analgesics, and topical anesthetic drops usually control the pain. Topical treatments may include antibiotics for infection and corticosteroids for inflammation. If the surrounding tissue is involved, systemic antibiotics are used. Improvement should occur in 48 hours. The patient needs to adhere to the prescribed therapy for 7 to 14 days for complete resolution.

Wash hands before and after applying eardrops (otic drops). The drops should be at room temperature. Cold drops can cause vertigo due to stimulation of the semicircular canals, and heated drops can burn the tympanum. The tip of the dropper should not touch the ear during application to prevent contamination of the entire bottle of drops. Position the ear so that the drops can run into the canal. The patient should stay in this position for 2 minutes to allow the drops to spread. Sometimes you can place the drops onto a wick of cotton, then place the wick in the canal. Tell the patient not to push the cotton farther into the ear. Careful handling and disposal of material saturated with drainage are important. Teach the patient ways to reduce the risk for external otitis (Table 21.7).

CERUMEN AND FOREIGN BODIES IN EXTERNAL EAR CANAL

Impacted cerumen (earwax) can cause discomfort and decreased hearing. Other symptoms include tinnitus and vertigo. Remove an impaction by irrigating the canal with body-temperature solutions to soften the earwax. Special syringes may be used. These vary from a simple bulb syringe to special irrigating equipment. Place the patient in a sitting position with an emesis basin under the ear. Pull the auricle up and back, and direct the flow of solution above or below the impaction. Do not completely occlude the ear canal with the syringe tip. If irrigation does not remove the wax, use mild lubricant drops to soften the earwax. The HCP may need to remove severe impactions.

Attempts to remove a foreign object from the ear may result in pushing it farther into the canal. Vegetable matter in the ear tends to swell. This can create a secondary inflammation, making removal more difficult. Mineral oil or lidocaine drops can be used to kill an insect before removal under microscope guidance. The HCP should remove impacted objects.

Cleanse ears with a washcloth and finger. Avoid using cotton-tipped applicators. Penetration of the middle ear by a cotton-tipped applicator can cause serious injury to the TM and ossicles. Their use can also cause earwax to become impacted against the TM and impair hearing.

TRAUMA

Trauma to the external ear can cause injury to the subcutaneous tissue and result in a hematoma. If a hematoma is not aspirated, inflammation of the membranes of the ear cartilage (perichondritis) can result. Blows to the ear can cause conductive hearing loss if the ossicles in the middle ear are damaged or the TM is perforated. Head trauma that injures the temporal lobe of the cerebral cortex can impair the ability to understand the meaning of sounds.

MALIGNANCY OF EXTERNAL EAR

Skin cancers are the only common cancers of the ear. Precancerous actinic keratoses, rough sandpaper-like lesions on the upper border of the auricle, are associated with chronic sun exposure. They are often treated with liquid nitrogen. Cancers in the external ear canal include basal cell carcinoma in the pinna and squamous cell carcinoma in the ear canal. If left untreated, they can invade underlying tissue. Teach the patient about the dangers of sun exposure and the importance of using hats and sunscreen when outdoors. See Chapter 23 for more about skin cancer.

MIDDLE EAR AND MASTOID

OTITIS MEDIA

Acute Otitis Media

Acute otitis media is an infection of the tympanum, ossicles, and space of the middle ear. Swelling of the auditory tube from colds or allergies can trap bacteria, causing a middle ear infection. Pressure from the inflammation pushes on the TM, causing it to become red, bulging, and painful. Acute otitis media is usually a childhood disease. In children the auditory tube that normally drains fluid and mucus from the middle ear is shorter and narrower, and its position is flatter than in adults. Infection can be due to viruses or bacteria. Pain, fever, malaise, drainage, and reduced hearing are signs and symptoms of infection. Referred pain from the TMJ, teeth, gums, sinuses, or throat can also cause ear pain.

Oral antibiotics and eardrops are used if an infection is present. Surgical intervention is reserved for the patient who does not respond to medical treatment. A *myringotomy* involves an incision in the tympanum to release the increased pressure and exudate from the middle ear. A tympanostomy tube may be used short- or long-term for ventilation of the ear. Prompt treatment of an episode of acute otitis media can help prevent spontaneous perforation of the TM. If allergies are a causative factor, the patient may receive antihistamines and a nasal corticosteroid spray.

Otitis Media With Effusion

Otitis media with effusion is an inflammation of the middle ear with a collection of fluid in the middle ear space. The fluid

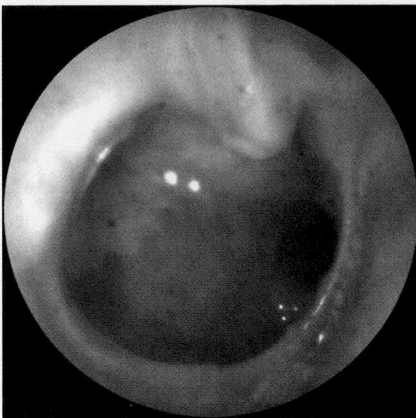

FIG. 21.3 Perforation of the tympanic membrane (TM). (From Flint P, Haughey B, Lund V, Niparko JK, eds: *Cummings otolaryngology: Head and neck surgery*, ed 5, St Louis, 2010, Mosby.)

may be thin, mucoid, or purulent. If the auditory tube does not open and allow equalization of atmospheric pressure, negative pressure within the middle ear pulls fluid from surrounding tissues. This problem commonly follows upper respiratory tract or chronic sinus infections, barotrauma (caused by pressure change), or otitis media.

Symptoms include a feeling of fullness of the ear, a "plugged" feeling or popping, and decreased hearing. The patient does not have pain, fever, or discharge from the ear. It is common to have otitis media with effusion for weeks to months after an episode of acute otitis media. It usually resolves without treatment but may recur.

Chronic Otitis Media and Mastoiditis

Repeated attacks of otitis media may lead to chronic otitis media, especially in adults who have a history of recurrent otitis media in childhood. Because the mucous membrane of the middle ear is continuous with the air cells of the mastoid bone, both can be involved in the chronic infectious process.

Chronic otitis media is characterized by a purulent exudate and inflammation that can involve the ossicles, auditory tube, and mastoid bone. It is often painless. Hearing loss, nausea, and episodes of dizziness can occur. Hearing loss is a complication from inflammatory destruction of the ossicles, a TM perforation, or accumulation of fluid in the middle ear space. A mass of epithelial cells and cholesterol in the middle ear (*cholesteatoma*) may develop. The cholesteatoma enlarges and can destroy the adjacent bones. Unless removed surgically, it can cause extensive damage to the ossicles and impair hearing.

Otoscopic examination of the TM may reveal changes in color and mobility or a perforation (Fig. 21.3). Culture and sensitivity tests of the drainage are necessary to identify the organisms involved so the patient may receive the appropriate antibiotic therapy. The audiogram may show a hearing loss as great as 50 to 60 dB if the ossicles have been damaged or separated. Sinus x-rays, MRI, or a CT scan of the temporal bone can assess for bone destruction and the presence of a mass.

❖ NURSING AND INTERPROFESSIONAL MANAGEMENT: CHRONIC OTITIS MEDIA

The goals of treatment are to clear the middle ear of infection, repair any perforations, and preserve hearing (Table 21.8). Otic

---

TABLE 21.8 Interprofessional Care

Chronic Otitis Media

Diagnostic Assessment
- History and physical examination
- Otoscopic examination
- Culture and sensitivity of middle ear drainage
- Mastoid x-ray

Management
- Ear irrigations
- Otic, oral, or parenteral antibiotics
- Analgesics
- Antiemetics
- Surgery
  - Tympanoplasty
  - Mastoidectomy

TABLE 21.9 Patient & Caregiver Teaching

After Ear Surgery

Include the following information in the teaching plan for the patient and caregiver after ear surgery.
1. Sleep on your back or the unoperated ear for 1 week.
2. Avoid air travel and sun exposure for 6 weeks.
3. If you need to cough or sneeze, keep your mouth open.
4. Blow your nose gently, without blocking either nostril.
5. Do not shampoo your hair for 5 days. Wear a shower cap when bathing.
6. No swimming. Keep your ear dry for 6 weeks.
7. You may resume strenuous activity and contact sports in 1 month.
8. Change your ear dressing daily as prescribed.
9. Report excess drainage or severe dizziness to the health care provider.

---

and systemic (oral and IV) antibiotic therapy is started based on the culture and sensitivity results. In many cases of chronic otitis media, antibiotic resistance is present. The patient may need to have frequent evacuation of drainage and debris in an outpatient setting.

Often chronic TM perforations do not heal with conservative treatment, and surgery is necessary. *Tympanoplasty (myringoplasty)* involves reconstruction of the TM and/or the ossicles. A *mastoidectomy* is often performed with a tympanoplasty to remove infected portions of the mastoid bone. Removal of tissue stops at the middle ear structures that appear capable of conducting sound. Sudden pressure changes in the ear and postoperative infections can disrupt healing or cause facial nerve paralysis.

Expect impaired hearing during the postoperative period if there is packing in the ear. A cotton ball dressing is used if an incision was made through the external auditory canal. Teach the patient to change the cotton packing as needed (Table 21.9). If a postauricular (behind the ear) incision was used and a drain is in place, place a dressing over that area. Then, place a soft outer dressing over the top of that dressing. This will prevent putting pressure on the auricle. Monitor the tightness of the outer dressing to prevent tissue necrosis and assess the amount and type of drainage. Keep the suture line dry.

OTOSCLEROSIS

Otosclerosis is a hereditary autosomal dominant disease. It is the most common cause of hearing loss in young adults. Spongy

TABLE 21.10 Interprofessional Care

Otosclerosis

Diagnostic Assessment
- History and physical examination
- Otoscopic examination
- Rinne test
- Weber test
- Audiometry
- Tympanometry

Management
- Hearing aid
- Surgery (stapedectomy or stapes prosthesis)
- Drug therapy
  - Calcium carbonate
  - Sodium fluoride with vitamin D

bone develops from the bony labyrinth, preventing movement of the footplate of the stapes in the oval window. This reduces the transmission of vibrations to the inner ear fluids and results in conductive hearing loss. Although otosclerosis is typically bilateral, one ear may show faster progression of hearing loss. The patient is often unaware of the problem until the loss becomes so severe that communication is difficult.

Otoscopic examination may reveal a reddish blush of the tympanum (Schwartz's sign) caused by the vascular and bony changes within the middle ear. Tuning fork tests (e.g., Rinne) and an audiogram show good hearing by bone conduction with poor hearing by air conduction (air-bone gap) (Table 21.6). Usually a difference of at least 20 to 25 dB between air and bone conduction levels of hearing occurs with otosclerosis.

The hearing loss associated with otosclerosis may be stabilized by giving oral sodium fluoride with vitamin D and calcium carbonate. These medications slow bone resorption and promote the calcification of bony lesions. Amplifying sound with a hearing aid can be effective because inner ear function is normal.

Interprofessional care of otosclerosis is outlined in Table 21.10. Microdrill or laser surgical treatment involves opening the footplate (stapedotomy) or replacing the stapes with a metal or Teflon substitute (prosthesis). These procedures are usually done with the patient under conscious sedation. The ear with poorer hearing is repaired first. The other ear may be operated on within a year. Immediately after surgery the patient often reports a significant improvement in hearing in the operative ear. Because blood and fluid accumulates in the middle ear during the postoperative period, the hearing level decreases initially, but it improves gradually with healing.

Nursing management of the patient undergoing surgery to correct otosclerosis is like that of the patient having a tympanoplasty. Place a cotton ball in the ear canal and cover the ear with a small dressing. The patient may have dizziness, nausea, and vomiting because of stimulation of the labyrinth during surgery. Disturbing the perilymph fluid can cause nystagmus. Teach the patient to avoid sudden movements that may bring on or worsen vertigo and actions that increase inner ear pressure, such as coughing, sneezing, lifting, bending, and straining during bowel movements.

INNER EAR PROBLEMS

Three manifestations that indicate disease of the inner ear are vertigo, sensorineural hearing loss, and tinnitus. Symptoms of vertigo arise from the vestibular labyrinth, while hearing loss and tinnitus arise from the auditory labyrinth. There is an overlap between manifestations of inner ear problems and central nervous system (CNS) disorders.

MÉNIÈRE'S DISEASE

Ménière's disease is a progressive disorder leading to an accumulation of endolymph in the membranous labyrinth. Although it usually affects only one ear, it can affect both. The cause is unknown. Genetic and environmental factors may play a role. Symptoms usually begin between 30 and 60 years of age. Women are more likely to be affected.[4]

The excess fluid and resulting pressure lead to hearing and balance problems, including episodic vertigo, tinnitus, and ear pressure or fullness. Progressive hearing loss occurs over time. The patient has significant disability because of sudden, severe attacks of vertigo with nausea, vomiting, and sweating. A sense of fullness in the ear, increasing tinnitus, and muffled hearing may precede an attack. The patient may have the feeling of being pulled to the ground ("drop attacks"). Some patients report feeling like they are whirling in space. Attacks may last hours or days and may occur several times a year. The clinical course of the disease is highly variable.

❖ NURSING AND INTERPROFESSIONAL MANAGEMENT: MÉNIÈRE'S DISEASE

Interprofessional care of Ménière's disease (Table 21.11) includes diagnostic tests to rule out other causes of the symptoms, including CNS disease. Results that suggest Ménière's disease include low-frequency sensorineural hearing loss on audiogram, 2 or more spontaneous episodes of vertigo, and abnormal vestibular tests.[5] A glycerol test may aid in diagnosis. The patient receives an oral dose of glycerol, followed by serial audiograms over 3 hours. Improvement in hearing or speech discrimination supports a diagnosis of Ménière's disease. This is attributed to the osmotic effect of glycerol pulling fluid from the inner ear.

No cure exists for Ménière's disease. Treatments aim to reduce the number and severity of vertigo attacks. During an acute attack, corticosteroids, antihistamines (e.g., diphenhydramine), anticholinergics (e.g., atropine), and benzodiazepines (e.g., lorazepam [Ativan]) can decrease the abnormal sensation and lessen nausea and vomiting.[4] Acute vertigo is treated symptomatically with bed rest, sedation, and antiemetics (e.g., prochlorperazine) or antivertigo drugs (e.g., meclizine) for motion sickness. Management between attacks may include diuretics, corticosteroids, a low-sodium diet, and stress reduction. Over time, most patients respond to the medications but must learn to live with the unpredictability of the attacks and the loss of hearing.

Frequent and incapacitating attacks are indications for surgical intervention. Decompression of the endolymphatic sac and shunting can reduce the pressure on the cochlear hair cells and prevent further damage and hearing loss. If relief is not achieved, a vestibular nerve section (cutting the nerve) may be done. When involvement is unilateral, surgical ablation of the labyrinth, resulting in the loss of vestibular and hearing cochlear function, is an option. Some patients with severe attacks of vertigo have shown improvement with the injection of gentamicin through the TM. This results in inner ear damage and a reduction in endolymph production.

TABLE 21.11 Interprofessional Care

Ménière's Disease

Diagnostic Assessment
- History and physical examination
- Studies (including speech discrimination, tone decay)
- Vestibular tests (including caloric test, positional test)
- Electronystagmography
- Glycerol test

Management
Acute Care
Drug Therapy
- Anticholinergics
- Antihistamines
- Antiemetics
- Benzodiazepines
- Corticosteroids

Surgical Therapy
- Endolymphatic sac decompression
- Endolymphatic shunt
- Labyrinthectomy
- Vestibular nerve section

Ambulatory Care
- Diuretics
- Corticosteroids
- Dietary restriction of sodium, caffeine, nicotine, and alcohol
- Stress reduction techniques

Plan nursing interventions to minimize vertigo and provide patient safety. During an acute attack, keep the patient in a quiet, darkened room in a comfortable position. Teach the patient to avoid sudden head movements and position changes and to close the eyes until vertigo stops. Avoid fluorescent or flickering lights and television as they may worsen symptoms. Make an emesis basin available because vomiting is common. To minimize the risk for falling, keep the side rails up and the bed in a low position when the patient is in bed. Teach the patient to call for help when getting out of bed. Give medications and fluids parenterally. Monitor intake and output. When the attack subsides, help the patient with ambulation because unsteadiness may remain.

Discharge teaching should emphasize ways to protect the patient from injury between attacks. Review with the patient the need to sit or lie down at the onset of any dizziness. Discuss home safety and measures to decrease fall risk. Teach the need to avoid swimming under water, using ladders, and being on high places until vertigo is under control. Encourage the patient to practice any balance therapy exercises daily.

BENIGN PAROXYSMAL POSITIONAL VERTIGO

Benign paroxysmal positional vertigo (BPPV) is a common cause of vertigo. About 50% of the cases of vertigo may be due to BPPV. In BPPV, free-floating debris in the semicircular canal causes vertigo with specific head movements, such as getting out of bed, rolling over in bed, and sitting up from lying down. The debris ("ear rocks") is composed of small crystals of calcium carbonate that come from the utricle in the inner ear. The utricle may have been injured by head trauma, infection, or degeneration from the aging process. However, for many patients, we do not know the cause.

Symptoms of BPPV include nystagmus, vertigo, light-headedness, loss of balance, and nausea. There is no hearing loss, and symptoms tend to be intermittent. The symptoms of BPPV may be confused with those of Ménière's disease. Diagnosis is based on the results of auditory and vestibular tests.

Although BPPV is bothersome, it is rarely serious unless a person falls. The Epley maneuver, or canalith repositioning procedure, is effective in providing symptom relief for many patients. This maneuver moves ear debris from areas in the inner ear that cause symptoms and into less sensitive areas where they do not cause these problems. It does not change the presence of debris but changes the location. A trained HCP can teach the patient how to perform the maneuver (Fig. 21.4).

ACOUSTIC NEUROMA

An acoustic neuroma is a unilateral benign tumor that occurs where the vestibulocochlear nerve (CN VIII) enters the internal auditory canal. Early diagnosis is important because the tumor can compress the trigeminal and facial nerves and arteries within the internal auditory canal. Symptoms usually begin between 40 and 60 years of age.

Early symptoms are associated with CN VIII compression and destruction. They include unilateral, progressive, sensorineural hearing loss; reduced touch sensation in the posterior ear canal; unilateral tinnitus; and mild, intermittent vertigo. Diagnostic tests include neurologic, audiometric, and vestibular tests; CT scans; and MRI.

Surgery to remove small tumors can preserve hearing and vestibular function. Large tumors (larger than 3 cm) and the surgery to remove them can leave the patient with permanent hearing loss and facial paralysis. Stereotactic radiosurgery may slow tumor growth and preserve the facial nerve. Teach the patient to report any clear, colorless discharge from the nose. This may be cerebrospinal fluid (CSF), which increases the risk for infection. Follow-up care after surgery is important to monitor hearing and for tumor recurrence.

HEARING LOSS AND DEAFNESS

Hearing disorders are a common cause of disability. Age is the strongest predictor of hearing impairment. In the United States, about 25% of those 65 to 74 and 50% of those 75 and older have hearing loss.[6] Causes of hearing loss are shown in Fig. 21.5.

Types of Hearing Loss

Conductive Hearing Loss. *Conductive hearing loss* occurs when conditions in the outer or middle ear impair the transmission of sound through air to the inner ear. Common causes of conductive hearing loss in adults include impacted cerumen, otitis media with effusion, TM perforation, otosclerosis, and narrowing of the external auditory canal.[1]

The audiogram shows better hearing through bone than through air (air-bone gap). The patient often speaks softly because hearing his or her own voice (which is conducted by bone) seems loud. This patient hears better in a noisy environment. The first step is to identify and treat the cause if possible. If correction of the cause is not possible, a hearing aid may help if the loss is greater than 40 to 50 dB.

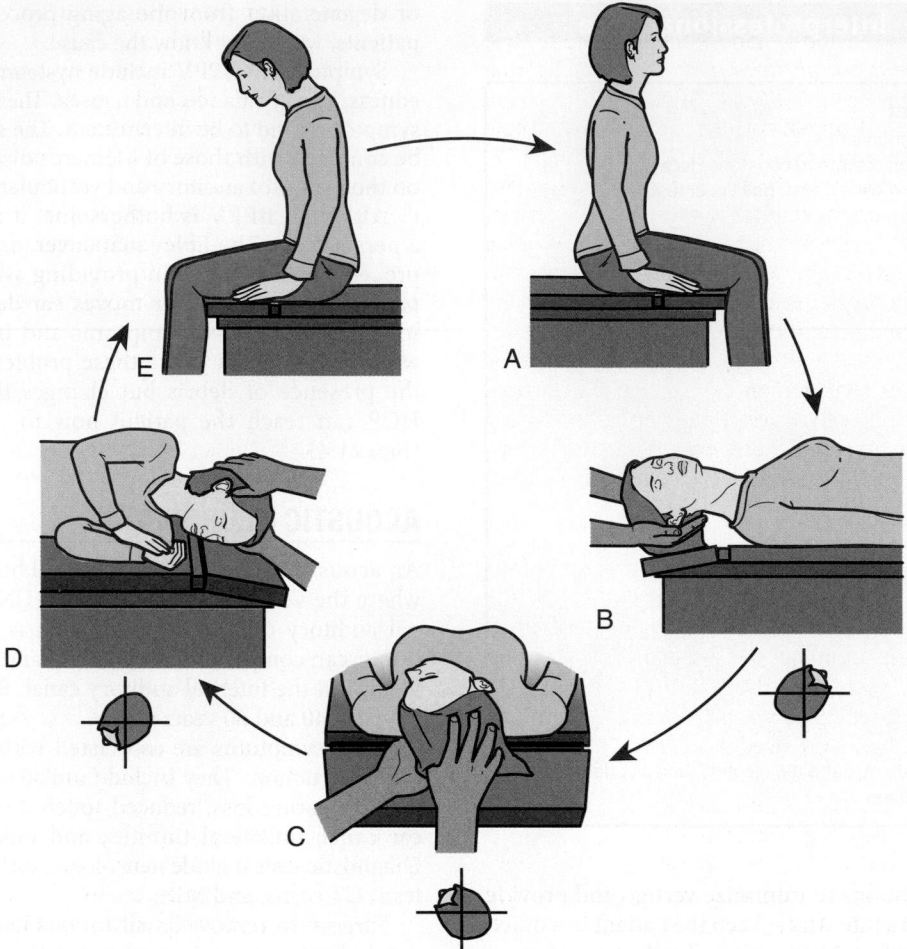

FIG. 21.4 Epley maneuver.

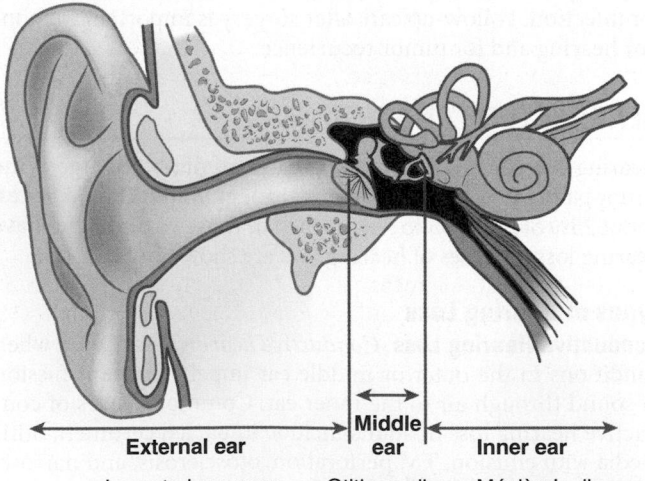

External ear	Middle ear	Inner ear
• Impacted cerumen	• Otitis media	• Ménière's disease
• Foreign bodies	• Serous otitis	• Noise-induced
• External otitis	• Otosclerosis	hearing loss
	• Tympanic	• Presbycusis
	membrane	• Ototoxicity
	trauma	
	• Cholesteatoma	
	• Acoustic neuroma	

FIG. 21.5 Causes of hearing loss.

Sensorineural Hearing Loss. *Sensorineural hearing loss* is caused by impairment of function of the inner ear or the vestibulo-cochlear nerve (CN VIII). Congenital and hereditary factors, noise exposure, aging (presbycusis), Ménière's disease, trauma, and ototoxicity can cause sensorineural hearing loss. The main problems are the ability to hear sound but not to understand speech and the lack of understanding of the problem by others. The ability to hear high-pitched sounds (including consonants) diminishes. Sounds become muffled and hard to understand. An audiogram shows a loss in decibel levels of the 4000-Hz range and eventually the 2000-Hz range. A hearing aid may help some patients, but it only makes sounds and speech louder, not clearer.

Mixed Hearing Loss. Mixed hearing loss occurs due to a combination of conductive and sensorineural causes. Careful evaluation is needed if corrective surgery for conductive loss is planned because the sensorineural hearing loss will still be present.

Central and Functional Hearing Loss. Central hearing loss involves an inability to interpret sound, including speech, because of a problem in the brain (CNS). A careful history is helpful because there are usually cases of deafness in the family. Refer the patient to a qualified hearing and speech service if indicated.

An emotional or a psychologic factor can cause functional hearing loss. The patient does not seem to hear or respond to pure-tone subjective hearing tests, but no physical reason for hearing loss can be found. Psychologic counseling may help.

Genetic Link

Heredity hearing loss is labeled non-syndromic or syndromic. Most persons have *non-syndromic hearing impairment,* in which hearing loss is the only primary problem. *GJB2* gene mutations are one of the most common causes of non-syndromic hearing loss. These result in changes in the production of the protein Connexin 26, which has a role in the cochlear function. Other genetic mutations increase the risk for ototoxicity or result in malformations of structures in the middle and/or inner ear. *Syndromic hearing impairment* is associated with other clinical abnormalities, such as malformations of the external ear or problems involving other organs. There are more than 400 syndromes that include hearing loss.

Classification of Hearing Loss. Hearing loss can be classified by the decibel level or loss as recorded on the audiogram. Normal hearing is in the 0- to 15-dB range. Most people with a hearing loss of 90 decibels or greater have been deaf since birth (congenitally deaf). Table 21.12 describes the levels of hearing loss.

Clinical Manifestations

Common early signs of hearing loss are answering questions inappropriately and not responding when not looking at the speaker (Table 21.3). Other behaviors that suggest hearing loss include straining to hear, cupping the hand around the ear, reading lips, and an increased sensitivity to slight increases in noise level. Often the patient is unaware of minimal hearing loss. Family and friends who get tired of repeating or talking loudly are often the first to notice the hearing loss. Pressure exerted by significant others is a significant factor in whether the patient seeks help for hearing impairment.

Sudden hearing loss, or sudden deafness, occurs as an unexplained, rapid loss of hearing (usually in one ear) either at once or over several days. It is a medical emergency, and the patient should see an HCP at once.

Tinnitus and Hearing Loss. *Tinnitus* is the perception of *sound* in the ears where no external source is present. It is "ringing in the ears" or "head noise" (see www.ata.org). Tinnitus is sometimes the first symptom of hearing loss, especially in older adults. It may be soft or loud, high pitched or low pitched.

Often, tinnitus occurs because of noise exposure. It also can be a drug side effect. More than 200 drugs are known to cause tinnitus.

❖ NURSING AND INTERPROFESSIONAL MANAGEMENT: HEARING LOSS AND DEAFNESS

Deafness is often called the "unseen handicap" because you may not realize the difficulty in communication with a deaf person until you begin a conversation with that person. You need to confirm a deaf person's understanding of health teaching. Descriptive visual aids can be helpful. If the significantly hearing-impaired person uses sign language to communicate, the Americans with Disabilities Act requires providing an interpreter when presenting significant information, such as for patient consent or discharge teaching.[7]

Interference in communication and interaction with others can be the source of many problems for the patient and caregiver. Often the patient refuses to admit or may be unaware of impaired hearing. Irritability is common because the patient must concentrate so hard to understand speech. The loss of clarity of speech in the patient with sensorineural hearing loss is most frustrating. The patient may hear what is said but not understand it. Withdrawal, depression, and accelerated cognitive decline are often associated with advancing hearing loss.[8]

❓ CHECK YOUR PRACTICE

Your newly assigned 68-yr-old female patient is being discharged today following a hip replacement. Before going to her room, you prepared the materials and information for her discharge. You sit down by her bed and start talking with her. She shakes her head and says, "No, no." You are perplexed until she flashes a bracelet that says *I am deaf.*

- How will you proceed?

◆ Health Promotion

◆ Environmental Noise Control. Noise is the most preventable cause of hearing loss. Fig. 21.6 lists the levels of environmental noise generated by common indoor and outdoor sounds. Sudden severe loud noise (acoustic trauma) and chronic exposure to loud noise (noise-induced hearing loss) can damage hearing. Acoustic trauma causes hearing loss by destroying the hair cells of the organ of Corti. Sensorineural hearing loss from increased and prolonged environmental noise, such as amplified sound, is occurring in young adults at an increasing rate. Amplified music (e.g., on smartphones) should not exceed 50% of maximum volume. Ear protection should be worn when firing a gun and during other recreational pursuits with high noise levels. Health teaching about avoiding continued exposure to noise levels greater than 70 dB is essential.

In work environments known to have high noise levels (more than 85 dB), people should wear ear protection. Occupational Safety and Health Administration (OSHA) standards mandate ear protection for workers in environments where the noise levels consistently exceed 85 dB. Periodic audiometric screening should be part of the health maintenance policies of industry. This provides baseline data on hearing to measure subsequent hearing loss.

Employees should take part in hearing conservation programs in work environments. Such programs should include noise exposure analysis, provision for control of noise exposure (hearing protectors), measurements of hearing, and employee-employer notification and education. Encourage young adults to keep amplified music at a reasonable level and limit their exposure time. Hearing loss caused by noise is not reversible

♥ PROMOTING POPULATION HEALTH

Promoting Healthy Hearing

- Wear ear protection during recreational and work activities involving high noise levels.
- Monitor your audio level and how long you use personal listening devices.
- Avoid exposure to excessively loud noise whenever possible.
- Undergo audiometric screening to detect hearing loss before it progresses.
- Avoid injury from cotton-tipped applicators and other cleaning materials.

TABLE 21.12 Classification of Hearing Loss	
Decibel (dB) Loss	**Meaning**
0–15	Normal hearing
16–25	Slight hearing loss
26–40	Mild impairment
41–55	Moderate impairment
56–70	Moderately severe impairment
71–90	Severe impairment
>90	Profound deafness

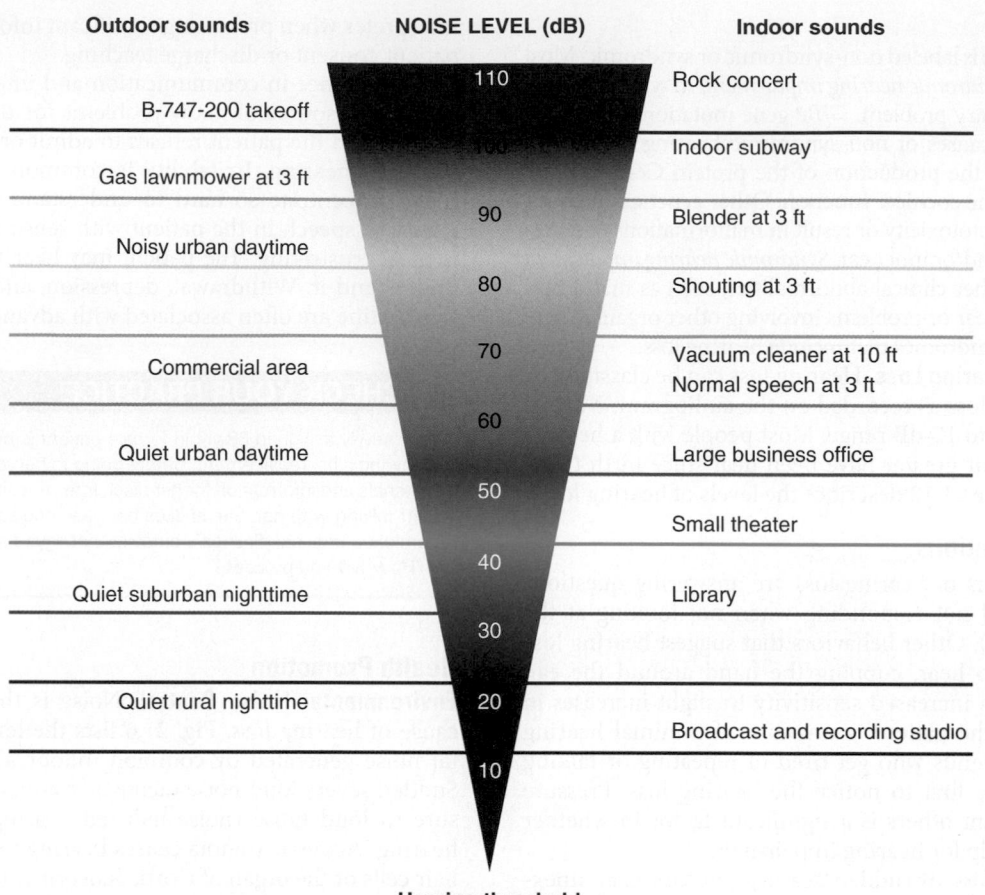

FIG. 21.6 Range of common environmental sounds.

Immunizations. Various viruses can cause deafness because of fetal damage and malformations affecting the ear. Promote childhood and adult immunizations, including the measles, mumps, and rubella (MMR) vaccine. Rubella infection during the first 8 weeks of pregnancy is associated with a high incidence of congenital rubella syndrome, which causes sensorineural deafness. Women of childbearing age should be tested for antibodies to these viral diseases. Women should avoid pregnancy for at least 3 months after being immunized. Immunization must be delayed if a woman is pregnant. Women who are susceptible to rubella can be vaccinated safely during the postpartum period.

Ototoxic Substances. Monitor the patient who is receiving ototoxic drugs or exposed to ototoxic agents for signs and symptoms of ototoxicity, including tinnitus, diminished hearing, and balance problems. If these symptoms develop, stopping the drug may prevent further damage and allow the symptoms to disappear.

Assistive Devices and Techniques

Hearing Aids. The patient with a suspected hearing loss should have a hearing assessment by a qualified audiologist. If a hearing aid is needed, it should be fitted by an audiologist or a speech and hearing specialist. Many types of hearing aids are available, each with advantages and disadvantages (Table 21.13). The conventional hearing aid serves as a simple amplifier. For the patient with bilateral hearing impairment, binaural hearing aids offer the best sound lateralization and speech discrimination.

The goal of hearing aid therapy is improved hearing with consistent use. Patients who are motivated and optimistic about using a hearing aid are more successful users. Determine the patient's readiness for hearing aid therapy, including acknowledgment of a hearing problem, the patient's feelings about wearing a hearing aid, the degree to which the hearing loss affects life, and any difficulties the patient has manipulating small objects such as putting a battery in a hearing aid.

Initially, use of a hearing aid should be restricted to quiet situations in the home. The patient must first adjust to voices (including the patient's own voice) and household sounds. The patient should try increasing and decreasing the volume as situations require. As the patient adjusts to the increase in sounds and background noise, they can progress to situations in which several people will be talking at once. Next, the environment is expanded to the outdoors and then a shopping mall or grocery store. Adjustment to different environments occurs gradually, depending on the patient.

When a hearing aid is not being worn, it should be placed in a dry, cool area where it will not be inadvertently damaged or lost. The battery should be disconnected or removed when not in use. Battery life averages 1 week, depending on the hearing

TABLE 21.13 Types of Hearing Aids

Type	Advantages	Disadvantages
Completely in the canal (mild to moderate hearing loss)	Smallest and least visible aid. Protected from sounds such as wind noise	Costly. No space for add-ons such as directional microphones or volume controls. Small, short-lived batteries
In the canal (mild to severe hearing loss)	More powerful than aids completely in the canal. Has adjustable features such as noise reduction	Small size of aid with added features may be hard to use for patients with visual loss or arthritis

Type	Advantages	Disadvantages
In the ear (mild to severe hearing loss)	Powerful amplification. Inserts and adjusts easily. Longer lasting batteries	Visible. May pick up wind noise readily
Behind the ear (all types of hearing loss)	Most powerful aid. Adjusts easily. Longest battery life	Largest, most visible aid. Newer models may be smaller and less obvious

aid, battery, and amount of use. Advise patients to buy only a month's supply at a time. Ear molds should be cleaned weekly or as needed. Toothpicks or pipe cleaners can easily clear a clogged ear tip.

An *implantable hearing device* or aid is available to patients who cannot or will not use traditional hearing aids or cochlear implants. Implanted hearing devices amplify sound and transmit the sound vibrations through the ear. The device does not have visible external components. There are 2 types of implantable hearing devices: fully implantable and partially implantable. Fully implantable devices are placed surgically, and nothing is visible externally. Partially implanted devices have an internal device that is implanted surgically and an external device that is worn behind or in the ear.

Speech Reading. *Speech reading,* or *lip reading,* can be helpful in increasing communication. It allows for about 40% understanding of the spoken word. The patient uses visual cues associated with speech, such as gestures and facial expressions, to help clarify the spoken message. In speech reading, many words look alike to the patient (e.g., rabbit, woman). Help the patient by using and teaching verbal and nonverbal communication techniques as described in Table 21.14.

TABLE 21.14 Communicating With Patients With Hearing Impairment

Nonverbal Aids
- Draw attention with hand movements.
- Have speaker's face in good light.
- Avoid light behind the speaker.
- Maintain eye contact.
- Avoid covering mouth or face with hands.
- Avoid chewing, eating, smoking while talking.
- Remove background noise.
- Move close to better ear.

Verbal Aids
- Speak normally and slowly. Do not shout.
- Do not exaggerate facial expressions.
- Do not overenunciate.
- Use simple sentences.
- Rephrase sentence. Use different words.
- Write name or difficult words.
- Speak in normal voice directly into better ear.

Sign Language. *Sign language* is a form of communication for people with profound hearing impairment. It involves gestures and facial features such as eyebrow motion and lip-mouth movements. Sign language is not universal. American Sign

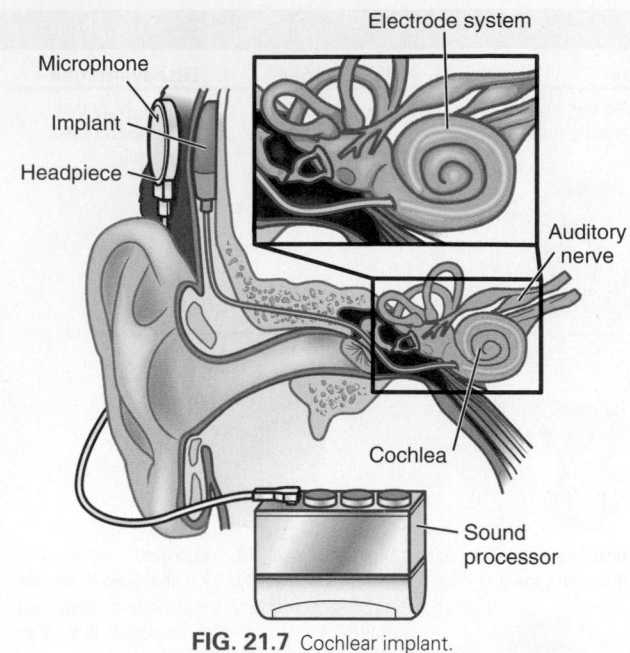

Electrode system
Microphone
Implant
Headpiece
Auditory nerve
Cochlea
Sound processor

FIG. 21.7 Cochlear implant.

TABLE 21.15 **Classification of Presbycusis**	
Type	**Hearing Change and Prognosis**
Cochlear	
Stiffening of basilar membrane, which interferes with sound transmission in the cochlea	Hearing loss increases from low to high frequencies. Speech discrimination affected with higher frequency losses. Helped by appropriate forms of amplification
Metabolic	
Atrophy of blood vessels in wall of cochlea with interruption of essential nutrient supply	Uniform loss for all frequencies accompanied by recruitment. Good response to hearing aid
Neural	
Degenerative changes in cochlea and spinal ganglion	Loss of speech discrimination. Amplification alone not sufficient
Sensory	
Atrophy of auditory nerve. Loss of sensory hair cells	Loss of high-pitched sounds. Little effect on speech understanding. Good response to sound amplification

Language (ASL) is used in the United States and the English-speaking parts of Canada.

Cochlear Implant. A *cochlear implant* may be used for some people with severe to profound sensorineural hearing loss in one or both ears.[9] The implant bypasses damaged or missing portions of the ear and directly activates cranial nerve VIII. The ideal candidate is one who has become deaf after acquiring speech and language. The system consists of (1) an external microphone placed behind the ear, (2) a speech processor, (3) a transmitter implanted under the skin that changes sounds into electrical impulses, and (4) electrodes placed within the cochlea that stimulate the auditory nerves in the ear (Fig. 21.7). The electrodes are inserted as far as possible into the cochlea. Cochlear implants send information that covers the entire range of sound frequencies. For patients with conductive and mixed hearing loss, the cochlear Baha system may be surgically implanted. The system works through direct bone conduction and integrates with the skull bone over time.

Extensive training and rehabilitation are essential to receive the most benefit from these implants. Besides providing sound to a person who heard none, cochlear implants improve lip-reading ability, allow self-monitoring of the loudness of speech, improve the sense of security, and decrease feelings of isolation.

Assistive Listening Devices. Many devices are available to help the hearing-impaired person. Direct amplification devices, amplified telephone receivers, alerting systems that flash when activated by sound, an infrared system for amplifying the sound of the television, and a combination FM receiver and hearing aid may be options based on patient needs. People with profound deafness may be aided by text-telephone alerting systems that flash when activated by sound, closed captioning on television, and a specially trained dog. The dogs are trained to alert their owners to specific sounds within the environment, thus increasing the person's safety and independence.

Gerontologic Considerations: Hearing Loss

Presbycusis, hearing loss associated with aging, includes the loss of peripheral auditory sensitivity, a decline in word recognition ability, and associated psychologic and communication issues. Because consonants (high-frequency sounds) help us recognize spoken words, the older person with presbycusis has a decreased ability to understand speech. Vowels are heard, but one cannot distinguish consonants in the high-frequency range. This may lead to confusion and embarrassment because of the difference in what was said and what was heard.

Degenerative changes in the inner ear cause presbycusis. Noise exposure is thought to be a common factor. Table 21.15 describes the classification of specific causes and associated hearing changes of presbycusis. Often a person may have more than one type of presbycusis. The prognosis for hearing depends on the cause of the loss. Sound amplification with the right device is often helpful in improving the understanding of speech. In other situations, an audiologic rehabilitation program can be valuable.

The older adult is often reluctant to use a hearing aid for sound amplification. Reasons cited most often include cost, appearance, insufficient knowledge about hearing aids, amplification of competing noise, and unrealistic expectations. Most hearing aids and batteries are small, and neuromuscular changes such as stiff fingers, enlarged joints, and decreased sensory perception often make the care and handling of a hearing aid frustrating for an older person. Some older adults may also tend to accept their losses as part of getting older and believe there is no need for improvement.

CASE STUDY
Ménière's Disease

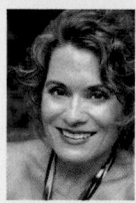

(© iStock.com/
EyeMark.)

Patient Profile

While R.S. is in the emergency department, she starts violently vomiting. She tells you that any movement is making her feel like she is "spinning like crazy." The HCP decides to admit her under observation with plans to administer an intratympanic injection of dexamethasone.

Objective Data

- Skin pale, extremely diaphoretic
- Heart rate 112 beats/min, respirations 22 breaths/min, BP 100/64

Interprofessional Care

- 1000 mg sodium diet as tolerated
- Ondansetron 2 mg IV now
- Lorazepam 1 mg IV every 6 hours
- Meclizine 25 mg PO every 6 hours

- Electronystagmogram and glycerol test
- Dextrose 5% with 0.45% NaCl at 75 mL/hr

Discussion Questions

1. Explain the etiology of Ménière's disease.
2. What clinical manifestations of Ménière's disease does R.S. exhibit?
3. Give the rationale for each treatment measure ordered.
4. *Priority Decision:* Based on the assessment data, what are the priority nursing diagnoses?
5. *Priority Decision:* What are the priority nursing interventions for R.S.?
6. *Delegation Decision:* Identify interventions for R.S. that can be delegated to unlicensed assistive personnel (UAP).
7. *Safety:* Identify an area of risk for injury to R.S. What actions will you take to ensure patient safety?
8. *Patient-Centered Care:* What teaching will you provide so R.S. can successfully self-manage her condition after discharge?
9. *Quality Improvement:* What outcomes would indicate interprofessional care was effective?

Answers available at *http://evolve.elsevier.com/Lewis/medsurg.*

BRIDGE TO NCLEX EXAMINATION

The number of the question corresponds to the same-numbered outcome at the beginning of the chapter.

1. In a patient with vertigo, the parts of the ear most likely involved are the *(select all that apply)*
   a. cochlea.
   b. ossicles.
   c. vestibule.
   d. semicircular canals.
   e. tympanic membrane.

2. A patient reports tinnitus and balance problems. The medication that may be responsible is
   a. digoxin.
   b. warfarin.
   c. furosemide.
   d. acetaminophen.

3. What assessment technique should the nurse use to assess an adult patient's tympanic membrane?
   a. Have the patient tilt the head toward the nurse.
   b. Stabilize the otoscope with your fingers on the patient's cheek.
   c. Pull the auricle down and back to straighten the auditory canal.
   d. Use a speculum slightly larger than the size of the patient's ear canal.

4. A normal finding the nurse would expect when assessing hearing would be
   a. absent cone of light.
   b. bluish purple tympanic membrane.
   c. fluid level at hairline in the tympanum.
   d. midline tone heard equally in both ears.

5. Common age-related changes in the auditory system include *(select all that apply)*
   a. drier cerumen.
   b. tinnitus in both ears.
   c. auditory nerve degeneration.
   d. atrophy of the tympanic membrane.
   e. greater ability to hear high-pitched sounds.

6. The nurse teaches a patient scheduled for an electronystagmography that the test involves
   a. measuring ear drum movement in response to pressure.

   b. recording eye movements associated with ear irrigation.
   c. placing an electrode on the eardrum and assessing for dizziness.
   d. wearing headphones and determining which sounds can be heard.

7. Care of the patient experiencing an acute attack of Ménière's disease includes *(select all that apply)*
   a. giving antiemetics as needed.
   b. implementing fall precautions.
   c. keeping the room dark and quiet.
   d. placing the patient on NPO status.
   e. ambulating in the hall independently.

8. The patient who has a conductive hearing loss
   a. hears better in a noisy environment.
   b. hears sound but does not understand speech.
   c. often speaks loudly because his or her own voice seems low.
   d. has clearer sound with a hearing aid if the loss is less than 30 dB.

9. Teach the patient who is newly fitted with bilateral hearing aids to *(select all that apply)*
   a. replace the batteries monthly.
   b. clean the ear molds weekly or as needed.
   c. clean ears with cotton-tipped applicators daily.
   d. disconnect or remove the batteries when not in use.
   e. initially restrict usage to quiet listening in the home.

10. Which strategies would *best* aid the nurse communicate with a patient who has a hearing loss *(select all that apply)*?
    a. Overenunciate speech.
    b. Speak normally and slowly.
    c. Exaggerate facial expressions.
    d. Raise the voice to a higher pitch.
    e. Write out names or difficult words.

1. c, d, 2. c, 3. b, 4. d, 5. a, b, c, 6. b, 7. a, b, c, 8. a, c, d, 9. d, e, 10. b, e

For rationales to these answers and even more NCLEX review questions, visit http://evolve.elsevier.com/Lewis/medsurg.

ⓔ EVOLVE WEBSITE/RESOURCES LIST

http://evolve.elsevier.com/Lewis/medsurg
Review Questions (Online Only)
Key Points
Answer Keys for Questions
- Rationales for Bridge to NCLEX Examination Questions
- Answer Guidelines for Case Study on pp. 378, 380, 381, 382, and 393

Conceptual Care Map Creator
Audio Glossary
Content Updates

REFERENCES

1. Eggermont J: *Hearing loss: Causes, prevention, and treatment*, Cambridge, 2017, Academic Press.
2. Hearing Loss Association of America Retrieved from *http://hearingloss.org*.
3. Popelka G, Moore B, Fay R, Popper A, eds: *Hearing aids*, Switzerland, 2016, Springer International Publishing.
4. Patel H, Isildak H: Ménière's disease, *Oper Tech Otolaryngol Head Neck Surg* 27:184, 2016.
5. Pullen R: Navigating the challenges of Ménière's disease, *Nursing* 47:38, 2017.
6. Quick statistics about hearing. Retrieved from *www.nidcd.nih.gov/health/statistics/quick-statistics-hearing*.
7. Communicating with people who are deaf or hard of hearing in hospital settings. Retrieved from *www.ada.gov/hospcombr.htm*.
8. Tremblay KL: Why is hearing loss a public health concern, *Hear J* 70:14, 2017.
9. National Institute on Deafness and Other Communication Disorders: Cochlear implants. Retrieved from *www.nidcd.nih.gov*.

*Evidence-based information for clinical practice.

22

Assessment: Integumentary System

Mariann M. Harding

*The greatest gift you can give another is the purity of
your attention.*

Richard Moss

ⓔ http://evolve.elsevier.com/Lewis/medsurg/

CONCEPTUAL FOCUS

Health Promotion   **Tissue Integrity**

LEARNING OUTCOMES

1. Describe the structures and functions of the integumentary system.
2. Link the age-related changes in the integumentary system to differences in assessment findings.
3. Obtain significant subjective and objective data related to the integumentary system from a patient.
4. Compare the critical components for describing primary and secondary lesions.
5. Perform a physical assessment of the integumentary system using appropriate techniques.
6. Specify the structural and assessment differences in light- and dark-skinned persons.
7. Distinguish normal from common abnormal findings of a physical assessment of the integumentary system.
8. Describe the purpose, significance of results, and nursing responsibilities related to diagnostic studies of the integumentary system.

KEY TERMS

alopecia, Table 22.8, p. 404
dermis, p. 396
epidermis, p. 395
erythema, Table 22.8, p. 404

hirsutism, Table 22.8, p. 404
intertriginous, p. 401
keloid, p. 404
keratinocytes, p. 395

melanocytes, p. 395
mole (nevus), Table 22.8, p. 404
pruritus, p. 401
sebaceous glands, p. 397

The integumentary system is the largest organ of the body. It is composed of the skin, hair, nails, and certain glands. The skin has 2 major layers: epidermis (outer layer) and dermis (inner layer). The subcutaneous tissue (layer) lies under the dermis (Fig. 22.1). The skin is as complex as any organ, but, unlike the others, it is readily visible. Being able to see and touch the skin helps you assess your patients. You can see abnormalities, understand their significance, and intervene early.

STRUCTURES AND FUNCTIONS OF SKIN AND APPENDAGES

Structures

Epidermis. The epidermis, the outer layer of the skin, is relatively thin, ranging from 0.05 mm on the eyelids to 0.1 mm on the soles.[1] There are no lymphatic or vascular structures in the epidermis. It is supported by passive circulation from the dermis.

The epidermis is divided into 5 distinct but interrelated layers. Two of the layers are the stratum corneum (the surface layer) and the stratum germinativum (deepest, basal layer) (Fig. 22.1).

Most epithelial cells are keratinocytes (90%). The remaining cells are melanocytes, Langerhans' cells, and Merkel cells.

Keratinocytes form in the basal layer. Initially, they are undifferentiated and shaped like columns. As they mature (keratinize), they move to the surface, where they flatten and die to form the outer skin layer (stratum corneum). Keratinocytes make a fibrous protein, keratin, which is vital to the skin's protective barrier function. The upward movement of keratinocytes from the basal layer to the outermost levels of the stratum corneum takes about 14 days. The keratinocytes stay there for another 14 days, allowing the epidermis to regenerate every 28 days. Thus each month you have a new layer of skin.

Many skin problems result from changes in this cell cycle. If dead cells slough off too rapidly, the skin appears thin and eroded. If new cells form faster than you shed old cells, the skin becomes scaly and thickened. Failure of the epidermis to function normally occurs with skin cancer and psoriasis (discussed in Chapter 23).

Melanocytes are found in the deep, basal layer. They contain melanin, a pigment that gives color to the skin and hair and protects the body from damaging ultraviolet (UV) sunlight.

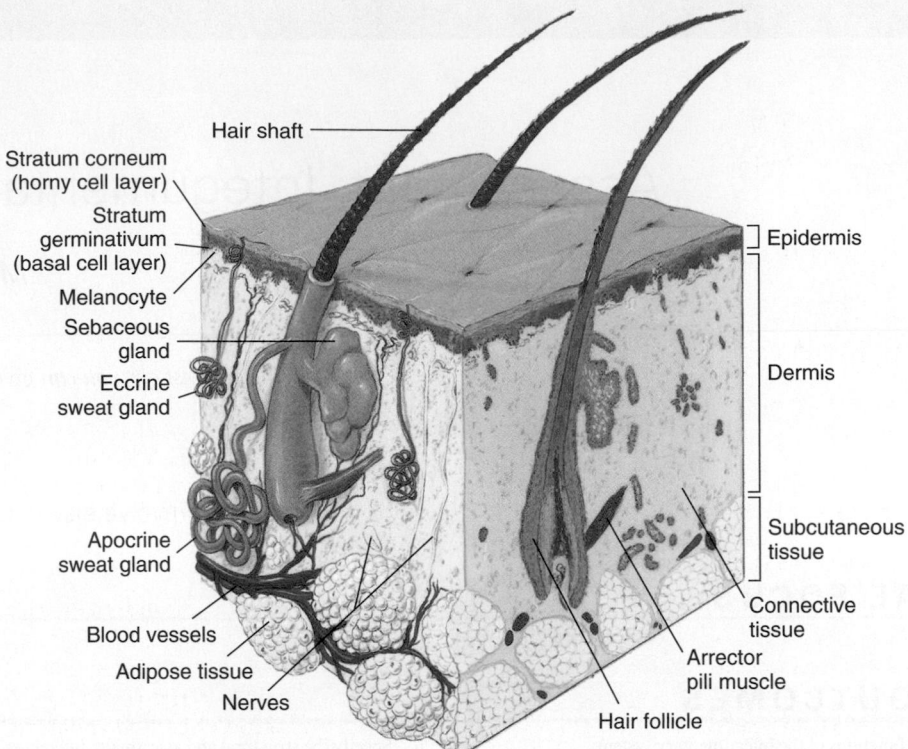

FIG. 22.1 Microscopic view of the skin in longitudinal section. (From Jarvis C: *Physical examination and health assessment,* ed 6, St Louis, 2012, Saunders.)

Sunlight and hormones stimulate the melanosome (within the melanocyte) to increase the production of melanin. People of all races have similar numbers of melanocytes. In darker skin, the melanosomes are larger and more numerous, thus producing more melanin.[2] This increased melanin forms a natural sun shield for dark skin and results in a decreased incidence of skin cancer. The distribution of melanocytes varies from one area of the body to another. For example, the face has more melanocytes than the abdomen.

Langerhans' cells are a type of dendritic cell (discussed in Chapter 13 on p. 191). They are immunocompetent cells that recognize antigens. When they are depleted, the skin cannot initiate an immune response. The Langerhans' cells in bioengineered skin grafts have been removed to prevent graft rejection. In skin diseases such as psoriasis and sarcoidosis, there are decreased numbers of Langerhans' cells. *Merkel cells* are found in the basal layer and are involved in the sensation of light touch. We use them when feeling the texture of an object and figuring out what it is.

The basement membrane zone is between the epidermis and dermis. This structure provides for the (1) exchange of fluids between the epidermis and dermis and (2) structural support for the epidermis. The basement membrane helps to secure the two layers together. Inflammation and separation of the epidermal and dermal layers result in the blisters seen with problems such as burns, full-thickness wounds, and mechanical trauma.

Dermis. The dermis is the connective tissue below the epidermis. Dermal thickness ranges from 0.3 mm on the eyelid to 3.0 mm on the back.[1] The dermis is very vascular, containing many blood vessels. It also contains nerves, lymphatic vessels, hair follicles, sebaceous glands, and specialized cells such as mast cells and macrophages that protect the body from external stimuli.

The dermis is made of 3 types of connective tissue: collagen, elastic fibers, and reticular fibers. Collagen forms the greatest part of the dermis. It gives the skin toughness and strength. The primary cell type in the dermis is the *fibroblast,* which makes collagen and elastin. Collagen is critical in wound healing.

The dermis has 2 layers: upper thin papillary layer and a deeper, thicker reticular layer. The papillary layer is arranged haphazardly in ridges, or papillae, which extend into the outer epidermal layer. These elevated surface ridges form fingerprints and footprints. The reticular layer forms the bulk of the dermis. It is made up of thick collagen bundles arranged parallel to the skin's surface.

Subcutaneous Tissue. The subcutaneous tissue lies below the dermis. It is made of loose connective tissue and fat cells that provide insulation, cushioning, temperature regulation, and energy storage. The subcutaneous tissue attaches the skin to underlying tissues, such as muscle and bone. The distribution pattern of subcutaneous tissue varies with gender, heredity, age, and nutritional status.

Skin Appendages. *Skin appendages* include the hair, nails, and glands (sebaceous, apocrine, and eccrine). These appendages are epidermal extensions that have their roots in the dermis. These structures receive nutrients, electrolytes, and fluids from the dermis. Hair and nails form from specialized keratin. Systemic diseases can affect the condition and health of both hair and nails.

Hair grows on most of the body except for the lips, palms of the hands, interdigital spaces, portions of the genitalia, and soles of the feet. The density and pattern of distribution varies depending on age, sex, and race. Hair color is a result of heredity and determined by the type and amount of melanin in the hair shaft. Hair grows about 1 cm per month. People lose about

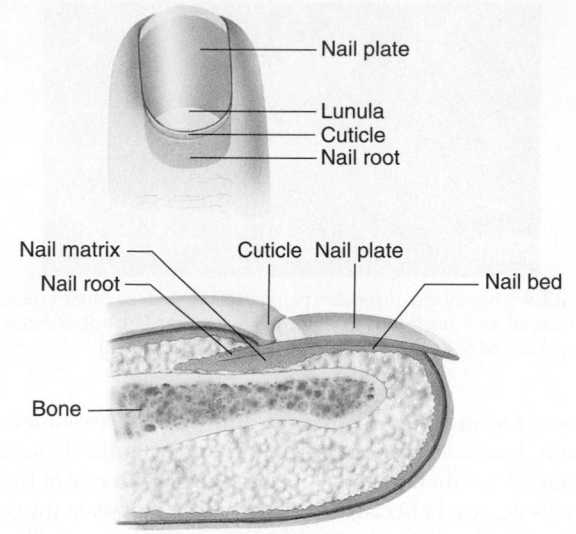

FIG. 22.2 Structure of a nail. (From Patton KT, Thibodeau GA, Douglas M: *Essentials of anatomy and physiology*, St Louis, 2014, Mosby.)

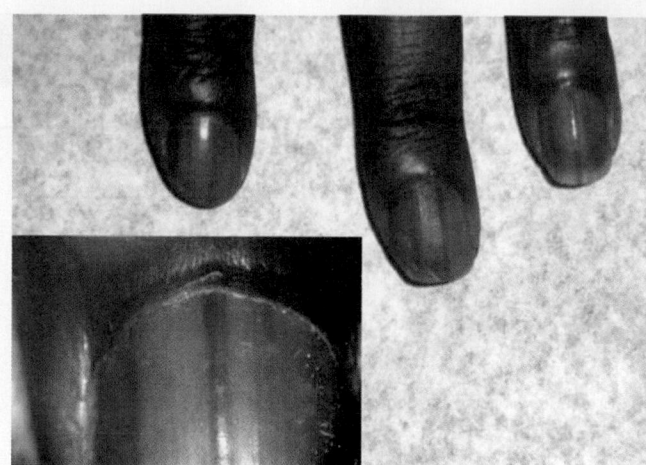

FIG. 22.3 Pigmented nail bands normally seen with dark skin color. (From Ball J, Dains J, Flynn J, et al: *Seidel's guide to physical examination*, ed 8, St Louis, 2014, Mosby.)

100 hairs each day.[3] Baldness, or *alopecia*, results when we do not replace lost hair.

Nails are made of heavily keratinized cells. The part of the nail that you can see is the nail body. The rest is the nail root. A fold of skin hides most of the nail root. The cuticle borders this skinfold. Nail growth begins in the nail root. The part of the nail root you can see is the *lunula*. This white, crescent-shaped area is the site of mitosis and nail growth (Fig. 22.2). Under the nail is an area of epidermis called the *nail bed*. The nail bed has many blood vessels. Nails grow slowly, but continuously. Fingernails grow much faster than toenails, at a rate of 0.5 to 2 mm per week.[1] It takes 3 to 6 months to replace a fingernail. A toenail may take 12 months or longer to replace. Nail color ranges from pink to yellow or brown depending on skin color. Color and texture variations in nails may be normal or represent an abnormal condition. Pigmented longitudinal bands *(melanonychia striata)* occur in the nail bed in 90% or more of people with dark skin[4] (Fig. 22.3).

There are 2 major types of glands in the skin: sebaceous and sweat (apocrine and eccrine) glands. Sebaceous glands secrete *sebum,* which is emptied into the hair follicles. Sebum waterproofs and lubricates the skin and promotes the absorption of fat-soluble substances. Sebum is somewhat bacteriostatic and fungistatic. These glands depend on sex hormones, particularly testosterone, to regulate sebum secretion and production. Actual production varies depending on age, sex, and testosterone and estrogen levels. Sebaceous glands are present on all areas of the skin except the palms and soles and dorsum of the feet. These glands are most abundant on the face, scalp, upper chest, and back.

The *apocrine sweat glands* are mainly found in the axillary, genital, and breast areas. They are always connected to a hair follicle. These glands enlarge and become active at puberty because of reproductive hormones. They secrete a thick milky substance that is naturally odorless. Odor occurs when skin surface bacteria alter the secretions.

The *eccrine sweat glands* are found on most of the body, except the lips, ear canals, nail beds, labia minora, glans penis, and prepuce. One square inch of skin has about 3000 eccrine sweat glands. Their main function is to cool the body by evaporation, excrete waste products, and moisturize surface cells. Sweat is a transparent watery solution composed of salts, ammonia, urea, and other wastes. In extreme situations, the body can make 2 to 4 L of sweat per hour or up to 12 liters in 24 hours. Heat, certain mental stimuli, and ingestion of hot, spicy foods stimulate sweat secretion.

Functions of Integumentary System

The skin's main function is to protect the underlying body tissues by serving as a barrier to the external environment. The skin acts as a barrier against invasion by bacteria and viruses and prevents excess water loss. The fat in the subcutaneous layer insulates the body and provides protection from trauma. Melanin screens and absorbs UV radiation.

The skin with its nerve endings and special receptors collects sensory information from environmental stimuli. These highly specialized nerve endings give information to the brain related to pain, heat and cold, touch, pressure, and vibration.

The skin controls heat regulation by responding to changes in internal and external temperature with vasoconstriction or vasodilation. The skin's excretory function and heat regulation are related. We lose between 600 and 900 mL of water daily through insensible water loss (invisible vaporization from the lungs and skin), which helps regulate body temperature. Sebum and sweat lubricate the skin surface. Endogenous synthesis of vitamin D, which is critical to calcium and phosphorus balance, occurs in the epidermis. Vitamin D is made in the epidermis when UV light acts on vitamin D precursor cells.

Gerontologic Considerations: Effects of Aging on Integumentary System

Many skin changes are associated with aging. Depending on a person's view of self, the normal, visible effects of aging on the skin and hair may have a profound psychologic effect. Having a youthful look may affect a person's self-image. The appearance of the signs of aging can be a threat to self-concept. Other changes in skin structure related to normal changes with aging can pose serious risk. Age-related changes of the integumentary system and differences in assessment findings are listed in Table 22.1.

Chronic UV exposure is the major contributor to the photoaging and wrinkling of skin.[5] Sun damage to the skin is

TABLE 22.1 Gerontologic Assessment Differences

Integumentary System

Changes	Differences in Assessment Findings
Skin	
Decreased subcutaneous fat, muscle laxity, degeneration of elastic fibers, collagen stiffening	Increased wrinkling, sagging breasts and abdomen, redundant flesh around eyes, slowness of skin to flatten when pinched (tenting)
Decreased extracellular water, surface lipids, and sebaceous gland activity	Dry, flaking skin with possible signs of excoriation caused by scratching
Decreased activity of apocrine and sebaceous glands	Dry skin with minimal to no perspiration, skin color uneven
Increased capillary fragility and permeability	Bruising
Increased focal melanocytes in basal layer with pigment accumulation	Solar lentigines on face and back of hands
Diminished blood supply	Decrease in rosy appearance of skin and mucous membranes. Skin cool to touch. Diminished awareness of pain, touch, temperature, peripheral vibration
Decreased proliferative capacity	Delayed wound healing
Decreased immunocompetence	Increase in neoplasms
Hair	
Decreased melanin and melanocytes	Gray or white hair
Decreased oil	Dry, coarse hair. Scaly scalp
Decreased hair density	Thinning and hair loss
Cumulative androgen effect; decreasing estrogen levels	Facial hirsutism, baldness
Nails	
Decreased peripheral blood supply	Thick, brittle nails with diminished growth
Increased keratin	Longitudinal ridging
Decreased circulation	Prolonged return of blood to nails on blanching

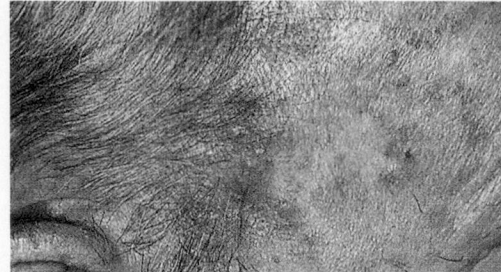

FIG. 22.4 Photoaging. Irregular pigmentation and keratoses occur on sun-damaged skin on forehead. (From Gawkrodger D, Ardern-Jones MR: *Dermatology,* ed 5, Edinburgh, 2012, Churchill Livingstone.)

Fewer melanocytes are present, and with decreased levels of melanin, hair color fades. Hormonal and vitamin deficiencies can cause dry, thin hair and alopecia. The growth rate of the hair and nails decreases because of atrophy. The nail plate thins, and nails become brittle and more prone to splitting and yellowing. Nails, especially the toenails, may thicken with age. With aging, the apocrine and eccrine sweat glands atrophy, causing dry skin and decreased body odor.

Benign neoplasms related to the aging process can occur. These growths include seborrheic keratoses, vascular lesions such as cherry angiomas, and skin tags. *Actinic keratoses* appear on areas of chronic sun exposure, especially in the person who has a fair complexion and light eyes (blue, green, or hazel). These premalignant cutaneous lesions place a person at increased risk for squamous cell and basal cell carcinomas.

ASSESSMENT OF INTEGUMENTARY SYSTEM

The general skin assessment begins with your first contact with the patient and continues throughout the examination. As you are meeting your patient for the first time, take a moment to note the overall condition of the patient's skin and hair. You will assess specific areas of the skin when examining other body systems, unless the chief complaint is a skin problem. Record a general statement about the skin's physical condition (Table 22.2). In addition, ask the health history questions presented in Table 22.3 when you note a skin problem.

cumulative (Fig. 22.4). The wrinkling of sun-exposed areas such as the face and hands is more marked than that of a sun-shielded area, such as the buttocks. A photoaged person is more susceptible to skin cancers because UV exposure decreases the ability to repair cellular damage. Chronic UV exposure from tanning beds causes the same damage as UV from the sun. Other factors that influence skin aging include diabetes, smoking, and alcohol use.

The junction between the dermis and epidermis flattens. This causes the two layers to lose their tight bond. Skin tears and other trauma become common as the epidermis slides separately from the dermis. Collagen fibers stiffen, elastic fibers degenerate, and the amount of subcutaneous tissue decreases. These changes, with the added effects of gravity, lead to wrinkling. Fewer free fatty acids in the epidermis results in dry, scaly, itchy skin. Dryness, combined with trauma caused by scratching, increases the risk for fissures (cracks) in the skin and secondary infections. Decreased subcutaneous fat increases the risk for traumatic injury, hypothermia, and skin shearing, which may lead to pressure ulcers.

CASE STUDY

Patient Introduction

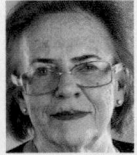

(© iStockphoto/ Thinkstock.)

D.A. is a 74-yr-old woman who comes to the medical clinic with concerns related to various "spots" on her face. She says they have been there for a while and she thought they were just "age spots." She became concerned after her friend was diagnosed with a malignant melanoma.

Discussion Questions

1. Which type of assessment should you perform: comprehensive, focused, or emergency?
2. What are the possible causes of D.A.'s facial lesions?
3. What questions would you ask D.A. to determine the possible causes?

You will learn more about D.A. and her condition as you read this chapter.

(See p. 401 for more information on D.A.)

TABLE 22.2 Normal Physical Assessment of Integumentary System

Skin	• Evenly pigmented. No petechiae, purpura, lesions, or excoriations
	• Warm, good turgor
Nails	• Pink, oval, adhere to nail bed with 160-degree angle
Hair	• Shiny and full; amount and distribution appropriate for age and gender
	• No flaking of scalp, forehead, or pinna

Subjective Data

Perform the interview using a sensitive and nonjudgmental attitude. The problem may be the result of poor hygiene or unhealthful behaviors. Some problems are highly visible and affect the patient's body image and self-concept. A thorough health history yields information about possible causes and the effect of the problem on the person's life.

Important Health Information

Past Health History. Past health history reveals previous trauma, surgery, or disease that involves the skin. Many diseases have skin manifestations (Table 22.4). Determine if the patient has noticed any problems such as jaundice (liver disease), delayed wound healing (diabetes), cyanosis (respiratory, cardiovascular disorder), or pallor (anemia). Obtain specific information related to food sensitivities, pet or drug allergies, and skin reactions to insect bites and stings. Note any history of chronic or unprotected exposure to UV light, including tanning bed use and radiation treatments.

Medications. A thorough medication history is important. Ask the patient about skin-related problems that occurred because of taking a medication. Many hormones, antibiotics, corticosteroids, and antimetabolites have side effects that manifest in the skin. Medications may contain fragrances and preservatives that can cause skin reactions. Document the use of medications specifically used to treat a primary skin problem, such as acne, or a secondary skin problem, such as itching. Record the drug's name, length of use, method of application, and effectiveness.

Surgery or Other Treatments. Determine if any surgical procedures, including cosmetic surgery, were done on the skin. Record any biopsy results. Note any treatments specific for a skin problem (e.g., phototherapy) or for a health problem (e.g., radiation therapy). Document any treatments undergone primarily for cosmetic purposes, such as tanning booth use, laser resurfacing, or cosmetic "peels."

Functional Health Patterns

Health Perception–Health Management Pattern. Ask the patient about health practices, such as self-care habits related to daily hygiene. Document the frequency of use and sun protection factor (SPF) of sunscreen products. Assess the use of personal care products (e.g., shampoos, moisturizing agents, cosmetics), including brand name, quantity, and frequency. Record a description of any current skin problem, including onset, symptoms, course, and treatment. Note any medications used for treating hair loss.

Obtain information about the family history of any skin diseases, including congenital and familial diseases (e.g., alopecia, psoriasis) and systemic diseases with skin manifestations (e.g., diabetes, thyroid disease, cardiovascular diseases, immune disorders). Note any family and personal history of skin cancer, particularly melanoma.

TABLE 22.3 Health History

Integumentary System

Health Perception–Health Management
- Describe your daily hygiene practices.
- What skin products are you now using?
- Describe any current skin condition, including onset, course, and treatment (if any).

Nutritional-Metabolic
- Describe any changes in the condition of your skin, hair, nails, and mucous membranes.
- Have you noticed any recent changes in the way sores or wounds heal?*
- Have you had any weight loss or dietary changes?*

Elimination
- Have you noticed recent changes in your skin related to excess sweating, dryness, or swelling?*

Activity-Exercise
- Do your leisure or work activities involve using any chemicals that might irritate your skin?*
- Do you do anything to protect yourself from the sun?*

Sleep-Rest
- Does your skin condition keep you awake or awaken you from sleep?*

Cognitive-Perceptual
- Do you have any unusual sensations of heat, cold, or touch?*
- Do you have any pain associated with your skin condition?*
- Do you have any joint pain?*

Self-Perception–Self-Concept
- How does your skin condition make you feel about yourself?

Role-Relationship
- Has your skin condition changed your relationships with others?*
- Have you changed your lifestyle because of your skin condition?*

Sexuality-Reproductive
- Has your skin condition changed your intimate relationships with others?*
- Has your birth control method (if used) caused a skin problem?*

Coping–Stress Tolerance
- Are you aware of any situation or stressor that changes your skin condition?*
- Do you think that stress plays a role in your skin condition?*
- How do you handle stress?

Value-Belief
- Are there any cultural beliefs that influence your thinking or feelings about your skin condition?*
- Are there any treatment options that you would be opposed to using?

*If yes, describe.

GENETIC RISK ALERT

- The primary risk factor leading to skin cancer and melanoma is environmental exposure to UV radiation. UV radiation damages DNA, causing an error in the genetic code and resulting in abnormal skin cells.[6]
- Inherited genetic factors can increase skin cancer risk. A person has an increased risk for developing melanoma if they have a first-degree relative (e.g., parent, full sibling) who had a melanoma.
- People with a fair complexion (light-colored skin that easily freckles, red or blond hair, and blue or light-colored eyes) have an increased risk for skin cancer.

TABLE 22.4 Diseases With Skin Manifestations

Systemic Problem	Skin Manifestations
Endocrine	
Addison's disease	Loss of body hair (especially axillary), generalized hyperpigmentation (accentuated in folds)
Androgen deficiency	Development of sparse hair. Marked reduction in sebum production
Androgen excess	Enlarged facial pores, male sex characteristics, acne, acceleration of coarse hair growth
Diabetes	Erythematous plaques of shins, delayed wound healing, neuropathy, acanthosis nigricans (velvety, dark skin on the neck and in skin folds)
Glucocorticoid excess (Cushing syndrome)	Atrophy, striae, epidermal thinning, telangiectasia, acne. Decreased subcutaneous fat over extremities. Thin, loose dermis. Impaired wound healing. Increased vascular fragility. Mild hirsutism. Excess collection of fat over clavicles, back of neck, abdomen, and face
Hypoparathyroidism	Opaque, brittle nails with transverse ridges. Coarse, sparse hair with patchy alopecia
Hypothyroidism	Cold, dry, pale to yellow skin. Generalized nonpitting edema. Dry, coarse, brittle hair. Brittle, slow-growing nails
Hyperpituitarism (acromegaly)	Coarsened skin, deepened lines. Increased oiliness and sweating, acne. Increased number of nevi, hyperpigmentation; hypertrichosis (excess hair growth)
Hyperthyroidism	Increased sweating, warm skin with persistent flush, thin nails, alopecia. Fine, soft hair
Reproductive Organs	
Paget's disease	Eczematous patch of nipple and areola
Primary syphilis	Chancre
Secondary syphilis	Generalized skin lesions, alopecia
Tertiary syphilis	Gummas
Gastrointestinal	
Cystic fibrosis	Abnormal sweat gland function
Deficiency of essential fatty acids	Scaly skin
Inflammatory bowel disease	Mouth ulcers, erythema nodosum
Liver disease and biliary tract obstruction	Jaundice, itching, pigmentary abnormalities, changes in nails and hair, spider angiomas, telangiectasia
Malabsorption syndrome	Acquired ichthyosis (dry, scaly skin)
Musculoskeletal and Connective Tissue	
Dermatomyositis	Edema; purplish-red upper eyelids; scaly, macular erythema over knuckles
Scleroderma	Leathery hardening and stiffness of skin
Systemic lupus erythematosus	Discoid lesions, maculopapular semiconfluent rash (butterfly rash), alopecia, mouth ulcers
Metabolic	
Nicotinic acid (niacin) deficiency	Redness of exposed areas of skin of hand or foot, face, or neck; infected dermatitis
Vitamin B_1 (thiamine) deficiency	Edema, redness of soles of feet
Vitamin B_2 (riboflavin) deficiency	Red fissures at corner of mouth, glossitis
Vitamin C deficiency	Petechiae, purpura, bleeding gums
Immune	
HIV infection	Kaposi sarcoma, eosinophilic folliculitis
Hodgkin's lymphoma	Pruritus, sensitive skin
Non-Hodgkin's lymphoma	Papules, nodules, plaques, pruritus
Cardiovascular	
Rheumatic heart disease	Petechiae, urticaria, nodules, erythema
Peripheral vascular disease	Loss of hair on hands and feet. Delayed capillary filling. Dependent rubor (redness), pain
Thromboangiitis obliterans (Buerger's disease)	Pallor or cyanosis, gangrene, ulceration
Venous ulcers	Leathery, brownish skin on lower leg; pruritus, concave lesion with edema. Scar tissue with healing
Respiratory	
Inadequate oxygenation due to respiratory disease	Cyanosis
Hematologic	
Anemia	Pallor, hyperpigmentation, pale mucous membranes, hair loss, nail dystrophy
Clotting disorders	Purpura, petechiae, ecchymosis
Renal	
Chronic kidney disease	Dry skin, pruritus, uremic frost, pallor, bruises
Neurologic	
Chronic sensory polyneuropathies Spinal cord trauma	Trophic changes in skin resulting from sensory denervation, pressure ulcers, anesthesia, paresthesias

Nutritional-Metabolic Pattern. Ask the patient about the condition of skin, hair, nails, and mucous membranes and whether they notice any changes related to diet. A diet history reveals the adequacy of nutrients essential to healthy skin and wound healing such as vitamins A, D, E, and C; dietary fat; and protein. Note any food allergies that cause a skin reaction. Ask obese patients if they have areas of chafing or a rash in intertriginous areas, where skin surfaces overlap and rub on each other (e.g., below the breasts, axillae, and groin). Skin in these areas is predisposed to skin tags (*acrochordons*) and candidiasis (yeast), intertrigo (bacteria, fungi, yeast), and erythrasma (bacteria) infections. Note any excess or absent sweating. Ask the patient about poor or delayed wound healing.

Elimination Pattern. Ask the patient about skin conditions, such as dehydration, edema, and pruritus (itching), which can indicate changes in fluid balance. If urinary or fecal incontinence is a problem, ask about the condition of the skin in the anal and perineal areas.

Activity-Exercise Pattern. Obtain information about environmental hazards in relation to hobbies and recreational activities, including exposure to known carcinogens, chemical irritants, and allergens. Ask the patient if any changes occur in the skin during exercise or other activities.

Sleep-Rest Pattern. Ask the patient about changes in sleep patterns caused by a skin condition. For example, pruritus can be distressing and interfere with normal sleep. Poor sleep and resulting tiredness can be reflected in a patient's face by dark circles under the eyes and a decreased firmness in the facial skin.

Cognitive-Perceptual Pattern. Determine the patient's perception of the sensations of heat, cold, pain, and touch. Note any discomfort associated with a skin condition, especially when observed in intact skin, or any reports of unusual skin sensations. Patients with neuropathy may describe numbness, tingling, or crawling sensations in their arms or legs. Ask about joint pain. Assess the mobility of the joints, since the patient's skin condition may cause changes in mobility.

Self-Perception–Self-Concept Pattern. Assess any feelings related to the patient's skin condition such as sadness, anxiety, despair, or altered body image. These feelings can occur with classic signs of aging or visible skin problems such as acne, rosacea, and psoriasis, which alter physical appearance.

Role-Relationship Pattern. Determine how the patient's skin condition affects relationships with family members, peers, and work associates. Ask the patient about the effect of environmental factors on the skin, such as occupational exposure to irritants, sun, and unusually cold or unhygienic conditions. Contact dermatitis caused by allergens and irritants is a common problem associated with occupation.

Sexuality-Reproductive Pattern. Tactfully assess the effect of the patient's skin condition on sexual activity. Note the reproductive status of the female patient relative to possible therapeutic interventions. For example, isotretinoin, used to treat acne, and topical fluorouracil, used to treat actinic keratoses, are teratogenic drugs that may cause abnormal fetal development. Pregnant women or women who could become pregnant should not use them.

Coping–Stress Tolerance Pattern. Assess the role that stress may play in creating or worsening the skin condition. Ask the patient what coping strategies are used to manage the skin condition.

Value-Belief Pattern. Ask about cultural or religious beliefs that could influence the patient's self-image as related to the skin condition. Assess values and beliefs that may influence or limit the choice of treatment options.

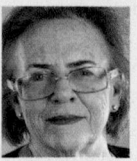
Answers available at *http://evolve.elsevier.com/Lewis/medsurg.*

Objective Data

Physical Examination. A physical examination of the skin begins with a systematic, general inspection and then a more specific assessment of problem areas. A normal range of differences exists in the skin, hair, and nails. Your assessment should note normal skin changes related to age, genetic factors, and environmental exposures from other changes. Look for changes in the color of the skin, turgor, temperature, dryness, thickness, and vascularity. General principles when assessing the skin are:

- Have a private examination room of moderate temperature with good lighting; a room with exposure to daylight is preferred.
- Ensure that the patient is comfortable and in a dressing gown that allows easy access to all skin areas.
- Perform a general inspection and then a lesion-specific examination.
- Use the metric system when taking measurements.
- Use the right terminology when reporting or documenting.

Clinical Photography. Photographs are an adjunct to documentation and promote communication among the interprofessional team. They are used to assess and monitor skin conditions and determine if the condition has improved or declined with treatment. They can be used to track moles and precancerous lesions and detect any changes early. Follow clinical agency protocol for obtaining a patient's consent to photograph lesions.

Inspection. Inspect the skin for general color and pigmentation, vascularity, bruising, and lesions or discolorations. The critical factor in assessment of skin color is change. A skin color that is normal for one patient can be a sign of a pathologic condition in another patient. The skin color depends on the amount of melanin (brown), carotene (yellow), oxyhemoglobin (red), and reduced hemoglobin (bluish red) present at a particular time. The most reliable areas to assess erythema, cyanosis, pallor, and jaundice are the areas of least pigmentation, such as the sclera, conjunctivae, nail beds, lips, and buccal mucosa. The true skin color is best seen in photo-protected areas such as the buttocks. Activity, sun (UV) exposure, emotions, cigarette smoking, and edema, as well as respiratory, renal, cardiovascular, and hepatic disorders, can all directly affect skin color.

In your general inspection, note the presence of body art such as piercings and tattoos. The nose, ears, eyebrows, lips, navel, and nipples are common sites of piercing. Examine tattoos and needle-track marks and note the location and characteristics of the surrounding skin area. Tattoo pigments deposited in the skin may cause itching, pain, and sensitivity for several weeks after the tattoo is placed.

Examine the skin for problems related to vascularity, including bruising and vascular and purpuric lesions such as *angioma* (benign tumor of blood or lymph vessels), *petechiae* (tiny, flat, purplish red pinpoint lesions on skin), *ecchymosis* (bruise larger than petechiae), or *purpura* (purple colored spots and patches characterized by ecchymosis or other small hemorrhages). Note the reaction to direct pressure on the lesion. If a lesion blanches on direct pressure and then refills, the redness is due to dilated blood vessels. If the discoloration stays, it is the result of subcutaneous or intradermal bleeding or a nonvascular lesion. Note any pattern of bruising such as discoloration in the shape of the hand or fingers or bruises at different stages of resolution. These may indicate other health problems or abuse and need further investigation.

Record the color, size, height, distribution, location, and shape of any lesions. Lesions may be primary or secondary lesions. *Primary skin lesions* develop on previously unaltered skin. The common characteristics of primary skin lesions are shown in Table 22.5. *Secondary skin lesions* are lesions that change with time or occur because of scratching or infection. Secondary skin lesions are shown in Table 22.6.

Skin lesions are usually described in terms related to the lesions' configuration (solitary or pattern in relation to other lesions) and distribution (arrangement of lesions over an area of skin) (Table 22.7). Note any unusual odors. Skin sites with lesions, such as rashes, may be colonized with yeast or bacteria, which can be associated with distinctive odors in areas where skin rubs together (Fig. 22.5).

Inspect all body hair. Note the distribution, texture, and quantity of hair. Changes in the normal distribution of body hair and growth may indicate an endocrine or vascular disorder. Carefully inspect the nails, including nail shape, thickness, curvature, and surface. Note any grooves, pitting, ridges, or detachment from nail bed. Changes in nail smoothness or thickness can occur with anemia, psoriasis, thyroid problems, decreased vascular circulation, and some infections.

Palpation. Palpate the skin to obtain information about temperature, turgor, moisture, and texture. Use the back of your hand to gauge skin temperature. The skin should be warm, not hot. Skin temperature increases when blood flow to the dermis increases. A localized temperature increase occurs with burns

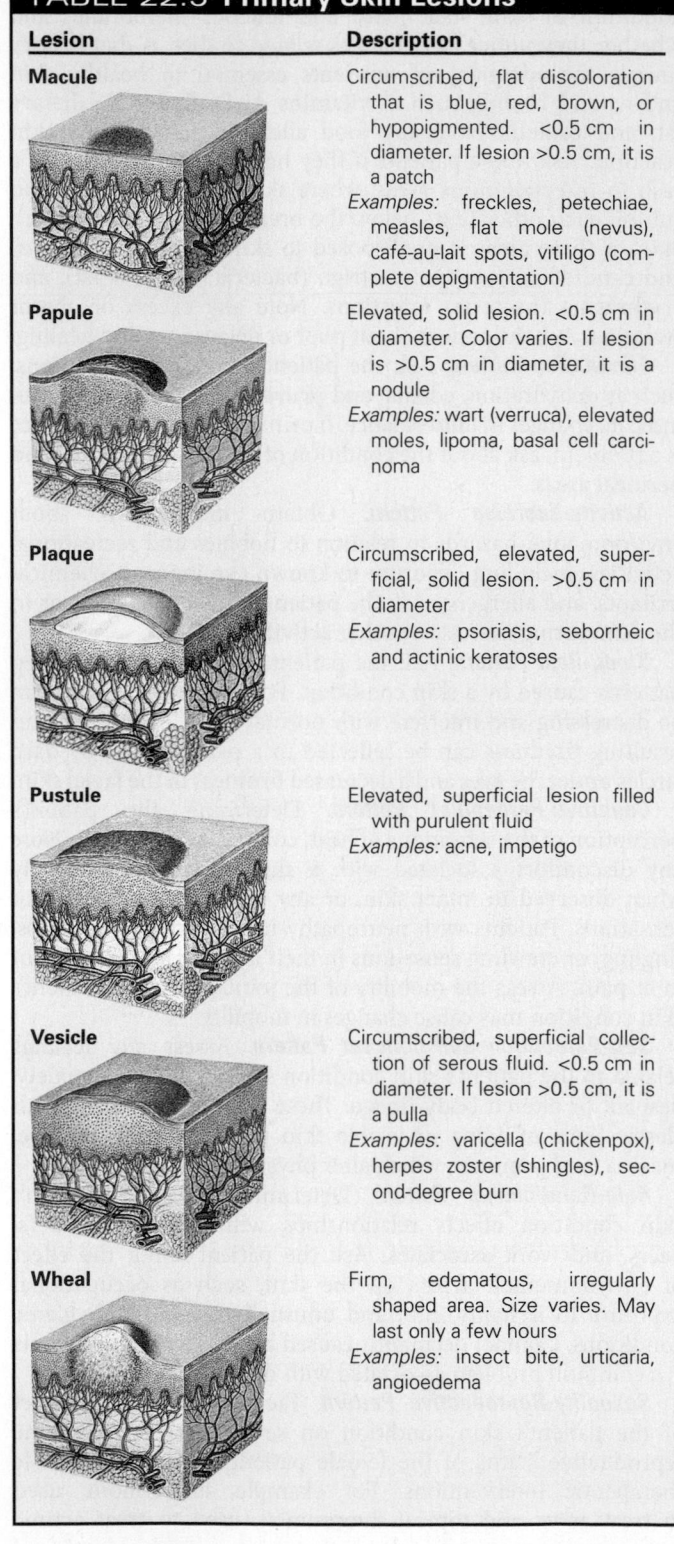

TABLE 22.5 **Primary Skin Lesions**	
Lesion	**Description**
Macule	Circumscribed, flat discoloration that is blue, red, brown, or hypopigmented. <0.5 cm in diameter. If lesion >0.5 cm, it is a patch *Examples:* freckles, petechiae, measles, flat mole (nevus), café-au-lait spots, vitiligo (complete depigmentation)
Papule	Elevated, solid lesion. <0.5 cm in diameter. Color varies. If lesion is >0.5 cm in diameter, it is a nodule *Examples:* wart (verruca), elevated moles, lipoma, basal cell carcinoma
Plaque	Circumscribed, elevated, superficial, solid lesion. >0.5 cm in diameter *Examples:* psoriasis, seborrheic and actinic keratoses
Pustule	Elevated, superficial lesion filled with purulent fluid *Examples:* acne, impetigo
Vesicle	Circumscribed, superficial collection of serous fluid. <0.5 cm in diameter. If lesion >0.5 cm, it is a bulla *Examples:* varicella (chickenpox), herpes zoster (shingles), second-degree burn
Wheal	Firm, edematous, irregularly shaped area. Size varies. May last only a few hours *Examples:* insect bite, urticaria, angioedema

and local inflammation. A generalized increase occurs when a person has a fever. A decreased body temperature may occur when shock or other circulatory problems, chilling, or infection are present.

Turgor refers to the elasticity of the skin. Assess turgor by gently pinching an area of skin under the clavicle or on the back of the hand. Skin with good turgor should move easily when

TABLE 22.6 Secondary Skin Lesions

Lesion	Description
Atrophy	Depression in skin resulting from thinning of the epidermis or dermis *Examples:* aged skin, striae
Excoriation	Area in which epidermis is missing, exposing the dermis *Examples:* abrasion, scratch
Fissure	Linear crack or break from the epidermis to the dermis. Dry or moist *Examples:* athlete's foot, chapping, eczema
Scale	Excess, dead epidermal cells made by abnormal keratinization and shedding *Examples:* flaking of skin after a drug reaction or sunburn
Scar	Abnormal formation of connective tissue that replaces normal skin *Examples:* surgical incision, healed wound
Ulcer	Loss of the epidermis and dermis. Crater-like, irregular shape. Heals with scarring *Examples:* pressure ulcer, chancre

TABLE 22.7 Lesion Distribution Terminology

Term	Description
Annular	Circular, begins in center and spreads to periphery (e.g., tinea corporis [ringworm])
Asymmetric	Unilateral distribution
Confluent	Merging together (e.g., urticaria [hives])
Discrete	Distinct individual lesions that are separate (e.g., acne)
Gyrate	Twisted, coiled spiral, snakelike
Grouped	Clusters of lesions (e.g., vesicles of contact dermatitis)
Localized	Clearly defined, limited areas of involvement (confined to one area)
Polycyclic	Annular lesions grow together (e.g., psoriasis)
Solitary	Single lesion
Symmetric	Bilateral distribution
Zosteriform	Linear arrangement along a dermatome area (e.g., herpes zoster)

flaking, scaling, or cracking. Skin generally becomes drier with increasing age.

Texture refers to the fineness or coarseness of the skin. The skin should feel smooth and firm with the surface evenly thin in most areas. Thickened callus areas are normal on the soles and palms and relate to weight bearing. Increased skin thickness is often work related and the result of excess pressure. Excess calluses on the soles of patients with neuropathy or diabetes predispose them to developing lesions.

Use a *focused assessment* to evaluate the status of previously identified skin problems and to monitor for signs of new problems. A focused assessment of the skin is presented in the following box. Assessment abnormalities of the skin are described in Table 22.8.

FOCUSED ASSESSMENT
Integumentary System

Use this checklist to make sure the key assessment steps have been done.

Subjective
Ask the patient about any of the following and note responses.

Hair loss (unusual or rapid)	Y	N
Changes in skin (e.g., lesions, bruising)	Y	N
Nail discoloration	Y	N

Objective: Diagnostic
Check the following for results and critical values.

Biopsy results	✓
Albumin	✓

Objective: Physical Examination
Inspect

Skin for color, integrity, scars, lesions, signs of breakdown	✓
Facial and body hair for distribution, color, quantity, hygiene	✓
Nails for shape, contour, color, thickness, cleanliness	✓
Dressings, if present	✓

Palpate

Skin for temperature, texture, moisture, thickness, turgor, mobility	✓

lifted and immediately return to its original position when released. In patients with dehydration and aging, a loss of turgor occurs and can cause tenting of the skin.

Skin moisture (dampness or dryness of the skin) increases in areas where skin rubs together. Skin moisture varies with environmental temperature, muscular activity, body weight, and body temperature. The skin should be intact with no

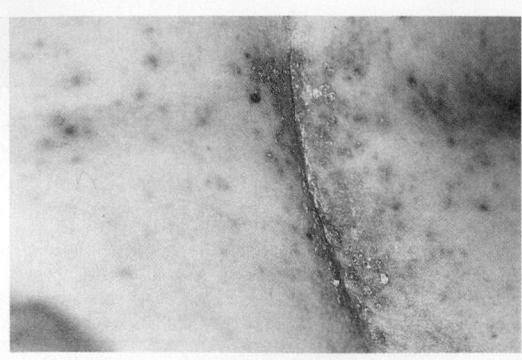

FIG. 22.5 Intertrigo. Rash in body folds with *Candida* infection. (From Graham-Brown R, Bourke J, Cunliffe T: *Dermatology: Fundamentals of practice*, Edinburgh, 2008, Mosby.)

Assessment of Dark Skin

The structures of dark skin are no different from those of lighter skin, but they are often harder to assess (Table 22.9). Color is easiest to assess in areas where the epidermis is thin, and pigmentation is not influenced by sun exposure, such as the lips, mucous membranes, nail beds, and protected areas (e.g., buttocks). Palmar and plantar surfaces are lighter than other skin areas in darker skinned persons. Rashes are often harder to see and may have to be palpated. Wrinkling is less apparent in those with dark skin.

Persons with dark skin are predisposed to certain skin and hair conditions. Keloid is an overgrowth of collagenous tissue at the site of a skin injury (e.g., ear piercing) (Fig. 22.6). *Vitiligo* is total loss of pigment in the affected area (Fig. 22.7). In *dermatosis papulosa nigra*, the person has small, pigmented wart-like

TABLE 22.8 Assessment Abnormalities

Integumentary System

Finding	Description	Possible Etiology and Significance
Alopecia	Loss of hair (localized or general)	Heredity, friction, rubbing, traction, trauma, stress, infection, inflammation, chemotherapy, pregnancy, emotional shock, tinea capitis, immunologic factors
Angioma	Tumor consisting of blood or lymph vessels	Normal increase in incidence with aging, liver disease, pregnancy, varicose veins
Carotenemia (carotenosis)	Yellow discoloration of skin, no yellowing of sclerae, most noticeable on palms and soles	Vegetables containing carotene (e.g., carrots, squash), hypothyroidism
Comedo (acne lesion)	Enlarged hair follicle plugged with sebum, bacteria, and skin cells; can be open (blackhead) or closed (whitehead)	Heredity, certain drugs, hormonal changes with puberty and pregnancy
Cyanosis	Slightly bluish gray or dark purple discoloration of the skin and mucous membranes caused by excess amounts of reduced hemoglobin in capillaries	Cardiorespiratory problems, vasoconstriction, asphyxiation, anemia, leukemia, and cancers
Cyst	Sac containing fluid or semisolid material	Obstruction of a duct or gland, parasitic infection
Ecchymosis	Large, bruise-like lesion caused by collection of extravascular blood in dermis and subcutaneous tissue	Trauma, bleeding disorders
Erythema	Redness occurring in patches of variable size and shape	Heat, certain drugs, alcohol, ultraviolet rays, any problem that causes dilation of blood vessels in the skin
Hematoma	Extravasation of blood of enough size to cause visible swelling	Trauma, bleeding disorders
Hirsutism	Male distribution of hair in women	Abnormality of ovaries or adrenal glands, decrease in estrogen level, familial trait
Hypopigmentation	Loss of pigmentation resulting in lighter patches than the normal skin	Chemical agents, nutritional factors, burns, inflammation, infection
Intertrigo	Dermatitis of overlying surfaces of the skin (Fig. 22.5)	Moisture, irritation, obesity; may be complicated by *Candida* infection
Jaundice	Yellow (in white patients) or yellowish brown (in dark-skinned patients) discoloration of the skin, best seen in the sclera, secondary to increased bilirubin in the blood	Liver disease, red blood cell hemolysis, pancreatic cancer, common bile duct obstruction
Keloid	Hypertrophied scar beyond wound margins (Fig. 22.6)	Predisposition more common in dark-skinned persons
Lichenification	Thickening of the skin with accentuated normal skin markings	Repeated scratching, rubbing, and irritation usually because of pruritus or neurosis
Mole (nevus)	Benign overgrowth of melanocytes	Defects of development; excess numbers and large, irregular moles; often familial
Petechiae	Pinpoint, discrete deposits of blood <1–2 mm in the extravascular tissues and visible through the skin or mucous membrane	Inflammation, marked vasodilation, blood vessel trauma, blood dyscrasia that results in bleeding tendencies (e.g., thrombocytopenia)
Telangiectasia	Visibly dilated, superficial, cutaneous small blood vessels, commonly found on face and thighs	Aging, acne, sun exposure, alcohol, liver failure, corticosteroids, radiation, certain systemic diseases, skin tumors
Tenting	Failure of skin to return immediately to normal position after gentle pinching	Aging, dehydration, cachexia
Varicosity	Increased prominence of superficial veins	Interruption of venous return (e.g., from tumor, incompetent valves, inflammation), commonly found on lower legs with aging
Vitiligo	Complete absence of melanin (pigment) resulting in chalky white patch (Fig. 22.7)	Autoimmune, familial, thyroid disease

TABLE 22.9 Nursing Assessment

Assessment Variations in Light- and Dark-Skinned Persons

Light Skin	Dark Skin
Cyanosis	
Grayish blue tone, especially in nail beds, earlobes, lips, mucous membranes, palms, and soles	Ashen or gray color most easily seen in the conjunctiva of the eye, mucous membranes, and nail beds
Ecchymosis	
Dark red, purple, yellow, or green color, depending on age of bruise	Purple to brownish black. Hard to see unless occurring in an area of light pigmentation
Erythema	
Reddish tone, possibly accompanied by increased skin temperature secondary to localized inflammation	Deeper brown or purple skin tone with evidence of increased skin temperature secondary to inflammation
Jaundice	
Yellowish color of skin, sclera, fingernails, palms, and oral mucosa	Yellowish green color most obviously seen in sclera of eye (do not confuse with yellow eye pigmentation, which may be seen in dark-skinned patients), palms, and soles
Pallor	
Pale skin color that may appear white or ashen; also seen on lips, nail beds, and mucous membranes	Lack of underlying red tone in brown or black skin. In lighter dark-skinned persons, yellowish brown skin. In darker dark-skinned persons, ashen or gray skin
Petechiae	
Lesions appearing as small, reddish purple pinpoints, best seen on abdomen and buttocks	Hard to see. May be seen in the buccal mucosa of the mouth or conjunctiva of the eye
Rash	
May be seen and felt with light palpation	Not easily seen. May be felt with light palpation
Scar	
Generally heals, showing narrow scar line	Higher incidence of keloid development, resulting in a thickened, raised scar (Fig. 22.6)

papules, often on the face (Fig. 22.8). *Nevus of Ota* is a slate-gray or blue-gray birthmark found on the forehead and face around the eye area. It may involve the sclera. *Traction alopecia* may be the result of trauma from hair rollers or from tight braiding of the hair (Fig. 22.9). The hair loss may be temporary or

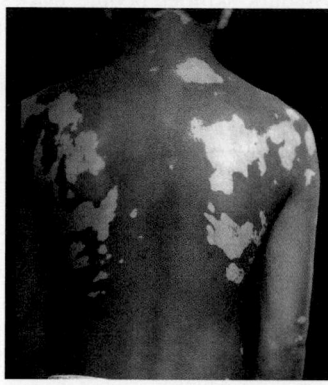

FIG. 22.7 Vitiligo. Total loss of pigment in the affected area. (From Graham-Brown R, Bourke J, Cunliffe T: *Dermatology: Fundamentals of practice,* Edinburgh, 2008, Mosby.)

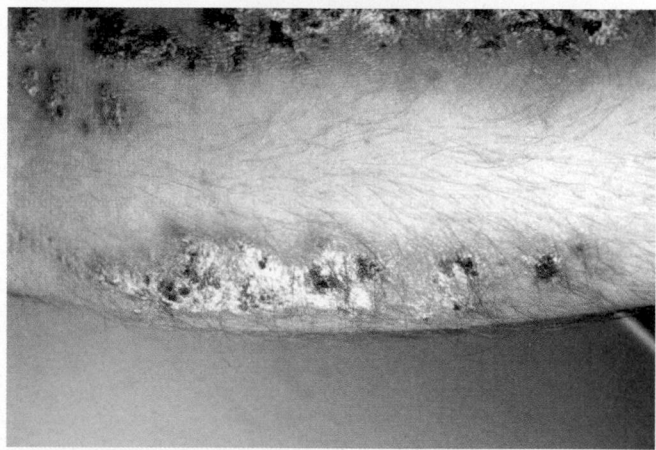

FIG. 22.8 Dermatosis papulosa nigra. Small, pigmented wart-like papules, often on the face. (From James W, Berger T, Elston D: *Andrews' diseases of the skin,* ed 12, Edinburgh, 2016, Elsevier.)

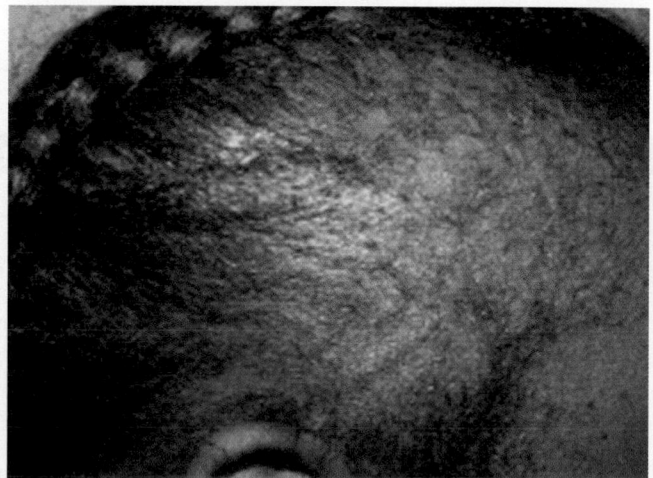

FIG. 22.9 Traction alopecia. Hair loss in scalp because of prolonged tension from hair rollers, braiding, or straightening combs. (From Ahanogbe I, Gavino A: Evaluation and management of the hair loss patient in the primary care setting, *Prim Care* 42:569, 2015.)

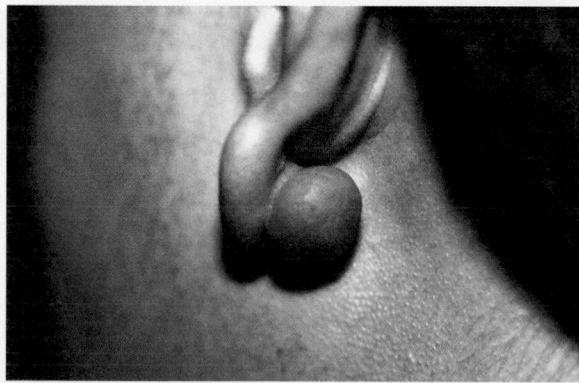

FIG. 22.6 Keloid. Hypertrophic scarring after skin injury, which is more common in dark-skinned persons. (From Kliegman RM et al: *Nelson textbook of pediatrics,* Philadelphia, 2011, Saunders.)

permanent. *Pseudofolliculitis* is an inflammatory response to ingrown hairs that occurs after shaving too closely in the beard area. The ingrown hairs result in pustules and papules.

Because of the darkness of the skin in some people, color may not be a reliable indicator of systemic conditions (e.g., flushed skin with fever). Cyanosis may be hard to detect because a normal bluish hue occurs in dark-skinned people. Dark skin rarely shows a blanch response, making it harder to identify pressure injuries.

DIAGNOSTIC STUDIES OF INTEGUMENTARY SYSTEM

Table 22.10 presents common diagnostic studies used for the integumentary system. The main diagnostic techniques related to skin problems are inspection of an individual lesion and a careful history related to the problem. If a definitive diagnosis cannot be made by these techniques, other tests may be needed. With *dermatoscopy*, the HCP uses a lighted instrument with optical magnification to see skin structures and colors not visible with the naked eye.[7] These hand-held screening devices (e.g., MelaFind) can help the HCP determine if a lesion should be biopsied.

Biopsy is one of the most common diagnostic tests used to evaluate a skin lesion. A biopsy is needed when cancer is suspected or a specific diagnosis is questionable. Techniques include punch, incisional, excisional, and shave biopsies. The method used depends on factors such as the site of the biopsy, cosmetic result desired, and type of tissue needed.

Other diagnostic procedures include stains and cultures for fungal, bacterial, and viral infections. Direct immunofluorescence is a special diagnostic technique used on biopsy specimens. It may be needed in certain conditions such as bullous diseases and systemic lupus erythematosus. Indirect immunofluorescence is done on blood samples.

CASE STUDY
Objective Data: Physical Examination

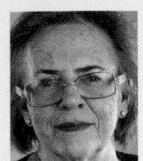
(© iStockphoto/ Thinkstock.)

- Physical examination findings of D.A.'s skin are as follows:
  - Complexion fair. Wrinkles around eyes, above upper lip, and on sides of cheeks bilaterally. Normal skin temperature and turgor.
  - Lesions: on upper right forehead measuring 2 × 3 mm; on left forehead near hairline measuring 1 × 2 mm; and on left lower cheek measuring 2 × 2.5 mm.

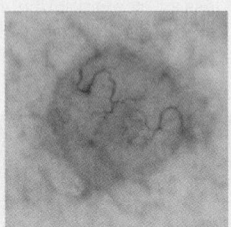

(Cheek lesion. From Bolognia JL, Schaffer JV, Duncan KO, et al: Dermatology essentials, Philadelphia, 2014, Saunders.)

- The lesions are slightly erythematous but do not blanch with direct pressure. Borders are distinct. The lesions on the forehead have minimal elevation noted on palpation. The lesion on the cheek is slightly elevated.
- No other skin lesions noted on rest of body.

Discussion Questions
1. Which physical assessment findings are of most concern to you?
2. What diagnostic studies do you think may be ordered for D.A.?

You will learn more about diagnostic studies related to the skin in the next section.
(See p. 407 for more information on D.A.)

Answers available at *http://evolve.elsevier.com/Lewis/medsurg.*

CASE STUDY
Objective Data: Diagnostic Studies

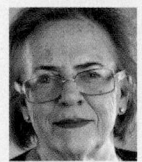
(© iStockphoto/ Thinkstock.)

The HCP examines the lesion via dermatoscopy and uses a Wood's lamp to rule out a fungal infection. The HCP suspects basal cell carcinoma.

Discussion Questions
1. Are these the diagnostic tests you expected the HCP to perform?
2. What, if any, other diagnostic studies would you expect to be ordered for D.A.?
3. What are the interprofessional team's priorities for D.A. at this time?

Answers available at *http://evolve.elsevier.com/Lewis/medsurg.*

TABLE 22.10 Diagnostic Studies Integumentary System

Study	Description and Purpose	Nursing Responsibility
Biopsy		
Excisional	Used when good cosmetic results and/or entire lesion removal desired. Skin closed with subcutaneous and skin sutures.	*Before:* Verify that consent form is signed (if needed).
Incisional	Wedge-shaped incision made in lesion too large for excisional biopsy. Useful when specimen needed is larger than shave or punch biopsy.	*During:* Help with site preparation, anesthesia, procedure, and hemostasis. Properly identify specimen.
Punch	Special punch biopsy instrument of appropriate size used. Instrument rotated to appropriate level to include dermis and some fat. Suturing depends on size and site. Provides full-thickness skin for diagnostic purposes.	*After:* Apply dressing, give postprocedure instructions to patient.
Shave	Single-edged razor blade used to shave off superficial lesions or small sample of a large lesion. Provides thin specimen for diagnostic purposes.	

TABLE 22.10 Diagnostic Studies Integumentary System—cont'd

Study	Description and Purpose	Nursing Responsibility
Microscopic Tests		
Culture	Test identifies fungal, bacterial, and viral organisms. For *fungi,* scraping or swab of skin performed. For *bacteria,* material obtained from intact pustules, bullae, or abscesses. For *viruses,* vesicle or bulla and exudate taken from base of lesion.	*Before:* Teach patient the purpose of test. *During:* Properly identify specimen. Follow instructions for storing specimen if not immediately sent to laboratory.
Immunofluorescence studies	Some skin diseases have specific, abnormal antibody proteins that can be identified by fluorescence studies. Can examine both skin tissue and serum.	*Before:* Teach patient the purpose of test. *During:* Help obtain specimen. For punch biopsy, place specimen in special fixative (e.g., Michel's) and not formalin.
Mineral oil slides	To check for infestations, place scrapings on slide with mineral oil and view microscopically.	*Before:* Teach patient the purpose of test. *During:* Prepare slide.
Potassium hydroxide (KOH)	Hair, scales, or nails examined for superficial fungal infection. Put specimen on glass slide and add 10%–20% concentration of KOH.	*Before:* Teach patient the purpose of test. *During:* Prepare slide.
Tzanck test (Wright's and Giemsa's stain)	Fluid and cells from vesicles examined. Used to diagnose herpes infections. Specimen put on slide, stained, and examined microscopically.	*Before:* Teach patient the purpose of test. *During:* Use sterile technique for collecting fluid.
Miscellaneous		
Patch test (Fig. 22.10)	Used to assess for allergic dermatitis and photoallergic reactions. Application of allergens to the patient's skin (usually on the back) for 48 hr. Test sites examined 48 hr later for a reaction, characterized by the presence of erythema, papules, and/or vesicles. May do additional readings beyond 48 hr.	*Before:* Teach patient the purpose of test and procedure. *After:* Tell patient to leave patches in place for 48 hr. During this time it is important not to wash the area or play vigorous sports because if the adhesive tape peels off, the process will need to be repeated. Do not expose the patches to sunlight or other sources of ultraviolet (UV) light.
Wood's lamp (black light)	Examination of skin with long-wave ultraviolet light causes specific substances to fluoresce (e.g., *Pseudomonas* organisms, fungal infections, vitiligo).	*Before:* Teach patient the purpose of test and procedure. Inform patient it is not painful. *During:* Darken room.

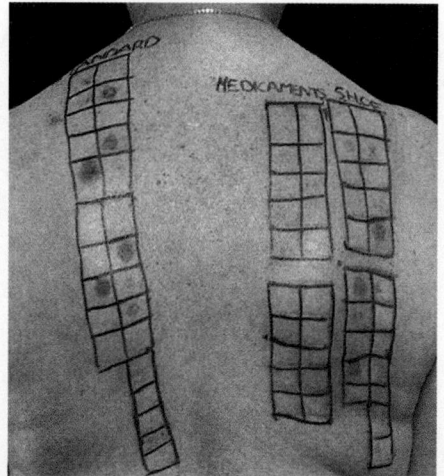

FIG. 22.10 Patch test. Results from applying possible allergens to the skin shows positive reactions in the sites labeled "standard" and "shoe." (From Graham-Brown R, Bourke J, Cunliffe T: *Dermatology: Fundamentals of practice,* Edinburgh, 2008, Mosby.)

■ BRIDGE TO NCLEX EXAMINATION

The number of the question corresponds to the same-numbered outcome at the beginning of the chapter.

1. The primary function of the skin is
   a. insulation.
   b. protection.
   c. sensation.
   d. absorption.

2. Age-related changes in the hair and nails include (*select all that apply*)
   a. oily scalp.
   b. scaly scalp.
   c. thinner nails.
   d. thicker, brittle nails.
   e. longitudinal nail ridging.

3. When assessing the nutritional-metabolic pattern in relation to the skin, the nurse asks the patient about
    a. joint pain.
    b. the use of moisturizing shampoo.
    c. recent changes in wound healing.
    d. self-care habits related to daily hygiene.

4. The nurse assessed the patient's skin lesions as firm, edematous, irregularly shaped with a variable diameter. They would be called
    a. wheals.
    b. papules.
    c. pustules.
    d. plaques.

5. During the physical examination of a patient's skin, the nurse would
    a. use a flashlight in a poorly lit room.
    b. note cool, moist skin as a normal finding.
    c. pinch up a fold of skin to assess for turgor.
    d. perform a lesion-specific examination first and then a general inspection.

6. Persons with dark skin are more likely to develop
    a. keloids.
    b. wrinkles.
    c. skin rashes.
    d. skin cancer.

7. On inspection of a patient's dark skin, the nurse notes a blue-gray birthmark on the forehead and eye area. This assessment finding is called
    a. vitiligo.
    b. intertrigo.
    c. Nevus of Ota.
    d. telangiectasia.

8. Diagnostic testing is recommended for skin lesions when
    a. a health history cannot be obtained.
    b. a more definitive diagnosis is needed.
    c. percussion reveals an abnormal finding.
    d. treatment with prescribed medication has failed.

1. b, 2. b, d, e, 3. c, 4. a, 5. c, 6. a, 7. c, 8. b

For rationales to these answers and even more NCLEX review questions, visit *http://evolve.elsevier.com/Lewis/medsurg*.

EVOLVE WEBSITE/RESOURCES LIST

http://evolve.elsevier.com/Lewis/medsurg
Review Questions (Online Only)
Key Points
Answer Keys for Questions
- Rationales for Bridge to NCLEX Examination Questions
- Answer Guidelines for Case Study on pp. 398, 401, and 406
Conceptual Care Map Creator
Audio Glossary
Content Updates

REFERENCES

1. Habif TP: *Clinical dermatology*, ed 6, St Louis, 2015, Mosby.
2. Gawkrodger D, Ardern-Jones M: *Dermatology*, ed 6, St Louis, 2016, Mosby.
3. Alikhan A, Hocker TL: *Review of dermatology*, St. Louis, 2016, Elsevier Health Sciences.
4. Bishop BE, Tosti A: *Melanonychias*, New York, 2017, Springer International Publishing.
*5. Tobin DJ: Introduction to skin aging, *J Tissue Viability* 26:37, 2017.
*6. Coit DG, Thompson JA, Algazi A, et al: Melanoma, *JNCCN* 14:450, 2016.
*7. Russo T, Piccolo V, Lallas A, Argenziano G: Recent advances in dermoscopy, *F1000Research* 5:184, 2016.

*Evidence-based information for clinical practice

23

Integumentary Problems

Mariann M. Harding

The world is not dangerous because of those who do harm, but because of those who look at it without doing anything.

Albert Einstein

http://evolve.elsevier.com/Lewis/medsurg/

CONCEPTUAL FOCUS

Cellular Regulation	Infection	Tissue Integrity
Coping	Pain	

LEARNING OUTCOMES

1. Specify health promotion practices related to environmental hazards.
2. Explain the etiology, clinical manifestations, and interprofessional and nursing management of skin cancers.
3. Relate the etiology, clinical manifestations, and interprofessional and nursing management of bacterial, viral, and fungal skin infections.
4. Describe the etiology, clinical manifestations, and interprofessional and nursing management of infestations and insect bites.
5. Discuss the etiology, clinical manifestations, and interprofessional and nursing management of allergic skin disorders.
6. Explain the etiology, clinical manifestations, and interprofessional and nursing management related to benign skin disorders.
7. Select appropriate nursing interventions to manage the patient with a skin problem.
8. Explain the indications and nursing management related to common cosmetic procedures and skin grafts.

KEY TERMS

acne vulgaris, Table 23.10, p. 421
actinic keratosis, p. 411
basal cell carcinoma (BCC), p. 413
cellulitis, Table 23.5, p. 415
cryosurgery, p. 424

curettage, p. 423
dysplastic nevi (DN), p. 414
herpes zoster, Table 23.6, p. 417
impetigo, Table 23.5, p. 415
lichenification, p. 425

melanoma, p. 413
psoriasis, p. 419
squamous cell carcinoma (SCC), p. 413
sun protection factor (SPF), p. 410

This chapter discusses common skin conditions and skin cancer. Impaired skin integrity affects many body functions. The skin reflects both physical and psychologic well-being. Having a small abrasion or cancerous lesion leaves underlying tissues unprotected from infection and chemical dangers. Lesions can be painful because the skin has many sensory nerve endings. Skin conditions are often highly visible, potentially affecting body image and causing distress.

ENVIRONMENTAL HAZARDS

Sun exposure comes with serious risk and results in permanent sun damage. Sunlight is made up of visible light and ultraviolet (UV) light. There are two types of UV light: UVA and UVB. Specific wavelengths (Table 23.1) have different effects on the skin. UVA light is responsible for tanning, UVB for sunburn. The damage caused by UV rays is cumulative. It results in degenerative changes in the dermis and premature aging (e.g., loss of elasticity, thinning, wrinkling, abnormal dryness). Prolonged and repeated sun exposure increases risk for actinic keratosis, basal and squamous cell cancers, and melanoma.

Patient teaching on sun protection is important. People often do not understand the serious risks of sun exposure. Following sun safety guidelines beginning early in life can help avoid the damaging effects of the sun and prevent the formation of skin cancer later in life. Fair-skinned persons and those with light-colored eyes should be especially cautious about excess sun exposure. They have less melanin and thus less natural protection.

Teach the patient ways to avoid the damaging effects of the sun. This includes wearing protective clothing, including sunglasses, a large-brimmed hat, and a darker colored, long-sleeved shirt of a tightly woven fabric or carrying an umbrella. The greatest risk is with midday sun, between the hours of 10:00 am and 2:00 pm, regardless of the latitude. This is when 80% of UV rays occur. Even on overcast days, serious sunburn can occur because up to 80% of the sun's UV rays can penetrate the clouds.

Warn people of the dangers of tanning booths and sun lamps, which emit UVA. Tanning booths increase the risk for sunburn, cataracts, and skin cancer.[1]

Sunscreens can filter both UVA and UVB wavelengths. The two types of topical sunscreens are chemical and physical. Chemical sunscreens are light creams or lotions designed to absorb or filter UV light, resulting in decreased UV light penetration. Physical sunscreens are thick, opaque, heavy creams that reflect UV radiation. Regular sunscreen use decreases the risk for developing melanoma.

The U.S. Food and Drug Administration (FDA) rates sunscreen products on their **sun protection factor (SPF)**. The SPF measures the effectiveness of a sunscreen in filtering and absorbing UV radiation. All sunscreen labels in the United States must say which rays they protect against. Products labeled with "broad spectrum" block both UVA and UVB.[2] Sunscreens with broad spectrum labeling must have an SPF of at least 15. Sunscreens with an SPF of 15 or more filter 92% of the UVB rays and make sunburn unlikely when applied appropriately.

People need to select the right sunscreen for their needs. The general recommendation is that everyone should use daily sunscreen with a minimum SPF of 15. Teach patients to look for the term *broad spectrum* on sunscreen packaging. Those who have a history of skin cancer or problems with sun sensitivity should use a product with an SPF of at least 30. Sunscreens should be applied 20 to 30 minutes before going outdoors, even in cloudy weather. The SPF value of all sunscreens decreases with time. Sunscreen should be reapplied every 2 hours. You should apply 1 ounce per total body application. The ears, toes, and lips also need sunscreen. Sunscreens are not "waterproof" and must be reapplied after swimming.

TABLE 23.1 Wavelengths of Sun and Effects on Skin

Wavelength	Effect
Long (ultraviolet A [UVA])	Can produce elastic tissue damage and actinic skin damage Contributes to formation of skin cancer
Middle (ultraviolet B [UVB])	Causes sunburn and cumulative effect of sun damage Major factor in development of skin cancer
Short (ultraviolet C [UVC])	Blocked by the atmosphere and does not reach earth

TABLE 23.2 Drug Therapy
Drugs That May Cause Photosensitivity

Categories	Examples
Antidepressants	amitriptyline, doxepin, venlafaxine
Antidysrhythmics	quinidine, amiodarone (Cordarone)
Antihistamines	diphenhydramine, chlorpheniramine, clemastine, cetirizine (Zyrtec)
Antimicrobials	tetracycline, sulfamethoxazole, azithromycin (Zithromax), ciprofloxacin (Cipro)
Antifungals	griseofulvin, ketoconazole
Antipsychotics	chlorpromazine, haloperidol
Chemotherapy	methotrexate, dacarbazine, fluorouracil
Diuretics	furosemide (Lasix), hydrochlorothiazide
Hypoglycemics	tolbutamide, glipizide (Glucotrol), glyburide
Nonsteroidal antiinflammatory drugs	diclofenac (Voltaren), piroxicam (Feldene), sulindac

EVIDENCE-BASED PRACTICE
Tanning Booths and Skin Cancer

You are a nurse working in a dermatology clinic. D.F., a 30-yr-old woman with fair skin and blue eyes, is completing her health history before her annual skin screening. She says she regularly visits an indoor tanning salon every other week. She tells you that being tan makes her feel "healthier and prettier."

Making Clinical Decisions

Best Available Evidence. There is a strong link between exposure to UVA from indoor tanning booth use and increased risk for skin cancer (melanoma and nonmelanoma). Melanoma causes less than 5% of skin cancers yet accounts for almost 75% of skin cancer deaths. Melanoma risk increases with the number of years, hours, and sessions of indoor tanning independent of outdoor exposure.

Clinician Expertise. You note that D.F. has the following skin cancer risk factors: fair skin, blue eyes, frequent use of tanning booths.

Patient Preferences and Values. After listening, D.F. tells you that she will consider reducing the frequency of her visits—going only when she has an important event to attend.

Implications for Nursing Practice

1. How would you respond to D.F. given the information that she has provided to you?
2. What resources can help address her view that a "tan looks healthy?"
3. What sun safety guidelines should she follow when outdoors to prevent skin cancer?

Reference for Evidence

Gershenwald JE, Halpern AC, Sondak VK: Melanoma prevention: avoiding indoor tanning and minimizing overexposure to the sun, *JAMA* 316(18):1913, 2016.
Tripp MK, Watson M, Balk SJ, et al.: State of the science on prevention and screening to reduce melanoma incidence and mortality, *CA Can J Clin* 66:460, 2016.

Certain drugs potentiate the sun's effects, even with brief exposure. The chemicals in these drugs absorb light when exposed to natural sunlight and release energy that harms cells and tissues. Common photosensitizing drugs are shown in Table 23.2. The manifestations of drug-induced photosensitivity (Fig. 23.1) are like those of a sunburn. These include swelling, erythema, vesicles, and papular, plaquelike lesions. Assess the photosensitivity of each individual drug. Teach patients who are taking these drugs about their photosensitizing effect and the need to protect the skin from photosensitivity reactions by using sunscreen products.

Teach patients to self-examine their skin monthly. They should have a periodic professional assessment of areas that are hard to see. The cornerstone of skin examination is the ABCDE rule. Examine skin lesions for *Asymmetry, Border* irregularity, *Color* change and variation, *Diameter* of 6 mm or more, and *Evolving* in appearance (Fig. 23.2). Emphasize that a persistent skin lesion that does not heal and lesions once flat and now raised, once small and recently growing, or changing in appearance are warning signs. Patients should consult their HCP at once if any lesions or moles show any clinical signs (ABCDEs).

SKIN CANCER

Skin cancer is the most commonly diagnosed cancer.[3] Skin cancers are either nonmelanoma or melanoma. The fact that

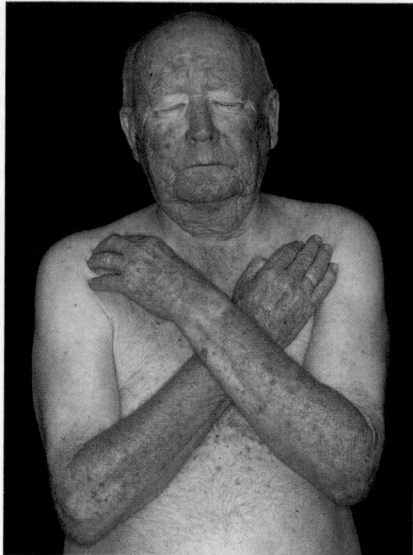

FIG. 23.1 Intense eruption in areas exposed to sunlight after patient started on hydrochlorothiazide. (From Habif TP: Clinical dermatology: A color guide to diagnosis and therapy, ed 5, St Louis, 2011, Mosby.)

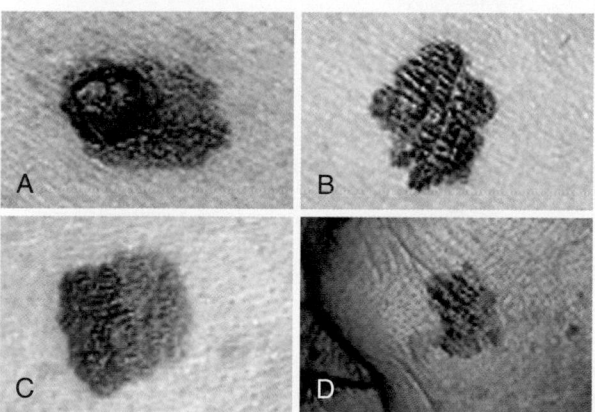

FIG. 23.2 The ABCDEs of melanoma. **A,** Asymmetry: one half unlike the other half. **B,** Border irregularity: edges are ragged, notched, or blurred. **C,** Color: varied pigmentation; shades of tan, brown, and black. **D,** Diameter: greater than 6 mm (diameter of a pencil eraser). **E,** (not pictured) Evolving; changing appearance (change in shape, size, color, or other characteristic noted over time). (From The Skin Cancer Foundation, New York, NY.)

TABLE 23.3 Fitzpatrick Classification of Skin Type		
Skin Type	Skin Color	Characteristics
I	White, freckles, very fair. Red or blond hair. Blue eyes	Always burns, never tans
II	White, fair. Red or blond hair. Blue, hazel, or green eyes	Usually burns, tans with difficulty
III	Cream white, fair. Any eye or hair color	Sometimes mild burn, gradually tan
IV	Brown, typical Mediterranean skin	Rarely burns, tans with ease
V	Deep brown, Middle Eastern skin types	Very rarely burns, tans very easily
VI	Black	Never burns, tans very easily

🌐 PROMOTING HEALTH EQUITY
Skin Problems

- Blacks, Asians, and Hispanics have a lower incidence of skin cancer than whites.
- Melanoma can occur in dark-skinned persons but often goes unrecognized until the advanced stages.
- Blacks and Asians are more likely to develop a keloid at the site of an injury.
- Skin cancer outcomes are poorer for ethnic minorities, those of low socioeconomic status, and the uninsured.

Dark-skinned persons are less susceptible to skin cancer because of their increased melanin, which acts like a sunscreen. However, there is still a risk, and they need to wear sunscreen. They often have melanomas on areas with less melanin, such as the palms, soles, mucous membranes, and under the nails. Since it is common for people with dark skin to have pigmented, longitudinal bands on their nails, assess and follow any nail discoloration.

NONMELANOMA SKIN CANCER

Nonmelanoma skin cancers (basal cell and squamous cell cancers) are the most common forms of skin cancer. More than 5.4 million new cases are diagnosed each year.[3] Nonmelanoma skin cancers do not develop from melanocytes. They develop in the basement membrane of the skin. Although there are few deaths from nonmelanoma skin cancer, they have the potential for severe local destruction, permanent disfigurement, and disability.

Nonmelanoma skin cancers usually develop in sun-exposed areas, such as the face, head, neck, back of the hands, and arms. The most common causative factor is sun exposure. There are some differences between basal and squamous cell cancers. Squamous cell cancers usually occur on the head and neck where there is the highest degree of UV radiation. Basal cell cancers do not follow that pattern and may occur in sun-protected areas.

Actinic Keratosis

Actinic keratosis (AK), also known as *solar keratosis,* is the most common precancerous skin lesion. They affect most of the older white population. Sun exposure is a key factor. AKs

skin lesions are so visible increases the chance of early detection and diagnosis. This can often lead to a highly favorable prognosis.

Risk Factors

Risk factors for skin cancer include (1) having fair skin, blond or red hair with blue eye color; (2) history of outdoor sunbathing; (3) living near the equator or at high altitudes; (4) family or personal history of skin cancer; (5) having an outdoor occupation; (6) spending a lot of time in outdoor recreation activities; and (7) indoor tanning.[4] The Fitzpatrick Classification of Skin Type can help you determine a person's skin complexion and how likely the person is to get skin cancer (Table 23.3). Patients treated with oral methoxsalen (psoralen) and psoralen plus ultraviolet A radiation (PUVA) have a higher risk.

appear most often on skin that has been exposed to the sun or to artificial UV light. They may spontaneously resolve if a person reduces exposure to sunlight.

The clinical appearance of AK can be highly varied. The typical lesion is an irregularly shaped, flat, slightly erythematous papule with indistinct borders and an overlying hard keratotic scale or horn (Table 23.4). Because AK is impossible to distinguish from squamous cell cancer, treatment should be aggressive. Nonsurgical procedures are the first-line treatment. Any lesion that persists should be evaluated for a biopsy.

TABLE 23.4 Premalignant and Malignant Conditions of the Skin

Etiology and Pathophysiology	Clinical Manifestations	Treatment and Prognosis
Actinic Keratosis • Actinic (sun) damage • Premalignant skin lesions • Common in older whites • Increase in number with age	• Flat or elevated, dry, hyperkeratotic scaly papule. Often multiple • May be rough or wartlike • Rough adherent scale on red base, which returns when removed • Often on erythematous sun-exposed area	• Cryosurgery. Topical application of fluorouracil, imiquimod (Aldara) or diclofenac (Solaraze), chemical peels, laser resurfacing, photodynamic therapy • Recurrence possible even with adequate treatment
Atypical or Dysplastic Nevi • Morphologically between common acquired nevi and melanoma • May be precursor of melanoma	• Often >5 mm. Irregular border, possibly notched. Frequently multiple • Varying colors of tan, brown, black, red, or pink within single mole • Central part often raised with flat edges • Most common site on back, but possible in uncommon mole sites such as scalp or buttocks (Fig. 23.5)	• Increased risk for melanoma • Careful monitoring of those with a familial tendency to melanoma or dysplastic nevi • Excisional biopsy for suspicious lesions
Basal Cell Carcinoma • Change in basal cells. No maturation or normal keratinization • Continuing division of basal cells and formation of enlarging mass • Related to excessive sun exposure, genetic skin type, x-ray radiation, scars, and some types of nevi	*Nodular and ulcerative:* • Small, slowly enlarging papule • Borders semitranslucent or "pearly" with overlying telangiectasia • Erosion, ulceration, and depression of center • Normal skin markings lost (Fig. 23.3) *Superficial:* • Erythematous, pearly, sharply defined, barely elevated plaques	• Surgical excision, electrodessication and curettage, cryosurgery, radiation therapy, laser therapy, and photodynamic therapy • Vismodegib (Erivedge) or sonidegib (Odomzo) for metastatic or recurrent locally invasive lesions • Fluorouracil and imiquimod for superficial lesions • Slow-growing tumor that invades local tissue • Metastasis rare, 90% cure rate with primary lesions
Cutaneous T-Cell Lymphoma • Origins in skin. Localized chronic, slowly progressing disease • Possibly related to environmental toxins and chemical exposure • Mycosis fungoides (MF) is most common form • Sézary syndrome is an advanced form of MF • Prevalence twice as high in men as in women	• Classic presentation involves 3 stages: patch (early), plaque, and tumor (advanced) • History of persistent macular eruption followed by gradual appearance of indurated erythematous plaques on trunk • Appears similar to psoriasis • Pruritus, lymphadenopathy	• Treatment usually controls symptoms but is not curative • Skin-directed treatment includes phototherapy with ultraviolet light, radiation therapy, corticosteroids, and topical nitrogen mustard, imiquimod, or retinoids • Interferon, systemic chemotherapy, extracorporeal photopheresis, romidepsin (Istodax), denileukin diftitox (Ontak), and vorinostat (Zolinza) for progressive disease • Disease course is unpredictable. 10% will have progressive disease
Melanoma • Neoplastic growth of melanocytes anywhere on skin, eyes, or mucous membranes • Classification according to major histologic mode of spread • Potential invasion and widespread metastases	• Irregular color, surface, and border • Variegated color, including red, white, blue, black, gray, brown • Flat or elevated. Eroded or ulcerated • Often <1 cm in size • Most common sites in males are back, then chest. In females are legs, then back (Fig. 23.2)	• Surgical excision and possible sentinel lymph node evaluation • Adjuvant therapy after surgery if lesion >1.5 mm in depth • Correlation between survival rate and depth of invasion • Poor prognosis unless diagnosed and treated early • Spreading by local extension, regional lymphatic vessels, and bloodstream
Squamous Cell Carcinoma • Frequent occurrence on previously damaged skin (e.g., from sun, radiation, scar) • Malignant tumor of squamous cell of epidermis. Invasion of dermis, surrounding skin	• Most common on sun-exposed areas such as face and hands • *Superficial:* Thin, scaly erythematous plaque without invasion into the dermis • *Early:* Firm nodules with indistinct borders, scaling, and ulceration • *Late:* Covering of lesion with scale or horn from keratinization, ulceration	• Surgical excision, cryosurgery, radiation therapy, electrosurgery, laser therapy, and photodynamic therapy • Untreated lesion may metastasize to regional lymph nodes and distant organs • Fluorouracil and imiquimod for noninvasive SCC • Chemotherapy for metastatic lesions • High cure rate with early detection and treatment

Basal Cell Carcinoma

Basal cell carcinoma (BCC) is a locally invasive cancer arising from epidermal basal cells. It is the most common type of skin cancer but the least deadly. BCC usually occurs in middle-aged to older adults. Most BCCs occur in the head and neck area (e.g., sun-exposed), followed by the trunk and extremities.[5]

Manifestations are described in Table 23.4. Some BCCs are pigmented, with curled borders and an opaque appearance. They may be hard to distinguish from melanoma. A tissue biopsy is needed to confirm the diagnosis. BCCs rarely metastasize (Fig. 23.3). However, untreated BCC may result in massive tissue destruction. Treatment depends on the tumor location and histologic type, size, history of recurrence, and patient characteristics (Table 23.4).

Squamous Cell Carcinoma

Squamous cell carcinoma (SCC) is a cancer arising from keratinizing epidermal cells. SCC can be aggressive and has the potential to metastasize. It may lead to death if not treated early and correctly. SCC often occurs at the base of an actinic keratosis or another lesion. The main risk factors are sun exposure and immunosuppression after organ transplantation.[6] Pipe, cigar, and cigarette smoking contribute to the formation of SCC on the mouth and lips. The manifestations of SCC are described in Table 23.4. A biopsy should always be done when a lesion is suspected to be SCC.

MELANOMA

Melanoma is a tumor arising from melanocytes, the cells that make melanin. It causes most skin cancer deaths. Unlike most cancers whose incidence is stable or decreasing, the incidence of melanoma is steadily rising.[1] More than 87,000 new cases are diagnosed every year in the United States and almost 10,000 people will die from the disease.[3] Melanoma can metastasize to any organ, including the brain and heart.

A combination of environmental and genetic factors is likely involved in the development of melanoma. UV radiation from the sun is the main cause of melanoma. Artificial sources of UV radiation, such as sunlamps and tanning booths, also play a role. UV radiation damages the deoxyribonucleic acid (DNA) in skin cells, causing "misspellings" (mutations) in their genetic code. This alters the cells. Although anyone can develop melanoma, the risk is greatest for people who have red or blond hair, blue or light-colored eyes, and light-colored skin that freckles easily. These people have less melanin and thus less protection from UV radiation. The use of immunosuppressive drugs and a history of dysplastic nevi also increase risk.

A person may have a genetic predisposition toward getting melanoma. Of those with melanoma, 5% to 10% have a first-degree relative (e.g., parent, full sibling) who had melanoma.[4] This risk increases significantly if multiple relatives have had melanoma. Mutated genes have been found in some families who have a high familial incidence of melanoma.

Cutaneous melanoma begins in the skin. There are 4 subtypes of melanoma: (1) superficial spreading melanoma, (2) nodular melanoma, (3) lentigo maligna melanoma, and (4) acral lentiginous melanoma.

Clinical Manifestations

Melanoma often occurs on the lower legs in women and on the trunk and head in men. About one fourth of melanomas occur in existing nevi or moles. About 20% occur in dysplastic nevi. Rarely, it occurs in the mouth, intestines, and eyes.

The cornerstone of skin examination is the ABCDE rule (Fig. 23.2). Because most melanoma cells continue to produce melanin, melanoma tumors are often deep brown or black (Table 23.4). Lesions showing any sudden or progressive change in the ABCDE rule need evaluated.

Interprofessional Care

One of the first steps in diagnosing a suspicious lesion is dermoscopic examination. Dermoscopy can help the HCP decide if a lesion should be biopsied. Biopsy is a critical tool for determining the type of lesion. A biopsy should be done using an excisional biopsy technique. Shave biopsy, shave excision, or electrocauterization should not be done because these techniques do not measure the depth of the lesion.

The most important prognostic factor is tumor thickness at the time of diagnosis. We use 2 methods to determine thickness. The *Breslow measurement* indicates the depth of the tumor in millimeters (Fig. 23.4). The *Clark level* indicates the depth of invasion of the tumor; the higher the number, the deeper the melanoma.

Treatment depends on the site of the original tumor and the stage of the cancer. Melanoma staging (stages 0 to IV) is based on tumor size (thickness), nodal involvement, and metastasis. In stage 0, melanoma is confined to one place (in situ) in the epidermis. Melanoma is nearly 100% curable by excision if diagnosed at stage 0. Unfortunately, those with deep tumors or disease that has already spread to lymph nodes often develop metastases. The 5-year survival rate for those with advanced disease is less than 10%.[7]

The initial treatment of melanoma is wide surgical excision. Melanoma that has spread to the lymph nodes or nearby sites usually requires additional (adjuvant) therapy with combinations of immunotherapy, targeted therapy, chemotherapy, and/or radiation therapy.

Immunotherapy can include cytokines (α-interferon, interleukin-2), PD-1 inhibitors, and CTLA-4 inhibitors. Cytokines enhance the production of many immune system cells, including T cells and B cells. Drugs that block PD-1 or CTLA-4 boost the immune response against melanoma cells.[7] PD-1 inhibitors include nivolumab (Opdivo) and pembrolizumab (Keytruda). They block PD-1, a protein on T cells that keeps T cells from attacking other cells in the body. Ipilimumab (Yervoy) blocks

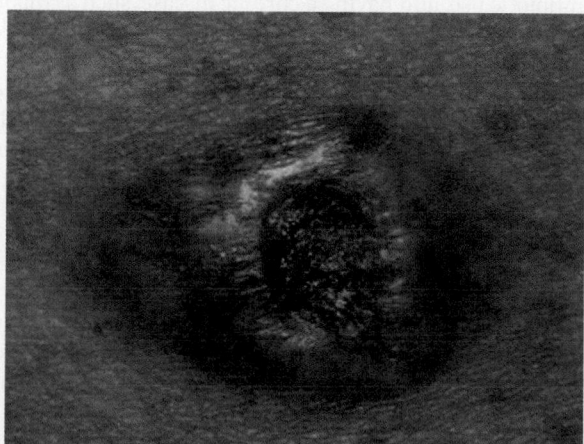

FIG. 23.3 Basal cell carcinoma. Rolled, well-defined border and central erosion. (From Goldman L, Schafer A: *Goldman-Cecil medicine*, ed 25, Philadelphia, 2016, Saunders.)

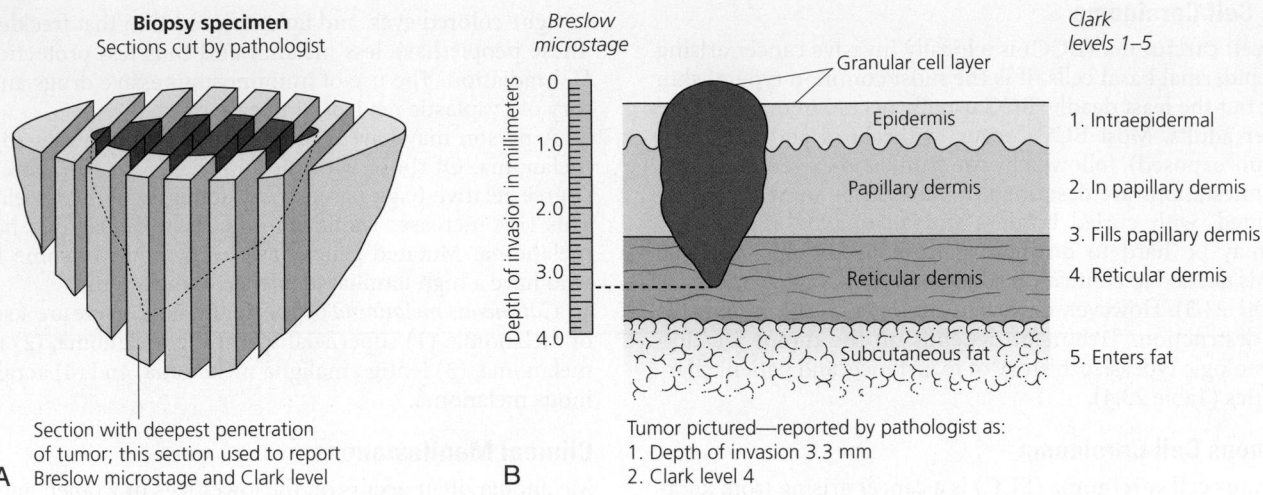

FIG. 23.4 A, Breslow measurement of tumor thickness. B, Clark level, showing tumor invasion. (From Habif TP: *Clinical dermatology: A color guide to diagnosis and therapy,* ed 6, St Louis, 2016, Mosby.)

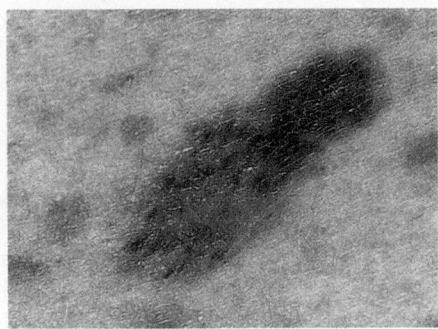

FIG. 23.5 Dysplastic nevus. Irregular border and color. (From Graham-Brown R, Bourke J, Cunliffe T: *Dermatology: Fundamentals of practice,* Edinburgh, 2008, Mosby.)

the action of CTLA-4, another protein that normally suppresses the action of T cells.

Targeted therapy for melanoma includes BRAF and MEK inhibitors. About half of all melanomas have mutations in the *BRAF* gene, which makes an altered BRAF protein that signals melanoma cells to proliferate. Vemurafenib (Zelboraf), dabrafenib (Tafinlar), trametinib (Mekinist), and cobimetinib (Cotellic) are drugs that target BRAF mutations.[7]

Chemotherapy is not as effective for melanoma as it is for most other cancers. It is usually used only with advanced disease. Drugs used includes dacarbazine, temozolomide, cisplatin, paclitaxel, carboplatin, and vincristine.[3] Radiation therapy has a role in treating lymph node and brain metastases.

Atypical or Dysplastic Nevus

Dysplastic nevi (DN), or atypical moles, are nevi that are larger than usual (greater than 5 mm across) with irregular borders and various shades of color (Fig. 23.5). DN may have the same ABCDE characteristics as melanoma, but they are less pronounced. About 5% of the white population have DN.[8] Those with DN have an increased risk for developing melanoma in a mole or elsewhere on the body. The more DN a person has, the higher the risk. Those with 10 or more DN have 12 times the risk for developing melanoma.

SKIN INFECTIONS AND INFESTATIONS

Bacterial Infections

The skin provides an ideal environment for bacterial growth with an abundant supply of nutrients, water, and warm temperature. Bacterial infection occurs when the balance between the host and microorganisms is changed. This can occur as a primary infection after a break in the skin. Or, a secondary infection can occur in already damaged skin or as a sign of a systemic disease (Table 23.5). Predisposing factors include the presence of excess moisture, obesity, having atopic dermatitis, systemic corticosteroid and antibiotic use, and having a chronic disease, such as diabetes.

Staphylococcus aureus and group A β-hemolytic streptococci are the major types of bacteria responsible for primary and secondary skin infections. Streptococci cause impetigo, erysipelas, cellulitis, and lymphangitis. *S. aureus* causes impetigo, folliculitis, cellulitis, and furuncles (Fig. 23.6). When an infection is present, the resulting drainage is infectious. Good skin hygiene and infection control practices are necessary to prevent the spread of the infection.

Viral Infections

Like viral infections anywhere in the body, viral infections of the skin are hard to treat. When a virus infects a cell, a skin lesion may develop. Lesions can also result from an inflammatory response to viral infections. Herpes simplex, herpes zoster (Fig. 23.7), and warts (Fig. 23.8) are the most common viral infections affecting the skin (Table 23.6).

TABLE 23.5 Common Bacterial Infections of the Skin

Etiology and Pathophysiology	Clinical Manifestations	Treatment and Prognosis
Carbuncle • Multiple, interconnecting furuncles	• Many pustules appearing in erythematous area • Most common at nape of neck	• Incision and drainage (possibly with packing), antibiotics, meticulous care of involved skin, frequent application of warm, moist compresses • Heal slowly with scar formation
Cellulitis • Inflammation of subcutaneous tissues • May be a primary infection or secondary complication • Often following break in skin • *Staphylococcus aureus* and streptococci usual causative agents • Deep inflammation of subcutaneous tissue from enzymes produced by bacteria	• Hot, tender, erythematous, and edematous area with diffuse borders • Chills, malaise, and fever (Fig. 23.6)	*Topical:* • Moist heat, immobilization, and elevation *Systemic:* • Systemic antibiotic therapy • Hospitalization if severe for IV antibiotic therapy (vancomycin, linezolid, ceftaroline fosamil, daptomycin) based on culture and sensitivity • Progression to gangrene possible if untreated
Erysipelas • Superficial cellulitis primarily involving the dermis • Group A β-hemolytic streptococci	• Red, hot, sharply demarcated plaque that is indurated and painful • Bacteremia possible • Most common on face and extremities • Toxic signs: fever, ↑ WBC count, headache, malaise	• Systemic antibiotics, usually penicillin • Hospitalization often needed
Folliculitis • Usually staphylococci • Present in areas subjected to friction, moisture, rubbing, or oil • Increased incidence in patients with diabetes mellitus	• Small pustule at hair follicle opening with minimal erythema • Development of crusting • Most common on scalp, beard, extremities in men • Tender to touch	• Antistaphylococcal soap (e.g., Hibiclens, Lever 2000, Dial) and water cleansing • Topical antibiotics (e.g., mupirocin) • Warm compresses of water or aluminum acetate solution • Usually heals without scarring • If lesions extensive and deep, possible scarring, loss of involved hair follicles, and treatment with systemic antibiotics
Furuncle • Deep infection with staphylococci around hair follicle • Often associated with severe acne or seborrheic dermatitis	• Tender erythematous area around hair follicle that is painful • Draining pus and core of necrotic debris on rupture • Most common on face, back of neck, axillae, breasts, buttocks, perineum, thighs	• Treatment is the same as for carbuncles
Furunculosis • Increased incidence in patients who are obese, diabetic, chronically ill, or regularly exposed to moisture, pressure	• Lesions as above • Malaise, regional adenopathy, elevated body temperature	*Topical:* • Incision and drainage of painful nodules • Warm, moist compresses to erythematous plaques • Measures to reduce surface staphylococci include antimicrobial cream to nares, armpits, and groin and antiseptic to entire skin • Meticulous personal hygiene *Systemic:* • Systemic antibiotic effective against MRSA pending culture and sensitivity results • Often recurrent with scarring
Impetigo • Group A β-hemolytic streptococci, staphylococci, or combination of both • Associated with poor hygiene • Primary or secondary infection. Contagious	• Vesiculopustular lesions that develop thick, honey-colored crust surrounded by erythema • Pruritic • Most common on face as primary infection	*Topical:* • Wound care with warm saline or aluminum acetate soaks followed by soap-and-water removal of crusts and application of topical antibiotic cream or ointment (mupirocin, retapamulin [Altabax]) • Meticulous hygiene essential *Systemic:* • Systemic antibiotics (e.g., cephalosporins, erythromycin, amoxicillin, clindamycin) for widespread infections or systemic manifestations

MRSA, Methicillin-resistant *S. aureus.*

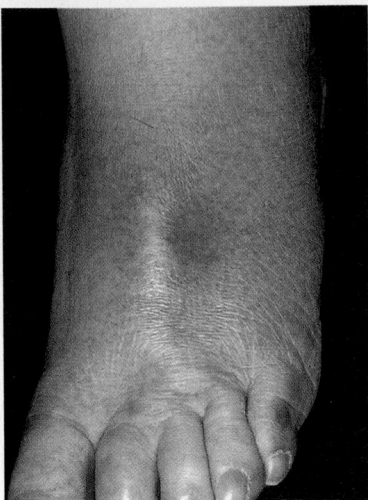

FIG. 23.6 Cellulitis with characteristic redness, tenderness, and edema. (From Habif TP: *Clinical dermatology: A color guide to diagnosis and therapy*, ed 5, St Louis, 2011, Mosby.)

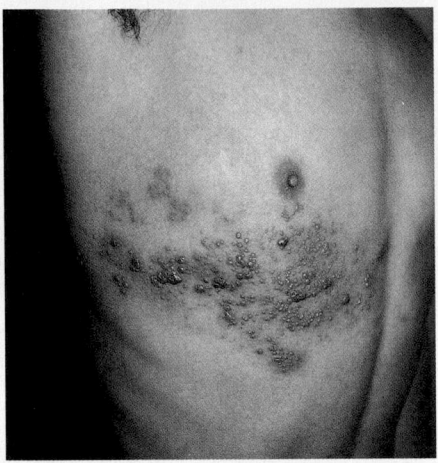

FIG. 23.7 Herpes zoster (shingles) on the anterior chest, classic dermatomal distribution. (From James WD, Berger T, Elston DMD: *Andrews' diseases of the skin*, ed 11, Philadelphia, 2011, Saunders.)

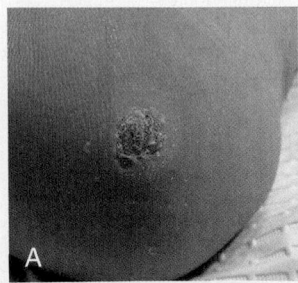 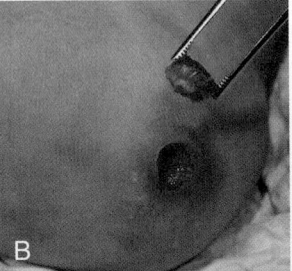

FIG. 23.8 Plantar wart. A, Keratotic lesion. B, After excision. (From Swartz MH: *Textbook of physical diagnosis: History and examination*, ed 6, Philadelphia, 2010, Saunders.)

Infestations and Insect Bites

There are many opportunities for exposure to *infestations* (harboring insects or worms) and insect bites (Table 23.7). In many instances, an allergy to the venom plays a key role in the reaction. In other cases, the clinical manifestations are a reaction to the eggs, feces, or body parts of the invading organism. Some

people react with a severe hypersensitivity (anaphylaxis), which can be life threatening. Anaphylaxis is discussed in Chapter 13.

Preventing insect bites by avoidance or using repellents is somewhat effective. Meticulous hygiene related to personal articles, clothing, bedding, and examination and care of pets, as well as careful choice of sexual partners, can reduce the incidence of infestations. Prompt, routine skin inspection is necessary in geographic areas where there is a risk for tick bite. Lyme disease, which is caused by a tick, is discussed in Chapter 64.

Fungal Infections

Because of the large number of fungi that are present everywhere, exposure to some pathologic varieties may occur. Skin, hair, and nails can become infected with fungi, including candidiasis and tinea unguium. Common fungal infections of the skin are described in Table 23.8. Most infections are harmless in healthy adults, but they can cause embarrassment and distress.

Fungal infections are easy to diagnose. A microscopic examination showing the appearance of hyphae (threadlike structures) in a skin scraping mounted in 10% to 20% potassium hydroxide (KOH) indicates a fungal infection. A Wood's light examination of hair infected with certain fungi will fluoresce blue to green.

ALLERGIC SKIN PROBLEMS

Patients often seek treatment for irritant or allergic dermatitis, two common types of contact dermatitis. *Irritant contact dermatitis* results from direct chemical injury to the skin. *Allergic contact dermatitis* is an antigen-specific, type IV delayed hypersensitivity response. The pathophysiology of allergic and contact dermatitis is discussed in Chapter 13. Skin problems associated with allergies and hypersensitivity reactions may present a challenge to the clinician (Table 23.9). A careful family history and discussion of exposure to possible offending agents can provide valuable data. Patch testing can help determine possible causative agents (see Fig. 22.10). The best treatment of allergic dermatitis is to avoid known irritants. The extreme pruritus and its potential for chronicity make it a frustrating problem for you and the patient, especially if we cannot determine the offending agent.

Cutaneous Drug Reactions

Stevens Johnson syndrome (SJS) and *toxic epidermal necrolysis* (TEN) are rare, life-threatening diseases. They are violent immune responses that often occur as a severe adverse reaction to either a medication or, more rarely, an infection. The result is the acute destruction of the epithelium of the skin and mucous membranes. SJS, SJS-TEN overlap, and TEN represent a spectrum of disease severity. SJS involves less than 10% of total body surface area, TEN involves more than 30% of total body surface area, and SJS-TEN overlap involves 10% to 29% of total body surface area.[8]

SJS/TEN typically occur 4 to 21 days after starting use of the offending drug. Systemic symptoms, including fever, cough, headache, anorexia, myalgia, and nausea, precede skin and mucous membrane findings by 1 to 3 days. Skin involvement starts as an erythematous, macular rash with purpuric centers. Over a period of hours to days, the rash merges to form blisters with sheet-like epidermal detachment (Fig. 23.9). The lesions usually start on the palms, soles, and trunk, then spread to the

TABLE 23.6 Common Viral Infections of the Skin

Etiology and Pathophysiology	Clinical Manifestations	Treatment and Prognosis
Herpes Simplex Virus (HSV) Types 1 and 2 • Oral or genital HSV infections serotyped as either HSV-1 or HSV-2 • Both are recurrent lifelong viral infections • Worsened by sunlight, trauma, menses, stress, and systemic infection • Contagious to those not previously infected • Transmitted by respiratory droplets or virus-containing fluid (e.g., saliva, cervical secretions) • Infection in one area readily transmitted to another site by contact	*First episode:* • Symptoms occurring 2 days to 2 weeks after contact • Painful local reaction • Single or grouped vesicles on erythematous base • Systemic symptoms (e.g., fever, malaise) possible or no symptoms possible *Recurrent:* • Recurrence in similar spot • Characteristic grouped vesicles on erythematous base	• Symptomatic • Soothing, moist compresses. Petroleum jelly to lesions • Scarring not usual result • Antiviral agents such as acyclovir (Zovirax), famciclovir (Famvir), and valacyclovir (Valtrex) • Vaccine not currently available, but is being researched, for HSV-1 or HSV-2
Herpes Zoster (Shingles) • Activation of the varicella-zoster virus • Incidence increases with age • Potentially contagious to anyone who has not had varicella or who is immunosuppressed	• Linear distribution along a dermatome of grouped vesicles and pustules on erythematous base resembling chickenpox (Fig. 23.7) • Usually unilateral on trunk, face, and lumbosacral areas • Burning, pain, and neuralgia preceding outbreak • Mild to severe pain during outbreak	*Topical:* • Wet compresses, silver sulfadiazine (Silvadene) to ruptured vesicles *Systemic:* • Antiviral agents (e.g., acyclovir, famciclovir, valacyclovir) within 72 hr to prevent postherpetic neuralgia • Analgesia. Mild sedation at bedtime • Gabapentin (Neurontin) to treat postherpetic neuralgia • Usually heals without complications, but scarring and postherpetic neuralgia possible • Vaccine (Zostavax) to prevent shingles one-time dose for adults ≥60 yr
Plantar Warts • Caused by human papillomavirus (HPV)	• Wart on bottom surface of foot, growing inward because of pressure of walking or standing (Fig. 23.8) • Painful when pressure applied • Interrupted skin markings • Cone shaped with black dots (thrombosed vessels) when wart removed	• Topical immunotherapy (imiquimod), cryosurgery, salicylic acid, duct tape
Verruca Vulgaris • Caused by HPV • May disappear spontaneously in 1-2 yr • Mildly contagious by autoinoculation • Specific response dependent on body part affected • Prevalence greater in youth and immunosuppressed	• Circumscribed, hypertrophic, flesh-colored papule limited to epidermis • Painful on lateral compression	• Multiple treatments, including surgery using blunt dissection with scissors or curette • Liquid nitrogen therapy • Blistering agent (cantharidin) • Keratolytic agent (salicylic acid) • CO_2 laser destruction

TABLE 23.7 Common Infestations and Insect Bites

Etiology and Pathophysiology	Clinical Manifestations	Treatment and Prognosis
Bedbugs • Cimicidae species • Feeding periodic, usually at night • Present in furniture, walls during day	• Wheal surrounded by vivid flare • Firm urticaria transforming into persistent lesion • Severe pruritus • Often grouped in threes appearing on uncovered parts of body	• Lesions usually require no treatment • Severe itching may require use of antihistamines or topical corticosteroids
Bees and Wasps • Hymenoptera species	• Intense, burning, local pain • Swelling and itching • Severe hypersensitivity may lead to anaphylaxis	• Cool compresses • Local application of antipruritic lotion • Antihistamines if indicated • Usually uneventful recovery

Continued

TABLE 23.7 Common Infestations and Insect Bites—cont'd

Etiology and Pathophysiology	Clinical Manifestations	Treatment and Prognosis
Pediculosis (Head Lice, Body Lice, Pubic Lice)		
• *Pediculus humanus* var. capitis, *Pediculus humanus* var. corporis, *Phthirus pubis* • Obligate parasites that suck blood, leave excrement and eggs on skin and hair, live in seams of clothing (if body lice) and in hair as nits. Transmission of pubic lice often by sexual contact	• Minute, red, noninflammatory • Points flush with skin. Progression to papular wheal-like lesions • Pruritus • Secondary excoriation, especially parallel linear excoriations in intrascapular region • Nits and eggs are firmly attached to hair shaft in head and body	• γ-Benzene hexachloride or pyrethrins to treat various parts of body • Spinosad (Natroba) topical suspension 0.9% to treat scalp and hair • Screen and treat close contacts (e.g., bed partners and playmates) as needed • Do not share head gear
Scabies		
• *Sarcoptes scabiei* • Mite penetrates stratum corneum, deposits eggs • Allergic reaction to eggs, feces, mite parts • Transmission by direct physical contact, sometimes by shared personal items • Rarely seen in dark-skinned people	• Severe itching, especially at night, usually not on face • Presence of burrows, especially in interdigital webs, flexor surface of wrists, genitalia, and anterior axillary folds • Erythematous papules (may be crusted), possible vesiculation, interdigital web crusting	• 5% permethrin topical lotion, 1 overnight application with second application 1 wk later, may yield 95% eradication • Treat all family members, treat environment with plastic covering for 5 days, launder all clothes and linen with bleach • Treat sexual partner • Antibiotics, if secondary infections present • Possible residual pruritus up to 4 wk after treatment • Recurrence possible if inadequately treated
Ticks		
• *Borrelia burgdorferi* (spirochete transmitted by ticks in certain areas) causes Lyme disease • Endemic areas include Northeast, Mid-Atlantic states, parts of Midwest and West (see Chapter 64)	• Spreading, ringlike rash 3–4 wk after bite (see Fig. 64.7) • Rash common in groin, buttocks, axillae, trunk, and upper arms and legs • Warm, itchy, or painful rash • Flu-like symptoms • Cardiac, arthritic, and neurologic manifestations possible • Unreliable laboratory test	• Oral antibiotics, such as doxycycline • IV antibiotics for arthritic, neurologic, and cardiac symptoms • Rest and healthy diet • Most patients recover

TABLE 23.8 Common Fungal Infections of the Skin and Nails

Etiology and Pathophysiology	Clinical Manifestations	Treatment and Prognosis
Candidiasis		
• Caused by *Candida albicans* • Also known as moniliasis • 50% of adults symptom-free carriers • Appears in warm, moist areas such as groin area, oral mucosa, and submammary folds • Immunosuppression (e.g., from HIV infection, chemotherapy, radiation, and organ transplantation) allows yeast to become pathogenic	*Mouth:* White, cheesy plaque, resembles milk curds *Vagina:* Vaginitis with red, edematous, painful vaginal wall, white patches. Vaginal discharge. Pruritus. Pain on urination and intercourse *Skin:* Diffuse papular erythematous rash with pinpoint satellite lesions around edges of affected area	• Azole antifungals (e.g., fluconazole, ketoconazole) or other specific medication such as vaginal suppository or oral lozenge • Sexual abstinence or use of condom • Skin hygiene to keep area clean and dry • Powder is effective on nonmucosal surfaces of skin to prevent recurrence
Tinea Corporis		
• Various dermatophytes, commonly called *ringworm*	• Typical annular (ringlike) scaly appearance, well-defined margins • Erythematous	• Cool compresses • Topical antifungals for isolated patches. Creams or solutions of miconazole, ketoconazole, clotrimazole, butenafine
Tinea Cruris		
• Various dermatophytes • Commonly called *jock itch*	• Well-defined scaly plaque in groin area • Does not affect mucous membranes	• Topical antifungal cream or solution
Tinea Pedis		
• Various dermatophytes • Commonly called *athlete's foot*	• Interdigital scaling and maceration • Scaly plantar surfaces sometimes with erythema and blistering • May be pruritic and painful	• Topical antifungal cream, gel, solution, spray, or powder
Tinea Unguium (Onychomycosis)		
• Various dermatophytes • Incidence increases with age	• Only few nails on one hand may be affected. Toenails more commonly affected • Scaliness under distal nail plate • Brittle, thickened, broken, or crumbling nails with yellowish discoloration	• Oral antifungal (terbinafine [Lamisil], itraconazole [Sporanox]) • Topical antifungal cream or solution (minimal effectiveness) if unable to tolerate systemic treatment • Thinning of toenails if needed • Nail avulsion (removal) is an option

TABLE 23.9 Common Allergic Conditions of the Skin

Etiology and Pathophysiology	Clinical Manifestations	Treatment and Prognosis
Allergic Contact Dermatitis • Type IV delayed hypersensitivity response (see Chapter 13) • Absorbed agent acts as antigen • Sensitization occurs after one or more exposures • Appearance of lesions 2–7 days after contact with allergen	• Red papules and plaques • Sharply circumscribed with occasional vesicles (see Fig. 13.10) • Usually pruritic • Area of dermatitis often takes shape of causative agent (e.g., metal allergy and bandlike dermatitis on ring finger).	• Topical or oral corticosteroids, antihistamines • Skin lubrication • Elimination of contact allergen • Avoidance of irritating affected area • Systemic corticosteroids if sensitivity severe
Atopic Dermatitis • Type 1 hypersensitivity response (see Chapter 13) • Genetically influenced, chronic, relapsing disease • Exaggerated by a skin response to environmental allergens • Associated with allergic rhinitis and asthma	• Multiple presentations, including acute, subacute, and chronic stages. All are pruritic • *Acute stage:* Bright erythema, oozing vesicles, with extreme pruritus (see Fig. 13.8) • *Subacute stage:* Scaly, light red to red-brown plaques • *Chronic stage:* Thickened skin with accentuation of skin markings (lichenification), possible hypopigmentation, or hyperpigmentation. Dry skin. Common in antecubital and popliteal space	• Lubrication of dry skin • Topical immunomodulators (pimecrolimus [Elidel], tacrolimus [Protopic]) • Reduction of stress reduces flares • Corticosteroids, phototherapy for severe inflammation and pruritus • Antibiotics for secondary infection as needed
Drug Reaction • May be caused by any drug that acts as antigen and causes hypersensitivity reaction • Certain drugs (e.g., penicillin) more likely to cause reactions • Not all reactions are allergic, some are intolerance (e.g., gastric upset)	• Rash of any morphology • Often red, macular and papular, semiconfluent, generalized rash with abrupt onset • Appearance as late as 14 days after cessation of drug. May be pruritic • Some reactions may be life threatening requiring immediate and intensive care	• Withdrawal of drug if possible • Antihistamines, topical or systemic corticosteroids may be necessary depending on severity of symptoms
Urticaria • Usually allergic phenomenon • Erythema and edema in upper dermis resulting from a local increase in permeability of capillaries (usually from histamine release)	• Spontaneously occurring, raised or irregularly shaped wheals, varying size, usually multiple • A single lesion usually resolves in 24 hr • Can occur anywhere on the body	• Removal of triggering agent, if known • Oral antihistamine therapy • Possibly systemic corticosteroids

face and extremities. They are extremely painful. Most people have mucosal lesions in the eye, mouth, and genital areas.

Identifying and stopping the offending drug(s) is the most important action in caring for a patient with SJS/TEN. The most common drugs involved include sulfonamides, carbamazepine, nonsteroidal antiinflammatory drugs, lamotrigine, allopurinol, phenytoin, and phenobarbital.[8] Immunotherapy may play a role in slowing disease progression and promoting skin repair.

The patient receives supportive care, often in an intensive care unit. Interventions focus on airway management, preserving renal function, maintaining fluid and electrolyte balance, and pain control. Fluid replacement is given to maintain urine output. Proper wound care helps prevent infection and promote healing. Dressing with petrolatum gauze or other nonadhesive material provides a barrier and offers moisture to help the skin repair. Because of painful oral lesions, most patients need parenteral or enteral nutrition to meet nutrition and caloric demands. Apply eyedrops, lubricating ointment, and antibiotic drops to those with conjunctivitis.

BENIGN SKIN PROBLEMS

Although the list of benign skin problems is extensive, some of the most commonly seen and distressing ones include acne vulgaris (Fig. 23.10), psoriasis, and seborrheic keratoses. Benign problems are outlined in Table 23.10.

Psoriasis is a chronic autoimmune disease. It is fairly common, affecting about 7.5 million Americans.[9] Men and women develop psoriasis at equal rates. The rate is highest in whites (3.6%).[10] It usually develops in those 15 to 35 years old. One third of people with psoriasis have at least one relative with the disease. It is associated with metabolic syndrome, heart disease, and type 2 diabetes. Up to 40% of people with psoriasis also have psoriatic arthritis. Psoriatic arthritis is discussed in Chapter 64.

The diagnosis of plaque psoriasis, the most common form, is based on the skin's appearance (Fig. 23.11). Lesions are distinct and appear as red, scaling papules that merge to form plaques. The affected area is normally rounded, with adherent silver scales that bleed easily when removed. Plaques are common on the knees, elbows, scalp, hands, feet, and lower back.[9] They are often pruritic and may be painful. Clinical presentation varies. While most have mild disease, some have psoriasis on much of their skin surface.

Treatment is tailored to meet a person's needs. This varies depending on the location of lesions, severity, patient preferences, and comorbidities. Goals range from improved quality of life to complete disease resolution. Psoriasis for most is more emotionally than physically disabling. It erodes the self-image. The person may be self-conscious and withdraws from social contacts.[8] Quality of life can diminish as people avoid activities. Depression is common.

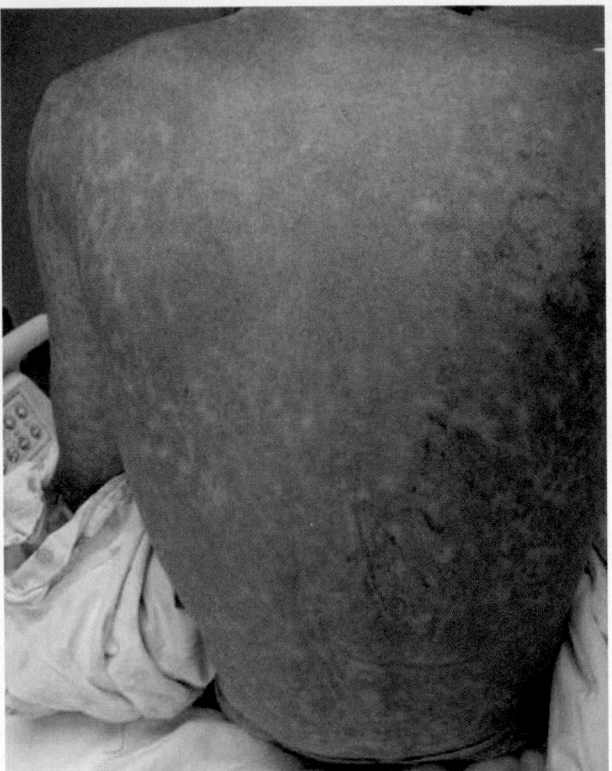

FIG. 23.9 Toxic epidermal necrolysis. (From *Ferri's clinical advisor 2018.* Dabiri, Ganary, MD, PhD; Rüenger, Thomas M., MD, PhD. Published January 1, 2018. Pages 1282.e2-1282.e3. © 2018.)

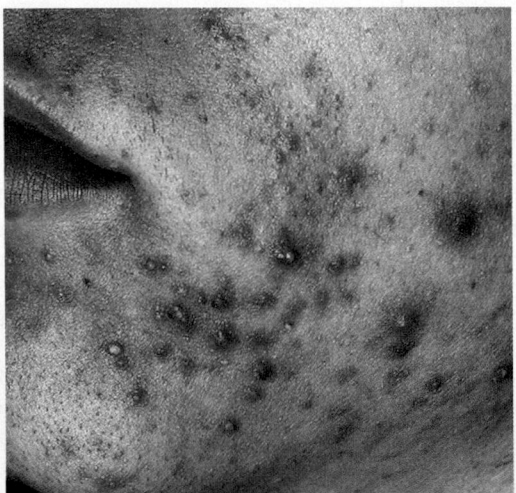

FIG. 23.10 Acne vulgaris. Papules and pustules. (From James WD, Berger T, Elston DMD: *Andrews' diseases of the skin*, ed 11, Philadelphia, 2011, Saunders.)

💊 **DRUG ALERT** Isotretinoin (Accutane)

- Used to treat acne (Table 23.10)
- Can cause serious damage to fetus
- Contraindicated in women who are pregnant or want to become pregnant
- Cannot donate blood during treatment and for 1 month after treatment ends
- May cause depression and suicidal ideation

INTERPROFESSIONAL CARE: SKIN PROBLEMS

Diagnostic Studies

A careful history is of prime importance in diagnosing skin problems. The HCP must be skilled at detecting any evidence that could lead to the cause of many different skin problems. After a careful history and physical examination, inspect individual lesions. The history, physical examination, and diagnostic test results guide therapy.

Interprofessional Therapy

Many different treatment methods are used in dermatology. Advances in this field have brought relief to many previously chronic, untreatable conditions. Many of the specific therapeutic treatments require specialized equipment. They are usually used by a dermatologist or specially trained nurse.

Phototherapy. Ultraviolet light (UVL) therapy is a part of treating many skin problems, including psoriasis, cutaneous T-cell lymphoma, atopic dermatitis, vitiligo, and pruritus. Light sources available include broadband UVB, narrowband UVB, and long-wave UV (UVA1). One form of phototherapy combines the use of the photosensitizing drug methoxsalen with UVA light (PUVA). With PUVA, patients receive methoxsalen and then are exposed to UVA.

Treatments are generally given 2 to 3 times a week. Side effects include nausea, itching, and erythema. Taking methoxsalen with food and milk may reduce nausea. Caution patients about the hazards of using methoxsalen and concurrent exposure to UV rays from sunlight or artificial UVL during therapy. Because of the risk for cataracts, patients receiving PUVA need to wear prescription goggles that block 100% of UVL. Teach patients to wear the eyewear for 24 hours after taking the medication when outdoors or near a bright window because UVA penetrates glass. Perform frequent skin assessments on all patients receiving phototherapy. The immunosuppressive effects of PUVA increase the risk for SCC, BCC, and melanoma.

Photodynamic therapy is a special type of phototherapy used to treat actinic keratosis and some skin cancers. This therapy uses a photosensitizing agent in a different way than other phototherapy treatments. The patient receives the photosensitizing agent IV or topically, depending on the area treated. Time is allowed for the drug to be absorbed by the target cells. Light is then applied to the area, causing the drug to react with oxygen. This starts a reaction that kills the cells.[11]

❓ **CHECK YOUR PRACTICE**

You are working in a dermatology clinic preparing a 64-yr-old woman for phototherapy to treat multiple actinic keratoses on her nose and both cheeks. She says the first lesion appeared a few years ago. She then started to worry about all the time she spent in her garden without sunscreen. She thought the lesions were just "age spots" and was unconcerned until a few started to grow and periodically bleed.

- What teaching will you do to get her ready for the procedure and to take care of herself after the procedure?

Radiation Therapy. The use of radiation therapy to treat BCC and SCC varies. The best candidates are those with lesions in challenging locations, such as the ear, nose, scalp, neck, and shin; those who may have trouble with wound healing; or those with medical comorbidities who cannot undergo surgery.[12]

TABLE 23.10 Common Benign Conditions of the Skin

Etiology and Pathophysiology	Clinical Manifestations	Treatment and Prognosis
Acne Vulgaris • Inflammatory disorder of sebaceous glands • More common in teenagers • May begin and persist into adulthood • Flare can occur with use of corticosteroids and androgen-dominant birth control pills and before menses.	• Noninflammatory lesions, including open comedones (blackheads) and closed comedones (whiteheads) • Inflammatory lesions, including papules and pustules • Most common on face, neck, and upper back (Fig. 23.10)	*Topical:* • Mechanical removal of multiple lesions with comedo extractor • Topical benzoyl peroxide, retinoids, or antimicrobials (clindamycin, erythromycin) *Systemic:* • Systemic antibiotics • Use of isotretinoin (Accutane) for severe nodulocystic acne may provide lasting remission. Pregnancy tests, monitor liver function, cholesterol, triglycerides, and for depression • Aim of treatment to suppress new lesions and minimize scarring • Spontaneous remission possible • Often improvement with exposure to sun
Acrochordons (Skin Tags) • Common after midlife • Appearance on neck, axillae, and upper trunk secondary to mechanical friction or redundant skin (associated with obesity)	• Small, skin-colored, soft, pedunculated papules • May become irritated	• No treatment medically necessary • Surgical removal when needed. Usually just snipping without anesthesia
Lentigo • Increased number of normal melanocytes in basal layer of epidermis from sun exposure and aging • Also called "liver spots" or "age spots"	• Hyperpigmented, brown to black macule or patch (flat lesion) on sun-exposed areas	• Evaluate carefully for progression • Treatment only for cosmetic purposes: liquid nitrogen, laser resurfacing • May recur • Biopsy when suspicious of melanoma
Lipoma • Benign tumor of adipose tissue, often encapsulated • Most common in 40- to 60-yr-old age group	• Rubbery, compressible, round mass of adipose tissue • Single or multiple • Variable in size, may be extremely large • Most common on trunk, back of neck, and forearms	• Usually no treatment • Biopsy to distinguish from liposarcoma • Excision usual treatment (when indicated)
Nevi (Moles) • Grouping of normal cells derived from melanocyte-like precursor cells	• Hyperpigmented areas that vary in form and color • Flat, slightly elevated, verrucoid, polypoid, dome-shaped, sessile, or papillomatous • Preservation of normal skin markings • Hair growth possible	• No treatment necessary except for cosmetic reasons • Skin biopsy for suspicious nevi
Psoriasis • Autoimmune chronic dermatitis that involves extremely rapid turnover of epidermal cells • Family predisposition • Usually develops before age 40	• Sharply demarcated silvery scaling plaques on reddish skin often on the scalp, elbows, knees, palms, soles, and fingernails (Fig. 23.11) • Itching, burning, pain • Localized or general, intermittent or continuous • Symptoms vary in intensity from mild to severe	• Goal to reduce inflammation and suppress rapid turnover of epidermal cells. No cure, but control is possible *Topical treatments:* • Corticosteroids, tazarotene, calcipotriene, anthralin, calcineurin inhibitors (tacrolimus) • Intralesional injection of corticosteroids for chronic plaques *Systemic treatments:* • Natural or artificial UVB. PUVA (UVA with topical or systemic photosensitizer [psoralen]) • Traditional and oral therapies: antimetabolite (methotrexate), retinoid (acitretin), apremilast (Otezla), immunosuppressant (cyclosporine) • Biologic therapies: adalimumab (Humira), etanercept (Enbrel), infliximab (Remicade), ustekinumab (Stelara), brodalumab (Siliq), certolizumab pegol (Cimzia), secukinumab (Cosentyx), golimumab (Simponi), guselkumab (Tremfya), ixekizumab (Taltz) for moderate to severe plaque disease
Seborrheic Keratoses • Benign, familial, exact etiology unknown • Usually occur after age 40, increase in number with age	• Irregularly round or oval, often verrucous papules or plaques • Well-defined shape, appearance of being stuck on • Increase in pigmentation with time • Usually multiple, may be itchy	• Removal by curettage or cryosurgery for cosmetic reasons or to eliminate source of irritation • Biopsy if unable to distinguish from melanoma

PUVA, Psoralen ultraviolet A; *UVA,* ultraviolet A; *UVB,* ultraviolet B.

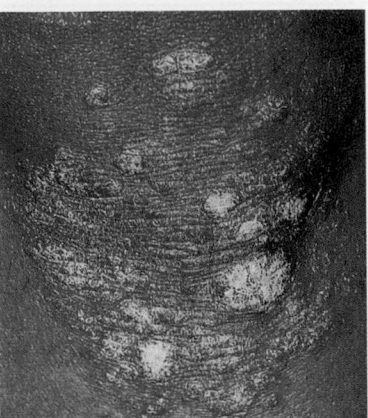

FIG. 23.11 Psoriasis. Characteristic inflammation and scaling. (From Habif TP: *Clinical dermatology: A color guide to diagnosis and therapy,* ed 5, St Louis, 2011, Mosby.)

TABLE 23.11 Skin Conditions Treated by Laser

- Acne scars
- Hair removal
- Hemangiomas
- Leg veins
- Pigment discoloration in epidermis
- Pigmented nevi
- Port wine stain
- Psoriasis
- Resurfacing of skin
- Rosacea
- Skin lesions
- Tattoo removal
- Vascular lesions
- Warts
- Wrinkles

Use is limited in those with melanoma to palliative pain control or treating brain metastases.

Radiation therapy requires multiple visits to a radiology department. It can produce permanent hair loss *(alopecia)* of the irradiated areas. Other adverse effects, depending on anatomic location and dose of radiation delivered, include telangiectasia, atrophy, hyperpigmentation, depigmentation, ulceration, hearing loss, ocular damage, atrophy, and mucositis. Careful shielding is necessary to prevent ocular lens damage if the irradiated area is around the eyes. See Chapter 15 for more on radiation therapy.

Total-body skin irradiation is one treatment for cutaneous T-cell lymphoma. Treatment follows a lengthy course and causes premature aging of the skin. Patients have varying degrees of permanent alopecia and radiation dermatitis with a transient loss of sweat gland function.

Laser Technology. Laser treatment is expanding rapidly as an efficient surgical tool for many types of skin problems (Table 23.11). Depending on the type of laser and the wavelength, lasers serve a wide variety of functions. Lasers can make measurable, repeatable, consistent zones of tissue damage. They can cut, coagulate, and vaporize tissue to some degree. Laser light does not accumulate in body cells and cannot cause cumulative cellular changes or damage. With less damage to surrounding tissue, there is a decreased risk for scarring.

The surgical use of laser energy requires a focusing device to produce a small, high-density spot of energy. Several types of lasers are available. The CO_2 laser, the most common, has many applications as a vaporizing and cutting tool for most tissues. The argon laser emits light that is primarily absorbed by hemoglobin. It helps in the treatment of vascular and other pigmented lesions. Other, less common lasers include copper and gold vapors and neodymium:yttrium-aluminum-garnet (Nd:YAG). Those who work with laser equipment must be familiar with facility policies and procedures on laser safety.

Drug Therapy

Antibiotics. Several topical and systemic antibiotics are used to treat skin problems. Sometimes they are used concurrently. Many common systemic antibiotics are not used topically because of the danger of allergic contact dermatitis. Common OTC topical antibiotics include bacitracin-neomycin-polymyxin (Neosporin), bacitracin, and polymyxin B. Some HCPs do not recommend Neosporin because of the risk for allergic contact dermatitis. Prescription topical antibiotics

include (1) mupirocin (for superficial *Staphylococcus* infections such as impetigo), (2) gentamicin (used for *Staphylococcus* and many gram-negative organisms), and (3) erythromycin (used for gram-positive cocci [staphylococci and streptococci] and gram-negative cocci and bacilli). Metronidazole is a common therapy for rosacea. Topical erythromycin and clindamycin are options for acne vulgaris.

Systemic infections require systemic antibiotics. They have a role in treating acne vulgaris and bacterial infections, such as erysipelas, cellulitis, abscesses, and certain wound infections. Frequently used oral drugs include penicillin, erythromycin, doxycycline, clindamycin, and linezolid. Vancomycin is the drug of choice for severe infections.[13] Give patients drug-specific instructions on the proper technique of taking or applying antibiotics.

Corticosteroids. Corticosteroids are effective in treating a wide variety of skin problems. They can be used topically, intralesionally, or systemically. Topical corticosteroids have local antiinflammatory and antipruritic effects. Since corticosteroids may alter the manifestations, try to diagnose a skin problem before applying a corticosteroid preparation.

The potency of a preparation depends on the concentration of active drug. With prolonged use, high-potency corticosteroids can cause adrenal suppression, especially if a large surface area is covered and occlusive dressings are used. Other side effects include skin atrophy from impaired cell mitosis, capillary fragility, rosacea eruptions, severe exacerbations of acne vulgaris, and bruising. In general, atrophy does not occur until a corticosteroid has been in use for 2 to 3 weeks. If drug use is stopped at the first sign of atrophy, recovery usually occurs in several weeks. Rebound dermatitis can occur when therapy is stopped. Tapering the use of high-potency topical corticosteroids when improvement is noted reduces the risk.

Low-potency corticosteroids such as hydrocortisone act more slowly. However, they can be used for a longer time without producing serious side effects. Low-potency corticosteroids are safe to use on the face and areas where skin may touch or rub together, such as the axillae and groin.

The most potent delivery system for a topical corticosteroid is an ointment form. Apply creams and ointments in thin layers and slowly massage into the site 1 to 3 times a day.

Intralesional corticosteroids are injected directly into or just beneath the lesion. This method provides a reservoir of medication with an effect lasting several weeks to months. Intralesional injection is common in the treatment of psoriasis, alopecia areata (patchy hair loss), cystic acne, hypertrophic scars, and keloids. Triamcinolone acetonide (Kenalog) is the most common drug used for intralesional injection.

Systemic corticosteroids can have remarkable results in the treatment of skin conditions. However, they often have undesirable systemic effects (see Chapter 49). Corticosteroids are helpful in short-term therapy for acute conditions such as contact dermatitis caused by poison ivy. Long-term therapy is reserved for those with severe disease such as bullous (blistering) disorders.

Antihistamines. Oral antihistamines are helpful in treating urticaria, angioedema, and pruritus that can occur in problems such as atopic dermatitis, allergic dermatitis, and other allergic cutaneous reactions. Several antihistamines may be tried before getting an acceptable effect. Antihistamines with sedative effects, such as hydroxyzine and diphenhydramine, may be better for pruritic conditions because the tranquilizing and sedative effects offer symptomatic relief. Warn the patient about sedative effects, a problem when driving or using heavy machinery. Antihistamines, such as loratadine (Claritin), fexofenadine (Allegra), and cetirizine (Zyrtec), bind to peripheral histamine receptors, giving antihistamine action without sedation. They are not effective for controlling pruritus. Use any antihistamines with caution in older adults because of their long half-life and anticholinergic effects.

Topical Fluorouracil. Fluorouracil is a topical cytotoxic agent with selective toxicity for sun-damaged cells. It is used to treat precancerous lesions (especially AK) and some skin cancers. Patient adherence is a consideration in the use of fluorouracil. The medication produces erythema, burning, and pruritus within 3 to 5 days. Painful, eroded areas over the damaged skin occur within 1 to 3 weeks, depending on skin thickness at the site. Reduce redness and pruritus by applying a low-potency topical corticosteroid 20 minutes after. There are 5 strengths (0.5%, 1%, 2%, 4%, and 5%). Treatment must continue with applications 1 or 2 times a day for 2 to 4 weeks. Healing may take up to 4 weeks after the medication is stopped.[8]

Adherence to therapy depends on your teaching. Tell the patient that they will look worse before they look better. Teach about the effect of the medication. Because fluorouracil is a photosensitizing drug, tell the patient to avoid sunlight during treatment. After treatment, skin should be smooth and free of AK. AK may recur in treated areas, and multiple courses of therapy may be necessary over the years for those with severely sun-damaged skin.

Immunomodulators. Topical immunomodulators, such as pimecrolimus (Elidel) and tacrolimus (Protopic), are used to treat atopic dermatitis, psoriasis, and rosacea.[14] They work by suppressing an overreactive immune system. The side effects are minimal and may include a transient burning or feeling of heat at the application site. Use may increase the risk for skin cancer and precancerous lesions.

The topical immunomodulator imiquimod (Aldara) is used to treat external genital warts, AK, and superficial BCC. It stimulates the production of α-interferon and other cytokines to enhance cell-mediated immunity. It boosts the immune response only where applied and is safe for transplant patients. Most patients using this cream experience skin reactions, including redness, swelling, blistering, peeling, itching, and burning. Dosing varies depending on the type of lesion treated and the strength of medication prescribed.[8]

Diagnostic and Surgical Therapy

Skin Scraping. Scraping with a scalpel blade can yield a sample of surface cells (stratum corneum) for microscopic inspection and diagnosis. The most common tests of skin scrapings are mineral oil examination for scabies and 10% to 20% potassium hydroxide (KOH) for fungus.

Electrodessication and Electrocoagulation. Electrical energy can be converted to heat with the tip of an electrode. The heat burns and destroys tissue. The major uses of these therapies are coagulation of bleeding vessels to obtain hemostasis and destruction of small *telangiectasias* (dilation of groups of superficial capillaries and venules). *Electrodessication* usually involves more superficial destruction. It uses a monopolar electrode. *Electrocoagulation* uses a bipolar electrode. It has a deeper effect, with better hemostasis, but an increased chance of scarring. While minor electrosurgery on patients with a pacemaker poses minimal risk, the electrical energy can affect both pacemakers and internal defibrillators.

Curettage. Curettage is the removal and scooping away of tissue using an instrument called a *curette*. A curette looks like a small spoon with very sharp edges. Although a curette is not usually strong enough to cut normal skin, it can remove many types of small, soft skin tumors and superficial lesions, such as warts, AK, seborrheic keratosis, and small BCCs and SCCs. The area to be curetted is anesthetized before the procedure. The HCP removes the lesion and then cauterizes the skin. The removed tissue is usually sent for biopsy. A dressing may be applied, and you will need to teach the patient wound care. A small scar and hypopigmentation can result.

Punch Biopsy. Punch biopsy is a common procedure used to obtain a tissue sample for histologic study or to remove small lesions (Fig. 23.12). The procedure is simple. The HCP marks the biopsy area and then anesthetizes it so that the anesthetic will not obscure the landmarks. The HCP rotates the punch into the skin and removes a small cylinder of skin. Hemostasis is

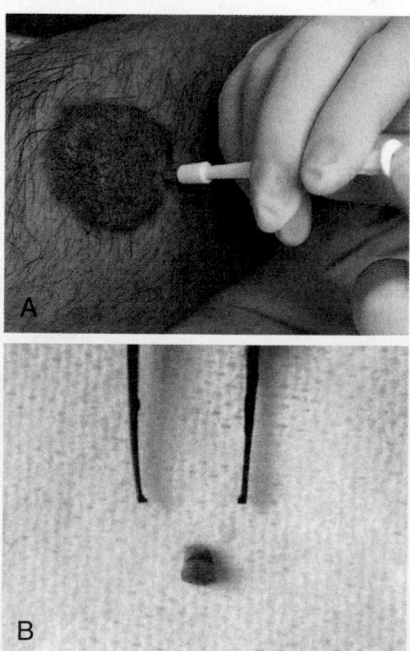

FIG. 23.12 Punch biopsy. **A,** Removal of skin for diagnostic purposes. **B,** Specimen obtained. (From Graham-Brown R, Bourke J, Cunliffe T: *Dermatology: Fundamentals of practice,* Edinburgh, 2008, Mosby.)

achieved with pressure or absorbable gelatin (Gelfoam) packing. Sites of 4 mm or larger are usually closed with sutures. Punch biopsies are not done below the knee if other sites are available. Circulatory changes can make evaluating the tissue sample more difficult.

Cryosurgery. Cryosurgery is the use of subfreezing temperatures to destroy epidermal lesions. Cryosurgery is used to treat common and genital warts, cutaneous tags, thin seborrheic keratoses, lentigines, AK, BCC, and SCC. Topical liquid nitrogen is the agent most commonly used for cryosurgery.[12] Damage occurs in treated tissue because of intracellular ice formation. It causes the cell to rupture during thaw, leading to cell death and necrosis. The degree of damage depends on the rate of cooling and the minimum temperature achieved.

Liquid nitrogen is applied topically (directly onto the lesion) with a direct spray or contact probe. Tell patients that they will feel a painful, stinging cold sensation. The lesion first becomes swollen and red, and it may blister. A scab forms and falls off in 1 to 3 weeks. The skin lesion sloughs along with the scab. Growth of new skin follows.

The size of an affected area may limit the use of cryotherapy. Other disadvantages include the potential for harming adjacent healthy tissue and the low temperature of liquid nitrogen destroying melanocytes, leaving an area of hypopigmentation resembling a scar.

Excision. Excision is an option if the lesion involves the dermis. Complete closure of the excised area usually results in a good cosmetic result.

A specific type of excision is *Mohs surgery,* which is the microscopically controlled removal of a skin cancer. In this procedure, the HCP removes tissue sections in thin horizontal layers. All the specimen's margins are examined to see if any cancer cells remain (Fig. 23.13). Any residual tumor not removed by the first surgical excision is removed in serial excisions performed the same day. Benefits of Mohs surgery are that it preserves normal tissue, produces the smallest possible wound, and can completely remove the cancer. Although it can be a lengthy procedure, it is done in an outpatient setting using local anesthesia.

❖ NURSING MANAGEMENT: SKIN PROBLEMS

◆ Ambulatory Care

Skin problems are not usually a primary reason for hospitalization. Nevertheless, many hospitalized patients have skin problems that need nursing intervention and patient education. Nursing interventions for skin conditions fall into broad categories. They apply to many problems in both inpatient and outpatient settings. A nursing care plan for the patient with chronic skin lesions (eNursing Care Plan 23.1) is available on the website for this chapter.

In your general teaching with the patient, stress the duration of the treatment and the need to follow package directions. Skin problems may be slow to resolve. Tell the patient to follow package directions when using OTC drugs. If the package insert says its use should not exceed 7 days, patients should heed this warning. Teach the patient to stop self-care and seek the help of an HCP if any systemic signs of inflammation or extensions of the skin problem (e.g., an increasing number of lesions, increased erythema, increased swelling) develop.

◆ **Wet Compresses.** For superficial skin problems that involve inflammation, itching, and infection, wet compresses are commonly used. They are appropriate for damaged, oozing skin. Wet compresses are a good way to remove crusts and scabs that are adhering to the wound surface. They provide comfort and treatment of conditions such as poison ivy, insect bites, and skin infections.

It is important to understand how to do a wet compress correctly. Unless there is a concern about water quality, tap water at room temperature is the best choice. If drinkable water is not available, use filtered, bottled, or sterile water. Depending on the problem, additives may be used. Common solutions include (1) saline, (2) Burow's solution (Domeboro powder [aluminum acetate; calcium acetate]), (3) acetic acid (vinegar), and (4) silver nitrate.[8] The temperature of the fluid should be tepid. However, when an anti-inflammatory effect is desired, the fluid should be cool.

The material you select for the compress should be 4 to 8 layers thick and slightly larger than the area that you are treating. Use gauze or any clean material (e.g., thin cotton sheeting, thermal underwear, tube socks). Ingenuity is sometimes needed when covering odd-shaped body parts. Do not use gauze sponges with fillers (abdominal pads). They will retain too much solution, and fibers can be left in the wound if the skin is open. Place the prescribed compress material into fresh solution and squeeze out excess fluid. Your goal is a wet compress—not damp but not dripping.

Wet compresses are applied continuously or intermittently. When used continuously, remove the compress and replace with a new one as needed. Do not add solution to a compress. This can change the fluid's concentration and damage the skin. They can be placed intermittently, for 10 to 30 minutes, several times a day. Careful monitoring of the skin is important. If the skin appears *macerated* (softens and turns white), stop the compresses for 2 to 3 days. Change and wash daily any material used repeatedly throughout the day. Protect the patient from discomfort and chilling. A water-resistant pad will help protect the mattress, linens, and furniture.

◆ **Baths.** Baths are an appropriate intervention when large areas of the body need treatment. Baths may be relaxing and will help decrease itching. Agents such as colloidal oatmeal (Aveeno) and

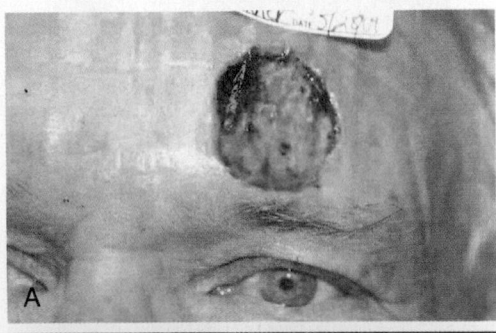
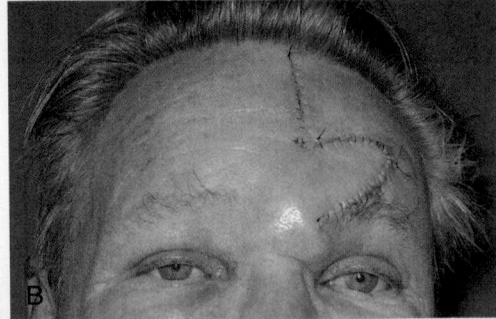

FIG. 23.13 **A,** Removal of melanoma by Mohs surgery. **B,** After plastic surgery using a skin flap to repair defect. (Courtesy Peter Bonner, Placitas, NM.)

sodium bicarbonate can be added directly to bath water. Fill the tub with tepid water to cover the affected areas. Depending on the severity of the problem and the patient's discomfort, have the patient soak for 15 to 20 minutes 3 or 4 times a day. Stress to the patient not to rub the skin dry with a towel but gently pat to prevent increased irritation and inflammation. Avoid adding oils as their use increases the risk for falls. To sustain the hydrating effect, apply cream, ointment emollients (moisturizers), or other prescribed topical agents after the bath. This helps seal the moisture in the hydrated cells and increases the absorption of any topical agents.

◆ **Hygienic Practices.** The patient's skin type, lifestyle, culture, age, and gender influence hygienic practices. The normal acidity of the skin and perspiration protect against bacterial overgrowth. Most soaps are alkaline and neutralize the skin surface, leading to a loss of protection. Using mild, moisturizing soaps and lipid-free cleansers and avoiding hot water and vigorous scrubbing can noticeably decrease local skin irritation and inflammation. Skin piercings in which jewelry has been inserted can be cared for with antibacterial soaps that do not contain sulfites.

In general, skin and hair must be washed often enough to remove excess oil and excretions and to prevent odor. Older persons should avoid harsh soaps and shampoos and frequent bathing because of the dryness of their skin and scalp. Using moisturizers right after a bath or shower (while the skin is still damp) seals in the moisture.

◆ **Topical Medications.** Topical medications are commonly used to treat skin problems. The effectiveness of topical therapy depends on which base the medication is prepared in. Table 23.12 summarizes the common agents used as bases for topical preparations and their therapeutic considerations. The base selected depends on the properties needed.

Creams are very versatile and most commonly prescribed. Ointments are more lubricating than creams and offer enhanced potency of the active ingredient. They may be too occlusive for conditions with lots of exudate or in body creases. Gels work well on the scalp, where other compounds may mat the hair, and for acute exudative conditions such as poison ivy. Lotions are also fine for the scalp but may cause stinging and drying when used in skinfolds. Pastes are good for protecting the skin but are messy. A limited number of foams are available.

TABLE 23.12 **Drug Therapy**
Common Bases for Topical Medications

Agent	Therapeutic Considerations
Cream	Emulsions of oil and water. Most common base for topical medications. Lubrication and protection
Gel	Nongreasy combination of propylene glycol and water. May contain alcohol
Lotion	Emulsions of water, alcohol, and/or oil. Cooling and drying. Some leave residual powder film after evaporation of water. Useful in subacute pruritic eruptions
Ointment	Oil with differing amounts of water added in suspension. Lubrication and prevention of dehydration. Petrolatum most common
Paste	Mixture of powder and ointment, used when drying effect necessary because moisture is absorbed
Powder	Promotion of dryness. Lubricates skinfold areas to prevent irritation. Base for antifungal preparations. Protect patient from inhaling

Apply topical medications as directed. Proper administration will yield best results and avoid waste. Some are very costly. As a rule, apply topical medication in a thin film to clean skin and spread evenly in a downward motion in the direction of hair growth. Thick creams will spread easier if the skin is still damp. If you are using a secondary dressing, you can apply the medication directly onto a dressing. Teach the patient and caregiver proper dosing, application technique, expected results, and common reactions.

Occlusion with a plastic wrap is an effective way to increase the absorption of topical corticosteroids or simple emollients. The plastic wrap traps perspiration against the outer layer of the epidermis. Applying preparations to moist skin increases absorption 10-fold. Use tape or stretch wraps to keep the plastic wrap in place. For conditions on the feet or lower legs, the patient can wear socks over the plastic wrap. Wraps applied multiple times daily are kept in place for 2 to 8 hours. Some patients choose to use the occlusion technique at bedtime. Occlusion is not appropriate in areas prone to infection, such as skin creases.

◆ **Control of Pruritus.** Many conditions cause *pruritus* (itching). This includes dry skin, almost any physical or chemical stimulus to the skin (such as drugs or insects), and any scaling skin disorder. The itch sensation is carried by the same nonmyelinated nerve fibers as pain and temperature. The patient will have pain rather than an itch if the epidermis is damaged or absent. It is important to figure out if itching preceded a skin lesion. Itching can lead to scratching that results in an excoriated and inflamed lesion.

Certain circumstances make itching worse. Teach the patient ways to help break the itch/scratch cycle. A cool environment may cause vasoconstriction and decrease itching. Hydration, wet compresses, and moisturizers (including antipruritic lotions) are normally helpful. Apply wet compresses for 30 to 60 minutes, pat the skin dry, and apply a lubricant or medication. Topical and injectable corticosteroids are sometimes used. Topically applied menthol, camphor, or phenol numb itch receptors. Systemic antihistamines may give relief. The main side effect of most antihistamines is sedation. This may be desirable because pruritus is often worse at night and can interfere with sleep. Adequate rest increases the patient's ability to tolerate itching, thereby decreasing skin damage from the resultant scratching. Have the patient avoid anything that causes vasodilation, such as heat or rubbing. Dry skin lowers the itch threshold and increases the itch sensation.

Lichenification is a thickening of epidermis with exaggerated markings resembling a washboard. It is caused by chronic scratching or rubbing of the skin. Lichenification is often associated with atopic dermatoses and other pruritic conditions. Although any area of the body may be affected, the hands, forearms, shins, and nape of the neck are common sites. Scratching may become a habit. Persistent scratching can cause excoriations. Treating the cause of the itching is the key to preventing lichenification.

◆ **Prevention of Spread.** Although most skin problems are not contagious, infection control precautions indicate wearing gloves when working with any open wounds or lesions with drainage. Not all infected drainage is purulent. Careful hand washing and properly disposing of soiled dressings are the best means of preventing the spread of infections or infestations. The most common contagious lesions include impetigo, streptococcal infections, staphylococcal infections (e.g., methicillin-resistant *S. aureus* [MRSA]), fungal infections, primary chancre, scabies, and pediculosis.

◆ **Prevention of Secondary Infections.** Open skin lesions are susceptible to invasion by other viral, bacterial, or fungal organisms. Meticulous hygiene, hand washing, and dressing changes are important to minimize the potential for secondary infections. Warn the patient about scratching lesions, which can cause excoriations and create a portal of entry for pathogens. Trim the patient's nails short to minimize trauma from scratching.

◆ **Specific Skin Care.** You are often in a position to teach patients skin care after simple surgical procedures, such as skin biopsy, excision, and cryosurgery. In general, your teaching should include dressing changes, use of topical antibiotics, and the signs and symptoms of infection. After a skin procedure, cleanse any oozing wound with a saline solution twice daily or as ordered by the HCP. Potable (safe, drinking water) is a safe alternative in some situations. Apply antibiotic or plain petrolatum ointment with a secondary dressing that is both absorbent and nonadherent.

Wounds that are kept moist and covered heal more rapidly and with less scarring. The initial crust that forms should be left undisturbed as a protective coating for the damaged skin beneath it. Healing crusts that have been moisturized and protected will separate naturally from healed epidermis.

A sutured wound may be covered with a variety of dressings. Sutures are generally removed in 4 to 14 days, depending on the placement site. Sometimes alternating sutures are removed after the third day. Incision lines may need daily cleansing, usually with plain water. If necessary, a topical antibiotic is applied and the wound either is covered with a dry dressing or left open to air. The patient may have some swelling and discomfort in the first 24 hours. Intermittent application of cold (ice packs) over the surgical dressing may reduce edema. Mild analgesics, such as acetaminophen, should control discomfort. Teach the patient how to distinguish normal inflammation from an infection. A slight red border during the first few days after a procedure is normal. Signs and symptoms of infection include redness that persists longer than a week or extends beyond a 1-cm border, a fever above 101° F, increased pain, pronounced swelling, and purulent drainage. If these occur, they should be reported to the HCP at once.

NURSING MANAGEMENT
Skin Conditions

- Assess patient's skin for acute and chronic skin problems.
- Assess patient's risk factors for skin problems.
- Document skin condition and risk factor assessment and develop a plan of care.
- Determine whether patient is taking drugs that increase photosensitivity.
- Teach about risks associated with sun exposure and methods for decreasing exposure to the sun.
- Administer prescribed therapies such as dressings and oral or topical medications.
- Teach about therapies used for skin disorders, including dressings, baths, and oral or topical medications used on an outpatient basis.
- Evaluate treatment for effectiveness and any adverse effects.

◆ **Psychologic Effects of Chronic Skin Problems.** Emotional stress can occur for those who suffer from chronic skin problems, such as psoriasis, atopic dermatitis, or acne. The sequelae of chronic skin problems could result in social and employment problems

with subsequent financial implications, a poor self-image, problems with sexuality, and increasing and progressive frustration. The usual lack of systemic illness coupled with the visibility of the skin lesions often presents a real problem to the patient.

Help the patient follow the prescribed regimen. Allow the patient to verbalize the "Why me?" question, even though there is no ready answer. Refer the patient to dermatology support groups. Many are listed on the American Academy of Dermatology website *(www.aad.org).* These groups are extremely helpful with patient support and education.

The location of lesions and scars is the determining factor with respect to their cosmetic implications. Facial scars are the most damaging psychologically because they are so visible. Creative use of cosmetics can do much to mask lesions and scarring. Consider individual sensitivity to product ingredients when selecting cosmetics. Oil-free, hypoallergenic cosmetics are available and may be beneficial for the allergic patient. Rehabilitative cosmetics are available to help camouflage and deemphasize such lesions as *vitiligo* (loss of pigmentation), *melasma* (tan to brown patches on the face), or healed postoperative wound sites. These commercially available products are opaque, smudge resistant, and water resistant.

COSMETIC PROCEDURES

A vast array of cosmetic procedures is available, including chemical peels, toxin injections, fillers, laser surgery, breast enlargement and reduction (see Chapter 51), face-lift, eyelid-lift, and liposuction. Common cosmetic topical procedures are outlined in Table 23.13. Other types of cosmetic procedures include the injection of botulinum toxin (Botox), deoxycholic acid (Kybella), calcium hydroxylapatite (Radiesse), collagen (Zyplast), and hyaluronic acid fillers (e.g., Restylane, Perlane, Juvéderm).[15] Transitory side effects may occur, such as mild redness, pain, swelling, and bruising. Uncommon side effects from cosmetic procedures include allergic reaction, infection, grayish skin discoloration, or lumps at the injection sites. Tell the patient that the procedure will need repeating at prescribed intervals to maintain the desired appearance.

The reasons for undergoing these procedures are as varied as the techniques. The most common reason that people incur the discomfort and financial expense (most are not covered by health insurance) of a cosmetic procedure is to improve their body image. If they feel better about themselves after having cosmetic procedures, they often act more confident and self-assured. Often social position and economic considerations are part of the decision. Increased longevity is providing a larger population to whom cosmetic procedures are appealing.

Regardless of the patient's reasons for seeking a cosmetic procedure, maintain a supportive, nonjudgmental attitude. If the patient wishes to change or enhance a body feature perceived as unattractive and has realistic expectations about the outcome, you should support this decision.

Elective Surgery
Laser Surgery. Laser surgery is used to treat congenital and acquired vascular lesions (cherry angiomas, spider leg veins, hemangiomas, port wine stains, and tattoo removal) and for skin resurfacing and hair removal. Lasers can reduce scarring and fine wrinkles around the lips or eyes and remove facial lesions (Table 23.11). Swelling, redness, and bruising are common after treatment. The treated areas usually are kept moist

TABLE 23.13 Common Cosmetic Topical Procedures

Tretinoin (Retin-A, Renova)	Chemical Peels (e.g., Beta-Hydroxy Acid, Jessner's Peel, TCA)	Microdermabrasion	α-Hydroxy Acids (e.g., Glycolic Acid, Lactic Acid)
Indications			
Improves appearance of photodamaged skin, especially fine wrinkling. Reduces actinic keratoses	Improves appearance of photodamaged skin, acne scarring, actinic and seborrheic keratoses	Smoothes appearance of photodamaged and wrinkled skin, acne scarring	Smoothes appearance of photodamaged and wrinkled skin, acne scarring
Description			
Initially applied every 2–3 days. Treatment stopped if severe inflammation occurs. Maximum response in 8–12 mo	Solution applied in varying amounts to the skin, causing a controlled burn with a loss of melanin	Epidermis and top dermal layer removed by applying aluminum oxide or baking soda crystals. Re-epithelialization of abraded surface then occurs	Low concentrations (<10%) in many skin care products consumers can apply to the skin. Higher concentrations (50%–70%) applied only by an HCP
Side Effects			
Erythema, swelling, flaking, pigmentation changes. Teratogenic. Increases phototoxicity if taking other photosensitive drugs	Moderate swelling and crusting for 1 wk. Redness for 6–8 wk. Pink tone possible for several mo. Photosensitivity	Light pink tone that resolves within 24 hr. Photosensitivity	Photosensitivity, slight irritation at lower concentrations, severe redness, oozing, and flaking skin possible with higher concentrations
Patient Teaching			
Apply at night since preparation is inactivated by light. Apply emollients, use sunscreen, use sun avoidance measures, avoid using abrasive or drying facial cleansers for severe sensitivity (e.g., excess irritation)	Use sunscreen. Avoid sun for 6 mo to prevent hyperpigmentation	Generous application of emollients and sunscreen	Use sunscreen and sun avoidance measures

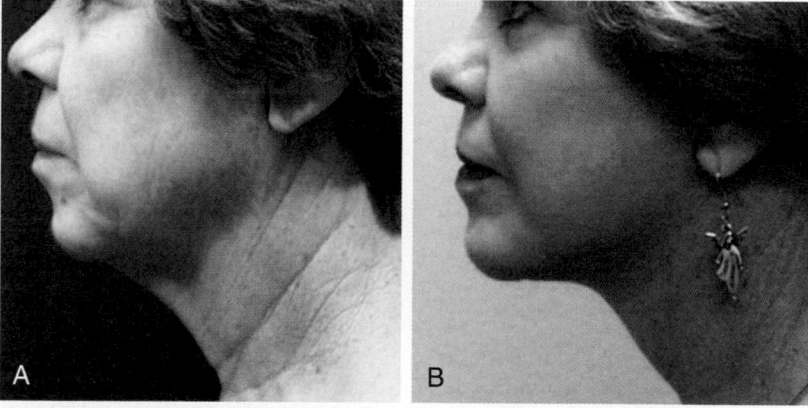

FIG. 23.14 Face-lift. A, Preoperative. B, Postoperative. (From Cuzalina A, Copty TV, Khan H: *Current therapy in oral and maxillofacial surgery*, St Louis, 2012, Elsevier.)

with ointment or occlusive dressings for the first few days. The patient must protect treated skin from the sun.

Face-Lift. A face-lift *(rhytidectomy)* is the lifting and repositioning of the lower two thirds of the face and neck to improve appearance (Fig. 23.14). Indications for this procedure include:

- Redundant soft tissue or scarring resulting from disease (e.g., acne scarring)
- Asymmetric redundancy of soft tissues (e.g., facial palsy)
- Redundant soft tissue resulting from trauma
- Preauricular lesions
- Redundant soft tissues resulting from *solar elastosis* (sagging of the skin from sun damage), changes in body weight, and the effects of gravity
- Restoration of body image

The surgical approach and lines of incisions vary according to the desired correction and the position of the hairline. Eyelid-lifts *(blepharoplasty)* can remove redundant tissue and possibly improve the field of vision. Preventing hematoma formation is the most important postoperative consideration. Ice packs are usually applied for the first 24 to 48 hours to reduce swelling and decrease the possibility of hematoma formation. Usually the pain is minimal. Antibiotics are used at the HCP's discretion. Complications can occur if the person smokes or is involved in vigorous exercise.

Liposuction. Liposuction is a technique for removing subcutaneous fat to improve facial and body contours. Although not a substitute for diet and exercise, it can be successful in removing areas of fat from almost any body area that is resistant to other techniques.

Liposuction is relatively free of complications. Possible contraindications include the use of anticoagulants, uncontrolled hypertension, diabetes, and poor cardiovascular status. Those under 40 years of age with good skin elasticity are the best candidates. However, patients over 40 can be treated successfully.

The procedure is usually done on an outpatient basis under local anesthesia. One or more sessions may be needed, depending on the size of the area. The HCP inserts a blunt-tipped cannula through a small incision and pushes into the fat to break it loose from the fibrous stroma. Multiple repeated thrusts disrupt the fat and create tunnels. The loosened fat is removed with a powerful suction. Afterward, firm pressure is applied to the wounds until drainage stops.[16] It may take several months for the results to be evident.

❖ NURSING MANAGEMENT: COSMETIC SURGERY

Many cosmetic surgical procedures are done in well-equipped day-surgery units or in dermatologist or plastic surgeon in-office surgery suites.

◆ Preoperative Management

A major consideration before surgery relates to informed consent and realistic expectations of what cosmetic surgery can accomplish. Although the HCP should provide this information, reinforce it and answer questions and concerns. For instance, a face-lift has little or no effect on deep wrinkling of the forehead and temples, deep nasolabial grooves, or vertical lip wrinkles. Before-and-after treatment photographs of similar cases are often useful in helping the patient to set realistic expectations.

Your teaching plan should include the timeframe for healing. Explain the oozing, crusting stage of an abrasive procedure so the patient can plan time off from work if necessary. Since wound healing may not be complete for 1 year, the patient should not expect complete results at once. The final result is affected by the patient's age, general state of health, and skin type and the extent (severity) of the condition being treated. Efforts should be made to correct or control any existing health problem before the procedure.

◆ Postoperative Management

Most cosmetic procedures are not extremely painful. Usually, mild analgesics are enough to keep the patient comfortable. Although infection is not a common problem after cosmetic surgery, assess the sites for signs of infection. Teach the patient signs and symptoms of infection. Stress that it is important to report them at once so that treatment can be started.

If the surgery involved a change in the skin's circulation, as in a face-lift, carefully monitor for adequate circulation. Warm, pink skin that blanches on pressure shows that adequate circulation is present in the surgical area. Supportive, compressive dressings and ice packs may be necessary early in the postoperative period.

SKIN GRAFTS

Uses

Skin grafts may be necessary to protect underlying structures or to reconstruct areas for cosmetic or functional purposes. They may be used to facilitate rapid closure and minimize complications. Ideally, wounds heal by primary intention. However, large wounds, surgically created wounds, trauma, and chronic wounds can result in extensive tissue destruction, making healing by primary intention impossible. In these cases, skin grafting may be necessary to close the defect. Improved surgical techniques make it possible to graft skin, bone, cartilage, fat, fascia, muscles, and nerves. For cosmetically pleasing results, the color, thickness, texture, and hair-growing nature of skin used for grafting should match the recipient site. See Chapter 24 for a discussion of skin grafting for patients with burn injuries.

Types

The two types of traditional skin grafts are free grafts and skin flaps. Free grafts are classified according to how they supply blood to the grafted skin. One method is to transfer the graft (epidermis and part or all the dermis) to the recipient site from the donor site. The *autograft* (from the patient's own body) or *isograft* (from an identical twin) revascularizes and becomes fixed to the new site. The other method of free skin grafting is by *reconstructive microsurgery*. With the use of an operating microscope, the HCP establishes circulation immediately in the graft by connecting blood vessels in the skin flap to vessels in the recipient site.

Skin flaps involve moving a section of skin and subcutaneous tissue from one part of the body to another without terminating the vascular attachment *(pedicle)*. Skin flaps are used to cover wounds with a poor vascular bed, provide padding when needed, and cover wounds over cartilage and bone. The patient may need intermediate flap placement if the recipient site is far removed from the donor site. For instance, a skin flap from the thigh to the head would require an intermediate graft. The flap is advanced to the recipient site when circulation is well established at the intermediate site. The patient's needs and the type of defect determine the type of flap and the route of transfer.

Soft tissue expansion is a technique for providing skin (1) for resurfacing of a defect, such as a burn scar; (2) for removal of a disfiguring mark (e.g., a tattoo); or (3) as a preliminary step in breast reconstruction. A subcutaneous tissue expander of a proper size and shape is placed under the skin, usually as an outpatient procedure. Weekly expansion with saline solution can be done in a health care setting or by the patient at home. This expansion procedure is repeated until the skin reaches the size needed for the repair. This may take from several weeks to 3 to 4 months. Once enough skin is available, the old incision is opened, the expander is removed, and the soft tissue is ready to be used as an advancement flap. The tissue expander next to a defect has the primary tissue characteristics, such as color and texture.

Engineered skin substitutes (e.g., Apligraf, Dermagraft, Integra) are gaining popularity. There are several available, each with its own indications and benefits. Some are two-layered membranes with both dermal and epidermal components. Others are only one layer. The skin is engineered from neonatal foreskins and cadavers. Skin substitutes do not contain structures such as blood vessels, hair follicles, sweat glands, or cells such as melanocytes, Langerhans cells, macrophages, and lymphocytes.[17] Engineered skin grafts have an extended shelf life. Some are cryopreserved, others shipped overnight as they are needed. Advantages include ready availability, the avoidance of a donor site, application in outpatient settings, minimal scarring, and less pain.

CASE STUDY

Melanoma and Dysplastic Nevi

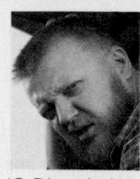

(© Dimedrol68/ iStock/Think stock.)

Patient Profile

G.L. is a 48-yr-old white, fair-skinned man who is a long-distance truck driver. In his leisure time, he enjoys swimming. He comes to the clinic because of a changing lesion on his left arm.

Subjective Data

- History of a basal cell cancer (BCC) on his left ear in the last 4 years
- Father treated for metastatic melanoma in the last 2 years
- First noted the lesion 1 month ago when it started changing size
- Anxious that removing the lesion will require extensive, disfiguring surgery

Objective Data

Physical Examination

- Has a 4-mm lesion, deep brown, scalloped with vaguely defined borders
- 5 dysplastic nevi found on back

Diagnostic Studies

- Excisional biopsy confirmed superficial spreading melanoma.
- Sentinel node biopsy results were negative.
- Diagnostic tests indicate melanoma stage I.

Discussion Questions

1. What risk factors for melanoma does he have?
2. What are the usual clinical manifestations associated with melanoma?
3. What is the prognosis for a patient with this stage of melanoma?
4. What treatment options are available for him?
5. **Priority Decision:** Based on the assessment data presented, what are the priority nursing diagnoses?
6. **Patient-Centered Care:** How would you help G.L. deal with his anxiety over the treatment outcomes?
7. **Priority Decision:** What is the priority of care for G.L.?
8. **Safety:** What would you include in his patient teaching plan to address future sun exposure?
9. **Evidence-Based Practice:** G.L. wants to know whether regularly applying sunscreen will reduce his risk for developing a second melanoma. How would you reply?

Answers available at *http://evolve.elsevier.com/Lewis/medsurg*.

BRIDGE TO NCLEX EXAMINATION

The number of the question corresponds to the same-numbered outcome at the beginning of the chapter.

1. Which safe sun practices would the nurse include in the teaching plan for a patient who has photosensitivity *(select all that apply)*?
   a. Wear protective clothing.
   b. Apply sunscreen liberally and often.
   c. Emphasize the short-term use of a tanning booth.
   d. Avoid exposure to the sun, especially during midday.
   e. Wear any sunscreen as long as it is bought at a drugstore.

2. When teaching a patient with melanoma about this disorder, the nurse recognizes that the patient's prognosis is *most* dependent on
   a. the thickness of the lesion.
   b. the degree of asymmetry in the lesion.
   c. the amount of ulceration in the lesion.
   d. how much the lesion has spread superficially.

3. The nurse determines that a patient with which disorder is *most* at risk for spreading the disease?
   a. Tinea pedis
   b. Impetigo on the face
   c. Candidiasis of the nails
   d. Psoriasis on the palms and soles

4. A mother and her two children have been diagnosed with pediculosis corporis at a health care center. An appropriate measure to treat this condition is
   a. applying pyrethrins to the body.
   b. topical application of griseofulvin.
   c. moist compresses applied frequently.
   d. administration of systemic antibiotics.

5. A common site for the lesions associated with atopic dermatitis is the
   a. buttocks.
   b. temporal area.
   c. antecubital space.
   d. plantar surface of the feet.

6. During the assessment of a patient, you note an area of red, sharply defined plaques covered with silvery scales that are mildly itchy on the patient's knees and elbows. You would describe this finding as
   a. lentigo.
   b. psoriasis.
   c. actinic keratosis.
   d. seborrheic keratosis.

7. In teaching a patient who is using topical corticosteroids to treat acute dermatitis, the nurse should tell the patient that *(select all that apply)*
   a. the cream form is the most efficient system of delivery.
   b. short-term use of topical corticosteroids usually does not cause systemic side effects.
   c. use a glove to apply small amounts of creams or ointments to prevent further infection.
   d. abruptly stopping the use of topical corticosteroids may cause the dermatitis to reappear.
   e. systemic side effects from topical corticosteroids are likely if the patient is malnourished.

8. Important patient teaching after a chemical peel includes
   a. avoidance of sun exposure.
   b. application of firm bandages.
   c. limitation of vigorous exercise.
   d. use of moist heat to relieve discomfort.

1. a, b, d, 2. a, 3. b, 4. a, 5. c, 6. b, 7. b, d, 8. a.

For rationales to these answers and even more NCLEX review questions, visit *http://evolve.elsevier.com/Lewis/medsurg*.

ⓔ EVOLVE WEBSITE/RESOURCE LIST

http://evolve.elsevier.com/Lewis/medsurg
Review Questions (Online Only)
Key Points
Answer Keys for Questions
- Rationales for Bridge to NCLEX Examination Questions
- Answer Guidelines for Case Study on p. 429

Nursing Care Plan
- eNursing Care Plan 23.1: Patient With Chronic Skin Lesions

Conceptual Care Map Creator
Audio Glossary
Supporting Media
- Animation
- Mohs Surgery

Content Updates

REFERENCES

*1. Tripp MK, Watson M, Balk SJ, et al: State of the science on prevention and screening to reduce melanoma incidence and mortality, *CA Can J Clin* 66:460, 2016.

2. US Food and Drug Administration: Sunscreen Innovation Act. Retrieved from *www.fda.gov/drugs/guidancecomplianceregulatoryinformation/ucm434782.htm*.

3. American Cancer Society: Skin cancer facts. Retrieved from *www.cancer.org/cancer/skin-cancer.html*.

4. Canavan T, Cantrell W: Recognizing melanoma: Diagnosis and treatment options, *TNP* 41:24, 2016.

*5. Verkouteren JA, Ramdas KH, Wakkee M, et al: Epidemiology of basal cell carcinoma: Scholarly review, *Br J Dermatol* 177:359, 2017.

*6. Green AC, Olsen CM: Cutaneous squamous cell carcinoma: An epidemiological review, *Br J Dermatol* 177:373, 2017.

*7. Coit DG, Thompson JA, Algazi A, et al: Melanoma, version 2.2016, NCCN clinical practice guidelines in oncology, *JCCN* 14:450, 2016.

8. Habif TP: *Clinical dermatology*, ed 6, St Louis, 2016, Saunders.

9. American Academy of Dermatology: Psoriasis. Retrieved from *www.aad.org/public/diseases/scaly-skin/psoriasis*.

*10. Cantrell W: Psoriasis and psoriatic therapies, *TNP* 42:35, 2017.

*11. Abrahamse H, Hamblin MR: New photosensitizers for photodynamic therapy, *Biochem J* 473:347, 2016.

*12. Stegman L: Electronic brachytherapy for nonmelanoma skin cancer, *Oncology Times* 39:38, 2017.

*13. Russo A, Concia E, Cristini F, et al: Current and future trends in antibiotic therapy of acute bacterial skin and skin-structure infections, *Clin Microbiol Infect* 22:S27, 2016.

14. Luger TA, McDonald I, Steinhoff M: *Clinical and basic immunodermatology*, New York, 2017, Springer.

*15. Costa CR, Kordestani R, Small KH, et al: Advances and refinement in hyaluronic acid facial fillers, *PRS* 138:233, 2016.

*16. Chia CT, Neinstein RM, Theodorou SJ: Evidence-based medicine: Liposuction, *PRS* 139:267, 2017.

17. Bryant R, Nix D: *Acute and chronic wound*, ed 5, St Louis, 2016, Mosby.

*Evidence-based information for clinical practice.

24

Burns

Cecilia Bidigare

Every life deserves a certain amount of dignity, no matter how poor or damaged the shell that carries it.

Rick Bragg

ⓔ http://evolve.elsevier.com/Lewis/medsurg/

CONCEPTUAL FOCUS

Coping	Nutrition	Tissue Integrity
Fluids and Electrolytes	Pain	
Infection	Perfusion	

LEARNING OUTCOMES

1. Relate the causes of burns to the prevention strategies for burn injuries.
2. Distinguish between partial-thickness and full-thickness burns.
3. Apply tools used to determine the severity of burns.
4. Compare the pathophysiology, clinical manifestations, complications, and interprofessional care throughout the 3 burn phases.
5. Compare the fluid and electrolyte shifts during the emergent and acute burn phases.
6. Outline the nutritional needs of the burn patient throughout the 3 burn phases.
7. Compare the various burn wound care techniques and surgical options for partial-thickness and full-thickness burn wounds.
8. Prioritize nursing interventions in the management of the burn patient's physiologic and psychosocial needs.
9. Examine the various physiologic and psychosocial aspects of burn rehabilitation.
10. Develop a plan of care to prepare the burn patient and caregiver for discharge.

KEY TERMS

burn, p. 431
carboxyhemoglobin, p. 433
chemical burns, p. 432
contracture, p. 448
cultured epithelial autograft (CEA), p. 447

debridement, p. 442
electrical burns, p. 433
escharotomy, p. 439
excision and grafting, p. 446
full-thickness burns, p. 434

partial-thickness burns, p. 434
smoke and inhalation injuries, p. 432
thermal burns, p. 432

The focus of this chapter is the care of patients who have a burn injury. A **burn** is an injury to the skin or other tissues of the body caused by heat, chemicals, electric current, or radiation. The resulting effects on tissue integrity are influenced by the temperature and type of burning agent, duration of contact, and type of tissue that is injured. The location of the injury, associated injuries, and age and general health of the patient influence the seriousness of the injury.

The patient with a burn injury may have a multitude of problems. There may be difficulty maintaining an airway and adequate circulation, affecting perfusion. Fluid and electrolyte imbalances are common. We must give attention to preventing malnutrition and infection. The patient often has fear, anger, guilt, and depression. The patient may have body image concerns, especially with facial and hand burns; anxiety about future therapy and surgery; and frustrations with ongoing pain.

An estimated 486,000 Americans seek medical care each year for burns.[1] Around 40,000 people are hospitalized, 60% receiving care in specialized burn centers. About 3275 Americans die annually as a direct result of their injuries. The highest fatality rates occur in children ages 4 years and younger and adults over age 65. Worldwide, over 11 million people need medical attention annually for burn injuries and about 180,000 die.[2] Although burn incidence in the United States has decreased over the past 20 years, international burn injuries still occur too often, mainly to those living in low- and middle-income counties. Most burn accidents are preventable. The focus of burn prevention has shifted from blaming victims to educating people in vulnerable communities to identify hazards and provide first aid.

Coordinated national prevention programs in higher income countries have focused on child-resistant lighters, tap water anti-scald devices, stricter building codes, having smoke detectors, and fire and burn safety education curriculums for schools.[3] As a nurse, you can advocate for and teach about burn risk-reduction strategies in the home and at work (Tables 24.1 and 24.2).

TABLE 24.1 Common Sources of Burn Injury

Home Hazards
Bathroom and Kitchen
- Hot water heaters set at 120°F (60°C) or higher
- Microwaved food
- Steam, hot grease or liquids from cooking

General Household
- Carelessness with cigarettes, matches, candles
- Heat lamps
- Fireplaces (e.g., gas, wood)
- Flammables (e.g., starter fluid, gasoline, kerosene)
- Frayed or defective wiring
- Multiple extension cords per outlet
- Open space heaters
- Outdoor grills (e.g., propane, charcoal)
- Radiators (e.g., home, automobile)

Occupational Hazards
- Cement
- Chemicals
- Combustible fuels
- Electricity from power lines
- Fertilizers, pesticides
- Hot metals
- Sparks from live electric sources
- Steam pipes
- Tar

 ## TABLE 24.2 Promoting Population Health

Strategies to Reduce Burn Injury

Chemical
- Store chemicals safely in approved containers and label clearly.
- Ensure safety of workers handling chemicals (education, protective eyewear, gloves, masks, clothing).

Electrical
- Avoid or repair frayed wiring.
- Avoid outdoor activities during electrical (i.e., lightning) storms.
- Ensure electrical power source is shut off before beginning repairs.
- Wear protective eyewear and gloves when making electrical repairs.

Flame or Contact
- Never smoke in bed.
- Use "child-resistant" lighters.
- Hold regular home fire exit drills.
- Never leave hot oil unattended while cooking.
- Never use gasoline or other flammable liquids to start a fire.
- Never leave candles unattended or near open windows or curtains.
- Consider a flame-retardant smoking apron for older or "at-risk" people.
- Exercise caution when microwaving food and beverages as they can get very hot.

Inhalation
- Install smoke and carbon monoxide detectors and change batteries annually (if appropriate).

Scald
- Use "anti-scald" devices with showerhead or faucet fixtures.
- Lower hot water temperature to the "lowest point" or 120°F (49°C).
- After running bath water, check temperature with back of hand or bath thermometer.
- Supervise bathing with small children, older adults, or anyone with impaired physical movement, physical sensation, or judgment.

TYPES OF BURN INJURY

Thermal Burns

Thermal burns, caused by flame, flash, scald, or contact with hot objects, are the most common type of burn injury (Fig. 24.1). The severity of the injury depends on the temperature of the burning agent and duration of contact time. Scald injuries often occur in bathrooms and kitchens. Flash, flame, or contact burns can occur while cooking, smoking, or burning leaves in the backyard.

Chemical Burns

Chemical burns are the result of contact with acids, alkalis, and organic compounds. In addition to skin damage, eyes can be injured if splashed. Acids are found in the home and at work. They include hydrochloric, oxalic, and hydrofluoric acid. Alkali burns can be more difficult to manage than acid burns since alkalis adhere to tissue, causing protein hydrolysis and melting. Alkalis are found in cement, oven and drain cleaners, and heavy industrial cleansers.[4] Organic compounds, including phenols (chemical disinfectants) and petroleum products (creosote and gasoline), produce contact burns and systemic toxicity.

Smoke and Inhalation Injury

Smoke and inhalation injuries from breathing noxious chemicals or hot air can damage the respiratory tract. Three types of smoke and inhalation injuries can occur: upper airway injury,

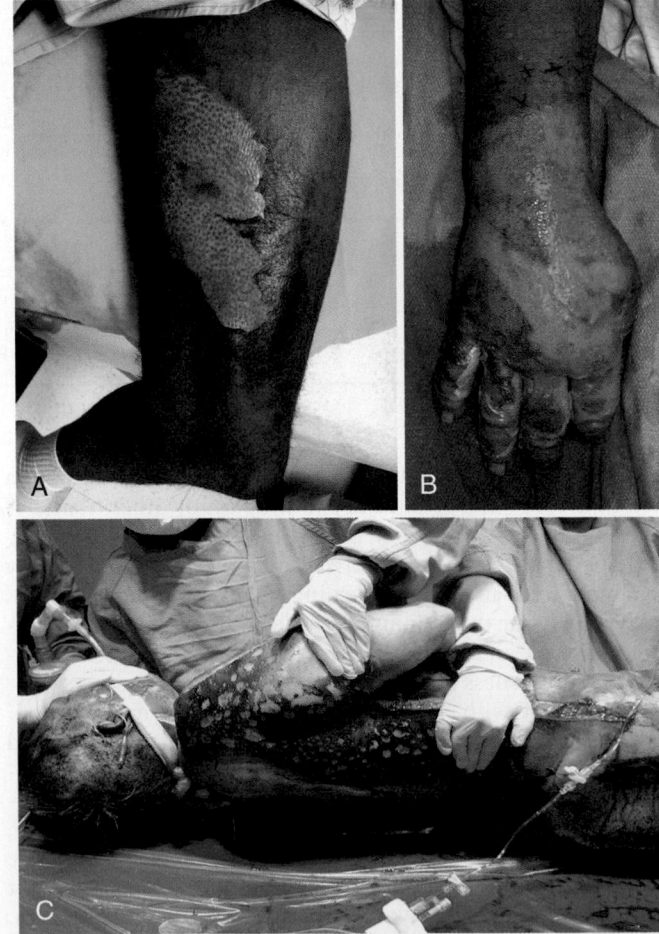

FIG. 24.1 Types of burn injury. **A,** Superficial, partial-thickness scald burn to thigh. **B,** Deep, partial-thickness flame burn to hand. **C,** Full-thickness flame burn to posterior chest and arm. (Courtesy Judy Knighton, Toronto, Canada.)

lower airway injury, and metabolic asphyxiation. Smoke inhalation injuries are a major predictor of mortality in burn patients. Rapid initial and ongoing assessment is critical. Airway compromise and pulmonary edema can quickly develop within hours of injury.[5]

Metabolic Asphyxiation. Most deaths at a fire scene are the result of inhaling certain smoke elements, primarily carbon monoxide (CO) or hydrogen cyanide. Oxygen delivery to or consumption by tissues is impaired, resulting in hypoxia. Death may occur if carboxyhemoglobin (i.e., hemoglobin combined with CO) blood levels are greater than 20%. CO and hydrogen cyanide poisoning may occur in the absence of burn injury to the skin.

Upper Airway Injury. Upper airway injury results from an inhalation injury to the mouth, oropharynx, and/or larynx. The injury may be caused by thermal burns or the inhalation of hot air, steam, or smoke. Mucosal burns of the oropharynx and larynx are manifested by redness, blistering, and edema (Table 24.3). The swelling can be massive and the onset rapid. Burns to the neck and chest may make breathing more difficult because of the burn eschar, which becomes tight and constricting. Edema from facial and neck burns can be lethal, as can internal pressure from edema narrowing the airway. Obstruction can occur quickly, presenting a true airway emergency.

Lower Airway Injury. An inhalation injury to the trachea, bronchioles, and alveoli is usually caused by breathing in toxic chemicals or smoke. Tissue damage is related to the duration of exposure to toxic fumes or smoke. Manifestations of lower airway lung injury are outlined in Table 24.3. Carefully assess the patient for facial burns, singed nasal hair, hoarseness, painful swallowing, darkened oral and nasal membranes, carbonaceous sputum, history of being burned in an enclosed space, and clothing burns around the neck and chest. Pulmonary edema may not appear until 12 to 48 hours after the burn. Then it may manifest as acute respiratory distress syndrome (ARDS) (see Chapter 67).

Electrical Burns

Electrical burns result from intense heat generated from an electric current. Direct damage to nerves and vessels, causing tissue anoxia and death, can occur. The severity of an electrical injury depends on the amount of voltage, tissue resistance,

current pathways, surface area in contact with the current, and length of time that the current flow was sustained (Fig. 24.2). Tissue densities offer various amounts of resistance to electric current. For example, fat and bone offer the most resistance. Nerves and blood vessels offer the least resistance. Current that passes through vital organs (e.g., brain, heart, kidneys) produces more life-threatening sequelae than that which passes through other tissues. In addition, electric sparks may ignite the patient's clothing, causing a flash injury.

As with inhalation injury, perform a rapid assessment of the patient with an electrical injury. Transfer to a burn center is indicated. The severity of an electrical injury can be hard to determine since most of the damage is below the skin.

Determining the electric current contact points and history of the injury may help reveal the likely path of the current and potential areas of injury. Contact with electric current can cause muscle contractions strong enough to fracture the long bones and vertebrae. Another reason to suspect long bone or spinal fractures is a fall resulting from the electrical injury. For this reason, consider cervical spine injury for all patients with electrical burns. Continue cervical spine immobilization during transport and diagnostic testing until injury is ruled out.

Electrical injury puts the patient at risk for dysrhythmias or cardiac arrest, severe metabolic acidosis, and myoglobinuria.[6] The electric shock can cause immediate heart standstill or ventricular fibrillation. Delayed dysrhythmias or arrest can occur without warning during the first 24 hours after injury. Whenever massive muscle and blood vessel damage occurs, myoglobin from injured muscle and hemoglobin from damaged red blood cells (RBCs) are released into the circulation. The myoglobin travels to the kidneys and can block the renal tubules. This can result in acute tubular necrosis (ATN) and acute kidney injury (see Chapter 46).

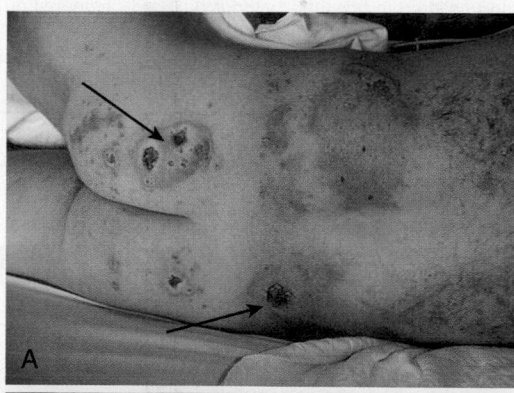
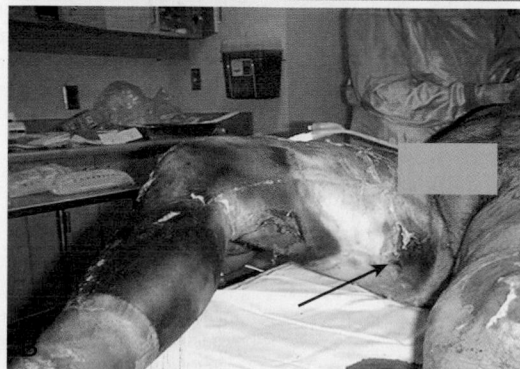

FIG. 24.2 Electrical injury produces heat coagulation of blood supply and contact area as electric current passes through the skin. **A,** Back and buttock *(arrows).* **B,** Leg *(arrow).* (Courtesy Judy Knighton, Toronto, Canada.)

TABLE 24.3 Manifestations of Burn-Related Lung Injury

Upper Airway
- Blisters, edema
- Copious secretions
- Difficulty swallowing
- Hoarseness
- Stridor
- Substernal and intercostal retractions
- Total airway obstruction

Lower Airway
- High degree of suspicion if patient was trapped in a fire in an enclosed space or clothing caught fire
- Altered mental status
- Carbonaceous sputum
- Dyspnea
- Facial burns or singed nasal or facial hair
- Hoarseness
- Wheezing

Cold Thermal Injury

Cold thermal injury, or frostbite, is discussed in Chapter 68.

CLASSIFICATION OF BURN INJURY

The treatment of burns is related to the severity of the injury.[7] Severity is determined by (1) depth of burn, (2) extent of burn calculated in percent of total body surface area (TBSA), (3) location of burn, and (4) age of the patient, preburn medical history, and circumstances or complicating factors. The American Burn Association (ABA) uses referral criteria to determine which burn injuries should be treated in burn centers (Table 24.4).[8] Patients with minor burn injuries can be managed in community hospitals.

TABLE 24.4 Burn Center Referral Criteria

Burn injuries that should be referred to a burn center include the following:

1. Partial thickness burns greater than 10% total body surface area (TBSA)
2. Burns that involve the face, hands, feet, genitalia, perineum, or major joints
3. Third-degree burns in any age-group
4. Electrical burns, including lightning injury
5. Chemical burns
6. Inhalation injury
7. Injury in patients with preexisting medical disorders that could complicate management, prolong recovery, or affect mortality
8. Any patient with burns and concomitant trauma (e.g., fractures) in which the burn injury poses the greatest risk for morbidity or mortality. In such cases, if the trauma poses the greater immediate risk, the patient may be initially stabilized in a trauma center before being transferred to a burn unit. Physician judgment will be necessary in such situations and should be in concert with the regional medical control plan and triage protocols
9. Burned children in hospitals without qualified personnel or equipment for the care of children
10. Burn injury in patients who will need special social, emotional, or rehabilitative intervention

Source: American Burn Association: Guidelines for the operation of burn centers. Retrieved from *http://ameriburn.org/wp-content/uploads/2017/05/burncenterreferralcriteria.pdf.*

Depth of Burn

Burn injury involves the destruction of the integumentary system. Table 24.5 compares the various burn classifications according to the depth of the burn injury. One system defines an injury by degrees as first, second, third, or fourth degree. The ABA recommends a more precise definition and classifies burns according to depth of skin destruction: **partial-thickness burns** and **full-thickness burns** (Fig. 24.3). If significant damage occurs to the dermis (i.e., a full-thickness burn), not enough skin cells remain to regenerate new skin. A permanent, alternative source of skin must be found.

Extent of Burn

Two common tools for determining the TBSA affected or the extent of a burn wound are the *Lund-Browder chart* (Fig. 24.4, *A*) and the *Rule of Nines* (Fig. 24.4, *B*). First-degree burns, equivalent to a sunburn, are not included when calculating TBSA. The Lund-Browder chart is considered more accurate because it considers the patient's age in proportion to relative body-area size. The Rule of Nines is often used for initial assessment of a burn patient because it is easy to remember. For irregular- or odd-shaped burns, the patient's hand (including the fingers) is 1% TBSA. Other tools include the *Sage Burn Diagram*, a free, Web-based tool for estimating TBSA burned (*www.sagediagram.com*). There are mobile applications (e.g., 3D Burn Report, Mersey Burns) that can estimate the percent of burn and fluid resuscitation needs.[9]

Location of Burn

The location of the burn injury influences the severity. Burns to the face and neck and circumferential burns to the chest or back may interfere with breathing because of obstruction from edema or leathery, devitalized burn tissue *(eschar)*. These burns may indicate possible smoke or inhalation injury.

Burns to the hands, feet, joints, and eyes are of concern because they make self-care difficult and may jeopardize future function. Burns to the hands and feet are challenging to manage because of superficial vascular and nerve supply systems that must be protected while the burn wounds are healing.

Burns of the ears and nose are at risk for infection as the skin is very thin and the underlying cartilage may be exposed. Burns

TABLE 24.5 Classification of Burn Injury Depth

Classification	Appearance	Possible Cause	Structures Involved
Partial-Thickness Skin Destruction			
Superficial (first-degree) burn	Erythema, blanching on pressure, pain and mild swelling, no vesicles or blisters (although after 24 hr skin may blister and peel)	Quick heat flash Superficial sunburn	Superficial epidermal damage with hyperemia. Tactile and pain sensation intact
Deep (second-degree) burn	Fluid-filled vesicles that are red, shiny, wet (if vesicles have ruptured). Severe pain caused by nerve injury. Mild to moderate edema	Chemicals Contact burns Electric current Flame Flash Scald Tar, cement	Epidermis and dermis involved to varying depths. Skin elements, from which epithelial regeneration occurs, remain viable
Full-Thickness Skin Destruction			
Third- and fourth-degree burns	Dry, waxy white, leathery, or hard skin. Visible thrombosed vessels. Insensitivity to pain because of nerve destruction. Possible involvement of muscles, tendons, and bones	Chemical Electric current Flame Scald Tar, cement	All skin elements and local nerve endings destroyed. Coagulation necrosis present. Surgical intervention required for healing

to the buttocks or perineum are at high risk for infection from urine or feces contamination. Circumferential burns to the extremities can cause circulation problems distal to the burn, with possible nerve damage to the affected extremity. Patients may develop compartment syndrome (see Chapter 62) from deep damage to muscles.

Patient Risk Factors

Any patient with preexisting heart, lung, or kidney disease has a poorer prognosis for recovery because of the increased demands placed on the body by a burn injury. The patient with diabetes or peripheral vascular disease is at high risk for delayed healing, especially with foot and leg burns.[10] General physical weakness from any chronic disease, including alcohol or drug use and malnutrition, makes it challenging for the patient to fully recover from a burn injury. The burn patient who has fractures, head injuries, or other trauma has a more difficult recovery.

PREHOSPITAL AND EMERGENCY CARE

At the scene of the injury, priority is given to removing the person from the source of the burn and stopping the burning process. Rescuers must protect themselves from being injured. In the case of electrical and chemical injuries, initial care involves removing the patient from contact with the electrical or chemical source.

Small thermal burns (10% or less of TBSA) should be covered with a clean, cool, tap water–dampened towel for the patient's comfort and protection until medical care is available. Cooling of the injured area (if small) within 1 minute helps minimize the depth of the injury. If the burn is large (greater than 10% TBSA) or an electrical or inhalation burn is suspected, and the patient is unresponsive, first focus your attention on CAB:

- *Circulation:* Check for presence of pulses and elevate the burned limb(s) above the heart to decrease pain and swelling.
- *Airway:* Check for patency, soot around nares and on the tongue, singed nasal hair, darkened oral or nasal membranes.
- *Breathing:* Check for adequacy of ventilation.

If the patient is responsive, your priorities would follow the order of the ABCs: airway, breathing, and circulation.

To prevent hypothermia, cool large burns for no more than 10 minutes. Do not immerse the burned body part in cool water because it may cause extensive heat loss. Never cover a burn with ice, since this can cause hypothermia and vasoconstriction of blood vessels, thus further reducing blood flow to the injury. Gently remove as much burned clothing as possible to prevent further tissue damage. Leave adherent clothing in place until the patient is transferred to a hospital. Wrap the patient in a dry, clean sheet or blanket to prevent further contamination of the wound and provide warmth.

Chemical burns are best treated by quickly removing any chemical particles or powder from the skin. Remove all clothing

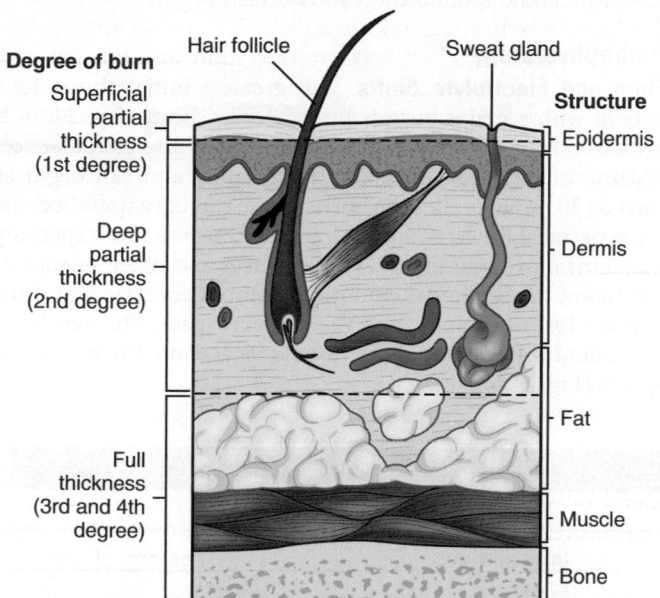

FIG. 24.3 Cross section of skin showing the depth of burn and structures involved.

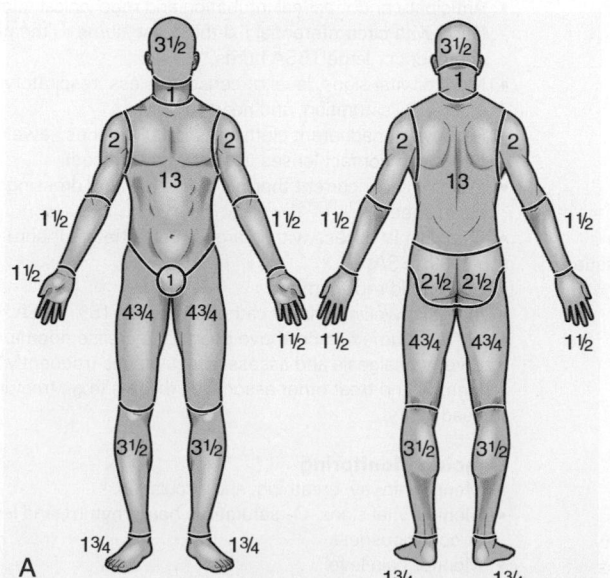

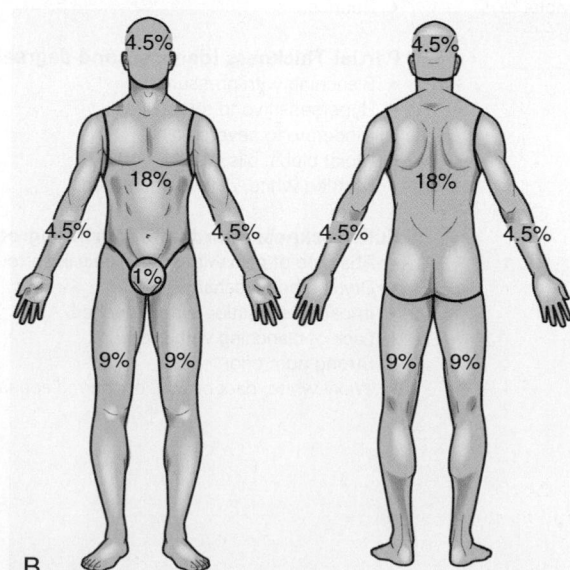

FIG. 24.4 A, Lund-Browder chart. By convention, areas of partial-thickness injury are colored in *blue* and areas of full-thickness injury in *red.* Superficial partial-thickness burns are not calculated. **B,** Rule of Nines chart.

containing the chemical because the burning process continues while the chemical is in contact with the skin. Flush the affected area with copious amounts of water to irrigate the skin from 20 minutes to 2 hours after exposure. Tap water is acceptable for flushing eyes exposed to chemicals. Tissue destruction may continue for up to 72 hours after contact with some chemicals.

Watch patients with inhalation injuries closely for signs of respiratory distress. These patients need to be treated quickly and efficiently if they are to survive. If CO poisoning is suspected, treat the patient with 100% humidified O_2. Patients who have both burns and an inhalation injury must be transferred to the nearest burn center.

Always remember that the burn patient may have sustained other injuries that could take priority over the burn itself. Persons involved in the prehospital phase of burn care must fully share the circumstances of the injury to emergency department (ED) staff. This is especially important if the patient was trapped in a closed space, exposed to hazardous chemicals or electricity, or had a possible traumatic injury (e.g., fall).

Prehospital and emergency care are outlined in tables that describe thermal burns (Table 24.6), inhalation injury (Table 24.7), electrical burns (Table 24.8), and chemical burns (Table 24.9).

PHASES OF BURN MANAGEMENT

Burn management can be organized chronologically into 3 phases: emergent (resuscitative), acute (wound healing), and rehabilitative (restorative). Overlap in care does exist.

For example, the emergent phase begins at the time of the burn injury, and care often begins prehospital or in the ED. Wound care is the primary focus of the acute phase, but wound care takes place in both the emergent and rehabilitation phases. Planning for rehabilitation begins on the day of the burn injury or admission to the burn center. Formal rehabilitation begins as soon as functional assessments can be done.

EMERGENT PHASE

The *emergent (resuscitative) phase* is the time needed to resolve the immediate, life-threatening problems resulting from the burn injury. This phase usually lasts up to 72 hours from the time the burn occurred. The main concerns are the onset of hypovolemic shock and edema formation. The emergent phase ends when fluid mobilization and diuresis begin.

Pathophysiology

Fluid and Electrolyte Shifts. The greatest initial threat to a patient with a major burn is hypovolemic shock (Fig. 24.5). It is caused by a massive shift of fluids out of the blood vessels because of increased capillary permeability and can begin as early as 20 minutes after the burn. As the capillary walls become more permeable, water, sodium, and plasma proteins (especially albumin) move into the interstitial spaces and other surrounding tissue. The colloidal osmotic pressure decreases with progressive loss of protein from the vascular space. This results in more fluid shifting out of the vascular space into the interstitial spaces (Fig. 24.6).

✚ TABLE 24.6 Emergency Management

Thermal Burns

Etiology	Assessment Findings	Interventions
• Flash flame • Hot liquids or solids • Hot surface • Open flame • Steam • Ultraviolet rays	**Partial-Thickness (superficial; first-degree) Burn** • Blanching with pressure • Minimal edema • Moderate to severe tenderness • Pain • Redness **Partial-Thickness (deep; second-degree) Burn** • Blanching with pressure • Hypersensitive to touch or air • Moderate to severe pain • Moist blebs, blisters • Mottled white, pink to cherry-red **Full-Thickness (third- and fourth-degree) Burns** • Absence of pain with severe pain in surrounding tissues • Dry, leathery eschar • Impaired sensation when touched • Lack of blanching with pressure • Strong burn odor • Waxy white, dark brown, or charred appearance	**Initial** • If unresponsive, assess circulation, airway, and breathing. • If responsive, monitor airway, breathing, and circulation. • Assess for inhalation injury. • Provide supplemental O_2 as needed. • Anticipate endotracheal intubation and mechanical ventilation with circumferential full-thickness burns to the neck and chest or large TBSA burns. • Monitor vital signs, level of consciousness, respiratory status, O_2 saturation, and heart rhythm. • Remove nonadherent clothing, shoes, watches, jewelry, glasses or contact lenses (if face was exposed). • Cover any concurrent thermal burns with dry dressings or clean sheet. • Establish IV access with 2 large-bore catheters if burn >15% TBSA. • Begin fluid replacement. • Insert indwelling urinary catheter if burn >15% TBSA. • Elevate burned limbs above heart to decrease edema. • Give IV analgesia and assess effectiveness frequently. • Identify and treat other associated injuries (e.g., fractures, head injury). **Ongoing Monitoring** • Monitor airway, breathing, and circulation. • Monitor vital signs, O_2 saturation, heart rhythm, and level of consciousness. • Monitor pain level. • Monitor urine output.

TBSA, Total body surface area.

✚ TABLE 24.7 Emergency Management
Inhalation Injury

Etiology	Assessment Findings	Interventions
• Exposure of respiratory tract to intense heat or flames • Inhalation of noxious chemicals, smoke, or CO • Occurs with being trapped in an enclosed space, being in an explosion, or having clothing catch fire	• Altered mental status, including confusion, coma • Carbonaceous sputum • Cherry-red skin color (CO levels >20%) • Coughing • Darkened oral or nasal membranes • Decreased O_2 saturation • Difficulty swallowing • Dysrhythmias • Increasing hoarseness • Irritation of upper airways or burning pain in throat or chest • Productive cough with black, gray, or bloody sputum • Rapid, shallow respirations • Restlessness, anxiety • Singed nasal or facial hair • Smoky breath	**Initial** • If unresponsive, assess circulation, airway, and breathing. • If responsive, monitor airway, breathing, and circulation. • Assess for concurrent thermal burn. • Provide 100% humidified O_2. • Anticipate endotracheal intubation and mechanical ventilation with significant inhalation injury. • Monitor vital signs, level of consciousness, O_2 saturation, and heart rhythm. • Obtain arterial blood gas, carboxyhemoglobin levels, and chest x-ray. • Remove nonadherent clothing, jewelry, glasses, or contact lenses (if face was exposed). • Establish IV access with 2 large-bore catheters if burn >15% TBSA. • Begin fluid replacement. • Insert indwelling urinary catheter if burn >15% TBSA. • Elevate burned limb(s) above heart to decrease edema. • Give IV analgesia and assess effectiveness frequently. • Identify and treat other associated injuries (e.g., fractures, pneumothorax, head injury). • Cover concurrent burned areas with dry dressings or clean sheet. • Anticipate need for fiberoptic bronchoscopy or intubation. **Ongoing Monitoring** • Monitor airway, breathing, and circulation. • Monitor vital signs, O_2 saturation, heart rhythm, and level of consciousness. • Monitor pain level. • Monitor urine output.

CO, Carbon monoxide; *TBSA*, total body surface area.

✚ TABLE 24.8 Emergency Management
Electrical Burns

Etiology	Assessment Findings	Interventions
• Defibrillator • Electric wires • Lightning • Utility wires	• Burn odor • Cardiac arrest • Depth and extent of wound difficult to see • Assume injury greater than what is seen • Decreased peripheral circulation in injured extremity • Dysrhythmias • Fractures or dislocations from force of current • Impaired touch sensation • Leathery, white, or charred skin • Location of contact points • Loss of consciousness • Minimal or absent pain • Neck or head injury if fall occurred • Thermal burns if clothing ignites	**Initial** • Remove patient from electrical source while protecting rescuer. • If unresponsive, assess circulation, airway, and breathing. • If responsive, monitor airway, breathing, and circulation. • Provide supplemental O_2 as needed. • Monitor vital signs, heart rhythm, level of consciousness, respiratory status, and O_2 saturation. • Remove nonadherent clothing, shoes, watches, jewelry, glasses or contact lenses (if face was exposed). • Cover burned areas with dry dressings or clean sheet. • Establish IV access with 2 large-bore catheters if burn >15% TBSA. • Begin fluid replacement. • Identify entrance and exit wounds. • Obtain arterial blood gas to assess acid-base balance. • Insert indwelling urinary catheter if burn >15% TBSA. • Elevate burned limb(s) above heart to decrease edema. • Give IV analgesia and assess effectiveness frequently. • Identify and treat other associated injuries (e.g., fractures, head injury, thermal burns). **Ongoing Monitoring** • Monitor airway, breathing, and circulation. • Monitor vital signs, O_2 saturation, heart rhythm, level of consciousness, and neurovascular status of injured limbs. • Monitor pain level. • Monitor urine output. • Monitor urine for development of myoglobinuria from muscle breakdown and hemoglobinuria from RBC breakdown. • Anticipate possible administration of $NaHCO_3$ to alkalinize the urine and maintain serum pH >6.0.

NaHCO₃, Sodium bicarbonate; *TBSA*, total body surface area.

✚ TABLE 24.9 Emergency Management

Chemical Burns

Etiology	Assessment Findings	Interventions
• Acids • Alkalis • Organic compounds	• Burning • Decreased muscle coordination (if organo-phosphate) • Discoloration of injured skin • Edema of surrounding tissue • Localized pain • Paralysis, redness, swelling of injured tissue • Respiratory distress if chemical inhaled • Tissue destruction continuing for up to 72 hr	**Initial** • If unresponsive, assess circulation, airway, and breathing before decon-tamination procedures. • If responsive, monitor airway, breathing, and circulation. • Provide supplemental O_2 as needed. • Brush dry chemical from skin before irrigation. • Remove nonadherent clothing, shoes, watches, jewelry, glasses or con-tact lenses (if face was exposed). • Flush chemical from wound and surrounding area with copious amounts of saline solution or water. • For chemical burn of the eye(s), flush from inner to outer corner of eye with water or lactated Ringer's (if available). • Cover burned areas with dry dressings or clean sheet. • Establish IV access with 2 large-bore catheters if burn >15% TBSA. • Begin fluid replacement. • Insert indwelling urinary catheter if burn >15% TBSA. • Elevate burned limb(s) above heart to decrease edema. • Give IV analgesia and assess effectiveness frequently. • Contact poison control center. **Ongoing Monitoring** • Monitor airway if exposed to chemicals. • Monitor pain level. • Monitor urine output. • Consider systemic impact of identified chemical. Monitor and treat accordingly. • Monitor pH of eye if exposed to chemicals.

TBSA, Total body surface area.

PATHOPHYSIOLOGY MAP

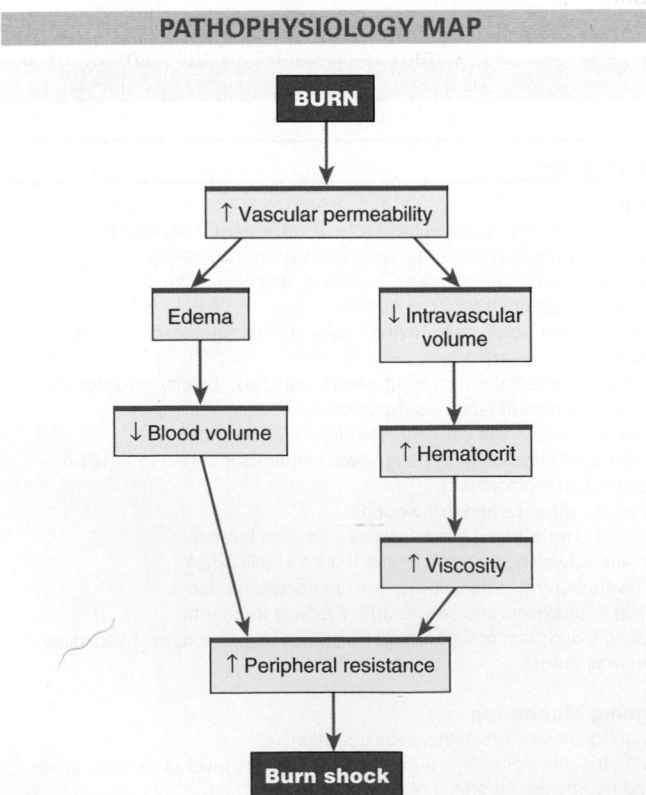

FIG. 24.5 At the time of major burn injury, there is increased capillary permeability. All fluid components of the blood begin to leak into the interstitium, causing edema and a decreased blood volume. Hematocrit increases, and the blood becomes more viscous. The combination of decreased blood volume and increased viscosity produces increased peripheral resistance. Burn shock, a type of hypovolemic shock, rapidly ensues and, if not corrected, can result in death.

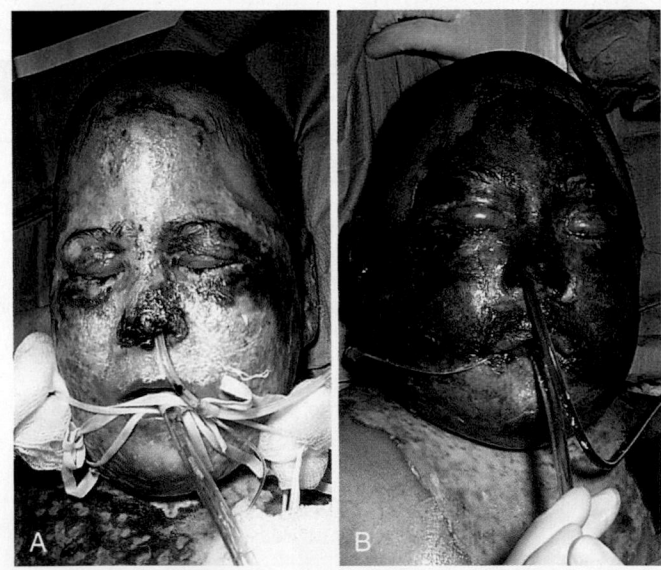

FIG. 24.6 A, Facial edema before fluid resuscitation. B, Facial edema after 24 hours. (Courtesy Judy Knighton, Toronto, Canada.)

Fluid moves to areas that normally have minimal to no fluid, a phenomenon termed *third spacing*. Examples of third spacing in burn injury are exudate and blister formation, as well as edema in unburned areas.

Other sources of fluid loss are insensible losses by evaporation from large, denuded body surfaces and the lungs. The normal insensible loss of 30 to 50 mL/hr is higher in the severely burned patient. The net result of the fluid shifts and losses is termed *intravascular volume depletion*. Signs of hypovolemic shock include decreased BP and increased heart rate. If hypovolemic shock is not corrected, refractory shock and death may result. (Shock is discussed in Chapter 66.)

The circulatory system is affected by the hemolysis of RBCs from circulating factors (e.g., oxygen free radicals) released at the time of the burn and the direct insult of the burn injury. Thrombosis in the capillaries of burned tissue causes loss of more circulating RBCs. A high hematocrit is often caused by hemoconcentration due to fluid loss. After fluid balance is restored, the hematocrit levels return to normal.

Major electrolyte shifts of sodium and potassium occur during this phase. A potassium shift develops first because injured cells and hemolyzed RBCs release potassium into the circulation. Sodium rapidly moves to the interstitial spaces and stays there until edema formation ends (Fig. 24.7).

Toward the end of the emergent phase, capillary membrane permeability is restored if fluid replacement is adequate. Interstitial fluid gradually returns to the vascular space (Fig. 24.7). Diuresis occurs, and the urine has a low specific gravity.

Inflammation and Healing. Burn injury to tissues and vessels causes coagulation necrosis. Neutrophils and monocytes accumulate at the site of injury. Fibroblasts and newly formed collagen fibrils appear and begin wound repair within the first 6 to 12 hours after injury. (The inflammatory response is discussed in Chapter 11.)

Immunologic Changes. A burn injury challenges the body's immune system. The skin barrier to invading organisms is destroyed. Bone marrow depression occurs and circulating levels of immunoglobulins decrease. Defects occur in the function of white blood cells (WBCs). The inflammatory cytokine cascade, triggered by tissue damage, impairs the function of lymphocytes, monocytes, and neutrophils. Thus the patient is at a greater risk for infection.

Clinical Manifestations

The patient with severe burns is likely to be in shock from hypovolemia. Often the areas of full-thickness and deep

partial-thickness burns are at first painless because the nerve endings have been destroyed. Superficial to moderate partial-thickness burns are very painful. Blisters, filled with fluid and protein, are common in partial-thickness burns. The patient with a larger burn may develop a paralytic ileus, with absent or decreased bowel sounds. Shivering may occur because of chilling that is caused by heat loss, anxiety, or pain.

The patient may be alert and able to answer questions shortly after admission or until intubated (if there is respiratory compromise). Patients are often frightened and need your calm reassurances. Give simple explanations of what to expect as you provide care. Unconsciousness or altered mental status in a burn patient usually results from hypoxia associated with smoke inhalation. Other possibilities include head trauma, substance use, or excess amounts of sedation or pain medication.

Complications

The three major organ systems most susceptible to complications during the emergent phase of burn injury are the cardiovascular, respiratory, and urinary systems.

Cardiovascular System. Cardiovascular complications include dysrhythmias and hypovolemic shock. These, if untreated, may progress to irreversible shock. Circulation to the extremities can be severely impaired by deep circumferential burns and subsequent edema formation, which act like a tourniquet. If untreated, ischemia, paresthesia, and necrosis can occur. An *escharotomy* (an incision through the full-thickness eschar) is often done to restore circulation to compromised extremities or improve chest expansion (Fig. 24.8).

Initially, blood viscosity increases because of the fluid loss. Microcirculation is impaired because of the damage to skin structures that contain small capillary systems. This results in a phenomenon termed *sludging*. Sludging is corrected by adequate fluid replacement.

Burn patients are at an increased risk for venous thromboembolism (VTE) if 1 or more of the following conditions are present: advanced age, obesity, extensive or lower extremity burns, concomitant lower extremity trauma, and prolonged immobility. VTE prophylaxis with anticoagulant drugs should be started, unless contraindicated.[11]

Respiratory System. The respiratory system is vulnerable to 2 types of injury: (1) upper airway burns and (2) lower airway

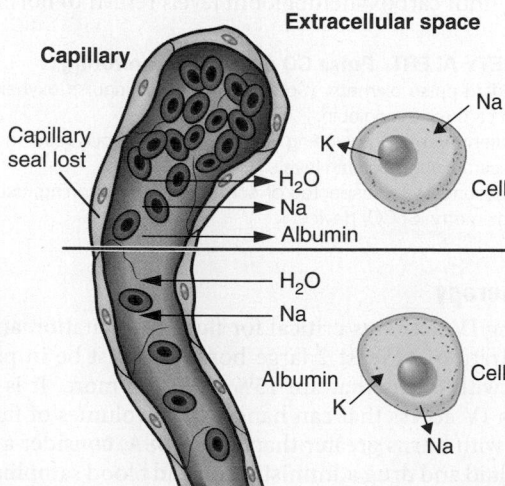

FIG. 24.7 The effects of burn shock are shown above the *purple line*. As the capillary seal is lost, interstitial edema develops. Cellular integrity is altered, with sodium (Na) moving into the cell in abnormal amounts and potassium (K) leaving the cell. The shifts after the resolution of burn shock are shown below the *blue line*. The water and sodium move back into the circulating volume through the capillary. Albumin stays in the interstitium. Potassium is transported into the cell and sodium is transported out as cellular integrity returns.

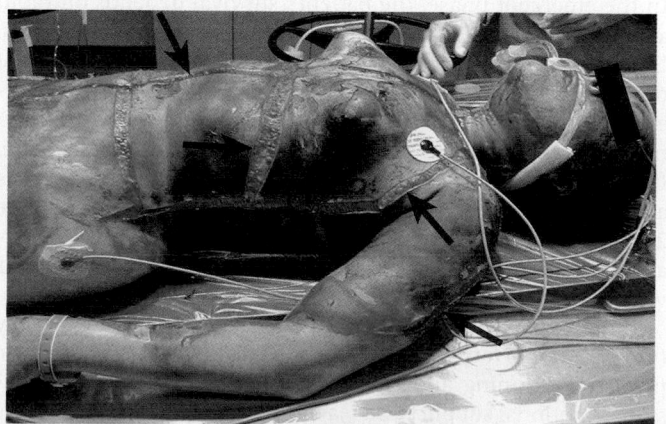

FIG. 24.8 Escharotomies of the anterior and lateral chest and arm (indicated by *arrows*). (Courtesy Judy Knighton, Toronto, Canada.)

injury (Table 24.3). Upper airway distress may occur with or without smoke inhalation, and airway injury at either level may occur in the absence of burn injury to the skin. (Smoke and inhalation injuries are discussed earlier in this chapter on pp. 432-433.)

The patient may need a fiberoptic bronchoscopy and carboxyhemoglobin blood levels to confirm a suspected inhalation injury. Look in the prehospital and ED notes to see if the patient was exposed to smoke or fumes. Examine any sputum for carbon. Watch for signs of respiratory distress, such as increased agitation, anxiety, restlessness, or a change in the rate or character of the patient's breathing, as symptoms may not be present at first.

In general, there is no correlation between the percentage TBSA burn (% TBSA) and the severity of inhalation injury. In a patient with inhalation injury, a chest x-ray may appear normal on admission, but changes can occur over the next 24 to 48 hours. Arterial blood gas (ABG) values may be within the normal range on admission and change over time.

Other Cardiopulmonary Problems. Patients with preexisting heart disease (e.g., myocardial infarction) or lung disease (e.g., chronic obstructive pulmonary disease [COPD]) are at an increased risk for complications. If fluid replacement is too vigorous, watch for early signs of heart failure or pulmonary edema. Invasive measures (e.g., hemodynamic monitoring) may be needed to monitor fluid resuscitation.

Patients with preexisting lung disease are more likely to develop a respiratory infection. Pneumonia, a common complication of major burns, is the leading cause of death in patients with an inhalation injury.[12]

Urinary System. The most common complication of the urinary system in the emergent phase is ATN. If your patient becomes hypovolemic, blood flow to the kidneys is decreased, causing renal ischemia. If this continues, acute kidney injury may develop.

With full-thickness and major electrical burns, myoglobin (from muscle cell breakdown) and hemoglobin (from RBC breakdown) are released into the bloodstream and block renal tubules. Carefully monitor the adequacy of fluid replacement because this can reverse the obstruction of the tubules.

❖ NURSING AND INTERPROFESSIONAL MANAGEMENT: EMERGENT PHASE

In the emergent phase, the patient's survival depends on rapid and thorough assessment and appropriate interventions. Usually the HCP and you make an initial assessment of the depth and extent of the burn and coordinate the actions of others on the health care team. In a community hospital, determine whether the patient needs inpatient or outpatient care. In the case of inpatient care, decide whether the patient stays at the hospital or must be transferred to a burn center (Table 24.4). Care mainly focuses on airway management, fluid therapy, and wound care (Table 24.10). Patients can improve or worsen, unpredictably.

Although physical therapy (PT) and occupational therapy (OT) are important in both the acute and rehabilitation phases, proper positioning and splinting begin on the day of admission. Emotional support and teaching of patients and caregivers begin on admission. A nursing care plan for the patient with burn injury (eNursing Care Plan 24.1) is available on the website for this chapter.

◆ Airway Management

Airway management often involves early endotracheal (preferably orotracheal) intubation.[14] Early intubation removes the need for emergency tracheostomy after respiratory problems have become apparent. In general, the patient with burns to the face and neck needs intubation within 1 to 2 hours after injury. Intubation is discussed in Chapter 65.

After intubation, the patient is placed on ventilatory support, with settings based on ABG results. Extubation may occur when the edema resolves. This is usually 3 to 6 days after burn injury unless severe inhalation injury exists. Chest escharotomy may be needed to relieve respiratory distress with circumferential, full-thickness burns of the neck and chest (Fig. 24.8).

A fiberoptic bronchoscopy should be done to assess the lower airway within 6 to 12 hours after injury if smoke inhalation is suspected. When intubation is not done, treatment of inhalation injury includes giving 100% humidified O_2. Place the patient in a high Fowler's position, unless contraindicated (e.g., spinal injury). Encourage deep breathing and coughing every hour. Reposition the patient every 1 to 2 hours. Provide suctioning and chest physiotherapy.

If severe respiratory distress (e.g., hoarseness, shortness of breath) develops, intubation and mechanical ventilation are started. Positive end-expiratory pressure (PEEP) may be used to prevent collapse of the alveoli and progressive respiratory failure (see Chapters 65 and 67). Bronchodilators may be given to treat severe bronchospasm. CO poisoning is treated by giving 100% O_2 until carboxyhemoglobin levels return to normal.

> **⚠ SAFETY ALERT Pulse CO Oximetry Monitoring**
> - Standard pulse oximetry (SpO_2) does not distinguish oxyhemoglobin from carboxyhemoglobin.
> - A patient with CO poisoning will have normal SpO_2 readings despite high carboxyhemoglobin levels.
> - For patients with suspected or confirmed CO poisoning, use a pulse CO oximetry (SpCO) device.

◆ Fluid Therapy

Obtaining IV access is critical for fluid resuscitation and drug administration. At least 2 large-bore IVs must be in place for patients with burns that are 15% TBSA or more. It is critical to obtain IV access that can handle large volumes of fluid. For patients with burns greater than 30% TBSA, consider a central line for fluid and drug administration and blood sampling (central lines are discussed in Chapter 16). An arterial line is often placed if frequent ABGs or invasive BP monitoring is needed.

Assess the extent of the burn wound using a standardized tool (Fig. 24.4). Then use a standardized formula to estimate the patient's fluid resuscitation needs. Fluid replacement is achieved with crystalloid solutions (usually lactated Ringer's), colloids (albumin), or a combination of the two. IV saline is usually started during the prehospital phase.

TABLE 24.10 Interprofessional Care

Burn Injury

Emergent Phase	Acute Phase	Rehabilitation Phase
Fluid Therapy (Table 24.11) • Assess fluid needs. • Begin IV fluid replacement. • Insert indwelling urinary catheter. • Monitor urine output.	**Fluid Therapy** • Continue to replace fluids, depending on patient's clinical response.	• Continue to teach patient and caregiver about wound care. • Continue to encourage and aid patient in resuming self-care. • Continue to prevent or minimize contractures. • Assess risk for scarring (surgery, physical and occupational therapy, splinting, pressure garments). • Discuss possible reconstructive surgery. • Prepare for discharge home or transfer to rehabilitation hospital. • Discuss possible need for home care nursing.
Wound Care • Start daily shower and wound care. • Debride as needed. • Assess extent and depth of burns. • Give tetanus toxoid or tetanus antitoxin.	**Wound Care** • Continue daily shower and wound care. • Continue debridement (if needed). • Assess wound daily and adjust dressing protocols as needed. • Observe for complications (e.g., infection).	
Pain and Anxiety • Assess and manage pain and anxiety.	**Early Excision and Grafting** • Provide temporary allografts. • Provide permanent autografts. • Care for donor sites.	
Physical and Occupational Therapy • Place patient in position that prevents contracture formation and reduces edema. • Assess need for splints.	**Pain and Anxiety** • Continue to assess for and treat pain and anxiety.	
Nutritional Therapy • Assess nutritional needs and begin feeding patient by most appropriate route as soon as possible.	**Physical and Occupational Therapy** • Begin daily therapy program for maintenance of range of motion. • Assess need for splints and anticontracture positioning. • Encourage and aid patient with self-care as possible.	
Respiratory Therapy • Assess oxygenation needs. • Provide supplemental O_2 as needed. • Intubate if needed. • Monitor respiratory status.	**Nutritional Therapy** • Continue to assess diet to support wound healing.	
Psychosocial Care • Provide support to patient and caregiver during initial crisis phase.	**Respiratory Therapy** • Continue to assess oxygenation needs. • Continue to monitor respiratory status. • Monitor for signs of complications (e.g., pneumonia).	
	Psychosocial Care • Provide ongoing support, counseling, and teaching to patient and caregiver about physical and emotional aspects of care and recovery. • Begin discharge planning.	
	Drug Therapy (Table 24.13) • Assess need for drugs (e.g., antibiotics). • Continue to monitor effectiveness and adjust dosage as needed.	

The Parkland (Baxter) formula for fluid replacement is the most common formula used (Table 24.11 or *www.mdcalc.com/parkland-formula-for-burns*). Remember that all formulas are estimates. Fluids are titrated based on the patient's response (e.g., hourly urine output, vital signs). Patients with an electrical injury have greater than normal fluid needs. They generally require an osmotic diuretic (mannitol [Osmitrol]) to increase their urine output and overcome high levels of hemoglobin and myoglobin in the urine. Too much fluid and overestimation of TBSA contribute to over-resuscitation of fluids or "fluid creep."[15] For the first 24 hours, the recommendation is 2 to 4 mL lactated Ringer's/kg/%TBSA burned.[16] Colloidal solutions (e.g., 5% albumin) may be given. However, they are often not started until 12 to 24 hours postburn when capillary permeability returns to normal or near normal. After this time, the plasma stays in the vascular space and expands the circulating volume. The replacement volume is calculated based on the patient's body weight and TBSA burned (e.g., 0.3 to 0.5 mL/kg/%TBSA burned).

Assess for the adequacy of fluid resuscitation hourly using clinical parameters. Urine output, the most often used parameter, and cardiac parameters are defined as follows:

• *Urine output:* 0.5 to 1 mL/kg/hr; 75 to 100 mL/hr for electrical burn patient with evidence of hemoglobinuria or myoglobinuria.
• *Cardiac parameters:* Mean arterial pressure (MAP) greater than 65 mm Hg, systolic BP greater than 90 mm Hg, heart rate less than 120 beats/min. MAP and BP are best measured by an arterial line. Manual BP measurement is often invalid because of edema and vasoconstriction.

CHECK YOUR PRACTICE

You are admitting a new burn patient who weighs 72 kg and has 45% TBSA burn.
• Outline the patient's fluid requirements over the first 24 hours.

TABLE 24.11 Fluid Resuscitation Formulas

Parkland (Baxter)*

4 mL lactated Ringer's solution per kilogram (kg) of body weight per percent of total body surface area (% TBSA) burned = Total fluid requirements for first 24 hr after burn

Application

½ of total in first 8 hr
¼ of total in second 8 hr
¼ of total in third 8 hr

Example

For a 70-kg patient with a 50% TBSA burn:

$$4 \text{ mL} \times 70 \text{ kg} \times 50 \text{ (\%TBSA) burned} = 14,000 \text{ mL in 24 hr}$$

½ of total in first 8 hr = 7000 mL (875 mL/hr)
¼ of total in second 8 hr = 3500 mL (437 mL/hr)
¼ of total in third 8 hr = 3500 mL (437 mL/hr)

American Burn Association Consensus Fluid Resuscitation

2–4 mL lactated Ringer's solution per kilogram (kg) of body weight per percent of total body surface area (% TBSA) burned = Total fluid requirements for first 24 hr after burn

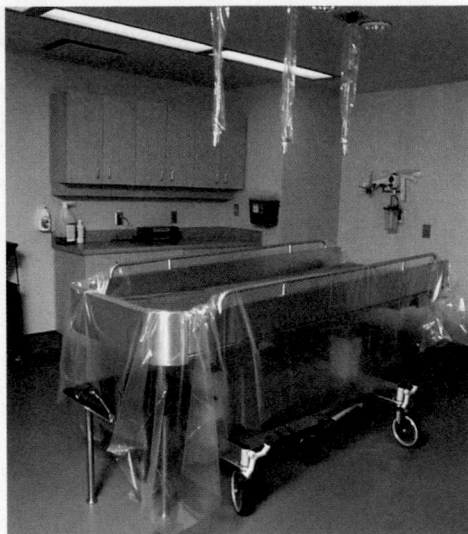

FIG. 24.9 Shower cart. Showering presents an opportunity for PT and wound care. (Courtesy Judy Knighton, Toronto, Canada.)

◆ Wound Care

Once a patent airway, effective circulation, and adequate fluid replacement have been achieved, priority is given to care of the burn wound. Partial-thickness burn wounds appear pink to cherry-red and are wet and shiny with serous exudate. These wounds may or may not have intact blisters; are painful when touched; and have only minor, localized sensation because nerve endings may have been destroyed in the burned dermis.

You can perform cleansing and gentle debridement (using scissors and forceps) on a shower cart (Fig. 24.9), in a regular shower, or on a patient's bed or stretcher. Extensive, surgical debridement is done in the operating room (OR) (Fig. 24.10). During debridement, necrotic skin is removed. Releasing escharotomies and fasciotomies are done in the emergent phase, usually in burn centers by physicians.

Patients find the first wound care to be both physically and mentally demanding. Provide emotional support and begin to build trust during this activity. A once-daily shower and dressing change in the morning, with an evening dressing change in the patient's room, are part of the routine in many burn centers. Others opt to shower the patient on admission and then perform all other dressing changes in the patient's room. Some of the newer antimicrobial dressings can be left in place from 3 to 14 days, reducing the frequency of dressing changes.

Infection can cause further tissue injury and possible sepsis. The source of infection in burn wounds is likely the patient's own flora, mostly from the skin, respiratory, and gastrointestinal (GI) systems.

Two approaches to burn wound treatment are (1) the open method and (2) the use of multiple dressing changes (closed method). In the *open method* the patient's burn is covered with a topical antimicrobial and has no dressing over the wound. This approach is usually limited to the care of facial burns. In the *multiple dressing change,* or *closed method,* sterile gauze dressings are impregnated with or laid over a topical antimicrobial (Fig. 24.11). These dressings are changed from every 12 hours to once every 14 days depending on the product. Most burn centers use the closed technique.

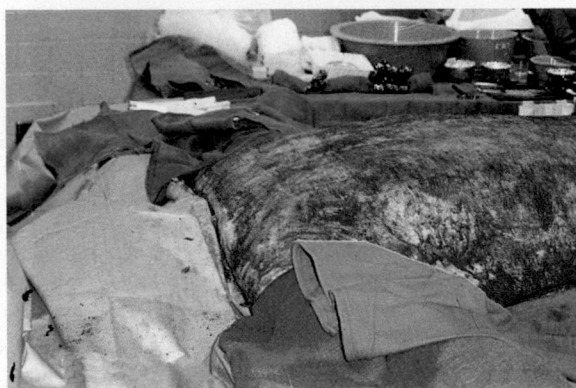

FIG. 24.10 Surgical debridement of full-thickness burns is necessary to prepare the wound for grafting. (Courtesy Judy Knighton, Toronto, Canada.)

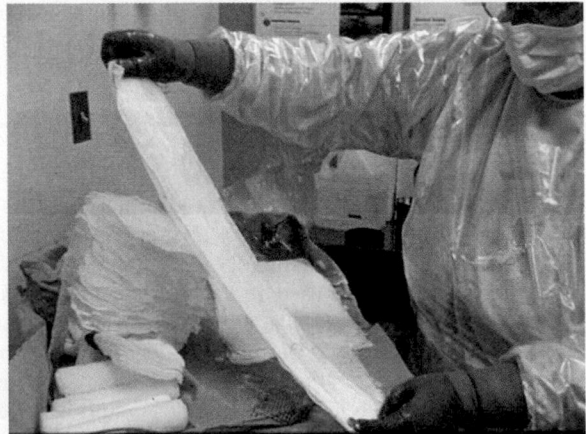

FIG. 24.11 Application of silver sulfadiazine cream to saline-moistened gauze. (Courtesy Judy Knighton, Toronto, Canada.)

When the patient's open burn wounds are exposed, always wear personal protective equipment (PPE) (e.g., disposable hats, masks, gowns, gloves). When removing contaminated dressings and washing wounds, use nonsterile, disposable gloves. Use sterile gloves when applying ointments and sterile dressings.

TABLE 24.12 Skin Grafts Used for Burn Injury

Graft Type	Source and Description	Coverage
Allograft (or homograft) (same species)	Cadaveric skin	Temporary (3 days to 2 wk)
Autografts		
Autograft	Patient's own skin	Permanent
Cultured epithelial autograft (CEA)–Epicel	Patient's own skin cell cultures	Permanent
Dermal Substitutes		
AlloDerm	Acellular dermal matrix derived from donated human skin	Permanent
Apligraf	Donated neonatal foreskin fibroblasts and keratinocytes in bovine collagen gel	Permanent
Biobrane	Semipermeable silicone membrane bonded to nylon fabric	Temporary (10–21 days)
Integra	Biodegradable dermal layer made of bovine collagen and glycosaminoglycan bonded to silicone membrane	Permanent
Matriderm	Bovine collagen and elastin matrix	Permanent
OrCel	Donated neonatal foreskin fibroblasts and keratinocytes in bovine collagen sponge	Permanent
Xenograft (or heterograft) (different species)	Porcine skin	Temporary (3 days to 2 wk)

In addition, prevent shivering by keeping the room warm (around 85°F [29.4°C]). Before leaving one patient, remove your PPE and wash your hands. Don new PPE before you treat another patient.

Permanent skin coverage is the primary goal for burn wound care. There is rarely enough unburned skin in the major (greater than 50% TBSA) burn patient for immediate skin grafting. In this situation, temporary wound closure methods are needed. *Allograft (homograft) skin* (from skin donor cadavers) is used, along with newer biosynthetic options. Treatment approaches vary among burn centers (Table 24.12).

◆ Other Care Measures

Certain parts of the body (e.g., face, eyes, hands, arms, ears, perineum) need vigilant nursing care. The face is highly vascular and can become very swollen. It is often covered with ointments and gauze but not wrapped to limit pressure on delicate facial structures. An eye exam should occur soon after admission for all patients with facial burns. Periorbital edema can temporarily prevent eye opening and is often frightening for the patient. Always check that the patient's eyelashes are not turned inward toward the eyeball. Provide assurance that the swelling is not permanent. Instill methylcellulose drops or artificial tears into the eyes for moisture and comfort. Apply antibiotic eye ointment for corneal burns or edema as ordered.

Keep the ears free from pressure because of their poor vascularization and tendency to become infected. Do not use pillows for the patient with ear burns. The pressure on the cartilage may cause chondritis. Also, the ear may stick to the pillowcase, causing pain and bleeding. Raise the patient's head using a rolled towel placed under the shoulders, being careful to avoid pressure necrosis. Follow the same strategy for the patient with neck burns to hyperextend the neck and prevent neck contracture.

Extend burned hands and arms and raise them on pillows or plastic-covered foam wedges to reduce edema. Ask the physical therapist (PT) and the HCP if splints should be applied to burned hands and feet to keep them in positions of function. Remove the splints often and inspect the skin and bony prominences to avoid areas of pressure from inappropriate or prolonged application. Elastic wraps may reduce edema.

Keep your patient's perineum as clean and dry as possible after each voiding or bowel movement. In addition to monitoring hourly urine outputs, an indwelling catheter prevents urine contamination of the perineal area. Regular once- or twice-daily perineal care is essential. Assess the need for an indwelling urinary catheter daily. Remove when it is no longer needed to limit the risk for a urinary tract infection. If your patient has frequent, loose stools, consider using a fecal diversion device.

Perform laboratory tests to monitor fluid and electrolyte balance. Draw ABGs to assess adequacy of ventilation and oxygenation in patients with suspected or confirmed inhalation or electrical injury.

Work with PT to perform range-of-motion (ROM) exercises during dressing changes and throughout the day. Movement aids the shift of the interstitial fluid back into the vascular bed. Active and passive exercise also maintains function and prevents skin and joint contractures. It may reassure the patient that movement is still possible.

❖ Drug Therapy

◆ **Analgesics and Sedatives.** Promote the use of analgesics for the patient's comfort. Early in the postburn period, IV pain medications should be given because (1) onset of action is fastest with this route; (2) oral drugs have a slower onset of action and are not as effective when GI function is slowed or impaired because of shock or paralytic ileus; and (3) IM injections are not absorbed well in burned or edematous areas, causing pooling of drugs in the tissues. Consequently, when fluid mobilization starts, the patient could be inadvertently overdosed from the interstitial accumulation of previous IM drugs.

Common drugs used for pain control are listed in Table 24.13. Opioids are the drug of choice for severe pain. When given appropriately, these drugs should provide adequate pain relief. Evaluate the pain management plan often since the patient's needs may change and tolerance to drugs may develop over time. Remember that the patient's pain level may not directly correlate with the extent and depth of burn. Analgesic needs vary from one patient to another. Consider a multimodal approach to pain control. Sedatives/hypnotics and antidepressants can be given with analgesics to control the anxiety, insomnia, or depression that patients may have (Table 24.13).

◆ **Tetanus Immunization.** All burn patients routinely receive tetanus toxoid because of the risk for anaerobic burn wound contamination. If the patient has not received an active immunization within 10 years before the burn injury, tetanus immunoglobulin should be considered. (Tetanus immunization is discussed in Table 68.6.)

TABLE 24.13 Drug Therapy

Burns

Drugs	Purpose
Analgesics	
morphine	Relieve pain
sustained-release morphine (MS Contin)	
hydromorphone (Dilaudid)	
sustained-release hydromorphone (Dilaudid CR)	
fentanyl (Sublimaze)	
oxycodone and acetaminophen (Percocet)	
nonsteroidal antiinflammatory (e.g., ketorolac)	
adjuvant analgesics (e.g., gabapentin [Neurontin])	
Anticoagulants	
enoxaparin (Lovenox)	Prevent venous thrombo-
heparin	embolism
Antidepressants	
citalopram (Celexa)	Reduce depression,
sertraline (Zoloft)	improve mood
Gastrointestinal Support	
aluminum hydroxide and magnesium hydroxide (Maalox)	Neutralize stomach acid
calcium carbonate and magnesium carbonate (Mylanta)	
esomeprazole (Nexium)	Decrease stomach acid
ranitidine (Zantac)	and risk for Curling's ulcer
nystatin	Prevent overgrowth of *Candida albicans* in oral mucosa
Nutritional Support	
Minerals: zinc, iron (ferrous sulfate)	Promote cell integrity and hemoglobin formation
Vitamins A, C, E, and multivitamins	Promote wound healing
Sedatives/Hypnotics	
lorazepam (Ativan)	Reduce anxiety
midazolam (Versed)	Provide short-acting amnesic effects
zolpidem (Ambien)	Promote sleep

◆ **Antimicrobial Agents**. After the wound is cleansed, topical antimicrobial agents may be applied (Fig. 24.11) and covered with a light dressing. Systemic antibiotics are not routinely used to control burn wound flora because the burn eschar has little or no blood supply, so little antibiotic is delivered to the wound. In addition, the routine use of systemic antibiotics increases the chance of developing multidrug-resistant organisms. Some topical burn agents penetrate the eschar and inhibit bacterial invasion of the wound. Silver-impregnated dressings can be left in place from 3 to 14 days, depending on the patient's clinical situation and the product. Silver sulfadiazine (Silvadene) and mafenide acetate (Sulfamylon) creams are also used.[17]

 SAFETY ALERT Drug Allergy Check
* Check the patient for any allergies to sulfa since many burn antimicrobial creams contain sulfa.

Sepsis is a leading cause of death in the patient with major burns and may lead to multiple organ dysfunction syndrome

(see Chapter 66). Systemic antibiotic therapy is started when the diagnosis of sepsis is made or when some other source of infection is identified (e.g., pneumonia).

Fungal infections may develop in the patient's mucous membranes (mouth and genitalia) because of systemic antibiotic therapy and low resistance. The offending organism is usually *Candida albicans*. Oral infection is treated with nystatin (Mycostatin) mouthwash. When a normal diet is resumed, yogurt or *Lactobacillus* (Lactinex) may be given to reintroduce the normal intestinal flora that was destroyed by antibiotic therapy.

◆ **Venous Thromboembolism Prophylaxis.** Burn patients are at risk for VTE. If there are no contraindications, it is recommended that low-molecular-weight heparin (enoxaparin) or low-dose unfractionated heparin be started as soon as it is considered safe. For burn patients who have a high bleeding risk, VTE prophylaxis with intermittent pneumatic compression devices and/or graduated compression stockings is used until the bleeding risk decreases and heparin can be started (Table 24.13). (VTE prophylaxis is discussed in Chapter 37.)

◆ **Nutritional Therapy**

Once fluid replacement needs have been addressed, nutrition takes priority in the initial emergent phase. Early and aggressive nutritional support within several hours of the burn injury can decrease complications and mortality, optimize burn wound healing, and minimize the negative effects of hypermetabolism and catabolism.[18] Nonintubated patients with a burn of less than 20% TBSA will usually be able to eat enough to meet their nutritional needs.

Intubated patients and those with larger burns need more support. Enteral feedings have almost entirely replaced parenteral feeding. Early enteral feeding, usually with smaller bore tubes, preserves GI function, increases intestinal blood flow, and promotes optimal conditions for wound healing. In general, begin the feedings slowly at a rate of 20 to 40 mL/hr and increase to the goal rate within 24 to 48 hours. If a large nasogastric tube is used, gastric residuals should be checked to rule out delayed gastric emptying. Assess bowel sounds every 8 hours.

A *hypermetabolic state* proportional to the size of the wound occurs after a major burn injury. Resting metabolic expenditure may be increased by 50% to 100% above normal in patients with major burns. Core temperature is increased. Catecholamines, which stimulate catabolism and heat production, are increased. Massive catabolism can occur and is characterized by protein breakdown and increased gluconeogenesis.

Failure to supply adequate calories and protein leads to malnutrition and delayed healing. Calorie-containing nutritional supplements are often given to meet the caloric needs.[19] Protein powder can be added to food and liquids. Supplemental vitamins may be started in the emergent phase, with iron supplements often given in the acute phase (Table 24.13).

ACUTE PHASE

The *acute phase* of burn care begins with the mobilization of extracellular fluid and subsequent diuresis. It ends when partial-thickness wounds are healed or full-thickness burns are covered by skin grafts. This may take weeks or months.

Pathophysiology

A healing burn injury causes many pathophysiologic changes in the body. Diuresis from fluid mobilization occurs, and the patient is less edematous. Bowel sounds return. The depth of the burn wounds may be more apparent as they "declare" themselves as partial or full thickness. The patient may now become more aware of the enormity of the situation and will benefit from emotional support and information.

Some healing begins as WBCs surround the burn wound and phagocytosis occurs. Necrotic tissue begins to slough. Fibroblasts lay down matrices of the collagen precursors that eventually form granulation tissue. A partial-thickness burn will heal, from both the wound edges and the dermal bed below, if kept free from infection and *desiccation* (dryness). However, full-thickness burn wounds, unless extremely small, must have the burn eschar surgically removed (excised) and skin grafts applied to heal. In some cases, healing time and length of hospitalization are decreased by early excision and grafting.

Clinical Manifestations

Partial-thickness wounds form eschar, which begins separating soon after injury. Once the eschar is removed, re-epithelialization begins at the wound margins and appears as red or pink scar tissue. Epithelial buds, from the hair follicles and glands in the dermal bed, eventually close the wound. Healing is spontaneous and usually occurs within 10 to 21 days.

Margins of full-thickness eschar take longer to separate. As a result, full-thickness burn wounds require surgical debridement and skin grafting to heal.

Laboratory Values

Because the body is trying to reestablish fluid and electrolyte balance in the initial acute phase, it is important to follow serum electrolyte levels closely.

Sodium. *Hyponatremia* can develop from excess GI suction and diarrhea. Manifestations include headache, irritability, confusion, vomiting, seizures, and even coma. The patient may develop, *dilutional hyponatremia,* called *water intoxication,* from excess water intake. To avoid this condition, offer the patient fluids other than water, such as juice or nutritional supplements.

Hypernatremia may occur after successful fluid resuscitation if large amounts of hypertonic solutions were used. Hypernatremia also may be caused by tube feedings or inappropriate fluid administration. Manifestations include changes in mental status, ranging from drowsiness, restlessness, confusion, and lethargy to seizures and coma. Sodium restrictions may be applied to IV fluids and enteral or oral feedings until levels return to safe limits.

Potassium. *Hyperkalemia* may occur if the patient has renal failure, adrenocortical insufficiency, or massive deep muscle injury (e.g., electrical burn). Large amounts of potassium are released from damaged cells. Dysrhythmias and arrest can occur with high potassium levels. The patient may have confusion, tetany, muscle cramps, paresthesias, and weakness.

Hypokalemia occurs with vomiting, diarrhea, prolonged GI suction, and IV therapy without potassium supplementation. Potassium is also lost through the patient's burn wounds. Besides dysrhythmias, the patient may have muscle weakness, paresthesia, decreased GI motility, and decreased reflexes (see Chapter 16).

Complications

Infection. A burn injury destroys the body's first line of defense, the skin. The burn wound is now colonized with the person's own organisms that were on the skin before the burn. The WBCs have functional defects, and the patient is immunosuppressed for many months after the burn injury.

If the levels of bacteria between the eschar and viable wound bed rise to greater than 10^5 per gram of tissue, the patient has a burn wound infection. Infection can convert partial-thickness burns to full-thickness wounds. Wound infections may be treated with systemic and local antibiotics based on wound culture and sensitivity results.

Localized inflammation, induration, and sometimes pus can be seen at the burn wound margins. Watch for signs and symptoms of infection, including hypothermia or hyperthermia, increased heart and respiratory rate, decreased BP, and decreased urine output. The patient may have mild confusion, chills, malaise, and loss of appetite. The WBC count is between 10,000/μL (10×10^9/L) and 20,000/μL (20×10^9/L).

The causative organisms of sepsis are usually gram-negative bacteria (e.g., *Pseudomonas, Proteus*), putting the patient at further risk for septic shock. If sepsis is suspected, obtain cultures from all possible sources, including the burn wound, blood, urine, sputum, oropharynx and perineal regions, and IV site. A lactate level is collected. Treatment begins with a bolus of normal saline IV and antibiotics.[20] Antibiotic therapy may be continued or changed based on the culture and sensitivity results. At this stage, the patient's condition is considered critical. Close monitoring of vital signs and mental status is needed.

Cardiovascular and Respiratory Systems. The same cardiovascular and respiratory complications present in the emergent phase continue into the acute phase of care. In addition, new problems might arise, requiring prompt intervention.

Neurologic System. Neurologically, the patient probably has no physical symptoms, unless severe hypoxia from respiratory injuries or complications from electrical injuries occur. Probable causes of neurologic complications include electrolyte imbalance, stress, cerebral edema, sepsis, sleep problems, and the use of analgesics and antianxiety drugs.

Some patients may have certain behaviors that are not completely understood. The patient may become extremely disoriented, withdraw or become combative, hallucinate, or have frequent nightmare-like episodes. Delirium is more acute at night and occurs more often in the older patient. Start appropriate nursing interventions to prevent delirium and use a screening tool to diagnose delirium (see Table 59.18). Orient and reassure a patient who is confused or agitated. This state is usually transient, lasting from a day or two to several weeks, but complications and sequelae can last for years and be serious.

Musculoskeletal System. The musculoskeletal system is particularly prone to complications during the acute phase. The involvement of both PT and OT is vitally important. As the burns begin to heal and scar tissue forms, the skin is less supple and pliant. ROM may be limited, and skin and joint contractures can occur. Because of pain, the patient prefers a flexed position for comfort. Have the patient stretch and move the burned body parts as much as possible. Consult with PT or OT about proper positioning and splinting to prevent or reduce contracture formation.

Gastrointestinal System. The GI system may develop complications during this phase. Sepsis can cause paralytic ileus. Diarrhea may result from the use of enteral feedings or antibiotics. Constipation can occur as a side effect of opioids, decreased mobility, and a low-fiber diet. *Curling's ulcer* is a type of gastroduodenal ulcer characterized by diffuse superficial lesions (including mucosal erosion). It is caused by a generalized stress response to decreased blood flow to the GI tract. The patient has increased gastric acid secretion.

Aim to prevent Curling's ulcer by feeding the patient as soon as possible after the burn injury. Antacids, H_2-histamine blockers (e.g., ranitidine), and proton pump inhibitors (e.g., omeprazole) are used prophylactically to neutralize stomach acids and inhibit histamine and the secretion of hydrochloric acid (Table 24.13). Patients with major burns may have occult blood in their stools during the acute phase and require close monitoring for bleeding.

Endocrine System. Watch for transient increases in the patient's blood glucose levels because of stress-mediated cortisol and catecholamine release. There is an increased mobilization of glycogen stores and gluconeogenesis. Subsequently, glucose is produced, along with an increase in insulin production. However, insulin's effectiveness is decreased because of relative insulin insensitivity. This results in a high blood glucose level. Hyperglycemia also may be caused by the increased caloric intake needed to meet some patients' metabolic requirements. When hyperglycemia occurs, check blood glucose levels and give insulin as ordered. Point-of-care testing of glucose can be done, but serum glucose testing is more accurate. As the patient's metabolic demands are met and less stress is placed on the entire system, this stress-induced condition is reversed.

❖ NURSING AND INTERPROFESSIONAL MANAGEMENT: ACUTE PHASE

The major therapeutic interventions in the acute phase are (1) wound care, (2) excision and grafting, (3) pain management, (4) PT and OT, and (5) nutritional therapy.

◆ Wound Care

The goals of wound care are to (1) prevent infection by cleansing and debriding the area of necrotic tissue that would promote bacterial growth and (2) promote wound re-epithelialization and/or successful skin grafting.

Wound care consists of ongoing observation, assessment, cleansing, debridement, and dressing reapplication. Nonsurgical debridement, dressing changes, topical antimicrobial therapy, graft care, and donor site care are done as often as needed, depending on the topical cream or dressing ordered. Enzymatic debriding agents made of natural ingredients, such as collagenase, may be used for *enzymatic debridement* of burn wounds, which speeds up the removal of dead tissue from the healthy wound bed.

Cleanse wounds with soap and water or normal saline-moistened gauze to gently remove the old antimicrobial agent and any loose necrotic tissue, scabs, or dried blood. During the debridement phase, cover the wound with topical antimicrobial creams (e.g., silver sulfadiazine) or silver-impregnated dressings. When the partial-thickness burn wounds have been fully debrided, a protective, coarse or fine-meshed, greasy-based (paraffin, petrolatum) gauze dressing is applied to protect the re-epithelializing keratinocytes as they resurface and close the open wound bed.

If grafting is done, protect the skin graft (discussed later) with the same greasy gauze dressings next to the graft, followed by saline-moistened middle dressing and dry gauze outer dressings. With facial grafts, the unmeshed sheet graft is left open, so it is possible for *blebs* (serosanguineous exudate) to form between the graft and recipient bed. Blebs prevent the graft from permanently attaching to the wound bed. The evacuation of blebs is best done by aspiration with a tuberculin syringe and only by those trained in this specialized skill. (Dressings are discussed in Table 11.9.)

◆ Excision and Grafting

Management of full-thickness burn wounds involves early removal (surgical excision) of the necrotic tissue, followed by application of split-thickness autograft skin.[21] This approach has improved the management and survival rate of burn patients. In the past, patients with major burns had low rates of survival because healing and wound coverage took so long that the patient usually died of sepsis or malnutrition.

Many patients, especially those with major burns, are taken to the OR for wound excision on day 1 or 2 (emergent phase). The wounds are covered with a biologic dressing or allograft for temporary coverage until permanent grafting can occur (Table 24.12).

During the procedure of excision and grafting, devitalized tissue (eschar) is excised down to the subcutaneous tissue or fascia, depending on the degree of injury. Surgical excision can result in massive blood loss. To decrease surgical blood loss, topical application of epinephrine or thrombin, injection of saline and epinephrine, application of extremity tourniquets, or application of a fibrin sealant (Artiss) is used.

Once hemostasis has been achieved, a graft is then placed on clean, viable tissue to achieve good adherence. Whenever possible, the freshly excised wound is covered with *autograft* (the person's own) skin (Table 24.12). Recently, fibrin sealant has been used to attach skin grafts to the wound bed. Grafts also can be stapled or sutured into place (Fig. 24.12, *A*). Negative pressure wound therapy dressings are often placed on top of skin grafts to optimize adherence of the graft to the excised wound bed.[22] A temporary allograft can be used to test the suitability of the recipient site to accept a graft. The allograft is then removed several days later in the OR and an autograft applied.

With early excision, function is restored, and scar tissue formation is minimized. Clots between the graft and wound keep the graft from adhering to the wound. Outer occlusive dressings apply just enough pressure to promote adherence of the graft to the wound bed and help control bleeding. Protect the grafted area from shearing, friction, and pressure. Facial, neck, and hand burns require skilled nursing care to identify and manage clots quickly for the best functional and aesthetic outcomes.

Donor skin is taken from the patient for grafting by means of a *dermatome*, which removes a thin split-thickness layer of skin from an unburned site (Fig. 24.12, *B*). The donor skin can be meshed to allow for greater wound coverage, or it may be applied as an unmeshed sheet for a better cosmetic result when grafting the face, neck, and hands. The donor site now becomes a new open wound.

The goals of donor site care are to promote rapid, moist wound healing; decrease pain at the site; and prevent infection. The choices of dressings for donor sites include transparent dressings (e.g., OpSite), xenograft, silver sulfadiazine, silver-impregnated dressings, calcium alginate, and hydrophilic foam dressings (Fig. 24.12, *C*). Nursing care of the donor site is specific to the dressing used. Several of the newer dressings decrease healing time, which allows earlier reharvesting of skin at the same site. The average healing time for a donor site is 10 to 14 days (Fig. 24.12, *D*).

◆ Cultured Epithelial Autografts.
In the patient with large body burns, only a limited amount of unburned skin may be available

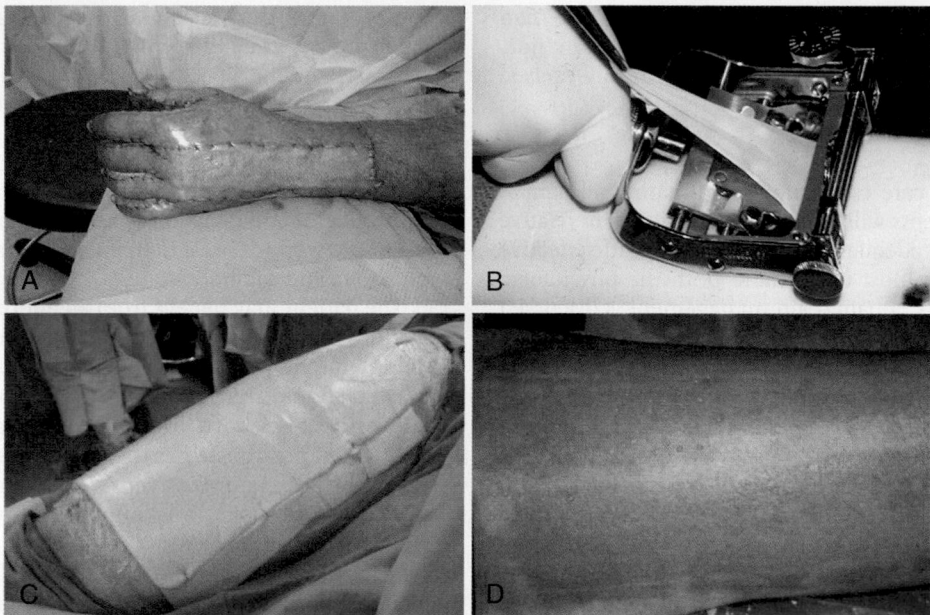

FIG. 24.12 **A,** Freshly applied split-thickness sheet skin graft to the hand. **B,** Split-thickness skin graft is harvested from a patient's thigh using a dermatome. **C,** Donor site is covered with a hydrophilic foam dressing after harvesting. **D,** Healed donor site. (Courtesy Judy Knighton, Toronto, Canada.)

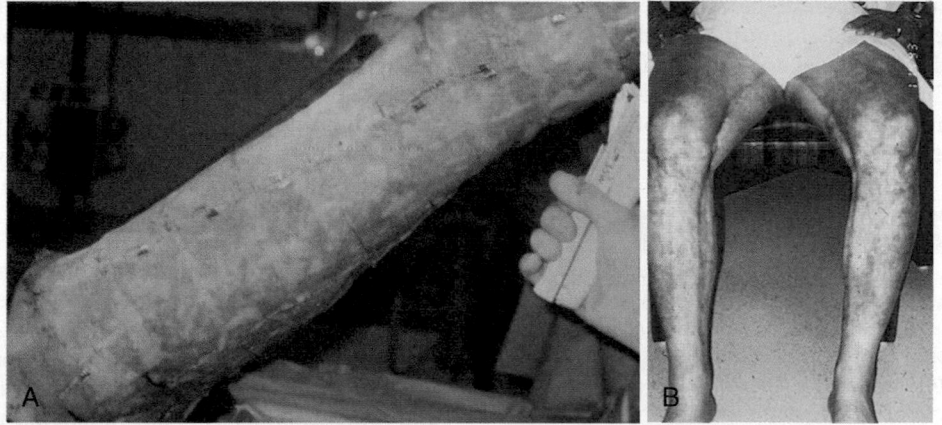

FIG. 24.13 Patient with cultured epithelial autograft (CEA). **A,** Intraoperative application of CEA. **B,** Appearance of healed CEA.

as donor sites for grafting, and some of that skin may not be suitable for harvesting. Cultured epithelial autograft (CEA) is a method of getting permanent skin from a person with limited skin available for harvesting. CEA is grown from biopsy samples obtained from the patient's unburned skin. This procedure is done in suitable patients in some burn centers as soon as possible. The specimens are sent to a commercial laboratory, where the biopsied keratinocytes are grown in a culture medium containing epidermal growth factor. After about 18 to 25 days, the keratinocytes have expanded up to 10,000 times and form sheets that we can use as skin grafts. The cultured skin is returned to the burn center, where it is placed on the patient's excised burn wounds (Fig. 24.13, *A*). CEA grafts generally form a seamless, smooth replacement skin tissue (Fig. 24.13, *B*). Problems related to CEA include a poor graft take because of thin epidermal skin, graft loss during healing, infection, and contracture development.

◆ **Dermal Substitutes.** Dermal substitutes act as a synthetic dermis and are covered by skin graft.[23] The Integra artificial skin

dermal regeneration template is an example of a skin replacement system. As with CEA, it is used in the treatment of life-threatening full-thickness or deep partial-thickness burn wounds when a conventional autograft is not available or advisable, as in older or high anesthetic-risk patients. It also has been successfully used in reconstructive burn surgery procedures. It must be applied within a few days postburn for greatest success.

Integra artificial skin has a bilayer membrane composed of acellular dermis and silicone. The wound is excised, the bilayer membrane is placed dermal layer down, and the wound is wrapped with dressings in the OR. The dermal layer functions as a biodegradable template that induces organized regeneration of new dermis by the body. The silicone layer stays intact for 3 weeks as the dermal layer degrades, and epidermal autografts become available. At this point, the silicone is removed during a second surgery and replaced by the patient's own epidermal autografts.

Another dermal replacement is AlloDerm, a cryopreserved allogenic dermis. Human allograft dermis, harvested from cadavers, is decellularized to make it immunogenic and then freeze-dried. Once thawed, AlloDerm is rehydrated in normal saline immediately before placement on a freshly excised wound.

◆ Pain Management

Many aspects of burn care cause pain. Eliminating all pain is difficult, but most patients will have acceptable levels of relative comfort if they receive adequate analgesia. To provide effective pain management, you must understand both the physiologic and psychologic aspects of pain. Pain management is discussed in Chapter 8.

Burn patients have 2 kinds of pain: (1) *continuous, background pain* that might be present throughout the day and night; and (2) *treatment-induced pain* associated with dressing changes, ambulation, and rehabilitation activities. The first line of pain treatment is drugs (Table 24.13). With background pain, frequent IV administration of an opioid (e.g., hydromorphone [Dilaudid]) provides a steady, therapeutic level of the drug. If tolerating food, slow-release, twice-daily opioids (e.g., morphine [MS Contin]) can be used. Patient-controlled analgesia (PCA) is used in some burn centers, with varying degrees of success. Anxiolytics (e.g., lorazepam [Ativan], midazolam) and adjuvant analgesics (e.g., gabapentin [Neurontin], pregabalin [Lyrica]), can enhance opioids. The use of these drugs can help reduce the opioid dosage and undesirable side effects.

Breakthrough doses of analgesia must be available regardless of the regimen used. Additional doses of opioids are usually given. For treatment-induced pain, premedicate with an analgesic, and possibly an anxiolytic, via the IV or oral route. For patients with an IV, a short-acting analgesic is often used.

❓ CHECK YOUR PRACTICE

Your patient with a burn injury is ordered fentanyl (Sublimaze) before a dressing change. The patient has multiple IV lines, and you are not sure which line to use to insert the drug. You know that mixing up IV lines can lead to serious drug errors.

• How would you determine which IV line to use to give the drug?

Some pain can be managed using nondrug strategies. Relaxation breathing, guided imagery, hypnosis, biofeedback, computerized gaming, and music therapy can help patients cope with pain (see Chapter 6).[24]

Remember, the more control the patient has in managing pain, the more successful the chosen strategies will be. Active participation in asking for time-outs and scheduling treatments and rest periods can help the patient manage feelings of anticipatory pain.

◆ Physical and Occupational Therapy

Continuous PT throughout burn recovery is imperative if the patient is to regain and maintain muscle strength and optimal joint function. A good time for exercise is during dressing changes, when bulky dressings are removed and patients are medicated for pain. Passive and active ROM should be performed on all joints. PT and OT may join the nurse and patient during dressing changes. Ensure that the patient with neck burns continues to sleep without pillows or with the head hanging slightly over the top of the mattress to encourage hyperextension.

Maintain the OT schedule for wearing custom-fitted splints, which are designed to keep joints in functional position. Check the splints often to ensure an optimal fit, with no undue pressure that may lead to skin breakdown or nerve damage.

◆ Nutritional Therapy

The goal of nutritional therapy during the acute burn phase is to provide adequate calories and protein to promote healing. When the wounds are still open, the burn patient is in a hypermetabolic and catabolic state.

The patient may benefit from an antioxidant protocol, which includes selenium, vitamin E, acetylcysteine, ascorbic acid, zinc, and a multivitamin. Meeting daily caloric requirements is crucial and should start within the first 1 to 2 days postburn. The daily estimated caloric needs must be regularly calculated by a dietitian and readjusted as the patient's condition changes (e.g., wound healing improves, sepsis develops). Monitor laboratory values (e.g., albumin, prealbumin, total protein, transferrin) on a regular basis.

If the patient is on mechanical ventilation or unable to eat enough calories by mouth, a small-bore feeding tube is placed, and enteral feedings are started. When the patient is extubated, contact the speech pathologist for a swallowing assessment before an oral diet is started. Encourage the patient to eat high-protein, high-carbohydrate foods to meet caloric goals. Ask caregivers to bring in favorite foods from home. Appetite is usually reduced, and you will need to reinforce whatever steps are taken to achieve adequate intake. Ideally, weight loss should not be more than 10% of preburn weight. Record the patient's daily caloric intake using calorie count sheets, which are reviewed by the dietitian. Weigh your patient weekly to evaluate progress.

REHABILITATION PHASE

The formal *rehabilitation phase* begins when the patient's wounds have nearly healed and they are engaging in some level of self-care. This may happen as early as 2 weeks or as long as 7 to 8 months after a major burn injury. Goals for the patient now are to (1) work toward resuming a functional role in society and (2) rehabilitate from any functional and cosmetic postburn reconstructive surgery that may be needed.

Pathophysiologic Changes and Clinical Manifestations

Burn wounds heal by either spontaneous re-epithelialization or skin grafting. Layers of keratinocytes begin rebuilding the tissue structure destroyed by the burn injury. Collagen fibers, present in the new scar tissue, help with healing and add strength to weakened areas. The new skin appears flat and pink. In about 4 to 6 weeks, the area becomes raised and hyperemic. If adequate ROM is not started, the new tissue will shorten, causing a contracture. Mature healing is reached in about 12 months, when suppleness has returned and the pink or red color has faded to a slightly lighter hue than the surrounding unburned tissue.

Tell patients who have more heavily pigmented skin that it will take longer for it to regain its color because many of the melanocytes have been destroyed. Often, the skin does not regain its original color, though this is impossible to predict. Provide teaching and emotional support to help the patient with grieving about these changes to his or her body. Cosmetic camouflage, the implantation of pigment within the skin, can help even out unequal skin tones and improve the patient's overall appearance and self-image.

Scarring has 2 characteristics: discoloration and contour. The discoloration of scars fades somewhat with time. However, scar tissue tends to develop altered contours. That is, it is no longer flat or slightly raised but becomes elevated and enlarged above the original burned area. Some burn care providers think that pressure can eventually help keep a scar flat. Gentle pressure is maintained on the healed burn with custom-fitted pressure garments and clear, thermoplastic face masks. Pressure garments and masks should never be worn over unhealed wounds. Once a wearing schedule has been set, they are removed only for short periods while bathing. Pressure garments are worn up to 23 hours a day for as long as 12 to 18 months.

The patient typically reports discomfort from itching where healing is occurring. Teach your patient about the application of water-based moisturizers and selective, short-term use of oral antihistamines (e.g., hydroxyzine [Atarax]) to help reduce the itching. Massage, cooling, emollients, gabapentin, antidepressants, and anesthetic creams also may help.[25]

As "old" epithelium is replaced by new cells, flaking occurs. The newly formed skin is extremely sensitive to trauma. Blisters and skin tears are likely to develop from slight pressure or friction. These newly healed areas can be hypersensitive or hyposensitive to cold, heat, and touch. Grafted areas are more likely to be hyposensitive until peripheral nerve regeneration occurs. Have patients protect healed burn areas from direct sunlight for about 3 months to prevent hyperpigmentation and sunburn injury. Tell them to always wear sunscreen when outside.

Complications

The most common complications during the rehabilitation phase are skin and joint contractures and hypertrophic scarring.[26] A *joint contracture* (an abnormal condition of a joint characterized by flexion and fixation) develops because of the shortening of scar tissue in the flexor tissues of a joint. Areas that are most susceptible to skin and joint contractures include the anterior and lateral neck areas, axillae, antecubital fossae, fingers, groin areas, popliteal fossae, knees, and ankles (Fig. 24.14). Some areas encompass major joints. Not only does the skin over these areas develop contractures, but the underlying tissues, such as the ligaments and tendons, tend to shorten during the healing process.

Carefully watch the patient for these potential problems. Encourage proper positioning, splinting, and exercise to minimize this complication. Tell the patient to continue with these strategies until the skin matures at around 1-year post healing. Rehabilitative therapy is aimed at the extension of body parts because the flexors are stronger than the extensors. Burned legs first may be wrapped with elastic (e.g., tensor, ACE) bandages to assist with circulation to leg-graft and donor sites before ambulation. Burned arms can be wrapped with a layer of tubular elastic gauze (e.g., Tubigrip). This interim pressure prevents blister formation, promotes venous return, and decreases pain and itchiness. Once the skin is completely healed and less fragile, custom-fitted pressure garments replace the elastic bandages and tubular gauze.

❖ NURSING AND INTERPROFESSIONAL MANAGEMENT: REHABILITATION PHASE

During the rehabilitation phase, encourage both the patient and caregiver to take part in care. Since the patient may go home with unhealed wounds, teach your patient and caregiver the skills for wound care. Before discharge, have them show you the proper dressing change. In addition, make sure they know when to contact the burn team (e.g., signs of infection, increased pain) and the need to keep outpatient visits to ensure good wound healing.

If needed, arrange home care nursing to assist with care. The newly discharged patient will need to know how to gently remove the dressings in the shower once daily, if a nonadherent, greasy gauze dressing is used or twice daily if a topical, antimicrobial cream is ordered. Teach that showering, not bathing, with mild soap and warm water keeps the wounds clean.

Give advice on scar management, moisturizing, and sun protection. Suggest using water-based creams that penetrate the dermis (e.g., Vaseline Intensive Rescue) on healed areas to keep the skin supple and moisturized. This will decrease itching and flaking. Sometimes antihistamines are used at bedtime if itching persists.

Base ongoing pain management and nutritional needs on individual patient status. Continue to encourage the patient to perform the PT and OT routines. Encourage and reassure the patient to maintain morale, particularly once the patient realizes that recovery can be slow. Rehabilitation may have to be a primary focus for at least the next 6 to 12 months.

Postburn reconstructive surgery is often done after a major burn. The need for further surgery is reviewed at the outpatient burn clinic appointments after discharge.

👤 Gerontologic Considerations: Burns

The older patient presents many challenges for the burn team.[27] The normal aging process puts the patient at risk for injury because of unsteady gait, limited eyesight, and decreased hearing. As people age, skin becomes drier and more wrinkled. Older adults have thinning of the dermal layer, a loss of elastic fibers, a reduction in subcutaneous adipose tissue, and a decrease in vascularity. As a result, the thinner dermis, with reduced blood flow, sustains deeper burns with poorer rates of healing.

Once injured, the older adult has more complications in the emergent and acute phases of burn resuscitation because of preexisting co-morbidities. For example, older patients with diabetes, heart failure, or COPD have morbidity and mortality rates exceeding those of healthy, younger patients. In older patients, pneumonia is a frequent complication, burn wounds and donor sites take longer to heal, and surgical procedures are not well tolerated. Weaning from a ventilator can be a challenge. Although usually self-limiting, delirium, if it develops, may be

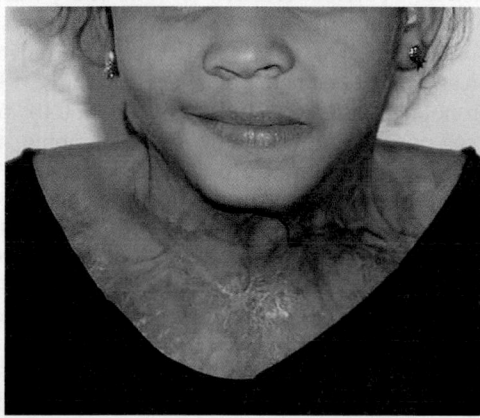

FIG. 24.14 Neck contracture. (Courtesy Linda Bucher, RN, PhD, CEN, CNE, Staff Nurse, Virtua Memorial Hospital, Mt. Holly, NJ.)

distressing.[28] It usually takes longer for these patients to rehabilitate to the point at which they can safely return home. For some, a return home to independent living may not be possible. As the population ages, developing strategies to prevent burn injuries in older adults is a priority.

EMOTIONAL/PSYCHOLOGIC NEEDS OF PATIENTS AND CAREGIVERS

Patients and caregivers have many emotional/psychologic needs during the often lengthy, unpredictable, and complex course of care. You have an important supportive and counseling role as patients struggle to get their lives back on track.

To manage the enormous range of emotional responses that the burn patient may have, assess the circumstances of the burn (e.g., cause, people involved), family relationships, and previous ways of coping with stress. At any time, the patient may have a variety of emotions, such as fear, anxiety, anger, guilt, and depression (Table 24.14).

Burn survivors often have thoughts and feelings that are frightening and disturbing, such as guilt about the burn incident, reliving the burn experience, fear of dying, concern about future therapy and surgery, frustrations with ongoing discomfort and treatment, and hopelessness about the future. During recovery, as more independence is expected from the patient, new fears may occur: "Can I really do this?" "Am I a desirable person?" "How can I go outside looking like this?" These challenges confront patients throughout their recovery and often for years to come.

A burn injury may adversely affect the person's self-esteem. Some may fear the loss of relationships because of perceived or actual physical disfigurement. In a society that values physical beauty, changes in body image can result in psychologic distress.

Open and frequent communication among the patient, caregivers, close friends, and burn team members is essential. Because of the tremendous psychologic impact of a burn injury, be particularly sensitive to the patient's emotions and concerns. Encourage the patient to discuss fears about loss of life as they once knew it, loss of function, temporary or permanent deformity and disfigurement, return to work and home life, and financial burdens resulting from a long and costly hospitalization and rehabilitation.[29]

Encourage appropriate independence and an eventual return to preburn activities, such as school or work. Peer counseling and informal interactions with other burn survivors may bring comfort and help to restore confidence. Reassure patients that their feelings during this period of adjustment are a normal reaction to an extraordinary life event. Their frustration and impatience are to be expected as they work to establish a new life. Help patients in adapting to a realistic, yet positive appraisal of their specific situation, emphasizing what they *can* do instead of what they *cannot* do.

Caregivers may share some or all these challenges and feelings. At times, they may feel helpless or too exhausted to help their loved one. Continued support from trusted and familiar burn team members is essential. Helping caregivers assist with aspects of the patient's care helps them to reconnect with their loved one and eases the transition home. Many burn survivors and their caregivers remark on the powerful learning experience of the burn and a renewed appreciation of life, despite the ongoing challenges of a prolonged recovery. You must acknowledge that their feelings are real and common. Most burn survivors speak of a real satisfaction with their postburn life and are more empowered as time goes on.

It is important to address individual spiritual and cultural needs because both have a role in treatment decisions and recovery. Pastoral care may be a helpful resource for the patient and caregiver. The need for support, information, and family involvement may vary among cultures. Identify what is important to your patient and caregiver and communicate that information in the patient's plan of care. Encourage the burn care team to be culturally aware of and sensitive to the patient's and caregiver's cultural needs.

The difficult issue of sexuality must be met with honesty. Acceptance of any changes in physical appearance is difficult at first for the patient and significant other. The nature of skin injury in itself can cause modifications in processing sexual stimuli.[30] Touch is an important part of sexuality, and immature scar tissue may make the sensation of touch unpleasant or may dull it. This may be only transient, but the patient and partner need to know that it is normal and receive anticipatory guidance from the burn team to avoid undue emotional strain.

Burn survivors may have preexisting mental health or substance use issues, any of which may have contributed to the burn incident.[31] The stress of the burn injury can precipitate a psychologic crisis. Assessment by a psychiatrist who can prescribe appropriate drugs, if needed, and offer counseling is often helpful. Early psychiatric intervention is essential if the patient has been previously treated for a psychiatric illness or if the injury was a suicide attempt. Many burn patients have posttraumatic stress disorder. A history of mental health issues can influence the length of hospitalization and time needed to prepare for discharge.[31] However, it has been noted that distress and trauma symptoms can act as a catalyst for positive posttraumatic growth. Coping styles and social support assist in these positive changes postburn.[32]

Psychologic care typically begins in the hospital, but links to community resources must be made before discharge to ensure continuity of treatment. A referral to a psychiatrist, psychologist, psychiatric advanced practice nurse (APN), mental health counselor, or social worker should be discussed if concerns are raised at burn clinic follow-up.

Caregiver and patient support groups may be beneficial in meeting the patient's and caregiver's emotional needs at any phase of the recovery process. Speaking with others who have had burn trauma can be beneficial, both in terms of confirming that the patient's feelings are normal and in sharing helpful

TABLE 24.14 **Common Emotional Responses**	
Emotion	**Possible Verbal Expression**
Anger	• Why did this happen to me? • The nurses enjoy hurting me. • I hope the person who did this to me dies.
Anxiety	• I feel out of control. • What's going to happen to me? • When will I look normal again?
Depression	• It is no use going on like this. • I do not care what happens to me. • I wish people would leave me alone.
Fear	• Will I die? • What will happen next? • Will I be disfigured? • Will my family and friends still love me?
Guilt	• If only I had been more careful. • I'm being punished because I did something wrong.
Hopefulness	• What do I need to do to survive this injury emotionally and return to my life/family/friends? • What am I meant to learn from this injury?

advice. The Phoenix Society *(www.phoenix-society.org)* is an international, highly respected burn survivors' support group. For many years the society has offered valuable support and resources (e.g., annual World Burn Congress conference) to burn survivors, caregivers, and burn team staff.

SPECIAL NEEDS OF NURSES

Warm, trusting, and mutually satisfying relationships often develop between burn patients and nursing staff during hospitalization and the long-term rehabilitation period. Sometimes the bond can be so strong that the patient has difficulty separating from the hospital and staff. The frequency and intensity of family contact can be rewarding as well as draining to you. You may find it difficult to cope with the deformities caused by the burn injury, odors, unpleasant sight of the wound, and reality of the pain that accompanies the burn and its treatment.

Do not hesitate to seek help from co-workers, a manager, or the employee assistance program should you feel the need.

In time, you will come to know that the specialized burn care you provide makes a critical difference in helping patients not only survive but also cope with and triumph over an intense and complex injury.

Ongoing support services or critical incident stress debriefings led by a psychiatrist, psychologist, psychiatric APN, or social worker may be helpful. Peer support groups (e.g., ABA, International Society for Burn Injuries) can serve a similar purpose by helping you cope with difficult feelings experienced when caring for burn patients. Because burn nursing is physically, psychologically, and intellectually demanding, it has many challenges and inherent rewards. Attention to your own self-care is important to maintain a positive attitude and healthy work-life balance. Time with family and friends and rest and relaxation at home are essential parts of self-care and a balanced life with purpose and meaning.

CASE STUDY

Burn Injury

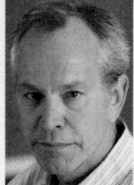

(© Comstock/
Thinkstock.)

Patient Profile

G.M., a 52-yr-old married white man, arrives at the ED with burns to his face, neck, chest, right arm and hand, and right foot. He was burning brush on his farm when the fire went out of control. He has an 18-gauge IV with NSS running at 100 mL/hr, and he is receiving 100% humidified O_2 by mask.

Subjective Data

- Reports blurry vision and trouble swallowing
- States his burns are painful and that he is scared
- States he is a "diabetic" and has "high blood pressure"

Objective Data

Physical Examination

- Is awake, alert, and oriented, but in some distress
- Eyes are red, irritated
- Voice is hoarse; nasal hair is singed
- Face is reddened with blisters noted on the nose and forehead
- Right arm, right hand, anterior chest, neck, and right foot have shiny, bright red, wet wounds
- Is shivering

Discussion Questions

1. ***Priority Decision:*** What are the priorities of care in the prehospital setting and ED? How should his airway, breathing, and circulation be managed?

2. ***Priority Decision:*** What factors place G.M. at high risk for an inhalation injury? What priority interventions can be anticipated?

3. ***Patient-Centered Care:*** What pain medications might be considered to relieve his pain?

4. Which of the criteria for burn center referral does G.M. meet for admission to the hospital burn unit?

5. What metabolic disturbances would be expected soon after G.M.'s admission? Explain the physiologic basis for these changes.

6. How might G.M.'s co-morbidities affect his burn care and rehabilitation?

7. ***Patient-Centered Care:*** What measures should be taken to support G.M.'s caregivers?

8. ***Priority Decision:*** Based on the assessment data presented, what are the priority nursing diagnoses?

9. ***Evidence-Based Practice:*** What are the most effective wound care strategies to manage G.M.'s burn wounds?

10. ***Patient-Centered Care:*** Prior to discharge what teaching should be provided to G.M. and his family so they can successfully manage his care at home?

11. ***Safety:*** To ensure G.M.'s safety at home, what interventions are necessary prior to discharge?

12. ***Quality Improvement:*** What outcomes will indicate that interprofessional care was effective?

Answers available at *http://evolve.elsevier.com/Lewis/medsurg.*

▌ BRIDGE TO NCLEX EXAMINATION

The number of the question corresponds to the same-numbered outcome at the beginning of the chapter.

1. Which prevention strategy would the nurse include when teaching about home fire safety?
   a. Set hot water temperature at 140° F.
   b. Use only hardwired smoke detectors.
   c. Encourage regular home fire exit drills.
   d. Do not allow older adults to cook unattended.

2. The injury that is *least* likely to result in a full-thickness burn is
   a. sunburn.
   b. scald injury.
   c. chemical burn.
   d. electrical injury.

3. When assessing a patient with a partial-thickness burn, the nurse would expect to find *(select all that apply)*
   a. blisters.
   b. exposed fascia.
   c. exposed muscles.
   d. intact nerve endings.
   e. red, shiny, wet appearance.

4. A patient is admitted to the burn center with burns to his head, neck, and anterior and posterior chest after an explosion in his garage. On assessment, the nurse auscultates wheezes throughout the lung fields. On reassessment, the wheezes are gone, and the breath sounds are greatly decreased. Which action is the *most* appropriate for the nurse to take *next*?
   a. Encourage the patient to cough and auscultate the lungs again.
   b. Obtain vital signs, oxygen saturation, and a STAT arterial blood gas.
   c. Document the findings and continue to monitor the patient's breathing.
   d. Anticipate the need for endotracheal intubation and notify the provider.

5. Fluid and electrolyte shifts that occur during the early emergent phase of a burn injury include
   a. adherence of albumin to vascular walls.
   b. movement of potassium into the vascular space.
   c. movement of sodium and water into the interstitial space.
   d. hemolysis of red blood cells from large volumes of rapidly administered fluid.

6. To maintain a positive nitrogen balance in a major burn, the patient must
   a. eat a high-protein, high-carbohydrate diet.
   b. increase normal caloric intake by about four times.
   c. eat at least 1500 calories/day in small, frequent meals.
   d. eat a gluten-free diet for the chemical effect on nitrogen balance.

7. A patient has 25% TBSA burn from a car fire. His wounds have been debrided and covered with a silver-impregnated dressing. The nurse's *priority* intervention for wound care would be to
   a. reapply a new dressing without disturbing the wound bed.
   b. observe the wound for signs of infection during dressing changes.
   c. apply cool compresses for pain relief in between dressing changes.
   d. wash the wound aggressively with soap and water three times a day.

8. Pain management for the burn patient is *most* effective when *(select all that apply)*
   a. a pain rating tool is used to monitor the patient's level of pain.
   b. painful dressing changes are delayed until the patient's pain is completely relieved.
   c. the patient is informed about and has some control over the management of the pain.
   d. a multimodal approach is used (e.g., sustained-release and short-acting opioids, NSAIDs, adjuvant analgesics).
   e. nonpharmacologic therapies (e.g., music therapy, distraction) replace opioids in the rehabilitation phase of a burn injury.

9. A therapeutic measure used to prevent hypertrophic scarring during the rehabilitation phase of burn recovery is
   a. applying pressure garments.
   b. repositioning the patient every 2 hours.
   c. performing active ROM at least every 4 hours.
   d. massaging the new tissue with water-based moisturizers.

10. A patient is recovering from second- and third-degree burns over 30% of his body, and the burn care team is planning for discharge. The *first* action the nurse should take when meeting with the patient would be to
   a. arrange a return-to-clinic appointment and prescription for pain medications.
   b. teach the patient and the caregiver proper wound care to be performed at home.
   c. review the patient's current health care status and readiness for discharge to home.
   d. give the patient written information and websites for information for burn survivors.

1. c, 2, 3, a, 4. d, 5. c, 6. a, 7. b, 8. a, c, d, 9. a, 10. c

For rationales to these answers and even more NCLEX review questions, visit *http://evolve.elsevier.com/Lewis/medsurg.*

ⓔ EVOLVE WEBSITE/RESOURCES LIST

http://evolve.elsevier.com/Lewis/medsurg
Review Questions (Online Only)
Key Points
Answer Keys for Questions
- Rationales for Bridge to NCLEX Examination Questions
- Answer Guidelines for Case Study on p. 451
- Answer Guidelines for Managing Care of Multiple Patients Case Study (Section 5) on p. 454
Student Case Study
- Patient With Burns
Nursing Care Plan
- eNursing Care Plan 24.1: Patient With a Thermal Burn Injury
Conceptual Care Map Creator
Audio Glossary
Content Updates

REFERENCES

1. American Burn Association: *Burn incidence and treatment in the US: 2016 fact sheet.* Retrieved from *http://ameriburn.org/who-we-are/media/burn-incidence-fact-sheet/.*
2. WHO International: *Burns fact sheet March 2018.* Retrieved from *www.who.int/news-room/fact-sheets/detail/burns.*
3. Grant EJ: Burn injuries: Prevention, advocacy, and legislation, *Clin Plast Surg* 44:451, 2017.
4. Roberts JR, Custalow CB, Thomsen TW: *Roberts and Hedges' clinical procedures in emergency medicine and acute care,* ed 7, Philadelphia, 2019, Elsevier.
5. Gupta K, Mehrotra M, Kumar P, et al: Smoke inhalation injury: Pathogenesis, diagnosis, and management, *Indian J Crit Care* Med 22:180, 2018.
6. Greenhalgh DG: *Burn care for general surgeons and general practitioners,* Wiesbaden, Germany, 2016, Springer.
7. Understanding burn care. Retrieved from *http://understandingburncare.org/burn-severity.html.*
8. American Burn Association Burn Center referral criteria. Retrieved from *www.ameriburn.org/wp-content/uploads/2017/05/burncenterreferral criteria.pdf*
9*. Wallis L, Fleming J, Hasselberg M, et al: A smartphone app and cloud-based consultation system for burn injury, *Emerg Care* 11:1, 2016.
10*. Sorg H, Tilkorn D, Hager S, et al: Skin wound healing: An update on the current knowledge and concepts, *European Surgical Res* 58:81, 2017.
11*. Pannucci C, Obi A, Timmins B, et al: Venous thromboembolism in patients with thermal injury: A review of risk assessment tools and current knowledge on the effectiveness and risks of mechanical and chemical prophylaxis, *Clin Plastic Surg* 44:573, 2017.
12*. Sutton T, Lenk I, Conrad P, et al: Severity of inhalation injury is predictive of alterations in gas exchange and worsened clinical outcomes, *J Burn Care Res* 38:390, 2017.
13. Alves dos Santos C, Souza-Junior V, Ferreira Lanza F, et al: Serious games in virtual environments for health teaching and learning, *Northeast Netw Nurs J* 18:702, 2017.
14. Deutsch C, Tan A, Smailes S, et al: The diagnosis and management of inhalation injury: An evidence-based approach, *Burns* 44:1040-1051, 2018.

15. Cartotto R, Greenhalgh D, Cancio C, et al: Burn state of the science: Fluid resuscitation, *J Burn Care Res* 38:e596-e604, 2017.

16. Ahuja R, Gibran N, Greenhalgh D, et al: ISBI practice guidelines for burn care, *Burns* 42:953, 2016.

17. Herndon DN: *Total burn care*, Edinburgh, 2018, Elsevier.

18. Berger M, Pantet O: Nutrition in burn injury: Any recent changes? *Curr Opin Crit Care* 22:285, 2016.

19. Clark A, Imran J, Madni T, et al : Nutrition and metabolism in burn patients, *Burns Trauma* 5:1, 2017.

20. Dellinger R, Schorr C, Levy M: A users guide to the 2016 surviving sepsis guidelines, *Crit Care Med* 45:381, 2017.

21. Ahuja R, Gibran N, Greenhalgh D, et al: ISBI practice guidelines for burn care, *Burns* 42:953, 2016.

22. Mushin O, Bogue J, Esquenazi M, et al: Use of a home vacuum-assisted closure device in the burn population is both cost-effective and efficacious, *Burns* 43:490, 2017.

23. Hussain A: Surgical treatment of acute burns, *Wounds UK* 14:30, 2018.

24. Najafi Ghezeljeh T, Mohades Ardebili F, Rafii F: The effects of massage and music on pain, anxiety and relaxation in burn patients, *Burns* 43:1034, 2017.

25. Parnell L: Itching for knowledge about wound and scar pruritus, *Wounds* 30:17, 2018.

26. Oosterwijk A, Mouton L, Schouten H, et al: Prevalence of scar contractures after burn: A systematic review, *Burns* 43:41, 2017.

27. Gregg D, Patil S, Singh K, et al: Clinical outcomes after burns in elderly patients over 70 years: A 17-year retrospective analysis, *Burns* 44:65, 2018.

28. Holmes E, Laughon S, Jones S: Retrospective analysis of neurocognitive impairment in older patients with burn injuries, *Psychosomatics* 58:386, 2017.

29. Jonathan B, Pius A, Richcane A: Study on acute burn injury survivors and the associated issues, *J Acute Dis* 3:206, 2016.

30. Kornhaber R, Haik J, Sayers J, et al: People with borderline personality disorder and burns: Some considerations for health professionals, *Issues Mental Health Nurs* 38:767, 2017.

31. Li F, Coombs D: Mental health history: A contributing factor for poorer outcomes in burn survivors, *Burns Trauma* 6:1, 2018.

32. Kruithof N, Traa M, Karabatzakis M, et al: Perceived changes in quality of life in trauma patients: A focus group study, *J Trauma Nurs* 25:177, 2018.

*Evidence-based information for clinical practice.

CASE STUDY
Managing Care of Multiple Patients

You are working the day shift on a medical-surgical unit and have been assigned to care for the following 5 patients. You have 1 UAP who is assigned to work with you. There are 15 other patients on the unit being cared for by an additional 3 RNs and 3 UAP.

Patients

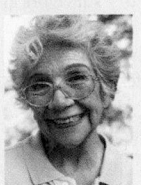

F.M., an 81-yr-old Hispanic woman, had pneumatic retinopexy surgery yesterday to repair a partial detached retina. She has a history of type 2 diabetes, hypothyroidism, and hypertension. She is scheduled to be discharged today, but the night nurse is concerned because her BP is elevated at 150/94 mm Hg.

(© Jack Hollingsworth/ Photodisc/Thinkstock.)

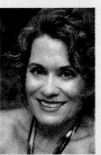

R.S., a 57-yr-old woman, is under observation with Ménière's disease. She continues to have extreme dizziness, tinnitus, and nausea. The HCP plans to administer an intratympanic injection of dexamethasone today.

(© iStock.com/EyeMark.)

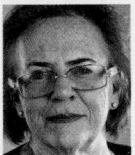

D.A., a 74-yr-old woman, is admitted to the hospital with complaints of chest tightness and shortness of breath. Her past medical history is negative except for a recent diagnosis of basal cell carcinoma (BCC) on her face. She was scheduled to have the BCC surgically removed tomorrow. The HCP suspects D.A.'s symptoms are caused by anxiety but first needs to rule out any coronary artery disease before surgery.

(© Stockphoto/ Thinkstock.)

G.L., a 48-yr-old white man, just arrived for admission. He is scheduled for surgical removal of melanoma lesions on his face at 1200. He is worried that the surgery will be disfiguring.

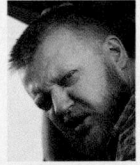

(© Dimedrol68/iStock/ Thinkstock.)

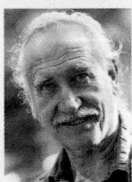

D.B., a 74-yr-old white man, was admitted 3 hours ago from the ED with partial thickness burns on his chest and arms (estimated to be 6% TBSA). He was burning leaves and branches using gasoline. The pile exploded and his clothes caught fire.

(© Stockphoto/ Thinkstock.)

Discussion Questions

1. **Priority Decision:** After receiving report, which patient should you see first? Provide rationale.
2. **Collaboration:** Which tasks could you delegate to the UAP *(select all that apply)*?
   a. Obtain vital signs on F.M.
   b. Take a blood pressure reading on D.B.
   c. Perform an admission assessment on G.L.
   d. Explain planned diagnostic testing to R.S.
   e. Obtain a 12-lead electrocardiograph on D.A.

3. **Priority Decision and Collaboration:** When you enter D.B.'s room, he tells you he is not feeling well. He says he has a headache and his legs are "cramping up." He is also somewhat confused as he is unaware that he is in the hospital. What initial action would be *most* appropriate?
   a. Administer acetaminophen for headache relief.
   b. Have the UAP obtain a STAT capillary blood glucose reading.
   c. Notify D.B.'s health care provider of his altered level of consciousness.
   d. Ask the UAP to obtain vital signs on D.B. while you review recent laboratory results.

Case Study Progression

D.B.'s vital signs are BP 154/88 mm Hg, heart rate is 112 bpm, respirations are 18 breaths/min, and temperature is 98°F (36.8°C). His most recent laboratory results reveal a serum sodium level of 128 mEq/L (128 mmol/L). You notify his HCP, who orders a normal saline IV to infuse at 100 mL/hr.

4. D.B. complains of thirst and asks for something to drink. Which fluids would be appropriate to give him *(select all that apply)*?
   a. Gatorade
   b. Tap water
   c. Cola soda
   d. Apple juice
   e. Orange juice
5. In addition to teaching F.M. how to administer postoperative eyedrops, you will also explain
   a. position and activity restrictions.
   b. how to change the dressing on her eye.
   c. the necessity for restricting fluid intake.
   d. that protective eyewear will no longer be required.
6. When giving report to your UAP regarding your assigned patients, you are asked by the UAP if there is a significant difference between D.A. and G.L.'s skin cancers. You reply based on knowledge that
   a. basal cell carcinoma is the deadliest form of skin cancer.
   b. melanoma typically appears as red, rough patches on the skin.
   c. melanoma can metastasize to any organ, including the brain and heart.
   d. basal cell carcinoma often occurs during the second and third decades of life.
7. **Management Decision:** Another RN offers to help you by providing care for F.M. Which observed action by the RN would require your immediate intervention?
   a. The RN assists F.M. to lie flat on her back.
   b. The RN gives F.M. oral medication for pain.
   c. The RN assures F.M. that retinal reattachment is usually successful.
   d. The RN explains to F.M. that she is at risk for detachment in the other eye.
8. **Priority Decision**: Which intervention has the *highest* priority for R.S.?
   a. Keeping the room dark and quiet.
   b. Placing an emesis basin at the bedside.
   c. Elevating the head of the bed to the height desired.
   d. Raising the side rails and having the bed in low position.

Answers available at *http://evolve.elsevier.com/Lewis/medsurg.*

Assessment: Respiratory System

Eugene Mondor

Do your little bit of good where you are; it's those little bits of good put together that overwhelm the world.

Desmond TuTu

ⓔ http://evolve.elsevier.com/Lewis/medsurg/

CONCEPTUAL FOCUS

Functional Ability   Gas Exchange

LEARNING OUTCOMES

1. Distinguish the structures and functions of the upper respiratory tract, lower respiratory tract, and chest wall.
2. Describe the process that initiates and controls inspiration and expiration.
3. Describe the process of oxygenation and ventilation.
4. Identify the respiratory defense mechanisms.
5. Describe the significance of arterial blood gas values in relation to respiratory function.
6. Relate the signs and symptoms of inadequate oxygenation to physical assessment findings.
7. Link age-related changes of the respiratory system to key differences in assessment findings.
8. Obtain significant subjective and objective assessment data related to the respiratory system.
9. Perform a physical assessment of the respiratory system using the appropriate techniques.
10. Distinguish normal from common abnormal findings in a physical assessment of a patient's respiratory system.
11. Describe the purpose, significance of results, and nursing responsibilities related to diagnostic studies of the respiratory system.

KEY TERMS

adventitious breath sounds, p. 467
chemoreceptor, p. 459
compliance, p. 458
crackles, Table 25.6, p. 468
dyspnea, p. 458

elastic recoil, p. 458
fremitus, p. 465
mechanical receptors, p. 459
oxygenation, p. 458
resistance, p. 458

surfactant, p. 457
tidal volume (V_T), p. 457
ventilation, p. 458
wheezes, Table 25.6, p. 468

The primary purpose of the respiratory system is gas exchange. This involves the transfer of oxygen (O_2) and carbon dioxide (CO_2) between the atmosphere and blood. While adequate perfusion is needed to distribute O_2 to the body tissues, adequate oxygenation depends on a healthy, functioning respiratory system.

STRUCTURES AND FUNCTIONS OF RESPIRATORY SYSTEM

The respiratory system is divided into 2 parts: the upper respiratory tract and the lower respiratory tract (Fig. 25.1).

Upper Respiratory Tract

The *upper respiratory tract* includes the nose, mouth, pharynx, epiglottis, larynx, and trachea. Air enters the respiratory tract through the nose. The nose is made of bone and cartilage. It is divided into 2 nares by the nasal septum. The inside of the nose is shaped into 3 passages by projections called *turbinates.* The turbinates increase the surface area of the nasal mucosa that warms and moistens the air as it enters the nose. The internal nose opens directly into the sinuses. The nasal cavity connects with the pharynx. It is a tubular passageway that is subdivided into 3 parts: the *nasopharynx, oropharynx,* and *laryngopharynx.*

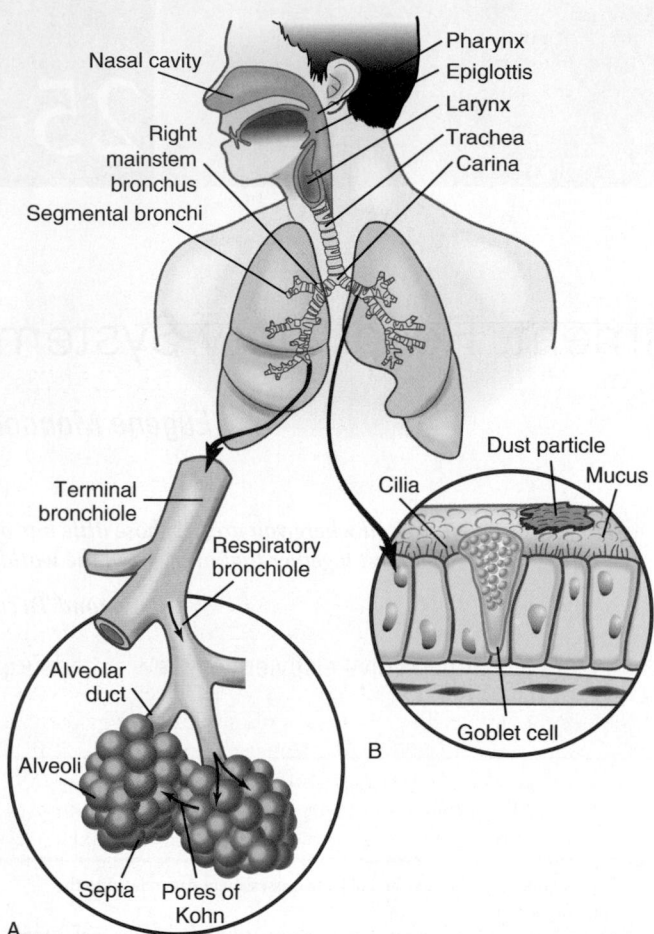

FIG. 25.1 Structures of the respiratory tract. **A,** Pulmonary functional unit. **B,** Ciliated mucous membrane. (Redrawn from Price SA, Wilson LM: *Pathophysiology: Clinical concepts of disease processes,* ed 6, St Louis, 2003, Mosby.)

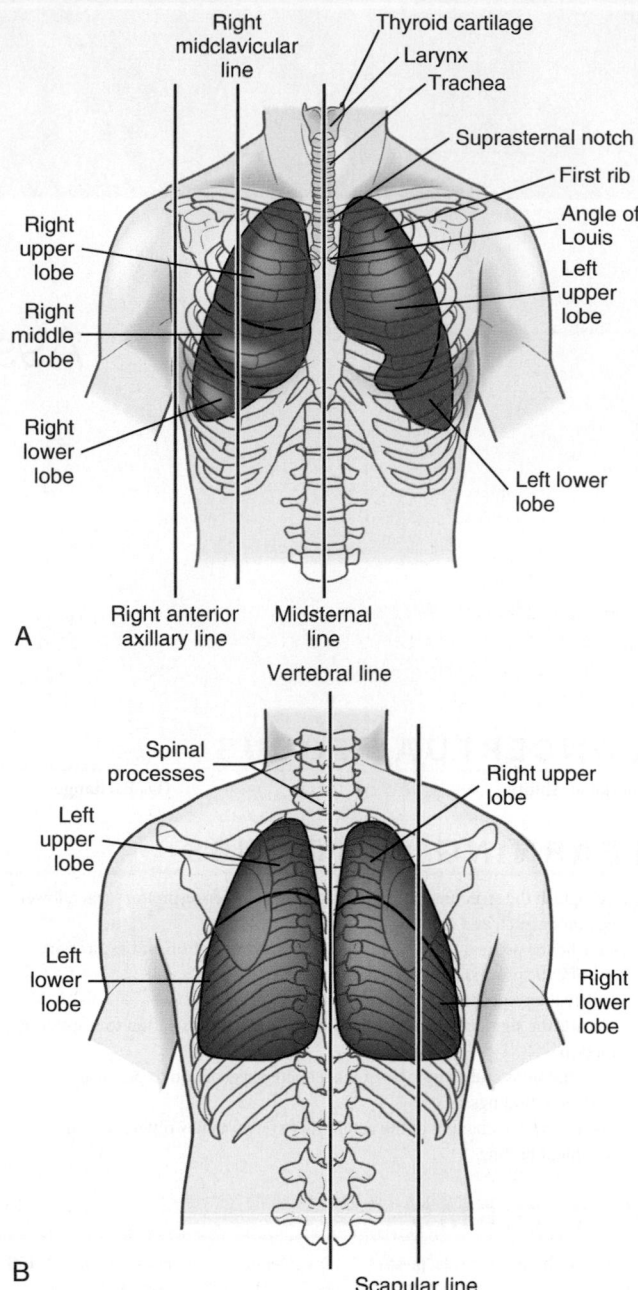

FIG. 25.2 Landmarks and structures of the chest wall. **A,** Anterior view. **B,** Posterior view. (Redrawn from Thompson JM, McFarland GK, Hirsch JE, et al: *Mosby's clinical nursing,* ed 5, St Louis, 2002, Mosby.)

The nose functions to protect the lower airway by warming and humidifying air and filtering small particles before air enters the lungs. The olfactory nerve, found within the mucosa of the upper part of the nasal cavity, is responsible for the sense of smell.[1]

Air moves through the oropharynx to the laryngopharynx. It then travels through the epiglottis to the larynx before moving into the trachea. The *epiglottis* is a small flap behind the tongue that closes over the larynx during swallowing. This prevents solids and liquids from entering the lungs. The vocal cords are in the larynx. Air passes through the glottis (the opening between the vocal cords) and into the trachea.

The trachea is a cylindrical tube about 5 in (10 to 12 cm) long and 1 in (1.5 to 2.5 cm) in diameter. U-Shaped cartilages keep the trachea open but allow the adjacent esophagus to expand for swallowing. The trachea bifurcates into the right and left mainstem bronchi at a point called the *carina.* The carina is located at the *angle of Louis,* which is at the level of the 4th and 5th thoracic vertebrae.[2] The carina is highly sensitive. Stimulation of this area during suctioning causes vigorous coughing.

Lower Respiratory Tract

Once air passes the carina, it is in the lower respiratory tract. The *lower respiratory tract* consists of the bronchi, bronchioles, alveolar ducts, and alveoli. Except for the right and left mainstem

bronchi, all lower airway structures are found within the lungs. The right lung is divided into 3 lobes (upper, middle, and lower) and the left lung into 2 lobes (upper and lower) (Fig. 25.2).

The mainstem bronchi, pulmonary vessels, and nerves enter the lungs through a slit called the *hilus.* The right mainstem bronchus is shorter, wider, and straighter than the left mainstem bronchus. That is why aspiration is more likely to occur in the right lung than in the left lung.

The mainstem bronchi subdivide several times to form the lobar, segmental, and subsegmental bronchi. Further divisions form the bronchioles. The most distal bronchioles are the respiratory bronchioles. The bronchioles are encircled by smooth muscles that constrict and dilate in response to various stimuli.

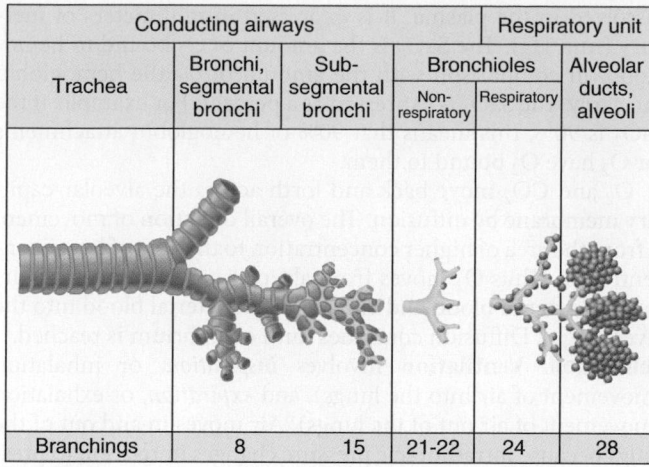

FIG. 25.3 Structures of lower airways. (Redrawn from Thompson JM, McFarland GK, Hirsch JE, et al: *Mosby's clinical nursing*, ed 5, St Louis, 2002, Mosby.)

Conducting airways					Respiratory unit
Trachea	Bronchi, segmental bronchi	Sub-segmental bronchi	Bronchioles		Alveolar ducts, alveoli
			Non-respiratory	Respiratory	
Branchings	8	15	21-22	24	28

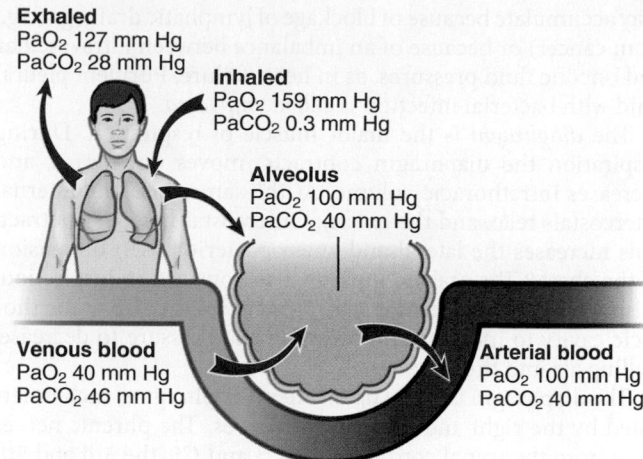

FIG. 25.4 Partial pressure of respiratory gases in normal respiration. The pressures are shown in inhaled and exhaled air from the lungs and at the level of the alveoli and pulmonary venous and arterial blood vessels.

The terms *bronchoconstriction* and *bronchodilation* refer to a decrease or increase in the diameter of the airways caused by contraction or relaxation of these muscles. Beyond the bronchioles lie the alveolar ducts and alveoli (Fig. 25.3).

The trachea and bronchi act as a pathway to conduct gases to and from the alveoli. The volume of air in the trachea and bronchi is called the *anatomic dead space* (V_D).[3] This air does not take part in gas exchange. In adults, a normal tidal volume (V_T), or volume of air exchanged with each breath, is about 500 mL (in a 150-lb man). Of each 500 mL inhaled, about 150 mL is V_D.

The alveoli are the terminal part of the respiratory tract (Fig. 25.3). *Alveoli* are small sacs in the lungs that are the primary site of gas exchange for O_2 and CO_2. The adult lung has over 300 million alveoli, each 0.3 mm in diameter. The alveoli are interconnected by pores of Kohn.[4] They allow movement of air from alveolus to alveolus (Fig. 25.1). Deep breathing promotes air movement through these pores and helps move mucus out of the respiratory bronchioles. Bacteria can also move through these pores, spreading infection to previously uninfected areas. Alveoli have a total volume of about 2500 mL with a surface area for gas exchange that is about the size of a tennis court.

Gases are exchanged across the alveolar-capillary membrane, where the alveoli come in contact with pulmonary capillaries (Fig. 25.4). In conditions such as pulmonary edema, excess fluid fills the interstitial space and alveoli, markedly reducing gas exchange.

Surfactant. Because alveoli are unstable, they have a natural tendency to collapse. Alveolar cells secrete surfactant. Surfactant is a lipoprotein that lowers the surface tension in the alveoli.[5] It reduces the amount of pressure needed to inflate the alveoli and makes them less likely to collapse. Normally, each person takes a slightly larger breath, termed a *sigh,* after every 5 or 6 breaths. This sigh stretches the alveoli and promotes surfactant secretion.

When there is not enough surfactant, the alveoli collapse. The term *atelectasis* refers to collapsed, airless alveoli. The postoperative patient is at risk for atelectasis because of the effects of anesthesia, decreased mobility, and pain, which can alter breathing and lung expansion. In acute respiratory distress syndrome (ARDS), lack of surfactant contributes to widespread atelectasis and collapse of lung tissue (see Chapter 67).

Blood Supply. The lungs have 2 different types of circulation: pulmonary and bronchial. Pulmonary circulation provides the lungs with blood that takes part in gas exchange. The pulmonary artery receives deoxygenated blood from the right ventricle of the heart and delivers it to pulmonary capillaries that lie directly alongside the alveoli. O_2–CO_2 exchange occurs at this point. The pulmonary veins return oxygenated blood to the left atrium, which then delivers it to the left ventricle, and into systemic circulation. Venous blood is collected from capillary networks of the body and returned to the right atrium by way of the superior and inferior vena cava.

Bronchial circulation starts with the bronchial arteries, which arise from the thoracic aorta. Bronchial circulation does not take part in gas exchange but provides O_2 to the bronchi and other lung tissues. Deoxygenated blood returns from the bronchial circulation through the azygos vein into the superior vena cava.[1]

Chest Wall

The chest wall is shaped, supported, and protected by 24 ribs (12 on each side). The thoracic cage, which consists of the ribs and sternum, protect the lungs and the heart from injury. The *mediastinum* is the space in the middle of the thoracic cavity. It contains the major organs of the chest, including the heart, aorta, and esophagus. The mediastinum physically separates the right and left lungs into 2 separate compartments.

The chest cavity is lined with a membrane called the *parietal pleura*. The lungs are lined with a membrane called the *visceral pleura*. The parietal and visceral pleurae join to form one continuous membrane. The visceral pleura does not have any sensory (pain) fibers or nerve endings. The parietal pleura has pain fibers. This is why irritation or inflammation of the parietal pleura can cause pain with each breath.

The *intrapleural space* is the space between the pleural layers. Normally this space contains 20 to 25 mL of fluid. This fluid serves 2 purposes: (1) it provides lubrication, allowing the pleural layers to slide over each other during breathing and (2) it increases unity between the pleural layers. This promotes expansion of the pleurae and lungs during inspiration.

Fluid drains from the pleural space via lymphatic circulation. Several pathologic conditions may cause the accumulation of greater amounts of fluid, termed a *pleural effusion*. Pleural fluid may accumulate because of blockage of lymphatic drainage (e.g., from cancer) or because of an imbalance between intravascular and oncotic fluid pressures, as in heart failure. Purulent pleural fluid with bacterial infection is called *empyema*.

The *diaphragm* is the major muscle of respiration. During inspiration the diaphragm contracts, moves downward, and increases intrathoracic volume. At the same time, the internal intercostals relax and the external intercostal muscles contract. This increases the lateral and anteroposterior (AP) dimension of the chest.[6] The scalene muscles also contract on inspiration, raising the first and second ribs. This causes the size of the thoracic cavity to increase and intrathoracic pressure to decrease, pulling air into the lungs.

The diaphragm is made up of 2 hemidiaphragms, each innervated by the right and left phrenic nerves. The phrenic nerves arise from the spinal cord between C3 and C5, the 3rd and 5th cervical vertebrae. Injury to the phrenic nerve results in hemidiaphragm paralysis on the side of the injury. Complete spinal cord injuries above the level of C3 result in total diaphragm paralysis and dependence on a mechanical ventilator.

Physiology of Respiration

Oxygenation. Oxygenation refers to the process of obtaining O_2 from the atmospheric air and making it available to the organs and tissues of the body. The lungs' ability to oxygenate arterial blood adequately is evaluated by partial pressure of O_2 in arterial blood (PaO_2), arterial O_2 saturation (SaO_2), and patient assessment (Table 25.1).

O_2 is carried in the blood in 2 forms: dissolved O_2 and hemoglobin-bound O_2. The PaO_2 represents the amount of O_2 dissolved in the plasma. It is expressed in millimeters of mercury (mm Hg). The SaO_2 is the amount of O_2 bound to hemoglobin in comparison with the amount of O_2 the hemoglobin can carry. The SaO_2 is expressed as a percent. For example, if the SaO_2 is 90%, this means that 90% of hemoglobin attachments for O_2 have O_2 bound to them.

O_2 and CO_2 move back and forth across the alveolar-capillary membrane by diffusion. The overall direction of movement is from the area of higher concentration to the area of lower concentration. Thus O_2 moves from alveolar gas (atmospheric air) into the arterial blood and CO_2 from the arterial blood into the alveolar gas. Diffusion continues until equilibrium is reached.

Ventilation. Ventilation involves *inspiration*, or inhalation (movement of air into the lungs), and *expiration*, or exhalation (movement of air out of the lungs). Air moves in and out of the lungs because intrathoracic pressure changes in relation to pressure at the airway opening. Contraction of the diaphragm and external intercostal and scalene muscles increases chest dimensions, thus decreasing intrathoracic pressure. Gas flows from an area of higher pressure (atmospheric) to one of lower pressure (intrathoracic). When dyspnea (shortness of breath) occurs, neck and shoulder muscles, as well as other accessory muscles of respiration, can aid the effort. Some conditions (e.g., phrenic nerve paralysis, rib fractures, neuromuscular disease) may limit diaphragm or chest wall movement. This causes the patient to breathe with smaller tidal volumes. As a result, the lungs do not fully inflate and gas exchange may be impaired.

In contrast to inspiration, expiration is passive. Elastic recoil is the tendency for the lungs to return to their original size after being stretched or expanded. The elasticity of lung tissue is due to the elastin fibers found in the alveolar walls and surrounding the bronchioles and capillaries. The elastic recoil of the chest wall and lungs allows the chest to passively decrease in size (volume). When intrathoracic pressure rises, air moves out of the lungs.

Exacerbations of asthma or chronic obstructive pulmonary disease (COPD) cause expiration to become an active, labored process (see Chapter 28). Abdominal, intercostal, and accessory muscles (e.g., scalene, trapezius) help expel air during labored breathing.

Compliance and Resistance. Compliance (distensibility) is a measure of the ease of expansion of the lungs. This is a product of the elasticity of the lungs and elastic recoil of the chest wall.[6] When compliance is decreased, it is harder for the lungs to inflate. This occurs with conditions that increase fluid in the lungs (e.g., pulmonary edema, ARDS, pneumonia), make lung tissue less elastic or distensible (e.g., pulmonary fibrosis, sarcoidosis), or restrict lung movement (e.g., pleural effusion). Compliance increases when there is destruction of alveolar walls and loss of tissue elasticity, as in COPD.

On the other hand, resistance refers to any obstacle to airflow during inspiration and/or expiration. The main factor affecting airway resistance is changes in the diameter (size) of the airways. For example, a patient with an acute asthma attack has narrowed airways, resulting in increased resistance. The presence of secretions in the bronchi also increases resistance. Secretions can partially occlude airways, making airways narrower. This makes it harder for patients to get air into their lungs. Giving bronchodilators decreases resistance by increasing the diameter of the bronchi, promoting air entry.

Changes in compliance and/or resistance can seriously affect both oxygenation and ventilation.

TABLE 25.1 **Manifestations of Inadequate Oxygenation**		
	ONSET	
Manifestations	**Early**	**Late**
Central Nervous System		
Unexplained apprehension	X	
Unexplained restlessness or irritability	X	
Unexplained confusion or lethargy	X	X
Combativeness		X
Coma		X
Respiratory		
Tachypnea	X	
Dyspnea on exertion	X	
Dyspnea at rest		X
Use of accessory muscles		X
Retraction of intercostal spaces on inspiration		X
Pause for breath between sentences, words		X
Cardiovascular		
Tachycardia	X	
Mild hypertension	X	
Dysrhythmias	X	X
Hypotension		X
Cyanosis		X
Cool, clammy skin		X
Other		
Diaphoresis	X	X
Decreased urine output	X	X
Unexplained fatigue	X	X

Control of Respiration

Located in the brainstem, the respiratory center (the medulla) responds to chemical and mechanical signals. The medulla sends impulses to the respiratory muscles through the spinal cord and phrenic nerves.

Chemoreceptors. A chemoreceptor is a receptor that responds to a change in the chemical composition ($PaCO_2$ and pH) of the fluid around it. Central chemoreceptors are found in the medulla. They respond to changes in the hydrogen ion (H^+) concentration.[7] An increase in the H^+ concentration (*acidosis*) causes the medulla to increase the respiratory rate and V_T. A decrease in H^+ concentration (*alkalosis*) has the opposite effect. Changes in $PaCO_2$ regulate ventilation primarily by their effect on the pH of the cerebrospinal fluid. When the $PaCO_2$ level is increased, more CO_2 is available to combine with H_2O and form carbonic acid (H_2CO_3). This lowers the cerebrospinal fluid pH and stimulates an increase in respiratory rate. The opposite process occurs with a decrease in $PaCO_2$ level.

Peripheral chemoreceptors are found in the carotid bodies at the bifurcation of the common carotid arteries and in the aortic bodies above and below the aortic arch.[8] The peripheral chemoreceptors respond to decreases in PaO_2 and pH and to increases in $PaCO_2$. These changes also stimulate the respiratory center.

In a healthy person, an increase in $PaCO_2$ or a decrease in pH causes an immediate increase in the respiratory rate. The $PaCO_2$ does not vary more than about 3 mm Hg if lung function is normal. Conditions such as COPD change lung function and may result in chronically elevated $PaCO_2$ levels. In these instances, the patient is not sensitive to further increases in $PaCO_2$ as a stimulus to breathe and may be maintaining ventilation largely because of a hypoxic drive from the peripheral chemoreceptors (see Chapter 28).

Mechanical Receptors. Mechanical receptors are found in the conducting upper airways, chest wall, diaphragm, and capillaries of the alveoli. They are stimulated by a variety of physiologic factors, such as irritants, muscle stretching, and alveolar wall distortion. The 3 major types of mechanical receptors are irritant, stretch, and juxtacapillary (J) receptors.[9]

Irritant receptors are found in the conducting airways. These receptors are sensitive to inhaled particles and aerosols and, when stimulated, initiate the cough reflex. Signals from stretch receptors, in the smooth muscle of the airways, aid in the control of respiration. As the lungs inflate, stretch receptors activate the inspiratory center to inhibit further lung expansion. This is called the *Hering-Breuer reflex,* and it prevents overdistention of the lungs. Stimulation of J receptors, found in the capillaries of the alveoli, occurs with increased pulmonary capillary pressure. This causes rapid, shallow respiration (tachypnea) seen in pulmonary edema.

Respiratory Defense Mechanisms

Respiratory defense mechanisms are efficient in protecting the lungs from inhaled particles, microorganisms, and toxic gases. The defense mechanisms include air filtration, mucociliary clearance system, cough reflex, reflex bronchoconstriction, and alveolar macrophages.

Filtration of Air. Nasal hairs filter inspired air. In addition, the abrupt changes in direction of airflow that occur as air moves through the nasopharynx and larynx increase air turbulence. This causes particles and bacteria to contact the mucosa lining these structures. Most large particles (greater than 5 μm) are less dangerous because they are removed in the nasopharynx or bronchi and do not reach the alveoli.

The velocity of airflow slows greatly after it passes the larynx, facilitating the deposition of smaller particles (1 to 5 μm). They settle out the way that sand does in a river, a process termed *sedimentation.* Particles less than 1 μm in size are too small to settle in this manner and are deposited in the alveoli. An example of small particles that can build up is coal dust, which can lead to pneumoconiosis (see Chapter 27).

Mucociliary Clearance System. Below the larynx, the mucociliary clearance system, also called the *mucociliary escalator,* is responsible for the movement of mucus. Goblet cells and submucosal glands continually secrete mucus at a rate of about 100 mL/day. This mucus forms a blanket that contains the impacted particles and debris from distal lung areas (Fig. 25.1). Secretory immunoglobulin A (IgA) in the mucus helps protect against bacteria and viruses.

Cilia cover the airways from the level of the trachea to the respiratory bronchioles (Fig. 25.1). Each ciliated cell has about 200 cilia. They beat rhythmically about 1000 times per minute in the large airways, moving mucus toward the mouth. We normally swallow the mucus without noticing.

The ciliary beat is slower further down the tracheobronchial tree. As a result, we remove particles that penetrate more deeply into the airways less rapidly. Dehydration, smoking, inhalation of high O_2 concentrations, infection, and drugs, such as atropine, anesthetics, alcohol, or cocaine, impair ciliary action. Patients with COPD and cystic fibrosis often have repeated lower respiratory tract infections. These conditions are associated with destroyed cilia, resulting in impaired secretion clearance, a chronic productive cough, and chronic colonization by bacteria. These lead to frequent respiratory tract infections.

Cough Reflex. The cough is a protective reflex that clears the airway by a high-pressure, high-velocity flow of air. It is a backup for mucociliary clearance, especially when this clearance mechanism is overwhelmed or ineffective. Coughing is effective in removing secretions only above the subsegmental level (large or main airways). Secretions below this level must be moved upward by the mucociliary mechanism before we can remove them by coughing.

Reflex Bronchoconstriction. *Reflex bronchoconstriction* is another defense mechanism. In response to the inhalation of large amounts of irritating substances (e.g., dusts, aerosols), the bronchi constrict to prevent entry of the irritants. A person with hyperreactive airways, such as a person with asthma, may have bronchoconstriction after inhalation of triggers, such as cold air, perfume, or other strong odors.

Alveolar Macrophages. Because there are no ciliated cells below the level of the respiratory bronchioles, the primary defense mechanism at the alveolar level is alveolar macrophages. *Alveolar macrophages* rapidly phagocytize inhaled foreign particles, such as bacteria. The debris is moved to the level of the bronchioles for removal by the cilia or removed from the lungs by the lymphatic system. Particles (e.g., coal dust, silica) that cannot be adequately phagocytized tend to remain in the lungs for indefinite periods and can stimulate inflammatory responses (see Chapter 27). Because alveolar macrophage activity is impaired by cigarette smoke, the smoker who is employed in an occupation with heavy dust exposure (e.g., mining, foundries) is at an especially high risk for lung disease.

Gerontologic Considerations: Effects of Aging on Respiratory System

Age-related changes in the respiratory system can be divided into alterations in structure, defense mechanisms, and respiratory

TABLE 25.2 Gerontologic Assessment Differences

Respiratory System

Changes	Differences in Assessment Findings
Structures	
Chest wall stiffening	Barrel chest appearance, kyphotic posture, ↓ chest wall movement, ↓ deep breathing, ↓ cough effectiveness
Costal cartilage calcification	
↑ Anteroposterior diameter	
↓ Elastic recoil	↓ Vital capacity, ↑ residual volume, ↑ functional residual capacity
↓ Chest wall compliance	
↓ Functioning alveoli	Decreased breath sounds, particularly at lung bases
↓ Respiratory muscle strength	↓ PaO$_2$ and SaO$_2$, normal pH and PaCO$_2$
Defense Mechanisms	
↓ Cell-mediated immunity	↓ Cough effectiveness, ↓ secretion clearance, thickened mucus
↓ Specific antibodies	
↓ Cilia function	↑ Risk for upper respiratory aspiration, infection, influenza, pneumonia
↓ Cough force	
↓ Alveolar macrophage function	Respiratory infections may be more severe and last longer
↓ Sensation in pharynx	
Respiratory Control	
↓ Response to hypoxemia	Slight ↓ PaO$_2$ and ↑ PaCO$_2$ before respiratory rate changes
↓ Response to hypercapnia	↓ Ability to maintain acid-base balance
	Significant hypoxemia or hypercapnia may develop from relatively small incidents
	Retained secretions, excessive sedation, or positioning that impairs chest expansion may substantially change PaO$_2$ or SpO$_2$ values

control (Table 25.2). Structural changes include calcification of the costal cartilages, which can interfere with chest expansion. The outward curvature of the spine is marked, especially with osteoporosis, and the lumbar curve flattens. Therefore the chest may appear barrel shaped, and the older person may need to use accessory muscles to breathe. Respiratory muscle strength progressively declines after age 50. Overall, the lungs in the older adult are harder to inflate.

Within the lung, the number of functional alveoli decreases and they become less elastic. Small airways in the lung bases close earlier in expiration. Therefore more inspired air is distributed to the lung apices and ventilation is less well matched to perfusion, lowering the PaO$_2$. As a result, older adults have less tolerance for exertion and dyspnea can occur if their activity exceeds their normal exercise.

In older adults, *respiratory defense mechanisms* are less effective because of a decline in both cell-mediated and humoral immunity (ability to produce antibodies). The alveolar macrophages are less effective at phagocytosis. An older patient has a less forceful cough and fewer and less functional cilia. Mucous membranes tend to be drier. Retained mucus predisposes the older adult to respiratory tract infections. Formation of secretory IgA, an important defense mechanism, is decreased. Swallowing is slower because of transit time in the pharyngeal area, and there is reduced sensation in the pharynx. Consequently, the older adult is at greater risk for aspiration.

The aging process alters respiratory control, resulting in a more gradual response to changes in blood O$_2$ or CO$_2$ level. The

PaO$_2$ may drop to a slightly lower than normal level, and the PaCO$_2$ may rise to a level slightly higher than normal before the respiratory rate changes.

The extent of these changes in people of the same age varies greatly. For example, the older adult who has a significant smoking history, is obese, and has a chronic illness is at greater risk for adverse outcomes.

ASSESSMENT OF RESPIRATORY SYSTEM

Determining a patient's needs related to the respiratory system requires an accurate health history and a thorough physical examination. A respiratory assessment can be done as part of a comprehensive physical examination or as a focused respiratory examination. Use judgment in determining whether all or part of the history and physical examination will be completed, based on your immediate assessment of the patient's degree of respiratory distress. If respiratory distress is severe, only obtain pertinent information and defer a thorough assessment until the patient's condition stabilizes.

CASE STUDY

Patient Introduction

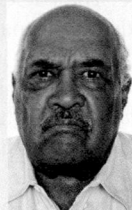

(© Fuse/Thinkstock.)

F.T. is a 70-yr-old black man who comes to the emergency department (ED) with nausea, fatigue, and increased shortness of breath, which started 3 days ago. He says that he started using his albuterol inhaler every 4 hours 2 days ago, and while it worked initially, it is no longer helping. He can walk only a few feet in his apartment before he becomes short of breath. He sleeps in a recliner in the living room. He has noticed some swelling to his hands and feet and has been having trouble urinating.

Discussion Questions

1. What are the possible causes of F.T.'s shortness of breath?
2. Does F.T. need to be admitted to the hospital or is his condition stable and he can be seen by an HCP in a few hours?
3. What questions would be a priority during the subjective assessment?

You will learn more about F.T. and his condition as you read through this assessment chapter.

(See p. 464 for more information on F.T.)

Subjective Data
Important Health Information

Past Health History. It is important to determine the frequency of upper respiratory problems (e.g., colds, sore throats, sinus problems, allergies) and whether seasonal changes influence these problems. Ask about a history of lower respiratory problems, such as asthma, COPD, pneumonia, and tuberculosis (TB).

Ask the patient with allergies about possible precipitating factors or triggers, such as medications, pollen, smoke, mold, or pet exposure. Record the characteristics and severity of the allergic reaction, such as runny nose, wheezing, scratchy throat, or chest tightness. Determine the frequency of asthma exacerbations.

Because respiratory symptoms are often manifestations of problems that involve other body systems, it is important to ask about a history of other health problems. For example, the patient with heart problems may have dyspnea (shortness of breath) because of heart failure. The patient with

TABLE 25.3 Health History

Respiratory System

Health Perception–Health Management

- Describe your daily activities. Have breathing problems prevented you from doing activities that you used to be able to do?* Are your breathing problems better, worse, or about the same compared with 6 months ago?
- How do your breathing problems affect your self-care abilities?
- Have you ever smoked? Do you smoke now? If so, what have you smoked? Cigarettes? Cigars? Pipes? Electronic cigarettes?
- If yes, how many cigarettes each day and for how long? Are you interested in stopping smoking? Are there aids we can tell you about that would assist your quitting? Would you be willing to come back for a visit so that we can explore your quitting? If you stopped smoking, did you do so because of your health?* How did you stop?
- Have you ever used chewing tobacco?
- Have you ever smoked street drugs?*
- Do you get the flu shot yearly? When was your last flu shot? Have you had a Pneumovax vaccination?
- What equipment helps you manage your respiratory problems? How often do you use it? Does it help? Cause problems?
- Do you feel that your respiratory problem is getting better or worse?

Nutritional-Metabolic

- Have you recently lost weight because of trouble eating related to your respiratory problem? How much weight have you lost? Have you lost this weight voluntarily?
- Do any foods affect your breathing?* Sputum production?*

Elimination

- Does your breathing problem make it hard for you to get to the toilet?*
- Are you inactive because of shortness of breath to the point that you have incontinence?* Constipation?*

Activity-Exercise

- Are you ever short of breath during exercise?* At rest?*
- Do you get too short of breath to do the things you want to do?*
- Is your home 1 story? 2 stories? How many steps from the street to your door?
- Can you walk up a flight of steps without stopping?
- Are you able to maintain your typical activities of daily living? If not, what are you able to do independently? What do you need help with? What have you had to give up?
- What do you do when you get short of breath? Does this help? How long does it take you to recover after you have been short of breath?

Sleep-Rest

- Do breathing problems cause you to wake up during the night?*
- Can you lie flat at night? If not, how many pillows do you use?

- Do you need to sleep upright in a chair?*
- Are you or your partner aware of any snoring?
- Do you awaken in the morning feeling rested?
- Do you ever wake up in the morning with a headache?*
- Do you fall asleep easily during the day?*

Cognitive-Perceptual

- Do you have any pain associated with breathing?* On a scale from 0 to 10, with 0 being "no pain" and 10 being "the worst pain you can imagine," where would you rate your pain? Does it hurt more on inspiration?* Expiration?* Or both?*
- If you are having pain with breathing, describe the pain.
- Has the pain gotten better, worse, or stayed about the same over the past 6 months?
- Do you ever feel restless, irritable, or confused without a reason?*
- Do you have difficulty remembering things?*

Self-Perception–Self-Concept

- Describe how your respiratory problems have changed your life.
- If you use O_2, do you ever go out without bringing it with you? How often does this occur? Why?

Role-Relationship

- Has your respiratory problem caused any problems in your work, family, or social relationships?*

Sexuality-Reproductive

- Has your respiratory problem caused a change in your sexual activity?*
- Have you and your partner talked about ways to minimize your breathing problems during sexual activity?

Coping–Stress Tolerance

- On a daily/weekly basis, how often do you leave your home?
- Do you feel under any stress right now?
- Does stress influence your breathing?*
- Do you notice if your emotions have any effect on your respiratory problems?
- Are you aware of any respiratory support groups in your area?

Value-Belief

- What do you think causes/has caused your respiratory problem(s)?
- How are you feeling right now?
- Do you think the things you have been told to do for your respiratory problems help? If not, why?
- What are you looking for/expecting from the HCP today, in terms of your breathing problem(s)?

*If answer is "yes" to any of the above questions, ask the patient to describe.

human immunodeficiency virus (HIV) infection may have frequent respiratory tract infections because of compromised immune function.

Medications. Take a thorough medication history, including the names of prescription and over-the-counter (OTC) medications and nonprescription (illicit) substances. Ask about the dose (if known), frequency, length of time taken, any side effects, and the reason for taking the medication. Assess for overuse of short-term bronchodilators as a key indicator of symptom control. Cough is a common side effect of angiotensin-converting enzyme (ACE) inhibitors. Encourage the patient to bring all medication bottles and any inhalers to each visit with an HCP.

If the patient is using O_2 for a breathing problem, record the fraction of inspired O_2 concentration (FIO_2), flow rate (liters per minute), method of administration, number of hours used

per day, and effectiveness of the therapy. Assess safety practices, including the patient's cognitive and physical ability related to using O_2 and any metered-dose inhalers.

Surgery or Other Treatments. Find out if the patient has been hospitalized for a respiratory problem. Note the dates, therapy (including surgery), and status of the problem. Determine if the patient has ever been intubated because of a respiratory problem. Ask about the use of and response to respiratory treatments, such as a nebulizer, humidifier, airway clearance modalities (see Chapter 28), high-frequency chest wall oscillation, postural drainage, and percussion.

Functional Health Patterns. Health history questions to ask a patient with a respiratory problem are outlined in Table 25.3.

Health Perception–Health Management Pattern. Ask the patient if there has been a perceived change in health status within the last several days, months, or years. In COPD, lung function declines slowly over many years. The patient may not notice this decline because they have been altering activity to accommodate reduced tolerance. If an upper respiratory tract infection is superimposed on a chronic problem, dyspnea and decreased exercise tolerance may occur very quickly. In asthma, symptoms may occur or worsen during exercise, in the presence of mold, or with changes in temperature or air pollution.

Explore common manifestations of respiratory problems (e.g., cough, dyspnea). Describe the course of the patient's illness, including when it began, type of symptoms, and factors that worsen or relieve these symptoms. Because of the chronic nature of respiratory problems, the patient may relate a change in symptoms (rather than the onset of new symptoms) when describing the present illness. For example, increased shortness of breath or increased purulence of sputum may suggest an acute exacerbation of COPD.

If a cough is present, assess its quality. For example, a loose-sounding cough occurs with secretions. A dry, hacking cough may mean an airway irritation or obstruction. A harsh, barky cough suggests upper airway obstruction from inhibited vocal cord movement due to subglottic edema. Assess whether the cough is strong enough to clear secretions. Note whether it is productive or nonproductive of secretions. Determine if the cough is acute or chronic (longer than 3 weeks in duration) or if it first began with an upper respiratory tract infection. The pattern and cause of the cough are determined by asking questions such as: What has been the pattern of coughing? Has it been regular or paroxysmal (i.e., sudden, periodic onset) or related to a time of day, the weather, certain activities, talking, or deep breathing? Any change over time? Do you clear your throat a lot? What have you tried to relieve the coughing? Did you try any prescription or OTC drugs?

If the patient has a productive cough, evaluate the following characteristics of sputum: amount, color, consistency, and odor. Quantify the amount of sputum per day. Note any recent increases or decreases in the amount. Sputum is normally clear or slightly whitish. If a patient is a cigarette smoker, the sputum is usually clear to gray with occasional specks of brown. The patient with COPD may have clear, whitish, or slightly yellow sputum, especially in the morning on rising. If the patient reports any change from baseline color, suspect pulmonary complications. Note any changes in consistency of sputum to thick, thin, or frothy and pink tinged. These changes may indicate dehydration, postnasal drip or sinus drainage, or possible pulmonary edema. Normally sputum should be odorless. A foul odor or exceptionally bad breath or taste in the mouth suggests an infectious process. Ask the patient if sputum production increases or decreases with changes in position (e.g., increased with lying down) or activity.

When assessing phlegm, determine if the patient has a history of spitting or coughing up blood *(hemoptysis)*. Hemoptysis can range from a slight streaking of blood in the sputum to massive coughing up of blood. The patient may not be able to tell between hemoptysis and *hematemesis* (vomiting blood). Hemoptysis occurs with a variety of conditions such as pneumonia, TB, lung cancer, and severe bronchiectasis.

Assess for a history of any difficulty breathing. For example, *wheezes* are musical sounds that can be audible. Wheezing indicates some degree of airway obstruction, such as asthma, foreign body aspiration, and emphysema. Assess for any history of family exposure to *Mycobacterium tuberculosis*.

🧬 GENETIC RISK ALERT

- Respiratory problems that have a strong genetic link include cystic fibrosis, COPD from α_1-antitrypsin deficiency, and asthma.
- If people have a family history of these respiratory problems, they have a greater risk for developing them.
- Although cigarette smoking is a major risk factor for COPD, only a minority of cigarette smokers develop symptomatic disease. The risk for COPD related to cigarette smoking is genetically related.
- Determine if there is a family history of any respiratory problems that may have genetic or familial tendencies.

Smoking is the most important risk factor for COPD and lung cancer. Ask about cigarette use and find out about the use of any tobacco products. This includes cigars, pipes, chewing tobacco, electronic cigarettes (e-cigarettes), and hookah (instrument for vaporizing and smoking flavored tobacco). Find out about exposure to secondhand smoke. Determine if the patient has tried to quit using tobacco products, including using prescription, OTC, and herbal remedies.

Discuss current and past smoking habits. Quantify smoking habits in *pack-years*. Do this by multiplying the number of cigarettes smoked per day by the number of years smoked. For example, a person who smoked 20 cigarettes per day for 15 years has a 15 pack-year history.

Assess if the patient received immunizations for influenza (flu) and pneumococcal pneumonia. Patients should receive an influenza vaccine yearly in the fall. Recommendations for pneumococcal vaccines are shown in Table 27.5.

Ask where the patient has lived and traveled. Risk factors for TB include prior residence in China, India, Africa, the former Soviet Republics, Latin America, or any developing country. Other TB risk factors include exposure to people with high rates of TB transmission, such as the homeless, injection drug users, and people with HIV infection. Risk factors for fungal lung infections include those exposed to bird and rodent feces or polluted water, those working closely with the soil, and immunocompromised patients. Ask the patient about the use of equipment to manage respiratory symptoms (e.g., home O$_2$ equipment, inhalers, devices for sleep apnea). Find out the type of equipment used, cleaning of the device, frequency of use, its effect, and any side effects. Have patients show you the use of their inhalers. Many patients do not use these devices correctly (see Chapter 28).

Nutritional-Metabolic Pattern. Weight loss can be a symptom of respiratory disease. Determine if weight loss was intentional, and, if not, if food intake is changed by anorexia (from medications), fatigue (from hypoxemia, increased work of breathing), or feeling full quickly (from lung hyperinflation). Anorexia, weight loss, and chronic malnutrition are common in patients with COPD, lung cancer, TB, and chronic severe infection (bronchiectasis). Assess fluid intake. Dehydration can cause sputum to thicken and obstruct the airway. Rapid weight gain from fluid retention may impair gas exchange.

Elimination Pattern. Healthy elimination habits depend on a healthy balance between activity and rest. Activity intolerance secondary to dyspnea could result in incontinence, when unable to reach a toilet when needed. Dyspnea can be the cause of limited mobility, which can cause constipation. Ask the patient with dyspnea about frequency, urgency, and elimination patterns (e.g., day vs night). People with a chronic cough, especially women, may have urinary incontinence during paroxysms of coughing.

TABLE 25.4 Dyspnea Rating Scale

Modified Borg Rating Scale for Perceived Dyspnea

Rate	Description
0	Nothing at all
0.5	Very, very slight shortness of breath
1	Very mild shortness of breath
2	Mild shortness of breath
3	Mild shortness of breath or breathing difficulty
4	Somewhat severe
5	Strong or hard breathing
6	
7	Severe shortness of breath or very hard breathing
8	
9	Extremely severe
10	Shortness of breath so severe you need to stop

From Hillegass E: *Essentials of cardiopulmonary physical therapy*, ed 4, Philadelphia, 2017, Saunders.

Activity-Exercise Pattern. Determine if dyspnea limits activity. Assess whether the patient's residence (e.g., number of steps, levels) poses any problems. Ask the patient about the perceived degree of the dyspnea (Table 25.4). For example, can the patient walk up 1 flight of stairs without stopping because of dyspnea? Is dyspnea associated with any activity better, worse, or about the same in the last few days? Months? Determine if the patient has difficulty breathing in a certain position, or if dyspnea is relieved by assuming a different position (e.g., tripod position in COPD).

Discuss whether the patient can carry out activities of daily living without dyspnea or other respiratory symptoms. If unable, record the amount and type of care the patient needs. Immobility and sedentary habits are risk factors for hypoventilation leading to atelectasis or pneumonia.

Sleep-Rest Pattern. Determine if the patient wakes up at night because of pulmonary problems. The patient with asthma or COPD may awaken with chest tightness, wheezing, or coughing. This suggests a need for adjunct therapy or other medication changes. The patient with heart disease (e.g., heart failure) may sleep with the head elevated on several pillows to avoid respiratory problems brought on by lying flat (*orthopnea*). Excess weight interferes with normal ventilation and may cause sleep apnea (see Chapter 7). Extremely obese persons may hypoventilate while awake or asleep. Manifestations of sleep apnea include snoring, insomnia, abrupt awakenings, daytime drowsiness, and early morning headaches. Night sweats may be a sign of TB.

Cognitive-Perceptual Pattern. Because hypoxia can cause neurologic symptoms, ask the patient about apprehension, restlessness, irritability, and memory changes. These can indicate inadequate cerebral oxygenation (Table 25.1). Assess the patient's cognitive ability to cooperate with treatment. Hypoxemia interferes with the ability to learn and retain information. Failure or inability to take part in needed therapy may result in worsening of respiratory problems. For this reason, teaching may be more effective if the caregiver is present during teaching sessions to provide reinforcement later.

Ask about any discomfort or pain with breathing. Explore reports of chest pain carefully to rule out heart involvement. Problems such as pleurisy, fractured ribs, and costochondritis cause chest pain. Careful assessment of the patient having pain with breathing, such as onset, exact location of the pain, and factors that make the pain better or worse, can help establish a diagnosis.

Self-Perception–Self-Concept Pattern. Dyspnea limits activity, impairs ability to fulfill normal roles, and often alters self-esteem. A patient may be reluctant to appear in public with a highly visible nasal cannula and O_2 equipment. A barrel chest, clubbed fingers, pursed-lip breathing, and frequent expectoration of sputum or throat clearing can be embarrassing and can lead to social isolation. Explore with the patient any body image concerns. Referral to a support group or pulmonary rehabilitation program may be beneficial in developing a support system and coping strategies.

Role-Relationship Pattern. Acute and chronic respiratory problems can seriously affect performance in work or other activities. Discuss the impact of medications, O_2 therapy, and special routines (e.g., pulmonary hygiene for cystic fibrosis) on the patient's family, job, and social life.

Review the nature of the patient's work and frequency and intensity of exposure to fumes, toxins, asbestos, coal, fibers, or silica. Ask whether symptoms are worse in specific situations (e.g., home vs. work environments). Hobbies, such as woodworking (sawdust) or pottery (silica), and animal exposure (allergies) can cause respiratory problems. Because of hyperreactive airways, exposure to fumes, smoke, and other chemicals may trigger an attack in the patient with asthma.

Sexuality-Reproductive Pattern. Most patients can continue to have satisfactory sexual relationships despite marked physical limitations. In a tactful manner, ask whether breathing difficulties have caused changes in sexual activity. If so, discuss positions that decrease dyspnea during sexual activity and alternative strategies for sexual fulfillment. For example, patients may need to perform good pulmonary hygiene (bronchodilators, coughing, deep breathing) before intimacy. They may need to use O_2 therapy equipment during intercourse just like they would with any strenuous physical activity.

Coping–Stress Tolerance Pattern. Dyspnea causes anxiety, and anxiety worsens dyspnea. The result is a vicious cycle—the patient avoids activities that cause dyspnea, becoming more deconditioned and more dyspneic. The outcome is often physical and leads to social isolation. Assess how often the patient leaves home and interacts with others. Referral to a support group or pulmonary rehabilitation program may be helpful.

The chronic nature of many respiratory problems, such as COPD and asthma, can cause prolonged stress. Ask about the patient's coping strategies to manage this stress.

Value-Belief Pattern. Determine the patient's adherence to his or her treatment program. Explore possible reasons for lack of adherence, including conflict with cultural beliefs, financial constraints (e.g., costs of prescriptions), or failure to understand benefit. Correct misinformation and provide up-to-date information about respiratory conditions and medication management. Including the patient and caregiver in the planning of care can improve adherence.

Objective Data

Physical Examination. Vital signs are important data to collect before examining the respiratory system.

Nose. Inspect the nose for patency, inflammation, deformities, symmetry, and discharge. Check each nare for air patency with respiration while briefly occluding the other nare. Tilt the patient's head backward and push the tip of the nose upward

CASE STUDY

Subjective Data

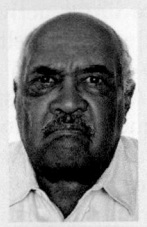

(© Fuse/ Thinkstock.)

A focused subjective assessment of F.T. revealed the following information:

PMH: COPD, hypertension, heart failure, benign prostatic hyperplasia. No history of allergies.

Medications: Metoprolol (Toprol XL) 50 mg daily PO, furosemide 20 mg PO daily, finasteride (Proscar) 5 mg/day PO, Advair inhaler (fluticasone and salmeterol) 2 puffs twice daily, and albuterol inhaler 2 puffs every 4hr PRN. Uses O₂ @ 3L/min via nasal cannula at home for the past 10 years.

Health Perception–Health Management: States he usually manages his COPD well with the Advair inhaler and occasional use of the albuterol inhaler. He thinks he caught a cold from his granddaughter last week. Increasing difficulty breathing, even with albuterol. Has a history of 30 pack-years of smoking, quitting 5 years ago.

Nutritional-Metabolic Pattern: Eating and drinking very little over past 2 to 3 days.

Elimination: Voiding small amounts of dark, concentrated urine (mostly at night).

Activity-Exercise: At present, cannot walk 100 feet without feeling short of breath. Cannot walk up 1 flight of stairs (21 steps) to get in or out of his apartment without stopping to catch his breath.

Sleep-Rest: Difficulty sleeping. Last night he slept upright in his recliner.

Cognitive-Perceptual: Denies any pain associated with shortness of breath. Feels slightly irritable because of lack of sleep.

Coping–Stress Tolerance: Does not know how he will manage to get groceries or clean his apartment. His daughter lives an hour away and has 3 children in school.

Discussion Questions

1. Of the information provided, which subjective assessment findings are of most concern to you?
2. From the information provided from F.T., what other information would you ask him about his condition (time permitting)?
3. What type of assessment would be most appropriate for F.T.: comprehensive, focused, or emergency?
4. F.T. cannot use his inhaler appropriately while he is talking with you. Is this a good time to teach him about the proper use of his inhaler?
5. What will you include in the physical assessment? What would you think will be priorities in your physical assessment?

You will learn about the physical assessment of the respiratory system in the next section.

(See p. 467 for more information on F.T.)

Answers available at *http://evolve.elsevier.com/Lewis/medsurg.*

gently. With a nasal speculum and a good light, inspect the interior of the nose. The mucous membrane should be pink and moist, with no evidence of edema (bogginess), exudate, or bleeding. Inspect the nasal septum for deviation, perforations, and bleeding. Some septal deviation is normal in an adult. Inspect the turbinates for polyps, which are abnormal, finger-like projections of swollen nasal mucosa. Polyps may result from long-term irritation of the mucosa (e.g., from allergies). Assess any discharge for color and consistency. Purulent and malodorous discharge could occur with a foreign body. Watery discharge could be related to allergies or from cerebrospinal fluid. Bloody discharge could be from trauma or dryness. Thick mucosal discharge could mean an infection.

Mouth and Pharynx. Using a good light source, inspect the interior of the mouth for color, lesions, masses, gum retraction, bleeding, and poor dentition. Inspect the tongue for symmetry and lesions. Observe the pharynx by pressing a tongue blade gently against the middle of the back of the tongue. If the oropharynx is tight, have the patient yawn, since this usually allows more structures to be visible. The pharynx should be smooth and moist, with no evidence of exudate, ulcerations, swelling, or postnasal drip. Note the color, symmetry, and any enlargement of the tonsils. Stimulate the gag reflex by placing a tongue blade along the side of the pharynx, at the back of the tongue. A normal response (gagging) means that cranial nerves IX (glossopharyngeal) and X (vagus) are intact and that the airway is protected.

Neck. Inspect the neck for symmetry and tender or swollen areas. Palpate the lymph nodes while the patient is sitting erect with the neck slightly flexed. Progression of palpation is from the nodes around the ears, to the nodes at the base of the skull, and then to those under the angles of the mandible to the midline. The patient may have small, mobile, nontender nodes (*shotty nodes*), which are not a sign of a pathologic condition. Tender, hard, or fixed nodes may indicate disease. Describe the location and characteristics of any palpable nodes.

Thorax and Lungs. Picture imaginary lines on the chest to help identify abnormalities (Fig. 25.2). Describe abnormalities in terms of their location relative to these lines (e.g., 2 cm lateral from the right midclavicular line).

Chest examination is best done in a well-lit, warm room with measures taken to ensure the patient's privacy. Expose the patient's chest. Perform all physical assessment maneuvers (inspection, palpation, percussion, auscultation) on either the anterior or the posterior chest first rather than moving from anterior to posterior or vice versa with each maneuver. It is best to begin on the posterior chest, particularly with female patients, since you can obtain more information without interference from breast tissue. If the patient tires or you are interrupted, you will obtain baseline data with the most information from examining the posterior chest.

When assessing the *posterior chest*, ask the patient to lean forward with arms folded. This position moves the scapulae away from the spine, exposing more of the area you need to examine. When assessing the *anterior chest*, have the patient sit upright or position the patient supine with the head of the bed elevated to 30 degrees (semi-Fowler's position). The patient may need to lean forward for support on the bedside table to facilitate breathing.

Inspection. First, observe the patient's appearance and note any evidence of respiratory distress, such as tachypnea or use of accessory muscles. Next, determine the shape and symmetry of the chest. Chest movement should be equal on both sides, and the anterior-posterior (AP) diameter should be less than the side-to-side or transverse diameter. Normal AP ratio is 1:2. An increase in AP diameter (e.g., barrel chest) may be due to normal aging or result from lung hyperinflation. Look for abnormalities in the sternum (e.g., *pectus carinatum* [a prominent protrusion of the sternum]) and *pectus excavatum* (an indentation of the lower sternum above the xiphoid process). Note any spinal curvature. Spinal curvatures that affect breathing include kyphosis, scoliosis, and kyphoscoliosis.

Observe the respiratory rate, depth, and rhythm. The normal adult respiratory rate is 12 to 20 breaths/min. Inspiration (I) should take half as long as expiration (E) (I/E ratio = 1:2). Observe for abnormal breathing patterns, such as *Kussmaul* (rapid, deep breathing), *Cheyne-Stokes* (abnormal respirations characterized by alternating periods of apnea and deep, rapid breathing), or *Biot's* (irregular breathing with apnea every 4 to 5 cycles) respirations.

Skin color provides clues to respiratory status. Cyanosis, a late sign of hypoxemia, is best seen in light-skinned patients as a bluish tinge to the mucous membranes, lips, and palms of the hands. In dark-skinned persons, cyanosis may be seen as a gray or white discoloration in the conjunctivae or around the mouth. Causes of cyanosis include hypoxemia or decreased cardiac output. Inspect the fingers for evidence of long-standing hypoxemia, known as *clubbing*. It is an increase in the angle between the base of the nail and the fingernail to 180 degrees or more. Clubbing usually accompanied by an increase in the depth, bulk, and sponginess of the end of the finger.

Palpation. Determine tracheal position by gently placing the index fingers on either side of the trachea just above the suprasternal notch and gently pressing backward. Normal tracheal position is midline; deviation to the left or right is abnormal. Tracheal deviation occurs away from the side of a tension pneumothorax or a neck mass, but toward the side of a pneumonectomy or lobar atelectasis.

Symmetry of chest expansion and extent of movement are determined at the level of the diaphragm. Place your hands over the lower anterior chest wall along the costal margin and move them inward until the thumbs meet at midline. Ask the patient to breathe deeply. Observe the movement of the thumbs away from each other. Normal expansion is 1 in (2.5 cm). Hand placement on the posterior side of the chest is at the level of the tenth rib. Move the thumbs until they meet over the spine (Fig. 25.5). You can check expansion anteriorly or posteriorly. It is not necessary to check both.

Normal chest movement is equal. Unequal expansion occurs when air entry is limited by conditions involving the lung (e.g., atelectasis, pneumothorax) or the chest wall (e.g., incisional pain). Equal but decreased expansion occurs in conditions that produce a hyperinflated or barrel chest or in neuromuscular diseases (e.g., amyotrophic lateral sclerosis, spinal cord lesions). Movement may be absent or unequal over a pleural effusion, an atelectasis, or a pneumothorax.

Fremitus is the vibration of the chest wall made by vocalization. You can feel tactile fremitus by placing the palmar surface of your hands against the patient's chest with the fingers hyperextended. Ask the patient to repeat a phrase, such as "boy-oh-boy," "toy boat," or "blue balloons," in a deeper, louder-than-normal voice. At the same time, move your hands from top to bottom on the patient's chest (Fig. 25.6). As you palpate, simultaneously compare vibrations (right side vs. left side, from top to bottom). Tactile fremitus is most intense by the sternum and between the scapulae because these areas are closest to the major bronchi. Fremitus is less intense farther away from these areas.

Note any increase, decrease, or absence of fremitus. Increased fremitus occurs when the lung becomes filled with fluid or is denser. As the patient's voice moves through a dense tissue or fluid, you can feel that the vibration is increased. This happens with pneumonia, lung tumors, thick bronchial secretions, and above a pleural effusion (the lung is compressed upward). Fremitus is decreased if the hand is farther from the lung (e.g., pleural effusion) or the lung is hyperinflated (e.g., barrel chest). Absent fremitus may occur with pneumothorax or atelectasis. The anterior of the chest is harder to palpate for fremitus because of the large muscles and breast tissue.

Percussion. Percussion is used to assess the density or aeration of the lungs. Percussion sounds are described in Table 25.5. (The technique for percussion is described in Chapter 3 and Fig. 3.3.)

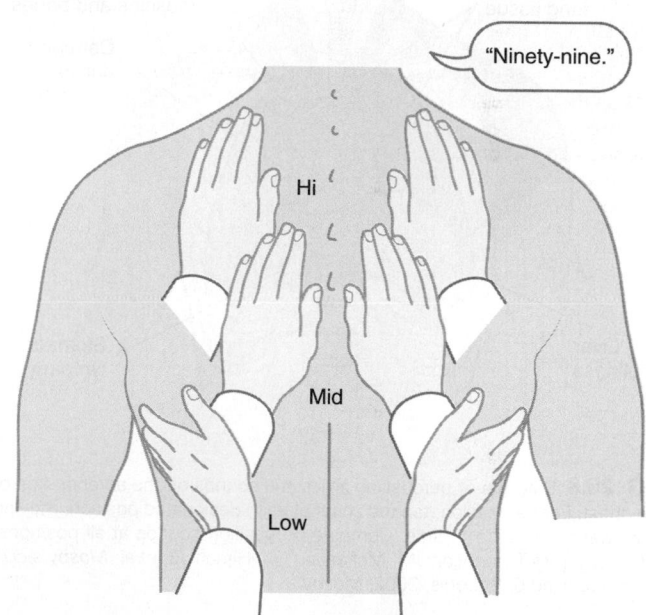

"Ninety-nine."

FIG. 25.6 Hand position for tactile fremitus. Place the palms of the hands in the position designated as "*low*" on the right and left sides of the chest. Compare the intensity of vibrations. Continue for all positions in each sequence.

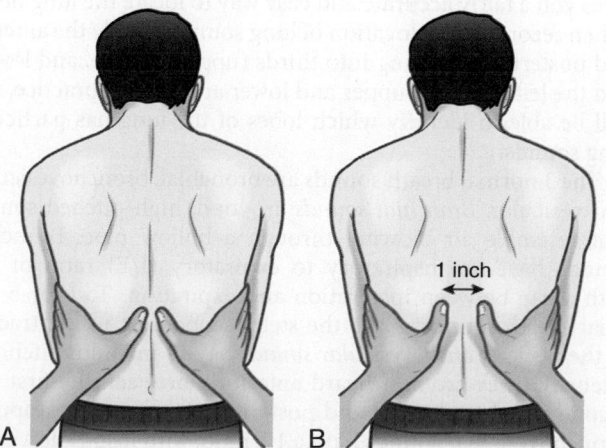

FIG. 25.5 Estimation of thoracic expansion. **A,** Exhalation. **B,** Maximal inhalation.

TABLE 25.5 Percussion Sounds

Sound	Description
Dull	Sound with medium-intensity pitch and duration heard over areas of "mixed" solid and lung tissue, such as top area of liver, partially consolidated lung tissue (pneumonia), or fluid-filled pleural space
Flat	Soft, high-pitched sound of short duration heard over very dense tissue where air is not present, such as posterior chest below level of diaphragm
Hyperresonance	Loud, lower pitched sound than normal resonance heard over hyperinflated lungs, such as in chronic obstructive pulmonary disease and acute asthma
Resonance	Low-pitched sound heard over normal lungs
Tympany	Drum-like, loud, empty quality sound heard over pneumothorax

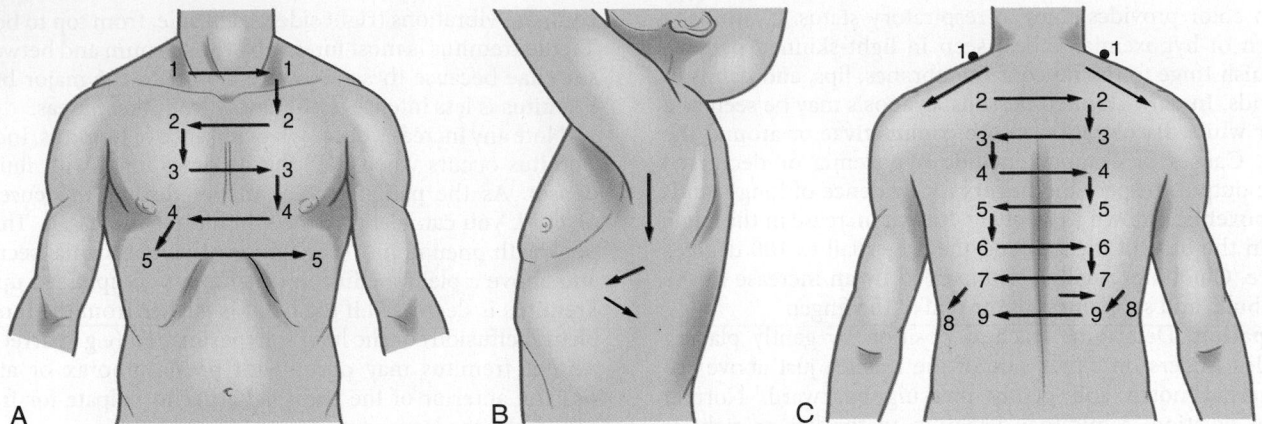

FIG. 25.7 Sequence for auscultation of the chest. **A,** Anterior sequence. **B,** Lateral sequence. **C,** Posterior sequence. Place the stethoscope at each position and listen to at least 1 complete inspiratory and expiratory cycle. Keep in mind that with a female patient the breast tissue will modify the completeness of the anterior examination.

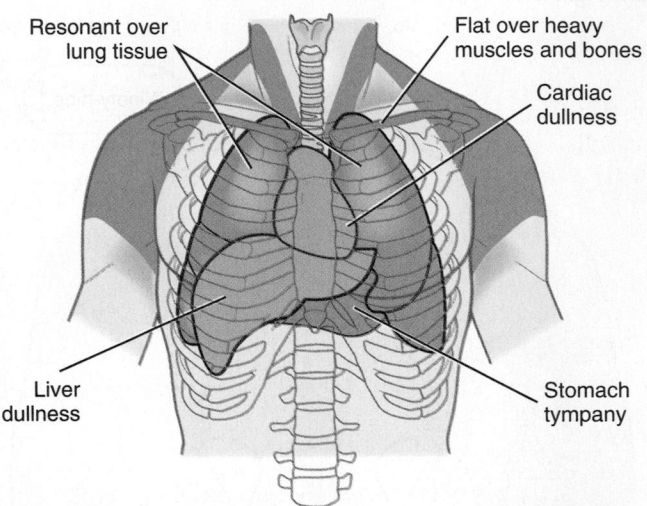

FIG. 25.8 Diagram of percussion areas and sounds on the anterior side of the chest. For percussion, tap the chest at each designated position, moving downward from side to side. Compare percussion sounds at all positions. (Redrawn from Thompson JM, McFarland GK, Hirsch JE, et al: *Mosby's clinical nursing*, ed 5, St Louis, 2002, Mosby.)

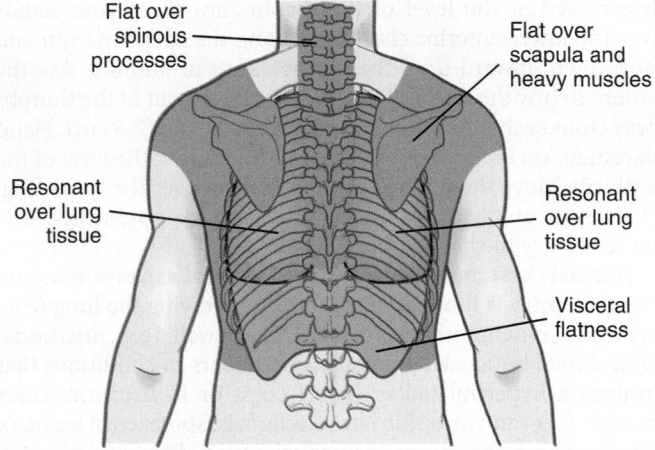

FIG. 25.9 Diagram of percussion areas and sounds on the posterior side of the chest. Percussion proceeds from the lung apices to the lung bases while comparing sounds in opposite areas of the chest. (Redrawn from Thompson JM, McFarland GK, Hirsch JE, et al: *Mosby's clinical nursing*, ed 5, St Louis, 2002, Mosby.)

The anterior chest is percussed with the patient in a semi-sitting or supine position. Starting above the clavicles, percuss downward, intercostal space by intercostal space (Fig. 25.7). The area over lung tissue should be resonant, except for the area of cardiac dullness (Fig. 25.8). To percuss the posterior chest, have the patient sit leaning forward with arms folded. The posterior chest should be resonant over lung tissue to the level of the diaphragm (Fig. 25.9).

Auscultation. During chest auscultation, have the patient breathe slowly and a little more deeply than normal through the mouth. Auscultation should proceed from the lung apices to the bases, comparing opposite areas of the chest. If the patient is in mild respiratory distress or you think the patient will tire easily, start at the bases. Place the stethoscope over lung tissue, not over bony prominences. At each placement of the stethoscope, listen to at least 1 cycle of inspiration and expiration. Visualize the location of normal breath sounds by using a lung model (Fig. 25.10).

Lung sounds are heard anteriorly from a line drawn perpendicular from the sternum lateral to the midclavicular line.

From the xiphoid process, palpate inferiorly (down) 2 ribs in the midaxillary line and around to the posterior chest. This gives you a fairly accurate and easy way to locate the lung fields. When recording the location of lung sounds, divide the anterior and posterior right lung into thirds (upper, middle, and lower) and the left lung into upper and lower areas. With practice, you will be able to identify which lobes of the lung has particular lung sounds.

The 3 normal breath sounds are bronchial, bronchovesicular, and vesicular. *Bronchial sounds* are loud, high-pitched sounds that resemble air blowing through a hollow pipe. Bronchial sounds have an inspiratory to expiratory (I/E) ratio of 2:3, with a gap between inspiration and expiration. To hear bronchial breath sounds, place the stethoscope next to the trachea in the neck. *Bronchovesicular sounds* have a medium pitch and intensity. They are best heard anteriorly between the first and second intercostal space and posteriorly between the scapulae. Bronchovesicular sounds have a 1:1 ratio, with inspiration equal to expiration. *Vesicular sounds* are relatively soft, low-pitched, gentle, rustling sounds. They are heard over all lung areas except

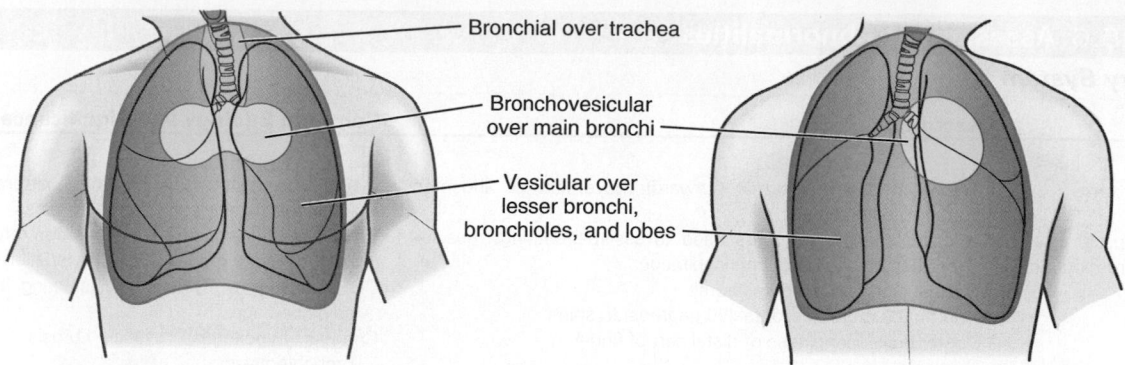

FIG. 25.10 Normal auscultatory sounds. (Redrawn from Beare PG, Myers JL: *Adult health nursing*, ed 3, St Louis, 1998, Mosby.)

Labels on figure:
Bronchial over trachea
Bronchovesicular over main bronchi
Vesicular over lesser bronchi, bronchioles, and lobes

the major bronchi. Vesicular sounds have a 3:1 ratio, with inspiration 3 times longer than expiration.

We classify breath sounds into 2 main categories: normal and abnormal (adventitious). There are a variety of terms that have been inconsistently used to describe abnormal breath sounds. Adventitious breath sounds include crackles (fine and coarse), wheezes, stridor, and pleural friction rub (Table 25.6). A *focused assessment* is used to evaluate the status of previously identified respiratory problems and to monitor for signs of new problems. A focused assessment of the respiratory system is shown in the box on this page.

As you begin your assessment of lung sounds, first note the air entry, which may be adequate, slightly decreased, or decreased. Absent air entry in any part of the lung is an assessment finding that you should report at once. Next, listen for the breath sounds and the presence of normal and adventitious sounds. Are the normal breath sounds where you would expect to hear them? Focus your assessment on the characteristics of

any abnormal sound, including the location, pitch (e.g., high, low), duration of sound, and whether the sound is heard on inspiration, expiration, or both.

Assessment abnormalities of the thorax and lungs are outlined in Table 25.6. A record of the normal physical assessment of the respiratory system is shown in Table 25.7. Chest examination findings in common pulmonary problems are described in Table 25.8. Age-related changes in the respiratory system and assessment findings are outlined in Table 25.2.

CASE STUDY

Objective Data: Physical Examination

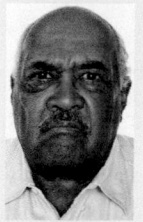

(© Fuse/Thinkstock.)

Physical examination findings of F.T. are as follows:
Temperature: 38°C (100.4°F), apical pulse 110 (irregular), respiratory rate 30 (regular, shallow, slightly labored), BP 170/90. Sitting on edge of bed with arms resting on bedside table. Skin color normal for race with no signs of cyanosis. Using accessory muscles in neck and shoulders. Trachea midline. Barrel-shaped chest; chest expansion minimal but equal. Prolonged expiration. Slight clubbing noted. Edema: 3+ pitting edema of both lower legs and feet, bilaterally. Lungs: adequate air entry at apices bilaterally with fine crackles; decreased air entry to right middle lobe and both bases with coarse crackles. Slight expiratory wheeze heard throughout all lung fields. Cough: moist, productive, with yellow-tinged sputum.

You decide to check F.T.'s O₂ saturation (SpO₂). His SpO₂ is 87% on room air.

Discussion Questions

1. What physical assessment findings are of most concern to you?
2. Identify 3 interventions that may be implemented immediately.
3. With F.T.'s physical assessment information, what diagnostic studies would you expect to be ordered?
(See p. 475 for more information on F.T.)

Answers available at *http://evolve.elsevier.com/Lewis/medsurg*.

FOCUSED ASSESSMENT
Respiratory System

Use this checklist to make sure the key assessment steps have been done.

Subjective
Ask the patient about any of the following and note responses.

Shortness of breath	Y	N
Pain with breathing	Y	N
Cough	Y	N
Sputum production (color, quantity)	Y	N
Wheezing	Y	N

Objective: Physical Examination

Observe
Respirations: Rate, quality, and pattern
Accessory muscle use
Mouth or nose breathing

Inspect
Neck for position of trachea
Shape, symmetry, and movement of chest wall
Skin and nails for integrity and color

Palpate
Chest and back for abnormalities (i.e. masses)

Auscultate
Lung sounds (anterior and posterior)

Objective: Diagnostic
Check the following diagnostic tests for abnormal results.
Arterial blood gases
Chest x-ray
Hemoglobin
Hematocrit

TABLE 25.6 Assessment Abnormalities

Respiratory System

Finding	Description	Common Etiology and Significance
Inspection		
Abdominal paradox	Inward (rather than normal outward) movement of abdomen during inspiration	Inefficient and ineffective breathing pattern. Nonspecific indicator of severe respiratory distress
Accessory muscle use. Intercostal retractions	Neck and shoulder muscles used to assist breathing; muscles between ribs pull in during inspiration	COPD, asthma exacerbation, secretion retention. Indicates severe respiratory distress/failure, hypoxemia
↑ AP diameter	AP chest diameter equal to lateral. Slope of ribs more horizontal (90 degrees) to spine	COPD, asthma, cystic fibrosis, lung hyperinflation, advanced age
Clubbing	↑ Depth, bulk, sponginess of distal part of finger	Chronic hypoxemia, cystic fibrosis, lung cancer, bronchiectasis
Cyanosis	Bluish color of skin best seen in lips and on the palpebral conjunctiva (inside the lower eyelid)	Reflects 5–6 g of hemoglobin not bound with O_2. ↓ O_2 transfer in lungs, ↓ cardiac output. Nonspecific, unreliable indicator
Kussmaul respirations	Regular, rapid, and deep respirations. Fruity odor to breath	Metabolic acidosis. Increases CO_2 excretion
Pursed-lip breathing	Exhalation through mouth with lips pursed together to slow exhalation	COPD, asthma. Suggests ↑ breathlessness. Strategy taught to slow expiration, ↓ dyspnea
Splinting	Voluntary ↓ in tidal volume to ↓ pain on chest expansion	Thoracic or abdominal incision, chest trauma, pleurisy
Tachypnea	Rate >20 breaths/min	Fever, anxiety, hypoxemia, restrictive lung disease. Magnitude of ↑ above normal rate reflects increased work of breathing
Tripod position. Inability to lie flat	Leaning forward with arms and elbows supported on overbed table	COPD, asthma exacerbation, pulmonary edema. Indicates moderate to severe respiratory distress
Palpation		
Altered chest movement	Unequal or equal but decreased movement of 2 sides of chest with inspiration	Unequal movement caused by atelectasis, pneumothorax, pleural effusion, splinting. Equal but decreased movement caused by barrel chest, restrictive disease, neuromuscular disease
Altered tactile fremitus	Increase or decrease in vibrations	↑ In pneumonia, pulmonary edema. ↓ in pleural effusion, lung hyperinflation. Absent in pneumothorax, atelectasis
Tracheal deviation	Leftward or rightward movement of trachea from normal midline position	Nonspecific indicator of change in position of mediastinal structures. Medical emergency if caused by tension pneumothorax (trachea deviates to side opposite collapsed lung)
Percussion		
Dullness	Medium-pitched sound over areas that normally make a resonant sound	↑ Density (pneumonia, large atelectasis), ↑ fluid in pleural space (pleural effusion)
Hyperresonance	Loud, lower pitched sound over areas that normally make a resonant sound	Lung hyperinflation (COPD), lung collapse (pneumothorax), air trapping (asthma)
Auscultation		
Absent breath sounds	No sound heard over entire lung or area of lung	Pneumothorax, pleural effusion, mainstem bronchi obstruction, large atelectasis, pneumonectomy, lobectomy
Bronchophony, whispered pectoriloquy	Spoken or whispered syllable more distinct than normal on auscultation	Pneumonia
Coarse crackles	Louder, discontinuous, low-pitched sounds caused by air passing through airway intermittently occluded by mucus, unstable bronchial wall. May be heard on inspiration, expiration, or both. Similar sound to blowing through straw under water	Excess fluid within the lungs, heart failure, pulmonary edema, pneumonia with severe congestion, COPD
Egophony	Spoken "E" similar to "A" on auscultation because of altered transmission of voice sounds	Pneumonia, pleural effusion
Fine crackles	Short, discontinuous, high-pitched sounds heard just before the end of inspiration. Result of rapid equalization of gas pressure when collapsed alveoli or terminal bronchioles suddenly snap open. Similar sound to that made by rolling hair between fingers	Interstitial edema (early pulmonary edema), alveolar filling (pneumonia), loss of lung volume (atelectasis), early phase of heart failure, idiopathic pulmonary fibrosis
Pleural friction rub	Creaking or grating sound from roughened, inflamed pleural surfaces rubbing together. Evident during inspiration, expiration, or both. No change with coughing. Often uncomfortable, especially on deep inspiration	Pleurisy, pneumonia, pulmonary infarct
Stridor	Continuous musical or crowing sound of constant pitch. Result of partial obstruction of larynx or trachea	Croup, epiglottitis, vocal cord edema after extubation, foreign body
Wheezes	Continuous high-pitched squeaking or musical sound caused by rapid vibration of bronchial walls. First evident on expiration but possibly evident on inspiration as obstruction of airway increases. May be audible without stethoscope	Bronchospasm (caused by asthma), airway obstruction (caused by foreign body, tumor), COPD

DIAGNOSTIC STUDIES OF RESPIRATORY SYSTEM

Numerous diagnostic studies are available to assess the respiratory system. Tables 25.9 through 25.17 describe common studies. Select studies are described in more detail here.

Two methods are used to assess the efficiency of gas transfer in the lung and tissue oxygenation: (1) pulse oximetry and (2) analysis of *arterial blood gases* (ABGs) (Table 25.9). These are primarily used to assess for hypoxia. For the patient with normal or near-normal cardiac function, assessing PaO_2 or SaO_2 is usually enough to determine the level of oxygenation. With either one, we can also use CO_2 monitoring to assess for hypercapnia to determine patient's oxygenation and ventilatory status. The patient with impaired cardiac output or hemodynamic instability (e.g., altered level of consciousness, changes in heart rate and rhythm, low BP) may have inadequate tissue O_2 delivery and/or abnormal O_2 consumption. For these patients, we can evaluate a mixed venous blood gas.

Oximetry

Arterial O_2 saturation can be monitored noninvasively and continuously using a *pulse oximetry* probe on the finger, toe, ear, forehead, or bridge of the nose. The abbreviation SpO_2 is used to indicate the O_2 saturation of hemoglobin as measured by pulse oximetry. SpO_2 and heart rate are displayed on the monitor as digital readings. Normal SpO_2 values are 94% to 99% (Table 25.10).

In many inpatient areas, SpO_2 is assessed with each routine vital sign check. Oximetry is also used during exercise testing and when adjusting flow rates during O_2 therapy. Pulse oximetry is especially valuable in perioperative and critical care situations, in which anesthesia, sedation, or decreased consciousness may mask hypoxia. Changes in SpO_2 can be detected and treated quickly (Table 25.9).

Values obtained by pulse oximetry are less accurate if the SpO_2 is less than 70%.[10] At this level the oximeter may display a value that is ±4% of the actual value. For example, if the SpO_2 reading is 70%, the actual value can range from 66% to 74%. Pulse oximetry is inaccurate if hemoglobin variants (e.g., carboxyhemoglobin, methemoglobin) are present. Other factors that can alter the accuracy of pulse oximetry include motion, low perfusion, anemia, cold extremities, bright fluorescent lights, intravascular dyes, thick acrylic nails, and dark skin color. If there is doubt about the accuracy of the SpO_2 reading, obtain an ABG analysis to verify the values.

Arterial Blood Gases

ABGs are obtained to determine oxygenation status and acid-base balance. ABG analysis includes measurement of the PaO_2, $PaCO_2$ (the partial pressure of CO_2 in arterial blood), acidity (pH), bicarbonate (HCO_3^-), and SaO_2. Normal values for ABGs are shown in Table 25.11.

Blood for ABG analysis can be obtained by arterial puncture or from an arterial catheter, which is usually inserted into the radial or femoral artery. Both techniques allow only intermittent analysis, but an arterial catheter permits ABG sampling without repeated arterial punctures. The normal PaO_2 decreases with advancing age. It varies in relation to the distance above sea level. At higher altitudes, the barometric pressure is lower, resulting in a lower inspired O_2 pressure and a lower PaO_2.

TABLE 25.7 Normal Physical Assessment of the Respiratory System

Nose	• Symmetric with no deformities • Nasal mucosa pink, moist with no edema, exudate, blood, or polyps • Nasal septum straight (slight nasal deviation possible) • Nares patent bilaterally
Oral mucosa	• Light pink, moist, no exudate or ulcerations
Pharynx	• Smooth, moist, and pink
Neck	• Trachea midline
Chest	• AP diameter 1:2 • Respirations nonlabored at 12–20 breaths/min • Breath sounds vesicular without crackles or wheezes • Excursion equal bilaterally with no increase in tactile fremitus

---

TABLE 25.8 Chest Examination Findings in Respiratory Problems

Problem	Inspection	Palpation	Percussion	Auscultation
Asthma exacerbation	Prolonged expiration, tripod position, pursed lips	↓ Movement	Hyperresonance	Wheezes, ↓ breath sounds ominous sign (severely decreased air movement)
Atelectasis	No change unless involves entire segment, lobe	If small, no change If large, ↓ movement, ↓ fremitus	Dull over affected area	Fine crackles (may disappear with deep breaths) Absent sounds if large
COPD	Barrel chest, cyanosis, tripod position, use of accessory muscles	↓ Movement	Hyperresonant or dull if consolidation	Crackles, wheezes, distant breath sounds
Pleural effusion	Tachypnea, use of accessory muscles	↑ Movement ↑ Fremitus above effusion Absent fremitus over effusion	Dull	Decreased or absent over effusion, egophony above effusion
Pneumonia	Tachypnea, use of accessory muscles, duskiness or cyanosis	↑ Fremitus over affected area	Dull over affected areas	*Early:* Bronchial sounds *Later:* Fine and/or coarse crackles, egophony, whispered pectoriloquy
Pulmonary edema	Tachypnea, labored respirations, cyanosis, pink-tinged sputum	↓ Movement or normal movement	Dull or normal depending on amount of fluid	Fine or coarse crackles
Pulmonary fibrosis	Tachypnea	↓ Movement	Normal	Crackles or sounds like Velcro being pulled apart

TABLE 25.9 Diagnostic Studies: Oxygenation

Study	Description and Purpose	Nursing Responsibility
Arterial blood gases (ABGs)	Arterial blood is obtained through puncture of radial or femoral artery or through arterial catheter. Done to assess acid-base balance, oxygenation/ventilation status, need for and/or change in O_2 therapy, or change in ventilator settings. See Table 25.11 for reference values.	*Before:* Indicate whether patient is using O_2 (flow rate in L/min). Avoid change in O_2 therapy or interventions (e.g., suctioning, position change) for 15 min before obtaining sample. *During:* Assist with positioning (e.g., palm up, wrist slightly hyperextended if radial artery is used). Collect blood in heparinized syringe. To ensure accurate results, expel all air bubbles. *After:* Apply pressure to radial artery for at least 5 min after specimen is obtained to prevent hematoma at the arterial puncture site. Send sample to lab promptly for analysis.
O_2 Monitoring **Oximetry**	Monitors arterial or venous O_2 saturation. Probe attaches to finger, toe, earlobe, bridge of the nose for SpO_2 monitoring or is in a pulmonary artery catheter for SvO_2 monitoring. Used for intermittent or continuous monitoring and exercise testing. *Normal SpO_2:* 94%–100% *Normal SvO_2:* 60%–80%	*During:* Apply probe. When interpreting SpO_2 and SvO_2 values, first assess patient status and presence of factors that can alter accuracy of pulse oximeter reading. For SpO_2, these include motion, low perfusion, cold extremities, bright lights, acrylic nails, dark skin color, carbon monoxide, and anemia. For SvO_2, these include change in O_2 delivery or O_2 consumption.
CO_2 Monitoring **End-tidal CO_2 ($PetCO_2$) (capnography)**	Assesses the level of CO_2 in exhaled air. Graphically displays partial pressure of CO_2. Expired gases are sampled from patient's airway and analyzed by a CO_2 sensor to measure exhaled CO_2. Sensor may be attached to an adaptor on endotracheal or tracheostomy tube. A nasal cannula with a sidestream capnometer can be used in patients without an artificial airway. Can be a diagnostic measure to detect lung disease and for monitoring patients. Normal difference between $PaCO_2$ and $PetCO_2$ is 2–5 mm Hg ($PaCO_2$: 35–45 mm Hg; $PetCO_2$: 40–50 mm Hg).	*Before:* Teach patient and caregiver about purpose of capnography monitoring, emphasizing the benefit of continuous monitoring. *During:* Make sure that sensor is properly attached. Record data per agency policy.

SvO_2, venous O_2 saturation.

TABLE 25.10 Normal and Critical Values for PaO_2 and SpO_2

PaO_2 (mm Hg)	SpO_2 (%)	Significance	Manifestations	Management
80–100	≥94	Normal value	Asymptomatic	• Routine assessment of patient
60–79	90	Mild hypoxemia	Restlessness, tachycardia, dysrhythmias, dyspnea, hypertension	• Assess patient condition as needed • Supplemental O_2 may be needed
40–59	88	Moderate hypoxemia	Confusion, lethargy, dysrhythmias, hypotension, respiratory distress, accessory muscle use	• O_2 required • Escalate level of care. Obtain critical care consult • Monitor frequently for sudden deterioration in condition
<40	75	Severe hypoxemia	Cyanosis, coma, respiratory and/or cardiac arrest possible	• High FIO_2, intubation, mechanical ventilation • Continuous patient assessment and evaluation

TABLE 25.11 Normal Arterial Blood Gas Values

Laboratory Value	Sea Level BP 760 mm Hg	1 Mile Above Sea Level BP 629 mm Hg
pH	7.35–7.45	7.35–7.45
PaO_2†	80–100 mm Hg	65–75 mm Hg
SaO_2†	>95%	>95%
$PaCO_2$	35–45 mm Hg	35–45 mm Hg
HCO_3^-	22–26 mEq/L (mmol/L)	22–26 mEq/L (mmol/L)

BP, Barometric pressure; *HCO_3^-,* bicarbonate; *PaO_2,* partial pressure of O_2 in arterial blood; *$PaCO_2$,* partial pressure of arterial CO_2; *SaO_2,* arterial O_2 saturation.

TABLE 25.12 Normal Venous Blood Gas Values

Venous Blood Gases	
Mixed Venous Blood Gases	
pH	7.31–7.41
PvO_2	38–42 mm Hg
SvO_2	60%–80%‡
$PvCO_2$	38–55 mm Hg
HCO_3^-	22–26 mEq/L (mmol/L)

$PvCO_2$, Partial pressure of CO_2 in venous blood; *PvO_2,* partial pressure of O_2 in venous blood; *SvO_2,* venous O_2 saturation.

TABLE 25.13 Sputum Studies

Study	Description and Purpose	Nursing Responsibility
Acid-fast bacteria (AFB) smear and culture	2 different tests used to assess sputum for acid-fast bacilli (e.g., *Mycobacterium tuberculosis*). In AFB smear (a rapid test), sputum sample spread thinly on glass slide, treated with a fluorochrome stain, and examined under a microscope for AFB. Culture for AFB may take up to 6 wk.	*During:* Obtain specimen in early morning after mouth care because secretions collect during night. Have patient expectorate sputum into container after coughing deeply. If unsuccessful, try increasing oral fluid intake unless fluids are restricted. Can collect sputum in sterile container (sputum trap) during suctioning via endotracheal tube or by aspirating secretions from the trachea. If patient cannot produce specimen, bronchoscopy may be needed (Fig. 25.11). *After:* Send specimen to laboratory promptly for analysis.
Culture and sensitivity	Diagnose bacterial infection, select antibiotic, and evaluate treatment. Sputum specimen collected in a sterile container. Takes 48–72 hr for results.	
Cytology	Determines presence of abnormal cells that may indicate cancer. Single sputum specimen collected in special container with fixative solution.	
Gram stain	Sputum staining allows for classification of bacteria into gram-negative and gram-positive types. Results guide therapy until culture and sensitivity results are complete.	

TABLE 25.14 Interpreting Tuberculin Skin Testing

Types of Responses	Consider Positive in the Following Groups
Positive Reactions	
≥5-mm induration	• HIV-infected people • People who had recent contact with a person with TB disease • People with fibrotic lesions on chest x-ray consistent with prior TB • Patients with organ transplants • Immunosuppressed persons (e.g., taking the equivalent of ≥15 mg/day of prednisone for ≥1 mo)
≥10-mm induration	• Recent immigrants (<5 yr) from high-prevalence countries • Injecting drug users • Residents and employees of high-risk congregate settings • Mycobacteriology laboratory personnel • People with clinical conditions (e.g., diabetes mellitus, end-stage kidney disease) that place them at high risk
≥15-mm induration	• Any person (including those with no known risk factors for TB)

False Reactions	Possible Causes
False-negative reactions (do not react even though infected)	• Anergy, immunosuppression • Recent TB infection (within 8–10 wk of exposure) • Overwhelming TB infection • Very old TB infection (many years) • Recent live virus vaccination (e.g., measles, chickenpox)
False-positive reactions (react even though not infected)	• Nontuberculous mycobacteria (e.g., *Mycobacterium avium-intracellulare* [MAI] or *Mycobacterium avium* complex [MAC]) • Previous BCG vaccine

Source: Centers for Disease Control and Prevention: Tuberculosis (TB) fact sheet: Tuberculin skin testing. Retrieved from *www.cdc.gov/tb/publications/factsheets/testing/skintesting.htm.*

CO₂ Monitoring

CO_2 can be monitored using transcutaneous CO_2 ($PtCO_2$) and end-tidal CO_2 ($PetCO_2$) capnography. Transcutaneous measurement of CO_2 is a noninvasive method of estimating arterial pressure of CO_2 ($PaCO_2$) using an electrode placed on the skin.[11]

$PetCO_2$ is the noninvasive measurement of alveolar CO_2 during exhalation when CO_2 concentration is at its peak. It is used to monitor and assess trends in the patient's ventilatory status. Expired gases are sampled from the patient's airway and are analyzed by a CO_2 sensor that uses infrared light to measure exhaled CO_2. The sensor may be attached to an adaptor on the endotracheal tube or the tracheostomy tube. A nasal cannula with a sidestream capnometer can be used in patients without an artificial airway. Capnography is usually presented as a graph of expiratory CO_2 plotted against time.[12]

In the past, capnography was mainly used during and after surgery and in critical care units. Today's $PetCO_2$ monitors are portable and practical for use in emergency departments and on inpatient units.

Mixed Venous Blood Gases

The pulmonary artery (PA) catheter is a flow-directed catheter. When it is positioned correctly, the tip of the catheter lies in the pulmonary artery. Blood drawn from a PA catheter is called a mixed venous blood gas (SvO_2), because (1) it consists of venous blood that has returned to the right side of the heart from all parts of the body and (2) it samples blood just before blood enters the lungs to be oxygenated. Normal SvO_2 is 60% to 80%. Other normal mixed venous values are given in Table 25.12.

SvO_2 can be monitored intermittently by obtaining a blood sample from the PA catheter or continuously via a fiberoptic sensor as part of a specific central line with SpO_2 monitoring capability. Changes in SvO_2 provide an early warning of a change in cardiac output or tissue O_2 delivery. A decrease in SvO_2 suggests that less O_2 is being delivered to the tissues or that more O_2 is being consumed.

Sputum Studies

Observe the patient's sputum for color, volume, viscosity, and presence or absence of blood. We can obtain a sputum sample by expectoration, tracheal suction, or bronchoscopy. When the patient is unable to expectorate spontaneously, sputum may be collected by inhaling an irritating aerosol, usually hypertonic saline. This is called *sputum induction*.

Specimens may be examined for culture and sensitivity to identify an infecting organism (e.g., *Mycobacterium*) or to confirm a diagnosis (e.g., cancer). Table 25.13 describes common sputum tests and specific responsibilities when obtaining samples.

TABLE 25.15 Diagnostic Studies

Respiratory System

Study	Description and Purpose	Nursing Responsibility
Radiology		
Chest x-ray	Used to screen, diagnose, and evaluate changes in respiratory system. Most common views are anteroposterior (AP) and lateral.	*Before:* Have patient undress to waist, put on gown, and remove any metal between neck and waist.
Computed tomography (CT) scan	Diagnose suspicious lesions difficult to assess (e.g., mediastinum, hilum, pleura) by conventional x-ray. Common types are helical or spiral CT (contrast medium usually used) and high-resolution CT scan (contrast medium not used). Spiral CT used to diagnose a pulmonary embolism.	*Before:* Before contrast medium used, evaluate renal function. Assess if patient is allergic to shellfish, since the contrast is iodine based. Patient may need to be NPO 4 hr prior to study. *During:* Warn patient that contrast injection may cause a feeling of being warm and flushed. Patient must lie completely still during scan. *After:* Encourage patient to drink fluids to avoid renal problems with any contrast.
Magnetic resonance imaging (MRI)	Used for in-depth diagnosis of lesions difficult to assess by CT scan (e.g., lung apex) and for differentiating vascular from nonvascular structures. An IV contrast agent (gadolinium) may be given.	*Before:* Oral and/or IV contrast injection may be used. Check for pregnancy, allergies, and renal function before test. Have patient remove all metal objects. Remove metallic foil patches. Contraindicated for persons with implanted metallic devices or other metal fragments unless noted to be MRI safe. Ask about any history of surgical insertion of staples, plates, dental bridges, or other metal appliances. Patient may need to be fasting. Assess for claustrophobia and the need for antianxiety medication. *During:* Patient must lie completely still during scan.
Positron emission tomography (PET) scan	Glucose-containing nuclear tracer substance injected and taken up by metabolically active cells. Follow-up scan shows different-colored tissues based on metabolic rate. Because cancer cells have an increased uptake of glucose, "hot spots" reflecting increased glucose consumption indicate the presence of active cancer. Used to distinguish benign and cancerous lung nodules.	*Before:* Obtain IV access to inject the tracer substance. Patients should be NPO, except for water and medications, for at least 4 hr prior. Hold glucose-containing IV solutions and change to normal saline. Check blood glucose levels. The glucose level must be between 60–140 mg/dL (3.3–7.8 μmol/L) for accurate glucose metabolic activity. *During:* Patient must lie completely still during scan. *After:* Encourage fluids to excrete radioactive substance.
Pulmonary angiogram	Visualize pulmonary vasculature and locate obstruction or pathologic conditions (e.g., pulmonary embolus). Contrast medium injected through a catheter threaded into pulmonary artery or right side of heart. Series of x-rays taken after contrast medium is injected into pulmonary artery.	*Before:* Assess for allergies, especially to contrast dye. Have patient fast 6–12 hours before. Give sedative and other drugs, as ordered. *After:* Check pressure dressing site after procedure. Monitor BP, pulse, and circulation distal to injection site. Place compression device over site. Maintain IV and/or oral fluid intake.
Ventilation-perfusion (V/Q) scan	Assesses ventilation and perfusion of lungs. IV radioisotope given to assess perfusion. To assess ventilation, patient inhales a radioactive gas (xenon or krypton) that outlines alveoli. Normal scans show homogeneous radioactivity. Decreased or absent radioactivity suggests lack of perfusion or airflow. Ventilation without perfusion suggests a pulmonary embolus.	Same as for chest x-ray. *After:* No precautions needed afterward because the gas and isotope transmit radioactivity for only a brief interval.
Endoscopy		
Bronchoscopy (Fig. 25.11)	Flexible fiberoptic scope used for diagnosis, biopsy, specimen collection, or assessment of changes. It may be done to suction mucous plugs, lavage lungs, or remove foreign objects.	*Before:* Obtain signed consent. Have patient be NPO for 6–12 hr before the test. Give sedative as ordered. *After:* Keep patient NPO until gag reflex returns. Monitor for recovery from sedation. Blood-tinged mucus is not abnormal. If biopsy was done, monitor for hemorrhage and pneumothorax.
Lung biopsy	Specimens may be obtained by transbronchial or percutaneous biopsy or via transthoracic needle aspiration (TTNA), video-assisted thoracoscopic surgery (VATS), or open lung biopsy. Transbronchial biopsy and VATS can be done in the bronchoscopy suite. TTNA is done under CT guidance in radiology department. Open lung and VATS are done in the OR. Tests used to obtain specimens for laboratory analysis.	*Before:* Obtain signed consent. Same as bronchoscopy if procedure done with bronchoscope, and same as thoracotomy if open lung biopsy done. *After TTNA:* Check breath sounds q4hr for 24 hr and report any respiratory distress. Check incision site for bleeding. A chest x-ray should be done after TTNA or transbronchial biopsy to check for pneumothorax. *After VATS:* A chest tube may be placed postprocedure until lung has reexpanded. Monitor breath sounds to follow chest reexpansion. Encourage deep breathing for lung reinflation.
Mediastinoscopy	Scope inserted through a small incision in suprasternal notch and advanced into mediastinum to inspect and biopsy lymph nodes. Used to diagnose lung cancer, non-Hodgkin's lymphoma, granulomatous infections, and sarcoidosis.	*Before:* Obtain signed consent. Prepare patient for surgical intervention. Performed in OR using a general anesthetic. *After:* Monitor as for bronchoscopy.

TABLE 25.15 Diagnostic Studies—cont'd

Respiratory System

Study	Description and Purpose	Nursing Responsibility
Thoracentesis (Fig. 25.12)	Used to obtain specimen of pleural fluid for diagnosis, remove pleural fluid, or instill medication. Obtain chest x-ray after procedure to check for pneumothorax.	*Before:* Explain procedure and obtain signed consent. *During:* Usually done in patient's room. Position patient upright with elbows on an overbed table and feet supported. Tell patient not to talk or cough during procedure. *After:* Observe for signs of hypoxia and pneumothorax, and verify breath sounds in all fields. Encourage deep breaths to expand lungs. Send labeled specimens to laboratory promptly for analysis.
Pulmonary Function Tests	Used to evaluate lung function. Involves use of spirometer to assess air movement as patient performs prescribed respiratory maneuvers (Tables 25.16 and 25.17).	*Before:* Avoid scheduling immediately after mealtime. Avoid administration of inhaled bronchodilator 6 hr before. Assess for respiratory distress. *During:* Assess for respiratory distress. *After:* Assess for respiratory distress. Provide rest after procedure.
Exercise Testing	Used to diagnose and determine exercise capacity. A *complete test* involves walking on a treadmill while monitoring expired O_2 and CO_2, respiratory rate, heart rate, and heart rhythm. In a *modified test* (desaturation test), only SpO_2 is monitored.	*Before:* Have patient wear comfortable shoes. *During:* Encourage patient to hold handlebars on treadmill and walk as quickly as possible.
6-Min walk test	Used to measure functional capacity and response to treatment in patients with heart or lung disease. Pulse oximetry usually monitored during walk. Distance walked measured and used to monitor progression of disease or improvement after rehabilitation.	*During:* Patient walks as far as possible during 6 min, stopping when short of breath and continuing when able. Continually assess and observe patient tolerance to test.

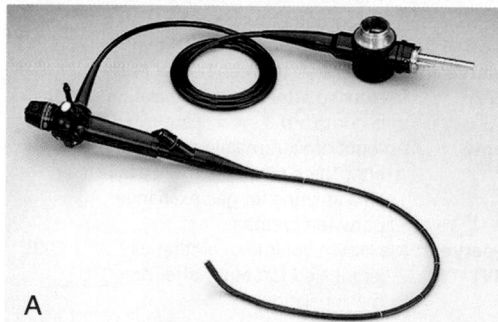
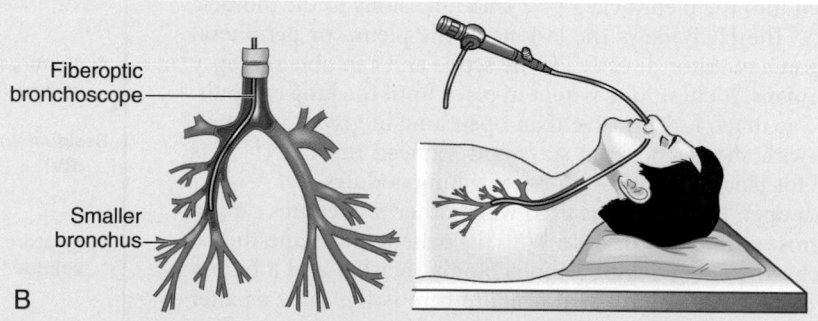

FIG. 25.11 Fiberoptic bronchoscope. **A,** The transbronchoscopic balloon-tipped catheter and the flexible fiberoptic bronchoscope. **B,** The catheter is introduced into a small airway and the balloon inflated with 1.5 to 2 mL of air to occlude the airway. Bronchoalveolar lavage is done by injecting and withdrawing 30-mL aliquots of sterile saline solution, gently aspirating after each instillation. Specimens are sent to the laboratory for analysis. (*A,* Courtesy Olympus America Inc, Melville, NY.)

Labels in Fig. B: Fiberoptic bronchoscope; Smaller bronchus

Skin Tests

Skin tests may be done to test for allergic reactions (see Chapter 13) or exposure to TB bacilli or fungi. Skin tests involve the intradermal injection of an antigen. Table 25.14 discusses how to interpret tuberculin skin testing. For example, a positive result on a TB skin test means that the patient has been exposed to the antigen. It does not mean that the patient has TB. A negative result means either no exposure or a depression of cell-mediated immunity, which occurs in HIV infection.

Our responsibilities are similar for all skin tests. First, to prevent a false-negative reaction, be sure that the injection is intradermal and not subcutaneous. After the injection, circle the site(s) and tell the patient not to remove the marks. When charting administration of the antigen, draw a diagram of the forearm and hand, and label the injection site. The diagram is especially helpful when the patient receives more than 1 test.

When reading test results, use a good light. If an induration is present, use a marking pen to indicate the periphery on all 4 sides of the induration. As the pen touches the raised area, make a mark. Then determine the diameter of the induration in millimeters. Do not measure reddened, flat areas.

Endoscopy

Bronchoscopy. *Bronchoscopy* is a procedure in which the bronchi are visualized through a fiberoptic tube (Fig. 25.11). Bronchoscopy may be used for diagnostic purposes (obtain biopsy specimens) and for treatment (e.g., to remove mucous plugs, foreign bodies). Laser therapy, electrocautery, cryotherapy, and stents may be placed through a bronchoscope to achieve patency of an airway that has been partially or nearly fully obstructed by tumors (Table 25.15).

Bronchoscopy can be done in an outpatient procedure room, in a surgical suite, or at the bedside in the critical care unit or on a medical-surgical unit. The patient may be positioned supine, in low-Fowler's, or even be seated. The HCP inserts the bronchoscope through the nose or mouth. Depending on the approach, the nasopharynx or oropharynx is anesthetized with local anesthetic spray. The bronchoscope is coated with water-soluble lubricant and inserted down into the airways. Small amounts (30 mL) of sterile saline may be injected through the scope and withdrawn and examined for cells, a technique termed *bronchoalveolar lavage* (BAL). Bronchoscopy can be done through the endotracheal tube of a mechanically ventilated patient.

Lung Biopsy

Lung biopsy may be done (1) transbronchially, (2) percutaneously or via transthoracic needle aspiration (TTNA), (3) by video-assisted thoracic surgery (VATS), or (4) as an open lung biopsy (Table 25.15). The purpose of a lung biopsy is to obtain tissue, cells, and/or fluid for evaluation. Specimens can be cultured or examined for cancer cells.

Transbronchial biopsy involves passing a forceps or needle through the bronchoscope for a specimen. A combination of transbronchial lung biopsy and BAL is used to distinguish infection and rejection in lung transplant recipients. A percutaneous or TTNA biopsy involves inserting a needle through the chest wall, usually under bedside ultrasound or CT guidance. Because of the risk for a pneumothorax, a chest x-ray is done after TTNA.

In VATS, a rigid scope with a lens is passed through a trocar placed into the pleura via 1 or 2 small incisions in the thoracic cavity. The HCP views the lesions in the pleura or peripheral lung on a monitor directly via the scope and can obtain biopsy specimens. A chest tube is kept in place until the lung expands. VATS is much less invasive than open lung biopsy. It is associated with shorter hospital stays and reduced mortality.[13] It is ideal for pleural biopsy and resecting lung nodules.

An open lung biopsy is used when other procedures cannot diagnose pulmonary disease. With the patient under anesthesia, the chest is opened with a thoracotomy incision and a biopsy specimen is obtained. Postprocedure care is the same as after thoracotomy (see Chapter 27).

Thoracentesis

Thoracentesis is the insertion of a large-bore needle through the chest wall into the pleural space to obtain specimens for diagnostic evaluation, remove pleural fluid, or instill medication (Fig. 25.12). The patient is positioned sitting upright, leaning on an overbed table with feet supported. The skin is cleansed and a local anesthetic (lidocaine) is injected subcutaneously. A percutaneous catheter may be left in to allow further drainage of fluid (Table 25.15).

Pulmonary Function Tests

Pulmonary function tests (PFTs) measure lung volumes and airflow. The results of PFTs can diagnose pulmonary disease, monitor disease progression, assess response to bronchodilators, and evaluate disability. Airflow measurement is obtained by trained personnel using a spirometer. The patient inserts a mouthpiece, takes as deep a breath as possible, and exhales as hard, as fast, and for as long as possible. Verbal coaching is given to ensure that the patient continues blowing out until exhalation is complete.

Computer software calculates the patient's percent of predicted values, that is, how well the performance compares with

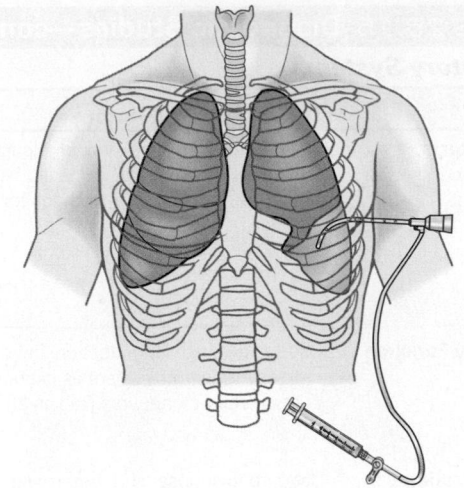

FIG. 25.12 Thoracentesis. A catheter is positioned in the pleural space to remove accumulated fluid.

TABLE 25.16 **Lung Volumes and Capacities**		
Parameter	**Definitions**	**Normal Value***
Volumes		
Tidal volume (V_T)	Volume of air inhaled and exhaled with each breath. Only a small proportion of total capacity of lungs	0.5 L
Expiratory reserve volume (ERV)	Additional air that can be forcefully exhaled after normal exhalation is complete	1.0 L
Residual volume (RV)	Amount of air remaining in lungs after forced expiration. Air available in lungs for gas exchange between breaths	1.5 L
Inspiratory reserve volume (IRV)	Maximum volume of air that can be inhaled forcefully after normal inhalation	3.0 L
Capacities		
Total lung capacity (TLC)	Maximum volume of air that lungs can contain (TLC = IRV + V_T + ERV + RV)	6.0 L
Functional residual capacity (FRC)	Volume of air remaining in lungs at end of normal exhalation (FRC = ERV + RV). Increase or decrease possible with lung disease	2.5 L
Vital capacity (VC)	Maximum volume of air that can be exhaled after maximum inspiration (VC = IRV + V_T + ERV). Higher VC for men (generally)	4.5 L
Inspiratory capacity (IC)	Maximum volume of air that can be inhaled after normal expiration (IC = V_T + IRV)	3.5 L

*Normal values vary with patient's height, weight, age, race, and gender.

an average based on age, gender, race, and height.[14] Normal values are 80% to 120% of the predicted value. Normal values for PFTs are shown in Tables 25.16 and 25.17.

Spirometry may be done before and after giving a bronchodilator to determine the patient's response. This helps gauge the reversibility of airway obstruction (e.g., asthma). A positive

TABLE 25.17 Pulmonary Function Airflow

Measure	Description	Normal Value*
Forced vital capacity (FVC)	Amount of air that can be quickly and forcefully exhaled after maximum inspiration	>80% of predicted
Forced expiratory volume in first second of expiration (FEV$_1$)	Amount of air exhaled in first second of FVC. Grades severity of airway obstruction	>80% of predicted
FEV$_1$/FVC ratio	Dividing value for FEV$_1$ by value for FVC. Useful in differentiating obstructive and restrictive pulmonary dysfunction	*Age <50:* ≥75% of predicted *Age ≥50:* ≥70% of predicted
Forced midexpiratory flow rate (FEF$_{25\%-75\%}$)	Measurement of airflow rate in middle half of forced expiration. Early indicator of disease of small airways	*Age <50:* ≥75% of predicted *Age ≥50:* ≥70% of predicted
Maximal voluntary ventilation (MVV)	Deep breathing as rapidly as possible for specified period. Fairly nonspecific test that gives information about exercise capacity. Used in conjunction with exercise stress test	About 170 L/min
Peak expiratory flow rate (PEFR)	Maximum airflow rate during forced expiration. Aids in monitoring bronchoconstriction in asthma. Can be measured with peak flow meter	Up to 600 L/min

*Normal values vary with patient's height, age, race, and gender.

bronchodilator response is an increase of greater than 200 mL or 12% in FEV$_1$ after administering a bronchodilator.

Home spirometry may be used to monitor lung function in people with asthma, cystic fibrosis, or COPD, as well as before and after lung transplantation or other thoracic surgeries. A peak flow meter is the hand-held instrument used at home. The person blows through it forcefully and quickly after taking a deep breath. Spirometry changes can warn of early lung transplant rejection or infection. Data from a peak flow meter provide important feedback to patients with asthma so that they can learn to change activities and medications in response to changes in peak expiratory flow rates.

More specific pulmonary function parameters can be directly assessed at the bedside in a high-acuity or critical care unit to determine the need for or weaning and extubation from mechanical ventilation (see Table 65.13).

CASE STUDY

Objective Data: Diagnostic Studies

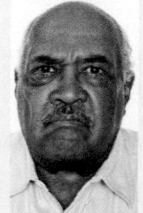

(© Fuse/Thinkstock.)

The HCP orders the following diagnostic studies for F.T.:
- Pulse oximetry
- Chest x-ray
- 12-lead electrocardiogram (ECG)
- CBC, basic metabolic panel (electrolytes, BUN, creatinine)
- ABGs
- Sputum for culture and sensitivity

F.T.'s SpO$_2$ is 87% on O$_2$ @ 3/L min via nasal cannula. The chest x-ray shows a slightly enlarged heart and bilateral consolidation to both lower lobes. The 12-lead ECG reveals sinus tachycardia, rate 110, with no ST segment elevation or depression and no T-wave inversion. The ABGs show compensated respiratory alkalosis with hypoxemia. The WBC is 17,350/μL and potassium 2.9 mEq/L. Sputum results are pending. F.T. is admitted to the medical nursing unit.

Discussion Questions

1. Of the diagnostic test results, is anything abnormal?
2. Which results concern you most?
3. What do you think is the cause of F.T.'s problems?
4. What patient teaching can you do with F.T. as he is waiting to be admitted to the hospital unit?
5. What is the interprofessional team's top priority for F.T. at this time?

You will learn more about the upper and lower respiratory problems and chronic obstructive pulmonary disease (COPD) in the next 3 chapters.

Answers available at *http://evolve.elsevier.com/Lewis/medsurg.*

▌ BRIDGE TO NCLEX EXAMINATION

The number of the question corresponds to the same-numbered learning outcome identified at the beginning of this chapter.

1. The key anatomic landmark that separates the upper respiratory tract from the lower respiratory tract is the
   a. carina.
   b. larynx.
   c. trachea.
   d. epiglottis.

2. A patient asks, "How does air get into my lungs?" The nurse bases her answer on knowledge that air moves into the lungs because of
   a. positive intrathoracic pressure.
   b. contraction of the accessory abdominal muscles.
   c. stimulation of the respiratory muscles by the chemoreceptors.
   d. a decrease in intrathoracic pressure from an increase in thoracic cavity size.

3. The nurse can *best* determine adequate arterial oxygenation of the blood by assessing
   a. heart rate.
   b. hemoglobin level.
   c. arterial oxygen partial pressure.
   d. arterial carbon dioxide partial pressure.

4. Defense mechanisms that help protect the lung from inhaled particles and microorganisms include the (*select all that apply*)
   a. cough reflex.
   b. mucociliary escalator.
   c. alveolar macrophages.
   d. reflex bronchoconstriction.
   e. alveolar capillary membrane.

5. A student nurse asks the RN what can be measured by arterial blood gas (ABG). The RN tells the student that the ABG can measure *(select all that apply)*
   a. acid-base balance.
   b. oxygenation status.
   c. acidity of the blood.
   d. bicarbonate (HCO_3^-).
   e. compliance and resistance.

6. To detect early signs or symptoms of inadequate oxygenation, the nurse would examine the patient for
   a. dyspnea and hypotension.
   b. apprehension and restlessness.
   c. cyanosis and cool, clammy skin.
   d. increased urine output and diaphoresis.

7. During the respiratory assessment of an older adult, the nurse would expect to find *(select all that apply)*
   a. a vigorous reflex cough.
   b. increased chest expansion.
   c. increased residual volume.
   d. decreased lung sounds at base of lungs.
   e. increased anteroposterior (AP) chest diameter.

8. When assessing subjective data related to the respiratory health of a patient with emphysema, the nurse asks about *(select all that apply)*
   a. date of last chest x-ray.
   b. dyspnea during rest or exercise.
   c. pulmonary function test results.
   d. ability to sleep through the entire night.
   e. prescription and over-the-counter medication.

9. When auscultating the chest of an older patient in mild respiratory distress, it is *best* to
   a. begin listening at the apices.
   b. begin listening at the lung bases.
   c. begin listening on the anterior chest.
   d. Ask the patient to breathe through the nose with the mouth closed.

10. Which respiratory assessment finding does the nurse interpret as abnormal?
    a. Inspiratory chest expansion of 1 inch
    b. Symmetric chest expansion and contraction
    c. Resonance (to percussion) over the lung bases
    d. Bronchial breath sounds in the lower lung fields

11. The nurse is preparing the patient for a diagnostic procedure to remove pleural fluid for analysis. The nurse would prepare the patient for which test?
    a. Thoracentesis
    b. Bronchoscopy
    c. Pulmonary angiography
    d. Sputum culture and sensitivity

1. a, 2. d, 3. c, 4. a, b, c, d, 5. a, b, c, d, 6. b, 7. c, d, e, 8. b, d, e, 9. b, 10. d, 11. a

For rationales to these answers and even more NCLEX review questions, visit *http://evolve.elsevier.com/Lewis/medsurg.*

EVOLVE WEBSITE/RESOURCES LIST

http://evolve.elsevier.com/Lewis/medsurg
Review Questions (Online Only)
Key Points
Answer Keys for Questions
- Rationales for Bridge to NCLEX Examination Questions
- Answer Guidelines for Case Study on pp. 460, 464, 467, and 475
Conceptual Care Map Creator
Audio Glossary
Supporting Media
- Animations
  - Inhalation
  - Oxygenation
  - Pulse Oximetry
  - Respiration Cycle
  - Respiratory System Overview
- Audio
  - Bronchial Breath Sounds
  - Bronchovesicular Breath Sounds
  - High-Pitched Crackles
  - High-Pitched Wheeze
  - Low-Pitched Crackles
  - Low-Pitched Wheeze
  - Pleural Friction Rub
  - Stridor
  - Vesicular Breath Sounds
Content Updates

REFERENCES

1. Patton KT, Thibodeau GA: *Essentials of anatomy and physiology,* ed 9, St Louis, 2016, Mosby.
2. Tatco V, Smith D: Carina. Retrieved from *https://radiopaedia.org/articles/carina.*
3. Meriam-Webster Dictionary: Anatomic dead space. Retrieved from: *www.merriam-webster.com/medical/anatomical%20dead%20space.*
4. Goel A, Gaillard F: *Pores of Kohn.* Retrieved from *https://radiopaedia.org/articles/pores-of-kohn.*
5. Stacy KM: Pulmonary anatomy and physiology. In: Urden LD, Stacy KM, Lough ME (ed): *Critical care nursing: Diagnosis and management,* ed 8, St Louis, 2018, Mosby.
6. DeWit SC, Stromberg HK, Dallred CV: *Medical-surgical nursing: Concepts and practice,* ed 3, St Louis, 2017, Mosby.
*7. Whitten C: Don't withhold oxygen from that CO_2 retainer. Retrieved from *https://airwayjedi.com/2016/01/09/dont-withhold-oxygen-from-that-co2-retainer/.*
8. Rhoades RA, Bell DR: *Medical physiology: Principles for clinical medicine,* ed 5, Philadelphia, 2018, Wolters-Kluwer.
9. Pathway Medicine: J receptors. Retrieved from *www.pathwaymedicine.org/j-receptors.*
10. Wilson SF, Giddens JF: *Health assessment for nursing practice,* ed 6, St Louis, 2017, Mosby.
*11. Horvath CM, Brutsche MH, Baty F, et al: Transcutaneous versus blood carbon dioxide monitoring during acute noninvasive ventilation in the emergency department, *Swiss Med Wkly* 146:w14373, 2016.
12. Luehrs P: Continuous end-tidal carbon dioxide monitoring. In Wiegand, DL (ed): *AACN procedure manual for high acuity, progressive, and critical care,* ed 7, St Louis, 2017, Saunders.
13. Jarrar D: Video-assisted thoracic surgery (VATS). Retrieved from *https://emedicine.medscape.com/article/1970013-overview.*
14. Mottram CD: *Ruppel's manual of pulmonary function testing,* ed 11, St Louis, 2017, Mosby.

*Evidence-based information for clinical practice.

26

Upper Respiratory Problems

Eugene Mondor

You really can change the world if you care enough.

Marian Wright Edelman

http://evolve.elsevier.com/Lewis/medsurg/

CONCEPTUAL FOCUS

Cellular Regulation
Functional Ability

Gas Exchange
Immunity

Infection
Sensory Perception

LEARNING OUTCOMES

1. Describe the clinical manifestations and nursing and interprofessional management of problems of the nose.
2. Discuss the clinical manifestations and nursing and interprofessional management of problems of the paranasal sinuses.
3. Describe the clinical manifestations and nursing and interprofessional management of problems of the pharynx and larynx.
4. Relate the nursing and interprofessional management of the patient who has a tracheostomy.

5. Identify the steps involved in performing tracheostomy care and suctioning a patient with a tracheostomy.
6. Outline the risk factors for and clinical manifestations of head and neck cancer.
7. Discuss the nursing and interprofessional management of patients requiring surgery for head and neck cancer.
8. Explain essential components of discharge teaching for the patient going home with a permanent tracheostomy after total laryngectomy for cancer.

KEY TERMS

allergic rhinitis, p. 480
decannulation, p. 493
deviated septum, p. 477
epistaxis, p. 478

laryngectomy, p. 494
laryngitis, p. 487
nasal polyps, p. 486
pharyngitis, p. 486

rhinoplasty, p. 478
sinusitis, p. 485
surgical cricothyroidotomy, p. 488
tracheostomy, p. 488

Disorders of the upper respiratory system, including the nose, sinuses, pharynx, and larynx, and the care of those undergoing surgery for head and neck cancers are the focus of this chapter. The primary concern with these problems is the impact on ventilation and oxygen (O_2) availability. Upper airway problems can negatively affect sleep and impair the ability to obtain and maintain nutrition. Sinus and upper respiratory tract infections, allergies, and oral problems can change the senses of both smell and taste. The patient with head and neck cancer often has depression and changes in body image and sexuality.

PROBLEMS OF NOSE AND PARANASAL SINUSES

DEVIATED SEPTUM

Deviated septum is a deflection of the normally straight nasal septum. Although up to 80% of adults may have septa that are slightly off center, the diagnosis of deviated septum is generally reserved for those whose septa are severely shifted.[1] Trauma to the nose, either at birth or later in life, is the most common cause

of deviated septum.[2] Deviated septum can interfere with both airflow and sinus drainage through the narrowed passageway.

Symptoms vary depending on the degree of deviation. Minor septal deviations can range from asymptomatic to nasal congestion and frequent sinus infections. Manifestations of severe septal deviation include facial pain, nosebleeds (*epistaxis*), and obstruction to nasal breathing.

The diagnosis of deviated septum is made during physical examination with a nasal speculum. The medical management of minor septal deviation focuses on symptom control. For nasal inflammation and congestion, use saline rinses and decongestants to clear nasal passages and analgesics for pain relief. For severe septal deviation, a nasal septoplasty, done under local or general anesthetic, reconstructs and properly aligns the deviated septum.

NASAL FRACTURE

Nasal fracture is the most common facial fracture and the third most common fracture of any bone.[3] They often occur from blunt trauma, including fights, automobile accidents, falls, and sports injuries. Using protective sports equipment and safeguarding against falls can prevent many nasal fractures.

There is no universally accepted classification system for nasal fractures. We can classify nasal fractures according to the fracture pattern (e.g., impacted, comminuted) or based on direction of injury (e.g., lateral, frontal). *Simple fractures* may be unilateral or bilateral and typically have little or no displacement. Powerful frontal blows can cause *complex fractures*, which may involve damage to adjacent facial structures, such as the teeth or eyes. Patients with complex nasal fractures should be evaluated for injury to the cervical spine, orbital bone, or mandible.[4] Complications include airway obstruction, nosebleeds, meningeal tears causing cerebrospinal fluid (CSF) leakage, septal hematoma, and cosmetic deformity.

Diagnosis of a nasal fracture is based on health history and physical assessment. Although facial deformity with a nasal fracture is common, a nosebleed may be the only manifestation. Other manifestations include localized pain, crepitus on palpation, swelling, difficulty breathing out of the nostrils, and bruising.

Assess the patient's ability to breathe through each side of the nose. Note the presence of edema, bleeding, or hematoma. Periorbital bruising involving both eyes is called *raccoon eyes*. It suggests a basilar skull fracture (see Chapter 56). Inspect the nose internally for evidence of septal deviation, clear drainage, edema, or bleeding.

Clear or pink-tinged persistent drainage after control of bleeding suggests a possible CSF leak. Checking this fluid for glucose at the bedside to help confirm the presence of CSF is not recommended because the result is highly unreliable. If needed, send a specimen to the laboratory to determine the fluid type.

Goals of nursing management are to maintain a patent airway, reduce edema and pain, prevent complications, and provide emotional support. The best way to maintain the airway is to keep the patient sitting upright. Apply ice to the face and nose in 10- to 20-minute intervals to help reduce edema and bleeding. Give analgesia as ordered to control pain. Acetaminophen is preferred over nonsteroidal antiinflammatory drugs (NSAIDs) or acetylsalicylic acid (ASA; aspirin) for the first 48 hours to avoid prolonging clotting time and increasing the risk for bleeding. Nasal stuffiness may be relieved with nasal decongestants, saline nasal sprays, and a humidifier. The patient should avoid hot showers and alcohol for the first 48 hours to prevent an increase in swelling. Encourage the patient to quit or decrease smoking to help tissue healing.

When a fracture is confirmed, the goals are to realign the fracture using closed or open reduction.[5] Simple fractures are often reduced with manual manipulation. With complex nasal fractures, considerable swelling of soft tissues occurs. It may be necessary to wait to repair the fracture until after the edema subsides, which may be 5 to 10 days. Antibiotics should be considered for any nasal fracture with disruption to the mucosa.

Surgical options include septoplasty and rhinoplasty. Septoplasty is done to correct a deviated septum. Patients have rhinoplasty for several reasons. Both procedures help maintain a patent airway, restore function of the nose, and help reestablish the patient's cosmetic appearance. The presence of septal hematoma increases the patient's risk for deformity and infection, which may require drainage and antibiotic therapy.

RHINOPLASTY

Rhinoplasty, surgical reconstruction of the nose, is done to improve airway function when trauma or developmental deformities result in nasal obstruction or for cosmetic reasons. When caring for rhinoplasty patients before surgery, assess the patient's expectations of the surgery. Actual or perceived changes in body image (e.g., deformed or enlarged nose) can affect self-esteem and interactions with others. The HCP can use digital photographs to show patients their projected appearance after surgery. These images can help patients decide whether to undergo rhinoplasty.

Most rhinoplasty is an outpatient procedure using regional or general anesthesia. Nasal tissue is added or removed, and the nose may be lengthened or shortened. Plastic implants are sometimes used to reshape the nose. Incisions are typically inside the nose and hidden. Sonic rhinoplasty incorporates the use of an ultrasonic device to gently aspirate bone, enabling a refined cosmetic result.[6]

After surgery, nasal packing may be inserted to apply pressure and prevent bleeding or septal hematoma formation. An external plastic splint protects and supports the new shape of the nose during the healing process. If present, nasal packing is usually removed 1 or 2 days after surgery. The splint may be left in place for 1 to 2 weeks.

❖ NURSING MANAGEMENT: NASAL SURGERY

Before surgery, teach patients to notify the HCP about any medications that they take at home. Aspirin-containing drugs and NSAIDs may need to be stopped for 5 days to 2 weeks preoperatively to reduce the risk for bleeding. Encourage smoking cessation to promote postoperative wound healing. During the immediate postoperative period, nursing interventions include (1) ensuring patency of the airway, (2) continuous assessment of respiratory status, (3) monitoring for airway obstruction, (4) pain management, and (5) observation of the surgical site for edema, bleeding, and signs and symptoms of infection.

Teaching is important because the patient must be able to detect complications at home. The patient typically has temporary nasal and/or facial edema and bruising. Cold compresses and elevation of the head can help minimize swelling and discomfort. Teach about activity restrictions aimed at preventing bleeding and injury (no nose blowing, swimming, heavy lifting, strenuous exercise). Sometimes swelling may be slow to resolve, delaying the achievement of a full cosmetic result for up to 1 year.

EPISTAXIS

Epistaxis (nosebleed) most often occurs in adults over age 50. Nosebleeds can be caused by trauma, hypertension, low humidity, upper respiratory tract infections, allergies, sinusitis, foreign bodies, chemical irritants (e.g., street drugs), overuse of decongestant nasal sprays, facial or nasal surgery, anatomic malformation, and tumors.[7] Conditions that prolong bleeding time or change platelet counts may predispose a patient to nosebleeds. Bleeding time may be prolonged if the patient takes aspirin, NSAIDs, warfarin, or other anticoagulant drugs.

About 90% of nosebleeds occur in the anterior part of the nasal cavity and are easily visualized. Anterior bleeding can be self-treated and usually stops spontaneously.

Posterior bleeding occurs more often with older adults secondary to other health problems (e.g., hypertension). Since posterior nosebleeds are closer to the throat, it is often hard to determine how much blood loss has occurred. Posterior bleeding may need medical treatment.

❖ Interprofessional and Nursing Care

Use simple first aid measures to control nosebleeds. These include (1) place the patient in a sitting position, leaning slightly forward with head tilted forward; (2) apply direct pressure by squeezing the entire soft lower part of the nose (nostrils) together for 5 to 15 minutes; and (3) reassure and calm the patient. If bleeding does not stop within 15 minutes, seek medical assistance.

Medical management involves trying to find the location of the bleed. For anterior bleeds, a pledget (nasal tampon) impregnated with anesthetic solution (lidocaine) and/or vasoconstrictive agents (epinephrine) may be placed into the nasal cavity. Absorbable materials, such as oxidized cellulose (surgical), gelatin foam (Gelfoam), or a gelatin-thrombin combination (Floseal), are another option. Packing for anterior bleeds can stay in place for 48 to 72 hours. Silver nitrate may be used to chemically cauterize a specific bleeding point. Thermal cauterization is reserved for more severe bleeding and may require the use of local or general anesthesia.[8]

It may be harder to find the location of a posterior bleed. Posterior bleeds often need packing. Packing with compressed nasal sponges (e.g., Merocel) or epistaxis balloons (e.g., Rapid Rhino) is preferred over the use of traditional Vaseline ribbon gauze because of the ease of placement. Packing is inserted into the nares and advanced along the floor of the nasal cavity. The sponge expands with moisture to fill the nasal cavity and tamponade bleeding. The epistaxis balloon is inflated with air to achieve the same pressure effect (Fig. 26.1). In the absence of a specific nasal device, a size 10F, 12F, or 14F Foley catheter with a 30-mL balloon may be used. A nasal sling (folded 2 × 2–inch gauze pad) may be gently taped under the nares to absorb drainage. If packing does not stop the bleeding, arterial embolization may be needed.

Nasal sponges, packing, and balloons can impair respiratory status. Closely monitor the level of consciousness, heart rate and rhythm, respiratory rate, and O_2 saturation (SpO_2) using pulse oximetry. Observe for any signs of difficulty breathing or swallowing. Because of the increased risk for complications due to location of the injury, all patients with posterior packing should be admitted to a monitored unit for close observation.

Nasal packing is painful because sufficient pressure must be applied to stop the bleeding. The patient should receive appropriate analgesia. Nasal packing predisposes patients to infection from bacteria (e.g., *Staphylococcus aureus*) present in the nasal cavity. Antibiotics effective against staphylococci may be prescribed.

Nasal packing for posterior bleeds may be left in place for 2 to 3 days. Before removal, pre-medicate the patient for pain because

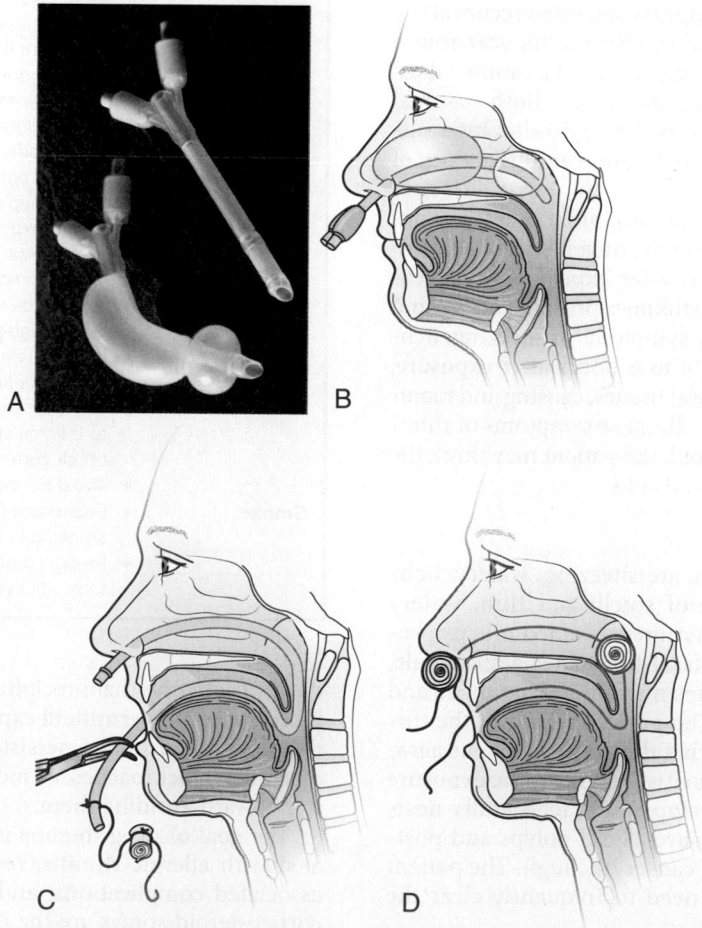

FIG. 26.1 **A,** Epistaxis balloon. The balloon is inflated after insertion. (Courtesy Boston Medical, Westborough, Mass.) **B,** Epistaxis balloon in proper position in nares. (From Roberts JR, Hedges JR: *Clinical procedures in emergency medicine,* ed 5, Philadelphia, 2009, Saunders.) **C,** Method for placing posterior nasal pack. Catheter is passed through the bleeding side of the nose and pulled out through the mouth with a hemostat. Strings are tied to the catheter, and the pack is pulled up behind the soft palate and into the nasopharynx. **D,** Nasal pack in position in the posterior nasopharynx. Dental roll at the nose helps maintain correct position.

this procedure is uncomfortable. After packing removal, cleanse the nares gently and lubricate them with water-soluble jelly.

Before discharge teach the patient and caregiver about follow-up care. Review how to use saline nasal spray and/or a humidifier. Have the patient sneeze with the mouth open and avoid the use of aspirin-containing products or NSAIDs. Teach the patient to avoid vigorous nose blowing, engaging in strenuous activity, and lifting and straining for 4 to 6 weeks.

ALLERGIC RHINITIS

Allergic rhinitis is inflammation of the nasal mucosa, often in response to a specific allergen. Allergic rhinitis can be classified according to the causative allergen (seasonal or perennial) or the frequency of symptoms (episodic, intermittent, or persistent). *Episodic* refers to symptoms related to sporadic exposure to allergens not typically encountered in the patient's normal environment, such as exposure to animal dander when visiting another person's home. *Intermittent* means that the symptoms are present less than 4 days a week or less than 4 weeks per year. *Persistent* means that symptoms are present more than 4 days a week and for more than 4 weeks per year.

Seasonal rhinitis usually occurs in the spring and fall. It is caused by allergy to pollens from trees, flowers, grasses, or weeds. Attacks may last for several weeks during times when pollen counts are high; then it disappears and often recurs at the same time the next year. *Perennial rhinitis* occurs year-round from exposure to environmental allergens, such as animal dander, dust mites, cockroaches, fungi, and molds. Both seasonal and perennial rhinitis can be classified as episodic, intermittent, or persistent, depending on the duration and frequency of symptoms.

Sensitization to an allergen occurs with initial allergen exposure, which results in the production of antigen-specific immunoglobulin E (IgE) (see Fig. 13.6). After exposure, mast cells and basophils release histamine, cytokines, prostaglandins, and leukotrienes. These cause the early symptoms of sneezing, itching, rhinorrhea, and congestion.[9] 4 to 8 hours after exposure, inflammatory cells infiltrate the nasal tissues, causing and maintaining the inflammatory response. Because symptoms of rhinitis are like those of the common cold, the patient may think the condition is a continuous or repeated cold.

Clinical Manifestations

Manifestations of allergic rhinitis are sneezing; watery, itchy eyes and nose; decreased sense of smell; and thin, watery nasal discharge that can lead to a more sustained mucus production and nasal congestion. Nasal turbinates appear pale, boggy, and swollen. The turbinates may fill the air space and press against the nasal septum. The posterior ends of the turbinates can become so enlarged that they obstruct sinus aeration or drainage and result in sinusitis. With chronic exposure to allergens, the patient may develop a headache, stuffy nose, nasal congestion, and sinus pressure. Nasal polyps and postnasal drip are the most common causes of cough. The patient may report hoarseness and the need to frequently clear the throat.

❖ Interprofessional and Nursing Care

The key step to managing allergic rhinitis is identifying and avoiding triggers of allergic reactions (Table 26.1). Teach the patient to take note when allergic reactions occur and keep a

TABLE 26.1 Patient & Caregiver Teaching

Avoiding Allergens in Allergic Rhinitis

Include the following instructions when teaching a patient or caregiver about allergic rhinitis:

What to Avoid	Specific Approaches
House dust	• Focus on the bedroom. Remove carpeting. Limit furniture.
	• Put the pillows and mattress in airtight vinyl bags.
	• Limit clothing in the bedroom to items worn often. Place clothing in airtight, zipper-sealed vinyl clothes bags.
	• Install a high-efficiency particulate air (HEPA) filter.
	• Close the air-conditioning vent into room.
	• Use blinds rather than draperies.
House dust mites	• Wash bedding in hot water (140° F [60° C]).
	• Wear a mask when vacuuming.
	• Install a filter on the outlet port of vacuum cleaner.
	• Avoid sleeping or lying on upholstered furniture.
	• Keep house temperature and conditions cool and dry.
Mold spores	• The 3 *D*s that promote growth of mold spores are darkness, dampness, and drafts.
	• Ventilate closed rooms and open doors. Consider adding windows to dark rooms and keeping a small light on in closets.
	• Basement light with a timer that provides light several hours a day may decrease mold growth.
	• Avoid places where humidity is high (e.g., basements, clothes hampers, greenhouses, barns). Dehumidifiers are rarely helpful.
Pet allergens	• Remove pets from interior of home.
	• Clean living area thoroughly.
	• Do not expect instant relief. Symptoms usually do not improve significantly for 1 to 2 months after pet removal.
Pollens	• Stay inside with doors and windows closed during high-pollen season.
	• Install an air conditioner with an air filter. Wash filters weekly during high-pollen season.
	• Use your car's air conditioner "recirculation" feature (circulates air inside the car, while shutting off air coming into the vehicle from the outside).
	• Avoid having plants, especially in the bedroom.
Smoke	• Encourage family and friends to refrain from smoking (if possible) or to go outdoors to smoke.
	• Presence of a smoker will sabotage any symptom reduction program.

diary of activities that precipitate the reaction. Patients are often more aware of intermittent exposure to an allergen, such as pets, than they are of a more persistent exposure to allergens, such as dust mites, cockroaches, or mold. Identifying triggers is the first step toward avoiding them.

The goal of drug therapy is to reduce inflammation associated with allergic rhinitis, reduce nasal symptoms, minimize associated complications, and maximize quality of life. Nasal corticosteroid sprays are the first-line and most effective treatment for allergic rhinitis.[10] Appropriate oral medication options include H_1-antihistamines, decongestants, and leukotriene receptor antagonists (LTRAs). Intranasal medications include antihistamines, anticholinergics, corticosteroids, cromolyn, and decongestants (Table 26.2).[11]

TABLE 26.2 Drug Therapy

Rhinitis and Sinusitis

Drug	Mechanism of Action	Side Effects	Nursing Actions
Anticholinergic *Nasal Spray* ipratropium bromide (Atrovent)	Blocks nasal cholinergic receptors, reducing nasal secretions in the common cold and nonallergic rhinitis.	Nasal dryness and irritation, nosebleeds may occur. Does not cause systemic side effects.	• May reduce the need for other rhinitis medications.
Antihistamines **First-Generation Agents (Oral)** brompheniramine chlorpheniramine (Chlor-Trimeton) clemastine (Tavist) dexchlorpheniramine diphenhydramine (Benadryl)	Bind with H₁ receptors on target cells, blocking histamine release. Relieve acute symptoms of allergic response (itching, sneezing, rhinorrhea).	Cross blood-brain barrier, often causing sedation and somnolence. Can cause paradoxic stimulation (restlessness, nervousness, insomnia). Anticholinergic side effects (e.g., palpitations, dry mouth, constipation, urinary hesitancy).	• Warn patient that operating machinery and driving may be dangerous because of sedative effect. • Teach patient to report palpitations, change in heart rate, change in bowel or bladder habits. • Teach patient not to use alcohol with antihistamines because of additive depressant effect. • Rapid onset of action, no drug tolerance with prolonged use.
Second-Generation Agents (Oral) cetirizine (Zyrtec) desloratadine (Clarinex) fexofenadine (Allegra) levocetirizine (Xyzal) loratadine (Claritin)	Same as above.	Limited affinity for brain H₁ receptors. Cause minimal sedation, few effects on psychomotor activities or bladder function.	• Teach patient to expect few, if any, side effects. • More expensive than traditional antihistamines. • Rapid onset of action, no drug tolerance with prolonged use.
Second-Generation Agents (Intranasal) azelastine (Astelin) olopatadine (Patanase)	Blocks histamine release and reduces nasal congestion.	Headache, bitter taste, somnolence, nasal irritation.	• Longer use increases risk for rebound vasodilation, which can increase congestion.
Corticosteroids **Nasal Spray** beclomethasone budesonide (Rhinocort) ciclesonide (Omnaris) flunisolide fluticasone (Flonase) fluticasone mometasone (Nasonex) triamcinolone	Inhibits inflammatory response of allergic rhinitis. Decreases mucosal inflammation and facilitates drainage of sinuses. Systemic effects may occur with higher than recommended doses.	At recommended dose, systemic side effects unlikely due to low systemic absorption. Mild transient nasal irritation, mucosal drying, nosebleeds. In rare instances, localized fungal infection with *Candida albicans*.	• Adherence important. Teach patient to use on regular basis and not PRN. • Teach patient to clear nasal passages before use. • Reinforce that spray acts to decrease inflammation and it may take several days or 1–2 wks to achieve maximum effects. • Stop use if nasal infection develops.
Decongestants **Oral** pseudoephedrine (Sudafed)	Stimulates adrenergic receptors and promotes vasoconstriction of superficial vessels in the nose and reduces nasal congestion.	CNS stimulation, causing insomnia, excitation, headache, irritability, increased blood and ocular pressure, dysuria, palpitations, tachycardia.	• Tolerance variable. • Advise patient of adverse reactions. • Patient to inform HCP if preexisting cardiovascular disease, hypertension, diabetes, glaucoma, benign prostatic hyperplasia, hepatic or renal disease present before starting therapy. • Rebound nasal congestion may occur with chronic overusage.
Intranasal (Nasal Spray) oxymetazoline phenylephrine	Same as above.	Same as above.	• Teach patient that these drugs should not be used for >3 days or >3 or 4 times/day. • Rebound nasal congestion may occur. • Addiction possible.
Leukotriene Receptor Antagonists (LTRAs) and Inhibitors **Antagonists** montelukast (Singulair) zafirlukast (Accolate) **Inhibitors** zileuton (Zyflo)	Suppress leukotriene activity, thereby inhibiting airway edema, bronchoconstriction, mucus production, and inflammation (see Fig. 11.2).	Well tolerated. May cause headaches, dizziness, rash, altered liver function, GI changes. *Zafirlukast and zileuton:* Monitor PT levels if patient is taking warfarin.	• Monitor liver function tests periodically while on therapy. Stop if elevated. • Give on empty stomach. • Do not stop therapy without consulting HCP. • Do not use for acute attacks.

Continued

TABLE 26.2 Drug Therapy—cont'd

Rhinitis and Sinusitis

Drug	Mechanism of Action	Side Effects	Nursing Actions
Mast Cell Stabilizer ***Nasal Spray*** cromolyn spray	Suppresses release of histamine and other inflammatory mediators from mast cells.	Minimal side effects. Occasional nasal irritation.	• Reinforce that spray prevents symptoms. • Begin 1 wk before pollen season starts and use throughout pollen season. • For isolated allergy, use prophylactically before exposure to allergen. • When used to treat chronic rhinitis, antihistamine and/or nasal decongestant may be used at the same time.
Combination Cold Medications hydrocodone, pseudoephedrine (Rezira oral solution) hydrocodone, chlorpheniramine, pseudoephedrine (Zutripro oral solution)	Hydrocodone suppresses cough. Mechanism of action of chlorpheniramine and pseudoephedrine discussed above.	See individual drugs above.	• Potential for misuse with repeated use. • Avoid in patients with head injury, increased ICP, acute abdominal conditions. • Do not use at the same time, or, within 14 days of MAOI drugs. • Increased risk for sedation when used with CNS depressants and/or benzodiazepines.

PT, prothrombin time; *ICP*, intracranial pressure; *MAOI*, monoamine oxidase inhibitor.

Second-generation antihistamines are used before first-generation antihistamines because of their nonsedating effects. Teach patients taking antihistamines to have adequate fluid intake to reduce adverse symptoms. Nasal corticosteroid sprays decrease inflammation with little absorption in the systemic circulation. Therefore systemic side effects are rare. If monotherapy does not relieve symptoms, a 2-drug combination, such as an oral H_1-antihistamine and an intranasal corticosteroid, may be helpful.

DRUG ALERT   **Antihistamines**
- First-generation antihistamines (e.g., chlorpheniramine [Chlor-Trimeton]) can cause drowsiness and sedation.
- Warn patients that operating machinery and driving may be dangerous because of the sedative effect.

DRUG ALERT   **Pseudoephedrine (Sudafed)**
- Large doses may cause tachycardia and palpitations, especially in patients with heart disease.
- Overdose in those over 60 years of age may result in central nervous system depression, seizures, and hallucinations.

Immunotherapy (allergy shots) may be used when a specific, unavoidable allergen is identified, and drugs are not tolerated or are ineffective in controlling symptoms. Immunotherapy involves controlled exposure to small amounts of the known allergen through frequent (at least weekly) injections with the goal of decreasing sensitivity. Sublingual or intranasal administration of allergen immunotherapy may an option for select patients. Immunotherapy is discussed in Chapter 13.

ACUTE VIRAL RHINOPHARYNGITIS

Acute viral rhinopharyngitis (nasopharyngitis, common cold) is an infection of the upper respiratory tract. It is the most prevalent infectious disease, with the average adult contracting 1 to 3 colds per year. More than 200 different viruses can cause a common cold. Most are caused by the coronavirus and are mild and self-limiting. Other viruses, such as human respiratory syncytial virus (RSV) and enterovirus, can cause a common cold.

The viruses are contagious. They spread by airborne droplets emitted by the infected person while breathing, talking, sneezing, or coughing. Because they can survive on inanimate objects for up to 3 days, transmission also occurs by direct hand contact. Frequency of the infection increases in winter months when people stay indoors and overcrowding is more common. Other factors that increase susceptibility include fatigue, physical and emotional stress, allergies affecting the nose and throat, and a compromised immune status. Exercise may reduce the number of upper respiratory tract infections.

Symptoms typically begin 2 or 3 days after infection. They may include runny nose, watery eyes, nasal congestion, sneezing, cough, sore throat, fever, headache, and fatigue. Patients are contagious 1 to 2 days before symptom onset and remain contagious until symptoms have subsided. Symptoms may last 2 to 14 days, with typical recovery in 7 to 10 days.

❧ COMPLEMENTARY & ALTERNATIVE THERAPIES
Echinacea

Scientific Evidence
- Echinacea may slightly reduce the incidence of the common cold.
- Taking echinacea does not appear to reduce the duration of a common cold.

Nursing Implications
- Echinacea is considered safe when used on a short-term basis in recommended doses.
- Caution patients with autoimmune disorders or a tendency toward allergic reactions about using this herb.

Source: Retrieved from *www.nccih.nih.gov/health/echinacea/ataglance.htm*.

COMPLEMENTARY & ALTERNATIVE THERAPIES
Zinc

Scientific Evidence
- Zinc is available in 2 forms: oral zinc (e.g., lozenges, tablets, syrup) and intranasal zinc (e.g., swabs, gels).
- When given within 24 hrs of onset of symptoms, zinc lozenges may reduce the duration of cold symptoms.

Nursing Implications
- Intranasal zinc can cause an irreversible loss of the sense of smell.
- Long-term zinc use, especially in high doses, can cause copper deficiency and may increase the risk for urinary tract problems and reduce immune function.
- Zinc may interact with drugs, including antibiotics and penicillamine.

Source: Retrieved from *www.nccih.nih.gov/health/zinc.*

❖ Interprofessional and Nursing Care

Interventions are directed at relieving symptoms. Rest, oral fluids, antipyretics, and analgesics are recommended. Warm salt water gargles, ice chips, lozenges, or sprays may help ease a sore throat. Petroleum jelly soothes a raw nose. Saline nasal spray reduces nasal congestion. Antihistamine and decongestant therapy reduce postnasal drip and decreases the severity of cough, nasal obstruction, and nasal discharge. Caution patients to use intranasal decongestant sprays for no more than 3 days to prevent rebound congestion from occurring. Cough suppressants, for irritating, bothersome coughs, may be used, but may not be effective. Patients may ask about vitamin C, echinacea, and zinc products. There is inconclusive evidence to support treatment with these therapies.

Complications include acute bronchitis, sinusitis, otitis media, tonsillitis, and pneumonia. Antibiotics have no effect on viruses. They are an option only if complications are present. Refer to an HCP if there is no improvement in symptoms within 10 to 14 days.

Teach patients to recognize the manifestations of a secondary bacterial infection, such as a temperature higher than 103° F (39.4° C); tender, swollen glands; severe sinus or ear pain; or significantly worsening symptoms. Green, purulent nasal drainage during the later stages of a cold is not uncommon and not always indicative of bacterial infection. In the patient with lung disease, signs of infection include a change in consistency, color, or volume of the sputum. Because infection can progress rapidly, teach the patient with chronic respiratory disease to immediately report sputum changes, increased shortness of breath, and chest tightness.

During the cold season, teach patients with a chronic illness or a compromised immune system to avoid crowded situations and those with obvious cold symptoms. Frequent hand washing and avoiding hand-to-face contact can help prevent direct spread.

INFLUENZA

Influenza (flu) is a highly contagious respiratory illness that causes significant morbidity and mortality. Millions of Americans (about 5% to 20% of U.S. population) contract influenza each year. The flu season begins in September and continues through April of each year, peaking between December to February. More than 310,000 people were hospitalized for flu-related complications in 2016.[12] Although the exact number of flu-related deaths is not known, it is estimated that influenza is responsible for 3000 - 49,000 deaths annually, depending on the strain.[13] Vaccination of high-risk groups may help prevent many of these deaths.

Etiology and Pathophysiology

We classify influenza viruses into 4 serotypes (A, B, C, D). Only A and B cause significant illness in humans. Influenza A is subtyped based on the presence of 2 surface proteins: hemagglutinin (H) and neuraminidase (N). The H antigens enable the virus to enter the cell, and the N antigens facilitate cell-to-cell transmission. As a result, we name influenza A viruses according to their H and N type (e.g., H3N2).

Influenza A is the most common and most virulent flu virus. It can infect a variety of animals as well as humans. More than 100 types of influenza A are found in birds (avian flu), pigs (swine flu), horses, seals, and dogs. When the virus mutates (changes), this allows it to infect different species. When a new viral strain reaches humans, people do not have immunity and the virus can spread quickly around the globe, causing a *pandemic*. For example, type A H1N1 influenza (swine flu) emerged in 2009 and had never been seen in humans before, resulting in a worldwide pandemic. The reemergence of a viral strain that has not circulated for many years can also trigger a pandemic. *Epidemics* are more localized outbreaks, often occurring yearly, caused by variants of already circulating strains of the influenza virus.

Influenza B and C viruses only infect humans. They are not divided into subtypes. Outbreaks of influenza B can cause regional epidemics, but the disease it produces is milder than that caused by influenza A. Influenza C causes mild illness and does not cause epidemics or pandemics. Influenza D only occurs in animals.

Influenza is communicable between humans primarily through infected droplets, inhalation of aerosolized particles, and, to a lesser extent, through direct contact with contaminated surfaces. The virus has an incubation period of 1 to 4 days, with peak transmission risk starting 1 day before onset of symptoms and continuing for 5 to 7 days after a person first becomes sick.[14]

Clinical Manifestations

For some patients, it may be hard to tell between the common cold and flu (Table 26.3). The onset of flu is abrupt. There may be chills, fever, and generalized myalgia, often accompanied by a headache, cough, sore throat, and fatigue. Assessment findings are usually minimal, with normal breath sounds on chest auscultation. In uncomplicated cases, symptoms often subside within 7 days.

Common complications include pneumonia, which can be either primary influenza [viral] pneumonia or secondary bacterial pneumonia, and ear or sinus infections. Dyspnea and diffuse crackles are signs of pulmonary complications. Some patients, especially older adults, have weakness or lethargy that may last for weeks. The patient who develops secondary bacterial pneumonia usually has gradual improvement of influenza symptoms, then worsening cough and purulent sputum. Treatment with antibiotics is usually effective if started early.

Diagnostic Studies

Influenza is often diagnosed based on the patient's health history and physical assessment and the knowledge of other cases of influenza in the community.

TABLE 26.3 Comparison of Common Cold and Influenza

Manifestations and Treatment	Common Cold (Viral Rhinitis)	Influenza
Symptom onset	Appear gradually	Abrupt onset. Within 3–6 hr
Fever	Rare	Characteristically high 102–104° F (38.9–40° C]). Lasts 3–4 days
Headache	Uncommon, but may occur	Common (can be severe)
General aches and pains	Slight	Often severe myalgia
Fatigue and weakness	Sometimes. Usually mild	Usual. Starts early and can last up to 2–3 wks
Exhaustion	Uncommon	Usual at beginning of illness
Stuffy nose	Common	Sometimes
Sneezing	Common	Sometimes
Sore throat	Common	Sometimes
Chest discomfort, cough	Common. Mild to moderate hacking cough	Common
Complications	Sinus congestion. Earache	Bronchitis, pneumonia, acute respiratory failure, ARDS. Can be life-threatening
Prevention	Hand washing. Avoid close contact with anyone who has a cold	Hand washing. Annual vaccination. Antiviral drugs. Avoid close contact with anyone who has the flu
Treatment	Temporary relief of symptoms: rest, hydration, decongestants, acetaminophen or ibuprofen for headache, aches, and pains	Antiviral drugs if given within 24–48 hrs of onset. Rest, hydration, acetaminophen or ibuprofen for headache, aches, and pains

Adapted from CDC Centers for Disease Control and Prevention. Retrieved from *www.cdc.gov/flu/about/qa/coldflu.htm.*

TABLE 26.4 Types of Influenza Immunization

Trivalent (TIV) or Quadrivalent (QIV) Inactivated Influenza Vaccine	Live Attenuated Influenza Vaccine (LSIV)
Trivalent: Protects against 3 different types of influenza virus (2-type A; 1-type B)	Made from weakened influenza virus
Quadrivalent: Protects against 4 different types of influenza virus (2-type A; 2-type B)	
Given by injection	Given as an intranasal spray into both nostrils
Approved for use in people ≥6 mo of age	Approved for healthy people ages 2–49 yrs
	• Children 2–8 yrs and have not had influenza vaccine before need 2 doses (second dose 4 weeks after first dose)
	• Children >9 yrs need 1 dose
Should NOT be used in:	Should NOT be used in:
• Infants <6 mo in age	• Children <2 yrs or adults >50 yrs
• Serious allergy/reaction to previous influenza vaccine	• Pregnant women or women who plan to become pregnant
• Guillain-Barré syndrome diagnosed within previous 6 wks	
Can be used in people at increased risk:	Prior to receiving the vaccination, please inform your HCP if you or the person you are caring for have any of the following:
• People of any age with chronic medical conditions	• Immunodeficiency
• Residents of nursing homes and long-term care facilities	• Children or adolescents receiving aspirin or other salicylates
• People who are immunocompromised	• Medical conditions that increase the risk for complications from influenza (chronic heart, lung, liver, kidney, or CNS disorders) diabetes; hemoglobinopathies)
• Pregnant women	• HCPs of high-risk patients because of risk for viral transmission from vaccine (should not care for high-risk patients for 7 days after vaccination)
Most common side effects are injection site reactions, such as pain, redness, and swelling	Adverse effects are rare. When effects do occur, may resemble mild flu with runny nose, nasal congestion, cough, and headache

Viral cultures, once considered the gold standard for diagnosing influenza, have decreased in popularity with the emergence of other rapid testing methods. We can obtain a viral culture from a throat swab, nasopharyngeal swab, expectorated sputum, ET tube sample, or bronchoscopy (bronchial wash). A viral culture can identify which virus (A, B, or another respiratory virus) and which viral strains are present.

Rapid influenza diagnostic tests (RIDTs) can help in the diagnosis by detecting the virus in secretions from the respiratory tract. Depending on the method, the test may be completed in the HCP's office with results available in as little as 5 minutes. The test can help distinguish influenza from other viral and bacterial infections with similar manifestations that may be serious but are treated differently. RIDTs are best used within the first 48 hours of the onset of symptoms. The main disadvantages of the rapid flu test are that it will miss some cases or occasionally be positive when a person does not actually have the flu. Always evaluate test results considering the patient's clinical condition.

❖ **Interprofessional and Nursing Care**

The most effective strategy for managing influenza is prevention. Two types of flu vaccines are available: inactivated and live attenuated (Table 26.4). Receiving a flu vaccine results in the production of antibodies against the viruses in the vaccine.

The influenza vaccine is changed on a yearly basis, depending on the virus strains the Centers for Disease Control and

Prevention (CDC) determines as being most likely to cause illness in the upcoming flu season. The best time to receive the vaccine is in September or October (before flu exposure) because it takes 2 weeks for full protection to occur. However, the vaccine can be given at any time during the flu season.

> **⚠ SAFETY ALERT Influenza Vaccination**
> - Advocate for vaccination of all people older than 6 months of age, especially those at high risk (e.g., health care workers, residents of long-term care facilities).
> - Give high priority to groups, such as health care workers, who can transmit influenza to high-risk persons.

Vaccinating healthy people decreases the incidence and risk for transmitting influenza to those who have less ability to cope with the effects of this illness. Many people do not get receive the vaccination despite the obvious benefits. Current vaccines are highly purified, and reactions are extremely rare. Soreness at the injection site is the most reported adverse effect. Contraindications are a history of severe allergic reactions to previous flu vaccine. Patients with anaphylactic hypersensitivity to eggs should discuss the vaccine with their HCP, as alternatives for vaccinating patients with egg allergies are now available.

The primary nursing goals are relief of symptoms and prevention of secondary infection. Unless the patient with influenza is at high risk or complications develop, supportive therapy is often all the patient needs. Rest, hydration, analgesics, and antipyretics can provide symptom relief. Older adults and those with a chronic illness may need hospitalization.

There are several antiviral medications we can use to treat shorten the duration of influenza symptoms and reduce the risk for complications. Zanamivir (Relenza), oseltamivir (Tamiflu), and peramivir (Rapivab) are neuraminidase inhibitors that prevent the virus from being released and spreading to other cells.[15] Zanamivir is given using an inhaler, oseltamivir is available as an oral capsule, and peramivir is given IV. The newest drug is baloxavir marboxil (Xofluza). It is a PA endonuclease inhibitor that works by inhibiting viral replication. Patients receive 1 oral dose. Do not give Xofluza with dairy products or calcium-fortified drinks.

Treatment with antiviral medication should be started as soon as possible in hospitalized patients with influenza, those with severe or complicated illness, or those at high risk for complications. For maximum benefit in the treatment of influenza, therapy should begin within 2 days of the onset of symptoms, but it can be started later based on clinical judgment.

SINUSITIS

Sinusitis affects 1 in every 7 adults. It develops when inflammation or swelling of the mucosa blocks the openings (ostia) in the sinuses, through which mucus drains into the nose (Fig. 26.2). *Rhinosinusitis*, which may accompany sinusitis, is concurrent inflammation or infection of the nasal mucosa. Nasal polyps, foreign bodies, deviated septa, or tumors can cause obstruction of mucus drainage. Secretions that accumulate behind the blocked ostia provide a rich medium for growth of bacteria, viruses, and fungi, all of which may cause infection.

Viral sinusitis may follow an upper respiratory tract infection in which the virus penetrates the mucous membrane and decreases ciliary function. Viral infections usually resolve without treatment in less than 14 days. If symptoms worsen

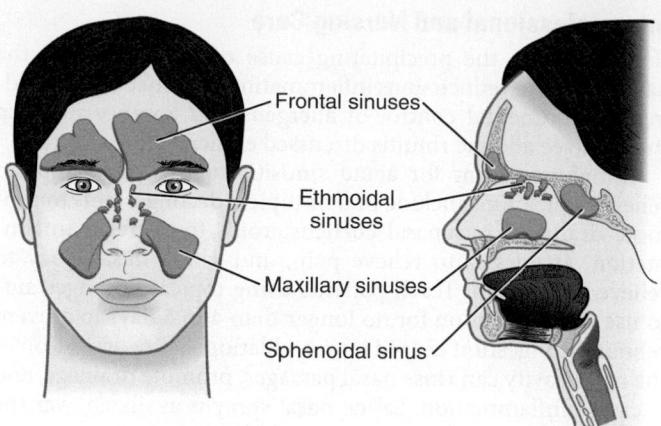

FIG. 26.2 Location of the sinuses.

after 3 to 5 days or last for longer than 10 days, a secondary bacterial infection may be present. Only 5% to 10% of patients with viral sinusitis develop a bacterial infection and need antibiotic therapy.

Streptococcus pneumoniae, Haemophilus influenzae, and *Moraxella catarrhalis* are the most common causes of bacterial sinusitis.[7] Fungal sinusitis is uncommon. It usually occurs in patients who are debilitated or immunocompromised.

Sinusitis can be classified as acute, subacute, or chronic.[16] *Acute sinusitis* typically begins within 1 week of an upper respiratory tract infection and lasts less than 4 weeks. *Subacute sinusitis* is present when symptoms progress over 4 to 12 weeks. *Chronic sinusitis* (lasting longer than 12 weeks) is a persistent infection usually associated with allergies and nasal polyps. Chronic sinusitis generally results from repeated episodes of acute sinusitis that result in irreversible loss of the normal ciliated epithelium lining the sinus cavity.

Clinical Manifestations

Acute sinusitis causes significant pain over the affected sinus, purulent nasal drainage, nasal obstruction, congestion, fever, and malaise. The patient may appear acutely ill. Inspect the nasal mucosa and palpate the paranasal sinuses for pain. Findings that indicate acute sinusitis include edematous mucosa, discolored purulent nasal drainage, enlarged turbinates, tenderness over the involved frontal and/or maxillary sinuses, and *halitosis* (bad breath). Recurrent headaches are common and may change in intensity with position changes or when secretions drain.

The symptoms of chronic sinusitis are often nonspecific. The patient is rarely febrile. The patient may have facial or dental pain, nasal congestion, and increased drainage. Severe pain and purulent drainage are often absent. Some symptoms mimic those seen with allergies. X-rays or CT scan of the sinuses may help confirm the diagnosis. CT scans may show the sinuses are filled with fluid or a thickened mucous membrane. Nasal endoscopy with a flexible scope may be used to examine the sinuses, obtain a specimen for culture, and restore normal drainage.

As many as 50% of patients with moderate to severe asthma have chronic sinusitis. The exact link between these diseases is unclear. Postnasal drip associated with sinusitis may trigger asthma by stimulating bronchoconstriction. Gastroesophageal reflux disease (GERD) and smoking may increase the risk for a person with asthma developing sinusitis. Appropriate treatment of sinusitis often causes a reduction in asthma symptoms.

❖ Interprofessional and Nursing Care

If allergies are the precipitating cause of sinusitis, teach the patient ways to reduce sinus inflammation and infection, including environmental control of allergens and appropriate drug therapy (see allergic rhinitis discussed earlier in this chapter).

Initial treatment for acute sinusitis focuses on symptom relief. Medications include oral or topical decongestants to promote drainage, intranasal corticosteroids to decrease inflammation, analgesics to relieve pain, and saline nasal spray to relieve congestion. Teach patients using topical decongestants to use the medication for no longer than 4 to 5 days to prevent rebound congestion caused by vasodilation. Saline irrigation of the nasal cavity can rinse nasal passages, promote drainage, and decrease inflammation. Saline nasal spray is available over the counter.

If symptoms worsen or last longer than 1 week, antibiotic therapy may be prescribed. Amoxicillin is the first-line drug of choice. It is taken for 10 to 14 days to prevent the formation of antibiotic-resistant organisms.[17] If symptoms do not resolve, the antibiotic should be changed to amoxicillin with clavulanate, a fluoroquinolone, or a 2nd or 3rd generation cephalosporin.

With chronic sinusitis, mixed bacterial flora is often present and infections are hard to eliminate. Broad-spectrum antibiotics may be used for 4 to 6 weeks. Patient and caregiver teaching for acute and chronic sinusitis is shown in Table 26.5.

Medical therapy may not relieve the symptoms of some patients with persistent, recurrent, or chronic sinus illnesses. These patients may need nasal endoscopic surgery to relieve blockage caused by hypertrophy or septal deviation. This is usually done as an outpatient procedure using local anesthesia. Propel, a self-expanding implant, can be placed directly in the sinus during surgery. Propel helps maintain patency to the sinus cavity after surgery and provide local corticosteroid delivery directly to the sinus lining before dissolving after 30 days.

OBSTRUCTION OF NOSE AND SINUSES

Nasal Polyps

Nasal polyps are soft, painless, benign (noncancerous) growths that form slowly in response to repeated inflammation of the sinus or nasal mucosa. They are most common in adults over age 40 and are twice as likely to occur in men than women.[18] Polyps, which appear as chronic yellow, gray, or pink semitransparent projections in the naris, can exceed the size of a grape.

Small polyps are typically asymptomatic. Manifestations of larger polyps include nasal obstruction, nasal discharge (usually clear mucus), and speech distortion. Topical and systemic corticosteroids are primary therapies used to shrink nasal polyps. Endoscopic or laser surgery can remove nasal polyps, but recurrence is common.

Foreign Bodies

A variety of foreign bodies may potentially lodge in the upper respiratory tract of adults, but these are rare occurrences. Some situations may be the result of trauma or found in patients with mental illness. Foreign bodies may be inorganic or organic. Inorganic foreign bodies, such as plastic or metal objects, may cause no symptoms and be incidentally discovered on routine examination. Organic foreign bodies, such as food, may cause a local inflammatory reaction and nasal discharge, which may become purulent and foul smelling if the object stays in the nasal cavity for an extended time. Foreign bodies can cause pain, difficulty breathing, and nasal bleeding.

Foreign bodies should be removed from the nose through the route of entry. Sneezing or blowing the nose with the opposite nostril closed may be effective in removing the foreign object. Avoid irrigating the nose or pushing the object backward, since these could cause aspiration and airway obstruction. If sneezing or blowing the nose does not remove the object, consult an HCP.

▌ PROBLEMS OF PHARYNX

ACUTE PHARYNGITIS

Acute pharyngitis is an acute inflammation of the pharyngeal walls. It may include the tonsils, palate, and uvula. It can be caused by a viral, bacterial, or fungal infection. Viral pharyngitis accounts for about 90% of cases. Bacterial pharyngitis ("strep throat") usually results from group A β-hemolytic streptococci and accounts for 5% to 10% of cases.

Fungal pharyngitis, such as candidiasis, can develop with the prolonged use of antibiotics or inhaled corticosteroids. It can also occur in immunosuppressed patients, especially those with human immunodeficiency virus (HIV) infection. Other causes of pharyngitis include dry air, smoking, GERD, allergy and postnasal drip, ET intubation, chemical fumes, and cancer.

Clinical Manifestations

Symptoms of acute pharyngitis range in severity from a "scratchy" throat to pain so severe that swallowing is difficult. Because both viral and streptococcal infections appear as a red and edematous pharynx (with or without patchy exudates), it may be hard to distinguish between them.

TABLE 26.5   Patient & Caregiver Teaching

Acute or Chronic Sinusitis

Include the following instructions when teaching the patient and caregiver about management of sinusitis:

1. Get plenty of rest to help body fight infection and promote recovery.
2. Keep well hydrated by drinking 6 to 8 glasses of water per day to loosen secretions.
3. Take hot showers. Use a steam inhaler (15-minute vaporization of boiled water), bedside humidifier, or nasal saline spray to promote secretion drainage.
4. Apply warm, damp towels around nose, cheeks, and eyes to ease facial pain.
5. Sleep with head elevated to help sinuses drain and reduce congestion.
6. Report a temperature of 100.4° F (38° C) or higher, which indicates infection.
7. Follow prescribed medication plan:
   - Take analgesics to relieve pain.
   - Take decongestants/expectorants to relieve swelling.
   - Take antibiotics (as prescribed) for infection. Be sure to take entire prescription and report continued symptoms or a change in symptoms.
   - Use nasal sprays to relieve congestion.
8. Perform nasal saline washes once or twice a day to wash sinuses.
9. Do not smoke and avoid exposure to smoke (will irritate and will worsen symptoms).
10. If allergies predispose to sinusitis, follow instructions about environmental control, drug therapy, and immunotherapy to reduce the inflammation and prevent sinus infection.

Four classic manifestations present in bacterial pharyngitis include: (1) fever greater than 100.4° F (38° C); (2) anterior cervical lymph node enlargement; (3) tonsillar or pharyngeal exudate; and (4) absence of cough.[19] However, appearance is not always diagnostic. When 2 or 3 of these criteria are present, a rapid antigen detection test and/or a throat culture can help establish the cause and direct treatment. White, irregular patches on the oropharynx suggest fungal infection with *Candida albicans*.

❖ Interprofessional and Nursing Care

The goals of nursing management are infection control, symptom relief, and prevention of secondary complications.

For viral pharyngitis, antibiotics are not recommended. For bacterial pharyngitis caused by group A β-hemolytic streptococci, penicillin is the drug of choice. This antibiotic must be taken several times a day for a full 10 days to prevent complications, such as rheumatic fever. For patients allergic to penicillin, erythromycin and clindamycin are appropriate substitutes.[20] Other antibiotics, such as azithromycin (Zithromax) or a 1st generation cephalosporin, are options. Most people with streptococcal infections are contagious until they have been on antibiotics for 24 to 48 hours. Repeat throat cultures after antibiotic therapy are not required.

Candida infections are treated with nystatin, an antifungal antibiotic. Teach patients to swish the preparation in their mouths for as long as possible before swallowing it. Treatment should continue until symptoms are gone. Patients taking inhaled corticosteroids are at risk for infection with *Candida* organisms. Thoroughly rinsing the mouth with water after using corticosteroids can prevent this infection.

Teach patients to use ibuprofen or acetaminophen for pain relief. Encourage the patient to increase fluid intake. For symptom relief, have patients to gargle with warm salt water (½ tsp of salt in 8 oz of water); drink warm or cold liquids; and suck on popsicles, hard candies, or throat lozenges. Cool, bland liquids and gelatin will not irritate the pharynx. Citrus juices are often irritating. Encourage the patient to use a cool mist vaporizer or humidifier.

PERITONSILLAR ABSCESS

Peritonsillar abscess is a complication of tonsillitis. It is most often caused by group A β-hemolytic streptococci. The abscess causes pain, swelling, and blockage of the throat (when severe), threatening airway patency. The patient may have a high fever, chills, leukocytosis, difficulty swallowing, and a muffled voice. Treatment consists of IV antibiotic therapy and needle aspiration or incision and drainage of the abscess. In some cases an emergency tonsillectomy is done or an elective tonsillectomy is scheduled after the infection has subsided.

PROBLEMS OF LARYNX AND TRACHEA

LARYNGEAL POLYPS

Laryngeal polyps develop on the vocal cords from vocal abuse (e.g., excessive talking, singing) or irritation (e.g., intubation, cigarette smoking). The most common sign is hoarseness. Polyps are treated conservatively with voice rest and adequate hydration. Large polyps may cause dysphagia, dyspnea, and stridor and may need surgically removed. Polyps are usually benign but may be removed because they can become cancerous.

ACUTE LARYNGITIS

Acute **laryngitis** is swelling and inflammation of the voice box (larynx). A virus (e.g., flu, common cold) is the most common cause. Other causes include inflammatory or infectious conditions of the upper respiratory tract (e.g., tonsillitis, acute bronchitis), overuse of one's voice (e.g., yelling loudly at a concert or a sporting event), exposure to smoke-filled environments, or chemical inhalation.

The classic hallmark signs of acute laryngitis include a tingling or burning sensation at the back of the throat, a persistent need to clear the throat, and hoarseness, which may be accompanied by complete loss of voice. The patient may have a low-grade fever, persistent cough, or feeling of fullness in the throat. Symptoms will appear suddenly, increase in severity over 2 to 3 days, then gradually subside over the next 7 to 10 days as the condition improves. It usually resolves within 21 days.

Diagnosis of acute laryngitis is made based on the history, clinical presentation, and changes in voice. Treatment for acute laryngitis is supportive. The patient is strongly encouraged to limit use of the larynx. This includes no talking or singing, which realistically is almost impossible to do. Patients will want to whisper when communicating but whispering places increased strain on the vocal cords that may worsen the pain. Acetaminophen, cough suppressants, throat lozenges, and use of a humidifier are helpful for throat discomfort.

Have the patient increase fluid intake. They should avoid caffeine and alcohol, which may worsen a sore throat. Encourage smoking cessation. If a bacterial cause is known, such as acute bronchitis or tonsillitis, antibiotics should help resolve the condition. If symptoms last longer than 3 weeks, patients should return to their HCP for further investigation and treatment.

AIRWAY OBSTRUCTION

Acute airway obstruction is a medical emergency. Airway obstruction can be caused by aspiration of food or a foreign body, allergic reactions, edema and inflammation caused by infections or burns, peritonsillar or retropharyngeal abscesses, cancer, laryngeal or tracheal stenosis, and trauma.

Airway obstruction may be partial or complete. The presentation of an airway obstruction often depends on the cause of the obstruction and/or location of the blockage. For example, objects lodged within the larynx may cause voice hoarseness or complete airway obstruction. Tracheal obstruction may produce wheezing. Objects lodged within the lower respiratory system (e.g., bronchus) may produce a cough or decreased air entry on the affected side.

Manifestations include choking, stridor, use of accessory muscles, suprasternal and intercostal retractions, flaring nostrils, wheezing, restlessness, tachycardia, cyanosis, and change in level of consciousness.[21] Prompt assessment and treatment are essential because partial obstruction may quickly progress to complete obstruction. Complete airway obstruction can result in permanent brain damage or death if not corrected within 3 to 5 minutes.

Your immediate priority is to ensure the patient has a patent airway. Interventions to reestablish a patent airway include the obstructed airway (Heimlich) maneuver (see Appendix A), cricothyroidotomy, ET intubation, or tracheostomy. Unexplained partial airway obstruction or recurrent symptoms indicate the need for more tests, including a chest x-ray, laryngoscopy, and rigid bronchoscopy.

TRACHEOSTOMY

A **tracheostomy** is a surgically created stoma (opening) in the anterior part of the trachea (Fig. 26.3, *A*). A tracheostomy may be done to (1) establish a patent airway, (2) bypass an upper airway obstruction, (3) facilitate removal of secretions, (4) permit long-term mechanical ventilation, and (5) assist with weaning from mechanical ventilation.[22]

The tracheostomy tube is shorter in length and slightly wider in diameter than an ET tube. This makes it easier to keep the tube clean and facilitates better oral and bronchial hygiene.

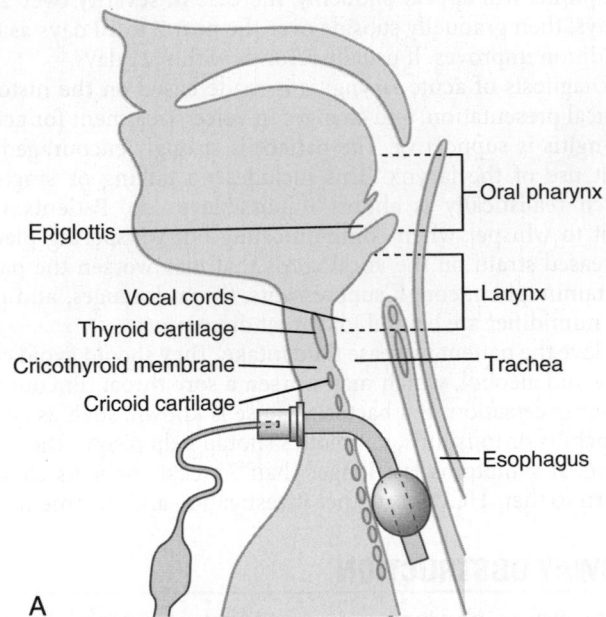

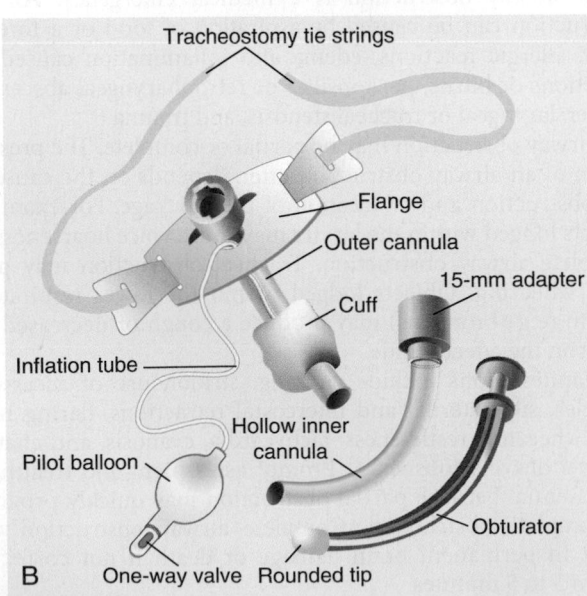

FIG. 26.3 Tracheostomy tube. **A,** Placement of a tracheostomy tube. **B,** Parts of a tracheostomy tube.

A tracheostomy (compared to an ET tube) may increase patient comfort because no tube is present in the mouth. There is also less risk for long-term damage to vocal cords.

A variety of tracheostomy tubes are available to meet specific patient needs (Table 26.6). All tracheostomy tubes have a faceplate, or *flange*, which rests against the neck, and an *obturator*, which is used to help insert the tube. Many tracheostomy tubes have an *outer cannula* (which keeps the airway patent), and an *inner cannula* (which can be disposable or nondisposable and removed for cleaning) (Fig. 26.3).

Cuffed and *uncuffed* tracheostomy tubes are available. A tracheostomy tube with an inflated cuff (balloon) is used the most, especially if the patient needs mechanical ventilation. The cuff, inflated via the *balloon inflation port* on the tracheostomy tube, ensures the patient receives the volume of air delivered by the ventilator, and helps decrease the risk for aspiration. Cuffless tubes are primarily used for patients with longer term tracheostomies, when mechanical ventilation is not required and the risk for aspiration has decreased. They make talking and eating easier.

The outer and/or inner cannula may be *fenestrated* or *non-fenestrated*. A *fenestrated tube* has an opening (a hole) on the dorsal surface of the tube. This tube promotes spontaneous breathing. For example, with the use of a cuffed, fenestrated tracheostomy tube, when the cuff is deflated and the inner cannula removed, air can pass from the lungs up through the opening in the tracheostomy tube through the vocal cords and larynx, into the upper airway, and out the mouth and nose. This allows the patient to breathe spontaneously and speak with the tracheostomy tube in place. When the cuff is reinflated and the inner cannula reinserted, air cannot pass from the lungs through the vocal cords.

Most patients who need mechanical ventilation first have an ET tube, because we can quickly insert one an emergency. Care of the patient with an ET tube is discussed in Chapter 65. When swelling, trauma, or upper airway obstruction prevents ET intubation, an emergent **surgical cricothyroidotomy** (also known as a cricothyrotomy) is needed. This procedure, which can be completed in minutes, involves making an incision through the skin and cricothyroid membrane on the anterior surface of the neck.

Most surgical tracheostomies are done in the operating room using general anesthesia. The HCP makes a horizontal incision on the anterior part of the trachea. After inserting the tracheostomy tube, the HCP sutures the incision and applies a sterile dressing.

A newer surgical technique is the *percutaneous tracheostomy*. Using local anesthesia, sedation, and under video-assisted guidance, the ET tube is withdrawn up to the level of the glottis. A needle is placed between the second and third tracheal rings, into the middle of the trachea. A dilator is then placed over the top of the needle. The HCP makes the opening progressively larger (with increasingly larger dilators) until the hole is big enough for insertion of the tracheostomy tube. Percutaneous tracheostomy approaches have less risk for bleeding and fewer postoperative complications.[23] Both surgical and percutaneous tracheostomies may be done at the patient's bedside in the emergency department or ICU.

❖ NURSING MANAGEMENT: TRACHEOSTOMY

◆ Acute Care

Before the tracheostomy procedure (and time permitting), explain the purpose of the procedure to both the patient and

TABLE 26.6 Nursing Management of Tracheostomies

Tube and Characteristics	Nursing Management

Tracheostomy tube with cuff and pilot balloon (Fig. 26.3, *B*)
When properly inflated, low-pressure, high-volume cuff distributes cuff pressure over large area, minimizing pressure on tracheal wall.
	Procedure for cuff inflation
	• Mechanically ventilated patient:
	  • *Minimal occlusion volume (MOV) technique* recommended. Place stethoscope over lateral neck (beside trachea). Inflate cuff by slowly injecting air into the cuff until no leak (sound) is heard at peak inspiratory pressure (end of ventilator inspiration).
	  • *Minimal leak technique (MLT).* Involves inflating the cuff to minimal occlusion pressure and then withdrawing 0.1–0.5 mL of air. No longer recommended due to risk for silent aspiration.
	  • *Spontaneously breathing patient:* Inflate cuff by slowly injecting air into the cuff until no sound is heard after deep breath or during inhalation with bag-valve-mask. If using MLT, remove 0.1–0.5 mL of air while maintaining seal. MLT should not be used if there is risk for aspiration.
	  • *Immediately after cuff inflation (both groups):* Verify pressure is within accepted range (20–30 cm H_2O, 15–22 mmHg) with a manometer. Record cuff pressure and volume of air used for cuff inflation in chart.
	Care of patients with an inflated cuff:
	• Monitor and record cuff pressure q8hr. Cuff pressure should be 20–30 cm H_2O (15–22 mm Hg) to allow adequate tracheal capillary perfusion. If needed, remove or add air to the pilot tubing using a syringe and stopcock. Afterward, verify cuff pressure is within accepted range with manometer.
	• Report inability to keep the cuff inflated or need to use progressively larger volumes of air to keep cuff inflated. Potential causes include tracheal dilation at the cuff site or a crack or slow leak in the housing of the 1-way inflation valve. If the leak is due to tracheal dilation, the HCP may cannulate the patient with a larger tube.

Fenestrated tracheostomy tube (Shiley, Portex) with cuff, inner cannula, and decannulation plug (Fig. 26.6) When nonfenestrated inner cannula is removed, cuff deflated, and decannulation plug inserted, air flows around tube, through fenestration in outer cannula, and up over vocal cords. Patient can then speak. A fenestrated inner cannula can be used to facilitate cleaning.	• If possible, assess risk for aspiration before removing inner cannula. A speech pathologist may be able to assist if available. Deflate cuff. Note coughing. • *Never* insert decannulation plug in tracheostomy tube until cuff is deflated and nonfenestrated inner cannula removed. Otherwise, patient will be prevented from breathing (no air inflow). This will precipitate a respiratory arrest. • Assess for signs of dyspnea and/or respiratory distress when a fenestrated cannula is first used. If this occurs, remove the cap, insert a nonfenestrated inner cannula, reinflate the cuff, and notify the HCP. • A nonfenestrated inner cannula must be used to suction patient to prevent tracheal damage from suction catheter passing through fenestrated openings. • Cuff management as described above.
Talking tracheostomy tube (Portex with cuff, 2 external tubings) Has 2 tubings, one leading to cuff and second to opening above the cuff. When port is connected to air source, air flows out of opening and up over the vocal cords.	• Patient must be awake, alert, and hemodynamically stable. • Must be able to tolerate cuff deflation and exhale around the tracheostomy tube. • When patient desires to speak, deflate cuff, and connect port to compressed air (or O_2). Be certain to identify correct tubing. If gas enters the cuff, it will overinflate and rupture, requiring an emergency tube change. Use lowest flow (typically 4–6 L/min) that results in speech. Patient may not tolerate high flows. • Give O_2 via tracheal collar or O_2 adaptor on speaking valve. • Observe for any signs of dyspnea and/or respiratory distress. • Disconnect flow when patient does not want to speak to prevent mucosal dehydration. • Cuff management as described above.
Tracheostomy tube (Bivona Fome-Cuf) with foam-filled cuff Cuff is filled with plastic foam. Before insertion, cuff is deflated. After insertion, cuff self-inflates. Pilot tubing is not capped. Does not require cuff pressure monitoring. Patient cannot speak with this tube.	• Before insertion, withdraw all air from the cuff using a 20-mL syringe. Cap pilot balloon tubing to prevent reentry of air. • After tracheostomy is inserted, remove cap from pilot tubing, allowing cuff to passively reinflate. Cuff is always inflated on this tube. • Do not inject air into tubing or cap pilot balloon tubing while it is in patient. Air will flow in and out in response to pressure changes (head turning). Place tag on tubing to alert staff not to cap or inflate cuff. • Tube tends to collect moisture and secretions while patient is on the ventilator. • Deflate cuff daily via pilot balloon to evaluate integrity of cuff. Assess ability to easily deflate cuff. Difficulty deflating cuff indicates a need for tube change. If aspirate returns with air, cuff is no longer intact. • Tube can be used for up to 1 month in patients on home mechanical ventilation. • Good choice for patients who need an inflated cuff at home, since teaching about cuff pressure is simplified.

caregiver. If the patient is having the tracheostomy in the operating room, follow all hospital policies and procedures for preparing the patient for surgery (see care of the preoperative patient in Chapter 17).

If the procedure is being done at the patient's bedside, ensure all appropriate personnel, including respiratory therapist, are present. Emergency resuscitation equipment, including a bag-valve-mask (BVM), should be readily available and functional.

Record vital signs, including heart rate, respiratory rate and rhythm, BP, and SpO2. Ensure an existing IV line is patent and that bedside suction is working. Help assemble and set up all necessary equipment. Position the patient supine. Give analgesia and sedation as ordered by the HCP, ensuring correct identification of times and dosages. Monitor patient response to analgesia and/or sedatives. Observe patient's tolerance to the procedure.

Immediately after the procedure, the tracheostomy cuff (balloon) is inflated. We use several different methods to confirm tracheostomy tube placement: (1) auscultation of the patient's chest for air entry, (2) end-tidal CO_2 capnography, and (3) passage of a suction catheter through the tracheostomy tube. After placement is confirmed, the ET tube (if present) is removed.

TABLE 26.7 **Complications of Tracheostomy**
Closely monitor patients with a tracheostomy for the following potential complications:
• Air leak
• Airway obstruction
• Altered body image
• Aspiration
• Bleeding
• Fistula formation
• Impaired cough
• Infection: wound or respiratory tract
• Subcutaneous emphysema
• Tracheal necrosis
• Tracheal stenosis
• Tube displacement

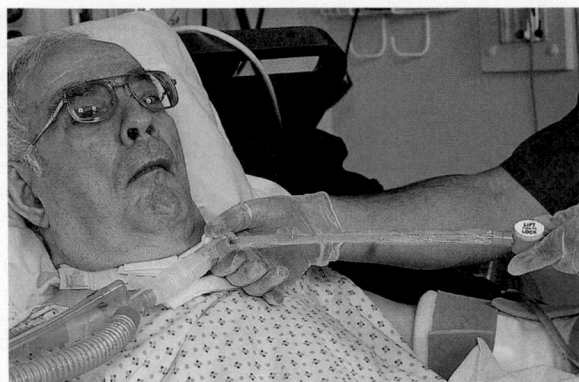

FIG. 26.4 Suctioning tracheostomy with closed system suction catheter. (From Potter PA, Perry AG: *Basic nursing: Essentials for practice*, ed 7, St Louis, 2011, Mosby.)

The tracheostomy tube is sutured and secured in place with cotton tracheostomy ties, tracheostomy tapes, or Velcro straps.

Monitor and record the patient's heart rate, respiratory rate, BP, and SpO_2. SpO_2 readings should remain stable. Note and record the mechanical ventilator settings, including mode, FIO_2, and positive end-expiratory pressure (PEEP). (Care of the patient receiving mechanical ventilation is discussed in Chapter 65.) Observe the amount of blood at the tracheostomy insertion site. Notify the HCP if bleeding persists. A chest x-ray should be obtained after the procedure. Many different complications can occur because of tracheostomy (Table 26.7). You must be aware of them, especially airway obstruction, bleeding, and infection.

There is considerable variation in the care of a patient with a new tracheostomy. In some places, it is the nurse who is primarily responsible; in others, it is a shared responsibility between nursing and respiratory therapy. You need to be familiar with your agency's policies and procedures. The following discussion highlights general guidelines when caring for a patient with a tracheostomy during the first few days after the procedure.

At a minimum, you must assess the tracheostomy site every shift. Confirm the patency of the tracheostomy tube. Observe the site for any redness, inflammation, edema, ulceration, or signs of infection. Sterile dressing changes should be done every 12 hours. Clean around the stoma with normal saline and apply a sterile pre-cut dressing around the tracheostomy tube site. You can complete dressing changes more often based on your assessment.

Because an inflated tracheostomy cuff exerts pressure on the tracheal mucosa, it is important to inflate the cuff with the least volume of air needed to obtain an airway seal. We can measure cuff inflation pressure with a hand-held cuff manometer. Monitor the pressure at least every 8 hours. Cuff inflation pressure should not exceed 20 to 25 cm H_2O. Higher pressures may compress tracheal capillaries, limit blood flow, and predispose the patient to tracheal necrosis. The minimal occlusion volume (MOV) is one way we often use to inflate the tracheostomy cuff (Table 26.6). Routine cuff deflation is not recommended.[24]

Suction the airway via the tracheostomy tube as needed (Fig. 26.4 and Table 26.8). Try to avoid suctioning through the newly created tracheostomy in the first few hours after the procedure, as this may aggravate discomfort and promote bleeding. Suctioning may be done using sterile glove and catheter technique, or an existing in-line suction catheter. Each time the patient is suctioned, note and record the amount, color, clarity, and patient tolerance to the procedure. At first, patients should receive humidified air to compensate for the loss of the upper airway to warm and moisturize secretions. Humidification is essential to keep secretions thin and decrease formation of mucous plugs.

If the inner cannula is disposable, replace as per manufacturer and agency guidelines. Clean a nondisposable inner cannula at least every shift. Cleaning removes mucus from the inside of the tube to prevent airway obstruction (Table 26.9).

Change the tracheostomy tapes after the first 24 hours and then as needed (Fig. 26.5 and Table 26.9). A 2-person technique, 1 person to stabilize the tracheostomy and the other to change the tapes, is best practice to ensure that the tracheostomy does not become accidentally dislodged during the procedure. In some places, the HCP and/or respiratory therapist may complete this task. At the end of the procedure, place 2 fingers underneath the tapes to ensure they are not too tight around the neck.

When turning and repositioning the patient, take care not to dislodge the tracheostomy tube. Because tube replacement may be difficult in the immediate postoperative period, several precautions are required, including (1) keep a replacement tube of equal or smaller size at the bedside, readily available for emergency reinsertion; (2) do not change tracheostomy tapes for at least 24 hours after the surgical procedure; and (3) if needed, the HCP performs the first tube change usually no sooner than 7 days after the tracheostomy.

If the tube is accidentally dislodged, immediately call for help. While waiting for the HCP, a respiratory therapist, or other designated individual to arrive, several options may be used (depending on your nursing scope of practice and specific agency policies and procedures). It is essential that you know and understand your role and scope of practice for care of the patient with a tracheostomy.

Immediately call for help. Quickly assess the patient's level of consciousness, ability to breathe, and the presence or absence of any respiratory distress. If respiratory distress is present, you can quickly use a hemostat to spread the opening where the tube was displaced. Insert the obturator in the replacement (spare) tracheostomy tube, lubricate with saline, and insert the tube into the stoma. Once the tube is inserted, remove the obturator at once so that air can flow through the tube. Another option is to insert a suction catheter to allow passage of air and serve as a guide for insertion. Thread the tracheostomy tube over the

TABLE 26.8 Suctioning a Tracheostomy

Assess the need for suctioning hourly. Indications include visible coughing, coarse crackles or wheezes over large airways, moist cough, increase in peak inspiratory pressure on mechanical ventilator, and restlessness or agitation. Neurologic patients may not show any signs and/or symptoms of the need to be suctioned, so suctioning once per shift (at minimum) is recommended. Do not suction routinely.

1. If suctioning is indicated, explain procedure to patient.
2. Collect necessary sterile equipment: suction catheter (no larger than half the lumen of the tracheostomy tube), sterile water, cup, and personal protective equipment (PPE). If a closed tracheal suction system is used, the catheter is enclosed in a plastic sleeve and reused (Fig. 26.4). No other equipment is needed.
3. Check suction source and regulator. Adjust suction pressure to no greater than 125 mm Hg pressure with tubing occluded.
4. Assess heart rate and rhythm, respiratory rate and SpO$_2$ to provide baseline for detecting changes in patient condition during suctioning.
5. Wash hands and put on PPE.
6. Use sterile technique to open package, fill cup with sterile water, put on sterile gloves, and connect catheter to suction tubing. Designate one hand as contaminated for (1) connecting and disconnecting the tubing at the suction catheter, (2) using the manual bag-valve-mask (BVM), and (3) operating the suction control. Suction sterile water through the catheter to test the system.
7. Provide preoxygenation for a minimum of 30 seconds by (1) adjusting ventilator to deliver 100% O$_2$ or (2) using a reservoir-equipped BVM connected to 100% O$_2$. The method chosen depends on whether the patient is attached to a mechanical ventilator or has a tracheostomy tube in place but is spontaneously breathing and receiving supplemental O$_2$. The patient who has a long-term chronic tracheostomy and is not acutely ill may be able to tolerate suctioning without using a BVM.
8. Gently insert catheter *without suction* to the point at which the patient coughs. Do *not* insert the catheter until you meet resistance (this is the carina, and repeated trauma with suction catheter can promote bleeding). Apply suction as you slowly begin to withdraw the catheter.
9. Apply continuous suction for no more than 10 to 15 seconds.
10. Observe the patient during the suctioning procedure. Immediately stop suctioning and remove the suction catheter from the patient's trachea if the patient becomes bradycardic or hypotensive, a dysrhythmia occurs, or SpO$_2$ decreases to less than 90%. A vagal response may have occurred.
11. After each suction pass, wait at least 30 seconds before suctioning again. Always hyperoxygenate for at least 30 seconds (via mechanical ventilator or BVM with 5 or 6 breaths) in between each suctioning pass.
12. Repeat procedure until airway is clear. Limit insertion of suction catheter to as few times as possible. If airway is not clear after 3 suction passes, allow the patient to rest before additional suctioning.
13. Return O$_2$ concentration to prior setting.
14. Rinse catheter. If using the in-line suction catheter (via mechanical ventilation), ensure that normal saline used to flush out the suction catheter does not enter the patient's airway. For disposable suction catheters, dispose of catheter by wrapping it around fingers of gloved hand and pulling glove over catheter. Discard equipment in proper waste container.
15. Suction the oropharynx or use mouth suction.
16. Reassess heart rate and rhythm and SpO$_2$. Auscultate to assess changes in lung sounds.
17. Record time, amount, and character of secretions and patient response to suctioning.

TABLE 26.9 Tracheostomy Care

The following are general guidelines for basic tracheostomy care. Become familiar with the specific policies and/or procedures in your agency:

1. Explain procedure to patient.
2. Use tracheostomy care kit or collect necessary sterile equipment (e.g., suction catheter, 1 pair sterile gloves, 1 pair nonsterile gloves, water basin, tracheostomy ties, tube brush or pipe cleaners, 4 × 4–inch gauze pads, sterile water or normal saline, tracheostomy dressing [optional]). NOTE: Clean rather than sterile technique is used at home.
3. Place patient in semi-Fowler's position.
4. Assemble needed materials on bedside table next to patient.
5. Wash hands. Put on PPE.
6. Auscultate chest sounds. If wheezes or coarse crackles are present, suction the patient if unable to cough up secretions (Table 26.8). Remove soiled dressing and clean gloves.
7. Open sterile equipment, pour sterile H$_2$O or normal saline into 2 compartments of sterile container or 2 basins, and put on sterile gloves. NOTE: Hydrogen peroxide (3%) is only used if an infection is present. If it is used, rinse the inner cannula and skin with sterile H$_2$O or normal saline afterward to prevent trauma to tissue.
8. If present, unlock and remove inner cannula. Many tracheostomy tubes do not have inner cannulas. Care for these tubes includes all steps except for inner cannula care.
9. Replace a disposable inner cannula with a new cannula. With a nondisposable cannula:
   • Immerse inner cannula in sterile solution and clean inside and outside of cannula using tube brush or pipe cleaners.
   • Rinse cannula in sterile solution. Remove from solution and shake to dry.
   • Insert inner cannula into outer cannula with the curved part downward, and lock in place.
10. Remove dried secretions from stoma using 4 × 4–inch gauze pad soaked in sterile water or saline. Gently pat area around the stoma dry. Be sure to clean under the tracheostomy flange (faceplate), using cotton swabs to reach this area.
11. Place dressing around tube (Fig. 26.5). Use a pre-cut tracheostomy dressing or unlined gauze. Do not cut the gauze because threads may be inhaled or wrap around the tracheostomy tube. Change the dressing as needed. Wet dressings promote infection and stoma irritation.
12. Change tracheostomy tapes, using a 2-person change technique. Tie tracheostomy tapes securely with room for 2 fingers between tapes and skin (Fig. 26.5). To prevent accidental tube removal, secure the tracheostomy tube by gently applying pressure to the flange of the tube during the tape changes. *Do not change tracheostomy tapes for 24 hours after the tracheostomy procedure.*
13. Some patients prefer tracheostomy tapes made of Velcro, which are easier to adjust.
14. Repeat care 3 times/day and as needed.

catheter and remove the suction catheter. Trying to reinsert will be easier if the stoma tract is mature or older than 1 week.

If the tube cannot be replaced because of tract immaturity (less than 1 week old) or other circumstances, immediately place the patient in semi-Fowler's position to decrease dyspnea.

Cover the stoma with a sterile dressing and provide ventilation with the BVM over the nose and mouth. If a patient has had a total laryngectomy, there will be complete separation between the upper airway and trachea. Ventilate this patient through the tracheostomy stoma. Severe dyspnea may progress to respiratory arrest.

❓ CHECK YOUR PRACTICE

You are caring for a patient who had a surgically created tracheostomy 6 hours ago. While suctioning the patient, he coughs, dislodging the tracheostomy tube.
• What should you do?

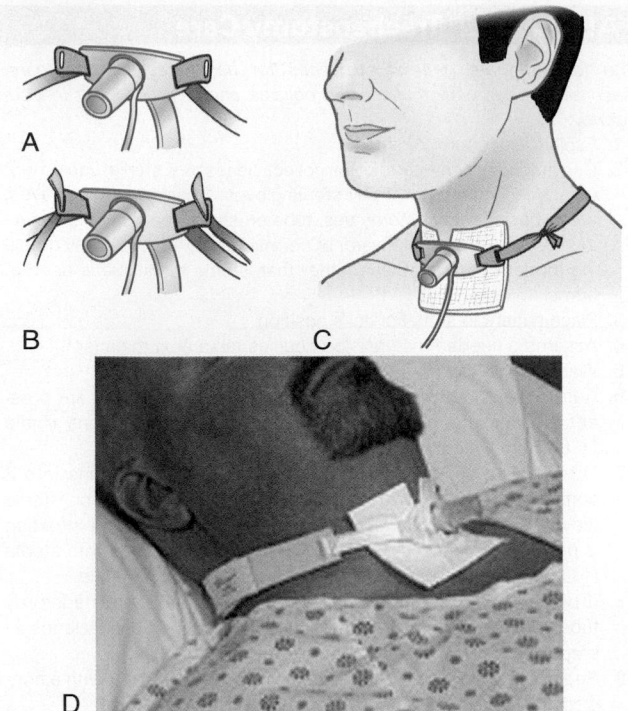

FIG. 26.5 Changing tracheostomy tapes. **A**, A slit is cut about 1 in (2.5 cm) from the end. The slit end is put into the opening of the cannula. **B**, A loop is made with the other end of the tape. **C**, The tapes are tied together with a double knot on the side of the neck. **D**, A Velcro tracheostomy tube holder. (*D*, Courtesy Dale Medical Products.)

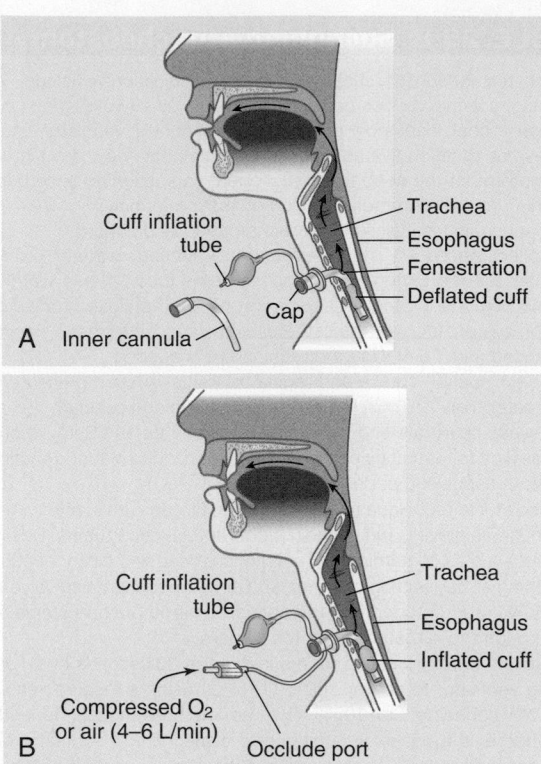

FIG. 26.6 Speaking tracheostomy tubes. **A**, Fenestrated tracheostomy tube with cuff deflated, inner cannula removed, and tracheostomy tube capped to allow air to pass over the vocal cords. **B**, Speaking tracheostomy tube. One tube is used for cuff inflation. The second tube is connected to a source of compressed air or O_2. When the port on the second tube is occluded, air flows up over the vocal cords, allowing speech with an inflated cuff.

◆ Chronic Care

Some patients will never be able to be weaned from mechanical ventilation and will need a tracheostomy for life. Care of the patient with a long-term tracheostomy includes all the same care as patients with a new tracheostomy. This includes observing the tracheostomy site, cleaning the inner cannula, suctioning, and changing tracheostomy tapes.

The tracheostomy tube should be changed around 1 month after the first tube change and every 1 to 3 months thereafter. When a tracheostomy has been in place for several months, the healed tract should be well formed. Changing the tracheostomy tube is important as it permits assessment of the stoma and cleaning of the tube. The patient may be taught to observe for signs and symptoms of infection and how to change the tube at home using a clean technique. Engaging patients to take part in their care may help decrease the incidence of complications, including infection, and promote an overall feeling of well-being.

◆ Swallowing Dysfunction

An inflated tracheostomy tube cuff may result in swallowing problems by interfering with the normal function of muscles used to swallow. Therefore, for long-term tracheostomy patients, it is important to evaluate the patient's swallowing ability and risk for aspiration.

A speech therapist is often the one who assesses the patient's ability to swallow. Using different consistencies of thickened fluids, the patient is evaluated for aspiration and/or microaspiration under videofluoroscopy or with a fiberoptic endoscopy. If the patient can swallow without aspiration when the cuff is deflated, the cuff may be left deflated or a cuffless tube

substituted. At this time, patients may be allowed varying levels of thickened fluids and soft foods.

◆ Speech With a Tracheostomy Tube

Several techniques promote speech in the patient with a tracheostomy. When the patient needs mechanical ventilation, provide the patient with a paper and pencil, a white board, or cellular phone for texting. A communication board with pictures of common needs is convenient for patients who may speak other languages. A visual alphabet for spelling words is useful for patients who are weak or have difficulty writing.

The spontaneously breathing patient may be able to talk with a tracheostomy. Several options are available depending upon the type of tracheostomy. For example, if the patient is at low risk for aspiration, (1) remove the inner cannula (if non-fenestrated), (2) deflate the cuff, and (3) place the cap on the tube (Fig. 26.6). When the tracheostomy cuff is deflated, exhaled air can flow upward over the vocal cords. When a fenestrated cannula is first used, frequently assess the patient for signs and symptoms of respiratory distress. If the patient is unable to tolerate the procedure, remove the cap, insert a non-fenestrated cannula, and reinflated the cuff. Monitor for improvement in patient condition.

The Passy-Muir valve is a simple device that attaches to the hub of the tracheostomy tube (Fig. 26.7). With the cuff deflated, the valve redirects airflow through the vocal cords. On inspiration, the valve on the device opens, allowing the patient to inhale. When the patient exhales, the valve closes and air flows

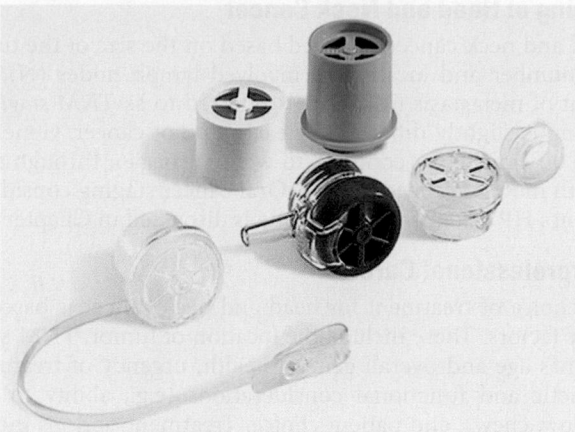

FIG. 26.7 Passy-Muir speaking tracheostomy valve. The valve is placed over the hub of the tracheostomy tube after the cuff is deflated. Multiple options are available and can be used for ventilated and nonventilated patients. The 1-way valve allows air to enter the lungs during inspiration and redirects air upward over the vocal cords into the mouth during expiration. (Courtesy Passy-Muir, Irvine, CA.)

upward around the tracheostomy and through the vocal cords. The patient exhales through the nose and mouth instead of through the tracheostomy, allowing speech. The patient may initially be able to tolerate only short periods of use until they become accustomed to exhaling through the mouth. Remove the valve immediately if there are any signs and symptoms of respiratory distress. Advocating for the use of speaking devices may help improve self-care and increase self-esteem for the patient with a long-term tracheostomy.

◆ Decannulation

Removal of the tracheostomy from the trachea is known as decannulation. Removal is possible when the primary condition for which the patient initially received a tracheostomy has been resolved. In addition, the patient needs to (1) be hemodynamically stable; (2) have a stable, intact respiratory drive; (3) be able to adequately exchange air, and (4) independently expectorate secretions.

Immediately prior to decannulation, explain to the patient what will occur. Monitor and record vital signs. Suction the patient prior to decannulation through the tracheostomy. Clear the mouth of any oral secretions. Loosen and/or cut the tracheostomy tapes, and remove any visible sutures holding the tracheostomy in place. Most importantly, ensure that the tracheostomy cuff is deflated. Pull the tracheostomy tube outward in one smooth motion. Stop if you meet any resistance and notify the appropriate personnel immediately.

After the tracheostomy tube is removed, care involves applying a sterile occlusive dressing and monitoring the site for bleeding. The dressing must be changed if it gets soiled or wet. If necessary, close the stoma with tape strips. Monitor the patient's respiratory status and O_2 saturation for any evidence of airway compromise or difficulty breathing. Apply an alternative method of O_2 delivery (e.g., nasal prongs) if needed. Teach the patient to splint the stoma with the fingers when coughing, swallowing, or speaking. Epithelial tissue begins to form in 24 to 48 hours, and the opening closes within 4 or 5 days. Surgical intervention to close the tracheostomy is usually not needed.

NURSING MANAGEMENT
Suctioning and Tracheostomy Care

Suctioning and tracheostomy care are complex nursing activities. Every nurse who performs suctioning and tracheostomy care is responsible for knowing the scope of practice and policies and procedures of the agency in which they work for all health care personnel. Collaborate with respiratory therapy staff, who will play a key role in the patient's care.

For unstable patients:
- Assess for the need for suctioning.
- Suction the ET or tracheostomy tube.
- Assess for adverse effects during suctioning, such as dysrhythmias.
- Evaluate the patient's respiratory status after suctioning.
- Maintain appropriate cuff inflation pressure at 20 to 25 cm H_2O or use minimal leak technique to maintain cuff pressure.
- Assess tracheostomy site at least once per shift for any signs of inflammation or infection.
- Replace the tracheostomy tube or ventilate the patient with a bag-valve-mask device after accidental tracheostomy dislodgment if needed.
- Assess swallowing ability and risk for aspiration.
- Develop plan to avoid aspiration in a patient with a tracheostomy.
- Teach patient and caregiver about home tracheostomy care.
- Delegate care of the stable patient to the licensed practical/vocational nurse (LPN/VN):
  - Determine the need for suctioning
  - Suction the tracheostomy
  - Evaluate patient status after suctioning
  - Provide tracheostomy care using sterile technique
  - Notify the RN of any changes in the patient's respiratory status
- Oversee the UAP in providing oral care to patient with a tracheostomy.
- Collaborate with the respiratory therapist:
  - Ensure proper equipment is available for suctioning and tracheotomy care
  - Measure tracheal cuff pressures
  - Replace tracheostomy tube after accidental dislodgement
  - Assist with bronchoscopy
  - Assist with decannulation

HEAD AND NECK CANCER

Head and neck cancer is classified according to the area where it occurs. These cancers may involve the nasal cavity and paranasal sinuses, nasopharynx, oropharynx, larynx, oral cavity, and/or salivary gland. (Cancer of the oral cavity is discussed in Chapter 41.) Most head and neck cancers arise from squamous cells that line the mucosal surfaces of the head and neck.

More than 52,000 new cases of head and neck cancer are diagnosed each year in the United States.[25] Tobacco use causes 85% of head and neck cancers. Excess alcohol consumption is another major risk factor. Head and neck cancer most often occurs in people over age 50 and twice as often in men compared to women. Head and neck cancers in those younger than 50 years are often associated with human papillomavirus (HPV) infection. Other risk factors include exposure to the sun, asbestos, industrial carcinogens, marijuana use, radiation therapy to the head and neck, and poor oral hygiene.[26]

Unfortunately, most patients have locally advanced disease at the time of diagnosis. Disability from both the disease and subsequent treatment is significant because of the potential loss of voice, adverse effects from chemotherapy and/or radiation, disfigurement, and social concerns.

Clinical Manifestations

The early manifestations of head and neck cancer vary with the location of the tumor. For example, patients with pharyngeal cancer may have what feels like a lump in the throat or a sore throat that does not get better with treatment. Some have white or red patches in the mouth or a change in the quality of the voice. Hoarseness that lasts more than 2 weeks may be a symptom of early laryngeal cancer.

Other manifestations may include ear pain or ringing in the ears, swelling or lumps in the neck, constant coughing, and coughing up blood. Swelling of the jaw can cause dentures to fit poorly or become uncomfortable. Unintentional weight loss and difficulty with chewing, swallowing, moving the tongue or jaw, and breathing are typically late symptoms. A partially or fully obstructed airway is often a late manifestation of head and neck cancer.

Diagnostic Studies

Early detection is key to patient survival. Physical assessment involves a focused assessment of the ears, nose, throat, mouth, and neck. Thoroughly examine the mouth, including the area under the tongue and dentures, with a flashlight. There may be thickening of the normally soft and pliable oral mucosa. Inspect the floor of the mouth and tongue. *Leukoplakia* (white patch) or *erythroplakia* (fiery red patch) may be present. Both leukoplakia and carcinoma in situ (localized to a defined area) may precede invasive carcinoma by many years. Palpate the lymph nodes in the neck.

If lesions are suspected, the HCP will examine upper airways may be examined using indirect pharyngoscopy and laryngoscopy (which involves using a laryngeal mirror). The larynx and vocal cords are visually inspected for lesions and tissue mobility. Typically, multiple biopsy specimens are obtained to help determine the extent of the disease. A CT scan or MRI may be done to detect local and regional spread. Positron emission tomography (PET) scanning is also used in diagnosis. The interprofessional care of head and neck cancer is outlined in Table 26.10.

TABLE 26.10 Interprofessional Care

Head and Neck Cancer

Diagnostic Assessment
- History and physical examination
- Indirect pharyngoscopy and laryngoscopy
- Endoscopy
- Biopsy
- Chest x-ray
- Barium swallow

Management
- Surgery
  - Vocal cord stripping
  - Laser surgery
  - Cordectomy
  - Partial or total laryngectomy
  - Pharyngectomy
  - Lymph node removal with neck dissection
  - Tracheostomy
  - Reconstructive procedures
- Radiation therapy
- Chemotherapy
- Targeted therapy
- Respiratory therapy
- Physical therapy
- Occupational therapy
- Speech therapy

Staging of Head and Neck Cancer

Head and neck cancer is staged based on the size of the tumor (T), number and location of involved lymph nodes (N), and extent of metastasis (M). This is referred to as *TNM staging*.[27] Staging is slightly different for each type of cancer. Generally, stage 0 is in situ, or confined to where it began, through stage 4, with more advanced disease. Oral cancer staging considers a patient's HPV status. TNM staging is discussed in Chapter 15.

Interprofessional Care

The choice of treatment for head and neck cancer is based on many factors. These include the location of tumor, TNM stage, patient's age and overall general health, urgency of treatment, cosmetic and functional considerations (e.g., ability to talk, swallow, chew), and patient choice. Treatment options include surgery, radiation therapy, chemotherapy, targeted therapy, or any combination of these modalities.[28]

Surgical Therapy. Surgery is often the first-line treatment option for head and neck cancers. Some patients may be treated with surgery alone. For other patients, combining surgery with radiation therapy and/or chemotherapy may be appropriate. Depending on the location and stage of cancer, surgical options include:
- *Vocal cord stripping:* Removal of outer layers of tissue on the vocal cords. This approach may be used for a biopsy or to treat some stage 0 cancers confined to the vocal cords. Vocal cord stripping rarely affects speech.
- *Laser surgery:* An endoscope with a laser is inserted down the throat, and the tumor can be vaporized or removed.
- *Cordectomy:* Removal of part or all the vocal cords. There may be changes in tone of voice. Removing part of a vocal cord may lead to a hoarse voice. If both vocal cords are removed, speech will no longer be possible.
- *Partial or total laryngectomy:* Removal of part or all the larynx. A total laryngectomy will change airflow in and out of the lungs and normal voice production will not be possible (Fig. 26.8).
- *Pharyngectomy:* Removal of part or all the throat.
- *Tracheostomy:* A tracheostomy is done to create an alternate pathway for breathing by creating a stoma in the trachea. *Lymph node removal:* Head and neck cancer sometimes spreads to the lymph nodes. The amount of tissue and number of lymph nodes that are removed depend on how far the cancer has spread.
- *Neck dissection surgery:* There are 3 main types:
  - *Radical neck dissection:* Removal of all the tissue on the side of the neck from the mandible to the clavicle. This includes the muscle, nerve, salivary gland, and major blood vessels.
  - *Modified radical neck dissection:* This is the most common type of neck dissection for cancer. All lymph nodes are removed. Less neck tissue is taken out than in radical dissection. This surgery may spare the nerves in the neck and, sometimes, the blood vessels or muscle.
  - *Selective neck dissection:* If cancer has not spread far, fewer lymph nodes are removed. The muscle, nerve, and blood vessels in the neck may be saved.

After extensive surgery to remove head and neck cancer, reconstructive operations can help restore both the structure and function of the affected areas.

Radiation Therapy. Radiation therapy can be delivered by either external-beam therapy or internal implants (brachytherapy). Brachytherapy is a concentrated and localized method of

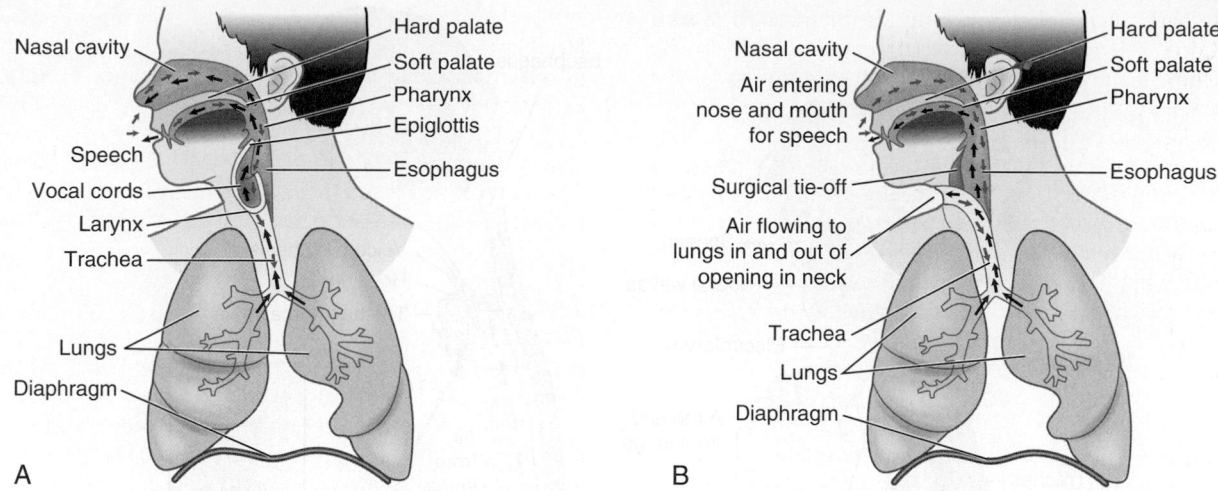

FIG. 26.8 Airflow in and out of the lungs after total laryngectomy. There is no anatomic connection between the nose, mouth, and throat. Inhaled and exhaled air enters the lungs through a surgically created stoma (hole) in the neck.

delivering radiation that involves placing a radioactive source near or into the tumor. The goal is to deliver high doses of radiation to the target area while limiting exposure of surrounding tissues. Thin, hollow, plastic needles are inserted into the tumor area, and radioactive seeds are placed in the needles. The seeds emit continuous radiation. Radiation therapy and brachytherapy are discussed in Chapter 15.

Radiation therapy is often preferred for patients with early head and neck cancer because it offers the patient good results with voice preservation. Some patients refuse surgical intervention for advanced lesions because of the extent of the procedure and potential risks involved. In this situation, radiation therapy is used as the sole treatment or in combination with chemotherapy. Other patients may opt for surgery and a combination of either radiation and/or chemotherapy treatments.

Chemotherapy and Targeted Therapy. Chemotherapy is used in combination with radiation therapy for patients with stage 3 or 4 head and neck cancers. Chemotherapy agents currently recommended include cisplatin, 5-fluorouracil, carboplatin, docetaxel (Taxotere), paclitaxel, methotrexate, and bleomycin.[29]

Cetuximab (Erbitux), a targeted therapy, is used with chemotherapy to treat patients with late-stage head and neck cancer. The drug targets epidermal growth factor receptor (EGFR), a specific protein within cancer cells, and stops the cells from growing. Targeted therapy is discussed in Chapter 15 and Table 15.13.

Nutritional Therapy. Many patients with head and neck cancer are malnourished even before treatment begins. Treatment modalities increase the risk for malnutrition. For example, after radical neck surgery, the patient may be unable to consume nutrients orally because of swelling, the location of sutures, or difficulty with swallowing. Side effects from chemotherapy and radiation therapy can impair the patient's ability to maintain adequate nutrition. Painful oral mucositis often leads to breaks in treatment if the patient is relying solely on oral intake for nutrition.

A thorough nutritional assessment and prophylactic placement of a gastrostomy tube in high-risk patients are vital to maintaining adequate nutrition. Enteral nutrition may be started before initiating treatment to obtain and maintain optimal nutritional status needed for tissue repair. (Enteral nutrition is described in Chapter 39.) Elevate the head of the bed while the patient is eating. Observe for feeding intolerance and adjust the amount, time, and/or formula if nausea, vomiting, diarrhea, or distention occurs. Teach the patient and caregiver about the enteral feedings.

Patients who are not candidates for or who refuse enteral feedings need to be monitored closely for weight loss. Antiemetics or analgesics given before meals can reduce nausea and mouth pain. Bland foods are easier for patients to tolerate. Patients can increase caloric intake by adding dry milk to foods during preparation, eating foods high in calories, and using oral supplements. It is helpful to add mild sauces and gravy to food. This adds calories and moistens food so that it is more easily swallowed. Expect swallowing problems when the patient resumes eating after surgery. The type and degree of difficulty varies depending on the surgical procedure. Videofluoroscopic swallowing studies may be used to evaluate the safety of swallowing postoperatively. When the patient can successfully swallow with low or no risk for aspiration, small amounts of thickened liquids or pureed foods may be given with the patient in high-Fowler's position. Avoid thin, watery fluids because they are hard to swallow and increase the risk for aspiration. Closely monitor and observe for any signs or symptoms of respiratory distress and/or choking when eating resumes. Oral suctioning may be done to prevent aspiration.

Physical Therapy. After surgery for head and neck cancer, the physical therapist will help teach the patient how to use the upper extremities to assist with support and movement of the head. In the immediate postoperative period, the patient should begin an exercise program to maintain strength and movement in the shoulders and neck. Without exercise, the patient could be left with a "frozen" shoulder and limited range of neck motion. The patient should continue the exercise program after discharge to prevent future functional disabilities.

Speech Therapy. Preoperatively, a speech therapist should meet with the patient and caregiver to discuss any effect that surgery will have on the voice and potential adaptations or voice restoration options. The International Association of Laryngectomees, an association of laryngectomy patients, focuses on helping patients reestablish speech. Local groups, such as "Lost Chord" or "New Voice," often have volunteers to visit patients before surgery.

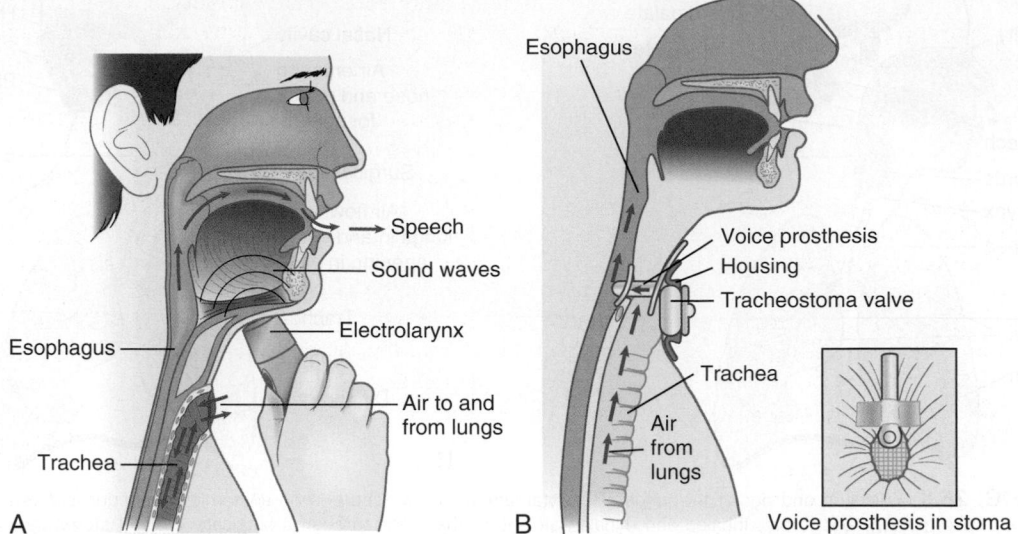

FIG. 26.9 A, The sound waves created by the electrolarynx allow the person to speak. B, The Blom-Singer voice prosthesis and valve.

Three major approaches are used to restore oral communication: (1) electrolarynx, (2) tracheoesophageal puncture (TEP) voice restoration, and (3) esophageal speech. An *electrolarynx* is a hand-held, battery-powered device that creates speech with the use of sound waves (Fig. 26.9, *A*). This option allows for speech immediately after surgery. It needs little maintenance and is easy to learn. The primary disadvantage of the electrolarynx is the mechanical sound quality, which many patients find unacceptable.

In *transesophageal puncture (TEP)*, a fistula is created in the tracheoesophageal wall that diverts pulmonary air across the pharyngoesophageal mucosa for phonation when the tracheostoma is occluded. A 1-way prosthetic valve is placed in the tract. The valve prevents aspiration of food or saliva from the esophagus into the tracheostomy. To speak, the patient manually blocks the stoma with the finger. Air moves from the lungs, through the prosthesis, into the esophagus, and out the mouth. Speech is made by the air vibrating against the esophagus and is formed into words by moving the tongue and lips. A common voice prosthesis is the Blom-Singer prosthesis (Fig. 26.9, *B*). TEP offers the best speech quality with the highest degree of patient satisfaction.

Esophageal speech depends upon air that is introduced into the esophagus and then expelled past the pharyngoesophageal segment, the vibratory source for sound production. The primary disadvantages of developing esophageal speech are the length of time needed to learn the technique and the reduction in voice quality.

❖ NURSING MANAGEMENT: HEAD AND NECK CANCER

◆ Nursing Assessment

Table 26.11 presents subjective and objective data to obtain from a person with head and neck cancer.

◆ Nursing Diagnoses

Nursing diagnoses for the patient with head and neck cancer include:
- Impaired airway clearance
- Risk for aspiration

TABLE 26.11 Nursing Assessment

Head and Neck Cancer

Subjective Data
Important Health Information

Past health history: Positive family history; prolonged tobacco use (cigarettes, pipes, cigars, chewing tobacco, smokeless tobacco); prolonged, heavy alcohol use; poor intake of fruits and vegetables
Medications: Prolonged use of over-the-counter medication for sore throat, decongestants

Functional Health Patterns

Health perception–health management: Does not take part in preventive health measures, long history of alcohol and tobacco use
Nutritional-metabolic: Mouth ulcer that does not heal, change in fit of dentures, change in appetite, sudden or unexplained weight loss, swallowing difficulty (e.g., sensation of lump in throat, pain with swallowing, aspiration when swallowing)
Activity-exercise: Fatigue with minimal exertion
Cognitive-perceptual: Sore throat, pain on swallowing, referred ear pain

Objective Data
Respiratory

Hoarseness, change in voice quality, chronic laryngitis, nasal voice, palpable neck mass and lymph nodes (tender, hard, fixed), tracheal deviation; dyspnea, stridor (late sign)

Gastrointestinal

White (leukoplakia) or red (erythroplakia) patches inside mouth, ulceration of mucosa, asymmetric tongue, exudate in mouth or pharynx, mass or thickening of mucosa

Possible Diagnostic Findings

Mass on direct or indirect laryngoscopy; tumor on soft tissue x-ray, CT scan, or MRI; positive biopsy

---

- Difficulty coping
- Impaired communication

More information on nursing diagnoses and the care of the patient with head and neck cancer is presented in eNursing Care Plan 26.2 on the website for this chapter.

Planning

The overall goals are that the patient will have (1) a patent airway, (2) an acceptable body image, (3) no complications related to therapy, (4) adequate nutritional intake, (5) minimal to no pain, and (6) the ability to communicate.

Nursing Implementation

Health Promotion. Most head and neck cancers can be prevented. The development of head and neck cancer is closely related to personal habits, mainly tobacco use and excess alcohol use. Poor oral hygiene and HPV infection are also risk factors for head and neck cancer.

Include information about risk factors in health teaching. Encourage good oral hygiene. Teach patients about safe sex practices to prevent HPV infection (e.g., use condoms, encourage monogamous relationships, choose a partner who has had no or few previous partners). If cancer has been diagnosed, tobacco and alcohol cessation are still important. The chance of a cure, by any treatment modality, for a patient with head and neck cancer who continues to smoke and use alcohol is decreased. Also, the risk for a second primary cancer is significantly increased. Give patients information about smoking cessation programs and techniques for success. If needed, refer to an alcohol treatment program. Smoking cessation and treatment of alcohol use are discussed in Chapter 10.

Acute Care. Teach the patient and caregiver about the type of treatment to be performed, care needed, and reason for treatment and care. Help prepare them to deal with the psychological impact of the diagnosis of cancer, change in physical appearance, possible need for enteral feedings, and use of other communication methods because of loss of voice.

Care plans should include assessment of the patient's support system. The patient may not have someone to help after discharge or may have a job that cannot be continued, leaving the patient unemployed.

Surgical Therapy. Preoperatively assess the patient's physical and psychosocial needs. Physical preparation is the same as for any major surgery, with an emphasis on oral hygiene. Assess knowledge and understanding of the planned surgical procedure and clarify misinformation or misunderstanding as needed. When possible, include the caregiver in preoperative teaching.

Tailor teaching to the planned surgical procedure. For example, include information about expected changes in speech after a laryngectomy. Alphabet boards, writing materials, pictorial guides, laptops, and hand signals are useful methods for communicating. Programmable speech-generating devices allow use of recorded messages that are matched with a graphic representing each message. Integration of newer technology into patient care enhances the patient's ability to communicate basic needs after surgery.

INFORMATICS IN PRACTICE

Communication Devices for Patient With Laryngectomy

- Assisting with communication will improve a patient's quality of life after a laryngectomy.
- Use a tablet or smartphone and download a text-to-speech application. These applications allow the patient to type in text, and then a computer voice says the text aloud.
- You can teach the patient how to use a keyboard-based communication program. The patient types on a traditional keyboard and generates speech that is transmitted through hand-held speakers.

Immediately after surgery, nursing care priorities include airway management, wound care, nutrition, communication, and psychosocial issues related to body image changes. Maintaining a patent airway is essential. Inflammation in the surgical area may compress the trachea. Keep the patient in a semi-Fowler's position to decrease edema and limit tension on suture lines.

Give analgesic drugs as needed for pain control. Because patients may not be able to speak, have them nonverbally rate their pain (e.g., visual pain scale) to help assess the effectiveness of the medication. (Pain management is discussed in Chapter 8.) Monitor vital signs frequently. Be alert for hemorrhage, as many of the structures in the head and neck area are very vascular. Pay careful attention to heart rate, blood pressure, SpO_2, and the patient's hemoglobin value.

The patient with a laryngectomy needs frequent suctioning via the tracheostomy tube. Secretions typically change in amount and consistency over time. The patient may initially have a large amount of blood-tinged secretions that gradually diminish and thicken. Maintain adequate fluid intake (IV, enteral) and humidification of inspired gases to keep secretions liquid and mucous membranes moist. Encourage deep breathing and coughing.

Pressure dressings, packing, or drainage tubes may be present, depending on the type of surgical procedure. Do not change any dressing unless you have a specific order from the HCP. If skin flaps are used, dressings are typically not present. This allows better visualization of the flap and avoids excess pressure on tissue. Skin flaps must initially be checked hourly for color and any change in size or edema. Doppler ultrasound may be used to determine the presence of a pulse, depending upon the location of the skin flap. Hemovac, Jackson-Pratt, and Penrose drains are some of the drainage devices that may be used.

Drainage may initially be bloody, then serosanguineous, and gradually decrease in volume over 24 to 48 hours. Monitor patency of drainage tubes every hour in the first few hours after surgery, then every 4 hours to ensure proper functioning. If tubing becomes obstructed, fluid will accumulate under the skin flap and predispose the patient to formation of hematomas or seromas, impair wound healing, and increase the risk for infection. After drainage tubes are removed, closely monitor the area to detect any swelling. Closely monitor incision sites for signs of infection.

The patient may have a nasogastric tube inserted during surgery to remove gastric contents via intermittent suction for the first 24 to 48 hours until peristalsis returns. Because the nasogastric tube lies close to internal incision lines, do not manipulate or move the tube. When bowel sounds return, start enteral feedings slowly and advance to meet nutritional needs.

Radiation Therapy. Dry mouth (*xerostomia*), a frequent and annoying problem, typically occurs within a few weeks of treatment. The patient's saliva decreases in volume and becomes thick. This change may be temporary or permanent. Pilocarpine hydrochloride (Salagen) is often effective in increasing saliva production.

CHECK YOUR PRACTICE

Your 64-yr-old male patient with oral cancer has been receiving radiation therapy for 3 weeks. He has developed xerostomia and oral mucositis. He asks if you have any suggestions to help relieve his symptoms.
- How would you respond?

Once patients can have foods or fluids by mouth, they can get symptom relief by increasing fluid intake, chewing sugarless gum or sugarless candy, using nonalcoholic mouth rinses (baking soda, glycerin solutions), and using artificial saliva. Teach patients to always carry a water bottle with them. Fluoride gels or treatments can help prevent dental deterioration caused by xerostomia.

Oral mucositis can cause irritation, ulceration, and pain. Teach the patient on oral care basics, including the use of a soft toothbrush and regular flossing. Empty fluoride gel trays, along with bite blocks, athletic mouth guards, or gauze pads, can be worn during radiation treatments. This prevents radiation scatter to the tongue and cheek from metal work in the mouth. Warm bland rinses, like those with salt and baking soda, 4 to 6 times daily may be helpful. Sucking on ice chips can also help with the pain. Patients should avoid commercial mouthwashes and hot, spicy, or acidic foods because they are irritating.

Skin over the irradiated area often becomes reddened and sensitive to touch. Teach patients to use only prescribed lotions and skin products while undergoing radiation therapy and to not use any lotions within 2 hours before treatment. Skin care for patients having radiation therapy is discussed in Chapter 15.

Fatigue is a common side effect of radiation therapy as well as chemotherapy. Encourage patients to walk 15 to 30 minutes each day since regular exercise can give them more energy. Teach patients to do activities that are most important to them and to rest during periods of low energy. Identify support systems and encourage patients to ask for help.

Stoma Care. Should the patient have a stoma after surgery, teach the patient proper care of the stoma. The patient should wash the area around the stoma daily with a moist cloth. A nasal wash spray (e.g., Alkalol) can be used every 1 to 2 hours to keep the stoma moist and prevent crusting. Dried secretions can be removed with tweezers. If a laryngectomy tube is in place, the patient must remove the entire tube at least daily and clean it in the same manner as a tracheostomy tube. The inner cannula may have to be removed and cleaned more often. A scarf or loose shirt can hide the stoma.

The patient should cover the stoma when coughing (because mucus may be expectorated) and during any activity (e.g., shaving, applying makeup) that may lead to inhalation of foreign materials. Because water can easily enter the stoma, the patient should wear a plastic collar when taking a shower. Swimming is contraindicated. Initially, humidification is given with mechanical ventilation or, after extubation, with a tracheostomy mask. After discharge, the patient can use a bedside humidifier.

Psychosocial Needs. Psychosocial care of the patient with head and neck cancer is of utmost importance. Issues concerning depression, change in body image, and sexuality are common. Although changes are discussed before surgery, the patient may not be psychologically prepared for the extent of these changes. If the patient has a significant other, this person's reaction to the patient's altered appearance is important. Acceptance by another person can promote an improved self-image.

Depression may occur for many reasons: inability to speak because of surgical procedure and/or presence of ET or tracheostomy tube, altered physical appearance due to the surgery and edema, loss of independence and reliance upon others, and feelings of helplessness and hopelessness. Depression also may be related to concern about the prognosis.

Allow the patient and caregiver to express their feelings and emotions. Convey acceptance to help patients regain positive feelings about their body image and self-concept. Encourage participation in support groups. Information about available groups can be obtained through the local branch of the American Cancer Society. A psychiatric referral may be needed for the patient who has prolonged or severe depression.

Surgery and surgical devices such as tracheostomy and gastrostomy tubes may dramatically affect body image. Xerostomia and fatigue can physically affect sexuality. It may be hard for the patient to talk about sexual problems because of changes in communication. Help the patient and partner by allowing them to talk about their sexuality and how surgery and treatment may affect their relationship. Helping the patient see that sexuality involves much more than appearance may relieve some anxiety.

◆ **Ambulatory Care.** The patient may be discharged with a tracheostomy and a nasogastric or gastrostomy feeding tube. Some patients initially need a home health care referral and assessment to evaluate the patient's or caregiver's ability to perform self-care activities. Both patient and caregiver need to learn how to manage tubes and whom to call if there are problems. Provide pictorial instructions for tracheostomy care, suctioning, stoma and skin care, and enteral feeding as appropriate. Encouraging the patient to take part in self-care is an important part of rehabilitation.

Teach the patient the importance of wearing a Medic Alert bracelet or other identification that alerts emergency personnel of the possible changes in breathing status because of surgery. Because the patient no longer breathes through the nose, the ability to smell smoke and taste food is often lost. Teach the patient to install smoke and carbon monoxide detectors in the home. Encourage preparation of food that is colorful, attractive, and nutritious because taste may be decreased due to the loss of smell and radiation therapy. Refer to a dietitian as needed.

The patient can resume exercise, recreation, and sexual activity when able. Most patients can return to work 1 to 2 months after surgery. However, many never return to full-time employment. The changes that follow a total laryngectomy can be upsetting. Loss of speech, loss of the ability to taste and smell, inability to produce audible sounds (including laughing and weeping), and the presence of a permanent tracheal stoma that produces undesirable mucus are often overwhelming to patients.

◆ **Evaluation**

Expected outcomes for the patient with head and neck cancer who is treated surgically are that the patient will:

- Have effective coughing and secretion clearance
- Swallow oral foods without aspiration
- Uses effective coping strategies
- Use techniques to effectively communicate

CASE STUDY
Laryngeal Cancer

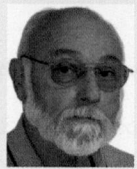

(© iStockphoto/
Thinkstock.)

Patient Profile

M.R., a 69-yr-old retired baker, was admitted to the hospital for influenza. He told his HCP that he has "a cough that just won't go away," difficulty swallowing, and "a sore throat that really hasn't gotten better" over the past year. His wife passed away 6 years ago. He has 3 adult children; 1 daughter lives in the same city. He has a history of hypertension, smoking, alcohol use, gastroesophageal reflux disease (GERD), and type 2 diabetes.

Subjective Data

- States that his symptoms worsened in the past 3 months
- Has used various cough and cold remedies over the past 6 months to relieve symptoms without relief
- Has lost weight because of decrease in appetite and difficulty swallowing
- Has smoked 3 packs of cigarettes a day for the past 50 yrs
- Consumes 4 to 6 cans of beer a day

Objective Data
Physical Examination

- *Vital signs:* Temperature 102.4° F (39.1° C), heart rate 99 beats/min (pulse strong, regular), respiratory rate 24 breaths/min (short, shallow, slightly labored), BP 176/84 (cuff), SpO₂ 87% on room air
- *Inspection:* Awake and alert, appears gray, malnourished, dehydrated. Small, irregular white patches on the sides of oral cavity
- *Palpation:* Enlarged cervical nodes bilaterally (nontender)
- *Auscultation:* Adequate and clear air entry to upper lung fields; slightly decreased air entry to bases with occasional fine crackles on expiration

Diagnostic Studies

- Chest x-ray: lung fields clear
- Laryngoscopy: mass in subglottic area (requires further evaluation)
- CT scan: subglottic lesion with lymph node involvement
- Diagnosis: laryngeal cancer

Interprofessional Care

- *Surgery:* suggests a total laryngectomy
- *Oncology:* suggests radiation and chemotherapy postoperatively

- *Gastroenterology:* percutaneous gastrostomy tube preoperatively for enteral feeding
- *Dietary:* explain nutritional options with/without ET tube/tracheostomy
- *Physical therapy:* visit pre-surgery to explain postoperative exercise routine
- *Social worker:* determine social supports available postoperatively

Discussion Questions

1. What assessment information suggests that M.R. is at risk for laryngeal cancer?
2. **Priority Decision:** What are your priority teaching strategies for M.R. before his total laryngectomy? Postoperative teaching priorities?
3. How would you explain the gastrostomy tube to M.R.?
4. Is there anything in his history that may affect wound healing after surgery?

Progression of Case

M.R. is transferred to the clinical unit after 24 hours in ICU. He is awake, alert, but slightly confused. Vital signs are stable. BP 168/94. Large surgical dressing on neck with 3 Jackson-Pratt drains. Tracheostomy tube in place. Receiving O₂ via tracheal mask. Enteral feeding at 30 mL/hr via gastrostomy tube. Foley catheter patent, draining a moderate amount of amber urine. M.R. is picking at his surgical drains, and when you try to reassure him, he just starts waving his hands at you.

5. **Collaboration:** What information would you want to know from the ICU nurse who has just transported M.R. to the clinical unit?
6. **Priority Decision:** Based on the assessment data presented, what are your priority nursing diagnoses? Are there any collaborative problems?
7. **Evidence-Based Practice:** How could you best meet M.R.'s communication needs during the first few postoperative days?
8. Four hours after transfer to the clinical unit, M.R. is tearful and is staring at the wall. What should you do?
9. **Patient-Centered Care:** What teaching is required to help him assume self-care after his surgery? What precautions should he take because of his stoma?

Answers available at *http://evolve.elsevier.com/Lewis/medsurg.*

BRIDGE TO NCLEX EXAMINATION

The number of the question corresponds to the same-numbered outcome at the beginning of the chapter.

1. A patient is seen in the clinic for a nosebleed, which is controlled by placement of anterior nasal packing. During discharge teaching, the nurse teaches the patient to
   a. use aspirin for pain relief.
   b. remove the packing later that day.
   c. avoid vigorous nose blowing and strenuous activity.
   d. insert more packing into the nose if rebleeding occurs.

2. A patient with allergic rhinitis reports severe nasal congestion; sneezing; and watery, itchy eyes and nose at various times of the year. When teaching the patient about how to control these symptoms, the nurse teaches the patient to
   a. avoid all intranasal sprays and oral antihistamines.
   b. limit the usage of nasal decongestant spray to 10 days.
   c. use oral decongestants at bedtime to prevent symptoms during the night.
   d. keep a diary of when the allergic reaction occurs and what precipitates it.

3. A patient is seen at the clinic with fever, muscle aches, sore throat with yellowish exudate, and headache. The nurse anticipates that the interprofessional management will include *(select all that apply)*
   a. antiviral agents to treat influenza.
   b. treatment with antibiotics starting ASAP.
   c. a throat culture or rapid strep antigen test.
   d. supportive care, including cool, bland liquids.
   e. comprehensive history to determine possible cause.

4. The *best* method for determining the risk for aspiration in a patient with a tracheostomy is to
   a. consult a speech therapist for swallowing assessment.
   b. have the patient drink plain water and assess for coughing.
   c. ask the patient to rate the perceived degree of swallowing difficulty.
   d. assess for sputum changes 48 hours after the patient drinks small amount of blue dye.

5. Which nursing action would be of *highest priority* when suctioning a patient with a tracheostomy?
   a. Auscultating lung sounds after suctioning is complete
   b. Giving antianxiety medications 30 minutes before suctioning
   c. Instilling 5 mL of normal saline into the tracheostomy tube before suctioning
   d. Assessing the patient's oxygen saturation before, during, and after suctioning

6. When planning health care teaching to prevent or detect early head and neck cancer, which people would be the *priority* to target (*select all that apply*)?
   a. 65-year-old man who has used chewing tobacco most of his life
   b. 45-year-old rancher who uses snuff to stay awake while driving his herds of cattle
   c. 21-year-old college student who drinks beer on weekends with his fraternity brothers
   d. 78-year-old woman who has been drinking liquor since her husband died 15 years ago
   e. 22-year-old woman who has been diagnosed with human papilloma virus of the cervix

7. While in the recovery room, a patient with a total laryngectomy is suctioned and has bloody mucus with some clots. Which nursing interventions would apply? (*select all that apply*)
   a. Notify the health care provider at once.
   b. Place the patient in semi-Fowler's position.
   c. Use a bag-valve-mask (BVM) and begin rescue breathing for the patient
   d. Instill 10 mL of normal saline into the tracheostomy tube to loosen secretions.
   e. Continue patient assessment, including O_2 saturation, respiratory rate, and breath sounds.

8. Appropriate discharge teaching for the patient with a permanent tracheostomy after a total laryngectomy for cancer would include (*select all that apply*)
   a. encouraging regular exercise such as swimming.
   b. washing around the stoma daily with a moist washcloth.
   c. encouraging participation in postlaryngectomy support group.
   d. providing pictures and "hands-on" instruction for tracheostomy care.
   e. teaching how to hold breath and trying to gag to promote swallowing reflex.

1. c, 2. d, 3. c, d, e, 4. a, 5. d, 6. a, b, 7. b, e, 8. b, c, d

For rationales to these answers and even more NCLEX review questions, visit *http://evolve.elsevier.com/Lewis/medsurg.*

EVOLVE WEBSITE/RESOURCES LIST

http://evolve.elsevier.com/Lewis/medsurg
Review Questions (Online Only)
Key Points
Answer Keys for Questions
- Rationales for Bridge to NCLEX Examination Questions
- Answer Guidelines for Case Study on p. 499
Student Case Study
- Patient With Head and Neck Cancer/Laryngectomy With Tracheostomy
Nursing Care Plans
- eNursing Care Plan 26.1: Patient With a Tracheostomy
- eNursing Care Plan 26.2: Patient Having Total Laryngectomy and/or Radical Neck Surgery
Conceptual Care Map Creator
Supporting Media
- Animation
- Tracheotomy
Audio Glossary
Content Updates

REFERENCES

1. American Academy of Otolaryngology: Deviated septum. Retrieved from *https://www.enthealth.org/nose-landing-page/*.
2. Paton KT, Thibodeau GA: *Anatomy and physiology,* ed 9, St Louis, 2016, Mosby.
3. Haraldson SJ: Nasal fracture. Retrieved from *https://emedicine.medscape.com/article/84829-overview*.
4. Good VS, Kirkwood PL: *Advanced critical care nursing,* ed 2, St Louis, 2018, Elsevier.
5. Rothrock JC: *Alexander's care of the patient in surgery,* ed 16, St Louis, 2019, Elsevier.
6. Shiffman MA, DiGiuseppe A: *Advanced aesthetic rhinoplasty: Art, science, and new clinical technologies,* New York, 2013, Springer (Classic).
7. DeWit SC, Stromberg HK, Dallred C: *Medical-surgical nursing: Concepts and practice,* ed 3, St Louis, 2017, Elsevier.
8. Nguyen QA: Epistaxis treatment and management. Retrieved from *https://emedicine.medscape.com/article/863220-treatment*.
9. Sheikh J: Allergic rhinitis. Retrieved from *https://emedicine.medscape.com/article/134825-overview#a5*.
*10. Scadding GK, Kariyawasam HH, Scadding G, et al: BSACI guideline for the diagnosis and management of allergic and non-allergic rhinitis, *Clin Exp Allergy,* 47:856, 2017.
11. American Academy of Asthma, Allergy and Immunology: Hay fever and allergy medications. Retrieved from *www.aaaai.org/conditions-and-treatments/library/allergy-library/hay-fever-medications*.
12. Centers for Disease Control and Prevention: Seasonal influenza-associated hospitalizations in the United States. Retrieved from *www.cdc.gov/flu/about/qa/hospital.htm*.
13. Centers for Disease Control and Prevention: Estimating seasonal influenza-associated deaths in the United States. Retrieved from *www.cdc.gov/flu/about/disease/us_flu-related_deaths.htm*.
14. University of California Irvine Health: How long is the flu contagious? Retrieved from *www.ucirvinehealth.org/blog/2017/02/flu-contagious*.
15. US Food and Drug Administration: Influenza (flu) antiviral drugs and related information. Retrieved from *www.fda.gov/drugs/drugsafety/informationbydrugclass/ucm100228.htm*.
*16. Hanson C, Lepule K: Management of acute and chronic sinusitis, *S Afr Pharm J* 84:45, 2017.
*17. Arina AM, Chan MM: Current concepts in adult acute rhinosinusitis, *Am Fam Physician* 94:97, 2016.
18. Newson L: Nasal polyps. Retrieved from *https://patient.info/health/nasal-polyps-leaflet*.
19. Hermann J: Say ahh: Acute pharyngitis diagnosis and management. Retrieved from *http://contemporaryclinic.pharmacytimes.com/journals/issue/2017/december2017/Say-Ahh-Acute-Pharyngitis-Diagnosis-and-Management*.
20. Carrillo-Marquez MA: Bacterial pharyngitis treatment and management. Retrieved from *https://emedicine.medscape.com/article/225243-treatment*.

*21. Lynch J, Crawley SM: Management of airway obstruction, *BJA Education* 18:46, 2018.

22. Urden LD, Stacy KM, Lough ME: *Critical care nursing: Diagnosis and management*, ed 8, St. Louis, 2018, Elsevier.

*23. Mehta C, Mehta Y: Percutaneous tracheostomy, *Ann Card Anaesth* 20:S19, 2017.

24. Salisbury NHS Foundation Trust: Tracheostomy cuffs—Management of. Retrieved from *www.icid.salisbury.nhs.uk/CLINICALMANAGEMENT/ ENT/Pages/Themanagementoftracheostomycuffs CPr.aspx*.

25. American Cancer Society: Key statistics for oral and oropharyngeal cancers. Retrieved from *www.cancer.org/cancer/oral-cavity-and- oropharyngeal-cancer/about/key-statistics.html*.

26. American Society of Clinical Oncology Cancer.Net: Head and neck cancer: Risk factors and prevention. Retrieved from *www.cancer.net/ cancer-types/head-and-neck-cancer/risk-factors-and-prevention*.

27. Cancer Treatment Centers of America: TNM system for head and neck cancer. Retrieved from *www.cancercenter.com/head-and-neck-cancer/ stages/*.

28. Australian Government Cancer Australia: Head and neck cancer treatment options. Retrieved from *https://head-neck-cancer.canceraustralia. gov.au/treatment*.

29. Cancer Treatment Centers of America: Head and neck cancer drug information. Retrieved from *www.cancercenter.com/head-and-neck-cancer/ diagnostics-and-treatments/tab/drug-information/*.

*Evidence-based information for clinical practice.

27

Lower Respiratory Problems

Eugene Mondor

To know even one life has breathed easier because you have lived, that is to have succeeded.

Ralph Waldo Emerson

http://evolve.elsevier.com/Lewis/medsurg/

CONCEPTUAL FOCUS

Cellular Regulation	Functional Ability	Infection
Clotting	Gas Exchange	

LEARNING OUTCOMES

1. Compare and contrast the clinical manifestations and nursing and interprofessional management of patients with acute bronchitis and pertussis.
2. Distinguish among the types of pneumonia and their etiology.
3. Describe the pathophysiology, clinical manifestations, diagnostic studies, and interprofessional and nursing management of patients with pneumonia.
4. Describe the pathogenesis, classification, clinical manifestations, complications, diagnostic abnormalities, and interprofessional and nursing management of patients with tuberculosis.
5. Describe the causes, clinical manifestations, and nursing and interprofessional management of patients with pulmonary fungal infections.
6. Explain the pathophysiology, clinical manifestations, and nursing and interprofessional management of a patient with a lung abscess.
7. Identify the causative factors, clinical manifestations, and nursing and interprofessional management of patients with environmental lung diseases.
8. Describe the etiology, risk factors, pathophysiology, clinical manifestations, and interprofessional and nursing management of lung cancer.
9. Compare and contrast the pathophysiology, clinical manifestations, and nursing and interprofessional management of fractured ribs, flail chest, and pneumothorax.
10. Describe the purpose, function, and nursing responsibilities related to chest tubes and chest drainage systems.
11. Explain the types of chest surgery and appropriate preoperative and postoperative care.
12. Describe the etiology, clinical manifestations, and nursing and interprofessional management of patients with restrictive lung disorders.
13. Describe the pathophysiology, clinical manifestations, and nursing and interprofessional management of pulmonary embolism, pulmonary hypertension, and cor pulmonale.
14. Discuss the use of lung transplantation as a treatment for pulmonary disorders, emphasizing nursing and interprofessional management of the postoperative lung transplant patient.

KEY TERMS

acute bronchitis, p. 502	lung abscess, p. 515	pulmonary edema, p. 532
community-acquired pneumonia (CAP), p. 504	pertussis, p. 503	pulmonary embolism (PE), p. 532
cor pulmonale, p. 535	pleural effusion, p. 531	pulmonary hypertension, p. 534
empyema, p. 531	pleurisy (pleuritis), p. 531	tension pneumothorax, p. 525
flail chest, p. 524	pneumoconiosis, p. 516	thoracentesis, p. 530
hemothorax, p. 525	pneumonia, p. 503	thoracotomy, p. 529
hospital-acquired pneumonia (HAP), p. 504	pneumothorax, p. 524	tuberculosis (TB), p. 509

A variety of problems affect the lower respiratory system. This chapter discusses lower respiratory tract diseases that influence the concept of gas exchange. It focuses on infectious, environmental, oncologic, traumatic, restrictive, and vascular problems that impair gas exchange. Gas exchange is related with multiple concepts, as a problem has profound consequences because of the need of adequate oxygenation for life.

LOWER RESPIRATORY TRACT INFECTIONS

Lower respiratory tract infection is both a common and serious occurrence. It is the reason for thousands of clinic and emergency department (ED) visits and hospital admissions each year. In the United States, pneumonia and influenza cause more than 57,000 deaths annually.[1]

ACUTE BRONCHITIS

Acute bronchitis is a self-limiting inflammation of the bronchi in the lower respiratory tract. It is the reason for 10% of all clinic visits and 100 million ED visits per year.[2] Most acute bronchial infections are caused by viruses. Air pollution, dust, inhalation of chemicals, smoking, chronic sinusitis, and asthma are other triggers.

Cough, which is the most common symptom, may last for up to 3 weeks. It is the main reason for seeking medical care. Clear sputum is often present, although some patients have purulent sputum. The presence of colored (e.g., green) sputum is not a reliable indicator of bacterial infection. Other symptoms may include headache, fever, malaise, hoarseness, myalgias, dyspnea, and chest pain.

Diagnosis is based on the assessment. Assessment may reveal normal breath sounds or crackles or wheezes, usually on expiration and with exertion. *Consolidation* (which occurs when fluid accumulates in the lungs), suggestive of pneumonia, is absent with bronchitis. Chest x-rays are normal and not needed unless pneumonia or some other pulmonary disorder is suspected.

The goal of treatment is to relieve symptoms and prevent pneumonia. Treatment is supportive. It includes cough suppressants (e.g., dextromethorphan), encouraging oral fluid intake, and using a humidifier. Throat lozenges, hot tea, and honey may help relieve cough. β_2-Agonist (bronchodilator) inhalers are useful for patients with wheezes or underlying pulmonary conditions. Antibiotics are not prescribed for viral infections because they have side effects and promote antibiotic resistance. Antibiotics may be given to patients with underlying chronic conditions who have a prolonged infection associated with systemic symptoms.

Encourage patients not to smoke, to avoid secondhand smoke, and to wash their hands often. If the acute bronchitis is due to an influenza virus, treatment with antiviral drugs may be started. If patients with acute bronchitis develop a fever, have difficulty breathing, or have symptoms last longer than 4 weeks, they should see their HCP.

PERTUSSIS

Pertussis is a highly contagious infection of the respiratory tract caused by the gram-negative bacillus *Bordetella pertussis*. The bacteria attach to the cilia of the respiratory tract and release toxins that damage the cilia, causing inflammation and swelling. The incidence of pertussis has been steadily increasing in the United States since the 1980s. The largest increase is seen in adults. We think that immunity from childhood tetanus, diphtheria, and pertussis vaccine (Tdap) vaccination may decrease over time, allowing a milder (but still contagious) infection. The Centers for Disease Control and Prevention (CDC) currently recommends that all adolescents (11 years and older) and adults who have not received a dose of Tdap receive a one-time vaccination as soon as possible.[3]

Manifestations of pertussis occur in stages. The first stage, lasting 1 to 2 weeks, manifests as a mild upper respiratory tract infection (URI) with a low-grade or no fever, runny nose, watery eyes, generalized malaise, and mild, nonproductive cough. The second stage, from the second to tenth week of infection, is characterized by paroxysms of cough. The last stage lasts 2 to 3 weeks. It is characterized by a less severe cough and weakness.

♥ PROMOTING POPULATION HEALTH

Preventing Respiratory Diseases

- Wash hands often to prevent and avoid spreading infections.
- Avoid cigarette smoking and exposure to environmental smoke.
- Get a pneumococcal vaccine and yearly flu vaccine as directed by the HCP.
- Avoid exposure to allergens, indoor pollutants, and ambient air pollutants.
- Wear proper personal protective equipment when working in an occupation with prolonged exposure to dust, fumes, or gases.

The hallmark characteristic of pertussis is uncontrollable, violent coughing. Inspiration after each cough produces the typical "whooping" sound as the patient tries to breathe in air against an obstructed glottis. The "whoop" is often not present in teens and adults (especially those who have been vaccinated). Like acute bronchitis, the coughing is more frequent at night. Vomiting may occur with coughing. Unlike acute bronchitis, the cough with pertussis may last from 6 to 10 weeks.

In the community, diagnosis is primarily by history and examination. In the clinical setting, the CDC recommends nasopharyngeal cultures, polymerase chain reaction (PCR) of nasopharyngeal secretions, or serology testing.[4] The treatment is macrolide (erythromycin, azithromycin [Zithromax]) antibiotics to minimize symptoms and prevent spread of the disease. For the patient who cannot take macrolides, trimethoprim/sulfamethoxazole is used. The patient is infectious from the beginning of the first stage through the third week after onset of symptoms or until 5 days after antibiotic therapy has been started. Routine and droplet precautions are required for hospitalized patients. Patients should not use cough suppressants and antihistamines as they are ineffective and may induce coughing episodes. Corticosteroids and bronchodilators are also not helpful. The CDC recommends postexposure antibiotics to those who have had close contact with the patient.

PNEUMONIA

Pneumonia is an acute infection of the lung parenchyma. Despite remarkable progress in the development of antibiotics to treat pneumonia, pneumonia is still associated with significant morbidity and mortality. The CDC reports that pneumonia and influenza are the 8th leading cause of death in the United States.[5]

Etiology

Normally, various defense mechanisms protect the airway distal to the larynx from infection. Mechanisms that create a mechanical barrier to microorganisms entering the tracheobronchial tree include air filtration, epiglottis closure over the trachea, cough reflex, mucociliary escalator mechanism, and reflex bronchoconstriction (see Chapter 25). Immune defense mechanisms include secretion of immunoglobulins A and G and alveolar macrophages.

Pneumonia is more likely to occur when defense mechanisms become incompetent or are overwhelmed by the virulence or quantity of infectious agents. A weakened cough or epiglottal reflex may allow aspiration of oropharyngeal contents into the lungs. Tracheal intubation bypasses normal filtration processes and interferes with the cough reflex and mucociliary escalator mechanism. Air pollution, cigarette smoking, viral URIs, and normal changes that occur with aging can impair the mucociliary mechanism. Chronic diseases can suppress the immune system's ability to inhibit bacterial growth. The risk factors for pneumonia are listed in Table 27.1.

Pathogens that cause pneumonia reach the lung in 3 ways:

1. *Aspiration* of normal flora from the nasopharynx or oropharynx. Many organisms that cause pneumonia are normal inhabitants of the pharynx in healthy adults.
2. *Inhalation* of microbes present in the air. Examples include *Mycoplasma pneumoniae* and fungal pneumonias.
3. *Hematogenous spread* from a primary infection elsewhere in the body. Examples are streptococci and *Staphylococcus aureus* from infective endocarditis.

TABLE 27.1 Risk Factors for Pneumonia

- Abdominal or chest surgery
- Age >65 years
- Air pollution
- Altered consciousness: alcoholism, head injury, seizures, anesthesia, drug overdose, stroke
- Bed rest and prolonged immobility
- Chronic diseases: chronic lung and liver disease, diabetes, heart disease, cancer, chronic kidney disease
- Debilitating illness
- Exposure to bats, birds, rabbits, and farm animal droppings (excrement)
- Immunosuppressive disease and/or therapy (corticosteroids, cancer chemotherapy, HIV infection, immunosuppressive therapy after organ transplant)
- Inhalation or aspiration of noxious substances
- Intestinal and gastric feedings via nasogastric or nasointestinal tubes
- IV drug use
- Malnutrition
- Recent antibiotic therapy
- Resident of a long-term care facility
- Smoking
- Tracheal intubation (endotracheal intubation, tracheostomy)
- URI

TABLE 27.2 Organisms Causing Pneumonia

Community-Acquired Pneumonia

- *Chlamydophila pneumoniae*
- *Chlamydophila psittaci*
- *Coxiella burnettii*
- Gram-negative bacilli
- Fungi
- Influenzae
- Influenza A and B
- *Klebsiella pneumoniae*
- *Legionella pneumophila**
- MRSA*
- *Moraxella catarrhalis*
- *Mycobacterium tuberculosis*
- *Mycoplasma pneumoniae*
- Oral anaerobes (e.g., alcoholism, IV drug use)
- *Pseudomonas aeruginosa*
- Respiratory viruses
- *S. pneumoniae**

Hospital-Acquired Pneumonia

- *Acinetobacter* species†
- *Enterobacter* species
- *Escherichia coli*†
- *H. influenzae*
- *Klebsiella pneumoniae*†
- *Proteus* species
- *Pseudomonas aeruginosa*†
- *S. aureus*
- *S. pneumoniae*

*Most common cause of community-acquired pneumonia (CAP).
†Most common causes of hospital-acquired pneumonia (HAP).

Classifications of Pneumonia

There is no universally accepted classification system for pneumonia. Some suggest classifying pneumonia according to the causative pathogens (e.g., bacterial, viral, fungal, etc.), characteristics of the disease, or radiographic appearance on chest x-ray. The most widely recognized and effective way to classify pneumonia is as either *community-acquired* or *hospital-acquired* pneumonia. This classification helps the HCP identify the most likely cause (Table 27.2) and the choice of antimicrobial therapy.
Community-Acquired Pneumonia. Community-acquired pneumonia (CAP) is an acute infection of the lung occurring in patients who have not been hospitalized or lived in a long-term care facility within 14 days of the onset of symptoms. The decision to treat the patient at home or admit to hospital is based on several factors. These include the patient's age, vital signs, mental status, presence of co-morbid conditions, and current physiologic condition. We can use tools such as the expanded CURB-65 scale (Table 27.3) to supplement clinical judgment.
Hospital-Acquired Pneumonia. Hospital-acquired pneumonia (HAP), also known as *nosocomial pneumonia*, is pneumonia in a nonintubated patient that begins 48 hours or longer after admission to hospital and was not present at the time of admission. *Ventilator-associated pneumonia (VAP)*, a type of HAP, refers to pneumonia that occurs more than 48 hours after endotracheal intubation.[6] VAP is discussed in Chapter 65. Both HAP and VAP are associated with longer hospital stays, increased associated costs, sicker patients, and increased risk for morbidity and mortality.

Once the diagnosis of CAP, HAP, or VAP is made, treatment is started based on known risk factors, early versus late onset, presentation, underlying medical conditions, hemodynamic stability, and the likely causative pathogen. *Empiric antibiotic therapy*, the initiation of treatment before a definitive diagnosis or causative agent is confirmed, should be started as soon as pneumonia is suspected. Empiric antibiotic therapy is based on the knowledge of drugs known to be effective for the likely cause. Antibiotic therapy can be adjusted once the results of sputum cultures identify the exact pathogen.

TABLE 27.3 Assessing Pneumonia Severity Using Expanded CURB-65

The **Expanded CURB-65 scale** may be used as a supplement to clinical judgment to determine the severity of pneumonia and if patients need to be hospitalized.

Identifying the Level of Risk
Patients receive 1 point for each of the following indicators:

- **C:** Confusion (compared to baseline)
- **U:** BUN >20 mg/dL
- **R:** Respiratory rate ≥30 breaths/min
- **B:** Systolic blood pressure <90 mm Hg or diastolic blood pressure ≤60 mm Hg
- **65:** ≥Age 65 yr
- **LDH:** >230 μ/L
- **Albumin:** <3.5 g/dL
- **Platelet count:** <100 × 10^9/L

Scoring and Decision Making

Score	Perceived Risk	Location
0–2	Low	Outpatient
3–4	Intermediate	In patient
5–8	High	ICU

Source: Liu J, Xu F, Zhou H, et al: Expanded CURB-65: A new score system predicts severity of community-acquired pneumonia with superior efficiency, *Sci Rep* 6:22911, 2016.

Types of Pneumonia

There are several types of pneumonia. *Viral pneumonia* is the most common type of pneumonia. It occurs in one third of all pneumonia cases. It may be mild and self-limiting or cause potentially life-threatening problems, such as acute respiratory failure in influenza. Patients with *bacterial pneumonia* may be extremely unwell and need hospital admission. *Mycoplasma pneumonia*, which has traits of both bacteria and viruses, is often referred to as "atypical" pneumonia. It is mild and occurs in persons younger than 40 years of age. Aspiration, necrotizing, and opportunistic pneumonia deserve further attention.

Aspiration Pneumonia. *Aspiration pneumonia* results from the abnormal entry of material from the mouth or stomach into the trachea and lungs. Conditions that increase the risk for aspiration include decreased level of consciousness (e.g., seizure, anesthesia, head injury, stroke, alcohol intake), difficulty swallowing, and insertion of nasogastric (NG) tubes with or without enteral feeding. With loss of consciousness, the gag and cough reflexes are depressed and aspiration is more likely to occur.

The aspirated material (food, water, vomitus, oropharyngeal secretions) triggers an inflammatory response. The most common form of aspiration pneumonia is a primary bacterial infection. Typically, the sputum culture shows more than 1 organism, including aerobes and anaerobes, since they both make up the flora of the oropharynx.

Until cultures are done and results obtained, initial antibiotic therapy is based on an assessment of probable cause, severity of illness, and patient factors (e.g., malnutrition, current use of antibiotic therapy). For patients who aspirate in hospitals, antibiotic coverage should include both gram-negative organisms and methicillin-resistant *Staphylococcus aureus* (MRSA). Aspiration of acidic gastric contents causes *chemical (noninfectious) pneumonitis,* which may not need antibiotic therapy. However, secondary bacterial infection can occur 48 to 72 hours later.

Necrotizing Pneumonia. *Necrotizing pneumonia* is a rare complication of bacterial lung infection. It causes the lung tissue to turn into a thick, liquid mass. In some situations, cavitation occurs. This often happens with CAP. Although we do not know the exact pathophysiologic mechanisms involved, causative organisms include *Staphylococcus, Klebsiella,* and *Streptococcus.* Lung abscesses often occur. Signs and symptoms include immediate respiratory insufficiency and/or failure, leukopenia, and bleeding into the airways.[7] Treatment includes long-term antibiotic therapy and possible surgery.

Opportunistic Pneumonia. *Opportunistic pneumonia* is inflammation and infection of the lower respiratory tract in immunocompromised patients. Persons at risk include those with altered immune responses. This can include people with severe protein-calorie malnutrition or immunodeficiencies (e.g., human immunodeficiency virus [HIV] infection) and those receiving radiation therapy, chemotherapy, and any immunosuppressive therapy, including long-term corticosteroid therapy. In addition to the risk for bacterial and viral pneumonia, the immunocompromised person may develop an infection from organisms that do not normally cause disease, such as *Pneumocystis jiroveci* (formerly *carinii*) or cytomegalovirus (CMV).

P. jiroveci pneumonia (PJP) rarely occurs in the healthy person. It is the most common form of pneumonia in people with HIV disease. The onset is slow and subtle with symptoms of fever, tachypnea, tachycardia, dyspnea, nonproductive cough, and hypoxemia. The chest x-ray usually shows diffuse bilateral infiltrates. In widespread disease, the lungs have massive consolidation. PJP can be life-threatening, causing acute respiratory failure and death. Infection can spread to other organs, including the liver, bone marrow, lymph nodes, spleen, and thyroid. Bacterial and viral pneumonias first must be ruled out

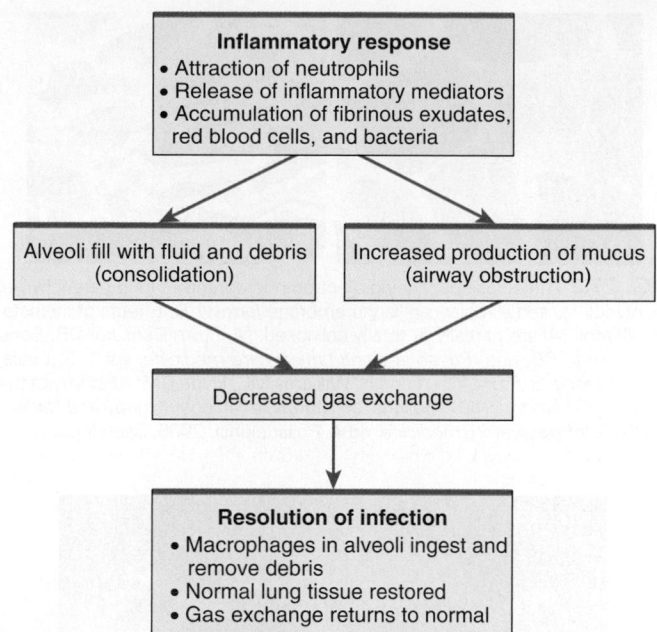

because of the vague presentation of PJP. Although the causative agent is fungal, PJP does not respond to antifungal agents. Treatment consists of a course of trimethoprim/sulfamethoxazole (Bactrim, Septra) either IV or orally depending on the severity of disease and the patient's response.

CMV, a herpesvirus, can cause viral pneumonia. Most CMV infections are asymptomatic or mild. Severe disease can occur in people with an impaired immune response. CMV is one of the most important life-threatening infectious complications after hematopoietic stem cell transplantation.[8] Antiviral medications (e.g., ganciclovir [Cytovene], foscarnet [Foscavir], cidofovir) and high-dose immunoglobulin are used for treatment.

Pathophysiology

Specific pathophysiologic changes related to pneumonia vary according to the offending pathogen. Almost all pathogens trigger an inflammatory response in the lungs (Fig. 27.1). Inflammation, characterized by an increase in blood flow and vascular permeability, activates neutrophils to engulf and kill the offending pathogens. As a result, the inflammatory process attracts more neutrophils, edema of the airways occurs, and fluid leaks from the capillaries and tissues into alveoli. Normal O_2 transport is affected, leading to manifestations of hypoxia (e.g., tachypnea, dyspnea, tachycardia).

Atelectasis, the absence of gas or air in 1 or more areas of the lung, may occur with pneumonia. It rarely causes any adverse effects except shortness of breath (Fig. 27.2). On the other hand, *consolidation,* a feature typical of bacterial pneumonia, occurs when the normally air-filled alveoli become filled with water, fluid, and/or debris (Fig. 27.3). This can potentially obstruct airflow, impair gas exchange, and cause the signs and symptoms associated with bacterial infection. Over time and with appropriate antibiotic therapy, macrophages lyse and process the debris. This allows lung tissue to recover and gas exchange to return to normal.

Clinical Manifestations

The most common presenting symptoms of pneumonia are cough, fever, chills, dyspnea, tachypnea, and pleuritic chest

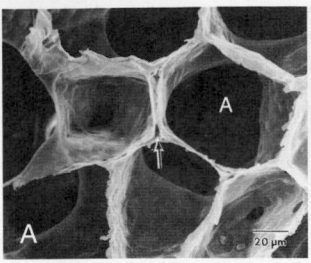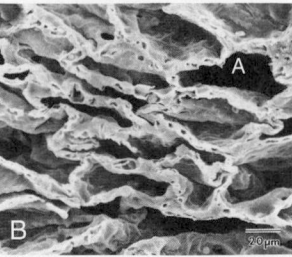

FIG. 27.2 Atelectasis. Scanning electron micrograph of lung parenchyma. **A,** Alveoli *(A)* and alveolar-capillary membrane *(arrow).* **B,** Effects of atelectasis. Alveoli *(A)* are partially or totally collapsed. (*A,* From Dantzker DR, Bone RC, George RB, eds: *Pulmonary and critical care medicine,* vol 1, St Louis, 1993, Mosby. *B,* From Albertine KH, Williams MC, Hyde DM: Anatomy of the lungs. In RJ Mason, VC Broaddus, JF Murray, et al, eds: *Murray and Nadel's textbook of respiratory medicine,* ed 4, Philadelphia, 2005, Saunders.)

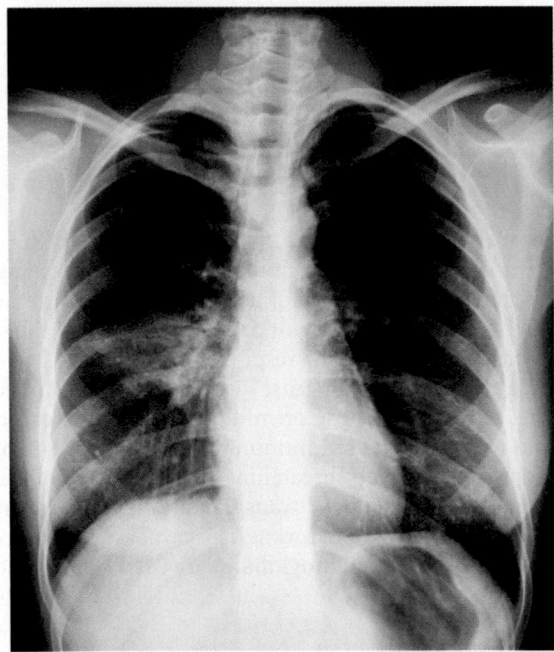

FIG. 27.3 Chest x-ray examination of patient with acute bacterial pneumonia. (© *iStock*.com/stockdevil.)

pain. The cough may or may not be productive. Sputum may be green, yellow, or even rust colored (bloody). Viral pneumonia may initially be seen as influenza, with respiratory symptoms appearing and/or worsening 12 to 36 hours after onset.

The older or debilitated patient may not have classic symptoms of pneumonia. Confusion or stupor (possibly related to hypoxia) may be the only finding. Hypothermia, rather than fever, also may be seen in the older adult. Nonspecific manifestations include diaphoresis, anorexia, fatigue, myalgias, and headache.

On assessment, fine or coarse crackles may be auscultated over the affected region. If consolidation is present, bronchial breath sounds, egophony (an increase in the sound of the patient's voice), and increased fremitus (vibration of the chest wall made by vocalization) may be present. Patients with pleural effusion may have dullness to percussion over the affected area.

Complications

A major problem today is pneumonia caused by multidrug-resistant (MDR) pathogens. Common culprits include MRSA

and gram-negative bacilli. Risk factors for MDR pneumonia include advanced age, immunosuppression, history of antibiotic use, and prolonged mechanical ventilation. Antibiotic susceptibility tests can identify MDR pathogens. The virulence of these pathogens can severely limit the available and appropriate antimicrobial therapy. MDR pathogens increase the morbidity and mortality associated with pneumonia. (See Chapter 14 for more about MDR pathogens.)

Other complications from pneumonia develop more often in older adults and those with underlying chronic diseases. These include:

- *Atelectasis*
- *Pleurisy,* an inflammation of the pleura.
- *Pleural effusion,* or fluid in the pleural space. In most cases, the effusion is sterile and is reabsorbed in 1 to 2 weeks. Sometimes, effusions require aspiration by thoracentesis.
- *Bacteremia,* bacterial infection in the blood, is more likely to occur in infections with *Streptococcus pneumoniae* and *Haemophilus influenzae.*
- *Pneumothorax* can occur when air collects in the pleural space, causing the lungs to collapse.
- *Acute respiratory failure* is one of the leading causes of death in patients with severe pneumonia. Failure occurs when pneumonia damages the lungs' ability to exchange O_2 and CO_2 across the alveolar-capillary membrane.
- *Sepsis/septic shock* can occur when bacteria within alveoli enter the bloodstream. Severe sepsis can lead to shock and multisystem organ dysfunction syndrome (MODS) (see Chapter 66).

Lung abscess is not a common complication of pneumonia. However, it may occur with pneumonia caused by *S. aureus* and gram-negative organisms. *Empyema,* the accumulation of purulent exudate in the pleural cavity, occurs in less than 5% of cases. It requires antibiotic therapy and drainage of the exudate by a chest tube or open surgical drainage.[9] Pleurisy, pleural effusion, atelectasis, lung abscess, and pneumothorax are discussed later in this chapter.

Diagnostic Studies

The common diagnostic procedures for pneumonia are outlined in Table 27.4. History, physical examination, and chest x-ray often give enough information to make immediate decisions about early treatment. Chest x-ray often shows patterns characteristic of the infecting pathogen and is important in diagnosing pneumonia. X-ray may also show pleural effusions. A thoracentesis and/or bronchoscopy with washings may be used to obtain fluid samples from patients not responding to initial therapy.

Arterial blood gases (ABGs) may be obtained to assess for hypoxemia (partial pressure of O_2 in arterial blood [PaO$_2$] less than 80 mm Hg), hypercapnia (partial pressure of carbon dioxide in arterial blood [PaCO$_2$] greater than 45 mm Hg), and acidosis (pH less than 7.35). Leukocytosis occurs in most patients with bacterial pneumonia. The white blood cell (WBC) count is usually greater than 15,000/μL (15 × 10^9/L) with the presence of bands (immature neutrophils).

Ideally, a sputum specimen for culture and Gram stain to identify the organism is obtained before beginning antibiotic therapy. However, antibiotic administration should not be delayed if a specimen cannot be obtained. Delays in antibiotic therapy can increase the risk for morbidity and mortality. Blood cultures are done for patients who are seriously ill.

TABLE 27.4 Interprofessional Care

Pneumonia

Diagnostic Assessment

- History and physical examination
- Chest x-ray
- Sputum: Gram stain, culture and sensitivity test
- Pulse oximetry or arterial blood gases (if indicated)
- CBC, white blood cell differential, and routine blood chemistries (if indicated)
- Blood cultures (if indicated)

Management

- Increased fluid intake (at least 3 L/day), IV fluids
- Balance between activity and rest
- O_2 therapy
- Physiotherapy
- VTE prophylaxis
- Critical care management, with mechanical ventilation as needed

Drug Therapy

- Appropriate antibiotic therapy (Table 27.6)
- Antipyretics
- Analgesics
- Nonsteroidal antiinflammatory drugs (if no contraindications)

TABLE 27.5 Pneumococcal Vaccines

Vaccine*	Recommendations for Use
Pneumococcal conjugate vaccine (PCV13, Prevnar 13)[†]	• All children <2 yrs • All adults ≥65 yrs • Anyone 2–64 yrs old with certain medical conditions (e.g., sickle cell disease, asplenia, immunodeficiencies, HIV infection, chronic renal failure, leukemia, cancer, long-term immunosuppressive therapy, CSF leaks, cochlear implant[s])
Pneumococcal polysaccharide vaccine (PPSV23, Pneumovax 23)[†]	• All adults ≥65 yrs • Anyone 2–64 yrs old with certain long-term health problems (e.g., heart disease, lung disease, diabetes, alcoholism, cirrhosis, sickle cell disease, CSF leaks, cochlear implant) • Anyone 2–64 yrs with a disease or condition that weakens the immune system or taking drugs that lower the body's resistance to infection (e.g., HIV infection; lymphoma or leukemia; kidney failure; damaged or no spleen; multiple myeloma; receiving immunosuppressive chemotherapy, radiation therapy, or long-term corticosteroids; after organ or bone marrow transplantation) • Adults 19–64 yrs who smoke cigarettes or have asthma

*For more details on scheduling of pneumococcal vaccinations, see *www.cdc.gov/vaccines/vpd/pneumo/hcp/recommendations.html*.
[†]As their names imply, PCV13 and Prevnar 13 protect against 13 types of pneumococcal bacteria, and PPSV23 and Pneumovax 23 protect against 23 types of pneumococcal bacteria. The vaccinations have different mechanisms of action.

Serum levels of C-reactive protein (CRP), kallistatin, and procalcitonin are currently being explored as sources of information to help distinguish pneumonia from other types of heart and respiratory failure.[10]

Interprofessional Care

Pneumococcal vaccine is used to prevent *S. pneumoniae* infection (Table 27.5). Prompt treatment with the appropriate antibiotic is essential. Antibiotics are highly effective for both bacterial and mycoplasma pneumonia. In uncomplicated cases, the patient responds to drug therapy within 48 to 72 hours. Signs of improvement include decreased temperature, improved breathing, and reduced chest discomfort. Abnormal physical findings can last more than 7 days. A repeat chest x-ray may be done in 6 to 8 weeks to assess for resolution.

Supportive measures are tailored to the patient's needs. These may include O_2 therapy to treat hypoxemia, analgesics to relieve chest pain, and antipyretics (e.g., aspirin, acetaminophen) for fever. Although cough suppressants, mucolytics, bronchodilators, and corticosteroids are often prescribed as adjunctive therapy, the use of these drugs is debatable. However, they may be prescribed for patients with underlying chronic conditions.

Tailor rest and activity to each patient's tolerance. Benefits of mobility include improved diaphragm movement and chest expansion, mobilization of secretions, and prevention of venous stasis.

Currently, no definitive treatment exists for most viral pneumonias. Care is generally supportive. In most circumstances, viral pneumonia is self-limiting and will often resolve in 3 to 4 days. Antiviral therapy may be used to treat pneumonia caused by influenza (e.g., oseltamivir, zanamivir) or a few other viruses (e.g., acyclovir [Zovirax] for herpes simplex virus).[11]

Drug Therapy. Once the pneumonia is classified, the HCP selects empiric therapy based on the likely pathogen (Table 27.2). Table 27.6 presents the drug therapy for bacterial CAP.

For all types of pneumonia, empiric antibiotic therapy is based on whether the patient has risk factors for MDR pathogens. The prevalence and resistance patterns of MDR pathogens vary among localities and agencies. Therefore the antibiotic regimen must be adapted to local patterns of antibiotic resistance. Multiple regimens exist, but all should initially include antibiotics that are effective against both resistant gram-negative and resistant gram-positive organisms.

Clinical improvement usually occurs in 3 to 5 days. Patients who deteriorate or do not respond to therapy need aggressive reevaluation to assess for noninfectious causes, complications, coexisting infectious processes, or pneumonia caused by an MDR pathogen.

IV antibiotic therapy should be switched to oral therapy as soon as the patient is hemodynamically stable, is improving clinically, is able to ingest oral medication, and has a functioning gastrointestinal (GI) tract. Stable patients do not need to be observed in the hospital and can be discharged to home on oral antibiotics. Total treatment time for patients with CAP should be a minimum of 5 days. The patient should be afebrile for 48 to 72 hours before stopping treatment. However, you need to emphasize the importance of completing the full course of antibiotic treatment. Longer treatment time may be needed if initial therapy was not active against the identified pathogen or complications occur.

Nutritional Therapy. Hydration is important in the supportive treatment of pneumonia to prevent dehydration and to thin and loosen secretions. Carefully monitor fluid intake. If the patient is an older adult, has heart failure (HF), or has a known preexisting respiratory condition, IV administration of fluids and electrolytes may be needed.

Weight loss may occur in patients with pneumonia because of increased metabolic needs and difficulty eating due to shortness of breath or nonspecific abdominal symptoms. Small, frequent meals are easier for dyspneic patients to tolerate. Offer foods high in calories and nutrients.

TABLE 27.6 Drug Therapy
Bacterial Community-Acquired Pneumonia

Patient Variable	Treatment Options
Outpatient	
Previously healthy No recent antibiotic therapy in past 3 months and no risk for drug-resistant *Staphylococcus pneumoniae* (DRSP)	Macrolide *OR* doxycycline
Co-morbidities (e.g., COPD; diabetes; chronic heart, liver, lung, or renal disease; cancer; use of antibiotics in past 3 months)	Respiratory fluoroquinolone *OR* β-Lactam plus macrolide (doxycycline may be substituted for macrolide)
Regions with ≥25% macrolide-resistant *S. pneumoniae*	Respiratory fluoroquinolone *OR* β-Lactam plus macrolide
Inpatient	
Medical unit	Respiratory fluoroquinolone *OR* β-Lactam plus macrolide
ICU Acute respiratory failure, septic shock, intubation and mechanical ventilation	β-Lactam plus either azithromycin or respiratory fluoroquinolone
Special Considerations	
• Community-acquired methicillin-resistant *Staphylococcus aureus* (CA-MRSA)	Add vancomycin or linezolid (Zyvox)
• *Pseudomonas* infection	Antipneumococcal, antipseudomonal β-lactam plus either ciprofloxacin or levofloxacin *OR* Antipneumococcal, antipseudomonal β-lactam plus aminoglycoside and azithromycin *OR* Antipneumococcal, antipseudomonal β-lactam plus an aminoglycoside and an antipneumococcal fluoroquinolone
• *Pseudomonas* infection in patient with penicillin allergy	Substitute aztreonam for the above β-lactam
Types of Antibiotics	
Antipneumococcal, antipseudomonal β-lactams	imipenem/cilastatin, meropenem (Merrem), cefepime (Maxipime), piperacillin/tazobactam (Zosyn)
β-Lactams	High-dose amoxicillin, amoxicillin/clavulanate (Augmentin), cefpodoxime, ceftriaxone, cefuroxime (Ceftin)
Fluoroquinolones	moxifloxacin (Avelox, Vigamox), levofloxacin, gemifloxacin (Factive)
Macrolides	erythromycin, azithromycin (Zithromax), clarithromycin (Biaxin)

Source: Infectious Diseases Advisor: Community acquired pneumonia guidelines. Retrieved from *www.infectiousdiseaseadvisor.com/clinical-charts/community-acquired-pneumonia-guidelines/article/419038/*.

❖ NURSING MANAGEMENT: PNEUMONIA

◆ Nursing Assessment
Table 27.7 presents subjective and objective data to obtain from a patient with pneumonia.

◆ Nursing Diagnoses
Nursing diagnoses for the patient with pneumonia may include:
- Impaired gas exchange
- Impaired breathing
- Fluid imbalance
- Hyperthermia
- Activity intolerance

Additional information on nursing diagnoses and interventions for the patient with pneumonia is presented in eNursing Care Plan 27.1 on the website for this chapter.

TABLE 27.7 Nursing Assessment
Pneumonia

Subjective Data
Important Health Information
Past health history: Lung cancer, COPD, diabetes, chronic debilitating disease, malnutrition, altered consciousness, immunosuppression, exposure to chemical toxins, dust, or allergens
Medications: Antibiotics, corticosteroids, chemotherapy, or any immunosuppressants
Surgery or other treatments: Recent abdominal or chest surgery, splenectomy, endotracheal intubation, or any surgery with general anesthesia. Enteral feedings

Functional Health Patterns
Health perception–health management: Cigarette smoking, alcohol use; recent URI, malaise
Nutritional-metabolic: Anorexia, nausea, vomiting. Chills
Activity-exercise: Prolonged bed rest or immobility. Fatigue, weakness. Dyspnea, cough (productive or nonproductive). Nasal congestion
Cognitive-perceptual: Pain with breathing, chest pain, sore throat, headache, abdominal pain, muscle aches

Objective Data
General
Fever, restlessness, or lethargy. Splinting of affected area

Respiratory
Tachypnea, pharyngitis, asymmetric chest movements or retraction, decreased excursion, nasal flaring. Use of accessory muscles (neck, abdomen). Crackles, friction rub on auscultation, dullness on percussion over consolidated areas, increased tactile fremitus on palpation. Pink, rusty, purulent, green, yellow, or white sputum (amount may be scant to copious)

Cardiovascular
Tachycardia

Neurologic
Changes in mental status, ranging from confusion to delirium

Possible Diagnostic Findings
Leukocytosis. Abnormal ABGs with ↓ or normal PaO_2, ↓ or normal $PaCO_2$, and ↑ or normal pH initially, and later ↓ PaO_2, ↑ $PaCO_2$, and ↓ pH. Positive sputum on Gram stain and culture. Patchy or diffuse infiltrates, abscesses, pleural effusion, or pneumothorax on chest x-ray

Planning

The overall goals are that the patient with pneumonia will have (1) clear breath sounds, (2) normal breathing patterns, (3) no signs of hypoxia, (4) normal chest x-ray, (5) normal WBC count, and (6) absence of complications related to pneumonia.

Nursing Implementation

Health Promotion. To reduce the risk for pneumonia, teach patients to practice good health habits, such as frequent hand washing, proper nutrition, adequate rest, regular exercise, and coughing or sneezing into the elbow rather than hands. Avoiding cigarette smoke is one of the most important health-promoting behaviors. If possible, avoid exposure to people with URIs. If a URI occurs, it requires prompt attention with supportive measures (e.g., rest, fluids). If symptoms persist for longer than 7 days, the person should seek medical care. Identifying patients at risk (Table 27.1) and taking measures to prevent pneumonia are priority interventions. Encourage those at risk for pneumonia (e.g., chronically ill, older adult) to obtain both influenza and pneumococcal vaccines (Table 27.5).

Acute Care. Although many patients with pneumonia are treated on an outpatient basis, the nursing care plan for a patient with pneumonia (eNursing Care Plan 27.1) applies to both patients at home and hospitalized patients. Essential nursing care for patients with pneumonia includes monitoring physical assessment parameters, providing treatment, and monitoring the patient's response to treatment. Prompt collection of specimens and initiation of antibiotics are critical. O_2 therapy, hydration, nutritional support, breathing exercises, early ambulation, and therapeutic positioning are part of nursing care. Working with respiratory therapy to monitor the patient's condition and with physical therapy for postural drainage and chest percussion is essential.

Place the patient with altered consciousness in positions (e.g., side-lying, upright) that will prevent or minimize the risk for aspiration. Turn and reposition patients at least every 2 hours to promote adequate lung expansion and mobilization of secretions. Encourage and assist with ambulation and positioning into a chair. In the ICU, strict adherence to all aspects of the ventilator bundle (see Table 67.8), a group of interventions aimed at reducing the risk for VAP, significantly reduces VAP.

For the patient who has difficulty swallowing and needs aid in eating, drinking, and taking medication to prevent aspiration, elevate the patient's head-of-bed to at least 30 degrees and have the patient sit up for all meals. Assess for a gag reflex before giving food or fluids. Patients who have orogastric or NG tubes are at risk for aspiration pneumonia (see Chapter 39). Although feeding tubes are small, any interruption in the integrity of the lower esophageal sphincter can allow reflux of gastric contents. To prevent aspiration, elevate the head of the bed to at least 30 degrees (see Table 39.11).

Patients with impaired mobility from any cause need help with turning and moving as well as encouragement to breathe deeply at frequent intervals. Observe the patient's skin and all pressure points for any evidence of redness or breakdown, especially the sacrum and coccyx. Treat pain to a comfort level that permits the patient to deep breathe and cough yet remain awake and alert and achieve optimum mobility. Early mobilization, the use of an incentive spirometer, and twice-daily oral hygiene with chlorhexidine swabs significantly reduce the incidence of pneumonia in postoperative patients.[12]

Practice strict medical asepsis and adherence to infection control guidelines to reduce the incidence of health care–associated infection (HAI). Staff and visitors should wash their hands on entering and leaving the patient's room. Staff must wash or use sanitizing hand gel before and after providing care and on removing gloves. Use strict sterile aseptic technique when suctioning the patient's trachea, and use caution when handling ventilator circuits, tracheostomy tubing, and nebulizer circuits that can become contaminated from patient secretions. Avoid inappropriate use of antibiotics to prevent the development of MDR organisms.

Ambulatory Care. Teach the patient about the importance of taking every dose of the prescribed antibiotic, any drug-drug and food-drug interactions for the prescribed antibiotic, and the need for adequate rest to promote recovery. Tell the patient to drink plenty of liquids (at least 6 to 10 glasses/day, unless contraindicated) and to avoid alcohol and smoking. A cool mist humidifier or warm bath may help the patient breathe easier. Tell patients that it may be several weeks before their usual vigor and sense of well-being return. Explain that a follow-up chest x-ray may be done in 6 to 8 weeks to evaluate resolution of pneumonia. The older adult or chronically ill patient may have a prolonged period of convalescence.

Teaching should include information about available influenza and pneumococcal vaccines. Patients can receive the pneumococcal vaccine and influenza vaccine at the same time but not in the exact same location. The vaccines cannot be mixed into 1 injection.

Evaluation

The expected outcomes are that the patient with pneumonia will have:

- Effective respiratory rate, rhythm, and depth of respirations
- Lungs clear to auscultation
- Absence of infection

TUBERCULOSIS

Tuberculosis (TB) is an infectious disease caused by *Mycobacterium tuberculosis*. It usually involves the lungs, but can infect any organ, including the brain, kidneys, and bones. About one third of the world's population are infected with TB.[13] The incidence of TB worldwide declined until the mid-1980s. We are now seeing increasing rates of TB. This is attributed to HIV disease and the emergence of drug-resistant strains of *M. tuberculosis*. TB is the leading cause of mortality in patients with HIV infection. Though the prevalence of TB in the United States has steadily declined, we do not think it is currently possible to eradicate TB in the United States.[14]

TB occurs disproportionately in the poor, underserved, and minorities. People most at risk include the homeless, residents of inner-city neighborhoods, foreign-born people, those living or working in institutions (long-term care facilities, prisons, shelters, hospitals), IV injecting drug users, overcrowded living conditions, less than optimal sanitation, and those with poor access to health care. Immunosuppression from any cause (e.g., HIV infection, cancer, long-term corticosteroid use) increases the risk for active TB infection.

Once a strain of *M. tuberculosis* develops resistance to the most potent first-line antitubercular drugs (isoniazid [INH] and rifampin [Rifadin]), it is defined as *multidrug-resistant tuberculosis (MDR-TB)*.[15] Extensively drug-resistant TB (XDR-TB)

🌐 PROMOTING HEALTH EQUITY

Tuberculosis

- Of the reported TB cases in the United States, most occur in racial and ethnic minorities.
- Asians have the highest TB rate of any ethnic group in the United States. Hispanics and blacks have the second and third highest TB rates.
- Of all the TB cases in the United States, 66% occur in foreign-born people. This rate is 13 times higher than in U.S.-born people.
- The percent of foreign-born people with MDR-TB increased from 31% in 1993 to 90% in 2013.

Source: Centers for Disease Control and Prevention: Health disparities in TB. Retrieved from www.cdc.gov/tb/topic/populations/healthdisparities/default.htm.

occurs when the organism is also resistant to any of the fluoroquinolones plus any injectable antibiotic agent.[16] Resistance results from several problems, including incorrect prescribing, lack of public health case management, patient nonadherence to the prescribed regimen, and lack of funding for education and prevention.

Etiology and Pathophysiology

M. tuberculosis is a gram-positive, aerobic, acid-fast bacillus (AFB). It is usually spread from person to person by airborne droplets expectorated when breathing, talking, singing, sneezing, and coughing. A process of evaporation leaves small droplet nuclei, 1 to 5 μm in size, suspended in the air for minutes to hours. Another person then inhales the bacteria. Humans are the only known reservoir for TB. TB is not highly infectious, as transmission usually requires close contact and frequent or prolonged exposure. The disease cannot be spread by touching, sharing food utensils, kissing, or any other type of physical contact.

Factors that influence transmission include the (1) number of organisms expelled into the air, (2) concentration of organisms (small spaces with limited ventilation would mean higher concentration), (3) length of time of exposure, and (4) immune system of the exposed person. Once inhaled, these small droplets lodge in bronchioles and alveoli. A local inflammatory reaction occurs, and the focus of infection is established. This is called the *Ghon lesion* or *focus*. It represents a calcified TB granuloma, the hallmark of a primary TB infection.[17] The formation of a granuloma is a defense mechanism aimed at walling off the infection and preventing further spread. Replication of the bacillus is inhibited, and the infection is stopped.

Most immunocompetent adults infected with TB can completely kill the mycobacteria. Some people have the mycobacteria in a nonreplicating dormant state. Of these persons, 5% to 10% develop active TB infection when the bacteria begin to multiply months or years later. While *M. tuberculosis* is aerophilic (O_2 loving) and has an affinity for the lungs, the infection can spread through the lymphatic system and find favorable environments for growth in other organs. These include the cerebral cortex, spine, epiphyses of the bone, liver, kidneys, lymph nodes, and adrenal glands.

Classification

Several systems can be used to classify TB. The American Thoracic Society classifies TB based on development of the disease (Table 27.8). TB also can be classified according to (1) its

TABLE 27.8 Classification of Tuberculosis

Class	Exposure or Infection	Description
0	No TB exposure	No TB exposure, not infected (no history of exposure, negative tuberculin skin test)
1	TB exposure, no infection	TB exposure, no evidence of infection (history of exposure, negative tuberculin skin test)
2	Latent TB infection, no disease	TB infection without disease (positive reaction to tuberculin skin test, negative bacteriologic studies, no x-ray findings compatible with TB, no clinical evidence of TB)
3	TB, clinically active	TB infection with clinically active disease (positive bacteriologic studies or both a significant reaction to tuberculin skin test and clinical or x-ray evidence of current disease)
4	TB, but not clinically active	No current disease (history of previous episode of TB or abnormal, stable x-ray findings in a person with a positive reaction to tuberculin skin test. Negative bacteriologic studies if done. No clinical or x-ray evidence of current disease)
5	TB suspect	TB suspect (diagnosis pending). Person should not be in this classification for >3 mo

Source: American Thoracic Society.

presentation (primary, latent, or reactivated) and (2) whether it is pulmonary or extrapulmonary.

Primary TB infection occurs when the bacteria are inhaled and start an inflammatory reaction. Most people mount effective immune responses to encapsulate these organisms for the rest of their lives, preventing the initial infection from progressing to disease. If the initial immune response is not adequate, the body cannot contain the organisms. As a result, the bacteria replicate and *active TB disease* results. When active disease develops within the first 2 years of infection, it is called *primary TB*. People co-infected with HIV are at greatest risk for developing active TB.

Post-primary TB, or *reactivation TB,* is defined as TB disease occurring 2 or more years after the initial infection. If the site of TB is pulmonary or laryngeal, the person is infectious and can transmit the disease to others.

Latent TB infection (LTBI) occurs in a person who does not have active TB disease (Table 27.9). People with LTBI have a positive skin test but are asymptomatic. They cannot transmit the TB bacteria to others but can develop active TB disease at some point. Immunosuppression, diabetes, poor nutrition, aging, pregnancy, stress, and chronic disease can reactivate the disease. Treatment of LTBI (discussed later in this chapter) is as important as primary TB.

Clinical Manifestations

Symptoms of pulmonary TB usually do not develop until 2 to 3 weeks after infection or reactivation. The primary manifestation is an initial dry cough that often becomes productive with mucoid or mucopurulent sputum. Active TB disease may initially present with constitutional symptoms (e.g., fatigue, malaise, anorexia, unexplained weight loss, low-grade fevers,

TABLE 27.9 Latent Tuberculosis Infection (LTBI) Compared to Tuberculosis Disease

LTBI	TB Disease
Has no symptoms	Has symptoms that may include: • Bad cough that lasts ≥3 wk • Pain in the chest • Coughing up blood or sputum • Weakness or fatigue • Weight loss, no appetite • Chills • Fever • Sweating at night
Does not feel sick	Usually feels sick
Cannot spread TB bacteria to others	May spread TB bacteria to others
Usually has a skin test or blood test result showing TB infection	Usually has a skin test or blood test result showing TB infection
Has a normal chest x-ray and a negative sputum smear	May have an abnormal chest x-ray or positive sputum smear or culture
Needs treatment for latent TB infection to prevent active TB disease	Needs treatment for active TB disease

Source: CDC: Latent TB infection and TB disease. Retrieved from *www.cdc.gov/tb/topic/basics/tbinfectiondisease.htm.*

night sweats). Dyspnea is a late symptom that may signify considerable pulmonary disease or a pleural effusion. Hemoptysis, which occurs in less than 10% of patients with TB, is also a late symptom.

Sometimes TB has a more acute, sudden presentation. The patient may have a high fever, chills, generalized flu-like symptoms, pleuritic pain, a productive cough, and acute respiratory failure. Auscultation of the lungs may be normal or reveal adventitious sounds, such as crackles.

Immunosuppressed (e.g., HIV-infected) people and older adults are less likely to have fever and other signs of an infection. In patients with HIV, classic manifestations of TB, such as fever, cough, and weight loss, may be wrongly attributed to PJP or other HIV-associated opportunistic diseases. Respiratory problems in patients with HIV must be carefully investigated to determine the cause. A change in cognitive function may be the only initial presenting sign of TB in an older person.

The manifestations of extrapulmonary TB depend on the organs infected. For example, renal TB can cause dysuria and hematuria. Bone and joint TB may cause severe pain. Headaches, vomiting, and lymphadenopathy may be present with TB meningitis.

Complications

Properly treated, pulmonary TB typically heals without complications, except for scarring and residual cavitation within the lung. Significant pulmonary damage, although rare, can occur in patients who are poorly treated or who do not respond to TB treatment.

Miliary TB is widespread dissemination of the mycobacterium. The bacteria spread through the bloodstream to several distant organs. The infection is characterized by a large amount of TB bacilli and may be fatal if untreated. It can occur with primary disease or reactivation of LTBI. Manifestations slowly progress over a period of days, weeks, or even months. Symptoms vary depending on the organs that are affected.

Fever, cough, and lymphadenopathy are present. Hepatomegaly and splenomegaly may occur.

Pleural TB, a specific type of extrapulmonary TB, can result from either primary disease or reactivation of a latent infection. Chest pain, fever, cough, and presence of a unilateral pleural effusion are common. A pleural effusion is caused by bacteria in the pleural space, which trigger an inflammatory reaction and a pleural exudate of protein-rich fluid. Empyema is less common than effusion but may occur from large numbers of tubercular organisms in the pleural space. Diagnosis is confirmed by AFB cultures and a pleural biopsy.

Because TB can infect organs throughout the body, various acute and long-term complications can result. TB in the spine (Pott's disease) can lead to destruction of the intervertebral disc and adjacent vertebrae. Central nervous system (CNS) TB can cause severe bacterial meningitis. Abdominal TB can lead to peritonitis, especially in HIV-positive patients. The kidneys, adrenal glands, lymph nodes, and urogenital tract can be affected.

❖ Diagnostic Studies

◆ **Tuberculin Skin Test.** The tuberculin skin test (TST) (Mantoux test) using purified protein derivative (PPD) is the standard method to screen people for *M. tuberculosis.* The test is given by injecting 0.1 mL of PPD intradermally on the ventral surface of the forearm. The test is read by inspection and palpation 48 to 72 hours later for the presence or absence of induration. Induration, a palpable, raised, hardened area or swelling (not redness) at the injection site means the person has been exposed to TB and has developed antibodies.[18] Antibody formation occurs 2 to 12 weeks after initial exposure to the bacteria. Any indurated area present is measured and recorded in millimeters. Based on the size of the induration and the risk factors, an interpretation is made according to CDC standards for determining a positive test reaction. Because the immunocompromised patient may have a decreased response to TST, smaller induration reactions (5 mm or larger) are considered positive. See Table 25.14 for guidelines in interpreting responses to the TST.

Two-step testing with the Mantoux TST should be used for baseline or initial screening. If the initial test is positive, the person needs further evaluation for active disease. If the first test is negative, a second TST is done 1 to 3 weeks later. Some people with LTBI or who were previously infected with TB may have a false negative result with the first TST. Repeating the TST may stimulate (boost) the body's ability to react to tuberculin in future tests.[18] A positive reaction to a subsequent test could be a new infection or the result of the boosted reaction to an old infection. Two-step testing is recommended for initial testing for health care workers and for those who have a decreased response to allergens. A previously negative 2-step TST ensures that any future positive results can be accurately interpreted as being caused by a new infection.

Interferon-γ Release Assays. Interferon-γ (INF-γ) release assays (IGRAs) are another screening tool for TB. IGRAs are blood tests that detect INF-γ release from T cells in response to *M. tuberculosis.*[19] Examples of IGRAs include QuantiFERON-TB Gold In-Tube test (QFT-GIT) and the T-SPOT.TB test. Test results are available in a few hours.

IGRAs offer several advantages over the TST in that they require only 1 patient visit, are not subject to reader bias, have no booster phenomenon, and are not affected by prior bacillus Calmette-Guérin (BCG) vaccination. The cost of an IGRA

TABLE 27.10 Interprofessional Care

Pulmonary Tuberculosis

Diagnostic Assessment
- History and physical examination
- Tuberculin skin test (TST)
- QuantiFERON-TB Gold In-Tube test (QFT-GIT) or T-SPOT.TB test
- Chest x-ray
- Bacteriologic studies
- Sputum smear for acid-fast bacilli (AFB)
- Sputum culture

Management
- Long-term treatment with antimicrobial drugs (Tables 27.11 and 27.12)
- Follow-up AFB smears, cultures, and chest x-rays
- Follow-up care, addressing needs and concerns of patient and close contacts, and involving community health care workers and social workers

is much higher than the TST. Current guidelines suggest that both tests are viable options and that choice should be based on context and reasons for testing. Neither IGRAs nor TST can tell between LTBI and active TB infection. LTBI can only be diagnosed by excluding active TB.

Chest X-ray. Although the chest x-ray findings are important, it is not possible to make a diagnosis of TB solely on chest x-ray findings. The chest x-ray may appear normal in a patient with TB. Findings suggestive of TB include upper lobe infiltrates, cavitary infiltrates, lymph node involvement, and pleural and/or pericardial effusion. Other diseases, such as sarcoidosis, can mimic the appearance of TB.

Bacteriologic Studies. Culture is the gold standard for diagnosing TB. Three consecutive sputum specimens are needed, each collected at 8- to 24-hour intervals, with at least 1 early morning specimen. The initial test involves a microscopic examination of stained sputum smears for AFB. A definitive diagnosis of TB requires mycobacterial growth, which can take up to 6 weeks. Treatment is needed pending the culture results for patients in whom suspicion of TB is high. Samples for other suspected TB sites can be collected from gastric washings, cerebrospinal fluid (CSF), or fluid from an effusion or abscess.

Interprofessional Care

Most patients with TB are treated on an outpatient basis (Table 27.10). Many people can continue to work and maintain their lifestyles with few changes. Patients with sputum smear–positive TB are considered infectious for the first 2 weeks after starting treatment. Advise these patients to restrict visitors and avoid travel on public transportation and trips to public places. Teach them the importance of good hand washing and oral hygiene. Hospitalization may be needed for the severely ill or debilitated.

Drug Therapy

Active TB Disease. The mainstay of TB treatment is drug therapy (Table 27.11). Promoting and monitoring adherence are critical for treatment to be successful. Because of the growing prevalence of MDR-TB, it is important to manage the patient with active TB aggressively. Drug therapy is divided into 2 phases: initial and continuation (Table 27.12). In most circumstances the treatment regimen for patients with previously untreated TB consists of a 3-month initial phase with 4 drugs (isoniazid, rifampin, pyrazinamide, and ethambutol). If drug susceptibility test results show that the bacteria are

TABLE 27.11 Drug Therapy

Tuberculosis

Drug	Common Side Effects
aminoglycosides	Hepatitis, GI toxicity
• amikacin	Prolongation of QT interval
• capreomycin (Capastat)	Ototoxicity, nephrotoxicity
bedaquiline (Sirturo)	Hepatotoxicity, nausea
ethambutol (Myambutol)	Headache, blurred vision, ocular toxicity (decreased red-green color discrimination)
fluoroquinolones	GI problems, neurologic effects (dizziness, headache), rash
• levofloxacin	
• moxifloxacin (Avelox, Vigamox)	
isoniazid	Hepatotoxicity, asymptomatic elevation of aminotransferases (ALT, AST) Vomiting, confusion, headaches
pyrazinamide	Hepatotoxicity, arthralgias, hyperuricemia
rifabutin (Mycobutin)	Hepatotoxicity, thrombocytopenia, neutropenia Orange discoloration of bodily fluids (sputum, urine, sweat, tears) Nausea, vomiting, loss of appetite
rifampin (Rifadin)	Hepatotoxicity, thrombocytopenia, Orange discoloration of bodily fluids (sputum, urine, sweat, tears) Anorexia, nausea, abdominal discomfort
rifapentine (Priftin)	Like those of rifampin
streptomycin	Ototoxicity, neurotoxicity, nephrotoxicity

ALT, Alanine transaminase; *AST,* aspartate aminotransferase; *MDR-TB,* multidrug resistant tuberculosis.

TABLE 27.12 Drug Therapy

Tuberculosis Treatment Regimens

Initial Phase	Continuation Phase
Option 1	
4-drug regimen consisting of isoniazid, rifampin, pyrazinamide, ethambutol Given daily for 56 doses (8 wk) *OR* 5 days/wk DOT for 40 doses (8 wk)	isoniazid, rifampin daily for 126 doses (18 wk) *OR* 5 days/wk DOT for 90 doses (18 wk)
Option 2	
4-drug regimen consisting of isoniazid, rifampin, pyrazinamide, ethambutol Given daily for 56 doses (8 wk) *OR* 5 days/wk DOT for 40 doses (8 wk)	isoniazid, rifampin 3 times weekly for 54 doses (18 wk)
Option 3	
4-drug regimen consisting of isoniazid, rifampin, pyrazinamide, ethambutol Given 3 times weekly for 24 doses (8 wk)	isoniazid, rifampin 3 times weekly for 54 doses (18 wk)
Option 4	
4-drug regimen consisting of isoniazid, rifampin, ethambutol, pyrazinamide Given daily for 14 doses (2 wk) then twice weekly for 12 doses	isoniazid, rifampin twice weekly for 36 doses (18 wk)

Source: Official American Thoracic Society/CDC/Infectious Diseases Society of America: Clinical practice guidelines: Treatment of drug susceptible tuberculosis. Retrieved from *www.cdc.gov/tb/topic/treatment/tbdisease.htm.*
DOT, Directly observed therapy.

susceptible to all drugs, ethambutol may be stopped. If the patient develops a toxic reaction to the primary drugs, other drugs can be used, including rifabutin and rifapentine (Priftin). If pyrazinamide cannot be included in the initial phase (because of liver disease, pregnancy, etc.), the remaining 3 drugs are used for the initial phase.

 DRUG ALERT Isoniazid

- Alcohol may increase risk for hepatotoxicity.
- Teach patient to avoid drinking alcohol during treatment.
- Monitor for signs of hepatitis before and while taking drug.

Sensitivity testing guides the treatment for MDR-TB. MDR-TB therapy in the initial phase typically includes 5 drugs: 1 or 2 first-line agents, a fluoroquinolone, an injectable antibiotic, and 1 or more second-line agents, for at least 6 months after sputum culture is negative. This is followed by at least 4 drugs, minus the injectable antibiotic, for 18 to 24 months. Two newer drugs, bedaquiline (Sirturo) and Delamanid (Deltyba), are used in combination with other drugs to treat MDR-TB and XDR-TB.

Directly observed therapy (DOT) involves providing the antitubercular drugs directly to patients and watching as they swallow the medications. To ensure adherence, it is the preferred strategy for all patients with TB, especially for those at risk for nonadherence.[20] Nonadherence is a major factor in the emergence of MDR-TB and treatment failures. Many people do not adhere to the treatment program despite understanding the disease process and value of treatment. DOT is an expensive but essential public health measure. The risk for reactivation of TB and MDR-TB is increased in patients who do not complete the full course of therapy. In many areas, the public health nurse administers DOT at a clinic site.

When DOT is not used, fixed-dose combination drugs may enhance adherence. Combinations of isoniazid and rifampin and of isoniazid, rifampin, and pyrazinamide are available to simplify therapy. The therapy for people with HIV follows the same therapy options outlined in Table 27.12. However, alternative regimens in any HIV-infected patient that include once-weekly isoniazid plus rifapentine continuation dosing or twice-weekly isoniazid plus rifampin or rifabutin, should not be used if CD4⁺ counts are less than 100/μL.

Teaching patients about the adverse effects of these drugs and when to seek prompt medical attention is critical. The major side effect of isoniazid, rifampin, and pyrazinamide is nonviral hepatitis. Baseline liver function tests (LFTs) are done at the start of treatment and monitored closely (e.g., every 2 to 4 weeks), especially if results are abnormal.

Latent Tuberculosis Infection. In people with LTBI, drug therapy helps prevent a TB infection from developing into active TB disease. Because a person with LTBI has fewer bacteria, treatment is much easier. Usually only 1 drug is needed. Drug therapy regimens for LTBI are outlined in Table 27.13.

The standard treatment regimen for LTBI is 9 months of daily isoniazid. It is an effective and inexpensive drug that the patient can take orally. While the 9-month regimen is more effective, adherence issues may make a 6-month regimen preferable. For patients with HIV and those with fibrotic lesions on chest x-ray, isoniazid is given for 9 months. An alternative 3-month regimen of isoniazid and rifapentine may be used for otherwise healthy patients who are not presumed to be infected with MDR bacilli. Four-month therapy with rifampin may be indicated if the patient is resistant to isoniazid. Because of severe liver injury

and deaths, the CDC does not recommend the combination of rifampin and pyrazinamide for treatment of LTBI.

Bacille Calmette-Guérin Vaccine. Bacille Calmette-Guérin (BCG) vaccine is a live, attenuated strain of *Mycobacterium*

TABLE 27.13 Drug Therapy
Latent Tuberculosis Infection Regimens

Drugs	Duration (mo)	Interval	Minimum Doses
isoniazid	9	Daily	270
		Twice weekly*	76
isoniazid	6	Daily	180
		Twice weekly*	52
isoniazid and rifapentine	3	Once weekly*	12
rifampin	4	Daily	120

Source: Centers for Disease Control and Prevention: Treatment regimens for latent TB infection, 2017. Retrieved from *www.cdc.gov/tb/topic/treatment/ltbi.htm.*

*Use directly observed therapy (DOT).

bovis. The vaccine is given to infants in parts of the world with a high prevalence of TB. In the United States, it is typically not used because of the low risk for infection, the vaccine's variable effectiveness against adult pulmonary TB, and potential interference with TB skin test reactivity. The BCG vaccination can result in a false-positive TST. IGRA results are not affected. The BCG vaccine should be considered only for select persons who meet specific criteria (e.g., health care workers who are continually exposed to patients with MDR-TB and when infection control precautions are not successful).

❖ NURSING MANAGEMENT: TUBERCULOSIS

◆ Nursing Assessment

Ask the patient about a previous history of TB, chronic illness, or any immunosuppressive disease or medications. Obtain a social and occupational history to determine risk factors for transmission of TB. Assess the patient for productive cough, night sweats, fever, weight loss, pleuritic chest pain, and abnormal lung sounds. If the patient has a productive cough, early morning is the ideal time to collect sputum specimens for an AFB smear.

◆ Nursing Diagnoses

Nursing diagnoses for the patient with TB may include:
- Impaired breathing
- Impaired airway clearance
- Risk for infection
- Lack of knowledge

◆ Planning

The overall goals are that the patient with TB will (1) have normal pulmonary function, (2) adhere to the therapeutic regimen, (3) take appropriate measures to prevent the spread of the disease, and (4) have no recurrence of disease.

◆ Nursing Implementation

Health Promotion. The ultimate goal is to eradicate TB worldwide. Screening programs in known risk groups are of value in detecting persons with TB. Treatment of LTBI reduces the number of TB carriers in the community. The person with a positive TST should have a chest x-ray to assess for active TB disease. People with a diagnosis of TB must be reported to the public health authorities for identification and assessment of contacts and risk to the community.

Programs to address the social determinants of TB are needed to decrease transmission of TB. Reducing HIV infection, poverty, overcrowded living conditions, malnutrition, smoking, and drug and alcohol use can help minimize TB infection rates. Improving access to health care and education is important.

◆ Acute Care.
Patients admitted to the ED or directly to the nursing unit with respiratory symptoms should always be assessed for the possibility of TB. Those strongly suspected of having TB should (1) be placed on airborne isolation; (2) receive a medical workup, including chest x-ray, sputum smear, and culture; and (3) receive appropriate drug therapy. Airborne infection isolation is needed for the patient with pulmonary or laryngeal TB until the patient is not infectious. *Airborne infection isolation* refers to isolation of patients infected with organisms spread by the airborne route. Patients are in a single-occupancy room with negative pressure and airflow of 6 to 12 exchanges per hour.

High-efficiency particulate air (HEPA) masks are worn whenever entering the patient's room. These masks are highly effective at protecting from small droplets 5 μm or less in diameter. Several types of HEPA masks are currently available. To ensure proper mask size, health care professionals should be "fit tested" with significant changes in weight gain or loss, with any facial and/or dental changes (e.g., Botox injections), and each time there is a new brand or model of mask. Otherwise, yearly mask "fit testing" is acceptable. To be effective, the mask must be molded to fit tightly around the nose and mouth.

Teach patients to cover the nose and mouth with paper tissues every time they cough, sneeze, or produce sputum. The tissues should be thrown into a paper bag and disposed of with the trash or flushed down the toilet. Emphasize careful hand washing after handling sputum and soiled tissues. If patients need to be out of the negative-pressure room, they must wear a standard isolation mask to prevent exposure to others. Minimize prolonged visitation to other parts of the hospital.

Identify and screen close contacts of the person with TB. Anyone testing positive for TB infection will need further evaluation and treatment for either LTBI or active TB disease.

◆ Ambulatory Care.
Patients who respond clinically are discharged home (even with positive cultures) if their household contacts have already been exposed and the patient is not posing a risk to others. A sputum specimen for AFB smear and culture should be obtained at a minimum of monthly intervals until 2 consecutive specimens are negative on culture. More frequent AFB smears may be useful to assess the early response to treatment and provide an indication of infectiousness. Negative cultures are needed to declare the patient not infectious.

Teach the patient how to minimize exposure to close contacts and household members. Homes should be well ventilated, especially the areas where the infected person spends a lot of time. While still infectious, the patient should sleep alone, spend as much time as possible outdoors, and minimize time in congregate settings or on public transportation.

It is important to teach the patient and caregiver about adherence with the prescribed regimen. Most treatment failures occur because the patient does not take the drug, stops taking it too soon, or takes it irregularly. Strategies to improve adherence include teaching and counseling, reminder systems, incentives or rewards, contracts, and DOT.

Notifying the public health department is required. The public health nurse is responsible for follow-up on household contacts and assessment of the patient for adherence. If adherence is an issue, the public health agency may be responsible for DOT. Most patients can be considered adequately treated when the therapy regimen has been completed and there is evidence of negative cultures, overall improvement in patient condition, and improvement on chest x-ray.

Because about 5% of patients have relapses, teach the patient to recognize the symptoms that occur with recurrent TB. If these symptoms occur, the patient should seek immediate medical attention. Teach the patient about factors that could reactivate TB, such as immunosuppressive therapy, cancer, and prolonged debilitating illness. If the patient has any of these events, the HCP must be told so that TB can be closely monitored for reactivation. In some situations, it is necessary to put the patient on anti-TB therapy. Because smoking is associated with poor outcomes in TB, patients should be encouraged to quit. Provide patients with teaching and resources to help them stop smoking.

Adherence to Tuberculosis Treatment Program

You are a nurse working in an outpatient health clinic with C.J., a 42-yr-old man diagnosed 2 months ago with active TB. He is on DOT. You notice C.J. has started to miss or has been late for his clinic appointments. He tells you it is hard to make his appointments as a new job requires long work hours. He asks if he needs to continue with his visits to get his drugs. He says he is "feeling better" and will take the drugs on his own.

Making Clinical Decisions

Best Available Evidence. Guidelines for effective case management of patients with TB include patient education, field/home visits, patient reminders, and incentives. TB clinic attendance and treatment completion rates are higher when patients take part in DOT compared to self-administered therapy. When appointments are missed, phone calls, Web-based videos, or home visits will engage patients, resulting in improved clinic attendance and treatment completion.

Clinician Expertise. You know that patient-centered care includes being responsive to patients' changing needs. You know that patients may stop attending clinics and taking their drugs when feeling well again. This can lead to treatment failure, the need to restart therapy, and multidrug resistance.

Patient Preferences and Values. C.J. tells you he has a busy job and does not always remember his appointment dates. He would like to self-administer his drugs.

Implications for Nursing Practice

1. What information would you give C.J. about the importance of DOT?
2. Your clinic has interest in starting a reminder system for clinic appointments. What strategy would you recommend?
3. How will you know if C.J. is adhering to the prescribed drug treatment program?

References for Evidence

1. Centers for Disease Control and Prevention: Tuberculosis: General considerations for treatment of TB disease. Retrieved from *www.cdc.gov/tb/publications/factsheets/treatment/treatmenthivnegative.pdf*.
2. Nahid P, Dorman SE, Alipanah N: Official American Thoracic Society/CDC/Infectious Diseases Society of America clinical practice guidelines: Treatment of drug-susceptible tuberculosis, *Clin Infect Dis* 63:e147, 2016.

◆ **Evaluation**

The expected outcomes are that the patient with TB will have:
- Resolution of the disease
- Normal pulmonary function
- Absence of any complications
- No further transmission of TB

ATYPICAL MYCOBACTERIA

There are more than 30 varieties of acid-fast mycobacteria that do not cause TB but cause pulmonary disease, lymphadenitis, skin or soft tissue disease, or disseminated disease. Atypical mycobacteria are not airborne or transmitted by droplets. They can be found in tap water, soil, bird feces, and house dust.

Pulmonary symptoms include cough, shortness of breath, weight loss, fatigue, and blood-tinged sputum. People who are immunosuppressed (e.g., HIV/AIDS) or have chronic pulmonary disease are most susceptible. We cannot distinguish this type of pulmonary disease from TB clinically and radiologically. A culture is required. Treatment is similar to that for TB.

PULMONARY FUNGAL INFECTIONS

Pulmonary fungal pneumonia is an infectious process in the lungs caused by endemic (native and common) or opportunistic fungi (Table 27.14). *Endemic* fungal pathogens cause infection in healthy people and in immunocompromised people in certain geographic locations in the United States. For example, *Coccidioides*, which causes coccidioidomycosis, is a fungus found in the soil of dry, low-rainfall areas.[21] It is endemic in many areas of the southwestern United States. *Opportunistic* fungal infections occur in immunocompromised patients (e.g., those receiving chemotherapy, immunosuppressive drugs) and in patients with HIV and cystic fibrosis. These pulmonary fungal infections can be life-threatening.

Pulmonary fungal infections are acquired by inhaling spores. They are not transmitted from person to person. The patient does not have to be placed in isolation. The manifestations are like those of bacterial pneumonia. Skin testing, serology, and biopsy methods aid in identifying the infecting organism.

The choice of antifungal agent is made based on the pathogen identified on culture or most likely suspected. Amphotericin B is the standard therapy for treating serious systemic fungal infections. It must be given IV to achieve adequate blood and tissue levels because the GI tract does not absorb it well. Less serious infections can be treated with oral antifungals, such as ketoconazole, fluconazole (Diflucan), voriconazole (Vfend), and itraconazole (Sporanox). Effectiveness of therapy can be monitored with fungal serology titers.

LUNG ABSCESS

Etiology and Pathophysiology

A **lung abscess** is necrosis of lung tissue. It typically results from bacteria aspirated from the oral cavity in patients with periodontal disease. They can also result from IV drug use, cancer, pulmonary emboli, TB, and various parasitic and fungal diseases. The abscess usually develops slowly, beginning with an enlarging area of infection that becomes necrotic and eventually forms a cavity filled with purulent material. Abscesses usually contain more than 1 type of microbe, most often reflecting the anaerobic flora of the mouth.

The area of the lung most often affected due to aspiration is the posterior segment of the upper lobes. The abscess may erode into the bronchial system, causing the production of foul-smelling or sour-tasting sputum. It may grow toward the pleura and cause pleuritic pain. Multiple small abscesses, sometimes referred to as *necrotizing pneumonia,* can occur within the lung.

TABLE 27.14 **Fungal Infections of the Lung**	
Infection	**Organism**
Endemic Fungal Infections	
Blastomycosis	*Blastomyces dermatitidis*
Coccidioidomycosis	*Coccidioides immitis*
Histoplasmosis	*Histoplasma capsulatum*
Opportunistic Fungal Infections	
Aspergillosis	*Aspergillus niger, Aspergillus fumigatus*
Candidiasis	*Candida albicans*
Cryptococcosis	*Cryptococcus neoformans*

Clinical Manifestations and Complications

Manifestations usually occur slowly over a period of weeks to months, especially if anaerobic organisms are the cause. Symptoms of abscess caused by aerobic bacteria develop more acutely and resemble bacterial pneumonia. The most common is cough-producing purulent sputum (often dark brown) that is foul smelling and foul tasting. Hemoptysis is common, especially when an abscess ruptures into a bronchus. Other manifestations include fever, chills, prostration, night sweats, pleuritic pain, dyspnea, anorexia, and weight loss.

Lung assessment reveals dullness to percussion and decreased breath sounds on auscultation over the involved segment of lung. Bronchial breath sounds may be transmitted to the periphery if the communicating bronchus becomes patent and the segment begins to drain. Crackles may be present in the later stages as the abscess drains.

The infection can spread through the bloodstream and cause several possible complications. Pulmonary abscess, bronchopleural fistula, bronchiectasis, and empyema from perforation of the abscess into the pleural cavity can occur.[22]

Diagnostic Studies

A chest x-ray is often the only test needed to diagnose a lung abscess. The presence of a single cavitary lesion with an air-fluid level and local infiltrate confirms the diagnosis. CT scanning may be helpful if the cavitation is not clear on chest x-ray. If there is drainage via the bronchus, sputum will contain the microorganisms that are present in the abscess. However, expectorated sputum samples are contaminated with oral flora, making it hard to determine the responsible organism(s).

Bronchoscopy may be used to (1) avoid oropharyngeal contamination, (2) collect a specimen if drainage is delayed, or (3) investigate for an underlying cancer. Pleural fluid and blood cultures may be useful to identify the offending organisms. Although nonspecific, an elevated neutrophil count from a complete blood count (CBC) may indicate an infectious process. Necrotic pulmonary lesions also can be caused by lung infarction, pulmonary embolism, and sarcoidosis.

❖ Interprofessional and Nursing Care

Monitor the patient's vital signs, level of consciousness, and respiratory status for any signs of hypoxemia. Note any signs and symptoms of respiratory distress. Apply O_2 as needed. IV antibiotic therapy should be started as soon as possible. Clindamycin is first-line therapy for its effectiveness against *Staphylococcus* and anaerobic organisms. Parenteral antibiotics are switched to oral antibiotics once the patient shows clinical and chest x-ray signs of improvement.

Because of the need for prolonged antibiotic therapy, the patient must be aware of the importance of continuing the medication for the prescribed period. To avoid the risk for a secondary or worsening infection, all antibiotics should be taken as directed for the entire prescribed period. Sometimes the patient is asked to return periodically during the course of antibiotic therapy for repeat cultures and sensitivity tests to ensure that the infecting organism is not becoming resistant to the antibiotic. When antibiotic therapy is complete, the patient is reevaluated.

Teach the patient how to cough effectively (see Table 28.21). Chest physiotherapy and postural drainage are not recommended because they may promote movement of microorganisms into other bronchi, extending infection. Rest, optimal nutrition, and adequate fluid intake are supportive measures to promote recovery. If dentition is poor and dental hygiene is not adequate, encourage the patient to obtain dental care. Collaborate with the social worker to evaluate available options for dental care if the patient has limited resources.

If the patient does not adequately respond to antibiotic treatment, percutaneous drainage of the abscess may be done. A small catheter, guided by CT or ultrasound, may be placed to drain the abscess. Surgery is sometimes done when reinfection of a large cavitary lesion occurs, when an empyema develops, or to establish a diagnosis when there is evidence of an underlying problem, such as cancer. The usual procedure in such cases is a lobectomy. A pneumonectomy may be needed for multiple abscesses.

ENVIRONMENTAL LUNG DISEASES

Environmental or occupational lung diseases result from inhaled dust or chemicals. The extent of lung damage is influenced by the toxicity of the inhaled substance, amount and duration of exposure, and individual susceptibility. Environmentally induced lung disease includes pneumoconiosis, chemical pneumonitis, and hypersensitivity pneumonitis.

Pneumoconiosis is a general term for a group of lung diseases caused by inhalation and retention of mineral or metal dust particles. The literal meaning of *pneumoconiosis* is "dust in the lungs." We classify these diseases according to the origin of the dust (e.g., silicosis, asbestosis, berylliosis). For example, silicosis occurs from inhaling silica from sand and rock. Coal worker's pneumoconiosis (CWP), also known as *black lung,* is caused by inhaling large amounts of coal dust. It is an occupational hazard for underground coal miners. The inhaled substance is ingested by macrophages, which releases substances that cause cell injury and death. Fibrosis occurs from tissue repair after inflammation. Breathing problems become evident after many years of repeated exposure, resulting in diffuse *pulmonary fibrosis* (excess connective tissue).

Asbestos is a group of minerals composed of microscopic fibers. For many years, asbestos was used for insulation and to help fireproof buildings. When disturbed, asbestos releases tiny filament particles into the air. Once inhaled, the tiny fibers become deposited within the lung. Asbestosis is chronic inflammation of the lung, and people with repeated exposure are at a greater risk for disease. Lung cancer, either squamous cell carcinoma or adenocarcinoma, is the most frequent cancer associated with asbestos exposure. There is a lapse of at least 15 to 19 years between first exposure and development of lung cancer. Mesothelioma, both pleural and peritoneal, is associated with asbestos exposure.

Chemical pneumonitis results from exposures to toxic chemical fumes. There are 2 types of chemical pneumonitis: acute and chronic. Acutely, there is diffuse lung injury characterized by pulmonary edema. Chronically, the clinical picture is that of *bronchiolitis obliterans* (obstruction of the bronchioles due to inflammation and fibrosis). It is usually associated with a normal chest x-ray or one that shows hyperinflation.

Hypersensitivity pneumonitis, or extrinsic allergic alveolitis, is a form of parenchymal lung disease seen when a person inhales antigens to which they are allergic. There are acute, subacute, and chronic forms. Examples include bird fancier's lung (exposure to particles in feathers and droppings of birds), and farmer's lung (inhalation of hay dust particles).

Clinical Manifestations

Symptoms of many environmental lung diseases may not occur until at least 10 to 15 years after the initial exposure to the inhaled irritant. Manifestations common to all pneumoconioses include dyspnea, cough, wheezing, and weight loss. Pulmonary function studies often show reduced vital capacity. A chest x-ray often reveals lung involvement specific to the primary problem. CT scans have been useful in detecting early lung involvement.

Cor pulmonale, a condition in which the right side of the heart fails, is a late complication, especially in conditions characterized by diffuse pulmonary fibrosis. COPD is the most common complication of environmental lung disease. Other associated disorders include acute pulmonary edema, lung cancer, mesothelioma, and TB. Appearance of these symptoms and complications are often the reason the patient seeks health care.

❖ Interprofessional and Nursing Care

The best approach to managing environmental lung diseases is to prevent or decrease environmental and occupational exposure. Teach those at risk about the use of appropriate personal protective equipment. Wearing masks and using well-designed, effective ventilation systems are appropriate for some occupations and household activities. Inhalation of smoke by nonsmokers has led to regulations requiring a smoke-free workplace. Periodic inspections and monitoring of workplaces by agencies such as the Occupational Safety and Health Administration (OSHA) and the National Institute for Occupational Safety and Health (NIOSH) reinforce employers' obligations to provide a safe work environment. NIOSH is responsible for workplace safety and health regulations in the United States.

Encourage regular medical check-ups. Early diagnosis is essential to halting the disease process. Strategies are directed toward preventing disease progression and monitoring, improving or controlling respiratory symptoms. They depend on the cause and severity of the condition. Strategies may include O_2 therapy, IV fluid, inhaled bronchodilators, corticosteroids, nonsteroidal antiinflammatory drugs (NSAIDs), intubation and mechanical ventilation, percussion therapy, and pulmonary rehabilitation. Patients should be immunized against pneumococcal pneumonia and influenza. Discontinuing exposure to the offending inhalant and smoking cessation may or may not be effective in stopping disease progression.

LUNG CANCER

Lung cancer is the leading cause of cancer-related deaths in the United States.[23] Lung cancer accounts for 26% of all cancer deaths, more than those caused by breast and colon cancer combined. In 2019, it is estimated that 234,000 new cases of lung cancer will be diagnosed, and 154,000 Americans will die. Although lung cancer is associated with a high mortality and low cure rate, advances in medical treatment are improving the response to treatment.

Etiology

Smoking causes 80% to 90% of all lung cancers.[24] There is no safe form of tobacco or tobacco product. Smokeless tobacco, pipes and cigars, hookah and waterpipe, bidis, and kreteks all pose significant risk for lung cancer to those who use them.[25]

Tobacco smoke contains over 7000 chemicals, of which 250 are harmful. Of the harmful substances in tobacco smoke, 69 interfere with normal cell development and are linked to lung cancer. Exposure to tobacco smoke causes changes in the bronchial epithelium, which usually returns to normal with smoking cessation. The risk for lung cancer gradually decreases with smoking cessation, reaching that of nonsmokers within 10 to 15 years of quitting.

The risk for developing lung cancer is directly related to total exposure to tobacco smoke. This is measured by total number of cigarettes smoked in a lifetime, age of smoking onset, depth of inhalation, tar and nicotine content, and the use of unfiltered cigarettes. Both smokers and nonsmokers can develop lung cancer. Sidestream smoke (smoke from burning cigarettes, cigars) has the same carcinogens found in mainstream smoke (smoke inhaled and exhaled by the smoker). This exposure to secondhand smoke creates a health risk for nonsmoking adults and children.

Other common causes of lung cancer include high levels of pollution, radiation (especially radon exposure), and asbestos. Heavy or prolonged exposure to industrial agents, such as ionizing radiation, coal dust, nickel, uranium, chromium, formaldehyde, and arsenic, can increase the risk for lung cancer, especially in smokers.[26]

Marked variations exist in a person's tendency to develop lung cancer. Differences in lung cancer incidence, risk factors, and survival exist between men and women (see Gender Differences box). Genetic, hormonal, and molecular influences may contribute to these differences.

GENDER DIFFERENCES

Lung Cancer

Men
- Have a 1 in 15 chance of developing lung cancer (smokers and nonsmokers)
- Diagnosed with lung cancer more than women
- Die from lung cancer more than women
- Male smokers are 10 times more likely to develop lung cancer than nonsmokers
- Lung cancer incidence and deaths are decreasing in men

Women
- Have a 1 in 17 chance of developing lung cancer (smokers and nonsmokers)
- Lung cancer incidence and deaths are increasing in women
- Develop lung cancer after fewer years of smoking than men
- Develop lung cancer at a younger age than men
- Nonsmoking women are at greater risk for developing lung cancer than nonsmoking men
- Women with lung cancer live, on the average, 12 months longer than men.

Pathophysiology

Most primary lung tumors are believed to arise from mutated epithelial cells. The growth of mutations, which are caused by carcinogens, is influenced by various genetic factors. Once underway, tumor development is promoted by epidermal growth factor. These cells grow slowly, taking 8 to 10 years for a tumor to reach 1 cm in size, the smallest lesion detectable on x-ray. Lung cancers occur primarily in the segmental bronchi or beyond and usually occur in the upper lobes of the lungs (Fig. 27.4).

Primary lung cancers are categorized into 2 broad subtypes (Table 27.15): non–small cell lung cancer (NSCLC) (85%) and small cell lung cancer (SCLC) (15%).[27] Lung cancers metastasize primarily by direct extension and through the blood and lymph system. The common sites for metastasis are the lymph nodes, liver, brain, bones, and adrenal glands.

Paraneoplastic Syndrome. Lung cancers can cause *paraneoplastic syndrome*. Paraneoplastic syndrome may be caused by hormones, cytokines, enzymes (secreted by tumor cells) or antibodies (made by the body in response to the tumor) that destroy healthy cells. Sometimes the symptoms of paraneoplastic syndrome manifest even before the cancer is diagnosed.

Examples of paraneoplastic syndrome include hypercalcemia, syndrome of inappropriate antidiuretic hormone secretion (SIADH), adrenal hypersecretion, polycythemia, and Cushing syndrome. SCLCs are most often associated with paraneoplastic syndrome. These conditions may stabilize with treatment of the underlying cancer. SIADH, adrenal hypersecretion, and Cushing syndrome are discussed in Chapter 49.

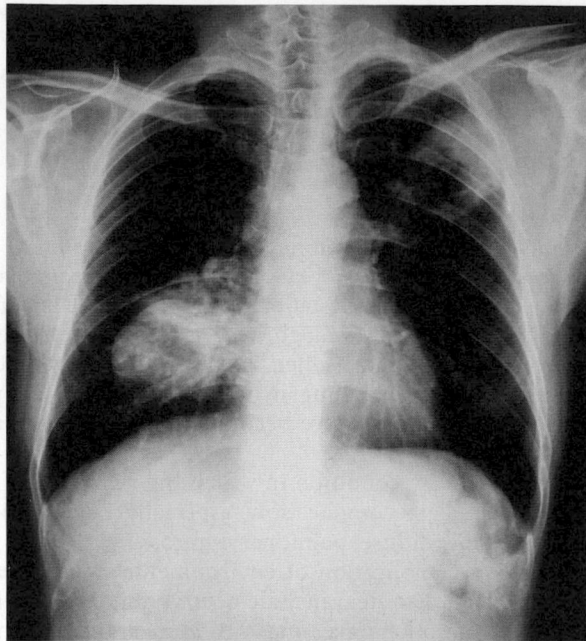

FIG. 27.4 Lung cancer lesion. (© iStock.com/Sutthaburawonk.)

Clinical Manifestations

The manifestations of lung cancer are usually nonspecific and appear late in the disease process. Symptoms may be masked by a chronic cough attributed to smoking or smoking-related lung disease. Manifestations depend on the type of primary lung cancer, its location, and extent of metastatic spread. Lung cancer often presents as a lobar pneumonia that does not respond to treatment.

The most common symptom and often the one that is reported first is a persistent cough. The patient may report dyspnea or wheezing. Blood-tinged sputum may be present because of bleeding caused by the cancer. Chest pain, if present, may be localized or unilateral, ranging from mild to severe.

Later manifestations include nonspecific systemic symptoms, such as anorexia, nausea and vomiting, fatigue, and weight loss. Hoarseness may be present due to laryngeal nerve involvement. Dysphagia, unilateral paralysis of the diaphragm, and superior vena cava obstruction may occur because of intrathoracic spread of the cancer. Lymph nodes are often palpable in the neck or axillae. Mediastinal involvement may lead to pericardial effusion, cardiac tamponade, and dysrhythmias.

Diagnostic Studies

A chest x-ray is the first diagnostic test done for patients with suspected lung cancer. The x-ray may be normal or identify a lung mass or infiltrate (Fig. 27.4). Evidence of metastasis to the ribs or vertebrae and a pleural effusion may be seen on chest x-ray. CT scanning is used to further evaluate the lung mass. CT scans can identify the location and extent of masses in the chest, any mediastinal involvement, and lymph node enlargement.

Sputum cytologic studies can identify cancer cells, but sputum samples are rarely used in diagnosing lung cancer because cancer cells are not always present in the sputum. A definitive diagnosis requires a biopsy. Cells for biopsy can be obtained by CT-guided needle aspiration, bronchoscopy, mediastinoscopy, or video-assisted thoracoscopic surgery (VATS). If a

TABLE 27.15 Types of Primary Lung Cancer

Type	Growth Rate	Characteristics	Response to Therapy
Non–Small Cell Lung Cancer (NSCLC)			
Adenocarcinoma	Moderate	• Accounts for 40% of lung cancers • Most common lung cancer in United States • Most common cancer in people who have not smoked • Found in peripheral areas of lung • Often has no manifestations until widespread metastasis is present	• Surgical resection may be tried depending on staging • Does not respond well to chemotherapy
Large cell (undifferentiated) cancer	Rapid	• Accounts for 10% of lung cancers • Composed of large cells that are anaplastic • Often arise in bronchi • Is highly metastatic via lymphatics and blood	• Surgery is not usually done because of high rate of metastases • Tumor may be radiosensitive but often recurs
Squamous cell cancer	Slow	• Accounts for 25%–30% of lung cancers • Centrally located • Causes early symptoms of nonproductive cough and hemoptysis • Does not have a strong tendency to metastasize	• Surgical resection may be tried • Adjuvant chemotherapy and radiation • Depending on the staging, life expectancy is better than for SCLC
Small Cell Lung Cancer (SCLC)			
Small cell cancer	Very rapid	• Accounts for about 10%–15% of lung cancers • Very aggressive form of lung cancer • Spreads early via lymphatics and bloodstream • Frequent metastasis to brain • Associated with endocrine problems	• Chemotherapy mainstay of treatment; more responsive to chemotherapy than NSCLC • Radiation used as adjuvant therapy and palliative measure • Overall poor prognosis

TABLE 27.16 Interprofessional Care

Lung Cancer

Diagnostic Assessment
- History and physical examination
- Chest x-ray
- Bronchoscopy
- Cytologic study of bronchial washings or pleural space fluid
- Transbronchial or percutaneous fine-needle aspiration
- CT scan, MRI, PET
- Mediastinoscopy
- Video-assisted thoracoscopic surgery (VATS)

Management
- Surgery (segmental or wedge resection, lobectomy, pneumonectomy)
- Radiation therapy
- Chemotherapy
- Targeted therapy and immunotherapy
- Prophylactic cranial radiation
- Bronchoscopic laser therapy
- Photodynamic therapy
- Airway stenting
- Radiofrequency ablation

TABLE 27.17 Staging of Non–Small Cell Lung Cancer

Stages		Characteristics
0		Cells found in respiratory airway, alveoli
I		Tumor is small and localized to lung. No lymph node involvement
	A	Tumor <3 cm
	B	Tumor 3–4 cm and invading main airway, visceral pleura.
II		Increased tumor size, some lymph node involvement
	A	Tumor 4–5 cm with invasion of main airway, visceral pleura, lymph nodes on same side of chest
	B	Tumor 5–7 cm involving the bronchus and lymph nodes on same side of chest OR Tumor 5–7 cm with visceral and parietal pleura, diaphragm, phrenic nerve involvement
III		Increased spread of tumor
	A	Tumor ≤5 cm or smaller spread to the nearby structures (chest wall, pleura, pericardium) and regional lymph nodes
	B	Extensive tumor >5 cm involving heart, trachea, esophagus, mediastinum, malignant pleural effusion, contralateral lymph nodes, scalene or supraclavicular lymph nodes
	C	Tumor >5 cm and more than one tumor in a different lobe of the lung
IV		Distant metastasis

thoracentesis is done to relieve a pleural effusion, the fluid is analyzed for cancer cells.

Accurate assessment of lung cancer is critical for staging and determining appropriate treatment. Bone scans and CT scans of the brain, pelvis, and abdomen are used to determine if metastatic disease is present. A complete history and physical examination, CBC with differential, chemistry panel, liver function tests, and renal function tests are ordered. In some situations, pulmonary function tests will be done. MRI and/or positron emission tomography (PET) may be used to evaluate and stage lung cancer. Table 27.16 outlines the diagnostic assessment of lung cancer.

Staging. Staging of NSCLC is done using the TNM staging system (see Table 15.5). Under the TNM system, cancer is grouped into 4 stages with A or B subtypes. A simplified version of staging of NSCLC is shown in Table 27.17. Patients with stages I, II, and IIIA disease may be surgical candidates. However, stage IIIB or IV disease is usually inoperable and has a poor prognosis.

Staging of SCLC by TNM has not been useful because this cancer is aggressive and is always considered systemic. The stages of SCLC are *limited* and *extensive*. *Limited* means that the tumor is only on 1 side of the chest and regional lymph nodes. *Extensive* SCLC means that the cancer extends beyond the limited stage. Most patients with SCLC have extensive disease at time of diagnosis.

Screening for Lung Cancer. The American College of Chest Physicians recommends screening for high-risk patients.[28] Adults ages 55 to 77 with a history of smoking (30 pack-year smoking history or currently smoke) or who quit smoking but less than 15 years ago should have annual screening for lung cancer. Screening is done using low-dose CT. Several other groups have endorsed these guidelines, including the American Cancer Society.[29]

Interprofessional Care

Surgical Therapy. Surgical resection is the treatment of choice in NSCLC stages I to IIIA without mediastinal involvement. Resection gives the best chance for a cure. Factors that affect survival include the size of the primary tumor and preexisting co-morbidities. For other NSCLC stages, patients may have surgery in conjunction with radiation therapy, chemotherapy, and targeted therapy. Many NSCLCs are not resectable at the time of diagnosis.

Surgical procedures include segmental or wedge resection procedures, lobectomy (removal of 1 or more lobes of the lung), or pneumonectomy (removal of 1 entire lung). VATS may be used to treat lung cancers near the outside of the lung. Surgery is generally not done for SCLC because of its rapid growth and dissemination at the time of diagnosis.

When the tumor is considered operable, the patient's cardiopulmonary status must be evaluated to determine the ability to have surgery. Pulmonary function studies, ABGs, and anesthesia and critical care consults are often done before surgery to assess the patient's cardiopulmonary status.

Radiation Therapy. Radiation therapy may be used as treatment for both NSCLC and SCLC. Radiation therapy may be given as curative therapy, palliative therapy (to relieve symptoms), or adjuvant therapy in combination with surgery, chemotherapy, or targeted therapy.

Radiation therapy may be used as primary therapy in the person who is unable to tolerate surgical resection because of co-morbidities. Radiation therapy relieves symptoms of dyspnea and hemoptysis from bronchial obstructive tumors and treats superior vena cava syndrome. It can treat pain from metastatic bone lesions or brain metastasis. Radiation before surgery can reduce the tumor mass before surgical resection. Complications of radiation therapy include esophagitis, skin irritation, nausea and vomiting, anorexia, and radiation pneumonitis (see Chapter 15).

Stereotactic body radiotherapy (SBRT), also called *stereotactic radiosurgery (SRS)*, is a newer lung cancer treatment. It is a type of radiation therapy that uses high doses of radiation delivered to tumors outside the CNS. SBRT uses special positioning procedures and radiology techniques to deliver a higher dose of radiation to the tumor and expose only a small part of healthy lung. It does not destroy the tumor, but damages tumor DNA. Therapy is given over 1 to 3 days. SBRT provides an option for patients with early-stage lung cancers who are not surgical candidates for other medical reasons.

Chemotherapy. Chemotherapy is the main treatment for SCLC. In NSCLC, chemotherapy may be used in the treatment of nonresectable tumors or as adjuvant therapy to surgery. We use a variety of chemotherapy drugs and multidrug protocols. Chemotherapy for lung cancer typically consists of combinations of 2 of the following drugs: etoposide (VP-16), carboplatin, cisplatin, paclitaxel (Taxol), vinorelbine (Navelbine), docetaxel (Taxotere), gemcitabine (Gemzar), and pemetrexed (Alimta).

Targeted Therapy. Targeted therapy uses drugs that block the growth of molecules involved in specific aspects of tumor growth (see Chapter 15). Because this type of therapy inhibits growth rather than directly killing cancer cells, targeted therapy may be less toxic than chemotherapy. One type of targeted therapy for patients with NSCLC inhibits tyrosine kinase, an enzyme associated with speeding up molecular reactions. Tyrosine kinase inhibitors, which block signals for growth in the cancer cells, include cetuximab (Erbitux), erlotinib (Tarceva), afatinib (Gilotrif), gefitinib (Iressa), osimertinib (Tagrisso), and necitumumab (Portrazza).

Another type of kinase inhibitor is used to treat patients with NSCLC who have an abnormal anaplastic lymphoma kinase *(ALK)* gene. Drugs in this class include crizotinib (Xalkori), brigatinib (Alunbrig), and ceritinib (Zykadia). These drugs directly inhibit the kinase protein made by the *ALK* gene that is responsible for cancer development and growth.

Another type of targeted therapy used to treat lung cancer inhibits the growth of new blood vessels (angiogenesis) by targeting vascular endothelial growth factor. Bevacizumab (Avastin) is an angiogenesis inhibitor.

Immunotherapy. Nivolumab (Opdivo), atezolizumab (Tecentriq), and pembrolizumab (Keytruda) are drugs that target PD-1, a protein on T cells that normally helps keep these cells from attacking other cells in the body. By blocking PD-1, these drugs boost the immune response against cancer cells. This can shrink some tumors or slow their growth. Nivolumab and pembrolizumab can be used in people with metastatic NSCLC whose cancer has progressed after other treatments and with tumors that express PD-1.

Other Therapies

Prophylactic Cranial Irradiation. Patients with SCLC have early metastases, especially to the CNS. Most chemotherapy does not penetrate the blood-brain barrier. As a result, after successful systemic treatment, the patient is at risk for brain metastases. Prophylactic radiation can decrease the incidence of brain metastases and may improve survival rates in patients with limited SCLC.[30]

Bronchoscopic Laser Therapy. Bronchoscopic laser therapy makes it possible to remove obstructing bronchial lesions. The laser's thermal energy is transmitted to the target tissue. It is a safe and effective treatment of endobronchial obstructions from tumors. Symptoms of airway obstruction are relieved due to thermal necrosis and shrinkage of the tumor. The procedure may be repeated as needed.

Photodynamic Therapy. Photodynamic therapy (PDT) is a form of treatment for early-stage lung cancers that uses a combination of a drug and a specific type of light. Cancer cells are killed when the drug, known as a photosynthesizer, is exposed to a specific wavelength of light. Porfimer (Photofrin) is the most used photosynthesizer. After an IV injection, it selectively concentrates in tumor cells in the esophagus and outer layers of the airways. After a set time (usually 48 hours), the tumor is exposed to laser light via bronchoscopy, activating the drug and causing cell death. Necrotic tissue is removed with bronchoscopy a few days later. This process can be repeated as needed. PDT can affect nutrient delivery to cancer cells and stimulate the immune system to attack the cancer cells.

Airway Stenting. Stents are used alone or in combination with other techniques for relief of dyspnea, cough, or respiratory insufficiency. The stent is inserted during a bronchoscopy. The advantage of an airway stent is that it supports the airway wall against collapse or external compression and can delay extension of tumor into the airway lumen. At this time, we do not know which patients will benefit most from airway stents.

Radiofrequency Ablation. Radiofrequency ablation therapy is used to treat small NSCLC lung tumors that are near the outer edge of the lungs. This therapy is an alternative to surgery in patients who cannot or elect not to have surgery. A thin, needle-like probe is inserted through the skin into the tumor. CT scans are used to guide placement. An electric current is then passed through the probe, which heats and destroys tumor cells. Local anesthesia is used for this outpatient procedure.

❖ NURSING MANAGEMENT: LUNG CANCER

◆ Nursing Assessment

It is important to determine the patient and caregiver's understanding of the current medical condition, diagnostic tests (those completed as well as those planned), diagnosis or potential diagnosis, treatment options, and prognosis. Assess the patient's level of anxiety and support provided by the patient's significant others. Subjective and objective data that should be obtained from a patient with lung cancer are described in Table 27.18.

◆ Nursing Diagnoses

Nursing diagnoses for the patient with lung cancer may include:
- Impaired airway clearance
- Impaired breathing
- Impaired gas exchange
- Anxiety

◆ Planning

The overall goals are that the patient with lung cancer will have (1) adequate airway clearance, (2) effective breathing patterns, (3) adequate oxygenation of tissues, (4) minimal to no discomfort, and (5) a realistic outlook about treatment and prognosis.

◆ Nursing Implementation

◆ Health Promotion.
The best way to halt the epidemic of lung cancer is to prevent people from smoking, help smokers stop smoking, and decrease exposure to environmental pollutants. Because most smokers start in the teenage years, prevention of teen smoking has the most significant role in reducing the incidence of lung cancer. A wealth of material is available to the smoker who is interested in smoking cessation. (See Chapter 10.)

Modeling healthy behavior by not smoking, promoting smoking cessation programs, and actively supporting education and policy changes related to smoking are important nursing activities. Many changes have occurred because of the

---

TABLE 27.18 Nursing Assessment
Lung Cancer

Subjective Data
Important Health Information
Past health history: Exposure to secondhand smoke, airborne carcinogens (e.g., asbestos, radon, hydrocarbons), or other pollutants. Urban living environment. Chronic lung disease (e.g., TB, COPD, bronchiectasis). History of cancer.
Medications: Cough medicines, bronchodilators, expectorants, or other respiratory medications

Functional Health Patterns
Health perception–health management: Smoking history, including what was smoked, amount per day, and number of years. Family history of lung cancer. Frequent respiratory tract infections
Nutritional-metabolic: Anorexia, nausea, vomiting, weight loss, dysphagia (late). *Activity-exercise:* Fatigue. Persistent cough (productive or nonproductive). Dyspnea at rest or with exertion, hemoptysis (late symptom)
Cognitive-perceptual: Chest pain or tightness, shoulder and arm pain, headache, bone pain (late symptom)

Objective Data
General
Fever, nose and/or throat infection, neck and axillary lymphadenopathy, paraneoplastic syndrome (e.g., syndrome of inappropriate ADH secretion)

Integumentary
Edema of neck and face (superior vena cava syndrome), digital clubbing. Jaundice (liver metastasis).

Respiratory
Wheezing, hoarseness, stridor, dyspnea on exertion (unilateral diaphragm paralysis), pleural effusions (late signs)

Cardiovascular
Pericardial effusion, cardiac tamponade, dysrhythmias (late signs)

Neurologic
Confusion, disorientation, unsteady gait (brain metastasis)

Musculoskeletal
Pathologic fractures, muscle wasting (late)

Possible Diagnostic Findings
Observance of lesion on chest x-ray, CT scan, or PET scan. MRI findings of vertebral, spinal cord, or mediastinal invasion. Positive sputum or bronchial washings for cytologic studies. Positive fiberoptic bronchoscopy and biopsy findings

ADH, Antidiuretic hormone; *PET,* positron emission tomography.

---

recognition that secondhand smoke is a health hazard. Laws prohibit smoking in most public places and limit public smoking to designated areas. Most hospital environments are now completely smoke free, prohibiting smoking by employees and patients. A new trend is for hospitals to refuse employment to anyone testing positive for nicotine.

◆ Acute Care.
Care of the patient with lung cancer initially involves support and reassurance during diagnostic evaluation. It is important to recognize the multiple stressors that occur when someone receives a lung cancer diagnosis. The stress response is a normal and adaptive response but can become detrimental when stress is overwhelming and intense.

Patients have the stress of their symptoms, including dyspnea and cough. Diagnostic and therapeutic interventions provide more stress by placing patients in unfamiliar environments with unusual and perhaps painful procedures. Emotional stressors include waiting for test results and awareness of the high mortality rate associated with lung cancer and the causal effect of cigarette smoking. Worries about role performance and ability to care for their family while undergoing cancer treatment provide further stress. Carefully assess the patient since each will have unique stressors. The insight gained will help the patient and caregiver cope with the stress of both illness and treatment.

Care of the patient undergoing chest surgery is discussed later in this chapter on pp. 529–530. Care of the patient undergoing radiation therapy and chemotherapy is discussed in Chapter 15. Individualized care depends on the plan for treatment. Assessment and intervention in symptom management are pivotal, as is teaching the patient to recognize signs and symptoms that may indicate progression or recurrence of disease. Teach signs and symptoms to report (e.g., hemoptysis, dysphagia, chest pain, hoarseness).

Provide patient comfort, teach methods to reduce pain, monitor for side effects of prescribed drugs, foster appropriate coping strategies for both the patient and caregiver, assess smoking cessation readiness, and help the patient access resources to deal with the illness.

? CHECK YOUR PRACTICE

You are completing discharge teaching with a 72-yr-old woman who had a lobectomy for NSCLC. She tells you, "I'm not going to give up smoking my cigarettes because I am just going to die anyhow. I might as well enjoy smoking while I still can."
• How would you respond?

◆ **Ambulatory Care.** Counseling patients on smoking cessation and prevention is essential in decreasing morbidity and mortality risks associated with lung cancer. Encourage the patient and family to provide a smoke-free environment. This may include smoking cessation for multiple family members. If the treatment plan includes home O_2, the teaching plan must include the safe use of O_2.

For many patients with lung cancer, little can be done to significantly prolong their lives. Radiation therapy and chemotherapy can provide palliative relief from distressing symptoms. Constant pain may become a major problem. Measures used to relieve pain are discussed in Chapter 8. Care of the patient with cancer is discussed in Chapter 15. The palliative care team should be involved as the patient and family move toward the end of life (see Chapter 9). The team can provide information about disability, financial planning, and community resources for end-of-life care, such as hospice and home care.

◆ Evaluation

The expected outcomes are that the patient with lung cancer will:
• Have adequate breathing patterns
• Maintain adequate oxygenation
• Have minimal to no pain
• Convey feelings openly and honestly, with a realistic attitude about prognosis

OTHER TYPES OF LUNG TUMORS

SCLC and NSCLC account for 95% of lung tumors. The other 5% include:
• *Hamartomas,* the most common benign tumor, is a slow-growing congenital tumor composed of fibrous tissue, fat, and blood vessels.
• *Mucous gland adenoma* is a benign tumor arising in the bronchi that consists of columnar cystic spaces.
• *Mesotheliomas* are either malignant or benign and start in the visceral pleura. Malignant mesotheliomas are associated with exposure to asbestos. Benign mesotheliomas are localized lesions.

Secondary metastases from other cancers can occur. Cancer cells from another part of the body reach the lungs through the pulmonary capillaries or lymphatic network. The main cancers that spread to the lungs often start in the breast, GI, or genitourinary tract.

CHEST TRAUMA AND THORACIC INJURIES

Traumatic injuries to the chest contribute to many deaths. Chest injuries range from simple rib fractures to cardiorespiratory arrest. We describe the primary mechanisms of injury responsible for chest trauma as either blunt trauma or penetrating trauma.

Blunt trauma occurs when the chest strikes or is struck by an object. The impact can cause shearing and compression of chest structures. The external injury may appear minor, but internally organs may have been severely damaged. Rib and sternal fractures can lacerate lung tissue. In a high-velocity impact, shearing forces can result in laceration or tearing of the aorta. Compression of the chest may result in contusion, crush injury, and organ rupture.

Penetrating trauma is an injury in which a foreign object impales or passes through the body tissues, creating an open wound. Examples include knife wounds, gunshot wounds, and injuries with other sharp objects. Emergency care of the patient with a chest injury is outlined in Table 27.19. The most common chest emergencies and their management are described in Table 27.20.

FRACTURED RIBS

Rib fractures are the most common type of chest injury from blunt trauma. Ribs 5 through 9 are most often fractured because they are the least protected by chest muscles. A fractured rib that is splintered or displaced can damage the pleura, lungs, heart, and other internal organs.

Manifestations of fractured ribs include pain at the site of injury, especially during inspiration and with coughing. The patient splints the affected area and takes shallow breaths to try to decrease the pain. Atelectasis and pneumonia may develop because of decreased chest wall movement and retained secretions.

The goal of treatment is to decrease pain so that the patient can breathe adequately and clear secretions. Strapping the chest with tape or using a thoracic binder is not recommended. These limit chest expansion and predispose the person to atelectasis. NSAIDs, opioids, and thoracic nerve blocks can be used to reduce pain and assist with deep breathing and coughing. Patient teaching should emphasize deep breathing, coughing, incentive spirometry, and appropriate use of pain medications.

✚ TABLE 27.19 Emergency Management

Chest Trauma

Etiology	Assessment Findings	Interventions
Blunt • Assault with blunt object • Crush injury • Explosion • Fall • Motor vehicle collision • Pedestrian accident • Sports injury **Penetrating** • Arrow • Gunshot • Knife • Stick	**Respiratory** • Audible air escaping from chest wound • Cough with or without hemoptysis • Cyanosis of mouth, face, nail beds, mucous membranes • Decreased breath sounds on side of injury • Decreased O$_2$ saturation • Dyspnea, respiratory distress • Frothy secretions • Tracheal deviation **Cardiovascular** • Asymmetric BP values in arms • Chest pain • Decreased BP • Distended neck veins • Dysrhythmias • Muffled heart sounds • Narrowed pulse pressure • Rapid, thready pulse **Surface Findings** • Abrasions • Asymmetric chest movement • Bruising • Contusions • Lacerations • Open chest wound • Subcutaneous emphysema	**Initial** • If unresponsive, immediately assess circulation, airway, and breathing. • If responsive, monitor airway, breathing, and circulation. • Apply high-flow O$_2$ to keep SpO$_2$ >90%. • Establish IV access with 2 large-bore catheters. Begin IV fluid resuscitation as appropriate. • Remove clothing to assess injury. • Cover sucking chest wound with nonporous dressing taped on 3 sides (vent dressing). • Stabilize impaled objects with bulky dressings. *Do not remove object.* • Assess for life-threatening injuries and treat appropriately. • Place patient in a semi-Fowler's position if breathing is easier *after* cervical spine injury has been ruled out. • Give small amounts of analgesia as needed for pain and to help with breathing. • Prepare for emergency needle decompression if tension pneumothorax or cardiac tamponade present. **Ongoing Monitoring** • Monitor level of consciousness, vital signs, O$_2$ saturation, cardiac rhythm, respiratory status, and urine output. • Anticipate intubation for respiratory distress. • Release vent dressing if tension pneumothorax develops after sucking chest wound is covered.

✚ TABLE 27.20 Emergency Management

Chest Injuries

Injury and Description	Manifestations	Intervention
Cardiac Tamponade Blood rapidly collects in pericardial sac, compresses myocardium because pericardium does not stretch, and prevents ventricles from filling.	Muffled, distant heart sounds, hypotension, neck vein distention, increased central venous pressure	Medical emergency. Pericardiocentesis with surgical repair as appropriate.
Flail Chest Fracture of 2 or more adjacent ribs in 2 or more places with loss of chest wall stability (Fig. 27.5).	Paradoxical movement of chest wall, respiratory distress. May be associated hemothorax, pneumothorax, pulmonary contusion	O$_2$ as needed to maintain O$_2$ saturation, analgesia. Stabilize flail segment with positive pressure ventilation (intubation and mechanical ventilation as needed). Treat associated injuries. Possible surgical fixation.
Hemothorax Blood in the pleural space, may or may not occur in conjunction with pneumothorax.	Dyspnea, decreased or absent breath sounds, dullness to percussion, decreased Hgb, shock (depending on blood volume lost)	Chest tube insertion with chest drainage system. Autotransfusion of collected blood, treatment of hypovolemia as needed with IV fluid, packed red blood cells.
Pneumothorax Air in pleural space (Fig. 27.6).	Dyspnea, decreased movement of involved chest wall, decreased or absent breath sounds on the affected side, hyperresonance to percussion	Chest tube insertion with chest drainage system.
Tension Pneumothorax Air in pleural space that does not escape Increased air in the pleural space shifts organs and increases intrathoracic pressure (Fig. 27.6).	Cyanosis, air hunger, extreme agitation, subcutaneous emphysema, neck vein distention, hyperresonance to percussion, tracheal deviation away from affected side (late sign)	Medical emergency: needle decompression followed by chest tube insertion with chest drainage system.

FLAIL CHEST

Flail chest results from the fracture of 3 or more consecutive ribs, in 2 or more separate places, causing an unstable segment (Fig. 27.5). It also can be caused by fracture of the sternum and several consecutive ribs. The resulting instability of the chest wall causes paradoxical movement during breathing. The affected (flail) area moves in the opposite direction with respect to the intact part of the chest. During inspiration, the affected part is sucked in, and during expiration, it bulges out. This paradoxical chest movement prevents adequate ventilation and increases the work of breathing. The underlying injured lung may be contused, aggravating hypoxemia.

A flail chest is usually apparent on physical examination. The patient has rapid, shallow respirations and tachycardia. Movement of the thorax is asymmetric and uncoordinated. The patient may ventilate poorly and try to splint the chest to assist with breathing. Observation of abnormal chest cavity movement, palpation for crepitus near the rib fractures, and chest x-ray all assist in the diagnosis.

Initial therapy consists of ensuring adequate ventilation and supplemental O2 therapy. The goal is to promote lung expansion and ensure adequate oxygenation. Analgesia can help promote adequate respiration. Although many patients can be managed without mechanical ventilation, intubation and ventilation may be needed. In cases of extreme chest trauma, surgical fixation of the flail segment may be done. The lung parenchyma and fractured ribs heal with time. Some patients continue to have intercostal pain several weeks after the flail chest has resolved.

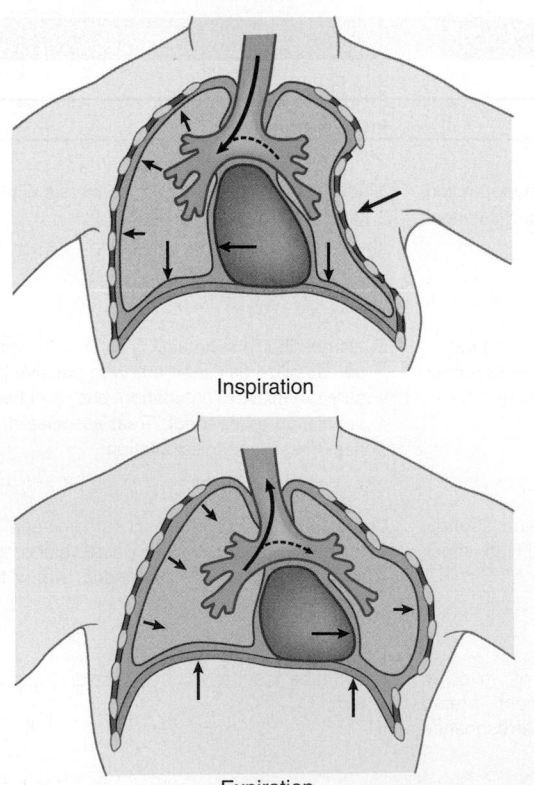

Inspiration

Expiration

FIG. 27.5 Flail chest causes paradoxical respiration. On inspiration, the flail section moves inward with mediastinal shift to the uninjured side. On expiration, the flail section bulges outward with mediastinal shift to the injured side.

PNEUMOTHORAX

A pneumothorax is caused by air entering the pleural cavity. Normally, negative (subatmospheric) pressure exists between the visceral pleura (surrounding the lung) and parietal pleura (lining the chest cavity), known as the *pleural space*. The pleural space has a few milliliters of lubricating fluid to reduce friction when the tissues move. When air enters this space, the change to positive pressure causes a partial or complete lung collapse (Fig. 27.6). As the volume of air in the pleural space increases, lung volume decreases.

Pneumothorax can be classified as *open* (air entering through an opening in the chest wall) or *closed* (no external wound). Penetrating trauma allows air to enter the pleural space through an opening in the chest wall (Fig. 27.6). A penetrating chest wound may be referred to as a *sucking chest wound*, since air enters the pleural space through the chest wall during inspiration. A pneumothorax should be suspected after any trauma to the chest wall.

If a pneumothorax is small, mild tachycardia and dyspnea may be the only manifestations. If the pneumothorax occupies a large area, respiratory distress may be present, including short, shallow, rapid respirations; dyspnea; air hunger; and O2 desaturation. On auscultation, breath sounds are absent over the affected area. Time permitting, a chest x-ray will show air or fluid in the pleural space and reduction in lung volume.

Types of Pneumothorax

Spontaneous Pneumothorax. A spontaneous pneumothorax typically occurs due to the rupture of small blebs (air-filled sacs) on the surface of the lung. These blebs can occur in healthy, young people or from lung disease, such as COPD, asthma, cystic fibrosis, and pneumonia. Smoking increases the risk for bleb formation. Other risk factors include being tall and thin, male gender, family history, and previous spontaneous pneumothorax.

Iatrogenic Pneumothorax. *Iatrogenic pneumothorax* can occur due to laceration or puncture of the lung during medical procedures. For example, transthoracic needle aspiration, subclavian catheter insertion, pleural biopsy, and transbronchial lung biopsy all have the potential to injure the lung. Barotrauma from excessive ventilatory pressure during manual or mechanical ventilation can rupture alveoli, creating a pneumothorax. Esophageal procedures may result in a pneumothorax. For example, tearing of the esophageal wall during insertion of a gastric tube can allow air from the esophagus to enter the mediastinum and pleural space.

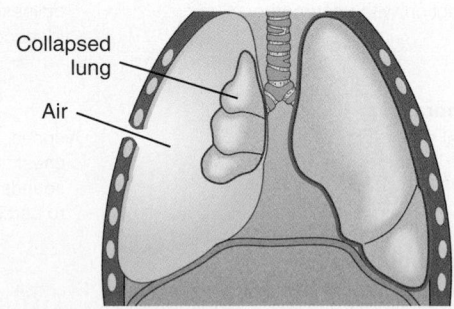

Collapsed lung

Air

FIG. 27.6 Open pneumothorax resulting from collapse of lung due to disruption of chest wall and outside air entering.

Tension Pneumothorax. Tension pneumothorax occurs when air enters the pleural space but cannot escape. The continued accumulation of air in the pleural space causes increasingly elevated intrapleural pressures. This results in compression of the lung on the affected side and pressure on the heart and great vessels, pushing them away from the affected side (Fig. 27.7). The mediastinum shifts toward the unaffected side, compressing the "good" lung, which further compromises oxygenation. As the pressure increases, venous return decreases and cardiac output falls.

Tension pneumothorax may result from either an open or a closed pneumothorax. In an open chest wound, a flap may act as a one-way valve. Thus air can enter on inspiration but cannot escape. Tension pneumothorax can occur with mechanical ventilation and resuscitative efforts. It can also occur if chest tubes are clamped or become blocked in a patient with a pneumothorax. Unclamping the tube or relieving the obstruction may correct this situation.

Tension pneumothorax is a medical emergency. It affects both the respiratory and cardiovascular systems. Manifestations include severe dyspnea, marked tachycardia, tracheal deviation, decreased or absent breath sounds on the affected side, neck vein distention, cyanosis, and profuse diaphoresis. If the tension in the pleural space is not relieved, the patient is likely to die from inadequate cardiac output or severe hypoxemia.

Hemothorax. Hemothorax is an accumulation of blood in the pleural space from injury to the chest wall, diaphragm, lung, blood vessels, or mediastinum. When it occurs with pneumothorax, it is called a *hemopneumothorax*. The patient with a traumatic hemothorax needs immediate insertion of a chest tube for evacuation of the blood. Recovered blood can be reinfused for a short time after the injury. (Autotransfusion is discussed in Chapter 30.)

Chylothorax. *Chylothorax* is the presence of lymphatic fluid in the pleural space. The thoracic duct is disrupted either traumatically or from cancer, allowing lymphatic fluid to fill the pleural space. This milky white fluid is high in lipids. Normal lymphatic flow through the thoracic duct is 1500 to 2500 mL/day. This amount can be increased up to 10-fold after ingestion of fats. Some cases heal with conservative treatment (chest drainage, bowel rest, dietary modifications). Octreotide may reduce the flow of lymphatic fluid. Surgery (thoracic duct ligation) and pleurodesis (the artificial production of adhesions between the parietal and visceral pleura) are options for refractory cases.

Interprofessional Care

Treatment of a pneumothorax depends on its severity, underlying cause, and hemodynamic stability of the patient. If the patient is stable and has minimal air and/or fluid accumulated in the intrapleural space, no treatment may be needed since the condition may resolve spontaneously.

Emergency treatment consists of covering the wound with an occlusive dressing that is secured on 3 sides (vent dressing). During inspiration, as negative pressure is created in the chest, the dressing pulls against the wound, preventing air from entering the pleural space. During expiration, as the pressure rises in the pleural space, the dressing is pushed out and air escapes through the wound and from under the dressing. If the object that caused the open chest wound is still in place, do not remove it. Stabilize the impaled object with a bulky dressing. Wait until an HCP is present or arrange transport to the nearest medical facility.

The most definitive and common treatment of pneumothorax and hemothorax is to insert a chest tube and connect it to water-seal drainage. Repeated spontaneous pneumothorax may need surgical treatment with a partial pleurectomy, stapling, or pleurodesis to promote adherence of the pleurae to one another. Tension pneumothorax is a medical emergency, requiring urgent needle decompression followed by chest tube insertion to water-seal drainage.

CHEST TUBES AND PLEURAL DRAINAGE

If enough fluid or air accumulates in the pleural space, the normally negative subatmospheric pressure becomes positive and the lungs collapse. Inserting a chest tube can drain the pleural space, reestablish negative pressure, and allow for proper lung expansion.

Chest tubes are about 20 in (51 cm) long and vary in size from 12F to 40F. The size inserted depends on the patient's condition. Large (36F to 40F) tubes are used to drain blood, medium (24F to 36F) tubes are used to drain fluid, and small (12F to 24F) tubes are used to drain air. Pigtail tubes are very small (10F to 14F) tubes with a curly end designed to keep them in place. Pigtail tubes are a safe and effective alternative to larger-bore chest tubes for treatment of pneumothorax.

Chest Tube Insertion

Insertion of a chest tube can take place in the ED, the operating room, or at the patient's bedside. Time permitting, a chest x-ray is used to confirm the affected side. The patient is positioned with the arm raised above the head on the affected side to expose the midaxillary area, the standard site for insertion. Elevate the patient's head 30 to 60 degrees, when possible, to lower the diaphragm and reduce the risk for injury.

The area is cleansed with an antiseptic solution. The HCP infiltrates the chest with a local anesthetic and makes a small incision over a rib. The chest tube is advanced up and over the top of the rib to avoid the intercostal nerves and blood vessels that are behind the rib inferiorly (Fig. 27.8). Once inserted, the HCP secures (sutures) the tube in place and closes the incision with sutures. The tube is connected to a pleural drainage system (Fig. 27.9). The wound is covered with an occlusive dressing. Most HCPs prefer

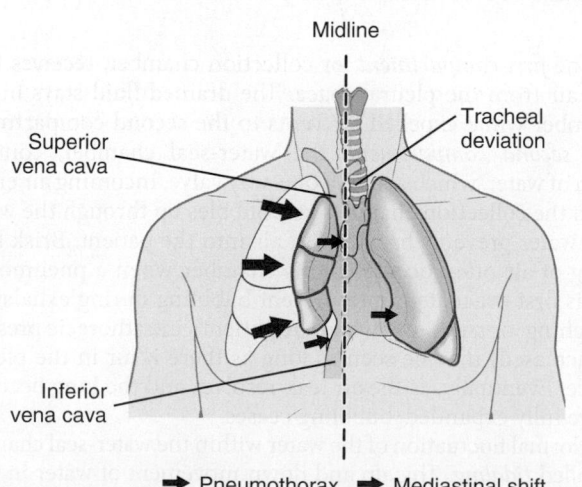

Midline

Tracheal deviation

Superior vena cava

Inferior vena cava

→ Pneumothorax   → Mediastinal shift

FIG. 27.7 Tension pneumothorax. As pleural pressure on the affected side increases, mediastinal displacement ensues, causing respiratory and cardiovascular compromise. Tracheal deviation is an external (but late) manifestation of the mediastinal shift.

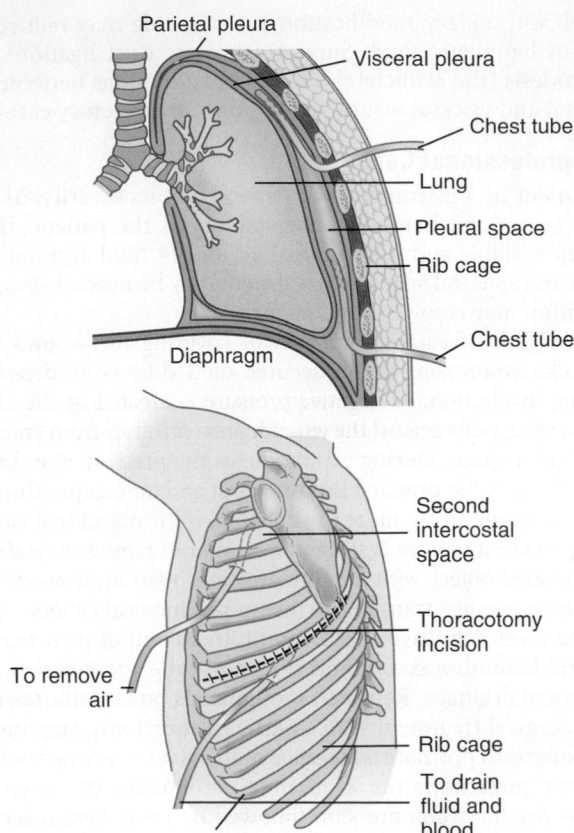

FIG. 27.8 Placement of chest tubes.

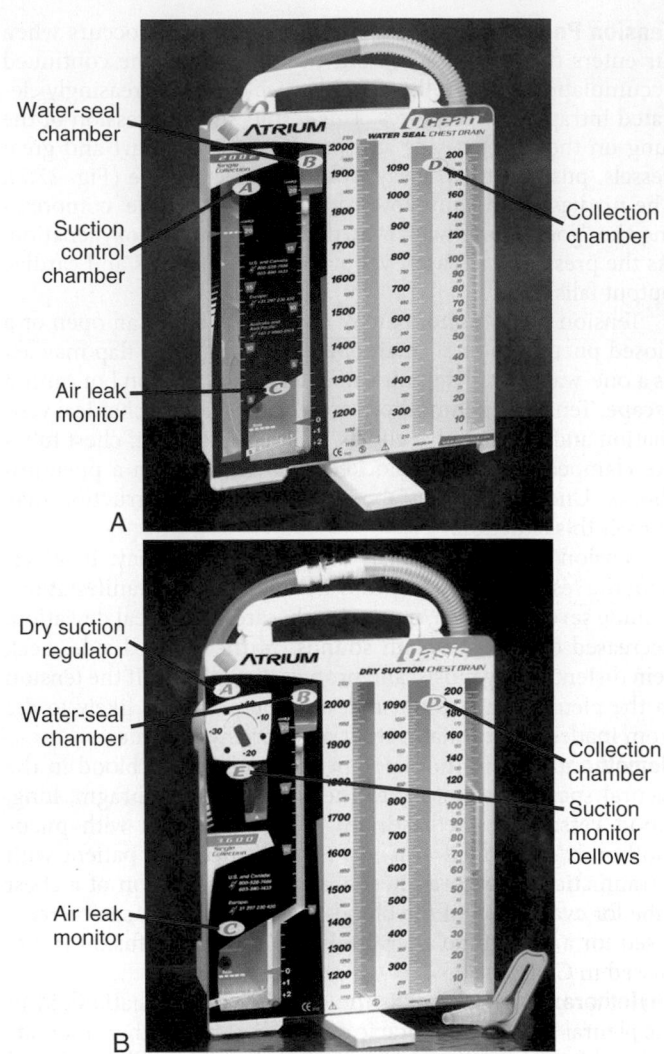

FIG. 27.9 Chest drainage unit. Both units have 3 chambers: (1) collection chamber; (2) water-seal chamber; and (3) suction control chamber. Suction control chamber requires a connection to a wall suction source that is dialed up higher than the prescribed suction for the suction to work. **A,** Water suction. This unit uses water in the suction control chamber to control the wall suction pressure. **B,** Dry suction. This unit controls wall suction by using a regulator control dial. (From Atrium Medical Corporation, Hudson, NH.)

to seal the wound around the chest tube with petroleum (airtight) gauze. Proper tube placement is confirmed by chest x-ray.

The insertion of a chest tube and its presence in the pleural space are painful. Monitor the patient's comfort frequently and use appropriate pain-relieving interventions.

Flutter or Heimlich Valve

A flutter valve (also called the *Heimlich valve*) is used to remove air from the pleural space (Fig. 27.10). This device consists of a one-way rubber valve within a rigid plastic tube. It is attached to the external end of the chest tube. It has 2 nozzles. The inlet nozzle allows the air to pass in the valve through the chest drainage tube attached to it. The outlet nozzle allows the air to pass to the environment or a collecting device during expiration. During inspiration, when pressure in the chest decreases, the valve closes. During expiration, when intrathoracic pressure increases, the valve closes.

The flutter valve can be used for small to moderate-sized pneumothorax. It also allows for patient mobility. The smaller drainage bag can be hidden under the clothes while the patient ambulates. Drainage bags attached to the flutter valve must have a vent to the atmosphere to prevent a tension pneumothorax. This is done by simply cutting a small slit in the top of any drainage bag that does not have a built-in vent. Patients may go home with a flutter valve in place.

Pleural Drainage

A chest tube is usually attached to a drainage device or chamber to collect fluid, air, and/or blood from the chest cavity. Several different disposable chest drainage units are currently available. All drainage units have 3 basic compartments (Fig. 27.9).

The *first compartment,* or collection chamber, receives fluid and air from the pleural space. The drained fluid stays in this chamber while expelled air vents to the second compartment. The *second compartment,* the water-seal chamber, contains 2 cm of water, which acts as a one-way valve. Incoming air enters from the collection chamber and bubbles up through the water. The water prevents backflow of air into the patient. Brisk bubbling of air often occurs in this chamber when a pneumothorax is first evacuated. Intermittent bubbling during exhalation, coughing, or sneezing (when the patient's intrathoracic pressure is increased) may be seen as long as there is air in the pleural space. Eventually, as the air leak resolves and the lung becomes more fully expanded, bubbling ceases.

Normal fluctuation of the water within the water-seal chamber is called *tidaling.* This up and down movement of water in concert with respiration reflects intrapleural pressure changes during inspiration and expiration. If tidaling stops suddenly, assess the chest tube as this may signify an occluded chest tube. As the lung reexpands, tidaling gradually slows then eventually stops.

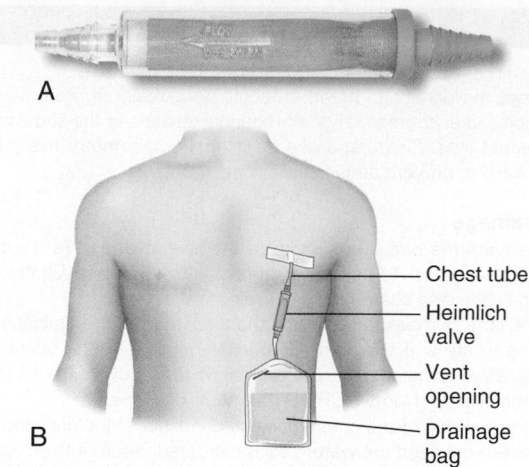

FIG. 27.10 A, Heimlich chest drain valve is a specially designed flutter valve that is used in place of a chest drainage unit for small uncomplicated pneumothorax with little or no drainage and no need for suction. The valve allows for escape of air but prevents the reentry of air into the pleural space. B, Placement of valve between chest tube and vented drainage bag, which can be worn under a person's clothes. (A, Courtesy and © Becton, Dickinson and Company.)

The *third compartment*, the suction control chamber, applies suction to the chest drainage unit. There are 2 main types of suction control: water and dry. The water suction control chamber uses a column of water to control the amount of suction from the wall regulator.

The chamber is typically filled with 20 cm of water. The amount of suction applied to the chest drainage unit is regulated by the amount of water in this chamber and not by the amount of suction applied to the system. An increase in wall suction does not result in an increase in negative pressure to the system because any excess suction merely draws in air through the vent on top of the third chamber. The suction pressure is usually ordered to be –20 cm H_2O. Higher pressures (–40 cm H_2O) are sometimes needed to evacuate the pleural space. Lower pressure (–10 cm H_2O) may be used for frail and older patients at risk for tissue damage with higher pressures. When the negative pressure generated by the suction source exceeds the set –20 cm H_2O, air from the atmosphere enters the chamber through a vent on top of the chest drainage unit and the air bubbles up through the water, causing a suction-breaker effect. As a result, excess pressure is relieved.

To start suction, adjust (increase) the vacuum source until gentle bubbling is present in the third chamber. Excessive bubbling does not increase the amount of suction but does increase the rate of evaporation of the water and the amount of noise made by the device.

Dry suction chest drainage systems do not contain water. They often have a visual alert that shows if the suction is working. It uses either a restrictive device or a regulator to dial the desired negative pressure; this is internal in the chest drainage system. To increase the suction pressures, turn the dial on the drainage system. Increasing the vacuum source does not increase the pressure. When decreasing suction, depress the manual vent to reduce excess vacuum to the lower prescribed level.

A variety of disposable plastic chest drainage systems are available. Manufacturers include directions for set-up and use with each unit.

❖ NURSING MANAGEMENT: CHEST DRAINAGE

General guidelines for nursing care of the patient with chest tubes and water-seal drainage systems are shown in Table 27.21.

Clamping of chest tubes during transport or when the tube is accidentally disconnected is no longer advocated. The danger of rapid accumulation of air in the pleural space, causing tension pneumothorax, is far greater than that of a small amount of atmospheric air that enters the pleural space. If a chest tube becomes disconnected, the immediate priority is to reestablish the water-seal system. In some agencies, when disconnection occurs, the chest tube is immersed in sterile water to act as a water seal until a new system can be set up and chest drainage reestablished. It is important to know the unit protocol, the clinical situation (whether an air leak exists), and HCP preference before any chest tube clamping occurs.

Chest tubes may be momentarily clamped to change the drainage apparatus or to check for air leaks. Appearance of a new air leak warrants assessment of the drainage system to identify whether the air leak is coming from the patient or the system. Again, you must be familiar with the policies and procedures of your agency about specific clinical situations when you may clamp a chest tube.

Closely monitor the patient for complications associated with chest tube placement and drainage. If volumes from 1 to 1.5 L of fluid and/or blood are removed rapidly, reexpansion pulmonary edema or severe, symptomatic hypotension can occur. Subcutaneous emphysema can occur from air leaking into the tissue surrounding the chest tube insertion site. A "crackling" sensation will be felt when palpating the skin. A small amount of subcutaneous air is harmless and will be reabsorbed. However, severe subcutaneous emphysema can cause drastic swelling of the head and neck with potential airway compromise.

Meticulous sterile technique during dressing changes can reduce the incidence of infected chest tube insertion sites. Nursing care and patient teaching can minimize the risk for atelectasis and shoulder stiffness. Encourage coughing, deep breathing, incentive spirometer use, and range-of-motion exercises. Inspect the integrity of the chest tube system. Monitor the color and amount of drainage hourly in the first few hours after chest tube insertion. Drainage greater than 200 mL in the first hour, development of subcutaneous emphysema, or any signs and symptoms of respiratory distress should be reported to the HCP at once.

TABLE 27.21　Chest Tubes and Water-Seal Drainage

Set-Up and Insertion

1. Make sure patient is aware of the procedure and informed consent is obtained.
2. Gather equipment.
   - Thoracotomy or chest tube insertion tray
   - Chest drainage unit (CDU)
   - Chest tube
   - Bottle of sterile water
   - 1% lidocaine
   - Suction tubing and collection container
   - Occlusive dressing
3. Prepare CDU.
   - *Wet suction:* Add sterile water to 2-cm mark in water-seal chamber and to 20-cm mark (or as ordered) in suction control chamber.
   - *Dry suction:* Add sterile water to the fill line of the air leak meter. Attach suction tubing and increase suction until the bellows-like float moves across the display window.
4. Position and support the patient to minimize movement during procedure.

Drainage System

1. Keep all tubing loosely coiled below chest level. Tubing should drop straight from bed or chair to drainage unit. Do not let it be compressed.
2. Keep all connections between chest tubes, drainage tubing, and the drainage collector tight, and tape all connections.
3. Observe for air fluctuations (tidaling) and bubbling in the water-seal chamber.
   - If tidaling (rising with inspiration and falling with expiration in the spontaneously breathing patient) is not seen, the drainage system is blocked, the lungs are reexpanded, or the system is attached to suction.
   - If bubbling increases, there may be an air leak in the drainage system or a leak from the patient (bronchopleural leak).
4. If the chest tube is connected to suction, disconnect from wall suction to check for tidaling.
5. Suspect a system leak when bubbling is continuous.
   - Retape tubing connections.
   - Ensure that dressing is air occlusive.
   - If leak persists, briefly clamp the chest tube at the patient's chest. If the leak stops, the air is coming from the patient*
   - If the air leak persists, briefly and methodically move the clamps down the tubing away from the patient until the air leak stops. The leak will then be present between the last 2 clamp points. If the air leak persists all the way to the drainage unit, replace the unit.*
6. High fluid levels in the water seal indicate residual negative pressure.
   - The chest system may have to be vented by using the high-negativity release valve available on the drainage system to release residual pressure from the system.
   - Do not lower water-seal column when wall suction is not operating or when patient is on gravity drainage.

Patient's Clinical Status

1. Monitor the patient's clinical status. Assess vital signs, lung sounds, and pain.
2. Assess for reaccumulation of air and fluid in the chest (↓ or absent breath sounds), significant bleeding (>100 mL/hr), infection at chest tube insertion site (drainage, erythema, fever, ↑ WBCs), or poor wound healing. Notify HCP for management plan.

3. Evaluate for subcutaneous emphysema at chest tube site.
4. Encourage the patient to breathe deeply periodically to promote lung expansion and encourage range-of-motion exercises to the shoulder on the affected side. Encourage use of incentive spirometry every hour while awake to prevent atelectasis or pneumonia.

Chest Drainage

1. Never elevate the drainage system to the level of the patient's chest because this will cause fluid to drain back into the lungs. Change the unit if the collection chamber is full. Do not try to empty it.
2. Mark the time of measurement and the fluid level on the drainage unit according to the unit standards. Report any change in the quantity or characteristics of drainage (e.g., clear yellow to bloody) to the HCP and record the change. Notify HCP if >100 mL/hr drainage.
3. Check the position of the chest drainage container. If the drainage system is overturned and the water seal is disrupted, return it to an upright position and encourage the patient to take a few deep breaths, followed by forced exhalations and cough maneuvers.
4. If the drainage system breaks, place the distal end of the chest tubing connection in a sterile water container at a 2-cm level as an emergency water seal.
5. Position tubing so that drainage flows freely.

Monitoring Wet Versus Dry Suction Chest Drainage Systems

Suction Control Chamber in Wet Suction System

1. Keep the suction control chamber at the right water level by adding sterile water as needed to replace water lost to evaporation.
2. Keep the cover over the suction control chamber in place to prevent more rapid evaporation of water and to decrease the noise of the bubbling.
3. After filling the suction control chamber to the ordered suction amount (generally 20 cm H_2O suction), connect the suction tubing to the wall suction.
4. Dial the wall suction regulator until there is continuous gentle bubbling in the suction control chamber (generally 80 to 120 mm Hg). Vigorous bubbling is not necessary and will increase the rate of evaporation.
5. If there is no bubbling in the suction control chamber, (1) there is no suction, (2) suction is not high enough, or (3) the pleural air leak is so large that suction is not high enough to evacuate it.

Suction Control Chamber in Dry Suction System (see manufacturer's directions)

1. After connecting patient to system, turn the dial on the chest drainage system to amount ordered (generally −20 cm H_2O pressure), connect suction tubing to wall suction source, and increase the suction until the float appears in the window of the CDU.
2. If ordered to decrease suction, turn the dial down, depress the high-negativity vent, and assess for a rise in the water level of the water-seal chamber.

Chest Tube Dressings

1. Change dressing according to unit protocol and HCP preference.
2. Remove old dressing carefully. Assess the site for inflammation or infection and culture site as needed.
3. Cleanse the site according to protocol, maintaining strict sterile asepsis.
4. Redress with occlusive dressing. Some HCPs prefer the use of petroleum gauze dressing around the tube to prevent air leak. Date the dressing and document dressing change.

*As per agency policy and procedures.

◆ Chest Tube Removal

Chest tubes are removed when the lungs are reexpanded and fluid drainage has ceased or is minimal. In some centers, suction is discontinued, and the chest drain is allowed to drain by gravity for 24 hours before the tube is removed. Give the patient pain medication about 30 to 60 minutes before tube removal.

Gather dressing supplies, including petroleum jelly and dry gauze dressing. Explain the procedure to the patient. In most settings, the tube is removed by the HCP or an advanced practice nurse. The suture is cut, and with the patient holding his or her breath or bearing down (Valsalva maneuver), the tube is removed. The site is immediately covered with the airtight dressing to prevent air from entering the pleural space. The pleura will seal off, and the wound usually heals in a few days. A chest x-ray is done 30 to 60 minutes after chest tube removal to evaluate for pneumothorax or fluid accumulation. Observe the wound for drainage and reinforce the dressing if needed. Monitor and record vital signs. Assess the patient for respiratory distress, which may signify a recurrence of the original problem.

CHEST SURGERY

Chest surgery is done for various reasons, including lung, heart, vascular, and esophageal disorders. The most common types of chest surgery are described in Table 27.22.

Surgical Procedures

Thoracotomy. A thoracotomy is a surgical incision into the chest to gain access to the heart, lungs, esophagus, thoracic aorta, or anterior spine. Two common approaches to a thoracotomy are the median sternotomy and lateral thoracotomy. The median sternotomy involves splitting the sternum. It is primarily used for surgery involving the heart. The lateral thoracotomy incision can be done using a posterolateral or anterolateral incision. The *posterolateral incision* is used for most surgeries involving the lung. The incision is made from front to back at the level of the 4th, 5th, or 6th intercostal space. Strong mechanical retractors are used to separate the ribs and gain access to the lung. The

TABLE 27.22 Chest Surgeries

Type	Description	Indications
Decortication Removal or stripping of thick, fibrous membrane from visceral pleura	• Need chest tubes postoperatively	Empyema or other inflammatory process unresponsive to conservative management
Exploratory Thoracotomy Incision into thorax to look for injured or bleeding tissues	• Need chest tubes postoperatively	Chest trauma
Lobectomy Removal of 1 lobe of lung	• Most common lung surgery • Lung tissue expands to fill up space left by resected lobe • Need chest tubes postoperatively	Lung cancer, bronchiectasis, TB, advanced emphysema, benign lung tumors, fungal infections
Lung Volume Reduction Surgery **Bronchoscopic procedure**	• Used to place one-way valves in airways leading to the diseased parts of the lung • Valves let air out, but not in, thus collapsing a certain segment of lungs	Advanced emphysema, α_1-antitrypsin emphysema
Open surgical procedure	• Involves reducing lung volume by multiple wedge excisions or VATS • Removes most diseased lung tissue	Emphysema, limited NSCLC
Pneumonectomy Removal of entire lung	• Done when lobectomy or segmental resection will not remove all diseased lung • Fluid will gradually fill space where lung was removed • May have chest tube postoperatively • Position patient on operative side to promote expansion of remaining lung	Lung cancer (most common)
Segmental Resection Removal of 1 or more lung segments	• Indicated for a patient unable to handle more extensive surgery • Remaining lung tissue expands to fill space • Need chest tubes postoperatively	Lung cancer, bronchiectasis
Thoracotomy (Not Involving Lungs) Incision into thorax for surgery on other organs	• Postoperative care related to thoracotomy and reason for surgical procedure • Need chest tubes postoperatively	Hiatal hernia repair, open heart surgery, esophageal surgery, tracheal resection, thoracic aorta repair
Video-Assisted Thoracic Surgery Video-assisted technique with a rigid scope with a distal lens inserted into pleura and image shown on a monitor screen	• Allows HCP to manipulate instruments passed into pleural space through separate small intercostal incisions • Done under general anesthesia in operating room • May need chest tube postoperatively	Lung biopsy, lobectomy, resection of nodules, repair of fistulas
Wedge Resection Removal of small, localized lesion that occupies only part of a segment	• Most conservative approach • Done to remove small peripheral nodules or for patients unable to handle more extensive surgery • Need chest tubes postoperatively	Lung biopsy, excision of small nodules

anterolateral incision is made in the 4th or 5th intercostal space from the sternal border to the midaxillary line. This procedure is often done for surgery or trauma victims, mediastinal operations, and wedge resections of the upper and middle lobes of the lung.

Video-Assisted Thoracic Surgery. *Video-assisted thoracoscopic surgery* (VATS) is a widely used, minimally invasive surgical approach. It provides a real-time 2-dimensional video image of the inside of the chest cavity. It is used for diagnosis and treatment of diseases of the pleura, pulmonary masses and nodules, mediastinal masses, and interstitial lung disease. Through incisions just large enough to insert the instruments, the HCP can inspect the chest cavity, biopsy suspicious areas, obtain samples of fluids for analysis, and remove tissue.

VATS is increasingly being used for patients with chest trauma. The HCP can examine, diagnose, and manage injuries in both blunt and penetrating trauma, including injuries to the diaphragm. A chest tube is placed in the pleural space through 1 or more of the incisions at the end of the procedure, secured with sutures, and connected to a drainage unit in the usual manner.

The advantages of VATS include less discomfort, faster return to normal activity level, reduced length of hospital stay, lower postoperative morbidity risk, and fewer complications.[31] Patients who have marginal respiratory reserve or are too debilitated to tolerate an open thoracotomy approach may benefit from the VATS procedure.

Preoperative Care

Assess the patient's cardiopulmonary status to determine their ability to tolerate the surgery and provide a baseline reference for postoperative care. Diagnostic studies may include chest x-ray, electrocardiogram (ECG), ABGs, pulmonary function studies, blood urea nitrogen (BUN), serum creatinine, blood glucose, serum electrolytes, prothrombin time/international normalized ratio (PT/INR), activated partial thromboplastin time (aPTT), and CBC. An anesthesia consult is usually completed.

The patient should be in the best possible health and, if applicable, stop smoking before elective surgery. Anxiety associated with anticipated surgery makes smoking cessation more difficult. Provide encouragement, support, and teaching about various methods to help stop smoking before surgery (see Chapter 10).

Teach the patient what to expect after surgery. Include the use of O$_2$, the chance of intubation, administration of blood and IV fluids, and the purpose and function of chest tubes. Reassure the patient that adequate medication will be used to reduce pain. Explain how to use patient-controlled analgesia (PCA), if planned. Preoperative teaching should always include exercises for effective deep breathing and use of incentive spirometry. If the patient practices these techniques before surgery, they will be easier to perform after surgery. Show the patient how to splint the incision with a pillow to promote deep breathing. Teach and have the patient provide a return demonstration of range-of-motion exercises on the surgical side (similar to those for the mastectomy patient [see Fig. 51.8]).

The thought of losing part of a vital organ is often frightening. Reassure the patient that the lungs have a large degree of functional reserve. Even after the removal of 1 lung, enough lung tissue is left to maintain adequate oxygenation. Be available to answer the patient and caregiver's questions. Answer questions openly and honestly. Encourage the expression of concerns, feelings, and questions.

Postoperative Care

The thoracotomy incision is the most painful surgical incision for patients and one of the most difficult for nurses to manage. Pain after a thoracotomy is typically intense because respiratory muscles are cut during surgery. For most chest surgeries, chest tubes are placed in the pleural space to allow for lung reexpansion. In a pneumonectomy, chest tubes may or may not be placed in the space from which the lung was removed. Adequate pain management is a priority to prevent respiratory compromise. The use of PCA, epidural infusions, and intercostal nerve blocks allows patients to breathe deeply, cough, and move the arm and shoulder on the operative side.

Nursing care priorities in the postoperative period include assessment of respiratory function, including observation of respiratory rate and effort, breath sounds, sputum volume and color, and chest tube function and drainage. Daily chest x-rays are often ordered. Assessment of pain, monitoring of temperature, and observation of the surgical site are similar to care provided for other postoperative patients (see Chapter 19). Care after thoracotomy is presented in eNursing Care Plan 27.2 (available on the website for this chapter).

Thoracentesis

Thoracentesis is aspiration of intrapleural fluid for diagnostic and therapeutic purposes. For a thoracentesis, the patient may sit on the edge of a bed and lean forward over a bedside table. A chest x-ray or ultrasound images are used to determine the optimal puncture site. The skin is cleansed with an antiseptic solution and injected with a local anesthetic. The thoracentesis needle is inserted into the intercostal space (see Fig. 25.12). Fluid is aspirated with a syringe, or tubing is connected to the needle to allow fluid to drain into a sterile container. After the fluid is removed, the needle is withdrawn, and a bandage is applied over the insertion site.

Usually no more than 1000 to 1200 mL of pleural fluid is removed at one time. Rapid removal of a large volume can result in hypotension, hypoxemia, or reexpansion pulmonary edema. A chest x-ray may be done after the procedure to assess for complications, such as pneumothorax. During and after the procedure, monitor vital signs and pulse oximetry. Observe the patient for respiratory distress.

RESTRICTIVE RESPIRATORY DISORDERS

Disorders that impair the ability of the chest wall and diaphragm to move with respiration are called *restrictive respiratory disorders*. There are 2 categories: *extrapulmonary conditions*, in which the lung tissue is normal, and *intrapulmonary conditions*, in which the cause is the lung or pleura. Examples of extrapulmonary and intrapulmonary conditions that alter respiratory functioning are listed in Table 27.23. These disorders are further described in their respective chapters.

Pulmonary function tests are the best means of distinguishing between restrictive and obstructive respiratory disorders. The hallmark characteristic of a restrictive lung disorder is a reduced total lung capacity (TLC). The hallmark characteristic of an obstructive disorder is reduced forced expiratory volume (FEV$_1$). Mixed obstructive and restrictive disorders sometimes occur together. For example, a patient may have both asthma (an obstructive problem) and pulmonary fibrosis (a restrictive problem).

TABLE 27.23 Common Causes of Restrictive Lung Disease

Intrapulmonary Causes
Pleural Disorders
- Pleural effusion
- Pleurisy (pleuritis)
- Pneumothorax

Parenchymal Disorders
- Acute respiratory distress syndrome (ARDS)
- Atelectasis
- Interstitial lung diseases
- Pneumonia

Extrapulmonary Causes
Central Nervous System
- Head injury, central nervous system lesion (e.g., tumor, stroke)
- Opioid and barbiturate overdose

Neuromuscular System
- Amyotrophic lateral sclerosis
- Guillain-Barré syndrome
- Muscular dystrophy
- Myasthenia gravis

Chest Wall
- Kyphoscoliosis
- Obesity-hypoventilation syndrome (Pickwickian syndrome)

ATELECTASIS

Atelectasis is a lung condition characterized by collapsed, airless alveoli. There may be decreased or absent breath sounds and dullness to percussion over the affected area. The most common cause of atelectasis is obstruction of the small airways with secretions. This is common in bedridden patients and in postoperative abdominal and chest surgery patients. Normally the pores of Kohn (see Fig. 25.1) provide collateral passage of air from one alveolus to another. Deep inspiration opens the pores effectively. For this reason, deep-breathing exercises, coughing, incentive spirometry, and early mobility are important to prevent atelectasis and treat the patient at risk. (The prevention and treatment of atelectasis are discussed in Chapter 19.)

PLEURISY

Pleurisy (pleuritis) is an inflammation of the pleura. It can be caused by infectious diseases, cancer, autoimmune disorders, chest trauma, GI disease, and certain medications. The inflammation usually subsides with adequate treatment of the primary disease. The pain of pleurisy is typically abrupt, sharp in onset, and worse with inspiration. The patient's breathing is shallow and rapid to avoid unnecessary movement of the pleura and chest wall. A pleural friction rub may occur. This is the sound heard over areas where inflamed visceral pleura and parietal pleura rub over one another during inspiration. This sound, like a squeaking door, is usually loudest at peak inspiration. It may be heard during exhalation as well.

Treatment of pleurisy is aimed at treating the underlying disease and providing pain relief. Teach the patient to splint the rib cage when coughing. If the pain is severe, intercostal nerve blocks may be considered.

PLEURAL EFFUSION

Types

The pleural space normally holds 5 to 15 mL of fluid that acts as a lubricant between the chest wall (parietal pleura) and lungs (visceral pleura). Pleural effusion is an abnormal collection of fluid in this space. It is not a disease but a sign of disease. A balance among hydrostatic pressure, oncotic pressure, and capillary membrane permeability governs movement of fluid in and out of the pleural space. Fluid accumulation can be due to increased pulmonary capillary pressure, decreased oncotic pressure, increased pleural membrane permeability, or obstruction of lymphatic flow.

We classify pleural effusions as transudative or exudative depending on the protein content. A *transudate* occurs primarily in noninflammatory conditions. It is an accumulation of protein-poor, cell-poor fluid. The fluid is clear, pale yellow. These effusions are caused by (1) increased hydrostatic pressure found in HF or (2) decreased oncotic pressure (from hypoalbuminemia) found in chronic liver or renal disease. An *exudative effusion* results from increased capillary permeability due to an inflammatory reaction. They most often occur with an infection or cancer (called a malignant effusion).

An empyema is the collection of purulent fluid in the pleural space. It is often caused by pneumonia, TB, lung abscess, and infected surgical wounds of the chest. Treatment options include antibiotic therapy (to eradicate the causative organism), percutaneous drainage, chest tube insertion, VATS, intrapleural fibrinolytic therapy (instilled through the chest tube) to dissolve fibrous adhesions, decortication, and open window thoracostomy.

Clinical Manifestations

Common manifestations of pleural effusion are dyspnea, cough, and occasional sharp, non-radiating chest pain that is worse on inhalation. Physical examination of the chest may show decreased movement of the chest on the affected side, dullness to percussion, and decreased breath sounds over the affected area. A chest x-ray and CT reveal the volume and location of the effusion. Indications of an empyema include the manifestations of pleural effusion as well as fever, night sweats, cough, and weight loss.

Interprofessional Care

The management of pleural effusions is to treat the underlying cause. For example, adequate treatment of HF with diuretics and sodium restriction may result in a decreased incidence of pleural effusion. The treatment of malignant effusions is more difficult. These effusions often reoccur and reaccumulate quickly after thoracentesis.

Chemical pleurodesis is done to obliterate the pleural space and prevent reaccumulation of effusion fluid. This procedure first requires chest tube drainage of the effusion. Once the fluid is drained, a chemical slurry is instilled into the pleural space. Talc is the most effective agent for pleurodesis. Other agents that can be used include doxycycline and bleomycin. The chest tube is clamped for 8 hours while the patient is turned in different positions to allow the chemical to contact the entire pleural space. After 8 hours the chest tube is unclamped and attached to a drainage unit. Chest tubes are left in place until fluid drainage is less than 150 mL/day and no air leaks are noted. Fever and chest pain are the most common side effects associated with pleurodesis.

INTERSTITIAL LUNG DISEASES

Interstitial lung disease (ILD), also called *diffuse parenchymal lung disease,* refers to more than 200 lung disorders in which the tissue between the air sacs of the lungs (the interstitium) is affected by inflammation or scarring (fibrosis).[32] Most ILDs are extremely rare. Many times, the cause is unknown. Two common ILDs of unknown cause are idiopathic pulmonary fibrosis and sarcoidosis. Other ILDs are caused by inhalation of occupational and environmental toxins, certain medications, radiation therapy, connective tissue disorders, cancer, and infection. Treatment is aimed at reducing exposure to the causative agent and/or treating the underlying disease process. Although scarring is irreversible, treatment with corticosteroids and immunosuppressant drugs can minimize progression. A lung transplant may be an option for some patients.

IDIOPATHIC PULMONARY FIBROSIS

Idiopathic pulmonary fibrosis (IPF) is a chronic, progressive disorder characterized by chronic inflammation and formation of scar tissue in the connective tissue. Risk factors include a history of cigarette smoking and exposure to wood and metal dust. IPF affects more men than women. It typically first appears between the ages of 50 and 70 years. There is no known cure for IPF.

Manifestations include exertional dyspnea; dry, nonproductive cough; clubbing of the fingers; and inspiratory crackles. Fatigue, weakness, anorexia, and weight loss may occur as the disease progresses. Chest x-ray findings are generally nonspecific. Pulmonary function tests may be abnormal, with evidence of restriction (reduced vital capacity) and impaired gas exchange. Open lung biopsy using VATS often helps to confirm the pathology and is considered the gold standard for diagnosis.

The course of IPF is variable and the prognosis is poor. The 5-year survival rate is 30% to 50% after diagnosis. Many people diagnosed with IPF are first treated with a corticosteroid (prednisone), sometimes in combination with other drugs that suppress the immune system (e.g., methotrexate, cyclosporine). Kinase inhibitor drugs, which block multiple pathways that involved with scarring, include nintedanib (Ofev) and pirfenidone (Esbriet).

O_2 therapy and pulmonary rehabilitation should be prescribed for all patients. Lung transplantation may be an option for those who meet the criteria. (Lung transplantation is discussed later in this chapter on p. 537.)

SARCOIDOSIS

Sarcoidosis is a chronic, multisystem granulomatous disease of unknown cause that primarily affects the lungs. The disease may also involve the skin, eyes, liver, kidney, heart, and lymph nodes. Those at higher risk include blacks and those with a family history of sarcoidosis.

Signs and symptoms vary depending on what organs are affected. Pulmonary symptoms include dyspnea, cough, and chest pain. Many patients do not have symptoms.

Staging and treatment decisions are based on pulmonary function and disease progression. Some patients have a spontaneous remission. Treatment is aimed at suppressing the inflammatory response. Patients are followed every 3 to 6 months with pulmonary function tests, chest x-ray, and CT scan to monitor disease progression.

TABLE 27.24 **Causes of Pulmonary Edema**

- Acute respiratory distress syndrome (ARDS)
- Altered capillary permeability of lungs: aspiration, inhaled toxins, inflammation (e.g., pneumonia), severe hypoxia, near-drowning
- Anaphylactic (allergic) reaction
- Hypoalbuminemia: nephrotic syndrome, liver disease, nutritional disorders
- Left ventricular (heart) failure
- Lymph system cancer (e.g., non-Hodgkin's lymphoma)
- Overhydration with IV fluids
- O_2 toxicity
- Unknown causes: neurogenic condition, opioid overdose, reexpansion pulmonary edema, high altitude

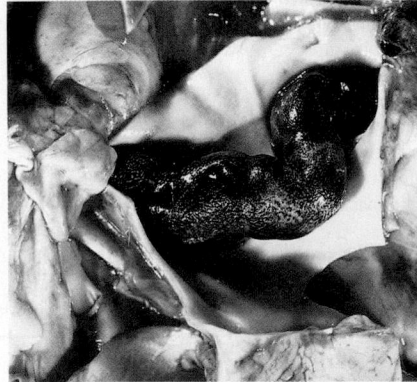

FIG. 27.11 Large embolus from the femoral vein lying in the main left and right pulmonary arteries. (From the teaching collection of the Department of Pathology, University of Texas Southwestern Medical School, Dallas, TX. In Kumar V, Abbas AK, Aster JC, Fausto N, eds: *Robbins and Cotran pathologic basis of disease,* ed 8, Philadelphia, 2010, Saunders.)

VASCULAR LUNG DISORDERS

PULMONARY EDEMA

Pulmonary edema is an abnormal accumulation of fluid in the alveoli and interstitial spaces of the lungs. It is a complication of various heart and lung diseases (Table 27.24). In severe cases, pulmonary edema can be a life-threatening medical emergency. The most common cause of pulmonary edema is left-sided HF. (HF is discussed in Chapter 34.)

PULMONARY EMBOLISM

Etiology and Pathophysiology

Pulmonary embolism (PE) is the blockage of 1 or more pulmonary arteries by a thrombus, fat or air embolus, or tumor tissue. The word *embolus* derives from a Greek word meaning "plug" or "stopper." *Emboli* are mobile clots that generally do not stop moving until they lodge at a narrowed part of the circulatory system. A PE consists of material that gains access to the venous system and then to the pulmonary circulation. The embolus travels with blood flow through ever-smaller blood vessels until it lodges and obstructs perfusion of the alveoli (Fig. 27.11). The lower lobes of the lung are most often affected.

Most PEs arise from deep vein thrombosis (DVT) in the deep veins of the legs. *Venous thromboembolism (VTE)* is the preferred term to describe the spectrum of pathologic conditions from DVT to PE (see Table 37.7). Other sites of origin of PE include femoral or iliac veins, right side of the heart (atrial fibrillation), and pelvic veins (especially after surgery or childbirth). Upper extremity DVT sometimes occurs in the presence of central venous catheters or arterial lines. These cases may resolve with the removal of the catheter. A *saddle embolus* refers to a large thrombus lodged at an arterial bifurcation.

Less common causes include fat emboli (from fractured long bones), air emboli (from improperly administered IV therapy), bacterial vegetation on heart valves, amniotic fluid, and cancer. Risk factors for PE include immobility or reduced mobility, surgery within the last 3 months (especially pelvic and lower extremity surgery), history of VTE, cancer, obesity, oral contraceptives, hormone therapy, cigarette smoking, prolonged air travel, HF, pregnancy, and clotting disorders.

Clinical Manifestations

The signs and symptoms of PE are varied and nonspecific, making diagnosis difficult. Manifestations depend on the type, size, and extent of emboli. Small emboli may go undetected or cause vague, transient symptoms. Symptoms may begin slowly or appear suddenly. Dyspnea is the most common presenting symptom, occurring in 85% of patients with PE. Mild to moderate hypoxemia may occur. Other manifestations include tachypnea, cough, chest pain, hemoptysis, crackles, wheezing, fever, accentuation of pulmonic heart sound, tachycardia, and syncope. Massive PE may cause a sudden change in mental status, hypotension, and feelings of impending doom.

Complications

About 10% of patients with massive PE die within the first hour. Treatment with anticoagulants significantly reduces mortality.

Complications include pulmonary infarction and pulmonary hypertension. *Pulmonary infarction* (death of lung tissue) is most likely when there is: (1) occlusion of a large or medium-sized pulmonary vessel (more than 2 mm in diameter), (2) insufficient collateral blood flow from the bronchial circulation, or (3) preexisting lung disease. Infarction results in alveolar necrosis and hemorrhage. Sometimes the necrotic tissue becomes infected and an abscess may develop. Concomitant pleural effusion is frequent.

Pulmonary hypertension results from hypoxemia or from involvement of more than 50% of the area of the normal pulmonary bed. As a single event, a PE rarely causes pulmonary hypertension. Recurrent PEs gradually reduce capillary bed blood flow and eventually cause pulmonary hypertension. Dilation and hypertrophy of the right ventricle can develop due to pulmonary hypertension. Depending on the degree of pulmonary hypertension and how quickly it develops, outcomes can vary, with some patients dying within months of the diagnosis and others living for decades.

Diagnostic Studies

D-dimer is a laboratory test that measures the amount of cross-linked fibrin fragments. These fragments are the result of clot degradation and are rarely found in healthy people. The disadvantage of D-dimer testing is that it is neither specific (many other conditions cause elevation) nor sensitive, because up to 50% of patients with a small PE have normal results. Patients with suspected PE and an elevated D-dimer level but normal venous ultrasound may need a spiral CT or lung scan.

A *spiral (helical) CT scan* (also known as CT angiography or CTA) is the most common test to diagnose PE. An IV injection of contrast media is needed to view the pulmonary blood vessels. The scanner continuously rotates around the patient while obtaining views (slices) of the pulmonary vasculature. This allows visualization of all anatomic regions of the lungs. Computer software reconstructs the data to give a 3-dimensional picture and assist in seeing PEs.

If a patient cannot have contrast media, a ventilation-perfusion (V/Q) scan is done. The V/Q scan has 2 parts. It is most accurate when both are done:

1. *Perfusion scanning* involves IV injection of a radioisotope. A scanning device images the pulmonary circulation.
2. *Ventilation scanning* involves inhalation of a radioactive gas, such as xenon. Scanning reflects the distribution of gas through the lung. The ventilation portion requires the patient's cooperation. It may not be possible to perform in the critically ill patient, especially if the patient is intubated.

ABG analysis is important but not diagnostic. The PaO_2 may be low because of inadequate oxygenation from occluded pulmonary vasculature preventing matching of perfusion to ventilation. The pH is often normal unless respiratory alkalosis develops because of prolonged hyperventilation or to compensate for lactic acidosis caused by shock. Abnormal findings may be seen on a chest x-ray (atelectasis, pleural effusion) and ECG (ST segment and T wave changes), but they are not diagnostic for PE. Serum troponin levels and b-type natriuretic peptide (BNP) levels are often increased but not diagnostic.

Interprofessional Care

To reduce mortality risk, treatment is started as soon as PE is suspected (Table 27.25). The goals are to (1) provide adequate tissue perfusion and respiratory function, (2) prevent further growth or extension of thrombi in the lower extremities, (3) prevent embolization from the upper or lower extremities to the pulmonary vascular system, and (4) prevent further recurrence of PE.

TABLE 27.25 Interprofessional Care

Acute Pulmonary Embolism

Diagnostic Assessment
- History and physical examination
- Chest x-ray
- Continuous ECG monitoring
- Arterial blood gases
- Spiral (helical) CT scan
- Ventilation-perfusion (V/Q) lung scan
- D-dimer level
- Troponin level, b-natriuretic peptide level

Management
- Supplemental O_2, intubation if needed
- Monitor hemoglobin, assess patient for bleeding
- Monitor activated partial thromboplastin time and international normalized ratio levels
- Balance activity and rest
- Inferior vena cava filter
- Pulmonary embolectomy in life-threatening situation

Drug Therapy
- Fibrinolytic agent
- Unfractionated heparin IV
- Low-molecular-weight heparin (e.g., enoxaparin [Lovenox])
- Warfarin (Coumadin) for long-term therapy
- Analgesia

Immediate assessment should focus on the patient's cardiopulmonary status, which can vary according to the size and location of the PE. O_2 should be given by mask or cannula when hypoxemia is present. The concentration of FIO_2 is titrated based on ABG analysis. In some situations, endotracheal intubation and mechanical ventilation are needed to maintain adequate oxygenation and ventilation. Respiratory measures, including turning, coughing, deep breathing, and incentive spirometry, are important to help prevent or treat atelectasis. If manifestations of shock are present, IV fluids and vasopressor agents are given as needed to support circulation (see Chapter 66). If HF is present, diuretics are used (see Chapter 34). Pain from pleural irritation or reduced coronary blood flow is treated with opioids.

Drug Therapy. Immediate anticoagulation is required for patients with PE. Subcutaneous administration of low-molecular-weight heparin (LMWH) (e.g., enoxaparin [Lovenox]) or fragmin [Dalteparin] or fondaparinux) is the recommended treatment for patients with acute PE. LMWH is safer and more effective than unfractionated heparin.[33] Advantages of LMWH over unfractionated heparin include greater bioavailability, subcutaneous administration, once daily dosing, and longer duration of therapeutic effect. Monitoring the aPTT is not necessary or useful with LMWH. Unfractionated IV heparin can be as effective but is hard to titrate to therapeutic levels.

Warfarin (Coumadin), an oral anticoagulant, should also be started at the time of diagnosis.[34] Warfarin should be given for at least 3 months and then reevaluated. Alternatives to warfarin include apixaban (Eliquis), dabigatran (Pradaxa), and edoxaban (Savaysa). Anticoagulant therapy may be contraindicated if the patient has complicating factors, such as liver problems causing changes in the clotting, overt bleeding, a history of hemorrhagic stroke, heparin-induced thrombocytopenia (HIT), or other blood dyscrasias.

Some HCPs use direct thrombin inhibitors (see Table 37.10) in the treatment of PE. Similarly, fibrinolytic agents, such as tissue plasminogen activator (tPA) or alteplase (Activase), may help dissolve the PE and the source of the thrombus in the pelvis or deep leg veins, thereby decreasing the risk for recurrent emboli. Fibrinolytic therapy is discussed in Chapter 33.

Surgical Therapy. Hemodynamically unstable patients with massive PE in whom thrombolytic therapy is contraindicated may be candidates for pulmonary embolectomy. Embolectomy, the removal of emboli, can be achieved through a diagnostic imaging (vascular catheter) or surgical approach. It can help decrease right ventricular afterload. Surgical outcomes have improved in recent years, in part due to rapid diagnosis and enhanced surgical procedures.

Percutaneous catheter embolectomy or endovascular ultrasound delivered thrombolysis are newer, moderately invasive procedures for PE. In patients who are at high risk and patients for whom anticoagulation is contraindicated, an inferior vena cava (IVC) filter may be the treatment of choice. This device, inserted percutaneously through the femoral vein, is placed at the level of the renal veins in the inferior vena cava. Once inserted, the filter expands and prevents migration of large clots into the pulmonary system. Complications associated with this device are rare but include misplacement, migration, and perforation.

❖ **NURSING MANAGEMENT: PULMONARY EMBOLISM**

Prevention of PE begins with prevention of DVT. Nursing measures aimed at prevention of PE are similar to those for prophylaxis of VTE (see Chapter 37). These include the use of intermittent pneumatic compression devices, early ambulation, and anticoagulant medications.

The prognosis of a patient with PE is good if therapy is started immediately. Keep the patient on bed rest in a semi-Fowler's position to facilitate breathing. Assess the patient's cardiopulmonary status with careful monitoring of vital signs, cardiac rhythm, pulse oximetry, ABGs, and lung sounds. Apply O_2 therapy as ordered. Maintain a patent IV line for medications and fluid therapy. Monitor laboratory results to ensure therapeutic ranges of INR (for warfarin) and aPTT (for IV heparin). Monitor platelet counts for thrombocytopenia and the development of HIT. Observe the patient for complications of anticoagulant and fibrinolytic therapy (e.g., bleeding, hematomas, bruising). Provide appropriate interventions related to immobility and fall precautions once the patient is permitted out of bed.

The patient may be anxious because of pain, inability to breathe, and fear of death. Carefully explain the situation and the medications. Provide emotional support and reassurance to help relieve the patient's anxiety.

Patient teaching about long-term anticoagulant therapy is essential. Anticoagulant therapy continues for at least 3 months. Patients with large or recurrent emboli may be treated indefinitely with anticoagulants. INR levels are drawn at intervals and warfarin dosage is adjusted. Some patients are monitored by nurses in an anticoagulation clinic.

Long-term management of PE is similar to that for the patient with VTE (see discussion of VTE in Chapter 37). Discharge planning is aimed at preventing worsening of the condition and avoiding complications and recurrence. Reinforce the need for the patient to return to the HCP for regular follow-up examinations.

PULMONARY HYPERTENSION

Pulmonary hypertension is characterized by elevated pulmonary artery pressure from an increase in resistance to blood flow through the pulmonary circulation. Normally the pulmonary circulation is characterized by low resistance and low pressure. In pulmonary hypertension the pulmonary pressures are high, with the mean pulmonary artery pressure greater than 25 mm Hg at rest (normal is 12 to 16 mm Hg) or greater than 30 mm Hg with exercise.

The World Health Organization (WHO) has identified 5 classes of pulmonary hypertension.[35] Each group is based on cause of the disorder.

Group 1: Attributed to medication, specific diseases, genetic (inherited) link, or idiopathic

Group 2: Related to left-sided HF

Group 3: Related to the lungs and hypoxemia

Group 4: Related to the cardiovascular system and thromboembolic occlusion

Group 5: Multifactorial (and often unclear) origins with hematologic or metabolic involvement

Pulmonary hypertension can occur as a primary disease *(idiopathic pulmonary arterial hypertension)* or as a secondary complication of a respiratory, heart, autoimmune, liver, or connective tissue disorder *(secondary pulmonary arterial hypertension).*

PATHOPHYSIOLOGY MAP

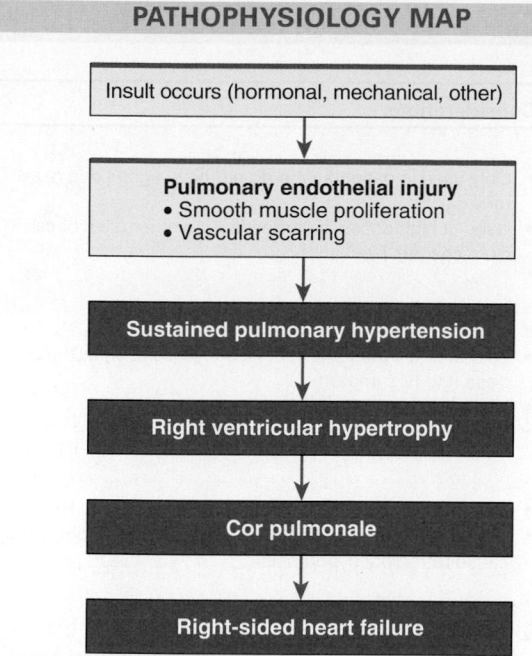

FIG. 27.12 Pathogenesis of pulmonary hypertension and cor pulmonale.

IDIOPATHIC PULMONARY ARTERIAL HYPERTENSION

Idiopathic pulmonary arterial hypertension (IPAH) is pulmonary hypertension that occurs without an apparent cause. It was previously known as *primary pulmonary hypertension* (PPH). If untreated, IPAH can rapidly progress, causing right-sided HF and death within a few years. Although new drug therapy has greatly improved survival, the disease is not curable.

Etiology and Pathophysiology

The cause of IPAH is unknown. It is related to connective tissue diseases, cirrhosis, and HIV. The exact relationship between these disorders and IPAH is unclear. Similarly, the pathophysiology of IPAH is poorly understood. We think that some type of insult (e.g., hormonal, mechanical) to the pulmonary endothelium may occur, causing a cascade of events leading to vascular scarring, endothelial dysfunction, and smooth muscle proliferation (Fig. 27.12). IPAH affects females more than males.

Clinical Manifestations and Diagnostic Studies

The classic symptoms are dyspnea on exertion and fatigue. Exertional chest pain, dizziness, and syncope may occur. These are related to the inability of cardiac output to increase in response to increased O_2 demand. Abnormal heart sounds may be heard, including an S_3. Eventually, as the disease progresses, dyspnea occurs at rest. Pulmonary hypertension increases the workload of the right ventricle and causes right ventricular hypertrophy (a condition called *cor pulmonale*) and eventually HF.

Right-sided cardiac catheterization is the definitive test to diagnose any type of pulmonary hypertension. It gives an accurate measurement of pulmonary artery pressures, cardiac output, and pulmonary vascular resistance. Confirmation of IPAH requires a thorough workup to exclude conditions that may cause secondary pulmonary hypertension. Diagnostic evaluation often includes ECG, chest x-ray, pulmonary function tests, echocardiogram, and CT scan.

The mean time between onset of symptoms and the diagnosis is about 2 years. By the time patients become symptomatic, the disease is already in the advanced stages and the pulmonary artery pressure is 2-3 times normal values.

❖ Interprofessional and Nursing Care

Early recognition is essential to interrupt the vicious cycle responsible for progression of the disease. Encourage patients to report unexplained shortness of breath, syncope, chest discomfort, and edema of the feet and ankles to their HCP.

Although IPAH has no cure, treatment can relieve symptoms, improve quality of life, and prolong life. Drug therapy consists of agents that promote vasodilation of the pulmonary blood vessels, reduce right ventricular overload, and reverse remodeling (Table 27.26). Diuretics are used to manage peripheral edema. Anticoagulants are beneficial in pulmonary complications related to thrombus formation. Because hypoxia is a potent pulmonary vasoconstrictor, low-flow O_2 gives symptomatic relief. The goal is to keep O_2 saturation 90% or greater.

Surgical interventions include pulmonary thromboendarterectomy (PTE), in which clots are removed from the pulmonary arteries. It is a technically demanding procedure and is done only at certain centers. Atrial septostomy (AS) is a palliative procedure that involves the creation of an intraatrial right-to-left shunt to decompress the right ventricle. It is used for a select group of patients awaiting lung transplantation. Lung transplantation is an option for patients who do not respond to drug therapy and progress to severe right-sided HF. Recurrence of the disease has not been reported in persons who had a transplant.

SECONDARY PULMONARY ARTERIAL HYPERTENSION

Secondary pulmonary arterial hypertension (SPAH) occurs when another disease causes a chronic increase in pulmonary artery pressures. The specific primary disease pathology can cause anatomic or vascular changes that cause the pulmonary hypertension. SPAH can develop due to parenchymal lung disease, left ventricular dysfunction, intracardiac shunts, chronic PE, or systemic connective tissue disease.

The symptoms can reflect the underlying disease, but some are directly attributable to SPAH, including dyspnea, fatigue, lethargy, and chest pain. The initial physical findings can include right ventricular hypertrophy and signs of right-sided HF (increased pulmonic heart sound, S_4 heart sound, peripheral edema, hepatomegaly).

Diagnosis of SPAH is like that of IPAH. Treatment of SPAH consists of treating the underlying primary disorder. When irreversible pulmonary vascular damage has occurred, therapies used for IPAH are started. A PTE may offer a cure for patients with chronic pulmonary hypertension caused by PE.

COR PULMONALE

Cor pulmonale is enlargement of the right ventricle caused by a primary disorder of the respiratory system. Almost any disorder that affects the respiratory system can cause cor pulmonale. The most common cause is COPD. Pulmonary hypertension is

TABLE 27.26 Drug Therapy

Pulmonary Hypertension

Drug	Mechanism of Action	Considerations
Calcium Channel Blockers diltiazem (Cardizem, Cardizem LA, Cartia XT, Tiazac) nifedipine (Procardia)	• Act on vascular smooth muscle, causing dilation • Lower pulmonary artery pressure	• Only used in patients who do not have right-sided heart failure (HF) • Used at high doses in comparison to other uses of calcium channel blockers
Endothelin Receptor Antagonists ambrisentan (Letairis) bosentan (Tracleer) macitentan (Opsumit)	• Binds to endothelin-1 receptors and blocks the constriction of pulmonary arteries • Promotes relaxation of pulmonary arteries and decrease pulmonary artery pressure	• Given orally • For patients with New York Heart Association (NYHA) class II to IV symptoms • Hepatotoxic • Monitor liver function tests monthly
Phosphodiesterase (Type 5) Enzyme Inhibitors sildenafil (Revatio) tadalafil (Adcirca)	• Promote selective smooth muscle relaxation in lung vasculature	• Given orally • Contraindicated in patients taking nitroglycerin, since may cause refractory hypotension
Vasodilators (Inhaled) iloprost (Ventavis) treprostinil (inhaled) (Tyvaso)	• Synthetic analogs of prostacyclin (PGI$_2$) • Dilate systemic and pulmonary arterial vasculature	• For patients with NYHA class III or IV HF • Given 6–9 times a day using a disk inserted into a nebulizer • Can cause orthostatic hypotension. Do not give to patients with systolic BP <85 mm Hg.
Vasodilators (Parenteral) adenosine (Adenocard) epoprostenol (Flolan, Veletri) treprostinil (Remodulin)	• Prostacyclin analog • Promote pulmonary vasodilation and reduce pulmonary vascular resistance	• Given IV to patients who do not respond to calcium channel blockers or have NYHA class III or IV right-sided HF • Given by continuous IV (central line) or continuous subcutaneous route • Half-life of epoprostenol is short. Potential clinical deterioration from abrupt withdrawal if infusion disrupted

usually a preexisting condition in the person with cor pulmonale. Overt HF may be present. Fig. 27.12 outlines the cause and pathogenesis of pulmonary hypertension and cor pulmonale.

Clinical Manifestations and Diagnostic Studies

Manifestations are subtle and often masked by symptoms of the pulmonary condition. Common symptoms include exertional dyspnea, tachypnea, cough, and fatigue. Physical signs include evidence of right ventricular hypertrophy on ECG and an increase in intensity of S$_2$. Chronic hypoxemia leads to polycythemia and increased total blood volume and viscosity of the blood. Polycythemia is often present in cor pulmonale from COPD.

If HF accompanies cor pulmonale, manifestations, including peripheral edema, weight gain, distended neck veins, full, bounding pulse, and enlarged liver, may occur. We use various laboratory tests and imaging studies to confirm the diagnosis of cor pulmonale (Table 27.27).

❖ Interprofessional and Nursing Care

Early identification is essential before changes to the heart occur that may be irreversible. Management is directed at determining the cause and treating the underlying problem (Table 27.27).

Long-term O$_2$ therapy, the mainstay of treatment to correct the hypoxemia, reduces vasoconstriction and pulmonary

TABLE 27.27 Interprofessional Care

Cor Pulmonale

Diagnostic Assessment
- History and physical examination
- Arterial blood gases, SpO$_2$
- Serum and urine electrolytes
- b-Type natriuretic peptide (BNP)
- ECG
- Chest x-ray
- Echocardiography
- CT scan, MRI
- Cardiac catheterization

Management
- O$_2$ therapy
- Low-sodium diet

Drug Therapy
- Bronchodilators
- Diuretics
- Vasodilators (if indicated)
- Calcium channel blockers (if indicated)
- Inotropic agents

hypertension. All other interventions are tailored for each patient. If fluid, electrolyte, and/or acid-base imbalances are present, they must be corrected. Diuretics may help decrease plasma volume and reduce the workload on the heart but must be used with extreme caution. In some cases, decreases in fluid volume from diuresis can worsen heart function. Bronchodilator therapy is needed if the underlying respiratory problem is due to an obstructive disorder.

Other treatments may include vasodilator therapy, calcium channel blockers, anticoagulants, digitalis, and phlebotomy. All have varying degrees of success. Chronic management of cor pulmonale from COPD is like that described for COPD (see Chapter 28).

LUNG TRANSPLANTATION

Lung transplantation has become an important alternative option for patients with end-stage lung disease. Unfortunately, the limiting factor for this therapy is the lack of donors. A variety of pulmonary disorders are potentially treatable with lung transplantation (Table 27.28). Better patient selection criteria, improvements in surgical techniques, enhanced methods of immunosuppression, and excellent postoperative care have resulted in improved survival rates.

Preoperative Care

Patients being considered for lung transplantation need to undergo extensive evaluation. Absolute contraindications for lung transplant include cancer within past 2 years (some types of skin cancer are excluded), chronic active hepatitis B or C, HIV, untreatable advanced dysfunction of another major organ system (e.g., liver or renal failure), current smoker, poor nutritional status, poor rehabilitation potential, and significant psychosocial problems. The patient and family must be able to cope with a complex postoperative regimen (e.g., strict adherence to immunosuppressive therapy, continuous monitoring for early signs of infection, prompt reporting of manifestations of infection). Many transplant centers require preoperative outpatient pulmonary rehabilitation to maximize physical conditioning.

In the United States, the United Network for Organ Sharing (UNOS) is a private, non-profit organization that works with the federal government to manage organ transplantation. UNOS designates recipients of donor lungs based on a lung allocation score (LAS). The LAS helps to prioritize waiting list recipients based on the urgency of need and expected posttransplant survival expectations.

Patients who are accepted as transplant candidates must always carry a pager in case a donor organ becomes available. They must be prepared to be at their transplant center at a moment's notice. Patients may be encouraged to limit their travel within a certain geographic region to facilitate rapid transportation to a transplant center.

TABLE 27.28 Common Indications for Lung Transplantation

- α_1-Antitrypsin deficiency
- Chronic obstructive pulmonary disease (COPD)
- Cystic fibrosis
- Idiopathic pulmonary arterial hypertension
- Idiopathic pulmonary fibrosis

Surgical Procedure

Four types of transplant procedures are available: single-lung transplantation, bilateral lung transplantation, heart-lung transplantation, and transplantation of lobes from a living-related donor.

Single-lung transplantation involves a thoracotomy incision on the side of the chest. The opposite lung is ventilated while the diseased lung is excised and the donor lung implanted. Three anastomoses are done: bronchus, pulmonary artery, and pulmonary veins. In *bilateral lung transplantation,* the incision is made across the sternum and the donor lungs are implanted separately. A median sternotomy incision is used for a *heart-lung transplant* procedure. *Lobar transplantation* from living donors is reserved for those who urgently need transplantation and are unlikely to survive until a donor becomes available. Most of these recipients are patients with cystic fibrosis, and donors are their parents or relatives. Once anastomosis is complete, the lung is gently reinflated, perfusion is reestablished, chest tubes are inserted, and the surgical incision is closed.

Postoperative Care

Early postoperative care often includes ventilatory support, hemodynamic management, IV fluid therapy, immunosuppression, nutritional support, detection of early rejection, and prevention or treatment of complications, including infection. Once hemodynamic stability has been achieved, the patient is often transferred from the ICU to a high-acuity observation or surgical unit. Maintaining accurate fluid balance is vital after surgery.

Lung transplant recipients are at high risk for multiple complications. Infections are the leading cause of death at all time points after lung transplant. Bacterial bronchitis and pneumonia are the most common infections. CMV, fungi, viruses, and mycobacteria are also causative agents. Noninfectious issues may include VTE, diaphragmatic dysfunction, and cancer.

Immunosuppressive therapy usually includes a 3-drug regimen of tacrolimus, mycophenolate mofetil (CellCept), and prednisone. The mechanisms of action of these drugs are discussed in Table 13.17 and Fig. 13.13.) Drug levels are monitored on a regular basis. Lung transplant recipients usually receive higher levels of immunosuppressive therapy than other organ recipients.

Acute rejection is fairly common in lung transplantation. It typically occurs in the first 5 to 10 days after surgery. Signs of rejection include low-grade fever, fatigue, dyspnea, dry cough, and O_2 desaturation. Accurate diagnosis of rejection is by transtracheal biopsy. Treatment consists of high doses of IV corticosteroids for 3 days, followed by high doses of oral prednisone. In patients with persistent or recurrent acute rejection, antilymphocyte therapy may be useful.

Bronchiolitis obliterans (BOS) is a manifestation of chronic rejection in lung transplant patients. BOS is characterized by airflow obstruction that progresses over time. The onset is often subacute, with gradual development of exertional dyspnea, nonproductive cough, wheezing, and/or low-grade fever. Airway obstruction is not responsive to bronchodilators and corticosteroid therapy. Although not proven effective, additional immunosuppressive agents may be used to treat chronic rejection. Because acute rejection is a major risk factor for BOS, preventing acute rejection is key to decreasing the incidence of chronic rejection.

Before discharge, the patient needs to be able to perform self-care activities, including medication management and activities of daily living, and to know when to call the transplant team. Patients are taught pulmonary clearance measures, including aerosolized bronchodilators, chest physiotherapy, and deep-breathing and coughing techniques, to help minimize complications. Home spirometry is useful in monitoring trends in lung function. Teach patients to keep medication logs, laboratory results, and spirometry records. Patients are placed in an outpatient rehabilitation program to improve physical endurance.

After discharge, the transplant team follows patients for transplant-related issues. Patients return to their HCP for health maintenance and routine illnesses. As transplant procedures become more frequent, transplant patients will return to hospitals for other routine procedures. Coordination of care among the transplant team, inpatient team, and primary care team is essential for ongoing successful management of these patients. (Organ transplantation, histocompatibility, rejection, and immunosuppressive therapy are discussed in Chapter 13.)

CASE STUDY

Pneumonia and Lung Cancer

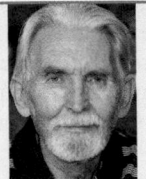

(© iStockphoto/
Thinkstock.)

Patient Profile

J.H. is a 52-yr-old white man who comes to the ED with shortness of breath. He has not seen an HCP for many years.

Subjective Data

- Has a 38 pack-year history of cigarette smoking
- Has had 25-lb weight loss despite a normal appetite in the past few months
- Admits to a "smoker's cough" for the past 2 to 3 years; recently coughing up blood
- Is married and the father of 3 adult children

Objective Data

Physical Examination

- Thin, pale man who looks older than stated age
- Height 6 ft (182.9 cm); weight 135 lb (61.2 kg)
- Intermittently confused and anxious
- Lung auscultation reveals coarse crackles on left side that clear with cough; right side has decreased breath sounds
- Chest wall has limited excursion on right side
- Vital signs: temperature 102.6° F (39.2° C), heart rate 120, respiratory rate 36, BP 98/54; short, shallow respirations

Diagnostic Studies

- Arterial blood gases: pH 7.51, PaO$_2$ 62 mm Hg, PaCO$_2$ 30 mm Hg, HCO$_3^-$ 22 mEq/L, O$_2$ saturation 88% (room air)

- Chest x-ray: consolidation of the right lung, especially in the base with mass around right bronchus; pleural effusion on the right side
- Bronchoscopy with biopsy of mass: small cell lung cancer

Interprofessional Care

- Diagnosis: pneumonia with small cell lung cancer
- Follow-up with patient and family to consider treatment options

Discussion Questions

1. How would you classify J.H.'s pneumonia? Why is this important?
2. What is your analysis of J.H.'s arterial blood gas results?
3. *Priority Decision:* Based on the assessment data presented, what are the priority nursing diagnoses? Are there any collaborative problems?
4. *Priority Decision:* What are the priority nursing interventions for J.H.?
5. *Collaboration:* Identify activities that can be delegated to unlicensed assistive personnel (UAP).
6. *Patient-Centered Care:* You are planning a meeting with J.H. and his family to discuss their needs. The HCP tells you that J.H. is terminally ill. Who will you include in this meeting?
7. *Evidence-Based Practice:* J.H.'s children tell you that they are worried they will get lung cancer, since their father has it and they grew up around his secondhand smoke. They want to know what kind of screening is available for them. How will you respond?
- What is the goal if radiation therapy is used for J.H.?
- *Patient-Centered Care:* What issues should be addressed in your teaching of J.H. and his wife as you prepare him for discharge and care at home?

Answers available at *http://evolve.elsevier.com/Lewis/medsurg.*

BRIDGE TO NCLEX EXAMINATION

The number of the question corresponds to the same-numbered outcome at the beginning of the chapter.

1. When caring for a patient with acute bronchitis, the nurse will *prioritize* interventions by
   a. auscultating lung sounds.
   b. encouraging fluid restriction.
   c. administering antibiotic therapy.
   d. teaching the patient to avoid cough suppressants.

2. Which patients have the greatest risk for aspiration pneumonia? *(select all that apply)*
   a. Patient with seizures
   b. Patient with head injury
   c. Patient who had thoracic surgery
   d. Patient who had a myocardial infarction
   e. Patient who is receiving nasogastric tube feeding

3. An appropriate nursing intervention to assist a patient with pneumonia manage thick secretions and fatigue would be to
   a. perform postural drainage every hour.
   b. provide analgesics as ordered to promote patient comfort.
   c. administer O$_2$ as prescribed to maintain optimal O$_2$ levels.
   d. teach the patient how to cough effectively and expectorate secretions.

4. A patient with TB has been admitted to the hospital and is placed on airborne precautions and in an isolation room. What should the nurse teach the patient? *(select all that apply)*
   a. Expect routine TB testing to evaluate the infection.
   b. No visitors will be allowed while in airborne isolation.
   c. Adherence to precautions includes coughing into a paper tissue.
   d. Take all medications for full length of time to prevent multidrug-resistant TB.
   e. Wear a standard isolation mask if leaving the airborne infection isolation room.

5. A patient has been receiving high-dose corticosteroids and broad-spectrum antibiotics for treatment of an infection after a traumatic injury. The nurse plans care for the patient knowing that the patient is most susceptible to
   a. candidiasis.
   b. cryptococcosis.
   c. histoplasmosis.
   d. coccidioidomycosis.

6. When caring for a patient with a lung abscess, what is the nurse's *priority* intervention?
   a. Postural drainage
   b. Antibiotic administration
   c. Obtaining a sputum specimen
   d. Patient teaching about home care

7. You are caring for patients exposed to a chlorine leak from a local factory. The nurse would closely monitor these patients for
   a. pulmonary edema.
   b. anaphylactic shock.
   c. respiratory alkalosis.
   d. acute tubular necrosis.

8. The nurse receives an order for a patient with lung cancer to receive influenza vaccine and pneumococcal vaccines. The nurse will
   a. call the health care provider to question the order.
   b. give both vaccines at the same time in different arms.
   c. give the pneumococcal vaccine and obtain a nasal influenza vaccine.
   d. give the flu shot and tell the patient to come back in 1 week to have the pneumococcal vaccine.

9. The nurse identifies a flail chest in a trauma patient when
   a. multiple rib fractures are determined by x-ray.
   b. a tracheal deviation to the unaffected side is present.
   c. paradoxical chest movement occurs during respiration.
   d. there is decreased movement of the involved chest wall.

10. The nurse notes tidaling of the water level in the water-seal chamber in a patient with closed chest tube drainage. The nurse should
    a. continue to monitor the patient.
    b. check all connections for a leak in the system.
    c. lower the drainage collector further from the chest.
    d. clamp the tubing at a distal point away from the patient.

11. After a pneumonectomy, an appropriate nursing intervention is
    a. monitoring chest tube drainage and functioning.
    b. positioning the patient on the unaffected side or back.
    c. doing range-of-motion exercises on the affected upper limb.
    d. auscultating frequently for lung sounds on the affected side.

12. A *priority* nursing intervention for a patient who has just undergone a chemical pleurodesis for recurrent pleural effusion is
    a. giving ordered analgesia.
    b. monitoring chest tube drainage.
    c. sending pleural fluid for laboratory analysis.
    d. monitoring the patient's level of consciousness.

13. When planning care for a patient at risk for pulmonary embolism, the nurse *prioritizes*
    a. maintaining the patient on bed rest.
    b. using intermittent pneumatic compression devices.
    c. encouraging the patient to cough and deep breathe.
    d. teaching the patient how to use the incentive spirometer.

14. Which statement(s) describe(s) the management of a patient following lung transplantation (*select all that apply*)?
    a. High doses of O_2 are administered around the clock.
    b. Using a home spirometer will help to monitor lung function.
    c. Immunosuppressant therapy usually involves a 3-drug regimen.
    d. Most patients have an acute rejection episode within the first 2 days.
    e. A lung biopsy is done using a transtracheal method if rejection is suspected.

1. a, 2. a, b, e, 3. d, 4. c, d, e, 5. a, 6. b, 7. a, 8. b, 9. c, 10. a, 11. c, 12. a, 13. b, 14. b, c, e

For rationales to these answers and even more NCLEX review questions, visit *http://evolve.elsevier.com/Lewis/medsurg*.

EVOLVE WEBSITE/RESOURCES LIST

http://evolve.elsevier.com/Lewis/medsurg
Review Questions (Online Only)
Key Points
Answer Keys for Questions
- Rationales for Bridge to NCLEX Examination Questions
- Answer Guidelines for Case Study on p. 538
Student Case Studies
- Patient With Lung Cancer
- Patient With Pulmonary Embolism and Respiratory Failure
Nursing Care Plans
- eNursing Care Plan 27.1: Patient With Pneumonia
- eNursing Care Plan 27.2: Patient After Thoracotomy
Conceptual Care Map Creator
Audio Glossary
Content Updates

REFERENCES

1. Centers for Disease Control and Prevention: *Deaths and mortality*. Retrieved from *www.cdc.gov/nchs/fastats/deaths.htm*.
*2. Harris AM, Hicks LA, Qaseem A: Appropriate antibiotic use for acute respiratory tract infection in adults: Advice for high-value care from the American College of Physicians and the CDC, *Ann Intern Med* 164:425, 2016.
*3. Centers for Disease Control and Prevention: Diphtheria, tetanus and pertussis vaccine recommendations. Retrieved from *www.cdc.gov/vaccines/vpd/dtap-tdap-td/hcp/recommendations.html*.
4. Centers for Disease Control and Prevention: Pertussis: diagnosis conformation. Retrieved from *www.cdc.gov/pertussis/clinical/diagnostic-testing/diagnosis-confirmation.html*.
5. Centers for Disease Control and Prevention: Leading causes of death. Retrieved from *www.cdc.gov/nchs/fastats/leading-causes-of-death.htm*.
6. Cunha BA: Hospital-acquired pneumonia and ventilator-associated pneumonia. Retrieved from *www.emedicine.medscape.com/article/234753-overview*.

7. Skidmore BD, Arteaga VA. Necrotizing pneumonia: diagnosis and treatment options, *Southwest J Pulm Crit Care* 15:274, 2017.

*8. Ljungman P, Lazarus HM: Optimal management approach to prevent cytomegalovirus infection in patients undergoing allogeneic hematopoietic cell transplantation, *The Hematologist* 15:4, 2018.

*9. Shen KR, Bribriesco A, Crabtree T, et al: The American Association for Thoracic Surgery consensus guidelines for the management of empyema, *J Cardiovasc Thorac Surg* 153:e129, 2016.

*10. Khan F, Martin-Loeches I: The significance of clinical scores and biological markers in disease severity, mortality prediction, and justifying hospital admissions in patients with community acquired pneumonia, *Community Acquir Infect* 3:36, 2016.

11. Mosenifar, Z: Viral pneumonia medication. Retrieved from *www.emedicine.medscape.com/article/300455-medication*.

12. Ruscic KJ, Grabitz SD, Rudolph MI, et al: Prevention of respiratory complications of the surgical patient, *Curr Opin Anaesthesiol* 30:399, 2017.

13. World Health Organization: Tuberculosis. Retrieved from *www.euro.who.int/en/health-topics/communicable-diseases/tuberculosis/tuberculosis-read-more*.

*14. CDC: Burden of TB in the United States. Retrieved from *www.cdc.gov/features/burden-tb-us/index.html*.

15. Lange C, Chesov D, Hevckendorf J, et al: Drug-resistant tuberculosis: an update on disease burden, diagnosis and treatment, *Respirology* 23:656, 2018.

16. Sloan DJ, Lewis JM: Management of multidrug resistant TB: Novel treatments and their expansion to low resource settings, *T Roy Soc Trop Med Hyg* 3:163, 2016.

17. Sharma R, Gaillard F: Ghon lesion. Retrieved from *www.radiopaedia.org/articles/ghon-lesion*.

18. Centers for Disease Control and Prevention: Tuberculin skin testing. Retrieved from *www.cdc.gov/tb/publications/factsheets/testing/skintesting.htm*.

*19. Lewinsohn DM, Leonard MK, LoBue PA, et al: Official American Thoracic Society/Infectious Diseases Society of America/CDC clinical practice guidelines: Diagnosis of tuberculosis in adults and children, *Clin Infect Dis* 64:111, 2017.

*20. World Health Organization Guidelines for treatment of drug-susceptible tuberculosis and patient care (2017 update). Retrieved from *www.who.int/tb/publications/2017/dstb_guidance_2017/en/*.

*21. Reyes-Montes MDR, Perez-Huitron MA, Ocana-Monroy JL, et al: The habitat of *Coccidioides* spp. and the role of animals as reservoirs and disseminators in nature, *BMC Infect Dis* 16:550, 2016.

22. Sethi S: Lung abscess. Retrieved from *www.merckmanuals.com/en-ca/professional/pulmonary-disorders/lung-abscess/lung-abscess*.

23. American Cancer Society: Key statistics for lung cancer. Retrieved from *www.cancer.org/cancer/non-small-cell-lung-cancer/about/key-statistics.html*.

24. American Lung Association: Lung cancer fact sheet. Retrieved from *www.lung.org/lung-health-and-diseases/lung-disease-lookup/lung-cancer/resource-library/lung-cancer-fact-sheet.html*.

25. National Cancer Institute: Harms of cigarette smoking and health benefits of quitting. Retrieved from *www.cancer.gov/about-cancer/causes-prevention/risk/tobacco/cessation-fact-sheet*.

26. Chandra AM: Cigarette smoking is the main cause of lung cancer. Retrieved from *www.healthxchange.sg/cancer/lung-cancer/cigarette-smoking-main-cause-lung-cancer*.

27. Lung Cancer.org: Types and staging of lung cancer. Retrieved from *www.lungcancer.org/find_information/publications/163-lung_cancer_101/268-types_and_staging*.

*28. Mazzone PJ, Silvestri GA, Patel S, et al: Screening for lung cancer: chest guideline and expert panel report, *Chest* 153:954, 2018.

*29. American Cancer Society: Lung cancer screening guidelines. Retrieved from *www.cancer.org/health-care-professionals/american-cancer-society-prevention-early-detection-guidelines/lung-cancer-screening-guidelines.html*.

*30. Groen HJM, Dingemans AMC, Belderbos J, et al: Prophylactic cranial irradiation versus observation in radically treated stage III non-small cell lung cancer, *J Clin Oncol* 35:s8502, 2017.

31. Simoglou C, Gymnopoulos D: Video-assisted thoracoscopic surgery, *Scientific Chronicles* 22:150, 2017.

32. Lee J: Overview of interstitial lung disease. Retrieved from *www.merckmanuals.com/en-ca/professional/pulmonary-disorders/interstitial-lung-diseases/overview-of-interstitial-lung-disease*.

33. Ryan J: Pulmonary embolism: New treatments for an old problem, *Emerg Medicine* 8:87, 2016.

34. Ouellette DR: Pulmonary embolism treatment and management. Retrieved from *https://emedicine.medscape.com/article/300901-treatment#d9*.

35. Pulmonary Hypertension Association: Types of pulmonary hypertension. Retrieved from *https://phassociation.org/patients/aboutph/types-of-ph/*.

*Evidence-based information for clinical practice.

28

Obstructive Pulmonary Diseases

Eugene Mondor

Kindness is a breath of fresh air to someone who feels they are suffocating.

Franklin D. Roosevelt

http://evolve.elsevier.com/Lewis/medsurg/

CENCEPTUAL FOCUS

Fatigue	Gas Exchange	Self-Management
Functional Ability	Infection	

LEARNING OUTCOMES

1. Describe the etiology, pathophysiology, and clinical manifestations of asthma.
2. Explain the difference between an acute asthma exacerbation and status asthmaticus.
3. Describe the interprofessional and nursing management of the patient with asthma.
4. Identify the classifications of drugs used in the treatment of asthma and chronic obstructive pulmonary disease (COPD).
5. Describe the etiology, pathophysiology, clinical manifestations, and interprofessional care of the patient with COPD.
6. Relate the indications for O_2 therapy, methods of delivery, and complications of O_2 administration.
7. Explain the nursing management of the patient with COPD.
8. Describe the pathophysiology, clinical manifestations, and interprofessional and nursing management of the patient with cystic fibrosis.
9. Describe the pathophysiology, clinical manifestations, and interprofessional and nursing management of the patient with bronchiectasis.

KEY TERMS

α_1-antitrypsin deficiency (AATD), p. 561
asthma, p. 542
bronchiectasis, p. 580
chest physiotherapy (CPT), p. 571
chronic bronchitis, p. 560

chronic obstructive pulmonary disease (COPD), p. 560
cor pulmonale, p. 563
cystic fibrosis (CF), p. 576
emphysema, p. 560

O_2 toxicity, p. 567
postural drainage, p. 571
pursed-lip breathing (PLB), p. 570
status asthmaticus, p. 545

Imagine needing to consciously think about every breath that you take each minute, each hour, and every day of your life. You are tired and weak and have not been sleeping well. Your appetite is poor. The stress of living with these symptoms makes you feel anxious and depressed. You have been absent from work and are having some financial problems. Many people with obstructive lung disease have this experience.

The obstructive pulmonary diseases are the most common chronic lung diseases. They are characterized by increased resistance to airflow because of airway obstruction or airway narrowing. There are 4 major types of obstructive lung disease: asthma, chronic obstructive pulmonary disease (COPD), cystic fibrosis (CF), and bronchiectasis.

Asthma causes inflammation with variable degrees of airflow obstruction. Between acute exacerbations, or attacks, the patient with asthma is often asymptomatic with normal lung function. On the other hand, in COPD there is progressive limitation in airflow that is not fully reversible. The limitation in expiratory airflow in COPD is generally more constant day-to-day and worsens over time. Emphysema and chronic bronchitis are 2 related respiratory conditions often responsible for COPD.[1]

The pathophysiology of asthma and the response to therapy differs from COPD. However, patients with asthma who have less responsive airflow obstruction are hard to tell from COPD patients. In fact, some patients share features of both asthma and COPD. This is known as asthma-COPD overlap syndrome.[2] It is characterized by significantly worse respiratory signs and symptoms, an increased number of hospitalizations, and a much poorer quality of life than asthma or COPD alone.[3]

CF is an inherited genetic disorder. It produces airway obstruction because of changes in exocrine glandular secretions, resulting in increased mucus production. There are about 30,000 people in the United States living with CF, with 52.7% being adults.[4]

Bronchiectasis is characterized by dilated bronchioles, making it hard to clear secretions. It most often results from poorly treated or untreated pulmonary infections, immune system problems, or genetic factors.

ASTHMA

Asthma is a heterogenous disease characterized by bronchial hyperreactivity with reversible expiratory airflow limitation. Signs and symptoms can be variable. They often include episodes of wheezing, breathlessness, chest tightness, and cough, particularly at night or in the early morning. These episodes are associated with widespread, variable airflow obstruction that is usually reversible, either spontaneously or with treatment. The clinical course of asthma is unpredictable, ranging from periods of adequate control to attacks with poor control of symptoms.

Asthma affects around 20.4 million adult Americans.[5] It is a major public health concern, with more than 1.7 million emergency department (ED) visits each year.[5] After a long period of an increasing incidence of asthma, the mortality and use of health care services for asthma have decreased over the past 10 years. Unfortunately, more than 3600 people still die each year from asthma.[5]

Risk Factors for Asthma and Triggers of Asthma Attacks

Risk factors for asthma and triggers of asthma attacks can be related to the patient (e.g., genetic factors) or the environment (e.g., pollen) (Table 28.1). Important factors and triggers are discussed in this section.

Nose and Sinus Problems. Most patients with asthma have a history of allergic rhinitis. Treatment of allergic rhinitis usually improves the symptoms of asthma. Acute and chronic sinusitis, especially bacterial rhinosinusitis, may worsen asthma. Patients with asthma often have chronic sinus problems that cause inflammation of the mucous membranes and can trigger an

TABLE 28.1 Triggers of Asthma Attacks

Air Pollutants
- Aerosol sprays
- Cigarette smoke
- Exhaust fumes
- Oxidants
- Perfumes
- Sulfur dioxides

Allergen Inhalation
- Animal dander (e.g., cats, mice, guinea pigs)
- Cockroaches
- House dust mite
- Molds
- Pollens

Drugs
- Aspirin
- β-Adrenergic blockers
- Nonsteroidal antiinflammatory drugs

Food Additives
- Beer, wine, dried fruit, shrimp, processed potatoes
- Monosodium glutamate
- Sulfites (bisulfites and metabisulfites)
- Tartrazine

Occupational Exposure
- Agriculture, farming
- Industrial chemicals and plastics
- Laundry detergents
- Metal salts
- Paints, solvents
- Wood and vegetable dusts

Viral or Bacterial Infection
- Sinusitis, allergic rhinitis
- Viral URI

Other Factors
- Exercise and cold, dry air
- Gastroesophageal reflux disease (GERD)
- Hormones, menses
- Stress

asthma attack. Sinusitis must be treated and large nasal polyps removed for an asthma patient to have good control. (Sinusitis is discussed in Chapter 27.)

Respiratory Tract Infections. Respiratory tract infections are often a major trigger of an acute asthma attack. Acute infection can decrease the diameter of the airways and induce airway hyperresponsiveness. Viral-induced changes in epithelial cells, the accumulation of inflammatory cells, edema of airway walls, and exposure of airway nerve endings contribute to altered respiratory function. These changes may exacerbate asthma.

Allergens. Allergens cause varying degrees of allergic reactions in susceptible persons. Indoor and outdoor allergens, such as cockroaches, furry animals, fungi, pollen, and molds, can trigger asthma attacks. However, their role in the actual development of asthma is not as clear.[6]

Cigarette Smoke. The Centers for Disease Control and Prevention (CDC) estimates that 21% of asthma patients smoke.[7] In a person with asthma, smoking is associated with a faster decline of lung function, increased disease severity, more frequent visits to the HCP, and a decreased response to treatment. The smoke exhaled by a smoker, known as secondhand smoke, is also a risk factor.

Air Pollutants. Various air pollutants, such as wood smoke or vehicle exhaust, can trigger asthma attacks. In heavily industrialized or densely populated areas, climate conditions often lead to concentrated pollution in the atmosphere, especially with thermal inversions and stagnant air masses. News sources report ozone alert days. Patients with breathing problems should minimize outdoor activity during these times.

Occupational Factors. *Occupational asthma* is the most common job-related respiratory disorder. These irritants cause a change in the responsiveness of the airways. However, the development of symptoms may not occur until the patient has had months to years of exposure. These agents are diverse and include wood dusts, laundry detergents, metal salts, chemicals, paints, solvents, and plastics. Often, people with occupational asthma give a history of arriving at work feeling well but gradually develop symptoms, which may become progressively worse, by the end of the day.

Exercise. Asthma that is induced or worse during physical exertion is called exercise-induced asthma (EIA) or exercise-induced bronchospasm (EIB). Typically, symptoms of EIA are pronounced during activities in which there is exposure to cold, dry air. For example, swimming in an indoor heated pool is less likely to cause symptoms than downhill skiing. Airway obstruction may occur due to changes in the airway mucosa caused by hyperventilation during exercise, with either cooling or rewarming of air and capillary leakage in the airway wall. EIB occurs after vigorous exercise, not during it (e.g., jogging, aerobics, walking briskly, climbing stairs).

Drugs and Food Additives. Some people with asthma have what we call the *asthma triad*: nasal polyps, asthma, and sensitivity to aspirin and nonsteroidal antiinflammatory drugs (NSAIDs). Some persons with asthma who use salicylic acid (e.g., aspirin) or NSAIDs develop wheezing within 2 hours. In addition, there is usually profound rhinorrhea, congestion, tearing, and even angioedema. Avoiding salicylic acid and NSAIDs is required. Teach the patient to read labels. Salicylic acid is in many OTC drugs and some foods, beverages, and flavorings. Under the care of an allergist, daily administration of the drug can desensitize some patients.

β-Adrenergic blockers in oral form (e.g., metoprolol [Toprol-XL]) or topical eye drops (e.g., timolol [Timoptic]) may trigger an asthma attack because they can cause bronchospasm. Angiotensin-converting enzyme (ACE) inhibitors (e.g., lisinopril) may cause a dry, hacking cough in susceptible persons, making asthma symptoms worse. Asthma attacks can occur after the use of sulfite-containing preservatives found in topical ophthalmic solutions, IV corticosteroids, and some inhaled bronchodilator solutions.

Food and drug additives that may trigger asthma in the susceptible person are tartrazine (yellow dye no. 5) and sulfiting agents. They are widely used as preservatives and sanitizing agents. Sulfiting agents are in fruits, beer, and wine. They are used in salad bars to protect vegetables from oxidation. Food allergies triggering asthma reactions in adults are rare. Avoidance diets are not recommended until testing has proven an allergy is present.

Gastroesophageal Reflux Disease. Gastroesophageal reflux disease (GERD) is more common in people with asthma than in the general population. GERD can worsen asthma symptoms because reflux may trigger bronchoconstriction and cause aspiration. Asthma drugs may worsen GERD symptoms. β_2-Agonists used to treat asthma (especially when given orally) relax the lower esophageal sphincter. This allows stomach contents to reflux into the esophagus and be aspirated into the lungs. Effective treatment for GERD can improve nocturnal asthma control, improve quality of life, and prevent asthma symptoms in some patients. (GERD is discussed in Chapter 41.)

Genetics. Asthma has an inherited component, but the genetics are complex. Numerous genes may be involved in the development of asthma. They are likely responsible for varying responses among patients to different types of asthma drugs. Atopy, the genetic predisposition to develop an allergic (immunoglobulin E [IgE]–mediated) response to common allergens, is a major risk factor for asthma.

Immune Response. The *hygiene hypothesis* suggests that a newborn baby's immune system must be conditioned so that it will function properly during infancy and the rest of life. People who have a lower incidence of asthma were exposed to certain infections early in life, used fewer antibiotics, were around other children (e.g., siblings, day care), or lived in rural settings or with pets. People for whom these factors are not present in childhood have a higher incidence of asthma.

Psychological Factors. Asthma is not a psychosomatic disease. However, many people with asthma report that symptoms worsen with stress. An asthma attack caused by any triggering event can produce panic, stress, and anxiety. These emotions, and other psychological factors, can cause bronchoconstriction through stimulation of the cholinergic reflex pathways. Extreme behavioral expressions (e.g., crying, laughing, anger, fear) can lead to hyperventilation and hypocapnia, which can cause airway narrowing.

Pathophysiology

The main pathophysiologic process in asthma is persistent but variable inflammation of the airways. Airflow is limited because inflammation results in bronchoconstriction, airway hyperresponsiveness (hyperreactivity), and edema of the airways. Exposure to allergens or irritants initiates the inflammatory cascade (Fig. 28.1). A variety of inflammatory cells are involved, including mast cells, macrophages, eosinophils, neutrophils, T and B lymphocytes, and epithelial cells of the airways.

As the inflammatory process begins, mast cells (found beneath the basement membrane of the bronchial wall) degranulate and release multiple inflammatory mediators (Fig. 28.2). IgE antibodies are linked to mast cells, and the allergen crosslinks the IgE. As a result, inflammatory mediators, such as leukotrienes, histamine, cytokines, prostaglandins, and nitric oxide, are released. Inflammatory mediators have effects on the (1) blood vessels, causing vasodilation and increasing capillary permeability (runny nose); (2) nerve cells, causing itching; (3) smooth muscle cells, causing bronchial spasms and airway narrowing; and (4) goblet cells, causing mucus production (Fig. 28.3). This whole process is sometimes referred to as the *early-phase response* in asthma. Clinically, it occurs within 30 to 60 minutes after exposure to an allergen or irritant.

Symptoms can recur 4 to 6 hours after the early response because of the influx of many inflammatory cells, which are set in motion by the initial response. At this later time, the patient may develop symptoms again or worsening of symptoms. This is called the *late-phase response*. It occurs in about 50% of people with asthma. In the late-phase response, more inflammatory cells are recruited and activated, with continuing inflammation of the airways. Thus bronchoconstriction with symptoms lasts for 24 hours or more. Corticosteroids are effective in treating inflammation in this phase.

Chronic inflammation may cause structural changes in the bronchial wall, known as *remodeling*. A progressive loss of lung function occurs that therapy cannot fully reverse. The changes in structure may include fibrosis of the subepithelium, hypertrophy of the smooth muscle of the airways, mucus hypersecretion, continued inflammation, and *angiogenesis* (proliferation of new blood vessels).[8] We think remodeling explains why some persons have persistent asthma and limited response to therapy.

PATHOPHYSIOLOGY MAP

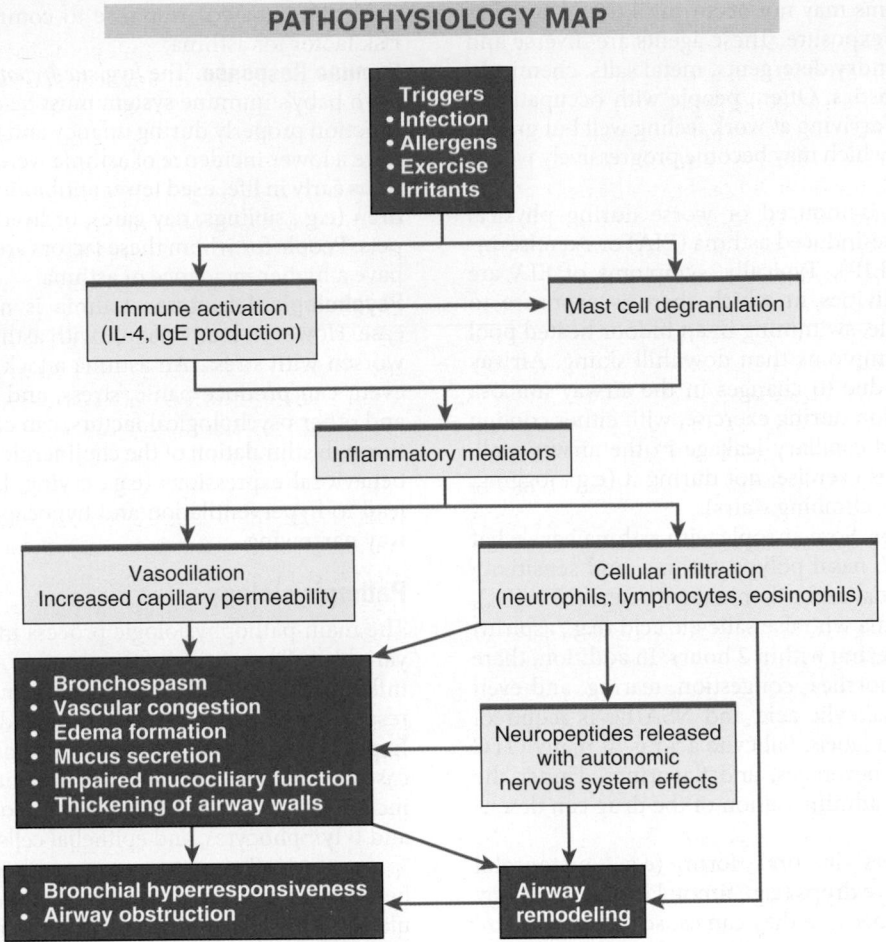

Triggers
- Infection
- Allergens
- Exercise
- Irritants

Immune activation (IL-4, IgE production)

Mast cell degranulation

Inflammatory mediators

Vasodilation
Increased capillary permeability

Cellular infiltration
(neutrophils, lymphocytes, eosinophils)

- Bronchospasm
- Vascular congestion
- Edema formation
- Mucus secretion
- Impaired mucociliary function
- Thickening of airway walls

Neuropeptides released with autonomic nervous system effects

- Bronchial hyperresponsiveness
- Airway obstruction

Airway remodeling

FIG. 28.1 Pathophysiology of asthma. (Adapted from McCance KL, Huether SE, Brashers, VL, Rote, NS, editors: *Pathophysiology: The biologic basis for disease in adults and children*, ed 7, St Louis, 2015, Elsevier.)

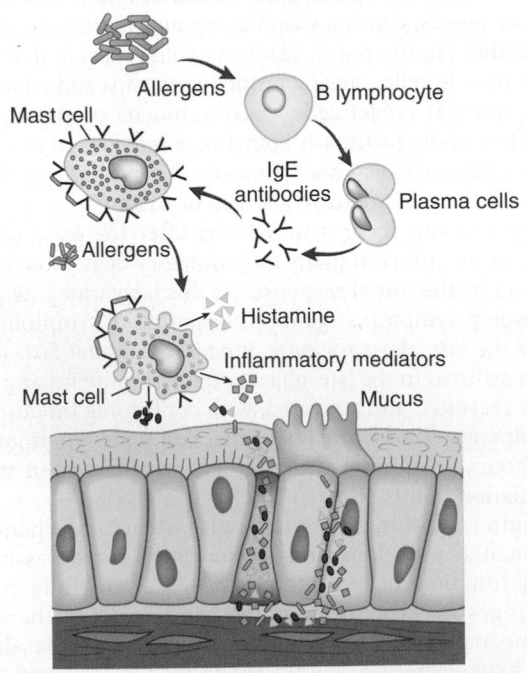

Allergens

Mast cell

B lymphocyte

IgE antibodies

Plasma cells

Allergens

Histamine

Inflammatory mediators

Mast cell

Mucus

FIG. 28.2 Allergic asthma is triggered when an allergen cross-links *IgE* receptors on mast cells, which are then activated to release histamine and other inflammatory mediators (early-phase response). A late-phase response may occur due to further inflammation.

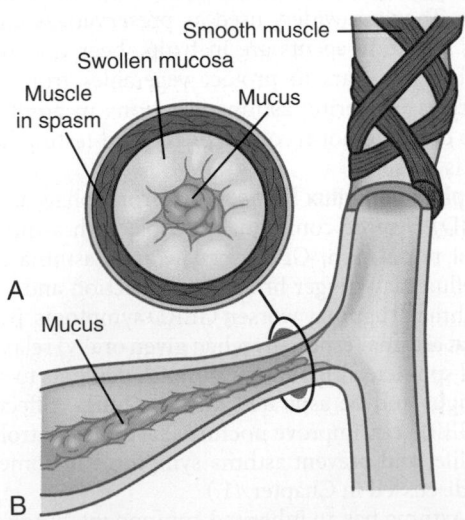

Smooth muscle

Swollen mucosa

Muscle in spasm

Mucus

A

Mucus

B

FIG. 28.3 Factors causing expiratory obstruction in asthma. A, Cross section of a bronchiole occluded by muscle spasm, swollen mucosa, and mucus in the lumen. B, Longitudinal section of a bronchiole. (Redrawn from Price SA, Wilson LM: *Pathophysiology: Clinical concepts of disease processes*, ed 6, St Louis, 2003, Mosby.)

Clinical Manifestations

The characteristic manifestations are wheezing, cough, dyspnea, and chest tightness after exposure to a risk factor or trigger. Normally the bronchioles constrict during expiration. However, in asthma, the airways become narrower than usual because of bronchospasm, edema, and mucus. As a result, it takes longer for the air to move out of the bronchioles (airflow obstruction). This causes the characteristic wheezing, air trapping, and hyperinflation of the lungs. As a result, expiration may be prolonged.

The most common finding during an acute asthmatic event is wheezing on auscultation. For wheezing to occur, the patient must be able to move enough air to make the sound. Wheezing usually occurs first on exhalation. As asthma progresses, the patient may wheeze during inspiration and expiration.

However, wheezing is an unreliable sign to gauge the severity of an attack. Many patients with minor attacks wheeze loudly. Others with severe attacks do not wheeze. The patient with a severe asthma attack may wheeze only during forced expiration or have no audible wheezing because of the marked reduction in airflow.

Decreased or absent breath sounds may signal a significant decrease in air movement resulting from exhaustion and an inability to generate enough muscle force to breathe. Severely decreased breath sounds, often referred to as the "silent chest," are an ominous sign. It means severe airway obstruction and impending respiratory failure.

> ⚠️ **SAFETY ALERT Silent Chest**
> - If the patient has been wheezing, then there is an absence of a wheeze (e.g., silent chest) and the patient is obviously struggling, this is a life-threatening situation. The patient may need mechanical ventilation.

Hyperventilation occurs during an asthma attack as lung receptors respond to increased lung volume from trapped air and airflow limitation. Decreased perfusion and ventilation of the alveoli and increased alveolar gas pressure lead to ventilation-perfusion abnormalities in the lungs. The patient is hypoxemic early on with decreased $PaCO_2$ and increased pH (respiratory alkalosis) because they are is hyperventilating. As the airflow limitation worsens with air trapping, the patient works much harder to breathe. The $PaCO_2$ normalizes as the patient tires, and then it increases to produce respiratory acidosis. This is an ominous sign of respiratory failure.

In some patients with asthma, cough is the only symptom. This is termed *cough variant asthma*. Bronchospasm is not present or may not be severe enough to cause airflow obstruction or wheezing, but it can increase bronchial tone and cause irritation with stimulation of the cough receptors. The cough may be nonproductive or with secretions. Sputum may be thick, tenacious, and gelatinous, which makes removal difficult.

The examination of the patient with asthma may be normal, especially between attacks. A runny nose, swollen nasal passages, and nasal polyps may be seen. The patient may have eczema and hives, which have been linked to asthma.

> ❓ **CHECK YOUR PRACTICE**
> Your patient with a history of asthma was admitted to the ED in acute respiratory distress. He has been receiving therapy and seems to be responding. You notice he is no longer wheezing.
> - Should you consider this finding a sign that he is doing better?

Asthma Classifications

There are several sets of guidelines for classifying asthma. Each set of guidelines has a slightly different perspective about asthma and how to classify the severity when attacks occur. Asthma severity is used to guide treatment decisions. Current guidelines focus on (1) assessing the severity of the disease at diagnosis and initial treatment and then (2) monitoring periodically to control the disease. All groups endorse the use of short-acting bronchodilators for an acute asthma attack and the importance of an "asthma action plan" to help prevent future attacks from occurring. They promote patient education and adherence to prescribed therapy. Many HCPs use the 2007 the National Heart, Lung, and Blood Institute classification of asthma severity (Table 28.2). It describes asthma as intermittent, mild persistent, moderate persistent, or severe persistent.

Complications

Asthma is characterized by an unpredictable and variable course. Asthma attacks range from minor interferences in breathing to life-threatening episodes. Depending on a person's response, asthma can rapidly progress from normal breathing to an acute, severe attack or a life-threatening medical emergency within a few minutes.

While asthma attacks may have an abrupt onset, most of the time, symptoms occur more gradually. Attacks may last for a few minutes to several hours. Between attacks, the patient may be asymptomatic with normal or near-normal spirometry, depending on the severity of disease. In some people, compromised pulmonary function (indicated by abnormal spirometry results) may lead to a state of continuous symptoms and chronic debilitation. Pneumonia, tension pneumothorax, status asthmaticus, and acute respiratory failure can occur.

Status Asthmaticus. A life-threatening medical emergency, status asthmaticus is the most extreme form of an acute asthma attack. It is characterized by hypoxia, hypercapnia, and acute respiratory failure.[9] The patient is unresponsive to treatment with bronchodilators and corticosteroids. The patient may have chest tightness, a severely marked increase in shortness of breath, or suddenly be unable to speak. Hypotension, bradycardia, and respiratory and/or cardiac arrest may occur if we do not recognize that the patient's condition is getting worse.

The patient must be immediately intubated, and mechanical ventilation started. Hemodynamic monitoring of the patient is critical. Analgesia and sedation are essential. Continuous analgesic infusions (e.g., ketamine, morphine) and sedation with drugs such as propofol (Diprivan) help decrease work of breathing (WOB) and facilitate patient synchrony with the ventilator. In some circumstances, neuromuscular blocking agents may be used. Inhaled anesthetics, such as isoflurane or halothane, are an option for those not responding to conventional treatment. IV magnesium sulfate, which has a bronchodilator effect, may be given to patients with a very low FEV_1 (forced expiratory volume in 1 second) or peak flow (less than 40% of predicted or personal best) or those who do not respond to initial treatment.

Diagnostic Studies

The tests we use to diagnose asthma are shown in Table 28.3. In general, the HCP should consider a diagnosis of asthma if various indicators (e.g., manifestations, health history, peak flow variability, spirometry) are positive.

Underdiagnosis of asthma is common. A detailed history is important to determine if a person has had similar attacks,

TABLE 28.2 Classification of Asthma Severity

Components of Severity	Intermittent	Mild	Moderate	Severe
		PERSISTENT		
		Mild	Moderate	Severe
Impairment				
Symptoms	≤2 days/wk	>2 days/wk, not daily	Daily	Continuous
Nighttime awakenings	≤2/mos	3–4/mos	>1/wk, not nightly	Often 7/wk
SABA use for symptoms	≤2 days/wk	>2 days/wk, not daily	Daily	Several times per day
Interference with normal activity	None	Minor limitation	Some limitation	Extremely limited
Lung function*	Normal FEV$_1$ between attacks FEV$_1$ >80% FEV$_1$/FVC normal	FEV$_1$ >80% predicted FEV$_1$/FVC normal	FEV$_1$ 60%–80% predicted FEV$_1$/FVC reduced by 5%	FEV$_1$ <60% predicted FEV$_1$/FVC reduced by 5%
Risk				
Attacks requiring oral corticosteroids	0–1/yr	≥2/yrs even in the absence of impairment		

Consider severity and interval since last attack. ⟶
Frequency and severity may fluctuate over time. ⟶
Relative annual risk for exacerbation may be related to FEV$_1$. ⟶

Recommended Step for Initiating Treatment	Step 1	Step 2	Step 3†	Step 4 or 5†

Reevaluate asthma control in 2–6 wk and adjust therapy as needed

Guidelines for Using Table

- Assign patients to the most severe step in which any feature occurs. Clinical features may overlap across steps. Determine level of severity by assessment of both impairment and risk. Assess impairment by patient's recall of previous 2–4 wk spirometry results.
- A person's classification should change over time with treatment. After treatment, the focus switches to the level of control, not the classification of severity.
- Patients at any level of severity of chronic asthma can have mild, moderate, or severe asthma attacks. Some patients with intermittent asthma have severe and life-threatening attacks separated by long periods of normal lung function and no symptoms.

Source: Adapted from National Asthma Education and Prevention Program, National Heart, Lung, and Blood Institute: *Expert Panel Report 3: Guidelines for the diagnosis and management of asthma,* NIH pub no 08-4051, Bethesda, MD, 2007, National Institutes of Health.
ercent predicted values for FEV$_1$ or ratio of FEV$_1$/FVC. Normal FEV$_1$/FVC: 8–19 yr, 85%; 20–39 yr, 80%; 40–59 yr, 75%; 60–80 yr, 70%.
†Consider short-term corticosteroid therapy.

TABLE 28.3 Interprofessional Care

Asthma

Diagnostic Assessment

- History and physical examination
- Spirometry, including response to bronchodilator therapy
- Peak expiratory flow rate (PEFR)
- Chest x-ray
- Measurement of oximetry
- Allergy skin testing (if indicated)
- Blood level of eosinophils and IgE (if indicated)

Management

- Identify and avoid or eliminate triggers
- Patient and caregiver teaching
- Drug therapy (Tables 28.6 and 28.7 and Figs. 28.4 and 28.5)
- Asthma action plan (Fig. 28.9)
- Desensitization (immunotherapy) if indicated
- Assess for control (e.g., Asthma Control Test [ACT])*

Acute Attacks

- SaO$_2$ monitoring
- ABGs
- Inhaled β$_2$-adrenergic agonists
- Inhaled anticholinergics
- O$_2$ by nasal cannula or mask
- IV or oral corticosteroids
- IV fluids
- IV magnesium
- Intubation and assisted ventilation

*See www.asthmacontroltest.com.

which are often precipitated by a known trigger. Because wheezing and cough occur with a variety of disorders (e.g., COPD, GERD, vocal cord problems, heart failure), it is important to determine if asthma or some other disease process is the cause of these problems. A comparison of asthma and COPD is shown in Table 28.4.

The peak expiratory flow rate (PEFR) measured by the peak flow meter (at home or in a health care setting) is a test of lung function (see Table 25.17). PEFR measurements can help predict an asthma attack or monitor the severity of disease. Test results depend on the patient's age, gender, and height. Since types of peak flow meters vary, PEFR should be compared with the patient's own previous best measurements using their own meter.

Spirometry is usually normal between asthma attacks if the patient has no other underlying pulmonary disease. However, the patient with asthma may show an obstructive pattern including a decrease in forced vital capacity (FVC), FEV$_1$, PEFR, and FEV$_1$ to FVC ratio (FEV$_1$/FVC) (see Table 25.16).

When spirometry is scheduled, the patient must stop taking any bronchodilator drugs for 6 to 12 hours before the test. Spirometry can be done before and after the administration of a bronchodilator to determine the degree of the response. This helps determine reversibility of airway obstruction, which is critical information for diagnosing asthma. A positive (favorable) response to the bronchodilator is an increase of more than 200 mL and an increase of more than 12% between preadministration and postadministration values.[10]

We can use a hand-held, point-of-care device to measure fractional exhaled nitric oxide (FENO). FENO levels are

TABLE 28.4 Comparison of Asthma and COPD*

	Asthma	COPD
Clinical Features		
Age	Usually <40 yr (onset)	Usually 40–50 yr (onset)
Smoking history	Not causal	Often long history (>10–20 pack-years)
Health and family history	Presence of allergy, rhinitis, eczema. Family history of asthma	Infrequent allergies. May have exposure to environmental pollutants. With α_1-antitrypsin deficiency, family history of lung or liver disease without smoking history
Clinical symptoms	Intermittent, vary day to day, worse at night or early morning	Slowly progressive and persistent
Dyspnea	Absent except in attacks or poor control	Dyspnea during exercise
Sputum	Infrequent	Often
Disease course	Stable (with attacks)	Progressive worsening (with exacerbations)
Diagnostic Study Results		
ABGs	Normal between or during attacks	Between exacerbations in advanced COPD • Often low-normal pH and PaO_2 • High-normal $PaCO_2$ with normal to high HCO_3^- (compensated respiratory acidosis)
pH	↑ Early in attack, then ↓ if prolonged or severe attack	N→↓
PaO_2	↓	N→↓
$PaCO_2$	↓ Early in attack, then ↑ if prolonged or severe attack	N→↑
Chest x-ray	May show hyperinflation	Hyperinflation. May have cardiac enlargement, flattened diaphragm
Lung volumes	Often normalizes	Never normalizes
• Total lung capacity	Increased	Increased
• Residual volume	Increased	Increased
• FEV_1	Decreased or normal	Decreased
• FEV_1/FVC	Normal to decreased	Decreased (<70%)

*Patients may have features of both asthma and COPD.

increased in people with asthma associated with eosinophilic-induced airway inflammation. FENO may be used to gauge loss of asthma control and attacks, assess a patient's adherence to therapy, or determine if more inhaled or oral antiinflammatory medication is needed.[11]

Increased serum eosinophil counts and IgE levels are highly suggestive of atopy. Allergy skin testing may be used to determine sensitivity to specific allergens. However, a positive skin test does not necessarily mean that the allergen is causing the asthma attack. On the other hand, a negative allergy test does not mean that the asthma event is not allergy related. (Allergy testing is discussed in Chapter 13.)

A chest x-ray in an asymptomatic patient with asthma is usually normal. A routine chest x-ray is usually not done unless other manifestations, such as fever, chills, or upper airway stridor, are present. It can show if something else is causing symptoms similar to those of asthma (e.g., pneumonia, foreign body in the airway.)

A sputum specimen for culture and sensitivity may be done to rule out bacterial infection, especially if the patient has purulent sputum, a history of upper respiratory tract infection (URI), a fever, or an increased white blood cell (WBC) count. However, most asthma attacks are viral, and sputum cultures are rarely done on an outpatient basis.

Interprofessional Care

The goal of care is to achieve and maintain control of the disease. Once the patient is diagnosed, guidelines provide direction about medications (based on steps) the patient needs (Fig. 28.4). The HCP will step up the medication therapy as asthma symptoms worsen and step down the medication as the patient achieves control (Table 28.5). The level of control is determined by the patient's medication use, symptoms, and PEFR or FEV_1.

During an acute attack, signs and symptoms, medication use, and PEFR or FEV_1 measurements can be used to help identify the severity of an asthma attack and guide us in providing the most appropriate treatment. The goal is to achieve rapid control of the symptoms and return the patient to their daily functioning at the best possible level. Management of acute asthma attacks is shown in Fig. 28.5.

Patients with mild or moderate asthma attacks are often seen in the community at an outpatient clinic. These attacks occur no more than twice per week, with minimal interference in day-to-day activity. The patient is alert, oriented, and speaks in sentences. The patient may describe chest tightness, varying degrees of difficulty breathing, and a slight increase in the use of asthma drugs. O_2 saturation is usually greater than 90% on room air and PEFR greater than 50% of predicted or personal best.

Inhaled bronchodilators and oral corticosteroids are the mainstays of treatment for mild to moderate asthma attacks. Monitor the patient's vital signs. Most improve within 60 minutes of starting therapy. Teach the patient the importance of a follow-up appointment with the HCP. Oral corticosteroids will be part of the discharge plan for a moderate attack and, based on the patient's history and HCP preference, sometimes for a mild attack. If the patient's condition is slow to respond, does not respond, or the HCP suspects that some other condition may be occurring or contributing to the acute attack, the patient should be transferred to an acute care facility.

In a severe attack the patient is still alert and oriented, but may be tachycardic, tachypneic, and focused on breathing. Respiratory rates greater than 30 breaths/min may be present. Accessory muscle use may be seen. The patient may be agitated from hypoxemia. If not immediately audible, auscultation of the lungs may reveal inspiratory or expiratory wheezing. The patient often sits forward to maximize diaphragmatic movement. Time permitting, percussion of the lungs indicates hyperresonance. PEFR is 50% or less of predicted or of personal best. Symptoms may re-occur, sometimes daily, and there is interference with activities of daily living (ADLs).

A severe acute attack is usually frightening enough for patients to go to the ED. In many cases, a severe attack will warrant hospital admission. Management of the patient with

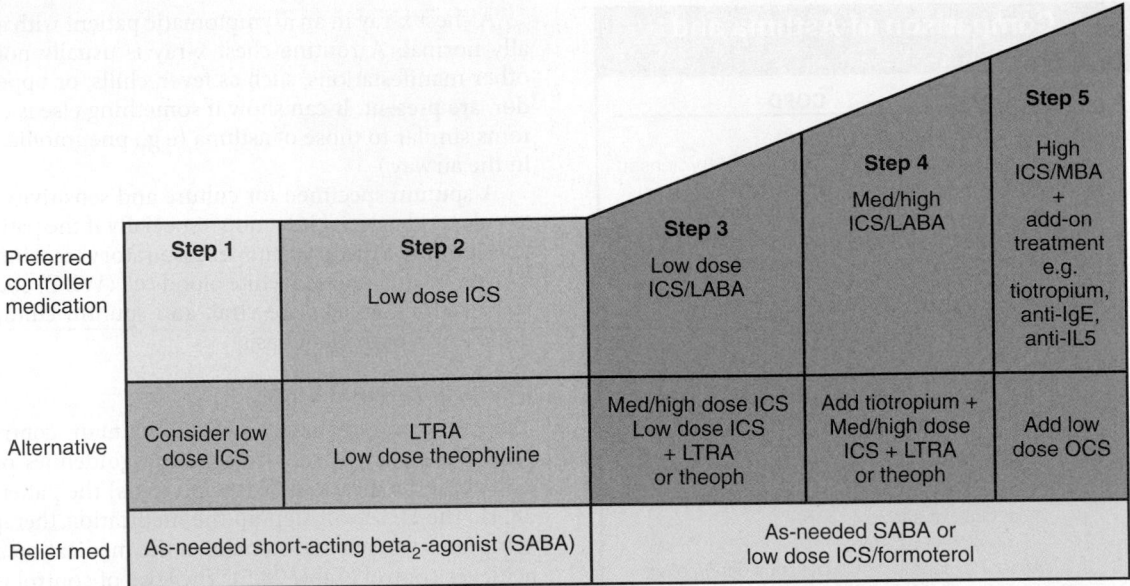

	Step 1	Step 2	Step 3	Step 4	Step 5
Preferred controller medication		Low dose ICS	Low dose ICS/LABA	Med/high ICS/LABA	High ICS/MBA + add-on treatment e.g. tiotropium, anti-IgE, anti-IL5
Alternative	Consider low dose ICS	LTRA Low dose theophyline	Med/high dose ICS Low dose ICS + LTRA or theoph	Add tiotropium + Med/high dose ICS + LTRA or theoph	Add low dose OCS
Relief med	As-needed short-acting beta₂-agonist (SABA)		As-needed SABA or low dose ICS/formoterol		

FIG. 28.4 Stepwise approach to asthma treatment. (Modified from GINA evidence-based strategy document, 2018. Retrieved from *https://ginasthma.org*.)

TABLE 28.5 Components of Asthma Control

Components of Control	CLASSIFICATION OF ASTHMA CONTROL		
	Well Controlled	**Not Well Controlled**	**Very Poorly Controlled**
Impairment			
Symptoms	≤2 days/wk	>2 days/wk	Throughout the day
Nighttime Awakenings	≤2/mo	1–3/wks	≥4/wks
Interference with normal activity	None	Some limitation	Extremely limited
SABA use	≤2 days/wk	>2 days/wk	Several times/day
FEV₁ or PEFR	>80% predicted/personal best	60%–80% predicted/personal best	<60% predicted/personal best
Risk			
Attacks requiring oral corticosteroids	0–1/yr	≥2/yr	≥2/yr
Progressive loss of lung function	Consider severity and interval since last attack. ⟶		
Treatment-related adverse effects	Evaluation requires long-term follow-up. ⟶ Can vary in intensity from none to very troublesome and worrisome. Level of intensity does not correlate to specific levels of control but should be considered in the overall assessment of risk. ⟶		
Recommended Action for Treatment (based on assessment of control)	• Maintain current step. • Regular follow-up every 1–6 mos to maintain control. • Consider step down if well controlled for at least 3 mo.	• Step up one step. • Reevaluate in 2–6 wk. • For side effects, consider alternative treatment options.	• Consider oral corticosteroids. • Step up 1 or 2 steps and reevaluate in 2 wk. • For side effects, consider alternative treatment options.

Source: Adapted from National Asthma Education and Prevention Program, National Heart, Lung, and Blood Institute: *Expert Panel Report 3: Guidelines for the diagnosis and management of asthma,* NIH pub no 08-4051, Bethesda, MD, 2007, National Institutes of Health.

a severe attack focuses on correcting hypoxemia and continually observing and/or improving ventilation. Supplemental O_2 is given by nasal cannula or mask to achieve a PaO_2 of at least 60 mm Hg or O_2 saturation greater than 93%. O_2 monitoring should be continuous with pulse oximetry.

Bedside PEFR may be used to monitor airflow obstruction. Serial PEFR results, oximetry, and measurement of arterial blood gases (ABGs) give information about the severity of the attack and the response to therapy. Obtaining a PEFR during a severe asthma attack is usually not possible. However, if it can be obtained and is less than 200 L/min, it indicates severe obstruction in all but very small adults.

Careful monitoring of the patient's heart rate, respiratory rate and rhythm, and BP are essential. Bronchodilators and oral corticosteroids will be part of the treatment plan. The "silent chest" is an ominous clinical finding. It often signals impending respiratory failure. Immediate notification of the HCP is required.

Drug Therapy

Drug therapy for asthma can be complex and overwhelming for many practitioners, including you. It is important to understand the intended purpose, desired effect, side effects, and when to use different drugs. Asthma drugs are divided into 2 general

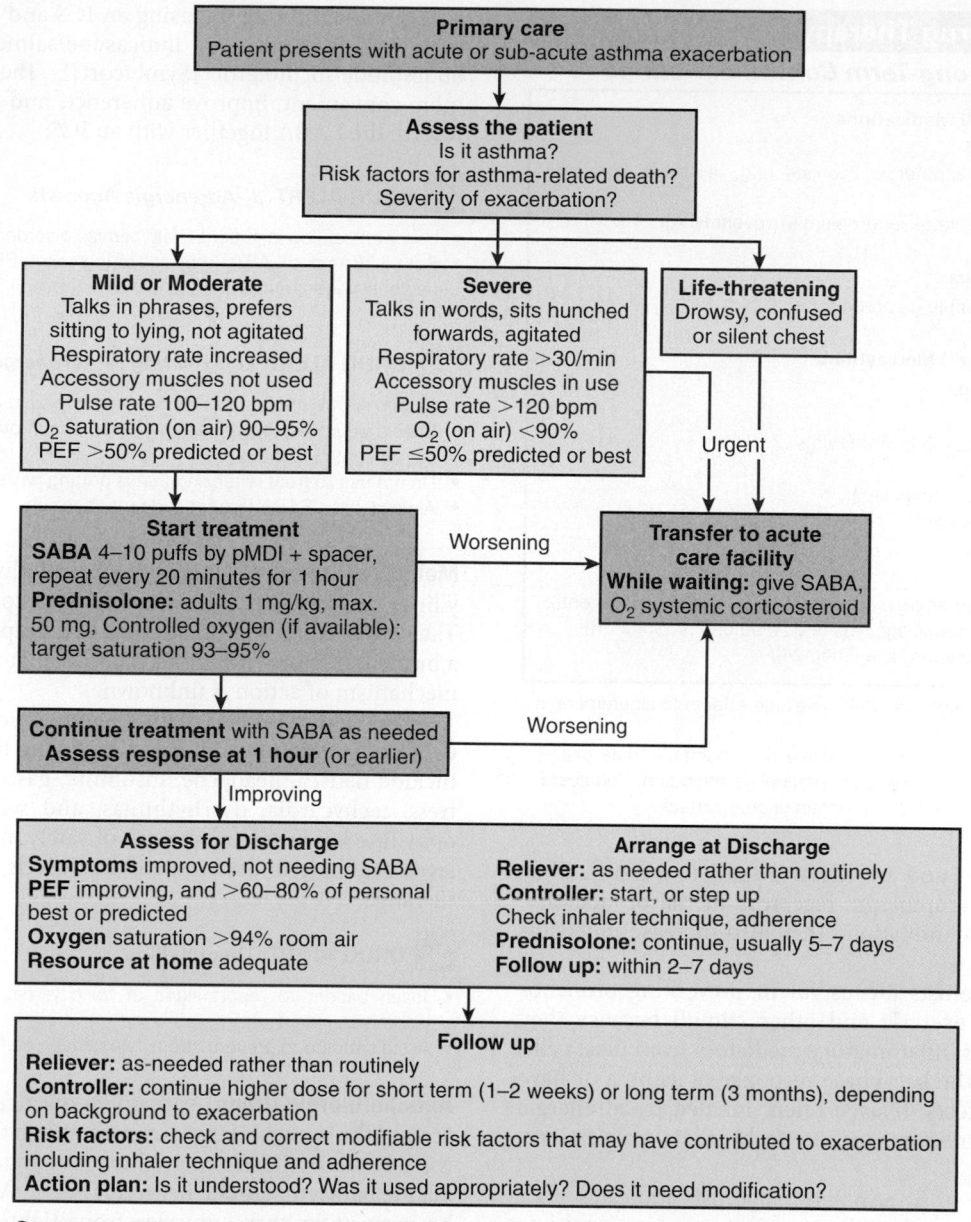

Primary care
Patient presents with acute or sub-acute asthma exacerbation

Assess the patient
Is it asthma?
Risk factors for asthma-related death?
Severity of exacerbation?

Mild or Moderate
Talks in phrases, prefers
sitting to lying, not agitated
Respiratory rate increased
Accessory muscles not used
Pulse rate 100–120 bpm
O_2 saturation (on air) 90–95%
PEF >50% predicted or best

Severe
Talks in words, sits hunched
forwards, agitated
Respiratory rate >30/min
Accessory muscles in use
Pulse rate >120 bpm
O_2 (on air) <90%
PEF ≤50% predicted or best

Life-threatening
Drowsy, confused
or silent chest

Urgent

Start treatment
SABA 4–10 puffs by pMDI + spacer,
repeat every 20 minutes for 1 hour
Prednisolone: adults 1 mg/kg, max.
50 mg, Controlled oxygen (if available):
target saturation 93–95%

Worsening

**Transfer to acute
care facility**
While waiting: give SABA,
O_2 systemic corticosteroid

Continue treatment with SABA as needed
Assess response at 1 hour (or earlier)

Worsening

Improving

Assess for Discharge
Symptoms improved, not needing SABA
PEF improving, and >60–80% of personal
best or predicted
Oxygen saturation >94% room air
Resource at home adequate

Arrange at Discharge
Reliever: as needed rather than routinely
Controller: start, or step up
Check inhaler technique, adherence
Prednisolone: continue, usually 5–7 days
Follow up: within 2–7 days

Follow up
Reliever: as-needed rather than routinely
Controller: continue higher dose for short term (1–2 weeks) or long term (3 months), depending
on background to exacerbation
Risk factors: check and correct modifiable risk factors that may have contributed to exacerbation
including inhaler technique and adherence
Action plan: Is it understood? Was it used appropriately? Does it need modification?

O_2: oxygen; PEF: peak expiratory flow; SABA: short-acting beta$_2$-agonist (doses are for salbutamol)

FIG. 28.5 Management of patient with acute asthma attack. (Modified from GINA evidence-based strategy document, 2018. Retrieved from *https://ginasthma.org*.)

types: (1) *quick relief*, or *rescue medications,* to treat attacks, and (2) long-term control medications (Table 28.6).

The patient's medical history, medication plan, and severity of attack helps the HCP determine which types of drugs are best suited to control asthma symptoms. Current guidelines all suggest a stepwise approach to drug therapy. Common drugs used in asthma therapy are discussed in Table 28.7.

The mainstay of asthma treatment is inhalation of short-acting β$_2$-adrenergic agonist (SABA) bronchodilators. All patients need a quick-relief or "rescue" medication. Short-acting SABAs, such as albuterol (ProAir HFA, Proventil HFA, Ventolin HFA), are the most effective rescue drugs for asthma.

In patients with a moderate to severe attack, inhaled ipratropium (Atrovent) is used in conjunction with a SABA. Combivent is a combination of both ipratropium and albuterol.

Oral and, in some situations, IV corticosteroids may be given to patients who do not initially respond to SABA alone.

Patients with asthma who have frequent attacks also must be on a long-term ("controller") medication. Inhaled corticosteroids (ICSs) (e.g., fluticasone [Flovent Diskus or HFA]) are the most effective long-term controllers to treat inflammation. Some ICSs are used in combination with long-acting bronchodilators (LABAs) to gain better asthma control.

Bronchodilators. The 3 classes of bronchodilator drugs used in asthma therapy are β$_2$-adrenergic agonists (also referred to as β$_2$-agonists), methylxanthines and derivatives, and anticholinergics.

β$_2$-Adrenergic Agonist Drugs. These drugs may be SABAs or LABAs. Because inhaled SABAs are the most effective drugs for relieving acute bronchospasm (as seen in an acute attack), they are known as *rescue medications.* These drugs have an onset of

TABLE 28.6 Drug Therapy

Quick Relief vs. Long-Term Control of Asthma

Quick-Relief ("Rescue") Medications
Bronchodilators
Short-acting inhaled β₂-adrenergic agonists (e.g., albuterol [Proventil HFA])
Anticholinergics (inhaled) (e.g., ipratropium [Atrovent HFA])*

Antiinflammatory Drugs
Corticosteroids (systemic) (e.g., prednisone)†

Long-Term ("Controller") Medications
Antiinflammatory Drugs
Corticosteroids
• Inhaled (e.g., fluticasone [Flovent Diskus or HFA])
• Oral (e.g., prednisone)
LTMAs (e.g., montelukast [Singulair])
Anti–IgE (omalizumab [Xolair])

Bronchodilators
Long-acting inhaled β₂-adrenergic agonists (e.g., salmeterol [Serevent])
Long-acting oral β₂-adrenergic agonists (e.g., albuterol [VoSpire ER])
Methylxanthines (e.g., theophylline [Theo-24])

*Used as alternative if patient has intolerable side effects to albuterol or in ED for severe attacks.
†Considered quick-relief drugs when used in a short burst (3–10 days) at the start of therapy or during a period of gradual deterioration. Corticosteroids are not used for immediate relief of an ongoing attack.

action within minutes and are effective for 4 to 8 hours. They act by stimulating β-adrenergic receptors in the bronchioles, thus producing bronchodilation. They also increase mucociliary clearance.

β₂-Adrenergic agonists are useful in preventing bronchospasm triggered by exercise and other stimuli because they prevent the release of inflammatory mediators from mast cells. They do not inhibit the late-phase response of asthma or have antiinflammatory effects. If used often, inhaled β₂-adrenergic agonists may cause tremors, anxiety, tachycardia, palpitations, and nausea.

Too frequent use of β₂-adrenergic agonists indicates poor asthma control, may mask asthma severity, and may lead to reduced drug effectiveness. The use of SABAs should be limited to less than 2 times weekly. SABA inhalers should last for months. SABAs are not to be used for long-term control. They should not be used alone for recurrent, repeated asthma attacks. Use of long-term bronchodilators with inhaled corticosteroids or other drugs can achieve this goal better if prescribed and used properly.

LABAs, including salmeterol (Serevent Diskus) and formoterol (Foradil), are effective for 12 hours. LABAs are added to a daily dose of ICSs for long-term control of moderate to severe persistent asthma and prevention of symptoms, particularly at night. When LABAs are added to a patient's daily regimen of corticosteroids, they decrease the need for SABAs and allow patients to achieve better asthma control with a lower dosage of ICSs.

LABAs should never be used alone as asthma therapy. They should only be used if the patient is on an ICS. Tell patients that these drugs should not be used to treat acute symptoms or to obtain quick relief from bronchospasm. Teach the patient that these drugs are used only once every 12 hours.

Combination therapy using an ICS and a LABA is available in several inhalers (e.g., fluticasone/salmeterol [Advair] and budesonide/formoterol [Symbicort]). The combinations are more convenient, improve adherence, and ensure that patients receive the LABA together with an ICS.

 DRUG ALERT *β₂-Adrenergic Agonists*

• Use with caution in patients with cardiac disorders.
• Both SABAs and LABAs may cause increased BP and heart rate, central nervous system stimulation, and dysrhythmias.

 DRUG ALERT *Long-Acting β₂-Adrenergic Agonists (LABAs)*

• Should not be the first or only drug used to treat asthma.
• Should be added to the treatment plan only if other controller medicines do not control asthma.
• Do not use to treat wheezing that is getting worse.
• Always use a SABA to treat sudden wheezing.

Methylxanthines. Sustained-release methylxanthine (theophylline) preparations are not a first-line controller medication. They are used only as an alternative therapy. Methylxanthine is a bronchodilator with mild antiinflammatory effects. The exact mechanism of action is unknown.

The main problems with theophylline are the high incidence of interaction with other drugs and the side effects. These include nausea, headache, insomnia, gastrointestinal (GI) distress, tachycardia, dysrhythmias, and seizures. Because theophylline has a narrow margin of safety, monitor serum blood levels regularly to determine if drug levels are within therapeutic range.

 DRUG ALERT *Theophylline*

• Teach patient to report signs of toxicity: nausea, vomiting, seizures, insomnia.
• Avoid caffeine to prevent intensifying adverse effects.

Anticholinergic Drugs. Anticholinergic drugs affect the muscles around the bronchi (large airways). When the lungs are irritated, these bands of muscle can tighten, causing bronchoconstriction via the parasympathetic nervous system. Anticholinergics work by preventing these muscles from tightening. Consequently, these drugs promote bronchodilation.

Anticholinergic drugs are less effective than equivalent doses of SABAs in asthma. However, they are more effective in COPD patients. Therefore short-acting anticholinergic drugs are not used in the routine management of asthma, except for in severe acute asthma attacks.

Antiinflammatory Drugs

Corticosteroids. Chronic inflammation is a key component of asthma. Corticosteroids are antiinflammatory drugs that reduce bronchial hyperresponsiveness, block the late-phase response, and inhibit migration of inflammatory cells. Corticosteroids are more effective in improving asthma control than any other long-term drug.

To gain prompt control in acute attacks, oral corticosteroids are used. ICSs must be used for 1 to 2 weeks before maximum therapeutic effects can be seen. Some ICSs (e.g., fluticasone, budesonide [Pulmicort Flexhaler]) begin to have a therapeutic effect in 24 hours. Long-term, maintenance doses of oral corticosteroids may be needed to control asthma in patients with severe chronic asthma. ICSs must be used on a fixed schedule.

TABLE 28.7 Drug Therapy
Asthma and Chronic Obstructive Pulmonary Disease (COPD)

Drug	Route of Administration	Comments
Anticholinergics		
Short Acting (SAMA)		
ipratropium (Atrovent HFA)	Nebulizer, MDI	Approved for COPD. May provide additive benefit to SABA in moderate to severe asthma attacks (used in ED with no benefit beyond that). Use in asthma as alternative for patients with intolerable side effects with SABA. Temporary blurred vision with eye contact. Use cautiously in patients with narrow-angle glaucoma or prostatic enlargement
Long Acting (LAMA)		
aclidinium bromide (Tudorza, Pressair)	DPI	Approved only for COPD. Do not give with other anticholinergics. Not for acute relief of bronchospasm. Dosed twice daily
revefenacin (Yupelri)	Nebulizer	Approved only for COPD. Dosed once daily as maintenance treatment. Do not give with other anticholinergics. Use cautiously in patients with narrow-angle glaucoma
tiotropium (Spiriva HandiHaler)	DPI	Approved only for COPD. Blurred vision if powder comes in contact with eyes. Must not use ipratropium while on tiotropium. Patients with COPD must use SABA or short-acting anticholinergics for quick-relief medication. Maximum effect 1 wk after starting drug. Dosed once daily
umeclidinium (Incruse Ellipta)	DPI	Approved only for COPD. Dosed once daily as maintenance treatment of airflow obstruction
β₂-Adrenergic Agonists		
Inhaled: Short Acting (SABA)		
albuterol (Proventil HFA, Ventolin HFA, Proair HFA, AccuNeb, VoSpire ER [oral only])	Nebulizer, MDI, oral tablets, including extended release. NOTE: Oral tablets not for acute use, only long acting	Use with caution in patients with cardiac disorders because β-agonists may cause ↑ BP and heart rate, CNS stimulation/excitation, and ↑ risk for dysrhythmias. Has rapid onset of action (1–3 min). Duration of action is 4–8 hr. Ventolin HFA is the only albuterol MDI with a counter
levalbuterol (Xopenex, Xopenex HFA)	Nebulizer, MDI	Too frequent use can result in loss of effectiveness. Efficacy no better than other SABAs
Inhaled: Long Acting (LABA)	*In asthma:* Never use as monotherapy. Use in combination with ICSs. *In COPD:* Can be used as monotherapy. Not used for rapid relief of dyspnea	
arformoterol (Brovana)	Nebulizer	See formoterol. For chronic COPD use
formoterol (Foradil Aerolizer, Perforomist)	DPI, nebulizer (Performist)	Can affect blood glucose levels. Use with caution in patients with diabetes
indacaterol (Arcapta Neohaler)	DPI	Only once-daily LABA. For chronic COPD use. Not intended to treat asthma
olodaterol (Striverdi Respimat)	MDI	2 puffs daily. Less expensive than other LABAs
salmeterol (Serevent Diskus)	DPI	Not to exceed 2 puffs q12hr. Not used for acute attacks. Has a counter
Corticosteroids		
hydrocortisone (Solu-Cortef)	IV	Alternate-day therapy minimizes side effects. Oral dose should be taken in morning with food or milk. When given in high dosages, observe for GI distress. Long-term therapy requires vitamin D and calcium supplements to prevent osteoporosis. Discontinue gradually to prevent adrenal insufficiency. If symptoms recur during tapering, notify HCP
methylprednisolone (Medrol, Solu-Medrol)	Oral, IV	
prednisone	Oral	
Inhaled		
beclomethasone (Qvar)	MDI	Not recommended for acute asthma attack. May not see effects until after at least 2 weeks of regular treatment
budesonide (Pulmicort Flexhaler)	DPI	Same as above
ciclesonide (Alvesco)	MDI	Oral candidiasis and other localized oropharyngeal effects (e.g., hoarseness). Fewer side effects than other ICSs because of small particle size with minimal activation in oropharynx
fluticasone (Flovent HFA, Flovent Diskus, Arnuity Ellipta)	MDI, DPI	Not recommended for acute asthma attack. Rinse mouth with water or mouthwash after use to prevent oral fungal infections. Use of spacer device with MDI may decrease incidence of oral candidiasis. May not see effects until after at least 2 wks of regular treatment
mometasone (Asmanex Twisthaler)	DPI	Not recommended for acute asthma attack. May not see effects until after at least 2 wks of regular treatment
Leukotriene Modifiers		
Leukotriene Receptor Blocker		
montelukast (Singulair)	Oral tablets, chewable tablets, oral granules	Not used to treat acute asthma episodes
zafirlukast (Accolate)	Oral tablets	Take at least 1 hr before or 2 hrs after meals. Affects metabolism of erythromycin and theophylline. Not used to treat acute asthma episodes

Continued

TABLE 28.7 **Drug Therapy**

Asthma and Chronic Obstructive Pulmonary Disease (COPD)—cont'd

Drug	Route of Administration	Comments
Leukotriene Inhibitor zileuton (Zyflo, Zyflo CR)	Oral tablets	Monitor liver enzymes. May interfere with metabolism of warfarin and theophylline. Not used to treat acute asthma episodes
Methylxanthines *IV agent:* aminophylline (second-line therapy) *Oral:* theophylline	Oral tablets, IV, elixir, sustained-release tablets	Wide variety of response to drug metabolism exists. Half-life is ↓ by smoking and ↑ by heart failure and liver disease. Cimetidine, ciprofloxacin, erythromycin, and other drugs may rapidly ↑ theophylline levels. Taking drug with food or antacids may help GI effects. Use limited to situations in which other long-term bronchodilators not available or not affordable
Monoclonal Antibodies ***Anti-IgE*** omalizumab (Xolair)	Subcutaneous	Only for moderate to severe, persistent, allergic asthma with symptoms not adequately controlled by ICSs. Not for acute bronchospasm. Give only under direct medical supervision biweekly or monthly, depending on IgE levels and weight. Observe patient for a minimum of 2 hrs after giving because anaphylaxis can occur
Anti-Interleukin 5 mepolizumab (Nucala)	Subcutaneous	Only used for maintenance in patients with severe asthma attacks despite receiving current asthma medications. Given once every 4 wks by health care professional
reslizumab (Cinqair)	IV only	
Phosphodiesterase Inhibitor Type 4 (PDE-4) roflumilast (Daliresp)	Oral	Only used in severe COPD to reduce exacerbation frequency. Not to be used for acute bronchospasm. GI symptoms occur within 6 mos of starting therapy. Teach patients to report any psychiatric symptoms (e.g., anxiety, depression, suicidal thoughts). Do not use with theophylline
Combination Agents ***SAMA/SABA*** ipratropium/albuterol (Combivent Respimat, DuoNeb)	Nebulizer (DuoNeb), inhalation spray (Combivent Respimat)	Patients must be careful not to overuse. Respimat is an inhaler, but propellant free, unlike an MDI. Respimat is independent of inspiratory flow. Has dose indicator
ICS/LABA budesonide/formoterol (Symbicort)	MDI	Has a counter
fluticasone/salmeterol (Advair Diskus or HFA)	DPI, MDI	Has a counter. Comes in 3 strengths
fluticasone/vilanterol (Breo Ellipta)	DPI	Dose once daily
mometasone furoate/formoterol fumarate (Dulera)	MDI	Not for relief of acute bronchospasm
LAMA/LABA umeclidinium/vilanterol (Anoro Ellipta)	DPI	Anticholinergic/LABA for COPD. Not for relief of acute bronchospasm

When ICSs are used, asthma can usually be controlled without significant systemic side effects since little systemic drug absorption occurs from these drugs. However, ICSs at the highest dosage levels have been associated with side effects (e.g., easy bruising, decreased bone mineral density). Oropharyngeal candidiasis, hoarseness, and dry cough are local side effects caused by inhalation of corticosteroids. These problems can be reduced or prevented by using a spacer with the metered-dose inhaler (MDI) and by gargling with water or mouthwash after each use. Using a spacer or holding device can help get more medication into the lungs.

Women, especially postmenopausal women, who have asthma and use corticosteroids should take adequate amounts of calcium and vitamin D and take part in regular weight-bearing exercise. (Osteoporosis is discussed in Chapter 63.)

Leukotriene Modifiers. Leukotrienes are inflammatory mediators produced from arachidonic acid metabolism. They are potent bronchoconstrictors. Some leukotrienes cause airway edema and inflammation, contributing to the symptoms of asthma. Leukotriene modifying agents (LTMAs) block the release of some substances from mast cells and eosinophils, thereby producing both bronchodilator and antiinflammatory effects. LTMAs include leukotriene receptor blockers (zafirlukast [Accolate], montelukast [Singulair]) and leukotriene synthesis inhibitors (zileuton [Zyflo CR]). These drugs interfere with the synthesis or block the action of leukotrienes.

LTMAs do not reverse bronchospasm in acute asthma attacks. They are used only for prophylactic and maintenance therapy. One advantage of these drugs is that they are taken orally.

Anti-IgE. Omalizumab (Xolair) is a monoclonal antibody to IgE that decreases circulating free IgE levels. Omalizumab prevents IgE from attaching to mast cells, thus preventing the release of chemical mediators. This drug is indicated for patients with moderate to severe asthma, or those not controlled with ICSs alone. Omalizumab is given subcutaneously every 2 to 4 weeks. The drug has a risk for anaphylaxis, so patients must receive the medication in an HCP's office where this potential emergency can be treated.

Anti-Interleukin 5. Mepolizumab (Nucala) and reslizumab (Cinqair) are monoclonal antibodies to interleukin-5 (IL-5). IL-5 is a major cytokine involved in the inflammatory response in asthma by promoting eosinophil activity. By inhibiting IL-5, these drugs inhibit the production and survival of eosinophils. They are used for patients who have a history of severe asthma attacks despite using current asthma medication.

Nonprescription Combination Drugs. Several nonprescription combination drugs are available OTC. They are usually combinations of a bronchodilator (ephedrine) and an expectorant (guaifenesin). Often patients seek OTC drugs because they are less expensive than prescription medication. Many people consider these drugs safe because they can be obtained without a prescription. In general, they should be avoided due to their potential side effects.

Inhalers containing epinephrine may be available. These agents are advertised as drugs to relieve bronchospasm. Those containing ephedrine and epinephrine are potentially dangerous because they stimulate the central nervous and cardiovascular systems, causing nervousness, heart palpitations and dysrhythmias, tremors, insomnia, and increased BP. Many respiratory products containing ephedrine are behind the counter at pharmacies or need a prescription. This limited access is to prevent the diversion of ephedrine to the production of methamphetamine. Many OTC products have been reformulated with phenylephrine, instead of ephedrine, which works well topically but has modest effects in the oral form.

It is important to teach patients about the dangers associated with nonprescription combination drugs. These drugs are high risk and possibly unsafe to a patient with underlying heart problems because tachycardia and hypertension often occur. For the patient who insists on taking these drugs, caution them to read and follow the directions on the label.

Inhalation Devices for Drug Delivery. Many asthma drugs are given by inhalation because the onset of action is faster and systemic side effects are reduced. Inhalation devices include MDIs, dry powder inhalers (DPIs), and nebulizers.

Inhalers. MDIs are small, hand-held, pressurized devices that deliver a measured dose of drug with each activation. The dosing is usually 1 or 2 puffs. Depending on the specific MDI, a spacer or holding chamber (e.g., AeroChamber, InspirEase [Fig. 28.6]) is used to reduce the amount of drug delivered to the oropharynx and improve the amount of drug delivered to the lungs. Spacers also help people who have hand-breath coordination problems.

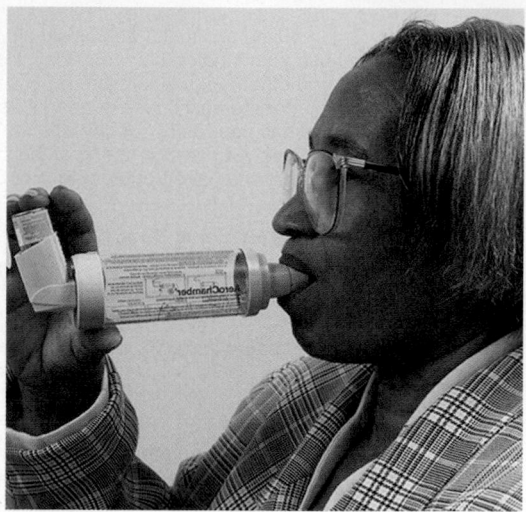

FIG. 28.6 Example of an AeroChamber spacer used with a metered-dose inhaler. (From Potter PA, Perry AG, Stockert P, et al: *Fundamentals of nursing,* ed 9, St Louis, 2017, Mosby.)

TABLE 28.8 Problems Using a Metered-Dose Inhaler (MDI)

- Not coordinating activation with inspiration
- Activating MDI in the mouth while breathing through nose
- Inspiring too rapidly
- Not holding the breath for 10 sec (or as close to 10 sec as possible)
- Holding MDI upside down or sideways
- Inhaling more than 1 puff with each inspiration
- Not shaking MDI before use (if indicated)
- Not waiting enough time between each puff
- Not opening mouth wide enough (if using open mouth technique), causing medication to bounce off teeth, tongue, or palate
- Not having adequate strength to activate MDI
- Not being able to understand and follow directions

International law mandates all MDIs have an ozone-friendly propellant that is a hydrofluoroalkane (HFA). This propellant is nontoxic, evaporates almost instantly once it forces medicine out of the MDI canister, and is not harmful to the patient. The number of times an MDI must be primed and the frequency of priming vary widely, so read the package insert with the patient.

The patient who needs to use several MDIs is often unclear about the order in which to take the medications. Historically it was recommended that SABAs be used first to open the airway and improve the delivery of subsequent medication. However, this recommendation is not evidence based. It is also a potential source of confusion to patients because SABAs are usually used on an as-needed basis.

One of the major problems with metered-dose drugs is the potential for overuse (more than 2 canisters per month) rather than seeking needed medical care (Table 28.8). As the patient has more asthmatic symptoms, they may use the β_2-adrenergic agonist MDI much more often. β_2-Adrenergic agonists help by relieving bronchospasm. They do not treat the inflammatory response. Therefore teach the patient the correct therapeutic use of these drugs.

Another problem is technique. Any MDI is effective only if taken properly. Review MDI technique during each visit as a standard part of care. The patient needs to know the correct way

Using an inhaler seems simple, but most patients do not use it the right way. When you use your inhaler the wrong way, less medicine gets to your lungs. (Your physician may give you other types of inhalers.)

For the next 2 weeks, read these steps aloud as you do them or ask someone to read them to you. Ask your physician or nurse to check how well you are using your inhaler.

Use your inhaler in one of the three ways pictured below (**A** or **B** is best, but **C** can be used if you have trouble with **A** or **B**).

Steps for Using Your Inhaler

Getting ready
1. Take off the cap and shake the inhaler.
2. Breathe out all the way.
3. Hold your inhaler the way your doctor said (**A, B,** or **C** below).

Breathe in slowly
4. As you start breathing in **slowly** through your mouth, press down on the inhaler **one** time. (If you use a holding chamber, first press down on the inhaler. Within 5 seconds, begin to breathe in slowly.)
5. Keep breathing in **slowly,** as deeply as you can.

Hold your breath
6. Hold your breath as you count to 10 slowly, if you can.
7. For inhaled quick-relief medicine (β_2-agonists), wait about 1 minute between puffs. There is no need to wait between puffs for other medicines.

A. Hold inhaler 1 to 2 inches in front of your mouth (about the width of two fingers).

B. Use a spacer/holding chamber. These come in many shapes and can be useful to any patient.

C. Put the inhaler in your mouth.

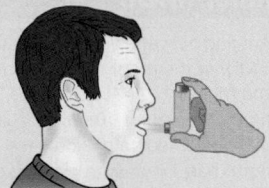 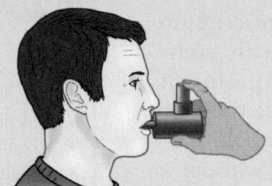 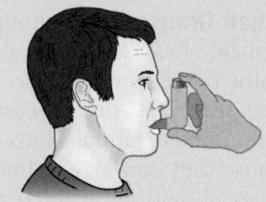

Clean Your Inhaler as Needed

Look at the hole where the medicine sprays out from your inhaler. If you see "powder" in or around the hole, clean the inhaler. Remove the metal canister from the L-shaped plastic mouthpiece. Rinse only the mouthpiece and cap in warm water. Let them dry overnight. In the morning, put the canister back inside. Put the cap on.

Know When to Replace Your Inhaler

For medicines you take each day (an example): Say your new canister has 200 puffs (number of puffs is listed on canister) and you are told to take 8 puffs per day.

$$8 \text{ puffs per day}\overline{)\frac{25 \text{ days}}{200 \text{ puffs in canister}}}$$

So this canister will last 25 days. If you started using this inhaler on May 1, replace it on or before May 25. You can write the date on your canister.

For **quick-relief medicine take as needed** and count each puff.

Do not put your canister in water to see if it is empty as water may enter MDI and impair inhaler.

FIG. 28.7 How to use your metered-dose inhaler correctly.

to determine whether the MDI is empty and how to effectively clean and care for the device (Fig. 28.7).

DPIs are simpler to use than MDIs. The DPI contains dry, powdered medication and is breath activated (Fig. 28.8). No propellant is used. Instead, an aerosol is created when the patient inhales through a reservoir containing a dose of powder.

DPIs have several advantages over MDIs: (1) less manual dexterity is needed, (2) there is no need to coordinate device puffs with inhalation, and (3) no spacer is needed. Disadvantages are that some common drugs are not yet available in DPIs, and the medication may clump if exposed to humidity. Since the medicine is delivered only by the patient's inspiratory effort, patients with a low FEV_1 (less than 1 L) may not be able to inspire the medication. Table 28.9 describes how to effectively use a DPI.

Differences between MDIs and DPIs are described in Table 28.10. Aerosolized medication delivery systems, when used with comparable drug doses, provide equivalent efficacy. Therefore patients should use the device best suited to their needs.

Nebulizers. Nebulizers are small machines used to convert drug solutions into mists. The mist can be inhaled through a face mask or mouthpiece held between the teeth. Nebulizers are usually used for those who have severe asthma or difficulty with the MDI inhalation. They do not provide better delivery of medication than a spacer with an inhaler.

Nebulizers are usually powered by a compressed air or O_2 generator. At home, the patient may have an air-powered compressor. In the hospital, wall O_2 or compressed air powers the nebulizer.

Aerosolized medication orders must include the medication, dose, diluent, and whether it is to be nebulized with O_2 or compressed air. The advantage of nebulization therapy is that it is easy to use. Medications that are routinely nebulized include albuterol and ipratropium.

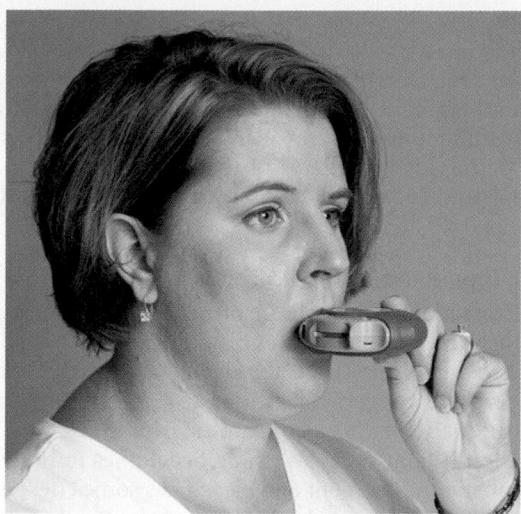

FIG. 28.8 Example of a dry powder inhaler (DPI). (From Potter PA, Perry AG, Stockert P, et al: *Fundamentals of nursing,* ed 9, St Louis, 2017, Mosby.)

TABLE 28.9 Patient Teaching

How to Use a Dry Powder Inhaler (DPI)

Include the following instructions when teaching a patient to use a DPI:
1. Remove mouthpiece cap or open the device according to manufacturer's instructions. Check for dust or dirt. If there is an external counter, note the number of doses left.
2. Load the medicine into the inhaler or engage the lever to allow the medicine to become available. Some DPIs re held upright while loading. Others are held sideways or in a horizontal position.
3. Do not shake your medicine.
4. Tilt your head back slightly and breathe out, getting as much air out of your lungs as you can. Do not breathe into your inhaler because this could affect the dose.
5. Close your lips tightly around the mouthpiece of the inhaler.
6. Breathe in deeply and quickly. This will ensure that the medicine moves down deeply into your lungs. You may not taste or sense the medicine going into your lungs.
7. Hold your breath for 10 seconds or as long as you can to disperse the medicine into your lungs.
8. If there is an external counter, note the number of doses left. It should be 1 less than the number in step 1 above.
9. Do not keep your DPI in a humid place, such as a shower room, because the medicine may clump.

The patient is placed in an upright position that allows for most efficient breathing to ensure adequate penetration and deposition of the aerosolized medication. The patient must breathe slowly and deeply through the mouth and hold each inspiration for 2 to 3 seconds. Deep diaphragmatic breathing helps ensure delivery of the medication. Tell the patient to breathe normally in between large, inhaled breaths. After treatment, have the patient cough effectively.

To reduce the potential for bacterial growth, review cleaning procedures for home respiratory equipment with the patient. An effective home-cleaning method is to wash the nebulizer daily in soap and water, rinse it with water, and soak it for 20 to 30 minutes in a 1:1 white vinegar–water solution, followed by a water rinse and air drying.

Patient Teaching Related to Drug Therapy. One of the major factors determining success in asthma management is the correct administration of drugs. The drug regimen can be

TABLE 28.10 Comparison of Metered-Dose and Dry Powder Inhalers

	Metered-Dose Inhaler (MDI)	Dry Powder Inhaler (DPI)
Shake before use	May be needed for some (e.g., albuterol), but not for others (Read package insert)	No
Inspiration	Slow	Rapid
Spacer	May be used with inhaled corticosteroids or for more effective delivery (Read package insert)	Not used
Counting device	Many have an external device, but some do not	Most preloaded forms include counter
Inhalations/dose	Often 2/dose	Often 1/dose
Cleaning	Use water for plastic case	Avoid moisture

confusing and complex. When teaching patients about their medications, include the name, purpose, dosage, method of administration, and when to use. It is essential that the patient understand the difference between rescue and controller medications, the importance of monitoring their response to therapy, and, most importantly, when to recognize that symptoms are not improving and help is required. Review side effects, appropriate action if side effects occur, and how to properly prime, use, and clean devices. Some patients may benefit from keeping a diary to record medication use, wheezing, or coughing, PEFR, side effects of drugs, and activity level. This information will help the HCP adjust the medication if needed.

Several factors can affect the correct use of inhalation devices. These include advanced age, changes in physical dexterity (e.g., arthritis in hands, coordination), psychologic state (e.g., cognition), affordability, convenience, and administration time and preference.

Poor adherence with medication therapy is a major challenge in the long-term management of chronic asthma. Lack of adherence often occurs when the patient is symptom free and does not use the long-term therapy (e.g., ICS) regularly because no immediate benefit is felt. The patient does not realize that ICSs are needed to treat the ongoing inflammatory process.

Explain the importance and purpose of taking the long-term therapy regularly, emphasizing that maximum improvement may take 1 week or longer. Tell the patient that without regular use, swelling in the airways may progress and asthma will likely worsen over time. Collaborate with social services to help lower income patients obtain medications.

Make sure that patients understand exactly how to use their inhaler device (Fig. 28.7). Give them printed instructions. At every clinic visit or hospitalization, reassess the patient's inhaler technique. If package inserts are available, you can review them before teaching the patient.

❖ NURSING MANAGEMENT: ASTHMA

◆ Nursing Assessment

If a patient is not in acute distress, obtain a detailed health history, including information about triggers and what has helped alleviate asthma attacks in the past. Subjective and objective data that should be obtained from a patient with asthma are outlined in Table 28.11.

TABLE 28.11 Nursing Assessment

Asthma

Subjective Data

Important Health Information

Past health history: Allergic rhinitis, sinusitis, or skin allergies. Previous asthma attack and hospitalization or intubation. Symptoms worsened by triggers in the environment. GERD. Occupational exposure to chemical irritants (e.g., paints, dust)

Medications: Adherence to medication, inhaler technique. Use of antibiotics. Pattern and amount of short-acting β_2-adrenergic agonist used per week. Medications that may trigger an attack in susceptible persons, such as aspirin, NSAIDs, β-adrenergic blockers

Functional Health Patterns

Health perception–health management: Family history of allergies or asthma. Recent URI or sinus infection

Activity-exercise: Fatigue, decreased or absent exercise tolerance. Dyspnea, cough (especially at night), productive cough with yellow or green sputum or sticky sputum. Chest tightness, feelings of suffocation, air hunger, talking in short sentences or words or phrases, sitting upright to breathe

Sleep-rest: Awakened from sleep because of cough or breathing difficulties, insomnia

Coping–stress tolerance: Emotional distress, stress in work environment or home

Objective Data

General

Restlessness or exhaustion, confusion, upright or forward-leaning body position

Integumentary

Diaphoresis, cyanosis (circumoral, nail bed), eczema

Respiratory

Nasal discharge, nasal polyps, mucosal swelling. Crackles, decreased or absent breath sounds, and wheezes (inspiratory, expiratory, or both) on auscultation. Hyperresonance on percussion. Sputum (thick, white, tenacious), ↑ work of breathing with use of accessory muscles. Intercostal and supraclavicular retractions. Tachypnea with hyperventilation. Prolonged expiration

Cardiovascular

Tachycardia, pulsus paradoxus, jugular venous distention, hypertension or hypotension, premature ventricular contractions

Possible Diagnostic Findings

Abnormal ABGs during attacks, ↓ O_2 saturation, serum and sputum eosinophilia, ↑ serum IgE, positive skin tests for allergens, chest x-ray showing hyperinflation with attacks, abnormal pulmonary function tests showing ↓ flow rates; FVC, FEV_1, PEFR, and FEV_1/FVC ratio that improve between attacks and with bronchodilators

◆ Nursing Diagnoses

Nursing diagnoses for the patient with asthma may include:
- Impaired breathing
- Activity intolerance
- Anxiety
- Lack of knowledge

Additional information on nursing diagnoses and interventions is presented in eNursing Care Plan 28.1 on the website for this chapter.

◆ Planning

The overall goals are that the patient with asthma will achieve asthma control, as evidenced by (1) minimal symptoms during the day and night, (2) acceptable activity levels (including exercise), (3) maintaining greater than 80% of personal best PEFR, (4) few or no adverse effects of therapy, (5) no acute attacks of asthma, and (6) adequate knowledge to carry out the plan of care.

◆ Nursing Implementation

◆ **Health Promotion.** Your role in preventing asthma attacks or decreasing their severity focuses primarily on teaching both the patient and caregiver. Teach the patient to identify and avoid known personal triggers for asthma (e.g., cigarette smoke, pet dander) and irritants (e.g., cold air, aspirin, foods, cats, indoor air pollution) (Table 28.1). Washing bedclothes in hot water or cooler water with detergent and bleach has some effect on allergen levels. Avoiding furred animals is suggested, but pet allergens are impossible to avoid. Pet allergens can be found in many public areas for months even after removal of the animal. Many people are allergic to cockroach remains and the dried droppings, so measures to avoid or control cockroaches are partly effective in removing allergens.

When cold air cannot be avoided, dressing properly with scarves or using a mask helps reduce the risk for an asthma attack. Aspirin and NSAIDs should be avoided if they are known to trigger an attack. Many OTC drugs contain aspirin. Teach the patient to read the labels carefully. Nonselective β-blockers (e.g., propranolol [Inderal]) are contraindicated because they inhibit bronchodilation. Selective β-blockers (e.g., atenolol [Tenormin]) should be used with caution. Desensitization (immunotherapy) may be partially effective in decreasing the patient's sensitivity to known allergens (see Chapter 13).

Prompt diagnosis and treatment of URIs and sinusitis may prevent an asthma attack. If occupational irritants are involved, the patient may need to consider changing jobs. Those who are obese often find that weight loss improves asthma control. Encourage the patient to maintain a fluid intake of 2 to 3 L/day, adequate nutrition, and plenty of rest. If exercise is planned or if the patient has asthma only with exercise, the HCP can suggest a medication regimen for pretreatment or long-term control of symptoms to prevent bronchospasm.

◆ **Acute Care.** A major goal in asthma care is to maximize the patient's ability to safely manage acute asthma using an asthma action plan developed in conjunction with the HCP (Fig. 28.9). Action plans are important for all people with asthma, especially those who have frequent, acute attacks. They are based on the patient's asthma symptoms and PEFR. The action plan dictates what symptoms or PEFR necessitates a change in asthma management to gain control.

The patient can take 2 to 4 puffs of a SABA every 20 minutes, up to 3 times, as a rescue plan. Depending on the response (e.g., alleviation of symptoms, improved PEFR), continued SABA use and/or oral corticosteroids may be a part of the home management plan. If symptoms persist or if the patient's PEFR is less than 50% of the personal best, the HCP or emergency medical services must be contacted at once.

When the patient is in the health care agency with an acute attack, it is important to monitor the patient's respiratory and cardiovascular systems. This includes (1) monitoring heart rate and rhythm, respiratory rate and WOB, and BP; (2) monitoring pulse oximetry, PEFR, and ABGs; and (3) auscultating lung sounds.

Asthma Action Plan

For: _____ Doctor: _____ Date: _____

Doctor's Phone Number _____ Hospital/Emergency Department Phone Number _____

GREEN ZONE

Doing Well

- No cough, wheeze, chest tightness, or shortness of breath during the day or night
- Can do usual activities

And, if a peak flow meter is used,

Peak flow: more than _____
(80 percent or more of my best peak flow)

My best peak flow is: _____

Take these long-term control medicines each day (include an antiinflammatory).

Medicine	How much to take	When to take it
_____	_____	_____
_____	_____	_____
_____	_____	_____
_____	_____	_____

| Before exercise | ☐ _____ | ☐ 2 or ☐ 4 puffs _____ | 5 minutes before exercise |

YELLOW ZONE

Asthma Is Getting Worse

- Cough, wheeze, chest tightness, or shortness of breath, or
- Waking at night due to asthma, or
- Can do some, but not all, usual activities

-Or-

Peak flow: _____ to _____
(50 to 79 percent of my best peak flow)

First → Add: quick-relief medicine—and keep taking your GREEN ZONE medicine.

_____
(short-acting beta₂-agonist)
☐ 2 or ☐ 4 puffs, every 20 minutes for up to 1 hour
☐ Nebulizer, once

Second → If your symptoms (and peak flow, if used) return to GREEN ZONE after 1 hour of above treatment:

☐ Continue monitoring to be sure you stay in the green zone.

-Or-

If your symptoms (and peak flow, if used) do not return to GREEN ZONE after 1 hour of above treatment:

☐ Take: _____ ☐ 2 or ☐ 4 puffs or ☐ Nebulizer
(short-acting beta₂-agonist)

☐ Add: _____ mg per day For _____ (3–10) days
(oral steroid)

☐ Call the doctor ☐ before/ ☐ within _____ hours after taking the oral steroid.

RED ZONE

Medical Alert!

- Very short of breath, or
- Quick-relief medicines have not helped, or
- Cannot do usual activities, or
- Symptoms are same or get worse after 24 hours in Yellow Zone

-Or-

Peak flow: less than _____
(50 percent of my best peak flow)

Take this medicine:

☐ _____ ☐ 4 or ☐ 6 puffs or ☐ Nebulizer
(short-acting beta₂-agonist)

☐ _____ mg
(oral steroid)

Then call your doctor NOW. Go to the hospital or call an ambulance if:

- You are still in the red zone after 15 minutes AND
- You have not reached your doctor.

DANGER SIGNS

- **Trouble walking and talking due to shortness of breath**
- **Lips or fingernails are blue**

→ ■ Take ☐ 4 or ☐ 6 puffs of your quick-relief medicine AND

■ Go to the hospital or call for an ambulance _____ NOW!
(phone)

FIG. 28.9 Asthma action plan. (Source: National Heart, Lung, and Blood Institute, Bethesda, MD.)

Give drugs as ordered. Louder wheezing may actually occur in airways that are responding to therapy as airflow increases. As improvement continues and airflow increases, breath sounds increase and wheezing decreases. The disappearance of most bronchospasm, resolution of edema and cellular infiltration of airway mucosa, and the elimination of viscous mucous plugs may take several days to improve. As a result, therapy must be continued even after clinical improvement. Always evaluate the patient's response to therapy.

An important nursing goal during an acute attack is to decrease the patient's anxiety and sense of panic. Position the patient comfortably (usually sitting, in semi- to high-Fowler's position) to maximize chest expansion. A calm, quiet, reassuring attitude may help the patient relax. A technique called "talking

TABLE 28.12 Patient Teaching
Pursed-Lip Breathing (PLB)

Teach the patient how to do PLB using the following guidelines:
1. Use PLB before, during, and after any activity causing you to be short of breath.
2. Inhale slowly and deeply through the nose.
3. Exhale slowly through pursed lips, as if whistling.
4. Relax your facial muscles without puffing your cheeks—like whistling—while you are exhaling.
5. Make breathing out (exhalation) 3 times as long as breathing in (inhalation).
6. The following activities can help you get the "feel" of PLB:
   - Blow through a straw in a glass of water with the intent of forming small bubbles.
   - Blow a lit candle enough to bend the flame without blowing it out.
   - Steadily blow a table-tennis ball across a table.
   - Blow a tissue held in the hand until it gently flaps.
7. Practice 8-10 repetitions of PLB 3 or 4 times a day.

down" can help the patient remain calm. In talking down, you gain eye contact with the patient. In a firm, calm voice, coach the patient to use pursed-lip breathing. Pursed-lip breathing keeps the airways open by maintaining positive pressure (Table 28.12). Stay with the patient until the respiratory rate has slowed.

When the acute attack subsides, provide rest and a quiet, calm environment. When the patient is less exhausted, can breathe easier, and beginning to recover, try to obtain a health history and do a physical assessment. If caregivers are present, they may be able to provide information about the patient's health history. This information is important in planning and implementing an individualized nursing care plan.

◆ **Ambulatory Care.** Control of symptoms can be achieved by teaching the patient about drug therapy and monitoring. Review the written asthma action plan. As part of the plan, the patient must measure PEFR at least daily. PEFR monitoring, when done correctly, is a reliable, objective measurement of asthma control (Table 28.13). Some patients may not perceive changes in their

TABLE 28.13 Patient Teaching
How to Use Your Peak Flow Meter

Include the following instructions when teaching the patient to use a peak flow meter:

Why Use a Peak Flow Meter?
- Peak flow meters are used to check your asthma the way that BP cuffs are used to check BP. A peak flow meter is a device that measures how well air moves out of your lungs.
- During an asthma episode, the airways of the lungs usually begin to narrow slowly. The peak flow meter may tell you if there is narrowing in the airways hours, sometimes even days, before you have any asthma symptoms.
- By taking your medicines early (before symptoms), you may be able to stop the episode quickly and avoid a severe asthma episode.
- The peak flow meter is used to help you and your HCP:
- Learn what makes your asthma worse.
- Decide if your treatment plan is working well.
- Decide when to add or stop medicine.
- Decide when to seek emergency care.

How to Use Your Peak Flow Meter
Complete the following 5 steps with your peak flow meter:
1. Move the indicator to the bottom of the numbered scale.
2. Stand up.
3. Take a deep breath, filling your lungs completely.
4. Place the mouthpiece in your mouth and close your lips around it. Do not put your tongue inside the hole.
5. Blow out as hard and fast as you can in a single blow.
   - Write down the number you get. But if you cough or make a mistake, do not write down the number. Perform the action again.
   - Repeat steps 1 through 5 two more times. Write down the best of the 3 blows in your asthma diary.

Find Your Personal Best Peak Flow Number
- Your personal best peak flow number is the highest peak flow number you can achieve over a 2-week period when your asthma is under good control. Good control is when you feel good and do not have any asthma symptoms.
- Each patient's asthma is different. Your best peak expiratory flow rate (PEFR) may be higher or lower than the peak flow of someone of your height, weight, and gender. This means that it is important for you to find your own personal best peak flow number, which is the basis for your treatment plan.

- To find your personal best peak flow number, take peak flow readings:
  - At least twice a day for 2-3 weeks, between 12 noon and 2 PM when your peak flow is the highest
  - 15 to 20 minutes after taking inhaled short-acting β_2-agonist (SABA) for quick relief
  - As instructed by your HCP

The Peak Flow Zone System
Once you know your personal best peak flow number, your HCP will put the peak flow numbers into zones that are set up like a traffic light. This will help you know what to do when your peak flow number changes. For example:

Green Zone (more than __ L/min [80% of your personal best number]) signals good control. No asthma symptoms are present. Take your medicines as usual.

Yellow Zone (between __ and __ L/min [50% to <80% of your personal best number]) signals caution. If you stay in the yellow zone after several measures of peak flow, take an inhaled SABA. If you continue to register peak flow readings in the yellow zone, your asthma may not be under good control. Ask your HCP if you need to change or increase your daily medicines.

Red Zone (<__ L/min [<50% of your personal best number]) signals a medical alert. Take an inhaled SABA (quick-relief medicine) right away. Call your HCP and ask what to do or go directly to the ED.

Use the Diary to Keep Track of Your Peak Flow
- Record your personal best peak flow number and peak flow zones in your asthma diary.
- Measure your peak flow when you wake up, *before* taking medicine. Write down your peak flow number in the diary every day, or as instructed by your HCP.

Actions to Take When Peak Flow Numbers Change
- PEFR goes between __ and __ L/min (50% to <80% of personal best, yellow zone).
  ACTION: Take an inhaled SABA (quick-relief medicine) as prescribed by your HCP.
- PEFR increases ≥20% when measured before and after taking an inhaled SABA (quick-relief medicine).
  ACTION: Talk to your HCP about adding more medicine to control your asthma better (e.g., an antiinflammatory medication).

Source: Adapted from National Asthma Education and Prevention Program, National Heart, Lung, and Blood Institute: *Expert Panel Report 3: guidelines for the diagnosis and management of asthma*, NIH pub no 08-4051, Bethesda, Md, 2007, National Institutes of Health.

breathing and may have a significant decrease in lung function without any symptoms other than a change in PEFR.

If a patient's PEFR is within the green zone (usually 80% to 100% of the patient's personal best), the patient should remain on their usual medications. A PEFR within the yellow zone (usually 50% to 80% of personal best) indicates caution. A PEFR in the red zone (50% or less of personal best) indicates a serious problem. In other words, something is triggering the patient's asthma (e.g., viral infection).

Consequently, the written asthma action plan needs to clearly identify the step-up increase in medications during the acute phase of an infection. For example, the patient can use different strategies, such as using the SABA more often. Although it may happen, it is unusual for a patient's PEFR to drop from the green zone to the red zone quickly. Usually the patient has time to make changes in medications, avoid triggers, and notify the HCP. The dose is stepped down once the symptoms subside.

❓ CHECK YOUR PRACTICE

A 32-yr-old man is admitted to the ED for an acute attack of asthma. It is his third admission in the past 2 months. He had been watching his 6-yr-old son play soccer when his attack started. He says to you, "I am just not a good father. My son is going to think I am just a 'sicky.' I can't play sports . . . can't . . . even . . . watch him . . . without something happening."
• How would you respond to this man?

It is important to involve the patient's caregivers. They should know where to find the patient's medications. Teach them how to decrease the patient's anxiety if an asthma attack occurs. When the patient is stabilized or controlled, the caregiver can gently remind the patient about monitoring daily PEFR by asking questions, such as "What zone are you in?" or "How's your peak flow today?" A patient and caregiver teaching guide for the patient with asthma is shown in Table 28.14.

Good nutrition is important. Physical exercise (e.g., swimming, walking, stationary cycling) within the patient's limit of tolerance is beneficial. It may require pretreatment with a SABA. Uninterrupted sleep is an important goal. If patients with asthma report lack of sleep because of asthma symptoms, their asthma is not under good control and their plan should be reevaluated.

INFORMATICS IN PRACTICE
Home Monitoring of Asthma

• To reduce the rate of hospital readmissions, the patient with asthma may be discharged with a home monitoring system. These systems provide an easy and inexpensive approach to remotely monitoring lung function.
• Asthma home monitoring usually consists of PEFR, pulse oximetry, vital signs, and lung sounds. This information is sent to the HCP so that problems are quickly detected.
• As part of your discharge planning, help the patient obtain a system and review its use.

Validated questionnaires (e.g., Asthma Control Test [ACT] available at *www.asthmacontroltest.com*) can be used to assess quality-of-life in asthma patients. Patients with asthma may have frequent absences from school or work and psychological issues, such as stress, anxiety, despair, and depression.

TABLE 28.14 Patient & Caregiver Teaching
Asthma

Include the following information in a teaching plan for the patient with asthma and the caregiver. It will help to improve the patient's quality of life and promote lifestyle changes that support successful living with asthma.

What Is Asthma?
• Basic anatomy and physiology of lung
• Pathophysiology of asthma
• Relationship of pathophysiology to signs and symptoms
• Measurement and correlation of spirometry and peak expiratory flow rate

What Is Good Asthma Control?
• Personal ideas of good control
• Use Asthma Control Test available at www.asthmacontroltest.com

Obstacles to Asthma Treatment and Control
• Discuss with patient and caregiver about possible obstacles (e.g., denial, poor perception of asthma severity by patient)

Environmental and Trigger Control
• Identify triggers and preventive measures (use trigger diary)
• Avoiding allergens and other triggers
• Need to maintain good hydration

Medications
• Types (include mechanism of action)
• Use of preventive and maintenance (e.g., antiinflammatory) agents
• Write out medication list and schedule
• Asthma Action Plan (Fig. 28.9)
• Correct use of inhalers, spacer, and nebulizer

Pursed-Lip Breathing (Table 28.12)
Correct Use of Peak Flow Meter (Table 28.13)
Asthma Action Plan (Fig. 28.9)
• Peak flow zones
• Individualize asthma action plan with HCP and patient
• Early recognition of infection
• Building a partnership with your HCP
• Questions patients may have about asthma, but patient cannot reach the HCP

For more information, visit the American Lung Association website at *www.lung.org/lung-disease/asthma.*

An increased number of older adults have asthma. This is a special concern because they have more complicated health issues than younger patients with asthma. Issues that face older adults are hypertension, heart disease, costly medications, and difficulty accessing the health care system. Keep these factors in mind when implementing a management plan for older adults.

Disparities in socioeconomic status and access to proper health care, as well as cultural beliefs about asthma may be part of the reason blacks and Hispanics have higher rates of poorly controlled asthma. Seek to explore and eliminate any potential barriers to health care. Use culturally appropriate resources and educational material in languages other than English to help improve knowledge about asthma and asthma control for these persons.

Relaxation therapies (e.g., yoga, meditation, relaxation techniques, breathing techniques) may help a patient relax respiratory muscles and decrease the respiratory rate. (Chapter 6 discusses relaxation breathing and other relaxation strategies.)

A healthy emotional outlook is also important in preventing asthma attacks. Asthma support groups are available online and around the country.

◆ Evaluation

The expected outcomes are that the patient with asthma will
- Maintain patent airway with removal of excessive secretions
- Have normal (for the patient) breath sounds and respiratory rate
- Report decreased anxiety with increased control of breathing
- Correctly use medications
- Express confidence in ability to manage asthma

CHRONIC OBSTRUCTIVE PULMONARY DISEASE

Chronic obstructive pulmonary disease (COPD) is a preventable, treatable, but often progressive disease characterized by persistent airflow limitation. COPD is associated with an enhanced chronic inflammatory response in the airways and lungs, primarily caused by cigarette smoking and other noxious particles and gases. COPD exacerbations and other coexisting illnesses or co-morbidities may contribute to the overall severity of the disease.

Previous definitions of COPD have included such terms as *chronic bronchitis* and *emphysema*. Neither term is part of the current definition of COPD. **Chronic bronchitis** is the presence of cough and sputum production for at least 3 months in each of 2 consecutive years. It is an independent disease that may precede or follow the development of airflow limitation. **Emphysema**, the destruction of alveoli without fibrosis, describes one of several structural abnormalities in COPD patients.

An estimated 16 million adults in the United States have COPD.[12] The number of people with COPD is greatly underestimated because the disease is usually not diagnosed until it is moderately advanced. COPD is the third leading cause of death in the United States, causing more than 120,000 deaths each year.[12]

GENDER DIFFERENCES
COPD

Men
- COPD is more common in men.
- The number of men with COPD is not increasing.
- Have a poorer response to O_2 therapy compared with women.

Women
- The number of women with COPD is increasing.
- The increase is likely due to more women smoking and increased susceptibility (e.g., smaller lungs and airways).
- More women die from COPD than men.
- Women with COPD have a lower quality of life, more exacerbations, and increased dyspnea, compared with men.

Risk Factors for COPD

Many factors affect the development and progression of COPD. The following discussion addresses the most common risk factors.

Cigarette Smoking. The major risk factor for developing COPD is cigarette smoking. COPD affects about 20% of smokers.[13] COPD should be considered in any person who is over the age of 40 with a smoking history of 10 or more pack-years.

TABLE 28.15 Effects of Tobacco Smoke on Respiratory System

Area of Defect	Acute Effects	Long-Term Effects
Respiratory mucosa		
• Nasopharyngeal	↓ Sense of smell	Cancer
• Tongue	↓ Sense of taste	Cancer
• Vocal cords	Hoarseness	Chronic cough, cancer
• Bronchus and bronchioles	Bronchospasm, cough	Chronic bronchitis, asthma, cancer
Cilia	Paralysis, sputum accumulation, cough	Chronic bronchitis, cancer
Mucous glands	↑ Secretions, ↑ cough	Hyperplasia and hypertrophy of glands, chronic bronchitis
Alveolar macrophages	↓ Function	↑ Incidence of infection
Elastin and collagen fibers	↑ Destruction by proteases ↓ Function of antiproteases (α_1-antitrypsin) ↓ Synthesis and repair of elastin	Emphysema

Cigarette smoke has several direct effects on the respiratory tract (Table 28.15). The irritating effect of smoke causes hyperplasia of cells, including goblet cells, thereby increasing mucus production. Hyperplasia reduces airway diameter and makes it harder to clear secretions. Smoking reduces the ciliary activity and may cause actual loss of cilia. Smoking causes abnormal dilation of the distal air space with destruction of alveolar walls. Many cells develop large, atypical nuclei, which are considered a precancerous condition. Smoking causes chronic, enhanced inflammation of various parts of the lung with structural changes and repair (called *remodeling*). The reasons for the inflammatory response are not clearly understood. Genetics may be involved since patients who have never smoked can develop COPD.

Cigarette smoking causes oxidative stress and an imbalance between proteases that break down connective tissue in the lung and antiproteases that protect the lungs. These changes increase with more severe disease and persist even after the patient has stopped smoking. (See Chapter 10 for more details about cigarette smoking.)

Passive smoking is the exposure of nonsmokers to cigarette smoke, also known as *environmental tobacco smoke* (ETS) or secondhand smoke. In adults, ETS is associated with decreased pulmonary function, increased respiratory symptoms, and severe lower respiratory tract infections (e.g., pneumonia). ETS is associated with increased risk for nasal sinus cancer and lung cancer.

Infection. Infections are a risk factor for developing COPD. Severe recurring respiratory tract infections in childhood have been associated with reduced lung function and increased respiratory symptoms in adulthood. It is unclear whether the development of COPD is related to recurrent infections in adults. People who smoke and have human immunodeficiency virus (HIV) infection have an accelerated development of COPD.[14] Tuberculosis is also a risk factor for COPD development.[15]

Asthma. Patients with COPD may have asthma. Asthma may be a risk factor for the development of COPD. There is a considerable pathologic and functional overlap between these disorders (Table 28.4), particularly among older adults, who may have components of both diseases. We call this *asthma-COPD overlap syndrome.*[3]

Air Pollution. High levels of urban air pollution are harmful to people with existing lung disease. However, the effect of outdoor air pollution as a risk factor for the development of COPD is unclear. Another risk factor is exposure to coal and other biomass fuels that are used for indoor heating and cooking. Many people who have never smoked have significant risk because of cooking with these fuels in poorly ventilated areas.

Occupational Chemicals and Dusts. If a person has intense or prolonged exposure to various dusts, vapors, irritants, or fumes in the workplace, symptoms of lung impairment consistent with COPD can develop. If a person has occupational exposure and smokes, the risk for COPD increases.

Aging. Although aging is often considered a risk factor for COPD, the evidence is unclear. Does the aging process lead to COPD, or is COPD a result of the cumulative exposures that occur over a lifetime? Normal aging results in loss of elastic recoil, stiffening of the chest wall, and decrease in exercise tolerance. The lungs gradually lose their elastic recoil. The thoracic cage becomes stiff and rigid, and the ribs are less mobile. The shape of the rib cage gradually changes because of the increased residual volume (RV), causing it to enlarge and become more rounded. Decreased chest compliance and elastic recoil of the lungs caused by aging affect the mechanical aspects of ventilation and increase the WOB. The number of functional alveoli decrease as peripheral airways lose supporting tissues. Over time, the surface area for gas exchange decreases, and the PaO_2 decreases. Changes in the elasticity of the lungs reduce the ventilatory reserve. These changes are similar to those seen in the patient with COPD.

Genetics. An intriguing question is why some smokers develop COPD and others do not. The fact that a small number of smokers get COPD strongly suggests genetic factors play a major role in who develops COPD. Because of the genetic-environmental interaction, 2 people may have the same smoking history, but only 1 develops COPD. To date, only 1 genetic factor has been clearly identified.

Alpha-1 Antitrypsin Deficiency (AATD). Alpha-1(α1) antitrypsin deficiency (AATD) is an autosomal recessive disorder that may affect the lungs or liver. AATD is a genetic risk factor for COPD.[16] α1-Antitrypsin (AAT) is a serum protein made by the liver and normally found in the lungs. The main function of AAT, an α_1-protease inhibitor, is to protect normal lung tissue from attack by proteases during inflammation related to smoking and infections. Severe AATD leads to premature bullous emphysema in the lungs. About 3% of all people diagnosed with COPD may have undetected AAT deficiency. Smoking hastens the disease process in these patients.

Pathophysiology

COPD is characterized by chronic inflammation of the airways, lung parenchyma (respiratory bronchioles and alveoli), and pulmonary blood vessels (Fig. 28.10). The pathogenesis of COPD is complex and involves many mechanisms. The defining feature of COPD is airflow limitation not fully reversible during forced exhalation. This is caused primarily by loss of elastic recoil and airflow obstruction, attributable to mucus hypersecretion, mucosal edema, and bronchospasm.

🧬 GENETICS IN CLINICAL PRACTICE

α_1-Antitrypsin Deficiency (AATD)

Genetic Basis
- Autosomal recessive disorder.
- Mutations in *SERPINA1* gene (found on chromosome 14) cause AAT deficiency.
- Gene provides instructions for the liver to make the protein AAT, which protects the lungs and liver from powerful proteolytic enzymes.
- Without enough functional AAT, proteolytic enzymes destroy alveoli and cause lung disease.

Incidence
- Occurs in 1 in 1700 to 3500 live births in the United States
- People of northern European descent most affected

Genetic Testing
- DNA testing is available.
- Screening of siblings is useful
- Serum assay is available to measure the amount of AAT

Clinical Implications
- AAT deficiency can cause lung and liver disease.
- Onset of disease is between ages 20 and 40 yrs.
- Treatment includes AAT replacement therapy.
- Disease predisposes to early-onset emphysema.

As the disease progresses, abnormalities in airflow limitation, air trapping, and gas exchange worsen. In severe COPD, pulmonary hypertension and systemic manifestations occur. COPD has an uneven distribution of pathologic changes. Severely impaired and/or destroyed areas of lung tissue exist alongside areas of relatively normal lung.

The inflammatory process most often starts with inhalation of noxious particles and gases (e.g., cigarette smoke). The abnormal inflammatory process causes tissue destruction and disrupts the normal defense mechanisms and repair process of the lung. We do not clearly understand the mechanisms for the enhanced inflammatory response. It may be genetically determined.

The predominant inflammatory cells in COPD are neutrophils, macrophages, and lymphocytes. This pattern of inflammatory cells is different from that in asthma, in which eosinophils, mast cells, neutrophils, lymphocytes, and macrophages are the main culprits. Inflammatory cells attract other inflammatory mediators (e.g., leukotrienes) and proinflammatory cytokines (e.g., tumor necrosis factor).

The inflammatory process may be magnified by oxidants, which are made by cigarette smoke and other inhaled particles and released from the inflammatory cells. Oxidants adversely affect the lungs as they inactivate antiproteases (which prevent the natural destruction of the lungs), stimulate mucus secretion, and increase fluid in the lungs. The result of the inflammatory process is structural changes in the lungs.

After the inhalation of oxidants in tobacco or air pollution, the activity of proteases (which break down the connective tissue of the lungs) increases and the antiproteases (which protect against the breakdown) are inhibited. Therefore the natural balance of protease/antiprotease is tipped in favor of destruction of the alveoli and loss of the lungs' elastic recoil.

Inability to expire air is a main characteristic of COPD. The main site of the airflow limitation is in the smaller airways. As the peripheral airways become obstructed, air is progressively

PATHOPHYSIOLOGY MAP

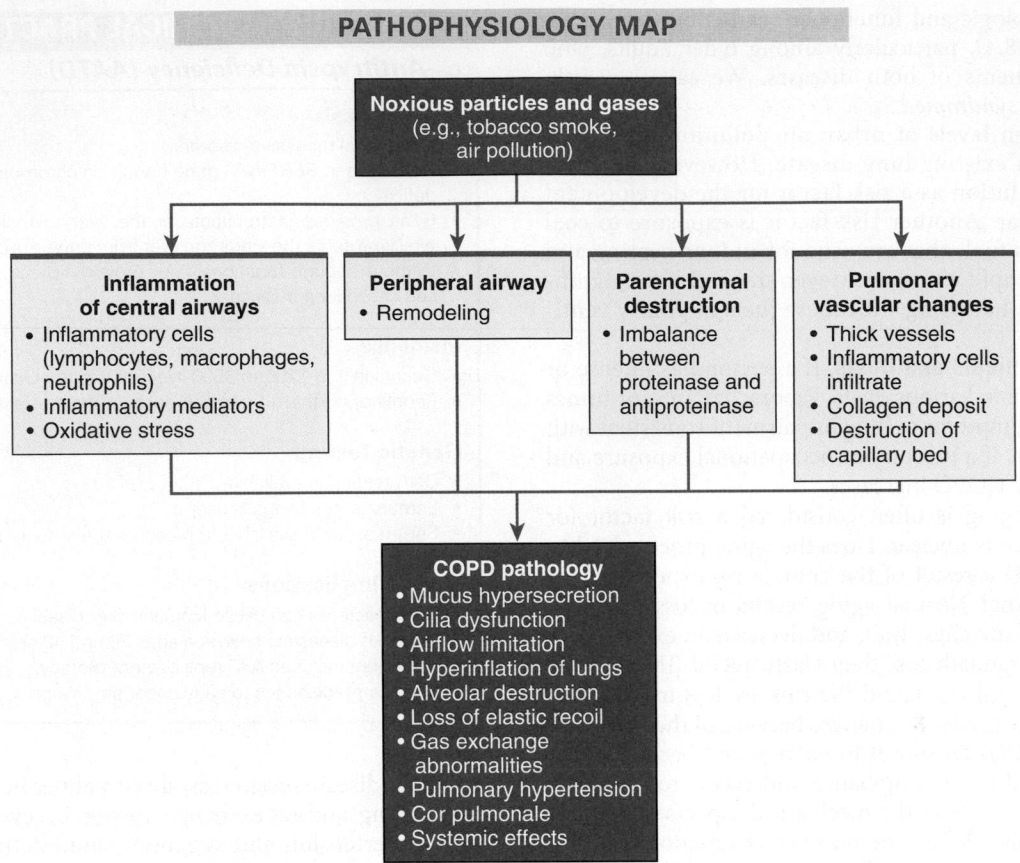

FIG. 28.10 Pathophysiology of chronic obstructive pulmonary disease *(COPD)*.

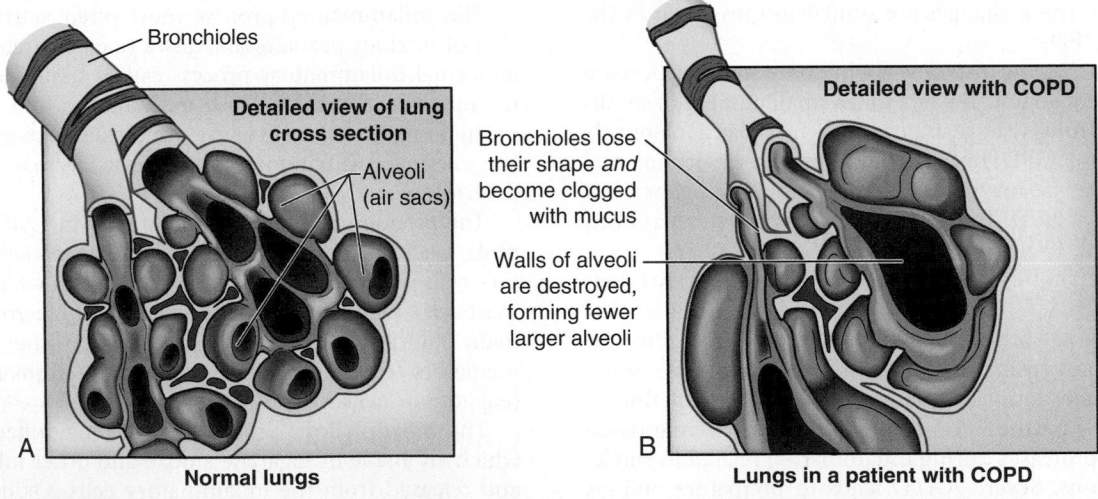

FIG. 28.11 A, Normal lungs showing bronchioles and alveoli. B, Changes in the bronchioles and alveoli in the lungs of a patient with chronic obstructive pulmonary disease *(COPD)*.

trapped during expiration. The volume of residual air becomes greatly increased in severe COPD as alveolar attachments (similar to rubber bands) to small airways are destroyed. As air is trapped in the lungs, the chest hyperexpands and becomes barrel shaped, because the respiratory muscles are not able to function effectively. Functional residual capacity (FRC) is increased. The residual air, combined with the loss of elastic recoil, makes passive expiration of air difficult. The patient is now trying to breathe in when the lungs are in an "overinflated" state. Thus, the patient becomes dyspneic with limited exercise capacity.

Typically, the patient does not have problems with hypoxemia at rest until late in the disease. Initially, hypoxemia may develop during exercise and the patient may benefit from supplemental O_2. Gas exchange abnormalities result in hypoxemia and hypercapnia (increased CO_2) as the disease worsens. As the air trapping increases, walls of alveoli are destroyed (Fig. 28.11). Bullae (large air spaces in the parenchyma) and blebs (air spaces next to pleurae) can form.

Bullae and blebs are not effective in gas exchange because they do not contain the capillary bed that normally surrounds each alveolus. Therefore a significant ventilation-perfusion (V/Q) mismatch and hypoxemia result. Peripheral airway obstruction also results in V/Q imbalance and, combined with respiratory muscle impairment, leads to CO_2 retention, particularly in severe forms of the disease.

Excess mucus production, resulting in a chronic productive cough, is a feature of persons with predominant chronic bronchitis. However, not all COPD patients have sputum production. When present, excess mucus production is multifactorial, including (1) an increased number of mucus-secreting goblet cells, (2) enlarged submucosal glands, (3) dysfunction of cilia, and (4) stimulation from inflammatory mediators.

In addition to lung disease, COPD is a systemic disease. Chronic inflammation is an underlying problem for many patients. Common systemic diseases, including osteoporosis, diabetes, and metabolic syndrome, have been seen with COPD. Cardiovascular diseases are common.

Pulmonary vascular changes resulting in mild to moderate pulmonary hypertension may occur late in the course of COPD. The small pulmonary arteries vasoconstrict due to hypoxia. As the disease advances, the structure of the pulmonary arteries changes, resulting in thickening of the vascular smooth muscle. Because of the loss of alveolar walls and the capillaries surrounding them, pressure in the pulmonary circulation increases. Pulmonary hypertension may progress and lead to hypertrophy of the right ventricle of the heart. The right ventricle dilates and may eventually lead to right-sided heart failure.

Classification of COPD

COPD can be classified as mild, moderate, severe, and very severe (Table 28.16). An FEV_1/FVC ratio of less than 70% establishes the diagnosis of COPD. The severity of obstruction (as shown by FEV_1) determines the stage of COPD. The management of COPD is based on the patient's symptoms, classification, and exacerbation history.

Clinical Manifestations

The manifestations of COPD typically develop slowly. A clinical diagnosis of COPD should be considered in any patient who has chronic cough or sputum production, dyspnea, and a history of exposure to risk factors for the disease (e.g., tobacco smoke, occupational dusts). It is sometimes hard to distinguish COPD from asthma, especially if the person has a history of cigarette smoking. However, some clinical features are different (Table 28.4).

A chronic intermittent cough, which is often the first symptom to develop, may be present as the disease becomes apparent to the patient. Patients often dismiss the cough as they associate it with smoking or environmental exposures. The cough may be productive. Significant airflow limitation may exist without cough or sputum. Typically, dyspnea is progressive, usually occurs with exertion, and is present every day.

Patients may report chest heaviness, not being able to take a deep breath, gasping, increased effort to breathe, and air hunger. Patients tend to ignore symptoms and rationalize that "I'm getting older" or "I'm out of shape." They change behaviors to avoid dyspnea, such as taking the elevator instead of the stairs. Patients will seek out medical care only when dyspnea is severe or when shortness of breath significantly impairs their ability to complete ADLs.

In late stages of COPD, dyspnea may be present at rest. As more alveoli become overdistended, increasing amounts of air

TABLE 28.16 Classification of COPD Severity*

Classification is based on postbronchodilator FEV_1

Classification	Level of Severity	FEV_1 Results
GOLD 1	Mild	FEV_1 ≥80% predicted
GOLD 2	Moderate	FEV_1 50%–80% predicted
GOLD 3	Severe	FEV_1 30%–50% predicted
GOLD 4	Very severe	FEV_1 <30% predicted

Adapted from Global Initiative for COPD: 2018 Global strategy for prevention, diagnosis, and management of COPD. Retrieved from *www.goldcopd.org*.
*A diagnosis of COPD is made when a patient has a FEV_1/FVC <70%.

are trapped. This causes the diaphragm to flatten, and the patient must work harder to breathe. Effective abdominal breathing is decreased because of the flattened diaphragm from overinflated lungs. The patient becomes more of a chest breather, relying on the intercostal and accessory muscles. However, chest breathing is not particularly efficient, especially over long periods.

Wheezing and chest tightness may be present but may vary by time of the day or from day to day, especially in patients with more severe disease. Chest tightness, which often follows activity, may feel similar to muscle contractions.

The person with advanced COPD often has fatigue, weight loss, and anorexia. Even with adequate caloric intake, the patient may still lose weight. Fatigue is a highly prevalent symptom that affects the patient's ADLs. During physical examination, a prolonged expiratory phase is observed. Decreased breath sounds and/or wheezes are auscultated in all lung fields. Because the anteroposterior diameter of the chest is increased ("barrel chest") from the chronic air trapping, the patient may need to breathe louder than normal for breath sounds to be heard with a stethoscope. The patient may sit upright with arms supported on a fixed surface, such as an overbed table (*tripod position*). The patient may naturally purse lips on expiration (pursed-lip breathing) and use accessory muscles, such as those in the neck, to aid with inspiration. Edema in the ankles may be the only clue to right-sided heart involvement (cor pulmonale).

Over time, hypoxemia (PaO_2 less than 60 mm Hg or O_2 saturation less than 88% on room air) may develop with hypercapnia ($PaCO_2$ over 45 mm Hg). The bluish-red color of the skin results from polycythemia and cyanosis. Polycythemia develops from increased production of red blood cells as the body tries to compensate for chronic hypoxemia. Hemoglobin concentrations may reach 20 g/dL (200 g/L) or more. However, the person may have lowered hemoglobin and hematocrit because of chronic anemia.

Complications

Primary complications that can occur in patients with COPD include pulmonary hypertension, cor pulmonale, acute exacerbations, and acute respiratory failure.

Pulmonary Hypertension and Cor Pulmonale. Cor pulmonale results from pulmonary hypertension, which is caused by diseases affecting the lungs or pulmonary blood vessels (Fig. 28.12). It is a late manifestation of COPD. Once the patient develops cor pulmonale, the prognosis worsens. Not all patients with COPD develop cor pulmonale.

PATHOPHYSIOLOGY MAP

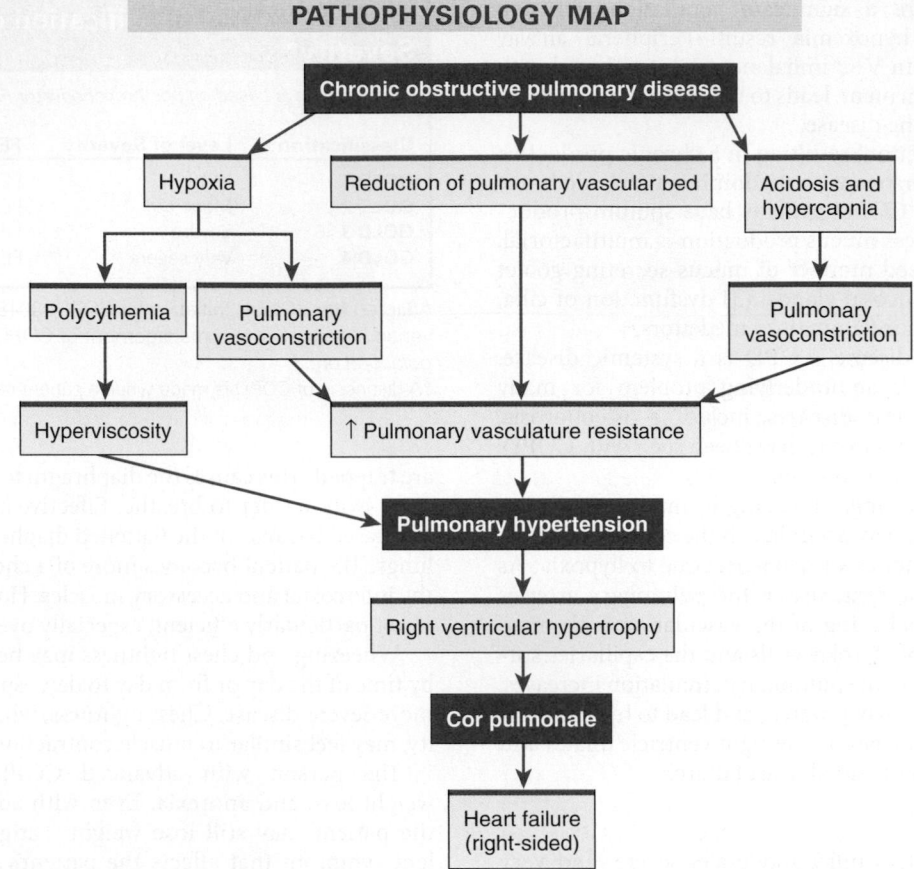

FIG. 28.12 Mechanisms involved in the pathophysiology of pulmonary hypertension and cor pulmonale from COPD.

In COPD, pulmonary hypertension is caused primarily by constriction of the pulmonary vessels in response to alveolar hypoxia. Chronic hypoxia stimulates erythropoiesis, which causes polycythemia. This results in increased viscosity of the blood. These patients have increased pulmonary vascular resistance, and, as a result, develop pulmonary hypertension.

Normally the right ventricle and pulmonary circulatory system are low-pressure systems compared with the left ventricle and systemic circulation. When pulmonary hypertension (pressure within the lungs increases), the pressures on the right side of the heart must increase to push blood into the lungs. Eventually, because the pressure in the lungs is so high, right-sided heart failure develops.

Dyspnea is the most common symptom of chronic cor pulmonale. Lung sounds are normal, or crackles may be heard in the bases of the lungs bilaterally. Heart sound changes may include the presence of S_3 and S_4 and systolic murmurs.[17] Other manifestations of right-sided heart failure may develop. These include distended neck veins, hepatomegaly with right upper quadrant tenderness, peripheral edema, and weight gain.

Typically, the patient has large pulmonary vessels on chest x-ray and increased pressure on right-sided heart catheterization. Echocardiogram may show right-sided heart enlargement. b-Type natriuretic peptide (BNP) levels, which are used to diagnose heart failure, may be high. Normally BNP levels are used to distinguish cardiac from respiratory causes of dyspnea, but in cor pulmonale the cause of the heart failure is the lung disease.

Treatment of cor pulmonale is initially targeted at managing the underlying cause, including COPD. Continuous low-flow,

long-term O_2 therapy is often part of care. Diuretics may be given if left heart failure or pulmonary edema are present but must be used with caution.[18] In some cases, decreases in fluid volume from diuresis can worsen heart function. Long-term anticoagulation therapy is started to help decrease the risk for venous thromboembolism (VTE). (Cor pulmonale is discussed in Chapter 27.)

Acute Exacerbations. An exacerbation of COPD is an acute event characterized by a worsening of the patient's respiratory symptoms. Exacerbations are signaled by an acute change in the patient's usual dyspnea, cough, and/or sputum (e.g., something different from the usual daily patterns). The main causes of exacerbations are bacterial or viral infections.[19] Exacerbations are common and increase in frequency (on average 1 or 2 per year) as the disease progresses. As the severity of COPD increases, COPD exacerbations are associated with poorer outcomes.

Assess patients for the classic manifestations of exacerbation, including increased dyspnea, increased sputum volume, or increased sputum purulence. They may have malaise, insomnia, fatigue, depression, confusion, decreased exercise tolerance, increased wheezing, or fever.

Exacerbations may be treated at home or in the hospital, depending on severity. The severity is determined by the patient's medical history leading up to the exacerbation, current symptoms, hemodynamic stability, O_2 requirements, WOB, ABGs, and the presence of coexisting diseases.

Your observations will help determine the severity of the exacerbation and whether the patient is treated as an inpatient or outpatient. Assess for new symptoms or worsening of usual symptoms. Be alert for signs of severity, such as use of accessory muscles, central cyanosis, edema in the lower extremities, unstable BP, right-sided heart failure, and altered alertness. Assess the patient's ABGs for respiratory acidosis and worsening hypoxemia, indicating an "acute-on-chronic" respiratory failure. Determine the number of exacerbations per year and if treatment occurred in the home or hospital. The presence of other co-morbid conditions often complicates exacerbations.

SABAs and oral systemic corticosteroids are the typical therapies for exacerbations. SABAs with short-acting anticholinergics are an option. Drug administration by MDI or nebulizer works equally well, although sicker patients often prefer the nebulizer. Antibiotics are given if the exacerbation was caused by a bacterial infection (e.g., pneumonia).

Therapies in the hospital are similar to home management, except supplemental O_2 therapy titrated by ABG measurement may be used. Attempts are made to use noninvasive mechanical methods (e.g., continuous positive airway pressure [CPAP] or bi-level positive airway pressure [Bi-PAP] to support ventilation rather than invasive ventilatory support [e.g., intubation and mechanical ventilation]). Small doses of diuretics maybe used for those with heart failure.

Teach the patient and caregiver early recognition of the 3 primary manifestations of exacerbations (increased dyspnea, increased sputum volume, or increased sputum purulence) to promote early treatment. This may prevent hospitalization and possible acute respiratory failure.

Acute Respiratory Failure. Patients with severe COPD who have severe exacerbations are at risk for acute respiratory failure. All too often, COPD patients wait too long to contact their HCP when they first develop symptoms suggestive of an exacerbation. Similarly, suddenly stopping a bronchodilator or corticosteroid medication may cause respiratory failure. (Respiratory failure is discussed in Chapter 67.)

Diagnostic Studies

A history and physical examination are extremely important in a diagnostic workup. Spirometry confirms the diagnosis in those suspected of having COPD. Spirometry confirms the presence of airflow obstruction and determines the severity of COPD.

In spirometry, the patient receives a SABA. Post-bronchodilator values are compared with a normal reference value. A diagnosis of COPD is made when the FEV_1/FVC ratio is less than 70%.[20] The value of FEV_1 provides a guideline for the degree of severity of COPD. The lower the FEV_1, the more obstructed are the airways.

Other diagnostic studies that may be done are outlined in Table 28.17. Chest x-rays are not diagnostic but often show a flat diaphragm because of hyperinflated lungs. Patients often have exercise-induced hypoxemia. A physical or respiratory therapist may do a 6-minute walk test. Pulse oximetry readings are taken when the patient is walking and at rest. If values of O_2 saturation are 88% or lower when at rest and the patient is breathing room air, they qualify for supplemental O_2.

Validated questionnaires such as the COPD Assessment Test (CAT) *(www.catestonline.org)* and Clinical COPD Questionnaire (CCQ) *(www.ccq.nl)* are recommended for a comprehensive assessment of symptoms.

ABGs are usually monitored in patients hospitalized with acute COPD exacerbations. ABGs alone are not diagnostic of COPD but help identify the severity of the exacerbation by assessing abnormalities in oxygenation and ventilation. In early

TABLE 28.17 Interprofessional Care
Chronic Obstructive Pulmonary Disease (COPD)

Diagnostic Assessment
- History and physical examination
- Spirometry
- Chest x-ray
- Serum α_1-antitrypsin levels
- ABGs
- 6-Minute walk test
- COPD Assessment Test (CAT)* or Clinical COPD Questionnaire (CCQ)†

Management
- Cessation of cigarette smoking
- Drug therapies (Tables 28.7 and 28.18)
- Airway clearance techniques
- Breathing exercises and retraining
- Hydration of 2 to 3 L/day (if not contraindicated)
- Immunizations:
  - Influenza yearly
  - Pneumococcal vaccine
- Long-term O_2 (if indicated)
- Progressive plan of exercise, especially walking and upper body strengthening
- Pulmonary rehabilitation program
- Nutritional supplementation
- Treatment of complications
  - Cor pulmonale
  - Acute exacerbations
  - Acute respiratory failure
- Surgical therapy
  - Lung volume reduction
  - Bullectomy
  - Lung transplantation

*See *www.catestonline.org.*
†See *www.ccq.nl.*

stages, there may be a normal or only slightly decreased PaO_2 and a normal $PaCO_2$. In the later stages of COPD, typical findings are a low-normal pH, high-normal or above-normal $PaCO_2$, and high-normal bicarbonate (HCO_3^-). This may indicate either partially or fully compensated respiratory acidosis. The patient has chronically retained CO_2 and the kidneys have conserved HCO_3^- to increase the pH to within the normal range.

An ECG may be normal or show signs of right heart failure. An echocardiogram or (MUGA) (cardiac blood pool) scan (see Table 31.7) can be used to evaluate heart function. Sputum for culture and sensitivity may be done if an infection, such as pneumonia, is suspected.

Interprofessional Care

Most patients with COPD are treated as outpatients. They are hospitalized for an acute exacerbation of COPD or complications, such as pneumonia, heart failure, or acute respiratory failure.

Evaluate the patient's exposure to environmental or occupational irritants and determine ways to control or avoid them. For example, teach the patient to avoid, if possible, smoke-filled rooms and air pollutants. The patient with COPD is extremely susceptible to lung infections. The patient with COPD should receive influenza immunization yearly. The pneumococcal vaccine is recommended for all smokers ages 19 or older and all patients with COPD. Guidelines for pneumococcal vaccine are outlined in Table 27.5.

Smoking Cessation. Stopping cigarette smoking in any person with COPD at any level of severity is the most important intervention that can affect the natural progression of COPD. After a person stops smoking, the accelerated decline in pulmonary function found with smoking slows to almost nonsmoking levels. The sooner the smoker stops, the less pulmonary function is lost and the sooner the symptoms decrease, especially cough and sputum production. Smoking cessation is discussed in Chapter 10 and in Tables 10.4 to 10.6.

Drug Therapy. Drugs for COPD can reduce symptoms, increase exercise capacity, improve overall health, and reduce the number and severity of exacerbations. Like asthma, they are given in a stepwise fashion according to the level of airflow obstruction determined from spirometry (FEV_1) and symptoms. Medications are stepped up but usually not stepped down, as in asthma, because in COPD continual symptoms are present (Table 28.18). The inhaled route of medication is preferred and used on a regular or as-needed basis.

Bronchodilator drug therapy relaxes smooth muscles in the airway and improves the ventilation of the lungs, thus reducing the degree of breathlessness. Patients with COPD do not respond as dramatically to bronchodilator therapy as those with asthma. However, bronchodilator therapy reduces dyspnea and increases FEV_1.

Bronchodilator drugs commonly used are β_2-adrenergic agonists, anticholinergic agents, and, to a much lesser extent, methylxanthines (Table 28.7). The choice of bronchodilator depends on the patient's response. They are given on a scheduled or as-needed basis. When the patient has mild COPD or fewer symptoms, a SABA is used. Albuterol or ipratropium may be used alone, but combining bronchodilators improves their effect and decreases the risk for adverse effects. Albuterol and ipratropium can be nebulized together (DuoNeb) or delivered by inhalation spray (Combivent Respimat).

In the moderate stage of COPD (FEV_1 less than 60%), a LABA is often part of the medication treatment plan. Unlike asthma, they can be used in COPD as monotherapy. Salmeterol and formoterol are widely used LABAs. A SABA may still be used as a "rescue" for dyspnea.

In COPD patients with FEV_1 of less than 60%, regular treatment with ICS is often prescribed with a LABA. Examples of

combinations of ICSs with LABAs are fluticasone/salmeterol (Advair) and budesonide/formoterol (Symbicort).

Inhaled long-acting anticholinergics, LABAs, and ICSs all reduce COPD exacerbations. However, in COPD, unlike asthma, ICSs are not used as monotherapy because of the concerns about side effects. Some patients with COPD are on triple therapy with Advair and tiotropium. Oral corticosteroids should not be used for long-term therapy in COPD but are effective for short-term use to treat acute exacerbations.

The use of long-acting theophylline in the treatment of COPD is controversial because it interacts with many drugs. A low dose of theophylline with an ICS may help a few patients with COPD who do not respond to other inhaled medications.

Roflumilast (Daliresp) is an oral medication used to decrease the frequency of exacerbations in patients with severe COPD and chronic bronchitis. This drug is a phosphodiesterase inhibitor. It is an antiinflammatory drug that suppresses the release of cytokines and other inflammatory mediators and inhibits the production of reactive O_2 radicals.

New drug delivery devices are becoming available at a rapid pace. One example is Respimat. It is an easy-to-use, hand-held device that provides a high deposition of drug to the lungs and low mouth and throat deposition. Respimat simplifies coordination between activation of the medication and inhalation without propellant. It is independent of inspiratory flow. Combivent and Spiriva Respimats are examples.

Surgical Therapy. Various surgical procedures are used to help manage severe COPD. However, it is important to remember that not all patients with severe COPD are candidates for surgery.

One type of surgery is *lung volume reduction surgery* (LVRS). The goal of LVRS is to reduce the size of the lungs by removing some of the diseased lung tissue, so that the remaining healthy lung tissue can perform better. Reducing the diseased lung tissue by about 30% results in decreased airway obstruction and increased room for the remaining normal alveoli (small air sacs at the end of each bronchiole) to expand and function.[21] Besides improving lung and chest wall mechanics, LVRS can allow the diaphragm to return to its normal shape. This allows the patient to breathe more efficiently.

Another type of surgical procedure is *bronchoscopic lung volume reduction surgery*. It involves placing 1-way valves, by bronchoscopy, in the airways leading to the diseased parts of the lung. By completely occluding a specific lobe of the lung, this collapses a certain segment of the lung and produces a result similar to LVRS.[22] Pneumothorax is a common complication. An a *bullectomy*, 1 or more very large bullae are removed. Removal of bullae help decrease WOB.

A lung transplant benefits certain patients with advanced COPD. Although single-lung transplant is the most commonly used technique because of a shortage of donors, bilateral transplantation can be done. (Lung transplantation is discussed in Chapter 27.)

Interprofessional Care: Respiratory Care

Oxygen Therapy. O_2 therapy is often used in the treatment of COPD and other problems associated with hypoxemia. O_2 is a colorless, odorless, tasteless gas that constitutes 21% of the atmosphere. Giving supplemental O_2 increases the partial pressure of O_2 (PO_2) in inspired air. Used clinically, it is considered a prescribed medication. It is the only one that has been linked to improved survival of COPD patients.

TABLE 28.18 Drug Therapy

Medication Guidelines

The treatment guidelines are based on the FEV_1 results.

FEV_1 Results	Treatment Guidelines
FEV_1 60%–80% predicted (with respiratory symptoms)	Treatment with inhaled bronchodilators may be used
FEV_1 <60% predicted (with respiratory symptoms)	Treat with inhaled bronchodilators: anticholinergics or long-acting β_2-agonist
	OR
	Monotherapy with long-acting inhaled anticholinergics or long-acting β_2-agonist
	OR
	Combination therapy with long-acting inhaled anticholinergics, long-acting β_2-agonist, or inhaled corticosteroids

O_2 is usually given to treat hypoxemia caused by many other problems, such as shock, pneumonia, and pulmonary emboli. O_2 therapy must be tailored to meet each patient's unique circumstances and physiologic needs. For most patients, the goal of O_2 therapy is to keep the SaO_2 greater than 90% during rest, sleep, and exertion or the PaO_2 greater than 60 mm Hg. These goals may be modified for the patient with moderate to severe COPD. For example, based upon the patient's condition, the HCP may accept an SaO_2 an PaO_2 greater than 88%.

Methods of Administration. There are various methods of administering O_2 (Table 28.19). The device used depends on the patient's underlying condition, fraction of inspired O_2 (FIO_2) needed by the patient and delivered by the device, humidification requirements, patient cooperation, comfort, cost, and financial resources.

O_2 delivery systems are classified as low- or high-flow systems. Most methods of O_2 delivery are low-flow devices that provide O_2 in concentrations that vary with the person's respiratory pattern. Low-flow devices pull in a proportion of room air. This makes the range of FIO_2 known, but the exact FIO_2 hard to determine. Nasal prongs and non-rebreather masks are examples of low-flow O_2 systems. High-flow O_2 delivery devices deliver fixed concentrations of O_2 (e.g., 28%, 35%) independent of the patient's respiratory pattern. The Venturi mask and mechanical ventilators are examples of a high-flow O_2 delivery systems.

Humidification and Nebulization. O_2 obtained from O_2 cylinders or wall systems is dry. Dry O_2 has an irritating effect on mucous membranes and dries secretions. Therefore it is important that O_2 be humidified. Humidification involves the addition of sterile distilled water, attached to the O_2 delivery device, to prevent breathing dry air. For example, a common device used for humidification when the patient has a cannula or a mask is a small plastic jar filled with distilled water called a *bubble-through humidifier*. It is attached to the O_2 source by a flowmeter.

Complications of Oxygen Therapy

Combustion. O_2 supports combustion and increases the rate of burning, so it is important to prohibit smoking or have open flames in the area in which O_2 is being used. A "No Smoking" sign should be prominently displayed on the patient's door. Caution the patient against smoking cigarettes with an O_2 cannula in place as it can easily ignite and cause significant burns and life-threatening airway issues.

CO_2 narcosis. Chemoreceptors in the respiratory center that control the drive to breathe respond to CO_2 and O_2. Normally, an increase in CO_2 in the blood is a major stimulant of the respiratory center. Over time, some COPD patients with hypercapnia develop a tolerance for high CO_2 levels (the respiratory center loses its sensitivity to high CO_2 levels). For these people, a major "drive" to breathe is hypoxemia. As a result, there is concern about the dangers of giving O_2 to COPD patients and reducing their drive to breathe.

However, the "hypoxic drive" is complex and involves other factors, including ventilation and perfusion. Plus, not all patients with COPD retain CO_2. So, the thought is that it is better to give O_2 to a patient who needs it because the danger of not giving O_2 to a patient far outweighs the risk.

Pulse oximetry and/or ABGs are used as a guide to determine the FIO_2 needed by each patient. Safe administration of O_2 can be achieved by gradually increasing the concentration of O_2 with close monitoring of both PaO_2 and $PaCO_2$. High-flow O_2 devices may be used to have tighter regulation of the FIO_2. Once again, the goal is a pulse O_2 saturation (SpO_2) of at least 90% or a PaO_2 of at least 60 mm Hg. Always remember to assess the patient's mental status and vital signs before starting O_2 therapy and frequently thereafter.

O_2 toxicity. Pulmonary O_2 toxicity may result from prolonged exposure to a high level of O_2 (PaO_2). High concentrations of O_2 can result in a severe inflammatory response because of O_2 free radical damage to alveolar-capillary membranes. This causes severe pulmonary edema, shunting of blood, and hypoxemia. Although it is rare, patients can develop acute respiratory distress syndrome (ARDS) (see Chapter 67).

Preventing O_2 toxicity is important. The amount of O_2 applied should be enough to maintain the PaO_2 within a normal or acceptable range for that patient. Monitor ABGs often to evaluate the effectiveness of therapy and guide the tapering of supplemental O_2. The most important rule you can follow is to provide FIO_2 at the lowest possible level, while still maintaining acceptable SaO_2 and PaO_2 values for every patient.

NURSING MANAGEMENT
Oxygen Administration

- Assess need for adjustments in O_2 flow rate.
- Evaluate response to O_2 therapy.
- Monitor patient for signs of adverse effects of O_2 therapy.
- Teach patient and caregivers about home O_2 use.
- Oversee UAP:
  - Use pulse oximetry to measure O_2 saturation and report level to RN.
  - Assist patient with adjustment of O_2 delivery devices (e.g., nasal cannula, face mask).
  - Report to RN any change in patient condition.
- Collaborate with respiratory therapist:
  - Assist RN with choosing optimal O_2 delivery device (e.g., nasal cannula or simple face mask).
  - Make sure equipment is clean and replaced as needed.
  - Check accuracy of O_2 delivery and assess need for adjustments in O_2 flow rate.
- Evaluate patient response to O_2 therapy.

Infection. Infection can be a complication of O_2 administration. Heated nebulizers present the highest risk. The constant use of humidity supports bacterial growth. The most common organism is *Pseudomonas aeruginosa*. Disposable equipment that operates as a closed system, such as the Ballard closed suctioning system, should be used. Each agency has a policy on the frequency of equipment changes based on the type of O_2 equipment used.

Oxygen Therapy at Home. Short-term home O_2 therapy (up to 30 days) may be needed for the patient in whom hypoxemia persists after discharge from the hospital. For example, a patient with underlying COPD who develops a serious respiratory tract infection may need continued O_2 therapy to treat hypoxemia for several weeks after discharge from the hospital. Home health care personnel can measure the patient's oxygenation status after an acute episode to determine if the O_2 is still needed.

Patients may receive O_2 only during exercise and/or sleep. Evaluate the need for O_2 during these periods with a 6-minute walk test or overnight oximetry. Improved survival occurs in patients with COPD who receive long-term O_2 therapy (LTOT)

TABLE 28.19 Methods of Oxygen Administration

Description	Nursing Interventions

Low-Flow Delivery Devices
Nasal Cannula

- Most commonly used device.
- O_2 delivered via plastic nasal prongs.
- Safe and simple method
- Allows some freedom of movement. Patient can eat, talk, or cough while wearing device.
- Used for a patient requiring low O_2 concentrations.
- Obtains O_2 concentrations of 24% (at 1 L/min) to 44% (at 6 L/min).

- Stabilize nasal cannula when caring for a restless patient.
- Amount of O_2 inhaled depends on room air and patient's breathing pattern.
- Most patients with COPD can tolerate 2 L/min via cannula.
- Assess patient's nares and ears for skin breakdown. May need to pad cannula where it sits on ears.
- If flow rates are >5 L/min, nasal membranes may dry and place patient at risk for nose bleeding.

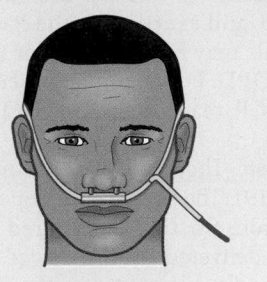
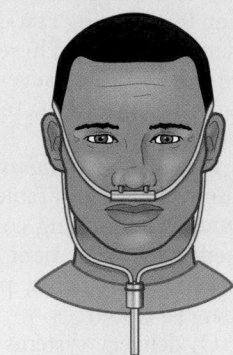

Simple Face Mask

- Covers patient's nose and mouth.
- Used only for short periods, especially when transporting patients.
- Longer use is typically not tolerated because of tight seal and heat generated around nose and mouth from mask.
- Achieves O_2 concentrations of 35%–50% with flow rates of 6–12 L/min.
- Mask provides adequate humidification of inspired air.

- Wash and dry under mask q4h and PRN.
- Mask must fit snugly.
- Nasal cannula may be used while patient is eating.
- Watch for pressure necrosis at top of ears from elastic straps if patient wears for a longer time. Gauze or other padding may alleviate this problem.

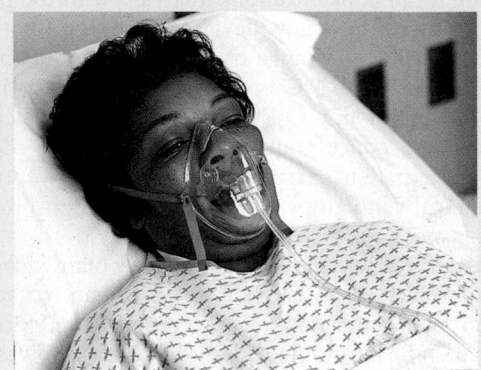

Partial and Non-Rebreather Masks

- Used for short-term (24 hr) therapy for patients needing higher O_2 concentrations (60%–90% at 10–15 L/min).
- O_2 flows into reservoir bag and mask during inhalation.
- Bag allows patient to rebreathe about first third of exhaled air (rich in O_2) in conjunction with flowing O_2.
- Vents stay open on partial mask only. Some agencies prefer this over non-rebreather as a safety issue.

- O_2 flow rate must be sufficient to keep bag from deflating during inspiration to avoid CO_2 buildup and rebreathing of CO_2.
- If deflation occurs, increase flowrate on flowmeter on wall to keep bag inflated.
- Mask should fit snugly.
- With non-rebreather masks, make sure valves are open during expiration and closed during inhalation to prevent decrease in FIO_2 or build-up in CO_2.
- Monitor patient closely, since more advanced interventions may be needed such as CPAP, BiPAP, or intubation with mechanical ventilation.

Oxygen-Conserving Cannula

- Generally indicated for long-term O_2 therapy at home (e.g., pulmonary fibrosis, pulmonary hypertension).
- Looks like a "moustache" (Oxymizer) or "pendant" type.
- Cannula has a built-in reservoir that ↑ O_2 concentration and allows patient to use lower flow, usually 30%–50%, which increases comfort, lowers cost, and can be increased with activities.
- Can deliver O_2 up to 8 L/min.

- May cause necrosis over tops of ears. Tubing can be padded.
- Cannula cannot be cleaned. Manufacturer recommends changing cannula every week.
- More expensive than standard cannulas and may need evaluation with ABGs and oximetry to determine correct flow for patient.
- Cannula is highly visible.

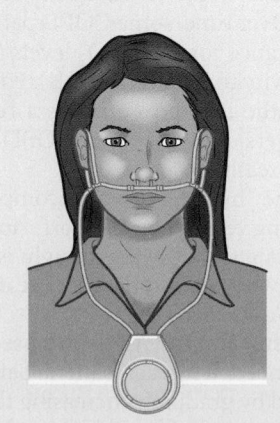

Pendant-type O_2-conserving cannula.

TABLE 28.19 Methods of Oxygen Administration

Description	Nursing Interventions

High-Flow Delivery Devices

Tracheostomy Collar

- Collar attaches to neck with elastic strap and can deliver humidity and O_2 via tracheostomy.
- Some O_2 concentration is lost into atmosphere because collar does not fit tightly.
- Venturi device can be attached to flowmeter and thus can deliver exact amounts of O_2 via collar.

- Secretions collect inside collar and around tracheostomy. Remove collar and clean at least q4hr and PRN to prevent aspiration of fluid and infection.
- Because condensation occurs in tubing, periodically drain tubing distal to tracheostomy.

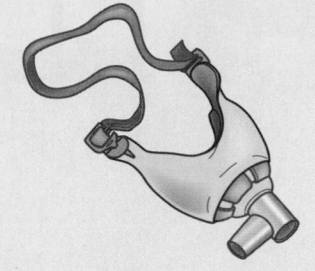

Tracheostomy T-Piece

- Almost identical to tracheostomy collar, but it has a T-connector attached to an O_2 blender.
- T-piece allows an inline catheter (e.g., Ballard catheter) to be connected for suctioning.
- Tight fit allows better O_2 and humidity delivery than tracheostomy collar.

- Because T-piece connectors can disconnect easily, monitor closely.
- T-piece connector may pull on a patient's tracheostomy tube, causing irritation and potential tissue damage. Monitor this closely.

Venturi Mask

- Mask can deliver precise, high-flow rates of O_2.
- Lightweight plastic, cone-shaped mask Masks are available for delivery of 24%, 28%, 31%, 35%, 40%, and 50% O_2.
- Method is especially helpful for giving low, constant O_2 concentrations to patients with COPD.
- Adaptors can increase humidification.

- Entrainment device on mask must be changed to deliver higher concentrations of O_2.
- Air entrainment ports must not be occluded.
- Uncomfortable.
- Must be removed when patient eats.
- Patient can talk but voice may be muffled.

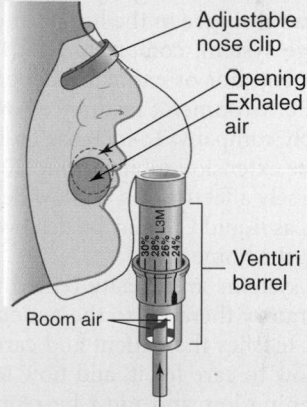

Adjustable nose clip

Opening Exhaled air

Venturi barrel

Room air

High-Flow Nasal Cannula

- Blends O_2 with compressed air to generate FIO_2 up to 1.0 at flow rate of up to 60 L/min.
- Active heated humidifier capable of providing 100% body humidity.
- Soft and flexible nasal prongs.
- More comfortable than mask.

- Nasal cannula must be smaller than 50% of nares to allow flow during exhalation and flush out end-expiratory CO_2.
- Patients can eat and drink with device in place.
- Well tolerated.
- Patient may describe feeling of always having to blow nose ("rainout") due to humidification.

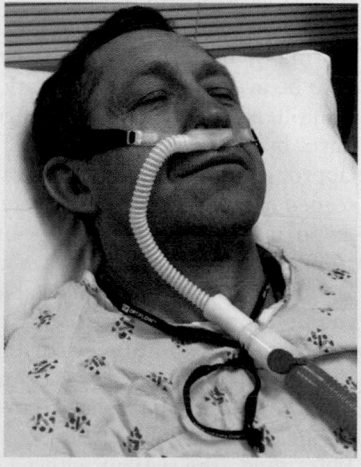

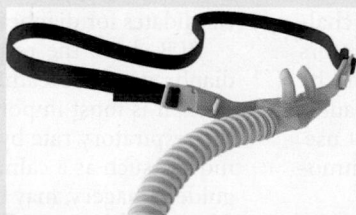

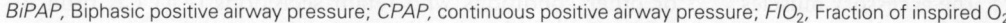

BiPAP, Biphasic positive airway pressure; CPAP, continuous positive airway pressure; FIO_2, Fraction of inspired O_2.

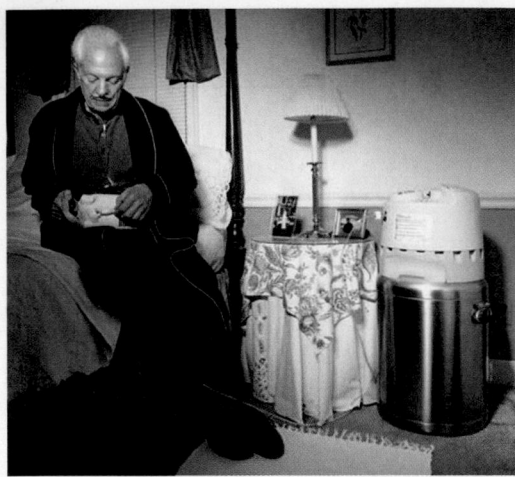

FIG. 28.13 A portable liquid O_2 unit can be refilled from a liquid O_2 reservoir unit. (Courtesy Nellcor Puritan Bennett, Pleasanton, CA.)

(more than 15 hr/day) to treat hypoxemia. Periodic reevaluations for the patient who is using LTOT is needed. The patient is reevaluated every 30 to 90 days during the first year of therapy and annually after that if the patient stays stable.

Nasal cannulas, including O_2 conservation systems, deliver O_2 from a central source in the home. The source may be a liquid O_2 storage system, compressed O_2 in tanks or cylinders, or an O_2 concentrator or extractor, depending on the patient's activity level, environment, insurance coverage, and proximity to an O_2 supply company. To increase mobility in the home, the patient can use extension tubing (up to 50 ft) with some devices without adversely affecting the O_2 flow delivery. Small, portable systems, such as liquid O_2, may be used with the patient who is active outside the home.

Home O_2 systems are usually rented from a company that sends a respiratory therapist to the patient's home (Fig. 28.13). The therapist teaches the patient and caregiver how to use the O_2 system, how to care for it, and how to recognize when the supply is running low and must be reordered. A patient and caregiver teaching guide for the use of O_2 at home is shown in Table 28.20.

Encourage the patient who uses home O_2 to remain active and travel normally. If travel is by car, arrangements can be made for O_2 to be available at the destination point. O_2 supply companies can often help with these arrangements. If a patient wishes to travel by bus, train, or airplane, the patient should inform the appropriate people when reservations are made that O_2 will be needed for travel. If there is a potential for the patient to become hypoxic, O_2 needs for flying can be determined by a pulmonary function test, a 6-minute walk test, hypoxic challenge test, or predictive formula.[23] Portable O_2 concentrators are a ready source of renewable O_2 and can be available by recharging at home or with a direct current (DC) (e.g., auto) power supply. Several are approved by airlines for in-flight use. The patient should contact the airline to determine accommodations and policies for in-flight O_2.

Breathing Retraining. The patient with COPD often has dyspnea with an increased respiratory rate. The accessory muscles of breathing in the neck and upper part of the chest are used excessively to promote chest wall movement. These muscles are not designed for long-term use and as a result the patient has increased fatigue.

TABLE 28.20 Patient & Caregiver Teaching

Home Oxygen Use

The company that provides the prescribed O_2 therapy equipment will teach the patient about equipment care. The following are some general instructions that you may include when teaching the patient and caregiver about the use of home O_2:

Decreasing Risk for Infection
- Brush teeth or use mouthwash several times a day.
- Wash nasal cannula (prongs) with a liquid soap and thoroughly rinse once or twice a week.
- Replace cannula every 2 to 4 weeks.
- If you have a cold, replace the cannula after your symptoms pass.
- Always remove secretions that are coughed out.
- If you use an O_2 concentrator, daily unplug the unit and wipe down the cabinet with a damp cloth and dry it.
- Ask the company providing the equipment how often to change the filter.

Safety Issues
- Post "No Smoking" warning signs outside the home.
- O_2 will not "blow up," but it will increase the rate of burning, since it is combustible.
- Do not allow smoking in the home, and do not smoke yourself while wearing O_2. Nasal cannulas and masks can catch fire and cause serious burns to face and airways.
- Do not use flammable liquids such as paint thinners, cleaning fluids, gasoline, kerosene, oil-based paints, or aerosol sprays while using O_2.
- Do not use blankets or fabrics that carry a static charge, such as wool or synthetics.
- Inform the staff at your electric company if you are using a concentrator. In case of a power failure, they will know the medical urgency of restoring your power.

Adapted from www.YourLungHealth.org.

Two main types of breathing retraining exercises are (1) pursed-lip breathing and (2) diaphragmatic breathing. The purpose of **pursed-lip breathing (PLB)** is to prolong exhalation, which prevents bronchiolar collapse and air trapping. PLB is simple, easy to teach and learn, and it gives the patient more control over breathing, especially during exercise and periods of dyspnea (Table 28.12). Patients should be taught to use "just enough" positive pressure with pursed lips because excessive resistance may increase the WOB.

Diaphragmatic (abdominal) breathing focuses on using the diaphragm instead of the accessory muscles of the chest to (1) achieve maximum inhalation and (2) slow the respiratory rate. However, the use of diaphragmatic breathing in patients with COPD may increase the WOB and dyspnea. Patients with moderate to severe COPD with marked hyperinflation may be poor candidates for diaphragmatic breathing.

PLB slows the respiratory rate and is easier to learn than diaphragmatic breathing. In the setting of extreme acute dyspnea, it is most important to focus on helping the patient slow the respiratory rate by using the principles of PLB. Other techniques, such as a calm demeanor, positive encouragement, and guided imagery, may be used to reduce dyspnea.

Airway Clearance Techniques. Many patients with COPD or other conditions who retain secretions (e.g., CF, bronchiectasis) need help to adequately clear their airways. Airway clearance techniques (ACTs) loosen mucus and secretions so they can be cleared by coughing. There are a variety of techniques. These include effective coughing, chest physiotherapy, airway clearance devices, and high-frequency chest ventilation. Respiratory therapists, physical therapists, and nurses can perform these techniques.

ACTs are especially beneficial in patients who have a COPD exacerbation. They are often used in conjunction with other treatments. Typically, the patient receives bronchodilator therapy through an inhaled device (e.g., nebulization) before ACT. Then the ACT is used, followed by effective coughing (e.g., huff coughing).

Effective Coughing. Many patients with COPD have developed ineffective coughing patterns that do not adequately clear the airways of sputum. They fear developing bronchospasm, or spastic coughing, resulting in increased dyspnea. Although other techniques (e.g., chest physiotherapy) are used to loosen secretions and mucus, the patient must cough effectively to bring the secretions to the central airways to expectorate them.

Huff coughing is an effective forced expiratory technique that you can easily teach the patient. Before starting, ensure that the patient is breathing deeply from the diaphragm. Place the patient's hands on the lower lateral chest wall and then ask the patient to breathe deeply through the nose. You should feel the patient's hands move outward, which represents a breath from the diaphragm. Guidelines for effective huff coughing are shown in Table 28.21.

Chest Physiotherapy. Chest physiotherapy (CPT) is mainly used for patients with excessive bronchial secretions who have difficulty clearing them (e.g., CF, bronchiectasis). CPT consists of postural drainage, percussion, and vibration. CPT should be done by a properly trained person. Complications associated with improperly performed CPT include fractured ribs, bruising, hypoxemia, and discomfort. CPT may be stressful for some patients. Some may develop hypoxemia and bronchospasms.

Postural drainage. Postural drainage is the use of positioning techniques that drain secretions from specific segments of the lungs and bronchi into the trachea. The postural drainage positions used depend on the areas of lung that are involved. This is determined by patient assessment, chest x-rays, chest auscultation, and, when possible, patient preference. For example, some patients with left lower lobe involvement need postural drainage of only the affected region. A person with CF may need postural drainage of all segments.

The purpose of various positions in postural drainage is to drain each segment toward the larger airways. The patient who cannot tolerate a head-down position may use a side-lying position. Aerosolized bronchodilators and hydration therapy are usually given before postural drainage. The chosen postural drainage position is maintained for about 5 minutes during percussion and vibration. A common order is 2 to 4 times a day. In acute situations, postural drainage may be done as often as every 4 hours. Schedule the procedure at least 1 hour before meals or 3 hours after meals.

Beds are available that can rotate and percuss in various postural drainage positions. These are quite effective. Some positions for postural drainage (e.g., Trendelenburg) should not be used on the patient with traumatic brain injury, chest trauma, hemoptysis, heart disease, pulmonary embolus, or any other situation in which the patient's condition is not stable.

Percussion. *Percussion* is performed in the appropriate postural drainage position with the hands in a cuplike position, with the fingers and thumbs closed (Fig. 28.14). The cupped

TABLE 28.21 Patient & Caregiver Teaching

Effective Huff Coughing

When teaching effective huff coughing:
1. Help the patient assume a sitting position with head slightly flexed, shoulders relaxed, knees flexed, forearms supported by pillow, and, if possible, feet on the floor.

Then teach the patient to:
2. Inhale slowly through the mouth while breathing deeply from the diaphragm.
3. Hold the breath for 2 to 3 seconds.
4. Forcefully exhale quickly as if one is fogging up a mirror with one's breath (thus creating a "huff"). This moves the secretions to larger airways.
5. Repeat the "huff" 1 or 2 more times while refraining from a "regular" cough.
6. Cough when mucus is felt in the breathing tubes.
7. Rest for 5 to 10 regular breaths.
8. Repeat the huffs (3 to 5 cycles) until you feel you have cleared mucus or you become tired.

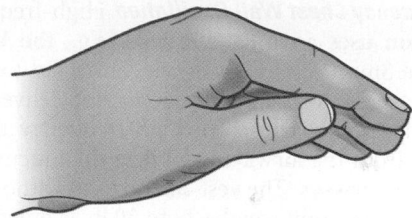

FIG. 28.14 Cupped-hand position for percussion. The hand should be cupped as though scooping up water.

hand should create an air pocket between the patient's chest and the hand. Both hands are cupped and used in an alternating rhythmic fashion. If it is done correctly, a hollow sound should be heard. The air-cushion impact facilitates the movement of thick mucus. For patient comfort, place a thin towel over the area to be percussed. The patient may choose to wear a T-shirt or hospital gown.

Vibration. *Vibration* is accomplished by tensing the hand and arm muscles repeatedly and pressing mildly with the flat of the hand on the affected area while the patient slowly exhales a deep breath. Vibrations promote movement of secretions to larger airways. Commercially available mechanical chest vibrators are available for hospital and home use.

Airway Clearance Devices. Various *airway clearance devices* are available to help mobilize secretions. They are easier to tolerate than CPT and take less time than CPT sessions. These devices include the Flutter, Acapella, and TheraPEP Therapy System. These devices use positive expiratory pressure (PEP). They may provide greater benefit to patients with COPD than other ACTs.

The Flutter mucus clearance device is a hand-held device. It is shaped like a small, fat pipe. It provides PEP treatment for patients with mucus-producing conditions. The Flutter has a mouthpiece, a high-density stainless-steel ball, and a cone that holds the ball. When the patient exhales through the Flutter, the steel ball moves, which causes oscillations (vibrations) in the airways and loosens mucus to allow improved expectoration. The patient must be upright as the angle at which the Flutter is held is critical.

The Acapella is another small hand-held device that combines the benefits of both PEP and airway vibrations to mobilize

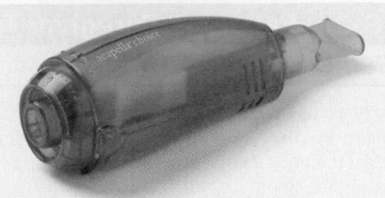

FIG. 28.15 Acapella airway clearance device. (Courtesy Smiths Medical North America.)

secretions (Fig. 28.15). It can be used in any setting, since patients are free to sit, stand, or recline.

TheraPEP Therapy System can provide sustained PEP and while delivering aerosols so that the patient can inhale and exhale through it. TheraPEP has a mouthpiece attached to tubing connected to a small cylindric resistor and a pressure indicator. The pressure indicator gives visual feedback about the pressure that the patient needs to hold in an exhalation to receive the PEP.

High-Frequency Chest Wall Oscillation. High-frequency chest wall oscillation uses an inflatable vest (e.g., the Vest Airway system or the SmartVest) with hoses connected to a high-frequency pulse generator. The pulse generator delivers air to the vest, which vibrates the chest. The high-frequency airwaves dislodge mucus from the airways, mobilize the mucus, and move it toward larger airways. The vest can be used without the aid of another person. The unit weighs 23 to 30 lb, is quiet, comes in a suitcase, and is portable.

Nutritional Therapy. Many COPD patients in the advanced stages are underweight with loss of muscle mass and cachexia. Weight loss is a predictor of a poor prognosis and increased frequency of COPD exacerbations.[23] Malnutrition is multifactorial, including increased inflammatory mediators, increased metabolic rate due to the ventilatory effort, and lack of appetite. Other factors that contribute to malnutrition include taste changes caused by chronic mouth breathing, excessive sputum, fatigue, anxiety, depression, increased energy needs, numerous infections, and side effects of multiple medications.

To decrease dyspnea and conserve energy, the patient should rest for at least 30 minutes before eating and use a bronchodilator before meals. Teach the patient to avoid exercise and treatments for at least 1 hour before and after eating. If a patient desaturates while eating, supplemental O_2 by nasal cannula may be helpful. Encourage activity, such as walking or getting out of bed during the day, to stimulate appetite. Sensations of bloating and feeling full after consuming small amounts can be attributed to swallowing air while eating, side effects of medication (especially corticosteroids and theophylline), and the abnormal position of the diaphragm relative to the stomach in association with hyperinflation of the lungs.

Getting the patient to eat adequate amounts of nutritionally sound foods may be difficult even though well-balanced meals are available. Give the patient or those responsible for meal preparation printed information that can make mealtime easier and more nutritious (Table 28.22).

Underweight patients with COPD need extra protein and calories. They may need 25 to 45 kcal/kg body weight and more than 1.5 g of protein/kg body weight to maintain their weight. The patient with malnutrition may need up to 2.5 g of protein/kg of body weight to begin restoring muscle mass.

TABLE 28.22 Nutritional Therapy

Maximizing Food Intake in COPD

Sometimes it is hard for patients with COPD to consume adequate amounts of nutrients. Teach the patients to make mealtimes easier and more nutritious by increasing calories and protein without increasing the amount of food eaten.

- Eat high-calorie foods first.
- Limit liquids at mealtimes.
- Rest before meals.
- Try more frequent meals and snacks.
- Increase calories by adding margarine, butter, mayonnaise, sauces, gravies, and peanut butter to foods.
- Keep favorite foods and snacks on hand.
- Try cold foods, which can make you feel less full than hot foods.
- Keep ready-prepared meals available for times when you have increased shortness of breath.
- Eat larger meals when you are not as tired.
- Avoid foods that you know cause gas (e.g., cabbage, beans, cauliflower).
- Add skim milk powder (2 Tbsp) to regular milk (8 oz) to add protein and calories.
- Use milk or half-and-half instead of water when making soups, cereals, instant puddings, cocoa, or canned soups.
- Add grated cheese to sauces, vegetables, soups, and casseroles.
- Choose dessert recipes that contain egg (e.g., sponge cake, angel food cake, egg custard, bread pudding, rice pudding).

Source: Grodner M, Escott-Stump S, Dorner S: *Nutritional foundations and clinical applications: A nursing approach,* ed 6, St Louis, 2016, Mosby.

A diet high in calories and protein, moderate in carbohydrate, and moderate to high in fat is recommended. It can be divided into 5 or 6 small meals a day.[24] Offer high-protein, high-calorie nutritional supplements between meals. The dietitian is an excellent resource to determine what combination of nutrients and what supplements are best for the patient. (Nutritional supplements are discussed in Chapter 39.)

Gerontologic Considerations: COPD

Older adults have physiologic changes, including reduced lean body mass, decreased respiratory muscle strength, increased dyspnea, and lower exercise tolerance that may increase the burden of disease from COPD. This may lead to a higher incidence of acute exacerbations, which require hospitalization. Smoking cessation is a key intervention but can be hard to achieve.

COPD is often complicated by the presence of co-morbidities, such as heart disease, serious infections, osteoporosis, psychological problems (depression, anxiety), impaired cognition, and lung cancer. The presence of co-morbidities can make it harder for patients to cope with the stress of an exacerbation. Assessment of co-morbidities can aid in ensuring comprehensive and safe management, especially during an exacerbation.

Older adults may have difficulty handling the increased secretions during an acute COPD exacerbation. Drugs used to manage the acute exacerbation can complicate disease management and increase the chance of adverse events. Assess for potential drug-drug interactions, especially in patients being treated for coexisting co-morbidities.

Some drugs used to treat common disorders, such as hypertension, can worsen COPD symptoms. If possible, nonspecific β-blockers should be avoided since they can block the $β_2$ receptors in the airway and cause bronchoconstriction. Similarly, ACE inhibitors may cause a dry cough or worsen a present cough. In some circumstances, it may not always be possible to eliminate these drugs.

Older adults may not be adherent to drug therapies due to cognitive impairment and complexity of the multiple medications at different times of the day. An attempt to simplify the medication regimen with written large-font action plans can be an important intervention in patients with poor memory and vision impairment. Arthritis in the hands can hinder the person from using proper technique for MDIs. Review MDI technique during clinic visits and have DPI or spacers prescribed (if possible) because they are easier to use. Long-term use of ICSs has the potential of causing local and systemic side effects, including cataracts, glaucoma, and osteoporosis. Monitoring of ocular pressures, bone densitometry, and using the lowest possible ICS dose is recommended.

Older patients with COPD generally have impaired quality of life. An important role for us is to focus on ways to improve quality of life. Psychologic and emotional support becomes imperative to help patients achieve successful outcomes. In the later stages of COPD, palliative and hospice care can help manage symptoms and improve the quality of the rest of their lives, which is important.

❖ NURSING MANAGEMENT: COPD

◆ Nursing Assessment

Subjective and objective data that should be obtained from a person with COPD are outlined in Table 28.23.

◆ Nursing Diagnoses

The nursing diagnoses for the patient with COPD may include:
- Impaired breathing
- Activity intolerance
- Impaired nutritional status
- Difficulty coping

Additional information on nursing diagnoses and interventions is presented in eNursing Care Plan 28.2 available on the website for this chapter.

◆ Planning

The overall goals are that the patient with COPD will have (1) relief from symptoms, (2) ability to perform ADLs and improved exercise tolerance, (3) no complications related to COPD, (4) knowledge and ability to implement a long-term treatment plan, (5) prevention of disease progression, and (6) overall improved quality of life.

◆ Nursing Implementation

◆ Health Promotion.
The incidence of COPD would decrease dramatically if people would not begin smoking or would stop smoking. Counseling the patient in smoking cessation is vital. It is the only way to slow the progression of COPD. As health care professionals, nurses who smoke should reevaluate their own smoking behavior and its relationship to their health. Nurses and other HCPs who smoke should be aware that the odor of smoke is obvious on their clothes and hair. It can be offensive or tempting to patients.

Early diagnosis and treatment of respiratory tract infections and exacerbations of COPD help prevent progression of the disease. People with COPD should avoid others who are sick, practice good hand-washing techniques, take drugs as prescribed, exercise regularly, and maintain a healthy weight. Avoiding or

controlling exposure to occupational and environmental pollutants and irritants is another preventive measure to maintain healthy lungs. Patients with COPD should have influenza and pneumococcal pneumonia vaccines.

Families with a history of COPD, as well as AATD, should be aware of the genetic nature of the disease. They may want to consider consulting a pulmonologist about regular spirometry

---

TABLE 28.23 Nursing Assessment
Chronic Obstructive Pulmonary Disease

Subjective Data

Important Health Information

Past health history: Long-term exposure to chemical pollutants, respiratory irritants, occupational fumes, dust; recurrent respiratory tract infections; previous hospitalizations

Medications: Use of O_2 and duration of O_2 use, bronchodilators, corticosteroids, antibiotics, anticholinergics, OTC drugs, illicit substances

Functional Health Patterns

Health perception–health management: Smoking (pack-years, including passive smoking, willingness to stop smoking, and previous attempts); what was smoked (e.g., cigarettes, pipes, cigars, e-cigarettes, hookahs, etc.); family history of respiratory disease (especially α_1-antitrypsin deficiency)

Nutritional-metabolic: Anorexia, weight loss or gain

Activity-exercise: Increasing dyspnea and/or increase in sputum volume or purulence; fatigue, ability to perform ADLs; swelling of feet; progressive dyspnea, especially on exertion; ability to walk up 1 flight of stairs without stopping; wheezing; recurrent cough; sputum production (especially in the morning); orthopnea

Elimination: Constipation, gas, bloating

Sleep-rest: Insomnia; sitting up position for sleeping, paroxysmal nocturnal dyspnea

Cognitive-perceptual: Headache, chest or abdominal soreness

Coping–stress tolerance: Anxiety, depression

Objective Data

General

Debilitation, restlessness, assumption of upright position

Integumentary

Cyanosis (bronchitis), pallor or ruddy color, poor skin turgor, thin skin, digital clubbing, easy bruising; peripheral edema (cor pulmonale)

Respiratory

Rapid, shallow breathing; inability to speak; prolonged expiratory phase; pursed-lip breathing; wheezing; crackles, decreased or bronchial breath sounds; ↓ chest excursion and diaphragm movement; use of accessory muscles; hyperresonant or dull chest sounds on percussion

Cardiovascular

Tachycardia, dysrhythmias, jugular venous distention, distant heart tones, right-sided S_3 (cor pulmonale), edema (especially in feet)

Gastrointestinal

Ascites, hepatomegaly (cor pulmonale)

Musculoskeletal

Muscle atrophy, ↑ anteroposterior diameter (barrel chest)

Possible Diagnostic Findings

Abnormal ABGs (compensated respiratory acidosis, ↓ PaO_2 or SaO_2, ↑ $PaCO_2$), polycythemia, pulmonary function tests showing expiratory airflow obstruction (e.g., low FEV_1, low FEV_1/FVC, large RV), chest x-ray showing flattened diaphragm and hyperinflation or infiltrates

screening, even if they do not have symptoms. Genetic counseling may be appropriate for the patient with AATD deficiency who is planning to have children.

◆ **Acute Care.** The patient with COPD needs hospitalization for acute exacerbations of COPD, brought on by pneumonia or heart failure and associated complications, such as cor pulmonale and respiratory failure. Once the crisis has been resolved, reassessment of the degree and severity of any underlying problems is needed. The information obtained will help in planning care going forward and may assist with changes in the treatment plan that will be needed after discharge.

◆ **Ambulatory Care.** The interprofessional team works together to individualize the treatment plan for COPD patients. By far the most important aspect in the long-term care of the patient with COPD is teaching. A large part of your role is to teach patients self-management of their disease. A patient and caregiver teaching guide is shown in Table 28.24.

Pulmonary Rehabilitation. Pulmonary rehabilitation can be done in an inpatient or outpatient setting or in the home. Components of pulmonary rehabilitation vary, but usually include exercise training, smoking cessation, nutrition counseling, and education. Physical therapists or nurses who have experience in respiratory care are often responsible for managing pulmonary rehabilitation centers. Pulmonary rehabilitation indicated for any degree of airway obstruction or GOLD classification. It works best if the patient starts when COPD is in a moderate stage, but even patients who have advanced COPD can benefit. Pulmonary rehabilitation relieves dyspnea and fatigue, improves emotional function, and enhances the sense of control that people have over their COPD.

Pulmonary rehabilitation may be inaccessible to some because of disability, transportation, geographic location, or cost. One alternative program to in-person pulmonary rehabilitation uses the Internet or gaming technology. However, the HCP must approve these types of programs to ensure safety.

INFORMATICS IN PRACTICE
E-Mail and Texting for COPD Patients

- Sometimes patients with COPD or those who use O_2 therapy have difficulty speaking because of shortness of breath.
- Encourage your patient to use typed messages, such as e-mail, to communicate.
- Texting and instant messaging family and friends are good alternatives to having phone conversations.

Activity Considerations. The patient with severe COPD typically uses upper thoracic and neck muscles to breathe rather than the diaphragm. Thus the patient has difficulty performing upper extremity activities, particularly those that require raising the arm above the head. Exercise training leads to energy conservation, which is an important part in COPD rehabilitation. Exercise training of the upper extremities may improve muscle function and help to reduce dyspnea.

Often the patient is already using some alternative energy-saving practices for ADLs. Explore alternative methods of hair care, shaving, showering, and reaching.

An occupational therapist may help with ideas in these areas. Assuming a tripod posture (elbows supported on a table, chest in fixed position) and placing a mirror on the table while using an electric razor or hair dryer conserves much more energy

---

TABLE 28.24 Patient & Caregiver Teaching
Chronic Obstructive Pulmonary Disease

Include the following information in the teaching plan to assist the patient with COPD and the caregiver to improve quality of life through promoting lifestyle practices that support successful living with COPD:

What Is COPD?
- Basic anatomy and physiology of lung
- Basic pathophysiology of COPD
- Signs and symptoms of COPD, exacerbation
- How to tell COPD from the common cold, flu, pneumonia
- Tests to assess breathing

Breathing and Airway Clearance Exercises
- Pursed-lip breathing (Table 28.12)
- Airway clearance technique: huff cough (Table 28.21)

Energy Conservation Techniques
- Daily activities (e.g., waking up, bathing, grooming, shopping, traveling)
- Consult with physical therapist and occupational therapist

Medications
Types (include mechanism of action and types of devices)
- Establishing medication schedule
- Correct use of inhalers, spacer, and nebulizer
- Reason for use of O_2 equipment
- Guide for home O_2 use and equipment

Psychosocial/Emotional Issues
Open discussion (sharing with patient and/or caregiver)
- Concerns about interpersonal relationships (e.g., intimacy)
- Problems with emotions (e.g., depression, anxiety, panic)
- Dependency
Treatment decisions and end-of-life issues
- Support and rehabilitation groups

COPD Management Plan
Nurse and patient develop and write up COPD management plan that meets individual needs.
- Focus on self-management
- Need to report changes
- Cause of acute exacerbations
- Recognition of signs and symptoms of respiratory infection, heart failure
- Reduce risk factors, especially smoking cessation
- Exercise program of walking and arm strengthening
- Yearly follow-up

Healthy Nutrition (Table 28.22)
- Ways to lose weight (if overweight)
- Ways to gain weight (if underweight)
- Consultation with dietitian

For more information, see American Lung Association at www.lung.org/lung-disease/copd.

---

than when the patient stands in front of a mirror to shave or blow-dry hair.

If the patient uses home O_2 therapy, O_2 should be used during hygiene because these tasks are energy consuming. Encourage the patient to make a schedule and plan daily and weekly activities, leaving plenty of time for rest periods. In severe COPD, the patient should try to sit as much as possible when performing activities. Another energy-saving tip is to exhale when pushing, pulling, or exerting effort during an activity and inhale during rest.

Regular physical exercise is important for patients with COPD. To ensure long-term adherence, the exercise plan must be individualized and easy to perform. Walking or other endurance exercises (e.g., cycling) combined with strength training are the best interventions to strengthen muscles and improve the patient's endurance. Teach the patient coordinated walking with slow, pursed-lip breathing. Many patients with moderate or severe COPD are anxious and fearful of walking or performing exercise. Both patients and their caregivers need support while they build the confidence they need to walk, perform daily exercises, or help with these activities.

Developing exercise endurance is very important. If it takes longer than 5 minutes to return to baseline, the patient has most likely "overdone it" and should proceed at a slower pace during the next exercise period. Keeping a diary or log of the exercise program may help. Stationary cycling can be used either alone or with walking. Cycles and treadmills are particularly good when weather prevents walking outside.

Fatigue, sleep problems, and dyspnea are common problems. Of these symptoms, dyspnea seems to be the one that most affects the patient's ability to carry out daily activities. Therefore focus your interventions on improving dyspnea, which should then improve the patient's overall functional performance.

Patients often ask whether moving to a warmer or drier climate will help. In general, such moves are generally not beneficial. Discourage moves to places with an elevation of 4000 ft or more because of the lower partial pressure of O_2 found in the air at higher elevations. A disadvantage of moving may be that a person leaves a job, friends, and familiar environment, which could be psychologically stressful. This may outweigh any advantage gained from being in a different climate.

EVIDENCE-BASED PRACTICE

Physical Activity and COPD

You are working as a nurse in a pulmonary clinic with R.P., a 71-yr-old man who was recently discharged from the hospital with a new diagnosis of COPD. He tells you he has been inactive for most of the past 8 months because his breathing seems to worsen with any type of physical activity.

Making Clinical Decisions

Best Available Evidence. Patients with COPD who take part in regular moderate physical activity (e.g., brisk walking) have fewer severe flare-ups and are less likely to be readmitted to the hospital. Physical activity improves lung function and lessens depressive symptoms. The season of the year and temperature can be barriers to outdoor exercise.

Clinician Expertise. Physical inactivity is common in patients with COPD. You are aware that inactivity may place R.P. at a greater risk for functional decline and readmission.

Patient Preference and Values. R.P. tells you that he misses taking walks every day with his wife and dog. He is wondering if he would be able to resume this activity at a slower pace.

Implications for Practice

1. What important factors will you discuss with R.P. about physical activity and COPD?
2. How would you assess R.P.'s willingness and motivation to engage in physical activity?
3. How would you involve the interprofessional team members to assist R.P. in regular physical activity?

Reference for Evidence

Kantorowski A, Wan ES, Homsy D, et al.: Determinants and outcomes of change in physical activity in COPD, *ERJ Open Res* 4:1, 2018.

Psychosocial Considerations. Coping is a challenge for the COPD patient and family. As the disease progresses, patients with COPD are often confronted with many lifestyle changes that may involve decreased ability to care for themselves, decreased energy for social activities, and loss or change in a job.

When a patient with COPD is first diagnosed or has complications that require hospitalization, expect a variety of emotional responses. Emotions often expressed include denial, anger, frustration from increased dependence, and loneliness from social isolation. Guilt may result if the disease was caused primarily by cigarette smoking.

Patients experience many losses as the disease progresses. Because many patients have depression and anxiety, assess for both. Ask patients if they "feel down or blue" most of the time. Do they appear anxious about being able to control their breathlessness or know what to do if they have an exacerbation? Are they showing concern over more difficulty in self-care activities, such as bathing? How is the family coping with the patient's disease? The patient with COPD may benefit from stress management techniques (e.g., massage, muscle relaxation).

It is important to convey a sense of understanding and caring to the patient. Teach patients about COPD and their treatment, which can provide a sense of control. It is important to include caregivers in the teaching so they can help the patient cope physically and emotionally. Support groups at local American Lung Association chapters (e.g., the Better Breathers Club), hospitals, and clinics can be helpful.

Consultation with a mental health therapist may be needed for proper screening and diagnosis of depression or other mental health problems. Cognitive and behavioral therapy along with COPD teaching may improve the quality of life. Drugs may be used to treat both depression and anxiety. Buspirone (BuSpar), used to treat anxiety, has few respiratory effects. Benzodiazepines should be avoided because they may depress the respiratory drive and may be habit forming. When the patient becomes anxious because of dyspnea, the use of pursed-lip breathing and SABAs may be appropriate.

Sexuality and Sexual Activity. Modifying sexual activity can contribute to healthy psychologic well-being. First, assess the patient's concerns related to sexuality and functioning. Ask open-ended questions to determine if the patient wants or is willing to discuss concerns. You could ask, "How has your breathing problem affected how you see yourself as a person?" Another question could be, "How does your shortness of breath affect your desire for intimacy with your partner?" These types of questions give the patient an opening to discuss concerns.

Dyspnea, the predominant symptom in COPD, should not be a major problem with success in sexual functioning, except for patients in severe late stages. If the patient can walk up 2 flights of stairs or walk briskly, they likely have enough energy for sexual activity. Using an inhaled bronchodilator before sexual activity can help ventilation. The patient may find these suggestions helpful: (1) plan sexual activity during the part of the day when breathing is best, which is usually late morning or early afternoon (plus older men often achieve an erection more easily in the morning); (2) use slow pursed-lip breathing; (3) refrain from sexual activity after eating or drinking alcohol; (4) choose less stressful positions during intercourse (missionary position for men is the worst); and (5) use O_2 if prescribed.

Most patients with COPD are older. Many of the sexual performance issues experienced by the patient with COPD are changes related to aging. You can teach the patient the "normalcy" of the changes. The patient with coexisting heart disease should obtain advice from an HCP related to appropriate levels of activity. Open communication between partners about their needs and expectations and any changes that may be needed is important.

Sleep. Adequate sleep is extremely important to maintain quality of life and productivity. Most patients with COPD have sleep problems. Hyperinflation of the lungs and reduction in ventilation can result in severe drops in O_2 saturation (down to 60% or less) during sleep. This leads to an increased workload on the heart. Hypercapnia may contribute to more frequent awakening. The net result is sleeping poorly and waking up unrefreshed and fatigued.

Current tobacco use, depression, and anxiety are all common in COPD and lead to more trouble sleeping. β_2-Agonists may cause restlessness and insomnia. Postnasal drip or nasal congestion may cause coughing and wheezing at night. Nasal saline sprays or rinses before sleep and in the morning may help. If the patient is prescribed O_2 therapy, using it at night may decrease insomnia. If the patient is a restless sleeper, snores, stops breathing while asleep, and tends to fall asleep during the day, the patient may need testing for sleep apnea (see Chapter 7).

End-of-Life Considerations. The trajectory of COPD is a gradual decline in health characterized by increasing exacerbations that are associated with an increased risk for death. In the later, severe stages of this disease, palliative, end-of-life, and hospice care are important components of care for the patient with advanced COPD.

Patients need to know that symptoms can be managed, but COPD cannot be cured. End-of-life issues and advance directives are important topics for discussion in the latter stages of COPD. This may be hard for the patient and family to consider because of the uncertainty of the disease.

◆ Evaluation

The expected outcomes are that the patient with COPD will
- Maintain a patent airway by effectively coughing
- Have an effective rate, rhythm, and depth of respirations
- Have clear breath sounds
- Return to pre-exacerbation baseline respiratory function
- Have $PaCO_2$ and PaO_2 values that return to normal for the patient

CYSTIC FIBROSIS

Cystic fibrosis (CF) is an autosomal recessive, multisystem disease characterized by altered transport of sodium and chloride ions in and out of epithelial cells. This defect primarily affects the lungs, GI tract (pancreas and biliary tract), and reproductive tract.

The first signs and symptoms typically occur in childhood, but some patients are not diagnosed until they are adults. The severity and progression of the disease vary. With early diagnosis and improvements in therapy, the prognosis of patients with CF has significantly improved. The median predicted survival in 1970 was 16 years of age. Today it has increased to more than 37.5 years.[25]

Etiology and Pathophysiology
Genetic Link. CF is an autosomal recessive disorder. The CF gene is found on chromosome 7, which makes a protein called *CF transmembrane conductance regulator (CFTR)*. The CFTR

ETHICAL/LEGAL DILEMMAS
Advance Directives

Situation

L.H., an 84-yr-old man with end-stage COPD, is admitted to the hospital in respiratory failure. He is intubated in the ED and placed on a ventilator. L.H. sometimes responds by opening his eyes. His advanced personal directive (AD) was drawn up 5 years ago, and copies were given to his wife and HCP at that time. His wife brings the documents to the critical care unit and tells you that the hospital must stop treating her husband, and as per his request, allow him to die. However, the patient's oldest son is threatening the hospital with a lawsuit if the staff does not provide full care to his father.

Ethical/Legal Points for Consideration

- A Living Will, one form of AD, permits persons to state their own preferences and refusals should the person become terminally ill or be in a situation in which there is no hope of recovery and the person is not able to speak for themselves.
- The Durable Power of Attorney for Health Care, another form of AD, permits persons to identify a proxy to make health care decisions in the event the person is incapacitated.
- The National POLST Paradigm is an approach to end-of-life planning that emphasizes documenting patients' wishes about the care they receive.[1]
- AD laws vary from state to state concerning the need for witnesses and designating the proxy.
- Some families are deeply divided about decisions for their loved ones, and conflicts often arise when feelings of remorse or guilt and money and/or property are involved. This situation requires you to notify the HCP, engage social work and spiritual care, and ask for a family conference. In some circumstances, a consult from the ethics committee may be needed.
- HCPs are obligated to follow the patient's ADs when a patient is no longer able to speak for himself or herself.
- In your scope of nursing practice, you need to (1) be informed about the decision-making laws and regulations in your state, (2) make AD documents available to patients, (3) teach patients and families about ADs, (4) determine if all involved HCPs are aware of the ADs, (5) assist the patient and family in communicating with the HCP when a "no code" or "DNR" (do not resuscitate) order is requested, and (6) assist the conflicted family in obtaining appropriate counseling when needed.

Discussion Questions

1. What should you do next with the information provided by L.H.'s wife?
2. The HCP has asked that you organize a family conference. How should you address the needs of each member of this family in L.H.'s plan of care?
3. What resources can you use to facilitate decision making in this situation?
4. What would be your approach to L.H.'s plan of care?

Reference

Physician Orders for Life Sustaining Treatment (POLST) Program. Retrieved from *www.polst.org.*

---

protein localizes to the epithelial surface of the airways, GI tract, and ducts of the liver, pancreas, and sweat glands. Under normal conditions, CFTR regulates sodium and chloride movement in and out of epithelial cells. However, mutations in the *CFTR* gene change this protein in such a way that the channels are blocked. As a result, cells that line the passageways of the lungs, pancreas, intestines, and other organs make secretions that are low in sodium chloride content (thus low in water content),

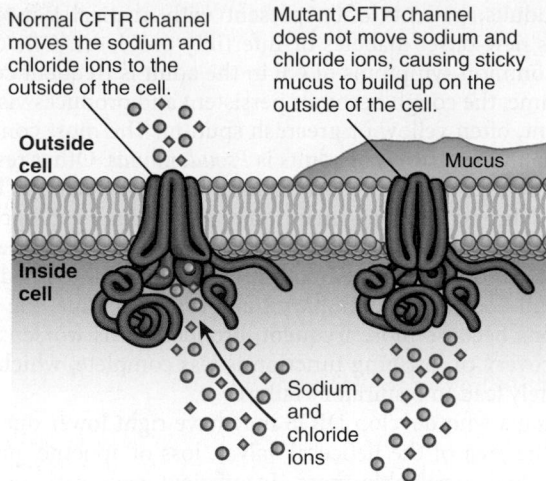

Normal CFTR channel moves the sodium and chloride ions to the outside of the cell.

Mutant CFTR channel does not move sodium and chloride ions, causing sticky mucus to build up on the outside of the cell.

Outside cell

Mucus

Inside cell

Sodium and chloride ions

FIG. 28.16 People with cystic fibrosis inherit a defective gene on chromosome 7 called *cystic fibrosis transmembrane conductance regulator (CFTR)*. The protein made by this gene normally helps sodium and chloride move in and out of cells. If the protein does not work correctly, the movement of sodium and chloride is blocked, and an abnormally thick sticky mucus is produced on the outside of the cell.

making mucus abnormally thick and sticky (Fig. 28.16). This mucus plugs up the ducts in these organs, causing scarring in the organs and resulting in organ failure. The high concentrations of sodium and chloride in the sweat of the patient with CF result from decreased chloride reabsorption in the sweat duct.

GENETICS IN CLINICAL PRACTICE

Cystic Fibrosis (CF)

Genetic Basis
- Autosomal recessive disorder
- Caused by mutations in CF transmembrane regulator *(CFTR)* gene on chromosome 7
- *CFTR* gene provides the instructions for making the protein that controls the channel that transports sodium and chloride
- There are more than 17,000 different mutations of the *CFTR* gene
- Mutations in the *CFTR* gene disrupt the function of the channels, preventing them from regulating the flow of sodium, chloride, and water across cell membranes

Incidence
- In the United States, 1 in 3000 white births
- Less common in other ethnic populations (1 in 15,000 blacks, 1 in 9200 Hispanics, 1 in 30,000 Asian Americans)
- One in 20 to 25 whites are carriers of the gene

Genetic Testing
- Blood-based DNA testing is available for disease and carrier states.
- All 50 states require CF screening for all newborns.
- Testing is usually done in children if CF is suspected or if parents are possible carriers.
- In parents who are known carriers, amniocentesis or chorionic villus sampling in pregnant women may be useful for prenatal testing.

Clinical Implications
- CF has a wide range of clinical expression of disease.
- Most people who have a child with CF are not aware of a family history of disease.
- CF screening should be offered to all people of reproductive age regardless of family history.

The hallmark of CF is its effect on the airways. CF can affect both upper and lower respiratory tracts. URI manifestations may include chronic sinusitis and nasal polyposis. CF progresses from being a disease of the small airways (*chronic bronchiolitis*) to involvement of the larger airways that causes destruction of lung tissue. The mucus lining the airways becomes dehydrated and tenacious due to defects in chloride secretion and sodium absorption. Cilia motility is decreased, allowing mucus to adhere to the airways. The bronchioles become obstructed with thick secretions, leading to scarring of the airways (bronchiectasis), air trapping, and hyperinflation of the lungs.

CF is characterized by a persistent, chronic airway infection that cannot be cured. *P. aeruginosa* is by far the most common organism in adults. Other organisms include *Staphylococcus aureus, H. influenzae,* and less often, but more seriously, *Burkholderia cepacia.* Antibiotic resistance develops after multiple exposure to antibiotics. Pulmonary inflammation is associated with the chronic infection and can cause a decrease in respiratory function, further narrowing the lumen of the airways. Inflammatory mediators (e.g., interleukins, oxidants, proteases released by neutrophils) are increased and contribute to disease progression.

Lung disorders that initially occur are chronic bronchiolitis and bronchiectasis (Fig. 28.17). Over a long period, pulmonary vascular remodeling occurs because of local hypoxia and arteriolar vasoconstriction. Pulmonary hypertension, enlarged pulmonary arteries, and cor pulmonale occur in the later phases of the disease. Blebs and large cysts in the lung are severe manifestations of lung destruction. Pneumothorax may occur. Hemoptysis is caused by proliferation of capillaries in response to chronic infection. During exacerbations, erosion of these capillaries occurs. Hemoptysis may range from scant streaking to major bleeding, which can be fatal.

Pancreatic insufficiency is caused by mucous plugging of the pancreatic exocrine ducts. This results in atrophy of the gland and progressive fibrotic cyst formation. The pancreas's exocrine function may be completely lost. Because of this dysfunction, pancreatic enzymes, such as lipase, amylase, and proteases (trypsin, chemotrypsin), are not made in sufficient amounts to allow for absorption of nutrients. Malabsorption of fat, protein, and fat-soluble vitamins (A, D, E, and K) occurs. Fat malabsorption results in steatorrhea. Protein malabsorption results in failure to grow and gain weight. Osteopenia and osteoporosis are common. They are related to malnutrition, malabsorption of vitamin D, insufficient testosterone levels, and chronically elevated inflammatory cytokines.[26]

We believe CF-related diabetes mellitus (CFRD) is caused by underdevelopment of pancreatic islet cells (in utero) and destruction of islet cells over the person's lifetime. CFRD is unique because it has characteristics of both type 1 and type 2 diabetes. The pancreas in people with CF makes insulin, but they make it too late to fully respond to carbohydrate intake.

Persons with CF often have other GI problems, including GERD, gallstones, and pancreatitis. The liver and gallbladder can be damaged by mucus deposits in the ducts. Liver enzymes may become chronically elevated, with cirrhosis developing over time. Portal hypertension can occur. Distal intestinal obstruction syndrome (DIOS) results from an intermittent obstruction, often in the terminal ileum at the point of the ileocecal junction. It is caused by thickened, dehydrated stool and mucus. The patient may appear to have a small bowel obstruction. DIOS develops because of chronic malabsorption related

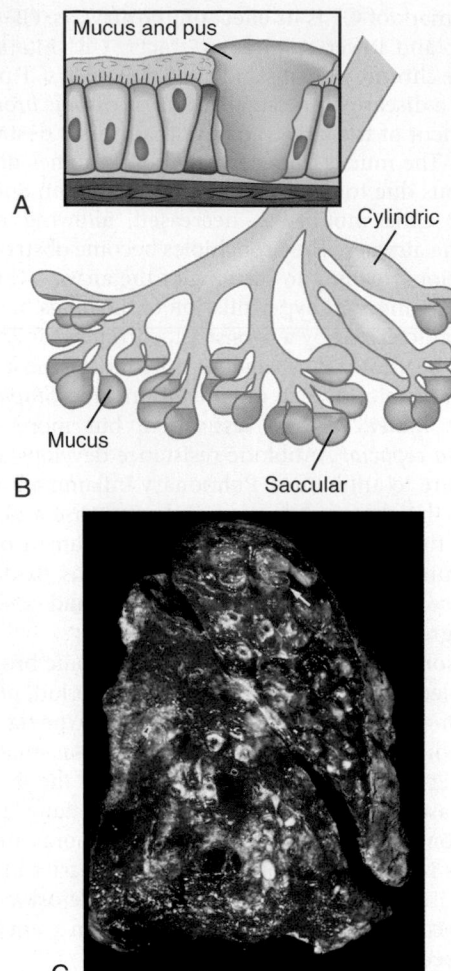

FIG. 28.17 Pathologic changes in bronchiectasis. **A,** Longitudinal section of bronchial wall where chronic infection has caused damage. **B,** Collection of purulent material in dilated bronchioles, leading to persistent infection. **C,** Bronchiectasis in a patient with cystic fibrosis who underwent lung transplantation. Cut surfaces of lung show markedly distended peripheral bronchi filled with mucopurulent secretions. (*C,* From Kumar V, Abbas AK, Aster JC, et al: *Robbins and Cotran pathologic basis of disease,* ed 8, Philadelphia, 2010, Saunders.)

to exocrine dysfunction, under- or over-dosing of pancreatic replacement enzyme supplementation, dehydration, and swallowing of mucus.

Clinical Manifestations

The manifestations vary depending on the severity of the disease. The disease severity may vary greatly, both within families and among different families. Mutations do not affect carriers.

The median age at diagnosis of CF is 6 to 8 months of age. Two thirds are diagnosed in the first year of life.[27] Currently every state has mandatory newborn screening for CF, which has allowed for early intervention. An initial finding of meconium ileus in the newborn infant prompts the diagnosis in 20% of people with CF. Other signs that suggest a CF diagnosis in childhood are acute or persistent respiratory symptoms (wheezing, coughing, frequent pneumonia), failure to thrive or malnutrition, steatorrhea (large, oily, frequent bowel movements), bronchiectasis, and family history. Without treatment, a large, protuberant abdomen may develop with an emaciated appearance of the extremities. Both males and females have delayed puberty.

In adults, patients often present with atypical symptoms, such as new-onset diabetes or infertility problems. One of the most common symptoms of CF in the adult is frequent cough. With time, the cough becomes persistent and produces viscous, purulent, often yellow or greenish sputum. The most common bacteria in the airways of adults is *Pseudomonas*. Other respiratory problems include recurring lung infections, such as bronchiolitis, bronchitis, and pneumonia. As the disease progresses, periods of clinical stability are interrupted by exacerbations characterized by increased cough, weight loss, increased sputum, and decreased pulmonary function. Over time, the exacerbations become more frequent, bronchiectasis worsens, and the recovery of lost lung function is less complete, which may ultimately lead to respiratory failure.

Patients who develop DIOS may have right lower quadrant pain (the area of the ileocecal valve), loss of appetite, nausea, emesis, and a palpable mass. Insufficient pancreatic enzyme release causes the typical pattern of protein and fat malabsorption with a person being thin with a low body mass index (BMI) and frequent bulky, foul-smelling stools.

Both males and females have delayed puberty. Some women with CF have difficulty conceiving. The cervical mucus may be thickened. During exacerbations, menstrual irregularities and secondary amenorrhea are common. Most women with CF can become pregnant. Most pregnancies result in viable infants.

Nearly all men with CF have reproductive issues because their vas deferens fails to develop in utero, so there is no transport of sperm from storage in the testes to the penile urethra. However, they make sperm normally, and with assisted reproductive technology, can father a child.

Complications

Complications in CF include CFRD and bone, sinus, and liver disease. With advanced lung disease, digital clubbing occurs. Respiratory failure and cor pulmonale caused by pulmonary hypertension are late complications of CF. Pneumothorax, a rare but serious complication, is caused by the formation of bullae and blebs. A small amount of blood in sputum is common in the CF patient because of chronic lung infection. Massive hemoptysis, though, is also rare but can be life-threatening.

Diagnostic Studies

The diagnostic criteria for CF include a combination of clinical presentation, family history, laboratory, and genetic testing. The sweat glands of CF patients secrete normal volumes of sweat, but sodium chloride cannot be absorbed from sweat as it moves through the sweat duct. As a result, 4 times the normal amount of sodium and chloride is excreted in sweat. This abnormality usually does not directly affect the person's general health, but helps confirm a diagnosis of CF.

The sweat chloride test is the gold standard for diagnosis of CF. It is done with the pilocarpine iontophoresis method.[28] Pilocarpine is placed on the skin and carried by a small electric current to stimulate sweat production. This part of the process takes about 5 minutes. The patient will feel a slight tingling or warmth. Next, the area (usually an arm) is wrapped in plastic to help facilitate sweating. The sweat is collected on filter paper or gauze and then analyzed for sweat chloride concentrations. The test takes about 1 hour. Sweat chloride values above 60 mmol/L are considered positive for the diagnosis of CF. A second sweat chloride test is done at the same time (1 test in each arm) to confirm the diagnosis.

Genetic testing is often used if the results from a sweat chloride test are uncertain. A blood sample or cells taken inside the cheek (buccal smear) are sent to a laboratory that specializes in genetic testing. Most laboratories test for only the most common mutations of the CF gene. Because more than 1700 mutations cause CF, screening for all mutations is hard and done only at a specialty laboratory.

Interprofessional Care

An interprofessional team should be involved in the care of a patient with CF. The Cystic Fibrosis Foundation provides funding for and accredits more than 120 CF care centers nationwide. The high quality of specialized care available throughout the care center network has led to the improved length and quality of life for people with CF. These care centers offer the best care, treatments, and support for those with CF. The teams at these care centers include a nurse, physician, respiratory therapist, physical therapist, dietitian, social worker, and often a nurse practitioner.

Management of pulmonary problems in CF aims at relieving airway obstruction and controlling infection. Drainage of thick bronchial mucus is assisted by aerosol and nebulization treatments of drugs used to dilate the airways, liquefy mucus, and promote clearance.

The abnormal viscosity of CF secretions is increased by concentrated deoxyribonucleic acid (DNA) from neutrophils involved in chronic infection. Agents that degrade the DNA in CF sputum (e.g., inhaled dornase alfa [Pulmozyme]) increase airflow and reduce the number of acute exacerbations. Inhaled hypertonic saline (7%) increases osmolality, allowing water to collect on airway surfaces. It is effective in clearing mucus and decreases the frequency of exacerbations. Some patients also need bronchodilators (e.g., β_2-adrenergic agonists) to control bronchospasm, but the long-term benefit is not known.

ACTs are critical since the normal ciliary motion in CF airways is impaired. CPT (including postural drainage with percussion and vibration) and high-frequency chest wall oscillation loosen mucus. Clearance is achieved by specialized expiratory techniques aimed at using airflow to remove the loosened secretions. Examples include PEP devices (Fig. 28.15), breathing exercises, pursed-lip breathing (Table 28.12), and huff coughing (Table 28.21). Persons with CF may prefer a certain technique or device that works well for them in a daily routine. No clear evidence exists that any ACT is better than the others.

Most patients with CF die of complications from lung infection. Standard treatment of infections includes antibiotics for exacerbations in conjunction with airway clearance. Early intervention with antibiotics is useful. Antibiotic choice should be based on sputum culture results. They may be given for 10 days to 3 weeks or longer. Some need chronic suppressive therapy. Prolonged high-dose therapy (larger doses, more frequent dosing) may be needed because many drugs are abnormally metabolized and rapidly excreted in the patient with CF.

If home support and resources are adequate, the CF patient and caregiver may be able to administer IV antibiotic therapy at home independently. The usual treatment is 2 antibiotics with different mechanisms of action (e.g., cephalosporin and an aminoglycoside). The patient with cor pulmonale or hypoxemia may need home O_2 therapy.

Oral agents used for mild exacerbations (e.g., increased cough and sputum) include a semisynthetic penicillin, trimethoprim/sulfamethoxazole (to treat *S. aureus*) or oral quinolones, especially ciprofloxacin (to treat *P. aeruginosa*). The quinolones are used with caution because of the rapid development of resistant strains.

Most patients have *Pseudomonas* infection, which can be hard to treat over time because the organism develops resistance to antibiotics. *Pseudomonas* can form a biofilm that protects the organism from antibiotics. One commonly used antibiotic to treat patients with chronic *Pseudomonas* infection is aerosolized tobramycin (TOBI). It is given twice a day, every day, every other month. Azithromycin used longer than 6 months decreases the frequency of pulmonary exacerbations, especially in those infected with *Pseudomonas*. It is also thought to act as an antiinflammatory.

Patients with a large pneumothorax need chest tube drainage, perhaps repeatedly. Sclerosing of the pleural space or partial pleural stripping and pleural abrasion may be done for recurrent episodes of pneumothorax. With massive hemoptysis, bronchial artery embolization is done. CF has become a leading reason for lung transplantation.

The management of pancreatic insufficiency includes pancreatic enzyme replacement of lipase, protease, and amylase (e.g., pancrelipase [Pancreaze, Creon, Zenpep]) taken before each meal and snack. Adequate intake of fat, calories, protein, and vitamins is important. Fat-soluble vitamins (A, D, E, and K) must be supplemented, since they are malabsorbed. Use of caloric supplements improves nutritional status. Dietary salt is indicated whenever sweating is excessive, such as during hot weather, when fever is present, or from intense physical activity. Hyperglycemia may need insulin treatment.

If the patient develops DIOS with partial or complete bowel obstruction, every attempt is made to manage the condition medically. Options include prokinetic agents (e.g., macrolide antibiotics, metoclopramide), mucolytics (oral N-acetylcysteine), stimulant laxatives, lactulose, and polyethylene glycol (PEG) electrolyte solution (MiraLAX, GoLYTELY).[29] Careful monitoring of bowel habits and patterns is essential for CF patients. If DIOS does not resolve with medical treatment, surgery may be done to prevent the development of ischemic bowel.

Ivacaftor (Kalydeco), a CFTR modulator, is used to treat patients who have mutations in a specific *CFTR* gene. It is not effective in patients with CF who have 2 copies (homozygous) of the *F508* mutation in the *CFTR* gene (the most common mutation that results in CF). If a patient's genotype is unknown, a CF mutation test should be done to detect the presence of a CFTR mutation. Combinations drugs, such as ivacaftor/lumacaftor (Orkambi), are used to treat CF patients with specific gene mutations. All patients diagnosed with CF should have CFTR genotyping. This will help determine if they carry a mutation that would be appropriate for CFTR modulator therapy.

❖ NURSING MANAGEMENT: CYSTIC FIBROSIS

◆ Nursing Assessment

Subjective and objective data that should be obtained from the patient with CF are presented in Table 28.25.

◆ Nursing Diagnoses

Nursing diagnoses for the patient with CF may include:
- Impaired airway clearance
- Impaired respiratory system function
- Impaired nutritional status
- Difficulty coping

TABLE 28.25   Nursing Assessment

Cystic Fibrosis

Subjective Data

Important Health Information

Past health history: Recurrent respiratory and sinus infections, persistent cough with excessive sputum production
Medications: Use of and compliance with bronchodilators, antibiotics

Functional Health Patterns

Health perception–health maintenance: Family history of cystic fibrosis, diagnosis of cystic fibrosis in childhood, genetic testing in offspring
Nutritional-metabolic: Dietary intolerances, voracious appetite, weight loss, heartburn
Elimination: Intestinal gas. Large, frequent bowel movements, constipation
Activity-exercise: Fatigue, ↓ exercise tolerance, amount and type of exercise. Dyspnea, cough, excessive mucus or sputum production, coughing up blood, airway clearance techniques
Cognitive-perceptual: Abdominal pain
Sexuality-reproductive: Delayed menarche, menstrual irregularities, problems conceiving or fathering a child
Coping–stress tolerance: Anxiety, depression, problems adapting to diagnosis

Objective Data

General

Restlessness; failure to thrive

Integumentary

Cyanosis (circumoral, nail bed), digital clubbing; salty skin

Eyes

Scleral icterus

Respiratory

Sinus congestion, postnasal drip, persistent runny nose. Decreased breath sounds, adventitious breath sounds (crackles, wheezes). Sputum (thick, light or dark, tenacious), ↑ WOB, use of accessory muscles of respiration, barrel chest, hemoptysis (rare)

Cardiovascular

Tachycardia

Gastrointestinal

Protuberant abdomen; abdominal distention; foul, fatty stools

Possible Diagnostic Findings

Abnormal ABGs and pulmonary function tests; abnormal sweat chloride test, chest x-ray, fecal fat analysis

◆ Planning

The overall goals are that the patient with CF will have (1) adequate airway clearance, (2) absence of respiratory infection, (3) adequate nutritional support to maintain appropriate BMI, (4) ability to perform ADLs, (5) recognition and treatment of complications related to CF, and (6) active participation in planning and implementing an achievable treatment plan.

◆ Nursing Implementation

Acute care for the patient with CF includes relief of bronchoconstriction, airway obstruction, and airflow limitation. Interventions include aggressive CPT, antibiotics, and O_2 therapy in severe disease. Good nutrition is important.

Aerobic exercise is effective in clearing the airways. Important needs to consider when planning an aerobic exercise program for the patient with CF are (1) meeting increased nutritional demands of exercise, (2) observing for dehydration, and (3) drinking large amounts of fluid and replacing salt losses.

As these persons continue into adulthood, you can help them in gaining independence by helping them assume responsibility for their care and life goals. An important issue to discuss is sexuality. Delayed development of secondary sex characteristics and irregular menses are common. The issue of marrying and having children is difficult. Genetic counseling is an appropriate suggestion for the couple considering having children. Another concern is the uncertainty surrounding the shortened life span of the parent with CF.

Other crises and life transitions that must be dealt with in the young adult include persisting with employment goals, developing motivation to achieve, learning to cope with the treatment program, and adjusting to the need for dependence if health fails. Disclosing the CF diagnosis to friends, potential spouses, or employers may pose significant emotional, social, psychological, and financial challenges.

CF imposes a significant emotional and financial burden on the patient and family. In many situations, the cost of drugs, special equipment, and health care poses considerable financial hardship. The burden of living with a chronic disease at a young age can be emotionally overwhelming. There is a higher incidence of depression among persons with CF than their unaffected peers. Issues related to costs of health care, burden of self-care, career choices, fertility, and decreased life expectancy, may lead to depression. Community resources are available to help patients and caregivers. The Cystic Fibrosis Foundation can be a source of information and support.

BRONCHIECTASIS

Etiology and Pathophysiology

Bronchiectasis is characterized by permanent, abnormal dilation of medium-sized bronchi. It is the result of inflammatory changes that destroy elastic and muscular structures supporting the bronchial wall. There is a continuing cycle of inflammation, airway damage, and remodeling, enhanced by the accumulation of neutrophils in the airways. Airways can become colonized with microorganisms (e.g., *Pseudomonas*), which causes the bronchial walls to weaken and pockets of infection to form (Fig. 28.17).

When the walls of the bronchial system are injured, the mucociliary mechanism is damaged, allowing bacteria and mucus to accumulate within the pockets. Bacteria attract neutrophils, which enhances inflammation and causes edema. Stasis of thickened mucus occurs due to impaired clearance of mucus by the cilia. This results in a reduced ability to clear mucus from the lungs and decreased expiratory airflow.

A variety of problems can result in bronchiectasis. CF is the main cause of bronchiectasis in children. In adults, the main cause is bacterial infections of the lungs. A wide variety of infectious agents initiate bronchiectasis. It can follow a single episode of severe pneumonia or infection that was either not treated or received delayed treatment. Other causes are obstruction of an airway with mucus plugs or generalized impairment of pulmonary defenses. Several systemic diseases, such as inflammatory bowel disease, rheumatoid arthritis, or immune disorders (e.g., acquired immunodeficiency syndrome [AIDS]) are associated with bronchiectasis.

Clinical Manifestations

The hallmark is persistent cough with consistent production of thick, tenacious, purulent sputum. In rare situations, some patients with severe disease and upper lobe involvement may have no sputum production and little cough. Recurrent infections injure blood vessels. Large connections (anastomoses) may develop between blood vessels in the lungs, and hemoptysis may occur. In severe cases the bleed can be life-threatening. Other manifestations are pleuritic chest pain, dyspnea, wheezing, clubbing of digits, weight loss, and anemia. On auscultation, adventitious sounds can be heard (e.g., crackles, wheezes).

Diagnostic Studies

A person who presents with a chronic productive cough with copious purulent sputum (which may be blood streaked) should be suspected of having bronchiectasis. A CT scan is the gold standard for diagnosing bronchiectasis.[30]

Chest x-rays may show nonspecific abnormalities. Spirometry usually shows an obstructive pattern, including a decrease in FEV_1 and FEV_1/FVC. Sputum may give information about the presence of active infection and the severity of impairment. Patients often have *H. influenzae, S. aureus,* or *P. aeruginosa,* with the latter leading to more frequent exacerbations and rapid decline in lung function. A complete blood cell count and AAT level may be done.

❖ INTERPROFESSIONAL AND NURSING MANAGEMENT: BRONCHIECTASIS

Bronchiectasis is hard to treat. Therapy is aimed at treating acute flare-ups and preventing a decline in lung function. Antibiotics are the mainstay of treatment. They are often given for a minimum of 14 days. Antibiotics may be given orally, IV, or inhaled (nebulizer). Choice of antibiotic primarily depends on culture results or most likely organism. The patient needs to understand the importance of taking prescribed drugs to obtain maximum effectiveness. Long-term antibiotic therapy is given to patients who have symptoms that recur a few days after stopping antibiotics. Concurrent bronchodilator therapy with SABAs, LABAs, or anticholinergics can prevent bronchospasm and stimulate mucus clearance. Some patients receive oral and inhaled corticosteroids.

One important goal is to promote drainage and removal of mucus. Various ACTs can be used to facilitate secretion removal. CPT with postural drainage is widely used. Direct hydration of the respiratory system may help with the expectoration of secretions. Hyperosmolar agents (e.g., hypertonic saline) given by nebulizer can liquefy secretions. At home, a steamy shower can be effective.

Teach the patient and caregiver manifestations to report to the HCP. These include increased sputum production, increasing dyspnea, fever, chills, and chest pain. Teach patients when to contact the HCP if hemoptysis occurs. Some patients may periodically expectorate a "spot" of blood that is usual for them and do not require urgent attention. However, if the patient expectorates a moderate to large amount of blood, they should contact the HCP at once. In the acute care setting, elevate the head of the bed, and place the patient in a side-lying position with the suspected bleeding side down. Closely monitor vital signs and respiratory status.

Maintaining hydration is important to liquefy secretions. Unless contraindicated, teach the patient to drink at least 2 to 3 L of fluid daily. To achieve this, tell the patient to increase intake by 1 glass per day until they reach that goal. Have the patient use low-sodium fluids, thereby avoiding systemic fluid retention. Rest is important to prevent overexertion.

Good nutrition is important but may be difficult to maintain because the patient is often anorexic. Oral hygiene to cleanse the mouth and remove dried sputum crusts may improve the patient's appetite. Offer foods that are appealing, in smaller quantities and more often since they may increase the patient's desire to eat.

Surgical resection of parts of the lungs, which was common in the past, has largely been replaced by more effective supportive and antibiotic therapy. For select patients who are disabled in spite of maximal therapy, lung transplantation may be an option. Massive hemoptysis may require surgical resection.

CASE STUDY

Chronic Obstructive Pulmonary Disease

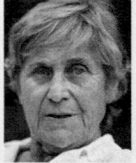
(© iStockphoto/Thinkstock.)

Patient Profile

H.M. is a 68-yr-old white, married, retired female police officer. She has been in the hospital for 6 days with an acute COPD exacerbation and will be discharged tomorrow.

Subjective Data

- Before admission, had 4 days of exceptional shortness of breath and increased volume of sputum, which turned greenish
- Increased Ventolin HFA use (at home) to 5 or 6 times a day for dyspnea
- Described having "jitters" and "racing heart"
- Had 3 or 4 COPD exacerbation in the past year that were managed at home
- 30 pack-year history of smoking; smokes half a pack per day now to "clear out lungs" in the morning
- Eats a regular diet but "gets full fast"
- Cannot climb 1 flight of stairs without stopping; walks down the flat driveway 10 yards without difficulty
- Awakens 2-3 times per night coughing and short of breath

Objective Data

Physical Examination

- Weight 129 lb, height 5 ft 8 in, BMI 20 kg/m²
- Temperature 37.8° C (100° F), pulse 86 (regular), respiratory rate 28 (shallow, slightly labored), BP 136/76 mm Hg
- Increased anteroposterior diameter of chest (barrel shaped)
- Slight use of accessory (neck) muscles with breathing
- Distant breath sounds with occasional expiratory wheezes
- 1+ non-pitting edema (ankles and feet bilaterally)

Diagnostic Studies

- Last spirometry: decreased FEV_1 (48%) and FEV_1/FVC (62%)
- ABG on admission: pH 7.34, $PaCO_2$ 59 mm Hg, HCO_3^- 27 mEq/L, PaO_2 68 mm Hg
- ABG (24 hours after admission): pH 7.30, $PaCO_2$ 63 mm Hg, HCO_3^- 29 mEq/L, PaO_2 64 mm Hg
- WBC: 14,000/μL on admission
- Chest x-ray: hyperinflation, flat diaphragm, no sign of pneumonia
- Sputum: negative (no organisms present)

Continued

CASE STUDY

Chronic Obstructive Pulmonary Disease—cont'd

Interprofessional Care

- GOLD 3 (severe) COPD with acute exacerbation
- O_2 2 L via nasal catheter while in hospital
- Prednisone 40 mg/day PO for 5 days
- Levofloxacin 750 mg/day PO for 10 days
- Ipratropium HFA MDI 2 puffs 4 times a day
- At discharge: Advair Diskus 250/50 one inhalation q12hr

Discussion Questions

1. What classic manifestations indicate the patient had a COPD exacerbation?
2. What are some likely causes of her COPD?
3. What symptoms in H.M. indicate the overuse of inhalers? Which drug would cause the symptoms described?

4. ***Patient-Centered Care:*** What is one suggestion you could make to H.M. that could halt the progression of her lung disease?
5. Why would H.M. "feel full fast" when eating? What could you do to minimize this issue?
6. Interpret the ABGs. What is your impression of each ABG? In comparing both ABGs, do you see a pattern?
7. ***Priority Decision:*** Based on the assessment data presented, what are the priority nursing diagnoses?
8. ***Evidence-Based Practice:*** H.M.'s son has been trying to convince his mother to quit smoking for many years without success. He asks you to tell his mother the results of her spirometry to convince her it is time to quit. Will this approach work?
9. ***Priority Decision:*** What are nursing priorities for discharge planning and teaching?
10. Develop a conceptual care map for H.M.

Answers available at *http://evolve.elsevier.com/Lewis/medsurg.*

■ BRIDGE TO NCLEX EXAMINATION

The number of the question corresponds to the same-numbered outcome at the beginning of the chapter.

1. A patient is concerned that he may have asthma. Of the symptoms that he describes to the nurse, which ones suggest asthma or risk factors for asthma? *(select all that apply)*
   a. Allergic rhinitis
   b. Prolonged inhalation
   c. Cough, especially at night
   d. Gastric reflux or heartburn
   e. History of chronic sinusitis

2. Which findings indicate that a patient is developing status asthmaticus? *(select all that apply)*
   a. PEFR <300 L/min
   b. Positive sputum culture
   c. Unable to speak in complete sentences
   d. Lack of response to conventional treatment
   e. Chest x-ray shows hyperinflated lungs and a flattened diaphragm

3. Which statement indicates the patient with asthma requires further teaching about self-care?
   a. "I use my corticosteroid inhaler when I feel short of breath."
   b. "I get a flu shot every year and see my HCP if I have an upper respiratory tract infection."
   c. "I use my inhaler before I visit my aunt who has a cat, but I only visit for a few minutes because of my allergies."
   d. "I walk 30 minutes every day but sometimes I have to use my bronchodilator inhaler before walking to prevent me from getting short of breath."

4. Which medications would be *most* appropriate to administer to a patient experiencing an acute asthma attack? *(select all that apply)*
   a. montelukast (Singulair)
   b. inhaled hypertonic saline
   c. albuterol (Proventil HFA)
   d. ipratropium (Atrovent HFA)
   e. salmeterol (Serevent Diskus)

5. The plan of care for the patient with chronic obstructive pulmonary disease (COPD) should include *(select all that apply)*
   a. exercise such as walking.
   b. high flow rate of O_2 administration.
   c. low-dose chronic oral corticosteroid therapy.
   d. use of peak flow meter to monitor the progression of COPD.
   e. breathing exercises, such as pursed-lip breathing that focus on exhalation.

6. The major advantage of a Venturi mask is that it can
   a. deliver up to 80% O_2.
   b. provide continuous 100% humidity.
   c. deliver a precise concentration of O_2.
   d. be used while a patient eats and sleeps.

7. Which guideline should the nurse include when teaching a patient how to use a metered-dose inhaler (MDI)?
   a. After activating the MDI, breathe in as quickly as you can.
   b. Estimate the amount of remaining medicine in the MDI by floating the canister in water.
   c. Disassemble the plastic canister from the inhaler and rinse both pieces under running water every week.
   d. To determine how long the canister will last, divide the total number of puffs in the canister by the puffs needed per day.

8. Which treatments would the nurse expect to implement in the management plan of a patient with cystic fibrosis? *(select all that apply)*
   a. Sperm banking
   b. IV corticosteroids on a chronic basis
   c. Airway clearance techniques (e.g., Acapella)
   d. GoLYTELY given as needed for severe constipation
   e. Inhaled tobramycin to combat *Pseudomonas* infection

9. A patient who has bronchiectasis asks the nurse, "What conditions would warrant a call to the clinic?"
   a. Blood clots in the sputum
   b. Sticky sputum on a hot day
   c. Increased shortness of breath after eating a large meal
   d. Production of large amounts of sputum on a daily basis

1. a, c, d, e, 2. a, c, d, 3. a, 4. c, d, 5. a, c, d, e, 6. c, 7. d, 8. a, c, d, e, 9. a

For rationales to these answers and even more NCLEX review questions, visit *http://evolve.elsevier.com/Lewis/medsurg.*

ⓔ EVOLVE WEBSITE/RESOURCES LIST

REFERENCES

1. Patton KT, Thibodeau GA: *Anatomy and physiology*, ed 9, St Louis, 2016, Elsevier.
*2. Leung JM, Sin DD: Asthma-COPD overlap syndrome: Pathogenesis, clinical features, and therapeutic targets, *BMJ* 358:j3772, 2017.
*3. Hines KL, Peebles RJ: Management of the asthma-COPD overlap syndrome: A review of the evidence, *Curr Allergy Asthma Rep* 17:15, 2017.
4. Cystic Fibrosis Foundation: 2016 Patient registry annual data report. Retrieved from *www.cff.org/Research/Researcher-Resources/Patient-Registry/2016-Patient-Registry-Annual-Data-Report.pdf*.
5. Centers for Disease Control and Prevention (CDC): Fast Facts: Asthma. Retrieved from *www.cdc.gov/nchs/fastats/asthma.htm*.
*6. Guibas GV, Matioudakis AG, Tsoumani M, et al: Relationship of allergy with asthma: There are more than the allergy "eggs" in the asthma "basket," *Front Pediatr* 5:92, 2017.
7. Centers for Disease Control and Prevention: Percentage of people with asthma who smoke. Retrieved from *www.cdc.gov/asthma/asthma_stats/people_who_smoke.htm*.
8. Fehrenbach H, Wagner C, Wegmann M: Airway remodeling in asthma: What really matters, *Cell Tissue Res* 367:551, 2017.
9. Saaden CK: Status asthmaticus. Retrieved from *https://emedicine.medscape.com/article/2129484-overview*.
10. Sim YS, Lee JH, Lee WY, et al: Spirometry and bronchodilator test, *Tuberc Respir Dis* 80:105, 2017.
*11. Sato S, Saito J, Fukuhara A, et al: The clinical role of fractional exhaled nitric oxide in asthma control, *Ann Allergy Asthma Immunol* 119:5421, 2017.
12. CDC: Chronic obstructive pulmonary disease. Retrieved from *www.cdc.gov/copd/index.html*.
*13. Terzikhan N, Verhamme KM, Hofman A, et al: Prevalence and incidence of COPD in smokers and non-smokers: The Rotterdam study, *Eur J Epidemiol* 31:785, 2016.
*14. Bigna JJ, Kenne AM, Asangbeh SL, et al: Prevalence of COPD in the global population with HIV: A systematic review and meta-analysis, *Lancet* 6:PE193, 2017.
15. Yakar HI, Gunen H, Pehlivan E, et al: The role of tuberculosis in COPD, *Int J Chron Obstruct Pulmon Dis* 12:323, 2017.
*16. Fahndrich S, Biertz F, Karch A, et al: Cardiovascular risk in patients with alpha-1-antitrypsin deficiency, *Respir Res* 18:171, 2017.
17. Leong D: Cor pulmonale: Overview of cor pulmonale management. Retrieved from *www.emedicine.medscape.com/article/154062-overview#a4*.
18. Shah SJ: Cor pulmonale. Retrieved from *www.merckmanuals.com/en-ca/professional/cardiovascular-disorders/heart-failure/cor-pulmonale*.
19. Viniol C, Vogelmeier CF: *Exacerbations of COPD, Eur Respir Rev* 27(147), 2018.
20. Lange P, Halpin DM, O'Donnell, et al: Diagnosis, assessment, and phenotyping of COPD: Beyond FEV_1, *Int J Chron Obstruct Pulmon Dis* 11:3, 2016.
21. American Lung Association: Surgery for COPD. Retrieved from *www.lung.org/lung-health-and-diseases/lung-disease-lookup/copd/diagnosing-and-treating/surgery.html*.
*22. Darwiche K, Karpf-Wissel R, Eisenmann S, et al: Bronchoscopic lung volume reduction with endobronchial valves in low-FEV 1 patients, *Respiration* 92:414, 2016.
23. Ergan B, Akgun M, Pacilli AMG, et al: Should I stay or should I go? COPD and Air Travel. Retrieved from *http://err.ersjournals.com/content/27/148/180030*.
*24. Hsieh MJ, Yang TM, Tsai YH: Nutritional supplementation in patients with chronic obstructive pulmonary disease, *JFMA* 115:595, 2016.
25. Henderson W: Life expectancy when you're living with cystic fibrosis. Retrieved from *https://cysticfibrosisnewstoday.com/2017/05/24/living-cf-life-expectancy/*.
26. Henderson W. Cystic fibrosis can lead to osteopenia and osteoporosis. Retrieved from: *https://cysticfibrosisnewstoday.com/2017/03/22/cystic-fibrosis-can-lead-osteopenia-osteoporosis/*.
27. Sharma GD: Cystic fibrosis clinical presentation. Retrieved from *https://emedicine.medscape.com/article/1001602-clinical*.
*28. Willems P, Weeks S, Meskal A, et al: Biological variation of chloride and sodium in sweat obtained by pilocarpine iontophoresis in adults: How sure are you about sweat test results? *Lung* 195:214, 2017.
*29. Green J, Gilchrist FJ, Carroll W: Interventions for treating distal intestinal obstruction syndrome (DIOS) in cystic fibrosis. Retrieved from *www.cochranelibrary.com/cdsr/doi/10.1002/14651858.CD012798/epdf/full*.
30. Smith MP: Diagnosis and management of bronchiectasis, *CMAJ* 189:E828, 2017.

*Evidence-based information for clinical practice.

CASE STUDY

Managing Care of Multiple Patients

You are assigned to care for the following 4 patients on a medical-surgical unit. You are sharing 1 UAP with another RN.

Patients

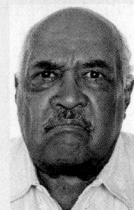

F.T. is a 70-yr-old man with a history of COPD who was admitted yesterday with bilateral lower lobe pneumonia. He is receiving O_2 at 2 L/min via nasal cannula and IV antibiotics. His last pulse oximetry reading was 92%.

(© Fuse/
Thinkstock.)

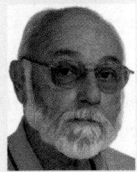

M.R. is a 69-yr-old man who is 3 days postoperative following a total laryngectomy with tracheostomy for treatment of laryngeal cancer. He is receiving intermittent feeding via a percutaneous endoscopic gastrostomy (PEG) tube and last received pain medication 4 hours ago.

(© iStockphoto/
Thinkstock.)

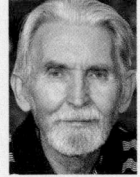

J.H. is a 52-yr-old man admitted with right lower lobe pneumonia. A bronchoscopy with biopsy showed small cell lung cancer. He is intermittently confused and anxious with rapid, shallow respirations. He and his family are currently considering his treatment options.

(© iStockphoto/
Thinkstock.)

H.M. is a 68-yr-old woman admitted 6 days ago with a COPD exacerbation. She has not been able to ambulate much because of her shortness of breath. She is on oral prednisone and ipratropium. She is being discharged later today. She is to start Advair Diskus and chronic O_2 therapy at home after discharge.

(© iStockphoto/
Thinkstock.)

Discussion Questions

1. **Priority Decision:** After receiving report, which patient should you see first? Provide a rationale for your decision.
2. **Collaboration:** Which morning tasks can you delegate to the UAP (select all that apply)?
   a. Take vital signs and a pulse oximetry reading on F.T.
   b. Assess M.R.'s pain level and show him how to administer his feeding.
   c. Assist H.M. with AM care and gather belongings in anticipation of discharge.
   d. Provide coffee for J.H.'s family as they await a family meeting with the HCP.
   e. Teach F.T. how to do pursed-lip breathing and titrate O_2 to obtain pulse oximetry >95%.

3. **Priority Decision and Collaboration:** While you are assessing J.H., the UAP tells you that H.M. is reporting chest pain and worsening shortness of breath. M.R. is requesting pain medication. What should you do *first*?
   a. Ask the UAP to get H.M.'s vital signs while you give M.R. pain medication.
   b. Ask the UAP to increase H.M.'s O_2 to 4 L/min while you assess M.R.'s pain.
   c. Ask the UAP to obtain a stat 12-lead ECG on H.M. while you perform a focused assessment.
   d. Ask the UAP to have another RN give M.R. his pain medication while you go directly to H.M.'s room.

Case Study Progression

After assessing H.M., you notify her HCP. A stat 12-lead ECG is done, and a blood sample is drawn to check cardiac enzymes. H.M.'s chest pain is not relieved by sublingual nitroglycerin. You then give 4 mg IV morphine. H.M. states that her pain is "a little better" but continues to report dyspnea. The 12-lead ECG and cardiac enzyme results are all within normal limits.

4. Because of H.M.'s reduced mobility, you recognize that she is at risk for developing _____ and anticipate the HCP will order which tests to determine the cause of her current symptoms?
   a. BNP and echocardiogram
   b. D-dimer and spiral CT scan
   c. CBC and abdominal flat-plate x-ray
   d. Serum electrolytes and renal ultrasound
5. While the charge nurse goes with H.M. to the radiology department, you turn your attention back to your remaining 3 patients. Before giving M.R.'s 8 AM enteral feeding, you find his PEG tube clogged. Which action should you take *next*?
   a. Flush the tube with warm water, using a back-and-forth motion.
   b. Obtain an x-ray to confirm the tube is still placed in the stomach.
   c. Notify the HCP so that surgery to insert new tube can be scheduled.
   d. Instill 30 mL of cranberry juice into the tube and recheck in 1 hour.
6. When preparing F.T.'s AM medications, you note that he is scheduled to receive the following antibiotics at 8 AM: levofloxacin 750 mg in 150 mL normal saline over 90 minutes (once daily) and cefazolin 1 gram in 100 mL normal saline over 30 minutes (every 8 hrs). He has only one IV site. Which action is *most* appropriate?
   a. Obtain a second peripheral IV site.
   b. Call the HCP to change the administration times.
   c. Check with pharmacy to see if they can be mixed together in the same IV bag.
   d. Administer the cefazolin first because it takes the least amount of time to infuse.
7. **Management Decision:** J.H.'s son calls you on the telephone to ask about his father's current condition and long-term prognosis. Which initial response would be *most* appropriate?
   a. Ask the person calling what the code word is to identify himself or herself as family.
   b. Tell the caller that you are not allowed to discuss any information over the telephone.
   c. Empathize with the son's need to know his father's long-term prognosis.
   d. Ask J.H.'s son what the HCP has told him to clarify his understanding of the situation.

Answers available at *http://evolve.elsevier.com/Lewis/medsurg.*

Assessment: Hematologic System

Sandra Irene Rome

We choose our destiny in the way we treat others.

Vivian, in "Wit"

ℯ http://evolve.elsevier.com/Lewis/medsurg/

CONCEPTUAL FOCUS

Clotting	Gas Exchange	Pain
Functional Ability	Infection	Perfusion

LEARNING OUTCOMES

1. Describe the structures and functions of the hematologic system.
2. Distinguish among the different types of blood cells and their functions.
3. Explain the process of hemostasis.
4. Link the age-related changes in the hematologic system to differences in findings of hematologic studies.
5. Obtain significant subjective and objective assessment data related to the hematologic system from a patient.
6. Perform a physical assessment of the hematologic system using the appropriate techniques.
7. Distinguish normal from common abnormal findings of a physical assessment of the hematologic system.
8. Describe the purpose, significance of results, and nursing responsibilities related to diagnostic studies of the hematologic system.

KEY TERMS

ecchymoses, p. 597	hemolysis, p. 587	petechiae, p. 597
erythropoiesis, p. 587	leukopenia, p. 602	reticulocyte, p. 587
fibrinolysis, p. 590	neutropenia, p. 602	thrombocytopenia, p. 603
hematopoiesis, p. 585	pancytopenia, p. 602	thrombocytosis, p. 603

Hematology is the study of blood and blood-forming tissues. This includes the bone marrow, blood, spleen, and lymph system. You need a basic knowledge of hematology to be able to evaluate several important concepts in the clinical setting. A functioning hematologic system is needed to support the patient's ability to transport oxygen (O_2) and carbon dioxide (CO_2), maintain intravascular volume, coagulate blood, and combat infections.

STRUCTURES AND FUNCTIONS OF HEMATOLOGIC SYSTEM

Bone Marrow

Blood cell production (hematopoiesis) occurs within the bone marrow. *Bone marrow* is the soft material that fills the central core of bones. There are 2 types of bone marrow, yellow (adipose) and red (hematopoietic). Red marrow actively makes blood cells. In adults, red marrow is found primarily in the flat and irregular bones, such as the ends of long bones, pelvic bones, vertebrae, sacrum, sternum, ribs, flat cranial bones, and scapulae.

All 3 types of blood cells (red blood cells [RBCs], white blood cells [WBCs], and platelets) develop from a common hematopoietic stem cell in the bone marrow. The hematopoietic *stem cell* is best described as an immature blood cell that can self-renew and differentiate into hematopoietic precursor cells. Several types of blood cells form as the cells mature and differentiate (Fig. 29.1).

The bone marrow responds by a negative feedback system to the need for specific blood cells by increasing that cell's production. Various factors or cytokines (e.g., erythropoietin, granulocyte colony-stimulating factor [G-CSF], stem cell factor, thrombopoietin) stimulate the bone marrow. This results in differentiation of the stem cells into one of the committed

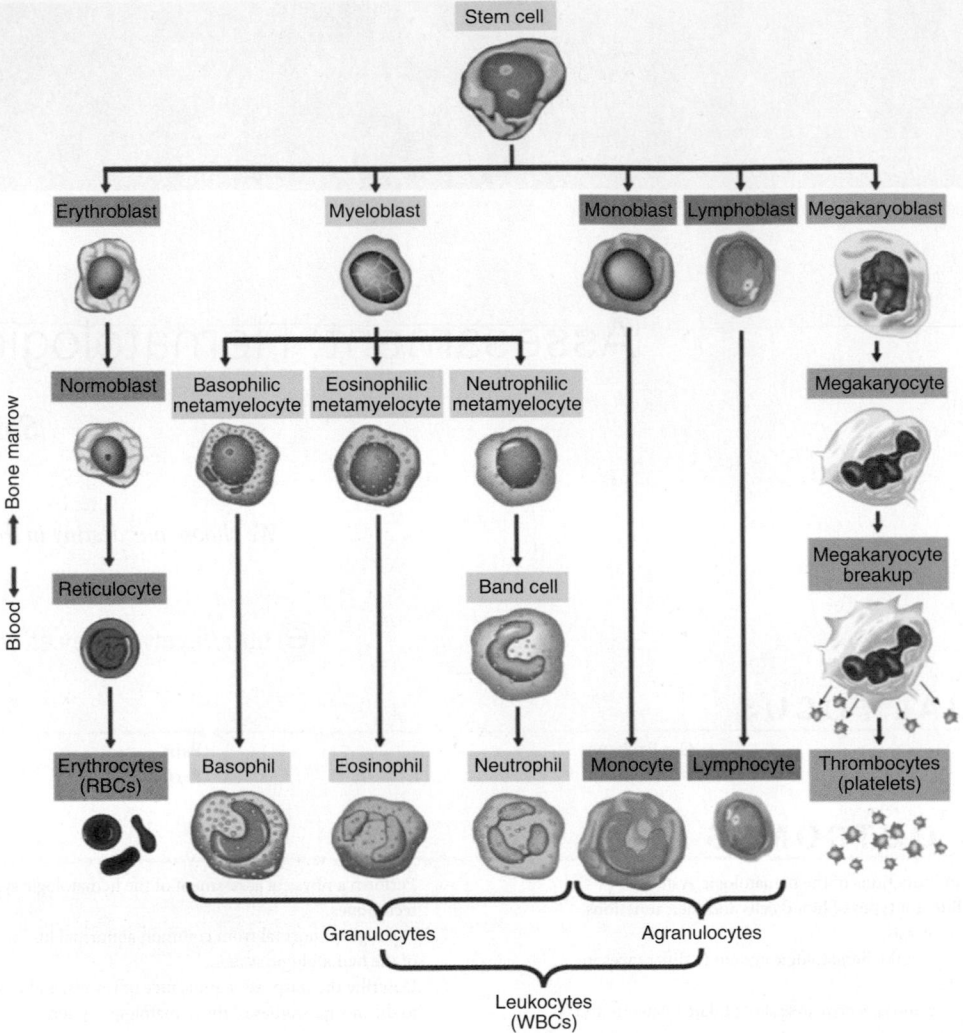

FIG. 29.1 Development of blood cells.

hematopoietic cells (e.g., RBC). For example, when tissue hypoxia occurs, the kidney secretes erythropoietin. It circulates to the bone marrow and causes proerythroblasts to differentiate in the bone marrow.[1]

Blood

Blood is a type of connective tissue that has 3 major functions: transportation, regulation, and protection (Table 29.1). Blood has 2 major components: plasma and blood cells. In an adult weighing between 150 and 180 lb, the volume of blood is usually between 4.7 and 5.5 L (5 to 6 quarts).

Plasma. About 55% of blood is plasma[1] (Fig. 29.2). Plasma is composed mainly of water. It also contains proteins, electrolytes, gases, nutrients (e.g., glucose, amino acids, lipids), and waste. The term *serum* refers to plasma minus its clotting factors. Plasma proteins include albumin, globulin, and clotting factors (mostly fibrinogen). Albumin is a protein that helps maintain oncotic pressure in the blood.[1] The liver makes most plasma proteins. The exception is antibodies (immunoglobulins). They are made by plasma cells.

Blood Cells. About 45% of the blood (Fig. 29.2) is composed of formed elements, or blood cells. The 3 types of blood cells are *erythrocytes* (RBCs), *leukocytes* (WBCs), and *thrombocytes*

TABLE 29.1	**Functions of Blood**
Function	**Examples**
Protection	• Maintaining homeostasis of blood coagulation • Combating invasion of pathogens and other foreign substances
Regulation	• Fluid and electrolyte balance • Acid-base balance • Body temperature • Maintaining intravascular oncotic pressure
Transportation	• O_2 from lungs to cells • Nutrients from GI tract to cells • Hormones from endocrine glands to tissues and cells • Metabolic waste products (e.g., CO_2, NH_3, urea) from cells to lungs, liver, and kidneys

(platelets). The primary function of RBCs is O_2 transportation. WBCs help protect the body from infection. Platelets promote blood coagulation.

Erythrocytes. The primary functions of RBCs include transport of gases (both O_2 and CO_2) and assistance in maintaining acid-base balance. RBCs are flexible cells with a unique

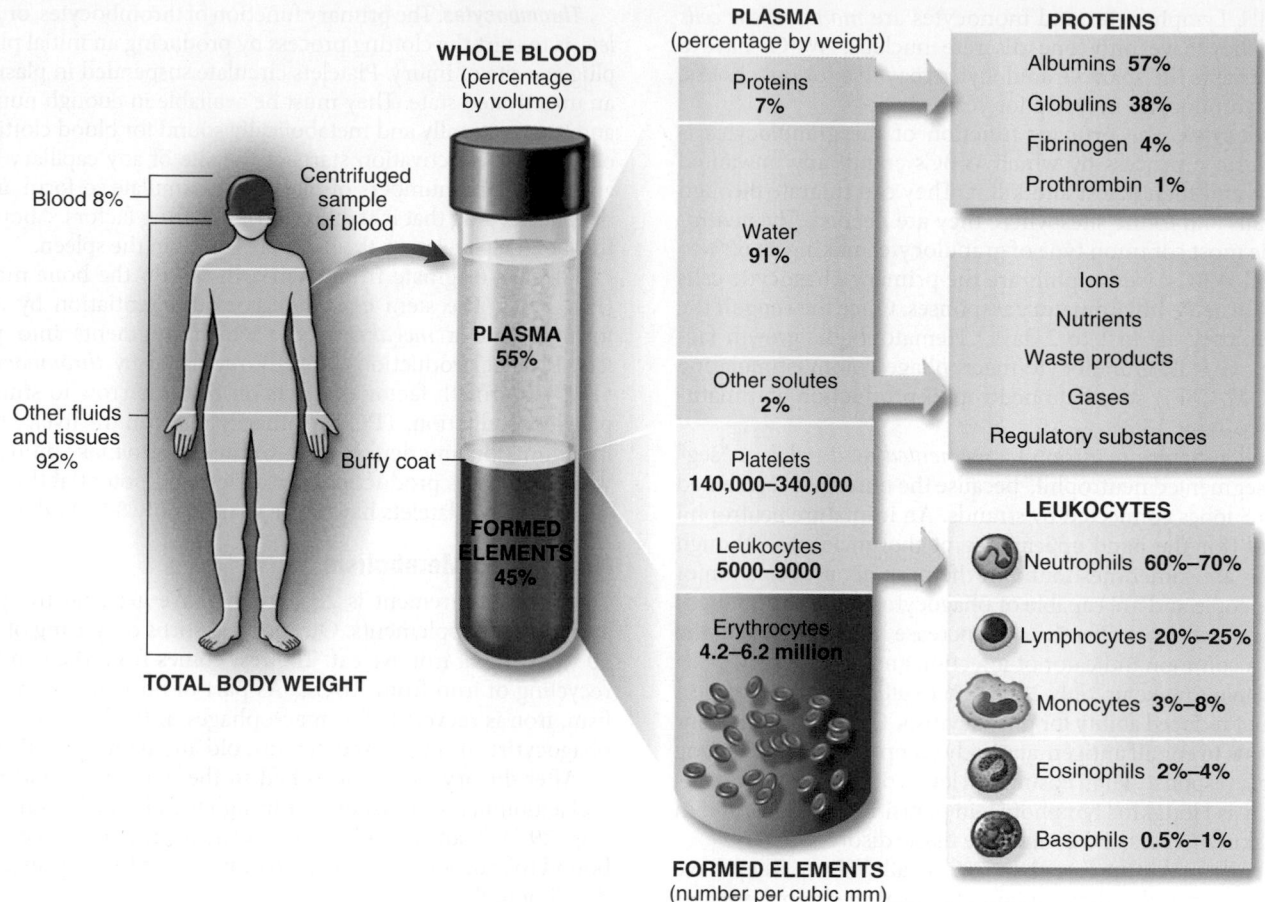

FIG. 29.2 Blood components in a healthy adult. Normally, 45% of the blood is composed of blood cells and 55% is composed of plasma. (From Patton KT, Thibodeau GA: Structure & function of the body, ed 15, St Louis, 2016, Mosby.)

biconcave shape. This flexibility allows the cell to change its shape so that it can easily pass through tiny capillaries. The cell membrane is thin to facilitate diffusion of gases.

RBCs are primarily composed of a large molecule called *hemoglobin*. Hemoglobin is a complex protein-iron compound composed of heme (an iron compound) and globin (a simple protein). It binds with O_2 and CO_2. As RBCs circulate through the capillaries surrounding alveoli within the lung, O_2 attaches to iron on the hemoglobin. We refer to this O_2-bound hemoglobin as *oxyhemoglobin*. It gives arterial blood its bright red appearance. As RBCs flow to body tissues, O_2 detaches from the hemoglobin and diffuses from the capillary into tissue cells. CO_2 diffuses from tissue cells into the capillary, attaches to the globin part of hemoglobin, and is transported to the lungs for removal. Hemoglobin also acts as a buffer and plays a role in maintaining acid-base balance. This buffering function is described in Chapter 16.

Erythropoiesis (the process of RBC production) is regulated by cellular O_2 requirements and general metabolic activity. Erythropoiesis is stimulated by hypoxia and controlled by *erythropoietin,* a glycoprotein growth factor made and released primarily by the kidney. Erythropoietin stimulates the bone marrow to increase RBC production. We make about 2.5 million RBCs per second. The normal life span of RBCs is about 120 days. The availability of nutrients influences erythropoiesis. Many essential nutrients are needed for erythropoiesis. These include protein, iron, folate (folic acid), cobalamin (vitamin B_{12}), riboflavin (vitamin B_2), pyridoxine (vitamin B_6),

pantothenic acid, niacin, ascorbic acid (vitamin C), copper, and vitamin E. Endocrine hormones, such as thyroxine, corticosteroids, and testosterone, also affect RBC production. For example, hypothyroidism is often associated with anemia.[1]

Several distinct cell types evolve during RBC maturation (Fig. 29.1). The **reticulocyte** is an immature RBC. Reticulocytes can develop into mature RBCs within 48 hours of release into the circulation. A mature RBC lacks a nucleus and cannot undergo mitotic division. Assessing the number of reticulocytes is a useful way to evaluate the rate and adequacy of RBC production.[1]

Hemolysis (destruction of RBCs) by monocytes and macrophages removes abnormal, defective, damaged, and old RBCs from circulation. Hemolysis normally occurs in the bone marrow, liver, and spleen. Because one of the components of RBCs is bilirubin, hemolysis of these cells results in increased bilirubin the body must process. When hemolysis occurs by normal mechanisms, the liver conjugates and excretes all the bilirubin in bile.

Leukocytes. Leukocytes (WBCs) appear white when separated from blood. Like the RBCs, WBCs originate from stem cells within the bone marrow (Fig. 29.1). They may eventually reside in the thymus or secondary lymphoid tissues, such as the spleen, lymph nodes, and Peyer patches. There are several types of WBCs. Each has a different function. WBCs that have granules in the cytoplasm are *granulocytes* (also known as *polymorphonuclear leukocytes*). Granulocytes include neutrophils, basophils, and eosinophils.

WBCs that do not have granules in the cytoplasm are *agranulocytes.* They include lymphocytes, monocytes, and natural killer cells. Lymphocytes and monocytes are *mononuclear cells* because they have only one discrete nucleus. WBCs have a widely variable life span. Granulocytes may live for only hours. Some T lymphocytes may live for years.

Granulocytes. The primary function of the granulocytes is *phagocytosis,* a process by which WBCs engulf any unwanted organism and then digest and kill it. They can migrate through vessel walls and to the sites where they are needed. The *neutrophil* is the most common type of granulocyte, making up 60% to 70% of all WBCs. Neutrophils are the primary phagocytic cells involved in acute inflammatory responses. Once they engulf the pathogen, they die in 1 to 2 days.[1] Hematopoietic growth factors (e.g., G-CSF, granulocyte-macrophage colony-stimulating factor [GM-CSF]) stimulate neutrophil production and maturation (see Table 13.3).

We call a mature neutrophil a *segmented neutrophil,* or "seg" or "polysegmented neutrophil," because the nucleus is segmented into 2 to 5 lobes connected by strands. An immature neutrophil is a *band* (for the band appearance of the nucleus). Although band cells are sometimes found in the peripheral circulation of normal people and are capable of phagocytosis, the mature neutrophil is much more effective. An increase in neutrophils in the blood is a common indicator of infection and tissue injury.

Eosinophils make up only 2% to 4% of all WBCs. They have a similar but reduced ability for phagocytosis. One of their primary functions is to engulf antigen-antibody complexes formed during an allergic response. High eosinophil levels occur with some cancers, such as Hodgkin's lymphoma, in parasitic infections, and in various skin diseases and connective tissue disorders.[1]

Basophils make up less than 2% of all WBCs. They have cytoplasmic granules that contain chemical mediators, such as heparin and histamine. A basophil responds to stimulation by an antigen or by tissue injury by releasing substances from the granules. This is part of the response seen in allergic and inflammatory reactions. *Mast cells* are like basophils, but they reside in connective tissues. They play a key role in inflammation, permeability of blood vessels, and smooth muscle contraction.

Lymphocytes. Lymphocytes make up 20% to 25% of the WBCs in the blood.[1] They form the basis of the cellular and humoral immune responses. Two lymphocyte subtypes are B cells and T cells. T-cell precursors originate in the bone marrow. They migrate to the thymus gland for further differentiation into T cells. *Natural killer (NK) cells* are lymphocytes that kill virus-infected cells and activate T cells and phagocytes. They do not need prior exposure to antigens. Dendritic cells are the primary phagocytic cells in the peripheral organs and skin. Most lymphocytes briefly circulate in the blood and reside in lymphoid and other tissues. Details of lymphocyte function are discussed in Chapter 13.

Monocytes. Monocytes, the other type of agranular WBC, make up about 3% to 8% of the total WBCs.[1] Monocytes are potent phagocytic cells that ingest small or large masses of matter, such as bacteria, dead cells, tissue debris, and old or defective RBCs. These cells are present in the blood for only a brief time before they migrate into the tissues and become macrophages. In addition to macrophages that have differentiated from monocytes, tissues also have resident macrophages. These resident macrophages have special names (e.g., Kupffer cells in the liver, osteoclasts in the bone, alveolar macrophages in the lung). They protect the body from pathogens at these entry points and are more phagocytic than monocytes. Macrophages interact with lymphocytes to facilitate humoral and cellular immune responses.

Thrombocytes. The primary function of thrombocytes, or *platelets,* is to start the clotting process by producing an initial platelet plug at a site of injury. Platelets circulate suspended in plasma in an unactivated state. They must be available in enough numbers and be structurally and metabolically sound for blood clotting to occur. Platelet activation starts at the site of any capillary damage. Increasing numbers of platelets accumulate to form an initial platelet plug that is stabilized with clotting factors. About one third of the platelets in the body are stored in the spleen.

Platelets originate from stem cells within the bone marrow (Fig. 29.1). The stem cell undergoes differentiation by transforming into a *megakaryocyte,* which fragments into platelets. Platelet production is partly regulated by *thrombopoietin* (TPO), a growth factor that acts on bone marrow to stimulate platelet production. TPO is primarily made in the liver. During inflammation, interleukin 6 (IL-6) causes us to make more TPO, which increases production of platelets and potential thrombosis. Typically, platelets have a life span of only 8 to 11 days.

Normal Iron Metabolism

Our iron requirement is 25 mg daily. We get iron from food and dietary supplements. Our body absorbs only 1 mg of every 10 to 20 mg of iron we eat. The rest comes from the continued recycling of iron from RBCs.[1] As part of normal iron metabolism, iron is recycled after macrophages in the liver and spleen phagocytize, or ingest and destroy, old and damaged RBCs.

After dietary iron is absorbed in the duodenum and proximal jejunum, it is transported through the plasma by transferrin (Fig. 29.3). Transferrin is made in the liver. How much iron is bound to transferrin is a reliable indicator of the iron supply for developing RBCs.

About two thirds of total body iron is bound to heme in RBCs (hemoglobin) and muscle cells (myoglobin). The other one third of iron is stored as ferritin and hemosiderin (degraded form of ferritin) in the bone marrow, spleen, liver, and macrophages (Fig. 29.3). When we do not replace stored iron, hemoglobin production is reduced. Normally there is very little iron loss except from blood loss. We lose about 3% daily in urine, sweat, bile, and epithelial cells in the gastrointestinal (GI) tract.

Normal Clotting Mechanisms

Hemostasis describes the arrest of bleeding. This process is important in minimizing blood loss when various body structures are injured. The sequence of events includes (1) vascular injury and subendothelial exposure, (2) adhesion, (3) activation, (4) aggregation, (5) platelet plug formation, and (6) clot retraction and dissolution.

Vascular Injury and Subendothelial Exposure. When a blood vessel is injured, an immediate local vasoconstrictive response occurs. Vasoconstriction reduces the leakage of blood from the vessel by restricting the vessel size and pressing the endothelial surfaces together. The latter reaction enhances vessel wall stickiness and keeps the vessel closed after vasoconstriction subsides. Vascular spasm may last for 20 to 30 minutes. This allows time for the body to activate the platelet response and plasma clotting factors. The platelet response and plasma clotting factors are triggered by endothelial injury and the release of substances such as thromboxane A_2 (TXA$_2$). Platelets begin to fill endothelial gaps.[1]

Adhesion. The loss of endothelial cells exposes adhesive glycoproteins, such as collagen and von Willebrand factor (vWF), to which more platelets adhere. The stickiness is termed *adhesiveness.* The formation of clumps is termed *aggregation* or *agglutination.*

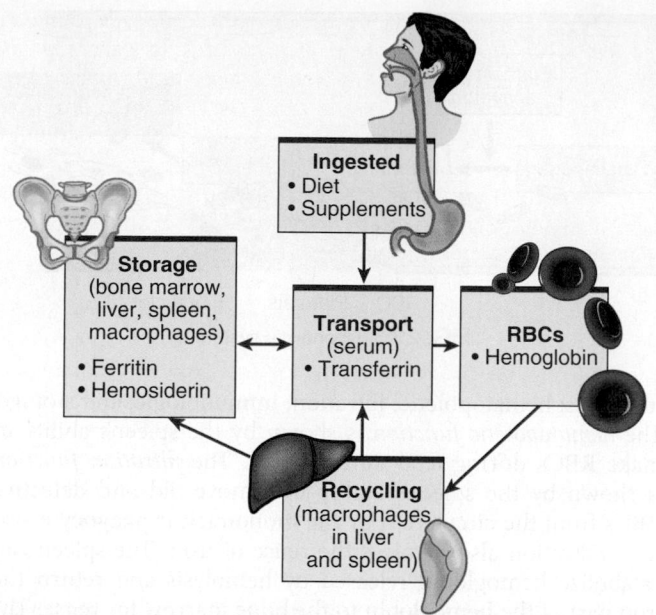

FIG. 29.3 Normal iron metabolism. Iron is ingested in the diet or from supplements. Macrophages break down ingested RBCs. Iron is returned to blood bound to transferrin or stored as ferritin or hemosiderin.

Activation. The interaction described previously causes the platelets to undergo an activation process. This leads to changes in platelet shape. The platelets then can bind adhesive proteins, including fibrinogen and vWF. Release of various platelet granules (including adenosine phosphate [ADP]) recruits and activates other platelets, clotting factors, and growth factors. As Fig. 29.4 shows, platelet lipoproteins stimulate necessary conversions in the clotting process.

Aggregation. Platelet aggregation is stimulated by TXA_2 and ADP, which induce fibrinogen receptors on the platelet. The formation of a visible fibrin clot on the platelet plug is the conclusion of a complex series of reactions involving different clotting (coagulation) factors. We label plasma clotting factors with both names and Roman numerals (Table 29.2).

Plasma proteins circulate in inactive forms until stimulated to start clotting through 1 of 2 pathways, intrinsic or extrinsic (Fig. 29.4). The *intrinsic pathway* is activated by collagen exposure from endothelial injury when the blood vessel is damaged. The *extrinsic pathway* is activated when tissue factor or tissue thromboplastin is released extravascularly from injured tissues.

Regardless of how we begin to clot, coagulation ultimately follows the same final common pathway of the clotting cascade. Thrombin, in the common pathway, is the most powerful enzyme in the coagulation process (Fig. 29.4). It converts fibrinogen to fibrin, which is an essential part of a blood clot.

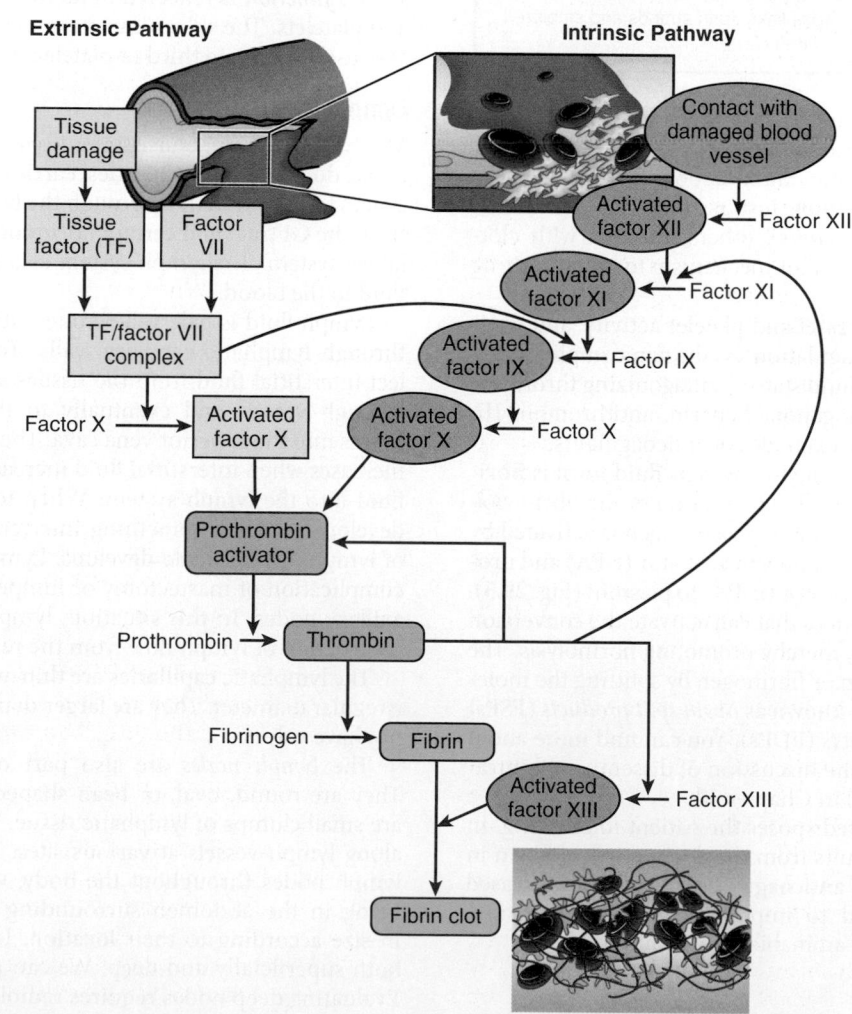

FIG. 29.4 Coagulation mechanism showing steps in the intrinsic pathway and extrinsic pathway as they would occur in the test tube.

TABLE 29.2 Coagulation Factors

Coagulation Factor	Action
I Fibrinogen	Source of fibrin to form a clot. Made in liver
II Prothrombin	Converted to thrombin, which then activates fibrinogen into fibrin as well as factors V, VII, VIII, XI, XIII, protein C, platelets
III Tissue factor, tissue thromboplastin	Released from damaged endothelial cells and activates the extrinsic pathway by reacting with factor VII
IV Calcium	Required cofactor at several points in the coagulation cascade
V Proaccelerin (labile) factor	Binds with factor X to activate prothrombin
VI	Not in use (obsolete)
VII Stable factor, proconvertin	Forms a complex with factor III and activates factors IX and X
VIII Antihemophilic factor	Works with factor IX and calcium to activate factor X
IX Christmas factor	Together with factor VIII, activates factor X
X Stuart factor	Activates conversion of factor II (prothrombin) to thrombin
XI Plasma thromboplastin antecedent	Activates factor IX when calcium is present
XII Hageman factor	Activates factor XI, which starts the intrinsic pathway
XIII Fibrin-stabilizing factor	Cross-links fibrin strands and stabilizes fibrin clot

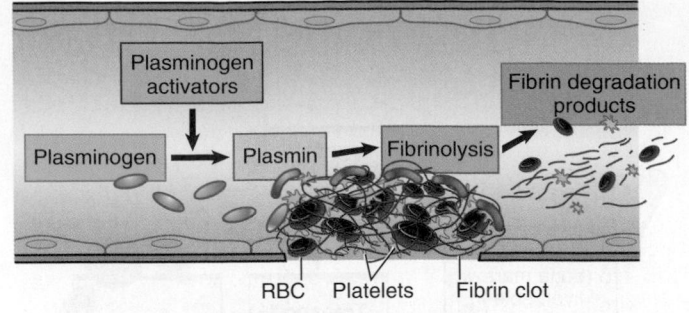

FIG. 29.5 Fibrinolytic system.

Platelet Plug Formation. The final blood clot is a meshwork of protein strands that stabilizes the platelet plug and traps other cells, such as RBCs, phagocytes, and microorganisms.

Clot Retraction and Dissolution. Just as some blood elements foster coagulation (*procoagulants*), others interfere with clotting (*anticoagulants*). This counter mechanism to blood clotting keeps blood in its fluid state.

Antithrombin activity, vessel and platelet activity, and fibrinolysis contribute to anticoagulation. As the name implies, antithrombins keep blood in a fluid state by antagonizing thrombin, a powerful coagulant. Endogenous heparin, antithrombin III, protein C, and protein S are examples of anticoagulants.

The second means of keeping blood in its fluid form is **fibrinolysis**, a process resulting in the dissolution of the fibrin clot. The fibrinolytic system starts when plasminogen is activated by substances such as tissue plasminogen activator (t-PA) and urokinase-like plasminogen activator (u-PA) to plasmin (Fig. 29.5). Thrombin is 1 of the substances that can activate the conversion of plasminogen to plasmin, thereby promoting fibrinolysis. The plasmin attacks either fibrin or fibrinogen by splitting the molecules into smaller elements known as *fibrin split products* (FSPs) or *fibrin degradation products* (FDPs). You can find more about FSPs in Table 29.8 and in the discussion of disseminated intravascular coagulation (DIC) in Chapter 30.

Excessive fibrinolysis predisposes the patient to bleeding. In this situation, bleeding results from the destruction of fibrin in platelet plugs or from the anticoagulation effects of increased FSPs. Increased FSPs lead to impaired platelet aggregation, reduced prothrombin, and an inability to stabilize fibrin.

Spleen

The spleen is the largest lymphoid organ. It is found in the upper left quadrant of the abdomen. The spleen has 4 major

functions: hematopoietic, filtration, immunologic, and storage. The *hematopoietic function* is shown by the spleen's ability to make RBCs during fetal development. The *filtration function* is shown by the spleen's ability to remove old and defective RBCs from the circulation by the mononuclear phagocyte system. Filtration also involves the reuse of iron. The spleen can catabolize hemoglobin released by hemolysis and return the iron part of the hemoglobin to the bone marrow for reuse. The spleen plays a vital role in filtering circulating bacteria, especially encapsulated organisms such as gram-positive cocci. The spleen's rich supply of lymphocytes, monocytes, and stored immunoglobulins plays a role in *immunologic function*. The *storage function* is reflected in its role as a storage site for RBCs and platelets. The spleen can store more than 300 mL of blood. We store about one third of platelets in the spleen.

Lymph System

The lymph system, consisting of lymph fluid, lymphatic capillaries, ducts, and lymph nodes, carries fluid from the interstitial spaces to the blood. It is through the lymph that proteins and fat from the GI tract and certain hormones can return to the circulatory system. The lymph system also returns excess interstitial fluid to the blood.

Lymph fluid is pale yellow interstitial fluid that has diffused through lymphatic capillary walls. The lymphatic vessels collect interstitial fluid from the tissues and transport it as lymph through vessels and eventually to the thoracic duct, which drains into the superior vena cava. The formation of lymph fluid increases when interstitial fluid increases, thereby forcing more fluid into the lymph system. When too much interstitial fluid develops or when something interferes with the reabsorption of lymph, *lymphedema* develops. Lymphedema may occur as a complication of mastectomy or lumpectomy with dissection of axillary nodes. In this situation, lymphedema is caused by the obstruction of lymph flow from the removal of lymph nodes.

The lymphatic capillaries are thin-walled vessels that have an irregular diameter. They are larger than blood capillaries and do not have valves.

The *lymph nodes* are also part of the lymphatic system. They are round, oval, or bean shaped. Structurally, the nodes are small clumps of lymphatic tissue. They are found in groups along lymph vessels at various sites. There are more than 200 lymph nodes throughout the body, with the greatest number being in the abdomen surrounding the GI tract. They vary in size according to their location. Lymph nodes are situated both superficially and deep. We can palpate superficial nodes. Evaluating deep nodes requires radiologic examination.[2] A primary function of lymph nodes is filtration of pathogens and foreign particles that are carried by lymph to the nodes.

Liver

The liver has metabolic, secretory, vascular, and storage functions. It makes all the procoagulants that are essential to hemostasis and blood coagulation and secretes bilirubin and bile. It stores iron that exceeds tissue needs, which can occur with frequent blood transfusions or diseases that cause iron overload. *Hepcidin,* made by the liver, is a key regulator of iron balance. Iron overload or inflammation stimulates hepcidin synthesis. Hepcidin inhibits the release of stored iron from enterocytes (in the intestines) and macrophages. So, when iron is deficient, hepatocytes make less hepcidin. This results in the release of stored iron and an increase in dietary absorption. Other functions of the liver are described in Chapters 38 and 43.

Gerontologic Considerations: Effects of Aging on Hematologic System

Aging leads to a decrease in bone marrow mass and cellularity and an increase in bone marrow fat.[3] 90% of the marrow space is occupied by hematopoietic tissue at birth. This is reduced to 50% at age 30 and 30% at age 70.[4] Although the older adult can still maintain adequate blood cell levels, the reduced reserve capacity leaves the older adult more vulnerable to possible problems with clotting, transporting O_2, and fighting infection, especially during periods of increased demand. This contributes to an older adult having a decreased ability to compensate for an acute or chronic illness.

Hemoglobin levels may begin to decrease in both men and women after middle age, with low-normal levels seen in most older people. Total serum iron, total iron-binding capacity, and intestinal iron absorption are all decreased in older adults. The RBC plasma membranes are more fragile. This may account for a slight increase in mean corpuscular volume (MCV) and a slight decrease in mean corpuscular hemoglobin concentration (MCHC) of RBCs in some older adults. While iron deficiency may cause low hemoglobin levels, other factors, such as GI bleeding, renal disease, testosterone deficiency, or bone marrow dysfunction, should be ruled out.[5] In 30% to 40% of cases, there is no specific cause of anemia. This is called "unexplained anemia in the elderly."[6] Cytokine levels may be high, but the amount of inflammation is not enough to increase hepcidin levels.[4] Healthy older patients are not able to make reticulocytes in response to hemorrhage or hypoxemia as well as younger adults. This is likely due to a blunted response to erythropoietin.[4]

Aging generally does not affect the total WBC count and differential. There may be a slight increase in neutrophils and a decrease in lymphocytes. However, the function of lymphocytes decreases, blunting the response to infection.[1] During an infection, the older adult may have only a minimal elevation in the total WBC count. This suggests decreased bone marrow reserve of granulocytes in older adults and reflects the possible impaired stimulation of hematopoiesis. Older adults are at higher risk for developing neutropenia from treatments.[6]

The number of platelets is unaffected by the aging process, but functionally they may have increased adhesiveness. Clotting factors increase with age. Thus aging is associated with an increased chance of clotting problems, such as venous thromboembolism.[3] Changes in vascular integrity related to aging can manifest as easy bruising.

Table 29.3 outlines the effects of aging on hematologic studies. Immune changes related to aging are detailed in Chapter 13.

TABLE 29.3 Gerontologic Assessment Differences

Effects of Aging on Hematologic Studies

Study	Changes
CBC Studies	
Hemoglobin (Hgb)	Usually normal in women; possibly slight ↓ in men
Mean corpuscular hemoglobin concentration (MCHC)	May be slightly ↓
Mean corpuscular volume (MCV)	May be slightly ↑
Platelets	Unchanged; possible ↑ in adhesiveness
White blood cell (WBC) count	Decreased response to infection
Clotting Studies	
D-dimers	↑
Erythrocyte sedimentation rate (ESR)	↑ Significantly
Factors V, VII, IX	May be ↑
Fibrinogen	May be ↑
Partial thromboplastin time	May be ↓
Iron Studies	
Erythropoietin	May be ↑
Ferritin	↑
Serum iron	↓
Total iron-binding capacity	↓

ASSESSMENT OF HEMATOLOGIC SYSTEM

Much of the evaluation of the hematologic system is based on a thorough health history and presenting signs and symptoms.

Subjective Data

Important Health Information

Past Health History. Determine if the patient has had prior hematologic problems. Ask about problems with anemia, bleeding problems, and blood disorders. Ask about related medical conditions, such as malabsorption or liver (e.g., hepatitis, cirrhosis), kidney, or spleen problems. Patients may have received a solid organ transplant, may have lost a spleen to traumatic injury, or may have a history of IV drug or alcohol use that affects their risk for hematologic problems. A history of recent or recurrent infections or problems with blood clotting is important to note.

Medications. A complete medication history is an important part of a hematologic assessment. Ask about the use of vitamins, herbal products, or dietary supplements. Many medications may interfere with normal hematologic function.[3] Those on long-term anticoagulant therapy, such as warfarin, are at risk for bleeding problems. Chemotherapy drugs used to treat cancer (see Chapter 15) and antiretroviral agents used to treat human immunodeficiency virus (HIV) infection (see Chapter 14) may cause bone marrow depression. A patient previously treated with chemotherapy agents, particularly alkylating agents, has a higher risk for developing a secondary cancer of leukemia or lymphoma.

Surgery or Other Treatments. Ask the patient about specific surgical procedures. This includes splenectomy, tumor removal, prosthetic heart valve placement, surgical excision of the

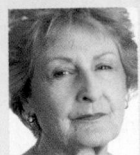
duodenum (where iron absorption occurs), partial or total gastrectomy (which removes parietal cells, thus reducing intrinsic factor needed for the absorption of cobalamin [vitamin B_{12}]), gastric bypass (the duodenum may be bypassed and parietal cell surface area decreased), and ileal resection (where cobalamin absorption takes place). Assess how wound healing progressed postoperatively and if and when any bleeding problems occurred in relation to the surgery. Discuss wound healing and bleeding as responses to injuries (including minor trauma) and dental extractions. Determine the number of previous blood transfusions and any complications with administration. The risk for transfusion reactions and iron overload increases with the number of blood transfusions.

Functional Health Patterns. Key questions to ask a patient with a hematologic problem are outlined in Table 29.4.

Health Perception–Health Management Pattern. Ask the patient to describe the usual and present state of health. Gather complete demographic data, including age, gender, race, and ethnic background. Ask if there is any family history of hematologic problems.

GENETIC RISK ALERT

- Hematologic problems with a strong genetic link include sickle cell anemia, hemophilia, thalassemia, and hemochromatosis.
- People with a family history of these problems have a much greater risk for developing them.
- Leukemia, pernicious anemia, and clotting disorders may have a genetic predisposition.

When taking a family health history, ask about jaundice, anemia, cancer, RBC disorders, such as sickle cell disease, and bleeding disorders, such as hemophilia and clotting disorders.

Assess risk factors, such as alcohol and cigarette use, that may disrupt the hematologic system. Alcohol is caustic to the GI mucosa and can cause damage that results in GI bleeding,

esophageal varices, and decreased absorption of cobalamin and other nutrients.

Chronic alcohol users often have vitamin deficiencies. Alcohol exerts a damaging effect on platelet function and the liver, where we make clotting factors. Consequently, bleeding problems can develop and should be expected in cases of known chronic alcohol use. Illicit drug use is important to determine, since many of these drugs may affect hematopoiesis.

Cigarette smoking increases low-density lipoprotein (LDL) cholesterol and levels of CO_2, leading to hypoxia and changing the anticoagulant properties of the endothelium. Smoking increases platelet reactivity, plasma fibrinogen, hematocrit, and blood viscosity.

Nutritional-Metabolic Pattern. Obtain the patient's weight. Determine if the patient has had anorexia, nausea, vomiting, or oral discomfort. A dietary history may give clues about the cause of anemia. Iron, cobalamin, and folic acid are needed for the development of RBCs. Iron and folic acid deficiencies are associated with inadequate intake of foods such as meat, fish, eggs, leafy green vegetables, legumes, citrus fruits, and whole-grain and enriched breads, cereals, and rice. A diet with foods high in iron may offset folic acid deficiencies.[7]

Hematemesis (bright red, brown, or black vomitus) is a manifestation of an underlying problem and always needs investigating. Peptic ulcer disease is a common cause of hematemesis.

Explore any changes in the skin's texture, color, or temperature. Ask about bleeding gum tissue or bleeding from anywhere on the body. Ask about any lumps or swelling in the neck, armpits, or groin. Specifically, ask what the lumps feel like (i.e., hard or soft, tender or nontender) and if they are mobile or fixed. Primary lymph tumors are usually not painful. A nontender, consistently swollen lymph node may be a sign of a cancer, such as Hodgkin's or non-Hodgkin's lymphoma. Enlarged, tender lymph nodes are usually associated with an acute infection.[8] Explore any reports of fever. Determine if the patient currently has a fever, recurring fevers, chills, or night sweats.

Ask patients if they have a history of heart or lung diseases. Cardiovascular problems, such as valvular disease or hypertension, may predispose patients to hemolysis. Many medications used to treat cardiovascular disease can cause problems with hematopoietic cell production or coagulation. Lung problems that lead to hypoxemia may cause chronic stimulation of erythropoietin and result in *polycythemia* (excess RBCs).

Elimination Pattern. Ask if there has been blood in the urine or stool or if black, tarry stools have occurred. Ask the patient if they have had a recent stool tested for occult blood or colonoscopy.

Activity-Exercise Pattern. Because fatigue is a prominent symptom in many hematologic problems, ask about feelings of tiredness. Determine any weakness or feelings of heavy extremities. Assess for apathy, malaise, dyspnea, or palpitations. Note any change in the patient's ability to perform regular exercise and/or activities of daily living (ADLs), especially as they relate to a history of falling.

Sleep-Rest Pattern. Determine whether the patient feels rested after a night's sleep. Fatigue secondary to a hematologic problem often does not resolve after sleep.

Cognitive-Perceptual Pattern. Assess for any *arthralgia* (joint pain) that may be caused by a hematologic problem. Pain in the joint may occur with an autoimmune disorder, such as

TABLE 29.4 Health History
Hematologic System

Health Perception–Health Management

- Do you have any problem performing daily activities because of a lack of energy?*
- Do you smoke cigarettes or drink alcohol?*
- Do you take any prescribed or over-the-counter medications?*
- Are you taking any herbs?* Home remedies?*
- Have you in the past or are you currently consuming illegal drugs? What agents? What route? How often? When did you last use?
- Have you ever received a blood transfusion?*
- Is there any family history of anemia, cancer, bleeding, or clotting problems?*
- Have you had any surgeries?*

Nutritional-Metabolic

- Do you have any problems with eating, chewing, or swallowing?*
- Have you had any mouth sores, sore tongue, swollen or sore gums, oral bleeding?*
- What kind of diet do you follow? If a vegetarian, do you eat eggs, milk products, fish?
- How has your appetite been?
- Have you had any changes in your weight in the past year?*
- Do you take any vitamins, nutritional supplements, or iron?*
- Is nausea and vomiting a problem for you?*
- Have you ever had any unusual bleeding or bruising?*
- Have there been recent changes in the condition or color of your skin?*
- Have you had night sweats or cold intolerance?*
- Have you noticed any swelling in your armpits, neck, or groin?*

Elimination

- Have you had black or tarry stools?* Have you had light, clay-colored stools?*
- Have you noticed any blood or dark "tea color" in your urine?*
- Has your urine had a foul odor or cloudiness?
- Have you had any decrease in urine output?*
- Do you ever have diarrhea or change in bowel patterns?*

Activity-Exercise

- Do you have any shortness of breath at rest? With activity?*
- Do you have any limitations in joint motion?* Have any of your joints been swollen?*
- Do you have a problem with unsteady gait? Have you fallen recently?*
- Do you exercise regularly? What type and how often?*
- After activity, do you ever notice bleeding or bruising?*

Sleep-Rest

- Have you had excessive fatigue recently?*
- Are you more tired than usual?*
- Do you feel rested on awakening? If no, explain.

Cognitive-Perceptual

- Have you had any numbness or tingling?*
- Have you had any problems with your vision, hearing, or taste?*
- Have you noticed any changes in your mental function?*
- Do you have any pain, such as bone, joint, or abdominal pain, or abdominal fullness?*
- Do you have pain when moving your joints?*
- Have your muscles been sore or achy recently?*

Self-Perception–Self-Concept

- Does your health problem make you feel differently about yourself?*
- Do you have any physical changes that cause you distress?*

Role-Relationship

- Does your occupation bring you into contact with hazardous substances?*
- Has your present illness caused a change in your roles and relationships?*

Sexuality-Reproductive

- Has your hematologic problem caused any sexual or intimacy problems that concern you?*
- *Women:* When was your last menses? Do you consider your cycle normal? How long does your bleeding usually last? Have you had any increase in cramping or clotting?* Have there been any changes in the amount of flow?*
- *Men:* Do you ever have impotence?*
- Have you had unprotected sex in the past 6 months?* Was your partner someone new or a person with whom you have had a long-term sexual relationship?

Coping–Stress Tolerance

- Do you have a support system to help you when needed?
- What coping strategies do you use when your symptoms are worse?
- Do you have any specific symptoms when you feel stressed?*

Value-Belief

- Do you have any personal or religious objection to receiving blood or blood products?*
- Do you have any conflicts between your planned therapy and your value-belief system?*

*If yes, describe.

---

rheumatoid arthritis. It may occur with gout from increased uric acid production due to hematologic cancer or hemolytic anemia. Aching bones may result from pressure of expanding bone marrow with diseases such as leukemia. *Hemarthrosis* (blood in a joint) occurs in the patient with bleeding disorders and can be painful.

Note any paresthesias, numbness, and tingling as they may be related to a hematologic disorder. Assess for any changes in vision, hearing, taste, or mental status.

Self-Perception–Self-Concept Pattern. Determine the effect of the health problem on the patient's perception of self and personal abilities. Assess the effect of certain problems, such as bruising, petechiae, and lymph node swelling, on the patient's personal appearance.

Role-Relationship Pattern. Ask the patient about any past or present occupational or household exposures to radiation or chemicals. If such exposure has occurred, determine the type, amount, and duration of the exposure.

A person who has been exposed to radiation, as a treatment modality or by accident, has a higher incidence of certain hematologic problems. The same is true of a person who has been exposed to certain chemicals (e.g., benzene, lead, naphthalene, phenylbutazone). These chemicals are often used by potters, dry cleaners, and people in occupations that use adhesives. Ask the patient about a history in the military. Many Vietnam War veterans were exposed to a dioxin-containing defoliant (Agent Orange), which is linked with leukemia and lymphoma. Assess the effect of the present illness on the patient's usual roles and responsibilities.

Sexuality-Reproductive Pattern. Take a careful menstrual history from women, including the age at which menarche and menopause began, duration and amount of bleeding, incidence of clotting and cramping, and any associated problems. Ask men if they have any problems related to impotence or prolonged erections. Ask the patient about sexual behavior that may increase the risk for HIV infection.

Coping–Stress Tolerance Pattern. The patient with a hematologic problem often needs help with ADLs. Ask the patient if adequate support is available to meet daily needs. Determine the patient's usual methods of handling stress. In the patient with platelet disorders or hemophilia, the potential for hemorrhage can be so frightening that usual life patterns may be drastically curtailed, affecting the person's quality of life.

Value-Belief Pattern. Treatment for some hematologic problems involves blood transfusions or a bone marrow transplant. Determine if these treatments conflict with the patient's value-belief system, including the patient's cultural and religious beliefs related to blood and blood transfusions. Notify the HCP if you identify any conflicts.

Objective Data

Physical Examination. A complete physical examination is needed to accurately examine all systems that affect or are affected by the hematologic system. A patient's presenting symptoms may not immediately point to a hematologic problem (Tables 29.5). For example, paresthesias of the lower extremities may not appear to be a hematologic problem, but when combined with other findings and risk factors, may indicate cobalamin deficiency and resulting pernicious anemia. Although you should perform a full physical examination on patients suspected of a hematologic disorder, certain aspects of that examination are specifically relevant. These include skin, lymph nodes, spleen, and liver.

Lymph Node Assessment. Assess lymph nodes symmetrically and take note of location, size (in centimeters), degree of fixation (e.g., movable, fixed), tenderness, and texture. Examine superficial lymph nodes with light palpation (Fig. 29.6). To assess superficial lymph nodes, lightly palpate the nodes using the pads of the fingers. Then gently roll the skin over the area and concentrate on feeling for lymph node enlargement. We cannot palpate deep lymph nodes. They are evaluated by radiologic examination.

Ordinarily, lymph nodes are not palpable in adults. If a node is palpable, it should be small (0.5 to 1 cm), mobile, firm, and nontender to be considered a normal finding. A node that is tender, hard, fixed, or enlarged (regardless if it is tender or not) is an abnormal finding and needs further investigation. Tender nodes are usually a result of inflammation. Hard or fixed nodes suggest cancer.[8]

Develop a sequence when examining the lymph nodes. A convenient sequence is to start at the head and neck. First, palpate the preauricular, posterior auricular, occipital, tonsillar, submandibular, submental, superficial cervical, posterior cervical chain, deep cervical chain, and supraclavicular nodes. Next, palpate the axillary lymph nodes and pectoral, subscapular, and lateral groups of nodes. Then examine the epitrochlear nodes, found in the antecubital fossa between the biceps and triceps muscles. Last, palpate the inguinal lymph nodes, found in the groin.

Palpation of Liver or Spleen. The liver and spleen are normally not detectable by palpating the abdomen. An enlarged liver or spleen may be detectable by percussion or palpation. Measure the degree of liver enlargement by the number of fingerbreadths it extends below the rib border. The spleen may be harder to detect because of its deep location in the left abdomen. Specific techniques for palpating the liver and spleen are described in Chapter 38.

Skin Assessment. Skin assessment may be a valuable source of information about the hematologic system. Examine the skin over the entire body in a systematic manner (e.g., starting with the face and oral cavity and moving downward over the body). In patients with RBC disorders, the skin may be pale or pasty or it may have a cyanotic tinge in severe anemia. Erythrocytosis often causes small vessel occlusions causing a purple, mottled appearance of the face, nose, fingers, or toes. Color changes in dark-skinned persons are best assessed in the sclera, conjunctiva, buccal mucosa, tongue, lips, nail beds, and palms.[8] *Clubbing of the fingers* (discussed in Chapter 25) can be seen with chronic anemia. Skin examination is discussed in Chapter 22.

CASE STUDY

Subjective Data

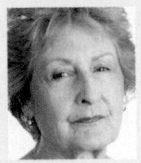

(© Lisa F. Young/iStock.)

A focused subjective assessment of A.J. revealed the following information:

Past Medical History: History of mild osteoarthritis. No surgical history. Prefers to take care of self with "natural therapy" and has not seen an HCP for 5 years, except for the recent sinus infection.

Medications: Metamucil 1 Tbsp/day PO; vitamins C, E, and D with calcium.

Health Perception–Health Management: A.J. denies family or personal history of anemia, cancer, or bleeding disorders. She believes she comes from a family with great genes for longevity because they "eat organic foods." She admits to drinking 1 glass of red wine with her evening meal "because it's good for your heart." She is a nonsmoker and cannot understand her gradual increase in shortness of breath with exertion. She says she really can't do anything anymore without having to stop and catch her breath. She says, "It's tough getting old."

Nutritional-Metabolic: A.J. and her husband eat a lot of pasta "because it is cheap." She uses a lot of garlic for flavoring and the "health benefit of it." Although not a vegetarian, she eats little meat.

Elimination: Denies black or tarry stool. Occasional constipation. No problems with urination. Urine without odor.

Activity-Exercise: A.J. is having a hard time performing ADLs without having to stop and catch her breath. Denies dyspnea at rest. States joints are stiff on arising in morning and after sitting but able to get around OK and work at her secretarial job. States her walking is steady but weak. No history of falling.

Sleep-Rest: Typically sleeps 8 to 9 hr/night with no trouble falling asleep. She still feels tired and needs to nap during her lunch break and during her days off.

Cognitive-Perceptual: Denies any numbness or tingling. Admits to being a little hard-of-hearing but can still see "pretty good."

Value-Belief: Prefers natural therapies over traditional medication.

Discussion Questions

1. What subjective assessment findings are of most concern to you?
2. Based on these subjective assessment findings, what type of physical assessment should you perform?
3. What should you include in the physical assessment? For what would you be looking?
4. How will you individualize the physical assessment based on the information from A.J. and her husband?

You will learn more about the physical examination of the hematologic system in the next section.
(See p. 598 for more information on A.J.)

Answers available at *http://evolve.elsevier.com/Lewis/medsurg.*

TABLE 29.5 Assessment Abnormalities

Hematologic System

Finding	Description	Possible Etiology and Significance
Abdomen		
Distended abdomen	A larger than normal abdominal profile. May be soft or firm, tender or nontender, and accompanied by other symptoms, such as nausea, vomiting, or rebound tenderness	Lymphoma may manifest as abdominal adenopathy, mass(es), or bowel obstruction
Hepatomegaly	Palpable liver	Leukemia, cirrhosis, or fibrosis secondary to iron overload from sickle cell disease or thalassemia
Splenomegaly	Palpable spleen	Anemia, thrombocytopenia, leukemia, lymphomas, leukopenia, mononucleosis, malaria, cirrhosis, trauma, portal hypertension
Eyes		
Blurred vision, diplopia, visual field cuts	Decreased visual acuity or areas of blindness (field cuts)	Anemia, extreme leukocytosis, polycythemia, hyperviscosity may cause visual abnormalities. Thrombocytopenia may cause intraocular hemorrhage with visual abnormalities. Excessive clotting may cause thromboses in circulation to the brain that cause visual field cuts
Conjunctival pallor	Paleness. Decreased or absence of coloration in the conjunctiva	Low Hgb level (anemia)
Jaundiced sclera	Yellow appearance of sclera	Accumulation of bile pigment resulting from rapid or excessive hemolysis or liver disease or infiltration
Heart and Chest		
Altered blood pressure	*Hypertension:* >140/90 mm Hg	May occur initially as a compensatory mechanism for anemia
	Hypotension: <90 mm Hg systolic or >40 mm Hg drop from baseline	Infectious process, blood loss, compromised cardiovascular compensatory mechanisms
	Orthostasis: heart rate >20 beats/min increase or blood pressure >20 mm Hg decrease from baseline when moving from a lying position to either sitting or standing	Common with anemia, especially if also accompanied by low blood volume
Low O_2 saturation	O_2-carrying capacity as reflected by O_2 saturation by pulse oximetry	O_2 saturation may be decreased in cases of severe anemia
Palpitations	Feeling the heartbeat, flutter, or pound in chest	Anemia, fluid volume overload, hypotension with impending syncope, hypertension, dysrhythmias
Sternal tenderness	Abnormal sensitivity to touch or pressure on sternum	Leukemia resulting from increased bone marrow cellularity, causing increase in pressure and bone erosion. Multiple myeloma because of stretching of periosteum
Tachycardia	Heart rate >100 beats/min	Compensatory mechanism in anemia to increase cardiac output
Lymph Nodes		
Lymphadenopathy	Lymph nodes enlarged (>1 cm). May be tender to touch	Infection, foreign infiltrations, systemic disease such as leukemia, lymphoma, Hodgkin's lymphoma, metastatic cancer
Mouth		
Gingival and mucous membrane changes	Pallor, gingival and mucosal ulceration, swelling, or bleeding	Low Hgb level (anemia), neutropenia thrombocytopenia. Inability of impaired leukocytes to combat oral infections. Gingival hyperplasia may be present with some types of leukemia
Smooth tongue	Tongue surface smooth and shiny. Mucosa thin and red from decreased papillae	Pernicious anemia, iron-deficiency anemia
Musculoskeletal System		
Arthralgia	Joint pain	Sickle cell disease from hemarthrosis (bleeding into joints)
Bone pain	Pain in pelvis, ribs, spine, sternum	Multiple myeloma related to enlarged tumors that stretch periosteum. Bone invasion by leukemia cells, bone demineralization resulting from various cancers, sickle cell disease
Joint swelling	Fluid-filled spaces surrounding joints	Occurs with hemophilia and sickle cell anemia as hemarthrosis causes inflammation
Nervous System		
Headache, nuchal rigidity	Pain in the cranium, potentially involving one area or extending from frontal area to back of neck	Generalized headache is a common manifestation of mild to moderate anemia. Severe headache with or without visual changes may signal intracranial hemorrhage due to thrombocytopenia

Continued

TABLE 29.5 Assessment Abnormalities

Hematologic System—cont'd

Finding	Description	Possible Etiology and Significance
Paresthesias of feet and hands, ataxia	Numbness sensation and extreme sensitivity in central and peripheral nerves. Impaired muscle movement	Cobalamin (vitamin B_{12}) deficiency or folate deficiency
Weakness	Lacking physical strength or energy	Low Hgb level (anemia)
Nose		
Epistaxis	Spontaneous bleeding from nares	May occur with low platelet counts, especially if patient bends down for a long time, tries to lift a heavy item, or performs an intense Valsalva maneuver
Skin		
Chloroma	A tumor arising from myeloid tissue and containing a pale green pigment	Acute myelogenous leukemia that has infiltrated the skin
Cyanosis	Bluish discoloration of skin and mucous membranes	Anemia, excess concentration of deoxyhemoglobin in blood
Excoriation	Scratch or abrasion of skin	Scratching from intense pruritus
Flushing	Transient, episodic redness of skin (usually around face and neck)	Increase in Hgb (polycythemia), congestion of capillaries. Flushing of palms of hands or soles of feet sign of anemia
Jaundice	Yellow appearance of skin and mucous membranes	Accumulation of bile pigment caused by rapid or excessive hemolysis or liver damage
Leg ulcers	Prominent on the malleoli on the ankles	Sickle cell disease
Pallor of skin or nail beds	Paleness. Decreased or absence of skin coloration	Low Hgb level (anemia)
Plasmacytoma	Tumor arising from abnormal plasma cells	Multiple myeloma that has infiltrated tissue
Pruritus	Unpleasant cutaneous sensation that provokes the desire to rub or scratch skin	Hodgkin's lymphoma, cutaneous lymphomas, infiltrative leukemias, increased bilirubin

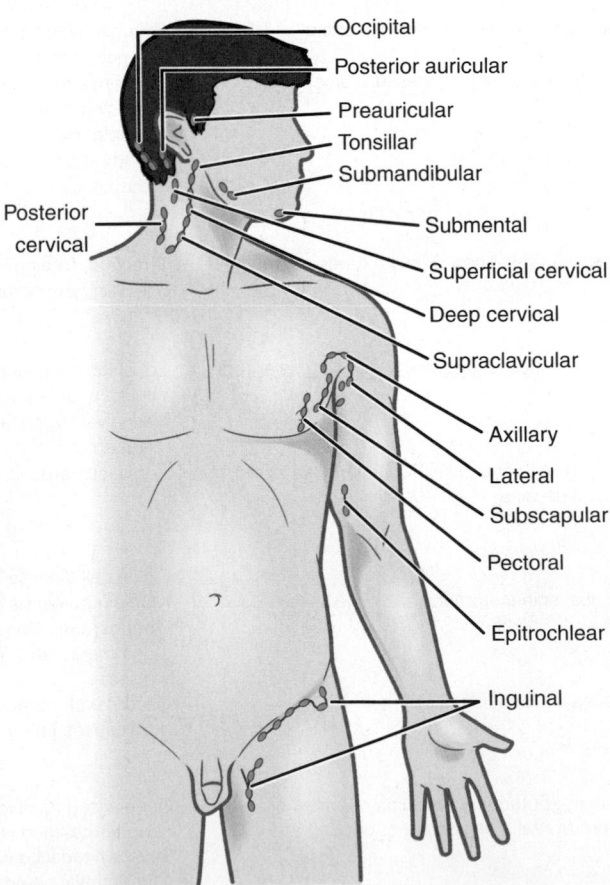

FIG. 29.6 Palpable superficial lymph nodes.

WBC disorders may cause infectious or cancerous skin lesions. These may occur anywhere and have a variable distribution pattern.

Look for findings that can indicate bleeding disorders. Assess for petechiae (small purplish red pinpoint lesions), ecchymoses (bruising), and *spider nevus* (a form of *telangiectasia*) (Table 29.6). The location of petechiae can indicate an accumulation of blood in the skin or mucous membranes. Small vessels leak under pressure, and the platelet numbers are not enough to stop the bleeding. Petechiae are more likely to occur where clothing constricts the circulation. In general, skin and mucosal bleeding means a platelet disorder, while spontaneous bleeding into joints or muscles means a coagulation factor problem.

A *focused assessment* is used to assess the status of previously identified hematologic problems and to monitor for signs of new problems. A focused assessment of the hematologic system is shown in the box on p. 598.

TABLE 29.6 Assessment Abnormalities

Vascular Skin Lesions

Finding	Description	Possible Etiology and Significance
Angioma 	Benign tumor. Consists consisting of blood or lymph vessels	Most are congenital. May disappear spontaneously
Ecchymosis (bruise) 	Hemorrhagic spots of varied size, Flat. Round or irregular	Decreased platelets or clotting factors resulting in hemorrhage into skin. Vascular abnormalities. Break in blood vessel walls from trauma
Petechiae 	Pinpoint, flat, round area >2 mm. Purple, dark red, or brown	Same as above
Purpura 	Flat purple or reddish discoloration. <5 mm. Do not blanche.	Same as above

Continued

TABLE 29.6 Assessment Abnormalities

Vascular Skin Lesions—cont'd

Finding	Description	Possible Etiology and Significance
Spider nevus (Spider angioma) 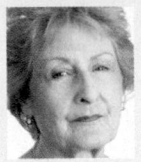	Has a round, red, central part and branching radiations resembling a spider's web. Usually found on face, neck, or chest	High estrogen levels as in pregnancy or liver disease
Telangiectasia	Fine, irregular red lines	Permanently dilated small blood vessels. Usually caused by sun damage or aging. May be seen with varicose veins, scleroderma, rosacea.

Figures from Ball JW, et al: *Seidel's guide to physical examination,* ed 9, St Louis, 2019, Mosby.

CASE STUDY

Objective Data: Physical Examination

(© Lisa F. Young/iStock.)

Physical examination findings of A.J. are as follows:
BP 100/70 (lying), 88/60 (standing); apical pulse 110 (lying), 124 (standing), but regular in rhythm. Respiratory rate 26, temperature 96.8° F (36° C), O₂ saturation 90% on room air. No jugular venous distention. Weight 106 lb (48 kg). Height 5 ft 1 in. Skin pale and 2 ecchymoses on her arms and 1 on her left lower leg. A few scattered petechiae on both ankles. No jaundice noted. Conjunctivae pale. Tongue smooth and shiny. Lungs clear but diminished breath sounds in the bases bilaterally. No visible bleeding. No enlarged lymph nodes, spleen, or liver noted. General weakness with dyspnea on exertion. No numbness or tingling or peripheral edema.

Discussion Questions

1. Which physical assessment findings are of most concern to you?
2. Based on the results of the subjective and physical assessment findings, what diagnostic studies do you think may be ordered for A.J.?

You will learn more about diagnostic studies in relation to the hematologic system in the next section.
(See p. 604 for more information on A.J.)

Answers available at *http://evolve.elsevier.com/Lewis/medsurg.*

DIAGNOSTIC STUDIES OF HEMATOLOGIC SYSTEM

The most direct means of evaluating the hematologic system is through laboratory analysis (Tables 29.7, 29.8, 29.9, and 29.10) and other diagnostic studies (Table 29.11).[9]

Laboratory Studies

Complete Blood Count. The complete blood count (CBC) involves several laboratory tests (Table 29.7). In addition to the CBC, a *peripheral smear* may be done. The smear is used to look

FOCUSED ASSESSMENT

Hematologic System

Use this checklist to make sure the key assessment steps have been done.

Subjective
Ask the patient about any of the following and note responses.

Unusual bleeding or bruising	Y	N
Black, tarry stool	Y	N
Blood in vomitus	Y	N
Swelling in neck, armpits, or groin	Y	N
Dark-colored urine	Y	N
Fatigue	Y	N
Heart palpitations	Y	N

Objective: Diagnostic
Check the following laboratory results for critical values.

CBC	✓
WBC count with differential	✓
Clotting: PT, INR, aPTT, platelets	✓
Hgb, Hct	✓

Objective: Physical Examination
Inspect

Skin for lesions or color changes	✓

Auscultate

BP for change or orthostasis	✓

Palpate

Pulse for tachycardia	✓
Liver and spleen for enlargement	✓
Lymph nodes for lymphadenopathy	✓

aPTT, Activated partial thromboplastin time; *INR,* international normalized ratio; *PT,* prothrombin time.

TABLE 29.7 Diagnostic Studies

Complete Blood Count Studies

Study	Description and Purpose	Reference Intervals
Hemoglobin (Hgb)	Measures gas-carrying capacity of RBC	*Female:* 12–16 g/dL (120–160 g/L) *Male:* 14–18 g/dL (140–180 g/L)
Hematocrit (Hct)	Measure of packed cell volume of RBCs expressed as a percentage of the total blood volume	*Female:* 37%–47% (0.37–0.47) *Male:* 42%–52% (0.42–0.52)
Total RBC count (erythrocyte count)	Number of circulating RBCs per volume of blood	*Female:* $4.2–5.4 \times 10^6/\mu L$ ($4.2\text{-}5.4 \times 10^{12}/L$) *Male:* $4.7–6.1 \times 10^6/\mu L$ ($4.7\text{-}6.1 \times 10^{12}/L$)
Red cell indices		
Mean corpuscular volume (MCV) $MSV = \dfrac{Hct \times 10}{RBC \times 10^6}$	Determination of relative size of RBCs. Low MCV reflection of microcytosis. High MCV reflection of macrocytosis	80–95 fL
Mean corpuscular hemoglobin (MCH) $MCH = \dfrac{Hgb \times 10}{RBC \times 10^6}$	Measurement of average weight of Hgb/RBCs. Low MCH indicates microcytosis or hypochromia. High MCH indicates macrocytosis	27–31 pg
Mean corpuscular hemoglobin concentration (MCHC) $MCHC = \dfrac{Hgb \times 100}{Hct}$	Evaluates RBC saturation with Hgb. Low MCHC indicates hypochromia. High MCHC occurs with spherocytosis	32%–36% (0.32–0.36)
RBC morphology	Examination of shape and size of RBCs	No variation in RBC morphology
Reticulocyte count	Number of immature red blood cells released from the bone marrow into the blood	0.5%–2.0% of RBC
WBC count	Total number of WBCs	$5000–10,000/\mu L$ ($5–10 \times 10^9/L$)
WBC differential	Determines whether each kind of WBC is present in proper proportion. Determine absolute value of each type of WBC by multiplying the percentage of cell type by total WBC count and dividing by 10	*Segmented neutrophils:* 55%–70% (0.55–0.70) *Banded neutrophils:* 0–8% (0–0.08) *Eosinophils:* 1%–4% (0.01–0.04) *Basophils:* 0.5%–1% (0.005–0.01) *Lymphocytes:* 20%–40% (0.20–0.40) *Monocytes:* 2%–8% (0.02–0.08)
Platelet count	Number of circulating platelets	$150,000–400,000 \times 10^3/L$ ($150–400 \times 10^9/L$)

TABLE 29.8 Diagnostic Studies

Clotting Studies

Study	Description and Purpose	Reference Intervals
Activated clotting time (ACT)	Evaluates intrinsic coagulation status. More accurate than aPTT. Used during dialysis, coronary artery bypass procedure, arteriograms	70–120 sec
Activated partial thromboplastin time (aPTT)	Assesses intrinsic coagulation by measuring factors I, II, V, VIII, IX, X, XI, XII. Higher in patients receiving heparin	30–40 sec
Antithrombin (antithrombin III)	Naturally occurring protein made by liver that inhibits coagulation by inactivating thrombin and other factors. Lower in DIC and hypercoagulable disorders	17–30 mg/dL (170–300 mg/L) or 80%–120% of standard
Bleeding time	Duration of bleeding after a standardized superficial puncture wound of the skin measuring the integrity of the platelet plug	1–9 min
Capillary fragility test (tourniquet test, Rumpel-Leede test)	Reflects capillary integrity when pressure is applied to various areas of the body. Positive test indicates thrombocytopenia, toxic vascular reactions	<2 petechiae or negative
D-dimer	Assay to measure a fragment of fibrin that forms because of fibrin degradation and clot lysis. Used as an adjunctive measure in diagnosis of hypercoagulable conditions (e.g., DIC, pulmonary embolism)	<250 ng/mL (<250 mcg/L)
Fibrin split products (FSPs) or fibrin degradation products (FDPs)	Reflects degree of fibrinolysis and predisposition to bleed (if present). Screening test for DIC. High levels associated with DIC, advanced cancer, severe inflammation	<10 mcg/mL (<10 mg/L)
Fibrinogen (factor I)	Reflects level of fibrinogen. Increase is a possible sign of enhancement of fibrin formation, making patient hypercoagulable. Decrease means the patient may be predisposed to bleeding.	200–400 mg/dL (2–4 g/L)
International normalized ratio (INR)	Standardized system of reporting prothrombin time (PT) based on a reference calibration model. Calculated by comparing patient's PT with a control value	0.8–1.1
Plasminogen	Assesses for deficiency of plasminogen in patients who have multiple thromboembolic episodes	2.4–4.4 units/mL
Platelet count	Number of circulating platelets	$150,000–400,000 \times 10^3/L$ ($150–400 \times 10^9/L$)
Prothrombin time (PT)	Assesses extrinsic coagulation by measuring factors I, II, V, VII, X	11–12.5 sec
Thrombin time	Reflects adequacy of thrombin and time to clot. Prolonged thrombin time means that coagulation is inadequate secondary to decreased thrombin activity	10–15 sec

DIC, Disseminated intravascular coagulation.

TABLE 29.9 ABO and Rh Blood Groups

Blood Type	ANTIGENS PRESENT ON RBC		ANTIBODIES POSSIBLY PRESENT IN PLASMA		Percent of General Population
	A or B	Rh (D)	A or B	Rh (D)	
O	—	—	A, B	Rh	35
O+	—	Rh	A, B	—	7
A	A	—	B	Rh	35
A+	A	Rh	B	—	7
B	B	—	A	Rh	8
B+	B	Rh	A	—	2
AB	A, B	—	—	Rh	4
AB+	A, B	Rh	—	—	2

TABLE 29.10 Diagnostic Studies

Miscellaneous Blood Studies

Study	Description and Purpose	Normal Values
Bilirubin	Measures degree of RBC hemolysis or liver's inability to excrete normal quantities of bilirubin. Increase in indirect bilirubin with hemolysis. Increase in direct bilirubin with obstructive problems (e.g., gallstones, liver tumor)	*Total:* 0.3–1.0 mg/dL (5.1–17.0 µmol/L) *Direct:* 0.1–0.3 mg/dL (1.7–5.1 µmol/L) *Indirect:* 0.2–0.8 mg/dL (3.4–12.0 µmol/L)
Blood smear (peripheral blood smear)	Reviews color, size, shape, quantity of cells in peripheral blood. Provides significant amount of information about problems affecting RBCs, WBCs, or platelets	Normal quantity of each cell type, normal size, shape and color of RBCs, normal WBC differential count and platelets
Coombs test	Differentiation among types of hemolytic anemias. Detection of immune antibodies and Rh factor	Negative
• Direct	Detects antibodies that are attached to RBCs	Negative
• Indirect	Detects circulating antibodies against red cells in serum	Negative
Cobalamin (vitamin B_{12})	Level of cobalamin available for production of new RBCs	160–950 pg/mL (118–701 pmol/L)
Erythrocyte sedimentation rate (ESR)	Measures sedimentation or settling of RBCs in 1 hr. Inflammatory process cause a change in plasma proteins, resulting in aggregation of RBCs and making them heavier. The faster the sedimentation rate, the higher the ESR	<20 mm/hr (some gender variation)
Erythropoietin	Measures degree of hormonal stimulation to bone marrow to stimulate the release of RBCs	5–25 mU/mL (5–30 U/L)
Ferritin	Major iron storage protein. Is normally present in blood in concentrations directly related to iron storage	10–300 ng/mL (10–300 mcg/L)
Folic acid (folate)	Amount of folic acid (folate) available for RBC production	5–25 ng/mL (11–57 nmol/L)
Haptoglobin	A serum glycoprotein that binds to Hgb released into the bloodstream by hemolysis. Decreased with red cell hemolysis. Increased with infection, inflammation, cancer	50–220 mg/dL
Hemoglobin (Hgb) electrophoresis	Proteins involved in development of Hgb molecule have a definitive pattern of separation on electrophoresis. This pattern is changed with abnormal Hgb synthesis (e.g., thalassemia) or sickle cell anemia (where Hgb S is increased)	Normal Hb A1: >95% Hb A2: 2%–3% Hb F: 0.8%–2% Hb S: 0 Hb C: 0
Homocysteine	An intermediate amino acid formed during the metabolism of the essential amino acid methionine. Rapidly metabolized through pathways that require cobalamin (vitamin B_{12}) and folic acid. Increased in cobalamin and folic acid deficiency	*Normal:* 4–14 µmol/L
Iron • Iron total	Reflects amount of iron combined with proteins in serum. Accurate indicator of status of iron storage and use	*Male:* 80–180 mcg/dL (14–32 µmol/L) *Female:* 60–160 mcg/dL (11–29 µmol/L)
• (Total) iron-binding capacity (TIBC)	Measures all proteins available for binding iron. Transferrin represents the largest quantity of iron-binding proteins. Therefore TIBC is an indirect measure of transferrin, an evaluation of the amount of extra iron that can be carried	250–460 mcg/dL (45–82 µmol/L)
Lactic dehydrogenase (LDH)	Intracellular enzyme present in almost all body tissues. Levels rise in response to cell damage. Increased levels confirm diagnosis of injury or disease. Used as a nonspecific marker of hematologic cancer growth and response to treatment	100–190 U/L
Methylmalonic acid (MMA)	Indirect test for cobalamin (vitamin B_{12}). MMA metabolism requires cobalamin. Decreased levels with cobalamin deficiency. Helps distinguish cobalamin deficiency from folic acid deficiency	<3.6 µmol/mmol creatinine
Microglobulin (beta₂ microglobulin)	Protein found on the surface of all cells. Increased in cancers such as lymphoma, leukemia, or multiple myeloma. May be used as a tumor marker	*Blood:* 0.7–1.8 mcg/mL *Urine:* ≤300 mcg/L *Spinal fluid:* ≤2.4 mg/L
Serum protein electrophoresis (SPEP)	Separates proteins in blood on basis of electric charge. Helps detect hyperglobulinemic states, such as in multiple myeloma or some lymphomas	Normal banding pattern of albumin and globulins. Increase in any protein (*protein spike*) is abnormal
Transferrin	Largest of proteins that bind to iron. Increased in most people with iron-deficiency anemia	*Male:* 215–365 mg/dL (2.15–3.65 g/L) *Female:* 250–380 mg/dL (2.5–3.8 g/L)
Transferrin saturation (%)	Decreased in iron-deficiency anemia. Increased in hemolytic and megaloblastic anemia	*Male:* 20%–50% *Female:* 15%–50%

TABLE 29.11 Diagnostic Studies

Hematologic System

Study	Description and Purpose	Nursing Responsibility
Molecular, Cytogenetic, and Gene Analysis Studies		
Cancer genomics (genotyping) **Cell surface immunophenotyping (flow cytometry)** **Chromosomal karyotyping** **Fluorescence in situ hybridization (FISH)**	Assesses for genetic or chromosomal abnormalities of cancer cells. Uses peripheral blood (e.g., leukemia), biopsy specimen (bone marrow, lymph node, tissue), or CSF. Used to confirm diagnosis and determine treatment modalities and prognosis	*Before:* Explain purpose of testing to patient. HCP will provide specific significance.
Procedures		
Bone marrow biopsy (Fig. 29.7)	Technique involves removal of bone marrow through a locally anesthetized site to evaluate status of blood-forming tissue. Used to diagnose and monitor aplastic anemia, multiple myeloma, myelodysplastic syndromes, leukemia, and some lymphomas	*Before:* Explain procedure to patient. Obtain signed consent form. Perform a surgical time-out before procedure. Analgesics may be given to enhance patient comfort and cooperation. *After:* Apply pressure dressing. Assess biopsy site for bleeding and apply pressure as needed. Tenderness at the puncture site for a few days may be normal. Assess for infection.
Lumbar puncture (LP)	Done to obtain CSF for testing for cancer, infection, and degenerative brain diseases. May be used to give chemotherapy to the central nervous system	*During:* Help position patient and provide support. *After:* Watch site for bleeding and signs of infection. Spinal headaches may occur. Follow postprocedure orders for how long the patient should lie flat. Encourage the patient to drink fluids.
Lymph node biopsy • Closed (needle) or fine needle • Open	Used to obtain lymph tissue for histologic examination to determine diagnosis and therapy Done at the bedside or in an outpatient area. An extremely small needle is used to reduce risk for tracking cancer cells through normal subcutaneous tissue Done in operating room or procedure area using either local or general anesthesia. After making an incision, the lymph node and surrounding tissue are excised whenever possible	*Before:* Explain procedure to patient. Obtain signed consent form. *After:* Watch site for bleeding and monitor vital signs, especially if platelet count is low. Change sterile dressing as ordered. Inspect wound for healing and infection.
Radioisotope Studies		
Bone scan	Radioactive isotope is injected IV and taken up by the bones. Uniform uptake is normal. Increased uptake seen in osteomyelitis, certain fractures, and bone cancer	*Before:* Patient may be asked to drink 4–6 glasses of water and then void before imaging (to see pelvic bones). Obtain IV access for injection of isotope.
SPECT scan (single-photon emission computed tomography)	Radioactive isotope is injected IV. Images from radioactive emissions used to evaluate the structures, such as spleen, liver, bone, and possible tumors. Patient is not a source of radioactivity	*Before:* Obtain IV access for injection of isotope. *After:* Have the patient drink fluids to aid in the excretion of the isotope.
Radiologic Studies		
Computed tomography (CT) scan	Noninvasive radiologic examination using computer-assisted x-ray evaluates the lymph nodes. Contrast medium used in abdominal studies of liver or spleen. Spiral (helical) CT scans used to evaluate lymph nodes	*Before:* Assess for iodine sensitivity if contrast medium used. IV and/or oral contrast may be given prior to procedure, depending on the area being studied. Patient may need to be NPO for 4 hr. *After:* Have patient drink fluids to avoid renal problems with any contrast.
Liver, spleen, or abdominal ultrasound	Noninvasive probe is lubricated and slid across the abdomen to detect density and borders of the abdominal organs. Can detect irregular borders, masses, vascular structure, fluid collections, and biliary tree	*During:* Patients must be comfortable lying flat and having probe compress abdomen.
Magnetic resonance imaging (MRI)	Noninvasive procedure produces sensitive images of soft tissue (central nervous system, neck and back, bones and joints, heart, breasts). An IV contrast agent (gadolinium) may be given. Provides a better contrast between normal tissue and pathologic tissue than CT	*Before:* Oral and/or IV contrast injection may be used. Check for pregnancy, allergies, and renal function before test. Have patient remove all metal objects. Ask about any history of surgical insertion of staples, plates, dental bridges, or other metal appliances. Remove metallic foil patches. Patient may need to be fasting. Assess for claustrophobia and the need for antianxiety medication. *During:* Patient must lie completely still during scan.

Continued

TABLE 29.11 Diagnostic Studies

Hematologic System—cont'd

Study	Description and Purpose	Nursing Responsibility
Positron emission tomography (PET)	Glucose-containing nuclear tracer substance is injected and taken up by metabolically active cells. Follow-up scan shows different-colored tissues based on metabolic rate. Because cancer cells have an increased uptake of glucose, "hot spots" reflecting increased glucose consumption indicate the presence of active cancer. CT scanning may be done in conjunction or images fused.	*Before:* Obtain IV access to inject the tracer substance. Patients should be NPO, except for water and medications, for at least 4 hr prior. Hold glucose-containing IV solutions and change to normal saline. Check the blood glucose levels as high levels may interfere with test. May need bowel preparation depending on area being studied. *After:* Encourage fluids to excrete radioactive substance.
Skeletal x-ray	X-rays done as a bone survey to detect lytic lesions associated with multiple myeloma. Bone scans do not identify lesions in this condition because there is no uptake of radioactive isotopes due to lack of blood supply.	No specific nursing responsibilities.
Urine Studies		
Bence Jones protein (free kappa and lambda light chains)	An electrophoretic measurement used to detect Bence Jones protein, which is found in most cases of multiple myeloma. May be present in some other hematologic disorders and metastatic cancers. Negative finding is normal.	*During:* Obtain random urine specimen early in the morning. If a 24-hr urine collection is done, discard first specimen, and collect all urine voided during the 24 hr, keeping on ice or refrigerated. Remind patient not to put toilet paper in urine collection container.

at the *morphology* (shape and appearance) of the blood cells and may help with the diagnosis. For example, many immature *blast* WBCs may indicate acute leukemia.

Although the status of each cell type is important, diseases or treatment of diseases can disrupt the entire system. When the entire CBC is suppressed, a condition termed pancytopenia (marked decrease in the number of RBCs, WBCs, and platelets) exists.

Red Blood Cells. The total RBC count is reported as RBC × $10^6/\mu L$. However, the total RBC count is not fully reliable in determining the adequacy of RBC function. We must evaluate other data, such as hemoglobin, hematocrit, and RBC indices. Normal values of some RBC tests are different for men and women because normal values are based on body mass. Men usually have a larger body mass than women.

The *hemoglobin (Hgb) value* is reduced in cases of anemia, hemorrhage, and hemodilution, such as that occurring with excess fluid volume. Increased hemoglobin is found in polycythemia or in states of hemoconcentration, which can develop from volume depletion (dehydration). Reductions and elevations of the hematocrit value and RBC count occur with the same conditions that raise and lower the hemoglobin value.

The *hematocrit (Hct) value* is determined by spinning blood in a centrifuge. This causes RBCs and plasma to separate. The RBCs, being the heavier elements, settle to the bottom (Fig. 29.2). The hematocrit value is the percent of RBCs compared with the total blood volume. The hematocrit value generally is 3 times the hemoglobin value.

RBC indices are special indicators that reflect RBC volume, color, and hemoglobin saturation (Table 29.7).[9] These parameters give insight into the cause of anemia. The significance of these parameters is discussed more in Chapter 30.

White Blood Cells. The WBC count gives two different sets of information. The first is a total count of WBCs in 1 μL of peripheral blood. A WBC count over 10,000/μL is associated with infection, inflammation, tissue injury or death, and cancer

(e.g., leukemia, lymphoma). Although the degree of WBC elevation does not necessarily predict the severity of illness, it can give clues to the cause. Extremely high WBC counts (e.g., greater than 25,000/μL) occur with certain types of leukemia. A WBC count less than 5000/μL (leukopenia) is associated with bone marrow depression, severe or chronic illness, and other types of leukemia.

The second aspect of the WBC count, the *differential count,* measures the percent of each type of WBC. The WBC differential gives valuable clues in determining the cause of illness. When infections are severe, we release more granulocytes from the bone marrow as a compensatory mechanism. To meet the increased demand, many young, immature polymorphonuclear neutrophils *(bands)* are released into circulation. More mature neutrophils are called *polymorphonuclear segmented neutrophils (segs).* Together, bands and segs make up the *absolute neutrophil count* (ANC). The usual laboratory procedure is to report the WBCs in order of maturity, with the less mature forms on the left side of the written report. That is why we call the presence of many immature cells a *"shift to the left."*

The WBC differential is very important because it is possible for the total WBC count to be essentially normal despite a marked change in 1 type of WBC. For example, a patient may have a normal WBC count of 8800/μL, but the differential count may show that the proportion of lymphocytes is only 10%. This is an abnormal finding that needs further investigation.

When the bone marrow does not make enough neutrophils, neutropenia occurs. Neutropenia is a condition in which the ANC is less than 1000 cells/μL. Severe neutropenia is associated with an ANC of less than 500 cells/μL. You calculate the ANC by multiplying the total WBC count by the percentage of neutrophils. Neutropenia results from many disease processes, such as leukemia, or from bone marrow depression (see Chapter 30). It is associated with a high risk for infection and death from sepsis.

Platelet Count. The platelet count is the number of platelets per microliter of blood. Normal platelet counts are between 150,000 and 400,000/μL. Counts below 100,000/μL signify a condition termed thrombocytopenia. Bleeding may occur with thrombocytopenia. Spontaneous hemorrhage is possible once platelet counts fall below 10,000/μL, depending on the clinical situation.[6] A more extensive description of clotting studies is given in Table 29.8.

Thrombocytosis is defined as too many platelets. It occurs with inflammation and some cancers (see Chapter 30). The most likely complication of thrombocytosis is excessive clotting.

Blood Typing and Rh Factor. Blood group antigens (A and B) are found only on RBC membranes. They form the basis for the ABO blood typing system. The presence or absence of 1 or both of the 2 inherited antigens is the basis for the 4 blood groups: A, B, AB, and O. Blood group A has A antigens, group B has B antigens, group AB has both antigens, and group O has neither A nor B antigens. Each person has antibodies in the serum termed *anti-A* and *anti-B* that react with A or B antigens. These antibodies are found when the corresponding antigen is absent from the RBC surface. For example, B antibodies are found in the serum of people with blood group A (Table 29.9).

Blood reactions based on ABO incompatibilities result from intravascular hemolysis of the RBCs. RBCs *agglutinate* (or clump) when a serum antibody is present to react with the antigens on the RBC membrane. For example, agglutination would occur in the blood of a person with type A blood if he or she receives blood transfused from a person with B antigens (i.e., type B or AB). The anti-B antibodies in the type A blood would react with the B antigens, starting the process that results in RBC hemolysis. Blood component compatibilities for transfusions are outlined in Table 30.32.

The *Rh system* is based on a third antigen, D, which is also on the RBC membrane. Rh-positive people have the D antigen, while Rh-negative people do not. Rh-positive blood is indicated with a "+" after the ABO group (e.g., AB+). Rh status is determined by a Coombs test (Table 29.10).

Because of transfusion therapy or during childbirth, a Rh-negative person may be exposed to Rh-positive blood. After exposure during childbirth, a Rh-negative mother forms an antibody, anti-D, which acts against Rh antigens (Rh-positive people normally have no anti-D). In future pregnancies the mother's anti-D antibodies can cross the placenta and attack the RBCs of a Rh-positive fetus, causing hemolysis of the RBCs. A pregnant Rh-negative woman should receive Rho(D) immune globulin (RhoGAM) injections to prevent anti-D antibodies from forming.

Iron Metabolism. The laboratory tests used to evaluate iron metabolism include serum iron, total iron-binding capacity (TIBC), serum ferritin, and transferrin saturation. Tests for nutritional deficiencies leading to defective RBC production may be done (Table 29.10).[9]

Serum iron is a measurement of the amount of protein-bound iron circulating in the serum. TIBC gives a measurement of all proteins that act to bind or transport iron between the tissues and bone marrow. Although this indirect measurement is a general reflection of the amount of transferrin present in the circulation, it overestimates transferrin levels by 16% to 20% because it measures other proteins that can bind iron. These alternative proteins bind iron only when transferrin is more than half saturated. TIBC varies inversely with tissue iron stores. It is higher when iron stores are low and lower when iron stores are high.

Transferrin saturation is a better indicator of the availability of iron for erythropoiesis than serum iron. Unlike serum iron, the iron bound to transferrin is readily available for the body to use. You calculate transferrin saturation by dividing serum iron by TIBC and multiplying by 100. For example, a patient with a serum iron level of 100 mcg/dL and a TIBC of 300 mcg/dL would have a transferrin saturation of about 33%.

Under normal conditions, the serum ferritin concentration correlates closely with body iron stores. In normal patients, 1 ng/mL of ferritin corresponds to 8 to 10 mg of stored iron.

Biopsies

Biopsy procedures specific to hematologic assessment are bone marrow examination and lymph node biopsy. In general, these procedures are done when a peripheral blood smear is nonspecific. Furthermore, a biopsy provides information that is needed for diagnosis and treatment planning.

Bone Marrow Examination. Bone marrow examination is important in evaluating many hematologic problems. It may involve aspiration only or aspiration with biopsy (Table 29.11). The benefits gained from bone marrow examination are (1) a full evaluation of hematopoiesis and (2) the ability to get specimens for cytopathologic and chromosomal analysis. The preferred site for both aspiration and biopsy of bone marrow is the posterior iliac crest. A physician, nurse practitioner, or physician's assistant can perform a bone marrow aspiration and biopsy. The patient may receive local anesthesia and sedation to minimize anxiety and pain.

For bone marrow aspiration, the skin over the puncture site is cleansed with a bactericidal agent. The skin, subcutaneous tissue, and periosteum are injected with a local anesthetic agent. Once the area is anesthetized, a bone marrow needle is inserted through the cortex of the bone. The stylet of the needle is then removed, the hub is attached to a 10-mL syringe, and 0.2 to 0.5 mL of the fluid marrow is aspirated (Fig. 29.7). The patient will have pain when the periosteum is penetrated and with aspiration. Although the pain will last only a few seconds, it can be quite uncomfortable. After the marrow aspiration, the needle is removed. Pressure is applied over the aspiration site to ensure hemostasis, then the site is covered with a sterile pressure dressing.

Although complications of bone marrow aspiration are minimal, there is a chance of damaging underlying structures. Other complications include hemorrhage (if the patient is thrombocytopenic) and infection (if the patient is leukopenic).

Monitor the patient's vital signs until stable and assess the site for excess drainage or bleeding. If bleeding is present, have the patient lie on that side for 30 to 60 minutes to keep pressure on the site. If the bed is too soft, have the patient lie on a rolled towel to provide more pressure. You may give analgesics for postprocedure pain. Soreness over the puncture site for 3 to 4 days after the procedure is normal.

Lymph Node Biopsy. Lymph node biopsy involves obtaining lymph tissue for histologic examination to determine the diagnosis and help plan therapy. This may be done by either an open biopsy or a closed (needle) biopsy.

If the results from a needle biopsy are negative, it may only mean that the cancer cells were not part of the tissue in the biopsy specimen. However, a positive finding may be enough evidence for confirming a diagnosis. This technique is rarely used to confirm an initial diagnosis because larger specimens, such as excisional biopsies are usually needed to perform cytopathologic tests.

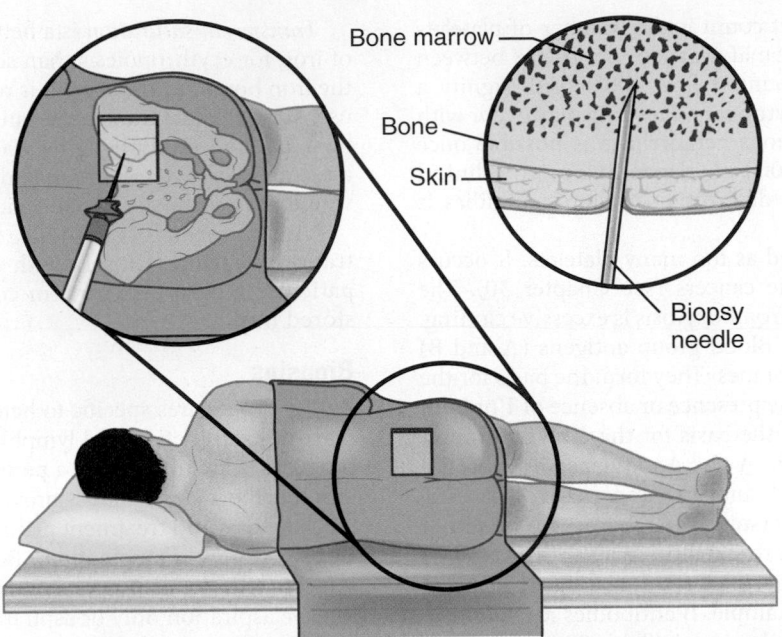

Bone marrow

Bone

Skin

Biopsy needle

FIG. 29.7 Bone marrow aspiration from the posterior iliac crest.

Molecular Cytogenetics and Gene Analysis

Testing for specific genetic or chromosomal variations in hematologic conditions is often helpful in diagnosis and staging (Table 29.11). These results help determine treatment options and prognosis. If a large number of abnormal cells are circulating in the blood, such as in acute leukemia, these tests may be done on peripheral blood. However, testing is usually done on samples from bone marrow, lymph node biopsies, and sometimes cerebrospinal fluid (CSF).[9] For example, fluorescence in situ hybridization (FISH) identifies genetic defects using nucleic probes that are complementary to a targeted region of deoxyribonucleic acid (DNA). It can identify an abnormal extra chromosome 8, which is common in certain leukemias. Chromosomal karyotyping allows each set of chromosomes to be painted different colors. This helps identify normal from abnormal banding patterns.[9] It can be used to identify the translocation of chromosome 22 to 9 in the Philadelphia chromosome of chronic myelogenous leukemia. More information on genetics is available in Chapter 12.

CASE STUDY

Objective Data: Diagnostic Studies

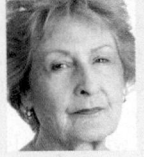

(© Lisa F. Young/iStock.)

The HCP orders the following diagnostic studies for A.J.:
- CBC, basic metabolic panel (electrolytes, BUN, creatinine), PT/PTT
- Arterial blood gases
- Chest x-ray

A.J.'s CBC reveals an Hgb of 5.9 g/dL, Hct of 18.2%, WBC of 2600/μL (2.6 × 10⁹/L), platelet count of 72,000/μL, PT = 18 sec, aPTT = 37. The arterial blood gases and chest x-ray are normal. The HCP orders more blood work, including a WBC differential and RBC indices and admits her to the hospital for further evaluation.

Discussion Questions

1. Are these the diagnostic studies that you expected to be ordered?
2. Which diagnostic study results are abnormal?
3. Which diagnostic study results are of most concern to you? What other studies may be ordered on admission?

This case study is continued in Chapter 30 on p. 652.

Answers available at *http://evolve.elsevier.com/Lewis/medsurg.*

▌ BRIDGE TO NCLEX EXAMINATION

The number of the question corresponds to the same-numbered outcome at the beginning of the chapter.

1. A person who lives at a high altitude may normally have an increased Hgb and RBC count because
   a. high altitudes cause vascular fluid loss, leading to hemoconcentration.
   b. hypoxia caused by decreased atmospheric O₂ stimulates erythropoiesis.
   c. the function of the spleen in removing old RBCs is impaired at high altitudes.
   d. impaired production of platelets leads to proportionally higher red cell counts.

2. Cancer arising from granulocytic cells in the bone marrow will have the primary effect of causing
   a. risk for hemorrhage.
   b. altered oxygenation.
   c. decreased production of antibodies.
   d. decreased phagocytosis of bacteria.

3. An anticoagulant such as warfarin that interferes with prothrombin production will alter the clotting mechanism during
   a. platelet aggregation.
   b. activation of thrombin.
   c. the release of tissue thromboplastin.
   d. stimulation of factor activation complex.

4. When reviewing laboratory results of an older patient with an infection, the nurse would expect to find
   a. mild leukocytosis.
   b. decreased platelet count.
   c. increased hemoglobin and hematocrit levels.
   d. decreased erythrocyte sedimentation rate (ESR).
5. Significant information from the patient's health history that relates to the hematologic system includes
   a. jaundice.
   b. bladder surgery.
   c. early menopause.
   d. multiple pregnancies.
6. While assessing the lymph nodes, the nurse should
   a. apply gentle, firm pressure to deep lymph nodes.
   b. palpate the deep cervical and supraclavicular nodes last.
   c. lightly palpate superficial lymph nodes with the pads of the fingers.
   d. use the tips of the second, third, and fourth fingers to apply deep palpation.
7. If a lymph node is palpated, what is a normal finding?
   a. Hard, fixed nodes
   b. Firm, mobile nodes
   c. Enlarged, tender nodes
   d. Hard, nontender nodes

8. Nursing care for a patient immediately after a bone marrow biopsy and aspiration includes *(select all that apply)*
   a. giving analgesics as needed.
   b. preparing to start a blood transfusion.
   c. giving preprocedure and postprocedure antibiotic medications.
   d. having the patient lie still to keep the sterile pressure dressing intact.
   e. monitoring vital signs and assessing the site for excess drainage or bleeding.
9. You are taking care of a male patient who has the following laboratory values from his CBC: WBC $6.5 \times 10^3/\mu L$, Hgb 13.4 g/dL, Hct 40%, platelets $50 \times 10^3/\mu L$. What are you *most* concerned about?
   a. The patient is neutropenic.
   b. The patient has an infection.
   c. There is an increased risk for bleeding.
   d. Fall risk precautions are needed due to anemia.

1. b, 2. d, 3. b, 4. a, 5. a, 6. c, 7. b, 8. a, d, e, 9. c

For rationales to these answers and even more NCLEX review questions, visit *http://evolve.elsevier.com/Lewis/medsurg.*

ⓔ EVOLVE WEBSITE/RESOURCES LIST

http://evolve.elsevier.com/Lewis/medsurg
Review Questions (Online Only)
Key Points
Answer Keys for Questions
- Rationales for Bridge to NCLEX Examination Questions
- Answer Guidelines for Case Studies on pp. 592, 594, 598, and 604

Conceptual Care Map Creator
Audio Glossary
Content Updates

REFERENCES

1. Huether SE, McCance KL: *Understanding pathophysiology*, ed 6, St Louis, 2017, Mosby.
2. Bickley LS, Szilagyi PG, Hoffman RM: *Bates' guide to physical examination and history taking*, ed 12, Philadelphia, 2017, Wolters Kluwer.
3. Lichtman MA, Kaushansky K, Prchal JT, et al: *Williams manual of hematology*, ed 9, New York, 2017, McGraw-Hill.
4. Kaushansky K, Lichtman MA, Prchal J, et al: *Williams hematology*, ed 9, New York, 2016, McGraw-Hill.
5. Bain BJ, Bates, I, Laffan MA: *Dacie and Lewis practical haematology*, ed 12, Philadelphia, 2017, Elsevier.
6. Hoffman R, Benz EJ, Silberstein LE, et al: *Hematology: Basic principles and practice*, ed 7, Philadelphia, 2018, Elsevier.
7. Academy of Nutrition and Dietetics: Food and nutrition topics. Retrieved from *www.eatright.org.*
8. Ball JW, Dains JE, Flynn JA, et al: *Seidel's guide to physical examination*, ed 9, St Louis, 2019, Mosby.
9. Pagana KD, Pagana TJ: *Mosby's manual of diagnostic and laboratory tests*, ed 6. St Louis, 2018, Mosby.

30

Hematologic Problems

Sandra Irene Rome

The capacity to care is what gives life its most deepest significance.

Pablo Casals

http://evolve.elsevier.com/Lewis/medsurg/

CONCEPTUAL FOCUS

Cellular Regulation

Clotting

Fatigue

Functional Ability

Gas Exchange

Immunity

Infection

Pain

Perfusion

LEARNING OUTCOMES

1. Describe the general clinical manifestations and complications of anemia.
2. Distinguish the etiologies, clinical manifestations, diagnostic findings, and interprofessional and nursing management of iron-deficiency, megaloblastic, and aplastic anemias.
3. Explain the nursing management of anemia from blood loss.
4. Describe the pathophysiology, clinical manifestations, and interprofessional and nursing management of anemia caused by increased erythrocyte destruction.
5. Describe the pathophysiology and nursing and interprofessional management of polycythemia.
6. Explain the pathophysiology, clinical manifestations, and interprofessional and nursing management of various types of thrombocytopenia.
7. Describe the types, clinical manifestations, diagnostic findings, and interprofessional and nursing management of hemophilia and von Willebrand disease.
8. Explain the pathophysiology, diagnostic findings, and interprofessional and nursing management of disseminated intravascular coagulation.
9. Describe the etiology, clinical manifestations, and interprofessional and nursing management of neutropenia.
10. Describe the pathophysiology, clinical manifestations, and interprofessional and nursing management of myelodysplastic syndrome.
11. Compare and contrast the distinguishing clinical and laboratory findings of the major types of leukemia.
12. Explain the nursing and interprofessional management of acute and chronic leukemias.
13. Compare Hodgkin's lymphoma and non-Hodgkin's lymphomas in terms of clinical manifestations, staging, and interprofessional and nursing management.
14. Describe the pathophysiology, clinical manifestations, and interprofessional and nursing management of multiple myeloma.
15. Describe the spleen disorders and related interprofessional care.
16. Describe the nursing management of the patient receiving transfusions of blood and blood components.

KEY TERMS

anemia, p. 606

aplastic anemia, p. 614

disseminated intravascular coagulation (DIC), p. 628

hemochromatosis, p. 619

hemolytic anemia, p. 615

hemophilia, p. 626

Hodgkin's lymphoma, p. 640

iron-deficiency anemia, p. 609

leukemia, p. 634

lymphomas, p. 640

megaloblastic anemias, p. 612

multiple myeloma, p. 645

myelodysplastic syndrome (MDS), p. 634

neutropenia, p. 631

non-Hodgkin's lymphomas (NHLs), p. 642

pernicious anemia, p. 612

polycythemia, p. 620

sickle cell disease (SCD), p. 616

thalassemia, p. 611

thrombocytopenia, p. 622

There are a wide range of blood conditions and cancers. Because blood has so many essential functions, when hematologic problems occur the patient is affected in multiple ways. Patients with anemia and hematologic cancer may have to cope with fatigue. Compromised immunity and the risk for infection is a concern among patients with hematologic cancer and a common side effect of therapy. Pain is a common symptom associated with cancer and sickle cell disease. Clotting is an important protective mechanism that allows us to maintain homeostasis when injury occurs. Excessive clotting can impair perfusion, while inadequate clotting can lead to blood loss and fluid volume deficits. This chapter will discuss the interprofessional and nursing care of common hematologic problems and their associated concepts.

ANEMIA

Definition and Classification

Anemia is a deficiency in the number of erythrocytes (red blood cells [RBCs]), the quantity or quality of hemoglobin, and/or volume of packed RBCs (hematocrit). It is a common condition

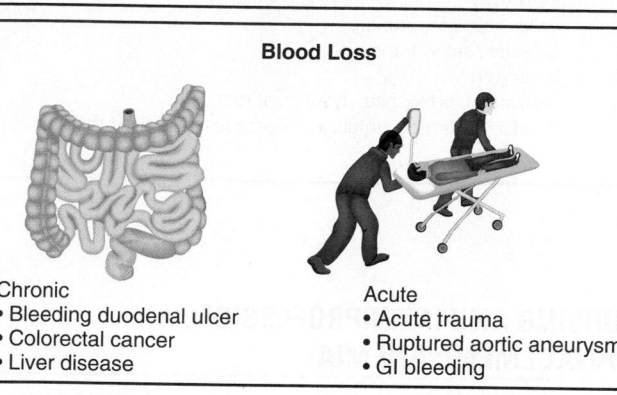

Decreased RBC Production

Deficient nutrients
• Iron
• Cobalamin
• Folic acid

Decreased erythropoietin

Decreased iron availability

Blood Loss

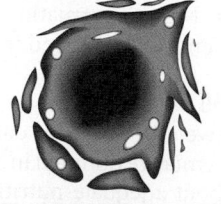

Chronic
• Bleeding duodenal ulcer
• Colorectal cancer
• Liver disease

Acute
• Acute trauma
• Ruptured aortic aneurysm
• GI bleeding

Increased RBC Destruction

Hemolysis
• Sickle cell disease
• Medication (e.g., methyldopa [Aldomet])
• Incompatible blood
• Trauma (e.g., cardiopulmonary bypass)

FIG. 30.1 Causes of anemia.

TABLE 30.2 Etiologic Classification of Anemia

Decreased RBC Production

Decreased Hemoglobin Synthesis
• Iron deficiency
• Sideroblastic anemia (decreased porphyrin)
• Thalassemia (decreased globin synthesis)

Decreased Number of RBC Precursors
• Aplastic anemia and inherited disorders (e.g., Fanconi syndrome)
• Anemia of myeloproliferative diseases (e.g., leukemia) and myelodysplasia
• Chronic diseases or disorders
• Medications and chemicals (e.g., chemotherapy, lead)
• Radiation

Defective DNA Synthesis
• Cobalamin (vitamin B_{12}) deficiency
• Folic acid deficiency

Blood Loss

Acute
• Blood vessel rupture
• Splenic sequestration crisis
• Trauma

Chronic
• Gastritis
• Menstrual flow
• Hemorrhoids

Increased RBC Destruction (Hemolytic Anemias)

Acquired (Extrinsic)
• Antibodies against RBCs
• Infectious agents (e.g., malaria) and toxins
• Physical destruction
• Extracorporeal circulation
• Disseminated intravascular coagulopathy (DIC)
• HELLP syndrome (hemolysis, high liver enzymes, low platelets associated with pregnancy)
• Prosthetic heart valves
• Thrombotic thrombocytopenic purpura (TTP)
• Widespread cancer

Hereditary (Intrinsic)
• Abnormal hemoglobin (sickle cell disease)
• Enzyme deficiency (glucose-6-phosphate dehydrogenase [G6PD])
• Membrane abnormalities (paroxysmal nocturnal hemoglobinuria, hereditary spherocytosis)

TABLE 30.1 Morphologic Classification of Anemia

Morphology	Etiology
Normocytic, normochromic (normal size and color) MCV 80–95 fL, MCH 27–31 pg	Acute blood loss, hemolysis, chronic kidney disease, chronic disease, cancers, endocrine disorders, starvation, aplastic anemia, sickle cell anemia, pregnancy
Microcytic, hypochromic (small size, pale color) MCV <80 fL, MCH <27 pg	Iron-deficiency anemia, vitamin B_6 deficiency, copper deficiency, thalassemia, lead poisoning
Macrocytic (megaloblastic), normochromic (large size, normal color) MCV >95 fL, MCH >31 pg	Cobalamin (vitamin B_{12}) deficiency, folic acid deficiency, liver disease (including effects of alcohol use)

MCH, Mean corpuscular hemoglobin; *MCV,* mean corpuscular volume.

with many diverse causes, such as blood loss, impaired production of RBCs, or increased destruction of RBCs (Fig. 30.1). Because RBCs transport O_2, RBC disorders can lead to tissue hypoxia. This hypoxia accounts for many of the signs and symptoms of anemia. Anemia is not a specific disease. It is a manifestation of a pathologic process.

We diagnose anemia based on a complete blood count (CBC), reticulocyte count, and peripheral blood smear. Once we identify anemia, further investigation is done to determine its specific cause.[1]

Anemia can result from primary hematologic problems or develop as a secondary consequence of diseases or disorders of other body systems. We classify the types of anemia according to either *morphology* (cellular characteristic) or *etiology* (cause). Morphologic classification is based on RBC size and color (Table 30.1). Etiologic classification is related to the clinical conditions causing the anemia (Table 30.2).[2] Although the morphologic system is the most accurate means of classifying anemias, it is easier to discuss patient care by focusing on the cause of the anemia.

⊕ PROMOTING HEALTH EQUITY

Hematologic Problems

• Sickle cell disease has a high incidence among African Americans.
• Thalassemia has a high incidence among blacks and people of Mediterranean origin.
• Tay-Sachs disease has the highest incidence in families of Eastern European Jewish origin, especially the Ashkenazi Jews.
• Pernicious anemia has a high incidence among Scandinavians and blacks.

TABLE 30.3 Manifestations of Anemia

Body System	SEVERITY OF ANEMI		
	Mild (Hgb 10–12 g/dL [100–120 g/L])	**Moderate** (Hgb 6–10 g/dL [60–100 g/L])	**Severe** (Hgb <6 g/dL [<60 g/L])
Cardiovascular	Palpitations	Increased palpitations, "bounding pulse"	Tachycardia, increased pulse pressure, systolic murmurs, intermittent claudication, angina, HF, myocardial infarction
Eyes	None	None	Icteric conjunctiva and sclera, retinal hemorrhage, blurred vision
Gastrointestinal	None	None	Anorexia, hepatomegaly, splenomegaly, difficulty swallowing, sore mouth
General	None or mild fatigue	Fatigue	Sensitivity to cold, weight loss, lethargy
Integument	None	None	Pallor, jaundice, pruritus
Mouth	None	None	Glossitis, smooth tongue
Musculoskeletal	None	None	Bone pain
Pulmonary	Exertional dyspnea	Dyspnea	Tachypnea, orthopnea, dyspnea at rest
Neurologic	None	"Roaring in the ears"	Headache, vertigo, irritability, depression, impaired thought processes

Clinical Manifestations

The manifestations of anemia are caused by the body's response to tissue hypoxia. Specific manifestations vary depending on how fast the anemia has evolved, its severity, and any coexisting disease. We often use hemoglobin (Hgb) levels to determine the severity of anemia.

Mild anemia (Hgb 10 to 12 g/dL [100 to 120 g/L]) may exist without causing symptoms. If symptoms develop, it is because the patient has an underlying disease or has a compensatory response to heavy exercise. Symptoms include palpitations, dyspnea, and mild fatigue.

In moderate anemia (Hgb 6 to 10 g/dL [60 to 100 g/L]), there is an increase in cardiopulmonary symptoms. The patient may have them while resting, as well as with activity.

In severe anemia (Hgb less than 6 g/dL [60 g/L]), the patient has many manifestations involving multiple body systems (Table 30.3).

Integumentary Manifestations. Skin manifestations include pallor, jaundice, and pruritus. Pallor results from reduced amounts of hemoglobin and reduced blood flow to the skin. Jaundice occurs when hemolysis of RBCs causes increased concentration of serum bilirubin. Hemolysis also causes pruritus because of increased serum and skin bile salt concentrations. Check the sclera of the eyes and mucous membranes for jaundice because they reflect skin changes more accurately, especially in a dark-skinned person.

Cardiopulmonary Manifestations. Cardiopulmonary manifestations of severe anemia result from the heart and lungs trying to provide adequate amounts of oxygen (O_2) to the tissues. Cardiac output is maintained by increasing the heart rate and stroke volume. The low viscosity of the blood contributes to the development of systolic murmurs and bruits. In extreme cases or when concomitant heart disease is present, angina pectoris and myocardial infarction (MI) may occur if myocardial O_2 needs cannot be met. Heart failure (HF), cardiomegaly, pulmonary and systemic congestion, ascites, and peripheral edema may develop if the heart is overworked for an extended period.

❖ NURSING AND INTERPROFESSIONAL MANAGEMENT: ANEMIA

This section discusses general management of anemia. Specific care related to various types of anemia is discussed later in this chapter. More information on the nursing care of the patient with anemia is presented in eNursing Care Plan 30.1.

◆ Nursing Assessment

Subjective and objective data you should obtain from a patient with anemia are outlined in Table 30.4. Assess the patient's knowledge about adequate nutritional intake and adherence to safety precautions to prevent cardiopulmonary stress, falls, and injury.

◆ Nursing Diagnoses

Nursing diagnoses for the patient with anemia include:
- Fatigue
- Impaired nutritional intake
- Ineffective tissue perfusion

◆ Planning

The overall goals are that the patient with anemia will (1) assume normal activities of daily living, (2) maintain adequate nutrition, and (3) develop no complications related to anemia.

◆ Nursing Implementation

Correcting the cause of the anemia is the goal of therapy. The many causes of anemia necessitate different nursing interventions specific to the patient's needs. Acute interventions may include blood transfusions, drug therapy (e.g., erythropoietin, vitamin supplements), and O_2 therapy to stabilize the patient. Dietary and lifestyle changes (described in sections on specific types of anemia) can reverse some anemias.

For the patient with fatigue, encourage alternate rest and activity periods. Help the patient prioritize activities to accommodate energy levels. Arrange physical activities (e.g., avoid activity right after meals) to reduce competition for O_2 supply to vital functions. Aid with regular physical activities (e.g.,

TABLE 30.4 Nursing Assessment
Anemia

Subjective Data	**Objective Data**
Important Health Information	**General**
Past health history: Recent blood loss or trauma; chronic liver, endocrine, or renal disease (including dialysis); GI disease (malabsorption syndrome, ulcers, gastritis, or hemorrhoids); inflammatory disorders (especially Crohn's disease); smoking, exposure to radiation or chemical toxins (arsenic, lead, benzenes, copper); infectious diseases (HIV) or recent travel with possible exposure to infection; angina, myocardial infarction; history of falling	Lethargy, apathy, general lymphadenopathy, fever
	Integumentary
	Pale skin and mucous membranes; blue, pale white, or icteric sclera; cheilitis (inflammation of the lips); poor skin turgor; brittle, spoon-shaped fingernails; jaundice; petechiae; ecchymoses; nose or gingival bleeding; poor healing; dry, brittle, thinning hair
Medications: Use of vitamin and iron supplements; aspirin, anticoagulants, oral contraceptives, phenobarbital, penicillins, nonsteroidal antiinflammatory drugs, omeprazole, phenacetin, phenytoin, sulfonamides, herbal products	**Respiratory**
	Tachypnea
Surgery or other treatments: Recent surgery, small bowel resection, gastrectomy, prosthetic heart valves, chemotherapy, radiation therapy	**Cardiovascular**
Dietary history: General dietary patterns, alcohol consumption	Tachycardia, systolic murmur, dysrhythmias; postural hypotension, widened pulse pressure, bruits (especially carotid); intermittent claudication, ankle edema
Functional Health Patterns	**Gastrointestinal**
Health perception–health management: Family history of anemia; malaise	Hepatosplenomegaly; glossitis; beefy, red tongue; stomatitis; abdominal distention; anorexia
Nutritional-metabolic: Nausea, vomiting, anorexia, weight loss; dysphagia, dyspepsia, heartburn; night sweats, cold intolerance	**Neurologic**
Elimination: Hematuria, decreased urine output; diarrhea, constipation, flatulence, tarry stools, bloody stools	Headache, roaring in the ears, confusion, impaired judgment, irritability, ataxia, unsteady gait, paralysis, loss of vibration sense
Activity-exercise: Fatigue, muscle weakness and decreased strength; dyspnea, orthopnea, cough, hemoptysis; palpitations; shortness of breath with activity	**Possible Diagnostic Findings**
Cognitive-perceptual: Headache; abdominal, chest, and bone pain; painful tongue; paresthesias of feet and hands; pruritus; changes in vision, taste, or hearing; vertigo; hypersensitivity to cold; dizziness	↓ RBCs, ↓ Hgb; ↓ Hct; ↑ or ↓ reticulocytes, ↑ or ↓ MCV; possible ↓ serum iron, ferritin, folate, or cobalamin (vitamin B$_{12}$); heme-positive stools; ↓ serum erythropoietin level; ↑ or ↓ LDH, bilirubin, transferrin (Table 30.6)
Sexuality-reproductive: Menorrhagia, metrorrhagia; recent or current pregnancy; male impotence	

ambulation, transfers, personal care) to minimize fatigue and risk for injury from falls. Monitor the patient's cardiorespiratory response to activity (e.g., tachycardia, dysrhythmias, dyspnea, diaphoresis, pallor, respiratory rate).

Determine, in collaboration with the dietitian, the number of calories and type of nutrients needed to meet nutritional requirements. Provide information about nutritional needs and how to meet them to increase the patient's intake of essential nutrients. Encourage increased intake of foods listed in Table 30.5 that are high in the nutrients needed for erythropoiesis.[2,3]

Gerontologic Considerations: Anemia

Modest changes in RBC mass occur in older adults. Healthy older men have a modest decline in Hgb of about 1 g/dL after age 70, in part because of the decreased production of testosterone. Only a minimal decrease in Hgb (about 0.2 g/dL) occurs in healthy women older than age 70.[1]

Anemia is not a normal finding in older adults. However, the prevalence increases starting from the seventh decade of life. For many, anemia is related to an underlying cause, such as iron deficiency, bleeding, chronic disease/inflammation, renal insufficiency, or a hematologic problem. For those with no identifiable cause, it may be due to cytokine dysregulation with aging.[3]

Manifestations of anemia in older adults may include pallor, confusion, ataxia, fatigue, and worsening cardiovascular and respiratory problems. Unfortunately, anemia may go unrecognized in older adults because we mistake these manifestations for normal aging changes or overlook them because of another health problem. By recognizing signs of anemia, you can play a key role in the care of older adults with anemia.

ANEMIA CAUSED BY DECREASED ERYTHROCYTE PRODUCTION

Normally RBC production (termed *erythropoiesis*) is in equilibrium with RBC destruction and loss. This balance ensures that an adequate number of RBCs is always available. The normal life span of an RBC is 120 days. There are 3 problems that lead to decreased RBC production: (1) decreased hemoglobin synthesis from iron-deficiency anemia, thalassemia, and sideroblastic anemia; (2) defective deoxyribonucleic acid (DNA) synthesis in RBCs (e.g., cobalamin deficiency, folic acid deficiency) may lead to megaloblastic anemias; and (3) diminished availability of erythrocyte precursors may result in aplastic anemia and anemia of chronic disease (Table 30.2).

IRON-DEFICIENCY ANEMIA

Iron-deficiency anemia is the most common nutritional disorder in the world. Those most susceptible to iron-deficiency anemia are the very young, those on poor diets, and women in their reproductive years.[4] Normally, we lose 1 mg of iron daily in urine, bile, sweat, sloughing of epithelial cells from the skin and intestinal mucosa, and minor bleeding.[2]

Etiology

Iron-deficiency anemia may develop because of inadequate dietary intake, malabsorption, blood loss, or hemolysis. Normal dietary iron intake is usually enough to meet the needs of men and older women. It may be inadequate for people with higher iron needs (e.g., menstruating or pregnant women).

TABLE 30.5 Nutritional Therapy

Nutrients for Erythropoiesis

Role in Erythropoiesis	Food Sources
Amino Acids (Protein)	
Heme and plasma membrane synthesis and structure	Eggs, meat, milk and milk products (cheese, ice cream), poultry, fish, legumes, nuts, soy
Cobalamin (Vitamin B$_{12}$)	
Synthesis of DNA, RBC maturation, facilitates folate metabolism	Meat, eggs, enriched grain products, milk and dairy foods, fish (especially salmon)
Copper	
Mobilizes iron from tissues to plasma	Shellfish, whole grains, beans, nuts, potatoes, organ meats, dark leafy greens, dried fruits
Folic Acid	
Synthesis of DNA and RNA, RBC maturation	Green leafy vegetables, enriched grain products and breakfast cereals, orange juice, peanuts, avocado
Iron	
Hemoglobin synthesis	Lean beef, turkey, pork and chicken, fish, legumes, dark green leafy vegetables, whole-grain and enriched bread and cereals, beans
Niacin	
RBC maturation	Peanut butter, beef, poultry, fish, avocado; enriched and fortified grains
Pantothenic Acid (Vitamin B$_5$)	
Heme synthesis	Meats, vegetables, cereal grains, legumes, eggs, milk
Pyridoxine (Vitamin B$_6$)	
Heme synthesis	Beef, pork, chicken, fish, fortified cereals, potatoes, bananas, nuts, beans
Riboflavin (Vitamin B$_2$)	
Oxidative reactions	Milk and dairy foods, enriched bread and other grain products, lean meats, eggs, green leafy vegetables
Vitamin C (Ascorbic Acid)	
Maintains iron in its ferrous form, aids in iron absorption	Citrus fruits, green leafy vegetables, strawberries, potatoes, kiwi fruit, tomatoes, green and red bell peppers
Vitamin E	
Heme synthesis. Protection against oxidative damage to RBCs	Vegetable oils, salad dressings, margarine, wheat germ, whole-grain products, seeds, nuts, peanut butter

Iron malabsorption may occur after certain types of gastrointestinal (GI) surgery and in malabsorption syndromes. Iron absorption occurs in the duodenum. So, malabsorption may occur after a surgical procedure that involves removal or bypass of the duodenum. Or, it may occur if disease of the duodenum alters or destroys the absorption surface.

Blood loss is a major cause of iron deficiency in adults. The major sources of chronic blood loss are from the GI and genitourinary (GU) systems. GI bleeding is often not obvious. It may exist for a considerable time before the problem is identified.

Loss of 50 to 75 mL of blood from the upper GI tract is enough for stools to appear black (*melena*). The black color results from the iron in the RBCs.

Common causes of GI blood loss are peptic ulcer, gastritis, esophagitis, diverticula, hemorrhoids, and cancer. GU blood loss occurs primarily from menstrual bleeding. The average monthly menstrual blood loss is about 45 mL and causes the loss of about 22 mg of iron. Postmenopausal bleeding can contribute to anemia in susceptible older women. In addition to anemia of chronic kidney disease, dialysis treatment may cause iron-deficiency anemia because of the blood lost in the dialysis equipment and frequent blood sampling.

Clinical Manifestations

In the early course of iron-deficiency anemia, the patient may not have any symptoms. As the disease becomes chronic, any of the general manifestations of anemia may develop (Table 30.3). In addition, specific manifestations may occur related to iron-deficiency anemia. Pallor is the most common finding. *Glossitis* (inflammation of the tongue) is the second most common. Another finding is *cheilitis* (inflammation of the lips). The patient may report headache, paresthesias, and a burning sensation of the tongue, all of which are caused by lack of iron in the tissues.

Diagnostic Studies

Laboratory abnormalities characteristic of iron-deficiency anemia are shown in Table 30.6. Other diagnostic studies (e.g., stool occult blood test) are done to determine the cause of the iron deficiency. Endoscopy and colonoscopy may detect GI bleeding. A bone marrow biopsy may be done if other tests are inconclusive.

Interprofessional and Nursing Management

The main goal is to treat the underlying problem that is causing iron loss or reduced intake (e.g., malnutrition, alcoholism) or poor absorption of iron. We also direct efforts toward replacing iron (Table 30.7). Teach the patient which foods are good sources of iron (Table 30.5). If nutrition is already adequate, increasing iron intake by dietary means may not be enough. The patient may need oral, or occasionally, parenteral iron supplements. If the iron deficiency is from acute blood loss, the patient may need a transfusion of packed RBCs.

Drug Therapy. Oral iron is a good option because it is inexpensive and convenient. Many iron preparations are available. When giving iron, consider the following factors:

1. Iron is absorbed best from the duodenum and proximal jejunum. So, enteric-coated or sustained-release capsules, which release iron farther down in the GI tract, are counterproductive and expensive.
2. The daily dose should provide 150 to 200 mg of elemental iron. This can be taken in 3 or 4 daily doses, with each tablet or capsule of the iron preparation containing between 50 and 100 mg of iron (e.g., a 325-mg tablet of ferrous sulfate contains 65 mg of elemental iron).[3]
3. Iron is best absorbed in an acidic environment. For this reason and to avoid binding the iron with food, iron should be taken about an hour before meals, when the duodenal mucosa is most acidic. Taking iron with vitamin C (ascorbic acid) or orange juice, which contains ascorbic acid, enhances iron absorption. Gastric side effects, however, may necessitate taking iron with meals.

TABLE 30.6 Laboratory Results in Anemia

Etiology of Anemia	Hgb/Hct	MCV	Reticulocytes	Serum Iron	TIBC	Transferrin	Ferritin	Bilirubin	Serum B12	Folate
Acute blood loss	↓	N or ↓	N or ↑	N	N	N	N	N	N	N
Aplastic anemia	↓	N or slight ↑	↓	N or ↑	N or ↑	N	N	N	N	N
Chronic blood loss	↓	↓	N or ↑	↓	↑	N	N	N or ↓	N	N
Chronic disease	↓	N or ↓	N or ↓	↓	↓	N	N	N or ↓	N	N
Cobalamin deficiency	↓	↑	N or ↓	N or ↑	N	Slight ↑	↑	N or slight ↑	↓	N
Folic acid deficiency	↓	↑	N or ↓	N or ↑	N	Slight ↑	↑	N or slight ↑	N	↓
Hemolytic anemia	↓	N or ↑	↑	N or ↑	N or ↓	N	N or ↑	↑	N	↓
Iron deficiency	↓	↓	N or slight ↓ or ↑	↓	↑	N or ↓	N or ↑	↑	N	N
Sickle cell anemia	↓	N	↑	N or ↑	N or ↓	N	N	↑	N	N
Thalassemia major	↓	N or ↓	↑	↑	↓	↓	N or ↑	↑	N	↓

MCV, Mean corpuscular volume; *N*, normal; *TIBC*, total iron-binding capacity.

TABLE 30.7 Interprofessional Care

Iron-Deficiency Anemia

Diagnostic Assessment
- History and physical examination
- Hgb and Hct (hematocrit) levels
- RBC count, including morphology
- Reticulocyte count
- Serum iron
- Serum ferritin
- Serum transferrin
- Total iron-binding capacity (TIBC)
- Stool examination for occult blood

Management
- Identification and treatment of underlying cause
- Drug therapy
- Oral: ferrous sulfate or ferrous gluconate
- IM or IV: iron dextran, sodium ferrous gluconate, iron sucrose
- Nutritional therapy (Table 30.5)
- Transfusion of packed RBCs

4. Undiluted liquid iron may stain the patient's teeth. Therefore it should be diluted and ingested through a straw.

5. GI side effects may occur, including heartburn, constipation, and diarrhea. Have the patient stay upright for 30 minutes after taking oral forms. If side effects develop, the dose and type of supplement may be adjusted. For example, many people who need supplemental iron cannot tolerate ferrous sulfate because of the effects of the sulfate base. However, ferrous gluconate may be a better substitute. Tell patients that iron preparations will cause their stools to become black because the GI tract excretes excess iron. Constipation is common. The patient should start on stool softeners and laxatives, if needed, when started on iron.

 DRUG ALERT Iron
- Some IV iron preparations have a risk for an allergic reaction, so monitor the patient accordingly.
- Oral iron should be taken about 1 hr before meals.
- Vitamin C (ascorbic acid) enhances iron absorption.

In some situations, it may be necessary to give iron parenterally. Parenteral use of iron is indicated for malabsorption, intolerance of oral iron, a need for iron beyond oral limits, or poor patient adherence in taking the oral preparations of iron.

Parenteral iron can be given IM or IV. Sodium ferrous gluconate and iron sucrose are alternatives and may carry less risk for life-threatening anaphylaxis.[3]

Because IM iron solutions may stain the skin, use separate needles for withdrawing the solution and injecting the medication. Use a Z-track injection technique.

Reassess the Hgb and RBC count to evaluate the response to therapy. Stress adherence with dietary and drug therapy. To replenish the body's iron stores, the patient needs to take iron therapy for 2 to 3 months after the Hgb level returns to normal. Monitor patients who need lifelong iron supplementation for potential liver problems related to the iron storage.

THALASSEMIA

Etiology

Thalassemia is a group of diseases involving inadequate production of normal hemoglobin, which decreases RBC production. Thalassemia is due to an absent or reduced globulin protein. α-Globin chains are absent or reduced in α-thalassemia, and β-globin chains are absent or reduced in β-thalassemia. Hemolysis also occurs as most erythroblasts are destroyed by mononuclear phagocytes in the marrow.[2] Thalassemia is commonly found in members of ethnic groups whose origins are near the Mediterranean Sea and equatorial or near-equatorial regions of Southeastern Asia, the Middle East, India, Pakistan, China, Southern Russia, and Africa.[3]

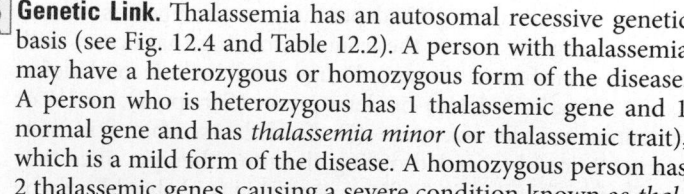 **Genetic Link.** Thalassemia has an autosomal recessive genetic basis (see Fig. 12.4 and Table 12.2). A person with thalassemia may have a heterozygous or homozygous form of the disease. A person who is heterozygous has 1 thalassemic gene and 1 normal gene and has *thalassemia minor* (or thalassemic trait), which is a mild form of the disease. A homozygous person has 2 thalassemic genes, causing a severe condition known as *thalassemia major*.[3]

Clinical Manifestations

The patient with thalassemia minor is often asymptomatic. The patient has mild to moderate anemia with *microcytosis* (small cells) and *hypochromia* (pale cells), mild splenomegaly, bronzed color of the skin, and bone marrow hyperplasia.[2]

Thalassemia major is a life-threatening disease in which growth, both physical and mental, is often slowed. The person with thalassemia major is pale and displays other general symptoms of anemia (Table 30.3). The symptoms develop in childhood by 2 years of age and can cause growth and developmental deficits. Jaundice from the hemolysis of RBCs is prominent. There is pronounced splenomegaly, since the spleen continuously tries to remove the damaged red cells. Hepatomegaly and cardiomyopathy may occur from iron deposition.

INFORMATICS IN PRACTICE

Using the Internet to Access Information on Unfamiliar Diseases

- If you are assigned to take care of a patient with a disease or disorder that you are not familiar with, such as thalassemia, access a reputable source on the Internet, such as the National Institutes of Health, and do a quick search.
- Within minutes, you can learn the pathophysiology of thalassemia or other disease, treatment options, complications that you will need to monitor, and recommended medical and nursing interventions.
- Using this readily available information will help you deliver high-quality, evidence-based care.

As the bone marrow responds to the reduced O_2-carrying capacity of the blood, RBC production is stimulated. The marrow becomes packed with immature erythroid precursors that die. This stimulates further erythropoiesis, leading to chronic bone marrow hyperplasia and expansion of the marrow space. This may cause thickening of the cranium and maxillary cavity. Thrombocytosis after spleen dysfunction and/or removal may occur.

Cardiac complications from iron overload, lung disease, and hypertension also contribute to early death. Endocrine problems (diabetes, growth retardation, hypogonadism), osteoporosis, pulmonary hypertension, and thrombosis may be present.[1]

Interprofessional Care

The laboratory abnormalities of thalassemia major are outlined in Table 30.6. No specific drug or diet therapies are effective in treating thalassemia. Thalassemia minor does not need treatment because the body adapts to the reduction of normal hemoglobin.

Thalassemia major is managed with blood transfusions or exchange transfusions in conjunction with chelating agents that bind to iron. Transfusions are given to keep the Hgb level around 10 g/dL (100 g/L), depending on the manifestations.[1] Chelating agents reduce the iron overloading that occurs with chronic transfusion therapy. Drugs used include oral deferasirox (Exjade, JadeNu) or deferiprone (Ferriprox), or IV or subcutaneous deferoxamine (Desferal).[1] Ascorbic acid supplements may be needed during chelation therapy, since they increase urine excretion of iron. Ascorbic acid should only be taken with chelation therapy because it increases the absorption of dietary iron. It is given, along with folic acid, if there is evidence of hemolysis. Zinc supplements may be needed since zinc is reduced with chelation therapy. Iron supplements should not be given.

Because RBCs are sequestered in the enlarged spleen, the patient may need a splenectomy. Hepatic, heart, and lung function are monitored and treated as needed.

Although hematopoietic stem cell transplantation (HSCT) is the only cure for patients with thalassemia, the risk of this procedure may outweigh its benefits. With proper iron chelation therapy, patients are living longer.

TABLE 30.8 Causes of Megaloblastic Anemia

Cobalamin (Vitamin B$_{12}$) Deficiency
- Chronic alcoholism
- Dietary deficiency
- Deficiency of gastric intrinsic factor
  - Celiac disease
  - Gastrectomy
  - Gastric bypass
  - *Helicobacter pylori*
  - Pernicious anemia
- Increased requirement (pregnancy)
- Intestinal malabsorption

Folic Acid Deficiency
- Chronic alcoholism
- Chronic hemodialysis (folic acid lost during dialysis)
- Dietary deficiency (e.g., leafy green vegetables, citrus fruits)
- Drugs interfering with absorption or use of folic acid
  - Methotrexate
  - Antiseizure drugs (e.g., phenobarbital, phenytoin)
- Increased requirement (pregnancy)
- Malabsorption syndromes
  - Celiac disease
  - Crohn's disease
  - Small bowel resection

Drug-Induced Suppression of DNA Synthesis
- Alkylating agents
- Folate antagonists
- Metabolic inhibitors

Inborn Errors
- Defective folate metabolism
- Defective transport of cobalamin

Erythroleukemia

MEGALOBLASTIC ANEMIAS

Megaloblastic anemias are a group of disorders caused by impaired DNA synthesis and characterized by the presence of large RBCs. When DNA synthesis is impaired, defective RBC maturation results. The RBCs are large *(macrocytic)* and abnormal. We call them *megaloblasts*. Macrocytic RBCs are easily destroyed because they have fragile cell membranes. Most megaloblastic anemias result from cobalamin (vitamin B$_{12}$) and folic acid deficiencies. They can also occur from congenital disorders, suppression of DNA synthesis by drugs, inborn errors of cobalamin and folic acid metabolism, and *erythroleukemia* (malignant blood disorder characterized by a proliferation of erythropoietic cells in bone marrow) (Table 30.8).[5]

Cobalamin Deficiency

The most common cause of cobalamin deficiency is pernicious anemia. It is caused by an absence of *intrinsic factor* (IF). Pernicious anemia is a disease of insidious onset. It begins in middle age or later (usually after age 40), with 60 years being the most common age at diagnosis. Pernicious anemia occurs most often in persons of Northern European ancestry (particularly Scandinavians) and blacks.[1]

Etiology

Normally, the parietal cells of the gastric mucosa secrete a protein termed *IF*. IF is required for cobalamin (extrinsic factor) absorption. Cobalamin is normally absorbed in the distal ileum. Without IF, cobalamin will not be absorbed. In pernicious anemia, the gastric mucosa is not secreting IF because of either gastric mucosal atrophy or autoimmune destruction of parietal cells. In the autoimmune process, antibodies are directed against the gastric parietal cells and/or IF itself. Because parietal cells also secrete hydrochloric acid (HCl), in pernicious anemia there is a decrease in HCl in the stomach. An acid environment in the stomach is required for the secretion of IF.

Cobalamin deficiency can occur in patients who have had GI surgery (e.g., gastrectomy, gastric bypass); patients who have had a small bowel resection involving the ileum; and patients with Crohn's disease, ileitis, celiac disease, diverticula of the small intestine, or chronic atrophic gastritis (Table 30.8). In these cases, cobalamin deficiency results from the loss of IF-secreting gastric mucosal cells or impaired absorption of cobalamin in the distal ileum. Cobalamin deficiency also occurs with excess alcohol or hot tea ingestion, smoking, long-term users of H_2-histamine receptor blockers and proton pump inhibitors, and those who are strict vegetarians.[2]

There is a familial predisposition for pernicious anemia, so evaluate patients who have a positive family history of pernicious anemia for symptoms. Although the disease cannot be prevented, early detection and treatment can lead to reversal of symptoms.

Clinical Manifestations

General manifestations of anemia related to cobalamin deficiency develop because of tissue hypoxia (Table 30.3). GI manifestations include a sore, red, beefy, and shiny tongue; anorexia, nausea, and vomiting; and abdominal pain. Typical neuromuscular manifestations include weakness, paresthesias of the feet and hands, reduced vibratory and position senses, ataxia, muscle weakness, and impaired thought processes ranging from confusion to dementia. Because cobalamin deficiency–related anemia has an insidious onset, it may take several months for manifestations to develop.

Diagnostic Studies

Laboratory data reflective of cobalamin-deficiency anemia are outlined in Table 30.6. The RBCs appear large (macrocytic) and have abnormal shapes. This structure contributes to RBC destruction because the cell membrane is fragile. Serum cobalamin levels are low.

Serum folate levels are reviewed. If they are normal and cobalamin levels are low, it suggests that megaloblastic anemia is due to a cobalamin deficiency. A serum test for anti-IF antibodies may be done that is specific for pernicious anemia. Patients with pernicious anemia have an increased risk for gastric cancer. They may undergo an upper GI endoscopy and biopsy of the gastric mucosa at the time of diagnosis and at appropriate intervals afterward.

Testing of serum methylmalonic acid (MMA) (high in cobalamin deficiency) and serum homocysteine (high in both cobalamin and folic acid deficiencies) helps determine the cause of this type of anemia.

❖ Interprofessional and Nursing Management

If IF is lacking or if absorption in the ileum is impaired, the patient will not be able to absorb cobalamin regardless of how much they ingest. For this reason, increasing dietary cobalamin does not correct this anemia. Parenteral vitamin B_{12}

(cyanocobalamin, hydroxocobalamin) or intranasal cyanocobalamin (Nascobal) is needed. Without cobalamin administration, the patient will die in 1 to 3 years. A typical treatment schedule consists of 1000 mcg/day of cobalamin IM for 2 weeks and then weekly until the hemoglobin is normal and then monthly for life.

High-dose oral cobalamin and sublingual cobalamin are options for those in whom GI absorption is intact.

The nursing measures discussed in eNursing Care Plan 30.1 for the patient with anemia are appropriate for the patient with cobalamin-deficiency anemia. In addition to these measures, assess for neurologic difficulties that are not fully corrected by replacement therapy. Implement measures to reduce the risk for injury from the decreased sensitivity to heat and pain related to neurologic impairment. Protect the patient from falling, burns, and trauma. In some people, the neuromuscular complications may not be reversible and physical therapy may be needed.

Folic Acid Deficiency

Folic acid (folate) deficiency also causes megaloblastic anemia. Folic acid is needed for DNA synthesis leading to RBC formation and maturation. Common causes of folic acid deficiency are listed in Table 30.8.

The manifestations of folic acid deficiency are similar to those of cobalamin deficiency. The disease develops insidiously. The patient's symptoms may be attributed to other coexisting problems (e.g., cirrhosis, esophageal varices). GI problems may include stomatitis, cheilosis, dysphagia, flatulence, and diarrhea. Thiamine deficiency, which is often present with folate deficiency, can cause neurologic symptoms.[2]

The diagnostic findings for folic acid deficiency are shown in Table 30.6. The serum folate level is low (normal is 5 to 25 ng/mL [11 to 57 nmol/L]), with a normal serum cobalamin level.

We treat folic acid deficiency with replacement therapy. The usual dosage is 1 mg/day by mouth. The patient with malabsorption or chronic alcoholism may need up to 5 mg/day. The duration of treatment depends on the reason for the deficiency. Teach the patient to eat foods high in folic acid (Table 30.5). The nursing measures discussed in eNursing Care Plan 30.1 for the patient with anemia are appropriate for the patient with folic acid deficiency anemia.

ANEMIA OF CHRONIC DISEASE

Anemia of chronic disease (also called *anemia of inflammation*) can be caused by cancer, autoimmune and infectious disorders (human immunodeficiency virus [HIV], hepatitis, malaria), HF, or chronic inflammation. Bleeding episodes can contribute to anemia of chronic disease.

Anemia of chronic disease is associated with an underproduction of RBCs and mild shortening of RBC survival. The RBCs are usually normocytic, normochromic, and hypoproliferative. The anemia is usually mild. It can become more severe if the underlying disorder is not treated.

This type of anemia, which usually develops after 1 to 2 months of disease activity, has an immune basis. The cytokines released in these conditions, particularly interleukin-6 (IL-6), cause an increased uptake and retention of iron within macrophages (see Fig. 29.3). This leads to a diversion of iron from circulation into storage sites with subsequent limited iron available for erythropoiesis. There is reduced RBC life span, suppressed production of erythropoietin, and an ineffective bone marrow response to erythropoietin. We think cytokine dysregulation may be the cause of this type of anemia in elderly and obese patients when no other cause can be found.[6]

For any chronic disease, other factors may contribute to the anemia. For example, with renal disease, the primary factor causing anemia is decreased erythropoietin, a hormone made in the kidneys that stimulates erythropoiesis. With impaired renal function, erythropoietin production is decreased (see Chapter 46).

Anemia of chronic disease must first be recognized and distinguished from anemia of other causes. High serum ferritin and increased iron stores distinguish it from iron-deficiency anemia. Normal folate and cobalamin blood levels distinguish it from megaloblastic anemias from folate and cobalamin deficiencies.

The best treatment of anemia of chronic disease is to correct the underlying disorder. If the anemia is severe, blood transfusions may be needed, but they are not recommended for long-term treatment. Erythropoietin therapy is used for anemia related to renal disease (see Chapter 46) and cancer and its therapies (see Chapter 15). Its use is limited, though, because of the increased risk for thromboembolism and death in some patients.

APLASTIC ANEMIA

Aplastic anemia is a disease in which the patient has peripheral blood *pancytopenia* (decrease of all blood cell types—RBCs, white blood cells [WBCs], and platelets) and hypocellular bone marrow. The spectrum can range from a moderate condition managed with erythropoietin or blood transfusions to very severe with potentially fatal hemorrhage and sepsis. The incidence of aplastic anemia is rare, with an annual rate of 2 to 5 new cases per million per year.[3]

Etiology

About 70% of aplastic anemias are due to autoimmune activity by autoreactive T lymphocytes.[3] The cytotoxic T cells target and destroy the patient's own hematopoietic stem cells. Other anemias may be acquired from toxic injury to bone marrow stem cells or result from an inherited stem cell defect (Table 30.9).

Clinical Manifestations

Aplastic anemia can manifest abruptly (over days) or insidiously over weeks to months. It can vary from mild to very severe. The patient may have symptoms caused by suppression of any or all bone marrow elements. General manifestations of anemia, such as fatigue and dyspnea, as well as cardiovascular and cerebral

---

TABLE 30.9 Causes of Aplastic Anemia

- Chemical agents and toxins (e.g., benzene, insecticides, arsenic, alcohol)
- Drugs (e.g., alkylating agents, antiseizure drugs, antimetabolites, antimicrobials, gold, nonsteroidal antiinflammatory drugs, antithyroid medications, allopurinol)
- Immune suppression of stem cells by autoreactive T-lymphocytes
- Inherited stem cell defect (e.g., Fanconi anemia)
- Radiation
- Toxic injury to bone marrow stem cells
- Viral and bacterial infections

---

responses, may be seen (Table 30.3). The patient with neutropenia (low neutrophil count) is susceptible to infection and is at risk for septic shock and death. Thrombocytopenia is manifested by a predisposition to bleeding (e.g., petechiae, bruising, nosebleeds).

Diagnostic Studies

Laboratory studies confirm the diagnosis. Because aplastic anemia affects all marrow elements, hemoglobin, WBC, and platelet values are decreased. Other RBC indices are generally normal (Table 30.6). The condition is therefore classified as a normocytic, normochromic anemia. The reticulocyte count is low.

We can further evaluate aplastic anemia by assessing various iron studies. The serum iron and total iron-binding capacity (TIBC) may be high as initial signs of erythropoiesis suppression. Bone marrow biopsy, aspiration, and pathologic examination may be done. The marrow in aplastic anemia is hypocellular with increased yellow marrow (fat content).

❖ Interprofessional and Nursing Management

Management of aplastic anemia is based on identifying and removing the causative agent (when possible) and providing supportive care until the pancytopenia reverses. Nursing interventions appropriate for the patient with pancytopenia from aplastic anemia are discussed in eNursing Care Plan 30.1 for anemia, eNursing Care Plan 30.2 for thrombocytopenia, and eNursing Care Plan 30.3 for neutropenia (available on the website for this chapter). Nursing actions are directed at preventing complications from infection and hemorrhage.

The prognosis of severe untreated aplastic anemia is poor. However, advances in medical management, including HSCT and immunosuppressive therapy with antithymocyte globulin (ATG), steroids, and cyclosporine or cyclophosphamide, have improved outcomes significantly.[7] ATG is a horse serum that contains polyclonal antibodies against human T cells. ATG and cyclosporine are discussed in Chapter 13. Eltrombopag (Promacta), an oral thrombopoietin receptor agonist, can increase platelet counts. High-dose cyclophosphamide, alemtuzumab, or androgens may be helpful in select patients who do not respond to other therapies.[1]

The treatment of choice for adults younger than 55 years of age who do not respond to the immunosuppressive therapy and who have a human leukocyte antigen (HLA)–matched, half-matched, or unrelated donor, is an HSCT.[7] The best results occur in younger patients who have not had previous blood transfusions. Prior transfusions increase the risk for graft rejection. HSCT is discussed in Chapter 15.

For older adults without a donor, the treatment of choice is immunosuppression with ATG and cyclosporine, steroids, and eltrombopag.[3] Patients who need ongoing supportive blood transfusion should be on an iron-binding agent to prevent iron overload.

ANEMIA CAUSED BY BLOOD LOSS

An acute or chronic problem can cause anemia from blood loss.

ACUTE BLOOD LOSS

Acute blood loss occurs because of sudden hemorrhage. Causes of acute blood loss include trauma, complications of surgery, and conditions or diseases that disrupt vascular integrity. There

TABLE 30.10 Manifestations of Acute Blood Loss

VOLUME LOST*		
%	mL	Manifestations
10	500	None or rare vasovagal syncope
20	1000	No detectable signs or symptoms at rest. Tachycardia with exercise and slight postural hypotension
30	1500	Normal supine blood pressure and pulse at rest. Postural hypotension and tachycardia with exercise
40	2000	BP, central venous pressure, and cardiac output below normal at rest; air hunger; rapid, thready pulse and cold, clammy skin
50	2500	Shock, lactic acidosis, and potential death

*Based on an adult with a total blood volume of 5 L.

are 2 clinical concerns in such situations. First, a sudden reduction in the total blood volume can lead to hypovolemic shock. Second, if the acute loss is more gradual, the body maintains its blood volume by slowly increasing the plasma volume. Although this preserves circulating fluid volume, the number of RBCs available to carry O_2 is significantly decreased.

Clinical Manifestations

The manifestations of anemia from acute blood loss are caused by the body's attempts to maintain an adequate blood volume and meet O_2 requirements. Table 30.10 outlines the manifestations of patients with varying degrees of blood volume loss. It is essential to understand that the signs and symptoms the patient has are more important than the laboratory values. For example, an adult with a bleeding peptic ulcer who had a 750-mL hematemesis (15% of a normal total blood volume) within the past 30 minutes may have postural hypotension but have normal values for hemoglobin and hematocrit. Over the next 36 to 48 hours, most of the blood volume deficit will be replaced by the movement of fluid from the extravascular into the intravascular space. Only then will the hemoglobin and hematocrit reflect the blood loss.

Assess the patient's expression of pain. Internal hemorrhage may cause pain because of tissue distention, organ displacement, and nerve compression. Pain may be localized or referred. In the case of retroperitoneal bleeding, the patient may not have abdominal pain. Instead the patient may have numbness and pain in a lower extremity from compression of the lateral cutaneous nerve, which is in the region of the first to third lumbar vertebrae. The major complication of acute blood loss is shock (see Chapter 66).

Diagnostic Studies

When blood volume loss is sudden, plasma volume has not yet had a chance to increase. The loss of RBCs is not reflected in laboratory data, and values may seem normal or high for 2 to 3 days. However, once the plasma volume is replaced, the RBC mass is less concentrated. Then, RBC, hemoglobin, and hematocrit levels are low and reflect the actual blood loss.

❖ Interprofessional and Nursing Management

Interprofessional care is initially concerned with (1) replacing blood volume to prevent shock and (2) finding the source of

the hemorrhage and stopping the blood loss. IV fluids used in emergencies include dextran, hetastarch, albumin, and crystalloid electrolyte solutions, such as lactated Ringer's solution. The amount of infusion varies with the solution used. Blood transfusions (packed RBCs) can be used depending on the volume lost. If a large volume of blood is lost, platelets, plasma, and cryoprecipitate may be needed because large volumes of RBCs dilutes the patient's own coagulation system. (See more on managing shock in Chapter 66.)

The body needs 2 to 5 days to make more RBCs in response to increased erythropoietin. The patient may need supplemental iron because the availability of iron affects the marrow production of RBCs. When anemia exists after acute blood loss, dietary sources of iron will probably not be enough to maintain iron stores. Therefore oral or parenteral iron preparations are given.

In the case of trauma, it may be impossible to prevent blood loss. For the postoperative patient, carefully monitor the blood loss from various drainage tubes and dressings and implement appropriate actions. The nursing care for the patient with anemia resulting from acute blood loss will likely include giving blood products (described at the end of this chapter on pp. 647–651).

The anemia should begin to correct itself once the source of hemorrhage is found, blood loss is controlled, and fluid and blood volumes are replaced. There should be no need for long-term treatment of this type of anemia.

CHRONIC BLOOD LOSS

The sources of chronic blood loss are similar to those of iron-deficiency anemia (e.g., bleeding ulcer, hemorrhoids, menstrual and postmenopausal blood loss). The effects of chronic blood loss are usually related to the depletion of iron stores and considered an iron-deficiency anemia. Management of chronic blood loss anemia involves identifying the source and stopping the bleeding. Supplemental iron may be needed.

ANEMIA CAUSED BY INCREASED ERYTHROCYTE DESTRUCTION

The third major cause of anemia is hemolytic anemia, a condition caused by the destruction or hemolysis of RBCs at a rate that exceeds production. Hemolysis can occur because of problems intrinsic or extrinsic to the RBCs. *Intrinsic hemolytic anemias,* which are usually hereditary, result from defects in the RBCs themselves (Table 30.2).

More common are the *acquired hemolytic anemias.* In this type of anemia, the RBCs are normal, but external factors are causing damage (Table 30.2). Macrophages, particularly those in the spleen, liver, and bone marrow, destroy RBCs that are old, defective, or moderately damaged. Fig. 30.2 shows the sequence of events involved in extravascular hemolysis.

The patient with hemolytic anemia has the general manifestations of anemia and specific manifestations related to this type of anemia (Table 30.3). Jaundice is likely because the increased destruction of RBCs causes an elevation in bilirubin levels. The spleen and liver may enlarge because of their hyperactivity, which is related to macrophage phagocytosis of the defective RBCs.

In all causes of hemolysis, a major focus of treatment is to maintain renal function. When RBCs are hemolyzed, the

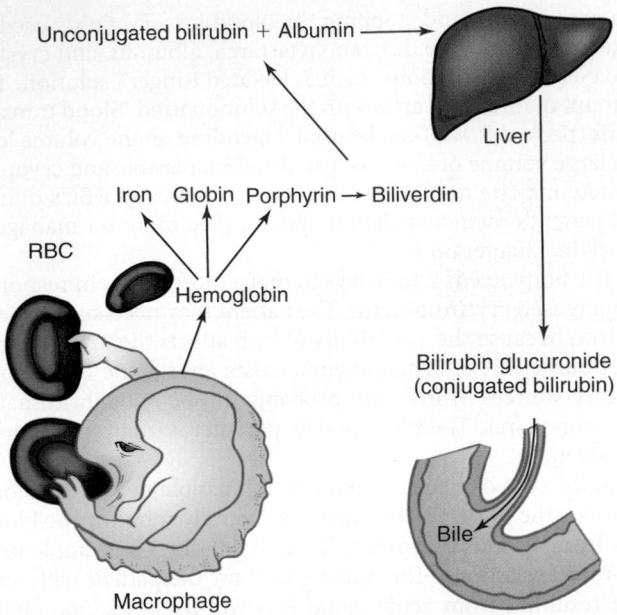

FIG. 30.2 Sequence of events in extravascular hemolysis.

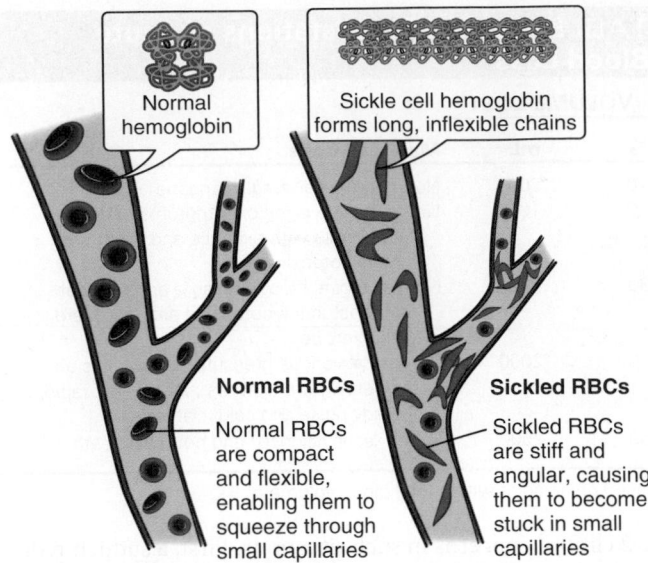

FIG. 30.3 In sickle cell, the hemoglobin forms long inflexible chains and alters the shape of the red blood cells (RBCs). The sickled RBCs can become stuck in the capillaries and occlude the blood flow.

hemoglobin molecule is released and filtered by the kidneys. The accumulation of hemoglobin molecules can obstruct the renal tubules and lead to acute tubular necrosis (see Chapter 46).

SICKLE CELL DISEASE

Sickle cell disease (SCD) is a group of inherited, autosomal recessive disorders characterized by an abnormal form of hemoglobin in the RBC. Because this is a genetic disorder, SCD is usually found during routine neonatal screening. Although median survival can now exceed 45 years old, the disease often results in irreversible damage of the lungs, kidneys, brain, retina, or bones that significantly affects patients' quality of life.[8]

Etiology and Pathophysiology

Genetic Link. In SCD, the abnormal hemoglobin, *hemoglobin S* (Hgb S), results from the substitution of valine for glutamic acid on the β-globin chain of hemoglobin (see Fig. 12.3). Hgb S causes the RBC to stiffen and elongate, taking on a sickle shape in response to low O_2 levels (Fig. 30.3).

Types of SCD disorders include sickle cell anemia, sickle cell–thalassemia, sickle cell Hgb C disease, and sickle cell trait. *Sickle cell anemia* is the most severe of the SCD syndromes. It occurs when a person is homozygous for hemoglobin S (Hgb SS), meaning the person has inherited Hgb S from both parents. *Sickle cell–thalassemia* and *sickle cell Hgb C* occur when a person inherits Hgb S from one parent and another type of abnormal hemoglobin (such as thalassemia or Hgb C) from the other parent. Both these forms of SCD are less common and less severe than sickle cell anemia. *Sickle cell trait* occurs when a person is heterozygous for hemoglobin S (Hgb AS). This means the person has inherited hemoglobin S from one parent and normal hemoglobin (Hgb A) from the other parent. Sickle cell trait is typically a mild to asymptomatic condition.

🧬 GENETICS IN CLINICAL PRACTICE

Sickle Cell Disease[9]

Genetic Basis
- Autosomal recessive disorder
- Mutation in β-globin *(HBB)* gene found on chromosome 11
- Various versions of β-globin result from different mutations in the *HBB* gene
- Hgb S variant involves substitution of valine for glutamic acid in the β-globin gene

Incidence
- Most common inherited blood disorder in the United States
- Affects about 100,000 Americans
- Occurs in about 1 of every 365 African American births
- Occurs in about 1 of every 16,300 Hispanic American births
- Affects people of Mediterranean, Caribbean, Arabian, and East Indian descent
- 1 in 13 African American babies is born with sickle cell trait

Genetic Testing
- DNA testing is available
- Electrophoresis of hemoglobin and sickling screening test are most often used

Clinical Implications
- Sickle cell trait is the carrier state for SCD and is a mild type of SCD
- If both parents have the trait, there is a 1 in 4 chance that their baby will have SCD
- Genetic counseling is recommended for people with a family history of SCD so they can understand the risks for transmitting the genetic mutation

Sickling Episodes. The major pathophysiologic event of SCD is the sickling of RBCs (Fig. 30.3). Sickling episodes are most often triggered by low O_2 tension in the blood. Hypoxia or deoxygenation of the RBCs can be caused by viral or bacterial infection, high altitude, emotional or physical stress, surgery, and blood loss. Infection is the most common precipitating factor. Other events that can trigger or sustain a sickling episode include dehydration, increased hydrogen ion concentration (acidosis), increased plasma osmolality, decreased plasma volume, and low body temperature. A sickling episode can also occur without an obvious cause.

Sickled RBCs become rigid and take on an elongated, crescent shape (Fig. 30.3). Sickled cells cannot easily pass through capillaries or other small vessels and can cause vascular occlusion, leading to acute or chronic tissue injury. The resulting hemostasis promotes a self-perpetuating cycle of local hypoxia, deoxygenation of more RBCs, and more sickling. Circulating sickled cells are hemolyzed by the spleen, leading to anemia. At first, sickling is reversible with reoxygenation. It eventually becomes irreversible because of cell membrane damage from recurrent sickling. Vaso-occlusive phenomena and hemolysis are the clinical hallmarks of SCD.

Sickle cell crisis is a severe, painful, acute exacerbation of RBC sickling, causing a vaso-occlusive crisis. As sickled cells impair blood flow, vasospasm occurs, further restricting blood flow. Severe capillary hypoxia causes changes in membrane permeability, leading to plasma loss, hemoconcentration, thrombi, and further circulatory stagnation. Tissue ischemia, infarction, and necrosis eventually occur from lack of O_2. Shock is a possible life-threatening consequence of sickle cell crisis because of severe O_2 depletion of the tissues and a reduction of the circulating fluid volume. Sickle cell crisis can begin suddenly and persist for days to weeks.

The frequency, extent, and severity of sickling episodes are highly variable and unpredictable. They depend on the percent of Hgb S present. People with sickle cell anemia have the most severe form because the RBCs have a high percent of Hgb S.

Clinical Manifestations

The effects of SCD vary from person to person, the severity of which may be due to genetic variants. Many people with sickle cell anemia are in reasonably good health most of the time. However, they may have chronic health problems and pain because of organ tissue hypoxia and damage (e.g., involving the kidneys or liver).

The typical patient is anemic but asymptomatic except during sickling episodes. Because most people with sickle cell anemia have dark skin, pallor is easier to detect by examining the mucous membranes. The skin may have a grayish cast. Because of the hemolysis, jaundice is common, and patients are prone to gallstones (cholelithiasis).

The main symptom associated with sickling is pain. The pain severity can range from trivial to excruciating. During sickle cell crisis, the pain is severe because of ischemia of tissue. The episodes can affect any area of the body or several sites simultaneously. The back, chest, extremities, and abdomen are affected most often. Pain episodes are often accompanied by other manifestations, such as fever, swelling, tenderness, tachypnea, hypertension, nausea, and vomiting.

Complications

With repeated episodes of sickling, there is gradual involvement of all body systems, especially the spleen, lungs, kidneys, and brain. Organs that need large amounts of O_2 are most often affected and form the basis for many of the complications of SCD (Fig. 30.4). Infection is a major cause of morbidity and mortality in patients with SCD. One reason for this is the failure of the spleen to phagocytize foreign substances as it becomes infarcted and dysfunctional (usually by 2 to 4 years of age) from the sickled RBCs. The spleen becomes small because of repeated scarring, a phenomenon termed *autosplenectomy.*

Pneumonia is the most common infection and often is of pneumococcal origin. Infections can be so severe that they cause an aplastic and hemolytic crisis and gallstones. *Aplastic crisis* can be so severe that it causes a temporary shutdown of RBC production in the bone marrow.

Acute chest syndrome is a term used to describe acute pulmonary complications that include pneumonia, tissue infarction, and fat embolism. It is characterized by fever, chest pain, cough, lung infiltrates, and dyspnea. Pulmonary infarctions may cause pulmonary hypertension, MI, and cor pulmonale. The heart may become ischemic and enlarged, leading to HF. Retinal vessel obstruction may result in hemorrhage, scarring, retinal detachment, and blindness. The increased blood viscosity and the lack of O_2 can injure the kidneys. Renal failure may occur. Pulmonary embolism or stroke can result from thrombosis and infarction of cerebral blood vessels. Bone changes may include osteoporosis and osteosclerosis after infarction. Chronic leg ulcers can result from the hypoxia and are especially prevalent around the ankles. *Priapism* (persistent penile erection) may occur if penile veins become occluded.

Diagnostic Studies

A peripheral blood smear may reveal sickled cells and increased, abnormal reticulocytes. Hemoglobin electrophoresis may be done to determine the amount of hemoglobin S and SCD from other variants.

Because of the accelerated RBC breakdown, the patient has characteristic findings of hemolysis (jaundice, high serum bilirubin levels) and abnormal laboratory test results (Table 30.6). Skeletal x-rays show bone and joint deformities and flattening. MRI can diagnose a stroke caused by blocked cerebral vessels from sickled cells. Doppler studies can assess for deep vein thromboses (DVT). A chest x-ray can diagnose infection or organ malfunction.

❖ Interprofessional and Nursing Management

Interprofessional care for a patient with SCD is directed toward (1) preventing sequelae from the disease; (2) alleviating the manifestations from the complications of the disease; (3) minimizing end-organ damage; and (4) continuously assessing for and promptly treating serious sequelae, such as acute chest syndrome, that can lead to immediate death.[8]

A patient in sickle cell crisis may need hospitalization. O_2 therapy treats hypoxia and controls sickling. Assess for any changes in respiratory status and encourage incentive spirometry. Rest can reduce metabolic requirements. DVT prophylaxis (using anticoagulants) should be prescribed. Fluids are given to reduce blood viscosity and maintain renal function. Priapism is managed with pain medication, fluids, and nifedipine (Procardia). If it does not resolve within a few hours, a urologist may be called.[10]

Transfusion therapy is indicated when an aplastic crisis occurs. Aggressive RBC exchange transfusion programs may be implemented for patients who have frequent crises or serious complications, such as acute chest syndrome. These patients, like those with thalassemia major, may need iron chelation therapy to reduce transfusion-produced iron overload.

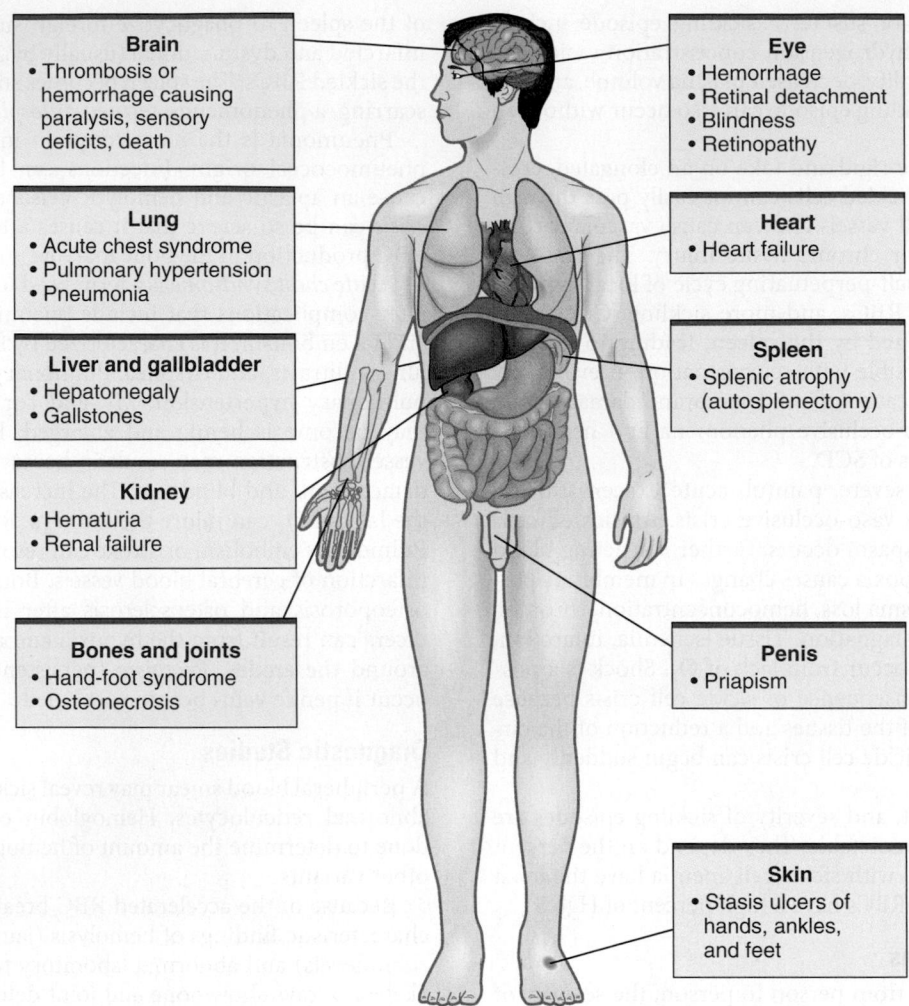

Brain
- Thrombosis or hemorrhage causing paralysis, sensory deficits, death

Lung
- Acute chest syndrome
- Pulmonary hypertension
- Pneumonia

Liver and gallbladder
- Hepatomegaly
- Gallstones

Kidney
- Hematuria
- Renal failure

Bones and joints
- Hand-foot syndrome
- Osteonecrosis

Eye
- Hemorrhage
- Retinal detachment
- Blindness
- Retinopathy

Heart
- Heart failure

Spleen
- Splenic atrophy (autosplenectomy)

Penis
- Priapism

Skin
- Stasis ulcers of hands, ankles, and feet

FIG. 30.4 Clinical manifestations and complications of sickle cell disease. (Modified from McCance KL, Huether SE: *Pathophysiology: The biologic basis for disease in adults and children,* ed 7, St Louis, 2014, Mosby.)

❓ CHECK YOUR PRACTICE

A 21-year-old African American woman was just admitted to the emergency department (ED) after a ski trip to Colorado. She is in excruciating pain in her chest and abdomen. She is short of breath and her O₂ saturation is 86%. Your examination reveals that her heart rate is 110 bpm and respiratory rate 28/minute. She has crackles in the lungs. She has had 6 previous ED admissions for sickle cell crises.
- What are your priorities for her nursing care?

Undertreatment of sickle cell pain is a major problem. Lack of understanding can lead HCPs to underestimate the severity of acute and chronic pain. SCD patients may develop tolerance, and larger doses of pain medication may be needed to reduce pain to a tolerable level. During an acute crisis, optimal pain control usually includes large doses of continuous (rather than as-needed) opioid analgesics, along with breakthrough analgesia, often in the form of patient-controlled analgesia (PCA). Morphine and hydromorphone are the drugs of choice.

Because patients may be having different types and sites of pain, as well as acute and chronic pain, a holistic approach should be used that addresses the pain and its impact on the patient's quality of life (see Chapter 8).[8] In addition to opioids, adjunctive measures, such as nonsteroidal antiinflammatory agents, antineuropathic pain drugs (e.g., antidepressants, antiseizure drugs), local anesthetics, or nerve blocks may be used. Occupational and physical therapy can optimize functioning. Referral to social and chaplain services can help address social, emotional, and spiritual needs.

Infection is a frequent complication. Any febrile illness in a patient with SCD is an emergency. Infections, such as chronic leg ulcers, may be treated with rest, antibiotics, warm saline soaks, mechanical or enzyme debridement, and grafting, if needed. Patients with acute chest syndrome are treated with broad-spectrum antibiotics, O₂ therapy, fluid therapy, and possibly exchange transfusion. Blood transfusions are done sparingly between crises since patients develop antibodies to RBCs and iron overload. Because chronic hemolysis results in increased use of folic acid stores, the patient should take an oral folic acid supplement.

Hydroxyurea (Hydrea) is the only medication that is clinically beneficial. This drug increases the production of hemoglobin F (fetal hemoglobin) and alters the adhesion of sickled RBCs to the endothelium. The increase in Hgb F is accompanied by a reduction in hemolysis, an increase in hemoglobin concentration, and a decrease in sickled cells and painful crises.[10] Dietary supplementation with oral glutamine, an amino acid, can reduce the number and frequency of pain crises and hospitalizations.[11]

HSCT is the only available treatment that can cure some patients with SCD but is not widely available. The selection of appropriate recipients, scarcity of appropriate donors, risk, and cost-effectiveness limit its use. (HSCT is discussed in Chapter 15.) Gene therapy approaches are under investigation.[8]

Patient teaching and support are important in the long-term care of the patient with SCD. The patient and caregiver must understand the basis of the disease and the reasons for supportive care and ongoing pertinent screening tailored to SCD manifestations. Teach the patient ways to avoid crises. Review steps to avoid dehydration and hypoxia, such as avoiding high altitudes and seeking medical attention quickly to counteract problems, such as upper respiratory tract infections. Teach patients to maintain adequate fluid intake. Immunizations, such as pneumococcal, *H. influenzae*, influenza, and hepatitis, should be given. Screening for retinopathy should begin at age 10. Each person with SCD should have a reproductive life plan.[10] Teaching about pain control is needed because the pain during a crisis may be severe and often requires considerable analgesia. Minor pain episodes that are not associated with infection or other symptoms that need medical attention can sometimes be managed at home.

ACQUIRED HEMOLYTIC ANEMIA

Acquired hemolytic anemia results from hemolysis of RBCs from extrinsic factors. These factors include (1) physical destruction, (2) antibody reactions, and (3) infectious agents and toxins (Table 30.2).[3]

Physical destruction of RBCs results from the exertion of extreme force on the cells. Traumatic events causing disruption of the RBC membrane include hemodialysis, extracorporeal circulation used in cardiopulmonary bypass, and prosthetic heart valves. In addition, the force needed to push blood through abnormal vessels, such as those that have been burned, irradiated, or affected by vascular disease (e.g., diabetes), may physically damage RBCs.

RBCs can be fragmented and destroyed as they try to pass through abnormal arterial or venous microcirculation. The RBCs are sheared as they try to pass by excess platelet aggregation and/or fibrin polymer formation, such as is seen in thrombotic thrombocytopenic purpura (TTP) and disseminated intravascular coagulation (DIC) (discussed later in this chapter).

Antibodies may destroy RBCs by the mechanisms involved in antigen-antibody reactions. In blood transfusion reactions, the recipient's antibodies attack and hemolyze donor cells. Autoimmune antibody reactions occur when people develop antibodies against their own RBCs. This can be an idiopathic (no prior hemolytic history) or from other autoimmune diseases (e.g., systemic lupus erythematosus [SLE]), leukemia, lymphoma, or medications (penicillin, ibuprofen, metformin, chlorpromazine, procainamide).

Infectious agents cause hemolysis in 3 ways: (1) by invading the RBC and destroying its contents (e.g., parasites, such as in malaria), (2) by releasing hemolytic substances (e.g., *Clostridium perfringens*), and (3) by generating an antigen-antibody reaction (e.g., *Mycoplasma pneumoniae*). Various agents may be toxic to RBCs and cause hemolysis. These hemolytic toxins involve chemicals, such as oxidative drugs, arsenic, lead, copper, and bee stings or spider bites.

Laboratory findings in hemolytic anemia are shown in Table 30.6. Treatment and management of acquired hemolytic anemias involve general supportive care until the causative agent can be eliminated or at least made less injurious to the RBCs. Because a hemolytic crisis is a potential consequence, be ready to institute appropriate emergency therapy. This includes aggressive hydration and electrolyte replacement to reduce the risk for kidney injury caused by hemoglobin (from RBC lysis) clogging the kidney tubules and subsequent shock. Supportive care may include giving corticosteroids and blood products or removing the spleen.

The patient with chronic hemolytic anemia may need folate replacement. To suppress the RBC destruction, immunosuppressive agents may be used, such as glucocorticoids or rituximab (Rituxan), which is a monoclonal antibody to B-cell CD20. For severe cases associated with hemolysis, thrombocytopenia, and acute kidney injury, plasma exchange and eculizumab (Soliris), a monoclonal antibody to complement protein C5, are options.[12]

OTHER RED BLOOD CELL DISORDERS

HEMOCHROMATOSIS

Hemochromatosis is an iron overload disorder. Although a genetic defect is the most common cause, it may occur with diseases such as sideroblastic anemia. It also may be caused by liver disease and the chronic blood transfusions used to treat thalassemia and SCD.

Genetic Link

The genetic disorder *(hereditary hemochromatosis)* is an autosomal recessive disorder characterized by increased intestinal iron absorption and, as a result, increased tissue iron deposition.

GENETICS IN CLINICAL PRACTICE[13]

Hemochromatosis

Genetic Basis
- Autosomal recessive disorder
- Caused by mutations in the *HAMP, HFE, HFE2, SLC40A1,* and *TFR2* genes
- These genes play a key role in regulating the absorption, transport, and storage of iron
- Mutations in these genes impair the control of iron absorption during digestion and change the distribution of iron to other parts of the body, resulting in iron accumulation in tissues and organs

Incidence
- Most common genetic disease in people of European ancestry
- The C282Y mutation of the *HFE* gene is the most common
- About 4 to 5 of every 1000 whites carry 2 copies of the *HFE* gene; 1 of every 10 carries one copy
- Affects 1 in 200 to 500 in the United States
- Very low prevalence in other ethnic populations

Genetic Testing
- DNA testing is available and recommended for all first-degree relatives of people with the disease
- American Hemochromatosis Society recommends genetic testing regardless of family history

Clinical Implications
- Most Americans who have the gene mutation do not know it until diseases becomes apparent
- Clinical expression is variable and depends on dietary iron, blood loss, and other modifying factors
- Early treatment can prevent serious complications
- If untreated, progressive iron deposits can lead to multiple organ failure

The normal range for total body iron is 40 mg/kg in women and 50 mg/kg in men. People with hemochromatosis accumulate iron at an increased rate and may exceed total iron concentrations of 50 g.[1]

Symptoms usually do not develop until after age 40 years in men and after 50 years in women.[13] Early symptoms are nonspecific and include fatigue, arthralgia, impotence, abdominal pain, and weight loss. Later, the excess iron accumulates in the liver and causes liver enlargement and eventually cirrhosis. Excess iron is deposited in the liver, pancreas, heart, joints, and endocrine glands, resulting in diabetes, skin pigment changes (bronzing), heart problems (e.g., cardiomyopathy), arthritis, and testicular atrophy. Physical examination reveals an enlarged liver and spleen and pigmentation changes in the skin.

Laboratory values show a high serum iron, TIBC, and serum ferritin. Testing for known genetic mutations confirms the diagnosis. Liver biopsy can quantify the amount of iron and establish the degree of organ damage.

The goal of treatment is to remove excess iron from the body and minimize any symptoms the patient may have. Iron removal is achieved by removing 500 mL of blood each week for 2 to 3 years until the iron stores in the body are depleted. Then blood is removed less often to maintain iron levels within normal limits.

Iron chelating agents may be used. Deferoxamine, which chelates and removes accumulated iron via the kidneys, can be given IV or subcutaneously. Deferasirox and deferiprone are oral agents that chelate iron. Chelating agents form a complex with iron and promote its excretion from the body.[1] Iron accumulation can be reduced by dietary changes, such as avoiding vitamin C and iron supplements, uncooked seafood, and iron-rich foods.

Management of organ involvement (e.g., diabetes, HF) is the same as conventional treatment for these problems. The most common causes of death are cirrhosis, liver failure, liver cancer, and HF. With early diagnosis and treatment, life expectancy is normal. However, many cases go undetected and untreated.

POLYCYTHEMIA

Polycythemia is the production and presence of increased numbers of RBCs. The increase in RBCs can be so great that blood circulation is impaired because of the increased blood viscosity *(hyperviscosity)* and volume *(hypervolemia)*.

Etiology and Pathophysiology

The 2 types of polycythemia are primary polycythemia, or polycythemia vera, and secondary polycythemia (Fig. 30.5). Their causes and pathogenesis differ, although their complications and manifestations are similar.

Primary Polycythemia. *Polycythemia vera* is a chronic myeloproliferative disorder. It involves not only RBCs, but also WBCs and platelets, with an increased production of all these blood cells. This leads to enhanced blood viscosity and blood volume and congestion of organs and tissues with blood. Splenomegaly and hepatomegaly are common. Patients have hypercoagulopathies that predispose them to clotting. The disease develops insidiously and follows a chronic, vacillating course. The median age at diagnosis is 60 years old, with a slight male predominance.

Genetic Link. Polycythemia vera is associated with mutations in the Janus kinase-2 *(JAK2)* gene. The *JAK2* gene provides instructions for making a protein that promotes proliferation of cells, especially blood cells from hematopoietic stem cells. Polycythemia vera begins with 1 or more DNA mutations of a single hematopoietic stem cell. Most cases of polycythemia vera are not inherited. They are associated with genetic changes that are somatic, which means they are acquired during a person's lifetime and are present only in certain cells.

Secondary Polycythemia. *Secondary polycythemia* can be either hypoxia driven or hypoxia independent. In hypoxia-driven secondary polycythemia, hypoxia stimulates erythropoietin (EPO) production in the kidneys, which in turn stimulates RBC production. The need for O_2 may result from high altitude, lung disease, cardiovascular disease, alveolar hypoventilation, defective O_2 transport, or tissue hypoxia.

EPO levels may return to normal once the hemoglobin stabilizes at a higher level. In this situation, secondary polycythemia is a physiologic response in which the body tries to compensate for a problem, rather than a pathologic response. Hypoxia-driven secondary polycythemia is discussed in Chapter 28.

In hypoxia-independent secondary polycythemia, cancer or benign tumor tissue makes EPO. Serum EPO levels often stay increased in these situations. Splenomegaly does not occur with secondary polycythemia.

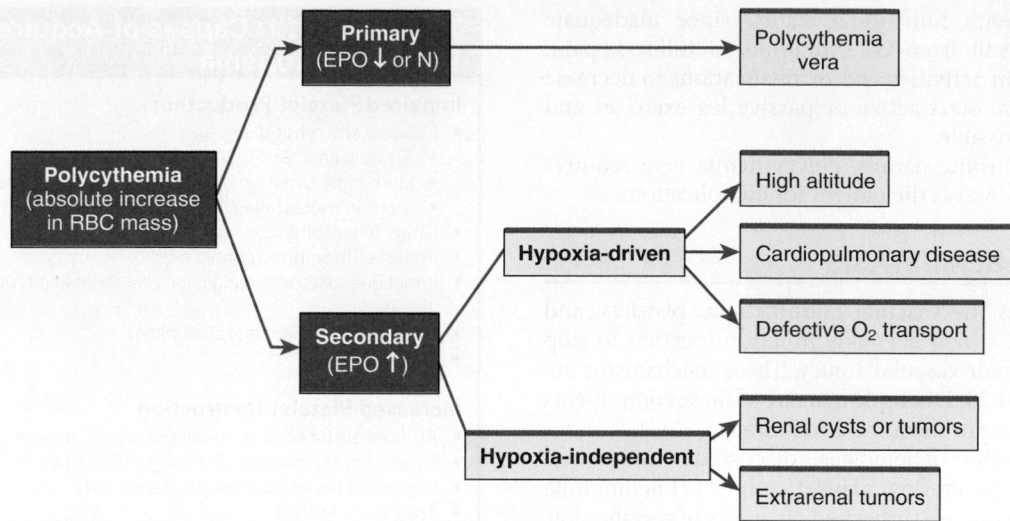

FIG. 30.5 Differentiating between primary and secondary polycythemia. *EPO,* Erythropoietin; *N,* normal.

Clinical Manifestations and Complications

Circulatory manifestations of polycythemia vera occur because of the hypertension caused by hypervolemia and hyperviscosity. They are often the first manifestations and include headache, vertigo, dizziness, tinnitus, and visual changes. Generalized pruritus (often exacerbated by a hot bath) may be a striking symptom and is related to histamine release from an increased number of basophils. Paresthesias and *erythromelalgia* (painful burning and redness of the hands and feet) may be present. The patient may have angina, HF, intermittent claudication, and thrombophlebitis, which may be complicated by embolization. These manifestations are caused by blood vessel distention, impaired blood flow, circulatory stasis, thrombosis, and tissue hypoxia from the hypervolemia and hyperviscosity. The most common serious acute complication is stroke from a thrombosis.

Hemorrhagic phenomena caused by either vessel rupture from overdistention or inadequate platelet function may result in petechiae, bruising, nosebleeds, or GI bleeding. Hemorrhage can be acute and catastrophic. Hepatomegaly and splenomegaly from organ engorgement may contribute to satiety and fullness. The patient may have pain from peptic ulcer caused either by increased gastric secretions or liver and spleen engorgement. *Plethora* (ruddy complexion) may be present. Uric acid is one of the products of RBC destruction. As RBC destruction increases, uric acid production increases, leading to hyperuricemia and gout.

Although the incidence is low, myelofibrosis and leukemia develop in some patients with polycythemia vera. These disorders may be caused by the chemotherapeutic drugs used to treat the disease, or they may be caused by a disorder in the stem cells that progresses to erythroleukemia. The major cause of morbidity and mortality from polycythemia vera is related to thrombosis (e.g., stroke).

Diagnostic Studies

The laboratory manifestations seen in a patient with polycythemia vera include (1) high hemoglobin and RBC count with microcytosis; (2) low to normal EPO level (secondary polycythemia has a high level); (3) high WBC count with basophilia and neutrophilia; (4) high platelet count (thrombocytosis) and platelet dysfunction; (5) high leukocyte alkaline phosphatase, uric acid, and cobalamin levels; and (6) high histamine levels.[3] Bone marrow examination in polycythemia vera shows hypercellularity of RBCs, WBCs, and platelets.

❖ Interprofessional and Nursing Management

Treatment is directed toward reducing blood volume and viscosity and bone marrow activity. Phlebotomy is the mainstay of treatment. The aim of phlebotomy is to reduce the hematocrit and keep it less than 45%.[14] Generally, at the time of diagnosis 300 to 500 mL of blood may be removed every few days until the hematocrit is reduced to acceptable levels.[14] Phlebotomy then may be needed every 2 to 3 months, reducing the blood volume by about 500 mL each time. A person managed with repeated phlebotomies eventually becomes deficient in iron, although this effect is rarely symptomatic. Avoid iron supplementation. Hydration therapy can reduce the blood's viscosity.

Myelosuppressive agents, such as hydroxyurea, busulfan (Myleran), and chlorambucil (Leukeran), may be given.[3] Ruxolitinib (Jakafi), which inhibits the expression of the *JAK2* mutation, is given to patients who have not responded to hydroxyurea.[14] Other therapies include anagrelide (Agrylin), which can reduce the platelet count and inhibit platelet aggregation. Low-dose aspirin is used to prevent clotting. α-Interferon (α-IFN) and pegylated interferon are given to women of childbearing age or those with intractable pruritus. Allopurinol (Zyloprim) may reduce the number of acute gouty attacks.[3]

When acute exacerbations of polycythemia vera develop, you have several nursing responsibilities. Depending on the agency's policies, you may either assist with or perform the phlebotomy. Assess fluid intake and output during hydration therapy to avoid fluid overload (which worsens circulatory congestion) or fluid deficit (which makes the blood even more viscous). If myelosuppressive agents are used, give the drugs as ordered, observe the patient, and teach the patient about the side effects of the drugs.

Assess the patient's nutritional status, since inadequate food intake can result from GI symptoms of fullness, pain, and dyspepsia. Begin activities and/or medications to decrease thrombus formation. Start active or passive leg exercises and ambulation when possible.

Because of its chronic nature, polycythemia vera requires ongoing evaluation. Assess the patient for complications.

PROBLEMS OF HEMOSTASIS

Hemostasis involves the vascular endothelium, platelets, and coagulation factors, which normally function together to stop hemorrhage and repair vascular injury. These mechanisms are described in Chapter 29. Disruption in any of these components may result in bleeding or thrombotic disorders.

Three major disorders of hemostasis discussed in this section are (1) thrombocytopenia (low platelet count), (2) hemophilia and von Willebrand disease (inherited disorders of specific clotting factors), and (3) DIC.

THROMBOCYTOPENIA

Etiology and Pathophysiology

Thrombocytopenia is a reduction of platelets below 150,000/μL (150 × 10⁹/L). Acute, severe, or prolonged decreases from this normal range can result in abnormal hemostasis that presents as prolonged bleeding from minor trauma or spontaneous bleeding without injury.

Platelet disorders occur because of impaired production, increased destruction, or abnormal distribution (Table 30.11).[15] While they can be inherited (e.g., Wiskott-Aldrich syndrome), most are acquired. A common cause of acquired disorders is the ingestion of certain drugs.[1] Although some drugs are directly myelosuppressive (e.g., chemotherapy, ganciclovir), the usual mechanism of drug-related thrombocytopenia is accelerated platelet destruction caused by antibodies. Antibodies attack the platelets when the drug binds to the platelet surface.

Some drugs can affect platelet aggregation. Aspirin doses as low as 81 mg can alter platelet aggregation. Normal function is restored when new platelets are made.

Immune Thrombocytopenia. The most common acquired thrombocytopenia is a syndrome of abnormal destruction of circulating platelets termed *immune thrombocytopenia* (ITP). ITP is an acquired immune disorder in which the thrombocytopenia results from antiplatelet antibodies, impaired platelet production, and T-cell–mediated destruction of platelets.[16] In ITP, platelets are coated with antibodies. These platelets function normally; however, when they reach the spleen, these antibody-coated platelets are mistaken as foreign and destroyed by macrophages. Decreased platelet production contributes to ITP. Sometimes autoimmune disease (such as SLE) or infection, such as *Helicobacter pylori* or viral infection (HIV), contributes to this disorder.[16]

Platelets normally survive 8 to 10 days. However, in ITP, platelet survival is shortened. Generally, the syndrome presents as an acute condition in children and a chronic condition in adults.

Thrombotic Thrombocytopenic Purpura. *Thrombotic thrombocytopenic purpura* (TTP) is an uncommon syndrome characterized by hemolytic anemia, thrombocytopenia, neurologic abnormalities, fever (in the absence of infection),

TABLE 30.11 Causes of Acquired Thrombocytopenia

Impaired Platelet Production
- Cancers and other disorders
  - Aplastic anemia
  - Leukemia, lymphoma, myeloma, myelodysplastic disorders
  - Marrow metastases by solid tumors
- Drugs (chemotherapy, others)
- Immune thrombocytopenia (ITP)
- Infections, bacterial, fungal, or viral (hepatitis C virus, HIV, cytomegalovirus)
- Nutritional deficiencies, alcoholism
- Radiation

Increased Platelet Destruction
- Artificial surfaces (e.g., cardiopulmonary bypass, hemodialysis)
- Disseminated intravascular coagulation (DIC)
- Heparin-induced thrombocytopenia (HIT)
- Pregnancy-related
- Thrombotic microangiopathy
  - Thrombotic thrombocytopenic purpura (TTP)
  - Atypical Hemolytic Uremic Syndromes (aHUS)

Abnormal Platelet Distribution
- Dilution (massive blood transfusion, fluids)
- Splenic sequestration

and renal abnormalities. Not all features are present in all patients. Because it is almost always associated with hemolytic-uremic syndrome (HUS), TTP is often referred to as *TTP-HUS*. The disease is associated with enhanced aggregation of platelets, which form microthrombi that deposit in arterioles and capillaries.

In most cases, TTP is caused by the deficiency of a plasma enzyme (ADAMTS13) that breaks down the von Willebrand clotting factor (vWF) into normal size. vWF is the most important protein-mediating platelet adhesion to damaged endothelial cells. Without the enzyme, unusually large amounts of vWF attach to activated platelets, promoting platelet aggregation.

TTP occurs primarily in previously healthy adults, with a slight female predominance. The syndrome may be idiopathic (thought to be due to an autoimmune disorder against ADAMTS13) or due to certain drug toxicities (e.g., chemotherapy, cyclosporine, quinine, oral contraceptives, valacyclovir, clopidogrel [Plavix]), pregnancy or preeclampsia, infection, or a known autoimmune disorder, such as SLE or scleroderma.[3] TTP is a medical emergency because bleeding and clotting occur at the same time.

Heparin-Induced Thrombocytopenia. One of the risks associated with the use of heparin is the development of the life-threatening condition called *heparin-induced thrombocytopenia* (HIT), also called *heparin-induced thrombocytopenia and thrombosis syndrome* (HITTS). Typically, patients develop thrombocytopenia 5 to 10 days after the onset of heparin therapy. HIT should be suspected if the platelet count falls by more than 50% or falls to below 150,000/μL. As many as 5% of patients on heparin therapy develop HIT.[3,17]

Although the major problem of HIT is venous thrombosis, arterial thrombosis can occur. DVT and pulmonary emboli most often result as a complication of the thromboses. Other complications include arterial vascular infarcts, resulting in

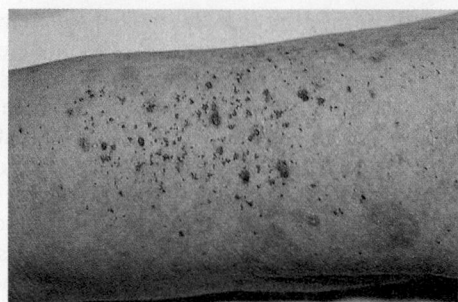

FIG. 30.6 Acute immune thrombocytopenic purpura often presents with purpuric lesions. (From Forbes CD, Jackson WF: *Colour atlas and text of clinical medicine,* ed 3, London, 2003, Mosby.)

TABLE 30.12 Laboratory Results in Thrombocytopenia and DIC

Laboratory Test	ITP	TTP	HIT	DIC
Platelets	↓↓↓↓	↓↓↓	↓↓	↓↓↓
Hemolysis				
Haptoglobin	N	↓	N	↓
Hgb	N	↓↓	N	N or ↓
Indirect bilirubin	N	↑	N	N or ↑
LDH	N	↑↑↑	N	↑
Reticulocytes	N	↑	N	N or ↑
Schistocytes	N	↑↑↑	N or ↑	N or ↑
Coagulopathy				
PT	N	N	N	↑
aPTT	N	N	N	↑
D-dimer	N	N or ↑	↑	↑↑
Other tests	ITP IgG assay, platelet activation/ function assay, *Helicobacter pylori*, hepatitis C, HIV, bone marrow biopsy	ADAMTS13 Urinalysis (for proteinuria, hematuria), Creatinine	Platelet activation/ function assay, PF4-heparin complex (antigen assay)	

skin necrosis, stroke, and end-organ damage (e.g., kidneys). Symptoms of bleeding are unusual because the platelet count rarely drops below 20,000/μL.

In HIT, platelet destruction and vascular endothelial injury are the 2 major responses to an immune-mediated response to heparin. Platelet factor 4 (PF4) (protein made and released by platelets) binds to heparin. This PF4-heparin complex then binds to the platelet surface, leading to further platelet activation and release of more PF4, thus creating a positive feedback loop. Antibodies are created against the PF4-heparin-platelet complex. They are removed prematurely from circulation, leading to thrombocytopenia and platelet-fibrin thrombi.

Clinical Manifestations

Many patients with thrombocytopenia are asymptomatic. The most common symptom is bleeding, usually mucosal or cutaneous. Mucosal bleeding may manifest as nosebleeds and gingival bleeding. Large bullous hemorrhages may appear on the buccal mucosa because of the lack of vessel protection by the submucosal tissue.

Bleeding into the skin is seen as petechiae, purpura, or superficial ecchymoses. *Petechiae* are small, flat, red or reddish brown microhemorrhages (see Table 29.6). When the platelet count is low, RBCs may leak out of the blood vessels and into the skin to cause petechiae. When there are many petechiae, we call the resulting reddish skin *purpura* (Fig. 30.6). Purplish lesions caused by hemorrhage are termed *ecchymoses.* Pain and tenderness are sometimes present.

The major complication of thrombocytopenia is hemorrhage. The hemorrhage may be insidious or acute and internal or external. It may occur in any area of the body, including the joints, retina, and brain. Cerebral hemorrhage may be fatal. Insidious hemorrhage may be first detected by discovering the anemia that accompanies blood loss. Be aware of manifestations that reflect internal blood loss, including weakness, fainting, dizziness, tachycardia, abdominal pain, and hypotension. Prolonged bleeding after routine procedures, such as venipuncture or IM injection, may indicate thrombocytopenia.

Because thrombocytopenia can be accompanied by vascular thromboses, signs and symptoms of vascular ischemic problems may occur (see Chapter 37). For example, subtle confusion, headache, or even serious manifestations, such as seizures and coma due to TTP-related thrombosis, may occur. Because signs and symptoms may be subtle, astute and thorough assessment of the patient is essential.

Diagnostic Studies

The platelet count is decreased in thrombocytopenia. Any reduction below 150,000/μL (150 × 10⁹/L) may be termed *thrombocytopenia.* However, prolonged bleeding from trauma or injury does not usually occur until platelet counts are less than 50,000/μL (50 × 10⁹/L).[1] When the count drops below 20,000/μL (20 × 10⁹/L), spontaneous, life-threatening hemorrhages (e.g., intracranial bleeding) can occur. Platelet transfusions are generally not recommended until the count is below 10,000/μL (10 × 10⁹/L) unless the patient is actively bleeding.[3]

The patient's history and clinical examination, along with comparisons of laboratory parameters, help to determine the cause of the thrombocytopenia. Table 30.12 compares the types of thrombocytopenia.

Laboratory tests that assess secondary hemostasis or coagulation, such as the prothrombin time (PT) and aPTT, can be normal even in severe thrombocytopenia. If they are increased, this may point toward DIC.

Specific assays, such as ITP antigen-specific assay, platelet activation/function assay, or PF4-heparin complex for HIT, can be done to assist with the diagnosis. In TTP, testing for deficiency of ADAMTS13 is not always diagnostic, so an increase of lactate dehydrogenase (LDH) may help establish the diagnosis. When thrombocytopenia occurs with anemia characterized by altered RBC morphology, including *spherocytes* (small, globular, completely hemoglobinated RBCs), fragmented cells (schistocytes), and pronounced reticulocytosis, a diagnosis of TTP should be suspected. These findings are partially a result of intravascular fibrin deposition causing a "slicing" of RBCs. In TTP, thrombocytopenia may be severe, but coagulation studies are normal.

TABLE 30.13 Interprofessional Care

Thrombocytopenia

Diagnostic Assessment
- History and physical examination
- Bone marrow aspiration and biopsy
- CBC, including platelet count
- Specific laboratory studies (Table 30.12)

Management

Immune Thrombocytopenic Purpura
- Corticosteroids
- IV immunoglobulin (IVIG)
- Anti-Rh$_o$(D)
- Rituximab (Rituxan)
- Romiplostim (Nplate)
- Eltrombopag (Promacta)
- Splenectomy
- Immunosuppressives (e.g., cyclosporine)
- Platelet transfusions
- Epsilon-aminocaproic acid (Amicar)

Thrombotic Thrombocytopenic Purpura
- Identification and treatment of cause
- Plasmapheresis (plasma exchange)
- Corticosteroids
- Rituximab (Rituxan)
- Immunosuppressives (e.g., cyclophosphamide)
- Splenectomy

Heparin-Induced Thrombocytopenia
- Direct thrombin inhibitor (argatroban [Acova])
- Indirect thrombin inhibitor (fondaparinux [Arixtra])
- Synthetic thrombin inhibitor (bivalirudin)
- Plasmapheresis (plasma exchange)
- Warfarin (Coumadin)
- Thrombolytic agents

Decreased Platelet Production
- Identification and treatment or removal of cause
- Corticosteroids
- Platelet transfusions

Bone marrow examination may be done to rule out production problems as the cause of thrombocytopenia (e.g., leukemia, aplastic anemia, other myeloproliferative disorders) or when other tests are inconclusive. When destruction of circulating platelets is the cause, bone marrow analysis shows *megakaryocytes* (precursors of platelets) to be normal or increased, even though circulating platelets are reduced. The absence or decreased number of megakaryocytes on bone marrow biopsy is consistent with thrombocytopenia caused by decreased bone marrow production (e.g., aplastic anemia).

Interprofessional Care

Interprofessional care of thrombocytopenia differs based on the cause. Removal or treatment of the underlying cause or disorder is sometimes sufficient. The patient with thrombocytopenia should avoid aspirin and other drugs that affect platelet function or production. The following sections discuss management strategies for the different causes of thrombocytopenia (Table 30.13).

Immune Thrombocytopenic Purpura. Multiple therapies are used to manage the patient with ITP. If the patient is asymptomatic,

therapy may not be used unless the patient's platelet count is below 30,000/μL.[1] Corticosteroids (e.g., prednisone, methylprednisolone) are used initially to treat ITP because of their ability to suppress the phagocytic response of splenic macrophages. This alters the spleen's recognition of platelets and increases the life span of the platelets. Corticosteroids depress antibody formation and reduce capillary leakage.

High doses of IV immunoglobulin (IVIG) and a component of IVIG, anti-Rh$_o$(D) (anti-D, WinRho), may be used in the patient who is unresponsive to corticosteroids or splenectomy or for whom splenectomy is not an option. We think that one way these agents work is by competing with the antiplatelet antibodies for macrophage receptors in the spleen. Rituximab (Rituxan) may be used for its ability to lyse activated B cells, thus reducing the immune recognition of platelets. Romiplostim (Nplate) and eltrombopag (Promacta) are used for patients with chronic ITP who had an insufficient response to the other treatments. These drugs are thrombopoietin receptor agonists, thus increasing platelet production.[1]

Splenectomy may be needed if the patient does not respond to treatment. Two thirds of patients benefit from splenectomy, resulting in a sustained remission.[3] The effectiveness of splenectomy is based on 4 factors. First, the spleen has an abundance of the macrophages that sequester and destroy platelets. Second, structural features of the spleen enhance the interaction between antibody-coated platelets and macrophages. Third, some antibody synthesis occurs in the spleen, so antiplatelet antibodies decrease after splenectomy. Fourth, the spleen normally sequesters around one third of the platelets, so its removal increases the number of platelets in circulation.

Immunosuppressive therapy (e.g., cyclosporine) may be used in refractory cases (Table 30.13).[1] Platelet transfusions may increase platelet counts in cases of life-threatening hemorrhage. Platelets should not be given prophylactically because of the risk for antibody formation. The usual indication for giving platelets is for a platelet count less than 10,000/μL or if there is expected bleeding before a procedure. Epsilon-aminocaproic acid (EACA, Amicar), an antifibrinolytic agent, may treat severe bleeding.[3]

Thrombotic Thrombocytopenic Purpura. TTP may be treated in a variety of ways. The first step is to treat the underlying disorder (e.g., infection) or remove the causative agent, if known. If untreated, TTP usually results in irreversible renal failure and death. Plasma exchange (plasmapheresis) (see Chapter 13) can aggressively reverse platelet consumption by supplying the appropriate vWF and enzyme (ADAMTS13) and removing the large vWF molecules that bind with platelets. Treatment should be continued daily until the patient's platelet counts normalize and hemolysis has ceased. Corticosteroids may be given with this treatment.[3]

Rituximab is used for patients who are refractory to plasma exchange. It decreases the level of inhibitory ADAMTS13 IgG antibodies. Other immunosuppressants, such as cyclosporine or cyclophosphamide, are options. Splenectomy may be considered in patients who are refractory to plasma exchange or immunosuppression. Platelet administration is generally contraindicated because this may lead to new vWF-platelet complexes and increased clotting.[3]

Heparin-Induced Thrombocytopenia. All forms of heparin must be stopped when HIT is first recognized. This includes heparin flushes for vascular catheters.

To maintain anticoagulation, the patient should be started on a direct thrombin inhibitor, such as argatroban. Fondaparinux (Arixtra), a factor Xa inhibitor (indirect thrombin inhibitor), or bivalirudin (a synthetic thrombin inhibitor) may be used.[17] Warfarin should be started only when the platelet count has reached 150,000/μL. If the clotting is severe, the most commonly used treatment modalities are plasmapheresis to clear the platelet-aggregating IgG from the blood, protamine sulfate to interrupt the circulating heparin, thrombolytic agents to treat the thromboembolic events, and surgery to remove clots. Platelet transfusions are not effective because they may enhance thromboembolic events.[3]

Patients who have had HIT should never receive heparin or low-molecular-weight heparin (LMWH) again. This should be clearly marked in the patient's medical record.

Thrombocytopenia From Decreased Platelet Production. The management of acquired thrombocytopenia is based on finding the cause and treating the disease or removing the causative agent. If the precipitating factor is unknown, the patient may receive corticosteroids. Platelet transfusions are given if life-threatening hemorrhage develops.

Often acquired thrombocytopenia is caused by another underlying condition (e.g., aplastic anemia, leukemia) or therapy used to treat another problem. For example, in acute leukemia all blood cell types may be depressed. Plus, the patient may receive chemotherapeutic drugs that cause bone marrow suppression. If the patient can be supported throughout the course of chemotherapy-induced thrombocytopenia, the thrombocytopenia will also resolve.

❖ NURSING MANAGEMENT: THROMBOCYTOPENIA

◆ Nursing Assessment

Subjective and objective data that should be obtained from a patient with thrombocytopenia are outlined in Table 30.14.

◆ Nursing Diagnoses

The main nursing diagnosis for the patient with thrombocytopenia is risk for bleeding.

◆ Planning

The overall goals are that the patient with thrombocytopenia will (1) have no bleeding, (2) maintain vascular integrity, and (3) manage home care to prevent any complications related to an increased risk for bleeding.

◆ Nursing Implementation

◆ **Health Promotion.** Discourage the use of over-the-counter (OTC) medications known to be causes of acquired thrombocytopenia and reduced platelet function. Some have aspirin as an ingredient. Aspirin reduces platelet adhesiveness, thus contributing to bleeding.

Encourage persons to have a complete medical evaluation if manifestations of bleeding tendencies (e.g., prolonged nosebleeds, petechiae) develop. Observe for early signs of thrombocytopenia in the patient receiving cancer chemotherapy drugs.

◆ **Acute Care.** The goal during acute episodes of thrombocytopenia is to prevent or control hemorrhage (see eNursing Care Plan 30.2 on the website for this chapter). In the patient with thrombocytopenia, bleeding is usually from superficial sites. Deep bleeding (into muscles, joints, and abdomen) usually occurs only when clotting factors are decreased. Stress that a minor nosebleed or

---

TABLE 30.14 Nursing Assessment

Thrombocytopenia

Subjective Data

Important Health Information

Past health history: Recent hemorrhage, excessive bleeding, or viral illness; HIV infection; cancer (especially leukemia or lymphoma); aplastic anemia; SLE; cirrhosis; exposure to radiation or toxic chemicals; DIC

Medications: Many medications, including chemotherapy agents, valproic acid (Depakote), furosemide (Lasix), gold, nonsteroidal antiinflammatory drugs, penicillin

Functional Health Patterns

Health perception–health management: Family history of bleeding problems; malaise

Nutritional-metabolic: Bleeding gingiva; coffee-ground or bloody vomitus; easy bruising

Elimination: Hematuria, dark or bloody stools

Activity-exercise: Fatigue, weakness, fainting; nosebleeds, hemoptysis; dyspnea

Cognitive-perceptual: Pain and tenderness in bleeding areas (e.g., abdomen, head, extremities); headache

Sexuality-reproductive: Menorrhagia, metrorrhagia

Objective Data

General

Fever, lethargy

Integumentary

Petechiae, bruising, purpura

Gastrointestinal

Splenomegaly, abdominal distention; heme-positive stools

Possible Diagnostic Findings

Platelet count <150,000/μL (150 × 10⁹/L), prolonged bleeding time, ↓ hemoglobin and hematocrit; normal or ↑ megakaryocytes in bone marrow examination

---

new petechiae may indicate potential hemorrhage and to notify the HCP.

Bleeding from the posterior nasopharynx may be hard to detect because the blood may be swallowed. If you cannot avoid a subcutaneous injection, use a small-gauge needle and apply direct pressure for at least 5 to 10 minutes after the injection. An ice pack may be helpful. Avoid IM injections. Help the patient understand the importance of adhering to self-care measures that reduce the risk for bleeding (Table 30.15).

Note that many of these disorders may be accompanied by vascular clotting, and appropriate assessment and management should be taken (see Chapter 37). As bleeding occurs, RBCs and coagulation factors are consumed along with platelets. It is important to monitor all blood cell and coagulation studies.

In a woman with thrombocytopenia, menstrual blood loss may exceed the usual amount and duration. Counting sanitary napkins used during menses is another important intervention to detect excess blood loss. Blood loss of 50 mL will completely soak a sanitary napkin. Suppression of menses with hormonal agents may be needed during predictable periods of thrombocytopenia (e.g., during chemotherapy and HSCT) to reduce blood loss from menses.

Closely monitor the platelet count, coagulation studies, hemoglobin, and hematocrit. Together these give vital information about potential or actual bleeding.

TABLE 30.15 Patient & Caregiver Teaching

Thrombocytopenia

Include the following instructions when teaching a patient or caregiver the precautions to take when the platelet count is low.

1. Notify your HCP of any symptoms of bleeding. These include:
   - Black, tarry, or bloody bowel movements
   - Black or bloody vomit, sputum, or urine
   - Bleeding from the mouth or anywhere in the body
   - Bruising or small red or purple spots on the skin
   - Difficulty talking, sudden weakness of an arm or leg, confusion
   - Headache or changes in how well you can see
2. Ask your HCP about restrictions in your normal activities, such as vigorous exercise or lifting weights. Generally, walking is safe. Wear sturdy shoes or slippers. If you are weak and at risk for falling, get help or supervision when getting out of bed or chair.
3. Do not blow your nose forcefully; gently pat it with a tissue if needed. For a nosebleed, keep your head up and apply firm pressure to the nostrils and bridge of your nose. If bleeding continues, place an ice bag over the bridge of your nose and the nape of your neck. If you are unable to stop a nosebleed after 10 minutes, call your HCP.
4. Do not bend down with your head lower than your waist.
5. Prevent constipation by drinking plenty of fluids. Do not strain when having a bowel movement. Your HCP may prescribe a stool softener. Do not use a suppository, an enema, or a rectal thermometer without the permission of your HCP.
6. Shave only with an electric razor. Do not use blades.
7. Do not tweeze your eyebrows or other body hair.
8. Do not puncture your skin, such as getting tattoos or body piercing.
9. Do not use any medication that can prolong bleeding, such as aspirin. Other medications and herbs can have similar effects. If you are unsure about any medication, ask your HCP or pharmacist about it in relation to your thrombocytopenia.
10. Use a soft-bristle toothbrush to prevent injuring the gums. Flossing is usually safe if done gently using the thin tape floss. Do not use alcohol-based mouthwashes since they can dry your gums and increase bleeding.
11. Women who are menstruating should keep track of the number of pads that are used per day. When you start using more pads per day than usual or bleed more days, notify your HCP. Do not use tampons; only use sanitary pads.
12. Ask your HCP before you have any invasive procedures done, such as a dental cleaning, manicure, or pedicure.

TABLE 30.16 Types of Hemophilia

Type	Inheritance Pattern
Hemophilia A Factor VIII	Recessive sex-linked (transmitted by female carriers, displayed almost exclusively in men)
Hemophilia B Factor IX	Recessive sex-linked (transmitted by female carriers, displayed almost exclusively in men)
von Willebrand Disease vWF, variable factor VIII deficiencies and platelet dysfunction	Autosomal dominant, seen in both genders Recessive (in severe forms of the disease)

vWF, von Willebrand factor.

HEMOPHILIA AND VON WILLEBRAND DISEASE

Hemophilia is an X-linked recessive genetic disorder caused by a defective or deficient coagulation factor. The 2 major types of hemophilia, which can occur in mild to severe forms, are *hemophilia A* (classic hemophilia, factor VIII deficiency) and *hemophilia B* (Christmas disease, factor IX deficiency). *von Willebrand disease* is a related disorder involving a deficiency of the von Willebrand coagulation protein. Factor VIII is made in the liver and circulates as a complex with vWF.

Hemophilia A is 4 times as common as hemophilia B.[18] Although rare, there are cases of *acquired hemophilia A*, which is due to the development of antibodies against the body's own factor VIII. von Willebrand disease is the most common congenital bleeding disorder.[19]

 Genetic Link. The inheritance patterns of hemophilia and von Willebrand disease are compared in Table 30.16. (X-linked genetic disorders are discussed in Chapter 12 and Table 12.2.)

GENETICS IN CLINICAL PRACTICE[1,3]

Hemophilia A and B

Genetic Basis
- X-linked recessive disorder
- *Hemophilia A:* Caused by mutations in the *F8* gene that provides instructions for making coagulation factor VIII
- *Hemophilia B:* Caused by mutations in the *F9* gene that provides instructions for making coagulation factor IX
- Mutations in the *F8* or *F9* gene lead to the production of an abnormal version or reduced amounts of coagulation factors

Incidence
- *Hemophilia A:* 1 in 5000 to 10,000 male births
- *Hemophilia B:* 1 in 25,000 to 30,000 male births

Genetic Testing
- DNA testing is available

Clinical Implications
- Female carriers transmit the genetic defect to 50% of their sons, 50% of their daughters are carriers
- Males with hemophilia do not transmit the genetic defect to their sons, but all their daughters are carriers
- Though rare, female hemophilia can occur if a male with hemophilia mates with a female carrier
- Replacement therapy is available for factors VIII and IX

The proper administration of platelet transfusions is an important nursing responsibility. This is discussed under Blood Component Therapy later in this chapter.

◆ **Ambulatory Care.** Monitor the patient with ITP who is receiving treatment for the response to therapy. Teach the person with acquired thrombocytopenia to avoid causative agents when possible (Table 30.11). If the patient cannot avoid causative agents (e.g., chemotherapy), teach them to avoid injury or trauma during these periods and to be aware of the signs and symptoms of bleeding caused by thrombocytopenia (Table 30.15).

Patients with either ITP or acquired thrombocytopenia should have planned periodic medical evaluations to assess and treat situations in which exacerbations and bleeding are likely to occur. Address the impact of either an acute or a chronic condition on the patient's quality of life.

◆ Evaluation

The expected outcomes are that the patient with thrombocytopenia will
- Have no evidence of bleeding or bruising
- State needed knowledge and skills to manage disease process

Clinical Manifestations and Complications

The manifestations of hemophilia A and B are similar. All manifestations relate to bleeding, and any bleeding episode in persons with hemophilia may lead to a life-threatening hemorrhage. Manifestations and complications related to hemophilia include (1) slow, persistent, prolonged bleeding from minor trauma and small cuts; (2) delayed bleeding after minor injuries (the delay may be several hours or days); (3) uncontrollable hemorrhage after dental extractions or irritation of the gingiva with a hard-bristle toothbrush; (4) nosebleeds, especially after a blow to the face; (5) GI bleeding from ulcers and gastritis; (6) hematuria and potential renal failure from GU trauma and splenic rupture resulting from falls or abdominal trauma; (7) bruising and subcutaneous hematomas (Fig. 30.7) and possible compartment syndrome; (8) neurologic signs, such as pain, anesthesia, and paralysis, which may develop from nerve compression caused by hematoma formation; and (9) hemarthrosis (bleeding into the joints) (Fig. 30.8), which may lead to joint injury and deformity severe enough to cause crippling (most often in knees, elbows, and ankles).[1]

In children, these manifestations may lead to the diagnosis. In adults, these may be the first sign of a newly diagnosed mild form of the disease that escaped detection through a childhood free of major injuries, dental procedures, or surgeries.

Diagnostic Studies

Laboratory studies are done to determine the type of hemophilia present. Any factor deficiency within the intrinsic system (factor VIII, IX, XI, or XII or vWF) will yield the laboratory results outlined in Table 30.17.

Interprofessional Care

The goals of interprofessional care are to prevent and treat bleeding. Care for persons with hemophilia or von Willebrand disease requires (1) preventive care, (2) the use of replacement therapy during acute bleeding episodes and as prophylaxis, and (3) the treatment of the complications of the disease and its therapy. Today, most patients can expect almost normal life spans free of bloodborne illnesses because of improved preparation of replacement products, improved screening of blood donor populations, and use of recombinant replacement factors.[1,3]

Replacement of deficient clotting factors is the primary means of supporting a patient with hemophilia. Replacement therapy may be given before surgery and dental care as a prophylactic measure. Table 30.18 lists examples of replacement therapy. Fresh frozen plasma, once commonly used for replacement therapy, is rarely used today.

For mild hemophilia A and certain subtypes of von Willebrand disease, desmopressin acetate (DDAVP), a synthetic

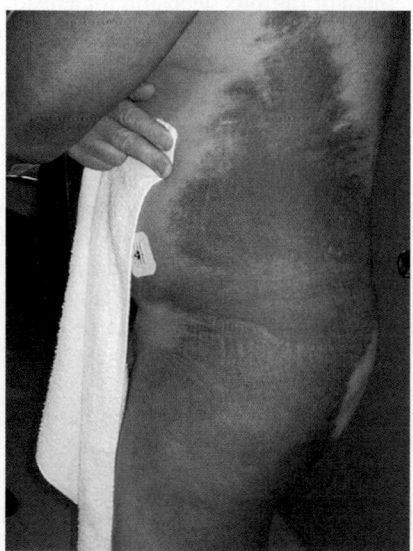

FIG. 30.7 Severe ecchymoses in a person with hemophilia after a fall. (Courtesy Peter Bonner.)

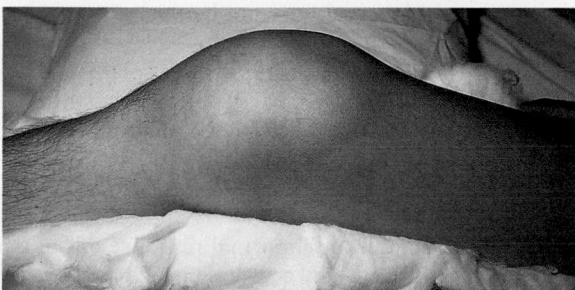

FIG. 30.8 Acute hemarthrosis of the knee is a common complication of hemophilia. (From Forbes CD, Jackson WF: *Colour atlas and text of clinical medicine*, ed 3, London, 2003, Mosby.)

TABLE 30.17 Laboratory Results in Hemophilia

Test	Results
Bleeding time	Prolonged in von Willebrand disease because of structurally defective platelets. Normal in hemophilia A and B because platelets not affected
Factor assays	Reductions of factor VIII in hemophilia A, factor IX in hemophilia B, vWF in von Willebrand disease
Partial thromboplastin time	Prolonged because of deficiency in intrinsic clotting system factor
Platelet count	Normal. Adequate platelet production
Prothrombin time	Normal. No involvement of extrinsic system
Thrombin time	Normal. No impairment of thrombin-fibrinogen reaction

vWF, von Willebrand factor.

TABLE 30.18 Drug Therapy

Replacement Factors for Hemophilia

Factor VIII	Factor IX	Von Willebrand	For Patients Who Have Inhibitors
Advate	Alphanine	Vonvendi	NovoSeven (factor VIIa)
Afstyla	Alprolix		
Alphanate	Bebulin VH		Autoplex T
Eloctate	BeneFIX		FEIBA (factor VIII inhibitor bypassing activity)
Hemofil M	Mononine		
Humate-P	Profilnine SD		
Koāte-DVI	Rixubis		
Kogenate FS			
Monoclate			
Obizur*			
Xyntha			

*For acquired hemophilia A.

analog of vasopressin, may be used to stimulate an increase in factor VIII and vWF. This drug acts on platelets and endothelial cells to cause the release of vWF, which then binds with factor VIII, thus increasing its concentration. It can be given IV, subcutaneously, or by intranasal spray. Beneficial effects (e.g., decreased bleeding time) of DDAVP when given IV are seen within 30 minutes and can last for more than 12 hours. Because the effect of DDAVP is short lived, the patient must be closely monitored and repeated doses may be needed. It is an appropriate therapy for minor bleeding episodes and dental procedures. The intranasal form may be used as home therapy for some patients with mild to moderate forms of the disease.

Antifibrinolytic therapy (tranexamic acid [Cyklokapron] and EACA) inhibits fibrinolysis by inhibiting plasminogen activation in the fibrin clot, thus enhancing clot stability. These agents stabilize clots in areas of increased fibrinolysis, such as the oral cavity, and in patients with difficult episodes of nosebleeds and menorrhagia. Topical thrombin and fibrin sealants may be used for mucosal bleeding.

Complications of the treatment of hemophilia include development of inhibitors to factors VIII or IX, transfusion-transmitted infectious disorders (hepatitis, HIV), allergic reactions, and thrombotic complications with the use of factor IX because it contains activated coagulation factors. Patients with vWF may develop antibodies against vWF concentrates, the infusion of which could cause life-threatening anaphylaxis. Thus replacement factors for these patients should not contain vWF.

The most common problems with acute management are starting factor replacement therapy too late and stopping it too soon. Minor bleeding episodes should be treated for at least 72 hours. Surgery and traumatic injuries may need longer therapy. Chronically, development of inhibitors to the factor products has occurred and needs individualized expert patient management. Designated treatment centers in the United States and many other countries provide interprofessional care of hemophilia and related disorders. Gene transfer therapy has been used on an experimental basis to treat hemophilia.[1]

❖ NURSING MANAGEMENT: HEMOPHILIA

◆ Nursing Implementation

◆ **Health Promotion.** Because of the hereditary nature of hemophilia, referral of affected persons for genetic counseling before reproduction is an important measure. This is especially important because many persons with hemophilia live into adulthood. Reproductive concerns and long-term effects are issues that you should include in the patient's care plan.

◆ **Acute Care.** Interventions are related primarily to controlling bleeding and include the following:

1. Stop the topical bleeding as quickly as possible. Apply direct pressure or ice, pack the area with Gelfoam or fibrin foam, and apply topical hemostatic agents, such as thrombin.
2. Give the specific coagulation factor to raise the patient's level of the deficient coagulation factor. Monitor the patient for signs and symptoms, such as hypersensitivity.
3. When joint bleeding occurs, in addition to giving replacement factors, it is important to use the "RICE" protocol. Rest the involved joint to prevent crippling deformities from hemarthrosis, ice the joint for 20 minutes every 3 to 4 hours, compress/wrap the joint, and elevate.[1] Give analgesics to reduce severe pain. Do not use aspirin and aspirin-containing compounds. As soon as bleeding ceases,

encourage mobilization of the affected area through range-of-motion exercises and physical therapy. Avoid weight bearing until all swelling has resolved and muscle strength has returned. Orthotics may be prescribed.

4. Manage any life-threatening complications that may develop because of hemorrhage or side effects from coagulation factors. Examples include nursing interventions to prevent or treat airway obstruction from hemorrhage into the neck and pharynx, recognition of compartment syndrome in an extremity, and early assessment and treatment of intracranial bleeding.

◆ **Ambulatory Care.** Home management is a primary consideration for the patient with hemophilia because the disease follows a progressive, chronic course. The quality and length of life may be significantly affected by the patient's knowledge of the illness and how to live with it. Refer the patient and caregiver to a local chapter of the National Hemophilia Foundation to encourage associations with others who are dealing with the problems of hemophilia.[18] Provide ongoing assessment of the patient's adaptation to the illness. Psychosocial support and assistance should be readily available as needed.

Most of the long-term care measures are related to patient teaching. Teach the patient to recognize disease-related problems and to learn which problems can be resolved at home and which require hospitalization. Immediate medical attention is needed for severe pain or swelling of a muscle or joint that restricts movement or inhibits sleep and for a head injury, swelling in the neck or mouth, abdominal pain, hematuria, melena, and skin wounds in need of suturing.

Teach the patient to perform daily oral hygiene without causing trauma. Understanding how to prevent injuries is another consideration. Teach the patient to take part only in noncontact sports (e.g., golf) and to wear gloves when doing household chores to prevent cuts or abrasions from knives, hammers, and other tools. The patient should wear a Medic Alert tag to ensure that HCPs know about the hemophilia in case of an accident. Many patients or their caregivers can be taught to self-administer the factor replacement therapies at home.

◆ Evaluation

The overall expected outcomes are similar to those for the patient with thrombocytopenia (see p. 626).

DISSEMINATED INTRAVASCULAR COAGULATION

Disseminated intravascular coagulation (DIC) is a serious bleeding and thrombotic disorder that results from abnormally initiated and accelerated clotting. Subsequent decreases in clotting factors and platelets ensue, which may lead to uncontrollable hemorrhage. The term DIC can be misleading because it suggests that blood is only clotting. However, there is profuse bleeding that results from the aggregation of platelets and clotting factors. DIC is always caused by an underlying disease or condition. That underlying problem must be treated for the DIC to resolve.

Etiology and Pathophysiology

DIC is not a disease. It is an abnormal response of the normal clotting cascade stimulated by a disease process or disorder.[2,3] The diseases and disorders known to predispose a patient to DIC are listed in Table 30.19. DIC can occur as an acute, catastrophic condition, or it may exist at a subacute or chronic level.

Each condition may have 1 or multiple triggering mechanisms to start the clotting cascade. For example, tumors and traumatized or necrotic tissue release tissue factors into circulation. Endotoxin from gram-negative bacteria activates several steps in the coagulation cascade.

Tissue factor is released at the site of tissue injury and by some cancers, such as leukemia, and enhances normal coagulation mechanisms. Abundant intravascular thrombin, the most powerful coagulant, is made (Fig. 30.9). It catalyzes the conversion of fibrinogen to fibrin and enhances platelet aggregation. There is widespread fibrin and platelet deposition in capillaries and arterioles, resulting in thrombosis. This process can lead to multiorgan failure.

In addition, clotting inhibitory mechanisms, such as antithrombin III (AT III) and protein C, are depressed. Excess clotting activates the fibrinolytic system, which in turn breaks down the newly formed clot, creating fibrin split products (FSPs). These products have anticoagulant properties and inhibit normal blood clotting. As FSPs accumulate and clotting factors are depleted, the blood loses its ability to clot. A stable clot cannot be formed at injury sites, which predisposes the patient to hemorrhage.

Chronic and subacute DIC is most often seen in patients with long-standing illnesses, such as cancer or autoimmune disease. Occasionally these patients have subclinical disease manifested only by laboratory abnormalities. However, the clinical spectrum ranges from easy bruising to hemorrhage, and from hypercoagulability to thrombosis.

Clinical Manifestations

DIC has both bleeding and thrombotic manifestations. Multiple factors cause bleeding manifestations of DIC (Fig. 30.9). They result from consumption and depletion of platelets and coagulation factors, as well as clot lysis and formation of FSPs that have anticoagulant properties. Bleeding in a person with no history or obvious cause should be questioned because it may be one of the first manifestations of acute DIC.

Bleeding manifestations include manifestations in the (1) skin, such as pallor, petechiae, purpura, oozing blood, venipuncture site bleeding, hematomas, and occult hemorrhage; (2) respiratory system (e.g., tachypnea, hemoptysis, and orthopnea); (3) cardiovascular system, such as tachycardia and hypotension; (4) GI tract, such as upper and lower GI bleeding, abdominal distention, and bloody stools; (5) urinary tract (e.g., hematuria); (6) neurologic system, such as vision changes, dizziness, headache, mental status changes, and irritability; and (7) musculoskeletal system (e.g., bone and joint pain).

Thrombotic manifestations are a result of fibrin or platelet deposition in the microvasculature (Fig. 30.9). These manifestations affect the (1) skin (e.g., cyanosis, ischemic tissue necrosis, hemorrhagic necrosis) (Fig. 30.10); (2) respiratory system (e.g., tachypnea, dyspnea, pulmonary emboli, and acute respiratory distress

TABLE 30.19 Risk Factors for DIC

Acute DIC

Cancers
- Acute leukemia
- Metastatic solid tumors

Hemolytic processes
- Acute hemolysis from infection or immunologic disorders
- Transfusion of mismatched blood

Obstetric conditions
- Abruptio placentae
- Amniotic fluid embolism
- HELLP syndrome
- Septic abortion or pregnancy

Septicemia (bacterial, viral, fungal, parasitic)

Shock
- Anaphylactic
- Cardiogenic
- Hemorrhagic

Tissue damage
- Acute anoxia (e.g., after cardiac arrest)
- Extensive burns and trauma

- Fulminant hepatitis
- Heatstroke
- Postoperative damage, especially after extracorporeal membrane oxygenation
- Prosthetic devices
- Severe head injury
- Snakebites
- Transplant rejections
- Vascular disorders (e.g., aortic aneurism)

Subacute DIC

Cancer
- Metastatic cancer
- Myeloproliferative/lymphoproliferative cancers

Obstetric
- Retained dead fetus

Chronic DIC
- Cancer
- Liver disease
- SLE

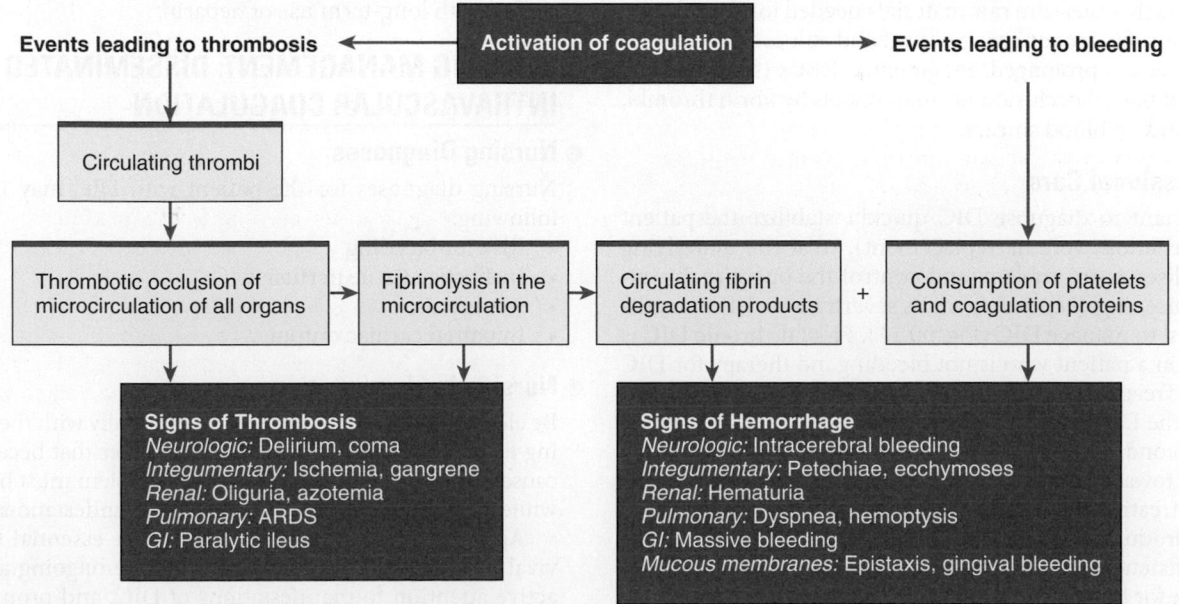

FIG. 30.9 Sequence of events that occur during DIC.

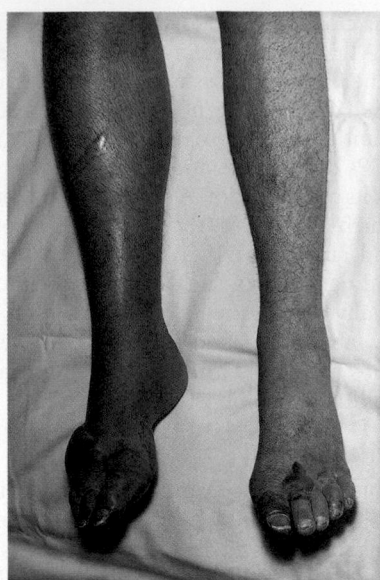

FIG. 30.10 Gangrene resulting from severe DIC. (From Howard MR, Hamilton PJ: *Haematology: An illustrated colour atlas*, ed 4, London, 2013, Churchill Livingstone.)

TABLE 30.20 Laboratory Results in Acute DIC

Test	Finding in Acute DIC
Screening Tests	
Prothrombin time (PT)	Prolonged
Partial thromboplastin time (PTT)	Prolonged
Activated partial thromboplastin time (aPTT)	Prolonged
Fibrinogen	Reduced
Platelets	Reduced
Thrombin time	Prolonged
Special Tests	
Antithrombin III (AT III)	Reduced
D-dimers (cross-linked fibrin fragments)	Increased
Factor assays (prothrombin and factors V, VIII, X, XIII)	Reduced but may give misleading results, since V and VIII rise with inflammation
Fibrin split products (FSPs)	Increased
Peripheral blood smear	Schistocytes present
Plasminogen, tissue plasminogen activator	Reduced
Proteins C and S	Reduced

syndrome [ARDS]); (3) cardiovascular system (e.g., ECG changes, venous distention); (4) GI tract (e.g., abdominal pain, paralytic ileus); and (5) kidney damage and oliguria, leading to failure.

Diagnostic Studies

Tests to diagnose acute DIC are listed in Table 30.20. As more clots are made in the body, more breakdown products from fibrinogen and fibrin are formed. These are termed *fibrin split products* (FSPs), and they interfere with blood coagulation by (1) coating the platelets and interfering with platelet function; (2) interfering with thrombin and thus disrupting coagulation; and (3) attaching to fibrinogen, which interferes with the polymerization process necessary to form a stable clot. D-dimer, a polymer resulting from the breakdown of fibrin (and not fibrinogen), is a specific marker for the degree of fibrinolysis. In general, tests that measure raw materials needed for coagulation (e.g., platelets, fibrinogen) are reduced and values that measure clotting times are prolonged. Fragmented RBCs (schistocytes), indicative of partial occlusion of small vessels by fibrin thrombi, may be found on blood smears.

Interprofessional Care

It is important to diagnose DIC quickly, stabilize the patient (e.g., oxygenation, volume replacement), treat the underlying causative disease or problem, and control the ongoing thrombosis and bleeding. Depending on its severity, a variety of methods are used to manage DIC (Fig. 30.11). First, if chronic DIC is diagnosed in a patient who is not bleeding, no therapy for DIC is needed. Treatment of the underlying disease may be enough to reverse the DIC (e.g., chemotherapy when DIC is caused by cancer). Second, when the patient with DIC is bleeding, therapy is directed toward providing support with needed blood products while treating the primary disorder.

Blood products are given cautiously based on specific component deficiencies to patients who have serious bleeding, are at high risk for bleeding (e.g., surgery), or require invasive procedures. Blood product support with platelets, cryoprecipitate,

and fresh frozen plasma (FFP) is usually reserved for a patient with life-threatening hemorrhage.[20] Therapy stabilizes a patient, prevents exsanguination or massive thrombosis, and permits institution of definitive therapy to treat the underlying cause. Cryoprecipitate replaces factor VIII and fibrinogen and is given if the fibrinogen level is below 100 mg/dL (1 g/L).[1] FFP is given only to patients with significant bleeding and a prolonged PT and aPTT. It replaces all clotting factors except platelets and is a source of antithrombin.

A patient with thrombosis is often treated by anticoagulation with heparin or LMSH. Heparin is used in the treatment of DIC only when the benefit (reduce clotting) outweighs the risk (further bleeding). Antithrombin III (ATnativ) may be useful in fulminant DIC, although it increases the risk for bleeding. Chronic DIC does not respond to oral anticoagulants. It is controlled with long-term use of heparin.

❖ NURSING MANAGEMENT: DISSEMINATED INTRAVASCULAR COAGULATION

◆ Nursing Diagnoses

Nursing diagnoses for the patient with DIC may include the following:

- Risk for bleeding
- Ineffective tissue perfusion
- Acute pain
- Impaired cardiac output

◆ Nursing Implementation

Be alert to the development of DIC, especially with the precipitating factors listed in Table 30.19. Remember that because DIC is caused by an underlying disease, that problem must be managed while providing supportive care for the manifestations of DIC.

Appropriate nursing interventions are essential to the survival of a patient with acute DIC. Astute ongoing assessment, active attention to manifestations of DIC, and prompt administration of prescribed therapies are crucial. Table 30.14 and

Therapy

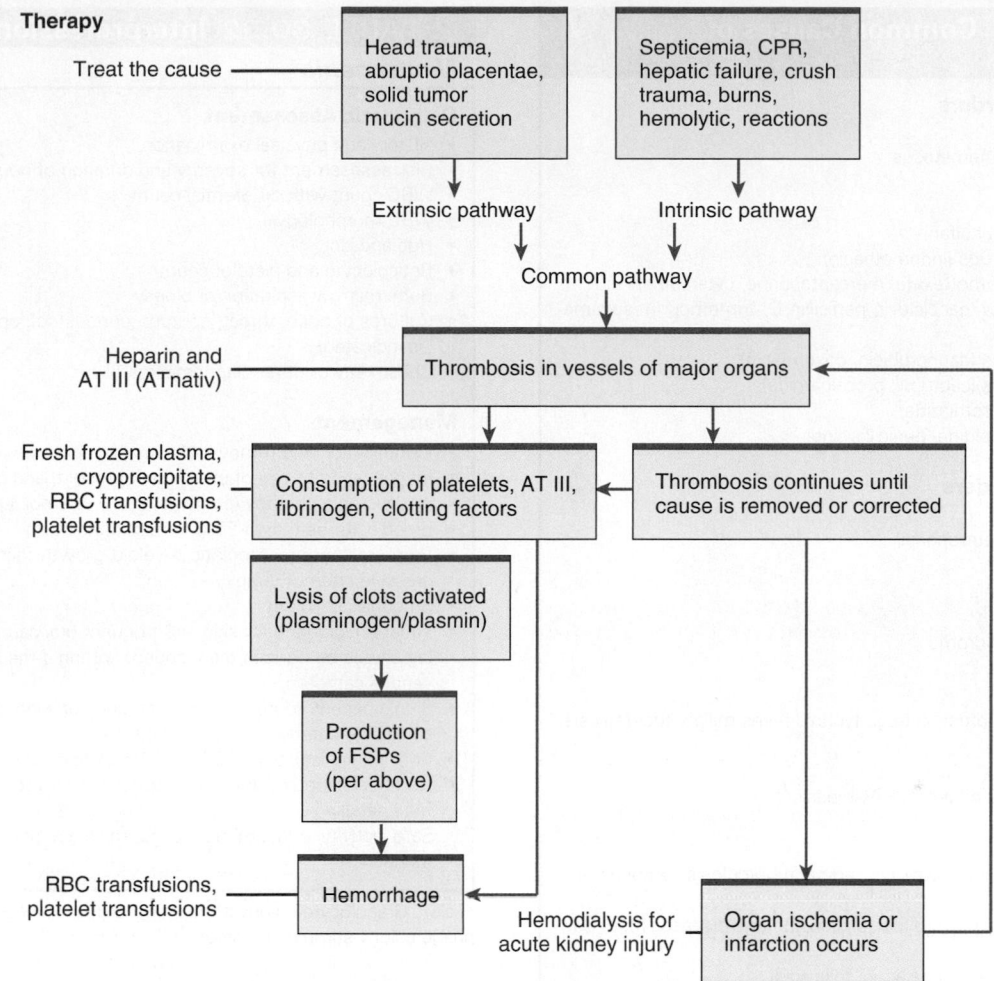

Treat the cause ——— Head trauma, abruptio placentae, solid tumor mucin secretion

Septicemia, CPR, hepatic failure, crush trauma, burns, hemolytic, reactions

Extrinsic pathway

Intrinsic pathway

Common pathway

Heparin and AT III (ATnativ) ——— Thrombosis in vessels of major organs

Fresh frozen plasma, cryoprecipitate, RBC transfusions, platelet transfusions

Consumption of platelets, AT III, fibrinogen, clotting factors

Thrombosis continues until cause is removed or corrected

Lysis of clots activated (plasminogen/plasmin)

Production of FSPs (per above)

RBC transfusions, platelet transfusions ——— Hemorrhage

Hemodialysis for acute kidney injury

Organ ischemia or infarction occurs

FIG. 30.11 Sites of action for therapies in DIC. *AT III,* Antithrombin III; *FSPs,* fibrin split products.

eNursing Care Plan 30.2 (available on the website for this chapter) provide assessments and interventions appropriate for the patient with DIC.

Early detection of bleeding and clotting, both occult and overt, must be a primary goal. Assess for signs of external bleeding (e.g., petechiae, oozing at IV or injection sites), signs of internal bleeding (e.g., increased heart rate, changes in mental status, increasing abdominal girth, pain), and any signs that microthrombi may be causing clinically significant organ damage (e.g., decreased renal output). Minimize tissue damage and protect the patient from sources of bleeding. Give blood products and medications correctly. Blood product transfusion is discussed later in this chapter on pp. 647–651.

NEUTROPENIA

Leukopenia refers to a decrease in the total WBC count (granulocytes, monocytes, and lymphocytes). *Granulocytopenia* is a deficiency of granulocytes, which include neutrophils, eosinophils, and basophils. The neutrophilic granulocytes (neutrophils), which play a key role in phagocytizing pathogenic microbes, are closely monitored in clinical practice as an indicator of a patient's risk for infection. A reduction in neutrophils is termed **neutropenia**. Some clinicians use the terms granulocytopenia and neutropenia interchangeably because the largest constituency of granulocytes is the neutrophils.

The *absolute neutrophil count* (ANC) is determined by multiplying the total WBC count by the percent of neutrophils. *Neutropenia* is defined as ANC less than 1000 cells/μL (1 × 10^9/L). Normally, neutrophils range from 2200 to 7700 cells/μL. *Severe neutropenia* is defined as an ANC less than 500 cells/μL.[21]

In considering the clinical significance of neutropenia, it is important to know whether the decrease in the neutrophil count was gradual or rapid, the degree of neutropenia, and the duration. The faster the drop and the longer the duration, the greater the chance of life-threatening infection, sepsis, and death. Other factors and co-morbid conditions, such as immune disorders (e.g., HIV), being older than 60, having an existing infection, being in the hospital, and having chronic obstructive pulmonary disease, can increase the risk for a serious infection.[22]

Neutropenia is a clinical consequence that occurs with a variety of conditions or diseases (Table 30.21). It can be an expected effect, a side effect, or an unintentional effect of certain drugs. The most common cause of neutropenia is the use of chemotherapy and immunosuppressive therapy in the treatment of cancer and autoimmune disease. A term we use to describe the lowest point of neutropenia (and other blood cells) in a patient treated with chemotherapy is *nadir.*

Clinical Manifestations

The patient with neutropenia is predisposed to infection with opportunistic pathogens and nonpathogenic organisms from

TABLE 30.21 Common Causes of Neutropenia

Autoimmune Disorders
- Felty syndrome
- Systemic lupus erythematosus

Drugs
- Alkylating agents (busulfan)
- Antiinflammatory drugs (indomethacin)
- Antimetabolites (methotrexate, mercaptopurine, cytarabine)
- Antimicrobial agents (ganciclovir, penicillin G, trimethoprim/sulfamethoxazole)
- Antitumor antibiotics (daunorubicin, doxorubicin)
- Cardiovascular drugs (captopril, procainamide)
- Diuretics (hydrochlorothiazide)
- Miscellaneous (ticlopidine, penicillamine)

Hematologic Disorders
- Aplastic anemia
- Congenital (cyclic neutropenia)
- Fanconi syndrome
- Idiopathic neutropenia
- Leukemia
- Myelodysplastic syndrome

Infections
- Fulminant bacterial infection (e.g., typhoid fever, miliary tuberculosis)
- Parasitic
- Rickettsial
- Viral (e.g., hepatitis, influenza, HIV, measles)

Others
- Bone marrow infiltration (e.g., carcinoma, tuberculosis, lymphoma)
- Hemodialysis
- Hypersplenism (e.g., portal hypertension, storage diseases [e.g., Gaucher disease])
- Nutritional deficiencies (cobalamin, folic acid)
- Severe sepsis

TABLE 30.22 Interprofessional Care

Neutropenia

Diagnostic Assessment
- History and physical examination
- Risk assessment for severity and duration of neutropenia
- WBC count with differential count
- WBC morphology
- Hgb and Hct
- Reticulocyte and platelet count
- Bone marrow aspiration or biopsy
- Cultures of nose, throat, sputum, urine, stool, obvious lesions, blood (as indicated)
- Chest x-ray or other diagnostic tests

Management
- Identification and removal of cause of neutropenia (if possible)
- Identification of site of infection (if present) and causative organism
- Antimicrobial therapy (prophylactically or empiric)
- Blood cultures drawn STAT, before antibiotics
- Prophylactic hematopoietic myeloid growth factors after myelosuppressive chemotherapy
- Strict hand hygiene
- Patient hygiene (daily skin and frequent oral care; chlorhexidine bathing should be done in the inpatient setting if the patient has a central venous catheter)
- Single-patient room, positive-pressure or high-efficiency particulate air (HEPA) filtration, depending on risk
- Community isolation and home precautions (if outpatient)
- Nutritional therapy (dietary instruction) on foods to avoid and safe food handling
- Safe activity and ambulation to maintain physical and pulmonary function

G-CSF, Granulocyte colony-stimulating factor; *GM-CSF,* granulocyte-macrophage colony-stimulating factor.

the normal body flora. When the WBC count is low or immature WBCs are present, normal phagocytic mechanisms are impaired. The classic manifestations of inflammation—redness, heat, and swelling—may not occur. WBCs are the major component of pus. Therefore, in the patient with neutropenia, pus formation (e.g., as a visible skin lesion or as lung infiltrates on a chest x-ray) is absent.

⚠ SAFETY ALERT Neutropenia
- A low-grade fever in neutropenic patients is of great significance because it may indicate infection and lead to septic shock and death unless treated promptly.
- Neutropenic fever (≥100.4°F [38°C] and/or new signs or symptoms suggesting infection and a neutrophil count <500/μL) is a medical emergency.[22]
- Blood cultures should be drawn STAT and antibiotics started within 1 hr.

When fever occurs in a neutropenic patient, it is assumed to be caused by infection and requires immediate attention. The immunocompromised, neutropenic patient has little or no ability to fight infection. So, minor infections can lead rapidly to sepsis and death. The mucous membranes of the throat and mouth, skin, perineal area, and pulmonary system are common entry points for pathogenic organisms in susceptible hosts.

Manifestations related to infection at these sites include sore throat and dysphagia, ulcerative lesions of the pharyngeal and buccal mucosa, diarrhea, rectal tenderness, vaginal itching or discharge, shortness of breath, and nonproductive cough. Any report of minor pain or any other symptom by the patient may be significant and should be reported to the HCP at once. These seemingly minor problems can progress to fever, chills, sepsis, septic shock, and death if not recognized and treated early.

Systemic infections caused by bacterial, fungal, and viral organisms are common in patients with neutropenia. The patient's own flora (normally nonpathogenic) contributes significantly to life-threatening infections. Organisms known to be common sources of infection include gram-positive coagulase-negative *Staphylococcus* and *Staphylococcus aureus* and gram-negative *E. coli, Klebsiella, Enterobacter,* and *Pseudomonas aeruginosa.*[22] Fungi involved include *Candida* (usually *C. albicans*) and *Aspergillus* organisms. Viral infections caused by reactivation of herpes simplex and zoster are common after prolonged periods of neutropenia, such as in HSCT patients.[23]

Diagnostic Studies

The primary diagnostic tests for assessing neutropenia are the peripheral WBC count and bone marrow aspiration and biopsy (Table 30.22). A total WBC count of less than 4000/μL (4 × 10^9/L) reflects leukopenia. However, only a differential count can confirm the presence of neutropenia (neutrophil count less than 1000/μL [1 × 10^9/L]). If the differential WBC count reflects an absolute neutropenia of 500 to 1000/μL (0.5 to 1.0 × 10^9/L), the patient is at moderate risk for a bacterial infection. An absolute neutropenia of less than 500/μL (0.5 × 10^9/L) places the patient at severe risk. Patients with acute leukemia who present with a high WBC may in fact have neutropenia, because most of the WBCs are ineffective leukemia blasts cells.

A peripheral blood smear assesses for immature forms of WBCs (e.g., bands). The hematocrit level, reticulocyte count, and platelet count are done to evaluate bone marrow function. Review the patient's recent past and current drug history. If the cause of neutropenia is unknown, a bone marrow aspiration and biopsy is done to examine cellularity and cell morphology. Other studies may be done to assess spleen and liver function.

❖ Interprofessional and Nursing Management

The nursing and interprofessional care of neutropenia includes (1) determining the cause of the neutropenia, (2) instituting antibiotic therapy promptly, (3) identifying the offending organisms if an infection has developed, (4) giving hematopoietic growth factors prophylactically after chemotherapy, and (5) implementing protective practices (e.g., strict hand washing, skin and oral hygiene) (Table 30.22).[24]

Sometimes, the cause of the neutropenia can be easily treated (e.g., nutritional deficiencies). However, neutropenia can be a side effect that must be tolerated as a necessary step in therapy (e.g., chemotherapy, radiation therapy). In some situations, the neutropenia resolves when the primary disease or disorder is treated.

NURSING MANAGEMENT
Caring for the Patient With Neutropenia

All members of the health care team have important roles in preventing infection in the patient with neutropenia. Careful hand washing is an important preventive measure. It should be done before, during, and after patient care by everyone caring for the patient.

- Determine the type of isolation precautions that need to be started, if any.
- Assess patient for signs and symptoms of infection.
- Screen visitors for infectious diseases.
- Place the patient on a neutropenic diet to protect them from bacteria found in some foods.
- Obtain cultures of sputum, throat, lesions, wounds, urine, and feces.
- Give antibiotics and hematopoietic growth factors.
- Teach patient and visitors about hand washing.
- Provide teaching about how to avoid infection, including the need for skin care and oral hygiene.
- Teach the patient and caregivers about signs and symptoms of infection and what to do if they occur.

Monitor the neutropenic patient for signs and symptoms of infection (e.g., any fever 100.4°F [38°C] or greater) and early septic shock. Early identification of a potentially infective organism depends on obtaining cultures from various sites. Serial blood cultures (at least 2) or 1 from a peripheral site and 1 from a venous access device should be done promptly and antibiotics started within 1 hour.

Giving broad-spectrum antibiotics is usually by the IV route because of the rapidly lethal effects of infection. However, some oral antibiotics are highly effective and routinely used for prophylaxis against infection in some neutropenic patients. The use of a third- or fourth-generation cephalosporin with broad microorganism coverage (e.g., cefepime, ceftazidime) or a carbapenem (e.g., imipenem/cilastatin [Primaxin]) will be started and augmented depending on the patient's response and/or results of the diagnostic tests.

Begin therapy promptly and observe the patient for side effects of antimicrobial agents. Ongoing febrile episodes or a change in the patient's assessment requires a call to the HCP for assessment, or more cultures, diagnostic tests, or antimicrobial therapies. The longer the neutropenia, the greater the risk is for a fungal infection. Antifungal therapy is started whenever a culture is positive, or in patients who do not become afebrile with broad-spectrum antibiotic coverage.

Cultures of sputum, throat, lesions, wounds, urine, and feces may part of patient surveillance. Depending on the clinical situation, it may be necessary to do CT scans, bronchoscopy with bronchial brushings, or lung biopsy to diagnose the cause of pneumonic infiltrates. Invasive diagnostic studies are often contraindicated because of the concern of introducing infection and the fact that these patients are also often thrombocytopenic. Despite these many tests, the causative organism is found in only 20% to 30% of neutropenic patients. Thus the priority is to obtain the blood cultures and begin the antibiotic at once. Ongoing monitoring is essential as early identification and appropriate management can prevent death from sepsis.[25]

Myeloid growth factors (see Table 15.15) can be used to prevent neutropenia or to reduce its severity and duration.[24] Once neutropenia has occurred, these agents are generally not as effective.

Keep the following care principles in mind: (1) the patient's normal flora is the most common source of microbial colonization and infection; (2) transmission of organisms from humans most often occurs by direct contact with the hands; (3) air, food, water, and equipment provide opportunities for infection transmission; and (4) HCPs, visitors, and other patients with infections also can be sources of infection transmission under certain conditions.

Hand washing is the single most important preventive measure to minimize the risk for infection in the neutropenic patient. Strict hand washing by staff and visitors using an antiseptic hand wash before and after contact is the major method to prevent transmission of harmful pathogens.

Separate immunocompromised patients from those who are infected or have conditions that increase the probability of transmitting infections (e.g., poor hygiene caused by lack of understanding or cognitive dysfunction). Often patients can be managed on an outpatient basis if the patient and caregiver can monitor for fever and other signs of infection and then report promptly to a nearby health care facility (Table 30.23).[1,21] If the patient is hospitalized, a private room should be used. High-efficiency particulate air (HEPA) filtration is an air-handling method with a high-flow filtering system that can reduce or eliminate the number of aerosolized pathogens in the environment used for hematopoietic stem cell transplant patients. Care routines in a HEPA environment are the same as care in any other private room. Neutropenic precaution guidelines may be used, such as prophylactic antibiotics and antifungals. Teach the patient and caregiver to avoid potentially hazardous foods, such as raw and undercooked meats and eggs and soft cheeses with molds.[1] The nursing measures discussed in eNursing Care Plan 30.3 (available on the website for this chapter) are important in the treatment of the patient with neutropenia.

Do not overlook quality-of-life issues for the patient with neutropenia. Fatigue, malaise, a decrease in functioning, and social isolation require coaching on safe activity.

TABLE 30.23   Patient & Caregiver Teaching

Neutropenia

Include the following instructions when teaching a patient or caregiver the precautions to take when the neutrophil count is low:

1. WASH YOUR HANDS frequently and make sure those around you wash their hands frequently, especially if they help with your care. You may also use an antibacterial hand gel.
2. Notify your nurse or HCP if you have any of the following:
   Fever ≥100.4° F (38° C)*
   Chills or feeling hot
   Redness, swelling, discharge, or new pain on or in your body
   Changes in urination or bowel movements
   Cough, sore throat, mouth sores, or blisters
3. If you are at home, take your temperature as directed and follow instructions on what to do if you have a fever.
4. Avoid crowds and people with colds, flu, or infections. If you are in a public area, wear a mask and use hand sanitizing gel frequently.
5. Avoid uncooked meats, seafood, or eggs and unwashed fruits and vegetables. Ask your HCP about specific dietary guidelines for you.
6. Bathe or shower daily. Use a moisturizer to prevent skin from drying and cracking.
7. Maintain some daily activity as instructed by your health care team. This may include walking and moderate exercise while avoiding crowds.
8. Brush your teeth with a soft toothbrush 4 times daily. You may floss once daily if it does not cause excessive pain or bleeding. Avoid alcohol-based mouthwashes.
9. Do not garden or clean up after pets. You may feed and pet your dog or cat if you wash your hands well after handling.

*Need to verify cut-off temperature with HCP.

MYELODYSPLASTIC SYNDROME

Myelodysplastic syndrome (MDS) is a group of related hematologic disorders characterized by peripheral blood cytopenias (from ineffective blood cell production) and changes in the cellularity of the bone marrow with dysplastic changes. In MDS, *hematopoiesis* is disorderly and ineffective. The estimated incidence is 4.9 per 100,000 people per year in the United States. Although it can occur in all age-groups, the highest prevalence is in people over 80 years of age, at which point the rate increases to 59.8 per 100,000.[26]

Etiology and Pathophysiology

The etiology of MDS is unknown. People who have received radiation therapy, had chemotherapy with alkylating agents (e.g., chlorambucil, cyclophosphamide, melphalan), or were exposed to industrial solvents (e.g., benzene) have a higher risk for developing MDS than people who have not had these exposures. About 50% of MDS patients have an overt chromosome abndormality.[1,3] Rarely, genetic disorders are responsible for the disease.

We refer to MDS as a *clonal disorder because* some bone marrow stem cells continue to function normally, while others do not. The abnormal clone of the stem cells is usually found in the bone marrow. Eventually, it may be found in the circulation.

Sometimes, one type of MDS transforms into another. Depending on the subtype, MDS may progress to acute myelogenous leukemia (AML).[26] In contrast to AML, in which the leukemic cells show little normal maturation, the clonal cells in MDS always display some degree of maturity. Disease progression is slower than in AML, and sometimes treatment is not needed.

Clinical Manifestations

Manifestations result from neoplastic transformation of the immature hematopoietic stem cells in the bone marrow. MDS often presents as infection and bleeding caused by inadequate numbers of ineffectively functioning circulating granulocytes or platelets. It may be found in the older adult during testing for the symptoms of anemia, thrombocytopenia, or neutropenia. It may be diagnosed incidentally from a routine CBC. During the advanced stage of MDS, life-threatening anemia, thrombocytopenia, and neutropenia occur.

Diagnostic Studies

Bone marrow biopsy with aspirate analysis is essential for both the diagnosis and classification of the specific type of MDS. The patient with MDS has peripheral cytopenia and changes in the bone marrow (hypocellular or hypercellular). Laboratory data and bone marrow studies help rule out other causes of the dysplasia, such as nonmalignant disorders, cobalamin and folate deficiencies, and infections.

❖ Interprofessional and Nursing Management

Treatment of MDS is based on the premise that the aggressiveness of treatment should match the aggressiveness of the disease. This is based on the amount and type of dysplasia in the bone marrow, specific genetic mutations, anticipated patient tolerance, and patient preference.[26] Supportive treatment consists of hematologic monitoring (serial bone marrow and peripheral blood examinations), antibiotic therapy, or transfusions with blood products along with iron chelators to prevent iron overload.

Low-risk patients often can be treated with EPO, myeloid growth factors, and thrombopoietin.[26] Some patients are treated with intensive chemotherapy and/or HSCT. Azacitidine (Vidaza) and decitabine (Dacogen) are drugs that help restore normal growth control and differentiation of hematopoietic cells and reduce the frequency of transformation of MDS to acute leukemia. Side effects include myelosuppression, nausea, vomiting, constipation or diarrhea, renal dysfunction, and injection site redness.

Other treatments for MDS include lenalidomide (Revlimid), cytarabine with or without antitumor antibiotics (anthracyclines), antithymocyte globulin, and cyclosporine.[25,26] Chemotherapy and allogeneic HSCT are used in appropriate patients with high-risk features to treat bone marrow dysfunction of MDS and restore it with normal hematopoiesis.

Nursing care of a patient with MDS is like that of a patient with manifestations of anemia, thrombocytopenia, and neutropenia. (See eNursing Care Plan 30.1 for the patient with anemia, eNursing Care Plan 30.2 for the patient with thrombocytopenia, and eNursing Care Plan 30.3 for the patient with neutropenia. The eNursing Care Plans are available on the website for this chapter.)

LEUKEMIA

Leukemia is the general term used to describe a group of cancers affecting the blood and blood-forming tissues of the bone marrow, lymph system, and spleen. Leukemia occurs in all age-groups. It results in an accumulation of dysfunctional cells because of a loss of regulation in cell division. An estimated 62,130 new cases are diagnosed each year. Leukemias account for 29% of all childhood cancers. Of those, 76% are lymphoid

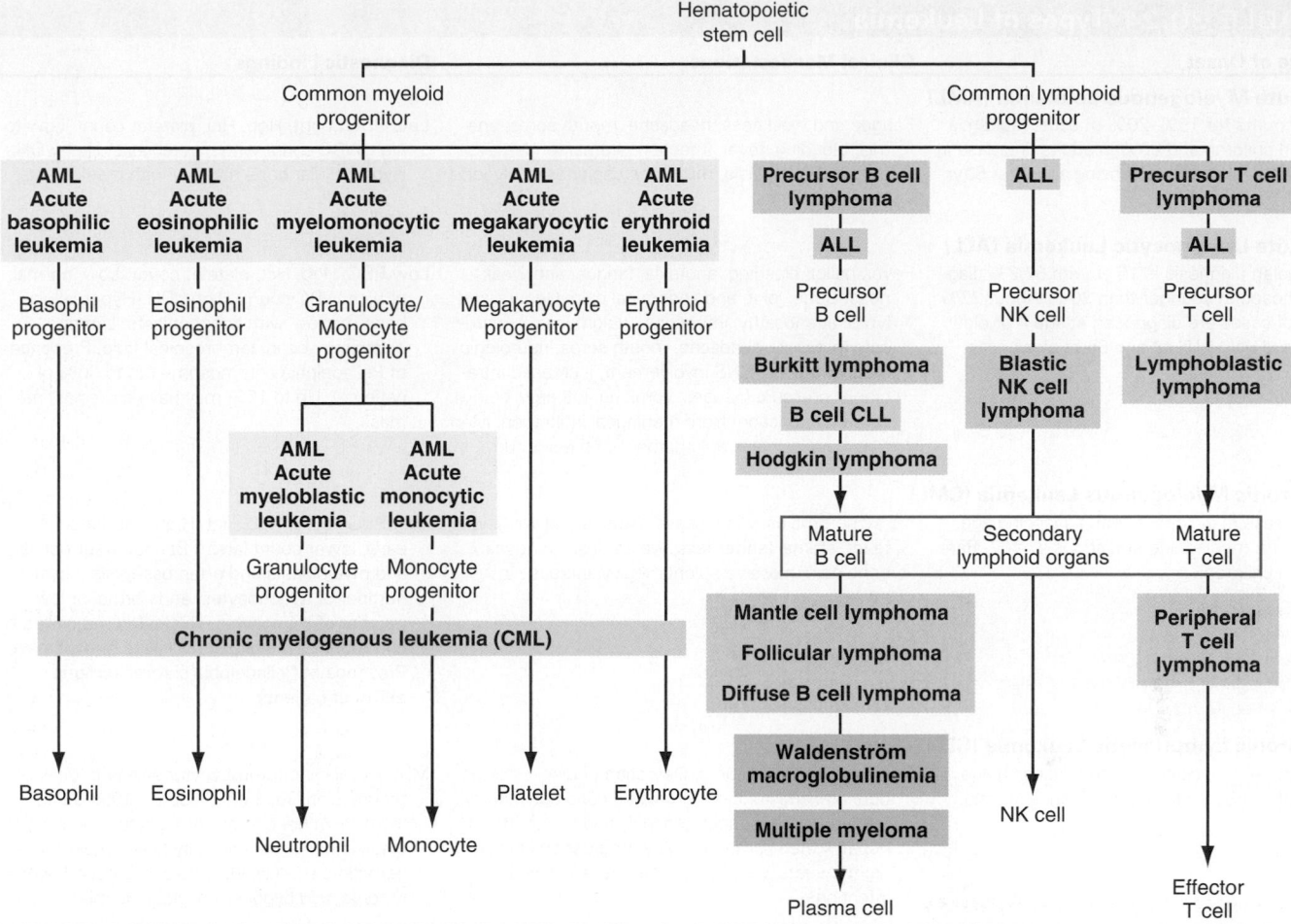

FIG. 30.12 Origins of leukemias, lymphomas, and myeloma. Differentiation pathways of blood-forming cells and the point at which the malignant clone originates. (Modified from Huether SE, McCance KL, editors: *Understanding pathophysiology,* ed 7, St Louis, 2017, Elsevier.)

leukemias.[27] Leukemia follows a progressive course that is eventually fatal if untreated. However, progress in successful cancer treatments has been most rapid for hematopoietic and lymphoid cancers in the past 3 decades.[27]

Etiology and Pathophysiology

Leukemia has no single cause. It is now known that all cancers, including leukemia, begin as a mutation in the DNA of certain cells. Most leukemias result from a combination of factors, including genetic and environmental influences. Abnormal genes *(oncogenes)* can cause many types of cancers, including leukemias (see Chapter 15). Chemical agents (e.g., benzene), chemotherapeutic agents (e.g., alkylating agents, topoisomerase II inhibitors), viruses, radiation, and immunologic deficiencies have all been associated with the development of leukemia. Depending on the type of leukemia, other potential causes are exposure to pesticides (farmworkers), smoking, and obesity.[3]

Although ribonucleic acid (RNA) retroviruses cause several leukemias in animals, a viral cause for a human leukemia has been established for only some patients with adult T-cell leukemia/lymphoma. This form of leukemia is endemic in southwestern Japan and parts of the Caribbean and is caused by the human T-cell leukemia virus, type 1 (HTLV-1).[28] Leukemia occurs more often in those with certain congenital or inherited abnormalities (e.g., Down syndrome). Chronic lymphocytic leukemia has a familial trend.[3]

Classification

Leukemia is classified based on acute versus chronic disease and on the type of WBC involved. The terms *acute* and *chronic* refer to cell maturity and nature of disease onset. Acute leukemia is characterized by the clonal proliferation of immature hematopoietic cells. The leukemia develops after malignant transformation of a single type of immature hematopoietic cell, followed by cellular replication and expansion of that malignant clone (Fig. 30.12). Chronic leukemias involve more mature forms of the WBC. The disease onset is more gradual.

Leukemia classified by the type of leukocyte involved is described as myelogenous or lymphocytic origin. By combining the acute and chronic categories with the cell type involved, one can identify 4 major types of leukemia: acute lymphocytic leukemia (ALL), acute myelogenous leukemia (AML), chronic myelogenous (granulocytic) leukemia (CML), and chronic lymphocytic leukemia (CLL). Other defining features of these leukemic subtypes are shown in Table 30.24.

Acute Myelogenous Leukemia. AML represents about one third of all leukemias, and it makes up about 80% of the acute leukemias in adults.[3,29] Its onset is often abrupt and dramatic.

TABLE 30.24 Types of Leukemia

Age of Onset	Clinical Manifestations	Diagnostic Findings
Acute Myelogenous Leukemia (AML)		
Accounts for 15%–20% of acute leukemia in children and 80% in adults. Increase in incidence with advancing age after 60 yr.	Fatigue and weakness, headache, mouth sores, anemia, bleeding, fever, infection, sternal tenderness, gingival hyperplasia, mild hepatosplenomegaly (one third of patients)	Low RBC count, Hgb, Hct, platelet count. Low to high WBC count with myeloblasts. High LDH. Hypercellular bone marrow with myeloblasts.
Acute Lymphocytic Leukemia (ALL)		
Median diagnosis is 15 yr with 57.2% diagnosed at younger than 20 yr. About 27% of cases are diagnosed at age 4 or older and only 11% at age 65 or older.	Fever, pallor, bleeding, anorexia, fatigue, and weakness. Bone, joint, and abdominal pain. Generalized lymphadenopathy, infections, weight loss, hepatosplenomegaly, headache, mouth sores, neurologic manifestations: CNS involvement, increased intracranial pressure (nausea, vomiting, lethargy, cranial nerve dysfunction) from meningeal infiltration. Men may have painless enlargement of the scrotum.	Low RBC, Hgb, Hct, platelet count. Low, normal, or high WBC count. High LDH. Hypercellular bone marrow with lymphoblasts. Lymphoblasts may be in cerebrospinal fluid. Presence of Philadelphia chromosome (up to 30% of patients). Up to 15% may have a mediastinal mass.
Chronic Myelogenous Leukemia (CML)		
Increase in incidence with advancing age, with median age at diagnosis of 67. Rare in children.	No symptoms early in disease. Fatigue and weakness, fever, sternal tenderness, weight loss, joint pain, bone pain, massive splenomegaly, increase in sweating.	Low RBC count, Hgb, Hct. High platelet count early, lower count later. ↑ Banded neutrophils and myeloblasts and often basophils, normal number of lymphocytes, and normal or low number of monocytes. Nucleated red cells are common. Low leukocyte alkaline phosphatase. Presence of Philadelphia chromosome in ≥90% of patients.
Chronic Lymphocytic Leukemia (CLL)		
Increase in incidence with advancing age after 65 yr, with predominance in men.	Frequently no symptoms. Detection of disease often during examination for unrelated condition, chronic fatigue, anorexia, splenomegaly and lymphadenopathy, hepatomegaly. May progress to fever, night sweats, weight loss, fatigue, and frequent infections.	Mild anemia and thrombocytopenia with disease progression. Total WBC count >100,000/µL. Increase in peripheral lymphocytes and lymphocytes in bone marrow. May have autoimmune hemolytic anemia, idiopathic thrombocytopenic purpura, and hypogammaglobulinemia.

A patient may have serious infections and abnormal bleeding from the onset of the disease.

AML is characterized by uncontrolled proliferation of myeloblasts, the precursors of granulocytes. There is hyperplasia of the bone marrow. The manifestations are usually related to replacement of normal hematopoietic cells in the marrow by leukemic myeloblasts and, to a lesser extent, to infiltration of other organs and tissue (Table 30.24).

Acute Lymphocytic Leukemia. ALL is the most common type of leukemia in children and accounts for about 20% of acute leukemia cases in adults.[3,30] In ALL, immature small lymphocytes proliferate in the bone marrow. Most are of B-cell origin. Most patients have fever at the time of diagnosis. Signs and symptoms may appear abruptly with bleeding or fever, or they may be insidious with progressive weakness, fatigue, bone and/or joint pain, and bleeding tendencies.

Central nervous system (CNS) manifestations are especially common in ALL and are a serious problem. Infiltration into other tissues and lymph nodes can occur.[3]

Chronic Myelogenous Leukemia. CML is caused by excessive development of neoplastic granulocytes in the bone marrow. These granulocytes are in all stages of development. They move into the peripheral blood in massive numbers and infiltrate the liver and spleen.[31]

The natural history of CML is a chronic stable phase followed by the development of a more acute, aggressive phase referred to as the *blastic phase*. The chronic phase of CML can last for several years. It usually can be well controlled with treatment.

Even with treatment, the chronic phase of the disease eventually progresses to the accelerated phase, ending in a blastic phase. Once CML transforms to an acute or blastic phase, it must be treated more aggressively, similar to an acute leukemia.

Genetic Link. The *Philadelphia chromosome* originates from the translocation between the *BCR* gene on chromosome 22 and the *ABL* gene on chromosome 9. The protein that is encoded by the newly created *BCR-ABL* gene on the Philadelphia chromosome interferes with normal cell cycle events, such as the regulation of cell proliferation.

The Philadelphia chromosome, which is present in about 90% or more of patients with CML, is a diagnostic hallmark of CML.[31] In addition, its presence is an important indicator of residual disease or relapse after treatment. However, the presence of the Philadelphia chromosome is not specific to diagnose CML. It is also found in ALL and occasionally in AML.

Chronic Lymphocytic Leukemia. CLL is the most common leukemia in adults in Western countries.[32] CLL is characterized by the production and accumulation of functionally inactive but long-lived, small, mature-appearing lymphocytes. B cells are usually involved. The lymphocytes infiltrate the bone marrow, spleen, and liver. Lymph node enlargement (lymphadenopathy) is present throughout the body.

Complications are rare in early-stage CLL but may develop as the disease advances. Pressure on nerves from enlarged lymph nodes causes pain and even paralysis. Mediastinal node enlargement leads to pulmonary symptoms. Because CLL is usually a disease of older adults, treatment decisions must be

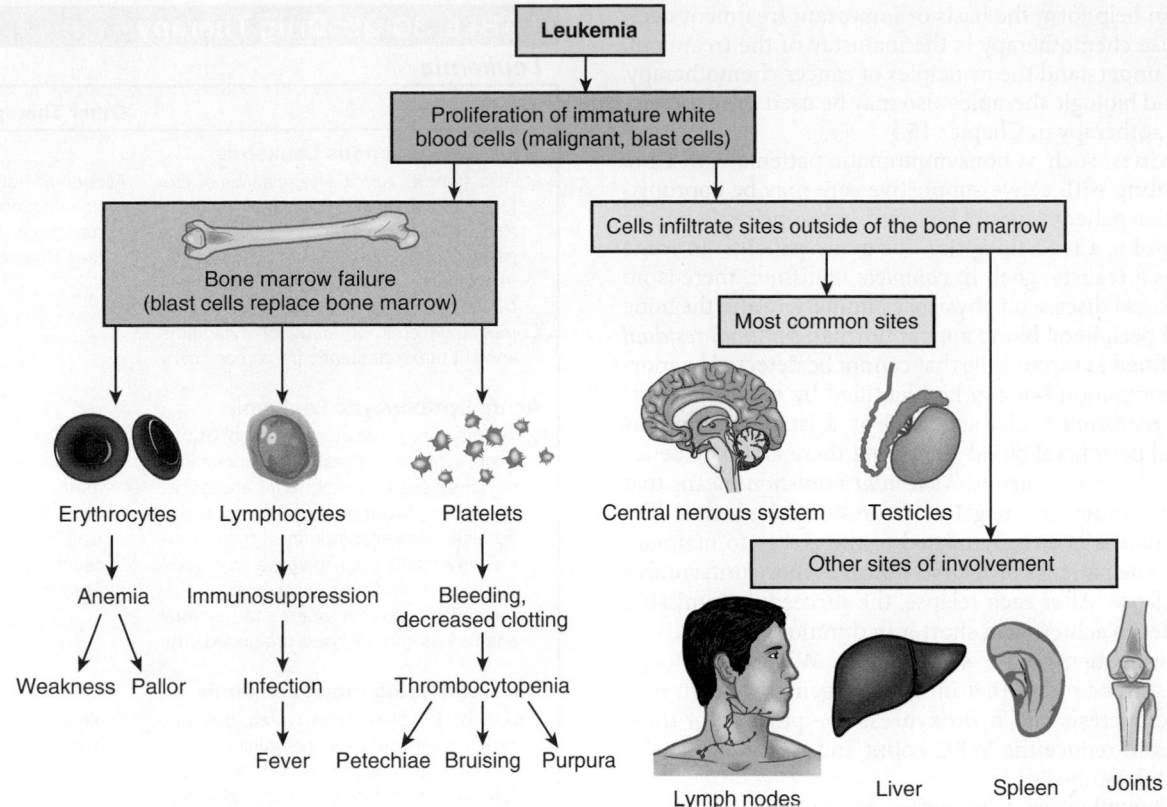

FIG. 30.13 Pathophysiology of leukemia. (Modified from McKinney ES, James SR, Murray SS, et al: *Maternal-child nursing,* Philadelphia, 2000, Saunders.)

made by considering the progression of the disease and the side effects of treatment. Many patients in the early stages of CLL do not need treatment. Others are followed closely and receive treatment only when the disease progresses. About one-third need immediate treatment at the time of diagnosis.

Other Leukemias. Occasionally the subtype of leukemia cannot be identified. The cancerous leukemic cells may have lymphoid, myeloid, or mixed characteristics. Often these patients do not respond to treatment and have a poor prognosis. Other rare types include hairy cell and biphenotypic (both abnormal myeloid and lymphoid clones) leukemias.

Overlap Between Leukemia and Lymphoma. Overlap exists between leukemia and non-Hodgkin's lymphoma (NHL) because both involve proliferation of lymphocytes or their precursors (Fig. 30.12). A leukemia-like picture with peripheral lymphocytosis and bone marrow involvement may be present in about 15% of adults with some types of NHL.[3] Patients with more extensive nodal involvement (especially mediastinal), fewer circulating abnormal cells, and fewer blast forms in the marrow are considered to have lymphoma. A prominent leukemic phase is less common in aggressive lymphomas, except Burkitt's, lymphoblastic lymphomas, and those classified as "double hit," meaning they have a double oncogene mutation.[3,33]

Clinical Manifestations

The manifestations of leukemia are varied (Table 30.24). They relate to problems caused by bone marrow failure and the formation of leukemic infiltrates (Fig. 30.13). Bone marrow failure results from (1) bone marrow overcrowding by abnormal cells and (2) inadequate production of normal marrow elements.

The patient is predisposed to anemia, thrombocytopenia, and decreased number and function of WBCs.

As leukemia progresses, fewer normal blood cells are made. The abnormal WBCs continue to accumulate because they do not go through the normal cell life cycle to death *(apoptosis).* The leukemic cells may infiltrate the patient's organs, leading to problems such as splenomegaly, hepatomegaly, lymphadenopathy, bone pain, meningeal irritation, and oral lesions. Solid masses resulting from collections of leukemic cells, called *chloromas,* can occur. A high leukemic white count in the peripheral blood (more than 100,000 cells/μL) can cause the blood to thicken and potentially block circulatory pathways. This is called *leukostasis.* It can be life threatening.

Diagnostic Studies

Peripheral blood evaluation and bone marrow examination are the primary methods of diagnosing and classifying the types of leukemia. Morphologic, histochemical, immunologic, and cytogenetic methods are used to identify leukemic cell types, stage of development, and significant genetic mutations. Knowing the type of leukemia is important because each type has a different prognosis and treatment options. For example, in CML, the finding of the Philadelphia chromosome is an important diagnostic indicator. It is also sometimes present in ALL and affects the treatment as well.[30,31] Other studies, such as lumbar puncture and PET/CT scans, can detect leukemic cells outside of the blood and bone marrow.

Interprofessional Care

Once a diagnosis of leukemia has been made, care focuses on the initial goal of attaining remission. Age and cytogenetic analysis often help form the basis of important treatment decisions. Because chemotherapy is the mainstay of the treatment, you need to understand the principles of cancer chemotherapy. Radiation and biologic therapies also may be used. (See the section on chemotherapy in Chapter 15.)

In some cases, such as nonsymptomatic patients with CLL, watchful waiting with active supportive care may be appropriate. Although a patient may not be cured, attaining remission or disease control is a realistic option for many patients. In some cases, cure is a realistic goal. In *complete remission*, there is no evidence of overt disease on physical examination, and the bone marrow and peripheral blood appear normal. *Minimal residual disease* is defined as tumor cells that cannot be detected by morphologic examination but can be identified by molecular testing. *Partial remission* is characterized by a lack of symptoms and a normal peripheral blood smear, but there is still evidence of disease in the bone marrow. *Molecular remission* means that all molecular studies are negative for residual leukemia. The patient's prognosis is directly related to the ability to maintain a remission. The patient's prognosis becomes more unfavorable with each relapse. After each relapse, the succeeding remission may be harder to achieve and shorter in duration.

Sometimes patients have such a high WBC count (e.g., 100,000 cells/μL or more) that initial emergent treatment may include leukapheresis and hydroxyurea. The purpose of these treatments is to reduce the WBC count and risk for leukemia cell–induced thrombosis.

Stages of Chemotherapy. Chemotherapy is often divided into 3 stages: induction, postinduction or postremission (consolidation), and maintenance.

Induction Therapy. The first stage, *induction therapy*, is the attempt to bring about a remission. Induction is aggressive treatment that seeks to destroy leukemic cells in the tissues, peripheral blood, and bone marrow to eventually restore normal hematopoiesis on bone marrow recovery. During induction therapy, a patient may become critically ill because the bone marrow is severely depressed by the chemotherapeutic agents. Nursing interventions focus on neutropenia, thrombocytopenia, and anemia. Common chemotherapy agents for induction of AML include cytarabine and an antitumor antibiotic (anthracycline), such as daunorubicin, idarubicin, or mitoxantrone.[29] After 1 course of induction therapy, around 70% of newly diagnosed patients younger than 60 achieve complete remission. It is assumed that leukemic cells persist undetected after induction therapy. This could lead to relapse within a few months without further therapy.[29]

Postinduction or Postremission Therapy. Terms used to describe postinduction or postremission chemotherapy include *intensification* and *consolidation*. *Intensification therapy*, or high-dose therapy, may be given immediately after induction therapy for several months. Other drugs that target the cell in a different way than those given during induction may be added.

Consolidation therapy is started after a remission is achieved. It may consist of 1 or 2 more courses of the same drugs given during induction or involve high-dose therapy (intensive consolidation). The purpose of consolidation therapy is to eliminate remaining leukemic cells that may not be clinically or pathologically evident.

Maintenance Therapy. *Maintenance therapy* may be used and involves treatment with lower doses of the same drugs used in induction or other drugs given every few weeks for a prolonged period. Like consolidation or intensification, the goal is to keep

TABLE 30.25 **Drug Therapy**	
Leukemia	
Drug Therapy	**Other Therapy**
Acute Myelogenous Leukemia	
arsenic trioxide, azacitidine, cladribine, clofarabine, cytarabine, daunorubicin, decitabine, enasidenib, etoposide, fludarabine, gemtuzumab ozogamicin, idarubicin, midostaurin, mitoxantrone, thioguanine, tretinoin, venetoclax Combination chemotherapy of cytarabine and antitumor antibiotic (most common)	Allogeneic hematopoietic stem cell transplant (HSCT) (see Chapter 15)
Acute Lymphocytic Leukemia	
blinatumomab, clofarabine, cyclophosphamide, cytarabine, dasatinib, daunorubicin, dexamethasone, doxorubicin, etoposide, imatinib, inotuzumab ozogamicin, L-asparaginase, 6-mercaptopurine, methotrexate, nelarabine, pegaspargase, ponatinib, prednisone, rituximab, vincristine Combination chemotherapy of several agents is common over a prolonged time	Cranial radiation therapy, intrathecal methotrexate or cytarabine, allogeneic HSCT, CAR-T cell therapy (see Chapter 15)
Chronic Myelogenous Leukemia	
bosutinib, dasatinib, hydroxyurea, imatinib, nilotinib, omacetaxine, ponatinib Combination chemotherapy with any of the following: busulfan, cytarabine, daunorubicin, etoposide, L-asparaginase, 6-mercaptopurine, methotrexate, mitoxantrone, prednisone, vincristine	Radiation, HSCT, α-interferon, leukapheresis
Chronic Lymphocytic Leukemia	
Alemtuzumab, chlorambucil, bendamustine, cyclophosphamide, fludarabine, ibrutinib, idelalisib, lenalidomide, obinutuzumab, ofatumumab, pentostatin, prednisone, rituximab, venetoclax, vincristine	Radiation, splenectomy, colony-stimulating factors, allogeneic HSCT

the body free of leukemic cells. This is often used with ALL and extends for several years.[30]

Drug Therapy Regimens. The therapeutic agents used to treat leukemia vary. Table 30.25 gives examples of treatment regimens used in various types of leukemia.

Combination therapy is the mainstay of treatment for leukemia. The 3 purposes for using multiple drugs are to (1) decrease drug resistance, (2) minimize the drug toxicity by using multiple drugs with varying toxicities, and (3) interrupt cell growth at multiple points in the cell cycle.

Some therapeutic drugs are aimed at small molecules that promote the growth and differentiation of leukemic cells. For example, all-*trans* retinoic acid, which treats acute promyelocytic leukemia (a type of AML), causes normal differentiation of the promyelocytes which has arrested in this type of leukemia by the translocation of the *PML* gene on chromosome 15 to the *RARA* gene on chromosome 17 (t15;17).[29] Midostaurin is a multikinase inhibitor that inhibits this growth pathway in AML patients with the *FLT3* mutation.[29] Imatinib (Gleevec) and other tyrosine-kinase inhibitors target the BCR-ABL protein that is present in nearly all patients with CML and some patients with ALL.[30,31] This drug kills only cancer cells, leaving healthy cells alone.

The use of specific targeted therapy in the form of monoclonal antibodies is an important treatment modality in hematopoietic cancers, but cures with these therapies alone are rare (see Table 15.13 and Fig. 15.16). Rituximab binds to the B-cell antigen (CD20) and is a treatment for CLL.[32] Alemtuzumab (Campath), a treatment for CLL, binds to CD52, a panlymphocyte antigen present on both T and B cells.[32]

Other Treatments. In addition to chemotherapy, corticosteroids and radiation therapy have a role in the treatment of the patient with leukemia. Total body radiation may be used to prepare a patient for bone marrow transplantation. Radiation may be restricted to certain areas (fields,) such as the liver and spleen, or other organs affected by infiltrates. In ALL, prophylactic intrathecal methotrexate or cytarabine is given to decrease the chance of CNS involvement, which is common in this type of leukemia. When CNS leukemia does occur, cranial radiation is an option. Immunotherapy and targeted therapy, such as monoclonal antibodies and chimeric antigen receptor (CAR) T cells, may be indicated for specific leukemias. (Immunotherapy and targeted therapy are discussed in Chapter 15.)

Hematopoietic Stem Cell Transplantation. HSCT is another type of therapy used for patients with different forms of leukemia. The goal of HSCT is to eliminate all leukemic cells from the body using combinations of chemotherapy with or without total body irradiation. This treatment eradicates the patient's hematopoietic stem cells, which are then replaced with those of an HLA-matched sibling, HLA-half-matched relative, volunteer donor (allogeneic), or identical twin (syngeneic). (HSCT is discussed in Chapter 15.)

The primary complications for patients with allogeneic HSCT are graft-versus-host disease (GVHD), relapse of leukemia, and infection and sepsis. Because HSCT has serious associated risks, the patient must weigh the significant risks for treatment-related death or treatment failure (relapse) with the hope of cure.

❖ NURSING MANAGEMENT: LEUKEMIA

◆ Nursing Assessment

Subjective and objective data that should be obtained from a patient with leukemia are outlined in Table 30.26.

◆ Nursing Diagnoses

Nursing diagnoses for the patient with leukemia include those for anemia (see p. 608), thrombocytopenia (see p. 625), and neutropenia (see eNursing Care Plan 30.3, available on the website).

◆ Planning

The overall goals are that the patient with leukemia will (1) understand and adhere to the treatment plan; (2) have minimal side effects and complications associated with both the disease and its treatment; and (3) establish realistic hope and goals, feeling supported during periods of treatment, relapse, or remission.

◆ Nursing Implementation

◆ **Acute Care.** The nursing role during acute phases of leukemia is extremely challenging because the patient has many physical and psychosocial needs. As with other forms of cancer, the diagnosis of leukemia can evoke great fear and be equated with death. It may be viewed as a hopeless, horrible disease with many painful

---

TABLE 30.26 Nursing Assessment

Leukemia

Subjective Data

Important Health Information

Past health history: Exposure to chemical toxins (e.g., benzene, arsenic), radiation, or viruses (HTLV-1); chromosome abnormalities (Down syndrome, Klinefelter syndrome, Fanconi syndrome), immunologic deficiencies; organ transplantation; frequent infections; bleeding tendencies

Medications: Chemotherapy

Surgery or other treatments: Radiation exposure; prior radiation and chemotherapy for cancer

Functional Health Patterns

Health perception–health management: Family history of leukemia; malaise

Nutritional-metabolic: Mouth sores, weight loss; chills, night sweats; nausea, vomiting, anorexia, dysphagia, early satiety; easy bruising

Elimination: Hematuria, decreased urine output; diarrhea, dark or bloody stools

Activity-exercise: Fatigue with progressive weakness; dyspnea, nosebleeds, cough

Cognitive-perceptual: Headache; muscle cramps; sore throat; generalized sternal tenderness, bone, joint, abdominal pain; paresthesias, numbness, tingling, visual changes

Sexuality-reproductive: Prolonged menses, menorrhagia, metrorrhagia, impotence

Objective Data

General

Fever, generalized lymphadenopathy, lethargy

Integumentary

Pallor or jaundice; petechiae, ecchymoses, purpura, reddish brown to purple cutaneous infiltrates, macules, and papules

Cardiovascular

Tachycardia, systolic murmurs

Gastrointestinal

Gingival bleeding and hyperplasia; oral ulcerations, herpes and *Candida* infections; perirectal irritation and infection; hepatomegaly, splenomegaly

Neurologic

Seizures, disorientation, confusion, decreased coordination, cranial nerve palsies, papilledema

Musculoskeletal

Muscle wasting, bone pain, joint pain

Possible Diagnostic Findings

Low, normal, or high WBC count with shift to the left (↑ blast cells) and neutropenia; anemia; ↓ hematocrit and hemoglobin, thrombocytopenia, specific chromosome abnormalities; hypercellular bone marrow aspirate or biopsy with myeloblasts, lymphoblasts, and markedly ↓ normal cells

HTLV-1, Human T-cell leukemia virus, type 1.

---

and undesirable consequences. The treatment and prognosis of each patient with leukemia are driven by many factors, such as age and type of leukemia. Therefore you must understand the patient's type of leukemia, prognosis, treatment plan, and goals. By doing this, you can help the patient realize that, although the future may be uncertain, one can have a meaningful quality of life while in remission or with disease control and that, in some cases, there is reasonable hope for cure.

The family needs help adjusting to the stress of this abrupt onset of serious illness and the losses imposed by the sick role (e.g., dependence, withdrawal, changes in role responsibilities, changes in body image). The diagnosis of leukemia often brings with it the need to make difficult decisions at a time of profound stress for the patient and family.

Patients may have co-morbid conditions that affect treatment decisions. Important nursing interventions include (1) maximizing the patient's physical functioning, (2) teaching patients that acute side effects of treatment are usually temporary, and (3) encouraging patients to discuss their quality-of-life issues.

You are an important advocate in helping the patient and family understand the complexities of treatment decisions and manage the side effects and toxicities. This may include making sure the HCP addresses fertility concerns. A patient may need a long hospitalization or may need to temporarily relocate to an appropriate treatment center. This situation can lead a patient to feel deserted and isolated at a time when support is most needed. You have contact with a patient many hours a day and can help reverse feelings of abandonment and loneliness by balancing the demanding technical needs with a humanistic, caring approach. The needs of the patient with leukemia are best met by an interprofessional team (e.g., psychiatric and oncology clinical nurse specialists, case managers, dietitians, chaplains, and social workers).

From a physical care perspective, you are challenged to make astute assessments and plan care to help the patient manage the severe side effects of chemotherapy. The life-threatening results of bone marrow suppression (neutropenia, thrombocytopenia, and anemia) require aggressive nursing interventions. Other critical aspects of care include anticipating, monitoring for, and helping to treat emergencies, such as DIC, tumor lysis syndrome, leukostasis, and cytokine release syndrome. Complications of chemotherapy may affect the patient's GI tract, nutritional status, skin and mucosa, cardiopulmonary status, liver, kidneys, and neurologic system. (Nursing interventions related to chemotherapy are discussed in Chapter 15.)

Review all drugs being given, including the mechanism of action, purpose, routes of administration, doses, potential side effects, safe handling considerations, and toxic effects. Assess laboratory data reflecting the effects of the drugs and sequelae of the disease. Unlike treatments for solid tumors, chemotherapy is given to patients with leukemia even if they have severe myelosuppression, since the underlying disorder is causing the problem and will not resolve unless treated. Quality nursing care significantly affects patient survival and comfort during aggressive chemotherapy.

◆ **Ambulatory Care.** Ongoing care for the patient with leukemia is necessary to monitor for signs and symptoms of disease control or relapse. For a patient receiving long-term or maintenance chemotherapy, the fatigue of long-term chronic disease management can become discouraging. Teach the patient and caregiver the importance of continued diligence in disease management and the need for follow-up care. Review the drugs, self-care measures, and when to seek medical attention.

The goals of rehabilitation for long-term survivors of leukemia are to manage the physical, psychologic, social, and spiritual consequences and delayed effects from the disease and its treatment. Assistance may be needed to reestablish the various relationships that are a part of the patient's life. Involving the patient in survivor networks and support groups or services may help the patient adapt to living after a life-threatening illness. Exploring national and community resources (e.g., American

TABLE 30.27 Comparison of Hodgkin's and Non-Hodgkin's Lymphoma

	Hodgkin's Lymphoma	Non-Hodgkin's Lymphoma
Cellular origin	B lymphocytes	B lymphocytes (88%) T or natural killer lymphocytes (12%)
Extent of disease	Localized to regional but may be more widespread. Spreads to adjacent tissues	Disseminated, can spread to other areas of the body
B symptoms (fever, drenching night sweats, weight loss)	Common	Uncommon
Extranodal involvement	Rare	Common

Cancer Society, Leukemia & Lymphoma Society) may reduce the financial burden and the feelings of dependence. Provide resources for spiritual support.

Vigilant follow-up care helps to ensure that we recognize and treat the cancer survivor's unique needs. Often these needs may need a referral or consultation. For example, physical therapy personnel may develop an exercise program to prevent post-treatment deficits caused by drug-induced peripheral neuropathy. Most patients should receive a pneumococcal vaccine and an annual influenza vaccine.

◆ **Evaluation**

The expected outcomes are that the patient with leukemia will
- Cope effectively with the diagnosis, treatment regimen, and prognosis
- Have no complications related to the disease or its treatment
- Feel supported throughout treatment

LYMPHOMAS

Lymphomas are cancers originating in the bone marrow and lymphatic structures resulting in the proliferation of lymphocytes. Lymphomas make up 4% to 5% of all cancers in the United States.[27] Two major types of lymphoma are Hodgkin's lymphoma and non-Hodgkin's lymphoma (NHL). A comparison of these 2 types of lymphoma is shown in Table 30.27.

HODGKIN'S LYMPHOMA

Hodgkin's lymphoma, also called *Hodgkin's disease,* makes up about 10% of all lymphomas. It is characterized by proliferation of abnormal giant, multinucleated cells, called *Reed-Sternberg cells,* or it's variant, *Hodgkin cells* (mononucleated), which proliferate in the lymph nodes.[3] The disease has a bimodal age-specific incidence, occurring most frequently in persons from 15 to 30 years of age and above 55 years of age.[34] Each year, about 8260 new cases of Hodgkin's lymphoma are diagnosed, with around 1070 deaths.[27] Long-term survival exceeds 80% for all stages.[34]

Etiology and Pathophysiology

Although the cause of Hodgkin's lymphoma is unknown, we think several key factors play a role in its development. The main

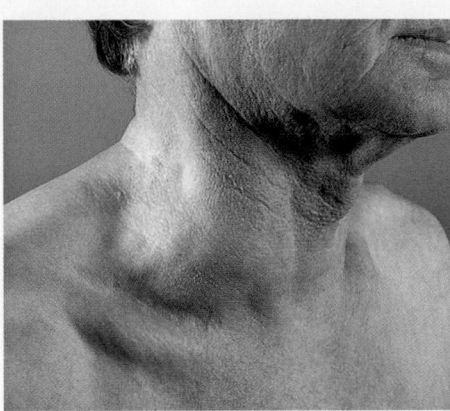

FIG. 30.14 Enlarged cervical lymph node in the neck of a man with Hodgkin lymphoma. (From Howard MR, Hamilton PJ: *Haematology: An illustrated colour atlas,* ed 4, London, 2013, Churchill Livingston.)

interacting factors include infection with Epstein-Barr virus (EBV), genetic predisposition, and exposure to occupational toxins. The incidence of Hodgkin's lymphoma is increased in those with HIV infection.[1]

The disease likely starts in a single location (it starts in cervical lymph nodes in 60% to 70% of patients) and then spreads along adjacent lymphatics.[3] However, in recurrent disease, it may spread more diffuse. It eventually infiltrates other organs, especially lungs, spleen, and liver. When the disease begins above the diaphragm, it stays confined to lymph nodes for a variable time. Disease originating below the diaphragm often spreads to extralymphoid sites, such as the liver. There are 5 histologic subtypes. Nodular sclerosis is the most common.[1]

Clinical Manifestations

The onset of symptoms in Hodgkin's lymphoma is usually gradual. The initial development is most often enlargement of cervical, axillary, or inguinal lymph nodes (Fig. 30.14). A mediastinal node mass is the second most common location. The nodes are movable and nontender. Enlarged nodes are not painful unless they exert pressure on adjacent nerves.

The patient may notice weight loss, fatigue, weakness, fever, chills, tachycardia, or night sweats. A group of initial findings, including fever (over 100.4° F [38° C]), drenching night sweats, and weight loss (exceeding 10% in 6 months), are termed *B symptoms.* They correlate with a worse prognosis. After having even small amounts of alcohol, patients with Hodgkin's lymphoma may have a rapid onset of pain at the site of disease. The cause for the alcohol-induced pain is unknown. Generalized pruritus without skin lesions may develop. Cough, dyspnea, stridor, and dysphagia may all reflect mediastinal node involvement.

In more advanced disease, there may be hepatomegaly and splenomegaly. Anemia results from increased destruction and decreased production of RBCs. Other physical signs vary depending on where the disease is located. For example, intrathoracic involvement may lead to superior vena cava syndrome. Enlarged retroperitoneal nodes may cause palpable abdominal masses or interfere with renal function. Jaundice may occur from liver involvement. Spinal cord compression leading to paraplegia may occur with extradural involvement. Bone pain occurs from bone involvement.

Diagnostic and Staging Studies

Peripheral blood analysis, excisional lymph node biopsy, bone marrow examination, and radiologic studies are important means of evaluating Hodgkin's lymphoma. Abnormalities in the CBC, such as a microcytic hypochromic anemia, are variable and not diagnostic. Leukopenia and thrombocytopenia may develop, but they are usually a consequence of treatment, advanced disease, or superimposed hypersplenism. Other blood studies may show increased erythrocyte sedimentation rate, high leukocyte alkaline phosphatase from liver and bone involvement, hypercalcemia from bone involvement, and hypoalbuminemia from liver involvement.

Radiologic evaluation can help define all sites and determine the clinical stage of the disease. PET and CT scans are used to stage and then assess the response to therapy and to distinguish residual tumor from fibrotic masses after treatment. These scans may show increased uptake (by PET) and masses, such as renal displacement caused by retroperitoneal node enlargement, abdominal or mediastinal lymph node enlargement, and liver, spleen, bone, and brain infiltration.

❖ Interprofessional and Nursing Management

Using all the information from the various diagnostic studies, HCPs determine a clinical stage of disease (Fig. 30.15).[34] The final staging is based on the clinical stage (extent of the disease), presence of B symptoms, and other unfavorable prognostic features. Treatment depends on the nature and extent of the disease. The terms used in staging involve an A or B classification, depending on whether systemic symptoms are present at diagnosis, and a Roman numeral (I to IV) that reflects the location and extent of the disease.[34]

Once the stage of Hodgkin's lymphoma is determined, management focuses on selecting a treatment plan. The standard for chemotherapy is the ABVD regimen: doxorubicin (**A**driamycin), **b**leomycin, **v**inblastine, and **d**acarbazine. Patients with favorable early-stage disease receive 2 to 4 cycles of chemotherapy.[3] Patients with early-stage disease but unfavorable prognostic features (e.g., B symptoms) or intermediate-stage disease receive 4 to 6 cycles of chemotherapy. Advanced-stage Hodgkin's lymphoma is treated more aggressively using 6 to 8 cycles of chemotherapy. A common regimen is BEACOPP (**b**leomycin, **e**toposide, doxorubicin [**A**driamycin], **c**yclophosphamide, vincristine [**O**ncovin], **p**rocarbazine, and **p**rednisone).[3,34] The role of involved-site radiation as a supplement to chemotherapy varies depending on the extent of disease and the presence of resistant disease after chemotherapy.[34] Response to therapy is determined by PET and CT scans and other diagnostic tests (e.g., bone marrow biopsy).

A variety of chemotherapy regimens and newer agents, such as brentuximab vedotin, nivolumab, bendamustine, and pembrolizumab are used to treat patients who have relapsed or refractory disease.[34] Ideally, once remission is obtained, a curative option may be intensive chemotherapy with the use of autologous or allogeneic HSCT.[34] HSCT has allowed patients to receive higher, potentially curative doses of chemotherapy while reducing life-threatening leukopenia (see Chapter 15). Combination chemotherapy works well because, as in leukemia, the drugs used have an additive antitumor effect without increasing side effects. As with

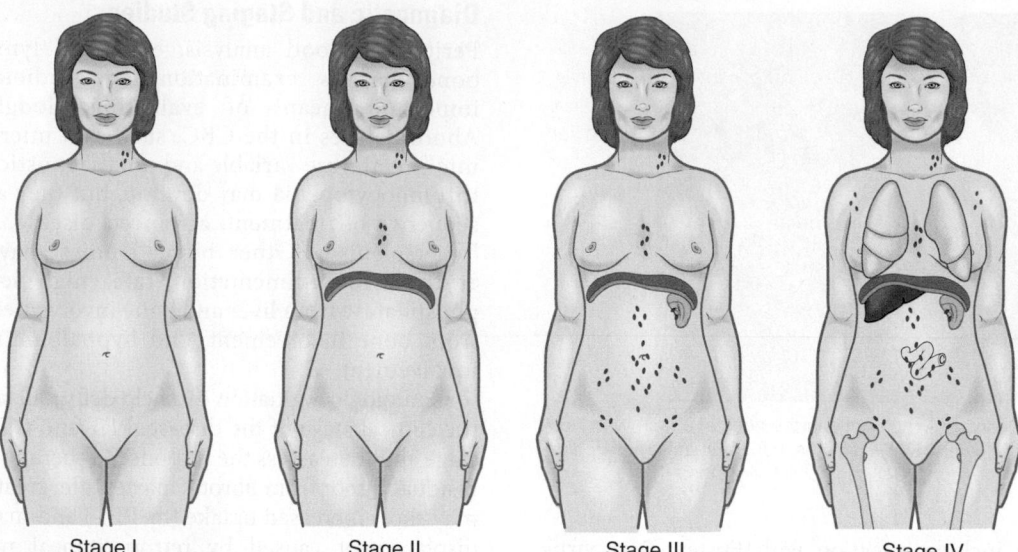

Stage I	Stage II	Stage III	Stage IV

FIG. 30.15 Staging system for Hodgkin's lymphoma and non-Hodgkin's lymphoma. *Stage I*, Involvement of single lymph node (e.g., cervical node). *Stage II*, Involvement of 2 or more lymph nodes on one side of diaphragm. *Stage III*, Lymph node involvement above and below the diaphragm. *Stage IV*, Involvement outside of diaphragm (e.g., liver, bone marrow). The stage is followed by the letter *A* (absence) or *B* (presence) to indicate significant systemic symptoms (e.g., fever, night sweats, weight loss).

leukemia, therapy must be aggressive. Potentially life-threatening problems are an issue in the attempt to achieve a remission.

Maintenance chemotherapy does not contribute to increased survival after achieving complete remission. Occasionally, single drugs may be given palliatively to those who cannot tolerate intensive combination therapy. A serious consequence of the treatment for Hodgkin's lymphoma is the later development of secondary cancers and potential long-term toxicities from the treatment, such as endocrine (hypothyroidism), heart, and lung dysfunction. Secondary solid tumor cancers may occur 10 years after treatment for Hodgkin's lymphoma.[34] The most common secondary cancers are lung and breast cancer, especially with radiation therapy. Patients should have close follow-up and screening for early detection of these problems.

The nursing care for Hodgkin's lymphoma is based on managing problems related to the disease (e.g., pain caused by a tumor, superior vena cava syndrome), pancytopenia, and other side effects of therapy. Because the survival of patients with Hodgkin's lymphoma depends on their response to treatment, supporting the patient through the consequences of treatment is extremely important.

Psychosocial considerations are as important as they are with leukemia. However, the prognosis for Hodgkin's lymphoma is better than that for many forms of cancer. Address the physical and spiritual consequences of the patient's disease. Fertility issues may be of concern because this disease is often seen in adolescents and young adults. Help to ensure that these issues are addressed soon after diagnosis. Evaluating patients for long-term effects of therapy is important because delayed consequences of disease and treatment may not be apparent for many years. Secondary cancers and delayed effects are discussed in Chapter 15.

EVIDENCE-BASED PRACTICE
Exercise and Hematologic Cancer

You are a nurse caring for G.R., a 59-yr-old male patient with non-Hodgkin's lymphoma who is receiving chemotherapy. Due to a decrease in red blood cells and platelets, he was told to rest and avoid the high level of physical exercise he once enjoyed. He misses his active lifestyle and now admits to you that he is "somewhat depressed."

Making Clinical Decisions

Best Available Evidence. Aerobic exercise, especially walking and stretching, to maintain mobility may improve physical functioning, fatigue, and depression in patients with hematologic cancers.

Clinician Expertise. You know recommendations to decrease intensive physical exercise may diminish quality of life for many patients, especially for people who are used to being physically active.

Patient Preferences and Values. G.R. is considering joining a neighborhood bicycling club so that he can "feel better."

Implications for Nursing Practice

1. Why is intensive exercise contraindicated in someone who is getting chemotherapy or acutely ill?
2. What precautions would you discuss with G.R. before he increases his exercise level?
3. How would you involve G.R. in monitoring his fatigue?
4. As G.R. seeks ways to improve his quality of life, how would you support him?

Reference for Evidence

Berger AM, Mooney K: Cancer-related fatigue, NCCN clinical practice guidelines, version 2,.2017. Retrieved from *www.nccn.org*.

NON-HODGKIN'S LYMPHOMA

Non-Hodgkin's lymphomas (NHLs) are a broad group of cancers of primarily B, T, natural killer (NK), histiocytic, and dendritic cells.[33] They affect persons of all ages. There are over 75 types. They are categorized by the level of differentiation (maturity), cell of origin, immunophenotype (cell surface markers), and genetic and clinical features.[33,35] The most common subtypes in the United States are diffuse large B-cell lymphoma, follicular lymphoma, marginal zone lymphoma, mantle cell lymphoma, and peripheral T-cell lymphoma not otherwise specified.[33] A simplified example of the classification system is shown in Table 30.28.[33,35]

A variety of presentations and courses occur, from indolent (slowly developing) to rapidly progressive disease. NHL is the most commonly occurring hematologic cancer. It causes 3% to 4% of cancer-related deaths. Each year about 72,240 new cases of NHL are diagnosed and 20,140 deaths occur.[27]

Etiology and Pathophysiology

As with Hodgkin's lymphoma, the cause of NHL is usually unknown. NHLs may result from chromosomal translocations, infections, environmental factors, and immunodeficiency states. Chromosomal translocations have a key role in the pathogenesis of many NHLs. Viruses and bacteria implicated in the pathogenesis of NHL, include HTLV-1, EBV, human herpesvirus 8, hepatitis B and C, *H. pylori, Chlamydophila psittaci, Campylobacter jejuni,* and *Borrelia burgdorferi.*[3] Environmental factors linked to the development of NHL include chemicals (e.g., pesticides, herbicides, solvents, organic chemicals, wood preservatives). NHL is more common in people who have inherited immunodeficiency syndromes, have used immunosuppressive agents (e.g., to prevent rejection after an organ transplant or to treat autoimmune disorders), or received chemotherapy or radiation therapy.

NHL does not have a hallmark feature that parallels the Hodgkin or Reed-Sternberg cell of Hodgkin's lymphoma. However, all NHLs involve lymphocytes arrested in various stages of development and may mimic a leukemia. For example, small lymphocytic lymphoma (SLL) and CLL result from malignant proliferation of small B lymphocytes, with most CLL disease within the bone marrow versus the lymph nodes. Some NHLs can begin outside the lymph nodes.

TABLE 30.28 Classification of Non-Hodgkin's Lymphoma*

B-Cell Lymphomas
- Burkitt's lymphoma
- Diffuse large B-cell lymphoma (DLBCL)
- Follicular lymphoma
- Mantle cell lymphoma
- Marginal zone B-cell lymphoma (MALT)
- Plasmablastic lymphoma
- Small lymphocytic lymphoma/chronic lymphocytic leukemia

T-Cell and NK-Cell Lymphomas
- Anaplastic large T-cell lymphoma
- Extranodal NK/T cell lymphoma
- Lymphoblastic lymphoma
- Mycosis fungoides and Sézary syndrome
- Peripheral T-cell lymphoma, not otherwise specified (NOS)

Posttransplant Lymphoproliferative Disorders (PTLD)
- Infectious mononucleosis-like PTLD

Histocytic and Dendritic Cell Tumors
- Langerhans cell histiocytosis

*This is only a partial list.

Diffuse large B-cell lymphoma, the most common aggressive lymphoma, starts in the lymph nodes, usually in the neck or abdomen. Burkitt's lymphoma is the most aggressive disease. We think it begins in B-cell blasts in the lymph nodes.

Clinical Manifestations

The method of spread can be unpredictable. Most patients have widespread disease at the time of diagnosis (Fig. 30.16). The primary manifestation is painless lymph node enlargement. The lymphadenopathy can wax and wane in indolent disease. Because the disease has usually spread, other symptoms are present depending on where the disease is present (e.g., hepatomegaly with liver involvement, neurologic symptoms with CNS disease). NHL can manifest in nonspecific ways, such as an airway obstruction, hyperuricemia and renal failure from tumor lysis syndrome, pericardial tamponade, and GI symptoms. Patients with high-grade lymphomas may have lymphadenopathy and B symptoms, such as fever, night sweats, and weight loss.

Diagnostic and Staging Studies

Diagnostic studies used for NHL resemble those used for Hodgkin's lymphoma. However, because NHL is more often in extranodal sites, more diagnostic studies may be done. These include an MRI or lumbar puncture to rule out CNS disease, a bone marrow biopsy to determine bone marrow infiltration, or a barium enema or upper endoscopy to look for GI involvement. Clinical staging, as described for Hodgkin's lymphoma, helps guide therapy (Fig. 30.15). Establishing the precise histologic subtype through biopsy is extremely important. NHL is classified based on morphologic, genetic, immunophenotypic (cell surface antigens, CD20, CD52), and clinical features. In early NHL, the CBC may be normal, but some lymphomas manifest in a "leukemic" phase.

Treatment is guided by the cell type, cytogenetic studies, and clinical behavior: *indolent* (low grade), aggressive (high grade), or *highly aggressive* (very high grade). Other factors, known as the International Prognostic Index (IPI), may be considered for each subtype. These include the clinical stage, number of extranodal sites, serum LDH, WBC count, and patient's age and performance status.[33,35] Immunologic, cytogenetic, and molecular studies are used for making therapeutic decisions and assessing prognosis. Other studies might include blood tests for tumor lysis; screening for hepatitis, HIV, and other infections; skin biopsies; bone marrow biopsies; and lumbar punctures. The prognosis for NHL is based on the histopathology.

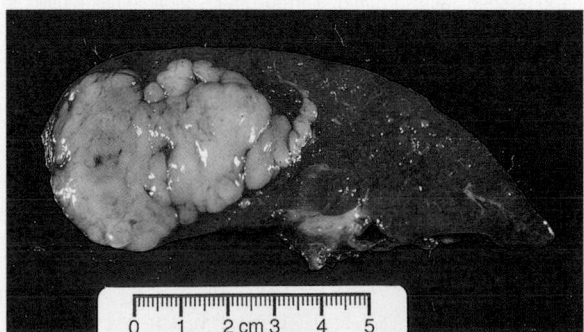

FIG. 30.16 Non-Hodgkin's lymphoma involving the spleen. The presence of an isolated mass is typical. (From Cotran RS, Kumar V, Abbas AK: *Robbins pathologic basis of disease,* ed 6, Philadelphia, 1999, Saunders.)

❖ Interprofessional and Nursing Management

Treatment for NHL involves chemotherapy, biotherapy, radiation, and sometimes phototherapy and topical therapy (Table 30.29).[35] Ironically, more aggressive lymphomas (diffuse large B cell) are generally more responsive to treatment. In contrast, indolent lymphomas (e.g., follicular lymphomas) have a naturally long course but are hard to effectively treat.[33]

Patients with low-grade (indolent) lymphoma may live 10 years or more without treatment. However, some early therapies can be well tolerated and may reduce the time to progression of the disease. Those that have an infectious basis, such as *H. pylori* gastric lymphomas, may be treated with antibiotic or antiviral therapy. HSCT may help in certain subtypes of aggressive or refractory lymphomas. Chimeric antigen receptor (CAR) T-cell immunotherapy may be used.

Rituximab, a monoclonal antibody against the CD20 antigen on the surface of normal and malignant B cells, is used to treat NHL in combination with other agents. Once bound to the cells, rituximab causes lysis and cell death. Numerous chemotherapy combinations are used to try to overcome the resistant nature of this disease. Targeted therapies are becoming more prevalent (Table 30.29).

 DRUG ALERT Rituximab (Rituxan)
- Monitor patient for signs of severe hypersensitivity infusion reactions, especially with first infusion.
- Manifestations may include hypotension, bronchospasm, dysrhythmias, angioedema, and cardiogenic shock.
- Screen for history of hepatitis because the drug may reactivate hepatitis.

Another therapy for some types of NHL is the monoclonal antibody ibritumomab tiuxetan (Zevalin). It contains a radioactive particle that can kill cancer cells. The therapy targets the CD20 antigen, which is on the surface of mature B cells and B-cell tumors. Targeting allows for the delivery of the radiation directly to the cancer cells. Side effects include pancytopenia. Use radiation precautions in caring for these patients. Teach patients about safety issues and how to minimize the risk for radiation exposure to staff and others.

In general, T-cell lymphomas are harder to treat. They are often treated aggressively up front, often followed by an HSCT. Cutaneous T-cell lymphomas may be treated with topical corticosteroids or topical chemotherapy for limited-stage disease. For more diffuse disease, treatment may include methotrexate, α-interferon, brentuximab vedotin, or other drugs.[35]

The nursing care for NHL is similar to that for Hodgkin's lymphoma. It is based on managing problems related to the disease (e.g., pain caused by the tumor, spinal cord compression, tumor

---

TABLE 30.29 Treatment of Non-Hodgkin's Lymphoma *

Recommended Therapies	Common Chemotherapy Combinations
Indolent (Low Grade) Follicular Lymphoma, Marginal Zone B-Cell Lymphoma, Mucosa-Associated Lymphoid Tissue (MALT)	
• Observation until disease progression for asymptomatic patients with low-volume tumors and normal blood counts • External beam irradiation for local, limited disease • Single-agent rituximab, obinutuzumab • Single-agent chemotherapy (bendamustine, chlorambucil, cyclophosphamide, idelalisib) • Rituximab with another agent (bendamustine, fludarabine, lenalidomide) • Combination chemotherapy (R-CHOP or other) • Radioimmunotherapy • Hematopoietic stem cell transplant (HSCT)	**R-CHOP: r**ituximab, **c**yclophosphamide, doxorubicin **h**ydrochloride, vincristine (**O**ncovin), **p**rednisone **R-CVP: r**ituximab, **c**yclophosphamide, **v**incristine, **p**rednisone **RFND: r**ituximab, **f**ludarabine, mitoxantrone (**N**ovantrone), **d**examethasone ± rituximab
Aggressive (Intermediate or High Grade) Mantle Cell, Diffuse Large B-Cell, T-Cell, Natural Killer Cell Lymphomas	
• Combination chemotherapy with localized radiation if needed • Aggressive combination chemotherapy for 3–8 cycles with rituximab with local radiation if needed • Intrathecal chemotherapy if needed • Single agent or other combination treatment, depending on subtype and response (e.g., acalabrutinib, alemtuzumab, asparaginase, belinostat, bendamustine, bortezomib, brentuximab vedotin, cladribine, gemcitabine, ibrutinib, lenalidomide, oxaliplatin, romidepsin, venetoclax) • HSCT	**CHOP** ± rituximab (see above) **ICE** (or "RICE" with rituximab): **i**fosfamide, **c**yclophosphamide, **e**toposide **R-EPOCH: r**ituximab, **e**toposide, **p**rednisone, vincristine (**O**ncovin), **c**yclophosphamide, doxorubicin **h**ydrochloride **ESHAP ± R: e**toposide, methylprednisolone (**S**olu-Medrol), **h**igh-dose cytarabine (**A**ra-C), cisplatin (**P**latinol), with or without **r**ituximab **Hyper-CVAD ± R:** hyperfractionated **c**yclophosphamide, **v**incristine, doxorubicin (**A**driamycin), **d**examethasone alternating with high-dose methotrexate and cytarabine with or without rituximab **DHAP ± R: d**examethasone, **h**igh-dose cytarabine (**A**ra-C), cisplatin (**P**latinol), with or without **r**ituximab
Highly Aggressive (e.g., Burkitt's Lymphoma)	
• Aggressive combination chemotherapy for 3–8 cycles • HSCT	**R-EPOCH: r**ituximab, **e**toposide, **p**rednisone, vincristine (**O**ncovin), **c**yclophosphamide, doxorubicin **h**ydrochloride **Hyper-CVAD ± R** (see above) **CODOX-M: c**yclophosphamide, vincristine (**O**ncovin), **dox**orubicin, high-dose **m**ethotrexate, with or without rituximab (includes intrathecal methotrexate)

*The acronym for some drug regimens use the trade name of chemotherapy agents. In some cases, the trade name drug has been discontinued, and the drug currently used is the generic version.

lysis syndrome), pancytopenia, and other side effects of therapy. However, because NHL can be more extensive and involve specific organs (e.g., CNS, spleen, liver, GI tract, bone marrow), it is important to understand the subtype and extent of the disease. For example, a patient with known involvement of the colon may report acute abdominal pain. The patient would likely have abdominal guarding and an enlarged and tympanic abdomen. This could indicate a bowel perforation and be considered a medical emergency. A patient with a Burkitt's NHL beginning chemotherapy would be at high risk for tumor lysis syndrome and would need frequent laboratory studies and monitoring, as well as strict documentation of intake and output. Cancer-related therapies and side effects are discussed in Chapter 15.

The patient undergoing external beam radiation therapy has special nursing needs. The skin in the radiation field needs special care. Concepts related to safety issues with radiation therapy are important to include in the plan of care (see Chapter 15).

Psychosocial considerations are important. Help the patient and family understand the disease, treatment, and expected and potential side effects. Some aggressive treatments need close follow-up and even inpatient admission. Fertility issues may be of concern in young patients. As in Hodgkin's lymphoma, evaluation of patients with NHL for long-term effects of therapy is important because the delayed consequences of disease and treatment may not become apparent for many years.

MULTIPLE MYELOMA

Multiple myeloma, or *plasma cell myeloma*, is a condition in which cancerous plasma cells proliferate in the bone marrow and destroy bone. Multiple myeloma accounts for about 1.8% of all cancers and for about 17% of all hematologic cancers.[27] The disease is more common in men than women and more common in blacks than whites.[3] It generally occurs between the ages of 65 and 74 years old, with an average onset age of 69 years.[36] Because of the variety of treatments that can be provided throughout the course of the disease, over 40% of patients have more than a 10-year survival rate.[1]

Etiology and Pathophysiology

The cause of multiple myeloma is unknown. It is possible that exposure to organic chemicals (such as benzene), herbicides, and insecticides may play a role. Viral infections, such as HIV, may influence the risk for developing multiple myeloma.[37]

The disease process involves excess production of plasma cells. Normal plasma cells are activated B cells, which make immunoglobulins (antibodies) that normally protect the body. In multiple myeloma, instead of a variety of plasma cells making antibodies to fight different infections, myeloma tumors make monoclonal antibodies. *Monoclonal* means they are all of one kind, making them ineffective and even harmful. Not only do they not fight infections, but they infiltrate the bone marrow. These monoclonal proteins (called *M proteins*) are made up of 2 light chains and 2 heavy chains. *Bence Jones proteins* are the light chain part of these monoclonal antibodies. They may show up in the urine in many patients with multiple myeloma.[1]

Furthermore, plasma cell production of excess, abnormal amounts of cytokines (interleukins [ILs]; IL-4, IL-5, and IL-6) plays a key role in the pathologic process of bone destruction. As myeloma protein increases, normal plasma cells are reduced. This further compromises the body's normal immune response.

Proliferation of cancerous plasma cells and the overproduction of immunoglobulin and proteins may result in the end-organ effects of myeloma on the bone marrow, bone, and kidneys and possibly the spleen, lymph nodes, liver, and even heart muscle.

Clinical Manifestations

Multiple myeloma develops slowly and insidiously. The patient often does not have symptoms until the disease is advanced. Skeletal pain is the major manifestation. Pain in the pelvis, spine, and ribs is particularly common and triggered by movement. Diffuse osteoporosis develops as the myeloma protein destroys bone. Osteolytic lesions are seen in the skull, vertebrae, long bones, and ribs. Vertebral destruction can lead to collapse of vertebrae with ensuing compression of the spinal cord. Loss of bone integrity can lead to the development of pathologic fractures.

Bony degeneration causes calcium loss from bones, eventually causing hypercalcemia. Hypercalcemia may cause renal, GI, or neurologic problems, such as polyuria, anorexia, confusion, and heart problems. A serum *hyperviscosity syndrome* leading to cerebral, lung, renal, and other organ dysfunction can occur in some patients. Even without hyperviscosity, high protein levels caused by the myeloma protein can result in renal tubular obstruction, interstitial nephritis, and renal failure. The patient may have anemia, thrombocytopenia, neutropenia, and immune dysfunction from the replacement of normal bone marrow with plasma cells. Neurologic problems may be caused by regional myeloma cell growth compressing the spinal cord or cranial nerves, or by perineuronal or perivascular deposition of the abnormal protein.[1,38]

Diagnostic Studies

Evaluating multiple myeloma involves laboratory, radiologic, and bone marrow examination. M protein is often found in the blood and urine. Possible findings include pancytopenia, hypercalcemia, Bence Jones protein in the urine, and a high serum creatinine.

Skeletal bone surveys, MRI, and/or PET and CT scans show distinct areas of destroyed bone; generalized thinning of the bones; or fractures, especially in the vertebrae, ribs, pelvis, and bones of the thigh and upper arms. Bone marrow analysis shows significantly increased numbers of plasma cells in the bone marrow. The simplest measure of staging and prognosis in multiple myeloma is based on blood levels of 2 markers: β_2-microglobulin and albumin. In general, higher levels of β_2-microglobulin and lower levels of albumin are associated with a poorer prognosis. Cytogenetic studies of the bone marrow plays a role in prognostic stratification. For example, deletion of chromosome 17p13 is considered a high risk (poor prognostic) feature.[36]

❖ Interprofessional and Nursing Management

Interprofessional care involves managing both the disease and its symptoms. The current treatment options include corticosteroids, chemotherapy, immunotherapy, targeted therapy, and HSCT.[36] Multiple myeloma is seldom cured. Treatment can relieve symptoms, produce remission, and prolong life. Control of pain and prevention of pathologic fractures are goals of management.

Bisphosphonates, such as pamidronate and zoledronic acid, inhibit bone breakdown and are used to treat skeletal pain and hypercalcemia. They inhibit bone resorption without inhibiting bone formation and mineralization. They are given monthly by IV infusion. A major focus of nursing care relates to patient safety due to the bone involvement and sequelae from bone breakdown. Because of the potential for pathologic fractures, use caution when moving and ambulating the patient. A slight twist or strain in the wrong area (e.g., a weak area in the patient's bones) may cause a fracture.

> ### 💊 DRUG ALERT Zoledronic Acid (Zometa)
> - Make sure the patient is adequately hydrated before giving drug.
> - Renal toxicity may occur if IV infusion of drug is given in less than 15 min.
> - Patients should have a dental exam prior to first dose and ongoing monitoring for osteonecrosis of the jaw.[36]

Kyphoplasty is sometimes used to control spine vertebral disease. *Kyphoplasty* is a minimally invasive procedure (usually done in an interventional radiology area) that injects cement to stabilize the vertebral compression.

Chemotherapy includes a corticosteroid (dexamethasone or prednisone) plus 2 chemotherapy agents, such as bortezomib and lenalidomide or bortezomib and cyclophosphamide. The goal is to reduce the number of plasma cells. Initial treatment depends on whether the patient is a future bone marrow transplant candidate and predicted tolerance of therapy. High-dose chemotherapy followed by HSCT has evolved as the standard of care in eligible patients.[36]

Immunotherapy and targeted therapy are options. Immunomodulator drugs (described in Chapter 15) include thalidomide, lenalidomide, and pomalidomide. Proteosome inhibitors include bortezomib, carfilzomib, and ixazomib. Panobinostat is a drug that affects enzymes that promote cancer cell growth. Daratumumab is a monoclonal antibody against CD38, a protein which is found on the surface of myeloma cells.

Other drugs can treat some complications of multiple myeloma. For example, IV furosemide promotes renal excretion of calcium. Although tumor lysis is rare, once chemotherapy is started, allopurinol may be given to prevent any renal damage from uric acid accumulation (from cell breakdown). Because of the myeloma proteins, the patient is at risk for renal dysfunction and electrolyte and fluid imbalances.

Ambulation and adequate hydration are used to treat hypercalcemia, dehydration, and potential renal damage. Weight bearing helps the bones resorb some calcium. Maintaining adequate hydration helps minimize problems from hypercalcemia and prevent protein precipitates from causing renal tubular obstruction. IV fluids may be given to maintain a urine output of 1.5 to 2 L/day if the patient does not already have renal compromise.

In some patients, the levels of plasma proteins are so high that it causes a hyperviscosity of the blood leading to neurologic changes, renal insufficiency, and other problems related to lack of blood flow. In this instance plasmapheresis is used.

Pain management requires innovative and knowledgeable nursing interventions. Analgesics, such as nonsteroidal antiinflammatory drugs, acetaminophen, or an acetaminophen/opioid combination, may be more effective than opioids alone in diminishing bone pain. Braces, especially for the spine, may help control pain. As in any pain management situation, assess the patient and implement measures to control pain (see Chapter 8). Peripheral neuropathy is common with several therapies for multiple myeloma and can contribute to discomfort, the inability to do basic activities of daily living, and the risk for injury from falling.

Patients are at risk for DVT related to chemotherapy and immobility and should have preventive measures employed.[36]

Assessment and prompt treatment of infection are important in the care of patients with multiple myeloma. Recurrent infections may be due to a decrease in the production of normal immunoglobulins, the ineffectiveness of the overproduced and abnormal immunoglobulins, corticosteroids, and/or neutropenia because of the bone marrow infiltration or side effects of treatment.

The patient's psychosocial needs require sensitive, skilled management. Help the patient and significant others adapt to changes fostered by chronic illness and adjust to the losses related to the disease process, while helping to maximize functioning and quality of life. The patient with multiple myeloma may have remissions and exacerbations. Patients may be on dialysis because of myeloma-induced renal failure. Acute care is needed at various times during the illness.

The final, acute phase is unresponsive to treatment and usually short in duration. Help the patient and family navigate needed resources, such as palliative or hospice care, social services, and spiritual care, as appropriate.

DISORDERS OF THE SPLEEN

Many illnesses can affect the spleen. Most can cause some degree of *splenomegaly* (enlarged spleen) (Table 30.30).[2] However, an enlarged spleen may be present in some people without any evidence of disease. The term *hypersplenism* refers to the occurrence of splenomegaly and peripheral cytopenias (anemia, leukopenia, and thrombocytopenia).[2] The degree of splenic enlargement varies with the disease. For example, massive splenic enlargement may occur with infectious mononucleosis, chronic myelogenous leukemia, and thalassemia major.

TABLE 30.30 Common Causes of Splenomegaly

Congestion
- Acquired hemolytic anemia
- Cirrhosis of the liver
- HF (portal hypertension)
- Portal or splenic vein thrombosis
- Sickle cell disease
- Thalassemia

Infections and Inflammations
- Autoimmune diseases: systemic lupus erythematosus, rheumatoid arthritis
- Bacterial infections: endocarditis, splenic abscess, syphilis, tuberculosis, Rocky Mountain spotted fever, typhoid fever
- Fungal infections: histoplasmosis, systemic candidiasis
- Parasitic infections: malaria, trypanosomiasis, schistosomiasis, leishmaniasis
- Viral infections: human immunodeficiency virus, cytomegalovirus, mononucleosis

Infiltrative Diseases and Tumors or Cysts
- Acute and chronic leukemia
- Amyloidosis
- Gaucher disease
- Lymphomas
- Polycythemia vera
- Other primary or secondary tumors and cysts
- Sarcoidosis

Mild splenic enlargement occurs with HF and SLE. The normal spleen holds 350 mL of blood. About one third of the platelet mass is stored in the spleen.

When the spleen enlarges, its normal filtering and storage capacity increases. Consequently, there is often a reduction in the number of circulating blood cells as they engorge the spleen. In addition, there are unusual findings in the peripheral smear, such as pitted or pocked RBCs or Howell-Jolly bodies. These findings aid in diagnosing a malfunctioning spleen. A slight to moderate enlargement of the spleen is usually asymptomatic and found during routine examination of the abdomen. While massive splenomegaly can be well tolerated, the patient may have abdominal discomfort and early satiety. Other techniques to assess the size of the spleen include radionuclide colloid liver-spleen scan, CT or PET scan, MRI, and ultrasound scan.[3]

Occasionally a splenectomy is done as part of the evaluation or treatment of splenomegaly. Another major reason for splenectomy is splenic rupture. The spleen may rupture from trauma; inadvertent tearing during other surgical procedures; and diseases, such as mononucleosis, malaria, and lymphoid tumors. After a splenectomy, there can be a dramatic increase in peripheral RBC, WBC, and platelet counts.

Nursing responsibilities for patients with spleen disorders vary depending on the problem. Splenomegaly may be painful. The patient may need analgesics; care in moving, turning, and positioning; and evaluation of lung expansion because spleen enlargement may impair diaphragmatic excursion. If anemia, thrombocytopenia, or leukopenia develops from splenic enlargement, institute nursing measures to support the patient and prevent life-threatening complications. After a splenectomy, observe the patient for hemorrhage and shock.

After splenectomy, immunologic deficiencies may develop, such as low IgG levels. Patients have a lifelong risk for infection, especially from encapsulated organisms, such as *Pneumococcus* species. This risk is reduced by immunization with pneumococcal vaccine.[3]

BLOOD COMPONENT THERAPY

Blood component therapy is often used to manage hematologic diseases. Many therapeutic and surgical procedures depend on blood product support. However, blood component therapy only temporarily supports the patient until the underlying problem is resolved. Because transfusions are not free from hazards, they should be used only if needed.

Avoid developing a complacent attitude about this common but potentially dangerous therapy. Make sure that the HCP has discussed the risks, benefits, and alternatives with the patient and that this is recorded in the medical record.

Traditionally, the term *blood transfusion* meant the administration of whole blood. Blood transfusion now has a broader meaning because of the ability to give specific components of blood, such as platelets, packed RBCs, or plasma. Usually, a specific component is ordered. Whole blood is rarely used except in cases of massive hemorrhage, severe coagulopathy, shock, or in military settings (Table 30.31).[1]

Administration Procedure

Blood components may be given through a 22-gauge IV needle, cannula, or catheter. Smaller gauges, such as 25-gauge, may be used in neonates.[39] Larger sizes (e.g., 18- or 16-gauge) in adults may be preferred if rapid transfusions are given or if the

---

ETHICAL/LEGAL DILEMMAS
Religious Beliefs

Situation

W.D., an 81-yr-old woman with dementia, is transferred from a nursing home to a hospital because of GI bleeding from an unknown cause. Some of her family members tell you that she is a Jehovah's Witness and must not receive blood products. If she does not have exploratory surgery and transfusions, the surgeon believes that she will die.

Ethical/Legal Points for Consideration

- Competent adults have the right to make health care decisions, including the right to refuse treatment, based on their religious beliefs.
- If the patient is determined to be incompetent and a guardian has been appointed, the guardian has the legal right to make the consent or refusal.
- If the HCP believes that the treatment is essential to preserve life and health and there is no legal decision maker, a request is made for a legal determination of whether the patient is incapable of consent or refusal. If the judge agrees, the patient is made a ward of the court for this issue. Usually the HCP is directed to make a decision based on the patient's best interests.

Discussion Questions

1. What resources do you have available to consult about religious practices?
2. How could you determine if the family were acting in W.D.'s best interest or their own?
3. What nonblood alternatives are available for Jehovah's Witnesses?

---

infusion is sluggish. Smaller needles can be used for platelets, albumin, and clotting factor replacement. Verify the patency of the venous access before requesting the blood component from the blood bank. Most blood product administration tubing is of a "Y type" with a macroaggregate filter (170 to 260 microns; filters out particulate). One arm of the Y is for the isotonic saline solution and the other arm of the Y for the blood product. You may use infusion pumps or syringes approved for blood administration according to agency policy.[39]

> **! SAFETY ALERT Blood Transfusions**
> - Do not use dextrose solutions, lactated Ringer's solution, or any other solution other than 0.9% sodium chloride for giving blood because they will cause RBC hemolysis.
> - Exceptions to the above restrictions may be appropriate, such as in trauma situations. These solutions, approved by the FDA, include ABO-compatible plasma and 5% albumin. Follow agency policy.[39]
> - Do not give any additives, including medications, in the same tubing as the blood unless you first clear the tubing with saline solution.

After obtaining the blood or blood components from the blood bank, make a positive identification of the blood product and recipient. Improper product-to-patient identification is the most common cause of hemolytic transfusion reactions, thus placing a great responsibility on nurses to carry out the identification procedure appropriately. Follow the policy and procedures at your agency. Most have a dual-checking system with 2 licensed persons checking the patient identification with the labeled blood component. The blood bank is responsible for typing and crossmatching the donor's blood with the recipient's blood. The result of any needed compatibility testing should be on the product bag or tag.

Table 30.32 outlines blood component compatibilities for transfusions.[37,39] ABO compatibility is not a prerequisite for platelet transfusions. However, after multiple platelet

TABLE 30.31 Common Blood Products

Description	Special Considerations	Indications for Use
Albumin Prepared from plasma. Can be stored for 5 yr. Available in 5% or 25% solution. Heat treated and does not transmit viruses.	Albumin 25% expands the blood volume by about 3.5 times, Hyperosmolar solution acts by moving water from extravascular to intravascular space.	Hypovolemic shock, hypoalbuminemia, after large-volume paracentesis, replacement in plasmapheresis.
Cryoprecipitates and Commercial Concentrates Prepared from fresh frozen plasma. 10–15 mL/bag. Can be stored for 1 yr. Once thawed, must be used within 5 days.	See also Table 30.18.	Replacement for fibrinogen deficiency, usually due to DIC, severe liver disease, or massive transfusion. Has other clotting factors, especially factor VIII, factor XIII, and von Willebrand factor.
Fresh Frozen Plasma Liquid portion of whole blood is separated from cells and frozen. 1 unit contains about 250 mL. Rich in clotting factors but contains no platelets. Can be stored for up to 1 yr, depending on storage. Must be used within 24 hr after thawing.	Use in treating hemorrhagic shock is being replaced by pure preparations, such as albumin and plasma expanders.	Bleeding caused by deficiency in clotting factors (e.g., DIC, hemorrhage, massive transfusion, liver disease, vitamin K deficiency, excess warfarin).
Frozen RBCs Prepared from RBCs using glycerol for protection and frozen. Can be stored for 10 yr.	Must be used within 24 hr of thawing. Successive washings with saline solution remove most WBCs and plasma proteins.	Autotransfusion. Stockpiling or rare donors for patients with alloantibodies.
Packed RBCs Prepared from whole blood by sedimentation or centrifugation. 1 unit contains 250–350 mL. Can be stored up to 42 days depending on processing (anticoagulants and preservatives).	Use of RBCs for treatment allows remaining components of blood (e.g., platelets, albumin, plasma) to be used for other purposes. Less danger of fluid overload. Preferred RBC source because they are more component specific. Leukocyte depletion (leukoreduction) by filtration, washing, or freezing is frequently used, Decreases non-hemolytic febrile or mild allergic reactions in patients who receive frequent transfusions. Reduces transmission of cytomegalovirus.	Severe or symptomatic anemia, acute blood loss. 1 unit of RBCs can be expected to increase Hgb by 1 g/dL or Hct by 3% in a typical adult. 1 unit can replace a blood loss of 500 mL.
Platelets Prepared from fresh whole blood. An apheresed single donation is usually 200–400 mL in volume. May be pooled from multiple donors.	Can obtain multiple units from 1 donor by plateletpheresis. Can be kept at room temperature in the blood bank under gentle agitation for 1–5 days depending on type of collection and storage bag used. For patients who receive frequent transfusions and become refractory, may give leukocyte reduced, HLA, or type specific to prevent alloimmunization to HLA antigens.	Bleeding caused by thrombocytopenia. May be contraindicated in thrombotic thrombocytopenic purpura and HITT except in life-threatening hemorrhage. Average corrected count increment is 10 × 10^9/L. Failure to have an increase may be due to fever, sepsis, splenomegaly, or DIC or development of antibodies (refractory).

DIC, Disseminated intravascular coagulation; *HITT,* heparin-induced thrombocytopenia and thrombosis; *HLA,* human leukocyte antigen.

TABLE 30.32 Blood Component Compatibilities for Transfusions

Recipient's Type	DONOR PRODUCT			
	Packed Red Blood Cells	Plasma	Platelets	Cryoprecipitate
O+	O+, O–	All groups	O, B, A, AB	Any group is safe to transfuse
O–	O–			
A+	A+, A–, O+, O–	A, AB	A, AB, B, O	
A–	A–, O–			
B+	B+, B–, O+, O–	B, AB	B, AB, A, O	
B–	B–, O–			
AB+	All groups	Only AB	Any group	
AB–	AB–, B–, A–, O–			

transfusions, a patient may develop anti-HLA antibodies to the transfused platelets. With the use of lymphocyte typing to match HLA types of the donor and recipient, multiple platelet transfusions can be given with fewer complications to those who develop antibodies to platelets. The patient may be premedicated with an antihistamine (e.g., diphenhydramine) and hydrocortisone to decrease the chance of reacting to platelet transfusions if there is a history of reactions.[39]

NURSING MANAGEMENT
Blood Transfusions

Role of Nursing Personnel
Registered Nurse (RN)
- Complete a baseline physical assessment of the patient as a basis to assess changes during and after the transfusion.
- Ensure that the IV line has an appropriate needle, catheter, or cannula, and that it is patent.
- Double-check patient identification and blood product identification data with another licensed nurse (consider state nurse practice act and agency policy).
- Adjust infusion rate of transfusion according to patient needs, provider's order, and agency policy.
- Assess patient for signs of transfusion reactions.
- Delegate UAP to take vital signs as directed.
- Evaluate for therapeutic effect of blood product (improvement in CBC, increased blood pressure, decreased bleeding).
- Monitor for signs of circulatory overload (e.g., shortness of breath) if the transfusion is given rapidly.

Role of Other Team Members
Blood Bank Personnel
- Responsible for typing and crossmatching the donor's blood with the recipient's blood.
- Note the result of the compatibility testing on the product bag or tag.
- When handing off the blood or blood component to nursing personnel, ensure that a positive identification is made with product and patient's information.

Take the patient's vital signs before beginning the transfusion so that you have a baseline measure. If the patient has abnormal vital signs (e.g., high fever), call the HCP to clarify if you should give the blood component. Start the blood as soon as it is brought to the patient. Do not refrigerate it on the nursing unit. If the blood is not started within 30 minutes, return it to the blood bank for storage. During the first 15 minutes or 50 mL of blood infusion, stay with the patient. If there are any untoward reactions, they are most likely to occur during this time. The rate of infusion during this period should be no more than 2 mL/min. Do not infuse packed RBCs quickly except in an emergency. Rapid infusion of cold blood may cause the patient to become chilled. If rapid replacement of large amounts of blood is needed, a blood-warming device may be used. Other blood components, such as fresh frozen plasma and platelets, may be given over 15 to 30 minutes. Refer to your agency's policy and procedure.

After the first 15 minutes, vital signs are usually retaken. The rate of infusion is determined by the prescriber's orders, the patient's clinical condition, and the product being infused. Observe the patient periodically throughout the transfusion (e.g., every 30 minutes) and up to 1 hour after the transfusion. Most patients not in danger of fluid overload can tolerate the infusion of 1 unit of packed RBCs over 2 hours. The transfusion

should not take more than 4 hours to give because of the increased risk for bacterial growth in the product once it is out of refrigeration.

Blood Transfusion Reactions

A *blood transfusion reaction* is an adverse reaction to blood transfusion therapy. It can range in severity from mild symptoms to a life-threatening condition. Because complications of transfusion therapy may be significant, careful evaluation of the patient is needed. Common signs and symptoms are associated with more than 1 type of adverse reaction. Blood transfusion reactions can be classified as acute or delayed[1,39] (Tables 30.33 and 30.34).

CHECK YOUR PRACTICE

Your 82-yr-old male patient with severe iron-deficiency anemia is receiving his second unit of packed RBCs. He received his first transfusions without any problems. He is now reporting chills and feels like his heart is racing.
- What should you do?

If a transfusion reaction occurs, take the following steps: (1) stop the transfusion; (2) maintain a patent IV line with saline solution; (3) notify the blood bank and the HCP immediately; (4) recheck identifying tags and numbers; (5) monitor vital signs and urine output; (6) treat symptoms per HCP order; (7) save the blood bag and tubing and send them to the blood bank for examination; (8) collect required blood and urine specimens at intervals based on the hospital policy to evaluate for hemolysis; and (9) document on transfusion reaction form and patient chart. The blood bank and laboratory are responsible for identifying the type of reaction.

A transfusion reaction is a *serious reportable event* (SRE) and a *sentinel event*. These events are discussed in Chapter 1.

Acute Transfusion Reactions. The most common cause of hemolytic reactions is transfusion of ABO-incompatible blood (Table 30.33). This is an example of a type II cytotoxic hypersensitivity reaction (see Chapter 13). Severe hemolytic reactions are rare. Mislabeling specimens and giving blood to the wrong person cause most acute hemolytic reactions. This again points to the importance of using proper patient identifiers when drawing blood samples and when giving medications and blood products.

Delayed Transfusion Reactions. Delayed transfusion reactions include delayed hemolytic reactions (discussed previously), infections, and iron overload (Table 30.34).

Autotransfusion

Autotransfusion, or autologous transfusion, involves removing whole blood from a person and transfusing that blood back into the same person. This avoids problems of incompatibility, allergic reactions, and disease transmission. Methods of autotransfusion include:
- *Autologous donation* or *elective phlebotomy* (predeposit transfusion). A person donates blood before a planned surgical procedure. The blood can be frozen and stored for up to 10 years. Usually the blood is stored without being frozen and given to the person within a few weeks of donation. This technique is especially beneficial to the patient with a rare blood type or for any patient who may be expected to need limited blood product support during a major surgical procedure (e.g., elective orthopedic surgery).

TABLE 30.33 Acute Transfusion Reactions

Cause	Manifestations	Management	Prevention
Acute Hemolytic Reaction			
Infusion of ABO-incompatible whole blood, RBCs, or components containing as little as 10 mL of RBCs. Antibodies in the recipient's plasma attach to antigens on transfused RBCs, causing RBC destruction.	Reactions usually develop in first 15 min. Fever with or without chills; back, abdominal, chest or flank pain; infusion site pain, tachycardia, dyspnea, tachypnea, hypotension, hemoglobinuria, acute jaundice, dark urine, bleeding, acute kidney injury, shock, cardiac arrest, DIC, death.	• Treat shock and DIC if present. • Draw blood samples for serologic testing slowly to avoid hemolysis from the procedure. Send urine specimen to the laboratory. • Maintain BP with IV colloid solutions. Give diuretics as prescribed to maintain urine flow. • Insert indwelling urinary catheter or measure voided amounts to monitor hourly urine output. Dialysis may be needed if renal failure occurs. • Do not transfuse more RBC-containing components until blood bank has provided newly crossmatched units.	Verify and document patient identification from sample collection to component infusion (e.g., visually compare label on sample collection and blood component with patient identification).
Febrile, Nonhemolytic Reaction			
Sensitization to donor WBCs (most common), platelets, or plasma proteins.	Sudden chills, rigors, and fever (rise in temperature of >1°C), headache, vomiting.	Give antipyretics as prescribed (acetaminophen). Do not restart transfusion unless HCP orders.	Consider leukocyte-reduced blood products (filtered, washed, or frozen) for patients with a history of 2 or more such reactions. Give acetaminophen or diphenhydramine 30 min before transfusion.
Mild Allergic Reaction			
Sensitivity to foreign plasma proteins. More common in people with history of allergies.	Flushing, itching, pruritus, urticaria (hives).	• Give antihistamine, corticosteroid, epinephrine, as ordered. • If symptoms are mild and transient, transfusion may be restarted slowly with HCP's order. • Do not restart transfusion if fever or pulmonary symptoms develop.	Treat prophylactically with antihistamines or steroids. Consider washed RBCs and platelets.
Anaphylactic and Severe Allergic Reaction			
Sensitivity to donor plasma proteins. Infusion of IgA proteins to IgA-deficient recipient who has developed IgA antibody.	Anxiety, abdominal pain, urticaria, dyspnea, wheezing, progressing to cyanosis, bronchospasm, hypotension, shock, and possible cardiac arrest.	• Start CPR, if indicated. Administer O$_2$. • Have epinephrine ready for injection. • Antihistamines, corticosteroids, β$_2$-agonists may be given. • Do not restart transfusion.	Transfuse extensively washed RBC products from which all plasma has been removed. Use blood from IgA-deficient donor. Use autologous components.
Circulatory Overload Reaction			
Fluid given faster than the circulation can accommodate. People with cardiac or renal disease at risk.	Cough, dyspnea, pulmonary congestion, adventitious breath sounds, headache, hypertension, tachycardia, distended neck veins.	• Place patient upright with feet in dependent position. • Obtain chest x-ray STAT if ordered. • Administer prescribed diuretics, O$_2$, morphine.	Adjust transfusion volume and flow rate based on patient size and clinical status. Have blood bank divide future units into smaller aliquots for better spacing of fluid infused.
Sepsis			
Transfusion of bacterially infected blood components.	Rapid onset of chills, rigors, high fever, vomiting, diarrhea, marked hypotension, or shock.	• Obtain culture of patient's blood. • Treat septicemia as directed—antibiotics, IV fluids, vasopressors,	Collect, process, store, and transfuse blood products according to blood banking standards and complete the transfusion within 4 hr of starting time.
Transfusion-Related Acute Lung Injury (TRALI) Reaction			
Reaction between transfused antileukocyte antibodies and recipient's leukocytes, causing pulmonary inflammation and capillary leak.	Fever, chills, hypotension, tachypnea, frothy sputum, dyspnea, hypoxemia, respiratory failure. Noncardiogenic pulmonary edema. Leading cause of transfusion-related deaths. Arises within 1–6 hr of transfusion.	• Draw blood for arterial blood gases and HLA or antileukocyte antibodies. Obtain chest x-ray STAT. • Provide O$_2$ and administer corticosteroids (diuretics of no value) as ordered. • Start CPR if needed and provide ventilatory and BP support if needed.	Provide leukocyte-reduced products. Identify donors who are implicated in TRALI reactions and do not allow them to donate.

TABLE 30.33 Acute Transfusion Reactions—cont'd

Cause	Manifestations	Management	Prevention
Massive Blood Transfusion Reaction			
Can occur with replacement of 10 or more RBC units within 24 hr. RBC transfusions do not contain clotting factors, albumin, and platelets.	Hypothermia and cardiac dysrhythmias (from rapid infusion of large quantities of cold blood). Citrate toxicity and hypocalcemia (from the use of citrate as a storage solution). Hypocalcemia (citrate binds calcium). Hyperkalemia or hypokalemia.	• When patients receive massive transfusions of blood products, monitor clotting status and electrolyte levels.	Use blood-warming equipment. Infuse 10% calcium gluconate with citrated blood products. Because of dilution effect on coagulation due to massive RBC transfusion, platelets and plasma will also be given.

DIC, disseminated intravascular coagulation; *HLA,* human leukocyte antigen; *IgA,* immunoglobulin A.

TABLE 30.34 Delayed Transfusion Reactions

Manifestations	Prevention and Management
Delayed Hemolytic	
Fever, mild jaundice, decreased hemoglobin. Occurs as early as 3 days or as late as several months posttransfusion as the result of destruction of transfused RBCs by alloantibodies not detected during crossmatch.	Generally, no acute treatment is needed. Hemolysis may be severe enough to warrant further transfusions.
Hepatitis B*	
Increased liver enzymes (AST and ALT), anorexia, malaise, nausea and vomiting, fever, dark urine, jaundice. Usually resolves spontaneously within 4–6 wk. Chronic carrier state can develop and result in permanent damage to the liver.	Hepatitis B virus can be detected in donated blood by the presence of hepatitis B surface antigen (HBsAg). Treat symptomatically.
Hepatitis C*	
Similar to hepatitis B, but symptoms are usually less severe. Chronic liver disease and cirrhosis may develop.	Before testing of anti-HCV in donated blood, accounted for 90%–95% of all posttransfusion hepatitis. Treat with direct-acting antivirals and symptomatically.
Iron Overload	
Excess iron is deposited in heart, liver, pancreas, and joints, causing dysfunction. HF, dysrhythmias, impaired thyroid and gonadal function, diabetes, arthritis, cirrhosis. Occurs in patients receiving >20 units for chronic anemia (e.g., sickle cell anemia, β-thalassemia) over time.	May be prevented by deferoxamine, which chelates and removes accumulated iron via the kidneys, given IV or subcutaneously. Deferasirox and deferiprone, oral agents that chelate iron, may be used. Phlebotomy may be used.
Other	
Cytomegalovirus (CMV), HIV, human herpesvirus type 6 (HSV-6), Epstein-Barr virus (EBV), human T cell leukemia virus, HTLV-1, and malaria. Most recent threats have been agents that primarily affect animals but have been transmitted to the blood supply through the food supply, or vectors, such as mosquitoes or ticks. These include *Plasmodium* species (malaria), dengue fever virus, West Nile virus, *Trypanosoma cruzi* (Chagas' disease), *Babesia* species (babesiosis), human herpesvirus 8 (KS virus), and variant Creutzfeldt-Jakob disease ("mad cow disease").	Treatment based on the cause. Ways of detecting some agents are now used, such as the nucleic acid test for West Nile virus, Zika virus, HIV, and *T. cruzi.* Donor screening has been the only available method to reduce the risk for donor-contaminated blood for others. Leukocyte-reduced components may reduce virus transmission. Patients may be monitored serologically (e.g., CMV titers are followed for allogeneic stem cell transplant patients).

*New cases of transfusion-related hepatitis B and C are not common.
ALT, Alanine aminotransferase; *AST,* aspartate aminotransferase; *HCV,* hepatitis C virus; *CMV,* cytomegalovirus; *HTLV-1,* human T-cell leukemia virus, type 1; *KS,* Kaposi sarcoma.

- *Autotransfusion.* A method for replacing blood volume that involves safely and aseptically collecting, filtering, and returning the patient's own blood lost during a major surgical procedure or from a traumatic injury. It is an important way to safely replace volume and stabilize bleeding patients. Autotransfusion collection devices are most often used with surgery. Some allow blood to be automatically and continuously reinfused. Others require collecting the blood for a time (usually no longer than 4 hours) and then reinfusing it. Drainage after the first 24 hours or drainage that is suspected to contain pathogens is generally not reinfused. Anticoagulants may be added before reinfusion. Clots that develop after blood is filtered through the collection system can sometimes prevent reinfusion of the blood. Sometimes the collected blood is depleted of its normal coagulation factors. So, monitoring coagulation studies in the patient receiving an autotransfusion is important.[1]

CASE STUDY

Leukemia

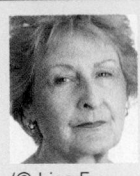

(© Lisa F. Young/iStock.)

Patient Profile

A.J. is a 63-yr-old white woman who is brought to the ED by her husband (see the Chapter 29 case study). She has become progressively weaker and was admitted for further evaluation.

Subjective Data

- Progressive weakness over the last couple of weeks
- Has had a recent sinus infection that resolved after 2 courses of antibiotics
- Reports periodic shortness of breath
- Has noticed a lot of bruising lately

Objective Data

Physical Examination

- Has scattered petechiae on both ankles and 2 ecchymoses on her arms and 3 on her left lower leg
- Her skin is very pale
- BP 100/70 (lying), 88/60 (standing), temperature 96.8°F (36°C), respiratory rate 26/min, apical pulse 110/min (lying), 124/min (standing), O₂ saturation 90% on room air

Laboratory Results

- Hct 18.2%
- Hgb 5.9 g/dL, WBC count 2600/µL (2.6 × 10⁹/L)
- Platelet count 72,000/µL (72 × 10⁹/L)
- Peripheral blood smear shows that 80% of the WBCs are blasts
- PT 18 sec, aPTT 37 sec
- LDH 560 units/L

Bone Marrow Biopsy

- Multiple myeloblasts (>50%)

Interprofessional Care

- Consultation with a hematologist-oncologist
- 2 units of packed red blood cells
- *Diagnosis:* acute myelogenous leukemia

Discussion Questions

1. What components of the laboratory test results and bone marrow biopsy suggest acute leukemia?
2. How is acute myelogenous leukemia treated?
3. What is A.J.'s prognosis?
4. What are the life-threatening problems that can occur because of this disease and treatment? How can you anticipate and assess for these problems?
5. *Priority Decision:* Based on the assessment data presented, what are the priority nursing diagnoses? Are there any collaborative problems?
6. *Priority Decision:* What are the priority nursing interventions for A.J.?
7. *Patient-Centered Care:* What are the priorities for patient teaching with a newly diagnosed adult with leukemia?
8. Collaboration: What members of the interprofessional team are likely to be involved in A.J.'s care?
9. *Evidence-Based Practice:* A.J. becomes fatigued after starting chemotherapy. She wants to know if she can still work and do household chores even if she is so fatigued. What is your best advice for her?
10. Develop a conceptual care map for A.J.

Answers available at *http://evolve.elsevier.com/Lewis/medsurg.*

BRIDGE TO NCLEX EXAMINATION

The number of the question corresponds to the same-numbered outcome at the beginning of the chapter.

1. In a severely anemic patient, the nurse would expect to find
   a. cyanosis and cardiomegaly.
   b. pulmonary edema and fibrosis.
   c. dyspnea at rest and tachycardia.
   d. ventricular dysrhythmias and wheezing.

2. When obtaining assessment data from a patient with a microcytic, hypochromic anemia, the nurse would ask the patient about
   a. folic acid intake.
   b. dietary intake of iron.
   c. a history of gastric surgery.
   d. a history of sickle cell anemia.

3. Nursing interventions for a patient with severe anemia related to peptic ulcer disease include (*select all that apply*)
   a. instructions for high-iron diet.
   b. taking vital signs every 8 hours.
   c. monitoring stools for occult blood.
   d. teaching self-injection of erythropoietin.
   e. administration of cobalamin (vitamin B₁₂) injections.

4. The nursing management of a patient in sickle cell crisis includes (*select all that apply*)
   a. monitoring CBC.
   b. optimal pain management and O₂ therapy.
   c. blood transfusions if needed and iron chelation.
   d. rest as needed and deep vein thrombosis prophylaxis.
   e. administration of IV iron and diet high in iron content.

5. A complication of the hyperviscosity of polycythemia is
   a. thrombosis.
   b. cardiomyopathy.
   c. pulmonary edema.
   d. disseminated intravascular coagulation (DIC).

6. When caring for a patient with thrombocytopenia, the nurse instructs the patient to
   a. dab his or her nose instead of blowing.
   b. be careful when shaving with a safety razor.
   c. continue with physical activities to stimulate thrombopoiesis.
   d. avoid aspirin because it may mask the fever that occurs with thrombocytopenia.

7. The nurse would expect that a patient with von Willebrand disease undergoing surgery would be treated with administration of vWF and
   a. thrombin.
   b. factor VI.
   c. factor VII.
   d. factor VIII.

8. DIC is a disorder in which
   a. the coagulation pathway is genetically altered, leading to thrombus formation in all major blood vessels.
   b. an underlying disease depletes hemolytic factors in the blood, leading to diffuse thrombotic episodes and infarcts.
   c. a disease process stimulates coagulation processes with resultant thrombosis, as well as depletion of clotting factors, leading to diffuse clotting and hemorrhage.
   d. an inherited predisposition causes a deficiency of clotting factors that leads to overstimulation of coagulation processes in the vasculature.

9. Priority nursing actions when caring for a hospitalized patient with a new-onset temperature of 102.2° F (39° C) and severe neutropenia include *(select all that apply)*
   a. starting the prescribed antibiotic STAT.
   b. drawing peripheral and central line blood cultures.
   c. ongoing monitoring of the patient's vital signs for septic shock.
   d. taking a full set of vital signs and notifying the physician immediately.
   e. administering transfusions of WBCs treated to decrease immunogenicity.

10. Because myelodysplastic syndrome arises from the pluripotent hematopoietic stem cell in the bone marrow, laboratory results the nurse would expect to find include a(n)
    a. excess of T cells.
    b. excess of platelets.
    c. deficiency of granulocytes.
    d. deficiency of all cellular blood components.

11. The most common type of leukemia in adults in western countries is
    a. acute myelocytic leukemia.
    b. acute lymphocytic leukemia.
    c. chronic myelocytic leukemia.
    d. chronic lymphocytic leukemia.

12. Multiple drugs are often used in combinations to treat leukemia and lymphoma because
    a. there are fewer toxic and side effects.
    b. the chance that one drug will be effective is increased.
    c. the drugs are more effective without causing side effects.
    d. the drugs work by different mechanisms to maximize killing of cancer cells.

13. The nurse is aware that a major difference between Hodgkin's lymphoma and non-Hodgkin's lymphoma is that
    a. Hodgkin's lymphoma occurs only in young adults.
    b. Hodgkin's lymphoma is considered potentially curable.
    c. non-Hodgkin's lymphoma can manifest in multiple areas.
    d. non-Hodgkin's lymphoma is treated only with radiation therapy.

14. A patient with multiple myeloma becomes confused and lethargic. The nurse would expect that these clinical manifestations may be explained by diagnostic results that indicate
    a. hyperkalemia.
    b. hyperuricemia.
    c. hypercalcemia.
    d. CNS myeloma.

15. When reviewing a patient's hematologic laboratory values after a splenectomy, the nurse would expect to find
    a. RBC abnormalities.
    b. increased WBC count.
    c. decreased hemoglobin.
    d. decreased platelet count.

16. Complications of transfusions that can be decreased by using leukocyte depletion or reduction of RBC transfusion are
    a. chills and hemolysis.
    b. leukostasis and neutrophilia.
    c. fluid overload and pulmonary edema.
    d. transmission of cytomegalovirus and fever.

1. c, 2. b, 3. a, c, 4. a, b, c, d, 5. a, 6. a, 7. d, 8. c, 9. a, b, c, d, 10. d, 11. d, 12. d, 13. c, 14. c, 15. b, 16. d

For rationales to these answers and even more NCLEX review questions, visit *http://evolve.elsevier.com/Lewis/medsurg.*

EVOLVE WEBSITE/RESOURCES LIST

http://evolve.elsevier.com/Lewis/medsurg

Review Questions (Online Only)

Key Points

Answer Keys for Review Questions
- Rationales for Bridge to NCLEX Examination Questions
- Answer Guidelines for Case Study on p. 652
- Answer Guidelines for Managing Care of Multiple Patients Case Study (Section 7) on p. 655

Student Case Studies
- Patient With Chronic Myelogenous Leukemia Including End-of-life Care
- Patient With Sickle Cell Anemia

Nursing Care Plans
- eNursing Care Plan 30.1: Patient With Anemia
- eNursing Care Plan 30.2: Patient With Thrombocytopenia
- eNursing Care Plan 30.3: Patient With Neutropenia

Conceptual Care Map Creator
- Conceptual Care Map for Case Study on p. 652

Audio Glossary

Content Updates

REFERENCES

1. Hoffman R, Benz EJ, Silberstein LE, et al: *Hematology: Basic principles and practice*, ed 7, Philadelphia, 2018, Elsevier.
2. Huether SE, McCance KL: *Understanding pathophysiology*, ed 6, St Louis, 2017, Mosby.
3. Lichtman MA, Kaushansky K, Prchal JT, et al: *Williams manual of hematology*, ed 9, New York, 2017, McGraw-Hill.
4. World Health Organization. Anemia policy brief. Retrieved from *www.who.int/nutrition/topics/globaltargets_anaemia_policybrief.pdf.*
*5. Green R, Mitra AD: Megaloblastic anemias: Nutritional and other causes, *Med Clin N Am* 101:297, 2017.
*6. Fraenkel PG: Anemia of inflammation: A review, *Med Clin N Am* 101:285, 2017.
*7. Kumar R, Bonfim C, George B: Hematopoietic cell transplantation for aplastic anemia, *Curr Opin Hematol* 24:509, 2017.
*8. Thein MS, Igbineweka NE, Thein SL: Sickle cell disease in the older adult, *Pathology* 49:1, 2017.
9. Centers for Disease Control: Sickle cell disease. Retrieved from *www.cdc.gov/ncbddd/sicklecell/data.html.*
*10. National Heart, Lung, and Blood Institute. Evidence-based management of sickle cell disease: Expert panel report. Retrieved from: *www.nhlbi.nih.gov/health-topics/evidence-based-management-sickle-cell-disease.*
*11. Wilmore DW: FDA approval of glutamine for sickle cell disease, *J Parenter Enteral Nutr* 41:912, 2017.
*12. Zhang K, Lu Y, Harley KT, et al: Atypical hemolytic uremic syndrome: A brief review, *Hematol Reports* 9:7053, 2017.
13. The National Institute of Diabetes and Digestive and Kidney Diseases: Hemochromatosis. Retrieved from *www.niddk.nih.gov/health-information/liver-disease/hemochromatosis.*

*14. Mesa R, Jamieson C, Bhatia R, et al: Myeloproliferative neoplasms, NCCN clinical practice guidelines, version 2.2018. Retrieved from *www.nccn.org*.

*15. Sverdlin D, Peters-Watral B: Atypical hemolytic uremic syndrome, *Clin J Oncol Nurs* 21:481, 2017.

*16. Lambert MP, Gernsheimer TB: Clinical updates in adult immune thrombocytopenia, *Blood* 129:2829, 2017.

*17. Arepally GM: Heparin-induced thrombocytopenia, *Blood* 129:2864, 2017.

18. National Hemophila Foundation. Retrieved from *www.hemophilia.org*.

19. Castaman G, Linari S: Diagnosis and treatment of von Willebrand Disease and rare bleeding disorders, *J Clin Med* 6:45, 2017.

20. Squizzato A, Hunt BJ, Kinasewitz GT, et al: Supportive management strategies for disseminated intravascular coagulation, *Thromb Haemost* 115:896, 2016.

21. White L, Ybarra M: Neutropenic fever, *Hematol Oncol Clin N Am* 31:981, 2017.

*22. Freifeld AG, Bow EJ, Sepkowitz KA, et al: Clinical practice guideline for the use of antimicrobial agents in neutropenic patients with cancer: 2010 Update by the Infectious Diseases Society of America, *Clin Infect Dis* 52:e56, 2011. (Classic)

*23. Baden LR, Swaminathan S: Prevention and treatment of cancer-related infections, NCCN clinical practice guidelines, version 1.2018. Retrieved from *www.nccn.org*.

*24. Crawford J, Becker PS: Myeloid growth factors, NCCN clinical practice guidelines, version 2.2017. Retrieved from *www.nccn.org*.

*25. Rhodes A, Evans LE, Alhazzani W, et al: Surviving sepsis campaign: International guidelines for management of sepsis and septic shock: 2016, *Intensive Care Med* 43:304, 2017.

*26. Greenberg PL, Stone RM: Myelodysplastic syndromes, NCCN clinical practice guidelines, version 1.2018. Retrieved from *www.nccn.org*.

27. Siegel RL, Miller KD, Jemal A: Cancer statistics, 2017, *CA Cancer J Clin* 67:7, 2017.

28. The Lymphoma Research Foundation. Adult T-cell leukemia/lymphoma. Retrieved from *www.lymphoma.org*.

*29. O'Donnell MR, Tallman MS: Acute myeloid leukemia, NCCN clinical practice guidelines, version 3.2017. Retrieved from *www.nccn.org*.

*30. Brown PA: Acute lymphoblastic leukemia, NCCN clinical practice guidelines, version 5.2017. Retrieved from *www.nccn.org*.

*31. Radich JP, Deininger M: Chronic myeloid leukemia, NCCN clinical practice guidelines, version 2.2018. Retrieved from *www.nccn.org*.

*32. Wierda WG, Byrd JC: Chronic lymphocytic leukemia/small lymphocytic lymphoma, NCCN clinical practice guidelines, version 2.2018. Retrieved from *www.nccn.org*.

*33. Zelenetz AD, Gordon LI: B-cell lymphomas, NCCN clinical practice guidelines, version 7.2017. Retrieved from *www.nccn.org*.

*34. Hoppe RT, Advani RH: *Hodgkin lymphoma, NCCN clinical practice guidelines, version 1.2018.* Retrieved from *www.nccn.org*.

*35. Horwitz SM, Ansell S: *T-cell lymphomas, NCCN clinical practice guidelines, version 1.2018.* Retrieved from *www.nccn.org*.

*36. Kumar SK, Callander NS: *Multiple myeloma, NCCN clinical practice guidelines, version 3.2018.* Retrieved from *www.nccn.org*.

37. International Myeloma Foundation. Retrieved from *www.nccn.org*.

*38. Bertolotti P, Pierre A, Rome S, et al. Evidence-based guidelines for preventing and managing side effects of multiple myeloma, *Semin Oncol Nurs* 33:332, 2017.

39. Fung MK, Eder AF, Spitalnik SL, et al: *Technical manual: Standards for blood banks and transfusion services,* ed 19, Bethesda, MD, 2017, AABB.

*Evidence-based information for clinical practice.

CASE STUDY

Managing Care of Multiple Patients

You are working on the oncology unit and have been assigned to care for the following 4 patients. You have 1 UAP who is assigned to help you, and there are 2 other RNs on your clinical unit.

Patients

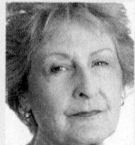
(© Lisa F. Young/iStock.)

A.J. is a 63-yr-old white woman admitted with severe anemia (Hgb 5.9 g/dL and Hct 18.2%). Her WBC count is 2600/µL and platelet count is 72,000/µL. She prefers to take care of herself with "natural therapy" and has not seen an HCP for 5 years. A.J. is having difficulty performing ADLs without having to stop and catch her breath. She received 2 units of RBCs. After a further workup, she is diagnosed with acute myelocytic leukemia (AML). She starts chemotherapy tomorrow.

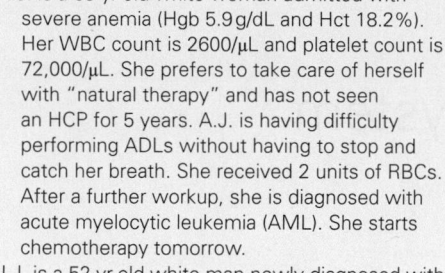
(© g-stockstudio/ iStock/Thinkstock.)

J.J. is a 52-yr-old white man newly diagnosed with acute lymphocytic leukemia (ALL). His most recent vital signs are BP 100/70, temperature 102.2°F (39°C), respiratory rate 26/min, pulse 110. Laboratory results reveal Hgb 6.9 g/dL, Hct 20%, WBC count 120,000/µL (120 × 10⁹/L), and platelet count 25,000/µL (25 × 10⁹/L). He is admitted for blood transfusions and induction therapy.

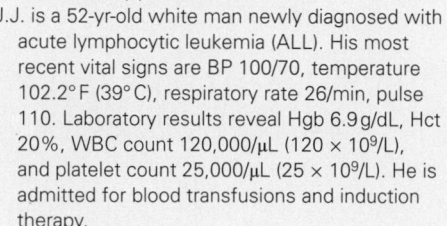
(© Studio Grand Ouest/ iStock/Thinkstock.)

P.H. is a 45-yr-old woman who is currently receiving chemotherapy for treatment of ovarian cancer. She is admitted with fever and chills. Her WBC count is 2200/µL (2.2 × 10⁹/L), with an absolute neutrophil count (ANC) of 400/µL (0.4 × 10⁹/L). She will begin IV antibiotic therapy. Her most recent vital signs are BP 118/60, temperature 99.2°F (37.3°C), respiratory rate 20/min, pulse 98.

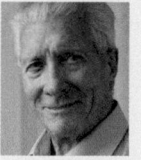
(© Ridofranz/ iStock.)

G.L. is a 67-yr-old man who came to the ED yesterday evening with abdominal pain. A CT scan of the abdomen revealed several masses in his lymphatic system. The HCP suspects non-Hodgkin's lymphoma and admits him for a diagnostic workup. He currently rates his pain as a 3 on a scale of 0 to 10.

Discussion Questions

1. **Priority Decision:** After receiving report, which patient should you see first? Provide a rationale for your decision.
2. **Collaboration:** Which tasks could you delegate to the UAP *(select all that apply)*?
   a. Assist A.J. to a chair after completing her AM care.
   b. Obtain the first unit of blood for J.J. from the blood bank.
   c. Explain the importance of isolation to P.H. and her family.
   d. Ask A.J. why she has not received regular medical care for 5 years.
   e. Assess G.L. for other clinical manifestations of non-Hodgkin's lymphoma.

3. **Priority and Delegation Decision:** When you enter J.J.'s room, you find him somewhat confused and lethargic. His family states he had just had a severe coughing episode. What initial action would be the *most* appropriate?
   a. Perform a focused neurologic examination.
   b. Call respiratory therapy to give him a breathing treatment.
   c. Have the UAP stay with J.J. while you page the HCP STAT.
   d. Ask his family members if they have a copy of his living will.

Case Study Progression

J.J.'s HCP orders a repeat CBC and an emergency CT scan of the head. Your supervisor makes arrangements for another RN to accompany J.J. to the CT scan while you prepare to administer the first unit of RBCs.

4. The HCP orders ferrous sulfate 325 mg TID for A.J. You teach A.J. to take her iron *(select all that apply)*
   a. at breakfast time in the morning.
   b. with orange juice to increase absorption.
   c. 1 hour before meals to facilitate absorption.
   d. 2 hours after eating to minimize side effects.
   e. whenever she feels tired or is short of breath with activity.
5. When teaching P.H.'s family about neutropenic precautions, you stress that the *most* important intervention to prevent infection is
   a. hand hygiene.
   b. wearing a mask.
   c. keeping P.H. in a private room.
   d. limiting the number of visitors in her room.
6. G.L. asks you to explain the diagnostic testing he can expect to undergo related to the suspected lymphoma. Which tests will you explain to him *(select all that apply)*?
   a. PET scan
   b. Bone marrow biopsy
   c. Peripheral blood smear
   d. Excisional lymph node biopsy
   e. Lymphangiography of internal lymph nodes
7. **Management Decision:** An RN from the float pool arrives to accompany J.J. to CT scan at the same time the UAP arrives with the first unit of packed RBCs. Which intervention would be *most* appropriate?
   a. Put the unit of RBCs in the refrigerator to start when J.J. returns to the floor.
   b. Ask the RN to verify the correct unit of RBCs with you and start the infusion.
   c. Give the RN an SBAR report and ask her to start the blood on the way to CT scan.
   d. Ask the RN if she would prefer to give the blood or hold it for J.J.'s return to the unit.

Answers available at *http://evolve.elsevier.com/Lewis/medsurg*.

31

Assessment: Cardiovascular System

Debra Hagler and Diana Rabbani Hagler

The purpose of human life is to serve, and to show compassion and the will to help others.

Albert Schweitzer

ⓔ http://evolve.elsevier.com/Lewis/medsurg/

CONCEPTUAL FOCUS

Health Promotion
Nutrition

Perfusion

LEARNING OUTCOMES

1. Discern the anatomic location and function of the pericardial layers, atria, ventricles, and valves.
2. Relate the coronary circulation to the areas of heart muscle supplied by the major coronary arteries.
3. Distinguish the structure and function of arteries, veins, capillaries, and endothelium.
4. Describe the mechanisms involved in the regulation of blood pressure.
5. Relate the various waveforms on a normal electrocardiogram to the associated cardiac events.
6. Obtain significant subjective and objective assessment data related to the cardiovascular system from a patient and/or caregiver.
7. Perform a physical assessment of the cardiovascular system using the appropriate techniques.
8. Distinguish normal from abnormal findings of a physical assessment of the cardiovascular system.
9. Link the age-related changes of the cardiovascular system to the differences in assessment findings.
10. Describe the purpose, significance of results, and nursing responsibilities related to diagnostic studies of the cardiovascular system.

KEY TERMS

action potential, p. 657
afterload, p. 659
arterial blood pressure, p. 660
cardiac index (CI), p. 658
cardiac output (CO), p. 658
cardiac reserve, p. 659
coronary angiography, p. 675

diastole, p. 657
diastolic blood pressure (DBP), p. 660
ejection fraction (EF), p. 674
heaves, p. 666
Korotkoff sounds, p. 660
mean arterial pressure (MAP), p. 660
murmur, p. 661

point of maximal impulse (PMI), p. 666
preload, p. 659
pulse pressure, p. 660
systole, p. 658
systolic blood pressure (SBP), p. 660

STRUCTURES AND FUNCTIONS OF CARDIOVASCULAR SYSTEM

Heart

Structure. The heart is a 4-chambered hollow muscular organ normally about the size of a fist. It lies within the thorax in the mediastinal space that separates the right and left pleural cavities. The heart is composed of 3 layers: a thin inner lining, the *endocardium;* a layer of muscle, the *myocardium;* and an outer layer, the *epicardium.* The heart is covered by a fibroserous sac called the *pericardium.* This sac consists of 2 layers: the inner *(visceral)* layer of the pericardium (part of the epicardium) and the outer *(parietal)* layer. A small amount of pericardial fluid (around 10 to 15 mL) lubricates the space between the pericardial layers *(pericardial space)* and prevents friction between the surfaces as the heart contracts.

The septum vertically divides the heart. The interatrial septum creates a right and left atrium. The interventricular septum creates a right and left ventricle. The thickness of the wall of each chamber is different. The atrial myocardium is thinner than that

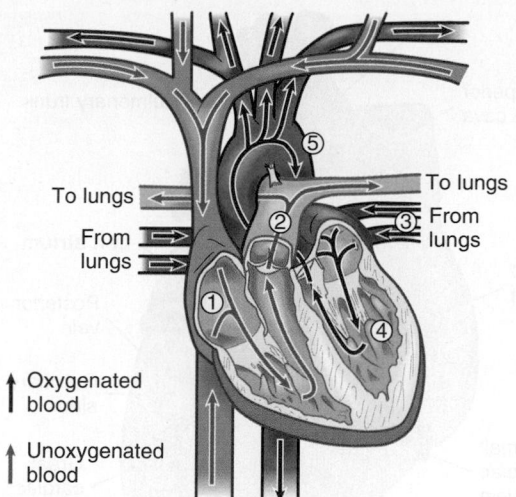

FIG. 31.1 Schematic representation of blood flow through the heart. *Arrows* show direction of flow. *1,* The right atrium receives venous blood from the inferior and superior venae cava and the coronary sinus. The blood then passes through the tricuspid valve into the right ventricle. *2,* With each contraction, the right ventricle pumps blood through the pulmonic valve into the pulmonary artery and to the lungs. *3,* Oxygenated blood flows from the lungs to the left atrium by way of the pulmonary veins. *4,* It then passes through the mitral valve and into the left ventricle. *5,* As the heart contracts, blood is ejected through the aortic valve into the aorta and thus enters the systemic circulation.

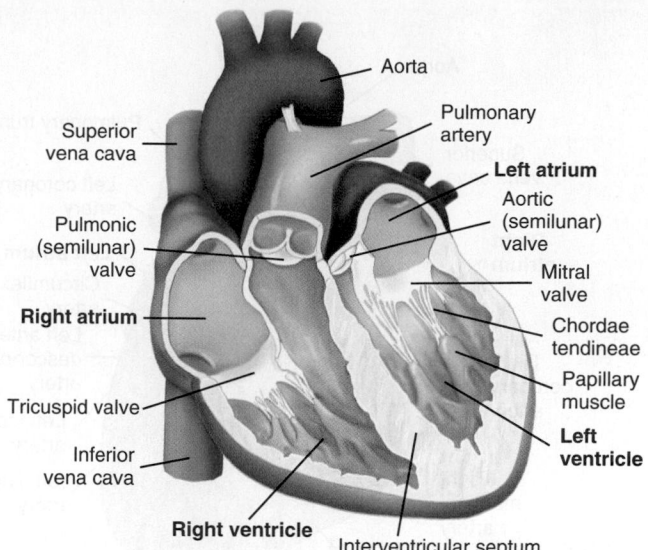

FIG. 31.2 Anatomic structures of the heart and heart valves.

of the ventricles. The left ventricular wall is 2 to 3 times thicker than the right ventricular wall. The thickness of the left ventricle is needed to make the force needed to pump the blood into the systemic circulation.[1]

Blood Flow Through Heart. The blood flow through the heart is shown in Fig. 31.1.

Heart Valves. The 4 valves of the heart keep blood flowing in a forward direction. The cusps of the mitral and tricuspid valves are attached to thin strands of fibrous tissue called *chordae tendineae* (Fig. 31.2). Chordae are anchored in the papillary muscles of the ventricles. This support system prevents the eversion of the leaflets into the atria during ventricular contraction. The pulmonic and aortic valves (also known as *semilunar valves*) prevent blood from regurgitating into the ventricles at the end of each ventricular contraction.

Blood Supply to Myocardium. The myocardium has its own blood supply, the *coronary circulation* (Fig. 31.3). Blood flow into the 2 major coronary arteries occurs primarily during **diastole** (relaxation of the myocardium). The left coronary artery arises from the aorta and divides into 2 main branches: the left anterior descending artery and left circumflex artery. These arteries supply the left atrium, left ventricle, interventricular septum, and part of the right ventricle. The right coronary artery also arises from the aorta, and its branches supply the right atrium, right ventricle, and part of the posterior wall of the left ventricle. In 90% of people, the atrioventricular (AV) node and the bundle of His receive blood supply from the right coronary artery. For this reason, blockage of this artery often causes serious defects in cardiac conduction.

The divisions of coronary veins parallel the coronary arteries. Most of the blood from the coronary system drains into the coronary sinus (a large channel), which empties into the right atrium near the entrance of the inferior vena cava.[1]

Conduction System. The conduction system consists of specialized tissue responsible for creating and transporting the

electrical impulse, or **action potential.** This impulse starts depolarization of the heart cells and leads to heart muscle contraction (Fig. 31.4, *A*). The electrical impulse normally begins in the sinoatrial (SA) node (pacemaker of the heart). Impulses from the SA node travel through interatrial pathways to depolarize the atria, resulting in a contraction.

The electrical impulse travels from the atria to the AV node through internodal pathways. The signal then moves through the bundle of His and the left and right bundle branches. The left bundle branch has 2 divisions: anterior and posterior. The action potential moves through the walls of both ventricles via *Purkinje fibers.* The ventricular conduction system delivers the impulse within 0.12 second. This triggers a synchronized right and left ventricular contraction and ejection of blood into the pulmonary and systemic circulations.

Last, repolarization occurs when the contractile and conduction pathway cells regain their resting polarized condition. Heart muscle cells have a compensatory mechanism that makes them unresponsive or refractory to restimulation during the action potential. During ventricular contraction, there is an *absolute refractory period* during which heart muscle does not respond to any stimuli. After this period, heart muscle gradually recovers its excitability, and a *relative refractory period* occurs by early diastole.

Electrocardiogram. The electrical activity of the heart can be detected on the body surface using electrodes. It is recorded on an electrocardiogram (ECG). We use the letters *P, QRS, T,* and *U* to name the separate waveforms (Fig. 31.4, *B*). The first waveform, the P wave, begins with the firing of the SA node. It represents depolarization of the atria. The QRS complex represents depolarization from the AV node throughout the ventricles. There is a delay of impulse transmission through the AV node that accounts for the time between the beginning of the P wave and the beginning of the QRS wave. The T wave represents repolarization of the ventricles. The U wave, if seen, may represent repolarization of the Purkinje fibers. A large U wave may occur with hypokalemia.[2]

Intervals between these waves (PR, QRS, and QT intervals) reflect the time it takes for the signal to travel from 1 area of the heart to another. We can measure these time intervals. Changes

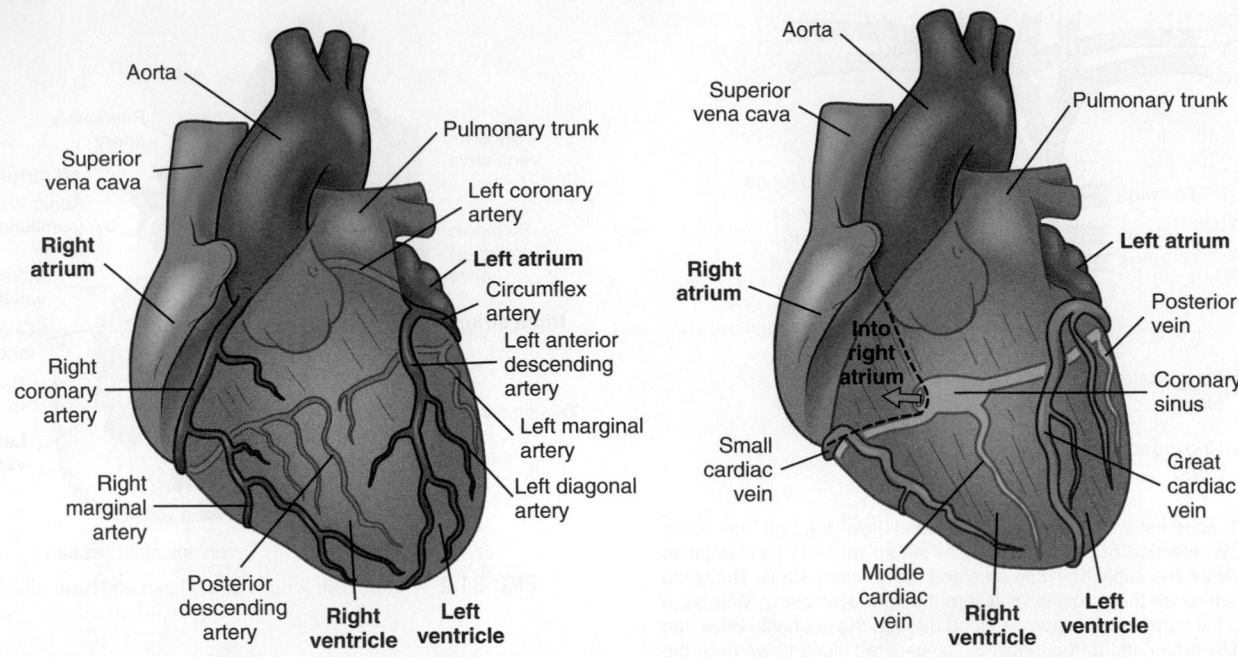

FIG. 31.3 Coronary arteries and veins.

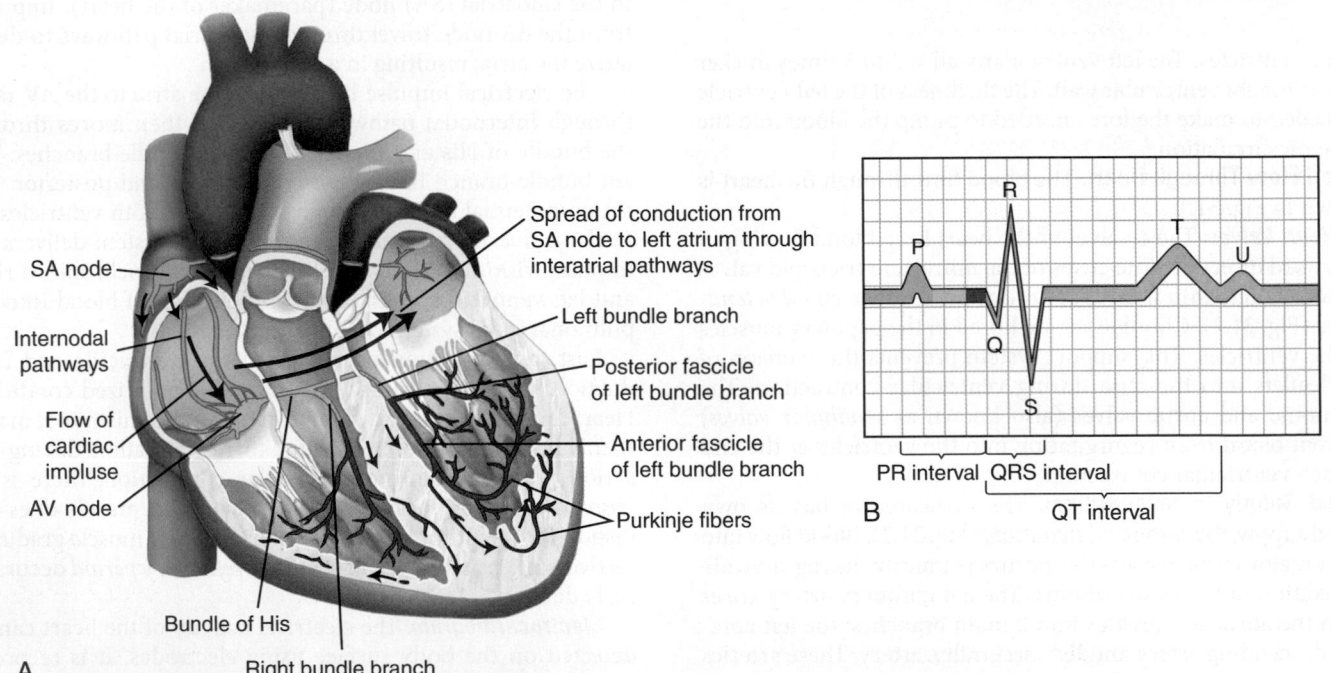

FIG. 31.4 A, Conduction system of the heart. *AV,* Atrioventricular; *SA,* sinoatrial. B, The normal electrocardiogram (ECG) pattern. The P wave represents depolarization of the atria. The QRS complex indicates depolarization of the ventricles. The T wave represents repolarization of the ventricles. The U wave, if present, may represent repolarization of the Purkinje fibers, or it may be associated with hypokalemia. The PR, QRS, and QT intervals reflect the time it takes for the impulse to travel from one area of the heart to another.

from these time references often indicate pathologic conditions. See Chapter 35 for a complete discussion of ECG monitoring.

Mechanical System. *Depolarization* triggers mechanical activity. **Systole,** contraction of the heart muscle, results in ejection of blood from the ventricles. Relaxation of the heart muscle, *diastole,* allows for filling of the ventricles. **Cardiac output (CO)** is the amount of blood pumped by each ventricle in 1 minute. It is

calculated by multiplying the amount of blood ejected from the ventricle with each heartbeat: *stroke volume* (SV) times heart rate (HR) per minute:

$$CO = SV \times HR$$

For the normal adult at rest, CO is maintained in the range of 4 to 8 L/min. **Cardiac index (CI)** is the CO divided by the body surface area (BSA). The CI reflects the relative CO for the body size. The normal CI is 2.8 to 4.2 L per minute per meter squared (L/min/m^2).[3]

Factors Affecting Cardiac Output. Numerous factors can affect either the HR or SV and thus the CO. The HR, which is controlled primarily by the autonomic nervous system, can reach as high as 180 beats/min for short periods without harmful effects. With rapid HRs, there is less time for diastolic filling and perfusion of the coronary arteries. The factors affecting the SV are preload, contractility, and afterload. Increasing preload, contractility, and afterload increases the workload of the heart muscle, resulting in increased O$_2$ demand.

The Frank-Starling law states that, to a point, the more the myocardial fibers are stretched, the greater their force of contraction. The volume of blood stretching the ventricles at the end of diastole, before the next contraction, is called preload. Preload can be increased by conditions such as hypertension, aortic valve disease, and hypervolemia. Preload is decreased when a rapid HR or hypovolemia reduces ventricular filling during diastole. Contractility can be increased by epinephrine and norepinephrine released by the sympathetic nervous system. Increasing contractility raises the SV by increasing ventricular emptying. [3]

Afterload is the peripheral resistance against which the left ventricle must pump. Afterload depends on the size of the ventricle, wall tension, and arterial BP. If the arterial BP is elevated, the ventricles meet increased resistance to ejection of blood, increasing the work demand. Eventually this results in *ventricular hypertrophy,* an enlargement of the heart muscle without an increase in CO or the size of chambers. Although we often think of afterload as affecting left heart function, both right and left ventricles work against resistance. The right ventricle pumps against the afterload of pulmonary arterial resistance.

Cardiac Reserve. The cardiovascular system must respond to many situations in health and illness (e.g., exercise, stress, hypovolemia). The ability to respond to these demands by altering CO is termed cardiac reserve.

Vascular System

Blood Vessels. The 3 major types of blood vessels are the arteries, veins, and capillaries. Arteries, except for the pulmonary artery, carry oxygenated blood away from the heart. Veins, except for the pulmonary veins, carry deoxygenated blood toward the heart. Small branches of arteries and veins are arterioles and venules, respectively. Blood circulates from the left side of the heart into arteries, arterioles, capillaries, venules, and veins, and then back to the right side of the heart.

Arteries and Arterioles. The arterial system differs from the venous system by the amount and type of tissue that make up arterial walls (Fig. 31.5). The large arteries have thick walls composed mainly of elastic tissue. This elastic property cushions the impact of the pressure created by ventricular contraction and provides recoil that propels blood forward into the circulation. Large arteries contain some smooth muscle. Examples of large arteries are the aorta and pulmonary artery.

Arterioles have more smooth muscle and little elastic tissue. Arterioles serve as the major control of arterial BP and distribution of blood flow. They respond readily to local conditions such as low oxygen (O$_2$) and increasing levels of carbon dioxide (CO$_2$) by dilating or constricting.

The innermost lining of the arteries is the endothelium. The endothelium maintains hemostasis, promotes blood flow, and,

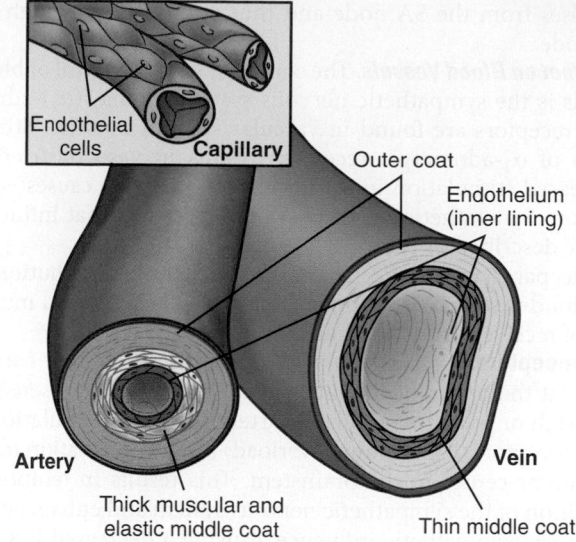

FIG. 31.5 Comparative thickness of layers of the artery, vein, and capillary.

under normal conditions, inhibits blood coagulation. When the endothelial surface is disrupted (e.g., rupture of an atherosclerotic plaque), the coagulation cascade is initiated and results in the formation of a fibrin clot.

Capillaries. The thin capillary wall, made up of endothelial cells, has no elastic or muscle tissue (Fig. 31.5). The exchange of cellular nutrients and metabolic end products takes place through these thin-walled vessels. Capillaries connect the arterioles and venules.

Veins and Venules. Veins are large-diameter, thin-walled vessels that return blood to the right atrium (Fig. 31.5). The venous system is a low-pressure, high-volume system. The larger veins have semilunar valves at intervals to maintain the blood flow toward the heart and to prevent backward flow. The amount of blood in the venous system is affected by several factors. These include arterial flow, compression of veins by skeletal muscles, changes in thoracic and abdominal pressures, and right atrial pressure.

The largest veins are the *superior vena cava,* which returns blood to the heart from the head, neck, and arms, and the *inferior vena cava,* which returns blood to the heart from the lower part of the body. Pressure in the right side of the heart affects these large vessels. Elevated right atrial pressure can cause distended neck veins or liver engorgement because of resistance to blood flow.

Venules are smaller vessels made up of a small amount of muscle and connective tissue. Venules collect blood from the capillary beds and channel it to the larger veins.

Regulation of Cardiovascular System

Autonomic Nervous System. The autonomic nervous system consists of the sympathetic nervous system and parasympathetic nervous system (see Chapter 55).

Effect on Heart. Stimulation of the sympathetic nervous system increases the HR, speed of impulse conduction through the AV node, and force of atrial and ventricular contractions. This effect is mediated by specific sites in the heart called *beta (β)-adrenergic receptors,* which are receptors for norepinephrine and epinephrine.

In contrast, stimulation of the parasympathetic system (mediated by the vagus nerve) slows the HR by decreasing the impulses from the SA node and thus conduction through the AV node.

Effect on Blood Vessels. The source of neural control of blood vessels is the sympathetic nervous system. Alpha$_1$ (α_1)-adrenergic receptors are found in vascular smooth muscles. Stimulation of α_1-adrenergic receptors results in vasoconstriction. Decreased stimulation to α_1-adrenergic receptors causes vasodilation. Sympathetic nervous system receptors that influence BP are described in Table 32.1.

The parasympathetic nerves have selective distribution in the blood vessels. For example, blood vessels in skeletal muscle do not receive parasympathetic input.

Baroreceptors. *Baroreceptors* in the aortic arch and carotid sinus (at the origin of the internal carotid artery) are sensitive to stretch or pressure within the arterial system. Stimulation of these receptors (e.g., volume overload) sends information to the vasomotor center in the brainstem. This results in temporary inhibition of the sympathetic nervous system and enhancement of the parasympathetic influence, causing a decreased HR and peripheral vasodilation. Decreased arterial pressure causes the opposite effect.

Chemoreceptors. *Chemoreceptors* are found in the aortic and carotid bodies and the medulla. They can cause changes in respiratory rate and BP in response to increased arterial CO_2 pressure (hypercapnia) and, to a lesser degree, decreased plasma pH (acidosis) and arterial O_2 pressure (hypoxia). Chemoreceptors in the medulla stimulate the vasomotor center to increase BP.[3]

Blood Pressure

The **arterial blood pressure** is a measure of the pressure exerted by blood against the walls of the arterial system. **The systolic blood pressure (SBP)** is the peak pressure exerted against the arteries when the heart contracts. The **diastolic blood pressure (DBP)** is the residual pressure in the arterial system during ventricular relaxation (or filling).

The main factors influencing BP are CO and *systemic vascular resistance* (SVR):

$$BP = CO \times SVR$$

SVR is the force opposing the movement of blood. This force is created primarily in small arteries and arterioles. Normal BP is SBP <120 mm Hg and DBP <80 mm Hg[4] (see Chapter 32).

Measurement of Arterial Blood Pressure. We can measure BP by using invasive and noninvasive techniques. The invasive technique consists of catheter insertion into an artery. The catheter is attached to a transducer, and the pressure is measured directly (see Chapter 65).

Noninvasive, indirect measurement of BP can be done with a sphygmomanometer and stethoscope. The sphygmomanometer consists of an inflatable cuff and a pressure gauge. The BP is measured by auscultating for sounds of turbulent blood flow through a compressed artery (termed **Korotkoff sounds**). The brachial artery is the recommended site for taking a BP.

After placing the right size cuff on the upper arm, inflate the cuff to a pressure 20 to 30 mm Hg above the SBP. This causes blood flow in the artery to cease. If the SBP is not known, estimate the pressure by palpating the brachial pulse and inflating the cuff until the pulse ceases. The pressure noted at this time is the estimated SBP. Inflate the BP cuff 20 to 30 mm Hg above this number.

As you lower the pressure in the cuff, listen to the artery for Korotkoff sounds. There are 5 phases of Korotkoff sounds. The first phase is a tapping sound caused by the spurt of blood into the constricted artery as the pressure in the cuff is gradually deflated. This sound is the SBP. The fifth phase occurs when the sound disappears, which is the DBP.[5]

BP is recorded as the ratio of SBP to DBP (e.g., 120/80 mm Hg). Sometimes, an *auscultatory gap* occurs, which is a loss of sound between the SBP and DBP. Proper BP technique (e.g., using the correct cuff size, positioning arm at heart level) is essential for correct readings (see Table 32.12).

Another noninvasive way to measure BP indirectly is an automated device that uses oscillometric measurements to assess BP. Though this method does not involve auscultation, the same attention to proper technique is essential for accuracy.

We can assess SBP and pulse using a Doppler ultrasonic flowmeter. The hand-held transducer is positioned over the artery (identified by audible, pulsatile sounds). The cuff is applied above the artery, inflated until the sounds disappear, and then inflated another 20 to 30 mm Hg beyond that point. The cuff is then slowly deflated. The point where sounds return is the SBP.

Pulse Pressure and Mean Arterial Pressure. Pulse pressure is the difference between the SBP and DBP. It is normally about one third of the SBP. If the BP is 120/80 mm Hg, the pulse pressure is 40 mm Hg. An increased pulse pressure due to an increased SBP may occur during exercise or in people with atherosclerosis of the larger arteries. A decreased pulse pressure may occur with heart failure (HF) or hypovolemia.

Another measurement related to BP is **mean arterial pressure (MAP)**. The MAP refers to the average pressure within the arterial system that is felt by organs in the body. It is not the average of the DBP and SBP, because the length of diastole exceeds that of systole at normal HRs. MAP is calculated as follows:

$$MAP = (SBP + 2\,DBP) \div 3$$

A person with a BP of 120/60 mm Hg has an estimated MAP of 80 mm Hg. A MAP greater than 60 mm Hg is needed to perfuse the vital organs of an average person under most conditions. When the MAP is low for a period of time, vital organs are underperfused and will become ischemic.

Gerontologic Considerations: Effects of Aging on the Cardiovascular System

One of the greatest risk factors for cardiovascular disease (CVD) is age. CVD is the leading cause of death in adults older than age 65. The most common cardiovascular problem is coronary artery disease (CAD) due to atherosclerosis. Many of the physiologic changes in the cardiovascular system of older adults are a result of the combined effects of the aging process, disease, environmental factors, and lifetime health behaviors rather than just age alone.[6]

Age-related changes in the cardiovascular system and differences in assessment findings are found in Table 31.1. With increased age, the amount of collagen in the heart increases and elastin decreases. These changes affect the heart muscle's ability to stretch and contract.[6] One of the major changes in the cardiovascular system is the response to physical or emotional stress. In times of increased stress, CO and SV decrease due to reduced contractility and HR response. Aging does not really affect the resting supine HR. When the patient changes positions (e.g., sits upright), the sympathetic nerve pathway results in a blunted (reduced) HR response.[7]

TABLE 31.1 Gerontologic Assessment Differences

Cardiovascular System

Changes	Differences in Assessment Findings
Chest Wall	
Kyphosis	Altered chest landmarks for palpation, percussion, and auscultation. Distant heart sounds
Heart	
Myocardial hypertrophy, ↑collagen and scarring, ↓elastin	↓ Cardiac reserve, HF. S_4 may be present
Downward displacement	Difficulty in isolating apical pulse.
↓ CO, HR, SV in response to exercise or stress	↓ Response to exercise and stress. Slowed recovery from activity
Cellular aging and fibrosis of conduction system	↓ Amplitude of QRS complex and slight lengthening of PR, QRS, and QT intervals. Irregular cardiac rhythms, ↓maximal HR, ↓ HR variability
Valvular rigidity from calcification, sclerosis, or fibrosis, impeding complete closure of valves	Systolic murmur (aortic or mitral) possible without a sign of cardiovascular disease
Blood Vessels	
Arterial stiffening caused by loss of elastin in arterial walls, thickening of intima of arteries, and progressive fibrosis of media	↑ In SBP and possible ↑ or ↓ in DBP. Possible widened pulse pressure. Pedal pulses diminished. Intermittent claudication
Venous tortuosity increased	Inflamed, painful, or cordlike varicosities. Dependent edema

Heart valves become thicker and stiffer from lipid accumulation, degeneration of collagen, and fibrosis. The aortic and mitral valves are most often affected. These changes result in either regurgitation of blood when the valve should be closed or narrowing of the orifice of the valve (*stenosis*) when the valve should be open. The turbulent blood flow across the affected valve results in a murmur.

Numbers of pacemaker cells in the SA node and conduction cells in the internodal tracts, bundle of His, and bundle branches decrease with age. These changes contribute to the development of sinus and atrial dysrhythmias and heart blocks. Many older adults have an abnormal resting ECG that shows increases in the PR, QRS, and/or QT intervals.[7]

The autonomic nervous system control of the cardiovascular system changes with aging. The number and function of β-adrenergic receptors in the heart decrease with age. So, the older adult not only has a decreased response to physical and emotional stress but also is less sensitive to β-adrenergic agonist drugs. Exercise results in a much smaller increase in CO for older adults than for younger adults.[7]

With age, arteries and veins thicken and become less elastic. Arteries increase their sensitivity to vasopressin (antidiuretic hormone). Both changes increase SBP with a decreased or unchanged DBP, increasing the pulse pressure. Valves in the large leg veins do not return the blood to the heart as effectively, often resulting in dependent edema.[6]

Orthostatic hypotension may be related to drugs and/or decreased baroreceptor function. *Postprandial hypotension*

(decrease in BP of at least 20 mm Hg that occurs within 75 minutes after eating) may occur in otherwise healthy older adults. Both orthostatic and postprandial hypotension may be related to falls in older adults. Despite the changes associated with aging, the heart can function adequately under most circumstances.

CASE STUDY

Patient Introduction

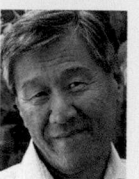

(© Jupiterimages/Banana-Stock/Thinkstock.)

L.P., a 63-yr-old Asian American man, is brought to the hospital by ambulance at 6 AM after reporting chest tightness, shortness of breath (SOB), and "heart pounding" (palpitations). The paramedics started an IV and O_2 at 2 L/min via nasal cannula. They obtained a 12-lead ECG and gave him 4 chewable baby ASA and a nitroglycerin tablet. L.P. is pain free on arrival to the emergency department, but still has palpitations.

Discussion Questions

1. Is L.P.'s condition stable or unstable?
2. What are the possible causes of L.P.'s chest tightness, SOB, and palpitations?
3. What type of assessment is most appropriate for L.P.: emergency, focused, or comprehensive? On what basis did you make that decision?
4. What assessment questions will you ask him?

You will learn more about L.P. and his condition as you read through this assessment chapter.
(See p. 664 for more information on L.P.)

Answers available at *http://evolve.elsevier.com/Lewis/medsurg*.

ASSESSMENT OF CARDIOVASCULAR SYSTEM

Subjective Data

A careful health history and physical examination will help you distinguish symptoms that reflect a cardiovascular problem from problems of other body systems. Explore and record all cues that alert you to the possibility of underlying CVD.

Important Health Information

History of Present Illness. Ask the patient what problem has brought him or her to seek health care. Fully explore all symptoms the patient reports.

Past Health History. Many illnesses affect the cardiovascular system directly or indirectly. Ask the patient about a history of angina, diabetes, alcohol and tobacco use, anemia, rheumatic fever, streptococcal throat infections, congenital heart disease, stroke, hypertension, thrombophlebitis, dysrhythmias, and varicosities. Fully explore any symptoms the patient may have. Ask about shortness of breath, fatigue, dizziness with position changes, syncope, edema, intermittent claudication, and palpitations.

Assess for allergies to drugs, food, or the environment. Determine whether the patient has ever had a drug reaction or an allergic or anaphylactic reaction. Ask specifically about any allergic reaction to contrast media.

Medications. Assess the patient's current and past use of medications. Include over-the-counter (OTC) and prescription drugs and herbal supplements. For example, aspirin prolongs the blood clotting time and is in some drugs used to treat cold symptoms. Record the dose and time last taken for each. Assess for noncardiac drugs that can adversely affect the cardiovascular system (Table 31.2).

TABLE 31.2 Potential Cardiovascular Effects of Select Noncardiac Drugs

Drug Classification	Examples	Cardiovascular Effects
Anticancer agents	daunorubicin doxorubicin	Dysrhythmias, cardiomyopathy
Antipsychotics	chlorpromazine haloperidol	Dysrhythmias, orthostatic hypotension
Corticosteroids	cortisone prednisone	Hypotension, edema, potassium depletion
Hormone therapy, oral contraceptives	estrogen + progestin (Prempro)	MI, thromboembolism, stroke, hypertension
Nonsteroidal antiinflammatory drugs (NSAIDs)	celecoxib (Celebrex) diclofenac ibuprofen	MI, stroke, hypertension, HF
Psychostimulants	amphetamines cocaine	Tachycardia, angina, MI, hypertension, dysrhythmias
Tricyclic antidepressants	amitriptyline doxepin (Silenor)	Dysrhythmias, orthostatic hypotension

Surgery or Other Treatments. Ask the patient about specific treatments, past surgeries, or hospital admissions related to cardiovascular problems. Explore any admissions or procedures performed for cardiovascular symptoms. Note whether a baseline ECG or a chest x-ray has been done.

Functional Health Patterns. The strong correlation between lifestyle and cardiovascular health supports the need to review each functional health pattern. Key questions to ask a person with a cardiovascular problem are listed in Table 31.3.

Health Perception–Health Management Pattern. Ask the patient about the presence of major cardiovascular risk factors. These include abnormal serum lipids, hypertension, sedentary lifestyle, diabetes, obesity, and tobacco use. Estimate the number of pack-years of tobacco use (number of packs smoked per day multiplied by the number of years the patient has smoked). Note the patient's attitude about tobacco use and attempts and methods used to stop. Record the type of alcohol used, amount, frequency, and any changes in the reaction to it. Note any use of habit-forming or recreational drugs.

🧬 GENETIC RISK ALERT

Coronary Artery Disease
- Specific genetic links, especially related to lipoprotein genes, have been found for some families with CAD.
- The clustering of CAD in families is strong if there is early age of onset affecting several relatives.

Cardiomyopathy
- Autosomal dominant mutations can cause hypertrophic cardiomyopathy.
- X-linked and autosomal dominant mutations can cause dilated cardiomyopathy.

Hypertension
- Hypertension results from a complex interplay between genetic and environmental factors.
- Lifestyle choices (e.g., smoking, lack of exercise) may trigger genetic tendencies to hypertension.

Genomic studies have found over 60 common genetic variants highly associated with CAD.[8] Confirmed illnesses of blood relatives can highlight any genetic or familial tendencies toward CAD, hypertension, varicosities, bleeding, diabetes, atherosclerosis, and stroke. Note any family members who had heart disease at an early age (<50 years of age for men; <55 years of age for women). Last, assess for family health history of noncardiac problems such as lung, kidney, or liver disease and obesity, because they can affect the cardiovascular system.

Nutritional-Metabolic Pattern. Being underweight or overweight may indicate potential cardiovascular problems. Assess the patient's weight history (e.g., over the past year) in relation to height. Determine the amount of salt and saturated fats in the patient's typical diet. In addition to food habits, which may be influenced by culture, explore the patient's attitudes and plans about diet and weight management.

Elimination Pattern. The patient taking diuretics may report increased voiding and/or nocturia. Ask about any history of incontinence or constipation, including use of drugs (prescribed and OTC) for constipation. Teach patients with heart problems to avoid straining (*Valsalva maneuver*) during a bowel movement. Ask patients if they have swelling of the lower extremities and if it resolves when their feet are elevated.

Activity-Exercise Pattern. The benefit of exercise for cardiovascular health is clear, with aerobic exercise being most beneficial. Record the types, duration, intensity, and frequency of exercise. Ask about symptoms during exercise (e.g., chest pain, shortness of breath, claudication) that may indicate a cardiovascular problem.

Sleep-Rest Pattern. Cardiovascular problems often disrupt sleep. *Paroxysmal nocturnal dyspnea* (attacks of shortness of breath, especially at night that awaken the patient) and *Cheyne-Stokes respiration* (periods of very shallow breaths to alternating periods of apnea and deep, rapid breathing) are associated with HF. Note the number of pillows needed to sleep or the need to sleep upright in a chair (*orthopnea*) and whether this has changed recently.

Sleep apnea is associated with an increased risk for life-threatening dysrhythmias, especially in patients with HF. Nocturia, a common finding with cardiovascular patients, interrupts normal sleep patterns.

Cognitive-Perceptual Pattern. Ask both the patient and caregiver about cognitive-perceptual problems. Cardiovascular problems such as dysrhythmias, hypertension, and stroke may cause difficulties with syncope, language, and memory. Report pain associated with the cardiovascular system (e.g., chest pain, claudication).

Self-Perception–Self-Concept Pattern. Acute cardiovascular events may affect the patient's self-perception. Invasive diagnostic procedures often lead to body image concerns. When CVD is chronic, the patient may describe an inability to "keep up" previous levels of activity, affecting quality of life.

Role-Relationship Pattern. Gender, race, and age are all related to cardiovascular health. The patient's marital status, role

TABLE 31.3 Health History

Cardiovascular System

Health Perception–Health Management

- Do you practice any measures to decrease risk factors for heart disease?*
- Have you noticed an increase in heart symptoms such as chest pain or dyspnea?*
- Does your heart problem cause you to be less able to care for yourself?*
- Do you foresee any potential self-care problems because of your heart problem?*
- Have you ever used tobacco? If yes, in what form, how much, and for how long? Have you tried to quit? If yes, what methods have you tried? Are you interested in more information about quitting?
- How often and how much alcohol do you drink?

Nutritional-Metabolic

- Describe your usual daily diet, including salt, fat, and liquid intake.
- What is your present weight? What was your weight 1 year ago? If different, explain.
- Does eating cause fatigue or shortness of breath?*

Elimination

- Do your feet or ankles ever swell?* If yes, how far up your legs? Does it go away after sleeping all night?
- Have you ever taken drugs to help you get rid of excess fluid or to relieve constipation?*
- Are you having any problems related to urination?*
- Do you ever strain to have a bowel movement?

Activity-Exercise

- Are your daily activities or exercise limited because of your heart problem?*
- When were you last able to comfortably perform your usual activities or exercise?
- Do you have any discomfort or symptoms because of exercise or any activity?*
- Can you comfortably walk and talk at the same time?
- How often do you attend activities outside your home?
- What was your most strenuous activity in the last few weeks compared with 6 months ago?

Sleep-Rest

- How many pillows do you sleep on at night? Has this changed recently?*
- Do you ever wake up suddenly and feel as if you cannot catch your breath?*
- Do you have a history of sleep apnea?*

- Do you ever sleep in a chair at night? Is yes, how often?
- How many times a night do you awaken to urinate?

Cognitive-Perceptual

- Do you ever have dizziness or fainting?*
- Do you ever find it hard to express yourself or to remember things?*
- Do you have any pain (e.g., chest pain, leg pain with activity) because of your heart problem?*

Self-Perception–Self-Concept

- Have your perceptions of yourself changed since you were diagnosed with heart disease?*
- How has your heart disease affected the quality of your life?

Role-Relationship

- Has this illness affected any of the roles that you play in your daily life?*
- How has your heart disease affected your significant others?

Sexuality-Reproductive

- Has your heart disease caused a change in your sexual activity?*
- Do you have any heart-related symptoms during sexual activity?*
- Do any of your drugs affect your ability to take part in sexual activities?*
- *Females:* Are you currently taking oral contraceptives, hormonal therapy, or drug therapy for breast cancer?
- *Males:* Are you taking any drugs to treat erectile dysfunction?

Coping–Stress Tolerance

- Describe your normal coping mechanisms during times of stress or anxiety.
- To whom or where would you turn during a time of stress? Are these people or services helping you now?*
- Do you practice any stress reduction techniques?*
- Do you have a history of depression?*
- Do you feel capable of handling your present health situation?
- Do you have any heart symptoms (e.g., chest pain, palpitations) during times of stress or anger?*

Values-Beliefs

- What influence have your values or beliefs had during your illness?
- Do you feel any conflicts between your values or beliefs and the plan of care?*
- Describe any cultural or religious beliefs that may influence the management of your heart problem.

*If yes, describe.

in the household, employment status, number of children and their ages, living environment, and caregivers help you to identify strengths and support systems in the patient's life. Assess the patient's satisfaction with life roles, since this may alert you to possible areas of stress or conflict.

Sexuality-Reproductive Pattern. Ask the patient about the effect of the cardiovascular problem on sexual activity. Because some patients fear sudden death during sexual intercourse, they may change their sexual behavior. Fatigue, chest pain, or shortness of breath may limit sexual activity. Erectile dysfunction (ED) may be a symptom of peripheral vascular disease and/or a side effect of some drugs used to treat CVD (e.g., β-blockers, diuretics). Ask male patients about the use of drugs for ED (phosphodiesterase inhibitors, e.g., sildenafil [Viagra]). These drugs are contraindicated if the patient is taking a nitrate because the combination can cause significant hypotension.[9]

Ask female patients if they use oral contraceptives, hormone therapy (HT) for symptoms of menopause, or drug therapy for breast cancer. Women who smoke tobacco and use oral contraceptives are at increased risk for blood clots (e.g., venous thromboembolism). Similarly, there is an increased risk for CVD with the use of HT and selective estrogen-receptor modulators (e.g., tamoxifen).[9]

Coping–Stress Tolerance Pattern. Ask the patient to identify sources of stress and the usual methods of coping with stress. Potentially stressful areas include health concerns, marital relationships, family and friends, occupation, and finances.

Work-related stress, depression, and inadequate social support are risk factors for CVD and heart events. Ask the patient about each of these factors. Information about support systems such as family, extended family and friends, counselors, or religious groups can give vital insight when planning care.

Values-Belief Pattern. Individual values and beliefs, which are greatly affected by culture, may play a key role in the real or potential conflict that a patient faces when dealing with CVD. Some patients may attribute their illness to punishment from God; others may think that a "higher power" can help them. Information about a patient's values and beliefs will help you provide support during periods of crisis.

CASE STUDY
Subjective Data

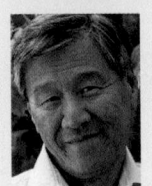

(@ Jupiterimages/ Banana-Stock/ Thinkstock.)

A focused subjective assessment of L.P. revealed the following information:

- ***Past Medical History:*** History of hypertension, mitral valve prolapse with mild regurgitation, HF, and type 2 diabetes.
- ***Oral Medications:*** Lisinopril (Prinivil) 10 mg/ day, metoprolol (Lopressor) 50 mg twice daily, ASA 81 mg/day , furosemide 40 mg/day, and glipizide (Glucotrol) 5 mg/day.
- ***Health Perception–Health Management:*** L.P. denies any history of chest pain or CAD. He reports feeling fine until this morning when he awoke and developed SOB, chest tightness, and palpitations while walking to the bathroom. He thought he was having a heart attack, so his wife called 911. Denies smoking or alcohol intake. SOB and chest tightness are now gone, but he continues to feel palpitations.
- ***Elimination:*** Denies edema or nocturia. States he takes Lasix in the morning and typically "passes urine until lunchtime."

Discussion Questions

1. Which subjective assessment findings are of most concern to you?
2. How will you individualize the assessment based on his age, ethnic/ cultural background, and condition?
3. Is this an appropriate time to teach him about the proper use of nitro- glycerin tablets? Why or why not?
4. What should you include in your physical assessment?

You will learn more about the physical examination of the cardiovascular system in the next section. (See p. 667 for more information on L.P.)

Answers available at *http://evolve.elsevier.com/Lewis/medsurg.*

Objective Data
Physical Examination

Vital Signs. Observe the patient's general appearance and obtain vital signs. Measure BP bilaterally. Readings can vary from 5 to 15 mm Hg between arms. Use the arm with the highest BP for later measurements. Obtain an orthostatic (postural) BP and HR while the patient is supine, sitting with legs dangling, and standing. SBP should not decrease more than 20 mm Hg from the supine to the standing position. HR should not increase more than 20 beats/min from the supine to the standing position.

Peripheral Vascular System

Inspection. Inspect the skin for color, hair distribution, and venous pattern. Check the extremities for edema, dependent rubor, clubbing of the nail beds, varicosities, and lesions such as stasis ulcers. Edema in the legs can be caused by gravity, varicosities, or right-sided HF.

Inspect the large neck veins (internal and external jugular) while gradually moving the patient from a supine position to an upright (30 to 45 degrees) position. Distention and prominent pulsations of the neck veins, referred to as *jugular venous disten- tion,* can be caused by right-sided HF.

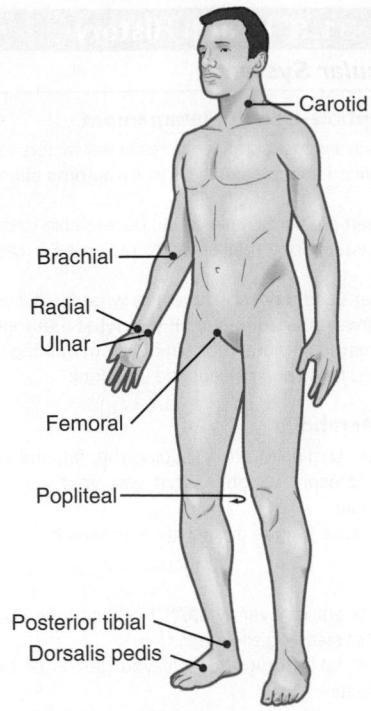

FIG. 31.6 Common sites for palpating arteries.

Palpation. Palpate the upper and lower extremities for temperature, moisture, pulses, and edema bilaterally to assess for symmetry. Look for edema by depressing the skin over the tibia or medial malleolus for 5 seconds. Normally, there is no depression after you release pressure. If pitting edema is present, grade it from 1+ (mild pitting, slight brief indentation) to 4+ (very deep pitting, indentation that lasts a long time).

Palpate the pulses in the neck and extremities for rhythm and force of arterial blood flow. Palpate each carotid pulse sep- arately to avoid vagal stimulation and dysrhythmias. Compare the characteristics of the arteries in the right and left extremities simultaneously to determine symmetry.

When palpating the arteries identified in Fig. 31.6, rate the force of the pulse using the following scale:

0 = Absent
1+ = Weak
2+ = Normal
3+ = Increased, full, bounding

Note the rigidity (hardness) of the artery. The normal pulse feels like a tap, but a narrowed or bulging vessel wall vibrates. The term for a palpable vibration is *thrill.*

Capillary refill is used to assess arterial flow to the extremi- ties. Position the patient's hands near the level of the heart and squeeze a nail bed briefly to produce blanching. Color should return to the nail bed in less than 2 seconds with normal tissue perfusion and CO.

Auscultation. An artery that is narrowed or has a bulging wall may create turbulent blood flow. This abnormal flow can cause a buzzing or humming termed a *bruit,* heard with the bell of the stethoscope over the vessel. Auscultate major arteries such as the carotid arteries, abdominal aorta, and femoral arteries as part of the initial cardiovascular assessment. Abnormalities of the peripheral vascular system are described in Table 31.4.

TABLE 31.4 Assessment Abnormalities

Cardiovascular System

Finding*	Description	Possible Etiology* and Significance
Inspection		
Central cyanosis	Bluish or purplish tinge in central areas such as tongue, conjunctivae, inner surface of lips	Inadequate O_2 saturation of arterial blood because of pulmonary or cardiac disorders (e.g., congenital defects)
Clubbing of nail beds	Obliteration of normal angle between base of nail and skin	Endocarditis, congenital defects, prolonged O_2 deficiency
Color changes in extremities with postural change	Pallor, cyanosis, mottling of skin after limb elevation. Dependent rubor (reddish blue discoloration). Glossy skin	Chronic decreased arterial perfusion
Jugular venous distention	Distended neck (jugular) veins with patient sitting at 30- to 45-degree angle	High right atrial pressure, right-sided HF
Peripheral cyanosis	Bluish or purplish tinge in extremities or in nose and ears	Reduced blood flow from HF, vasoconstriction, cold environment
Splinter hemorrhages	Small red to black streaks under fingernails	Infective endocarditis (infection of endocardium, usually in area of cardiac valves)
Ulcers	*Venous:* Necrotic crater-like lesion usually found on lower leg at medial malleolus. Characterized by slow wound healing	Poor venous return, varicose veins, incompetent venous valves
	Arterial: Pale ischemic base, well-defined edges usually found on toes, heels, lateral malleoli	Arteriosclerosis, diabetes
Varicose veins	Visible dilated, discolored, tortuous vessels in lower extremities	Incompetent valves in vein
Palpation		
Pulse		
<60 beats/min	Bradycardia	Rest or sleeping, SA or AV node damage, athletic conditioning, side effect of drugs (e.g., β-blockers), hypothyroidism
>100 beats/min	Tachycardia	Exercise, anxiety, shock, need for increased cardiac output, hyperthyroidism
Absent	Lack of pulse	Atherosclerosis, trauma, embolus
Bounding	Sharp, brisk, pounding pulse	Hyperkinetic states (e.g., anxiety, fever), anemia, hyperthyroidism
Displaced point of maximal impulse (apical pulse)	Palpate (or auscultate) the point of maximal impulse below the fifth ICS and to the left of the MCL	Cardiac enlargement because of coronary artery disease, HF, cardiomyopathy
Irregular	Regularly irregular or irregularly irregular. Skipped beats	Dysrhythmias
Pulsus alternans	Regular rhythm, but strength of pulse varies with each beat	HF, cardiac tamponade
Rigidity	Stiffness or inflexibility of vessel wall	Atherosclerosis
Thready	Weak, slowly rising pulse easily obliterated by pressure	Blood loss, decreased cardiac output, aortic valve disease, peripheral arterial disease
Thrill	Vibration of vessel or chest wall	Aneurysm, aortic regurgitation, arteriovenous fistula
Extremities		
Abnormal capillary refill	Blanching of nail bed for ≥2 sec after release of pressure	Possible reduced arterial capillary perfusion, anemia
Asymmetry in limb circumference	Measurable swelling of involved limb	Venous thromboembolism, varicose veins, lymphedema
Cold extremities	Hands and/or feet cold to touch. External covering needed for comfort	Intermittent claudication, peripheral arterial disease, low cardiac output, severe anemia
Pitting edema of lower extremities or sacral area	Visible finger indentation after application of firm pressure, weight gain, tightening of clothing (including shoes), marks or indentations from constricting garments	Interruption of venous return to heart, right-sided HF
Unusually warm extremities	Hands and feet warmer than normal	Thyrotoxicosis
Auscultation		
3rd heart sound (S_3)	Extra heart sound, low pitched, heard in early diastole. Similar to sound of a gallop	Left ventricular failure. Volume overload. Mitral, aortic, or tricuspid regurgitation. Hypertension (possible)
4th heart sound (S_4)	Extra heart sound, low pitched, heard in late diastole. Similar to sound of a gallop	Forceful atrial contraction from resistance to ventricular filling (e.g., in left ventricular hypertrophy, aortic stenosis, hypertension, coronary artery disease)
Arterial bruit	Turbulent flow sound in peripheral artery	Arterial obstruction or aneurysm
Heart murmurs	Turbulent sounds occurring between normal heart sounds. Characterized by loudness, pitch, shape, quality, duration, timing	Heart valve disorder, abnormal blood flow patterns
Pericardial friction rub	High-pitched, scratchy sound heard during S_1 and/or S_2 at the apex. Heard best with patient sitting and leaning forward, and while holding breath at the end of expiration	Pericarditis
Pulse deficit	Apical heart rate exceeding peripheral pulse rate	Dysrhythmias, most often atrial fibrillation/flutter or premature ventricular contractions

*Limited to common abnormal assessment findings and etiologic factors. (Further discussion of conditions listed may be found in Chapters 32 to 37, 65, and 66.)

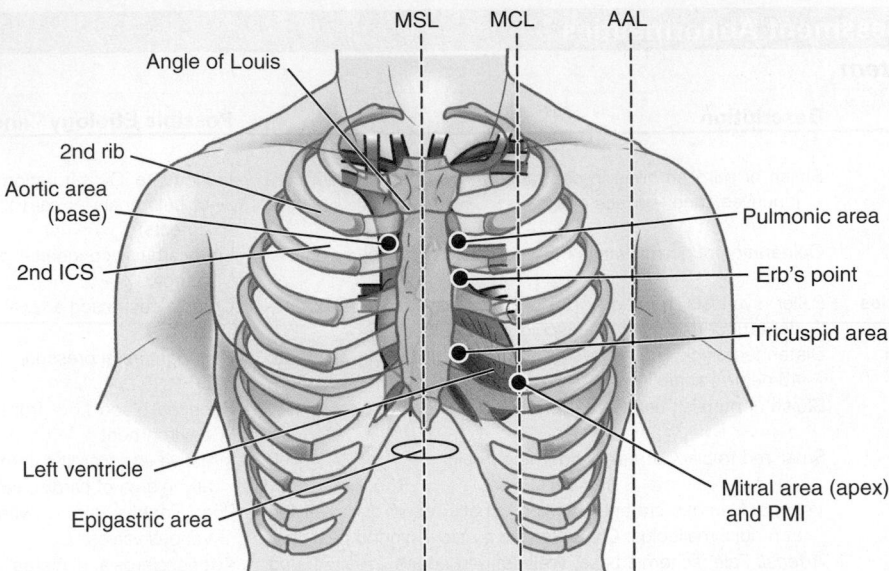

FIG. 31.7 Orientation of the heart within the thorax and cardiac auscultatory areas. *Red lines* indicate the midsternal line *(MSL)*, midclavicular line *(MCL)*, and anterior axillary line *(AAL)*. *ICS,* Intercostal space; *PMI,* point of maximal impulse.

Thorax

Inspection and palpation. Begin examining the thorax with a general inspection and palpation. Next, inspect and palpate the areas where the heart valves project their sounds by finding the intercostal spaces (ICSs). The raised notch, the *angle of Louis,* is where the manubrium and body of the sternum join at the level of the second rib. It is palpable in the midline of the sternum. Palpate for the 2nd ICS then count each ICSs to find specific auscultatory areas (Fig. 31.7).

Locate the following auscultatory areas: aortic area in the second ICS to the right of the sternum, pulmonic area in the second ICS to the left of the sternum, tricuspid area in the fifth left ICS close to the sternum, and mitral area in the left midclavicular line at the fifth ICS. A fifth auscultatory area is *Erb's point,* located at the third left ICS near the sternum. Normally, we cannot feel pulsations in these areas unless the patient has a thin chest wall.

A heart valve disorder may be present if you feel abnormal pulsations or thrills. Next, inspect and palpate the epigastric area on either side of the midline just below the xiphoid process. In a thin person, you may see pulsations from the abdominal aorta. Normally, you can palpate it here. Next, inspect the precordium, which is over the heart, for heaves. Heaves are sustained lifts of the chest wall in the precordial area that you can see or palpate. They may be caused by left ventricular hypertrophy. Normally no pulsations are seen or felt here.

When the patient is supine, palpate the mitral valve area for the **point of maximal impulse (PMI)** (also called the *apical pulse*). This reflects the pulsation of the apex of the heart. The PMI lies medial to the midclavicular line in the 4th or 5th ICS. If you can palpate the PMI, record its position in relation to the midclavicular line and ICSs. If the PMI is below the fifth ICS and left of the midclavicular line, the heart may be enlarged.

Auscultation. Normal heart sounds are made by the movement of blood through the heart valves. These sounds can be heard through a stethoscope placed on the chest wall. The first heart sound (S_1) is associated with closure of the tricuspid

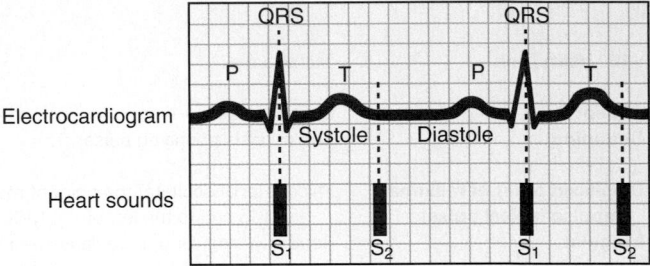

FIG. 31.8 Relationship of electrocardiogram, cardiac cycle, and heart sounds.

and mitral valves. It has a soft lubb sound. The second heart sound (S_2) is associated with closure of the aortic and pulmonic valves. It has a sharp dupp sound. S_1 signals the beginning of systole. S_2 signals the beginning of diastole (Fig. 31.8). Listen to the auscultatory areas in sequence (Fig. 31.7).

S_1 and S_2 are heard best with the diaphragm of the stethoscope because they are high pitched. Extra heart sounds (S_3 or S_4), if present, are heard best with the bell of the stethoscope because they are low pitched. Have the patient lean forward while sitting to enhance the sounds from the second ICSs (aortic and pulmonic areas). Place the patient in a left side-lying position to enhance the sounds at the mitral area.

When auscultating the apical area, simultaneously palpate the radial pulse. Determine whether the rhythm is regular or irregular while listening and feeling. If the apical and radial pulses are not equivalent, count the apical pulse while a second person simultaneously counts the radial pulse for 1 full minute. A difference between the 2 numbers, called a *pulse deficit,* can indicate dysrhythmias.

Normally no sound is heard between S_1 and S_2. An exception to this is a normal splitting of S_2, which is best heard at the pulmonic area during inspiration. Splitting of S_2 can be abnormal if it is heard during expiration or if it is constant (fixed) during the respiratory cycle. Describe any sounds heard in addition to S_1 and S_2.

The S$_3$ heart sound is a low-intensity vibration of the ventricular walls usually associated with decreased compliance of the ventricles during filling. An S$_3$ heart sound may be normal (physiologic) in young adults. It is pathologic in patients with left-sided HF or mitral valve regurgitation. S$_3$ is heard closely after S$_2$ and is known as a *ventricular gallop*.

The S$_4$ heart sound is a low-frequency vibration caused by atrial contraction. It precedes S$_1$ of the next cycle and is known as an *atrial gallop*. An S$_4$ heart sound may be normal in older adults with no evidence of heart disease. It is pathologic in patients with CAD, cardiomyopathy, left ventricular hypertrophy, or aortic stenosis.

Murmurs, if heard, are graded on a 6-point Roman numeral scale based on loudness and recorded as a ratio. I/VI means a murmur that is barely audible with the stethoscope, heard only in a quiet room and then not easily. VI/VI means a murmur that we can hear with the stethoscope lifted just off the chest wall.

Pericardial friction rubs are sounds that occur when inflamed surfaces of the pericardium (pericarditis) move against each other. They are high-pitched, scratchy sounds that may be intermittent and may last several hours to days. Friction rubs are heard best at the apex with patients upright, leaning forward, and holding their breath after expiration.[5]

Record the characteristics of any abnormal sounds. This includes the timing (during systole or diastole), location (the anatomic site on the chest where it is heard the loudest), position (heard best when the patient is supine, sitting and leaning forward, or in the left side-lying position), and any other findings (irregular apical pulse or palpable chest wall heaves) associated with the sound.

Abnormal assessment findings are described in Table 31.4. A method of recording data from the cardiovascular assessment is shown in Table 31.5.

A *focused assessment* is used to evaluate the status of previously identified cardiovascular problems and to monitor for signs of new problems. A focused assessment of the cardiovascular system is outlined in the box on this page.

CASE STUDY

Objective Data: Physical Examination

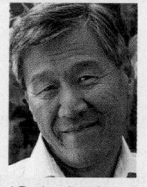
(© Jupiterimages/ Banana-Stock/ Thinkstock.)

Physical examination findings of L.P. are as follows:
- BP 100/54, apical-radial pulse 154, pulse irregular, respiratory rate 20, temperature 98.2° F (36.8° C), O$_2$ saturation 94% on room air
- Awake, alert, and oriented ×3
- Lungs clear on auscultation; systolic murmur present
- Heart monitor shows atrial fibrillation with a rapid ventricular response
- +1 pedal pulses bilaterally
- No peripheral edema, jugular venous distention, or heaves noted

Discussion Questions

1. Which physical assessment findings are of most concern to you?
2. Based on the results of the subjective and physical assessment findings, what diagnostic studies do you think will be ordered for L.P.?

You will learn more about diagnostic studies related to the cardiovascular system in the next section.

(See p. 676 for more information on L.P.)

Answers available at *http://evolve.elsevier.com/Lewis/medsurg*.

TABLE 31.5 Normal Physical Assessment of Cardiovascular System

Inspection	No pallor or cyanosis. PMI not visible. No JVD with patient at 45-degree angle
Palpation	Skin warm. Capillary refill <2 sec. PMI palpable in 4th ICS at left MCL. No thrills or heaves. Slight palpable pulsations of abdominal aorta in epigastric area. Carotid and extremity pulses 2+ and equal bilaterally. No pedal or sacral edema
Auscultation	S$_1$ and S$_2$ heard. Apical-radial pulse rate equal, 72, and regular. No murmurs or extra heart sounds

ICS, Intercostal space; *JVD,* jugular venous distention; *MCL,* midclavicular line; *PMI,* point of maximal impulse.

FOCUSED ASSESSMENT
Cardiovascular System

Use this checklist to remind you of the key assessment steps.

Subjective
Ask the patient about the following and note responses.

Chest pain, discomfort	Y	N
Palpitations	Y	N
Shortness of breath (especially when lying down or at rest)	Y	N
Edema in legs or any part of body	Y	N
Leg pain during exercise	Y	N
Excess urination at night	Y	N

Objective: Diagnostic
Check the following for critical values or changes.

Cardiac biomarkers	✓
Hematocrit, hemoglobin, platelets	✓
Glucose, electrolytes, BUN, creatinine	✓
Electrocardiogram	✓
Chest x-ray	✓

Objective: Physical Examination
Inspect and Palpate

Anterior chest wall for pulsations and heaves	✓
Pulses for symmetry, quality, and rhythm	✓

Auscultate

Bilateral blood pressures	✓
Heart for rate, rhythm, and sounds	✓

DIAGNOSTIC STUDIES OF CARDIOVASCULAR SYSTEM

Numerous diagnostic tests are available to assess the cardiovascular system. Tables 31.6, 31.7, and 31.8 describe common serology studies, diagnostic studies, and interventional study procedures. Select studies are discussed in more detail next.

Blood Studies

Many blood studies provide information about the cardiovascular system. For example, some reflect the O$_2$-carrying capacity (red blood cell count and hemoglobin) and coagulation properties (clotting times) of the blood. See Chapter 29 and Tables 29.7, 29.8, and 29.10 about hematology studies.

Cardiac Biomarkers. When cells are injured, they release their contents, including enzymes and other proteins, into the

TABLE 31.6 Serology Studies

Cardiovascular System

Study	Reference Interval*	Description and Purpose
Biomarkers		
b-Type natriuretic peptide (BNP)	<100 pg/mL (100 pmol/L)	Peptide that causes natriuresis. High in HF. Levels increased after nesiritide (Natrecor) infusion and for 1 month after cardiac surgery.
CK-MB	Concentrations <4%–6% of total creatine kinase (CK)	Tests for myocardial cell injury. High levels highly indicative of MI. Serum levels increase within 3–6 hr after MI, peak after 12–24 hours, normalize within 48 hours. Explain purpose of serial sampling.
Copeptin	<10 pmol/L	Reflects arginine vasopressin (AVP) concentration. High levels highly indicative of MI. Higher in men, after exercise, and with stress. Influenced by fasting and water load.
C-reactive protein (CRP)	High-sensitivity (hs) CRP assay. *Lowest risk:* <1 mg/dL *Moderate risk:* 1–3 mg/dL *High risk:* >3 mg/dL	Marker of inflammation. May help predict risk for cardiac disease and cardiac events such as an acute MI. High in bacterial infections and inflammatory disorders.
Homocysteine	4–14 µmol/L Levels may increase with age	Amino acid made during protein catabolism. Risk factor for cardiovascular disease. Associated with vitamin B_{12} and folate deficiencies.
NT-Pro-BNP	*≤74 yr:* 124 pg/mL *>75 yr:* 449 pg/mL	Helps to assess severity of HF. Levels are higher in women and patients with renal insufficiency.
Troponin (cardiac)	*Troponin T (cTnT)* <0.1 ng/mL (<0.1 mcg/L) *Troponin I (cTnI)* *Negative:* <0.03 ng/mL (<0.03 mcg/L)	Contractile proteins released after an MI. Both troponin T and troponin I test for cardiac injury/ischemia. Serial sampling needed: draw 3 sets of troponins 3–6 hours apart.
Lipids		
Cholesterol	<200 mg/dL (<5.2 mmol/L) (varies with age and gender)	A blood lipid associated with arteriosclerosis. High level is a risk factor for cardiovascular heart disease. Can obtain in a nonfasting or fasting state.
Lipoprotein (a) (Lp[a])	<30 mg/dL (<0.3 g/L)	High levels indicate an increased risk for atherosclerosis, MI, and stroke. Can obtain in a nonfasting or fasting state.
Lipoprotein-associated phospholipase A_2 (Lp-PLA$_2$)	*Low risk:* ≤151 ng/mL *Moderate risk:* 152–194 ng/mL *High risk:* ≥195 ng/mL	Indicates inflammation and increased risk for CAD. Serum levels are measured by the PLAC test. Can obtain in a nonfasting or fasting state.
Lipoproteins (HDL, LDL)	HDL Recommended *Male:* >45 mg/dL *Female:* >55 mg/dL *Low risk for CAD:* ≥60 mg/dL *High risk for CAD:* <40 mg/dL LDL <130 mg/dL *Moderate risk for CAD:* 130–159 mg/dL *High risk for CAD:* >160 mg/dL	There are marked day-to-day fluctuations, so more than 1 level is needed for accurate diagnosis. Can be obtained in a nonfasting or fasting state. Assess risk for heart disease by dividing the total cholesterol level by the HDL level and obtaining a ratio. *Low risk:* Ratio <3 *Average risk:* Ratio 3–5 *Increased risk:* Ratio >5
Triglycerides	*Male:* 40–160 mg/dL *Female:* 35–135 mg/dL	Mixtures of fatty acids. Elevations are associated with cardiovascular disease and diabetes. Avoid alcohol for 24 hr before testing. Can obtain in a nonfasting or fasting state.

*Reference ranges for the laboratory tests vary by agency because of differences in equipment and reagents used.

circulation. These *biomarkers* are useful in the diagnosis of acute coronary syndrome (ACS) (Table 31.6). Interpreting biomarker level results requires you to consider the time elapsed from the onset of symptoms. Other data (patient symptoms, history, and ECG changes) complete the diagnostic picture for the patient with suspected ACS.

Cardiac-specific troponin is a heart muscle protein released into circulation after injury or infarction. Two subtypes, cardiac-specific troponin T (cTnT) and cardiac-specific troponin I (cTnI), are specific to heart muscle. Normally the level in the blood is very low, so a rise in level is diagnostic of myocardial infarction (MI) or injury. cTnT and cTnI are detectable within hours (on average 4 to 6 hours) of MI or injury, peak at 10 to 24 hours, and can be detected for up to 10 to 14 days. Troponin is the biomarker of choice in the diagnosis of ACS. High-sensitivity troponin (hs-cTnT, hs-cTnI) assays may provide even

earlier detection of a heart event.[10] Fig. 33.15 shows the changes in cardiac markers related to an MI.

Copeptin, a substitute marker for arginine vasopressin (AVP), can be detected immediately in patients with an acute MI. Considering both troponin and copeptin levels together may provide increased sensitivity for rapidly diagnosing acute MI.[10] High circulating copeptin levels are associated with increased mortality in patients with HF.[11]

Creatine kinase (CK) enzymes are found in a variety of organs and tissues and occur as 3 isoenzymes. These isoenzymes are specific to skeletal muscle (CK-MM), brain and nervous tissue (CK-BB), and the heart (CK-MB). CK-MB rise is specific for MI or injury. Levels begin to increase 3 to 6 hours after symptom onset, peak in 12 to 24 hours, and return to baseline within 12 to 48 hours after MI.[12] In some acute care settings, CK is no longer used for diagnosis of acute MI.[13]

TABLE 31.7 Diagnostic Studies

Cardiovascular System

Study	Description and Purpose	Nursing Responsibility
Electrocardiography (ECG)		
12-lead ECG	Electrodes are placed on the chest and extremities, allowing the ECG machine to record cardiac electrical activity from 12 different views. A resting 12-lead ECG can identify conduction problems, dysrhythmias, position of heart, cardiac hypertrophy, pericarditis, myocardial ischemia or infarction, pacemaker activity, and effectiveness of drug therapy at one point in time.	*Before:* Prepare skin and apply electrodes and leads. Place patient supine (or with head of bed elevated, if short of breath). Tell patient that no discomfort is involved and to lie still to decrease motion artifact. *During:* Ensure the patient lies still to decrease motion artifact.
ECG event monitor or loop recorder	Records rhythm changes that are not frequent enough to be recorded in 1 24-hr period. Can aid in diagnosing the cause of chest pain, palpitations, shortness of breath, and syncope. It allows more freedom than a regular Holter monitor. Some units have electrodes that attach to the chest and have a loop of memory that captures the onset and end of an event. Other types are placed directly on patient's wrist, chest, or fingers and have no loop of memory but record the patient's ECG in real time. Recordings may be transmitted over the phone to a receiving unit.	*Before:* Teach how to use equipment for recording and transmitting events. Teach patient about skin preparation for lead placement or steady skin contact to ensure quality tracings. Tell patient to start recording when symptoms begin or as soon after as possible.
ECG Holter monitoring	Recording of ECG rhythm for 24–48 hr to correlate with symptoms and activities recorded in diary. Encourage normal patient activity to simulate conditions that produce symptoms. Electrodes are placed on chest. A recorder stores information until it is recalled, printed, and analyzed for any rhythm changes.	*Before:* Prepare skin and apply electrodes and leads. Explain importance of keeping an accurate diary of activities and symptoms. Tell patient there is no bathing and showering during monitoring. Skin irritation may develop from electrodes. If device has an event marker, teach patient to push that button when experiencing symptoms.
Signal-averaged ECG (SAECG)	A high-resolution ECG that can identify electrical activity called late potentials, indicating a patient is at risk for developing ventricular dysrhythmias (e.g., ventricular tachycardia).	Same as for 12-lead ECG.
Functional		
6-minute walk test	Distance patient can walk on a flat surface in 6 min. Used to measure response to treatments and determine functional capacity for activities of daily living. Can help assess response to therapy for chronic cardiopulmonary conditions. Useful in those who are debilitated or unable to perform treadmill or exercise bike testing. May be a better measure of fitness for older adults than exercise testing.	*Before:* Tell patient to wear comfortable shoes. Inform patient to carry or pull O_2 if used routinely. *During:* Encourage patient to walk as quickly as possible.
Exercise or stress testing	Provides information on cardiac function and exercise tolerance. A common protocol uses 3-min stages at set speeds and elevation of treadmill belt. The patient can exercise to either predicted peak HR (calculated by subtracting the person's age from 220) or peak exercise tolerance, at which time the test is ended. The test is ended for chest discomfort, significant changes in vital signs from baseline, or significant ECG changes (e.g., ischemia, dysrhythmias). Vital signs and ECG are monitored. The ECG is monitored after exercise for ischemia and rhythm changes or, if ECG changes occurred with exercise, for return to baseline. Important in the diagnosis of CAD. An exercise bike may be used if the patient is unable to walk on the treadmill.	*Before:* Tell patient to wear comfortable clothes and shoes that can be worn for walking or running. Tell patient to report any symptoms. β-Blockers may be held 24 hr before the test because they blunt the HR and limit the patient's ability to achieve maximal HR. Caffeine is held for 24 hr. Patients must refrain from smoking and strenuous exercise for 3 hr before test. Obtain baseline vital signs and 12-lead-ECG. *During:* Monitor vital signs and ECG during each stage of exercise and after until all vital signs and ECG changes have returned to normal or baseline. Monitor patient's response throughout procedure for any signs of distress (e.g., angina, shortness of breath).
Noninvasive hemodynamic monitoring	Obtained using a continuous finger cuff or by thoracic bioreactance method. Possible to obtain repeated measurements of stroke volume, cardiac output, and systemic BP.	Minimal to no risk. Patients who need hemodynamic monitoring are likely to be in perioperative settings, critical care units, and emergency departments. See Chapter 65 for complete information on hemodynamic monitoring.
Imaging		
Chest x-ray	Patient is placed in 2 upright positions to examine lung fields and heart size. The 2 common positions are lateral and posteroanterior (PA) (Fig. 31.9). Helps with the diagnosis of HF and pulmonary edema and visualization of heart size and contour.	*Before:* Ask about frequency of recent x-rays and chance of pregnancy. Provide lead shielding to areas not being viewed. Remove jewelry or metal objects that may obstruct the view of heart and lungs.

Continued

TABLE 31.7 Diagnostic Studies—cont'd

Cardiovascular System

Study	Description and Purpose	Nursing Responsibility
Cardiac computed tomography (CT); electron beam CT (EBCT)	Cardiac CT is heart-specific imaging technology with or without IV contrast medium used to evaluate heart anatomy, coronary circulation, and blood vessels. EBCT, or ultrafast CT, uses a scanning electron beam to quantify calcification in coronary arteries and heart valves (Fig. 31.11). IV contrast may be used if calcium scoring is below threshold level. Primarily used for risk assessment in asymptomatic patients and to assess for heart disease in patients with atypical symptoms potentially related to cardiac causes.	*Before:* Assess for contrast allergy. Explain that patient may feel a warm sensation, salty taste after IV contrast injection, nausea. *During:* Patient must lie still during test.
Cardiovascular magnetic resonance imaging (CMRI)	Noninvasive imaging technique obtains information about heart tissue, EF, aneurysms, cardiac output, and patency of proximal coronary arteries. Measures regurgitant fraction that may determine valve repair or replacement. It does not involve ionizing radiation and is an extremely safe procedure. Provides images in multiple planes with uniformly good resolution.	*Before:* Check for pregnancy, allergies, and renal function before test. Have patient remove all metal objects. Remove metallic foil patches. Patient may need to be fasting. Assess for claustrophobia and the need for antianxiety medication Contraindicated for persons with implanted metallic devices or other metal fragments unless noted to be MRI safe. Ask about any history of surgical insertion of staples, plates, dental bridges, or other metal appliances. *During:* Patient must lie completely still during test.
Coronary CT angiography (CTA)	Use of CT with injected IV contrast medium to obtain images of coronary vessels and diagnose CAD. Used to evaluate chest pain and monitor the progression of coronary vascular disease.	*Before:* Assess for contrast allergy. Obtain IV access. Remove metal objects before test. The patient may need to fast for several hours prior. A β-blocker may be given before the test to control HR. *During:* Patients must have a regular heart rhythm for accurate testing.
Echocardiogram • Contrast • M-mode • 2-dimensional • Color-flow imaging (duplex) • Real-time 3-dimensional • Pharmacologic echocardiogram	Ultrasound transducer is placed in 4 positions on the chest to record sound waves bounced off the heart. Records direction and flow of blood through the heart and transforms it to audio and graphic data. Measures valve abnormalities, congenital heart defects, wall motion, EF, and heart function. IV contrast agent may be used to enhance images (Fig. 31.10). Pharmacologic Echocardiogram is a substitute for the exercise stress test in persons unable to exercise. IV adenosine, dobutamine, or dipyridamole is given over several minutes or regadenoson (Lexiscan) is given as a single bolus over 10 sec while echocardiogram is performed to detect wall motion abnormalities.	*Before:* Place patient in a left side-lying position. Tell patient about procedure and sensations (pressure and mechanical movement from head of transducer). May be difficult to obtain in patients with COPD due to large amount of air between heart and chest cavity. *Pharmacologic echocardiogram:* *Before:* Obtain baseline vital signs and IV access for injection of drugs. *During:* Monitor vital signs until baseline achieved. Monitor patient for signs and symptoms of distress or side effects (e.g., shortness of breath, dizziness, nausea). Aminophylline may be given to prevent or reverse side effects of dipyridamole.
Exercise (stress) nuclear imaging	Purpose of test is to identify cardiac symptoms and rhythm changes and simulate in a safe environment. Nuclear imaging images are taken at rest. Injection is given at maximum HR (usually 85% of age-predicted maximum) on bicycle or treadmill. Patient then continues exercise for 1 min to circulate the radioactive isotope. Scanning is done 15–60 min after exercise. A resting scan is done 60–90 min after initial infusion or 24 hr later.	*Before:* Tell patient to eat only a light meal between scans. Certain drugs may need to be held for 1–2 days before the scan. Patients should not have caffeine 12 hr prior. Obtain IV access. *During:* If targeted maximum HR is not achieved with exercise, test may be changed to pharmacologic imaging.
Magnetic resonance angiography (MRA)	Used for imaging vascular occlusive disease and abdominal aortic aneurysms. Same as MRI but with use of gadolinium as IV contrast medium.	*Before:* Contraindications include allergies to contrast medium and implanted metallic devices or other metal fragments unless noted to be MRA safe. Discuss any implants before scan. Obtain IV access.
Multigated acquisition (MUGA) (cardiac blood pool) scan	Small amount of the patient's blood is removed, mixed with a radioactive isotope (e.g., Technetium-99m (^{99m}Tc sestamibi), and reinjected IV. With the ECG used for timing, images are obtained during the cardiac cycle. Indicated for patients with MI, HF, or valve disease. Can evaluate the effect of various cardiac or cardiotoxic drugs on the heart and the cardiac EF.	*Before:* Explain procedure to patient. Obtain IV access for removal of blood sample and reinjection of isotope. Start ECG monitoring.
Nuclear imaging	Study involves IV injection of radioactive isotopes (^{99m}Tc sestamibi [Cardiolite]). Radioactive uptake is counted over the heart by scintillation camera. It supplies information about heart contractility, myocardial perfusion, and acute injury.	*Before:* Women must remove bras to decrease breast artifact. Obtain IV access for injection of isotopes. Explain that radioactive isotope used is a small, diagnostic amount and will lose most of its radioactivity in a few hours. Tell patient that they will be lying still on back with arms extended overhead for 20 min. *During:* Repeat scans are done within a few minutes to hours after the injection.

TABLE 31.7 Diagnostic Studies—cont'd

Cardiovascular System

Study	Description and Purpose	Nursing Responsibility
Pharmacologic nuclear imaging	Regadenoson, dipyridamole, or adenosine are given to produce vasodilation for patients unable to tolerate exercise. Vasodilation increases blood flow to well-perfused coronary arteries. Scanning procedure is same. Aminophylline may be given to prevent or reverse side effects of dipyridamole (e.g., shortness of breath, dizziness, nausea). Dobutamine is used if vasodilators are contraindicated.	*Before*: Tell patient to avoid caffeine products and theophylline (for regadenoson or dipyridamole testing) for 12 hr before procedure. Hold calcium channel blockers and β-blockers for 24 hr before the test. *During*: Observe patient for any side effects (e.g., shortness of breath, dizziness, nausea).
Positron emission tomography (PET)	Highly sensitive in distinguishing viable and nonviable heart tissue. Uses 2 radionuclides. Nitrogen-13-ammonia is injected IV first and scanned to evaluate myocardial perfusion. A second radioactive isotope, fluoro-18-deoxyglucose, is then injected and scanned to show myocardial metabolic function. In the normal heart, both scans match, but in an ischemic or damaged heart, they differ. The patient may or may not be stressed. A baseline resting scan is usually done for comparison.	*Before:* Obtain IV access to inject the tracer substance. Patients should be NPO, except for water and medications, for at least 4 hr prior. If exercise is part of testing, patient needs to fast and refrain from tobacco and caffeine for 24 hr before test. Hold glucose-containing IV solutions and change to normal saline. Check blood glucose levels. The glucose level must be between 60–140 mg/dL (3.3–7.8 μmol/L) for accurate glucose metabolic activity. *During*: Patient must lie completely still during scan. *After:* Encourage fluids to excrete radioactive substance.
Single-photon emission computed tomography (SPECT)	Used to determine size or risk for infarction and to determine infarction size. Small amounts of a radioactive isotope (e.g., 99mTc tetrofosmin [Myoview], thallium-201) are injected IV and recordings are made of the radioactivity emitted over a specific area of the body. Circulation of the isotope can detect coronary artery blood flow, intracardiac shunts, motion of ventricles, EF, and size of the heart chambers.	*Before:* Short fasting period may be needed. Obtain IV access for injection of isotope. Remove all jewelry from chest wall. Start ECG monitoring. *During*: Patient must lie completely still during scan. *After:* Encourage fluids to excrete radioactive substance.
Stress echocardiogram	Combination of exercise test and echocardiogram. Differences in left ventricular wall motion and thickening before and after exercise are evaluated with ultrasound. Postexercise images are taken within 1 min of stopping exercise.	*Before:* Prepare patient for treadmill or exercise bicycle. Tell patient of importance of timely return to examination table for imaging after exercise.
Transesophageal echocardiogram (TEE)	A probe with an ultrasound transducer at the tip is swallowed while the HCP controls angle and depth. As it passes down the esophagus, it sends back clear images of heart size, wall motion, valve abnormalities, endocarditis vegetation, and possible source of thrombi without interference from lungs or chest ribs. A contrast medium may be injected IV for evaluating direction of blood flow if an atrial or ventricular septal defect is suspected. Doppler ultrasound and color-flow imaging can be used concurrently.	*Before:* Tell patient to fast for at least 6 hr before test. Remove dentures. *During:* IV sedation is given and throat locally anesthetized. A bite block is placed in the mouth. Monitor vital signs, specifically O₂ saturation and BP. Perform suctioning as needed during procedure. *After:* Patient may not eat or drink until gag reflex returns. Monitor patient until sedation resolves. Sore throat is temporary. A designated driver is needed if test is done in the outpatient department.

C-Reactive Protein. C-reactive protein (CRP) is made by the liver during periods of acute inflammation. An increased level of CRP is linked with the presence of atherosclerosis and the first occurrence of a heart event. The CRP level may predict the risk for future heart events in patients with MI.[14]

Homocysteine. Homocysteine (Hcy) is an amino acid made during protein catabolism. High Hcy levels can be either hereditary or from dietary deficiencies of vitamin B₆, vitamin B₁₂, or folate. They are linked to a higher risk for CVD, peripheral vascular disease, and stroke. Hcy testing is recommended for patients with a familial predisposition for early CVD or a history of CVD in the absence of common risk factors.[14]

Cardiac Natriuretic Peptide Markers. There are 3 natriuretic peptides: (1) atrial natriuretic peptide (ANP) from the atrium, (2) b-type natriuretic peptide (BNP) from the ventricles, and (3) c-type natriuretic peptide from endothelial and renal epithelial cells. BNP is the marker of choice for distinguishing between a cardiac or respiratory cause of dyspnea. N-terminal pro-brain natriuretic peptide (NT-pro-BNP) is secreted in the ventricles and is more sensitive but less specific than BNP

as a diagnostic marker of HF.[12] When DBP increases (e.g., HF), BNP and NT-pro-BNP are released and increase natriuresis (excretion of sodium in the urine). ANP and BNP are also discussed in Chapter 32 on p. 680 and in Chapter 34 on p. 638.

Serum Lipids. Serum lipids consist of triglycerides, cholesterol, and phospholipids (Table 31.6). These *lipoproteins* circulate in the blood bound to protein. A lipid panel usually measures cholesterol, triglyceride, low-density lipoprotein (LDL), and high-density lipoprotein (HDL).

Triglycerides, the main storage form of lipids, make up about 95% of fatty tissue. Cholesterol, a structural part of cell membranes and plasma lipoproteins, is a precursor of corticosteroids, sex hormones, and bile salts. In addition to being absorbed from food in the gastrointestinal tract, cholesterol can be synthesized in the liver. Phospholipids contain glycerol, fatty acids, phosphates, and a nitrogenous compound. Although formed in most cells, phospholipids usually enter the circulation as lipoproteins synthesized by the liver. Apoproteins are water-soluble proteins that combine with most lipids to form lipoproteins.

TABLE 31.8 Interventional and Invasive Studies

Cardiovascular System

Study	Description and Purpose	Nursing Responsibility
Cardiac catheterization; coronary angiography	Involves insertion of catheter into heart via a vein (for right side of heart) and/or an artery (for left side of heart). Procedure is done to evaluate chest pain and obtain information about the aorta, inferior vena cava, pulmonary artery and veins. Measures pressures within the heart chambers. Contrast medium is injected to help see structures and motion of heart. With coronary angiography, contrast medium is injected directly into coronary arteries to evaluate patency and collateral circulation.	See Table 31.9.
Electrophysiology study (EPS)	Invasive study to record intracardiac electrical activity using catheters (with multiple electrodes) inserted via the femoral or jugular veins into right side of heart. Catheter electrodes record the electrical activity in different heart structures. Can induce and stop dysrhythmias. Insertion of a pacemaker or implantable cardioverter defibrillator (ICD) or ablation of a dysrhythmia pathway may be done during or right after the EPS. See Chapter 35 for more details.	*Before:* Antidysrhythmic drugs may be stopped several days before study. Keep patient NPO 6–8 hr before test. Give premedication to promote relaxation if ordered. Obtain IV access. IV sedation often used during procedure. *After:* Assess vital signs often. Monitor ECG continuously per agency protocol. Patient will be on bedrest for 6–8 hr after procedure.
Fractional flow reserve (FFR)	During cardiac catheterization, a specialized wire is inserted into coronary arteries to measure pressure and flow. Information is used to determine need for angioplasty or stenting on nonsignificant blockages.	Same as for cardiac catheterization.
Invasive hemodynamic monitoring	Invasive and minimally invasive bedside hemodynamic monitoring is done using intraarterial, pulmonary artery, and central vein catheters. Monitors arterial BP, stroke volume variation, pulmonary artery pressure, pulmonary artery wedge pressure, cardiac output, and central venous pressure. Used to evaluate cardiovascular status and response to treatment.	Patients who need invasive hemodynamic monitoring are critically ill and are monitored in critical care units. See Chapter 65 for complete information on hemodynamic monitoring.
Intravascular ultrasound (IVUS)	During cardiac catheterization a small ultrasound probe is introduced into coronary arteries. Used to assess blood vessel patency, size and consistency of plaque, arterial walls, and effectiveness of intracoronary artery treatment.	Same as for cardiac catheterization.
Peripheral arteriography and venography	Peripheral vessel blood flow is assessed by injecting contrast media into appropriate arteries or veins (arteriography and venography). Serial x-ray studies done to detect atherosclerotic plaques, occlusion, aneurysms, venous abnormalities, or traumatic injury. See Table 37.9 for more peripheral vascular diagnostic studies.	*Before:* Assess for contrast allergy. Explain that patient may feel a warm sensation, salty taste after contrast injection. Patient may have nausea. Give mild sedative, if ordered. *During:* Observe patient for allergic reaction to contrast media. *After:* Inspect insertion site for bleeding or swelling. Check extremity with puncture site for pulsation, warmth, color, and motion. Encourage fluids to excrete radioactive substance.

Different classes of lipoproteins contain varying amounts of the naturally occurring lipids. These include:

1. *Chylomicrons:* primarily exogenous triglycerides from dietary fat
2. *Low-density lipoproteins (LDLs):* mostly cholesterol with moderate amounts of phospholipids
3. *High-density lipoproteins (HDLs):* about 50% protein and 50% phospholipids and cholesterol
4. *Very-low-density lipoproteins (VLDLs):* primarily endogenous triglycerides with moderate amounts of phospholipids and cholesterol

Elevations in triglycerides and LDL are strongly associated with CAD. An increased HDL level is associated with a decreased risk of CAD. HDLs serve a protective role by mobilizing cholesterol from tissues.

Although a relationship exists between high serum cholesterol levels and CAD, a measure of total cholesterol alone is not enough for an assessment of CAD. A risk assessment is calculated by comparing the total cholesterol to HDL ratio over time. An increase in the ratio means increased risk. This provides more information than either value alone.

Plasma levels of apolipoprotein A-I (apo A-I) (the major HDL protein) and the ratio of apo A-I to apolipoprotein B (apo B) (the major LDL protein) are stronger predictors of CAD than the HDL cholesterol level alone. Measurements of these lipoproteins can be useful in identifying patients at risk for CAD.

Lipoprotein (a), or Lp(a), has been studied for its role as a risk factor for CAD. Increased levels of Lp(a), especially with increased levels of lactate dehydrogenase (LDH), have been linked with the progression of atherosclerosis, especially in women.

Lipoprotein-associated phospholipase A_2 (Lp-PLA$_2$) is an inflammatory enzyme expressed in atherosclerotic plaques. High levels of Lp-PLA$_2$ are related to an increased risk for CAD, especially in black women.[14]

TABLE 31.9 Nursing Management

Care of the Patient Undergoing Cardiac Catheterization

Preprocedure

- Assess for allergies, especially to contrast dye.
- Perform baseline assessment, including vital signs, pulse oximetry, heart and breath sounds, neurovascular assessment of extremities (e.g., distal pulses, skin temperature, skin color, sensation).
- Withhold food and fluids for 6–12 hours before.
- Assess baseline laboratory values (e.g., cardiac biomarkers, creatinine).
- Teach patient and caregiver about procedure and postprocedure care. Explain the use of local anesthesia at insertion site, placement of catheter, flushed feeling when dye is injected, and possible fluttering sensation of heart as catheter is passed.
- Give sedative and other drugs, as ordered.

Postprocedure

- Perform assessment and compare to baseline: vital signs, pulse oximetry, and heart and breath sounds. Note hypotension or hypertension and signs of pulmonary emboli (e.g., respiratory difficulty).
- Assess neurovascular status, including peripheral pulses, color, and sensation, of extremity per agency protocol.
- Place compression device over arterial site to achieve hemostasis, if indicated.
- Observe insertion site for hematoma and bleeding every 15 min for the first hour, then according to agency policy
- Monitor ECG for dysrhythmias or other changes (e.g., ST segment elevation).
- Monitor patient for chest pain and other sources of pain or discomfort.
- Maintain bedrest as ordered after femoral access.
- Maintain IV and/or oral fluid intake and monitor urine output.
- Teach patient and caregiver about discharge care, including signs and symptoms to report to HCP (e.g., site complications, return of chest pain), and any activity restrictions.

Electrocardiography

Electrocardiogram. The basic P, QRS, and T waveforms (Fig. 31.4, *B*) are used to assess heart activity. Deviations from the normal sinus rhythm can indicate problems in heart function. There are many types of ECG monitoring, including a resting 12-lead ECG, ambulatory ECG monitoring, and exercise or stress testing (Table 31.7). Continuous ambulatory ECG (Holter monitoring) provides diagnostic information over a period of time. See Chapter 35 for a complete discussion of ECG monitoring.

Event Monitor or Loop Recorder. An event monitor or loop recorder is used to record less frequent ECG events. An event monitor is a portable unit that uses electrodes to store ECG data. There are 2 types, external and implantable. External loop recorders are worn for a month. They require electrodes continuously placed on the skin. They must be activated by the patient when symptoms occur. A disadvantage of external recorders is that, if symptoms occur for only a brief time, they may be over before the patient puts on the device and triggers it to record. Likewise, if patients are extremely symptomatic (e.g., syncopal), they may not be physically able to trigger the ECG recording. These devices can be perform a routine pacemaker check over the phone.

An implantable loop recorder is used for patients who may have serious yet infrequent dysrhythmias. This small recorder is implanted through a small incision into the chest wall. It continuously monitors heart activity. It keeps recordings if the patient uses a remote device when symptoms occur or automatically if the HR exceeds or goes below a set rate.

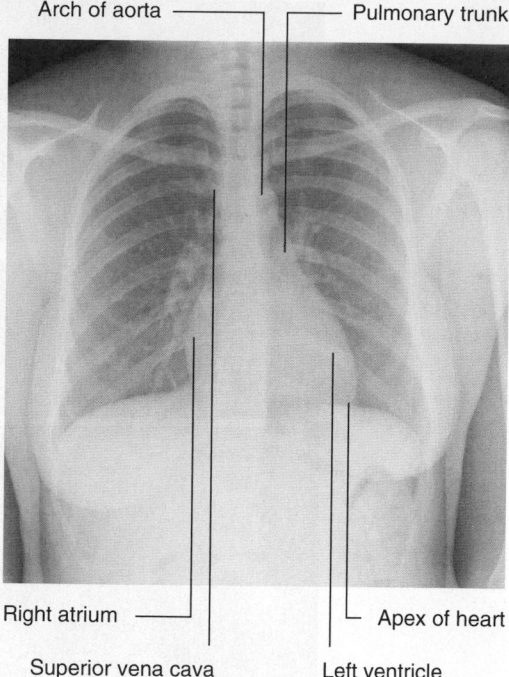

FIG. 31.9 Chest x-ray: standard posterior-anterior view. (From Drake RL, Vogl AW, Mitchell AWM: *Gray's anatomy for students,* ed 2, Philadelphia, 2010, Churchill Livingstone.)

Functional Studies

Exercise or Stress Testing. Heart symptoms often occur only with activity because of the demand on the coronary arteries to supply more O_2. Exercise testing can evaluate the heart's response to physical stress. This helps to assess CVD and set limits for exercise programs. Exercise testing is used for persons who can walk unassisted or use a bicycle. It is also helpful for those with normal ECGs that limit diagnostic interpretation (e.g., pacemakers) (Table 31.7). ECG and BP are monitored throughout the exercise period for signs of cardiac stress.

6-Minute Walk Test. A general test of cardiac fitness, often used with older adults, is measuring the distance the patient can walk on a flat surface in 6 minutes. The test can provide a baseline for determining response to treatment and physical therapy.

Noninvasive Hemodynamic Monitoring. Noninvasive hemodynamic monitoring provides information about cardiovascular status changes without the risks of inserting and maintaining invasive devices. SV, CO, and systemic BP are measured using a continuous finger cuff or by thoracic bioreactance.[15] Monitoring stroke volume and CO during complex surgical procedures allows the anesthesia provider to titrate fluids and vasoactive drugs.

Imaging

Chest X-Ray. A radiographic picture of the chest can show heart shape and size and anatomic changes in individual chambers (Fig. 31.9). The chest x-ray records any displacement or enlargement of the heart, extra fluid around the heart (pericardial effusion), and pulmonary congestion (Table 31.7).

Echocardiography. The echocardiogram uses ultrasound (US) waves to record the movement of the structures of the heart. In the normal heart, US waves directed at the heart are reflected back in typical patterns. *Contrast echocardiography* involves the addition of an IV contrast agent (e.g., agitated saline) to help

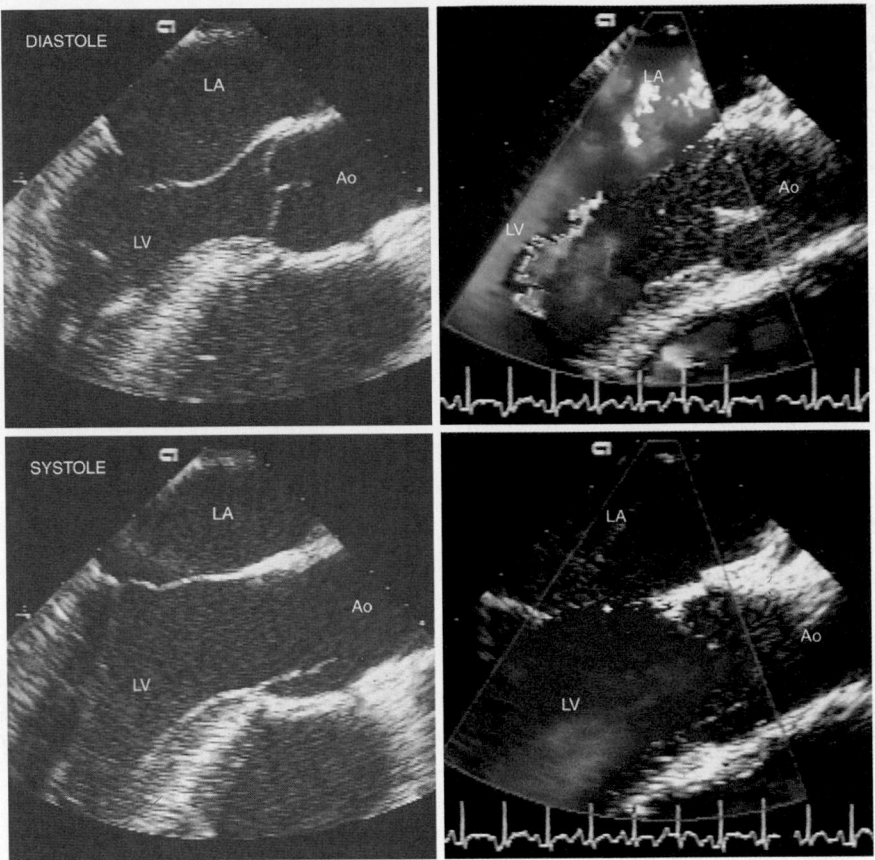

FIG. 31.10 Long-axis images of the aortic and mitral valve with the depth adjusted to optimize evaluation of valve anatomy and motion. The 2-D images *(left)* in diastole *(top)* and systole *(bottom)* show normal aortic and mitral opening and closure. The color flow images *(right)* show normal left ventricular inflow with no aortic regurgitation in diastole *(top)* and normal antegrade flow in the left ventricular outflow tract and no mitral regurgitation in systole *(bottom)*. (From Otto C: *Textbook of clinical echocardiography*, ed 3, St Louis, 2004, Saunders.)

define the images, especially in technically difficult patients (e.g., obese).

The echocardiogram provides information about abnormalities of (1) valvular structures and motion, (2) heart chamber size and contents, (3) ventricular and septal motion and thickness, (4) pericardial sac, and (5) ascending aorta. The **ejection fraction (EF)**, or the percentage of end-diastolic blood volume that is ejected during systole, can be measured. The EF provides information about the function of the left ventricle during systole.

Two common types of echocardiograms are the *motion-mode (M-mode) echocardiogram* and the *two-dimensional (2-D) echocardiogram*. In the M-mode, a single US beam is directed toward the heart, recording the motion of the intracardiac structures and detecting wall thickness and chamber size. The 2-D echocardiogram sweeps the US beam through an arc, producing a cross-sectional view. This shows correct spatial relationships among the structures.

Doppler technology allows for sound evaluation of the flow or motion of the scanned object (heart valves, ventricular walls, blood flow). *Color-flow imaging (duplex)* is the combination of 2-D echocardiography and Doppler technology (Fig. 31.10). It uses color changes to show the speed and direction of blood flow. Pathologic conditions, such as valvular leaks and congenital defects, can be diagnosed more effectively.

Real-time three-dimensional (3-D) ultrasound is a technology that uses multiple 2-D echo images with computer technology to provide a reconstruction of the heart. This technique gives information about the structures of the heart and how these structures change during the cardiac cycle.

Stress echocardiography combines the information from a stress test with the information from an echocardiogram. A digital computer compares images before and after exercise, revealing wall motion and function. For those persons unable to exercise, IV drugs are used. These include dobutamine, which produces pharmacologic stress on the heart and dipyridamole (Persantine), which vasodilates healthy arteries. Unhealthy arteries do not respond as well, which is seen on the echocardiogram.

Transesophageal echocardiography (TEE) provides more precise echocardiography of the heart than surface 2-D echocardiography by removing interference from the chest wall and lungs (Table 31.7). The TEE uses a flexible endoscope with a US transducer in the tip for imaging of the heart and great vessels. The scope is passed into the esophagus to the level of the heart. M-mode, 2-D, Doppler, and color-flow imaging can be obtained.

TEE is used often in an outpatient setting for evaluation of mitral valve disease and for identification of endocarditis vegetation, thrombus before cardioversion, or the source of heart emboli. In addition, TEE is used in the operating room to assess intraoperative heart function and in the emergency department to detect suspected aortic dissection.

The risks of TEE are low. However, complications include perforation or tearing of the esophagus, hemorrhage, dysrhythmias, vasovagal reactions, and transient hypoxemia. TEE is contraindicated if the patient has a history of esophageal disorders, dysphagia, or radiation therapy to the chest wall. Patients need sedation during a TEE.

Cardiac Computed Tomography. Cardiac CT is a heart-imaging test that uses CT technology with or without IV contrast (dye) to see the heart anatomy, coronary circulation, and great blood vessels (e.g., aorta, pulmonary veins, artery). This technology is often called *multidetector CT (MDCT) scanning*. Types of CT scans used to diagnose heart disease include coronary CT angiography (CTA) and calcium-scoring CT scan (Table 31.7).

Coronary CTA is a noninvasive test. It can be done faster than a cardiac catheterization with less risk and discomfort to the patient. Patients must have a normal sinus rhythm for this test. Although the use of coronary CTA is increasing, cardiac catheterization is the gold standard to diagnose CAD. Further, when a cardiac catheterization is done, procedures (e.g., angioplasty, stent placement) can be done if coronary blockages are found. Last, the radiation exposure during a cardiac catheterization is less than the exposure during a CTA.

The calcium-scoring CT scan is used to find calcium deposits in plaque in the coronary arteries. The most common method used is the electron beam CT (EBCT) (Fig. 31.11). It can detect early coronary calcification before symptoms develop and confirm CAD in patients with suspected CAD. The amount of coronary calcium is a predictor of future cardiac events. The calcium score can be used in the risk analysis of patients without known CVD.

Cardiovascular Magnetic Resonance Imaging. Cardiovascular magnetic resonance imaging (CMRI) can detect and find areas of MI in a 3-D view. It is sensitive enough to find even small MIs that are not apparent with single-photon emission computed tomography (SPECT). CMRI aids in the final diagnosis of MI and the assessment of EF. It plays a role in prediction of recovery from MI and in the diagnosis of congenital heart and aortic disorders and CAD. One major advantage of CMRI is that it does not require any radiation to the patient.

Patients with coronary stents can undergo CMRI 6 weeks after stent placement. In patients with older model pacemakers and ICDs, CMRI is discouraged because the magnets can change the function of the devices. However, when there is a strong clinical need and the benefits outweigh the risks, CMRI can be done at centers experienced in this procedure. Many newer models of pacemakers and ICDs are approved for use with MRI.

Nuclear Cardiology. One of the most common nuclear imaging tests is the multigated acquisition (MUGA) or cardiac blood pool scan. This test provides information on wall motion during systole and diastole, heart valves, and EF (Table 31.7).

Perfusion imaging is used with exercise testing to determine whether the coronary blood flow changes with increased activity. Stress perfusion imaging may show an abnormality even when a resting image is normal. This procedure is used to diagnose CAD, make a prognosis in existing CAD, distinguish viable heart muscle from scar tissue, and determine the potential for success of various interventions (e.g., coronary artery bypass surgery, percutaneous coronary intervention) (see Chapter 33).

Exercise stress perfusion imaging is an option if a patient cannot exercise. IV regadenoson (Lexiscan), dipyridamole, or adenosine (Adenocard) can be given to dilate the coronary arteries and simulate the effect of exercise. After the drug takes effect, the isotope is injected, and the imaging is done.

SPECT uses technetium, thallium, or sestamibi as an imaging agent (isotope). Both obese patients and women with large breasts can have artifact, which can lead to false-positive results. Patients with severe multivessel coronary disease or blockages in their left main coronary artery may have false-negative results.

Positron emission tomography (PET) stress testing is increasingly being used due to its high sensitivity for revealing myocardial ischemia and viability. This type of myocardial perfusion imaging is often performed using rubidium-82. This agent allows for quicker studies with lower radiation exposure and better diagnostic quality.[16]

Interventional and Invasive Studies

Cardiac Catheterization. Cardiac catheterization is a common procedure. It provides information about CAD, coronary spasm, congenital and valvular heart disease, and ventricular function. Cardiac catheterization is also used to measure intracardiac pressures and O2 levels, as well as CO and EF. With injection of contrast media and fluoroscopy, the coronary arteries can be seen, chambers of the heart can be outlined, and wall motion assessed (Table 31.8).

Cardiac catheterization is done by inserting a radiopaque catheter into the right and/or left side of the heart. For the right side of the heart, the HCP inserts a catheter into the femoral, internal jugular, subclavian, or antecubital vein. Pressures are recorded as the catheter is moved into the vena cava, right atrium, right ventricle, and pulmonary artery. The catheter is then moved until it is wedged or lodged in position. This blocks the blood flow and pressure from the right side of the heart and looks ahead through the pulmonary capillary bed to the pressure in the left side of the heart (*pulmonary artery wedge pressure*). This pressure assesses the function of the left side of the heart.

Left-sided heart catheterization is done by inserting a catheter into a radial, femoral, or brachial artery. The catheter is passed in a retrograde manner up to the aorta, across the aortic valve, and into the left ventricle.

Coronary angiography is done with a left-sided heart catheterization. The catheter is positioned at the origin of the

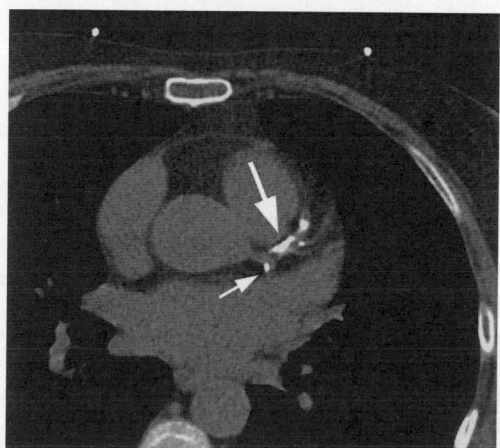

FIG. 31.11 Examples of coronary calcification of the left anterior descending coronary artery *(large arrow)* and left circumflex artery *(small arrow)* as seen on electron beam computed tomography. (From Libby P, Bonow R, Zipes D, et al: *Braunwald's heart disease: A textbook of cardiovascular medicine*, ed 8, St Louis, 2008, Saunders.)

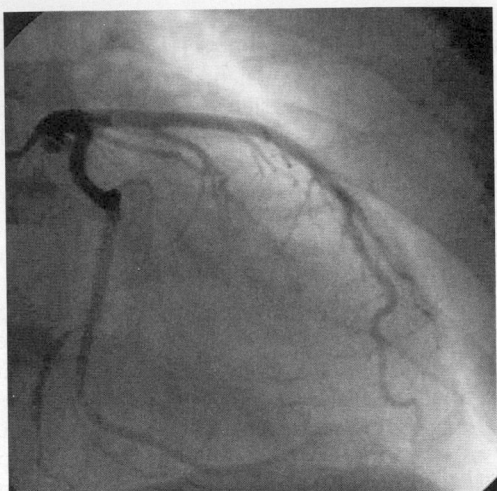

FIG. 31.12 Angiogram showing a normal left coronary and circumflex artery. (From Drake RL, Vogl AW, Mitchell AWM: *Gray's anatomy for students*, ed 2, Philadelphia, 2010, Churchill Livingstone.)

coronary arteries (Fig. 31.3), and contrast medium is injected into the arteries. Patients often feel a temporary flushed sensation with dye injection. The images show the location and severity of any coronary blockages (see Figs. 31.12 and 33.7).

Complications of cardiac catheterization include bleeding or hematoma at the puncture site; allergic reactions to the contrast media; looping or kinking of the catheter; infection; thrombus formation; aortic dissection; dysrhythmias; MI; stroke; and puncture of the ventricles, septum, or lung tissue.

Intravascular Ultrasound. Intravascular ultrasound (IVUS), or intracoronary ultrasound (ICUS), is an invasive procedure done in the catheterization laboratory with coronary angiography. The 2-D or 3-D US images provide a cross-sectional view of the arterial walls of the coronary arteries. In IVUS, a miniature transducer attached to a small catheter is moved to the artery to be studied. Once it is in the artery, US images are obtained. The health of the arterial layers is assessed, including the composition, location, and thickness of any plaque. IVUS can evaluate vessel response to treatments such as stent placement and atherectomy, as well as any complications that

may have occurred during the procedure. Patients often have IVUS in addition to angiography or a coronary intervention. Thus nursing care after is similar to that of patient after a cardiac catheterization.

Electrophysiology Study. The electrophysiology study (EPS) records and manipulates the heart's electrical activity using electrodes placed inside the heart chambers. It provides information on SA node, AV node, and ventricular conduction. It is particularly helpful in determining the source and treatment of dysrhythmias. Patients with symptomatic tachydysrhythmias are at risk for sudden cardiac death. Information from an EPS helps to make a correct diagnosis and guides treatment decisions (Table 31.8). In EPS, catheters are inserted like a right-sided heart catheterization. Thus nursing care after EPS is similar to that of a patient after a cardiac catheterization.

CASE STUDY

Objective Data: Diagnostic Studies

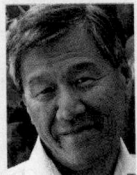

(© Jupiterimages/ Banana-Stock/ Thinkstock.)

The HCP orders the following initial diagnostic studies for L.P.:
- 12-lead ECG
- CBC, basic metabolic panel (glucose, electrolytes, BUN, creatinine)
- PTT, PT, INR
- Pro-BNP
- Troponin, CK-MB
- TSH, free T$_4$
- Chest x-ray

The ECG shows atrial fibrillation with a rapid ventricular response. L.P.'s initial troponin and CK-MB levels are within normal limits. Chest x-ray, CBC, and coagulation studies are all within normal limits. The potassium level is 3.1 mEq/L and pro-BNP is high (1204 pg/mL). The HCP orders 250 mL NSS IV bolus; an oral dose of potassium, a loading dose of IV diltiazem followed by a continuous infusion, and weight-based heparin to be started in the emergency department. L.P. will be admitted to the progressive care unit and will have a consult with a cardiologist.

Discussion Questions

1. Are these the diagnostic studies that you expected to be ordered?
2. Which diagnostic study results are abnormal?
3. Which diagnostic study results are of most concern to you?

Answers available at *http://evolve.elsevier.com/Lewis/medsurg*.

■ BRIDGE TO NCLEX EXAMINATION

The number of the question corresponds to the same-numbered outcome at the beginning of the chapter.

1. A patient with a tricuspid valve disorder has impaired blood flow between the
   a. vena cava and right atrium.
   b. left atrium and left ventricle.
   c. right atrium and right ventricle.
   d. right ventricle and pulmonary artery.

2. A patient has a severe blockage in his right coronary artery. Which heart structures are *most* likely to be affected by this blockage *(select all that apply)*?
   a. AV node
   b. Left ventricle
   c. Coronary sinus
   d. Right ventricle
   e. Pulmonic valve

3. The part of the vascular system responsible for hemostasis is the
   a. thin capillary vessels.
   b. endothelial layer of the arteries.
   c. elastic middle layer of the veins.
   d. smooth muscle of the arterial wall.

4. When a person's blood pressure rises, the homeostatic mechanism to compensate for an elevation involves stimulation of
   a. baroreceptors that inhibit the sympathetic nervous system, causing vasodilation.
   b. chemoreceptors that inhibit the sympathetic nervous system, causing vasodilation.
   c. baroreceptors that inhibit the parasympathetic nervous system, causing vasodilation.
   d. chemoreceptors that stimulate the sympathetic nervous system, causing an increased heart rate.

5. A P wave on an ECG represents an impulse arising at the
   a. SA node and repolarizing the atria.
   b. SA node and depolarizing the atria.
   c. AV node and depolarizing the atria.
   d. AV node and spreading to the bundle of His.

6. Which subjective data related to the cardiovascular system should be obtained from the patient (select all that apply)?
   a. Annual income
   b. Smoking history
   c. Religious preference
   d. Number of pillows used to sleep
   e. Blood for basic laboratory studies

7. Which heart valve sound is heard best at the left midclavicular line at the level of the fifth ICS?
   a. Aortic
   b. Mitral
   c. Tricuspid
   d. Pulmonic

8. When assessing a patient, you note a pulse deficit of 23 beats. This finding may be caused by
   a. dysrhythmias.
   b. heart murmurs.
   c. gallop rhythms.
   d. pericardial friction rubs.

9. An expected finding in the assessment of an 81-year-old patient is
   a. a narrowed pulse pressure.
   b. diminished carotid artery pulses.
   c. difficulty isolating the apical pulse.
   d. an increased heart rate in response to stress.

10. Which nursing responsibilities are priorities when caring for a patient returning from a cardiac catheterization (select all that apply)?
    a. Monitoring vital signs and ECG
    b. Checking the catheter insertion site and distal pulses
    c. Helping the patient to ambulate to the bathroom to void
    d. Telling the patient that he will be sleepy from the general anesthesia
    e. Teaching the patient about the risks of the radioactive isotope injection

1. c, 2. a, b, 3. b, 4. a, 5. b, 6. b, c, d, 7. b, 8. a, 9. c, 10. a, b

For rationales to these answers and even more NCLEX review questions, visit *http://evolve.elsevier.com/Lewis/medsurg*.

EVOLVE WEBSITE/RESOURCES LIST

http://evolve.elsevier.com/Lewis/medsurg
Review Questions (Online Only)
Key Points
Answer Keys for Questions
- Rationales for Bridge to NCLEX Examination Questions
- Answer Guidelines for Case Studies on pp. 661, 664, 667, and 676
Conceptual Care Map Creator
Audio Glossary
Supporting Media
- Animations
- Auscultation of Heart Valves
- Blood Flow: Circulatory System
- Cardiac Cycle During Systole and Diastole
- Pulse Variations
- Audio
- Diastolic Murmur
- Fourth Heart Sound (S$_4$)
- Murmurs: Blowing, Harsh or Rough, and Rumble
- Murmurs: High, Medium, and Low
- S$_1$ at Various Locations
- S$_2$ at Various Locations
- Single S$_1$
- Single S$_2$
- Systolic Murmur
- Third Heart Sound (S$_3$)
Content Updates

REFERENCES

1. Patton KT, Thibodeau GA: *The human body in health and disease*, ed 7, St Louis, 2018, Elsevier.
2. Wesley K: *Huszar' ECG and 12-lead interpretation*, ed 5, St Louis, 2017, Elsevier.
3. Huether S, McCance K: *Understanding pathophysiology*, ed 6, St Louis, 2017, Elsevier.
4. American Heart Association: Understanding blood pressure readings. Retrieved from *www.heart.org/HEARTORG/Conditions/HighBloodPressure/AboutHighBloodPressure/Understanding-Blood-Pressure-Readings_UCM_301764_Article.jsp*.
5. Wilson SF, Giddens JF: *Health assessment for nursing practice*, ed 6, St Louis, 2017, Elsevier.
*6. Parikh JD, Hollingsworth KG, Wallace D, et al: Left ventricular functional, structural and energetic effects of normal aging: Comparison with hypertension, *PLoS One* 12, 2017. Retrieved from *https://doi.org/10.1371/journal.pone.0177404*.
7. Fajemiroye JO, Cunha LC, Saavedra-Rodríguez R, et al: Aging-induced biological changes and cardiovascular diseases, *Biomed Res Int*, 2018. Retrieved from *www.hindawi.com/journals/bmri/2018/7156435/*.
8. Girelli D, Piubelli C, Martinelli N, et al: A decade of progress on the genetic basis of coronary artery disease, *Eur J Intern Med* 41:10, 2017.
9. Clayton BD, Willihnganz MJ: *Basic pharmacology for nurses*, ed 17, St Louis, 2017, Elsevier.
*10. Ricci F, Di Scala R, Massacesi C, et al: Ultra-sensitive copeptin and cardiac troponin in diagnosing non-ST-segment elevation acute coronary syndromes—The COPACS study, *AJM* 129:105, 2016.
*11. Zhang P, Wu X, Li G, et al: Prognostic role of copeptin with all-cause mortality after heart failure: A systematic review and meta-analysis, *Ther Clin Risk Manag* 13:49, 2017.
12. Pagana KD, Pagana TJ, Pagana TN: *Mosby's diagnostic and laboratory test reference*, ed 13, St Louis, 2017, Elsevier.
*13. Alvin MD, Jaffe AS, Ziegelstein RC, et al: Eliminating creatine kinase–myocardial band testing in suspected acute coronary syndrome, *JAMA Intern Med* 177:1508, 2017.
*14. Rusnak J, Fastner C, Behnes M, et al: Biomarkers in stable coronary artery disease, *Curr Pharm Biotechnol* 18:456, 2017.
15. Renner J, Grünewald M, Bein B: Monitoring high-risk patients: Minimally invasive and non-invasive possibilities, *Best Pract Res Clin Anaesthesiol* 30:201, 2016.
16. Waterstram-Rich KM, Gilmore DA: *Nuclear medicine and PET/CT: Technology and techniques*, ed 8, St Louis, 2017, Elsevier.

*Evidence-based information for clinical practice.

32

Hypertension

Pamela Wilkerson and Melissa Hutchinson

By doing what you love, you inspire and awaken the hearts of others.

Satsuki Shibuya

ⓔ http://evolve.elsevier.com/Lewis/medsurg/

CONCEPTUAL FOCUS

Adherence

Fluids and Electrolytes

Perfusion

Self-Management

LEARNING OUTCOMES

1. Relate the pathophysiologic mechanisms associated with primary hypertension to the clinical manifestations and complications.
2. Choose appropriate strategies for the prevention of primary hypertension.
3. Describe the interprofessional care for primary hypertension, including drug therapy and lifestyle modifications.

4. Explain the interprofessional care of the older adult with primary hypertension.
5. Prioritize the nursing management of the patient with primary hypertension.
6. Describe the nursing and interprofessional care of a patient with a hypertensive crisis.

KEY TERMS

blood pressure (BP), p. 678

hypertension, p. 678

hypertensive crisis, p. 695

orthostatic hypotension, p. 692

elevated blood pressure, p. 681

primary hypertension, p. 681

secondary hypertension, p. 681

systemic vascular resistance (SVR), p. 679

Hypertension, or high blood pressure (BP), is one of the most important modifiable risk factors that can lead to the development of cardiovascular disease (CVD). As BP increases so does the risk for myocardial infarction (MI), heart failure (HF), stroke, and renal disease. Hypertension-induced retinopathy can impair vision. This chapter discusses the nursing and interprofessional care of patients with or at risk for hypertension. Providing comprehensive care will require you to collaborate with many members of the health care team. Patient education is key to hypertension management. Proper nutrition and exercise are important health promotion behaviors.

Current guidelines reveal that around 46% of adults in the United States meet criteria for the general diagnosis of hypertension. Heart disease, often directly related to hypertension, accounts for 23.7% of all deaths each year in the United States.[1,2] The National Health and Nutrition Examination Survey (NHANES) tracks prevention, treatment, and control of hypertension.[3] Data from NHANES showed that 83% of people 20 years of age and older with hypertension were aware that they had high BP. Of those, 76% were receiving treatment; 48%, though, did not currently have their BP well controlled.[4]

The American College of Cardiology Foundation and the American Heart Association (AHA) provide performance measures for hypertension management that address the treatment and control of BP to target goals. Target goals have been updated with new information from the evidence-based Guideline for the Prevention, Detection, Evaluation, and Management of High Blood Pressure in Adults: A Report of the American College of Cardiology/AHA Task Force on Clinical Practice Guidelines and the Systolic Blood Pressure Intervention Trial (SPRINT). Target goals take age and comorbidities into consideration when recommending treatment options.[5]

National guidelines are designed to apply to all racial and ethnic groups. However, specific groups have a higher incidence of risk factors (see boxes on Promoting Health Equity and Gender Differences).[5,6]

NORMAL REGULATION OF BLOOD PRESSURE

Blood pressure (BP) is the force exerted by the blood against the walls of the blood vessel. It must be adequate to maintain tissue perfusion during activity and rest. Maintaining normal BP and tissue perfusion requires the integration of both systemic factors and local peripheral vascular effects. BP is mainly a function of cardiac output (CO) and systemic vascular resistance (Fig. 32.1).

PROMOTING HEALTH EQUITY
Hypertension

All Ethnicities
- There are 3 factors associated with decreased prevalence of hypertension for all ethnicities: People born outside the United States, living in a household that does not speak English in the home, or living in a household with limited time living in the United States

Blacks
- Have the highest prevalence of hypertension in the world
- Are more likely to have resistant hypertension
- Develop hypertension at a younger age than other ethnicities with higher average blood pressure
- Have a higher incidence of hypertension among women than among men
- Have more nocturnal nondipping BP than whites, which is associated with an increase in CVD
- Hypertension is more aggressive and results in more severe end-organ damage
- Have the highest death rate resulting from hypertension
- Make less renin and do not respond well to renin-inhibiting drugs
- Have better BP control with calcium channel blockers and diuretics, especially with monotherapy
- Have a higher risk for angioedema with ACE inhibitors than whites

Hispanics
- Are less likely to receive treatment for hypertension than whites and blacks
- Have lower rates of BP control than whites and blacks
- Have lower levels of awareness of hypertension and its treatment than whites and blacks

GENDER DIFFERENCES
Hypertension

Men
- Before early middle age, hypertension is more common in men.

Women
- Hypertension is 2 to 3 times more common in women who take oral contraceptives than in women who do not.
- A history of preeclampsia may be an early sign of risk for CVD.
- After age 64, hypertension is more common in women. Part of the rise in BP in women is attributed to menopause-related factors, such as estrogen withdrawal, overproduction of pituitary hormones, and weight gain
- It is harder to control hypertension in older women (ages 70 to 79) than in women ages 50 to 69, despite having similar rates of treatment.

CO is the total blood flow through the systemic or pulmonary circulation per minute. It is described as the stroke volume (SV) or the amount of blood pumped out of the left ventricle per beat (about 70 mL) multiplied by the heart rate (HR).

Systemic vascular resistance (SVR) is the force opposing the movement of blood within the blood vessels. The radius of the small arteries and arterioles is the principal factor determining SVR. As arteries narrow, resistance to blood flow increases. As arteries dilate, resistance to blood flow decreases. A small change in the radius of the arterioles creates a significant change in the SVR. If SVR is increased and CO stays constant or increases, arterial BP will increase.

The mechanisms that regulate BP can affect either CO or SVR or both. Regulation of BP is a complex process involving both short-term (seconds to hours) and long-term (days to weeks) mechanisms. Short-term mechanisms, including the sympathetic nervous system (SNS) and vascular endothelium, are active within a few seconds. Long-term mechanisms include renal and hormonal processes that regulate arteriolar resistance and blood volume. In a healthy person, these regulatory mechanisms work in response to the body's demands.

Sympathetic Nervous System

The nervous system, which reacts within seconds after a drop in BP, increases BP by activating the SNS. Increased SNS activity increases HR, and cardiac contractility produces widespread vasoconstriction in the peripheral arterioles and promotes the release of renin from the kidneys. The net effect of SNS activation is to increase BP by increasing both CO and SVR.

Specialized nerve cells called *baroreceptors* are found in the carotid arteries and arch of the aorta. These cells sense changes in BP and send this information to the vasomotor centers in the brainstem. The brainstem sends this information through complex networks of neurons that excite or inhibit efferent nerves. SNS efferent nerves innervate cardiac and vascular smooth muscle cells. Under normal conditions, a low level of continuous SNS activity maintains vascular tone. BP may be reduced by the withdrawal of SNS activity or by stimulation of the parasympathetic nervous system (PNS). The PNS decreases the HR (via the vagus nerve) and thereby decreases CO.

The neurotransmitter norepinephrine (NE) is released from SNS nerve endings. NE activates receptors in the sinoatrial

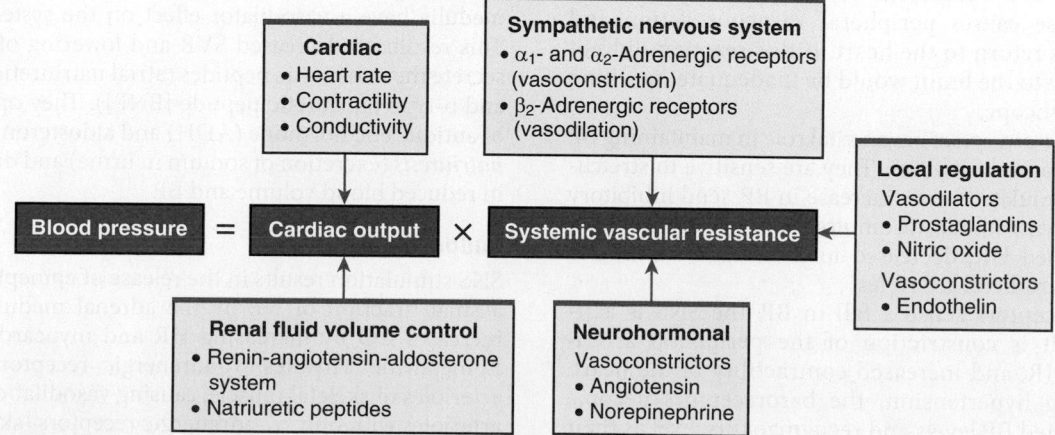

FIG. 32.1 Factors influencing BP. Hypertension develops when one or more of the BP-regulating mechanisms are defective.

TABLE 32.1 Sympathetic Nervous System Receptors Affecting BP

Receptor	Location	Response When Activated
α_1	Vascular smooth muscle	Vasoconstriction
	Heart	Increased contractility (positive inotropic effect)
α_2	Presynaptic nerve terminals	Inhibition of norepinephrine release
	Vascular smooth muscle	Vasoconstriction
β_1	Heart	Increased contractility (positive inotropic effect)
		Increased heart rate (positive chronotropic effect)
		Increased conduction (positive dromotropic effect)
	Juxtaglomerular cells of the kidney	Increased renin secretion
β_2	Smooth muscle of blood vessels in heart (e.g., coronary arteries), lungs (e.g., bronchi), and skeletal muscle	Vasodilation
Dopamine receptors	Primarily renal blood vessels	Vasodilation

node, myocardium, and vascular smooth muscle. The response to NE depends on the type of receptors present. SNS receptors are classified as α_1, α_2, β_1, and β_2 (Table 32.1). The smooth muscle of the blood vessels has α-adrenergic and β_2-adrenergic receptors. α-Adrenergic receptors found in the peripheral vasculature cause vasoconstriction when stimulated by NE. β_1-Adrenergic receptors in the heart respond to NE and epinephrine with increased HR (chronotropic), increased force of contraction (inotropic), and increased speed of conduction (dromotropic). β_2-Adrenergic receptors are activated mainly by epinephrine released from the adrenal medulla and cause vasodilation (Fig. 32.1).

The sympathetic vasomotor center interacts with many areas of the brain to maintain normal BP under various conditions. It is activated during times of pain, stress, and exercise. The SNS response causes an appropriate increase in CO and BP to adjust to the body's increased O_2 demands. During postural change from lying to standing, there is a transient decrease in BP. The vasomotor center is stimulated, and the SNS response causes peripheral vasoconstriction and increased venous return to the heart. If this reaction did not occur, blood flow to the brain would be inadequate, resulting in dizziness or syncope.

Baroreceptors. *Baroreceptors* have a vital role in maintaining BP stability during normal activities. They are sensitive to stretching and, when stimulated by an increase in BP, send inhibitory impulses to the sympathetic vasomotor center. SNS inhibition results in decreased HR, decreased force of contraction, and vasodilation in peripheral arterioles.

When baroreceptors sense a fall in BP, the SNS is activated. The result is constriction of the peripheral arterioles, increased HR, and increased contractility of the heart. In long-standing hypertension, the baroreceptors become adjusted to elevated BP levels and recognize this level as their new "normal."

Vascular Endothelium

The vascular endothelium is a single-cell layer that lines the blood vessels. The endothelium is very active and responsible for several critical functions. These include platelet adhesion, coagulation regulation, immune function, and regulating fluid control within the vessel and extravascular space. The endothelium can cause adhesion and aggregation of neutrophils and stimulate smooth muscle growth.

The endothelium is essential to the regulation and maintenance of vasodilating and vasoconstricting substances. Endothelium-derived vasoactive substances include *nitric oxide* (NO) and *prostacyclin*, which are both vasodilators. Another product of the endothelium is *endothelin* (ET), which is a potent vasoconstrictor (Fig. 32.1). Cardiovascular risk factors, such as smoking and diabetes, can reduce functional endothelial cells. This can cause arterial tone changes (through either excessive constriction or dilation), which is an early warning signal of CVD.

Renal System

The kidneys contribute to BP regulation by controlling sodium excretion and extracellular fluid (ECF) volume (see Chapter 44). Sodium retention results in water retention, which causes an increase in ECF volume. This action increases the venous return to the heart and SV. Together these increase CO and BP.

The renin-angiotensin-aldosterone system (RAAS) plays an essential role in BP regulation (Fig. 32.1). The juxtaglomerular apparatus in the kidney secretes renin in response to SNS stimulation, decreased blood flow through the kidneys, or decreased serum sodium concentration. Renin is an enzyme that converts angiotensinogen to angiotensin I. Angiotensin I is then converted to angiotensin II (A-II) by angiotensin-converting enzyme (ACE). A-II increases BP by 2 different mechanisms (see Fig. 44.4). First, A-II is a potent vasoconstrictor and increases SVR. This results in an immediate increase in BP. Second, over a period of hours or days, A-II increases BP indirectly by stimulating the adrenal cortex to secrete aldosterone.

A-II acts at a local level within the heart and blood vessels. These effects include vasoconstriction and tissue growth that result in remodeling of the vessel walls, which can be due to or caused by endothelial dysfunction. These changes are linked to the development of primary hypertension and the long-term effects of hypertension (e.g., atherosclerosis, renal disease, cardiac hypertrophy).

Prostaglandins (PGE_2 and PGI_2) secreted by the renal medulla have a vasodilator effect on the systemic circulation. This results in decreased SVR and lowering of BP. Heart cells secrete the natriuretic peptides (atrial natriuretic peptide [ANP] and b-type natriuretic peptide [BNP]). They oppose the effects of antidiuretic hormone (ADH) and aldosterone. This results in *natriuresis* (excretion of sodium in urine) and diuresis, resulting in reduced blood volume and BP.

Endocrine System

SNS stimulation results in the release of epinephrine along with a small fraction of NE by the adrenal medulla. Epinephrine increases CO by increasing HR and myocardial contractility. Epinephrine activates β_2-adrenergic receptors in peripheral arterioles of skeletal muscle, causing vasodilation. In peripheral arterioles with only α_1-adrenergic receptors (skin and kidneys), epinephrine causes vasoconstriction.

A-II stimulates the adrenal cortex to release aldosterone. Aldosterone stimulates the kidneys to retain sodium and water, which increases blood volume and CO (see Fig. 44.4).

Increased blood sodium and osmolarity levels stimulates the release of ADH from the posterior pituitary gland. ADH increases the ECF volume by promoting the reabsorption of water in the distal and collecting tubules of the kidneys. The resulting increase in blood volume causes an increase in CO and BP.

HYPERTENSION

Classification of Hypertension

Table 32.2 shows the BP classifications for people 18 years of age and older. Normal blood pressure is defined as a systolic BP (SBP) < 120 mm Hg and a diastolic BP (DBP < 80 mm Hg. Elevated blood pressure is defined as an SBP between 120 -129 mm Hg and a DBP < 80 mm Hg. *Hypertension (stage 1)* is defined as an SBP between 130-139 mm Hg and a DBP between 80-89 mm Hg. *Hypertension (stage 2)* is defined as an SBP > 140 mm Hg and a DBP > 90 mm Hg.[5] If either the SBP or DBP is outside of a range, the higher measurement determines the classification. For example, 115/86 would be classified as hypertension stage 1 even though the SBP is within normal limits. SBP increases with age. DBP rises until around 55 years old and then declines. BP classification is based on 2 or more readings, accurately performed on both arms, on 2 separate occasions.

Etiology

Hypertension can result from either primary or secondary causes.

Primary Hypertension. Primary hypertension *(essential* or *idiopathic)* is elevated BP without an identified cause. It accounts for 90% to 95% of all cases of hypertension. Although the exact reason for primary hypertension is unknown, there are multiple contributing factors. These include changes in endothelial function related to either vasoconstricting or vasodilating agents, increased SNS activity, overproduction of sodium-retaining hormones, increased sodium intake, greater than ideal body weight, age, family history, ethnicity, diabetes, tobacco use, and excess alcohol intake.

Secondary Hypertension. Secondary hypertension is elevated BP with a specific cause that often can be identified and corrected (Table 32.3). Secondary hypertension can become resistant, causing cardiovascular complications if left untreated. This type of hypertension accounts for 5% to 10% of hypertension in adults. Secondary hypertension should be suspected in people

who suddenly develop high BP, especially if it is severe. Findings that suggest secondary hypertension relate to the underlying cause. For example, an abdominal bruit heard over the renal arteries may indicate renal disease. It is often present in patients with obstructive sleep apnea. Treatment is aimed at removing or treating the underlying cause. Secondary hypertension is a contributing factor to hypertensive crisis (discussed later in this chapter).

Pathophysiology of Primary Hypertension

BP rises with any increase in CO or SVR. As hypertension progresses from elevated to stage 1, increases in both blood volume and CO are often present, leading to an increase in SVR. As hypertension progresses, SVR rises, and CO returns to normal. The hemodynamic hallmark of hypertension is a persistently increased SVR. This persistent elevation in SVR may occur in several ways. Table 32.4 shows factors that relate to the development of primary hypertension or contribute to its consequences. Abnormalities of any of the mechanisms involved in maintaining normal BP can result in hypertension (Fig. 32.1).

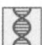 **Genetic Link**

Different sets of genes may regulate BP at various times throughout the life span.[2] Genetic variations are associated with the development of hypertension. For example, genetic abnormalities have been associated with a rare form of hypertension characterized by excess levels of potassium. Several genetic variants of substances on the endothelium affect BP and the development of hypertension by influencing the body's sensitivity to salt. When endothelial surface proteins are activated, proinflammatory properties are stimulated, impairing the endothelial cells' ability to activate vasodilatory effects, which leads to hypertension.

Research is currently ongoing to understand the complicated role that endothelial dysfunction and genetics play in the formation and progression of hypertension. We currently recommend screening of children and siblings of persons with hypertension and strongly advising them to adopt healthy lifestyles to minimize their risk for developing hypertension.

Water and Sodium Retention. Excess sodium intake is linked to the development of hypertension. Although most people consume a high-sodium diet, only 1 in 3 will develop hypertension. When sodium is restricted in people with hypertension, their BP usually falls. This suggests that some degree of sodium sensitivity may exist for high sodium intake to trigger the development of hypertension. A high sodium intake may

---

TABLE 32.2 **Classification of Hypertension**

Category	SBP (mm Hg)		DBP (mm Hg)
Normal	<120	and	<80
Elevated	120–129	and	<80
Hypertension, stage 1	130–139	or	80–89
Hypertension, stage 2	≥140	or	≥90

Source: Whelton PK, Carey RM, Aronow WS, et al: 2017 ACC/AHA/AAPA/ ABC/ACPM/AGS/APhA/ASH/ASPC/NMA/PCNA guideline for the prevention, detection, evaluation, and management of high blood pressure in adults: A report of the American College of Cardiology/AHA Task Force on Clinical Practice Guidelines, *Journal of the American College of Cardiology* 71:e127, 2018.
DBP, Diastolic blood pressure; *SBP,* systolic blood pressure.

TABLE 32.3 **Common Causes of Secondary Hypertension**

- Cirrhosis
- Coarctation or congenital narrowing of the aorta
- Drug-related: estrogen replacement therapy, oral contraceptives, corticosteroids, nonsteroidal antiinflammatory drugs (e.g., cyclooxygenase-2 inhibitors), SNS stimulants (e.g., cocaine, monoamine oxidase)
- Endocrine disorders (e.g., pheochromocytoma, Cushing syndrome, thyroid disease)
- Neurologic disorders (e.g., brain tumors, quadriplegia, traumatic brain injury)
- Pregnancy-induced hypertension
- Renal disease (e.g., renal artery stenosis, glomerulonephritis)
- Sleep apnea

activate a number of systemic mechanisms. Fig. 32.2 shows the relationships among salt intake, BP, and changes in the structure of the heart.

In clinical practice, there is not an easy or straightforward test to identify people whose BP will rise with even a small increase in salt intake *(salt sensitive)* versus those who can ingest large amounts of sodium without much change in BP *(salt resistant)*. The effect of sodium on BP has a strong genetic component. The effect of sodium is more significant in blacks and middle-aged and older adults. This can increase the potential of renal dysfunction, endothelial dysfunction, and HF in these persons.[7,8]

TABLE 32.4   Risk Factors for Primary Hypertension

Risk Factor	Description
Age	• Systolic BP rises progressively with age. • After age 50, SBP >140 mm Hg is a more important cardiovascular risk factor than diastolic BP
Alcohol	• Excess alcohol intake is strongly associated with hypertension • Moderate intake of alcohol has cardioprotective properties; males should limit their daily intake of alcohol to 2 drinks per day, and 1 drink per day for females
Diabetes	• Hypertension is more common in patients with diabetes • When hypertension and diabetes coexist, complications (e.g., target organ disease) are more severe
Elevated serum lipids	• ↑ Levels of cholesterol and triglycerides are primary risk factors for atherosclerosis • Hyperlipidemia is more common in people with hypertension
Ethnicity	• The incidence of hypertension is 2 times higher in blacks than in whites (See Promoting Health Equity box on p. 679.)

Excess dietary sodium	• High sodium intake can
	   • Contribute to hypertension in salt-sensitive patients
	   • Decrease the effectiveness of certain antihypertensive drugs

Family history	• History of a close blood relative (e.g., parents, sibling) with hypertension is associated with an ↑ risk for developing hypertension
Gender	• Hypertension is more prevalent in men in young adulthood and early middle age • After age 64, hypertension is more prevalent in women (See Gender Differences box on p. 679)
Obesity	• Weight gain is associated with ↑ frequency of hypertension • Risk increases with central abdominal obesity
Sedentary lifestyle	• Regular physical activity can help control weight and reduce cardiovascular risk • Physical activity may ↓ BP
Socioeconomic status	• Hypertension is more prevalent in lower socioeconomic groups and among the less educated
Stress	• People exposed to repeated stress may develop hypertension more often than others • People who develop hypertension may respond differently to stress than those who do not develop hypertension
Tobacco use	• Smoking tobacco greatly ↑ risk for CVD • People with hypertension who smoke tobacco are at even greater risk for CVD

Altered Renin-Angiotensin-Aldosterone Mechanism. High plasma renin activity (PRA) increases the conversion of angiotensinogen to angiotensin I (see Fig. 44.4). This change in the RAAS may contribute to the development of hypertension. Any rise in BP inhibits the release of renin from the renal juxtaglomerular cells. Based on this feedback loop, we would expect low levels of PRA in patients with primary hypertension. However, only about 30% have low PRA, 50% have normal levels, and 20% have high PRA. These normal or high PRA levels may be related to excess renin secretion from ischemic nephrons.

Stress and Increased Sympathetic Nervous System Activity. We have long recognized that factors such as anger, fear, and pain influence BP. Physiologic responses to stress, which are typically protective, may persist to a pathologic degree, resulting in a prolonged increase in SNS activity. Increased SNS stimulation produces increased vasoconstriction, increased HR, and increased renin release. Increased renin activates the RAAS, leading to elevated BP. People with high levels of repeated psychological stress develop hypertension more than those who have less stress.

Insulin Resistance and Hyperinsulinemia. Defects in glucose, insulin, and lipoprotein metabolism are common in primary hypertension. These defects are not present in secondary hypertension and do not improve when primary hypertension is treated. Insulin resistance is a risk factor in the development of hypertension and CVD. High insulin levels stimulate SNS activity and impair nitrous oxide–mediated vasodilation. Other pressor effects of insulin include vascular hypertrophy and increased renal sodium reabsorption.

Endothelial Dysfunction. Endothelial dysfunction is a marker for CVD, including primary hypertension. Hypertension can manifest as a prolonged vasoconstriction response or as a reduced vasodilator response. High levels of ET may cause prolonged vasoconstriction. Vasodilation effects can be altered by oxygen free radicals, which impair the bioavailability of NO. This leads to cellular dysfunction and an imbalance of the vasodilation and vasoconstriction mechanisms in the endothelium.

Clinical Manifestations

Hypertension is often called the "silent killer" because it is often asymptomatic until it becomes severe and target organ disease occurs. A patient with severe hypertension may have a variety of symptoms secondary to the effects on blood vessels in the various organs and tissues or to the increased workload of the heart. These secondary symptoms include fatigue, dizziness, palpitations, angina, and dyspnea.

In the past, we thought headaches and nosebleeds were symptoms of hypertension. Unless BP is very high, these symptoms are no more frequent in people with hypertension than in the general population. However, patients with hypertensive crisis (discussed later in the chapter) may have severe headaches, dyspnea, anxiety, and nosebleeds.[9]

Complications

The most common complications of hypertension are *target organ diseases* occurring in the heart (hypertensive heart disease), brain (cerebrovascular disease), peripheral vessels (peripheral vascular disease), kidneys (nephrosclerosis), and eyes (retinal damage) (Fig. 32.3).

Hypertensive Heart Disease

Coronary Artery Disease. Hypertension is a significant risk factor for coronary artery disease (CAD). The mechanisms

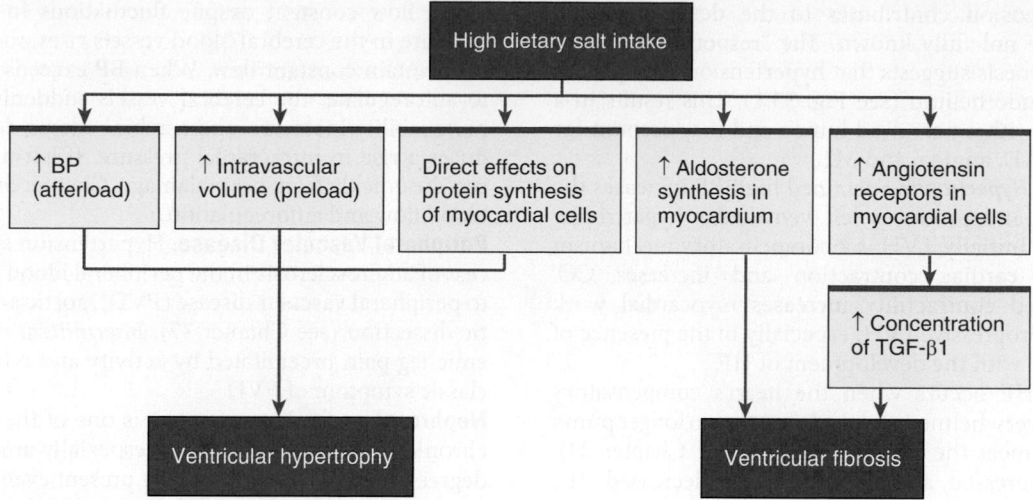

High dietary salt intake

↑ BP (afterload)

↑ Intravascular volume (preload)

Direct effects on protein synthesis of myocardial cells

↑ Aldosterone synthesis in myocardium

↑ Angiotensin receptors in myocardial cells

↑ Concentration of TGF-β1

Ventricular hypertrophy

Ventricular fibrosis

FIG. 32.2 Proposed link among salt intake, blood pressure, and changes in the heart. High dietary salt intake exerts hypertrophic effects on the left (and potentially also on the right) ventricle. Ventricular fibrosis can also result from the high salt intake through mechanisms mediated by the renin-angiotensin-aldosterone system (RAAS). Transforming growth factor-β1 (TGF-β1) is a multifunctional cytokine with fibrogenic properties. Overproduction of TGF-β1 (in part mediated by angiotensin II) results in fibrosis and ventricular dysfunction. (Modified from Frisoli TM, Schmieder RE, Grodzicki T, et al: Salt and hypertension: Is salt dietary reduction worth the effort? *Am J Med* 125:433, 2012.)

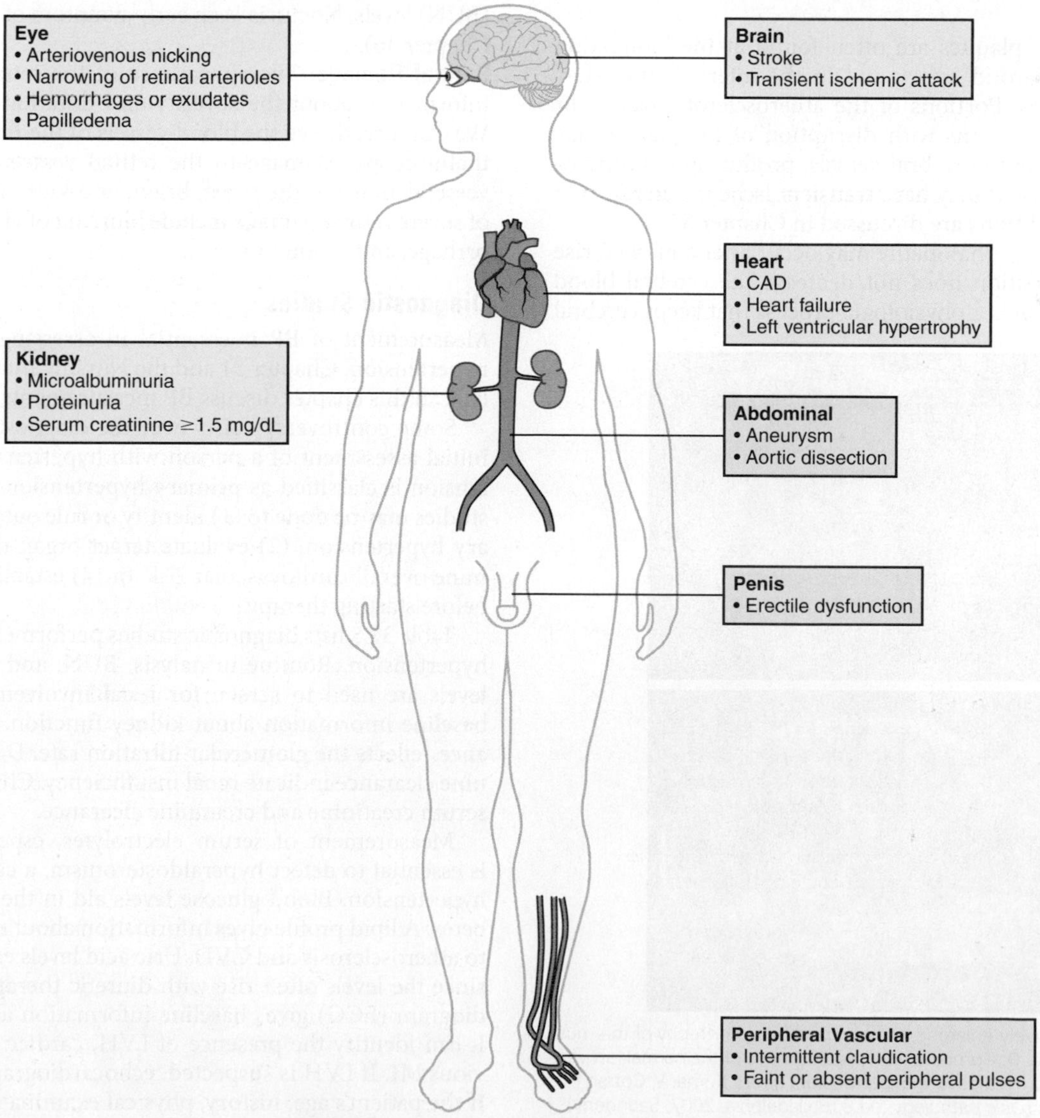

Eye
- Arteriovenous nicking
- Narrowing of retinal arterioles
- Hemorrhages or exudates
- Papilledema

Brain
- Stroke
- Transient ischemic attack

Heart
- CAD
- Heart failure
- Left ventricular hypertrophy

Kidney
- Microalbuminuria
- Proteinuria
- Serum creatinine ≥1.5 mg/dL

Abdominal
- Aneurysm
- Aortic dissection

Penis
- Erectile dysfunction

Peripheral Vascular
- Intermittent claudication
- Faint or absent peripheral pulses

FIG. 32.3 Common complications of hypertension.

by which hypertension contributes to the development of atherosclerosis are not fully known. The "response-to-injury" theory of atherogenesis suggests that hypertension disrupts the coronary artery endothelium (see Fig. 33.1). This results in a rigid arterial wall with a narrowed lumen and may account for the high rate of CAD, angina, and MI.

Left Ventricular Hypertrophy. Sustained high BP increases the cardiac workload and produces left ventricular hypertrophy (LVH) (Fig. 32.4). Initially, LVH is a compensatory mechanism that strengthens cardiac contraction and increases CO. However, increased contractility increases myocardial work and O_2 demand. Progressive LVH, especially in the presence of CAD, is associated with the development of HF.

Heart Failure. HF occurs when the heart's compensatory mechanisms are overwhelmed and the heart can no longer pump enough blood to meet the body's demands (see Chapter 34). Contractility is depressed, and SV and CO are decreased. The patient may have shortness of breath on exertion, paroxysmal nocturnal dyspnea, and fatigue.

Cerebrovascular Disease. Atherosclerosis is the most common cause of cerebrovascular disease. Hypertension is a significant risk factor for cerebral atherosclerosis and stroke. Even in mildly hypertensive people, the risk for stroke is 4 times higher than in normotensive people. Adequate BP control decreases the risk for stroke.

Atherosclerotic plaques are often found at the bifurcation of the common carotid artery and in the internal and external carotid arteries. Portions of the atherosclerotic plaque or the blood clot that forms with disruption of the plaque may break off and travel to cerebral vessels, producing a thromboembolism. The patient may have transient ischemic attacks or a stroke. These conditions are discussed in Chapter 57.

Hypertensive encephalopathy may occur after a marked rise in BP if autoregulation does not decrease the cerebral blood flow. *Autoregulation* is a physiologic process that keeps cerebral blood flow constant despite fluctuations in BP. Typically, as pressure in the cerebral blood vessels rises, the vessels constrict to maintain constant flow. When BP exceeds the body's ability to autoregulate, the cerebral vessels suddenly dilate, capillary permeability increases, and cerebral edema develops. This produces a rise in intracranial pressure. If left untreated, patients can die quickly from brain damage. Chapter 56 reviews cerebral blood flow and autoregulation.

Peripheral Vascular Disease. Hypertension speeds up the process of atherosclerosis in the peripheral blood vessels. This leads to peripheral vascular disease (PVD), aortic aneurysm, and aortic dissection (see Chapter 37). *Intermittent claudication* (ischemic leg pain precipitated by activity and relieved by rest) is a classic symptom of PVD.

Nephrosclerosis. Hypertension is one of the leading causes of chronic kidney disease (CKD), especially among blacks. Some degree of renal disease is usually present even with mild hypertension. Renal disease results from ischemia caused by the narrowing of the renal blood vessels. This leads to atrophy of the tubules, destruction of the glomeruli, and eventual death of nephrons. Initially intact nephrons can compensate, but these changes may eventually lead to renal failure. Laboratory signs of renal disease are albuminuria, proteinuria, microscopic hematuria, and high serum creatinine and blood urea nitrogen (BUN) levels. Nocturia is an early symptom of renal disease (see Chapter 46).

Retinal Damage. The appearance of the retina gives essential information about the severity and duration of hypertension. We can directly see the blood vessels of the retina with an ophthalmoscope. Damage to the retinal vessels indicates related vessel damage in the heart, brain, and kidneys. Manifestations of severe retinal damage include blurring of vision, retinal hemorrhage, and vision loss.

Diagnostic Studies

Measurement of BP is essential in assessing and monitoring hypertension. Chapter 31 and the Nursing Management section later in this chapter discuss BP measurement.

Some controversy exists over the diagnostic workup in the initial assessment of a person with hypertension. Most hypertension is classified as primary hypertension. Basic laboratory studies may be done to (1) identify or rule out causes of secondary hypertension, (2) evaluate target organ disease, (3) determine overall cardiovascular risk, or (4) establish baseline levels before starting therapy.

Table 32.5 lists diagnostic studies performed in a person with hypertension. Routine urinalysis, BUN, and serum creatinine levels are used to screen for renal involvement and provide baseline information about kidney function. Creatinine clearance reflects the glomerular filtration rate. Decreases in creatinine clearance indicate renal insufficiency. Chapter 44 discusses serum creatinine and creatinine clearance.

Measurement of serum electrolytes, especially potassium, is essential to detect hyperaldosteronism, a cause of secondary hypertension. Blood glucose levels aid in the diagnosis of diabetes. A lipid profile gives information about risk factors related to atherosclerosis and CVD. Uric acid levels establish a baseline since the levels often rise with diuretic therapy. An electrocardiogram (ECG) gives baseline information about heart status. It can identify the presence of LVH, cardiac ischemia, or previous MI. If LVH is suspected, echocardiography is often done. If the patient's age, history, physical examination, or severity of

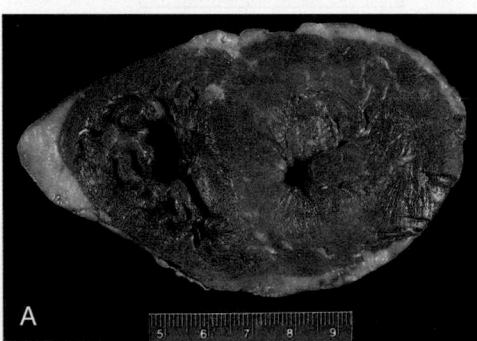
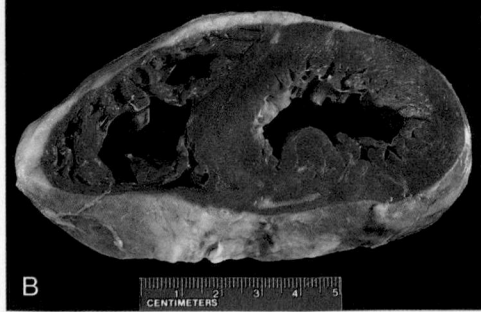

FIG. 32.4 A, Massively enlarged heart caused by hypertrophy of the muscle in the left ventricle. B, Compare with the thickness of the normal left ventricle. The patient had from severe hypertension. (From Kumar V, Cotran RS, Robbins SL: *Robbins basic pathology,* ed 8, Philadelphia, 2007, Saunders.)

TABLE 32.5 Interprofessional Care

Hypertension

Diagnostic Assessment
- History and physical examination, including an ophthalmic examination
- Fasting blood glucose
- Routine urinalysis
- Basic metabolic panel with eGFR
- Complete blood count
- Serum lipid profile (total lipids, triglycerides, HDL and LDL cholesterol, total-to-HDL cholesterol ratio)
- Serum uric acid, calcium, and magnesium
- 12-Lead ECG

Optional
- 24-hour urinary creatinine clearance
- Echocardiography
- Liver function studies
- Serum thyroid-stimulating hormone (TSH)

Management
- Periodic BP monitoring
  - Home BP monitoring
  - Ambulatory BP monitoring
  - Every 3 to 6 months by an HCP once goal BP is achieved and stabilized
- Nutritional therapy
  - Restrict salt and sodium
  - Restrict cholesterol and saturated fats
  - Maintain adequate intake of potassium and calcium
  - Weight management
- Regular, moderate physical activity
- Tobacco cessation (see Tables 10.4 through 10.6)
- Moderation of alcohol intake
- Stress management techniques (see Chapter 6)
- Antihypertensive drugs (Tables 32.7, 32.8 and 32.9)
- Patient and caregiver teaching

eGFR, Estimated glomerular filtration rate.

hypertension points to a secondary cause, further diagnostic testing is needed.

Ambulatory Blood Pressure Monitoring. Some patients have elevated BP readings in a clinical setting and normal readings when BP is measured elsewhere. This phenomenon is referred to as *"white coat"* hypertension. Ambulatory BP monitoring (ABPM) is one method for diagnosing white coat hypertension. It is a noninvasive, fully automated system that measures BP at preset intervals over a 12- to 24-hour period. The equipment is worn continuously for 24 hours, and results are reviewed by the provider. The monitoring equipment includes a BP cuff and a microprocessing unit that fits into a pouch worn on a shoulder strap or belt. Tell patients to hold their arm still by their side when the device is taking a reading. Have them keep a diary of activities that may affect BP. Other potential applications for ABPM include suspected antihypertensive drug resistance, hypotensive symptoms with antihypertensive therapy, episodic hypertension, or SNS dysfunction.

BP has diurnal variability expressed as sleep-wakefulness difference. For day-active people, BP is highest in the early morning, decreases during the day, and is lowest at night. BP at night (during sleep) usually drops by 10% or more from daytime (awake) BP.[5] ABPM verifies the presence of diurnal variability.

Some patients with hypertension do not show a typical nocturnal dip in BP. They are referred to as "nondippers." Patients at highest risk for CVD are "reverse dippers." These patients have an increase in nighttime systolic BP. Current research is focused on using drugs to optimize cardioprotective effects and convert nondippers and reverse dippers to dippers.

Interprofessional Care

Table 32.5 summarizes the interprofessional care for a patient with hypertension. Goals include achieving and maintaining goal BP and reducing cardiovascular risk and target organ disease. Lifestyle modifications are a part of therapy for all patients with elevated blood pressure and hypertension.

Lifestyle Modifications. Lifestyle modifications are directed toward reducing the patient's BP and overall cardiovascular risk. The AHA's "Life's Simple 7" steps support ways to modify and improve health. These are (1) manage blood pressure, (2) control cholesterol, (3) reduce blood sugar, (4) get active, (5) eat better, (6) lose weight, and (7) stop smoking. Other modifications by the taskforce on hypertension address sodium restrictions and alcohol intake. Tools used by the AHA are available online at *www.heart.org/HEARTORG/Conditions/My-Life-Check---Lifes-Simple-7_UCM_471453_Article.jsp#.Wm1uaainHIU.*

Weight Reduction. Persons who are overweight have an increased incidence of hypertension and increased risk for CVD. Weight reduction has a significant effect on lowering BP in many people. The effect is seen with even moderate weight loss. A rule of thumb is for every 1 kg of weight lost, BP will decrease by 1 mm Hg. When a person decreases caloric intake, sodium and fat intake are usually also reduced. Although reducing the fat content of the diet has not shown any sustained benefits in BP control, it may slow the progress of atherosclerosis and reduce overall CVD risk (see Chapter 33). Weight reduction through a combination of calorie restriction and moderate physical activity is recommended for overweight patients with hypertension (see Chapter 40).

DASH Eating Plan. The DASH (Dietary Approaches to Stop Hypertension) eating plan stresses fruits, vegetables, fat-free or low-fat milk and milk products, whole grains, fish, poultry, beans, seeds, and nuts. Compared with the typical American diet, the plan has less red meat, salt, sweets, added sugars, and sugar-containing beverages. The DASH eating plan significantly lowers BP and reduces low-density lipoprotein (LDL) cholesterol.[7]

Dietary Sodium Reduction. Healthy adults should restrict sodium intake to 2300 mg/day or less. Blacks, people middle aged and older, and those with hypertension, diabetes, or CKD should restrict sodium to 1500 mg/day or less.[7] This involves avoiding foods known to be high in sodium. The AHA calls 6 food groups that are the highest sodium sources throughout the United States the "Salty Six." They recommend not adding salt and reducing intake of foods in these groups: bread products, lunch meat and cured meats, pizza, soup, sandwiches, and poultry (see Table 34.8).

Most adults exceed the recommended limits for sodium. Average sodium intake is around 4200 mg/day in men and 3300 mg/day in women.[8] The patient and caregiver, especially the person who prepares the meals, need to learn about low-sodium diets. Teaching should include reading labels of over-the-counter (OTC) drugs, prepared and packaged foods, and health products (e.g., toothpaste containing baking soda) to identify hidden sources of sodium. Review the patient's typical diet to identify foods high in sodium.

Sodium restriction may be enough to control BP in some patients. This may allow for lower drug dosages. Further, moderate sodium restriction lessens the risk for hypokalemia associated with diuretic therapy. However, the response differs between patients who are salt sensitive or salt resistant.

The significance of other dietary elements for the control of hypertension is not certain. Increased levels of dietary potassium and calcium are associated with lower BP in the general population and those with hypertension. People with hypertension should receive adequate intake of these from food sources. Calcium supplements are not recommended to lower BP.

Moderation of Alcohol Intake. Excess alcohol intake is strongly associated with hypertension. Drinking 3 or more alcoholic drinks a day is a risk factor for CVD and stroke. Men should limit their intake of alcohol to no more than 2 drinks per day and women and lighter weight men to no more than 1 drink per day; 1 drink is defined as 12 oz of regular beer, 5 oz of wine (12% alcohol), or 1.5 oz of 80-proof distilled spirits. Excess alcohol intake that results in cirrhosis is a frequent cause of secondary hypertension.

Physical Activity. A physically active lifestyle is essential to promote good health. The AHA and American College of Sports Medicine recommend that adults perform a moderate-intensity aerobic physical activity for at least 30 minutes most days (i.e., more than 5 days per week) with a goal of at least 150 minutes per week. Exercise goals can be achieved by performing shorter periods of exercise that last at least 10 minutes, several times during a day. Combinations of moderate and vigorous activity are acceptable (e.g., walking briskly for 30 minutes on 2 days of the week and jogging for 20 minutes on 2 other days).[10]

Differences in physical activity guidelines exist for adults age 18 to 65 years, adults over 65 years, and adults age 50 to 64 years with functional limitations. The differences relate to the definition of moderate and vigorous aerobic activity. For adults ages 18 to 65, walking briskly at a pace that noticeably increases the pulse defines moderate-intensity aerobic activity. Jogging at a pace that substantially increases the pulse and causes rapid breathing is an example of vigorous activity for this age group. For all other adults, individual fitness levels guide aerobic intensity.[10]

All adults should perform muscle-strengthening activities using the major muscles of the body at least twice a week. This helps to maintain or increase muscle strength and endurance. Flexibility and balance exercises are recommended at least twice a week for older adults, especially for those at risk for falls.[11] Moderate-intensity activities can lower BP, promote relaxation, and decrease or control body weight. Regular activity of this type can reduce SBP by 4 to 9 mm Hg.[5]

Physical activity is more likely to become a habit if it is safe and enjoyable, fits easily into one's daily schedule, and is inexpensive. Many shopping malls open early in the morning, offering a warm, safe, flat area for walking. Some health clubs offer special "off-peak" rates to encourage physical activity among older adults. Some health insurance carriers offer health club discounts as a benefit to encourage member fitness. Cardiac rehabilitation programs offer supervised exercise and education about cardiovascular risk factor reduction.

Help people with hypertension to increase their physical activity by explaining the need for physical activity, describing the types of physical activities, and aiding in starting an exercise plan. Advise sedentary people to increase activity levels gradually. Those with CVD or other serious health problems need a thorough examination and possibly a stress test before beginning an exercise program.

Avoiding Tobacco Products. Nicotine contained in tobacco causes vasoconstriction and increases BP, especially in people with hypertension. Smoking tobacco is a major risk factor for CVD. The cardiovascular benefits of stopping tobacco use are seen within a year in all age-groups. Strongly encourage everyone, especially patients with hypertension, to avoid tobacco use. Advise those who continue to use tobacco products to monitor their BP during use. Chapter 10 discusses tobacco use and smoking cessation.

Managing Risk Factors. Risk factors can be related to social determinants of health and psychosocial risk factors. These factors can contribute to the risk for developing CVD, and to a poorer prognosis and clinical course in patients with CVD. Social determinants of health are defined by the World Health Organization as "the conditions in which people are born, grow, live, work, and age, and the wider set of forces and systems shaping the conditions of daily life."[12] These factors include socioeconomic status, resources to meet daily needs, emotional and social support systems, stress at work and in family life, educational preparation, access to health care, safe housing, exposure to crime and violence, and negative emotions, such as depression and hostility. Often, these risk factors are clustered. For example, rates of depression tend to be higher in people with job stress or without access to safe housing.

These risk factors have direct effects on the cardiovascular system by activating the SNS and stress hormones. A wide variety of pathophysiologic responses can occur, including hypertension and tachycardia, inflammation, endothelial dysfunction, increased platelet aggregation, insulin resistance, and central obesity.[12]

Social determinants of health and psychosocial risk factors can contribute to CVD indirectly by their impact on lifestyle behaviors and choices. Screening for risk factors is essential so appropriate referrals can be given to help the patient and family. Referrals might include counseling, behavioral interventions, such as community or religious support systems, social work assistance for finding resources, such as fresh fruits and vegetables, or information on housing assistance. Once basic needs are met, options that can be beneficial might include relaxation

training, stress management courses, support groups, and exercise training for people who are not in acute psychologic distress.[13]

Drug Therapy. The following are recommendations for antihypertensive drug therapy from the 2017 High Blood Pressure Clinical Practice Guidelines[5]:

- In patients 65 years or older with an average SBP of more than 130 mm Hg who are ambulatory and living in a community setting, rather than living in a care facility, treatment goals should be to obtain an SBP < 130 mmHg.
- In patients 65 years or older with an average SBP of more than 130 mm Hg who live in a care facility, and/or have multiple comorbidities or limited life expectancy, treatment should be based on patient preference, clinical experiences, and team input.
- In patients over 18 years old with hypertension, known CVD or other risk factors, a BP of 130/80 mm Hg is the goal of treatment.
- In all other patients without CVD or other risk factors, a BP of less than 130/80 mm Hg may be reasonable.

Drugs currently available for treating hypertension have 2 primary actions: (1) decrease the volume of circulating blood and (2) reduce SVR (Tables 32.6, 32.7, and 32.8).[5]

TABLE 32.6 Drug Therapy
Antihypertensive Agents

Drug	Mechanism of Action	Nursing Considerations
Adrenergic Inhibitors		
Central-Acting α-Adrenergic Agonist		
clonidine (Catapres) clonidine patch (Catapres-TTS)	Reduce sympathetic outflow from central nervous system Reduce peripheral sympathetic tone, produces vasodilation, decreases SVR and BP	Sudden discontinuation may cause withdrawal syndrome, including rebound hypertension, tachycardia, headache, tremors, apprehension, sweating Chewing gum or hard candy may relieve dry mouth Alcohol and sedatives increase sedation Transdermal patch may be related to fewer side effects and better adherence
guanabenz guanfacine (Tenex)	Same as clonidine	Same as clonidine, but not available in the transdermal formulation
methyldopa	Same as clonidine	Teach patient about daytime sedation and avoiding hazardous activities Taking a single daily dose at bedtime minimizes the sedative effect
α₁-Adrenergic Blockers		
doxazosin (Cardura) prazosin (Minipress) terazosin	Block α₁-adrenergic effects, producing peripheral vasodilation (decreases SVR and BP) Beneficial effects on lipid profile	Reduced resistance to the outflow of urine in benign prostatic hyperplasia Take at bedtime to reduce risk associated with orthostatic hypotension
phentolamine	Blocks α₁-adrenergic receptors, resulting in peripheral vasodilation (decreases SVR and BP)	Used in the short-term management of pheochromocytoma Used locally to prevent necrosis of skin and subcutaneous tissue after extravasation of adrenergic drug No oral formulation
β-Adrenergic Blockers		
Cardioselective Blockers		
acebutolol (Sectral) atenolol (Tenormin) betaxolol bisoprolol esmolol (Brevibloc) metoprolol (Lopressor)	Block β₁-adrenergic receptors (Table 32.1) Reduce BP by blocking β-adrenergic effects Decrease CO and reduce sympathetic vasoconstrictor tone Decrease renin secretion by kidneys	Monitor pulse and BP regularly Use with caution in patients with diabetes because may depress the tachycardia associated with hypoglycemia and adversely affect glucose metabolism Drug of choice for patients with a history of an MI or HF Less effective BP reduction in black patients Esmolol is for IV use only Lose cardioselectivity at higher doses
Non-Cardioselective Blockers		
nadolol (Corgard) pindolol propranolol (Inderal)	Block β₁- and β₂-adrenergic receptors (Table 32.1) Reduce BP by blocking β₁- and β₂-adrenergic effects	Same as cardioselective, except may cause bronchospasm, especially in patients with a history of asthma

TABLE 32.6 Drug Therapy

Antihypertensive Agents—cont'd

Drug	Mechanism of Action	Nursing Considerations
Mixed α- and β-Blockers		
carvedilol (Coreg) labetalol	α_1-, β_1-, and β_2-adrenergic blocking properties producing peripheral vasodilation and decreased heart rate (Table 32.1) Reduce CO, SVR, and BP	Same as β-blockers IV form is available for hypertensive crisis in hospitalized patients Keep patient supine during IV administration Assess patient tolerance of upright position (severe orthostatic hypotension) before allowing upright activities (e.g., commode)
Angiotensin Inhibitors		
Angiotensin-Converting Enzyme (ACE) Inhibitors		
benazepril (Lotensin) captopril enalapril (Vasotec) fosinopril lisinopril (Zestril) moexipril perindopril quinapril (Accupril) ramipril (Altace) trandolapril (Mavik)	Inhibit ACE, reduce conversion of angiotensin I to angiotensin II (A-II) Inhibit A-II–mediated vasoconstriction	Aspirin and NSAIDs may reduce effectiveness Adding a diuretic enhances effect, but should not be used with potassium-sparing diuretics Can cause an increase in serum creatinine Inhibit breakdown of bradykinin, which may cause a dry, hacking cough that can occur at any point during treatment, even years later Captopril may be given orally for hypertensive crisis
Angiotensin II Receptor Blockers (ARBs)		
azilsartan (Edarbi) candesartan (Atacand) eprosartan (Teveten) irbesartan (Avapro) losartan (Cozaar) olmesartan (Benicar) telmisartan (Micardis) valsartan (Diovan)	Prevent action of A-II and produce vasodilation and increased Na^+ and water excretion	Full effect on BP may not be seen for 3–6 wk Do not affect bradykinin levels, therefore an acceptable alternative to ACE inhibitors in people who develop a dry cough In patients with kidney disease, ACE inhibitors and ARBs should not be used together due to adverse renal effects
Calcium Channel Blockers		
Non-Dihydropyridines		
diltiazem extended release (Cardizem LA) verapamil intermediate release (Calan) verapamil timed-release (Verelan PM)	Inhibit movement of Ca^{++} across cell membrane, resulting in vasodilation Cardioselective resulting in a decrease in heart rate and slowing of AV conduction	Use with caution in patients with HF Grapefruit juice may increase serum concentrations and toxicity of certain calcium channel blockers; avoid concurrent use Used for supraventricular tachydysrhythmias Avoid in patients with second- or third-degree AV block or left ventricular systolic dysfunction
Dihydropyridines		
amlodipine (Norvasc) clevidipine (Cleviprex) felodipine isradipine nicardipine sustained release nifedipine long acting (Procardia XL) nisoldipine (Sular)	Cause vascular smooth muscle relaxation resulting in decreased SVR and arterial BP	More potent peripheral vasodilators Clevidipine is for IV use only; solution must be changed every 12 hrs Use of sublingual short-acting nifedipine in hypertensive emergencies is unsafe and not effective Serious adverse events (e.g., stroke, acute MI) have occurred IV nicardipine is available for hypertensive crisis in hospitalized patients; change peripheral IV infusion sites every 12 hrs
Direct Vasodilators		
fenoldopam (Corlopam)	Activates dopamine receptors, resulting in systemic and renal vasodilation	IV use only for hypertensive crisis in hospitalized patients Use cautiously in patients with glaucoma Patient should remain flat for 1 hr after administration
hydralazine	Reduces SVR and BP by direct arterial vasodilation	IV use for hypertensive crisis in hospitalized patients Twice-daily oral dosage Not used as monotherapy because of side effects Contraindicated in patients with CAD
minoxidil	Reduces SVR and BP by direct arterial vasodilation	Reserved for treatment of severe hypertension associated with renal failure and resistant to other therapy Once- or twice-daily dosage
nitroglycerin	Relaxes arterial and venous smooth muscle, reducing preload and SVR At a low dose, venous dilation predominates; at a higher dose, arterial dilation is present	IV use for hypertensive crisis in hospitalized patients with myocardial ischemia Given by continuous IV infusion with pump or control device
sodium nitroprusside	Direct arterial vasodilation reduces SVR and BP	IV use for hypertensive crisis in hospitalized patients Given by continuous IV infusion with pump or control device Arterial BP monitoring BP recommended Wrap IV solutions with an opaque material to protect from light Stable for 24 hrs then metabolized to cyanide, then thiocyanate Monitor thiocyanate levels with prolonged use (>3 days) or doses $\geq$4 mcg/kg/min

TABLE 32.7 Drug Therapy

Diuretic Agents

Drug	Mechanism of Action	Nursing Considerations
Aldosterone Receptor Blockers		
spironolactone (Aldactone) eplerenone (Inspra)	Inhibit the Na$^+$-retaining and K$^+$-excreting effects of aldosterone in the distal and collecting tubules	Monitor for orthostatic hypotension and hyperkalemia Do not combine with potassium-sparing diuretics or potassium supplements Use with caution in patients on ACE inhibitors or angiotensin II blockers Classified as potassium-sparing diuretics
Loop Diuretics		
bumetanide (Bumex) furosemide (Lasix) torsemide (Demadex)	Inhibit NaCl reabsorption in the ascending limb of the loop of Henle Increase excretion of Na$^+$ and Cl$^-$ More potent diuretic effect than thiazides, but shorter duration of action	Monitor for orthostatic hypotension and electrolyte abnormalities Remain effective despite renal insufficiency Diuretic effect increases at higher doses Less effective for hypertension
Thiazide and Related Diuretics		
chlorothiazide chlorthalidone hydrochlorothiazide indapamide metolazone (Zaroxolyn)	Inhibit NaCl reabsorption in the distal convoluted tubule Increase excretion of Na$^+$ and Cl$^-$ Initial decrease in ECF Sustained decrease in SVR Lower BP moderately in 2–4 wk	Monitor for orthostatic hypotension, hypokalemia, and alkalosis May potentiate cardiotoxicity of digoxin by producing hypokalemia Dietary sodium restriction reduces the risk for hypokalemia NSAIDs can decrease diuretic and antihypertensive effect and potentially cause renal impairment Teach patient to supplement with potassium-rich foods
Potassium-Sparing Diuretics		
amiloride (Midamor) triamterene (Dyrenium)	Reduce K$^+$ and Na$^+$ exchange in the distal and collecting tubules Reduce excretion of K$^+$, H$^+$, Ca^{++}, and Mg^{++}	Monitor for orthostatic hypotension and hyperkalemia Contraindicated in patients with renal failure Use with caution in patients on ACE inhibitors or angiotensin II blockers Avoid potassium supplements
Renin Inhibitors		
Aliskiren hemifumarate (Tekturna)	Directly inhibits renin, thus reducing the conversion of angiotensinogen to angiotensin I	May cause angioedema of the face, extremities, lips, tongue, glottis, and/or larynx Not to be used in pregnancy

ECF, extracellular fluid.

Fig. 32.5 shows the various sites and methods of action of antihypertensive agents. Drugs used in the treatment of hypertension include:

- *Adrenergic-inhibiting agents* act by decreasing the SNS effects that increase BP. Adrenergic inhibitors include drugs that work centrally on the vasomotor center and peripherally to inhibit norepinephrine release or to block the adrenergic receptors on blood vessels.
- *Angiotensin-converting enzyme (ACE) inhibitors* prevent the conversion of angiotensin I to angiotensin II and reduce angiotensin II (A-II)–mediated vasoconstriction and sodium and water retention.
- *A-II receptor blockers (ARBs)* prevent angiotensin II from binding to its receptors in the walls of the blood vessels.
- *Calcium channel blockers (CCB)* increase sodium excretion and cause arteriolar vasodilation by preventing the movement of extracellular calcium into cells.
- *Direct vasodilators* decrease the BP by relaxing the vascular smooth muscle and reducing SVR.
- *Diuretics* promote sodium and water excretion, reduce plasma volume, and reduce the vascular response to catecholamines.

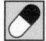 **DRUG ALERT Doxazosin (Cardura)**

- Use caution when giving the first dose. It is best to give the first dose at bedtime to reduce the first dose BP drop.
- Syncope occasionally occurs 30 to 90 min after the first dose, a too-rapid increase in dose, or addition of another antihypertensive agent to therapy.
- Drug interactions (severe low BP) can occur with patients taking phosphodiesterase inhibitors, such as sildenafil (Viagra) or tadalafil (Cialis).

The preferred first-line therapy for patients with stage 1 hypertension includes nonpharmacologic treatment and 1 first-line pharmacologic drug. The 3 preferred 3 first-line drugs are a thiazide diuretic, a calcium channel blocker, and an ACE inhibitor or ARB. For most patients, a diuretic should be the first drug ordered.[5] Patients with stage 2 hypertension will receive nonpharmacologic treatment and 2 antihypertensive agents from difference classifications. If a drug is not tolerated or is contraindicated, then a drug from another class is used.

Once antihypertensive therapy is started, patients should return for follow-up and dosage adjustments at monthly intervals until the goal BP is reached. More frequent visits are needed for patients with stage 2 hypertension or with co-morbidities.

TABLE 32.8 Drug Therapy
Combination Therapy for Hypertension

Combinations	Trade Names
Angiotensin-Converting Enzyme Inhibitors and Diuretics	
benazepril/hydrochlorothiazide	Lotensin HCT
enalapril/hydrochlorothiazide	Vaseretic
lisinopril/hydrochlorothiazide	Zestoretic
Angiotensin II Receptor Blockers and Calcium Channel Blockers	
olmesartan/amlodipine	Azor
telmisartan/amlodipine	Twynsta
valsartan/amlodipine	Exforge
Angiotensin II Receptor Blockers and Diuretics	
candesartan/hydrochlorothiazide	Atacand HCT
losartan/hydrochlorothiazide	Hyzaar
olmesartan medoxomil/hydrochlorothiazide	Benicar HCT
valsartan/hydrochlorothiazide	Diovan HCT
Angiotensin II Receptor Blocker, Diuretic, and Calcium Channel Blocker	
amlodipine/hydrochlorothiazide/valsartan	Exforge HCT
β-Blockers and Diuretics	
metoprolol/hydrochlorothiazide	Lopressor HCT
nadolol/bendroflumethiazide	Corzide
olmesartan medoxomil/amlodipine/ hydrochlorothiazide	Tribenzor
Calcium Channel Blocker and Angiotensin-Converting Enzyme Inhibitor	
amlodipine/benazepril	Lotrel
Diuretics and Diuretics	
spironolactone/hydrochlorothiazide	Aldactazide
triamterene/hydrochlorothiazide	Dyazide, Maxzide

After BP is at goal and stable, follow-up visits can usually be at 3- to 6-month intervals. Comorbidities (e.g., HF), associated diseases (e.g., diabetes), and the need for ongoing monitoring (e.g., laboratory testing) influence the frequency of visits.

Patient and Caregiver Teaching Related to Drug Therapy. Side effects of antihypertensive therapy are common and may be so severe or undesirable that the patient does not adhere to the therapy.[5] Telling the patient about side effects that may reduce with time may help the person to continue with therapy. The number or severity of side effects may relate to the dose. It may be necessary to change the drug or decrease the dose. Advise the patient to report all side effects to the HCP.

A common side effect of several of the antihypertensive drugs is orthostatic hypotension. It results from a change in the autonomic nervous system's mechanisms for regulating BP, which are needed for position changes. Consequently, the patient may feel dizzy and faint when assuming an upright position after sitting or lying down. Table 32.12 (later in this chapter) presents specific measures to control or decrease orthostatic hypotension.

Sexual problems may occur with many antihypertensive drugs. This can be a significant reason that patients do not adhere to the treatment plan. Problems can range from reduced libido to erectile dysfunction. Rather than discussing a sexual problem with an HCP, the patient may decide just to stop therapy.

Approach the patient on this sensitive subject and encourage discussion of any sexual problems. The sexual problems may be easier for the patient to discuss once you explain that the drug may be the source of the problem.

Changing to another antihypertensive drug can decrease or relieve these side effects. Encourage the patient to discuss sexual issues with the HCP. If the patient is reluctant to do so, offer to alert the HCP to the side effects that the patient has. There are many options for treating hypertension, and a plan that is acceptable to the patient should be the goal.

Some unpleasant side effects result from a drug's therapeutic effect, but these can be decreased. For example, diuretics cause dry mouth and frequent voiding. Sugarless gum or hard candy may help ease the dry mouth. Taking diuretics earlier in the day may limit frequent voiding during the night and preserve sleep.

Resistant Hypertension. Carefully explore all reasons why a patient may not be at goal BP (Table 32.9). *Resistant hypertension* is the failure to reach goal BP in patients who are taking full doses of an appropriate 3-drug therapy regimen that includes a diuretic. Resistant hypertension carries a 2- to 6-fold increase in complications including MI and stroke over other hypertensive patients. Treatments focus on identifying potential factors that could contribute to hypertension, assessing adherence, and evaluating alternative drug combinations. Overactive renal nerves can be a cause of resistant hypertension. Percutaneous catheter-based radiofrequency ablation of the renal nerves (known as *renal denervation*) may help lower BP and SNS activity in patients with resistant hypertension. But, we need more evidence to support this treatment as a standard of care.

❖ NURSING MANAGEMENT: PRIMARY HYPERTENSION

◆ Nursing Assessment

Table 32.10 presents subjective and objective data to obtain from a patient with hypertension.

TABLE 32.9 Causes of Resistant Hypertension

- **Causes of pseudoresistant hypertension:**
  - Improper BP measurements (i.e., inappropriate BP cuff size)
  - Inadequate drug doses
  - Inappropriate drug therapy
  - Poor adherence to drug regimen (e.g., due to side effects, finances)
  - White coat syndrome
- **Volume overload**
  - Excess salt intake
  - Volume retention from kidney disease
  - Inadequate diuretic therapy
  - Drug-induced
  - Corticosteroids
  - Cyclosporine and tacrolimus (Prograf)
  - Erythropoietin
  - Illegal drugs (e.g., cocaine, amphetamines)
  - Licorice
  - Nonsteroidal antiinflammatory drugs
  - Oral contraceptives
  - OTC dietary or herbal supplements and drugs (e.g., ma huang, bitter orange)
  - Sympathomimetics (e.g., decongestants, diet pills)
- **Associated conditions**
  - Excess alcohol intake
  - Increasing obesity

Source: Brandani L: Resistant hypertension: A therapeutic challenge, *J Clin Hypertens* 20:76, 2018.

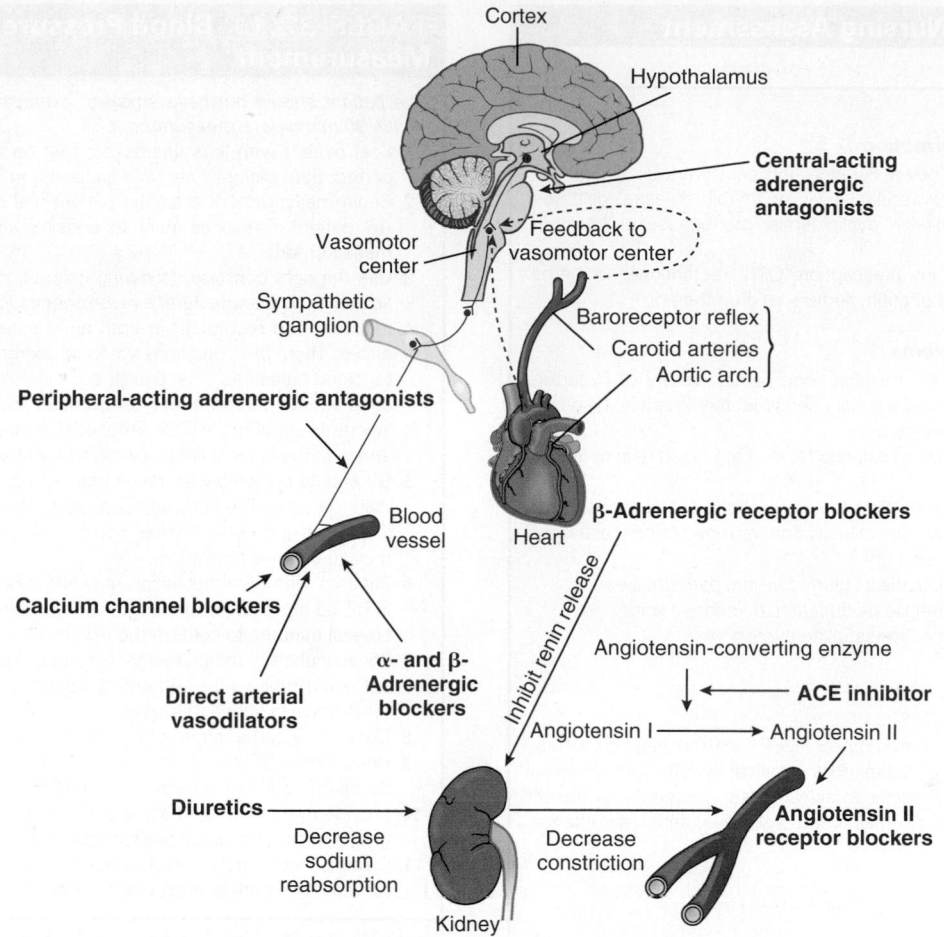

FIG. 32.5 Site and method of action of various antihypertensive drugs (*bold type*). (From US Department of Health and Human Services: Seventh report of the Joint National Committee on Prevention, Detection, Evaluation, and Treatment of High Blood Pressure [JNC 7], Washington, DC, 2003, National Institutes of Health.)

◆ Nursing Diagnoses

Nursing diagnoses and collaborative problems for the patient with hypertension include:

- Altered blood pressure
- Ineffective tissue perfusion
- Impaired sexual function
- Potential complication: stroke, MI

◆ Planning

Nursing care focuses on the priority problems of maintaining BP at a level that decreases complications and supporting the patient to manage what may be a complicated drug regimen with many side effects. The overall goals for the patient with hypertension are that the patient will (1) achieve and maintain the goal BP; (2) have minimal side effects of therapy; and (3) manage and cope with this condition.

◆ Nursing Implementation

◆ Health Promotion.
Primary prevention of hypertension is a cost-effective approach. Current recommendations for primary prevention include lifestyle modifications that prevent or delay the rise in BP in at-risk people. Following the DASH diet and reducing sodium can lower BP. This diet is recommended for primary prevention in the general population. Dietary changes

by the food industry (e.g., reducing the amount of salt in processed foods) may be useful.

The National Heart, Lung, and Blood Institute provides web-based educational materials in several languages for HCPs, patients, and the public to raise awareness about the dangers of high BP. Search available publications at *https://catalog.nhlbi.nih.gov/*.

Individual Patient Evaluation. Hypertension is usually discovered through routine screening for insurance, employment, and military physical examinations. You are in an ideal position to assess for the presence of hypertension, identify the risk factors for hypertension and CAD, and teach patients about these conditions. In addition to BP measurement, a health assessment should include such factors as age, gender, and race; diet history (including salt and alcohol intake); weight patterns; tobacco use; and family history of CVD, stroke, renal disease, and diabetes. Note all drugs taken, prescribed, OTC, and recreational. Last, ask the patient about a history of high BP and the results of any treatment.

Blood Pressure Measurement. Proper size and correct placement of the BP cuff are critical for accurate measurement (Table 32.11). Place the cuff snugly around the patient's bare upper arm with the midline of the bladder of the cuff (usually marked on the cuff by the manufacturer) placed in line with the brachial artery. Place the patient's arm at the level of the heart

TABLE 32.10 Nursing Assessment

Hypertension

Subjective Data
Important Health Information
- *Past health history:* Known duration and past workup of high BP; cardiovascular, cerebrovascular, renal, or thyroid disease; diabetes; pituitary disorders; obesity; dyslipidemia; menopause or hormone replacement status
- *Medications:* Use of any prescription, OTC, recreational, or herbal drugs or products; use of antihypertensive drug therapy

Functional Health Patterns
- *Health perception–health management:* Family history of hypertension or CVD; tobacco use, alcohol use; sedentary lifestyle; health literacy; readiness for change
- *Nutritional-metabolic:* Usual salt and fat intake; weight gain or loss
- *Elimination:* Nocturia
- *Activity-exercise:* Fatigue; dyspnea on exertion, palpitations, exertional chest pain; intermittent claudication, muscle cramps; usual pattern and type of exercise
- *Cognitive-perceptual:* Dizziness; blurred vision; paresthesias
- *Sexual-reproductive:* Erectile dysfunction, decreased libido
- *Coping–stress tolerance:* Stressful life events

Objective Data
Cardiovascular
- SBP consistently >130 mm Hg or DBP >80 mm Hg; orthostatic changes in BP and HR; bilateral BPs significantly different; abnormal heart sounds; laterally displaced apical pulse; decreased or absent peripheral pulses; carotid, renal, or femoral bruits; peripheral edema

Gastrointestinal
- Obesity (BMI ≥30 kg/m²); abnormal waist-hip ratio

Neurologic
- Mental status changes

Possible Diagnostic Findings
- Abnormal serum electrolytes (especially potassium); ↑ BUN, creatinine, glucose, cholesterol, and triglyceride levels; proteinuria, albuminuria, microscopic hematuria; evidence of ischemic heart disease and left ventricular hypertrophy on ECG; evidence of structural heart disease and left ventricular hypertrophy on echocardiogram; evidence of arteriovenous nicking, retinal hemorrhages, and papilledema on funduscopic examination

TABLE 32.11 Blood Pressure Measurement

The patient should not have smoked, exercised, or ingested caffeine within 30 min before measurement.

1. Seat patient with legs uncrossed, feet on the floor, and back supported. Bare patient's arm and support it at heart level.
2. Begin measurement after the patient has rested quietly for 5 min. Ask patient to relax as much as possible and not to talk during the measurement.
3. Use the right cuff size, following instructions for fit and placement according to manufacturer's recommendations.
4. Measure and record BP in both arms initially and note any differences. There are conditions when an extremity should not be used for blood pressures. These exclusions include, but are not limited to, deep venous thrombosis, arteriovenous fistula or graft, peripherally inserted central line (PICC), lymphedema, and limb ischemia. Use the arm with the highest BP and verify the reference point is at the heart.
5. BP should preferably be taken with an oscillometric device, rather than manually. The accuracy of oscillometric devices may be limited if patients are hypertensive, hypotensive, or have heart dysrhythmias (e.g., atrial fibrillation).
6. Patients with atrial fibrillation may HR variations causing variations in BP, so it is recommended to take 3 different measurements over several minutes to confirm the BP.
7. For auscultatory measurement, estimate SBP by palpating the radial pulse and inflating the cuff until the pulse disappears. Inflate the cuff 20–30 mm Hg above this level.
8. Deflate the cuff at a rate of 2–3 mm Hg/sec.
9. Record the SBP and DBP. Note the SBP when the first of 2 or more Korotkoff sounds are heard and the DBP when sound disappears.
10. Provide the patient (verbally and in writing) with the BP reading, BP goal, and recommendations for follow-up.
11. Clean BP cuffs between patients according to the agencies policy for reusable medical equipment cleaning.

Source: Whelton PK, Carey RM, Aronow WS, et al: 2017 ACC/AHA/AAPA/ABC/ACPM/AGS/APhA/ASH/ASPC/NMA/PCNA guideline for the prevention, detection, evaluation, and management of high blood pressure in adults: A report of the American College of Cardiology/AHA Task Force on Clinical Practice Guidelines, *Journal of the American College of Cardiology* 71:e127, 2018.

! SAFETY ALERT Blood Pressure Measurement
- If using the forearm rather than the upper arm for BP measurement, document the site.
- BP cuffs that are too small or too large will result in readings that are falsely high or low, respectively.
- If bilateral BP measurements are not equal, record this finding and use the arm with the highest BP for all future measurements.

during BP measurement. For BP measurements taken in the sitting position, raise and support the arm at the level of the heart. For measurements taken in a supine position, raise and support (e.g., with a small pillow) the arm at heart level. If the arm is resting on the bed, it will be below heart level.

BP can be measured using the auscultatory (oscillatory) method.[14] Note any differences in measurements between each arm. Atherosclerosis in the subclavian artery can cause a falsely low reading on the side where the narrowing occurs.

If neither upper arm can be used to measure the BP (e.g., the presence of IV lines, fistula), or if a maximum size BP cuff does not fit the upper arm, use the forearm. In this case, position the proper size cuff midway between the elbow and the wrist. Auscultate Korotkoff sounds over the radial artery or use a Doppler device to note SBP. Use of an oscillometric device on the forearm is acceptable. Forearm and upper arm BPs are not interchangeable.[14]

Assess for orthostatic (or postural) changes in BP and HR in older adults, people taking antihypertensive drugs, and patients who report symptoms consistent with reduced BP on standing (e.g., light-headedness, dizziness, syncope). Measure serial BP and HR with the patient in the supine, sitting, and standing positions. First, have the patient lie down for 5 minutes then measure BP and HR. Help the patient to a standing position and measure the BP and HR both 1 minute and 3 minutes after standing. Record all 3 measurements, noting the patient's position and corresponding measurement. Usually, the SBP decreases slightly (less than 10 mm Hg) on standing, while the DBP and pulse increase slightly. **Orthostatic hypotension** occurs when a patient moves from a supine to standing position, and there is a decrease of 20 mm Hg or more in SBP, a decrease of 10 mm Hg or more in DBP, and/or an increase in the HR of 20 beats/min. Document any lightheadedness or dizziness during the procedure, which is considered an abnormal finding.[15] Common causes of orthostatic hypotension include dehydration and inadequate vasoconstrictor mechanisms related to disease or drug therapy.

Some people have a wide gap between the first Korotkoff sound and subsequent beats. This is called the *auscultatory gap*. Failure to inflate the cuff high enough may result in an inaccurate SBP, one that is too low for the patient.

In acute care settings, BP measurement is usually done to assess vital signs, volume status, and effects of drugs, rather than to diagnose hypertension. Trends in BP are more important than a single value. Inform the HCP of any patient with a persistent elevated BP. These patients should be evaluated for hypertension.[5]

Verifying how blood pressures are obtained at home is important when assessing for potential hypertension. Ensure that the home machine has been validated for accuracy and the patient records measurements to review later and measures the pressure at the same time of day for consistency. Confirming office BP readings with blood pressures obtained at home can help determine average BP.

Screening Programs. Screening programs in the community are widely used to identify persons who have a high BP. At the time of the BP measurement, give each person a written, numeric value of the reading. Explain why further evaluation is needed.

NURSING MANAGEMENT
Caring for the Patient With Hypertension

You will need to collaborate with many health care team members to deliver, delegate, and coordinate care based on the patient's status.
- Develop and conduct hypertension screening programs.
- Assess patients for hypertension risk factors and develop risk modification plans.
- Teach patients about lifestyle management and drug therapy.
- Monitor for adverse effects of antihypertensive drugs.
- Evaluate the effectiveness of lifestyle management and drug therapy in decreasing BP to acceptable levels.
- Teach about home BP monitoring, including the correct use of automatic BP monitors. Check that the device chosen by the patient meets the Association for the Advancement of Medical Instrumentation standards *(www.dableducational.org/sphygmomanometers/devices_1_clinical.html#ClinTable)*.
- Make appropriate referrals to other HCPs, such as dietitians or stress management programs.
- Monitor for complications of hypertension, such as CAD, HF, cerebrovascular disease, PVD, and renal disease.
- Assess the patient with a hypertensive crisis for evidence of target organ disease (e.g., encephalopathy, renal insufficiency, cardiac decompensation).
- Manage the patient with hypertensive urgency or emergency, including giving drugs and evaluating for resolution of the crisis.
- Oversee UAP:
- Obtain accurate BP readings in outpatient and inpatient settings.
- Report high or low BP readings at once to RN.
- Check postural BPs as directed.

Collaborate With Other Team Members
Dietitian
- Obtain a diet history from the patient.
- Teach the components of the DASH diet.
- Provide instructions for dietary changes as needed.

Physical Therapist
- Assess patient's current level of fitness.
- Develop an exercise plan with the patient.

Focus efforts on (1) controlling BP in persons already identified as having hypertension; (2) identifying and controlling BP in at-risk groups, such as blacks, obese people, and blood relatives of people with hypertension; (3) screening those with limited access to health care; and (4) connecting persons with a HCP and/or health insurance if needed.

Cardiovascular Risk Factor Modification. Teaching about CVD risk factors is appropriate for all persons. Modifiable CVD risk factors include hypertension, obesity, diabetes, tobacco use, and physical inactivity. Discuss lifestyle modifications based on identified risk factors. Table 32.12 discusses general information and health-promoting behaviors for patients with hypertension.

◆ **Ambulatory Care.** Your primary role in the long-term management of hypertension is to assist the patient to reach the goal BP and adhere to the treatment plan. Your actions include

TABLE 32.12 Patient & Caregiver Teaching
Hypertension

When teaching the patient and/or caregiver about hypertension, include the following information:

General Instructions
- Give patient the BP reading and explain what it means (e.g., high, low, goal, borderline).
- Encourage patient to monitor BP at home and teach the patient to call the HCP if BP exceeds high or low limits set by HCP.
- Hypertension is usually asymptomatic, and symptoms (e.g., nosebleeds) do not reliably indicate BP levels.
- Long-term therapy and follow-up care are necessary to treat hypertension. Therapy involves lifestyle changes (e.g., weight management, sodium reduction, smoking cessation, regular physical activity) and, in most cases, drugs to regulate the BP.
- Therapy will not cure but should control, hypertension.
- Controlled hypertension usually results in an excellent prognosis.
- Explain the potential dangers of uncontrolled hypertension (e.g., stroke, heart attack).

Instructions Related to Medication Therapy
- Be specific about the names, actions, dosages, and side effects of prescribed drugs.
- Help the patient plan regular and convenient times for taking medications and measuring BP.
- Do not stop drugs abruptly since withdrawal may cause a severe hypertensive reaction.
- Do not double up on a dose when a dose is missed.
- If BP increases or decreases, do not change the dose of the drug without consulting the HCP.
- Do not take any drugs belonging to someone else.
- Supplement diet with foods high in potassium (e.g., citrus fruits, green leafy vegetables) if taking potassium-wasting diuretics.
- Avoid hot baths, excess amounts of alcohol, and strenuous exercise within 3 hours of taking drugs that promote vasodilation.
- Many drugs cause orthostatic hypotension. Reduce the effects of orthostatic hypotension by rising slowly from the bed, sitting on the side of the bed for a few minutes, standing slowly, and beginning to move if no symptoms develop (e.g., dizziness, lightheadedness). Do not stand still for prolonged periods, do leg exercises to increase venous return, or sleep with the head of the bed raised. Do lie or sit down when dizziness occurs.
- Some drugs cause sexual problems (e.g., erectile dysfunction, decreased libido). Consult with the HCP about changing drugs or dosages if sexual problems develop.
- Some side effects may decrease with time (e.g., fatigue, diarrhea).
- Be careful about taking potentially high-risk OTC drugs, such as high-sodium antacids, NSAIDs, appetite suppressants, and cold and sinus medications. Read warning labels and consult with a pharmacist.

evaluating therapeutic effectiveness, detecting and reporting any adverse treatment effects, assessing and enhancing adherence, and patient and caregiver teaching.

Home BP Monitoring. Most patients with known or suspected hypertension should monitor their BP at home. Home BP monitoring reduces the white coat effect. The readings are often lower than those taken in the office setting and are a better predictor of CVD risk. Home BP readings may help achieve patient adherence by reinforcing the need to remain on therapy. However, some patients become overly concerned with the BP readings. Provide information that will help patients understand what their goal or target BP is and why.

CHECK YOUR PRACTICE

You are making a home visit for a 78-yr-old woman who is recovering from a hip replacement after she fractured her femur. She currently takes a combination of lisinopril/hydrochlorothiazide. The patient's daughter (her caregiver) tells you that her BP that morning was 150/88 and then she took it 2 more times and it was the same. They are both worried and anxious that something is wrong because they heard that a BP over 120/80 is very bad.
- What should you do? What teaching would you provide?

Patient teaching is critical to ensure accuracy. Tell patients to buy an oscillometric BP monitor that uses a cuff for the upper arm or wrist. The patient should bring the BP monitor to the office to verify proper cuff size, the accuracy of the device, and the patient's technique.

Teach the patient to obtain a BP according to the steps in Table 32.11. Tell the patient to measure BP in the nondominant arm, or arm with the higher BP if there is a known difference between arms. Tell the patient to measure BP first thing in the morning (if possible, before taking any drugs) and at night before going to bed. Have the patient record all BP measurements and bring the record to office visits.

For clinical decision making (e.g., changes in dosage, starting a new drug), tell patients to take BP readings as described for 1 week. Stable, normotensive patients should measure morning and evening BP for at least 1 week every 3 months. Devices that have memory or printouts of the readings are convenient for reporting.[5]

INFORMATICS IN PRACTICE

Monitoring Blood Pressure

- Smartphone and computer applications can help patients manage their care, including BP self-monitoring, medication history, and appointment tracking. Patients can enter a variety of variables including SBP and DBP, HR, time of day, arm or wrist used, and position (e.g., lying, sitting).
- Remote BP monitoring using telehealth technology can be used with those who have limited access to health care services.
- Reports can be used to evaluate BP control.

Patient Adherence. A significant problem in the long-term management of the patient with hypertension is poor adherence to the treatment plan. The reasons for nonadherence are complicated and can include inadequate patient teaching, low health literacy, unpleasant drug side effects, the BP returns to normal range with the therapy, the high cost of drugs, and lack of insurance.

It is important to determine the reasons why a patient is not adhering to treatment. Assess the patient's diet, activity level, and lifestyle as other indicators of adherence. Develop a plan with the patient and caregiver to improve adherence. The plan should be compatible with the patient's habits, cultural beliefs, and lifestyle. Active patient participation increases the chance of adherence to the plan. Measures include involving the patient in choosing drugs that are affordable and involving caregivers to help increase patient adherence.

Substituting combination drugs for multiple drugs once the BP is stable may promote adherence. They reduce the number of pills that the patient must take each day and may reduce costs. Combination drugs are shown in Table 32.8.

It is important to help the patient and caregiver understand that hypertension is a chronic illness that cannot be cured. Stress that it can be controlled with drug therapy, diet changes, physical activity, periodic follow-up, and other relevant lifestyle modifications.

◆ Evaluation

The overall expected outcomes are that the patient with hypertension will
- Achieve and maintain goal BP as defined for the person
- Understand, accept, and implement the treatment plan
- Report minimal side effects of drug therapy

Gerontologic Considerations: Hypertension

The prevalence of hypertension increases with age. The lifetime risk for developing hypertension is around 90% for normotensive men and women over age 55. Older adults are more likely to have white coat hypertension.[5]

The pathophysiology of hypertension in the older adult involves several age-related physical changes: (1) loss of elasticity in large arteries from atherosclerosis, (2) increased collagen content and stiffness of the myocardium, (3) increased peripheral vascular resistance, (4) decreased adrenergic receptor sensitivity, (5) blunting of baroreceptor reflexes, (6) decreased renal function, and (7) decreased renin response to sodium and water depletion.

In the older adult who is taking antihypertensive drugs, absorption of some agents may be altered because of decreased blood flow to the gut. Metabolism and excretion may be prolonged.

Current recommendations for target BP goals in people older than 65 years of age who live independently are no different for other independent living adults under 65 years old. Care should be taken to assess for orthostatic hypotension and acute kidney injury in patients over 65 years old. Older adults who have multiple comorbidities and do not live independently (i.e., skilled facility) should have gradual titrations of antihypertensives to minimize complications.[5]

Orthostatic hypotension often occurs in older adults because of varying degrees of impaired baroreceptor reflexes. Orthostatic hypotension in this age group is often associated with volume depletion or chronic disease states, such as decreased renal and hepatic function or electrolyte imbalance.

Older adults may have postprandial drops in BP. The most significant decrease occurs about 1 hour after eating. BP returns to preprandial levels 3 to 4 hours after eating. Drugs should be started at low doses and increased slowly to reduce the chance of orthostatic hypotension. Measure BP and HR in the supine, sitting, and standing positions at every visit.

After CVD, arthritis is the second most prevalent disease in older adults. Older adults most often take prescription and OTC nonsteroidal antiinflammatory drugs (NSAIDs). Nonselective NSAIDs (e.g., ibuprofen) and selective NSAIDs (e.g., celecoxib) can cause loss of BP control and HF. There is the potential for adverse renal effects and/or hyperkalemia when NSAIDs are used with ACE inhibitors, ARBs, or aldosterone antagonists.

HYPERTENSIVE CRISIS

Hypertensive crisis is a term used to indicate either a hypertensive urgency or emergency. A hypertensive crisis occurs at systolic BP greater than 180 mm Hg and/or diastolic BP greater than 120 mm Hg. BPs often can be greater than 220/140 mm Hg. Difference between hypertensive urgency and emergency are the presence of target organ damage and the type of treatment the patient will receive.

Hypertensive emergencies have evidence of target organ disease. It most often requires hospitalization for immediate, controlled reduction of BP. Without prompt treatment, a hypertensive emergency can produce severe problems. These include encephalopathy, intracranial or subarachnoid hemorrhage, HF, MI, renal failure, dissecting aortic aneurysm, and retinopathy.[16] Untreated hypertensive emergencies have a 1-year mortality rate of more than 79%, so prompt recognition and treatment are essential to decrease the threat to organ function and life.

Hypertensive urgency has no clinical evidence of target organ disease. Hospitalization may not be needed to correct the BP. Hypertensive urgency is much more common than hypertensive emergency. It may be associated with chronic, stable complications such as stable angina, chronic HF, or prior MI or cerebrovascular accident with no threat of an acute event.

A hypertensive crisis occurs more often in patients with a history of hypertension who have not adhered to their medication regimens or who have been undermedicated. Rapidly increasing BP can cause shearing of the endothelial surface due to turbulent blood flow within the vessels leading to further vascular damage and the release of more vasoconstricting substances. A vicious cycle of BP elevation follows, leading to life-threatening damage to target organs.

Hypertensive crisis related to cocaine or crack use is a frequent problem. Other drugs, such as amphetamines, phencyclidine (PCP), and lysergic acid diethylamide (LSD), can cause a hypertensive crisis that may be complicated by drug-induced seizures, stroke, MI, or encephalopathy. Table 32.13 lists causes of hypertensive crisis.

Clinical Manifestations

A hypertensive emergency often presents as *hypertensive encephalopathy*, a syndrome in which a sudden rise in BP is associated with a severe headache, nausea, vomiting, seizures, confusion, and coma. The manifestations of encephalopathy are the result of increased

cerebral capillary permeability, which can lead to cerebral edema and disruption in cerebral function. On retinal examination, exudates, hemorrhages, and/or papilledema are found (Fig. 32.6).

Renal insufficiency ranging from minor injury to complete renal failure can occur. Rapid cardiac decompensation ranging from unstable angina to MI and pulmonary edema is possible. Patients can have chest pain and dyspnea. Aortic dissection can develop and will cause sudden, severe chest and back pain with reduced or absent pulses in the extremities.

◆ Interprofessional and Nursing Management

Hypertensive emergencies require hospitalization, IV administration of antihypertensive drugs, and intensive monitoring. BP level alone is not the major factor in deciding the treatment for a hypertensive crisis. The link between elevated BP and signs of new or progressive target organ disease determines the seriousness of the situation.

When treating hypertensive emergencies, we often use the mean arterial pressure (MAP instead of BP readings to guide and evaluate therapy. Calculate the MAP as follows:

$$MAP = (SBP + 2\,DBP) \div 3$$

The initial goal is to decrease MAP by no more than 20% to 25% or to decrease MAP to 110 to 115 mm Hg. If the patient is clinically stable, drugs can be titrated to gradually lower BP over the next 24 hours. Lowering the BP too quickly or too much may decrease cerebral, coronary, or renal perfusion. A rapid decrease could cause a stroke, MI, or renal failure.

> ### ? CHECK YOUR PRACTICE
>
> A 68-yr-old male patient presents to the emergency department with a BP 210/118 and reporting a severe headache and vomiting. You know that his BP is dangerously high and must be lowered.
> - Calculate his MAP.
> - What treatments would you expect to be ordered for this patient?

Patients with aortic dissection require special consideration. These patients should have their SBP lowered to less than 100 to 120 mm Hg as soon as possible (if tolerated). Another exception is patients with acute ischemic stroke. Their BP is lowered to allow the use of thrombolytic agents. Last, an elevated BP in the

TABLE 32.13 Causes of Hypertensive Crisis

- Acute aortic dissection
- Exacerbation of chronic hypertension
- Head injury
- Monoamine oxidase inhibitors are taken with tyramine-containing foods
- Pheochromocytoma
- Preeclampsia, eclampsia
- Rebound hypertension (from abrupt withdrawal of some antihypertensive drugs, such as clonidine or β-blockers)
- Recreational drug use (cocaine, amphetamines)
- Renovascular hypertension

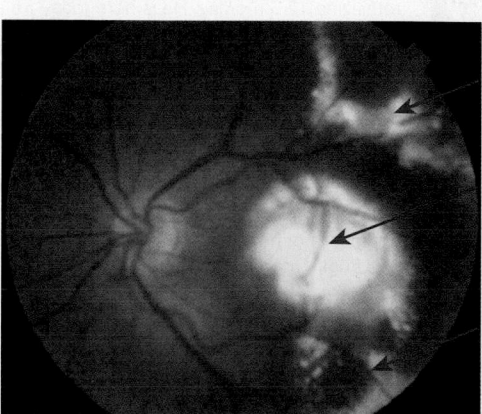

FIG. 32.6 Massive retinal exudates (indicated by *arrows*) from hypertensive retinopathy. To see what a normal retina looks like on ophthalmoscopic examination, see Fig. 20.7. (From Kliegman RM, Behrman RE, Jenson HB, Stanton B: *Nelson textbook of pediatrics*, ed 18, Philadelphia, 2011, Saunders.)

immediate poststroke period may be a compensatory response to improve cerebral perfusion to ischemic brain tissue. There is no evidence supporting the use of antihypertensive drugs in these patients (see Chapter 57).[5]

IV agents used for hypertensive emergencies include vasodilators (e.g., sodium nitroprusside, fenoldopam, nicardipine), adrenergic inhibitors (e.g., phentolamine, labetalol, esmolol), and the calcium channel blocker clevidipine (Cleviprex). Sodium nitroprusside is the most effective IV drug to treat hypertensive emergencies. Oral agents may be given along with IV ones to help make an earlier transition to long-term therapy.

> **DRUG ALERT Labetalol**
> - Teach patient not to stop the drug abruptly.
> - Abrupt cessation may precipitate angina or HF.

Antihypertensive drugs given IV have a rapid (within seconds to minutes) onset of action. Assess the patient's BP and HR every 2 to 3 minutes during their initial administration. Use an arterial line (see Chapter 65) or an automated, noninvasive BP machine to monitor the BP. Titrate the drug according to MAP or BP as ordered. Monitor the ECG for dysrhythmias and signs of ischemia or MI. Use extreme caution in treating the patient with CAD or cerebrovascular disease. Measure urine output hourly to assess renal perfusion. Patients receiving IV agents may be on bed rest. Getting up (e.g., to use the commode) may cause severe cerebral ischemia and fainting.

Ongoing assessment is essential to evaluate the effectiveness of and the patient's response to therapy. Monitor cardiac, lung, and renal systems for decompensation caused by the severe elevation in BP (e.g., angina, pulmonary edema, renal failure).

Frequent neurologic checks, including the level of consciousness, pupillary size and reaction, and movement of extremities, help detect any changes in the patient's condition. The neurologic changes are often like those of a stroke. However, a hypertensive crisis does not show focal or lateralizing signs often seen with a stroke. In a stroke, focal impairments affect a specific region of the body, such as weakness in the left arm or right leg. Lateralizing signs are restricted to one side of the body, such as weakness of an arm or leg.

Hypertensive urgencies usually do not need IV drugs but can be managed with oral agents. The patient with hypertensive urgency may not need hospitalization but will need follow-up. The initial decision for oral antihypertensive agents should be made based on the underlying cause of the hypertensive urgency, the patient characteristics, and comorbidities. Some of the most commonly used oral drugs are captopril, labetalol, clonidine (Catapres), and amlodipine (Norvasc) (Table 32.6).[16] The disadvantage of oral drugs is the inability to regulate the dosage moment to moment, as can be done with IV therapy. A patient with hypertensive urgency who is not hospitalized should have outpatient follow-up care within 24 hours.

Once the hypertensive crisis is resolved, it is essential to determine the cause. The patient will need appropriate management and teaching to avoid future crises.

> **DRUG ALERT Clonidine (Catapres)**
> - Teach patient to change positions slowly to limit orthostatic hypotension.
> - Avoid hazardous activities since the drug may cause drowsiness.
> - Do not stop abruptly as this may cause rebound hypertension.

Not every patient with an elevated BP and no target organ disease will need emergent drug therapy or hospitalization. Allowing the patient to sit for 20 or 30 minutes in a quiet environment may significantly reduce BP. Oral drugs may be started or adjusted. Other interventions include encouraging the patient to share any concerns or fears, answering questions about hypertension, and reducing any adverse stimuli (e.g., excess noise) in the environment.

CASE STUDY

Primary Hypertension

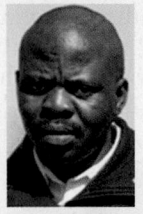

(© iStockphoto/Thinkstock.)

Patient Profile

R.L. is a 45-yr-old black man with no history of hypertension. At a screening clinic 2 months ago, his BP was 150/95 mm Hg. His HCP has followed him for the past month. During this time, he has been taking hydrochlorothiazide 12.5 mg/day. He is here today for a follow-up visit.

Subjective Data
- Father died of stroke at age 60
- Mother is alive but has hypertension and a history of MI
- States that he feels fine and is not a "hyper" person
- Smokes 1 pack of cigarettes daily for the past 28 yrs
- Drinks "about 2" 6-packs of beer on most Friday and Saturday nights
- Has heard that BP drugs "make you impotent"

Objective Data

Physical Examination
- Mild retinopathy (retinal arteriolar narrowing on ophthalmoscopic examination)
- BP: 166/108 mm Hg (highest of 2 readings, 2 min apart)
- Sustained apical impulse palpable in the 4th intercostal space just lateral to the midclavicular line

Diagnostic Studies
- ECG: mild left ventricular hypertrophy
- Urinalysis: protein 30 mg/dL (0.3 g/L)
- Serum creatinine level: 1.6 mg/dL (141 mmol/L)

Interprofessional Care
- Low-sodium, DASH diet
- Hydrochlorothiazide 25 mg/day oral (dose increase)
- Nicardipine sustained-release 30 mg oral twice daily (second drug added)

Discussion Questions
1. What risk factors for hypertension does R.L. have?
2. What evidence of target organ disease is present?
3. ***Patient-Centered Care:*** What misconceptions about hypertension should be corrected?
4. ***Priority Decision:*** Based on the assessment data, what are the priority nursing diagnoses? What are the collaborative problems?
5. ***Evidence-Based Practice:*** R.L. wants to know the most effective nonpharmacologic strategies to lower his BP. What would you tell him?
6. ***Patient-Centered Care:*** What lifestyle preferences should be addressed in R.L.'s plan of care?
7. ***Collaboration:*** What referrals may be indicated?
8. ***Safety:*** What safety precautions should be considered when changing R.L.'s antihypertensive therapy?
9. ***Quality Improvement:*** What outcomes would indicate that interprofessional care was successful?

Answers available at *http://evolve.elsevier.com/Lewis/medsurg.*

BRIDGE TO NCLEX EXAMINATION

The number of the question corresponds to the same-numbered outcome at the beginning of the chapter.

1. Which BP-regulating mechanism(s) can result in the development of hypertension if defective? *(select all that apply)*
   a. Release of norepinephrine
   b. Secretion of prostaglandins
   c. Stimulation of the sympathetic nervous system
   d. Stimulation of the parasympathetic nervous system
   e. Activation of the renin-angiotensin-aldosterone system

2. While obtaining subjective assessment data from a patient with hypertension, the nurse recognizes that a modifiable risk factor for the development of hypertension is
   a. A low-calcium diet.
   b. Excess alcohol intake.
   c. A family history of hypertension.
   d. Consumption of a high-protein diet.

3. In teaching a patient with hypertension about controlling the illness, the nurse recognizes that
   a. All patients with elevated BP need drug therapy.
   b. Obese persons must achieve a normal weight to lower BP.
   c. It is not necessary to limit salt in the diet if taking a diuretic.
   d. Lifestyle modifications are needed for all persons with elevated BP.

4. A *priority* consideration in the management of the older adult with hypertension is to
   a. Prevent primary hypertension from converting to secondary hypertension.
   b. Recognize that the older adult is less likely to adhere to the drug therapy regimen than a younger adult.
   c. Ensure that the patient receives larger initial doses of antihypertensive drugs because of impaired absorption.
   d. Use precise technique in assessing the BP of the patient because of the possible presence of an auscultatory gap.

5. A patient with newly discovered high BP has an average reading of 158/98 mm Hg after 3 months of exercise and diet modifications. Which management strategy will be a *priority* for this patient?
   a. Drug therapy will be needed because the BP is still not at goal.
   b. BP monitoring should continue for 3 months to confirm a diagnosis of hypertension.
   c. Lifestyle changes are less important since they were not effective, and drugs will be started.
   d. More changes in the patient's lifestyle are needed for a longer time before starting drug therapy.

6. A patient is admitted to the hospital in a hypertensive emergency (BP 244/142 mm Hg). Sodium nitroprusside is started to treat the elevated BP. Which management strategies would be *most* appropriate for this patient? *(select all that apply)*
   a. Measuring hourly urine output
   b. Continuous BP monitoring with an arterial line
   c. Decreasing the MAP by 50% within the first hour
   d. Maintaining bed rest and giving tranquilizers to lower the BP
   e. Assessing the patient for signs and symptoms of heart failure and changes in mental status

1. a, c, e, 2. b, 3. d, 4. d, 5. a, 6. a, b, e

For rationales to these answers and even more NCLEX review questions, visit *http://evolve.elsevier.com/Lewis/medsurg*.

ⓔ EVOLVE WEBSITE/RESOURCES LIST

http://evolve.elsevier.com/Lewis/medsurg
Review Questions (Online Only)
Key Points
Answer Keys for Questions
- Rationales for Bridge to NCLEX Examination Questions
- Answer Guidelines for Case Study on p. 696
Student Case Study
Patient With Hypertension and Stroke
Conceptual Care Map Creator
Audio Glossary
Content Updates

REFERENCES

1. Centers for Disease Control and Prevention: High blood pressure facts. Retrieved from *www.cdc.gov/bloodpressure/facts.htm*.
2. Benjamin EJ, Blaha MJ, Chiuve SE, et al: Heart disease and stroke statistics—2017 update: A report from the American Heart Association, *Circulation* 135:e146, 2017.
3. Centers for Disease Control and Prevention: National Health and Nutrition Examination Survey (NHANES). Retrieved from *www.cdc.gov/nchs/nhanes/index.htm*.
4. Merai R, Siegel C, Rakotz M, et al: CDC grand rounds: A public health approach to detect and control hypertension, *MMWR Morb Mortal Wkly Rep* 65:1261, 2016.
*5. Whelton PK, Carey RM, Aronow WS, et al: 2017 ACC/AHA/AAPA/ABC/ACPM/AGS/APhA/ASH/ASPC/NMA/PCNA guideline for the prevention, detection, evaluation, and management of high blood pressure in adults: A report of the American College of Cardiology/AHA Task Force on Clinical Practice Guidelines, *Journal of the American College of Cardiology* 71:e127, 2018.
*6. McKibben RA, Al Rifai M, Mathews LM, et al: Primary prevention of atherosclerotic cardiovascular disease in women, *Curr Cardiovascular Risk Reports* 10:1, 2016.
7. National Heart, Lung, and Blood Institute: DASH eating plan. Retrieved from *www.nhlbi.nih.gov/health-topics/dash-eating-plan*.
8. Kirabo A: A new paradigm of sodium regulation in inflammation and hypertension, *Am J Physiol Regul Integr Comp Physiol* 313:R706, 2017.
9. American Heart Association: What are the symptoms of high blood pressure? Retrieved from *http://www.heart.org/HEARTORG/Conditions/HighBloodPressure/SymptomsDiagnosisMonitoringofHighBloodPressure/What-are-the-Symptoms-of-High-Blood-Pressure_UCM_301871_Article.jsp*.
*10. Haskell WL, Lee I-M, Pate RR, et al: Physical activity and public health: Updated recommendations for adults from the American College of Sports Medicine and the American Heart Association, *Circulation* 116:1081, 2007. (Classic)
*11. Nelson ME, Rejeski WJ, Blair SN, et al: Physical activity and public health in older adults: Recommendation from the American College of Sports Medicine and the American Heart Association, *Circulation* 116:1094, 2007. (Classic)
12. International health constitution of the World Health Organization, *Bulletin of the World Health Organization* 80:983, 2002. (Classic)
13. Rozanski A, Blumenthal JA, Davidson KW, et al: The epidemiology, pathophysiology, and management of psychosocial risk factors in cardiac practice, *J Am Coll Cardiol* 45:637, 2005. (Classic)
*14. AACN Clinical Resources Task Force: AACN practice alert: Non-invasive blood pressure monitoring. Retrieved from *www.aacn.org/~/media/aacn-website/clincial-resources/practice-alerts/nibpadult2016pa.pdf*.
15. CDC's STEADI Tools and Resources: Measuring orthostatic changes. Retrieved from *www.cdc.gov/steadi/pdf/measuring_orthostatic_blood_pressure-a.pdf*.
16. Ipek E, Oktay AA, Krim SR: Hypertensive crisis: An update on clinical approach and management, *Curr Opin Cardiol* 32:397, 2017.

*Evidence-based information for clinical practice.

33

Coronary Artery Disease and Acute Coronary Syndrome

Rose Shaffer

I have witnessed the softening of the hardest hearts with a warm smile.

Goldie Hawn

CONCEPTUAL FOCUS

Adherence	Glucose Regulation	Sexuality
Clotting	Pain	
Fatigue	Perfusion	

LEARNING OUTCOMES

1. Relate the etiology and pathophysiology of coronary artery disease (CAD), chronic stable angina, and acute coronary syndrome (ACS) to the clinical manifestations of each disorder.
2. Describe the nursing role in the promotion of therapeutic lifestyle changes in patients at risk for CAD.
3. Distinguish the precipitating factors, clinical manifestations, and interprofessional and nursing care of the patient with CAD and chronic stable angina.
4. Explain the clinical manifestations, diagnostic studies, complications, and interprofessional and nursing care of the patient with ACS.
5. Outline drug therapy used to treat patients with CAD, chronic stable angina, and ACS.
6. Prioritize key components to include in the rehabilitation of patients recovering from ACS and coronary revascularization procedures.
7. Distinguish the precipitating factors, manifestations, and interprofessional and nursing care of patients who are at risk for or have had sudden cardiac death.

KEY TERMS

acute coronary syndrome (ACS), p. 717
angina, p. 708
atherosclerosis, p. 698
chronic stable angina, p. 708
collateral circulation, p. 699

coronary artery disease (CAD), p. 698
coronary revascularization, p. 714
metabolic equivalent (MET), p. 728
myocardial infarction (MI), p. 718
percutaneous coronary intervention (PCI), p. 714

Prinzmetal's angina, p. 709
silent ischemia, p. 708
stent, p. 714
sudden cardiac death (SCD), p. 730
unstable angina (UA), p. 717

Cardiovascular disease (CVD) is the leading cause of death both globally and in the United States.[1] Coronary artery disease (CAD) is the most common type of CVD. CAD was an underlying cause of death in about 1 of every 7 deaths.[2] Patients with CAD may be asymptomatic or develop chronic stable angina (chest pain). CAD may evolve to more serious conditions of unstable angina (UA) and myocardial infarction (MI), which are referred to as acute coronary syndrome (ACS).

Conceptually, CAD has a profound effect on perfusion. The process of perfusion is based on the heart's ability to generate enough cardiac output (CO) to distribute blood to all body tissues. CAD negatively affects cardiac function, resulting in impaired CO and decreased perfusion. This chapter discusses the care of patients with CAD, chronic stable angina, and ACS and measures to promote optimal perfusion.

CORONARY ARTERY DISEASE

Coronary artery disease (CAD) is a type of blood vessel disorder that we consider in the general category of atherosclerosis. The term **atherosclerosis** comes from 2 Greek words: *athere,* meaning "fatty mush," and *skleros,* meaning "hard."[3] This combination means that atherosclerosis begins as soft deposits of fat that harden with age. That is why many refer to atherosclerosis as "hardening of the arteries." It can occur in any artery in the body. When the *atheromas* (fatty deposits) form in the coronary arteries, the disease is called CAD. The terms *arteriosclerotic heart disease (ASHD), cardiovascular heart disease (CVHD), ischemic heart disease (IHD), coronary heart disease (CHD),* are other terms used to describe CAD. They are often used interchangeably.

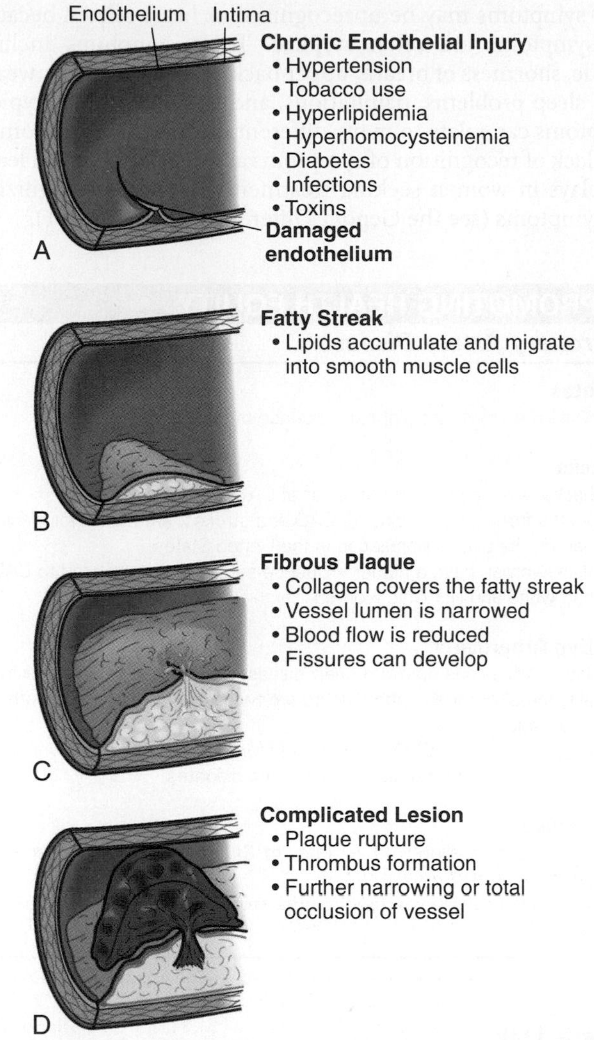

Chronic Endothelial Injury
- Hypertension
- Tobacco use
- Hyperlipidemia
- Hyperhomocysteinemia
- Diabetes
- Infections
- Toxins

Damaged endothelium

Endothelium Intima

A

Fatty Streak
- Lipids accumulate and migrate into smooth muscle cells

B

Fibrous Plaque
- Collagen covers the fatty streak
- Vessel lumen is narrowed
- Blood flow is reduced
- Fissures can develop

C

Complicated Lesion
- Plaque rupture
- Thrombus formation
- Further narrowing or total occlusion of vessel

D

FIG. 33.1 Pathogenesis of atherosclerosis. **A,** Damaged endothelium. **B,** Fatty streak and lipid core formation. **C,** Fibrous plaque covers the lipid core. **D,** Complicated lesion: Plaque rupture with thrombus formation.

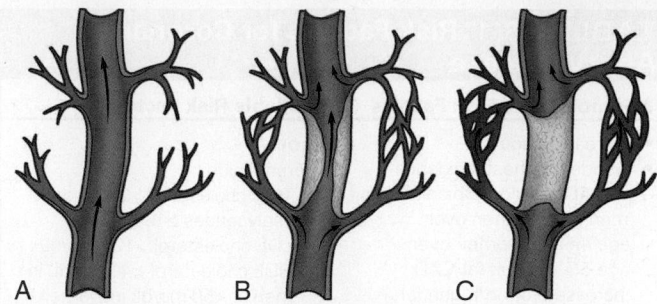

FIG. 33.2 Vessel occlusion with collateral circulation. **A,** Open, functioning coronary artery. **B,** Partial coronary artery closure with collateral circulation being established. **C,** Total coronary artery occlusion with collateral circulation bypassing the occlusion to supply blood to the myocardium.

of development in atherosclerosis are (1) fatty streak, (2) fibrous plaque, and (3) complicated lesion.

Fatty Streak. Fatty streaks, the earliest lesions of atherosclerosis, are lipid-filled smooth muscle cells. As streaks of fat develop within the smooth muscle cells, a yellow tinge appears. Fatty streaks can be seen in the coronary arteries by age 20. They involve an increasing amount of surface area as one ages. Treatment that lowers low-density lipoprotein (LDL) cholesterol may slow this process (Fig. 33.1, *B*).

Fibrous Plaque. The *fibrous plaque* stage is the beginning of progressive changes in the endothelium of the arterial wall. These changes can appear in the coronary arteries by age 30 and increase with age.

Normally, the endothelium repairs itself immediately. This does not occur in the person with CAD. LDLs and growth factors from platelets stimulate smooth muscle proliferation and thickening of the arterial wall. Once endothelial injury has taken place, lipoproteins (carrier proteins within the bloodstream) transport cholesterol and other lipids into the arterial intima. Collagen covers the fatty streak and forms a fibrous plaque with a grayish or whitish appearance. These plaques can form on one side of the artery or in a circular fashion involving the entire lumen. The borders can be smooth or irregular with rough, jagged edges. The result is a narrowing of the vessel lumen and reduced blood flow to the distal tissue (Fig. 33.1, *C*).

Complicated Lesion. The last stage in the development of the atherosclerotic lesion is the most dangerous. As the fibrous plaque grows, continued inflammation can result in plaque instability, ulceration, and rupture. Once the integrity of the artery's inner wall is compromised (plaque rupture), platelets accumulate in large numbers, leading to a thrombus (platelet aggregation and adhesion is the body's attempt to "heal" the ruptured area). The thrombus may adhere to the wall of the artery, leading to further narrowing or total occlusion of the artery. Activation of the exposed platelets causes expression of glycoprotein IIb/IIIa receptors that bind fibrinogen. This, in turn, leads to more platelet aggregation and adhesion, further enlarging the thrombus. At this stage, the plaque is referred to as a *complicated lesion* (Fig. 33.1, *D*).

Collateral Circulation. Normally, some arterial anastomoses or connections, called collateral circulation, exist within the coronary circulation. Two factors contribute to the growth and extent of collateral circulation: (1) inherited predisposition to develop new blood vessels (*angiogenesis*) and (2) presence of chronic ischemia (poor blood flow). When plaque blocks the normal flow of blood through a coronary artery and the resulting *ischemia* is chronic, increased collateral circulation may develop (Fig. 33.2). When blockages in coronary arteries occur

Etiology and Pathophysiology

Atherosclerosis is the major cause of CAD. It is characterized by lipid deposits within the intima of the artery. Endothelial injury and inflammation play a key role in the development of atherosclerosis.

The endothelium (inner lining of the vessel wall) is normally nonreactive to platelets and leukocytes, as well as coagulation, fibrinolytic, and complement factors. Damage to the endothelial lining can result from tobacco use, hyperlipidemia, hypertension, toxins, diabetes, high homocysteine levels, and infection causing a local inflammatory response (Fig. 33.1, *A*).[3]

C-reactive protein (CRP), a protein made by the liver, is a nonspecific marker of inflammation. CRP levels rise when there is systemic inflammation, such as rheumatoid arthritis or inflammatory bowel disease. CRP and levels of lipoprotein(a), which has proinflammatory properties, are increased in many patients with CAD (see Table 31.6). CRP and lipoprotein(a) are not a part of a routine risk assessment for CAD. They can be used in patients with an intermediate- or high-risk suspicion of CAD.[4]

Developmental Stages. CAD is a progressive disease that develops in stages over many years. When the patient becomes symptomatic, the disease process usually is well advanced. The stages

TABLE 33.1 Risk Factors for Coronary Artery Disease

Nonmodifiable Risk Factors	Modifiable Risk Factors

• Increasing age
• Gender (highest incidence of CAD is among middle-aged men, but for men over age 45 and women over age 55, the risk for CAD increases for both genders)
• Ethnicity (more common in white than black men)
• Genetic predisposition and family history of heart disease
	Major
	• Serum lipids:
	  • Total cholesterol >200 mg/dL
	  • Triglycerides ≥150 mg/dL*
	  • LDL cholesterol >130 mg/dL
	  • HDL cholesterol <40 mg/dL in men or <50 mg/dL in women*
	• BP >120/80 mm Hg*
	• Diabetes*
	• Tobacco use
	• Physical inactivity
	• Obesity: Waist circumference ≥102 cm (≥40 in) in men and ≥88 cm (≥35 in) in women*
	
	Contributing
	• Psychosocial risk factors (e.g., depression, hostility)
	• High homocysteine levels
	• Substance abuse

*3 or more of these risk factors meet the criteria for metabolic syndrome (discussed in Chapter 40).

slowly over a long time, there is a greater chance of collateral circulation developing, so the heart muscle may still receive an adequate amount of blood and oxygen (O_2) except during increased workload on the heart, such as exercise.

However, with rapid-onset CAD (e.g., familial hypercholesterolemia) or coronary spasm, there is not enough time to develop collateral circulation. When this happens, reduced blood flow results in more severe ischemia or infarction.

Risk Factors for Coronary Artery Disease

Many risk factors have been associated with CAD. We group them as nonmodifiable and modifiable (Table 33.1). *Nonmodifiable risk factors* are age, gender, ethnicity, family history, and genetics. *Modifiable risk factors* include high serum lipids, high BP, tobacco use, physical inactivity, obesity, diabetes, metabolic syndrome, psychologic states, and high homocysteine level.

Nonmodifiable Risk Factors

Age, Gender, Ethnicity, and Genetics. The incidence of CAD is highest among middle-aged men, however, the risk for CAD increases for men over age 45 and women over age 55.[4] Heart disease is often diagnosed about 10 years later in women than men. One possible reason for this may be the cardioprotective effects of estrogen. But, interestingly, hormone replacement therapy does not protect women after menopause and may be harmful.[4] Because women are older at the time of CAD diagnosis, they are more likely to have co-morbidities (e.g., hypertension, diabetes). Women are more likely than men to die after their first MI. CAD is present in black women at rates higher than their white or Hispanic counterparts.[4] (See Promoting Health Equity box for more differences in CAD among ethnic groups.)

Most women do not consider CAD their greatest health risk.[4] Despite efforts to increase awareness that more women die from heart disease than from breast cancer (e.g., the American Heart Association's Go Red for Women campaign), heart disease kills almost 10 times more women than breast cancer. It is the leading cause of death in women. When women present to the HCP,

their symptoms may be unrecognized as heart related because the symptoms are often atypical. These symptoms include fatigue, shortness of breath, upper back pain, indigestion, weakness, sleep problems, palpitations, and anxiety.[5] These atypical symptoms can relate to many different diseases and syndromes. This lack of recognition of symptoms as a cardiac problem leads to delays in women seeking treatment and HCPs recognizing the symptoms (see the Gender Differences box on p. 701).

🌐 PROMOTING HEALTH EQUITY
Coronary Artery Disease

Whites
• White men have the highest incidence of CAD.

Blacks
• Blacks have an early age of onset of CAD.
• Deaths from CVDs, including CAD and strokes, are higher for blacks than for the overall population in the United States.
• Black women have a higher incidence and death rate related to CAD than white and Hispanic women.

Native Americans
• Native Americans die from heart disease earlier than expected. Mortality rates for those under age 65 are twice as high as those of other Americans.
• Major modifiable CVD risk factors for Native Americans include tobacco use, hypertension, obesity, and diabetes.

Hispanics
• Hispanics have slightly lower rates of CAD than either non-Hispanic whites or blacks.
• Hispanics have lower death rates from CAD than non-Hispanic whites.

🧬 Genetic Link

Genetic predisposition is a key factor in the occurrence of CAD. Family history is a risk factor for CAD and MI. Often patients with angina or MI can name a parent or sibling who died of CAD.

The genetic basis of CAD/MI is complex and poorly understood. We estimate that the genetic contribution to CAD is as high as 40% to 60%. This proportion relates mainly to genes that control known risk factors (e.g., lipid metabolism).[6] (See Genetics in Clinical Practice box.)

Major Modifiable Risk Factors

High Serum Lipids. A high serum lipid level is a major risk factors for CAD (see Table 31.6). The risk for CAD is associated with a total serum cholesterol level greater than 200 mg/dL (5.2 mmol/L), an LDL greater than 130 mg/dL (3.4 mmol/L), a high-density lipoprotein (HDL) level less than 40 mg/dL (1.0 mmol/L) in men and less than 50 mg/dL (1.3 mmol/L) in women, and/or a fasting triglyceride level greater than 150 mg/dL (1.7 mmol/L).

For the body to be able to use and transport lipids, they must become soluble in blood by combining with proteins. Lipids combine with proteins to form lipoproteins. Lipoproteins are vehicles for fat mobilization and transport. They vary in composition. The 3 major lipoproteins are HDLs, LDLs, and very-low-density lipoproteins (VLDLs).[7]

HDLs contain more protein by weight and fewer lipids than any other lipoprotein. HDLs carry lipids away from arteries to the liver for metabolism. This process of HDL transport

GENDER DIFFERENCES

Coronary Artery Disease and Acute Coronary Syndrome

Men	Women
• First heart event is more often MI than angina.	• First heart event is more often UA than MI.
• Report more typical signs and symptoms of angina and MI.	• Fewer women have the "classic" signs and symptoms of UA or MI.
• Receive more evidence-based therapies (e.g., aspirin, statins, diagnostic catheterization, PCI) when acutely ill from CAD (e.g., MI).	• Fatigue is often the first symptom of ACS.
• Mortality rates from CAD have decreased more rapidly for men than women.	• Experience the onset of heart disease about 10 years later than men.
• Have larger diameter coronary arteries. Vessel diameter is inversely related to risk for restenosis after interventions.	• More women with MI die of sudden cardiac death before reaching the hospital.
• After age 55, the incidence of MI in men and women equalizes.	• Before menopause, have higher HDL cholesterol levels and lower LDL cholesterol levels. After menopause LDL levels and risk for MI increase.
• Develop more collateral circulation.	• Report more disability after a heart event.
• Standard screening for risk for sudden cardiac death is more predictive in men.	• Seek medical care later in the CAD process, most likely because of lack of recognition of atypical symptoms.
	• Have more "silent" MIs compared with men.
	• Those who have an MI are more likely to have a fatal heart event within 1 year than men.
	• Women who have coronary artery bypass graft surgery have a higher mortality rate and more complications after surgery.
	• Ae undertreated with guideline-based recommendations, leading to worse outcomes and increased rates of readmission, reinfarction, and death in the first year after MI.

GENETICS IN CLINICAL PRACTICE

Familial Hypercholesterolemia

Genetic Basis

• Autosomal dominant disorder
• Exists in both heterozygous (most common) and homozygous forms
• Mutation in low-density lipoprotein receptor (LDLR) gene
• Gene codes for low-density lipoprotein (LDL) receptor that binds to LDLs
• LDLs are the primary carriers of cholesterol in the blood. By removing LDLs from the bloodstream, the LDL receptors play a critical role in regulating cholesterol levels
• High cholesterol levels are a result of defective function of the LDL receptors
• Person has high serum LDLs throughout life

Incidence

• Heterozygotes: 1 in 500
• Homozygotes: rare

Genetic Testing

• DNA testing is available

Clinical Implications

• Develop severe atherosclerosis in early to middle years
• A serum lipid profile measures total cholesterol, triglycerides, LDLs, and high-density lipoproteins (HDLs)
• Homozygous familial hypercholesterolemia is much more severe. Cholesterol levels may exceed 600 mg/dL
• Develop xanthomas (fatty growths on the skin [e.g., around eyes, over joints])
• Treatment includes low-fat diet, exercise, and lipid-lowering drugs (e.g., PCSK9 inhibitors)

prevents lipid accumulation within the arterial walls.[7] Therefore high serum HDL levels are desirable and lower the risk for CAD. Premenopausal women usually have higher HDL levels than men. This may be related to the protective effects of natural estrogen. After menopause, women's HDL levels decrease to levels near those of men. In general, HDL levels are higher in women, decrease with age, and are low in those with CAD.

Physical activity, eating more healthy fats, losing excess weight, moderate alcohol intake, and quitting smoking help increase HDL levels.

LDLs contain more cholesterol than any of the lipoproteins and have an attraction for arterial walls. High LDL levels correlate closely with an increased incidence of atherosclerosis and CAD. This is why low serum LDL levels are desirable. We cannot routinely calculate LDL if the triglycerides are higher than 400 mg/dL (> 4.35 mmol/L). VLDLs have a higher concentration of triglycerides and can deposit cholesterol directly on the walls of arteries.

Triglycerides are the most common type of fat in the blood. A certain amount of triglycerides is needed for bodily function, but high triglyceride levels may increase the risk for CAD. Certain diseases (e.g., type 2 diabetes, chronic kidney disease [CKD]), drugs (e.g., corticosteroids, hormone therapy) and genetic disorders have been associated with high triglyceride levels. Lifestyle factors that can contribute to high levels include high alcohol intake, high intake of refined carbohydrates and simple sugars, and physical inactivity. When a high triglyceride level is combined with a high LDL level, a smaller, denser LDL particle is formed, which favors deposition on arterial walls. People with insulin resistance often have this pattern.

Guidelines for treating high LDL cholesterol are based on a person's 10-year and lifetime risk for having heart disease or stroke. The following data generate a risk score: (1) age, (2) gender, (3) race, (4) use of tobacco, (5) diabetes, (6) systolic BP, (7) diastolic BP, (8) use of BP drugs, (9) total cholesterol level, and (10) HDL cholesterol level. A 10-year risk calculator is available at *www.cvriskcalculator.com*.

The 2013 American College of Cardiology (ACC)/American Heart Association (AHA) Cholesterol Guideline[8] does not promote treating LDL to target goals as had been recommended in earlier guidelines. However, the 2017 American Association of Clinical Endocrinologists (AACE) guideline endorses treating LDL to specific target goals.[9] The AACE guideline states that those with no cardiac risk factors are considered at low risk for the development of CAD. Their LDL goal is <130 mg/dL. Those with 2 or less risk factors and a 10-year risk of < 10% (moderate risk) should be treated to an LDL target of < 100 mg/dL. Those at high risk (>2 risk factors and a 10-year risk of 10-20%; or diabetes or CKD stage 3 to 4 with no other risk factors) should be treated to an LDL of < 100 mg/dL. Those at very high risk for developing CAD (recent hospitalization for ACS, established CAD, carotid disease or peripheral vascular disease; diabetes, CKD stage 3 to 4 with 1 or more risk factors) should be treated to an LDL target of < 70 mg/dL.[9]

Hypertension. Hypertension increases the risk for CAD, stroke, peripheral vascular disease, heart failure (HF), and death. In postmenopausal women, hypertension is associated with a higher incidence of CAD than in men and premenopausal women.

According to the most recent published hypertension guidelines, a normal BP is defined as < 120 mm Hg/< 80 mm Hg. BP is classified as elevated (BP 120-129 mm Hg/< 80 mm Hg); stage 1 hypertension (BP 130-139 mmHg/80-89 mm Hg); or stage 2 hypertension (BP >140 mm Hg/ > 90 mm Hg).[10]

The cause of hypertension in 90% of those affected is unknown, but it is usually controllable with lifestyle changes and medications.[11] Lifestyle changes are a part of therapy for all people with elevated BP and hypertension. Those with stage 1 or 2 hypertension usually need drug therapy, often more than 1 drug, to reach therapeutic goals (see Table 32.6).[10] Teach patients the importance of achieving and maintaining target BP goals.

The shearing stress of an elevated BP causes endothelial injury that increases the rate of atherosclerosis. Atherosclerosis, in turn, causes narrowed, thickened arterial walls and decreases the distensibility and elasticity of vessels. More force is needed to pump blood through diseased arteries. This increased force is reflected in a higher BP. This added workload results in left ventricular (LV) hypertrophy and decreased stroke volume with each contraction. See Chapter 32 for a complete discussion of hypertension.

Tobacco Use. A third major risk factor in CAD is tobacco use. The risk for developing CAD is much higher in those who smoke tobacco or use smokeless tobacco than in those who do not. Further, tobacco smoking decreases estrogen levels, placing premenopausal women who smoke at greater risk for CAD.

Nicotine in tobacco smoke causes catecholamine (i.e., epinephrine, norepinephrine) release. These neurohormones cause an increased heart rate (HR), peripheral vasoconstriction, and increased BP. These changes increase the heart's workload. Tobacco smoke is related to an increase in LDL level, a decrease in HDL level, and release of toxic O_2 radicals. All of these add to vessel inflammation and thrombosis.

Carbon monoxide, found in tobacco smoke, affects the O_2-carrying capacity of hemoglobin by reducing the sites available for O_2 transport. Thus the effects of an increased cardiac workload and the O_2-depleting effect of carbon monoxide significantly decrease the O_2 available to the heart muscle. We also believe that carbon monoxide is a chemical irritant that injures the endothelium.

The benefits of smoking cessation are dramatic and almost immediate. CAD mortality rates drop to those of nonsmokers within 12 months. However, nicotine is highly addictive, and people usually need intensive intervention to quit. Individual and group counseling, nicotine replacement therapy, and smoking cessation drugs (e.g., bupropion, varenicline) are examples of smoking cessation strategies. (See Chapter 10, Tables 10.4 through 10.6 for information on smoking cessation.)

Nonsmokers exposed to secondhand tobacco smoke increase their risk for CAD by 25% to 30%.[1] People who live in the same house as the person who smokes should encourage that person to quit. This reinforces the person's effort and decreases the risk for ongoing exposure to environmental smoke. Pipe and cigar smokers, who often do not inhale, have an increased risk for CAD similar to those exposed to secondhand smoke. The few studies on electronic cigarettes suggest they increase HR and BP through systemic absorption of nicotine.[12]

Physical Inactivity. Physical inactivity is the fourth major modifiable risk factor for CAD. Physical inactivity implies a lack of adequate physical exercise on a regular basis. The ACC and the AHA recommend 30 to 60 minutes of exercise, such as brisk walking at least 5 days per week.[13]

How physical inactivity predisposes a person to CAD is still unclear. Physically active people have increased HDL levels. Exercise improves thrombolytic activity, thus reducing the risk for clot formation. Exercise may help with the development of collateral circulation in the heart.

Exercise training for those who are physically inactive reduces the risk for CAD through more efficient lipid metabolism, increased HDL production, and more efficient O_2 extraction by the muscles. This decreases the heart's workload. For people with CAD, regular physical activity may reduce symptoms, improve functional capacity, and improve other risk factors, such as insulin resistance and glucose intolerance.

Obesity. The death rate from CAD is higher in obese persons. Obesity is defined as a body mass index (BMI) of greater than 30 kg/m^2 and a waist circumference more than 40 inches for men and more than 35 inches for women. We calculate BMI by dividing a person's weight (in kilograms) by the square of the height in meters (see Fig. 40.6).

The increased risk for CAD is proportional to the degree of obesity. Obese persons may make increased levels of LDLs and triglycerides, which are strongly related to atherosclerosis. Obesity is often linked with hypertension and insulin resistance. People who tend to store fat in the abdomen (an "apple" figure) rather than in the hips and buttocks (a "pear" figure) have a higher incidence of CAD (see Table 40.6).

Contributing Modifiable Risk Factors

Diabetes Mellitus. The incidence of CAD is 2 to 4 times greater among people who have diabetes, even those with well-controlled blood glucose levels. The patient with diabetes manifests CAD more often and at an earlier age. There is no age difference between males or females with diabetes in the onset of symptoms of CAD.

Undiagnosed diabetes is often discovered when a person has an MI. The person with diabetes has an increased tendency toward endothelial dysfunction. This may account for the development of fatty streaks in the arteries. Patients with diabetes also have changes in lipid metabolism and tend to have high cholesterol and triglyceride levels. Management of diabetes should include lifestyle changes and drug therapy to achieve a glycosylated hemoglobin (A1C or Hb A1C) level of less than 7%.[13]

Metabolic Syndrome. Metabolic syndrome refers to a cluster of risk factors for CAD whose underlying pathophysiology may be related to insulin resistance. These risk factors include central obesity, hypertension, abnormal serum lipids, and a high fasting blood glucose (see Table 40.12). These interrelated risk factors appear to promote the development of CAD. Chapter 40 discusses metabolic syndrome.

Psychologic States. Certain behaviors and lifestyles may contribute to the development of CAD. One type of behavior, referred to as type A, includes perfectionism and a hardworking, driven personality. The type A personality often suppresses anger and hostility, has a sense of time urgency, is impatient, and creates stress and tension. This person may be more prone to MIs than one with a type B personality, who is more easygoing, takes upsets in stride, knows personal limitations, takes time to relax, and is not an overachiever. However, the relationship between behaviors and the risk for CAD/MI is controversial and complex.

Psychologic risk factors thought to increase the risk for CAD include depression, acute and chronic stress (e.g., poverty, serving as a caregiver), anxiety, hostility and anger, and lack of social support.[14] Stressful states contribute to the development and progression of CAD. Sympathetic nervous system (SNS) stimulation and its effect on the heart are the physiologic mechanisms by which stress predisposes a person to the development of CAD. SNS stimulation causes an increased release of catecholamines (i.e., epinephrine, norepinephrine), which may contribute to endothelial injury, inflammation, and platelet activation.[14] SNS stimulation also increases HR and the force of myocardial contraction, which increases myocardial O_2 demand. Stress-induced mechanisms can cause elevated lipid and glucose levels and changes in blood coagulation, which contribute to the development of atherosclerosis.

Homocysteine. High blood levels of homocysteine are linked to an increased risk for CAD and other CVDs.[13] Homocysteine is made by the breakdown of the essential amino acid methionine, which is found in dietary protein. High homocysteine levels may contribute to atherosclerosis by (1) damaging the inner lining of blood vessels, (2) promoting plaque buildup, and (3) changing the clotting mechanism to make clots more likely to occur. Although folic acid lowers homocysteine levels, research has not shown that reducing homocysteine levels lowers the risk of CAD.[15]

Substance Use. The use of illegal drugs, such as cocaine and methamphetamine, can produce coronary artery spasm resulting in myocardial ischemia and chest pain. Most patients with drug-induced chest pain initially cannot be distinguished from those with CAD. They often have sinus tachycardia, high BP, and chest pain. Chest pain occurs because of increased myocardial O_2 demand from the increased HR and contractility and coronary vasoconstriction.[16] An MI can occur because of coronary spasm. Serum cardiac biomarkers and an electrocardiogram (ECG) help determine if the patient is experiencing ACS. A drug screen may be helpful to identify what precipitated the cardiac event.

❖ INTERPROFESSIONAL AND NURSING CARE: CORONARY ARTERY DISEASE

◆ Health Promotion

Management of CAD risk factors may prevent, modify, or slow disease progression. In the United States, there has been a gradual decline in CAD-related deaths over the past 35 years. This relates to people's efforts to become healthier and advances in the treatment of CAD. Prevention and early treatment of heart disease must involve a multifaceted approach and must be ongoing throughout the life span. In fact, healthy lifestyle behaviors should begin in childhood.

◆ Identifying High-Risk Persons. Clinical signs of CAD are not apparent in the early stages of the disease. Therefore it is critical to identify people at risk for CAD. Risk screening involves obtaining a thorough health history. Ask the patient about a family history of heart disease in parents and siblings, especially a premature history of CAD (under age 55 for males and under age 65 for females).[13] Note the presence of any cardiovascular symptoms. Assess environmental factors, such as eating habits, type of diet, and level of exercise, to elicit lifestyle patterns. Include a psychosocial history to determine tobacco use, alcohol intake, recent stressful events (e.g., loss of a spouse), and psychologic state (e.g., anxiety, depression, anger). The place and type of employment provide vital information on the kind of activity performed, exposure to pollutants or toxins, and degree of stress associated with work.

Identify the patient's attitudes and beliefs about health and illness. This gives insight to how disease and lifestyle changes may affect the patient. It also can reveal misconceptions about heart disease. Knowing the patient's educational background and health literacy helps determine teaching needs. If the patient has prescribed drugs, it is important to know the names and dosages and if the patient adheres to the drug regimen.

◆ Managing High-Risk Persons. Recommend preventive measures for all persons at risk for CAD. The person with nonmodifiable risk factors (e.g., age, gender, ethnicity) can still reduce the risk for CAD by controlling the additive effects of modifiable risk factors. For example, a young person with a family history of heart disease can decrease the risk for CAD by maintaining an ideal body weight, getting adequate physical exercise, reducing intake of saturated fats, and avoiding tobacco and illicit drug use.

Encourage people who have modifiable risk factors to make lifestyle changes to reduce their risk for CAD. You can play a key role in teaching health-promoting behaviors (Table 33.2). For highly motivated persons, just knowing how to reduce their risk may be all the information they need to start.

For people who are less motivated to take charge of their health, the idea of reducing risk factors may be so remote that they are unable to perceive a threat of CAD. Few people want to make lifestyle changes, especially in the absence of symptoms. First, help them to clarify their personal values. Then, discuss risk factors and have them identify their individual risks. This can help them set realistic goals and choose which risk factor(s) to change first. Some people are reluctant to change until they begin to have symptoms or have an MI. Others, having had an MI, may find the idea of changing lifelong habits still unacceptable. Help them review options and respect their decisions.

◆ Physical Activity

A regular physical activity program should be designed and implemented to improve physical fitness by following the FITT formula (Table 33.3): Frequency (how often), Intensity (how hard), Type (isotonic), and Time (how long). Everyone should aim for at least 30 minutes of moderate physical activity on most days of the week. Examples of moderate physical activity include brisk walking, hiking, biking, and swimming. The AHA encourages people to increase their daily physical activity and lower the chance of developing heart disease simply by walking. Adding weight training to an exercise program 2 days a week can help treat metabolic syndrome and improve muscle strength. Regular physical activity helps with weight reduction, reduces systolic BP, and can help increase HDL cholesterol.

◆ Nutritional Therapy

Dietary recommendations focus on ways to lower LDL cholesterol. They emphasize a decrease in saturated fat and cholesterol and an increase in complex carbohydrates (e.g., whole grains,

TABLE 33.2 Patient & Caregiver Teaching

Reducing Risk Factors for Coronary Artery Disease

Include the following instructions when teaching risk reduction for coronary artery disease:

Risk Factor	Health-Promoting Behaviors	Risk Factor	Health-Promoting Behaviors
Hypertension	• Monitor home-based BP and obtain regular checkups. • Take prescribed drugs for BP control. • Reduce salt intake. • Stop tobacco use. Avoid exposure to environmental tobacco (secondhand) smoke. • Control or reduce weight. • Perform physical activity daily.	**Psychologic state**	• Increase awareness of behaviors that are harmful to health. • Change patterns that add to stress (e.g., get up 30 min earlier so that breakfast is not eaten on way to work). • Set realistic goals for self. • Reassess priorities in light of identified risk factors. • Learn effective stress management strategies (see Chapter 6). • Seek professional help if feeling depressed, angry, anxious, etc. • Plan time for adequate rest and sleep (see Chapter 7).
High serum lipids	• Reduce total fat intake. • Reduce saturated fat intake. • Take prescribed drugs for lipid reduction. • Adjust total caloric intake to achieve and maintain ideal body weight. • Engage in daily physical activity. • Increase amount of complex carbohydrates, fiber, and vegetable proteins in diet. • Follow-up with HCP for regular lipid panel assessments.		
Tobacco use (see Chapter 10)	• Begin a tobacco cessation program. • Change daily routines associated with tobacco use to reduce desire to smoke. • Substitute other activities for smoking. • Ask caregivers to support efforts to stop smoking. • Avoid exposure to environmental tobacco smoke.	**Obesity use** (see Chapter 40)	• Change eating patterns and habits. • Reduce caloric intake to achieve body mass index of 18.5 to 24.9 kg/m². • Increase physical activity to increase caloric expenditure. • Avoid fad and crash diets, which are not effective over time. • Avoid large, heavy meals. Consider smaller, more frequent meals.
		Diabetes use (see Chapter 48)	• Follow the recommended diet. • Control or reduce weight. • Take prescribed drugs for diabetes. • Monitor blood glucose levels regularly and follow up with HCP regularly.
Physical inactivity	• Develop and maintain at least 30 minutes of moderate physical activity daily (minimum 5 days a week). • Increase activities to a fitness level.		

TABLE 33.3 Patient & Caregiver Teaching

FITT Activity Guidelines for CAD, Chronic Stable Angina, and ACS

Include the following information in the teaching plan for the patient with chronic stable angina and acute coronary syndrome and the caregiver:

Warm-Up/Cool-Down

Perform mild stretching for 3–5 min before the physical activity and 5 min after the activity. Do not start or stop activity abruptly.

Frequency

Perform physical activity on most days of the week.

Intensity

The patient's HR determines the activity intensity. If an exercise stress test has not been performed, the HR of the patient recovering from an MI should not exceed 20 beats/min over the resting HR.

Type of Physical Activity

Select physical activity that is regular, rhythmic, and repetitive, using large muscles to build up endurance (e.g., walking, cycling, swimming, rowing).

Time

Physical activity sessions should be at least 30 min long. Begin slowly at personal tolerance (perhaps only 5–10 min) and build up to 30 min.

fruit, vegetables) and fiber (Tables 33.4 and 33.5). Fat intake should be about 25% to 35% of total calories, with most coming from monounsaturated and polyunsaturated fats. Red meat, egg yolks, and whole milk products are major sources of saturated fat and cholesterol. They should be reduced or eliminated from diets. With a high serum triglyceride level, alcohol and simple sugars should be reduced or eliminated.

Omega-3 fatty acids reduce triglyceride levels and can slow the progression of CAD. They do not affect LDL levels. The AHA recommends eating fatty fish twice a week. Examples of fatty fish include salmon, tuna, and mackerel. Other foods that contain omega-3 fatty acids include soybean oils, canola, walnuts, and flaxseed.[17] Omega-3 fatty acids can be hard to get by diet alone. The HCP may recommend dietary supplements.

◆ Lipid-Lowering Drug Therapy

An estimated 28.5 million American adults over age 20 have cholesterol levels of 240 mg/dL (6.2 mmol/L) or greater.[1] Treatment of high cholesterol focuses mostly on lowering LDL cholesterol. A complete lipid profile should be done every 5 years beginning at age 20.[9] Middle-aged adults should be screened every 1 to 2 years. If multiple risk factors are present, more frequent testing is recommended.[9] Guidelines recommend the following groups of people receive statin therapy: (1) patients with known CVD, (2) patients with primary elevations of LDL cholesterol levels of 190 mg/dL or greater (e.g., familial hypercholesterolemia), (3)

TABLE 33.4 Nutritional Therapy
Therapeutic Lifestyle Changes to Diet

Dietary Recommendations	Recommended Daily Intake

Combined total fat calories from:
• *Saturated fats:* Limit fats that are usually solid at room and refrigerator temperature (e.g., lard, butter, whole-milk products, fatty cuts of meat, bacon)
• *Trans fats:* Mainly in foods made with hydrogenated vegetable oils, such as many hard margarines and shortenings
• *Unsaturated fats:* In oils that are usually liquid at room and refrigerator temperature (e.g., olive, corn, sunflower, soybean). There are 2 types of unsaturated fats:
  • *Monounsaturated fats:* In greatest amounts in foods from plants, including olives, avocadoes, and canola, sunflower, and peanut oils.
  • *Polyunsaturated fats:* Found mostly in nuts, seeds, fish, seed oils, and oysters. Omega-3 fatty acid is a type of polyunsaturated fat that may help reduce the risk of CAD.
	25%–35% of total daily calories (including <7% from saturated fat)

Cholesterol	<200 mg
Plant stanols or sterols (e.g., margarines, nuts, seeds, legumes, vegetable oils)*	2 g
Dietary soluble fiber*	10–25 g of soluble fiber
Total calories	Only enough calories to reach or maintain a healthy weight

Physical Activity

In addition to diet, teach the patient to get at least 30 min of a moderate intensity physical activity, such as brisk walking, on most, and preferably all, days of the week.

*Diet options for additional lowering of low-density lipoprotein (LDL).

COMPLEMENTARY & ALTERNATIVE THERAPIES
Lipid-Lowering Agents

Agent	Evidence for Use
Berberine	Possibly effective for reducing total cholesterol, low-density lipoproteins (LDLs), triglycerides
Garlic	Conflicting evidence. Possibly effective for reducing total cholesterol and LDL over short periods
Green tea	Possibly effective for reducing total cholesterol
Flaxseed	Conflicting evidence on the efficacy for reducing total cholesterol
Omega-3 fatty acids (fish oil)	Effective for reducing cholesterol and triglyceride levels
Black psyllium	Possibly effective for reducing total cholesterol and LDL
Plant sterols	Likely effective for reducing total cholesterol and LDL
Red yeast rice	Likely effective for reducing total cholesterol, LDL, and triglycerides. Red yeast rice contains a chemical similar to statins.
Soy	Possibly effective for slight reduction in total cholesterol and LDL

Source: Sahebkar A, Serban MC, Gluba-Brzózka A, et al: Lipid-modifying effects of nutraceuticals: an evidence-based approach, *Nutrition* 32:1179, 2016; Siscovick DS, Barringer TA, Fretts AM, et al: Omega-3 polyunsaturated fatty acid (fish oil) supplementation and the prevention of clinical cardiovascular disease, *Circulation*, 2017.

TABLE 33.5 Nutritional Therapy
Tips to Make Diet and Lifestyle Changes

General Tips
1. Know your calorie needs to achieve and maintain a healthy weight.
2. Know the calorie content of the foods and beverages you eat.
3. Track your weight, physical activity, and calorie intake.
4. Prepare and eat smaller, more frequent meals.
5. Track your activities and, whenever possible, decrease sedentary activities (e.g., watching television, computer time).
6. Incorporate physical movement into daily activities (e.g., take stairs and extra steps whenever possible).
7. Do not smoke or use tobacco products.
8. If you drink alcohol, do so in moderation (i.e., no more than 1 drink for women or 2 drinks for men a day).

Tips Related to Food Choices and Preparation
1. Use the Nutrition Facts panel on food labels and ingredients list when choosing foods to buy.
2. Use fresh or frozen vegetables and fruits in place of canned vegetables and fruits.
3. Replace high-calorie foods with fresh fruits and vegetables.
4. Increase fiber intake by eating beans (legumes), whole-grain products, fruits, and vegetables.
5. Use liquid vegetable oils in place of solid fats.
6. Limit beverages and foods high in added sugars (e.g., sucrose, glucose, fructose, maltose, dextrose, corn syrups, concentrated fruit juice, honey).
7. Choose foods made with whole grains (e.g., whole wheat, oats, rye, barley, brown rice, wild rice, buckwheat).
8. Avoid pastries and high-calorie bakery products (e.g., muffins, doughnuts).
9. Select milk and dairy products that are either fat free or low fat.
10. Reduce salt intake by
    • Comparing the sodium content of similar products (e.g., different brands of tomato sauce) and choosing products with less sodium.
    • Choosing versions of processed foods with reduced salt, including cereals, canned products, and baked goods.
    • Limiting condiments (e.g., soy sauce, ketchup).
11. Use lean cuts of meat and remove skin from poultry before cooking or eating.
12. Avoid processed meats that are high in saturated fat and sodium (e.g., deli meats).
13. Grill, bake, or broil fish, meat, and poultry.
14. Incorporate plant-based meat substitutes into recipes (e.g., soy, tofu, quinoa).
15. Consume whole vegetables and fruits in place of juices.

Source: U.S. Department of Health and Human Services: Your guide to lowering your cholesterol with TLC. Retrieved from *www.nhlbi.nih.gov/files/docs/public/heart/chol_tlc.pdf*.

patients 40 to 75 years old with diabetes and LDL cholesterol levels between 70 and 189 mg/dL, and (4) patients 40 to 75 years old with LDL cholesterol levels between 70 and 189 mg/dL and a 10-year risk for CVD of at least 7.5%.[8,18]

Drug therapy should continue for a lifetime unless the patient becomes intolerant. In that case, the patient should switch to another drug. The patient must fully understand the rationale and goals of treatment, as well as the safety and side effects of lipid-lowering drugs.

Concurrent diet change is essential to reduce the need for drug therapy. Treatment also includes weight loss, if overweight, and increased physical activity. Serum lipid levels should be reassessed after 6 weeks of therapy. If they are still high, changes in drug therapy (Table 33.6) and more dietary options (see the Complementary & Alternative Therapies box) may be considered.

◆ Drugs That Restrict Lipoprotein Production

HMG-CoA Reductase Inhibitors (Statins). The statin drugs are the most widely used lipid-lowering drugs (Table 33.6). These drugs inhibit the synthesis of cholesterol in the liver. An unexplained result of inhibiting cholesterol synthesis is an increase in hepatic LDL receptors. This allows the liver to remove more LDL from the blood. In addition, statins cause a minor increase in HDL and lower CRP levels. The statins are not equal in reducing LDL levels. Rosuvastatin (Crestor) is the most potent statin currently available. Serious adverse effects of these drugs are rare and include liver damage and myalgia (muscle ache or weakness without breakdown of skeletal muscle) that can progress to rhabdomyolysis (breakdown of skeletal muscle). Liver enzymes are initially monitored and rechecked with any increase in dosage. The creatine kinase isoenzyme, CK-MM (found in skeletal muscle), is assessed if symptoms of myopathy (e.g., muscle aches, weakness) occur.

 DRUG ALERT Simvastatin (Zocor)

- Increased risk for rhabdomyolysis when used with fibric acid derivatives (e.g., gemfibrozil [Lopid]), niacin (Niaspan), or erythromycin.
- Manifestations of rhabdomyolysis include high creatine kinase levels and muscle pain.
- Prothrombin times may increase in patients taking warfarin (Coumadin).

Niacin. Niacin, a water-soluble B vitamin, is effective in lowering LDL and triglyceride levels by interfering with their synthesis (Table 33.6). Niacin, at high doses, increases HDL levels better than many other lipid-lowering drugs. Unfortunately, side effects are common. They may include severe flushing, pruritus, gastrointestinal (GI) symptoms, and orthostatic hypotension.

 DRUG ALERT Niacin (Niaspan)

- Teach the patient that flushing (especially of face and neck) may occur within 20 minutes after taking drug and last for 30 to 60 minutes.
- Premedicate with aspirin or NSAID 30 minutes before taking to reduce flushing.
- Use of extended-release niacin may decrease side effects.

Fibric Acid Derivatives. The *fibric acid derivatives* (Table 33.6) work by aiding the removal of VLDLs. They are very effective for lowering triglycerides and increasing HDL levels. They have no effect on LDLs. Although most patients tolerate the drugs well, GI irritability is common. These drugs should be used with caution when combined with statin medications due to increased risk for myopathy.

 DRUG ALERT Gemfibrozil (Lopid)

- May increase the risk for bleeding in patients taking warfarin (Coumadin)
- Increases the risk of hypoglycemia in patients taking repaglinide (Prandin)

◆ Drugs That Increase Lipoprotein Removal

Bile Acid Sequestrants. Bile-acid sequestrants increase conversion of cholesterol to bile acids in the liver and decrease hepatic cholesterol (Table 33.6). The primary effect is a decrease in total cholesterol and LDL levels. These drugs have been associated with side effects related to taste and a variety of upper and lower GI symptoms. These include belching, heartburn, nausea, abdominal pain, and constipation. Bile-acid sequestrants decrease absorption of many other drugs (e.g., warfarin, thiazides, thyroid hormones, β-adrenergic blockers

[β-blockers]). Separating the time of giving these drugs from that of other drugs by at least 2 hours decreases this adverse effect.[7]

Proprotein Convertase Subtilisin/Kexin 9 (PCSK9) Inhibitors. PCSK9 inhibitors are a newer class of cholesterol-lowering drugs (Table 33.6). PCSK9 reduces the number of receptors on the liver that remove LDL cholesterol from the blood. By blocking PCSK9's ability to work, more receptors are available and can get rid of LDL, thus decreasing circulating LDL levels. Evolocumab (Repatha) and alirocumab (Praluent) are 2 PCSK9 inhibitors. They are given subcutaneously every 2 weeks. Evolocumab may be given every 4 weeks at a higher dose, depending on patient preference. They are not a first-line therapy. They are used in addition to diet and maximum statin therapy for adults with familial hypercholesterolemia and for patients intolerant of statin drugs. They also can be used for patients with CAD who need added LDL lowering because of inadequate treatment with statins.[7]

◆ Drugs That Decrease Cholesterol Absorption. Ezetimibe (Zetia) selectively inhibits the absorption of dietary and biliary cholesterol across the intestinal wall (Table 33.6). It serves as an adjunct to dietary changes, especially for patients with primary hypercholesterolemia. When it is combined with a statin, either as a combination drug (e.g., ezetimibe and simvastatin [Vytorin]) or as 2 separate drugs (ezetimibe and a statin), even greater reductions in LDLs occur.

◆ Antiplatelet Therapy

Low-dose aspirin (81 mg) is recommended for people who have CAD. For people at risk but without known CAD, low-dose aspirin is recommended for adults 50 to 59 years old who have a calculated 10-year CVD risk of 10% or more, are not at increased risk for bleeding (e.g., history of GI bleeding), have a life expectancy of at least 10 years, and are willing to take low-dose aspirin for at least 10 years. For adults 60 to 69 years old who have a calculated 10-year CVD risk of 10% or more, the decision to take low-dose aspirin is an individual one made in conjunction with the HCP. Adults who have no contraindications (e.g., history of bleeding), have a life expectancy of at least 10 years, and are willing to take low-dose aspirin daily for at least 10 years are more likely to benefit. Currently there is not enough evidence to recommend low-dose aspirin for primary prevention in those younger than 50 or older than 70.[19] Clopidogrel (Plavix) is an option for people who are aspirin intolerant.[15]

Gerontologic Considerations: Coronary Artery Disease

The incidence of heart disease is greatly increased in older adults and the leading cause of death in older persons. In the older adult, CAD is often a result of the complex interaction of nonmodifiable risk factors (e.g., age) and lifelong modifiable risk behaviors (e.g., inactivity, tobacco use). Strategies to reduce CAD risk and to treat CAD are effective in this age-group.

Aggressive treatment of hypertension and hyperlipidemia helps stabilize plaques in the coronary arteries. Tobacco cessation helps to decrease the risk for CAD at any age. Similarly, encourage the older patient to consider a planned program of physical activity. Physical activity improves activity performance, endurance, and ability to tolerate stress. Positive psychologic benefits can include increased self-esteem, emotional well-being, and improved body image. For the older adult who is obese, making modest dietary changes and slowly increasing physical activity (e.g., walking) results in more positive benefits than aiming for a significant weight loss.

TABLE 33.6 Drug Therapy

Hyperlipidemia

Drug	Mechanism of Action	Side Effects	Nursing Considerations
Restrict Lipoprotein Production			
Fibric Acid Derivatives			
fenofibrate (Tricor) gemfibrozil (Lopid)	Decrease hepatic synthesis and secretion of VLDL. Reduce triglycerides by ↓ VLDL ↓ LDL ↓ Triglycerides ↑ HDL	Rashes, mild GI problems (e.g., nausea, diarrhea), high liver enzymes	May ↑ effects of warfarin (Coumadin) and some antihyperglycemic drugs. When used in combination with statins, may increase adverse effects of statins, especially myopathy.
HMG-CoA Reductase Inhibitors (Statins)			
atorvastatin (Lipitor) fluvastatin (Lescol XL) lovastatin pitavastatin (Livalo) pravastatin (Pravachol) rosuvastatin (Crestor) simvastatin (Zocor)	Block synthesis of cholesterol and increase LDL receptors in liver ↓ LDL ↓ Triglycerides ↑ HDL (small amount)	Rash, GI problems, high liver enzymes, myopathy, rhabdomyolysis	Well tolerated with few side effects. Monitor liver enzymes and creatine kinase (if muscle weakness or pain occurs).
Niacin			
Niacin (Niaspan)	Inhibits synthesis and secretion of VLDL and LDL ↓ LDL ↓ Triglycerides ↑ HDL	Flushing and pruritus in upper torso and face, GI problems (e.g., nausea and vomiting, dyspepsia, diarrhea), orthostatic hypotension	Most side effects subside with time. Taking aspirin or NSAID 30 min before drug may prevent flushing. Take drug with food. Decreased liver function may occur with high doses.
Omega-3 Fatty Acid			
icosapent ethyl (Vascepa) (contains eicosapentaenoic acid [EPA]) omega-3 acid ethyl esters (Lovaza) (contains eicosapentaenoic acid [EPA] and docosahexaenoic acid [DHA])	Inhibits synthesis and/or secretion of triglycerides ↓ Triglycerides ↑ HDL	Arthralgia Anaphylaxis, rash, taste changes, GI problems (e.g., constipation, vomiting)	Used for patients with severe hypertriglyceridemia (levels ≥ 500 mg/dL) Used for patients with high triglycerides. Give with meals and do not open or dissolve capsules
Increase Lipoprotein Removal			
Bile-Acid Sequestrants			
cholestyramine (Prevalite) colesevelam (Welchol) colestipol (Colestid)	Binds with bile acids in intestine, forming insoluble complex and excreted in feces Binding results in removal of LDL and cholesterol ↓ LDL	Unpleasant quality to taste, GI problems (e.g., indigestion, constipation, bloating)	Effective and safe for long-term use. Side effects lessen with time. Interferes with absorption of many drugs (e.g., digoxin, thiazide diuretics, warfarin, some antibiotics [e.g., penicillins])
Proprotein Convertase Subtilisin/Kexin 9 (PCSK9) Inhibitors			
alirocumab (Praluent) evolocumab (Repatha)	Inactivate PCSK9 protein ↓ LDL	Injection-site reactions, muscle pain, limb pain, and fatigue	Used with diet and maximum statin therapy to treat familial hypercholesterolemia and for those who need further LDL lowering or for those who are statin intolerant Drugs are given by injection every 2–4 wks (evolocumab may be given every 4 wks at a higher dose)
Decrease Cholesterol Absorption			
Cholesterol Absorption Inhibitor			
ezetimibe (Zetia)	Inhibits the intestinal absorption of cholesterol ↓ LDL ↑ HDL	Infrequent, but may include headache and mild GI distress	When used with a statin, further reduces LDL. Should not be used by patients with liver impairment

TABLE 33.7 Select Conditions Influencing Myocardial O₂ Needs

Decreased O₂ Supply	Increased O₂ Demand or Consumption
Cardiac	
• Coronary artery atherosclerosis	• Aortic stenosis
• Coronary artery spasm	• Cardiomyopathy
• Coronary artery thrombosis	• Dysrhythmias
• Dysrhythmias	• Left ventricular hypertrophy
• Heart failure	• Tachycardia
• Valve disorders	
Noncardiac	
• Anemia	• Anxiety
• Asthma	• Hypertension
• Chronic obstructive pulmonary disease	• Hyperthermia
• Hypovolemia	• Hyperthyroidism
• Hypoxemia	• Physical exertion
• Pneumonia	• Substance (stimulant) abuse (e.g., cocaine, amphetamines)
• Substance (stimulant) abuse (e.g., cocaine, amphetamines)	

TABLE 33.8 PQRST Assessment of Angina

Use the following memory aid to obtain information from the patient who has chest pain:

	Factor	Questions to Ask Patient
P	Precipitating events	What events or activities precipitated the pain or discomfort (e.g., argument, exercise, resting)?
Q	Quality of pain	What does the pain or discomfort feel like (e.g., pressure, dull, aching, tight, squeezing, heaviness)?
R	Region (location) and radiation of pain	Can you point to where the pain or discomfort is located? Does the pain or discomfort radiate to other areas (e.g., back, neck, arms, jaw, shoulder, elbow)?
S	Severity of pain	On a scale of 0 to 10, with 0 indicating no pain and 10 being the most severe pain you could imagine, what number would you give the pain or discomfort?
T	Timing	When did the pain or discomfort begin? Has it changed since this time? Have you had pain/discomfort like this before?

When planning a physical activity program, recommend: (1) longer warm-up periods, (2) longer periods of low-level activity, and/or (3) longer rest periods between sessions. Heat intolerance results from a decreased ability to sweat efficiently. Teach the patient to avoid physical activity in temperature extremes and to maintain a moderate pace. The older adult should exercise a minimum of 30 minutes on most days of the week as able.

Encouraging the older patient to adopt a healthy lifestyle may increase the quality of life and reduce the risk for CAD and fatal heart events. Older adults face many of the same challenges as younger persons when it comes to making lifestyle changes. Older adults are more likely to consider change either (1) when hospitalized or (2) when symptoms (e.g., chest pain) are the result of CAD and not normal aging (see Table 31.1). First, assess for the readiness to change and health literacy. Then, help the patient select the lifestyle changes most likely to produce the greatest reduction in risk for CAD.

CHRONIC STABLE ANGINA

CAD is a chronic and progressive disease. Patients may be asymptomatic for many years but may eventually develop chronic stable chest pain. When the demand for myocardial O₂ exceeds the ability of the coronary arteries to supply the heart with O₂, *myocardial ischemia* occurs. Angina, or chest pain, is the clinical manifestation of myocardial ischemia. It is caused by either an increased demand for O₂ or a decreased supply of O₂ (Table 33.7). The most common reason for angina to develop is significant narrowing of 1 or more coronary arteries by atherosclerosis. This leads to insufficient blood flow to the heart muscle. For ischemia to occur from an atherosclerotic plaque, the artery is usually blocked (stenosed) 70% or more (50% or more for the left main coronary artery).[20]

Chronic stable angina refers to chest pain that occurs intermittently over a long period of time with a similar pattern of onset, duration, and intensity of symptoms. It is often provoked by physical exertion, stress, or emotional upset. It is important to get an accurate assessment of the angina symptoms (Table 33.8). When asked, some patients may deny feeling pain, but

describe a pressure, heaviness, or discomfort in the chest. This discomfort is often described as a squeezing, heavy, tight, or suffocating sensation. It may be associated with other symptoms, such as dyspnea or fatigue. Chronic angina pain usually does not change with position or breathing.

Although most angina pain occurs substernally, it may radiate to other locations, including the jaw, neck, shoulders, and/or arms. Many people with angina describe a feeling of indigestion or a burning sensation in the epigastric region. The sensation may be felt between the shoulder blades (Fig. 33.3). Often, people who describe pain between the shoulder blades or indigestion type pain dismiss it as not being heart related. Some patients, especially women and older adults, report atypical symptoms of angina, including dyspnea, nausea, mid-epigastric discomfort, and/or fatigue.[13] We refer to this as an *angina equivalent*.

The pain of chronic stable angina usually lasts for only a few minutes. It often subsides when the precipitating factor is resolved (e.g., by resting, calming down, using sublingual nitroglycerin [SL NTG]) (Table 33.9). Pain at rest is unusual and may indicate UA. With ischemia, the 12-lead ECG often shows ST segment depression and/or T wave inversion. These changes represent inadequate supply of blood and O₂ to the heart muscle. ST depression is significant if it is at least 1 mm (1 small box) below the isoelectric line in at least 2 contiguous (neighboring) leads. In a normal heart, the isoelectric line should be flat (see Fig. 35.10). The ECG changes return to baseline when adequate blood flow is restored, and pain is relieved.

Chronic stable angina is controlled with drugs on an outpatient basis. Because chronic stable angina is often predictable, drugs are timed to provide peak effects during the time of day when angina is likely to occur. For example, if angina occurs when rising, the patient can take medication as soon as awakening and wait 30 minutes to 1 hour before engaging in activity. A comparison of the major types of angina is outlined in Table 33.10.

Silent ischemia refers to ischemia that occurs in the absence of any subjective symptoms. Patients with diabetes have an increased prevalence of silent ischemia. This is likely due to

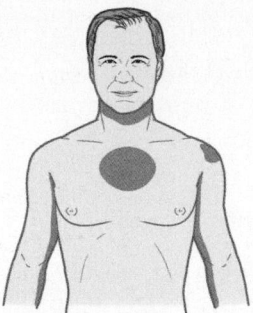
- Mid sternum
- Left shoulder and down both arms
- Neck and arms

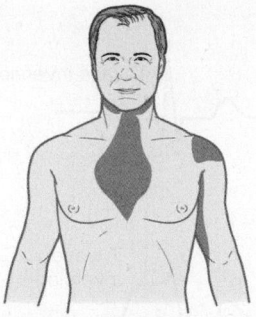
- Substernal radiating to neck and jaw
- Substernal radiating down left arm

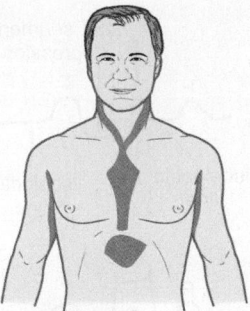
- Epigastric
- Epigastric radiating to neck, jaw, and arms

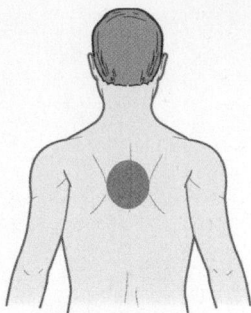
- Intrascapular

FIG. 33.3 Common locations and patterns of pain during angina or MI.

TABLE 33.9 Precipitating Factors of Angina

Physical Exertion
- Increases HR, reducing the time the heart spends in diastole (the time of greatest coronary blood flow), resulting in an increase in myocardial O_2 demand
- Isometric exercise of the arms (e.g., raking, lifting heavy objects, snow shoveling) can cause exertional angina

Temperature Extremes
- Increase the workload of the heart
- Blood vessels constrict in response to a cold stimulus
- Blood vessels dilate and blood pools in the skin in response to a hot stimulus

Strong Emotions
- Stimulate the sympathetic nervous system, activating the stress response
- Increase the workload of the heart

Consumption of Heavy Meal (e.g., holiday meals)
- Can increase the workload of the heart
- During the digestive process, blood is diverted to the GI system, reducing blood flow in the coronary arteries

Tobacco Use and Environmental Tobacco Smoke
- Decrease available O_2 by increasing the level of carbon monoxide
- Nicotine stimulates catecholamine release, causing vasoconstriction and an increased HR

Sexual Activity
- Increases the cardiac workload and sympathetic stimulation
- In a person with CAD, the extra cardiac workload may precipitate angina

Stimulants (e.g., cocaine, amphetamines)
- Increase HR and BP and increases myocardial O_2 demand
- Stimulate vasoconstriction and decreases myocardial O_2 supply
- May precipitate dysrhythmias

Circadian Rhythm Patterns
- Manifestations of CAD tend to occur in the early morning after awakening

TABLE 33.10 Comparison of Major Types of Angina

Type	Etiology	Characteristics
Chronic stable angina	Myocardial ischemia (usually from CAD) caused by an O_2 supply/demand mismatch	• Episodic pain lasting a few minutes • Provoked by exertion or stress • Relieved by rest or nitroglycerin
Prinzmetal's angina	Coronary vasospasm	• Occurs primarily at rest • Triggered by smoking and increased levels of some substances (e.g., histamine, epinephrine, cocaine) • May occur in presence or absence of CAD • Treatment may include long-acting nitrates and/or calcium channel blockers
Microvascular angina	Myocardial ischemia from microvascular disease affecting the small, distal branches of coronary arteries	• More common in women • Triggered by activities of daily living (e.g., shopping, work) vs. physical exercise (exertion) • Treatment may include nitroglycerin
Unstable angina	Rupture of unstable plaque, exposing thrombogenic surface	• New-onset angina • Chronic stable angina that increases in frequency, duration, or severity • Occurs at rest or with minimal exertion • Lasts more than 10 min

diabetic neuropathy affecting the nerves that innervate the cardiovascular system. When patients are monitored and silent ischemia occurs, ECG changes are revealed (e.g., ST depression and/or T wave inversion) (Fig. 33.4, *A*). Ischemia with pain or without pain has the same prognosis.

Prinzmetal's Angina

Prinzmetal's angina *(variant angina)* is a rare form of angina that often occurs at rest and not with increased physical demand. It is sometimes seen in patients with a history of migraine headaches, Raynaud's phenomenon, and heavy smoking. It is usually due to spasm of a major coronary artery. Strong contraction (spasm) of smooth muscle in the coronary artery results from increased intracellular calcium.[21] The spasm may occur in the presence or absence of CAD.

Factors contributing to coronary artery spasm include increased levels of certain substances (e.g., alcohol, cocaine), exposure to medications that narrow blood vessels (e.g.

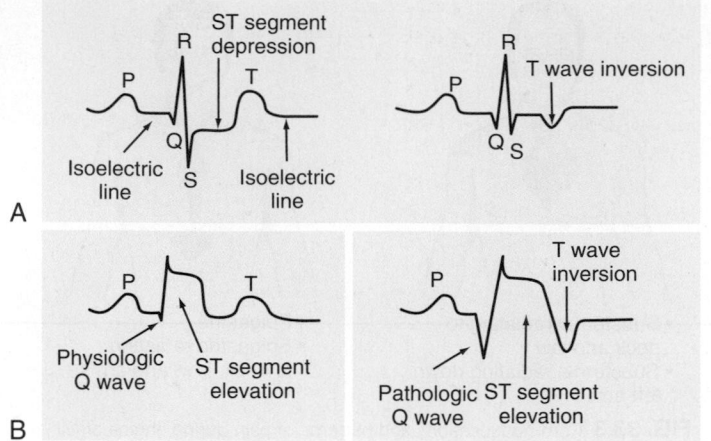

FIG. 33.4 ST segment, T wave, and Q wave changes associated with myocardial ischemia (**A**), injury coronary spasm (**B**), and infarction (**C**). (From Bucher L, Melander S: *Critical care nursing,* Philadelphia, 1999, Saunders.)

sumatriptan [Imitrex]), or cold weather exposure. When spasm occurs, the patient has angina and transient ST segment elevation (not usually associated with an MI) (Fig. 33.4, *B*). The pain may occur during rapid-eye-movement (REM) sleep when myocardial O_2 consumption increases between midnight and early morning or at rest. The pain may be relieved by moderate exercise, with SL NTG, or it may disappear spontaneously. Cyclic, short bursts of pain at the same time each day may occur with this type of angina. Calcium channel blockers and/or nitrates are an option. Stopping the use of any offending substances is recommended.[22]

Microvascular Angina

In *microvascular angina,* chest pain occurs in the absence of significant CAD or coronary spasm of a major coronary artery. In these patients, chest pain is related to myocardial ischemia associated with atherosclerosis or spasm of the small distal branch vessels of the coronary microcirculation. This is known as *coronary microvascular disease* (MVD). MVD is often used interchangeably with the term *syndrome X.* It is more common in women. Often the angina is prolonged and brought on by physical exertion. These patients usually have positive stress test results and an inconsistent response to nitrates.[22] Prevention and treatment of coronary MVD follow the same recommendations as for CAD.

INTERPROFESSIONAL AND NURSING CARE: CHRONIC STABLE ANGINA

Chronic stable angina can progress or develop into UA or ACS. Therefore any change in the usual pattern of angina should be evaluated. A patient with chronic stable angina may be admitted with a change in the angina pattern. Until an assessment and diagnostic studies are completed, it may be unclear if the patient is having typical chronic stable angina, UA, or an MI.

The goal of treatment for a patient admitted with angina is to decrease O_2 demand and/or increase O_2 supply. Nursing care focuses on the priority problems of managing acute pain and anxiety while increasing O_2 delivery to the myocardium. The overall goals for a patient who presents with angina include (1) relief of pain, (2) immediate and appropriate treatment, (3) preservation of heart muscle if an MI is suspected, (4) effective coping with illness-associated anxiety, (5) participation in a rehabilitation plan, and (6) reduction of risk factors.

Acute Care

If your patient has angina, perform the following measures: (1) position patient upright unless contraindicated and apply supplemental O_2, (2) assess vital signs, (3) place patient on continuous ECG monitor, (4) obtain a 12-lead ECG, (5) provide prompt pain relief, first with NTG, followed by an IV opioid analgesic, if needed, (6) obtain cardiac biomarkers, (7) assess heart and breath sounds, and (8) obtain a chest x-ray. The patient may be anxious and may have pale, cool, clammy skin. The BP and HR may be high. Auscultation of the heart may reveal an atrial (S_4) or a ventricular (S_3) gallop. A new systolic murmur heard during an angina attack may indicate ischemia of a papillary muscle of the mitral valve, causing mitral regurgitation (the mitral valve does not close properly). The murmur may be transient and disappear when symptoms resolve.

Ask the patient to describe the pain and to rate it on a scale of 0 to 10 before and after treatment to evaluate the effectiveness of the interventions. It is important to use the same words the patient uses to describe the symptoms (e.g., tightness, pressure). Assess for other signs of pain, such as restlessness; ECG changes; high HR, respiratory rate, or BP; clutching of the bed linens; or other nonverbal cues. Support and reassure the patient. Use a calm approach to help reduce the patient's anxiety during an angina attack. If the chest pain is not related to an ACS, the patient may be discharged within 1 or 2 days. Further testing may be done during the hospitalization or as an outpatient.

> ### ❓ CHECK YOUR PRACTICE
>
> A visitor finds you in the hallway and tells you that her father is having chest pain. The patient is not assigned to you.
> • How would you proceed?

Patient Teaching

Reassure the patient with a history of angina that a long, active life is possible. Preventing angina or at least reducing the frequency of angina is key, so teaching is important. Emphasize the importance of risk factor modification to slow the progression of CAD (Tables 33.1 and 33.11). Give the patient information about CAD, angina, precipitating factors for angina (Table 33.9) and medications to treat angina (Table 33.11).

You can provide patient teaching in a variety of ways. One-on-one contact between you and the patient is often the most effective approach. Time spent providing daily care (e.g., giving drugs) offers many teachable moments. Teaching aids, such as DVDs, heart models, and printed information, are important resources for patient and caregiver teaching (see Chapter 4).

Help the patient to identify factors that precipitate angina (Table 33.9). Tell the patient how to avoid or control these factors. For example, teach the patient to avoid exposure to extremes of weather and eating large, heavy meals. Tell the patient to rest for 1 to 2 hours after a heavy meal because blood shifts to the GI tract to aid digestion and absorption.

Help the patient to identify personal risk factors for CAD and ways to reduce modifiable risk factors (Table 33.2). Teach the patient and caregiver about diets low in salt and saturated fats (Tables 33.4 and 33.5). Maintaining ideal body weight is important in controlling angina because excess weight increases the heart's workload.

It is important that the patient has a regular, individualized program of physical activity that conditions rather than stresses the heart. For example, tell patients that walking briskly on a flat surface at least 30 minutes a day, most days of the week is recommended.

If needed, arrange for counseling to assess the psychologic adjustment of the patient and caregiver to the diagnosis of CAD and the resulting angina. Many patients feel a threat to identity, self-esteem, and the usual roles in society. These emotions are normal and real.

Drug Therapy

Drug therapy for chronic stable angina aims to reduce symptoms of and the risk for MI and death. The most common medications to optimize myocardial perfusion in chronic stable angina include nitrates, angiotensin-converting enzyme (ACE) inhibitors, β-blockers, and calcium channel blockers (Table 33.11 and Fig. 33.5). Aspirin (previously discussed) is given in the absence of contraindications (Table 33.12).

Short-Acting Nitrates. Short-acting nitrates are first-line therapy for an acute episode of angina. Nitrates produce their principal effects by the following mechanisms:

Dilating peripheral blood vessels: This results in decreased SVR, venous pooling, and decreased venous blood return to the heart (preload). Therefore myocardial O_2 demand is decreased because of the reduced cardiac workload.

Dilating coronary arteries and collateral vessels: This may increase blood flow to the ischemic areas of the heart. However, when the coronary arteries are severely atherosclerotic, coronary dilation is hard to achieve.

Sublingual Nitroglycerin. SL NTG tablets or translingual spray (Nitrolingual) usually relieves pain in about 5 minutes and lasts about 30 to 40 minutes. The recommended dose of NTG is 1 tablet taken sublingually (SL) or 1 to 2 metered sprays on or under the tongue for symptoms of angina. If symptoms are unchanged or worse after 5 minutes, the patient should repeat NTG every 5 minutes for a maximum of 3 doses. Teach the patient to contact the emergency response system (e.g., 911) if symptoms have not resolved completely after 3 doses.

Teach the patient the proper storage and use of NTG. It should be always easily accessible to the patient. Store the tablets away from light and heat sources, including body heat, to protect them from degradation. Tablets are packaged in light-resistant bottles with metal caps. Once opened, the tablets lose potency. They should be replaced every 6 months.

TABLE 33.11 Treatment of Chronic Stable Angina and Acute Coronary Syndrome

Strategies for the patient with chronic stable angina should address all the treatment elements and related patient teaching in the following mnemonic:

Element	Treatment
A	Antiplatelet/anticoagulant therapy
	Antianginal therapy
	ACE inhibitor/angiotensin receptor blocker
B	β-Blocker
	BP control
C	Cigarette smoking cessation
	Cholesterol (lipid) management
	Calcium channel blockers
	Cardiac rehabilitation
D	Diet (weight management)
	Diabetes management
	Depression screening
E	Education
	Exercise
F	Flu vaccination

Modified from Smith SC, Benjamin EJ, Bonow RO, et al: AHA/ACCF secondary prevention and risk reduction therapy for patients with coronary and other atherosclerotic vascular disease: 2011 update, *J Am Coll Cardiol* 58:2432, 2011.

Tell the patient to sit down and place the NTG tablet under the tongue and allow it to dissolve. If using the spray, the patient should direct it on or under the tongue, not inhale it. SL NTG tablets should cause a tingling sensation when taken; otherwise it may be outdated. Warn the patient that a headache, dizziness, or flushing may occur. Caution the patient to change positions slowly after NTG use because orthostatic hypotension may occur.

Teach the patient and caregiver the proper use of NTG. Patients can use NTG prophylactically before starting an activity that is known to cause angina (e.g., emotionally stressful situation, sexual intercourse). In these cases, the patient can take a tablet or spray 5 to 10 minutes before beginning the activity. Tell the patient to report any changes in the usual pattern of pain, such as increasing frequency, nighttime angina, or angina at rest.

Long-Acting Nitrates. Oral nitrates, such as isosorbide dinitrate (e.g., Isordil) and isosorbide mononitrate, are longer acting than SL or translingual NTG. They are used to reduce the frequency of angina attacks and to treat Prinzmetal's angina. The main side effect is headache from the dilation of cerebral blood vessels. Tell patients to take acetaminophen (Tylenol) to relieve the headache. Over time, the headaches may decrease, but the antianginal effects are still present.

Orthostatic hypotension is a complication of all nitrates. Monitor BP after the first dose, since the venous dilation that occurs may cause a drop in BP, especially in volume-depleted patients. Finally, tolerance to long-acting NTG can develop. To limit this, patients may have a scheduled 10- to 14-hour nitrate-free period every day. Remind patients that taking a long-acting NTG preparation should not keep them from using translingual or SL NTG if chest pain develops.

Nitroglycerin Ointment. Nitropaste is a 2% NTG topical ointment dosed by the inch. It is placed on the upper body or arm, over a flat muscular area that is free of hair and scars. Once absorbed, it prevents angina for 3 to 6 hours. The ointment

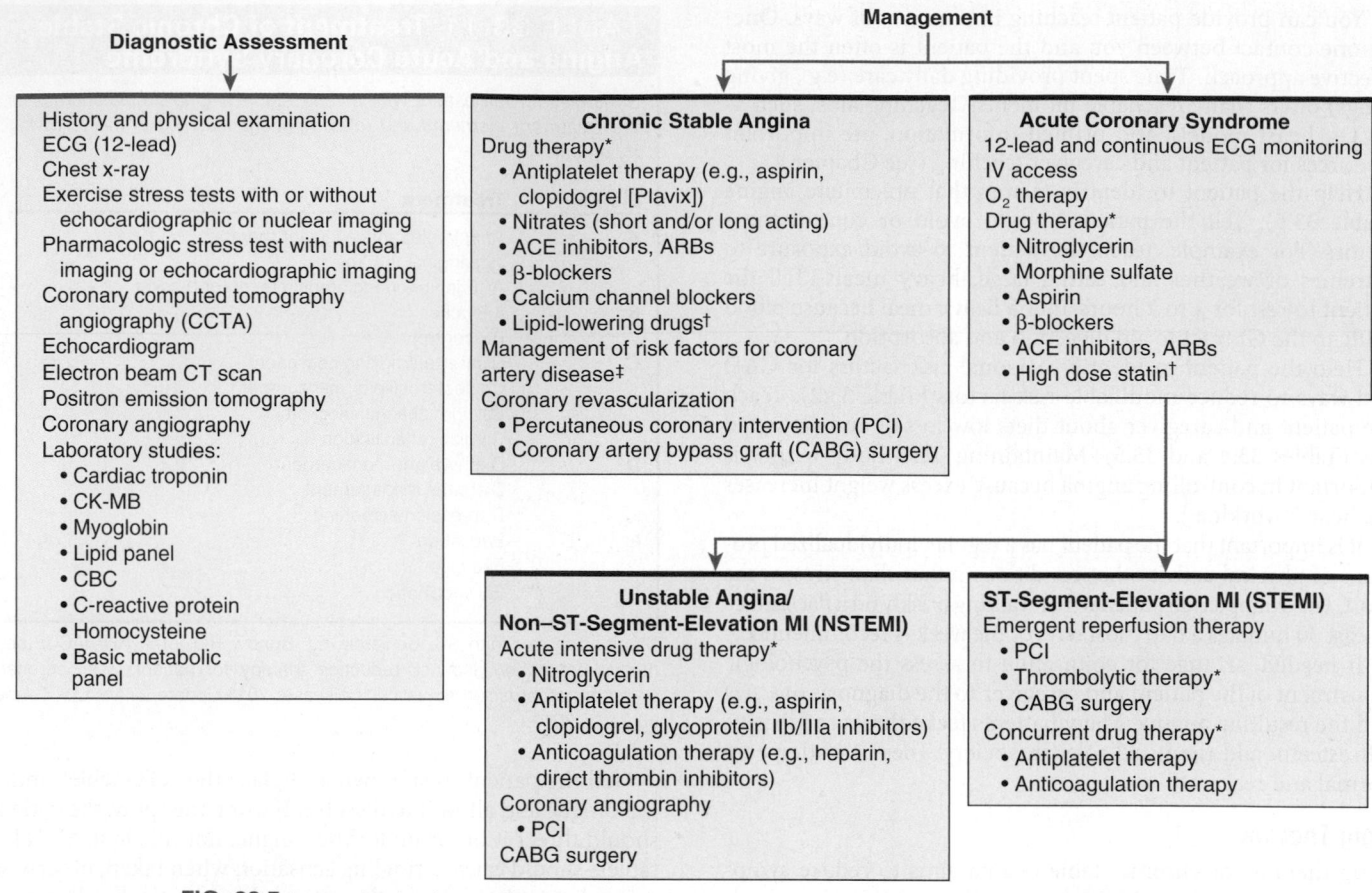

FIG. 33.5 Interprofessional care: Chronic stable angina and acute coronary syndrome. *Table 33.12. †Table 33.6. ‡Tables 33.2, 33.4, and 33.5.

should be wiped off each evening to allow for a 10- to 14-hour nitrate-free interval to prevent nitrate tolerance.

Transdermal Controlled-Release Nitrates. Currently 2 systems are available for transdermal NTG drug delivery: silicone gel and polymer matrix. These systems allow timed release of NTG over a 24-hour period. These preparations may be removed in the evening to allow for a 10- to 14-hour nitrate-free interval to reduce the risk for NTG tolerance.

DRUG ALERT Nitrates

- Keep NTG tablets in a dark, airtight container to maintain potency.
- Tell patients to sit down before using short-acting nitrates.
- SL NTG must be placed under the tongue.
- Spray translingual NTG onto or under the tongue.
- Tell patient not to combine NTG with drugs used for erectile dysfunction (e.g., sildenafil [Viagra]) as severe hypotension can occur.
- Monitor for orthostatic hypotension after administration.
- Headaches are common after taking any NTG preparation.
- Caregivers should use gloves to apply and remove NTG ointment or transdermal patches to avoid contact with drug.
- Never cardiovert or defibrillate over NTG ointment or a transdermal patch.
- When using long-acting nitrates, provide a 10- to 14-hour nitrate-free period.
- Remind patient when using long-acting nitrates that short acting nitrates can still be used, if needed.

Angiotensin-Converting Enzyme (ACE) Inhibitors and Angiotensin Receptor Blockers (ARBs). Patients with chronic stable angina who have an ejection fraction (EF) of 40% or less, diabetes, hypertension, or CKD should take an ACE inhibitor

(e.g., lisinopril [Zestril]) indefinitely, unless contraindicated. Patients with chronic stable angina and a normal EF, diabetes, and 1 other CAD risk factor should also take an ACE inhibitor to decrease the risk for MI, stroke, and death.[23]

These drugs result in vasodilation and reduced blood volume. Most important, they can prevent or reverse ventricular remodeling in patients who have had an MI (see p. 725). For patients who are intolerant of ACE inhibitors (e.g., cough, angioedema), angiotensin receptor blockers (ARBs) (e.g., losartan [Cozaar]) are used. ACE inhibitors and ARBs are also discussed later in the chapter and in Chapter 32 and Table 32.6.

β-Adrenergic Blockers. β-Blockers are given for relief of angina symptoms in patients with chronic stable angina. Patients who have LV dysfunction or elevated BP or had an MI should start and continue β-blockers indefinitely, unless contraindicated. These drugs decrease myocardial contractility, HR, SVR, and BP, all of which reduce the myocardial O_2 demand and relieve angina symptoms. β-Blockers that reduce the risk for death in patients with LV dysfunction, HF, or MI include carvedilol (Coreg), metoprolol succinate (Toprol XL), and bisoprolol.[13]

β_1-Receptors are found in the heart. β_2 Receptors are found in blood vessels, lungs, and liver. Some β-blockers are called cardioselective β-blockers because they only block β_1 receptors (e.g., atenolol [Tenormin], metoprolol [Lopressor]). Some β-blockers, referred to as nonselective β-blockers, block both β_1 and β_2 receptors (e.g., nadolol [Corgard], propranolol [Inderal]). Some β-blockers block α_1, β_1, and β_2 receptors (e.g., carvedilol [Coreg], labetalol [Trandate]).

TABLE 33.12 Drug Therapy

Chronic Stable Angina and Acute Coronary Syndrome

Drug	Mechanism of Action and Comments
Angiotensin-Converting Enzyme (ACE) Inhibitors (See Table 32.6)	
benazepril (Lotensin) captopril enalapril (Vasotec) lisinopril (Zestril) quinapril (Accupril) ramipril (Altace)	• Prevents conversion of angiotensin I to angiotensin II, resulting in vasodilation • May prevent or limit ventricular remodeling • Decreases endothelial dysfunction • Useful with HF, decreased LV function, tachycardia, MI, hypertension, diabetes, and chronic kidney disease
Angiotensin II Receptor Blockers (See Table 32.6)	
candesartan (Atacand) irbesartan (Avapro) losartan (Cozaar) olmesartan (Benicar) valsartan (Diovan)	• Inhibits binding of angiotensin II to angiotensin I receptors, resulting in vasodilation • Used for patients intolerant of ACE inhibitors
Anticoagulant Agents (See Table 37.10)	
Direct Thrombin Inhibitors	
bivalirudin (Angiomax) argatroban	• Direct inhibition of the clotting factor thrombin • Used during PCI procedure
Low-Molecular-Weight Heparin†	
dalteparin (Fragmin) enoxaparin (Lovenox)	• Binds to antithrombin III, enhancing its effect • Heparin–antithrombin III complex inactivates activated factor X and thrombin. • Prevents conversion of fibrinogen to fibrin
Unfractionated Heparin†	
heparin	• Prevents conversion of fibrinogen to fibrin and prothrombin to thrombin
Vitamin K Antagonist†	
warfarin (Coumadin)	• Interferes with hepatic synthesis of vitamin K–dependent clotting factors • Used for patients with atrial fibrillation or those at risk for thromboembolism (large anterior wall infarctions or ventricular aneurysms) • Closely monitor for bleeding when taking with antiplatelet drugs
Antiplatelet Agents	
aspirin	• Inhibits cyclooxygenase, which in turn produces thromboxane A_2, a potent platelet activator • Should be given as soon as ACS is suspected, unless truly allergic
cangrelor (Kengreal)	• Inhibits platelet aggregation • Given IV • Approved for use in patients having PCI during procedure
clopidogrel (Plavix)	• Inhibits platelet aggregation • Alternative for patients who cannot take aspirin • Used in combination with low-dose aspirin to treat ACS with or without PCI and after elective PCI
prasugrel (Effient)	• Inhibits platelet aggregation • Used as an alternative to clopidogrel in combination with aspirin for patient with ACS who had PCI • Not indicated to treat ACS without PCI or for use after elective PCI

Drug	Mechanism of Action and Comments
ticagrelor (Brilinta)	• Inhibits platelet aggregation • Alternative for patient who cannot take aspirin • Used in combination with low-dose aspirin to treat ACS with or without PCI • Effectiveness may be decreased by aspirin dosages >100 mg/day
vorapaxar (Zontivity)	• Inhibits platelet aggregation • Increases risk for bleeding, including life-threatening and fatal bleeding (boxed warning) • Must not be used in people who have had a stroke, transient ischemic attack (TIA), or bleeding in the head, because the risk for bleeding in the head is too great
Glycoprotein IIb/IIIa Inhibitors	
abciximab (ReoPro) eptifibatide (Integrilin) tirofiban (Aggrastat)	• Prevents the binding of fibrinogen to platelets, thereby blocking platelet aggregation • May be used in combination with aspirin for patients with ACS or during PCI
β-Adrenergic Blockers (See Table 32.6)	
atenolol (Tenormin) carvedilol (Coreg) metoprolol (Lopressor) nadolol (Corgard)	• Inhibits sympathetic nervous stimulation of the heart • Reduces heart rate, contractility, and BP • Reduces ischemia • Decreases afterload • Cardioselective β-blockers include atenolol and metoprolol
Calcium Channel Blockers (See Table 32.6)	
amlodipine (Norvasc) diltiazem (Cardizem) felodipine nicardipine (Cardene) verapamil (Calan) nifedipine (Procardia)	• Prevents calcium entry into vascular smooth muscle cells and myocytes (cardiac cells) • May prevent or control coronary vasospasm • Promotes coronary and peripheral vasodilation • Reduces HR, contractility, and BP
Nitrates (See Table 32.6)	
Sublingual nitroglycerin (Nitrostat) Translingual spray nitroglycerin (Nitrolingual) nitroglycerin ointment Transdermal nitroglycerin isosorbide dinitrate (Isordil) isosorbide mononitrate IV nitroglycerin	• Promotes peripheral vasodilation, decreasing preload and afterload • Promotes coronary artery vasodilation • May prevent or control coronary vasospasm
Opioid	
morphine	• Functions as an analgesic and sedative • Acts as a vasodilator to reduce preload and myocardial O_2 consumption
Thrombolytic Agents	
reteplase (Retavase) alteplase (Activase) tenecteplase (TNKase)	• Breaks up fibrin meshwork in clots • Used only in ST-segment-elevation MI when access to a hospital with PCI capability is not available

β-Blockers have many side effects that can be poorly tolerated. These include bradycardia, hypotension, wheezing from bronchospasm, and GI effects. Many patients report weight gain, depression, fatigue, and sexual dysfunction. Absolute contraindications to using β-blockers include severe bradycardia and acute decompensated HF. Patients with asthma should avoid β-blockers, especially nonselective ones. They are used cautiously in patients with diabetes since they mask signs of hypoglycemia. β-Blockers should not be stopped abruptly without medical supervision, as this may result in an increase in the number and intensity of angina attacks.

Calcium Channel Blockers. If β-blockers are contraindicated, are poorly tolerated, or do not control anginal symptoms, calcium channel blockers are used. Their main effects are: (1) systemic vasodilation with decreased SVR, (2) decreased myocardial contractility, (3) coronary vasodilation, and (4) decreased HR. They are used to treat Prinzmetal's angina.

There are 2 groups of calcium channel blockers. The dihydropyridines (e.g., amlodipine [Norvasc], nifedipine [Procardia]) have more vasodilatory effects. The nondihydropyridines (e.g., verapamil [Calan], diltiazem [Cardizem]) have a greater effect on decreasing HR and contractility.

Side effects include fatigue, headache, dizziness, flushing and peripheral edema. The nondihydropyridines enhance the action of digoxin by increasing serum digoxin levels. Digoxin levels are closely monitored after starting these agents. Teach the patient the signs and symptoms of digoxin toxicity. Verapamil can cause severe constipation by relaxing GI smooth muscle and slowing peristalsis, especially in older adults.[7]

Lipid-Lowering Drugs. A moderate or high dose of a lipid-lowering drug is given, unless contraindicated (Table 33.6). Patients with chronic stable angina are encouraged to follow a diet low in saturated fat and cholesterol.

Sodium Current Inhibitor. Ranolazine (Ranexa), a sodium current inhibitor, is used to treat chronic angina in patients who have not had an adequate response with other antianginal medications. Although it is approved as a first-line agent, it is usually added to the medication regimen only when the angina is not well controlled. Ranolazine does not affect the BP or HR, but it can prolong the QT interval. Use it very cautiously in patients with a long QT interval or who are taking other QT-prolonging drugs (e.g., fluoxetine [Prozac]).[7] Common side effects include dizziness, nausea, constipation, and headache.

Diagnostic Studies

When a patient describes new-onset chest pain and CAD is suspected or when a patient with chronic stable angina has a change in the angina pattern, a variety of studies are done (Fig. 33.5). After a detailed health history and physical examination, a 12-lead ECG is done and compared with a previous ECG to look for changes that may indicate an ACS. Laboratory tests (e.g., cardiac biomarkers) are used to determine if the patient is experiencing an ACS. Other laboratory tests may be done (e.g., lipid profile, CRP) to identify risk factors for CAD. A chest x-ray is done to look for cardiac enlargement, aortic calcifications, and pulmonary congestion. An echocardiogram can detect resting LV wall motion abnormalities, which may suggest CAD.

If the ECG and cardiac biomarkers are negative, an exercise stress test with or without echocardiography or nuclear imaging may be done either during the hospitalization or as an outpatient. For patients with physical limitations in walking, a pharmacologic (adenosine [Adenocard]) or dipyridamole stress test with nuclear imaging, or a pharmacologic (dobutamine) stress echocardiogram are options. Stress testing usually does not detect coronary blockages less than 70%.[13] Besides stress testing, other tests may be done if the ECG and cardiac biomarkers are negative. Electron beam computed tomography (EBCT) or coronary computed tomography angiography (CCTA or CTA) testing may be done if there is no evidence of an ACS and the patient remains free of chest pain. See Table 31.7 for more about these studies.

Cardiac Catheterization. For patients with increasing angina symptoms, a cardiac catheterization is the gold-standard test to identify and localize CAD. It is also recommended if the ECG shows ST-T wave changes (not ST elevation) and/or cardiac biomarkers are positive. This procedure should be done only if the patient is a candidate for percutaneous or surgical coronary revascularization.

If a coronary blockage is amenable to treatment, coronary revascularization with percutaneous coronary intervention (PCI) may be recommended. PCI may be done at the same time as the cardiac catheterization. During PCI, a catheter with a deflated balloon tip is inserted into the blocked coronary artery. The deflated balloon is positioned inside the blockage and inflated. This compresses the plaque against the artery wall, resulting in vessel dilation and a larger vessel diameter. This procedure is called *balloon angioplasty*.

Intracoronary stents are usually placed after a balloon angioplasty. A stent is an expandable mesh-like structure designed to keep the vessel open. It provides support to the arterial wall (Figs. 33.6 and 33.7). There are 2 types of stents: bare metal (BMS) and drug-eluting (DES). A DES is coated with a drug (e.g., everolimus, zotarolimus) to reduce the risk for overgrowth of the intimal lining (*neointimal hyperplasia*) within the stent. This is the primary cause of in-stent restenosis (ISR). This risk is lower with the use of a DES.

Because stents are thrombogenic, drugs are used to prevent platelet aggregation within the stent and acute stent thrombosis. Drugs commonly used during PCI are unfractionated heparin (UH) or low-molecular-weight heparin (LMWH), a direct thrombin inhibitor (e.g., bivalirudin [Angiomax]), and/or a glycoprotein IIb/IIIa inhibitor (e.g., eptifibatide [Integrilin]) (Table 33.12). After PCI, the patient receives dual antiplatelet therapy

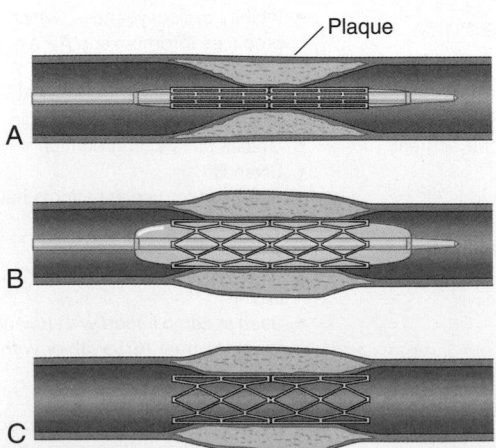

FIG. 33.6 Placement of a coronary artery stent. **A,** The stent is positioned at the site of the lesion. **B,** The balloon is inflated, expanding the stent. The balloon is then deflated and removed. **C,** The implanted stent is left in place.

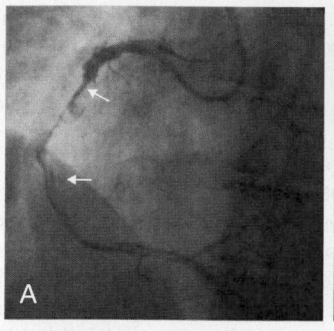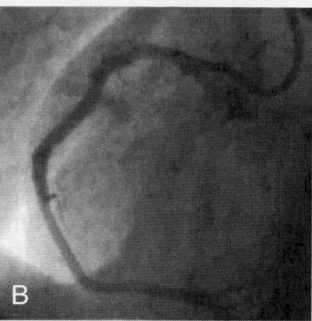

FIG. 33.7 **A,** A thrombotic occlusion of the right coronary artery is seen *(arrows).* **B,** Right coronary artery is opened and blood flow restored following angioplasty and placement of a 4-mm stent. (From Zipes DB, Libby P, Bonow RO, Braunwald E: *Braunwald's heart disease: A textbook of cardiovascular medicine,* ed 7, St Louis, 2005, Saunders.)

(DAPT) (e.g., aspirin [indefinitely] and ticagrelor or clopidogrel [Plavix]) until the intimal lining grows over the stent and provides a smooth vascular surface.

After DES placement, DAPT is used for a minimum of 12 months. The duration of DAPT for patients with a BMS is a minimum of 1 month after PCI. With the newer generation stents, 3 to 6 months of DAPT is enough to prevent stent thrombosis. Aspirin must continue forever.[24]

Potential complications from cardiac catheterization with PCI include abrupt closure from coronary artery dissection or rupture, vascular injury at the artery access site (e.g., femoral, radial), acute MI from acute stent thrombosis or from plaque dislodging and blocking the vessel distal to the catheter, stent embolization, failure to cross the blockage with a balloon or stent, coronary spasm, dye allergy, renal compromise, bleeding (e.g., retroperitoneal bleeding when the femoral artery is used or vascular access-site bleeding), infection, stroke, and emergent coronary artery bypass graft (CABG) surgery. The risk for dysrhythmias during and after the procedure is always present, so patients should be on a cardiac monitor afterwards.

More PCIs are done in the United States than CABGs.[1] PCI may not be a feasible option for all patients (e.g., patients with 3-vessel CAD [3 different coronary arteries] and/or significant left main coronary artery disease).[25] Coronary revascularization with CABG surgery may be recommended after cardiac catheterization.

Before and after cardiac catheterization and PCI, patients need frequent interventions (see Nursing Management: Cardiac Catheterization and PCI box and Table 31.9). Respiratory therapy may give prescribed therapies (e.g., nebulizer treatments) depending on the patient's past medical history.

Coronary Surgical Revascularization

In patients with chronic stable angina, coronary revascularization with CABG surgery is recommended for patients who (1) fail medical management, (2) have left main coronary artery or 3-vessel disease, (3) are not candidates for PCI (e.g., blockages are long or difficult to access), or (4) have failed PCI and continue to have chest pain. CABG also may be an option for patients with diabetes, LV dysfunction, and/or CKD.[25] CABG surgery and PCI are considered palliative treatment for CAD and not a cure. Lifestyle changes and medications may help slow the progression of the CAD and reduce the risk for recurrent events.

Traditional Coronary Artery Bypass Graft Surgery. CABG surgery consists of the placement of arterial or venous grafts to

NURSING MANAGEMENT
Percutaneous Coronary Intervention

Preprocedure
- Assess for allergies, especially to contrast dye.
- Perform baseline assessment, including vital signs, pulse oximetry, heart and breath sounds, neurovascular assessment of extremities (e.g., distal pulses, skin temperature, skin color, sensation).
- Assess baseline laboratory values (e.g., cardiac biomarkers, creatinine).
- Give drugs before the procedure and stop drugs not needed for the procedure (e.g., systemic heparin is stopped right before the cardiac catheterization).
- Teach patient and caregiver about procedure and postprocedure care.

Postprocedure
- Perform assessment and compare to baseline: vital signs, pulse oximetry, heart and breath sounds, neurovascular assessment of extremity used for procedure, assessment of catheter insertion site for hematoma, bleeding, and bruit.
- Assess neurovascular status of involved extremity every 15 min for the first hour, then according to agency policy.
- Check for bleeding at catheter insertion site every 15 min for the first hour, then according to agency policy.
- Report changes in neurovascular status of involved extremity or any bleeding.
- Monitor ECG for dysrhythmias or other changes (e.g., ST segment elevation or depression).
- Monitor patient for chest pain and other sources of pain or discomfort (e.g., back, vascular access site).
- Monitor IV infusions of antianginals (e.g., nitroglycerin) and antiplatelet medications (e.g., eptifibatide).
- Teach patient and caregiver about discharge drugs (e.g., aspirin, clopidogrel, lipid lowering drugs).
- Teach patient and caregiver about discharge care, including signs and symptoms to report to HCP (e.g., access site complications, return of chest pain).

Unlicensed Assistive Personnel (UAP)
- Oversee UAP:
  - Take vital signs and report increases or decreases in HR or BP to RN.
  - Report patient descriptions of chest pain, shortness of breath, and/ or any other discomfort or distress to RN.
  - Report changes in neurovascular status of the involved extremity or any bleeding to the RN.
  - Help with oral hygiene and hydration, meals, and toileting.
  - Record oral intake and urine output as ordered.

provide blood from the aorta or a branch of a major artery that originates from the aorta (e.g., internal mammary artery) to the heart muscle distal to blocked coronary arteries. The procedure may involve one or more grafts using the internal mammary (thoracic) artery (IMA or ITA), saphenous vein, and/or radial artery (Fig. 33.8). The gastroepiploic artery, and/ or inferior epigastric artery can be used as conduits but are not used as often due to the time and difficulty in harvesting those arteries.

CABG surgery requires a sternotomy (opening of the chest cavity) and *cardiopulmonary bypass* (CPB). During CPB, blood is diverted from the patient's heart to a machine where it is oxygenated and returned (via a pump) to the patient. This allows the HCP to operate on a quiet, nonbeating, bloodless heart while perfusion to vital organs is maintained. CPB is associated with postoperative neurologic dysfunction, renal problems, and systemic inflammatory response syndrome (SIRS).[25]

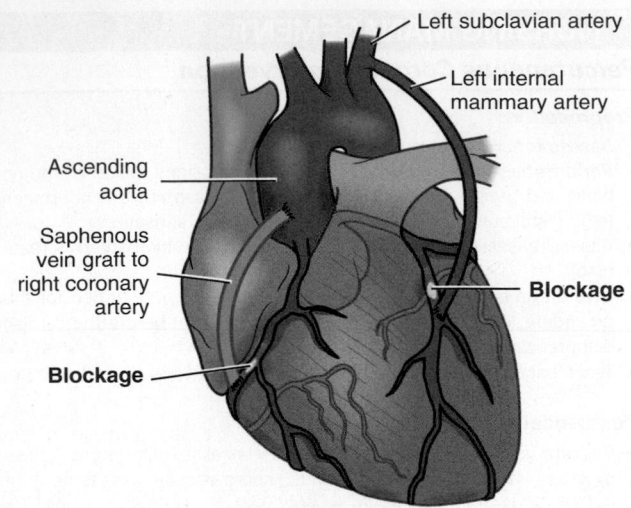

Left subclavian artery

Left internal mammary artery

Ascending aorta

Saphenous vein graft to right coronary artery

Blockage

Blockage

FIG. 33.8 Proximal end of the left internal mammary artery (LIMA) is left attached to the subclavian artery and the distal end of the LIMA is grafted (sutured) into the LAD artery below the blockage. Proximal end of the saphenous vein is grafted (sutured) to the aorta, and the distal end is grafted (sutured) into the right coronary artery below the area of blockage.

The IMA is the most common artery used for bypass graft. The proximal part is left attached to its origin (the subclavian artery). The distal end of the IMA is dissected from the chest wall. Next, it is *anastomosed* (sutured) to the coronary artery distal to the blockage. It usually is used to bypass the left anterior descending (LAD) artery because the LAD supplies blood to the largest part of the heart muscle (anterior wall). The IMA tends to have longer patency rates than saphenous veins (Fig. 33.8).

Saphenous veins can be used for bypass grafts. The HCP endoscopically removes the saphenous vein from one or both legs. A section is sutured into the ascending aorta near the native coronary artery opening and then anastomosed to the coronary artery distal to the blockage (Fig. 33.8). Saphenous vein grafts are more prone to develop diffuse intimal hyperplasia. This contributes to future stenosis and graft occlusion. The use of antiplatelet and statin therapy after surgery helps maintain vein graft patency.

The radial artery, another potential graft, is a thick muscular artery prone to spasm. Perioperative calcium channel blockers and long-acting nitrates can control the spasms. Patency rates are not as good as the IMA but are better than saphenous veins. Serious extremity complications (e.g., hand ischemia, wound infection) are rare after removal of the radial artery. Paresthesia and impaired sensation are common side effects after radial artery harvest.[26]

Women have higher periprocedural mortality and morbidity rates than men. This has been attributed to the late treatment of CAD in women because women first present with CAD at an older age and have more co-morbidities at the time of surgery. Other factors include smaller diameter coronary vessels, smaller body surface area, and the fact that women are less likely to be referred for catheterization.[25]

Minimally Invasive Direct Coronary Artery Bypass. *Minimally invasive direct coronary artery bypass* (MIDCAB) offers patients with disease of the LAD or right coronary artery an approach to surgical treatment that does not involve a sternotomy and CPB. The technique requires several small incisions between the ribs or a mini-thoracotomy. A thoracoscope or robotic assistance

may be used to dissect the IMA from the chest wall, but usually it is done via direct visualization.[26] A mechanical stabilizer immobilizes the operative site. The IMA is then sutured to the LAD or right coronary artery. Some patients undergo hybrid procedures in which they have a MIDCAB for the LAD artery and undergo a PCI of a second or third artery later.

Off-Pump Coronary Artery Bypass. The *off-pump coronary artery bypass* (OPCAB) procedure uses a median sternotomy to access all coronary vessels. OPCAB is performed on a beating heart (no CPB) using mechanical stabilizers. OPCAB is associated with less blood loss, less renal dysfunction, less postoperative atrial fibrillation, and fewer neurologic complications.[25] Worldwide, less than 30% of CABG procedures are OPCAB procedures.[26]

Totally Endoscopic Coronary Artery Bypass. Totally endoscopic coronary artery bypass (TECAB) uses a robotic technology to perform CABG surgery. Several instrument ports in the chest are required. This procedure is done without the use of CPB or with the use of CPB using femoral access. TECAB is used for limited bypass grafting. The benefits include smaller incisions, decreased blood loss, less pain, and shorter recovery time.[26]

Transmyocardial Laser Revascularization. *Transmyocardial laser revascularization* is an indirect revascularization procedure. It is used for patients with advanced CAD who are not candidates for traditional CABG surgery and who have persistent angina despite maximum medical therapy. The procedure involves the use of a high-energy laser to create channels in the heart muscle to allow blood flow to ischemic areas. The procedure can be done using a left thoracotomy approach. It is used as an adjunctive therapy when bypass grafts cannot be placed to help reduce angina symptoms. It also can be used in combination with CABG surgery.[26]

Postoperative Care After CABG Surgery

Care after CABG surgery is provided in the intensive care unit (ICU) for the first 24 to 36 hours. Ongoing and intensive monitoring of the patient's hemodynamic status is critical. The patient will have many invasive lines for monitoring heart status and other vital functions (see Chapter 65). These include (1) hemodynamic monitoring (e.g., CO), (2) an arterial line for continuous BP monitoring, (3) pleural and mediastinal chest tubes for chest drainage, (4) continuous ECG monitoring, (5) an endotracheal tube connected to mechanical ventilation, (6) epicardial pacing wires for emergency pacing of the heart, (7) a urinary catheter to monitor urine output, and (8) a nasogastric tube for gastric decompression. Most patients are extubated within 6 hours and transferred to a step-down unit within 24 to 48 hours for continued monitoring.

Many of the postoperative complications that develop after CABG surgery relate to the use of CPB. Major complications of CPB are systemic inflammation, bleeding and anemia from damage to red blood cells and platelets, fluid and electrolyte imbalances, infections, and hypothermia (because blood is cooled as it passes through the CPB machine). Focus your care on assessing the patient for bleeding (e.g., chest tube drainage, incision sites), monitoring hemodynamics, checking fluid status, replacing blood and electrolytes as needed, and restoring temperature (e.g., warming blankets).

Postoperative dysrhythmias, especially atrial dysrhythmias (e.g., atrial fibrillation [AF]), are common. The incidence of postoperative AF after CABG surgery is 20% to 40%.[26] β-Blockers should be started or restarted as soon as possible after surgery (unless contraindicated) to reduce the incidence of AF.[25]

Discharge may be delayed in patients who develop AF in order to begin anticoagulation therapy, especially if using warfarin. (See Chapter 35 for information on treatment of AF.)

Nursing care for the patient with a CABG includes wound care for the patient's surgical sites (e.g., leg, chest, arm). Chest incisions are often closed with skin adhesive and do not need dressings after 24 hours. Management of the chest wound is similar to that of other chest surgeries (see Chapter 27). Care of the leg incision is minimal since endoscopy is used to harvest the vein.

Care of a radial artery harvest site includes monitoring sensory and motor function of the hand. The patient with radial artery harvest should take a calcium channel blocker and/or a long-acting nitrate for around 3 months to reduce the incidence of arterial spasm at the arm or anastomosis site.

Other nursing interventions include strategies to manage pain and prevent venous thromboembolism (e.g., early ambulation, sequential compression device) and respiratory complications (e.g., incentive spirometry, splinting during coughing and deep-breathing exercises). (See Chapter 19 for care of the postoperative patient.)

Patients may have some cognitive dysfunction. This includes impairment of memory, concentration, language comprehension, and social integration. Depression and anxiety are common. Patients may cry or become teary. *Postoperative cognitive dysfunction* (POCD) can manifest days to weeks to months after surgery but usually improves within a few months after surgery. However, it may become a chronic disorder.[27] POCD is discussed in Chapter 19.

In the older patient (> age 80), elective CABG is generally well tolerated. Many patients have multiple preoperative co-morbidities, so the incidence of postoperative complications (e.g., dysrhythmias, stroke, POCD, infection) is higher. Although the benefits of treatment may outweigh risks in this group, morbidity and mortality are higher than in younger persons.[25]

Postoperative nursing care of the patient with a MIDCAB, OPCAB, or TECAB procedure is similar to that for CABG surgery patients. The recovery time is shorter with these procedures. Patients often resume routine activities sooner than patients who have CABG surgery. Pain control is important regardless of the procedure. Patients generally report higher levels of pain with a thoracotomy incision than a sternotomy incision.

Alternative Therapies for Refractory Chronic Stable Angina

For patients with refractory angina, *enhanced external counterpulsation* (EECP) may be used. EECP consists of placing inflatable BP cuffs around the legs. The cuffs sequentially inflate during diastole and deflate during systole from the calves to the thighs. This action increases venous return and augments diastolic BP. This increases coronary perfusion, improves LV diastolic filling, and helps with collateral circulation. Patients get treatments 5 days a week for a total of 35 treatments. EECP is contraindicated in patients with decompensated HF, severe peripheral arterial disease, and severe aortic insufficiency.[13]

ACUTE CORONARY SYNDROME

When chest pain from ischemia is prolonged and not immediately reversible, acute coronary syndrome (ACS) may develop. ACS includes the spectrum of non-ST elevation acute coronary syndrome (*UA and non–ST-segment-elevation myocardial infarction* [NSTEMI]), and *ST-segment-elevation myocardial infarction*

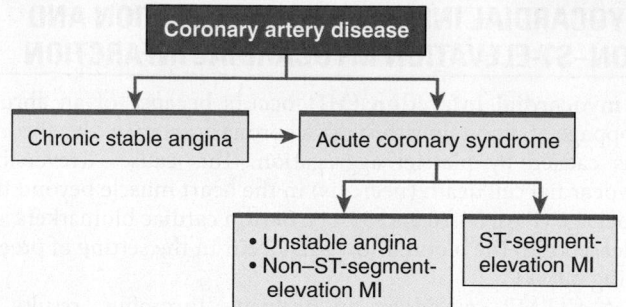

FIG. 33.9 Relationships among coronary artery disease, chronic stable angina, and acute coronary syndrome.

(STEMI) (Fig. 33.9). When patients first present with chest pain, ST-elevations on the 12-lead ECG most likely indicate a STEMI (Fig. 33.4, *B*). The ECG should be compared to a previous ECG whenever possible. ST elevation represents myocardial injury that is potentially reversible, but, if not treated, will likely evolve to permanent necrosis (tissue death) of the myocardium. Patients with UA or NSTEMI may or may not have ST segment depression and/or T wave inversion on the ECG. For patients with chest pain who do not have ST segment elevation or ST-T wave changes on the ECG, it is difficult to distinguish between UA and NSTEMI until we evaluate serum cardiac biomarkers.[15]

On the cellular level, the heart muscle becomes hypoxic within the first 10 seconds of a total coronary occlusion. Heart cells are deprived of O_2 and glucose needed for aerobic metabolism and contractility. Anaerobic metabolism begins, and lactic acid accumulates. In ischemic conditions, heart cells are viable for about 20 minutes. Irreversible heart damage starts after 20 minutes if there is no collateral circulation (Fig. 33.2).[21] With restoration of blood flow (reperfusion), aerobic metabolism resumes, contractility is restored, and cellular repair begins.

ACS is caused by the decline of a once-stable atherosclerotic plaque. The previously stable plaque ruptures, releasing the lipid core into the vessel. This causes platelet aggregation and thrombus formation. The vessel may be partially blocked by a thrombus (manifesting as UA or NSTEMI) or totally blocked by a thrombus (manifesting as STEMI). We are not sure what causes the plaque to suddenly become unstable. Systemic inflammation (described earlier) may play a role. Patients with suspected ACS need immediate hospitalization.

UNSTABLE ANGINA

Unstable angina (UA) is chest pain that is new in onset, occurs at rest, or occurs with increasing frequency, duration, or less effort than the patient's chronic stable angina pattern. The pain usually lasts 10 minutes or more.

The patient with chronic stable angina may develop UA, or UA may be the first clinical sign of CAD. Unlike chronic stable angina, UA is unpredictable and must be treated immediately. The patient with previously diagnosed chronic stable angina describes a significant change in the pattern of angina. It occurs with increasing frequency and is easily provoked by minimal exertion, during sleep, or even at rest. The patient without previously diagnosed angina describes chest pain that has progressed rapidly in the past few hours, days, or weeks, often ending in pain at rest. ECG changes that may be seen with UA include ST depression and/or T wave inversion (Fig. 33.4, A). These changes are referred to as ischemic changes.

MYOCARDIAL INFARCTION: ST-ELEVATION AND NON–ST-ELEVATION MYOCARDIAL INFARCTION

A **myocardial infarction (MI)** occurs because of an abrupt stoppage of blood flow through a coronary artery with a thrombus caused by platelet aggregation. This causes irreversible myocardial cell death (necrosis) in the heart muscle beyond the blockage (Figs. 33.10 and 33.11). Serum cardiac biomarkers are released into the blood. Most MIs occur in the setting of preexisting CAD.[13]

A STEMI, caused by an occlusive thrombus, results in ST-elevation in the ECG leads facing the area of infarction (Figs. 33.12 and 33.13). ST segment elevation is significant if it is 1 mm or more above the isoelectric line in at least 2 contiguous (neighboring) leads except in V_2 and V_3, where the ST elevation must be 2 mm or more.[28]

A STEMI is an emergency. To limit the infarct size, the artery must be opened within 90 minutes of presentation to restore blood and O_2 to the heart muscle and limit the infarct size. This can be done either by PCI or with thrombolytic (fibrinolytic) therapy. PCI is the first-line treatment, if available. It confirms which artery has the occlusive thrombus so it can be opened with a balloon and stent (Fig. 33.6). Thrombolytic therapy is done in hospitals that do not have a catheterization laboratory for PCI. If the patient does not seek treatment quickly, the STEMI will evolve.

NSTEMI, caused by a nonocclusive thrombus, does not cause ST segment elevation on the 12-lead ECG. The ECG may or may not show ST depression and/or T wave inversion in the leads facing the area of infarction. NSTEMI patients usually undergo catheterization within 12 to 72 hours. Thrombolytic therapy is not indicated for NSTEMI.

With either NSTEMI or STEMI, an echocardiogram may show *hypokinesis* (worsening myocardial contractility) or *akinesis* (absent myocardial contractility) in the necrotic area(s). The degree of LV dysfunction depends on the area of the heart involved and size of the infarction.

The acute MI process evolves over time, from hours to a few days. The earliest tissue to become ischemic is the subendocardium (the innermost layer of tissue in the heart muscle). If ischemia persists, it takes around 4 to 6 hours for the entire thickness of the heart muscle to necrose. If the thrombus is not completely blocking the artery, the time to complete necrosis may be as long as 12 hours.

Most MIs affect the LV and are usually described based on the location of damage (e.g., anterior, inferior, lateral, septal, or posterior wall infarction). The location of the MI and ECG changes correlate with the involved coronary artery (Table 33.13). For example, in most people, the right coronary artery supplies blood to the inferior and posterior LV walls. Blockage of the right coronary artery results in an inferior wall and/or posterior wall MI. Anterior wall infarctions result from blockages in the LAD artery. Blockages in the left circumflex artery usually cause lateral wall MIs. Damage can occur in more than 1 location, especially if more than 1 coronary artery is involved (e.g., anterolateral MI). Right ventricular MIs are much less common and treated differently from LV MIs. Suspect a right ventricular MI in patients who have a left inferior wall STEMI.[28]

The degree of collateral circulation influences the severity of the MI (Fig. 33.2). Not everyone develops collateral circulation. A person with a long history of CAD may develop good

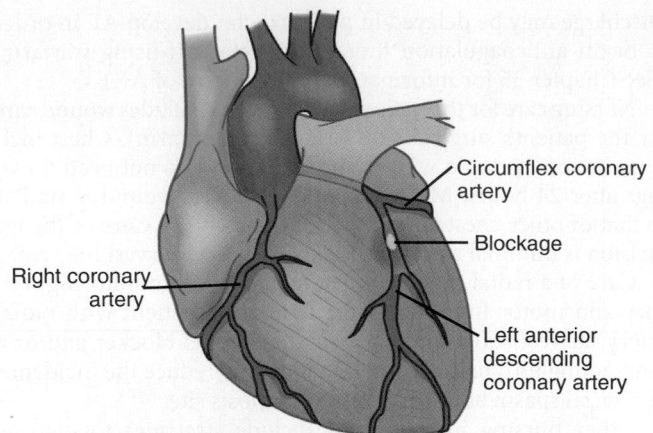

FIG. 33.10 Occlusion of the LAD coronary artery, resulting in acute MI.

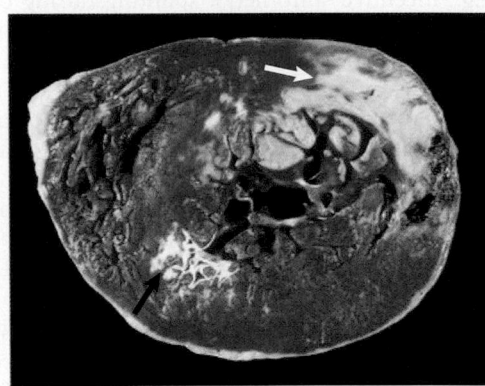

FIG. 33.11 Acute MI in the posterolateral wall of the left ventricle. This is shown by the absence of staining in the areas of necrosis *(white arrow)*. Note the scarring from a previous anterior wall MI *(black arrow)*. (From Kumar V, Abbas AK, Aster JC, et al: *Robbins and Cotran pathologic basis of disease,* ed 8, Philadelphia, 2010, Saunders.)

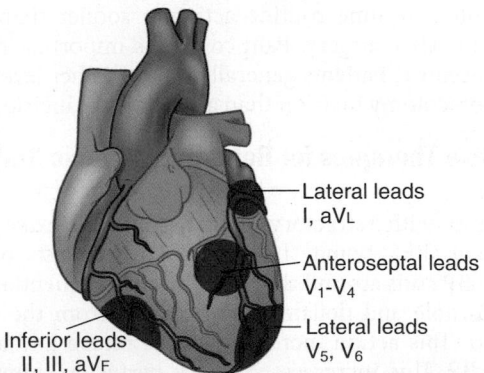

FIG. 33.12 Definitive ECG changes occur in leads that face the area of ischemia, injury, or infarction. Reciprocal changes may occur in leads facing opposite the area of ischemia, injury, or infarction.

collateral circulation to provide the area surrounding the infarction site with an adequate blood supply. This is one reason why a younger person may have a more serious first MI than an older person with the same degree of blockage.

Women who have MIs are often undertreated with guideline-based recommendations, leading to worse outcomes and increased rates of readmission, reinfarction, and death in the first year after MI.[5]

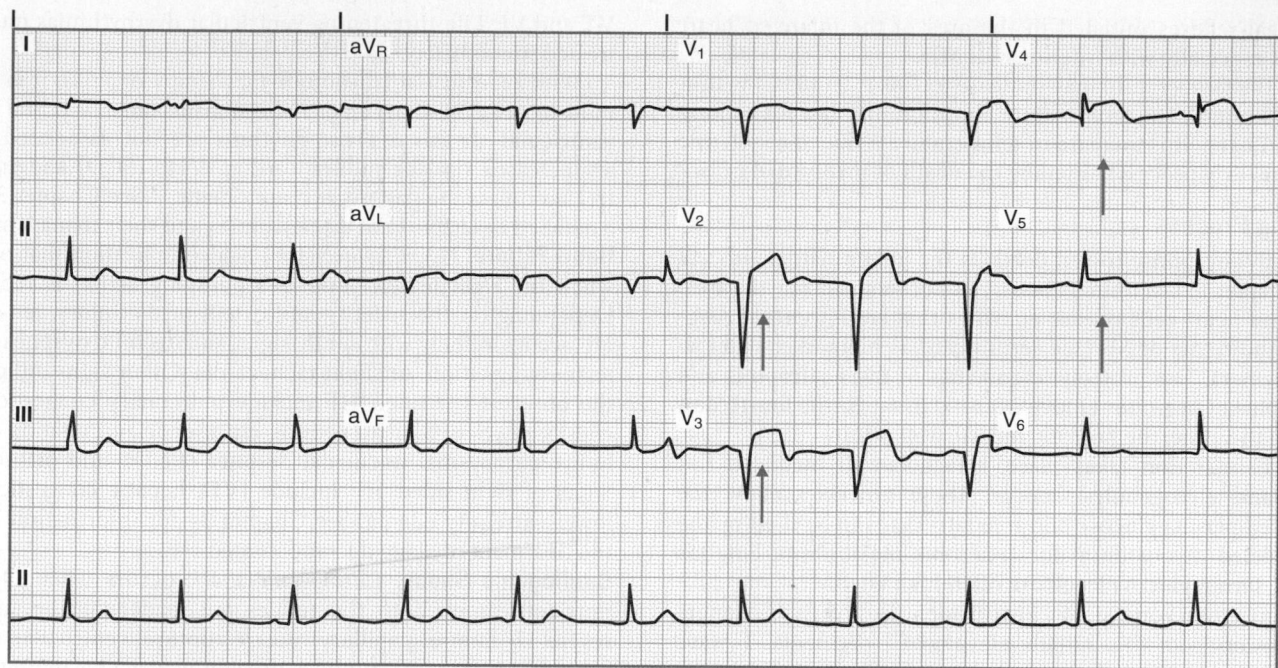

FIG. 33.13 ECG findings with anteroseptal lateral wall MI. Normally, leads I, aVL, and V₁ to V₃ have a positive R wave. Note the pathologic Q waves in these leads and the ST segment elevation in leads V₂ to V₆ (arrows).

TABLE 33.13 ECG Evidence in Acute Coronary Syndrome

| Left Ventricle Involvement | ECG EVIDENCE | | |
	Leads Facing Area	Leads Opposite Area (Reciprocal Changes)	Associated Coronary Artery
Septal wall	V₁, V₂	II, III, aVF	LAD
Anterior wall	V₃, V₄	II, III, aVF	LAD
Lateral wall, low	V₅, V₆	II, III, aVF	LAD or circumflex
Lateral wall, high	I, aVL	II, III, aVF	Circumflex
Inferior wall	II, III, aVF	I, aVL, V₅, V₆	Right coronary artery, posterior descending coronary artery

---

Clinical Manifestations of Myocardial Infarction

Pain. Severe chest pain not relieved by rest, position change, or nitrate administration may mean the patient is having an MI. Persistent and unlike any other pain, it is usually described as a heavy, pressure, tight, burning, constricted, or crushing feeling. Common locations are the substernal or epigastric area. The pain may radiate to the neck, lower jaw, and arms or to the back (Fig. 33.3). When epigastric pain is present, the patient may relate it to indigestion, take antacids without relief, and therefore delay seeking treatment. It may occur while the patient is active or at rest, asleep, or awake. It often occurs in the early morning hours. It usually lasts for 20 minutes or longer and is more severe than chronic angina pain.

Not everyone who has an MI has classic symptoms. Some patients may not have pain but may have "discomfort," weakness, nausea, indigestion, or shortness of breath. Some women may have atypical discomfort, shortness of breath, or fatigue. Patients with diabetes may have silent (asymptomatic) MIs because of cardiac neuropathy or have atypical symptoms (e.g., shortness of breath). An older patient may have a change in mental status (e.g., confusion), shortness of breath, pulmonary edema, dizziness, or a dysrhythmia.

Sympathetic Nervous System Stimulation. During the initial phase of MI, the ischemic heart cells release catecholamines (norepinephrine and epinephrine) that are normally found in these cells. This results in diaphoresis, increased HR and BP, and vasoconstriction of peripheral blood vessels. On physical examination, the patient's skin may be ashen, clammy, and cool to touch.

Cardiovascular Manifestations. In response to the release of catecholamines, BP and HR may be high initially. Later, the BP may drop because of decreased CO. If severe enough, this may result in decreased renal perfusion and urine output. Crackles, if present, may persist for several hours to several days, suggesting LV dysfunction. Jugular venous distention (JVD), hepatic engorgement, and peripheral edema may mean right ventricular dysfunction.

Examination may reveal abnormally distant heart sounds. Other abnormal sounds suggesting LV dysfunction are S₃ and S₄. A loud holosystolic murmur may occur with a ventricular septal defect, papillary muscle rupture, or mitral valve dysfunction (mitral regurgitation).

Nausea and Vomiting. The patient may have nausea and vomiting. These symptoms can result from reflex stimulation of the vomiting center by the severe pain. They can also result from vasovagal reflexes initiated in the area of the infarcted heart muscle, especially with inferior wall MIs.

Fever. The temperature may increase to 100.4° F (38° C) within 24 to 48 hours. The temperature elevation may last for as long as 4 to 5 days. This increase in temperature is due to a systemic inflammatory process caused by the death of myocardial cells.

Healing Process

The body's response to cell death is the inflammatory process (see Chapter 11). Within 24 hours, leukocytes infiltrate the area. The dead heart cells release enzymes that are important diagnostic indicators of MI (see serum cardiac biomarkers later in this chapter). The proteolytic enzymes of the neutrophils and macrophages begin to remove necrotic tissue by the fourth day. During this time, the necrotic muscle wall is thin.

Once infarction takes place, catecholamine-mediated lipolysis and glycogenolysis occur. These processes allow the increased plasma glucose and free fatty acids to be used by the O_2-depleted myocardium for anaerobic metabolism. For this reason, serum glucose levels are often high after MI.

The necrotic zone of a STEMI is identified by ECG changes (e.g., lowering of the initially elevated ST segments, T wave inversion and/or a pathologic Q wave) within 1 or 2 days. At this point, the neutrophils and monocytes have cleared the necrotic debris from the injured area, and the collagen matrix that will eventually form scar tissue is laid down.

At 10 to 14 days after MI, the new scar tissue is still weak. The heart muscle is vulnerable to increased stress during this time. At the same time, the patient's activity level may be increasing, so special caution and assessment are necessary. By 6 weeks after MI, scar tissue has replaced necrotic tissue and the injured area is considered healed. Often the scarred area is less compliant than the surrounding area. This condition may be manifested by abnormal wall motion on an echocardiogram or nuclear imaging (e.g., hypokinesis, akinesis), LV dysfunction, altered conduction patterns, dysrhythmias, or HF. The scarred area may become an irritable focus for life-threatening dysrhythmias causing sudden cardiac death (SCD) years later (see section on SCD on pp. 730–731).

These changes in the infarcted heart muscle also cause changes in the unaffected areas. To try to compensate for the damaged muscle, the normal myocardium hypertrophies and dilates. This process is called *ventricular remodeling*. Remodeling of normal myocardium can lead to the development of late HF, especially in the person with atherosclerosis of other coronary arteries and/or an anterior MI. ACE inhibitor drugs are given to limit ventricular remodeling.

Complications of Myocardial Infarction

Dysrhythmias. Any condition that affects the heart cells' sensitivity to nerve impulses (e.g., ischemia, electrolyte imbalances, SNS stimulation) can cause dysrhythmias that adversely affect the damaged heart muscle. Dysrhythmias are the most common complication after an MI. They occur in 80% to 90% of patients. Ventricular tachycardia (VT) and ventricular fibrillation (VF) are the most common cause of death in patients in the prehospital period.

After MI, bradycardias (e.g., complete heart block) develop when key areas of the conduction system are destroyed (e.g., infarction involves the sinus or atrioventricular node). VT or VF most often occurs within the first 4 hours after the onset of pain. Premature ventricular contractions (PVCs) may precede VT and VF. Life-threatening ventricular dysrhythmias must be treated immediately.

With reperfusion (thrombolytic therapy or PCI), it is common to see PVCs, asymptomatic nonsustained VT, and idioventricular rhythms. These rhythms are not associated with an increased risk for sudden cardiac death (SCD) and are not treated unless the patient is symptomatic.[28] See Chapter 35 for a detailed description of dysrhythmias and their management.

Heart Failure. *Heart failure* (HF) is a complication that occurs when the right or left ventricle's pumping action is reduced. Depending on the severity and extent of the injury, left-sided HF occurs initially with subtle signs, such as mild dyspnea, restlessness, agitation, or slight tachycardia. Other signs indicating the onset of left-sided HF include pulmonary congestion on chest x-ray, S_3 or S_4 heart sounds, crackles on auscultation of the lungs, paroxysmal nocturnal dyspnea (PND), and orthopnea. Signs of right-sided HF include JVD, hepatic congestion, or lower extremity edema. See Chapter 34 for information about the treatment of acute decompensated HF.

Cardiogenic Shock. *Cardiogenic shock* occurs when O_2 and nutrients supplied to the tissues are inadequate because of severe LV failure, papillary muscle rupture, ventricular septal rupture, LV free wall rupture, or right ventricular infarction.[28] This occurs less often when STEMI is treated early and rapidly with PCI or thrombolytic therapy. Cardiogenic shock, associated with a high death rate, requires aggressive management. This includes control of dysrhythmias, intraaortic balloon pump (IABP) therapy, and support of contractility with vasoactive drugs. Goals of therapy are to maximize O_2 delivery, reduce O_2 demand, and prevent complications (e.g., acute kidney injury). Cardiogenic shock is discussed in Chapter 66.

Papillary Muscle Dysfunction or Rupture. *Papillary muscle dysfunction* may occur if the infarcted area includes or is near the papillary muscle that attaches to the mitral valve (see Fig. 31.2). Suspect papillary muscle dysfunction if you hear a new systolic murmur suggestive of mitral regurgitation at the cardiac apex. An echocardiogram confirms the diagnosis.

Papillary muscle rupture is a rare and life-threatening complication. It causes acute and massive mitral valve regurgitation with no time for the heart to compensate. Dyspnea, pulmonary edema, and decreased CO result from the backup of blood in the left atrium. This condition aggravates an already damaged LV by reducing CO even further. The patient undergoes rapid clinical decline. Treatment includes afterload reduction with nitroprusside (Nipride) and/or IABP therapy and immediate cardiac surgery with mitral valve repair or replacement. (See Chapter 36 for discussion of valve disorders.)

Left Ventricular Aneurysm. *Left ventricular aneurysm* results when the infarcted heart wall is thin and bulges out during contraction. This can develop within a few days, weeks, or months. It is more common with anterior MIs.[28] The patient with a ventricular aneurysm may develop HF, dysrhythmias, and angina. Besides ventricular rupture, which is usually fatal, ventricular aneurysms can hide thrombi that can lead to an embolic stroke. Anticoagulation therapy is recommended for these patients unless contraindicated.

Ventricular Septal Wall Rupture and Left Ventricular Free Wall Rupture. A new loud systolic murmur heard in patients with acute MI may signal ventricular septal wall rupture. Depending on the size of the defect and degree of right and LV dysfunction, HF and cardiogenic shock may occur. The patient must undergo emergency repair, either surgically or percutaneously. The defect can quickly expand and lead to hemodynamic compromise.[28]

LV free wall rupture is an emergent clinical situation. Rapid hemodynamic compromise and death ensues if not treated immediately. Although this is a rare complication, death rates are high. Free wall rupture is seen more often in patients after their first MI, patients with anterior MIs, older adults, and women.[28]

Pericarditis. *Acute pericarditis,* an inflammation of the visceral and/or parietal pericardium, may occur 2 or 3 days after an acute MI. Pericarditis is characterized by mild to severe chest pain that increases with inspiration, coughing, and movement of the upper body. Sitting in a forward position often relieves the pain. The pain is usually different from pain associated with an MI.

Assess the patient with suspected pericarditis for the presence of a friction rub over the pericardium. The sound is best heard with the diaphragm of the stethoscope at the mid to lower left sternal border. It may be persistent or intermittent. Fever may be present. The patient may have hypotension and/or a narrow pulse pressure if it is accompanied by significant pericardial effusion or cardiac tamponade. Asymptomatic pericardial effusions are common after STEMI.[28]

Diagnosis of pericarditis can be made with the 12-lead ECG. Typical ECG changes include diffuse ST segment elevations in many leads (with STEMI, ST elevation occurs in the leads facing the infarcted wall). This reflects the inflammation of the pericardium. Treatment includes pain relief with high doses of aspirin (e.g., 650 mg every 4 to 6 hours). Nonsteroidal antiinflammatory drugs (NSAIDs) and corticosteroids are avoided in the first 4 weeks after MI because they can interfere with myocardial scar formation.[21,28] Pericarditis is discussed in Chapter 36.

Dressler Syndrome. *Dressler syndrome* is pericarditis and fever that develop 1 to 8 weeks after MI. Although the cause is unclear, it may be an autoimmune reaction to the necrotic heart muscle. The patient has chest pain, fever, malaise, a pericardial friction rub, and arthralgia. A pericardial effusion may be present. Laboratory findings include a high white blood cell count and sedimentation rate. High-dose aspirin is the treatment of choice.

DIAGNOSTIC STUDIES: ACUTE CORONARY SYNDROME

In addition to the patient's history of pain, risk factors, and health history, the primary diagnostic studies used to determine whether a person has UA or an MI (STEMI or NSTEMI) include a 12-lead ECG and serum cardiac biomarkers.

Electrocardiogram Findings

The ECG is one of the primary tools to diagnose UA or an MI (STEMI or NSTEMI). Whenever possible, it should be compared to a previous ECG. Changes in the QRS complex, ST segment, and T wave caused by injury, ischemia, and infarction can develop slowly or quickly with UA and MI. The pattern of ECG changes among the 12 leads provides information on the coronary artery involved in ACS (Table 33.13).

The ECG must be read carefully since changes can be absent or subtle at first. For this reason, serial 12-lead ECGs are done. For diagnostic and treatment purposes, it is important to distinguish between STEMI and NSTEMI/UA. STEMI patients usually have a complete coronary occlusion. ST elevation in the leads facing the infarcted wall is seen first on the 12-lead ECG

(Figs. 33.4, *B*, 33.12, and 33.13 and Table 33.13). ST segment elevation is significant if it is 1 mm or more above the isoelectric line in at least 2 contiguous leads. Within a few hours to days, the ST segments begin to lower, with T wave inversion and pathologic Q waves developing in the same leads (Fig. 33.4, *C*). The Q wave is the first negative deflection after a P wave (Fig. 33.4, *A*). A pathologic Q wave is defined as a deep Q wave, greater than or equal to one-third the height of the R wave in the same lead. The pathologic Q wave will remain on the ECG forever. T wave inversion may persist for months after a STEMI. With early reperfusion, Q waves may not develop.

Patients with NSTEMI or UA usually have transient thrombosis or incomplete coronary occlusion. ECG changes with UA or an NSTEMI include ST depression and/or T wave inversion in the leads facing the area of infarction (Figs. 33.4, 33.12, 33.14, and Table 33.13). Both groups of patients may present with angina and have the same ECG changes. The only way to tell if the patient is experiencing an NSTEMI or UA is by drawing cardiac biomarkers. The biomarkers will be high in the NSTEMI patient but normal in the patient with UA. These patients do not develop pathologic Q waves on the ECG.

Because MI is a dynamic process that evolves over time, serial ECGs are done to show the evolution of ischemia, injury, infarction, and resolution of the infarction.

Serum Cardiac Biomarkers

Serum cardiac biomarkers are proteins released into the blood from necrotic heart muscle after an MI (see Table 31.6). These biomarkers are important in the diagnosis of MI. The onset, peak, and duration of levels of these biomarkers are shown in Fig. 33.15.

Cardiac-specific troponin has 2 subtypes: cardiac-specific troponin T (cTnT) and cardiac-specific troponin I (cTnI). These biomarkers are highly specific indicators of MI and have greater sensitivity and specificity for myocardial injury than creatine kinase MB (CK-MB). Serum levels of cTnI and cTnT increase 4 to 6 hours after the onset of MI, peak at 10 to 24 hours, and return to baseline over 10 to 14 days. Sets of serial cardiac biomarkers are drawn over 24 hours (e.g., every 6 hours × 3). The presence of biomarkers helps distinguish between UA (negative biomarkers) and NSTEMI (positive biomarkers). A newer high-sensitivity troponin test is available that provides more rapid detection of cardiac necrosis at an earlier time than traditional troponin assays, allowing for a quicker diagnosis.

CK levels begin to rise about 6 hours after an MI, peak at about 18 hours, and return to normal within 24 to 36 hours. The CK enzymes are fractionated into bands. The CK-MB band is specific to heart muscle cells and helps to quantify myocardial damage. CK-MB is a less sensitive marker for myocardial injury compared to troponin.[15] Therefore troponin is the best biomarker for diagnosis of acute MI.[28]

Myoglobin is released into the circulation within 2 hours after an MI and peaks in 3 to 15 hours. Although it is one of the first serum cardiac biomarkers to appear after an MI, it lacks cardiac specificity. It has a limited role in diagnosing MI.

Cardiac Catheterization

The patient with a STEMI must undergo cardiac catheterization within 90 minutes of presentation or receive thrombolytic therapy within 30 minutes in agencies without PCI capability. The goal is to open the totally occluded artery and limit the infarction size. The patient with UA or NSTEMI usually undergoes

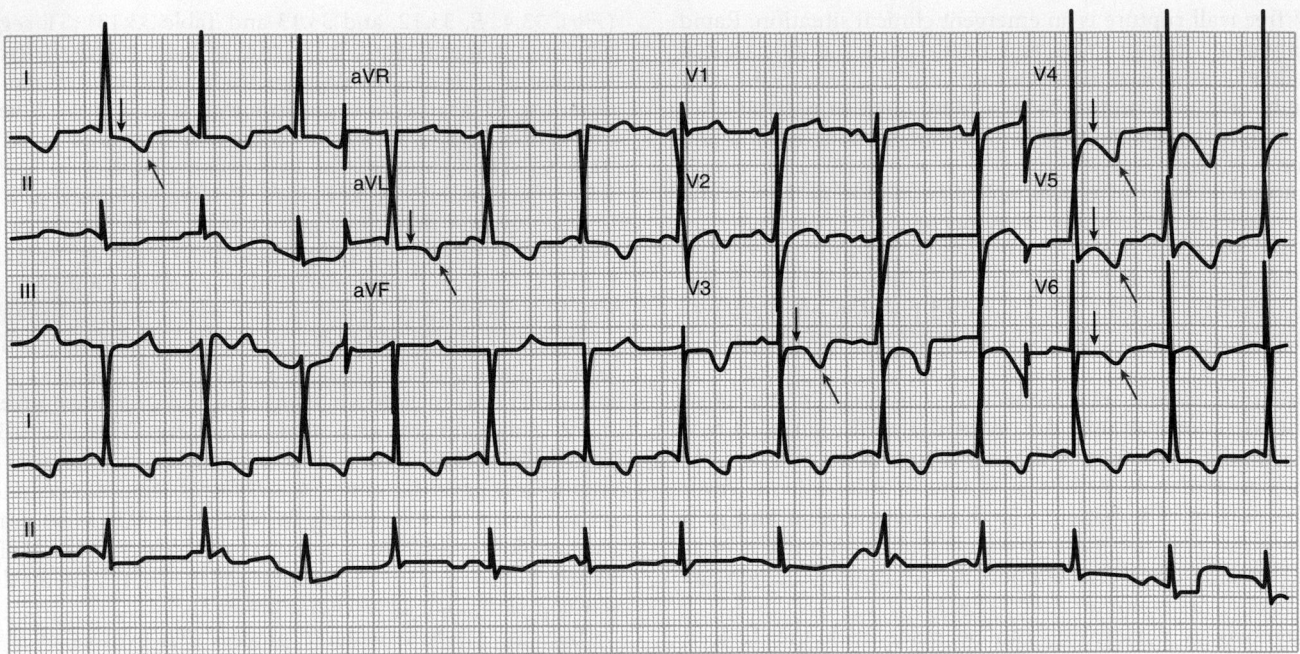

FIG. 33.14 ECG findings with anterior and lateral ischemia or an NSTEMI. Note the ST depression in the lateral leads (lead I, aVL, V5 and V6 [black arrows]) and the T wave inversion in I, aVL, V5 and V6 [red arrows]. These leads face the lateral wall. Note the ST depression in 2 anterior leads (V3 and V4 [black arrows]) and the T wave inversion in V3 and V4 [red arrows]. These leads face the anterior wall.

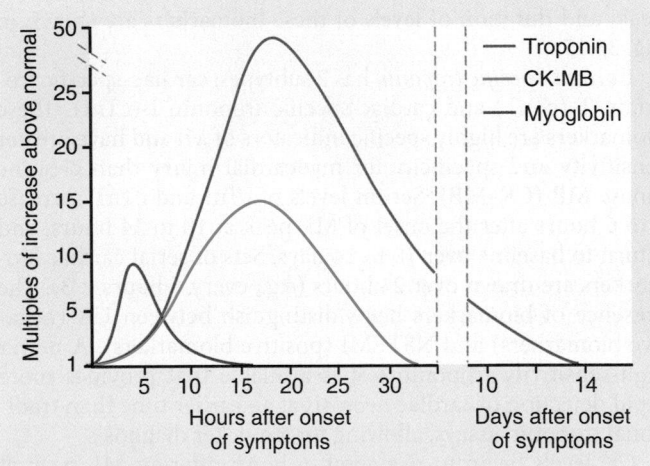

FIG. 33.15 Serum cardiac biomarkers found in the blood after MI.

cardiac catheterization during the hospitalization to diagnose and evaluate the extent of the disease. Guidelines suggest that it is reasonable to do cardiac catheterization on stable but high-risk patients with UA or NSTEMI within 12 to 72 hours after presentation.[15] If appropriate, a PCI is performed at this time. Depending on the findings and many factors, some patients may be treated with medical therapy and some patients may be referred for CABG surgery.

INTERPROFESSIONAL CARE: ACUTE CORONARY SYNDROME

It is extremely important to quickly diagnose and treat a patient with ACS to preserve heart muscle. Initial management of the patient with chest pain most often occurs in the ED. Table 33.14

presents the emergency care of the patient with chest pain. Obtain a 12-lead ECG and start continuous ECG monitoring. Position the patient in an upright position unless contraindicated and start O_2 by nasal cannula to keep O_2 saturation above 93%. Obtain IV access for drug administration. Give SL NTG and 162 to 325 mg of chewable aspirin if not given before arrival at the ED. Morphine is given for pain unrelieved by NTG. A high-dose statin (e.g., atorvastatin [Lipitor]) is given.

If the ECG shows ST elevation, the patient is taken directly for cardiac catheterization in PCI-capable hospitals. Thrombolytic therapy is started if the patient is unable to be quickly transported to a PCI-capable hospital. If the ECG shows ST depression and/or T wave inversion, the patient is usually transferred to an ICU or telemetry unit for ongoing care. Dysrhythmias are treated according to agency protocols. Serial cardiac biomarkers are drawn until the peak level drops off. UA and NSTEMI patients are started on heparin. Some patients with UA or NSTEMI start on glycoprotein IIb/IIIa inhibitors (e.g., eptifibatide [Integrilin]) either before catheterization or at the time of PCI. Glycoprotein IIb/IIIa inhibitors may be used during PCI for STEMI patients. Fig. 33.5 shows the interprofessional care of ACS.

Emergent PCI

Emergent PCI is the first line of treatment for patients with confirmed STEMI (i.e., ST-elevation on the ECG and positive cardiac biomarkers). The goal is to open the blocked artery within 90 minutes of arrival to an agency that has an interventional cardiac catheterization laboratory to limit the infarction size. In this case, the patient undergoes a cardiac catheterization to locate and assess the severity of the blockage(s), determine the presence of collateral circulation, and evaluate LV function. During the procedure, a bare metal stent (BMS) or drug-eluting

✚ TABLE 33.14 Emergency Management

Chest Pain

Etiology	Assessment Findings	Interventions
Cardiovascular • Aortic aneurysm • Aortic valve disease • Dysrhythmia • MI • Myocardial ischemia • Pericarditis **Respiratory** • Costochondritis • Pleurisy • Pneumonia • Pneumothorax, hemothorax • Pulmonary edema • Pulmonary embolus **Chest Trauma** • Cardiac tamponade • Flail chest • Great vessel injury • Hemothorax • Pulmonary contusion • Rib/sternal fracture **Gastrointestinal** • Cholecystitis • Esophagitis • GERD • Hiatal hernia • Peptic ulcer **Others** • Acute anxiety • Drugs (e.g., cocaine) • Strenuous exercise • Stress	• Pain in chest, neck, jaw, arm, or shoulder • Cold, clammy skin • Diaphoresis • Nausea and vomiting • Epigastric pain • Indigestion, heartburn • Dyspnea, tachypnea • Weakness • Anxiety • Feeling of impending doom • Tachycardia, bradycardia • Irregular HR, murmurs • Palpitations • Dysrhythmias • Decreased or increased BP • Narrowed pulse pressure • Unequal BP readings in upper extremities • Syncope, loss of consciousness • Decreased O_2 saturation • Decreased or absent breath sounds • Pericardial friction rub	**Initial** • If unresponsive, assess circulation, airway, and breathing. • If responsive, monitor airway, breathing, and circulation (ABC). • Position patient upright unless contraindicated. • Give O_2 by nasal cannula or nonrebreather mask. • Obtain baseline vital signs, including O_2 saturation. • Auscultate heart and breath sounds. • Obtain 12-lead ECG. • Insert 2 IV catheters. • Assess pain using PQRST mnemonic (Table 33.8). • Medicate for pain as ordered (e.g., nitroglycerin, morphine). • Start continuous ECG monitoring and identify underlying rhythm. • Obtain baseline blood work (e.g., cardiac biomarkers, CBC, basic metabolic panel, coagulation studies). • Obtain portable chest x-ray. • Assess for contraindications for antiplatelet, anticoagulant, or thrombolytic therapy, or PCI as appropriate. • Give aspirin for heart-related chest pain unless contraindicated. • Give a high-dose statin. • Give antidysrhythmic drugs for life-threatening dysrhythmias. **Ongoing Monitoring** • Monitor ABCs, vital signs, level of consciousness, heart and breath sounds, heart rhythm, and O_2 saturation. • Assess and record response to drugs (e.g., decrease in chest pain) and remedicate or titrate drugs (e.g., nitroglycerin) as needed. • Provide reassurance and emotional support to patient and caregiver. • Explain all interventions and procedures to patient and caregiver in simple terms. • Anticipate need for intubation if respiratory distress is evident. • Prepare for CPR and defibrillation if cardiac arrest is evident. • Anticipate need for transcutaneous pacing for symptomatic bradycardia or heart block.

stent (DES) is inserted into the blocked coronary artery (Figs. 33.6 and 33.7). PCI should not be done on a noninfarct artery during the same urgent procedure if the patient is hemodynamically stable.[28] Patients with severe LV dysfunction may require IABP therapy and/or inotropes (e.g., dobutamine). A small percent of patients may need emergent CABG surgery.

The advantages of PCI (compared to CABG surgery) include (1) it allows for faster reperfusion to limit infarction size; (2) it provides an alternative to surgical intervention; (3) it is performed with local anesthesia; (4) the patient is ambulatory shortly after the procedure; (5) the length of hospital stay is about 3 to 4 days after MI compared with the 4 to 6 days with CABG surgery, thus reducing hospital costs; and (6) the patient can return to work several weeks sooner after PCI, compared with a 6- to 8-week convalescence after CABG.

Complications of PCI that may lead to emergent CABG include dissection or rupture of the coronary artery, abrupt artery closure, acute stent thrombosis, and failure to cross the blockage with a balloon or stent. There is a risk that the infarction could be extended if a part of the plaque dislodges and blocks the vessel distal to the catheter.

In stent restenosis, ISR is a potential problem whenever stents are placed in a coronary artery. ISR is the build-up of scar tissue inside the stent (referred to as neointimal hyperplasia). ISR usually occurs within a few months to a year after stent placement.

Stent thrombosis is the other potential problem with stents, so DAPT is required up to 12 months post procedure.

❓ CHECK YOUR PRACTICE

Your patient underwent an emergent PCI 2 days ago for a STEMI. You are about to give him his morning medications, which include clopidogrel and aspirin. The patient asks you if he will need to take these medications forever.

• What would you tell the patient?

Thrombolytic Therapy

Thrombolytic (fibrinolytic) therapy is indicated only for patients with a STEMI. Advantages include availability and rapid administration in agencies that do not have an interventional cardiac catheterization laboratory or when one is too far away to transfer the patient quickly. Patients who are admitted to non–PCI-capable hospitals can be moved to a PCI-capable hospital if the first medical contact to balloon inflation (PCI) time can be done within 120 minutes.[28] Treatment of STEMI with thrombolytic therapy aims to limit the infarction size by dissolving the thrombus in the coronary artery to reperfuse the heart muscle. The goal is to give the thrombolytic within 30 minutes of the patient's arrival to the ED.

TABLE 33.15 Contraindications for Thrombolytic Therapy

Absolute Contraindications

- Active internal bleeding or bleeding diathesis (excluding menstruation)
- History of intracranial hemorrhage
- Intracranial or intraspinal surgery within 2 mo
- Known structural or vascular abnormality (e.g., arteriovenous malformation)
- Known intracranial cancer (primary or metastatic)
- Recent (within past 3 mo) ischemic stroke
- Severe uncontrolled hypertension
- Significant closed-head or facial trauma within past 3 mo
- Suspected aortic dissection
- For streptokinase, prior treatment within the past 6 mo

Relative Contraindications

- Active peptic ulcer disease
- Current use of oral anticoagulants
- Dementia
- History of chronic, severe, poorly controlled hypertension
- Known intracranial pathology not covered in absolute contraindications
- Major surgery (<3 wks)
- Noncompressible vascular punctures
- Pregnancy
- Prior ischemic stroke (>3 mo ago)
- Recent (within 2-4 wks) internal bleeding
- Significant hypertension on presentation (SBP >180 mm/Hg or DBP >110 mm/Hg)
- Traumatic or prolonged (>10 min) cardiopulmonary resuscitation

Source: O'Gara PT, Kushner FG, Ascheim DD, et al: 2013 ACCF/AHA guideline for the management of ST-elevation myocardial infarction: A report of the ACCF/AHA Task Force on Practice Guidelines, *Circulation* 127:e362, 2013.

Indications and Contraindications. All thrombolytics (e.g., tenecteplase, alteplase) are given IV (Table 33.12). The cost, efficacy, and ease of administration guide the choice of a thrombolytic agent. Although these drugs have different pharmacokinetics, they all open the blocked artery by lysis of the thrombus. Because thrombolytics lyse the pathologic clot, they may also lyse other clots (e.g., a postoperative site). Therefore patient selection is important because minor or major bleeding can be a complication of therapy.

Inclusion criteria for thrombolytic therapy are (1) chest pain less than 12 hours with 12-lead ECG findings consistent with acute STEMI and (2) no absolute contraindications (Table 33.15). Patients with chest pain lasting 12 to 24 hours with ECG changes supporting STEMI may be considered for thrombolytic therapy.[28]

Procedure. Each hospital has a protocol for giving thrombolytic therapy, but 2 steps should be completed before thrombolytic therapy is started: (1) draw blood to obtain baseline laboratory values and (2) start 2 or 3 lines for IV therapy. Perform all other invasive procedures before giving the thrombolytic agent to reduce the risk for bleeding.

Depending on the drug selected, therapy is given in 1 IV bolus or over time (30 to 90 minutes). Note the time at which therapy begins and monitor the patient during and after the thrombolytic. Assess heart rhythm, vital signs, and pulse oximetry. Assess the heart and lungs often to evaluate the patient's response to therapy. Regularly assess for changes in neurologic status that may indicate cerebral bleeding.

When reperfusion occurs (e.g., a blocked coronary artery is opened and blood flow is restored to the heart muscle), several clinical signs can be seen. The most reliable sign is the return of the ST segment to baseline on the ECG. Other signs include resolution of chest pain and an early, rapid rise of the serum cardiac biomarkers within 3 hours of therapy, peaking within 12 hours. These levels increase as the necrotic heart cells release proteins into the circulation after perfusion is restored to the area. The presence of *reperfusion dysrhythmias* (e.g., accelerated idioventricular rhythm) is a less reliable sign of reperfusion. These dysrhythmias are generally self-limiting and do not require aggressive treatment. (See Chapter 35 for management of dysrhythmias.)

A major concern with thrombolytic therapy is reocclusion of the artery. The site of the thrombus is unstable, and formation of another clot or spasm of the artery may occur. Therefore IV heparin therapy is started. If another clot develops, the patient will describe similar chest pain symptoms and ECG changes will return. Patients receiving thrombolytic therapy should be moved to an agency with PCI capabilities as soon as possible so PCI can be performed if thrombolytic therapy fails.

The major complication with thrombolytic therapy is bleeding. Ongoing nursing assessment is essential. Minor bleeding (e.g., surface bleeding from IV sites or gingival bleeding) is expected and controlled by applying manual pressure followed by a pressure dressing or ice packs.

> **⚠ SAFETY ALERT** Thrombolytic Therapy
> - Minor or major bleeding can occur with thrombolytic drugs.
> - Place 2 or 3 IV lines before thrombolytic therapy is started.
> - If signs and symptoms of major bleeding occur (e.g., drop in BP, increase in HR, sudden change in the patient's mental status, blood in the urine or stool), stop the drug and notify the HCP.

Drug Therapy

When a patient presents with suspected ACS, antiplatelet therapy (e.g., chewable aspirin for UA patients plus clopidogrel or ticagrelor [for STEMI and NSTEMI patients]), IV NTG, and atorvastatin are drug treatments of choice. Since STEMI patients are taken directly to cardiac catheterization, systemic anticoagulation with either subcutaneous LMWH or IV UH is used only for UA and NSTEMI patients. Glycoprotein IIb/IIIa inhibitors may be given if PCI is anticipated. DAPT should continue for 1 year after an MI whether the patient receives a stent or not. Aspirin should never be stopped. Oral β-blockers are given within the first 24 hours if there are no contraindications (e.g., HF, heart block, hypotension). Calcium channel blockers are used if the patient cannot tolerate β-blockers. These drugs must be used cautiously after MI because they can decrease contractility. ACE inhibitors are added after an MI if there are no contraindications. Nitrates may be used for persistent chest pain.

Table 33.12 and Fig. 33.5 present drug therapy for patients with chronic stable angina and ACS. These drugs are discussed on p. 713. Drugs specifically used to treat ACS are discussed in this section.

IV Nitroglycerin. IV NTG is used in the initial treatment of the patient with ACS. SL NTG can be used until the IV NTG is prepared. The goal of therapy is to reduce angina pain and improve coronary blood flow. IV NTG decreases preload and afterload while increasing the myocardial O_2 supply. The onset of action is immediate. Titrate NTG to eliminate chest pain. Because hypotension is a common side effect, closely monitor BP. Patients who become hypotensive may be volume depleted and may benefit from an IV fluid bolus. Closely assess for volume overload after the bolus (e.g., crackles on lung auscultation).

Morphine. Morphine is the drug of choice for chest pain that is unrelieved by NTG. As a vasodilator, it decreases cardiac workload by lowering myocardial O_2 consumption, reducing contractility, and decreasing BP and HR. In addition, morphine can help reduce anxiety and fear. In rare situations, morphine can depress respirations. Monitor patients for signs of bradypnea or hypotension, which are conditions to avoid in myocardial ischemia and infarction.

β-Adrenergic Blockers. β-blockers decrease myocardial O_2 demand by reducing HR, BP, and contractility. The use of these drugs in patients who are not at risk for complications of MI (e.g., cardiogenic shock, bradycardia, hypotension) reduces the risk for reinfarction and the development of HF. Therapy continues indefinitely.

Angiotensin-Converting Enzyme Inhibitors and Angiotensin Receptor Blockers. ACE inhibitors should be started within the first 24 hours if the BP is stable and there are no contraindications. They are continued indefinitely in patients recovering from STEMI or NSTEMI, with HF, or an EF of 40% or less. The use of ACE inhibitors can help prevent ventricular remodeling and prevent or slow the progression of HF. For patients who cannot tolerate ACE inhibitors (e.g., angioedema, cough), ARBs should be considered.

Antidysrhythmic Drugs. Dysrhythmias are the most common complications after an MI. In general, they are self-limiting and not treated aggressively unless they are life threatening (e.g., sustained ventricular tachycardia). Chapter 35 discusses the drugs used in the treatment of dysrhythmias.

Lipid-Lowering Drugs. A lipid panel is done on all patients with ACS. Patients with ACS or CAD should receive lipid-lowering drugs indefinitely, unless contraindicated (Table 33.6).

Stool Softeners. After an MI, the patient may be predisposed to constipation because of bed rest and opioid drugs. Stool softeners (e.g., docusate sodium [Colace]) prevent straining and the resultant vagal stimulation from the *Valsalva maneuver*. Vagal stimulation produces bradycardia and can provoke dysrhythmias. A laxative may be used, if needed.

Nutritional Therapy

Initially, patients may be NPO (nothing by mouth) except for water until stable (e.g., pain free, nausea resolved). Advance the diet as tolerated to a low-salt, low-saturated-fat, and low-cholesterol diet (Tables 33.4 and 33.5).

❖ NURSING MANAGEMENT: ACUTE CORONARY SYNDROME

◆ Nursing Assessment

Table 33.16 presents the subjective and objective data to obtain from a patient with ACS.

◆ Nursing Diagnoses

Nursing diagnoses for the patient with ACS may include:
- Impaired cardiac output
- Acute pain
- Anxiety
- Activity intolerance

More information on nursing diagnoses of patients with ACS is presented in eNursing Care Plan 33.1 available on the website for this chapter.

TABLE 33.16 Nursing Assessment

Acute Coronary Syndrome

Subjective Data

Important Health Information

Past health history: Previous history of CAD, chest pain/angina, MI, valve disease (e.g., aortic stenosis), heart failure, or cardiomyopathy. Hypertension, diabetes, anemia, lung disease, hyperlipidemia

Medications: Use of antiplatelets, anticoagulants, nitrates, ACE inhibitors, β-blockers, calcium channel blockers, antihypertensive drugs, lipid-lowering drugs, over-the-counter drugs (e.g., vitamin and herbal supplements)

History of present illness: Description of events related to current illness (Table 33.9), including any self-treatments and response

Functional Health Patterns

Health perception–health management: Family history of heart disease. Sedentary lifestyle, tobacco use, exposure to environmental smoke

Nutritional-metabolic: Indigestion, heartburn, nausea, belching, vomiting

Elimination: Urinary urgency or frequency, straining at stool

Activity-exercise: Palpitations, dyspnea, dizziness, weakness

Cognitive-perceptual: Substernal chest pain or pressure (squeezing, constricting, aching, sharp, tingling), radiation to jaw, neck, shoulders, back, or arms (Table 33.8)

Coping–stress tolerance: Stressful lifestyle, depression; anger, anxiety. Feeling of impending doom

Objective Data

General

Anxious, fearful, restless, distressed

Integumentary

Cool, clammy, pale skin

Cardiovascular

Tachycardia or bradycardia, pulsus alternans (alternating weak and strong heartbeats), pulse deficit, dysrhythmias (especially ventricular), murmur, S_3, S_4, ↑ or ↓ BP

Possible Diagnostic Findings

Positive serum cardiac biomarkers, ↑ serum lipids; ↑ WBC count. Positive exercise or pharmacologic stress test and thallium scans. Pathologic Q wave, ST segment elevation, and/or ST-T wave abnormalities on ECG. Cardiac enlargement, calcifications, or pulmonary congestion on chest x-ray. Abnormal wall motion with stress echocardiogram or resting echocardiogram. Positive coronary angiography.

◆ Planning

Nursing care focuses on the priority problems of acute pain and decreased CO. The immediate goals for a patient with ACS include (1) relief of pain, (2) quick and appropriate treatment, and (3) preservation of heart muscle. During the hospitalization, the overall goals include: (1) effective coping with illness-associated anxiety, (2) participation in a rehabilitation plan, and (3) reduction of risk factors. The Joint Commission has identified a core measure set in the management of patients with an acute MI (AMI) to reflect standards of evidence-based care.

◆ Nursing Implementation

Acute Care. When the patient is admitted to the intensive care or telemetry unit, monitor vital signs and pulse oximetry frequently (e.g., every hour) during the first few hours after admission and closely thereafter, according to agency protocol. Start continuous ECG monitoring. Obtain serial 12-lead ECGs, and draw serial cardiac biomarkers Maintain bed rest and limit activity for 12 to 24 hours, with a gradual increase in activity unless contraindicated.

For patients with UA and NSTEMI, heparin (UH or LMWH) is recommended to prevent microemboli from forming and causing further chest pain. DAPT (e.g., aspirin and clopidogrel or ticagrelor [Brilinta]) (Table 33.12) also is recommended for NSTEMI patients (with or without a stent). UA patients receive aspirin alone unless they have a stent placed; then DAPT is used. Cardiac catheterization is an option for both UA and NSTEMI patients once the patient is stabilized and angina is controlled or if angina returns or increases in severity. Depending on the results, options include medical management, PCI, or CABG surgery.

For patients with STEMI, reperfusion therapy is started as soon as possible. *Reperfusion therapy* includes emergent PCI (preferred, for PCI-capable hospitals) or thrombolytic therapy (in hospitals not capable of performing PCI). The goal in the treatment of STEMI is to save as much heart muscle as possible. Technical advances in PCI technology have almost eliminated CABG surgery as the primary treatment for patients with STEMI unless there is another reason to perform surgery (e.g., ventricular septal rupture, papillary muscle rupture).

◆ **Pain.** Provide NTG, morphine, and supplemental O_2 as needed to eliminate or reduce chest pain. Ongoing evaluation and documentation of the effectiveness of the interventions is important. Once pain is relieved, some patients interpret the absence of pain as an absence of heart disease. Provide information about the importance of continued therapy to limit myocardial damage.

◆ **Monitoring.** Maintain continuous ECG monitoring while the patient is in the ED and ICU and after transfer to a step-down unit. Treat life-threatening dysrhythmias quickly. During the initial period after MI, ventricular fibrillation is the most common lethal dysrhythmia. In many patients, premature ventricular contractions or ventricular tachycardia (VT) precedes this dysrhythmia. Isolated PVCs are not usually treated. VT may or may not be treated depending on whether it is sustained VT or nonsustained VT and depending on the patient's hemodynamic status. Using the bedside ST segment monitor, assess the patient's ST segments for reinfarction or ischemia (ST segments will shift above or below the baseline of the ECG). Silent ischemia, noted only by ST segment changes, can occur without subjective symptoms (e.g., chest pain). Notify the HCP if you see ST segment changes with or without clinical symptoms. (See Chapter 35 for a complete discussion of ECG monitoring.)

Perform a physical assessment to detect changes from the patient's baseline findings. Assess heart and breath sounds and for signs of early HF (e.g., dyspnea, tachycardia, pulmonary congestion, distended neck veins). In addition to routine vital signs, monitor intake and output.

Assessment of the patient's oxygenation status is important. If a nasal cannula is used to deliver O_2, check the nares for irritation or dryness, which can cause considerable discomfort.

◆ **Rest and Comfort.** It is important to promote rest and comfort for the patient with any degree of heart damage. Bed rest may be ordered for the first few days after a large MI. A patient with an uncomplicated MI (e.g., angina resolved, no signs of complications) may rest in a chair within 8 to 12 hours after the event. Prolonged bed rest is not recommended. The use of the bathroom, a commode, or a bedpan is based on patient preference and hemodynamic status.

TABLE 33.17 Phases of Rehabilitation After Acute Coronary Syndrome

Phase I: Hospital
- Occurs while the patient is still hospitalized
- Activity level depends on severity of angina or MI
- Patient may first sit up in bed or chair, perform range-of-motion exercises and self-care (e.g., washing, shaving), and progress to walking in hallway and limited stair climbing
- Attention focuses on management of chest pain, anxiety, dysrhythmias, and complications

Phase II: Early Recovery
- Begins after the patient is discharged
- Usually lasts from 2-12 weeks and is held in an outpatient facility but may be done in the home
- Activity level is gradually increased under the supervision of the cardiac rehabilitation team and with ECG monitoring
- Team may suggest that physical activity (e.g., walking program) be started at home
- Information about risk factor reduction is provided at this time

Phase III: Late Recovery
- Long-term maintenance program
- Individual physical activity programs are designed and implemented at home, a local gym, or the rehabilitation center
- Patient and caregiver restructure lifestyles and roles
- Therapeutic lifestyle changes should become lifelong habits
- Medical supervision recommended

When sleeping or resting, the body requires less work from the heart than it does when active. It is important to plan nursing and other interventions to ensure adequate rest periods free from interruption. Comfort measures that can promote rest include a quiet environment, use of relaxation techniques (e.g., music therapy, guided imagery), and assurance that staff is nearby and responsive to the patient's needs.

It is important that the patient understand the reasons why activity is limited. Gradually increase the patient's heart workload through more demanding physical tasks. Before discharge, it is important that the patient achieve an activity level adequate for home care. Cardiac rehabilitation should be discussed and encouraged as an outpatient. Table 33.17 outlines the phases of cardiac rehabilitation.

◆ **Anxiety.** A degree of anxiety is present in all patients with ACS. Your role is to identify the source of anxiety and assist the patient in reducing it. If the patient is afraid of being alone, allow a caregiver to sit by quietly and check the patient frequently. If a source of anxiety is fear of the unknown, explore these concerns with the patient. For anxiety caused by lack of information, provide teaching based on the patient's stated need and level of understanding. Answer the patient's questions with clear, simple explanations.

❓ CHECK YOUR PRACTICE

You are walking in the hallway with a 64-yr-old woman who had an MI 3 days ago. She is scheduled for discharge tomorrow. She is visibly anxious and irritable, wringing her hands, and talking very fast. She tells you, "My heart is pounding." You do not know if she is anxious or about to have another MI.
- What should you do?

TABLE 33.18 Psychosocial Responses to Acute Coronary Syndrome

Anger and Hostility
- Is often expressed as, "Why did this happen to me?"
- May be directed at family, staff, or medical regimen

Anxiety and Fear
- Fears long-term disability and death
- Overtly displays apprehension, restlessness, insomnia, tachycardia
- Less overtly displays increased verbalization, projection of feelings to others, hypochondriasis
- Fears activity
- Fears recurrent chest pain, heart attacks, and sudden death

Denial
- May have history of ignoring signs and symptoms related to heart disease
- Minimizes severity of health condition
- Ignores activity restrictions
- Avoids discussing illness or its significance

Dependency
- Totally reliant on staff
- Unwilling to perform tasks or activities unless approved by HCP
- Always wants to be monitored by ECG
- Hesitant to leave the intensive care or telemetry unit or hospital

Depression
- Mourns loss of health, altered body function, and changes in lifestyle
- Realizes seriousness of situation
- Begins to worry about future implications of health problem
- Shows manifestations of withdrawal, crying, apathy
- May be more evident after discharge

Realistic Acceptance
- Focuses on optimum rehabilitation
- Plans changes compatible with altered cardiac function
- Actively engages in lifestyle changes to address modifiable risk factors

It is important to start teaching at the patient's level rather than to present a prepackaged program. For example, patients generally are not ready to learn about the pathology of CAD. The earliest questions usually relate to how the disease affects perceived control and independence. Examples include:
- When will I leave the intensive care unit?
- When can I be out of bed?
- When will I be discharged?
- When can I return to work?
- How many changes will I have to make in my life?
- Will this happen again?

Tell the patient that more complete teaching will begin once the patient is feeling stronger. Often the patient may not be able to ask the most serious concern of ACS patients: Am I going to die? Even if a patient denies this concern, it is helpful for you to start a conversation by remarking that fear of dying is a common concern among most patients who have had ACS. This gives the patient "permission" to talk about an uncomfortable and fearful topic.

◆ **Emotional and Behavioral Reactions.** Patients' emotional and behavioral reactions vary, but often follow a predictable response pattern (Table 33.18). Your role is to understand what the patient is currently experiencing and to support the use of constructive coping styles.

Assess the support structure of the patient and caregiver. Determine how you can help maximize the support system. Often the patient is separated from the most significant support system at the time of hospitalization. Talk with the caregiver(s) about the patient's progress. Allow the patient and caregivers to interact as necessary and support the caregivers who will provide the necessary assistance to the patient. Open visitation is helpful in decreasing anxiety and increasing support for the patient with ACS.[29] It is important for you to help the patient identify additional support systems (e.g., spiritual care, Mended Hearts) that can assist during the hospital stay and/or after discharge.

◆ **Patient Teaching.** Patient teaching is needed at every stage of the patient's hospitalization and recovery (e.g., ED, telemetry unit, home). Give patients and caregivers the tools they need to make informed decisions about their health. For teaching to be meaningful, the patient must be aware of the need to learn. Careful assessment of the patient's health literacy and learning needs helps you set realistic goals (see Chapter 4).

The timing of the teaching is important. When patients and caregivers are in crisis, they may not be ready to learn new information. Answer the patient's questions in simple, brief terms. The answers often need repetition. When the shock accompanying a crisis subsides, the patient and caregiver are better able to focus on new and more detailed information.

Limit your use of medical terms. For example, you are caring for a patient with UA who asks you why he has chest tightness when he climbs stairs. Begin by explaining that the heart is a muscle that works as a pump. Like all muscles, it needs O_2 to work (or pump) properly. When blood vessels supplying the heart muscle with O_2 are blocked by fat and cholesterol, less O_2 is available to the muscle. As a result, the pump cannot work well. Tell the patient that the chest tightness (angina) is the heart's message that it is having trouble doing its work. Use a model of the heart to support what you are explaining.

Anticipatory guidance involves preparing the patient and caregiver for what to expect during recovery and rehabilitation. By learning what to expect, the patient gains a sense of control.

The idea of perceived control is operationalized as the process by which the patient makes decisions by cutting back. Cutting back is one way of reducing the psychologic and physiologic losses after ACS (or any other life-changing event). For example, a middle-aged man who smokes 2 packs of cigarettes a day, is 20 lb overweight, and gets no physical exercise may feel overwhelmed. He may decide that he can live with a weight reduction plan and will get more exercise (although perhaps not daily) but that it is not possible for him to quit smoking. He believes that because he is changing 2 of his 3 risk factors, he will be healthier. Ideally, the tobacco risk factor should be a priority for this patient. If the information about risks and effects of tobacco use is not accepted, you must respect the patient's choices.

In addition to teaching the patient and caregiver what they wish to know, several types of information are essential in achieving optimal health. Table 33.19 presents a teaching guide for the patient with ACS and the caregiver.

◆ **Physical Activity.** Physical activity, an integral part of rehabilitation, is necessary for optimal physiologic functioning and psychologic well-being. It has a direct, positive effect on maximal O_2 uptake, increasing CO, decreasing blood lipids, decreasing BP, increasing blood flow through the coronary arteries, increasing muscle mass and flexibility, improving the

TABLE 33.19 Patient & Caregiver Teaching

Acute Coronary Syndrome

Include the following information in the teaching plan for the patient with acute coronary syndrome and the caregiver:

- Signs and symptoms of angina and MI and what to do should they occur (e.g., how to take nitroglycerin)*
- When and how to seek help (e.g., contact 911)*
- Anatomy and physiology of the heart and coronary arteries
- Cause and effect of CAD
- Definition of terms (e.g., CAD, angina, MI, heart failure)
- Identification of and plan to decrease risk factors* (Tables 33.1, 33.2, 33.4, and 33.5)
- Reasons for tests and treatments (e.g., ECG monitoring, blood work, angiography), activity limitations and rest, diet, and drugs*
- Appropriate expectations about recovery (anticipatory guidance)
- Resumption of work, physical activity, sexual activity
- Measures to promote recovery and health (e.g., cardiac rehabilitation)
- Importance of the gradual, progressive resumption of activity*

*Identified by patients as most important to learn before discharge.

TABLE 33.20 Energy Expenditure in Metabolic Equivalents (METs)

Low-Energy Activities (<3 METs or <3 cal/min)
Activities in Hospital
- Eating
- Resting supine
- Washing hands, face

Activities Outside Hospital
- Driving a car
- Painting, seated
- Sewing by machine
- Sweeping floor

Moderate-Energy Activities (3–6 METs or 3–5 cal/min)
Activities in Hospital
- Showering
- Sitting on bedside commode
- Using bedpan
- Walking at 3–4 mph

Activities Outside Hospital
- Cycling at 5.5 mph on level ground
- Going up a flight of stairs
- Golfing
- General gardening
- Ironing, standing
- Painting, standing

High-Energy Activities (6–8 METs or 6–8 cal/min)
- Mowing lawn using walking mower
- Performing carpentry
- Walking 5 mph

Very-High-Energy Activities (>9 METs or >9 cal/min)
- Cross-country skiing
- Cycling at >13 mph
- Running at >6 mph
- Shoveling heavy snow

psychologic state, and assisting in weight loss and control. A regular schedule of physical activity, even after many years of sedentary living, is beneficial.

One method of identifying levels of physical activity is by using **metabolic equivalent (MET)** units: 1 MET is the amount of O_2 needed by the body at rest—3.5 mL of O_2 per kilogram per minute, or 1.4 cal/kg of body weight per minute. The MET determines the energy costs of various exercises (Table 33.20).

In the hospital, the activity level is gradually increased so that by the time of discharge the patient can tolerate moderate-energy activities of 3 to 6 METs. Many patients with UA or an uncomplicated MI are in the hospital for 3 or 4 days. By day 2, the patient can walk in the hallway and begin climbing a few steps. Because of the short hospital stay, it is critical to give the patient specific guidelines for physical activity so that overexertion will not occur. Tell the patient to always "listen to what your body is saying"—the most important aspect of recovery.

Teach patients that 30 to 60 minutes of moderate-intensity aerobic activity (e.g., brisk walking) at least 5 days a week is recommended by the AHA. For patients who have been hospitalized for a coronary event (e.g., PCI, UA, NSTEMI, STEMI), they must "work up" to 30 minutes of exercise per day. An exercise stress test may be ordered after hospitalization to assess for chest pain with activity and help guide physical activity. The patient who has been physically inactive and just starting an exercise program should do so under supervision whenever possible. Cardiac rehabilitation, either in a group setting or home-based setting, is recommended.[15,28]

Teach patients to check their HR. Some patients may use technology (e.g., cell phone applications, fitness trackers) to check their HR. The patient should know the limits within which to exercise. Tell the patient that the heart rate should return to the resting HR within a few minutes of stopping the exercise. Tell the patient to stop exercising and rest if chest pain or shortness of breath occurs. The key factor is the patient's response to physical activity in terms of symptoms rather than absolute HR, especially since many patients are taking β-blockers and may not be able to reach a target HR. This point cannot be overstressed. Basic physical activity guidelines for patients after ACS follow the FITT formula (Table 33.3).

The basic categories of physical activity are isometric (static) and isotonic (dynamic). Most daily activities are a mixture of the two. *Isometric activities* involve the development of tension during muscular contraction but produce little or no change in muscle length or joint movement. Lifting, carrying, and pushing heavy objects are isometric activities. These activities are associated with the Valsalva maneuver and may cause a vasovagal response. Because the HR and BP change rapidly during isometric work, isometric exercises should be limited.

Isotonic activities involve changes in muscle length and joint movement with rhythmic contractions at relatively low muscular tension. Walking, jogging, swimming, bicycling, and jumping rope are examples of activities that are mostly isotonic. Isotonic exercise can put a safe, steady load on the heart and lungs and improve the circulation to other organs.

Women who have an MI often have poor adherence to a regular physical activity program.[4] Women often are the caregivers for everyone else and do not take good care of themselves. They may prioritize a physical activity program as less important than caring for others. Often women describe continued fatigue. Another factor linked to poor adherence to a physical activity program after MI is depression. Depression is common among patients with CAD, especially in women.[4] Routinely screen for depression in patients with CAD/ACS and recommend referral for treatment as appropriate.

◆ **Cardiac Rehabilitation.** *Cardiac rehabilitation* is the restoration of a person to an optimal state of function in 6 areas: (1) physiologic, (2) psychologic, (3) mental, (4) spiritual, (5) economic, and (6) vocational.

Discuss participation in an outpatient cardiac rehabilitation program with patients who have had UA, an MI, a PCI, or CABG surgery (Table 33.17). These programs are helpful, but not all patients choose or are able to take part in them due to cost, location, and travel limitations. Home-based cardiac rehabilitation programs can provide an alternative. Physical activity guidelines are developed for the patient and staff to maintain ongoing contact (e.g., telehealth, exercise logs, Internet). Maintaining contact with the patient is a key to the success of these programs.

Many patients recover physically from ACS or CABG surgery but do not attain psychologic well-being. All patients should be referred to an outpatient or home-based cardiac rehabilitation program because exercise-based cardiac rehabilitation is a Class I recommendation from the ACC/AHA for any patient with HF or who had a cardiac event.[13,15,20] Despite the proven beneficial effects of cardiac rehabilitation, it is often not recommended, and participation is less than optimal.

In considering rehabilitation, the patient must recognize that CAD is a chronic disease. It is not curable. Therefore basic changes in lifestyle must be made to promote recovery and future health. Tell patients that recovery takes time and resuming physical activity after ACS or heart surgery is slow and gradual. However, with appropriate and adequate supportive care, recovery is more likely.

◆ **Resuming Sexual Activity.** It is important to include sexual counseling for heart patients and their partners. This often-neglected area of discussion may be difficult for both the patient and HCP to approach. However, the patient's concern about resumption of sexual activity after hospitalization for ACS often produces more stress than the physiologic act. Most patients change their sexual behavior because they are concerned about sexual inadequacy, death during intercourse, and impotence. A concerned and knowledgeable HCP can clarify any misconceptions with specific counseling.

Before providing guidelines on resumption of sexual activity, it is important to know the patient's physiologic status, physiologic effects of sexual activity, and psychologic effects of having an MI. Sexual activity for most middle-aged men and women with their usual partners is considered a moderate-energy activity equivalent to climbing 2 flights of steps or walking briskly.[30]

You may be uncertain of how and when to begin counseling about resumption of sex. It is helpful to consider sex as a physical activity and to discuss or explore feelings in this area when discussing other physical activities. One helpful approach is, "Many people who have had a heart attack wonder when they will be able to resume sexual activity. Has this been of concern to you?" You may also state, "Sexual activity, like other forms of activity, should be gradually resumed after MI. If your ability to perform sexually is concerning you, the energy you use is likely no more than climbing 2 flights of steps or walking briskly." Facilitate discussion by providing the patient with reading material on resumption of sexual activity. Say something such as, "If resuming sexual activity has been of concern to you, this information should be helpful." This type of nonthreatening statement brings up the topic, allows the patient to explore personal feelings, and gives the patient an opportunity to raise questions with you or another HCP. Common guidelines are outlined in Table 33.21.

TABLE 33.21 Patient & Partner Teaching

Sexual Activity After Acute Coronary Syndrome

Include the following information in the teaching plan for the patient and his/her partner after an acute coronary syndrome:

- Resume sexual activity at a level that relates to sexual activity before experiencing ACS.
- Physical training may improve the physiologic response to intercourse. Encourage daily physical activity during recovery.
- Consumption of food and alcohol should be reduced before intercourse is anticipated (e.g., waiting 3–4 hr after eating a large meal before engaging in sexual activity).
- Familiar surroundings and a familiar partner reduce anxiety.
- Masturbation may be a useful sexual outlet and may reassure the patient that sexual activity is still possible.
- Avoid hot or cold showers just before and after intercourse.
- Foreplay is desirable because it allows a gradual increase in HR before orgasm.
- Positions during intercourse are a matter of individual choice.
- Orogenital sex places no undue strain on the heart.
- A relaxed atmosphere free of fatigue and stress is optimal.
- Prophylactic use of nitrates to decrease chest pain during sexual activity may be suggested.
- Use of erectile agents (e.g., sildenafil) is contraindicated if taking nitrates in any form.
- Avoid anal intercourse because of the chance of inducing a vasovagal response.

Tell the patient that the inability to perform sexually after MI is common and that sexual dysfunction usually disappears after several attempts. Reinforce the idea that patience and understanding usually solve the problem. However, many male patients may be interested in using drugs to correct erectile dysfunction. Warn the patient that these drugs are not to be used with nitrates because severe hypotension, and even death, have been reported. Tell patients to discuss the use of these drugs with their HCP.

It is common for a patient who has chest pain on physical exertion to have some angina during sexual stimulation or intercourse. The patient may take NTG prophylactically if he is not using erectile dysfunction medications. Tell the patient to delay sex after a heavy meal or excess alcohol intake, when extremely tired or stressed, or with unfamiliar partners. Patients should avoid anal intercourse because of the chance of eliciting a vasovagal response.

Tell the patient that resumption of sex depends on the patient and partner's emotional readiness and on the HCP's assessment of the extent of recovery. It is generally safe to resume sexual activity 7 to 10 days after an uncomplicated MI. However, some HCPs think that the patient should decide when to resume sex. Others think patients must be asymptomatic during moderate-energy activities before resuming sexual activity.[30]

◆ **Evaluation**

The expected outcomes are that the patient with ACS will
- Maintain stable signs of adequate cardiac output
- Have relief of pain and/or shortness of breath
- Report decreased anxiety and increased sense of self-control
- Achieve a realistic program of activity that balances physical activity with energy-conserving activities
- Describe the disease process, measures to reduce risk factors, and rehabilitation activities necessary to manage the therapeutic regimen

SUDDEN CARDIAC DEATH

Sudden cardiac death (SCD) is a sudden, unexpected death resulting from a variety of cardiac causes. Around 350,000 adults experience SCD yearly.[1]

Etiology and Pathophysiology

SCD is defined as sudden unexpected death occurring within 1 hour of symptom onset. In SCD, a sudden disruption in heart function from a life-threatening dysrhythmia produces an abrupt loss of CO and cerebral blood flow. The affected person may or may not have a known history of heart disease. CAD is the main cause of SCD in the United States, especially in adults over 35 years of age.[31] Black women have a higher incidence of SCD as the first manifestation of CAD than white women.[5] SCD is the initial manifestation of CAD or structural heart disease in up to 50% of people; however, SCD can occur without evidence of CAD.[31]

Acute ventricular dysrhythmias (e.g., ventricular tachycardia, ventricular fibrillation) cause most cases of SCD. With the use of implantable cardioverter-defibrillators (ICDs), the incidence

of SCD from VT and VF is declining.[31] These dysrhythmias may or may not be associated with an acute MI. Many SCD survivors have a history of a prior (old) MI.

Besides patients with CAD, patients with LV dysfunction and structural heart disease are at risk for SCD. Structural heart disease includes LV hypertrophy, myocarditis, and hypertrophic cardiomyopathy. Hypertrophic cardiomyopathy is a risk factor for SCD, especially in young, athletic people.

Some cases of SCD (especially in people less than age 45) occur in the absence of structural heart disease, LV dysfunction or CAD. These involve changes in the conduction system (e.g., prolonged QT syndrome, Wolff-Parkinson-White syndrome complicated by atrial fibrillation, Brugada syndrome).

Clinical Manifestations and Complications

Some people have symptoms within 1 hour of an SCD event, such as angina, palpitations, dizziness, or lightheadedness. People who experience SCD because of CAD fall into 2 groups: (1) those who had a prior (old) MI and (2) those who had an acute MI. SCD is more common in people who had a prior (old) MI. Those who had a prior MI and survive SCD are at risk for another SCD event because of the continued electrical instability from the scarred heart muscle that caused the first event to occur. They are usually referred for an ICD. Patients who have SCD associated with an acute MI undergo at least 40 days of maximal medical therapy to see if there is recovery in the EF before an ICD can be implanted.[32]

Most SCD patients have a lethal ventricular dysrhythmia that is associated with a high incidence of recurrence. It is difficult to know who is at high risk for SCD. However, LV dysfunction (EF < 30%) is the most commonly used tool to help guide decisions about ICD implantation.[31]

❖ Interprofessional and Nursing Care

People who survive an SCD event need a diagnostic workup to determine whether they had an acute MI. Serial analysis of cardiac biomarkers and ECGs are done to rule out ACS. Because some people with SCD have undiagnosed CAD, cardiac catheterization is done to identify if significant CAD (e.g., greater than 70% stenosis in multiple coronary arteries) was the cause of the SCD event. PCI or CABG surgery may be indicated because significant CAD may be a reversible cause of SCD.

If no reversible cause is identified and the EF is low normal, it is useful to know if these patients are likely to have a recurrence. Assessment of dysrhythmias in these patients may include obtaining an electrophysiology study (EPS).[32] EPS is done under fluoroscopy. Pacing electrodes are placed in various intracardiac areas and stimuli are selectively used in an attempt to reproduce life-threatening dysrhythmias. See Chapters 31 and 35 for a discussion of EPS.

For patients with syncope with the suspected cause of ventricular dysrhythmias, an outpatient wearable monitor (e.g., Holter monitor) can be used for up to 48 hours or a Mobile Cardiac Outpatient Telemetry (MCOT) (e.g., CardioNet) may be worn up to 30 days. An implantable cardiac monitor (e.g., LINQ) may be implanted and left in place up to 3 years.

The most common approach to preventing a recurrence of SCD is the use of an ICD. It has been shown that an ICD improves survival.[31,32] (See Chapter 35 for a discussion of ICDs.) Drug therapy with amiodarone may be used with an ICD to decrease episodes of ventricular dysrhythmias if the patient is receiving multiple ICD shocks from the dysrhythmias.

Some patients at risk for SCD (e.g., during the time when a patient with an MI and low EF must wait at least 40 days on maximum medical therapy to see if there is improvement in LV function) are recommended to use a wearable cardioverter-defibrillator (e.g., LifeVest) as a bridge to ICD or heart transplantation.[33] The wearable cardioverter-defibrillator is a personal external defibrillator that has 2 main parts: a garment and monitor. The garment is worn under clothing and has electrodes that continuously record the patient's ECG. The monitor is worn around the waist or from a shoulder strap. If the patient has ventricular tachycardia or ventricular fibrillation, the device sounds an alarm to confirm that the patient is unresponsive. If the patient is conscious, the patient can press 2 buttons to stop the shock. If the patient does not respond, the device warns bystanders that a shock is about to be delivered. If the dysrhythmia continues and the patient still does not respond, a treatment shock is delivered through the electrodes.[33]

Teaching people about the care of SCD victims and the actions to take can save lives. Rapid cardiopulmonary resuscitation (CPR) and defibrillation with an automatic external defibrillator (AED), combined with early advanced cardiac life support, has improved long-term survival rates for a witnessed arrest due to ventricular dysrhythmias.

When caring for these patients, be alert to the patient's psychosocial adaptation to this sudden "brush with death." Many patients develop a "time bomb" mentality. They fear the recurrence of cardiac arrest and may become anxious, angry, and depressed. Their caregivers are likely to have the same feelings. Patients and caregivers may need to deal with other issues, such as driving restrictions, role reversal, and change in occupation. The grief response varies among patients and caregivers. Be attuned to the specific needs of the patient and caregiver. Teach them accordingly while providing emotional support.

CASE STUDY

Myocardial Infarction

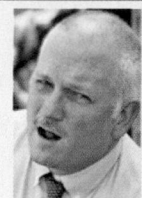

(© iStockphoto/Thinkstock.)

Patient Profile

D.M., a 51-yr-old, white, small business owner, is rushed to the ED by ambulance with crushing, substernal chest pain that radiates down his left arm. He reports dizziness and nausea.

Subjective Data

- Short of breath, nauseous
- History of chronic stable angina and hypertension
- States he is "borderline diabetic"
- Overweight, but recently lost 10 lb
- Rarely exercises
- Has 3 teenage children who are causing "problems"
- Recently lost his best friend and business partner, who died from cancer

Objective Data

Physical Examination

- Diaphoretic
- BP 165/100 mm Hg, pulse rate 120/min, respiratory rate 26/min

Diagnostic Studies

- 12-lead ECG shows sinus tachycardia with occasional premature ventricular contractions and ST elevation in leads II, III, aVF, V5, V6 consistent with an inferolateral wall MI
- High cardiac-specific troponin I level
- Total cholesterol 350 mg/dL (9.1 mmol/L)
- Hb A1C 9.0%

Interprofessional Care

- ED: Notify the cardiac catheterization laboratory of patient with STEMI:
  - O2 2 L/min via nasal cannula, titrate to keep O2 saturation above 93%
  - Continuous ECG monitoring
  - 2 IV access sites
  - Aspirin 325 mg (chewable)
  - Atorvastatin (Lipitor) 80 mg PO
  - Eptifibatide (Integrilin) IV (this should *not* delay the patient getting to the cardiac catheterization laboratory)

- Weight-based heparin IV (only used if the patient does not go directly to cardiac catheterization)
- SL NTG until an IV line is placed, then titrate nitroglycerin IV to relieve chest pain; hold for systolic BP below 100 mm Hg
- Morphine 2 mg IV q5–15 min as needed for chest pain unrelieved by NTG
- Vital signs (including pulse oximetry) every 10 minutes
- Prepare patient for cardiac catheterization with possible PCI

Discussion Questions

1. Which coronary artery(ies) is (are) most likely occluded in D.M.'s coronary circulation?
2. Explain the pathogenesis of CAD. What risk factors contribute to its development? What risk factors were present in D.M.'s life?
3. What is angina? How does chronic stable angina differ from angina associated with acute coronary syndrome?
4. Explain the pathophysiologic basis for the clinical manifestations that D.M. exhibited.
5. Explain the significance of the results of the laboratory tests and the 12-lead ECG findings.
6. Give a rationale for each treatment measure ordered for D.M.
7. **Priority Decision:** Based on the assessment data presented, what are the priority nursing diagnoses? Identify any collaborative problems.
8. **Priority Decision:** What are the priority nursing interventions for D.M. before PCI? Immediately after his PCI?
9. **Collaboration:** Identify activities that can be delegated to unlicensed assistive personnel (UAP).
10. **Evidence-Based Practice:** Two days after an uncomplicated PCI and the placement of 2 stents, D.M. wants to know what the most effective strategies are to prevent another MI. Based on his clinical situation, what would you tell him?
11. **Quality Improvement:** What outcomes would show that the interdisciplinary care was successful?
12. Develop a conceptual care map for D.M.

Answers and a corresponding conceptual care map available at *http://evolve.elsevier.com/Lewis/medsurg.*

BRIDGE TO NCLEX EXAMINATION

The number of the question corresponds to the same-numbered outcome at the beginning of the chapter.

1. In teaching a patient about coronary artery disease, the nurse explains that the changes that occur in this disorder include *(select all that apply)*
   a. diffuse involvement of plaque formation in coronary veins.
   b. abnormal levels of cholesterol, especially low-density lipoproteins.
   c. accumulation of lipid and fibrous tissue within the coronary arteries.
   d. development of angina due to a decreased blood supply to the heart muscle.
   e. chronic vasoconstriction of coronary arteries leading to permanent vasospasm.

2. After teaching about ways to decrease risk factors for CAD, the nurse recognizes that further instruction is needed when the patient says
   a. "I can keep my blood pressure normal with medication."
   b. "I would like to add weight lifting to my exercise program."
   c. "I can change my diet to decrease my intake of saturated fats."
   d. "I will change my lifestyle to reduce activities that increase my stress."

3. A hospitalized patient with a history of chronic stable angina tells the nurse that she is having chest pain. The nurse bases his actions on the knowledge that ischemia
   a. will always progress to myocardial infarction.
   b. can be relieved by rest, nitroglycerin, or both.
   c. is often associated with vomiting and extreme fatigue.
   d. indicates that irreversible myocardial damage is occurring.

4. The nurse is caring for a patient who is 2 days post MI. The patient reports that she is experiencing chest pain when she takes a deep breath. Which action would be a *priority*?
   a. Notify the provider STAT and obtain a 12-lead ECG.
   b. Obtain vital signs and auscultate for a pericardial friction rub.
   c. Apply high-flow O_2 by face mask and auscultate breath sounds.
   d. Medicate the patient with as-needed analgesic and reevaluate in 30 minutes.

5. A patient is admitted to the ICU with a diagnosis of NSTEMI. Which drugs(s) would the nurse expect the patient to receive? *(select all that apply)*
   a. Oral statin therapy
   b. Antiplatelet therapy
   c. Thrombolytic therapy
   d. Prophylactic antibiotics
   e. Intravenous nitroglycerin

6. A patient is recovering from an uncomplicated MI. Which rehabilitation guideline is a *priority* to include in the teaching plan?
   a. Refrain from sexual activity for a minimum of 3 weeks.
   b. Plan a diet program that aims for a 1- to 2-lb weight loss per week.
   c. Begin an exercise program that aims for at least 5 30-minute sessions per week.
   d. Consider the use of erectile agents and prophylactic NTG before engaging in sexual activity.

7. The most common finding in people at risk for sudden cardiac death is
   a. aortic valve disease.
   b. mitral valve disease.
   c. left ventricular dysfunction.
   d. atherosclerotic heart disease.

1. b, c, d; 2. b; 3. b; 4. b; 5. a, b, e; 6. c; 7. c

For rationales to these answers and even more NCLEX review questions, visit *http://evolve.elsevier.com/Lewis/medsurg.*

ⓔ EVOLVE WEBSITE/RESOURCES LIST

http://evolve.elsevier.com/Lewis/medsurg
Review Questions (Online Only)
Key Points
Answer Keys for Questions
- Rationales for Bridge to NCLEX Examination Questions
- Answer Guidelines for Case Study on p. 731

Student Case Study
- Patient With Coronary Artery Disease and Acute Coronary Syndrome

Nursing Care Plan
- eNursing Care Plan 33.1: Patient With Acute Coronary Syndrome

Conceptual Care Map Creator
- Conceptual Care Map for Case Study on p. 731

Audio Glossary
Content Updates

REFERENCES

1. World Health Organization: Cardiovascular diseases. Retrieved from *www.who.int/mediacentre/factsheets/fs317/en/.*
2. Benjamin EJ, Blaha MJ, Chiuve SE, et al: Heart disease and stroke statistics—2017 update: A report from the AHA, *Circulation* 135:e146, 2017.
3. Lilly LS: *Pathophysiology of heart disease: A collaborative project of medical students and faculty,* ed 6, Philadelphia, 2016, Wolters Kluwer.
*4. McSweeney JC, Rosenfeld AG, Abel WM, et al: Preventing and experiencing ischemic heart disease as a woman: State of the science: A scientific statement from the AHA, *Circulation* 133:1302, 2016.
*5. Mehta LS, Beckie TM, DeVon HA, et al: Acute myocardial infarction in women: A scientific statement from the AHA, *Circulation* 133:916, 2016.
6. Girelli D, Piubelli C, Martinelli N, et al: A decade of progress on the genetic basis of coronary artery disease, *Euro J Int Med* 1:10, 2017.
7. Brenner GM, Stevens CW: *Pharmacology e-book,* ed 5, Philadelphia, 2018, Elsevier.
*8. Stone NJ, Robinson JG, Lichtenstein AH, et al: 2013 ACC/AHA guideline on the treatment of blood cholesterol to reduce atherosclerotic cardiovascular risk in adults: A report of the ACC/AHA Task Force on Practice Guidelines, *Circulation* 129:S1, 2014. (Classic)

*9. Jellinger PS, Handelsman Y, Rosenblit PD, et al: American Association of Clinical Endocrinologist and American College of Endocrinology guidelines for management of dyslipidemia and prevention of cardiovascular disease, *Endocr Pract* 23:S1, 2017.

*10. Whelton PK, Carey RM, Aronow WS, et al: 2017 ACC/AHA/AAPA/ABC/ACPM/AGS/APhA/ASH/ASPC/NMA/PCNA guideline for the prevention, detection, evaluation, and management of high blood pressure in adults: A report of the ACC/AHA Task Force on Clinical Practice Guidelines, *Journal of the American College of Cardiology* 71:e127, 2018.

*11. James PA, Oparil S, Carter BL, et al: 2014 Evidence-based guideline for the management of high blood pressure in adults: Report from the panel members appointed to the Eighth Joint National Committee, *JAMA* 311:507, 2014. (Classic)

*12. Bhatnagar A, Whitsel LP, Ribisl KM, et al: Electronic cigarettes: A policy statement from the AHA, *Circulation* 130:1418, 2014. (Classic)

*13. Fihn SD, Blankenship JC, Alexander KP, et al: ACC/AHA/AATS/PCNA/SCAI/STS focused update of the guideline for the diagnosis and management of patients with stable ischemic heart disease: A report of the ACC/AHA Task Force on Practice Guidelines and the American College of Physicians, AATS, PCNA, SCAI, and STS, *Circulation* 130:1749, 2014. (Classic)

14. Bottaccioli AG: The role of stress and emotions in cardiovascular disease. In *Integrative cardiology: A new therapeutic vision*, New York, 2017, Springer.

*15. Amsterdam EA, Wenger NK, Brindis RG, et al: 2014 ACC/AHA guideline for the management of patients with non–ST-elevation acute coronary syndromes: A report of the ACC/AHA Task Force on Practice Guidelines, *Circulation* 130:e344, 2014. (Classic)

16. Havakuk O, Rezkalla SH, Kloner RA: The cardiovascular effects of cocaine, *JACC* 70:101, 2017.

17. American Heart Association: Fish and omega-3 fatty acids. Retrieved from *www.heart.org/en/healthy-living/healthy-eating/eat-smart/fats/fish-and-omega-3-fatty-acids*.

*18. Naylor M, Vasan R: Recent update to the US cholesterol treatment guidelines: A comparison with international guidelines, *Circulation* 133:1795, 2016.

*19. Bibbins-Domingo K, Grossman DC, Curry SJ, et al: Aspirin use for the primary prevention of cardiovascular disease and colorectal cancer: U.S. Preventive Services Task Force recommendation statement, *Ann Intern Med* 164:836, 2016.

*20. Levine GN, O'Gara PT, Bates ER, et al: 2015 ACC/AHA/SCAI focused update on primary PCI for patients with ST-elevation myocardial infarction: An update of the 2011 ACCF/AHA/SCAI guideline for PCI and the 2013 ACCF/AHA guideline for the management of ST-elevation myocardial infarction, *Circulation* 133:1135, 2016.

21. Mann DL, Zipes DP, Libby P, et al: *Braunwald's heart disease: A textbook of cardiovascular medicine*, ed 10, St Louis, 2015, Saunders. (Classic)

*22. Naderi S: Microvascular coronary dysfunction: An overview, *Curr Atheroscler Rep* 20:7, 2018.

*23. The Heart Outcomes Prevention Evaluation (HOPE) Study Investigators: Effects of an angiotensin-converting-enzyme inhibitor, ramipril, on cardiovascular events in high-risk patients, *N Engl J Med* 342:145, 2000. (Classic)

*24. Levine GN, Bates ER, Bittl JA, et al: 2016 ACC/AHA guideline focused update on duration of dual antiplatelet therapy in patients with coronary artery disease: A report of the ACC/AHA Task Force on Clinical Practice Guidelines, *Circulation* 134:e123, 2016.

*25. Hillis LD, Smith PK, Anderson JL, et al: 2011 ACCF/AHA guideline for coronary artery bypass graft surgery: A report of the ACC Foundation/AHA Task Force on Practice Guidelines, *Circulation* 124:e652, 2011. (Classic)

26. Cohn LH: *Cardiac surgery in the adult*, ed 8, New York, 2012, McGraw-Hill.

27. Sauër AC, Veldhuijzen DS, Ottens TH, et al: Association between delirium and cognitive change after cardiac surgery, *Brit J Anaesth* 119:308, 2017.

*28. O'Gara PT, Kushner FG, Ascheim DD, et al: 2013 ACCF/AHA guideline for the management of ST-elevation myocardial infarction: A report of the ACC Foundation/AHA Task Force on Practice Guidelines, *Circulation* 127:e362, 2013. (Classic)

29. American Association of Critical-Care Nurses: Family presence: Visitation in the adult ICU. Retrieved from *www.aacn.org/clinical-resources/practice-alerts/family-presence-visitation-in-the-adult-icu*.

*30. Levine GN, Steinke EE, Bakaeen FG, et al: Sexual activity and cardiovascular disease: A scientific statement from the AHA, *Circulation* 125:1058, 2012. (Classic)

31. Mitrani RD, Myerburg RJ: Ten advances defining sudden cardiac death, *Trends Cardiovasc Med* 26:23, 2016.

*32. Al-Khatib SM, Stevenson WG, Ackerman MJ, et al: 2017 AHA/ACC/HRS guideline for management of patients with ventricular arrhythmias and the prevention of sudden cardiac death: a report of the ACC Foundation/AHA Task Force on Clinical Practice Guidelines and the Heart Rhythm Society, *Circulation* 138:e272, 2018. Retrieved from *www.ahajournals.org/doi/pdf/10.1161/CIR.0000000000000549*.

33. Ferrick AM, Tian D, Vudathaneni V, et al: Wearable cardioverter defibrillators, *Cardiology in Review* 24:282, 2016.

*Evidence-based information for clinical practice.

34

Heart Failure

Vera Barton-Maxwell

There is no exercise better for the heart than reaching down and lifting people up.

John Holmes

e http://evolve.elsevier.com/Lewis/medsurg/

CONCEPTUAL FOCUS

Fatigue	Functional Ability	Self-Management
Fluids and Electrolytes	Hormonal Regulation	

LEARNING OUTCOMES

1. Compare the pathophysiology of heart failure with reduced ejection fraction (HFrEF) and heart failure with preserved ejection fraction (HFpEF).
2. Relate the compensatory mechanisms involved in heart failure (HF) to the development of acute decompensated heart failure (ADHF) and chronic HF.
3. Describe appropriate nursing and interprofessional care to manage the patient with ADHF.
4. Describe appropriate nursing and interprofessional care to manage the patient with chronic HF.
5. Discuss advanced therapeutic options for patients with stage D HF.
6. Describe the indications for heart transplantation and the nursing care of heart transplant recipients.

KEY TERMS

acute decompensated heart failure, p. 738
cardiac resynchronization therapy, p. 741
heart failure (HF), p. 734

heart failure with reduced ejection fraction (HFrEF), p. 734
heart failure with preserved ejection fraction (HFpEF), p. 734

heart transplantation, p. 750
orthopnea, p. 740
paroxysmal nocturnal dyspnea (PND), p. 740
pulmonary edema, p. 739

HEART FAILURE

Heart failure (HF) is a complex clinical syndrome that develops in response to myocardial insult. It results in the inability of the heart to provide sufficient blood to meet the oxygen (O_2) needs of tissues and organs. The decreased cardiac output leads to decreased tissue perfusion, impaired gas exchange, fluid volume imbalance, and decreased functional ability. This chapter discusses the nursing and interprofessional care of patients with HF.

The *percentage* of the total blood volume in the left ventricle (LV) at the end of diastole that is pumped out of the LV with the next systole is called the left ventricular ejection fraction (LVEF). HF manifestations occur due to a defect in either ventricular systolic function/LV contraction (heart failure with reduced ejection fraction [HFrEF]) and/or a defect in ventricular diastolic function/filling (heart failure with preserved ejection fraction [HFpEF]).[1]

HF is associated with many cardiovascular diseases (CVDs), particularly long-standing hypertension (HTN), coronary artery disease (CAD), and myocardial infarction (MI). HF is increasing in incidence and prevalence. This is partially due to better survival after cardiac events and the aging population. HF is primarily a disease of older adults. The incidence is similar in men and women.[2]

HF is a major health problem in the United States. The number of people diagnosed with HF has increased from 5.7 million (2009–2012) to 6.5 million (2011–2014). That number is projected to rise 46% by 2030.[2] HF is the most common reason for hospital admission in adults over the age of 65. This places a significant economic burden on the health care system.[1] The complex, progressive nature of HF often results in poor outcomes, such as hospital readmissions. Around 25% of patients discharged with a primary diagnosis of HF are readmitted within 30 days. The total cost of HF care exceeds $40 billion annually, with over half of these costs spent on hospitalizations.[2]

Etiology

HTN and CAD are the primary risk factors for HF. HTN is a modifiable risk factor that should be aggressively treated and managed. Long-term treatment of HTN reduces the incidence of HF by 50%.[1] Co-morbidities. such as diabetes, metabolic syndrome, advanced age, tobacco use, and vascular disease, contribute to the development of HF. Other causes of HF include congenital abnormalities (e.g., septal defects), infiltrative cardiomyopathies (e.g., sarcoidosis), infections and inflammatory processes (e.g., viral myocarditis), persistent dysrhythmias, and toxins (e.g., alcohol, drug use, chemotherapy).[3]

Any interference with the normal mechanisms regulating cardiac output (CO) may cause HF. CO depends on (1) preload, (2) afterload, (3) myocardial contractility, and (4) HR. These factors affect stroke volume (SV), which is the amount of blood pumped per heartbeat. Thus the equation: CO = SV × HR. Preload and afterload are discussed in Chapter 31. Any changes in these factors can lead to decreased ventricular function and HF.

The major causes of HF are divided into 2 subgroups: (1) primary causes (Table 34.1) and (2) precipitating causes (Table 34.2). Precipitating causes often increase the workload of the heart, resulting in an acute condition and decreased heart function.

Genetic Link

Several different forms of heart disease are passed down in families. Research suggests that 1 form of HF partially depends on a genetic predisposition. Mutations in more than 30 genes can cause the familial form of cardiomyopathy, a group of diseases that weaken the heart muscle. These genes provide the instructions for cardiomyocyte (heart muscle cell) proteins. The body's largest known protein, *titin*, responds to such a mutated gene. Titin mutations impair sarcomere function and disrupt chemical signaling, which negatively affects ventricular structure and stability.[5] Specific genes and gene mutations are linked to the development of HTN and CAD, known risk factors for HF (see Chapters 32, 33, and 36). Research into the effects of gene mutations on the incidence of HF is ongoing.

Pathophysiology

HF is a complex clinical syndrome that develops in response to myocardial injury and results in decreased heart function. Manifestations of HF are the result of neurohormonal compensatory mechanisms activated in response to myocardial dysfunction, leading to *remodeling* of myocardial structure and function (Fig. 34.1).

Left-Sided Heart Failure. The most common form of HF, left-sided HF, results either from the inability of the LV to (1) empty adequately during systole or (2) fill adequately during diastole. We can further classify left-sided HF as HFrEF (systolic HF), HFpEF (diastolic HF), or a combination of the two.

Heart Failure With Reduced EF (Systolic Failure). HFrEF results from an inability of the heart to pump blood effectively. The hallmark of HFrEF is a decrease in the LVEF. Normal LVEF is 55% to 65%. Patients with HFrEF generally have an LVEF < 40%. It can be as low as 5% to 10%. HFrEF is caused by impaired contractile function (e.g., MI), increased afterload (e.g., HTN), cardiomyopathy, and mechanical abnormalities (e.g., valvular heart disorders).[3]

The LV in HFrEF loses the ability to generate enough pressure to eject blood forward through the aorta. Over time, the LV becomes dilated and hypertrophied. The weakened heart muscle cannot generate adequate SV, which impairs CO. Because the LV cannot effectively push blood forward, end diastolic volumes and pressures in the LV increase. When the LV fails, blood backs up into the left atrium (LA). This causes fluid accumulation in the lungs. The increased pulmonary hydrostatic pressure causes fluid leakage from the pulmonary capillary bed into the interstitium and then the alveoli. This results in pulmonary congestion and edema (Fig. 34.2, *A* through *D*). Fortunately, there are many therapies that reduce morbidity and mortality in HFrEF.

Heart Failure With Preserved EF (Diastolic Failure). HFpEF results from the inability of the ventricles to relax and fill during diastole. About 50% of patients with HF have HFpEF. HTN is the primary cause of HFpEF.[1] Other risk factors include older

TABLE 34.1 Primary Causes of Heart Failure

- Cardiomyopathy (e.g., viral, postpartum, substance use)
- Congenital heart defects (e.g., ventricular septal defect)
- CAD, including MI
- HTN, including hypertensive crisis
- Hyperthyroidism
- Myocarditis
- Pulmonary HTN
- Rheumatic heart disease
- Valvular disorders (e.g., mitral stenosis)

TABLE 34.2 Common Precipitating Causes of Heart Failure

Cause	Mechanism
Anemia	↓ O_2-carrying capacity of the blood stimulating ↑ in CO to meet tissue demands, leading to increase in cardiac workload and increase in size of LV
Bacterial endocarditis	*Infection:* ↑ metabolic demands and O_2 requirements
	Valvular dysfunction: causes stenosis or regurgitation
Dysrhythmias	May ↓ CO and ↑ workload and O_2 requirements of myocardial tissue
Hypervolemia	↑ Preload causing volume overload on the RV
Hypothyroidism	Indirectly predisposes to ↑ atherosclerosis. Severe hypothyroidism decreases myocardial contractility.
Infection	↑ O_2 demand of tissues, stimulating ↑ CO
Nutritional deficiencies	May ↓ cardiac function by ↑ myocardial muscle mass and myocardial contractility
Obstructive sleep apnea	Frequent nighttime apnea results in ↑ afterload, intermittent hypoxia, and ↑ sympathetic nervous system activity.
Paget's disease	↑ Workload of the heart by ↑ vascular bed in the skeletal muscle
Pulmonary embolism	↑ Pulmonary pressure resulting from obstruction leads to pulmonary HTN, ↓ CO.
Thyrotoxicosis	Changes the tissue metabolic rate, ↑ HR and workload of the heart

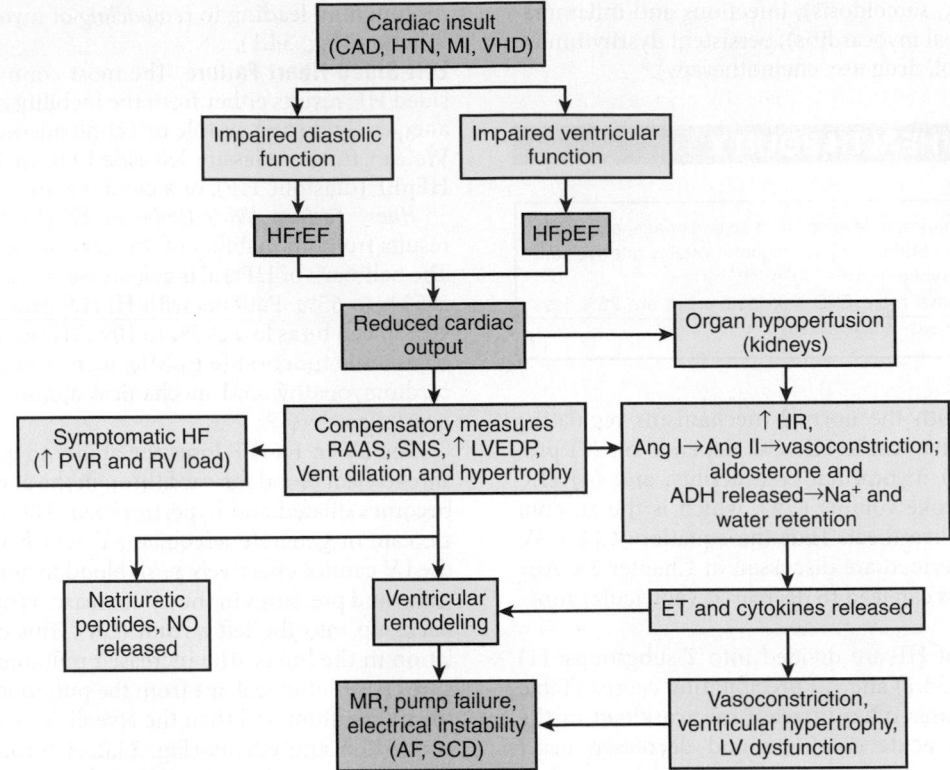

FIG. 34.1 Pathophysiology of HF. *Ang I,* Angiotensin I; *Ang II,* angiotensin II; *ADH,* Antidiuretic hormone; *ET,* endothelin; *HFpEF,* HF with preserved ejection fraction; *HFrEF,* HF with reduced ejection fraction; *LVEDP,* left ventricular end-diastolic pressure; *MR,* mitral regurgitation; *NO,* nitric oxide; *PVR,* pulmonary vascular resistance; *RAAS,* renin-angiotensin-aldosterone system; *SCD,* sudden cardiac death; *SNS,* sympathetic nervous system; *VHD,* valvular heart disease.

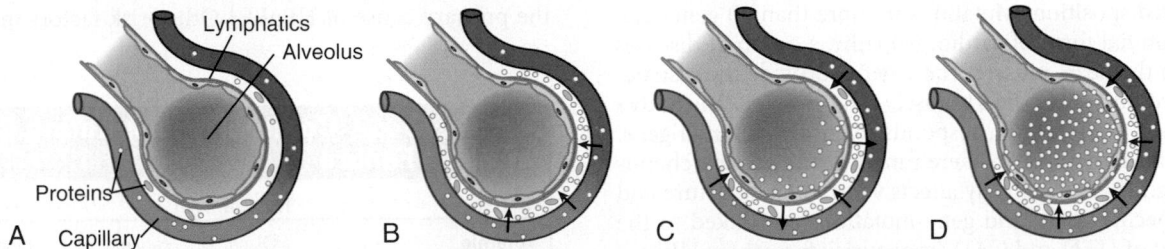

FIG. 34.2 As pulmonary edema progresses, it inhibits O_2 and CO_2 exchange at the alveolar-capillary interface. **A,** Normal relationship. **B,** Increased pulmonary capillary hydrostatic pressure causes fluid to move from the vascular space into the pulmonary interstitial space. **C,** Lymphatic flow increases to try to pull fluid back into the vascular or lymphatic space. **D,** Failure of lymphatic flow and worsening of left-sided HF result in further movement of fluid into the interstitial space and into the alveoli. (Modified from Urden LD, Stacy KM, Lough ME: *Critical care nursing: Diagnosis and management,* ed 6, St Louis, 2010, Mosby.)

age, female gender, diabetes, and obesity (see Gender Differences box). In HFpEF, the LV is generally stiff and noncompliant, resulting in high filling pressures. Decreased filling of the ventricles results in decreased SV. The eventual result of HFpEF is the same as that of HFrEF, a reduced CO leading to fluid congestion. The diagnosis of HFpEF is based on (1) signs and symptoms of HF, (2) normal LVEF, and (3) evidence of LV diastolic dysfunction by echocardiography or cardiac catheterization. Therapies are targeted at reducing underlying risk factors, treating co-morbidities, and reducing symptoms.[6]

Borderline HFpEF describes HF patients with LVEF 41% to 49%. Characteristics and therapies are like those for patients with HFpEF.[1] The patient with ventricular failure of any type may have low BP, low CO, and poor renal perfusion. Poor exercise tolerance and heart dysrhythmias are common. The patient may arrive at this point acutely from an MI or chronically from worsening cardiomyopathy or HTN. In both acute and chronic causes of HF, the body's response to low CO is to mobilize its compensatory mechanisms to maintain CO and BP.[3]

Right-Sided Heart Failure. Right-sided HF occurs when the right ventricle (RV) does not pump effectively. When the RV fails, fluid backs up into the venous system. This causes movement of fluid into the tissues and organs (e.g., peripheral edema, abdominal ascites, hepatomegaly, jugular venous distention [JVD]).

The most common cause of right-sided HF is left-sided HF. As the LV fails, fluid backs up into the pulmonary system, causing increased pressures in the lungs. The RV must work harder to push blood to the pulmonary system. Over time, this increased workload weakens the RV and gradually it fails. Other causes of right-sided HF (independent of the function of the LV) include RV infarction, pulmonary embolism, and *cor pulmonale* (RV dilation and hypertrophy caused by pulmonary disease) (see Chapter 27).

Biventricular Failure. Biventricular failure includes both LV and RV dysfunction, the inability of both ventricles to pump effectively. Because of decreased contractility, fluid build-up and systemic venous engorgement occur. Inadequate CO results in decreased perfusion to vital organs.[3]

Compensatory Mechanisms. HF can have an abrupt onset as with acute MI, or it can be a subtle process resulting from slow, progressive changes. The overloaded heart uses compensatory mechanisms to try to maintain adequate CO. The main compensatory mechanisms include (1) neurohormonal responses: renin-angiotensin-aldosterone system (RAAS) and the sympathetic nervous system (SNS); (2) ventricular dilation; and (3) ventricular hypertrophy.

Neurohormonal Response

Renin-angiotensin-aldosterone system. The renin-angiotensin-aldosterone system (RAAS) is a regulatory system that works to maintain normal homeostasis. The goal of RAAS activation is augmentation of preload and ventricular contractility to maintain CO. RAAS activation promotes retention of fluid and sodium. The juxtaglomerular apparatus in the kidneys senses decreased renal perfusion from a falling CO. In response, the kidneys release renin, which converts angiotensinogen to angiotensin I (see Chapter 44 and Fig. 44.4). Angiotensin I is next converted to angiotensin II by a converting enzyme made in the lungs. Angiotensin II is a potent vasoconstrictor that stimulates renal water and sodium retention and the release of aldosterone from the adrenal gland. Aldosterone acts in the nephron to stimulate sodium retention and potassium excretion and promoting myocardial fibrosis in the failing heart.

Continuous activation of the RAAS and SNS in HF leads to increased levels of antidiuretic hormone (ADH). ADH regulates water retention by stimulating renal tubular reabsorption. It is released in response to arterial low pressure/under filling via baroreceptor signals. It causes vasoconstriction and increases BP and central venous pressure (CVP). The consequences are fluid congestion and hyponatremia.[7] Chronic activation of the RAAS can cause harmful effects, such as cardiac myocyte apoptosis (programmed cell death), hypertrophy, and fibrosis. These cause the burdensome signs and symptoms that develop with HF.[8]

Sympathetic nervous system. Baroreceptors sense low arterial pressure, stimulating the SNS to try to maintain CO. Catecholamines (epinephrine and norepinephrine) are released. Stimulation of β-adrenergic receptors increases

HR (*chronotropy*) and ventricular contractility (*inotropy*). Ultimately, chronic SNS stimulation increases myocardial O_2 demand on the already weakened heart.

Continuous activation of the neurohormonal responses (RAAS and SNS) in HF leads to high levels of ADH, endothelin, and proinflammatory cytokines. Together, these factors further increase in the heart's workload, intensify ventricular dysfunction, and force ventricular remodeling.[3,7]

Peptides and Cytokines. Endothelin, a vasoconstrictor peptide made by the vascular endothelial cells, is stimulated by hypoxia, ischemia, neurohormones, and inflammatory cytokines. Although endothelin stimulates contraction in most smooth muscles, it has the opposite effect on the heart, acting as a negative inotrope. This serves to decrease ventricular contractility in the failing heart.

Proinflammatory cytokines are released by myocytes in response to heart injury (e.g., MI, HF). Two cytokines, tumor necrosis factor (TNF) and interleukin-1 (IL-1), further depress heart function by exerting a negative inotropic effect, causing myocyte hypertrophy and apoptosis. Over time, a systemic inflammatory response also occurs.[9] High levels of endothelin and proinflammatory cytokines result in an increase in the heart's workload, progressive LV dysfunction, myocyte hypertrophy, and *ventricular remodeling*.[3,8]

Ventricular Adaptations

Dilation. *Dilation* is an enlargement of the heart chambers (Fig. 34.3, *A*). It occurs when pressure in the heart chambers (usually the LV) is elevated over time. The heart muscle fibers stretch in response to the volume of blood in the heart at the end of diastole. According to the *Frank-Starling Law,* the strength of the heart's contraction is directly proportional to its diastolic expansion. The implication is that increased preload (a greater influx of blood into the ventricle during diastole) will cause a more forceful contraction. This increased contraction initially leads to increased CO and maintains BP and perfusion. Dilation starts as an adaptive mechanism to cope with increasing blood volume. However, excessive preload exhausts the Frank-Starling mechanism, cardiac muscle fibers are overstretched, and further increases in preload no longer increase CO.

Hypertrophy. *Hypertrophy* is an adaptive increase in the muscle mass and heart wall thickness as a slow response to overwork and strain (Fig. 34.3, *B*). It occurs slowly because it takes time for this increased muscle tissue to develop. Initially, the increased contractile power of the muscle fibers leads to an increase in CO and maintains tissue perfusion. Over time, hypertrophic heart muscle has poor contractility, needs more O_2 to perform work, has poor coronary artery circulation (tissue becomes ischemic more easily), and is prone to dysrhythmias.

Remodeling. Pathologic ventricular *remodeling* is an actual change in the structure (dimensions, mass, shape) of the heart. Ventricular remodeling in HF occurs over time in response to pressure or volume overload and/or cardiac injury and the subsequent compensatory mechanisms. These include neurohormonal, ET, and cytokine activation and ventricular adaptations, including dilatation and hypertrophy. This altered shape of the ventricles eventually leads to increased ventricular mass, increased wall tension, increased O_2 consumption, and impaired contractility. The actual shape of the heart becomes less elliptical and more spherical. Although the ventricles become larger, they become less effective pumps. The LVEF further declines due to loss of mechanical advantage from altered

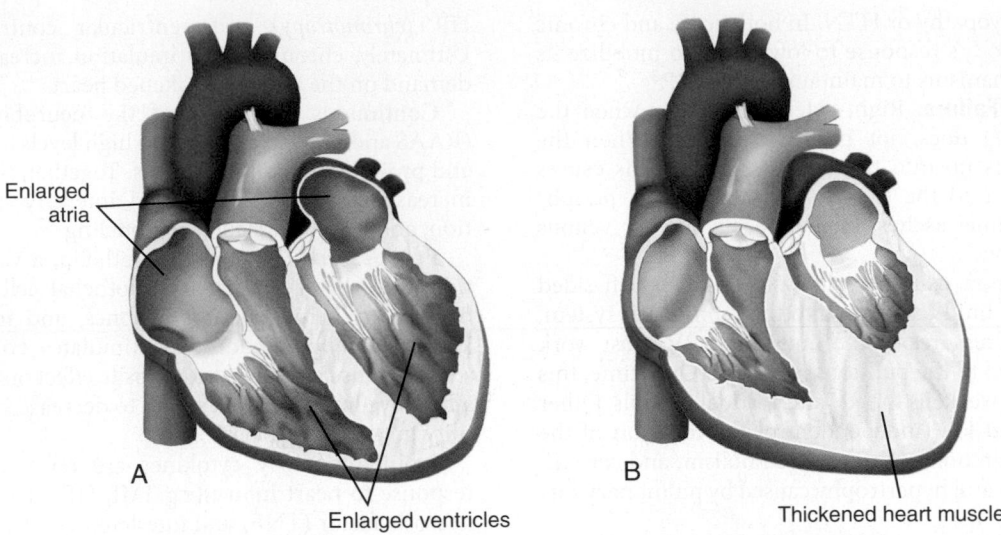

FIG. 34.3 A, Dilated heart chambers. B, Hypertrophied heart chambers.

ventricular geometry. Increases in angiotensin II, aldosterone, and cytokines stimulate collagen synthesis leading to fibrosis and further impaired pumping ability.[10] Ventricular remodeling is a risk factor for life-threatening dysrhythmias and sudden cardiac death (SCD). Drug therapies to prevent or reverse remodeling and decrease mortality are recommended. These include ACE inhibitors, β-adrenergic blockers (β-blockers), and aldosterone antagonists.

Beneficial Counterregulatory Mechanisms. The body tries to maintain balance through several beneficial counterregulatory processes. Natriuretic peptides (atrial natriuretic peptide [ANP] and brain [b-type] natriuretic peptide [BNP]) are hormones made by the heart muscle. ANP is released from the atria and BNP is released from the ventricles in response to increased blood volume and ventricular wall stretching.[11]

The natriuretic peptides have beneficial renal, cardiovascular, and hormonal effects. Renal effects include: (1) increased glomerular filtration rate and diuresis and (2) excretion of sodium (natriuresis). Cardiovascular effects include vasodilation and decreased BP. Hormonal effects include (1) inhibition of aldosterone and renin secretion and (2) interference with ADH release. The combined effects of ANP and BNP help to counter the adverse effects of the SNS and RAAS.[11] We can measure serum BNP levels. High serum BNP corresponds proportionately with fluid retention and is a predictor of mortality in HF.

Nitric oxide (NO) and prostaglandin are counterregulatory substances released from the vascular endothelium in response to the compensatory mechanisms activated in HF. NO and prostaglandin work to relax the arterial smooth muscle, resulting in vasodilation and decreased afterload.[10]

Compensated HF occurs when compensatory mechanisms succeed in maintaining an adequate CO that is needed for tissue perfusion. *Decompensated HF* occurs when these mechanisms can no longer maintain adequate CO and inadequate tissue perfusion results.

Classifications of Heart Failure

New York Heart Association Classes of Heart Failure. The New York Heart Association (NYHA) Functional Classification places patients in 1 of 4 categories (I–IV) based on physical activity limitation due to symptom burden.[1] NYHA class designation changes based on worsening or improving symptoms.

The Stages of Heart Failure. The American College of Cardiology Foundation and the American Heart Association (ACCF/AHA) more recently developed a staging system (A–D) that emphasizes the evolution and progression of HF as well as treatment strategies.[1] This system identifies people at risk for developing HF who do not currently have heart disease (stage A). This classification encourages clinicians to actively address the patient's risk factors and treat any existing conditions to prevent further disease progression. This staging system is progressive and unidirectional. Patients advance to a higher (worse) stage as the disease progresses. Table 34.3 compares the NYHA classification and ACC/AHA staging system.

Clinical Manifestations: Acute Decompensated Heart Failure

Acute decompensated heart failure (ADHF) is an increase (usually sudden) in symptoms of HF with a decrease in functional status, often requiring rapid escalation of therapy and hospital admission. ADHF is the most common cause of hospitalization for older Americans.[12] The presentation of ADHF typically includes symptoms and signs related to pulmonary congestion and volume overload. Neurohormonal activation leads to impaired regulation of sodium excretion through the kidneys that results in sodium and fluid accumulation. The lungs become less compliant. There is increased resistance in the small airways. To help compensate, the lymphatic system increases its flow to help maintain a constant volume of the pulmonary extravascular fluid (Fig. 34.1, *A* and *B*). This early stage is clinically associated with a mild increase in the respiratory rate (RR) and a decrease in partial pressure of O_2 in arterial blood (PaO_2).

If pulmonary venous pressure continues to increase, the increase in intravascular pressure causes more fluid to move into the interstitial space than the lymphatics can remove resulting in *interstitial edema* (Fig. 34.1, *C*). Tachypnea develops, and the patient becomes symptomatic (e.g., short of breath). If the pulmonary venous pressure increases further, the alveoli lining cells are disrupted, and fluid moves into the alveoli (*alveolar edema*). This is accompanied by a worsening of the arterial

TABLE 34.3 Comparison of ACCF/AHA Stages of Heart Failure and NYHA Functional Classifications

ACCF/AHA Stages of Heart Failure (HF)	NYHA Functional Classifications
A At high risk for HF, but without structural heart disease or symptoms of HF	None
B Structural heart disease, but without signs or symptoms of HF	I No limitation of physical activity. Ordinary physical activity does not cause symptoms of HF.
C Structural heart disease with prior or current symptoms of HF	I No limitation of physical activity. Ordinary physical activity does not cause symptoms of HF.
	II Slight limitation of physical activity. Comfortable at rest, but ordinary physical activity results in symptoms of HF.
	III Marked limitation of physical activity. Comfortable at rest, but less than ordinary activity causes symptoms of HF.
	IV Unable to carry on any physical activity without symptoms of HF, or symptoms of HF at rest
D Refractory HF requiring specialized interventions	IV Unable to carry on any physical activity without symptoms of HF, or symptoms of HF at rest

Reprinted with permission. *Circulation* 128:e240-e327, 2013. © 2013 American Heart Association, Inc.
ACCF, American College of Cardiology Foundation; *AHA*, American Heart Association; *NYHA*, New York Heart Association.

TABLE 34.4 Clinical Profile in Acute Decompensated Heart Failure

		CONGESTION (WET)	
		No	**Yes**
LOW PERFUSION (COLD)	**No**	**Dry-Warm** • PAWP normal • CO normal • Signs and symptoms: none	**Wet-Warm** • PAWP ↑ • CO normal • Signs and symptoms: dyspnea, edema, orthopnea
	Yes	**Dry-Cold** • PAWP ↓ or normal • CO ↓ • Signs and symptoms: edema, hypotension, cool extremities	**Wet-Cold** • PAWP ↑ • CO ↓ • Signs and symptoms: altered mental status, decreased O_2 saturation, reduced urine output, shock

PAWP, Pulmonary artery wedge pressure.

blood gas values (i.e., lower PaO_2, increased $PaCO_2$, progressive respiratory acidosis).

ADHF can manifest as **pulmonary edema**. This is an acute, life-threatening situation, in which the lung alveoli become filled with serosanguineous fluid (Fig. 34.1, *D*). The most common cause of pulmonary edema is left-sided HF. Other causes of pulmonary edema are listed in Table 27.24.

Manifestations of pulmonary edema include acute manifestations of left HF, such as dyspnea, *orthopnea*, and *paroxysmal nocturnal dyspnea*. JVD is often present and is the most sensitive and specific sign for elevated LV filling pressures. Coughing may provide an early clue to developing pulmonary edema in patients with chronic HF. The patient is usually anxious and pale and may be cyanotic. The RR is often > 30 breaths per minute. You may see use of accessory respiratory muscles. Pink, frothy sputum may be present in patients with severe disease. Auscultation of the lungs may reveal crackles and wheezes throughout. The absence of crackles does not rule out ADHF as many patients with a history of chronic HF develop increased lymphatic drainage of the alveolar edema. The patient's HR is often rapid, and an abnormal S_3 or S_4 heart sound may be heard (Table 31.4). BP may be high or decreased depending on the severity of the HF. Hypotension indicates severe LV systolic dysfunction and the

chance of cardiogenic shock. Cool extremities occur with low CO and poor perfusion. Skin pallor or mottling may be present. They result from peripheral vasoconstriction and shunting of blood to the central circulation. Sometimes, hoarseness may be present because of compression of the recurrent laryngeal nerve from an enlarged LA (Ortner sign).

Patients with ADHF are categorized into 1 of 4 groups based on hemodynamic and clinical status: dry-warm, dry-cold, wet-warm, and wet-cold (Table 34.4).[1] The most common presentation in patients with ADHF is the wet and warm patient. A patient is "wet" due to volume overload (e.g., congestion, dyspnea) but "warm" due to adequate perfusion (warm skin, positive pulses).

❓ CHECK YOUR PRACTICE

You are assigned to a patient with ADHF who was admitted to the HF unit. Your assessment reveals that the patient has bilateral crackles in the mid-lower lung fields and dyspnea on exertion (e.g., moving from the bed to the commode). The patient's skin is warm, and pulses are present in all extremities. Your preceptor asks you to categorize your patient based on the classification systems in Tables 34.3 and 34.4.
• In what NYHA class would you place your patient?
• In what ACCF/AHA stage would you place your patient?
• What ADHF clinical profile does your patient best fit?

Clinical Manifestations: Chronic Heart Failure

Chronic HF is a progressive syndrome characterized by reduced CO and increased venous pressure, associated with underlying molecular changes that result in the death of cardiac muscle cells. The compensatory mechanisms in response to this reduced CO include neurohormonal and hemodynamic reactions to maintain major organ perfusion through vasoconstriction and SNS stimulation, an inflammatory response involving cytokines, and ventricular remodeling. These physiologic responses are responsible for the manifestations of chronic HF. Many therapies for chronic HF work by counteracting these mechanisms. Table 34.5 lists the manifestations of right-sided and left-sided chronic HF.

Fatigue. Fatigue following usual daily activities can be an early symptom of chronic HF. As the falling CO cannot sustain

TABLE 34.5 Manifestations of Heart Failure

Right-Sided Heart Failure	Left-Sided Heart Failure
Signs	
• Right ventricular heaves	• Left ventricular heaves
• ↑ HR	• ↑ HR
• Murmurs	• Pulsus alternans (alternating
• Jugular venous distention	pulses: strong, weak)
• Edema (e.g., pedal, scrotum,	• PMI displaced inferiorly and
sacrum)	left of the midclavicular line (LV
• Weight gain	hypertrophy)
• Ascites	• ↓ PaO$_2$, slight ↑ PaCO$_2$ (poor O$_2$
• Anasarca (massive general-	exchange)
ized body edema)	• Crackles (pulmonary edema)
• Hepatomegaly (liver enlarge-	• S$_3$ and S$_4$ heart sounds
ment)	• Pleural effusion
	• Changes in mental status
	• Restlessness, confusion
	• Shallow respirations up to
	32–40/min
	• Dry, hacking cough
	• Frothy, pink-tinged sputum
	(advanced pulmonary edema)
Symptoms	
• Fatigue	• Weakness, fatigue
• Anxiety, depression	• Anxiety, depression
• Right upper quadrant pain	• Dyspnea
• Anorexia and GI bloating	• Paroxysmal nocturnal dyspnea
• Nausea	• Orthopnea
	• Nocturia

PaCO$_2$, Partial pressure of CO$_2$ in arterial blood; *PaO$_2$*, partial pressure of O$_2$ in arterial blood; *PMI*, point of maximal impulse.

activities, fatigue eventually limits activities. Anemia, common in HF, is another potential cause of fatigue.

Dyspnea. Dyspnea is the most common manifestation of chronic HF. It is caused by increased pulmonary pressures from interstitial and alveolar edema. Dyspnea can occur early in the HF disease process with mild exertion. As HF progresses, dyspnea develops with less exertion until dyspnea occurs at rest.

Orthopnea, or dyspnea in the recumbent position, suggests HF. Orthopnea occurs due to redistribution of fluid from the lower extremities into the lungs while in a supine position. The dyspnea is usually relieved with sitting up. Asking the patient about the number of pillows used under the head while sleeping or about sleeping in a recliner can reveal adaptive behaviors that aid breathing.

Paroxysmal nocturnal dyspnea (PND) is episodic, sudden dyspnea that wakes a patient at night. PND is caused by fluid accumulation in the lungs entering the alveoli while the patient is supine. The patient can awaken in a panic with feelings of suffocation and a strong desire to sit or stand to aid breathing.

Cough. A chronic, nonproductive cough that is worse in the recumbent position is often associated with pulmonary congestion and can be a sign of HF. Other potential causes of cough include gastric conditions, medications (e.g., ACE inhibitors due to increased bradykinin levels), and pulmonary conditions.

Tachycardia. Tachycardia is an early sign of HF. One of the body's first responses to compensate for a reduced CO is to increase the HR via activation of the SNS. At first, this compensatory response has a favorable effect on CO. But over time, persistent tachycardia is harmful and may worsen HF and the

accompanying manifestations. Adequate HR control in patients with chronic HF has been associated with better clinical outcomes, including decreased hospitalizations and mortality.[1]

Palpitations. Palpitations, or an irregular heartbeat, can occur due to dysrhythmias that occur with chronic HF. Atrial fibrillation (AF) is the most common of these dysrhythmias. Patients may report a fast or irregular heartbeat, a fluttering sensation, or "skipped beats" that may be intermittent. Palpitations may be accompanied by dyspnea, lightheadedness, or near syncope if the dysrhythmia further decreases CO.

Edema. Edema is a common sign of HF. It may occur in dependent body areas (peripheral edema), liver (hepatomegaly), abdominal cavity (ascites), and lungs (pulmonary edema and pleural effusion). If the patient is in bed, dependent sacral and scrotal edema may develop. Pressing the edematous skin with the finger may leave a depression (*pitting edema*). Accumulation of extravascular fluid in the lower extremities can indicate volume overload and be a sign of ADHF. It is important to note that not all lower extremity edema is a result of HF. Hypoproteinemia, renal insufficiency, cellulitis, venous stasis, cirrhosis, and certain drugs can cause peripheral edema.

Changes in Urine Output. Urine output may be decreased because of decreased renal perfusion. HF patients often develop resistance to diuretics, which can result in a drop in urinary output. *Nocturia* is the tendency to urinate excessively during the night due to increased renal perfusion in the supine position.

Skin Changes. A low CO can result in decreased perfusion to the skin of the extremities resulting in *mottling*, a blue or gray coloring. A coolness or clammy feeling to touch can occur with poor perfusion. Because tissue capillary O$_2$ extraction is increased with chronic HF, the skin may appear dusky. Chronic edema can result in pigment changes. The skin can become dry from overdiuresis. It is important to recognize integumentary signs of other conditions, such as venous stasis, peripheral arterial disease, and cellulitis.

Neurologic Manifestations. Dizziness, lightheadedness, near syncope, or syncope can occur due to reduced CO and hypoperfusion to the brain or dysrhythmias that often occur with chronic HF. Hypotension secondary to HF medications and hypovolemia are common causes of neurologic symptoms in chronic HF.

Mental Status and Behavioral Changes. Cerebral hypoperfusion may occur because of hypoxia to the brain from decreased CO. The patient or caregiver may report confusion, forgetfulness, inattentiveness, and restlessness. A thorough assessment is needed to evaluate for possible confounding conditions, including psychologic disorders (especially depression and anxiety) or neurologic disorders, such as stroke or transient ischemic attack (TIA). Around 1 in 5 patients with HF have clinical depression, which confers a twofold risk of mortality and higher readmission rates.[13] Patients with psychologic disorders have poorer adherence to treatment plans. All HF patients should be screened for depression or coexisting mental health conditions.

Sleep Problems. Snoring and daytime sleepiness can indicate sleep apnea, a common confounding condition with chronic HF. Sleep apnea screening questions include those about daytime sleepiness and falling asleep, feeling rested in the morning, frequent nighttime awakenings, and history and results of a sleep study. Alternatively, insomnia could be due to psychologic issues, including anxiety or depression, or due to excessive daytime napping. The need to void often with nocturia may disturb the patient's rest.

Chest Pain. Chest pain or angina can be the result of the reduced CO associated with HF compounded with CAD. Chest pain in HF can also occur due to myocardial stretch from volume overload. Careful questioning and assessment will help distinguish among the many potential causes for chest pain in the patient with chronic HF.

Weight Changes. Many factors contribute to weight changes. Progressive weight gain in the patient with chronic HF may indicate fluid retention. Renal failure may contribute to fluid retention. Abdominal fullness from ascites and hepatomegaly often causes anorexia and nausea. As HF advances, the patient may have cardiac *cachexia* with muscle wasting and fat loss. This can be masked by the patient's edematous condition and may not be evident until the edema subsides.

Complications of Heart Failure

Pleural Effusion. *Pleural effusion,* fluid between the 2 tissue layers (pleura) that cover the lung and line the chest wall, is a common complication in HF. Increased capillary hydrostatic pressure in the systemic or pulmonary circulation from HF causes fluid leakage into the pleural space. Pleural effusions may result in symptoms of dyspnea, cough, and chest pain. Pleural effusion is discussed in Chapter 27.

Dysrhythmias and Dyssynchronous Contraction. Both atrial and ventricular dysrhythmias are common in HF. Structural changes, including myocardial stretch, fibrosis, and chamber dilatation, alter the electrical paths of the heart. Early and delayed depolarizations, both common in HF, can trigger dysrhythmias. AF is quite common in patients with HF, and the prevalence increases as the severity of HF increases. AF occurs when numerous sites in the atria fire spontaneously and rapidly, and organized atrial depolarization (contraction) no longer occurs. Loss of "atrial kick" during systole may contribute to decreased CO and worsening HF symptoms.

AF promotes thrombus formation within the atria. Thrombi can break loose and form emboli, placing patients at significant risk for stroke. Treatment with anticoagulation should be a priority if there are no significant contraindications. Treatment with drugs to achieve HR control is important. Restoring normal sinus rhythm with cardioversion and ablation may be considered. Atrial fibrillation is discussed in Chapter 35.

An enlarged LV and very low LVEF also increase the risk for thrombus formation in the LV. Anticoagulant therapy may be considered for patients with these problems.

Patients with HF are at risk for dangerous ventricular dysrhythmias (e.g., ventricular tachycardia [VT], ventricular fibrillation [VF]). SCD (sudden loss of cardiac function due to a fatal ventricular tachyarrhythmia), is a major cause of death in the HF population. Patients with HFrEF are at greatest risk for SCD. Guidelines recommend implantation of a prophylactic implantable cardioverter-defibrillator (ICD) for patients with an LVEF < 35%, who are NYHA Class II or III.[1] SCD is discussed in Chapter 33. Dysrhythmias are discussed in Chapter 35.

Ventricular remodeling can lead to dyssynchrony in ventricular contractions. One ventricle may contract prior to the other ventricle, leading to suboptimal ventricular filling (preload), reduced force of ventricular contraction (systole), and severe mitral regurgitation (MR). This worsens HF symptoms. **Cardiac resynchronization therapy (CRT)** in the form of implantable cardiac devices can significantly improve morbidity and mortality for these patients. Many HF patients receive a combination ICD and CRT device, discussed later in the chapter.

Hepatomegaly. HF can lead to severe hepatomegaly. The liver becomes congested with venous blood from right HF or ADHF. The hepatic congestion can lead to impaired liver function. Eventually liver cells die, fibrosis occurs, and cirrhosis can develop (see Chapter 43).

Cardiorenal Syndrome. Reduction in CO results in decreased renal perfusion, decreased glomerular filtration rate, and increased serum creatinine. Neurohormonal activation causes sodium and water retention, worsening HF symptoms and renal function. Impaired renal function with HF is an independent risk factor for HF morbidity and mortality.

Anemia. The primary cause of anemia in chronic HF is chronic kidney insufficiency due to the renal vasoconstriction that often occurs with HF. This vasoconstriction results in reduced erythropoietin production in the kidney, leading to anemia. Excessive cytokine production also can reduce erythropoietin secretion. The anemia itself can worsen cardiac function due to increased cardiac workload through tachycardia, fluid retention, and increased SV. Because anemia can reduce renal blood flow, it adds further stress to the heart and worsens fatigue and other manifestations of chronic HF.

Diagnostic Studies

Diagnosing HF can be challenging. Signs and symptoms are not highly specific and may mimic many other medical conditions (e.g., anemia, lung disease). Diagnostic tests for ADHF and chronic HF are outlined in Table 34.6. A primary goal in diagnosis is to find the underlying cause of HF.

An echocardiogram is a valuable, noninvasive diagnostic tool used in patients with HF. The echocardiogram gives information about chamber size and function, LVEF, heart valve function, wall thickness and motion, presence of effusion or thrombus, and intracardiac and pulmonary pressures. This test helps to distinguish between HFrEF and HFpEF. Other useful tests include 12-lead ECG, ambulatory heart monitors, chest x-ray, 6-minute walk test, multigated acquisition (MUGA) scan, cardiopulmonary exercise stress test, cardiac MRI, and cardiac catheterization/angiogram. Polysomnography studies for obstructive sleep apnea may be done. An endomyocardial biopsy may be done as part of a heart catheterization to evaluate for infective or infiltrative disease in acutely ill patients who develop unexplained, new-onset HF unresponsive to usual care.

Laboratory studies aid in the diagnosis of HF. In general, BNP and N-terminal prohormone of BNP (NT-proBNP) levels correlate positively with the degree of LV failure.[11] Levels are temporarily higher in patients receiving nesiritide (Natrecor) and may be high in patients with chronic, stable HF. So, it is important you know the baseline levels. Increases in BNP or NT-proBNP levels can be caused by conditions other than HF, including pulmonary embolism, renal failure, and acute coronary syndrome.

Interprofessional Care: Acute Decompensated Heart Failure

Mortality and readmission rates for ADHF remain unacceptably high. Professional HF organizations have developed quality improvement initiatives, such as "Get with the Guidelines" and the Acute Decompensated HF Registry (ADHERE), to help clinicians and agencies improve HF outcomes.[1]

Goals of therapy for the patient hospitalized with ADHF include (1) symptom relief; (2) optimizing volume status; (3) supporting oxygenation, ventilation, CO, and end organ

TABLE 34.6 Interprofessional Care

Heart Failure

Both ADHF and Chronic HF	ADHF	Chronic HF
Diagnostic Assessment		
• History and physical examination	• Measure LV function	• Cardiopulmonary exercise stress test
• Determine underlying cause	• Hemodynamic monitoring	• 6-minute walk test
• Serum chemistries, cardiac biomarkers, BNP or NT-proBNP level (see Table 31.6), liver function tests, thyroid function tests, CBC, lipid profile, kidney function tests, urinalysis	• Endomyocardial biopsy in select patients	• Sleep studies in select patients
• Chest x-ray		
• 12-lead ECG		
• 2-dimensional echocardiogram (see Table 31.7)		
• Nuclear imaging studies (see Table 31.7)		
• Cardiac catheterization (see Table 31.8)		
Management		
• Treatment of underlying cause	• High-Fowler's position	• Cardiac resynchronization therapy with biventricular pacing and internal cardioverter-defibrillator
• Drug therapy (Table 34.7)	• Noninvasive positive pressure ventilation	
• Circulatory assist devices (e.g., ventricular assist device)	• Circulatory assist device: intraaortic balloon pump	• Heart transplantation
• Daily weights	• Endotracheal intubation and mechanical ventilation	• Rest-activity periods
• Sodium- and possibly fluid-restricted diet	• Vital signs, urine output at least q1hr until stable	• Dietitian consult
• O_2 by mask or nasal cannula if indicated	• Continuous ECG and pulse oximetry monitoring	• Physical/occupational therapy consult
	• Hemodynamic monitoring (e.g., intraarterial BP, PAWP, CO)	• Cardiac rehabilitation
	• Cardioversion (e.g., atrial fibrillation)	• Home health nursing care (e.g., telehealth monitoring)
	• Ultrafiltration	• Palliative and end-of-life care

BNP, b-type natriuretic peptide; *LVAD,* left ventricular assist device; *NT-proBNP,* N-terminal prohormone of BNP; *PAWP,* pulmonary artery wedge pressure.

perfusion; (4) identifying and addressing the cause of the ADHF; (5) avoiding complications; (6) providing patient teaching addressing factors that precipitated HF exacerbation; and (7) discharge planning.

Patients with ADHF need ongoing monitoring and assessment of vital signs, O_2 saturation, weight, mentation, ECGs, and indicators of volume overload and decreased organ perfusion. Assessment findings indicating fluid volume overload include edema, ascites, JVD, a positive hepatojugular reflux test, an S_3 heart sound, crackles, hypoxia, and worsening renal function.

Stable patients with ADHF may be treated in the emergency department (ED) or admitted to a telemetry unit. Assess these patients every 4 hours (e.g., vital signs, pulse oximetry) for adequate oxygenation. Record intake, output, and daily weights to evaluate fluid status. If the patient has dyspnea, place in a high-Fowler's position with the feet horizontal in the bed or dangling at the bedside. This position helps decrease venous return because of the pooling of blood in the extremities. This position also increases the thoracic capacity, allowing for improved breathing.

If unstable, these patients are managed in an intensive care unit (ICU). In addition to continual ECG and O_2 saturation monitoring, vital signs and urine output are assessed at least hourly. Indicators of decreased perfusion include hypotension, decreased urine output, cool extremities, altered mentation, heart murmur, dysrhythmias, and worsening renal and liver function tests. The patient may have hemodynamic monitoring, including arterial BP and pulmonary artery pressures. If a pulmonary artery (PA) catheter is placed, CO and pulmonary artery wedge pressure (PAWP) are routinely monitored. PAWP is an indirect measurement of LA filling pressure measured from the tip of the PA catheter when inflated in a capillary artery. A normal PAWP is 6 to 15 mm Hg. Patients with ADHF

may have a PAWP as high as 30 mm Hg. Therapies are adjusted to maximize CO and reduce PAWP. Hemodynamic monitoring is discussed in Chapter 65.

Supplemental O_2 is provided to help increase the PaO_2. O_2 therapy is discussed in Chapter 28. In severe pulmonary edema, the patient may need noninvasive positive pressure ventilation (e.g., bilevel positive airway pressure [BiPAP]) or intubation and mechanical ventilation. BiPAP also decreases preload. Ventilatory support is discussed in Chapter 65.

Nonpharmacologic Therapies. *Ultrafiltration,* or *aquapheresis,* is an option for the patient with volume overload when diuretics have not been effective.[1] It can rapidly remove intravascular fluid volume and excess sodium from the patient's blood while maintaining hemodynamic stability. Hemodialysis can be used for volume overload with concomitant renal failure. They are discussed in Chapter 46.

Implantation of CRT, a biventricular pacemaker, may be considered for patients with ADHF who meet specific criteria and do not respond to more traditional therapies.

In the ICU, *mechanical cardiac assist devices* are used temporarily to manage patients with worsening HF. The intraaortic balloon pump (IABP) is a device that increases coronary blood flow to the heart muscle and decreases the heart's workload through a process called *counterpulsation.* The IABP is useful in hemodynamically unstable patients because it can decrease pulmonary artery pressures and systemic vascular resistance (SVR), leading to improved CO. Ventricular assist devices (VADs) can help maintain the pumping action of a weakened heart. A VAD is a surgically implanted mechanical pump. IABPs and VADs are discussed in Chapter 65.

Drug Therapy. Drug therapy is essential in treating ADHF (Table 34.7).

TABLE 34.7 Drug Therapy
Heart Failure

Drug	Mechanism of Action
Anticoagulants (see Table 37.10)	• Prevent thromboembolism • Recommended for patients with an ejection fraction <20% and/or atrial fibrillation
Antidysrhythmic Drugs (see Table 35.9)	• Prevent or treat dysrhythmias
β-Adrenergic Blockers (see Table 32.6) bisoprolol (Zebeta) carvedilol (Coreg) metoprolol succinate (Toprol XL)	• Promote reverse remodeling • Decrease afterload • Inhibit SNS • Reverse cardiac remodeling • Reduce mortality and morbidity in patients with chronic HF
Diuretics (see Table 32.7) ***Loop Diuretics*** bumetanide (Bumex) furosemide (Lasix)	• Block absorption of sodium and chloride in the kidneys at the loop of Henle • Increase urine output • Decrease fluid volume • Decrease preload • Decrease pulmonary venous pressure • Relieve symptoms of fluid congestion
Thiazide Diuretics hydrochlorothiazide metolazone (Zaroxolyn)	• Affect electrolyte reabsorption at the distal renal tubule resulting in sodium and chloride excretion • Increased urine output (milder diuretic effect than loop diuretics) • Decrease blood pressure
Aldosterone Antagonists (Potassium-Sparing Diuretics) eplerenone (Inspra) spironolactone (Aldactone)	• Inhibit aldosterone that causes sodium and water retention and antiinflammatory responses in HF • Prevent potassium loss by inhibiting sodium and potassium exchange in the distal tubule • Mild diuretic effect • Reduce mortality and HF hospitalizations in patients with chronic HF
Morphine morphine (MS Contin, Duramorph, Embeda, Kadian)	• Binds to opioid receptors • May decrease the chemoreceptor response to hypoxia, and/or cause vasodilation reducing pulmonary congestion • Reduces anxiety
Neprilysin-Angiotensin Receptor Inhibitors sacubitril/valsartan (Entresto)	• Sacubitril inhibits neprilysin, decreasing natriuretic degradation which promotes diuresis, natriuresis • Valsartan selectively blocks angiotensin II receptors • Lower blood pressure • Dilate venules and arterioles • Improve renal blood flow • May decrease mortality and hospitalizations in patients with chronic HF

Drug	Mechanism of Action
Positive Inotropes ***β-Adrenergic Agonists**** dobutamine dopamine	• Increase contractility (positive inotropic effect) • Increase CO • May reduce PAWP • May cause dysrhythmias • Increase myocardial O_2 demand
Digitalis Glycoside digoxin	• Weak positive inotrope mostly at higher doses • Reduce effects of RAAS and SNS • May reduce HF symptoms and hospitalization if added to standard therapy for chronic HF
Phosphodiesterase Inhibitor* milrinone	• Produce mild vasodilation • Increase SV and CO • Promote vasodilation
Renin-Angiotensin-Aldosterone System Inhibitors (see Table 32.6) ***ACE Inhibitors*** benazepril (Lotensin) captopril (Capoten) enalapril (Vasotec) ***Angiotensin II Receptor Blockers*** losartan (Cozaar) valsartan (Diovan)	• Dilate venules and arterioles • Reduce afterload and SVR • Improve renal blood flow • May relieve HF symptoms • Promote reverse remodeling • May reduce morbidity, mortality, and HF hospitalizations in patients with chronic HF
Selective SA Node Inhibitor ivabradine (Corlanor)	• Selectively inhibits the I f-current in the SA node • Decreases heart rate • May reduce CVD death and HF hospitalizations in patients with HFrEF in sinus rhythm with a HR ≥70 bpm • Used only for patients with chronic HF
Vasodilators isosorbide dinitrate/ hydralazine (BiDil) neseritide (Natrecor)* nitrates (e.g., nitroglycerin [Nitro-Bid], isosorbide dinitrate [Isordil]) nitroprusside (Nitropress)*	• Reduce afterload • Dilate the arterioles of the kidneys, leading to increased renal perfusion and fluid loss • Decrease BP • Decrease preload • Neseritide may reduce PAWP • May relieve HF symptoms (e.g., dyspnea) • Isosorbide dinitrate/hydralazine, fixed dose, may reduce morbidity and mortality in blacks with HFrEF and NYHA Class III–IV symptoms

*Used for ADHF only.

Diuretics. Diuretics are the first line for treating patients with volume overload. They decrease sodium reabsorption at various sites within the kidneys, enhancing sodium and water loss. Decreasing intravascular volume with diuretics reduces volume returning to the LV (preload). This allows for more efficient LV pumping, decreased pulmonary vascular pressures, and improved alveolar gas exchange. IV administration of loop diuretics (e.g., furosemide) by bolus or infusion is preferred. We evaluate effectiveness by increased urine output, decreased symptoms, and fluid weight loss. Serum potassium and magnesium levels are continually monitored.

Vasodilators. Vasodilators are used to treat ADHF in the absence of hypotension. IV nitroglycerin (NTG) is a primary venodilator that reduces circulating blood volume. It also improves coronary artery blood flow by dilating the coronary arteries. So, NTG reduces preload, slightly reduces afterload (in high doses), and increases myocardial O_2 supply. Tolerance often develops with continued IV use, requiring higher doses. When titrating IV NTG, monitor BP often (every 5 to 10 minutes) to avoid hypotension. Patients on IV vasodilators may have an indwelling arterial line or continuous noninvasive blood pressure monitoring.

Sodium nitroprusside (Nitropress) is a potent IV arterial vasodilator that reduces both preload and afterload, thus improving myocardial contraction, increasing CO, and reducing pulmonary congestion. Complications of therapy include hypotension and, at high doses, thiocyanate (cyanide) toxicity. It is given in an ICU.

DRUG ALERT Sodium Nitroprusside (Nitropress)

- Record baseline BP and continuously monitor during administration.
- Arterial BP monitoring is recommended during drug infusion.
- Too rapid rate of IV infusion can reduce BP too quickly and cause hypotension.
- Headache, dizziness, nausea, agitation, and restlessness can occur.
- Monitor thiocyanate (drug by-product) levels if infusion is greater than 3 mcg/kg/min, as toxicity can occur.

IV nesiritide is a recombinant form of BNP used for short-term treatment of ADHF after a failed response to IV diuretics.[1] As a venous and arterial vasodilator, its main effects include a reduction in PAWP and decrease in dyspnea. Because the primary adverse effect is symptomatic hypotension, BP is carefully monitored.

Morphine. Morphine dilates pulmonary and systemic blood vessels, reducing preload and afterload. It is often given in small IV boluses for the dyspnea associated with ADHF. Cautious use and close monitoring are advised. Morphine has serious adverse effects, including respiratory depression, which can require mechanical ventilation.

Positive Inotropes. Inotropic drugs increase myocardial contractility and are used for patients with evidence of cardiogenic shock or with low CO. Drugs include β-agonists (e.g., dopamine, dobutamine, norepinephrine [Levophed]) and phosphodiesterase inhibitors (milrinone). β-Agonists are used as a short-term treatment of ADHF. In addition to increasing myocardial contractility and SVR, dopamine dilates the renal blood vessels and enhances urine output. Unlike dopamine, dobutamine is a selective β-agonist that works mainly on the β₁-receptors in the heart and does not increase SVR. Effectiveness of inotropes is evaluated by assessing for improved CO, BP, urine output, and reduced filling pressures.

DRUG ALERT Dopamine

- Monitor IV site. Tissue necrosis and sloughing can occur with drug extravasation.
- High doses may produce ventricular dysrhythmias.

Milrinone has both inotropic and vasodilator properties. Milrinone improves myocardial contractility, increases CO, and reduces BP (decreases afterload). Like dopamine and dobutamine, this drug is available only for IV use. Adverse effects include dysrhythmias, thrombocytopenia, and hepatotoxicity.

Digitalis is a weaker positive inotrope that can be added if symptoms persist after other medications have been started. Digoxin can mildly increase contractility but also increases myocardial O_2 consumption. It can optimize heart rate, especially in those with atrial fibrillation. We monitor digoxin levels and make dose adjustments based on renal function. Serum potassium and magnesium levels must be maintained.

Current evidence recommends the use of inotropic therapy only for the short-term management of patients with ADHF who have not responded to conventional drug therapy (e.g., diuretics, vasodilators, morphine).[1] Continuous cardiac monitoring is necessary with all positive inotropic drugs as they can cause life-threatening dysrhythmias.

SAFETY ALERT Infusion Pumps

- To control the rate and assist with titration, use an infusion pump whenever you are giving IV vasodilators and inotropes.
- Ideally, pumps that have drug libraries can help to avoid rates and dosages that are out of the safe range for the drug.

Interprofessional Care: Chronic Heart Failure

The evolution of evidence-based medication and device therapies over the last few decades has dramatically improved the potential for better patient outcomes with chronic HF. The Heart Failure Society of America (HFSA) and the AHA have regularly published and updated guidelines on therapies for HF. Specialized inpatient, transitional, and ambulatory HF units have emerged. These units are staffed with interprofessional HF teams (Table 34.6).

Chronic HF therapies are tailored to the individual patient based on co-morbid conditions. The goals of chronic HF therapies include (1) optimal symptom management, (2) mortality and morbidity benefit, (3) minimizing side effects, and (4) monitoring responses to therapies. Specifically, these therapies treat the underlying cause and contributing factors, maximize CO, improve ventricular function, improve quality of life (QOL), and preserve target organ function.

In a person with HF, the blood may not be adequately oxygenated, resulting in reduced O_2 saturation. The use of supplemental O_2 improves saturation and helps meet tissue O_2 needs. This helps to relieve patient dyspnea and fatigue. Ongoing pulse oximetry monitors the need for and effectiveness of O_2 therapy.

Physical and emotional rest allows the patient to conserve energy and decreases the need for more O_2. The degree of rest recommended depends on the severity of HF. A patient with severe HF may be on bed rest. A patient with mild to moderate HF can be ambulatory with restricted activity. Urge the patient to take part in prescribed activities, allowing for adequate recovery periods. A structured exercise program, such as cardiac rehabilitation, should be considered for all patients with chronic HF. These programs are associated with decreased hospitalizations, reduced mortality, improved QOL, and less depression.[1,14]

Drug Therapy. The cornerstone of drug therapy in chronic HF is neurohormonal blockade. The result of neurohormonal blockade is decreased plasma aldosterone levels, decreased SNS activity, vasodilation, and sodium and water excretion. Each class of evidence-based medications has been shown to decrease mortality and morbidity in patients with chronic HFrEF. Recommendations for HFpEF primarily address symptoms and co-morbid conditions. Drug therapy for chronic HF is outlined in Table 34.7.

Evidenced-Based Medications for HFrEF

ACE inhibitors. ACE inhibitors are first-line drugs for chronic HFrEF. They decrease mortality, morbidity, hospitalizations, and symptoms in patients with HFrEF.[1] ACE inhibitors block the RAAS by inhibiting the conversion of angiotensin I to angiotensin II. They reduce afterload and SVR and inhibit the development of ventricular remodeling by inhibiting ventricular hypertrophy.

Major side effects include symptomatic hypotension, intractable cough, hyperkalemia, angioedema (allergic reaction involving edema of the face and airways), and renal insufficiency (when used in high doses). Aging and renal insufficiency slow the metabolism of ACE inhibitors and may lead to increased serum drug levels. We monitor renal function and serum potassium levels. Examples of ACE inhibitors are listed in Table 34.7. More information about ACE inhibitors is found in Chapter 32.

 DRUG ALERT Captopril

- Severe hypotension and hyperkalemia may occur.
- Monitor patient for first-dose hypotension (first-dose syncope).
- Skipping doses or discontinuing the drug can result in rebound HTN.
- Angioedema, a rare adverse effect, can develop suddenly and be life-threatening.

Angiotensin II receptor blockers. For patients who are unable to tolerate ACE inhibitors, angiotensin II receptor blockers (ARBs) (see Table 32.6) are recommended.[1] They prevent the vasoconstrictor and aldosterone-secreting effects of angiotensin II by binding to the angiotensin II receptor sites. ARBs promote afterload reduction and vasodilation. The side effects are similar to those of ACE inhibitors except that ARBs do not typically cause a cough. Angioedema is less common. Monitoring is similar to that for ACE inhibitors.

Neprilysin-angiotensin receptor inhibitors. Sacubitril/valsartan (Entresto) is a combination of a neprilysin inhibitor (sacubitril) and an ARB (valsartan). This drug provides dual blockade of the RAAS and the natriuretic peptide system. Sacubitril, a recombinant form of BNP, inhibits neprilysin, an enzyme that degrades natriuretic peptides. Sacubitril inhibition allows for more available circulating BNP. This results in decreased SVR, afterload, and CVP and increased natriuresis and diuresis. This drug is an alternative to ACE inhibitors and ARBs in patients meeting criteria with symptomatic HFrEF and reduces death and hospitalization. Patients are monitored for hypotension, renal insufficiency, and angioedema.[15]

Aldosterone antagonists. Spironolactone (Aldactone) and eplerenone (Inspra) are potassium-sparing diuretics that inhibit aldosterone activation. These drugs work by binding to receptors at the aldosterone-dependent sodium-potassium exchange site in the distal renal tubule, where they have a mild diuretic effect.

They may prolong survival in patients with HFrEF.[1] It is critical to carefully monitor serum potassium levels and renal function in patients taking aldosterone antagonists.

 DRUG ALERT Spironolactone (Aldactone)

- Monitor potassium levels during treatment.
- Use with caution in patients taking digoxin, since hyperkalemia may reduce the effects of digoxin.
- Teach patient to avoid foods high in potassium (e.g., bananas, oranges).
- Assess male patients for gynecomastia, a common side effect of long-term use of spironolactone.

β-adrenergic blockers. β-Blockers directly block the negative effects of the SNS (e.g., increased HR) on the failing heart. Three β-blockers decrease mortality in patients with HFrEF: metoprolol succinate (Toprol XL), bisoprolol (Zebeta), and carvedilol (Coreg). These β-blockers may also increase LVEF. The improvement in LVEF is dose-related, so the highest tolerated dose should be given.[1] However, because β-blockers can reduce myocardial contractility, care must be taken in patients with volume overload. They are usually started at low dose, then the dosage is increased every 2 weeks as tolerated. Major side effects include worsening of HF symptoms, hypotension, fatigue, and bradycardia.

 DRUG ALERT Carvedilol (Coreg)

- Obtain standing BP 1 hr after dosing to assess tolerance.
- Overdose can cause profound bradycardia, hypotension, bronchospasm, and cardiogenic shock.
- Abrupt withdrawal may result in sweating, palpitations, and headaches.

Ivabradine (Corlanor). Ivabradine selectively inhibits a particular sodium/potassium current in the SA node, resulting in a decreased HR. It can decrease hospitalizations in patients with HFrEF who are in sinus rhythm with an HR greater than 70 bpm and have symptoms despite optimal doses of other medications. Monitor patients for bradycardia and lightheadedness.[15]

Hydralazine/isosorbide dinitrate combination (Bidil). This drug is a fixed combination of the vasodilator hydralazine and isosorbide dinitrate. It can significantly reduce mortality and improve LVEF and exercise tolerance by reducing afterload through blood vessel vasodilation. The drug is specifically effective in blacks with HFrEF already receiving optimal doses of other evidence-based medications.[1] Although non-black patients do not see the same benefit, it may be used in any patient with HFrEF already on evidence-based medication. Major side effects include hypotension and headache. Like other nitrates, it should not be used with phosphodiesterase inhibitors, such as sildenafil (Viagra).

Digitalis. Digitalis (digoxin), a weak positive inotrope, acts primarily as a neurohormonal modulator that reduces the effects of the SNS and suppresses renin secretion from the kidneys. Low-dose digitalis decreases HF hospitalizations and symptoms in patients who are still symptomatic despite standard HF therapies.[1,12] No mortality benefit has been found. Better outcomes occur with digoxin serum levels of <0.9 ng/ml. Higher serum doses are associated with increased mortality rate and digoxin toxicity. Dose should be based on body mass, renal function, and concomitant medications. The usual maintenance dose in HF is 0.125 mg daily. Monitor renal function and serum potassium levels of all patients taking digitalis. Concerns about digoxin toxicity are abated by the subtherapeutic dosing in HF.

Medications for Symptom Management

Diuretics. Diuretics reduce symptoms of fluid overload and congestion in both HFrEF and HFpEF. Diuretics reduce edema, pulmonary venous pressure, and preload (see Table 32.7). These drugs act on the kidney by promoting excretion of sodium and water. Loop diuretics (e.g., furosemide (Lasix) and bumetanide [Bumex]) act on the ascending loop of Henle to promote sodium, chloride, and water excretion. Problems in using loop diuretics include low serum potassium levels, ototoxicity, and possible allergic reaction in patients sensitive to sulfa-type drugs. Thiazide diuretics inhibit sodium reabsorption in the distal tubule, promoting excretion of sodium and water. They also can severely lower potassium levels.

In chronic HF, the lowest effective dose of diuretic should be used. Side effects of diuretics include dehydration, hypotension, orthostasis, renal dysfunction, and electrolyte abnormalities. Diuretic resistance can occur in HF patients, necessitating dosing augmentation and the addition of different diuretic classes.

Device Therapy. Patients with HFrEF may benefit from implantable cardiac devices. HF patients must be on appropriate therapies before becoming a candidate for device therapy. Patients with an LVEF < 35% are at significant risk for SCD. An ICD is recommended for primary prevention of SCD in these patients.[1] In patients with a LVEF <35%, neurohormonal effects and cardiac remodeling can result in dyssynchronous contraction of the LV and RV, contributing to poor ventricular filling and reduced CO. CRT is recommended for these patients.[1] With CRT, an extra pacing lead is placed through the coronary sinus to a coronary vein of the LV. This lead coordinates right and left ventricular contractions (Fig. 34.4). Patients with symptomatic HFrEF often need both CRT and an ICD. Combination implantable devices are available. (Pacemakers and defibrillators are discussed in Chapter 35.) Mechanical assist devices available to sustain HF patients with deteriorating function and those awaiting cardiac transplant will be discussed later in the chapter.

> **❓ CHECK YOUR PRACTICE**
>
> Your patient is scheduled for a biventricular pacemaker for her worsening HF. She currently has a demand pacemaker and asks you why she needs this new one.
> - How would you respond to her question?

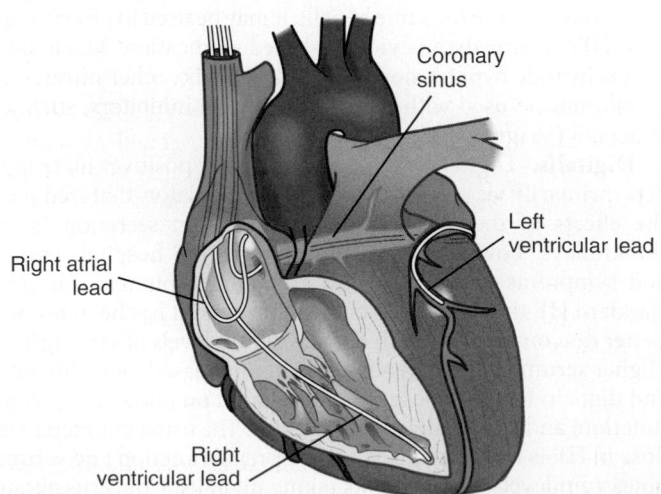

FIG. 34.4 Placement of pacing leads in cardiac resynchronization therapy.

Labels: Coronary sinus; Left ventricular lead; Right atrial lead; Right ventricular lead

Remote Monitoring of Physiologic Data

Implanted ICD and CRT devices can be used for remotely monitoring HF patients. Physiologic parameters of worsening HF known to change prior to symptom emergence can predict HF decompensation and help with clinical decision making. Information from these devices can be retrieved electronically via secure websites. Examples of parameters we can remotely follow are BP, weight, HR trends (can evaluate adequacy of beta blockade, increasing HR can indicate worsening HF), HR variability (HRV, a reduction is associated with higher risk for exacerbation and hospitalization), patient activity level, dysrhythmias, and intrathoracic impedance (an indicator of intrathoracic fluid level providing early detection of impending ADHF).[16] Implantable hemodynamic monitoring is also possible. A pulmonary artery sensor can be implanted in the pulmonary artery during a right heart catheterization. It can provide information about HR, systolic, diastolic, and mean pulmonary artery pressure. Detection of early hemodynamic and fluid status changes can allow for proactive management to reduce fluid overload, which decreases hospitalizations in patients with HFrEF.[17]

Nutritional Therapy

Poor adherence to a low-sodium diet and failure to take prescribed medications as directed are the most common reasons for readmissions of HF patients to the hospital. It is critical that you accurately assess a patient's diet and teach both the patient and caregiver about the importance of diet.

Take a detailed diet history. Determine not only what foods the patient eats, but also when, where, and how often the patient dines out. Assess the cultural value of food. Use this information to help the patient in making appropriate dietary choices when developing an individualized and culturally sensitive diet plan. The AHA website has helpful dietary guidelines for HF patients.

HF guidelines vary with regard to sodium restriction in HF management. There is agreement that excess sodium may worsen HF symptoms and facilitate an exacerbation. A low sodium intake may lead to higher adverse event rates in later stages of HFrEF. The degree of sodium restriction depends on the severity of the HF and the effectiveness of diuretic therapy. Generally, sodium intake is restricted to 2 grams per day (Table 34.8). Teach the patient what foods are low and high in sodium content and how to read labels. Review how to find sodium content per serving and the number of servings per package (Fig. 34.5). Teach ways to enhance food flavors without the use of salt (e.g., substituting lemon juice, various spices). Discuss the high sodium content of most restaurant foods.

Fluid restrictions are not often prescribed for the patient with mild to moderate HF. However, fluid restrictions may be needed for stage D HF patients with persistent fluid retention despite appropriate sodium restriction.

To monitor fluid status, tell patients to weigh themselves at the same time each day. To ensure valid trending, this should be before breakfast, using the same scale, and wearing the same type of clothing. For patients with visual limitations, suggest scales with larger numbers or an audible response. Tell patients to call the HCP about a weight gain of 3 lb (1.4 kg) over 2 days or a 3- to 5-lb (2.3-kg) gain over a week.[12]

❖ NURSING MANAGEMENT: HEART FAILURE

◆ Nursing Assessment

Subjective and objective data that you should obtain from a patient with HF are shown in Table 34.9. Carefully review the

TABLE 34.8 Nutritional Therapy

Low-Sodium Diets

General Principles

- Do not add salt or seasonings containing sodium when preparing foods.*
- Do not use salt at the table.*
- 1 tsp of salt equals 2.3 g of sodium.
- Avoid high-sodium foods (e.g., canned soups, processed meats, cheese, frozen meals).
- Limit milk products to 2 cups daily.

Sample Menu Plans for 2400-mg Sodium Diet

Breakfast	Sodium (mg)
⅔ cup bran cereal	161
(⅔ cup Shredded Wheat cereal)†	3
1 slice whole-wheat bread	149
1 medium banana	1
6 oz fruit yogurt, fat free	85
1 cup fat-free milk	126
2 Tbsp jelly	5
Coffee, 8 oz	5

Lunch	
Chicken breast sandwich	
2 slices (3 oz) chicken breast, skinless	65
2 slices whole wheat bread	299
1 slice (¾ oz) American cheese	328
(1 slice [¾ oz] Swiss cheese, natural)†	54
Large-leaf romaine lettuce	1
2 slices tomato	90
1 Tbsp mayonnaise, low fat	90
1 medium peach	7

Dinner	
¾ cup vegetarian spaghetti sauce	459
(6 oz no-salt-added tomato paste)†	260
1 cup spaghetti	1
3 Tbsp parmesan cheese	349
Spinach salad	
1 cup fresh spinach leaves	24
¼ cup fresh carrots (grated)	10
¼ cup fresh mushrooms (sliced)	1
2 Tbsp vinaigrette dressing	0
½ cup canned pears, juice pack	4
½ cup corn, cooked from frozen	4

Snack	
⅓ cup almonds	4
¼ cup dried apricots	3
6 oz fruit yogurt, fat free	85

*1 tsp of salt equals 2.3 g of sodium.
†Substitutes to reduce to 1500-mg sodium diet.

TABLE 34.9 Nursing Assessment

Heart Failure

Subjective Data

Important Health Information

Past health history: CAD (including recent MI), HTN, cardiomyopathy, valvular or congenital heart disease, diabetes, hyperlipidemia, renal disease, thyroid or lung disease, rapid or irregular heart rate
Medications: Use of and adherence with any heart drugs. Use of diuretics, estrogens, corticosteroids, NSAIDs, OTC drugs, herbal supplements

Functional Health Patterns

Health perception–health management: Fatigue, depression, anxiety
Nutritional-metabolic: Usual sodium intake. Nausea, vomiting, anorexia, stomach bloating. Weight gain, ankle swelling
Elimination: Nocturia, decreased daytime urine output, constipation
Activity-exercise: Dyspnea, orthopnea, cough (e.g., dry, productive). Palpitations, dizziness, fainting
Sleep-rest: Number of pillows used for sleeping. Paroxysmal nocturnal dyspnea, insomnia, sleep apnea
Cognitive-perceptual: Chest pain or heaviness. RUQ pain, abdominal discomfort. Behavioral changes, visual changes

Objective Data

Integumentary

Cool, diaphoretic skin. Cyanosis or pallor. Peripheral edema (right-sided HF)

Respiratory

Tachypnea, crackles, wheezes. Frothy, blood-tinged sputum

Cardiovascular

Tachycardia, S_3, S_4, murmurs. Pulsus alternans. PMI displaced inferiorly and posteriorly, lifts and heaves, jugular venous distention

Gastrointestinal

Abdominal distention, hepatosplenomegaly, ascites

Neurologic

Restlessness, confusion, decreased attention or memory

Possible Diagnostic Findings

Altered serum electrolytes (especially Na^+ and K^+), ↑ BUN, creatinine, or liver function tests. ↑ NT-proBNP or BNP. Chest x-ray showing cardiomegaly, pulmonary congestion, and interstitial pulmonary edema. Echocardiogram showing increased chamber size, decreased wall motion, decreased LVEF or normal LVEF with evidence of diastolic dysfunction (abnormal relaxation/filling). Atrial and ventricular enlargement on ECG. ↓ O_2 saturation

problems as they may exacerbate HF, affecting the plan of care and the timing and choice of therapies. For example, a patient with sleep apnea may not use a continuous positive airway pressure device at night. This can worsen pulmonary or systemic HTN and lead to an exacerbation of HF.

◆ **Nursing Diagnoses**

Nursing diagnoses for the patient with HF include:

- Impaired gas exchange
- Impaired cardiac output
- Fluid imbalance
- Activity intolerance

Additional information on nursing diagnoses and interventions for the patient with HF is presented in eNursing Care Plan 34.1 on the website for this chapter.

patient's current prescription and over-the-counter (OTC) drugs. Chronic HF patients often take multiple other medications for co-existing conditions and underlying CVD. OTC medications known to pose significant risk to people with HF include nonsteroidal antiinflammatory drugs (NSAIDs), higher-than-prescribed aspirin doses, ephedrine, pseudoephedrine, and diet pills. NSAIDs can contribute to sodium retention and an exacerbation of HF.

Review the patient's dietary habits to identify issues related to an exacerbation of HF. Explore the patient's chronic health

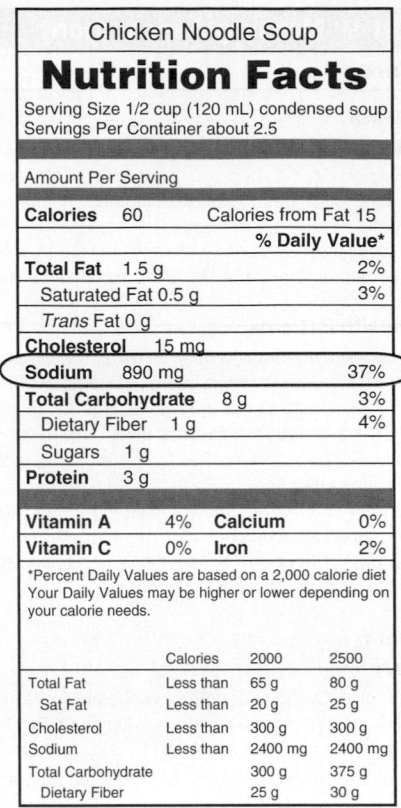

FIG. 34.5 Typical nutrition label. Note that a single serving (½ cup) provides more than one third of the daily recommended intake of sodium.

Planning

Nursing care focuses on the priority problems of decreased CO, impaired oxygenation, fluid overload, intolerance of physical activity and managing a complex medication regimen. The overall goals for the patient with HF include (1) decrease in symptoms (e.g., shortness of breath, fatigue); (2) decrease in peripheral edema; (3) increase in exercise tolerance; (4) adherence with the treatment plan, including appropriate evidence-based medication and device therapies; and (5) no complications related to HF.

Nursing Implementation

Health Promotion. Communication and joint decision making among the patient, caregiver, and interprofessional team are integral to high-quality, patient-centered care. Currently, the emphasis is on aggressively identifying and treating risk factors in the patient with stage A HF to prevent or slow the progression to symptomatic HF.[18] By identifying patients with obesity, metabolic syndrome, diabetes, HTN, and hyperlipidemia as already having stage A HF, goals related to a heart-healthy lifestyle can be given deserved urgency. Recommended lifestyle modifications begin with weight management, diet, and regular exercise. Often, medications are needed. Encourage patients to get influenza and pneumococcal vaccinations. Patients with valvular disease that may be contributing to HF should be evaluated for valve repair or replacement procedures. Coronary revascularization procedures should be considered in patients with CAD. Antidysrhythmic drugs or pacing therapy may be indicated for patients with serious dysrhythmias or conduction disturbances.

Acute Care. Many persons with HF have 1 or more episodes of ADHF. Common precipitating factors to HF hospitalization include respiratory infections, dysrhythmias, acute coronary syndrome, uncontrolled HTN, and nonadherence to medications and/or diet. Patients with ADHF are usually admitted through the ED, stabilized, then cared for in an ICU, intermediate care unit, or specialized HF unit with continuous ECG monitoring capability.

Successful HF care depends on several important principles: (1) HF is a progressive disease; (2) treatment plans are established with QOL goals; (3) symptom management depends to a significant degree on adherence to self-management protocols (e.g., daily weights, diet, exercise, recognizing signs and symptoms of decompensation); and drug and device therapies; (4) precipitating factors, etiologies, and contributing comorbid conditions must be addressed; (5) complex care needs often require care in multiple settings, increasing risk for fragmented care; and (6) support systems are essential to the success of the entire treatment plan.

Ambulatory Care. Transitional care programs and protocols are designed to ensure coordination and continuity of health care as patients transfer between care settings. Programs that include comprehensive discharge planning, collaboration among providers, and planned, prompt follow-up with HCPs have shown reduced readmission rates.[19]

Goals of ambulatory HF care include symptom management, QOL maintenance, morbidity and mortality benefit from therapy, identifying and mitigating factors precipitating ADHF and hospitalization, and closely monitoring responses to and potential side effects of therapies. HF is a chronic and progressive condition that will require lifelong therapies. It is important to include the patient and caregiver(s) in the overall care plan. Help them develop a clear action plan for response to increased signs and symptoms of impending exacerbation. A patient and caregiver guide for the patient with HF is shown in Table 34.10.

Effective home health (HH) care can prevent future hospitalizations by providing ongoing assessments (e.g., monitoring vital signs and weight, evaluating response to therapies) and followup.[19] HH nurses often use individualized care protocols coordinated with the patient and HCP. The protocols allow the nurse and patient to identify signs and symptoms of worsening HF (e.g., weight gain, increased dyspnea). Many agencies offer specialized HF programs. Telehealth and device remote monitoring technology (e.g., electronic scale, BP cuff, pulse oximeter) can collect physiologic and symptom data (Fig. 34.6).[15,16] Results can be sent to the HCP via telephone or secure website. In response to collected data, therapeutic interventions, such as a temporary increase in diuretic therapy, can be implemented to improve functional capacity and prevent rehospitalization.

Teach the patient the basic mechanism of action of medications and signs of drug toxicity in easily understood terms. Effective self-care includes proper technique in taking a pulse (for a full minute) and use of home BP monitor and device remote monitoring equipment. The patient should understand specific HCP instructions on when to hold heart rate–lowering medications, such as β-blockers and digoxin. If patients are taking diuretic and/or potassium supplement medications, teach them the signs and symptoms of hypokalemia and hyperkalemia, including weakness, fatigue, constipation, and muscle cramping.

Exercise training (e.g., CR) can improve symptoms of chronic HF. Exercise for patients with HF has been found to be safe and to improve overall sense of well-being. It has been associated

---

TABLE 34.10 Patient & Caregiver Teaching

Heart Failure

Include the following instructions when teaching the patient and caregiver about the management of heart failure:

Dietary Therapy

- Consult the diet plan and list of permitted and restricted foods.
- Adhere to specific sodium restriction guidelines outlined by your HCP.
- Examine labels to determine sodium content. Also examine the labels of over-the-counter drugs, such as laxatives, cough medicines, and antacids for sodium content.
- Avoid using salt when preparing foods or adding salt to foods.
- Weigh yourself at the same time each day, preferably in the morning, using the same scale and wearing similar clothes.
- Eat small, frequent meals.

Activity Program

- Increase walking and other activities gradually, provided they do not cause fatigue or dyspnea.
- Consider a cardiac rehabilitation program.
- Avoid extremes of heat and cold.

Ongoing Monitoring

- Know the signs and symptoms of worsening HF, including increasing dyspnea, cough, orthopnea, PND, weight gain, edema, fluid retention, fatigue, and tiredness with physical activity.
- Recall the symptoms when illness began. Reappearance of previous symptoms may indicate a recurrence.
- Report at once any of the following to the HCP:
  - Weight gain of 3 lb (1.4 kg) in 2 days, or 3–5 lb (2.3 kg) in a week
  - Difficulty breathing, especially with activity or when lying flat
  - Waking up breathless at night
  - Frequent dry, hacking cough, especially when lying down
  - Fatigue, weakness
  - Swelling of ankles, feet, or abdomen. Swelling of face or difficulty breathing (if taking ACE inhibitors)
  - Nausea with abdominal swelling, pain, and tenderness
  - Dizziness or fainting

- Follow up with HCP on regular basis.
- Consider joining a local support group with your family members and/or caregiver(s).

Health Promotion

- Obtain annual influenza vaccination.
- Obtain pneumococcal vaccine (see Table 27.5 for guidelines on pneumococcal vaccination).
- Develop plan to reduce risk factors (e.g., BP control, tobacco cessation, blood glucose/Hb A1C control, weight reduction).

Rest

- Plan a regular daily rest and activity program.
- After exertion, such as exercise and ADLs, plan a rest period.
- Consider shorter working hours or schedule rest period during working hours.
- Avoid emotional upsets. Share any concerns, fears, feelings of depression, etc. with HCP.

Drug Therapy

- Take each drug as prescribed.
- Develop a system (e.g., daily chart, weekly pillbox) to ensure drugs are taken.
- Count pulse rate each day before taking drugs (if appropriate). Know the limits that your HCP wants for your pulse rate.
- Take BP at determined intervals (if appropriate). Know your target BP limits.
- Know signs and symptoms of orthostatic hypotension and how to prevent them (see Table 32.12).
- If taking anticoagulants, know signs and symptoms of internal bleeding (bleeding gums, increased bruises, blood in stool or urine) and what to do.
- Know your INR and target range if taking warfarin (Coumadin) and how often to have blood checked.

ACE, Angiotensin-converting enzyme; *INR,* international normalized ratio.

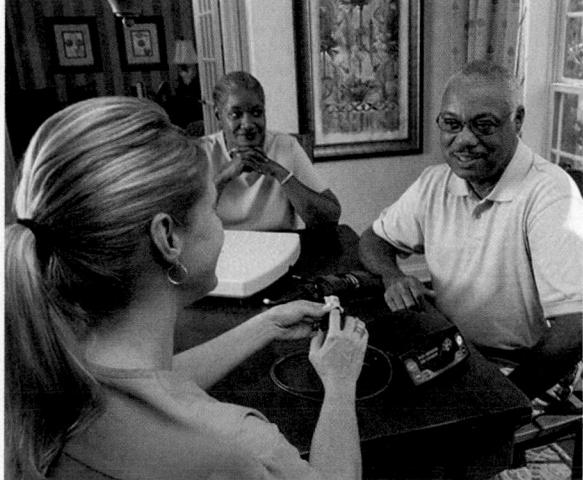

FIG. 34.6 Home-based telehealth monitoring unit. (Used with permission from Honeywell HomMed.)

with reduced mortality.[1,14] Tailor exercise programs based on what the patient most enjoys doing. Teach the patient about the importance of rest periods, especially after exertion, and energy-conserving behaviors. Changes may be needed if environmental conditions involve an increased cardiac workload

(e.g., frequent climbing of stairs). Consultation with a physical therapist or occupational therapist may be appropriate.

Mechanical Circulatory Support Devices in End-Stage Heart Failure. Therapeutic options for stage D HF patients include: (1) chronic inotropic therapy, (2) mechanical circulatory support (MCS) devices, (3) palliative care and hospice that may or may not include ICD deactivation, and (4) heart transplant. MCS devices can be beneficial to carefully selected patients for short-term management, long-term and bridge-to-transplant management, or as destination therapy.[12] Patients who are ineligible for heart transplant may be candidates for lifelong MCS. Short-term MCS include IABP, extracorporeal membrane oxygenation (ECMO), and various continual flow pumps. The limitations of bed rest and the risk for infection and vascular complications prevent long-term use of these devices.

Long-term MCS devices include LV assist devices (VADs), including percutaneous devices (PVAD) and transplanted devices (LAVDs, BiVADs) (see Chapter 65). VADs provide highly effective long-term support and have become standard care in many heart transplant centers. The heart pump runs via a driveline that exits the abdominal wall and attaches to a system controller with patient specific settings. VADs operate on AC current or batteries (Fig. 34.7). Morbidity and mortality is significantly reduced if MCS is started before onset of severe right HF and systemic organ failure.[12]

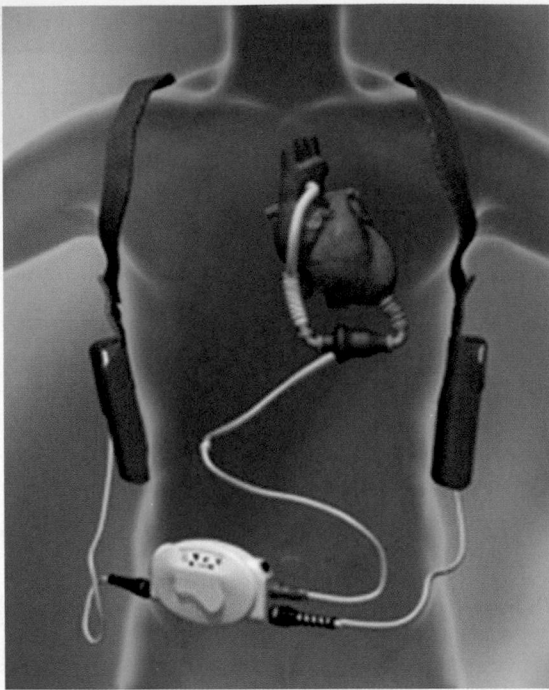

FIG. 34.7 Left ventricular assist device. (Reprinted with the permission of Thoratec Corp.)

TABLE 34.11 Common Indications and Contraindications for Heart Transplantation
Indications
• End-stage HF refractory to medical care
• Severe, decompensated, inoperable, valvular heart disease
• Recurrent life-threatening dysrhythmias not responsive to maximal interventions, including defibrillators
• Any other heart abnormalities that severely limit normal function and/or have a mortality risk of more than 50% within 2 years
Absolute Contraindications
• Chronologic age over 70 years or physiologic age over 65 years
• Life-threatening illness (e.g., cancer) that will limit survival to <5 years despite therapy
• Advanced cerebral or peripheral vascular disease not amenable to correction
• Active infection, including HIV infection
• Severe pulmonary disease that will likely result in the patient being ventilator-dependent after transplant
Relative Contraindications
• Severe obesity
• Psychologic impairment
• Active substance use (e.g., alcohol, drugs, tobacco)
• Uncontrolled diabetes with vascular and neurologic complications
• Irreversible liver or kidney dysfunction not explained by HF
• Evidence of noncompliance with accepted medical practices
• Lack of social support network that can make long-term commitment for patient's welfare
• Unrealistic expectations by the patient or caregiver about transplant, its risks, and its benefits

◆ **Palliative and End-of-Life Care.** HF mortality rates are still high. One in 5 persons with HF die within a year of diagnosis. The estimated 5-year survival rate is worse than for most types of cancer. Repeated hospitalizations and ED visits for ADHF can be predictive of end-stage HF.[1,15,19]

The ACCF and AHA provide guidelines for patients with end-stage HF (stage D).[1] End-of-life discussions and management are emphasized, including advanced directives and information about advanced HF therapies (e.g., VADs, heart transplants), palliative care, and hospice.

Palliative care may be appropriate earlier in the course of the illness in conjunction with other therapies intended to prolong life. Palliative nursing care of the HF patient emphasizes (1) unifying the patient, family, and health care team in formulating a plan of care; (2) aggressive symptom management; (3) avoiding therapies that are no longer appropriate or effective and may prolong suffering; (4) integrating emotional and spiritual support for patient and family; and (5) determining when a patient may be ready to consider hospice care.

Patients with advanced CVD are eligible for hospice when (1) an HCP certifies that a life expectancy of 6 months or less is expected assuming the disease takes its normal course, (2) the patient has received optimal medical treatment and is not a candidate for further invasive procedures, and (3) the patient is assessed at NYHA Class IV. End-stage HF patients who meet hospice criteria are often referred late or not at all. Challenges in referring these patients to hospice include (1) difficulties with accurate life expectancy prediction, (2) reluctance to accept a DNR order due to multiple resuscitation survivals and implantable devices, and (3) a lack of patient and family understanding as to the chronic and terminal nature of HF.[20,21]

End-of-life nursing care of HF patients includes ongoing assessment and evaluation of interventions for effectiveness. Strategies include patient and caregiver support, drug therapies, and nondrug therapies. Palliative and end-of-life care are discussed in Chapter 9.

◆ **Evaluation**

The expected outcomes are that the patient with HF will
• Maintain adequate O_2/CO_2 exchange at the alveolar-capillary membrane to meet O_2 needs of the body
• Maintain adequate blood pumped by the heart to meet metabolic demands of the body
• Reduction or absence of edema and stable baseline weight
• Achieve a realistic program of activity that balances physical activity with energy-conserving activities

HEART TRANSPLANTATION

Heart transplantation is the transfer of a healthy donor heart to a patient with a diseased heart. It is done to treat a variety of terminal or end-stage heart conditions (Table 34.11). In the United States, about 3000 patients are awaiting heart transplants. However, an average of only 2000 hearts become available. The 1-year transplant survival rate is 85% to 90%, while the 3-year survival rate is about 75%.[22,23] A heart transplant is a gold standard therapy for some patients in end-stage HF.

Criteria for Selection

A careful selection process ensures that hearts are distributed fairly and to those who will benefit most from the donor heart. The United Network for Organ Sharing (UNOS) oversees a system to allocate donor organs. UNOS and transplantation are discussed in Chapter 13.

Indications and contraindications for a heart transplant are outlined in Table 34.11. Once a person meets the criteria for a transplant, an exhaustive physical examination and diagnostic workup are done. Heart function, vascular and immune systems are assessed. The patient and caregiver undergo a comprehensive psychologic evaluation that assesses coping skills, support systems, and commitment to follow a rigorous life-long regimen. The complexity of the transplant process may be overwhelming to a patient without an adequate support system and understanding of the needed lifestyle changes.

Donor and recipient matching is based on body and heart size and an immunologic assessment. That assessment includes ABO blood type, antibody screen, panel of reactive antibody (PRA) level, and human leukocyte antigen typing.

ETHICAL/LEGAL DILEMMAS
Competence

Situation

M.T., a 60-yr-old man, has been awaiting heart transplantation for 6 months. He has been in the ICU for 1 month since he needed a VAD for his failing heart. He recently had a stroke, which is a complication of the device. It left him paralyzed on his right side. He is only able to answer yes/no questions by shaking his head. He has needed mechanical ventilation since his stroke. For the past 2 weeks, he has needed hemodialysis because of renal failure. Recently, when you suction him, he turns his head away from you and bites down on the endotracheal tube. Although he does not have an advance directive, his wife and daughter tell you that, on many occasions before these events, he expressed that he would not want to live if he lost his independence. His wife and daughter request to have the mechanical ventilator withdrawn.

Ethical/Legal Points for Consideration

- Decisional capacity for informed consent related to treatment decisions involves 4 elements: (1) information provided about possible treatment options must be understood by patients, (2) patients must have the capacity to deliberate about the treatment choices and their consequences, (3) patients' treatment decisions must be freely chosen and made without coercion, and (4) patients must be able to communicate their decisions.
- Legal competence, as determined by the courts, has a low threshold. The ability to respond to questions by signaling a yes or no may be enough to prove understanding of the questions, ability to discriminate between choices, and ability to communicate choices, providing that the answers make sense and are appropriate. Review how your state defines legal competence.
- Next of kin are the legal decision makers in the absence of advance directives if the patient is unable to make decisions for himself. Decisional capacity should be tested without assuming it is absent.
- Some courts have accepted past assertions of preferences, past behavior, and assertions of their parties as evidence to support end-of-life preferences in the absence of advance directives.
- Know your agency's policies and the local jurisdiction's laws and regulations about informed consent and end-of-life decision making.

Discussion Questions

1. What would you do next given M.T.'s behavior and the information you obtained from his wife?
2. What are your feelings and concerns about caring for a patient for whom withdrawal of treatment will result in death?

A person accepted as a transplant candidate is placed on a transplant list. This may happen quickly during an acute illness or after a longer period. Stable patients may wait at home and receive ongoing medical care. If unstable, a patient may be hospitalized for more intensive therapy. Unfortunately, the overall waiting period for a new heart is long. Many patients die while waiting for a transplant.

Surgical Procedure

The transplant donor is someone who has irreversible brain injury. A surgical team goes to the hospital of the donor to remove donated organs after the declaration of brain death. The retrieved organs are transported on ice until they can be implanted. For the heart, this is optimally less than 4 hours. Often the donor heart is flown to the recipient's hospital. The donor heart is then implanted into the recipient using 1 of 2 approaches. In the biatrial approach, the recipient's damaged heart is removed at the midatrial level and the donor heart connected at the LA, pulmonary artery, aorta, and RA. In the bicaval approach, the RA of the recipient's heart (with the SA node and atrial conduction intact) is preserved and then the donor heart is connected. Cardiopulmonary bypass is needed during the surgical procedure to maintain oxygenation and perfusion to vital organs.

Posttransplantation

After cardiac transplant, a variety of complications can occur, including a risk for SCD. Acute rejection is an immediate posttransplant complication, and immunosuppressive therapy is the key in posttransplant management. In the first year after transplantation, the major causes of death are infection and acute rejection.

Most immunosuppressive regimens include corticosteroids, calcineurin inhibitors (tacrolimus), and antiproliferative drugs (mycophenolate mofetil). The mechanisms of action and side effects of these and other immunosuppressants are discussed in Chapter 13 and Table 13.17. Because of the use of immunosuppressive therapy, infection is a primary concern after transplant surgery. On a long-term basis, immunosuppressive therapy increases the risk for cancers, especially lymphomas, and cardiac vasculopathy (accelerated CAD).[23]

To detect rejection, an endomyocardial biopsy is done on a weekly basis for the first month, monthly for the next 6 months, and yearly thereafter. In this procedure, the HCP inserts a catheter into the jugular vein and moves it into the RV. The catheter uses a bioptome, a device with 2 small cups that can be closed, to remove small samples of heart muscle for analysis.[23]

Nursing management throughout the posttransplant period focuses on promoting patient adaptation to the transplant process, monitoring heart function, managing lifestyle changes, and providing ongoing teaching of the patient and caregiver.

CASE STUDY
Heart Failure

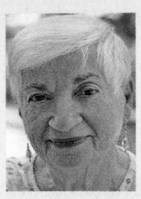

(© iStockphoto/Thinkstock.)

Patient Profile

J.E. is a 70-yr-old Hispanic woman who was admitted to the intermediate care unit with a report of increasing shortness of breath, fatigue, and weight gain.

Subjective Data

- History of HTN for 20 yrs
- History of MI at 58 yrs of age
- Has increasing shortness of breath, fatigue, and an unexplained 11-lb weight gain during the past 2 wks
- Had a respiratory tract infection 2 wks ago; has persistent cough and edema in legs
- Cannot climb a flight of stairs without getting short of breath
- Sleeps with head elevated on 3 pillows
- Lives alone, does not always remember to take medication

Objective Data

Physical Examination

- Moderate respiratory distress, use of accessory muscles, respiratory rate 36 breaths/min
- Systolic heart murmur
- Bilateral crackles in all lung fields
- Cyanotic lips and extremities
- Skin cool and diaphoretic

Diagnostic Studies

- Chest x-ray results: cardiomegaly with right and left ventricular hypertrophy; fluid in lower lung fields
- Echocardiogram results: ejection fraction 20%

Interprofessional Care

- Furosemide (Lasix) 40 mg IV twice daily
- Potassium 40 mEq PO twice daily
- Enalapril (Vasotec) 5 mg/day PO
- Nesiritide (Natrecor) 2 mcg/kg IV bolus followed by a continuous infusion of 0.01 mcg/kg/min
- Continuous ECG monitoring
- Diet: 2-gram sodium diet
- Titrate O_2 to keep O_2 saturation >93%
- Monitor intake and output, and daily weights
- Serum electrolytes; cardiac biomarkers q8hr × 3

Discussion Questions

1. Explain the pathophysiology of J.E.'s heart disease and symptoms.
2. What clinical manifestations of ADHF did J.E. exhibit?
3. What is the significance of the findings of the diagnostic studies?
4. How would a serum NT-proBNP be beneficial in the diagnosis of ADHF?
5. Provide the rationale for each of the HCP's orders prescribed for J.E.
6. **Priority Decision:** Based on the assessment data presented, what are the priority nursing diagnoses? Identify any collaborative problems.
7. **Priority Decision:** What are your priority nursing interventions for J.E.?
8. **Collaboration:** Which interventions could be delegated to UAP or other members of the interprofessional team?
9. **Patient-Centered Care:** What priority patient teaching measures should be instituted to prevent recurrence of ADHF and prepare J.E. for discharge?
10. **Evidence-Based Practice:** J.E. asks you why it is so important to "watch her salt." She tells you that food tastes better with salt. How would you respond to her?
11. Develop a conceptual care map for J.E.

Answers and a corresponding concept map available at *http://evolve.elsevier.com/Lewis/medsurg.*

■ BRIDGE TO NCLEX EXAMINATION

The number of the question corresponds to the same-numbered outcome at the beginning of the chapter.

1. Which statements accurately describe heart failure with preserved ejection fraction (HFpEF)? *(select all that apply)*
   a. Uncontrolled hypertension is the primary cause.
   b. Left ventricular ejection fraction may be within normal limits.
   c. The pathophysiology involves ventricular relaxation and filling.
   d. Multiple evidence-based therapies have been shown to decrease mortality.
   e. Therapies focus on symptom control and treatment of underlying conditions.

2. What compensatory mechanism involved in both chronic heart failure and acute decompensated heart failure leads to fluid retention and edema?
   a. Ventricular dilation
   b. Ventricular hypertrophy
   c. Increased systemic blood pressure
   d. Renin-angiotensin-aldosterone activation

3. The nurse is caring for a patient with acute decompensated heart failure who is receiving IV dobutamine. Why would this drug be prescribed? *(select all that apply)*
   a. It dilates renal blood vessels.
   b. It will increase the heart rate.
   c. Heart contractility will improve.
   d. Dobutamine is a selective β-agonist.
   e. It increases systemic vascular resistance.

4. A patient with chronic heart failure and atrial fibrillation is treated with low-dose digitalis and a loop diuretic. What does the nurse need to do to prevent complications of this drug combination? *(select all that apply)*
   a. Monitor serum potassium levels.
   b. Teach the patient how to take a pulse rate.
   c. Withhold digitalis if pulse rhythm is irregular.
   d. Keep an accurate measure of intake and output.
   e. Teach the patient about dietary potassium restrictions.

5. A barrier to hospice referrals for patients with stage D heart failure is
   a. family member refusal.
   b. scarcity of hospice facilities.
   c. history of pacemaker placement.
   d. difficulty in estimating prognosis.

6. Patients are at risk for which complications in the first year after heart transplantation? *(select all that apply)*
   a. Cancer
   b. Infection
   c. Rejection
   d. Vasculopathy
   e. Sudden cardiac death

1. b, c, e. 2. d. 3. c. 4. a, b. 5. d. 6. b, c, e

For rationales to these answers and even more NCLEX review questions, visit *http://evolve.elsevier.com/Lewis/medsurg.*

EVOLVE WEBSITE/RESOURCES LIST

REFERENCES

*1. Yancy CW, Jessup M, Bozkurt B, et al: 2013 ACCF/AHA guideline for the management of heart failure: executive summary: a report of the American College of Cardiology Foundation/AHA Task Force on Practice Guidelines, *Circulation* 128:1810, 2013. (Classic)

2. Benjamin EJ, Blaha MJ, Chieve SE, et al: Heart disease and stroke statistics—2017 update: A report from the AHA, *Circulation* 135:e146, 2017.

3. Reddy Y, Lewis G, Shoh S, et al: Heart failure pathophysiology, *Circ Heart Fail* 10:e003862, 2017.

*4. Pandey A, Omar W, Ayers ML, et al: Sex and race differences in lifetime risk of heart failure with preserved ejection fraction and heart failure with reduced ejection fraction, *Circulation* 137:117, 2018.

*5. Tayal U, Prasad S, Cook SA: Genetics and genomics of dilated cardiomyopathy and systolic heart failure, *Gen Med* 9:20, 2017.

*6. Redfield MM: Heart failure with preserved ejection fraction, *New Engl J Med* 375:1868, 2016.

*7. Lueder T, Kotecha D, Ator D, et al: Neurohormonal blockade in heart failure, *Card Fail Rev* 3:19, 2017.

*8. Hartupee J, Mann DL: Neurohormonal activation in heart failure with reduced ejection fraction, *Natl Rev Cardiol* 14:30, 2017.

*9. Zhang Y, Bauersachs J, Langer H: Immune mechanisms in heart failure, *Eur J Heart Fail* 19:1379, 2017.

*10. Chirinos J, Akers S, Trieu L, et al: Heart failure, left ventricular remodeling and circulating nitric oxide metabolism, *J AM Heart Assoc* 5:3004133, 2016.

*11. Silver MA, Maisal A, Yancy CW, et al: BNP Consensus Panel 2004: A clinical approach for the diagnostic, prognostic, screening, treatment monitoring, and therapeutic roles of natriuretic peptides in cardiovascular diseases, *Conges Heart Fail* 10:1, 2004. (Classic)

*12. Lindenfeld J, Albert N, Boehmer JP, et al: HFSA 2010 comprehensive heart failure practice guidelines, *J Card Fail* 16:e1, 2010. (Classic)

*13. Gathright EC, Goldstein CM, Josephson RA, et al: Depression increases the risk of mortality in patients with heart failure: A meta-analysis, *J Psychosom Res* 94:82, 2017.

14. Volterrani M, Iellamo F: Cardiac rehabilitation in patients with heart failure: New perspectives in exercise training, *Card Fail Rev* 2:63, 2016.

*15. Yancy CW, Jessup M, Bozkurt B, et al: 2017 ACC/AHA/HFSA focused update of the 2013 ACCF/AHA guidelines for the management of heart failure: A report of the ACC/AHA Task Force on Clinical Practice Guidelines, *Circ* 136:e137, 2017.

16. Abraham W, Perl L: Implantable hemodynamic monitoring for heart failure patients, *J Am Col Card* 70:389, 2017.

*17. Abraham WT, Adamson PB, Bourge RC, et al: Wireless pulmonary artery hemodynamic monitoring in chronic heart failure: A randomized controlled trial, *Lancet* 377:658, 2011. (Classic)

18. Schocken DD, Benjamin EJ, Fonarow G, et al: Prevention of heart failure: A scientific statement from the AHA Councils on Epidemiology and Prevention, Clinical Cardiology, Cardiovascular Nursing, and High Blood Pressure Research, *Circulation* 117:2544, 2008. (Classic)

*19. Desai AS: Intensive management to reduce hospitalizations in patients with heart failure, *Circulation* 133:1704, 2016.

20. Kavalieratos D, Gelfman L, Tycon L, et al: Palliative care in heart failure: Rationale, evidence, and future priorities, *J Am Col Card* 70:1919, 2017.

*21. Hamel A, Gaugler J, Porta C, et al: Complex decision making in heart failure: a systematic review and thematic analysis, *J Card Nurs* 33:225, 2017.

22. Stehlik J, Edwards LB, Kucheryavaya AY, et al.: The registry of the International Society of Heart and Lung Transplantation: Twenty Eighth Adult Heart Transplant Report—2011, *J Heart Lung Tran* 30:1078, 2011. (Classic)

*23. Wilhelm M: Long term outcomes following heart transplantation: A current perspective, *J Thorac Dis* 7:549, 2015. (Classic)

*Evidence-based information for clinical practice.

35

Dysrhythmias

Kimberly Day

All I ever wanted was to reach out and touch another human being not just with my hands but with my heart.

Tahereh Mafi

http://evolve.elsevier.com/Lewis/medsurg

CONCEPTUAL FOCUS

Fluids and Electrolytes   Perfusion

LEARNING OUTCOMES

1. Examine the nursing care of patients needing continuous electrocardiographic (ECG) monitoring.
2. Distinguish the clinical characteristics and ECG patterns of normal sinus rhythm, common dysrhythmias, and pacemaker rhythms.
3. Describe the nursing and interprofessional management of patients with common dysrhythmias.
4. Compare and contrast defibrillation and cardioversion, including indications for use and physiologic effects.
5. Describe the nursing and interprofessional management of patients with pacemakers and implantable cardioverter-defibrillators.
6. Select appropriate interventions for patients undergoing electrophysiologic testing and radiofrequency catheter ablation therapy.

KEY TERMS

asystole, p. 768
atrial fibrillation, p. 763
atrial flutter, p. 763
automatic external defibrillator (AED), p. 769

cardiac pacemaker, p. 771
complete heart block, p. 766
dysrhythmias, p. 754
premature atrial contraction (PAC), p. 762

premature ventricular contraction (PVC), p. 766
telemetry monitoring, p. 757
ventricular fibrillation (VF), p. 768
ventricular tachycardia (VT), p. 767

This chapter describes basic principles of electrocardiographic monitoring and the recognition and treatment of common dysrhythmias. Adequate perfusion requires the heart to generate sufficient cardiac output (CO) to distribute blood to the body tissues. Abnormal heart rhythms, called **dysrhythmias**, can directly decrease CO by changing stroke volume and heart rate (HR). For example, tachycardia from a fever may decrease CO and cause hypotension. Your ability to recognize normal heart rhythms and dysrhythmias is an essential nursing skill.[1] Prompt recognition of a dysrhythmia and assessment of the patient's response to the rhythm is critical to maintaining adequate perfusion.

RHYTHM IDENTIFICATION AND TREATMENT

Conduction System

Four properties of heart cells allow the conduction system to start an electrical impulse, send it through the heart tissue, and stimulate muscle contraction (Table 35.1). The heart's conduction system consists of specialized neuromuscular tissue found throughout the heart (see Fig. 31.4, *A*). A normal impulse starts in the sinoatrial (SA) node in the upper right atrium near the entrance of the vena cava. It spreads over the atrial myocardium

via interatrial and internodal pathways, causing atrial contraction. The impulse then travels to the atrioventricular (AV) node, through the bundle of His, and down the left and right bundle branches to the Purkinje fibers, which transmit the impulse to the ventricles.

Nervous Control of the Heart

The autonomic nervous system plays a vital role in the rate of impulse formation, speed of conduction, and strength of cardiac contraction. The parts of the autonomic nervous system that affect the heart are the vagus nerve fibers of the parasympathetic nervous system and the nerve fibers of the sympathetic nervous system.

Stimulation of the vagus nerve slows firing of the SA node and slows impulse conduction of the AV node. This decreases heart rate. Stimulation of the sympathetic nerves increases SA node firing, AV node impulse conduction, and cardiac contractility. This increases heart rate.[2,3]

Electrocardiographic Monitoring

The *electrocardiogram* (ECG) is a graphic tracing of the electrical impulses produced in the heart. The waveforms on the ECG represent the electrical activity of depolarization and

TABLE 35.1 Properties of Heart Cells

Property	Definition
Automaticity	Ability to initiate an impulse spontaneously and continuously
Excitability	Ability to be electrically stimulated
Conductivity	Ability to transmit an impulse along a membrane in an orderly manner
Contractility	Ability to respond mechanically to an impulse

repolarization produced by the movement of ions across the membranes of heart cells (see Fig. 31.4, *B*).

The membrane of a heart cell is semipermeable. This allows it to maintain a high concentration of potassium and a low concentration of sodium inside the cell. Outside the cell, a high concentration of sodium and a low concentration of potassium exist. The inside of the cell, when at rest or in the polarized state, is negative compared with the outside. When a cell or groups of cells are stimulated, the cell membrane changes its permeability. This allows sodium to move rapidly into the cell, making the inside of the cell positive compared with the outside *(depolarization)*. A slower movement of ions across the membrane restores the cell to the polarized state, called *repolarization*. Fig. 35.1 describes the phases of the cardiac action potential.[1,2]

A 12-lead ECG view of the heart is helpful in assessing dysrhythmias. Six of the leads measure electrical forces in the frontal plane. These are bipolar (positive and negative) leads I, II, and III and unipolar (positive) leads aVR, aVL, and aVF (Fig. 35.2, *A* and *B*). The remaining 6 unipolar leads (V_1 through V_6) measure the electrical forces in the horizontal plane (precordial leads) (Fig. 35.2, *C*). The 12-lead ECG may show changes suggesting structural changes, conduction changes, damage (e.g., ischemia, infarction), electrolyte imbalance, or drug toxicity. Fig. 35.3 is an example of a normal 12-lead ECG.

We can use one or more ECG leads to continuously monitor a patient. The most common leads used are leads II and V_1 (Fig. 35.4). A modified chest lead (MCL_1) is used when only 3 leads are available for monitoring. MCL_1 is similar to V_1. Accurate interpretation of an ECG depends on the correct placement of the leads on the patient. The monitoring leads used are determined by the patient's clinical status.[4,5]

The ECG monitor continuously displays the heart rhythm. Paper attached to the monitor records the ECG (i.e., rhythm strip) to provide a record of the patient's rhythm. It allows for measurement of complexes and intervals and for assessment of dysrhythmias.

To correctly interpret an ECG, measure time and voltage on the ECG paper. ECG paper consists of large (heavy lines) and small (light lines) squares (Fig. 35.5). Each large square consists of 25 smaller squares (5 horizontal and 5 vertical). Horizontally, each small square (1 mm) represents 0.04 second. This means

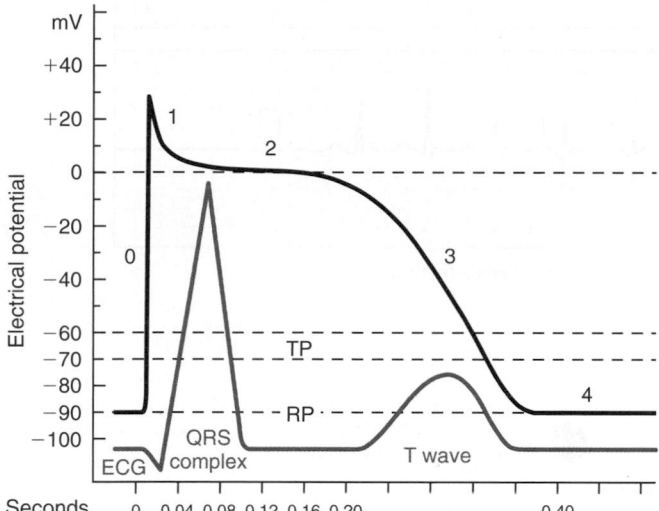

FIG. 35.1 Phases of the cardiac action potential. The electrical potential, measured in millivolts (mV), is indicated along the vertical axis of the graph. Time, measured in seconds (sec), is indicated along the horizontal axis. The action potential has 5 phases, labeled *0* through *4*. Each phase represents a specific electrical event or combination of electrical events. Phase 0 is the upstroke of rapid depolarization and corresponds with ventricular contraction. Phases 1, 2, and 3 represent repolarization. Phase 4 is known as complete repolarization (or the polarized state) and corresponds to diastole. *RP*, Resting membrane potential; *TP*, threshold membrane potential.

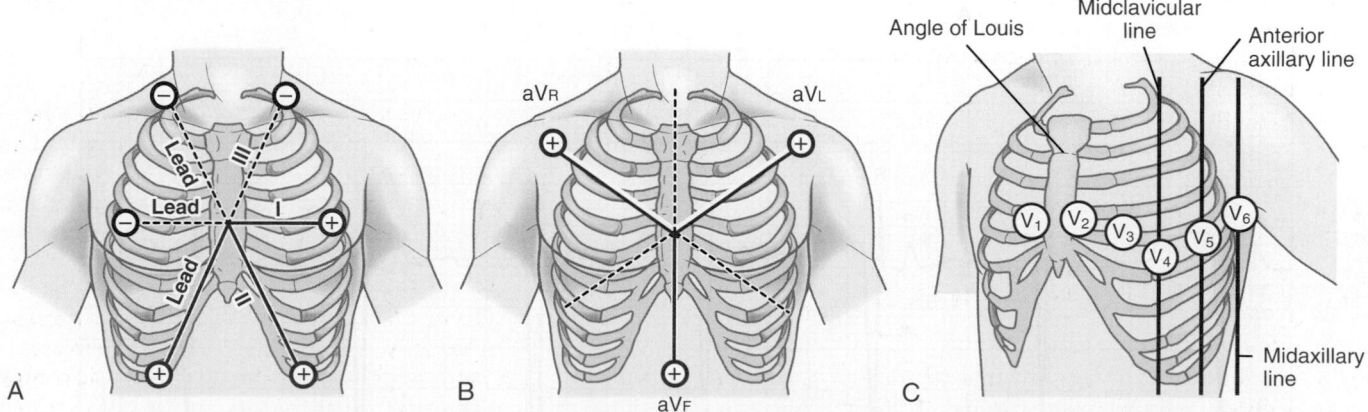

FIG. 35.2 **A**, Limb leads I, II, and III. These bipolar leads are placed on the extremities. Shown are the angles from which these leads view the heart. **B**, Limb leads aVR, aVL, and aVF. These unipolar leads use the center of the heart as their negative electrode. **C**, Placement for the unipolar chest leads: V_1, 4th intercostal space at the right sternal border; V_2, 4th intercostal space at the left sternal border; V_3, halfway between V_2 and V_4; V_4, 5th intercostal space at the left midclavicular line; V_5, 5th intercostal space at the left anterior axillary line; V_6, 5th intercostal space at the left midaxillary line.

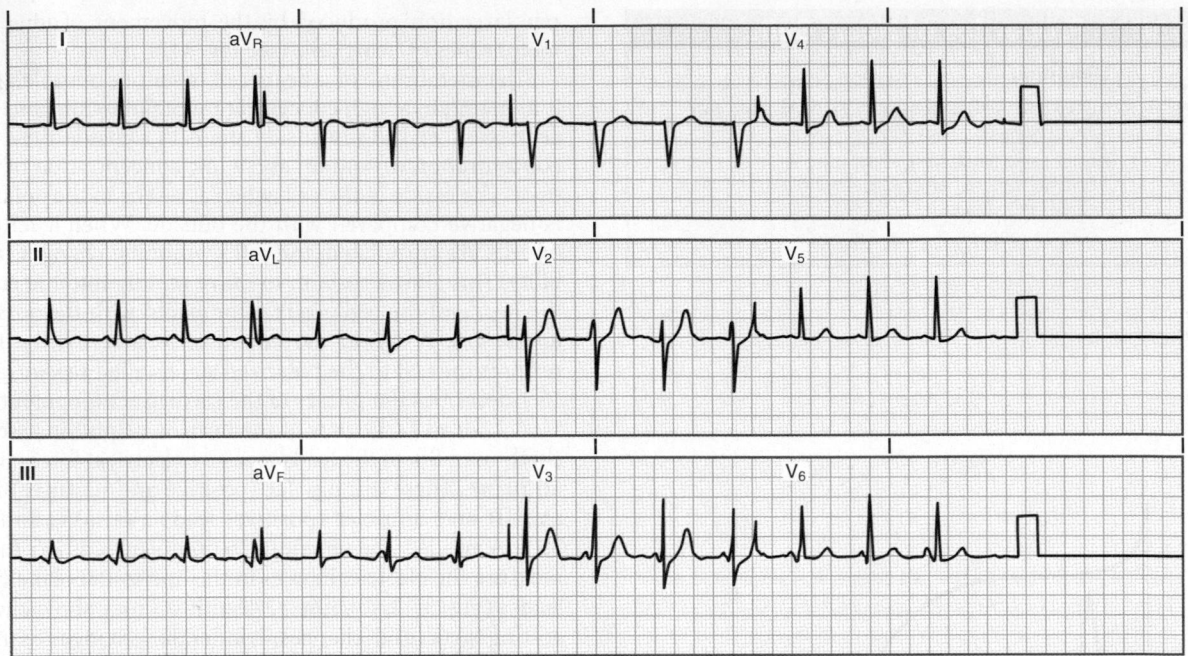

FIG. 35.3 12-lead electrocardiogram showing a normal sinus rhythm.

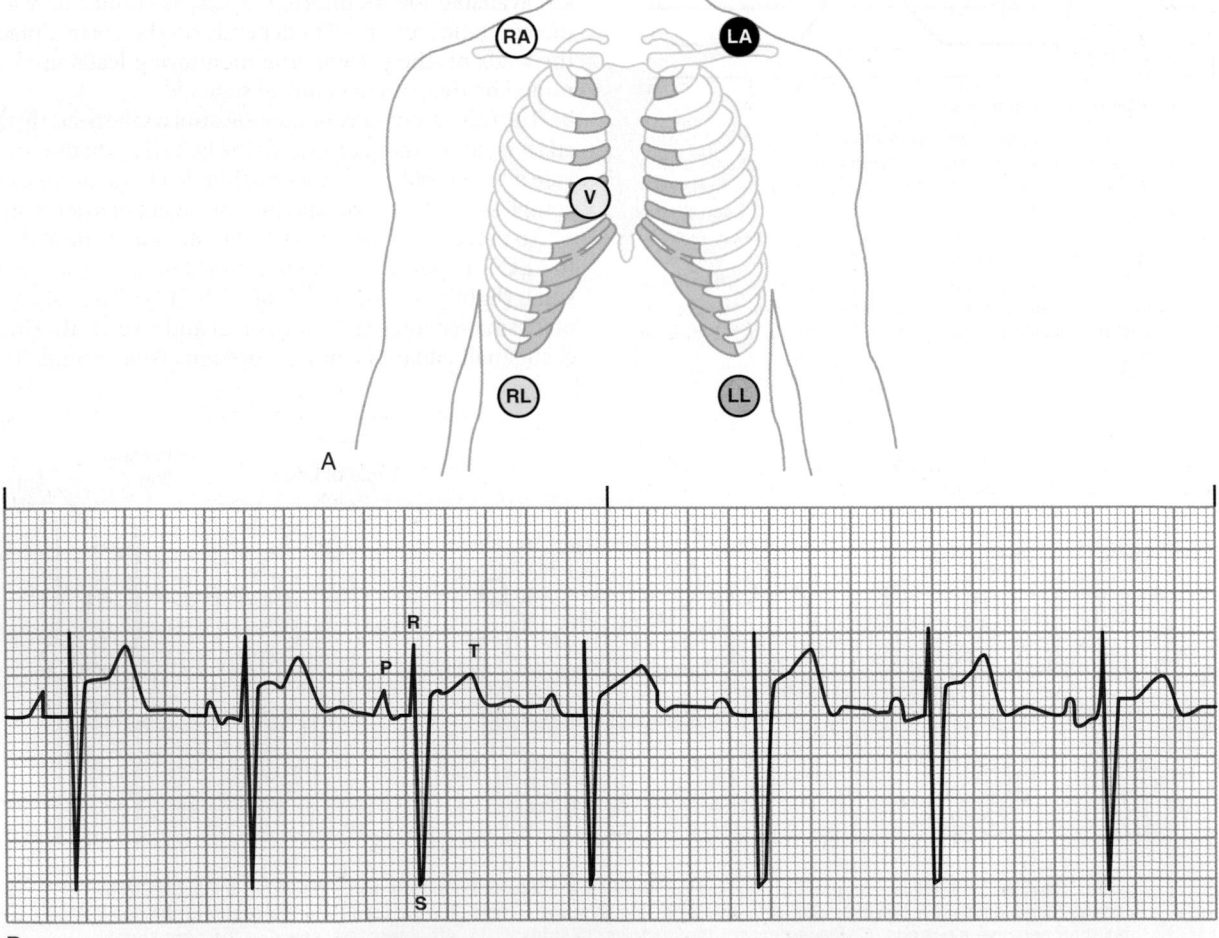

FIG. 35.4 A, Lead placement for V₁ using a 5-lead system. B, Typical ECG tracing in lead V₁. *V,* Chest lead; *LA,* left arm; *LL,* left leg; *RA,* right arm; *RL,* right leg.

that 1 large square equals 0.20 second and that 300 large squares equal 1 minute. Vertically, each small square (1 mm) represents 0.1 millivolt (mV). This means that 1 large square equals 0.5 mV. Use these squares to calculate the HR and measure time intervals for the different ECG complexes.

You can use a variety of methods to calculate the HR from an ECG. The most accurate way is to count the number of QRS complexes in 1 minute. However, because this method is time consuming, you can use a simpler process. Note that every 3 seconds a marker appears on the ECG paper (Fig. 35.5). Count the number of QRS complexes in 6 seconds and multiply that number by 10. This is the estimated number of beats per minute (Fig. 35.6).

Another method to calculate the HR is to count the number of small squares between 1 R-R interval. Divide this number into 1500 to get the HR. Last, you can count the number of large squares between 1 R-R interval and divide this number into 300 to get the HR (Fig. 35.6). All these methods are more accurate when the rhythm is regular.[1,2]

Another way to measure distances on the ECG strip is to use calipers. Often a P or R wave will not fall directly on a light or heavy line. Place the fine points of the calipers exactly on the parts you need to measure and then move to another part of the strip for a more precise time measurement.

Fig. 35.7 shows the components of a normal ECG tracing. Table 35.2 describes ECG waveforms and intervals, normal durations, and possible sources of changes in each. Table 35.3 presents a systematic approach to assessing a heart rhythm.

ECG leads consist of an electrode pad fixed with electrical conductive gel. Before placing these on the patient, properly prepare the skin. Clip excess hair on the chest wall with scissors. Gently rub the skin with dry gauze until slightly pink. If the skin is oily, wipe with alcohol first. If the patient is diaphoretic, apply a skin protectant before placing the electrode.

Artifact is a distortion of the baseline and waveforms seen on the ECG (Fig. 35.8). It is hard to accurately interpret heart rhythm when artifact is present. You will see artifact on the monitor when leads and electrodes are not secure, the conductive gel is becoming dry, and there is muscle activity (e.g., shivering, ambulating) or electrical interference. If artifact occurs, check the connections in the equipment. Replace the electrodes if the conductive gel has dried out.

Telemetry Monitoring. Telemetry monitoring is the observation of a patient's HR and rhythm at a site distant from the patient. This technology can help rapidly identify dysrhythmias, ischemia, or infarction. There are 2 types of systems for telemetry monitoring. The first type is a centralized monitoring system. It requires you or a telemetry technician to continuously observe a group of patients' ECGs at a central location. The second system of telemetry monitoring does not require constant surveillance. These systems have the capability of detecting and storing data. Advanced alarm systems provide different levels of detection of dysrhythmias, ischemia, or infarction.

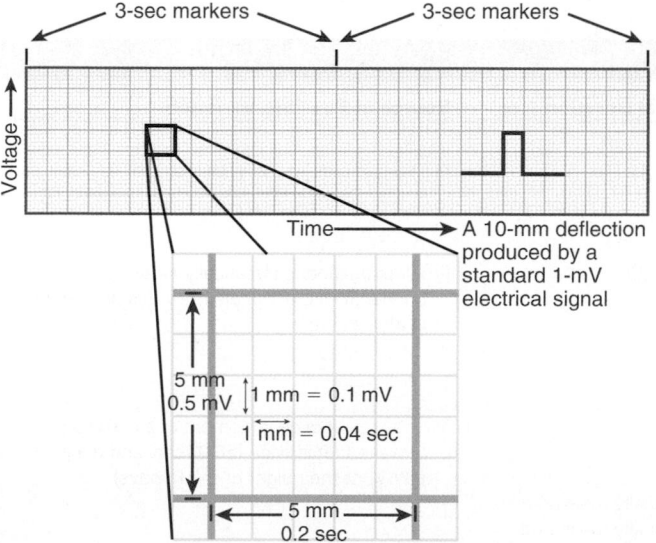

FIG. 35.5 Time and voltage on the electrocardiogram; 6-sec strip. (Modified from Wesley K: *Basic dysrhythmias and acute coronary syndromes,* ed 4, St Louis, 2011, Mosby JEMS.)

INFORMATICS IN PRACTICE
Wireless ECG Monitoring

- Wireless ECG monitoring systems continuously monitor and interpret the findings, sending an alert when a patient's rhythm and/or measurements fall outside of set parameters.
- Early detection of abnormal heart rhythms allows you time to assess the patient for signs of hemodynamic instability (e.g., chest pain, hypotension, palpitations, dyspnea) and determine the need to intervene (e.g., call the rapid response team).
- These systems can automatically save the pre-event portion of the ECG while continuing to record the post-event portion and send all the information to the HCP.
- Computerized monitoring systems are not fail-proof. Frequently assess all monitored patients for signs of hemodynamic instability.

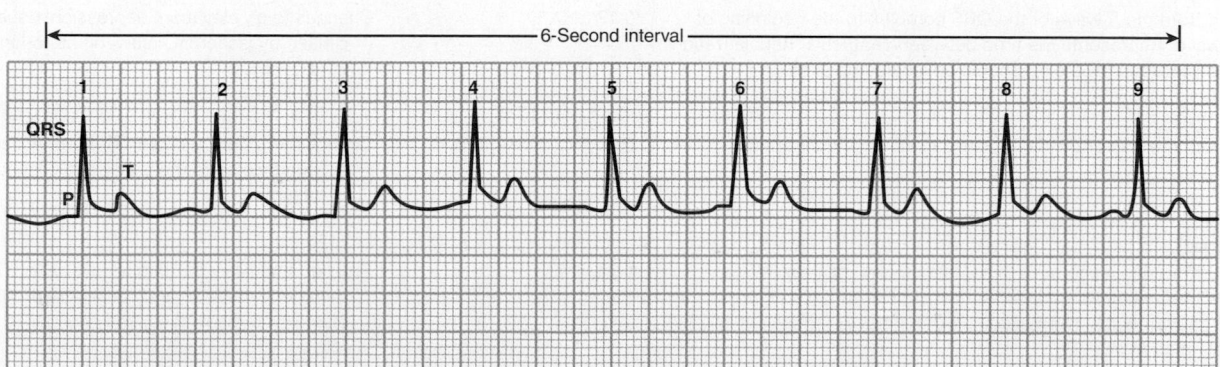

FIG. 35.6 When the rhythm is regular, heart rate can be easily determined by counting the number of "R" waves. The estimated heart rate is 90 beats/min. NOTE: Recorded from lead II.

Electrophysiologic Mechanisms of Dysrhythmias

Dysrhythmias result from disorders of impulse formation, impulse conductions, or both. The heart has specialized cells in the SA node, atria, AV node, bundle of His, and Purkinje fibers (His-Purkinje system), which can fire (discharge) spontaneously. This is termed *automaticity*. Normally, the SA node is the natural pacemaker of the heart. It spontaneously fires 60 to 100 times per minute (Table 35.4). A secondary pacemaker from another site may fire in 2 ways. If the SA node fires more slowly than a secondary pacemaker, the electrical signals from the secondary pacemaker may "escape." The secondary pacemaker will then fire automatically at its intrinsic rate. These secondary pacemakers may start from the AV node at a rate of 40 to 60 times per minute or the His-Purkinje system at a rate of 20 to 40 times per minute.

Another way that secondary pacemakers can start is when they fire more rapidly than the normal pacemaker of the SA node. *Triggered beats* (early or late) may come from an *ectopic focus* or *accessory pathway* (area outside the normal conduction pathway) in the atria, AV node, or ventricles. This results in a dysrhythmia, which replaces the normal sinus rhythm.

The impulse started by the SA node or an ectopic focus is conducted to the heart cells. The property of myocardial tissue that allows it to be depolarized by a stimulus is called *excitability*. The level of excitability is determined by the length of time after depolarization before the tissues can be restimulated. The recovery period after stimulation is the *refractory phase* or period. The *absolute refractory phase* or period occurs when excitability is zero and the heart cannot be stimulated. The *relative refractory period* occurs slightly later in the cycle, and excitability is more likely. In states of *full excitability,* the heart is completely recovered. Fig. 35.9 shows the relationship between the refractory period and ECG.

If conduction is depressed and some areas of the heart are blocked (e.g., by infarction), the unblocked areas are activated earlier than the blocked areas. When the block is unidirectional,

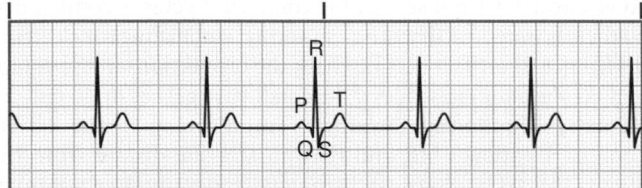

FIG. 35.7 Normal sinus rhythm. NOTE: Recorded from lead II.

TABLE 35.2 ECG Waveforms and Intervals*

Description	Normal Duration (sec)	Source of Possible Variation
P Wave		
Represents time for the passage of the electrical impulse through the atrium causing atrial depolarization (contraction). Should be upright	0.06–0.12	Problem in conduction within atria
PR Interval		
Measured from beginning of P wave to beginning of QRS complex. Represents time taken for impulse to spread through the atria, AV node and bundle of His, bundle branches, and Purkinje fibers, to a point immediately before ventricular contraction	0.12–0.20	Problem in conduction usually in AV node, bundle of His, or bundle branches but can be in atria as well
QRS Complex		
Q wave: First negative (downward) deflection after the P wave, short and narrow, not present in several leads	<0.03	MI may result in development of a pathologic Q wave that is wide (≥0.03 sec) and deep (≥25% of the height of the R wave)
R wave: First positive (upward) deflection in the QRS complex	Not usually measured	
S wave: First negative (downward) deflection after the R wave	Not usually measured	
QRS Interval		
Measured from beginning to end of QRS complex. Represents time taken for depolarization (contraction) of both ventricles (systole)	<0.12	Problem in conduction in bundle branches or in ventricles
ST Segment		
Measured from the S wave of the QRS complex to the beginning of the T wave. Represents the time between ventricular depolarization and repolarization (diastole). Should be isoelectric (flat)	0.12	Changes (e.g., elevation, depression) usually caused by ischemia, injury, or infarction
T Wave		
Represents time for ventricular repolarization. Should be upright	0.16	Changes (e.g., tall, peaked; inverted) usually caused by electrolyte imbalances, ischemia, or infarction
QT Interval†		
Measured from beginning of QRS complex to end of T wave. Represents time taken for entire electrical depolarization and repolarization of the ventricles. Normal adult women have slightly longer QT intervals than men.	0.34–0.43	Problems usually affecting repolarization more than depolarization and caused by drugs, electrolyte imbalances, and changes in heart rate

*Heart rate influences the duration of these intervals, especially the PR and QT intervals (e.g., QT interval shortens in duration as heart rate increases).
†A corrected QT interval (QTc) is calculated to account for the influence of heart rate.

TABLE 35.3 Approach to Assessing Heart Rhythm

When assessing a heart rhythm, use a consistent and systematic approach. One such approach includes the following:

1. Look for the P wave. Is it upright or inverted? Is there 1 for every QRS complex or more than 1? Are atrial fibrillatory or flutter waves present?
2. Evaluate the atrial rhythm. Is it regular or irregular?
3. Calculate the atrial rate.
4. Measure the duration of the PR interval. Is it normal duration or prolonged? Is the duration consistent before each QRS?
5. Evaluate the ventricular rhythm. Is it regular or irregular?
6. Calculate the ventricular rate.
7. Measure the duration of the QRS complex. Is it normal duration or prolonged?
8. Assess the ST segment. Is it isoelectric (flat), elevated, or depressed?
9. Measure the duration of the QT interval. Correct for heart rate (cQT) to determine if it is normal or prolonged.*
10. Note the T wave. Is it upright or inverted?

Other questions to consider include:

1. What is the dominant or underlying rhythm and/or dysrhythmia?
2. What is the clinical significance of your findings?
3. What is the treatment for the particular rhythm?

*A website for calculating the cQT interval for heart rate can be found at *www.mdcalc.com/corrected-qt-interval-qtc.*

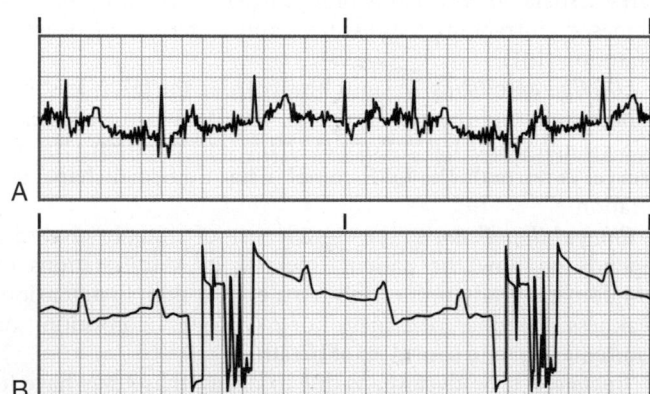

FIG. 35.8 Artifact. **A,** Muscle tremor. **B,** Loose electrodes.

TABLE 35.4 Intrinsic Rates of the Conduction System

Part of Conduction System	Rate
SA node and atria	60–100 times/min
AV node and bundle of His	40–60 times/min
Bundle branches and Purkinje fibers	20–40 times/min

this uneven conduction may allow the initial impulse to reenter areas that were previously not excitable but have recovered. The reentering impulse may be able to depolarize the atria and ventricles, causing a premature beat or rapid rhythm.

Evaluation of Dysrhythmias

Dysrhythmias occur as the result of various abnormalities and disease states. Assess the heart rhythm, any changes in rhythm, and the patient's clinical status. Determining the cause of dysrhythmias is a priority. The cause influences the patient's treatment. Table 35.5 presents common causes of dysrhythmias.

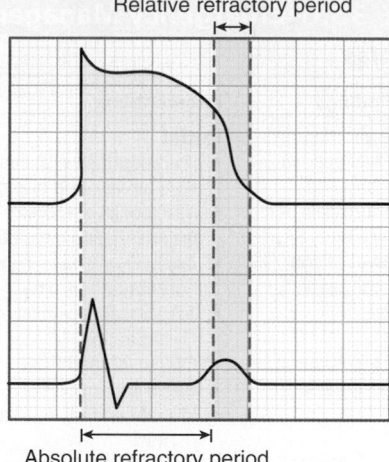

FIG. 35.9 Absolute and relative refractory periods correlated with the heart muscle's action potential and with an ECG tracing. (Modified from Urden LD, Stacy KM, Lough ME: *Critical care nursing: Diagnosis and management,* ed 6, St Louis, 2010, Mosby.)

TABLE 35.5 Common Causes of Dysrhythmias

Heart Conditions
- Accessory pathways
- Cardiomyopathy
- Conduction defects
- Heart failure
- Myocardial ischemia, infarction
- Valve disease

Other Conditions
- Acid-base imbalances
- Alcohol
- Caffeine, tobacco
- Connective tissue disorders
- Drowning
- Drug effects (e.g., antidysrhythmic drugs, stimulants, β-blockers) or toxicity
- Electric shock
- Electrolyte imbalances (e.g., hyperkalemia, hypocalcemia)
- Emotional crisis
- Herbal supplements (e.g., areca nut, wahoo root bark, yerba maté)
- Hypoxia
- Metabolic conditions (e.g., thyroid dysfunction)
- Sepsis, shock
- Toxins

Dysrhythmias occurring in nonmonitored settings present management challenges. If the patient becomes symptomatic (e.g., chest pain, syncope), determination of the rhythm by heart monitoring is a high priority. Activate the emergency response system (ERS). Table 35.6 outlines the emergency care of the patient with a dysrhythmia.

In addition to continuous ECG monitoring during hospitalization, several other tests can assess dysrhythmias and the effectiveness of antidysrhythmic drug therapy. An electrophysiologic study, Holter monitoring, event monitoring (or loop recorder), exercise treadmill testing, and signal-averaged ECG can be done on an inpatient or outpatient basis (see Tables 31.7 and 31.8 for nursing care related to these tests).

An *electrophysiologic study* (EPS) can identify the causes of heart blocks, tachydysrhythmias (dysrhythmias with rates greater than 100 beats/min), bradydysrhythmias (dysrhythmias

✚ TABLE 35.6 Emergency Management

Dysrhythmias

Assessment Findings	Interventions
• Irregular rate and rhythm; tachycardia, bradycardia • Chest, neck, shoulder, back, jaw, or arm pain • Cold, clammy skin • Decreased level of consciousness, confusion • Decreased or increased BP • Decreased O_2 saturation • Decreased peripheral pulses • Diaphoresis • Dizziness, syncope • Dyspnea • Extreme restlessness, anxiety • Feeling of impending doom • Nausea and vomiting • Numbness, tingling of arms • Pallor • Palpitations • Weakness and fatigue	**Initial** • If unresponsive, assess circulation, airway, and breathing (CAB). • If responsive, monitor airway, breathing, and circulation (ABC). • Apply O_2 via nasal cannula or nonrebreather mask. • Take baseline vital signs, including O_2 saturation. • Obtain 12-lead ECG. • Begin continuous ECG monitoring. • Identify underlying rate and rhythm. • Identify dysrhythmia. • Establish IV access. • Obtain baseline laboratory studies (e.g., CBC, electrolytes). **Ongoing Monitoring** • Monitor ABCs, vital signs, level of consciousness, O_2 saturation, and heart rhythm. • Anticipate need for antidysrhythmic drugs and analgesics. • Anticipate need for intubation if respiratory distress occurs. • Anticipate need to begin advanced cardiovascular life support (e.g., CPR, defibrillation, transcutaneous pacing).

with rates less than 60 beats/min), and syncope. An EPS study can locate accessory pathways and determine the effectiveness of antidysrhythmic drugs.

The Holter monitor continuously records the ECG while the patient is ambulatory and performing daily activities. The patient keeps a diary and records activities and any symptoms. Events in the diary are correlated with any dysrhythmias seen on the ECG. Use of event monitors has improved the evaluation of dysrhythmias in outpatients. Event monitors are recorders that the patient activates only when he or she has symptoms. New technology using smart phone apps can obtain and save ECG recordings and even detect some dysrhythmias (e.g., Kardia at *https://itunes.apple.com/us/app/aliveecg/id579769143?mt=8*).

Exercise treadmill testing evaluates the patient's heart rhythm during exercise. Any exercise-induced dysrhythmias or ECG changes that occur can be evaluated for treatment.

The signal-averaged ECG identifies *late potentials,* which suggest that the patient may be at risk for developing serious ventricular dysrhythmias. (See Chapter 31 for a discussion of diagnostic procedures for assessment of the cardiovascular system and related nursing care.)

Overview of Cardiac Rhythms

Figs. 35.10 to 35.21 give examples of the ECG tracings of common normal cardiac rhythms and dysrhythmias. Table 35.7 presents the characteristics of each.

Normal Cardiac Rhythms

Normal Sinus Rhythm. Normal *sinus rhythm* refers to a rhythm that starts in the SA node at a rate of 60 to 100 beats/min and

follows the normal conduction pathway (Fig. 35.10). The P wave is normal, precedes each QRS complex, and has a normal shape and duration. The PR interval is normal. The QRS complex has a normal shape and duration. Normal sinus rhythm implies that cardiac electrical activity is normal.

Sinus Arrhythmia. In *sinus arrhythmia,* the conduction pathway is the same as that in sinus rhythm, but the SA node fires irregularly. This often results from changes in intrathoracic pressure during breathing. The HR increases slightly during inspiration and decreases slightly during exhalation. It remains 60 to 100 beats/min. It is common in healthy adults.

Types of Dysrhythmias

Sinus Bradycardia. In *sinus bradycardia,* the conduction pathway is the same as that in sinus rhythm, but the SA node fires at a rate less than 60 beats/min (Fig. 35.11, *A*). *Symptomatic bradycardia* refers to a HR that is less than 60 beats/min and causes the patient to have symptoms of inadequate perfusion (e.g., fatigue, dizziness, chest pain, syncope).

Clinical Associations. Sinus bradycardia may be a normal sinus rhythm in aerobically trained athletes and in some people during sleep. It also occurs in response to carotid sinus massage, Valsalva maneuver, hypothermia, increased intraocular pressure, vagal stimulation, and certain drugs (e.g., β-blockers, calcium channel blockers). Common disease states associated with sinus bradycardia are hypothyroidism, increased intracranial pressure, and inferior myocardial infarction (MI).

ECG Characteristics. In sinus bradycardia, the HR is less than 60 beats/min and rhythm is regular. The P wave precedes each QRS complex and has a normal shape and duration. The PR interval is normal. The QRS complex has a normal shape and duration.

Clinical Significance. The significance of sinus bradycardia depends on how the patient tolerates it. Manifestations of symptomatic bradycardia include pale, cool skin; hypotension; weakness; angina; dizziness or syncope; confusion or disorientation; and shortness of breath.

Treatment. If bradycardia is due to drugs, these may have to be held, stopped, or reduced. For the patient with symptoms, treatment consists of giving IV atropine (anticholinergic drug). If atropine is ineffective, transcutaneous pacing or a dopamine or epinephrine infusion are options. The patient may need a permanent pacemaker.

Sinus Tachycardia. The conduction pathway is the same in *sinus tachycardia* as that in normal sinus rhythm. The discharge rate from the sinus node increases because of vagal inhibition or sympathetic stimulation. The sinus rate is 101 to 180 beats/min (Fig. 35.11, *B*).[2]

Clinical Associations. Sinus tachycardia is associated with physiologic and psychologic stressors, such as exercise, fever, pain, hypotension, hypovolemia, anemia, hypoxia, hypoglycemia, myocardial ischemia, heart failure (HF), hyperthyroidism, anxiety, and fear. It can be an effect of drugs, such as epinephrine, norepinephrine (Levophed), atropine, caffeine, theophylline, or hydralazine. In addition, many over-the-counter cold remedies have active ingredients (e.g., pseudoephedrine) that can cause tachycardia.

ECG Characteristics. In sinus tachycardia, the HR is 101 to 180 beats/min and rhythm is regular.[2] The P wave is normal and precedes each QRS complex. The PR interval is normal. The QRS complex has a normal shape and duration.

TABLE 35.7 Characteristics of Common Dysrhythmias

Pattern	Rate and Rhythm	P Wave	PR Interval	QRS Complex
Normal sinus rhythm (NSR)	60–100 beats/min and regular	Normal	Normal	Normal
Sinus bradycardia	<60 beats/min and regular	Normal	Normal	Normal
Sinus tachycardia	101–180 beats/min and regular	Normal	Normal	Normal
Premature atrial contraction (PAC)		Abnormal shape	Normal	Normal (usually)
Paroxysmal supraventricular tachycardia (PSVT)	151–220 beats/min and regular	Abnormal shape, may be hidden in the preceding T wave	Normal or shortened	Normal (usually)
Atrial flutter	*Atrial:* 200–350 beats/min and regular *Ventricular:* > or <100 beats/min and may be regular or irregular	Flutter (F) waves (saw-toothed pattern); more flutter waves than QRS complexes; may occur in a 2:1, 3:1, 4:1, etc., pattern	Not measurable	Normal (usually)
Atrial fibrillation	*Atrial:* 350–600 beats/min and irregular *Ventricular:* > or <100 beats/min and irregular	Fibrillatory (f) waves	Not measurable	Normal (usually)
Junctional dysrhythmias	40–180 beats/min and regular	Inverted, may be hidden in QRS complex, or behind the S wave	Shortened, if present	Normal (usually)
First-degree AV block	Normal and regular	Normal	>0.20 sec	Normal
Second-degree AV block				
• Type I (Mobitz I, Wenckebach heart block)	*Atrial:* Normal and regular *Ventricular:* Slower and irregular	Normal	Progressive lengthening (longer, longer, longer, drop, now you have a Wenckebach)	Normal QRS width, with pattern of 1 nonconducted (blocked) QRS complex
• Type II (Mobitz II heart block)	*Atrial:* Usually normal and regular *Ventricular:* Slower and regular or irregular	More P waves than QRS complexes (e.g., 2:1, 3:1)	Normal or prolonged but consistent for every QRS	Widened QRS, preceded by ≥2 P waves, with nonconducted (blocked) QRS complex
Third-degree AV block (complete heart block)	*Atrial:* Regular but may appear irregular due to P waves hidden in QRS complexes *Ventricular:* 20–60 beats/min and regular	Normal, but no connection with QRS complex	Inconsistent	Normal or widened, no relationship with P waves
Premature ventricular contraction (PVC)	Underlying rhythm can be any rate, regular or irregular rhythm, PVCs occur at variable rates	Not usually visible, hidden in the PVC	Not measurable	Wide and distorted
Ventricular tachycardia (VT)	150–250 beats/min and regular or irregular	Not usually visible	Not measurable	Wide and distorted
Accelerated idioventricular rhythm	40–100 beats/min and regular	Not usually visible	Not measurable	Wide and distorted
Ventricular fibrillation (VF)	Not measurable and irregular	Absent	Not measurable	Not measurable

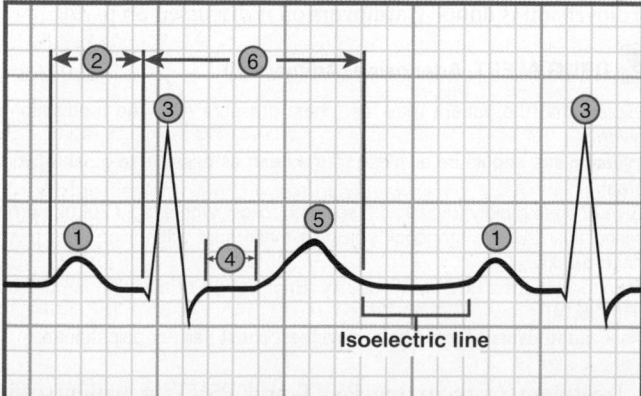

FIG. 35.10 The ECG tracing as seen in normal sinus rhythm. *1,* P wave; *2,* PR interval; *3,* QRS complex: Q wave, R wave, S wave; *4,* ST segment; *5,* T wave; *6,* QT interval. Isoelectric (flat) line or baseline represents the absence of electrical activity in the heart cells. (See Table 35.2 for timing of intervals.)

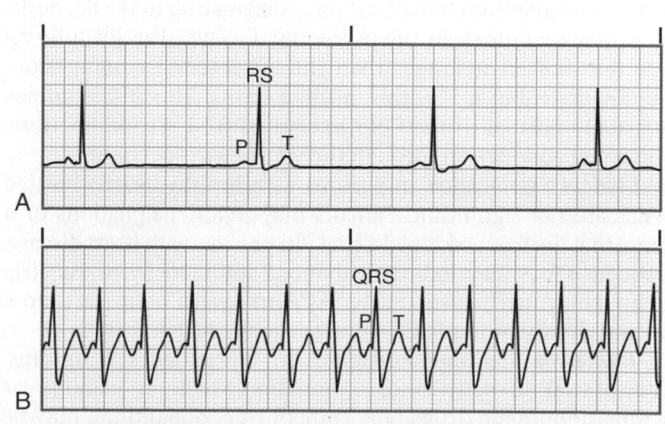

FIG. 35.11 A, Sinus bradycardia. B, Sinus tachycardia.

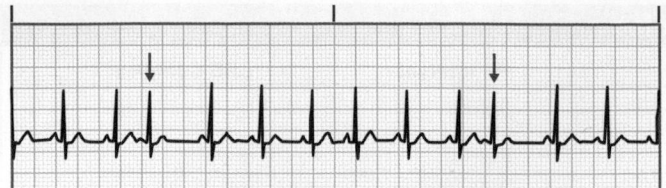

FIG. 35.12 Premature atrial contractions *(arrows).*

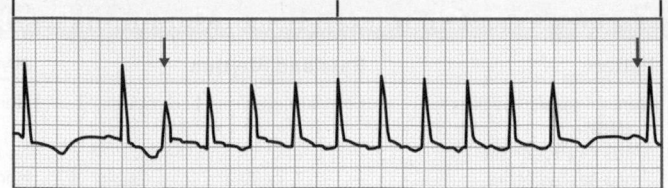

FIG. 35.13 Paroxysmal supraventricular tachycardia (PSVT). *Arrows* indicate beginning and ending of PSVT.

Clinical Significance. The clinical significance of sinus tachycardia depends on the patient's tolerance of the increased HR. The patient may have dizziness, dyspnea, and hypotension because of decreased CO. An increased HR increases myocardial oxygen (O₂) consumption. Angina or an increase in infarction size may occur with sinus tachycardia in those with coronary artery disease (CAD) or an acute MI.

Treatment. The underlying cause of tachycardia guides the treatment. For example, if the patient has tachycardia from pain, effective pain management is important to treat the tachycardia. In clinically stable patients, vagal maneuvers can be tried. IV β-blockers (e.g., metoprolol), adenosine (Adenocard), or calcium channel blockers (e.g., diltiazem) can reduce HR and decrease myocardial O₂ consumption. Clinically unstable patients may need synchronized cardioversion. Cardioversion is discussed on p. 770.

Premature Atrial Contraction. A **premature atrial contraction (PAC)** is a contraction starting from an ectopic focus in the atrium (i.e., a location other than the SA node) sooner than the next expected sinus beat. The ectopic signal starts in the left or right atrium and travels across the atria by an abnormal pathway. This creates a distorted P wave (Fig. 35.12). At the AV node, it may be stopped (nonconducted PAC), delayed (lengthened PR interval), or conducted normally. If the signal moves through the AV node, in most cases it is conducted normally through the ventricles.

Clinical Associations. In a normal heart, a PAC can result from emotional stress or physical fatigue, or from caffeine, tobacco, or alcohol use. A PAC can also result from hypoxia, electrolyte imbalances, hyperthyroidism, chronic obstructive pulmonary disease (COPD), and heart disease, including CAD and valvular disease.

ECG Characteristics. HR varies with the underlying rate and frequency of the PAC. The rhythm is irregular. The P wave has a different shape from that of a P wave originating in the SA node, or it may be hidden in the preceding T wave. The PR interval may be shorter or longer than the PR interval coming from the SA node, but it is within normal limits. The QRS complex is usually normal. If the QRS interval is 0.12 second or more, abnormal conduction through the ventricles is occurring.

Clinical Significance. In persons with healthy hearts, isolated PACs are not significant. Patients may report palpitations or a sense that the heart "skipped a beat." In persons with heart disease, frequent PACs may indicate enhanced automaticity of the atria or a reentry mechanism. Such PACs may warn of or start more serious dysrhythmias (e.g., supraventricular tachycardia).

Treatment. Treatment depends on the patient's symptoms. Withdrawal of sources of stimulation, such as caffeine or sympathomimetic drugs (e.g. epinephrine, dopamine), may be needed. β-Blockers may be used to decrease PACs.

Paroxysmal Supraventricular Tachycardia. *Paroxysmal supraventricular tachycardia* (PSVT), also known as supraventricular tachycardia (SVT) or atrial tachycardia, is a dysrhythmia starting in an ectopic focus anywhere above the bifurcation of the bundle of His (Fig. 35.13). Identifying the ectopic focus is often hard even with a 12-lead ECG since it requires recording the dysrhythmia as it starts.

PSVT occurs because of a reentrant phenomenon (reexcitation of the atria when there is a 1-way block). Usually a PAC triggers a run of repeated premature beats. *Paroxysmal* refers to an abrupt onset and ending. A brief period of *asystole* (absence of all cardiac electrical activity) may follow the termination. AV block may prevent some of the impulses from being conducted to the ventricles. PSVT can occur with Wolff-Parkinson-White (WPW) syndrome or "preexcitation" with extra conduction or accessory pathways.

Clinical Associations. In the normal heart, PSVT is associated with overexertion, emotional stress, deep inspiration, and stimulants, such as caffeine and tobacco. PSVT is also associated with rheumatic heart disease, digitalis toxicity, CAD, and cor pulmonale.

ECG Characteristics. In PSVT, the HR is 151 to 220 beats/min. The rhythm is regular or slightly irregular. The P wave may have an abnormal shape or be hidden in the preceding T wave. The PR interval may be shortened or normal. The QRS complex is usually normal.

Clinical Significance. The significance of PSVT depends on the associated symptoms. A prolonged episode and HR greater than 180 beats/min will cause decreased CO because of reduced stroke volume. Manifestations include hypotension, palpitations, dyspnea, and angina.

Treatment. Treatment for PSVT includes vagal stimulation and drug therapy. Common vagal maneuvers include Valsalva, carotid massage, and coughing. IV adenosine is the drug of choice to convert PSVT to a normal sinus rhythm (Fig. 35.14). This drug has a short half-life (10 seconds) and is well tolerated.[6] IV β-blockers and calcium channel blockers (e.g., diltiazem, verapamil) are options. If the patient becomes hemodynamically unstable, synchronized cardioversion is done.[7] Cardioversion is discussed on p. 770.

DRUG ALERT Adenosine (Adenocard)

- Explain that the patient may feel chest pressure after the medication is given.
- Injection site should be as close to the heart as possible (e.g., antecubital area).
- Give IV dose rapidly (over 1 to 2 sec) and follow with a rapid 20-mL normal saline flush. Use a stopcock setup to make sure adenosine gets to the heart quickly.
- Monitor patient's ECG continuously. Brief period of asystole is common (Fig. 35.14).
- Assess the patient for flushing, dizziness, chest pain, or palpitations.

Treatment of recurring PSVT and PSVT in patients with WPW syndrome includes radiofrequency catheter ablation of the accessory pathway.[7] Catheter ablation therapy is discussed on p. 773.

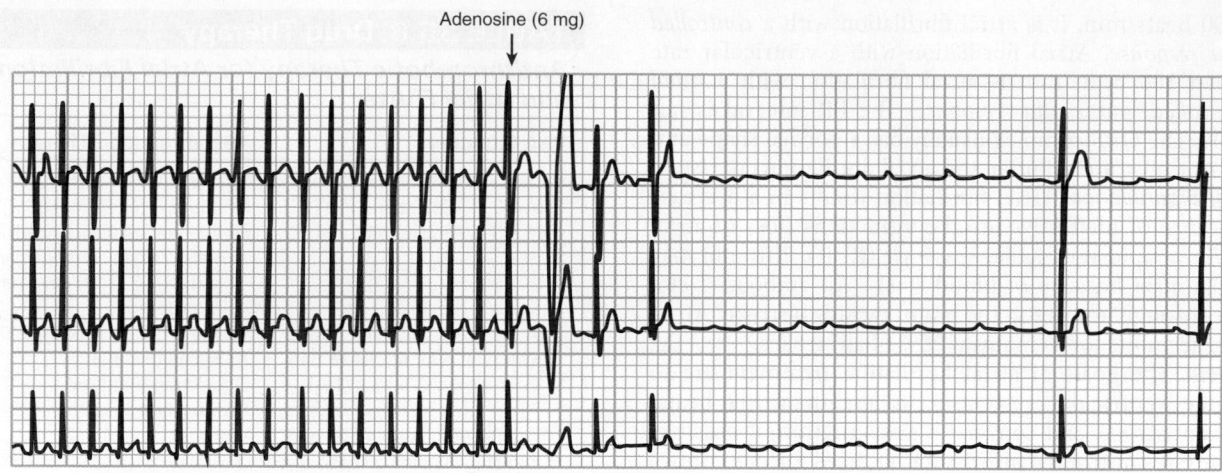

FIG. 35.14 Administration of adenosine rapid IV push. Note that SVT is followed by a brief period of asystole before the return to normal sinus rhythm. This is a common occurrence after adenosine.

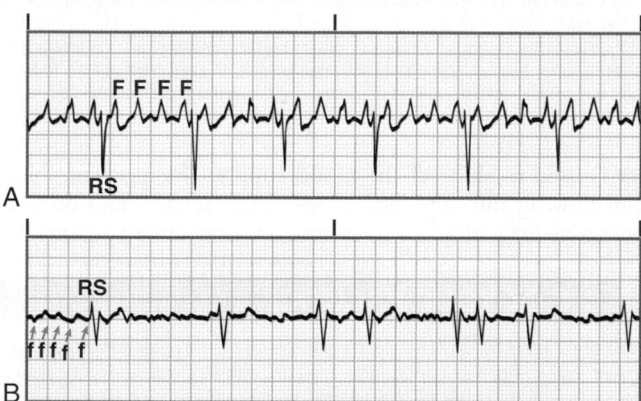

FIG. 35.15 A, Atrial flutter with a 4:1 conduction (4 flutter *[F]* waves to each QRS complex). B, Atrial fibrillation with a controlled ventricular response. Note the chaotic fibrillatory *(f)* waves *(arrows)* between the RS complexes. NOTE: Recorded from lead V₁.

Atrial Flutter. Atrial flutter is an atrial tachydysrhythmia identified by recurring, regular, sawtooth-shaped flutter waves that originate from a single ectopic focus in the right atrium or, less often, the left atrium (Fig. 35.15, *A*).

Clinical Associations. Atrial flutter rarely occurs in a healthy heart. It is associated with CAD, hypertension, mitral valve disorders, pulmonary embolus, chronic lung disease, cor pulmonale, cardiomyopathy, hyperthyroidism, and the use of drugs, such as digoxin, quinidine, and epinephrine.

ECG Characteristics. Atrial rate is 200 to 350 beats/min. The ventricular rate varies based on the conduction ratio. In 2:1 conduction, the ventricular rate is typically around 150 beats/min. Atrial and ventricular rhythms are usually regular. The atrial flutter waves represent atrial depolarization followed by repolarization. The PR interval is variable and not measurable. The QRS complex is usually normal. There is usually some AV block in a fixed ratio of flutter waves to QRS complexes because the AV node can delay signals from the atria.

Clinical Significance. The high ventricular rates (greater than 100 beats/min) and loss of the atrial "kick" (atrial contraction coordinated with ventricular contraction) that are associated

with atrial flutter decrease CO. This can cause serious problems, such as HF, especially in the patient with underlying heart disease. Patients with atrial flutter have an increased risk for stroke because thrombi (clots) can form in the atria from the stasis of blood. Warfarin or another anticoagulant is given to prevent stroke in patients who have atrial flutter.[8] (See Chapter 37 for discussion of anticoagulation therapy.)

Treatment. The primary goal in treatment of atrial flutter is to slow the ventricular response by increasing AV block. Drugs used to control ventricular rate include calcium channel blockers and β-blockers. Electrical cardioversion may be done to convert the atrial flutter to sinus rhythm in an emergency (i.e., when the patient is clinically unstable) and electively. Antidysrhythmic drugs can convert atrial flutter to sinus rhythm (e.g., ibutilide [Corvert]) or to maintain sinus rhythm (e.g., amiodarone, flecainide).[6,8]

Radiofrequency catheter ablation in an EPS laboratory is the treatment of choice for atrial flutter.[8] The procedure involves placing a catheter in the right atrium. Low-voltage, high-frequency electrical energy is then used to ablate (or destroy) the ectopic foci. This should restore normal sinus rhythm. (Catheter ablation is discussed on p. 773.)

Atrial Fibrillation. Atrial fibrillation is characterized by a total disorganization of atrial electrical activity because of multiple ectopic foci. It results in loss of effective atrial contraction (Fig. 35.15, *B*). The dysrhythmia may be paroxysmal (i.e., beginning and ending spontaneously) or persistent (lasting more than 7 days).[1] Atrial fibrillation is the most common, clinically significant dysrhythmia with respect to morbidity and mortality rates and economic impact. Its prevalence increases with age.[8]

Clinical Associations. Atrial fibrillation usually occurs in a patient with underlying heart disease, such as CAD, valvular heart disease, cardiomyopathy, hypertensive heart disease, HF, and pericarditis. It often develops acutely with thyrotoxicosis, alcohol intoxication, caffeine use, electrolyte problems, stress, and heart surgery.

ECG Characteristics. During atrial fibrillation, the atrial rate may be as high as 350 to 600 beats/min. Chaotic, fibrillatory waves replace the P waves. Ventricular rate varies, and the rhythm is usually irregular. When the ventricular rate is between

60 and 100 beats/min, it is atrial fibrillation with a *controlled ventricular response*. Atrial fibrillation with a ventricular rate greater than 100 beats/min is atrial fibrillation with a *rapid (or uncontrolled) ventricular response*. The PR interval is not measurable. The QRS complex usually has a normal shape and duration. At times, atrial flutter and atrial fibrillation coexist.[1]

Clinical Significance. Atrial fibrillation results in a decrease in CO because of ineffective atrial contractions (loss of atrial kick) and/or a rapid ventricular response (RVR). Thrombi may form in the atria because of blood stasis. An embolized clot may move through arteries to the brain, causing a stroke. Atrial fibrillation accounts for as many as 20% of all strokes.[9]

Treatment. The goals of atrial fibrillation treatment are to decrease the ventricular response (to less than 100 beats/min), prevent stroke, and convert to sinus rhythm, if possible. Ventricular rate control is a priority. Drugs used for rate control include calcium channel blockers (e.g., diltiazem), β-blockers (e.g., metoprolol), amiodarone, and digoxin (Lanoxin).

Some patients need drug or electrical conversion of atrial fibrillation to a normal sinus rhythm (e.g., reduced exercise tolerance with rate control drugs, contraindications to warfarin). The most common antidysrhythmic drug used for conversion to and maintenance of sinus rhythm is amiodarone.[8]

Electrical cardioversion may convert atrial fibrillation to a normal sinus rhythm. If a patient is in atrial fibrillation for longer than 48 hours, anticoagulation therapy with warfarin is needed for 3 to 4 weeks before the cardioversion.[1,8] Anticoagulation therapy continues for several weeks after because the procedure can cause the clots to dislodge, placing the patient at risk for stroke. A transesophageal echocardiogram may be done to rule out clots in the atria. If no clots are present, anticoagulation therapy may not be needed before the cardioversion.

If drugs or cardioversion does not convert atrial fibrillation to normal sinus rhythm, the patient needs long-term anticoagulation therapy (Table 35.8). Warfarin is often used, and we monitor for therapeutic levels (e.g., international normalized ratio [INR]). Alternatives to warfarin are available that do not require routine laboratory testing. Examples include dabigatran (Pradaxa), apixaban (Eliquis), and rivaroxaban (Xarelto).[8] See Chapter 37 for discussion of anticoagulation therapy.

For symptomatic patients with atrial fibrillation refractory to drugs or electrical conversion, radiofrequency catheter ablation (similar to procedure for atrial flutter), AV nodal ablation, and the Maze procedure are further options. AV nodal ablation involves the destruction of the AV node and insertion of a permanent ventricular pacemaker.[8]

The Maze procedure is a surgical intervention that stops atrial fibrillation by interrupting the ectopic foci that are causing the dysrhythmia. Incisions are made in both atria, and *cryoablation* (cold therapy) is used to stop the formation and conduction of ectopic signals and restore normal sinus rhythm.

Left atrial appendage occlusion. The left atrial appendage (LAA) is a pouch that extends off the left atrium. The LAA is known to trigger atrial fibrillation. It is a common source of blood clots in patients with atrial fibrillation. LAA occlusion is a treatment strategy to prevent blood clot formation in patients who have atrial fibrillation. Removing or occluding the LAA can decrease the incidence of strokes.

A special stapler can be used to remove the LAA. Or, the LAA can be occluded manually with sutures or an LAA occlusion device (e.g., Amplatzer, Lariat, Watchman). These devices are positioned around the LAA and then closed, like a clamp

TABLE 35.8 **Drug Therapy**	
Antithrombotic Therapy for Atrial Fibrillation and Atrial Flutter	
Risk Category	**Recommended Therapy**
Mechanical heart valve	Warfarin (target INR 2.5–3.5)
CHA_2DS_2-VASc* score of 0	No therapy recommended
CHA_2DS_2-VASc score of 1	No therapy recommended. An oral anticoagulant or aspirin (e.g., 81–325 mg/day) may be considered
CHA_2DS_2-VASc score of ≥2 or a history of prior stroke or transient ischemia attack (TIA)	Warfarin (target INR 2.0–3.0) Apixaban (Eliquis) Dabigatran (Pradaxa) Rivaroxaban (Xarelto)
CHA_2DS_2-VASc score of ≥2 and end-stage kidney disease or on hemodialysis	Warfarin

Source: Heidenreich PA, Solis P, Estes N, et al: 2016 ACC/AHA clinical performance and quality measures for adults with atrial fibrillation or atrial flutter, *J Am Coll Cardiol* 68:525, 2016.
*The CHA_2DS_2-VASc score for nonvalvular atrial fibrillation stroke risk can be calculated at *www.mdcalc.com/cha2ds2-vasc-score-for-atrial-fibrillation-stroke-risk/*.
CHA_2DS_2-VASc, Congestive heart failure; hypertension; age ≥75 (doubled); diabetes; prior stroke, transient ischemic attack, thromboembolism (doubled); vascular disease; age 65–74; sex, *INR*, international normalized ratio.

that is used to shut off the blood supply. This prevents blood from flowing into and out of the LAA. LAA occlusion is an alternative for patients who cannot use oral anticoagulants.[10]

> **? CHECK YOUR PRACTICE**
>
> You are caring for a 72-yr-old female patient who was admitted with chest pain. She has continuous EGG monitoring. You are concerned because you think her ECG tracing is hard to interpret and she may be in atrial fibrillation. Your preceptor tells you that there is a lot of artifact present.
> • What can you do to improve the ECG tracing?
> • How would you determine the patient's rhythm?

Junctional Dysrhythmias. *Junctional dysrhythmias* start in the area of the AV node to the bundle of His known as the AV junction. They result because the SA node does not fire or the signal is blocked. When this occurs, the AV node becomes the pacemaker of the heart. The impulse from the AV node usually moves in a retrograde (backward) fashion. This produces an abnormal P wave that occurs just before or after the QRS complex or is hidden in the QRS complex. The impulse usually moves normally through the ventricles. Junctional premature beats may occur. They are treated in a manner similar to that for PACs. Other junctional dysrhythmias include junctional escape rhythm (Fig. 35.16), accelerated junctional rhythm, and junctional tachycardia. Their treatment depends on the patient's tolerance of the rhythm and the patient's clinical condition.

Clinical Associations. Junctional dysrhythmias are often associated with CAD, HF, cardiomyopathy, electrolyte imbalances, inferior MI, and rheumatic heart disease. Certain drugs (e.g., digoxin, nicotine, amphetamines, caffeine) can also cause junctional dysrhythmias.

ECG Characteristics. In junctional escape rhythm, the HR is 40 to 60 beats/min. It is 61 to 100 beats/min in accelerated

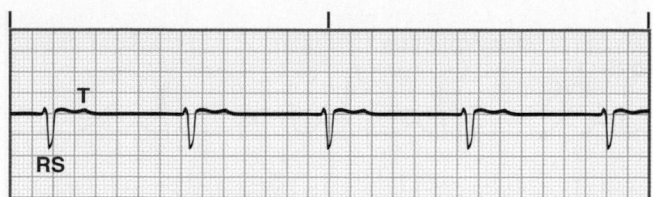

FIG. 35.16 Junctional escape rhythm. P wave is hidden in the RS complex. Note: Recorded from lead V$_1$.

junctional rhythm and 101 to 180 beats/min in junctional tachycardia. The rhythm is regular. The P wave is abnormal in shape and inverted, or it may be hidden in the QRS complex (Fig. 35.16). The PR interval is less than 0.12 second when the P wave precedes the QRS complex. The QRS complex is usually normal.

Clinical Significance. Junctional escape rhythms serve as a safety mechanism when the SA node has not been effective. Escape rhythms like this should not be suppressed. Accelerated junctional rhythm is due to sympathetic stimulation to improve CO. Junctional tachycardia indicates a more serious problem. This rhythm may reduce CO, causing the patient to become hemodynamically unstable (e.g., hypotensive).

Treatment. Treatment varies according to the type of junctional dysrhythmia. If a patient has symptoms with a junctional escape rhythm, atropine can be used. If accelerated junctional rhythm or junctional tachycardia are caused by drug toxicity, the drug is stopped. In the absence of digitalis toxicity, β-blockers, calcium channel blockers, and amiodarone are used for rate control. Cardioversion is not done.

First-Degree AV Block. *First degree AV block* is a type of AV block in which every impulse is conducted to the ventricles, but the time of AV conduction is prolonged (Fig. 35.17, *A*). After the impulse moves through the AV node, the ventricles usually respond normally.

Clinical Associations. First-degree AV block is associated with increasing age, MI, CAD, rheumatic fever, hyperthyroidism, electrolyte imbalances (e.g., hypokalemia), vagal stimulation, and drugs, such as digoxin, β-blockers, calcium channel blockers, and flecainide.

ECG Characteristics. In first-degree AV block, the HR is normal. The rhythm is regular. The P wave is normal. The PR interval is prolonged (greater than 0.20 second). The QRS complex usually has a normal shape and duration.

Clinical Significance. First-degree AV block is usually not serious. Patients are asymptomatic.

Treatment. There is no treatment for first-degree AV block. Treatment of associated conditions may be considered. Monitor patients for changes in heart rhythm (e.g., more serious AV block).

Second-Degree AV Block, Type I. *Type I second-degree AV block (Mobitz I or Wenckebach heart block)* includes a gradual lengthening of the PR interval. AV conduction time is increasingly prolonged until an atrial impulse is nonconducted and a QRS complex is blocked (missing) (Fig. 35.17, *B*). Type I AV block most often occurs in the AV node, but it can occur in the His-Purkinje system.

Clinical Associations. Type I AV block may result from drugs, such as digoxin or β-blockers. It may be associated with CAD and other diseases that can slow AV conduction.

ECG Characteristics. Atrial rate is regular, but ventricular rate may be slower because of nonconducted or blocked QRS

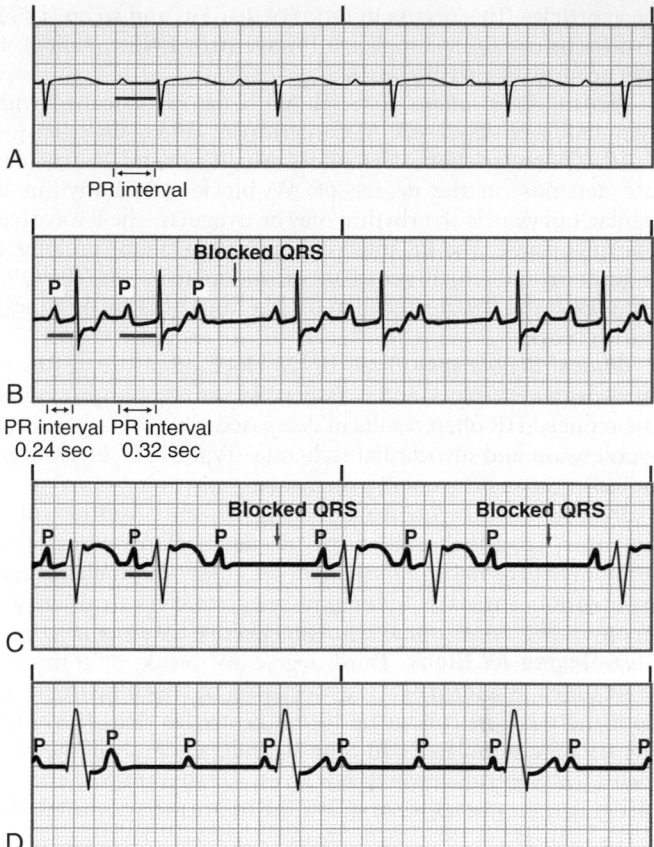

FIG. 35.17 Heart block. A, First-degree AV block with a PR interval of 0.40 sec. B, Second-degree AV block, type I, with progressive lengthening of the PR interval until a QRS complex is blocked. C, Second-degree AV block, type II, with constant PR intervals and variable blocked QRS complexes. D, Third-degree AV block. Note that there is no relationship between P waves and QRS complexes.

complexes resulting in bradycardia. Once a ventricular beat is blocked, the cycle repeats itself with progressive lengthening of the PR intervals until another QRS complex is blocked. Think of the phrase, "longer, longer, longer, drop, now you have a Wenckebach." The rhythm appears on the ECG in a pattern of grouped beats. Ventricular rhythm is irregular. The P wave has a normal shape. The QRS complex has a normal shape and duration.

Clinical Significance. Type I AV block is usually a result of myocardial ischemia or inferior MI. It is generally transient and well tolerated. However, in some patients (e.g., acute MI) it may be a warning sign of a more serious AV conduction problem (e.g., complete heart block).

Treatment. A symptomatic patient may need atropine or a temporary pacemaker to increase HR, especially if the patient has had an MI. If the patient is asymptomatic, observe the rhythm closely and have a transcutaneous pacemaker on standby. Bradycardia is more likely to become symptomatic when hypotension, HF, or shock is present.

Second-Degree AV Block, Type II. In *type II second-degree AV block (Mobitz II heart block)*, a P wave is nonconducted without progressive PR lengthening. This usually occurs when a block in 1 of the bundle branches is present (Fig. 35.17, *C*). On conducted beats, the PR interval is constant. Type II second-degree AV block is a more serious type of block because a certain number of impulses from the SA node are not conducted to the ventricles. This occurs in ratios of 2:1, 3:1, and so on (i.e., 2 P waves to one QRS complex, 3 P waves to 1 QRS complex). It may occur with varying ratios.

Clinical Associations. Type II AV block is associated with rheumatic heart disease, CAD, anterior MI, and drug toxicity.

ECG Characteristics. Atrial rate is usually normal. Ventricular rate depends on the degree of AV block. Atrial rhythm is regular, but ventricular rhythm may be irregular. The P wave has a normal shape. The PR interval may be normal or prolonged in duration and remains constant on conducted beats. The QRS complex is usually greater than 0.12 second because of bundle branch block.

Clinical Significance. Type II AV block often progresses to third-degree AV block and is associated with a poor prognosis. The reduced HR often results in decreased CO with subsequent hypotension and myocardial ischemia. Type II AV block is an indication for a permanent pacemaker.

Treatment. Transcutaneous pacing or the insertion of a temporary pacemaker may be needed before inserting a permanent pacemaker if the patient becomes symptomatic (e.g., hypotension, angina).[1,11] (Temporary pacemakers are discussed on pp. 772–773.) Atropine is not an effective treatment.

Third-Degree AV Block. Third-degree AV block, or **complete heart block**, is a form of AV dissociation in which no impulses from the atria are conducted to the ventricles (Fig. 35.17, *D*). The atria are stimulated and contract independently of the ventricles. The ventricular rhythm is an escape rhythm. The ectopic pacemaker may be above or below the bifurcation of the bundle of His.

Clinical Associations. Third-degree AV block is associated with severe heart disease, including CAD, MI, myocarditis, cardiomyopathy, and some systemic diseases, such as scleroderma. Some drugs can cause third-degree AV block, such as digoxin, β-blockers, and calcium channel blockers.

ECG Characteristics. The atrial rate is usually a sinus rate of 60 to 100 beats/min. The ventricular rate depends on the site of the block. If it is in the AV node, the rate is 40 to 60 beats/min. If it is in the His-Purkinje system, it is 20 to 40 beats/min. Atrial and ventricular rhythms are regular but unrelated to each other. The P wave has a normal shape. The PR interval is variable. There is no relationship between the P wave and the QRS complex. The QRS complex is normal if the escape rhythm starts at the bundle of His or above. It is widened if the escape rhythm starts below the bundle of His.

Clinical Significance. Third-degree AV block usually results in reduced CO with subsequent ischemia, HF, and shock. Syncope from third-degree AV block may result from severe bradycardia or even periods of asystole.

Treatment. Symptomatic patients need a transcutaneous pacemaker until a temporary transvenous pacemaker can be inserted.[1,11] (Types of temporary pacemakers are discussed on pp. 772–773.) The use of drugs such as dopamine and epinephrine is an interim measure to increase HR and support BP until temporary pacing is started.[11] Patients need a permanent pacemaker as soon as possible. Atropine is not an effective treatment.

Premature Ventricular Contractions. A **premature ventricular contraction (PVC)** is a contraction coming from an ectopic focus in the ventricles. It is the premature (early) occurrence of a QRS complex. A PVC is wide and distorted in shape compared with a QRS complex coming down the normal conduction pathway (Fig. 35.18). PVCs that have the same shape are *unifocal*

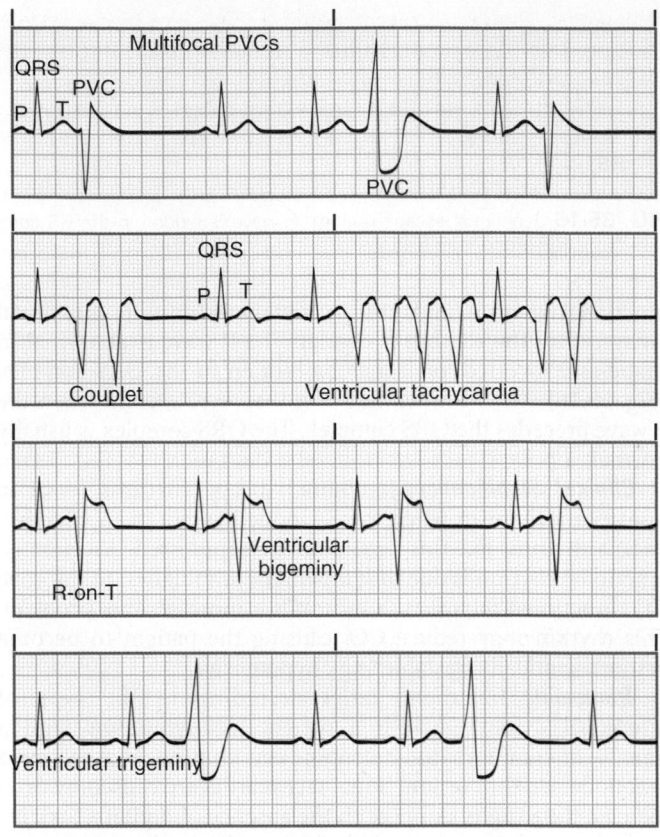

FIG. 35.18 Various types of premature ventricular contractions (PVCs).

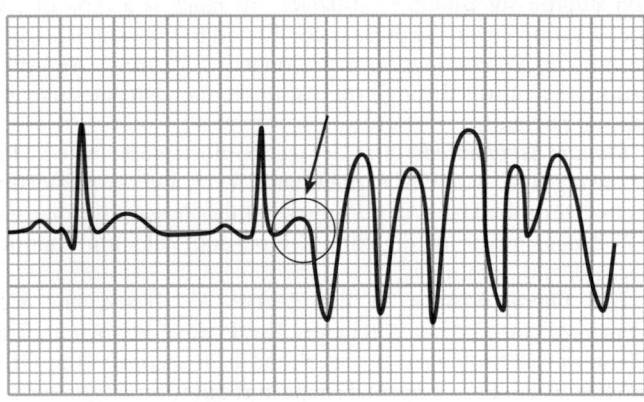

FIG. 35.19 R-on-T phenomenon. The "shock" occurred on the T wave leading to ventricular tachycardia.

PVCs. PVCs that arise from different foci appear different in shape from each other. These are *multifocal* PVCs. When every other beat is a PVC, the rhythm is called *ventricular bigeminy*. When every third beat is a PVC, it is called *ventricular trigeminy*. We call 2 consecutive PVCs a *couplet*.

Ventricular tachycardia (VT) occurs when there are 3 or more consecutive PVCs. *R-on-T phenomenon* occurs when a PVC falls on the T wave of a preceding beat (Fig. 35.19). This is especially dangerous because the PVC is firing during the relative refractory phase of ventricular repolarization. Excitability of the heart cells increases during this time, and the risk for the PVC to start VT or ventricular fibrillation (VF) is great.

Clinical Associations. PVCs are associated with stimulants, such as caffeine, alcohol, nicotine, aminophylline, epinephrine, and isoproterenol. They are also associated with electrolyte imbalances, hypoxia, fever, exercise, and emotional stress. Disease states associated with PVCs include MI, mitral valve prolapse, HF, cardiomyopathy, and CAD.

ECG Characteristics. HR varies according to intrinsic rate and number of PVCs. Rhythm is irregular because of premature beats. The P wave is rarely visible. It is usually lost in the QRS complex of the PVC. Retrograde conduction may occur with the P wave seen after the ectopic beat. The PR interval is not measurable. The QRS complex is wide and distorted in shape, lasting more than 0.12 second. The T wave is generally large and opposite in direction to the major direction of the QRS complex.

Clinical Significance. PVCs are usually not harmful in a patient with a normal heart. PVCs in CAD or acute MI indicate ventricular irritability. PVCs may reduce the CO and lead to angina and HF for those with heart disease, so assess the patient's physiologic response. Take the patient's apical-radial pulse rate and determine the pulse deficit, since PVCs often do not generate a sufficient ventricular contraction to result in a peripheral pulse.

Treatment. Treatment relates to the cause of the PVCs (e.g., O₂ therapy for hypoxia, electrolyte replacement). Assessing the patient's hemodynamic status is important to determine if treatment with drug therapy is needed. Drug therapy includes β-blockers, lidocaine, or amiodarone.

Accelerated Idioventricular Rhythm.
An *accelerated idioventricular rhythm* (AIVR) can develop when the intrinsic pacemaker (SA node or AV node) rate becomes less than that of a ventricular ectopic pacemaker. The rate is between 40 and 100 beats/min.

Clinical Associations. It is most often associated with acute MI and reperfusion of the myocardium after thrombolytic therapy or percutaneous coronary interventions (e.g., angioplasty). It can occur with digitalis toxicity.

Treatment. In the setting of acute MI, AIVR is usually self-limiting and well tolerated, and it needs no treatment. If the patient becomes symptomatic (e.g., hypotensive, chest pain), atropine is an option. Temporary pacing may be needed. Drugs that suppress ventricular rhythms (e.g., amiodarone) should not be used since they can further reduce the HR.

Ventricular Tachycardia.
A run of 3 or more PVCs defines **ventricular tachycardia (VT)**. It occurs when an ectopic focus or foci fire repeatedly and the ventricle takes control as the pacemaker. Different forms of VT exist, depending on QRS configuration. *Monomorphic* VT (Fig. 35.20, *A*) has QRS complexes that are the same in shape, size, and direction. *Polymorphic* VT occurs when the QRS complexes gradually change back and forth from one shape, size, and direction to another over a series of beats. *Torsades de pointes* (French for "twisting of the points") is polymorphic VT associated with a prolonged QT interval of the underlying rhythm (Fig. 35.20, *B*).

VT may be sustained (longer than 30 seconds) or nonsustained (less than 30 seconds). The development of VT is an ominous sign. It is a life-threatening dysrhythmia because of decreased CO and the possible development of VF, which is lethal.

Clinical Associations. VT is associated with MI, CAD, significant electrolyte imbalances, cardiomyopathy, long QT syndrome, drug toxicity, and central nervous system disorders. It can occur in patients who have no evidence of heart disease.

ECG Characteristics. Ventricular rate is 150 to 250 beats/min. Rhythm may be regular or irregular. AV dissociation may be present, with P waves occurring independently of the QRS complex. The atria may be depolarized by the ventricles in a retrograde fashion. The P wave is usually buried in the

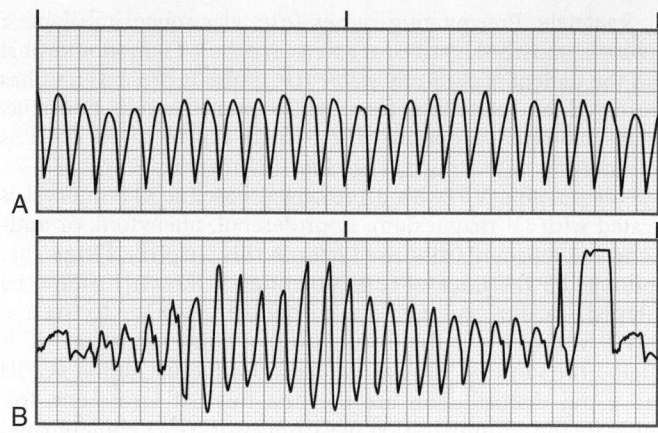

FIG. 35.20 Ventricular tachycardia. **A**, Monomorphic. **B**, Torsades de pointes (polymorphic).

QRS complex. The PR interval is not measurable. The QRS complex appears distorted and wide (greater than 0.12 second in duration). The T wave is in the opposite direction of the QRS complex (Fig. 35.20).

Clinical Significance. VT can be stable (patient has a pulse) or unstable (patient is pulseless). Sustained VT causes a severe decrease in CO because of decreased ventricular diastolic filling times and loss of atrial contraction. This results in hypotension, pulmonary edema, decreased cerebral blood flow, and cardiopulmonary arrest. VT must be treated quickly, even if it occurs only briefly and stops abruptly. Episodes may recur if prophylactic treatment is not started. VF may develop.

ETHICAL/LEGAL DILEMMAS
Scope and Standards of Practice

Situation

A young woman is admitted to the intensive care unit (ICU) after having several episodes of nonsustained VT credited to a history of viral cardiomyopathy. While she is being stabilized, she codes (pulseless VT) and needs intubation. A nurse anesthetist tries to intubate her 3 times unsuccessfully. There is an unforeseen delay in the arrival of the anesthesiologist. P.F., an ICU nurse who is a paramedic certified in advanced trauma life support (ATLS) and advanced cardiovascular life support (ACLS), tries to intubate the patient and does so successfully. The next day the nursing supervisor questions P.F. about intubating the patient since this is not within the scope of practice for an ICU nurse.

Ethical/Legal Points for Consideration

- The RN *Scope of Practice*, including rules and regulations that guide practice, are defined by individual state boards of nursing and can vary from state to state.
- Individual agencies have policies and procedures that describe the scope of practice for nurses. These can be more restrictive than those of the state.
- P.F. has had training, education, and certification beyond the usual nursing role.
- The life-threatening situation is an extenuating circumstance.
- Negligence may have been a factor if P.F., who is a nurse with training and experience, had not acted.

Discussion Questions

1. What would you have done in this situation?
2. How would you respond to the nursing supervisor?
3. What are the legal ramifications for P.F. in this situation?
4. What are the ethical issues in this situation?

Treatment. Precipitating causes (e.g., electrolyte imbalances, ischemia) must be identified and treated. If the VT is monomorphic and the patient is clinically stable (i.e., pulse is present) and has preserved left ventricular function, IV procainamide, lidocaine, or amiodarone are options. These drugs can be given if VT is polymorphic with a normal baseline QT interval.

Polymorphic VT with a prolonged baseline QT interval is treated with IV magnesium, isoproterenol, phenytoin, or anti-tachycardia pacing (discussed later in this chapter). Drugs that prolong the QT interval (e.g., dofetilide [Tikosyn]) should be stopped. Cardioversion is used if drug therapy is ineffective.

VT without a pulse is a life-threatening situation. It is treated the same as VF. Cardiopulmonary resuscitation (CPR) and rapid defibrillation are the first lines of treatment, followed by the administration of vasopressors (e.g., epinephrine) and antidysrhythmics (e.g., amiodarone) if defibrillation is unsuccessful.[11]

❓ CHECK YOUR PRACTICE

You are assigned to a 69-yr-old male patient on a telemetry unit who is recovering from colon surgery. He has a history of 2 MIs and he has 3 coronary stents in place. You hear his ECG monitor alarm and see what looks like ventricular tachycardia on the screen.
- What should you do?

Ventricular Fibrillation. Ventricular fibrillation (VF) is a severe derangement of the heart rhythm characterized on ECG by irregular waveforms of varying shapes and amplitude (Fig. 35.21). This represents the firing of multiple ectopic foci in the ventricle. Mechanically, the ventricle is simply "quivering," with no effective contraction, and so no CO occurs. VF is a lethal dysrhythmia.

Clinical Associations. VF occurs in acute MI and myocardial ischemia and in chronic diseases such as HF and cardiomyopathy. It may occur during cardiac pacing or cardiac catheterization procedures because of catheter stimulation of the ventricle. It may also occur with coronary reperfusion after thrombolytic therapy. Other causes are electric shock, hyperkalemia, hypoxemia, acidosis, and drug toxicity.

ECG Characteristics. HR is not measurable. Rhythm is irregular and chaotic. The P wave is not visible. The PR interval and the QRS interval are not measurable.

Clinical Significance. VF results in an unresponsive, pulseless, and apneic state. If VF is not treated quickly, the patient will not recover.

Treatment. Treatment consists of immediate initiation of CPR and ACLS with the use of defibrillation and definitive drug therapy (e.g., epinephrine, amiodarone). There should be no delay in starting chest compressions and using a defibrillator once available.

Asystole. Asystole is the total absence of ventricular electrical activity. Occasionally, P waves are seen. No ventricular contraction occurs because depolarization does not occur. Patients are unresponsive, pulseless, and apneic. Asystole is a lethal dysrhythmia that needs immediate treatment. VF may masquerade as asystole. Always assess the rhythm in more than 1 lead. The prognosis of a patient with asystole is extremely poor.

Clinical Associations. Asystole is usually a result of advanced heart disease, a severe cardiac conduction system problem, or end-stage HF.

Clinical Significance. Generally, the patient with asystole has end-stage heart disease or has a prolonged arrest and cannot be resuscitated.

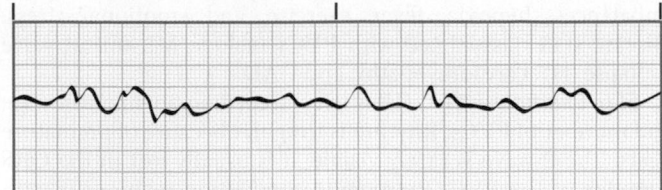

FIG. 35.21 Ventricular fibrillation.

Treatment. Treatment consists of CPR with ACLS measures. These include definitive drug therapy with epinephrine and intubation.

Pulseless Electrical Activity. *Pulseless electrical activity* (PEA) is a situation in which organized electrical activity is seen on the ECG, but there is no mechanical heart activity and the patient has no pulse. It is the most common dysrhythmia seen after defibrillation. Prognosis is poor unless the underlying cause is quickly identified and treated. Common causes of PEA include hypovolemia, hypoxia, metabolic acidosis, hyperkalemia, hypokalemia, hypoglycemia, hypothermia, toxins (e.g., drug overdose), cardiac tamponade, thrombosis (e.g., MI, pulmonary embolus), tension pneumothorax, and trauma. Treatment begins with CPR, followed by drug therapy (e.g., epinephrine) and intubation. Correcting the underlying cause is critical to prognosis.

Sudden Cardiac Death. The term *sudden cardiac death* (SCD) refers to death from a cardiac cause. Most SCDs result from ventricular dysrhythmias, specifically VT or VF. SCD is discussed in Chapter 33.

Prodysrhythmia. Antidysrhythmic drugs can cause life-threatening dysrhythmias similar to those for which they are treating. We call this a *prodysrhythmia*. The patient who has severe left ventricular dysfunction is the most susceptible to prodysrhythmias. Digoxin and class IA, IC, and III antidysrhythmic drugs can cause a prodysrhythmic response.[6] The first several days of drug therapy are the vulnerable period for developing prodysrhythmias. For this reason, many patients start oral antidysrhythmic drugs in a monitored hospital setting.

INTERPROFESSIONAL AND NURSING CARE: DYSRHYTHMIAS

Antidysrhythmic Drug Therapy

Table 35.9 shows antidysrhythmic drugs by their primary effects on the heart cells and the ECG.

Before giving any *antidysrhythmic drug*, perform a thorough assessment with a complete physical assessment, health history, and medication history. Assess for contraindications, cautions, and drug interactions. Obtain a baseline ECG. Assess vital signs, heart and lung sounds, and pulse rate, rhythm, and quality. Assess for signs and symptoms associated with decreased CO because of the dysrhythmia, such as restlessness, syncope, chest pain, dyspnea, and crackles. Review laboratory studies, including electrolytes, and liver and kidney function tests.

When giving antidysrhythmics, closely monitor the ECG and vital signs, especially BP and pulse rate. Continue to perform an ongoing physical assessment. Monitor laboratory studies as needed. Give specific instructions for each drug. Teach the patient that oral forms are often better tolerated if taken with food and fluids to help decrease GI upset. Tell patients to avoid alcohol, caffeine, and tobacco.

TABLE 35.9 Drug Therapy
Antidysrhythmic Drugs

Drug	Effects on the Action Potential	Effects on ECG
Class I: Sodium Channel Blockers	Decrease impulse conduction in the atria, ventricles, and His-Purkinje system	
Class IA	Delay repolarization	Widened QRS and prolonged QT interval
disopyramide (Norpace)		
procainamide		
quinidine		
Class IB	Accelerate repolarization	Little or no effect on ECG
lidocaine		
mexiletine		
phenytoin (Dilantin)		
Class IC	Decrease impulse conduction	Pronounced prodysrhythmic actions, widened QRS, prolonged QT interval
flecainide		
propafenone (Rythmol)		
Class II: β-Adrenergic Blockers	Decrease automaticity of the SA node, slow impulse conduction in AV node, reduce atrial and ventricular contractility	Bradycardia, prolonged PR interval, AV block
esmolol (Brevibloc)		
metoprolol (Lopressor)		
propranolol (Inderal)		
Class III: Potassium Channel Blockers	Delay repolarization, resulting in prolonged duration of action potential and refractory period	Prolonged PR and QT intervals, widened QRS, bradycardia
amiodarone		
dofetilide (Tikosyn)		
ibutilide (Corvert)		
sotalol* (Betapace)		
Class IV: Calcium Channel Blockers	Decrease automaticity of SA node, delay AV node conduction; reduce myocardial contractility	Bradycardia, prolonged PR interval, AV block
diltiazem (Cardizem)		
verapamil		
Other Agents		
adenosine (Adenocard)	Decrease conduction through AV node, reduce automaticity of SA node	Prolonged PR interval, AV block
digoxin (Lanoxin)		
dronedarone (Multaq)†	Suppress atrial dysrhythmias though mechanism is unknown	Prolonged QT interval
magnesium	Decrease impulse conduction through AV node	AV block

*Sotalol has both class II and class III properties.
†Dronedarone has class I through IV properties.

Defibrillation

Defibrillation is the treatment of choice to end VF and pulseless VT. It is most effective when the myocardial cells are not anoxic or acidotic. Rapid defibrillation (within 2 minutes) is critical to a successful patient outcome. Defibrillation involves the passage of an electric shock through the heart to depolarize the myocardial cells. The goal is that after repolarization, the SA node will be able to resume the role of pacemaker.

Defibrillators deliver energy using a monophasic or biphasic waveform. Monophasic defibrillators deliver energy in 1 direction. Biphasic defibrillators deliver energy in 2 directions (Fig. 35.22). The shocks delivered are at lower energies and with fewer post-shock dysrhythmias than monophasic defibrillators.

We measure the output of a defibrillator in *joules,* or watts per second. The recommended energy for initial shocks in defibrillation depends on the type of defibrillator. Biphasic defibrillators deliver the first and any successive shocks using 120 to 200 joules. Recommendations for monophasic defibrillators include an initial shock at 360 joules. After the first shock, start CPR immediately beginning with chest compressions.

We can perform rapid defibrillation using a manual or automatic device (Fig. 35.23). Manual defibrillators require you to interpret heart rhythms, determine the need for a shock, and deliver a shock. An **automatic external defibrillator (AED)** can detect heart rhythms and tell the user to deliver a shock using hands-free defibrillator pads. Proficiency in AED use is part of the basic life support course for health care professionals. Be familiar with the operation of the type of defibrillator used in your clinical setting.

The following general steps are taken for defibrillation: (1) continue CPR until the defibrillator is charged; (2) turn the defibrillator on, and select the proper energy level; (3) check to see that the synchronizer switch is turned off (discussed later); (4) apply conductive materials (e.g., defibrillator gel pads) to the chest, one to the right of the sternum just below the clavicle, and the other to the left of the apex; (5) charge the defibrillator using the button on the defibrillator or the paddles; (6) position the paddles firmly on the chest wall over the conductive material (Fig. 35.22); (7) call and look to see that everyone is "all clear" to ensure that staff are not touching the patient or the bed at the time of discharge; and (8) deliver the charge by depressing buttons on both paddles simultaneously.

Hands-free, multifunction defibrillator pads are available. We place them on the chest as described earlier. Hands-free pads decrease the risk for injury compared to paddles. Connect the cables from the pads to the defibrillator. Charge and discharge the defibrillator using buttons on the defibrillator. It is still essential to ensure that all staff are clear before discharging the defibrillator.

> **! SAFETY ALERT Defibrillation and Cardioversion**
> - Check that the synchronizer switch is OFF for defibrillation.
> - Turn the synchronizer switch ON for a cardioversion.
> - Never apply defibrillator pads over a pacemaker or implantable cardioverter-defibrillator.
> - Be certain that personnel are "all clear" before discharging the device.

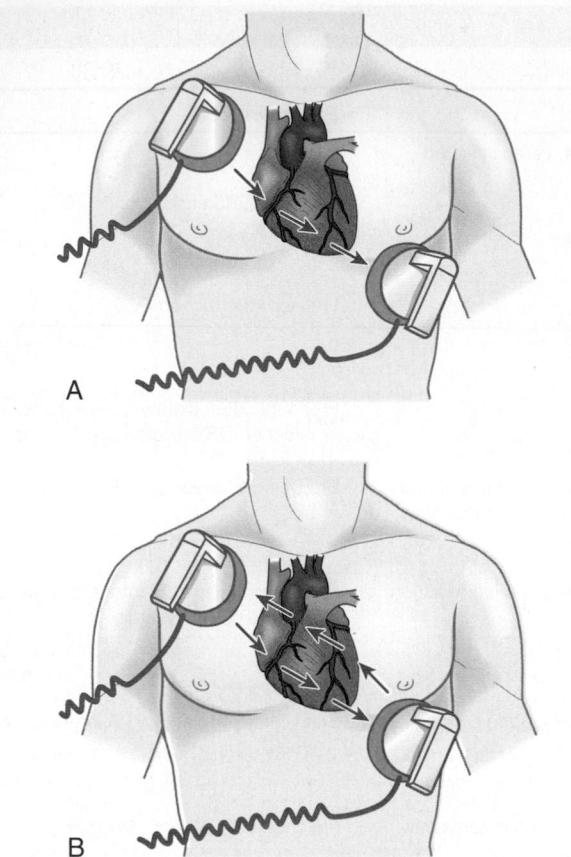

FIG. 35.22 Paddle placement and current flow in monophasic defibrillation (A) and biphasic defibrillation (B).

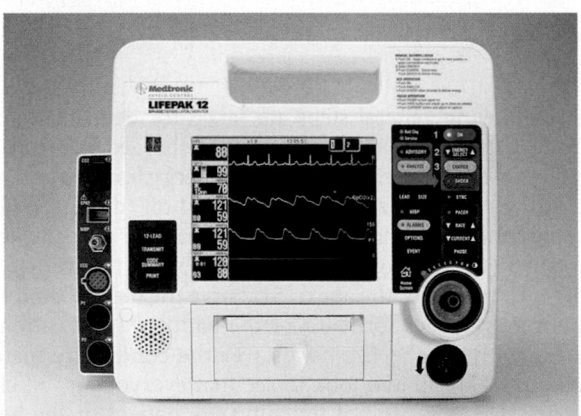

FIG. 35.23 LifePak contains a monitor, defibrillator, and transcutaneous pacemaker. (Courtesy Medtronic Physio-Control, Redmond, Wash.)

Synchronized Cardioversion. *Synchronized cardioversion* is the therapy of choice for the patient with ventricular tachydysrhythmias (e.g., VT with a pulse) or supraventricular tachydysrhythmias (e.g., atrial flutter with a rapid ventricular response). A synchronized circuit in the defibrillator delivers a shock on the R wave of the QRS complex of the ECG. The synchronizer switch must be turned on when performing cardioversion.

The procedure for synchronized cardioversion is the same as for defibrillation with a few exceptions (Table 35.10). If synchronized cardioversion is done on a nonemergency basis (i.e., the patient is awake and hemodynamically stable), we sedate the patient with IV agents (e.g., midazolam, fentanyl) beforehand.

TABLE 35.10 Nursing Management

Assisting With Cardioversion

Preprocedure
- Obtain 12-lead ECG and initiate ECG monitoring.
- Perform baseline assessment, including vital signs, pulse oximetry, noting any manifestations of the dysrhythmia.
- Withhold food and fluids per institution policy.
- Assess baseline laboratory values (e.g., cardiac biomarkers, electrolytes).
- Teach patient and caregiver about procedure and postprocedure care.
- Remove all metallic objects, dentures, and transdermal patches. Clipping or removing chest hair may be needed.
- Establish IV access.
- Give sedative and other drugs, as ordered.

Postprocedure
- Maintain patent airway and administer O_2 as needed.
- Monitor ECG for dysrhythmias or other changes (e.g., ST segment elevation).
- Perform assessment and compare to baseline: vital signs, pulse oximetry, and heart and breath sounds.
- Assess level of consciousness and reorient as needed.
- Administer IV dysrhythmic and analgesic medications as ordered.
- Assess for burns and provide skin care.

Strict attention to maintaining the patient's airway is critical. If a patient with supraventricular tachycardia or VT with a pulse becomes hemodynamically unstable, synchronized cardioversion should be done as quickly as possible. Start the initial energy for synchronized cardioversion at 50 to 100 joules (biphasic defibrillator) and 100 joules (monophasic defibrillator) and increase if needed. If the patient becomes pulseless or the rhythm changes to VF, turn the synchronizer switch off and perform defibrillation.

Implantable Cardioverter-Defibrillator. The *implantable cardioverter-defibrillator* (ICD) is an important technology for patients who (1) have survived SCD, (2) have spontaneous sustained VT, (3) have syncope with inducible VT or VF during EPS, or (4) are at high risk for future life-threatening dysrhythmias (e.g., have cardiomyopathy). The use of ICDs has significantly decreased mortality rates in these patients.[12]

The ICD consists of a lead system placed via a subclavian vein to the endocardium. A battery-powered pulse generator is implanted subcutaneously, usually over the pectoral muscle on the patient's nondominant side. The pulse generator is similar in size to a pacemaker. Most systems are single-lead systems (Fig. 35.24). The ICD sensing system monitors the HR and rhythm and identifies VT or VF. After the sensing system detects a lethal dysrhythmia, the device delivers a 25-joule or less shock to the patient's heart. If the first shock is unsuccessful, the device recycles and can continue to deliver shocks.

In addition to defibrillation capabilities, ICDs have *antitachycardia* and *antibradycardia pacing* capabilities. These devices use algorithms that detect dysrhythmias and determine the appropriate response. They can start *overdrive pacing* of supraventricular tachycardia and VT, sparing the patient painful defibrillator shocks. They can provide backup pacing for bradydysrhythmias that may occur after defibrillation. Nursing care of the patient undergoing ICD placement is similar to the care of a patient undergoing permanent pacemaker implantation (see p. 771).

Patients with structural or congenital cardiac anomalies may receive a totally subcutaneous ICD (S-ICD).[13] The S-ICD pulse

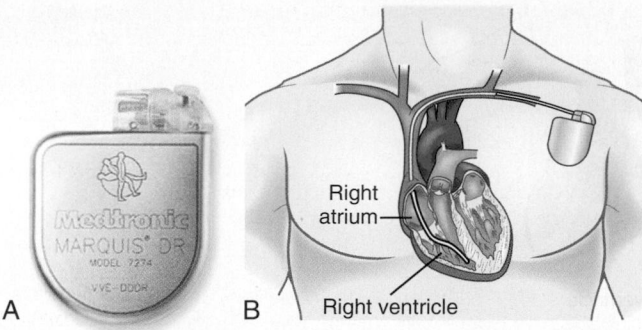

FIG. 35.24 A, The implantable cardioverter-defibrillator (ICD) pulse generator from Medtronic, Inc. (Courtesy Medtronic, Inc., Minneapolis, Minn.) B, The ICD is placed in a subcutaneous pocket over the pectoral muscle. A single-lead system is placed transvenously from the pulse generator to the endocardium. The single lead detects dysrhythmias and delivers an electric shock to the heart muscle.

generator is placed under the skin on the left side of the chest with the electrode under the skin above the sternum. The system delivers a shock if it detects VT or VF. Since the S-ICD does not have any electrodes implanted in the heart, it has no pacing capability.[13]

Teaching the patient who is receiving an ICD and the caregiver is extremely important. Patients may have a variety of emotions, including fear of body image change, fear of recurrent dysrhythmias, expectation of pain with ICD discharge (described as a feeling of a blow to the chest), and anxiety about going home. Encourage patients and caregivers to take part in local or online ICD support groups.[14] Table 35.11 presents a teaching guide for the patient with an ICD and the caregiver.

Pacemakers

The artificial **cardiac pacemaker** is an electronic device used to pace the heart when the normal conduction pathway is damaged. The basic pacing circuit consists of a power source (battery-powered pulse generator) with programmable circuitry, 1 or more pacing leads, and the myocardium. The electrical signal (stimulus) travels from the pulse generator, through the leads, to the wall of the myocardium. The heart muscle is "captured" and stimulated to contract (Fig. 35.25).

Current pacemakers are small, sophisticated, and physiologically precise. They pace the atrium and/or 1 or both ventricles. Most pacemakers are *demand pacemakers*. This means that they sense the heart's electrical activity and fire only when the HR drops below a preset rate. Demand pacemakers have 2 distinct features: (1) a sensing device that inhibits the pacemaker when the HR is adequate and (2) a pacing device that triggers the pacemaker when no QRS complexes occur within a preset time.[1]

In addition to antibradycardia pacing, devices now include antitachycardia and overdrive pacing. *Antitachycardia pacing* involves the delivery of a stimulus to the ventricle to end tachydysrhythmias (e.g., VT). Overdrive pacing involves pacing the atrium at rates of 200 to 500 impulses per minute to try to stop atrial tachycardias (e.g., atrial flutter with a rapid ventricular response).[15,16]

Permanent Pacemaker. A *permanent pacemaker* is totally implanted within the body (Fig. 35.26). The power source is placed subcutaneously, usually over the pectoral muscle on the patient's nondominant side. The pacing leads are placed

---

TABLE 35.11 Patient & Caregiver Teaching

Implantable Cardioverter-Defibrillator (ICD)

Include the following information in the teaching plan for a patient receiving an ICD and the patient's caregiver:

1. Follow up with your HCP for routine checks of the function of the ICD. This is often done by interrogating the device using a telephone.
2. Report any signs of infection at incision site (e.g., redness, swelling, drainage) or fever to your HCP at once.
3. Keep incision dry for 4 days after insertion or as instructed.
4. Avoid lifting arm on ICD side above shoulder until approved.
5. Discuss resuming sexual activity with your HCP. It is usually safe to resume sexual activity once your incision is healed.
6. Do not drive until cleared by your HCP. This decision is usually based on the ongoing presence of dysrhythmias, the frequency of ICD firings, your overall health, and state laws about drivers with ICDs.
7. Avoid direct blows to ICD site.
8. Avoid large magnets and strong electromagnetic fields because these may interfere with the device.
9. You should not have an MRI unless the ICD is approved as MRI safe or there is a protocol in place for patient safety during the procedure.
10. Travel is not restricted. Tell security (e.g., airport, train station, public buildings) of presence of ICD because it may set off the metal detector. If hand-held screening wand is used, it should not be placed directly over the ICD. Manufacturer information may vary about the effect of metal detectors on the function of the ICD.
11. Do not stand near antitheft devices in doorways of stores and public buildings. You should walk through them at a normal pace.
12. If your ICD fires once, call your HCP right away. If you feel sick or if it fires more than once, contact the emergency response system.
13. You should always wear a Medic Alert ID device.
14. Always carry the ICD identification card and a current list of your drugs.
15. Consider joining an ICD support group (e.g., *www.icdsupportgroup. org/*).
16. Caregivers should learn cardiopulmonary resuscitation (CPR).

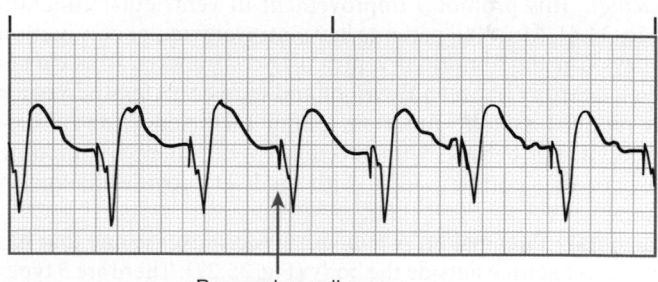

Pacemaker spike

FIG. 35.25 Ventricular capture (depolarization) secondary to signal *(pacemaker spike)* from pacemaker lead in the right ventricle.

transvenously to the right atrium and/or 1 or both ventricles and attached to the power source. Common reasons for insertion of a permanent pacemaker are found in Table 35.12.

New technology and research are focused on miniaturized, leadless permanent pacemakers. Single-component devices have the battery, sensors, electronics, and stimulating electrodes in a small capsule that is placed in the ventricle using a deflatable sheath. A multicomponent device has a small "seed" that is placed in a cardiac chamber. It acts as an energy transducer while an outside piece beams ultrasound (or radio waves) to the seed. The seed converts the energy to a pacing pulse.[15] The lack of a transvenous lead and subcutaneous pulse generator is

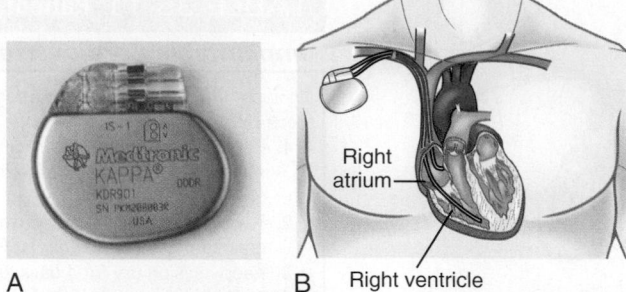

A   B   Right ventricle

Right
atrium

FIG. 35.26 A, A dual-chamber rate-responsive pacemaker from Medtronic, Inc., is designed to treat patients with chronic heart problems in which the heart beats too slowly to support the body's circulation needs. (Courtesy Medtronic, Inc., Minneapolis, Minn.) B, Pacing leads in both the atrium and the ventricle enable a dual-chamber pacemaker to sense and pace in both heart chambers.

TABLE 35.12 Indications for Permanent Pacemakers

- Acquired AV block
- Second-degree AV block
- Third-degree AV block
- Atrial fibrillation with a slow ventricular response
- Bundle branch block
- Cardiomyopathy
  - Dilated
  - Hypertrophic
- HF
- SA node dysfunction
- Symptomatic bradycardia with unknown cause
- Tachydysrhythmias (e.g., ventricular tachycardia)

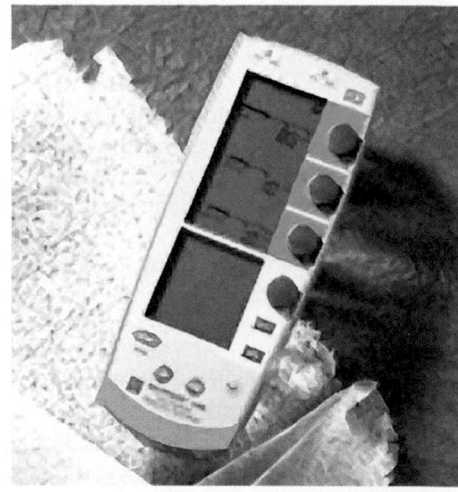

FIG. 35.27 Temporary external, dual-chamber demand pacemaker. (Courtesy Medtronic, Inc., Minneapolis, Minn.)

TABLE 35.13 Common Indications for Temporary Pacemakers

- Maintain adequate HR and rhythm during special circumstances
  - During surgery and postoperative recovery
  - During cardiac catheterization or coronary angioplasty
  - With drug therapy that may cause bradycardia
  - Before implantation of a permanent pacemaker
- Prophylaxis after open heart surgery
- Acute anterior MI with second- or third-degree AV block or bundle branch block
- Acute inferior MI with symptomatic bradycardia and AV block
- EPS to evaluate patient with bradydysrhythmias and tachydysrhythmias

a major shift in cardiac pacing.[16] Other research is focusing on making permanent pacemakers without batteries.

Cardiac Resynchronization Therapy. *Cardiac resynchronization therapy* (CRT) is a pacing technique that resynchronizes the heart cycle by pacing both ventricles *(biventricular pacing).* This promotes improvement in ventricular function (Fig. 34.4). Most HF patients have intraventricular conduction delays causing abnormal ventricular contraction. This causes dyssynchrony between the right and left ventricles and results in reduced systolic function, pump inefficiency, and worsened HF. For patients with severe left ventricular dysfunction, devices that combine CRT with an ICD provide maximum therapy.[15,16]

Temporary Pacemaker. A *temporary pacemaker* is one that has the power source outside the body (Fig. 35.27). There are 3 types of temporary pacemakers: transvenous, epicardial, and transcutaneous. Table 35.13 lists common reasons for temporary pacing.

A *transvenous pacemaker* consists of a lead or leads that are threaded transvenously to the right atrium and/or right ventricle and attached to the external power source (Fig. 35.28). Most of these pacemakers are inserted in the ED or ICU in emergency situations. They provide a bridge to insertion of a permanent pacemaker or until the underlying cause of the dysrhythmia is resolved.

Epicardial pacing involves attaching an atrial and ventricular pacing lead to the epicardium during heart surgery. The leads are passed through the chest wall and attached to the external power source. Epicardial pacing leads are placed prophylactically in case a bradydysrhythmia or tachydysrhythmia occurs in the early postoperative period.[15,16]

A *transcutaneous pacemaker* (TCP) can provide adequate HR and rhythm to the patient in an emergency. Placement of a TCP is a noninvasive, temporary procedure used until a transvenous pacemaker can be inserted or more definitive therapy is available.[1,11]

The TCP consists of a power source and a rate- and voltage-control device that attaches to 2 large, multifunction electrode pads. Position 1 pad on the anterior part of the chest, usually on the V_4 lead position, and the other pad on the back between the spine and left scapula at the level of the heart (Fig. 35.29). When programming the TCP, use the lowest current that results in a ventricular contraction (capture) to minimize patient discomfort.

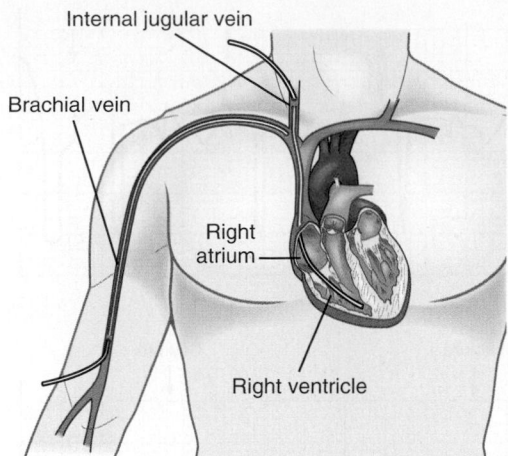

FIG. 35.28 Temporary transvenous pacemaker catheter insertion. A single lead is positioned in the right ventricle through the brachial, subclavian, jugular, or femoral vein.

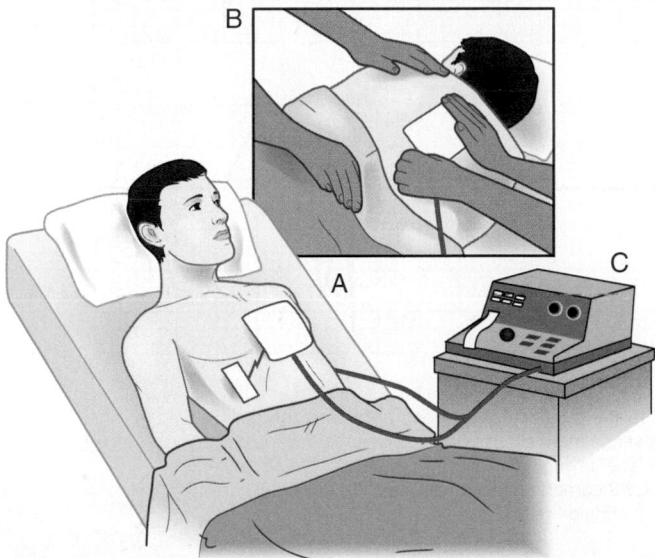

FIG. 35.29 Transcutaneous pacemaker. Pacing electrodes are placed on the patient's anterior (A) and posterior (B) chest walls and attached to an external pacing unit (C).

Before starting TCP therapy, it is important to tell the patient what to expect. Explain that the muscle contractions created by the pacemaker when the current passes through the chest wall are uncomfortable. Reassure the patient that the TCP is temporary, and that it will be replaced by a transvenous pacemaker as soon as possible. Whenever possible, provide analgesia and/or sedation while the TCP is in use.

Monitoring of Patients With Pacemakers. Patients with temporary or permanent pacemakers are ECG monitored to evaluate the status of the pacemaker. Pacemaker malfunction involves a failure to sense, a failure to capture, or a failure to pace. *Failure to sense* occurs when the pacemaker does not recognize spontaneous atrial or ventricular activity, and it fires inappropriately (Fig. 35.30, A). This can result in the pacemaker firing during the excitable period of the cardiac cycle, resulting in VT. Failure to sense is caused by fibrosis around the tip of the pacing lead, battery failure, sensing set too high, or dislodgment of the electrode.

Failure to capture occurs when the electrical charge to the myocardium is insufficient to produce atrial or ventricular contraction (Fig. 35.30, B). This can result in serious bradycardia or asystole. Failure to capture is caused by pacer lead damage, battery failure, dislodgment of the electrode, electrical charge set too low, or fibrosis at the electrode tip.

Failure to pace occurs when the pacemaker does not initiate an electrical stimulus when it should fire (Fig. 35.30, C). This can happen from a wire fracture, lead displacement, oversensing, or electrical interference. Table 35.14 describes pacemaker troubleshooting.

Complications of invasive temporary (i.e., transvenous) or permanent pacemaker insertion include infection and hematoma formation at the insertion site, pneumothorax, failure to sense or capture, perforation of the atrial or ventricular septum by the pacing lead, and appearance of "end-of-life" battery power on testing the pacemaker. Several measures can prevent or assess for complications. These include prophylactic IV antibiotic therapy before and after insertion, postinsertion chest x-ray to check lead placement and to rule out a pneumothorax, careful observation of insertion site, and continuous ECG monitoring of the patient's rhythm.

After pacemaker insertion, the patient can be out of bed once stable. Have the patient limit arm and shoulder activity on the operative side to prevent dislodging the newly implanted pacing leads. Observe the insertion site for signs of bleeding and check that the incision is intact. Note any temperature elevation or pain at the insertion site and treat as ordered. Most patients are discharged by the next day if stable.

Table 35.15 outlines patient and caregiver teaching for the patient with a pacemaker. The patient with a newly implanted pacemaker and the caregiver may have questions about activity restrictions and concerns about body image. The goals of pacemaker therapy include enhancing physiologic functioning and quality of life. Emphasize this to the patient and caregiver and provide specific advice on activity restrictions.

After discharge, patients need to check pacemaker function on a regular basis. This can include outpatient visits to a pacemaker clinic or home monitoring using telephone transmitter devices. Another method to evaluate pacemaker performance is noninvasive program stimulation. This procedure is done on an outpatient basis in the EPS laboratory.

Radiofrequency Catheter Ablation Therapy

Radiofrequency catheter ablation therapy uses electrical energy to "burn" or ablate areas of the conduction system. Ablation therapy is done after EPS has identified the source of the dysrhythmia. An electrode-tipped ablation catheter ablates accessory pathways or ectopic sites in the atria, AV node, and ventricles. Catheter ablation is a definitive treatment for tachydysrhythmias. It is the nonpharmacologic treatment of choice for atrial dysrhythmias resulting in rapid ventricular rates and AV nodal reentrant tachycardia refractory to drug therapy.[8]

The ablation procedure is an effective treatment with a low complication rate. Nursing care of the patient after ablation therapy is similar to that of a patient undergoing cardiac catheterization (see Chapter 31 and Table 31.9).

SYNCOPE

Syncope is a brief lapse in consciousness accompanied by a loss in postural tone (fainting). The causes of syncope can

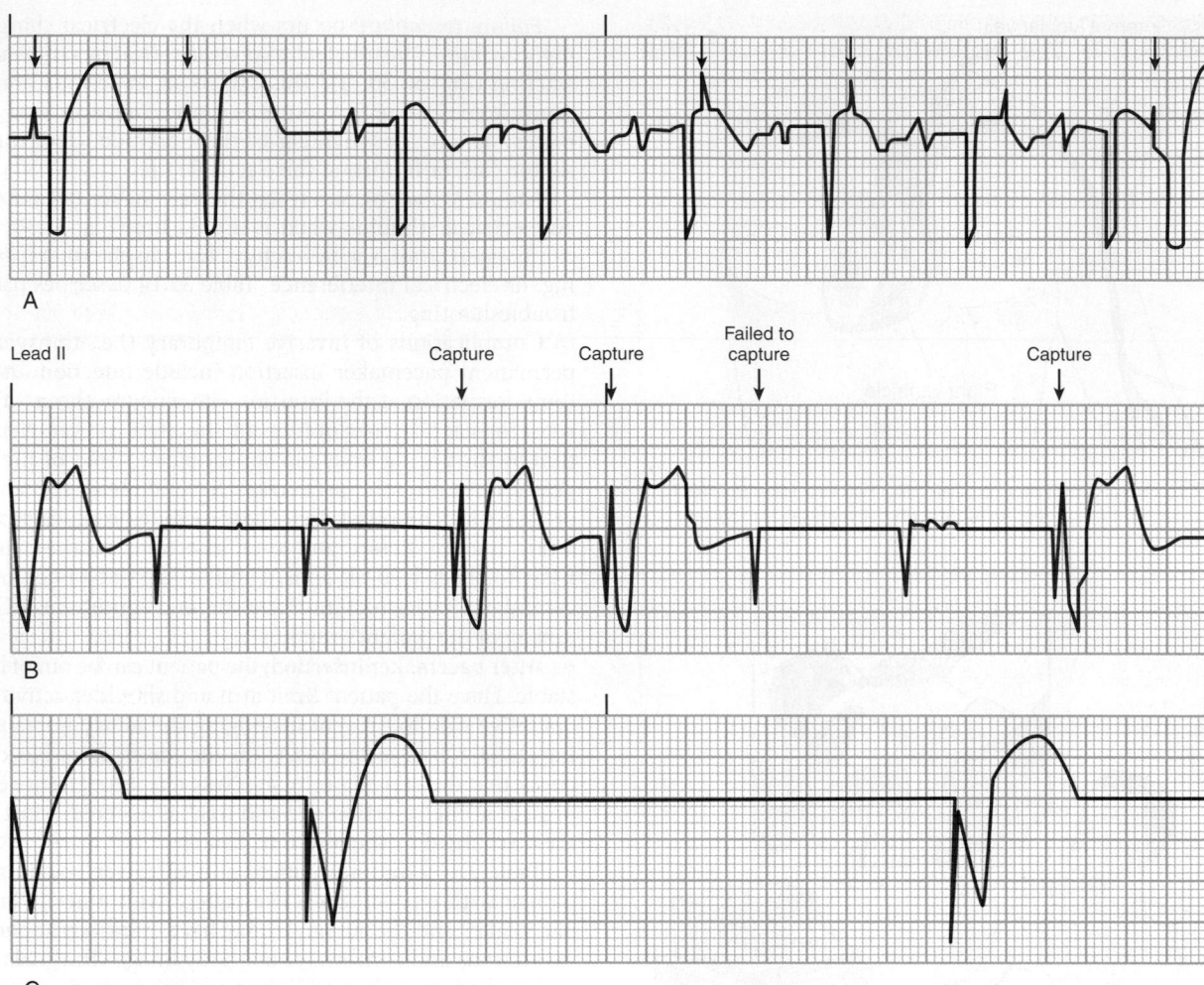

FIG. 35.30 Causes of pacemaker malfunction. **A,** Failure to sense: the pacemaker does not sense the patient's own cardiac rhythm and initiates an electrical impulse. Failure to sense manifests as pacer spikes that fall too closely to the patient's own rhythm, earlier than the programmed rate (see *arrows*). **B,** Failure to capture: a pacer spike is noted but is not followed by a P wave (atrial pacemaker) or a QRS complex (ventricular pacemaker). **C,** Failure to pace: the pacemaker fails to initiate an electrical stimulus when it should fire.

TABLE 35.14 Nursing Management

Troubleshooting Pacemakers

Problem	Potential Solution
Identified initial concern about pacemaker function	• Monitor continuous ECG and patient's vital signs while troubleshooting pacemaker problems • Call emergency response services if needed • Contact HCP immediately if basic troubleshooting does not work, as patient could have a lead wire displaced or a defective lead wire
Temporary pacemaker not firing	• Check to make sure all connections are hooked up correctly and tight • Ensure that hands-free pads have contact with the skin (shave excess hair, dry off perspiration) • Check that the generator has power (plug in the equipment or use a new battery each time)
Temporary pacemaker not capturing	• Check connections • Check for generator power • Turn up the milliamps on the generator, look for capture and set 10 milliamps above capture • Place patient on left side to promote contact of the transvenous pacing wire with the epicardium
Temporary pacemaker not sensing patient's underlying rhythm	• Check connections • Check for generator power • Turn up sensitivity • Place patient on left side
Permanent pacemaker not working	• Contact HCP • Contact pacemaker company for service if requested by HCP

TABLE 35.15 Patient & Caregiver Teaching

Pacemaker

Include the following information in the teaching plan for a patient with a pacemaker and the patient's caregiver:

1. Maintain follow-up care with your HCP to begin regular pacemaker function checks. This is often done by checking the device using a telephone.
2. Report any signs of infection at incision site (e.g., redness, swelling, drainage) or fever to your HCP at once.
3. Keep incision dry for 4 days after implantation, or as ordered.
4. Avoid lifting arm on pacemaker side above shoulder until approved by your cardiologist.
5. Avoid direct blows to pacemaker site.
6. Avoid close proximity to high-output electric generators since these can interfere with the function of the pacemaker.
7. You should not have an MRI unless the pacemaker is approved as MRI safe or there is a protocol in place for patient safety during the procedure.
8. Microwave ovens are safe to use and do not interfere with pacemaker function.
9. Avoid standing near antitheft devices in doorways of department stores and public libraries. You should walk through them at a normal pace.
10. Travel is not restricted. Tell security (e.g., airport, train station, public buildings) of presence of pacemaker because it may set off the metal detector. If hand-held screening wand is used, it should not be placed directly over the pacemaker. Manufacturer information may vary about the effect of metal detectors on the function of the pacemaker.
11. Monitor pulse and tell your HCP if heart rate drops below predetermined rate.
12. Always carry your pacemaker information card and a current list of drugs.
13. Always wear a Medic Alert ID device.
14. Consider joining a pacemaker support group (e.g., *www.pacemakerclub.com/*).

be cardiovascular or noncardiovascular. The most common cause of syncope is cardioneurogenic syncope, or "vasovagal" syncope (e.g., carotid sinus sensitivity). Other cardiovascular causes relate to dysrhythmias (e.g., tachycardias, bradycardias), prosthetic valve malfunction, pulmonary emboli, and HF. Noncardiovascular causes vary and include stress, hypoglycemia, dehydration, stroke, and seizure.[17]

A diagnostic workup for a patient with syncope from a suspected heart cause begins with ruling out structural and ischemic heart disease. This is done with echocardiography and stress testing. EPS is used to diagnose atrial and ventricular tachydysrhythmias and conduction problems causing bradydysrhythmias, all of which can cause syncope. These problems can be treated with antidysrhythmic drug therapy, pacemakers, ICDs, and/or catheter ablation therapy.

A patient without structural heart disease or in whom EPS testing is not diagnostic may have a *head-up tilt-test*. Normally, an upright position results in gravity displacing 300 to 800 mL of blood to the lower extremities. Specialized nerve fibers called mechanoreceptors are found throughout the vascular system. These respond to the increased blood volume by starting a reflex increase in sympathetic stimulation and decrease in parasympathetic output. The end results are a slight increase in HR and diastolic BP, and a slight decrease in systolic BP.[17,18]

In cardioneurogenic syncope, the increase in venous pooling that occurs in the upright position reduces venous return to the heart. This results in a sudden, compensatory increase in ventricular contraction. The brain mistakenly thinks this is a hypertensive state and stops sympathetic stimulation. This produces a paradoxical vasodilation and bradycardia (vasovagal response). The end results are bradycardia, hypotension, cerebral hypoperfusion, and syncope.

In the head-up tilt-test the patient is placed on a table supported by a belt across the torso and feet. Baseline ECG, BP, and HR are obtained in the horizontal position. Next, the table is tilted 60 to 80 degrees and the patient is kept in this upright position for 20 to 60 minutes. ECG and HR are recorded continuously. BP is measured every 3 minutes throughout the test.

If the patient's BP and HR responses are abnormal and clinical symptoms occur (e.g., faintness), the test is positive. If after 30 minutes there is no response, the table is returned to the horizontal position and an IV infusion of low-dose isoproterenol may be started to try to provoke a response.

Other diagnostic tests for syncope can include various recording devices (e.g., Holter monitor or event monitor/loop recorder, discussed in Chapter 31 and Table 31.7), blood volume determination, hemodynamic testing, and autonomic reflex testing. About 30% of those who have 1 episode of syncope have a recurrence. The underlying cause of syncope and the patient's age and co-morbidities affect the patient's treatment and prognosis.[17,18]

CASE STUDY

Dysrhythmia and Cardiac Arrest

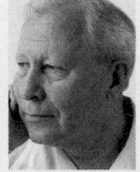
(© iStockphoto/ Thinkstock.)

Patient Profile

J.M., a 68-yr-old white, retired postal worker, was admitted to the telemetry unit with a diagnosis of acute decompensated heart failure (ADHF). He had a cardiac arrest (pulseless ventricular tachycardia [VT]) and was successfully defibrillated after 1 shock. He was transferred to the cardiac care unit. J.M. is awake but lethargic and responds appropriately to questions.

Subjective Data

- History of hypertension, CAD, 2 MIs, and chronic HF
- Reports shortness of breath at rest and in an upright position

Objective Data

Physical Examination

- Appears weak, anxious
- BP 102/60 mm Hg, pulse 70/min, respirations 26/min
- Lungs: bilateral coarse crackles in the bases
- Heart: S_3 gallop at apex

Diagnostic Studies

- Echocardiogram: severe left ventricular dysfunction with ejection fraction of 24%
- Serum potassium: 2.9 mEq/L (2.9 mmol/L)
- Serum cardiac biomarkers: negative
- Serum b-type natriuretic peptide (BNP): 1852 pg/mL

CASE STUDY—cont'd

Dysrhythmia and Cardiac Arrest

Interprofessional Care

- Continuous ECG monitoring

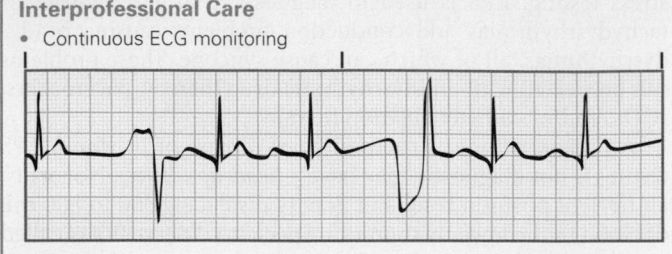

- Amiodarone infusion
- Cardiac rehabilitation consult
- Dietary consult

Discussion Questions

1. Why is J.M. at risk for sudden cardiac death?
2. Explain the reason for using amiodarone after cardiac arrest.
3. What methods are used to assess the effectiveness of the antidysrhythmic therapy?
4. Interpret the rhythm strip.
5. Explain the significance of the diagnostic studies and other interprofessional care orders.
6. Why would J.M. be a candidate for CRT and an ICD?
7. **Priority Decision:** Based on the assessment data provided, what are the priority nursing diagnoses?
8. **Priority Decision:** What are the priority nursing interventions for J.M.?
9. **Collaboration:** Which tasks could be delegated to UAP?
10. **Evidence-Based Practice:** Once J.M. is stable, he is scheduled for the insertion of a CRT/ICD. On your rounds, he asks you why he needs 2 devices. How would you respond?

Answers available at *http://evolve.elsevier.com/Lewis/medsurg.*

BRIDGE TO NCLEX EXAMINATION

The number of the question corresponds to the same-numbered outcome at the beginning of the chapter.

1. A patient admitted with syncope has continuous ECG monitoring. An examination of the rhythm strip reveals the following: atrial rate 74 beats/min and regular; ventricular rate 62 beats/min and irregular; P wave normal shape; PR interval lengthens progressively until a P wave is not conducted; QRS normal shape. The *priority* nursing intervention would be to
   a. give epinephrine 1 mg IV push.
   b. prepare for synchronized cardioversion.
   c. observe for symptoms of hypotension or angina.
   d. apply transcutaneous pacemaker pads on the patient.

2. The ECG monitor of a patient in the cardiac care unit after an MI shows ventricular bigeminy with a rate of 50 beats/min. The nurse would
   a. perform defibrillation.
   b. administer IV amiodarone.
   c. prepare for temporary pacemaker insertion.
   d. assess the patient's response to the dysrhythmia.

3. In the patient with supraventricular tachycardia, which assessment indicates decreased cardiac output?
   a. Hypertension and dyspnea
   b. Chest pain and palpitations
   c. Abdominal distention and tachypnea
   d. Bounding pulses and a systolic murmur

4. The nurse prepares a patient for synchronized cardioversion knowing that cardioversion differs from defibrillation in that
   a. defibrillation delivers a lower dose of electrical energy.
   b. cardioversion is a treatment for atrial bradydysrhythmias.
   c. defibrillation is synchronized to deliver a shock during the QRS complex.
   d. patients should be sedated if cardioversion is done on a nonemergency basis.

5. Which patient teaching points should the nurse include when providing discharge instructions to a patient with a new permanent pacemaker and the caregiver? *(select all that apply)*
   a. Avoid or limit air travel.
   b. Take and record a daily pulse rate.
   c. Obtain and wear a Medic Alert ID device at all times.
   d. Avoid lifting arm on the side of the pacemaker above shoulder.
   e. Do not use a microwave oven because it interferes with pacemaker function.

6. Important teaching for the patient scheduled for a radiofrequency catheter ablation procedure includes explaining that
   a. ventricular bradycardia may be induced and treated during the procedure.
   b. catheter will be placed in both femoral arteries to allow double-catheter use.
   c. the procedure will destroy areas of the conduction system that are causing rapid heart rhythms.
   d. general anesthetic will be given to prevent the awareness of any "sudden cardiac death" experiences.

1. c, 2. d, 3. b, 4. d, 5. b, c, d, 6. c

For rationales to these answers and even more NCLEX review questions, visit *http://evolve.elsevier.com/Lewis/medsurg.*

Ⓔ EVOLVE WEBSITE/RESOURCES LIST

http://evolve.elsevier.com/Lewis/medsurg
Review Questions (Online Only)
Key Points
Answer Keys for Questions
- Rationales for Bridge to NCLEX Examination Questions
- Answer Guidelines for Case Study on p. 775
Case Study
- Patient With Atrial Fibrillation
Conceptual Care Map Creator
Audio Glossary
Content Updates

REFERENCES

1. Sole ML, Klein DG, Moseley MJ: *Introduction to critical care nursing*, ed 7, St Louis, 2017, Elsevier.
2. Wesley K: *Huszar's ECG and 12-lead interpretation*, ed5, St Louis, 2017, Elsevier.
3. Franciosi S, Perry FK, Roston TM, et al: The role of the autonomic nervous system in arrhythmias and sudden cardiac death, *Auton Neurosci-Basic* 205:1, 2017.
*4. American Association of Critical-Care Nurses: AACN practice alert: Ensuring accurate ST-segment monitoring. Retrieved from *www.aacn.org/~/media/aacn-website/clincial-resources/practice-alerts/stsegmentmonitoring.pdf*.
*5. American Association of Critical-Care Nurses: AACN practice alert: Accurate dysrhythmia monitoring in adults. Retrieved from *www.aacn.org/clinical-resources/practice-alerts/dysrhythmia-monitoring*.
6. Clayton BD, Willihnganz MJ: *Basic pharmacology for nurses*, ed 17, St Louis, 2017, Elsevier.
*7. Page RL, Joglar JA, Caldwell MA, et al: 2015 ACC/AHA/HRS guideline for the management of adult patients with supraventricular tachycardia, *Circulation* 133:e471, 2016.
*8. Heidenreich PA, Solis P, Estes NA, et al: 2016 ACC/AHA clinical performance and quality measures for adults with atrial fibrillation or atrial flutter, *J Am Coll Cardiol* 68:525, 2016.
*9. Center for Disease Control: Atrial fibrillation fact sheet. Retrieved from *www.cdc.gov/dhdsp/data_statistics/fact_sheets/fs_atrial_fibrillation.htm*.
10. American College of Cardiology: Left atrial appendage closure. Retrieved from *www.acc.org/latest-in-cardiology/articles/2016/09/20/06/41/left-atrial-appendage-closure-in-2016*.
*11. Sinz E, Navarro K, Soderberg ES: *Advanced cardiovascular life support: Provider manual 2015*, Dallas, 2015, American Heart Association. (Classic)
12. Mulpuru SK, Madhavan M, McLeod CJ: Cardiac pacemakers: Function, troubleshooting, and management, *J Am Coll Cardiol* 69:189, 2017.
13. Boersma L, Barr C, Knops R: Implant and midterm outcomes of the subcutaneous implantable cardioverter-defibrillator registry, *J Am Coll Cardiol* 70:830, 2017.
14. ICD Support Group. Retrieved from *www.icdsupportgroup.org/board/*.
15. Madhavan M, Mulpuru SK, McLeod C, et al: Advances and future directions in cardiac pacemakers, *J Am Coll Cardiol* 69:211, 2017.
*16. Reddy VY, Miller MA, Neuzil P, et al: Cardiac resynchronization therapy with wireless left ventricular endocardial pacing: the SELECT-LV study, *J Am Coll Cardiol* 69:2119, 2017.
*17. Shen WK, Sheldon RS, Benditt DG: 2017 ACC/AHA/HRS guideline for the evaluation and management of patients with syncope, *Circulation* 136:e25, 2017.
18. Cleveland Clinic: Syncope. Retrieved from *https://my.clevelandclinic.org/health/diseases/17536-syncope*.

*Evidence-based information for clinical practice.

36

Inflammatory and Structural Heart Disorders

Patricia Keegan

*A kind heart is a fountain of gladness, making
everything in its vicinity freshen into smiles.*

Washington Irving

ⓔ http://evolve.elsevier.com/Lewis/medsurg

CONCEPTUAL FOCUS

Fatigue
Functional Ability

Inflammation
Perfusion

LEARNING OUTCOMES

1. Describe the pathophysiology, clinical manifestations, and interprofessional and nursing management of the patient with infective endocarditis or pericarditis.
2. Describe the pathophysiology, clinical manifestations, and interprofessional and nursing management of the patient with myocarditis.
3. Distinguish the etiology, pathophysiology, and clinical manifestations of rheumatic fever and rheumatic heart disease.
4. Describe the interprofessional and nursing management of the patient with rheumatic heart disease.
5. Describe the pathophysiology, clinical manifestations, and interprofessional and nursing management of patients with various types of valvular heart disease.
6. Relate the pathophysiology, clinical manifestations, and interprofessional and nursing management of patients with different types of cardiomyopathy.

KEY TERMS

aortic regurgitation (AR), p. 790
aortic stenosis (AS), p. 789
cardiac tamponade, p. 783
cardiomyopathy (CMP), p. 794
chronic constrictive pericarditis, p. 784
dilated cardiomyopathy, p. 794

hypertrophic cardiomyopathy, p. 795
infective endocarditis (IE), p. 778
mitral valve prolapse (MVP), p. 789
myocarditis, p. 785
pericardiocentesis, p. 784
pericarditis, p. 782

regurgitation, p. 788
rheumatic fever (RF), p. 785
rheumatic heart disease, p. 785
stenosis, p. 788

This chapter describes the pathophysiology and management of patients with select inflammatory and structural heart problems. Conceptually, these problems can adversely affect perfusion. Inflammatory, infectious, and structural problems result in impaired cardiac output (CO), which leads to decreased tissue perfusion and impaired gas exchange. The patient may have pain, hyperthermia, and decreased functional and cognitive ability. The nurse plays a key role in providing patients with the education needed to manage problems and their effects.

INFLAMMATORY DISORDERS OF HEART

INFECTIVE ENDOCARDITIS

Infective endocarditis (IE) is a disease of the endocardial layer of the heart. The *endocardium* is the innermost layer of the heart (Fig. 36.1) and heart valves. IE most often affects the aortic and mitral valves. In the United States, there are around 40,000 to 50,000 new cases of IE per year.[1] The 1-year mortality of IE has not changed in the past 20 years.[1]

Classification

We often classify IE based on the cause (e.g., IV drug use IE [IVDA IE], fungal IE) or site of involvement (e.g., prosthetic valve endocarditis [PVE]). In the past, we have described IE as subacute or acute. The *subacute form* affects those with preexisting valve disease over a period of months. In contrast, the *acute form* affects those with healthy valves and appears as a rapidly progressive illness.

Etiology and Pathophysiology

IE occurs when blood flow allows organisms to contact and infect previously damaged heart valves or other endothelial surfaces. About 30% of cases are caused by *Staphylococcus aureus*.[1] Other bacterial causes include *Streptococcus viridans* and coagulase-negative staphylococci. The organisms make biofilms, which protect the organisms from immune defenses and make antimicrobials less effective.[2]

Persons with a variety of underlying cardiac and noncardiac conditions can develop IE (Table 36.1). Patients are stratified into categories of high, moderate, or low risk for developing

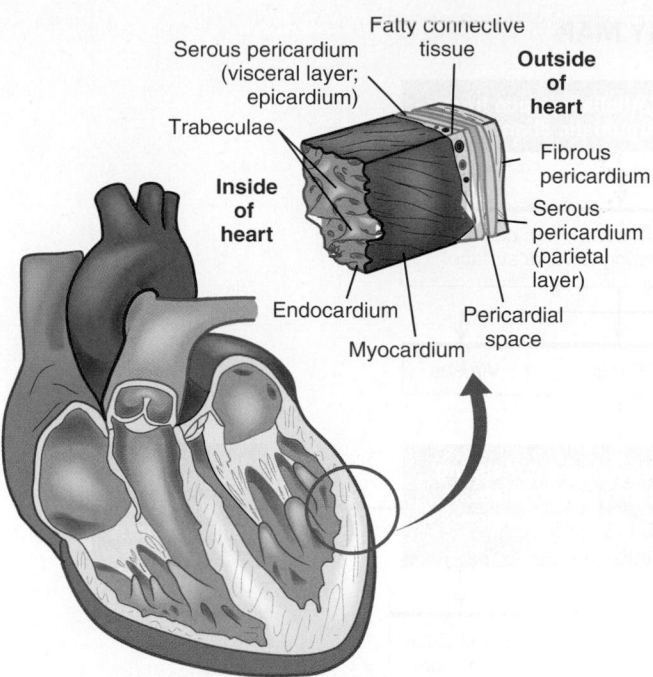

FIG. 36.1 Layers of the heart muscle and pericardium. The section of the heart wall shows the fibrous pericardium, the parietal and visceral layers of the serous pericardium (with the pericardial sac between them), the myocardium, and the endocardium. (Modified from Patton KT, Thibodeau GA: *The human body in health and disease,* ed 5, St Louis, 2010, Mosby.)

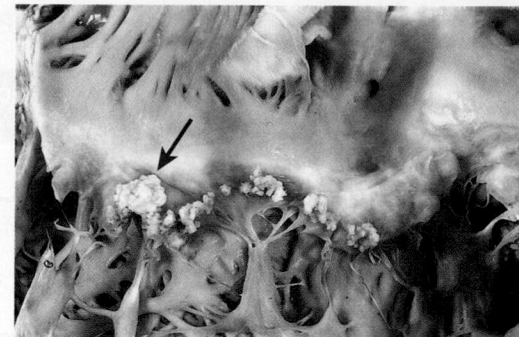

FIG. 36.2 Bacterial IE of the mitral valve. The valve is covered with large, irregular vegetations *(arrow).* (From Damjanov I, Linder J: *Pathology: A color atlas,* St Louis, 2000, Mosby.)

TABLE 36.1 Common Risk Factors for Endocarditis

Cardiac Conditions
- Acquired valve disease (e.g., mitral valve prolapse with regurgitation, calcified aortic stenosis)
- Cardiomyopathy
- Congenital heart disease
- Heart lesions (e.g., ventricular septal defect, asymmetric septal hypertrophy)
- Marfan's syndrome
- Pacemaker
- Prior IE
- Prosthetic heart valve(s)
- Rheumatic heart disease (e.g., mitral valve regurgitation)

Noncardiac Conditions
- Hospital-acquired bacteremia
- IV drug use

Procedure-Associated Risks
- Intravascular devices (e.g., central venous catheter)
- Procedures listed in Table 36.2

IE or having a poor outcome.[2] Rheumatic heart disease used to be the most common cause of IE. Now, it accounts for less than 20% of cases. The main risk factors for IE include (1) aging (more than 50% of older people have calcified aortic stenosis), (2) IV drug use, (3) having a prosthetic valve, (4) use of intravascular devices resulting in health care–associated infections (e.g., methicillin-resistant *S. aureus* [MRSA]), and (5) renal dialysis.[1]

IE typically develops in 3 stages: (1) bacteremia, (2) adhesion, and (3) vegetation.[1] *Vegetations,* the primary lesions of IE, consist of fibrin, leukocytes, platelets, and microbes that stick to the valve surface or endocardium (Fig. 36.2). The loss of parts of these fragile vegetations into the circulation results in *emboli.* Up to 30% of persons with IE develop embolization.[3] This occurs when left-sided heart vegetation moves to various organs (e.g., brain, kidneys, spleen) and to the extremities, causing limb infarction. Right-sided heart lesions move to the lungs, resulting in pulmonary emboli.

The infection may spread locally and damage the valves or their supporting structures. This causes dysrhythmias, valve dysfunction, and invasion of the myocardium, leading to heart failure (HF), sepsis, and heart block (Fig. 36.3).

Clinical Manifestations

The manifestations of IE are nonspecific and can involve multiple organ systems. Most patients have fever.[3] Fever may be low grade or may be absent in older adults or those who are immunocompromised. Other symptoms include chills, weakness, malaise, fatigue, and anorexia. Patients may have arthralgias, myalgias, back pain, abdominal discomfort, weight loss, headache, and clubbing of fingers in subacute forms of IE.[4]

Vascular signs include *splinter hemorrhages* (black longitudinal streaks) in the nail beds. Petechiae from microembolization of vegetative lesions can occur on the conjunctivae, lips, buccal mucosa, and palate and over the ankles, feet, and antecubital and popliteal areas. *Osler's nodes* (painful, tender, red or purple, pea-size lesions) are found on the fingertips or toes. *Janeway's lesions* (flat, painless, small, red spots) may be seen on the fingertips, palms, soles of feet, and toes. Eye examination may show hemorrhagic retinal lesions called *Roth's spots.*

Most patients have a new or worsening systolic murmur. Murmurs are usually absent in tricuspid IE because right-sided heart sounds are too low to be heard. HF is common, occurring in up to 80% of patients with aortic valve IE and 50% of those with mitral valve IE.[3]

Septic embolism is a potential complication of IE. Embolic events occur in more than half of patients.[3] The central nervous system (CNS) is the most often affected organ system, followed by extremities, spleen, and kidney.

Diagnostic Studies

The health history is important in assessing IE. Ask patients if they have had any recent (within the past 3 to 6 months) dental, urologic, surgical, or gynecologic procedures, including obstetric delivery. Note any history of IVDA, heart disease, recent heart catheterization, heart surgery, intravascular device

PATHOPHYSIOLOGY MAP

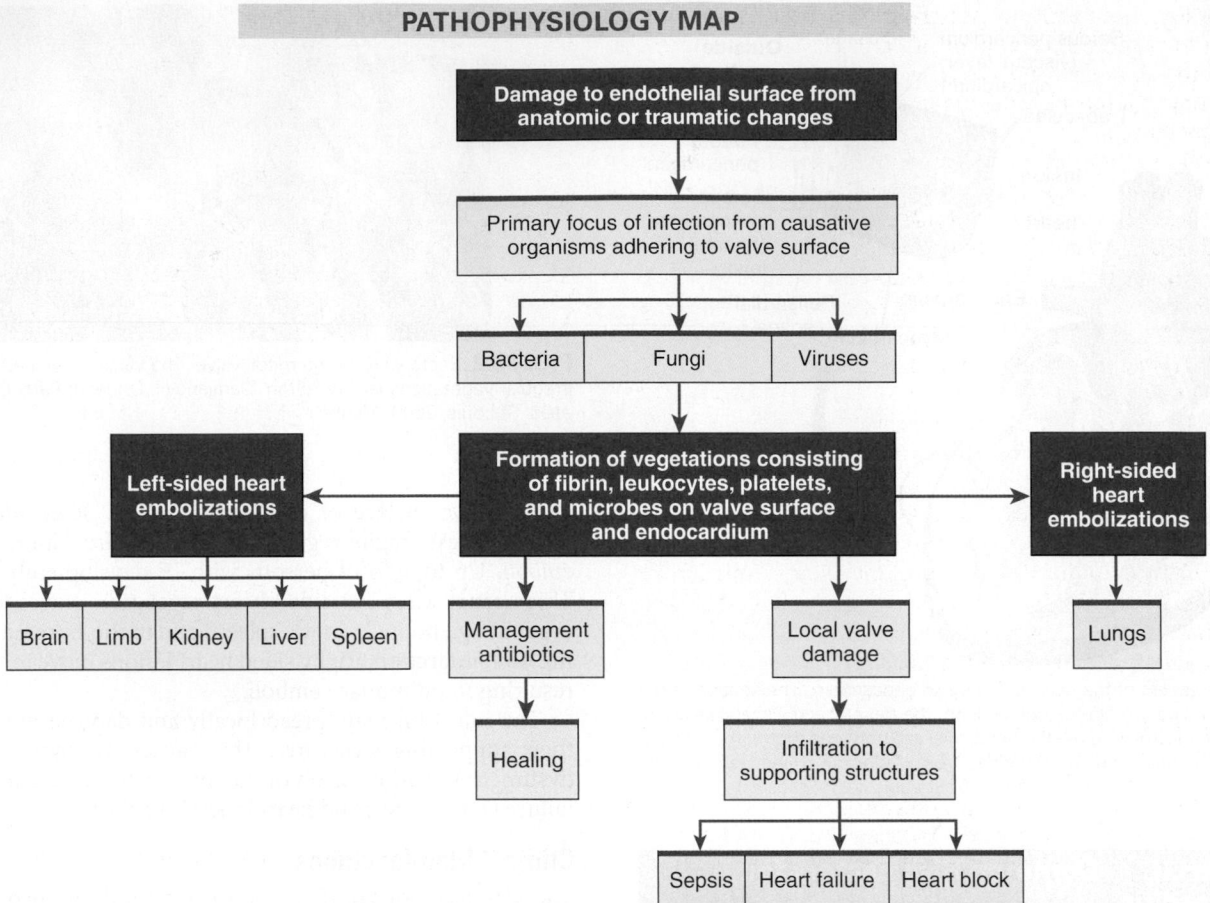

FIG. 36.3 Pathogenesis of IE.

placement, renal dialysis, or infections (e.g., skin, respiratory, urinary tract).

Three blood cultures drawn over a period of 1 hour from 3 different sites will be positive in most patients with IE.[4] Culture-negative IE is associated with antibiotic usage within the previous 2 weeks or results from a pathogen not easily detected by standard cultures A mild leukocytosis occurs in acute IE. The erythrocyte sedimentation rate (ESR) and C-reactive protein (CRP) levels may be increased. Echocardiography can show vegetations.

Guidelines for the diagnosis of IE are based on the Duke Criteria. The patient must have 2 major criteria and 1 minor criterion, or 1 major and 3 minor, or 5 minor criteria. Major criteria include positive blood cultures, typical microorganism for IE from 2 separate blood cultures, evidence of endocardial involvement, and new valvular vegetation. Minor criteria include predisposing heart condition or IV drug use, vascular phenomena, immunologic phenomena, microbiologic evidence, or echocardiographic findings consistent with IE but not meeting major criteria.[5]

A chest x-ray may show *cardiomegaly* (an enlarged heart). An electrocardiogram (ECG) may show first- or second-degree atrioventricular (AV) block because the heart valves lie close to conductive tissue, especially the AV node.

Interprofessional Care

Prophylactic Treatment. Situations and conditions that require antibiotic prophylaxis are detailed in Table 36.2.

TABLE 36.2 Antibiotic Prophylaxis to Prevent Endocarditis

Target Groups for Prophylactic Antibiotics

People with the following heart conditions should receive prophylactic antibiotics when they have the conditions or procedures listed below:

- Prosthetic heart valve or prosthetic material used to repair heart valve
- History of infectious IE
- Congenital heart disease (CHD)
  - Unrepaired cyanotic CHD (including palliative shunts and conduits)
  - Repaired congenital heart defect with prosthetic material or device for 6 mo after the procedure
  - Repaired CHD with residual defects at the site or next to the site of prosthetic patch or prosthetic device
- Heart transplant recipients who develop heart valve disease

Conditions or Procedures Requiring Antibiotic Prophylaxis

When the target groups have the following conditions or procedures, they need prophylactic antibiotics:

- Oral
  - Dental manipulation involving the gums or roots of the teeth
  - Dental manipulation involving puncture of the oral mucosa
- Respiratory
  - Respiratory tract incisions (e.g., biopsy)
  - Tonsillectomy and adenoidectomy
- Surgical procedures that involve infected skin, skin structures, or musculoskeletal tissue

Source: Nishimura RA, Otto CM, Bonow RO, et al: 2014 AHA/ACC guidelines for the management of patients with valvular heart disease: executive summary—A report of the American College of Cardiology/AHA Task Force on Practice Guidelines, *Circulation* 129:2440, 2014.

Drug Therapy. Accurately identifying the causative organism is the key to successful treatment of IE. Long-term treatment is needed to kill dormant bacteria within the valvular vegetations. Complete removal of the organism generally takes weeks. Relapses are common.[5]

Antibiotic therapy is based on blood culture results. The effectiveness of therapy is assessed with subsequent blood cultures. Cultures that stay positive indicate inadequate or inappropriate antibiotics, an aortic root or myocardial abscess, or the wrong diagnosis (e.g., an infection elsewhere). It is reasonable to obtain 2 sets of blood cultures every 24 to 48 hours until the infection is cleared.[3] After completion of antibiotics, follow-up echocardiogram and inflammatory markers are done at 1, 3, 6, and 12 months.[4]

Fungal IE and PVE respond poorly to antibiotic therapy alone. Early valve replacement followed by prolonged (6 weeks or more) antibiotics is needed in these situations. Valve replacement surgery (discussed later in this chapter) is done in 50% to 60% of cases of IE. Three reasons to perform surgery are for valve dysfunction leading to HF, to prevent embolization, or for uncontrolled infection.[4]

Fever that persists after treatment has been started is managed with aspirin, acetaminophen, fluids, and rest. Complete bed rest is usually not needed unless the temperature stays elevated or there are signs of HF. IE with HF responds poorly to drug therapy and valve replacement, so it can be life threatening.

 SAFETY ALERT Communicating Test Results
- If blood culture results for a patient diagnosed with IE show that the organism is not susceptible to the ordered antibiotic, immediately notify the HCP.
- A National Patient Safety Goal stresses the importance of communicating critical test results to the right HCP in a timely manner.

❖ NURSING MANAGEMENT: INFECTIVE ENDOCARDITIS

◆ Nursing Assessment

Subjective and objective data to obtain from a patient with IE are found in Table 36.3. Assess vital signs together with heart sounds to detect a murmur, a change in a preexisting murmur, and extra sounds (e.g., S_3).

Arthralgia (joint pain) and myalgias are common. Assess the patient for joint tenderness, decreased range of motion (ROM), and muscle tenderness. Examine the patient for petechiae, splinter hemorrhages, and Osler's nodes. Complete a general systems assessment to determine any hemodynamic or embolic complications.

◆ Nursing Diagnoses

Nursing diagnoses for the patient with IE include:
- Impaired cardiac output
- Activity intolerance

More information on nursing diagnoses and interventions for the patient with IE is in eNursing Care Plan 36.1 on the website for this chapter.

◆ Planning

The overall goals for the patient with IE include (1) normal or baseline heart function, (2) ability to perform activities of daily living (ADLs) without fatigue, and (3) an understanding of the treatment plan to prevent recurrence.

TABLE 36.3 Nursing Assessment

Infective Endocarditis

Subjective Data

Important Health Information

Past health history: Valvular, congenital, or syphilitic heart disease, including valve repair or replacement. Previous IE, childbirth, staphylococcal or streptococcal infections, hospital-acquired bacteremia

Medications: Immunosuppressive therapy

Surgery or other treatments: Recent obstetric or gynecologic procedures. Invasive procedures, including catheterization, cystoscopy. Recent dental or surgical procedures, GI procedures (e.g., endoscopy)

Functional Health Patterns

Health perception–health management: IV drug use, alcohol use. Malaise

Nutritional-metabolic: Weight gain or loss, anorexia. Chills, diaphoresis

Elimination: Bloody urine

Activity-exercise: Exercise intolerance, generalized weakness, fatigue. Cough, dyspnea on exertion, orthopnea, palpitations

Sleep-rest: Night sweats

Cognitive-perceptual: Chest, back, or abdominal pain. Headache, joint tenderness, muscle tenderness

Objective Data

General

Fever

Integumentary

Osler's nodes on extremities, splinter hemorrhages under nail beds, Janeway's lesions on fingertips, palms, soles of feet, and toes. Petechiae of skin, mucous membranes, or conjunctivae. Purpura, peripheral edema, finger clubbing

Respiratory

Tachypnea, crackles

Cardiovascular

Dysrhythmia, tachycardia, new murmurs, S_3, S_4. Retinal hemorrhages

Possible Diagnostic Findings

Leukocytosis, anemia, ↑ ESR, ↑ CRP and cardiac biomarkers. Positive blood cultures, hematuria. Echocardiogram showing chamber enlargement, valvular dysfunction, and vegetations. Chest x-ray showing cardiomegaly and pulmonary infiltrates. ECG showing ischemia and conduction defects. Signs of systemic embolization or pulmonary embolism

---

◆ Nursing Implementation

◆ Health Promotion.

Teaching the patient at high risk for IE (Tables 36.1 and 36.2) helps reduce the incidence and recurrence of IE. Tell the patient to avoid people with infections, especially upper respiratory tract infections, and to report cold, flu, and cough symptoms. Stress the importance of avoiding excessive fatigue, planning rest periods, using good oral hygiene, and scheduling regular dental visits.[5]

Tell the patient to inform HCPs scheduling invasive procedures about the history of IE, as prophylactic antibiotic therapy may be needed. Refer the patient with a history of IVDA for drug rehabilitation.

Ambulatory Care. A patient with IE has many problems that need nursing management. IE generally requires treatment with antibiotics for 4 to 6 weeks. After initial treatment in the hospital, the patient may continue treatment at home if hemodynamically stable and adherent. Assess the home setting for adequate support. Patients who receive outpatient IV antibiotics need vigilant home nursing care.

Assessment findings are often nonspecific (Table 36.3). Tell the patient and caregiver about the importance of monitoring body temperature. Persistent temperature elevations may mean that the antibiotic is ineffective. Patients are at risk for life-threatening complications, such as stroke, pulmonary edema, and HF. Teach patients and caregivers to recognize signs and symptoms of these complications (e.g., change in mental status, dyspnea, chest pain, unexplained weight gain).

The patient needs adequate periods of physical and emotional rest. Bed rest may be needed when the patient has fever or complications (e.g., heart damage). Otherwise, the patient may perform moderate activity. To prevent problems related to decreased mobility, have the patient to wear elastic compression stockings, perform ROM exercises, and deep breathe and cough every 2 hours. The patient may have anxiety and fear. You must recognize this and begin strategies to help the patient cope with the illness.

Monitor laboratory data, including blood cultures, to determine antibiotic effectiveness. Assess IV lines for patency and signs of complications (e.g., phlebitis). Give antibiotics as prescribed. Monitor the patient for any adverse drug reactions.

Teach the patient and caregiver the nature of the disease and on how to reduce the risk for reinfection. Explain the relationship of follow-up care, good nutrition and dental care, and prompt treatment of common infections (e.g., colds) to stay healthy. Teach the patient about symptoms to report that may indicate another infection (e.g., fever, fatigue, chills). Finally, explain the importance of prophylactic antibiotic therapy before certain invasive procedures (Table 36.2).

◆ **Evaluation**

The expected outcomes are that the patient with IE will
- Maintain adequate tissue and organ perfusion
- Maintain normal body temperature
- Report an increase in physical and emotional comfort

ACUTE PERICARDITIS

Pericarditis is a condition caused by inflammation of the pericardial sac (pericardium), often with fluid accumulation. The pericardium is composed of the inner serous membrane (visceral pericardium) and the outer fibrous (parietal) layer (Fig. 36.1). The pericardial space between these 2 layers normally holds 10 to 15 mL of serous fluid. The pericardium anchors the heart, provides lubrication to decrease friction between heart contractions, and helps to prevent excess dilation of the heart during diastole.

Etiology and Pathophysiology

Common causes of acute pericarditis are listed in Table 36.4. Most often the cause of acute pericarditis is *idiopathic* (unknown) or viral.[6] The coxsackievirus B is the most commonly identified virus.[7]

There are 3 types of pericarditis: acute, subacute, and chronic. Acute pericarditis develops rapidly, causing the pericardial sac to become inflamed and leak fluid (pericardial effusion). The characteristic pathologic finding in acute pericarditis is inflammation. There is an influx of neutrophils, increased pericardial vascularity, and eventually fibrin deposition on the epicardium (Fig. 36.4). Subacute pericarditis occurs weeks to months after

an event. We refer to pericarditis lasting more than 6 months as chronic.[7]

Myocardial infarction (MI) causes 5% to 8% of acute pericarditis cases. Post-MI syndrome (Dressler syndrome) pericarditis can occur 4 to 6 weeks after transmural MI (see Chapter 33). This syndrome is more common after a large anterior infarct.[6] Viral pericarditis is often seen after respiratory or GI illness.[6]

Clinical Manifestations

Clinical symptoms include progressive, severe, sharp chest pain.[6] The pain is generally worse with deep inspiration and when lying flat. Sitting up and leaning forward relieves the pain.

TABLE 36.4 Common Causes of Pericarditis

Infectious
- Bacterial: Pneumococci, staphylococci, streptococci, *Neisseria gonorrhoeae*, *Legionella pneumophila*, *Mycobacterium tuberculosis*, septicemia from gram-negative organisms
- Fungal: Histoplasma, *Candida* species
- Viral: Coxsackie A and B virus, echovirus, adenovirus, mumps, hepatitis, Epstein-Barr, varicella zoster, human immunodeficiency virus
- Others: Toxoplasmosis, Lyme disease

Noninfectious
- Acute MI
- Cancers: Lung, breast, leukemia, Hodgkin's lymphoma, non-Hodgkin's lymphoma
- Dissecting aortic aneurysm
- Myxedema
- Radiation
- Renal failure
- Trauma: Thoracic surgery, pacemaker insertion, cardiac diagnostic procedures

Hypersensitive or Autoimmune
- Dressler syndrome
- Drug reactions (e.g., procainamide, hydralazine)
- Postpericardiotomy syndrome
- Rheumatic fever
- Rheumatologic diseases: Rheumatoid arthritis, systemic lupus erythematosus, systemic sclerosis (scleroderma), ankylosing spondylitis

---

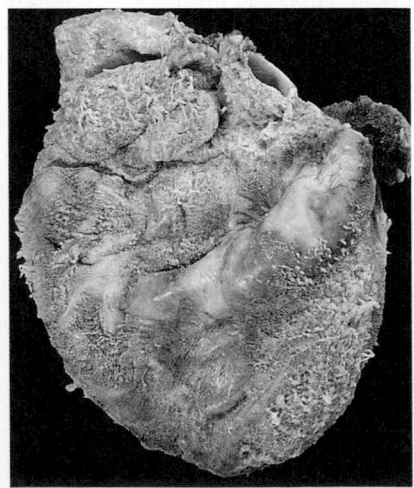

FIG. 36.4 Acute pericarditis. Note shaggy coat of fibers covering surface of heart. (From Damjanov I, Linder J: *Pathology: A color atlas*, St Louis, 2000, Mosby.)

The pain may radiate to the neck, arms, or left shoulder, making it hard to distinguish from angina. One distinction is that the pain from pericarditis can be referred to the trapezius muscle (shoulder, upper back). Dyspnea is related to the patient's breathing in rapid, shallow breaths to avoid chest pain. Fever and anxiety may worsen dyspnea.

The hallmark finding in acute pericarditis is the *pericardial friction rub*. The rub is a scratching, grating, high-pitched sound believed to result from friction between the roughened pericardial and epicardial surfaces. It is best heard with the stethoscope at the lower left sternal border of the chest with the patient leaning forward. Since it is hard to tell a pericardial friction rub from a pleural friction rub, ask the patient to hold their breath. If you still hear the rub, it is cardiac. Pericardial friction rubs may be hard to identify because they are often intermittent.

Complications

The major complications are pericardial effusion and cardiac tamponade. *Pericardial effusion* is a build-up of fluid in the pericardium. It can occur rapidly (e.g., chest trauma) or slowly (e.g., tuberculosis pericarditis). Large effusions compress nearby structures. Pulmonary tissue compression can cause cough, dyspnea, and tachypnea. Phrenic nerve compression can cause hiccups. Compression of the laryngeal nerve may result in hoarseness. Heart sounds are generally distant and muffled. BP is usually maintained.

Cardiac tamponade develops as the pericardial effusion volume increases and compresses the heart. The speed of fluid accumulation affects the severity of clinical signs. Cardiac tamponade can occur acutely (e.g., rupture of heart, trauma) or subacutely (e.g., from renal failure, cancer).

The patient with cardiac tamponade may report chest pain and is often confused, anxious, and restless. As the compression of the heart increases, there is decreased CO, muffled heart sounds, narrowed pulse pressure, tachypnea, and tachycardia. Neck veins are markedly distended because of increased jugular venous pressure. *Pulsus paradoxus,* if present, is a large decrease in systolic BP during inspiration (Table 36.5). In a patient with a slow onset of a cardiac tamponade, dyspnea may be the only manifestation.

Diagnostic Studies

The ECG is useful in diagnosing acute pericarditis, with changes noted in 90% of cases. The most sensitive ECG changes include diffuse (widespread) ST segment elevations. This reflects the abnormal repolarization from the pericardial inflammation. These changes are different from the ST changes seen in MI. In myocardial ischemia, there are usually localized ST segment changes. In acute pericarditis serial ECGs do not show evolving changes, such as those with MI.

An echocardiogram can determine the presence of a pericardial effusion or cardiac tamponade. Doppler imaging and color M-mode can assess diastolic function and diagnose constrictive pericarditis (discussed later in the chapter). A CT scan and MRI can visualize the pericardium and pericardial space. Chest x-ray findings are generally normal, but a large pericardial effusion may appear as cardiomegaly (Fig. 36.5).

Common laboratory findings include leukocytosis and increased CRP and ESR. Troponin levels may be increased in patients with ST segment elevation and acute pericarditis, which could indicate concurrent heart damage. Fluid obtained during pericardiocentesis or tissue from a pericardial biopsy may be studied to determine the cause of the pericarditis.

Interprofessional Care

Management is aimed at identifying and treating the underlying problem and symptoms (Table 36.6). Antibiotics treat

---

TABLE 36.5 Measurement of Pulsus Paradoxus

1. Position the patient in a semirecumbent position.
2. Have patient breathe normally.
3. Using a manually operated BP cuff, measure systolic BP.
4. Inflate BP cuff at least 20 mm Hg above systolic BP.
5. Deflate cuff slowly until you hear sounds throughout the respiratory cycle (inspiration and expiration) and note the pressure.
6. Determine the difference between the measurements taken in steps 4 and 5. This will equal the amount of paradox:

Sounds heard on expiration at	110 mm Hg
Sounds heard throughout cycle at	−82 mm Hg
Amount of paradox	28 mm Hg

The difference is normally <10 mm Hg. If the difference is >10 mm Hg, cardiac tamponade may be present.

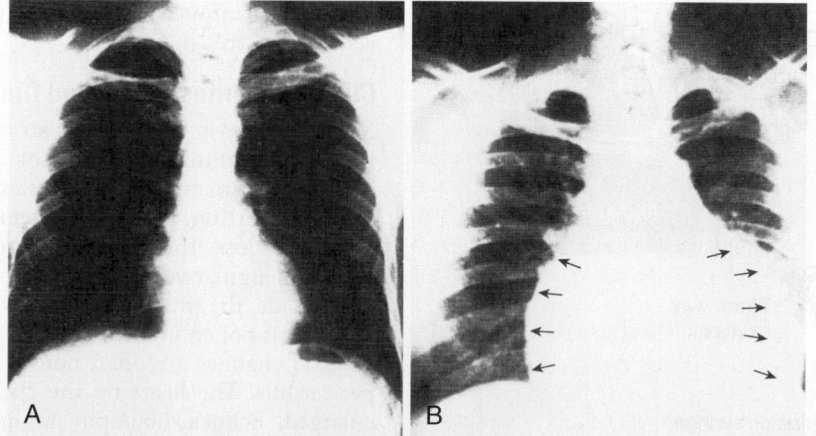

FIG. 36.5 A, X-ray of a normal chest. B, Pericardial effusion is present, and the cardiac silhouette is enlarged with a globular shape *(arrows)*. (From Guzzetta CE, Dossey BM: *Cardiovascular nursing: Holistic practice,* St Louis, 1992, Mosby.)

bacterial pericarditis, and nonsteroidal antiinflammatory drugs (NSAIDs) (e.g., salicylates [aspirin], ibuprofen) control the pain and inflammation. Corticosteroids are used for patients with pericarditis from systemic lupus erythematosus, patients already taking corticosteroids for autoimmune conditions, or patients who do not respond to NSAIDs. They are used cautiously because of their many side effects (see Chapter 49). Colchicine, an antiinflammatory drug used for gout, may help patients who have recurrent pericarditis.[6]

Pericardiocentesis is usually done for pericardial effusion with acute cardiac tamponade, purulent pericarditis, or suspected cancer. Hemodynamic support for the patient before the procedure may include giving volume expanders and inotropic agents (e.g., dopamine) and stopping any anticoagulants. The procedure is done rapidly and safely using a percutaneous approach guided by echocardiography (Fig. 36.6). A needle is inserted into the pericardial space to remove fluid for analysis and relieve heart pressure. Complications include dysrhythmias, further cardiac tamponade, pneumomediastinum, pneumothorax, myocardial laceration, and coronary artery laceration.

A *pericardial window* is a surgical procedure for diagnosis or drainage of excess fluid. Cutting a "window," or part of the pericardium, allows the fluid to drain continuously into the peritoneum or chest.

TABLE 36.6 Interprofessional Care

Acute Pericarditis

Diagnostic Assessment	Management
• History and physical examination (assess for pericardial friction rub, pulsus paradoxus)	• Treatment of underlying disease
• Laboratory: CRP, ESR, white blood cell count	• Bed rest
• ECG	• Drug therapy
• Chest x-ray	• NSAIDs
• Echocardiogram	• Corticosteroids
• CT scan	• Pericardiocentesis (for tamponade)
• MRI	• Pericardial window (for tamponade or ongoing pericardial effusion)
• Pericardiocentesis, pericardial window	
• Pericardial biopsy	

CRP, C-reactive protein; *ESR,* erythrocyte sedimentation rate.

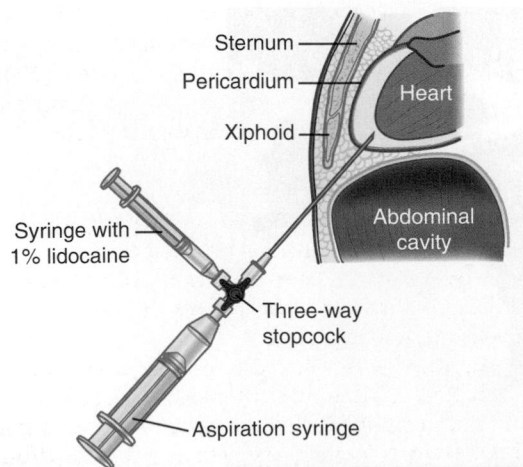

Sternum
Pericardium
Heart
Xiphoid
Syringe with 1% lidocaine
Abdominal cavity
Three-way stopcock
Aspiration syringe

FIG. 36.6 Pericardiocentesis performed under sterile conditions in conjunction with ECG and hemodynamic measurements.

❖ NURSING MANAGEMENT: ACUTE PERICARDITIS

Managing the patient's pain and anxiety during acute pericarditis is your key nursing consideration. Assess the pain to distinguish angina (myocardial ischemia) (see Table 33.8) from the pain of pericarditis. Pericarditis pain is usually found in the precordium or left trapezius region and has a sharp quality that increases with inspiration. Pain is often relieved when the patient sits up or leans forward and is worse when lying flat.

Pain relief measures include keeping the patient on bed rest with the head of the bed raised to 45 degrees and providing an overbed table for support. Antiinflammatory drugs can help control the pain. Give these drugs with food or milk. Tell the patient to avoid alcohol because of the risk for GI bleeding. Other drugs, such as a proton pump inhibitor (e.g., pantoprazole, omeprazole), can reduce stomach acid.

Provide simple, complete explanations of procedures and possible causes of the pain to help reduce anxiety. These explanations are particularly important when the patient is undergoing testing and for the patient who has previously had angina or an MI.

The patient with acute pericarditis is at risk for cardiac tamponade and decreased CO. Monitor for manifestations of tamponade and prepare for possible pericardiocentesis.

❓ CHECK YOUR PRACTICE

You are assigned to a 58-yr-old male patient who had an MI 3 days ago. He has now developed pericarditis. When you are making rounds, you assess that the patient is slightly confused and has prominent neck veins. His heart rate is 118 beats/min.
• What should you do next?

CHRONIC CONSTRICTIVE PERICARDITIS

Etiology and Pathophysiology

Chronic constrictive pericarditis results from fibrotic thickening and rigidity of the pericardium, usually after an episode of acute pericarditis. It is characterized by fibrin deposition and pericardial effusion. Reabsorption of the effusion slowly follows, with progression to fibrous scarring, thickening of the pericardium from calcium deposits, and eventual destruction of the pericardial space. The fibrotic, thickened, and adherent pericardium encases the heart and prevents adequate atrial and ventricular stretch.

Clinical Manifestations and Diagnostic Studies

Manifestations of chronic constrictive pericarditis occur over time. They mimic HF and cor pulmonale. Decreased CO accounts for many of the manifestations. These include dyspnea on exertion, peripheral edema, ascites, fatigue, anorexia, and weight loss. The most prominent finding on physical examination is jugular venous distention (JVD). Unlike with cardiac tamponade, the presence of pulsus paradoxus (greater than 10 mm Hg) is not common.[6]

ECG changes are often nonspecific in chronic constrictive pericarditis. The heart on the chest x-ray may be normal or enlarged. Echocardiography findings may show a thickened pericardium but without a large pericardial effusion. CT and MRI can measure pericardial thickness and assess diastolic filling patterns.

❖ Interprofessional and Nursing Care

The treatment of choice for symptomatic chronic constrictive pericarditis is a *pericardiectomy*. This involves complete resection of the pericardium through a median sternotomy with the use of cardiopulmonary bypass (see Chapter 33). Some patients show immediate improvement, but others may take weeks. The prognosis improves when the patient has surgery before becoming clinically unstable.

MYOCARDITIS

Etiology and Pathophysiology

Myocarditis is a focal or diffuse inflammation of the myocardium. Causes include viruses, bacteria, fungi, radiation therapy, and pharmacologic and chemical factors. Coxsackie A and B viruses are the most common causative agents. Autoimmune disorders (e.g., polymyositis) have been linked with the development of myocarditis. It also may be idiopathic.

When the myocardium becomes infected, the causative agent invades the myocytes and causes cellular damage and necrosis. This activates the immune response. Cytokines and O_2 free radicals are released. As the infection progresses, an autoimmune response is activated. This causes further destruction of myocytes. Myocarditis results in heart dysfunction. Dilated cardiomyopathy can occur (discussed later in this chapter).[8]

Clinical Manifestations

The features of myocarditis vary from a benign course without any overt symptoms to progressive HF, dysrhythmias, or sudden cardiac death (SCD).[8] Fever, fatigue, malaise, myalgias, pharyngitis, dyspnea, lymphadenopathy, and nausea and vomiting are early manifestations of the viral illness.

Early cardiac signs appear 7 to 10 days after viral infection because pericarditis often accompanies myocarditis. These include pleuritic chest pain with a pericardial friction rub and effusion. Late cardiac signs relate to the development of HF and include an S_3 heart sound, crackles, JVD, syncope, peripheral edema, and angina.

Diagnostic Studies and Interprofessional Care

The ECG changes with myocarditis are often nonspecific but reflect associated pericardial involvement (e.g., diffuse ST segment changes). Dysrhythmias and conduction problems may be present. Laboratory findings are often inconclusive. They may include mild to moderate leukocytosis and atypical lymphocytes, elevated viral titers, and increased ESR, CRP levels, and levels of cardiac biomarkers, such as troponin. The virus is generally present in tissue and pericardial fluid samples only during the first 8 to 10 days of illness.

Endomyocardial biopsy provides histologic confirmation of myocarditis.[8] A biopsy is most diagnostic during the first 6 weeks of acute illness, when lymphocytic infiltration and myocyte damage are present. Nuclear scans, echocardiography, and MRI are used to assess heart function.

Treatment consists of managing symptoms. Angiotensin-converting enzyme (ACE) inhibitors and β-adrenergic receptor blockers (β-blockers) are used if the heart is enlarged or to treat HF (see Chapter 34). Diuretics reduce fluid volume and preload. If the patient is not hypotensive, IV drugs such as nitroprusside and milrinone reduce afterload and improve CO by decreasing systemic vascular resistance. Digoxin (Lanoxin) improves heart contractility and reduces HR. It is used cautiously in patients with myocarditis because of increased sensitivity to the adverse effects (e.g., dysrhythmias) and the potential toxicity. Anticoagulation reduces the risk for clot formation from blood stasis in patients with a low ejection fraction (EF).

 DRUG ALERT Digoxin (Lanoxin)

- Use cautiously in patients with myocarditis.
- Myocarditis predisposes to drug-related dysrhythmias and toxicity.

Myocarditis with an autoimmune basis is treated with immunosuppressive agents. These drugs reduce heart inflammation and damage. However, the use of these drugs for the treatment of myocarditis is controversial because they may lead to recurrence.[8] In some instances, antivirals may be used as adjunct therapy to treat myocarditis.

General supportive measures include O_2 therapy, bed rest, and restricted activity. In cases of severe HF, intraaortic balloon pump therapy and ventricular assist devices (VAD) may be needed (see Chapters 34 and 65).

❖ NURSING MANAGEMENT: MYOCARDITIS

Focus your interventions on improving CO and managing the signs and symptoms of HF. Select nursing measures to decrease cardiac workload. These include placing the patient in a semi-Fowler's position, spacing activity and rest periods, and providing a quiet environment. Carefully monitor drugs that increase the heart's contractility and decrease preload, afterload, or both. Evaluate the effectiveness of your interventions on an ongoing basis.

The patient may be anxious about the diagnosis of myocarditis. Assess the level of anxiety, take measures to decrease anxiety, and keep the patient and caregiver informed about the therapeutic plan.

The patient who receives immunosuppressive therapy is at increased risk for infection. Monitor for complications and provide the patient with proper infection control procedures.

Although most patients recover spontaneously, some develop dilated cardiomyopathy (discussed later in this chapter). If severe HF occurs, the patient may need a heart transplant.

RHEUMATIC FEVER AND RHEUMATIC HEART DISEASE

Rheumatic fever (RF) is an acute inflammatory disease that can involve all the heart layers. RF occurs most often between the ages of 5 and 15.[9] Rheumatic heart disease is a chronic scarring and deformity of the heart valves resulting from RF.

Etiology and Pathophysiology

RF occurs as a complication 2-3 weeks after a group A streptococcal pharyngitis. Signs of RF appear to be from an abnormal immune response to bacterial antigens.[9] RF affects the heart, skin, joints, and CNS. Rheumatic heart disease, caused by RF, primarily affects young adults.

RF has declined in developed countries because of the effective use of antibiotics to treat streptococcal infections. However, it is an important public health problem in developing countries.[9] Risk factors include age, gender, and environmental factors.[10]

Cardiac Lesions and Valve Deformities. About 50% of RF episodes are *rheumatic pancarditis,* involving all layers of the heart (endocardium, myocardium, and pericardium) (Fig. 36.1).[11]

Rheumatic IE is found mainly in the valves, with swelling and erosion of the valve leaflets. Vegetation forms from deposits of fibrin and blood cells in areas of erosion. The lesions initially create thickening of the valve leaflets, fusion of commissures and chordae tendineae, and fibrosis of the papillary muscle. Valve leaflets may become calcified, resulting in stenosis. The less mobile valve leaflets may not close properly, resulting in regurgitation. The mitral and aortic valves are most often affected.

Nodules, called *Aschoff's bodies,* are formed by a reaction to inflammation with swelling and destruction of collagen fibers. As the Aschoff's bodies age, they become more fibrous, and scar tissue forms in the myocardium. Rheumatic pericarditis develops and affects both layers of the pericardium. The layers become thick and covered with a fibrinous exudate. A serosanguineous pericardial effusion may develop. When healing occurs, fibrosis and adhesions develop that partially or completely destroy the pericardial sac. Damage to the heart begins during the first attack of RF. Recurrent infections cause further structural damage.

Extracardiac Lesions. The systemic lesions of RF involve the skin, joints, and CNS. Painless subcutaneous nodules, arthralgias or arthritis, and chorea may develop.

Clinical Manifestations

Jones criteria are used to diagnose acute RF.[9] The presence of 2 major criteria or 1 major and 2 minor criteria plus evidence of a preceding group A streptococcal infection indicate a high probability of acute RF (Table 36.7).

TABLE 36.7 Revised Jones Criteria for Diagnosing Rheumatic Fever*

Major Criteria
- Carditis: Clinical and/or subclinical
- Arthritis
  - Monoarthritis or polyarthritis
  - Polyarthralgia
- Erythema marginatum
- Subcutaneous nodules
- Sydenham's chorea

Minor Criteria
- Monoarthralgia
- Fever
- Laboratory findings: ↑ ESR and/or ↑ CRP
- ECG findings: Prolonged PR interval after accounting for age variability (unless carditis is a major criterion)

Evidence of Group A Streptococcal Infection
- Laboratory findings
  - ↑ Antistreptolysin-O titer, positive throat culture, or positive rapid antigen test for group A streptococci

Modified from Gewitz MH, Baltimore RS, Tani LY, et al: Revision of the Jones criteria for the diagnosis of acute rheumatic fever in the era of Doppler echocardiography: A scientific statement from the AHA, *Circulation* 131:1806, 2015.
*Criteria apply to initial episode of rheumatic fever in moderate- or high-risk populations as defined by an all-age prevalence of rheumatic heart disease of ≥1 per 1000 population per year.

Major Criteria. *Carditis* is the most important manifestation of RF. It results in 3 signs: (1) heart murmur or murmurs of mitral or aortic regurgitation, or mitral stenosis; (2) heart enlargement and HF from myocarditis; and (3) pericarditis resulting in muffled heart sounds, chest pain, pericardial friction rub, or signs of effusion.

Monoarthritis or *polyarthritis* is the most common finding in RF, occurring in up to 75% of patients.[9] The inflammatory process affects the synovial membranes of the joints. This causes swelling, heat, redness, tenderness, and limitation of motion. The larger joints, particularly the knees, ankles, elbows, and wrists, are most often affected.

Sydenham's chorea is the major CNS manifestation.[9] It is characterized by involuntary movements, especially of the face and limbs; muscle weakness; and speech and gait problems.

Erythema marginatum lesions are a less common feature of RF. They only occur in less than 10% of RF patients.[10] The bright pink, nonpruritic, maplike macular lesions occur mainly on the trunk and proximal extremities. They intensify with heat (e.g., warm bath). *Subcutaneous nodules* associated with severe carditis are small, hard, painless swellings found over extensor surfaces of joints, particularly the knees, wrists, and elbows.

Minor Criteria. Minor clinical manifestations (Table 36.7) are helpful in diagnosing the disease. The minor criteria confirm the presence of RF when only 1 major criterion is present.

Evidence of Infection. In addition to the major and minor criteria, there must be evidence of a preceding group A streptococcal infection. Table 36.7 lists the various laboratory tests used to confirm evidence of infection.

Complications

Chronic rheumatic carditis results from changes in valve structure months to years after an episode of RF. Rheumatic IE can result in fibrous tissue growth in valve leaflets and chordae tendineae with scarring and contractures. The mitral valve is most often involved. The aortic and tricuspid valves may be affected.

Diagnostic Studies and Interprofessional Care

No single diagnostic test exists for RF. An echocardiogram may show valvular insufficiency and pericardial fluid or thickening.[11] A chest x-ray may show an enlarged heart. The most consistent ECG change is a prolonged PR interval from delayed AV conduction.

Treatment consists of drug therapy and supportive measures (Table 36.8). Antibiotic therapy does not change the course of the acute disease or the development of carditis. It eliminates residual group A streptococci in the tonsils and pharynx and prevents the spread of organisms to close contacts. Salicylates, NSAIDs, and corticosteroids are the antiinflammatory agents most widely used to control the fever and joint manifestations.[10]

TABLE 36.8 Interprofessional Care

Rheumatic Fever

Diagnostic Assessment	Management

- History and physical examination
- Laboratory studies (Table 36.7)
  - Chest x-ray
  - Echocardiogram
  - ECG
	- Bed rest or limited activity
	- Drug therapy
	  - Antibiotics
	  - NSAIDs
	  - Salicylates
	  - Corticosteroids

❖ NURSING MANAGEMENT: RHEUMATIC FEVER AND RHEUMATIC HEART DISEASE

◆ Nursing Assessment

Table 36.9 presents the subjective and objective data to obtain from a patient with RF and rheumatic heart disease.

Inspect the patient's skin for subcutaneous nodules and erythema marginatum. Palpate for subcutaneous nodules over all bony surfaces and along extensor tendons of the hands and feet. The nodules range in size from 1 to 4 cm and are hard, painless, and freely movable. Erythema marginatum can occur on the trunk and inner aspects of the upper arm and thigh. Assess for these bright pink maculae in good light because the rash is hard to see, especially in dark-skinned patients.

◆ Nursing Diagnoses

Nursing diagnoses for the patient with RF and rheumatic heart disease include:

- Impaired cardiac output
- Activity intolerance

TABLE 36.9 Nursing Assessment

Rheumatic Fever and Rheumatic Heart Disease

Subjective Data

Important Health Information

Past health history: Recent streptococcal infection, history of RF or rheumatic heart disease

Functional Health Patterns

Health perception–health management: Family history of rheumatic fever. Malaise
Nutritional-metabolic: Anorexia, weight loss
Activity-exercise: Palpitations, generalized weakness, fatigue, impaired coordination
Cognitive-perceptual: Chest pain, widespread joint pain and tenderness (especially large joints)

Objective Data

General

Fever

Integumentary

Subcutaneous nodules and erythema marginatum

Cardiovascular

Tachycardia, pericardial friction rub, muffled heart sounds, murmurs, peripheral edema

Neurologic

Chorea (involuntary, purposeless, rapid motions; facial grimaces)

Musculoskeletal

Signs of monoarthritis or polyarthritis, including swelling, heat, redness, limitation of motion (especially of knees, ankles, elbows, shoulders, wrists)

Possible Diagnostic Findings

Cardiomegaly on chest x-ray. Prolonged PR interval on ECG. Valve abnormalities, chamber dilation, and pericardial effusion on echocardiogram. ↑ Antistreptolysin-O titer, positive throat culture, positive rapid antigen test for group A streptococci, ↑ ESR, ↑ CRP, leukocytosis

◆ Planning

The goals for a patient with RF and rheumatic heart disease include (1) normal or baseline heart function, (2) resumption of daily activities without joint pain, and (3) ability to manage the long-term antibiotic therapy.

◆ Nursing Implementation

◆ **Health Promotion.** Early detection and immediate treatment of group A streptococcal pharyngitis can prevent RF. Treatment with oral penicillin V (Penicillin-VK) or amoxicillin for 10 days is recommended.[9] If the patient is allergic to penicillin, a narrow-spectrum cephalosporin (e.g., cephalexin), clindamycin (Cleocin), or azithromycin (Zithromax) is used.[12] Therapy requires strict adherence to the full course of treatment. Teach people in the community to seek prompt medical care for symptoms of streptococcal pharyngitis.

◆ **Acute Care.** Give antibiotics as prescribed to treat the streptococcal infection. Teach the patient that completing the full course of antibiotics is vital to successful treatment.

Promote optimal rest to reduce cardiac workload and the body's metabolic needs. Position painful joints for proper alignment and apply heat for comfort. Give salicylates, NSAIDs, and corticosteroids as prescribed for joint pain.

After the acute symptoms subside, the patient without carditis can walk. The patient with carditis with HF may be restricted to bed rest (see Chapter 34 for care of a patient with HF). Stress the importance of gentle activities during recovery.

❓ CHECK YOUR PRACTICE

Your 28-yr-old male patient is recovering from carditis after RF. As you are preparing him for discharge from the hospital, he is pacing the floor and seems quite upset. You ask him to sit down so you can talk. He tells you, "I'm a cardiac cripple. I'll never be able to play ball with my sons or go skiing again. I might as well just go to bed and stay there."
- What are the key elements to include in your teaching plan?

◆ **Ambulatory Care.** The aim of secondary prevention is to stop the recurrence of RF. Prior history of RF makes the patient more susceptible to a second attack after a streptococcal infection. The best prevention is treatment with prophylactic antibiotics. Patients with RF without carditis need prophylaxis until age 20 and for a minimum of 5 years. Patients with rheumatic carditis and residual heart disease (e.g., persistent valve disease) need lifelong prophylaxis.[12]

Teach the patient with a history of RF about the disease process and the need for ongoing antibiotic prophylaxis. Teach the patient about good nutrition, hygienic practices, and adequate rest. Caution the patient about the possible development of heart valve disease. Tell the patient to seek medical care for symptoms, such as excessive fatigue, dizziness, palpitations, unexplained weight gain, or exertional dyspnea.[12]

◆ Evaluation

The expected outcomes are that the patient with RF and rheumatic heart disease will

- Be able to perform ADLs with minimal fatigue and pain
- Adhere to treatment regimen
- Express confidence in managing disease
- Use measures to prevent complications

VALVULAR HEART DISEASE

Two AV valves (mitral and tricuspid) and 2 semilunar valves (aortic and pulmonic) control blood flow through the heart (see Fig. 31.1). Valvular heart disease is defined by the valves affected and the type of dysfunction: stenosis or regurgitation (Fig. 36.7).

The pressure on either side of an open valve is normally equal. However, in a stenotic valve, the valve opening is smaller. The forward flow of blood is impaired. This creates a difference in pressure on the 2 sides of the open valve. The amount of stenosis (constriction or narrowing) is seen in the pressure differences (i.e., the higher the difference, the greater the stenosis). When regurgitation occurs (referred to as *incompetence* or *insufficiency*), there is incomplete closure of the valve. This results in the backward flow of blood.

Congenital heart conditions are the most common cause of valve disorders in children and adolescents. Aortic stenosis and mitral regurgitation (MR) often occur in older adults who have some form of heart disease. Other causes of valve disease in adults are related to acquired immunodeficiency syndrome and the use of some antiparkinsonian drugs.[12]

MITRAL VALVE STENOSIS

Etiology and Pathophysiology

Worldwide, the most common cause of mitral stenosis is rheumatic heart disease.[13] Rheumatic mitral stenosis is widespread in developing countries. Less common causes are congenital mitral stenosis, rheumatoid arthritis, radiation exposure, and systemic lupus erythematosus. Rheumatic IE causes scarring of the valve leaflets and the chordae tendineae. Contractures and adhesions develop between the commissures (the junctional

areas). The stenotic mitral valve takes on a "fish mouth" shape because of the thickening and shortening of the mitral valve structures. Severe mitral annular calcification is another cause in the aging population.

These deformities block the blood flow and create a pressure difference between the left atrium and left ventricle during diastole. As a result, left atrial pressure and volume increase, causing higher pulmonary vasculature pressure. The overloaded left atrium places the patient at risk for atrial fibrillation. In chronic mitral stenosis, pressure overload occurs in the left atrium, pulmonary bed, and right ventricle.

Clinical Manifestations

The main symptom of mitral stenosis is exertional dyspnea caused by reduced lung compliance (Table 36.10). Heart sounds include a loud first heart sound and a low-pitched, diastolic murmur (best heard at the apex with the stethoscope). Less often, patients may have hoarseness (from atrial enlargement pressing on the laryngeal nerve), hemoptysis (from pulmonary hypertension), and chest pain (from decreased CO and coronary perfusion). Emboli can form in the left atrium from atrial fibrillation and cause a stroke.[13] Fatigue and palpitations from atrial fibrillation may occur.

MITRAL VALVE REGURGITATION

Etiology and Pathophysiology

Mitral valve function depends on intact mitral leaflets, mitral annulus, chordae tendineae, papillary muscles, left atrium, and left ventricle. A defect in any of these structures can cause regurgitation. MR may result from problems with the leaflets or from the surrounding structures. In primary (degenerative) MR, a problem with the leaflets causes the regurgitation. In secondary

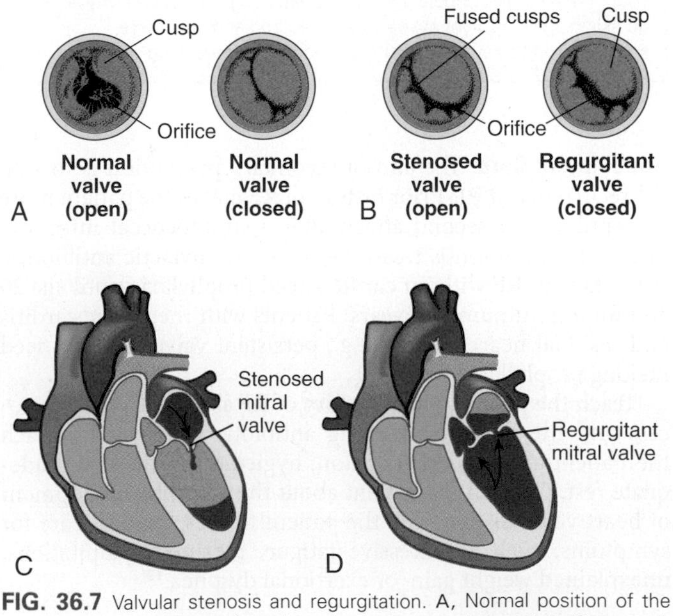

FIG. 36.7 Valvular stenosis and regurgitation. **A,** Normal position of the valve leaflets, or cusps, when the valve is open and closed. **B,** Open position of a stenosed valve *(left)* and closed position of regurgitant valve *(right)*. **C,** Hemodynamic effect of mitral stenosis. The stenosed valve is unable to open sufficiently during left atrial systole, inhibiting left ventricular filling. **D,** Hemodynamic effect of mitral regurgitation. The mitral valve does not close completely during left ventricular systole, letting blood reenter the left atrium. At the same time, blood is moving forward through the aortic valve. (From McCance KL, Huether SE: *Pathophysiology: The biologic basis for disease in adults and children,* ed 6, St Louis, 2010, Mosby.)

TABLE 36.10 **Manifestations of Valvular Heart Disease**	
Type	**Manifestations**
Mitral valve prolapse	Palpitations, dyspnea, chest pain, activity intolerance, syncope, holosystolic murmur
Mitral valve regurgitation	*Acute:* Generally poorly tolerated. New systolic murmur with pulmonary edema. Cardiogenic shock develops rapidly
	Chronic: Weakness, fatigue, exertional dyspnea, palpitations, S_3 gallop, holosystolic murmur
Mitral valve stenosis	Dyspnea on exertion, hemoptysis, fatigue. Atrial fibrillation on ECG. Palpitations. Loud, accentuated S_1. Low-pitched, diastolic murmur
Aortic valve regurgitation	*Acute:* Abrupt onset of profound dyspnea, chest pain, left ventricular failure and cardiogenic shock
	Chronic: Fatigue, exertional dyspnea, orthopnea, PND. Water-hammer pulse, heaving precordial impulse, decreased or absent S_1, S_3, or S_4. Soft high-pitched diastolic murmur, Austin Flint murmur
Aortic valve stenosis	Angina, syncope, dyspnea on exertion, HF, normal or soft S_1, decreased or absent S_2, systolic murmur, prominent S_4
Tricuspid and pulmonic stenosis	*Tricuspid:* Peripheral edema, ascites, hepatomegaly. Diastolic low-pitched murmur with increased intensity during inspiration
	Pulmonic: Fatigue, loud midsystolic murmur

PND, Paroxysmal nocturnal dyspnea.

(functional) MR, myocardial disease causes the regurgitation.[13] Most cases of MR are caused by MI, chronic rheumatic heart disease, mitral valve prolapse, ischemic papillary muscle dysfunction, and IE. MI with left ventricular failure increases the risk for rupture of the chordae tendineae and acute MR.

MR allows blood to flow backward from the left ventricle to the left atrium because of incomplete valve closure during systole. Both the left ventricle and left atrium must work harder to preserve an adequate CO. In acute MR, the sudden increase in pressure and volume transmits back to the pulmonary bed. This results in pulmonary edema and, if not treated, cardiogenic shock. In chronic MR, the added volume results in left atrial enlargement, left ventricular dilation and hypertrophy, and, finally, a decrease in CO.

Clinical Manifestations

The nature of its onset determines the clinical course of MR (Table 36.10). Patients with acute MR have thready peripheral pulses and cool, clammy extremities. A low CO may mask a new systolic murmur. Rapid assessment (e.g., heart catheterization) and intervention (e.g., valve repair or replacement) are critical.

Patients with chronic MR may remain asymptomatic for many years. Early symptoms of left ventricular failure may include weakness, fatigue, palpitations, and dyspnea. These gradually progress to orthopnea, paroxysmal nocturnal dyspnea, and peripheral edema. Increased left ventricular volume leads to an audible third heart sound (S_3), even with normal left ventricular function. The murmur is a loud holosystolic murmur at the apex radiating to the left axilla. Patients with asymptomatic MR must be monitored carefully.

Treatment for MR depends on the cause of the regurgitation. Primary MR typically requires valve repair or replacement before significant left ventricular failure or pulmonary hypertension develop.[14] Medical management includes standard HF therapy.[13]

MITRAL VALVE PROLAPSE

Etiology and Pathophysiology

Mitral valve prolapse (MVP) is an abnormality of the mitral valve leaflets and the papillary muscles or chordae that allows the leaflets to prolapse, or buckle, back into the left atrium during systole (Fig. 36.8). MVP affects 2% to 3% of the general population.[15]

The use of the term *prolapse* can be misleading because it is used even when the valve is working normally. MVP is usually benign, but serious complications can occur, including MR, IE, SCD, HF, and cerebral ischemia.

Genetic Link

Although the cause of MVP is unknown, there is an increased familial incidence. The genetic inheritance is often autosomal dominant (see Chapter 12). MVP in this group results from a connective tissue defect affecting only the valve, or as part of Marfan's syndrome or other hereditary conditions that affect collagen structure.

Clinical Manifestations

MVP has a broad range of severity. Most patients are asymptomatic for their entire lives. About 10% of those with MVP become symptomatic. A characteristic of MVP is a regurgitation murmur that is louder during systole. MVP does not alter S_1 or S_2 heart sounds. Severe MR is an uncommon but serious complication of MVP.

M-mode and 2-D echocardiography are used to confirm MVP. Dysrhythmias, such as premature ventricular contractions, paroxysmal supraventricular tachycardia, and ventricular tachycardia, may cause palpitations, light-headedness, and syncope. IE may occur in patients with MR associated with MVP.

Patients may have chest pain.[15] The cause of the chest pain may be the result of abnormal tension on the papillary muscles. Chest pain episodes tend to occur in clusters, especially during periods of emotional stress. Dyspnea, palpitations, and syncope sometimes accompany the chest pain and do not respond to antianginal treatment (e.g., nitrates). β-Blockers may control palpitations and chest pain. Encourage the patient to stay hydrated, exercise regularly, and avoid caffeine.

Most patients with MVP have a benign, manageable course. For those who do develop symptomatic MR, no current therapy delays the need for valve surgery.[16] A teaching plan for patients with MVP is outlined in Table 36.11.

AORTIC VALVE STENOSIS

Etiology and Pathophysiology

Congenital aortic stenosis (AS) is generally found in childhood, adolescence, or young adulthood. In older adults, AS is a result of RF or degeneration, similar to coronary artery disease. AS is the

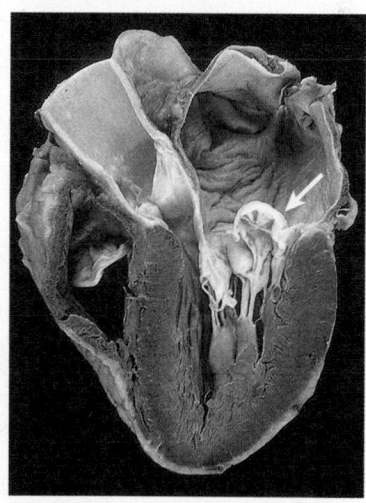

FIG. 36.8 Mitral valve prolapse. In this valvular abnormality, the mitral leaflets have prolapsed back into the left atrium. There is hooding *(arrow)*. The left ventricle is on the right. (From Kumar V, Abbas AK, Aster JC, et al: *Robbins and Cotran pathologic basis of disease,* ed 8, Philadelphia, 2010, Saunders.)

TABLE 36.11 Patient & Caregiver Teaching

Mitral Valve Prolapse

Include the following information in the teaching plan for a patient with mitral valve prolapse (MVP) and the patient's caregiver:

- Take drugs as prescribed (e.g., β-blockers to control palpitations, chest pain).
- Adopt healthy eating habits.
- Avoid caffeine because it is a stimulant and may worsen symptoms.
- If you use diet pills or other over-the-counter drugs, check for common ingredients that are stimulants (e.g., caffeine, ephedrine), since these can worsen symptoms.
- Begin, or maintain, an exercise program to achieve optimal health.
- Contact the HCP or emergency response system (ERS) if symptoms develop or worsen (e.g., palpitations, fatigue, shortness of breath, anxiety).

most frequent degenerative valve disorder, affecting 3% of people over 65 years of age.[17] In rheumatic valve disease, fusion and calcification cause the valve leaflets to stiffen and retract, resulting in stenosis. AS due to rheumatic heart disease accompanies mitral valve disease. Isolated AS is usually nonrheumatic.

AS causes obstruction of blood flow from the left ventricle to the aorta during systole. The result is left ventricular hypertrophy and increased myocardial O_2 consumption because of the increased myocardial mass. As the disease progresses and compensation fails, reduced CO leads to decreased tissue perfusion, pulmonary hypertension, and HF. Left untreated, severe AS has a poor prognosis.[18]

Clinical Manifestations

Manifestations of AS (Table 36.10) develop when the valve orifice becomes about one-third its normal size. They include the classic triad of angina, syncope, and exertional dyspnea, reflecting left ventricular failure.[17] Auscultation often reveals a normal or soft S_1, a decreased or absent S_2, and a crescendo-decrescendo systolic murmur, with radiation to the carotids.

Some patients may be asymptomatic. The prognosis is poorer for patients with symptoms and those whose valve obstruction is not fixed. Nitroglycerin is used cautiously to treat angina, since the drug can significantly reduce BP and worsen chest pain.

 DRUG ALERT Nitroglycerin

- Use cautiously in patients with AS since significant hypotension may occur.
- The drug can worsen chest pain due to the decrease in preload and drop in BP.

AORTIC VALVE REGURGITATION

Etiology and Pathophysiology

Aortic regurgitation (AR) may be the result of primary disease of the aortic valve leaflets, the aortic root, or both.[19] Trauma, IE, or aortic dissection can cause acute AR, which is a life-threatening emergency. Chronic AR generally results from rheumatic heart disease, a congenital bicuspid aortic valve, syphilis, a connective tissue problem, or a postsurgical cause.[19]

AR causes retrograde (backward) blood flow from the ascending aorta into the left ventricle during diastole. This results in volume overload. The left ventricle initially compensates for chronic AR by dilation and hypertrophy. Myocardial contractility eventually declines, and blood volume in the left atrium and pulmonary bed increases. This leads to pulmonary hypertension and right ventricular failure.

Clinical Manifestations

Patients with acute AR have sudden signs of cardiovascular collapse (Table 36.10). The patient develops severe dyspnea, chest pain, and hypotension indicating left ventricular failure and cardiogenic shock, a life-threatening emergency.

Patients with chronic, severe AR develop a *water-hammer pulse* (strong, quick beat that collapses immediately). Heart sounds may include a soft or absent S_1, S_3, or S_4 and a soft, high-pitched diastolic murmur.

The patient with chronic AR generally is asymptomatic for years.[19] Exertional dyspnea, orthopnea, and paroxysmal nocturnal dyspnea develop only after considerable heart dysfunction has occurred (Table 36.10). Angina occurs less often than in AS.

TRICUSPID AND PULMONIC VALVE DISEASE

Etiology and Pathophysiology

Tricuspid regurgitation (TR) can be primary or secondary. Primary TR is less common and is typically due to IE. Secondary TR is caused by right ventricular (RV) dilatation from pulmonary hypertension, cor pulmonale, or pulmonary outflow tract obstruction. The patient does not show JVD, enlarged liver, and peripheral edema until regurgitation is severe. Diagnosis is made by history and physical as well as echocardiogram. The prognosis is poor for severe TR.

Tricuspid stenosis is almost always caused by RF. Signs and symptoms include a fluttering discomfort in the neck, fatigue, and possible right upper quadrant pain.

Pulmonary regurgitation is often asymptomatic. A crescendo-decrescendo murmur is present. Potential causes include pulmonary hypertension, surgical repair of tetralogy of Fallot (TOF), or congenital valve disease. It can cause RV dilation.

Pulmonic stenosis is almost always a congenital part of TOF. It results in right ventricular hypertension and hypertrophy (Table 36.10). It is largely asymptomatic. When symptoms develop, they are similar to those of AS (syncope, dyspnea, angina). Symptoms typically do not present until adulthood.

DIAGNOSTIC STUDIES: VALVULAR HEART DISEASE

Diagnosis of valvular heart disease includes information from the history and physical examination and a variety of tests (Table 36.12). An echocardiogram shows valve structure, function, and heart chamber size. Transesophageal echocardiography

TABLE 36.12 Interprofessional Care

Valvular Heart Disease

Diagnostic Assessment
- History and physical examination
- Chest x-ray
- Complete blood count
- ECG
- Echocardiography (Doppler and transesophageal)
- Heart catheterization

Management
Conservative Therapy
- Prophylactic antibiotic therapy (Table 36.2)
  - Rheumatic fever
  - IE
- Sodium restriction
- Drug therapy to treat or control HF
  - Vasodilators* (e.g., nitrates, ACE inhibitors)
  - Positive inotropes (e.g., digoxin)
  - Diuretics
  - β-Blockers
- Anticoagulation therapy (see Table 37.10)
- Antidysrhythmic drugs (see Table 35.9)
- Percutaneous transluminal balloon valvuloplasty
- Percutaneous valve replacement

Surgical Therapy
- Valve repair
  - Annuloplasty
  - Commissurotomy (valvulotomy)
  - Valvuloplasty
- Valve replacement

*Use cautiously in patients with aortic stenosis.

and Doppler color-flow imaging help diagnose and monitor valvular heart disease progression. Real-time 3-D echocardiography can help assess mitral valve and congenital heart disease.

Chest x-ray shows the heart size, altered pulmonary circulation, and valve calcification. An ECG identifies HR, rhythm, and any ischemia or ventricular hypertrophy. Heart catheterization detects pressure changes in the heart chambers, records pressure differences across the valves, and measures the size of valve openings.

INTERPROFESSIONAL CARE: VALVULAR HEART DISEASE

Conservative Therapy

Overall treatment focuses on preventing exacerbations of HF, acute pulmonary edema, thromboembolism, and recurrent RF and IE (Table 36.12). HF is treated with vasodilators, positive inotropes, β-blockers, diuretics, and a low-sodium diet (see Chapter 34).

Atrial dysrhythmias are common. They are treated with calcium channel blockers, β-blockers, antidysrhythmic drugs, or electrical cardioversion (see Chapter 35). Anticoagulant therapy is used in patients with atrial fibrillation to prevent systemic or pulmonary emboli.

Percutaneous Transluminal Balloon Valvuloplasty

An alternative treatment for some patients with valvular heart disease is *percutaneous transluminal balloon valvuloplasty* (PTBV). During PTBV, the fused commissures are split open. Balloon valvuloplasty treats mitral, tricuspid, pulmonic, and AS. [14]

The PTBV procedure is done in the heart catheterization laboratory. It involves threading a balloon-tipped catheter from the femoral artery or vein to the stenotic valve. The balloon is inflated to separate the valve leaflets. A single- or double-balloon technique may be used. Using a single Inoue balloon with hourglass shape allows sequential inflation. This technique is the most popular because it is easy and has good results with few complications (Fig. 36.9).

Like PTBV, the Sapien Transcatheter Heart Valve (THV) is used for select patients with AS. The THV is inserted through the femoral artery and moved to the heart. It is released and expanded with a balloon in the location of the aortic valve. This procedure is limited to patients who are eligible for surgery but who are at high risk for surgical complications (e.g., those with multiple co-morbidities).

Surgical Therapy

The decision for valve repair or replacement depends on the patient's symptoms using the New York Heart Association classification system for functional disability (see Table 34.3). [14] The procedure used depends on the (1) valves involved, (2) pathology and severity of the disease, and (3) patient's clinical condition.

Valve Repair. Valve repair is preferred over replacement when clinically appropriate. Repair has a lower operative mortality rate than valve replacement. It is often used in mitral or tricuspid valve disease. [14] Although repair avoids the risks of replacement, it may not restore total valve function.

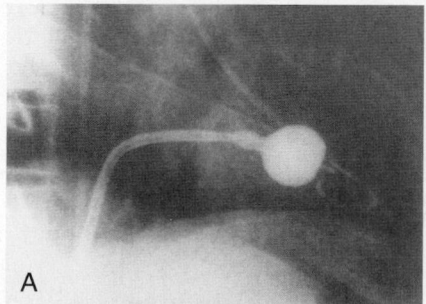
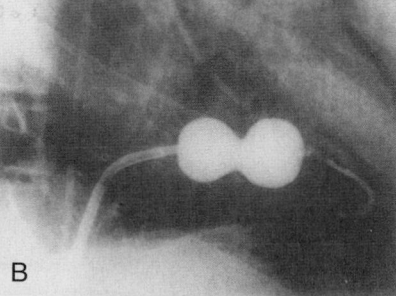
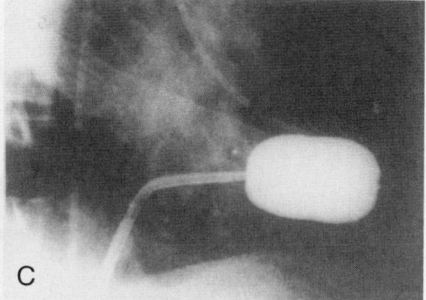

FIG. 36.9 Mitral valvuloplasty performed by the Inoue technique. The catheter is placed in the mitral valve and the distal part of the Inoue balloon inflated (**A**). The balloon is then pulled back in the mitral valve and inflated for 10 to 15 sec under fluoroscopic control (**B**) until the waist of the balloon is no longer visible (**C**) and the balloon falls back into the left atrium. (From Crawford MH, DiMarco JP, Paulus WJ: *Cardiology*, ed 3, Edinburgh, 2010, Mosby.)

Open surgical *valvuloplasty* involves repair of the valve by suturing the torn leaflets, chordae tendineae, or papillary muscles. It is primarily used to treat mitral or tricuspid regurgitation.

Minimally invasive valve surgery involves a mini-sternotomy or parasternal approach. It may include robotic and thoracoscopic surgical systems. Advantages include shorter lengths of stay, fewer blood transfusions, less pain, and lower risk for sternal infection and postoperative atrial fibrillation.

For patients with mitral or tricuspid regurgitation, further valve repair or reconstruction using annuloplasty is an option. *Annuloplasty* involves reconstruction of the annulus, with or without the aid of prosthetic rings.

Valve Replacement. Valve replacement may be needed for mitral, aortic, tricuspid, and pulmonic valve disease. A wide variety of prosthetic valves are available. Desirable valves are nonthrombogenic, are durable, and create minimal stenosis. Valves are either mechanical or biologic (tissue) valves (Fig. 36.10).

Mechanical valves are made from artificial materials. They consist of combinations of metal alloys, pyrolytic carbon, and Dacron. *Biologic valves* are made from bovine, porcine,

and human (cadaver) heart tissue. They usually contain some human-made materials. A "decellularizing" process removes the cadaver cells from the valve to lower the risk for tissue rejection. Biologic valves are asymmetric in shape. They produce a more natural pattern of blood flow compared with mechanical valves.

Mechanical valves are more durable and last longer than biologic valves. However, they have an increased risk for thromboembolism. Patients need long-term anticoagulation therapy, which increases the risk of bleeding.[13] Anticoagulation therapy is not needed with biologic valves because of their low thrombogenicity. However, they are less durable and tend to cause early calcification, tissue degeneration, and stiffening of the leaflets. Both valve types are subject to leaking and risk of IE.

Transcatheter therapies are another option for treating valvular heart disease. They are used to treat patients at high risk for surgery who have aortic or mitral bioprosthetic valve failure. Transcatheter pulmonary valve replacement is approved for use in pediatric and adult patients with pulmonary valve disease caused by congenital heart disease.

Transcatheter aortic valve replacement (TAVR) is an option for patients with severe, symptomatic AS who are at intermediate risk or higher for surgical aortic valve replacement (SAVR).[20] Symptomatic AS has a poor prognosis if left untreated. The procedure is ideally done using a transfemoral approach. The evaluation for TAVR includes echocardiogram, coronary CT angiogram, heart catheterization, and pulmonary function testing.[21] Imaging can determine valve size and plan the procedure. Currently, there are 2 TAVR valves in the United States. The Edwards Sapien 3 valve is made of bovine pericardial tissue. It is a balloon expandable valve (Fig. 36.10).[22] The CoreValve transcatheter aortic valve is a self-expanding valve made of porcine pericardial tissue (Fig. 36.11, *D*).[23]

Long-term anticoagulation is needed for those patients with biologic valves who have atrial fibrillation. Some patients with biologic valves or annuloplasty with prosthetic rings may need anticoagulation the first few months after surgery until the suture lines are covered by endothelial cells (endothelialized).

The choice of valves depends on many factors. A mechanical valve may be best for a younger patient because it is more durable. If a patient cannot take an anticoagulant (e.g., women of childbearing age), a biologic valve is considered. Frail patients with co-morbidities should be referred to a qualified heart team for a full evaluation before considering surgery.[20] Encourage patients to discuss short- and long-term consequences of valve choices with their HCPs.[21]

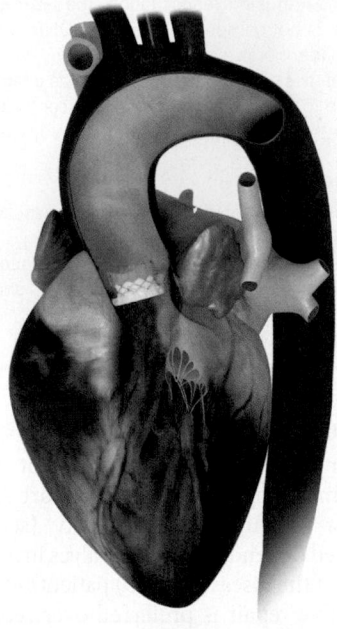

FIG. 36.10 Edwards Sapien 3 Transcatheter Heart Valve. (Courtesy Edwards Lifesciences LLC, Irvine, CA.)

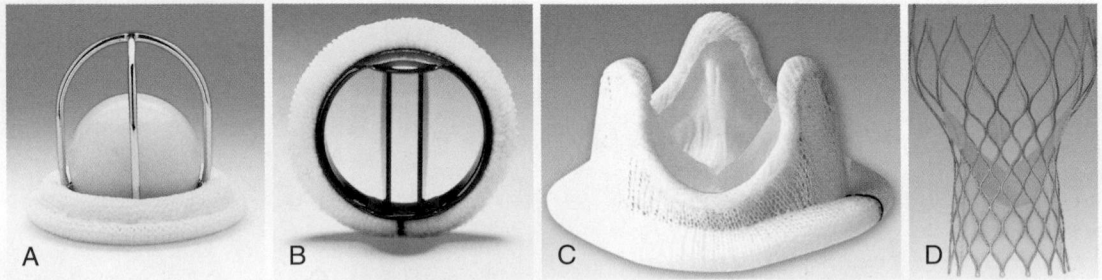

FIG. 36.11 Types of prosthetic heart valves. **A,** Starr-Edwards caged ball valve. **B,** St. Jude bi-leaflet valve. **C,** Carpentier-Edwards porcine valve. **D,** CoreValve transcatheter aortic valve (CV26 Hero), Medtronic 2015. (*A, B,* and *C,* From Bonow RO, Mann DL, Zipes DP, et al: *Braunwald's heart disease: A textbook of cardiovascular medicine,* ed 9, Philadelphia, 2012, Saunders.)

Heart Surgery Videos

Many patients prefer to watch recorded videos instead of reading educational pamphlets. For a patient facing heart surgery, these formats can be effective tools to teach the patient and caregiver what to expect before and after the procedure.
- Remember that the recorded video is not the teacher.
- Beforehand, discuss what the video presentation will cover.
- Encourage the patient and caregiver to write down questions or note what they do not understand.
- After the patient and caregiver view the material, answer any questions they have. Reinforce important information.

❖ NURSING MANAGEMENT: VALVULAR DISORDERS

◆ Nursing Assessment

Table 36.13 presents the subjective and objective data to obtain from a patient with valve disease.

◆ Nursing Diagnoses

Nursing diagnoses for the patient with valvular heart disease include:
- Impaired cardiac output
- Activity intolerance
- Fluid imbalance

More information on nursing diagnoses and interventions is in eNursing Care Plan 36.2, available on the website for this chapter.

◆ Planning

The overall goals for the patient with valve disease include (1) normal heart function, (2) improved activity tolerance, and (3) an understanding of the disease process and health maintenance measures.

◆ Nursing Implementation

◆ Health Promotion. Encouraging early treatment of streptococcal infections and providing prophylactic antibiotics for patients with a history of RF are critical to prevent acquired rheumatic valve disease. The patient at risk for IE and any patient with certain heart conditions must receive prophylactic antibiotics (Table 36.2). Teach the person with a history of RF, IE, or congenital heart disease the symptoms of valvular heart disease to report.

◆ Acute Care and Ambulatory Care. A patient with progressive valvular heart disease may need outpatient care or hospitalization for management of HF, IE, embolic disease, or dysrhythmias. HF is the most common reason for ongoing medical care.

Design activities considering the patient's limitations. An appropriate exercise plan can increase cardiac tolerance, but activities that cause fatigue and dyspnea should be limited. Tell the patient to avoid strenuous physical exercise because damaged valves may not handle the increased CO demand. Develop your patient's care plan to emphasize conserving energy, setting priorities, and taking planned rest periods. Discourage tobacco use. Consider a referral to a vocational counselor if the patient has a physically or emotionally demanding job.

Perform ongoing cardiac assessments to monitor the effectiveness of drugs. Teach the actions and side effects of drugs to increase adherence. The patient must understand the importance of prophylactic antibiotic therapy to prevent IE (Table 36.2).

When valvular heart disease can no longer be managed medically, surgery is needed (see Chapter 33 for the care of a patient having heart surgery). The patient on anticoagulants (e.g., warfarin) after surgery for valve replacement must have the international normalized ratio (INR) checked regularly to determine proper dosage and adequacy of therapy. INR values of 2.5 to 3.5 are therapeutic for patients with mechanical valves.

A teaching guide related to anticoagulation therapy is found in Table 37.14. Teach the patient to follow up with an HCP regularly and when to seek urgent medical care. Tell the patient to notify the HCP of any signs of infection, HF, or bleeding and any planned invasive or dental work. Last, encourage patients to wear a Medic Alert device or bracelet and carry the manufacturer's valve information card.

◆ Evaluation

The expected outcomes are that a patient with valvular heart disease will
- Maintain adequate tissue and organ perfusion
- Achieve fluid balance
- Achieve optimal level of activity
- Describe disease process and measures to prevent complications

TABLE 36.13 Nursing Assessment
Valvular Heart Disease

Subjective Data
Important Health Information
Past health history: RF, IE; congenital defects, heart attack, chest trauma, cardiomyopathy; syphilis, Marfan's syndrome, streptococcal infections

Functional Health Patterns
Health perception–health management: IV drug use, fatigue
Activity-exercise: Palpitations, generalized weakness, activity intolerance, dizziness, fainting, dyspnea on exertion, cough, hemoptysis, orthopnea
Sleep-rest: Paroxysmal nocturnal dyspnea
Cognitive-perceptual: Angina or atypical chest pain

Objective Data
General
Fever

Integumentary
Diaphoresis, flushing, cyanosis, clubbing, peripheral edema

Respiratory
Crackles, wheezes, hoarseness

Cardiovascular
Abnormal heart sounds, including murmurs, S_3, and S_4. Dysrhythmias, including atrial fibrillation, premature ventricular contractions. Tachycardia. ↑ or ↓ in pulse pressure, hypotension, water-hammer or thready peripheral pulses

Gastrointestinal
Ascites, hepatomegaly, unexplained weight gain

Possible Diagnostic Findings
Cardiomegaly on chest x-ray. ECG abnormalities specific to involved valve. Echocardiogram (valve disorders, chamber dilation), heart catheterization (abnormal valves, chamber pressures, CO, and blood flow, depending on involved valve)

CARDIOMYOPATHY

Cardiomyopathy (CMP) is a group of diseases that directly affect myocardial structure or function. CMP is classified as primary or secondary. *Primary CMP* refers to those conditions in which the cause is idiopathic. The heart muscle is the only part of the heart involved, and other heart structures are unaffected. In *secondary CMP*, the cause of the myocardial disease is known and is due to another disease process. Common causes of secondary CMP are listed in Table 36.14.

Three major types of CMP are dilated, hypertrophic, and restrictive. Each type has its own pathogenesis, clinical presentation, and treatment protocols (Tables 36.15 and 36.16). CMP that leads to cardiomegaly and HF is the main reason for heart transplants.

Takotsubo cardiomyopathy is a transient heart syndrome that mimics acute coronary syndrome. Patients often have chest pain, ST segment elevation on ECG, and elevated cardiac biomarkers consistent with an MI. However, when the patient undergoes heart catheterization, there is no significant coronary artery disease. It is an acute, stress-related syndrome that is more common in postmenopausal women. Most patients recover rapidly without lasting symptoms.[24]

DILATED CARDIOMYOPATHY

Etiology and Pathophysiology

Dilated cardiomyopathy is the most common type of CMP, with a prevalence of 5 to 8 cases per 100,000 people in the United States. It causes HF in 25% to 40% of cases and occurs more often in middle-aged blacks and men. Dilated CMP often follows an infectious myocarditis. Some evidence links dilated CMP with an autoimmune process or genetic causes.[25] Alcohol-related dilated CMP has its own unique presentation and treatment.[21] Other common causes of dilated CMP are listed in Table 36.14.

Dilated CMP appears with diffuse inflammation and rapid degeneration of heart fibers. This results in ventricular dilation, impaired systolic function, atrial enlargement, and blood stasis in the left ventricle. SCD from dysrhythmias is a leading cause of death in idiopathic dilated CMP.[26] Ventricular dilation causes *cardiomegaly* (Fig. 36.12) and contractile dysfunction. In contrast to HF, the walls of the ventricles do not hypertrophy.

Clinical Manifestations

The signs and symptoms of dilated CMP may develop acutely after an infection or slowly over time. Most people eventually develop HF. Symptoms can include decreased exercise capacity, fatigue, dyspnea at rest, paroxysmal nocturnal dyspnea, and orthopnea. As the disease progresses, the patient may have a

---

TABLE 36.14 Causes of Cardiomyopathy

Dilated
- Cardiotoxic agents: alcohol, cocaine, doxorubicin
- Coronary artery disease
- Genetic (autosomal dominant)
- Hypertension
- Metabolic problems
- Muscular dystrophy
- Myocarditis
- Pregnancy
- Valve disease

Hypertrophic
- Aortic stenosis
- Genetic (autosomal dominant)
- Hypertension

Restrictive
- Amyloidosis
- Cancer
- Endomyocardial fibrosis
- Post-radiation therapy
- Sarcoidosis
- Ventricular thrombus

TABLE 36.15 Types of Cardiomyopathy

	Dilated	Hypertrophic	Restrictive
Cardiac Output	Decreased	Normal or decreased	Normal or decreased
Cardiomegaly	Moderate to severe	Mild to moderate	Mild
Contractility	Decreased	Increased or decreased	Normal or decreased
Dysrhythmias	Sinus tachycardia, atrial and ventricular dysrhythmias	Atrial and ventricular dysrhythmias	Atrial and ventricular dysrhythmias
Major Manifestations	Fatigue, weakness, palpitations, dyspnea	Exertional dyspnea, fatigue, angina, syncope, palpitations	Dyspnea, fatigue
Outflow Tract Obstruction	None	Increased	None
Valvular Incompetence	Atrioventricular (AV) valves, especially mitral	Mitral valve	AV valves

---

TABLE 36.16 Interprofessional Care

Cardiomyopathy

Diagnostic Assessment
- History and physical examination
- ECG
- b-Type natriuretic peptide (BNP)
- Chest x-ray
- Echocardiogram
- Nuclear imaging studies
- Heart catheterization
- Endomyocardial biopsy

Management
- Drug therapy
  - Nitrates (except in hypertrophic cardiomyopathy)
  - β-Blockers
  - Antidysrhythmics
  - ACE inhibitors
  - Diuretics
  - Digitalis (except in hypertrophic CMP unless used to treat atrial fibrillation)
  - Anticoagulants (if indicated)
- VAD
- Cardiac resynchronization therapy
- Implantable cardioverter-defibrillator
- Surgical repair
- Heart transplant
- Cardiac rehabilitation
- Palliative and hospice care

dry cough, palpitations, abdominal bloating, nausea, vomiting, and anorexia. Signs can include an abnormal S_3 and/or S_4, dysrhythmias, heart murmurs, pulmonary crackles, edema, weak peripheral pulses, pallor, hepatomegaly, and JVD. Decreased blood flow through an enlarged heart promotes stasis and blood clot formation and may lead to systemic embolization.

Diagnostic Studies

The diagnosis of dilated CMP is based on the patient's history and exclusion of other causes of HF. Doppler echocardiography is usually the basis for diagnosing dilated CMP. Echocardiography can assess EF. EF less than 20% is associated with a 50% mortality rate within 1 year. The chest x-ray may show cardiomegaly with signs of pulmonary venous hypertension and pleural effusion. The ECG may show tachycardia, bradycardia, and dysrhythmias with conduction problems. Laboratory studies may show increased b-type natriuretic peptide (BNP) levels if HF is present.

Heart catheterization confirms or rules out coronary artery disease. An endomyocardial biopsy done at the time of the right-sided heart catheterization will identify any infectious organisms or other causes of disease.

❖ Interprofessional and Nursing Care

Interventions focus on controlling HF by enhancing heart contractility and decreasing preload and afterload. This is similar to the management of chronic HF. Treatment guidelines are based on the specific stage of disease progression (see Table 34.3). Treatment of patients with Class IV (stage D) HF is more palliative than curative.

Several different types of drugs are available to manage HF (see Table 34.7). Nitrates (e.g., nitroglycerin) and diuretics (e.g., furosemide) decrease preload. ACE inhibitors reduce afterload. β-Blockers (e.g., metoprolol [Lopressor]) and aldosterone antagonists (e.g., spironolactone [Aldactone]) control the neurohormonal stimulation that occurs in HF. Dysrhythmias are treated with the appropriate antidysrhythmic (see Chapter 35). Anticoagulation therapy reduces the risk for systemic embolization from clots that form in the heart chambers.

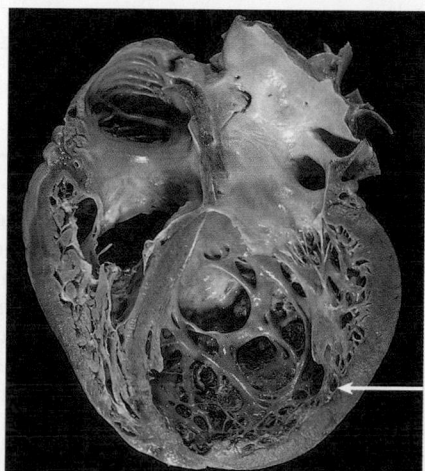

FIG. 36.12 Dilated cardiomyopathy. The dilated left ventricular wall has thinned *(arrow)*, and the chamber size and volume are increased. (From Kumar V, Abbas AK, Aster JC, et al: *Robbins and Cotran pathologic basis of disease*, ed 8, Philadelphia, 2010, Saunders.)

Drug and nutritional therapy and cardiac rehabilitation may help (1) lessen symptoms of HF and (2) improve CO and quality of life. A patient with secondary dilated CMP is treated for the underlying disease process. For example, teach the patient with alcohol-related dilated CMP to abstain from alcohol. (See Chapter 10 for more on alcohol use.)

Unfortunately, dilated CMP does not respond well to therapy and patients have multiple episodes of HF. Patients may be hospitalized for infusions of dobutamine or milrinone, followed by aggressive diuresis. Sometimes these treatments are done in an outpatient setting or in the home under nursing supervision. After treatment, many patients see an improvement in symptoms for several weeks. Medical management is based on clinical guidelines for HF.[27] Statins may be helpful (see Table 33.6).

Patients may benefit from nondrug therapies. A VAD allows the heart to rest and recover from acute HF. It may also serve as a bridge to a heart transplant. Other options include cardiac resynchronization therapy and an implantable cardioverter-defibrillator (ICD) (see Chapter 34).

The patient with terminal or end-stage CMP may consider a heart transplant. A permanent, implantable VAD, known as *destination therapy,* is an option for patients with advanced disease who are not candidates for a heart transplant (see Chapter 34). Currently, about 50% of heart transplants are done to treat CMP. Heart transplant recipients have a good prognosis. However, donor hearts are hard to obtain, and many patients with dilated CMP die before receiving a heart.

Patients with dilated CMP are very ill and have a grave prognosis. Your expert nursing care is critical. Observe for signs and symptoms of worsening HF, dysrhythmias, embolus formation, and drug effectiveness. The goals of therapy are to keep the patient at an optimal level of functioning and out of the hospital. Always include caregivers when planning a patient's care. Encourage caregivers to learn cardiopulmonary resuscitation (CPR). Teach them when and how to access emergency care.

Home health and hospice nursing can provide the patient and caregiver with palliative care. This includes strategies to maximize and maintain functional status or end-of-life care to prepare for a peaceful death.

HYPERTROPHIC CARDIOMYOPATHY

Etiology and Pathophysiology

Hypertrophic cardiomyopathy is asymmetric left ventricular hypertrophy without ventricular dilation.[28] In one form of the disease, the septum between the 2 ventricles becomes enlarged and blocks the blood flow from the left ventricle. We call this *hypertrophic obstructive cardiomyopathy* (HOCMP) or *asymmetric septal hypertrophy* (ASH).

Hypertrophic CMP occurs less often than dilated CMP. It is more common in men than in women. It is usually diagnosed in young adults and, most often, in active, athletic persons. Hypertrophic CMP is the most common cause of SCD in otherwise healthy young people. It accounts for 3% of deaths in young competitive athletes.[29] There is a link between genetic mutations and HOCMP. MYH7 and MYBPC3 are the 2 most common genes involved. They are found in about 50% of cases of HOCMP.[29]

Early identification is important (Table 36.14). The 4 main characteristics of hypertrophic CMP are (1) massive ventricular hypertrophy; (2) rapid, forceful contraction of the left ventricle; (3) impaired relaxation (diastole); and (4) obstruction to aortic outflow (not present in all patients). Ventricular hypertrophy is associated with a thickened intraventricular septum and ventricular wall (Fig. 36.13). The result is poor filling of the stiff ventricle. Decreased ventricular filling and obstruction to outflow can result in decreased CO, especially during exertion.

Clinical Manifestations

Patients with hypertrophic CMP may be asymptomatic or may have exertional dyspnea, fatigue, angina, and syncope. The most common symptom is dyspnea caused by an elevated left ventricular diastolic pressure. Fatigue occurs because of the resulting decrease in CO and in exercise-induced flow obstruction. Angina can occur and is often caused by the increased left ventricular mass or compression of the small coronary arteries by the hypertrophic ventricular myocardium. The patient may have syncope from obstruction to aortic outflow during increased activity. This results in decreased CO and cerebrovascular circulation. Syncope also can be caused by dysrhythmias, such as supraventricular tachycardia, atrial fibrillation, ventricular tachycardia, and ventricular fibrillation (see Chapter 35).

Diagnostic Studies

Clinical findings on examination may be unremarkable. On chest palpation the apical impulse can be exaggerated and displaced to the left. Auscultation may reveal an S_4 and a systolic murmur between the apex and sternal border at the fourth intercostal space. ECG findings usually show ventricular hypertrophy, ST-T wave abnormalities, prominent Q waves in the inferior or precordial leads, and dysrhythmias (see Chapter 35).

The echocardiogram is the main diagnostic tool used to confirm hypertrophic CMP. It may show wall motion abnormalities and diastolic dysfunction. Heart catheterization and nuclear stress testing may help diagnose and guide the treatment of hypertrophic CMP.

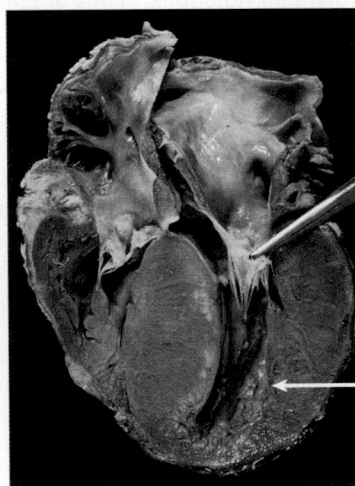

FIG. 36.13 Hypertrophic cardiomyopathy. There is marked left ventricular hypertrophy *(arrow)*, with decreased chamber size and volume. (From Kumar V, Abbas AK, Aster JC, et al: *Robbins and Cotran pathologic basis of disease,* ed 8, Philadelphia, 2010, Saunders.)

❖ Interprofessional and Nursing Care

Goals of care are to improve ventricular filling by reducing ventricular contractility and relieving left ventricular outflow obstruction. These can be achieved with β-blocker (e.g., metoprolol) or calcium channel blocker (e.g., verapamil) therapy. Digitalis is considered if needed to treat atrial fibrillation. Amiodarone or sotalol (Betapace) are effective antidysrhythmic drugs. However, their use does not prevent SCD. Patients at risk for SCD need a cardioverter-defibrillator (see Chapter 35).

AV pacing is helpful for patients with hypertrophic CMP and outflow obstruction. When the ventricles are paced from the apex of the right ventricle, septal depolarization occurs first. This allows the septum to move away from the left ventricular wall and reduces the degree of obstruction of the outflow tract.

Some patients with severe symptoms unresponsive to therapy may be candidates for surgical treatment of their hypertrophied septum. A *ventriculomyotomy and myectomy* involves cutting into the thickened septal muscle and removing some of the ventricular muscle. Most patients have an improvement in symptoms and exercise tolerance after surgery.

An alternative nonsurgical procedure to reduce symptoms and the left ventricular outflow obstruction is alcohol-induced *percutaneous transluminal septal myocardial ablation* (PTSMA). This procedure consists of injecting alcohol into the first septal artery branching off the left anterior descending artery to cause ischemia and septal wall infarction. Ablation of the septal wall decreases the obstruction to flow, and the patient's symptoms decrease. The procedure can improve HF symptoms and exercise capacity.[29] Potential complications of PTSMA include conduction problems (e.g., heart block) and MI.

Nursing interventions for hypertrophic CMP focus on relieving symptoms, observing for and preventing complications, and providing emotional support. Focus your teaching on helping patients plan to avoid strenuous activity and dehydration. Any activity that causes an increase in systemic vascular resistance (thus increasing the obstruction to forward flow) is dangerous. Rest and elevation of the feet to improve venous return to the heart can help manage chest pain. Vasodilators, such as nitroglycerin, may worsen the chest pain by decreasing venous return and further increasing obstruction of blood flow from the heart.

RESTRICTIVE CARDIOMYOPATHY

Etiology and Pathophysiology

Restrictive cardiomyopathy is the least common type of CMP. It is a disease of the myocardium that impairs diastolic filling and stretch. Systolic function stays unchanged. Although the specific cause of restrictive CMP is unknown, several pathologic processes may be involved in its development. Myocardial fibrosis, hypertrophy, and infiltration produce stiffness of the ventricular wall with loss of ventricular compliance. Secondary causes of restrictive CMP include amyloidosis, endocardial fibrosis, sarcoidosis, and radiation to the thorax. With restrictive CMP, the ventricles are resistant to filling and demand high diastolic filling pressures to maintain CO.

Clinical Manifestations and Diagnostic Studies

Classic manifestations of restrictive CMP are fatigue, exercise intolerance, and dyspnea. These occur because the heart cannot increase CO by increasing the HR without further compromising ventricular filling. Other symptoms may include angina, orthopnea, syncope, and palpitations. The patient may have signs of HF, including dyspnea, peripheral edema, weight gain, ascites, hepatomegaly, and JVD.

The chest x-ray may be normal, or it may show cardiomegaly from atrial enlargement. Pleural effusions and pulmonary congestion may occur as the patient progresses to HF. The ECG may show mild tachycardia at rest. The most common dysrhythmias are supraventricular (atrial fibrillation) or AV block. Echocardiography may show a left ventricle that is normal size with a thickened wall, slightly dilated right ventricle, and dilated atria. Endomyocardial biopsy, CT scan, and nuclear imaging may help in the diagnosis.

❖ Interprofessional and Nursing Care

There is no specific treatment for restrictive CMP. Interventions are aimed at improving diastolic filling and the underlying disease process. Treatment includes conventional therapy for HF and dysrhythmias. Heart transplant may be an option. Nursing care is similar to the care of a patient with HF. As in the treatment of patients with hypertrophic CMP, teach the patient to avoid situations that impair ventricular filling and increase systemic vascular resistance, such as strenuous activity and dehydration.

Nursing care of a patient with CMP includes individualized teaching based on the patient's manifestations. All patients with CMP are at risk for IE from any procedure that may cause bacteremia. Teach the patient about the need for prophylactic antibiotics (Table 36.2). A guide for patient and caregiver teaching is outlined in Table 36.17.

TABLE 36.17 Patient & Caregiver Teaching

Cardiomyopathy

Include the following information in the teaching plan for a patient with cardiomyopathy and the patient's caregiver.

1. Take all drugs as prescribed and regularly follow up with HCP.
2. Follow a low-sodium diet (if prescribed) and read all product labels (food and over-the-counter drugs) for sodium content.
3. Drink 6 to 8 glasses of water a day unless fluids are restricted.
4. Achieve and maintain a reasonable weight and avoid large meals.
5. Avoid alcohol, caffeine, diet pills, and over-the-counter cold medicines that may contain stimulants.
6. Balance activity and rest periods.
7. Avoid heavy lifting or vigorous isometric exercises and check with HCP for exercise guidelines.
8. Use stress management techniques: relaxation breathing, guided imagery.
9. Report any signs of HF to HCP, including weight gain, edema, shortness of breath, and increased fatigue.
10. Encourage caregivers to learn CPR because of the potential for cardiac arrest (see Appendix A).
11. Access emergency response system (ERS) according to the HCP's instructions.

CASE STUDY

Valvular Heart Disease

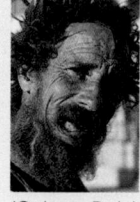
(© JennaDub/ iStock/ Thinkstock.)

Patient Profile

R.B., a 50-yr-old white man, is admitted to the hospital for acute decompensated HF due to valvular heart disease.

Subjective Data

- History of IV drug use
- Reports current regular alcohol intake of 1 pint of whiskey per day
- States, "I'm short of breath all the time. I can't sleep when I lay down."
- Describes chest pain with minimal exertion
- Recently unemployed
- States, "I'm always tired."
- States, "The drugs are too expensive. I can't afford them."
- Smokes a pack of cigarettes a day for past 35 years

Objective Data

Physical Examination

- Third heart sound (S₃)
- Loud holosystolic murmur of mitral regurgitation
- Missing all teeth from periodontal disease
- Vital signs: temperature 99.0° F (37.2° C); apical-radial pulse equal at 110 beats/min, irregular; respirations 24; BP 104/58

Diagnostic Studies

- ECG shows atrial fibrillation with a rapid ventricular response
- Chest x-ray shows pulmonary congestion and cardiomegaly
- Transesophageal echocardiography shows left atrial and ventricular hypertrophy and mitral and aortic regurgitation. EF 30%

Discussion Questions

1. Identify the cause and course of R.B.'s disease based on his history and current examination.
2. Distinguish between mitral and aortic regurgitation.
3. What medical treatments or surgical procedures will R.B. probably need as his condition worsens?
4. *Priority Decision:* Identify the priority nursing interventions for R.B.
5. *Safety:* What safety precautions should be initiated for R.B.?
6. *Collaboration:* Identify the tasks that you could delegate to unlicensed assistive personnel (UAP).
7. *Evidence-Based Practice:* R.B. asks you why he needs to be on "blood thinners" after his valves are replaced. How would you respond?

Answers are available at *http://evolve.elsevier.com/Lewis/medsurg.*

BRIDGE TO NCLEX EXAMINATION

The number of the question corresponds to the same-numbered outcome at the beginning of the chapter.

1. Which signs and symptoms should the nurse expect to find when assessing a patient with infective endocarditis who uses IV cocaine? *(select all that apply)*
   a. Retinal hemorrhages
   b. Splinter hemorrhages
   c. Presence of Osler's nodes
   d. Painless nodules over bony prominences
   e. Erythematous macules on the palms and soles

2. *Priority* nursing management for a patient with myocarditis includes interventions related to
   a. meticulous skin care.
   b. antibiotic prophylaxis.
   c. tight glycemic control.
   d. oxygenation and ventilation.

3. When teaching a patient about the long-term consequences of rheumatic fever, the nurse should discuss the possibility of
   a. valvular heart disease.
   b. pulmonary hypertension.
   c. superior vena cava syndrome.
   d. hypertrophy of the right ventricle.

4. Which is a *priority* nursing intervention for a patient during the acute phase of rheumatic fever?
   a. Giving IV antibiotics as prescribed
   b. Managing pain with opioid analgesics
   c. Encouraging fluid intake for hydration
   d. Performing frequent active range-of-motion exercises

5. A patient is diagnosed with mitral stenosis and new-onset atrial fibrillation. Which interventions could the nurse delegate to unlicensed assistive personnel (UAP)? *(select all that apply)*
   a. Obtain and record daily weight.
   b. Determine apical-radial pulse rate.
   c. Observe for overt signs of bleeding.
   d. Teach the patient how to get a Medic Alert device.
   e. Obtain and record vital signs, including pulse oximetry.

6. The nurse is caring for a patient newly admitted with heart failure secondary to dilated cardiomyopathy. Which intervention would be a *priority*?
   a. Encourage caregivers to learn CPR.
   b. Consider a consultation with hospice for palliative care.
   c. Monitor the patient's response to prescribed medications.
   d. Arrange for the patient to enter a cardiac rehabilitation program.

1. a, b, c, e. 2. d. 3. a. 4. a. 5. a, c, e. 6. c.

For rationales to these answers and even more NCLEX review questions, visit *http://evolve.elsevier.com/Lewis/medsurg.*

ⓔ EVOLVE WEBSITE/RESOURCES LIST

REFERENCES

*1. Cahill T, Baddour L, Habib G, et al: Challenges in infective endocarditis, *JACC* 69:324, 2017.

*2. Thornhill M, Jones S, Predergast B, et al. Quantifying IE risk in patients with predisposing cardiac conditions, *Eur Heart Journal* 39:586, 2018.

3. Wojda T, Cornejo K, Lin A, et al: Septic embolism: A potentially devastating complication of infective endocarditis. Retrieved from *www.intechopen.com/books/contemporary-challenges-in-endocarditis/septic-embolism-a-potentially-devastating-complication-of-infective-endocarditis.*

4. Cahill T, Predergast B: Infective endocarditis, *The Lancet* 387:882, 2016.

*5. Baddour LM, Wilson WR, Bayer AS, et al: Infective endocarditis in adults: Diagnosis, antimicrobial therapy, and management of complications, *Circulation* 132:e215, 2015. (Classic)

6. Rahman A, Sarawat A: Pericarditis, *Am Family Physician* 46:810, 2017.

7. Doctor N, Shah A, Coplan B, et al: Acute pericarditis, *Prog Cardiovasc Dis* 59:349, 2017.

8. Fung G, Luo H, Qiu Y, et al: Myocarditis, *Circ Res* 118:496, 2016.

9. Carapetis JR, Beaton A, Cunningham MW, et al: Acute rheumatic fever and rheumatic heart disease, *Nat Rev Dis Primers* 2:150, 2016.

10. Sika-Paotonu D, Beaton A, Raghu A, et al: *Acute rheumatic fever and rheumatic heart disease*, Oklahoma City, 2017, University of Oklahoma Press.

*11. Gewitz MH, Baltimore RS, Tani LY, et al: Revision of the Jones criteria for the diagnosis of acute rheumatic fever in the era of Doppler echocardiography: A scientific statement from the AHA, *Circulation* 131:1806, 2015. (Classic)

12. Wallace, M: Antibiotics for rheumatic fever. Retrieved from *https://emedicine.medscape.com/article/236582.*

13. Holmes K, Gibbison B, Vohra H: Mitral valve and mitral valve disease, *BJA Education* 17:1, 2017.

*14. Nishimura RA, Otto CM, Bonow RO, et al: 2014 AHA/ACC guideline for the management of patients with valvular heart disease: Executive summary: A report of the American College of Cardiology/AHA Task Force on Practice Guidelines, *Circulation* 129:2440, 2014. (Classic)

15. Jelani Q: Mitral valve prolapse. Retrieved from *https://emedicine.medscape.com/article/155494.*

16. Deeling F, Rong J, Larson M, et al: The evolution of mitral valve prolapse: Insights from the Framingham Heart Study, *Circulation* 133:1688, 2016.

17. Kamperidis V, Delgado V, van Mieghem N, et al: Diagnosis and management of aortic valve stenosis in patients with heart failure, *Euro Journal HF* 18:469, 2016.

18. Marquis-Gravel G, Redfors B, Leon MN, et al: Medical treatment of aortic stenosis, *JASE* 124:1766, 2016.

19. Wang SS: Aortic regurgitation. Retrieved from *https://emedicine.medscape.com/article 150490*.

*20. Nishimura RA, Otto CM, Bonow RO, et al: 2017 ACC/AHA focused update of the 2014 guidelines for the management of patients with valvular heart disease, *Circulation* 135:e1159, 2017.

*21. Bonow RO, Brown AS, Gillam C, et al: AUC for treatment of patients with severe aortic stenosis, *JASE* 31:117, 2018.

22. Edwards Lifesciences: TAVR with the Sapien 3 Valve. Retrieved from *https://tavrbyedwards.com/*.

23. Medtronic; Evolut TAVR Platform, CoreValve® Transcatheter Aortic Valve Implantation (TAVI) platform. Retrieved from *www.medtronic.com/us-en/healthcare-professionals/therapies-procedures/cardiovascular/transcatheter-aortic-valve-replacement.html*.

24. Lyon A, Bossone E, Schneider B, et al: Current state of knowledge on Takotsubo syndrome, *Eur J Heart Fail* 18:8, 2016.

25. Pinto Y, Elliott P, Arbustini E, et al: Proposal for a revised definition of DCM, *Eur Heart J* 37:1850, 2016.

*26. Al-Zaiti SS, Fallavollita JA, Cantry JM, et al: Electrocardiographic predictors of sudden and non-sudden cardiac death in patients with ischemic cardiomyopathy, *Heart Lung* 43:527, 2014. (Classic)

27. Bozkurt B, Colvin M, Cook J, et al: Current diagnostic and treatment strategies for specific DCM, *Circulation* 134:e579, 2016.

28. Hensley N, Deitrich J, Nyhan D, et al: Hypertrophic cardiomyopathy: A review, *Anesth Analg* 120:554, 2015. (Classic)

29. Marian A, Brunwald E: Hypertrophic cardiomyopathy: Genetics, pathogenesis, clinical manifestations, diagnosis, and therapy, *Circ Res* 121:749, 2017.

*Evidence-based information for clinical practice.

37

Vascular Disorders

Kimberly Day

Be the reason someone believes in the goodness of people.

Karen Salmansohn

http://evolve.elsevier.com/Lewis/medsurg

CONCEPTUAL FOCUS

Clotting
Glucose Regulation

Perfusion
Tissue Integrity

LEARNING OUTCOMES

1. Relate the etiology and pathophysiology of peripheral artery disease (PAD) to the major risk factors.
2. Describe the clinical manifestations and interprofessional and nursing management of the patient with PAD of the lower extremities.
3. Plan appropriate nursing and interprofessional management for the patient with acute arterial ischemic disorders of the lower extremities.
4. Distinguish the pathophysiology, clinical manifestations, and nursing and interprofessional management of the patient with thromboangiitis obliterans (Buerger's disease) and Raynaud's phenomenon.
5. Distinguish the pathophysiology, clinical manifestations, and interprofessional and nursing management of patients with different types of aortic aneurysms.
6. Select appropriate nursing interventions for a patient undergoing an aortic aneurysm repair.

7. Describe the pathophysiology, clinical manifestations, and interprofessional and nursing management of the patient with aortic dissection.
8. Evaluate the risk factors predisposing patients to develop superficial vein thrombosis or venous thromboembolism (VTE).
9. Distinguish between the clinical characteristics of superficial vein thrombosis and VTE.
10. Outline the interprofessional and nursing management of patients with superficial vein thrombosis and VTE.
11. Prioritize the key aspects of nursing management for the patient receiving anticoagulant therapy.
12. Relate the pathophysiology and clinical manifestations to the interprofessional care of patients with varicose veins, chronic venous insufficiency, and venous leg ulcers.

KEY TERMS

acute arterial ischemia, p. 805
aneurysm, p. 807
aortic dissection, p. 812
chronic venous insufficiency (CVI), p. 823
critical limb ischemia, p. 802
deep vein thrombosis (DVT), p. 813

intermittent claudication, p. 801
peripheral artery disease (PAD), p. 800
post-thrombotic syndrome (PTS), p. 815
superficial vein thrombosis, p. 813
thromboangiitis obliterans (Buerger's disease), p. 806

varicose veins, p. 821
venous thromboembolism (VTE), p. 813
venous thrombosis, p. 813
Virchow's triad, p. 814

Problems of the vascular system include disorders of the arteries, veins, and lymphatic vessels. These problems can result in decreased perfusion to the peripheral tissues, causing ischemia. Patients often have pain and difficulties with mobility and taking part in activities of daily living. Education is a key part of management. Proper nutrition, smoking cessation, and exercise are important health promotion behaviors. Following measures to promote safety, especially for those on anticoagulant therapy, is critical.

We classify arterial disorders as atherosclerotic, aneurysmal, and nonatherosclerotic vascular diseases. Atherosclerotic vascular disease is divided into coronary, cerebral, peripheral, mesenteric, and renal artery disease.[1] This chapter discusses peripheral artery disease, aortic aneurysm and dissection, and venous diseases.

PERIPHERAL ARTERY DISEASE

Peripheral artery disease (PAD) involves thickening of artery walls. This results in a progressive narrowing of the arteries of the upper and lower extremities. PAD prevalence increases with age. It typically becomes symptomatic between ages 50 and 70 years. In people with diabetes, PAD occurs earlier. In the United States, about 8.5 million people over age 40 have PAD, with higher prevalence in blacks.[2,3]

PAD is strongly related to other types of cardiovascular disease (CVD) and their risk factors. Patients with PAD have a significantly higher risk for mortality (in general), CVD mortality, major coronary events, and stroke.[3] PAD is a marker of advanced systemic atherosclerosis. Patients with PAD are more likely to have coronary artery disease (CAD) and/or cerebral artery disease.

Unfortunately, many people in the United States are unaware of PAD and its risk factors. PAD remains underdiagnosed and undertreated.

Etiology and Pathophysiology

The leading cause of PAD is *atherosclerosis,* a gradual thickening of the *intima* (the innermost layer of the arterial wall) and *media* (middle layer of the arterial wall). This results from cholesterol and lipids deposited within the vessel walls and leads to narrowing of the artery (see Fig. 33.1). Although the exact cause of atherosclerosis is unknown, inflammation and endothelial injury play a major role (see Chapter 33). Atherosclerosis often affects certain segments of the arterial tree. These include the coronary, carotid (see Chapter 57), and lower extremity arteries.

Other risk factors for PAD are similar, but not identical, to those for CAD. Important risk factors for PAD are tobacco use (most important), diabetes, hypertension, high cholesterol, and age over 60.[2] The presence of multiple risk factors dramatically increases the risk for PAD, especially in blacks.[2] Symptoms occur when vessels are 60% to 75% blocked.

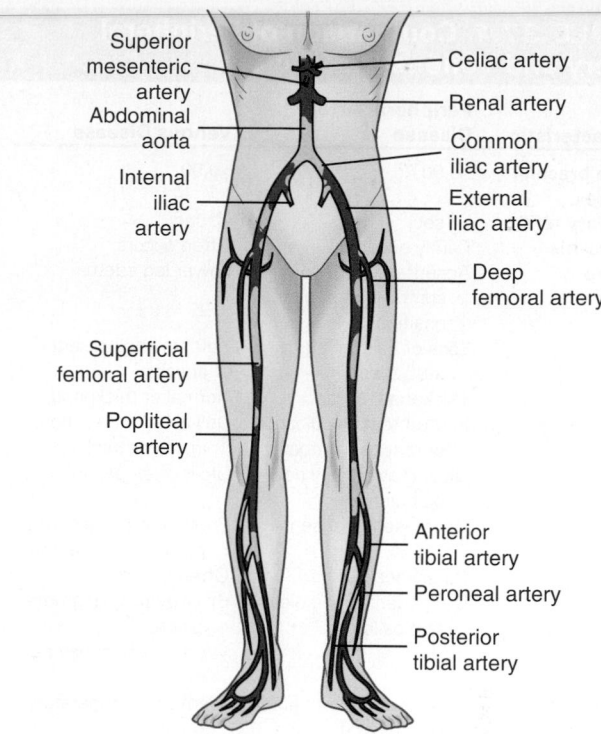

FIG. 37.1 Common anatomic locations of atherosclerotic lesions (shown in *yellow*) of the abdominal aorta and lower extremities.

Clinical Manifestations

The severity of PAD symptoms depends on the site and extent of the blockage and the amount of collateral circulation. The classic symptom of lower extremity PAD is **intermittent claudication.** This ischemic muscle pain is caused by exercise, resolves within 10 minutes or less with rest, and is reproducible. The ischemic pain is due to the buildup of lactic acid from anaerobic metabolism. Once the patient stops exercising, the lactic acid clears, and the pain subsides. PAD of the iliac arteries causes claudication in the buttocks and thighs. Calf pain indicates femoral or popliteal artery involvement.

As many as one third of patients with PAD report classic symptoms. Others have no symptoms or present with atypical leg symptoms (e.g., burning, heaviness, pressure, soreness, tightness, weakness) in atypical locations (e.g., ankle, foot, hamstring, hip, knee, shin). PAD involving the internal iliac arteries may result in erectile dysfunction.

Paresthesia (numbness or tingling) in the toes or feet may result from nerve tissue ischemia. True peripheral neuropathy occurs more often in patients with diabetes (see Chapter 48) and in those with long-standing ischemia. Neuropathy causes severe shooting or burning pain in the extremity. It does not follow particular nerve roots and may be present near ulcerated areas. Gradual, reduced blood flow to neurons causes loss of pressure and deep pain sensations. So, patients may not notice lower extremity injuries.

The limb's appearance gives vital information about reduced blood flow. The skin becomes thin, shiny, and taut. The lower legs lose their hair. Pedal, popliteal, or femoral pulses are decreased or absent. Pallor (blanching of the foot) develops when the leg is elevated (*elevation pallor*). Conversely, *reactive hyperemia* (redness of the foot) develops when the limb is in a dependent position (*dependent rubor*) (Table 37.1).

PERIPHERAL ARTERY DISEASE OF THE LOWER EXTREMITIES

Lower extremity PAD may affect the iliac, femoral, popliteal, tibial, or peroneal arteries, or any combination of these arteries (Fig. 37.1). The femoral popliteal area is the most common site in nondiabetic patients. Patients with diabetes tend to develop PAD in the arteries below the knee. Those with advanced PAD often have multiple arterial occlusions.

TABLE 37.1 Comparison of Peripheral Artery and Venous Disease

Characteristic	Peripheral Artery Disease	Venous Disease
Ankle-brachial index	≤0.90	>0.90
Capillary refill	>3 sec	<3 sec
Dermatitis	Rarely occurs	Often occurs
Edema	Absent unless leg constantly in dependent position	Lower leg edema
Hair	Loss of hair on legs, feet, toes	Hair may be present or absent
Nails	Thickened, brittle	Normal or thickened
Pain	Intermittent claudication or rest pain in foot	Dull ache or heaviness in calf or thigh
	Ulcer may or may not be painful	Ulcer often painful
Peripheral pulses	Decreased or absent	Present, may be hard to palpate with edema
Pruritus	Rarely occurs	Often occurs
Skin color	Dependent rubor, elevation pallor	Bronze-brown pigmentation
		Varicose veins may be visible
Skin temperature	Cool, temperature gradient down the leg	Warm, no temperature gradient
Skin texture	Thin, shiny, taut	Skin thick, hardened, and indurated
Ulcer		
• Location	Tips of toes, foot, or lateral malleolus	Near medial malleolus
• Margin	Rounded, smooth, looks "punched out"	Irregularly shaped
• Drainage	Minimal	Moderate to large amount
• Tissue	Black eschar or pale pink granulation	Yellow slough or dark red, "ruddy" granulation

TABLE 37.2 Interprofessional Care

Peripheral Artery Disease

Diagnostic Assessment
- Health history and physical examination, including palpation of peripheral pulses
- Doppler ultrasound studies
- Segmental BPs
- ABI (Table 37.3)
- Duplex imaging
- Angiography
- Magnetic resonance angiography

Management
- CVD risk factor modification
  - Tobacco cessation
  - Regular physical exercise
  - Achieve or maintain ideal body weight
  - Follow Dietary Approaches to Stop Hypertension (DASH) diet
  - Tight glucose control with diabetes, including Hb A1C monitoring
  - Tight BP control
  - Treatment of hyperlipidemia and hypertriglyceridemia (see Table 33.6)
  - Antiplatelet agent (aspirin, clopidogrel [Plavix])
  - ACE inhibitors (see Table 32.6)
- Treatment of claudication symptoms
  - Structured walking or exercise program
  - Cilostazol or pentoxifylline
- Nutritional therapy
- Physical/occupational therapy
- Proper foot care (see Table 48.21)

Surgical Therapy
- Percutaneous transluminal balloon angioplasty with or without stent
- Percutaneous transluminal atherectomy
- Percutaneous transluminal cryoplasty
- Peripheral artery bypass surgery
- Patch graft angioplasty, often in conjunction with bypass surgery
- Endarterectomy (for localized stenosis; rarely done as a stand-alone procedure)
- Thrombolytic therapy or mechanical clot extraction therapy (for acute ischemia only)
- Sympathectomy (for pain management only)
- Amputation

As PAD progresses and involves multiple arterial segments, continuous pain develops at rest. *Rest pain* most often occurs in the foot or toes. It is worse with limb elevation. Rest pain occurs when blood flow is insufficient to meet basic metabolic requirements of the distal tissues. Rest pain occurs more often at night because cardiac output tends to drop during sleep and the limbs are at the level of the heart. Patients often try to achieve pain relief by gravity, dangling the leg over the side of the bed or sleeping in a chair.

Critical limb ischemia (CLI) is a condition characterized by chronic ischemic rest pain lasting more than 2 weeks, nonhealing arterial leg ulcers, or gangrene of the leg from PAD. Patients with PAD who have diabetes, heart failure (HF), and a history of a stroke are at increased risk for CLI.[3]

Complications

Lower extremity PAD progresses slowly. Prolonged ischemia leads to atrophy of the skin and underlying muscles. Minor trauma to the feet (e.g., stubbing one's toe, blister from shoes) can result in delayed healing, wound infection, and tissue necrosis, especially in the patient with diabetes. Arterial (ischemic) ulcers most often occur over bony prominences on the toes, feet, and lower legs (Table 37.1). Nonhealing arterial ulcers and gangrene are the most serious complications. If PAD develops over an extended period, collateral circulation may prevent gangrene.

Amputation may be needed if adequate blood flow is not restored or if severe infection occurs. Uncontrolled pain and severe, spreading infection are indicators for amputation in people who are not candidates for revascularization.

Diagnostic Studies

Various tests assess blood flow and the vascular system (Table 37.2). Doppler ultrasound with duplex imaging maps blood flow throughout the entire region of an artery. When palpating a peripheral pulse is hard because of severe PAD, Doppler ultrasound can determine the degree of blood flow. A palpable pulse and a Doppler pulse are not equivalent, and the terms are not interchangeable.

Segmental BPs are obtained using Doppler ultrasound and a sphygmomanometer at the thigh, below the knee, and at ankle level while the patient is supine. A drop in segmental BP of greater than 30 mm Hg suggests PAD. Angiography and magnetic resonance angiography show the location and extent of PAD (see Table 31.7).

The *ankle-brachial index* (ABI) is a PAD screening tool. It is done using a hand-held Doppler. The ABI is calculated by

TABLE 37.3 Interpreting Ankle-Brachial Index Results

Ankle-Brachial Index (ABI)	Clinical Significance
>1.30	Noncompressible arteries
1.00–1.30	Normal ABI
0.91–0.99	Borderline ABI
≤0.90	Abnormal ABI
Classification of PAD Severity	
0.90–0.71	Mild PAD
0.70–0.41	Moderate PAD
≤0.40	Severe PAD

dividing the ankle systolic BPs (SBPs) by the higher of the left and right brachial SBPs. PAD guidelines recommend uniform reporting of ABI results (Table 37.3).[3] Calcified and stiff arteries in older patients and those with diabetes often show a falsely elevated ABI.

Interprofessional Care

Table 37.2 outlines the interprofessional care for a patient with PAD.

Risk Factor Modification. The first treatment goal for patients with PAD is to reduce CVD risk factors regardless of the severity of symptoms. Encourage risk factor modification with both drug therapy and lifestyle changes (see Tables 33.2 to 33.5). Hypertension is another well-known risk factor for PAD progression. Encourage reducing dietary sodium and following the Dietary Approaches to Stop Hypertension (DASH) diet. Chapter 32 discusses hypertension.

Tobacco cessation is essential to reduce the risk for CVD events, PAD progression, and death. This is a complex, difficult process with a high incidence of relapse. Suggest comprehensive tobacco cessation strategies (see Tables 10.3 to 10.6).

Diabetes is a major risk factor for PAD and increases the risk for amputation. Patients with diabetes should maintain a glycosylated hemoglobin (A1C) below 7.0% and, optimally, as near as possible to 6.0%.[5] Chapter 48 discusses diabetes.

Support aggressive lipid management for all patients with PAD. Both dietary interventions and drug therapy are needed. Statins (e.g., simvastatin [Zocor]) and a fibric acid derivative (gemfibrozil [Lopid]) may be used (see Table 33.6).

Drug Therapy. Angiotensin-converting enzyme (ACE) inhibitors (e.g., ramipril [Altace]) can reduce PAD symptoms. Antiplatelet agents are critical for reducing the risks for CVD events and death. Oral antiplatelet therapy should include low-dose aspirin therapy. Aspirin-intolerant patients may take clopidogrel (Plavix) daily. Combination antiplatelet therapy with aspirin and clopidogrel may be used by select high-risk patients. Anticoagulants (e.g., warfarin [Coumadin]) are not recommended for prevention of CVD events in patients with PAD.

 DRUG ALERT Clopidogrel (Plavix) and Omeprazole (Prilosec)

- Antiplatelet effect of clopidogrel is reduced by about half when given with omeprazole.
- This reduced effect increases the risk for myocardial infarction (MI) and stroke.

Two drugs are available to treat intermittent claudication: cilostazol and pentoxifylline. Cilostazol, a phosphodiesterase inhibitor, inhibits platelet aggregation and increases vasodilation.

Pentoxifylline, a xanthine derivative, improves the flexibility of RBCs and WBCs and decreases fibrinogen concentration, platelet adhesiveness, and blood viscosity. It is not as effective as cilostazol. Cilostazol is usually stopped within 3 months due to side effects.[3]

 DRUG ALERT Cilostazol

- Contraindicated in patients with HF.

Exercise Therapy. A supervised exercise program is recommended as part of the initial treatment for all patients with intermittent claudication. Exercise should be done for 30 to 45 min/day, at least 3 times/week, for a minimum of 3 months. Although walking is most commonly prescribed, other modes of exercise (e.g., cycling) improve walking ability and quality of life.[3]

Encouraging taking part in exercise is particularly important for women with PAD. Women have faster functional decline and greater mobility loss than men with PAD. Overall, patients with PAD who have higher levels of daily physical activity have better survival rates.[3,4]

Nutritional Therapy. Teach patients with PAD to maintain a body mass index (BMI) less than 25 kg/m² and a waist circumference less than 40 inches for men and less than 35 inches for women. Even modest, sustained weight loss of 3% to 5% yields important reductions in triglycerides, glucose, A1C, and the risk for developing type 2 diabetes. Greater weight loss has greater benefits.[5] Recommend a diet reduced in calories and salt for obese or overweight persons.[5]

Complementary and Alternative Therapies. Patients taking antiplatelet agents, nonsteroidal antiinflammatory drugs (NSAIDs) (e.g., ibuprofen), and anticoagulants (e.g., warfarin) should consult with their HCP before taking any dietary or herbal supplements because of potential interactions and bleeding risks.[6,7] See the Complementary & Alternative Therapies box on p. 818.

Care of the Leg With Critical Limb Ischemia. Optimal therapy for the patient with CLI is revascularization via bypass surgery using an *autogenous* (native) vein. An alternative is percutaneous transluminal angioplasty (PTA).[3,8] Patients with CLI who are not candidates for surgery or PTA may receive IV prostanoids (e.g., iloprost [Ventavis]). However, the FDA has not approved this drug for CLI treatment.[3,8] Patients with CLI should continue optimal drug therapy (e.g., statin, antiplatelet, ACE inhibitor, β-blocker) to reduce the risk for a CVD event.

Conservative management includes protecting the extremity from trauma, decreasing ischemic pain, preventing and controlling infection, and improving perfusion. Carefully inspect, cleanse, and lubricate feet to prevent skin cracking and infection. Avoid lubrication between the toes and soaking the patient's feet to prevent skin *maceration* (or breakdown). Keep the affected foot clean and dry. Cover any ulcers with a dry, sterile dressing. Deep ulcers are treated with a variety of wound care products. Healing is unlikely without increasing the blood flow.

Encourage the patient to wear soft, roomy, and protective footwear and avoid extremes of heat and cold. Keep the patient's heels free of pressure. Place a pillow under the calves so that the heels are off the mattress or use a commercially available heel protection device. Giving analgesics and placing the bed in the reverse Trendelenburg position may control pain and increase perfusion to the lower extremities.

Spinal cord stimulation may help manage pain for patients with CLI. Other promising strategies include growth factors and gene and stem cell therapy to stimulate blood vessel growth *(angiogenesis).* Unfortunately, almost half of the patients with CLI will die within 5 years.[8]

Interventional Radiology Catheter-Based Procedures.

Interventional radiology catheter-based procedures are alternatives to open surgery for treatment of lower extremity PAD. These procedures take place in a catheterization laboratory rather than in an operating room.

All these procedures are similar to angiography in that they involve the insertion of a specialized catheter into the femoral artery. The PTA procedure uses a catheter that has a balloon at the tip. The end of the catheter is moved to the narrowed (stenotic) area of the artery. The balloon is then inflated, compressing the atherosclerotic intimal lining.[3]

Stents, expandable metallic devices, are placed within the artery after the balloon angioplasty. The stent holds the artery open. Angioplasty balloons and peripheral stents may be coated with a drug (e.g., paclitaxel) to limit the growth of new tissue in the treated area and improve long-term patency rates.[3,9]

Atherectomy is the removal of the obstructing plaque. A directional atherectomy device uses a high-speed cutting disk that cuts long strips of the atheroma. Laser atherectomy uses ultraviolet energy to break up the atheroma. Other types of atherectomy catheters have a diamond-coated tip that rotates at a high speed (like a dental drill).

Cryoplasty combines PTA and cold therapy. A specialized balloon is filled with liquid nitrous oxide, which changes to gas as it enters the balloon. Expansion of the gas results in cooling to 14° F (−10° C). The cold temperature limits restenosis by reducing smooth muscle cell activity.

Nursing care is the same as for diagnostic angiography (see Tables 31.7 and 31.8). Antiplatelet agents are needed postprocedure to reduce the risk for restenosis. Long-term, low-dose aspirin therapy or clopidogrel is recommended.

Surgical Therapy.

Various surgical approaches can be used to improve blood flow beyond a blocked artery. When possible, peripheral artery bypass surgery is done with an autogenous vein to bypass (carry blood around) the lesion (Fig. 37.2).

Synthetic grafts are used for long routes, such as an axillary-femoral bypass. When a person's own vein is not available, human umbilical vein or a composite sequential bypass graft (native vein plus synthetic graft) can be used.[3] PTA with stenting also may be done in combination with bypass surgery.

Other surgical options include *endarterectomy* (opening the artery and removing the obstructing plaque) and *patch graft angioplasty* (opening the artery, removing plaque, and sewing a patch to the opening to widen the lumen). In-hospital mortality is higher in women undergoing revascularization than men, regardless of disease severity or procedure done.[4]

Amputation may be needed if tissue necrosis is extensive, gangrene or osteomyelitis develops, or all major arteries in the limb are blocked. We make every effort to preserve as much of the limb as possible to improve rehabilitation potential. Amputation is discussed in Chapter 62.

❖ NURSING MANAGEMENT: LOWER EXTREMITY PERIPHERAL ARTERY DISEASE

◆ Nursing Assessment

Table 37.4 presents subjective and objective data that you should obtain from a patient with PAD.

◆ Nursing Diagnoses

Nursing diagnoses for the patient with PAD may include:
- Ineffective tissue perfusion
- Activity intolerance

Additional information on nursing diagnoses and interventions for the patient with PAD of the lower extremities is presented in eNursing Care Plan 37.1 on the website for this chapter.

◆ Planning

Nursing care focuses on the priority problems of poor tissue perfusion and pain. The overall goals for the patient who has lower extremity PAD include (1) adequate tissue perfusion; (2) relief of pain; (3) increased exercise tolerance; (4) intact, healthy skin on the extremities; and (5) increased knowledge of disease and treatment plan.

◆ Nursing Implementation

◆ Health Promotion.

Assess the patient for and provide instructions on how to control CVD risk factors (see Table 33.2). Teach diet modification to reduce cholesterol, saturated fat, and refined sugars (see Tables 33.4 and 33.5). Teach proper foot care and injury prevention. Encourage patients with positive family histories of cardiac, diabetes, or vascular disease to obtain regular follow-up care.

◆ Acute Care.

After surgical or radiologic intervention, observe the patient in a recovery area. Check the operative extremity every 15 minutes initially and then hourly for color, temperature, capillary refill, presence of peripheral pulses, and sensation and movement. Immediately notify the HCP of any loss of palpable pulses or change in the Doppler sound over a pulse. Postoperative ABI measurements are not obtained as they place the patient at risk for graft thrombosis. Compare assessment findings with the patient's baseline and with findings in the opposite limb.

PAD patients with a history of chronic ischemic rest pain may have developed a tolerance to opioids. Thus aggressive pain management may be needed after surgery.

After the patient leaves the recovery area, continue to monitor extremity perfusion. Assess for complications, such as bleeding,

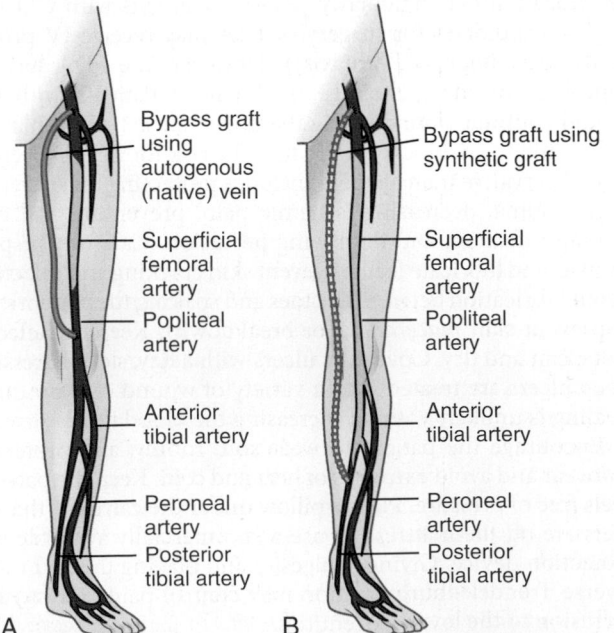

FIG. 37.2 A, Femoral-popliteal bypass graft around an occluded superficial femoral artery. B, Femoral-posterior tibial bypass graft around occluded superficial femoral, popliteal, and proximal tibial arteries.

Labels for A:
- Bypass graft using autogenous (native) vein
- Superficial femoral artery
- Popliteal artery
- Anterior tibial artery
- Peroneal artery
- Posterior tibial artery

Labels for B:
- Bypass graft using synthetic graft
- Superficial femoral artery
- Popliteal artery
- Anterior tibial artery
- Peroneal artery
- Posterior tibial artery

TABLE 37.4 Nursing Assessment

Peripheral Artery Disease

Subjective Data

Important Health Information

Past health history: Tobacco use, diabetes, hypertension, hyperlipidemia, hypertriglyceridemia, hyperuricemia, impaired renal function, obesity. ↑ High-sensitivity C-reactive protein, homocysteine, or lipoprotein (a) [Lp(a)] levels. Positive family history, sedentary lifestyle, stress

Functional Health Patterns

Health perception–health management: Family history of CVD. Tobacco use, including exposure to environmental smoke
Nutritional-metabolic: High sodium, saturated fat, and cholesterol intake. Elevated Hb A1C
Activity-exercise: Exercise intolerance
Cognitive-perceptual: Buttock, thigh, or calf pain that is precipitated by exercise and that subsides with rest (intermittent claudication) or progresses to pain at rest. Burning pain in feet and toes at rest. Numbness, tingling, sensation of cold in legs or feet. Progressive loss of sensation and deep pain in extremities
Sexuality-reproductive: Erectile dysfunction

Objective Data

Integumentary

Loss of hair on legs and feet. Thick toenails. Pallor with elevation. Dependent rubor. Thin, cool, shiny skin with muscle atrophy. Skin breakdown and arterial ulcers, especially over bony areas. Gangrene

Cardiovascular

Decreased or absent peripheral pulses. Feet cool to touch. Capillary refill >3 seconds. Bruits may be present at pulse sites.

Neurologic

Mobility or sensation impairment

Possible Diagnostic Findings

Arterial stenosis evident with duplex imaging, ↓ Doppler pressures, ↓ ABI, angiography shows peripheral atherosclerosis

---

hematoma, thrombosis, embolization, and compartment syndrome. A dramatic increase in pain, loss of previously palpable pulses, extremity pallor or cyanosis, numbness or tingling, or a cold extremity suggests graft or stent blockage. Report these findings to the HCP at once.

Do not place the patient in a knee-flexed position except for exercise. Turn the patient and position frequently with pillows to support the incision. On postoperative day 1, assist the patient out of bed several times. Walking even short distances is desirable. A walker may be helpful, especially for frail, older patients. Discourage prolonged sitting with legs lowered, since it may cause pain and edema, increase the risk for venous thrombosis, and place stress on the suture lines. Graduated compression stockings may help control leg edema. If edema develops, position the patient supine, and elevate the leg above heart level.

CHECK YOUR PRACTICE

You are caring for a 74-yr-old male patient who is recovering from left femoral-popliteal bypass graft surgery. When you respond to the patient's call bell, the patient reports severe pain in the operative leg. On assessment, you note that the dorsalis pedis and posterior tibial pulses are no longer palpable and the foot is cold to touch.
• What are your next actions?

Surgical site infection (SSI) is a serious complication. Careful postoperative assessment and wound care are important. SSIs are associated with early graft loss, longer hospitalizations, reoperation, and sepsis. If no complications occur, discharge occurs 3 to 5 days after surgery.

◆ **Ambulatory Care.** Assess for CVD risk factors. Be alert for opportunities to teach patients health promotion strategies. Continued tobacco use dramatically decreases the patency rates of grafts and stents and increases the risk for an MI or stroke.

Long-term antiplatelet therapy with aspirin or clopidogrel is used after surgery. Patients having distal peripheral bypass surgery (i.e., below the knee) using synthetic graft materials receive dual antiplatelet therapy (clopidogrel plus aspirin) for 1 to 3 months, followed by lifelong single antiplatelet therapy.[10]

Encourage supervised exercise training after revascularization. Explain that exercise decreases CVD risk factors, including hypertension, hyperlipidemia, obesity, and glucose levels. Teach foot care to all patients with PAD. Meticulous foot care is especially important in the patient with diabetes and PAD (see Table 48.21). Diabetic neuropathy increases the patient's risk for injury and results in delay in seeking treatment. Tell patients to inspect their legs and feet daily for changes in skin color or texture. Show patients how to check skin temperature and capillary refill and to palpate pulses. Stress reporting any changes in these findings or the development of ulceration or inflammation to the HCP.

Thick or overgrown toenails and calluses are potentially serious and need regular attention by an HCP (e.g., podiatrist). Patients who have poor eyesight, back problems, obesity, or arthritis may need help with foot care. Encourage patients to wear clean, all-cotton or all-wool socks and comfortable shoes with rounded (not pointed) toes and soft insoles. Tell patients to lace shoes loosely and to break in new shoes gradually (Table 37.5).

◆ **Evaluation**

The expected outcomes are that a patient with PAD of the lower extremities will have
• Adequate peripheral tissue perfusion
• Increased activity tolerance
• Effective pain management
• Knowledge of disease and treatment plan

ACUTE ARTERIAL ISCHEMIC DISORDERS

Etiology and Pathophysiology

Acute arterial ischemia is a sudden interruption in the arterial blood supply to a tissue, an organ, or an extremity that, if left untreated, can result in tissue death. It is caused by embolism, thrombosis of an atherosclerotic artery, or trauma. *Embolization* of a thrombus from the heart is the most frequent cause of acute arterial occlusion. Heart conditions in which thrombi can develop include infective endocarditis, mitral valve disease, atrial fibrillation, cardiomyopathies, and prosthetic heart valves. Noncardiac sources of emboli include aneurysms, ulcerated atherosclerotic plaque, recent endovascular procedures, and venous thrombi.

Thrombi that originate in the left side of the heart may dislodge and travel anywhere in the systemic circulation. Most emboli block an artery of the leg where vessels branch (e.g., iliofemoral, popliteal, tibial) or narrow. Sudden local thrombosis may occur at the site of an atherosclerotic plaque. Hypovolemia

TABLE 37.5 Patient & Caregiver Teaching

Peripheral Artery Bypass Surgery

Include the following information in the teaching plan for a patient undergoing peripheral artery bypass surgery and the patient's caregiver:

1. Reduce risk factors by stopping the use of all tobacco products, controlling blood glucose levels with diabetes and BP, lowering cholesterol and triglyceride levels, achieving or maintaining ideal body weight, and exercising regularly.
2. Provide teaching about the basic mechanism of action (why prescribed for patient) and side effects of drugs, such as antiplatelets, antihypertensives, lipid-lowering therapy, and pain medication.
3. Eat healthy—it is essential to recovery. Drink plenty of fluids, eat a well-balanced diet (e.g., foods high in protein, vitamins C and A, and zinc; high-fiber foods; fresh fruits and vegetables), eat fewer high-fat foods, and reduce salt intake.
4. Take part in a supervised exercise program or take a daily walk. In the beginning, take several short walks a day and rest between activities. Gradually increase your walking to 30 to 40 min/day, 3 to 5 days/wk.
5. Care for feet and legs. Inspect feet and wash them daily. Wear clean cotton or wool socks and well-fitting shoes. File toenails straight across. Avoid sitting with legs crossed, extreme hot and cold temperatures, and prolonged standing.
6. Follow routine postoperative wound care that includes keeping incision clean and dry; do not disturb Steri-Strips (if present).
7. Monitor for signs and symptoms of impaired healing or infection of the leg incision, and notify HCP if any of the following occur:
   - Prolonged drainage or pus from the incision
   - Increased redness, warmth, pain, or hardness along incision
   - Separation of wound edges
   - Temperature >100° F (37.8° C)
8. Keep all follow-up appointments with HCP.
9. Notify HCP at once of increased leg or foot pain or a change in the color or temperature of leg or foot.

(e.g., shock), hyperviscosity (e.g., polycythemia), and hypercoagulability (e.g., chemotherapy) predispose a person to thrombotic arterial occlusion.

Traumatic injury to an extremity may cause partial or total arterial blockage. Acute arterial occlusion may develop from arterial dissection in the carotid artery or aorta or from a procedure-related arterial injury (e.g., after angiography).

Clinical Manifestations

Manifestations of acute arterial ischemia include the *6 Ps: pain, pallor, pulselessness, paresthesia, paralysis,* and *poikilothermia* (adaptation of the limb to the environmental temperature, most often cool). If you detect these signs, immediately notify the HCP. Without immediate intervention, ischemia may progress to tissue necrosis and gangrene within a few hours.

Paralysis is a late sign of acute arterial ischemia and signals the death of nerves supplying the extremity. Foot drop occurs from nerve damage. Because nerve tissue is extremely sensitive to hypoxia, limb paralysis or ischemic neuropathy may persist even after revascularization.

Interprofessional Care

Early diagnosis and treatment are essential to keep the affected limb viable during acute arterial ischemia. Anticoagulant therapy with IV unfractionated heparin (UH) is started to prevent thrombus growth and inhibit further embolization. In patients undergoing embolectomy, UH should be followed by long-term anticoagulation (see discussion of anticoagulant options later in this chapter).

To restore blood flow, the thrombus is removed as soon as possible. Options consist of surgical thrombectomy (recommended procedure), percutaneous catheter-directed thrombolytic therapy, percutaneous mechanical thrombectomy with or without thrombolytic therapy, or surgical bypass.

Percutaneous catheter-directed thrombolytic therapy using alteplase or urokinase is recommended for acute arterial ischemia of less than 14 days. The HCP inserts a catheter into the femoral artery and moved it to the site of the clot, and the thrombolytic drug is continuously infused. Thrombolytic agents work by directly dissolving the clot over a period of 24 to 48 hours. (Chapter 33 discusses thrombolytic therapy.) Close monitoring is required to make sure the catheter does not move and the patient does not bleed from the site of the catheter insertion.

Surgical revascularization may be used in a patient with trauma (e.g., laceration of the artery) or with significant arterial blockage. Amputation is reserved for patients with ischemic rest pain and tissue loss in whom limb salvage is not possible. If the patient is at risk for further embolization from a persistent source (e.g., chronic atrial fibrillation), long-term anticoagulation is recommended.[6,10]

THROMBOANGIITIS OBLITERANS

Thromboangiitis obliterans (Buerger's disease) is a nonatherosclerotic, segmental, recurrent inflammatory disorder of the small and medium arteries and veins of the arms and legs. Rarely, cerebral, coronary, mesenteric, pulmonary, and/or renal arteries may be involved. The disease occurs mostly in men younger than 45 years of age with a long history of tobacco and/or marijuana use without other CVD risk factors (e.g., hypertension, hyperlipidemia, diabetes).[11]

In the acute phase of Buerger's disease, an inflammatory thrombus blocks the vessel. Over time, the thrombus becomes more organized and the inflammation in the vessel wall subsides.[11] During the chronic phase, thrombosis and fibrosis in the vessel cause tissue ischemia.

The symptoms of Buerger's disease often are confused with PAD and other autoimmune diseases (e.g., scleroderma). Patients may have intermittent claudication of the feet, hands, or arms. As the disease progresses, rest pain and ischemic ulcerations develop. Other signs and symptoms may include color and temperature changes of the limbs, paresthesia, superficial vein thrombosis, and cold sensitivity.

There are no laboratory or diagnostic tests specific to Buerger's disease. The diagnosis is based on age of onset; history; symptoms; involvement of distal vessels; presence of ischemic ulcerations; and exclusion of autoimmune disease, diabetes, thrombophilia (inherited tendency to clot), and other sources of emboli, such as atherosclerosis and aneurysm.[11]

The main treatment for Buerger's disease is the complete cessation of tobacco and marijuana use in any form. Use of nicotine replacement products is contraindicated.

Conservative management includes avoiding limb exposure to cold temperatures, a supervised walking program, antibiotics to treat any infected ulcers, and analgesics to manage the ischemic pain. Teach patients to avoid trauma to the extremities.

IV iloprost (Ventavis), a prostaglandin analog that promotes vasodilation, is used to manage rest pain, promote healing of ischemic ulcers, and decrease the need for amputation.[11] Surgical options include lumbar sympathectomy (transection of a nerve, ganglion, and/or plexus of the sympathetic nervous system), implanting a spinal cord stimulator, microsurgical flap and omental transfer, bypass surgery, and stem cell therapy.[11] Sympathectomy and a spinal cord stimulator can improve distal blood flow, reduce pain, and decrease the rate of amputation, but neither alters the inflammatory process. Bypass surgery typically is not an option because of the involvement of smaller, distal vessels. It may be used in select patients with severe ischemia. Stem cells can differentiate into specialized adult cells, with the potential to become any tissue in the human body. Stem cell therapy promotes ulcer healing, new blood vessel formation, and nerve cell regeneration.[11]

Painful ulcerations may require finger or toe amputations. Amputation below the knee may be needed in severe cases. The rate of amputation in those who continue tobacco or marijuana use after diagnosis is much higher than in those who stop.[11]

RAYNAUD'S PHENOMENON

Raynaud's phenomenon is an episodic vasospastic disorder of small cutaneous arteries, most often involving the fingers and toes. It occurs more often in women, especially those between 15 and 40 years of age. The pathogenesis of Raynaud's phenomenon is due to abnormalities in the vascular, intravascular, and neuronal mechanisms that cause vasodilation.[12]

Raynaud's phenomenon may occur in isolation (primary Raynaud's phenomenon) or with an underlying disease (e.g., thyroid conditions, scleroderma, systemic lupus erythematosus) (secondary Raynaud's phenomenon). Other contributing factors include the use of vibrating machinery or work in cold environments, exposure to heavy metals (e.g., lead), and high homocysteine levels.

Diagnosis is based on persistent symptoms for at least 2 years. Patients with Raynaud's phenomenon should have routine follow-up to monitor for development of connective tissue or autoimmune diseases.

Raynaud's phenomenon is characterized by vasospasm-induced color changes of fingers, toes, ears, and nose (white, blue, and red). Decreased perfusion results in pallor (white). The digits then appear cyanotic (bluish purple) (Fig. 37.3). These changes are followed by rubor (red), a hyperemic response when blood flow is restored. The patient usually describes coldness and numbness in the vasoconstrictive phase. This is followed by throbbing, aching pain, tingling, and swelling in the hyperemic phase. An episode usually lasts only minutes but may last for several hours. Exposure to cold, emotional upsets, tobacco use, and caffeine often bring on symptoms.

After frequent, prolonged attacks, the skin may become thickened and the nails brittle. Sometimes, complications include *punctate* (small hole) lesions of the fingertips and superficial gangrenous ulcers.

Patient teaching is the focus of nursing care for Raynaud's phenomenon. Focus your instructions on preventing episodes. Tell patients to avoid temperature extremes and wear loose, warm clothing as protection from the cold, including gloves when handling cold objects. The patient should stop using all tobacco products and avoid caffeine and other drugs that have vasoconstrictive effects (e.g., cocaine, amphetamines, ergotamine, pseudoephedrine). Provide patients with appropriate stress management strategies. Immersing hands in warm water often decreases the vasospasm.

Sustained-release calcium channel blockers (e.g., nifedipine [Procardia]) are the first-line drug therapy. They relax smooth muscles of the arterioles by blocking the influx of calcium into the cells. This reduces the frequency and severity of vasospastic attacks. If symptoms persist, other vasodilators (e.g., phosphodiesterase-5 inhibitors [sildenafil]) or topical nitroglycerin 2% ointment may be used. Calcium channel blockers can be taken with nitroglycerin topical ointment. Phosphodiesterase-5 inhibitors are not used with topical nitroglycerin due to risk for hypotension.[12]

Prompt intervention is needed for patients with digital ulceration or critical ischemia. Treatment options include prostacyclin infusion therapy (e.g., iloprost), antibiotics, analgesics, and surgical debridement of necrotic tissue. Botulinum toxin A and statins may lessen the severity of Raynaud's phenomenon.[12] Sympathectomy is done only in severe cases refractory to medical treatment where digit survival is threatened.

AORTIC ANEURYSMS

The aorta is the largest artery and supplies O_2, nutrients, and blood to all vital organs. One of the most common problems affecting the aorta is an aneurysm, which is a permanent, localized outpouching or dilation of the vessel wall. Aneurysms occur in men more often than in women and in whites more often than blacks. The incidence increases with age.[3,13] Aneurysms may occur in more than 1 location.

Etiology and Pathophysiology

Aortic aneurysms may involve the aortic arch and thoracic and/or abdominal aorta. Three fourths of aortic aneurysms occur in the abdominal aorta (Fig. 37.4) and one fourth in the thoracic aorta. Most abdominal aortic aneurysms (AAAs) occur below the renal arteries.

A variety of disorders are associated with aortic aneurysms. The main causes are classified as degenerative, congenital, mechanical (e.g., penetrating or blunt trauma), inflammatory (e.g., aortitis [Takayasu's arteritis]), or infectious (e.g., aortitis [*Chlamydia pneumoniae*, human immunodeficiency virus]).

Risk factors for aortic aneurysms include age, male gender, hypertension, CAD, family history, tobacco use, high cholesterol, lower extremity PAD, carotid artery disease, previous stroke, and obesity. Tobacco use is the most important modifiable risk factor.[1,13] The larger the aneurysm, the greater is the risk for rupture.

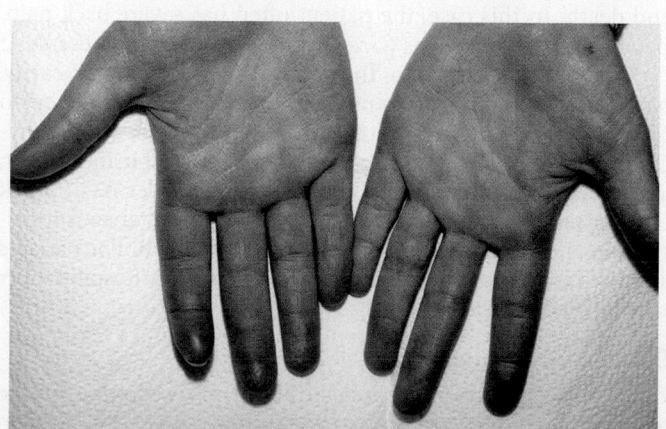

FIG. 37.3 Raynaud's phenomenon. (From James WD, Elston DM, Dirk M: *Andrews' diseases of the skin clinical atlas*, St Louis, 2018, Elsevier.)

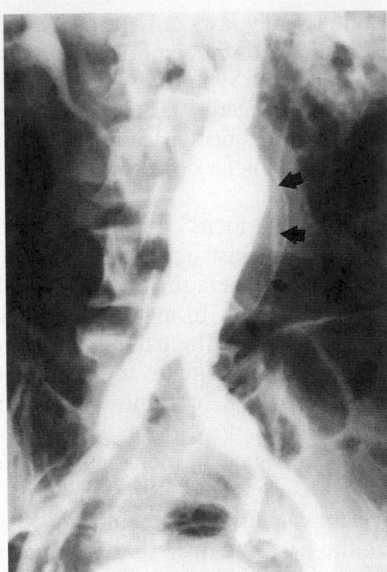

FIG. 37.4 Angiography showing fusiform abdominal aortic aneurysm. Note calcification of the aortic wall (arrows) and extension of the aneurysm into the common iliac arteries. (Courtesy Jo Menzoian, Boston, MA.)

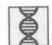 ## Genetic Link

Both aortic aneurysm and aortic dissection has a strong genetic component. The familial tendency is related to several congenital anomalies. Examples include bicuspid aortic valve, coarctation of the aorta, Turner syndrome, autosomal dominant polycystic kidney disease, specific collagen defects (e.g., Ehlers-Danlos syndrome), and premature breakdown of vascular elastic tissue (e.g., Marfan's syndrome).[1,13]

Classification

Aneurysms are classified as true or false aneurysms (Fig. 37.5, A to C). A *true aneurysm* is one in which the wall of the artery forms the aneurysm, with at least 1 vessel layer still intact. True aneurysms are subdivided into fusiform and saccular types. A *fusiform aneurysm* is circumferential and relatively uniform in shape. A *saccular aneurysm* is pouchlike with a narrow neck connecting the bulge to 1 side of the arterial wall.

A *false aneurysm,* or *pseudoaneurysm,* is not an aneurysm. It is a disruption of all arterial wall layers with bleeding that is contained by surrounding anatomic structures. False aneurysms may result from trauma, infection, peripheral artery bypass graft surgery (at the site of the graft-to-artery anastomosis), or arterial leakage after removal of cannulae (e.g., femoral artery catheters, intraaortic balloon pump devices).

Clinical Manifestations

Thoracic aortic aneurysms (TAAs) are often asymptomatic. When present, symptoms include deep, diffuse chest pain that may extend to the interscapular area. Ascending aorta and aortic arch aneurysms can cause (1) angina from decreased blood flow to the coronary arteries; (2) transient ischemic attacks from decreased blood flow to the carotid arteries; and (3) coughing, shortness of breath, hoarseness, and/or difficulty swallowing from pressure on the laryngeal nerve. If the aneurysm presses on the superior vena cava, decreased venous return can result in jugular venous distention and edema of the face and arms.

AAAs are often asymptomatic. They are often found during routine physical examinations or evaluations for an unrelated

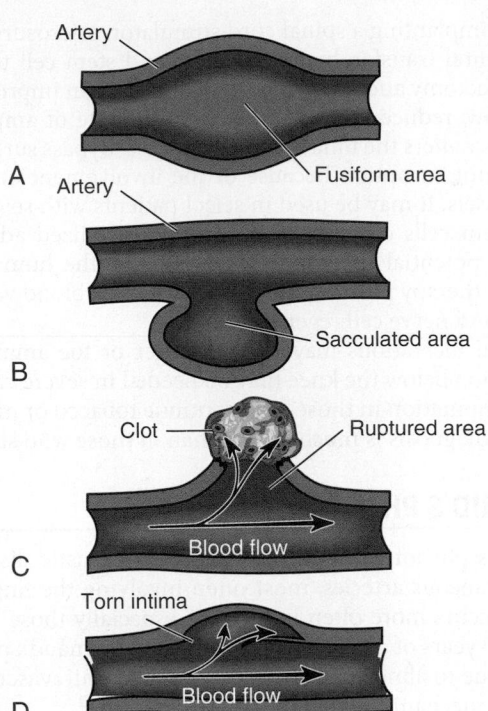

FIG. 37.5 A, True fusiform abdominal aortic aneurysm. B, True saccular aortic aneurysm. C, False aneurysm, or pseudoaneurysm. D, Aortic dissection.

problem (e.g., abdominal x-ray, CT scan). A pulsatile mass in the periumbilical area slightly to the left of the midline may be present. Bruits may be auscultated over the aneurysm. Physical findings may be hard to detect in obese persons.

AAA symptoms may mimic pain associated with abdominal or back disorders. Compression of nearby anatomic structures and nerves may cause symptoms, such as back pain, epigastric discomfort, altered bowel elimination, and intermittent claudication. Sometimes, aneurysms spontaneously embolize plaque, causing "blue toe syndrome" (patchy mottling of the feet and toes in the presence of palpable pedal pulses).

Complications

Aneurysm rupture is the most serious complication. It is more likely to occur in people who smoke tobacco.[13] If rupture occurs into the retroperitoneal space, bleeding may be controlled by surrounding anatomic structures, preventing exsanguination and death. In this case, the patient often has severe back pain. Back or flank ecchymosis (*Grey Turner sign*) may be present.

If rupture occurs into the thoracic or abdominal cavity, patients can die from massive hemorrhage. The patient who reaches the hospital will be in hypovolemic shock with tachycardia, hypotension, pale clammy skin, decreased urine output, altered level of consciousness, and abdominal tenderness. (Shock is discussed in Chapter 66.) In this situation, simultaneous resuscitation and immediate surgical repair are needed. For patients admitted to the hospital with a ruptured AAA, in-hospital mortality is high at 53%.[13]

Diagnostic Studies

Chest x-rays are done to reveal abnormal widening of the thoracic aorta. An abdominal x-ray may show calcification within the aortic wall. An ECG may rule out MI, since thoracic aneurysm or dissection symptoms can mimic angina.

Echocardiography assesses the function of the aortic valve. Ultrasound is useful for aneurysm screening and to monitor aneurysm size. A CT scan or MRI can diagnose and assess the location and severity of aneurysms. Angiography gives helpful information by using contrast imaging to map the entire aortic system. (Chapter 31 and Table 31.7 discuss angiography.)

Interprofessional Care

The main goal of interprofessional care is to prevent the rupture of an aneurysm. Early detection and prompt treatment are essential. Conservative medical therapy of small, asymptomatic AAAs (less than 5.4 cm) is the best practice.[13] This consists of risk factor modification (ceasing tobacco use, decreasing BP, optimizing lipid profile, gradually increasing physical activity).[13] Patients should receive medical management for hypertension, hyperlipidemia, diabetes, and other CVD risk factors. A statin and an ACE inhibitor could prove to be beneficial. Those with small aneurysms, 4.0 to 5.4 cm, should have monitoring of aneurysm size using ultrasound or CT every 6 to 12 months. Ultrasound monitoring every 3 years is done for patients with AAAs smaller than 4.0 cm in diameter.

Surgical repair is recommended in patients with asymptomatic aneurysms 5.5 cm in diameter or larger. Surgical intervention may occur sooner if the patient has a genetic disorder (e.g., Marfan's, Ehlers-Danlos syndrome), the aneurysm expands rapidly, the patient becomes symptomatic, or the risk for rupture is high.[13] A careful review of body systems is needed to identify any co-morbidities as they affect the patient's surgical risk. Correcting existing carotid or coronary artery blockages may be needed before aneurysm repair.

Surgical Therapy. For elective aneurysm repair surgery, the patient should be well hydrated with normal electrolytes, coagulation, and hematocrit. If the aneurysm ruptures, emergent surgery is required.

Open aneurysm repair (OAR) involves a large abdominal incision through which the surgeon (1) cuts into the diseased aortic segment, (2) removes any thrombus or plaque, (3) sutures a synthetic graft to the aorta proximal and distal to the aneurysm, and (4) sutures the native aortic wall around the graft to act as a protective cover (Fig. 37.6). For iliac artery aneurysms, a bifurcated graft replaces the entire diseased segment. With saccular aneurysms, it may be possible to excise only the bulbous lesion and repair the artery by primary closure (suturing the artery together) or applying an autogenous or synthetic patch graft.

All OARs require aortic cross-clamping proximal and distal to the aneurysm. Most resections are done in 30 to 45 minutes, then the clamps are removed and blood flow is restored. The risk for postoperative complications, such as acute kidney injury, increases in patients who have OAR of AAAs above the level of the renal arteries.

Endovascular Graft Procedure. Minimally invasive endovascular aneurysm repair (EVAR) is an alternative to OAR for select patients. Eligibility criteria include iliofemoral vessels that allow for safe graft insertion and vessels of sufficient length and width to support the graft.[13]

EVAR involves the placement of a sutureless aortic graft into the abdominal aorta inside the aneurysm via the femoral artery. Grafts are made of various materials, such as a Dacron cylinder consisting of several sections, and supported with multiple rings of flexible wire.

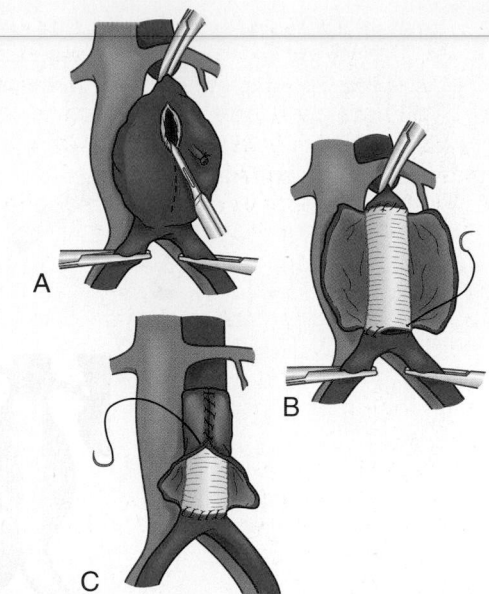

FIG. 37.6 Surgical repair of an abdominal aortic aneurysm. **A,** Incising the aneurysmal sac. **B,** Insertion of synthetic graft. **C,** Suturing native aortic wall over synthetic graft.

The main section of the graft is bifurcated. It is delivered through a femoral artery catheter. The second part of the graft is inserted through the opposite femoral artery. When all graft components are in place, they are deployed against the vessel wall by balloon inflation. The blood then flows through the endovascular graft, preventing further expansion of the aneurysm (Fig. 37.7).

Angiography is done afterward to check for any leaks and to confirm patency of all stent-graft components. The aneurysmal wall shrinks over time because the blood is diverted through the endograft.

Complications. EVAR is less invasive than OAR and requires a shorter hospital stay. EVAR also has fewer complications, such as paraplegia and death.

The most common complication of AAA repair is *endoleak,* the seepage of blood back into the old aneurysm. This may result from an inadequate seal at either graft end, a tear through the graft fabric, or leakage between overlapping graft segments. Repair may require coil embolization (insertion of beads) for hemostasis.

Other complications include aneurysm growth above or below the graft, aneurysm rupture, aortic dissection, bleeding, renal artery occlusion caused by stent migration, graft thrombosis, incisional site hematoma, and incisional infection. Patients undergoing EVAR need periodic imaging for the rest of their lives to monitor for an endoleak, document stability of the aneurysm sac, and determine the need for surgical intervention.

A potentially lethal complication in an emergency repair of a ruptured AAA is the development of *intraabdominal hypertension* (IAH) with associated *abdominal compartment syndrome*. Persistent IAH reduces blood flow to the viscera. Abdominal compartment syndrome refers to the impaired organ perfusion caused by IAH and resulting multisystem organ failure. IAH is confirmed by measuring the patient's intraabdominal pressure indirectly through a catheter and transducer system.

Treatment goals include control of situations that lead to IAH. Interventions include open (surgical) decompression,

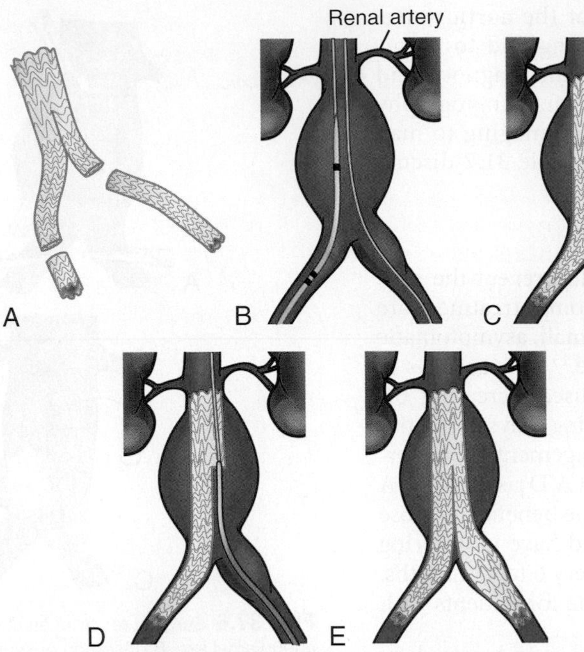

FIG. 37.7 Bifurcated (2-branched) endovascular stent grafting of an aneurysm. **A,** Insertion of a woven polyester graft covered by a tubular metal web (stent). **B,** The stent graft is inserted through a large blood vessel (e.g., femoral artery) using a delivery catheter. The catheter is positioned below the renal arteries in the area of the aneurysm. **C,** The stent graft is slowly released into the blood vessel. When the stent comes in contact with the blood vessel, it expands to a preset size. **D,** A second stent graft can be inserted in the opposite vessel, if needed. **E,** Fully deployed bifurcated stent graft.

percutaneous drainage, and percutaneous drainage combined with a thrombolytic infusion. Conservative measures, such as intubation, ventilation, patient positioning, gastric decompression, cautious fluid resuscitation, pain management, and temporary hemofiltration, are used.

❖ NURSING MANAGEMENT: AORTIC ANEURYSMS

◆ Nursing Assessment

Begin by performing a thorough history and physical assessment. Because atherosclerosis is a systemic disease, look for signs of coexisting cardiac, pulmonary, cerebral, and lower extremity vascular problems. Monitor the patient for signs of aneurysm rupture. These include diaphoresis; pallor; weakness; tachycardia; hypotension; abdominal, back, groin, or periumbilical pain; changes in level of consciousness; or a pulsating abdominal mass.

Establish baseline data to compare with later assessments. Pay special attention to the character and quality of the patient's peripheral pulses and renal and neurologic status. Before surgery, mark pedal pulse sites (dorsalis pedis, posterior tibial) with a single-use marker and document any skin lesions on the lower extremities.

◆ Planning

The overall goals for a patient undergoing aortic surgery include (1) normal tissue perfusion; (2) intact motor and sensory function; and (3) no complications related to surgical repair, such as thrombosis, infection, or rupture.

◆ Nursing Implementation
◆ Health Promotion. To promote overall health, encourage the patient to reduce CVD risk factors (see Table 33.2), including

controlling BP, ceasing tobacco use (see Chapter 10), and maintaining normal body weight and serum lipid levels. These measures also help ensure continued graft patency after surgical repair. Counsel the patient about taking part in moderate physical activity.

◆ Acute Care. Before surgery, provide emotional support and teaching to the patient and caregiver. Preoperative teaching includes a brief explanation of the disease process, the planned surgical procedure(s), preoperative routines, what to expect right after surgery (e.g., recovery room, tubes, drains), and usual postoperative timelines. Specific routines vary by agency and HCP. In general, aortic surgery patients have a bowel preparation and skin cleansing with an antimicrobial agent the day before surgery, have NPO after midnight the day of surgery, and receive IV antibiotics before the incision is made. Patients with a history of CVD should receive a β-blocker (e.g., metoprolol [Lopressor]). Scheduling a preoperative visit to the ICU may be helpful to the patient and caregiver.

After surgery, patients typically go to an ICU for 24 to 48 hours for close monitoring. When the patient arrives in the ICU, various devices are in place. These include an endotracheal tube for mechanical ventilation, an arterial line, a central venous pressure (CVP) catheter, peripheral IV lines, an indwelling urinary catheter, and a nasogastric (NG) tube. The patient needs continuous ECG and pulse oximetry monitoring. If the thorax is opened during surgery, chest tubes will be in place. The patient may have a lumbar catheter draining cerebrospinal fluid to prevent neurologic deficits. Pain medication is given via subcutaneous infusion into incision site (e.g., On-Q pain pump), epidural catheters, or IV patient-controlled analgesia (PCA).

In addition to the usual goals of care for a postoperative patient (e.g., maintaining adequate respiratory function, fluid and electrolyte balance, and pain control [see Chapter 19]), check for graft patency and renal perfusion. Watch for and intervene to limit or treat cardiac ischemia, dysrhythmias, infections, VTE, and neurologic complications. eNursing Care Plan 37.2 for the patient with an aneurysm repair or other aortic surgery is available on the website for this chapter.

Graft Patency. An adequate BP is important to maintain graft patency. Prolonged low BP may result in graft thrombosis. Give IV fluids and blood components as ordered to maintain adequate blood flow. Monitor CVP or PA pressures and urine output hourly in the immediate postoperative period to assess the patient's hydration and perfusion status.

Avoid severe hypertension, which may stress the arterial anastomoses, resulting in leakage of blood or rupture at the suture lines. Drug therapy with IV diuretics (e.g., furosemide) or IV antihypertensive agents (e.g., labetalol, metoprolol, hydralazine, sodium nitroprusside [Nipride]) may be indicated.

Cardiovascular Status. Myocardial ischemia or infarction may occur in the perioperative period because of decreased myocardial O_2 supply or increased myocardial O_2 demands. Dysrhythmias may occur because of electrolyte imbalances, hypoxemia, hypothermia, or myocardial ischemia. Nursing interventions include continuous ECG monitoring; frequent electrolyte and arterial blood gas determinations; O_2 administration, IV antidysrhythmic and antihypertensive drugs, and electrolytes as needed; adequate pain control; and resumption of cardiac drugs.

Infection. A prosthetic vascular graft infection is a rare but potentially life-threatening complication. Nursing interventions to prevent infection include giving a broad-spectrum antibiotic as prescribed. Assess temperature regularly, and promptly report elevations. Monitor laboratory results for a high WBC count, which may be the first sign of an infection. Ensure adequate nutrition and assess the surgical incision for signs of infection (e.g., redness, swelling, drainage). Keep surgical incisions clean and dry and perform wound care as prescribed.

Use good hand-washing and strict aseptic technique in the care of all peripheral, arterial, and CVP catheter insertion sites, since these are ports of entry for bacteria. Meticulous perineal care for the patient with an indwelling urinary catheter and early catheter removal are essential to minimize the risk for urinary tract infection.

Gastrointestinal Status. After OAR, postoperative ileus may develop because of anesthesia and the handling of the bowel during surgery. The intestines may become swollen and bruised, and peristalsis ceases for variable intervals. A retroperitoneal surgical approach decreases the risk for bowel complications.

An NG tube may be present and connected to low, intermittent suction to decompress the stomach, prevent aspiration of stomach contents, and decrease pressure on suture lines. Record the amount and character of the NG output. While the patient is NPO, provide frequent oral care. Ice chips or lozenges can help soothe a dry or irritated throat. Assess for bowel sounds every 4 hours. Note the passing of flatus as it signals returning bowel function. Encourage early ambulation since this will help the return of bowel function. A postoperative ileus rarely lasts beyond the 4th postoperative day.

If the blood supply to the bowel is disrupted during surgery, ischemia or infarction (death) of intestinal tissue may result. Manifestations of this rare, but serious, complication include absent bowel sounds, fever, abdominal distention and pain, diarrhea, and bloody stools. If bowel infarction occurs, immediate reoperation is needed to restore blood flow, with resection of the infarcted bowel.

Neurologic Status. Neurologic complications can occur after aortic surgery. When the ascending aorta and aortic arch are involved, assess the patient's level of consciousness, pupil size and response to light, facial symmetry, tongue position, speech, upper extremity movement, and quality of hand grasps). When the descending aorta is involved, perform a neurovascular assessment of the lower extremities. Record all assessments and report changes from baseline to the HCP immediately.

Peripheral Perfusion Status. The location of the aneurysm determines what type of peripheral perfusion assessment to do. Check and record all peripheral pulses hourly for several hours and then routinely (based on agency policy). When the ascending aorta and aortic arch are involved, assess the carotid, radial, and temporal artery pulses. For surgery of the descending aorta, assess the femoral, popliteal, posterior tibial, and dorsalis pedis pulses (see Fig. 31.6). You may need a Doppler to assess peripheral pulses. Check skin temperature and color, capillary refill time, and sensation and movement of the extremities.

Sometimes, lower extremity pulses may be absent for a short time after surgery because of vasospasm and hypothermia. A decreased or absent pulse together with a cool, pale, mottled, or painful extremity may indicate embolization or graft occlusion. Report these findings to the HCP at once. Graft occlusion requires reoperation if identified early. It is essential to compare your findings with the preoperative status to determine the cause of a decreased or absent pulse and the proper treatment. In some patients, pulses may have been absent before surgery because of coexistent PAD.

Renal Perfusion Status. The patient will have an indwelling urinary catheter after surgery. In the immediate postoperative period, record hourly urine output. Further evaluate renal function by monitoring daily BUN and serum creatinine levels. CVP pressures give vital information about hydration status. Maintain accurate fluid intake and output and record daily weights until the patient resumes a regular diet.

Decreased renal perfusion can occur from embolization of an aortic thrombus or plaque to 1 or both renal arteries. This causes ischemia of 1 or both kidneys. Hypotension, dehydration, prolonged aortic clamping during surgery, or blood loss can lead to decreased renal perfusion. Irreversible renal failure may occur after surgery, particularly in high-risk people (e.g., patients with diabetes). (Acute kidney injury is discussed in Chapter 46.)

◆ **Ambulatory Care.** Teach the patient and caregiver to gradually increase activities once home. Fatigue, poor appetite, and irregular bowel patterns are common. Have the patient avoid heavy lifting for 6 weeks after surgery. Report any redness, swelling, increased pain, drainage from incisions, or fever greater than 100° F (37.8° C) to the HCP.

Teach the patient and caregiver to look for changes in color or warmth of the extremities. Patients and caregivers can learn to palpate peripheral pulses to assess changes in their quality.

Sexual dysfunction in male patients is common after aortic surgery. A referral to a urologist and counseling may be useful if erectile dysfunction occurs.

◆ **Evaluation**

Expected outcomes are that the patient who undergoes aortic surgery will have:
- Patent arterial graft with adequate distal perfusion
- Adequate urine output
- No signs of infection

AORTIC DISSECTION

Aortic dissection, often misnamed *"dissecting aneurysm,"* is not a type of aneurysm. Rather, dissection results from the creation of a false lumen between the intima (inner lining) and the media (middle layer) of arterial wall (Figs. 37.5, *D,* and 37.8). Aortic dissection is classified based on the location of the dissection and duration of onset. *Type A dissection* affects the ascending aorta and arch, requiring emergency surgery. *Type B dissection* begins in the descending aorta, allowing for potential conservative management. We also describe dissections as acute (first 14 days), subacute (14 to 90 days), or chronic (greater than 90 days) based on symptom onset.[14,15]

Etiology and Pathophysiology

Nontraumatic aortic dissection is caused by weakened elastic fibers in the arterial wall. Chronic hypertension hastens this process. In aortic dissection, a tear develops in the inner layer of the aorta. Blood surges through this tear into the middle layer of the aorta, causing the inner and middle layers to separate (dissect). If the blood-filled channel ruptures through the outside aortic wall, aortic dissection is often fatal.

As the heart contracts, each pulsation increases the pressure on the damaged area and worsens the dissection. Extension of the dissection may cut off blood supply to the brain, kidneys, spinal cord, and extremities. The false lumen may remain patent, become thrombosed (clotted), rejoin the true lumen by way of a distal tear, or rupture.

Men are at a higher risk for developing aortic dissection than women.[15] Women who develop aortic dissection are older and more likely than men to present with HF, coma, or altered mental status.[15] Hypertension is the most important risk factor for aortic dissection.[15] Other predisposing factors include age, aortic diseases (e.g., aortitis, coarctation, arch hypoplasia), atherosclerosis, blunt trauma, tobacco use, cocaine or methamphetamine use, congenital heart disease (e.g., bicuspid aortic valve), connective tissue disorders (e.g., Marfan's syndrome), family history, history of heart surgery, and pregnancy.[15]

Clinical Manifestations

About 80% of patients with an acute Type A aortic dissection report an abrupt onset of severe anterior chest or back pain.

Patients with acute Type B aortic dissection are more likely to report pain in their back, abdomen, or legs. Pain location may overlap between Type A and B dissections. The pain may be described as "sharp" and "worst ever," or as "tearing," "ripping," or "stabbing."

Dissection pain can be distinguished from MI pain, which is more gradual in onset and has increasing intensity. As the dissection progresses, pain may follow the path of the dissection. Older patients are less likely to have an abrupt onset of pain and more likely to have hypotension and vague symptoms. Some patients have a painless aortic dissection, emphasizing the importance of the physical examination.

If the aortic arch is involved, the patient may have neurologic deficits. These include altered level of consciousness, weakened or absent carotid and temporal pulses, and dizziness or syncope. Type A aortic dissection usually disrupts blood flow in the coronary arteries and causes aortic valve insufficiency. When either subclavian artery is involved, the radial, ulnar, and brachial pulse quality and BP readings may be different between the left and right arms. As the dissection progresses down the aorta, the abdominal organs and lower extremities show evidence of decreased tissue perfusion.

Complications

A severe and life-threatening complication of an acute ascending aortic dissection is *cardiac tamponade*. This occurs when blood from the dissection leaks into the pericardial sac. Manifestations of tamponade include hypotension, narrowed pulse pressure, jugular venous distention, muffled heart sounds, and pulsus paradoxus (see Chapter 36).

An aorta weakened by dissection may rupture. Hemorrhage may occur into the mediastinal, pleural, or abdominal cavities. Aortic rupture typically results in exsanguination and death.

Aortic dissection can lead to occlusion of the blood supply to vital organs. Spinal cord ischemia leads to weakness and decreased sensation and rarely to complete lower extremity paralysis. Renal ischemia can lead to renal failure. Abdominal (mesenteric) ischemia can occur and cause abdominal pain, decreased bowel sounds, altered bowel function, and bowel necrosis.

Diagnostic Studies

Diagnostic studies to detect aortic dissection are similar to those for suspected aneurysms (Table 37.6). An ECG can help

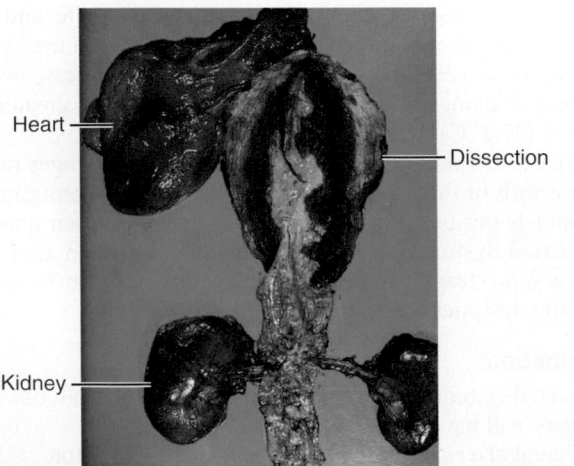

Heart

Dissection

Kidney

FIG. 37.8 Aortic dissection of the thoracic aorta. (From Damjanov I, Linder J, editors: *Anderson's pathology,* ed 10, St Louis, 1996, Mosby.)

TABLE 37.6 Interprofessional Care

Aortic Dissection

Diagnostic Assessment	Management
• Health history and physical examination	• Bed rest
• ECG	• Pain relief with opioids
• Chest x-ray	• Blood transfusion (if needed)
• CT scan	
• Transesophageal echocardiogram	***Drug Therapy (see Table 32.6)***
• MRI	• IV β-blockers
	• IV calcium channel blockers
	• ACE inhibitors
	Surgical Therapy
	• Endovascular aortic dissection repair
	• Open surgical repair

rule out cardiac ischemia. A chest x ray may show a widening of the mediastinum and pleural effusion. MRI, 3-D CT scanning, and transesophageal echocardiography (TEE) are equally reliable for the diagnosis of acute aortic dissection. A CT scan or MRI can give more detailed information on the severity of the dissection and related complications (e.g., pericardial effusions, carotid dissection). TEE is preferred in very unstable patients or those with contraindications to CT or MRI (e.g., those with metal implants, allergies to contrast material).[15]

Interprofessional Care

Patients with acute aortic dissection are managed in the ICU. The initial goals of therapy for acute aortic dissection without complications are heart rate (HR) and BP control and pain management. HR and BP control reduces aortic wall stress by decreasing SBP and myocardial contractility (Table 37.6). An IV β-blocker (e.g., esmolol [Brevibloc]) is titrated to a target HR under 60 beats/min or SBP between 100 and 110 mm Hg.

A calcium channel blocker (e.g., diltiazem) can be used to lower HR if a β-blocker is contraindicated. Reducing the HR, BP, and myocardial contractility limits extension of the dissection. Morphine decreases sympathetic nervous system stimulation and relieves pain. Supportive treatment for an acute aortic dissection serves as a bridge to surgery.

Conservative Therapy. The patient with an acute or chronic Type B aortic dissection without complications can be treated conservatively. Conservative treatment includes pain relief, HR and BP control, and CVD risk factor modification with close surveillance imaging with CT or MRI.

Endovascular Dissection Repair. Endovascular repair is a treatment option for acute Type B aortic dissections with complications (e.g., hemodynamic instability) and chronic Type B aortic dissection with complications (e.g., peripheral ischemia). Thoracic endovascular aortic repair (TEVAR) is similar to EVAR. Fewer postsurgical complications occur with TEVAR. However, TEVAR does not prevent the risk for renal failure, paraplegia, or stroke.[16] A lumbar spinal drain may be inserted to help decrease or prevent neurologic complications. If a lumbar drain is used, strict aseptic technique is essential to prevent infection.

Surgical Therapy. An acute Type A aortic dissection is a surgical emergency. Mortality rate is 50% within 48 hours of symptom onset. Otherwise, surgery is indicated when conservative therapy is ineffective or when complications (e.g., HF) occur. Open surgical repair is recommended for patients with a chronic dissection who have a connective tissue disorder or an aneurysm greater than 5.5 cm.[13,15]

The aorta is fragile after dissection. Surgery is delayed, when possible, to allow time for edema to decrease and to permit blood clotting in the false lumen. Surgery involves resection of the aortic segment with the intimal tear and replacement with a synthetic graft. Even with prompt surgical intervention, the in-hospital mortality is high.[15,16] Causes of death include aortic rupture, mesenteric ischemia, MI, sepsis, stroke, and multiorgan failure.

❖ NURSING MANAGEMENT: AORTIC DISSECTION

Preoperative nursing care includes keeping the patient in bed in a semi-Fowler's position and maintaining a quiet environment. These measures help to keep the HR and SBP at the lowest possible level that maintains vital organ perfusion (typically HR less than 60 beats/min; SBP between 100 and 120 mm Hg). Give opioids and sedatives as ordered. Manage pain and anxiety because they can cause elevations in the HR and SBP.

Titrating IV antihypertensive agents requires careful supervision, including continuous ECG and arterial BP monitoring. Monitor vital signs frequently, sometimes as often as every 2 to 3 minutes, until target HR and BP are reached. Look for changes in peripheral pulses and signs of increasing pain, restlessness, and anxiety. Postoperative care is similar to that after OAR (see earlier section on nursing management of aortic aneurysms).

In preparation for discharge, focus on patient and caregiver teaching. All patients with a history of aortic dissection require long-term health care to control HR and BP. Help patients understand that they need to take antihypertensive drugs daily for the rest of their lives. β-Blockers are used to control HR and BP and decrease myocardial contractility. ACE inhibitors (e.g., lisinopril [Zestril]) are given if the patient cannot tolerate β-blockers. It is important that patients understand the drug regimen and side effects (e.g., dizziness, depression, fatigue, erectile dysfunction). Tell the patient to discuss any side effects with the HCP before stopping any medication.

Follow-up with regularly scheduled MRIs or CTs is essential. The most common cause of death in long-term survivors is aortic rupture from redissection or aneurysm formation. Tell patients that if the pain or other symptoms return, they should activate the emergency response system (ERS) for immediate care.

▍ACUTE AND CHRONIC VENOUS DISORDERS

PHLEBITIS

Most hospitalized patients have an IV catheter inserted for fluids and/or drugs. *Phlebitis* is an acute inflammation of the walls of small cannulated veins of the hand or arm. Manifestations include pain, tenderness, warmth, erythema, swelling, and a palpable cord. Risk factors are mechanical irritation from the catheter, infusion of irritating drugs, and catheter location. Severe phlebitis is more likely to occur in areas of flexion (e.g., wrist and antecubital area). Avoid IV catheter insertion in this area whenever possible.

Phlebitis is rarely infectious and usually resolves quickly after catheter removal. If edema is present, elevate the extremity to promote reabsorption of fluid. Apply warm, moist heat and give oral NSAIDs (e.g., ibuprofen) or topical NSAIDs (e.g., diclofenac gel) to relieve pain and inflammation.

VENOUS THROMBOSIS

Venous thrombosis involves the formation of a *thrombus* (blood clot) with vein inflammation. It is the most common disorder of the veins. We classify it as either superficial vein thrombosis or deep vein thrombosis. Superficial vein thrombosis is the formation of a thrombus in a superficial vein, usually the greater or lesser saphenous vein. Deep vein thrombosis (DVT) involves a thrombus in a deep vein, most often the iliac and/or femoral veins. Venous thromboembolism (VTE) is the preferred terminology. It represents the spectrum from DVT to pulmonary embolism (PE) (Table 37.7). (Chapter 27 discusses PE.)

Superficial vein thrombosis is serious. Nearly 25% of patients with superficial vein thrombosis have a DVT or PE at the time of diagnosis. Further, these patients are at risk for developing recurrent VTE.

Etiology

The 3 key factors (called Virchow's triad) that cause venous thrombosis are (1) venous stasis, (2) damage of the endothelium (inner lining of the vein), and (3) hypercoagulability of the blood (Fig. 37.9). The patient at risk for developing VTE usually has predisposing conditions to these 3 disorders (Table 37.8).

TABLE 37.7 Comparison of Superficial Vein Thrombosis and Venous Thromboembolism

	Superficial Vein Thrombosis	Venous Thromboembolism (VTE)
Usual location	Typically, superficial leg veins (e.g., varicosities). Sometimes superficial arm veins.	Deep veins of arms (e.g., axillary, subclavian), legs (e.g., femoral), pelvis (e.g., iliac), vena cava, and pulmonary system.
Clinical findings	Tenderness, itchiness, redness, warmth, pain, inflammation, and induration along the course of superficial vein. Vein appears as a palpable cord. Edema rarely occurs.	Tenderness to pressure over involved vein, induration of overlying muscle, venous distention. Edema. May have mild to moderate pain, deep reddish color to area caused by venous congestion. Some have no obvious physical changes in the affected extremity.
Sequelae	If untreated, clot may extend to deeper veins and VTE may occur.	Embolization to lungs (PE) may occur and may result in death. Pulmonary hypertension and post-thrombotic syndrome with or without venous leg ulceration may develop.

Venous Stasis. Normal venous blood flow depends on the action of muscles in the extremities and the function of venous valves, which allow flow in one direction. *Venous stasis* occurs when the valves are dysfunctional or the muscles of the extremities are inactive. Venous stasis occurs most often in people who are obese or pregnant, have chronic HF or atrial fibrillation, have been traveling on long trips without regular exercise, have a prolonged surgical procedure, or are immobile for long periods (e.g., spinal cord injury, fractured hip, limb paralysis).[17]

Endothelial Damage. Damage to the endothelium of the vein may be caused by direct (e.g., surgery, intravascular catheterization, trauma, burns, prior VTE) or indirect (chemotherapy, diabetes, sepsis) injury. Damaged endothelium stimulates platelet activation and starts the coagulation cascade. This predisposes the patient to thrombus development.

Hypercoagulability of Blood. Blood hypercoagulability occurs in many disorders. These include severe anemias, polycythemia, cancers (e.g., breast, brain, pancreas, GI tract); nephrotic syndrome; high homocysteine levels; and protein C, protein S, and antithrombin deficiency.[17] A patient with sepsis is predisposed to hypercoagulability because of endotoxins released from bacteria. Some drugs (e.g., corticosteroids, estrogens) predispose a patient to thrombus formation.

Women who use tobacco, are of childbearing age and take estrogen-based oral contraceptives, are postmenopausal on oral hormone therapy, are over 35 years old, and have a family history of VTE are at a very high risk for VTE.[17] Women who use oral contraceptives with tobacco double their risk. Smoking causes hypercoagulability by increasing plasma fibrinogen and homocysteine levels and activating the intrinsic coagulation pathway.

Pathophysiology

Localized platelet aggregation and fibrin entrap RBCs, WBCs, and more platelets to form a thrombus. A frequent site of

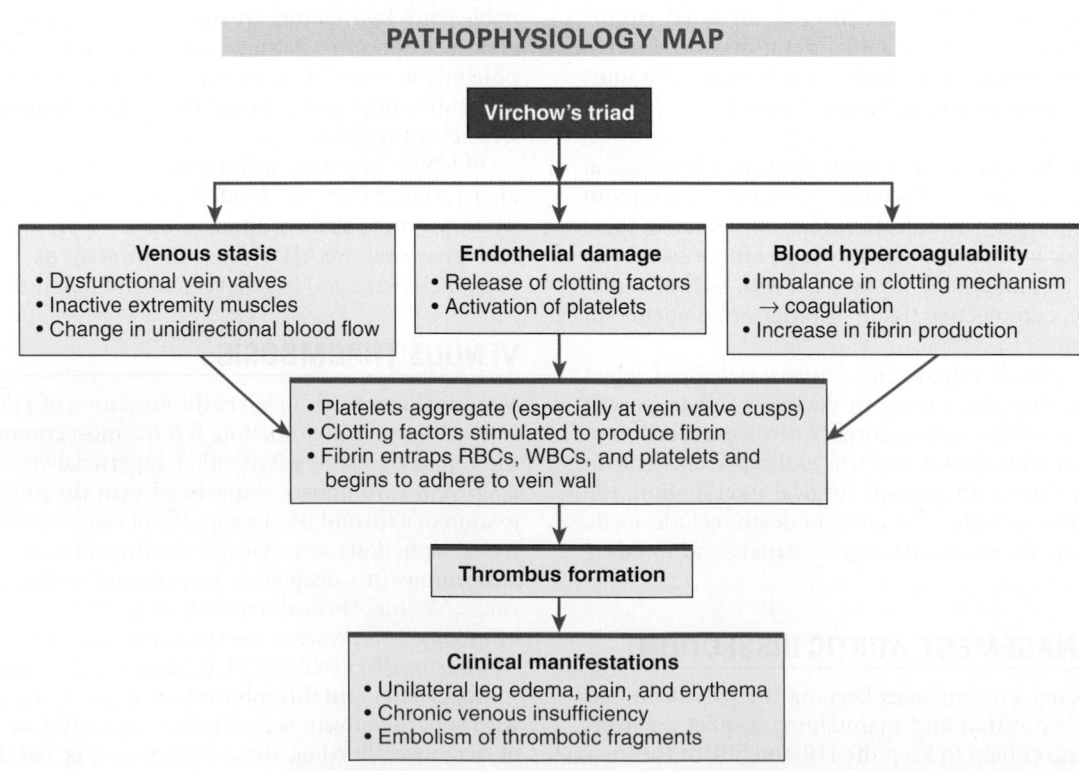

FIG. 37.9 Pathophysiology of venous thromboembolism.

TABLE 37.8 Risk Factors for VTE

Endothelial Damage
- Abdominal and pelvic surgery (e.g., gynecologic, urologic surgery)
- Caustic or hypertonic IV drugs
- Pelvis, hip, or leg fractures
- History of VTE
- Indwelling, peripherally inserted central vein catheter
- IV drug abuse
- Trauma

Venous Stasis
- Advanced age
- Atrial fibrillation
- Bed rest
- Chronic heart failure
- Fractured leg or hip
- Long trips without adequate exercise
- Obesity
- Orthopedic surgery (especially hip or lower extremity)
- Pregnancy and postpartum period
- Prolonged immobility
- Spinal cord injury or limb paralysis
- Stroke
- Varicose veins

Hypercoagulability of Blood
- Antiphospholipid antibody syndrome
- Antithrombin III deficiency
- Cancer (especially breast, brain, hepatic, pancreatic, GI)
- Dehydration or malnutrition
- Elevated (clotting) factor VIII or lipoprotein (a)
- Erythropoiesis-stimulating drugs (e.g., epoetin alfa [Procrit])
- High altitudes
- Hormone therapy
- High homocysteine levels
- Nephrotic syndrome
- Oral contraceptives, especially in women older than 35 years who use tobacco
- Polycythemia vera
- Pregnancy and postpartum period
- Protein C deficiency
- Protein S deficiency
- Sepsis
- Severe anemias
- Tobacco use

thrombus formation is the valve cusps of veins, where venous stasis occurs. As a thrombus enlarges, increased numbers of blood cells and fibrin collect behind it. This makes a larger clot with a "tail" that eventually blocks the lumen of the vein.

If a thrombus only partially blocks the vein, endothelial cells cover the thrombus and stop the thrombotic process. If the thrombus does not become detached, it undergoes lysis or becomes firmly organized and adherent within 5 to 7 days. The organized thrombus may detach and result in an embolus. Turbulence of blood flow is a major factor in embolization. The thrombus can become an embolus that flows through the venous circulation to the heart and lodges in the pulmonary circulation, becoming a PE.

Superficial Vein Thrombosis

Clinical Manifestations. The patient with superficial vein thrombosis may have a palpable, firm, subcutaneous cordlike vein (Table 37.7). The area surrounding the vein may be itchy, painful to the touch, reddened, and warm. A mild temperature elevation and leukocytosis may be present. Extremity edema may occur. Lower extremity superficial vein thrombosis often involves 1 or more varicose veins.

Risk factors include increased age, pregnancy, obesity, cancer, recent fracture(s), estrogen therapy, recent sclerotherapy (e.g., treatment for varicose veins), recent surgery or long-distance travel, hypercoagulability, and a history of chronic venous insufficiency (CVI), superficial vein thrombosis, or VTE.[18] It can occur in people with endothelial problems (e.g., Buerger's disease).

Interprofessional Care. Ultrasound is used to confirm the diagnosis (clot 5 cm or larger) and to rule out clot extension to a deep vein.[18] If the superficial vein thrombosis affects a very short vein segment (less than 5 cm) and is not near the saphenofemoral junction, anticoagulants may not be needed and oral NSAIDs can ease symptoms. Other interventions include telling the patient to wear graduated compression stockings or bandages, apply warm compresses, elevate the affected limb above the level of the heart, apply topical NSAIDS, and perform mild exercise, such as walking.

Venous Thromboembolism

Clinical Manifestations. The patient with lower extremity VTE may or may not have unilateral leg edema, pain, tenderness with palpation, dilated superficial veins, a sense of fullness in the thigh or the calf, paresthesias, warm skin, erythema, or a systemic temperature greater than 100.4° F (38° C) (Table 37.7). If the inferior vena cava is involved, both legs may be edematous and cyanotic. About 10% of VTEs involve the upper extremity veins and may extend into the internal jugular vein or superior vena cava.[17] If the superior vena cava is involved, similar symptoms may occur in the arms, neck, back, and face. Diagnosis of an initial VTE is based on the assessment combined with D-dimer testing and/or ultrasound.

Complications. The most serious complications of VTE are PE, chronic thromboembolic pulmonary hypertension, post-thrombotic syndrome, and phlegmasia cerulea dolens. Post-thrombotic syndrome (PTS) occurs in 8% to 70% of patients. It results from chronic inflammation and chronic venous hypertension. Chronic venous hypertension is caused by vein wall and vein valve damage (from acute inflammation and thrombus reorganization), venous valve reflux, and persistent venous (outflow) obstruction. Symptoms include pain, aching, fatigue, heaviness, sensation of swelling, cramps, pruritus, tingling, paresthesia, bursting pain with exercise, and venous claudication.[19]

Manifestations include persistent edema, spider veins (telangiectasia), venous dilation (ectasia), redness, cyanosis, increased pigmentation, eczema, pain during compression, atrophie blanche (white scar tissue), and *lipodermatosclerosis* (Fig. 37.10). Venous ulceration can occur with severe PTS. Signs of PTS typically begin within a few months to a few years of a VTE. Risk factors include persistent leg symptoms 1 month after VTE, proximal VTE location (e.g., near the iliofemoral junction), extensive VTE, recurrent ipsilateral (same side) VTE, residual thrombus, obesity, older age, poor INR control, daily tobacco use before pregnancy, increased D-dimer levels, elevated inflammatory markers, varicose veins, and asymptomatic VTE.[17-19]

Phlegmasia cerulea dolens (swollen, blue, painful leg) is a rare complication of a severe lower extremity VTE(s). It involve(s) the major leg veins, causing near-total occlusion of venous outflow. Patients typically have sudden, massive swelling; deep pain; and intense cyanosis of the extremity. If untreated, the venous obstruction causes arterial occlusion and gangrene, requiring amputation.

Diagnostic Studies. Table 37.9 presents the diagnostic studies used to determine the site or location and extent of a VTE.

Interprofessional Care

Prevention. All members of the interprofessional team have important roles in VTE prevention. VTE prevention is a core measure of high-quality health care in high-risk hospitalized patients developed by The Joint Commission (TJC) and the National Quality Forum. There are 3 VTE measures. TJC recommends that hospitals have a policy that addresses

VTE prevention on admission of all adult patients. In patients at risk for VTE, interventions used are based on bleeding and thrombosis risk, past medical history, current drugs, medical diagnoses, scheduled procedures, and patient preferences.

Early and aggressive mobilization is the easiest and most cost-effective method to decrease VTE risk. Patients on bed rest should change position at least every 2 hours. Unless contraindicated, teach patients to flex and extend their feet, knees, and hips at least every 2 to 4 hours while awake. Patients who can get out of bed need to be in a chair for meals and walk at least 4 to 6 times per day. Tell the patient and caregiver about the importance of these measures. Early and frequent ambulation is sufficient prophylaxis for patients at very low risk for VTE who

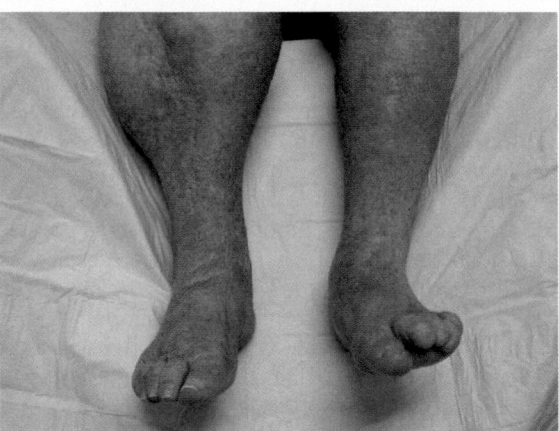

FIG. 37.10 Lipodermatosclerosis. Skin on lower leg becomes scarred, and the leg becomes tapered like an "inverted bottle." Hallmark signs are leathery skin, brown discoloration, changes in pigmentation, and circumferential or near circumferential scarring and shrinking of the extremity. (From Etufugh CN, Phillips TJ: Venous ulcers, *Clin Dermatol* 25[1]:125, 2007.)

had minor surgical procedures.[20] Anticoagulation and mechanical prophylaxis are not recommended for acutely ill medical patients at low risk for VTE.

Graduated compression stockings (e.g., thromboembolic deterrent [TED] hose) are a part of VTE prevention in hospitalized patients. VTE prevention is enhanced if the stockings are used along with anticoagulation. Proper stocking use means any toe hole is under the toes, the heel patch is over the heel, a thigh gusset is on the inner thigh (thigh length only), and there are no wrinkles. The stockings should not be rolled down, cut, or otherwise altered. If the stockings are not fitted and worn correctly, venous return is impeded. This can cause arterial ischemia, edema, skin breakdown, and VTE. Stockings are not recommended if the patient already has a VTE.[20]

Intermittent pneumatic compression devices (IPCs) use inflatable sleeves or boots to compress the calf and thigh and/or foot and ankle to improve venous return. The sleeves apply external pressure through an electric pump. IPCs may be used with graduated compression stockings. Ensure correct fit of IPCs by accurately measuring the extremities. IPCs will not be effective if they are not applied correctly, if the fit is incorrect, or if the patient does not wear the device continuously while at rest. The IPCS can be removed for bathing, skin assessment, and ambulation. IPCs are not worn when a patient has an active VTE because of the risk for PE.[20]

Drug Therapy. Anticoagulants are used routinely for VTE prevention and treatment. The regimen depends on the patient's VTE risk. The goal of anticoagulant therapy for VTE prevention is to prevent clot formation. The goals for treatment of a confirmed VTE are to prevent new clot development, spread of the clot, and embolization.[20]

The 3 major classes of anticoagulants available are (1) vitamin K antagonists (VKAs), (2) thrombin inhibitors (both indirect and direct), and (3) factor Xa inhibitors (Table 37.10).[21]

TABLE 37.9 Diagnostic Studies

VTE

Study	Description and Abnormal Findings
Blood Laboratory Studies	
ACT, aPTT, INR, bleeding time, Hgb, Hct, platelet count	Altered if patient has underlying blood dyscrasia (e.g., increased Hgb and Hct in patient with polycythemia)
D-dimer	Fragment of fibrin formed from fibrin degradation and clot lysis. High results suggest VTE. *Normal results:* <250 ng/mL (<250 mcg/L)
Fibrin monomer complex	Forms when concentration of thrombin exceeds that of antithrombin. Presence is evidence of thrombus formation and suggests VTE. *Normal results:* <6.1 mg/L
Noninvasive Venous Studies	
Duplex ultrasound	Combination of compression ultrasound with spectral and color flow Doppler. Veins examined for compressibility and intraluminal filling defects to help determine location and extent of thrombus (most widely used test to diagnose VTE).
Venous compression ultrasound	Evaluation of deep femoral, popliteal, and posterior tibial veins. *Normal finding:* Veins collapse with application of external pressure. *Abnormal finding:* Veins do not collapse with application of external pressure. Failure to collapse suggests a thrombus.
Invasive Venous Studies	
Computed tomography venography (CTV)	Uses spiral CT to evaluate veins in the pelvis, thighs, and calves after injection of contrast material. May be done simultaneously with CT angiography of pulmonary vessels for patients being evaluated for VTE.
Magnetic resonance venography	Uses MRI with specialized software to evaluate blood flow through veins. Can be done with or without contrast. Highly accurate for pelvic and proximal veins. Less accurate for calf veins. Can distinguish acute and chronic thrombus
Contrast venography (phlebogram)	X-ray determination of location and extent of clot using contrast media to outline filling defects. Identifies the presence of collateral circulation. Once the gold standard, but now rarely done

ACT, Activated clotting time.

TABLE 37.10 Drug Therapy
Anticoagulant Therapy

Drug	Route of Administration	Considerations
Vitamin K Antagonists (VKA)		
warfarin (Coumadin)	PO	INR used to monitor therapeutic levels.
		Give at the same time each day.
		Variations of certain genes (e.g., *CYP2CP, VKORC1*) may influence response to drug.
		Antidote: Vitamin K. For VKA-related bleeding, treatment with prothrombin complex concentrate (human) (Kcentra), IV vitamin K and/or fresh frozen plasma is recommended.
Thrombin Inhibitors: Indirect		
Low-Molecular-Weight Heparin (LMWH)		
dalteparin (Fragmin)	Subcutaneous	Routine coagulation tests typically not needed.
enoxaparin (Lovenox)		Monitor CBC count at regular intervals.
		Do not expel air bubble from prefilled syringe. If giving subcutaneously, inject deep into subcutaneous tissue (preferably into the abdominal fatty tissue or above the iliac crest), inserting the entire length of the needle. Hold skinfold during injection but release before removing needle. Do not aspirate. Do not inject IM. Do not rub site after injection. Rotate sites.
		Reduced dosage needed in patients with renal impairment. Use extreme caution in patients with a history of HIT.
		Antidote: Protamine neutralizes the effects of LMWH.
Unfractionated Heparin (UH)		
heparin sodium	Continuous IV	Therapeutic effects measured at regular intervals by the aPTT or ACT.
	Intermittent IV	Monitor CBC counts at regular intervals and titrate according to parameters.
	Subcutaneous	Follow administration guidelines for LMWH if giving subcutaneously.
		Antidote: Protamine neutralizes the effect of UH.
Factor Xa Inhibitors		
apixaban (Eliquis)	PO	All are approved for VTE prevention and treatment.
betrixaban (Bevyxxa)	PO	Routine coagulation tests not needed. Monitor CBC and creatinine at regular intervals.
edoxaban (Savaysa)	PO	May cause thrombocytopenia.
fondaparinux (Arixtra)	Subcutaneous	Do not expel air bubble before giving fondaparinux. Follow administration guidelines as described for
rivaroxaban (Xarelto)	PO	subcutaneous LMWHs.
		Antidote: Andexanet alfa (Andexxa) reverses the effects of rivaroxaban and apixaban.
Thrombin Inhibitors: Direct		
Hirudin Derivatives		
bivalirudin (Angiomax)	IV	Therapeutic effect measured by ACT or aPTT. Used in patients with HIT when anticoagulation is needed.
desirudin (Iprivask)	Subcutaneous	*Antidote:* None.
Synthetic Thrombin Inhibitors		
argatroban (Acova)	IV	Argatroban therapeutic effect measured by aPTT. No routine coagulation tests needed for dabigatran.
dabigatran (Pradaxa)	PO	Used in patients at risk for or with HIT, for VTE prevention in joint replacement surgery, stroke prevention in nonvalvular atrial fibrillation
		Antidote: Idarucizumab (Praxbind) neutralizes the effect of dabigatran only.

ACT, Activated clotting time; *HIT,* heparin-induced thrombocytopenia.

Anticoagulant therapy does not dissolve the clot. Clot lysis begins naturally through the body's intrinsic fibrinolytic system (see Chapter 29).

Vitamin K antagonists. The oral anticoagulant for long-term or extended anticoagulation is warfarin, a VKA. Warfarin inhibits activation of the vitamin K–dependent coagulation factors II, VII, IX, and X and the anticoagulant proteins C and S. (See the list of clotting factors in Table 29.2. Fig. 29.4 shows the clotting pathways.) Warfarin begins to take effect in 48 to 72 hours. It then takes several more days to achieve a maximum effect. Thus an overlap of a parenteral anticoagulant (e.g., UH or low-molecular-weight heparin [LMWH]) and warfarin typically is required for 5 days. The level of anticoagulation is monitored daily using the INR. The INR is a standardized system of reporting prothrombin time (PT) (Table 37.11). The antidote for

warfarin-related bleeding is vitamin K, prothrombin complex concentrate (human) (Kcentra), or fresh frozen plasma (FFP).

Take a careful history before starting warfarin. Do not give antiplatelet drug or NSAIDs with warfarin as these increase bleeding risk.[21] Many other drugs, vitamins, minerals, and dietary and herbal supplements interact with warfarin (see the Complementary & Alternative Therapies box). A diet that varies in vitamin K intake (e.g., green leafy vegetables) can make it hard to achieve and maintain a target INR level. Genetic variants in the genes *VKORC1* and cytochrome P450 2C9 (*CYP2C9*) may influence how some people respond to warfarin (see Table 12.5 and Fig. 12.7).

Thrombin inhibitors. There are 2 major classes of *indirect thrombin inhibitors*: UH and LMWHs. UH (e.g., heparin) affects both the intrinsic and common pathways of blood coagulation

TABLE 37.11 Blood Coagulation Tests

Test and Drugs Monitored	Normal Value	Therapeutic Value
Activated Clotting Time (ACT)	70–120 sec*	>300 sec
• Hirudin derivatives (e.g., bivalirudin [Angiomax])		
• Synthetic thrombin inhibitors (e.g., argatroban [Acova])		
• Unfractionated heparin (e.g., heparin [Hep-Lock])		
Activated Partial Thromboplastin Time (aPTT)	30–40 sec	46–70 sec
• Hirudin derivatives		
• Synthetic thrombin inhibitors		
• Unfractionated heparin		
Anti-Factor Xa		
• Factor Xa inhibitors (e.g., fondaparinux [Arixtra], rivaroxaban [Xarelto])	0 units/mL 0 units/mL	0.6–1.0 units/mL 0.2
• Low-molecular-weight heparin (e.g., enoxaparin [Lovenox])		1.5 units/mL
International Normalized Ratio (INR)	0.75–1.25	2–3
• Vitamin K antagonists (e.g., warfarin [Coumadin])		

*Varies based on type of system and test reagent or activator used.

🌿 COMPLEMENTARY & ALTERNATIVE THERAPIES
Herbal and Dietary Supplements That May Affect Clotting

Scientific Evidence
Many herbs and dietary supplements may affect blood clotting. These include bilberry, black cohosh, chamomile, chondroitin sulfate, dehydroepiandrosterone (DHEA), feverfew, garlic, ginger, ginkgo biloba, ginseng, goldenseal, grapeseed extract, green tea, horse chestnut seed extract, melatonin, niacin, omega-3 fatty acids, psyllium, red yeast rice extract, saw palmetto, soy, turmeric.

Nursing Implications
• Tell patients that taking these herbs or dietary supplements may increase their risk for bleeding.
• Caution patients with bleeding disorders about using these herbs and dietary supplements. Teach them to consult with their HCP before using these substances.

by way of the plasma antithrombin. Antithrombin inhibits thrombin-mediated conversion of fibrinogen to fibrin by affecting factors II (prothrombin), IX, X, XI, and XII (see Fig. 29.4).

Heparin can be given subcutaneously for VTE prevention or by continuous IV infusion for VTE treatment. When given IV, heparin requires frequent monitoring of clotting status as measured by activated partial thromboplastin time (aPTT) (Table 37.11). Protamine sulfate reverses the effect of heparin.

One serious side effect of heparin is *heparin-induced thrombocytopenia* (HIT). HIT is an immune reaction to heparin. It causes a severe, sudden reduction in the platelet count along with a paradoxical increase in venous or arterial thrombosis. HIT is diagnosed by measuring the presence of heparin antibodies in the blood. Treatment includes immediately stopping heparin therapy and, if further anticoagulation is needed, using a non-heparin anticoagulant (e.g., fondaparinux).[21] Another side effect of long-term heparin therapy is osteoporosis.

LMWHs (e.g., enoxaparin [Lovenox]) are derived from UH. They have more predictable dose response, longer half-life, and fewer bleeding complications than UH. LMWHs are less likely to cause HIT and osteoporosis. LMWHs typically do not require ongoing anticoagulant monitoring and dose adjustment. Their antiinflammatory properties may help prevent PTS and venous ulcer development.[21] Protamine neutralizes the effect of LMWH.

Direct thrombin inhibitors are classified as hirudin derivatives or synthetic thrombin inhibitors. Hirudin is made using recombinant deoxyribonucleic acid (DNA) technology. It binds specifically with thrombin and directly inhibits its function without causing plasma protein and platelet interactions. Hirudin derivatives (e.g., bivalirudin [Angiomax]) are given by continuous IV infusion. Bivalirudin is approved for patients with or at risk for HIT having a percutaneous coronary intervention. Anticoagulant activity is monitored using aPTT or activated clotting time (ACT) (Table 37.11). If bleeding occurs, there is no antidote for hirudin derivatives.

Argatroban, a synthetic direct thrombin inhibitor, hinders thrombin. Like bivalirudin, it is an alternative to heparin for the prevention and treatment of HIT and for patients with or at risk for HIT needing percutaneous coronary interventions. The effect of argatroban is not reversible. Its anticoagulant effect is monitored using aPTT or ACT.

Dabigatran (Pradaxa) is an oral direct thrombin inhibitor. It is used for VTE prevention after elective joint replacement, for stroke prevention in nonvalvular atrial fibrillation, and as a treatment for VTE. Idarucizumab (Praxbind) neutralizes the effect of dabigatran. Dabigatran has 5 major advantages compared to warfarin: rapid onset, no need to monitor anticoagulation, few drug-food interactions, lower risk for major bleeding, and predictable dose response.[21]

Factor Xa inhibitors. *Factor Xa inhibitors* inhibit factor Xa directly or indirectly, producing rapid anticoagulation. These include fondaparinux (Arixtra), rivaroxaban (Xarelto), apixaban (Eliquis), and edoxaban (Savaysa). All are used for both VTE prevention and treatment. Fondaparinux is given subcutaneously. It is contraindicated in patients with severe renal disease. Rivaroxaban, apixaban, and edoxaban are oral drugs. Although coagulation monitoring or dose adjustment is not needed, the drug's anticoagulant activity can be measured using anti-Xa assays (Table 37.11). If uncontrollable bleeding occurs, recombinant factor VIIa may be useful. Andexanet Alfa (Andexxa) reverses the effects of rivaroxaban and apixaban.

Anticoagulant therapy for VTE prevention. For VTE prevention in the hospitalized medical patient at risk for thrombosis who is not bleeding, low-dose UH, LMWH, or fondaparinux is used. If the patient is at low VTE risk, drug prophylaxis is not needed. Patients with moderate VTE risk (e.g., general, gynecologic, urologic surgery) should receive either UH or LMWH. Patients with high VTE risk (e.g., trauma) should receive UH or LMWH until discharge. Patients having abdominal or pelvic surgery for cancer or major orthopedic surgery (e.g., total knee or hip replacement) should receive VTE prophylaxis.[20]

Anticoagulant therapy for VTE treatment. Patients with confirmed VTE should receive initial treatment with either LMWH, UH, or an oral factor Xa drug. Oral VKA therapy may be an option. A therapeutic INR is maintained between 2.0 and 3.0 if VKA therapy is used. Active treatment of VTE should continue for at least 3 months and may continue longer in some patients.[20]

Patients with multiple co-morbidities, complex medical issues, or a very large VTE usually are hospitalized for treatment.

Parenteral administration of UH is the typical initial treatment. Depending on the presentation and home situation, patients may be safely and effectively managed as outpatients.

Thrombolytic therapy for VTE treatment. Another treatment option for patients with a thrombus is catheter-directed administration of a thrombolytic drug (e.g., urokinase, tPA). It dissolves the clot(s), reduces the acute symptoms, improves deep venous flow, reduces valvular reflux, and may help to decrease the incidence of PTS. Catheter-directed thrombolysis is an option for select patients who are at a low bleeding risk and present with an acute, extensive, symptomatic, proximal VTE. Systemic anticoagulation is needed before, during, and after catheter-directed thrombolysis. (Chapter 33 discusses thrombolytic therapy.)

�

CHECK YOUR PRACTICE

Your 55-yr-old female patient is admitted with an extensive VTE in her right leg. She is receiving weight-based IV heparin per agency protocol: 18 units/kg/hr. You receive the following critical laboratory result: aPTT 122 seconds.
• Describe your next actions.

Surgical and Interventional Radiology Therapies. A few patients with extensive, acute, proximal VTE who are not candidates for catheter-directed thrombolysis and/or interventional radiology therapies (due to bleeding risk) may have surgery.[3,16] Surgical options include open venous thrombectomy and inferior vena cava interruption. *Venous thrombectomy* involves the removal of a clot through a vein incision. Anticoagulant therapy is used after venous thrombectomy.

Vena cava interruption devices (e.g., Greenfield, Vena Tech, TrapEase filters) can be placed percutaneously through the right femoral or right internal jugular veins. The filter device is opened, and the spokes penetrate the vessel walls (Fig. 37.11). The filters act as a "sieve-type" device, allowing filtration of clots without interruption of blood flow. Complications after the insertion are rare but include air embolism, improper placement, migration of the filter, and perforation of the vena cava with retroperitoneal bleeding. Over time, clots can clog the filter and completely block the vena cava, requiring filter removal and replacement. A filter device is recommended with acute PE or proximal VTE of the leg in patients with active bleeding or if anticoagulant therapy is contraindicated or ineffective.

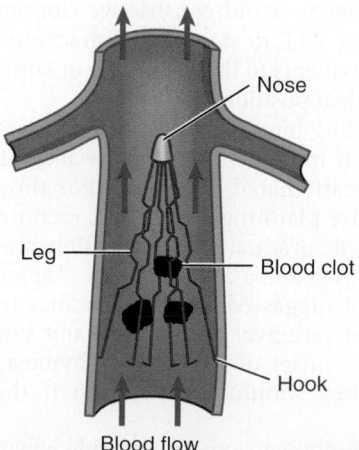

FIG. 37.11 Inferior vena cava interruption technique using Greenfield stainless steel filter to prevent pulmonary embolism. As blood travels up the vena cava, clots are trapped in the filter.

Percutaneous endovascular interventional radiology procedures can be used along with catheter-directed thrombolytic therapy, especially for severely symptomatic patients with iliocaval or iliofemoral obstruction.[17] The interventional radiology procedures are like those used in the treatment of lower extremity PAD. The difference is accessing an occluded vein instead of an artery. Options include mechanical thrombectomy, pharmaco-mechanical devices, and post-thrombus extraction, angioplasty, and/or stenting.[17] Anticoagulation therapy is recommended after an iliofemoral interventional radiology procedure. Postprocedure nursing care focuses on (1) maintaining catheter systems (if continuous infusions); (2) monitoring for bleeding, embolization, and impaired perfusion; and (3) VTE prevention teaching.[17]

❖ NURSING MANAGEMENT: VENOUS THROMBOEMBOLISM

◆ Nursing Assessment

Table 37.12 presents the subjective and objective data to obtain from a patient with VTE.

TABLE 37.12 Nursing Assessment
VTE

Subjective Data
Important Health Information (Table 37.8)

Past health history: Trauma to vein, intravascular catheter (e.g., peripherally inserted central catheter), varicose veins, pregnancy or recent childbirth, bacteremia, obesity, prolonged bed rest, irregular heartbeat (e.g., atrial fibrillation), COPD, HF, cancer, coagulation disorders and hypercoagulable states, systemic lupus erythematosus, MI, spinal cord injury, stroke, prolonged travel, recent bone fracture, dehydration
Medications: Use of estrogens (including oral contraceptives, hormone therapy), tamoxifen, raloxifene (Evista), corticosteroids, excessive amounts of vitamin E, erythropoiesis-stimulating drugs
Surgery or other treatments: Any recent surgery, especially orthopedic, gynecologic, GI, or urologic. Previous surgery involving veins. Central venous catheter

Functional Health Patterns

Health perception–health management: IV drug abuse, tobacco use, obesity
Activity-exercise: Inactivity
Cognitive-perceptual: Pain in area on palpation or ambulation

Objective Data
General

Fever, anxiety, pain

Integumentary

Increased size of extremity when compared with other side. Taut, shiny, warm skin, erythematous, tender to palpation. No physical changes in the affected extremity in some patients

Cardiovascular

Distention and warmth of superficial veins in affected area. Edema and cyanosis of extremities, neck, back, and face (if superior vena cava involvement)

Possible Diagnostic Findings

Leukocytosis, abnormal coagulation, anemia or ↑ hematocrit and RBC count, ↑ D-dimer level, positive venous compression on duplex ultrasound study; positive CT venogram, magnetic resonance venogram, or contrast venogram study

◆ Nursing Diagnoses

Nursing diagnoses and collaborative problems for the patient with VTE include:

- Acute pain
- Impaired tissue integrity
- Impaired physical mobility
- Risk for bleeding

◆ Planning

The overall goals for the patient with VTE include (1) pain relief, (2) decreased edema, (3) increased knowledge of disorder and treatment plan, (4) no skin ulceration, (5) no bleeding complications, and (6) no evidence of PE.

Nursing Implementation

◆ Acute Care. Focus your nursing care for the patient with VTE on preventing thrombi and reducing inflammation. Review with the patient any drugs, vitamins, minerals, and dietary and herbal supplements that may interfere with anticoagulant therapy (see the Complementary & Alternative Therapies box on p. 818). Depending on the anticoagulant ordered, monitor INR, aPTT, ACT, anti-factor Xa levels, complete blood count (CBC), creatinine, factor X levels, hemoglobin, hematocrit, platelet levels, and/or liver enzymes.[21] Monitor platelet counts for patients getting UH or LMWH to assess for HIT. Titrate doses of UH, warfarin, and direct thrombin inhibitors based on results of blood studies and agency protocols. Direct thrombin inhibitors may need adjustment for patients with renal or liver disease. Check the results of pertinent tests before starting, giving, or changing anticoagulant therapy.

Monitor for and reduce the risk for bleeding with anticoagulant therapy (Table 37.13). Bleeding risk is greater in people receiving LMWH or UH with an active gastroduodenal ulcer, prior bleeding history, low platelet count, hepatic or renal failure, rheumatic disease, cancer, or age greater than 85 years.[21] Patients receiving warfarin with an INR of 5.0 or more are at increased risk for bleeding. In case of anticoagulation above target goals, give reversal agents (e.g., protamine, vitamin K) or make dosage adjustments as prescribed.

 DRUG ALERT Anticoagulant Therapy

- Avoid IM injections.
- Observe closely for any signs of bleeding: hypotension, tachycardia, hematuria, melena, hematemesis, petechiae, bruising, oozing or visible bleeding from trauma site or surgical incision.
- Tell patients to report bleeding: black or bloody stools, bleeding gums, bloody urine or sputum, coffee-ground or bloody vomit, excessive bruising, nosebleeds, excessive menstrual bleeding.
- Assess for mental status changes, especially in the older patient, since this may indicate cerebral bleeding.
- Tell patients to avoid taking aspirin, NSAIDs, fish oil supplements, garlic supplements, ginkgo biloba, and certain antibiotics (e.g., sulfamethoxazole and trimethoprim [Bactrim]).

Early ambulation does not increase the short-term risk of a PE in patients with VTE. In addition, early ambulation after acute VTE results in a more rapid decrease in edema and limb pain, fewer PTS symptoms, and better quality of life. Teach the patient and caregiver the importance of physical activity. Help the patient ambulate several times a day. For patients with acute VTE with severe edema and limb pain, bed rest with limb elevation may initially be prescribed.

◆ Ambulatory Care. Focus discharge teaching on modifying VTE risk factors, monitoring laboratory values, dietary and drug instructions, and guidelines for follow-up. If appropriate,

---

▓▓ TABLE 37.13 **Nursing Management**

Patients Receiving Anticoagulants

Assessment

- Monitor vital signs as indicated.
- Examine urine and stool for overt and occult signs of blood.
- Inspect skin often, especially under any splinting devices.
- Evaluate platelet count for signs of heparin-induced thrombocytopenia.
- Evaluate appropriate laboratory coagulation tests for target therapeutic levels.
- Evaluate lower extremity for bruising or hematoma development if intermittent pneumatic compression device used.
- Perform assessments frequently for signs and symptoms of bleeding (e.g., hypotension, tachycardia) or clotting.
- Notify the HCP of any abnormalities in assessments, vital signs, or laboratory values.

Injections

- Avoid IM injections.
- Minimize venipunctures.
- Use small-gauge needles for venipunctures unless therapy requires a larger gauge.
- Apply manual pressure for at least 10 minutes (or longer if needed) on venipuncture sites.

Patient Care

- Avoid restrictive clothing.
- Apply moisturizing lotion to skin.
- Use electric razors, not straight razors.
- Perform physical care in a gentle manner.
- Tell patient not to forcefully blow nose.
- Avoid removing or disrupting established clots.
- Humidify O_2 source if supplemental O_2 is ordered.
- Use soft toothbrushes or foam swabs for oral care.
- Reposition the patient carefully at regular intervals.
- Limit tape application. Use paper tape as appropriate.
- Give stool softeners to avoid hard stools and straining.
- Lubricate tubes (e.g., suction catheter) adequately before insertion.
- Use support pads, mattresses, bed cradles, and therapeutic beds as indicated.
- Apply graduated compression stockings or intermittent pneumatic compression devices (if ordered) and with attention to proper size, application, and use.
- Perform risk for fall and skin breakdown assessments per agency policy and implement safety and preventive measures as needed.

---

suggest the patient stop smoking and avoid all nicotine products. Teach the patient to avoid constrictive clothing. Tell women with a history of VTE to stop oral contraceptives or hormone therapy. Teach patients to limit standing or sitting in a motionless, leg-dependent position.

When traveling long distances, tell patients to frequently exercise the calf muscles, take short walks, and drink nonalcoholic, noncaffeinated beverages. For those at high risk for VTE who are planning a long trip, recommend properly fitted, knee-high graduated compression stockings during travel to decrease edema and VTE risk. Aspirin or anticoagulant use is not suggested for long-distance travelers. Teach the patient and caregiver about signs and symptoms of PE, such as sudden onset of dyspnea, tachypnea, and pleuritic chest pain. They should contact ERS if these symptoms occur.

Review drug dosage, actions, and side effects; the need for routine blood tests; and what symptoms need immediate medical attention (Table 37.14). Devices are available for home monitoring of INR. Teach patients taking LMWH or fondaparinux

NURSING MANAGEMENT
Caring for the Patient With Venous Thromboembolism (VTE)

- Assess patients for VTE risk and monitor for VTE in at-risk patients.
- Teach patients who are at risk for VTE about preventive measures, such as increasing mobility, using graduated compression stockings and IPCs, and taking anticoagulant drugs.
- Measure patients for graduated compression stockings and/or IPCs.
- Assess for the use of dietary supplements or herbs that may affect the coagulation status before the start of anticoagulant therapy.
- Give prescribed oral, subcutaneous, and IV anticoagulants.
- Evaluate the effect of anticoagulant drugs by monitoring appropriate laboratory results and side effects of therapy.
- Assess for complications of VTE, including PE and chronic venous insufficiency.
- Teach the patient and caregiver the manifestations of PE and the need to contact the ERS if these occur.
- Provide discharge teaching about use of graduated compression stockings, anticoagulant drugs, diet, laboratory testing, and subcutaneous anticoagulant therapy (if needed).
- Teach safety precautions to prevent falls or other injuries that might result in bleeding.
- Discuss how to use pressure to stop bleeding and to contact ERS for persistent bleeding.
- Teach the patient about lifestyle measures to prevent VTE, including leg exercises, ambulation, and avoiding nicotine and oral contraceptives.
- Oversee the UAP:
  - Reposition patients who are on bed rest at least every 2 hrs.
  - Remind patients about the need to flex and extend the legs and feet at least every 2 hrs while in bed.
  - Help ambulatory patients to walk at least 4 to 6 times daily.
  - Help patients with putting on graduated compression stockings.
  - Apply IPCs.
- Collaborate with the physical therapist:
  - Assess patient's mobility status.
  - Develop exercise/muscle strengthening program as needed.
- Collaborate with the dietitian:
  - Assess patient's diet and nutritional status.
  - Provide diet teaching as needed.

TABLE 37.14 Patient & Caregiver Teaching
Anticoagulant Therapy

Include the following information in the teaching plan for a patient receiving anticoagulant therapy and the patient's caregiver:

1. Give reasons for and action of anticoagulant drug and how long therapy will last.
2. Take drug at the same time each day (preferably in afternoon or evening).
3. Depending on drug prescribed, obtain blood tests to assess therapeutic effect of the drug and whether change in dosage is needed.
4. Contact ERS immediately for any of the following adverse side effects of drug therapy:
   - Blood in urine or stool; or black, tarry stools
   - Vomiting blood, coffee-grounds emesis
   - Unusual bleeding from gums, skin, or nose, or heavy menstrual bleeding
   - Severe headaches or stomach pain
   - Chest pain, shortness of breath, palpitations (heart racing)
   - Weakness, dizziness, mental status changes
   - Cold, blue, or painful feet
5. Avoid any trauma or injury that may cause bleeding (e.g., vigorous brushing of teeth, contact sports, rollerblading, use of straight razor).
6. Avoid all aspirin-containing drugs and NSAIDs.
7. Limit alcohol intake to small to moderate amounts (12 oz beer, 4 oz wine, 1 oz hard liquor/day).
8. Wear a Medic Alert device saying what anticoagulant drug is being taken.
9. If taking warfarin (Coumadin), avoid frequent or dramatic changes in eating foods high in vitamin K (e.g., broccoli, spinach, kale, greens). Do not take supplemental vitamin K.
10. Consult with HCP before beginning or stopping any drug, vitamin, mineral, or dietary or herbal supplement (see Complementary & Alternative Therapies box on p. 818).
11. Inform all HCPs, including dentist, of anticoagulant therapy.
12. Correct dosing is essential. Provide supervision if patient has confusion or cognitive impairment.

and their caregivers how to give the drug subcutaneously. Active or young patients need to avoid contact sports and activities with high risk for trauma (e.g., skiing). Teach older patients about safety precautions to prevent falls (e.g., avoid use of throw rugs). Tell the patient and caregiver to apply pressure for 10 to 15 minutes if bleeding occurs (e.g., nosebleed).

A well-balanced diet is important. Teach patients taking warfarin to follow a consistent diet of foods containing vitamin K and to avoid any supplements containing vitamin K (e.g., vitamins, green tea). Tell the patient to avoid excess amounts of vitamin E and alcohol. Encourage proper hydration to prevent hypercoagulability of the blood, which may occur with dehydration.

The overweight patient needs to limit carbohydrates and total caloric intake and increase physical activity to achieve and maintain desired weight. Exercise may help patients with VTE and PTS.[17,20] Help the patient develop an exercise program with an emphasis on leg strength training and aerobic activity. An exercise program also improves the patient's quality of life.

Graduated compression stockings reduce symptomatic swelling in patients with a proximal VTE.[17,20] Alternatively, IPCs may be used for patients with significant edema and

moderate to severe PTS. The long-term use of graduated compression stockings may not prevent PTS development.

◆ Evaluation

The expected outcomes are that the patient with VTE will have
- Minimal to no pain
- Intact skin
- Increased knowledge of disorder and treatment plan
- No signs of hemorrhage or occult bleeding

VARICOSE VEINS

Varicose veins, or *varicosities,* are dilated (3 mm or larger in diameter), tortuous superficial veins often found in the saphenous vein system. Varicosities may be small and harmless or large and bulging. *Primary varicose veins* (idiopathic) are due to a weakness of the vein walls. They are more common in women. *Secondary varicose veins* result from direct injury, a previous VTE, or excessive vein distention. Secondary varicose veins may occur in the esophagus (esophageal varices), vulva, spermatic cords (varicoceles), and anorectal area (hemorrhoids), and as abnormal arteriovenous (AV) connections.

Congenital varicose veins result from chromosomal defects that cause abnormal development of the venous system.[22] *Reticular veins* are smaller varicose veins that appear flat, less tortuous, and blue-green in color. *Telangiectasias* (often called spider veins), are small visible vessels (generally less than 1 mm in diameter) that appear bluish black, purple, or red.

Etiology and Pathophysiology

Superficial veins in the lower extremities become dilated and tortuous in response to backward (retrograde) blood flow and increased venous pressure. Risk factors include family history of chronic venous disease, weak vein structure, female gender, tobacco use, increasing age, obesity, multiparity, history of VTE, venous obstruction resulting from extrinsic pressure by tumors, thrombophilia, phlebitis, previous leg injury, and occupations that require prolonged standing or sitting.[22,23]

In primary varicose veins, weak vein walls allow the vein valve ring to enlarge, so the leaflets no longer fit together properly (incompetent). Incompetent vein valves allow backward blood flow, particularly when the patient is standing. This results in increased venous pressure and further venous distention. High pressure in the superficial veins also can be caused by vein valve dysfunction in the deep veins or perforator veins (veins that perforate the deep fascia of muscles to connect the superficial veins to the deep veins).

Clinical Manifestations and Complications

Discomfort from varicose veins varies among people and tends to be worse after episodes of superficial vein thrombosis. Symptoms affect women more often than men.[23] The most common symptoms include a heavy, achy feeling or pain after prolonged standing or sitting, which is relieved by walking or limb elevation. Some patients feel pressure or an itchy, burning, tingling, throbbing, or cramp-like leg sensation. Swelling, restless or tired legs, fatigue, and nocturnal leg cramps may occur.

Superficial venous thrombosis is the most frequent complication of varicose veins. It may occur spontaneously or after trauma, surgical procedures, or pregnancy. Rare complications include rupture of the varicose veins resulting in external bleeding and skin ulcerations.

Diagnostic Studies and Interprofessional Care

Superficial varicose veins often can be diagnosed by careful physical examination. Duplex ultrasound imaging is the gold standard to evaluate venous anatomy, valvular competence, and venous obstruction.[22] Conservative treatment involves rest with limb elevation; graduated compression stockings; leg strengthening exercise, such as walking; and weight loss, if indicated.

Drug Therapy

Venoactive drugs, derived from plant extracts, are powerful antioxidants that work by stimulating release of chemicals within the vein walls to strengthen the circulation and reduce inflammation and edema. Several natural and synthetic venoactive agents have been used to treat varicose veins and advanced chronic venous disease. These include micronized purified flavonoid fraction, rutosides (e.g., horse chestnut seed extract [*Aesculus hippocastanum*]), proanthocyanidins (from grapes and apples), and *Ruscus* (butcher's broom).[23]

Therapeutic benefits of venoactive drugs include pain relief, edema reduction, and decreased leg cramping and restless legs. These drugs are widely used in Europe. They are not approved by the FDA. However, many are available over the counter as dietary or herbal supplements.

 DRUG ALERT Horse Chestnut Seed Extract (Aesculus hippocastanum)

- May interact with lithium and antidiabetes, antiplatelet, and anticoagulant drugs.
- Should not be taken by persons with liver or kidney disease or with a latex allergy.

Interventional and Surgical Therapies

Sclerotherapy involves the direct IV injection of a liquid or foam sclerosing substance (e.g., hypertonic saline, polidocanol, glycerin) that chemically ablates (destroys) the treated veins. Sclerotherapy can be used on telangiectasias, perforator veins, reticular veins, varicose veins 5 mm in diameter or smaller, and venous malformations (Fig. 37.12). This procedure is done in an office setting and causes minimal discomfort.

The most common complications of sclerotherapy are residual pigmentation, matting (new telangiectasias develop in the area), thrombophlebitis, and ulcers.[23] After injection, a graduated compression stocking or compression bandage is worn. Patients should not travel long distances during the first week after sclerotherapy to minimize the risk for a VTE.

Other noninvasive options include transcutaneous laser therapy for telangiectasias and high-intensity pulsed-light therapy for reticular veins. Transcutaneous laser or light therapy is used for patients in whom sclerotherapy is contraindicated or has been ineffective.[23] Vascular lasers work by heating the hemoglobin in the vessels, resulting in vessel sclerosis. Complications of these therapies include pain, blistering, hyperpigmentation, and superficial erosions.

A minimally invasive treatment option for saphenous vein reflux is endovenous ablation using thermal energy from radiofrequency or laser therapy. The HCP inserts a catheter into the vein to heat the vein wall, which then causes the vein to collapse. Complications include bruising, skin burns, hyperpigmentation, infection, paresthesia, superficial or deep vein thrombosis, and pulmonary embolism. Graduated compression stockings or bandages are worn afterwards. Endovenous thermal ablation may be done in combination with surgical ligation or phlebectomy.

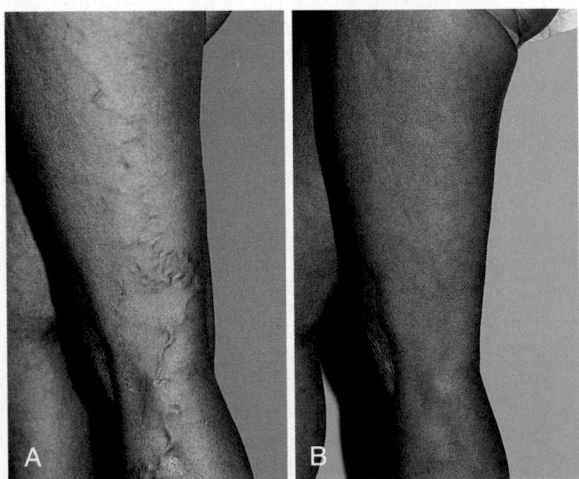

FIG. 37.12 A, Lateral aspect of varicose veins before treatment. B, Lateral aspect of varicose veins 2 years after initial treatment with sclerotherapy. (From Goldman MP, Guex JJ, Weiss RA: *Sclerotherapy: Treatment of varicose and telangiectatic leg veins*, ed 5, Philadelphia, 2011, Mosby.)

Surgical intervention is needed for recurrent superficial venous thrombosis or when symptoms cannot be controlled with other therapy. The traditional surgical intervention involves ligation of the entire vein (usually the greater saphenous vein) and removal of its incompetent branches. An alternative but time-consuming technique is *ambulatory phlebectomy*. This involves pulling the varicosity through a "stab" incision followed by excision of the vein. *Transilluminated powered phlebectomy* involves the use of a tissue resector to destroy clusters of varicosities and removes the pieces via aspiration. Complications include bleeding, bruising, and infection.

NURSING MANAGEMENT: VARICOSE VEINS

Prevention is a key factor related to varicose veins. Tell the patient to avoid sitting or standing for long periods, maintain ideal body weight, take precautions against injury to the extremities, avoid wearing constrictive clothing, and walk daily.

After vein ligation surgery, encourage the patient to deep breathe, which promotes venous return. Check the extremities regularly for color, movement, sensation, temperature, edema, and quality of pedal pulses. Some bruising and discoloration are normal. Elevate the legs 15 degrees to limit edema. Apply graduated compression stockings or bandages. Remove them every 8 hours for short periods and then reapply.

Long-term management of varicose veins is directed toward improving circulation and appearance, relieving discomfort, and avoiding complications and ulceration. Varicosities can recur in other veins after surgery. Teach the patient the proper use and care of custom-fitted graduated compression stockings. The patient should apply stockings in bed before rising in the morning.

Emphasize the importance of periodic positioning of the legs above the heart. The overweight patient may need help with weight loss. The patient with a job that requires long periods of standing or sitting needs to frequently flex and extend the hips, legs, and ankles and change positions. Remind patients to consult with their HCP before taking any dietary or herbal supplements to avoid drug interactions.

CHRONIC VENOUS INSUFFICIENCY AND VENOUS LEG ULCERS

Chronic venous insufficiency (CVI) describes abnormalities of the venous system that result in advanced signs and symptoms, such as edema, skin changes, and/or venous leg ulcers.[22] CVI can lead to *venous leg ulcers* (formerly called *venous stasis ulcers* or *varicose ulcers*). Although CVI and venous leg ulcers are not life-threatening diseases, they are painful, slow to heal, debilitating, and costly conditions that adversely affect patients' quality of life. They are a common problem in older adults.

Etiology and Pathophysiology

Both long-standing primary varicose veins and PTS can progress to CVI. *Ambulatory venous hypertension* causes serous fluid and RBCs to leak from the capillaries and venules into the tissue. This causes edema and chronic inflammatory changes. Enzymes in the tissue eventually break down RBCs, causing the release of *hemosiderin*, which causes a brownish skin discoloration. Over time, fibrous tissue replaces the skin and subcutaneous tissue around the ankle. This results in thick, hardened, contracted skin. Although the causes of CVI are known, the exact pathophysiology of venous leg ulcers is unknown.

Clinical Manifestations and Complications

In patients with CVI, the skin of the lower leg is leathery, with a characteristic brownish or "brawny" appearance from the hemosiderin deposition. Edema usually has been persistent for a prolonged period. Eczema with itching and scratching is often present (Table 37.1).

Venous ulcers classically occur above the medial malleolus (Fig. 37.13). The ulcer is often quite painful, particularly when edema or infection is present. Pain may be worse when the leg is in a dependent position. If the venous ulcer is untreated, the wound becomes wider and deeper, increasing the risk for infection.

Interprofessional and Nursing Care

Compression is essential for venous ulcer healing and preventing venous ulcer recurrence.[22,23] A variety of options are available for compression therapy. These include custom-fitted graduated compression stockings, elastic tubular support bandages, a Velcro wrap (CircAid), IPCs, and multilayer (3 or 4) bandage systems (e.g., Profore).[22,23] Evaluate patients individually when choosing a compression method. Before starting compression therapy, assess the arterial status to make sure that PAD is not present. An ABI of 0.4 or less suggests severe PAD, and the patient should not have any type of compression therapy.[3] Show how to correctly apply the compression therapy and have the patient "show back" the skill. Stockings should be worn daily to prevent recurrent leg ulcers. Tell the patient to replace stockings every 4 to 6 months.

Discuss activity guidelines and proper limb positioning. Tell patients with CVI to avoid standing or sitting for long periods, which decreases blood return from the lower extremities. Teach patients to frequently elevate their legs above the level of the heart to reduce edema. Encourage patients to begin a daily walking program once an ulcer heals. Tell the patient and caregiver to avoid trauma to the limbs. Teach proper foot and leg care to avoid more skin trauma.

Moist environment dressings are the basis of wound care. A variety of dressings are available. These include transparent film dressings, hydrocolloids, hydrogels, foams, alginates, gauze, and combination dressings. Dressing decisions should be based on wound characteristics, cost, best evidence, and clinician judgment. Chapter 11 and Table 11.9 discuss dressings.

Evaluate the nutritional status of a patient with a venous ulcer. A balanced diet with adequate protein, calories, and

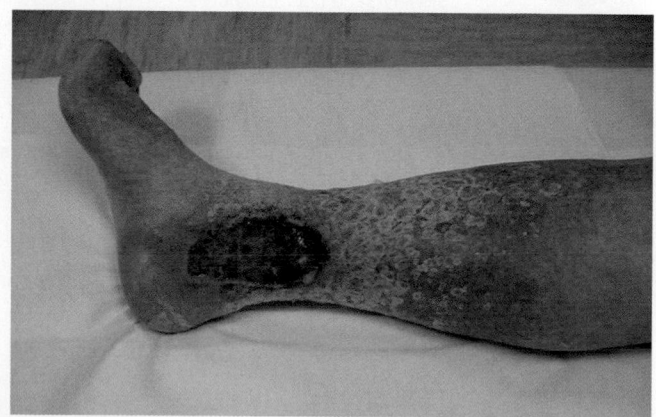

FIG. 37.13 Venous leg ulcer. (From Mosti G: Compression and venous surgery for venous leg ulcers, *Clin Plast Surg* 39:269, 2012.)

nutrients is essential. Foods high in protein (e.g., meat, beans, cheese, tofu), vitamin A (green leafy vegetables), vitamin C (citrus fruits, tomatoes, cantaloupe), and zinc (meat, seafood) are most important for healing. For patients with diabetes, maintaining normal blood glucose levels aids the healing process.

Though venous leg ulcers are colonized by bacteria, routine use of antibiotics is not indicated. Signs of infection include change in quantity, color, or odor of the drainage; pus; erythema of the wound edges; change in sensation around the wound; warmth around the wound; increased local pain, edema, or both; dark-colored granulation tissue; induration around the wound; delayed healing; and cellulitis. If signs of infection occur, obtain a wound culture. Culture results guide antibiotic therapy. The usual treatment for infection is wound debridement, wound excision, and systemic antibiotics.

If the ulcer does not heal with conservative therapy, drug therapy should be considered. Pentoxifylline or micronized purified flavonoid fraction (Daflon) is recommended with compression therapy to improve healing.[23] Pentoxifylline minimizes WBC activation and adhesion to capillary endothelium and decreases oxidative stress. Micronized purified flavonoid fraction acts on WBCs to decrease inflammation and edema.[23]

Other treatments are considered for large venous leg ulcers that do not respond to standard therapy after 4 to 6 weeks. These include coverage with a skin replacement or substitute, such as split-thickness skin grafts or artificial bioengineered skin.[22] (Chapter 24 discusses skin grafting.) Although grafts may aid with healing, they do not replace the need for lifelong compression therapy.

Patients with CVI have dry, flaky, itchy skin. Daily moisturizing decreases itching and prevents skin cracking. Contact dermatitis may result from contact with sensitizing products, such as topical antimicrobial agents (e.g., gentamicin); additives in bandages or dressings (e.g., adhesives); ointments containing lanolin, alcohols, or benzocaine; and over-the-counter creams or lotions with fragrance or preservatives. Assess wounds for signs of infection with each dressing change.

▓ NURSING MANAGEMENT
Caring for the Patient With Chronic Venous Insufficiency

Many patients with CVI and venous ulcers receive outpatient care. The registered nurse (RN) does the initial wound assessment, develops and implements the plan of care, and periodically evaluates the patient and venous ulcer. Routine wound care can be done by LPN/VNs and UAP depending on the state nurse practice act and agency policy.

- Assess the patient for increases in edema, eczema, and venous leg ulcers.
- Assess diet and nutritional status and make referrals as needed.
- Assess for the use of venoactive dietary supplements or herbs that may adversely affect co-morbid conditions and/or prescription drugs.
- Choose best options for compression therapy and wound care.
- Give prescribed analgesics, antibiotics, or other drugs.
- Apply compression therapy.
- Provide wound care for venous leg ulcers.
- Evaluate for the effectiveness of therapies and need for alternative approaches.
- Teach patient and caregiver about the manifestations, complications, and treatment of venous insufficiency.
- Oversee the UAP in providing care:
  - Aid patients in elevating legs to reduce edema and pain.
  - Apply graduated compression stockings.
- Collaborate with the dietitian:
  - Assess diet and nutritional status.
  - Provide diet education as needed.

CASE STUDY
Peripheral Artery Disease

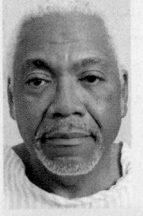
(© IPGGutenbergUKLtd/iStock/Thinkstock.)

Patient Profile

S.J., a 73-yr-old black man, is admitted to the hospital with rest pain in both legs and a nonhealing ulcer of the big toe on the right foot.

Subjective Data

- History of a myocardial infarction, stroke, hypertension, HF, and type 1 diabetes
- Underwent a left femoral-popliteal bypass 5 yrs ago
- Has a 45-pack-yr history of tobacco use
- Has been using insulin for 30 yrs
- Reports sudden, intense increase in right foot pain for past 2 hrs
- Has slept in recliner with right leg in dependent position for several months to decrease leg pain

Current Medications

- Furosemide (Lasix) 40 mg/day PO
- Isosorbide dinitrate/hydralazine hydrochloride (BiDil) 1 tablet every 8 hr
- Aspart (NovoLog) insulin with meals
- Glargine insulin 50 units/day subcutaneously
- Diltiazem sustained release (Cardizem LA) 240 mg/day PO
- Aspirin 325 mg/day PO
- Fish oil daily (self-prescribed)

Objective Data
Physical Examination

- BP 148/92 mm Hg, irregular apical HR 90/min, respiratory rate 22/min, temperature 97.9° F (36.6° C)
- Alert and oriented, anxious, with no apparent physical or mental deficits from stroke
- Has 1+ right femoral pulse, popliteal pulse by Doppler only, posterior tibial pulse by Doppler only, and dorsalis pedis pulse absent (not palpable or present by Doppler). Left leg pulses are 1+
- Right leg ABI: 0.20. Left leg ABI: 0.68
- Has a 2-cm necrotic ulcer on tip of right big toe
- Has thickened toenails. Shiny, thin skin on legs. No hair on both lower legs
- Right foot is very cool, pale, and mottled in color with decreased sensation
- No peripheral edema
- Bedside glucose measurement 298 mg/dL (last meal 4 hrs before admission)

Discussion Questions

1. Assess S.J.'s risk factors for PAD.
2. Distinguish S.J.'s signs and symptoms of chronic PAD and acute arterial ischemia.
3. Identify the possible cause(s) for the sudden, intense increase in right foot pain.
4. How would you interpret S.J.'s ABI findings?

Continued

CASE STUDY

Peripheral Artery Disease—cont'd

5. What other diagnostic tests can be done to assess the extent of his PAD?
6. Given the physical examination data, what initial drug(s) would you expect the HCP to prescribe?
7. What treatment modalities are possible for S.J.?
8. **Priority Decision:** Based on the assessment data presented, what are the priority nursing diagnoses?
9. **Priority Decision:** What are the priority nursing responsibilities in caring for S.J.?

10. **Collaboration:** Identify activities that can be delegated to UAP.
11. **Evidence-Based Practice:** When teaching S.J., what evidence-based advice would you give him about the use of dietary supplements, such as fish oil?
12. **Safety:** To ensure S.J.'s safety, what nursing interventions are necessary to initiate?

Answers available at *http://evolve.elsevier.com/Lewis/medsurg.*

■ BRIDGE TO NCLEX EXAMINATION

The number of the question corresponds to the same-numbered outcome at the beginning of the chapter.

1. A 50-year-old woman who weighs 95 kg has a history of tobacco use, high blood pressure, high sodium intake, and sedentary lifestyle. Which is the *most important* risk factor for peripheral artery disease (PAD) to address in the nursing plan of care?
   a. Salt intake
   b. Tobacco use
   c. Excess weight
   d. Sedentary lifestyle

2. When teaching a patient about rest pain with PAD, what should the nurse explain as the cause of the pain?
   a. Vasospasm of cutaneous arteries in the feet.
   b. Decrease in blood flow to the nerves of the feet.
   c. Increase in retrograde venous perfusion to the lower legs.
   d. Constriction in blood flow to leg muscles during exercise.

3. A patient with infective endocarditis develops sudden left leg pain with pallor, paresthesia, and a loss of peripheral pulses. What should be the nurse's *initial* action?
   a. Notify the HCP of the change in perfusion.
   b. Start anticoagulant therapy with IV heparin.
   c. Elevate the leg to improve the venous return.
   d. Position the patient in reverse Trendelenburg.

4. Which clinical manifestations can the nurse expect to see in both patients with Buerger's disease and patients with Raynaud's phenomenon? *(select all that apply)*
   a. Intermittent low-grade fevers
   b. Sensitivity to cold temperatures
   c. Gangrenous ulcers on fingertips
   d. Color changes of fingers and toes
   e. Episodes of superficial vein thrombosis

5. A patient is admitted to the hospital with a diagnosis of abdominal aortic aneurysm. Which signs and symptoms would suggest that the aneurysm has ruptured?
   a. Rapid onset of shortness of breath and hemoptysis
   b. Sudden, severe low back pain and bruising along his flank
   c. Gradually increasing substernal chest pain and diaphoresis
   d. Sudden, patchy blue mottling on feet and toes and rest pain

6. What are the *priority* nursing interventions 8 hours after an abdominal aortic aneurysm repair?
   a. Assessing nutritional status and dietary preferences
   b. Initiating IV heparin and monitoring anticoagulation
   c. Administering IV fluids and watching kidney function
   d. Elevating the legs and applying compression stockings

7. What is the *first* priority of interprofessional care for a patient with a suspected acute aortic dissection?
   a. Reduce anxiety.
   b. Monitor chest pain.
   c. Control blood pressure.
   d. Increase myocardial contractility.

8. Which patient is at *highest* risk for venous thromboembolism (VTE)?
   a. A 62-yr-old man with spider veins who is having arthroscopic knee surgery
   b. A 32-yr-old woman who smokes, takes oral contraceptives, and is planning a trip to Europe
   c. A 26-yr-old woman who is 3 days postpartum and received maintenance IV fluids for 12 hours during her labor
   d. An active 72-yr-old man at home recovering from transurethral resection of the prostate for benign prostatic hyperplasia

9. Which clinical findings should the nurse expect in a person with an acute lower extremity VTE? *(select all that apply)*
   a. Pallor and coolness of foot and calf
   b. Mild to moderate calf pain and tenderness
   c. Grossly decreased or absent pedal pulses
   d. Unilateral edema and induration of the thigh
   e. Palpable cord along a superficial varicose vein

10. Which treatment should the nurse anticipate for an otherwise healthy person with an initial VTE?
    a. IV argatroban as an inpatient
    b. IV unfractionated heparin as an inpatient
    c. Subcutaneous unfractionated heparin as an outpatient
    d. Subcutaneous low-molecular-weight heparin as an outpatient

11. Which instruction is a *key* aspect of teaching for the patient on anticoagulant therapy?
    a. Monitor for and report any signs of bleeding.
    b. Do not take acetaminophen (Tylenol) for a headache.
    c. Decrease your dietary intake of foods containing vitamin K.
    d. Arrange to have blood drawn twice a week to check drug effects.

12. The nurse is planning care and teaching for a patient with venous leg ulcers. What is the *most* important patient action in healing and control of this condition?
    a. Following activity guidelines.
    b. Using moist environment dressings.
    c. Taking horse chestnut seed extract daily.
    d. Applying graduated compression stockings.

1. b, 2. b, 3. a, 4. b, c, d, 5. b, 6. c, 7. c, 8. b, 9. b, d, 10. d, 11. a, 12. d

For rationales to these answers and even more NCLEX review questions, visit *http://evolve.elsevier.com/Lewis/medsurg.*

ⓔ EVOLVE WEBSITE/RESOURCES LIST

http://evolve.elsevier.com/Lewis/medsurg

Review Questions (Online Only)

Key Points

Answer Keys for Questions
- Rationales for Bridge to NCLEX Examination Questions
- Answer Guidelines for Case Study on p. 824
- Answer Guidelines for Managing Care of Multiple Patients Case Study (Section 8) on p. 827

Student Case Studies
- Patient With Abdominal Aortic Aneurysm
- Patient With Chronic Peripheral Artery Disease

Nursing Care Plans
- eNursing Care Plan 37.1: Patient With Peripheral Artery Disease of the Lower Extremities
- eNursing Care Plan 37.2: Patient After Surgical Repair of the Aorta

Conceptual Care Map Creator

Audio Glossary

Content Updates

REFERENCES

*1. Creager MA, Belkin B, Bluth EI, et al: 2012 ACCF/AHA/ACR/SCAI/SIR/STS/SVM/SVN/SVS key data elements and definitions for peripheral atherosclerotic vascular disease: a report of the ACCF/AHA Task Force on clinical data standards, *Circulation* 125:395, 2012. (Classic)

2. Centers for Disease Control and Prevention: Peripheral arterial disease (PAD) fact sheet. Retrieved from *www.cdc.gov/DHDSP/data_statistics/fact_sheets/fs_PAD.htm*.

*3. Gerhard-Herman M, Gornick H, Barrett C, et al: 2016 AHA/ACC guideline on the management of patients with lower extremity peripheral artery disease: Executive summary, *Circulation* 135:e686, 2017.

*4. Roumia M, Herbert H, Soukas P, et al: Sex differences in disease-specific health status measures in patients with symptomatic peripheral artery disease: Data from the PORTRAIT study, *Vasc Med* 22:103, 2017.

*5. American Diabetes Association: Standards of medical care in diabetes 2018. Retrieved from *http://care.diabetesjournals.org/content/41/Supplement_1*.

6. Di Minno A, Frigeri o B, Spadarella G, et al: Old and new anticoagulants: Food, herbal medicines, and drug interactions, *Blood Rev* 31:193, 2017.

7. Dowd F, Johnson B, Mariotti A: Use of herbs and herbal dietary supplements in dentistry. In *Pharmacology and therapeutics for dentistry*, ed 7, St Louis, 2017, Elsevier.

*8. Terra M, Conte M, Moll F, et al: Critical limb ischemia: Current trends and future directions, *JAHA* 5:002938, 2016.

9. Bunte M, Shisehbar M: Next generation endovascular therapies in peripheral artery disease, *Prog Cardiovasc Dis* 60:593, 2018.

*10. Hess C, Norgren L, Ansel G, et al: A structured review of antithrombotic therapy in peripheral artery disease with a focus on revascularization: A TASC initiative, *Circulation* 135:2534, 2017.

*11. Cacione D, Moreno D: Stem cell therapy for treatment of thromboangiitis obliterans (Buerger's disease), *Cochrane Database Syst Rev* 10:CD012794, 2018.

*12. Stringer T, Femia A: Raynaud's phenomenon: Current concepts of skin and systemic manifestations, *Dermatology* 36:498, 2018.

*13. Chaikof EL, Dalman RL, Eskandari MK, et al: The Society of Vascular Surgery practice guidelines on the care of patients with an abdominal aortic aneurysm, *J Vasc Surg* 67:1, 2017.

*14. Rylski B, Perez M, Beyersdorf F, et al: Acute non-A non-B aortic dissection: Incidence, treatment and outcome, *Eur J Cardiothorac Surg* 52:1111, 2017.

15. Gawinecka J, Schonrath F, von Eckardstein A: Acute aortic dissection: Pathogenesis, risk factors, and diagnosis, *Swiss Med Weekly* 147:1, 2017.

*16. Li FR, Wu X, Yuan J, et al: Comparison of thoracic endovascular aortic repair, open surgery, and best medical treatment for type B aortic dissection: A meta-analysis, *Int J Cardiol* 250:240, 2018.

*17. Hattab Y, Kung S, Fasanya A, et al: Deep venous thrombosis of the upper and lower extremity, *Crit Care Nurs Q* 40:230, 2017.

18. Evans N, Rachford E: Superficial vein thrombosis, *Vasc Med* 23:187, 2018.

*19. Wik H, Enden T, Ganima W, et al: Diagnostic scales for the post thrombotic syndrome, *Thromb Res* 164:110, 2018.

*20. Kearon C, Aki E, Orneals J, et al: Antithrombotic therapy for VTE disease: CHEST guideline and expert panel report, *CHEST* 149:315, 2016.

21. Burcham JR, Rosenthal LD: *Lehne's pharmacology for nursing care*, ed 10, St Louis, 2019, Elsevier.

*22. Ito T, Kukino R, Takahara M, et al: Guidelines for the management of lower leg ulcers/varicose veins, *J Dermatol* 43:853, 2016.

*23. Chen JC: Current therapy for primary varicose veins, *BC Med J* 59:418, 2017.

*Evidence-based information for clinical practice.

CASE STUDY
Managing Care of Multiple Patients

You are working on the cardiovascular stepdown unit and have been assigned to care for the following 6 patients. You have 1 LPN and 1 UAP assigned to help you.

Patients

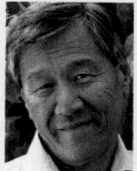
(© Jupiterimages/ Banana-Stock/ Thinkstock.)

L.P. is a 63-yr-old Asian American man who came to the ED with chest pain, shortness of breath, and palpitations. L.P.'s CK-MB and troponin levels are within normal limits. His ECG showed atrial fibrillation with a rapid ventricular response. He has been on IV diltiazem and IV heparin for 24 hr. Although his heart rate has decreased to 102 beats/min, the atrial fibrillation persists.

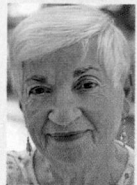
(© iStockphoto/ Thinkstock.)

J.E. is a 70-yr-old Hispanic woman admitted with increasing shortness of breath, fatigue, and weight gain. She has a systolic murmur and bilateral crackles. Her ejection fraction is 20%. She is receiving IV furosemide, oral potassium and enalapril (Vasotec), and a continuous infusion of nesiritide (Natrecor). She has O₂ at 6 L via nasal cannula to keep her O₂ saturation >93%. Normal initial set of cardiac enzymes.

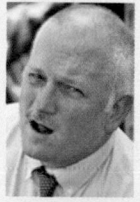
(© iStockphoto/ Thinkstock.)

D.M. is a 51-yr-old man who was admitted 2 days ago with a suspected inferolateral wall MI. His cardiac-specific troponin I level was high, and the ECG showed marked ST segment elevation in the inferior leads. Cardiac catheterization showed a 90% blockage of his left anterior descending (LAD) artery. Coronary angioplasty was done, and 2 stents inserted. He is now 2 days post-PTCA, has had no recurrence of his chest pain, and is to be discharged today.

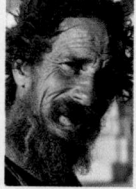
(© JennaDub/ iStock/ Thinkstock.)

R.B. is a 50-yr-old man admitted for HF due to valvular heart disease. He has a history of IV drug and alcohol use. He reports chest pain with minimal exertion. He has atrial fibrillation with a rapid ventricular response. His rhythm converted to normal sinus rhythm after receiving IV amiodarone. TEE shows left atrial and ventricular hypertrophy and mitral and aortic regurgitation.

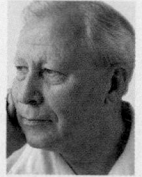
(© iStockphoto/ Thinkstock.)

J.M. is a 68-yr-old man admitted 3 days ago with a diagnosis of acute decompensated HF. He had a cardiac arrest (pulseless VT) and was successfully defibrillated after 1 shock. He underwent electrophysiology studies and implantation of an implantable cardiodefibrillator (ICD). He now is being treated for HF.

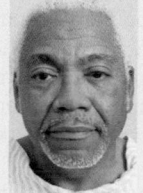
(© IPGGutenberg-UKLtd/iStock/ Thinkstock.)

S.J. is a 73-yr-old black man admitted with rest pain in both legs and a nonhealing ulcer of the big toe on the right foot. He has history of an MI, stroke, hypertension, and type 1 diabetes. He had a left femoral-popliteal bypass 5 years ago. His right foot is cool, pale, and mottled in color with decreased sensation. He has a 1+ right femoral pulse, right popliteal and posterior tibial pulses only obtained by Doppler, and his right dorsalis pedis pulse is absent (not palpable or present by Doppler). His left leg pulses are 1+. His right leg ABI: 0.20; left leg ABI: 0.68.

Discussion Questions

1. **Priority Decision:** After receiving report, which patient should you see first? Second? Provide a rationale for your decision.
2. **Collaboration:** Which tasks could you delegate to the LPN? *(select all that apply)*
   a. Monitor L.P.'s heparin infusion.
   b. Report changes in pain or sensation of S.J.'s legs.
   c. Teach D.M. about activity restriction after PTCA.
   d. Administer prescribed medications to R.B. and J.M.
   e. Hook up J.M. to 12-lead ECG and monitor for dysrhythmias.
3. **Priority Decision and Collaboration:** As you are assessing L.P., the LPN tells you that S.J. is diaphoretic and reports chest pain. Which initial action would be *most* appropriate?
   a. Ask the LPN to notify S.J.'s HCP.
   b. Have the LPN administer prescribed nitroglycerin to S.J.
   c. Leave L.P.'s room to perform a focused assessment on S.J.
   d. Finish assessing L.P. while the UAP obtains a 12-lead ECG on S.J.

Case Study Progression

S.J. rates his chest pain as a 9/10. His blood pressure is 110/70, heart rate 110, respiratory rate 26, and O₂ saturation 93% on room air. You obtain a 12-lead ECG and administer 0.4 mg SL nitroglycerin with minimal pain relief after 5 minutes. The 12-lead ECG shows new ST elevation in leads II, III, and aVF.

4. Which interventions would you expect the HCP to order for S.J.? *(select all that apply)*
   a. IV nitroglycerin
   b. IV morphine sulfate
   c. Emergent cardiac catheterization
   d. Furosemide 40 mg IV push STAT
   e. Increase the O₂ flow rate to 12 L/min
5. What would you include in teaching about ICDs with J.M. and his family?
   a. Avoid air travel.
   b. Avoid driving for 6 weeks.
   c. Avoid any sexual activity in case the ICD discharges.
   d. Avoid standing near antitheft devices in stores and public buildings.
6. J.E is receiving nesiritide. What information is the priority to monitor?
   a. Blood pressure
   b. Respiratory rate
   c. b-Natriuretic peptide (BNP) level
   d. Troponin and CK-MB laboratory values
7. **Priority Decision**: You are preparing to give morning medications. Which patient's medication should be given first?
   a. Oral potassium and enalapril to J.E.
   b. Oral metoprolol, aspirin, and clopidogrel to D.M.
   c. IV furosemide, oral enalapril and metoprolol to R.B.
   d. Subcut Novolog, oral diltiazem and furosemide to S.J.
8. **Management Decision:** You ask the UAP to take D.M.'s vital signs before and after having him walk 300 feet. When reviewing the patient's chart, you note record of the patient's walk but not his vital signs. What is your initial action?
   a. Report the incident to the charge nurse for follow-up.
   b. Talk to the UAP about why the vital signs were not recorded.
   c. Walk D.M. yourself again and take his vital signs pre- and post-activity.
   d. Ask the LPN to ambulate D.M. and obtain his vital signs before and after.

Answers and rationales available at *http://evolve.elsevier.com/Lewis/medsurg*.

38

Assessment: Gastrointestinal System

Kara Ann Ventura

We can't help everyone, but everyone can help someone.

Ronald Reagan

ⓔ http://evolve.elsevier.com/Lewis/medsurg

CONCEPTUAL FOCUS

Elimination
Fluids and Electrolytes

Nutrition

LEARNING OUTCOMES

1. Describe the structures and functions of the organs of the gastrointestinal tract.
2. Describe the structures and functions of the liver, gallbladder, biliary tract, and pancreas.
3. Distinguish the processes of ingestion, digestion, absorption, and elimination.
4. Explain the processes of biliary metabolism, bile production, and bile excretion.
5. Link the age-related changes of the gastrointestinal system to the differences in assessment findings.
6. Obtain significant subjective and objective assessment data related to the gastrointestinal system from a patient.
7. Perform a physical assessment of the gastrointestinal system using appropriate techniques.
8. Distinguish normal from abnormal findings of a physical assessment of the gastrointestinal system.
9. Describe the purpose, significance of results, and nursing responsibilities related to diagnostic studies of the gastrointestinal system.

KEY TERMS

absorption, p. 830
bilirubin, p. 832
borborygmi, Table 38.10, p. 842
cheilosis, Table 38.10, p. 841
deglutition, p. 829

digestion, p. 830
endoscopy, p. 846
hematemesis, Table 38.10, p. 841
Kupffer cells, p. 832
melena, Table 38.10, p. 842

pyorrhea, Table 38.10, p. 841
pyrosis, Table 38.10, p. 842
steatorrhea, Table 38.10, p. 842
tenesmus, Table 38.10, p. 842
Valsalva maneuver, p. 832

The gastrointestinal (GI) system, also called the *digestive system,* consists of the GI tract and its associated organs and glands. Included in the GI tract are the mouth, esophagus, stomach, small intestine, large intestine, rectum, and anus. The associated organs are the liver, pancreas, and gallbladder (Fig. 38.1). Problems that change physiologic processes or associated organs affect a person's ability to maintain nutritional status and eliminate waste.

STRUCTURES AND FUNCTIONS OF GASTROINTESTINAL SYSTEM

The GI tract extends around 30 ft (9 m) from the mouth to the anus. The GI tract is essentially a tube composed of 4 layers. From the inside to the outside, these layers are (1) mucosa lining; (2) submucosa connective tissue, which contains glands, blood vessels, and lymph nodes; (3) muscle; and (4) serosa. The muscular coat has 3 smooth muscle layers: the oblique (inner) layer, circular (middle) layer, and longitudinal (outer) layer.

Parasympathetic and sympathetic branches of the autonomic nervous system (ANS) innervate the GI tract. The parasympathetic (cholinergic) system is mainly excitatory. The sympathetic (adrenergic) system is mainly inhibitory. For example, parasympathetic stimulation increases peristalsis and sympathetic stimulation decreases it. Both sympathetic and parasympathetic afferent fibers relay sensory information.

The GI tract has its own nervous system: the enteric nervous system (ENS) or intrinsic nervous system. The ENS system regulates motility and secretion along the entire GI tract. The ENS is composed of 2 networks: (1) Meissner plexus in the

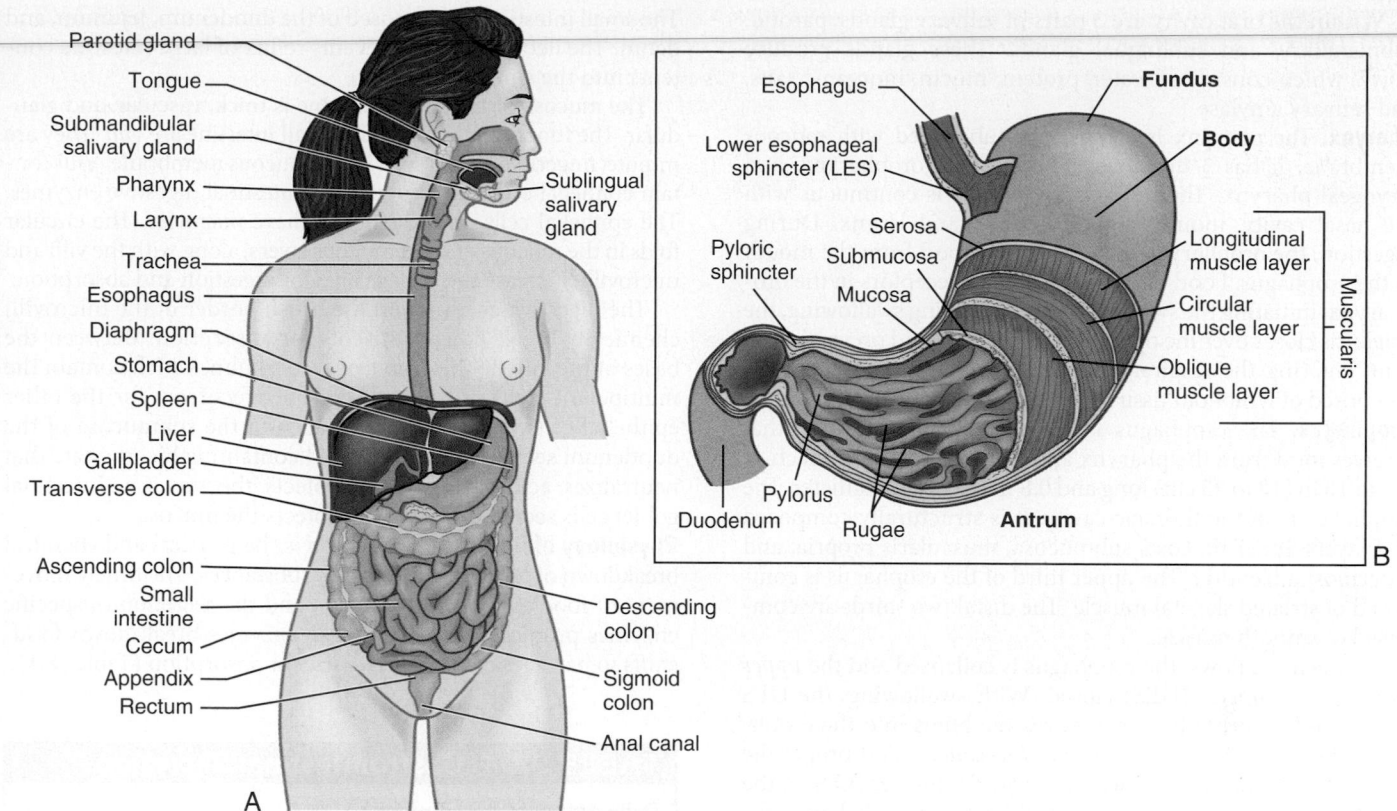

FIG. 38.1 A, Location of organs of the gastrointestinal system. B, Parts of the stomach.

submucosa and (2) Auerbach (myenteric) plexus between the muscle layers. The submucosal plexus controls secretion and is involved in many sensory functions. The myenteric plexus is the major nerve supply to the GI tract and controls GI movements. Although the ENS receives innervation from the ANS, it functions independently of the brain and spinal cord.

Circulation in the GI system is unique in that venous blood draining the GI tract organs empties into the portal vein, which then perfuses the liver. This allows the liver to clean the blood of bacteria and toxins from the GI tract. The celiac artery, superior mesenteric artery (SMA), and the inferior mesenteric artery (IMA) supply arterial blood to the GI tract. The stomach and duodenum receive their blood supply from the celiac axis. The distal small intestine to mid large intestine receives its blood supply from branches of the hepatic and SMA. The distal large intestine through the anus receives its blood supply from the IMA. The GI tract and accessory organs receive 25% to 30% of the cardiac output at rest and 35% or more after eating. Because such a large percent of the cardiac output perfuses these organs, the GI tract is a major source from which to divert blood flow during exercise, stress, or injury.

The peritoneum almost completely covers the abdominal organs. The 2 layers of the peritoneum are the *parietal layer,* which lines the abdominal cavity wall, and the *visceral layer,* which covers the abdominal organs. The peritoneal cavity is the potential space between the parietal and visceral layers. The 2 folds of the peritoneum are the mesentery and omentum. The mesentery attaches the small intestine and part of the large intestine to the posterior abdominal wall. It contains blood and lymph vessels. The omentum hangs like an apron from the stomach to the intestines. It contains fat and lymph nodes.

The main function of the GI system is to supply nutrients to body cells. This is accomplished through the processes of (1) *ingestion* (taking in food), (2) *digestion* (breaking down food), and (3) *absorption* (transferring food products into circulation). *Elimination* is the process of excreting the waste products of digestion.

Ingestion

Ingestion is the intake of food. *Appetite,* the desire to ingest food, influences how much food a person eats. An appetite center is found in the hypothalamus. Several factors, including hypoglycemia, an empty stomach, and a decrease in body temperature, stimulate appetite. The hormone *ghrelin* released from the stomach mucosa plays a role in appetite stimulation. Another hormone, *leptin,* is involved in appetite suppression. (See Chapter 40 for a discussion of ghrelin and leptin.) The sight, smell, and taste of food can stimulate appetite. Stomach distention, illness (especially accompanied by fever), hyperglycemia, nausea and vomiting, and certain drugs (e.g., amphetamines) inhibit appetite.

Deglutition, or swallowing, is the mechanical portion of ingestion. The organs involved in deglutition are the mouth, pharynx, and esophagus.

Mouth. The mouth consists of the lips and oral (buccal) cavity. The lips surround the opening of the mouth and function in speech. The hard and soft palates form the roof of the oral cavity. The oral cavity contains the teeth, used in *mastication* (chewing), and the tongue. The tongue is a solid muscle mass. It aids in chewing and moving food to the back of the throat for swallowing. The taste receptors (taste buds) are on the sides and tip of the tongue. The tongue is also important in speech.

Within the oral cavity are 3 pairs of salivary glands: parotid, submaxillary, and sublingual glands. These glands produce saliva, which consists of water, protein, mucin, inorganic salts, and salivary amylase.

Pharynx. The pharynx is a muscular tube lined with mucous membrane. It has 3 divisions: nasopharynx, oropharynx, and laryngeal pharynx. The mucous membrane is continuous with the nasal cavity, mouth, auditory tubes, and larynx. During ingestion, the oropharynx is the route for food from the mouth to the esophagus. Food or liquid stimulates receptors in the oropharynx, initiating the swallowing reflex. During swallowing, the epiglottis closes over the opening to the larynx and prevents food from entering the respiratory tract. The tonsils and adenoids, composed of lymphoid tissue, help the body prevent infection.

Esophagus. The esophagus is a hollow, muscular tube that receives food from the pharynx and moves it to the stomach. It is 7 to 10 in (18 to 25 cm) long and 0.8 in (2 cm) in diameter. The esophagus is in the thoracic cavity. It is structurally composed of 4 layers: inner mucosa, submucosa, muscularis propria, and outermost adventitia. The upper third of the esophagus is composed of striated skeletal muscle. The distal two thirds are composed of smooth muscle.

Between swallows, the esophagus is collapsed and the *upper esophageal sphincter* (UES) closed. With swallowing, the UES relaxes and a peristaltic wave moves the bolus into the esophagus. The muscular layers contract *(peristalsis)* and propel the food to the stomach. The *lower esophageal sphincter* (LES) at the distal end of the esophagus controls the opening of the esophagus into the stomach. It stays contracted except during swallowing, belching, or vomiting. The LES is an important barrier that normally prevents reflux of acidic gastric contents into the esophagus.

Digestion and Absorption

Stomach. The stomach's functions are to store food, mix food with gastric secretions, and empty contents in small boluses into the small intestine. The stomach absorbs only small amounts of water, alcohol, electrolytes, and certain drugs.

The stomach is usually J shaped and lies obliquely in the epigastric, umbilical, and left hypochondriac regions of the abdomen (Fig. 38.5 later in the chapter). It always contains gastric fluid and mucus. The 3 main parts of the stomach are the fundus (cardia), body, and antrum (Fig. 38.1). The pylorus is a small portion of the antrum proximal to the pyloric sphincter. The LES and pyloric sphincter guard the entrance to and exit from the stomach.

The stomach wall has 4 layers. The serous (outer) layer of the stomach is continuous with the peritoneum. The muscular layer consists of the longitudinal (outer) layer, circular (middle) layer, and oblique (inner) layer. The mucosal layer forms folds called rugae that have many small glands. In the fundus the glands contain (1) chief cells, which secrete pepsinogen and (2) parietal cells, which secrete hydrochloric (HCl) acid, water, and intrinsic factor. The secretion of HCl acid makes gastric juice acidic. This acidic pH helps protect us against ingested organisms. Intrinsic factor promotes cobalamin (vitamin B_{12}) absorption in the small intestine.

Small Intestine. The primary functions of the small intestine are digestion and absorption, the uptake of nutrients from the gut lumen to the bloodstream. The small intestine is a coiled tube about 23 ft (7 m) in length and 1 to 1.1 in (2.5 to 2.8 cm) in diameter. It extends from the pylorus to the ileocecal valve.

The small intestine is composed of the duodenum, jejunum, and ileum. The ileocecal valve prevents reflux of large intestine contents into the small intestine.

The mucosa of the small intestine is thick, vascular, and glandular. The functional units of the small intestine are *villi*. They are minute, fingerlike projections in the mucous membrane. Villi contain epithelial cells that produce the intestinal digestive enzymes. The epithelial cells on the villi also have *microvilli*. The circular folds in the mucous and submucous layers, along with the villi and microvilli, increase the surface area for digestion and absorption.

The digestive enzymes on the brush border of the microvilli chemically break down nutrients for absorption. Between the bases of the villi lie the crypts of Lieberkühn, which contain the multipotent stem cells. These are the precursors for the other epithelial cell types. Brunner's glands in the submucosa of the duodenum secrete an alkaline fluid containing bicarbonate that neutralizes acidic fluids and protects the mucosa. Intestinal goblet cells secrete mucus that protects the mucosa.

Physiology of Digestion. Digestion is the physical and chemical breakdown of food into absorbable substances. The timely movement of food through the GI tract and the secretion of specific enzymes promote digestion. These enzymes break down foodstuffs to particles of appropriate size for absorption (Table 38.1).

TABLE 38.1 Gastrointestinal Secretions

Daily Amount (mL)	Secretions/ Enzymes	Action
Salivary Glands		
1000–1500	Salivary amylase	Initiation of starch digestion
Stomach		
2500	HCl acid	Activation of pepsinogen to pepsin
	Intrinsic factor	Essential for cobalamin absorption in ileum
	Lipase	Fat digestion
	Pepsinogen	Protein digestion
Small Intestine		
3000	Aminopeptidases	Protein digestion
	Amylase	Carbohydrate digestion
	Enterokinase	Activation of trypsinogen to trypsin
	Lactase	Lactose to glucose and galactose
	Lipase	Fat digestion
	Maltase	Maltose to 2 glucose molecules
	Peptidases	Protein digestion
	Sucrase	Sucrose to glucose and fructose
Pancreas		
700	Amylase	Starch to disaccharides
	Chymotrypsin	Protein digestion
	Lipase	Fat digestion
	Trypsinogen	Protein digestion
Liver and Gallbladder		
1000	Bile	Emulsification of fats and aid in absorption of fatty acids and fat-soluble vitamins (A, D, E, K)

The process of digestion begins in the mouth, where food is chewed, mechanically broken down, and mixed with saliva. Saliva helps us swallow by lubricating food. Saliva contains amylase, which breaks down starches to maltose. Chewing and the sight, smell, thought, and taste of food stimulate the release of saliva. A person makes about 1 L of saliva each day. After swallowing, food moves through the esophagus to the stomach. No digestion or absorption occurs in the esophagus.

Both GI secretion and motility are under neural and hormonal control. Food entering the stomach and small intestine triggers the release of hormones into the bloodstream (Tables 38.2 and 38.3). These hormones play important roles in the control of HCl acid secretion, production and release of digestive enzymes, and motility.

In the stomach, muscle action mixes the food with gastric secretions to form *chyme,* which is now ready for absorption. Protein digestion begins with the release of pepsinogen from chief cells. The stomach's acidic environment results in the conversion of pepsinogen to its active form, pepsin. Pepsin begins the breakdown of proteins. There is minimal digestion of starches and fats. The stomach also serves as a reservoir for food, releasing it slowly into the small intestine. The length of time that food stays in the stomach depends on the composition of the food. The average meal stays in the stomach for 3 to 4 hours.

In the small intestine, the physical presence and chemical nature of chyme stimulates motility and secretion. Secretions involved in digestion include enzymes from the pancreas, bile from the liver, and enzymes from the small intestine (Table 38.1). Carbohydrates are broken down to monosaccharides, fats to glycerol and fatty acids, and proteins to amino acids. Enzymes on the brush border of the microvilli complete the digestion process. These enzymes break down disaccharides to monosaccharides and peptides to amino acids for absorption.

The absorption of most of the end products of digestion occurs in the small intestine. The movement of the villi enables these end products to come in contact with the absorbing membrane. Monosaccharides, fatty acids, amino acids, water, electrolytes, vitamins, and minerals are absorbed.

Elimination

Large Intestine. The large intestine is a hollow, muscular tube around 5 to 6 ft (1.5 to 1.8 m) long and 2 in (5 cm) in diameter. The 4 parts of the large intestine are shown in Fig. 38.2.

The most important functions of the large intestine are water and electrolyte absorption. The large intestine also forms feces and serves as a reservoir for the fecal mass until defecation occurs. Feces are composed of water (75%), bacteria, unabsorbed minerals, undigested foodstuffs, bile pigments, and desquamated (shed) epithelial cells. The large intestine secretes mucus, which acts as a lubricant and protects the mucosa.

Microorganisms in the colon contribute to digestion by (1) producing vitamin K and some B vitamins and (2) breaking down proteins that are not digested or absorbed in the small intestine into amino acids. Bacteria deaminate the amino acids, resulting in ammonia. Ammonia is carried to the liver, where it is converted to urea. Urea is excreted by the kidneys. Bacteria produce gas that escapes the colon through the anus, a phenomenon called *flatulence* or *flatus.* If an infection or antibiotics alter the normal microbiome, an overgrowth of pathogenic bacteria can occur and cause disease.

The movements of the large intestine are usually slow. However, propulsive (mass movements) peristalsis does occur. Food entering the stomach and duodenum triggers gastrocolic and duodenocolic reflexes, resulting in peristalsis in the colon. These reflexes are more active after the first daily meal and often result in bowel evacuation.

Defecation is a reflex action involving voluntary and involuntary control. Feces in the rectum stimulate sensory nerve endings that produce the desire to defecate. The reflex center for defecation is in the parasympathetic nerve fibers in the sacral part of the spinal cord. These fibers produce contraction of the rectum and relaxation of the internal anal sphincter. When a

TABLE 38.2 Phases of Gastric Secretion

Stimulus to Secretion	Secretion
Cephalic (nervous)	
Sight, smell, taste of food (before food enters stomach). Initiated in the CNS and mediated by the vagus nerve.	HCl acid, pepsinogen, mucus
Gastric (hormonal and nervous)	
Food in antrum of stomach, vagal stimulation.	Release of gastrin from antrum into circulation to stimulate gastric secretions and motility
Intestinal (hormonal)	
Presence of chyme in small intestine.	*Acidic chyme* (pH <2): Release of secretin, gastric inhibitory polypeptide, cholecystokinin into circulation to decrease HCl acid secretion
	Chyme (pH >3): Release of gastrin from duodenum to increase acid secretion

TABLE 38.3 Hormones Controlling GI Secretion and Motility

Hormone	Source	Activating Stimuli	Function
Gastrin	Gastric and duodenal mucosa	Stomach distention, partially digested proteins in pylorus	Stimulates gastric acid secretion and motility. Maintains lower esophageal sphincter tone.
Cholecystokinin	Duodenal mucosa	Fatty acids and amino acids in small intestine	Contracts gallbladder and relaxes sphincter of Oddi. Allows increased flow of bile into duodenum. Release of pancreatic digestive enzymes.
Gastric inhibitory peptide	Duodenal mucosa	Fatty acids and lipids in small intestine	Inhibits gastric acid secretion and motility.
Secretin	Duodenal mucosa	Acid entering small intestine	Inhibits gastric motility and acid secretion. Stimulates pancreatic bicarbonate secretion.

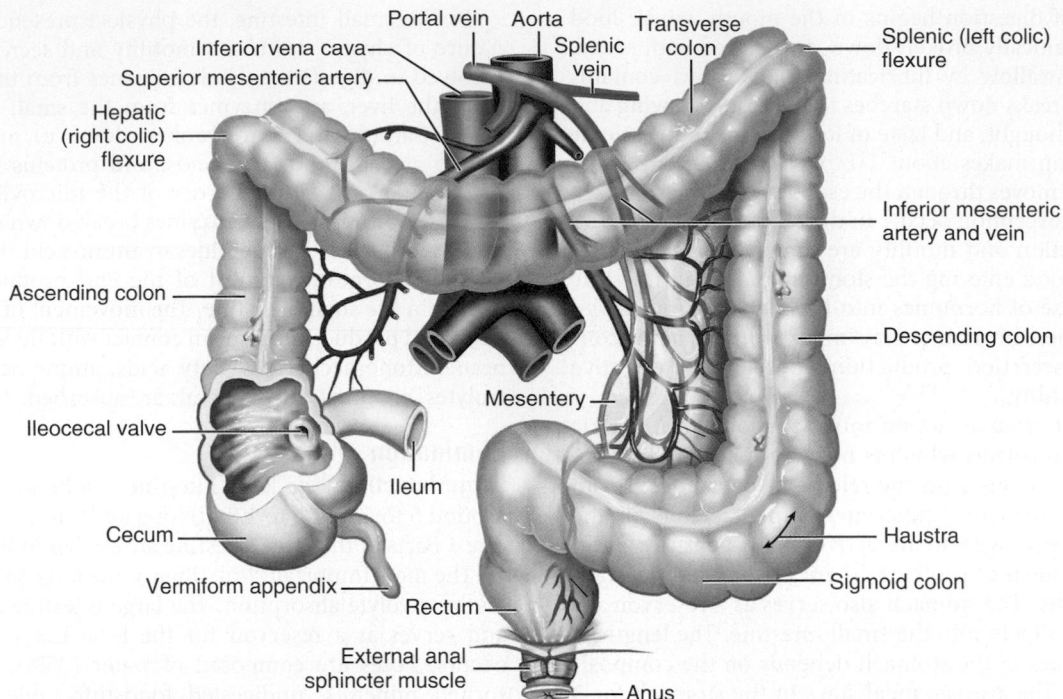

FIG. 38.2 Anatomic locations of the large intestine. (From Patton KT, Thibodeau GA: *Anatomy and physiology,* ed 8, St Louis, 2013, Mosby.)

person feels the desire to defecate, they can voluntarily relax the external anal sphincter. An acceptable environment for defecation is usually needed or the urge to defecate will be ignored. If defecation is suppressed for long periods, problems can occur, such as constipation or fecal impaction.

The Valsalva maneuver, often referred to as "bearing down," can promote defecation. During this maneuver, the person inspires deeply and holds the breath, closing the airway, while contracting abdominal muscles and bearing down. This increases both intraabdominal and intrathoracic pressures and reduces venous return to the heart. The heart rate temporarily decreases along with a decrease in cardiac output. This results in a transient drop in BP. When the patient relaxes, thoracic pressure falls, resulting in a sudden flow of blood into the heart, increased heart rate, and an immediate rise in BP. The Valsalva maneuver may be contraindicated in the patient with a head injury, eye surgery, heart problems, hemorrhoids, abdominal surgery, or liver cirrhosis with portal hypertension.

Liver, Biliary Tract, and Pancreas

Liver. The liver is the largest internal organ in the body, weighing around 3 lb (1.36 kg). It lies in the right epigastric region (Fig. 38.5 later in the chapter). Most of the liver is enclosed in peritoneum. It has a fibrous capsule that divides it into right and left lobes (Fig. 38.3).

The functional units of the liver are lobules. A lobule consists of rows of hepatic cells *(hepatocytes)* arranged in cords that radiate out from a central vein. Capillaries called *sinusoids* lie between the rows of hepatocytes. Sinusoids are lined with Kupffer cells, which carry out phagocytic activity, removing bacteria and toxins from the blood. The hepatic cells secrete bile into tiny canals called *canaliculi*. These merge with other canals to form larger, interlobular bile ducts, which unite into the 2 main left and right hepatic ducts.

The liver has a rich blood supply. The portal circulatory system brings blood to the liver from the stomach, intestines, spleen, and pancreas. About 25% of the blood supply comes from the hepatic artery, a branch of the celiac artery. The other 75% comes from the portal vein. The portal vein carries absorbed products of digestion directly to the liver. Once in the liver, the portal vein branches and comes in contact with each lobule.

The liver performs many functions and is essential for life. It has metabolic, secretory, vascular, and storage functions (Table 38.4). The hepatic cells constantly make bile. Bile consists of water, cholesterol, bile salts, electrolytes, fatty acids, and bilirubin. It provides the alkaline medium needed for the action of pancreatic lipase. Bile salts are needed for fat emulsification and digestion.

Bilirubin Metabolism. The liver constantly makes bilirubin, a pigment derived from the breakdown of hemoglobin (Fig. 38.4). When released into the bloodstream, it binds to albumin. This form of bilirubin is called *unconjugated*. It is insoluble in water and transported to the liver. In the liver, unconjugated bilirubin is conjugated with glucuronic acid and excreted in bile into the intestine. *Conjugated* bilirubin is soluble in water. In the intestines, bacterial action reduces bilirubin to stercobilinogen and urobilinogen. Stercobilinogen accounts for the brown color of stool. A small amount of urobilinogen is reabsorbed into the blood, where it is returned to the liver through the portal circulation. There, it is excreted again in the bile or entered into circulation and excreted by the kidneys.

Biliary Tract. The biliary tract consists of the gallbladder and ducts that connect the liver, gallbladder, and duodenum. The gallbladder is a pear-shaped sac found below the liver. The gallbladder's function is to concentrate and store bile. It holds around 45 mL of bile. The presence of fat in the upper duodenum triggers the release of cholecystokinin, which causes the gallbladder to contract and release bile.

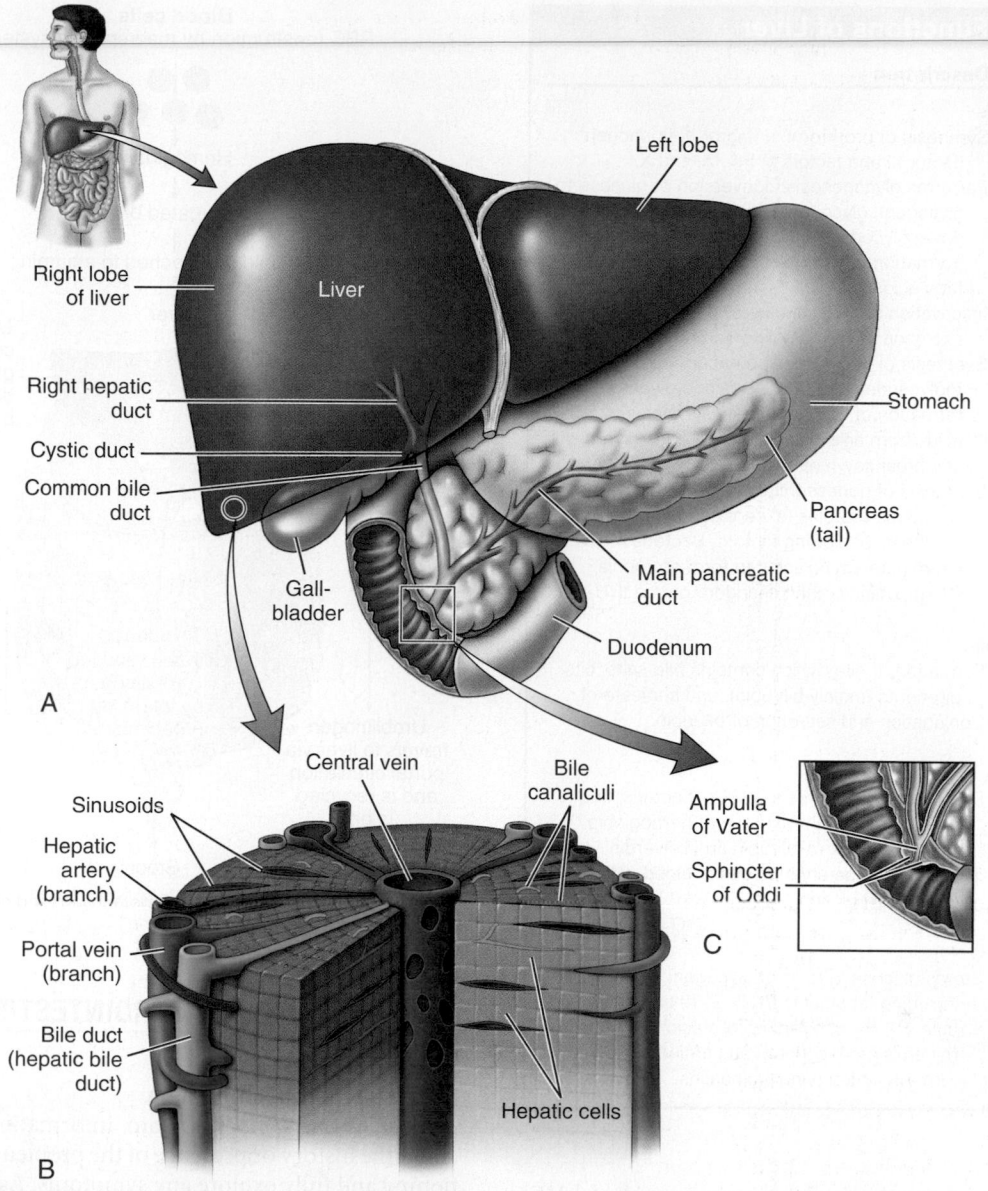

Central vein

Sinusoids

Hepatic artery (branch)

Portal vein (branch)

Bile duct (hepatic bile duct)

Bile canaliculi

Ampulla of Vater

Sphincter of Oddi

Hepatic cells

Left lobe

Right lobe of liver

Liver

Right hepatic duct

Cystic duct

Common bile duct

Gall-bladder

Stomach

Pancreas (tail)

Main pancreatic duct

Duodenum

A

B

C

FIG. 38.3 A, Gross structure of the liver, gallbladder, pancreas, and duct system. B, Liver lobule. C, Entrance of the common bile duct into the duodenum.

The hepatic ducts receive bile from the canaliculi in the liver lobules. The left and right hepatic ducts merge with the cystic duct from the gallbladder to form the common bile duct. Bile moves down the common bile duct to enter the duodenum at the ampulla of Vater (Fig. 38.3). The pancreatic duct also enters the duodenum at this point.

Pancreas. The pancreas is a long, slender gland lying behind the stomach and in front of the first and second lumbar vertebrae. It consists of a head, body, and tail. The peritoneum covers the anterior surface of the pancreas. The pancreas has lobes and lobules. The pancreatic duct extends along the gland and enters the duodenum through the common bile duct at the ampulla of Vater (Fig. 38.3).

The pancreas has both exocrine and endocrine functions. The exocrine function contributes to digestion through the production and release of enzymes (Table 38.1). The endocrine function occurs in the islets of Langerhans, whose β cells secrete insulin and amylin; α cells secrete glucagon; δ cells secrete somatostatin; and F cells secrete pancreatic polypeptide.

Gerontologic Considerations: Effects of Aging on Gastrointestinal System

The process of aging changes the functional ability of the GI system. Diet, alcohol intake, and obesity affect organs of the GI system, making it a challenge to separate the sole effects of aging from lifestyle. Many factors can lead to a decrease in appetite and make eating less pleasurable. Caries and periodontal disease can lead to loss of teeth. Taste buds decline in number and the sense of smell lessens, leading to decreased ability to taste. With less saliva, a very dry mouth (xerostomia) is common.[1]

Age-related changes in the esophagus include delayed emptying, resulting from smooth muscle weakness; reduced UES opening; and an incompetent LES. Although GI motility decreases with age, secretion and absorption are less affected.

TABLE 38.4 Functions of Liver

Function	Description
Metabolic Functions	
Blood clotting	Synthesis of prothrombin (factor I), fibrinogen (factor II) and factors V, VII, IX, and X.
Carbohydrate metabolism	Performs glycogenesis (conversion of glucose to glycogen), glycogenolysis (process of breaking down glycogen to glucose), gluconeogenesis (formation of glucose from amino acids and fatty acids).
Detoxification	Inactivation of drugs and harmful substances and excretion of their breakdown products.
Fat metabolism	Synthesis of lipoproteins, breakdown of triglycerides into fatty acids and glycerol, formation of ketone bodies, synthesis of fatty acids from amino acids and glucose, synthesis and breakdown of cholesterol.
Protein metabolism	Synthesis of nonessential amino acids, synthesis of plasma proteins (except gamma globulin), synthesis of clotting factors. Bacteria in colon deaminate amino acids to form ammonia (NH_3). which is then changed to urea (NH_4).
Secretory Functions	
Bile production	Formation of bile, which contains bile salts, bile pigments (mainly bilirubin), and cholesterol.
Bilirubin	Conjugation and secretion of bilirubin.
Vascular Functions	
Blood filtration	Breakdown of old RBCs, WBCs, bacteria, and other particles. Breakdown of hemoglobin from old RBCs to bilirubin and biliverdin.
Blood reservoir	Serves as temporary storage for blood within general circulation.
Storage Functions	
Storage	Stores glucose in form of glycogen; vitamins, including fat-soluble (A, D, E, K) and water-soluble (B_1, B_2, cobalamin, folic acid); fatty acids; minerals (iron, copper); and amino acids in form of albumin and β-globulins.

The older adult often has a decrease in intrinsic acid and HCl acid secretion *(hypochlorhydria).*[1]

Constipation affects 30% to 40% of adults over age 60.[2] Factors that may increase the risk for constipation include slower peristalsis, anorectal dysfunction, inactivity, decreased dietary fiber, inadequate fluid intake, and constipating medications. Neurologic, cognitive, and metabolic problems may play a role. See Chapter 42 for a detailed discussion of constipation.

The liver size decreases after 50 years of age but results of liver function tests stay within normal ranges. Age-related enzyme changes in the liver decrease the liver's ability to metabolize drugs and hormones.[1]

The size of the pancreas is unaffected by aging. It does undergo structural changes, such as fibrosis, fatty acid deposits, and atrophy. Gallbladder diseases increase with age.[3]

Older adults, especially those over 85, are at risk for decreased food intake. The inability to obtain food affects nutritional intake. Economic constraints may reduce the number of fresh fruits and vegetables consumed and thus the amount of fiber. Immobility limits the ability to prepare meals. Age-related changes in the GI system and differences in assessment findings are outlined in Table 38.5.

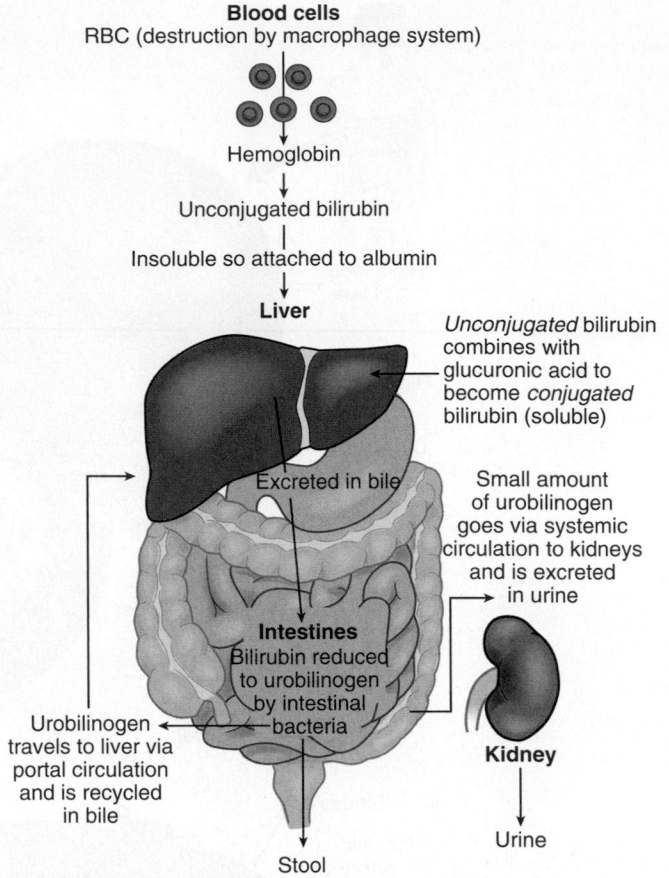

FIG. 38.4 Bilirubin metabolism and conjugation.

ASSESSMENT OF GASTROINTESTINAL SYSTEM

Subjective Data

Important Health Information

Past Health History. Obtain information from the patient about the history or presence of the problems related to GI functioning and fully explore any symptoms. Ask about any abdominal pain, nausea, vomiting, abdominal distention, jaundice, heartburn, dyspepsia, changes in appetite, hematemesis, indigestion, bloating, and trouble swallowing. Review the patient's bowel habits. Ask about diarrhea, constipation, melena, rectal bleeding and excessive gas, Document related conditions, such as food intolerance or allergies, lactose intolerance, and anemia. Ask the patient about a history or presence of diseases such as reflux, gastritis, hepatitis, colitis, gallstones, hemorrhoids, peptic ulcer, cancer, diverticuli, or hernias.

Ask the patient about weight history. Explore in detail any unexplained or unplanned weight loss or gain within the past 6 to 12 months. Discuss any history of chronic dieting and repeated weight loss and gain.

Medications. Assess the patient's past and current use of medications. Ask about the reason for taking the medication, its name, the dose and frequency, length of time taken, its effect, and any side effects. It is critical to include information about over-the-counter (OTC) medications, prescription drugs, herbal products, vitamins, probiotics, and nutritional supplements. Many medications cause side effects in the GI system. GI problems can affect drug absorption and effectiveness.

TABLE 38.5 Gerontologic Assessment Differences

Gastrointestinal System

Expected Aging Changes	Differences in Assessment Findings
Mouth	
Atrophy of gingival tissue	Poor-fitting dentures
Decreased taste buds, decreased sense of smell	Decreased sense of taste (especially salty and sweet)
Decreased volume of saliva	Dry oral mucosa
Gingival retraction	Loss of teeth, dental implants, dentures, difficulty chewing
Esophagus	
Lower esophageal sphincter pressure decreased, motility decreased	Epigastric distress, dysphagia, potential for hiatal hernia and aspiration
Abdominal Wall	
Decreased number and sensitivity of sensory receptors	Less sensitivity to surface pain
Thinner and less taut	More visible peristalsis, easier palpation of organs
Stomach	
Atrophy of gastric mucosa, decreased blood flow	Food intolerances, signs of anemia as result of cobalamin malabsorption, slower gastric emptying
Small Intestines	
Slightly decreased motility and secretion of most digestive enzymes	Indigestion, slowed intestinal transit, delayed absorption of fat-soluble vitamins
Liver	
Decreased protein synthesis, ability to regenerate decreased	Decreased drug and hormone metabolism
Decreased size and lowered position	Easier palpation because of lower border extending past costal margin
Large Intestine, Anus, Rectum	
Decreased anal sphincter tone and nerve supply to rectal area	Fecal incontinence
Decreased muscular tone, decreased motility	Flatulence, abdominal distention, relaxed perineal musculature
Increased transit time, decreased sensation to defecation	Constipation, fecal impaction
Pancreas	
Pancreatic ducts distended, lipase production decreased, pancreatic reserve impaired	Impaired fat absorption, decreased glucose tolerance

CASE STUDY

Patient Introduction

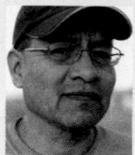

(© iStockphoto/Thinkstock.)

Patient Profile

L.C. is a 58-yr-old Native American man from a Pueblo tribe in northern New Mexico. L.C.'s wife and family drove 50 miles to take him to the Indian Health Service hospital. He comes into the emergency department (ED) doubled over with abdominal pain. He is grimacing and holding his abdomen with both arms. You are working as the triage nurse that morning.

Discussion Questions

1. What are the possible causes for L.C.'s acute abdominal pain?
2. Is his condition stable or is it an emergency?
3. What type of assessment should you do: comprehensive, focused, or emergency?
4. What assessment questions will you ask him?
5. How will you individualize the assessment based on his ethnic/cultural background?

You will learn more about L.C. and his condition as you read through this assessment chapter.

(See p. 838 for more information on L.C.)

Answers available at *http://evolve.elsevier.com/Lewis/medsurg.*

TABLE 38.6 Gastrointestinal Surgeries

Procedure	Description
Appendectomy	Removal of appendix
Cholecystectomy	Removal of gallbladder
Choledochojejunostomy	Opening between common bile duct and jejunum
Choledocholithotomy	Opening into common bile duct for removal of stones
Colectomy	Removal of colon
Colostomy	Opening into colon
Esophagoenterostomy	Removal of part of esophagus with segment of colon attached to remaining part
Esophagogastrostomy	Removal of esophagus and anastomosis of remaining part to stomach
Gastrectomy	Removal of stomach
Gastrostomy	Opening into stomach
Glossectomy	Removal of tongue
Hemiglossectomy	Removal of half of tongue
Herniorrhaphy	Repair of a hernia
Ileostomy	Opening into ileum
Mandibulectomy	Removal of mandible
Pyloroplasty	Enlargement and repair of pyloric sphincter area
Vagotomy	Resection of branch of vagus nerve

Many chemicals and drugs are potentially hepatotoxic (see *livertox.nih.gov*) and result in significant harm unless monitored closely. For example, chronic high doses of acetaminophen and nonsteroidal antiinflammatory drugs (NSAIDs) may be hepatotoxic. NSAIDs may predispose a patient to upper GI bleeding, with an increasing risk as the person ages. Other medications, such as antibiotics, may change the normal bacterial composition in the GI tract, resulting in diarrhea. Antacids and laxatives may affect medication absorption. Ask the patient about laxative or antacid use, including the kind and frequency.

Surgery or Other Treatments. Obtain information about hospitalizations for any problems related to the GI system. Record any abdominal or rectal surgery, including the year, reason for surgery, postoperative course, and blood transfusions. Terms related to common GI surgeries are listed in Table 38.6.

TABLE 38.7   Health History

Gastrointestinal System

Health Perception–Health Management
- Describe any measures used to treat GI symptoms such as diarrhea or constipation.
- Do you smoke?* Do you drink alcohol?*
- Are you exposed to any chemicals on a regular basis?* Have you been exposed in the past?*
- Have you recently traveled outside the United States?*

Nutritional-Metabolic
- Describe your usual daily food and fluid intake.
- Do you take any supplemental vitamins or minerals?*
- Have you had any changes in appetite or food tolerance?*
- Has there been any weight change in the past 6 to 12 months?*
- Are you allergic to any foods?*

Elimination
- Describe the frequency and time of day you have bowel movements. What is the consistency of the bowel movement?
- Do you use laxatives or enemas?* If so, how often?
- Have there been any recent changes in your bowel pattern?*
- Do you have any pain with bowel movements or pain relieved by bowel movements?
- Describe any skin problems caused by GI problems.
- Do you need any assistive equipment, such as ostomy equipment, raised toilet seat, commode?

Activity-Exercise
- Do you have limitations in mobility that make it hard for you to obtain and prepare food?*

Sleep-Rest
- Do you have any problem sleeping because of a GI problem?*
- Are you awakened by symptoms such as gas, abdominal pain, diarrhea, or heartburn?*

Cognitive-Perceptual
- Have you had any change in taste or smell that has affected your appetite?*
- Do you have any heat or cold sensitivity that affects eating?*
- Does pain interfere with food preparation, appetite, or chewing?*
- Do pain medications cause constipation, diarrhea, or appetite suppression?*

Self-Perception–Self-Concept
- Describe any changes in your weight that have affected how you feel about yourself.
- Have you had any changes in normal elimination that have affected how you feel about yourself?*
- Have any symptoms of GI disease caused physical changes that are a problem for you?*

Role-Relationship
- Describe the impact of any GI problem on your usual roles and relationships.
- Have any changes in elimination affected your relationships?*
- Do you live alone? Describe how your family or others assist you with your GI problems.

Sexuality-Reproductive
- Describe the effect of your GI problem on your sexual activity.

Coping–Stress Tolerance
- Do you have GI symptoms in response to stressful or emotional situations?*
- Describe how you deal with any GI symptoms that result.

Value-Belief
- Describe any culturally specific health beliefs about food and food preparation that may influence the treatment of your GI problem.

*If yes, describe.

Functional Health Patterns. Key questions to ask a patient with a GI problem are outlined in Table 38.7.

Health Perception–Health Management Pattern. Ask about the patient's health practices related to the GI system, such as maintaining normal body weight, proper dental care, adequate nutrition, and effective elimination habits.

Ask about recent foreign travel with possible exposure to hepatitis or parasitic infestation. Explore any sexual and drug use behaviors that may increase risk for hepatitis exposure. Determine whether the patient has received hepatitis A and B vaccination.

Assess the patient for habits that directly affect GI functioning. The intake of alcohol in large quantities or for long periods has detrimental effects on the stomach mucosa. Chronic alcohol exposure causes fatty infiltration of the liver and can cause damage, leading to cirrhosis and hepatocellular cancer. Obtain a history of cigarette smoking. Nicotine is irritating to the GI tract mucosa. Cigarette smoking is related to GI cancers (especially mouth and esophageal cancers), esophagitis, and ulcers. Smoking delays the healing of ulcers.

Family history is an important part of this health pattern. About one third of cases of colorectal cancer occur in patients with a family history. Because of the relationship between colorectal and breast cancer, ask about a history of either type of cancer in the family.

🧬 GENETIC RISK ALERT

Colorectal Cancer
- Colorectal cancer may run in families if first-degree relatives (parents, siblings) or many other family members (grandparents, aunts, uncles) had colorectal cancer. This is especially true when family members are diagnosed with colorectal cancer before age 50
- Genetic conditions associated with an increased risk for colorectal cancer include:
- Hereditary nonpolyposis colorectal cancer (HNPCC). It is caused by mutations in several different genes.
- Familial adenomatous polyposis (FAP). FAP is characterized by multiple polyps that are noncancerous at first but eventually develop into cancer if not treated. Most cases of FAP are due to mutations of the adenomatous polyposis coli (APC) gene.

Inflammatory Bowel Disease (IBD)
- People with IBD have a genetic predisposition or susceptibility to the disease.
- First-degree relatives have a 5- to 20-fold increased risk for developing IBD.

Nutritional-Metabolic Pattern. A thorough nutritional assessment is essential. Take a diet history and ask about both content and amount or portion size. Food preferences and preparation may vary by culture. Open-ended questions allow the patient to express beliefs and feelings about the diet. For example, you can say, "Please tell me about your food and beverage intake over the past 24 hours." A 24-hour dietary recall can be used to analyze the adequacy of the diet. Help the patient recall the preceding day's food intake, including early morning and nighttime intake, snacks, liquids, and vitamin supplements. You can then evaluate the diet in relation to recommended servings for dietary intake using a guide such as MyPlate (*www.choosemyplate.gov*). A 1-week recall may provide more information on usual dietary patterns. Compare weekday and weekend dietary intake patterns in relation to both the quality and quantity of food.

Ask the patient about the use of sugar and salt substitutes, caffeine intake, and amount of fluid and fiber intake. Note any changes in appetite, food tolerance, and weight. Anorexia and weight loss may indicate cancer or inflammation. Decreased food intake also can be the consequence of economic problems or depression.

Ask about food allergies and dietary intolerances, including lactose and gluten. Have the patient describe the allergic response and any GI symptoms.

Elimination Pattern. Elicit a detailed account of the patient's bowel elimination pattern. Note the frequency, time of day, and usual stool consistency. Ask about the presence of pain with bowel movements, if bowel movements relieve pain, and any recent changes in bowel patterns. Explore the use of laxatives and enemas, including type, frequency, and results.

Document the amount and type of fluid and fiber intake. These influence the frequency and consistency of stools. Inadequate fiber intake can be associated with constipation. Look for any association between a skin and GI problem. Food allergies can cause skin lesions, pruritus, and edema. Diarrhea can result in redness, irritation, and pain in the perianal area. External drainage systems, such as an ileostomy or ileal conduit, may cause local skin irritation.

Activity-Exercise Pattern. Activity and exercise affect GI motility. Immobility is a risk factor for constipation. Assess ambulatory status to determine if the patient can secure and prepare food. If the patient is unable to do these tasks, see if a family member or an outside agency is meeting this need. Note any limitation in the ability to feed oneself. Assess for access to a toilet. Identify the use of and access to supplies such as a commode or ostomy supplies.

Sleep-Rest Pattern. GI symptoms can interfere with the quality of sleep. Nausea, vomiting, diarrhea, indigestion, and bloating can produce sleep problems. Ask the patient if GI symptoms affect sleep or rest. For example, a patient with gastroesophageal reflux disease (GERD) may wake with burning epigastric pain.

A patient may have a bedtime ritual that involves a specific food or beverage. Herbal teas may be sleep inducing. Document individual routines and comply with these whenever possible to avoid sleeplessness. Hunger can prevent sleep, and a light, easily digested snack may be helpful.

Cognitive-Perceptual Pattern. Sensory changes can result in problems related to acquiring, preparing, and ingesting food. Changes in taste or smell can affect appetite and eating pleasure. Vertigo can make shopping or standing at a stove difficult and dangerous. Heat or cold sensitivity can make certain foods painful to eat. Problems in expressive communication limit the patient's ability to state personal dietary preferences.

Both acute and chronic pain influence dietary intake. Behaviors associated with pain include avoiding activity, fatigue, and disrupted eating patterns. For patients receiving opioid medications, assess for decreased appetite, constipation, nausea, and sedation.

Self-Perception–Self-Concept Pattern. Many GI and nutritional problems affect the patient's self-perception. Overweight and underweight persons may have problems related to self-esteem and body image. Repeated attempts to achieve a personally acceptable weight can be discouraging and depressing for some people. The way a person recounts a weight history can alert you to potential problems in this area.

The need for external devices to manage elimination, such as a colostomy or an ileostomy, may be challenging for some patients. The patient's willingness to engage in self-care and to discuss this situation provides you with valuable information related to body image and self-esteem.

The altered physical changes often associated with advanced liver disease can be disturbing for the patient. Jaundice and ascites cause significant changes in external appearance. Assess the patient's attitude about these changes.

Role-Relationship Pattern. Problems related to the GI system, such as cirrhosis, hepatitis, ostomies, obesity, and cancer, may affect the patient's ability to maintain usual roles and relationships. A person may need to leave a job or reduce work hours. Changes in body image and self-esteem can affect relationships.

Sexuality-Reproductive Pattern. Changes related to sexuality and reproductive status can result from problems of the GI system. For example, obesity, jaundice, and ascites could decrease the acceptance of a potential sexual partner. An ostomy can affect the patient's confidence related to sexual activity. Your sensitive questioning can identify potential problems.

Anorexia can affect the reproductive status of a female patient. Obesity leads to reduced fertility and increased miscarriage rates in women.

Coping–Stress Tolerance Pattern. Determine what is stressful for the patient and what coping mechanisms the patient uses. Factors outside the GI tract can influence its functioning. Both psychologic and emotional factors, such as stress and anxiety, influence GI functioning in many people. Stress can manifest as anorexia, nausea, epigastric and abdominal pain, or diarrhea. It can worsen some diseases of the GI system, such as peptic ulcer disease, irritable bowel syndrome, and IBD. However, never attribute GI symptoms solely to psychologic factors.

Value-Belief Pattern. Assess the patient's spiritual and cultural beliefs about food and food preparation. Whenever possible, respect these preferences. Determine if any value or belief could interfere with planned interventions. For example, if the patient with anemia is a vegetarian, you will need to consider how to increase dietary intake of iron-rich foods other than meat. Thoughtful assessment and consideration of the patient's beliefs and values usually increase adherence and satisfaction.

Objective Data
Physical Examination
Mouth

Inspection. Inspect the mouth for symmetry, color, and size. Observe for abnormalities such as pallor or cyanosis, cracking, ulcers, or fissures. The dorsum (top) of the tongue should have a thin white coating. The undersurface should be smooth. Observe for any lesions. Using a tongue blade, inspect the buccal mucosa and note the color, any areas of pigmentation, and any lesions. Dark-skinned persons normally have patchy areas of pigmentation. In assessing the teeth and gums, look for caries; loose teeth; abnormal shape and position of teeth;

CASE STUDY
Subjective Data

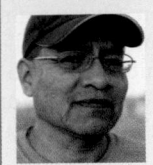

(© iStockphoto/ Thinkstock.)

A focused subjective assessment of L.C. revealed the following information:

- **Past Medical History:** Negative history for medical or surgical problems.
- **Medications:** None.
- **Health Perception–Health Management:** L.C. states he has not been feeling well for the past several weeks. He feels weak and is easily fatigued. Denies exposure to chemicals. No recent travel outside of the United States. Smokes 1 pack of cigarettes per day for 20 yrs. Drinks 3 to 4 bottles of beer per day.
- **Nutritional-Metabolic:** L.C. is 5 ft, 9 in tall and weighs 140 lb (BMI: 20.7 kg/m²). States has been losing weight over the past several months and does not have an appetite. No food allergies.
- **Elimination:** States has had alternating episodes of constipation and diarrhea. He noticed some bright red blood in stools. Has not had a bowel movement for 4 days.
- **Cognitive-Perceptual:** Rates pain as a 9 on a scale of 0 to 10. States pain comes and goes in waves. Prefers to lie still with knees flexed and drawn into his abdomen.

Discussion Questions

1. Which subjective assessment findings are of most concern to you?
2. Based on these subjective assessment findings, what should be included in the physical assessment? What would you be looking for?
3. What would be your priority assessment?

You will learn more about physical examination of the gastrointestinal system in the next section.
(See p. 840 for more information on L.C.)

Answers available at *http://evolve.elsevier.com/Lewis/medsurg.*

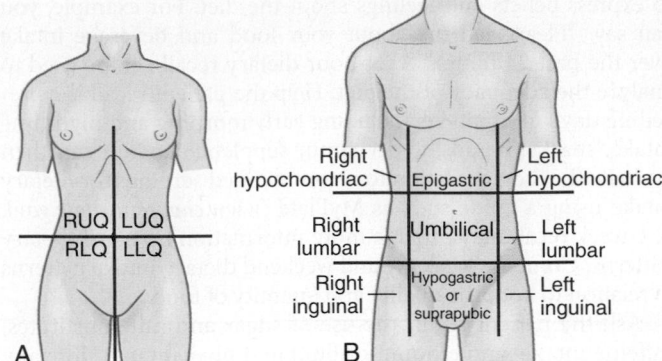

FIG. 38.5 **A**, Abdominal quadrants. **B**, Abdominal regions. *LLQ*, Left lower quadrant; *LUQ*, left upper quadrant; *RLQ*, right lower quadrant; *RUQ*, right upper quadrant.

and swelling, bleeding, discoloration, or gingival inflammation. Note any distinctive breath odor.

Inspect the pharynx by tilting the patient's head back and depressing the tongue with a tongue blade. Observe the tonsils, uvula, soft palate, and anterior and posterior pillars. Tell the patient to say "ah." The uvula and soft palate should rise and remain in the midline.

Palpation. Palpate any suspicious areas in the mouth. Note ulcers, nodules, indurations, and areas of tenderness. The mouth of the older adult needs careful assessment. Pay attention to dentures (e.g., fit, condition), the ability to swallow, and the tongue, and note any lesions. Ask the patient with dentures to remove them during an oral examination to allow for good visualization and palpation of the area.

Abdomen. We use 2 systems to anatomically describe the surface of the abdomen. One system divides the abdomen into 4 quadrants by a perpendicular line from the sternum to the pubic bone and a horizontal line across the abdomen at the umbilicus (Fig. 38.5, *A*, and Table 38.8). The other system divides the abdomen into 9 regions (Fig. 38.5, *B*). Only the epigastric, umbilical, and suprapubic or hypogastric regions are commonly assessed.

For the abdominal examination, good lighting should shine across the abdomen. The patient should be in the supine position and as relaxed as possible. To help relax the abdominal muscles, have the patient slightly flex the knees and raise the head of the bed slightly. The patient should have an empty bladder. Use warm hands when doing the abdominal examination to avoid eliciting muscle guarding. Ask the patient to breathe slowly through the mouth.

The standard approach for examining the abdomen is appropriate for an older adult. The abdomen may be thinner and laxer unless the patient is obese.

Inspection. Assess the abdomen for skin changes (color, texture, scars, striae, dilated veins, rashes, lesions), umbilicus (location and contour), symmetry, contour (flat, rounded [convex], concave, protuberant, distended), observable hernias or masses, and movement (pulsations, peristalsis). A normal aortic pulsation may be seen in the epigastric area. Look across the abdomen tangentially (across the abdomen in a line) for peristalsis. Peristalsis is not normally visible in an adult but may be visible in a thin person.

Auscultation. When you examine the abdomen, auscultate before percussion and palpation because these latter procedures may alter the bowel sounds. Use the diaphragm of the stethoscope to auscultate bowel sounds because they are relatively high pitched. Use the bell of the stethoscope to detect lower pitched sounds. Warm the stethoscope in your hands before auscultating to help prevent abdominal muscle contraction. Listen in the epigastrium and in all 4 quadrants. Start in the right lower quadrant because bowel sounds are normally present there. Listen for bowel sounds for at least 2 minutes. Do not count bowel sounds. Determine if they are normal, hypoactive, or hyperactive.

The frequency and intensity of bowel sounds vary depending on the phase of digestion. Normal sounds are relatively high pitched and gurgling. Stomach growling or loud gurgles *(borborygmi)* indicate hyperperistalsis. The bowel sounds are high pitched (rushes and tinkling) when the intestines are under tension, as in intestinal obstruction. Listen for decreased or absent bowel sounds. A perfectly "silent abdomen" is uncommon.[4] If you are patient and listen for several minutes, you will often find the bowel sounds are not absent but are hypoactive. If you do not hear bowel sounds, note the amount of time you listened in each quadrant without hearing bowel sounds.

Listen for vascular sounds. A *bruit*, best heard with the bell of the stethoscope, is a swishing or buzzing sound and indicates turbulent blood flow. Normally you should not hear aortic bruits.

Percussion. The purpose of percussing the abdomen is to estimate the size of the liver and determine the presence of fluid, distention, and masses. Sound waves vary according to the density of underlying tissues. Air produces a higher pitched, hollow sound termed *tympany*. Fluid or masses produce a

TABLE 38.8 Structures Located in Abdominal Regions

Right Upper Quadrant	Left Upper Quadrant	Right Lower Quadrant	Left Lower Quadrant
• Liver and gallbladder	• Left lobe of liver	• Lower pole of right kidney	• Lower pole of left kidney
• Pylorus	• Spleen	• Cecum and appendix	• Sigmoid flexure
• Duodenum	• Stomach	• Portion of ascending colon	• Part of descending colon
• Head of pancreas	• Body of pancreas	• Bladder (if distended)	• Bladder (if distended)
• Right adrenal gland	• Left adrenal gland	• Right ovary and fallopian tube	• Left ovary and fallopian tube
• Portion of right kidney	• Portion of left kidney	• Uterus (if enlarged)	• Uterus (if enlarged)
• Hepatic flexure of colon	• Splenic flexure of colon	• Right spermatic cord	• Left spermatic cord
• Portion of ascending and transverse colon	• Portion of transverse and descending colon	• Right ureter	• Left ureter

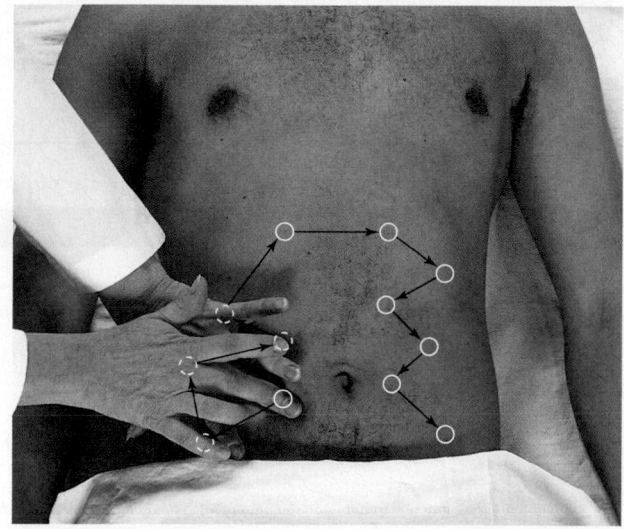

FIG. 38.6 Technique for percussion of the abdomen. Moving clockwise, percuss lightly in all 4 quadrants. (From Jarvis C: *Physical examination and health assessment,* ed 6, St Louis, 2012, Saunders.)

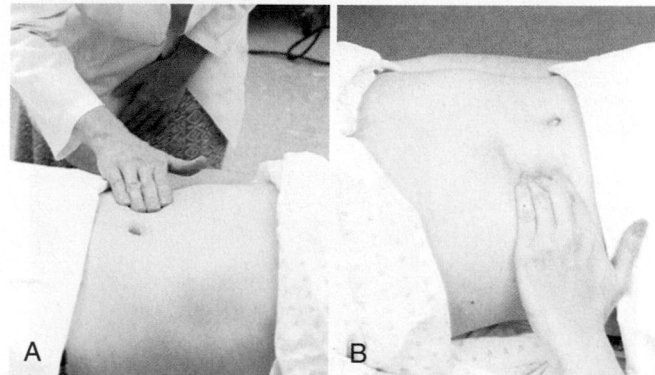

FIG. 38.7 A, Technique for light palpation of the abdomen. B, Technique for deep palpation.

short, high-pitched sound with little resonance termed *dullness.* Lightly percuss all 4 quadrants of the abdomen and assess the distribution of tympany and dullness (Fig. 38.6). Tympany is the predominant percussion sound of the abdomen.

To percuss the liver, start below the umbilicus in the right midclavicular line and percuss lightly upward until you hear dullness. This is the lower border of the liver. Next, start at the nipple line in the right midclavicular line and percuss downward between ribs to the area of dullness indicating the upper border of the liver. Measure the height or vertical space between the 2 borders to determine the size of the liver. The normal range of liver height in the right midclavicular line is 2.4 to 5 in (6 to 12.7 cm).

Palpation. Use palpation to assess the abdominal organs and detect any tenderness, distention, masses, or fluid. Palpation is important because it may reveal a tumor. Begin with light palpation. Palpate any areas in which the patient reports tenderness last.

Use *light palpation* to detect tenderness or cutaneous hypersensitivity, muscular resistance, masses, and swelling. Help the patient relax for deeper palpation. Keep your fingers together and press gently with the pads of the fingertips, depressing the abdominal wall about 0.4 in (1 cm). Use smooth movements and palpate all quadrants (Fig. 38.7, *A*).

Use *deep palpation* to delineate abdominal organs and masses (Fig. 38.7, *B*). Use the palmar surfaces of your fingers to press more deeply. Again, palpate all quadrants and note

the location, size, and shape of masses, as well as the presence of tenderness. During these maneuvers, observe the patient's facial expression because it will provide nonverbal cues of discomfort or pain.

An alternative method for deep abdominal palpation is the two-hand method. Place 1 hand on top of the other and apply pressure to the bottom hand with the fingers of the top hand. With the fingers of the bottom hand, feel for organs and masses. Practice both methods of palpation to determine which is most effective.

Check a problem area on the abdomen for rebound tenderness by pressing in slowly and firmly over the painful site. Withdraw the palpating fingers quickly. Pain on withdrawal of the fingers indicates peritoneal inflammation. Because assessing for rebound tenderness may produce pain and severe muscle spasm, it should be done at the end of the examination and only by an experienced practitioner.

To palpate the liver, place your left hand behind the patient to support the right eleventh and twelfth ribs (Fig. 38.8). The patient may relax on your hand. Press the left hand forward and place the right hand on the patient's right abdomen lateral to the rectus muscle. The fingertips should be below the lower border of liver dullness and pointed toward the right costal margin. Gently press in and up. The patient should take a deep breath with the abdomen so that the liver drops and is in a better position for palpation. Try to feel the liver edge as it comes down to the fingertips. During inspiration, the liver edge should feel firm, sharp, and smooth. Describe the surface and contour and any tenderness. If the patient has chronic obstructive pulmonary disease, large lungs, or a low diaphragm, the liver may be palpated 0.4 to 0.8 in (1 to 2 cm) below the right costal margin.

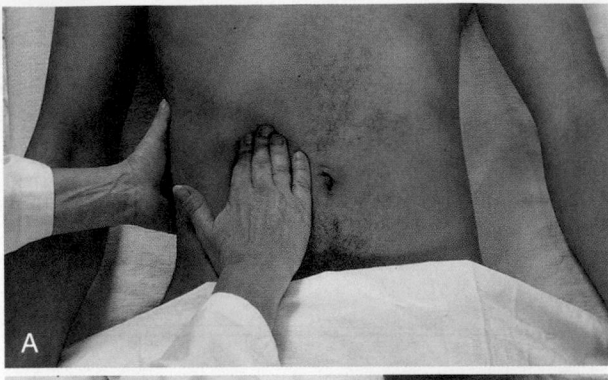

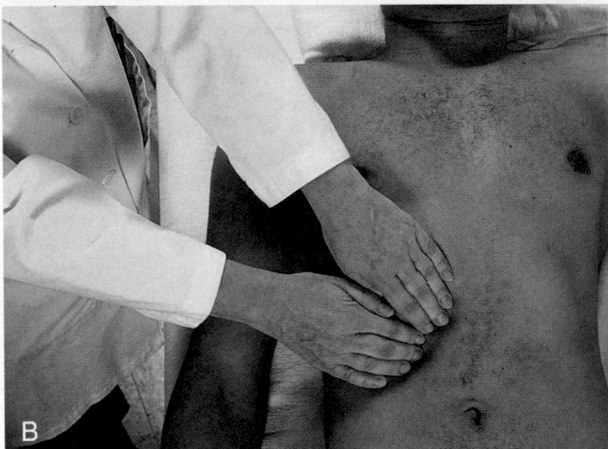

FIG. 38.8 A, Technique for liver palpation. B, Alternative technique to palpate liver with fingers hooked over the costal region. (From Jarvis C: *Physical examination and health assessment*, ed 6, St Louis, 2012, Saunders.)

To palpate the spleen, move to the patient's left side. Place your right hand under the patient, and support and press the patient's left lower rib cage forward. Place your left hand below the left costal margin and press it in toward the spleen. Ask the patient to breathe deeply. The fingertips can feel the tip or edge of an enlarged spleen. The spleen is normally not palpable. If it is palpable, do not continue because manual compression of an enlarged spleen may cause it to rupture.

Rectum and Anus. Inspect perianal and anal areas for color, texture, masses, rashes, erythema, fissures, and external hemorrhoids. Palpate any masses or unusual areas with a gloved hand.

For the digital examination of the rectum, place a gloved, lubricated index finger against the anus while having the patient gently bear down (Valsalva maneuver). Then, as the sphincter relaxes, insert the finger. Point the finger toward the umbilicus. Try to get the patient to relax. Insert the finger into the rectum as far as possible and palpate all surfaces. Assess any nodules, tenderness, or irregularities. Use the gloved finger to remove a stool sample and check it for occult blood. However, a single guaiac-based fecal occult blood test has limited sensitivity in detecting colorectal cancer.

Findings of a normal physical assessment of the GI system are given in Table 38.9. Table 38.10 outlines assessment abnormalities. Gerontologic differences in the GI system and differences in assessment findings are described in Table 38.5. A *focused assessment* is used to evaluate the status of previously identified GI problems and to monitor for signs of new problems. A focused assessment of the GI system is shown on this page.

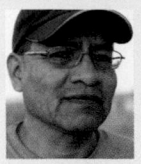
FOCUSED ASSESSMENT
Gastrointestinal System

Use this checklist to make sure the key assessment steps have been done.

Subjective
Ask the patient about any of the following and note responses.

Loss of appetite	Y	N
Abdominal pain	Y	N
Changes in stools (e.g., color, blood, consistency, frequency, pain)	Y	N
Nausea, vomiting	Y	N
Painful swallowing	Y	N

Objective: Diagnostic
Check the following results for critical values.

Endoscopy: colonoscopy, sigmoidoscopy, esophagogastroduodenoscopy	✓
CT scan	✓
Radiologic series: upper GI, lower GI	✓
Stool for occult blood or ova and parasites	✓
Liver function tests	✓

Objective: Physical Examination
Inspect

Skin for color, scars, petechiae, and other lesions.	✓
Abdominal contour for symmetry and distention	✓
Perianal area for intact skin, hemorrhoids	✓

Auscultate*

Bowel sounds	✓

Palpate

Abdominal quadrants using light touch	✓
Abdominal quadrants using a deep technique	✓

*NOTE: Perform auscultation before palpation.

DIAGNOSTIC STUDIES OF GASTROINTESTINAL SYSTEM

Tables 38.11 and 38.12 present common diagnostic studies of the GI system. Selected diagnostic studies are described in more detail in the following discussion.

For most diagnostic studies, make sure a signed consent form for the procedure has been completed and is in the medical record. The HCP doing the procedure is responsible for explaining the procedure and obtaining written consent. You have a key role in teaching patients about the procedures. When preparing the patient, it is important to ask about any known allergies to drugs, iodine, shellfish, or contrast media.

Many GI system diagnostic procedures require (1) measures to cleanse the GI tract and (2) ingestion or injection of a contrast medium or a radiopaque tracer. Often the patient has a series of GI diagnostic tests done. Monitor the patient closely to ensure adequate hydration and nutrition during the testing period.

Some diagnostic studies are especially difficult and uncomfortable for the older adult. Adjustments may be needed during the preparation, especially for those with certain health conditions (e.g., diabetes).[5] Make sure to consider any physical limitations when positioning the older patient during testing. Close monitoring is needed to avoid problems, such as dehydration from prolonged fluid restriction and diarrhea from bowel-cleansing procedures.

Radiologic Studies

Upper Gastrointestinal Series. An upper GI series with small bowel follow-through provides visualization of the oropharyngeal area, esophagus, stomach, and small intestine. The procedure consists of the patient swallowing contrast medium (a thick barium solution or gastrograffin) and then assuming different positions on the x-ray table. The movement of the contrast medium is observed with fluoroscopy, and a series of x-rays are taken. An upper GI series is useful in identifying esophageal strictures, polyps, tumors, hiatal hernias, foreign bodies, and ulcers.

Lower Gastrointestinal Series. The purpose of a lower GI series, or a barium enema, is to observe (using fluoroscopy) the colon filling with contrast medium and to observe (by x-ray) the filled colon. The patient receives an enema of contrast medium. This procedure identifies polyps, tumors, and other lesions in the colon. Adding air contrast after the barium provides better visualization (Fig. 38.9). Because the patient must retain the barium, an older or immobile patient may not tolerate it very well.

TABLE 38.9 Normal Physical Assessment of Gastrointestinal System

Mouth
- Moist and pink lips
- Pink and moist buccal mucosa and gingivae without plaques or lesions
- Teeth in good repair
- Protrusion of tongue in midline without deviation or twitches
- Pink uvula (in midline), soft palate, tonsils, and posterior pharynx
- Swallows smoothly without coughing or gagging

Abdomen
- Flat without masses or scars. No bruises
- Bowel sounds in all quadrants
- No abdominal tenderness; nonpalpable liver and spleen
- Liver 10 cm in right midclavicular line
- Generalized tympany

Anus
- Absence of lesions, fissures, and hemorrhoids
- Good sphincter tone
- Rectal walls smooth and soft
- No masses
- Stool soft, brown, and heme negative

TABLE 38.10 Assessment Abnormalities

Gastrointestinal System

Finding	Description	Possible Etiology and Significance
Mouth		
Acute marginal gingivitis	Friable, edematous, painful, bleeding gingivae	Irritation from ill-fitting dentures or orthodontic appliances, calcium deposits on teeth, food impaction
Candidiasis	White, curdlike lesions surrounded by erythematous mucosa	*Candida albicans*
Cheilitis	Inflammation of lips (usually lower) with fissuring, scaling, crusting	Often unknown
Cheilosis	Softening, fissuring, and cracking of lips at angles of mouth	Riboflavin deficiency
Geographic tongue	Scattered red, smooth (loss of papillae) areas on dorsum of tongue	Unknown
Glossitis	Reddened, ulcerated, swollen tongue	Exposure to streptococci, irritation, injury, vitamin B deficiencies, anemia
Herpes simplex	Benign vesicular lesion	Herpesvirus
Leukoplakia	Thickened white patches	Premalignant lesion
Pyorrhea	Recessed gingivae, purulent pockets	Periodontitis
Smooth tongue	Red, slick appearance	Cobalamin deficiency
Ulcer, plaque on lips or in mouth	Sore or lesion	Cancer, viral infections
Esophagus and Stomach		
Dyspepsia	Burning or indigestion	Peptic ulcer disease, gallbladder disease
Dysphagia	Difficulty swallowing, sensation of food sticking in esophagus	Esophageal problems, cancer of esophagus
Eructation	Belching	Gallbladder disease
Hematemesis	Vomiting of blood	Esophageal varices, bleeding peptic ulcer
Nausea and vomiting	Feeling of impending vomiting, expulsion of gastric contents through mouth	GI infections, common manifestation of many GI diseases; stress, fear, and pathologic conditions

TABLE 38.10 Assessment Abnormalities

Gastrointestinal System—cont'd

Finding	Description	Possible Etiology and Significance
Odynophagia	Painful swallowing	Cancer of esophagus, esophagitis
Pyrosis	Heartburn, burning in epigastric or substernal area	Hiatal hernia, esophagitis, incompetent lower esophageal sphincter
Abdomen		
Absence of liver dullness	Tympany on percussion	Air from viscus (e.g., perforated ulcer)
Absent bowel sounds	No bowel sounds on auscultation	Peritonitis, paralytic ileus, obstruction
Ascites	Accumulated fluid within abdominal cavity, eversion of umbilicus (usually)	Peritoneal inflammation, heart failure, metastatic cancer, cirrhosis
Borborygmi	Waves of loud, gurgling sounds	Hyperactive bowel as result of eating
Bruit	Humming or swishing sound heard through stethoscope over vessel	Partial arterial obstruction (narrowing of vessel), turbulent flow (aneurysm)
Distention	Excessive gas accumulation, enlarged abdomen, generalized tympany	Obstruction, paralytic ileus
Hepatomegaly	Enlargement of liver, liver edge >1–2 cm below costal margin	Metastatic cancer, hepatitis, venous congestion
Hernia	Bulge or nodule in abdomen, usually appearing on straining	Inguinal (in inguinal canal), femoral (in femoral canal), umbilical (herniation of umbilicus), or incisional (defect in muscles after surgery)
Hyperresonance	Loud, tinkling rushes	Intestinal obstruction
Masses	Lump on palpation	Tumors, cysts
Nodular liver	Enlarged, hard liver with irregular edge or surface	Cirrhosis, cancer
Rebound tenderness	Sudden pain when fingers withdrawn quickly	Peritoneal inflammation, appendicitis
Splenomegaly	Enlarged spleen	Chronic leukemia, hemolytic states, portal hypertension, some infections
Rectum and Anus		
Fissure	Ulceration in anal canal	Straining, irritation
Hemorrhoids	Thrombosed veins in rectum and anus (internal or external)	Portal hypertension, chronic constipation, prolonged sitting or standing, pregnancy
Mass	Firm, nodular edge	Tumor, cancer
Melena	Abnormal, black, tarry stool containing digested blood	Cancer, bleeding in upper GI tract from ulcers, varices
Pilonidal cyst	Opening of sinus tract, cyst in midline just above coccyx	Probably congenital
Steatorrhea	Fatty, frothy, foul-smelling stool	Chronic pancreatitis, biliary obstruction, malabsorption problems
Tenesmus	Painful and ineffective straining at stool. Sense of incomplete evacuation	Inflammatory bowel disease, irritable bowel syndrome, diarrhea secondary to GI infection (e.g., food poisoning)

TABLE 38.11 Diagnostic Studies

Gastrointestinal System

Study	Description and Purpose	Nursing Responsibility
Endoscopy		
Colonoscopy	Directly visualizes entire colon up to ileocecal valve with flexible fiberoptic scope. Patient's position is changed frequently during procedure to assist with advancement of scope to cecum. Used to diagnose or detect inflammatory bowel disease, polyps, tumors, and diverticulosis and dilate strictures. Procedure allows for biopsy and removal of polyps without laparotomy.	*Before:* Bowel preparation prior varies depending on HCP. Patient should avoid fiber for up to 72 hr prior, then either a clear or full liquid diet 24 hr before. Bowel cleansing should follow a split-dose regimen. The evening before the procedure, the patient should drink a cleansing solution. The second dose should begin 4–6 hr before the procedure. A split-dose regimen started early morning the day of a procedure provides better cleansing for patients scheduled in the afternoon. Encourage the patient to drink all the solution. Stools will be clear or clear yellow liquid when the colon is clean. Bisacodyl tablets or suppositories may be given before the cleansing solution to remove the bulk of the stool. Explain to patient that a flexible scope will be inserted while patient in side-lying position and sedation will be given. *After:* Patient may have abdominal cramps caused by stimulation of peristalsis because the bowel is constantly inflated with air during procedure. Teach patients about pain post-colonoscopy and the characteristics of this pain. Tell patients if pain lasts longer than 24 hr to notify HCP. Check vital signs. Observe for rectal bleeding and manifestations of perforation (e.g., malaise, abdominal distention, tenesmus).

TABLE 38.11 Diagnostic Studies

Gastrointestinal System—cont'd

Study	Description and Purpose	Nursing Responsibility
Endoscopic retrograde cholangiopancreatography (ERCP)	Fiberoptic endoscope (using fluoroscopy) is orally inserted into descending duodenum. Then common bile and pancreatic ducts are cannulated. Contrast medium is injected into ducts to allow for direct visualization of structures. Can be used to retrieve a gallstone from distal common bile duct, dilate strictures, biopsy, and diagnose pseudocysts.	*Before:* Explain procedure. Keep patient NPO 8 hr before. Ensure consent form is signed. Give sedation immediately before and during procedure. Give antibiotics if ordered. *After:* Check vital signs. Assess for perforation or infection. Pancreatitis is most common complication. Check for return of gag reflex.
Esophagogastroduodenoscopy (EGD)	Directly visualizes mucosal lining of esophagus, stomach, and duodenum with flexible endoscope. Test may use video imaging to visualize stomach motility. Detects inflammation, ulcerations, tumors, varices, or Mallory-Weiss tears. Biopsies may be taken. Varices can be treated with band ligation or sclerotherapy.	*Before:* Keep patient NPO for 8 hr. Ensure consent form is signed. Give preoperative medication if ordered. Explain to patient that local anesthesia may be sprayed on throat before insertion of scope and that patient will be sedated during procedure. *After:* Keep patient NPO until gag reflex returns. Gently tickle back of throat to determine reflex. Use warm saline gargles for relief of sore throat. Check temperature q15–30min for 1–2 hr (sudden temperature spike is sign of perforation).
Laparoscopy (peritoneoscopy)	Visualize peritoneal cavity and contents with laparoscope. Double-puncture peritoneoscopy permits better visualization of abdominal cavity, especially liver. Done in operating room. Can obtain biopsy specimen.	*Before:* Ensure consent form is signed. Keep patient NPO 8 hr. Give preoperative sedative medication. Ensure bladder and bowels are emptied. *After:* Observe for complications of bleeding and bowel perforation after the procedure.
Sigmoidoscopy	Directly visualizes rectum and sigmoid colon with lighted flexible endoscope. Sometimes a special table is used to tilt patient into knee-chest position. Used to detect tumors, polyps, inflammatory and infectious diseases, fissures, hemorrhoids.	*Before:* Bowel preparation similar to colonoscopy. Explain to patient knee-chest position, need to take deep breaths during insertion of scope, and possible urge to defecate as scope is passed. Encourage patient to relax and let abdomen go limp. *After:* Observe for rectal bleeding after polypectomy or biopsy.
Video capsule endoscopy	Patient swallows a vitamin-sized capsule with camera, which provides endoscopic visualization of GI tract (Fig. 38.11). Camera takes >50,000 images during test, relaying them to monitoring device that patient wears on a belt. Images then downloaded to computer. Used to look at areas of GI tract not accessible by upper and lower endoscopy.	*Before:* Keep patient NPO for 8 hr. May have bowel preparation similar to colonoscopy. After swallowing capsule, clear liquids resumed in 2 hr and food in 4 hr. *After:* 8 hr after swallowing device, patient returns to have monitoring device removed. Tell patient that capsule is disposable and will be present in a bowel movement.

Radiology

Cholangiography

• Magnetic resonance cholangiopancreatography (MRCP)	Use of MRI technology to obtain images of biliary and pancreatic ducts.	Same as MRI.
• Percutaneous transhepatic (PTC)	Under local anesthesia and monitored anesthesia care, a long needle is passed into liver (under fluoroscopy) and into bile duct. Bile is removed, and radiopaque contrast medium directly injected into biliary system. Used to determine filling of hepatic and biliary ducts.	*Before:* Assess patient's medications for contraindications, precautions, or complications with use of contrast medium. Keep patient NPO for 8–12 hr before test. Start prophylactic IV antibiotics 1 hr prior. *After:* Observe patient for signs of hemorrhage, bile leakage, and infection. Observe safety precautions until sedation wears off. Maintain bed rest for 6 hr.
• Surgical cholangiogram	Contrast medium is injected into common bile duct during surgery on biliary structures.	*Before:* Explain that anesthetic will be used. Assess patient's medications for contraindications, precautions, or complications with use of contrast medium.
Computed tomography (CT) scan	Noninvasive radiologic examination allows for exposures at different depths. Using oral and IV contrast medium accentuates density differences. Detects biliary tract, liver, and pancreatic disorders.	*Before:* Before contrast medium used, evaluate renal function. Assess if patient is allergic to shellfish since the contrast is iodine based. Patient may need to be NPO prior. *During:* Warn patient that contrast injection may cause a feeling of being warm and flushed. Patient must lie completely still during scan. *After:* Encourage patient to drink fluids to avoid renal problems with any contrast.

Continued

TABLE 38.11 Diagnostic Studies

Gastrointestinal System—cont'd

Study	Description and Purpose	Nursing Responsibility
Defecography	Uses fluoroscopy or MRI to assess the shape and position of the rectum during defecation. Using a lubricated small plastic tip, fill rectum and anus with barium. Oral barium allows small bowel to be visualized. The person then sits on a toilet-like seat attached to the x-ray table and is asked to push and empty the rectum. Images are taken while person is sitting at rest, straining, squeezing, and during defecation. Detects pelvic floor abnormalities.	*Before:* Keep patient NPO for 2 hr. 2 enemas are given 2 hr before, 15 min apart. Oral barium is given 1 hr before.
Gastric emptying breath test (GEBT)	Noninvasive test that measures CO_2 in a patient's breath. Used to diagnose delayed gastric emptying. Baseline breath test done. Then patient eats a special test meal that includes a scrambled egg mix and *Spirulina platensis,* a protein enriched with carbon-13. It is measured in breath samples collected at multiple time points after the meal.	*Before:* Teach patient to be NPO after midnight and that the test takes 4 hr. *During:* Can be done in any clinical setting. It does not require special training or special precautions related to radiation.
Lower GI or barium enema	Fluoroscopic x-ray examination of colon using contrast medium, which is given rectally (enema) (Fig. 38.9). Double-contrast or air-contrast barium enema is test of choice. Air is infused after the barium flows through transverse colon. Used to detect the presence of tumors, diverticula, and polyps.	*Before:* Give laxatives and enemas until colon is clear of stool evening before procedure. Follow clear liquid diet evening before procedure. Keep patient NPO for 8 hr before test. Teach patient about the barium enema. Explain that cramping and urge to defecate may occur during procedure and patient may be placed in various positions on tilt table. *After:* Give fluids, laxatives, or suppositories to help in expelling barium. Observe stool for passage of contrast medium. Tell patient that stool may be white for up to 72 hr.
Magnetic resonance imaging (MRI)	Noninvasive procedure using radiofrequency waves and a magnetic field. IV contrast medium (gadolinium) may be used. Used to detect hepatobiliary disease, hepatic lesions, and sources of GI bleeding and stage colorectal and other cancers.	*Before:* Check for pregnancy, allergies, and renal function. Have patient remove all metal objects. Ask about any history of surgical insertion of staples, plates, dental bridges, or other metal appliances. Remove metallic foil patches. Patient may need to be fasting. Assess for claustrophobia and the need for antianxiety medication. *During:* Patient must lie completely still during scan.
Nuclear imaging scans (scintigraphy)	Tracer doses of a radioactive isotope are injected IV, and a scanning device picks up radioactive emission, which is recorded on paper. Shows size, shape, and position of organ. Identifies functional disorders and structural defects.	*Before:* Tell patient that the substance used contains only traces of radioactivity and poses little to no danger. Schedule no more than 1 radionuclide test a day. Explain to patient need to lie flat during scanning.
• Gastric emptying studies	Assesses ability of stomach to empty solids. Patient eats cooked egg containing ^{99m}Tc and toast with water. Images are obtained at 0, 1, 2, and 4 hr later. Used to study gastric emptying disorders caused by ulcers, ulcer surgery, diabetes, cancer, or functional disorders.	Same as above.
• Hepatobiliary scintigraphy (HIDA)	Patient is given IV injection of ^{99m}Tc and positioned under camera to record distribution of tracer dose in liver, biliary tree, gallbladder, and proximal small intestine. Used to identify obstructions of bile ducts (gallstones, tumors), diseases of gallbladder, and bile leaks.	Same as above.
• Scintigraphy of GI bleeding	^{99m}Tc–labeled sulfur colloid or ^{99m}Tc labeling of the patient's own RBCs to determine the site of active GI blood loss. Sulfur colloid or patient's RBCs are injected, then images of abdomen taken at intermittent intervals.	Same as above.
Small bowel series	Contrast medium is ingested, and films taken every 30 min until medium reaches terminal ileum.	*Before:* Explain procedure, including the need to drink contrast medium and assume various positions on x-ray table. Keep patient NPO for at least 8 hr. Tell patient to avoid smoking after midnight. *After:* Take measures to prevent contrast medium impaction (fluids, laxatives). Tell patient that stool may be white for up to 72 hr.

TABLE 38.11 Diagnostic Studies

Gastrointestinal System—cont'd

Study	Description and Purpose	Nursing Responsibility
Upper gastrointestinal (GI) or barium swallow	Fluoroscopic x-ray study using contrast medium. Used to diagnose structural abnormalities of esophagus, stomach, and duodenum.	Same as for small bowel series.
Ultrasound	Noninvasive procedure using high-frequency ultrasound waves, which are passed into body structures and recorded as they are reflected. Used to show size and configuration of an organ.	
• Abdominal ultrasound	A conductive gel is applied to skin, and a transducer is placed on the area. Detects abdominal masses (tumors, cysts), gallstones, biliary and liver disease.	*Before:* Teach patient to be NPO for 8–12 hr. Air or gas can reduce quality of images. Food intake can cause gallbladder contraction, resulting in suboptimal study.
• Endoscopic ultrasound (EUS)	Small ultrasound transducer is installed on tip of endoscope. Because EUS transducer gets close to the organ(s) being examined, images obtained are more accurate and detailed than those provided by traditional ultrasound. Detects and stages esophageal, gastric, rectal, biliary, and pancreatic tumors and abnormalities.	Same as esophagogastroduodenoscopy (EGD).
• Ultrasound elastography (Fibroscan)	Transient elastography uses an ultrasound transducer to assess level of liver fibrosis. Used to monitor patients with chronic liver disease.	*Before:* Explain the need to lie in dorsal decubitus position with right arm in extreme abduction.
Virtual colonoscopy	Combines CT scanning or MRI with computer virtual reality software. Air is introduced via a tube placed in rectum to enlarge colon to enhance visualization. Images obtained while patient is on back and abdomen. Computer combines images to form 2-D and 3-D pictures that are viewed on monitor. Detects intestine and colon diseases, including polyps, cancer, diverticulosis, and lower GI bleeding.	*Before:* Bowel preparation similar to colonoscopy.

TABLE 38.12 Laboratory Studies

Gastrointestinal System

Test	Reference Interval	Description and Purpose
Blood Studies		
Amylase	60–120 U/L (30–220 U/L)	Enzyme secreted by pancreas. Important in diagnosing acute pancreatitis. Level of amylase peaks in 24 hr and then returns to normal in 48–72 hr
Gastrin	25–100 pg/mL when fasting	Hormone secreted by cells of the antrum of the stomach, the duodenum, and the pancreatic islets of Langerhans
Lipase	0–160 U/L	Enzyme secreted by pancreas. Important in diagnosing pancreatitis. Level stays higher longer than serum amylase in acute pancreatitis
Fecal Tests		
Fecal analysis	Note form, consistency, and color. Specimen examined for mucus, blood, pus, parasites, and fat content	Teach patient to keep diet free of red meat for 24–48 hr before occult blood test
Stool culture	Normal intestinal flora	Tests for the presence of bacteria, including *Clostridium difficile*

Virtual Colonoscopy. *Virtual colonoscopy* combines CT scanning or MRI to produce images of the colon and rectum less invasively. It requires radiation and prior cleansing of the colon but no sedation.

Compared to conventional colonoscopy, virtual colonoscopy provides a better view inside the colon that is narrow from inflammation or a growth.[6] If a polyp is found, it will have to be removed by conventional colonoscopy. Virtual colonoscopy may be less sensitive in obtaining information on the details and color of the mucosa and in detecting small (less than 10 mm) or flat polyps.

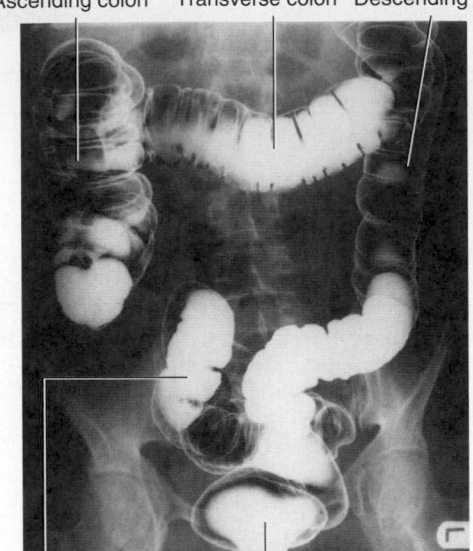

FIG. 38.9 Barium enema x-ray showing the large intestine. (From Drake RL, Vogl W, Mitchell AWM: *Gray's anatomy for students,* ed 3, Edinburgh, 2014, Churchill Livingstone.)

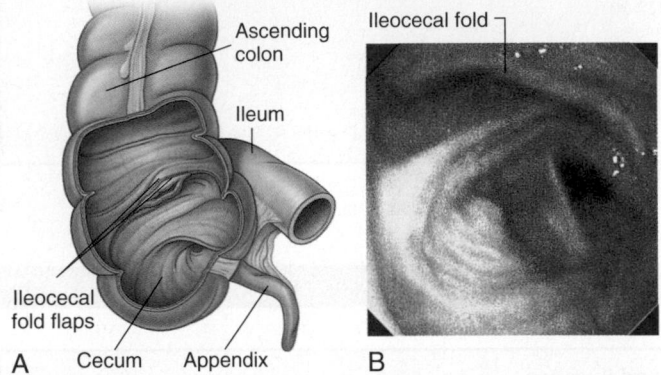

FIG. 38.10 **A,** Illustration showing the ileocecal junction and the ileocecal fold. **B,** Endoscopic image of the ileocecal fold. (From Drake RL, Vogl W, Mitchell AWM: *Gray's anatomy for students,* ed 3, Edinburgh, 2015, Churchill Livingstone.)

Endoscopy

Endoscopy refers to the direct visualization of a body structure through an endoscope. An endoscope is a fiberoptic instrument with a light and camera attached, allowing the ability to take video and still pictures (Fig. 38.10). Some endoscopes have a channel through which to pass instruments, such as biopsy forceps and cytology brushes.

Endoscopy can examine the esophagus, stomach, duodenum, and colon. *Endoscopic retrograde cholangiopancreatography* (ERCP) visualizes the pancreatic, hepatic, and common bile ducts. Endoscopy is often combined with diagnostic procedures, including biopsy, cytologic studies, invasive, and therapeutic

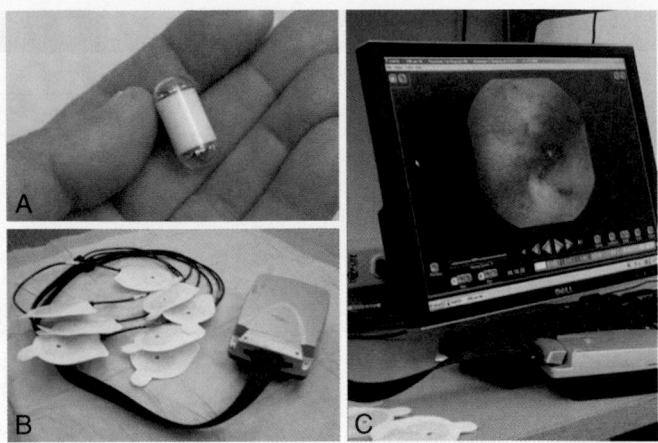

FIG. 38.11 Capsule endoscopy. **A,** The pill-sized video capsule has its own camera and light source. **B,** As it travels through the GI tract, it sends messages through sensing electrodes placed on the chest and abdomen to a data recorder worn on a waist belt. **C,** After the test, the images are viewed on a computer. (From Dye CE, Gaffney RR, Dykes TM, et al: Endoscopic and radiographic evaluation of the small bowel in 2012, *Am J Med* 125:1228e1, 2012.)

procedures. Examples include polypectomy, sclerosis or banding of varices, cauterization of bleeding sites, common bile duct stone removal, and balloon dilation.

The major complication of GI endoscopy is perforation through the structure being studied. Many endoscopic procedures require short-acting IV sedation. All endoscopic procedures require informed, written consent. Specific endoscopy procedures are discussed in Table 38.11.

Capsule endoscopy is a noninvasive approach to visualize the GI tract (Fig. 38.11). Colon capsule endoscopy is useful in diagnosing small bowel disease and monitoring inflammation in patients with IBD. Its sensitivity in detecting small lesions, colonic polyps, and colorectal cancer is under investigation.[7]

Liver Function Studies

Liver function tests (LFTs) are laboratory (blood) studies that reflect hepatic disease. Table 38.13 describes the most common LFTs.

Liver Biopsy

The purpose of a liver biopsy is to obtain hepatic tissue to use to establish a diagnosis of cancer or assess and stage fibrosis. It may be done to follow the progress of liver disease, such as chronic hepatitis.

The 2 types of liver biopsy are open and closed. The *open method* involves making an incision and removing a wedge of tissue. It is done in the operating room with the patient under general anesthesia, often with another surgical procedure. The *closed,* or *needle, biopsy* is a percutaneous procedure. It is often done with ultrasound or CT guidance. The HCP administers a local anesthetic, then inserts a needle between 6th and 7th or 8th and 9th intercostal spaces on the right side to obtain specimen of hepatic tissue. Table 38.14 outlines the nursing management of a patient undergoing a liver biopsy.

TABLE 38.13 Liver Function Tests

Test	Reference Interval	Description and Purpose
Bile Formation and Excretion		
Serum bilirubin		Measures liver's ability to conjugate and excrete bilirubin, distinguishing between unconjugated (indirect) and conjugated (direct) bilirubin in plasma
• Total	0.3–1.0 mg/dL (5.1–17 µmol/L)	Measures direct and indirect total bilirubin
• Direct	0.1–0.3 mg/dL (1.7–5.1 µmol/L)	Measures conjugated bilirubin. High in obstructive jaundice
• Indirect	0.2–0.8 mg/dL (3.4–12 µmol/L)	Measures unconjugated bilirubin. High in hepatocellular and hemolytic conditions
Urinary bilirubin	0 or negative	Measures urinary excretion of conjugated bilirubin
Hemostatic Function		
Prothrombin time (PT)	11–12.5 sec	Determination of prothrombin activity
Vitamin K	0.1–2.2 ng/mL (0.22–4.88 nmol/L)	Essential cofactor for many clotting factors
Lipid Metabolism		
Cholesterol (serum)	200 mg/dL (<5.2 mmol/L), varying with age	Synthesized and excreted by liver. High in biliary obstruction. Low in cirrhosis and malnutrition
Protein Metabolism		
α-Fetoprotein	<10 ng/mL (<10 mcg/L)	Sign of hepatocellular cancer
Ammonia	10–80 mcg/dL (6–47 µmol N/L)	Conversion of ammonia to urea normally occurs in liver. Increase can result in hepatic encephalopathy secondary to liver cirrhosis
Protein (serum)	• Albumin: 3.5–5.0 g/dL (35–50 g/L) • Globulin: 2.3–3.4 g/dL (23–34 g/L) • Total protein: 6.4–8.3 g/dL (64–83 g/L)	Measures serum proteins made by liver
Serum Enzymes		
Alanine aminotransferase (ALT)	4–36 U/L	High in liver damage and inflammation
Alkaline phosphatase (ALP)	30–120 U/L (0.5–2.0 µkat/L)	Originates from bone and liver. Serum levels rise when excretion is impaired because of obstruction in biliary tract
γ-Glutamyl transpeptidase (GGT)	Male and Female > 45: 8–38 U/L Female < 45: 5–27 U/L	Present in biliary tract, not in skeletal or heart muscle. High in hepatitis and alcoholic liver disease. More sensitive for liver dysfunction than ALP
Aspartate aminotransferase (AST)	0–35 U/L (0.0–0.58 µkat/L)	High in liver damage and inflammation

TABLE 38.14 Nursing Management

Care of the Patient Undergoing Liver Biopsy

Preprocedure
- Perform baseline assessment, including vital signs, pulse oximetry.
- Withhold food and fluids for 8–12 hr before.
- Check patient's coagulation status (prothrombin time, clotting or bleeding time).
- Give sedative and other drugs, as ordered
- Obtain type and crossmatch.
- Teach patient and caregiver about procedure and postprocedure care. Explain need to hold breath after expiration when needle is inserted.
- Ensure informed consent has been signed.

Postprocedure
- Check vital signs to detect internal bleeding q15min × 2, q30min × 4, q1hr × 4.
- Notify HCP of dyspnea, cyanosis, and restlessness, which may occur with pneumothorax.
- Keep patient lying on right side for minimum of 2 hr to splint puncture site. Then maintain bed rest for 12–14 hr, as ordered.
- Apply a small dressing over the needle insertion site.
- Teach patient and caregiver about discharge care including signs and symptoms to report to HCP (e.g., site complications) and any activity restrictions. Tell patient to avoid straining or coughing, which cause increased intraabdominal pressure.

CASE STUDY

Objective Data: Diagnostic Studies

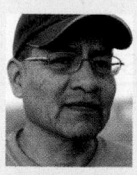
(© iStockphoto/ Thinkstock.)

The ED physician performs a rectal examination and finds a palpable mass. The following diagnostic tests are ordered:
- CBC
- Electrolytes
- Liver function tests
- Urinalysis
- CT scan of the abdomen
- Colonoscopy

The CBC reveals an Hgb of 6.8 g/dL and Hct of 20%. The WBC count is normal. The electrolytes, liver function tests, and urinalysis are within normal limits. The CT scan reveals pockets of gas and fluid in the ascending colon and 2 medium-sized tumors in the transverse colon.

Discussion Questions

1. Which diagnostic study results are of most concern to you?
2. With this information, what other diagnostic studies would you expect to be ordered for L.C.?
3. What are the interprofessional team's priorities for L.C. at this time?

Case study continued in Chapter 42 on p. 966.

Answers available at *http://evolve.elsevier.com/Lewis/medsurg.*

BRIDGE TO NCLEX EXAMINATION

The number of the question corresponds to the same-numbered outcome at the beginning of the chapter.

1. A patient is admitted to the hospital with a diagnosis of diarrhea with dehydration. The nurse recognizes that increased peristalsis resulting in diarrhea can be related to
   a. sympathetic inhibition.
   b. mixing and propulsion.
   c. sympathetic stimulation.
   d. parasympathetic stimulation.

2. A patient has a high blood level of indirect (unconjugated) bilirubin. One cause of this finding is that
   a. the gallbladder is unable to contract to release stored bile.
   b. bilirubin is not being conjugated and excreted into the bile by the liver.
   c. the Kupffer cells in the liver are unable to remove bilirubin from the blood.
   d. there is an obstruction in the biliary tract preventing flow of bile into the small intestine.

3. As gastric contents move into the small intestine, the bowel is normally protected from the acidity of gastric contents by the
   a. inhibition of secretin release.
   b. secretion of mucus by goblet cells.
   c. release of pancreatic digestive enzymes.
   d. release of gastrin by the duodenal mucosa.

4. A patient is jaundiced, and her stools are clay colored. This is *most* likely related to
   a. decreased bile flow into the intestine.
   b. increased production of urobilinogen.
   c. increased bile and bilirubin in the blood.
   d. increased production of cholecystokinin.

5. An 80-yr-old man states that, although he adds a lot of salt to his food, it still does not have much taste. The nurse's response is based on the knowledge that the older adult
   a. should not have any changes in taste.
   d. has a loss of taste buds, especially for sweet and salt.
   c. has some loss of taste but no problems chewing food.
   d. loses the sense of taste because the ability to smell is decreased.

6. When the nurse is assessing the health perception–health maintenance pattern as related to gastrointestinal function, an appropriate question to ask is
   a. "What is your usual bowel elimination pattern?"
   b. "What percentage of your income is spent on food?"
   c. "Have you traveled to a foreign country in the last year?"
   d. "Do you have diarrhea when you are under a lot of stress?"

7. During an examination of the abdomen the nurse should
   a. position the patient in the supine position with the bed flat and knees straight.
   b. listen for bowel sounds in the epigastrium and all four quadrants for 2 minutes.
   c. describe bowel sounds as absent if no sound is heard in a quadrant after 2 minutes.
   d. use the following order of techniques: inspection, palpation, percussion, auscultation.

8. Normal physical assessment findings of the gastrointestinal system are *(select all that apply)*
   a. nonpalpable spleen.
   b. borborygmi in upper right quadrant.
   c. tympany on percussion of the abdomen.
   d. liver edge 2 to 4 cm below the costal margin.
   e. finding of a firm, nodular edge on the rectal examination.

9. In preparing a patient for a colonoscopy, the nurse explains that
   a. a signed permit is not needed.
   b. sedation will be used during the procedure.
   c. one cleansing enema part of the required preparation.
   d. light meals should be eaten for 3 days before the procedure.

1. d, 2. b, 3. b, 4. a, 5. b, 6. c, 7. b, 8. a, c, 9. b

For rationales to these answers and even more NCLEX review questions, visit *http://evolve.elsevier.com/Lewis/medsurg*.

ⓔ EVOLVE WEBSITE/RESOURCES LIST

http://evolve.elsevier.com/Lewis/medsurg
Review Questions (Online Only)
Key Points
Answer Keys for Questions
- Rationales for Bridge to NCLEX Examination Questions
- Answer Guidelines for Case Studies on pp. 835, 838, 840, and 847

Conceptual Care Map Creator
Audio Glossary
Supporting Media
- Animation
- Rectal Examination

Content Updates

REFERENCES

1. Lichtenstein AH: Optimal nutrition for the older adults. In: Rippe JM: *Nutrition in lifestyle medicine*, New York, 2017, Humana Press.
*2. Emmanuel A, Mattace-Raso F, Neri MC, et al: Constipation in older people: A consensus statement, *Int J Clin Pract* 1:71, 2017.
3. Matsumoto T, Seno H: Updated trends in gallbladder and other biliary tract cancers worldwide, *Clin Gastroenterol Hepatol* 16:339, 2018.
4. Jarvis C: *Physical examination and health assessment*, ed 7, St Louis, 2016, Saunders.
*5. Ho SB, Hovsepians R, Gupta S: Optimal bowel cleansing for colonoscopy in the elderly patient, *Drugs Aging* 34:163, 2017.
6. National Digestive Diseases Information Clearinghouse: Virtual colonoscopy. Retrieved from *www.niddk.nih.gov/health-information/health-topics/diagnostic-tests/virtual-colonoscopy/Pages/diagnostic-test.aspx*.
7. Yu S, Sridhar S, Chamberlain SM: Capsule endoscopy: Diagnostic and therapeutic procedures in gastroenterology, New York, 2018, Springer.

*Evidence-based information for clinical practice.

39

Nutritional Problems

Mariann M. Harding

They may forget your name, but they will never forget how you made them feel.

Maya Angelou

ⓔ http://evolve.elsevier.com/Lewis/medsurg

CONCEPTUAL FOCUS

Functional Ability
Health Promotion

Nutrition

LEARNING OUTCOMES

1. Relate the essential components of a well-balanced diet to their impact on health outcomes.
2. Describe the etiology, clinical manifestations, and interprofessional and nursing management of malnutrition.
3. Describe the components of a nutritional assessment.

4. Explain the indications, complications, and nursing management related to the use of enteral nutrition.
5. Explain the indications, complications, and nursing management related to the use of parenteral nutrition.
6. Compare the etiology, clinical manifestations, and nursing management of eating disorders.

KEY TERMS

anorexia nervosa (AN), p. 866
bulimia nervosa (BN), p. 866
enteral nutrition (EN), p. 860

malabsorption syndrome, p. 852
malnutrition, p. 851
parenteral nutrition (PN), p. 863

refeeding syndrome, p. 864
tube feeding, p. 860

This chapter focuses on problems related to nutrition. A review of normal nutrition provides a basis for evaluating nutritional status. We need sufficient energy, protein, and other nutrients to maintain health. Many problems affect nutrition by changing the way we ingest, absorb, digest, and metabolize nutrients. These changes can lead to malnutrition, and health problems which affect functional status and quality of life. This makes it important for nurses to incorporate assessment and interventions aimed at promoting optimal nutrition.

NUTRITIONAL PROBLEMS

Nutrition is the sum of processes by which one takes in and uses nutrients. We view nutritional status on a continuum from undernutrition to normal nutrition to overnutrition. Any change in nutrient intake or use can cause nutritional problems. Nutritional problems occur in all ages, cultures, ethnic groups, and socioeconomic classes and across all educational levels.

Many factors influence nutritional status. A person establishes attitudes toward food and eating habits early. Dietary intake often reflects cultural or religious preferences. A person or family's financial status influences the type and amount of nutritious food they can buy.[1]

NORMAL NUTRITION

Nutrition is important for energy, growth, and maintaining and repairing body tissues. Optimal nutrition (in the absence of any underlying disease process) results from eating a balanced diet. The major components of the basic food groups are macronutrients (carbohydrates, fats, proteins), micronutrients (vitamins, minerals, electrolytes), and water. Optimal nutrition and daily physical activity are essential for a healthy lifestyle.

Body type, age, gender, medications, physical activity, and the presence or absence of disease influence a person's daily caloric requirements. Adjustments in caloric intake are necessary depending on changes in health status and daily activity level. There are several ways to estimate caloric need. The Mifflin–St. Jeor equation calculates daily adult energy (calorie) requirements based on resting metabolic rate (Table 39.1).[2] A simpler way to estimate daily calories needed is by kilocalories

TABLE 39.1 Estimating Daily Energy (Calorie) Requirements

Mifflin–St. Jeor Equation

For each gender, use the formula below to calculate energy expenditure:

Men: 10 × weight (kg) + 6.25 × height (cm) − 5 × age (yr) + 5
Women: 10 × weight (kg) + 6.25 × height (cm) − 5 × age (yr) − 161

To determine total daily calorie needs, the energy expenditure is multiplied by the appropriate activity factor, as follows:

1.200 = sedentary (little or no exercise)
1.375 = lightly active (light exercise/sports 1–3 days/wk)
1.550 = moderately active (moderate exercise/sports 3–5 days/wk)
1.725 = very active (hard exercise/sports 6–7 days a wk)
1.900 = extra active (very hard exercise/sports and physical job)

Example

Man: Weight 180 lb (82 kg); height 5 ft, 10 in (178 cm); age 50, very active

Energy expenditure = 10 (82) + 6.25 (178) − 5 (50) + 5 × 1.725 = 2911

Woman: Weight 150 lb (68 kg); height 5 ft, 6 in (168 cm); age 60; lightly active

Energy expenditure = 10 (68) + 6.25 (168) − 5 (60) −161 × 1.375 = 1745

TABLE 39.2 Nutritional Therapy

Foods High in Protein

Complete Proteins	Incomplete Proteins
• Eggs	• Grains (e.g., corn)
• Fish	• Legumes (e.g., navy beans, soybeans, peas)
• Meats	• Nuts (e.g., peanuts)
• Milk and milk products (e.g., cheese)	• Seeds (e.g., sesame seeds, sunflower seeds)
• Poultry	

per kilogram (kcal/kg). An average adult should consume 20 to 25 cal/kg body weight to lose weight, 25 to 30 cal/kg to maintain body weight, and 30 to 35 cal/kg to gain weight.[3] Energy needs may be greater during illness.

Carbohydrates, the body's main source of energy, yield about 4 cal/g. We classify them as either simple or complex, depending on the number of sugars they have. Simple carbohydrates come in 2 forms: monosaccharides (e.g., glucose, fructose), which are found in fruits and honey, and disaccharides (e.g., sucrose, maltose, lactose). They are found in foods such as table sugar, malted cereal, and milk.. Complex carbohydrates (polysaccharides) include starches, such as cereal grains, potatoes, and legumes.

Carbohydrates are the chief protein-sparing ingredient in a nutritionally sound diet. The Dietary Reference Intake (DRI) recommendations are that 45% to 65% of total calories should come from carbohydrates.[3] A person should take around 14 g of dietary fiber per 1000 calories eaten per day from fruits, vegetables, and whole grains. This equals roughly 28 to 30 g for a typical 2000-calorie diet. We should choose food and beverages with little added sugar or caloric sweeteners.

Fats are a major source of energy for the body. One gram of fat yields 9 calories. Fats are stored in adipose tissue and the abdominal cavity. They act as carriers of essential fatty acids and fat-soluble vitamins. Fats give us a feeling of satiety after eating. Fat intake should be no more than 20% to 35% of total calories.[3]

Fats can be divided into (1) potentially harmful (saturated fat and *trans* fat) and (2) healthier dietary fat (monounsaturated and polyunsaturated fat). One type of polyunsaturated fat, omega-3 fatty acids, may be especially beneficial to your heart. Omega-3 fatty acids (found in some types of fatty fish) appear to decrease the risk for coronary artery disease.[4]

Diets high in excess calories, usually in the form of fats, contribute to the development of obesity. We should consume less than 10% of calories from saturated fatty acids (about 20 g of saturated fat per day in a 2000-calorie diet) and choose foods with no *trans*-fatty acids.

Proteins are an essential part of a well-balanced diet. They are needed for tissue growth, repair, and maintenance; body

regulatory functions; and energy production. Ideally, 10% to 35% of daily caloric needs should come from protein.[3] The recommended daily protein intake is 0.8 to 1 g/kg of body weight. For the normal healthy person of average body size, this equals about 45 to 65 g of protein daily. One gram of protein yields 4 calories. Amino acids are the fundamental units of protein structure. We classify the 22 amino acids as essential or nonessential. The body can make nonessential amino acids if an adequate supply of protein is available. The body cannot make the 9 essential amino acids. Their availability depends totally on dietary sources. We obtain them from both animal and plant sources. *Complete proteins* contain all the essential amino acids. Proteins that lack one or more of the essential amino acids are *incomplete proteins*. Table 39.2 lists foods high in protein.

Vitamins are organic compounds needed in small amounts for normal metabolism. Vitamins function primarily in enzyme reactions that facilitate amino acid, fat, and carbohydrate metabolism. A diet consisting of foods from the 5 basic food groups is essential for obtaining the recommended dietary allowances of essential vitamins. Vitamins are divided into 2 categories: *water-soluble* vitamins (vitamin C and the B-complex vitamins) and *fat-soluble* vitamins (vitamins A, D, E, and K). Since the body stores excess fat-soluble vitamins, consuming too much can result in toxicity. There are upper limits for vitamins A, D, and E.

♥ PROMOTING POPULATION HEALTH

Health Impact of a Well-Balanced Diet

- Reduces risk for anemia
- Maintains normal body weight and prevents obesity
- Maintains good bone health and reduces risk for osteoporosis
- Lowers the risk for developing high cholesterol and type 2 diabetes
- Decreases the risk for heart disease, hypertension, and certain types of cancers

Mineral salts (e.g., magnesium, iron, calcium) make up about 4% of the total body weight. The body needs minerals to build and repair tissues, regulate body fluids, and assist in various functions. Minerals needed in amounts greater than 100 mg/day are *major minerals*. Minerals present in minute amounts are *trace elements*. Table 39.3 lists the major minerals and trace elements. Some minerals are stored and can be toxic if taken in excess amounts. The amount of minerals needed daily varies from a few micrograms of trace minerals to 1 g or more of the major minerals, such as calcium, phosphorus, and sodium. A well-balanced diet usually meets the daily requirements of minerals. However, deficiency and excess states can occur.

TABLE 39.3 Major Minerals and Trace Elements

Major Minerals	Trace Elements
• Calcium	• Chromium
• Chloride	• Copper
• Magnesium	• Fluoride
• Phosphorus	• Iodine
• Potassium	• Iron
• Sodium	• Manganese
• Sulfur	• Molybdenum
	• Selenium
	• Zinc

TABLE 39.4 Nutritional Therapy

Foods High in Iron

These foods provide 25%–39% of the Dietary Reference Intake (DRI) of iron.

Food	Selected Serving Size
Breads, Cereals, and Grain Products	
Farina, regular or quick cooked (enriched)	⅔ cup
Oatmeal, instant, fortified, prepared (enriched)	⅔ cup
Ready-to-eat cereals, fortified (enriched)	1 oz
Meat, Poultry, Fish, and Alternatives	
Beef liver, braised	3 oz
Chicken or turkey liver, braised	½ cup diced
Clams: steamed, boiled, or canned (drained)	3 oz
Oysters: baked, broiled, steamed, or canned (undrained)	3 oz
Pork liver, braised	3 oz
Soybeans, cooked	½ cup

VEGETARIAN DIET

There are many types of vegetarians and no strict definition of the word "vegetarian." The common element among all vegetarians is the exclusion of red meat from the diet. Many vegetarians are *vegans,* who are pure or total vegetarians and eat only plants, or *lacto-ovo-vegetarians.* They eat plants, dairy products, and eggs.

Without a well-planned diet, vegetarians can have vitamin or protein deficiencies. Plant protein, although a lesser quality than animal protein, fulfills most protein requirements. Combinations of vegetable protein foods (e.g., cornmeal, kidney beans) can increase the nutritional value. Milk made from soybeans or almonds is an excellent protein source and should be calcium fortified. Vegans and lacto-ovo-vegetarians are also at risk for iron deficiency. Table 39.4 lists examples of foods high in iron.

The primary deficiency for a strict vegan is lack of cobalamin (vitamin B$_{12}$).[5] We obtain cobalamin from animal protein, special supplements, or foods fortified with the vitamin. Vegans not using cobalamin supplements are susceptible to the development of megaloblastic anemia and the neurologic signs of cobalamin deficiency. Other deficiencies that may be present in a vegan diet include calcium, zinc, and vitamins A and D.

Culturally Competent Care: Nutrition

People have unique cultural heritages that may affect eating customs and nutritional status. Each culture has its own beliefs and behaviors related to food and the role that food plays in the cause and treatment of disease. Culture and religion can influence which foods are considered edible, how they are prepared, when they are eaten, and how and who prepares them. For example, some religions, such as Judaism and Islam, have specific laws about food. Assess the extent to which Jewish or Muslim patients adhere to Kosher or Halal dietary practices to ensure that we serve proper meals. The websites Kosher Quest *(www.kosherquest.org)* and the Islamic Food and Nutrition Council of America *(www.ifanca.org)* provide detailed information.

Assess the patient's diet history and implement needed dietary changes. Avoid cultural stereotyping by not making assumptions or generalizations about diet based on a person's cultural background. Dietary habits differ considerably within and among ethnic groups. Acculturation, the process by which immigrants adopt the lifestyle of a new culture, can affect dietary practices.

It is important to know whether the patient eats "traditional foods" associated with the culture. Assess the impact of eating traditional foods on health. For example, traditional foods eaten by some Asian Americans may be high in fiber and low in fat and cholesterol. The diet may be low in calcium because of limited dairy product intake. "Soul food," identified with some blacks, includes foods such as collard greens and vegetables prepared with pork; beans; fried meats; grits; and cornbread. This diet may increase the risk for diabetes and heart disease.

Considering cultural beliefs is important when planning and monitoring acceptance of dietary changes. Culture can influence the perception of body weight and size. Ask the patient or family about how culture affects dietary choices and weight maintenance. For example, in some cultures obesity does not carry the stigma that it does in Western cultures. This may make teaching about weight reduction harder. A Jewish patient who eats only Kosher food may find comfort in knowing that an enteral feeding formula is Kosher. Another example of culturally sensitive planning is adjusting meal plans for the Muslim patient observing Ramadan (the Islamic month of *fasting,* in which Muslims refrain from eating and drinking during daylight hours).

MALNUTRITION

Malnutrition is a deficit, excess, or imbalance of essential nutrients. It may occur with or without inflammation. Malnutrition affects body composition and functional status. Other terms used to describe malnutrition include *undernutrition* and *overnutrition.*

Undernutrition occurs when nutritional reserves are depleted, and nutrient and energy intake are not sufficient to meet daily needs or added metabolic stress.[6] *Overnutrition* refers to the ingestion of more food than is required for body needs, as in obesity.

Malnutrition is a problem in both developing and developed countries across the care continuum (community, hospital, long-term care). Prevalence rates for malnutrition in the hospital setting range from 30% to 50%.[7] The prevalence of malnutrition in older adults based on the Mini Nutritional Assessment (MNA) ranges from about 3% (community-dwelling older adults) to 30% (rehabilitation settings).[8]

Etiology

Several terms describe the types and causes of adult malnutrition. Older terms still used in some settings include *primary* or *secondary protein-calorie malnutrition* (PCM), *marasmus,* and *kwashiorkor.* Marasmus and kwashiorkor describe forms of malnutrition seen in children in developing countries. You should not use these terms to describe malnutrition in adults.

The following cause-based terms are the preferred ones to use in clinical practice settings, since they indicate the interaction and importance of inflammation on nutritional status (Fig. 39.1).[9]

- *Starvation-related malnutrition,* or primary PCM, occurs when nutritional needs are not met. In primary PCM, there is chronic starvation without inflammation (e.g., anorexia nervosa).
- *Chronic disease–related malnutrition,* or secondary PCM, is related to conditions that have sustained mild to moderate inflammation. This occurs when dietary intake does not meet tissue needs, although it would under normal conditions. Examples of conditions associated with this type of malnutrition include organ failure, cancer, rheumatoid arthritis, and obesity.
- *Acute disease–related or injury-related malnutrition* is related to acute disease or injury states with marked inflammatory response (e.g., major infection, burns, trauma, surgery).

Contributing Factors

Many factors contribute to the development of malnutrition, including socioeconomic factors, physical illnesses, incomplete diets, and drug-nutrient interactions. Table 39.5 lists conditions that increase the risk for malnutrition.

Socioeconomic Factors. Persons or families with limited financial resources may have *food insecurity* (inadequate access). Food insecurity is a major public health problem. It affects the overall quality of food that is available in both quantity and nutritional value. Those with food insecurity usually choose less expensive "filling" foods, which are more energy dense (high fat) and lack nutritional value. This type of diet increases the risk for nutrient deficiencies.

To help obtain food, people may use "safety net programs." These include food assistance programs; housing and energy subsidies; and in-kind contributions from relatives, friends, food pantries, or charitable organizations. Consult with social workers to help patients gain access to government and local programs, such as Meals on Wheels, that deliver nutritious meals to homebound people.

The "heat or eat" phenomenon is problematic, as those with limited economic resources struggle to pay household utility bills or put food on the table. Older adults on a fixed income have an added burden of deciding on whether to pay for medications or food. You and the dietitian can help patients in making food choices that meet nutritional requirements while staying within their limited resources.

Physical Illnesses. Malnutrition is a common consequence of illness, surgery, injury, or hospitalization. The hospitalized patient, especially the older adult, is at risk for becoming malnourished. Prolonged illness, major surgery, sepsis, draining wounds, burns, hemorrhage, fractures, and immobilization can all contribute to malnutrition. Undernutrition can worsen a pathologic condition. An existing deficiency state is likely to become more severe during illness.

Anorexia, nausea, vomiting, diarrhea, abdominal distention, and abdominal cramping may accompany gastrointestinal (GI) disease. Any combination of these symptoms interferes with normal food consumption and metabolism. In addition, a patient may restrict intake to a few foods or fluids that may not be nutritious out of fear of worsening an existing GI problem.

Malabsorption syndrome is the impaired absorption of nutrients from the GI tract. Decreases in digestive enzymes or in bowel surface area can quickly lead to a deficiency state. Many drugs have undesirable GI side effects and alter normal digestive and absorptive processes. For example, antibiotics can change the normal flora of the intestines. This decreases the body's ability to make biotin, a B-complex vitamin whose production depends on that gut flora.

Fever accompanies many illnesses, injuries, and infections, with a concomitant increase in the body's basal metabolic rate (BMR) and nitrogen loss. Each degree of temperature increase on the Fahrenheit scale raises the BMR by about 7%. Without an

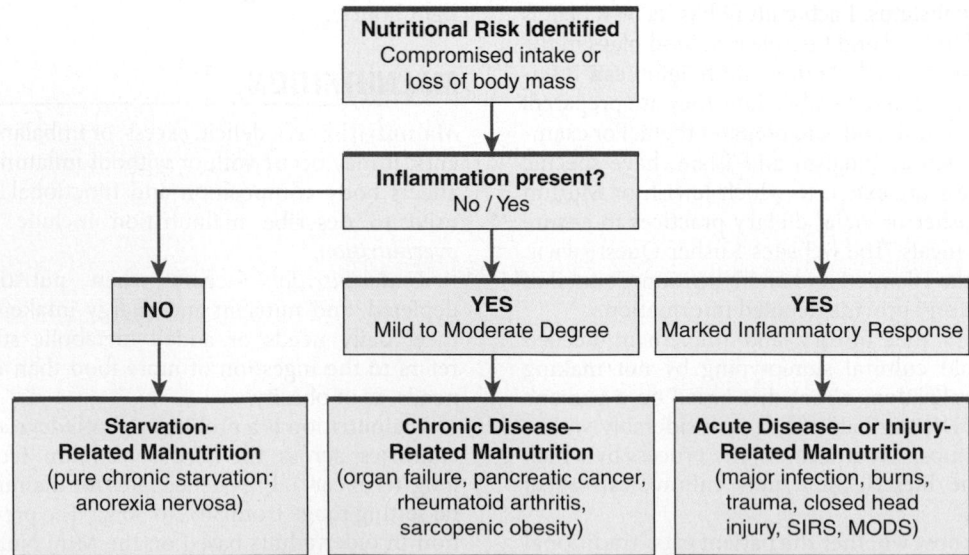

FIG. 39.1 Definitions of malnutrition. *MOD,* Multiple organ dysfunction; *SIRS,* systemic inflammatory response syndrome. (From Nix, S: *Williams' basic nutrition and diet therapy,* ed 15, St Louis, 2018, Elsevier.)

increase in caloric intake, the body uses protein stores to supply calories and protein depletion develops. After the body temperature returns to normal, the rate of protein breakdown and resynthesis may stay increased for several weeks.

Consider the nutritional requirements of a patient who is not overtly ill but having diagnostic studies. This patient may be nutritionally fit on entering the hospital but can become malnourished because of the dietary restrictions imposed by multiple diagnostic studies.

Incomplete Diets. Vitamin deficiencies are rare in most developed countries. When vitamin imbalances do occur, they usually involve several vitamins, rather than a single one. This may happen with a person with a pattern of alcohol and drug use, those who are chronically ill, and those who follow poor dietary practices. Persons who had surgery on the GI tract may be at risk for vitamin deficiencies. For example, resection of the terminal ileum poses a risk for deficiencies of fat-soluble vitamins. After a gastrectomy, patients need cobalamin supplements. Because intrinsic factor (normally made in the stomach) is not available to bind with cobalamin, cobalamin cannot be absorbed in the ileum. Followers of fad diets or poorly planned vegetarian diets are also at risk.

Manifestations of vitamin imbalances range from skin conditions to neurologic signs. The recommended dietary allowances for essential vitamins and manifestations of imbalances are outlined in Table 39.6.

Drug-Nutrient Interactions. A *drug-nutrient interaction* occurs when a drug affects the use of nutrients in the body. Many drug and food or beverage interactions may occur. Potential adverse interactions include incompatibilities, altered drug effectiveness, and impaired nutritional status. Many drugs have side effects, such as changes in taste, appetite, and nausea. Grapefruit juice can increase the absorption of some drugs, enhancing their effect. Drug-nutrient interactions can also occur with the use of herbs and dietary supplements. Monitor and prevent these potential interactions for patients in the hospital and at home.

Pathophysiology of Starvation

Knowing the pathophysiology of the starvation process will help you understand the physiologic changes that occur in malnutrition. Initially, the body selectively uses carbohydrates (glycogen) rather than fat and protein to meet metabolic needs. These carbohydrate stores, found in the liver and muscles, are minimal. They may be totally depleted within 18 hours. During the early phase of starvation, protein is used only in its normal participation in cellular metabolism.

However, once carbohydrate stores are depleted, the body converts skeletal protein to glucose for energy. Alanine and glutamine are the first amino acids used in *gluconeogenesis,* the process by which the liver forms glucose. The resulting plasma glucose allows metabolic processes to continue. When these amino acids are used as energy sources, the person may be in negative nitrogen balance (nitrogen excretion exceeds nitrogen intake).

Within 5 to 9 days, the body uses fat to supply much of the needed energy. In prolonged starvation, fat provides up to 97% of calories, conserving protein. Depletion of fat stores depends on the amount available. Fat stores are generally used up in 4 to 6 weeks. Once fat stores are gone, the body uses visceral and body proteins, including those in internal organs and plasma.

TABLE 39.5 Conditions That Increase the Risk for Malnutrition

- Chronic alcohol use
- Decreased mobility that limits access to food or its preparation
- Dementia
- Depression
- Drugs with antinutrient or catabolic properties (e.g., corticosteroids, antibiotics)
- Excessive dieting to lose weight
- Need for increased nutrients because of hypermetabolism or stress (e.g., infection, trauma, fever)
- No oral intake and/or receiving standard IV solutions for 10 days (adults) or for 5 days (older adults)
- Nutrient losses from malabsorption, dialysis, diarrhea, or wounds
- Swallowing disorders (e.g., head and neck cancer)

TABLE 39.6 Recommended Daily Vitamin Intake and Manifestations of Deficiencies

Vitamin	Dietary Reference Intake	Manifestations of Deficiencies
A (retinol)	*Men:* 900 mcg/retinol equivalents* *Women:* 700 mcg/retinol equivalents	Dry, scaly skin. Increased susceptibility to infection, night blindness, anorexia, eye irritation, keratinization of respiratory and GI mucosa, bladder stones, anemia, retarded growth
D	*Adults ages 19–70:* 600 IU *Adults age >70:* 800 IU	Muscular weakness, excessive sweating, diarrhea and other GI problems, bone pain, active or healed rickets, osteomalacia
E	*Adults:* 15 mg	Neurologic deficits
K	*Men:* 120 mcg *Women:* 90 mcg	Blood coagulation problems
B₁ (thiamine)	*Men:* 1.2 mg *Women:* 1.1 mg	Anorexia, fatigue, nervous irritability, constipation, paresthesias, insomnia
B₆ (pyridoxine)	*Men ages 19–50:* 1.3–1.7 mg *Men age >51:* 1.7 mg *Women ages 19–50:* 1.3–1.5 mg *Women age >51:* 1.5 mg	Seizures, dermatitis, anemia, neuropathy with motor weakness, anorexia
B₁₂ (cobalamin)	*Adults:* 2.4 mcg	Megaloblastic anemia, anorexia, glossitis, sore mouth and tongue, pallor, neurologic problems (e.g., depression, dizziness), weight loss, nausea, constipation
C	*Men:* 90 mg *Women:* 75 mg	Bleeding gums, loose teeth, easy bruising, poor wound healing, scurvy, dry, itchy skin
Folate (folic acid)	*Adults:* 400 mcg	Impaired cell division and protein synthesis, megaloblastic anemia, anorexia, fatigue, sore tongue, diarrhea, forgetfulness

*1 retinol equivalent = 10 international units vitamin A activity from β-carotene or 3.33 international units vitamin A activity from retinol.

They rapidly decrease because they are the only remaining body source of energy available.

If a malnourished patient has surgery, physical trauma, or an infection, the stress response is superimposed on the starvation response. The body uses protein stores for energy to meet the increased metabolic energy expenditure.

As protein depletion continues, liver function becomes impaired and protein synthesis decreases. The decrease in protein synthesis lowers plasma oncotic pressure. A major function of plasma proteins, primarily albumin, is to maintain the osmotic pressure of blood. When the oncotic pressure decreases, body fluids shift from the vascular space into the interstitial compartment. Eventually albumin leaks into the interstitial space along with the fluid. Edema becomes observable. Often edema in the patient's face and legs masks the underlying muscle wasting.

As the total blood volume decreases, the skin appears dry and wrinkled. As fluids shift to the interstitial space, ions also move. Sodium (the main extracellular ion) increases in amount within the cell. Potassium (the main intracellular ion) and magnesium shift to the extracellular space. The sodium-potassium exchange pump has high-energy needs, using 20% to 50% of all calories ingested. When the diet is extremely deficient in calories and essential proteins, the pump will fail. This leaves sodium inside the cell (along with water), and the cell expands.

The liver is the body organ that loses the most mass during protein deprivation. Fat gradually infiltrates the liver due to decreased synthesis of lipoproteins. Death will rapidly ensue if the person does not receive dietary protein and necessary nutrients.

Impact of Inflammation. Inflammation affects nutrient metabolism and is an important part of nutritional status. During the starvation process, there is a decreased BMR, sparing of skeletal muscle, and decreased protein breakdown. However, in inflammatory states, there are changes in the expression of proinflammatory (e.g., interleukin-6 [IL-6]) and antiinflammatory cytokines (e.g., IL-10). These cytokine changes result in increased protein and skeletal muscle breakdown, increased BMR, increased glucose turnover, decreased negative acute phase protein (albumin, prealbumin) production, and increased positive acute phase protein (e.g., C-reactive protein [CRP]) production.[10]

Clinical Manifestations and Diagnostic Studies

The manifestations of malnutrition range from mild to emaciation and death (Fig. 39.2). The most obvious signs are seen in the skin (dry and scaly skin, brittle nails, rashes, hair loss), mouth (crusting and ulceration, changes in tongue), muscles (decreased mass and weakness), and CNS (mental changes, such as confusion, irritability). The speed at which malnutrition develops depends on the quantity and quality of the protein intake, caloric value, illness, and person's age.

The manifestations result from numerous interactions at the cellular level. As protein intake declines, the muscles (the largest store of protein in the body) become wasted and flabby. This leads to weakness and fatigability. Decreased protein is available for tissue repair, causing delayed wound healing. The person is more susceptible to infections. Both humoral and cell-mediated immunity are deficient. Leukocytes decrease in the peripheral blood. Impaired phagocytosis occurs because of the lack of energy needed to drive the process. Many malnourished persons are anemic because they lack iron and folic acid (necessary building blocks for red blood cells [RBCs]).

The diagnosis of malnutrition is best determined by body composition, including a thorough history of weight loss,

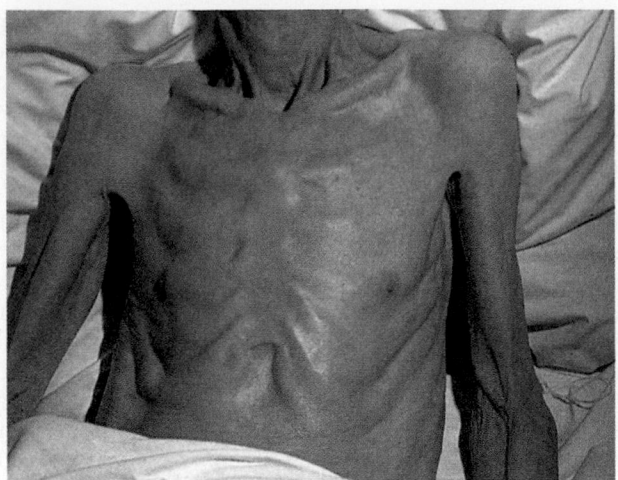

FIG. 39.2 Severe malnutrition results in wasting and extensive loss of adipose tissue. (From Kamal A, Brockelhurst JC: *Color atlas of geriatric medicine*, ed 2, St Louis, 1991, Mosby.)

nutrient intake, and measures of functional status. Obtain vital signs, height, and weight. Assess and document the patient's physical state and each body system. Table 39.7 outlines the assessment and findings of the patient with malnutrition.

Laboratory Studies. Serum albumin has a half-life of 20 to 22 days. In the absence of marked fluid loss (e.g., from hemorrhage or burns), the serum albumin value lags behind actual protein changes by more than 2 weeks. This makes albumin a poor indicator of acute changes in nutritional status. Prealbumin, a protein made by the liver, has a half-life of 2 days. It is a better indicator of recent or current nutritional status. However, the extent to which visceral proteins, including albumin and prealbumin, are true markers of malnutrition is questionable.

Albumin and prealbumin are *negative acute phase proteins*. This means that during an inflammatory response, the liver decreases synthesis of these proteins. So low or below normal levels of albumin and prealbumin may indicate an inflammatory state rather than accurately depicting nutritional status. One way to determine if low albumin and prealbumin levels are due to malnutrition is to measure CRP, a *positive acute phase protein*. CRP typically increases during inflammation. A high CRP and low albumin or prealbumin suggest that inflammation is driving the change in albumin and prealbumin levels.[11]

Serum electrolyte levels reflect changes taking place between the intracellular and extracellular spaces. The serum potassium level often increases. The RBC count and hemoglobin level indicate the presence and degree of anemia. The total lymphocyte count decreases with malnutrition. Calculate it by multiplying the percent of lymphocytes times the total white blood cell (WBC) count. Liver enzyme levels may increase with malnutrition. Serum levels of both fat-soluble and water-soluble vitamins usually decrease. Low serum levels of fat-soluble vitamins correlate with the presence of *steatorrhea* (fatty stools).

❖ NURSING AND INTERPROFESSIONAL MANAGEMENT: MALNUTRITION

◆ Nursing Assessment

As a nurse, you are responsible for nutritional screening across care settings. Nutritional screening identifies those who are malnourished or at risk for malnutrition. The Joint Commission

TABLE 39.7 Nursing Assessment

Malnutrition

Subjective Data

Important Health Information

- *Past health history:* Severe burns, major trauma, hemorrhage, draining wounds, bone fractures with prolonged immobility, chronic renal or liver disease, cancer, malabsorption syndromes, GI obstruction, infectious diseases, acute (e.g., trauma, sepsis) or chronic inflammatory condition (e.g., rheumatoid arthritis)
- *Medications:* Corticosteroids, chemotherapy, diet pills, dietary supplements, herbs
- *Surgery or other treatments:* Recent surgery, radiation

Functional Health Patterns

- *Health perception–health management:* Alcohol or drug use. Malaise, apathy
- *Nutritional-metabolic:* Increase or decrease in weight, weight problems. Increase or decrease in appetite, typical dietary intake, food preferences and aversions, food allergies or intolerance. Ill-fitting or absent dentures. Dry mouth, problems chewing or swallowing, bloating, or gas. ↑ Sensitivity to cold, delayed wound healing
- *Elimination:* Constipation, diarrhea, nocturia, decreased urine output
- *Activity-exercise:* Increase or decrease in activity patterns. Weakness, fatigue, decreased endurance
- *Cognitive-perceptual:* Pain in mouth. Paresthesias, loss of position and vibratory sense
- *Role-relationship:* Change in family (e.g., loss of a spouse), financial resources
- *Sexual-reproductive:* Amenorrhea, impotence, decreased libido

Objective Data

General

- Listless, cachectic, underweight for height

Eyes

- Pale or red conjunctivae, gray keratinized epithelium on conjunctiva (Bitot's spots). Dryness and dull appearance of conjunctivae and cornea, soft cornea. Blood vessel growth in cornea. Redness and fissuring of eyelid corners

Integumentary

- Dry, brittle, sparse hair with color changes and lack of luster, alopecia. Dry, scaly lips. Fever blisters, angular crusts and lesions at corners of mouth (cheilosis). Brittle, ridged nails. Decreased tone and elasticity of skin. Cool, rough, dry, scaly skin with brown-gray pigment changes. Reddened, scaly dermatitis, scrotal dermatitis. Slight cyanosis, peripheral edema

Respiratory

- Decreased respiratory rate, ↓ vital capacity, crackles, weak cough

Cardiovascular

- Increased or decreased heart rate, ↓ BP, dysrhythmias

Gastrointestinal

- Swollen, smooth, raw, beefy red tongue (glossitis), hypertrophic or atrophic papillae. Dental cavities, absent or loose teeth, discolored tooth enamel. Spongy, pale, receded gums with a tendency to bleed easily, periodontal disease. Ulcerations, white patches or plaques. Redness, swelling of oral mucosa. Distended, tympanic abdomen. Ascites, hepatomegaly, decreased bowel sounds, steatorrhea

Neurologic

- Decreased or loss of reflexes, tremor; irritability, confusion, syncope, peripheral neuropathy

Musculoskeletal

- Decreased muscle mass with poor tone, "wasted" appearance, bow-legs, knock-knees, beaded ribs, chest deformity, prominent bony structures

Possible Diagnostic Findings

- ↓ Hemoglobin and hematocrit, ↓ mean corpuscular volume (MCV), mean corpuscular hemoglobin (MCH), or mean corpuscular hemoglobin concentration (MCHC). Altered serum electrolyte levels, especially hyperkalemia. ↓ BUN and creatinine, ↓ serum albumin, transferrin, and prealbumin. ↑ CRP, ↓ lymphocytes, ↑ liver enzymes, ↓ serum vitamin levels

---

requires nutritional screening for all patients within 24 hours of admission, with a detailed nutrition assessment if a patient is at risk. Following a standard approach to nutritional screening, using valid and reliable tools, will accurately identify those at risk. Many nutritional screening and assessment tools are available. Hospital-specific screening tools review common admission assessment data, including history of weight loss, intake before admission, use of nutritional support, chewing or swallowing issues, and skin breakdown.

The Malnutrition Universal Screening Tool (Fig. 39.3) and Nutrition Risk Screening are common tools used with adults in acute care. The MNA assesses nutrition status in older adults. In long-term care, the Minimum Data Set (MDS) form is used to obtain nutrition information.[12] In home care settings, the Outcome and Assessment Information Set (OASIS) is used to collect information on diet, oral intake, dental health, swallowing problems, and any need for meal assistance.

If screening identifies a person at nutritional risk, perform a full nutritional assessment. A nutritional assessment is a comprehensive approach that includes medical, nutritional, and medication histories; physical examination; anthropometric measurements; and laboratory data (Table 39.8). Nutritional assessment provides the basis for nutritional intervention.

Obtain a complete diet history from the patient or caregiver. Assessing the foods eaten over the past week reveals a great deal about the patient's diet habits and knowledge of good nutrition. Often the patient's nutritional state is not the reason for seeking medical care. However, it may be a contributing factor to the disease and have an impact on management and recovery.

Anthropometric Measurements. Obtain height, weight, and girth measurements. Calculate the body mass index (BMI). We often use waist circumference and hip-to-waist ratio to assess nutritional status (see Chapter 40). Obtaining accurate measures of weight and height are critical. When possible, measure the patient's actual height rather than using the patient's self-report. Alternatives to standing height (stature) measurements include arm demi-span and knee-height measurements. The *arm demi-span* is the distance from a point on the midline at the suprasternal notch to the web between the middle and ring fingers with the arm horizontally outstretched. For persons confined to bed, using a Luft ruler is an alternative to standing height.

When assessing weight, obtain a detailed weight history, noting weight loss. Ask whether the weight loss was intentional or unintentional and the period over which it took place. A loss of more than 5% of usual body weight over 6 months (whether intentional or unintentional) is a critical indicator for further

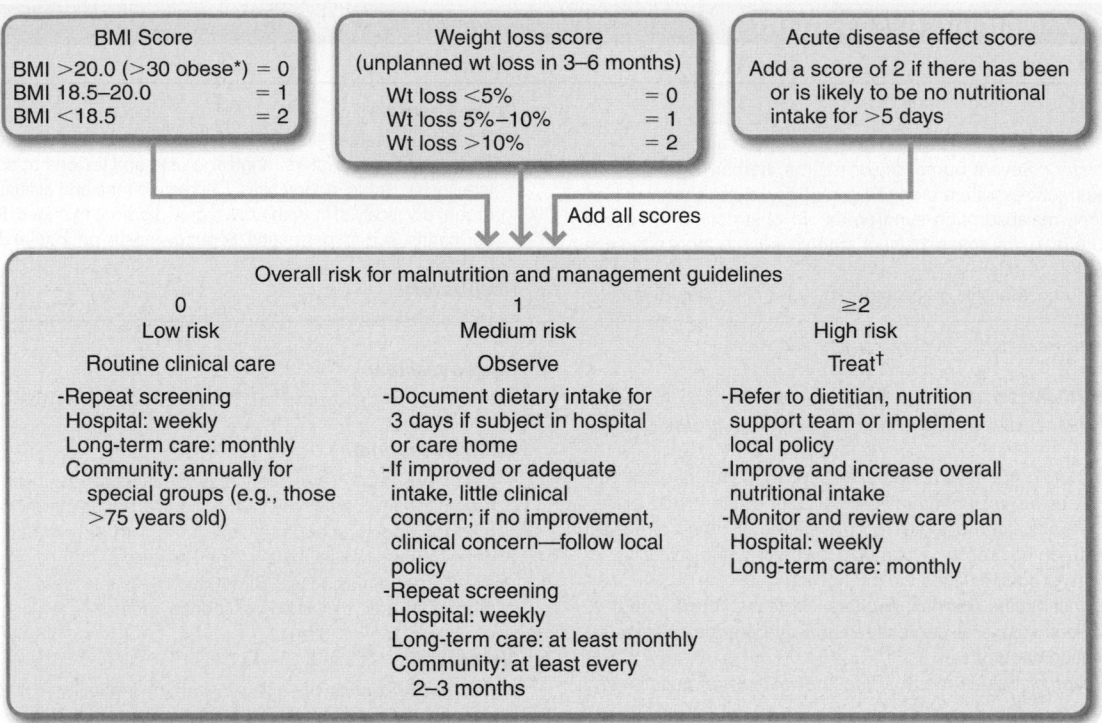

FIG. 39.3 The Malnutrition Universal Screening Tool (MUST) for adults. (Adapted from Mahan LK, Raymond JL: *Krause's food & the nutrition care process*, ed 14, St Louis, 2016, Saunders.)

TABLE 39.8 Components of Nutritional Assessment

Anthropometric Measurements
- Height and weight
- Body mass index (BMI)
- Rate of weight change
- Amount of weight loss

Physical Examination
- Physical appearance
- Muscle mass and strength
- Dental and oral health

Health History
- Personal and family history
- Acute or chronic illnesses
- Current medications, herbs, supplements
- Cognitive status, depression

Diet History
- Chewing and swallowing ability
- Changes in appetite or taste
- Food and nutrient intake
- Availability of food

Laboratory Data
- Glucose
- Electrolytes
- Lipid profile
- Blood urea nitrogen (BUN)
- Albumin, prealbumin, C-reactive protein

Functional Status
- Ability to perform basic and instrumental activities of daily living
- Handgrip strength
- Performance tests (e.g., timed walk tests)

assessment, especially in the older adult.[13] If an involuntary weight loss exceeds 10% of the usual weight, determine the reason. Unintentional weight loss is important to consider in the obese person. Latent malnutrition may be present despite excess body weight. Determine the patient's current weight in relation to ideal body weight.

Body mass index (BMI) is a measure of weight for height (see Fig. 40.6). A BMI of less than 18.5 kg/m² is considered underweight, normal weight is a BMI between 18.5 and 24.9 kg/m², and overweight is a BMI between 25 and 29.9 kg/m². A BMI of 30 kg/m² or greater is obese. BMIs outside the normal weight range are associated with increased morbidity and mortality.

Measure skinfold thickness at various sites (indicators of subcutaneous fat stores) and midarm muscle circumference (indicator of protein stores). The sites most reflective of body fat are those over the biceps and triceps, below the scapula, above the iliac crest, and over the upper thigh. The measures obtained are compared with standards for healthy persons of the same age and gender. Both skinfold thickness and midarm circumference may decrease in malnutrition. Shifts in hydration status influence these measurements. These measurements are most beneficial when done serially and by persons trained in anthropometry.

Functional Measurements. Functional assessment focuses on performance of activities of daily living (ADLs) tools. The tools used most often are the Katz Index and Lawton Scale.[14] Measuring muscle strength can assess physical functional status, an important outcome of nutrition status. Handgrip strength is measured with a hand dynamometer. Timed gait and chair stands are markers of lower extremity strength.

◆ Nursing Diagnoses

Nursing diagnoses for the patient with malnutrition include:
- Impaired nutritional status
- Impaired nutritional intake
- Fluid imbalance
- Risk for impaired tissue integrity

◆ Planning

The overall goals are that the patient with malnutrition will (1) achieve an appropriate weight, (2) consume a specified number of calories per day on an individualized diet, and (3) have no adverse consequences related to malnutrition or nutritional therapies.

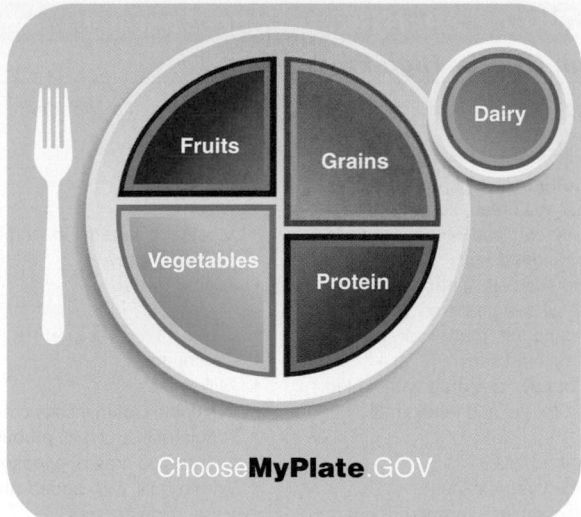

ChooseMyPlate.GOV

FIG. 39.4 MyPlate is the primary food group symbol that serves as a reminder to make healthy food choices and to build a healthy plate at mealtimes. It is a visual cue that shows the 5 food groups from which to select healthy foods. The plate is divided into 4 slightly different-sized quadrants, with fruits and vegetables taking up half the space and grains and protein making up the other half. The vegetables and grains portions are the largest portion. Next to the plate is a blue circle for dairy, which could be a glass of milk or a food, such as cheese or yogurt. For more information, see *www.choosemyplate.gov*. (From US Department of Agriculture, Center for Nutrition Policy and Promotion: *Guidance on use of USDA's MyPlate and statements about amounts of food groups contributed by foods on food product labels*, Washington, DC.)

◆ **Nursing Implementation**

◆ **Health Promotion.** It is part of your role to teach and reinforce healthy eating habits. Use MyPlate, the Dietary Guidelines for Americans, and Nutrition Facts food labels to promote healthy nutrition. The MyPlate approach is a visual guide for sensible meal planning. It helps Americans eat healthfully and make good food choices. MyPlate focuses on the proportions of 5 food groups (grains, protein, fruits, vegetables, and dairy) that you should eat at each meal (Fig. 39.4 and Table 39.9). At the health professionals' link at *www.choosemyplate.gov*, you can download daily food plans, sample menus, and tips for how to be physically active. These materials are valuable to use in patient teaching. MyPlate materials for older adults are available at *https://hnrca.tufts.edu/myplate/*.

There are many resources to help people eat a nutritious diet and maintain a healthy weight. Electronic and print sources are available for determining nutritional information in commonly consumed foods. Many food products have Nutrition Facts labels (Fig. 39.5). Consumer and health professional education materials on Nutrition Facts labels are available on the U.S. Food and Drug Administration (FDA) website (*www.fda.gov/Food/LabelingNutrition/ucm20026097.htm*).

Help the patient find reliable Internet sources that provide evidence-based food and nutrition recommendations. Interactive web-based programs and mobile device applications are available to track physical activity, calories, nutrients, and foods eaten. Mobile device applications help with making healthy eating choices easier. Some use built-in barcode scanners to scan foods quickly and give individual food items' nutrition facts. Users can compare items for their nutrition benefit and cost. Other applications give information on portion sizes

TABLE 39.9 Nutritional Therapy

MyPlate Tips for a Healthy Lifestyle

Making food choices for a healthy lifestyle can be as simple as using these 10 tips. Use the ideas in this list to (1) balance your calories, (2) choose foods to eat more often, and (3) cut back on foods to eat less often.

1. Balance calories	• Find out how many calories you need for a day as a first step in managing your weight. Go to *www.choosemyplate.gov* to find your calorie level. • Being physically active also helps you balance calories.
2. Enjoy your food, but eat less	• Take the time to enjoy your food as you eat it. • Eating too fast or when your attention is elsewhere may lead to eating too many calories. • Pay attention to hunger and fullness cues before, during, and after meals. Use them to recognize when to eat and when you have had enough.
3. Avoid over-sized portions	• Use a smaller plate, bowl, and glass. • Portion out foods before you eat. • When eating out, choose a smaller size portion, share a dish, or take home part of your meal.
4. Foods to eat more often	• Eat more vegetables, fruits, whole grains, and fat-free or 1% milk and dairy products. • These foods have the nutrients you need for health, including potassium, calcium, vitamin D, and fiber. • Make them the basis for meals and snacks.
5. Make half your plate fruits and vegetables	• Choose red, orange, and dark-green vegetables such as tomatoes, sweet potatoes, and broccoli, along with other vegetables, for your meals. • Add fruit to meals as part of main or side dishes or as dessert.
6. Switch to fat-free or low-fat (1%) milk	• They have the same amount of calcium and other essential nutrients as whole milk. • They have fewer calories and less saturated fat.
7. Make half your grains whole grains	• To eat more whole grains, substitute a whole-grain product for a refined product. • For example, eat whole-wheat bread instead of white bread, or brown rice instead of white rice.
8. Foods to eat less often	• Cut back on foods high in solid fats, added sugars, and salt. • Limit cakes, cookies, ice cream, candies, sweetened drinks, pizza, and fatty meats such as ribs, sausages, bacon, and hot dogs. • Use these foods as occasional treats, not everyday foods.
9. Compare sodium in foods	• Use the Nutrition Facts label (Fig. 39.4) to choose lower sodium versions of foods, such as soup, bread, and frozen meals. • Select foods labeled "low sodium," "reduced sodium," or "no salt added."
10. Drink water instead of sugary drinks	• Cut calories by drinking water or unsweetened beverages. • Soda, energy drinks, and sports drinks are a major source of added sugar and calories in American diets.

Source: US Department of Agriculture Center for Nutrition Policy and Promotion: Nutrition education series, DG Tips Sheet No 1, June 2011. Retrieved from *www.choosemyplate.gov* and *www.health.gov/dietaryguidelines*.

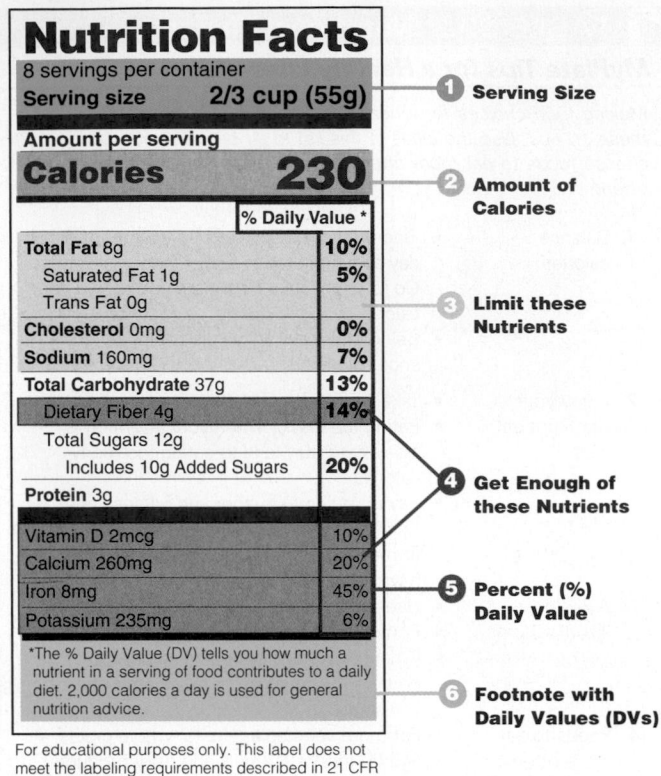

Nutrition Facts

8 servings per container

Serving size   **2/3 cup (55g)**   ① **Serving Size**

Amount per serving

Calories   **230**   ② **Amount of Calories**

	% Daily Value *
Total Fat 8g	**10%**
Saturated Fat 1g	**5%**
Trans Fat 0g	
Cholesterol 0mg	**0%**
Sodium 160mg	**7%**
Total Carbohydrate 37g	**13%**
Dietary Fiber 4g	**14%**
Total Sugars 12g	
Includes 10g Added Sugars	**20%**
Protein 3g	
Vitamin D 2mcg	10%
Calcium 260mg	20%
Iron 8mg	45%
Potassium 235mg	6%

③ **Limit these Nutrients**

④ **Get Enough of these Nutrients**

⑤ **Percent (%) Daily Value**

*The % Daily Value (DV) tells you how much a nutrient in a serving of food contributes to a daily diet. 2,000 calories a day is used for general nutrition advice.

⑥ **Footnote with Daily Values (DVs)**

For educational purposes only. This label does not meet the labeling requirements described in 21 CFR 101.9.

FIG. 39.5 Sample of a Nutrition Facts label. (From US Department of Health and Human Services, *Nutrition facts label,* Silver Spring, MD.)

and adjustments needed to reduce calories, sodium, or fat in the diet based on the user's height, weight, and activity level.

Acute Care. Collaborate with the HCP and dietitian to identify patients with malnutrition and implement appropriate interventions to meet the patient's nutritional needs. Assess nutritional state during your assessment of the patient's other physical problems. Identify risk factors for malnutrition and why they exist. With increased stress, such as surgery, severe trauma, and sepsis, the patient needs more calories and protein. Wound healing requires increased protein synthesis. The patient having major surgery who is malnourished or is at risk for malnutrition needs several weeks of increased protein and calorie intake preoperatively to promote healing postoperatively.

Teach the patient and caregiver the importance of good nutrition and the reason for recording the daily weight, intake, and output. Measure weight and height on admission, then routinely assess the person's weight. Daily weights give an ongoing record of body weight gain or loss. Rapid gains and losses are usually the result of shifts in fluid balance. In conjunction with accurate recording of food and fluid intake, body weight gives a clearer picture of the patient's fluid and nutritional state.

If the patient can take food by mouth, obtain a daily calorie count and diet diary to give an accurate record of food intake. You and the dietitian can help the patient and family in selecting high-calorie and high-protein foods (unless medically contraindicated). Table 39.10 gives examples of high-calorie, high-protein foods. Offering foods preferred by the patient enhances intake. Encourage the family to bring the patient's favorite foods from home.

Make sure the environment is conducive to eating. Provide a quiet environment. Offer oral hygiene and hand hygiene. Help the patient to a comfortable position and place the bedside table at the right height. Clear the bedside table of clutter. Place

TABLE 39.10 Nutritional Therapy

High-Calorie, High-Protein Diet

Suggestions for foods for a high-calorie, high-protein diet include:

Breads and Cereals
- Buttermilk biscuits, muffins, banana bread, zucchini bread
- Granola and other cereals with dried fruit
- Hot cereals (oatmeal, cream of wheat) prepared with milk, added fat (butter or margarine), and sugar
- Potatoes prepared with added fat (butter and whole milk)

Vegetables
- Fried vegetables
- Vegetables prepared with added fat (margarine, butter)

Fruits
- Canned fruit in heavy syrup
- Dried fruit

Meat
- Casseroles
- Fried meats
- Meats covered in cream sauces or gravy
- Peanut butter

Milk and Milk Products
- Ice cream
- Milkshakes
- Whipping cream, heavy cream
- Whole milk and milk products (yogurt, ice cream, cheese)
- Whole milk with added nutritional supplements

urinals, bedpans, and emesis basins out of sight. If needed, open cartons and packages. Protect mealtime from unnecessary interruptions by performing nonurgent care before or after mealtime.

The undernourished patient usually needs to have between-meal supplements. These may consist of items prepared in the dietary department or commercially prepared products. Eating these items provides extra calories, proteins, fluids, and nutrients. If the patient is unable to consume enough nutrition with a high-calorie, high-protein diet, consider adding oral liquid nutritional supplements.

Some patients may benefit from appetite stimulants, such as megestrol acetate or dronabinol (Marinol), to improve intake. Enteral nutrition (EN) may be an option in the patient who is still unable to take in enough calories (Fig. 39.6). Contraindications for EN include GI obstruction, prolonged ileus, severe diarrhea or vomiting, and enterocutaneous fistula. If EN is not possible, consider starting parenteral nutrition (PN).

Ambulatory Care. Many patients are discharged on a therapeutic diet. Discharge preparation for both the patient and caregiver is essential. Teach them about the cause of the undernourished state and ways to avoid the problem in the future. They need to be aware that undernourishment, whatever the cause, can recur and that adhering to their diet for a few weeks cannot fully restore a normal nutritional state. It may take many months to reach this goal.

Assess their ability to follow the dietary instructions considering past eating habits, religious and ethnic preferences, age, income, resources, and state of health. Emphasize the need for continual follow-up care to achieve and maintain rehabilitation. In your discharge planning, ensure proper follow-up, such as visits by the home health nurse and outpatient dietitian referrals.

Determine the need for nutritious meals and snacks after discharge from the hospital. If access to a dietitian is limited, you may be the main source of nutritional information. In your assessment, consider the availability and acceptability of community resources that provide meals, such as Meals on Wheels, senior congregate feeding sites, and the Supplemental Nutrition Assistance Program (SNAP). SNAP allows low-income households, regardless of age, to buy more food of a greater variety.

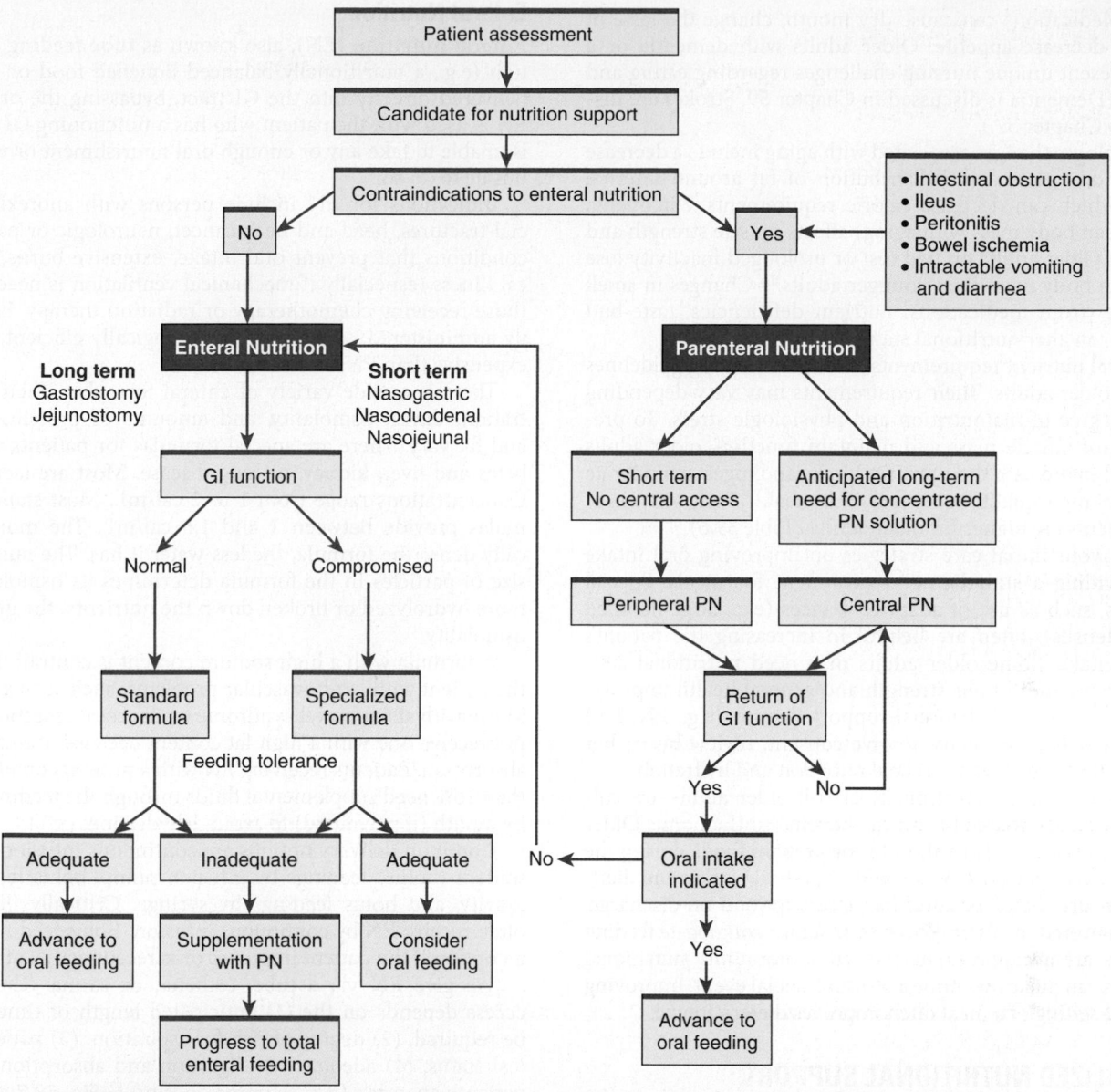

FIG. 39.6 Nutritional support algorithm. (Adapted from Ukleja A, Freeman KL, Gilbert K, ASPEN Board of Directors: Standards for nutrition support: Adult hospitalized patients, *Nutr Clin Pract* 25:403, 2010.)

Keeping a diet diary for 3 days at a time is one way to analyze and reinforce healthful eating patterns. These records are also helpful in the follow-up care. Encourage self-assessment of progress by having the patient weigh himself or herself once or twice a week and keep a weight record.

◆ Evaluation

The expected outcomes are that the patient who is malnourished will

- Achieve and maintain optimal body weight
- Consume a well-balanced diet
- Has no adverse outcomes related to malnutrition
- Maintain optimal physical functioning

Gerontologic Considerations: Malnutrition

Nutrition affects quality of life, functional status, and health in older adults. They are particularly vulnerable to malnutrition across care settings. You play a key role in assessing the physiologic, functional, environmental, dietary, psychologic, and

social factors related to nutritional risk in older adults. Older hospitalized adults with malnutrition are more likely to have poor wound healing, pressure injuries, infections, decreased muscle strength, postoperative complications, and increased morbidity and mortality risks. They are less able to regain body weight after periods of undernutrition due to illness or surgery.

Older adults may report little or no appetite, problems with eating or swallowing, inadequate servings of nutrients, and fewer than 2 meals per day. Limited incomes may cause them to restrict the number of meals or the dietary quality of meals eaten. Social isolation is a problem in older adults. Those who live alone may lose their desire to cook and report decreased appetite. Functional limitations may affect the ability to feed oneself, buy food, or cook and prepare meals. Some may lack transportation to buy food.

Chronic illnesses associated with aging can affect nutritional status. For example, depression and dysphagia (from a stroke) can affect intake. Poor oral health from gum disease, missing teeth, or dry mouth can impair the ability to chew and swallow food.[15] Medications can cause dry mouth, change the taste of food, or decrease appetite. Older adults with dementia or a stroke present unique nursing challenges regarding eating and feeding. (Dementia is discussed in Chapter 59. Strokes are discussed in Chapter 57.)

Physiologic changes associated with aging include a decrease in lean body mass and redistribution of fat around internal organs, which can decrease caloric requirements. Sarcopenia (loss of lean body mass with aging) affects muscle strength and function. Older adults on bed rest or prolonged inactivity lose more lean body mass than younger adults.[16] Changes in smell and taste (from medications, nutrient deficiencies, taste-bud atrophy) can alter nutritional status.

General nutrient requirements and healthy eating guidelines apply to older adults. Their requirements may vary depending on the degree of malnutrition and physiologic stress. To prevent loss of muscle mass and maintain function, older adults may need to increase their protein intake and ingest a moderate amount of high-quality protein at each meal.[17] Daily vitamin D requirements are higher for older adults (Table 39.6).

Focus your initial care strategies on improving oral intake and providing a stimulating environment for meals. Special strategies, such as use of adaptive devices (e.g., large-handled eating utensils), often are helpful in increasing the patient's dietary intake. Some older adults may need nutritional support therapies until their strength and general health improve. Before starting any nutritional support therapy (e.g., EN, PN) for an older patient unable to give consent, review his or her advance directives about artificial nutrition and hydration.

Malnourished or nutritionally at-risk older adults are vulnerable when discharged from the hospital to the home. Older adults may not be able to shop for or prepare foods during the initial recovery period. Consult with the social worker and dietitian to ensure the older adult has access to food on discharge. Home-delivered meals or groceries or senior congregate feeding programs are an appropriate referral. Community nutritional programs can make mealtime a pleasant, social event. Improving the social setting of a meal often improves dietary intake.

SPECIALIZED NUTRITIONAL SUPPORT

If patients are unable to maintain or achieve adequate nutritional status, nutritional support may be needed. For a decision-making plan related to nutritional support, see Fig. 39.6.

Some agencies have nutritional support teams composed of a physician, nurse, dietitian, and pharmacist. The team's function is to oversee the nutritional support of select inpatients and outpatients. The nutritional support nurse on that team is a key resource for issues about patients' nutrition and nutritional access.

Oral Feeding

Oral supplements are widely used as an adjunct to meals and fluid intake in the patient whose nutritional intake is deficient. They provide advanced nutrition and calories and are relatively inexpensive. These include milkshakes, puddings, or commercially available products (e.g., Carnation Instant Breakfast, Ensure, Boost). Oral liquid supplements have a role in improving the nutritional status of older adults. Do not use supplements as meal substitutes, use them as snacks between meals. In long-term care, using these beverages instead of water for oral medication administration increases caloric intake.

Enteral Nutrition

Enteral nutrition (EN), also known as tube feeding, is nutrition (e.g., a nutritionally balanced liquefied food or formula) delivered directly into the GI tract, bypassing the oral cavity. EN is used with the patient who has a functioning GI tract but is unable to take any or enough oral nourishment or when it is unsafe to do so.

Indications for EN include persons with anorexia, orofacial fractures, head and neck cancer, neurologic or psychiatric conditions that prevent oral intake, extensive burns, or critical illness (especially if mechanical ventilation is needed), and those receiving chemotherapy or radiation therapy. EN is easily administered, safer, more physiologically efficient, and less expensive than PN.

There is a wide variety of enteral formulas. Their concentration, flavor, osmolality, and amounts of protein, sodium, and fat vary. There are special formulas for patients with diabetes and liver, kidney, or lung disease. Most are lactose free. Concentrations range from 1 to 2 cal/mL. Most standard formulas provide between 1 and 1.5 cal/mL. The more calorically dense the formula, the less water it has. The number and size of particles in the formula determines its osmolality. The more hydrolyzed or broken down the nutrients, the greater the osmolality.

A formula with a high sodium content is contraindicated in the patient with cardiovascular problems, such as heart failure. Those with short bowel syndrome or ileocecal resection should not receive one with a high fat content because of impaired fat absorption. Patients receiving EN with a protein content greater than 16% need supplemental fluids through the feeding tube or by mouth (if permitted) to avoid dehydration.

Common delivery options are continuous infusion or intermittent (bolus) feedings by infusion pump, bolus feedings by gravity, and bolus feedings by syringe. Critically ill patients often receive EN by continuous infusion. Bolus feeding may be an option if the patient improves or is receiving EN at home.[17]

We give EN via a tube, catheter, or stoma. The type of access depends on the (1) anticipated length of time EN will be required, (2) degree of risk for aspiration, (3) patient's clinical status, (4) adequacy of digestion and absorption, and (5) patient's anatomy (e.g., extreme obesity).[12] Fig. 39.7 shows the locations of commonly used enteral feeding tubes.

Orogastric, Nasogastric, and Nasointestinal Tubes. Nasally and orally placed tubes (orogastric, nasogastric [NG], nasoduodenal, nasojejunal) are appropriate for short-term feeding (less than 4 weeks). Nasoduodenal and nasojejunal tubes are transpyloric tubes. They are used when pathophysiologic conditions call for feeding the patient below the pyloric sphincter. Placement into the small intestine decreases the chance of regurgitating gastric contents into the esophagus and aspiration.[17] However, the patient can still aspirate gastric secretions if the stomach is not emptying properly.

Polyurethane or silicone feeding tubes are long, small in diameter, soft, and flexible. This design decreases the risk for mucosal damage from prolonged placement. These tubes are radiopaque, making their position readily identified by x-ray. A stylet is used for tube placement in a comatose patient because the ability to swallow is not essential during insertion. A complication that can result from using a stylet is increased risk for perforation.

While smaller feeding tubes have many advantages over tubes with wider lumens, such as the standard decompression

NG tube, there are some disadvantages. Because of the small diameter and length, these tubes clog easily. They are harder to use for checking residual volumes. They are particularly prone to occlusion if you do not thoroughly crush and dissolve oral drugs before administration. Failure to flush the tubing before and after giving drugs or checking residual volume can cause tube occlusion. Vomiting or coughing can dislodge the tubes. They can become knotted or kinked. Problems with a tube may require removal and insertion of a new tube, which adds to cost and patient discomfort.

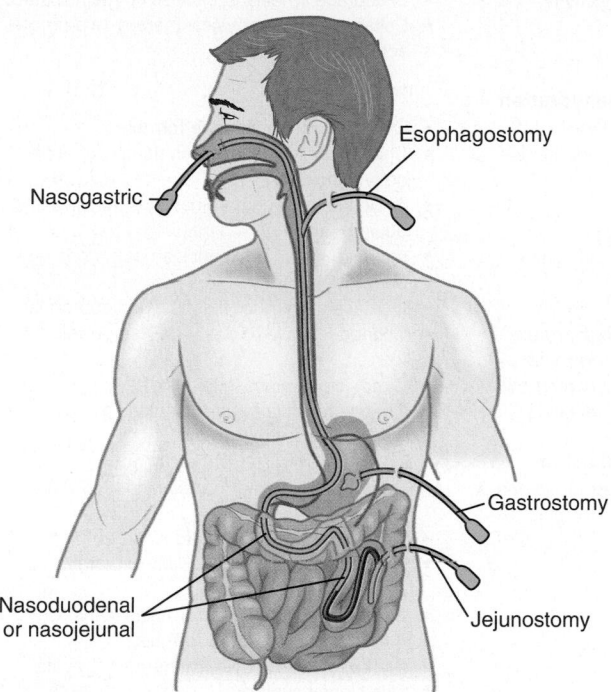

FIG. 39.7 Common enteral feeding tube placement locations.

Gastrostomy and Jejunostomy Tubes. If feedings are needed for an extended time, tubes can be placed in the stomach (gastrostomy) or small bowel (jejunostomy). A gastrostomy tube can be placed surgically, radiologically, or endoscopically (Fig. 39.7). The patient must have an intact, unobstructed GI tract. The esophageal lumen must be wide enough to pass the endoscope for percutaneous endoscopic gastrostomy (PEG) tube placement (Fig. 39.8). PEG tube and radiologically placed gastrostomy tube procedures have fewer risks than surgical placement. The procedure requires IV sedation and local anesthesia. IV antibiotics are given before the procedure.

For the patient with chronic reflux, feeding through a jejunostomy (J-tube) may be necessary to reduce the risk for aspiration. Jejunostomy tubes are placed either endoscopically or with open or laparoscopic surgery. Combination gastrojejunostomy (G-J) tubes allow for simultaneous gastric decompression and small bowel feeding. When a patient has a G-J tube, it is important to know which port is the gastric and which is the jejunal.

The tube is either premarked or marked at the skin insertion site. Enteral feedings can start within 24 hours after a surgically placed gastrostomy or jejunostomy tube without waiting for flatus or a bowel movement. Most other PEG tube feedings can start within 4 hours of insertion, although agency policies may vary.[17]

EN and Safety. You have a critical role in ensuring that EN is administered safely. Aspiration and dislodged tubes are important safety concerns. Nursing management of enteral feeding is addressed in Table 39.11.

Accidental tube removal can result in delayed feedings and potential discomfort with tube replacement. The management of common problems in patients receiving EN is outlined in Table 39.12. A nursing care plan for the patient receiving EN (eNursing Care Plan 39.1) is available on the website for this chapter.

Specific care and teaching related to feeding tubes and EN are discussed in the following section. Remember that is important

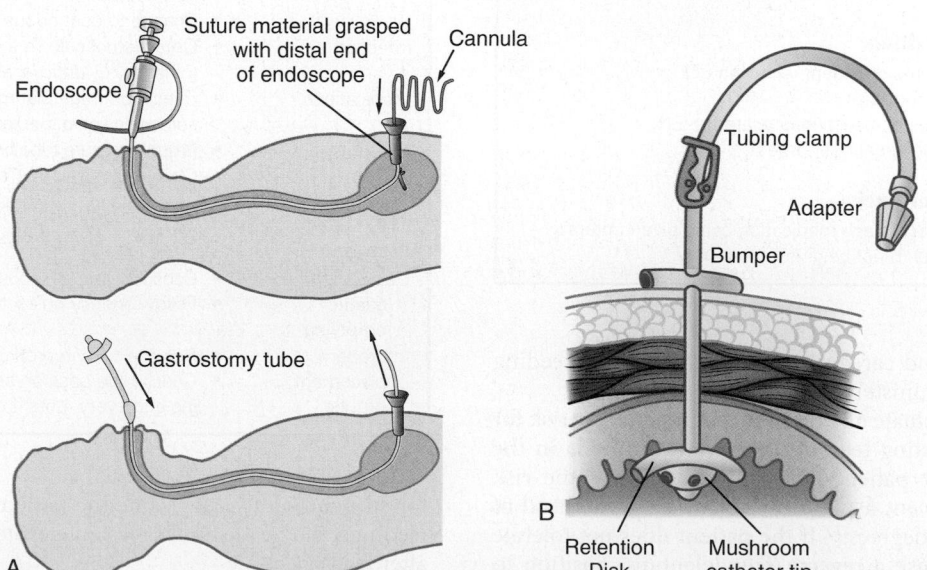

FIG. 39.8 Percutaneous endoscopic gastrostomy. **A,** Gastrostomy tube placement via percutaneous endoscopy. With use of endoscopy, a gastrostomy tube is inserted through the esophagus into the stomach and then pulled through a stab wound made in the abdominal wall. **B,** A retention disk and bumper secure the tube.

TABLE 39.11 Nursing Management

EN

Maintaining EN Infusions
- Check tube placement before feeding and before each medication administration.
- Assess for bowel sounds before feeding.
- Flush NG or gastrostomy tube as needed.
- Evaluate nutritional status of patient receiving enteral feedings.

Ensuring Patient Safety
- Give medications in the safest form possible.
  - Dilute viscous liquid medications.
  - Use liquid medications only if they are designated safe for enteral use.
  - Do not add medications to enteral feeding formula.
  - If using tablets, only use immediate-release forms.
  - Crush drugs to a fine powder and dissolve in 30–60 mL of purified water.
- Employ measures to decrease aspiration risk.
- Keep head of bed elevated to 30- to 45-degree angle.
- Check for GVR per agency policy.
- Assess regularly for complications related to tubes and enteral feedings (e.g., aspiration, diarrhea, abdominal distention, hyperglycemia, fecal impaction).
- Teach patient and caregiver about home EN and tube care.

Delegate to Licensed Practical/Vocational Nurse (LPN/VN)
- Insert NG tube for stable patient.
- Flush NG and gastrostomy tubes.
- Give bolus or continuous enteral feeding for stable patient.
- Remove NG tube.
- Give medications through NG or gastrostomy tube to stable patient.
- Provide skin care around gastrostomy or jejunostomy tubes.

Oversee Unlicensed Assistive Personnel (UAP)
- Provide oral care to patient with NG, gastrostomy, or jejunostomy tube.
- Weigh patient who is receiving EN.
- Keep the head of bed elevated 30–45 degrees.
- Report patient symptoms (e.g., nausea, diarrhea) that may indicate problems with EN to RN or LPN.
- Alert RN or LPN about infusion pump alarms.
- Empty drainage devices and measure output.

Collaborate With Dietitian
- Evaluate nutritional status of patient receiving EN.
- Select appropriate EN formula.
- Monitor for and manage complications related to EN.
- Teach patient and caregiver about home EN.

Collaborate With Pharmacist
- Select appropriate form of each medication being given enterally.
- Determine if medication must be given separately.

TABLE 39.12 Nursing Management

EN Problems

Problems and Causes	Management
Constipation	
Decreased fluid intake	• Increase fluid intake if not contraindicated. • Give total fluid intake of 30 mL/kg body weight.
Formula	• Change formula to one with more fiber content. • Give as-needed laxative.
Inactivity	• Encourage ambulation unless contraindicated. • Collaborate with physical therapy to promote activity.
Dehydration	
Diarrhea, vomiting	• Decrease rate or change formula. • Check drugs that patient is receiving, especially antibiotics. • Avoid bacterial contamination of formula and equipment.
Fluid intake	• Increase intake and check amount and number of feedings. • Increase amount of fluid intake if appropriate.
High-protein formula	• Change formula to one with less protein.
Hyperosmotic diuresis	• Check blood glucose levels often. • Change formula to one with less glucose.
Diarrhea	
Contaminated formula	• Refrigerate unused formula and record date opened. • Discard outdated formula. • Discard formula left standing for longer than manufacturer's guidelines. • 8 hrs for ready-to-feed formulas (cans) • 4 hrs for reconstituted formula • 24 hrs for closed-system enteral formulas • Use closed system.
Feeding too fast	• Dilute or decrease rate of feeding. • Change to continuous feedings. • Stop excess water boluses.
Formula	• Change to formula that has more fiber or is less hypertonic. • Change to continuous feedings.
Infection	• Obtain stool culture for fecal leukocyte determination, *C. difficile,* and/or toxin assay.
Medications	• Check for drugs that may cause diarrhea (e.g., sorbitol in liquid medications, antibiotics).
Tube moving distally	• Properly secure tube before beginning feeding. • Check placement before each bolus feeding or at least every 4 hrs if continuous feedings.
Vomiting	
Delayed gastric emptying	• Consult with HCP about use of prokinetic drug. • Follow agency policy to manage GRV.
Improper placement of tube	• Replace tube in proper position. • Check tube position before each bolus feeding and every 4 hrs if continuous feedings.

to teach the patient and caregiver how to care for the feeding tube and properly administer EN.

Aspiration Risk. Evaluate all enterally fed patients for risk for aspiration. Before starting feedings, ensure the tube is in the right position. Proper patient positioning decreases the risk for aspiration. To prevent aspiration, always keep the head of bed elevated 30 to 45 degrees.[17] If the patient does not tolerate a backrest elevation, use a reverse Trendelenburg position to elevate the head of the bed, unless contraindicated. If you need to lower the head of the bed for a procedure, quickly returning the patient to at least 30 degrees is critical. Follow agency policy

for suspending feeding while the patient is supine. With bolus feedings, the head should remain elevated for 30 to 60 minutes after feeding.

There is much disagreement about whether to check gastric residual volume (GRV) when giving feedings into the stomach. Some think an increased GRV increases the risk for aspiration.

Other research does not support the practice. Follow your agency policy for checking GRV. Common protocols call for checking GRV every 6 to 8 hours in non–critically ill patients and before each bolus feeding.

Other measures to decrease aspiration risk include giving feedings continuously, minimizing the use of sedation, and performing frequent oral suctioning, if needed. Promotility drugs, such as erythromycin or metoclopramide, improve gastric emptying and may reduce aspiration risk.

Tube Position. Obtain x-ray confirmation of newly inserted nasal or orogastric tubes to confirm proper position before starting feedings or medications. Smaller feeding tubes can pass directly into the bronchus on insertion without any obvious respiratory manifestations. Do not rely on the auscultation method to determine between gastric and respiratory or gastric and small bowel placement. Placing a tube under electromagnetic guidance reduces the risk for misplacement associated with blind insertion.[17] Capnography, a direct monitor of breath-to-breath CO_2 level, can determine tube placement in the respiratory tract. However, it still requires x-ray confirmation to verify location before feeding.[17]

Maintain proper placement of the tube after starting feedings. To determine if a tube is still in the proper position, mark the exit site of the tube at the time of the initial x-ray and check the tube external length at regular intervals.[17] Consider applying a nasal bridle in patients who try to pull out a tube or for whom taping the nose is difficult.

A small bowel tube may dislocate upward into the stomach, or the tube's tip can dislocate upward into the esophagus. If you see a significant increase in the external length, use other bedside tests to help determine whether the tube has become dislocated. These measures include assessing aspirate color and pH. Because each of these measures has limitations, confirm placement with more than one test. If you are checking GVR, watch for unexpected changes in volume. An increase in GVR may indicate displacement of a small intestine tube into the stomach.[18]

Site Care. Skin care around gastrostomy and jejunostomy tube sites is important because the action of digestive juices irritates the skin. Assess the skin around the feeding tube daily for signs of redness and maceration. Monitor bumper tension and routinely check for pressure injury.

To keep the skin clean and dry, initially rinse it with sterile water and dry it. Apply a dressing until the site is healed. After that, wash with mild soap and water. A protective ointment (zinc oxide, petroleum gauze) or a skin barrier (Karaya, Stomahesive) may be used on the skin around the tube. If the skin is irritated, consider using other types of drain or tube pouches. Consult a wound, ostomy, and continence nurse (WOCN) if problems occur.

Tube Patency. All enteral feedings require routine flushing. Flush feeding tubes in adults with 30 mL of warm tap water every 4 hours during continuous feedings or before and after each bolus feeding. Use sterile water in immunocompromised and critically ill patients. Always flush tubes between each medication and after all medications are given. Flush clogged tubes with warm water, using a back-and-forth motion. If that does not work, a pancreatic enzyme solution, an enzymatic declogging kit, or mechanical devices for clearing feeding tubes are options.[17]

Misconnection. An *enteral feeding misconnection* is an inadvertent connection between an enteral feeding system and

---

TABLE 39.13 Nursing Management
Decreasing Enteral Feeding Misconnections

The following are tips to help you decrease your risk for making an enteral feeding misconnection:

1. Teach visitors, LPN/VNs, and UAP to notify the nurse if an enteral feeding line becomes disconnected and not to reconnect any line.
2. Do not change or adapt IV or feeding devices because it may compromise the safety features incorporated into their design.
3. Do not use an IV pump or IV tubing to deliver an enteral feeding.
4. When making a reconnection or connecting any new device or infusion, trace lines back to their origins and ensure connections are secure.
5. When patient arrives on a new unit or setting or during shift hand-off, recheck connections and trace all tubes.
6. Route tubes and catheters that have different purposes in unique and standardized directions (e.g., route IV lines toward the patient's head and enteral lines toward the feet).
7. Label or color-code feeding tubes and connectors.
8. When there are multiple access points and/or several bags hanging, place proximal and distal labels on all tubings.
9. Check the patient's vital signs after making any connection.
10. Identify and confirm a solution's label, since a 3-in-1 PN solution can look like an enteral nutrition formulation bag. Label the bags with large, bold statements such as "WARNING! For Enteral Use Only—NOT for IV Use."
11. Make all connections under proper lighting conditions.

---

a nonenteral system, such as an IV line, a peritoneal dialysis catheter, or a tracheostomy tube cuff. With an enteral feeding misconnection, nutritional formula intended for the GI tract is given IV or into the respiratory tract. Severe patient injury and death can result from tubing misconnection. Table 39.13 gives tips to decrease the risk for enteral feeding misconnections.

Gerontologic Considerations: Enteral Nutrition

EN is used in the older patient to improve nutritional status. Because of physiologic changes associated with aging, the older adult is more vulnerable to complications associated with EN, especially fluid and electrolyte imbalances. Complications such as diarrhea can leave the patient dehydrated. Decreased thirst perception or impaired cognitive function decreases the patient's ability to seek needed fluids.

With aging, there is an increased risk for glucose intolerance. As a result, the older patient may be more susceptible to hyperglycemia from the high carbohydrate load of some EN formulas. The older adult with compromised cardiovascular function (e.g., heart failure) will have a decreased ability to handle large volumes of formula. If this happens, the patient may need a more concentrated formula (2.0 cal/mL). The older adult has an increased risk for aspiration caused by gastroesophageal reflux disease (GERD), delayed gastric emptying, hiatal hernia, or decreased gag reflex. Physical mobility, fine motor movement, and visual system changes associated with aging may contribute to problems managing EN in the home setting.

Parenteral Nutrition

Parenteral nutrition (PN) is the administration of nutrients directly into the bloodstream. PN is used when the GI tract cannot be used for the ingestion, digestion, and absorption of essential nutrients. Table 39.14 lists common reasons for the use of PN. PN is a relatively safe method of providing complete nutritional support.

TABLE 39.14 **Common Indications for PN**	
• Chronic severe diarrhea and vomiting	• Intractable diarrhea
• Complicated surgery or trauma	• Severe anorexia nervosa
• GI obstruction	• Severe malabsorption
• GI tract anomalies and fistulae	• Short bowel syndrome

Composition. PN is customized to meet the needs of each patient. The composition is reformulated as the patient's condition changes. This requires you to collaborate with the interprofessional team in delivering PN to the patient.

Commercially prepared PN base solutions are available. These base solutions contain dextrose and protein in the form of amino acids. The pharmacy adds prescribed electrolytes (e.g., sodium, potassium, chloride, calcium, magnesium, phosphate), vitamins, and trace elements (e.g., zinc, copper, chromium, selenium, manganese) to meet the patient's needs. A 3-in-1 or total nutrient admixture containing an IV fat emulsion, dextrose, and amino acids is widely used. Premixed PN solutions require mixing the dextrose and amino acid chambers prior to use. Standard electrolytes are available in some premixed solutions. Multivitamins can be added before use.[19]

Calories. Calories in PN mainly come from carbohydrates in the form of dextrose and by fat in the form of fat emulsion. Dextrose 100 to 150 g/day (1 g provides about 3.4 calories, as opposed to oral carbohydrates, which provide 4 calories) has a protein-sparing effect. Providing adequate nonprotein calories in the form of glucose and fat allows the use of amino acids for wound healing and not for energy. However, overfeeding can lead to metabolic complications. To minimize these problems, the recommended energy intake is 25 to 30 cal/kg/day in a nonobese patient.[19]

Fat-emulsion solutions of 10%, 20%, and 30% are available. Fat emulsions supply about 1 cal/mL (10% solution) or 2 cal/mL (20% solution). Fat emulsions primarily contain soybean or safflower triglycerides with egg phospholipids added as an emulsifier. They supply a large number of calories in a small amount of fluid. This is beneficial when the patient is at risk for fluid overload.

IV fat emulsions should provide up to 20% to 30% of total calories of PN. Most stable patients receive 1 g/kg/day. The maximum daily lipid dose is 2.5 g/kg/day. Critically ill patients may not tolerate this dose and may receive less than 1 g/kg/day. Serum triglyceride levels are done at the beginning of PN and then closely monitored. Give IV fat emulsions administered separately over 12 hours.[19] The infusion rate should not exceed 0.5 mL/kg/hr.

Fat emulsions are contraindicated in the patient with a problem with fat metabolism, such as hyperlipidemia. They are used cautiously in the patient at risk for fat embolism (e.g., fractured femur) and the patient with an allergy to eggs or soybeans.

Protein. Protein is provided at the rate of 1 to 1.5 g/kg/day depending on the patient's needs. In a nutritionally depleted patient who is under the stress of illness or surgery, protein requirements can exceed 150 g/day (2 g/kg/day) to ensure a positive nitrogen balance. Burn and multiple trauma patients may need more than 2 g/kg protein.[20] Protein needs may be lower than 1 g/kg and restricted in those with end-stage renal disease who are not on dialysis.

Electrolytes. The exact amount of electrolytes needed depends on the patient's health problem and on serum electrolyte levels. Assess individual requirements daily at the beginning of therapy and then several times a week as the treatment progresses. The following are ranges for average daily electrolyte requirements for adult patients without renal or liver impairment:

- Sodium: 1 to 2 mEq/kg
- Potassium: 1 to 2 mEq/kg
- Magnesium: 8 to 20 mEq
- Calcium: 10 to 15 mEq
- Phosphate: 20 to 40 mmol

Trace Elements and Vitamins. Zinc, copper, manganese, selenium, and chromium are added according to the patient's condition and needs. Monitor levels of these elements. The daily addition of a multivitamin preparation to the PN generally meets the vitamin requirements. The HCP may order additional amounts.

Methods of Administration. PN is given as central PN or peripheral parenteral nutrition (PPN). Central PN and PPN differ in nutrient content and tonicity, which is measured in milliosmoles (mOsm; the concentration of particles in a fluid).

Central Parenteral Nutrition. Central PN is indicated when long-term support is needed or when the patient has high protein and caloric requirements. We give central PN through a central venous catheter or a peripherally inserted central catheter (PICC) whose tip lies in the superior vena cava (see Chapter 16). Central PN solutions are hypertonic, measuring at least 1600 mOsm/L. The high glucose content ranges from 20% to 50%. Central PN must be infused in a large central vein so that rapid dilution can occur. The use of a peripheral vein for hypertonic, central PN solutions would cause irritation and thrombophlebitis.

Peripheral Parenteral Nutrition. PPN is given through a peripherally inserted catheter or vascular access device into a large vein. PPN is used when (1) nutritional support is needed for only a short time, (2) protein and caloric requirements are not high, (3) the risk for a central catheter is too great, or (4) to supplement inadequate oral intake.

Compared with central PN, PPN has fewer nutrients. While this makes PPN less hypertonic, it still has an osmolality of up to 800 mOsm/L. This increases the risk for phlebitis. Another potential complication is fluid overload. PPN requires large volumes of fluid, which many patients cannot tolerate.

❖ NURSING MANAGEMENT: PARENTERAL NUTRITION

Nursing management of patients receiving PN is outlined in Table 39.15 and eNursing Care Plan 39.2, available on the website for this chapter.

◆ Complications

Complications associated with PN are related to either the catheter or the PN infusion itself (Table 39.16).

Refeeding syndrome can occur any time a malnourished patient starts aggressive nutritional support. It is characterized by fluid retention and electrolyte imbalances (hypophosphatemia, hypokalemia, hypomagnesemia). Hypophosphatemia is the hallmark of refeeding syndrome. It is associated with serious outcomes, including dysrhythmias, respiratory arrest, and neurologic problems (e.g., paresthesias). Conditions that predispose patients to refeeding syndrome include long-standing malnutrition states, such as chronic alcohol use, vomiting and diarrhea, chemotherapy, and major surgery.

TABLE 39.15 Nursing Management
PN Infusions

Preparation of PN Solutions

- All PN solutions must be prepared by a pharmacist or trained technician using strict aseptic techniques under a laminar flow hood.
- Add nothing to PN solutions after they are prepared in the pharmacy.
- Limit number of people involved in preparing and administering PN to reduce risk for infection.
- PN solutions are ordered daily to adjust to the patient's current needs.
- PN solution label shows the nutrient content, all additives, time mixed, and expiration date and time.
- Solutions are good for 24 hrs and must be refrigerated until 30 min before use.

Maintaining PN Infusions

- Follow proper aseptic techniques to reduce infection risk.
- Use a 0.22-micron filter with parenteral solutions not containing fat emulsion and a 1.2-micron filter with solutions containing fat emulsion.
- Change filters and IV tubing with each new PN container or every 24 hr.
- Label tubing and filter with date and time they are put into use.
- If a multilumen catheter is present, use a dedicated line for PN.
- Do not draw blood from a line dedicated for PN unless absolutely necessary.
- Control the infusion rate. Give PN using an infusion pump.
- Set an alarm to alert for tubing obstruction.
- Periodically check the volume infused because pump malfunctions can change the rate.

Ensuring Patient Safety

- Before starting PN, check label and ingredients in solution to make sure they match what the HCP ordered.
- A second RN should verify infusion pump settings before beginning PN.
- Trace the administration tubing to the point of origin in the body at the start of the infusion and at all handoffs.
- Check the solution for leaks, color changes, particulate matter, clarity, and fat emulsions cracking (separating into layers). If present, promptly return it to the pharmacy for replacement.
- Discontinue a PN solution and replace it with a new solution if bag is not empty at the end of 24 hr. At room temperature, the solution (especially when containing fat emulsion) is a good medium for microorganism growth.
- If fat emulsions are infused separately from the PN solution, the preferred delivery method is a continuous low volume delivered over 12 hr.

Hyperglycemia

- Check glucose blood levels at bedside q4–6hr with glucose-testing meter.
- Maintain a glucose range of 140–180 mg/dL. Give sliding scale doses of insulin to keep the glucose level in normal range.

Hypoglycemia

- If a PN formula bag should empty before the next solution is available, a 10% or 20% dextrose solution (based on the amount of dextrose in the central PN solution) or 5% dextrose solution (based on the amount of dextrose in the peripheral PN solution) can be given to prevent hypoglycemia.

Catheter-Related Infections

- Carefully assess the catheter site for signs of inflammation and infection. Phlebitis can readily occur because of the hypertonic infusion. Catheter-related infection and septicemia can occur:
  - Local manifestations: erythema, tenderness, and exudate at the catheter insertion site
  - Systemic manifestations: fever, chills, nausea, vomiting, and malaise
- Immunosuppressed patients are at high-risk for infection. Note subtle signs in patients receiving chemotherapy, corticosteroids, or antibiotics, which can mask signs of infection.
- To reduce the risk for infection, catheters with antibiotic or antiseptic surfaces may be used.
- Follow agency policy for changing catheter dressings and other central line infection prevention measures (see Chapter 16).
- If you suspect an infection during a dressing change, send a culture specimen of the site and drainage and notify the HCP at once.
- If a catheter-related infection is suspected, blood cultures are drawn. A chest x-ray is taken to detect changes in pulmonary status.

Transitioning to Oral Nutrition

- Encourage oral nourishment and keep a careful record of intake. A general rule is that 60% of caloric needs should be met orally or through EN before discontinuing PN.
- Begin with clear liquids and advance as tolerated to a soft diet.

Assessing Effectiveness

- Monitor initial vital signs q4–8hr.
- Weigh patient daily as a measure of the patient's hydration status.
- Maintain accurate intake and output record.
- Determine the cause of any weight changes (e.g., fluid gained from edema, actual increase or decrease in tissue weight).
- Assess blood levels of glucose, electrolytes, and urea nitrogen.
- CBC and hepatic enzyme studies are obtained a minimum of 3 times per week until stable and then weekly as the patient's condition warrants.

TABLE 39.16 Complications of PN

Metabolic Problems	Catheter-Related Problems
• Altered renal function	• Air embolus
• Essential fatty acid deficiency	• Catheter-related sepsis
• Hyperglycemia, hypoglycemia	• Dislodgment
• Hyperlipidemia	• Hemorrhage
• Liver dysfunction	• Occlusion
• Refeeding syndrome	• Phlebitis
	• Pneumothorax, hemothorax, and hydrothorax
	• Thrombosis of vein

◆ Home Nutritional Support

Home PN or EN is an accepted mode of nutritional therapy for the person who does not need hospitalization but needs continued nutritional support. Some patients successfully receive home therapy for many months, even years. It is important for you to teach the patient and caregiver about catheter or tube care, proper technique in mixing and handling of the solutions and tubing, and side effects and complications.

Home nutritional therapies are expensive. Specific criteria must be met for expenses to be reimbursed. The discharge planning team must be involved early to help plan for such issues. Home nutritional support may be a burden for the patient and caregivers and affect quality of life. Tell the family about support groups, such as the Oley Foundation *(www.oley.org)*, that provide peer support and advocacy.

EATING DISORDERS

Eating disorders are psychiatric conditions associated with physiologic alterations and risk for death. The manifestations of eating disorders vary across gender, age, socioeconomic status, and race and ethnicity. Patients with eating disorders may be hospitalized for fluid and electrolyte problems; dysrhythmias; and nutritional, endocrine, and metabolic disorders. Menstrual problems may occur in women of childbearing age. Many of the nutritional problems associated with these disorders require you to implement a nutritional plan of care.

The 3 most common types of eating disorders are anorexia nervosa, bulimia nervosa, and binge-eating disorder. *Binge-eating disorder* is less severe than bulimia nervosa and anorexia nervosa. Those with binge-eating disorder do not have a distorted body image and are often overweight or obese.

Eating disorders also occur in some who are health conscious. For example, men with *bigorexia* or muscle dysmorphia (an extreme concern with becoming more muscular) may use steroids or other drugs to increase muscle mass. They may also use supplements and protein shakes to increase their body weight and mass.

The *female athlete triad* is a syndrome in which eating disorders, amenorrhea, and osteoporosis are present. The triad occurs in females taking part in sports that emphasize leanness and low body weight.

ANOREXIA NERVOSA

Anorexia nervosa (AN) is characterized by restricting energy intake, difficulties in maintaining an appropriate weight, an intense fear of gaining weight or being fat, and distorted body image.[21] People with AN generally restrict the number of calories and the types of food they eat. Some people exercise compulsively, purge via vomiting and laxatives, and/or binge eat. AN manifests as unwillingness to maintain a healthy weight, refusal to eat, continuous dieting, detailed food rituals, and avoiding social situations.[21] Common assessment findings include signs of malnutrition, extreme thinness, hypothermia, and muscle weakness (Fig. 39.9).

Diagnostic studies often show osteopenia or osteoporosis, iron-deficiency anemia, a high blood urea nitrogen level from marked intravascular volume depletion, and abnormal renal function. A lack of dietary potassium and potassium loss in the urine lead to potassium deficiency. Manifestations of potassium deficiency include muscle weakness, dysrhythmias, and renal failure. Leukopenia; hypoglycemia; and decreased sodium, magnesium, and phosphorus may be present.

Treatment involves a combination of nutritional support and psychiatric care. Nutritional care focuses on reaching and maintaining a healthy weight, normal eating patterns, and perception of hunger and satiety. The patient may be hospitalized if there are medical complications that cannot be managed in an outpatient therapy program. Nutritional repletion is closely supervised to ensure consistent and ongoing weight gains. Refeeding syndrome is a rare but serious complication of refeeding programs. The patient may need EN or PN.

Improved nutrition, however, is not a cure for AN. The underlying psychiatric issues must be addressed by identifying problematic personal and family interactions, followed by personal and family counseling.

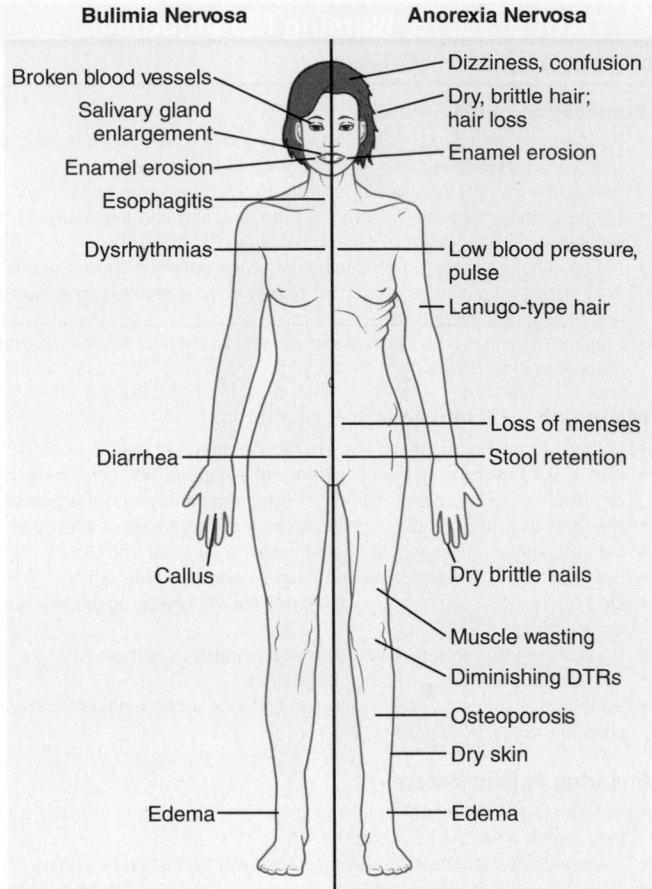

FIG. 39.9 Manifestations of anorexia nervosa and bulimia nervosa. (Modified from Mahan LK, Raymond JL: *Krause's food & the nutrition care process*, ed, 14, St Louis, 2016, Saunders.)

BULIMIA NERVOSA

Bulimia nervosa (BN) is a disorder characterized by episodes of binge eating with inappropriate compensatory behaviors to avoid weight gain (vomiting, laxative misuse, overexercise).[21] Like those with AN, the person with BN is concerned with body image and often goes to great lengths to conceal abnormal eating habits.[21] They may have normal weight for height, or their weight may fluctuate with bingeing and purging. There may have signs of frequent vomiting, such as macerated knuckles, swollen salivary glands, broken blood vessels in the eyes, and dental problems (Fig. 39.9). Abnormal laboratory values, including hypokalemia, metabolic alkalosis, and increased serum amylase, may occur from frequent vomiting.

The cause of BN is unclear. It is thought to be similar to that of AN. Some persons with BN report substance use, anxiety, affective disorders, and personality changes. Over time, problems associated with BN become increasingly hard to deal with effectively. A treatment combination of psychologic counseling (i.e., cognitive behavioral therapy) and nutritional counseling is essential.

Fluoxetine (Prozac) is the only FDA-approved antidepressant for treating BN. It may not be appropriate for all patients with BN. Education and emotional support for the patient and family are vital. Support groups, such as the National Association of Anorexia Nervosa and Associated Disorders (ANAD) *(www.anad.org)*, are helpful to those affected by these disorders.

CASE STUDY
Undernutrition

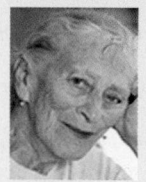

(© iStockphoto/Thinkstock.)

Patient Profile

M.S. is a 70-yr-old white woman who was recently admitted to the inpatient medical unit with a diagnosis of malnutrition.

Subjective Data
- Reports 30-lb weight loss in past 2 mo
- Recently had a thrombotic stroke with hemiparesis and dysphagia
- Has a history of rheumatoid arthritis
- Has had nothing by mouth for the past 24 hr and just started EN via PEG tube
- Lives with her daughter, who is at her bedside

Objective Data

Physical Examination
- Has left-sided weakness
- BP is 150/90 mm Hg
- 5 ft, 4 in tall, weight 100 lb
- PEG tube recently placed

Laboratory Results
- Serum albumin 2.9 g/dL
- Prealbumin 11.0 mg/dL
- C-reactive protein 0.9 mg/L

Discussion Questions

1. What are M.S.'s risk factors for malnutrition?
2. What is her BMI?
3. What are contributing factors to her developing dysphagia and malnutrition?
4. What should you include in a successful weight gain program for M.S.?
5. For which complications of EN could M.S. be at risk?
6. *Priority Decision:* What is the priority of the nursing care for M.S.?
7. *Priority Decision:* Based on the assessment data presented, what are the priority nursing diagnoses? Identify any collaborative problems.
8. *Collaboration:* Which interventions could be delegated to unlicensed assistive personnel (UAP)?
9. *Evidence-Based Practice:* M.S.'s daughter tells you that her mother's abdomen appears bloated and she wonders if she should massage it.
10. *Collaboration:* What is the interprofessional team's top priority at this time for M.S.?
11. *Safety:* To ensure M.S.'s safety, what nursing interventions are needed considering M.S.'s recent weight loss?

Answers available at *http://evolve.elsevier.com/Lewis/medsurg*

BRIDGE TO NCLEX EXAMINATION

The number of the question corresponds to the same-numbered outcome at the beginning of the chapter.

1. The percentage of daily calories for a healthy person consists of
   a. 50% carbohydrates, 25% protein, 25% fat, and <10% of fat from saturated fatty acids.
   b. 65% carbohydrates, 25% protein, 25% fat, and >10% of fat from saturated fatty acids.
   c. 50% carbohydrates, 40% protein, 10% fat, and <10% of fat from saturated fatty acids.
   d. 40% carbohydrates, 30% protein, 30% fat, and >10% of fat from saturated fatty acids.

2. Place in order the substrates the body uses for energy during starvation, beginning with 1 for the first component and ending with 4 for the last component.
   a. skeletal protein.
   b. glycogen.
   c. visceral protein.
   d. fat stores.

3. A complete nutritional assessment including anthropometric measurements is *most* important for the patient who
   a. has a BMI of 25.5 kg/m².
   b. reports episodes of nightly nocturia.
   c. reports a 5-year history of constipation.
   d. reports an unintentional weight loss of 10 lb in 2 months.

4. Which method is *best* to use when confirming initial placement of a blindly inserted small-bore NG feeding tube?
   a. X-ray
   b. Air insertion
   c. Observing patient for coughing
   d. pH measurement of gastric aspirate

5. A patient is receiving peripheral parenteral nutrition. The solution is completed before the new solution arrives on the unit. The nurse gives
   a. 20% intralipids.
   b. 5% dextrose solution.
   c. 0.45% normal saline solution.
   d. 5% lactated Ringer's solution.

6. A patient with anorexia nervosa shows signs of malnutrition. During initial refeeding, the nurse carefully assesses the patient for *(select all that apply)*
   a. hypokalemia.
   b. hypoglycemia.
   c. hypercalcemia.
   d. hypomagnesemia.
   e. hypophosphatemia.

1. a, 2. b, a, d, c, 3. d, 4. d, 5. b, 6. a, d, e

For rationales to these answers and even more NCLEX review questions, visit *http://evolve.elsevier.com/Lewis/medsurg*.

e EVOLVE WEBSITE/RESOURCES LIST

http://evolve.elsevier.com/Lewis/medsurg

Review Questions (Online Only)

Key Points

Answer Keys for Questions
- Rationales for Bridge to NCLEX Examination Questions
- Answer Guidelines for Case Study on p. 867

Nursing Care Plans
- eNursing Care Plan 39.1: Patient Receiving Enteral Nutrition
- eNursing Care Plan 39.2: Patient Receiving Parenteral Nutrition

Conceptual Care Map Creator

Audio Glossary

Content Updates

REFERENCES

*1. Dave JM, Thompson DI, Svendsen-Sanchez A, et al : Perspectives on barriers to eating healthy among food pantry clients, *Health Equity* 1:28, 2017.

2. Mifflin MD, St. Jeor ST, Hill LA, et al: A new predictive equation for resting energy expenditure in healthy individuals, *Am J Clin Nutr* 51:242, 1990. (Classic)

3. US Department of Health and Human Services, US Department of Agriculture: 2015-2020 Dietary guidelines for Americans, ed 8. Retrieved from *www.health.gov/dietaryguidelines/2015-scientific-report*.

*4. Elagizi A, Lavie CJ, Marshall K, et al: Omega-3 polyunsaturated fatty acids and cardiovascular health: A comprehensive review, *Prog Cardiovasc Dis* 61:76, 2018.

5. Moll R, Davis B: Iron, vitamin B_{12} and folate, *Medicine* 45:198, 2017.

6. Nix, S: *Williams' basic nutrition and diet therapy,* ed 15, St Louis, 2018, Elsevier.

*7. Sriram K, Sulo S, VanDerBosch G, et al: A comprehensive nutrition-focused quality improvement program reduces 30-day readmissions and length of stay in hospitalized patients, *JPEN* 41:384, 2017.

*8. Cereda E, Pedrolli C, Klersy C, et al: Nutritional status in older persons according to healthcare setting: A systematic review and meta-analysis of prevalence data using MNA®, *Clin Nutr* 35:1282, 2016.

9. White JV, Guenter P, Jensen G, et al: Consensus statement of the Academy of Nutrition and Dietetics/ASPEN: Characteristics recommended for the identification and documentation of adult malnutrition, *J Acad Nutr Diet* 112:730, 2012. (Classic)

10. Naisbitt C, Davies S: Starvation, exercise and the stress response, *Anaesth Intensive Care Med* 18:508, 2017.

*11. Bharadwaj S, Ginoya S, Tandon P, et al: Malnutrition: Laboratory markers vs nutritional assessment, *Gastroenterol Rep* 4:272, 2016.

12. Mahan LK, Raymond JL: *Krause's food & the nutrition care process,* ed 14, St Louis, 2016, Saunders.

*13. Park SY, Wilkens LR, Maskarinec G, et al: Weight change in older adults and mortality: The Multiethnic Cohort Study, *Int J Obes* 42:205, 2018.

14. Russell MK: Clinical assessment of undernutrition, *Adv Nutr Dietetics Nutr Suppl* 6:74, 2018.

*15. Hengeveld LM, Wijnhoven HA, Olthof MR, et al: Prospective associations of poor diet quality with long-term incidence of protein-energy malnutrition in community-dwelling older adults: The Health, Aging, and Body Composition Study, *Am J Clin Nutr* 107:155, 2018.

*16. Biolo G, Pišot R, Mazzucco S, et al: Anabolic resistance assessed by oral stable isotope ingestion following bed rest in young and older adult volunteers: Relationships with changes in muscle mass, *Clin Nutr* 36:1420, 2017.

*17. Cardon-Thomas DK, Riviere T, Tieges Z, et al: Dietary protein in older adults: Adequate daily intake but potential for improved distribution, *Nutrients* 9:184, 2017.

*18. Boullata JI, Carrera AL, Harvey L, et al: ASPEN safe practices for enteral nutrition therapy, *JPEN* 41:15, 2017.

*19. Mehta NM, Skillman HE, Irving SY, et al: Guidelines for the provision and assessment of nutrition support therapy in the pediatric critically ill patient: Society of Critical Care Medicine and ASPEN, *JPEN* 41:706, 2017.

*20. Guenter P, Worthington P, Ayers P, et al: Standardized competencies for parenteral nutrition administration: The ASPEN model, *Nutr Clin Pract* 33:295, 2018.

21. National Eating Disorders Association: Learn. Retrieved from: *www.nationaleatingdisorders.org/*.

*Evidence-based information for clinical practice.

40

Obesity

Mariann M. Harding

Helping one person might not change the whole world, but it could change the world for the one person.

Paul Shane Spear

ⓔ http://evolve.elsevier.com/Lewis/medsurg

CONCEPTUAL FOCUS

Coping
Functional Ability

Nutrition
Self-Management

LEARNING OUTCOMES

1. Discuss the epidemiology and etiology of obesity.
2. Explain the health risks associated with obesity.
3. Compare the classification systems for determining a person's body size.
4. Discuss nutritional therapy and exercise plans for the obese patient.
5. Distinguish among the bariatric surgical procedures used to treat obesity.

6. Describe the nursing and interprofessional management related to conservative and surgical therapies for obesity.
7. Describe the etiology, clinical manifestations, and nursing and interprofessional management of metabolic syndrome.

KEY TERMS

bariatric surgery, p. 879
body mass index (BMI), p. 875
extreme obesity, p. 875

lipectomy, p. 885
metabolic syndrome, p. 885
obese, p. 875

obesity, p. 869
overweight, p. 875
waist-to-hip ratio (WHR), p. 876

OBESITY

Obesity is an excessively high amount of body fat or adipose tissue (Fig. 40.1). Obesity is a global problem because it is a major risk factor for leading causes of death, including type 2 diabetes, heart disease, and certain cancers. Overweight persons often have a number of other problems, such as problems with mobility and sleeping, that affect health.

The consequences of obesity extend beyond the physical changes. Social stigma can take an emotional toll on a person's psychologic well-being. Many have problems related to altered body image, depression, and low self-esteem and withdraw from social interaction. Attitudes about obesity can create biases and discrimination against people who are obese. Obesity must be viewed and treated as a chronic disease similar to other chronic diseases, such as diabetes and hypertension.

Epidemiology of Obesity

The obesity problem is a public health crisis. After decades of rising obesity rates among adults, the rate of increase is beginning to slow, but rates are still far too high. Currently, about 40% of adults in the United States are obese. Significant geographic, racial and ethnic, and income disparities exist. Obesity rates are

highest in the South (Fig. 40.2) and among blacks, Hispanics, and lower income, less-educated Americans[1] (Fig. 40.3).

🌐 PROMOTING HEALTH EQUITY
Obesity

- Hispanics (47%) and blacks (46.8%) have the highest rates of obesity.
- Among women, blacks have the highest prevalence of being obese, with 17% having extreme obesity.
- Among men, Hispanics (43.1%) have the highest prevalence of being obese.
- Asian Americans have the lowest prevalence of being obese or extremely obese.

Obesity in adulthood is often a problem that begins in childhood or adolescence. One in 10 children becomes obese as early as age 2 to 5.[1] Reversing the childhood obesity crisis is key to addressing the overall obesity epidemic.

Etiology and Pathophysiology

Obesity is an increase in body weight beyond the body's physical requirements. This results in an abnormal increase and accumulation of fat cells. However, the processes leading to and sustaining the obese state are complex and still undergoing investigation.

In obesity, there is an increase in the number of adipocytes *(hyperplasia)* and an increase in their size *(hypertrophy)*. Adipocyte *hypertrophy* is a process by which adipocytes can increase their volume several thousand times to accommodate large increases in lipid storage. When storage of existing fat cells is exceeded, preadipocytes are triggered to become adipocytes. This process occurs primarily in the visceral (intraabdominal) and subcutaneous tissues. The process of *hyperplasia* of adipocytes is greatest from infancy through adolescence.

Most obese persons have *primary obesity,* which is excess calorie intake over energy expenditure for the body's metabolic demands. Others have *secondary obesity,* which can result from various congenital anomalies, chromosomal anomalies,

metabolic problems, central nervous system (CNS) lesions and disorders, or drugs (e.g., corticosteroids, antipsychotics).

The cause of obesity involves genetic and biologic factors that are influenced by environmental and psychosocial factors. While each of these factors can and should be considered individually, in reality they are interrelated.

Genetic Link

A genetic predisposition to obesity may be present in as many as 70% of those who are obese.[2] Several genes that are linked to obesity have been found. Genes appear to influence how calories are stored and energy released. "Energy-thrifty" genes, once protective against long periods when food was not available, are now maladaptive in societies in which food availability is no longer an issue. Genes may be responsible for why 2 people living in the same environment can vary considerably in body size.

A strong link exists between a gene known as *FTO* (fat mass and obesity-associated gene) and body mass index (BMI). Variants of this gene may explain why some people become overweight while others do not. People with a certain allele of the *FTO* gene appear to have an increased appetite, reduced satiety, and higher calorie intake.[2] More research is needed to better understand the role of genes in obesity.

Physiologic Regulatory Mechanisms in Obesity. Research has focused on the physiologic regulatory processes that control eating behavior, energy metabolism, and body fat metabolism. Knowing how appetite is triggered and energy is spent gives important information for understanding obesity and specific targets for the development of drugs.

The hypothalamus, gut, and adipose tissue synthesize hormones and peptides that stimulate or inhibit appetite (Fig. 40.4). The hypothalamus is a major site for regulating appetite. Neuropeptide Y, made in the hypothalamus, is a powerful appetite stimulant. When it is imbalanced, it leads to overeating and

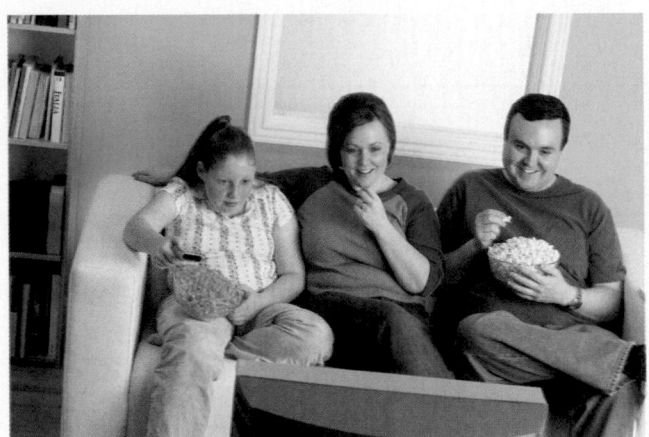

FIG. 40.1 The obesity epidemic has taken its toll on both adults and children in the United States. (© iStock.com/IPGGutenbergUKLtd.)

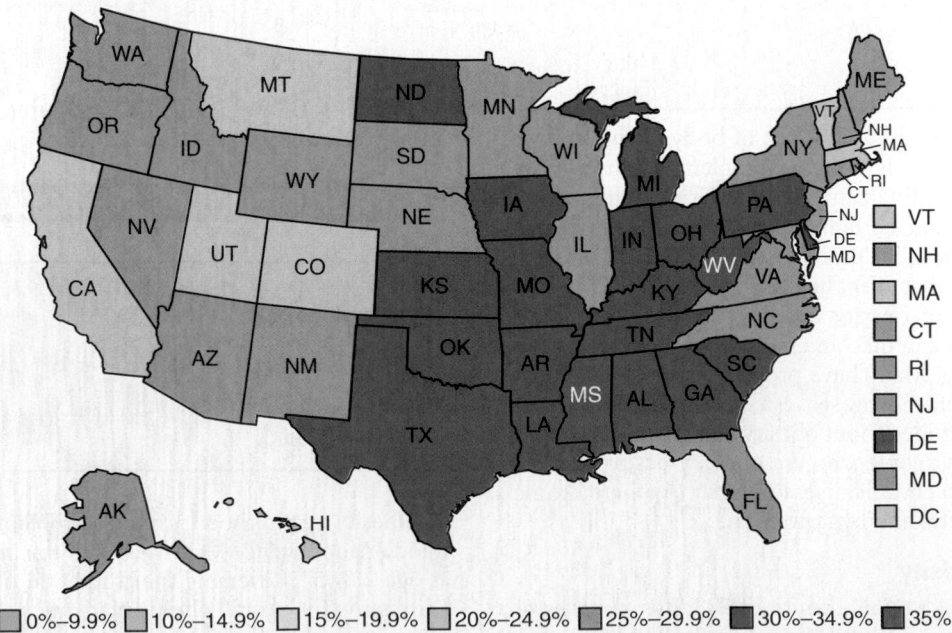

☐ 0%–9.9% ☐ 10%–14.9% ☐ 15%–19.9% ☐ 20%–24.9% ☐ 25%–29.9% ☐ 30%–34.9% ☐ 35%+

FIG. 40.2 Percent of obese adults (BMI >30 kg/m²) in the United States. Alabama, Arkansas, Louisiana, Mississippi, and West Virginia have the highest rates of obesity. Colorado has the lowest rate at 22.3%. 20 states have rates at or above 30%, 47 states have rates of at least 25%, and every state is above 20%. (Source: Trust for America's Health, Robert Wood Johnson Foundation. The state of obesity. 2017. Retrieved from *http://stateofobesity.org*.)

obesity. Hormones and peptides made in the gut and adipocyte cells affect the hypothalamus and have a critical role in appetite and energy balance (Table 40.1). When overeating develops at an early age and continues into adulthood, one's ability to sense fullness (satiety) is altered.

Leptin, secreted from adipocytes when they fill with fat, acts in the hypothalamus to suppress appetite and increase fat metabolism. A genetic deficiency of leptin causes extreme obesity. However, most obese persons have high leptin levels, suggesting they are leptin resistant. This may be due to a

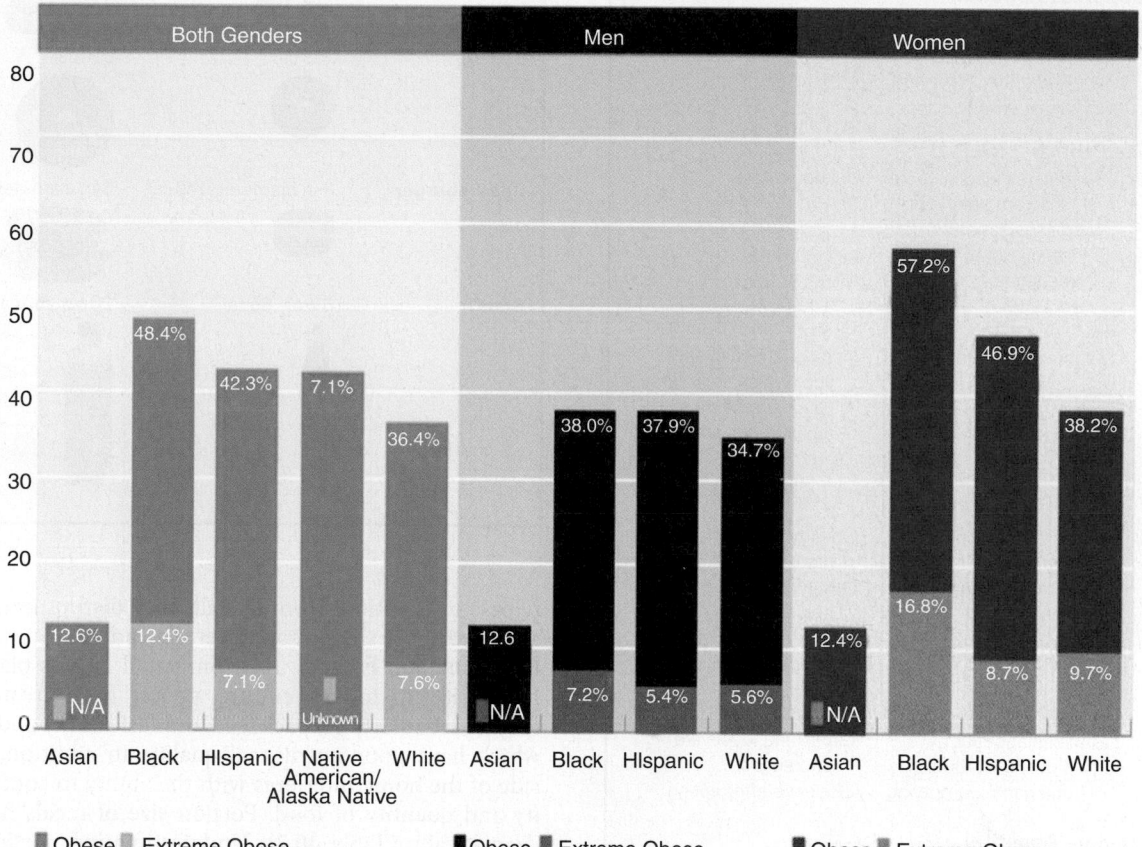

FIG. 40.3 Obesity affects some groups disproportionately. Among U.S. adults, black and Hispanic populations have higher rates of obesity than do white populations. (Source: Trust for America's Health, Robert Wood Johnson Foundation. The state of obesity. 2017. Retrieved from *http://stateofobesity.org*.)

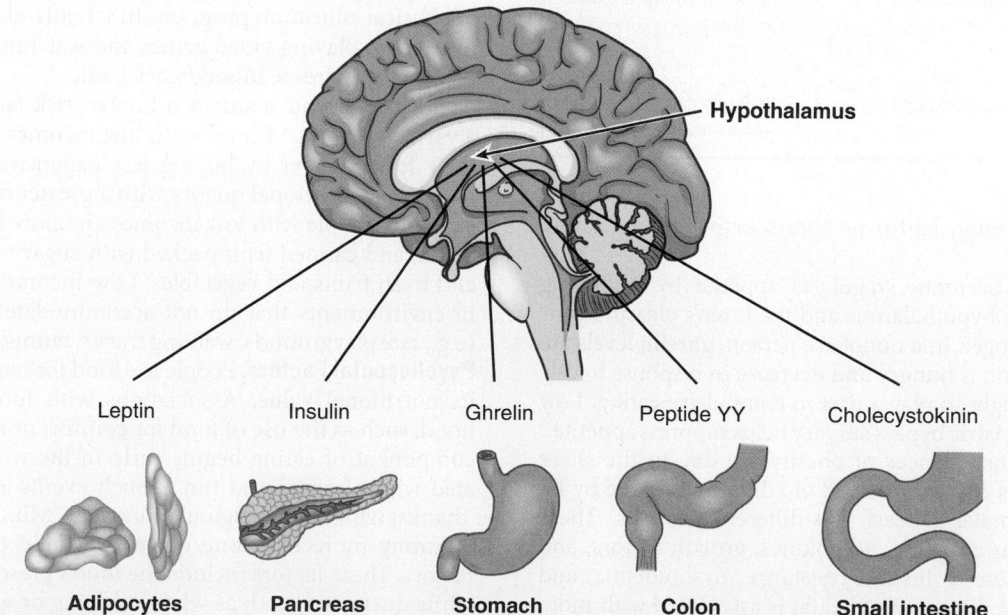

FIG. 40.4 Some of the common hormones and peptides that interact with the hypothalamus to control and influence eating patterns, metabolic activities, and digestion. Obesity disrupts this balance (Table 40.3).

TABLE 40.1 Hormones and Peptides in Obesity

Where Produced	Normal Function	Alteration in Obesity
Anorexins (Suppress Appetite)		
Cholecystokinin		
Small intestine	Inhibits gastric emptying Sends satiety signals to hypothalamus	Unknown role
Glucagon-Like Peptide-1 (GLP-1)		
Small intestine	Stimulates insulin secretion from pancreas Increases satiety (mediated by GLP-1 receptors in brain)	Unknown role
Insulin		
Pancreas	Decreases appetite	Increased insulin secretion, which stimulates ↑ liver synthesis of triglycerides and ↓ HDL production
Leptin		
Adipocytes	Suppresses appetite and hunger Regulates eating behavior	Obesity is associated with high levels Leptin resistance develops so obese people may lose the effect of appetite suppression
Peptide YY		
Colon	Inhibits appetite by slowing GI motility and gastric emptying	Circulating levels are decreased. ↓ Release after eating
Orexins (Stimulate Appetite)		
Ghrelin		
Stomach (primarily)	Stimulates appetite ↑ After food deprivation ↓ In response to food in the stomach	Normal postprandial decline does not occur, which can lead to increased appetite and overeating
Neuropeptide Y		
Hypothalamus	Stimulates appetite	Imbalance causes increased appetite

TABLE 40.2 Portion Sizes: 40 Years Ago vs. Today

	40 Yrs Ago	Today
Turkey sandwich	320 cal	820 cal
Bagel	333 cal	590 cal
Cheeseburger	3-in diameter, 140 cal	6-in diameter, 350 cal
Soda	6½ oz, 85 cal	20 oz, 250 cal

failure to make enough leptin receptors or producing faulty receptors.

Ghrelin, a gut hormone, regulates appetite by inhibiting leptin. It acts in the hypothalamus and the brain's pleasure centers to stimulate hunger. In a nonobese person, ghrelin levels are higher when a person is hungry and decrease in response to eating. Ghrelin is thought to play a part in compulsive eating. Low ghrelin levels after gastric bypass surgery helps suppress appetite.[3]

The 2 major consequences of obesity are due to the sheer increase in fat mass and production of adipokines made by fat cells. Adipocytes make at least 100 different proteins. These proteins, secreted as enzymes, adipokines, growth factors, and hormones, contribute to insulin resistance, dyslipidemia, and high blood pressure. Excess visceral fat is associated with more alterations of adipokines. This causes people with abdominal (android) obesity more complications of obesity.[4] An increased release of cytokines from fat cells may disrupt immune factors and predispose the person to certain cancers.

Environmental Factors. Environmental factors play a key role in obesity. In today's culture, people have greater access to food (particularly prepackaged and fast foods) and soft drinks, which have poor nutritional quality. In addition, eating outside of the home interferes with the ability to control the quality and quantity of food. Portion size of meals has increased dramatically (Table 40.2). Underestimating portion sizes and therefore caloric intake is common. Lack of physical exercise is another factor that contributes to weight gain and obesity. With increases in the use of technology, labor-saving devices, and cars, we expend less energy in our everyday lives. Elimination of physical education programs in schools, along with increased time spent playing video games and watching TV, has contributed to the increase in sedentary habits.

Socioeconomic status is a known risk factor for obesity in a variety of ways.[5] People with low incomes may try to stretch their food dollars by buying less expensive foods that often have poor nutritional quality with a greater caloric content. For example, people with low incomes are more likely to buy pasta, bread, and canned fruit packed with sugar rather than chicken and fresh fruits and vegetables. Low-income residents may live in environments that do not accommodate outdoor activities (e.g., safe playgrounds, walking tracks, tennis, swimming pools).

Psychosocial Factors. People use food for many reasons besides its nutritional value. Associations with food begin in childhood, such as the use of food for comfort or rewards. The social component of eating begins early in life when food is associated with pleasure and fun at such events as birthday parties, Thanksgiving, and religious holidays. "Mindless eating" refers to eating more than one normally would because of outside factors. These factors include the food's presentation and eating while distracted, such as when studying or watching television. Mindless eating leads to consuming unnecessary calories and an increase in body weight.

♥ PROMOTING POPULATION HEALTH

Health Impact of Maintaining a Healthy Weight

- Lowers the risk for hypertension and high cholesterol
- Increases chance for longevity and better quality of life
- Reduces the risk for developing type 2 diabetes
- Reduces the risk for heart disease, stroke, and gallbladder disease
- Reduces the risk for breathing problems, including sleep apnea and asthma
- Decreases the risk for developing osteoarthritis, low back pain, and certain types of cancers

HEALTH RISKS ASSOCIATED WITH OBESITY

Hippocrates wrote that "corpulence is not only a disease itself, but the harbinger of others," thus recognizing that obesity has major adverse effects on health. Many problems occur in obese people at higher rates than in people of normal weight (Fig. 40.5).

Mortality rates rise as obesity increases, especially when obesity is associated with visceral fat.[1] In addition to these problems, obese patients have a reduced quality of life. Fortunately, most of these conditions can improve if a person loses weight.

Cardiovascular Problems

Obesity is a significant risk factor for cardiovascular disease (CVD) and stroke in both men and women. Android obesity is the best predictor of these risks and is linked with increased low-density lipoproteins (LDLs), high triglycerides, and decreased high-density lipoproteins (HDLs).[6] Hypertension can occur because of increased circulating blood volume, abnormal vasoconstriction, increased inflammation (damaging blood vessels), and increased risk for sleep apnea (raises BP). Excess body fat can lead to chronic inflammation throughout the body, especially in blood vessels, thus increasing the risk for heart disease.

Diabetes

Obesity is a major risk factor for the development of type 2 diabetes. Hyperinsulinemia and insulin resistance, common features of type 2 diabetes, are also found in obesity. The term *diabesity* reflects the combined effects of diabetes and obesity.

Excess weight decreases the effectiveness of insulin. When insulin does not work effectively, too much glucose stays in the bloodstream. Thus more insulin is made to compensate. Pancreatic β cells (cells that make insulin) may get overworked and become worn out. Over time, the pancreas is no longer able to keep blood glucose in normal range. Adiponectin, a peptide that increases insulin sensitivity, is decreased in obese people.

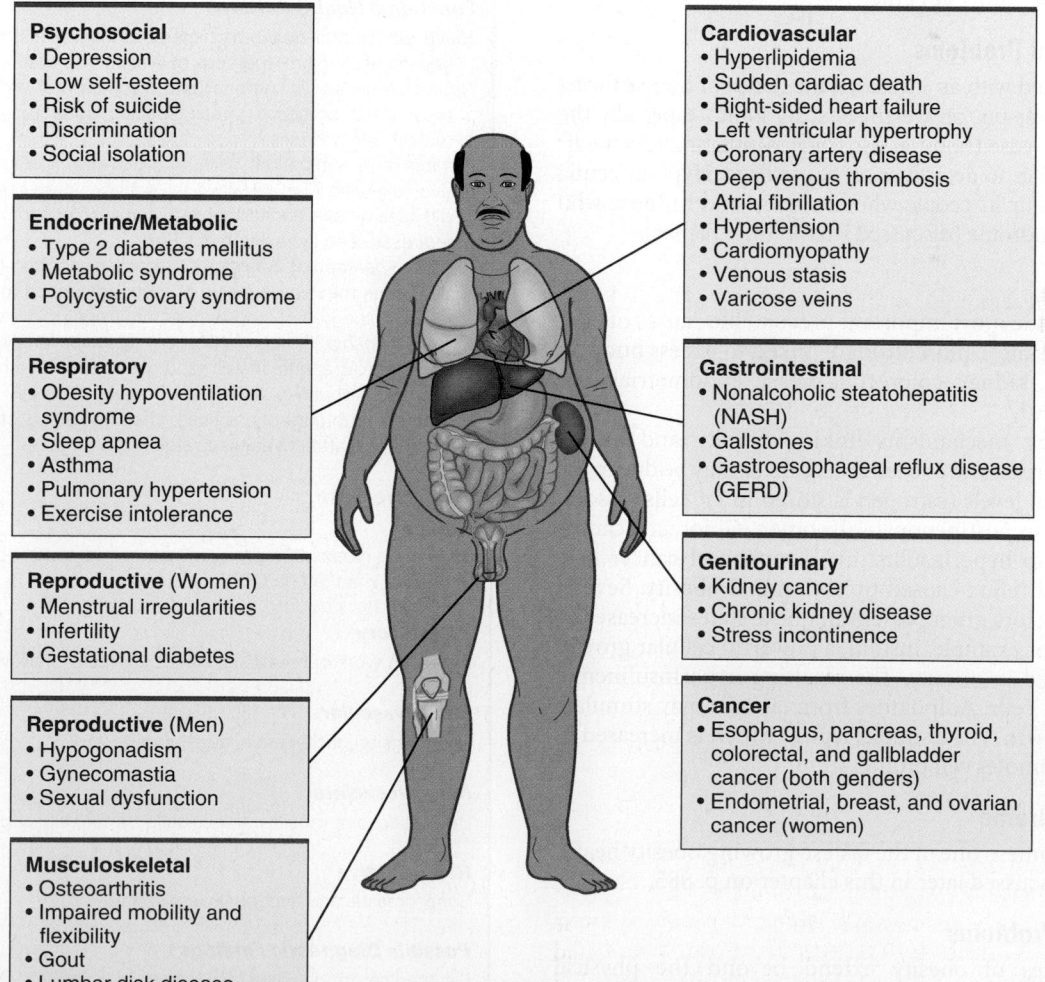

Psychosocial
- Depression
- Low self-esteem
- Risk of suicide
- Discrimination
- Social isolation

Endocrine/Metabolic
- Type 2 diabetes mellitus
- Metabolic syndrome
- Polycystic ovary syndrome

Respiratory
- Obesity hypoventilation syndrome
- Sleep apnea
- Asthma
- Pulmonary hypertension
- Exercise intolerance

Reproductive (Women)
- Menstrual irregularities
- Infertility
- Gestational diabetes

Reproductive (Men)
- Hypogonadism
- Gynecomastia
- Sexual dysfunction

Musculoskeletal
- Osteoarthritis
- Impaired mobility and flexibility
- Gout
- Lumbar disk disease
- Chronic low back pain

Cardiovascular
- Hyperlipidemia
- Sudden cardiac death
- Right-sided heart failure
- Left ventricular hypertrophy
- Coronary artery disease
- Deep venous thrombosis
- Atrial fibrillation
- Hypertension
- Cardiomyopathy
- Venous stasis
- Varicose veins

Gastrointestinal
- Nonalcoholic steatohepatitis (NASH)
- Gallstones
- Gastroesophageal reflux disease (GERD)

Genitourinary
- Kidney cancer
- Chronic kidney disease
- Stress incontinence

Cancer
- Esophagus, pancreas, thyroid, colorectal, and gallbladder cancer (both genders)
- Endometrial, breast, and ovarian cancer (women)

FIG. 40.5 Health risks associated with obesity.

Obesity complicates the management of type 2 diabetes by increasing insulin resistance and glucose intolerance. These factors make drug treatment for diabetes less effective.

Gastrointestinal and Liver Problems

Gastroesophageal reflux disease (GERD) and gallstones are more prevalent in obese people. Gallstones occur due to supersaturation of the bile with cholesterol. Nonalcoholic steatohepatitis (NASH) is a condition in which lipids are deposited in the liver, resulting in a fatty liver. NASH is associated with increased hepatic glucose production. NASH can eventually progress to cirrhosis and can be fatal. Weight loss can improve NASH.

Respiratory and Sleep Problems

The increased fat mass associated with obesity may lead to sleep apnea and obesity hypoventilation syndrome. The increased distribution of fat around the diaphragm causes reduced chest wall compliance, increased work of breathing, and decreased total lung capacity. Sleep apnea results from increased fat around the neck, leading to snoring and hypoventilation while sleeping. Weight loss can improve lung function.

Poor sleep and sleep deprivation may increase appetite. Sleep deprivation has been associated with obesity. Building up a sleep debt over a matter of days can impair metabolism and disrupt hormone levels. The level of leptin falls in people who are sleep deprived, thus promoting appetite.

Musculoskeletal Problems

Obesity is associated with an increased incidence of osteoarthritis because of the stress put on weight-bearing joints, especially the knees and hips. Increased body fat also triggers inflammatory mediators and contributes to deterioration of cartilage. Hyperuricemia and gout often occur in people who are obese and in those who have metabolic syndrome (discussed later in this chapter).

Cancer

Obesity is one of the most important preventable causes of cancer. The types of cancer most strongly linked to excess body fat are thyroid, liver, kidney, colorectal, breast, endometrial, and gallbladder cancer.[1,7]

The underlying mechanisms linking obesity and cancer remain unclear. Breast and endometrial cancer may be due to the increased estrogen levels (estrogen is stored in fat cells) associated with obesity in postmenopausal women. Colorectal cancer has been linked to hyperinsulinemia. Esophageal cancer may be related to acid reflux caused by abdominal obesity. Several hormones and factors often present in obese states increase the risk for cancer. For example, insulin, a powerful cellular growth factor, is increased in obesity. The resulting hyperinsulinemia may affect cancer cells. Adipokines from fat cells may stimulate or inhibit cell growth. For example, leptin, which is increased in obese people, promotes cell proliferation.

Metabolic Syndrome

Metabolic syndrome is one of the fastest-growing obesity health concerns. It is discussed later in this chapter on p. 885.

Psychosocial Problems

The consequences of obesity extend beyond the physical changes. Stigmatization of obese people, and in some cases discrimination, occurs in 3 important areas of living: employment, education, and health care. The social stigma associated with obesity has an emotional toll on a person's psychologic well-being. Many obese persons have low self-esteem, withdraw from social interaction, and have major depression.[8]

❖ NURSING AND INTERPROFESSIONAL MANAGEMENT: OBESITY

◆ Nursing Assessment

The first step in the treatment of obesity is to determine whether any physical conditions are present that may be causing or contributing to obesity. This requires a thorough history and physical examination (Table 40.3). Before you begin, examine your

---

TABLE 40.3 Nursing Assessment

Patients With Obesity

Subjective Data

Important Health Information

Past health history: Time of obesity onset; diseases related to metabolism and obesity, including hypertension, CVD, stroke, cancer, chronic joint pain, respiratory problems, diabetes, cholelithiasis, metabolic syndrome

Medications: Thyroid preparations, diet pills, herbal products

Surgery or other treatments: Prior weight-reduction procedures (bariatric surgery)

Functional Health Patterns

Health perception–health management: Family history of obesity; perception of problem; methods of weight loss tried

Nutritional-metabolic: Amount and frequency of eating; overeating in response to boredom, stress, specific times, or activities; history of weight gain and loss

Elimination: Constipation

Activity-exercise: Typical physical activity; drowsiness, somnolence; dyspnea on exertion, orthopnea, paroxysmal nocturnal dyspnea

Sleep-rest: Sleep apnea, use of CPAP

Cognitive-perceptual: Feelings of rejection, depression, isolation, guilt, or shame; meaning or value of food; adherence to prescribed reducing diets, degree of long-term commitment to a weight loss program

Role-relationship: Change in financial status or family relationships; personal, social, and financial resources to support a reducing diet

Sexuality-reproductive: Menstrual irregularity, heavy menstrual flow in women, birth control practices, infertility; effect of obesity on sexual activity and attractiveness to significant other

Objective Data

General

Body mass index $\geq 30\,kg/m^2$; waist circumference: woman >35 in (89 cm), man >40 in (102 cm)

Respiratory

Increased work of breathing; wheezing; rapid, shallow breathing

Cardiovascular

Hypertension, tachycardia, dysrhythmias

Musculoskeletal

Decreased joint mobility and flexibility; knee, hip, and low back pain

Reproductive

Gynecomastia and hypogonadism in men

Possible Diagnostic Findings

Elevated serum glucose, cholesterol, triglycerides; chest x-ray showing enlarged heart; ECG showing dysrhythmia; abnormal liver function test results

own personal beliefs and any potential biases related to obesity. If you associate obesity with a lack of willpower and overindulgence, you may convey your attitude to patients. They may experience shame in a setting that claims to be a caring one.

When assessing a person who is overweight or obese, be sensitive and nonjudgmental in asking specific and leading questions about weight, diet, and exercise (Table 40.4). In doing so, you can often obtain information that the patient may have withheld out of embarrassment or shyness. Patients need to understand the reason for questions asked about weight or dietary habits. You must be ready to respond to their concerns.

CHECK YOUR PRACTICE

You are working in the hypertension clinic, and the provider has asked you to do an assessment on a 54-yr-old man for referral to a weight loss program. He is 5 ft, 9 in and weighs 242 lb. His BP has been hard to control with drugs and diet. While you are trying to do an assessment (using the questions in Table 40.4), he interrupts you and asks you if he can leave. He angrily tells you, "I do not want to give up my favorite foods, quit drinking, or exercise. Do you understand that?"

• How would you respond to him?

Assess a patient's willingness to change and potential for change. If people are not ready for change, offer them the opportunity to return for further discussion when they are ready to discuss their weight again and make lifestyle changes.

When obtaining the history, explore genetic and endocrine factors, such as hypothyroidism, hypothalamic tumors, Cushing syndrome, hypogonadism in men, and polycystic ovary syndrome in women. Laboratory tests of liver function and thyroid function, a fasting glucose level, and a lipid panel (triglyceride level, LDL and HDL cholesterol levels) aid in evaluating the cause and effects of obesity. When no organic cause (e.g., hypothyroidism) is associated with obesity, the disorder should be considered a chronic, complex disease.

Assess for any co-morbid diseases associated with obesity (e.g., hypertension, sleep apnea). These obesity-related complications require special treatment.

TABLE 40.4 Assessing Patients With Obesity

When assessing patients with obesity and before selecting a weight loss strategy, ask the following questions:

• What is your history with weight gain and weight loss?
• Are other family members overweight?
• How has your body weight affected your health?
• What do you think contributes to your weight?
• What does food mean to you? How do you use food (e.g., to relieve stress, provide comfort)?
• Describe your motivation for losing weight.
• What have you already tried to lose weight? Was it successful? If not, why not?
• Would you like to manage your weight differently? If so, how?
• What sort of barriers do you think impede your weight loss efforts?
• Are there any major stresses that will make it hard to focus on weight control?
• How much time can you devote to exercise on a daily or weekly basis?
• Describe the support you have from family and/or friends for losing weight.

As part of the initial nursing physical examination, assess each body system with particular attention to the organ system in which the patient has expressed a problem or concern. Measurements used with the obese person may include height (without shoes), weight (obtain in a private location and in a gown, if possible), waist circumference, and BMI. Have the right equipment to take these measurements. Provide special chairs, examination tables, and scales that can accommodate an obese person.

◆ Classifications of Body Weight and Obesity

An important part of your patient assessment is to determine and classify a patient's body weight. Common assessment methods include BMI, waist circumference, waist-to-hip ratio (WHR), and body shape. The most widely used and endorsed measures are BMI and waist circumference. These measures are cost-effective, reliable, and easily used in all practice settings.

◆ **Body Mass Index.** The most common measure of obesity is the body mass index (BMI). BMI is calculated by dividing a person's weight (in kilograms) by the square of the height in meters (Fig. 40.6). Table 40.5 shows the classification of overweight and obesity by BMI. Persons with a BMI less than 18.5 kg/m² are considered underweight. A BMI between 18.5 and 24.9 kg/m² reflects a normal body weight. A BMI of 25 to 29.9 kg/m² is classified as being overweight. Those with values at 30 kg/m² or above are considered obese. The term extreme obesity (*morbid* or *severe obesity*) is used for those with a BMI greater than 40 kg/m².

$$\text{BMI (kg/m}^2) = \frac{\text{Weight (pounds)} \times 703}{\text{Height (inches)}^2}$$

Weight in Pounds

Height in Feet and Inches	120	130	140	150	160	170	180	190	200	210	220	230	240	250
4'6	29	31	34	36	39	41	43	46	48	51	53	56	58	60
4'8	27	29	31	34	36	38	40	43	45	47	49	52	54	56
4'10	25	27	29	31	34	36	38	40	42	44	46	48	50	52
5'0	23	25	27	29	31	33	35	37	39	41	43	45	47	49
5'2	22	24	26	27	29	31	33	35	37	38	40	42	44	46
5'4	21	22	24	26	28	29	31	33	34	36	38	40	41	43
5'6	19	21	23	24	26	27	29	31	32	34	36	37	39	40
5'8	18	20	21	23	24	26	27	29	30	32	34	35	37	38
5'10	17	19	20	22	23	24	26	27	29	30	32	33	35	36
6'0	16	18	19	20	22	23	24	26	27	28	30	31	33	34
6'2	15	17	18	19	21	22	23	24	26	27	28	30	31	32
6'4	15	16	17	18	20	21	22	23	24	26	27	28	29	30
6'6	14	15	16	17	19	20	21	22	23	24	25	27	28	29
6'8	13	14	15	17	18	19	20	21	22	23	24	25	26	28

☐ Underweight ☐ Normal weight ☐ Overweight
☐ Obese ☐ Extreme obesity

FIG. 40.6 Body mass index (BMI) chart. Healthy weight: BMI 18 to 24.9 kg/m²; overweight: BMI 25 to 29.9 kg/m²; obesity: BMI 30 kg/m². BMI = weight (kg)/height (m²).

TABLE 40.5 Classification of Overweight and Obesity

	BMI (kg/m²)	Obesity Class	DISEASE RISK RELATIVE TO NORMAL WEIGHT AND WAIST CIRCUMFERENCE	
			Men ≤40 in (102 cm) Women ≤35 in (89 cm)	**Men >40 in (102 cm) Women >35 in (89 cm)**
Underweight	<18.5	—	—	—
Normal	18.5–24.9	—	—	—
Overweight	25.0–29.9	—	Increased	High
Obesity	30.0–34.9	Class I	High	Very high
	35.0–39.9	Class II	Very high	Very high
Extreme obesity	≥40.0	Class III	Extremely high	Extremely high

Source: National Heart, Lung, and Blood Institute: Classification of overweight and obesity by BMI, waist circumference, and associated disease risks. Retrieved from *www.nhlbi.nih.gov/health/public/heart/obesity/lose_wt/bmi_dis.htm.*

Though BMI provides an overall assessment of fat mass, we must consider BMI in relation to the patient's age, gender, and body build. For example, a body builder may have a BMI associated with obesity, but because of a high muscle mass, the BMI would not be an accurate assessment. In contrast, in those who have lost body mass (e.g., older adults), the BMI would underestimate the degree of obesity. For this reason, other measures must be combined with the BMI for an accurate evaluation of a person's weight.

◆ **Waist Circumference.** *Waist circumference* is another way to assess and classify a person's weight. The average waist size has increased by more than 1 inch (from 37.6 inches to 38.8 inches) in the past decade. Health risks increase if the waist circumference is greater than 40 inches in men and greater than 35 inches in women.[9] People who have visceral fat with android obesity have an increased risk for CVD and metabolic syndrome (discussed later in this chapter).

◆ **Waist-to-Hip Ratio.** The waist-to-hip ratio (WHR) is another method used to assess obesity. This ratio describes the distribution of both subcutaneous and visceral adipose tissue. Calculate the WHR by dividing the waist measurement by the hip measurement. A WHR less than 0.8 is best. A WHR greater than 0.8 indicates more truncal fat, which puts a person at a greater risk for health complications.

◆ **Body Shape.** *Body shape* is another way of identifying those who are at a higher risk for health problems (Table 40.6). People with fat primarily in the abdominal area, an *apple-shaped body,* have *android obesity.* Those with fat distribution in the upper legs, a *pear-shaped body,* have *gynoid obesity.* Genetics has an important role in determining a person's body shape and weight.

◆ **Nursing Diagnoses**

Nursing diagnoses for the patient with obesity may include:
- Obesity
- Activity intolerance
- Impaired physical mobility
- Disturbed body image

◆ **Planning**

The overall goals are that the obese patient will (1) modify eating patterns, (2) take part in a regular physical activity program, (3) achieve and maintain weight loss to a specified level, and (4) minimize or prevent health problems related to obesity.

◆ **Nursing Implementation**

Obesity is one of the most challenging health problems. For most patients, successful weight management will be a hard,

TABLE 40.6 Relationship Between Body Shape and Health Risks

Body Shape	Characteristics	Health Risks
Android (apple)	• Fat primarily in abdominal area • Fat also distributed over upper body (neck, arms, shoulders) • Greater risk for obesity-related complications	• Heart disease • Diabetes • Breast cancer • Endometrial cancer • Visceral fat more active, causing ↓ insulin sensitivity • ↑ Triglycerides • ↓ HDL cholesterol • ↑ BP • ↑ Free fatty acid release into blood
Gynoid (pear)	• Fat mainly in the upper legs • Has a better prognosis but hard to treat	• Osteoporosis • Varicose veins • Cellulite • Subcutaneous fat traps and stores dietary fat • Trapped fatty acids stored as triglycerides

lifelong project. Obesity treatment begins with patients understanding their weight history and deciding on a plan that is best for them. It is rare to find an obese person who has not tried to lose weight. Some people have met with limited and temporary success, and others have met only with failure.

You are in a key position to help obese patients by (1) helping them explore and deal with their negative experiences and (2) teaching other health professionals about stigma and biases experienced by obese patients. Although health care for obese people has greater demands, HCPs often do not address these needs. HCPs are often reluctant to counsel patients about obesity for a variety of reasons, including (1) time constraints during appointments make it hard, (2) weight management may be viewed as professionally unrewarding, (3) reimbursement for weight management services is hard to obtain, and (4) many HCPs do not feel knowledgeable about giving weight loss advice.

Despite knowing benefits of weight loss, most people find the process tough. Achieving an "ideal" BMI is not necessary and may not be a realistic goal. Modest weight loss of even 3% to 5% of starting weight can have clinical benefits, and greater weight losses produce greater benefits.[10] In general, the average weight loss program (except for bariatric surgery) results in a 10% reduction of body weight. This average should not be considered a failure since it is associated with significant health benefits.[10]

Exploring a person's motivation for weight loss is essential for overall success. Using principles from motivational interviewing (see Chapter 4), you can help patients understand their desire to lose weight and gain confidence in achieving weight loss.

Focusing on the reasons for wanting to lose weight may help patients develop strategies for a weight loss program. Any supervised plan of care must be directed at 2 different processes: (1) successful weight loss, which requires a short-term energy deficit, and (2) successful weight control, which requires long-term behavior changes.

Together with other members of the interprofessional care team, you have a key role in planning for and managing the care of an obese patient. A holistic approach for weight loss must be used that includes nutritional therapy, exercise, behavior modification, and, for some, drugs or surgical intervention (Table 40.7). Combining more than one aspect supports more effective weight loss and weight control efforts. While teaching patients, stress healthy eating habits and adequate physical activity as lifestyle patterns to develop and maintain.

 PROMOTING POPULATION HEALTH

Maintaining a Healthy Weight

- Weigh yourself regularly.
- Consume 5 or more servings of fruits and vegetables daily.
- Choose whole grain foods, such as brown rice and whole wheat bread.
- Avoid highly processed foods made with refined white sugar, flour, and saturated fat.
- Avoid foods that are high in "energy density" or have a lot of calories in a small amount of food.
- Take part in physical activity:
  - 150 minutes of moderate-intensity aerobic activity (i.e., brisk walking) every week
  - Muscle-strengthening activities on 2 or more days a week

 Nutritional Therapy. There are no "magic" diets for weight loss. No one diet is superior for weight loss. All diets can work if they reduce caloric intake compared to expenditure and are one to which the patient will adhere.[11] The ability to adhere to a diet and degree of weight loss strongly depends on the patient's

motivation. Restricting dietary intake so that it is below energy requirements is a cornerstone for any weight loss or maintenance program. Table 40.8 presents an example of a 1200-calorie diet. It is best to recommend a dietary approach in which calorie restriction includes all food groups. In general, recommend a diet that includes adequate amounts of fruits and vegetables, gives enough bulk to prevent constipation, and meets daily vitamin A and vitamin C requirements. Lean meat, fish, and eggs provide sufficient protein and the B-complex vitamins. Patients will find it easier to incorporate such a change into their lifestyle and not become as bored with their food options.

A very-low-calorie diet plan that limits calories to a total of 800 or less per day may be prescribed if rapid weight loss is needed.[11] These diets are not sustainable on a long-term basis. They should be provided only by trained professionals in a medical care setting. Persons on very-low-calorie diets need frequent professional monitoring because the severe energy restriction places them at risk for multiple health complications.

Many people try to lose weight by following one of the many fad diets that offer the enticement of quick weight loss with little effort. Often, these quick weight-reduction diets (found in the popular media) advocate eliminating one category of foods (e.g., carbohydrates). Therefore these should be discouraged. Low-carbohydrate diets do produce a rapid weight loss but reduce the ability to get adequate amounts of fiber, vitamins, and minerals. Restrictive diets are hard to maintain on a long-term basis. The more restrictive the diet, the greater the demand for intense discipline in the face of an intense desire to eat foods not allowed on the diet.

The degree of success of any diet depends in part on the amount of weight to be lost. A moderately obese person will

TABLE 40.7 **Interprofessional Care**
Obesity

Diagnostic Assessment	Management

• History and physical examination
• Family history
• BMI, waist circumference, waist-to-hip ratio
• Assessment of health risks and co-morbidities
	• Management of co-morbidities
	• Lifestyle interventions
	  • Taking part in weight loss program
	  • Support groups
	  • Behavior modification
	  • Nutritional therapy
	  • Exercise
	  • Behavior modification
	  • Support groups
	• Drug therapy (Table 40.9)
	• Surgical therapy (Table 40.10)

TABLE 40.8 **Nutritional Therapy**
1200-Calorie–Restricted Weight-Reduction Diet

General Principles
1. Eat regularly. Do not skip meals.
2. Measure foods to determine the correct portion size.
3. Avoid concentrated sweets, such as sugar, candy, honey, pies, cakes, cookies, and regular sodas.
4. Reduce fat intake by baking, broiling, or steaming foods.
5. Maintain a regular exercise program for successful weight loss.

Sample Meal Plan

Meal	Exchanges	Menu Plan
Breakfast	1 meat	1 hard-boiled egg
	2 breads	1 slice toast
		¾ cup dry cereal (unsweetened)
	1 fruit	½ small banana
	1 fat	1 tsp margarine
	1 dairy	1 cup low-fat milk
	Beverage	Coffee
Lunch	2 meats	Cheese enchiladas (made with 2 oz
	2 breads	cheese, 2 corn tortillas, lettuce, chili
	Vegetable	sauce)
	1 fruit	Fresh grapes (12)
	Beverage	Diet soda
Dinner	2 meats	2 oz baked chicken
	1 bread	Corn on the cob with 1 tsp margarine
	1 fat	
	Vegetable	Tossed salad and 1 Tbsp salad dressing
	1 fruit	¾ cup strawberries
	1 milk	1 cup low-fat milk

obviously reach a weight goal more easily than a person with extreme obesity. Because men have a higher percent of lean body mass, they are often able to lose weight more quickly than women. Women have a higher percent of body fat, which is metabolically less active than muscle tissue. Postmenopausal women are particularly prone to weight gain, especially increased abdominal fat.

Setting a realistic and healthy goal, such as losing 1 to 2 lb per week, should be mutually agreed on at the beginning of a weight loss program. Trying to lose too much too fast usually results in a sense of frustration and failure for the patient. You can help patients understand that losing large amounts of weight in a short period causes skin and underlying tissue to lose elasticity and tone. Slower weight loss offers better cosmetic results.

Inevitably, the patient reaches plateau periods during which no weight is lost. These plateaus may last from several days to several weeks. Remind the patient that plateaus are normal occurrences during weight reduction. A weekly check of body weight is a good method of monitoring progress. Daily weighing is not recommended because of fluctuations that result from retained water (including urine) and feces. Teach the patient to record the weight at the same time of the day, wearing the same type of clothing.

EVIDENCE-BASED PRACTICE

Obesity Interventions and Faith-Based Organizations

J.W. is a 39-yr-old black woman who is 5 ft, 6 in tall and weighs 196 lb. You work in the clinic that she visits for health care. Your clinic is referring patients who would benefit from losing weight to community and hospital-based weight loss programs. She tells you she has been trying to lose weight by "watching what she eats" and that she is "not sure what else she can do." In further talks with her, you learn she is an active member of her neighborhood church.

Making Clinical Decisions

Best Available Evidence. Obesity is highest among racial and ethnic minority groups in the United States. Many faith-based organizations (FBOs) provide programs that have helped obese persons improve weight-related behaviors (e.g., increase in physical activity and fruit and vegetable intake) and lose weight. Successes in these programs have been more notable for females. Overall, programs that offer comprehensive and intensive behavioral interventions for weight loss are an option for weight management.

Clinician Expertise. You know it is important for J.W. to engage in a weight loss program that will help her to adopt and maintain healthy behaviors. You also know that FBOs can play a major role in providing health promotion programs in the black community.

Patient Preferences and Values. J.W. says she is interested in learning about a weight loss program at her church.

Implications for Nursing Practice

1. Why is it important to discuss with J.W. her motivation for starting a weight loss program at her church?
2. How will you help J.W. to set realistic short- and long-term goals related to weight loss? How may these goals differ?
3. At each clinic visit, how will you support J.W.'s efforts to lose weight?

References for Evidence

Lv N, Azar KM, Rosas LG, et al.: Behavioral lifestyle interventions for moderate and severe obesity: a systematic review, *Prev Med* 100:180, 2017.
Tucker CM, Wippold GM, Williams JL, et al.: A CBPR study to test the impact of a church-based health empowerment program on health behaviors and health outcomes of black adult churchgoers, *J Racial Ethn Health Disparities* 4:70, 2017.

There is no clear consensus on the number of meals a person on a diet should eat. Some advocate several small meals per day because the body's metabolic rate is temporarily increased right after eating. However, patients eating several small meals a day might consume more calories unless they carefully adhere to portion sizes and total daily calorie allotment.

When a person first starts a weight loss program, food portion sizes must be carefully determined to stay within the dietary guidelines. Portion sizes over the past 40 years have increased considerably (Table 40.2). Food portions can be weighed using a scale, or everyday objects can be used as a visual cue to determine portion sizes. The size of a woman's fist or a baseball is equivalent to a serving of vegetables or fruit. The recommended portion size of meat is 3 oz. This is about the size of a person's palm or a deck of cards. A serving of cheese is about the size of a thumb or 6 dice. The standard size for chopped vegetables is ½ cup, according to MyPlate guidelines (see Table 39.9). A portion size quiz is available at *www.nhlbi.nih.gov/health/educational/wecan/eat-right/portion-distortion.htm*.

Another aspect of the American diet to consider is which foods contribute the most calories—animal sources, fruits, grains, or vegetables. Two thirds or more of a person's diet should be plant-source foods, and the other one third or less should be from animal protein. Being aware of personal consumption habits and striving for the two-thirds to one-third ratio is a simple goal that one can achieve without weighing and measuring foods at every meal. Once this ratio is part of meal planning, the patient can gradually reduce portions as they gradually increase activity levels to achieve healthy weight loss. A list of healthy or low-calorie foods serves as a good reference and allows the patient to dine out on occasion. Furthermore, the patient who carefully follows the prescribed diet may not need to take vitamin supplements.

Encourage the appropriate fluid intake in the form of water. Alcoholic and sugary beverages should be limited or avoided, since they increase caloric intake and are low in nutritional value.

◆ **Exercise.** Exercise is an essential part of a weight loss program. Patients should exercise daily, preferably 30 minutes to an hour, with a goal of more than 10,000 steps per day.[11] There is no evidence that increased activity promotes an increase in appetite or leads to dietary excess. In fact, exercise has the opposite effect. The addition of exercise results in more weight loss than dieting alone and has a favorable effect on body fat distribution.

The type of exercise (e.g., high intensity versus low intensity) does not seem to affect overall weight loss. More intensive activity may result in weight loss with a reduced time commitment, making it preferable to some people. Exercise is especially important in supporting weight loss. Higher levels of physical activity, 200 to 300 minutes per week, are recommended to maintain weight loss or minimize weight regain in the long term.[11]

Explore ways to incorporate exercise in daily routines. It may be as simple as parking farther from their place of employment or taking the stairs versus an elevator. Encourage a person to use a pedometer to track progress toward meeting the 10,000 steps a day goal. However, success may be walking one third of the recommended steps with incremental increases over time. Patients can swim and cycle, which both have long-term benefits. Joining a health club can be another way of getting exercise. Stress to patients that engaging in weekend exercise only or in spurts of strenuous activity is not helpful and can be dangerous.

◆ **Behavior Modification.** The assumptions behind behavior modification are: (1) obesity is a learned disorder caused by overeating and (2) often the critical difference between an obese person and a person of normal weight is the cues that regulate eating behavior. Therefore most behavior-modification programs deemphasize the diet and focus on how and when to eat. Ideally, behavior intervention should begin with counseling sessions with a trained interventionist. Persons who are in a behavioral therapy program are more successful in maintaining their losses over an extended time than those who do not take part in such training.[12]

Various behavioral techniques for patients engaged in a weight loss program include (1) self-monitoring, (2) stimulus control, and (3) rewards. *Self-monitoring* may involve keeping a record of the type and time food was consumed, what the person was doing, and how the person was feeling when eating. By looking at the cues and events before eating, the person can identify areas in which to make behavior changes to break the chain of events and prevent overeating. These eating behaviors must be changed, or any weight loss will only be temporary.

Stimulus control is aimed at eliminating cues in the environment that trigger eating. For example, if the patient overeats while watching television, limiting eating to a certain area (e.g., kitchen table) can be an effective way to weaken the link between eating and television watching. The more often the person does not eat in front of the television, the less likely television watching will trigger overeating.

Rewards may be incentives for weight loss. Short- and long-term goals are useful benchmarks for earning rewards. It is important that the reward for a specified weight loss not be associated with food, such as dinner out or a favorite treat. Reward items do not need to have a monetary component. For example, time for a hot bath or an hour of pleasure reading would be an enjoyable reward for many people. Praise your patient's successes, even small ones, at every opportunity. Changing existing behaviors is hard.

◆ **Support Groups.** People who are on a weight management plan are often encouraged to join a group in which others are also trying to change their eating habits. Many self-help groups offer support and information on dieting tips. For example, Take Off Pounds Sensibly (TOPS) *(www.tops.org)* is the oldest nonprofit organization of this type. Behavior modification is an integral part of the program, along with nutrition education. Weight Watchers International *(www.weightwatchers.com)*, Jenny Craig *(www.jennycraig.com)*, and Nutrisystem *(www.nutrisystem.com)* are probably the most successful commercial weight-loss programs.[13] Weight Watchers offers a food plan that is nutritionally balanced and practical to follow. Group leaders, all of whom have successfully lost weight with Weight Watchers, teach members various behavior-modification techniques.

There are many commercial weight-reduction centers. Most programs are staffed by nurses and dietitians. These weight-reduction centers are cost prohibitive for those with limited financial resources. Most programs offer special prepackaged foods and supplements that a person must buy as part of the weight-reduction plan. The person only consumes these prescribed foods and drinks until an agreed-on amount of weight is lost. The person is encouraged to buy the same type of foods for the maintenance phase of the program, lasting from 6 months to 1 year. Behavior-modification training is part of these programs. People must learn how to adjust their diet once they are

no longer using the commercial products. This can be challenging for many. The person may regain weight lost once the restricted food program is completed.[13]

In recent years, many employers have begun weight loss programs at the workplace. The reason for such programs is that better health repays the cost of the programs through improved work performance, decreased absenteeism, less hospitalization, and lower insurance costs. Both employees and employers report benefiting from such programs.

◆ **Drug Therapy**

Drugs should never be used alone. Rather, drugs should be part of a comprehensive weight loss program that includes reduced-calorie diet, exercise, and behavior modification. They should be reserved for adults with a BMI of 30 kg/m^2 or greater (obese) or adults with a BMI of 27 kg/m^2 or greater (overweight) who have at least 1 weight-related condition, such as hypertension, type 2 diabetes, or dyslipidemia.[10,14] There are currently 5 obesity drugs for long-term management approved by the FDA (Table 40.9).

◆ **Appetite-Suppressing Drugs.** Sympathomimetic amines suppress appetite by increasing the availability of norepinephrine in the brain, thus stimulating the CNS. Sympathomimetics fall into 2 groups: amphetamines and nonamphetamines. Amphetamines have a much higher abuse potential than nonamphetamines. The FDA does not recommend or approve amphetamines for either short- or long-term weight loss.

We usually do not use nonamphetamines for weight loss because of the potential for abuse. If used, they should be used only short term (for 3 months or less). These drugs include phentermine (Adipex, Lomaira, Suprenza), diethylpropion (Tenuate), and phendimetrazine (Bontril). Adverse effects include palpitations, tachycardia, overstimulation, restlessness, dizziness, insomnia, weakness, and fatigue.

◆ **Nursing Interventions Related to Drug Therapy.** Drugs will not cure obesity. People must understand that without substantial changes in food intake and increased physical activity, they will gain weight when drug therapy is stopped.

As with any drug treatment, there are side effects (Table 40.9). Careful evaluation for other medical conditions can help determine which drugs, if any, would be advisable for a given patient. Many insurance companies do not cover the cost of weight loss drugs.

Your role related to drug therapy is to teach the patient about proper administration, side effects, and how the drugs fit into the overall weight loss plan. Changing drug dosages without consultation with the HCP can have detrimental effects. Stress that diet and exercise plans are the cornerstones of permanent weight loss. Finally, discourage patients from buying over-the-counter diet aids unless recommended by an HCP.

BARIATRIC SURGICAL THERAPY

Bariatric surgery, surgery on the stomach and/or intestines to help a person with extreme obesity lose weight, has become a viable option for treating obesity. Surgery is currently the only treatment that has a successful and lasting impact for sustained weight loss for those with extreme obesity.[15]

Criteria guidelines for bariatric surgery include having a BMI of 40 kg/m^2 or more or a BMI of 35 kg/m^2 or more with other significant co-morbidities (e.g., hypertension, type 2 diabetes, heart failure, sleep apnea).

TABLE 40.9 Drug Therapy

Obesity

Drug	Mechanism of Action	Nursing Considerations
bupropion/naltrexone (Contrave)	• *bupropion:* antidepressant • *naltrexone:* opioid antagonist	• Common side effects: nausea, constipation, headache, dizziness, insomnia, dry mouth • Suicidal thoughts and behaviors and neuropsychiatric reactions can occur • Can increase BP and heart rate. Should not be used in patients with uncontrolled hypertension • Can cause seizures. Must not be used in patients who have seizure disorder
liraglutide (Saxenda)	• Glucagon-like peptide 1 (GLP-1) agonist • Induces satiety	• Used to treat type 2 diabetes • Injected • Side effects: thyroid tumors, pancreatitis
lorcaserin (Belviq)	• Selective serotonin (5-HT) agonist • Suppresses appetite and creates a sense of satiety	• Side effects: headache, dizziness, fatigue, nausea, dry mouth, constipation
orlistat (Xenical, Allī [low-dose form available over the counter])	• Blocks fat breakdown and absorption in intestine • Inhibits the action of intestinal lipases, resulting in undigested fat excreted in feces	• Associated with stool leakage, flatulence, diarrhea, abdominal bloating, especially if a high-fat diet is consumed • Severe liver injury may occur • May need fat-soluble vitamin supplements
phentermine/topiramate ER (Qsmyia)	• *phentermine:* Sympathomimetic • *topiramate:* Decreases appetite	• Common side effects: dizziness, insomnia, dry mouth • Do not use in patients with glaucoma or hyperthyroidism • Must avoid pregnancy • Can increase heart rate. Should not be used in patients with uncontrolled hypertension or heart disease

Most people who undergo bariatric surgery successfully improve their overall quality of life. In addition to losing weight, outcomes include improved glucose control with improvement or reversal of diabetes, normalization of BP, decreased total cholesterol and triglycerides, decreased GERD, and decreased sleep apnea.[16]

Insurance coverage for bariatric surgery varies. Those who cover surgery often require extensive documentation. This often includes taking part in a supervised weight loss program for around 6 months and a psychologic evaluation.

Although overall mortality is very low, several complications can arise from surgery. Therefore, having surgery is carefully considered. Candidates for surgery must be screened for psychologic, physical, and behavioral conditions that have been associated with poor surgical outcomes. These include untreated depression, binge eating disorders, and drug and alcohol abuse that may interfere with a commitment to lifelong behavioral changes. Other contraindications to surgery include illnesses that are known to reduce life expectancy and are not likely to improve with weight reduction. These include advanced cancer; end-stage kidney, liver, and cardiopulmonary disease; severe coagulopathy; or inability to follow nutritional recommendations.

Bariatric surgeries fall into 1 of 3 broad categories: restrictive, malabsorptive, or a combination of malabsorptive and restrictive (Table 40.10 and Fig. 40.7). In *restrictive procedures,* the stomach is reduced in size (less food eaten). In *malabsorptive procedures,* the small intestine is shortened or bypassed (less food absorbed). Most procedures are done laparoscopically. These patients have fewer wound infections, shorter hospital stays, and a faster recovery period.

Restrictive Surgeries

Restrictive bariatric surgery reduces either the size of the stomach, which causes the patient to feel full more quickly, or the amount allowed to enter the stomach. In these surgeries, digestion is not altered, so the risk for anemia or cobalamin deficiency is low. The most common restrictive surgeries include adjustable gastric banding and sleeve gastrectomy.

Adjustable Gastric Banding. Laparoscopic *adjustable gastric banding* (AGB) involves limiting the stomach size with an inflatable band placed around the fundus of the stomach (Fig. 40.7, *A*). This restrictive procedure can be done using a Lap-Band or Realize Band system. The band is connected to a subcutaneous port that can be inflated or deflated (by fluid injection in the HCP's office) to change the stoma size to meet the patient's needs as weight is lost. The restrictive effect of the band creates a sense of fullness as the upper part of the stomach now accommodates less than the average stomach. The band then causes a delay in stomach emptying, providing patients with further satiety.

The procedure can be either modified or reversed at a later date, if needed. AGB is the preferred option for patients who are surgical risks because it is a less invasive approach. Because it is restrictive only, patients must follow a strict diet to lose weight and not regain weight.

Sleeve Gastrectomy (Gastric Sleeve). In the sleeve gastrectomy (gastric sleeve), about 75% of the stomach is removed, leaving a sleeve-shaped stomach (Fig. 40.7, *B*). Although the stomach is drastically reduced in size, its function is preserved. Removing most of the stomach results in the elimination of hormones made in the stomach that stimulate hunger, such as ghrelin.

Research is ongoing on a new procedure called *endoscopic sleeve gastroplasty.* It involves using an endoscope rather than making a surgical incision. When the endoscope reaches the stomach, the surgeon places sutures in the stomach, making it smaller and changing its shape.

Gastric Plication. Gastric plication is a minimally invasive weight-loss surgery that reduces the size of the stomach. It is done by folding the stomach wall inward, and then sutures are placed to secure the folded stomach wall. This reduces the stomach volume by as much as 70%. An advantage is reversibility, since there is no gastric resection.

TABLE 40.10 Surgical Therapy for Obesity

Description	Advantages	Disadvantages
Restrictive Surgery		
Adjustable Gastric Banding (AGB) (Lap-Band, Realize Band) (Fig. 40.7, A)		
• Inflatable band encircles stomach • Creation of gastric pouch with about 30 mL (1 oz) capacity • Later stretches to 60–90 mL (2–3 oz) • Upper gastric pouch connected by very narrow channel to lower section of stomach	• Food digestion occurs through normal process • Band can be adjusted to ↑ or ↓ restriction • Can be reversed • Absence of dumping syndrome • Lack of malabsorption • Low complication rate	• Some nausea and vomiting initially (eating too much too quickly) • Food intolerance, gastric dysmotility, regurgitation • Problems with adjustment device • Band may slip or erode into stomach wall • Gastric perforation or obstruction may occur, requiring surgery • Weight loss may be more limited than with other types of surgery
Sleeve Gastrectomy (Gastric Sleeve) (Fig. 40.7, B)		
• About 75% of stomach removed • Creation of sleeve-shaped stomach with 60–150 mL (2–5 oz) capacity	• Function of stomach preserved • No bypass of intestine • Avoids complications of obstruction, anemia, vitamin deficiencies	• Weight loss may be more limited than with other types of surgery • Leakage related to stapling • Irreversible
Gastric Plication		
• Adapted version of sleeve gastrectomy (gastric sleeve) • Sleeve created by suturing rather than removing stomach	• Minimal surgery compared to sleeve gastrectomy • No rerouting of intestines • Maintains natural nutrient absorption capabilities	• Requires hospital stay of 24–48 hr • Nausea common after procedure • Risks include stomach leakage from sutured areas, blockage of stomach from swelling or fold too tight
Intragastric Balloon		
• Involves placing a deflated balloon into stomach • Balloon then filled with saline and occupies space in stomach	• Most are placed endoscopically as an outpatient procedure • Does not require invasive surgery	• Can only be left in place for 6 mos • Once device is in stomach, patients may have nausea, vomiting, abdominal pain, indigestion, gastric ulcers
Malabsorptive Surgery		
Biliopancreatic Diversion (BPD) With or Without Duodenal Switch (Fig. 40.7, C)		
• 70% of the stomach removed horizontally • Anastomosis between stomach and intestine • Decreases the amount of small intestine available for nutrient absorption • Duodenal switch cuts the stomach vertically and is shaped like a tube	• Able to eat larger meals than with gastric bypass or banding procedures • Less food intolerance • Rapid weight loss • Greater long-term weight loss	• Abdominal bloating, diarrhea, foul-smelling gas (steatorrhea) • 3 or 4 loose bowel movements a day • Malabsorption of fat-soluble vitamins • Iron deficiency • Protein-calorie malnutrition • Dumping syndrome • Most complicated of weight loss surgeries
Combination of Restrictive and Malabsorptive Surgery		
Roux-en-Y Gastric Bypass (RYGB) (Fig. 40.7, D)		
• Surgery on stomach to create a pouch (restrictive) • Small gastric pouch connected to jejunum • Remaining stomach and first segment of small intestine are bypassed (malabsorptive)	• Better weight loss results than with restrictive procedures • Lower incidence of malnutrition and diarrhea • Rapid improvement of weight-related comorbidities • Good long-term results	• Leak at site of anastomosis • Anemia: iron deficiency, cobalamin deficiency, folic acid deficiency • Calcium deficiency • Dumping syndrome • Irreversible
Implanted Gastric Stimulation Device		
Maestro Rechargeable System (Fig. 40.8)		
• Device implanted into abdomen • Works like a pacemaker to deliver electrical impulses to vagus nerve, which tells brain when stomach is full	• Least invasive of weight loss surgeries • Procedure done on outpatient basis	• Device must be charged 1–2 times/wk • If battery completely drained, device needs to be reprogrammed • Side effects include nausea, vomiting, heartburn, belching, swallowing problems

Intragastric Balloons. Intragastric balloon weight-loss systems use a gastric balloon to occupy space in the stomach. The balloon does not change or alter the stomach's natural anatomy. It is designed to help patients feel more full, curb the appetite, and reduce food intake. Patients should follow a diet and exercise plan to help with weight loss efforts.

The balloons are less invasive than having gastric bypass surgery. Most are placed endoscopically, while the patient is under mild sedation. The HCP places the balloon into the stomach through the mouth. Once in place, the balloon is filled with saline so that it expands. The balloon can be filled with different amounts of saline (from 400 to 700 mL).

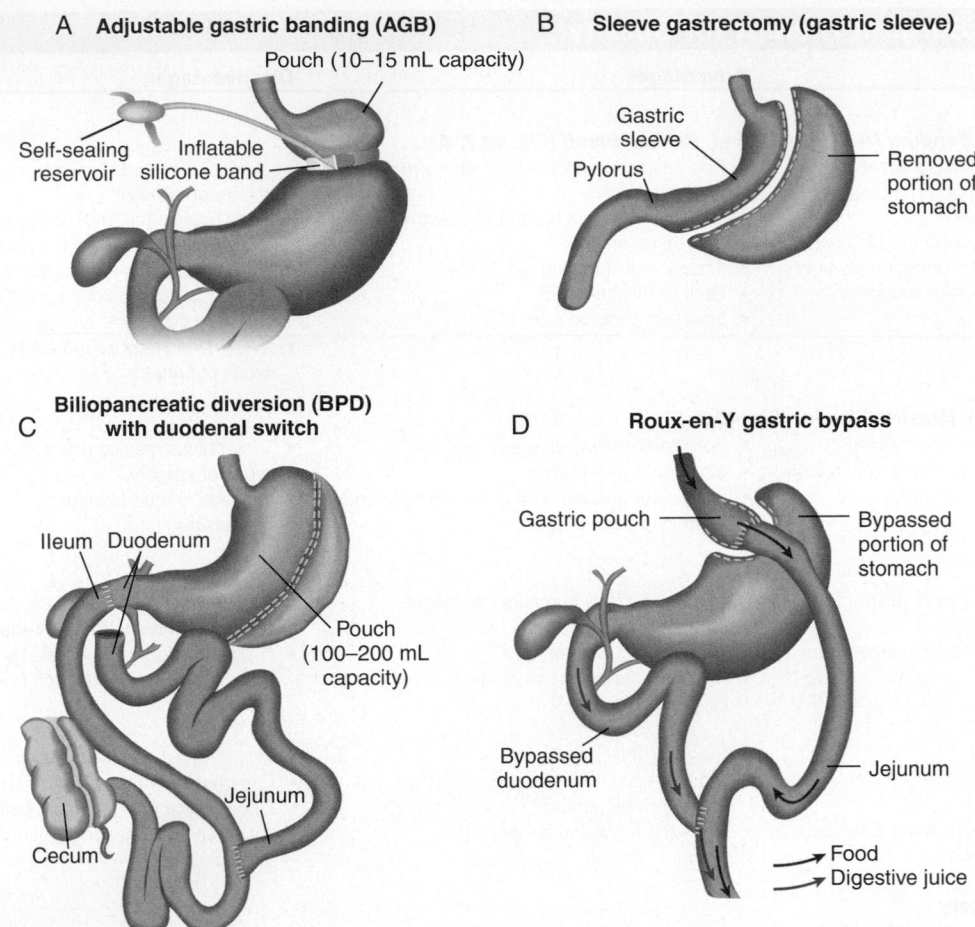

A   Adjustable gastric banding (AGB)

Pouch (10–15 mL capacity)

Self-sealing reservoir

Inflatable silicone band

B   Sleeve gastrectomy (gastric sleeve)

Gastric sleeve

Pylorus

Removed portion of stomach

C   Biliopancreatic diversion (BPD) with duodenal switch

Ileum   Duodenum

Pouch (100–200 mL capacity)

Cecum

Jejunum

D   Roux-en-Y gastric bypass

Gastric pouch

Bypassed portion of stomach

Bypassed duodenum

Jejunum

Food
Digestive juice

FIG. 40.7 Bariatric surgical procedures. **A,** Adjustable gastric banding (AGB) uses a band to create a gastric pouch. **B,** Sleeve gastrectomy involves creating a sleeve-shaped stomach by removing about 75% of the stomach. **C,** Biliopancreatic diversion (BPD) with duodenal switch procedure creates an anastomosis between the stomach and intestine. **D,** Roux-en-Y gastric bypass procedure involves constructing a gastric pouch whose outlet is a Y-shaped limb of small intestine.

With newer balloons, the patient swallows the balloon in a capsule that is attached to a microcatheter. The balloon is inflated with nitrogen gas through the microcatheter. After inflation, the catheter is detached and removed, leaving the balloon in the stomach.[17] When it is time to remove a balloon, it is first deflated and then removed using another endoscopic procedure.

Balloons should not be used in patients who have had gastrointestinal or bariatric surgery or who have inflammatory bowel disease, large hiatal hernia, delayed gastric emptying, or active *Helicobacter pylori* infection. Patients may have vomiting, nausea, abdominal pain, and feelings of indigestion. Other potential risks are gastric ulcers and balloon deflation.

Combination of Restrictive and Malabsorptive Surgery
Roux-en-Y Gastric Bypass. The Roux-en-Y gastric bypass (RYGB) procedure is a combination of restrictive and malabsorptive surgery. This surgical procedure is the most common bariatric procedure done in the United States. It is considered the gold standard among bariatric procedures. Overall, it has low complication rates, has excellent patient tolerance, and sustains long-term weight loss.

The RYGB involves creating a small gastric pouch and attaching it directly to the small intestine using a Y-shaped

limb of the small bowel (Fig. 40.7, *D*). After the procedure, food bypasses 90% of the stomach, the duodenum, and a small segment of jejunum.

A complication of the RYGB is *dumping syndrome,* in which gastric contents empty too rapidly into the small intestine, overwhelming its ability to digest nutrients. Symptoms can include vomiting, nausea, weakness, sweating, faintness, and, on occasion, diarrhea. Patients are discouraged from eating sugary foods after surgery to avoid dumping syndrome. Because sections of the small intestine are bypassed, poor absorption of iron can cause iron-deficiency anemia. Patients need to take a multivitamin with iron and calcium supplements. Chronic anemia caused by cobalamin deficiency may occur. This problem can usually be managed with parenteral or intranasal cobalamin.

Implantable Gastric Stimulation
An implantable gastric stimulation device (e.g., Maestro Rechargeable System) consists of a pacemaker-like electrical pulse generator, wire leads, and electrodes that are implanted in the abdomen (Fig. 40.8). The Maestro System works by sending intermittent electrical pulses to the vagus nerve, which is involved in regulating stomach emptying and signaling to the brain that the stomach feels empty or full. External controllers allow the patient to charge the device and allow HCPs to adjust

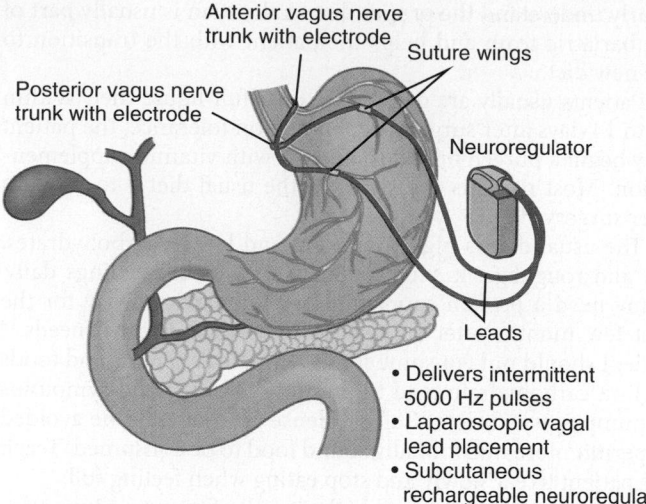

Anterior vagus nerve trunk with electrode

Suture wings

Posterior vagus nerve trunk with electrode

Neuroregulator

Leads

- Delivers intermittent 5000 Hz pulses
- Laparoscopic vagal lead placement
- Subcutaneous rechargeable neuroregulator

FIG. 40.8 The Maestro Rechargeable System is an electrical stimulator that is surgically implanted into the abdomen. It works by sending intermittent electrical pulses to the vagus nerve, which is involved in regulating stomach emptying and signaling to the brain that the stomach feels empty or full.

the device's settings to provide optimal therapy. Adverse events include nausea, heartburn, problems swallowing, belching, and chest pain.

❖ NURSING MANAGEMENT: PERIOPERATIVE CARE OF THE OBESE PATIENT

◆ Nursing Implementation

This section discusses general nursing considerations for the care of the obese patient who is having surgery. Special nursing considerations are described for the patient who is having bariatric surgery (Table 40.11). See Chapters 17 through 19 for more on care of the surgical patient.

◆ **Preoperative Care.** Special considerations are needed for the obese patient, especially the patient with extreme obesity, who is having surgery. Before surgery, interview the patient to identify past and current health information and any assistive devices currently in use (e.g., continuous positive airway pressure [CPAP] for sleep apnea). Co-morbidities related to obesity increase the risk for complications in the perioperative period. You may need to coordinate care with the patient's specialists.

Have a plan in place before the patients arrive so that they receive optimal care and do not feel like they are a burden to the nursing staff. You must have available appropriate-size hospital gowns, beds that accommodate an increased body size, and necessary patient transfer equipment. A larger BP cuff size is needed to avoid measurement errors. Ensure that an oversized BP cuff is available and placed in the patient's room.

Consider how the patient will be weighed and transported throughout the hospital. A wheelchair with removable arms that is large enough to safely accommodate the patient and pass easily through doorways should be available.

You may need to use alternative assessment techniques to perform assessment of heart, lung, and bowel sounds. For example, because of the large chest wall, breath and heart sounds are often distant. You can use an electronic stethoscope to amplify lung, heart, and bowel sounds.

Teach the patient proper coughing and deep breathing techniques and methods of turning and positioning to prevent

TABLE 40.11 Nursing Management
Care of the Patient Undergoing Bariatric Surgery

Preoperative

- Assess for use of assistive devices. Note any physical limitations or mobility issues.
- Perform baseline assessment, including vital signs, pulse oximetry, height, weight, BMI, skin condition, nutrition status, and heart, lung, and bowel sounds.
- Assess baseline laboratory values and diagnostic test results (e.g., pulmonary function tests).
- Teach patient and caregiver about procedure and postoperative care. Review proper coughing and deep breathing techniques, incentive spirometer use, and methods of turning and positioning to prevent pulmonary complications.
- Explain the need for frequent assessment and interventions to prevent VTE.
- Have available proper-sized hospital gowns, beds, BP cuffs, and transfer equipment.

Immediate Postoperative

- Perform assessment and compare to baseline: vital signs, pulse oximetry, and heart and lung sounds.
- Assess abdominal wound for the amount and type of drainage, condition of the incision, and signs of infection.
- Observe for anastomosis leak (tachycardia, fever, tachypnea, chest and abdominal pain).
- Help patient turn, cough and deep breath, and use incentive spirometer at least every 2 hrs.
- Protect the incision against any straining that accompanies turning and coughing.
- Give pain medications as needed.
- Position the patient upright at a minimum of a 45-degree angle.
- Maintain IV and/or oral fluid intake and monitor urine output.
- Institute measures to prevent VTE.
- Nutrition
  - Start with room temperature water and low-sugar clear liquids.
  - Teach the patient to avoid drinking with a straw.
  - Begin with 15 mL every 10–15 minutes, gradually increase to 90 mL every 30 min.
  - Move to a low-fat, full-liquid diet after 48 hrs if tolerating clear liquids.
  - Observe for dehydration (thirst, decreased urine output, headache, dizziness).

pulmonary complications after surgery. If possible, show how to use a spirometer before surgery. Spirometer use helps prevent and treat postoperative lung congestion. Practicing these strategies preoperatively can help the patient perform them correctly postoperatively. If the patient uses CPAP at home for sleep apnea, make arrangements for the use of a machine while the patient is hospitalized.

Excess adipose tissue may make obtaining venous access difficult. A longer IV catheter is helpful (longer than 1 in) to go through the overlying tissue to the vein. It is important that the cannula is far enough into the vein so it is not dislodged or infiltrated.

Special Considerations for Bariatric Surgery. Ensure that the patient scheduled for bariatric surgery understands the surgical procedure. Your teaching depends on the type of procedure and surgical approach (Table 40.10). Stress that we will frequently assess vital signs and general assessment to monitor for complications. Tell the patient that they will be assisted with ambulation soon after surgery and encouraged to cough and deep breathe to prevent pulmonary complications.

◆**Postoperative Care.** The initial postoperative care focuses on careful assessment and immediate intervention for cardiopulmonary complications, thrombus formation, anastomosis leaks, and electrolyte imbalances. The transfer from surgery may require many staff members. During the transfer, keep the patient's airway stabilized and give attention to managing the patient' pain. Maintain the patient's head at a 45-degree angle to reduce abdominal pressure and increase lung expansion.[18]

The body stores anesthetics in adipose tissue, thus placing patients with excess adipose tissue at risk for resedation. As adipose cells release anesthetics back into the bloodstream, the patient may become sedated after surgery. If this happens, be prepared to perform a head-tilt or jaw-thrust maneuver and keep the patient's oral and nasal airways open.

Diligence in turning and ambulation postoperatively will prevent complications from surgery. The patient will typically begin walking the evening after surgery and then at least 3 or 4 times each day. Assist the patient as needed. The patient may be reluctant to move or may not have the stamina to walk even a short distance. In either situation, you will need help moving an obese patient.

Obesity can cause a patient's breathing to become shallow and rapid. The extra adipose tissue in the chest and abdomen compresses the diaphragmatic, thoracic, and abdominal structures. This compression restricts the chest's ability to expand, preventing the lungs from working as efficiently as they would otherwise. The patient retains more CO_2 with less O_2 delivered to the lungs. This results in hypoxemia, pulmonary hypertension, and polycythemia.

After surgery, the risk for venous thromboembolism (VTE) is increased. Intermittent pneumatic compression devices or compression stockings with low-dose heparin decrease the risk for VTE. Active and passive range-of-motion exercises are a frequent part of daily care.[18]

Wound infection, dehiscence, and delayed healing are potential problems for all obese patients. Assess the patient's skin for any complications related to wound healing. Keep skinfolds clean and dry to prevent dermatitis and bacterial or fungal infections.

Special Considerations for Bariatric Surgery. Patients have considerable abdominal pain after bariatric surgery (Table 40.11). Give pain medications as needed during the immediate postoperative period (first 24 hours). Be aware that pain could be from an anastomosis leak rather than typical surgical pain. Abdominal wounds require frequent observation for the amount and type of drainage, condition of the incision, and signs of infection. Monitor vital signs to help identify problems, such as infection or anastomosis leak.

Give room temperature water and low-sugar clear liquids as soon as the patient is fully awake and there is no evidence of any anastomosis leaks. Begin with 15-mL increments every 10 to 15 minutes. Gradually increase intake to a goal of 90 mL every 30 minutes by postoperative day 1. Teach the patient to avoid gulping fluids or drinking with a straw to reduce the incidence of air swallowing. The patient who tolerates clear liquids may begin a low-fat, full-liquid diet on postoperative day 3.

◆**Ambulatory and Home Care**

Special Considerations for Bariatric Surgery. The patient who has undergone major surgical treatment for obesity has not been successful in the past in following or maintaining a prescribed diet. Now the patient must reduce oral intake because of the anatomic changes from the surgical procedure. The patient must clearly understand the proper diet. A dietitian is usually part of the bariatric team and helps the patient with the transition to the new diet.

Patients usually are discharged on a full-liquid diet. Within 10 to 14 days after surgery, depending on tolerance, the patient may begin a pureed or soft foods diet with vitamin supplementation. Most patients transition to the usual diet 4 to 6 weeks after surgery.[19]

The usual diet is high in protein and low in carbohydrates, fat, and roughage. It should consist of 6 small feedings daily. Many need a protein supplement once or twice a day for the first few months after surgery to meet their protein needs.[19] Patient should not consume fluids with meals. Fluids and foods high in carbohydrate tend to promote diarrhea and symptoms of dumping syndrome. Calorie-dense foods should be avoided to permit more nutritionally sound food to be consumed. Teach the patient to eat slowly and stop eating when feeling full.

Weight loss is considerable during the first 6 to 12 months. Although behavior modification is not necessarily an intended outcome with these surgical procedures, it becomes an unexpected secondary gain. For example, a person who has had bariatric surgery cannot overeat or binge eat without consequences (e.g., vomiting, abdominal pain). The patient may fail to lose weight if the stomach pouch is too large. An outlet that is much too small may result in the patient losing too much weight. Some patients have been known to overeat when they return home and gain rather than lose weight.

Stress the importance of long-term follow-up care, in part because of potential complications. Teach patients to inform the HCP of any changes in their physical or emotional condition. Nutritional deficiencies are expected after malabsorptive bariatric surgery, including anemia, vitamin deficiencies, and diarrhea. Patients should take multivitamins with folate, calcium, vitamin D, iron, and vitamin B_{12} for life.[20] Peptic ulcer formation, dumping syndrome, and small bowel obstruction may be seen late in the recovery and rehabilitation stage.

INFORMATICS IN PRACTICE
Use of Smart Phone for Weight Loss

- Phone apps (e.g., My Fitness Pal) are available to help track calories, weight, exercise, and eating patterns.
- Tracking systems give immediate access to nutritional information for better dietary decision making.
- Some apps can scan the barcode of foods in the grocery store and give nutritional information.
- Calorie tracker apps can be used to monitor daily calorie intake and keep a record of weight loss progress.
- With text messaging, a phone "buddy" can provide support when a person's will power is lacking.
- Share progress with friends and family. Some weight loss apps sync with social media accounts so that a person can share milestones on Twitter and Facebook.

Several potential psychologic problems may arise after surgery. Assess social functioning, self-esteem, sexual life, and activities of daily living in follow-up care. Some patients feel guilty that they had to achieve weight loss by surgical intervention rather than by the "sheer willpower" of reduced dietary intake and exercise. Be ready to provide support and assist the patient in moving away from such negative feelings.

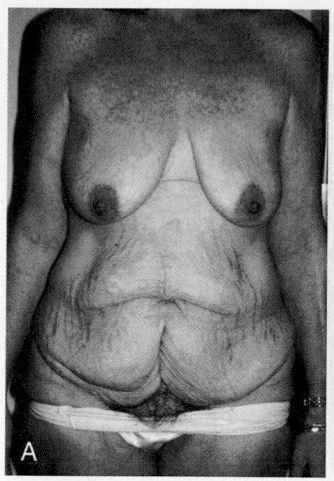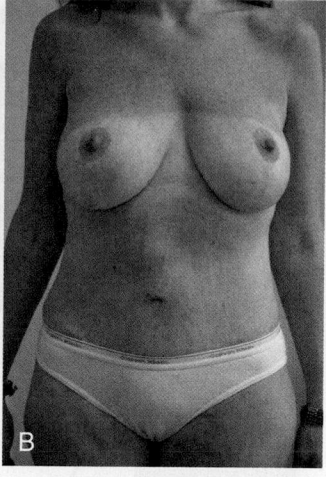

FIG. 40.9 A, Preoperative view of a 37-yr-old woman with massive weight loss who had gastric bypass surgery. B, Postoperative view 2½ years after abdominoplasty. She underwent breast surgery, thigh lift, back lift with excision of excess skin of the lower back and upper buttocks, and upper arm surgery. (From Shermak MA: Contouring the epigastrium, *Aesthet Surg J* 25:506, 2005.)

By 6 to 8 months after surgery, most patients have lost considerable weight and are able to see how much their appearance has changed. Help the patient adjust to a new body image. Massive weight loss may leave the patient with large quantities of flabby skin that can result in problems related to altered body image (Fig. 40.9). Discuss this possible outcome with the patient before surgery and again during the rehabilitation phase. Cosmetic surgery may alleviate this situation. Do not hesitate to encourage counseling for unresolved psychologic issues.

Often one result of bariatric surgery is the return of fertility in women. Pregnancy complications can result from anemia and nutritional deficiencies. Furthermore, depending on the type of surgery, intestinal obstructions and hernias may occur with pregnancy. Women must carefully consider the risk for pregnancy after bariatric surgery. In general, encourage women to postpone pregnancy for 12 to 18 months after bariatric surgery.

👤 CHECK YOUR PRACTICE

You are working in the bariatric surgery outpatient clinic. When you walk into the clinic room where a 36-yr-old woman is waiting for her follow-up visit, you find her distraught and crying. You ask her what is wrong. She responds, "I am a total failure. I have been fat all my life, and I had to have this horrible surgery to help me. Why couldn't I do it on my own?"
• What is an effective way for you to handle this situation?

◆ Evaluation

The expected outcomes are that the obese patient will
• Have long-term weight loss
• Have improvement in obesity-related co-morbidities
• Integrate healthy practices into daily routines
• Monitor for adverse side effects of surgical therapy
• Have an improved self-image

👤 Gerontologic Considerations: Obesity in Older Adults

The prevalence of obesity is increasing in older people. The number of obese older persons has markedly risen because of increases in both the total number of older persons and the percent of the older adults who are obese. Obesity is more common in older women than in older men. A decrease in energy expenditure is an important contributor to a gradual increase in body fat with age.

Obesity in older adults can worsen age-related declines in physical function and lead to frailty and disability. Obesity is associated with decreased survival. Those who are obese live 6 to 7 years less than people of normal weight.

Obesity worsens many changes associated with aging. Excess body weight places more demands on arthritic joints. The mechanical strain on weight-bearing joints can lead to premature immobility. Excess intraabdominal weight can cause problems with urinary incontinence. Excess weight may contribute to hypoventilation and sleep apnea.

Obesity affects the quality of life for older adults. Weight loss can improve physical functioning and obesity-related health complications. The same therapeutic approaches for obesity discussed earlier also apply to the older adult.

COSMETIC SURGICAL THERAPY

Lipectomy

Lipectomy (adipectomy) is done to remove unsightly flabby folds of adipose tissue (Fig. 40.9). There is no evidence that regeneration of adipose tissue occurs at the surgical sites. However, Stress to the patient that surgical removal does not prevent obesity from recurring, especially if lifetime eating habits stay the same. Although body image and self-esteem may improve with such procedures, these operations are not without complications. Do not underestimate the dangerous effects of anesthesia and the potential for poor wound healing in the obese patient.

Liposuction

Another cosmetic surgical procedure is liposuction, or suction-assisted lipectomy. It is used for cosmetic purposes and not for weight reduction. This surgical intervention helps improve facial appearance or body contours. A good candidate is a person who has achieved weight reduction and has excess fat under the chin, along the jaw line, in the nasolabial folds, over the abdomen, or around the waist and upper thighs. A long, hollow, stainless steel cannula is inserted through a small incision over the fatty tissue to be suctioned. This surgical procedure is not usually recommended for an older person because the skin is less elastic and will not accommodate the new underlying shape.

METABOLIC SYNDROME

Metabolic syndrome is a group of metabolic risk factors that increase a person's chance of developing CVD, stroke, and diabetes. About 1 in 3 adults have metabolic syndrome. The syndrome is more prevalent in those 60 years of age and older.[21]

Metabolic syndrome is a cluster of health problems, including obesity, hypertension, abnormal lipid levels, and high blood glucose. Metabolic syndrome is diagnosed if a person has 3 or more of the conditions listed in Table 40.12.

Etiology and Pathophysiology

The main underlying risk factor for metabolic syndrome is insulin resistance related to excess visceral fat (Fig. 40.10). Insulin resistance is the decreased ability of the body's cells to respond to the action of insulin. The pancreas compensates by secreting more insulin, resulting in hyperinsulinemia.

TABLE 40.12 Criteria for Metabolic Syndrome

Any 3 of the 5 measures are needed to diagnose metabolic syndrome:

Measure	Criteria
Waist circumference	≥40 in (102 cm) in men
	≥35 in (89 cm) in women
Triglycerides	>150 mg/dL (1.7 mmol/L)
	OR
	Drug treatment for high triglycerides
HDL cholesterol	<40 mg/dL (0.9 mmol/L) in men
	<50 mg/dL (1.1 mmol/L) in women
	OR
	Drug treatment for high cholesterol
BP	≥130 mm Hg systolic BP
	OR
	≥85 mm Hg diastolic BP
	OR
	Drug treatment for hypertension
Fasting blood glucose	≥100 mg/dL
	OR
	Drug treatment for elevated glucose

Source: National Heart, Lung, and Blood Institute: How is metabolic syndrome diagnosed? Retrieved from *www.nhlbi.nih.gov/health/health-topics/topics/ms/diagnosis.*

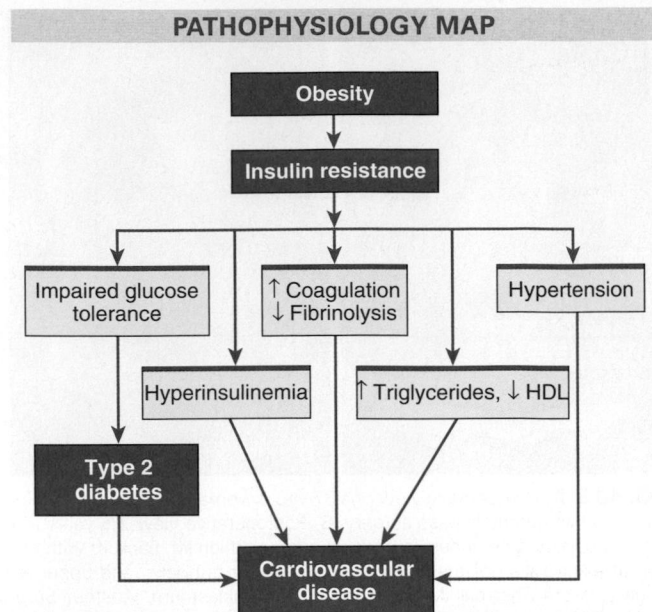

PATHOPHYSIOLOGY MAP

FIG. 40.10 Relationship among insulin resistance, obesity, diabetes, and CVD.

Other characteristics include hypertension, increased risk for clotting, and abnormalities in cholesterol levels. The net effect of these conditions is an increased prevalence of coronary artery disease.

Clinical Manifestations and Diagnostic Studies

The signs of metabolic syndrome are impaired fasting blood glucose, hypertension, abnormal cholesterol levels, and obesity. Medical problems develop over time if the condition is not addressed. Patients with this syndrome are at a higher risk for heart disease, stroke, diabetes, renal disease, and polycystic ovary syndrome. Patients who have metabolic syndrome and smoke are at an even higher risk.

❖ NURSING AND INTERPROFESSIONAL MANAGEMENT: METABOLIC SYNDROME

There is no specific management of metabolic syndrome. Interventions focus on reducing the major risk factors of CVD and type 2 diabetes: reducing LDL cholesterol, stopping smoking, lowering BP, losing weight, and reducing glucose levels. There are no specific medications for metabolic syndrome. Patients receive cholesterol-lowering and antihypertensive drugs as needed. Metformin (Glucophage) can lower glucose levels and enhance the cells' sensitivity to insulin. Obese patients may be candidates for bariatric surgery.

For long-term risk reduction, the person needs to maintain a healthy weight, increase physical activity, and follow healthy diet habits. You can help patients by giving information on healthy diets, exercise, and positive lifestyle changes. The diet, which should be low in saturated fats, should promote weight loss. Weight reduction and maintaining a lower weight are a priority in those with abdominal obesity and metabolic syndrome.

Because sedentary lifestyles contribute to metabolic syndrome, increasing regular physical activity will lower a patient's risk factors. In addition to helping with weight reduction, regular exercise decreases triglyceride levels and increases HDL cholesterol levels in those with metabolic syndrome.

CASE STUDY

Obesity

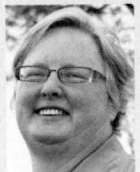

(© Thinkstock.)

Patient Profile

S.R. is a 48-yr-old white woman who comes to the clinic reporting hip pain.

Subjective Data

- States that it is "getting hard to get around"
- Reports gradual weight gain of 40 lbs over past 20 yrs
- Lives in a rural community with no sidewalks
- Spends her free time watching television
- Reports a history of type 2 diabetes, shortness of breath, hypertension, and osteoarthritis
- Had knee replacement surgery at age 46 for osteoarthritis
- Tried orlistat (Xenical) but hated the side effects

Objective Data

Physical Examination

- 5 ft, 6 in tall; weighs 230 lb; BMI 37 kg/m², waist circumference of 40 in
- Has obese, nontender, soft round, abdomen
- BP 160/100 mm Hg
- Moderate pain with range of motion of both hips

Laboratory Results

- Fasting blood glucose 250 mg/dL (13.9 mmol/L)
- Total cholesterol 205 mg/dL (5.3 mmol/L)
- Triglyceride 298 mg/dL (3.36 mmol/L)
- HDL cholesterol 31 mg/dL (0.8 mmol/L)
- LDL cholesterol 114 mg/dL

CASE STUDY
Obesity—cont'd

Interprofessional Care
- Referral to a community weight loss program
- Consultation with bariatric surgeon
- Diagnosed with bilateral osteoarthritis of the hips

Discussion Questions
1. What are S.R.'s risk factors for obesity?
2. Of the possible complications of obesity, which ones does S.R. have? Why did she develop them?

3. *Patient-Centered Care:* How would you help S.R. in designing a successful weight loss and weight management program?
4. *Collaboration:* How could a comprehensive community weight loss program be beneficial to S.R.?
5. What are S.R.'s risk factors for metabolic syndrome?
6. Is S.R. a candidate for bariatric surgery? Why or why not?
7. *Evidence-Based Practice:* S.R. tells you that she is not sure surgery will work for her. She asks you, "What is the best surgery for me?"

Answers available at *http://evolve.elsevier.com/Lewis/medsurg.*

BRIDGE TO NCLEX EXAMINATION

The number of the question corresponds to the same-numbered outcome at the beginning of the chapter.

1. Which statement *best* describes the etiology of obesity?
   a. Obesity primarily results from a genetic predisposition.
   b. Psychosocial factors can override the effects of genetics in causing obesity.
   c. Obesity is the result of complex interactions between genetic and environmental factors.
   d. Genetic factors are more important than environmental factors in the etiology of obesity.

2. Health risks associated with obesity include *(select all that apply)*
   a. colorectal cancer.
   b. rheumatoid arthritis.
   c. polycystic ovary syndrome.
   d. nonalcoholic steatohepatitis.
   e. systemic lupus erythematosus.

3. The obesity classification that is *most* often associated with cardiovascular health problems is
   a. primary obesity.
   b. secondary obesity.
   c. gynoid fat distribution.
   d. android fat distribution.

4. The *best* nutritional therapy plan for a person who is obese
   a. is high in animal protein.
   b. is fat-free and low in carbohydrates.
   c. restricts intake to under 800 calories per day.
   d. lowers calories with foods from all the basic groups.

5. This bariatric surgical procedure involves creating a gastric pouch that is reversible, and no malabsorption occurs. Which surgical procedure is this?
   a. Vertical gastric banding
   b. Biliopancreatic diversion
   c. Roux-en-Y gastric bypass
   d. Adjustable gastric banding

6. A patient with extreme obesity has undergone Roux-en-Y gastric bypass surgery. In planning postoperative care, the nurse anticipates that the patient
   a. may have severe diarrhea early in the postoperative period.
   b. will not be allowed to ambulate for 1 to 2 days postoperatively.
   c. will require nasogastric suction until the drainage is pale yellow.
   d. may have limited amounts of oral liquids during the early postoperative period.

7. Which criteria must be met for a diagnosis of metabolic syndrome? *(select all that apply)*
   a. Hypertension
   b. High triglycerides
   c. Elevated plasma glucose
   d. Increased waist circumference
   e. Decreased low-density lipoproteins

1. c, 2. a, c, d, 3. d, 4. d, 5. d, 6. d, 7. a, b, c, d

For rationales to these answers and even more NCLEX review questions, visit *http://evolve.elsever.com/Lewis/medsurg.*

EVOLVE WEBSITE/RESOURCES LIST

http://evolve.elsevier.com/Lewis/medsurg
Review Questions (Online Only)
Key Points
Answer Keys for Questions
- Rationales for Bridge to NCLEX Examination Questions
- Answer Guidelines for Case Study on p. 886
Student Case Study
- Patient With Obesity and Osteoarthritis
Conceptual Care Map Creator
Audio Glossary
Content Updates

REFERENCES

1. Centers for Disease Control and Prevention: Overweight and obesity. Retrieved from *www.cdc.gov/obesity/data/adult.html.*
*2. Albuquerque D, Nóbrega C, Manco L, et al: The contribution of genetics and environment to obesity, *BMJ* 123:73, 2017.
*3. Dimitriadis GK, Randeva MS, Miras AD: Potential hormone mechanisms of bariatric surgery, *Curr Obes Rep* 6:253, 2017.
*4. Shibata R, Ouchi N, Ohashi K, et al: The role of adipokines in cardiovascular disease, *J Cardiol* 70:329, 2017.
5. Robert Wood Johnson Foundation. The state of obesity. Retrieved from *https://stateofobesity.org/resources/.*
*6. Björnson E, Adiels M, Taskinen MR, et al : Kinetics of plasma triglycerides in abdominal obesity, *Curr Opin Lipidol* 28:11, 2017.

7. The link between obesity and cancer (editorial), *Lancet* 390:1716, 2017.

*8. Rotenberg KJ, Bharathi C, Davies H, et al: Obesity and the social withdrawal syndrome, *Eating Behaviors* 26:167, 2017.

9. Centers for Disease Control and Prevention: Assessing your weight. Retrieved from *www.cdc.gov/healthyweight/assessing/index.html.*

*10. Acosta A, Streett S, Kroh MD, et al: White paper AGA: POWER—Practice guide on obesity and weight management, education and resources, *Clin Gastroenterol Hepat* 515:631, 2017.

11. Bray GA, Frühbeck G, Ryan DH, et al: Management of obesity, *Lancet* 387:1947, 2016.

*12. Lv N, Azar KM, Rosas LG, et al: Behavioral lifestyle interventions for moderate and severe obesity: A systematic review, *Prev Med* 100:180, 2017.

13. Alfaris N, Minnick A, Hong P, et al: A review of commercial and proprietary weight loss programs. In: Mechanik J, Kushner R, eds: *Lifestyle medicine: A manual for clinical practice,* New York, 2016, Springer.

14. Igel LI, Kumar RB, Saunders KH, et al: Practical use of pharmacotherapy for obesity, *Gastroenterol* 152:1765, 2017.

*15. Gadde KM, Martin CK, Berthoud HR, et al: Obesity: Pathophysiology and management, *J Am Coll Cardiol* 71:69, 2018.

*16. Adams TD, Davidson LE, Litwin SE, et al: Weight and metabolic outcomes 12 years after gastric bypass, *NEJM* 377:1143, 2017.

17. Genco A, Maselli R, Casella G, et al: *Intragastric balloon treatment for obesity,* New York, 2016, Springer.

*18. Thorell A, MacCormick AD, Awad S, et al: Guidelines for perioperative care in bariatric surgery: Enhanced Recovery After Surgery (ERAS) Society recommendations, *World J Surg* 40:2065, 2016.

*19. Dagan SS, Goldenshluger A, Globus I, et al: Nutritional recommendations for adult bariatric surgery patients, *Adv Nutr* 8:382, 2017.

*20. Cooley M: Preventing long-term poor outcomes in the bariatric patient postoperatively, *DCCN* 36:30, 2017.

*21. Moore JX, Chaudhary N, Akinyemiju T: Metabolic syndrome prevalence by race/ethnicity and sex in the United States, *PCD* 14:24, 2017.

*Evidence-based information for clinical practice.

41

Upper Gastrointestinal Problems

Kara Ann Ventura

Anywhere I see suffering that is where I want to be, doing what I can.

Princess Diana

http://evolve.elsevier.com/Lewis/medsurg

CONCEPTUAL FOCUS

Fluids and Electrolytes	Pain	Stress
Nutrition	Sleep	Tissue Integrity

LEARNING OUTCOMES

1. Describe the etiology, complications, and interprofessional and nursing management of nausea and vomiting.
2. Relate the etiology, clinical manifestations, and interprofessional and nursing management of common oral inflammations and infections.
3. Describe the etiology, clinical manifestations, complications, and interprofessional and nursing management of oral cancer.
4. Explain the types, pathophysiology, clinical manifestations, complications, and interprofessional and nursing management of gastroesophageal reflux disease and hiatal hernia.
5. Relate the pathophysiology, clinical manifestations, complications, and interprofessional management of esophageal cancer, diverticula, achalasia, and esophageal strictures.
6. Distinguish between acute and chronic gastritis, including the etiology, pathophysiology, and interprofessional and nursing management.
7. Compare and contrast gastric and duodenal ulcers, including the etiology, pathophysiology, clinical manifestations, complications, and interprofessional and nursing management.
8. Describe the clinical manifestations and interprofessional and nursing management of stomach cancer.
9. Explain the common etiologies, clinical manifestations, and interprofessional and nursing management of upper gastrointestinal bleeding.
10. Identify common types of foodborne illnesses and nursing responsibilities related to food poisoning.

KEY TERMS

achalasia, p. 904	gastritis, p. 915	peptic ulcer disease (PUD), p. 904
Barrett's esophagus, p. 897	gastroesophageal reflux disease (GERD), p. 896	stomach (gastric) cancer, p. 911
dysphagia, p. 894	hiatal hernia, p. 900	stress-related mucosal disease (SRMD), p. 917
esophageal cancer, p. 901	Mallory-Weiss tear, p. 891	vomiting, p. 889
esophagitis, p. 897	nausea, p. 889	

Several upper gastrointestinal (GI) problems and the care of the patient undergoing upper GI surgery are discussed in this chapter. These include nausea and vomiting, oral and gastric cancers, gastroesophageal reflux, ulcerative disease, inflammatory and infectious bowel disorders, GI bleeding, and structural problems. Conceptually, patients with impaired GI function may have malnutrition from impaired nutritional intake. Many are at risk for altered fluid, electrolyte, and acid-base balance. Problems with eating, drinking, or talking may cause pain and impair the ability to communicate. Pain can disrupt sleep and cause fatigue. Difficulty swallowing increases the risk for aspiration.

NAUSEA AND VOMITING

Nausea and vomiting are the most common manifestations of GI disease. Although nausea and vomiting can occur independently, they are closely related and usually treated as one problem. Nausea is a feeling of discomfort in the epigastrium with a conscious desire to vomit. Vomiting is the forceful ejection of partially digested food and secretions (*emesis*) from the upper GI tract.

Etiology and Pathophysiology

Nausea and vomiting occur in a wide variety of GI disorders and in many conditions unrelated to GI disease. These include pregnancy; infection; central nervous system (CNS) problems (e.g., meningitis, tumor); cardiovascular disease (CVD) (e.g., myocardial infarction, heart failure); metabolic disorders (e.g. psychologic factors (e.g., stress, fear); and when the GI tract becomes overly irritated, excited, or distended. Patients may have nausea and vomiting after surgery with general anesthesia or as a drug side effect (e.g., chemotherapy, opioids). Women are more likely to have nausea and vomiting associated with anesthesia and motion sickness.[1]

A vomiting center in the medulla coordinates the multiple components involved in vomiting. This center receives input from various stimuli. Neural impulses reach the vomiting center via afferent pathways through branches of the autonomic nervous system. Receptors for these afferent fibers are found in the GI tract, kidneys, heart, and uterus. When stimulated, these receptors relay information to the vomiting (emetic) center, which then initiates the vomiting reflex (Fig. 41.1).

Vomiting is a complex act. It requires the coordinated activity of several structures: closure of the glottis, deep inspiration with contraction of the diaphragm in the inspiratory position, closure of the pylorus, relaxation of the stomach and lower esophageal sphincter (LES), and contraction of the abdominal muscles with increasing intraabdominal pressure. These simultaneous activities force the stomach contents up through the esophagus, into the pharynx, and out the mouth.

The chemoreceptor trigger zone (CTZ), found in the brainstem, responds to chemical stimuli from drugs, toxins, and labyrinthine stimulation (e.g., motion sickness). Once stimulated, the CTZ transmits impulses directly to the vomiting center. This action activates the autonomic nervous system, resulting in both parasympathetic and sympathetic stimulation. Sympathetic activation causes tachycardia, tachypnea, and diaphoresis. Parasympathetic stimulation causes relaxation of the LES, an increase in gastric motility, and a pronounced increase in salivation.

Clinical Manifestations

Nausea is subjective. *Anorexia* (lack of appetite) usually accompanies nausea. When nausea and vomiting occur over a long period, dehydration can develop rapidly. Water and essential electrolytes (e.g., potassium, sodium, chloride, hydrogen) are lost. As vomiting persists, the patient may have severe electrolyte imbalances, extracellular fluid volume loss, decreased plasma volume, and eventually circulatory failure.

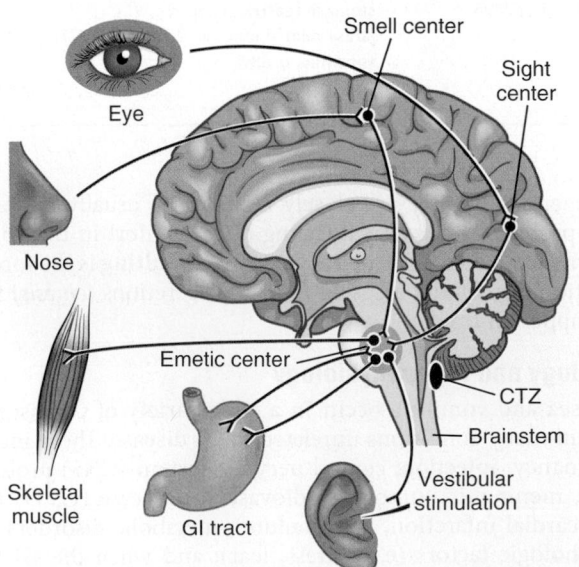

FIG. 41.1 Stimuli involved in the act of vomiting. *CTZ,* Chemoreceptor trigger zone. (Modified from McKenry L, Tessier E, Hogan M: *Mosby's pharmacology in nursing,* ed 22, St Louis, 2006, Mosby.)

Metabolic alkalosis can result from loss of gastric hydrochloric (HCl) acid. Metabolic acidosis can occur with vomiting of small intestine contents. However, metabolic acidosis is less common than metabolic alkalosis. Weight loss resulting from fluid loss can occur in a short time with severe vomiting.

Interprofessional Care

In managing nausea and vomiting, the goals of care are to determine and treat the underlying cause, recognize and correct any complications, and provide symptomatic relief.

Drug Therapy. The use of drugs to treat nausea and vomiting depends on the cause of the problem (Table 41.1). Many antiemetic drugs act in the CNS via the CTZ to block the neurochemicals that trigger nausea and vomiting. When the cause has not been determined, use drugs with caution. Using antiemetics before knowing the cause can mask the underlying disease process and delay diagnosis and treatment.

 DRUG ALERT Promethazine Injection

- Do not give into an artery or under the skin because of the risk for severe tissue injury.
- When given IV, it can leak out of the vein and cause severe damage to surrounding tissue.
- Deep muscle injection is the preferred route of injection administration.

5-HT$_3$ (Serotonin) receptor antagonists are effective in reducing chemotherapy-induced vomiting (CINV), postoperative nausea and vomiting (PONV), and nausea and vomiting related to migraine headache and anxiety. Dexamethasone is given with other antiemetics to manage acute and delayed CINV. Neurokinin-1 receptor antagonists (NK$_1$RAs) (e.g., aprepitant [Emend], rolapitant [Varubi]), can treat CINV and PONV.[2]

 DRUG ALERT Metoclopramide (Reglan)

- Chronic use or high doses carry the risk for tardive dyskinesia.
- Tardive dyskinesia is a neurologic condition characterized by involuntary and repetitive movements of the body (e.g., extremity movements, lip smacking).
- Tardive dyskinesia may persist after stopping the drug.

An oral cannabinoid (e.g., dronabinol) may be part of the regimen to manage CINV. Because of the potential for abuse as well as drowsiness and sedation, this is an option only when other therapies are not effective.

❖ NURSING MANAGEMENT: NAUSEA AND VOMITING

◆ Nursing Assessment

Each patient with a history of prolonged and persistent nausea or vomiting needs a thorough nursing assessment. You should have a basic understanding of the common conditions associated with nausea and vomiting and be able to identify the patient who is at high risk. Assess the patient for precipitating factors and describe the contents of the emesis. Table 41.2 presents subjective and objective data to obtain from a patient with nausea and vomiting.

When food is the precipitating cause of nausea and vomiting, help the patient identify the specific food. Determine when it was eaten, prior history with the food, and whether anyone else who ate the food is sick. Emesis containing

TABLE 41.1 Drug Therapy
Nausea and Vomiting

Drug	Mechanism of Action	Side Effects
Anticholinergics		
scopolamine transdermal	Block cholinergic pathways to vomiting center	Xerostomia, somnolence
Antihistamines		
dimenhydrinate (Dramamine) diphenhydramine hydroxyzine meclizine (Antivert)	Block histamine receptors that trigger nausea and vomiting	Dry mouth, hypotension, sedative effects, rashes, constipation
Cannabinoids		
dronabinol (Marinol) nabilone (Cesamet)	Inhibit vomiting control mechanism in the medulla oblongata	Xerostomia, amnesia, ataxia, confusion, coordination problems, dizziness, somnolence
Corticosteroids		
dexamethasone	Not well understood how it prevents nausea and vomiting	Hyperglycemia, insomnia, euphoria
5-HT$_3$ (Serotonin) Antagonists		
granisetron ondansetron (Zofran) palonosetron (Aloxi)	Block action of serotonin	Constipation, diarrhea, headache, fatigue, malaise, increased liver function tests
Phenothiazines		
chlorpromazine prochlorperazine promethazine Prokinetic	Act in the CNS level of the chemoreceptor trigger zone (CTZ). Block dopamine receptors that trigger nausea and vomiting	Dry mouth, hypotension, sedative effects, rashes, constipation
Metoclopramide (Reglan)	Inhibit action of dopamine. ↑ Gastric motility and emptying	CNS side effects ranging from anxiety to hallucinations, extrapyramidal side effects, including tremor and dyskinesias
Substance P/Neurokinin-1 Receptor Antagonists		
aprepitant (Emend) netupitant and palonosetron (Akynzeo) rolapitant (Varubi)	Block interaction of Substance P at NK-1 receptor	Headache, hiccups, fatigue, constipation, diarrhea, anorexia

partially digested food several hours after a meal indicates gastric outlet obstruction or delayed gastric emptying. The presence of fecal odor and bile after prolonged vomiting suggests intestinal obstruction below the level of the pylorus. Bile in the emesis suggests obstruction below the ampulla of Vater.

The color of the emesis helps determine the presence and source of any bleeding. Bright red blood occurs with active bleeding. This could be due to a **Mallory-Weiss tear** (disruption of the mucosal lining near the esophagogastric junction), esophageal varices, gastric or duodenal ulcer, or cancer. Vomitus with a "coffee-grounds" appearance is related to gastric bleeding. The blood changes to dark brown because of its interaction with HCl acid.

It is important to discern among vomiting, regurgitation, and projectile vomiting. *Regurgitation* is an effortless process in which partially digested food slowly comes up from the stomach. Retching or vomiting rarely occurs before it. *Projectile vomiting* is a forceful expulsion of stomach contents without nausea. It often occurs with brain and spinal cord tumors.

The timing of nausea and vomiting can help determine its cause. Early morning vomiting is common in pregnancy. Emotional stressors may elicit vomiting during or right after eating. Those with *cyclic vomiting syndrome* have recurring

episodes of nausea, vomiting, and fatigue that last from a few hours up to 10 days.

◆ Nursing Diagnoses

Nursing diagnoses for the patient with nausea and vomiting may include:
- Nausea
- Fluid imbalance
- Electrolyte imbalance
- Impaired nutritional intake

More information on nursing diagnoses and interventions are in eNursing Care Plan 41.1 (available on the website for this chapter).

◆ Planning

The overall goals are that the patient with nausea and vomiting will (1) have minimal or no nausea and vomiting, (2) have normal electrolyte levels and hydration status, and (3) return to a normal pattern of fluid balance and nutrient intake.

◆ Nursing Implementation

◆ **Acute Care.** Most people with nausea and vomiting are at home. When nausea and vomiting persist, the patient may need hospitalized to diagnose the underlying problem. Until we confirm

TABLE 41.2 Nursing Assessment

Nausea and Vomiting

Subjective Data

Important Health Information

Past health history: GI disorders, chronic indigestion, food allergies, pregnancy, infection, CNS problems, recent travel, eating disorders, metabolic disorders, cancer, CVD, renal disease
Medications: Antiemetics, digitalis, opioids, ferrous sulfate, aspirin, aminophylline, alcohol, antibiotics, chemotherapy. General anesthesia
Surgery or other treatments: Recent surgery

Functional Health Patterns

Nutritional-metabolic: Amount, frequency, character, and color of vomitus. Dry heaves. Anorexia, weight loss
Activity-exercise: Weakness, fatigue
Cognitive-perceptual: Abdominal tenderness or pain
Coping–stress tolerance: Stress, fear

Objective Data

General

Lethargy, sunken eyeballs

Integumentary

Pallor, dry mucous membranes, poor skin turgor

Gastrointestinal

Amount, frequency, character (e.g., projectile), content (undigested food, blood, bile, feces), and color of vomitus (red, coffee-grounds, green-yellow)

Urinary

Decreased output, concentrated urine

Possible Diagnostic Findings

Altered serum electrolytes (especially hypokalemia), metabolic alkalosis, abnormal upper GI findings on endoscopy or abdominal x-rays

---

a diagnosis, the patient is NPO and given IV fluids. The patient with persistent vomiting, a possible bowel obstruction, or paralytic ileus may need a nasogastric (NG) tube connected to suction to decompress the stomach. Secure the NG tube to prevent its movement in the nose and back of the throat, because this can stimulate nausea and vomiting.

With prolonged vomiting, there is a chance of dehydration and acid-base and electrolyte imbalances. Record intake and output, monitor vital signs, and assess for signs of dehydration. Provide physical and emotional support. Maintain a quiet, odor-free environment. Observe for changes in the patient's physical comfort and mentation. The risk for pulmonary aspiration is a concern when vomiting occurs in older or unconscious patients or in patients with conditions that impair the gag reflex. To prevent aspiration, put the patient who cannot manage self-care in a semi-Fowler's or side-lying position.

◆ **Nutritional Therapy.** The patient with severe vomiting needs IV fluid therapy with electrolyte and glucose replacement until able to tolerate oral intake. Start oral nutrition beginning with clear liquids once symptoms have subsided. A patient may be reluctant to resume fluid intake because of fear of symptoms recurring. Water is the initial fluid of choice for oral rehydration. Have the patient sip small amounts of fluid (5 to 15 mL) every 15 to 20 minutes. Other options include carbonated beverages with the carbonation removed at room temperature and

warm tea. Extremely hot or cold liquids are often hard to tolerate. Broth and sports drinks (e.g., Gatorade) are high in sodium, so give them with caution. Dry toast, crackers, and plain gelatin may be helpful.

As the patient's condition improves, provide a diet high in carbohydrates and low in fat. Bland foods, such as a baked potato, rice, cooked chicken, and cereal, are ideal. Many patients do not tolerate coffee, spicy foods, highly acidic foods, and those with strong odors. Tell the patient to eat food slowly and in small amounts to prevent overdistending the stomach. Liquids taken between meals rather than with meals reduce overdistention. Consult a dietitian about nutritious foods that the patient can tolerate.

> ### ❓ CHECK YOUR PRACTICE
>
> You are caring for a newly admitted 76-yr-old man who reports vomiting for the past 3 days. He says, "I cannot keep anything down, not even water."
> * What assessment do you need to perform?
> * What findings would show he is dehydrated?
> * What are your priority nursing interventions?

◆ **Ambulatory Care.** Teach the patient and caregiver (1) how to manage the unpleasant sensation of nausea, (2) methods to prevent nausea and vomiting, and (3) ways to maintain fluid and nutritional intake. Tell them to keep the immediate environment quiet, free of noxious odors, and well ventilated. Avoiding sudden changes of position and unnecessary activity are helpful. Encourage the use of relaxation techniques, frequent rest periods, effective pain management strategies, and diversional tactics. Cleansing the face and hands with a cool washcloth and providing mouth care between episodes increase the person's comfort level. When symptoms occur, stop all foods and drugs until the acute phase is over.

If you suspect a medication is the cause, notify the (HCP at once. The HCP can change the dose or prescribe a new drug. Tell the patient that stopping the drug without consulting the HCP may have adverse effects on the person's health. The patient should take an antiemetic drug only if prescribed by the HCP. Taking over-the-counter (OTC) drugs to relieve symptoms may make the problem worse.

Some patients find that acupressure or acupuncture at specific points is effective in reducing PONV.[3] Others use herbs, such as ginger and peppermint oil. Relaxation breathing exercises, changes in body position, or exercise may help some patients.

> ### 🌿 COMPLEMENTARY & ALTERNATIVE THERAPIES
>
> #### Ginger
>
> **Scientific Evidence**
> * May be effective for nausea and vomiting in pregnancy when used at recommended doses for short periods
> * May help CINV if used with antiemetic drugs
>
> **Nursing Implications**
> * Few adverse effects reported with short-term use
> * May interact with anticoagulants and increase risk for bleeding
> * Use with caution in people with gallbladder disease
>
> Source: *www.nccih.nih.gov/health/ginger*.

TABLE 41.3 Infections and Inflammation of the Mouth

Infection or Inflammation	Etiology	Manifestations	Treatment
Aphthous stomatitis (canker sore)	• Recurrent and chronic form of infection • Related to systemic disease, trauma, stress, or unknown causes	• Ulcers of mouth and lips, causing extreme pain • Ulcers surrounded by erythematous base	• Corticosteroids (topical or systemic) • Tetracycline oral suspension
Gingivitis	• Neglected oral hygiene, malocclusion, missing or irregular teeth, faulty dentistry • Eating soft rather than fibrous foods	• Inflamed gingivae and interdental papillae • Bleeding during tooth brushing • Development of pus, abscess formation with loosening of teeth (periodontitis)	• Prevention through health teaching, dental care, gingival massage, professional cleaning of teeth • Eat fibrous foods • Conscientious brushing habits with flossing
Herpes simplex (cold sore, fever blister) (see Table 23.6)	• Herpes simplex virus (type 1 or 2) • Predisposing factors of upper respiratory tract infections, excessive exposure to sunlight, food allergies, emotional tension, onset of menstruation	• Lip lesions, mouth lesions, vesicle formation (single or clustered) • Shallow, painful ulcers	• Spirits of camphor, corticosteroid cream, mild antiseptic mouthwash, viscous lidocaine • Remove or control predisposing factors • Antiviral agents (e.g., acyclovir [Zovirax], valacyclovir [Valtrex])
Oral candidiasis (moniliasis or thrush)	• *Candida albicans* (yeastlike fungus) • Debilitation • Prolonged high-dose antibiotic or corticosteroid therapy	• Pearly, bluish white "milk-curd" membranous lesions on mucosa of mouth and larynx • Sore mouth, yeasty halitosis	• Miconazole buccal tablets (Oravig) • Nystatin or amphotericin B as oral suspension or buccal tablets • Good oral hygiene
Parotitis (inflammation of parotid gland, surgical mumps)	• *Staphylococcus* species usually • *Streptococcus* species occasionally • Debilitation and dehydration with poor oral hygiene • Extended NPO status	• Pain in area of gland and ear • Absence of salivation • Purulent exudate from gland, erythema, ulcers	• Antibiotics, mouthwashes, warm compresses • Preventive measures, such as chewing gum, sucking on hard candy (lemon drops) • Adequate fluid intake
Stomatitis (inflammation of mouth)	• Trauma, pathogens, irritants (tobacco, alcohol) • Renal, liver, and hematologic diseases • Side effect of chemotherapy and radiation	• Excess salivation • Halitosis • Sore mouth	• Remove or treat cause • Oral hygiene with soothing solutions, topical medications • Soft, bland diet
Vincent's infection (acute necrotizing ulcerative gingivitis, trench mouth)	• Fusiform bacteria, Vincent spirochetes • Predisposing factors of stress, excessive fatigue, poor oral hygiene • Nutritional deficiencies (B and C vitamins)	• Painful, bleeding gingivae • Eroding necrotic lesions of interdental papillae • Ulcerations that bleed • Increased saliva with metallic taste, fetid mouth odor • Anorexia, fever, general malaise	• Physical and mental rest • Avoid smoking and alcohol • Soft, nutritious diet • Correct oral hygiene habits • Topical applications of antibiotics • Mouth irrigations with chlorhexidine and saline solutions

◆ **Evaluation**

The expected outcomes are that the patient with nausea and vomiting will

• Be comfortable, with minimal or no nausea and vomiting
• Have electrolyte levels within normal range
• Be able to maintain adequate intake of fluids and nutrients

Gerontologic Considerations: Nausea and Vomiting

The older adult with nausea and vomiting needs careful assessment and monitoring, especially during periods of fluid loss and rehydration therapy. They are more likely to have cardiac or renal problems that places them at greater risk for life-threatening fluid and electrolyte imbalances. Excess fluid and electrolytes replacement may have adverse consequences for a person with heart failure or renal disease. The older adult with a decreased level of consciousness has a high risk for aspirating. Close monitoring of the patient's physical status and level of consciousness during episodes of vomiting is important.

Older adults are particularly susceptible to the CNS side effects of antiemetic drugs. These drugs may cause confusion and increase fall risk. Doses should be reduced and efficacy closely evaluated. Use safety precautions for these patients (e.g., removing rugs that may cause slipping).

ORAL INFLAMMATION AND INFECTIONS

Inflammations and infections of the oral cavity are shown in Table 41.3. They may be due to specific mouth diseases or related to systemic disorders, such as leukemia or vitamin deficiency. The patient who is immunosuppressed (e.g., receiving chemotherapy for cancer) or using corticosteroid inhalant treatment for asthma is at risk for oral infections (e.g., candidiasis). Oral infections may predispose the patient to infections in other body organs. For example, the oral cavity is a potential reservoir for respiratory pathogens. Oral pathogens are associated with diabetes and heart disease.[4]

Managing these problems focuses on identifying the cause, eliminating infection, providing comfort measures, and maintaining nutritional intake. They can severely impair oral ingestion. Regular and good oral and dental hygiene reduces oral infections and inflammation.

ORAL CANCER

There are 2 types of oral cancer: *oral cavity cancer*, which starts in the mouth, and *oropharyngeal cancer*, which develops in the part of the throat just behind the mouth (the oropharynx). *Head and neck squamous cell carcinoma* (HNSCC) is a broad term used for cancers of the oral cavity, pharynx, and larynx. Most oral cancer lesions occur on the lower lip. Other common sites are the lateral border and undersurface of the tongue, labial commissure, and buccal mucosa. Annually 51,540 Americans are diagnosed with oral cancer. An estimated 10,030 people die from the disease.[5]

Oral cancer is more common after age 35. The average age at diagnosis is 65 years. It is 2 times more common in men than in women. The 5-year survival rate is 84% for localized cancer and 65% for all stages of oral cavity and pharynx cancer combined.[5] Lip cancer has the most favorable prognosis of any of the oral tumors. The visibility of lip lesions usually leads to an earlier diagnosis.

⊕ PROMOTING HEALTH EQUITY
Oral, Pharyngeal, and Esophageal Problems

Nausea and Vomiting
- Asian Americans, Middle Easterners, and blacks are more likely to have nausea and vomiting than whites

Cancers of Oral Cavity and Pharynx
- Incidence and mortality rates are higher in black men than in whites
- Death rates from oral cancer are decreasing in whites and increasing in nonwhites

Esophageal Cancer
- Highest incidence is in non-Hispanic white men
- Lowest incidence occurs in Asian Americans, Pacific Islanders, and Hispanics.

Stomach Cancer
- Asian Americans and Pacific Islanders, Hispanics, and blacks have higher rates of stomach cancer than non-Hispanic whites
- Asian Americans have higher survival rates than other ethnic groups

---

Etiology and Pathophysiology

Although the exact cause of oral cancer is unknown, there are predisposing factors (Table 41.4). Of those with oral cancer, 75% to 90% report either using tobacco or a history of frequent alcohol use. More than 30% of patients with cancer of the lip have outdoor occupations, showing that prolonged exposure to sunlight is a risk factor. Irritation from the pipe stem resting on the lip is a factor in pipe smokers. Human papillomavirus (HPV) contributes to 25% of oral cancer cases. HPV-associated oropharyngeal cancer is associated with multiple sexual partners, especially multiple oral sex partners.[6]

Clinical Manifestations

The common manifestations are shown in Table 41.4. Patients may report nonspecific symptoms such as chronic sore throat, sore mouth, and voice changes. *Leukoplakia*, called "smoker's patch," is a white patch on the mouth mucosa or tongue. It is a precancerous lesion, although less than 15% actually transform into cancer cells. The patch becomes *keratinized* (hard and leathery). This is described as hyperkeratosis. Leukoplakia is the result of chronic irritation, especially from smoking. *Erythroplasia* (erythroplakia), a red velvety patch on the mouth or tongue, is another precancerous lesion. More than 50% of cases of erythroplasia progress to squamous cell cancer. About 30% of patients with oral cancer have an asymptomatic neck mass.

Cancer of the lip usually appears as an indurated, painless ulcer on the lip. The first sign of cancer of the tongue is an ulcer or area of thickening. Soreness or pain of the tongue may occur, especially when eating hot or highly seasoned foods. Lesions are most likely to develop in the proximal half of the tongue. Some patients have limited tongue movement. Later symptoms include increased salivation, slurred speech, **dysphagia** (difficulty swallowing), toothache, and earache.

Diagnostic Studies

Diagnostic tests are done to identify oral dysplasia, which is a precursor to oral cancer (Table 41.5). Oral exfoliative cytologic study involves scraping the suspicious lesion and spreading the scraping on a slide for microscopic examination. The toluidine blue test is a screening test for oral cancer. When toluidine blue is applied topically to stain an area, cancer cells preferentially take up the dye. A negative cytologic smear or negative toluidine blue test does not necessarily rule out cancer. Once cancer is diagnosed, CT scan, MRI, and positron emission tomography (PET) are used for staging cancer.

TABLE 41.4 Types and Characteristics of Oral Cancer

Location	Predisposing Factors	Clinical Manifestations	Treatment
Lip	Constant overexposure to sun, ruddy and fair complexion, recurrent herpetic lesions, irritation from pipe stem, syphilis, immunosuppression	Indurated, painless ulcer	Surgical excision, radiation
Oral cavity	Poor oral hygiene, tobacco usage (pipe and cigar smoking, snuff, chewing tobacco), chronic alcohol intake, chronic irritation (jagged tooth, ill-fitting prosthesis, chemical or mechanical irritants), HPV	Leukoplakia, erythroplakia, ulcerations, sore spot, rough area, pain, dysphagia, a lump or thickening in the cheek A sore throat or a feeling that something is stuck Difficulty chewing and speaking (later signs)	Surgery (mandibulectomy, radical neck dissection, resection of buccal mucosa), internal and external radiation
Tongue	Tobacco, alcohol, chronic irritation, syphilis	Ulcer or area of thickening, soreness, or pain Limited tongue movement Increased salivation, slurred speech, dysphagia, toothache, earache (later signs)	Surgery (hemiglossectomy or glossectomy), radiation

Interprofessional Management: Oral Cancer

Management usually consists of surgery, radiation, chemotherapy, or a combination of these. The curative treatments are usually surgery and radiation.

Surgical Therapy. Surgery is the most effective treatment, especially for early-stage disease.[7] The procedure done depends on the location and extent of the tumor. Some patients with small tumors in the mouth and throat are candidates for minimally invasive robotic-assisted surgery. However, many of the operations are radical procedures involving extensive resections. Some examples are partial *mandibulectomy* (removal of the mandible), *hemiglossectomy* (removal of half of the tongue), *glossectomy* (removal of the tongue), resections of the buccal mucosa and floor of the mouth, and radical neck dissection.

Radical neck dissection includes wide excision of the primary lesion with removal of the regional lymph nodes, the deep cervical lymph nodes, and their lymphatic channels. The following structures are removed or transected depending on the extent of the primary lesion: sternocleidomastoid muscle and other closely associated muscles, internal jugular vein, mandible, submaxillary gland, part of the thyroid and parathyroid glands, and spinal accessory nerve. The patient usually has a tracheostomy. Drainage tubes inserted into the surgical area are connected to suction to remove fluid and blood. Head and neck surgery is described in more detail in Chapter 26.

Nonsurgical Therapy. Radiation therapy may be used alone to treat small cancers or when lesions cannot be removed. Patients usually do not have radiation before surgery because it is hard to remove radiated tissue. The tissue becomes fibrotic and heals slower. Most patients begin radiation about 6 weeks after surgery.

Chemotherapy can shrink lesions before surgery, decrease metastasis, sensitize cancer cells to radiation, or treat distant metastases. Common chemotherapy drugs include fluorouracil, cisplatin, carboplatin, paclitaxel, docetaxel, and hydroxyurea. A common combination is cisplatin and fluorouracil.[8] This combination is more effective than either drug alone. (Chemotherapy is discussed in Chapter 15.)

Palliative treatment is the best management when the prognosis is poor, the cancer is inoperable, or the patient decides against surgery. Palliation aims to treat the symptoms and make the patient more comfortable. If it becomes hard for the patient to swallow, placing a gastrostomy tube will allow for adequate nutritional intake. Give analgesic drugs freely. Frequent suctioning of the oral cavity is needed when swallowing becomes difficult. Other palliative and end-of-life nursing measures are discussed in Chapter 9.

Nutritional Therapy. Many patients are malnourished before surgery. They may need placement of a percutaneous endoscopic gastrostomy (PEG) and enteral nutrition (EN) before radiation treatment or surgery. After radical neck surgery, the patient may be unable to ingest nutrients orally because of mucositis, swelling, location of sutures, or difficulty swallowing. PN is given for the first 24 to 48 hours. After that time, EN is given via NG, gastrostomy, or jejunostomy tube. (See Chapter 39 for information on EN.) Cervical esophagostomy and pharyngostomy are options for some patients.

Assess for feeding tolerance and adjust the amount, time, and formula if nausea, vomiting, diarrhea, or distention occurs. Give small amounts of water when the patient can swallow. Observe for choking. Suctioning may be needed to prevent aspiration.

❖ NURSING MANAGEMENT: ORAL CANCER

◆ Nursing Assessment

Subjective and objective data to obtain from a patient with oral cancer are outlined in Table 41.6.

◆ Nursing Diagnoses

Nursing diagnoses for the patient with oral cancer may include the following:

- Impaired nutritional intake
- Acute pain
- Anxiety

◆ Planning

The overall goals are that the patient with cancer of the oral cavity will (1) have a patent airway, (2) be able to communicate, (3) have adequate nutritional intake to promote wound healing, and (4) have relief of pain and discomfort.

TABLE 41.5 Interprofessional Care

Oral Cancer

Diagnostic Assessment	Management
• History and physical examination	• Surgical therapy
• Biopsy	• Surgical excision of the tumor
• Oral exfoliative cytology	• Radical neck dissection
• Toluidine blue test	• Radiation therapy
• CT, MRI, PET scans	• Chemotherapy
	• Nutrition therapy

TABLE 41.6 Nursing Assessment

Oral Cancer

Subjective Data

Important Health Information

Past health history: Recurrent oral herpetic lesions, HPV infection or vaccination, syphilis, exposure to sunlight

Medications: Immunosuppressants

Surgery or other treatments: Removal of prior tumors or lesions

Functional Health Patterns

Health perception–health management: Alcohol and tobacco use, pipe smoking. Poor oral hygiene

Nutritional-metabolic: Reduced oral intake, weight loss, difficulty chewing food, increased salivation, intolerance to certain foods or temperatures of food

Cognitive-perceptual: Mouth or tongue soreness or pain, toothache, earache, neck stiffness, dysphagia, difficulty speaking

Objective Data

Integumentary

Indurated, painless ulcer on lip. Painless neck mass

Gastrointestinal

Areas of thickening or roughness, ulcers, leukoplakia, or erythroplakia on the tongue or oral mucosa. Limited tongue movement. Increased salivation, drooling. Slurred speech. Foul breath odor

Possible Diagnostic Findings

Positive exfoliative smear cytology (microscopic examination of cells removed by scraping), positive biopsy

◆ Nursing Implementation

You play a key role in the early detection and treatment of oral cancer. Identify patients at risk (Table 41.4) and provide information about predisposing factors. Review information about smoking cessation with the patient who smokes. Warn adolescents and teenagers about the danger of using snuff or chewing tobacco and electronic cigarettes. Smoking cessation is discussed in Chapter 10 and Tables 10.3 to 10.6.

Because early detection of oral cancer is important, teach the patient to report unexplained pain or soreness of the mouth, unusual bleeding, dysphagia, sore throat, voice changes, or swelling or lump in the neck. Refer any person with an ulcerative lesion that does not heal within 2 to 3 weeks to the HCP.

♥ PROMOTING POPULATION HEALTH

Health Impact of Good Oral Hygiene

- Improves quality of life
- Lowers risk for teeth loss
- Reduces pain and disability
- Aids in early detection of oral and craniofacial cancers
- Decreases cost of care needed from dental professionals
- Decreases risk for periodontal disease, gingivitis, and dental caries

Preoperative care for the patient who will have a radical neck dissection must consider the patient's physical and psychosocial needs. Physical preparation is the same as that for any major surgery, with special emphasis on oral hygiene. Explanations and emotional support should include information on postoperative communication and feeding. Explain the surgical procedure and ensure that the patient understands the information. See Chapter 26 and eNursing Care Plan 26.2 for more information about the nursing management of a patient undergoing a radical neck dissection.

◆ Evaluation

The expected outcomes are that the patient with oral cancer will
- Have no respiratory complications
- Be able to communicate
- Maintain an adequate nutritional intake to promote wound healing
- Have minimal pain and discomfort with eating, drinking, and talking

ESOPHAGEAL DISORDERS

GASTROESOPHAGEAL REFLUX DISEASE

Gastroesophageal reflux disease (GERD) is a chronic symptom of mucosal damage caused by reflux of stomach acid into the lower esophagus. GERD is not a disease but a syndrome. GERD is the most common upper GI problem. About 15 million Americans have GERD symptoms (heartburn or regurgitation) each day.[9]

Etiology and Pathophysiology

GERD has no one single cause (Fig. 41.2). GERD results when the reflux of acidic gastric contents into the esophagus overwhelms the esophageal defenses. Gastric HCl acid and pepsin secretions in refluxate cause esophageal irritation and

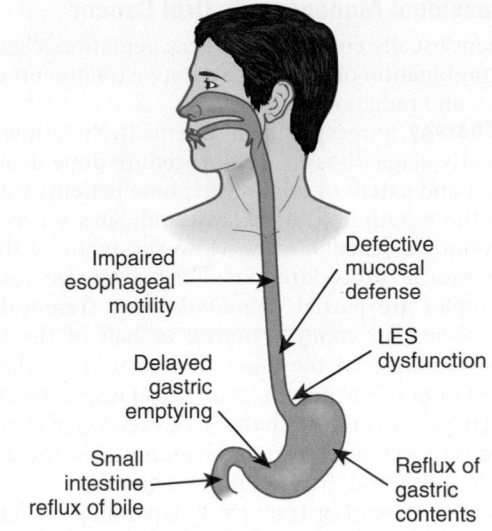

FIG. 41.2 Factors involved in the pathogenesis of GERD.

TABLE 41.7 Factors Affecting Lower Esophageal Sphincter Pressure

Decrease Pressure
- Alcohol
- Chocolate (theobromine)
- Drugs
  - Anticholinergics
  - β-Adrenergic blockers
  - Calcium channel blockers
  - Diazepam (Valium)
  - Morphine sulfate
  - Nitrates
- Progesterone
- Theophylline
- Fatty foods
- Nicotine
- Peppermint, spearmint
- Tea, coffee (caffeine)

Increase Pressure
- Bethanechol (Urecholine)
- Metoclopramide (Reglan)

inflammation (*esophagitis*). If it contains intestinal proteolytic enzymes (e.g., trypsin) and bile, this further irritates the esophageal mucosa. The degree of inflammation depends on the amount and composition of the gastric reflux and on the esophagus's mucosal defense mechanisms.

One of the primary factors causing GERD is an incompetent LES. Normally, the LES acts as an antireflux barrier. An incompetent LES lets gastric contents move from the stomach to the esophagus when the patient is supine or has an increase in intraabdominal pressure.

Decreased LES pressure can be due to certain foods and drugs (Table 41.7). Obesity is a risk factor. In an obese person the intraabdominal pressure is increased, which can worsen GERD. Cigarette and cigar smoking can contribute to GERD. Hiatal hernia, discussed in the next section, often causes GERD.

Clinical Manifestations

The symptoms of GERD vary from person to person. Persistent mild symptoms (i.e., more than twice a week) or moderate to severe symptoms once a week is considered GERD.

Heartburn (*pyrosis*) is the most common symptom. Heartburn is a burning, tight sensation felt intermittently beneath the lower sternum and spreading upward to the throat or jaw. It may occur after ingesting food or drugs that decrease the LES pressure or directly irritate the esophageal mucosa. An HCP should evaluate heartburn that occurs more than twice a

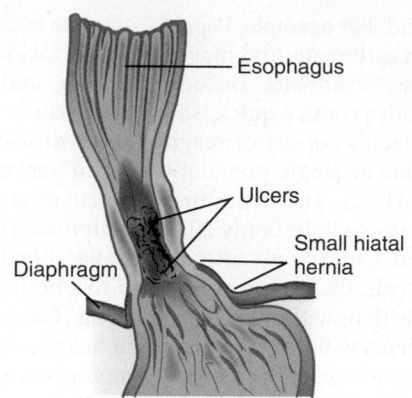

FIG. 41.3 Esophagitis with esophageal ulcerations.

week, is severe, is associated with dysphagia, or occurs at night and wakes a person from sleep. Older adults who report the recent onset of heartburn should receive medical evaluation.

GERD-related chest pain can mimic angina. It is described as burning; squeezing; or radiating to the back, neck, jaw, or arms. Chest pain is more common in older adults with GERD. Unlike angina, GERD-related chest pain is relieved with antacids.

Patients may have dyspepsia or regurgitation. *Dyspepsia* is pain or discomfort centered in the upper abdomen (mainly in or around the midline as opposed to the right or left hypochondrium). Regurgitation is often described as hot, bitter, or sour liquid coming into the throat or mouth.

A person with GERD may report respiratory symptoms, including wheezing, coughing, and dyspnea. Nighttime discomfort and coughing can awaken the person, resulting in disturbed sleep patterns. Otolaryngologic symptoms include hoarseness, sore throat, a *globus sensation* (sense of a lump in the throat), hypersalivation, and choking.

Complications

Complications of GERD are due to the direct local effects of gastric acid on the esophageal mucosa. **Esophagitis** (inflammation of the esophagus) is a common complication of GERD. Esophagitis with esophageal ulcerations is shown in Fig. 41.3. Repeated esophagitis may lead to scar tissue formation, stricture, and dysphagia.

Another complication of chronic GERD is **Barrett's esophagus (BE)** (esophageal metaplasia). *Metaplasia* is the reversible change from one type of cell to another type because of an abnormal stimulus. In BE, the flat epithelial cells in the distal esophagus change into columnar epithelial cells. These cell changes are primarily due to GERD. However, some people with no history of GERD develop BE.

About 5% to 20% of people with chronic GERD have BE.[10] Other risk factors include being over age 60, being male, being white, and having central obesity. BE is a precancerous lesion that increases the patient's risk for esophageal cancer. Because of this risk, those with BE undergo surveillance endoscopy or radiofrequency ablation as recommended.

Respiratory complications of GERD include cough, bronchospasm, laryngospasm, and cricopharyngeal spasm. These complications are due to gastric secretions irritating the upper air*way. Asthma, chronic bronchitis, and pneumonia may develop from aspiration into the respiratory system. Dental erosion, especially in the posterior teeth, may result from acid reflux into the mouth.

TABLE 41.8 Interprofessional Care

GERD and Hiatal Hernia

Diagnostic Assessment	Drug Therapy (Table 41.10)
• History and physical examination	• PPIs
• Upper GI endoscopy with biopsy and cytologic analysis	• H₂ receptor blockers
• Esophagram (barium swallow)	• Antacids
• Motility (manometry) studies	• Prokinetic drug therapy
• pH monitoring (laboratory or 24 hr ambulatory)	**Surgical Therapy**
• Radionuclide studies	• Nissen fundoplication
	• Toupet fundoplication
Management	**Endoscopic Therapy**
Conservative	• Intraluminal valvuloplasty
• Elevate head of bed on 4- to 6-in blocks	• Radiofrequency ablation
• Avoid reflux-inducing foods (fatty foods, chocolate, peppermint)	
• Avoid alcohol	
• Reduce or avoid acidic pH beverages (colas, red wine, orange juice)	

Drug Therapy (Table 41.10) uses H_2 receptor blockers.

Diagnostic Studies

GERD is often diagnosed based on symptoms and the patient's response to behavioral and drug therapies. Diagnostic tests are done when usual therapy is ineffective or when complications are suspected. Diagnostic studies done to determine the cause of the GERD are shown in Table 41.8.

Endoscopy is useful in assessing the LES competence and the degree of inflammation (if present), potential scarring, and strictures. Biopsy and cytologic specimens can distinguish stomach or esophageal cancer from BE. In addition, the degree of dysplasia (low grade versus high grade) is determined. Manometric studies measure pressure in the esophagus and LES and esophageal motility function. Ambulatory esophageal pH monitoring is an option for those with refractory symptoms and no evidence of mucosal inflammation. Radionuclide tests can detect reflux of gastric contents and the rate of esophageal clearance.

❖ NURSING AND INTERPROFESSIONAL MANAGEMENT: GERD

Most patients with GERD can successfully manage the condition through lifestyle modifications, drug therapy, and nutrition therapy. These approaches require patient teaching and adherence to therapies. When these therapies are ineffective, surgery is an option (Table 41.8).

◆ Lifestyle Modifications

Teach the patient with GERD to avoid factors that trigger symptoms. The head of the bed is elevated 30 degrees. This can be done using pillows or with 4- to 6-in blocks under the bed. The patient should not be supine for 2 to 3 hours after a meal. A patient and caregiver teaching guide is shown in Table 41.9.

Encourage patients who smoke to stop. If needed, refer the patient to community resources for help in stopping smoking. See Chapter 10 for more information related to smoking

TABLE 41.9 Patient & Caregiver Teaching

GERD

Include the following instructions when teaching the patient and caregiver about managing GERD:

1. Explain the reason for a low-fat diet.
2. Have the patient to eat small, frequent meals to prevent gastric distention.
3. Explain the reason for avoiding alcohol, smoking (causes an almost immediate, marked decrease in lower esophageal sphincter pressure), and beverages that contain caffeine.
4. Tell the patient to not lie down for 2–3 hr after eating, wear tight clothing around the waist, or bend over (especially after eating).
5. Have the patient avoid eating within 3 hr of bedtime.
6. Have the patient to sleep with head of bed elevated on 4- to 6-in blocks (gravity fosters esophageal emptying).
7. Provide information about drugs, including reason for their use and common side effects.
8. Discuss strategies for weight reduction if appropriate.
9. Encourage patient and caregiver to share concerns about lifestyle changes and living with a chronic problem.

cessation. If stress causes symptoms, discuss measures to cope with stress. (See Chapter 6 for stress management techniques.)

◆ Drug Therapy

Drug therapy for GERD focuses on decreasing the volume and acidity of reflux, improving LES function, increasing esophageal clearance, and protecting the esophageal mucosa (Table 41.10). Proton pump inhibitors (PPIs) and histamine (H_2) receptor blockers are the most common and effective treatments for symptomatic GERD.[11] The goal of HCl acid suppression treatment is to reduce the acidity of the gastric refluxate. Patients who are symptomatic with GERD but do not have esophagitis *(nonerosive GERD)* achieve symptom relief with PPIs and H_2 receptor blockers.

Both PPIs and H_2 receptor blockers are available in prescription or OTC preparations. Teach the patient about side effects. Tell the patient to take medications as prescribed and not to stop without checking with the HCP. Have patients contact the HCP if symptoms persist.

PPIs are more effective in healing esophagitis than H_2 receptor blockers. PPIs also decrease the incidence of esophageal strictures, a complication of chronic GERD. Therapy should start with once-daily dosing, taken before the first meal of the day. Long-term use of PPIs may be associated with decreased bone density, kidney disease, vitamin B_{12} and magnesium deficiency, and increased risk for dementia.[12]

 DRUG ALERT Proton Pump Inhibitors (PPIs)

- Long-term use or high doses may increase the risk for fractures of hip, wrist, and spine.
- Patients should take the lowest dose for the shortest duration needed to treat their condition.
- Use may increase the risk for *C. difficile* infection in hospitalized patients.[12]

H_2 receptor blockers reduce symptoms and promote esophageal healing in 50% of patients. The onset of action of H_2 receptor blockers is 1 hour. Depending on the specific drug, therapeutic effects last up to 12 hours. We can give famotidine, ranitidine, and cimetidine orally or IV. Nizatidine is only available orally. Some preparations combine an H_2 receptor blocker

with an antacid. For example, Pepcid Complete includes famotidine, calcium carbonate, and magnesium hydroxide.

Adjunctive treatments include antacids and prokinetic drugs. Antacids produce quick, short-lived relief of heartburn. Common antacids consist of magnesium hydroxide or aluminum hydroxide as single preparations or in various combinations (Table 41.10). The neutralizing effects of antacids taken on an empty stomach last only 20 to 30 minutes. They are most effective taken 1 to 3 hours after meals and at bedtime. When taken after meals, their effects may last 3 to 4 hours.

Antacids with or without alginic acid (e.g., Gaviscon) may be useful in patients with mild, intermittent heartburn. In patients with moderate to severe or frequent symptoms or patients with esophagitis, antacids are not effective in relieving symptoms or healing lesions. After an acute phase of bleeding, antacids may be given hourly, either orally or through the NG tube. If an NG tube is in place, periodically aspirate the stomach contents and test the pH level. If pH is less than 5, intermittent suction may be used, or the frequency or dosage of the antacid or antisecretory agent increased.

The type and dosage of antacid given depend on side effects and potential drug interactions. Antacids high in sodium are used cautiously in older adults and patients with CVD, liver, and renal disease. Patients with renal failure should not take magnesium preparations because of the risk for magnesium toxicity. An antacid combination of aluminum and magnesium decreases the side effects of both.

Antacids can interact unfavorably with many drugs. They enhance the effects of some drugs, like benzodiazepines and pseudoephedrine. In many instances, antacids decrease the absorption rates of other drugs, such as thyroid hormones, phenytoin, and tetracycline. Before antacid therapy begins, inform the HCP of any drugs that a patient is taking.

Prokinetics increase LES pressure and improve gastric emptying, which may result in a small improvement in regurgitation and vomiting. Common agents include cisapride, metoclopramide (Reglan), bethanechol, and baclofen. However, many have significant side effects, so their use is limited only to those with known delayed gastric emptying.[13]

◆ Nutritional Therapy

No specific diet is used to treat GERD. Some patients may need to avoid foods that decrease LES pressure, such as chocolate, peppermint, fatty foods, coffee, and tea (Table 41.7), which predispose them to reflux. Certain foods (e.g., tomato-based products, orange juice, cola, red wine) may irritate the esophagus.

Tell the patient to avoid late evening meals, nighttime snacking, and milk, especially at bedtime, since it increases gastric acid secretion. Small, frequent meals and drinking fluids between meals help prevent overdistention of the stomach. Increased saliva production by chewing gum and oral lozenges may help with mild symptoms. Recommend weight reduction if the patient is overweight.

◆ Surgical Therapy

Surgical therapy (*antireflux* surgery) is reserved for patients with complications, such as esophagitis, medication intolerance, stricture, BE, and persistent severe symptoms. The goal of surgical therapy is to reduce reflux by enhancing the integrity of the LES. Most surgical procedures are done laparoscopically. The fundus of the stomach is wrapped around the lower part of the esophagus to reinforce and repair the defective barrier. Nissen and Toupet fundoplications are common laparoscopic antireflux surgeries.

TABLE 41.10 Drug Therapy

GERD and Peptic Ulcer Disease (PUD)

Drug	Mechanism of Action	Side Effects
Proton Pump Inhibitors (PPIs)		
dexlansoprazole (Dexilant) esomeprazole (Nexium) lansoprazole (Prevacid) omeprazole (Prilosec) omeprazole and sodium bicarbonate (Zegerid) pantoprazole (Protonix) rabeprazole (Aciphex)	↓ HCl acid secretion by inhibiting the proton pump (H⁺-K⁺-ATPase) responsible for the secretion of H⁺ ↓ Irritation of the esophageal and gastric mucosa	Headache, abdominal pain, nausea, diarrhea, vomiting, flatulence
Histamine (H₂) Receptor Blockers		
cimetidine famotidine (Pepcid) nizatidine (Axid) ranitidine (Zantac)	Block the action of histamine on the H₂ receptors to ↓ HCl acid secretion ↓ Conversion of pepsinogen to pepsin ↓ Irritation of the esophageal and gastric mucosa	Headache, abdominal pain, constipation, diarrhea
Antacids, Acid Neutralizers		
Single Substance aluminum hydroxide (Amphojel) calcium carbonate (Tums) sodium bicarbonate (Alka-Seltzer) sodium citrate (Bicitra) *Aluminum and Magnesium* Gelusil, Maalox, Mylanta aluminum/magnesium trisilicate (Gaviscon)	Neutralize HCl acid Taken 1–3 hr after meals and at bedtime	*Aluminum hydroxide:* Constipation, phosphorus depletion with chronic use *Calcium carbonate:* Constipation or diarrhea, hypercalcemia, milk-alkali syndrome, renal calculi *Magnesium preparations:* Diarrhea, hypermagnesemia *Sodium preparations:* Milk-alkali syndrome if used with large amounts of calcium. Use with caution in patients on sodium restrictions
Cholinergic		
bethanechol (Urecholine)	↑ Lower esophageal sphincter pressure, improve esophageal emptying, increase gastric emptying	Lightheadedness, syncope, flushing, diarrhea, stomach cramps, dizziness
Cytoprotective		
sucralfate (Carafate)	Act to form a protective layer and serve as a barrier against acid, bile salts, and enzymes in the stomach	Constipation
Prokinetic		
metoclopramide (Reglan)	Block effect of dopamine ↑ Gastric motility and emptying Reduce reflux	CNS side effects ranging from anxiety to hallucinations Extrapyramidal side effects (tremor and dyskinesias similar to Parkinson's disease)
Prostaglandin (Synthetic)		
misoprostol (Cytotec)	Protect lining of stomach *Cytoprotective:* Increase production of gastric mucus and mucosal secretion of bicarbonate *Antisecretory:* ↓ HCl acid secretion	Abdominal pain, diarrhea, GI bleeding, uterine rupture if pregnant

Laparoscopic fundoplication is often an outpatient procedure. However, patients at risk for complications, including those with prior upper abdominal surgeries or co-morbidities (e.g., cardiac disease, obesity), may be hospitalized after the procedure. A small number of patients have complications, including gastric or esophageal injury, splenic injury, pneumothorax, perforation, bleeding, infection, and pneumonia.

After surgery, reflux symptoms should decrease. However, recurrence is possible. In the first month after surgery, the patient may report mild dysphagia caused by edema, but it should resolve. Teach the patient to report persistent symptoms, such as heartburn and regurgitation.

A LINX Reflux Management System is an option for patients who have symptoms despite maximum medical management. A LINX system is a ring of small, flexible magnets enclosed in titanium beads and connected by titanium wires. Once implanted laparoscopically into the LES, the ring strengthens the weak LES. Under resting (nonswallowing) conditions, the magnetic attraction between the beads helps keep a weak LES closed to prevent reflux. When the person swallows, the force of pressure associated with the movement of fluids or foods overwhelms the magnetic forces and the fluid or food passes to the stomach. Adverse events with the system include difficulty swallowing, nausea, and pain when swallowing food. Tell patients who have a LINX system not to have an MRI as it could cause serious harm.

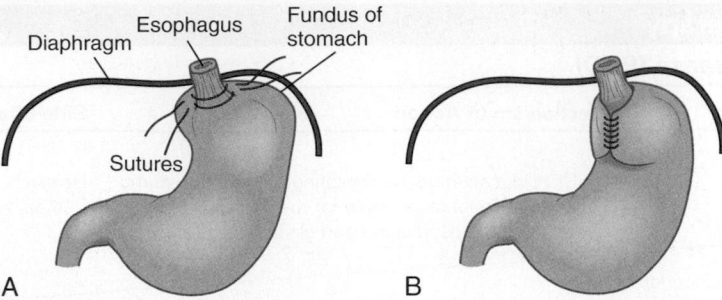

FIG. 41.4 Nissen fundoplication. **A,** Fundus of stomach is wrapped around distal esophagus. **B,** The fundus is then sutured to itself. (Modified from Doughty DB, Jackson DB: *Mosby's clinical nursing series: Gastrointestinal disorders,* St Louis, 1993, Mosby.)

◆ Endoscopic Therapy

Alternatives to surgical therapy include endoscopic mucosal resection (EMR) and radiofrequency ablation. The heat energy delivered through radiofrequencies creates lesions, which we think thicken the LES. For patients with high-grade dysplasia, EMR can be used as a diagnostic test to obtain biopsy samples. Biopsy results determine whether cancer is present.

HIATAL HERNIA

Hiatal hernia is herniation of part of the stomach into the esophagus through an opening, or hiatus, in the diaphragm. We also call it a *diaphragmatic hernia* or *esophageal hernia*. Hiatal hernias are the most common abnormality found on x-ray examination of the upper GI tract. They are common in older adults and occur more often in women.

There are 2 types of hiatal hernias (Fig. 41.4):
1. *Sliding:* The junction of the stomach and esophagus is above the diaphragm, and a part of the stomach slides through the hiatal opening in the diaphragm. This occurs when the patient is supine. The hernia usually goes back into the abdominal cavity when the patient is standing upright. This is the most common type.
2. *Paraesophageal* or *rolling:* The fundus and greater curvature of the stomach roll up through the diaphragm, forming a pocket alongside the esophagus. The esophagogastric junction stays in the normal position. Acute paraesophageal hernia is a medical emergency.

Etiology and Pathophysiology

Many factors contribute to the development of a hiatal hernia. Structural changes (weakening of the muscles in the diaphragm around the esophagogastric opening) occur with aging. Factors that increase intraabdominal pressure may predispose patients to developing a hiatal hernia. These include obesity, pregnancy, ascites, tumors, intense physical exertion, and heavy lifting on a continual basis.

Clinical Manifestations and Complications

Some people with hiatal hernia are asymptomatic. When present, manifestations of hiatal hernia are similar to those described for GERD on pp. 896-897.

Complications that may occur with hiatal hernia include GERD, esophagitis, hemorrhage from erosion, stenosis (narrowing of the esophagus), ulcerations of the herniated part of the stomach, strangulation of the hernia, and regurgitation with tracheal aspiration.

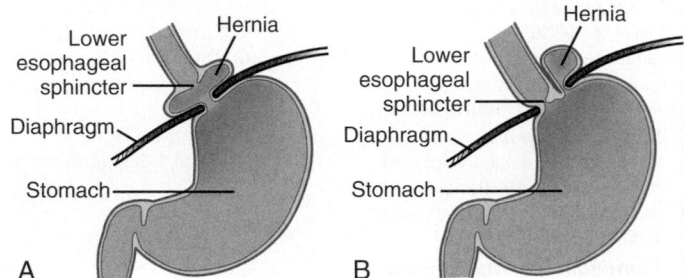

FIG. 41.5 **A,** Sliding hiatal hernia. **B,** Rolling or paraesophageal hernia.

Diagnostic Studies

An esophagram (barium swallow) may show the protrusion of gastric mucosa through the esophageal hiatus. Endoscopic visualization of the lower esophagus gives information on the degree of mucosal inflammation or other abnormalities. Other tests done are the same as those for GERD (Table 41.8).

NURSING AND INTERPROFESSIONAL MANAGEMENT: HIATAL HERNIA

Conservative therapy of hiatal hernia is similar to that described for GERD (pp. 897-898). Teach the patient to reduce intraabdominal pressure by eliminating constricting garments and avoiding lifting and straining.

Surgical approaches to hiatal hernias can include reduction of the herniated stomach into the abdomen, *herniotomy* (excision of the hernia sac), *herniorrhaphy* (closure of the hiatal defect), fundoplication, and *gastropexy* (attachment of the stomach below the diaphragm to prevent reherniation). The goals are to reduce the hernia, provide an acceptable LES pressure, and prevent movement of the gastroesophageal junction.

Surgery to repair hiatal hernia is often done laparoscopically by either Nissen or Toupet techniques (Fig. 41.5). The approach used (thoracic or abdominal) depends on the patient.

Gerontologic Considerations: GERD and Hiatal Hernia

The incidence of hiatal hernia and GERD increases with age. Hiatal hernia is associated with weakening of the diaphragm, obesity, kyphosis, or other factors (e.g., wearing girdles) that increase intraabdominal pressure. Older patients may take drugs known to decrease LES pressure (e.g., nitrates, calcium channel blockers, antidepressants). Other agents, such as nonsteroidal antiinflammatory drugs (NSAIDs) and potassium, can irritate the esophageal mucosa, causing *medication-induced esophagitis*.

Some older adults with hiatal hernia and GERD are asymptomatic or have less severe symptoms. The first sign may be a serious problem, such as esophageal bleeding from esophagitis or respiratory complications (e.g., aspiration pneumonia) due to aspiration of gastric contents.

The clinical course and management of GERD and hiatal hernia in the older adult are similar to those for the younger adult. Changes in lifestyle, including smoking cessation and elevating the head of the bed on blocks may be challenging for the older adult.

Laparoscopic procedures reduce the risk associated with surgical repair. An older patient with heart and lung problems may not be a good candidate for surgical intervention.

ESOPHAGEAL CANCER

Esophageal cancer is not common. However, the rates are increasing. In the United States, around 17,280 new cases are diagnosed and 15,850 deaths occur from esophageal cancer each year.[5] The overall 5-year survival rate is 19%.

Most esophageal cancers are adenocarcinomas. The others are squamous cell tumors. Adenocarcinomas arise from the glands lining the esophagus and resemble cancers of the stomach and small intestine. The incidence of esophageal cancer increases with age. Those between 65 and 75 are at greatest risk. The incidence is higher in men than in women.

Etiology and Pathophysiology

The cause of esophageal cancer is unknown. Key risk factors include BE, smoking, excess alcohol use, and obesity. For example, current smoking or a history of smoking is associated with a twofold higher risk for esophageal cancer. Those with injury to the esophageal mucosa (e.g., from occupational exposure to asbestos and cement dust) are at greater risk. *Achalasia,* a condition marked by delayed emptying of the lower esophagus, is associated with squamous cell cancer.

Most esophageal tumors occur in the middle and lower portions of the esophagus. The tumor usually appears as an ulcerated lesion. It may penetrate the muscular layer and extend outside the wall of the esophagus. Many patients have advanced disease at the time of diagnosis. The cancer spreads via the lymph system, with the liver and lung being common sites of metastasis.

Clinical Manifestations and Complications

By the time the patient has symptoms, the tumor is often advanced. Progressive dysphagia is the most common symptom. It may be described as a substernal feeling that food is not passing. Initially the dysphagia occurs only with meat, then with soft foods, and eventually with liquids.

Pain develops late. It occurs in the substernal, epigastric, or back areas and usually increases with swallowing. The pain may radiate to the neck, jaw, ears, and shoulders. If the tumor is in the upper third of the esophagus, symptoms, such as sore throat, choking, and hoarseness, may occur. Most patients lose weight. When esophageal stenosis (narrowing) is severe, regurgitation of blood-flecked esophageal contents is common.

Hemorrhage occurs if the cancer erodes through the esophagus and into the aorta. Esophageal perforation with fistula formation into the lung or trachea sometimes develops. The tumor may enlarge enough to cause esophageal obstruction, particularly in the later stages.

TABLE 41.11 Interprofessional Care
Esophageal Cancer

Diagnostic Assessment	Management
• History and physical examination	• Surgical therapy
• Endoscopy of esophagus with biopsy	• Esophagectomy
	• Esophagoenterostomy
	• Esophagogastrostomy
• Endoscopic ultrasonography	• Endoscopic therapy
• Esophagram (barium swallow)	• Dilation
• Bronchoscopy	• Endoscopic mucosal resection
• CT, MRI, PET scans	• Laser therapy
	• Photodynamic therapy
	• Radiofrequency ablation
	• Stent or prosthesis placement
	• Radiation therapy
	• Chemotherapy

Diagnostic Studies

Endoscopic biopsy is required to diagnose esophageal cancer. Endoscopic ultrasonography (EUS) is important in staging esophageal cancer. Esophagram (barium swallow) may show narrowing of the esophagus at the tumor site (Table 41.11).

Interprofessional Management

The treatment of esophageal cancer depends on the tumor's location and whether invasion or metastasis is present. Esophageal cancer usually has a poor prognosis because it is often diagnosed at an advanced stage. The best results occur with a multimodal approach, including surgery, endoscopic ablation, chemotherapy, and radiation therapy. Depending on the location and cancer spread, only chemotherapy and radiation may be used. Palliative therapy consists of restoring swallowing function and maintaining nutrition and hydration.

Surgical Therapy. The types of surgical procedures done are (1) removal of part or all of the esophagus *(esophagectomy)* with use of a Dacron graft to replace the resected part, (2) resection of a portion of the esophagus and anastomosis of the remaining portion to the stomach *(esophagogastrostomy),* and (3) resection of a portion of the esophagus and anastomosis of a segment of colon to the remaining portion *(esophagoenterostomy).* The surgical approaches may be open (thoracic, abdominal incision) or laparoscopic.

Minimally invasive esophagectomy (e.g., laparoscopic vagal nerve–sparing surgery) is being done more often. It has the advantage of using smaller incisions, decreasing intensive care unit (ICU) and hospital stays, and producing fewer pulmonary complications.

Endoscopic Therapy. Endoscopic therapy includes photodynamic therapy, EMR, and radiofrequency ablation. In photodynamic therapy, the patient receives an IV injection of porfimer sodium (Photofrin), a photosensitizer. Although most tissues absorb porfimer, cancer tissue absorbs it to a greater degree. The HCP directs light towards the cancerous area using a fiber passed through an endoscope. The light reacts with porfimer, starting a reaction that destroys the cancer cells. Patients must avoid direct sunlight for up to 6 weeks after the procedure.

EMR is an option for some small, very early stage cancers. It involves the removal of cancer tissue using an endoscope. Radiofrequency ablation uses electric currents to kill cancer cells by heating them.

Dilation, stent placement, or both can relieve obstruction. Dilation increases the lumen of the esophagus. It often relieves dysphagia and allows for improved nutrition. There are various types of dilators. Placement of stents or expandable stents may help when dilation is no longer effective. Stents allow food and liquid to pass through the stenotic area of the esophagus. Self-expandable metal stents are available with features to prevent stent migration and tumor ingrowth. Stents placed before surgery may help improve the patient's nutritional status.

Endoscopic laser therapy may be used in combination with dilation. Laser therapy can be repeated if obstruction recurs as the tumor grows. Sometimes these procedures are combined with radiation therapy.

Radiation Therapy. Depending on the type and stage of esophageal cancer, the patient may receive chemotherapy with or without radiation therapy. Concurrent therapy is given for palliation of symptoms, especially dysphagia, and to increase survival. Some patients receive radiation therapy before surgery.

Chemotherapy. Many different chemotherapy drugs can be used to treat esophageal cancer. The preferred regimens are carboplatin and paclitaxel, cisplatin with capecitabine (Xeloda), cisplatin and fluorouracil, and oxaliplatin with either fluorouracil or capecitabine. DCF (docetaxel, cisplatin, fluorouracil) is an option for metastatic disease. Other treatments include ECF (epirubicin [Ellence], cisplatin, fluorouracil) and irinotecan (Camptosar).[14] Chemotherapy is discussed in Chapter 15.

Targeted Therapy. Some esophageal cancers have too much HER-2 protein on their cell surfaces, which helps cancer cells to grow. Trastuzumab (Herceptin) is a drug that targets the HER-2 protein and kills the cancer cells. This drug can cause heart damage, so it is not given with other chemotherapy drugs that also cause heart damage, such as epirubicin.[14]

Ramucirumab (Cyramza), an angiogenesis inhibitor, binds to the receptor for *vascular endothelial growth factor* (VEGF), a compound that stimulates blood vessel growth. Thus it prevents VEGF from binding to the receptor and signaling the body to make more blood vessels. This can help slow or stop the growth and spread of cancer. Ramucirumab treats advanced cancers that start at the gastroesophageal junction. Targeted therapies are discussed in Chapter 15.

Nutritional Therapy. After esophageal surgery IV fluids are given. A jejunostomy, gastrostomy, or esophagostomy feeding tube may be placed to feed the patient depending on the type of surgery (e.g., esophagogastrectomy). A swallowing study is often done before allowing the patient to have oral fluids. When starting fluids, give water (30 to 60 mL) hourly and gradually progress to small, frequent, bland meals. Place the patient in an upright position for 2 hours after to prevent regurgitation. With EN, observe the patient for signs of intolerance to the feeding or leakage of the feeding into the mediastinum. Symptoms that indicate leakage are pain, increased temperature, and dyspnea. (EN is discussed in Chapter 39.)

❖ NURSING MANAGEMENT: ESOPHAGEAL CANCER

◆ Nursing Assessment

Ask the patient about a history of GERD, hiatal hernia, achalasia, BE, and tobacco and alcohol use. Assess the patient for progressive dysphagia and *odynophagia* (burning, squeezing pain while swallowing). Ask about the type of substances (e.g., meats, soft foods, liquids) that cause dysphagia. Assess the patient for pain (substernal, epigastric, or back areas), choking, heartburn, hoarseness, cough, anorexia, weight loss, and regurgitation.

◆ Nursing Diagnoses

Nursing diagnoses for the patient with esophageal cancer include:

- Chronic pain
- Impaired nutritional intake
- Impaired nutritional status
- Risk for aspiration
- Anxiety

◆ Planning

The overall goals are that the patient with esophageal cancer will (1) have relief of symptoms, including pain and dysphagia; (2) achieve optimal nutritional intake; and (3) have a quality of life appropriate to stage of disease and prognosis.

◆ Nursing Implementation

◆ Health Promotion. Counsel the patient with GERD, BE, or hiatal hernia about the importance of regular follow-up evaluation. Health counseling should focus on smoking cessation and reducing risk factors for GERD (Table 41.7). Maintaining good oral hygiene and dietary habits (e.g., intake of fresh fruits and vegetables) is important. Encourage patients to seek medical attention for any esophageal problems, especially dysphagia.

◆ Acute Care

Preoperative Care. The patient and caregiver usually react with shock, disbelief, and depression when given the diagnosis of esophageal cancer. Provide emotional and physical support, provide information, clarify test results, and maintain a positive attitude with respect to the patient's immediate recovery and long-term survival.

In addition to general preoperative teaching and preparation, pay attention to the patient's nutritional needs. Many are poorly nourished because of the inability to ingest adequate amounts of food and fluids. A high-calorie, high-protein diet is recommended. Some patients need a liquid form of this diet. Others may need IV fluid replacement or parenteral nutrition (PN). Teach the patient and caregiver how to keep an intake and output record and assess for signs of fluid and electrolyte imbalance. Some treatment protocols include preoperative radiation and chemotherapy.

Meticulous oral care is essential. Cleanse the mouth thoroughly, including the tongue, gingivae, and teeth or dentures. It may be necessary to use swabs or a gauze pad and to scrub the mouth, including the tongue. Milk of Magnesia with mineral oil helps remove crust formation.

Teaching should include information about chest tubes (with a planned open thoracic approach), IV lines, NG tubes, pain management, gastrostomy or jejunostomy feeding, turning, coughing, and deep breathing. (General preoperative care is discussed in Chapter 17.)

Postoperative Care. During the immediate postoperative period, the patient usually receives care in the ICU for 1 to 2 days. In addition to usual postoperative complications, dysrhythmias may result from the proximity of the pericardium to the surgical site. Other complications include anastomotic leaks, fistula formation, interstitial pulmonary edema, and acute respiratory distress related to the disruption of the mediastinal lymph nodes.

The patient usually has an NG tube in place for 5 to 7 days. The drainage may be bloody for 8 to 12 hours. The drainage gradually changes to greenish yellow. Assessing the drainage, maintaining the tube, and providing oral and nasal care are key nursing responsibilities. Do not irrigate the NG tube, reposition it, or reinsert it without consulting the HCP.

If the chest cavity is entered, postoperative drainage is achieved with chest tube insertion. Assess the amount and type of drainage. Notify the HCP of excess drainage (e.g., over 400 to 600 mL in 8 hours). Chest surgery and drainage tubes are discussed in Chapter 27.

Because of the location of the surgery and the patient' general condition, implement measures to prevent respiratory complications. Have the patient turn, cough and deep breathe, and use an incentive spirometer every 2 hours. Follow VTE prophylaxis measures and provide effective pain management. Position the patient in a semi-Fowler's or Fowler's position to prevent reflux and aspiration of gastric secretions. When the patient can drink fluids or eat, maintain the upright position for at least 2 hours after eating to assist with gastric emptying.

◆ **Ambulatory Care.** Many patients need long-term follow-up care after surgery for esophageal cancer. The patient may need chemotherapy and radiation treatment after surgery. Encourage and assist the patient in maintaining adequate nutrition. A permanent feeding gastrostomy may be needed. The patient usually is afraid and anxious about the cancer diagnosis. Know what the HCP has told the patient about the prognosis and provide appropriate counseling.

Referral to a palliative care or home health nurse may be needed. (See Chapter 15 for the care of the cancer patient and Chapter 9 for a discussion of palliative and end-of-life care.)

◆ **Evaluation**

The expected outcomes are that the patient with esophageal cancer will

- Maintain a patent airway
- Have relief of pain
- Be able to swallow comfortably and consume adequate nutritional intake
- Have a quality of life appropriate to stage of disease and prognosis

OTHER ESOPHAGEAL DISORDERS

Eosinophilic Esophagitis

Eosinophilic esophagitis (EoE) is characterized by swelling of the esophagus from an infiltration of *eosinophils*. People with EoE often have a personal or family history of other allergic diseases. The most common food triggers are milk, egg, wheat, rye, and beef. Environmental allergens, such as pollens, molds, cat, dog, and dust mite allergens, may be involved in the development of EoE.

Patients may have severe heartburn, difficulty swallowing, food impaction in the esophagus, nausea, vomiting, and weight loss. The diagnosis is based on symptoms and biopsy findings of eosinophils infiltrating esophageal tissue obtained from endoscopy.

Allergy skin testing helps to determine the person's allergens. A trial of avoiding the foods to which the person has positive allergy tests is the first treatment. Other common treatments include the use of PPIs (Table 41.10) and corticosteroids. Corticosteroids are used to treat EoE when avoiding allergic triggers does not relieve symptoms.

Corticosteroids may be used orally (prednisone) or as a topical therapy with inhaled corticosteroids (e.g., fluticasone

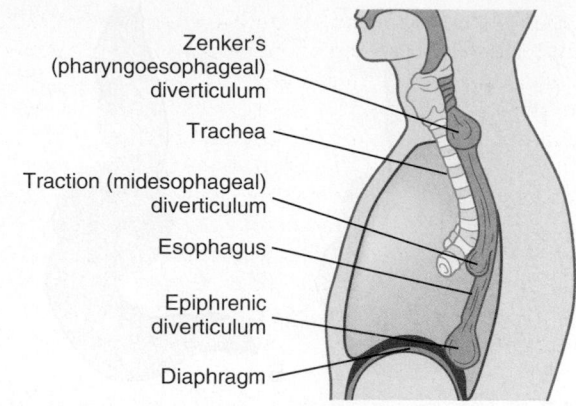

FIG. 41.6 Sites for esophageal diverticula. These hollow outpouchings may occur just above the upper esophageal sphincter (Zenker's), near the midpoint of the esophagus (traction), and just above the lower esophageal sphincter (epiphrenic). (Modified from Price SA, Wilson LM: *Pathophysiology: Clinical concepts of disease processes*, ed 6, St Louis, 2003, Mosby.)

[Flovent]). The patient takes a puff of fluticasone, and rather than inhaling it, swallows the medication. This directly delivers the drug to the esophagus. The most common side effect is a yeast infection of the throat (esophageal candidiasis).

Esophageal Diverticula

Esophageal diverticula are saclike outpouchings of 1 or more layers of the esophagus. They occur in 3 main areas: (1) above the upper esophageal sphincter *(Zenker's diverticulum)*, which is the most common location; (2) near the esophageal midpoint *(traction diverticulum)*; and (3) above the LES *(epiphrenic diverticulum)* (Fig. 41.6). Zenker's diverticula occur commonly in people older than 60 years.

Typical symptoms include dysphagia, regurgitation, chronic cough, aspiration, and weight loss. Food becomes trapped in the outpouches. This causes tasting sour food and smelling a foul odor. Complications include malnutrition, aspiration, and perforation. Endoscopy or barium studies can easily establish a diagnosis.

There is no specific treatment. Some patients find that they can empty the pocket of food that collects by applying pressure at a certain point on the neck. The diet may have to be limited to foods that pass more readily (e.g., blenderized foods). Surgical treatment may be needed if nutrition is disrupted. Endoscopic stapling diverticulotomy or diverticulostomy is associated with decreased complications compared with the open approaches. The most serious surgical complication is esophageal perforation.

Esophageal Structures

The most common cause of *esophageal strictures* (or narrowing) is chronic GERD. The ingestion of strong acids or alkalis, external beam radiation, and surgical anastomosis can also create strictures. Trauma, such as throat lacerations and gunshot wounds, can lead to strictures because of scar formation. Strictures can cause dysphagia and regurgitation, leading to weight loss.

Strictures can be dilated using mechanical *bougies* (dilating instruments) or balloons. Dilation may be done with or without endoscopy, or with fluoroscopy. Surgical excision with anastomosis is sometimes needed. The patient may have a temporary or permanent gastrostomy.

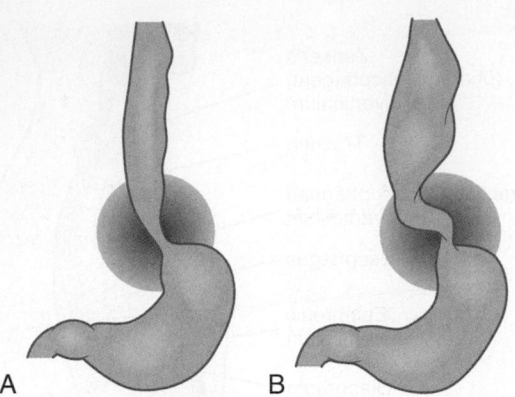

FIG. 41.7 Esophageal achalasia. **A,** Early stage, showing tapering of lower esophagus. **B,** Advanced stage, showing dilated, tortuous esophagus.

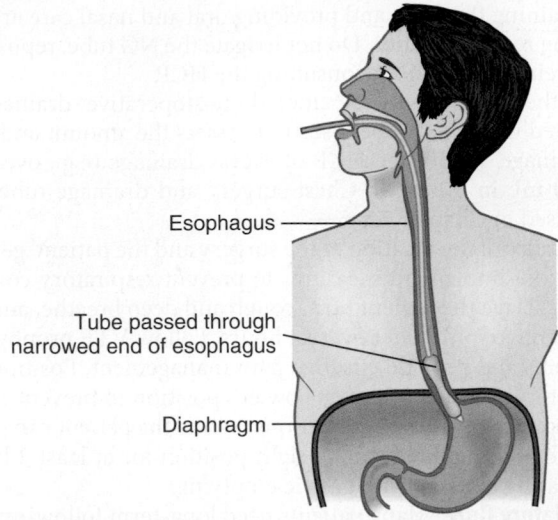

FIG. 41.8 Pneumatic dilation can treat achalasia by maintaining an adequate lumen and decreasing lower esophageal sphincter (LES) tone. (Modified from Price SA, Wilson LM: *Pathophysiology: Clinical concepts of disease processes,* ed 6, St Louis, 2003, Mosby.)

Achalasia

In achalasia, peristalsis of the lower two thirds (smooth muscle) of the esophagus is absent. Achalasia is a rare, chronic disorder. The exact cause is unknown. With achalasia, the pressure in the LES increases along with incomplete relaxation. Esophageal obstruction at or near the diaphragm occurs. Food and fluid accumulate in the lower esophagus. The result is dilation of the esophagus above the tapered affected segment of the lower esophagus (Fig. 41.7). There is a selective loss of inhibitory neurons, resulting in unopposed contraction of the LES.

The onset of achalasia is usually slow. Dysphagia is the most common symptom and occurs with both liquids and solids. Patients may report a globus sensation and/or substernal chest pain (similar to angina pain) during or right after a meal. About a third have nighttime regurgitation. *Halitosis* (foul-smelling breath) and the inability to eructate (belch) can occur. Patients may report symptoms of GERD and regurgitation of sour-tasting food and liquids, especially when they are lying down. Weight loss is common.

Diagnosis is made with esophagram (barium swallow), manometric evaluation (high-resolution manometry), and/or endoscopic evaluation. Treatment focuses on symptom management. The goals of treatment are to relieve dysphagia and regurgitation, improve esophageal emptying by disrupting the LES, and prevent the development of megaesophagus (enlargement of the lower esophagus).

Endoscopic pneumatic dilation involves dilating the LES muscle using balloons of progressively larger diameter (3.0, 3.5, and 4.0 cm) (Fig. 41.8). It is an outpatient procedure. If this is ineffective, the next option is a Heller myotomy, done laparoscopically. In this procedure, the HCP cuts through the muscles of the LES, allowing food to pass. Because GERD with esophagitis and stricture is a common complication, the patient often has anti-reflux surgery at the same time. The patient typically returns to usual activities 1 to 2 weeks afterward.

Medical therapy is less effective than invasive procedures. The injection of botulinum toxin endoscopically into the LES gives short-term relief of symptoms and improves esophageal emptying. It works by promoting relaxation of the smooth muscle. This treatment is used for older patients for whom surgery and pneumatic dilation may not be appropriate due to other chronic illnesses.

Nitrates (e.g., isosorbide dinitrate) and calcium channel blockers (e.g., nifedipine [Procardia]) relax the LES and may improve dysphagia. They are taken sublingually 10 to 30 minutes before meals. Side effects (e.g., headache), drug tolerance, and short duration of action limit their use. Symptomatic treatment consists of eating a semisoft diet, eating slowly, drinking fluid with meals, and sleeping with the head elevated.

Esophageal Varices

Esophageal varices are dilated, tortuous veins occurring in the lower part of the esophagus because of portal hypertension. Esophageal varices are a common complication of liver cirrhosis. They are discussed in Chapter 43.

DISORDERS OF THE STOMACH AND UPPER SMALL INTESTINE

PEPTIC ULCER DISEASE

Peptic ulcer disease (PUD) is a condition characterized by erosion of the GI mucosa from the digestive action of HCl acid and pepsin. Any part of the GI tract that is in contact with gastric secretions is susceptible to ulcer development. This includes the lower esophagus, stomach, duodenum, and margin of a gastrojejunal anastomosis after surgical procedures. PUD affects about 4.5 million people in the United States each year.[15]

Types

Peptic ulcers are classified as acute or chronic, depending on the degree and duration of mucosal involvement, and gastric or duodenal, according to the location. The *acute ulcer* (Fig. 41.9) is associated with superficial erosion and minimal inflammation. It is of short duration and resolves quickly when the cause is identified and removed. A chronic ulcer (Fig. 41.10) is one of long duration, eroding through the muscular wall with the formation of fibrous tissue. It is present continuously for many months or intermittently throughout the person's lifetime. Chronic ulcers are more common than acute erosions.

Although gastric and duodenal ulcers are both considered PUD, they are different in their incidence and presentation (Table 41.12).

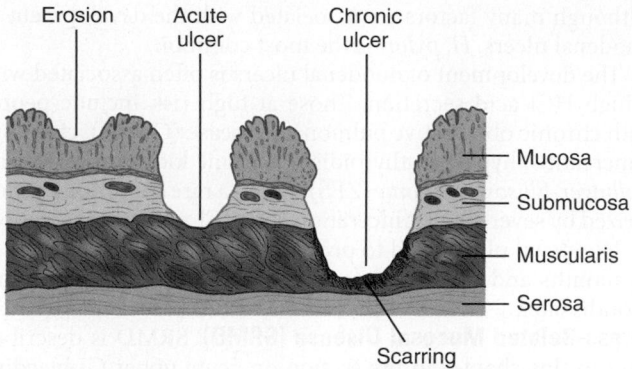

FIG. 41.9 Peptic ulcers, including an erosion, an acute ulcer, and a chronic ulcer. Both the acute ulcer and the chronic ulcer may penetrate the entire wall of the stomach. (Modified from Price SA, Wilson LM: *Pathophysiology: Clinical concepts of disease processes,* ed 6, St Louis, 2003, Mosby.)

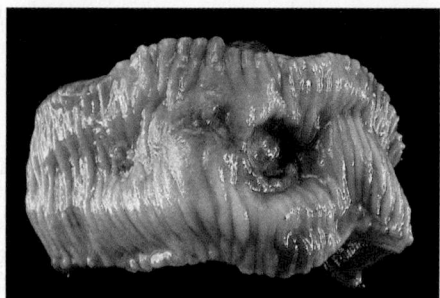

FIG. 41.10 Peptic ulcer of the duodenum. (From Kumar V, Abbas AK, Aster JC, Fausto N: *Robbins and Cotran pathologic basis of disease,* ed 8, Philadelphia, 2010, Saunders.)

Etiology and Pathophysiology

Peptic ulcers develop only in an acid environment. However, an excess of HCl acid is not necessary for ulcer development. Pepsinogen, the precursor of pepsin, changes to pepsin in the presence of HCl acid and a pH of 2 to 3. When food or antacids neutralize the stomach acid level or drugs block acid secretion, the pH increases to 3.5 or more. At a pH of 3.5 or more, pepsin has little or no proteolytic activity.

The pathophysiology of ulcer development is outlined in Fig. 41.11. The back diffusion of HCl acid into the gastric mucosa results in cellular destruction and inflammation. Histamine is released from the damaged mucosa. This results in vasodilation, increased capillary permeability, and further secretion of acid and pepsin. Fig. 41.12 shows the interrelationship between the mucosal blood flow and disruption of the gastric mucosal barrier. Several factors damage the mucosal barrier.

Helicobacter Pylori. The major risk factor for PUD is infection with *Helicobacter pylori.* 80% of gastric and 90% of duodenal ulcers are related to *H. pylori.* In the United States, *H. pylori* affects 20% of persons younger than 30 years and 50% of those older than 60 years. Infection likely occurs during childhood with transmission from family members to the child, possibly through a fecal-oral or oral-oral route. The rate is highest in black and Hispanic people.[15] Although most people with *H. pylori* never develop ulcers, it appears that those infected with *CagA*-positive strains are more likely to have PUD.[16]

In the stomach, the bacteria can survive a long time by colonizing the gastric epithelial cells within the mucosal layer. The bacteria make urease, which metabolizes urea-producing

TABLE 41.12 Comparison of Gastric and Duodenal Ulcers

Gastric Ulcers	Duodenal Ulcers
Lesion	
Superficial, smooth margins. Round, oval, or cone shaped	Penetrating (associated with deformity of duodenal bulb from healing of recurrent ulcers)
Location of Lesion	
Predominantly antrum, also in body and fundus of stomach	First 1–2 cm of duodenum
Gastric Secretion	
Normal to decreased	Increased
Incidence	
Greater in women	Greater in men, but increasing in women (especially postmenopausal)
Peak age 50–60 yr	Peak age 35–45 yr
Increased cancer risk	No increase in cancer risk
H. pylori infection in 80%	*H. pylori* infection in 90%
↑ With incompetent pyloric sphincter and bile reflux	Associated with other diseases (e.g., COPD, pancreatic disease, hyperparathyroidism, ZES, chronic renal failure)
Clinical Manifestations	
Burning or gaseous pressure in epigastrium	Burning, cramping, pressure-like pain across midepigastrium and upper abdomen. Back pain with posterior ulcers
Pain 1–2 hr after meals. If penetrating ulcer, aggravation of discomfort with food	Pain 2–5 hr after meals and midmorning, midafternoon, middle of night. Periodic and episodic. Pain relief with antacids and food
Recurrence Rate	
High	High

ammonium chloride and other damaging chemicals. Urease activates the immune response with both antibody production and the release of inflammatory cytokines. This leads to increased gastric secretion and causes tissue damage, leading to PUD.

Medication-Induced Injury. NSAID use is responsible for most non–*H. pylori* peptic ulcers. NSAIDs inhibit prostaglandin synthesis, increase gastric acid secretion, and reduce the integrity of the mucosal barrier. NSAID use in the presence of *H. pylori* further increases the risk for PUD. Patients taking corticosteroids or anticoagulants with NSAIDs have a higher risk for PUD.[15] Corticosteroids affect mucosal cell renewal and decrease its protective effects.

Lifestyle Factors. High alcohol intake is associated with acute mucosal lesions. Alcohol and smoking stimulate acid secretion. Coffee (caffeinated and decaffeinated) is a strong stimulant of gastric acid secretion. Smoking and psychologic distress, including stress and depression, can delay the healing of ulcers once they have developed.

Gastric Ulcers. Gastric ulcers can occur in any part of the stomach. They most often occur in the antrum. Gastric ulcers are less common than duodenal ulcers. Gastric ulcers are more prevalent in women and those over 50 years of age. Because of the peak incidence of gastric ulcers in older adults, the mortality rate from

PATHOPHYSIOLOGY MAP

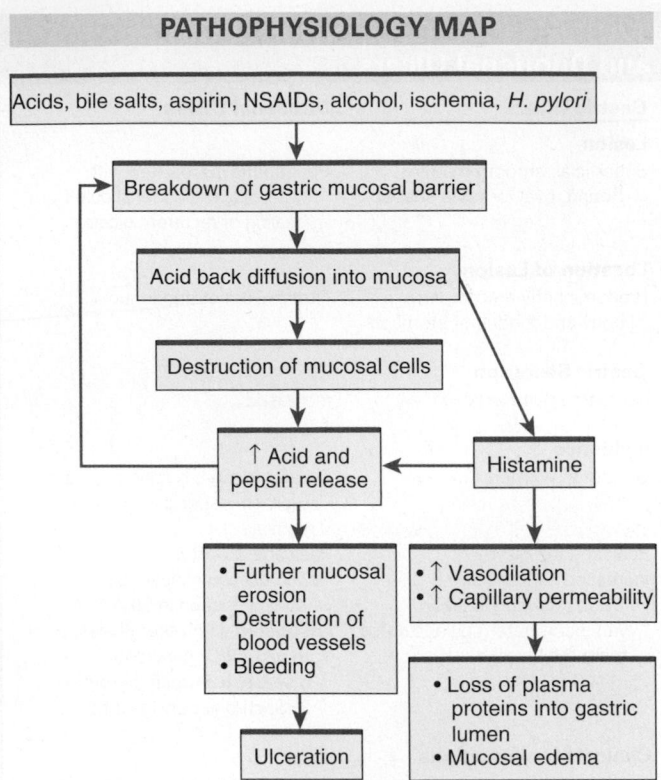

FIG. 41.11 Disruption of gastric mucosa and pathophysiologic consequences of back diffusion of acids.

PATHOPHYSIOLOGY MAP

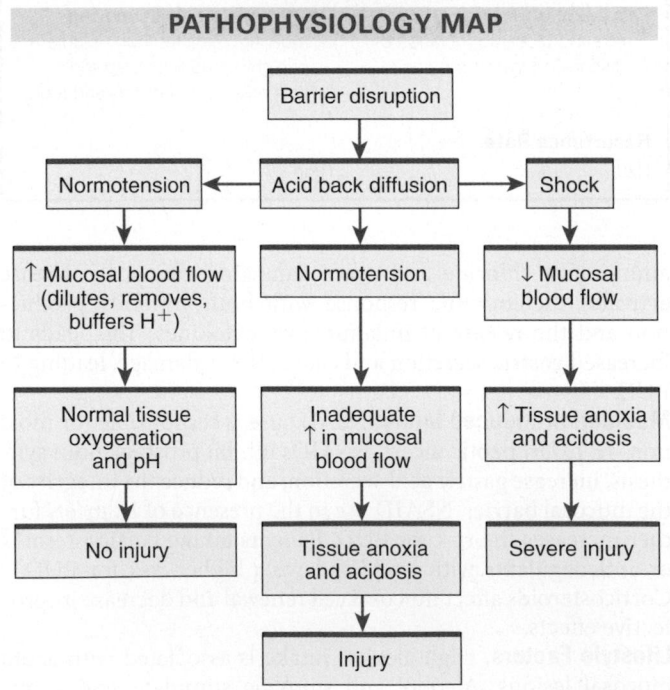

FIG. 41.12 Relationship between mucosal blood flow and disruption of the gastric mucosal barrier.

gastric ulcers is greater than that from duodenal ulcers. Gastric ulcers are more likely than duodenal ulcers to cause an obstruction. *H. pylori*, NSAIDs, and bile reflux are the main risk factors.
Duodenal Ulcers. Duodenal ulcers account for about 80% of all peptic ulcers. Duodenal ulcers occur at any age, but the incidence is especially high between 35 and 45 years of age.

Although many factors are associated with the development of duodenal ulcers, *H. pylori* is the most common.

The development of duodenal ulcers is often associated with a high HCl acid secretion. Those at high risk include people with chronic obstructive pulmonary disease (COPD), cirrhosis, pancreatitis, hyperparathyroidism, chronic kidney disease, and *Zollinger-Ellison syndrome* (ZES). ZES is a rare condition characterized by severe peptic ulceration and HCl acid hypersecretion.

Duodenal ulcers tend to occur continuously for a few weeks or months and then disappear for a time, only to recur some months later.
Stress-Related Mucosal Disease (SRMD). SRMD is described later in this chapter in the section on acute upper GI bleeding on p. 917.

Clinical Manifestations

In gastric ulcers, the discomfort is generally high in the epigastrium and occurs about 1 to 2 hours after meals. The pain is described as "burning" or "gaseous." If the ulcer has eroded through the gastric mucosa, food tends to worsen the pain. For some patients, the earliest symptoms are due to a serious complication, such as perforation.

In duodenal ulcers, symptoms occur when gastric acid comes in contact with the ulcers. With meal ingestion, food is present to help buffer the acid. Symptoms occur generally 2 to 5 hours after a meal. The pain is described as "burning" or "cramplike." It is most often in the midepigastric region beneath the xiphoid process. Duodenal ulcers can also cause back pain.

Some patients have bloating, nausea, vomiting, and early feelings of fullness. Not all patients with ulcers will have pain or discomfort. *Silent* peptic ulcers are more likely to occur in older adults and those taking NSAIDs. The presence or absence of symptoms is not related to the size of the ulcer or the degree of healing.

Diagnostic Studies

Endoscopy is the most accurate procedure to determine the presence and location of an ulcer.[15] It allows for direct viewing of the gastric and duodenal mucosa (Fig. 41.13). During endoscopy, tissue specimens are taken to determine if *H. pylori* is present and rule out stomach cancer. Endoscopy can also assess the degree of ulcer healing after treatment.

Several noninvasive and invasive tests are available to confirm *H. pylori* infection. The gold standard for diagnosing *H. pylori* infection is a biopsy of the antral mucosa with testing for urease (rapid urease testing). Urea is a by-product of the metabolism of *H. pylori* bacteria. Noninvasive tests include serology, stool, and breath testing. The urea breath and stool antigen tests can identify active infection. Stool tests are not as accurate as the urea breath test. Antibody tests for *H. pylori* can remain positive for years. They are not good for evaluating treatment results.

A barium contrast study may be used to diagnose gastric outlet obstruction or for ulcer detection in those who cannot undergo endoscopy. High fasting serum gastrin levels may show the presence of a possible gastrinoma (ZES). A secretin stimulation test can discern a gastrinoma from other causes of hypergastrinemia.

Laboratory tests, including a CBC, liver enzyme studies, serum amylase, and stool examination, may be done. A CBC may show anemia from ulcer bleeding. Liver enzyme studies help detect any liver problems (e.g., cirrhosis) that may complicate ulcer treatment. Stools are tested for blood. A serum amylase evaluates pancreatic function if we suspect posterior duodenal ulcer penetration of the pancreas.

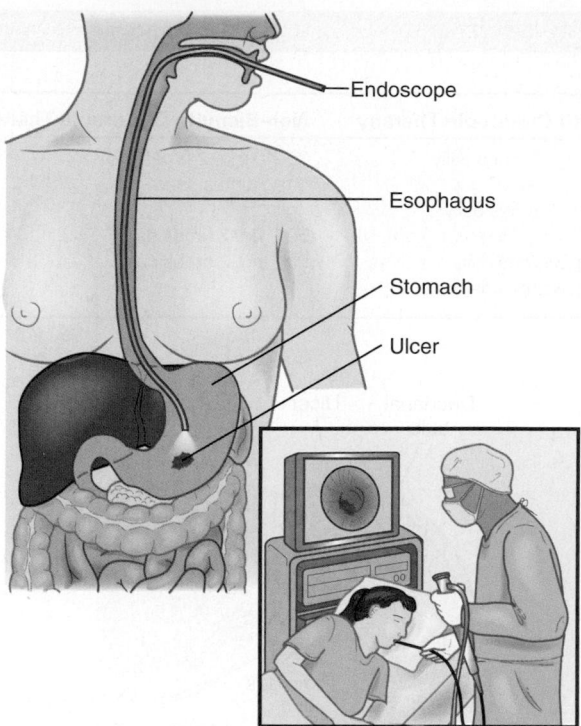

FIG. 41.13 Esophagogastroduodenoscopy (EGD) directly visualizes the mucosal lining of the stomach with a flexible endoscope. Ulcers or tumors can be directly seen and biopsies obtained.

Interprofessional Management

Conservative Care. Treatment begins after diagnostic studies confirm the presence of PUD (Table 41.13). The regimen consists of adequate rest, drug therapy, smoking cessation, dietary modifications (if needed), and long-term follow-up care. The aim of treatment is to decrease gastric acidity and enhance mucosal defense mechanisms.

Patients are generally treated in ambulatory care clinics. Pain disappears after 3 to 6 days, but ulcer healing is much slower. Complete healing may take 3 to 9 weeks, depending on ulcer size, treatment plan, and patient adherence. Endoscopic examination is the most accurate method to monitor ulcer healing. The usual follow-up endoscopic evaluation is done 3 to 6 months after diagnosis and treatment.

Aspirin and nonselective NSAIDs are stopped for 4 to 6 weeks. When aspirin must be continued, co-administration with a PPI, H_2 receptor blocker, or misoprostol may be prescribed. Patients receiving low-dose aspirin (LDA) for CVD and stroke risk who have a history of ulcer disease or complications may need to receive long-term treatment with a PPI. Enteric-coated aspirin decreases localized irritation but does not reduce the overall risk for GI bleeding.

Smoking has an irritating effect on the mucosa and delays mucosal healing. The patient should either stop or severely reduce smoking. (See Chapter 10 for ways to promote smoking cessation.) Adequate rest, both physical and emotional, is important for ulcer healing and may require some changes in the patient's daily routine. Avoiding or restricting alcohol use will enhance healing.

Drug Therapy. Medications are a key part of therapy (Table 41.10). Drug therapy focuses on reducing gastric acid secretion and, if needed, eliminating *H. pylori* infection. Patients with *H. pylori* infection need treatment with antibiotics and a PPI. After

the ulcer has healed, many patients can stop PPI therapy. Some may need to continue low-dose maintenance therapy.

Because ulcers often recur, interrupting or stopping therapy can have harmful results. Strict adherence to the prescribed drug regimen is important. Encourage the patient to adhere to therapy and continue with follow-up care as prescribed. Teach the patient and caregiver about each drug prescribed, why it is

TABLE 41.13 Interprofessional Care

Peptic Ulcer Disease

Diagnostic Assessment
- History and physical examination
- Upper GI endoscopy with biopsy
- Endoscopic ultrasound
- *H. pylori* testing of breath, urine, blood, tissue
- Complete blood cell count
- Liver enzymes
- Serum amylase
- Stool testing for blood

Management

Conservative Therapy
- Adequate rest
- Smoking and alcohol cessation
- Stress management (see Chapter 6)

Drug Therapy (Tables 41.10 and 41.14)
- Antibiotics for *H. pylori*
- PPIs
- Adjunctive therapy
  - H2-receptor blockers
  - Cytoprotective drugs
  - Antacids

Acute Exacerbation Without Complications
- NPO
- NG suction
- Adequate rest
- IV fluid replacement

Drug Therapy (Tables 41.10 and 41.14)
- Antibiotics for *H. pylori*
- PPIs
- Adjunctive therapy
  - H_2 receptor blockers
  - Cytoprotective drugs
  - Antacids
  - Sedatives

Acute Exacerbation With Complications (Hemorrhage, Perforation, Obstruction)
- NPO
- NG suction
- IV PPI
- Bed rest
- IV fluid replacement (lactated Ringer's solution)
- Blood transfusions
- Stomach lavage (possible)

Surgical Therapy
- Gastric outlet obstruction: Pyloroplasty and vagotomy
- Perforation: Simple closure with omentum graft
- Ulcer removal or reduction
  - Billroth I and II
  - Vagotomy and pyloroplasty

TABLE 41.14 Drug Therapy

H. pylori *Infection*

Drug Class	Drug	Triple Therapy	Bismuth Quadruple Therapy	Non-Bismuth Quadruple Therapy
Acid suppression	PPI	20–40 mg, 2 times daily	20–40 mg, 2 times daily	20–40 mg, 2 times daily
Standard antibiotics	Amoxicillin	1gram, 2 times daily		1 g, 2 times daily
	Bismuth compound		2 tablets, 2 times daily	
	Clarithromycin	500 mg, 2 times daily		500 mg, 2 times daily
	Metronidazole		500 mg, 3 times daily	500 mg, 2 times daily
	Tetracycline		500 mg, 4 times daily	

ordered, and the expected benefits. Review what to do if pain and discomfort recur or there is blood in vomitus or stools.

Antibiotic Therapy. Eradicating *H. pylori* is the most important part of treating PUD in patients positive for *H. pylori*. Antibiotic therapy is prescribed concurrently with a PPI for 14 days (Table 41.14). If the patient has a penicillin allergy, metronidazole is used instead of amoxicillin in the triple-drug regimen. Bismuth can be given alone or as part of a combination capsule (Pylera) containing bismuth, tetracycline, and metronidazole. Because of the existence of antibiotic-resistant organisms, a growing number of patients do not have *H. pylori* eradicated with a single round of therapy.

Proton Pump Inhibitors. PPIs are more effective than H₂ receptor blockers in reducing gastric acid secretion and promoting ulcer healing. PPIs are used in combination with antibiotics to treat ulcers caused by *H. pylori*.

Cytoprotective Drug Therapy. Sucralfate is used for short-term ulcer treatment. It provides mucosal protection for the esophagus, stomach, and duodenum. Sucralfate does not have acid-neutralizing capabilities. Since it is most effective at a low pH, give it at least 60 minutes before or after an antacid. Adverse side effects are minimal. It binds with cimetidine, digoxin, warfarin, phenytoin, and tetracycline, reducing their bioavailability.

Adjunct Drugs. H₂ receptor blockers and antacids may be used as adjunct therapy to promote ulcer healing. Antacids increase gastric pH by neutralizing HCl acid. As a result, they reduce the acid content of chyme reaching the duodenum. Some antacids (e.g., aluminum hydroxide) can bind to bile salts, thus decreasing the damaging effects of bile on the gastric mucosa.

Misoprostol is a synthetic prostaglandin analog prescribed to prevent gastric ulcers caused by NSAIDs and LDA. It has protective and some antisecretory effects on gastric mucosa. People who need chronic NSAID therapy, such as those with osteoarthritis, may benefit from its use. However, it can cause diarrhea and abdominal pain. It is teratogenic and must be used with caution in women of childbearing potential.

Tricyclic antidepressants (e.g., imipramine, doxepin) may be prescribed for some patients. They may contribute to overall pain relief through their effects on afferent pain fiber transmission. In addition, they have varying degrees of anticholinergic properties, which result in reduced acid secretion.

Anticholinergic drugs are sometimes used for PUD treatment. Anticholinergics are associated with several side effects, such as dry mouth, warm skin, flushing, thirst, tachycardia, dilated pupils, blurred vision, and urine retention.

Nutritional Therapy. There is no specific diet used to treat PUD. Patients should eat and drink foods and fluids that do not cause any distressing symptoms. Foods that may cause gastric

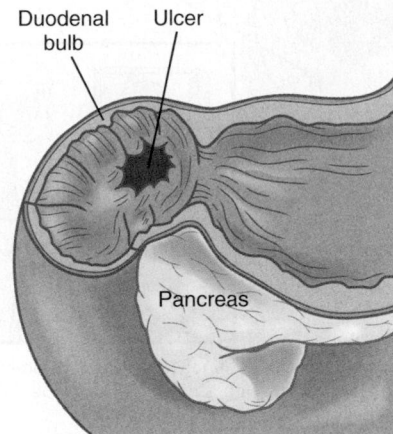

FIG. 41.14 Duodenal ulcer of the posterior wall penetrating the head of the pancreas, resulting in walled-off perforation.

irritation include pepper, carbonated beverages, broth (meat extract), and hot, spicy foods. Caffeine-containing beverages and foods can increase symptoms in some patients. Teach the patient to avoid alcohol use because it can delay healing.

Surgical Therapy. With the use of drug therapy and endoscopic therapy to treat PUD, surgery is used less often. Surgery is done on patients with complications that are unresponsive to medical management or concerns about stomach cancer. Gastric surgeries are described later in this chapter on p. 914.

Complications

The 3 major complications of chronic PUD are hemorrhage, perforation, and gastric outlet obstruction.[16] All these complications are considered emergency situations and may need surgical intervention.

Hemorrhage. Hemorrhage is the most common complication of PUD. Duodenal ulcers cause more upper GI bleeding episodes than gastric ulcers.

Perforation. Perforation is considered the most lethal complication of PUD. Perforation risk is highest with large penetrating duodenal ulcers (Fig. 41.14). However, the mortality rate associated with perforation of gastric ulcers is higher. The patient with gastric ulcers is older and often has concurrent medical problems, which accounts for the higher mortality rate.

With perforation, the ulcer penetrates the serosal surface with spillage of either gastric or duodenal contents into the peritoneal cavity. The contents entering the peritoneal cavity may contain air, saliva, food particles, HCl acid, pepsin, bacteria, bile, and pancreatic fluid and enzymes.

The manifestations of perforation are sudden and dramatic in onset. During the initial phase (0 to 2 hours after perforation), the patient has sudden, severe upper abdominal pain that quickly spreads throughout the abdomen. The pain radiates to the back and shoulders. Food or antacids do not relieve the pain. The abdomen appears rigid and boardlike as the abdominal muscles try to protect from further injury. The patient's respirations become shallow and rapid. The heart rate is elevated, and the pulse is weak. Bowel sounds are usually absent. Nausea and vomiting may occur.

If the condition is untreated, bacterial peritonitis may occur within 6 to 12 hours. The intensity of peritonitis is proportional to the amount and duration of the spillage through the perforation. It is hard to determine from symptoms alone whether a gastric or duodenal ulcer has perforated, because the manifestations of peritonitis are the same (see Chapter 42).

The immediate focus of managing a patient with a perforation is to stop the spillage of gastric or duodenal contents into the peritoneal cavity and restore blood volume. An NG tube can provide continuous aspiration and gastric decompression to stop spillage through the perforation. For duodenal aspiration, the tube is placed as near to the perforation site as possible to facilitate decompression.

Circulating blood volume is replaced with lactated Ringer's and albumin solutions. These solutions substitute for the fluids lost from the vascular and interstitial space as peritonitis develops. Blood replacement in the form of packed RBCs may be needed. A central venous pressure line and an indwelling urinary catheter may be inserted and monitored hourly. The patient with a history of heart disease needs ECG monitoring or placement of a pulmonary artery catheter for accurate assessment of left ventricular function. Broad-spectrum antibiotic therapy is started immediately to treat bacterial peritonitis.

Small perforations may spontaneously seal themselves and symptoms cease. Spontaneous sealing occurs because of fibrin production in response to the perforation. This can lead to fibrinous fusion of the duodenum or gastric curvature to adjacent tissue (mainly the liver) and strictures that can obstruct the flow of intestinal contents and the passage of stool.

Larger perforations need immediate surgical closure. Whether the patient has an open or laparoscopic repair depends on the location of the ulcer and HCP preference. The procedure involving the least risk to the patient is simple oversewing of the perforation and reinforcement of the area with a graft of omentum. Excess gastric contents are suctioned from the peritoneal cavity during the surgical procedure.

Gastric Outlet Obstruction. Both acute and chronic PUD can cause gastric outlet obstruction. Obstruction in the distal stomach and duodenum is the result of edema, inflammation, pylorospasm, or fibrous scar tissue formation. With obstruction the patient reports discomfort or pain that is worse toward the end of the day as the stomach fills and dilates. Belching or self-induced vomiting may provide some relief. Vomiting is common and often projectile. The vomitus may contain food particles that were ingested hours or days before. Constipation occurs because of dehydration and decreased diet intake from anorexia. Over time dilation of the stomach and visible swelling in the upper abdomen may occur.

The aim of therapy for obstruction is to decompress the stomach, correct any existing fluid and electrolyte imbalances, and improve the patient's general state of health. An NG tube is used as described previously. With continuous decompression for several days, the ulcer can begin healing and the

---

TABLE 41.15   Nursing Assessment

Peptic Ulcer Disease

Subjective Data

Important Health Information

Past health history: Chronic kidney disease, pancreatic disease, COPD, serious illness or trauma, hyperparathyroidism, cirrhosis of the liver, ZES

Medications: Aspirin, corticosteroids, NSAIDs

Surgery or other treatments: Complicated or prolonged surgery

Functional Health Patterns

Health perception–health management: Chronic alcohol use, smoking, caffeine use. Family history of PUD

Nutritional-metabolic: Weight loss, anorexia, nausea and vomiting, hematemesis, dyspepsia, heartburn, belching

Elimination: Black, tarry stools

Cognitive-perceptual:
- Duodenal ulcers: Burning, midepigastric or back pain occurring 2–5 hr after meals and relieved by food; nighttime pain common
- Gastric ulcers: High epigastric pain occurring 1–2 hr after meals. Food may precipitate or worsen pain.

Coping–stress tolerance: Acute or chronic stress

Objective Data

General

Anxiety, irritability

Gastrointestinal

Epigastric tenderness

Possible Diagnostic Findings

Anemia. Guaiac-positive stools. Positive blood, urine, breath, or stool tests for *H. pylori*. Abnormal upper GI endoscopic and barium studies

---

inflammation and edema will subside. Pain relief results from the decompression.

IV fluids and electrolytes are replaced according to the degree of dehydration, vomiting, and electrolyte imbalance shown by laboratory studies. A PPI or H_2 receptor blocker is used if the obstruction is due to an active ulcer. Balloon dilation can open a pyloric obstruction. Surgery may be needed to remove scar tissue.

❖ NURSING MANAGEMENT: PEPTIC ULCER DISEASE

◆ Nursing Assessment

Subjective and objective data to obtain from a patient with PUD are outlined in Table 41.15.

◆ Nursing Diagnoses

Nursing diagnoses related to PUD may include:
- Acute pain
- Lack of knowledge
- Nausea

Additional information on nursing diagnoses and interventions for the patient with PUD are in eNursing Care Plan 41.2 available on the website for this chapter.

◆ Planning

The overall goals are that the patient with PUD will (1) adhere to the prescribed therapeutic regimen, (2) see a reduction in or absence of discomfort, (3) have no signs of GI complications, (4) have complete healing of the peptic ulcer, and (5) make appropriate lifestyle changes to prevent recurrence.

◆Nursing Implementation

◆**Health Promotion.** You play an important role in identifying patients at risk for PUD. Early detection and effective treatment of ulcers are important aspects of reducing morbidity risks associated with PUD. Patients who are taking ulcerogenic drugs (e.g., NSAIDs, LDA) are at risk for PUD. Encourage patients to take these drugs with food. Teach patients to report symptoms related to gastric irritation, including epigastric pain, to their HCP.

◆**Acute Care.** During an acute exacerbation, the patient often reports increased pain, nausea, and vomiting. Some may have bleeding. Initially, many patients try to cope with the symptoms at home before seeking medical care.

During the acute phase, the patient may be NPO for a few days, have an NG tube connected to intermittent suction, and receive IV fluid replacement. Explain to the patient and caregiver the reasons for these therapies so they understand that the advantages far outweigh any temporary discomfort. Regular mouth care relieves the dry mouth. Cleaning and lubricating the nares facilitate breathing and decrease soreness. Analysis of gastric contents may include pH testing and analysis for blood, bile, or other substances. When the stomach is empty of gastric secretions, pain decreases and ulcer healing begins.

The volume of fluid lost, the patient's signs and symptoms, and laboratory test results (hemoglobin, hematocrit, electrolytes) determine the type and amount of IV fluids given. Take vital signs initially and then at least hourly to detect and treat shock. Give IV fluids as ordered and record intake and output.

Physical and emotional rest is helpful to ulcer healing. The patient's environment should be quiet and restful. Give pain medications as ordered. A mild sedative or tranquilizer has beneficial effects when the patient is anxious and apprehensive. Use good judgment before sedating a person who is becoming increasingly restless because the drug could mask the signs of shock from upper GI bleeding.

Hemorrhage. Changes in vital signs and an increase in the amount and redness of aspirate often signal massive upper GI bleeding. With bleeding, the patient's pain often decreases because the blood helps neutralize the acidic gastric contents. It is important to maintain the patency of the NG tube so that blood clots do not obstruct the tube. If the tube becomes blocked, the patient can develop abdominal distention. Use interventions similar to those described for upper GI bleeding on pp. 918–920.

Perforation. If the patient with an ulcer develops manifestations of a perforation, notify the HCP immediately. Take vital signs promptly and record them every 15 to 30 minutes. Temporarily stop all oral or NG drugs and feedings. If perforation exists, anything taken orally can add to the spillage into the peritoneal cavity and increase discomfort. Give IV fluid as ordered to replace the depleted plasma volume. Giving pain medications provides comfort.

Those with confirmed perforation will start on antibiotic therapy. If the perforation does not seal spontaneously, surgical closure is needed. Since surgery is done as soon as possible, there may not be time to prepare the patient and family.

Gastric Outlet Obstruction. Gastric outlet obstruction can happen at any time. It is most likely to occur in the patient whose ulcer is close to the pylorus. The onset of symptoms is usually gradual. Constant NG aspiration of stomach contents can help relieve symptoms. This allows edema and inflammation to subside and permits normal flow of gastric contents through the pylorus.

Regularly irrigate the NG tube with a normal saline solution per agency policy to assist proper functioning. It may be helpful to reposition the patient from side to side so that the tube tip is not constantly lying against the mucosal surface. Maintain accurate intake and output records, especially of the gastric aspirate.

To check for ongoing obstruction, clamp the NG tube intermittently and measure the gastric residual volume. The frequency and amount of time the tube is clamped are related to the amount of aspirate obtained and the patient's comfort level. A common method is to clamp the tube overnight (usually 8 to 12 hours) and measure the gastric residual volume in the morning. When the aspirate falls below 200 mL, it is within a normal range and the patient can begin oral intake of clear liquids. Oral fluids begin at 30 mL/hr and then gradually increase in amount. As the amount of gastric residual decreases, solid foods are added, and the tube removed.

If the patient has resumed oral feedings and you note symptoms of obstruction, promptly inform the HCP. Generally, all that is needed to treat the problem is to resume gastric aspiration so that the edema and inflammation resulting from the acute episode resolve. IV fluids with electrolyte replacement keep the patient hydrated during this period. If conservative treatment is not successful, surgery is done after the acute phase has passed.

◆**Ambulatory Care.** Patients with PUD have specific needs to prevent recurrence and complications. Teaching should cover aspects of the disease process, drugs, lifestyle changes (alcohol use, smoking), and regular follow-up care. Table 41.16 provides a patient and caregiver teaching guide for PUD.

Knowing the causes of PUD may motivate the patient to become involved in care and improve adherence to therapy. Work with the dietitian to elicit a dietary history and plan ways to incorporate any needed dietary modifications into the patient's home and work setting.

Teach the patient about prescribed drugs, including their actions, side effects, and dangers if omitted for any reason. Make

---

TABLE 41.16 Patient & Caregiver Teaching

Peptic Ulcer Disease (PUD)

Include the following instructions when teaching the patient and caregiver about management of PUD:

1. Avoiding foods that cause epigastric distress, such as acidic foods.
2. Avoid cigarettes. Smoking promoting ulcer development and delays ulcer healing.
3. Reduce or eliminate alcohol use.
4. Avoid OTC drugs unless approved by the HCP. Many preparations contain ingredients, such as aspirin, that should not be taken unless approved by the HCP. Check with the HCP about the use of NSAIDs.
5. Do not interchange brands of PPIs, antacids, or H_2 receptor blockers that you can buy OTC without checking with the HCP. This can lead to harmful side effects.
6. Take all medications as prescribed. This includes both antisecretory and antibiotic drugs. Not taking medications as prescribed can cause a relapse.
7. It is important to report any of the following:
   - Increased nausea or vomiting
   - Increased epigastric pain
   - Bloody emesis or tarry stools
8. Stress can be related to signs and symptoms of PUD. Learn and use stress management strategies (see Chapter 6).
9. Share concerns about lifestyle changes and living with a chronic illness.

sure the patient knows not to take OTC drugs (e.g., NSAIDs, LDA) unless approved by the HCP. Some H_2 receptor blockers and PPIs are available without a prescription. Tell the patient to check with the HCP before switching from a prescription to an OTC preparation to avoid side effects and incorrect dosing. Obtain information about the patient's psychosocial status. Knowledge of lifestyle, occupation, and coping behaviors can be helpful in planning care. The patient may be reluctant to talk about personal subjects, the stress at home or on the job, the usual methods of coping, or dependence on drugs or alcohol.

The patient may not be honest about habitual use of alcohol or cigarettes. Provide information about the negative effects of alcohol and cigarettes on PUD and ulcer healing. Changes such as smoking cessation and alcohol abstinence are hard for many people. The patient may do better in reducing, rather than totally eliminating, use of these substances. However, the goal is total cessation.

PUD is a chronic, recurring disorder. Teach patients with chronic PUD about potential complications, and what to do until they see the HCP. Emphasize the need for long-term follow-up care. Encourage the patient to seek immediate intervention if symptoms return. Some patients do not adhere to the plan of care and have repeated exacerbations. Patients quickly learn that they often have no discomfort when they omit prescribed drugs, smoke, or drink alcohol. Consequently, they make no or few changes in their lifestyle. After an acute exacerbation, the patient is likely to be more amenable to following the plan of care and open to suggestions for changes in lifestyle.

◆ Evaluation

Expected outcomes are that the patient with PUD will

- Have pain controlled without the use of analgesics
- States an understanding of the treatment plan
- Commit to self-care and management of the disease
- Have no complications (hemorrhage, perforation)

🧍 Gerontologic Considerations: Peptic Ulcer Disease

The morbidity and mortality rates associated with PUD in older adults are higher than for younger adults because of concurrent health problems and a decreased ability to withstand hypovolemia. Monitor older adults who use NSAIDs for osteoarthritis for PUD. In older patients, pain may not be the first symptom associated with an ulcer. For some patients the first sign is frank gastric bleeding or a decrease in hematocrit.

The treatment and management of PUD in older adults are similar to those in younger adults. The emphasis is on preventing gastritis and PUD. This includes teaching the patient to take NSAIDs and other gastric-irritating drugs with food, milk, or antacids. Teach the patient to avoid irritating substances, adhere to the PPI therapy as prescribed, and report abdominal pain or discomfort to the HCP.

STOMACH CANCER

Stomach (gastric) cancer is an adenocarcinoma of the stomach wall (Fig. 41.15). It accounts for more than 26,240 new cancer cases and 10,800 deaths annually.[5] The rate of stomach (particularly distal) cancer has been steadily declining in the United States. However, cancer in the proximal gastric and gastroesophageal junction is increasing.

Asian Americans, Pacific Islanders, Hispanics, and blacks have higher rates of stomach cancer than non-Hispanic whites. In the United States the incidence is higher in men than in women by a 2:1 ratio. Stomach cancer mostly affects older people. The average age of people at the time of diagnosis is 68.[5]

At the time of diagnosis, only 10% to 20% of patients have disease confined to the stomach. The 5-year survival rate in this group is 71%. However, more than 50% have advanced metastatic disease. The overall 5-year survival rate of all people with stomach cancer is about 31%.[5]

Etiology and Pathophysiology

While many factors are implicated in the development of stomach cancer, no single causative agent has been identified. Stomach cancer probably begins with a nonspecific mucosal injury because of infection (H. pylori), autoimmune-related inflammation, repeated exposure to irritants such as bile or NSAIDs, and tobacco use.

Stomach cancer has been associated with diets high in smoked foods, salted fish and meat, and pickled vegetables. Whole grains and fresh fruits and vegetables are associated with reduced rates of stomach cancer. Infection with H. pylori, especially at an early age, is a risk factor for stomach cancer. It is possible that H. pylori and resulting cell changes can induce a sequence of transitions from dysplasia to cancer. People with lymphoma of the stomach (mucosa-associated lymphoid tissue [MALT]) are at higher risk of stomach cancer.

Other predisposing factors include atrophic gastritis, pernicious anemia, adenomatous polyps, hyperplastic polyps, and *achlorhydria* (absent or low production of gastric HCl). Smoking and obesity both increase the risk for stomach cancer. Although first-degree relatives of patients with stomach cancer are at increased risk, only about 10% of stomach cancers have an inherited component.[17]

Stomach cancer spreads by direct extension and typically infiltrates rapidly to the surrounding tissue and liver. Seeding of tumor cells into the peritoneal cavity occurs late in the course of the disease.

Clinical Manifestations

Stomach cancers often spread to adjacent organs before any distressing symptoms occur. Manifestations include unexplained weight loss, indigestion, abdominal discomfort or pain, and signs and symptoms of anemia. The patient may report *early satiety,* or a sense of being full sooner than usual. Anemia is common. It is caused by chronic blood loss as the lesion erodes through the mucosa or from pernicious anemia (caused by loss of intrinsic factor). The person appears pale and weak. They

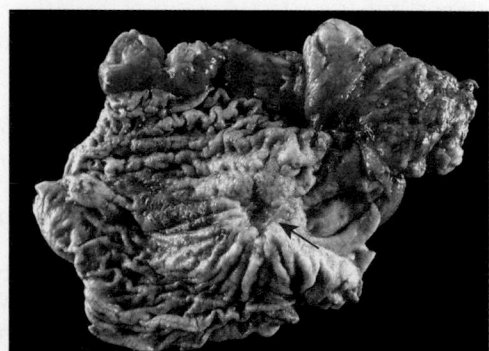

FIG. 41.15 Stomach cancer. Gross photograph showing an ill-defined, excavated central ulcer *(arrow)* surrounded by irregular, heaped-up borders. (From Kumar V, Abbas AK, Aster JC, Fausto N: *Robbins and Cotran pathologic basis of disease,* ed 8, Philadelphia, 2010, Saunders.)

TABLE 41.17 Interprofessional Care

Stomach Cancer

Diagnostic Assessment	Management
• History and physical examination	• Surgical therapy
• Endoscopy and biopsy	• Subtotal gastrectomy (Billroth I or II procedure)
• CT, MRI, PET scans	• Total gastrectomy with esophagojejunostomy
• Upper GI barium study	• Chemotherapy
• Exfoliative cytologic study	• Radiation therapy
• Endoscopic ultrasonography	• Targeted therapy
• CBC	
• Liver enzymes	
• Urinalysis	
• Stool examination	
• Serum amylase	
• Tumor markers	
• α-Fetoprotein	
• Carbohydrate antigen (CA)-19-9, CA-125, CA 72-4	
• Carcinoembryonic antigen (CEA)	

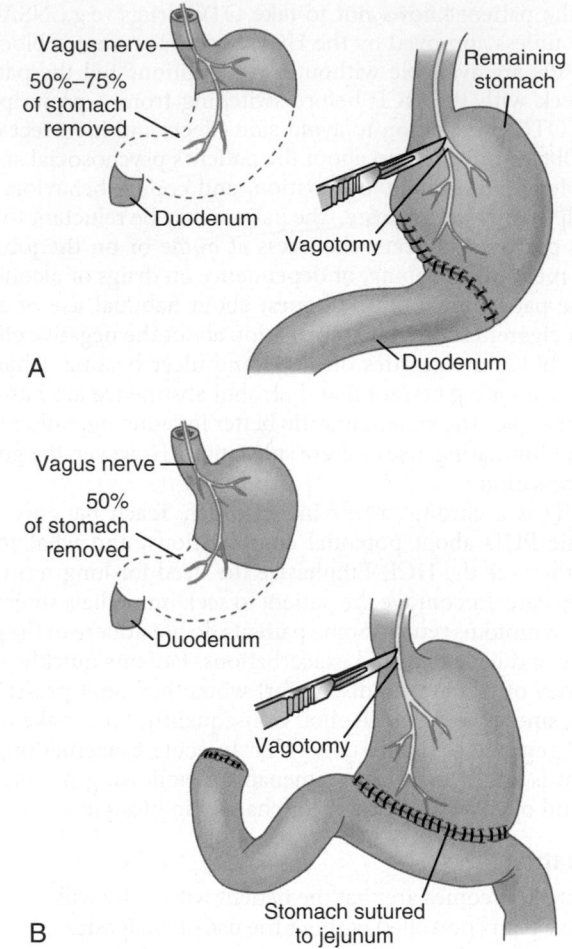

FIG. 41.16 A, Billroth I procedure (subtotal gastric resection with gastroduodenostomy anastomosis). B, Billroth II procedure (subtotal gastric resection with gastrojejunostomy anastomosis).

may report fatigue, weakness, dizziness, and, in extreme cases, shortness of breath. The stool may be positive for occult blood. Supraclavicular lymph nodes that are hard and enlarged suggest metastasis via the thoracic duct. The presence of ascites is a poor prognostic sign.

Diagnostic Studies

The diagnostic studies for stomach cancer are outlined in Table 41.17. Upper GI endoscopy is the best diagnostic tool. The stomach can be distended with air during the procedure, stretching the mucosal folds. Tissue biopsy and histologic examination are important in diagnosing stomach cancer.

Endoscopic ultrasound, CT, MRI, and PET scanning can be used to stage the disease. Laparoscopy is done to determine peritoneal spread.

Blood studies detect anemia and determine its severity. Increased liver enzymes and serum amylase levels may mean liver and pancreatic involvement. Stool examination provides evidence of occult or gross bleeding. The presence of tumor markers can help diagnose cancer.

Interprofessional Management

The treatment of choice for stomach cancer is surgical removal of the tumor. Preoperative management focuses on correcting nutritional deficits and treating anemia. Transfusions of packed RBCs correct the anemia. If gastric outlet obstruction occurs, gastric decompression may be needed before surgery.

Surgical Therapy. The surgical aim is to remove as much of the stomach as required to remove the tumor and a margin of normal tissue. The location and extent of the lesion, the patient's physical condition, and the HCP's preference determine the specific surgery used (e.g., open versus laparoscopic).

Lesions in the antrum or pyloric region are generally treated by either a Billroth I or II procedure (Fig. 41.16). When the lesion is in the fundus, a total gastrectomy with esophagojejunostomy is done (Fig. 41.17). When metastasis has occurred to adjacent organs, such as the spleen, ovaries, or bowel, the surgical procedure is extended as needed. If the tumor extends into the transverse colon, partial colon resection is done.

Chemotherapy and Radiation Therapy. A number of chemotherapy drugs can be used to treat stomach cancer. These include fluorouracil, capecitabine (Xeloda), carboplatin, cisplatin, docetaxel (Taxotere), epirubicin (Ellence), irinotecan (Camptosar), oxaliplatin (Eloxatin), and paclitaxel. Combination therapies are preferred as the drugs affect different phases of the cell cycle. Examples of combination therapy include ECF (epirubicin, cisplatin, fluorouracil) and docetaxel, irinotecan, oxaliplatin, or cisplatin with fluorouracil or capecitabine.[18] Intraperitoneal administration of chemotherapy agents may also be used to treat metastatic disease. Chemotherapy is discussed in Chapter 15.

Radiation therapy may be used together with chemotherapy to reduce the recurrence or as a palliative measure to decrease tumor mass and provide temporary relief of obstruction.

Targeted Therapy. Trastuzumab (Herceptin) and ramucirumab (Cyramza) are targeted therapies used to treat stomach cancer. About 20% of patients with stomach cancer have too much HER-2 on the surface of the cancer cells. Trastuzumab targets the HER-2 protein and kills the cancer cells. Ramucirumab binds to the receptor for VEGF and prevents VEGF from binding to the receptor, thus preventing the growth and spread of cancer. These drugs are used to treat esophageal cancer and were discussed on p. 902.

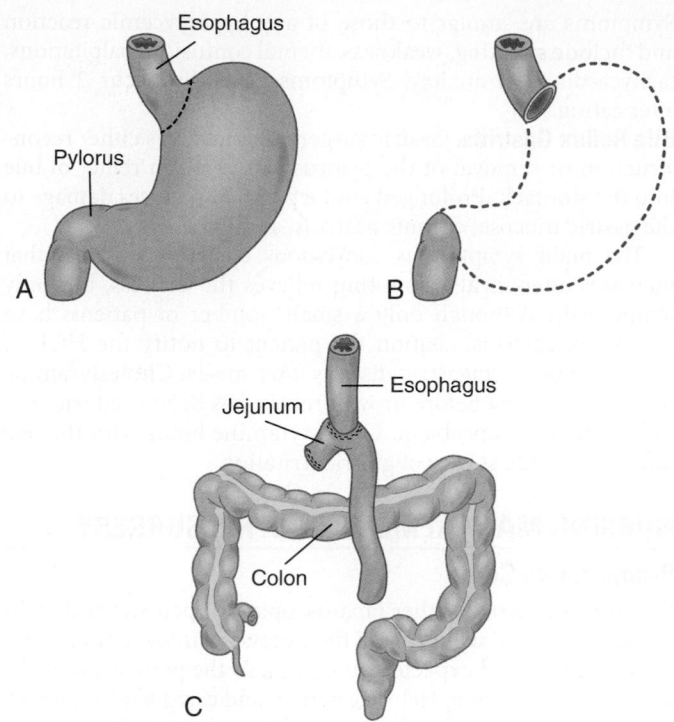

FIG. 41.17 Total gastrectomy for stomach cancer. **A**, Normal anatomic structure of the stomach. **B**, Removal of the stomach (total gastrectomy). **C**, Anastomosis of the esophagus with the jejunum (esophagojejunostomy).

❖ NURSING MANAGEMENT: STOMACH CANCER

◆ Nursing Assessment

The assessment of a person with stomach cancer is similar to that for PUD (Table 41.15). Important data to obtain from the patient and caregiver include a nutritional assessment, a psychosocial history, the patient's perceptions of the health problem and need for care, and a physical examination.

The nutritional assessment obtains information about appetite and changes in eating patterns over the previous 6 months. Determine the patient's normal weight and any recent weight changes. Unexplained weight loss and anorexia are common. Evaluate the patient's nutritional status. Cachexia may be present if oral intake has been reduced for an extended period. A malnourished patient does not respond well to chemotherapy or radiation therapy and is a poor surgical risk. The patient may report a history of vague abdominal symptoms, including dyspepsia and intestinal gas discomfort or pain. If the patient reports pain, explore where and when it occurs and how it is relieved.

Determine the patient's personal perception of the health problem and method of coping with hospitalization, diagnostic tests, and procedures. A possible diagnosis of cancer and a treatment plan that may include surgery, chemotherapy, or radiation treatment is stressful. If surgery is planned, assess the patient's expectations about surgery (cure or palliation) and how the patient has responded to previous surgical procedures.

◆ Nursing Diagnoses

Nursing diagnoses for the patient with stomach cancer include:
- Impaired nutritional intake
- Impaired nutritional status
- Acute pain
- Anxiety

◆ Planning

The overall goals are that the patient with stomach cancer will (1) have minimal discomfort, (2) achieve optimal nutritional status, and (3) maintain a degree of spiritual and psychologic well-being appropriate to the disease stage.

◆ Nursing Implementation

◆ **Health Promotion.** Your role in the early detection of stomach cancer focuses on identifying the patient at risk because of specific disorders such as *H. pylori* infection, pernicious anemia, and achlorhydria. Be aware of symptoms associated with stomach cancer and the significant findings on physical examination. Symptoms often occur late and mimic other conditions, such as PUD. Poor appetite, weight loss, fatigue, and persistent stomach distress are symptoms of stomach cancer. Encourage patients with a positive family history of stomach cancer to undergo diagnostic evaluation if anemia, PUD, or vague epigastric distress are present. It is important that you recognize the possibility of stomach cancer in a patient who is treated for PUD and does not get relief with prescribed therapy.

Acute Care. When diagnostic tests confirm cancer, the patient and family generally react with shock, disbelief, and depression. Provide emotional and physical support, provide information, clarify test results, and maintain a positive attitude with respect to the patient's immediate recovery and long-term survival.

Because of changes in appetite and early satiety, the patient may be malnourished. Surgery may be delayed until the patient is more physically able to withstand it. A positive nutritional state enhances wound healing and the ability to deal with infection and other possible postoperative complications. The patient may better tolerate several small meals a day than 3 regular meals. It may be challenging to persuade the patient to eat when he or she has no appetite and is depressed. Getting the patient's caregiver to help with meals and encourage intake may be beneficial. Diet may be supplemented by commercial liquid supplements and vitamins. If the patient is unable to ingest oral feedings, the HCP may prescribe EN or PN (see Chapter 39).

If needed, packed RBCs and fluid volume restoration may be given during the preoperative period. The preoperative teaching plan and the postoperative care of the patient having stomach cancer surgery is described in the next section on gastric surgery.

Radiation therapy or chemotherapy is used as an adjuvant to surgery or for palliation. Your role is to provide detailed instructions, reassure the patient, and ensure completion of the designated number of treatments. Start by assessing the patient's knowledge of these therapies. Teach the patient about skin care, need for nutrition and fluid intake, and the use of antiemetic drugs. Specific care of the patient receiving chemotherapy and radiation therapy is discussed in Chapter 15.

Ambulatory Care. When chemotherapy or radiation treatment is continuing after discharge, a referral to home health care may be beneficial. The home health nurse can help with recovery, determine the degree of patient adherence, and provide support to the patient and caregiver. Provide the patient with a list of community agencies (e.g., American Cancer Society) that are available before the patient goes home. Encourage the patient to adhere to the prescribed therapies, keep appointments for chemotherapy administration or radiation treatments, and keep the HCP informed of changes in physical condition. Recurrence of cancer is common, and patients need regular follow-up examinations and imaging assessments. Long-term management of the cancer patient is discussed in Chapter 15.

◆ Evaluation

Expected outcomes are that the patient with stomach cancer will
- Have no or minimal discomfort, pain, or nausea
- Achieve optimal nutritional status
- Maintain a degree of psychologic well-being appropriate to the disease stage

GASTRIC SURGERY

Gastric surgeries are done to treat stomach cancer, as well as polyps, perforation, chronic gastritis, and PUD. Surgeries include partial gastrectomy, gastrectomy, vagotomy, and pyloroplasty. Partial gastrectomy with removal of the distal two thirds of the stomach and anastomosis of the gastric stump to the duodenum is a *gastroduodenostomy* or *Billroth I* operation (Fig. 41.16, *A*). If the gastric stump is anastomosed to the jejunum, the surgery is a *gastrojejunostomy* or *Billroth II* operation (Fig. 41.16, *B*). A total gastrectomy involves resection of the lower esophagus, removal of the entire stomach, and anastomosis of the esophagus to the jejunum.

Vagotomy is the severing of the vagus nerve, either totally *(truncal)* or selectively *(highly selective vagotomy)*. These procedures decrease gastric acid secretion. *Pyloroplasty* consists of surgical enlargement of the pyloric sphincter to facilitate the easy passage of contents from the stomach. It is often done after vagotomy or to enlarge an opening that is constricted from scar tissue.

Postoperative Complications

As with all surgeries, acute postoperative bleeding at the surgical site can occur. Monitoring of patients is similar to that described later under acute upper GI bleeding. The most common long-term postoperative complications from gastric surgery are (1) dumping syndrome, (2) postprandial hypoglycemia, and (3) bile reflux gastritis.

Dumping Syndrome. *Dumping syndrome* is the direct result of surgical removal of a large part of the stomach and pyloric sphincter. Normally, gastric chyme enters the small intestine in small amounts. After surgery, the stomach no longer has control over the amount of gastric chyme entering the small intestine. Therefore a large bolus of hypertonic fluid enters the intestine and causes fluid to be drawn into the bowel lumen. This creates a decrease in plasma volume, distention of the bowel lumen, and rapid intestinal transit.

Symptoms begin within 15 to 30 minutes after eating. The patient usually describes feelings of generalized weakness, sweating, palpitations, and dizziness. These symptoms are due to the sudden decrease in plasma volume. The patient may have abdominal cramps, *borborygmi* (audible abdominal sounds made by hyperactive intestinal peristalsis), and the urge to defecate. These manifestations usually last less than 1 hour after eating. A short rest period after each meal reduces the chance of dumping syndrome.

Postprandial Hypoglycemia. *Postprandial hypoglycemia* is a variant of dumping syndrome. It is the result of uncontrolled gastric emptying of a bolus of fluid high in carbohydrate into the small intestine. The bolus of concentrated carbohydrate results in hyperglycemia and the release of excess amounts of insulin into the circulation. This results in reflex hypoglycemia.

Symptoms are similar to those of any hypoglycemic reaction and include sweating, weakness, mental confusion, palpitations, tachycardia, and anxiety. Symptoms generally occur 2 hours after eating.

Bile Reflux Gastritis. Gastric surgery that involves either reconstruction or removal of the pylorus can result in reflux of bile into the stomach. Prolonged contact with bile causes damage to the gastric mucosa, chronic gastritis, and PUD.

The main symptom is continuous epigastric distress that increases after meals. Vomiting relieves the distress, but only temporarily. Although only a small number of patients have bile reflux gastritis, caution the patient to notify the HCP of any continuous epigastric distress after meals. Cholestyramine (Questran), given before or with meals, has been used successfully to treat this problem. Cholestyramine binds with the bile salts that are the source of gastric irritation.

❖ NURSING MANAGEMENT: GASTRIC SURGERY

◆ Preoperative Care

Surgery can involve either laparoscopic or open surgical techniques. The HCP will provide the necessary information about the procedure and expected outcomes, so the patient can make an informed decision. Help the patient and caregiver by answering their questions. Teach them what to expect after surgery, including comfort measures, pain relief, coughing and breathing exercises, use of an NG tube, and IV fluid administration (see Chapter 17 for more on preoperative care).

◆ Postoperative Care

Postoperative care focuses on maintaining fluid and electrolyte balance, preventing respiratory complications, maintaining comfort, and preventing infection. Complications include atelectasis, pneumonia, anastomotic leak, deep vein thrombosis, pulmonary embolus, and bleeding. Morbidly obese patients have a higher risk for many postoperative complications.

After surgery, an NG tube is used for decompression. This decreases pressure on suture lines and allows edema and inflammation resulting from surgical trauma to resolve. Observe the gastric aspirate for color, amount, and odor. Small volumes of bloody drainage from the NG can be expected for the first 2 to 3 hours because bleeding at the anastomotic site is common. Report bright red bleeding that does not decrease after this period or bleeding that becomes excessive (more than 75 mL/hr) immediately to the HCP. The NG aspirate should gradually darken within the first 24 hours after surgery. Normally the color changes to yellow-green within 36 to 48 hours. After total gastrectomy, the NG tube does not drain a large quantity of secretions because removing the stomach has eliminated the reservoir capacity.

Observe the NG tube closely because blood easily clots and clogs the tube. Notify the HCP immediately if the tube stops draining or appears obstructed with blood. If the tube becomes clogged, the HCP may order periodic gentle irrigations with normal saline solution. It is essential that the NG suction is working and that the tube stays patent so that accumulated gastric secretions do not put a strain on the anastomosis. This can lead to distention of any remaining part of the stomach and result in (1) rupture of the sutures, (2) leakage of gastric contents into the peritoneal cavity, (3) hemorrhage, and (4) abscess formation. If the tube must be replaced or repositioned, call the HCP to perform this task because of the danger of perforating the gastric mucosa or disrupting the suture line.

While the NG tube is connected to suction, maintain IV therapy. Before the NG tube is removed, the patient begins clear liquids to determine the tolerance level. In a partial gastrectomy, the stomach may be aspirated within 1 or 2 hours to assess the amount remaining and its color and consistency. When fluids are well tolerated, the NG tube is removed. Solids are added gradually with the goal of resuming a normal diet.

Closely observe the patient for an anastomotic leak and notify the HCP at once if one is suspected. A leak occurs when there is a breakdown of the suture line in an anastomosis that allows gastric or intestinal contents to enter the abdomen or mediastinum. It requires immediate treatment to prevent sepsis and death. Signs and symptoms include tachycardia, dyspnea, fever, abdominal pain, anxiety, and restlessness.

Since most procedures are done laparoscopically, the risk for respiratory complications is reduced. In an open surgical approach, the incision is relatively high in the epigastrium and respiratory complications may occur. Respiratory assessment includes respiratory rate and rhythm, pulse rate and rhythm, and signs of pneumothorax (e.g., dyspnea, chest pain, cyanosis). Have the patient cough and deep breathe to expand the lungs. Pain may interfere with deep breathing and coughing. Encourage the patient to splint the area with a pillow. Splinting also protects the abdominal suture line from rupturing during deep breathing and coughing. Encourage early ambulation and frequent position changes.

Give pain medications as needed. Be aware that pain could be from an anastomosis leak rather than typical surgical pain. Abdominal wounds need frequent observation for the amount and type of drainage, condition of the incision, and signs of infection. Monitor vital signs to help identify problems such as infection, hemorrhage, or anastomosis leak. Implement measures to control nausea and vomiting. Measure and record the intake and output and obtain daily weights.

◆ **Nutritional Therapy.** Understanding the patient's surgery and the resulting anatomy is important. Long-term, many patients have malnutrition, metabolic bone disease, anemia, and weight loss. Nutrition interventions help minimize the occurrence of expected complications and maximize nutrient intake (Table 41.18). Start nutrition teaching as soon as the immediate postoperative period has passed. The dietitian usually provides dietary instructions. You must reinforce them. Following dietary measures will decrease symptoms and is essential to long-term adherence.

Postoperative wound healing may be impaired because of poor nutritional intake. Give potassium and vitamin supplements as ordered. For those who were malnourished preoperatively, a small bowel feeding tube may be placed intraoperatively. EN may be started on postoperative day 1 and adjusted depending on how oral intake is tolerated. Some may be discharged with nighttime tube feedings. PN is an option if the patient is not able to tolerate oral nutrition.

Pernicious anemia is a long-term complication of total gastrectomy and may occur after partial gastrectomy. It is due to the loss of intrinsic factor, which is made by the parietal cells. *Intrinsic factor* is essential for the absorption of cobalamin in the terminal ileum. Because it is essential for the growth and maturation of RBCs, the lack of cobalamin results in pernicious anemia and neurologic complications. The patient will require cobalamin replacement therapy (see Chapter 30). Patients should take multivitamins with folate, calcium, vitamin D, and iron for life.

TABLE 41.18 Nutritional Therapy
Postgastrectomy Dumping Syndrome

The amount of time these restrictions should be followed varies. The HCP decides the proper amount of time to remain on this prescribed diet according to the patient's clinical condition and progress.

Purposes
- Slow the rapid passage of food into the intestine
- Control symptoms of dumping syndrome (dizziness, sense of fullness, diarrhea, tachycardia), which sometimes occurs after a partial or total gastrectomy

Diet Principles
- Divide meals into 6 small feedings to avoid overloading the stomach and intestine at mealtimes.
- Do not take fluids with meals but at least 30–45 min before or after meals. This helps prevent distention or a feeling of fullness.
- Avoid concentrated sweets (e.g., honey, sugar, jelly, jam, candies, sweet pastries, and sweetened fruit) because they sometimes cause dizziness, diarrhea, and a sense of fullness.
- Protein consumption is unlimited to promote rebuilding of body tissues. Meat and eggs are specific foods to increase in the diet.
- Milk contains lactose, which may be hard to digest. Introduce milk and milk products slowly several weeks after surgery.
- Avoid carbonated beverages and foods that are gas forming to help prevent gastric distention.
- Low-roughage and raw foods are allowed as tolerated a few weeks after surgery.
- Increase complex carbohydrates (e.g., bread, vegetables, rice, potatoes) and fats to meet energy needs.

Because partial gastrectomy decreases the stomach's reservoir, patients must reduce their meal size accordingly. For the first few weeks after surgery, the patient should consume soft, bland foods with low fiber and high complex carbohydrates and protein content. Teach the patient to eat in small portions and not to drink fluids with meals. Simple sugars, lactose, and fried foods should be avoided. Teach the patient to avoid extreme temperatures in food and to chew food thoroughly.

To avoid hypoglycemic episodes, teach the patient to limit the amount of sugar consumed with each meal and eat small, frequent meals with moderate amounts of protein and fat. The immediate ingestion of sugared fluids or candy relieves hypoglycemic symptoms.

◆ **Ambulatory Care.** Patients who have had a total gastrectomy and are debilitated may need skilled care after discharge. For those going home, assist the patient and caregiver with symptom management. Make plans for pain relief, including comfort measures and the judicious use of analgesics. Teach wound care (if needed) to the primary caregiver. Dressings, special equipment, or special services may be needed. Collaborate with the dietitian to provide teaching about the diet that will optimize nutrition.

GASTRITIS

Gastritis, an inflammation of the gastric mucosa, is one of the most common problems affecting the stomach. Gastritis may be acute or chronic and diffuse or localized.

Etiology and Pathophysiology

Gastritis occurs as the result of a breakdown in the normal gastric mucosal barrier. This mucosal barrier normally protects the

TABLE 41.19 Causes of Gastritis

Drugs
- Aspirin
- Bisphosphonates
- Corticosteroids
- Digitalis
- Iron supplements
- Nonsteroidal antiinflammatory drugs (NSAIDs)

Diet
- Alcohol
- Large amounts of spicy, irritating foods

Microorganisms
- *H. pylori*
- Cytomegalovirus
- *Mycobacterium* species
- *Salmonella* organisms
- *Staphylococcus* organisms
- *Treponema pallidum* (syphilis)

Environmental Factors
- Radiation
- Smoking

Diseases/Disorders
- Burns
- Crohn's disease
- Large hiatal hernia
- Physiologic stress
- Reflux of bile and pancreatic secretions
- Renal failure
- Sepsis
- Shock

Other Factors
- Endoscopy procedures
- Nasogastric tube
- Psychologic stress

stomach tissue from the corrosive action of HCl acid and pepsin. When the barrier is broken, HCl acid and pepsin can diffuse back into the mucosa. This back diffusion results in tissue edema, disruption of capillary walls with loss of plasma into the gastric lumen, and possible hemorrhage.

Risk Factors. Risk factors and causes of gastritis are listed in Table 41.19. Some risk factors are discussed in this section.

Drug-Related Gastritis. Drugs contribute to the development of acute and chronic gastritis. NSAIDs and corticosteroids inhibit the synthesis of prostaglandins that are protective to the gastric mucosa. This makes the mucosa more susceptible to injury. Factors that increase the risk for NSAID-induced gastritis include being female; being over age 60; having a history of ulcer disease; taking anticoagulants, LDA, or corticosteroids; and having a chronic disorder, such as CVD. Some drugs such as digoxin and alendronate (Fosamax) have direct irritating effects on the gastric mucosa.

Diet. Dietary indiscretions can cause acute gastritis. After an alcoholic drinking binge, acute damage to the gastric mucosa can range from localized injury of superficial epithelial cells to destruction of the mucosa with mucosal congestion, edema, and hemorrhage. Prolonged damage induced by repeated alcohol use results in chronic gastritis. Eating large quantities of spicy, irritating foods can cause acute gastritis.

Helicobacter Pylori. A key cause of chronic gastritis is *H. pylori* infection. *H. pylori* infection causes acute gastritis in most infected persons. Chronic gastritis may develop in some. Prolonged inflammation leads to functional changes in the stomach and may cause stomach cancer. *H. pylori* was discussed earlier in this chapter on p. 905.

Other Risk Factors. Although not as common as *H. pylori*, other bacterial, viral, and fungal infections are associated with chronic gastritis. Gastritis can occur from reflux of bile salts from the duodenum into the stomach because of anatomic changes after surgical procedures (e.g., gastroduodenostomy, gastrojejunostomy). Prolonged vomiting may cause reflux of bile salts. Intense emotional responses and CNS lesions may cause inflammation of the mucosal lining from hypersecretion of HCl acid.

Autoimmune Gastritis. Autoimmune metaplastic atrophic gastritis (also called *autoimmune atrophic gastritis*) is an inherited condition in which there is an immune response directed against parietal cells. It most often affects women of northern European descent. Patients often have other autoimmune disorders. The loss of parietal cells leads to low chloride levels, inadequate production of intrinsic factor, cobalamin (vitamin B_{12}) malabsorption, and pernicious anemia. It is associated with an increased risk of stomach cancer.

Clinical Manifestations

The symptoms of *acute gastritis* include anorexia, nausea and vomiting, epigastric tenderness, and a feeling of fullness. Hemorrhage is often associated with alcohol use and at times, is the only symptom. Acute gastritis is self-limiting, lasting from a few hours to a few days. Complete healing of the mucosa is expected.

The manifestations of *chronic gastritis* are like those of acute gastritis. Some patients are asymptomatic. However, when parietal cells are lost because of atrophy, the source of intrinsic factor is also lost. *Intrinsic factor* is essential for cobalamin absorption. The lack of cobalamin results in pernicious anemia. Cobalamin deficiency anemia is discussed in Chapter 30.

Diagnostic Studies

Acute gastritis is usually diagnosed based on the patient's symptoms and a history of drug or alcohol use. Occasionally, an endoscopic examination with biopsy is required to make the diagnosis. Breath, urine, serum, stool, and gastric tissue biopsy tests are done to assess for *H. pylori* infection. A CBC may show anemia from blood loss or lack of intrinsic factor. Stools are tested for occult blood. Serum tests for antibodies to parietal cells and intrinsic factor may be done. A tissue biopsy can rule out gastric cancer.

❖ NURSING AND INTERPROFESSIONAL MANAGEMENT: GASTRITIS

◆ Acute Gastritis

Eliminating the cause and preventing or avoiding it in the future are generally all that is needed to treat acute gastritis. The plan of care is supportive and similar to that described for nausea and vomiting. If vomiting is present, rest, NPO status, and IV fluids may be prescribed. Antiemetics are given (Table 41.1). Monitor for dehydration. It can occur rapidly in acute gastritis with vomiting.

In severe cases of acute gastritis, an NG tube may be used to (1) monitor for bleeding, (2) lavage the precipitating agent from the stomach, or (3) keep the stomach empty and free of noxious stimuli. Clear liquids are resumed when symptoms have subsided. Reintroduce solids gradually.

If the patient is at risk for hemorrhage, frequently check vital signs and test the vomitus for blood. All the management strategies discussed in the section on upper GI bleeding apply to the patient with severe gastritis (see pp. 917–920).

Drug therapy focuses on reducing irritation of the gastric mucosa and providing symptomatic relief. H_2 receptor blockers (e.g., ranitidine, cimetidine) or PPIs (e.g., omeprazole) reduce gastric HCl acid secretion (Table 41.10). Teach the patient about the therapeutic effects of PPIs and H_2 receptor blockers.

❖ Chronic Gastritis

The treatment of chronic gastritis focuses on evaluating and eliminating the specific cause (e.g., cessation of alcohol use,

TABLE 41.20 **Types of Upper GI Bleeding**	
Type	**Manifestations**
Obvious bleeding	
• Hematemesis	Bloody vomitus appearing as fresh, bright red blood or "coffee-grounds" appearance (dark, grainy digested blood).
• Melena	Black, tarry stools (often foul smelling) caused by digestion of blood in the GI tract. Black appearance is from the presence of iron.
Occult bleeding	Small amounts of blood in gastric secretions, vomitus, or stools not apparent by appearance. Detectable by guaiac test

TABLE 41.21 **Causes of Upper GI Bleeding**	
Stomach and Duodenum	**Esophagus**
• Drug-induced	• Esophageal varices
• Corticosteroids	• Esophagitis
• NSAIDs	• Mallory-Weiss tear
• Salicylates	
• Erosive gastritis	**Systemic Diseases**
• Polyps	• Blood dyscrasias (e.g., leukemia, aplastic anemia)
• PUD	• Renal failure
• Stress-related mucosal disease	
• Stomach cancer	

abstinence from drugs, *H. pylori* eradication). Antibiotic combinations are used to eradicate *H. pylori* (Table 41.14). The patient with pernicious anemia needs lifelong cobalamin therapy (see Chapter 30).

The patient undergoing treatment for chronic gastritis may have to adapt to lifestyle changes and strictly adhere to a drug regimen. Some patients find a nonirritating diet consisting of 6 small feedings a day helpful. Smoking is contraindicated in all forms of gastritis. An interprofessional team approach in which the HCP, nurse, dietitian, and pharmacist provide consistent information and support will increase the patient's success in making these changes.

UPPER GASTROINTESTINAL BLEEDING

In the United States, 250,000 hospital admissions occur each year for upper GI bleeding.[19] About 60% of these are adults over age 65. Though the mortality rate is still around 2.5%, this rate has decreased over the past few decades due to advances in the prevention and treatment of upper GI bleeding.

Etiology and Pathophysiology

Although the most serious loss of blood from the upper GI tract is characterized by a sudden onset, insidious occult bleeding can be a major problem. The severity of bleeding depends on whether the origin is venous, capillary, or arterial. Types of upper GI bleeding are described in Table 41.20. Bleeding from an arterial source is profuse, and the blood is bright red because it has not been in contact with gastric HCl acid secretion. In contrast, coffee-grounds vomitus means that the blood has been in the stomach for some time. *Melena* (black, tarry stools) occurs with slow bleeding from an upper GI source. The longer the passage of blood through the intestines, the darker the stool color because of the breakdown of hemoglobin and release of iron.

Discovering the cause of the bleeding is not always easy. A variety of areas in the GI tract may be involved. Table 41.21 lists the common causes of upper GI bleeding.

Stomach and Duodenal Origin. Peptic ulcers, due to *H. pylori* infection and the use of NSAIDS, are the most common causes of upper GI bleeding. About 25% of people on chronic NSAIDs (e.g., ibuprofen) develop ulcer disease; of these, 2% to 4% will bleed. Even LDA is associated with a risk for GI bleeding. Many OTC preparations contain aspirin. Obtain a careful medication history whenever upper GI bleeding is suspected.

Stress-related mucosal disease (SRMD), also called *physiologic stress ulcers*, describes mucosal damage in the GI tract ranging from small single lesions to multiple gastric ulcers

and major bleeding. SRMD most often occurs in critically ill patients who have had severe burns, trauma, or major surgery. Patients with coagulopathy, liver disease, or organ failure and those receiving renal replacement therapy are at highest risk for SRMD.[20]

Esophageal Origin. Bleeding from the esophagus is likely due to chronic esophagitis, Mallory-Weiss tear, or esophageal varices. Chronic esophagitis can be caused by GERD, smoking, alcohol use, and the ingestion of drugs irritating to the mucosa. Esophageal varices most often occur from cirrhosis of the liver. Esophageal varices are discussed in Chapter 43.

Diagnostic Studies

Endoscopy is the primary tool for diagnosing the source (e.g., esophageal varices, PUD, gastritis) of upper GI bleeding. Angiography is used when endoscopy cannot be done or when bleeding persists after endoscopic therapy. Angiography requires preparation and setup time and may not be appropriate for a high-risk, unstable patient. In this procedure, a catheter is inserted into the femoral artery and advanced to the left gastric or superior mesenteric artery until the site of bleeding is found.

Laboratory studies include CBC, blood urea nitrogen (BUN), serum electrolytes, prothrombin time, partial thromboplastin time, liver enzymes, arterial blood gases (ABGs), and a type and crossmatch for possible blood transfusions. All vomitus and stools are tested for gross and occult blood.

Monitor the patient's laboratory studies to estimate the effectiveness of therapy. The hemoglobin and hematocrit values are not of immediate help in estimating the degree of blood loss, but they provide a baseline for guiding further treatment. The initial hematocrit may be normal and may not reflect the loss until 4 to 6 hours after fluid replacement, since initially the loss of plasma and RBCs is equal.

Assess the patient's BUN level. During a significant hemorrhage, GI tract bacteria break down proteins, resulting in increased BUN levels. An increased BUN level may also show renal hypoperfusion or renal disease.

Interprofessional Management

A massive upper GI hemorrhage is a loss of more than 1500 mL of blood or 25% of intravascular blood volume. Although 80% to 85% of patients with massive hemorrhage spontaneously stop bleeding, the cause must be identified and treatment started at once.

Emergency Assessment and Management. A complete history of events leading to the bleeding episode is deferred until emergency care has been started. To facilitate early intervention, focus your physical examination on identifying signs and symptoms of shock, such as tachycardia, weak pulse, hypotension, cool extremities, prolonged capillary refill, and apprehension. (Shock is discussed in Chapter 66.)

Urine output is one of the best measures of vital organ perfusion. An indwelling urinary catheter is inserted so that hourly output can be accurately assessed. Hemodynamic monitoring provides an accurate and quick assessment of blood flow and pressure in the cardiovascular system (see Chapter 65). A central venous pressure line may be used for fluid volume status assessment. If the patient has a history of valvular heart disease, coronary artery disease, or heart failure, a pulmonary artery catheter may be needed. Give supplemental O_2 to increase blood O_2 saturation.

The patient is at risk for perforation and peritonitis. Do a thorough abdominal examination. Note the presence of a tense, rigid, boardlike abdomen and the presence or absence of bowel sounds.

The type and amount of fluids infused are based on physical and laboratory findings. Generally, an isotonic crystalloid solution (e.g., lactated Ringer's solution) is started. Whole blood, packed RBCs, and fresh frozen plasma may be used for volume replacement in massive hemorrhage. When upper GI bleeding is less profuse, infusion of isotonic saline solution followed by packed RBCs restores the hematocrit more quickly and does not create complications related to fluid volume overload. (The use of blood transfusions and volume expanders is discussed in Chapter 30.)

Endoscopic Therapy. The first-line management of upper GI bleeding is endoscopy. Endoscopy within the first 24 hours of bleeding is important for diagnosis, determining the need for surgical intervention, and providing treatment.

The goal of endoscopic hemostasis is to coagulate or thrombose the bleeding vessel. Several techniques are used, including (1) mechanical therapy with clips or bands, (2) thermal ablation, and (3) injection (e.g., epinephrine, alcohol). Clips and bands directly compress the bleeding vessel. Thermal ablation cauterizes tissue through applying heat to the bleeding site. Common devices include neodymium:yttrium-aluminum-garnet (YAG) laser, monopolar or bipolar electrocoagulation, heater probes, and argon plasma coagulation (APC).[21]

For variceal bleeding, other strategies include variceal ligation, injection sclerotherapy, and balloon tamponade (see Chapter 43).

Surgical Therapy. Surgical intervention is needed when bleeding continues regardless of the therapy provided and when the site of the bleeding has been identified. Surgery may be done if the patient continues to bleed after rapid transfusion of up to 2000 mL of whole blood or is still in shock after 24 hours. The site of the hemorrhage determines the choice of surgery. Mortality rates increase considerably in older patients.

Drug Therapy. During the acute phase of upper GI bleeding, drugs are used to decrease bleeding, decrease HCl acid secretion, and neutralize the HCl acid that is present. Empiric PPI therapy with high-dose IV bolus and subsequent infusion to decrease acid secretion is often started before endoscopy (Table 41.10). Efforts are made to reduce acid secretion because the acidic environment can alter platelet function and interfere with clot stabilization. This may decrease the amount of bleeding and need for endoscopic therapy.

After an acute phase of bleeding, antacids may be given hourly, either orally or through the NG tube. If an NG tube is in place, the stomach contents should be aspirated and tested periodically for pH level. If pH is less than 5, intermittent suction

may be used or the frequency or dosage of the antacid or antisecretory agent increased.

❖ NURSING MANAGEMENT: UPPER GASTROINTESTINAL BLEEDING

◆ Nursing Assessment

A thorough nursing assessment is an essential first step as you begin care of the patient admitted with upper GI bleeding. The patient may not be able to give specific information about the cause of the bleeding until immediate physical needs are met. Perform an immediate nursing assessment while you are getting the patient ready for initial treatment. The assessment includes the patient's level of consciousness, vital signs, skin color, and capillary refill. Check the abdomen for distention, guarding, and peristalsis. Immediate determination of vital signs indicates whether the patient is in shock from blood loss and provides a baseline BP and pulse for monitoring the progress of treatment. Signs and symptoms of shock include low BP; rapid, weak pulse; increased thirst; cold, clammy skin; and restlessness. Monitor vital signs every 15 to 30 minutes. Inform the HCP of any significant changes.

Once the immediate interventions have begun, the patient or caregiver should answer the following questions: Is there a history of bleeding episodes? Has the patient received blood transfusions? Were there any transfusion reactions? Are there any other illnesses (e.g., liver disease, cirrhosis) or medications that may contribute to bleeding or interfere with treatment? Does the patient have a religious preference that prohibits the use of blood or blood products?

Subjective and objective data to obtain from the patient or caregiver are outlined in Table 41.22.

◆ Nursing Diagnoses

Nursing diagnoses for the patient with upper GI bleeding include:

- Impaired cardiac output
- Fluid imbalance
- Ineffective tissue perfusion
- Anxiety

◆ Planning

The overall goals are that the patient with upper GI bleeding will (1) have no further GI bleeding, (2) have the cause of the bleeding identified and treated, (3) return to a normal hemodynamic state, and (4) have minimal or no symptoms of pain or anxiety.

◆ Nursing Implementation

◆ Health Promotion. Although not all cases of upper GI bleeding can be prevented, you have an important role in identifying patients at high risk. Always consider the patient with a history of chronic gastritis, cirrhosis, or PUD at high risk. The patient who has had an upper GI bleeding episode is more likely to have another bleed. Patients on daily LDA to reduce CVD risk are at risk for upper GI bleeding, especially those over 60 years old with a history of PUD.

Teach the patient who takes regular doses of drugs that cause GI toxicity (peptic ulcer formation, bleeding), such as corticosteroids and NSAIDs, about the risk for GI bleeding. They may need to receive long-term treatment with a PPI, H_2 receptor blocker, or misoprostol. Taking these drugs with meals or snacks lessens their direct irritation.

TABLE 41.22 Nursing Assessment

Upper GI Bleeding

Subjective Data

Important Health Information

Past health history: Precipitating events before bleeding episode, prior bleeding episodes and treatment, PUD, esophageal varices, esophagitis, acute and chronic gastritis, stress-related mucosal disease
Medications: Aspirin, NSAIDs, corticosteroids, anticoagulants

Functional Health Patterns

Health perception–health management: Family history of bleeding, smoking, alcohol use
Nutritional-metabolic: Nausea, vomiting, weight loss, thirst
Elimination: Diarrhea. Black, tarry stools. Decreased urine output. Sweating
Activity-exercise: Weakness, dizziness, fainting
Cognitive-perceptual: Epigastric pain, abdominal cramps
Coping–stress tolerance: Acute or chronic stress

Objective Data

General

Fever

Integumentary

Clammy, cool, pale skin. Pale mucous membranes, nail beds, and conjunctivae. Spider angiomas, jaundice, peripheral edema

Respiratory

Rapid, shallow respirations

Cardiovascular

Tachycardia, weak pulse, orthostatic hypotension, slow capillary refill

Gastrointestinal

Red or coffee-grounds vomitus. Tense, rigid abdomen, ascites. Hypoactive or hyperactive bowel sounds. Black, tarry stools

Urinary

Decreased urine output, concentrated urine

Neurologic

Agitation, restlessness. Decreasing level of consciousness

Possible Diagnostic Findings

↓ Hematocrit and hemoglobin, hematuria. Guaiac-positive stools, emesis, or gastric aspirate. ↓ Levels of clotting factors, ↑ liver enzymes, abnormal endoscopy results

✚ TABLE 41.23 Emergency Management

Acute GI Bleeding

Assessment Findings	Interventions
Abdominal and GI Findings • Abdominal pain • Abdominal rigidity • Hematemesis • Melena • Nausea **Hypovolemic Shock** • ↓ BP • ↓ Pulse pressure • Tachycardia • Cool, clammy skin • ↓ Level of consciousness • ↓ Urine output (<0.5 mL/kg/hr) • Slow capillary refill	• Initial • If unresponsive, assess circulation, airway, and breathing. • If responsive, monitor airway, breathing, and circulation. • Establish IV access with large-bore catheter and start fluid replacement therapy. Insert a second large-bore catheter if shock present. • Give O₂ via nasal cannula or nonrebreather mask. • Initiate ECG monitoring. • Obtain blood for CBC, clotting studies, and type and crossmatch as appropriate. • Insert NG tube as needed. • Insert indwelling urinary catheter. • Give IV PPI therapy to decrease acid secretion. • Ongoing Monitoring • Monitor vital signs, level of consciousness, O₂ saturation, ECG, bowel sounds, and intake/output. • Assess amount and character of emesis. • Keep patient NPO. • Provide reassurance and emotional support to patient and caregiver.

Acute Care. Emergency management of acute GI bleeding is outlined in Table 41.23. Place IV lines, preferably 2, with a 16- or 18-gauge needle for fluid and blood replacement. Give fluid or blood replacement as ordered. An accurate intake and output record is essential so that the patient's hydration status can be assessed. Measure the urine output hourly. If a central venous pressure line or pulmonary artery catheter in place, record these readings every 1 to 2 hours. Use ECG monitoring to evaluate cardiac function. Close monitoring of vital signs, especially in the patient with CVD, is important because dysrhythmias may occur.

❓ CHECK YOUR PRACTICE

You are admitting a 71-yr-old man to the unit from the emergency department. He has a diagnosis of upper GI bleeding. He reports heartburn and pain (6 on a scale of 10) in the upper epigastric region and has just had a 250 mL coffee-grounds emesis.
• What assessment data do you need to obtain?
• What are the priority nursing interventions for this man?

Teach the at-risk patient to avoid known gastric irritants, such as alcohol and smoking, and to take only prescribed medications. OTC drugs can be harmful because they may contain ingredients (e.g., aspirin) that increase the risk for bleeding. Review how to test vomitus or stools for occult blood. Teach them to report positive results promptly to the HCP. Stress the importance of treating an upper respiratory tract infection promptly. Severe coughing or sneezing can increase pressure on the already fragile varices and may result in massive hemorrhage (see Chapter 43).

Patients with blood dyscrasias (e.g., aplastic anemia) or liver dysfunction or those who are taking chemotherapy drugs are at risk due to a decrease in clotting factors and platelets. Teach patients about their disease process, drugs, and increased risk for GI bleeding.

Observe the older adult or the patient with CVD closely for signs of fluid overload. However, volume overload and pulmonary edema are concerns in all patients who are receiving large amounts of IV fluids within a short time. Auscultate breath sounds and closely observe the respiratory effort. Keep the head of the bed elevated to provide comfort and prevent aspiration.

When an NG tube is present, pay special attention to keeping it in proper position and checking the aspirate for blood. Although gastric lavage (room temperature, cool, or iced) is used in some agencies, its effectiveness as a treatment for upper GI bleeding is questionable. When lavage is used, around 50 to

TABLE 41.24 Bacterial Food Poisoning

Type and Cause	Sources	Manifestations	Treatment and Prevention
Botulism Toxin from *Clostridium botulinum;* ingested toxin absorbed from gut and blocks acetylcholine at neuromuscular junction	Improperly canned or preserved food, home-preserved vegetables (most common), preserved fruits and fish, canned commercial products	*Onset:* 12–36 hr *GI:* Nausea, vomiting, abdominal pain, constipation, distention *Central nervous system:* Headache, dizziness, muscular incoordination, weakness, inability to talk or swallow, diplopia, breathing problems, paralysis, delirium, coma	*Treat:* Maintain ventilation, polyvalent antitoxin, guanidine hydrochloric acid (enhances acetylcholine release) *Prevent:* Correct processing of canned foods, boiling of suspected canned foods for 15 min before serving
Clostridial *Clostridium perfringens*	Meat or poultry dishes cooked at lower temperature (stew, pot pie), rewarmed meat dishes, gravies, improperly canned vegetables	*Onset:* 8–24 hr Diarrhea, nausea, abdominal cramps, vomiting (rare), midepigastric pain	*Treat:* Symptomatic, fluid replacement *Prevent:* Correct preparation of meat dishes. Serving food immediately after cooking or rapid cooling of food
Escherichia coli *E. coli* O157:H7	Contaminated beef, pork, milk, cheese, fish, cookie dough	*Onset:* 8 hr to 1 wk (varies by strain) Bloody stools, hemolytic uremic syndrome, abdominal cramping, profuse diarrhea	*Treat:* Symptomatic, fluid and electrolyte replacement *Prevent:* Correct preparation of food
Salmonella *Salmonella typhimurium* (grows in gut)	Improperly cooked poultry, pork, beef, lamb, and eggs	*Onset:* 8 hr to several days Nausea and vomiting, diarrhea, abdominal cramps, fever, and chills	*Treat:* Symptomatic, fluid and electrolyte replacement *Prevent:* Correct preparation of food
Staphylococcal Toxin from *Staphylococcus aureus*	Meat, bakery products, cream fillings, salad dressings, milk Skin and respiratory tract of food handlers	*Onset:* 30 min to 7 hr Vomiting, nausea, abdominal cramping, diarrhea	*Treat:* Symptomatic, fluid and electrolyte replacement, antiemetics *Prevent:* Immediate refrigeration of foods, monitoring food handlers

100 mL of fluid is instilled at a time into the stomach. The lavage fluid may be aspirated from the stomach or drained by gravity. When aspiration is the method used, it is important not to aspirate if you feel resistance. The tip of the NG tube may be up against the gastric mucosal lining. When resistance is a factor, use the gravity method.

Approach the patient in a calm manner to help decrease the level of anxiety. Use caution when giving sedatives for restlessness because it is one of the warning signs of shock and may be masked by the drugs.

Assess the stools for blood (black-tarry, bright red). Black, tarry stools are not usually associated with a brisk hemorrhage but are indicative of prolonged bleeding. Determine if menses or bleeding are possible sources of blood in the stools. When vomitus contains blood, but the stool contains no gross or occult blood, the hemorrhage is thought to be of short duration.

When beginning oral nourishment, observe the patient for symptoms of nausea and vomiting and a recurrence of bleeding. Feedings initially consist of clear fluids. They are given hourly until tolerance is determined. Gradually introduce foods if the patient has no signs of discomfort.

When hemorrhage is the result of chronic alcohol use, closely observe the patient for delirium tremens as alcohol withdrawal takes place. Symptoms indicating the onset of delirium tremens are agitation, uncontrolled shaking, sweating, and hallucinations. (Alcohol withdrawal is discussed in Chapter 10.)

Ambulatory Care. Teach the patient and caregiver how to avoid future bleeding episodes. Ulcer disease, drug or alcohol use, liver and respiratory diseases can all cause upper GI bleeding. Help the patient and caregiver to be aware of the consequences of not adhering to drug therapy.

Emphasize not to take any drugs (especially aspirin, NSAIDs) other than those prescribed by the HCP. Support the patient in smoking and alcohol cessation because they are sources of irritation and interfere with tissue repair. Long-term follow-up care may be needed because of possible recurrence. Teach the patient and caregiver what to do if an acute hemorrhage occurs in the future.

◆ **Evaluation**

The expected outcomes are that the patient with upper GI bleeding will

- Have no upper GI bleeding
- Maintain normal fluid volume
- Return to a normal hemodynamic state
- Understand potential risk factors and make lifestyle modifications

FOODBORNE ILLNESS

Foodborne illness (food poisoning) is a nonspecific term that describes acute GI symptoms such as nausea, vomiting, diarrhea, and cramping abdominal pain caused by the intake of contaminated food or liquids.[22] There are more than 250 foodborne illnesses. Each year 1 in 6 Americans, or 48 million, gets a foodborne illness. Of these, 128,000 are hospitalized and around 3000 die.[22]

Bacteria account for most foodborne illnesses. The most common source is raw foods that become contaminated during growing, harvesting, processing, storing, shipping, or final preparation. Bacteria multiply quickly when the temperature of food is between 40 and 140 degrees. So, bacteria can multiply if hot food is not kept hot enough or cold food not cold enough. The most common bacterial food poisonings are described in Table 41.24.

Focus interventions on preventing infection. Teaching includes correct food preparation and cleanliness, adequate cooking, and refrigeration (Table 41.25). For the hospitalized

TABLE 41.25 Patient & Caregiver Teaching

Preventing Food Poisoning

Include these instructions when teaching the patient and caregiver how to prevent food poisoning.

1. Cook all ground beef and hamburger thoroughly.
   - Use a digital instant-read meat thermometer to ensure thorough cooking (ground beef can turn brown before disease-causing bacteria are killed).
   - Cook ground beef until a thermometer inserted into several parts of the patty, including the thickest part, reads at least 160° F.
   - People who cook ground beef without using a thermometer can decrease their risk for illness by not eating ground beef patties that are still pink in the middle.
2. If you are served an undercooked hamburger or other ground beef product in a restaurant, send it back for further cooking. Ask for a new bun and a clean plate.
3. Avoid spreading harmful bacteria. Keep raw meat separate from ready-to-eat foods. Wash hands, counters, and utensils with hot soapy water after they touch raw meat. Never place cooked hamburgers or ground beef on the unwashed plate that held raw patties. Wash meat thermometers in between tests of patties that need more cooking.
4. Drink only pasteurized milk, juice, or cider. Commercial juice with an extended shelf-life that is sold at room temperature (e.g., juice in cardboard boxes, vacuum-sealed juice in glass containers) has been pasteurized. Juice concentrates are heated enough to kill pathogens.
5. Wash fruits and vegetables thoroughly, especially those you will not be cooking.
6. Do not eat raw food products that are supposed to be cooked. Follow package directions for cooking at proper temperatures.
7. People who are immunocompromised should avoid eating alfalfa sprouts until the safety of the sprouts can be ensured.

patient, emphasize correcting fluid and electrolyte imbalances from diarrhea and vomiting. With botulism, additional assessment and care related to neurologic symptoms are indicated (see Chapter 60).

***Escherichia coli* O157:H7 Poisoning.** Most strains of *Escherichia coli* are harmless and live in the intestines of healthy humans and animals. *E, coli* O157:H7 makes a powerful toxin and can cause severe illness with hemorrhagic colitis and kidney failure. In the very young and older adults, *E. coli* O157:H7 can be life threatening.

E. coli O157:H7 is found primarily in undercooked meats, particularly poultry and hamburger. *E. coli* outbreaks have occurred with contaminated leafy vegetables, fruits, and nuts. Infection can occur after drinking raw milk, unpasteurized or contaminated fruit juices and after swimming in or drinking sewage-contaminated water. Person-to-person contact in families, nursing homes, and child care centers is an important mode of transmission.

Illness starts 1 to 10 days after swallowing the organism and lasts 5 to 10 days. Manifestations include diarrhea (often bloody), vomiting, and abdominal cramping pain. The diarrhea is variable, ranging from mild to bloody. It may start out as watery but may progress to bloody. Systemic complications, including hemolytic uremia and thrombocytopenic purpura, and even death can occur.

Infection with *E. coli* O157:H7 is diagnosed by detecting the bacteria in the stool. All people who suddenly have diarrhea with blood should have a stool culture for *E. coli* O157:H7.

Treatment involves hydration to maintain blood volume. There is no evidence that antibiotic therapy improves the course of disease. We think that treatment with some antibiotics may precipitate kidney complications. Patients should avoid antidiarrheal agents, such as loperamide (Imodium). Other therapies may include dialysis and plasmapheresis.

A small number of patients, especially young children and older adults, develop hemolytic uremic syndrome (HUS). With HUS, the RBCs are destroyed and the kidneys fail. It is a life-threatening condition usually treated in an ICU. Blood transfusions and kidney dialysis are often needed. The mortality rate is around 5%. About one third of people with HUS have abnormal kidney function for years afterward. A few need long-term dialysis. Other long-term complications of HUS include hypertension, seizures, blindness, and paralysis.

CASE STUDY

Peptic Ulcer Disease

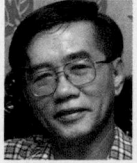

(© iStockphoto/Thinkstock.)

Patient Profile

F.H., a 40-yr-old male immigrant from Vietnam, has a 1-yr history of epigastric distress. Increasingly, it is not relieved by over-the-counter omeprazole (Prilosec). He is scheduled for an upper endoscopy this morning.

Subjective Data
- Reports increasing substernal pain, especially 2 to 3 hr after eating
- Currently avoids alcohol and is taking an over-the-counter PPI
- Smoking history of 1 pack of cigarettes per day for 20 yr
- Has had increasing fatigue with exercise
- Reports occasional black bowel movement
- Takes Chinese medicine for frequent back pain

Objective Data

Physical Examination
- Height 5 ft, 5 in tall and weight 140 lb

Diagnostic Studies
- Endoscopy reveals a duodenal ulcer
- Hgb 10.2 g/dL; Hct 30%
- Histology of biopsied tissue reveals *H. pylori* infection

Interprofessional Care
- omeprazole 20 mg twice daily × 10 days
- clarithromycin 500 mg twice daily × 10 days
- amoxicillin 1 gram twice daily × 10 days

Discussion Questions

1. Explain the pathophysiology of peptic ulcer disease.
2. What are the risk factors for duodenal ulcers? Which of these did F.H. have?
3. What is the pathophysiology of *H. pylori*?
4. ***Priority Decision:*** Based on the assessment data provided, what are the priority nursing diagnoses? Are there any collaborative problems?
5. ***Patient-Centered Care:*** How will you consider F.H.'s cultural preferences in planning care?
6. ***Priority Decision:*** What are the priority nursing interventions for F.H.?
7. What lifestyle interventions would you recommend for F.H.?
8. ***Evidence-Based Decision:*** F.H. asks you if the treatment will work and this will be the end of his problems. How will you respond?
9. ***Collaboration:*** What referrals may be indicated?

Answers available at *http://evolve.elsevier.com/Lewis/medsurg.*

BRIDGE TO NCLEX EXAMINATION

The number of the question corresponds to the same-numbered outcome at the beginning of the chapter.

1. M.J. calls the clinic and tells the nurse that her 85-yr-old mother has been nauseated all day and has vomited twice. Before the nurse hangs up and calls the HCP, she should tell M.J. to
   a. administer antiemetic drugs and assess her mother's skin turgor.
   b. give her mother sips of water and elevate the head of her bed to prevent aspiration.
   c. offer her mother large quantities of Gatorade to decrease the risk for sodium depletion.
   d. give her mother a high-protein liquid supplement to drink to maintain her nutritional needs.

2. The nurse explains to the patient with Vincent's infection that treatment will include
   a. tetanus vaccinations.
   b. viscous lidocaine rinses.
   c. amphotericin B suspension.
   d. topical application of antibiotics.

3. The nurse teaching young adults about behaviors that put them at risk for oral cancer includes
   a. discouraging use of chewing gum.
   b. avoiding use of perfumed lip gloss.
   c. avoiding use of smokeless tobacco.
   d. discouraging drinking of carbonated beverages.

4. Which instructions would the nurse include in a teaching plan for a patient with mild gastroesophageal reflux disease (GERD)?
   a. "The best time to take an as-needed antacid is 1 to 3 hours after meals."
   b. "A glass of warm milk at bedtime will decrease your discomfort at night."
   c. "Do not chew gum; the excess saliva will cause you to secrete more acid."
   d. "Limit your intake of foods high in protein because they take longer to digest."

5. A patient who has undergone an esophagectomy for esophageal cancer develops increasing pain, fever, and dyspnea when a full-liquid diet is started postoperatively. The nurse recognizes that these symptoms are *most* indicative of
   a. an intolerance to the feedings.
   b. extension of the tumor into the aorta.
   c. leakage of fluids into the mediastinum.
   d. esophageal perforation with fistula formation into the lung.

6. The pernicious anemia that may accompany gastritis is due to
   a. chronic autoimmune destruction of cobalamin stores in the body.
   b. progressive gastric atrophy from chronic breakage in the mucosal barrier and blood loss.
   c. a lack of intrinsic factor normally produced by acid-secreting cells of the gastric mucosa.
   d. hyperchlorhydria from an increase in acid-secreting parietal cells and degradation of RBCs.

7. The nurse is teaching the patient and family that peptic ulcers are
   a. caused by a stressful lifestyle and other acid-producing factors, such as *H. pylori*.
   b. inherited within families and reinforced by bacterial spread of *Staphylococcus aureus* in childhood.
   c. promoted by factors that cause oversecretion of acid, such as excess dietary fats, smoking, and alcohol use.
   d. promoted by a combination of factors that cause erosion of the gastric mucosa, including certain drugs and *H. pylori*.

8. An optimal teaching plan for an outpatient with stomach cancer receiving radiation therapy should include information about
   a. cancer support groups, alopecia, and stomatitis.
   b. nutrition supplements, ostomy care, and support groups.
   c. prosthetic devices, wound and skin care, and grief counseling.
   d. wound and skin care, nutrition, drugs, and community resources.

9. The teaching plan for the patient being discharged after an acute episode of upper GI bleeding includes information about the importance of (*select all that apply*)
   a. limiting alcohol intake to 1 serving per day.
   b. only taking aspirin with milk or bread products.
   c. avoiding taking aspirin and drugs containing aspirin.
   d. only taking drugs prescribed by the health care provider.
   e. taking all drugs 1 hour before mealtime to prevent further bleeding.

10. Several patients come to the urgent care center with nausea, vomiting, and diarrhea that began 2 hours ago while attending a large family reunion potluck dinner. You ask the patients specifically about foods they ingested containing
   a. beef.
   b. meat and milk.
   c. poultry and eggs.
   d. home-preserved vegetables.

1. b, 2. d, 3. c, 4. a, 5. c, 6. c, 7. d, 8. d, 9. c, d, 10. b

For rationales to these answers and even more NCLEX review questions, visit *http://evolve.elsevier.com/Lewis/medsurg*.

ⓔ EVOLVE WEBSITE/RESOURCES LIST

http://evolve.elsevier.com/Lewis/medsurg

Review Questions (Online Only)

Key Points

Answer Keys for Questions
- Rationales for Bridge to NCLEX Examination Questions
- Answer Guidelines for Case Study on p. 921

Student Case Studies
- Patient With Oral Cancer
- Patient With Peptic Ulcer Disease

Nursing Care Plans
- eNursing Care Plan 41.1: Patient With Nausea and Vomiting
- eNursing Care Plan 41.2: Patient With Peptic Ulcer Disease

Conceptual Care Map Creator

Audio Glossary

Content Updates

REFERENCES

*1. Matthews C: A review of nausea and vomiting in the anaesthetic and post anaesthetic environment, *J Perioper Pract* 27:224, 2017.

*2. Bošnjak SM, Gralla RJ, Schwartzberg L: Prevention of chemotherapy-induced nausea, *Support Care Cancer* 25:1661, 2017.

*3. Nguyen LA, Lee L: Complementary and alternative medicine for nausea and vomiting. In: Koch KL, Hasler WL, eds: *Nausea and vomiting*, New York, 2017, Springer.

*4. Dietrich T, Webb I, Stenhouse L, et al: Evidence summary: The relationship between oral and cardiovascular disease, *British Dental Jour* 222:381, 2017.

5. National Cancer Institute: SEER stat fact sheets. Retrieved from *http://seer.cancer.gov/statfacts/html*.

*6. de Martel C, Plummer M, Vignat J, et al: Worldwide burden of cancer attributable to HPV by site, country and HPV type, *Int J Cancer* 141:664, 2017.

7. The Oral Cancer Foundation. Surgery for oral cancer. Retrieved from *https://oralcancerfoundation.org/treatment/surgery/*.

8. American Cancer Society. Treating oral cancer. Retrieved from *www.cancer.org/cancer/oral-cavity-and-oropharyngeal-cancer/treating.html*.

9. American Gastroenterological Association. GERD. Retrieved from *www.gastro.org/patient-care/conditions-diseases/gerd*.

*10. Mansour NM, El-Serag HB, Anandasabapathy S: Barrett's esophagus: Best practices for treatment and post-treatment surveillance, *Ann Cardiothoracic Surg* 6:75, 2017.

*11. Sandhu DS, Fass R: Current trends in the management of gastroesophageal reflux disease, *Gut Liver* 12:7, 2018.

*12. Nehra AK, Alexander JA, Loftus CG, et al: Proton pump inhibitors: Review of emerging concerns, *Mayo Clinic Proc* 93:240, 2018.

*13. Gyawali CP, Fass R. Management of gastroesophageal reflux disease, *Gastroenterology* 154:302, 2018.

14. American Cancer Society. Treating esophageal cancer. Retrieved from *www.cancer.org/cancer/esophagus-cancer/treating.html*.

15. Prasad MA, Friedman LS, Anania FA: Peptic ulcer disease. In: Srinivasan S, Friedman L, eds:*Sitaraman and Friedman's essentials of gastroenterology*, ed 2, Oxford, United Kingdom, 2018, John Wiley & Sons Ltd.

16. Lanas A, Chan FK: Peptic ulcer disease, *Lancet* 390:613, 2017.

17. Gigek CO, Chen ES, Smith MA: Epigenetic alterations in stomach cancer. In: Patel V, Preedy VR, eds: *Handbook of nutrition, diet, and epigenetics*, New York, 2017, Springer.

18. American Cancer Society. Treating stomach cancer. Retrieved from *www.cancer.org/cancer/stomach-cancer/treating.html*.

*19. Abougergi MS: Epidemiology of upper gastrointestinal hemorrhage in the USA: Is the bleeding slowing down? *Digestive Diseases and Science* 63:1091, 2018.

*20. Barletta JF, Mangram AJ, Sucher JF, et al: Stress ulcer prophylaxis in neurocritical care, *Neurocrit Care* 19:1, 2017.

21. Rey JW, Hoffman A, Teubner D, et al: *Therapeutic endoscopy in the gastrointestinal tract*, New York, 2018, Springer.

22. National Digestive Diseases Information Clearinghouse. Bacteria and foodborne illness. Retrieved from *www.niddk.nih.gov/health-information/health-topics/digestive-diseases/foodborne-illnesses/Pages/facts.aspx*.

*Evidence-based information for clinical practice.

42

Lower Gastrointestinal Problems

Mariann M. Harding

In this life we cannot do great things. We can only do small things with great love.

Mother Teresa

http://evolve.elsevier.com/Lewis/medsurg

CONCEPTUAL FOCUS

Acid-Base Balance	Inflammation	Stress
Elimination	Nutrition	
Fluids and Electrolytes	Pain	

LEARNING OUTCOMES

1. Explain the common etiologies and interprofessional and nursing management of diarrhea, fecal incontinence, and constipation.
2. Describe common causes of acute abdominal pain and nursing management of the patient after a laparotomy.
3. Describe the interprofessional and nursing management of acute appendicitis, peritonitis, and gastroenteritis.
4. Compare and contrast the inflammatory bowel diseases of ulcerative colitis and Crohn's disease, including pathophysiology, clinical manifestations, complications, and interprofessional and nursing management.
5. Distinguish among small and large bowel obstructions, including causes, clinical manifestations, and interprofessional and nursing management.
6. Describe the clinical manifestations and interprofessional and nursing management of colorectal cancer.
7. Select nursing interventions to manage the care of the patient after bowel resection and ostomy surgery.
8. Distinguish between diverticulosis and diverticulitis, including clinical manifestations and interprofessional and nursing management.
9. Compare and contrast the types of hernias, including etiology and surgical and nursing management.
10. Describe the types of malabsorption syndromes and interprofessional care of celiac disease, lactase deficiency, and short bowel syndrome.
11. Describe the types, clinical manifestations, and interprofessional and nursing management of anorectal conditions.

KEY TERMS

anal fistula, p. 965
appendicitis, p. 937
celiac disease, p. 960
constipation, p. 929
Crohn's disease, p. 939
diarrhea, p. 924
diverticulitis, p. 957
fecal incontinence, p. 928

fistula, p. 958
gastroenteritis, p. 939
hemorrhoids, p. 963
hernia, p. 959
inflammatory bowel disease (IBD), p. 939
intestinal obstruction, p. 945
irritable bowel syndrome (IBS), p. 936
lactase deficiency, p. 962

ostomy, p. 952
paralytic ileus, p. 945
peritonitis, p. 938
short bowel syndrome (SBS), p. 962
steatorrhea, p. 960
ulcerative colitis (UC), p. 939

The wide variety of gastrointestinal (GI) problems discussed in this chapter include diarrhea, constipation, and fecal incontinence; inflammatory and infectious bowel problems; bowel trauma; bowel obstructions; colorectal cancer; abdominal and bowel surgery (including ostomy formation); and malabsorption problems. Conceptually, patients often have problems with impaired elimination and nutrition. Many have inflammation and pain and are at risk for altered fluid and electrolyte balance. Promoting optimal bowel habits and nutrition are common goals.

DIARRHEA

Diarrhea is the passage of at least 3 loose or liquid stools per day.[1] It may be acute, lasting 14 days or less, or persistent, lasting longer than 14 days. Chronic diarrhea lasts 30 days or longer.

Etiology and Pathophysiology

The primary cause of acute diarrhea is ingesting infectious organisms (Table 42.1). Viruses cause most cases of infectious diarrhea in the United States. While some viral infections can

TABLE 42.1 Causes and Manifestations of Acute Infectious Diarrhea

Type of Organism	Manifestations	Source of Infection/Susceptibility
Bacterial		
Campylobacter jejuni	• Diarrhea, abdominal cramps, and fever. Sometimes nausea and vomiting • Lasts about 7 days	• Undercooked poultry and unpasteurized milk • Most frequent in summer months
Clostridium difficile	• Watery diarrhea, fever, anorexia, nausea, abdominal pain	• Prolonged use of antibiotics followed by exposure to feces-contaminated surfaces • Spores on hands and environmental surfaces are extremely hard to kill
Clostridium perfringens	• Diarrhea, abdominal cramps, nausea, and vomiting • Occurs 6–24 hr after eating contaminated food and lasts about 24 hr	• Associated with meats, gravies, stews, dried or precooked foods • Can cause serious illness in anyone, especially older adults
Enterohemorrhagic Escherichia coli (e.g., E. coli O157:H7)	• Severe abdominal cramping, bloody diarrhea, and vomiting • Low-grade fever • Usually lasts 5–7 days	• Can cause serious illness, especially in older adults • May progress to life-threatening renal failure • Transmitted in water or food contaminated with infected feces
Enterotoxigenic E. coli	• Watery or bloody diarrhea, abdominal cramps • Nausea, vomiting, and fever may be present • Mean duration >60 hr	• Most common cause of traveler's diarrhea • Transmitted in water or food contaminated with infected feces
Salmonella	• Diarrhea, fever, and abdominal cramps • Lasts 4–7 days	• Reservoir is poultry, reptiles, and other animals (especially turtles, lizards, snakes, chicks, and young birds) • Can be transmitted by handling animals • Found in undercooked poultry, meat, and foods prepared with raw eggs
Shigella	• Diarrhea (sometimes bloody), fever, and stomach cramps • Usually lasts 5–7 days • Postinfection arthritis may occur	• Transmitted via fecal-oral route or in food or water contaminated with infected feces • Can contaminate recreational water
Staphylococcus	• Nausea, vomiting, abdominal cramps, and diarrhea • Usually mild • May cause illness in as little as 30 min • Lasts 1–3 days	• 25%–50% of people are carriers in mucous membranes, skin, or hair • Transmitted in food contaminated by food workers who are carriers or through contaminated milk and cheese
Parasitic		
Cryptosporidium	• Watery diarrhea • Lasts about 2 wks • May have abdominal cramps, nausea, vomiting, fever, dehydration, weight loss • May be fatal in those who are immunocompromised (e.g., AIDS)	• Lives in human intestines • Transmitted in stool of infected human or animal • Outer shell allows it to live for long periods outside of body and makes it resistant to chlorine • Common cause of waterborne disease (swimming pools, lakes, drinking water, food contaminated with feces)
Entamoeba histolytica	• Diarrhea, abdominal cramping • Only 10%–20% are ill, and symptoms are usually mild	• Fecally contaminated food, water, or hands • Most common in developing countries • In the United States, high-risk groups include travelers, recent immigrants, and homosexual men
Giardia lamblia	• Abdominal cramps, nausea, diarrhea • May interfere with nutrient absorption	• Highly contagious • Transmitted via fecal-oral route • Found in fresh lakes and rivers. Can be transmitted in swimming pools, water parks, and hot tubs
Viral		
Norovirus (Norwalk-like virus)	• Nausea, vomiting, diarrhea, stomach cramping • Rapid onset. Lasts 1–2 days	• Very contagious • Virus is present in stool and emesis
Rotavirus	• Fever, vomiting, and profuse watery diarrhea • Lasts 3–8 days	• Highly contagious • Transmitted mainly by fecal-oral route

be deadly, most are mild and last less than 24 hours. So, most patients rarely seek treatment.

Bacterial infection with *Escherichia coli* O157:H7, a type of enterohemorrhagic *E. coli*, is a common cause of bloody diarrhea in the United States. It is transmitted by undercooked beef or chicken contaminated with the bacteria or in fruits and vegetables exposed to contaminated manure. Other pathologic *E. coli* strains are endemic in developing countries and often cause traveler's diarrhea. *Giardia lamblia* is the most common intestinal parasite that causes diarrhea in the United States.

Infectious organisms attack the intestines in different ways. Some organisms (e.g., Rotavirus A, Norovirus, *G. lamblia*) change the secretion and/or absorption of enterocytes in the small intestine and do not cause inflammation. Other organisms (e.g., *Clostridium difficile*) impair absorption by destroying cells, causing inflammation in the colon, and producing toxins that cause damage.

Secretory diarrhea is a common result of bacterial or viral infections. It occurs when ingested pathogens survive in the GI tract long enough to absorb into the enterocytes. The resulting chain reaction changes cell permeability and causes the oversecretion of water and sodium and chloride ions into the bowel.

Organisms enter the body in contaminated food (e.g., *Salmonella* in undercooked eggs and chicken) or contaminated drinking water (*G. lamblia* in contaminated lakes or pools). Travelers often get diarrhea, especially if they travel to countries with poorer sanitation than their own. Infection can spread from person to person via the fecal-oral route. For example, adult day care workers can transmit infection from one resident to another if they do not wash their hands after changing soiled diapers or linens.

A person's age, gastric acidity, intestinal microflora, and immune status influence susceptibility to pathogenic organisms. Older adults are most likely to have life-threatening diarrhea. Since stomach acid kills ingested pathogens, taking drugs to decrease stomach acid (e.g., proton pump inhibitors [PPIs]) increases the chance that pathogens will survive.[2]

The healthy human colon contains short-chain fatty acids and bacteria, such as *E. coli*. These organisms aid in fermentation and provide a microbial barrier against pathogenic bacteria. Antibiotics kill the normal flora, making the person more susceptible to pathogenic organisms. For example, patients receiving broad-spectrum antibiotics (e.g., carbapenems, cephalosporins, piperacillin/tazobactam) are susceptible to pathogenic strains of *C. difficile*.[2] *C. difficile* infection (CDI) causes the most serious antibiotic-associated diarrhea and is a common cause of hospital-acquired GI illness in the United States.

People who are immunocompromised because of disease (e.g., human immunodeficiency virus [HIV]) or immunosuppressive drugs are susceptible to GI tract infection. Immunocompromised patients receiving jejunal enteral nutrition (EN) are especially prone to CDI and other foodborne infections. Jejunostomy and nasointestinal feedings, which bypass the stomach's acid environment, do not contain the poorly digestible fiber that normal colonic bacteria need for survival.

Diarrhea is not always due to infection. Drugs and specific food intolerances can cause diarrhea. Large amounts of undigested carbohydrate in the bowel, lactose intolerance, and certain laxatives (e.g., lactulose, sodium phosphate, magnesium citrate) produce osmotic diarrhea. *Osmotic diarrhea* results from rapid GI transit that prevents fluid and electrolyte absorption. Bile salts and undigested fats lead to excess fluid secretion into the GI tract. Diarrhea from celiac disease and short bowel syndrome result from malabsorption in the small intestine.

Clinical Manifestations

Infections that attack the upper GI tract (e.g., Norovirus, *G. lamblia*) usually produce large-volume, watery stools, cramping, and periumbilical pain (Table 42.1). Patients have either a low-grade or no fever and often have nausea and vomiting before the diarrhea begins. Infections of the colon and distal small bowel (e.g., *Shigella, Salmonella, C. difficile*) cause fever and frequent bloody diarrhea with a small volume.

Leukocytes, blood, and mucus may be present in the stool, depending on the causative agent. Severe diarrhea may cause life-threatening dehydration, electrolyte problems (e.g., hypokalemia), and acid-base imbalances (metabolic acidosis). CDI can progress to severe colitis and intestinal perforation.

Diagnostic Studies

Stool cultures are usually done only in patients who are very ill; have a fever, bloody diarrhea, or diarrhea lasting longer than 3 days; or were exposed during an outbreak.[1] Those with travelers' diarrhea lasting 14 days or longer should be evaluated

TABLE 42.2 Drug Therapy

Antidiarrheal Drugs

Drug	Mechanism of Action
bismuth subsalicylate (Pepto-Bismol)	Decreases secretions and has weak antibacterial activity. Used to prevent traveler's diarrhea
calcium polycarbophil (FiberCon)	Bulk-forming agent that absorbs excess fluid from diarrhea to form a gel. Used when intestinal mucosa cannot absorb fluid
diphenoxylate with atropine (Lomotil)	Opioid and anticholinergic. Decreases peristalsis and intestinal motility
loperamide (Imodium, Pepto Diarrhea Control)	Inhibits peristalsis, delays transit, increases absorption of fluid from stools
octreotide acetate (Sandostatin)	Suppresses serotonin secretion, stimulates fluid absorption from GI tract, decreases intestinal motility
paregoric (camphorated tincture of opium)	Opioid. Decreases peristalsis and intestinal motility

for parasitic infections. Stools are examined for blood, mucus, white blood cells (WBCs), and parasites. Cultures reliably identify infectious organisms. Multiple-pathogen stool tests can detect common viral, parasitic, and bacterial organisms from a single stool sample.

Blood cultures should be done in those with signs of sepsis or systemic infection (e.g., high fever) or who are immunocompromised.[1] The WBC count may be high. People with long-standing diarrhea can develop anemia from iron and folate deficiencies. Increased hematocrit, blood urea nitrogen (BUN), and creatinine levels are signs of fluid deficit.

In patients with chronic diarrhea, measuring stool electrolytes, pH, and osmolality helps determine whether the diarrhea is from decreased fluid absorption or increased fluid secretion. Measuring stool fat and undigested muscle fibers may show fat and protein malabsorption conditions. Some patients with secretory diarrhea have high serum levels of GI hormones, such as vasoactive intestinal polypeptide and gastrin.

Interprofessional Care

Treatment of diarrhea depends on the cause. Acute infectious diarrhea is usually self-limiting. The major concerns are preventing transmission, replacing fluid and electrolytes, and protecting the skin. Most patients tolerate oral fluids. Solutions containing glucose and electrolytes (e.g., Pedialyte) may be enough to replace losses from mild diarrhea. If losses are severe, it will be necessary to give parenteral fluids, electrolytes, vitamins, and nutrition. Teach the patient to avoid foods and drugs that cause diarrhea.

Antidiarrheal agents have limited short-term use. They coat and protect mucous membranes, absorb irritating substances, inhibit intestinal transit, decrease intestinal secretions, or decrease central nervous system stimulation of the GI tract (Table 42.2). Antidiarrheal agents are contraindicated in treating some infectious diarrheas because they potentially prolong exposure to the organism.[1] They are used cautiously in inflammatory bowel disease (IBD) because of the danger of causing *toxic megacolon* (colonic dilation greater than 5 cm).

Antibiotics rarely have a role in treating acute diarrhea. They are given only for certain infections or when the infected person is severely ill or immunosuppressed. The 2 antibiotics recommended for empiric therapy in adults are a fluoroquinolone, such as ciprofloxacin, and azithromycin.[1]

***Clostridium difficile* infection.** CDI is a particularly hazardous health care–associated infection (HAI). The risk for contracting CDI is highest in patients receiving antimicrobial, chemotherapy, gastric acid–suppressing, or immunosuppressive agents. *C. difficile* spores can survive for up to 70 days on objects, including commodes, telephones, bedside tables, and floors. Health care workers who do not adhere to strict infection control precautions can transmit *C. difficile* from patient to patient. Meticulous hand washing with soap and water is extremely important in limiting the spread of *C. difficile. Lactobacillus* probiotics may be used to prevent CDI or as an adjunct therapy to help prevent the risk for recurrent CDI.[3]

CDI is treated with either oral vancomycin (125 mg 4 times a day) or fidaxomicin (200 mg twice daily) for 10 days. All nonessential antibiotics, stool softeners, laxatives, and antidiarrheal agents should be stopped. Metronidazole is an option when patients are unable to be treated with vancomycin or fidaxomicin. Patients with severe, complicated CDI with shock, hypotension, ileus, or megacolon should receive vancomycin 500 mg 4 times daily orally with IV metronidazole. Patients with ileus can receive vancomycin via enema.

Recurrent CDI occurs in about 20% of patients. The risk increases with the use of additional antibiotics and CDI recurrences. *Fecal microbiota transplantation* (FMT) is emerging as the most effective treatment for recurrent CDI.[3] FMT reestablishes healthy intestinal flora by infusing fecal bacteria obtained from healthy donor stool into the patient's colon. To perform an FMT, feces obtained from the donor is pureed into a liquid, slurry consistency using saline, water, or pasteurized cow's milk. The donor stool is then placed in the GI tract via an enema, nasoenteral tube, or during colonoscopy. The major concern with FMT is the potential for transmitting infectious agents in the donor stool. Using feces from donors who have intimate physical contact with the recipient and careful screening minimize this risk. Most patients have diarrhea immediately after the procedure.

❖ NURSING MANAGEMENT: ACUTE INFECTIOUS DIARRHEA

◆ Nursing Assessment

Begin the nursing assessment with a thorough history and physical examination (Table 42.3). Ask the patient to describe their stool pattern and associated symptoms. Focus on the duration, frequency, character, and consistency of stool and the relationship to other symptoms, such as pain and vomiting. Ask about medical conditions that may cause diarrhea and whether the person is taking drugs, such as antibiotics and laxatives, which are known to cause diarrhea, decrease stomach acidity, or cause immunosuppression. Determine whether the patient has traveled to a foreign country or been at a day care facility recently and if other family members are ill. Ask about food preparation practices, food intolerances (e.g., milk), and changes in diet and appetite.

Assess for fever and signs of dehydration (dry skin, low-grade fever, orthostatic changes in pulse and BP, decreased and concentrated urine). Assess the abdomen for distention, pain, and guarding. Inspect the perineal skin for signs of redness and breakdown from the diarrhea.

TABLE 42.3 Nursing Assessment
Diarrhea

Subjective Data
Important Health Information
Past health history: Recent travel, hospitalization, infections, stress. Diverticulitis or malabsorption, metabolic disorders, IBD, IBS
Medications: Laxatives or enemas, magnesium-containing antacids, sorbitol-containing suspensions or elixirs, antibiotics, methyldopa, digitalis, colchicine; OTC antidiarrheal drugs
Surgery or other treatments: Stomach or bowel surgery, radiation

Functional Health Patterns
Health perception–health management: Chronic laxative use, malaise
Nutritional-metabolic: Ingestion of fatty and spicy foods, food intolerances. Anorexia, nausea, vomiting, weight loss. Thirst
Elimination: Increased stool frequency, volume, and looseness. Change in color and character of stools. Steatorrhea, abdominal bloating. Decreased urine output
Cognitive-perceptual: Abdominal tenderness, abdominal pain and cramping, tenesmus

Objective Data
General
Lethargy, sunken eyeballs, fever, malnutrition

Integumentary
Pallor, dry mucous membranes, poor skin turgor, perianal irritation

Gastrointestinal
Frequent soft to liquid stools that may alternate with constipation, altered stool color. Abdominal distention, hyperactive bowel sounds. Pus, blood, mucus, or fat in stools. Fecal impaction

Urinary
Decreased output, concentrated urine

Possible Diagnostic Findings
Abnormal serum electrolyte levels. Anemia, leukocytosis, eosinophilia, hypoalbuminemia. Positive stool cultures. Ova, parasites, leukocytes, blood, or fat in stool. Abnormal sigmoidoscopy or colonoscopy findings. Abnormal lower GI series

---

◆ Nursing Diagnoses

Nursing diagnoses for the patient with acute infectious diarrhea include:

- Diarrhea
- Fluid imbalance
- Electrolyte imbalance

For more information on nursing diagnoses and interventions for diarrhea, see eNursing Care Plan 42.1 on the website for this chapter.

◆ Planning

The overall goals are that the patient with diarrhea will have (1) cessation of diarrhea and resumption of normal bowel patterns; (2) normal fluid, electrolyte, and acid-base balance; (3) normal nutritional status; and (4) no perianal/perineal skin breakdown.

◆ Nursing Implementation

Consider all cases of acute diarrhea as infectious until the cause is known. Strict infection control precautions are needed to prevent the illness from spreading to others. Wash your hands with soap and water before and after contact with each patient and when handling body fluids of any kind. Flush vomitus and stool in the toilet. Teach the patient principles of hygiene, infection control, and the potential dangers of an illness that is infectious to themselves and others. Discuss proper food handling, cooking, and storage with the patient and caregiver (see Tables 41.24 and 41.25).

Viruses and *C. difficile* spores are extremely hard to kill. Alcohol-based hand cleaners and ammonia-based disinfectants are ineffective. Vigorous cleaning with soap and water does not kill everything. Immediately put patients with CDI in isolation. Ensure that visitors and all providers wear gloves and gowns. Give infected patients their own disposable stethoscopes and thermometers. Consider all objects in the room contaminated. Ensure surfaces and equipment are disinfected with a 10% bleach solution or a disinfectant labeled as *C. difficile* sporicidal.

FECAL INCONTINENCE

Etiology and Pathophysiology

Fecal incontinence is the involuntary passage of stool. It occurs when the normal structures that maintain continence are damaged or disrupted. Defecation is a voluntary action when the neuromuscular system is intact (see Chapter 38). Problems with motor function (contraction of sphincters and rectal floor muscles) and/or sensory function (ability to perceive the presence of stool or have the urge to defecate) can result in fecal incontinence. Contributing factors include altered bowel habits, weakness or disruption of the internal or external anal sphincter, damage to the pudendal nerve or other nerves that innervate the anorectum, and damage to the anal tissue (Table 42.4).

For women, obstetric trauma is the most common cause of sphincter disruption. Childbirth, aging, and menopause contribute to the development of fecal incontinence. Anorectal surgery can damage the sphincters and pudendal nerves. Radiation for prostate cancer decreases rectal compliance. Neurologic conditions, including stroke and multiple sclerosis, interfere with defecation.

People with normal functioning defecation can have incontinence if immobility prevents prompt access to a toilet or stool is accidentally discharged with diarrhea. Chronic constipation can lead to *fecal impaction*, a collection of hardened feces in the rectum or sigmoid colon that a person cannot expel. Incontinence occurs as liquid stool seeps around the hardened feces. Fecal impaction is a common problem in older adults with limited mobility. Constipated persons tend to strain during defecation. Straining contributes to incontinence because it weakens the pelvic floor muscles.

Diagnostic Studies and Interprofessional Care

The diagnosis and effective management of fecal incontinence require a thorough health history and physical examination. Ask the patient about the number of incontinent episodes per week, stool consistency and volume, and the degree that incontinence interferes with work and social activities. A rectal examination can reveal reduced anal canal muscle tone and contraction strength of the external sphincter, as well as detect internal prolapse, rectocele, hemorrhoids, masses, and fecal impaction. Other tests, such as anorectal manometry, anorectal ultrasonography, and anal electromyography, are done when symptoms persist after treating underlying problems or certain problems need further evaluation.[4]

TABLE 42.4 Common Causes of Fecal Incontinence

Anal Sphincter Weakness
- Anorectal infection
- Injury
  - Anorectal surgery for hemorrhoids, fistula, and fissures
  - Childbirth injury
  - Perineal trauma or pelvic fracture
- Internal sphincter thinning

Functional
- Physical or mobility impairments affecting toileting ability (e.g., frail older person who cannot get to the bathroom in time)

Inflammatory
- Inflammatory bowel disease
- Radiation

Neurologic Disease
- Brain tumor
- Congenital abnormalities (e.g., spina bifida, myelomeningocele)
- Dementia
- Diabetes
- Multiple sclerosis
- Neuropathy
- Spinal cord lesions
- Stroke

Pelvic Floor Dysfunction
- Fistula
- Rectal prolapse

Other
- Chronic constipation
- Denervation of pelvic muscles from chronic straining
- Diarrhea
- Fecal impaction

Treatment of incontinence depends on the cause. Maintaining normal stool consistency and a bowel management program are important. This includes regular defecation, a high-fiber diet, and increased intake of caffeine-free fluids. Dietary fiber supplements or bulk-forming laxatives, like psyllium (e.g., Metamucil), increase stool bulk, firm consistency, and promote the sensation of rectal filling. Patients may need to reduce the intake of foods that cause diarrhea and rectal irritation. Common triggers include caffeine, products containing artificial sweeteners, dairy products, high gas–producing vegetables (e.g., broccoli, cabbage, cauliflower), and vegetables containing insoluble fiber (e.g., lettuce, tomatoes, corn).

Fecal incontinence from fecal impaction usually resolves after manual removal of the hard feces and cleansing enemas. Antidiarrheal agents (e.g., loperamide) are useful in slowing intestinal transit.

Physical therapy and biofeedback training can improve awareness of rectal sensation, coordinate internal and external anal sphincters, and increase the strength of external sphincter contraction. Biofeedback training requires intact sensory and motor nerves and motivation to learn. It is a safe, painless, and effective treatment.[4]

Mild electrical stimulation of the sacral nerves targets communication problems between the brain and nerves that control the pelvic floor muscles and sphincters. Electrical stimulation can improve quality of life. Some patients may achieve complete continence.[4]

For patients who do not respond to conservative measures, treatment with dextranomer/hyaluronic acid gel (Solesta) may be used. In this treatment, the gel is injected into the deep submucosa of the patient's anal canal. It works by building up tissue in the anal area, narrowing the anal canal and allowing muscles to more adequately close. No anesthesia is given. Postinjection pain and bleeding may occur.

Surgery (e.g., sphincter repair procedures) is an option when other conservative treatments fail, the patient has a full-thickness prolapse, or the anal sphincter needs repair. A colostomy is sometimes needed.

❖ NURSING MANAGEMENT: FECAL INCONTINENCE

◆ Nursing Assessment

Fecal incontinence is embarrassing, uncomfortable, and irritating to the skin. Its unpredictable nature makes it hard to maintain school and work activities and hampers social or intimate contact. Be sensitive to the patient's feelings when discussing incontinence.

Ask about bowel patterns before the incontinence developed; current bowel habits; stool consistency, volume, and frequency; and symptoms, including pain during defecation and a feeling of incomplete evacuation *(tenesmus).* The Bristol Stool Scale is helpful to assess stool consistency. Assess whether the patient has a sensation of urgency to evacuate the bowel or sensation of passing flatus and leaking stool. Ask about daily activities (mealtimes and work), diet, and family and social activities and the degree that incontinence interferes with these activities.

Check the perineal area for irritation or breakdown. Patients who have fecal incontinence are at risk for *incontinence-associated dermatitis* (IAD).[4] IAD results from chemical irritants in the feces causing skin damage. Symptoms include redness, skin loss, and rash. The location of IAD is usually the perianal or perineal area, buttocks, or upper thighs. Fungal infection is common and seen as a dark red center surrounded by satellite lesions. Your assessment is important in distinguishing IAD from pressure injury development.

◆ Nursing Implementation

Regardless of the cause of fecal incontinence, bowel training is effective for many patients. Bowel elimination occurs at regular intervals in most people. Knowing the patient's usual bowel pattern can help you plan a bowel program that will achieve optimal stool consistency and establish predictable bowel elimination patterns. For the hospitalized patient, placement on a bedpan, help to a bedside commode, or walks to the bathroom at a regular time daily help to establish regular defecation. The best time to schedule elimination is within 30 minutes after breakfast.

If these techniques are not effective in reestablishing bowel regularity, administer bisacodyl, a glycerin suppository, or a small phosphate enema 15 to 30 minutes before the usual evacuation time. These preparations stimulate the anorectal reflex. Since stimulation will not occur unless the suppository or enema touches the rectal wall, first check for stool in the rectum and digitally remove it before inserting the laxative. Once a regular pattern is established, stop these drugs. Digital stimulation is another method for stimulating the anorectal reflex. It is often included in bowel programs for people with neurogenic bowels (e.g., from spinal cord injury). Irrigating the rectum and colon (usually with tap water) at regular intervals is another way to achieve continence in patients with neurogenic bowel.

Maintaining perineal skin integrity is a priority, especially in the bedridden patient. Feces can contaminate wounds, damage skin, cause bladder infections, and spread infections such as *C. difficile.* Fecal containment is essential. One way to contain stool is a stool management system (e.g., Flexi-Seal, DigniCare, Actiflo). These systems funnel liquid stool from the rectum into a containment system. Common features include a retention cuff that sits above the anal sphincter and soft tubing that extends from this cuff to a secure hub that allows a person to change the containment canister when it is full. A system can remain in place for weeks. Their use may decrease the risk for CDI, skin damage from exposure to stool, IAD, and pressure injuries. Do not use a rectal tube or urinary catheter as a stool catheter. They can reduce the responsiveness of the rectal sphincter and irritate or ulcerate the rectal mucosa.

Perform frequent skin assessments when using absorbent products. Incontinence pads are an option when the patient is in bed. Briefs should be used only during ambulation or when sitting in a chair. Make sure they are changed promptly after each episode of incontinence.

Use absorbent products in combination with a defined skin care program. This includes prompt cleansing, moisturizing, and skin protection. Cleanse the skin gently, using a skin cleanser rather than soap and water. Options include a cotton cloth moistened with a hydrating skin cleansing foam, incontinence clean-up cloths, or baby wipes. Avoid products that contain alcohol as they can cause drying of the skin and discomfort if skin is irritated. Pat the skin dry or use a blow dryer on a cool setting. Do not rub the skin dry. Apply a moisture barrier and, if needed, a skin barrier cream for more protection. For patients unable to care for themselves at home, you should teach caregivers how to maintain skin integrity.

Fecal incontinence is an overwhelming burden for most patients. Be sensitive to their fears. Teach them ways to reduce incontinence episodes and better cope with them when they do occur. Help patients identify food triggers that may worsen symptoms. Encourage them to avoid those foods and exercise after meals. Tell them to try to use bathrooms when they are available. Patients may be more confident when they use discreet, disposable briefs or pads. Have them wear dark-colored clothing that they can quickly remove for toileting. Ready access to a spare set of clothing and cleansing cloths is important.

CONSTIPATION

Constipation is characterized by difficult or infrequent bowel movements, often accompanied by excessive exertion during defecation or a feeling of incomplete evacuation.[5] Constipation is a symptom, not a disease. It can be acute, usually lasting less than 1 week, or chronic, lasting over 3 months.

Etiology and Pathophysiology

Risk factors associated with chronic constipation include a low-fiber diet, decreased physical activity, or ignoring the defecation urge. Ignoring the urge to defecate for a prolonged period can cause the muscles and mucosa of the rectum to become insensitive to the presence of feces. In addition, the prolonged retention of feces results in drying of stool due to water absorption. The harder and drier the feces, the harder it is to expel. Emotions, including anxiety, depression, and stress, affect the GI tract and can contribute to constipation.

Constipation occurs with diseases that slow GI transit and hamper neurologic function, such as diabetes, Parkinson's disease, and multiple sclerosis (Table 42.5). Many drugs, especially opioids, cause constipation (Table 42.6).[5]

Some people think they are constipated if they do not have a daily bowel movement. This can result in chronic laxative use and *cathartic colon syndrome,* a condition in which the colon becomes dilated and atonic (lacking muscle tone). Ultimately, the person cannot defecate without a laxative.

Clinical Manifestations

The clinical presentation varies from a mild discomfort to a more severe event mimicking an "acute abdomen." Stools are absent or hard, dry, and difficult to pass. Abdominal distention, bloating, increased flatulence, and increased rectal pressure may be present.

TABLE 42.5 Diseases Associated With Constipation

Colonic Disorders
- Cancer
- Diverticular disease
- Inflammatory bowel disease
- Intestinal stenosis
- Intussusception
- Luminal or extraluminal obstructing lesions
- Rectocele
- Prolapse

Systemic Disorders
Collagen Vascular Disease
- Amyloidosis
- Systemic lupus erythematosus
- Systemic sclerosis (scleroderma)

Metabolic/Endocrine
- Chronic renal failure
- Diabetes
- Hypercalcemia/hyperparathyroidism
- Hypokalemia
- Hypothyroidism
- Pheochromocytoma
- Pregnancy

Neurologic Disorders
- Autonomic neuropathy (from diabetes)
- Hirschsprung's megacolon
- Multiple sclerosis
- Neurofibromatosis
- Parkinson's disease
- Spinal cord lesions or injury
- Stroke

TABLE 42.6 Drugs Associated With Constipation

Cardiovascular	• Antihypertensives • Furosemide • Hypolipidemics (cholestyramine, colestipol, statins)
GI	• Antacids containing aluminum, calcium • Antidiarrheals • Proton-pump inhibitors • Supplements (e.g., bismuth, calcium, iron)
Central nervous system	• Antidepressants (tricyclics, selective serotonin reuptake inhibitors) • Antiepileptics (carbamazepine, phenytoin, clonazepam) • Antipsychotics (butyrophenones, phenothiazines, barbiturates) • Benzodiazepines
Other	• Analgesics (opiates and derivatives) • Antitussives (codeine, dextromethorphan)

Hemorrhoids are a common complication of chronic constipation. They result from venous engorgement caused by repeated *Valsalva maneuvers* (straining) and venous compression from hard, impacted stool. The Valsalva maneuver may have serious outcomes for patients with heart failure, cerebral edema, hypertension, and coronary artery disease. During straining, the patient inspires deeply and holds the breath while contracting abdominal muscles and bearing down. This increases both intraabdominal and intrathoracic pressures and reduces venous return to the heart. The heart rate temporarily decreases along with a decrease in cardiac output. This results in a transient drop in arterial pressure. When the patient relaxes, thoracic pressure falls, resulting in a sudden flow of blood into the heart, increased heart rate, and an immediate rise in arterial pressure. These changes may be fatal for the patient who cannot compensate for the sudden increased blood flow returning to the heart.

Rectal mucosal ulcers and fissures may occur from stool stasis or straining. Diverticulosis is another potential complication of chronic constipation. It is more common in older patients.

In the presence of *obstipation* (absolute constipation with no passage of gas or stool) or fecal impaction secondary to constipation, colonic perforation may occur. Perforation, which is life threatening, causes abdominal pain, nausea, vomiting, fever, and a high WBC count.

Diagnostic Studies and Interprofessional Care

In most patients, the diagnosis of constipation is based on findings from a thorough history and physical examination. The physical should include an abdominal examination, inspection of the perianal and rectal region, and a digital rectal examination. Concerning signs include a sudden, persistent change in bowel habits (>6 weeks) in those over 50 years, rectal bleeding or bloody stools, iron deficiency anemia, weight loss, significant abdominal pain, family or personal history of colorectal cancer (CRC) or inflammatory bowel disease and palpable mass.[5] If any of these are present, tests are needed to rule out serious disease, such as CRC. These may include abdominal x-rays, barium enema, and colonoscopy or sigmoidoscopy.

Increasing dietary fiber, fluid intake, and exercise can prevent many cases of constipation.[6] Laxatives (Table 42.7) and enemas are an option in treating constipation. All promote bowel movements, but each class works differently. Which one a patient receives depends on the severity and duration of the constipation and the patient's health. Daily bulk-forming laxatives (psyllium) can prevent constipation because they work like dietary fiber and do not cause dependence. In patients with chronic constipation who do not respond to diet and lifestyle modifications, osmotic laxatives are the next recommended treatment. Stimulant laxatives are given to patients who do not respond to osmotic laxatives. Enemas are fast acting and can give immediate treatment of constipation but must be used cautiously. Agents containing sodium phosphate and magnesium can cause electrolyte imbalances in older adults and patients with heart and kidney problems.

Other therapies target specific patient needs. Peripherally acting opioid receptor antagonists (e.g., methylnaltrexone, naldemedine, naloxegol) decrease constipation caused by opioid use. They do not block the analgesic effects of opioids. Biofeedback therapy may help patients who have constipation because of *anismus* (uncoordinated contraction of the anal sphincter during straining).

A patient with severe constipation related to bowel motility or mechanical disorders may need more intense treatment. Diagnostic studies include anorectal manometry, GI tract transit studies, balloon expulsion test, and defecography. A patient with unrelenting constipation may need a colostomy, ileostomy, or continent fecal diversion. These procedures are discussed later in this chapter.[6]

Nutritional Therapy. Diet is a key factor in preventing and treating constipation. Many patients have improved symptoms when they increase their dietary fiber intake. Dietary fiber is found in fruits, vegetables, and grains (Table 42.8). Wheat bran and prunes are especially effective for preventing and treating constipation. Whole wheat and bran are high in insoluble fiber.

Dietary fiber adds to the stool bulk directly by attracting water. Adequate fluid intake (2 L/day) is essential. Large, bulky stools move through the colon much more quickly than small stools. However, the recommended fluid intake may be contraindicated in a patient with heart disease or renal failure. Tell the patient that increasing fiber intake may initially increase gas production because of fermentation in the colon, but this effect decreases over several days.

TABLE 42.7 Drug Therapy

Constipation

Mechanism of Action	Indications	Example	Comments
Bulk Forming			
Absorbs water. Increases bulk, thereby stimulating peristalsis *Action:* Usually within 24 hr	Acute and chronic constipation, irritable bowel syndrome, diverticulosis	methylcellulose (Citrucel) psyllium (Metamucil, Konsyl, Hydrocil, Fiberall)	Contraindicated in patients with abdominal pain, nausea, and vomiting and those suspected of having appendicitis, biliary tract obstruction, or acute hepatitis. Must be taken with fluids (≥8oz). Best choice for initial treatment of constipation
Emollients			
Lubricate intestinal tract and soften feces, making hard stools easier to pass. Do not affect peristalsis *Action:* Softeners in 72 hr, lubricants in 8 hr	Acute and chronic constipation, fecal impaction, anorectal conditions	*Softeners:* docusate (Colace, Surfak) *Lubricants:* mineral oil (Fleet Mineral Oil Enema)	Can block absorption of fat-soluble vitamins, such as vitamin K, which may increase risk for bleeding in patients on anticoagulants
Prosecretory Agents			
Increases intestinal fluid secretion through direct action on epithelial cells, speeding colonic transit *Action:* Usually within 24 hr	Chronic idiopathic constipation, irritable bowel syndrome with constipation (women only)	linaclotide (Linzess) lubiprostone (Amitiza) plecanatide (Trulance)	Contraindicated in patients with history of mechanical GI obstruction. Can cause nausea and watery diarrhea
Saline and Osmotic Solutions			
Cause retention of fluid in intestinal lumen, reducing stool consistency and increasing volume *Action:* Within 15 min–3 hr	Chronic constipation, bowel preparation for diagnostic tests and surgery	lactulose magnesium salts (magnesium citrate, Milk of Magnesia) sodium phosphates (Fleet Enema, Phospho-soda) polyethylene glycol (MiraLAX, GoLYTELY)	May cause abdominal distention and diarrhea. Overuse of magnesium or sodium phosphates in older adults or those with renal failure can lead to fluid and electrolyte imbalances; least effective agents in this class
Stimulants			
Increases peristalsis and speeds colonic transit by irritating colon wall and stimulating enteric nerves *Action:* Usually within 12 hr	Acute constipation, bowel preparation for diagnostic tests and surgery	anthraquinones (cascara sagrada, senna) phenolphthalein: sennosides (Ex-Lax), bisacodyl (Correctol, Dulcolax)	Cause melanosis coli (brown or black pigmentation of colon). Most widely abused laxatives. Should not be used in patients with impaction or obstipation

EVIDENCE-BASED PRACTICE

Probiotics and Constipation

L.R. is an 82-yr-old woman with decreased mobility due to a recent hip fracture. During a check-up visit at the orthopedic clinic, L.R. states she is having discomfort due to constipation. She tells you she is following her discharge instructions, "drinking lots of water," and trying to increase fiber in her diet.

Making Clinical Decisions

Best Available Evidence. Quality of life decreases with increased severity in constipation symptoms. Many patients with constipation have modifiable risk factors related to their lifestyle. These include low-fiber diet, poor hydration, and/or sedentary lifestyle. In adults with constipation, there is an association between the use of probiotics, especially products containing *Bifidobacterium longum* and *Bifidobacterium lactis,* and significant improvements in gut transit time, stool frequency, and stool consistency.

Clinician Expertise. You know that diet, fluid intake, and activity can play a key role in treating and preventing constipation. You recently read about the potential benefit of probiotics in relieving constipation.

Patient Preferences and Values. L.R. asks if you know of anything else she can do as she does not want to take any more drugs.

Implications for Nursing Practice

1. What information would you share with L.R. about probiotics and constipation?
2. What data would you want from L.R. about her diet, activity, medications, and fluid intake?
3. Why is it important for you to know about alternative therapies? What is your role in supporting patients who want alternatives to drug therapy?

References for Evidence

Martinez-Martinez MI, Calabuig-Tulsa R, Cauli O: The effects of probiotics as a treatment for constipation in elderly people: A systematic review, *Arch Gerontol Geriatr* 71:142, 2017.

Serra J, Mascort-Roca J, Marzo-Castillejo M, et al.: Clinical practice guidelines for the management of constipation in adults: Part 2: Diagnosis and treatment, *Gastroenterol Hepatol* 40:303, 2017.

TABLE 42.8 Nutritional Therapy
High-Fiber Foods

	Fiber/Serving (g)	Serving Size	Calories/Serving
Vegetables			
Asparagus	3.5	½ cup	18
Beans			
• Navy	8.4	½ cup	80
• Kidney	9.7	½ cup	94
• Lima	8.3	½ cup	63
• Pinto	8.9	½ cup	78
• String	2.1	½ cup	18
Broccoli	3.5	½ cup	18
Carrots, raw	1.8	½ cup	15
Corn	2.6	½ medium ear	72
Peas, canned	6.7	½ cup	63
Potatoes			
• Baked	1.9	½ medium	72
• Sweet	2.1	½ medium	79
Squash, acorn	7.0	1 cup	82
Tomato, raw	1.5	1 small	18
Fruits			
Apple	2.0	½ large	42
Blackberries	6.7	¾ cup	40
Orange	1.6	1 small	35
Peach	2.3	1 medium	38
Pear	2.0	½ medium	44
Raspberries	9.2	1 cup	42
Strawberries	3.1	1 cup	45
Grain Products			
Bread, whole wheat	1.3	1 slice	59
Cereal			
• All Bran (100%)	8.4	⅓ cup	70
• Corn Flakes	2.6	¾ cup	70
• Shredded Wheat	2.8	1 biscuit	70
Popcorn	3.0	3 cups	62

TABLE 42.9 Nursing Assessment
Constipation

Subjective Data
Important Health Information
Past health history: Colorectal disease, neurologic dysfunction, bowel obstruction, environmental changes, cancer, IBD, diabetes
Medications: Aluminum and calcium antacids, antidepressants, hypolipidemics, antipsychotics, diuretics, opioids, iron, PPIs, antidiarrheals

Functional Health Patterns
Health perception–health management: Chronic laxative or enema use. Rigid beliefs about bowel function. Malaise
Nutritional-metabolic: Changes in diet or mealtime. Fiber and fluid intake. Anorexia, nausea
Elimination: Change in usual bowel patterns. Hard, difficult-to-pass stool, decrease in stool frequency and amount. Flatus, abdominal distention. Straining, tenesmus, rectal pressure. Fecal incontinence (if impacted)
Activity-exercise: Daily activity routine. Immobility, sedentary lifestyle
Cognitive-perceptual: Dizziness, headache, anorectal pain. Abdominal pain on defecation
Coping–stress tolerance: Acute or chronic stress

Objective Data
General
Lethargy

Integumentary
Anorectal fissures, hemorrhoids, abscesses

Gastrointestinal
Abdominal distention. Hypoactive or absent bowel sounds. Palpable abdominal mass. Fecal impaction. Small, hard, dry stool. Stool with blood

Possible Diagnostic Findings
Guaiac-positive stools. Abdominal x-ray showing stool in lower colon

❖ NURSING MANAGEMENT: CONSTIPATION

◆ Nursing Assessment

Determine the patient's usual defecation patterns and habits. Ask the patient about the onset and duration of symptoms; the shape and consistency of the stool; and any difficulty with evacuation. Is the patient straining during defecation? Is there a feeling of incomplete evacuation or the need to use fingering to expel the feces? Ask about diet, exercise, laxative use, and history that could contribute to problems with defecation. Table 42.9 outlines the subjective and objective data you should obtain from a patient with constipation.

◆ Nursing Implementation

Tailor the nursing management of constipation to your assessment of the patient's symptoms. Teach the patient about the role of diet, adequate fluid intake, and regular exercise in preventing and treating constipation (Table 42.10). Emphasize the importance of a high-fiber diet. Teach the patient to establish a regular time to defecate and not to suppress the urge to defecate. Discourage the use of laxatives and enemas.

Defecation is easiest when the person is sitting on a commode with the knees higher than the hips. The sitting position allows gravity to aid defecation, and flexing the hips straightens the angle between the anal canal and rectum so that stool flows out more easily. Place a footstool in front of the toilet to promote flexion of the hips. It is challenging to defecate while sitting on a bedpan. For a patient in bed, raise the head of the bed as high as the patient can tolerate.

The sights, odors, and sounds of defecation embarrass most people. Provide as much privacy as possible and use an odor eliminator. Encourage patients to maintain abdominal muscle tone. Prompt patients to contract abdominal muscles several times a day. Sit-ups and straight-leg raises can help improve abdominal muscle tone.

For the patient whose perceived constipation is related to rigid beliefs about bowel function, start a discussion about these concerns. Give appropriate information on normal bowel function and discuss the adverse consequences of overuse of laxatives and enemas.

ACUTE ABDOMINAL PAIN AND LAPAROTOMY

Etiology and Pathophysiology

Acute abdominal pain is pain of recent onset. It may signal a life-threatening problem, so it requires immediate attention. Causes include damage to organs in the abdomen and pelvis, which leads to inflammation, infection, obstruction, bleeding, and perforation (Fig. 42.1). Perforation of the GI tract results in irritation of the *peritoneum* (serous membrane lining the abdominal cavity) and peritonitis. Hypovolemic shock occurs from

TABLE 42.10 Patient & Caregiver Teaching

Constipation

Include the following instructions when teaching the patient and caregiver about management of constipation.

1. Eat Dietary Fiber

Eat 20 to 30 g of fiber per day. Gradually increase the amount of fiber eaten over 1 to 2 wk. Fiber softens hard stool and adds bulk to stool, promoting evacuation. Eat prunes or drink prune juice daily. Prunes stimulate defecation.

- Foods high in fiber: raw vegetables and fruits, beans, breakfast cereals (All Bran, oatmeal)
- Fiber supplements: Metamucil, Citrucel, FiberCon

2. Drink Fluids

Fluid softens hard stools. Drink 2 L per day. Drink water or fruit juices. Avoid caffeinated coffee, tea, and cola. Caffeine stimulates fluid loss through urination.

3. Exercise Regularly

Walk, swim, or bike at least 3 times per wk. Contract and relax abdominal muscles when standing or by doing sit-ups to strengthen muscles and prevent straining. Exercise stimulates bowel motility and moves stool through the colon.

4. Establish a Regular Time to Defecate

First thing in the morning or after the first meal of the day is the best time because people often have the urge to defecate at this time.

5. Do Not Delay Defecation

Respond to the urge to have a bowel movement as soon as possible. Delaying defecation results in hard stools and a decreased "urge" to defecate. Water is absorbed from stool by the intestine over time. The colon becomes less sensitive to the presence of stool in the rectum.

6. Record Your Bowel Elimination Pattern

Develop a habit of recording on your calendar when you have a bowel movement. Regular monitoring of bowel movement will help you identify a problem early.

7. Avoid Laxatives and Enemas

Do not overuse laxatives and enemas, because they cause dependence. People who overuse them become unable to have a bowel movement without them.

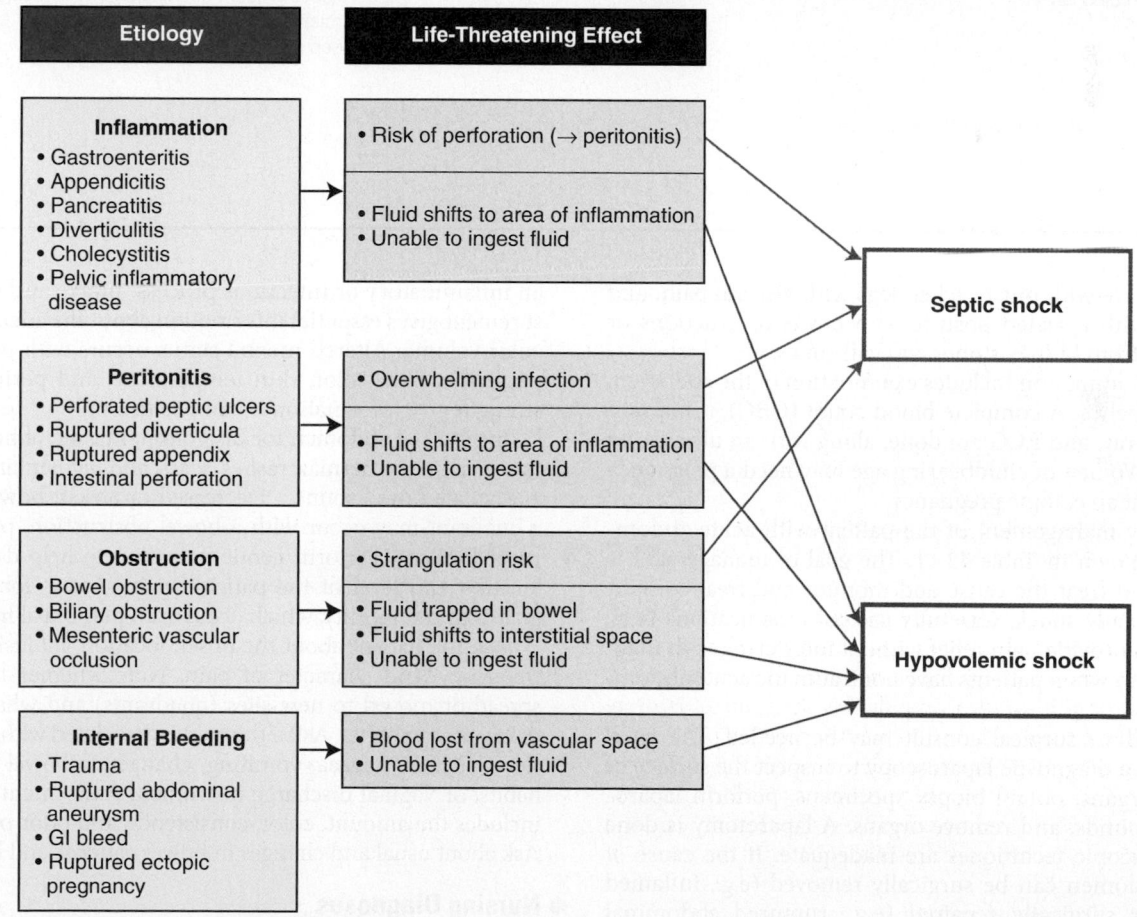

FIG. 42.1 Cause of acute abdominal pain and pathophysiologic sequelae.

bleeding or obstruction and peritonitis causing large amounts of fluid to move from the vascular space into the abdomen.

Clinical Manifestations

Pain is the most common symptom of an acute abdominal problem. The patient may have nausea, vomiting, diarrhea, constipation, flatulence, fatigue, fever, rebound tenderness, and bloating.

Diagnostic Studies and Interprofessional Care

Diagnosis begins with a complete history and physical examination. Description of the pain (frequency, timing, duration, location), accompanying symptoms, and sequence of symptoms (e.g., pain before or after vomiting) provide vital clues about the origin of the problem. Note the patient's position. The fetal posture is common with peritoneal irritation (e.g., appendicitis),

✚ TABLE 42.11 Emergency Management

Acute Abdominal Pain

Etiology	Assessment Findings	Interventions
Inflammation • Appendicitis • Cholecystitis • Diverticulitis • Gastritis • Inflammatory bowel disease • Pancreatitis • Pyelonephritis	**Abdominal and GI Findings** • Diffuse, localized, dull, burning, or sharp abdominal pain or tenderness • Rebound tenderness • Abdominal distention • Abdominal rigidity • Nausea and vomiting • Diarrhea • Hematemesis • Melena	**Initial** • Ensure patent airway. • Apply O_2 via nasal cannula or nonrebreather mask. • Establish IV access with large-bore catheter and infuse warm normal saline or lactated Ringer's solution. Insert another large-bore catheter if shock present. • Obtain blood for CBC and electrolyte levels. • Obtain blood for amylase level, pregnancy tests, clotting studies, and type and crossmatch as appropriate. • Insert indwelling urinary catheter. • Obtain urinalysis. • Insert NG tube as needed.
Vascular Problems • Mesenteric vascular occlusion • Ruptured aortic aneurysm	**Hypovolemic Shock** • ↓ BP • ↓ Pulse pressure • Tachycardia • Cool, clammy skin • ↓ Level of consciousness • ↓ Urine output (<0.5 mL/kg/hr)	**Ongoing Monitoring** • Monitor vital signs, level of consciousness, O_2 saturation, and intake/output. • Assess quality and amount of pain. • Assess amount and character of emesis. • Anticipate surgical intervention. • Keep patient NPO.
Gynecologic Problems • Pelvic inflammatory disease • Ruptured ectopic pregnancy • Ruptured ovarian cyst		
Infectious Disease • *Escherichia coli* O157:H7 • *Giardia* • *Salmonella*		
Other • Obstruction or perforation of abdominal organ • GI bleeding or ischemia • Myocardial infarction • Trauma		

a supine posture with outstretched legs with visceral pain, and restlessness with a seated posture with bowel obstructions or obstructions from kidney stones and gallstones.

Physical examination includes examination of the abdomen, rectum, and pelvis. A complete blood count (CBC), urinalysis, abdominal x-ray, and ECG are done, along with an ultrasound or CT scan. Women of childbearing age may need a pregnancy test to rule out an ectopic pregnancy.

Emergency management of the patient with acute abdominal pain is shown in Table 42.11. The goal of management is to identify and treat the cause and monitor and treat complications, especially shock. Carefully use pain medications (e.g., morphine) to provide pain relief without interfering with diagnostic accuracy when patients have nontraumatic acute abdominal pain.

An immediate surgical consult may be needed. The HCP may perform a diagnostic laparoscopy to inspect the surface of abdominal organs, obtain biopsy specimens, perform laparoscopic ultrasounds, and remove organs. A laparotomy is done when laparoscopic techniques are inadequate. If the cause of the acute abdomen can be surgically removed (e.g., inflamed appendix) or surgically repaired (e.g., ruptured abdominal aneurysm), surgery is considered definitive therapy.

❖ NURSING MANAGEMENT: ACUTE ABDOMINAL PAIN

◆ Nursing Assessment

For the patient with acute abdominal pain, take vital signs immediately and again at frequent intervals. Increased pulse and decreasing BP indicate impending shock. A fever suggests an inflammatory or infectious process. Intake and output measurement gives essential information about the adequacy of vascular volume. Altered mental status occurs with poor cerebral perfusion. Skin color, skin temperature, and peripheral pulse strength give information about perfusion.

Inspect the abdomen for distention, masses, abnormal pulsation, symmetry, hernias, rashes, scars, and pigmentation changes. Auscultate bowel sounds. Decreased or absent bowel sounds in a quadrant may occur with a bowel obstruction, peritonitis, or paralytic ileus. Perform gentle palpation to help determine the location and level of the patient's pain. Assess for involuntary guarding and rigidity, which occur with peritoneal irritation.

Ask the patient about the onset, location, intensity, duration, frequency, and character of pain. Note whether the pain has spread or moved to new sites (quadrants) and what makes the pain worse or better. Ask if the pain is associated with other symptoms, such as nausea, vomiting, changes in bowel and bladder habits, or vaginal discharge in women. Assessment of vomiting includes the amount, color, consistency, and odor of the emesis. Ask about usual and changes in bowel patterns and habits.

◆ Nursing Diagnoses

Nursing diagnoses for the patient with acute abdominal pain include:
- Acute pain
- Fluid imbalance
- Risk for infection

◆ Planning

The overall goals are that the patient with acute abdominal pain will have (1) relief of abdominal pain, (2) resolution of inflammation, (3) freedom from complications (especially hypovolemic shock), and (4) normal nutritional status.

◆ Nursing Implementation

General care for the patient with acute abdominal pain involves managing fluid and electrolyte imbalances, pain, and anxiety. Assess the quality and intensity of pain at regular intervals. Provide medication and other comfort measures. Maintain a calm environment and give information to help decrease anxiety. A nasogastric (NG) tube with low suction may decrease vomiting and relieve discomfort from gastric distention. Conduct ongoing assessments of vital signs, intake and output, and level of consciousness, which are key indicators of hypovolemic shock.

◆ Acute Care

Preoperative Care. Preoperative care includes the emergency care of the patient described in Table 42.11 and general care of the preoperative patient (see Chapter 17).

Postoperative Care. Postoperative care depends on the type of surgical procedure. See eNursing Care Plan 19.1, a general plan for the postoperative patient, on the website for Chapter 19.

After surgery, some patients will have an NG tube with low suction to empty the stomach and prevent gastric dilation. If the upper GI tract was entered, drainage from the NG tube may be dark brown to dark red for the first 12 hours. Later it should be light yellowish brown, or it may have a greenish tinge because of bile. If a dark red color continues or you see bright red blood, notify the HCP because of the risk for hemorrhage. "Coffee-grounds" granules in the drainage mean the blood has been changed by acidic gastric secretions.

Nausea and vomiting are common after a laparotomy and result from the surgery, decreased peristalsis, or pain medications. Antiemetics, such as ondansetron (Zofran), promethazine (Phenergan), and aprepitant (Emend), may be ordered. Monitor fluid and electrolyte status along with BP, heart rate, and respirations. See Chapter 41 for further discussion of managing nausea and vomiting.

Swallowed air and reduced peristalsis from decreased mobility, manipulation of the abdominal organs during surgery, and anesthesia can result in abdominal distention and gas pains. Early ambulation helps restore peristalsis, expel flatus, and reduce gas pain. Gradually, as intestinal activity increases, distention and gas pain disappear.

◆ Ambulatory Care.

Preparation for discharge begins soon after surgery. Teach the patient and caregiver about any modifications in activity, care of the incision, diet, and drug therapy. Initially the patient starts on clear liquids after surgery and then, if tolerated, progresses to a regular diet.

Early ambulation speeds recovery, but normal activities are resumed gradually, with planned rest periods. Patients generally have restrictions not to lift anything heavier than a few pounds. The patient and caregiver should be aware of any possible complications. Teach them to notify the HCP at once if fever is greater than 101°F (38.6°C), vomiting, pain, weight loss, incisional drainage, or changes in bowel function occur.

◆ Evaluation

The expected outcomes are that the patient with acute abdominal pain will:

- Have resolution of the cause of the acute abdominal pain
- Experience relief of abdominal pain and discomfort
- Be free from complications, especially hypovolemic shock and sepsis
- Have normal fluid, electrolyte, and nutritional status

ABDOMINAL TRAUMA

Etiology and Pathophysiology

Injuries to the abdominal area usually are a result of blunt trauma or penetrating injuries. Common injuries of the abdomen include lacerated liver, ruptured spleen, mesenteric artery tears, diaphragm rupture, urinary bladder rupture, great vessel tears, renal or pancreas injury, and stomach or intestine rupture.

Blunt trauma often occurs with motor vehicle accidents, direct blows, and falls. It may not be obvious because it does not leave an open wound. Both compression injuries (e.g., direct blow to the abdomen) and shearing injuries (e.g., rapid deceleration in a motor vehicle crash allowing some tissue to move forward while other tissues stay stationary) occur with blunt trauma. *Penetrating injuries* occur when a gunshot or stabbing produces an obvious, open wound into the abdomen.

When solid organs (liver, spleen) are injured, bleeding can be profuse, resulting in hypovolemic shock. When contents from hollow organs (e.g., bladder, stomach, intestines) spill into the peritoneal cavity, the patient is at risk for peritonitis. In addition, abdominal compartment syndrome can develop.

Abdominal compartment syndrome, or abdominal hypertension, is excessively high pressure in the abdomen. Anything that increases the volume in the abdominal cavity (e.g., edematous organs, bleeding) increases abdominal pressure. This high pressure restricts ventilation, potentially leading to respiratory failure. The high pressure decreases cardiac output, venous return, and arterial perfusion of organs. Decreased perfusion to the kidneys can lead to renal failure.

Clinical Manifestations

Careful assessment provides important clues to the type and severity of injury. Intraabdominal injuries are often associated with rib fractures, fractured pelvis, spinal injury, and thoracic injury. If the patient was in an automobile accident, a contusion or abrasion across the lower abdomen may indicate internal organ trauma due to seat belt use. Seat belts can produce blunt trauma to abdominal organs by pressing the intestine and pancreas into the spinal column.

Classic manifestations of abdominal trauma are (1) guarding and splinting of the abdominal wall (indicating peritonitis); (2) a hard, distended abdomen (occurs with intraabdominal bleeding); (3) decreased or absent bowel sounds; (4) abrasions or bruising over the abdomen; (5) abdominal pain; (6) hematemesis or hematuria; and (7) signs of hypovolemic shock (Table 42.12). Ecchymosis around the umbilicus (*Cullen's sign*) or flanks (*Grey Turner's sign*) may mean retroperitoneal hemorrhage. Loss of bowel sounds occurs with peritonitis. If the diaphragm ruptures, you can hear bowel sounds (if present) in the chest. Auscultation of bruits is indicative of arterial damage.

Diagnostic Studies

Laboratory tests include a baseline CBC and urinalysis. Even when bleeding, the patient will have normal hemoglobin and hematocrit because fluids are lost at the same rate as the red blood cells. Deficiencies are evident after fluid resuscitation begins. Blood in the urine may be a sign of kidney or bladder damage. Other laboratory work includes arterial blood gases, prothrombin time, electrolytes, BUN and creatinine, and type and crossmatch (in anticipation of possible blood transfusions). An abdominal CT scan and focused abdominal ultrasound are

✚ TABLE 42.12 **Emergency Management**

Abdominal Trauma

Etiology	Assessment Findings	Interventions
Blunt	**Hypovolemic Shock**	**Initial**
• Falls	• ↓ Level of consciousness	• If unresponsive, assess circulation, airway, and breathing.
• Motor vehicle collisions	• Tachypnea	• If responsive, monitor airway, breathing, and circulation.
• Pedestrian event	• Tachycardia	• Apply appropriate O₂ therapy.
• Assault with blunt object	• ↓ BP	• Control external bleeding with direct pressure or sterile pressure dressing.
• Crush injuries	• ↓ Pulse pressure	
• Explosions		• Establish IV access with 2 large-bore catheters and infuse normal saline or lactated Ringer's solution.
	Surface Findings	• Obtain blood for type and crossmatch and CBC.
Penetrating	• Abrasions or ecchymoses on abdominal wall, flank, or peritoneum	• Remove clothing.
• Knife	• Open wounds: lacerations, eviscerations, puncture wounds, gunshot wounds	• Stabilize impaled objects with bulky dressing—*do not remove*.
• Gunshot wounds	• Impaled object	• Cover protruding organs or tissue with sterile saline dressing.
• Impalement		• Insert indwelling urinary catheter if there is no blood at the meatus, pelvic fracture, or boggy prostate.
• Other missiles	**Abdominal and GI Findings**	• Obtain urine for urinalysis.
	• Nausea and vomiting	• Insert NG tube if no evidence of facial trauma.
	• Hematemesis	• Anticipate diagnostic peritoneal lavage.
	• Absent or decreased bowel sounds	
	• Hematuria	**Ongoing Monitoring**
	• Abdominal distention	• Monitor vital signs, level of consciousness, O₂ saturation, and urine output.
	• Abdominal rigidity	• Maintain patient warmth using blankets, warm IV fluids, or warm humidified O₂.
	• Abdominal pain with palpation	
	• Rebound tenderness	

the most common diagnostic methods, but the patient must be stable before going for CT.

Diagnostic peritoneal lavage can detect blood, bile, intestinal contents, and urine in the peritoneal cavity. It is generally used only for unstable patients to identify blood in the peritoneum.

❖ Interprofessional and Nursing Care

Emergency management of abdominal trauma is outlined in Table 42.12. Volume expanders or blood given if the patient is hypotensive. An NG tube with low suction will decompress the stomach and prevent aspiration. Frequent ongoing assessment is needed to monitor fluid status, detect deterioration in condition, and determine the need for surgery. The decision about whether to do surgery depends on clinical findings, diagnostic test results, and the patient's response to conservative management. Do not remove an impaled object until skilled care is available. Removal may cause further injury and bleeding.

CHRONIC ABDOMINAL PAIN

Chronic abdominal pain may originate from abdominal structures or be referred from a site with the same or a similar nerve supply. The pain is often described as dull, aching, or diffuse. Common causes of chronic abdominal pain include irritable bowel syndrome (IBS), peptic ulcer disease, chronic pancreatitis, hepatitis, pelvic inflammatory disease, adhesions, and vascular insufficiency.

Diagnosing the cause of chronic abdominal pain begins with a thorough history and description of specific pain characteristics, including severity, location, frequency, duration, and onset. The assessment includes factors that increase or decrease the pain, such as eating, defecation, and activities. Endoscopy, CT scan, MRI, laparoscopy, and barium studies may be done.

Treatment for chronic abdominal pain depends on the underlying cause.

IRRITABLE BOWEL SYNDROME

Irritable bowel syndrome (IBS) is a disorder characterized by chronic abdominal pain or discomfort and alteration of bowel patterns. Patients may have diarrhea or constipation, alternating periods of both.

IBS has no known organic cause. Psychologic stressors (e.g., depression, anxiety, panic disorders, posttraumatic stress disorder) are associated with the development and exacerbation of IBS. Patients often have a history of GI infections and adverse reactions to food. Dietary intolerances that may contribute to symptoms include gluten and fermentable oligo-, di-, and monosaccharides and polyols (FODMAPs).[7] Examples of oligosaccharides are wheat and rye products, some fruits and vegetables, onions, garlic, legumes, and nuts. The disaccharide lactose is found in milk and milk products. Fructose is a monosaccharide found in honey, apples, pears, and high-fructose corn syrup. Polyols are found in apples, pears, stone fruits, cauliflower, mushrooms, and artificial sweeteners, like sorbitol.[8]

IBS is diagnosed solely on symptoms. The Rome IV criteria for diagnosing IBS require the presence of abdominal pain and/or discomfort at least 1 day per week for 3 months that is associated with 2 or more of the following: related to defecation, change in stool frequency, or change in the stool form.[7] Depending on the stool patterns, IBS is categorized as IBS with constipation (IBS-C), IBS with diarrhea (IBS-D), IBS mixed, and IBS unsubtyped. Other common symptoms include abdominal distention, nausea, flatulence, bloating, urgency, mucus in the stool, and sensation of incomplete evacuation. Non-GI symptoms may include fatigue, headache, and sleep problems.

GENDER DIFFERENCES
Irritable Bowel Syndrome (IBS)

Men
- More likely to have IBS with diarrhea
- Less likely to admit to symptoms or seek help for them

Women
- Overall affects women 2 to 2.5 times more often than men
- More likely to have IBS with constipation
- Report more severe abdominal pain, gas, and bloating
- Have a lower quality of life with higher levels of fatigue and depression

The key to accurate diagnosis is a thorough history and physical examination. Ask patients to describe symptoms, health history (including psychosocial factors, such as stress and anxiety), family history, and drug and diet history. Determine if and how IBS symptoms interfere with school, work, or recreational activities. Diagnostic tests are used to rule out other disorders, such as colorectal cancer, IBD, endometriosis, and malabsorption disorders (lactose intolerance, celiac disease).

No single therapy is effective for all patients with IBS. Treatment may include dealing with psychologic factors, dietary changes, and drugs to regulate stool output and reduce discomfort. Patients may benefit from keeping a diary of symptoms, diet, and episodes of stress to help identify any factors that trigger the IBS symptoms. Cognitive behavior therapy and stress management techniques may help a patient cope. Participating in regular exercise reduces bloating and constipation and reduces stress-related symptoms.

Review with the patient foods that are high in FODMAPs and teach them to follow a low-FODMAP diet.[8] If dairy products tend to cause symptoms, yogurt may be the best option because of the lactobacillus bacteria it contains. Probiotics can improve symptoms. Tell the patient with flatulence to avoid common gas-producing foods, such as broccoli and cabbage. For those with constipation, encourage an intake of enough dietary fiber to produce soft, painless bowel movements.

Drug therapy focuses on the dominant bowel symptom and pain. The opioid agonist eluxadoline (Viberzi) decreases colonic contractions to reduce diarrhea and pain. It is contraindicated in those without a gallbladder. An option for women with IBS-D is alosetron (Lotronex). Because of serious side effects (e.g., severe constipation, ischemic colitis), it is available only in a restricted access program. Other treatments for IBS-D include loperamide, antidepressants, and antispasmodic medications (hyoscyamine, dicyclomine). Antispasmodics decrease GI motility and smooth muscle spasms, reducing pain and diarrhea.[8]

 DRUG ALERT Alosetron (Lotronex)

- Taking this drug can cause severe constipation and ischemic colitis (reduced blood flow to intestines).
- Teach the patient to stop the drug and contact the HCP if constipation, rectal bleeding, bloody diarrhea, or abdominal pain occurs.

Women with IBS-C may benefit from lubiprostone (Amitiza). Men or women with IBS-C can take linaclotide (Linzess). It is contraindicated in patients with a history of mechanical obstruction or prior bowel surgery.

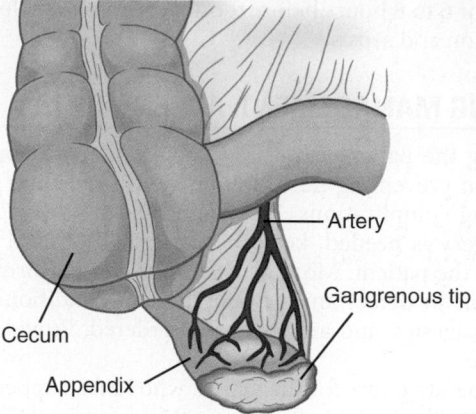

FIG. 42.2 In appendicitis the blood supply of the appendix is impaired by inflammation and bacterial infection, which may result in gangrene.

INFLAMMATORY DISORDERS

APPENDICITIS

Appendicitis is inflammation of the appendix, a narrow blind tube that extends from the inferior part of the cecum (Fig. 42.2). It is the most common reason for emergency abdominal surgery.

Etiology and Pathophysiology

About 7% of people will develop appendicitis sometime during their lifetime.[9] It is most common in those 10 to 30 years of age. A common cause of appendicitis is obstruction of the lumen by a fecalith (accumulated feces). Obstruction results in distention; venous engorgement; and the accumulation of mucus and bacteria, which can lead to gangrene, perforation, and peritonitis.

Clinical Manifestations

Diagnosis can be difficult because many patients do not have classic symptoms. Appendicitis typically begins with dull periumbilical pain, followed by anorexia, nausea, and vomiting. The pain is persistent and continuous, eventually shifting to the right lower quadrant and localizing at *McBurney's point* (halfway between the umbilicus and right iliac crest). A low-grade fever may develop. Further assessment reveals localized tenderness, rigidity, rebound tenderness, and muscle guarding. Coughing, sneezing, and deep inhalation worsen pain. The patient usually prefers to lie still, often with the right leg flexed. The older adult may report less severe pain, slight fever, and discomfort in the right iliac fossa.

Diagnostic Studies and Interprofessional Care

Patient examination includes a complete history, physical examination, and a differential WBC count. Most patients have a mildly to moderately high WBC count. A urinalysis is done to rule out genitourinary conditions that mimic appendicitis. CT scan is the preferred diagnostic procedure. However, ultrasound and MRI are options.

If there is a delay in diagnosis and treatment, the appendix can rupture and the resulting peritonitis can be fatal. The standard treatment of appendicitis is an immediate *appendectomy* (surgical removal of appendix).[9] If the inflammation is localized, surgery should be done as soon as the diagnosis is made. Antibiotics and fluid resuscitation are started before surgery.

If the appendix has ruptured and there is evidence of peritonitis or an abscess, giving parenteral fluids and antibiotic therapy for 6 to 8 hours before the appendectomy helps prevent dehydration and sepsis.

❖ NURSING MANAGEMENT: APPENDICITIS

Managing the patient who has manifestations of appendicitis focuses on preventing fluid volume deficit, relieving pain, and preventing complications. To ensure the stomach is empty in case surgery is needed, keep the patient NPO until the HCP evaluates the patient. Monitor vital signs and perform ongoing assessment to detect any deterioration in condition. Give IV fluids, analgesics, and antiemetics as ordered. Provide comfort measures.

Postoperative care for the patient who had an appendectomy is similar to the patient after a laparotomy (see p. 935). Patients are usually discharged within 24 hours after an uncomplicated laparoscopic appendectomy. Ambulation begins a few hours after surgery, and the diet is advanced as tolerated. Those who had a perforation usually have a longer length of stay and need IV antibiotic therapy. Most patients resume normal activities 2 to 3 weeks after surgery.

❓ CHECK YOUR PRACTICE

A 28-yr-old female patient comes to the emergency department with acute abdominal pain.
- What manifestations would make you suspect appendicitis is the cause of the patient's abdominal pain?

PERITONITIS

Etiology and Pathophysiology

Peritonitis results from a localized or generalized inflammatory process of the peritoneum. Causes of peritonitis are listed in Table 42.13. Primary peritonitis occurs when blood-borne organisms enter the peritoneal cavity. For example, the ascites that occurs with cirrhosis of the liver provides an excellent liquid environment for bacteria to flourish. Organisms can enter the peritoneum during peritoneal dialysis.

Secondary peritonitis is much more common. It occurs when abdominal organs perforate or rupture and release their contents (bile, enzymes, and bacteria) into the peritoneal cavity. Common causes include a ruptured appendix, perforated gastric or duodenal ulcer, severely inflamed gallbladder, and trauma from gunshot or knife wounds.

Intestinal contents and bacteria irritate the normally sterile peritoneum and produce an initial chemical peritonitis. Bacterial peritonitis develops a few hours later. The resulting inflammatory response leads to massive fluid shifts (peritoneal edema) and adhesions as the body tries to wall off the infection.

Clinical Manifestations

Abdominal pain is the most common symptom of peritonitis. A universal sign is tenderness over the involved area. Rebound tenderness, muscular rigidity, and spasm are other signs of peritoneal irritation. Patients may lie still and take only shallow breaths because movement worsens the pain. Abdominal distention, fever, tachycardia, tachypnea, nausea, vomiting, and altered bowel habits may be present. These manifestations vary, depending on the severity and acuteness of the underlying condition. Complications include hypovolemic shock, sepsis,

---

TABLE 42.13 Causes of Peritonitis

Primary
- Blood-borne organisms
- Cirrhosis with ascites
- Genital tract organisms

Secondary
- Appendicitis with rupture
- Blunt or penetrating trauma to abdominal organs
- Diverticulitis with rupture

- Ischemic bowel disorders
- Pancreatitis
- Perforated intestine
- Perforated peptic ulcer
- Peritoneal dialysis
- Postoperative (breakage of anastomosis)

TABLE 42.14 Interprofessional Care

Peritonitis

Diagnostic Assessment
- History and physical examination
- CBC, including WBC differential
- Serum electrolytes
- Abdominal x-ray
- Abdominal paracentesis and culture of fluid
- CT scan or ultrasound
- Peritoneoscopy

Management
Preoperative or Nonoperative
- NPO status
- IV fluid replacement
- NG to low-intermittent suction
- O_2 PRN
- Parenteral nutrition as needed

Drug Therapy
- Antibiotic therapy
- Analgesics (e.g., morphine)
- Antiemetics as needed

Postoperative
- NPO status
- NG to low-intermittent suction
- Semi-Fowler's position
- IV fluids with electrolyte replacement
- PN as needed
- Blood transfusions as needed

Drug Therapy
- Antibiotic therapy
- Sedatives and opioids
- Antiemetics as needed

---

intraabdominal abscess formation, paralytic ileus, and acute respiratory distress syndrome. Peritonitis can be fatal if treatment is delayed.

Diagnostic Studies and Interprofessional Care

A CBC is done to determine elevations in WBC count and hemoconcentration from fluid shifts (Table 42.14). Peritoneal aspiration may be done with the fluid analyzed for blood, bile, pus, bacteria, fungus, and amylase content. An abdominal x-ray may show dilated loops of bowel consistent with paralytic ileus, free air if perforation has occurred, or air and fluid levels if an obstruction is present. Ultrasound and CT scans may be useful in identifying ascites and abscesses. Peritoneoscopy may be helpful in the patient without ascites. It allows for direct examination of the peritoneum and the ability to obtain biopsy specimens for diagnosis.

Patients with milder cases of peritonitis or those who are poor surgical risks receive conservative care. Treatment consists of antibiotics, NG suction, analgesics, and IV fluid administration. Surgery is indicated to locate the cause of the inflammation, drain purulent fluid, and repair any damage (e.g., perforated organs).

❖ NURSING MANAGEMENT: PERITONITIS

◆ Nursing Assessment

Assessment of the patient's pain, including the location, is important and may help to determine the cause of peritonitis. Assess for the presence and quality of bowel sounds, increasing abdominal distention, abdominal guarding, nausea, fever, and manifestations of hypovolemic shock.

◆ Nursing Diagnoses

Nursing diagnoses for the patient with peritonitis include:
- Acute pain
- Fluid imbalance
- Impaired gas exchange
- Risk for infection

◆ Planning

The overall goals are that the patient with peritonitis will have (1) resolution of inflammation, (2) relief of abdominal pain, (3) freedom from complications (especially sepsis and hypovolemic shock), and (4) normal nutritional status.

◆ Nursing Implementation

The patient with peritonitis is extremely ill and needs skilled supportive care. Establish IV access so that you can give replacement fluids lost to the peritoneal cavity and have access for antibiotic therapy. Monitor the patient for pain and response to analgesics. You may position the patient with knees flexed to increase comfort. Sedatives may relieve anxiety and promote rest.

Accurate monitoring of intake and output and electrolyte status is essential to determine replacement therapy. Frequently monitor vital signs. Give antiemetics to decrease nausea and vomiting and prevent further fluid and electrolyte losses. Place the patient on NPO status. The patient may need an NG tube to decrease gastric distention and further leakage of bowel contents into the peritoneum. Give low-flow oxygen therapy as needed.

If the patient had an open surgical procedure, drains are inserted to remove purulent drainage and excess fluid. Postoperative care is similar to that for the patient who had a laparotomy (see p. 935).

GASTROENTERITIS

Gastroenteritis is an inflammation of the mucosa of the stomach and small intestine. Features of *acute gastroenteritis* are sudden diarrhea accompanied by nausea, vomiting, fever, and abdominal cramping. Viruses are the most common cause of gastroenteritis (Table 42.1).

Norovirus is a leading cause of foodborne outbreaks of acute gastroenteritis. Laboratory testing to identify norovirus is useful when a number of people simultaneously have gastroenteritis and there is a clear avenue for virus transmission, such as a shared location or food.

Most cases of gastroenteritis are self-limiting. Encourage oral fluids containing glucose and electrolytes (e.g., Pedialyte) to prevent and treat dehydration. Older adults and chronically ill patients may be unable to consume enough fluids to make up for fluid loss. If dehydration occurs, IV fluid replacement may be needed. Nursing management of the patient with gastroenteritis is the same as for the patient with acute diarrhea (see p. 927).

INFLAMMATORY BOWEL DISEASE

Inflammatory bowel disease (IBD) is a chronic inflammation of the GI tract characterized by periods of remission interspersed with periods of exacerbation. We classify IBD as either Crohn's disease or ulcerative colitis (UC) based on clinical manifestations (Table 42.15). As the name suggests, ulcerative colitis is usually limited to the colon. Crohn's disease can involve any segment of the GI tract from the mouth to the anus.

About 1.3 million Americans have IBD. It often begins during the teenage years and early adulthood. IBD has a second peak in the 6th decade. The incidence and frequency of IBD varies depending on geographic location and racial or ethnic background. The highest rates are in the Northern Hemisphere and industrialized nations.[10] The risk for having IBD is greater in urban compared with rural areas and those of white and Ashkenazic Jewish origin than in other racial and ethnic groups.[10] The strongest risk factor is family history. Many people with IBD have a family member with the disorder.

Etiology and Pathophysiology

We do not know the exact cause of IBD. IBD is an autoimmune disease involving an immune reaction to a person's own intestinal tract. We think that it results from an overactive, inappropriate, or sustained immune response to environmental and bacterial triggers, probably in a genetically susceptible person. The resulting inflammation causes widespread tissue destruction.

Environmental factors, such as diet, smoking, and stress, increase susceptibility by changing the environment of the GI microbial flora. We think that dietary factors unique to industrialized countries contribute to the development of IBD. High intake of refined sugar, total fats, polyunsaturated fatty acid (PUFA), and omega-6 fatty acids is associated with an increased risk for IBD. Eating fewer raw fruits, vegetables, omega-3–rich foods, and dietary fiber decrease risk.[11] Use of nonsteroidal antiinflammatory drugs (NSAIDs), antibiotics, and oral contraceptives are associated with increased risk.[12]

Genetic Link

IBD occurs more often in family members of people with IBD, especially monozygotic twins. To date, we have found over 200 genes associated with IBD. Certain genetic mutations are associated with Crohn's disease, others with UC, and many with both.

The number of gene variations suggests that IBD is a group of diseases that produce similar types of mucosal destruction. The path from genetic mutation to abnormal immune responses varies depending on which gene or genes are affected. Several of the genes are involved in protective functions of the intestines. Others have a role in the immune system, especially in the maturation and function of T cells.

TABLE 42.15 Comparison of Ulcerative Colitis and Crohn's Disease

Characteristic	Ulcerative Colitis	Crohn's Disease
Clinical		
Usual age at onset	Teens to mid-30s. After 60	Teens to mid-30s. After 60
Abdominal pain	Common, severe constant	Common, cramping
Diarrhea	Common	Common
Fever (intermittent)	During acute attacks	Common
Malabsorption and nutritional deficiencies	Minimal incidence	Common
Rectal bleeding	Common	Sometimes
Tenesmus	Common	Rare
Weight loss	Rare	Common, may be severe
Pathologic		
Location	Usually starts in rectum and spreads in a continuous pattern up the colon	Occurs anywhere along GI tract. Most common site is distal ileum
Cobblestoning of mucosa	Rare	Common
Depth of involvement	Mucosa	Entire thickness of bowel wall (transmural)
Distribution	Continuous areas of inflammation	Healthy tissue interspersed with areas of inflammation (skip lesions)
Pseudopolyps	Common	Rare
Small bowel involvement	Minimal	Common
Complications		
Cancer	Increased incidence of colorectal cancer after 10 yrs of disease	Increased incidence of small intestinal cancer. Increased incidence of colorectal cancer but less than with ulcerative colitis
C. difficile infection	Increased incidence and severity	Increased incidence and severity
Perforation	Common (because of toxic megacolon)	Common (because inflammation involves entire bowel wall)
Perianal abscess and fistulas	Rare	Common
Strictures	Occasional	Common
Toxic megacolon	More common	Rare

Genetic variation may explain differences in patient responses to drug therapies for IBD.

Many of the major genes related to Crohn's disease, including *NOD2*, *ATG16L1*, *IL23R*, and *IRGM*, are involved in immune system function. The proteins made from these genes help the immune system sense and respond appropriately to bacteria in the lining of the GI tract. *NOD2* gene changes are associated with a form of Crohn's disease that affects the ileum in persons of northern European descent. Changes in the *NOD2* gene trigger an abnormal immune response that allows bacteria to grow unchecked and invade intestinal cells. This causes chronic inflammation and digestive problems.[13]

IBD is more likely to occur in those with other genetic syndromes, including cystic fibrosis. An increased prevalence occurs in the presence of other inflammatory disorders with genetic susceptibility, such as psoriasis and multiple sclerosis.

Pattern of Inflammation in Ulcerative Colitis vs. Crohn's Disease. The pattern of inflammation differs between Crohn's disease and UC (Fig. 42.3). Crohn's disease can occur anywhere in the GI tract from the mouth to the anus. It most often involves the distal ileum and proximal colon. Segments of normal bowel can occur between diseased portions, so-called "skip" lesions. The inflammation in Crohn's disease involves all layers of the bowel wall. Typically, ulcerations are deep, longitudinal, and penetrate between islands of inflamed edematous mucosa, causing the classic cobblestone appearance. Strictures at the areas of inflammation can cause bowel obstruction. Since the inflammation goes through the entire wall, microscopic leaks can allow bowel contents to enter the peritoneal cavity and form abscesses or produce peritonitis. In active Crohn's disease, fistulas are common.

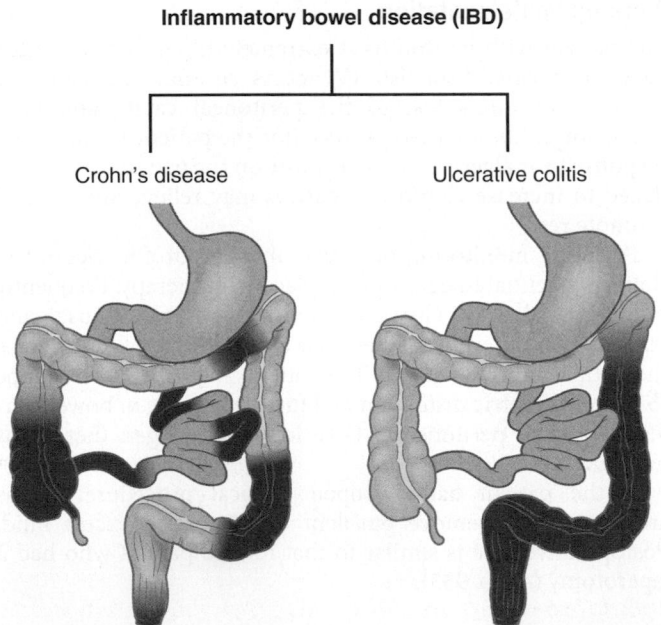

FIG. 42.3 Comparison of distribution patterns of Crohn's disease and ulcerative colitis.

UC usually starts in the rectum and moves in a continual fashion toward the cecum. Although mild inflammation may occur in the terminal ileum, UC is a disease of the colon and rectum. The inflammation and ulcerations occur in the mucosal layer, the innermost layer of the bowel wall. Fistulas and abscesses are rare since inflammation does not extend through

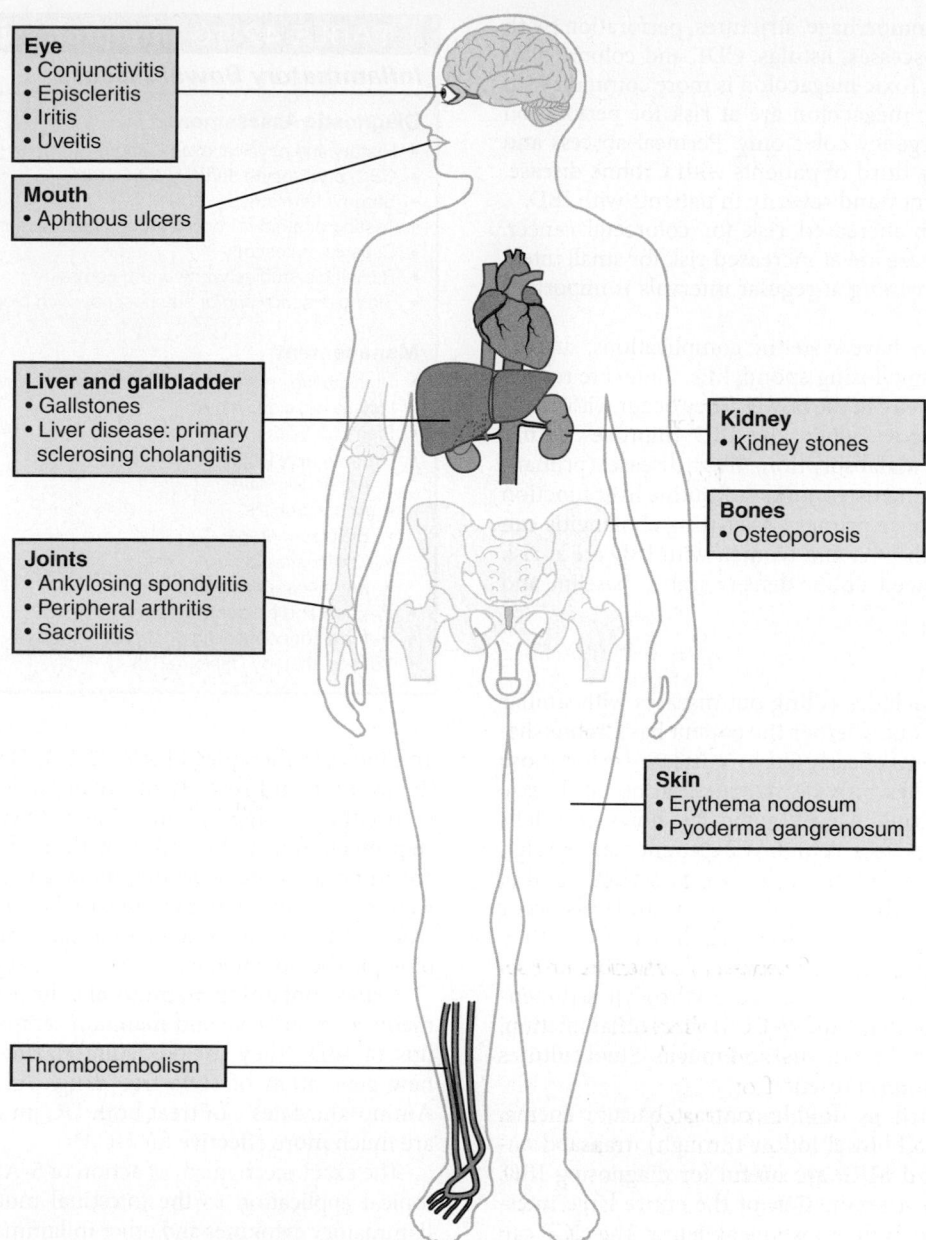

Eye
• Conjunctivitis
• Episcleritis
• Iritis
• Uveitis

Mouth
• Aphthous ulcers

Liver and gallbladder
• Gallstones
• Liver disease: primary
  sclerosing cholangitis

Kidney
• Kidney stones

Bones
• Osteoporosis

Joints
• Ankylosing spondylitis
• Peripheral arthritis
• Sacroiliitis

Skin
• Erythema nodosum
• Pyoderma gangrenosum

Thromboembolism

FIG. 42.4 Extraintestinal manifestations of IBD.

all bowel wall layers. Because water and electrolytes are not absorbed through inflamed mucosa, diarrhea with large fluid and electrolyte losses is common. Breakdown of cells results in protein loss through the stool. Areas of inflamed mucosa form *pseudopolyps,* tongue-like projections into the bowel lumen.

Clinical Manifestations

Both forms of IBD are chronic disorders with mild to severe acute exacerbations that occur at unpredictable intervals over many years. Although the manifestations of Crohn's disease and UC are similar (diarrhea, weight loss, abdominal pain, fever, fatigue), there are differences (Table 42.15).

In Crohn's disease, diarrhea and cramping abdominal pain are common symptoms. If the small intestine is involved, weight loss occurs from inflammation of the small intestine causing malabsorption. Rectal bleeding sometimes occurs with Crohn's disease, although not as often as with UC.

In UC, the primary problems are bloody diarrhea and abdominal pain. Pain may vary from the mild lower abdominal cramping associated with diarrhea to severe, constant pain associated with acute perforations. With *mild disease,* diarrhea may consist of no more than 4 semiformed stools daily that contain small amounts of blood. The patient may have no other manifestations. In *moderate disease,* the patient has increased stool output (up to 10 stools/day), increased bleeding, and systemic symptoms (fever, malaise, mild anemia, anorexia). In *severe disease,* diarrhea is bloody, contains mucus, and occurs 10 to 20 times a day. In addition, fever, rapid weight loss greater than 10% of total body weight, anemia, tachycardia, and dehydration are present.

Complications

Patients with IBD have both local (confined to the GI tract) and systemic (extraintestinal) complications (Fig. 42.4). GI tract complications include hemorrhage, strictures, perforation (with possible peritonitis), abscesses, fistulas, CDI, and colonic dilation (toxic megacolon). Toxic megacolon is more common with UC. Patients with toxic megacolon are at risk for perforation and may need an emergency colectomy. Perineal abscess and fistulas occur in up to a third of patients with Crohn's disease. CDI increases in frequency and severity in patients with IBD.

IBD is related to an increased risk for colorectal cancer. Those with Crohn's disease are at increased risk for small intestinal cancer. Cancer screening at regular intervals is important in persons with IBD.

People with IBD may have systemic complications, such as multiple sclerosis and ankylosing spondylitis. Some are related to the inflammatory activity in the bowel. They occur with active inflammation and improve when the IBD improves. Other complications include malabsorption, liver disease (primary sclerosing cholangitis), and osteoporosis. Routine liver function tests are important because primary sclerosing cholangitis can lead to liver failure. Both men and women with IBD are at risk for osteoporosis. They need a bone density scan at baseline and every 2 years.

Diagnostic Studies

The diagnosis of IBD includes ruling out diseases with similar symptoms and figuring out whether the patient has Crohn's disease or UC. The symptoms of early Crohn's disease are like those of IBS. Diagnostic studies provide information about disease severity and complications. A CBC typically shows iron-deficiency anemia from blood loss. A high WBC count may be a sign of toxic megacolon or perforation. Decreased serum sodium, potassium, chloride, bicarbonate, and magnesium levels occur due to fluid and electrolyte losses from diarrhea and vomiting. Hypoalbuminemia is present with severe disease because of poor nutrition or protein loss. Increased erythrocyte sedimentation rate, C-reactive protein, and WBCs reflect inflammation. The stool is examined for blood, pus, and mucus. Stool cultures can determine if infection is present.

Imaging studies, such as double-contrast barium enema, small bowel series (small bowel follow through), transabdominal ultrasound, CT, and MRI, are useful for diagnosing IBD. Colonoscopy allows for examination of the entire large intestine lumen and sometimes the most distal ileum. The HCP can determine the extent of inflammation, ulcerations, pseudopolyps, and strictures and obtain biopsy specimens for a definitive diagnosis. Since a colonoscope can enter only the distal ileum, capsule endoscopy (see Chapter 38) may be needed to diagnose Crohn's disease in the small intestine.

Interprofessional Care

The goals of treatment of IBD are to (1) rest the bowel, (2) control the inflammation, (3) combat infection, (4) correct malnutrition, (5) provide symptomatic relief, and (6) improve quality of life. There is no cure for IBD. Treatment relies on drugs to treat the inflammation and maintain remission (Table 42.16). Several drugs are available to treat IBD. Since the recurrence rate is high after surgical treatment of Crohn's disease, drugs are the preferred treatment. Hospitalization is needed if the patient does not respond to drug therapy, the disease is severe, or complications are suspected.

Drug Therapy. The goal of drug treatment in IBD is to induce and maintain remission. Five major classes of drugs are used: aminosalicylates, antimicrobials, corticosteroids, immunomodulators,

TABLE 42.16 Interprofessional Care

Inflammatory Bowel Disease

Diagnostic Assessment
- History and physical examination
- CBC, erythrocyte sedimentation rate
- Serum chemistries
- Testing of stool for occult blood and infection
- Capsule endoscopy
- Radiologic studies with barium contrast
- Sigmoidoscopy and/or colonoscopy with biopsy

Management
- High-calorie, high-vitamin, high-protein, low-residue, lactose-free (if lactase deficiency) diet
- Elemental diet or PN
- Drug therapy (Table 42.17)
  - Aminosalicylates
  - Antimicrobials
  - Biologic therapies
  - Corticosteroids
  - Immunosuppressants
- Physical and emotional rest
- Referral for counseling or support group
- Surgical therapy (Table 42.18)

and biologic therapies (Table 42.17). Drug choice depends on the location and severity of inflammation. Patients are treated with either a "step-up" or a "step-down" approach. With the step-up approach, the patient with mild symptoms begins with an aminosalicylate or antimicrobial and adds a more toxic medication (e.g., biologic therapies) when initial therapies do not work. The step-down approach uses immunosuppressant and biologic therapy first.[14]

Drugs containing 5-aminosalicylic acid (5-ASA) remain the mainstay to achieve and maintain remission and prevent flare-ups of IBD. They include sulfasalazine (Azulfidine) and the new generation of sulfa-free drugs (olsalazine, mesalamine). Aminosalicylates can treat both UC and Crohn's disease. They are much more effective for UC.[14]

The exact mechanism of action of 5-ASA is unclear. We think topical application to the intestinal mucosa suppresses proinflammatory cytokines and other inflammatory mediators. People can take aminosalicylates orally or rectally. Oral forms are available with different coatings that affect where the medication is released along the GI tract. This allows more effective treatment of specific symptoms. Rectal forms include suppositories and enemas. Rectal use offers the advantage of delivering the 5-ASA directly to the affected tissue. This is useful in treating inflammation in the rectum and/or large intestine. The combination of oral and rectal therapy is better than oral or rectal therapy alone.

Corticosteroids can help achieve remission in IBD. They are given for the shortest possible time because of the side effects associated with long-term use. Patients with disease in the left colon, sigmoid, and rectum benefit from suppositories, enemas, and foams because they deliver the corticosteroid directly to the inflamed tissue with minimal systemic effects. Oral prednisone is given to patients with mild to moderate disease who did not respond to either 5-ASA or topical corticosteroids. Those with severe inflammation may need a short course of IV corticosteroids. Corticosteroids must be tapered to very low levels when surgery is planned to prevent postoperative complications (e.g., infection, delayed wound healing, fistula formation).

TABLE 42.17 Drug Therapy

Inflammatory Bowel Disease

Class	Action	Examples
5-Aminosalicylates (5-ASA)	Decrease inflammation by suppressing proinflammatory cytokines and other inflammatory mediators	*Systemic:* balsalazide (Colazal), mesalamine (Pentasa), olsalazine (Dipentum), sulfasalazine (Azulfidine) *Topical:* 5-ASA enema (Rowasa), mesalamine suppositories
Antimicrobials	Prevent or treat secondary infection	ciprofloxacin (Cipro), clarithromycin (Biaxin), metronidazole (Flagyl)
Biologic therapies	Inhibit the cytokine tumor necrosis factor (TNF)	adalimumab (Humira), certolizumab pegol (Cimzia), golimumab (Simponi), infliximab (Remicade)
	Prevent migration of leukocytes from bloodstream to inflamed tissue	natalizumab (Tysabri), vedolizumab (Entyvio)
Corticosteroids	Decrease inflammation	*Systemic:* corticosteroids (prednisone, budesonide [Uceris]); hydrocortisone or methylprednisolone (IV for severe IBD) *Topical:* hydrocortisone suppository or foam (budesonide, Cortifoam) or enema (Cortenema)
Immunosuppressants	Suppress immune response	azathioprine, cyclosporine, methotrexate, 6-mercaptopurine

Immunosuppressants (6-mercaptopurine, azathioprine) are given for several reasons. They can maintain remission after corticosteroid therapy. Patients who do not respond to aminosalicylates, corticosteroids, or antibiotics; have side effects from corticosteroids; or have fistulas may benefit. These drugs require regular CBC monitoring because they can suppress the bone marrow and lead to inflammation of the pancreas or liver. They have a delayed onset of action and are not useful for acute flare-ups.

Methotrexate is most useful in patients with Crohn's disease who cannot stop corticosteroid use without a flare-up or in whom other drugs have been ineffective. Many patients have flu-like symptoms with use. Some develop bone marrow depression and liver dysfunction. Correct dosing is critical to minimize the risk for toxicity. Careful monitoring of the CBC and liver enzymes is essential. Advise women of childbearing age to avoid pregnancy because use causes birth defects and fetal death.

Biologics reduce IBD-related inflammation by blocking specific proteins that play a role in inflammation. There are 2 main classes: anti–tumor necrosis factor (TNF) agents and integrin receptor antagonists.

The anti-TNF agent infliximab (Remicade) is given IV to induce and maintain remission in patients with Crohn's disease and in patients with draining fistulas who do not respond to conventional drug therapy. The other anti-TNF agents are given subcutaneously.[15] The anti-TNF agents have similar side effects. The most common ones are upper respiratory and urinary tract infections, headaches, nausea, joint pain, and abdominal pain. More serious effects include reactivation of hepatitis and tuberculosis (TB); opportunistic infections; and cancers, especially lymphoma. Patients need to know the risks before starting therapy. They are tested for TB and hepatitis before treatment begins and cannot receive live virus immunizations. Teaching includes how to prevent infection and recognize early signs and symptoms (e.g., fever, cough, malaise, dyspnea).

Integrin receptor antagonists include natalizumab (Tysabri) and vedolizumab (Entyvio). They inhibit leukocyte adhesion by blocking α_4-integrin, an adhesion molecule. Use is limited to those who have not had an adequate response with other therapies (corticosteroids, immunosuppressants, anti-TNF agents). Both are given by IV infusion. Their use is associated with increased risk for infection, hepatotoxicity, and hypersensitivity reactions. Because of the risk for progressive multifocal leukoencephalopathy, natalizumab is available only through a restricted program.

The biologic agents do not work for everyone. They are costly and may produce allergic reactions. They are immunogenic, meaning that patients receiving them often make antibodies against them. Immunogenicity leads to acute infusion reactions and delayed hypersensitivity-type reactions. The drugs are most effective when given at regular intervals. Infusion reactions are more likely if a drug is stopped and then restarted.

Surgical Therapy

Ulcerative Colitis. Indications for surgery for UC are outlined in Table 42.18. Surgical procedures used include (1) total proctocolectomy with ileal pouch/anal anastomosis (IPAA) and (2) total proctocolectomy with permanent ileostomy. Since UC affects only the colon, a total proctocolectomy is curative. The most common surgical procedure for UC is a total proctocolectomy with IPAA. For more detail, see the discussion on bowel resection and ostomy surgery later in this chapter on p. 952.

Crohn's Disease. Surgery for Crohn's disease is usually done for complications such as strictures, obstructions, bleeding, and fistula (Table 42.18). Most patients with Crohn's disease eventually need surgery. The most common surgery involves resecting the diseased segments with reanastomosis of the remaining intestine. Unfortunately, the disease often recurs at the anastomosis site. Repeated removal of sections of the small intestine can lead to short bowel syndrome. *Short bowel syndrome (SBS)* occurs when either surgery or disease leaves too little small intestine surface area to maintain normal nutrition and hydration. Lifetime fluid boluses and parenteral nutrition (PN) may be needed. For more detail, see the discussion on short bowel syndrome later in this chapter on p. 962.

TABLE 42.18 Indications for Surgical Therapy for IBD

- Drainage of abdominal abscess
- Failure to respond to conservative therapy
- Fistulas
- Inability to decrease corticosteroids
- Intestinal obstruction
- Massive hemorrhage
- Perforation
- Severe anorectal disease
- Suspicion of cancer

The other common surgery for Crohn's disease is a stricture-plasty. This opens narrowed areas obstructing the bowel. Since the intestine stays intact, it reduces the risk for developing short-bowel syndrome and its associated complications. Recurrences at the site are uncommon.

Nutritional Therapy. An individualized diet is an important part of treating IBD. Patients with IBD need a balanced, healthy diet with enough calories, protein, and nutrients. Consult a dietitian about dietary recommendations. The goals of diet management are to (1) provide adequate nutrition without worsening symptoms, (2) correct and prevent malnutrition, (3) replace fluid and electrolyte losses, and (4) prevent weight loss.

Nutritional deficiencies are due to decreased oral intake, blood loss, and, depending on the location of the inflammation, impaired absorption. Patients may reduce food intake to reduce diarrhea. Inflammatory mediators reduce appetite. Blood loss and malabsorption lead to iron-deficiency anemia (see Chapter 30). The patient may need oral iron supplements. Parenteral or IV iron is an option for those who cannot tolerate oral iron or if anemia is severe. Zinc deficiency can result from ostomies or diarrhea. Zinc supplements may be needed.[16]

Disease of the terminal ileum reduces absorption of cobalamin and bile acids. Reduced cobalamin contributes to anemia. Those who develop anemia should receive cobalamin injections. Bile salts are important for fat absorption and contribute to osmotic diarrhea. Cholestyramine, an ion-exchange resin that binds unabsorbed bile salts, helps control diarrhea.

Drug therapy can contribute to nutritional problems. Patients taking sulfasalazine should take 1 mg folate (folic acid) daily.[16] Those receiving corticosteroids are prone to osteoporosis and need calcium supplements. Potassium supplements may be needed with corticosteroids.

During an acute exacerbation, patients with IBD may not be able to tolerate a regular diet. Liquid enteral feedings are preferred over PN because atrophy of the gut and bacterial overgrowth occur when the GI tract is not used. EN is high in calories and nutrients, lactose free, and easily absorbed. They help achieve remission and improve nutritional status. EN is discussed in Chapter 39.

There are no universal food triggers for IBD, but some may find that certain foods cause diarrhea. A food diary helps to identify problem foods to avoid. Patients are typically taught to then avoid or limit foods that cause GI distress or worsen symptoms.

❖ NURSING MANAGEMENT: INFLAMMATORY BOWEL DISEASE

◆ Nursing Assessment

Table 42.19 outlines the subjective and objective data you should obtain from a patient with IBD.

◆ Nursing Diagnoses

Nursing diagnoses for the patient with IBD include:

- Diarrhea
- Impaired nutritional status
- Difficulty coping
- Chronic pain

For more information on nursing diagnoses and interventions for IBD, see eNursing Care Plan 42.2 on the website for this chapter.

TABLE 42.19 Nursing Assessment
Inflammatory Bowel Disease

Subjective Data
Important Health Information
Past health history: Infection, autoimmune disorders
Medications: Antidiarrheal drugs

Functional Health Patterns
Health perception–health management: Family history of ulcerative colitis or Crohn's disease. Fatigue, malaise
Nutritional-metabolic: Nausea, vomiting; anorexia. Weight loss
Elimination: Diarrhea. Blood, mucus, or pus in stools
Cognitive-perceptual: Lower abdominal pain (worse before defecation), cramping, tenesmus

Objective Data
General
Intermittent fever, emaciated appearance, fatigue

Integumentary
Pale skin with poor turgor, dry mucous membranes. Skin lesions, anorectal irritation, skin tags, cutaneous fistulas

Gastrointestinal
Abdominal distention, hyperactive bowel sounds, abdominal cramps

Cardiovascular
Tachycardia, hypotension

Possible Diagnostic Findings
Anemia, leukocytosis. Electrolyte imbalance, hypoalbuminemia, vitamin, and trace metal deficiencies. Guaiac-positive stool. Abnormal sigmoidoscopy, colonoscopy, and/or barium enema findings

---

◆ Planning

The overall goals are that the patient with IBD will (1) have fewer and less severe acute exacerbations, (2) maintain normal fluid and electrolyte balance, (3) be free from pain or discomfort, (4) adhere to medical regimens, (5) maintain nutritional balance, and (6) have an improved quality of life.

◆ Nursing Implementation

◆ **Acute Care.** During the acute phase, focus your attention on hemodynamic stability, pain control, fluid and electrolyte balance, and nutritional support. Maintain accurate intake and output records. Monitor the number and appearance of stools. Assess for the presence of blood in stools and emesis. Give IV fluids, electrolytes, analgesics, and antiinflammatory drugs as prescribed. Monitor serum electrolytes, CBC, and vital signs, being alert for changes related to diarrhea and dehydration. If the patient has orthostatic hypotension, teach the patient to change position slowly and use safety precautions.

Help the patient stay clean, dry, and free of odor until the diarrhea is under control. Place a deodorizer in the room. Meticulous perianal skin care using plain water (no harsh soap) with a moisturizing skin barrier cream prevents skin breakdown. Dibucaine, witch hazel, sitz baths, and other soothing compresses or ointments may reduce perianal irritation and pain.

Calculate the adequacy of the daily calorie intake. Obtain a daily weight. Assess the abdomen, including bowel sounds, as needed. Consult with a dietitian about diet modifications and the need for nutritional supplements.

Postoperative care after surgical procedures for IBD is similar to that described later in this chapter in the intestinal and ostomy surgery section (see p. 952) and in the general nursing care plan for the postoperative patient (see eNursing Care Plan 19.1 on the website for Chapter 19).

◆ **Ambulatory Care.** IBD is a chronic illness. Assist the patient in accepting the chronicity of IBD and learning ways to cope with its recurrent, unpredictable nature. Teaching includes (1) the importance of rest and diet management, (2) perianal care, (3) drug action and side effects, (4) symptoms of recurrence of disease, (5) when to seek medical care, and (6) ways to reduce stress. Excellent teaching resources, written in easily comprehensible language are available from the Crohn's and Colitis Foundation of America (*www.crohnscolitisfoundation.org*).

It is important to establish rapport and encourage the patient to talk about self-care. Ask patients what you can do to promote their self-care. An explanation of all procedures and treatments helps to build trust, decrease apprehension, and increase self-control. Once you have established a therapeutic relationship, talk with smokers who have Crohn's disease about quitting since smoking is associated with more severe disease.

The patient and caregiver may need your help setting realistic short- and long-term goals. Patients may have severe fatigue, which limits their energy for physical activity. Rest is important. Patients may lose sleep because of frequent episodes of diarrhea and abdominal pain. Nutritional deficiencies and anemia worsen fatigue and leave the patient feeling weak. Teach them to schedule activities around rest periods.

Many patients have intermittent exacerbations and remissions of symptoms. Given the chronicity and uncertainty related to the frequency and severity of flares, the patient may have frustration, depression, and anxiety. Psychotherapy and behavioral therapies may help patients deal with their feelings about the disease and help to manage their symptoms. Because of the relationship between emotions and the GI tract, teach the patient ways to manage stress (see Chapter 6). Suggest the patient seek support through a local or online support group from the Crohn's and Colitis Foundation of America.

◆ **Evaluation**

The expected outcomes are that the patient with IBD will
- Have a decrease in the number of diarrhea stools
- Maintain body weight within a normal range
- Be free from pain and discomfort
- Use effective coping strategies

Gerontologic Considerations: Inflammatory Bowel Disease

A second peak in occurrence of IBD is in the 6th decade. The cause, natural history, and clinical course of IBD are similar to those seen in younger patients. However, in the older patient, proctitis and left-sided UC are more common. Diagnosis is sometimes difficult in older adults since IBD can be confused with CDI, diverticulitis, or colitis.

The interprofessional care of IBD is also similar; however, challenges exist. Drug therapy and surgery have an increased risk for adverse events, hospitalization, and mortality. Older adults are more prone to adverse events from corticosteroids. Immunosuppressant and biologic therapies have a higher risk for infection and cancer. Anemia and malnutrition are more common.[17] They are more vulnerable to volume depletion from diarrhea. Those with physical limitations may have trouble handling fecal urgency and multiple trips to the bathroom without help.

INTESTINAL OBSTRUCTION

Intestinal obstruction occurs when intestinal contents cannot pass through the GI tract. The obstruction may occur in the small (SBO) or large (LBO) intestine. It can be partial or complete, simple or strangulated. Partial obstructions do not completely occlude the intestinal lumen, allowing for some fluid and gas to pass through. They usually resolve with conservative treatment. A complete obstruction totally occludes the lumen and usually requires surgery. A simple obstruction has an intact blood supply; a strangulated one does not.

Types of Intestinal Obstruction

The causes of intestinal obstruction are either mechanical or nonmechanical.

Mechanical. In *mechanical obstruction,* there is a physical obstruction of the intestinal lumen. Most intestinal obstructions occur in the small intestine. Surgical adhesions are the most common cause of SBO.[18] They can occur within days of surgery or years later (Fig. 42.5). Other causes of SBO are hernia, cancer, strictures from Crohn's disease, and intussusception after bariatric surgery. The most common cause of LBO is colorectal cancer (malignant obstruction) followed by diverticular disease. Other causes include adhesions, ischemia, volvulus, and Crohn's disease.[19]

Nonmechanical. A *nonmechanical obstruction* occurs with reduced or absent peristalsis due to altered neuromuscular transmission of the parasympathetic innervation to the bowel. It may result from a neuromuscular or vascular disorder. Paralytic ileus (lack of intestinal peristalsis and bowel sounds) is the most common form of nonmechanical obstruction. It occurs to some degree after any abdominal surgery. It can be hard to know if a postoperative obstruction is due to paralytic ileus or adhesions. One clue is that bowel sounds usually return before postoperative adhesions develop. Other causes of paralytic ileus include peritonitis, inflammatory responses (e.g., acute pancreatitis, acute appendicitis), electrolyte abnormalities (especially hypokalemia), and thoracic or lumbar spinal fractures.

Pseudo-obstruction is a mechanical obstruction without any cause found on radiologic imaging. It is a GI motility disorder. There are several conditions associated with pseudo-obstruction. These include major surgery, electrolyte imbalance, neurologic conditions, medications, sepsis, cancer, trauma, and burns.[20]

Vascular obstructions are rare. They are the result of an interference with the blood supply to a part of the intestines. The most common causes are emboli and atherosclerosis of the mesenteric arteries. Emboli may originate from thrombi in patients who have chronic atrial fibrillation, diseased heart valves, and prosthetic valves. Venous thrombosis may occur in conditions of low blood flow, such as heart failure and shock.

Etiology and Pathophysiology

About 6 to 8 L of fluid enter the small intestine daily. Most of the fluid is absorbed before it reaches the colon. Around 75% of intestinal gas is swallowed air. When an obstruction occurs, fluid, gas, and intestinal contents accumulate proximal to the obstruction. Distention reduces fluid absorption and initially

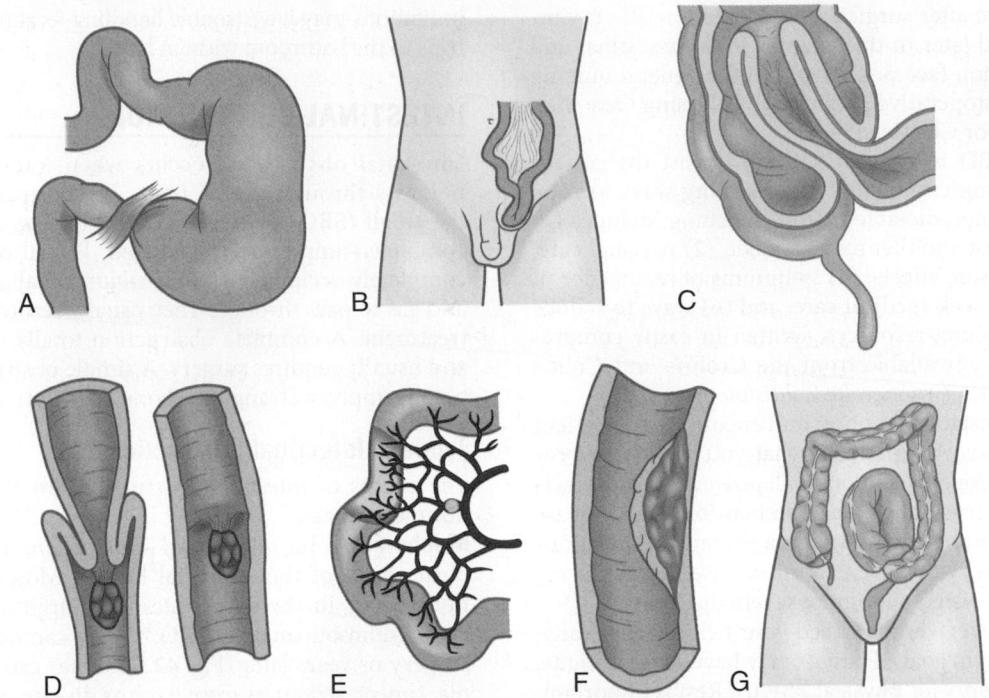

FIG. 42.5 Bowel obstructions. A, Adhesions. B, Strangulated inguinal hernia. C, Ileocecal intussusception. D, Intussusception from polyps. E, Mesenteric occlusion. F, Neoplasm. G, Volvulus of the sigmoid colon.

stimulates intestinal secretions. Distal to the obstruction, the bowel empties, and then collapses. As distention increases in the proximal bowel, intraluminal bowel pressure rises. The increased pressure leads to an increase in capillary permeability and extravasation of fluids and electrolytes into the peritoneal cavity. Eventually the intestinal muscle becomes fatigued, and peristalsis stops. Retention of fluids in the intestine and peritoneal cavity leads to a severe reduction in circulating blood volume. This leads to hypotension and hypovolemic shock.

If blood flow is inadequate, bowel tissue becomes ischemic, then necrotic, and the bowel may perforate. In the most dangerous situation the bowel becomes so distended that the blood flow stops, causing edema, cyanosis, and gangrene of a bowel segment. This is called *intestinal strangulation* or *intestinal infarction*. If not quickly corrected, the bowel will become necrotic and rupture, leading to infection, septic shock, and death.

The location of the obstruction determines the extent of fluid, electrolyte, and acid-base imbalances. If the obstruction is high (e.g., upper duodenum), metabolic alkalosis may result from the loss of gastric hydrochloric (HCl) acid through vomiting or NG intubation and suction. When the obstruction is in the small intestine, dehydration occurs rapidly. Dehydration and electrolyte imbalances do not occur early in large bowel obstruction. If the obstruction is below the proximal colon, solid fecal material accumulates until symptoms of discomfort appear.

Clinical Manifestations

The 4 hallmark clinical manifestations of an obstruction are abdominal pain, nausea and vomiting, distention, and constipation. The order and degree these appear vary by the cause, location, and type of obstruction (Table 42.20). Colicky abdominal pain is usually the first symptom. In SBO, the pain is often of sudden onset. It occurs at 4- to 5-minute intervals for proximal obstructions and less often for distal obstructions. The

TABLE 42.20 Manifestations of Small and Large Intestinal Obstructions

Manifestation	SMALL INTESTINE Proximal	SMALL INTESTINE Distal	Large Intestine
Onset	Rapid	Rapid	Gradual
Vomiting	Frequent and copious	Less frequent	Late or absent
Pain	Colicky, cramping, occurs at frequent intervals	Colicky, occurs more intermittently	Persistent, cramping
Bowel movement	Feces for a short time	Gradual constipation	Obstipation
Abdominal distention	Minimal	Increased	Increased

nature of the vomiting gives a clue to the level of obstruction. In a proximal obstruction, patients rapidly develop nausea and vomiting. It may be projectile and contain bile. Vomiting usually gives temporary relief from abdominal pain in higher obstructions. Vomiting from a more distal small bowel obstruction is more gradual in onset and more fecal and foul smelling. Bowel sounds may be high-pitched above the area of obstruction. Bowel sounds are usually absent with paralytic ileus.

Signs of LBO include abdominal distention, either obstipation or a marked change in bowel function, and lack of flatus. The patient has persistent, cramping abdominal pain. Bowel sounds are usually present and become progressively hypoactive. Vomiting is rare. Strangulation causes severe, constant pain that is rapid in onset.[19]

With both types, abdominal tenderness and rigidity occur. The patient appears acutely ill, with signs of dehydration and sepsis. These include tachycardia, dry mucous membranes, and hypotension. The patient's temperature may rise above 100°F (37.8°C).

Diagnostic Studies

Perform a thorough history and physical examination. Imaging can identify an obstruction and guide decisions about surgery. Abdominal x-rays, CT scan, or contrast enema may be done. Sigmoidoscopy or colonoscopy provides direct visualization of an LBO.

Blood tests include a CBC and blood chemistries. A high WBC count may mean strangulation or perforation. Increased hematocrit values may reflect hemoconcentration. Decreased hemoglobin and hematocrit values may mean bleeding from cancer or strangulation with necrosis. Serum electrolytes, BUN, and creatinine are monitored to assess the degree of dehydration. Metabolic alkalosis can develop from vomiting.

Interprofessional Care

Treatment of a bowel obstruction depends on the cause. If a strangulated obstruction or perforation is present, the patient will need emergency surgery to relieve the obstruction and survive. In some, especially those due to surgical adhesions, an obstruction may resolve without surgery.

Surgery may involve simply resecting the obstructed segment of bowel and anastomosing the remaining healthy bowel back together. Partial or total colectomy, colostomy, or ileostomy may be done when extensive obstruction or necrosis is present. Sometimes, an obstruction can be removed nonsurgically. Colonoscopy offers a means to remove polyps, dilate strictures, and remove and destroy tumors with a laser.

The initial treatment includes placing the patient on NPO status, providing IV fluid therapy with either normal saline or lactated Ringer's solution, and giving IV antiemetics. If needed, insert an NG tube for decompression and give ordered electrolyte replacement. Obtain blood cultures and start IV antibiotic therapy. Some patients need PN to allow bowel rest and improve nutritional status before surgery.

The treatment goal for a patient with a malignant obstruction is to regain patency and resolve the obstruction. Stents can be placed via endoscopic or fluoroscopic procedures. They are used for palliative purposes or as "a bridge to surgery," allowing a patient to avoid emergency surgery.[19] This gives the interprofessional team time to correct fluid volume problems and treat other problems, thus improving surgical outcomes. Corticosteroids with antiemetic properties that decrease edema and inflammation may be used with stent placement.

❖ NURSING MANAGEMENT: INTESTINAL OBSTRUCTION

◆ Nursing Assessment

Intestinal obstruction is a potentially life-threatening condition. Major concerns are preventing fluid and electrolyte deficiencies and early recognition of deterioration in the patient's condition (e.g., hypovolemic shock, sepsis, bowel strangulation). Nursing assessment begins with a detailed patient history and physical examination. Determine the location, duration, intensity, and frequency of abdominal pain.

Record the onset, frequency, color, odor, and amount of vomitus. Assess bowel function, including the passage of flatus. Auscultate for bowel sounds and document their character and location. Inspect the abdomen for scars, visible masses, and distention. Assess whether abdominal tenderness or rigidity is present. Measure the abdominal girth. Check for signs of peritoneal irritation (e.g., muscle guarding, rebound pain). If

the HCP decides to wait to see if the obstruction resolves on its own, assess the patient regularly. Notify the HCP of changes in vital signs, changes in bowel sounds, decreased urine output, increased abdominal distention, and pain.

Maintain a strict intake and output record, including emesis and tube drainage. A urinary catheter allows for hourly monitoring of urine output. Report if the urine output is less than 0.5 mL/kg of body weight per hour. This indicates inadequate vascular volume and the potential for acute kidney injury. Rising serum creatinine and BUN levels are other indicators of acute kidney injury.

◆ Nursing Diagnoses

Nursing diagnoses for the patient with intestinal obstructions include:

- Acute pain
- Fluid imbalance

◆ Planning

The overall goals are that the patient with an intestinal obstruction will have (1) relief of the obstruction and return to normal bowel function, (2) minimal to no discomfort, and (3) normal fluid and electrolyte and acid-base status.

◆ Nursing Implementation

Monitor the patient closely for signs of dehydration and electrolyte imbalances. Give IV fluids as ordered. Assess for signs and symptoms of fluid imbalance. Some patients, especially older adults, may not tolerate rapid fluid replacement. Monitor serum electrolyte levels closely. A patient with a high intestinal obstruction is more likely to have metabolic alkalosis. A patient with a low obstruction is at greater risk for metabolic acidosis. The patient is often restless and constantly changes position to relieve the pain. Provide comfort measures and promote a restful environment. Nursing care of the patient after surgery for an intestinal obstruction is similar to care of the patient after a laparotomy (see p. 935).

With an NG tube in place, oral care is extremely important. Vomiting leaves an unpleasant taste in the patient's mouth, and fecal odor may be present. The patient breathes through the mouth, drying the mouth and lips. Provide frequent oral care and water-soluble lubricant for the lips. Check the nose for signs of irritation from the NG tube. Clean and dry this area daily, apply water-soluble lubricant, and retape the tube. Check the NG tube every 4 hours for patency.

POLYPS OF LARGE INTESTINE

Colonic polyps arise from the mucosal surface of the colon and project into the lumen. They may be *sessile* (flat, broad based, and attached directly to the intestinal wall) or *pedunculated* (attached to the intestinal wall by a thin stalk). Polyps tend to be sessile when small and become pedunculated as they enlarge (Fig. 42.6). They may be found anywhere in the large intestine. As patients age, polyps are increasingly present in the proximal colon. Rectal bleeding and occult blood in the stool are the most common signs, but most patients with polyps are asymptomatic.

Types of Polyps

The most common types of polyps are hyperplastic and adenomatous. *Hyperplastic polyps* are noncancerous. They rarely grow larger than 5 mm and never cause clinical symptoms. Other benign polyps include inflammatory polyps, lipomas, and juvenile polyps.

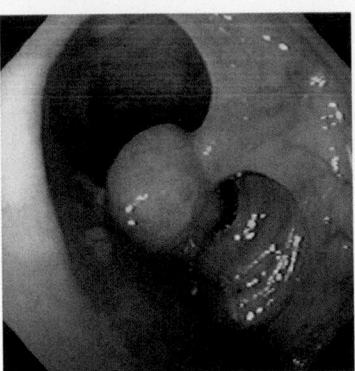

FIG. 42.6 Endoscopic image of pedunculated polyp in descending colon. (Courtesy David Bjorkman, MD, University of Utah School of Medicine, Department of Gastroenterology. In McCance KL, Huether SE: *Pathophysiology: The biologic basis for disease in adults and children*, ed 6, St Louis, 2010, Mosby.)

Adenomatous polyps are neoplastic and closely linked to colorectal adenocarcinoma. There are 3 types: tubular, tubulovillous, and villous. Villous or large adenomatous polyps are more likely to have cancers develop in them. Removing adenomatous polyps decreases the occurrence of colorectal cancer.

Genetic Link

Familial adenomatous polyposis (FAP) is the most common polyposis syndrome (see the Genetics in Clinical Practice box), causing 1% of all CRCs. FAP is a genetic disorder characterized by hundreds or sometimes thousands of polyps in the colon that appear during adolescence and early adulthood. They eventually become cancerous, usually by age 40. Since CRC is inevitable,

---

GENETICS IN CLINICAL PRACTICE

Familial Adenomatous Polyposis (FAP)

Genetic Basis
- Autosomal dominant FAP
  - Classic form of disease
  - Mutations in adenomatous polyposis coli *(APC)* gene
  - Normally this is a tumor suppressor gene involved in DNA repair
  - Normally this gene makes a protein that keeps polyps from developing in the colon
  - 50% of the offspring of a patient with FAP carry the *FAP* gene
- Autosomal recessive FAP
  - Autosomal recessive disorder
  - Mutations in the *mutY* homolog *(MUTYH)* gene
  - Normally this gene is involved in DNA repair
  - Characterized by fewer polyps, typically <100

Incidence
- Affects 1 in 7000 to 22,000 people
- Equally affects men and women

Genetic Testing
- DNA testing is available

Clinical Implications
- Anyone with a family history of FAP should undergo genetic testing during childhood
- If the FAP gene is present, colorectal screening begins at puberty, and annual colonoscopy begins at age 16
- Persons with a family history of FAP can benefit from genetic counseling

---

TABLE 42.21 Risk Factors for Colorectal Cancer

- Alcohol (≥4 drinks/wk)
- Cigarette smoking
- Family history of colorectal cancer (first-degree relative)
- Family or personal history of familial adenomatous polyposis (FAP)
- Family or personal history of hereditary nonpolyposis colorectal cancer (HNPCC) syndrome
- Obesity (body mass index ≥30 kg/m²)
- Personal history of colorectal cancer, inflammatory bowel disease, or diabetes
- Red meat (≥7 servings/wk)

---

the colon and rectum are removed, usually by age 25, by proctocolectomy with an IPAA or an ileostomy. Patients with classic FAP are at risk for cancers of the thyroid, stomach, small intestine, liver, and brain, so lifetime cancer surveillance is essential.

Diagnostic Studies and Interprofessional Care

Colonoscopy, sigmoidoscopy, barium enema, and virtual colonoscopy (CT or MRI colonography) are used to discover polyps. Colonoscopy is preferred because it allows evaluation of the total colon. All polyps are considered abnormal and should be removed *(polypectomy)*. Polyps can be removed during colonoscopy or sigmoidoscopy. They cannot be removed during barium enema and virtual colonoscopy. After polypectomy, watch the patient for rectal bleeding, fever, severe abdominal pain, and abdominal distention, which may indicate hemorrhage or perforation.

COLORECTAL CANCER

Of cancers that affect both men and women, colorectal cancer (CRC) is the third leading cause of cancer-related deaths and the third most common cancer in men and women. Annually about 140,250 people in the United States are diagnosed with CRC and 50,600 people die from CRC.[21]

CRC is more common in men than in women. The risk for CRC increases with age, with about 90% of new CRC cases detected in people older than 50. However, while the incidence of CRC in people over 50 years is decreasing, the number of cases in people aged 20 to 49 years is rising and expected to continue to do so.[22] This is thought to be related to diet, physical inactivity, and increasing rates of obesity.

PROMOTING HEALTH EQUITY

Colorectal Cancer

- Blacks are most likely to develop colorectal cancer (CRC).
- Blacks are more likely to die of CRC than any other ethnic group.
- Cancer may occur at an earlier age in blacks and Hispanics.
- Hispanics are the least likely to undergo CRC screening.

Etiology and Pathophysiology

Unlike some other cancers, no single risk factor accounts for most cases of CRC (Table 42.21). The risk is highest in those with first-degree relatives with CRC and people with IBD. About 20% of cases of CRC occur in patients with a family history of CRC. Hereditary forms of CRC, including FAP and hereditary nonpolyposis colorectal cancer (HNPCC) syndrome (Lynch syndrome), account for another 10% of cases.

About 30% to 50% of people with CRC have an abnormal *KRAS* gene. The *KRAS* gene, which is primarily involved in regulating cell division, belongs to a class of genes known as *oncogenes*. When mutated, oncogenes have the potential to cause normal cells to become cancerous.

🧬 GENETICS IN CLINICAL PRACTICE

Hereditary Nonpolyposis Colorectal Cancer (HNPCC) or Lynch Syndrome

Genetic Basis
- Autosomal dominant disorder
- Mutations in *MSH2, MLH1, MSH6,* or *PMS2* genes
- These genes are involved with the repair of mistakes in DNA replication

Incidence
- Affects 1 in 500 to 2000 people

Genetic Testing
- DNA testing is available

Clinical Implications
- Accounts for 3% to 5% of all CRC
- Depending on the genetic mutation, the risk for developing CRC is from 50% to 80%
- If colon polyps are present, they occur at an earlier age than do polyps in the general population and are more prone to become cancerous
- Have increased risk for stomach, brain, ovary, uterus, skin, urinary tract, small bowel, and bile ducts cancers
- People with HNPCC need to have a colonoscopy every year
- Women with HNPCC should undergo ovarian and endometrial cancer screening

---

Maintaining a healthy weight, being physically active, limiting alcohol use, not smoking, and eating a diet with large amounts of fruits, vegetables, and grains may decrease the risk for CRC.

CRC usually starts as a polyp on the inner lining of the colon or rectum that grows over a period of 10 to 20 years. Most polyps are adenomas, which arise from the cells that make mucus. As the tumor grows, the cancer invades and penetrates the wall of colon or rectum (Fig. 42.7). Eventually cancer cells gain access to the lymph nodes and vascular system and spread to distant sites. Since venous blood leaving the colon and rectum flows through the portal vein and the inferior rectal vein, the liver is a common site of metastasis. The cancer spreads from the liver to other sites, including the lungs, bones, and brain. CRC can also spread directly into adjacent structures.

Clinical Manifestations

CRC develops slowly, and symptoms do not appear until the disease is advanced. Common manifestations include iron-deficiency anemia, rectal bleeding, abdominal pain, and change in bowel habits.

Physical findings may include:
- *Early disease:* None or nonspecific findings (fatigue, weight loss)
- *More advanced disease:* Abdominal tenderness, palpable abdominal mass, hepatomegaly, ascites

Bleeding can occur with both right- and left-sided CRC. Bleeding on the right side is more common than on the left side. It is often unrecognized, and an early manifestation is often anemia. Hematochezia (fresh blood in the stool) is more often caused by left-sided CRC than right-sided CRC.

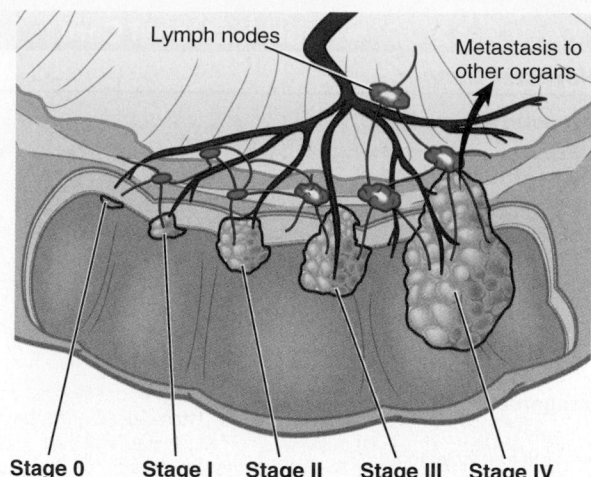

FIG. 42.7 The 5 stages of colorectal cancer. Stage 0 cancer has not grown beyond the mucosal layer. Stage I cancer has grown beyond the mucosa into the submucosa, but no lymph nodes are involved. Stage II cancer has grown beyond the submucosa into the muscle, but there is no lymph node involvement or metastasis. Stage III cancer is any tumor with lymph node involvement but no metastasis. Stage IV cancer is any tumor with lymph node involvement and metastasis.

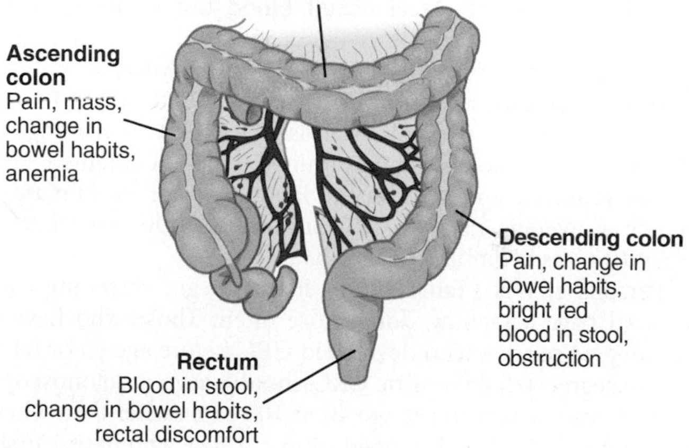

Transverse colon
Pain, obstruction, change in bowel habits, anemia

Ascending colon
Pain, mass, change in bowel habits, anemia

Descending colon
Pain, change in bowel habits, bright red blood in stool, obstruction

Rectum
Blood in stool, change in bowel habits, rectal discomfort

FIG. 42.8 Signs and symptoms of colorectal cancer by location of primary cancer. (Modified from McCance KL, Huether SE: *Pathophysiology: The biologic basis for disease in adults and children*, ed 6, St Louis, 2010, Mosby.)

Right-sided cancers are more likely to cause diarrhea. Left-sided cancers are usually detected later and could present with bowel obstruction (Fig. 42.8). Complications of CRC include obstruction, bleeding, perforation, peritonitis, and fistula formation.

Diagnostic Studies

Obtain a thorough history with close attention to family history (Table 42.22). Since symptoms of CRC do not become evident until the disease is advanced, there is an increased emphasis on screening. Beginning at age 45 and continuing until age 75, men and women at average risk for developing CRC should have screening tests to detect both polyps and cancer based on 1 of these testing schedules:
- Flexible sigmoidoscopy (every 5 years)
- Colonoscopy (every 10 years)

TABLE 42.22 Interprofessional Care

Colorectal Cancer

Diagnostic Assessment
- History and physical examination
- Digital rectal examination
- Testing of stool for occult blood
- CBC
- Liver function tests
- Barium enema
- Sigmoidoscopy and/or colonoscopy with biopsy
- Abdominal CT scan, ultrasound, or MRI
- Carcinoembryonic antigen (CEA) test

Management
- Surgery
  - Right hemicolectomy
  - Left hemicolectomy
  - Abdominal-perineal resection
  - Laparoscopic colectomy
- Chemotherapy
- Targeted therapy
- Radiation therapy

TABLE 42.23 TNM Classification of Colorectal Cancer

T	**Primary Tumor**
T_x	Cannot assess primary tumor because of incomplete information.
T_{is}	Carcinoma in situ. Cancer is in earliest stage and has not grown beyond mucosa layer.
T_1	Tumor has grown beyond mucosa into the submucosa.
T_2	Tumor has grown through submucosa into muscularis propria.
T_3	Tumor has grown through the muscularis propria into the pericolorectal tissues.
T_4	Tumor invades the visceral peritoneum or invades or adheres to adjacent organ or structure.
N	**Lymph Node Involvement**
N_x	Cannot assess lymph nodes.
N_0	No regional lymph node involvement is found.
N_1	Cancer is found in 1 to 3 nearby lymph nodes.
N_2	Cancer is found in 4 or more nearby lymph nodes.
M	**Metastasis**
M_x	Cannot assess presence of metastasis.
M_0	No distant metastasis seen.
M_1	Distant metastasis is present.

- Double-contrast barium enema (every 5 years)
- CT colonography (virtual colonoscopy) (every 5 years)
- Tests that primarily find cancer include:
  - High-sensitivity fecal occult blood test (FOBT) (every year), *or*
  - Fecal immunochemical test (FIT) (every year)
  - Stool DNA test (every 3 years)

Colonoscopy is the gold standard for CRC screening. It allows the entire colon to be examined, biopsies obtained, and polyps removed and sent to the laboratory for examination. People at average risk for CRC should undergo colonoscopy every 10 years beginning at age 45.

Persons at risk (Table 42.21) should begin screening earlier and have screening done more often. Those who have a first-degree relative who developed CRC before age 60 or have 2 first-degree relatives with CRC should have a colonoscopy every 5 years beginning at age 40 or 10 years earlier than when the youngest relative developed cancer. Those who have 1 first-degree relative who had CRC after age 60 should have a colonoscopy every 10 years beginning at age 40.[23]

Less favorable, but acceptable, screening methods include stool testing for fecal blood. The FOBT and FIT look for blood in the stool. Stool tests must be done yearly since tumor bleeding occurs at intervals and may easily be missed if a single test is done. Stool DNA tests (PreGen-Plus, Cologuard) can detect DNA mutations that may occur with CRC.

Once tissue biopsies confirm the diagnosis of CRC, the patient needs a CBC to check for anemia and liver function tests. A CT scan or MRI of the abdomen will be done to detect liver metastases, retroperitoneal and pelvic disease, and depth of penetration of tumor into the bowel wall. However, liver function tests may be normal even when metastasis has occurred.

Carcinoembryonic antigen (CEA) is a complex glycoprotein sometimes made by CRC cells. It may be used to monitor for disease recurrence after surgery or chemotherapy but is not a good screening tool because of the large number of false-positive findings. CEA levels also may be increased in noncolon cancers (e.g., gastric, pancreatic, breast, thyroid cancers) as well

TABLE 42.24 Classification System Used to Stage Colorectal Cancer

Stage*	TNM†	5-Yr Survival Rate (%)
0	$T_{is} N_0 M_0$	>96
I	$T_1 N_0 M_0$	92
	$T_2 N_0 M_0$	87
II	$T_3 N_0 M_0$	70–80
III	Any T, $N_{1-2} M_0$	53–84
IV	Any T, any N, M_1	12

*Staging system is shown in Fig. 42.7.
†See Table 42.23.

as some noncancerous conditions, like IBD, pancreatitis, cirrhosis, and chronic obstructive pulmonary disease.

Interprofessional Care

The prognosis and treatment of CRC correlates with pathologic staging of the disease. The most commonly used staging system is the tumor, node, metastasis (TNM) staging (Table 42.23). As with other cancers, prognosis worsens with greater size and depth of tumor, lymph node involvement, and metastasis (Table 42.24).

Surgical Therapy. Goals of surgical therapy include (1) complete resection of the tumor, (2) a thorough exploration of the abdomen to determine if the cancer has spread, (3) removing all lymph nodes that drain the area where the cancer is located, (4) restoring bowel continuity so that normal bowel function will return, and (5) preventing surgical complications.

Some polyps can be removed during colonoscopy, while others require surgery. Polypectomy during colonoscopy can be used to resect CRC in situ. It is considered successful when the resected margin of the polyp is free of cancer, the cancer is well differentiated, and there is no apparent lymphatic or blood vessel involvement.

The decision for surgical treatment depends on the staging and location of the cancer and the ability to restore normal bowel function and continence. Surgical removal of stage I cancer includes removing the tumor and at least 5 cm of intestine on either side of it, plus nearby lymph nodes. The remaining cancer-free ends are sewn back together (anastomosis). Laparoscopic surgery is sometimes used for stage I tumors, especially those in the left colon. Low-risk stage II tumors are treated with wide resection and reanastomosis. Chemotherapy is used after surgery for high-risk stage II tumors. Stage III tumors are treated with surgery and chemotherapy. Radiation and chemotherapy may be done before surgery to reduce tumor size.

When the tumor is not resectable or metastasis is present, palliative surgery can control hemorrhage or relieve a malignant bowel obstruction. Chemotherapy and radiation can control the spread and provide pain relief. A few patients with limited lung or liver metastases can achieve a cure after primary and metastatic tumor resection and chemotherapy. In rectal cancer, the location and size of the tumor determines the course of treatment. Local excision may be an option. If the tumor is in the distal rectum (1 to 2 cm from the anorectal junction) and the sphincters cannot be preserved, the patient will undergo an *abdominal-perineal resection (APR)*. An APR involves removing the entire rectum with the tumor, and the patient will have a permanent colostomy.

If the tumor is in the mid or proximal rectum, it may be possible to preserve the sphincters with a low anterior resection (LAR). A LAR involves removing the rectum and anastomosing the colon to the anal canal. A temporary ileostomy or colostomy may be done to divert stool and allow time for the anastomosis to heal. Another option if the anal sphincters remain is for the HCP to create an alternative reservoir with either a colonic J-pouch or coloplasty. A LAR is increasingly common because of advancements in laparoscopy and stapling techniques.

Chemotherapy and Targeted Therapy. Chemotherapy can be used to shrink the tumor before surgery, as an adjuvant therapy after colon resection, and as palliative treatment for nonresectable cancer. Adjuvant chemotherapy is recommended for patients with stage III tumors. Current protocols include varying doses of fluorouracil and leucovorin alone or in combination with oxaliplatin (Eloxatin) or irinotecan (Camptosar). The preferred protocol includes oxaliplatin. Oral fluoropyrimidines (e.g., capecitabine [Xeloda]) in combination with oxaliplatin are an alternative to fluorouracil/leucovorin.[24]

Several targeted therapies have a role in treating metastatic CRC. Angiogenesis inhibitors, which inhibit the blood supply to tumors, include aflibercept (Zaltrap), bevacizumab (Avastin), and ramucirumab (Cyramza). Cetuximab (Erbitux) and panitumumab (Vectibix) block the epidermal growth factor receptor. These drugs are often given with a combination chemotherapy regimen (e.g., fluorouracil/leucovorin/oxaliplatin).

Regorafenib (Stivarga) is a multikinase inhibitor that blocks several enzymes that promote cancer growth. It, or Lonsurf, a combination of trifluridine and tipiracil, are given to patients with metastatic CRC who are no longer responding to other therapies. Trifluridine impairs DNA function and angiogenesis. Tipiracil prevents the rapid metabolism of trifluridine, thus increasing its bioavailability.

Radiation Therapy. Some patients may receive radiation therapy as an adjuvant to surgery and chemotherapy or as a palliative measure for those with metastatic cancer. As a palliative measure, the primary goal is to reduce tumor size and provide symptomatic relief. Radiation therapy is described in Chapter 15.

TABLE 42.25 Nursing Assessment
Colorectal Cancer

Subjective Data

Important Health Information

Past health history: Previous breast or ovarian cancer, familial polyposis, villous adenoma, adenomatous polyps, IBD

Medications: Medications affecting bowel function (e.g., laxatives, antidiarrheal drugs)

Functional Health Patterns

Health perception–health management: Family history of colorectal, breast, or ovarian cancer; weakness, fatigue

Nutritional-metabolic: High-calorie, high-fat, low-fiber diet. Anorexia, nausea and vomiting, weight loss

Elimination: Change in bowel habits, alternating diarrhea and constipation, defecation urgency. Rectal bleeding, mucoid stools. Black, tarry stools. Increased flatus, decrease in stool caliber. Feelings of incomplete evacuation

Cognitive-perceptual: Abdominal and low back pain, tenesmus

Objective Data

General

Pallor, cachexia, lymphadenopathy (later signs)

Gastrointestinal

Palpable abdominal mass, distention, ascites, and hepatomegaly (liver metastasis)

Possible Diagnostic Findings

Anemia. Guaiac-positive stools, palpable mass on digital rectal examination. Positive sigmoidoscopy, colonoscopy, barium enema, or CT scan. Positive biopsy

❖ NURSING MANAGEMENT: COLORECTAL CANCER

◆ Nursing Assessment

Table 42.25 outlines the subjective and objective data you should obtain from a patient with CRC.

◆ Nursing Diagnoses

Nursing diagnoses for the patient with CRC include:
- Diarrhea or constipation
- Anxiety
- Difficulty coping

◆ Planning

The overall goals are that the patient with CRC will have (1) normal bowel elimination patterns, (2) quality of life appropriate to the disease progression, (3) relief of pain, and (4) feelings of comfort and well-being.

◆ Nursing Implementation

◆ Health Promotion. Encourage all persons over 45 to have regular CRC screening. Help identify those at high risk who need screening at an earlier age. Discuss with patients how taking part in cancer screening helps decrease mortality rates. Realize that barriers exist, including lack of accurate information and fear of diagnosis.

Endoscopic and radiographic procedures can only reveal polyps when the bowel has been adequately prepared. Provide teaching about bowel cleansing for outpatient diagnostic procedures and give cleansing preparations to inpatients (see more on diagnostic procedures in Chapter 38).

◆ **Acute Care.** Nursing care for the patient after a colon resection is discussed in depth in the next section. If enough healthy bowel remained that the HCP could reconnect the bowel ends, normal bowel function is maintained. Routine postoperative care is appropriate. Patients with more extensive surgery (e.g., APR) may have an open wound and drains (e.g., Jackson-Pratt, Hemovac) and a permanent ostomy. Postoperative care includes sterile dressing changes, care of drains, and patient and caregiver teaching about the ostomy. Ostomy care is discussed in the next section on pp. 954–957.

◆ **Ambulatory Care.** Psychologic support for the patient and caregiver dealing with the diagnosis of cancer is important. Discuss the patient's feelings about the prognosis and future screening. Patients need much emotional support. The special needs of the cancer patient are discussed in Chapter 15. You may need to address issues surrounding palliative care, end-of-life issues, and hospice (see Chapter 9).

Patients with CRC need to know how to manage changes that result from cancer and cancer treatment. Those who had sphincter-sparing surgery may have diarrhea and incontinence of feces and gas. They may need antidiarrheal drugs or bulking agents to control the diarrhea, but overuse can result in constipation. A consult with a dietitian or wound, ostomy, and continence nurse (WOCN) may help patients and caregivers understand how to manage food and fluid options. Ostomy rehabilitation, including teaching and ongoing support, should be available for all ostomy patients. Patients with skin changes from incontinence and/or radiation therapy will need help with managing these conditions.

◆ **Evaluation**

The expected outcomes for the patient with CRC are that the patient will
- Have minimal changes in bowel elimination patterns
- Achieve optimal nutritional intake
- Experience quality of life appropriate to disease progression
- Have feelings of comfort and well-being

BOWEL RESECTION AND OSTOMY SURGERY

Surgical resection of the bowel may be done to (1) remove cancer; (2) repair a perforation, fistula, or traumatic injury; (3) relieve an obstruction or stricture; and (4) treat an abscess, inflammatory disease, or hemorrhage. For example, if a person has stage III CRC, the HCP will remove the diseased part of the colon along with a certain margin of healthy tissue. It may be a prophylactic procedure for those with complications from IBD. Patients at high risk for CRC, such as those with FAP, and patients with UC may have a total colectomy and an ileostomy.

Depending on the problem being treated, the following surgical procedures may be done:
- *Total proctocolectomy with IPAA:* 2 surgeries, 8 to 12 weeks apart. The first includes colectomy, rectal mucosectomy, ileal pouch (reservoir) construction, ileoanal anastomosis, and temporary ileostomy. A diverting ileostomy is done, and an ileal pouch is created and anastomosed directly to the anus (Fig. 42.9). The second involves closure of the ileostomy to direct stool toward the new pouch.

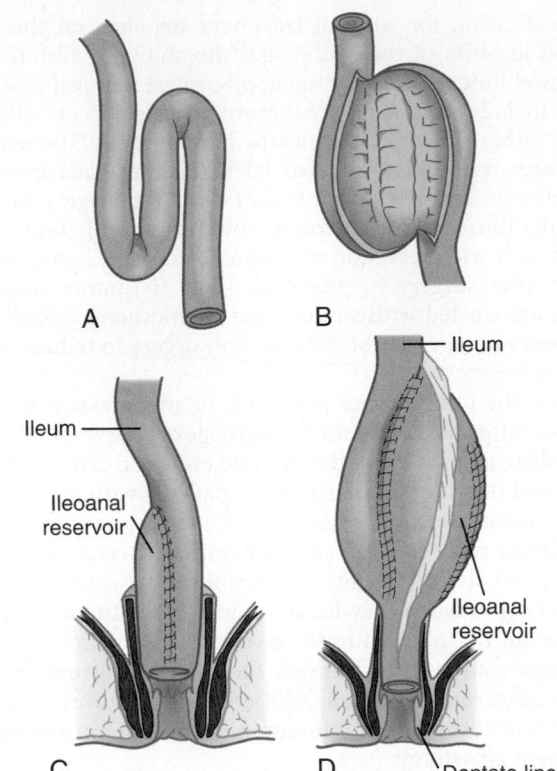

FIG. 42.9 Ileoanal pouch (reservoir). **A,** Formation of a pouch. **B,** Posterior suture lines completed. **C,** J-shaped configuration for ileoanal pouch (J-pouch). **D,** S-shaped configuration for ileoanal pouch (S-pouch).

- *Proctocolectomy with a permanent ileostomy:* Removal of the colon, rectum, and anus with closure of the anal opening. The end of the terminal ileum is brought out through the abdominal wall to form a permanent ileostomy.
- *Right hemicolectomy:* Removal of ascending colon and hepatic flexure with the ileum anastomosed to transverse colon.
- *Left hemicolectomy:* Removal of splenic flexure, descending colon, and sigmoid colon with the transverse colon anastomosed to rectum.
- *Anterior rectosigmoid resection:* Removal of part of descending colon, the sigmoid colon, and upper rectum with the descending colon anastomosed to remaining rectum.
- *Abdominal-perineal resection (APR):* Removal of the entire rectum with creation of a permanent colostomy.
- *Low anterior resection (LAR):* Removal of the rectum and with anastomosis of the colon to the anal canal. A temporary ileostomy or colostomy may be done to divert stool and allow time for the anastomosis to heal. After 8 to 12 weeks, the ostomy can be "taken down," and the ends of the colon surgically reconnected.

Ostomy. An **ostomy** is a surgically created opening on the abdomen that allows the discharge of body waste when the normal elimination route is no longer possible. The outermost part that is visible is a *stoma*. The stoma is the result of the large or small bowel being brought to the outside of the abdomen and sutured in place. When a stoma is created as a fecal diversion, feces will drain through the stoma instead of the anus.

Ostomies are named according to their location and type (Fig. 42.10). An ostomy in the ileum is an ileostomy. An ostomy in the colon is a colostomy. The ostomy is further characterized

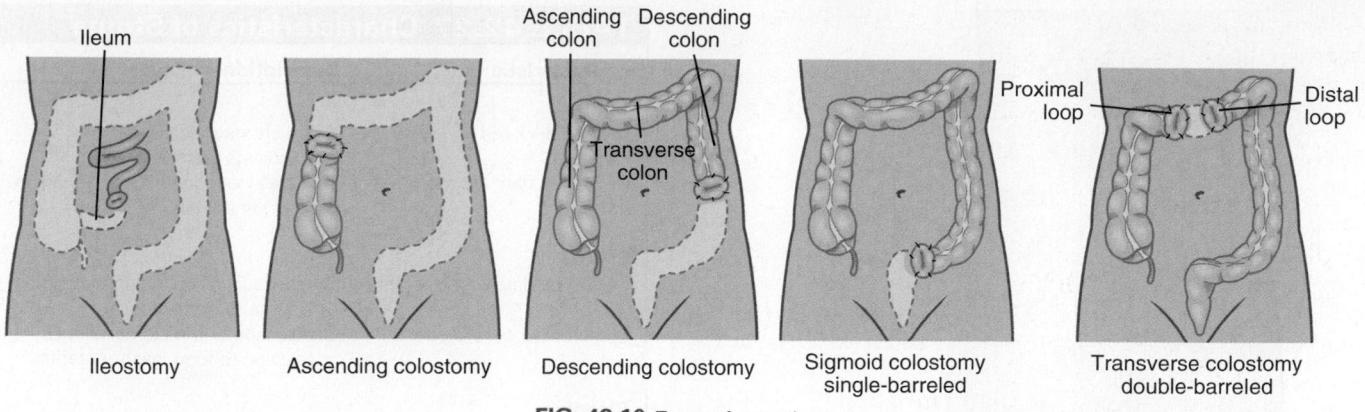

FIG. 42.10 Types of ostomies.

Characteristic	Ileostomy	COLOSTOMY		
		Ascending	**Transverse**	**Sigmoid**
Stool consistency	Liquid to semiliquid	Semiliquid	Semiliquid to semiformed	Formed
Fluid requirement	Increased	Increased	Possibly increased	No change
Bowel regulation	No	No	No	Yes, if there is a history of a regular bowel pattern
Pouch and skin barriers	Yes	Yes	Yes	Dependent on regulation
Indications for surgery	Ulcerative colitis, Crohn's disease, diseased or injured colon, familial polyposis, trauma, cancer	Perforating diverticulum in lower colon, trauma, rectovaginal fistula, inoperable tumors of colon, rectum, or pelvis	Same as for ascending	Cancer of the rectum or rectosigmoid area, perforating diverticulum, trauma

TABLE 42.26 Comparison of Ileostomy and Colostomy

by its anatomic site (e.g., ascending, transverse, sigmoid). The more distal the ostomy, the more functioning bowel remains and the more likely that the intestinal contents will resemble the feces that would have been eliminated from an intact colon and rectum. Ileostomy output will be a liquid to thin paste since it did not enter the colon. Patients have no control over ileostomy drainage; it is involuntary. An ileostomy drains frequently, and the patient must wear an ostomy appliance (pouch) to collect the drainage. In contrast, sigmoid colostomy output resembles normal formed stool. Some patients can regulate emptying time with colostomy irrigation and may not need to wear a pouch. See Table 42.26 for a comparison of colostomies and ileostomies.

Ostomies may be temporary or permanent. For example, the person with a draining fistula may need a temporary ostomy to prevent stool from reaching the diseased area. Cancer involving the rectum requires a permanent ostomy if all bowel distal to the ostomy is removed.

Permanent ostomies may be continent or traditional. *Continent ileostomies* (e.g., Koch pouch, Barnett Continent Ileal Reservoir) use 40 to 45 cm of the terminal ileum to fashion an internal pouch, nipple valve, and abdominal stoma. The pouch replaces the rectum as a reservoir for stool. It can hold around 500 mL of material. Continent ostomies are an option for patients who have had a prior APR with ileostomy for UC or FAP. Patients must be motivated and compliant. They must drain the pouch manually by inserting a catheter through the nipple valve. At first, this is done every 1 to 2 hours. As the pouch enlarges, the frequency decreases to 4 times daily and as needed.

They must keep the stool consistency relatively fluid by following a low-residue diet.

The major types of traditional ostomies include end, double-barreled, and loop ostomy.

End Stoma. An end stoma is made by dividing the bowel and bringing out the proximal end as a single stoma, making a colostomy or ileostomy. The distal part of the GI tract is surgically removed or the distal segment is oversewn and left in the abdominal cavity with its mesentery intact. If the distal bowel is removed, the stoma is permanent. When the distal bowel is oversewn and not removed, the procedure is called a *Hartmann's pouch* (Fig. 42.11). With a Hartmann's pouch, the potential exists for the bowel to be reanastomosed and the stoma closed (referred to as a *takedown*).

Loop Stoma. A loop stoma is made by bringing a loop of bowel to the abdominal surface and then opening the anterior wall of the bowel to provide fecal diversion. This results in 1 stoma with a proximal opening for feces and a distal opening for mucus drainage from the distal colon. An intact posterior wall separates the 2 openings. A plastic rod holds the loop of bowel in place for 7 to 10 days after surgery to prevent it from slipping back into the abdominal cavity (Fig. 42.12). A loop stoma is usually temporary.

Double-Barreled Stoma. To create a double-barreled stoma, the HCP divides the bowel and both the proximal and distal ends are brought through the abdominal wall as 2 separate stomas (Fig. 42.10). The proximal stoma is the functioning stoma. The distal, nonfunctioning stoma is a *mucus fistula*. A double-barreled stoma is usually temporary.

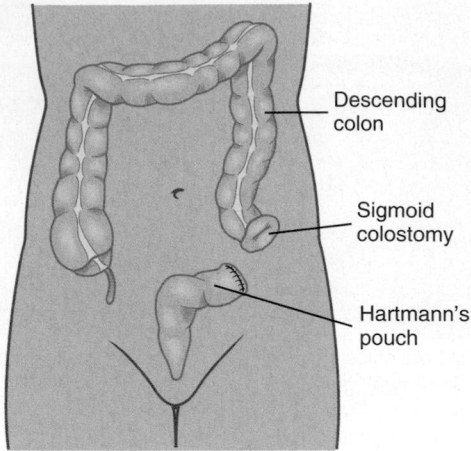

FIG. 42.11 Sigmoid colostomy. Distal bowel is oversewn and left in place to create Hartmann's pouch.

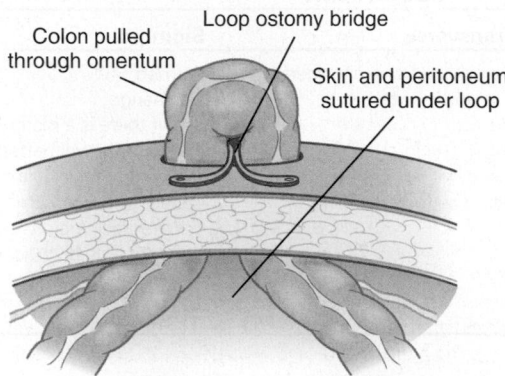

FIG. 42.12 Loop colostomy.

TABLE 42.27 **Characteristics of Stoma**

Characteristic	Description or Cause
Color	
Rose to brick-red	Viable stoma mucosa.
Pale	May indicate anemia.
Blanching, dark red to purple	Indicates inadequate blood supply to the stoma or bowel.
Edema	
Mild to moderate edema	Normal in initial postoperative period. Trauma to the stoma.
Moderate to severe edema	Obstruction of the stoma, allergic reaction to food, gastroenteritis.
Bleeding	
Small amount	Oozing from stoma mucosa when touched is normal because of its high vascularity.
Moderate to large amount	Could indicate lower GI bleeding, coagulation factor deficiency, stomal varices secondary to portal hypertension.

❖ NURSING MANAGEMENT: BOWEL RESECTION AND OSTOMY SURGERY

◆ Preoperative Care

Psychologic preparation and emotional support are particularly important as the person begins to cope with potential changes in body image and elimination. The patient and caregiver should understand the extent of surgery planned. It is normal for the patient and caregiver to have questions concerning the procedures. Provide the patient opportunities to share concerns and questions. This will enhance the patient's feelings of control and ability to cope.

Care that is unique to ostomy surgery includes (1) psychologic preparation for the ostomy, (2) educational preparation, and (3) selecting the best site for the stoma. Ideally, the management of patients facing ostomy surgery begins preoperatively. If available, a WOCN should visit with the patient and caregiver to determine the patient's ability to perform self-care, identify support systems, and determine any modifications that could promote learning during recovery.

A WOCN should choose the site where the ostomy will be and mark the abdomen before surgery. The site should be within the rectus muscle, on a flat surface, and in a place that the patient is able to see. Stomas placed outside the rectus muscle increase the chance of developing a hernia. A flat site makes it much easier to create a good seal and avoid leakage from the bag. Being able to see the stoma makes caring for it easier. Whenever possible, it should be discreetly hidden under clothing and appropriate for normal activities.

◆ Postoperative Care

If the patient's wound is closed or partially closed, assess the incision for suture integrity and signs and symptoms of wound inflammation and infection. A patient who has an open wound with packing needs meticulous care. Reinforce dressings and change them often during the first several hours postoperatively when drainage is likely to be profuse. Carefully assess all drainage for amount, color, and consistency. The drainage is usually serosanguineous.

Assess the wound regularly and record bleeding, excess drainage, and unusual odor. Monitor for edema, erythema, and drainage around the suture line, as well as fever and a high WBC count. Observe the skin around any drains for signs of inflammation. Keep the area around the drain clean and dry. Complications that can occur include delayed wound healing, hemorrhage, fistulas, and infections.

If an ostomy is present, assess the stoma and place a clear pouching system that protects the skin and contains drainage and odor. The stoma should be rosy pink to red and mildly swollen (Table 42.27). A dusky blue stoma indicates ischemia; a brown-black stoma indicates necrosis. Assess and document stoma color every 4 hours and ensure that there is no excess bleeding. Report any sustained color changes or bleeding to the HCP. Edema will resolve over the first 6 weeks.

The colostomy starts functioning when peristalsis returns. Record the volume, color, and consistency of the drainage. When a colostomy is done on a colon that was not cleaned out before surgery, stool will drain when peristalsis returns. If the bowel was cleansed preoperatively, it will not begin producing stool until a few days after the patient is eating again. Excessive amounts of gas are common during the first 2 weeks. Because this can be distressing to patients, assure them this is temporary.

In the first 24 to 48 hours after surgery, the amount of drainage from an ileostomy may be negligible. When peristalsis returns, ileostomy output may be as high as 1500 to 1800 mL/24 hr.

If the small bowel is shortened by surgery, drainage may be greater. This is because the patient has lost the absorptive functions provided by the colon and the delay provided by the ileocecal valve. Observe the patient for signs and symptoms of fluid and electrolyte imbalance, particularly potassium, sodium, and fluid deficits. Over a period of days to weeks, the proximal small bowel adapts and increases fluid absorption. Then, feces will thicken to a paste-like consistency and the volume decrease to around 500 mL/day. Patients, especially those with Crohn's disease, are at risk for developing a bowel obstruction during the first 30 days postoperatively.

After an IPAA, initially, patients may have 4 to 6 stools or more daily. Adaptation over the next 3 to 6 months will result in fewer bowel movements. The patient can control defecation at the anal sphincter.

After intraoperative manipulation of the anal canal, transient incontinence of mucus may occur. Have the patient start Kegel exercises about 4 weeks after surgery to strengthen the pelvic floor and sphincter muscles (see Table 45.18). Perianal skin care is important to protect the epidermis from mucous drainage and maceration. Teach the patient to gently clean the skin with a mild cleanser, rinse well, and dry thoroughly. A moisture barrier ointment and a perineal pad may be used. Some patients have phantom rectal pain or still feel as if they need to have a bowel movement. This is normal and often subsides over time. Be astute in distinguishing phantom sensations from perineal abscess pain.

◆ Colostomy Care

Two major aspects of nursing care for the patient with an ostomy are (1) patient and caregiver teaching about ostomy care and (2) emotional support as the patient copes with a radical change in body image. With shorter hospital stays, patient teaching should focus on the critical aspects that patients need to master. Teaching must include (1) basic skills about managing the ostomy (e.g., changing the pouch), (2) diet, and (3) how to get help for problems. Home care and outpatient follow-up may be helpful, especially if there is access to a WOCN. Patient and caregiver teaching is outlined in Table 42.28. Nursing care for the patient with an ostomy is discussed in eNursing Care Plan 42.3 on the website.

An appropriate pouching system is vital to protect the skin and provide dependable stool collection. Most pouching systems have an adhesive skin barrier and a pouch to collect the feces. Most skin barriers are made of pectin-based or karaya mediums with hydrocolloid properties. Adhesion occurs in 2 phases. First, the wafer's backing has adhesive material that forms an immediate bond with the skin. Second, the hydrocolloids interface with the moisture on the skin to form a tighter seal. Caulking strips or "paste" around the stoma may help ensure a secure seal.

If the abdominal stoma site has bends or creases, it is hard to get a good seal and the skin barrier will pull away faster. Since excess weight of collected stool pulls the wafer away from the skin, empty ostomy bags when one-third full.

Use a transparent pouch in the initial postoperative period so that you can easily assess stoma viability and pouch application by the patient. Each time the pouch is changed, assess the skin for irritation. If the peristomal skin is irritated and raw, more products may have to be applied. Do not allow feces to remain on the skin or irritation will quickly develop. If a pouch has failed, it must be changed at once.

TABLE 42.28 Patient & Caregiver Teaching
Ostomy Self-Care

Include the following points when teaching the patient and/or caregiver about self-care of an ostomy:

1. Explain what an ostomy is and how it functions.
2. Describe the underlying condition that resulted in the need for an ostomy.
3. Demonstrate and allow the patient and caregiver to practice the following activities:
   - Remove the old skin barrier, cleanse the skin, and correctly apply new skin barriers.
   - Apply, empty, clean, and remove the pouch.
   - Empty the pouch before it is one-third full to prevent leakage.
4. Irrigate the colostomy to regulate bowel elimination (optional).
5. Explain how to contact the wound, ostomy, and continence nurse (WOCN) with questions.
6. Describe how to obtain ostomy supplies.
7. Explain dietary and fluid management.
   - Identify a well-balanced diet and dietary supplements to prevent nutritional deficiencies.
   - Identify foods to avoid to reduce diarrhea or gas (see Table 42.29).
   - Promote fluid intake of least 3000 mL/day to prevent dehydration (unless contraindicated).
   - Increase fluid intake during hot weather, excess perspiration, and diarrhea to replace losses and prevent dehydration.
   - Describe symptoms of fluid and electrolyte imbalance.
   - Explain how to contact the dietitian with questions.
   - Explain how to recognize problems (fluid and electrolyte deficits, fever, diarrhea, skin irritation, stomal problems) and how to contact the HCP and/or WOCN.
8. Describe community resources to assist with emotional and psychologic adjustment to the ostomy.
9. Explain the importance of follow-up care.
10. Describe the ostomy's potential effects on sexual activity, social life, work, and recreation and ways to manage these changes.

NURSING MANAGEMENT
Ostomy Care

Although licensed practical/vocational nurses (LPN/VNs) and unlicensed assistive personnel (UAP) provide much of the ostomy care for patients with established ostomies, patients with new ostomies have complex needs and require frequent assessment, planning, intervention, and evaluation by a registered nurse (RN).

Role of Nursing Personnel
Registered Nurse (RN)
- Assess and document stoma and peristomal skin appearance.
- For patient with a new ostomy, assess patient's psychologic preparation for ostomy care.
- Choose appropriate ostomy pouching system for patient.
- Place ostomy pouching system for a new ostomy.
- Monitor the volume, color, and odor of the ostomy drainage.
- Develop plan of care for skin care around the ostomy.
- Teach ostomy care and skin care to patient and caregiver.
- Irrigate new colostomy, if indicated.
- Teach colostomy irrigation to patient and caregiver.
- Teach patient and caregivers about appropriate dietary choices (Table 42.29).
- Delegate to UAP:
  - Empty ostomy bag and measure liquid contents.
  - Place the ostomy pouching system for an established ostomy.
  - Assist stable patient with colostomy irrigation.

TABLE 42.29 Nutritional Therapy

Effects of Food on Stoma Output

Odor Producing	Gas Forming	Diarrhea Causing
Alcohol	Beans	Alcohol
Asparagus	Beer	Beer
Broccoli	Cabbage family	Cabbage family
Cabbage	Carbonated beverages	Coffee
Eggs	Cheeses (strong)	Fruits (raw)
Fish	Onions	Green beans
Garlic	Sprouts	Spicy foods
Onions		Spinach

A colostomy in the ascending and transverse colon has semiliquid stools. Have the patient use a drainable pouch. A drainable pouch may last up to 4 to 7 days. A colostomy in the sigmoid or descending colon has semiformed or formed stools. The patient can use a drainable pouch or choose a disposable, closed end pouch changed every day. Optional charcoal filters can deodorize and automatically release flatus. They are available for both drainable and nondrainable pouches.

Another option is colostomy irrigation. It may be used to stimulate emptying of the colon. Patients who irrigate may not need a regular pouch as they may be able to regulate when the colon empties. Regularity is possible only when the stoma is in the distal colon. The patient may need to wear only a pad or small pouch over the stoma as little or no spillage should occur between irrigations. Irrigation requires manual dexterity and adequate vision. People who irrigate regularly should have ostomy bags available in case they develop diarrhea.

Teach the patient about the importance of fluids and a healthy diet. The effect of food on stoma output is individual. Most patients with colostomies can eat anything they want. However, some choose to avoid certain foods because of possible increased gas, odor, or stoma output (Table 42.29). Teach patients to chew their food very well to reduce the chance of blockage.

The patient can resume activities of daily living within 6 to 8 weeks but should avoid heavy lifting. The patient's physical condition determines when they can resume sports. Swimming with an ostomy pouch intact is not a problem. The patient can bathe and shower with or without the pouching system in place because water does not harm the stoma.

◆ Ileostomy Care

Nursing care for a patient with an ileostomy is similar to that for a patient with a colostomy. Because the stool from an ileostomy is caustic to the skin, a secure pouching system is important. This is easier with stoma protrusion of at least 1 to 1.5 cm. When the stoma is flat, recessed, or in a crease, seepage occurs and results in altered skin integrity. The patient must wear a pouch at all times since regularity is not possible with an ileostomy. An open-ended, drainable pouch is best so drainage can be easily emptied. A drainable pouch usually lasts for 4 to 7 days.

Patients need to increase fluid intake to at least 2 to 3 L/day or more when there are excess fluid losses from heat and sweating. They may need to ingest added sodium. Patients must learn signs and symptoms of fluid and electrolyte imbalance so that they can take appropriate action.

The ileostomy patient is susceptible to obstruction because the lumen is less than 1 inch in diameter. It may narrow further at the point where the bowel passes through the fascia/muscle layer of the abdomen. Foods such as nuts, raisins, popcorn, coconut, mushrooms, olives, stringy vegetables, foods with skins, dried fruits, and meats with casings must be chewed extremely well before swallowing.

◆ Psychologic Adaptation to an Ostomy

The patient's response to a new ostomy is highly individualized. Some have minimal difficulty and view their ostomy positively. It may be curative if their presenting condition was UC or a step toward remission if the diagnosis was CRC. Other patients may have a grief reaction from the loss of a body part and a change in body image. They may be angry, depressed, or resentful. Anxiety and fear are normal. Concerns about stool leaking, odor, sounds of flatus, pouch reliability, and changes in normal lifestyle are all valid worries. Accurate information, emotional support, and mastering basic skills will help patients learn to live a full life with an ostomy and accept the changes in body appearance.

The patient's emotional state may limit the ability to take part in teaching and ostomy care. Discuss with the patient the psychologic impact of the stoma and its effect on body image and self-esteem. Help the patient identify ways of coping with depression and anxiety resulting from the illness, surgery, or postoperative problems. Support from the caregiver, family, and friends is vital. It reassures the patient of their value despite having the ostomy. Encourage patients to share their concerns and ask questions. Provide information in an easily understood manner and help patients develop confidence and competence in managing the stoma.

New ostomy patients will have questions on a variety of topics ranging from managing gas to intimacy to travel. Give the names and contact information for support groups. The Wound Ostomy Continence Nurses Society (www.wocn.org), local support groups, and United Ostomy Associations of America (www.ostomy.org) provide practical information about living with an ostomy. Online support groups are also available. Most hospitals have a visitor's program. These programs give the patient and caregiver an opportunity to talk with a person who has adjusted well to an ostomy and had some of the same feelings and concerns they have.

◆ Sexual Function

Help the patient understand if specific aspects of surgery and treatment have the potential for sexual dysfunction. Pelvic surgery can disrupt nerve and vascular supplies to the genitalia. Pelvic radiation can reduce blood flow to the pelvis by causing scarring in the small blood vessels. Chemotherapy can alter sexual function. The patient's overall physical health influences sexual desire. Generalized fatigue caused by illness can decrease desire. Understanding this information can help patients plan the timing of sexual activity.

Problems with sexual dysfunction depend on the surgical technique used. Unfortunately, any pelvic surgery that removes the rectum has the potential of damaging the parasympathetic nerve plexus. The HCP should discuss the possibility with the patient.

For men, the main concern may be erection and ejaculation. Erection depends on intact parasympathetic and nonadrenergic noncholinergic nerves as well as adequate blood supply. Sympathetic nerve damage in the presacral area can disrupt the ability to ejaculate. This can occur with the APR procedure. Sexual dysfunction may be temporary and resolve in 3 to 12

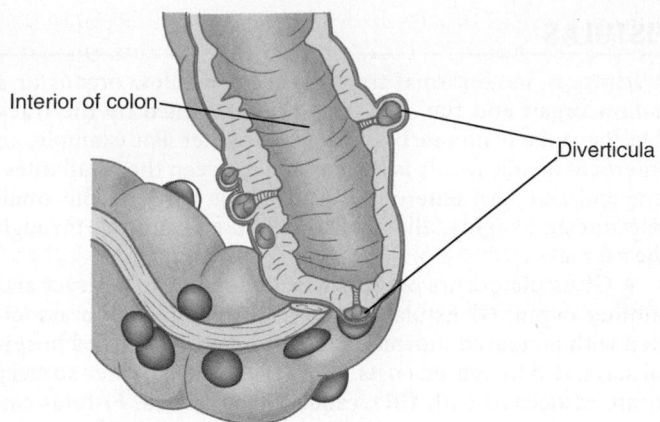

FIG. 42.13 Diverticula are outpouchings of the colon. When they become inflamed, the condition is diverticulitis. The inflammatory process can spread to the surrounding area in the intestine.

PATHOPHYSIOLOGY MAP

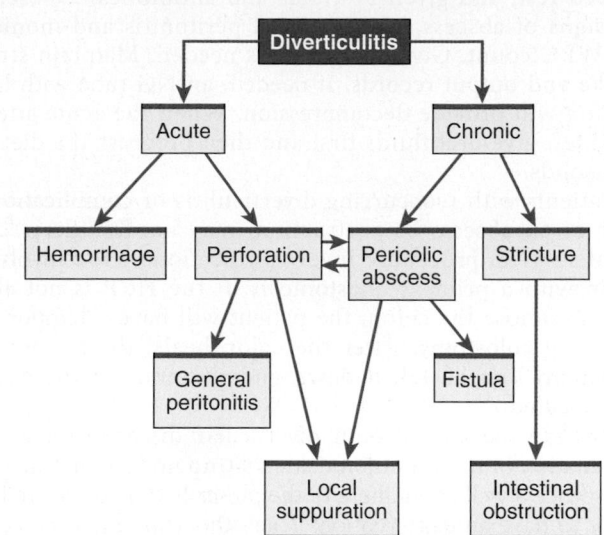

FIG. 42.14 Complications of diverticulitis.

months. Nerve-sparing surgical techniques are used when possible to preserve sexual function.

For women, nerve damage can result in vaginal dryness and decreased sensation in the vagina and clitoris, making arousal and achieving orgasm more challenging. Experimenting with positions and using lubrication may help. A woman with an ostomy can still become pregnant.

Sexual function and sexuality concerns affect most patients with an ostomy. The patient with a stoma may fear rejection by a partner or that others will not find them desirable. Discuss sexuality and sexual function. Help the patient realize that it takes time to adjust to the pouch and to body changes before feeling secure with sexual functioning.

Teach the patient to empty the pouch before sexual activities. Some may apply a smaller pouch during sexual activity. Women may consider wearing open panties, a short slip, or similar lingerie. Men may consider wearing a wrap or cummerbund around the midsection to secure the pouch. There are many types of pouch covers that patients can make or purchase.

DIVERTICULOSIS AND DIVERTICULITIS

Diverticula are saccular dilations or outpouchings of the mucosa that develop in the colon (Fig. 42.13). Diverticulosis is the presence of multiple noninflamed diverticula. **Diverticulitis** is inflammation of 1 or more diverticula, resulting in perforation into the peritoneum. Clinically, diverticular disease covers a spectrum from asymptomatic, uncomplicated diverticulosis to diverticulitis with complications, such as perforation, abscess, fistula, and bleeding. Diverticula are common, especially in older adults, but most people never develop diverticulitis.

Etiology and Pathophysiology

Diverticula may occur anywhere in the GI tract but are most common in the left (descending, sigmoid) colon. They seem to occur at weak points in the intestinal wall, such as where the blood vessels pass through the muscle layer. The cause is thought to include both genetic and environmental factors. We think the main contributing factors are constipation and a lack of dietary fiber. The disease is more prevalent in Western, industrialized populations, where people tend to consume diets low in fiber and high in refined carbohydrates. Diverticula are uncommon in vegetarians. Other risk factors are obesity, inactivity, smoking, excess alcohol use, and NSAID use.

Clinical Manifestations and Complications

Most patients with diverticulosis have no symptoms. Those with symptoms typically have abdominal pain, bloating, flatulence, and changes in bowel habits. In more serious situations, the diverticula bleed or diverticulitis develops. The most common signs and symptoms of diverticulitis are acute pain in the left lower quadrant, distention, decreased or absent bowel sounds, nausea, vomiting, and systemic symptoms of infection (fever, leukocytosis with a shift to the left). Older adults with diverticulitis may be afebrile, with a normal WBC count and little, if any, abdominal tenderness. Diverticulitis can cause erosion of the bowel wall and perforation into the peritoneum (Fig. 42.14). A localized abscess develops when the body walls off the perforated area. Peritonitis develops if it cannot be contained. Bleeding can be extensive but usually stops spontaneously.

Diagnostic Studies

Diverticular disease can be asymptomatic. It is typically found during routine sigmoidoscopy or colonoscopy. Diagnosis of diverticulitis is based on the history and physical examination (Table 42.30). The preferred diagnostic test is a CT scan with oral contrast. Abdominal and chest x-ray rule out other causes of acute abdominal pain.

❖ Interprofessional and Nursing Care

A high-fiber diet, mainly from fruits and vegetables with a decreased intake of fat and red meat, is the best way to prevent diverticular disease. High levels of physical activity seem to decrease the risk. Currently there is no evidence to support the theory that diverticulitis can be prevented by avoiding nuts and seeds.

In acute diverticulitis, the goal of treatment is to let the colon rest and the inflammation subside. Some patients can be managed at home with a clear liquid diet, bed rest, and analgesics. Hospitalization is needed if symptoms are severe, the patient is unable to tolerate oral fluids, there are systemic manifestations of infection (fever, significant leukocytosis), or the patient has co-morbid conditions (e.g., immunosuppression).

If hospitalized, the patient is kept on NPO status, placed on bed rest, and given IV fluids and antibiotics.[25] Observe for signs of abscess, bleeding, and peritonitis and monitor the WBC count. Give analgesics as needed. Maintain strict intake and output records. If needed, an NG tube with low suction will provide decompression. When the acute attack subsides, give oral fluids first and then progress the diet to semisolids.

Patients with reoccurring diverticulitis or complications, such as an abscess or obstruction, may need surgery. The usual surgical procedure involves resection of the involved colon with a primary anastomosis. If the HCP is not able to anastomose the colon, the patient will have a temporary diverting colostomy. After the colon heals, the temporary colostomy can be taken down and the ends of the colon reconnected.

Provide the patient with diverticular disease with a full explanation of the condition. Patients who understand the disease process well and adhere to the prescribed regimen are less likely to have an exacerbation. Teach them the importance of following a high-fiber diet (Table 42.8) and encourage a fluid intake of at least 2 L/day. The patient does not have to avoid nuts, seeds, and corn.

A patient with diverticular disease should avoid increased intraabdominal pressure because it may precipitate an attack. Factors that increase intraabdominal pressure are straining at stool, vomiting, bending, heavy lifting, and wearing tight, restrictive clothing. Weight reduction is important for the obese person with diverticular disease.

TABLE 42.30 Interprofessional Care

Diverticulosis and Diverticulitis

Diagnostic Assessment
- History and physical examination
- Testing of stool for occult blood
- CBC
- Urinalysis
- Barium enema
- Colonoscopy with biopsy
- Blood culture
- CT scan with oral contrast
- Abdominal and/or chest x-ray

Management

Conservative Therapy
- High-fiber diet
- Dietary fiber supplements
- Stool softeners
- Anticholinergics
- Clear liquid diet
- Weight reduction (if overweight)

Acute Care: Diverticulitis
- Antibiotic therapy
- NPO status
- IV fluids
- Analgesics
- NG suction
- Surgery
- Possible resection of involved colon
- Possible temporary colostomy

FISTULAS

A fistula is an abnormal tract between 2 hollow organs or a hollow organ and the skin. Fistulas are named by the track that they take from one body part to another. For example, an enterocutaneous fistula is an opening between the small intestine and skin. An enterovaginal fistula is between the small intestine and vagina, allowing stool and gas to drain through the vagina.

A GI fistula occurs between the lumen of the GI tract and another organ. GI fistulas are a serious complication associated with increased morbidity and mortality, extended hospital stays, and increased costs. Most fistulas occur after surgery or are associated with IBD, cancer, or radiation. Fistulas can form with diverticulitis, pancreatitis, and trauma.[26] Fistulas are classified as simple or complex and by the amount of output. A simple fistula has only one short, direct tract. A complex fistula is associated with an abscess, involves multiple organs, and may open into the base of a wound. High-output fistulas drain more than 500 mL/day, moderate-output fistulas drain 200 to 500 mL/day, and low-output fistulas drain less than 200 mL/day.

Fever and abdominal pain are early signs of a fistula. Other manifestations depend on the type of fistula. With an enterocutaneous fistula, there may be pus or intestinal contents draining through the skin opening. Patients with a colocutaneous (colon to skin) fistula may have stool or pus draining through the opening. If a colovesical (colon to urinary tract) fistula is present, manifestations include fecaluria (passing stool with urination), recurrent urinary tract infections, dysuria, and hematuria.

❖ Interprofessional and Nursing Care

A draining fistula can be disheartening for the patient and caregiver and a time-consuming challenge for HCPs. Managing a fistula requires (1) identifying the fistula tract, (2) maintaining fluid and electrolyte balance, (3) controlling infection, (4) protecting the surrounding skin, (5) managing output, and (6) providing nutritional support. Most fistulas heal spontaneously. Surgery may be needed to treat the complications.

Appropriate fluid and electrolyte replacement can be challenging, especially when the patient has a high-output fistula. Monitor the volume of fistula output as this guides replacement therapies and nutritional support. Assess the character of the drainage, noting the color, consistency, and odor. Monitor laboratory values. Low serum levels of potassium, magnesium, and phosphorus from the loss of GI fluids are common. Give IV fluids and electrolyte replacement as ordered. Keep an accurate intake and output record. Many patients are NPO as this reduces intestinal output. They may receive acid suppression with a proton-pump inhibitor and antimotility agents (e.g., loperamide). Cholestyramine and octreotide decrease GI secretions.[26] Measure vital signs frequently and be alert for signs of dehydration.

Malnutrition is a significant problem, particularly if the patient is NPO or has a small intestinal fistula. Consult a dietitian. High-calorie, high-protein PN or EN is needed to provide enough calories and protein to replace losses and support healing.[26] Many patients need trace element (e.g., copper, zinc, magnesium) and vitamin supplements.

Maintaining skin integrity and optimizing healing is essential. Consult a WOCN if available. Low-output fistulas may be managed with a simple absorbent dressing. A high-output enterocutaneous fistula often needs advanced techniques, including specialty pouches; barrier creams, powders, and sealants to protect the skin; and negative pressure wound therapy.

HERNIAS

A hernia is a protrusion of the viscus (e.g., the intestine) through an abnormal opening or a weakened area in the wall of the cavity in which it is normally contained. A hernia may occur in any part of the body, but it usually occurs within the abdominal cavity. *Reducible* hernias easily return into the abdominal cavity. Reducing can be done manually or may occur spontaneously when the person lies supine. *Irreducible*, or *incarcerated*, hernias cannot be placed back into the abdominal cavity. They have abdominal contents trapped in the opening. Strangulation occurs if the blood supply to the contents trapped in an irreducible hernia becomes compromised. The result is an acute intestinal obstruction. Gangrene and necrosis of the hernia contents are possible.

Types

An *umbilical hernia* occurs when the rectus muscle is weak (as with obesity) or the umbilical opening does not close after birth (Fig. 42.15, *A*). A *femoral hernia* occurs when there is a protrusion through the femoral ring into the femoral canal. It appears as a bulge below the inguinal ligament. Femoral hernias easily strangulate (Fig. 42.15, *B*).

The *inguinal hernia* is the most common type of hernia and occurs at the point of weakness in the abdominal wall where the spermatic cord (in men) or the round ligament (in women) emerges (Fig. 42.15, *C*).

Ventral or *incisional hernias* are due to weakness of the abdominal wall at the site of a previous incision. They occur most often in those who are obese, have had multiple surgical procedures in the same area, or have had inadequate wound healing because of poor nutrition or infection. Peristomal hernias are ventral hernias.

Clinical Manifestations

Pain is the classic symptom of a hernia. It may worsen with activities that increase intraabdominal pressure, such as lifting, coughing, and straining. A hernia may be readily visible, especially when the person tenses the abdominal muscles. If the hernia becomes strangulated, the patient will have severe pain and symptoms of a bowel obstruction, such as vomiting, cramping abdominal pain, and distention.

❖ Interprofessional and Nursing Care

Diagnosis of a hernia is usually based on history and physical examination findings. Ultrasound, CT, and MRI can help identify a hernia and determine the contents. Laparoscopic surgery is the treatment of choice. The surgical repair of a hernia, known as a *herniorrhaphy*, is usually an outpatient procedure. Reinforcing the weakened area with wire, fascia, or mesh is known as a *hernioplasty*. Emergency surgery is needed for strangulated hernias or inflamed, irreducible hernias. Surgery for strangulated hernias involves resecting the involved area with possible placement of a temporary colostomy.

After a hernia repair, the patient may have problems voiding. Measure intake and output. Observe for a distended bladder. Scrotal edema is a painful complication after an inguinal hernia repair. A scrotal support with application of an ice bag and elevating the scrotum may help relieve pain and edema. Encourage

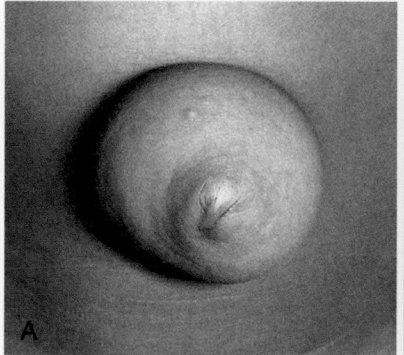
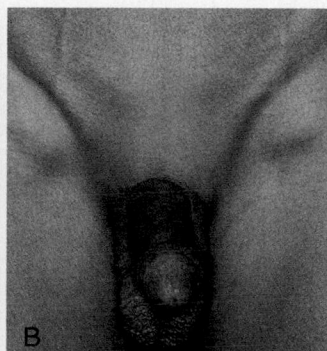
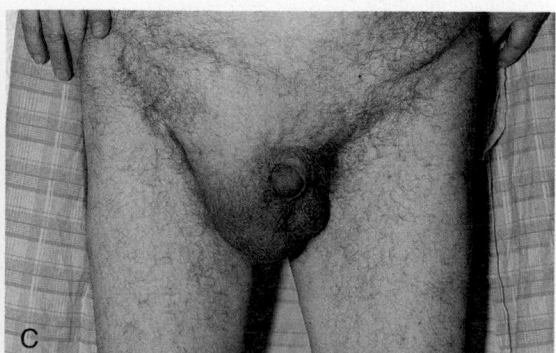

FIG. 42.15 A, Umbilical hernia. B, Femoral hernias (note swelling below the inguinal ligaments). C, Right inguinal hernia. (*A* and *B*, From Zitelli BJ, McIntire SC, Nowalk AJ: *Zitelli and Davis' atlas of pediatric physical diagnosis*, ed 6, Philadelphia, 2012, Saunders. *C*, From Swartz MH: *Textbook of physical diagnosis: History and examination*, ed 6, Philadelphia, 2010, Saunders.)

deep breathing, but not coughing. Teach patients to splint the incision and keep their mouths open when coughing or sneezing is unavoidable. The patient may be restricted from heavy lifting (>10 lb) for 6 to 8 weeks.

MALABSORPTION SYNDROME

Malabsorption results from impaired absorption of fats, carbohydrates, proteins, minerals, and vitamins. The stomach, small intestine, liver, and pancreas regulate normal digestion and absorption. Digestive enzymes ordinarily break down nutrients so that absorption can take place. Malabsorption may occur if this process is interrupted at any point. Several problems can cause malabsorption (Table 42.31). Lactose intolerance is the most common malabsorption disorder, followed by IBD, celiac disease, tropical sprue, and cystic fibrosis.

The most common signs of malabsorption are weight loss, diarrhea, and steatorrhea (bulky, foul-smelling, yellow-gray, greasy stools with putty-like consistency) (Table 42.32). Steatorrhea does not occur with lactose intolerance.

Tests to determine the cause of malabsorption include qualitative examination of stool for fat (e.g., Sudan III stain), a 72-hour stool collection for quantitative measurement of fecal fat, serologic testing for celiac disease, and fecal elastase testing to determine if there is pancreatic insufficiency. Near-infrared reflectance analysis (NIRA) for fecal fat is available at some centers in the United States.

Other diagnostic studies include a CT scan and endoscopy to obtain a small bowel biopsy specimen. A small bowel barium enema can identify abnormal mucosal patterns. Capsule endoscopy is useful in assessing the small intestine for changes in mucosal integrity and inflammation. Tests for carbohydrate malabsorption include the D-xylose test and the lactose tolerance test. Laboratory studies include a CBC, measurement of prothrombin time (to see if vitamin K absorption is adequate), serum vitamin A and carotene levels, serum electrolytes, cholesterol, and calcium. Treatment depends on the cause.

CELIAC DISEASE

Celiac disease is an autoimmune disease that causes damage to the small intestinal mucosa. It is triggered by ingesting gluten, a protein in wheat, barley, and rye.[27] It can occur at any age and has a wide variety of symptoms. *Celiac sprue* and *gluten-sensitive enteropathy* are other names for celiac disease.

Celiac disease is not the same disease as *tropical sprue*, a chronic disorder occurring primarily in tropical areas. Tropical sprue causes progressive disruption of jejunal and ileal tissue,

---

TABLE 42.31 Causes of Malabsorption

Bacterial Proliferation
- Parasitic infection
- Tropical sprue

Biochemical or Enzyme Deficiencies
- Biliary tract obstruction
- Chronic pancreatitis
- Cystic fibrosis
- Lactase deficiency
- Pancreatic insufficiency
- Zollinger-Ellison syndrome

Disturbed Lymphatic and Vascular Circulation
- Heart failure
- Ischemia
- Lymphangiectasia
- Lymphoma

Small Intestinal Mucosal Disruption
- Celiac disease
- Crohn's disease
- Whipple's disease

Surface Area Loss
- Billroth II gastrectomy
- Distal ileal resection, disease, or bypass
- Short bowel syndrome

TABLE 42.32 Manifestations of Malabsorption

Manifestations	Pathophysiology
Cardiovascular	
Hypotension	Dehydration
Peripheral edema	Protein malabsorption, protein loss in diarrhea
Tachycardia	Hypovolemia, anemia
Gastrointestinal	
Diarrhea	Impaired absorption of water, sodium, fatty acids, bile salts, and carbohydrates
Flatulence	Bacterial fermentation of unabsorbed carbohydrates
Glossitis, cheilosis, stomatitis	Deficiency of iron, riboflavin, cobalamin, folic acid, and other vitamins
Steatorrhea	Undigested and unabsorbed fat
Weight loss	Malabsorption of fat, carbohydrates, and protein leading to loss of calories. Marked reduction in caloric intake or increased use of calories
Hematologic	
Anemia	Impaired absorption of iron, cobalamin, and folic acid
Hemorrhagic tendency	Vitamin C deficiency. Vitamin K deficiency inhibiting production of clotting factors II, VII, IX, and X
Integumentary	
Brittle nails	Iron deficiency
Bruising	Vitamin K deficiency
Dermatitis	Fatty acid deficiency, zinc deficiency, niacin, and other vitamin deficiencies
Hair thinning and loss	Protein deficiency
Musculoskeletal	
Bone pain	Osteoporosis from impaired calcium absorption. Osteomalacia secondary to hypocalcemia, hypophosphatemia, inadequate vitamin D
Muscle wasting	Protein malabsorption
Tetany	Hypocalcemia, hypomagnesemia
Weakness, muscle cramps	Anemia, electrolyte depletion (especially potassium)
Neurologic	
Altered mental status	Dehydration
Night blindness	Thiamine deficiency, vitamin A deficiency
Paresthesias	Cobalamin deficiency
Peripheral neuropathy	Cobalamin deficiency

resulting in nutrition problems. It is treated with folic acid and tetracycline.

Celiac disease affects about 1 in 100 people worldwide.[28] First-degree relatives of someone with celiac disease have a 4% to 15% chance of developing the disorder. It is associated with other autoimmune diseases, particularly rheumatoid arthritis, type 1 diabetes, and thyroid disease. It is slightly more common in women. Symptoms often begin in childhood.

Etiology and Pathophysiology

Three factors necessary for developing celiac disease are genetic predisposition, gluten ingestion, and an immune-mediated response.

Genetic Link

About 90% to 95% of patients with celiac disease have human leukocyte antigen (HLA) allele HLA-DQ2. The other 5% to 10% have HLA-DQ8. However, not everyone with these genetic markers develops celiac disease, and some people with celiac disease do not have these HLA alleles.

As with other autoimmune diseases, the tissue destruction that occurs with celiac disease is the result of chronic inflammation. Gluten contains specific peptides called *prolamines*. Partial digestion of gluten releases the prolamine peptides, which are absorbed into the intestinal submucosa. In genetically susceptible persons, the peptides bind to HLA-DQ2 and/or HLA-DQ8 and activate an inflammatory response. Inflammation damages the microvilli and brush border of the small intestine, decreasing the amount of surface area available for nutrient absorption. Damage is most severe in the duodenum, probably because it has more exposure to gluten. The inflammation lasts as long as gluten ingestion continues.

Clinical Manifestations

Classic manifestations of celiac disease include foul-smelling diarrhea, abdominal pain, flatulence, abdominal distention, and malnutrition.[27] Some people have no obvious GI symptoms and may instead have atypical signs and symptoms. These include joint pain, osteoporosis, dental enamel hypoplasia, fatigue, peripheral neuropathy, and reproductive problems. An intensely pruritic, vesicular skin lesion, called *dermatitis herpetiformis*, is sometimes present and occurs as a rash on the buttocks, scalp, face, elbows, and knees.

Protein, fat, and carbohydrate absorption is affected. Weight loss, muscle wasting, and other signs of malnutrition may be present. Abnormal serum folate, iron, and cobalamin levels can occur. Iron-deficiency anemia is common. Patients may have lactose intolerance and need to refrain from lactose-containing products until the disease is under control. Inadequate calcium intake and vitamin D absorption can lead to decreased bone density and osteoporosis.

Diagnostic Studies

Early diagnosis and treatment can prevent complications. Screening is recommended for close relatives of patients known to have the disease, young patients with decreased bone density, those with anemia if other causes are ruled out, and certain autoimmune diseases.

Celiac disease is confirmed by a combination of findings from the history and physical examination, serology testing, and histologic analysis of small intestine biopsies.[27] Have the patient complete diagnostic testing before starting a gluten-free diet, since the diet will change the results. Serologic testing for immunoglobulin A (IgA) antitissue transglutaminase and IgA endomysial antibody offer good sensitivity and specificity. Histologic evidence is the gold standard for confirming the diagnosis. Biopsies show flattened mucosa and noticeable losses of villi. Genotyping involves testing for HLA-DQ2 and/or HLA-DQ8 antigens.

Interprofessional and Nursing Care

A gluten-free diet (Table 42.33) is the only effective treatment for celiac disease. Most patients need to stay on a gluten-free diet for the rest of their lives. Periodic nutrition evaluations and laboratory monitoring are done to monitor for anemia and malnutrition. The patient should undergo bone density screening every 2 to 3 years.[28]

Refer all patients for a dietary consultation. You can work with a dietitian to teach the patient how to eat a nutritionally adequate diet while staying within a budget. Teach the patient to avoid wheat, barley, oats, and rye products. Although pure oats do not contain gluten, wheat, rye, and barley can contaminate oat products during the milling process. Teach the patient to read medication and food labels. Some medications and many food additives, preservatives, and stabilizers contain gluten. The patient needs to know where to buy gluten-free products. Good sources are health food stores, many grocery stores, and through Internet sites.

Maintaining a gluten-free diet can be hard, particularly when traveling or eating in restaurants. Many with celiac disease describe feeling embarrassed or like a burden when having to discuss gluten-free menu options with restaurant staff or when dining in other's homes. Mobile phone users will find apps listing gluten-free menu options at popular restaurants helpful. Many restaurants now indicate which food choices are gluten

TABLE 42.33 Nutritional Therapy

Celiac Disease

Foods to Eat
- Butter
- Cheese, cottage cheese
- Coffee, tea, and cocoa
- Corn tortillas
- Eggs
- Flax, corn, and rice
- Fresh fruits
- Gluten-free flour breads, crackers, pasta, and cereals
- Meat, fish, poultry (not marinated or breaded)
- Peanut butter
- Potatoes
- Soy products
- Tapioca
- Unflavored milk
- Yogurt

Foods to Avoid
- Baked goods, including muffins, cookies, cakes, pies
- Barley
- Bread, including wheat bread, white bread, "potato" bread
- Flour
- Gluten stabilizers
- Oats
- Pasta, pizza, bagels
- Rye
- Wheat

free. The Celiac Sprue Association website (*www.csaceliacs.info*) and the Celiac Disease Foundation (*www.celiac.org*) provide suggestions for maintaining a gluten-free diet and living with celiac disease.

LACTASE DEFICIENCY

Lactase deficiency is a condition in which the lactase enzyme is deficient or absent. Lactase is the enzyme that breaks down lactose into 2 simple sugars: glucose and galactose. Primary lactase insufficiency is often a result of genetic factors. Certain ethnic or racial groups, especially those with Asian or African ancestry, develop low lactase levels in childhood. Less common causes include low lactase levels resulting from premature birth and congenital lactase deficiency, a rare genetic disorder. Lactose malabsorption can occur when conditions leading to bacterial overgrowth promote lactose fermentation in the small bowel or when intestinal mucosal damage interferes with absorption. The latter occurs with IBD and celiac disease.

Symptoms of lactose intolerance include bloating, flatulence, cramping abdominal pain, and diarrhea. Diarrhea results from the excess, undigested lactose in the small intestine attracting water molecules, which prevents them from being properly absorbed. Symptoms generally occur within 30 minutes to several hours after drinking a glass of milk or ingesting a milk product. Lactose intolerance is diagnosed with a lactose tolerance test, a lactose hydrogen breath test, or genetic testing.

Treatment consists of eliminating lactose from the diet by avoiding milk and milk products, and/or replacing lactase with commercially available preparations. A lactose-free diet generally results in prompt resolution of symptoms. Many lactose-intolerant persons are aware of their condition. They likely have been avoiding lactose-containing products and using lactose-free milk products. Lactase enzyme (Lactaid) is available as an over-the-counter (OTC) product. It breaks down the lactose present in ingested milk. A number of milk products treated with lactase enzyme are readily available.

The diet may gradually advance to a low-lactose diet as tolerated. Many lactose-intolerant persons may not have symptoms if they have lactose in small amounts. Cheese has less lactose than milk and ice cream. Live culture yogurt has less lactose because the bacteria help digest the lactose. Teach the patient to read labels to detect any hidden sources of milk products. Some people tolerate lactose better if taken with meals. Teach the patient that adhering to the diet is important. Since avoiding milk and milk products can lead to calcium deficiency, supplements may be needed to prevent osteoporosis.

SHORT BOWEL SYNDROME

Short bowel syndrome (SBS) is a condition in which the small intestine does not have enough surface area to absorb enough nutrients. This leaves the person unable to meet energy, fluid, electrolyte, and nutritional needs to stay healthy on a normal diet. Causes of SBS include diseases that damage the intestinal mucosa, surgical removal of too much small intestine (e.g., with Crohn's disease, cancer), and congenital defects.

SBS is likely to develop in patients with a loss of around 75% of the small intestine. The length and area of the remaining small intestine and the presence of the colon affect the patient's outcome. If the terminal ileum and ileocecal valve are intact, the remaining intestine undergoes adaptive changes that are most pronounced in the ileum. The villi and crypts increase in size, and the absorptive capacity of the remaining intestine increases. When the colon is present, fluid and electrolyte absorption increase. Those with an end jejunostomy often have little to no adaptation.

Clinical Manifestations

SBS results in reduced nutrient, fluid, and electrolyte absorption. This leads to dehydration, weight loss, diarrhea, malnutrition, vitamin deficiencies, and electrolyte imbalances. Other manifestations include abdominal pain, flatulence, and steatorrhea. The patient may develop lactase deficiency and bacterial overgrowth. Those who do not receive appropriate nutrition may have manifestations associated with specific deficiencies. For example, patients may have peripheral neuropathy from vitamin B_{12}, vitamin E, copper, or thiamine deficiencies or fatigue due to anemia from decreased folate or iron.[29]

Interprofessional Care

The treatment goals are that the patient will have fluid and electrolyte balance, normal nutritional status, and control of diarrhea. The main treatment is nutritional support involving PN, EN, medications, and a tailored diet. In the immediate period after massive bowel resection, patients receive PN to replace fluid, electrolyte, and nutrient losses and to rest the bowel. Those with severe resections will need PN indefinitely. EN and a normal diet are gradually resumed to stimulate the remaining intestine to function better. Some can eventually stop PN.

Refer the patient to a dietitian. The ideal diet is high in protein and complex carbohydrates and low in fat and concentrated sweets. Oral supplements of calcium, zinc, and multivitamins may be needed. Soluble fiber is encouraged if the colon is present. The patient should eat at least 6 small meals per day to increase the time of contact between food and the intestine. Oral intake may be supplemented with elemental nutrient formulas and tube feeding during the night. Patients with severe malabsorption may need PN (see Chapter 39).

Patients often take multiple medications to help control fecal output. PPIs, H_2 blockers, α-adrenergic receptor agonists (e.g., clonidine), or octreotide reduce excess fluid secretion. Opioid antidiarrheal drugs decrease intestinal motility (Table 42.2). For patients who have limited ileal resections, cholestyramine reduces diarrhea resulting from unabsorbed bile acids by increasing their excretion in feces. Bile acids stimulate intestinal fluid secretion and reduce colonic fluid absorption. Antibiotic therapy is used if bacterial overgrowth is contributing to diarrhea.

Three drugs have FDA approval for the treatment of SBS: somatropin, glutamine, and teduglutide (Gattex). Somatropin enhances intestinal adaption and increases the flow of water, electrolytes, and nutrients into the bowel. Glutamine improves intestinal absorption. Teduglutide increases the surface area of the intestine and improves intestinal absorption of fluids and nutrients.

Intestinal transplantation is done at a few specialized transplant centers in the United States. It is considered the only long-term treatment option for patients with intestinal failure who have significant complications from PN or nutrition failure. The leading cause of intestinal failure is SBS. Transplantation may include the intestine alone, liver and intestine, or multivisceral combinations (stomach, duodenum, jejunum, ileum, colon, and/or pancreas).

GASTROINTESTINAL STROMAL TUMORS

Gastrointestinal stromal tumors (GISTs) are a rare form of cancer that originates in cells found in the wall of the GI tract. These cells, known as *interstitial cells of Cajal,* help control the movement of food and liquid through the stomach and intestines. About 60% of GISTs are in the stomach; 25% are in the small intestine; and the rest are in the esophagus, colon, or peritoneum.[30] Most GISTs occur in people between the ages of 50 and 70. While the exact cause of GISTs is unknown, genetic mutations likely play a role. A few GISTs occur in people with familial mutations in either the KIT or platelet-derived growth factor receptor a (PDGFRa) or in those with neurofibromatosis type 1.[30]

The manifestations of GISTs depend on the part of the GI tract affected. Early manifestations are often subtle, including early satiety, fatigue, bloating, nausea or vomiting, and a change in bowel habits. Because these manifestations are like those of many other GI problems, early detection of the cancer is difficult. Later manifestations may include GI bleeding and obstruction caused by growth of the tumor. GISTs are often found during imaging for other problems. Diagnosis is based on histologic examination of biopsied tissue. Endoscopic ultrasound, CT, or MRI are used to determine the extent of disease.

Surgery offers the only permanent cure. Often, though, GISTs have metastasized by the time of diagnosis or commonly recur. GISTs are unresponsive to conventional chemotherapy. The discovery of genetic mutations led to the development of tyrosine kinase inhibitor drugs (e.g., imatinib mesylate [Gleevec], sunitinib, regorafenib [Stivarga]) that are effective against certain GISTs.[31]

ANORECTAL PROBLEMS

HEMORRHOIDS

Hemorrhoids are dilated hemorrhoidal veins. They may be internal (occurring above the internal sphincter) or external (occurring outside the external sphincter) (Figs. 42.16 and 42.17). In affected persons, hemorrhoids appear periodically, depending on the amount of anorectal pressure.

Etiology and Pathophysiology

Hemorrhoids develop because of increased anal pressure and weakening of the connective tissue that supports the hemorrhoidal veins. Weakened supporting tissue allows for downward displacement of the hemorrhoidal veins, causing them to dilate. Blood flow through the veins of the hemorrhoidal plexus is impaired. An intravascular clot in the venule results in a thrombosed external hemorrhoid. Many factors increase the risk for hemorrhoids, including pregnancy, constipation, straining to defecate, diarrhea, heavy lifting, prolonged standing and sitting, obesity, and ascites.[31]

Clinical Manifestations

Hemorrhoids are the most common reason for bleeding with defecation. Internal hemorrhoids most often cause painless bright red bleeding with stools, on the toilet paper, or dripping into the toilet water. If internal hemorrhoids become constricted, the patient will report pain. Internal hemorrhoids can prolapse into the anal canal or externally. Symptoms of prolapse include pressure with defecation and a protruding mass.

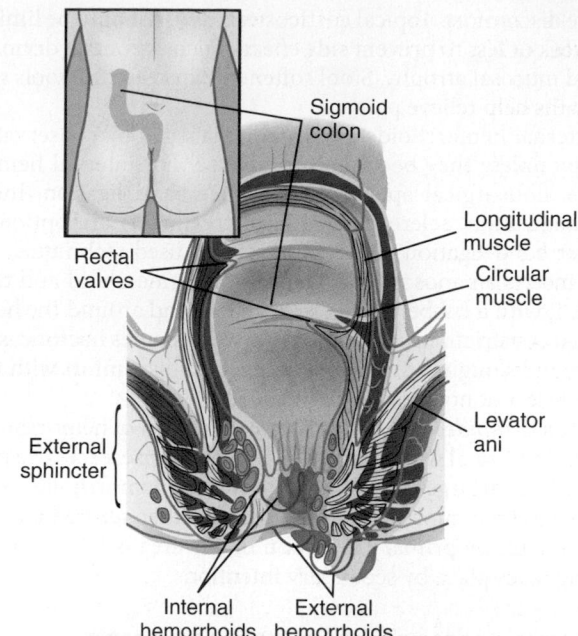

FIG. 42.16 Anatomic structures of the rectum and anus with external and internal hemorrhoids.

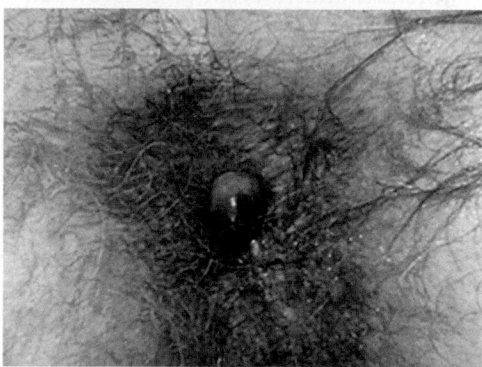

FIG. 42.17 Thrombosed external hemorrhoids. (From Townsend CM, Beauchamp RD, Evers BM, et al: *Sabiston textbook of surgery: The biological basis of modern surgical practice,* ed 19, Philadelphia, 2012, Saunders.)

External hemorrhoids are reddish blue and seldom bleed. There may be itching, burning, and edema. They usually do not cause pain unless thrombosis (blood clots) is present. Thrombosed hemorrhoids are a bluish-purple tinge and palpable at the anal orifice. They usually cause pain and inflammation. The clot can erode through the overlying stretched skin, causing bleeding with defecation. Constipation or diarrhea can worsen these symptoms.

Diagnostic Studies and Interprofessional Care

It is easy to diagnose external hemorrhoids visual inspection and digital examination. Digital examination, anoscopy, and sigmoidoscopy are used to diagnose internal hemorrhoids.

Therapy is based on the cause and the patient's symptoms. A high-fiber diet and increased fluid intake prevent constipation and reduce straining, which allows engorgement of the veins to subside. The resulting stool bulk may decrease stool leakage and itching. Ointments, such as dibucaine; creams, suppositories, and impregnated pads that contain antiinflammatory agents (e.g., hydrocortisone); or astringents and anesthetics (e.g., witch hazel, benzocaine), may shrink the mucous membranes and relieve discomfort. Topical corticosteroids use should be limited to 1 week or less to prevent side effects, such as contact dermatitis and mucosal atrophy. Stool softeners can keep the stools soft. Sitz baths help relieve pain.

External hemorrhoids are usually managed by conservative therapy unless they become thrombosed. For internal hemorrhoids, nonsurgical approaches (rubber band ligation, infrared coagulation, sclerotherapy, laser treatment) are options.[31] Rubber band ligation is the most widely used technique. The HCP inserts an anoscope to identify the hemorrhoid and then ligates it with a rubber band. The rubber band around the hemorrhoid constricts circulation. The tissue becomes necrotic, separates, and sloughs off. There is some local discomfort with this procedure, but no anesthetic is needed.

A *hemorrhoidectomy* is the surgical excision of hemorrhoids. Surgery is needed when there is marked prolapse, excessive pain or bleeding, or large or multiple thrombosed hemorrhoids. After removing the hemorrhoids, the tissue is either sutured and the wound heals by primary intention or the area is left open and healing takes place by secondary intention.

NURSING MANAGEMENT: HEMORRHOIDS

Conservative nursing management includes teaching ways to prevent constipation and to avoid prolonged standing or sitting and proper use of OTC drugs for hemorrhoidal symptoms. Teach the patient to seek medical care for severe symptoms of hemorrhoids (e.g., excessive pain and bleeding, prolapsed hemorrhoids). Sitz baths (15 to 20 minutes, 2 or 3 times each day) may help to reduce discomfort and swelling associated with hemorrhoids.

Nursing care after a hemorrhoidectomy focuses on pain control and promoting wound healing. Be aware that although the procedure is minor, the pain is severe and feared by many. There are several analgesic regimens, using a combination of medications. Most patients receive multimodal analgesia. This may involve an opioid and NSAID in conjunction with topical preparations that provide anesthesia or reduce internal sphincter spasms, such as topical lidocaine, 2% diltiazem, and glyceryl trinitrate.

The patient usually dreads the first bowel movement and often resists the urge to defecate. Give pain medication before the bowel movement to reduce discomfort. Stool softeners (e.g., docusate) and bulking agents are given to help form a soft, bulky stool that is easier to pass. If the patient does not have a bowel movement within 2 or 3 days, an oil-retention enema is given.

Sitz baths are started 1 or 2 days after surgery and continued for 1 to 2 weeks. A warm sitz bath provides comfort and keeps the anal area clean. A sponge ring in the sitz bath helps relieve pressure on the area. Initially, do not leave the patient alone because of the possibility of weakness or fainting. Teach the patient that pressure relief cushions are acceptable to ease discomfort when sitting. Tell the patient not to use a pressure relief ring or "doughnut" because they can reduce blood flow to the area.

The patient may have packing in the rectum to absorb drainage, with a T-binder to hold the dressing in place. Packing is usually removed on the first or second postoperative day. Assess for rectal bleeding, especially in patients taking clopidogrel or oral anticoagulants. The patient may be embarrassed when the dressing is changed. Provide as much privacy as possible.

Teach the patient care of the anal area, symptoms of complications (especially bleeding), and ways to avoid constipation and straining. Hemorrhoids may recur. Sometimes, anal strictures develop, requiring dilation. Regular checkups are important to prevent any further problems.

ANAL FISSURE

An *anal fissure* is a skin ulcer or a crack in the lining of the anal wall. Many times, the inciting event is trauma from passing hard stools. Other fissures are related to trauma (anal intercourse, foreign body insertion, such as endoscope), local infection (syphilis, gonorrhea, *Chlamydia,* herpes simplex virus, HIV), or inflammation. An anal fissure is acute when it is of recent onset (less than 6 weeks), and chronic if it has been present for a longer period. Chronic fissures have a characteristic appearance that includes perianal skin tag and fibrotic edges.[32]

Anal tissue ulcerates because of ischemia caused by a combination of high pressure in the internal anal sphincter and poor blood supply to the area. The ischemic tissue may ulcerate spontaneously or when traumatized by factors such as hard stools, which would not normally cause tissue breakdown. Ischemia must be corrected for a fissure to heal.

The hallmark of an anal fissure is severe anal pain. It tends to be worse with defecation and with direct pressure on the site (e.g., sitting). Acute fissures tend to bleed slightly. Patients may report red blood on the toilet paper. Constipation results because of fear of pain associated with bowel movements.

Anal fissures are easy to diagnose with a physical examination. Conservative care with fiber supplements, increased fluid intake, sitz baths, and topical analgesics is successful in most cases, especially if the fissure is acute. Topical preparations, including nitrates and calcium channel blockers, decrease rectal anal pressure and allow the fissure to heal without sphincter damage. Local injections of botulinum toxin can decrease rectal anal pressure. They are most effective when combined with nitrates. Pain is managed by softening stools with a bulk-producing agent (psyllium) or stool softener and warm sitz baths (15 to 20 minutes, 3 times per day).[32]

If conservative treatment fails, a lateral internal sphincterotomy is the recommended surgical procedure. It carries the risk for postoperative incontinence. Postoperative nursing care is the same as the care for the patient who had a hemorrhoidectomy.

ANORECTAL ABSCESS

An *anorectal abscess* is a collection of perianal pus (Fig. 42.18). The abscess results from obstruction of the anal glands, leading to infection and abscess formation. Abscess formation occurs with anal fissures, trauma, or IBD. The most common causative organisms are *E. coli,* staphylococci, and streptococci. Manifestations include local severe pain and swelling, foul-smelling drainage, tenderness, and fever. Sepsis can occur as a complication. Anorectal abscesses are diagnosed by rectal examination.

Anorectal abscesses require surgical drainage. Larger abscesses need packing afterward with impregnated gauze or placement of drains (e.g., Penrose) to promote drainage. The area then heals by granulation. Patients who have diabetes or cellulitis or are immunocompromised (e.g., chemotherapy) may need antibiotic therapy. Nursing care includes warm, moist heat applications and changing packing daily. The patient is usually more comfortable lying on the abdomen or side. A low-fiber

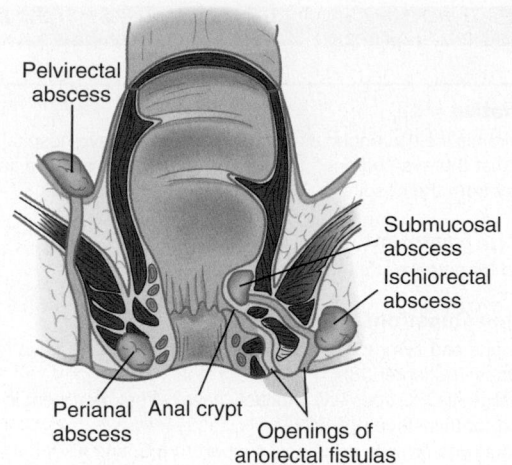

Pelvirectal abscess

Submucosal abscess

Ischiorectal abscess

Perianal abscess   Anal crypt

Openings of anorectal fistulas

FIG. 42.18 Common sites of anorectal abscesses and fistula formation.

diet is given. The patient may leave the hospital with the wound still open. Teach the patient about wound care and the importance of sitz baths, thorough cleaning after urinating or bowel movements, and follow-up visits with the HCP.

ANAL FISTULA

An **anal fistula** is an abnormal tunnel leading from the anus or rectum. It may extend to the outside of the skin, vagina, or buttocks and often precedes an abscess. Anal fistulas are a complication of Crohn's disease and may resolve when drug treatment achieves remission of the disease. About 50% of anal fistulas are due to anorectal abscess.

Feces may enter the fistula and cause an infection. There may be persistent, bloody or purulent discharge, or stool leakage from the fistula. The patient may need to wear a pad to avoid staining clothes.

Surgical treatment of an anal fistula depends on the location and nature of the fistula. In a fistulotomy, the HCP opens the fistula and healthy tissue is allowed to granulate in the wound. Care is the same as after a hemorrhoidectomy. Options for complex fistulas include ligation of the intersphincteric fistula tract (LIFT) or the use of rectal flaps, setons, plugs, or fibrin glue injections to seal the fistula.

ANAL CANCER

Anal cancer is uncommon in the general population, but the incidence is increasing. In the United States around 8200 people are diagnosed with anal cancer each year.[33] It mainly occurs in older adults, with the average age being in the early 60s. Human papillomavirus (HPV) is associated with about 80% of the cases of anal cancer. Those at high risk for anal cancer include smokers, HIV-positive homosexual men, people who are immunocompromised (e.g., posttransplant immunosuppression), and women with cervical, vaginal, or vulvar cancer.[33]

Rectal bleeding is the most common presenting sign. Other symptoms include rectal pain, fullness, and changes in bowel habits. Some patients have no symptoms, which leads to delayed diagnosis and treatment.

It is especially important to screen high-risk persons using digital rectal examination (DRE) and anal Pap tests. In an anal Pap test, the anal lining is swabbed and the cells examined to identify any cell changes (e.g., dysplasia, neoplasia). High-resolution anoscopy allows for visualization of the mucosa and biopsy. An endoanal *(endorectal) ultrasound* may be done.

Treatment of anal cancer depends on the size and depth of the lesions. Cancer therapy involves surgery or a combination of low-dose radiation and chemotherapy. Chemotherapy regimens include combinations of mitomycin, cisplatin, and fluorouracil.[33] Options for precancerous lesions are surgical removal or treatment with topical imiquimod (Aldara) and fluorouracil. If the tumor involves the rectum and is large enough to require removing the anal sphincters, the anus will be sutured shut and a permanent ostomy created.

PILONIDAL SINUS

A *pilonidal sinus* is a small tract under the skin between the buttocks in the sacrococcygeal area. It is thought to be of congenital origin. It may have several openings and is lined with epithelium and hair, hence the name *pilonidal* ("a nest of hair"). The skin is moist, and movement of the buttocks causes the short, wiry hair to penetrate the skin. If the irritated skin becomes infected, it forms a pilonidal cyst or abscess. There are no symptoms with a pilonidal sinus unless there is an infection. Then the patient may have pain and swelling at the base of the spine.

An abscess requires incision and drainage. The wound may be closed or left open to heal by secondary intention. The wound is packed, and sitz baths ordered. Nursing care includes warm, moist heat applications when an abscess is present. The patient is usually more comfortable lying on the abdomen or side. Teach the patient to avoid contaminating the dressing when urinating or defecating and to avoid straining whenever possible.

CASE STUDY

Colorectal Cancer

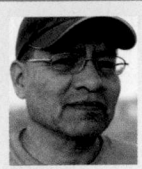

(©iStockphoto/
Thinkstock)

Patient Profile

L.C., a 58-yr-old Native American man, is from a Pueblo tribe in northern New Mexico. L.C.'s wife and family drove 50 miles to take him to the Indian Health Service hospital because of his deteriorating health (see the case study in Chapter 38 on p. 835).

Subjective Data

See the case study in Chapter 38 on p. 838.

Objective Data

Physical Examination

See the case study in Chapter 38 on p. 840.

Laboratory Tests

- CT scan and colonoscopy show 2 medium-sized tumors in the transverse colon

Interprofessional Care

Surgical Procedure

- Had a transverse hemicolectomy with lymph node biopsies
- Pathology results: Adenocarcinoma, has invaded the muscle wall of colon, 2 of 5 lymph nodes are positive for cancer

Postoperative

- Feels like his life has ended and does not want to leave hospital
- States that there is "no one" to take care of him at his home and he is far away from the hospital

Follow-Up Treatment

Scheduled for outpatient chemotherapy

Discussion Questions

1. What signs and symptoms of colorectal cancer did L.C. have (see the case study in Chapter 38)?
2. What stage of CRC does L.C. probably have? What treatment is recommended for this stage of CRC?
3. How could you provide emotional support to L.C. and his family?
4. ***Patient-Centered Care:*** What is a culturally sensitive way for you to support L.C. and his family in making decisions about his continued health care?
5. ***Priority Decision:*** Based on the assessment data, what are the priority nursing diagnoses? Are there any collaborative problems?
6. ***Priority Decision:*** What are the priority nursing interventions for L.C. at this stage of his illness?
7. ***Collaboration:*** What referrals may be indicated at this time?
8. ***Evidence-Based Practice:*** L.C. is worried that other members of his family may have colon cancer. What can you tell him about the recommendations for colorectal cancer screening?
9. ***Quality Improvement:*** What outcomes would indicate nursing interventions were successful?

Answers available at *http://evolve.elsevier.com/Lewis/medsurg.*

▌ BRIDGE TO NCLEX EXAMINATION

The number of the question corresponds to the same-numbered outcome at the beginning of the chapter.

1. The *most* appropriate therapy for a patient with acute diarrhea caused by a viral infection is to
   a. increase fluid intake.
   b. administer an antibiotic.
   c. administer an antimotility drug.
   d. quarantine the patient to prevent spread of the virus.

2. A 35-yr-old female patient is admitted to the emergency department with acute abdominal pain. Which medical diagnoses should you consider as possible causes of her pain? *(select all that apply)*
   a. Gastroenteritis
   b. Ectopic pregnancy
   c. Gastrointestinal bleeding
   d. Irritable bowel syndrome
   e. Inflammatory bowel disease

3. Assessment findings suggestive of peritonitis include *(select all that apply)*
   a. rebound tenderness.
   b. a soft, distended abdomen.
   c. dull, intermittent abdominal pain.
   d. shallow respirations with bradypnea.
   e. observing that the patient is lying still.

3. In planning care for the patient with Crohn's disease, the nurse recognizes that a major difference between ulcerative colitis and Crohn's disease is that Crohn's disease
   a. often results in toxic megacolon.
   b. causes fewer nutritional deficiencies than ulcerative colitis.
   c. often recurs after surgery, while ulcerative colitis is curable with a colectomy.
   d. is manifested by rectal bleeding and anemia more often than is ulcerative colitis.

4. The nurse performs a detailed assessment of the abdomen of a patient with a possible bowel obstruction, knowing that manifestations of an obstruction in the large intestine are *(select all that apply)*
   a. persistent abdominal pain.
   b. marked abdominal distention.
   c. diarrhea that is loose or liquid.
   d. colicky, severe, intermittent pain.
   e. profuse vomiting that relieves abdominal pain.

5. A patient with stage I colorectal cancer is scheduled for surgery. Patient teaching for this patient would include an explanation that
   a. chemotherapy will begin after the patient recovers from the surgery.
   b. both chemotherapy and radiation can be used as palliative treatments.
   c. follow-up colonoscopies will be needed to ensure that the cancer does not recur.
   d. a wound, ostomy, and continence nurse will visit the patient to identify the site for the ostomy.

6. The nurse determines a patient undergoing ileostomy surgery understands the procedure when the patient states
   a. "I should only have to change the pouch every 4 to 7 days."
   b. "The drainage in the pouch will look like my normal stools."
   c. "I may not need to wear a drainage pouch if I irrigate it daily."
   d. "Limiting my fluid intake should decrease the amount of output."

7. In contrast to diverticulitis, the patient with diverticulosis
   a. has rectal bleeding.
   b. often has no symptoms.
   c. usually develops peritonitis.
   d. has localized cramping pain.

8. A nursing intervention that is *most* appropriate to decrease postoperative edema and pain after an inguinal herniorrhaphy is to
   a. apply a truss to the hernia site.
   b. allow the patient to stand to void.
   c. support the incision during coughing.
   d. apply a scrotal support with an ice bag.

9. The nurse determines that the goals of dietary teaching have been met when the patient with celiac disease selects from the menu
   a. scrambled eggs and sausage.
   b. buckwheat pancakes with syrup.
   c. oatmeal, skim milk, and orange juice.
   d. yogurt, strawberries, and rye toast with butter.

10. What should a patient be taught after a hemorrhoidectomy?
    a. Take mineral oil before bedtime.
    b. Eat a low-fiber diet to rest the colon.
    c. Use oil-retention enemas to empty the colon.
    d. Take prescribed pain medications before a bowel movement.

1. a, 2. a, b, c, d, e, 3. a, e, 4. c, 5. a, b, 6. c, 7. a, 8. b, 9. d, 10. a, 11. d

For rationales to these answers and even more NCLEX review questions, visit *http://evolve.elsevier.com/Lewis/medsurg*.

EVOLVE WEBSITE/RESOURCES LIST

http://evolve.elsevier.com/Lewis/medsurg
Review Questions (Online Only)
Key Points
Answer Keys for Questions
- Rationales for Bridge to NCLEX Examination Questions
- Answer Guidelines for Case Study on p. 966

Student Case Study
- Patient With Ulcerative Colitis

Nursing Care Plans
- eNursing Care Plan 42.1: Patient With Acute Infectious Diarrhea
- eNursing Care Plan 42.2: Patient With Inflammatory Bowel Disease
- eNursing Care Plan 42.3: Patient With a Colostomy/Ileostomy

Conceptual Care Map Creator
Audio Glossary
Content Updates

REFERENCES

*1. Shane AL, Mody RK, Crump JA, et al: 2017 IDSA clinical practice guidelines for the diagnosis and management of infectious diarrhea, *Clin Infect Dis* 65:e45, 2017.

*2. Watson T, Hickok J, Fraker S, et al: Evaluating the risk factors for hospital-onset *Clostridium difficile* infections in a large healthcare system, *Clin Infect Dis* 66:1957-1959, 2018.

*3. McDonald LC, Gerding DN, Johnson S, et al: Clinical practice guidelines for *Clostridium difficile* infection in adults and children: 2017 Update by the IDSA and SHEA, *Clin Infect Dis* 66:e1, 2018.

4. Chabkraborty S, Bharucha AE: Fecal incontinence. In: Barden E, Shaker R, eds: *Gastrointestinal motility disorders*, New York, 2018, Springer.

*5. Serra J, Mascort-Roca J, Marzo-Castillejo M, et al: Clinical practice guidelines for the management of constipation in adults: Definition, etiology and clinical manifestations, *Gastroenterol Hepatol* 40:132, 2017.

6. Camilleri M, Ford AC, Mawe GM, et al: Chronic constipation, *Nat Rev Dis Primers* 3:1, 2017.

7. Weaver KR, Melkus GD, Henderson WA: Irritable bowel syndrome, *AJN* 117:48, 2017.

*8. Ireton-Jones C: The low FODMAP diet: Fundamental therapy in the management of IBS, *Curr Opin Clin Nutr Metab Care* 20:414, 2017.

9. Braslow B: Management of appendicitis. In: Khwaja KA, Diaz JJ (eds.), *Minimally invasive acute care surgery*, New York, 2018, Springer.

10. Centers for Disease Control and Prevention: Epidemiology of the IBD. Retrieved from *www.cdc.gov/ibd/ibd-epidemiology.htm*.

*11. Shivashankar R, Lewis JD: The role of diet in inflammatory bowel disease, *Curr Gastroenter Reports* 19:22, 2017.

*12. Shouval D, Rufo P: The role of environmental factors in the pathogenesis of IBD, *JAMA Pediatric* 171:999, 2017.

*13. Venema U, Werna TC, Voskuil MD, et al: The genetic background of inflammatory bowel disease: from correlation to causality, *J Pathol* 241:146, 2017.

14. Crohn's and Colitis Foundation: IBD medications. Retrieved from *www.ibdetermined.org/ibd-information/ibd-treatment/ibd-medication.aspx*.

*15. Bots S, Gecse K, Barclay M, et al: Combination immunosuppression in IBD, *Inflamm Bowel Dis* 24:539, 2018.

16. Flier LC, Welstead LA: Nutrition matters. In: Cohen R, ed: *Inflammatory bowel disease*, New York, 2017, Humana Press.

*17. John ES, Katz K, Saxena M, et al: Management of inflammatory bowel disease in the elderly, *Curr Treat Options Gastroenterol* 14:285, 2016.

*18. Reddy SR, Cappell MS: A systematic review of the clinical presentation, diagnosis, and treatment of small bowel obstruction, *Curr Gastroenterol Rep* 9:28, 2017.

19. Alavi K, Friel CM: Large bowel obstruction. In: Steele SR, Hull TL, Read TE, Saclarides TJ, Senagore AJ, Whitlow CB, eds: *The ASCRS textbook of colon and rectal surgery*, New York, 2016, Springer.

20. Toevs CC, Mazellan K, Kohr R: Ogilvie's syndrome, *Am Surg* 83:217, 2017.

21. American Cancer Society: Key statistics for colorectal cancer. Retrieved from *www.cancer.org/cancer/colon-rectal-cancer/about/key-statistics.html*.

*22. Ansa BE, Coughlin SS, Alema-Mensah E, et al: Evaluation of colorectal cancer incidence trends in the United States (2000–2014), *J Clin Med* 7:22, 2018.

23. American Cancer Society: Colorectal cancer screening guidelines. Retrieved from *www.cancer.org/cancer/colon-rectal-cancer/detection-diagnosis-staging/acs-recommendations.html*.

24. National Cancer Institute: Colon cancer treatment. Retrieved from *www.cancer.gov/types/colorectal/hp/colon-treatment-pdq#link/_125*.

*25. Ellison DL: Acute diverticulitis management, *Crit Care Nurs Clin North Am* 30:67, 2018.

*26. Ortiz LA, Zhang B, McCarthy MW, et al: Treatment of enterocutaneous fistulas, then and now, *Nutr Clin Pract* 32:508, 2017.

*27. Leonard MM, Sapone A, Catassi C, et al: Celiac disease and nonceliac gluten sensitivity, *JAMA* 318:647, 2017.

28. Celiac Disease Foundation: Celiac disease. Retrieved from *https://celiac.org/celiac-disease/understanding-celiac-disease-2/what-is-celiac-disease/*.

29. Boutte HJ, Rubin DC: Short bowel syndrome. In: Barden E, Shaker R, eds: *Gastrointestinal motility disorders*, New York, 2018, Springer.

*30. Nishida T, Blay JY, Hirota S, et al: The standard diagnosis, treatment, and follow-up of gastrointestinal stromal tumors based on guidelines, *Gastric Cancer* 19:3, 2016.

*31. American Society of Colon and Rectal Surgeons: Clinical practice guidelines for the management of hemorrhoids. Retrieved from *www.fascrs.org/physicians/clinical-practice-guidelines*.

32. American Society of Colon and Rectal Surgeons: Anal fissure, *Dis Colon Rectum* 61:293, 2018.

33. Eng C, Shridhar R, Chan E, et al: Anal cancer. *The American Cancer Society's Oncology in Practice: Clinical Management* 9:149, 2018.

*Evidence-based information for clinical practice.

43

Liver, Biliary Tract, and Pancreas Problems

Mary C. Olson

Never define yourself by your relationship status, income, or looks. It is your kindness, generosity, and compassion that counts.

Brigette Nicole

ⓔ http://evolve.elsevier.com/Lewis/medsurg

CONCEPTUAL FOCUS

Infection   Nutrition
Inflammation   Pain

LEARNING OUTCOMES

1. Distinguish among the types of viral hepatitis, including etiology, pathophysiology, clinical manifestations, and complications.
2. Describe the interprofessional and nursing management of the patient with viral hepatitis.
3. Describe the pathophysiology, clinical manifestations, complications, and interprofessional care of the patient with nonalcoholic fatty liver disease.
4. Explain the etiology, pathophysiology, clinical manifestations, complications, and interprofessional and nursing management of the patient with cirrhosis.
5. Describe the clinical manifestations and management of liver cancer.

6. Distinguish between acute and chronic pancreatitis related to pathophysiology, clinical manifestations, complications, interprofessional care, and nursing management.
7. Explain the clinical manifestations and interprofessional and nursing management of the patient with pancreatic cancer.
8. Describe the pathophysiology, clinical manifestations, and interprofessional care of gallbladder disorders.
9. Describe the nursing management of the patient undergoing surgical treatment of cholecystitis and cholelithiasis.

KEY TERMS

acute liver failure, p. 989
acute pancreatitis, p. 992
ascites, p. 982
asterixis, p. 984
cholecystitis, p. 998
cholelithiasis, p. 998
chronic pancreatitis, p. 996

cirrhosis, p. 980
esophageal varices, p. 982
gastric varices, p. 982
hepatic encephalopathy, p. 983
hepatitis, p. 968
hepatorenal syndrome, p. 984
jaundice, p. 971

nonalcoholic fatty liver disease (NAFLD), p. 979
nonalcoholic steatohepatitis (NASH), p. 979
paracentesis, p. 985
portal hypertension, p. 982
spider angiomas, p. 980

Nursing management of patients with a wide range of liver, pancreatic, and gallbladder problems is the focus of this chapter. These organs are closely positioned together anatomically and highly associated in their digestive functions. Liver and pancreatic problems can lead to altered nutrient absorption and use, causing malnutrition and impaired elimination. Inflammation may be present, with the patient having pain, nausea, and vomiting. Nursing care focuses on helping the patient and caregiver manage symptoms and develop ways to cope with the diagnosis and, sometimes, prognosis. Health promotion focuses on reducing risk through immunizations and avoiding substance use.

DISORDERS OF THE LIVER

HEPATITIS

Hepatitis is inflammation of the liver. Hepatitis is most often caused by viruses. It also can be caused by substances (e.g., alcohol, medications, chemicals), autoimmune diseases, and metabolic problems.

Viral Hepatitis

There are several types of viral hepatitis. We designate each type by a letter (A, B, C, D, E). The different types have similar

TABLE 43.1 Characteristics of Hepatitis Viruses

Incubation Period and Mode of Transmission	Sources of Infection	Infectivity
Hepatitis A Virus (HAV) *Incubation:* 15–50 days (average 28) • Fecal-oral (primarily fecal contamination and oral ingestion)	• Contaminated food, milk, water, shellfish • Crowded conditions (e.g., day care, nursing home) • Persons with subclinical infections, infected food handlers, sexual contact, IV drug users • Poor personal hygiene • Poor sanitation	• Most infectious during 2 wk before onset of symptoms • Infectious until 1–2 wk after the start of symptoms
Hepatitis B Virus (HBV) *Incubation:* 115–180 days (average 56–96) • Percutaneous (parenteral) or mucosal exposure to blood or blood products • Sexual contact • Perinatal transmission	• Contaminated needles, syringes, and blood products • HBV-infected mother (perinatal transmission) • Sexual activity with infected partners. Asymptomatic carriers • Tattoos or body piercing with contaminated needles	• Before and after symptoms appear • Infectious for months • Carriers continue to be infectious for life
Hepatitis C Virus (HCV) *Incubation:* 14–180 days (average 56) • Percutaneous (parenteral) or mucosal exposure to blood or blood products • High-risk sexual contact • Perinatal contact	• Blood and blood products • Needles and syringes • Sexual activity with infected partners, low risk	• 1–2 wk before symptoms appear • Continues during clinical course • 75%–85% go on to develop chronic hepatitis C and remain infectious
Hepatitis D Virus (HDV) Incubation: 2–26 wk • HBV must precede HDV • Chronic carriers of HBV always at risk	• Same as HBV • Can cause infection only when HBV is present	• Blood infectious at all stages of HDV infection
Hepatitis E Virus (HEV) *Incubation:* 15–64 days (average 26–42 days) • Fecal-oral route • Outbreaks associated with contaminated water supply in developing countries	• Contaminated water, poor sanitation • Found in Asia, Africa, and Mexico • Not common in United States but is increasing in some areas	• Not known • May be similar to HAV

manifestations, but their modes of transmission and disease course vary (Table 43.1). Some can lead to chronic liver disease. Other less common viruses can also cause liver disease. These include cytomegalovirus (CMV), Epstein-Barr virus (EBV), herpesvirus, coxsackievirus, and rubella virus.

Hepatitis A Virus. Hepatitis A is a self-limiting infection that can cause a mild flu-like illness and jaundice. In more severe cases, it can cause acute liver failure. Hepatitis A virus (HAV) is a ribonucleic acid (RNA) virus. It is transmitted primarily through the fecal-oral route. It often occurs in small outbreaks caused by fecal contamination of food or drinking water. Poor hygiene, improper handling of food, crowded situations, and poor sanitary conditions are contributing factors.

Transmission occurs between family members, institutionalized persons, and children in day care centers. Foodborne outbreaks are usually due to food contaminated by an infected food handler. People at increased risk for infection include drug users (both injection and noninjection drugs), men who have sex with men (MSM), and persons traveling to developing countries.

The greatest risk for transmission occurs before clinical symptoms appear. The virus is found in feces 1 to 2 weeks before the onset of symptoms and at least 1 week after the onset of illness (Fig. 43.1). This means it can be carried and transmitted by persons who have undetectable, subclinical infections. It is present only briefly in blood, usually less than 3 weeks. Fecal excretion can occur in infants for months.

Anti-HAV (antibody to HAV) immunoglobulin M (IgM) appears during the acute phase. Detection of hepatitis A IgM

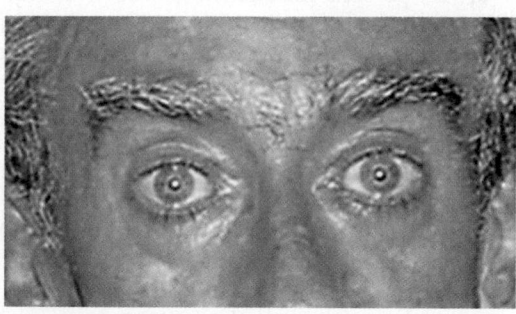

FIG. 43.1 Jaundiced patient. (From Butcher GP: *Gastroenterology: An illustrated colour text,* London, 2004, Churchill Livingstone.)

indicates acute hepatitis. Hepatitis A IgG without anti-HAV IgM indicates past infection. IgG antibody provides lifelong immunity (Fig. 43.2). HAV vaccination and thorough hand washing are the best measures to prevent outbreaks. In the United States, the incidence of infection has declined since we started vaccinating at-risk persons and children (beginning 12 to 24 months).[1]

Hepatitis B Virus. Hepatitis B virus (HBV) is a blood-borne pathogen that can cause either acute or chronic hepatitis. The incidence of HBV infection has decreased in areas where the use of the HBV vaccine is widespread.[2]

Asians and Pacific Islanders have an incidence of HBV of up to 8%. Perinatal transmission is the most common mode of transmission in this population and often results in chronic HBV infection.[2]

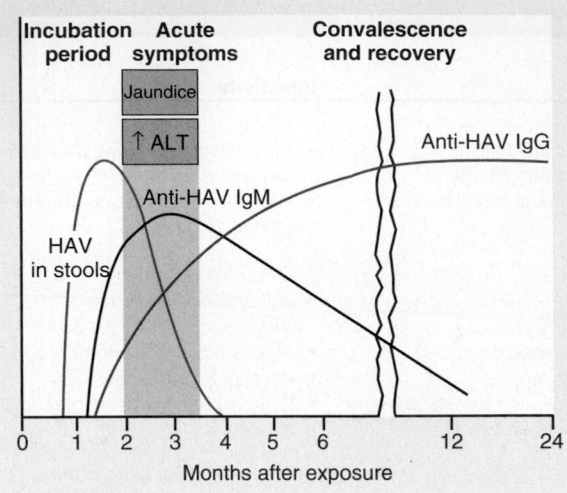

FIG. 43.2 Course of infection with hepatitis A virus *(HAV)*. *ALT,* Alanine aminotransferase. (From McCance KL, Huether SE: *Pathophysiology: The biologic basis for disease in adults and children,* ed 6, St Louis, 2010, Mosby.)

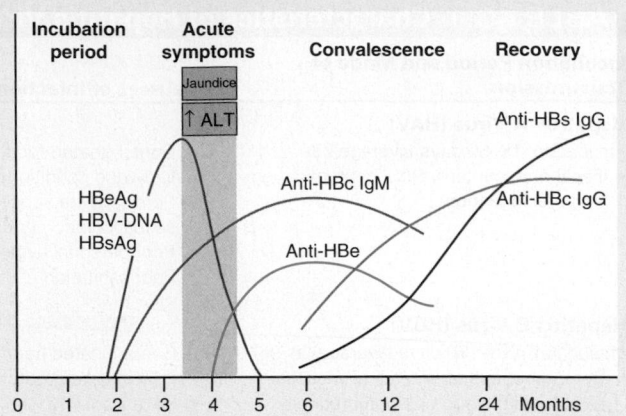

FIG. 43.3 Course of infection with hepatitis B virus *(HBV)*. *ALT,* Alanine aminotransferase; *anti-HBc,* antibody to hepatitis B core antigen; *anti-HBe,* antibody to HBeAg; *anti-HBs,* antibody to HBsAg; *HBeAg,* hepatitis B e antigen; *HBsAg,* hepatitis B surface antigen. (From McCance KL, Huether SE: *Pathophysiology: The biologic basis for disease in adults and children,* ed 6, St Louis, 2010, Mosby.)

HBV is a deoxyribonucleic acid (DNA) virus. It can be transmitted in several ways: (1) perinatally from mothers infected with HBV to their infants; (2) percutaneously (e.g., IV drug use, accidental needle-stick punctures); or (3) via small cuts on mucosal surfaces and exposure to infectious blood, blood products, or other body fluids (e.g., semen, vaginal secretions, saliva).

Sexual transmission is a common mode of HBV transmission. MSM (especially those practicing unprotected anal intercourse) are at an increased risk for HBV infection. Most believe that casual encounters, like hugging, kissing, and sharing utensils, do not transmit the disease.

Other at-risk persons include those who live with chronically HBV-infected persons, patients on hemodialysis, health care personnel, public safety workers, IV drug users, recipients of blood products, and Native Alaskans, Pacific Islanders, and Native Americans.

HBV has been detected in almost every body fluid. Infected semen, cervicovaginal secretions, and saliva contain much lower concentrations of HBV than blood, but the virus can be transmitted via these secretions. If gastrointestinal (GI) bleeding occurs, feces can be contaminated with the virus from the blood. There is no evidence of fecal-oral transmission. Organ and tissue transplantation is another potential source of infection. However, in some patients with acute hepatitis B, there is no readily identifiable risk factor.

HBV is a complex structure with 3 distinct antigens: surface antigen (HBsAg), core antigen (HBcAg), and e antigen (HBeAg). Each antigen, along with its corresponding antibody, may appear or disappear in serum depending on the phase of infection and immune response.

In most people who acquire HBV infection as an adult, the infection completely resolves without any long-term complications. In those who develop chronic HBV infections, the liver may range from a normal-appearing liver to severe liver inflammation and scarring (fibrosis). Around 25% of those who become chronically HBV-infected in childhood die from complications of chronic liver disease, including liver cancer.[3]

Screening for HBV usually includes identifying those at high risk for infection and testing the blood for the presence of hepatitis B surface antigen (HBsAg), hepatitis B antibody (anti-HBs),

and hepatitis B core antibody (anti-HBc). The presence of anti-HBs in the blood indicates immunity from the HBV vaccine or from past HBV infection (Fig. 43.3). HBsAg in the serum for 6 months or longer after infection indicates chronic HBV infection.

Hepatitis C Virus. Hepatitis C virus (HCV) causes a type of hepatitis that can result in both acute illness and chronic infection. Acute hepatitis C, which can be mild in presentation, can be hard to detect unless a diagnosis is made with laboratory testing. The most common causes of acute hepatitis C outbreaks are among injection drug users and MSM with HIV infection.

HCV is an RNA virus that is blood-borne and primarily transmitted percutaneously. The most common mode of HCV transmission is the sharing of contaminated needles and equipment among injection drug users. High-risk sexual behavior (e.g., unprotected sex, multiple partners), especially among MSM, is associated with increased risk for transmission.

After a needle-stick exposure or sharps exposure to HCV-positive blood, the transmission rate is 0.1%. The risk for perinatal HCV transmission is 4% to 7% per pregnancy. Persons who were given blood or blood products before 1992 (when blood product testing for HCV began) are at higher risk for chronic HCV infection and should be routinely tested.[4] Some patients with HCV infection cannot identify a source of infection.

Most patients usually develop chronic infection. However, because signs and symptoms of HCV infection are generally mild, most people are unaware of their infection. HCV is the most common cause of chronic liver disease and liver failure. About 20% to 30% develop cirrhosis and eventually liver failure and/or liver cancer.[4] Along with chronic HBV, HCV accounts for most cases of liver cancer. HCV hepatitis is the most common reason for liver transplantation in the United States.

Because of the 15- to 20-year delay between infection and the manifestations of liver damage, long-term effects of HCV infection pose important health care challenges.

Persons at risk for HCV infection are also at risk for HBV and HIV infections. About 30% to 40% of HIV-infected patients also have HCV. This high rate of co-infection is primarily related to IV drug use. Co-infection with HIV and HCV places the patient at greater risk for progression to cirrhosis.

People in the United States born between 1945 and 1965 and those at increased risk should be screened for HCV infection. This includes people who engage in high-risk sexual practices, injection drug users, those who may have had blood or blood products prior to 1992, and/or those who have abnormal liver function tests. A positive antibody test for HCV (anti-HCV) is usually enough for a diagnosis.[2] However, a positive viral load is needed to confirm active infection because anti-HCV can also indicate a past infection.

Hepatitis D Virus. Hepatitis D virus (HDV), also called *delta virus,* is uncommon in the United States. HDV is a defective single-stranded RNA virus that cannot survive on its own. It requires HBV surface Ag to serve as its outer shell. So, only those who are infected with HBV can be infected with HDV. It can be acquired at the same time as HBV or a person with HBV can be infected with HDV later. HDV is transmitted like HBV. It can cause a range of illness, from an asymptomatic chronic carrier state to acute liver failure. There is no vaccine for HDV. However, vaccination against HBV reduces the risk for HDV co-infection.[3]

Hepatitis E Virus. Like hepatitis A, the hepatitis E virus (HEV) is an RNA virus transmitted by the fecal-oral route. The usual mode of transmission is drinking contaminated water. HEV infection occurs primarily in developing countries, with epidemics reported in India, Asia, Mexico, and Africa. Only a few

cases of HEV have been reported in the United States. These have been primarily in persons who recently traveled to an HEV-endemic area. It is generally acute and self-resolving, but chronicity in immunosuppressed persons, such as liver transplant recipients, has been reported. Pregnant women may be affected severely, with reported mortality rates of up to 10%. An IgM antibody assay is available to test for acute hepatitis E.[3]

Pathophysiology

Liver. In viral hepatitis, hepatocytes become targets of the virus in one of 2 ways: through direct action of the virus (as in HCV infection) or through a cell-mediated immune response to the virus (as in HBV and HCV infection).[3]

During acute viral hepatitis, large numbers of infected hepatocytes are destroyed. The destruction of hepatocytes leads to a wide range of liver-related dysfunction. Bile production, coagulation, blood glucose, and protein metabolism can be affected. Detoxification and processing of drugs, hormones, and metabolites (e.g., ammonia from protein catabolism) may be disrupted.

After resolution of an acute infection, liver cells can regenerate. If no complications occur, the liver can resume its normal appearance and function. In certain cases, the acute hepatitis can become so severe and irreversible that people develop liver failure or die.

Chronic viral hepatitis can be insidious and silent, causing persistent and continual destruction of infected hepatocytes. Over time scar tissue can develop, which leads to fibrosis and compromised liver function. Fibrosis can lead to cirrhosis and liver failure. Cirrhosis is a generally irreversible condition that can increase one's risk for liver dysfunction, portal hypertension, and primary liver cancer. Cirrhosis is discussed later in this chapter.

Systemic Effects. In the early phases of hepatitis infection, antigen-antibody complexes between the virus and its corresponding antibody may form circulating immune complexes. The circulating immune complexes activate the complement system (see Chapter 11). The manifestations of this activation are rash, angioedema, arthritis, fever, and malaise. *Cryoglobulinemia* (abnormal proteins found in the blood), glomerulonephritis, vasculitis, and involvement of other organs can occur from immune complex activation.

Clinical Manifestations and Complications

The manifestations of the different viral hepatitis infections can be classified into acute hepatitis and chronic hepatitis (Table 43.2).

Acute Hepatitis. Many patients with acute hepatitis have no symptoms and may not even know they have been infected. However, others may have intermittent or ongoing anorexia, lethargy, nausea, vomiting, skin rashes, diarrhea or constipation, malaise, fatigue, myalgias, arthralgias, other flu-like symptoms, and right upper quadrant tenderness (caused by liver inflammation).

Although the acute phase of viral hepatitis varies depending on the type of hepatitis, it usually lasts from 1 to 6 months. During this time, the patient may have a decreased sense of smell and find food repugnant. Smokers may have distaste for cigarettes. Physical examination often reveals hepatomegaly, lymphadenopathy, abdominal tenderness, and sometimes splenomegaly. The acute phase is the period of maximal infectivity.

A patient in the acute phase of hepatitis may be *icteric* (jaundiced) or anicteric. Jaundice, a yellowish discoloration of body tissues, results from a change in normal bilirubin metabolism or disruption of the flow of bile into the hepatic or biliary duct systems. The types of jaundice are described in Table 43.3. The urine may appear darker due to excess bilirubin being excreted by the kidneys. If conjugated bilirubin cannot pass into the intestines from the liver because of obstruction or inflammation of the bile ducts, the stools will be clay colored.

Pruritus (intense generalized itching) sometimes accompanies jaundice. It occurs from the accumulation of bile salts beneath the skin. Itching can be intolerable to the patient.

As jaundice fades, the convalescent phase begins. The convalescent phase can last for weeks to months, with an average of 2 to 4 months. During this period, patients typically have malaise and easy fatigability. Hepatomegaly remains for several weeks. Splenomegaly (if present) subsides during this period.

Most patients with acute viral hepatitis recover completely. Almost all cases of acute hepatitis A resolve. However, some patients may have a relapse in the first 2 to 3 months after the infection. The disappearance of jaundice does not mean the patient has totally recovered. Some HBV infections and most HCV infections result in chronic hepatitis.

The overall mortality rate for acute hepatitis is less than 1%. The mortality rate is higher in older adults and those with underlying debilitating illnesses (including chronic liver disease).

Complications that can result from acute hepatitis are acute liver failure, chronic hepatitis, cirrhosis of the liver, portal hypertension, and liver cancer.

Acute Liver Failure. Sometimes, acute liver failure (fulminant hepatic failure) may occur, which is a serious condition with a poor prognosis. Manifestations include encephalopathy, GI bleeding, disseminated intravascular coagulation (DIC), fever with leukocytosis, renal manifestations (oliguria, azotemia), ascites, edema, hypotension, respiratory failure, hypoglycemia, bacterial infections, thrombocytopenia, and coagulopathies. Liver transplantation is usually the cure for these patients. Acute liver failure is discussed in this chapter on p. 989.

Chronic Hepatitis. Manifestations of chronic hepatitis are shown in Table 43.2. Chronic HBV is more likely to develop in infants born to infected mothers and in those who acquire the infection before age 5 than in those who acquire the virus after age 5.[3]

Problems with the patient's cellular immune response may be important in the development of the chronic HBsAg carrier state and the progression of acute HBV to chronic HBV. More than 50% of immunocompromised adults who are acutely infected with HBV progress to chronic infection.[3]

HCV infection is more likely than HBV to become chronic. As previously mentioned, many patients with chronic HCV infection develop chronic liver disease, cirrhosis, portal hypertension, and liver cancer. Risk factors for progression to cirrhosis include male gender, alcohol use, concomitant fatty liver disease, and excess iron deposition in the liver. In some patients, co-infection with HIV may cause complications or require treatment modification. Manifestations of chronic hepatitis include

---

TABLE 43.2 Manifestations of Hepatitis

Acute Hepatitis	Chronic Hepatitis
• Anorexia	• ALT, AST elevations (may be normal in some people)
• Clay-colored stools	• Ascites and lower extremity edema
• Dark urine	• Asterixis ("liver flap")
• Decreased sense of taste and smell	• Bleeding abnormalities (thrombocytopenia, easy bruising, prolonged clotting time)
• Diarrhea or constipation	• Fatigue, malaise
• Fatigue, lethargy, malaise	• Hepatic encephalopathy: confusion, difficulty concentrating, easy agitation
• Flu-like symptoms (e.g., headache)	• Hepatomegaly
• Hepatomegaly	• Increased bilirubin
• Jaundice	• Jaundice
• Low-grade fever	• Myalgias and/or arthralgias
• Lymphadenopathy	• Palmar erythema
• Myalgias and/or arthralgias	• Spider angiomas
• Nausea, vomiting	
• Pruritus	
• Right upper quadrant tenderness	
• Splenomegaly	
• Weight loss	

TABLE 43.3 Classification of Jaundice

	Hemolytic Jaundice	Hepatocellular Jaundice	Obstructive Jaundice
Causes	• Blood transfusion reactions, hemolytic anemia, sickle cell crisis	• Cirrhosis, hepatitis, liver cancer	• Cirrhosis, hepatitis, liver cancer • Common bile duct obstruction from stone(s), biliary strictures, pancreatic cancer, sclerosing cholangitis
Description	• Caused by increased breakdown of RBCs, which produces an increased amount of unconjugated bilirubin in blood • Liver is unable to handle increased load	• Results from liver's altered ability to take up bilirubin from blood or to conjugate or excrete it • In hepatocellular disease, damaged hepatocytes leak bilirubin	• Results from decreased or obstructed flow of bile through liver or biliary duct system • Obstruction may occur in intrahepatic or extrahepatic bile ducts • Intrahepatic obstructions are due to swelling or fibrosis of the liver's canaliculi and bile ducts
Diagnostic Findings			
Serum Bilirubin			
Unconjugated (indirect)	↑	↑	↑
Conjugated (direct)	Normal	↑ or ↓ (severe disease)	↑
Urine Bilirubin	Negative	↑	↑
Urobilinogen			
Stool	↑	Normal, ↓	↓
Urine	↑	Normal, ↑	↓

anemia and coagulation problems (easy bruising, bleeding). Since the liver produces clotting factors, clotting and bleeding times can be impaired or prolonged.

Skin manifestations may include spider angiomas, palmar erythema, and gynecomastia. Some patients have spleen, liver, or cervical lymph node enlargement.

In patients with severe liver damage, *hepatic encephalopathy* is a potentially life-threatening spectrum of neurologic, psychiatric, and motor disturbances. Hepatic encephalopathy results from the liver's inability to remove toxins (especially ammonia) from the blood. Hepatic encephalopathy is discussed later in this chapter on p. 983.)

Ascites, a common manifestation of hepatitis (especially chronic hepatitis), is the accumulation of excess fluid in the peritoneal cavity. Fluid accumulates due to reduced protein levels in the blood, which reduces the plasma oncotic pressure. Ascites is discussed later in this chapter on p. 982.

Diagnostic Studies

The only definitive way to distinguish among the types of viral hepatitis is by testing the patient's blood for the specific antigen or antibody. In some types of viral hepatitis, the blood can be tested for the viral load (viral level). Tests for the different types of viral hepatitis are outlined in Table 43.4. Many liver function tests show significant abnormalities, as shown in Table 43.5.

Several tests are available to determine the presence of HCV. The screening test for HCV infection is HCV antibody testing. Antibodies can be detected within 4 weeks of infection. If the antibody test is positive, HCV RNA testing is done to assess for chronic infection. A positive result confirms chronic infection. A few patients may have a false-positive HCV antibody result with a negative HCV RNA test. If recent HCV infection is suspected, HCV RNA testing is usually done because it may take several weeks or longer for HCV antibodies to develop.

HCV RNA testing may be used for immunocompromised patients (e.g., patient with HIV). Because of altered or delayed antibody response to HCV, these patients may not have detectable antibody levels even if they are infected with HCV.

Viral genotype testing is done in patients undergoing drug therapy for HBV or HCV infection. HBV has at least 8 different genotypes (A to H). In some centers, HBV genotyping is done before starting treatment. HBV genotype may be useful in predicting disease course and treatment outcomes. HBV core Ab (HBVcAb) IgG indicates that the patient has a history of HBV infection. HBV may reactivate in these patients if they become immunosuppressed.

HCV has 6 genotypes and more than 50 subtypes. In the United States, 75% of HCV infections are caused by HCV genotype 1. For patients who test positive for HCV, genotyping is done before drug therapy is started. The genotype determines the choice and duration of therapy. It is one of the strongest predictors of a patient's response to drug therapy.

A liver biopsy is done in acute hepatitis only if diagnosis is in doubt. In chronic hepatitis, a liver biopsy allows for histologic examination of liver cells and determination of the degree of inflammation, fibrosis, or cirrhosis that may be present. A patient who has a bleeding disorder may not be a candidate for a percutaneous liver biopsy because of the risk for bleeding. In these patients, a transjugular biopsy may be an alternative. This type of biopsy consists of obtaining liver tissue through a rigid cannula introduced into a hepatic vein, typically using jugular venous access.

Techniques for noninvasive assessment of liver fibrosis are increasingly replacing the need for liver biopsy. One option is the use of ultrasound elastography (e.g., FibroScan), which uses

TABLE 43.4 Diagnostic Studies

Viral Hepatitis

Virus	Tests	Significance
A	Anti-HAV immunoglobulin M (IgM)	Acute infection
	Anti-HAV immunoglobulin G (IgG)	Previous infection or immunization
		Not routinely done in clinical practice
B	HBsAg (hepatitis B surface antigen)	Marker of infectivity
		Present in acute or chronic infection
		Positive in chronic carriers
	Anti-HBs (hepatitis B surface antibody)	Indicates previous infection with HBV or immunization
	HBeAg (hepatitis B e antigen)	Indicates high infectivity
		Used to determine the clinical management of patients with chronic hepatitis B
	Anti-HBe (hepatitis B e antibody)	Indicates previous infection
		In chronic hepatitis B, indicates a low viral load and low degree of infectivity
	Anti-HBc (antibody to hepatitis B core antigen) IgM	Indicates acute infection
		Does not appear after vaccination
	Anti-HBc IgG	Indicates previous infection or ongoing infection with hepatitis B
		Does not appear after vaccination
	HBV DNA quantitation	Indicates active ongoing viral replication
		Best indicator of viral replication and effectiveness of therapy in patient with chronic hepatitis B
	HBV genotyping	Indicates the genotype of HBV
C	Anti-HCV (antibody to HCV)	Marker for acute or chronic infection with HCV
	HCV RNA quantitation	Indicates active ongoing viral replication
	HCV genotyping	Indicates the genotype of HCV
D	Anti-HDV	Present in past or current infection with HDV
	HDV Ag (hepatitis D antigen)	Present within a few days after infection
E	Anti-HEV IgM and IgG	Present 1 wk–2 mo after illness onset
	HEV RNA quantitation	Indicates active ongoing viral replication

A, Hepatitis A virus (HAV); *B,* hepatitis B virus (HBV); *C,* hepatitis C virus (HCV); *D,* hepatitis D virus (HDV); *E,* hepatitis E virus (HEV).

TABLE 43.5 Diagnostic Findings in Acute Hepatitis

Test	Abnormal Finding	Etiology
Alkaline phosphatase	Moderately ↑	Impaired excretory function of liver
γ-Glutamyl transpeptidase (GGT)	↑	Liver cell injury
Aminotransferases		
• Aspartate aminotransferase (AST)	↑ in acute phase Decreases as jaundice disappears	Liver cell injury
• Alanine aminotransferase (ALT)	↑ in acute phase Decreases as jaundice disappears	Liver cell injury
Prothrombin time	Prolonged	↓ prothrombin production by liver
Serum proteins		
• Albumin	Normal or ↓	Liver cell injury
• γ-Globulin	Normal or ↓	Impaired clearance from liver
Total bilirubin (serum)	Increased to about 8–15 mg/dL (137–257 µmol/L)	Liver cell injury
Urinary bilirubin	↑	Conjugated hyperbilirubinemia
Urinary urobilinogen	↑ 2–5 days before jaundice	Decreased urobilinogen reabsorption

TABLE 43.6 Interprofessional Care

Viral Hepatitis

Diagnostic Assessment
- History and physical examination
- Liver function tests (ALT, AST, alkaline phosphatase, bilirubin, γ-glutamyl transpeptidase [GGT])
- PT time and INR
- Hepatitis testing
  - *Hepatitis A:* Anti-HAV IgM, anti-HAV IgG, or HAV total antibody
  - *Hepatitis B:* HBsAg, anti-HBs, HBeAg, anti-HBe, anti-HBc IgM and IgG, HBV DNA quantitation, HBV genotyping
  - *Hepatitis C:* Anti-HCV, HCV RNA quantitation, HCV genotyping
  - *Hepatitis D:* Anti-HDV, HDV Ag
- FibroScan
- FibroSure (FibroTest)

Management
Acute and Chronic
- Well-balanced diet
- Vitamin supplements
- Rest (degree of strictness varies)
- Avoiding alcohol and drugs detoxified by liver

Chronic HBV and HCV
- Drug therapy (Table 43.7)

HAV, Hepatitis A virus; *HB,* hepatitis B; *HBeAg,* hepatitis B e antigen; *HBsAg,* hepatitis B surface antigen; *HBV,* hepatitis B virus; *HCV,* hepatitis C virus; *HDV Ag,* hepatitis D antigen; *HDV,* hepatitis D virus.

an ultrasound transducer to determine the degree of liver fibrosis.[5] FibroSure (FibroTest) is an example of one of several biomarkers that uses the results of serum tests to assess the extent of hepatic fibrosis.

Interprofessional Care

There is no specific treatment for acute viral hepatitis. Most patients are managed at home. Emphasis is on providing adequate nutrition and measures to rest the body and help the liver to regenerate and repair (Table 43.6). Rest reduces the metabolic demands on the liver and promotes liver cell regeneration. The degree of rest depends on the severity of symptoms, but usually alternating periods of activity and rest are adequate. Counseling should include the importance of avoiding alcohol and notifying contacts for testing and prophylaxis, if indicated.

In patients with chronic viral hepatitis, care may involve hepatologists, infectious disease specialists, pharmacists, dietitians, and mental health or substance use specialists. The role and extent of involvement of team members is based on the patient's specific needs.

Drug Therapy

Acute Hepatitis. There are no drug therapies for treating acute HAV infection. Treatment of acute HBV may be indicated only in patients with severe hepatitis and liver failure.

In acute hepatitis C, some patients may choose to be monitored for spontaneous clearance of the infection. For patients who choose treatment, one of the direct-acting antivirals (DAAs) may be used.[6] DAAs are discussed later in the section on chronic hepatitis.

Supportive drug therapy may include antihistamines for generalized itching and antiemetics for nausea. These drugs include promethazine (Phenergan) and ondansetron (Zofran).

COMPLEMENTARY & ALTERNATIVE THERAPIES

Milk Thistle (Silymarin)

Scientific Evidence
People have used milk thistle for liver disorders, including hepatitis, cirrhosis, and gallbladder problems.
- Clinical trials of milk thistle for liver diseases have mixed results.
- Silymarin was no better than placebo for chronic hepatitis C in people who had not responded to standard antiviral treatment.
- The 2008 Hepatitis C Antiviral Long-Term Treatment Against Cirrhosis (HALT-C) study found that patients with hepatitis C who used silymarin had fewer and milder symptoms of liver disease and better quality of life but no change in virus activity or liver inflammation.

Nursing Implications
- Well tolerated in recommended doses. Some people report GI side effects
- May lower blood glucose
- May interfere with the liver's cytochrome P450 enzyme system

Source: National Center for Complementary and Alternative Therapy: Milk thistle. Retrieved from *www.nccih.nih.gov/health/milkthistle/ataglance.htm.*

Chronic Hepatitis B. Drug therapy for chronic HBV focuses on decreasing the hepatitis B viral load and liver enzymes, and in turn, slowing the rate of disease progression. Long-term goals are preventing the development of cirrhosis, portal hypertension, liver failure, and liver cancer. Current drug therapies for chronic HBV do not eradicate the virus but suppress viral replication and prevent complications of infection. First-line therapies now include primarily nucleoside and nucleotide analogs (Table 43.7) and sometimes interferon therapy.[7]

TABLE 43.7 Drug Therapy

Viral Hepatitis B and C

Drug Class	Examples	Mechanism of Action	Indication
Immune modulator	pegylated interferon (Pegasys, PegIntron)	Has antiviral, antiproliferative, immune-regulating actions	Chronic hepatitis B and C*
Nucleoside and nucleotide analogs	entecavir (Baraclude) lamivudine (Epivir HBV) telbivudine (Tyzeka) tenofovir (Vemlidy, Viread)	Inhibits HBV DNA polymerase enzyme by competing with natural substrates. Prevents viral replication	Chronic hepatitis B
Direct-acting antivirals for hepatitis C			
• NS3/4A protease inhibitors	simeprevir (Olysio) glecaprevir† grazoprevir† paritaprevir† voxilaprevir†	Blocks viral protease enzyme. Prevents viral replication in genotype 1 HCV	Chronic hepatitis C
• NS5A inhibitors	daclatasvir (Daklinza) elbasvir† ledipasvir† ombitasvir† pibrentasvir† velpatasvir†	Blocks nonstructural protein 5A (NS5A) at early stage in RNA HCV replication	Chronic hepatitis C
• NS5B polymerase inhibitors	dasabuvir† sofosbuvir (Sovaldi)	Nucleotide inhibitor and non-nucleoside inhibitor of HCV polymerase. Prevent replication of RNA HCV	Chronic hepatitis C
Combination therapies	elbasvir + grazoprevir (Zepatier) ledipasvir + sofosbuvir (Harvoni) ombitasvir + paritaprevir + ritonvir‡ + dasabuvir (Viekira Pak) Pibrentasvir + glecaprevir (Mavyret) velpatasvir + sofosbuvir (Epclusa) velpatasvir + sofosbuvir + voxilaprevir (Vosevi)	Drugs are combined in single tablet. Drugs may be from the same or different classes.	Chronic hepatitis C

*Use of all oral or noninterferon therapies for chronic hepatitis C is preferred.
†Used only in combination therapy.
‡CYP3A inhibitor used to enhance the pharmacokinetics of the other agents.

Nucleoside and nucleotide analogs. Nucleoside and nucleotide analogs inhibit viral DNA replication. HBV reproduces by making copies of its viral DNA nucleosides and nucleotides. The nucleoside and nucleotide analog drugs mimic normal building blocks for DNA but are actually faulty viral DNA building blocks. Once they become incorporated into the viral DNA, they halt DNA synthesis.

Nucleoside and nucleotide analogs do not prevent all viral reproduction, but they can substantially lower the amount of virus in the body. These medications include lamivudine (Epivir), adefovir (Hepsera), entecavir (Baraclude), telbivudine (Tyzeka), and tenofovir (Viread). These oral medications are used to treat chronic HBV when there is evidence of significant active viral replication and liver inflammation.[7]

These drugs also reduce viral load, decrease liver damage, and decrease serum liver enzyme levels. Most patients with HBV need long-term treatment. When these drugs are stopped, many patients' (except those who have seroconverted) HBV DNA and liver enzyme levels return to pretreatment levels.

Severe exacerbations of hepatitis B can develop after ending treatment. If these drugs are stopped for any reason, closely monitor liver function for several months.

Interferon. Interferon is a naturally occurring immune protein made by the body during an infection to recognize and respond to pathogens. It has antiviral, antiproliferative, and immune-modulating effects. (Interferon is discussed in Chapter 13). Pegylated interferon (PEG-Intron, Pegasys) is given by subcutaneous injection.

The many side effects with interferon therapy, including flu-like symptoms (e.g., fever, malaise, fatigue), make adhering to therapy hard for some patients. Currently, the availability of better tolerated and more effective oral treatments limits interferon use. However, it is still among the first-line options recommended by hepatology societies.

Patients receiving interferon should have blood counts and liver function tests every 4 to 6 weeks. Depression is a side effect of interferon. Patients must be screened for depression and other mood disorders before starting interferon treatment and monitored frequently while on therapy.

Chronic Hepatitis C. Treatment of chronic hepatitis C is patient specific and based on the genotype of the HCV, severity of liver disease, and presence of other health problems (e.g., HIV). The goal of drug therapy is eradicating the virus and preventing HCV-related complications. Treatment for HCV primarily includes the use of DAAs (Table 43.7), which block proteins needed for HCV replication.

With DAAs, patients typically complete a 12-week regimen with oral drugs. Almost all (>95%) of those who complete treatment with the DAAs are now able to cure their chronic HCV infection.[6]

 DRUG ALERT Ribavirin (Rebetol, Ribasphere)

- May cause severe birth defects. During treatment, women taking the drug and women whose male partners are taking the drug must avoid pregnancy.
- Monitor hemoglobin and hematocrit as it may cause anemia.
- Used only for specific populations.

Many patients with HIV also have HCV. Patients who have stable HIV and intact immune systems (CD4$^+$ counts greater than 200/μL) receive HCV treatment with the goal of eradicating HCV and reducing the risk for progression to cirrhosis. HCV treatment may reduce CD4$^+$ counts and increase the patient's risk for anemia and leukopenia.

Patients with advanced fibrosis or cirrhosis can undergo drug therapy if liver decompensation (e.g., ascites, variceal rupture, jaundice, wasting, encephalopathy) is not present.

Nutritional Therapy. No special diet is needed in the treatment of viral hepatitis. Emphasis is placed on a well-balanced diet that the patient can tolerate. During acute viral hepatitis, adequate calories are important because the patient usually loses weight. If fat content is poorly tolerated because of decreased bile production, it should be reduced. Vitamin supplements, particularly B-complex and vitamin K, are often given. If anorexia, nausea, and vomiting are severe, IV solutions of glucose or supplemental enteral nutrition (EN) therapy may be used. Fluid and electrolyte balance must be maintained.

❖ NURSING MANAGEMENT: VIRAL HEPATITIS

◆ Nursing Assessment

Subjective and objective data that should be obtained from a person with hepatitis are outlined in Table 43.8.

◆ Nursing Diagnoses

Nursing diagnoses for the patient with viral hepatitis may include:

- Impaired nutritional intake
- Activity intolerance
- Risk for bleeding

Additional information on nursing diagnoses and interventions for the patient with hepatitis is presented in eNursing Care Plan 43.1 available on the website for this chapter.

◆ Planning

The overall goals are that the patient with viral hepatitis will (1) have relief of discomfort, (2) be able to resume normal activities, and (3) return to normal liver function without complications.

◆ Nursing Implementation

Health Promotion. Viral hepatitis is a public health problem. Your role is important in the prevention and control of this disease. It is helpful to understand the epidemiology of the different types of viral hepatitis when considering appropriate control measures. Preventive and control measures for hepatitis A, B, and C are outlined in Table 43.9.

A suggested guideline for general practice to prevent you from contracting viral hepatitis from diagnosed and undiagnosed patients and carriers is for you to wear disposable gloves, goggles, and gowns (sometimes) when fecal or blood contamination is likely in handling (1) soiled bedpans, urinals, and catheters and (2) when the patient's bed linens are soiled by body excreta or secretions.

Hepatitis A. Viral hepatitis outbreaks are usually due to HAV. Preventive measures include personal and environmental hygiene and health education to promote good sanitation. Hand washing is the most important precaution. Teach about careful hand washing after bowel movements and before eating.

Vaccination is the best protection against HAV. All children at 1 year of age should receive the vaccine. Adults at risk should

TABLE 43.8 Nursing Assessment
*Hepatitis**

Subjective Data
Important Health Information

Past health history: Hemophilia, cancer, exposure to infected persons, ingestion of contaminated food or water. Exposure to benzene, carbon tetrachloride, or other hepatotoxic agents. Crowded, unsanitary living conditions. Exposure to contaminated needles. Recent travel, organ transplant recipient, exposure to new drug regimens, hemodialysis, transfusion of blood or blood products before 1992. HIV status (if known)

Medications: Use and misuse of acetaminophen, new prescription, over-the-counter, or herbal medications or supplements

Functional Health Patterns

Health perception–health management: IV drug and chronic alcohol use. Malaise, distaste for cigarettes (in smokers), high-risk sexual behaviors

Nutritional-metabolic: Weight loss, anorexia, nausea, vomiting. Feeling of fullness in right upper quadrant

Elimination: Dark urine, light-colored stools, constipation or diarrhea, skin rashes, hives

Activity-exercise: Fatigue, arthralgias, myalgias

Cognitive-perceptual: Right upper quadrant pain and liver tenderness, headache, itching

Role-relationship: Exposure as health care worker, resident in long-term care institution, incarceration, homelessness

Objective Data
General

Low-grade fever, lethargy, lymphadenopathy

Integumentary

Rash or other skin changes, jaundice, icteric sclera, injection sites

Gastrointestinal

Hepatomegaly, splenomegaly

Possible Diagnostic Findings

Elevated liver enzyme levels. ↑ Serum total bilirubin, hypoalbuminemia, anemia, bilirubin in urine and increased urobilinogen, prolonged PT time, positive tests for hepatitis, including anti-HAV IgM, HBsAg, anti-HBs, HBeAg, anti-HBe, anti-HBc IgM and IgG, HBV DNA quantitation, anti-HCV, HCV RNA quantitation, anti-HDV, HDV Ag. Abnormal liver scan, abnormal results on liver biopsy

*Tailor history questions to the type of hepatitis.

HAV, Hepatitis A virus; *HBcAg,* hepatitis B core antigen; *HBeAg,* hepatitis B e antigen; *HBsAg,* hepatitis B surface antigen; *HBV,* hepatitis B virus; *HCV,* hepatitis C virus; *HDV Ag,* hepatitis D antigen; *HDV,* hepatitis D virus.

also receive the vaccine. These include people who travel to areas with increased rates of hepatitis A, MSM, injecting and noninjecting drug users, persons with clotting factor disorders (e.g., hemophilia), and persons with chronic liver disease.

HAV vaccine is inactivated HAV protein. There are 2 forms of HAV vaccine in the United States: Havrix and Vaqta. Primary immunization consists of 1 dose given IM in the deltoid muscle. A booster is recommended 6 to 12 months after the first dose to ensure adequate antibody titers and long-term protection. Primary immunization provides immunity within 30 days after 1 dose in more than 95% of those vaccinated.

Twinrix, a combined HAV and HBV vaccine, is available for people over 18 years of age. Immunization consists of 3 doses, given on a 0-, 1-, and 6-month schedule, the same

TABLE 43.9 Preventive Measures for Viral Hepatitis

Hepatitis A
General Measures
- Hand washing
- Proper personal hygiene
- Environmental sanitation
- Control and screening (signs, symptoms) of food handlers
- Serologic screening for those carrying virus
- Active immunization: HAV vaccine

Use of Immune Globulin
- Early administration (1–2 wk after exposure) to those exposed
- Prophylaxis for travelers to areas where hepatitis A is common if not vaccinated with HAV vaccine

Special Considerations for Health Care Personnel
- Wash hands after contact with a patient or removal of gloves
- Use infection control precautions

Hepatitis B and C
Percutaneous Transmission
- Screening of donated blood
- *HBV:* HBsAg
- *HCV:* Anti-HCV
- Use of disposable needles and syringes

Sexual Transmission
- Acute exposure: HBIG administration to sexual partner of HBsAg-positive person
- HBV vaccine series given to uninfected sexual partners
- Condoms used for sexual intercourse

General Measures
- Hand washing
- Avoid sharing toothbrushes and razors
- HBIG administration for one-time exposure (needle stick, contact of mucous membranes with infectious material)
- Active immunization: HBV vaccine

Special Considerations for Health Care Personnel
- Use infection control precautions
- Reduce contact with blood or blood-containing secretions
- Handle the blood of patients as potentially infective
- Dispose of needles properly
- Use needleless IV access devices when available

HAV, Hepatitis A virus; *HBIG,* hepatitis B immune globulin; *HBsAg,* hepatitis B surface antigen; *HBV,* hepatitis B virus; *HCV,* hepatitis C virus.

schedule as that used for the single HBV vaccine. Twinrix may be given to high-risk persons, including patients with chronic liver disease, users of illicit IV drugs, patients on hemodialysis, MSM, and people with clotting factor disorders who receive therapeutic blood products. The side effects of the vaccine are mild and usually limited to soreness and redness at the injection site.

Isolation is not needed for HAV infection. For a patient with HAV infection, use infection control precautions. Place the patient who is incontinent of stool or has poor personal hygiene in a private room.

Both hepatitis A vaccine and immune globulin (IG) are used to prevent HAV infection after exposure to an infected person *(postexposure prophylaxis).* The vaccine is used for preexposure prophylaxis. IG can be given either before or after exposure. IG gives temporary (1 to 2 months) passive immunity and is

effective for preventing hepatitis A if given within 2 weeks after exposure. IG is recommended for persons who do not have anti-HAV antibodies and were exposed by close (household, day care center) contact with persons who have HAV or foodborne exposure. Because patients with HAV are most infectious just before the onset of symptoms (the preicteric phase), those exposed through household contact or foodborne outbreaks should receive IG. Although IG may not prevent infection in all persons, it may lessen the illness to a subclinical infection. When hepatitis A occurs in a food handler, IG should be given to all other food handlers at the establishment. Patrons may need to receive IG.

Persons exposed to HAV who have received a dose of HAV vaccine more than 1 month previously or who have a history of laboratory-confirmed HAV infection do not need IG.

Hepatitis B. The best way to reduce HBV infection is to identify those at risk, screen them for HBV, and vaccinate those who are not infected. Teach those at high risk for contracting HBV to reduce risks by following good hygienic practices, including hand washing and using gloves when expecting contact with blood. Patients should not share razors, toothbrushes, and other personal items. Teach patients to use a condom for sexual intercourse. In addition, the partner should be vaccinated.

The HBV vaccine is the best means of prevention. The HBV vaccines (Recombivax HB, Engerix-B) contain HBsAg, which promotes the synthesis of specific antibodies directed against HBV. The vaccine is given in a series of 3 IM injections in the deltoid muscle. The second dose is given within 1 month of the first dose and the third dose within 6 months of the first. The vaccine is more than 95% effective. Minor reactions include transient fever and soreness at the injection site. The vaccine can be given in pregnancy.

The first dose of hepatitis B vaccine should be given at birth, with the vaccine series completed by age 6 to 18 months. Older children and adolescents who did not receive the hepatitis B vaccine should be vaccinated.[3] It is important to vaccinate adults who are in the at-risk groups and are not immune. Household members of the patient with HBV should be tested and vaccinated if they are HBsAg and antibody negative. Hepatitis vaccination is recommended for patients with chronic kidney disease before they start dialysis. Dialysis patients should routinely have their antibody titer levels checked to determine the need for revaccination.

For postexposure prophylaxis, the HBV vaccine series and hepatitis B immune globulin (HBIG) are given. HBIG has antibodies to HBV and confers temporary passive immunity. HBIG is prepared from plasma of donors with a high titer of anti-HBs. HBIG is recommended for postexposure prophylaxis in cases of needle stick, mucous membrane contact, or sexual exposure and for infants born to mothers who are positive for HBsAg. Ideally HBIG should be given within 24 hours of exposure. Giving antiviral therapy (e.g., tenofovir) to pregnant women in the third trimester with viral levels over 200,000 IU/mL can prevent the small risk for neonatal infection that may occur even with postnatal immunization and vaccination.

The Centers for Disease Control and Prevention (CDC) recommends following standard precautions for the patient with HBV (see Table 14.9). This includes using disposable needles and syringes and disposing of them in puncture-resistant units without recapping, bending, or breaking.

Hepatitis C. No vaccine is currently available for hepatitis C. Therefore it is important to identify those at high risk for contracting HCV and teach them how to reduce their risks. Primary measures to prevent HCV transmission include (1) screening of blood, organ, and tissue donors; (2) using infection control precautions; and (3) modifying high-risk behavior.

In the United States, there are many people who have undiagnosed hepatitis C. Therefore the CDC recommends universal screening for all persons born between 1945 and 1965.[4] The CDC does not recommend IG or antiviral agents (e.g., interferon) for postexposure prophylaxis for HCV infection (e.g., needle-stick exposure from an infected patient). After an acute exposure (e.g., needle stick), the person should have anti-HCV testing done. For the person exposed to HCV, baseline anti-HCV and ALT levels should be measured, with follow-up testing at 4 to 6 months. Testing for HCV RNA may be done after 4 to 10 weeks.[4]

◆ **Acute Care.** In patients with hepatitis, assess for the presence and degree of jaundice. In light-skinned persons, jaundice is usually seen first in the sclera of the eyes and later in the skin. In dark-skinned persons, jaundice is seen in the hard palate of the mouth and inner canthus of the eyes. The urine may have a dark brown or brownish red color from bilirubin excretion from the kidneys. Comfort measures to relieve itching, headache, and arthralgias are helpful.

? CHECK YOUR PRACTICE

You are caring for a 32-yr-old man who has acute hepatitis A. He has severe nausea and vomiting. He is admitted to the hospital for IV hydration and monitoring. The patient says, "I'm so weak and I feel like I'm going to vomit all the time. Isn't there something you can do to help me?"
- How would you handle this situation?
- What information and teaching will you give him?

Ensuring that the patient receives adequate nutrition is not always easy. The anorexia and distaste for food may cause nutritional problems. Assess the patient's tolerance of specific foods and eating pattern. Small, frequent meals may be preferable to 3 large ones and may help prevent nausea. Often a patient with hepatitis finds that anorexia is not as severe in the morning, so it is easier to eat a good breakfast than a large dinner. Include measures to stimulate the appetite, such as mouth care, antiemetics, and attractively served meals in pleasant surroundings, in the care plan. Drinking carbonated beverages and avoiding very hot or cold foods may help ease anorexia. Adequate fluid intake (2500 to 3000 mL/day) is important.

Rest is a critical factor in promoting hepatocyte regeneration. Assess the patient's response to the rest and activity plan. Modify it as needed based on liver function tests and symptoms.

Psychologic and emotional rest is as essential as physical rest. Limited activity may produce anxiety and restlessness in some patients. Diversion activities, such as reading and hobbies, may help a patient cope with the plan of care and ensure adequate rest.

◆ **Ambulatory Care.** Most patients with viral hepatitis are cared for at home. Assess the patient's knowledge of nutrition and provide any needed dietary teaching. Caution the patient about overexertion and the need to follow the HCP's advice about when to return to work. For patients who have fatigue, tell them to plan activities after periods of rest when energy levels are highest. Teach the patient and caregiver how to prevent transmission to other family members and symptoms to report to the HCP.

Assess the patient for any signs of complications. These include bleeding tendencies with increasing prothrombin (PT) time values, manifestations of encephalopathy, sudden increase in weight and abdominal girth (may indicate fluid retention and/or ascites), bloody or tarry stools, vomiting of blood, or elevated liver enzymes.

Teach the patient to have regular follow-ups for at least 1 year after the diagnosis of hepatitis. Because relapses occur with hepatitis B and C, teach the patient the symptoms of recurrence and the need for follow-up evaluations. All patients with chronic HBV or HCV should avoid alcohol as it can accelerate disease progression.

Note that patients who are positive for HBsAg (chronic carrier status) or HCV antibody cannot be blood donors.

◆ **Evaluation**

Expected outcomes are that the patient with hepatitis will
- Maintain food and fluid intake adequate to meet nutritional needs
- Avoid alcohol and other hepatotoxic agents
- Show gradual increase in activity tolerance
- Perform daily activities with scheduled rest periods

DRUG- AND CHEMICAL-INDUCED LIVER DISEASES

Alcohol use is the most frequent cause of both acute and chronic liver disease. It can cause injury and necrosis of liver tissue. Alcohol use can cause a spectrum of manifestations, ranging from mild elevation in liver enzymes to acute alcoholic hepatitis. It may also cause advanced fibrosis and cirrhosis, which usually occurs after decades of excess alcohol use. Patients may have serious liver disease caused by another chronic disease (e.g., chronic HCV infection) in combination with alcoholic liver disease, which can compound the problem.

Acute alcoholic hepatitis is a syndrome of hepatomegaly, jaundice, elevated liver enzymes (AST, ALT, alkaline phosphate), and low-grade fever with possible ascites and prolonged PT time. These manifestations may improve if alcohol intake ceases.

Even at the end-stage of cirrhosis, abstinence can result in significant reversal in some patients. If liver function does not recover after abstaining from alcohol for 6 months or longer, liver transplantation may be considered.

Chemical hepatotoxicity is liver injury caused by exposure to certain compounds (e.g., carbon tetrachloride, gold compounds). Some agents can cause hepatotoxicity, while others may induce cholestasis, necrosis, or liver cancer. Fortunately, because of the decreased use of these agents, the incidence of chemically induced liver toxicity has decreased since the 1980s.

Drug-induced liver injury (DILI) can present similarly to other forms of liver disease. The main cause of DILI is antimicrobial agents, especially amoxicillin-clavulanate. Many drugs (prescription, OTC, diet and herbal supplements) can cause an increase in liver enzymes and, in severe cases, jaundice and acute liver failure. The pattern of injury depends on the drug causing the reaction. The most common cause of acute liver failure is acetaminophen. In patients with chemical hepatotoxicity or DILI, all drugs identified as the cause of liver injury should be stopped.[3]

DRUG ALERT Acetaminophen (Tylenol)

- Safe when taken at recommended levels.
- Its prevalence in a variety of pain relievers, fever reducers, and cough medicines may mean that patients do not realize they are taking several drugs that all contain acetaminophen and overdose may occur.
- Acute liver failure can occur because of overdosing, either intentionally or unintentionally.
- The FDA has asked drug manufacturers to limit the strength of acetaminophen in prescription drug products to 325 mg per tablet, capsule, or other dosage unit, making these products safer.
- Combining the drug with alcoholic beverages increases the risk for liver damage.

AUTOIMMUNE, GENETIC, AND METABOLIC LIVER DISEASES

Autoimmune Hepatitis

Autoimmune hepatitis is a chronic inflammatory disorder of the liver in which the patient's own immune system attacks the liver. The cause of this condition is unknown. Autoimmune hepatitis is characterized by the presence of autoantibodies and high levels of serum immunoglobulins. It often occurs with other autoimmune diseases.

Most patients with autoimmune hepatitis are women. Laboratory tests useful in the diagnosis include antinuclear antibody (ANA), anti–smooth muscle antibody (ASMA), and antimitochondrial antibody (AMA) testing. A liver biopsy is often done to confirm the diagnosis and guide the treatment decision.[8]

Although autoimmune hepatitis can cause acute liver failure, the spectrum of disease is variable. Most patients develop chronic hepatitis. Untreated autoimmune hepatitis can progress to cirrhosis. Prednisone with or without azathioprine (Imuran) is the recommended treatment for active autoimmune hepatitis. Cyclosporine (Gengraf), tacrolimus (Prograf, FK506), budesonide (Entocort), methotrexate, mercaptopurine, and mycophenolate mofetil (CellCept) are options in those who do not respond to prednisone and azathioprine.[8] Mycophenolate is most often used for patients intolerant to azathioprine.

Wilson's Disease

Wilson's disease is an autosomal recessive disorder involving cellular copper transport. A defect in biliary excretion leads to accumulation of copper in the liver, causing progressive liver injury and cirrhosis. About 30 people per million have Wilson's disease. It usually appears between ages 5 and 35.[9]

Once cirrhosis occurs, copper leaks into the plasma, leading to multiple complications, including neurologic, hematologic, and renal disease. The hallmark of Wilson's disease is corneal Kayser-Fleischer rings. These are brownish red rings seen in the cornea near the limbus on eye examination. Low serum ceruloplasmin levels and markedly elevated copper concentrations from liver biopsy samples are present. Diagnosis is based on clinical findings, including the corneal rings and neurologic symptoms. First-degree relatives of patients with Wilson's disease should be screened for the disease.

The recommended first treatment of symptomatic patients or those with active disease is chelating agents, such as D-penicillamine (Cuprimine) or trientine (Syprine). They promote the excretion of urinary copper. Zinc acetate (Galzin), another therapy, interferes with copper absorption. Once we have reduced the amount of copper in the body, treatment focuses on preventing copper from building up again. Liver transplantation may be an option with severe liver damage.

Hemochromatosis

Hemochromatosis is a condition in which excess iron accumulates in the body. It is primarily caused by a genetic defect *(hereditary hemochromatosis)*. It also can be caused by liver disease and chronic blood transfusions used to treat thalassemia and sickle cell disease. Hemochromatosis is discussed in Chapter 30.

Primary Biliary Cholangitis

Primary biliary cholangitis (PBC), formerly known as primary biliary cirrhosis, is a chronic disease of the small bile ducts of the liver.[3] In PBC, there is a T cell–mediated attack of the small bile duct cells, resulting in loss of bile ducts and cholestasis (blockage of bile flow). Over time, this leads to liver fibrosis and cirrhosis.

Most patients diagnosed with PBC are middle-aged women. The disease is associated with other autoimmune disorders, such as rheumatoid arthritis, Sjögren's syndrome, and scleroderma. High serum alkaline phosphatase levels, AMAs, ANAs, and serum lipid levels occur in patients with PBC.

The goals of treatment are suppressing ongoing liver damage, preventing complications, and symptom management. Drugs for PBC include ursodeoxycholic acid (ursodiol [Actigall]), a bile acid, and obeticholic acid (Ocaliva). It decreases bile in the liver. Management focuses on preventing or minimizing malabsorption, skin disorders, such as itching and xanthomas (cholesterol deposits in the skin), hyperlipidemia, vitamin deficiencies, anemia, and fatigue. Cholestyramine is used to treat itching. Patients are monitored for progression to cirrhosis. Liver transplantation is an option for end-stage liver disease in patients with PBC.

Primary Sclerosing Cholangitis

Primary sclerosing cholangitis (PSC) is a disease of unknown cause characterized by chronic inflammation, fibrosis, and strictures (narrowing) of the medium and large bile ducts both inside and outside the liver.[3] Most patients with PSC also have ulcerative colitis or, less often, Crohn's disease. Complications of PSC can include cholangitis, cholestasis with jaundice, bile duct cancer, and cirrhosis.

Drug therapy has no proven benefit, although many HCPs use ursodiol. Treatment is directed at reducing the incidence of biliary complications and screening for bile duct and colorectal cancer, which is related to the high incidence of ulcerative colitis. Patients with advanced liver disease may need liver transplantation.

Nonalcoholic Fatty Liver Disease and Nonalcoholic Steatohepatitis

Nonalcoholic fatty liver disease (NAFLD) refers to a wide spectrum of liver diseases ranging from a fatty liver (steatosis) to nonalcoholic steatohepatitis (NASH) to cirrhosis. The term *nonalcoholic* is used because NAFLD and NASH occur in people who do not consume excess amounts of alcohol.

The fundamental characteristic of NAFLD is the accumulation of fatty infiltration in the hepatocytes. In NASH, the fat accumulation is associated with varying degrees of inflammation and fibrosis of the liver. If NASH is untreated, it can become a serious liver disease leading to cirrhosis, liver cancer, and liver failure.

Currently, NAFLD is increasing because of the growing number of people who are obese. NAFLD occurs in 90% to 95% of severely obese children and adults. NASH occurs in 8% to 20% of obese persons with NAFLD.[3] NAFLD should be considered in patients with risk factors, including obesity, diabetes, hyperlipidemia, and hypertension (also known as *metabolic syndrome*).

Elevated liver function tests (ALT, AST) are often the first sign of NAFLD. Ultrasound and CT scans can be used to diagnose NAFLD. Definitive diagnosis is by a liver biopsy.

There is no currently approved medication for NAFLD.[10] The goal of therapy is weight loss of at least 10% of body weight, if overweight or obese and exercise. Reducing risk factors, including hyperlipidemia, hypertension, and diabetes, is important.

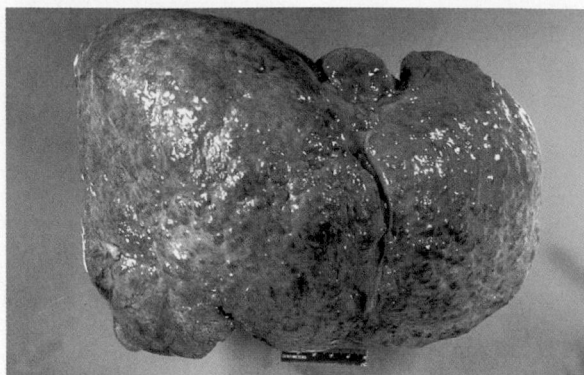

FIG. 43.4 Cirrhosis that developed from alcohol use. The characteristic diffuse nodularity of the surface is due to the combination of regeneration and scarring of the liver. (From Kumar V, Abbas AK, Aster JC, et al: *Robbins and Cotran pathologic basis of disease*, ed 8, Philadelphia, 2010, Saunders.)

⊕ PROMOTING HEALTH EQUITY
Liver, Pancreas, and Gallbladder Disorders

Hepatitis
- Hepatitis C has a higher incidence among blacks than whites.
- Hepatitis B has a higher incidence among Asian Americans and Pacific Islanders.
- Deaths caused by hepatitis C are more common in blacks.

Liver and Pancreatic Cancer
- Primary liver cancer has a highest incidence in Hispanics, followed by blacks and whites.
- Pancreatic cancer occurs more often among blacks than whites.

Gallbladder Disease
- Whites and Native Americans have a higher incidence of gallbladder disease than blacks or Asian Americans

---

CIRRHOSIS

Cirrhosis is the end stage of liver disease. Cirrhosis is characterized by extensive degeneration and destruction of the liver cells. This results in the replacement of liver tissue by fibrosis (scar tissue) and regenerative nodules that occur from the liver's attempt to repair itself (Fig. 43.4). The development of cirrhosis usually happens after decades of chronic liver disease.

Etiology and Pathophysiology

Any chronic liver disease, including disease from excess alcohol use and NAFLD, can cause cirrhosis. The most common causes of cirrhosis in the United States are chronic hepatitis C infection and alcohol-induced liver disease. In patients with alcohol-induced liver disease, controversy exists as to the degree to which malnutrition adds to the damage caused by the alcohol itself. Some cases of nutrition-related cirrhosis have resulted from extreme dieting, malabsorption, and obesity. Environmental factors and genetic predisposition may lead to the development of cirrhosis, regardless of dietary or alcohol intake.

Around 20% of patients with chronic hepatitis C and 25% of those with chronic hepatitis B develop cirrhosis.[3] Chronic inflammation and cell necrosis from viral hepatitis can result in progressive fibrosis and cirrhosis. Chronic hepatitis combined with alcohol use has a synergistic effect in accelerating liver damage.

Biliary causes of cirrhosis include primary biliary cholangitis (PBC) and primary sclerosing cholangitis (PSC). Both are described earlier in this chapter.

Cardiac cirrhosis includes a spectrum of hepatic problems that result from long-standing, severe, right-sided heart failure. It causes hepatic venous congestion, parenchymal damage, necrosis of liver cells, and fibrosis over time. Treatment is aimed at managing the patient's underlying heart failure.

In cirrhosis, the liver cells try to regenerate, but the regenerative process is disorganized. This results in abnormal blood vessel and bile duct architecture. The overgrowth of new and fibrous connective tissue distorts the liver's normal lobular structure, resulting in lobules of irregular size and shape with impeded blood flow. Eventually, irregular and disorganized liver regeneration, poor cellular nutrition, and hypoxia (from inadequate blood flow and scar tissue) result in decreased liver function.

Clinical Manifestations

Early Manifestations. Patients may be unaware of their liver condition because there are few symptoms in early-stage disease. If a person does have symptoms, these may include fatigue or an enlarged liver. Blood tests may show normal liver function (compensated cirrhosis). The diagnosis of cirrhosis is often made later when a patient presents with symptoms of more advanced liver disease.

Late Manifestations. Late manifestations result from liver failure and portal hypertension (Fig. 43.5). Jaundice, peripheral edema, and ascites develop gradually. Other late manifestations include skin lesions, hematologic problems, endocrine problems, and peripheral neuropathies (Fig. 43.6). In the advanced stages, the liver becomes small and nodular. Liver function is dramatically impaired.

Jaundice. Jaundice results from decreased ability to conjugate and excrete bilirubin into the small intestines (Table 43.3). There is an overgrowth of connective tissue in the liver, which compresses the bile ducts and leads to an obstruction. This results in an increase in the bilirubin in the vascular system, and jaundice occurs. The jaundice may be minimal or severe, depending on the degree of liver damage.

Skin Lesions. Various skin manifestations often occur with cirrhosis. Spider angiomas (*telangiectasia* or *spider nevi*) are small, dilated blood vessels with a bright red center point and spiderlike branches. They occur on the nose, cheeks, upper trunk, neck, and shoulders. *Palmar erythema* (a red area that blanches with pressure) occurs on the palms of the hands. Both lesions are due to an increase in circulating estrogen due to the damaged liver's inability to metabolize steroid hormones.

PATHOPHYSIOLOGY MAP

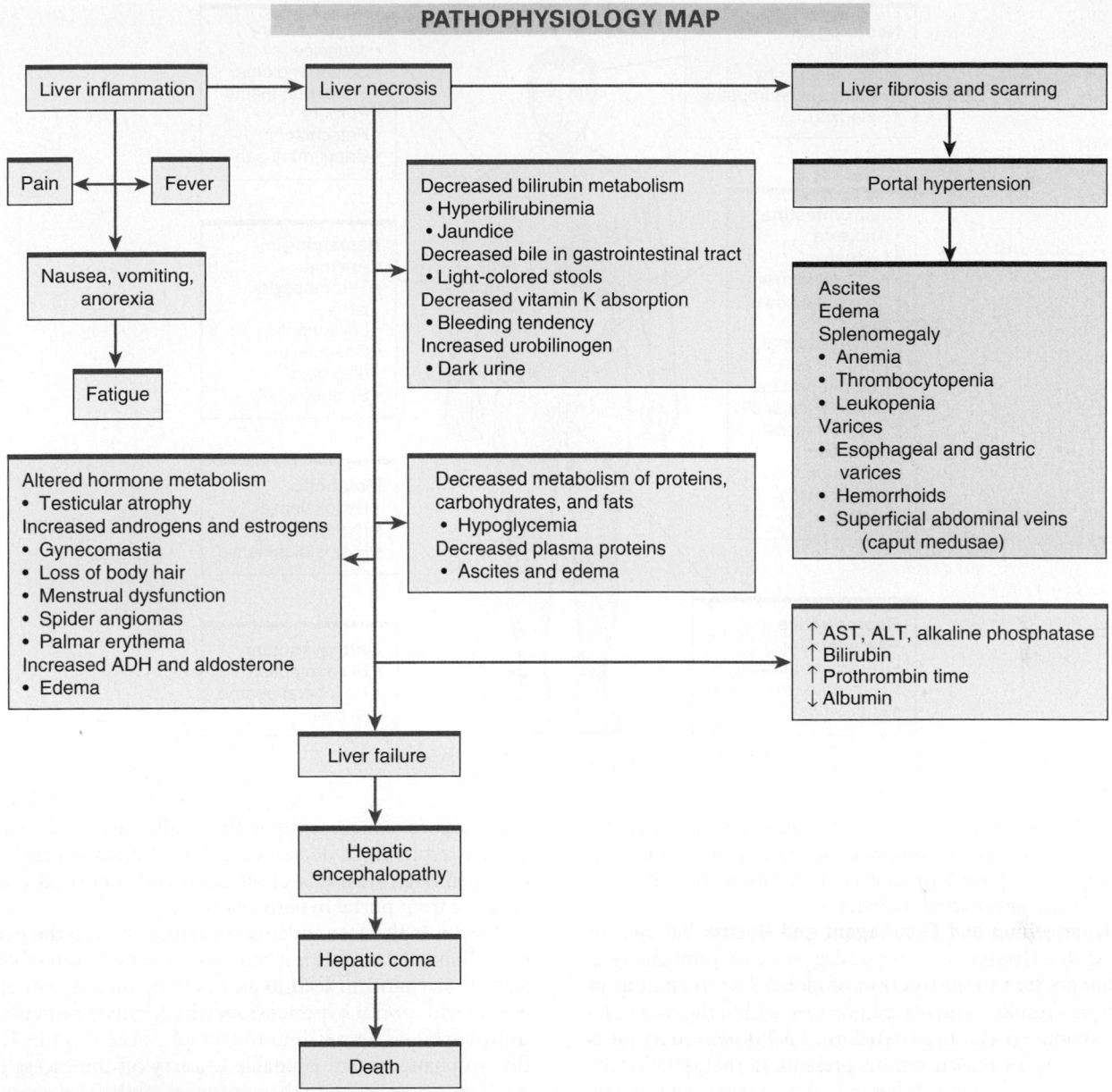

FIG. 43.5 Continuum of liver dysfunction in cirrhosis and resulting manifestations. (Adapted from Huether SE, McCance KL: *Understanding pathophysiology,* ed 5, St Louis, 2012, Mosby.)

Hematologic Problems. Hematologic problems include thrombocytopenia, leukopenia, anemia, and coagulation disorders. We think thrombocytopenia, leukopenia, and anemia are caused by the splenomegaly that results from backup of blood from the portal vein into the spleen (portal hypertension). Overactivity of the enlarged spleen results in increased removal of blood cells from circulation. Anemia can result from inadequate red blood cell (RBC) production and survival, poor diet, poor absorption of folic acid, and bleeding from varices.

The coagulation problems result from the liver's inability to make prothrombin and other factors essential for blood clotting. Manifestations of coagulation problems (bleeding tendencies) include epistaxis, purpura, petechiae, easy bruising, gingival bleeding, and heavy menstrual bleeding.

Endocrine Problems. The liver plays a vital role in the metabolism of hormones, such as estrogen and testosterone. In men with cirrhosis, gynecomastia (benign growth of the glandular tissue of the male breast), loss of axillary and pubic hair, testicular atrophy, and impotence with loss of libido may occur because of increased estrogen levels. Younger women with cirrhosis may develop amenorrhea, and older women may have vaginal bleeding. If the liver does not metabolize aldosterone properly, it can lead to hyperaldosteronism with sodium and water retention and potassium loss.

Peripheral Neuropathy. Peripheral neuropathy is a common finding in alcoholic cirrhosis. It is probably due to a dietary deficiency of thiamine, folic acid, and cobalamin. The neuropathy usually results in sensory and motor symptoms, but sensory symptoms may predominate.

Complications

Major complications of cirrhosis are portal hypertension, esophageal and gastric varices, peripheral edema, abdominal ascites, hepatic encephalopathy (mental status changes, including

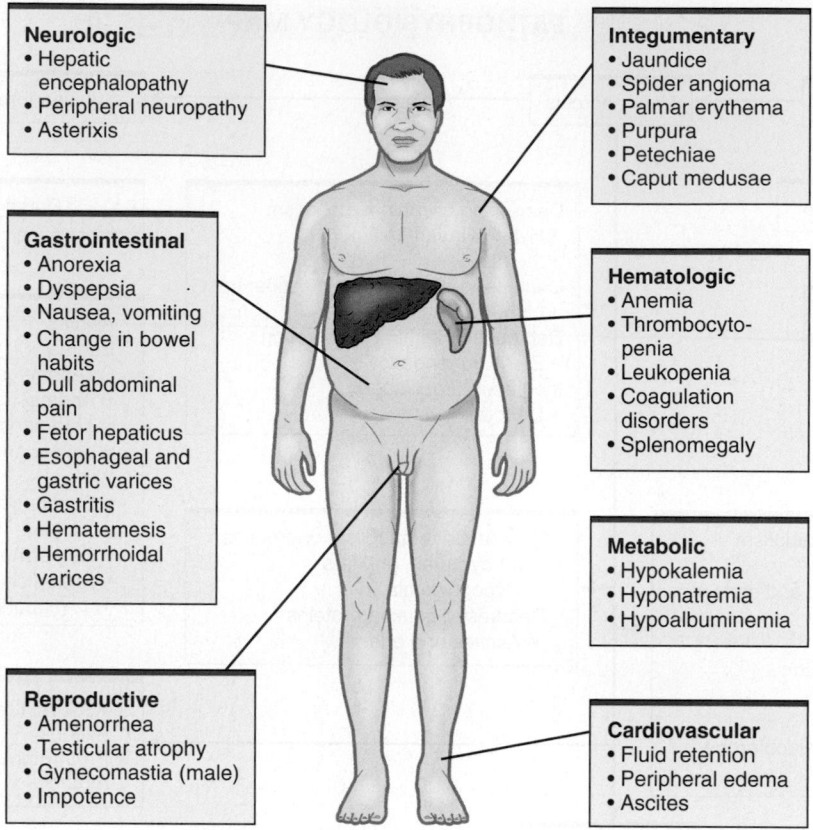

Neurologic
- Hepatic encephalopathy
- Peripheral neuropathy
- Asterixis

Integumentary
- Jaundice
- Spider angioma
- Palmar erythema
- Purpura
- Petechiae
- Caput medusae

Gastrointestinal
- Anorexia
- Dyspepsia
- Nausea, vomiting
- Change in bowel habits
- Dull abdominal pain
- Fetor hepaticus
- Esophageal and gastric varices
- Gastritis
- Hematemesis
- Hemorrhoidal varices

Hematologic
- Anemia
- Thrombocytopenia
- Leukopenia
- Coagulation disorders
- Splenomegaly

Metabolic
- Hypokalemia
- Hyponatremia
- Hypoalbuminemia

Reproductive
- Amenorrhea
- Testicular atrophy
- Gynecomastia (male)
- Impotence

Cardiovascular
- Fluid retention
- Peripheral edema
- Ascites

FIG. 43.6 Systemic manifestations of liver cirrhosis.

coma), and hepatorenal syndrome. Patients who are cirrhotic but who have no obvious complications have *compensated cirrhosis*. Those who have 1 or more complications of their liver disease have *decompensated cirrhosis*.

Portal Hypertension and Esophageal and Gastric Varices. In patients with cirrhosis, the liver undergoes structural changes. These changes lead to obstruction of blood flow in and out of the liver. This results in increased pressure within the liver's circulatory system (portal hypertension). Portal hypertension is characterized by increased venous pressure in the portal circulation, splenomegaly, large collateral veins, ascites, and gastric and esophageal varices.

As a way of reducing pressure, the body develops alternate circulatory pathways, referred to as *collateral circulation*. The collateral channels often form in the lower esophagus, anterior abdominal wall, parietal peritoneum, and rectum. Varicosities (distended veins) develop in areas where the collateral and systemic circulations communicate, resulting in esophageal and gastric varices, *caput medusae* (ring of varices around the umbilicus), and hemorrhoids.

Esophageal varices are a complex of tortuous, enlarged veins at the lower end of the esophagus. Gastric varices are found in the upper part of the stomach. These varices are fragile and do not tolerate high pressure, so they can bleed easily. Large varices are more likely to bleed. Esophageal varices can cause variceal hemorrhages with a 5-year mortality of 20%.[11] The patient may present with melena or hematemesis. Ruptured esophageal varices are the most life-threatening complication of cirrhosis and considered a medical emergency.

Peripheral Edema and Ascites. Peripheral edema occurs in the lower extremities and presacral area. Peripheral edema can occur before, concurrently with, or after ascites development. Edema results from decreased colloidal oncotic pressure from impaired liver synthesis of albumin and increased portacaval pressure from portal hypertension.

Ascites is the accumulation of serous fluid in the peritoneal or abdominal cavity. It is a common manifestation of cirrhosis. Several mechanisms lead to ascites. One mechanism of ascites occurs with portal hypertension, which causes proteins to shift from the blood vessels into the lymph space (Fig. 43.7). When the lymphatic system is unable to carry off the excess proteins and water, they leak into the peritoneal cavity. The osmotic pressure of the proteins pulls more fluid into the peritoneal cavity (Table 43.10).

A second mechanism of ascites formation is hypoalbuminemia resulting from the liver's decreased ability to synthesize albumin. The hypoalbuminemia results in decreased colloidal oncotic pressure.

A third mechanism of ascites is hyperaldosteronism, which occurs when the damaged hepatocytes metabolize aldosterone. The increased aldosterone level causes increased sodium reabsorption by the renal tubules. Sodium retention, combined with an increase in antidiuretic hormone in blood, leads to further water retention and edema. Edema decreases intravascular volume with decreased renal blood flow and glomerular filtration.

Ascites is manifested by abdominal distention with weight gain (Fig. 43.8). If the ascites is severe, the increase in abdominal pressure from the fluid accumulation may cause eversion of the umbilicus. Abdominal striae with distended abdominal wall veins may be present. Patients may have signs of dehydration (e.g., dry tongue and skin, sunken eyeballs, muscle weakness) and a decrease in urine output. Hypokalemia is common. It is

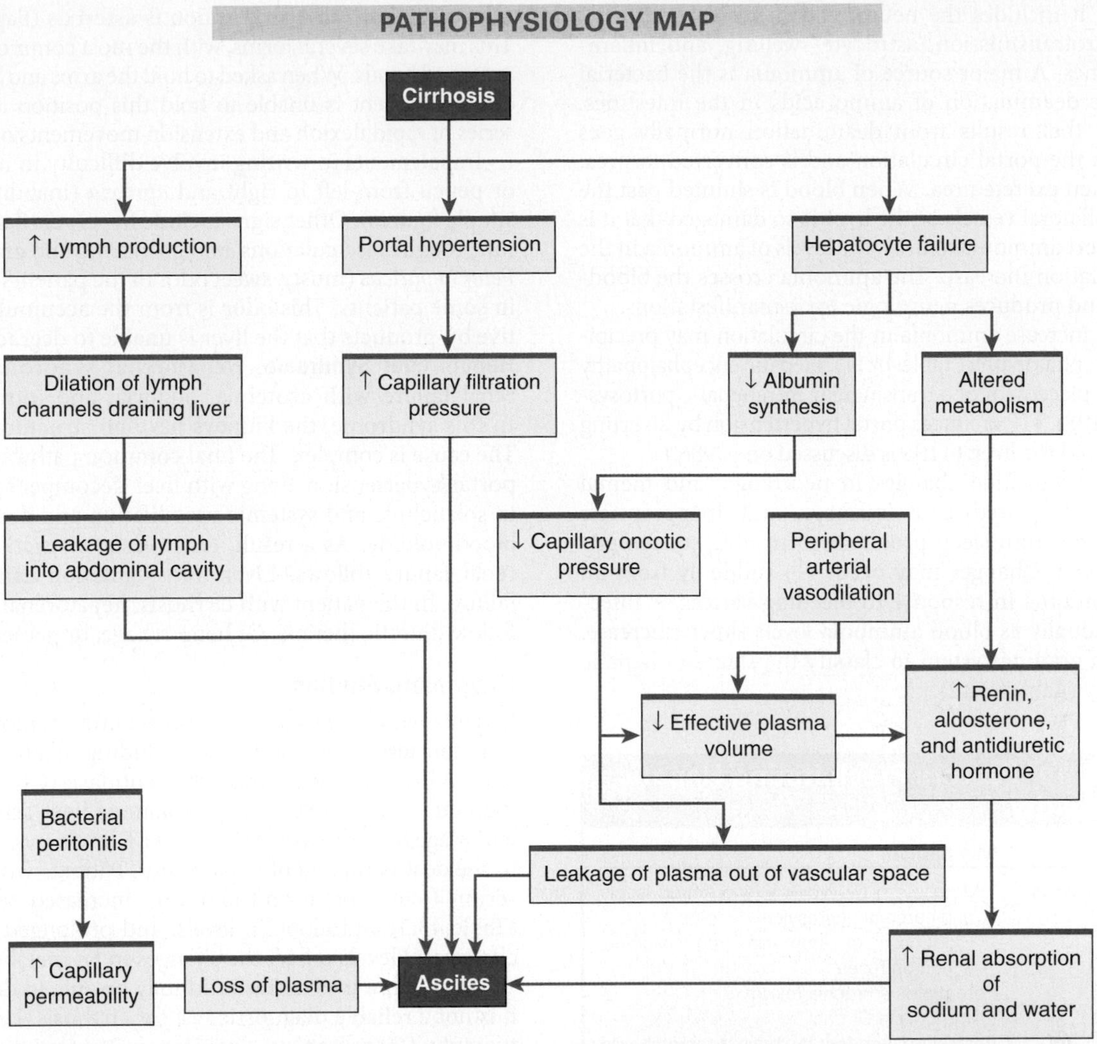

PATHOPHYSIOLOGY MAP

```
                            Cirrhosis

        ↑ Lymph production    Portal hypertension    Hepatocyte failure

    Dilation of lymph      ↑ Capillary filtration    ↓ Albumin      Altered
    channels draining         pressure               synthesis     metabolism
    liver

                                              ↓ Capillary oncotic   Peripheral
    Leakage of lymph                             pressure           arterial
    into abdominal cavity                                           vasodilation

                                                                                ↑ Renin,
                                                  ↓ Effective plasma            aldosterone,
                                                     volume                     and antidiuretic
    Bacterial                                                                   hormone
    peritonitis

                                           Leakage of plasma out of vascular space

    ↑ Capillary    Loss of plasma    Ascites                         ↑ Renal absorption
    permeability                                                          of
                                                                     sodium and water
```

FIG. 43.7 Mechanisms for development of ascites. (Adapted from Huether SE, McCance KL: *Understanding pathophysiology,* ed 5, St Louis, 2012, Mosby.)

TABLE 43.10 Factors Involved in Ascites

Factor	Mechanism
Decreased serum colloidal oncotic pressure	Impaired liver synthesis of albumin Loss of albumin into peritoneal cavity
Hyperaldosteronism	↑ Aldosterone secretion stimulated by ↓ renal blood flow ↓ Liver catabolism of circulating aldosterone
Impaired water excretion	↑ Antidiuretic hormone stimulated by ↓ renal blood flow
Increased flow of hepatic lymph	Leaking of protein-rich lymph from surface of cirrhotic liver
Portal hypertension	↑ Resistance of blood flow through liver

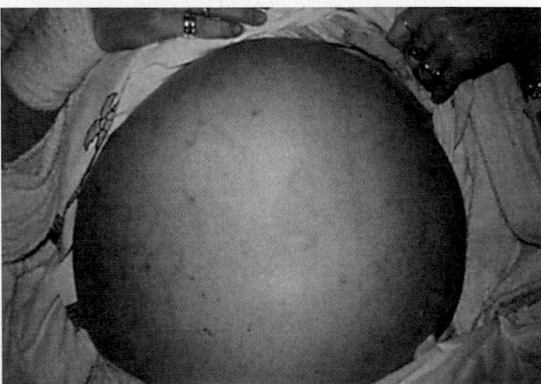

FIG. 43.8 Gross ascites. (From Butcher GP: *Gastroenterology: An illustrated colour text,* London, 2004, Churchill Livingstone.)

due to an excessive loss of potassium caused by hyperaldosteronism. Low potassium levels can also result from diuretic therapy used to treat the ascites.

Because of decreased immune function associated with cirrhosis, patients with ascites are at risk for *spontaneous bacterial peritonitis* (SBP). SBP is a bacterial infection of the ascitic fluid. In SBP, bacteria normally found in the intestines move into the peritoneal space. The bacteria most often responsible for the infection are a gram-negative enteric pathogen, such as *Escherichia coli*. SBP is a common complication of hospitalized patients with cirrhosis and ascites. Worsening vasodilation contributes to the development of SBP.[11]

Hepatic Encephalopathy. Hepatic encephalopathy is a neuropsychiatric manifestation of liver disease. The pathogenesis is multifactorial. It includes the neurotoxic effects of ammonia, abnormal neurotransmission, astrocyte swelling, and inflammatory cytokines. A major source of ammonia is the bacterial and enzymatic deamination of amino acids in the intestines. The ammonia that results from deamination normally goes to the liver via the portal circulation and is converted to urea. The kidneys then excrete urea. When blood is shunted past the liver via the collateral vessels or the liver is so damaged that it is unable to convert ammonia to urea, the levels of ammonia in the systemic circulation increase. The ammonia crosses the blood-brain barrier and produces neurologic toxic manifestations.

Factors that increase ammonia in the circulation may precipitate hepatic encephalopathy (Table 43.11). Hepatic encephalopathy can occur after placement of a transjugular intrahepatic portosystemic shunt (TIPS). TIPS reduces portal hypertension by diverting blood flow around the liver. (TIPS is discussed on p. 986.)

Manifestations include changes in neurologic and mental responsiveness; impaired consciousness; and inappropriate behavior, ranging from sleep problems to trouble concentrating to deep coma. Changes may occur (1) suddenly from an increase in ammonia in response to bleeding varices or infection or (2) gradually as blood ammonia levels slowly increase. We often use a grading system to classify the stages of hepatic encephalopathy (Table 43.12).

A characteristic manifestation is asterixis (flapping tremors). This may take several forms, with the most common involving the arms and hands. When asked to hold the arms and hands stretched out, the patient is unable to hold this position and performs a series of rapid flexion and extension movements of the hands.

Impairments in writing involve difficulty in moving the pen or pencil from left to right and *apraxia* (inability to construct simple figures). Other signs include hyperventilation, hypothermia, tongue fasciculations, and grimacing and grasping reflexes. *Fetor hepaticus* (musty, sweet odor of the patient's breath) occurs in some patients. This odor is from the accumulation of digestive by-products that the liver is unable to degrade.

Hepatorenal Syndrome. Hepatorenal syndrome is a type of renal failure with azotemia, oliguria, and intractable ascites. In this syndrome, the kidneys have no structural abnormality. The cause is complex. The final common pathway is likely to be portal hypertension along with liver decompensation, resulting in splanchnic and systemic vasodilation and decreased arterial blood volume. As a result, renal vasoconstriction occurs, and renal failure follows. Liver transplantation can reverse renal failure. In the patient with cirrhosis, hepatorenal syndrome can follow diuretic therapy, GI hemorrhage, or paracentesis.

Diagnostic Studies

Patients with cirrhosis have abnormalities in most of their liver function tests. Enzyme levels, including alkaline phosphatase, AST, ALT, and γ-glutamyl transpeptidase (GGT), are initially high due to their release from inflamed liver cells. However, in end-stage liver disease, AST and ALT levels may be normal due to the death and loss of hepatocytes. Patients will also have low serum total protein and albumin, increased serum bilirubin (Table 43.3) and globulin levels, and prolonged PT time. Low cholesterol levels reflect the changes in fat metabolism.

Although a liver ultrasound may be able to detect cirrhosis, it is not a reliable diagnostic test for cirrhosis. Ultrasound elastography (Fibroscan) is a noninvasive test used to quantify the degree of liver fibrosis. A liver biopsy, which may be done to identify liver cell changes, is the gold standard for a definitive diagnosis of cirrhosis.

Interprofessional Care

The goal of treatment is to slow the progression of cirrhosis and to prevent and treat any complications. Interprofessional care measures are listed in Table 43.13. Management of specific problems associated with cirrhosis is described next.

Ascites. Management of ascites focuses on sodium restriction, diuretics, and fluid removal.[12] Patients may need to limit sodium intake to 2 g/day. Very low sodium intake can result in reduced

---

TABLE 43.11 Factors Precipitating Hepatic Encephalopathy

Factor	Mechanism
Cerebral depressants (e.g., opioids)	↓ Metabolism by liver, causing ↑ drug levels and cerebral depression
Constipation	↑ Production of ammonia from bacterial action on feces
Dehydration	Potentiates ammonia toxicity
GI hemorrhage	↑ Ammonia in GI tract
Hypokalemia	Potassium needed by brain to metabolize ammonia
Hypovolemia	↑ Blood ammonia because of hepatic hypoxia. Impaired cerebral, hepatic, and renal function because of ↓ blood flow
↑ Metabolism	↑ Workload of liver
Infection	↑ Metabolic rate and cerebral sensitivity to toxins
Metabolic alkalosis	Facilitation of transport of ammonia across blood-brain barrier. Increased renal production of ammonia
Paracentesis	Loss of sodium and potassium ions. ↓ Blood volume
Uremia (renal failure)	Retention of nitrogenous metabolites

TABLE 43.12 Grading Scale for Hepatic Encephalopathy

Grade	Level of Consciousness	Intellectual Function	Neurologic Findings
0	Normal to minimal change	Subtle to no change in personality, behavior, memory, concentration	Asterixis absent. May have abnormal psychometric test
1	Lack of awareness, sleep disturbance	Short attention span, impaired computational skills, personality change, decrease in short-term memory, mild confusion, depression	Incoordination, asterixis may be absent
2	Lethargy, drowsiness	Disoriented to time, inappropriate behavior, deficits in executive function	Asterixis, abnormal reflexes
3	Somnolent, arousable	Disoriented to time, loss of meaningful conversation, marked confusion, incomprehensible speech	Asterixis, abnormal reflexes
4	Not arousable, comatose	Absent	Decerebrate. May be responsive to painful stimuli

TABLE 43.13 Interprofessional Care

Cirrhosis of the Liver

Diagnostic Assessment

- History and physical examination
- Liver function tests (ALT, AST, alkaline phosphatase, bilirubin, γ-glutamyl transpeptidase [GGT])
- Serum albumin
- Serum electrolytes
- PT time
- Complete blood count
- Liver biopsy (percutaneous needle)
- Liver ultrasound (e.g., FibroScan)
- Upper endoscopy (esophagogastroduodenoscopy)
- CT scan, MRI

Management

Conservative Therapy

- Rest
- B-complex vitamins
- Avoiding alcohol
- Minimizing or avoiding aspirin, acetaminophen, and NSAIDs

Ascites

- Low-sodium diet
- Diuretics
- Paracentesis (if needed)

Esophageal and Gastric Varices

- Endoscopic band ligation or sclerotherapy
- Balloon tamponade
- Transjugular intrahepatic portosystemic shunt (TIPS)

Drug Therapy

- Nonselective β-blocker (e.g., propranolol [Inderal])
- octreotide (Sandostatin)
- vasopressin

Hepatic Encephalopathy

Drug Therapy

- Antibiotics (rifaximin [Xifaxan])
- lactulose

---

nutritional intake and malnutrition. The patient is usually not on restricted fluids unless severe ascites develops. When caring for patients with ascites, accurately monitor fluid and electrolyte balance. An albumin infusion may help maintain intravascular volume and adequate urine output by increasing plasma colloid oncotic pressure.

Diuretic therapy is an important part of management. Often a combination of drugs that work at multiple sites of the nephron is more effective than a single agent. Spironolactone (Aldactone) is an effective diuretic, even in patients with severe ascites. Spironolactone is also an antagonist of aldosterone and is potassium sparing. Other potassium-sparing diuretics include amiloride (Midamor) and triamterene (Dyrenium). A high-potency loop diuretic (e.g., furosemide [Lasix]), is often used in combination with a potassium-sparing drug.

Tolvaptan (Samsca), a vasopressin-receptor antagonist, can correct hyponatremia, a common problem in patients with cirrhosis. It causes an increase in water excretion, resulting in an increase in serum sodium concentration.

A paracentesis is a sterile procedure in which a catheter is used to withdraw fluid from the abdominal cavity. This procedure can diagnose a medical condition or relieve pain, pressure, or difficulty breathing. In the patient with cirrhosis, this procedure is done for the person with impaired respiration or abdominal discomfort caused by severe ascites who does not respond to diuretic therapy. It is only a temporary measure of palliation because the fluid tends to reaccumulate rapidly.[12]

TIPS (discussed later in this section) is used to treat ascites that does not respond to diuretics. A peritoneovenous shunt is a surgical procedure that provides continuous reinfusion of ascitic fluid into the venous system. It is rarely used due to the high rate of complications.

Esophageal and Gastric Varices. The main therapeutic goal for esophageal and gastric varices is to prevent bleeding and variceal rupture by reducing portal pressure. The patient who has esophageal and/or gastric varices should avoid alcohol, aspirin, and nonsteroidal antiinflammatory drugs (NSAIDs).

All patients with cirrhosis should have an upper endoscopy (esophagogastroduodenoscopy [EGD]) to screen for varices. Patients with varices at risk for bleeding are often started on a nonselective β-blocker (nadolol [Corgard] or propranolol [Inderal]) to reduce the risk of hemorrhage. β-Blockers decrease high portal pressure, which decreases the risk for rupture.

When variceal bleeding occurs, the first step is to stabilize the patient and manage the airway. IV therapy is started and may include giving blood products. Care then moves toward stopping the bleeding, identifying the source, and applying interventions to prevent further bleeding. Management that involves a combination of drug therapy and endoscopic therapy is more successful than either approach alone.

Drug therapy for bleeding varices may include the somatostatin analog octreotide (Sandostatin) or vasopressin. Both produce vasoconstriction of the splanchnic arterial bed, decrease portal blood flow, and decrease portal hypertension. Currently, octreotide is used more often because it has fewer side effects than vasopressin.

At the time of endoscopy, band ligation or sclerotherapy of varices may be used to prevent rebleeding. Endoscopic variceal ligation (EVL, or "banding") is done by placing a small rubber band (elastic O-ring) around the base of the *varix* (enlarged vein). Sclerotherapy involves injecting a sclerosing solution into the swollen veins through a needle placed through the endoscope.

Balloon tamponade is an option when endoscopy does not control acute esophageal or gastric variceal hemorrhage. Balloon tamponade controls the hemorrhage by mechanical compression of the varices. Several types of tubes are available. The Sengstaken-Blakemore tube has 2 balloons, gastric and esophageal, with 3 lumens: 1 for the gastric balloon, 1 for the esophageal balloon, and 1 for gastric aspiration. Two other types of balloons are the Minnesota tube (a modified Sengstaken-Blakemore tube with an esophageal suction port above the esophageal balloon) and the Linton-Nachlas tube.

! SAFETY ALERT Balloon Tamponade
- Label each lumen to avoid confusion.
- Secure the tube to prevent movement of the tube that could result in occlusion of the airway.
- Deflate balloons for 5 minutes every 8 to 12 hr per agency policy to prevent tissue necrosis.

Supportive measures during an acute variceal bleed include giving fresh frozen plasma and packed RBCs, vitamin K, and proton pump inhibitors (PPIs; e.g., pantoprazole). Lactulose and rifaximin (Xifaxan) may be given to prevent hepatic encephalopathy from breakdown of blood and the release of ammonia in the intestine. Antibiotics are given to prevent bacterial infection.

Because of the high incidence of recurrent bleeding with each bleeding episode, continued therapy is necessary. Long-term management of patients who have had an episode of bleeding includes nonselective β-blockers, repeated band ligation of the varices, and portosystemic shunts in patients who develop recurrent bleeding.

Shunting Procedures. Nonsurgical and surgical methods of shunting blood away from the varices are available. Shunting procedures tend to be done more after a second major bleeding episode than during an initial bleeding episode. *Transjugular intrahepatic portosystemic shunt (TIPS)* is a nonsurgical procedure in which a tract (shunt) between the systemic and portal venous systems is created to redirect portal blood flow. A catheter is placed in the jugular vein and then threaded through the superior and inferior vena cava to the hepatic vein. The wall of the hepatic vein is punctured, and the catheter is directed to the portal vein. Stents are positioned along the passageway, overlapping in the liver tissue and extending into both veins.

This procedure reduces portal venous pressure and decompresses the varices, thus controlling bleeding. TIPS does not interfere with a future liver transplantation. Limitations of TIPS include the increased risk for hepatic encephalopathy (toxin-containing blood bypasses the liver) and stenosis of the stent.

TIPS is contraindicated in patients with severe hepatic encephalopathy, liver cancer, severe hepatorenal syndrome, and portal vein thrombosis.

Various surgical shunting procedures can decrease portal hypertension by diverting some of the portal blood flow while allowing adequate liver perfusion. Currently, the surgical shunts most often used are the portacaval shunt and the distal splenorenal shunt (Fig. 43.9).

Hepatic Encephalopathy. The goal of management of hepatic encephalopathy is to reduce ammonia formation. Lactulose, a drug that traps ammonia in the gut, reduces ammonia formation in the intestines. We can give it orally, as an enema, or through a nasogastric (NG) tube. The drug's laxative effect expels the ammonia from the colon. Antibiotics, such as rifaximin, also may be given, especially in patients who do not respond to lactulose. Regular and frequent bowel movements are necessary to minimize the ammonia buildup, so use measures to prevent constipation.

Control of hepatic encephalopathy also involves treatment of precipitating causes (Table 43.10). This includes lowering dietary protein intake, preventing and controlling GI bleeds, and, in the case of a bleed, removing the blood promptly from the GI tract to decrease the protein accumulation in the gut.

Drug Therapy. There is no specific drug therapy for cirrhosis. However, several drugs are used to treat symptoms and complications of advanced liver disease (Table 43.14).

Nutritional Therapy. The diet for the patient who has cirrhosis without complications is high in calories (3000 cal/day). It is high in carbohydrate content with moderate to low levels of fat. Protein restriction may be needed for some patients right after a severe flare of symptoms (i.e., episodic hepatic encephalopathy). However, protein restriction is rarely needed in patients with cirrhosis and persistent hepatic encephalopathy. For many, malnutrition is a more serious clinical problem than hepatic encephalopathy.[3]

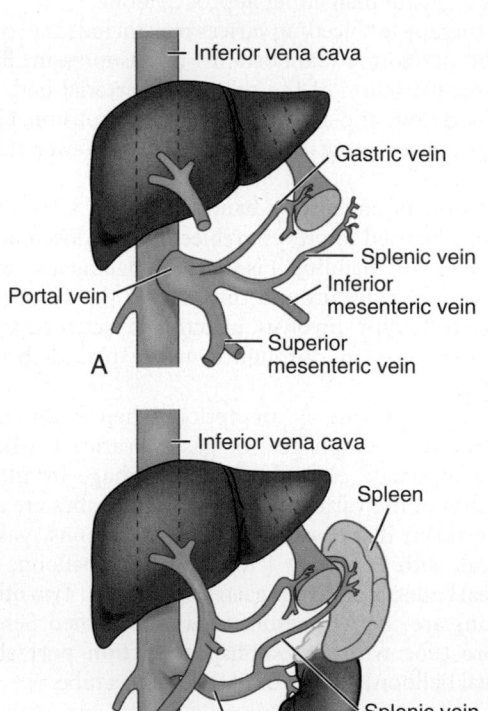

FIG. 43.9 Portosystemic shunts. **A,** Portacaval shunt. The portal vein is anastomosed to the inferior vena cava, diverting blood from the portal vein to the systemic circulation. **B,** Distal splenorenal shunt. The splenic vein is anastomosed to the renal vein. The portal venous flow stays intact while esophageal varices are selectively decompressed. (The short gastric veins are decompressed.) The spleen conducts blood from the high pressure of the esophageal and gastric varices to the low-pressure renal vein.

TABLE 43.14 **Drug Therapy**	
Cirrhosis	
Drug	**Mechanism of Action**
Diuretics	
furosemide (Lasix)	Acts on distal tubule and loop of Henle to ↓ reabsorption of sodium and water
spironolactone (Aldactone)	Blocks actions of aldosterone, potassium sparing
Other Therapy	
lactulose	Acidifies feces in bowel and traps ammonia, causing its elimination in feces
magnesium sulfate	Corrects hypomagnesemia that may occur with liver dysfunction
nadolol (Corgard) propranolol (Inderal)	Reduces portal venous pressure and esophageal variceal bleeding
neomycin sulfate rifaximin (Xifaxan)	↓ Bacterial flora, thus reducing ammonia formation
octreotide (Sandostatin) vasopressin	Hemostasis and control of bleeding in esophageal and gastric varices, constricts splanchnic arterial bed
PPIs (e.g., pantoprazole [Protonix])	↓ Gastric acidity
Vitamin K	Corrects clotting abnormalities from decreased vitamin K levels

A patient with alcoholic cirrhosis often has protein-calorie malnutrition. Oral nutritional supplements containing protein from branched-chain amino acids that are metabolized by the muscles may be needed. These supplements provide protein that the liver can more easily metabolize. Parenteral nutrition or EN are used with severe cases of malnutrition (see Chapter 39).

The patient with ascites and edema is placed on a low-sodium diet. The degree of sodium restriction depends on the patient's condition. Teach the patient and caregiver about the degree of restriction. Table salt is a well-known source of sodium. Other foods high in sodium include canned soups and vegetables, many frozen foods, salted snacks (e.g., potato chips), nuts, smoked meats and fish, crackers, breads, baking soda, olives, pickles, ketchup, and beer. Teach the patient to read labels for sodium content (see Fig. 34.5). Offer suggestions about how to make the diet more palatable. Seasonings, like garlic, parsley, onion, lemon juice, and spices may make food more appetizing. Collaborate with a dietitian about dietary strategies.

❖ NURSING MANAGEMENT: CIRRHOSIS

◆ Nursing Assessment

Subjective and objective data that should be obtained from a person with cirrhosis are outlined in Table 43.15.

◆ Nursing Diagnoses

Nursing diagnoses for the patient with cirrhosis may include:
- Impaired nutritional status
- Ineffective tissue perfusion
- Activity intolerance
- Fluid imbalance

Additional information on nursing diagnoses and interventions for the patient with cirrhosis is presented in eNursing Care Plan 43.2 available on the website for this chapter.

◆ Planning

The overall goals are that the patient with cirrhosis will (1) have relief of discomfort, (2) have minimal to no complications (ascites, esophageal varices, hepatic encephalopathy), and (3) return to as normal a lifestyle as possible.

◆ Nursing Implementation

◆ Health Promotion. Common risk factors for cirrhosis include alcohol use, malnutrition, viral hepatitis, biliary obstruction, obesity, and right-sided heart failure. Prevention and early treatment of cirrhosis focus on reducing or eliminating these risk factors. Urge patients to abstain from alcohol. Encourage those with chronic alcohol use to enroll in support programs that help patients maintain sobriety. (The treatment of alcohol use is discussed in Chapter 10.)

Adequate nutrition, especially for the person who uses alcohol and other people at risk for cirrhosis, is essential to promote normal liver regeneration. Identify and treat acute hepatitis early so that it does not progress to chronic hepatitis and cirrhosis. Bariatric surgery for morbidly obese persons reduces the incidence of NAFLD.

◆ Acute Care. Nursing care for the patient with cirrhosis focuses on conserving the patient's strength while maintaining muscle strength and tone. When the patient needs complete bed rest, implement measures to prevent pneumonia, thromboembolic problems, and pressure injuries. Modify the activity and rest

---

TABLE 43.15 Nursing Assessment

Cirrhosis

Subjective Data

Important Health Information

Past health history: Viral, toxic, or idiopathic hepatitis. Alcohol use, metabolic syndrome, chronic biliary obstruction and infection, severe right-sided heart failure

Medications: Adverse reaction to any medication. Use of anticoagulants, aspirin, NSAIDs, acetaminophen

Functional Health Patterns

Health perception–health management: Chronic alcohol use. Weakness, fatigue

Nutritional-metabolic: Anorexia, weight loss, dyspepsia, nausea and vomiting, gingival bleeding. Dry, yellow skin, bruising

Elimination: Dark urine, decreased urine output, light-colored or black stools, flatulence, change in bowel habits.

Cognitive-perceptual: Dull, right upper quadrant or epigastric pain. Numbness, tingling of extremities. Itching

Sexuality-reproductive: Impotence, amenorrhea

Objective Data

General

Fever, cachexia, wasting of extremities

Integumentary

Icteric sclera, jaundice, petechiae, ecchymoses, spider angiomas, palmar erythema, alopecia, loss of axillary and pubic hair, peripheral edema

Respiratory

Shallow, rapid respirations. Epistaxis

Gastrointestinal

Abdominal distention, ascites, distended abdominal wall veins, palpable liver and spleen, foul breath. Hematemesis. Black, tarry stools. Hemorrhoids

Neurologic

Altered mentation, asterixis

Reproductive

Gynecomastia, testicular atrophy, and impotence (men); loss of libido (men and women); amenorrhea or heavy menstrual bleeding (women)

Possible Diagnostic Findings

Anemia, thrombocytopenia; leukopenia. ↓ Serum albumin, potassium. Abnormal liver function studies. ↑ INR, ↓ platelets, ↑ ammonia, ↑ bilirubin levels. Abnormal abdominal ultrasound, CT, or MRI

---

schedule according to signs of improvement (e.g., decreasing jaundice, improvement in liver function studies).

Anorexia, nausea and vomiting, pressure from ascites, and poor eating habits all interfere with adequate intake of nutrients. Oral hygiene before meals may improve the patient's taste sensation. Make between-meal snacks available so that the patient can eat them at times when food is best tolerated. Offer preferred foods whenever possible. Explain the reason for any dietary restrictions to the patient and caregiver.

Nursing assessment and care should include the patient's physical status. Is jaundice present? Where is it seen—sclera, skin, hard palate? What is the progression of jaundice? If the pruritis accompanies jaundice, use measures to relieve itching. Cholestyramine or hydroxyzine (Atarax) may help. Other

TABLE 43.16 Nursing Management

Care of the Patient Undergoing Paracentesis

Preprocedure

- Have the patient void or insert an indwelling catheter.
- Obtain baseline vital signs and pulse oximetry. Weigh patient, inspect and palpate abdomen, and assess abdominal girth. Assess bladder for distention and determine last voiding.
- Assess baseline laboratory values (e.g., CBC, electrolytes, coagulation studies).
- Give any sedation or analgesia, if ordered.
- Teach patient to remain immobile during the procedure.
- Help the patient to a high-Fowler (sitting) position with feet on the floor.

Postprocedure

- Perform assessment and compare to baseline: vital signs, pulse oximetry, abdominal girth, abdominal pain. Note any signs of hypovolemia.
- Have the patient sit on the side of the bed or place in high-Fowler's position.
- Label and send the fluid for laboratory analysis.
- Check the dressing for bleeding and/or leakage of ascitic fluid.
- Give IV fluid and/or albumin as ordered.
- Measure any drainage and describe the collected fluid.
- Reweigh the patient and monitor intake and output.
- Maintain bedrest per agency protocol.

measures to relieve itching include baking soda or moisturizing bath oils (Alpha Keri), lotions containing calamine, antihistamines, soft or old linens, and control of the temperature (not too hot and not too cold). Keep the patient's nails short and clean. Teach patients to rub with their knuckles rather than scratch with their nails when they cannot resist scratching.

Note the color of urine and stools and assess for improvement or normalization of color. When jaundice is present, the urine is often dark brown, and the stool is gray or tan.

Edema and ascites require your assessment and intervention. Accurate calculation and recording of intake and output, daily weights, and measurements of extremities and abdominal girth help in the ongoing assessment of the location and extent of the edema. Mark the abdomen with a permanent marker so that you measure the girth at the same location each time.

Immediately before a paracentesis, have the patient void to prevent puncturing of the bladder during the procedure. Other nursing care associated with a paracentesis is outlined in Table 43.16.

Dyspnea is a frequent problem for the patient with severe ascites and can lead to pleural effusions. A semi-Fowler's or Fowler's position allows for maximal respiratory efficiency. Use pillows to support the arms and chest to increase the patient's comfort and ability to breathe.

Meticulous skin care is essential because the edematous tissues are prone to breakdown. Use an alternating-air pressure mattress or other special mattress. A turning schedule (minimum of every 2 hours) must be adhered to rigidly. Support the abdomen with pillows. If the abdomen is taut, cleanse it gently. The patient will tend to avoid moving because of abdominal discomfort and dyspnea. Range-of-motion exercises are helpful. Implement measures such as coughing and deep breathing to prevent respiratory problems. The lower extremities may be elevated. If scrotal edema is present, a scrotal support gives some comfort.

When the patient is taking diuretics, monitor serum sodium, potassium, chloride, and bicarbonate levels. Monitor renal function (blood urea nitrogen [BUN], serum creatinine) routinely and with any change in the diuretic dosage. Observe for signs of fluid and electrolyte imbalance, especially hypokalemia. Dysrhythmias, hypotension, tachycardia, and generalized muscle weakness may occur with hypokalemia. Muscle cramping, weakness, lethargy, and confusion may be present with hyponatremia from water excess.

Observe for and provide nursing care for any hematologic problems. These include bleeding tendencies, anemia, and increased susceptibility to infection.

Assess the patient's response to altered body image resulting from jaundice, spider angiomas, palmar erythema, ascites, and gynecomastia. The patient may have anxiety and embarrassment about these changes. Explain these phenomena and be a supportive listener. Provide nursing care with concern and encouragement to help the patient maintain his or her self-esteem.

CHECK YOUR PRACTICE

You are caring for a 69-yr-old male patient with advanced cirrhosis who just underwent banding for esophageal varices. The UAP tells you that the patient's BP is 80/60 mm Hg and he is hard to arouse.
- What is your concern?
- What would you do?

Bleeding Varices. If the patient has esophageal or gastric varices, observe for any signs of bleeding from the varices, such as hematemesis and melena. If hematemesis occurs, assess the patient for hemorrhage, call the HCP, and be ready to transfer the patient to the endoscopy suite and/or assist with equipment to control the bleeding. Maintain the patient's airway. Patients with bleeding varices are usually admitted to the intensive care unit (ICU).

Balloon tamponade is an option for patients who have bleeding that is unresponsive to band ligation or sclerotherapy. When balloon tamponade is used, explain to the patient and caregiver the use of the tube and how the balloon is inserted. Check the balloons for patency. It is usually the HCP's responsibility to insert the tube by either the nose or mouth. Then the gastric balloon is inflated with 250 mL of air, and the tube is retracted until resistance (lower esophageal sphincter) is felt. The tube is secured by placing a piece of sponge or foam rubber at the nostrils (nasal cuff). For continued bleeding, the esophageal balloon is then inflated. A sphygmomanometer is used to measure and maintain the desired pressure at 20 to 40 mm Hg. An x-ray verifies the balloon's position.

Nursing care includes monitoring for complications of rupture or erosion of the esophagus, regurgitation and aspiration of gastric contents, and occlusion of the airway by the balloon. If the gastric balloon breaks or is deflated, the esophageal balloon will slip upward, obstructing the airway and causing asphyxiation. If this happens, cut the tube or deflate the esophageal balloon. Keep scissors at the bedside. Minimize regurgitation by oral and pharyngeal suctioning and by keeping the patient in a semi-Fowler's position.

The patient is unable to swallow saliva because the inflated esophageal balloon occludes the esophagus. Encourage the patient to expectorate and provide an emesis basin and tissues. Frequent oral and nasal care offers relief from the taste of blood and irritation from mouth breathing.

ETHICAL/LEGAL DILEMMAS
Rationing

Situation

T.H., a 43-yr-old female patient with cirrhosis of the liver, is frequently admitted to the hospital. She has been told that her continued alcohol use will inevitably lead to her death. She now has GI bleeding and needs blood transfusions. She has a rare blood type that is hard to match. Should you ask for an ethics consultation?

Ethical/Legal Points for Consideration

- *Rationing*, or the controlled distribution of scarce resources, is a difficult ethical problem. The needs of an individual patient or group of patients are weighed against the needs of many patients, who may have a greater chance of recovery, and the availability of the necessary resources.
- Health interests can supersede the interests or rights of a person. For example, in anticipation of an anthrax attack, the government could confiscate all relevant antibiotics and restrict their use to treat the disease.
- Two individual rights that must be considered regarding rationing are the (1) constitutional right to privacy and (2) right to consent to or refuse medical procedures and therapy.
- The competent adult is the only person who may consent to or refuse treatment for his or her health care problems.
- If T.H. consents to a blood transfusion, an intervening party may be allowed to refuse that treatment only given substantial intervening circumstances and not as a threat to compel adherent future behavior.
- If involved parties cannot reach an agreement, legal intervention by way of a court order may become necessary.

Discussion Questions

1. Do you think patients with diseases that have a behavioral component, like substance use, deserve aggressive treatment?
2. Would you request an ethics committee consultation in T.H.'s case?

Hepatic Encephalopathy. Nursing care of the patient with hepatic encephalopathy focuses on maintaining a safe environment, sustaining life, and assisting with measures to reduce the formation of ammonia. Patients with hepatic encephalopathy may be confused and at risk for falls or other injuries. Assess the patient's (1) level of responsiveness (e.g., reflexes, pupillary reactions, orientation), (2) sensory and motor abnormalities (e.g., hyperreflexia, asterixis, motor coordination), (3) fluid and electrolyte imbalances, (4) acid-base imbalances, and (5) response to treatment measures.

Assess the neurologic status, including an exact description of the patient's behavior, at least every 2 hours. Plan your care of the patient based on the severity of the encephalopathy. In patients with altered levels of consciousness or whose airway may become compromised, have emergency equipment readily available. Any GI bleeding may worsen encephalopathy. Institute measures to prevent falls or injuries.

. Control factors known to precipitate encephalopathy as much as possible, including anything that may cause constipation (e.g., dehydration, opioid drugs). Measures to minimize constipation are important to reduce ammonia production. Give drugs, laxatives, and enemas as ordered. Encourage fluids, if not contraindicated. Assess the patient taking lactulose for diarrhea and excessive fluid and electrolyte losses.

◆ **Ambulatory Care.** The patient with cirrhosis may be faced with a prolonged course and the chance of life-threatening problems and complications. The patient and caregiver need to understand the importance of continual health care and medical supervision.

TABLE 43.17 Patient & Caregiver Teaching
Cirrhosis

When teaching the patient and caregiver about management of cirrhosis, do the following:
1. Explain that cirrhosis is a chronic illness and requires continual health care.
2. Teach the symptoms of complications and when to seek medical attention to enable prompt treatment.
3. Teach the patient to avoid potentially hepatotoxic over-the-counter drugs, because the diseased liver is unable to metabolize them.
4. Encourage abstinence from alcohol because continued use increases the rate of liver disease progression and risk for liver complications.
5. Teach the patient with esophageal or gastric varices to avoid aspirin and NSAIDs to prevent hemorrhage.
6. Teach the patient with portal hypertension and varices that straining at stool, coughing, sneezing, and retching and vomiting may increase the risk for variceal hemorrhage.

Supportive measures include proper diet, rest, avoiding potentially hepatotoxic OTC drugs, such as acetaminophen in high doses, and abstaining from alcohol. Abstinence from alcohol is important and results in improvement in most patients. However, some patients find abstinence extremely hard and need emotional support. Explore your own attitude toward the patient whose cirrhosis is from chronic alcohol use. Always provide care without being condescending or judgmental. Treat patients with respect and concern for their well-being (see Chapter 10).

Cirrhosis is a chronic disease, and people can live many years with symptoms and complications from cirrhosis. The patient is affected not only physically but also psychologically, socially, and economically. Major lifestyle changes may be needed, especially if chronic alcohol use is the primary cause. Provide information about community support programs, such as Alcoholics Anonymous, for help with chronic alcohol use.

Teach the patient and caregiver about complications and when to seek medical attention (Table 43.17). Include instructions about adequate rest periods, how to detect early signs of complications, skin care, drug therapy side effects, observation for bleeding, and protection from infection.

Referral to a community or home health nurse may help ensure patient adherence to prescribed therapy. Home care for the patient with cirrhosis focuses on helping the patient with activities of daily living while maintaining the highest level of wellness possible.

◆ **Evaluation**

Expected outcomes are that the patient with cirrhosis will
- Maintain food and fluid intake adequate to meet nutritional needs
- Maintain skin integrity with relief of edema and itching
- Have normal fluid and electrolyte balance
- Acknowledge and get treatment for a substance use problem

ACUTE LIVER FAILURE

Acute liver failure, or *fulminant hepatic failure*, is a potentially life-threatening clinical syndrome.[3] It is characterized by a rapid onset of severe liver dysfunction in someone with no history of liver disease. It is often accompanied by hepatic encephalopathy.

The most common cause of acute liver failure is drugs, usually acetaminophen. Other drugs that can cause acute liver failure include isoniazid, sulfa-containing drugs, and anticonvulsants. Drugs can cause hepatocyte damage by disrupting essential intracellular processes or causing an accumulation of toxic metabolic products. Other causes can include viral hepatitis, especially HBV. Hepatitis A is a less common cause.

Outcomes depend on the cause. Cerebral edema, cerebellar herniation, and brainstem compression are the most common causes of death. Treatment of cerebral edema is described in Chapter 56. Liver transplantation is associated with a significant survival benefit in patients with a low probability of spontaneous recovery.

Clinical Manifestations and Diagnostic Studies

Manifestations of acute liver failure include jaundice, coagulation abnormalities, and encephalopathy. Changes in cognitive function are often the first clinical sign. Patients are susceptible to a wide variety of complications, including cerebral edema, renal failure, hypoglycemia, metabolic acidosis, sepsis, and multiorgan failure.

Serum bilirubin is high, and the PT time is prolonged. Liver enzyme levels (AST, ALT) are often markedly increased. Other laboratory tests include blood chemistries (especially glucose, since hypoglycemia may be present and need correction), complete blood count (CBC), acetaminophen level, screening for other drugs and toxins, viral hepatitis serology (especially HAV and HBV), serum ceruloplasmin (enzyme synthesized in liver) and α_1-antitrypsin levels, iron levels, ammonia levels, and autoantibodies (ANAs and ASMAs).

CT or MRI can provide information about the liver size and contour, presence of ascites or tumors, and patency of the blood vessels.

◆ Interprofessional and Nursing Care

Since acute liver failure may progress rapidly, with hour-by-hour changes in consciousness, the patient is usually transferred to the ICU once the diagnosis is made. Planning for transfer to a transplant center should begin in patients with grade 1 or 2 encephalopathy because they may worsen rapidly. Early transfer is important because the risks involved with patient transport may increase or even prevent transfer if stage 3 or 4 encephalopathy develops (Table 43.12).

Renal failure is a frequent complication of liver failure. It may be due to dehydration, hepatorenal syndrome, or acute tubular necrosis. The frequency of renal failure may be even greater with acetaminophen overdose or other toxins with which direct renal toxicity occurs. Although few patients die of renal failure alone, it often increases the mortality risk and may worsen the prognosis. Protect renal function by maintaining adequate fluid balance, avoiding nephrotoxic agents (e.g., aminoglycosides, NSAIDs), and promptly identifying and treating infection.

Monitoring and management of hemodynamic and renal function, as well as glucose, electrolytes, and acid-base status, are critical. Conduct frequent neurologic evaluations for signs of increased intracranial pressure. Position the patient with the head elevated at 30 degrees. Avoid excessive patient stimulation. Maneuvers that cause straining or Valsalva-like movements may increase intracranial pressure (ICP). ICP monitoring is discussed in Chapter 56.

Assess the patient regularly for baseline level of consciousness and orientation and report any changes to the HCP. Avoid the use of any sedatives due to their effects on mental status. The effects can be confused with worsening encephalopathy. Only minimal doses of benzodiazepines should be used due to their delayed metabolism by the failing liver. Closely observe the patient to prevent injuries and pad bedrails to avoid injury from possible seizures. Monitor intake and output for renal function and provide good skin and oral care to avoid breakdown and infection.

Changes in level of consciousness may compromise nutritional intake. Many patients receive vitamin supplementation. Other factors, such as coagulation problems, may influence whether EN is started. An NG tube may be irritating to the nasal and esophageal mucosa and cause bleeding.

LIVER CANCER

Primary liver cancer starts in the liver. The most common types of liver cancer are hepatocellular carcinoma (HCC) (75% of cases) and intrahepatic cholangiocarcinoma (bile duct cancer). In 2018 there were about 40,710 cases of HCC and 28,920 HCC deaths in the United States. Worldwide liver cancer is the fifth most common cancer and second most common cause of cancer death.[13]

Liver cancer is the most common cause of death in patients with cirrhosis. Cirrhosis caused by hepatitis C is the most common cause of HCC in the United States, followed by NAFLD. About 2% of patient with cirrhosis develop liver cancer each year.

In primary liver cancer, lesions may be singular or numerous and nodular or diffusely spread over the entire liver. Some tumors infiltrate other organs, such as the gallbladder, or move into the peritoneum or the diaphragm. Primary liver cancer often metastasizes to the lung.

Metastatic cancer in the liver is more common than primary liver cancer (Fig. 43.10). The liver is a common site of metastatic

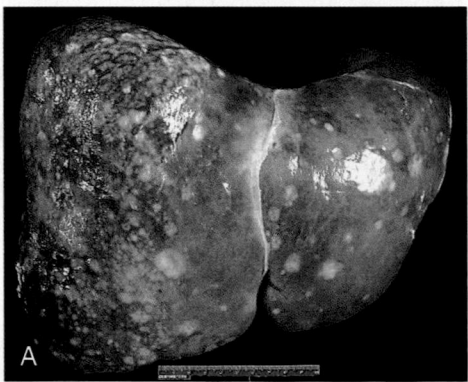

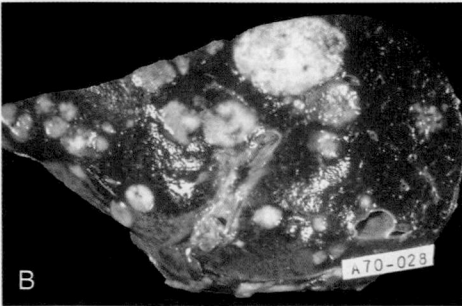

FIG. 43.10 Multiple hepatic metastases from a primary colon cancer. A, Gross specimen showing outside of liver. B, Liver section showing metastatic lesions. (A, From Kumar V, Abbas AK, Fausto N: *Robbins and Cotran pathologic basis of disease*, ed 7, Philadelphia, 2005, Saunders. B, From Kumar V, Abbas AK, Aster JC, et al: *Robbins and Cotran pathologic basis of disease*, ed 8, Philadelphia, 2010, Saunders.)

growth because of its high rate of blood flow and extensive capillary network. Cancer cells in other parts of the body are often carried to the liver via the portal circulation.

Clinical Manifestations and Diagnostic Studies

The manifestations of early liver cancer can be absent or subtle. They are often a result of the underlying cirrhosis rather than from the actual liver tumor(s). The patient may present with hepatomegaly, splenomegaly, fatigue, peripheral edema, ascites, and other complications from portal hypertension. In late stages, patients will often have fever/chills, jaundice, anorexia, weight loss, palpable mass, and right upper quadrant pain.

Diagnostic and screening for liver cancer are ultrasound, CT, and MRI. Recent advancements in MRI scanning have allowed for accurate diagnosis of liver cancers without the need for a percutaneous biopsy.[13] Sometimes, a biopsy may be done when the results of diagnostic imaging studies are inconclusive or tissue is needed to guide treatment. Risks of a biopsy include bleeding and potential tumor cell seeding along the needle tract. Therefore a biopsy is generally not done unless a diagnosis cannot be made by CT or MRI and clinical presentation. Serum α-fetoprotein (AFP) levels combined with ultrasound have a high rate of detection of early-stage HCC. (AFP is discussed in Chapter 15.)

❖ Interprofessional and Nursing Care

Prevention of liver cancer focuses on identifying and treating chronic hepatitis B and C viral infections. Treatment of chronic alcohol use may lower the risk for liver cancer. Screening for at-risk patients (e.g., those with cirrhosis) usually involves a combination of serum AFP and CT, MRI, or ultrasound imaging of the liver.

Treatment of liver cancer depends primarily on the stage of cancer: number, size, and location of tumors; involvement of any blood vessels; patient age and overall health; and extent of underlying liver disease. Surgical liver resection (partial hepatectomy) offers the best chance for a cure. However, only about 15% of people have enough healthy liver tissue for this to be an option. The underlying cirrhosis and portal hypertension often compromise liver function and may cause liver failure after surgery. Furthermore, many patients are diagnosed at an advanced stage of cancer when surgery is not an option. For those patients who have early-stage liver cancer and impaired liver function, liver transplantation offers a good prognosis.

Nonsurgical therapies include percutaneous ablation, chemoembolization, radioembolization, and sorafenib (Nexavar) oral therapy.[13] In ablation, a thin needle is inserted into the core of the tumor. Then various substances can be injected (ethanol, acetic acid) and the temperature of the probe (radiofrequency, microwave, cryotherapy) can be altered to destroy the tumor. This procedure can be done percutaneously, laparoscopically, or through an open incision. It is typically limited by the number, size, and location of liver tumors. It is usually offered to patients with early-stage liver cancer. Although complications are not common, they can include infection, bleeding, dysrhythmias, and skin burn.

In patients with multinodular HCC or intermediate-stage liver cancer, embolization of the tumors is another intervention. There are 2 options typically used: transarterial chemoembolization (TACE) or transarterial radioembolization (TARE). TACE and TARE are minimally invasive procedures done by interventional radiologists. A catheter is placed via the femoral artery or radial artery and advanced to the arterial blood supply of the tumors in the liver. Either a chemotherapy drug (TACE) or radioactive beads (TARE) along with embolizing agents are then injected into the arteries of the tumor(s) region. TACE works by shutting off the blood supply to the tumors and exposing liver tumor cells to the chemotherapy agent. TARE destroys the tumor(s) by slowly releasing radioactive material directly to the site of the tumor. It can take up to 3 months for complete results.

In patients with advanced HCC, sorafenib (Nexavar) is typically the first-line treatment. It is a kinase inhibitor, a type of targeted therapy, that blocks certain proteins (kinases) that play a role in tumor growth and cancer progression (see Table 15.13). This drug has the potential to slow tumor progression and prolong life.

Nursing interventions focus on keeping the patient as comfortable as possible. Since these patients have the same problems as any patient with advanced liver disease, the nursing interventions discussed for cirrhosis of the liver apply to these patients (see p. 987).

Although the prognosis for patients with liver cancer is poor, it is improving with early screening and surveillance programs for those with chronic hepatitis and/or cirrhosis. The cancer often progresses rapidly, with patients having complications from the advancing cancer and declining liver function. Without treatment, death may occur within 6 to 12 months, most often from hepatic encephalopathy or massive blood loss from GI bleeding.

LIVER TRANSPLANTATION

Liver transplantation has become an option for many people with end-stage liver disease or localized HCC. Liver disease related to chronic viral hepatitis is the leading reason for liver transplantation. Other reasons include congenital biliary abnormalities (biliary atresia), inborn errors of metabolism, sclerosing cholangitis, acute liver failure, and chronic end-stage liver disease. In 2018, 11,514 patients were listed for a liver transplant in the United States with 8250 patients undergoing a transplant.[3]

Liver transplant candidates must go through a rigorous transplant evaluation prior to being placed on the transplant list. This is done to confirm the diagnosis of end-stage liver disease and to assess for other co-morbid conditions (e.g., cardiovascular disease, chronic kidney disease) that may affect the patient's surgical outcome. The evaluation includes physical examination, laboratory tests (CBC, liver function tests), cardiac and pulmonary evaluations, endoscopy, CT scan, and psychologic testing. Potential recipients receive counseling about cigarette smoking and alcohol abstinence. Contraindications for liver transplant include severe extrahepatic disease, advanced HCC or other cancer, ongoing drug or chronic alcohol use, and inability to understand or adhere with the rigorous posttransplant care.

Liver transplantation is done using both deceased (cadaver) and live donor livers. The live donor liver transplant was first developed for children whose parents wanted to serve as donors. Today, some liver transplant centers are performing live liver transplant procedures for adults. In this procedure, the living person donates a part of his or her liver to another. However, live liver donation poses potential risks to the donor, including biliary problems, hepatic artery thrombosis, wound infection, postoperative ileus, and pneumothorax.

Because of the limited number of donor livers, when a liver becomes available for transplant it may be divided into 2 parts (split liver transplant) and implanted into 2 recipients. The decision to use a split donor liver is based on the donor's size and health. The recipients of the split liver generally are smaller than the donor. The success rate associated with split liver transplantation is somewhat lower than that associated with whole organ transplantation.

Postoperative complications of liver transplant include bleeding, infection, and rejection. However, the liver is subject to a less aggressive immunologic attack than other organs, like the kidneys. Transplants and immunosuppressive therapy are discussed in Chapter 13.

Immunosuppressive therapy generally involves a combination of corticosteroids, a calcineurin inhibitor (cyclosporine or tacrolimus), and an antiproliferative agent (e.g., azathioprine). Tacrolimus is superior to cyclosporine in liver transplantation. Standard immunosuppressive regimens often change over the course of the recipient's life. Corticosteroid withdrawal may be done and is relatively safe to do in liver transplant recipients.

About 80% of patients live more than 5 years after liver transplant. Long-term survival depends on the cause of liver failure (e.g., localized HCC, chronic hepatitis B or C, biliary disease). Patients who have liver disease from hepatitis B or C often have reinfection of the transplanted liver. For patients with hepatitis B, treatment after surgery with IV HBIG and a nucleoside or nucleotide analog (used to treat HBV infection) has reduced the rates of reinfection of the transplanted liver. For patients with HCV, treatment with the new direct-acting antivirals (DAAs) that can cure HCV infection has provided the opportunity to use HCV-positive liver grafts. The need for liver transplant may decrease in the HCV population. Research is ongoing to decide if DAAs should be started before or after transplant.

The patient who had a liver transplant needs highly skilled nursing care, either in an ICU or other specialized unit. Postoperative nursing care includes assessing neurologic status; monitoring for signs of hemorrhage; preventing pulmonary complications; electrolyte levels, and urine output; and monitoring for manifestations of infection and rejection. Common respiratory problems are pneumonia, atelectasis, and pleural effusions. To prevent these complications, encourage the patient to cough, deep breathe, use incentive spirometry, and frequently reposition. Measure the drainage from the Jackson-Pratt drain, NG tube, and T tube and note the color and consistency of the drainage at regular intervals.

The first 2 months after surgery are critical for monitoring for infection. Causes of infection can be viral, fungal, or bacterial. Fever may be the only sign of infection. Adhering to the medication regimen can be hard, especially in the beginning. Emotional support and teaching for the patient and caregiver are essential to the success of the patient with a liver transplant.

Gerontologic Considerations: Liver Disease in the Older Adult

The incidence of liver disease increases with age. The liver's size and metabolic breakdown of drugs decrease, and hepatobiliary function is changed. The liver has a decreased capacity to respond to injury. This especially applies to regeneration after injury. Transplanted livers take longer to regenerate in the older adult compared with the younger adult.

Older adults are particularly vulnerable to drug-induced liver injury. This is due to several factors, including the increased use of multiple prescription and OTC drugs, which can lead to drug interactions and potential drug toxicity. Age-related decreases in liver function result in decreased drug metabolism and a decreased ability to recover from drug-induced injury.

A growing number of older adults have chronic hepatitis C and the resulting cirrhosis. Antibodies to HCV and elevated liver enzymes may be found during a routine health assessment in asymptomatic patients.

Lifetime health behaviors may influence the development of chronic liver disease in the older adult. Chronic alcohol use and obesity can contribute to cirrhosis, fatty liver inflammation (NASH), and liver failure. Because of many older adults' concomitant cardiovascular and lung diseases and possible anticoagulant therapy, variceal bleeding can cause significant morbidity and mortality and needs immediate medical intervention. In the older adult with liver disease, hepatic encephalopathy is sometimes misdiagnosed as dementia and often overlooked.

Because older adults tend to have more co-morbid conditions, transplantation may have more risks for complications. Therefore older adults may not be good candidates for liver transplants.

DISORDERS OF THE PANCREAS

ACUTE PANCREATITIS

Acute pancreatitis is an acute inflammation of the pancreas. Spillage of pancreatic enzymes into surrounding pancreatic tissue causes autodigestion and severe pain. The degree of inflammation varies from mild edema to severe hemorrhagic necrosis.

Etiology and Pathophysiology

Many factors can cause injury to the pancreas. In the United States, the most common cause is gallbladder disease (gallstones), which is more common in women. The second most common cause is chronic alcohol use. This is more common in men.

Other less common causes include drug reactions, pancreatic cancer, and hypertriglyceridemia (serum levels over 1000 mg/dL).[14] Biliary sludge and microlithiasis, which is a mix of cholesterol crystals and calcium salts, can be present in patients with acute pancreatitis.

The most common pathogenic mechanism in acute pancreatitis is autodigestion of the pancreas (Fig. 43.11). The causative factors injure pancreatic cells or activate the pancreatic enzymes in the pancreas rather than in the intestine. This may be due to reflux of bile acids into the pancreatic ducts through an open or distended sphincter of Oddi. This reflux may be caused by blockage created by gallstones. Obstruction of pancreatic ducts results in pancreatic ischemia.

The exact mechanism by which chronic alcohol use predisposes a person to pancreatitis is not known. We think that alcohol increases the production of digestive enzymes in the pancreas.

The pathophysiologic involvement of acute pancreatitis is classified as either *mild pancreatitis* (also known as *edematous* or *interstitial pancreatitis*) or *severe pancreatitis* (also called *necrotizing pancreatitis*) (Fig. 43.12). In severe pancreatitis, about half the patients have permanent decreases in pancreatic endocrine and exocrine function. Patients with severe pancreatitis are at high risk for developing pancreatic necrosis, organ failure, and septic complications, resulting in an overall fatality rate of 5%.[14]

PATHOPHYSIOLOGY MAP

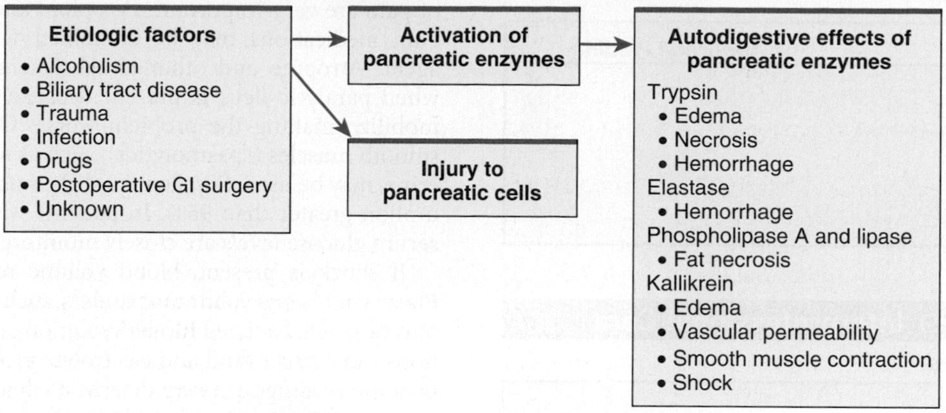

Etiologic factors	Activation of pancreatic enzymes	Autodigestive effects of pancreatic enzymes
• Alcoholism • Biliary tract disease • Trauma • Infection • Drugs • Postoperative GI surgery • Unknown	Injury to pancreatic cells	Trypsin • Edema • Necrosis • Hemorrhage Elastase • Hemorrhage Phospholipase A and lipase • Fat necrosis Kallikrein • Edema • Vascular permeability • Smooth muscle contraction • Shock

FIG. 43.11 Pathogenic process of acute pancreatitis.

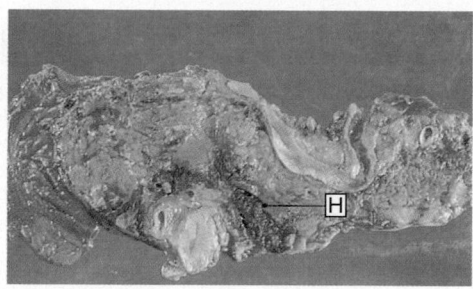

FIG. 43.12 In acute pancreatitis, the pancreas appears edematous and is often hemorrhagic *(H)*. (From Stevens A, Lowe J: *Pathology: Illustrated review in colour,* ed 2, London, 2000, Mosby.)

Clinical Manifestations

Abdominal pain is the main manifestation of acute pancreatitis. The pain is due to distention of the pancreas, peritoneal irritation, and obstruction of the biliary tract. The pain is usually in the left upper quadrant, but it may be mid-epigastric. It often radiates to the back due to the retroperitoneal location of the pancreas. The pain has a sudden onset. It is described as severe, deep, piercing, and continuous or steady. Eating worsens the pain. It often starts when the patient is recumbent. Pain is not relieved by vomiting and may be accompanied by flushing, cyanosis, and dyspnea. The patient may assume various positions involving flexion of the spine to try to relieve the severe pain.

Other manifestations include nausea and vomiting, low-grade fever, leukocytosis, hypotension, tachycardia, and jaundice. Abdominal tenderness with muscle guarding is common.

Bowel sounds may be decreased or absent. Paralytic ileus may occur and causes marked abdominal distention. The lungs are often involved with crackles present. Intravascular damage from circulating trypsin (a proteolytic enzyme) may cause areas of cyanosis or greenish to yellow-brown discoloration of the abdominal wall. Other areas of ecchymoses are the flanks (*Grey Turner' spots* or *sign,* a bluish flank discoloration) and the periumbilical area (*Cullen's sign,* a bluish periumbilical discoloration). These result from seepage of bloodstained exudate from the pancreas and may occur in severe cases.

Shock may occur from hemorrhage into the pancreas, toxemia from the activated pancreatic enzymes, or hypovolemia due to fluid shift into the retroperitoneal space (massive fluid shifts).

Complications

The severity of acute pancreatitis depends on the extent of pancreatic destruction. Acute pancreatitis can be life threatening. Some patients recover completely, others have recurring attacks, and others develop chronic pancreatitis.

Two significant local complications of acute pancreatitis are pseudocyst and abscess. A *pancreatic pseudocyst* is an accumulation of fluid, pancreatic enzymes, tissue debris, and inflammatory exudates surrounded by a wall next to the pancreas. Manifestations are abdominal pain, palpable epigastric mass, nausea, vomiting, and anorexia. The serum amylase level is often high. CT, MRI, and endoscopic ultrasound (EUS) may detect a pseudocyst. The cysts usually resolve spontaneously within a few weeks but may perforate, causing peritonitis or rupture into the stomach or the duodenum. Treatment options include surgical drainage, percutaneous catheter placement and drainage, and endoscopic drainage.

When a pseudocyst gets infected, a *pancreatic abscess* results from extensive necrosis in the pancreas. It may rupture or perforate into adjacent organs. Manifestations of an abscess include upper abdominal pain, abdominal mass, high fever, and leukocytosis. Pancreatic abscesses need prompt surgical drainage to prevent sepsis.

The main systemic complications of acute pancreatitis are cardiovascular and pulmonary (pleural effusion, atelectasis, pneumonia, and acute respiratory distress syndrome [ARDS]). The pulmonary complications are due to the passage of exudate containing pancreatic enzymes from the peritoneal cavity through transdiaphragmatic lymph channels. Enzyme-induced inflammation of the diaphragm occurs, with the result being atelectasis caused by reduced diaphragm movement. Trypsin can activate prothrombin and plasminogen, increasing the patient's risk for intravascular thrombi, pulmonary emboli, and DIC. Hypotension can occur from fluid shifts and sepsis.

Tetany, which can be caused by hypocalcemia, is a sign of severe disease. It is due in part to the combining of calcium and fatty acids during fat necrosis. We do not understand the exact mechanisms of how or why hypocalcemia occurs. Patients with severe acute pancreatitis are at risk for abdominal compartment syndrome from intraabdominal hypertension and edema.

Diagnostic Studies

The primary diagnostic tests for acute pancreatitis are serum amylase and lipase (Table 43.18). The serum amylase level is

TABLE 43.18 Diagnostic Findings
Acute Pancreatitis

Laboratory Test	Abnormal Finding
Serum amylase	↑
Serum lipase	↑
Urinary amylase	↑
Blood glucose	↑
Serum calcium	↓
Serum triglycerides	↑

TABLE 43.19 Interprofessional Care
Acute Pancreatitis

Diagnostic Assessment
- History and physical examination
- Serum amylase and lipase
- Blood glucose
- Serum calcium
- Serum triglycerides
- Flat plate of the abdomen
- Abdominal ultrasound
- Endoscopic ultrasound (EUS)
- MRCP
- ERCP
- Contrast-enhanced CT of pancreas
- Chest x-ray

Management
- NPO with NG tube to suction
- Albumin (if shock present)
- IV calcium gluconate (10%) (if tetany present)
- Lactated Ringer's solution

Drug Therapy
- Pain medication (e.g., morphine)
- PPI (e.g., omeprazole [Prilosec])
- Antibiotics (if necrotizing pancreatitis)

usually high early and stays high for 24 to 72 hours. Serum lipase level, which is high in acute pancreatitis, is an important test because other disorders (e.g., mumps, cerebral trauma, renal transplantation) may increase serum amylase levels. Other serum findings include an increase in liver enzymes, triglycerides, glucose, and bilirubin and a decrease in calcium.

Diagnostic evaluation of acute pancreatitis is directed at determining the cause. An abdominal ultrasound, x-ray, or contrast-enhanced CT scan may identify pancreatic problems. CT scan is the best imaging test for pancreatitis and related complications, such as pseudocysts and abscesses. ERCP is an option (although ERCP can cause acute pancreatitis), along with EUS, magnetic resonance cholangiopancreatography (MRCP), and angiography. Chest x-rays may show atelectasis and pleural effusions.

Interprofessional Care

Goals of interprofessional care for acute pancreatitis include (1) relief of pain, (2) prevention or alleviation of shock, (3) reduction of pancreatic secretions, (4) correction of fluid and electrolyte imbalances, (5) prevention or treatment of infections, and (6) removal of the precipitating cause, if possible (Table 43.19).
Conservative Therapy. Treatment of acute pancreatitis is focused on supportive care, including aggressive hydration, pain

management, management of metabolic complications, and minimization of pancreatic stimulation. Treatment and control of pain are very important. IV opioid analgesics may be given. Pain medications may be combined with an antispasmodic agent. Atropine and other anticholinergic drugs are avoided when paralytic ileus is present because they can decrease GI mobility, making the problem worse. Other drugs that relax smooth muscles (spasmolytics), such as nitroglycerin or papaverine, may be used. Supplemental O_2 is used to maintain O_2 saturation greater than 95%. In patients with severe pancreatitis, serum glucose levels are closely monitored for hyperglycemia.

If shock is present, blood volume replacements are used. Plasma or plasma volume expanders, such as dextran or albumin, may be given. Lactated Ringer's solution or other electrolyte solutions can correct fluid and electrolyte problems. Central venous pressure readings can help determine fluid replacement requirements. Vasoactive drugs, such as dopamine, may be needed to increase systemic vascular resistance in those with hypotension.

CHECK YOUR PRACTICE

You are a nurse working in the emergency department. Your patient is a 45-yr-old woman who reports acute abdominal pain in her left upper quadrant. She is diagnosed with acute pancreatitis. She tells you, "I've been waiting in this emergency room for 8 hours and I'm starving. Why can't I get something to eat? My pain is so bad; I think it's becoming worse because you won't give me food."
- How would you respond?
- What information and teaching would you give her?

It is important to reduce or suppress pancreatic enzymes to decrease stimulation of the pancreas and allow it to rest. This is achieved in several ways. First, the patient is NPO. Second, NG suction may be used to reduce vomiting and gastric distention and to prevent gastric acidic contents from entering the duodenum. Certain drugs are given to suppress gastric acid secretion (Table 43.20). With resolution of the pancreatitis, the patient resumes oral intake. For the patient with severe acute pancreatitis who does not resume oral intake, EN support may be started.

The inflamed and necrotic pancreatic tissue is a good medium for bacterial growth. In patients with acute necrotizing pancreatitis, infection is the leading cause of morbidity and mortality. Therefore it is important to prevent infections. Because many of the organisms come from the intestine, enteral feeding reduces the risk for necrotizing pancreatitis. Monitor the patient closely so that antibiotic therapy can be started early if necrosis and infection occur. Endoscopic- or CT-guided percutaneous aspiration with Gram stain and culture may be done.
Surgical Therapy. When the acute pancreatitis is related to gallstones, an urgent ERCP plus endoscopic *sphincterotomy* (severing of the muscle layers of the sphincter of Oddi) may be done. Laparoscopic cholecystectomy may follow ERCP to reduce the potential for recurrence. Surgical intervention may be needed when the diagnosis is uncertain and for patients who do not respond to conservative therapy.

Those with severe acute pancreatitis may need drainage of necrotic fluid collections. This is done surgically, under CT guidance, or endoscopically. Percutaneous drainage of a pseudocyst can be done, and a drainage tube left in place.
Drug Therapy. Several different drugs are used to prevent and treat problems associated with pancreatitis (Table 43.20). Currently, there are no drugs that cure pancreatitis.

TABLE 43.20 Drug Therapy
Acute and Chronic Pancreatitis

Drug	Mechanism of Action
Acute Pancreatitis	
Antacids	Neutralize gastric hydrochloric (HCl) acid secretion ↓ Production and secretion of pancreatic enzymes and bicarbonate
Antispasmodics (e.g., dicyclomine [Bentyl])	↓ Vagal stimulation, motility, pancreatic outflow (↓ volume and concentration of bicarbonate and enzyme secretion) Contraindicated in paralytic ileus
Carbonic anhydrase inhibitor (acetazolamide)	↓ Volume and bicarbonate concentration of pancreatic secretion
Morphine	Pain relief
PPIs (e.g., omeprazole [Prilosec])	↓ HCl acid secretion (HCl acid stimulates pancreatic activity)
Chronic Pancreatitis	
Insulin	Treat diabetes or hyperglycemia, if needed
Pancreatic enzyme products (pancrelipase [Pancrease, Zenpep, Creon, Viokace])	Replacement therapy for pancreatic enzymes

TABLE 43.21 Nursing Assessment
Acute Pancreatitis

Subjective Data
Important Health Information
Past health history: Biliary tract disease, alcohol use, abdominal trauma, duodenal ulcers, infection, metabolic disorders
Medications: Thiazides, NSAIDs
Surgery or other treatments: Surgical procedures on the pancreas, stomach, duodenum, or biliary tract. Endoscopic retrograde cholangiopancreatography (ERCP)

Functional Health Patterns
Health perception–health management: Chronic alcohol use, fatigue
Nutritional-metabolic: Nausea and vomiting, anorexia
Activity-exercise: Dyspnea
Cognitive-perceptual: Severe midepigastric or left upper quadrant pain that may radiate to the back, worsened by food and alcohol intake, unrelieved by vomiting

Objective Data
General
Restlessness, anxiety, low-grade fever

Integumentary
Flushing, diaphoresis, discoloration of abdomen and flanks, cyanosis, jaundice. Decreased skin turgor, dry mucous membranes

Respiratory
Tachypnea, basilar crackles

Cardiovascular
Tachycardia, hypotension

Gastrointestinal
Abdominal distention, tenderness, and muscle guarding. Decreased bowel sounds

Possible Diagnostic Findings
↑ Serum amylase and lipase, leukocytosis, hyperglycemia, hypocalcemia, abnormal ultrasound and CT scans of pancreas, abnormal ERCP or MRCP

Nutritional Therapy. Initially, the patient with acute pancreatitis is on NPO status to reduce pancreatic secretion. Depending on the severity of the pancreatitis, EN is started. Because of infection risk, parenteral nutrition is reserved for patients who cannot tolerate EN (see Chapter 39). If IV lipids are given, monitor blood triglyceride levels. In cases of moderate to severe pancreatitis, the patient may need enteral feeding via a jejunal feeding tube.

When food is allowed, small, frequent feedings are given. The diet is high in carbohydrate content because that is the least stimulating to the exocrine part of the pancreas. Suspect intolerance to oral foods when the patient reports pain, has increasing abdominal girth, or has increased serum amylase and lipase levels. Supplemental fat-soluble vitamins may be given.

❖ NURSING MANAGEMENT: ACUTE PANCREATITIS

◆ Nursing Assessment

Subjective and objective data that should be obtained from a person with acute pancreatitis are outlined in Table 43.21.

◆ Nursing Diagnoses

Nursing diagnoses for the patient with acute pancreatitis may include:
- Acute pain
- Fluid imbalance
- Electrolyte imbalance
- Impaired nutritional intake

Additional information on nursing diagnoses and interventions for the patient with acute pancreatitis is presented in eNursing Care Plan 43.3 available on the website for this chapter.

◆ Planning

The overall goals are that the patient with acute pancreatitis will have (1) relief of pain, (2) normal fluid and electrolyte balance, (3) minimal to no complications, and (4) no recurrent attacks.

◆ Nursing Implementation

◆ **Health Promotion.** The major factors involved in health promotion are (1) assessing the patient for predisposing and etiologic factors and (2) encouraging early treatment of these factors to prevent acute pancreatitis. Encourage the patient to cease alcohol intake, especially if they have had pancreatitis before. Recurrent attacks of pancreatitis may become milder or disappear if alcohol use is stopped. Encourage early diagnosis and treatment of biliary tract disease, such as gallstones.

◆ **Acute Care.** During the acute phase, it is important to monitor vital signs. Hypotension, fever, and tachypnea may compromise hemodynamic stability. Monitor the response to IV fluids. Closely monitor fluid and electrolyte balance. Frequent vomiting, along with gastric suction, may result in decreased chloride, sodium, and potassium levels.

Respiratory failure may develop in the patient with severe acute pancreatitis. Assess respiratory function (e.g., lung sounds, O_2 saturation levels). If ARDS develops, the patient may need intubation and mechanical ventilation support.

SAFETY ALERT Respiratory Distress in Acute Pancreatitis
- Assess for respiratory distress in the patient with severe acute pancreatitis.
- Listen to lung sounds and monitor O_2 saturation on a regular basis.

Because hypocalcemia can occur, observe for symptoms of tetany, including jerking, irritability, and muscular twitching. Numbness or tingling around the lips and in the fingers is an early sign of hypocalcemia. Assess the patient for a positive Chvostek's sign or Trousseau's sign (see Fig. 16.15). Give calcium gluconate (as ordered) to treat symptomatic hypocalcemia. Monitor serum magnesium levels since hypomagnesemia may develop.

Because abdominal pain is a primary symptom of pancreatitis, a major focus of your care is pain relief. Pain and restlessness can increase the metabolic rate and contribute to hemodynamic instability. Opioids may be used for pain relief. Assess and document the duration of pain relief. Comfortable positioning, frequent changes in position, and relief of nausea and vomiting help reduce the restlessness that usually accompanies the pain. Assuming positions that flex the trunk and draw the knees up to the abdomen may decrease pain. A side-lying position with the head elevated 45 degrees decreases tension on the abdomen and may help ease the pain.

For the patient who is on NPO status or has an NG tube, provide frequent oral and nasal care to relieve the dryness of the mouth and nose. Oral care is essential to prevent parotitis. If the patient is taking anticholinergics to decrease GI secretions, the mouth will be especially dry. If the patient is taking antacids to neutralize gastric acid secretion, they should be sipped slowly or inserted in the NG tube.

Observe for fever and other manifestations of infection in the patient with acute pancreatitis. Respiratory tract infections are common, which causes the patient to take shallow, guarded abdominal breaths. Measures to prevent respiratory tract infections include turning, coughing, deep breathing, and assuming a semi-Fowler's position.

Other important assessments are observation for signs of paralytic ileus, renal failure, and mental changes. Determine the blood glucose level to assess damage to the β cells of the islets of Langerhans in the pancreas.

If patients have surgery to drain necrotic fluid or treat a cyst, they may need special wound care for an anastomotic leak or a fistula. To prevent skin irritation, use skin barriers (e.g., Stomahesive, Karaya Paste), pouching, and drains. In addition to protecting the skin, pouching allows a more accurate determination of fluid and electrolyte losses and increases patient comfort. Sterile pouching systems are available. Consult with a clinical specialist or wound, ostomy, and continence nurse (WOCN).

Ambulatory Care. After acute pancreatitis, the patient may need home care follow-up. Because of loss of physical and muscle strength, physical therapy may be needed. Continued care to prevent infection and detect any complications is important. Counseling about abstinence from alcohol is important to prevent the patient from experiencing future attacks of acute pancreatitis and development of chronic pancreatitis. Because nicotine can stimulate the pancreas, smoking should be avoided.

Teach the patient and caregiver about the treatment plan, including the importance of taking the required medications and following the recommended diet. Dietary teaching should include fat restriction because fats stimulate the secretion of cholecystokinin, which then stimulates the pancreas. Encourage carbohydrates as they are less stimulating to the pancreas. Teach the patient to avoid crash and binge dieting because they can precipitate attacks.

Teach the patient and caregiver to recognize and report symptoms of infection, diabetes, or steatorrhea (foul-smelling, fatty stools). These changes indicate ongoing destruction of pancreatic tissue and pancreatic insufficiency. The patient may need exogenous enzyme supplementation.

◆ Evaluation

The expected outcomes are that the patient with acute pancreatitis will
- Have adequate pain control
- Maintain adequate fluid and electrolyte balance
- Be knowledgeable about the treatment plan to restore health
- Get help for alcohol use and smoking cessation (if needed)

CHRONIC PANCREATITIS

Chronic pancreatitis is a continuous, prolonged, inflammatory, and fibrosing process of the pancreas. The pancreas is progressively destroyed as it is replaced by fibrotic tissue. Strictures and calcifications may occur in the pancreas.

Etiology and Pathophysiology

Chronic pancreatitis can be due to chronic alcohol use; obstruction caused by gallstones, tumor, pseudocysts, or trauma; and systemic diseases (e.g., systemic lupus erythematosus), autoimmune pancreatitis, and cystic fibrosis. Some patients may not have an identifiable risk factor (idiopathic pancreatitis). Chronic pancreatitis may follow acute pancreatitis, but it may also occur in the absence of any history of an acute condition.

The most common cause of obstructive pancreatitis is inflammation of the sphincter of Oddi associated with gallstones. Cancer of the ampulla of Vater, duodenum, or pancreas can also cause this type of chronic pancreatitis.

The most common cause of nonobstructive pancreatitis (the most common type of chronic pancreatitis) is chronic alcohol use. There is inflammation and sclerosis, mainly in the head of the pancreas and around the pancreatic duct. In some people who drink alcohol, a genetic factor may predispose them to the direct toxic effect of the alcohol on the pancreas.

Clinical Manifestations

As with acute pancreatitis, a major manifestation of chronic pancreatitis is abdominal pain. The patient may have episodes of acute pain, but it usually is chronic (recurrent attacks at intervals of months or years). The attacks may become more frequent until they are almost constant, or they may decrease as pancreatic fibrosis develops. The pain is found in the same areas as in acute pancreatitis, but is usually described as a heavy, gnawing feeling or sometimes as burning and cramp-like. Food or antacids do not relieve the pain.

Other manifestations include symptoms of pancreatic insufficiency, including malabsorption with weight loss, constipation, mild jaundice with dark urine, steatorrhea, and diabetes. The steatorrhea may become severe, with voluminous, foul-smelling, fatty stools. Some abdominal tenderness may be present.

Chronic pancreatitis is associated with a variety of complications. These include pseudocyst formation, bile duct or duodenal obstruction, pancreatic ascites or pleural effusion, splenic vein thrombosis, pseudoaneurysms, and pancreatic cancer.

Diagnostic Studies

Confirming the diagnosis of chronic pancreatitis can be hard. The diagnosis is based on the patient's signs and symptoms, laboratory studies, and imaging. In chronic pancreatitis, serum amylase and lipase levels may be increased slightly or not at all, depending on the degree of pancreatic fibrosis. Serum bilirubin and alkaline phosphatase levels may be increased. There is usually mild leukocytosis and a high sedimentation rate.

ERCP can visualize the pancreatic and common bile ducts. Imaging studies, such as CT, MRI, MRCP, abdominal ultrasound, and EUS, can show a variety of changes, including calcifications, ductal dilation, pseudocysts, and enlargement of the pancreas.

Stool samples are examined for fecal fat content. Deficiencies of fat-soluble vitamins and cobalamin, glucose intolerance, and diabetes may occur in those with chronic pancreatitis. A secretin stimulation test can assess the degree of pancreatic dysfunction.

❖ Interprofessional and Nursing Care

When the patient with chronic pancreatitis has an acute attack, the therapy is identical to that for acute pancreatitis. At other times, the focus is on prevention of further attacks, relief of pain, and control of pancreatic exocrine and endocrine insufficiency. It sometimes takes frequent doses of analgesics (morphine, fentanyl patch [Duragesic]) to relieve the pain if dietary measures and enzyme replacement are not effective.

Diet, pancreatic enzyme replacement, and control of diabetes are ways to control the pancreatic insufficiency. Small, bland, frequent meals that are low in fat content are recommended to decrease pancreatic stimulation. Smoking is associated with accelerated progression of chronic pancreatitis. Teach the patient not to consume alcohol and caffeinated beverages. If the patient is dependent on alcohol, refer the patient to other resources as needed (see Chapter 10).

Pancreatic enzyme products, such as pancrelipase (Pancrease, Zenpep, Creon, Viokace), contain amylase, lipase, and trypsin. They are used to replace the deficient pancreatic enzymes. The enzymes are usually enteric coated to prevent their breakdown or inactivation by gastric acid. They are usually taken with meals and snacks. Teach the patient and caregiver to monitor stools for steatorrhea to help determine the effectiveness of the enzymes. Bile salts may be given to help with fat-soluble vitamin (A, D, E, and K) absorption and prevent further fat loss.

If diabetes develops, it is controlled with insulin (most often) or oral hypoglycemic agents. Teach the patient about testing blood glucose levels and drug therapy (see Chapter 48). While acid-neutralizing drugs (e.g., antacids) and acid-inhibiting drugs (e.g., H_2 receptor blockers, PPIs) may be given to control gastric acidity, they have little overall effect on patient outcomes. Antidepressants can reduce any neuropathic pain associated with chronic pancreatitis.

Treatment of chronic pancreatitis sometimes requires endoscopic therapy or surgery. When biliary disease is present or obstruction or pseudocyst develops, surgery may be needed. Surgical procedures can divert bile flow or relieve ductal obstruction. A choledochojejunostomy diverts bile around the ampulla of Vater, where there may be spasm or hypertrophy of the sphincter. In this procedure, the common bile duct is anastomosed into the jejunum. Another type of surgical diverting procedure is the Roux-en-Y pancreato-jejunostomy, in which the pancreatic duct is opened and an anastomosis made with the jejunum. Pancreatic drainage procedures can relieve ductal obstruction and are often done with ERCP. Some patients may have an ERCP with sphincterotomy and/or stent placement at the site of obstruction. These patients need follow-up procedures, such as ERCP, to either exchange or remove the stent.

PANCREATIC CANCER

There is a high mortality rate of pancreatic cancer with the incidence almost equal to the mortality rates. The median age at diagnosis is around 71 years of age.[15] Most pancreatic tumors are adenocarcinomas that begin in the epithelium of the ductal system. More than half of the tumors occur in the head of the pancreas. As the tumor grows, the common bile duct becomes obstructed and obstructive jaundice develops. Tumors starting in the body or the tail often remain silent until their growth is advanced. Most cancers have metastasized at the time of diagnosis. The signs and symptoms of pancreatic cancer are similar to those of chronic pancreatitis. The prognosis of a patient with cancer of the pancreas is poor. Most patients die within 5 to 12 months of diagnosis. The 5-year survival rate is only 8%.[15]

Etiology and Pathophysiology

The cause of pancreatic cancer is unknown. Risk factors for pancreatic cancer include chronic pancreatitis, diabetes, age, cigarette smoking, family history of pancreatic cancer, high-fat diet, and exposure to chemicals, such as benzidine. Blacks have a higher incidence of pancreatic cancer than whites. The most established risk factor is cigarette smoking. Smokers are 2 to 3 times more likely to develop pancreatic cancer than nonsmokers. The risk is related to both the duration and number of cigarettes smoked.

Clinical Manifestations

Common manifestations include abdominal pain (dull, aching), anorexia, rapid and progressive weight loss, nausea, and jaundice. The most common manifestations with cancer of the head of the pancreas are pain, jaundice, and weight loss. In general, pain is common and is related to the cancer's location. The pain is often in the upper abdomen or left hypochondrium and often radiates to the back. It is often related to eating and occurs at night. Extreme, unrelenting pain is related to extension of the cancer into the retroperitoneal tissues and nerve plexuses. Pruritus may accompany obstructive jaundice. Weight loss is due to poor digestion and absorption caused by lack of digestive enzymes from the pancreas.

Diagnostic Studies

Abdominal ultrasound or EUS, spiral CT scan, ERCP, MRI, and MRCP are the most often used diagnostic imaging techniques for pancreatic diseases, including cancer. EUS involves imaging the pancreas with the use of an endoscope positioned in the stomach and duodenum. EUS also allows for fine-needle aspiration of the tumor for pathologic examination. CT scan is often the first study and gives information on metastasis and vascular involvement of the tumor. ERCP allows visualization of the pancreatic duct and biliary system. With ERCP, pancreatic secretions and tissue can be obtained for biopsy and analysis of tumor markers. MRI, PET, PET/CT scans and MRCP may be done to confirm a cancer diagnosis and determine staging. They can also monitor progress and response to therapy.

Tumor markers are used both for diagnosing pancreatic cancer and monitoring the response to treatment. Cancer-associated antigen 19-9 (CA 19-9) is increased in pancreatic cancer. It is the most commonly used tumor marker. However, CA 19-9 also can be increased in gallbladder cancer or in benign conditions, such as acute and chronic pancreatitis, hepatitis, and biliary obstruction.

Interprofessional Care

Surgery is the most effective treatment for pancreatic cancer. Only 15% to 20% of patients have resectable tumors at the time of diagnosis. With the use of neoadjuvant chemotherapy (treatment before surgery), more patients can eventually become surgical candidates. The type of surgery depends on the size and location of the tumor. Pancreatic head tumors require the classic Whipple procedure or pancreaticoduodenectomy (Fig. 43.13). In the Whipple surgery, the proximal pancreas (proximal pancreatectomy), along with duodenum (duodenectomy), distal segment of the common bile duct and distal part of the stomach (partial gastrectomy) are removed together followed by a surgical anastomosis of the pancreatic duct, common bile duct, and stomach to the jejunum. Pancreatic body and/or tail tumors require a distal pancreatectomy procedure. Sometimes, a total pancreatectomy is done. It causes diabetes and the patient is dependent on exogenous insulin and pancreatic enzyme supplementation for life. If the pancreatic tumor cannot be removed surgically, palliative measures, such as a cholecystojejunostomy, to relieve biliary obstruction and/or endoscopically placed biliary stents, can be done.

Radiation therapy alone has little effect on survival but may be effective for pain relief. External radiation is most common, but implantation of internal radiation seeds into the tumor has been used. The current role of chemotherapy is limited and can have a significant side effect profile. Chemotherapy usually consists of fluorouracil and gemcitabine (Gemzar) either alone or in combination with agents such as capecitabine (Xeloda), paclitaxel (Abraxane), erlotinib (Tarceva), or irinotecan (Onivyde). Erlotinib is a targeted therapy drug (see Chapter 15).

❖ NURSING MANAGEMENT: PANCREATIC CANCER

Because the patient with pancreatic cancer has many of the same problems as the patient with pancreatitis, nursing care includes many of the same measures (see sections on acute and chronic pancreatitis on pp. 995 and 996). Provide symptomatic and supportive nursing care. This includes giving medications and providing comfort measures to relieve pain. Psychologic support is essential, especially during times of anxiety or depression.

Adequate nutrition is an important part of the nursing care plan. Frequent and supplemental feedings may be needed. Include measures to stimulate the appetite as much as possible and to manage anorexia, nausea, and vomiting. If the patient is undergoing radiation therapy, observe for adverse reactions, such as anorexia, nausea, vomiting, and skin irritation.

The prognosis for a patient with pancreatic cancer is poor. A significant part of the nursing care is helping the patient and caregiver cope with the diagnosis and prognosis. Chapter 9 provides information on palliative and end-of-life care.

DISORDERS OF THE BILIARY TRACT

CHOLELITHIASIS AND CHOLECYSTITIS

The most common disorder of the biliary system is cholelithiasis (stones in the gallbladder) (Fig. 43.14). The gallstones may lodge in the neck of the gallbladder or in the cystic duct. Cholecystitis (inflammation of the gallbladder wall) is usually associated with gallstones. They usually occur together, although a person can have gallstones without cholecystitis. Cholecystitis may present acutely or chronically.

Gallbladder disease is a common health problem in the United States. Up to 10% of American adults have cholecystitis caused by gallstones. The actual number is not known because many persons with stones are asymptomatic. *Cholecystectomy* (removal of the gallbladder) is among the most common surgical procedures done in the United States.

Gallstones are more common in women, especially multiparous women and women over 40 years of age. Postmenopausal

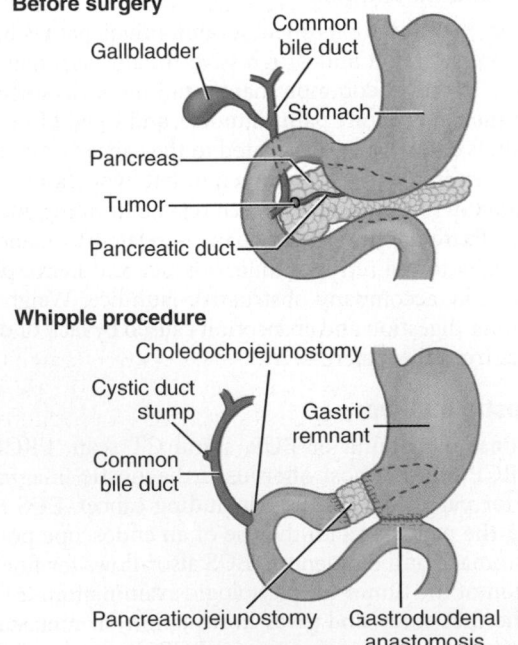

Before surgery

Gallbladder
Common bile duct
Stomach
Pancreas
Tumor
Pancreatic duct

Whipple procedure

Choledochojejunostomy
Cystic duct stump
Gastric remnant
Common bile duct
Pancreaticojejunostomy   Gastroduodenal anastomosis

FIG. 43.13 Whipple procedure or radical pancreaticoduodenectomy. This surgical procedure involves resecting the proximal pancreas, adjoining duodenum, distal part of the stomach, and distal part of the common bile duct. An anastomosis of the pancreatic duct, common bile duct, and stomach to the jejunum is done. (From Butcher GP: *Gastroenterology: An illustrated colour text*, London, 2004, Churchill Livingstone.)

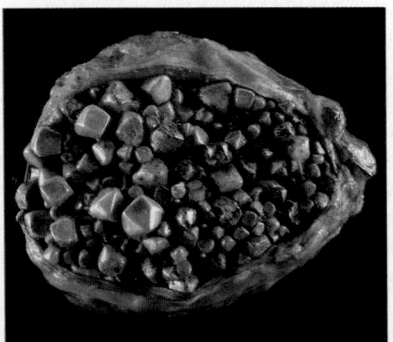

FIG. 43.14 Cholesterol gallstones in a gallbladder that was removed. (From Kumar V, Abbas AK, Aster JC, et al: *Robbins and Cotran pathologic basis of disease*, ed 8, Philadelphia, 2010, Saunders.)

women on estrogen replacement therapy and younger women on oral contraceptives are at an increased risk for gallbladder disease. Oral contraceptives affect cholesterol production and increase gallbladder cholesterol saturation. Other factors that increase the occurrence of gallbladder disease are a sedentary lifestyle, a familial tendency, and obesity. Obesity causes increased secretion of cholesterol in bile. The incidence of gallbladder disease is especially high in the Native American population.

GENDER DIFFERENCES
Cholelithiasis

Men
- Incidence is lower in men than in women.
- Gender differences in incidence decrease after age 50.

Women
- Pregnancy is the greatest risk factor for increased prevalence in women.
- Obesity increases the risk, especially for women.

Etiology and Pathophysiology

Cholelithiasis. The cause of gallstones is unknown. They develop when the balance that keeps cholesterol, bile salts, and calcium in solution is changed so that these substances precipitate. Conditions that upset this balance include infection and changes in cholesterol metabolism. In patients with gallstones, the bile secreted by the liver is supersaturated with cholesterol (lithogenic bile). The bile in the gallbladder then becomes supersaturated with cholesterol and precipitation of cholesterol occurs in the gallbladder.

Other components of bile that precipitate into stones are bile salts, bilirubin, calcium, and protein. Mixed cholesterol stones, which are mainly cholesterol, are the most common gallstones.

Changes in the composition of bile are significant in gallstone formation. Bile stasis leads to progression of the supersaturation and changes in the chemical composition of the bile (biliary sludge). Immobility, pregnancy, and inflammatory or obstructive lesions in the biliary system decrease bile flow. Hormonal factors during pregnancy may cause delayed emptying of the gallbladder, resulting in bile stasis.

The stones may stay in the gallbladder or migrate to the cystic duct or the common bile duct. They cause pain as they pass through the ducts, and they may lodge in the ducts and cause an obstruction. Small stones are more likely to move into a duct and cause obstruction. Table 43.22 describes the changes and manifestations that occur when the stones obstruct the common bile duct. If the blockage occurs in the cystic duct, the bile can continue to flow into the duodenum directly from the liver. However, when the bile in the gallbladder cannot escape, this stasis of bile may lead to cholecystitis.

Cholecystitis. Cholecystitis is most often associated with obstruction caused by gallstones or biliary sludge. Cholecystitis in the absence of obstruction (*acalculous cholecystitis*) occurs most often in older adults and in patients who are critically ill. Acalculous cholecystitis is also associated with prolonged immobility and fasting, prolonged parenteral nutrition, and diabetes. We think the main cause of this illness is bile stasis. Critically ill patients are more predisposed because of increased bile viscosity due to fever and dehydration and because of prolonged

TABLE 43.22 Manifestations of Obstructed Bile Flow

Manifestation	Etiology
Bleeding tendencies	Lack of or ↓ absorption of vitamin K, resulting in ↓ production of prothrombin
Clay-colored stools	No bilirubin reaching small intestine to be converted to urobilinogen
Dark amber to brown urine, which foams when shaken	↑ Water-soluble (conjugated) bilirubin elimination in urine
Fever and chills	Bacterial reflux from biliary tract to systemic circulation
Intolerance for fatty foods	No bile in small intestine for fat digestion
Jaundice	No bile flow into duodenum, bilirubin accumulates in blood
Pruritus	Deposition of bile salts in skin tissues
Steatorrhea	Undigested fatty components of food are eliminated in stool. Occurs because no bile in small intestine, thus preventing emulsion, digestion, and absorption of fat
Urobilinogen absent in urine	No bilirubin reaching small intestine to be converted to urobilinogen

absence of oral feeding resulting in a decrease or absence of cholecystokinin-induced gallbladder contraction. Other risk factors include adhesions, cancer, anesthesia, and opioids.

Once acalculous cholecystitis is present, secondary infection with enteric pathogens, including *E. coli, Enterococcus faecalis, Klebsiella, Pseudomonas,* and *Proteus,* is common. Perforation occurs in severe cases.

Inflammation is the major pathophysiologic condition. It may be confined to the mucous lining or involve the entire wall of the gallbladder. During an acute attack of cholecystitis, the gallbladder is edematous and hyperemic, and it may be distended with bile or pus. The cystic duct is also involved and may become occluded. The wall of the gallbladder becomes scarred after an acute attack. Decreased functioning will occur if large amounts of tissue become fibrotic.

Clinical Manifestations

Gallstones may produce a range of symptoms. The severity depends on whether the stones are stationary or mobile and whether obstruction is present. When a stone is lodged in the ducts or when stones are moving through the ducts, spasms may result in response to the stone. This sometimes causes severe pain, which is termed *biliary colic,* even though the pain is rarely colicky. The pain is more often steady. The pain can be excruciating and accompanied by tachycardia, diaphoresis, and prostration. The severe pain may last up to an hour, and when it subsides, there is residual tenderness in the right upper quadrant. The attacks of pain often occur 3 to 6 hours after a high-fat meal or when the patient lies down.

When total obstruction occurs, symptoms related to bile blockage occur (Table 43.22). If the common bile duct is obstructed, no bilirubin will reach the small intestine to be converted to urobilinogen. Thus the kidneys will excrete bilirubin, causing dark amber to brown urine.

Manifestations of cholecystitis vary from indigestion to moderate to severe pain, fever, chills, and jaundice. Initial symptoms of acute cholecystitis include indigestion and acute pain and tenderness in the right upper quadrant. Pain may be referred to the right shoulder and scapula. The pain may be accompanied by nausea and vomiting, restlessness, and diaphoresis. Inflammation results in leukocytosis and fever. Physical findings include right upper quadrant or epigastrium tenderness and abdominal rigidity. Chronic cholecystitis may present with a history of fat intolerance, dyspepsia, heartburn, and flatulence.

Complications

Complications of gallstones and cholecystitis include gangrenous cholecystitis, subphrenic abscess, pancreatitis, *cholangitis* (inflammation of biliary ducts), biliary cirrhosis, fistulas, and rupture of the gallbladder, which can cause bile peritonitis. In older adults and those with diabetes, gangrenous cholecystitis and bile peritonitis are the most common complications of cholecystitis. *Choledocholithiasis* (stone in the common bile duct) may occur, producing symptoms of obstruction.

Diagnostic Studies

Ultrasound is often used to diagnose gallstones (see Table 38.11). It is especially useful for patients with jaundice (because it does not depend on renal function) and for patients who are allergic to contrast medium. ERCP allows for visualization of the gallbladder, cystic duct, common hepatic duct, and common bile duct. Bile taken during ERCP is sent for culture to identify possible infecting organisms.

Percutaneous transhepatic cholangiography is the insertion of a needle directly into the gallbladder duct followed by injection of contrast materials. It is generally done after ultrasound shows a bile duct blockage.

Laboratory tests may reveal an increased WBC count because of inflammation. Serum enzymes (e.g., alkaline phosphatase, ALT, and AST), direct and indirect bilirubin levels, and urinary bilirubin levels may be increased if an obstructive process is present (Table 43.3). Serum amylase is increased if there is pancreatic involvement.

Interprofessional Care

Once gallstones become symptomatic, definitive surgical intervention with cholecystectomy is usually needed. However, in some cases, conservative therapy may be considered.

Conservative Therapy

Cholelithiasis. The treatment of gallstones depends on the stage of disease. Bile acids (cholesterol solvents), such as ursodeoxycholic acid (Ursodiol) and chenodeoxycholic acid (Chenodiol), are used to dissolve stones. However, the gallstones may recur. We usually do not treat gallstones with drugs because of the high use and success of laparoscopic cholecystectomy.

ERCP with endoscopic sphincterotomy (papillotomy) may be used to remove stones (Fig. 43.15). ERCP allows for visualization of the biliary system, dilation (balloon sphincteroplasty), and placement of stents and sphincterotomy. Special catheters with wire baskets or inflatable balloon tip may be used for stone removal.[16] When a stent is placed, it is generally removed or changed after a few months.

Extracorporeal shock-wave lithotripsy (ESWL) is an alternative treatment used when endoscopic approaches cannot remove stones. In ESWL, a lithotripter uses high-energy shock waves to disintegrate gallstones. It usually takes 1 to 2 hours to disintegrate the stones. After they are broken up, the fragments pass through the common bile duct and into the small intestine. Usually ESWL and oral dissolution therapy are used together.

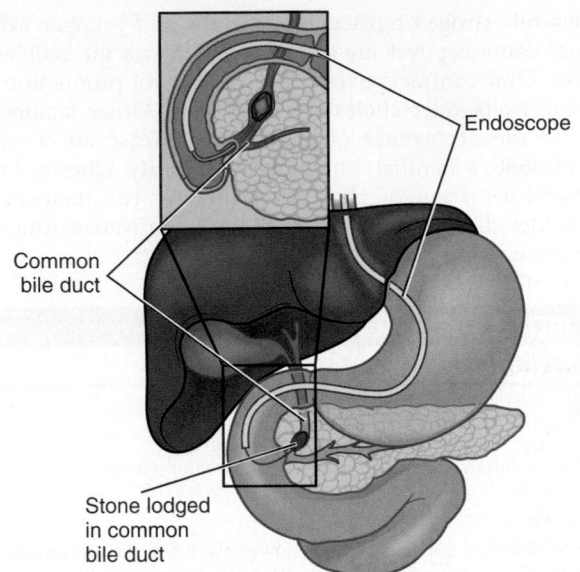

FIG. 43.15 During endoscopic sphincterotomy, an endoscope is advanced through the mouth and stomach until its tip sits in the duodenum opposite the common bile duct. *Inset,* After widening the duct mouth by incising the sphincter muscle, the HCP advances a basket attachment into the duct and snags the stone.

TABLE 43.23 Interprofessional Care
Cholelithiasis and Acute Cholecystitis

Diagnostic Assessment
- History and physical examination
- Ultrasound
- ERCP
- Percutaneous transhepatic cholangiography
- Liver function tests
- White blood cell count
- Serum bilirubin

Management
Conservative Therapy
- IV fluid
- NPO with NG tube, later progressing to low-fat diet
- Antiemetics
- Analgesics
- Fat-soluble vitamins (A, D, E, and K)
- Anticholinergics (antispasmodics)
- Antibiotics (for secondary infection)
- Transhepatic biliary catheter
- ERCP with sphincterotomy (papillotomy)
- Extracorporeal shock-wave lithotripsy

Dissolution Therapy
- ursodeoxycholic acid (ursodiol [Actigall])

Surgical Therapy
- Laparoscopic cholecystectomy
- Incisional (open) cholecystectomy

Cholecystitis. During an acute episode of cholecystitis, treatment focuses on pain control, control of infection with antibiotics, and maintaining fluid and electrolyte balance (Table 43.23). Treatment is supportive and focused on symptom management. If nausea and vomiting are severe, NG tube insertion and gastric decompression may be used to prevent further gallbladder stimulation. A cholecystostomy may be used to drain purulent material from the obstructed gallbladder. Opioids are given for pain management. Anticholinergics may be used to decrease GI secretions and counteract smooth muscle spasms.

Surgical Therapy. Laparoscopic cholecystectomy is the treatment of choice for symptomatic gallstones. About 90% of cholecystectomies are done laparoscopically. In this procedure, the gallbladder is removed through 1 to 4 small punctures in the abdomen. The HCP makes a small cut below the umbilicus and inserts a needle into the area. CO_2 gas is passed into the abdomen to expand the area, which allows the HCP to see the organs more clearly and gives more room to work. A laparoscope, which has a camera attached, and grasping forceps are inserted into the abdomen through the punctures. Using closed-circuit monitors to view the abdominal cavity, the HCP retracts and dissects the gallbladder and removes it with grasping forceps. This is a safe and routine procedure with minimal morbidity and quick recovery time.

Most patients have minimal postoperative pain and are discharged the day of surgery or the day after. They can usually resume normal activities and return to work within 1 week. The main complication is injury to the common bile duct. The few contraindications to laparoscopic cholecystectomy include peritonitis, cholangitis, gangrene or perforation of the gallbladder, portal hypertension, and serious bleeding disorders.

Some patients may need an incisional (open) cholecystectomy. This involves removing the gallbladder through a right subcostal incision. A T tube may be inserted into the common bile duct during surgery when a common bile duct exploration is part of the surgical procedure (Fig. 43.16). This ensures patency of the duct until the edema from the trauma of exploring and probing the duct has subsided. It also allows excess bile to drain while the small intestine is adjusting to receiving a continuous flow of bile.

Transhepatic Biliary Catheter. The transhepatic biliary catheter can be used preoperatively in biliary obstruction and in hepatic dysfunction from obstructive jaundice. It also can be inserted for palliative care when inoperable liver, pancreatic, or bile duct cancer obstructs bile flow. The catheter is used when endoscopic drainage has been unsuccessful. The catheter is inserted percutaneously and allows for decompression of obstructed extrahepatic bile ducts so that bile can flow freely. After placement of the catheter into the obstructed duct internally, the external catheter is connected to a drainage bag. Encourage patients to replace fluids lost in the drainage bag with electrolyte-rich drinks. Cleanse the skin around the catheter insertion site daily with an antiseptic. Observe for bile leakage at the insertion site and any signs or symptoms of sudden abdominal pain, nausea, fever, or chills that may signal an occluded or malfunctioning drain.

Drug Therapy. The most common drugs used in the treatment of gallbladder disease are analgesics, anticholinergics (antispasmodics), fat-soluble vitamins, and bile salts. Morphine may be used initially for pain management. Anticholinergics, such as atropine and other antispasmodics, may be used to relax the smooth muscle and decrease ductal tone.

The patient with chronic gallbladder disease or any biliary tract obstruction may need fat-soluble vitamin (A, D, E, and K) replacement. Bile salts may be given to help digestion and vitamin absorption.

Cholestyramine may provide relief from pruritus. Cholestyramine is a resin that binds bile salts in the intestine, increasing their excretion in the feces. It comes in powder form that is mixed with milk or juice. Side effects include nausea, vomiting, diarrhea or constipation, and skin reactions. Cholestyramine may bind with other medications, so check drug-to-drug interactions.

Nutritional Therapy. People have fewer gallbladder problems if they eat smaller, more frequent meals with some fat at each meal to promote gallbladder emptying. If obesity is a problem, a reduced-calorie diet is indicated. The diet should be low in saturated fats (e.g., butter, shortening, lard) and high in fiber and calcium. Rapid weight loss should be avoided because it can promote gallstone formation.

After a laparoscopic cholecystectomy, teach the patient to have liquids for the rest of the day and eat light meals for a few days. After an incisional cholecystectomy, the patient will progress from liquids to a regular diet once bowel sounds have returned. The amount of fat in the postoperative diet depends on the patient's tolerance of fat. A low-fat diet may be helpful if the flow of bile is reduced (usually only in the early postoperative period) or if the patient is overweight. Sometimes the patient must restrict fats for 4 to 6 weeks. Otherwise, no special diet is needed other than to eat nutritious meals and avoid excess fat intake.

❖ NURSING MANAGEMENT: GALLBLADDER DISEASE

◆ Nursing Assessment

Subjective and objective data that should be obtained from a person with gallbladder disease are outlined in Table 43.24.

◆ Nursing Diagnoses

Nursing diagnoses for the patient with gallbladder disease treated surgically may include:
- Acute pain
- Lack of knowledge

◆ Planning

The overall goals are that the patient with gallbladder disease will have (1) relief of pain and discomfort, (2) no complications postoperatively, and (3) no recurrent attacks of cholecystitis or gallstones.

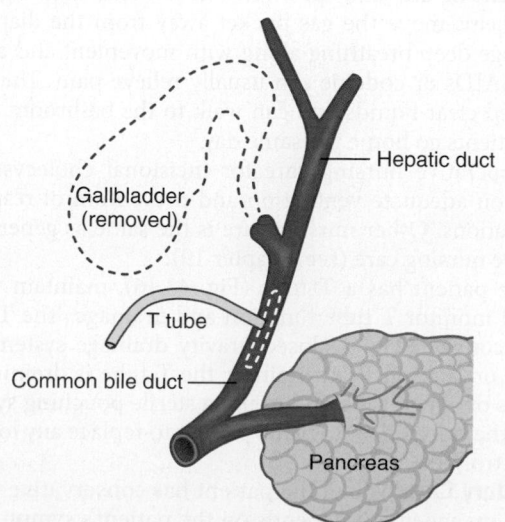

FIG. 43.16 Placement of T tube. *Dotted lines* show parts removed.

TABLE 43.24 Nursing Assessment

Cholecystitis or Cholelithiasis

Subjective Data

Important Health Information

Past health history: Obesity, multiparity, infection, cancer, extensive fasting, pregnancy
Medications: Estrogen or oral contraceptives
Surgery or other treatments: Abdominal surgery

Functional Health Patterns

Health perception–health management: Positive family history, sedentary lifestyle
Nutritional-metabolic: Weight loss, anorexia, indigestion, fat intolerance, nausea and vomiting, dyspepsia, chills
Elimination: Clay-colored stools, steatorrhea, flatulence. Dark urine
Cognitive-perceptual: Moderate to severe pain in right upper quadrant that may radiate to the back or scapula. Itching

Objective Data

General

Fever, restlessness

Integumentary

Jaundice, icteric sclera, diaphoresis

Respiratory

Tachypnea, splinting during respirations

Cardiovascular

Tachycardia

Gastrointestinal

Palpable gallbladder, abdominal guarding, and distention

Possible Diagnostic Findings

↑ Serum liver enzymes, alkaline phosphatase, and bilirubin. Absence of urobilinogen in urine, ↑ urinary bilirubin, leukocytosis. Abnormal gallbladder ultrasound

◆ **Nursing Implementation**

◆ **Health Promotion.** Be aware of predisposing factors for gallbladder disease in general health screening. Teach patients from ethnic groups in which the disease is more common, such as Native Americans, the early manifestations and to see their HCP if these manifestations occur. Patients with chronic cholecystitis may not have acute symptoms and may not seek help until jaundice and biliary obstruction occur. Earlier detection in these patients is important so that they can be managed with a low-fat diet and monitored more closely.

Acute Care. Nursing goals for the patient undergoing conservative therapy include (1) treat pain, (2) relieve nausea and vomiting, (3) provide comfort and emotional support, (4) maintain fluid and electrolyte balance and nutrition, and (5) observe for complications.

The patient with acute cholecystitis or gallstones often has severe pain. Give the drugs ordered to relieve the pain as needed before pain becomes severe. Observe for side effects of the drugs as part of the continued assessment. Nursing comfort measures, such as a clean bed, comfortable positioning, and oral care, are appropriate.

Some patients have more severe nausea and vomiting than others. For these patients, an NG tube and gastric decompression may be ordered. Eliminating intake of food and fluids prevents further stimulation of the gallbladder. Oral hygiene, care of nares, accurate intake and output measurements, and maintaining suction should be a part of the nursing care plan. For patients with less severe nausea and vomiting, antiemetics are usually adequate. When the patient is vomiting, provide comfort measures, such as frequent mouth rinses. Remove any vomitus at once from the patient's view. If itching occurs with jaundice, use measures to relieve itching. These can include antihistamines or other treatments as previously discussed.

Assess for progression of the symptoms and development of complications. Observe for signs of obstruction of the ducts by stones. These include jaundice; clay-colored stools; dark, foamy urine; steatorrhea; fever; and increased WBC count.

When manifestations of obstruction are present (Table 43.22), bleeding may result from decreased prothrombin production by the liver. Common sites to observe for bleeding are the mucous membranes of the mouth, nose, gingivae, and injection sites. When giving injections, use a small-gauge needle and apply gentle pressure after the injection. Know the patient's PT time and use it as a guide in the assessment process.

Assessment for infections includes monitoring vital signs. A temperature elevation with chills and jaundice may indicate choledocholithiasis.

Your care of the patient after ERCP with papillotomy includes assessment to detect complications, such as pancreatitis, perforation, infection, and bleeding. Monitor the patient's vital signs. Abdominal pain, fever, and increasing amylase and lipase may indicate acute pancreatitis. The patient should be on bed rest for several hours and should be NPO until the gag reflex returns. Teach the patient the need for follow-up if the stent is to be removed or changed.

Postoperative Care. Postoperative nursing care after a laparoscopic cholecystectomy includes monitoring for complications, such as bleeding, making the patient comfortable, and preparing the patient for discharge. Patients may report referred pain to the shoulder because of the CO_2 that the HCP uses to inflate the abdominal cavity during surgery. It may not be released or absorbed by the body. The CO_2 can irritate the phrenic nerve and diaphragm, causing some difficulty in breathing. Placing the patient in the Sims' position (on left side with right knee flexed) helps move the gas pocket away from the diaphragm. Encourage deep breathing along with movement and ambulation. NSAIDs or codeine can usually relieve pain. The patient is allowed clear liquids and can walk to the bathroom to void. Most patients go home the same day.

Postoperative nursing care for incisional cholecystectomy focuses on adequate ventilation and prevention of respiratory complications. Other nursing care is the same as general postoperative nursing care (see Chapter 19).

If the patient has a T tube (Fig. 43.16), maintain the system and monitor T-tube function and drainage. The T tube is usually connected to a closed gravity drainage system. If the Penrose or Jackson-Pratt drain or the T tube is draining large amounts of bile, it is helpful to use a sterile pouching system to protect the skin. Encourage the patient to replace any lost fluids and electrolytes.

Ambulatory Care. When the patient has conservative therapy, nursing management depends on the patient's symptoms and on whether surgical intervention is planned. Dietary teaching

TABLE 43.25 Patient & Caregiver Teaching
Postoperative Laparoscopic Cholecystectomy

Postoperative teaching should include:
1. Remove the bandages on the puncture sites the day after surgery and you can shower.
2. Notify your HCP if any of the following signs and symptoms occurs:
   - Redness, swelling, bile-colored drainage or pus from any incision
   - Severe abdominal pain, nausea, vomiting, fever, chills
3. You can gradually resume normal activities.
4. Return to work within 1 wk of surgery.
5. You can resume your usual diet, but a low-fat diet is usually better tolerated for several weeks after surgery.

is usually needed. The diet is usually low in fat. The patient may need to take fat-soluble vitamin supplements. If needed, review a weight-reduction diet. Teach the patient signs and symptoms of obstruction (e.g., stool and urine changes, jaundice, itching). Explain the importance of continued health care follow-up.

The patient who undergoes a laparoscopic cholecystectomy is discharged soon after the surgery, so home care and teaching are important (Table 43.25).

After an incisional cholecystectomy, tell the patient to avoid heavy lifting for 4 to 6 weeks. Usual sexual activities, including intercourse, can be resumed as soon as the patient feels ready, unless otherwise instructed by the HCP.

Sometimes the patient needs to remain on a low-fat diet for 4 to 6 weeks. If so, an individualized dietary teaching plan is needed. A weight-reduction program may be helpful if the patient is overweight. Most patients tolerate a regular diet with no problems but should avoid excess fats.

◆ Evaluation

The overall expected outcomes are that the patient with gallbladder disease will
- Appear comfortable and have pain relief
- State knowledge of activity level and dietary restrictions

GALLBLADDER CANCER

Gallbladder cancer is the sixth most common GI cancer in the United States.[17] Most gallbladder cancers are adenocarcinomas. They are often found incidentally as the patient is asymptomatic. The majority have advanced disease at the time of diagnosis.

The early symptoms are insidious and similar to those of chronic cholecystitis and gallstones, which makes the diagnosis difficult. Later symptoms are usually those of biliary obstruction.

Diagnosis and staging of gallbladder cancer are done using EUS, abdominal ultrasound, CT, MRI, and/or MRCP. Unfortunately, gallbladder cancer often is not detected until the disease is advanced. When it is found early, surgery can be curative. Several factors influence successful surgical outcomes, including the depth of cancer invasion, extent of liver involvement, venous or lymphatic invasion, and lymph node metastasis. Extended cholecystectomy with lymph node dissection has improved outcomes for those with gallbladder cancer.

When surgery is not an option, endoscopic stenting of the biliary tract can reduce obstructive jaundice. Adjuvant therapies, including radiation therapy and chemotherapy, may be used depending on the disease state. Overall, gallbladder cancer has a poor prognosis.

Nursing management involves palliative care with special attention to nutrition, hydration, skin care, and pain relief. Nursing care measures used for patients with cholecystitis and gallstones and for the patient with cancer (see Chapter 15) are appropriate.

CASE STUDY
Cirrhosis of the Liver

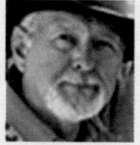
(© sbeagle/ iStock/ Thinkstock.)

Patient Profile

M.B., a 58-yr-old male rancher who lives in rural Wyoming, is admitted with a diagnosis of cirrhosis of the liver. He has been vomiting for 2 days and noticed blood in the toilet when he vomited. He lives 40 miles from the nearest hospital. He had one of his ranch hands drive him to the hospital. His medical history includes chronic hepatitis C, depression, and stage II chronic kidney disease.

Subjective Data
- Has been estranged from his 2 children since his divorce 3 years ago
- Has had cirrhosis for 12 yrs
- Acknowledges that he had been drinking heavily for 20 yrs but has been sober for the past 2 yrs
- Reports experiencing anorexia, nausea, and abdominal discomfort

Objective Data
Physical Examination
- Has moderate ascites
- Has jaundice of sclera and skin
- Has 4+ pitting edema of the lower extremities
- Liver and spleen are palpable

Laboratory Values
- Total bilirubin: 15 mg/dL (257 mmol/L)
- AST: 190 U/L (3.2 μkat/L)
- ALT: 210 U/L (3.5 μkat/L)
- Platelets: 45,000/μL
- eGFR: 62 mL/min
- ECG is below:

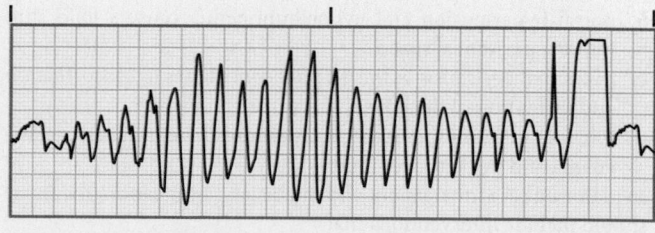

Discussion Questions
1. What are possible causes of cirrhosis? What type of cirrhosis does M.B. likely have?
2. Describe the pathophysiologic changes that occur in the liver as cirrhosis develops.

Continued

CASE STUDY

Cirrhosis of the Liver—cont'd

3. List M.B.'s clinical manifestations of liver failure. For each manifestation, explain the pathophysiologic basis.

4. Explain the significance of the results of his laboratory values and ECG findings.

5. If M.B. begins to show signs and symptoms of hepatic encephalopathy, what would you monitor? What measures would be used to control or decrease the encephalopathy?

6. What are possible causes of his GI bleeding?

7. *Priority Decision:* Based on the assessment data, what are the priority nursing diagnoses? Are there any collaborative problems?

8. *Priority Decision:* What are the priority nursing interventions for a patient at this stage of his illness?

9. *Evidence-Based Practice:* M.B. discusses his prognosis with you. He says, "There is no hope. I might as well keep drinking." How would you respond to his statement?

10. *Safety:* Given M.B.'s bleeding history and current laboratory values, identify areas of injury risk and specify actions you will take to ensure patient safety.

11. Develop a conceptual care map for M.B.

Answers and corresponding conceptual care map available at *evolve.elsevier.com/Lewis/medsurg.*

■ BRIDGE TO NCLEX EXAMINATION

The number of the question corresponds to the same-numbered outcome at the beginning of the chapter.

1. A patient with hepatitis A is in the acute phase. The nurse plans care for the patient based on the knowledge that
   a. itching is a common problem with jaundice in this phase.
   b. the patient is most likely to transmit the disease during this phase.
   c. gastrointestinal symptoms are not as severe in hepatitis A as they are in hepatitis B.
   d. extrahepatic manifestations of glomerulonephritis and polyarteritis are common in this phase.

2. A patient with acute hepatitis B is being discharged. The discharge teaching plan should include instructions to
   a. avoid alcohol for the first 3 weeks.
   b. use a condom during sexual intercourse.
   c. have family members get an injection of immunoglobulin.
   d. follow a low-protein, moderate-carbohydrate, moderate-fat diet.

3. A patient has been told that she has elevated liver enzymes caused by nonalcoholic fatty liver disease (NAFLD). The nursing teaching plan should include
   a. having genetic testing done.
   b. recommending a heart-healthy diet.
   c. the necessity to reduce weight rapidly.
   d. avoiding alcohol until liver enzymes return to normal.

4. The patient with advanced cirrhosis asks why his abdomen is so swollen. The nurse's response is based on the knowledge that
   a. a lack of clotting factors promotes the collection of blood in the abdominal cavity.
   b. portal hypertension and hypoalbuminemia cause a fluid shift into the peritoneal space.
   c. decreased peristalsis in the GI tract contributes to gas formation and distention of the bowel.
   d. bile salts in the blood irritate the peritoneal membranes, causing edema and pocketing of fluid.

5. In planning care for a patient with metastatic liver cancer, the nurse should include interventions that
   a. focus primarily on symptomatic and comfort measures.
   b. reassure the patient that chemotherapy offers a good prognosis.
   c. promote the patient's confidence that surgical excision of the tumor will be successful.
   d. provide information needed for the patient to make decisions about liver transplantation.

6. Nursing management of the patient with acute pancreatitis includes *(select all that apply)*
   a. administering pain medication.
   b. checking for signs of hypocalcemia.
   c. providing a diet low in carbohydrates.
   d. giving insulin based on a sliding scale.
   e. monitoring for infection, particularly respiratory tract infection.

7. A patient with pancreatic cancer is admitted to the hospital for evaluation of treatment options. The patient asks the nurse to explain the Whipple procedure that the surgeon has described. The explanation includes the information that a Whipple procedure involves
   a. creating a bypass around the obstruction caused by the tumor by joining the gallbladder to the jejunum.
   b. resection of the entire pancreas and the distal part of the stomach, with anastomosis of the common bile duct and the stomach into the duodenum.
   c. removal of part of the pancreas, part of the stomach, the duodenum, and the gallbladder, with joining of the pancreatic duct, the common bile duct, and the stomach into the jejunum.
   d. removal of the pancreas, the duodenum, and the spleen, and attachment of the stomach to the jejunum, which requires oral supplementation of pancreatic digestive enzymes and insulin replacement therapy.

8. The nurse caring for a patient with suspected acute cholecystitis would anticipate *(select all that apply)*
   a. ordering a low-sodium diet.
   b. administration of IV fluids.
   c. monitoring of liver function tests.
   d. administration of antiemetics for patients with nausea.
   e. insertion of an indwelling catheter to monitor urinary output.

9. Teaching in relation to home management after a laparoscopic cholecystectomy should include
   a. keeping the bandages on the puncture sites for 48 hours.
   b. reporting any bile-colored drainage or pus from any incision.
   c. using over-the-counter antiemetics if nausea and vomiting occur.
   d. emptying and measuring the contents of the bile bag from the T tube every day.

1. a, 2. b, 3. b, 4. b, 5. a, 6. a, b, e, 7. c, 8. b, c, d, 9. b.

For rationales to these answers and even more NCLEX review questions, visit *evolve.elsevier.com/Lewis/medsurg.*

EVOLVE WEBSITE/RESOURCES LIST

evolve.elsevier.com/Lewis/medsurg

Review Questions (Online Only)

Key Points

Answer Keys for Questions

- Rationales for Bridge to NCLEX Examination Questions
- Answer Guidelines for Case Study on p. 1003
- Answer Guidelines for Managing Care of Multiple Patients Case Study (Section 9) on p. 1006

Student Case Studies

- Patient With Acute Pancreatitis and Septic Shock
- Patient With Cholelithiasis/Cholecystitis
- Patient With Cirrhosis
- Patient With Hepatitis

Nursing Care Plans

- eNursing Care Plan 43.1: Patient With Acute Viral Hepatitis
- eNursing Care Plan 43.2: Patient With Cirrhosis
- eNursing Care Plan 43.3: Patient With Acute Pancreatitis

Conceptual Care Map Creator

- Conceptual Care Map for Case Study on p. 1003

Audio Glossary

Content Updates

REFERENCES

1. Centers for Disease Control and Prevention: Viral hepatitis—Hepatitis A information—United States. Retrieved from *www.cdc.gov/hepatitis/hav/index.htm.*
2. Centers for Disease Control and Prevention: Viral hepatitis—Hepatitis B information—United States. Retrieved from *www.cdc.gov/hepatitis/hbv/index.htm.*
3. Friedman LS, Martin P: *Handbook of liver disease,* ed 4, Philadelphia, 2018, Elsevier.
4. Centers for Disease Control and Prevention: Viral hepatitis—Hepatitis C information—United States. Retrieved from *www.cdc.gov/hepatitis/hcv/index.htm.*
5. Barr R: Shear wave liver elastography, *Abdom Radiol* 43:800, 2018.
*6. American Association for the Study of Liver Diseases: Recommendations for testing, managing, and treating hepatitis C—United States. Retrieved from *www.hcvguidelines.org/full-report/initial-treatment-hcv-infection.*
*7. Terrault N, Lok A, McMahon B, et al: Update on prevention, diagnosis, and treatment of chronic hepatitis B: AASLD 2018 hepatitis B guidance, *Hepatology* 67:4, 2018.
8. Liberal R, de Boer YS, Andrade RJ, et al: Expert clinical management of autoimmune hepatitis in the real world, *Aliment Pharmacol Ther* 45:723, 2017.
9. Kathawala M, Hirschfield GM: Insights into the management of Wilson's disease, *Therap Adv Gastroenterol* 10:889, 2017.
10. Lazaridis N, Tsochatzis E: Current and future treatment options in non-alcoholic steatohepatitis, *Expert Rev Gastroenterol Hepatol* 11:4 357, 2017.
*11. Garcia-Tsao G: Current management of the complications of cirrhosis and portal hypertension: Variceal hemorrhage, ascites, and spontaneous bacterial peritonitis, *Dig Dis* 34:382, 2016.
12. Tsochatzis E, Gerbes A: Hepatology snapshot: Diagnosis and treatment of ascites, *J Hepatol* 67:184, 2017.
*13. Heimbach J, Kulik L, Finn R, et al: AASLD guidelines for the treatment of hepatocellular carcinoma, *Hepatology* 67:358, 2018.
*14. Crockett S, Wani S, Gardner T, et al: American Gastroenterological Association Institute guideline on initial management of acute pancreatitis, *Gastroenterol* 154: 1096, 2018.
15. Munoz A, Chakravarthy D, Gong J, et al: Pancreatic cancer: Current status and challenges, *Curr Pharm Rep* 3:396, 2017.
*16. Doshi B, Yasuda I, Ryozawa S, et al: Current endoscopic strategies for managing large bile duct stones, *Dig Endosc* 30:59, 2018.
17. Rahman R, Simoes E, Schmaltz C, et al: Trend analysis and survival of primary gallbladder cancer in the United States: A 1973–2009 population-based study, *Cancer Med* 6:874, 2017.

CASE STUDY
Managing Care of Multiple Patients

You are working on the medical-surgical unit and have been assigned to care for the following 5 patients. You have 1 LPN and 1 UAP who are assigned to help you.

Patients

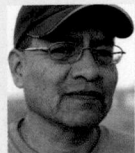

(© iStockphoto/ Thinkstock.)

L.C. is a 58-yr-old Native American man admitted from the ED with acute abdominal pain. A CT scan and colonoscopy showed 2 medium-sized tumors in the transverse colon. A hemicolectomy was done 4 days ago. The adenocarcinoma had spread to the muscle of the colon wall, and there were 2 positive lymph nodes. He is scheduled to be discharged today.

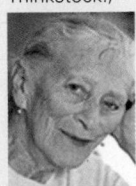

(© iStockphoto/ Thinkstock.)

M.S. is a 70-yr-old white woman who was recently admitted to the unit with generalized weakness and malnutrition. She is 5 ft, 4 in tall and weighs 100 lb, with a 30-lb weight loss in past 2 months. Her medical history includes a recent thrombotic stroke with hemiparesis and dysphagia. She has had nothing by mouth for the past 24 hours and just started EN via PEG tube.

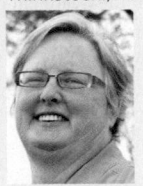

(© Christa Brunt/ iStock/ Thinkstock.)

S.R. is a 48-yr-old white woman admitted with hip pain. She has a history of type 2 diabetes, hypertension, and osteoarthritis. She is 5 ft, 6 in tall and weighs 230 lb. Her most recent BP was 160/110 mm Hg. Her morning laboratory results reveal high fasting blood glucose, total cholesterol, LDL cholesterol, and triglycerides. Her HDL cholesterol is low. Her cardiac enzymes and ECG are all within normal limits. She is scheduled to have a cardiac stress test at 10 AM.

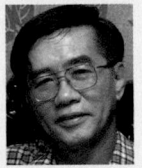

(© iStockphoto/ Thinkstock.)

F.H., a 40-yr-old male immigrant from Vietnam, has a 1-yr history of epigastric distress. He had an upper endoscopy a few weeks ago, which revealed a duodenal ulcer and *H. pylori*. He was started on omeprazole, clarithromycin, and amoxicillin for 10 days. He came to the ED yesterday with severe epigastric pain and melena. His Hgb is 8.2 g/dL and Hct is 26%. He was admitted and put on a pantoprazole (Protonix) continuous infusion and is scheduled for a repeat EGD today.

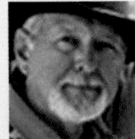

(© sbeagle/ iStock/ Thinkstock.)

M.B. is a 58-yr-old man admitted with a diagnosis of upper GI bleeding. He has been vomiting for 2 days and noticed blood in the toilet when he vomits. He has had cirrhosis for 12 yr and admits to drinking heavily for 20 yr but has been sober for the past 2 yr. He currently reports anorexia, nausea, and abdominal discomfort. He has moderate ascites, jaundice of sclera and skin, 4+ pitting edema of the lower extremities, and palpable liver and spleen. His bilirubin and liver enzymes are all high. His platelet and RBC counts are low.

Discussion Questions

1. *Priority Decision:* After receiving report, which patient should you see first? Provide a rationale for your decision.

2. *Collaboration:* Which tasks could you delegate to the LPN? *(select all that apply)*
   a. Administer a bolus enteral tube feeding to M.S.
   b. Assess L.C.'s dressing, pain level, and bowel sounds.
   c. Administer a scheduled dose of oral lactulose solution to M.B.
   d. Because she speaks Vietnamese, teach F.H.'s wife about his disease.
   e. Perform bedside glucometer reading and administer oral medications to S.R.

3. *Priority Decision:* Which diagnostic finding should you report to the health care provider immediately?
   a. Hemoglobin 7.9 g/dL and hematocrit 25% for F.H.
   b. Serum albumin 2.7 g/dL and prealbumin 11.2 g/dL for M.S.
   c. Cholesterol 250 mg/dL and triglycerides 202 mg/dL for S.R.
   d. Total bilirubin 3.2 mg/dL with positive urine bilirubin for M.B.

4. *Priority Decision:* As you are assessing M.B., the LPN informs you that F.H. just vomited a large amount of bright red blood. What initial action would be *most* appropriate?
   a. Have the LPN administer an antiemetic to F.H.
   b. Ask the LPN to notify F.H.'s health care provider.
   c. Leave M.B.'s room to perform a focused assessment on F.H.
   d. Ask the UAP to obtain a unit of packed RBCs from the blood bank.

Case Study Progression

When you enter F.H.'s room, he tells you that his pain actually feels somewhat relieved since he vomited. However, you note that his skin is cool and clammy, his BP is 90/54 mm Hg, and his heart rate is 116 bpm. You notify his HCP.

4. Which interventions would you expect the HCP to order for F.H.? *(select all that apply)*
   a. Stat hemoglobin and hematocrit
   b. Emergent endoscopy with band ligation
   c. Discontinue the pantoprazole (Protonix) infusion
   d. Start a second IV site and administer a 500 mL normal saline bolus
   e. Contact HCP and notify operating room that patient is unstable and needs surgery

5. *Priority Decision:* After giving a bolus feeding of enteral nutrition to M.S., it would be *most* important to
   a. assess for gastric residual.
   b. obtain an abdominal x-ray.
   c. keep head of bed elevated 30 to 45 degrees.
   d. record the total amount of fluid administered.

6. Which intervention to treat ascites would you expect the HCP to order for M.B.? *(select all that apply)*
   a. Paracentesis
   b. 2 g sodium diet
   c. Diuretic therapy
   d. 1800 mL/day fluid restriction
   e. Shunt insertion from peritoneum to heart

7. *Management Decision:* As you enter the nurse's station, you overhear derogatory comments made by the UAP to the LPN about S.R.'s weight. Which response would be *most* appropriate?
   a. Report the incident to charge nurse for follow-up.
   b. Talk to the UAP to discuss a possible HIPAA violation.
   c. Talk to S.R. about the impact of UAP's bias on the patient's self-image.
   d. Set up an in-service to teach staff members to recognize obesity as a disease process.

Answers and rationales available at *http://evolve.elsevier.com/Lewis/medsurg*.

44

Assessment: Urinary System

Teresa Turnbull

Wherever there is a human being, there is an opportunity for a kindness.

Seneca

ⓔ http://evolve.elsevier.com/Lewis/medsurg

CONCEPTUAL FOCUS

Elimination   Fluids and Electrolytes

LEARNING OUTCOMES

1. Identify the anatomic location and functions of the kidneys, ureters, bladder, and urethra.
2. Explain the physiologic events involved in the formation and passage of urine from glomerular filtration to voiding.
3. Obtain significant subjective and objective data related to the urinary system from a patient.
4. Link the age-related changes of the urinary system to the differences in assessment findings.
5. Perform a physical assessment of the urinary system using appropriate techniques.
6. Distinguish normal from abnormal findings of a physical assessment of the urinary system.
7. Describe the purpose, significance of results, and nursing responsibilities related to diagnostic studies of the urinary system.
8. Evaluate findings of a urinalysis.

KEY TERMS

costovertebral angle (CVA), p. 1015
creatinine, p. 1018
cystoscopy, Table 44.11, p. 1019

glomerular filtration rate (GFR), p. 1009
glomerulus, p. 1008
nephron, p. 1008

renal biopsy, Table 44.11, p. 1020
urinalysis, p. 1018

Adequate kidney function is essential to health. If a person has complete kidney failure and treatment is not provided, death is inevitable. This chapter discusses the structures and functions, assessment, and diagnostic studies of the urinary system.

STRUCTURES AND FUNCTIONS OF URINARY SYSTEM

The *upper urinary system* consists of 2 kidneys and 2 ureters. The *lower urinary system* consists of a urinary bladder and urethra (Fig. 44.1). Urine is formed in the kidneys, drains through the ureters to be stored in the bladder, and then passes out of the body through the urethra.

Kidneys

The kidneys are the principal organs of the urinary system. The primary functions of the kidneys are to (1) regulate the volume and composition of extracellular fluid (ECF) and (2) excrete waste products from the body. The kidneys also function to control BP, make erythropoietin, activate vitamin D, and regulate acid-base balance.

Macrostructure. The paired kidneys are bean-shaped organs located retroperitoneally (behind the peritoneum) on either side of the vertebral column at about the level of the twelfth thoracic (T12) vertebra to the third lumbar (L3) vertebra. Each kidney weighs 4 to 6 oz (113 to 170 g) and is about 5 in (12.5 cm) long. The right kidney, positioned at the level of the twelfth rib, is lower than the left. An adrenal gland lies on top of each kidney.

Each kidney is surrounded by a considerable amount of fat and connective tissue that cushions, supports, and helps the kidney maintain its position. A thin, smooth layer of fibrous membrane called the *capsule* covers the surface of each kidney. The capsule protects the kidney and serves as a shock absorber if this area is traumatized from a sudden force or strike. The

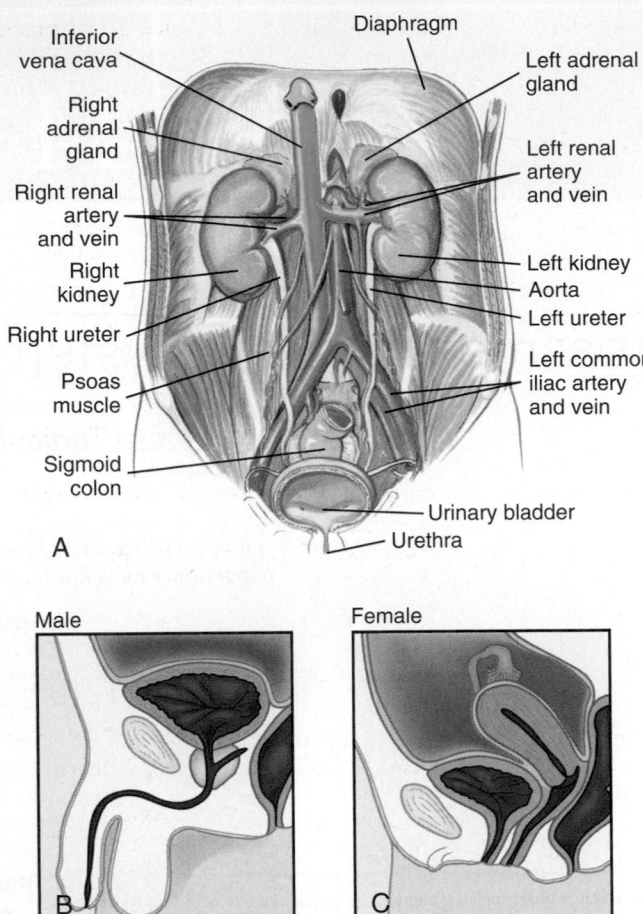

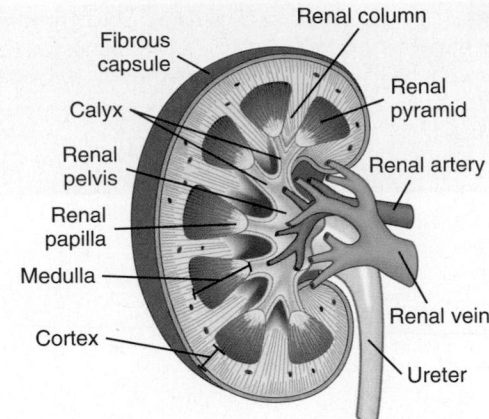

FIG. 44.2 Longitudinal section of the kidney.

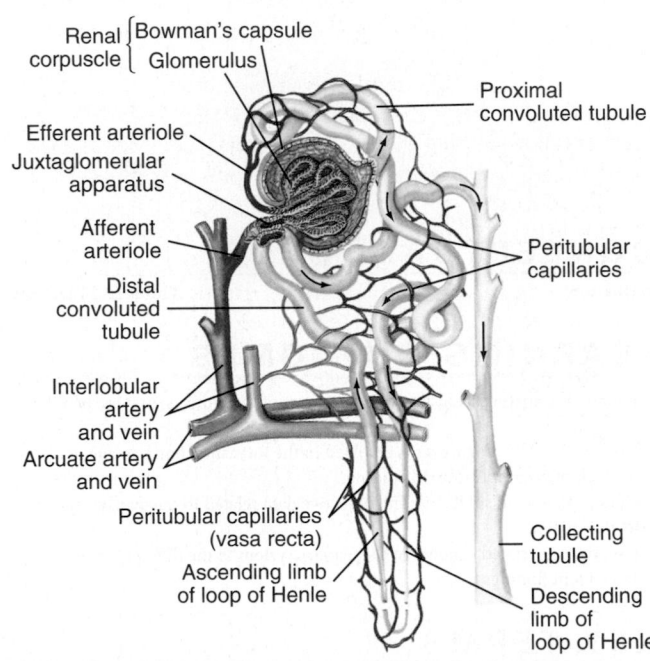

FIG. 44.1 Organs of the urinary system. **A,** Upper urinary tract in relation to other anatomic structures. **B,** Male urethra in relation to other pelvic structures. **C,** Female urethra.

FIG. 44.3 The nephron is the basic functional unit of the kidney. This illustration of a single nephron unit shows the surrounding blood vessels. (Modified from Thibodeau GA, Patton KT: *The human body in health and disease,* ed 4, St Louis, 2005, Mosby.)

hilus on the medial side of the kidney serves as the entry site for the renal artery and nerves and as the exit site for the renal vein and ureter.

The *parenchyma* is the actual tissue of the kidney (Fig. 44.2). The outer layer of the parenchyma is the *cortex,* and the inner layer is the *medulla.* The medulla consists of a number of pyramids. The apices (tops) of these pyramids are the *papillae,* through which urine passes to enter the calyces. The minor calyces widen and merge to form major calyces, which form a funnel-shaped sac called the *renal pelvis.* The minor and major calyces transport urine to the renal pelvis, from there it drains through the ureter to the bladder. The renal pelvis can store a small volume of urine (3 to 5 mL).

Microstructure. The nephron is the functional unit of the kidney. Each kidney has around 1 million nephrons. Each nephron is composed of the glomerulus, Bowman's capsule, and a tubular system. The tubular system consists of the proximal convoluted tubule, loop of Henle, distal convoluted tubule, and collecting tubules (Fig. 44.3). The glomerulus, Bowman's capsule, proximal tubule, and distal tubule are in the cortex of the kidney. The loop of Henle and collecting tubules are in the medulla. Several collecting tubules join to form a single collecting duct. The collecting ducts eventually merge into a pyramid that empties via the papilla into a minor calyx.

Blood Supply. Blood flow to the kidneys, around 1200 mL/min, accounts for 20% to 25% of the cardiac output. Blood reaches

the kidneys via the renal artery, which arises from the aorta and enters the kidney through the hilus. The renal artery divides into secondary branches and then into still smaller branches, each of which forms an afferent arteriole. The afferent arteriole divides into a capillary network, the glomerulus, which is a collection of up to 50 capillaries (Fig. 44.3). The capillaries of the glomerulus unite in the efferent arteriole. This efferent arteriole splits to form a capillary network, the peritubular capillaries, which surround the tubular system. All peritubular capillaries drain into the venous system. The renal vein empties into the inferior vena cava.

Physiology of Urine Formation. Urine formation is the outcome of a complex, multistep process of filtration, reabsorption, secretion, and excretion of water, electrolytes, and metabolic waste products. Although urine formation is the result of this process, the primary functions of the kidneys are to filter the blood and maintain the body's internal homeostasis.

Glomerular Function. Urine formation begins at the glomerulus, where blood is filtered. The glomerulus is a semipermeable membrane that allows filtration (Fig. 44.3). The hydrostatic pressure of the blood within the glomerular capillaries causes a portion of blood to be filtered across the semipermeable membrane into Bowman's capsule. There, the filtered portion of the blood (glomerular filtrate) begins to pass down to the tubule. Filtration is more rapid in the glomerulus than in ordinary tissue capillaries because the glomerular membrane is porous. The glomerular filtrate is similar in composition to blood except that it lacks blood cells, platelets, and large plasma proteins. Under normal conditions, capillary pores are too small to allow the loss of these large blood components. However, in many kidney diseases, capillary permeability increases, which allows plasma proteins and blood cells to pass into the urine.

The amount of blood filtered each minute by the glomeruli is expressed as the glomerular filtration rate (GFR). The normal GFR is about 125 mL/min. The peritubular capillary network reabsorbs most of the glomerular filtrate before it reaches the end of the collecting duct. Therefore only 1 mL/min (on average) is excreted as urine.

Tubular Function. The tubules and collecting ducts are responsible for the reabsorption of essential materials and excretion of nonessential ones (Table 44.1). They carry out these functions by reabsorption and secretion. *Reabsorption* is the passage of a substance from the lumen of the tubules through the tubule cells and into the capillaries. This process involves both active and passive transport mechanisms. Tubular *secretion* is the passage of a substance from the capillaries through the tubular cells into the lumen of the tubule. Reabsorption and secretion cause many changes in the composition of the glomerular filtrate as it moves through the entire length of the tubule.

In the proximal convoluted tubule, about 80% of the electrolytes are reabsorbed. Normally, this includes all glucose, amino acids, and small proteins. As reabsorption continues in the loop of Henle, water is conserved, which is important for concentrating the filtrate. The descending loop is permeable to water and moderately permeable to sodium, urea, and other solutes. In the ascending limb, chloride ions (Cl^-) are actively reabsorbed, followed by passive reabsorption of sodium ions (Na^+). About 25% of the filtered sodium is reabsorbed in the ascending limb.

Two important functions of the distal convoluted tubules are final regulation of water balance and acid-base balance. Antidiuretic hormone (ADH) is needed for water reabsorption in the kidney and is important in water balance. ADH makes the distal convoluted tubules and collecting ducts permeable to water. This allows water to be reabsorbed into the peritubular capillaries and eventually returned to the circulation.

Osmoreceptors in the anterior hypothalamus detect decreases in plasma osmolality. These osmoreceptors send neural input to *superoptic nuclei cells* in the hypothalamus. These superoptic nuclei cells have neuronal axons that end in the posterior pituitary gland and act to inhibit secretion of ADH. In the absence of ADH, the tubules are essentially impermeable to water. Thus any water in the tubules leaves the body as urine.

Aldosterone (released from the adrenal cortex) acts on the distal tubule to cause reabsorption of Na^+ and water. In exchange for Na^+, potassium ions (K^+) are excreted. The secretion of aldosterone is influenced by both circulating blood volume and plasma concentrations of Na^+ and K^+.

Acid-base regulation involves reabsorbing and conserving most of the bicarbonate (HCO_3^-) and secreting excess hydrogen ions (H^+). The distal tubule has different ways to keep the pH of ECF within a range of 7.35 to 7.45 (see Chapter 16).

Myocyte cells in the right atrium secrete a hormone, atrial natriuretic peptide (ANP), in response to atrial distention from an increase in plasma volume. ANP acts on the kidneys to increase sodium excretion. At the same time, ANP inhibits renin, ADH, and the action of angiotensin II on the adrenal glands, thereby suppressing aldosterone secretion. These combined effects of ANP result in the production of a large volume of dilute urine. ANP also causes relaxation of the afferent arteriole, thus increasing the GFR.

The renal tubules are also involved in calcium balance. The parathyroid gland releases parathyroid hormone (PTH) in response to low serum calcium levels. PTH maintains serum calcium levels by causing increased tubular reabsorption of calcium ions (Ca^{2+}) and decreased tubular reabsorption of phosphate ions (PO_4^{2-}). In kidney disease the effects of PTH may have a major effect on bone metabolism.

Vitamin D is a hormone that we obtain in the diet or synthesize by the action of ultraviolet radiation on cholesterol in the skin. These forms of vitamin D are inactive and go through 2 more steps to become metabolically active. The first step occurs in the liver; the second step occurs in the kidneys. Active vitamin D is essential for the absorption of calcium from the gastrointestinal (GI) tract. The patient with kidney failure (also called *renal failure*) will have a deficiency of the active metabolite of vitamin D and problems with calcium and phosphate balance (see Chapter 47).

In summary, the basic function of nephrons is to cleanse blood plasma of unnecessary substances. After the glomerulus has filtered the blood, the tubules select the unwanted from the wanted portions of tubular fluid. Essential constituents are returned to the blood, and dispensable substances pass into urine.

Other Functions of Kidneys. The kidneys participate in red blood cell (RBC) production and BP regulation. Erythropoietin is a hormone made in the kidneys and secreted in response to hypoxia and decreased renal blood flow. Erythropoietin stimulates RBC production in the bone marrow. A deficiency of erythropoietin occurs in kidney failure, leading to anemia.

Renin is important in the regulation of BP. Renin is made and secreted by the kidney's juxtaglomerular cells (Fig. 44.4). Renin is released into the bloodstream in response to decreased renal perfusion, decreased arterial BP, decreased ECF, decreased serum Na^+ concentration, and increased urinary

TABLE 44.1 Functions of Nephron Segments

Segment	Function
Glomerulus	Selective filtration
Proximal tubule	Reabsorption of 80% of electrolytes and water, glucose, amino acids, HCO_3^- Secretion of H^+ and creatinine
Loop of Henle	Concentration of filtrate Reabsorption of Na^+ and Cl^- in ascending limb and water in descending loop
Distal tubule	Reabsorption of water (regulated by ADH) and HCO_3^- Regulation of Ca^{2+} and PO_4^{2-} by parathyroid hormone Regulation of Na^+ and K^+ by aldosterone Secretion of K^+, H^+, ammonia
Collecting duct	Reabsorption of water (requires ADH)

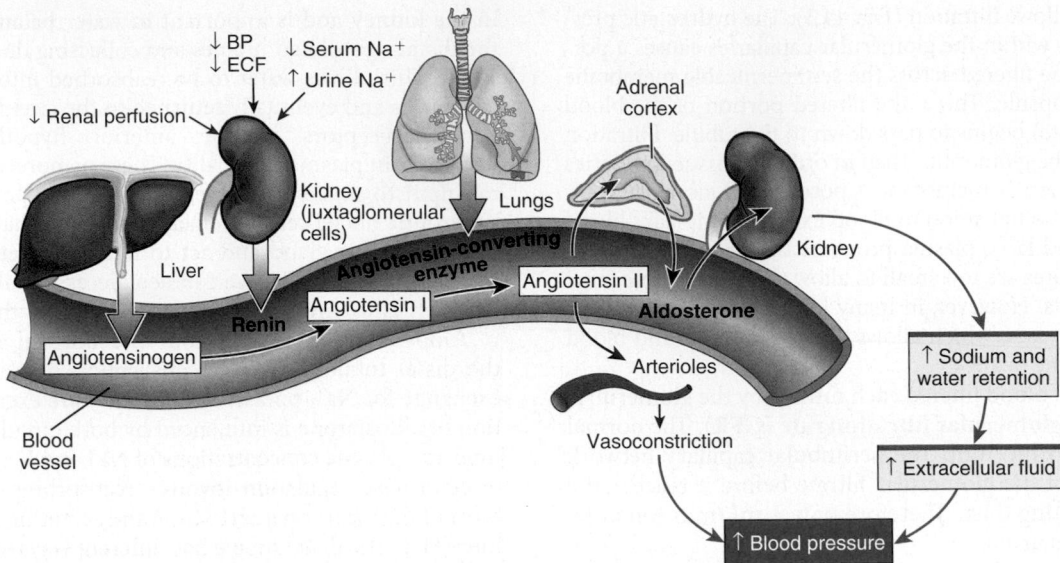

FIG. 44.4 Renin-angiotensin-aldosterone system. (Modified from Herlihy B, Maebius N: *The human body in health and disease,* ed 4, Philadelphia, 2011, Saunders.)

Na⁺ concentration. The plasma protein angiotensinogen (from the liver) is activated to angiotensin I by renin. Angiotensin I is then converted to angiotensin II by angiotensin-converting enzyme (ACE). ACE is found on the inner surface of all blood vessels, with especially high levels in the vessels of the lungs. Angiotensin II stimulates the release of aldosterone from the adrenal cortex. This causes Na⁺ and water retention, leading to increased ECF volume. Angiotensin II also causes increased peripheral vasoconstriction. An elevated BP inhibits renin release. Excessive renin production caused by impaired renal perfusion may be a contributing factor in causing hypertension (see Chapter 32).

Most body tissues synthesize prostaglandins (PGs) from the precursor arachidonic acid in response to appropriate stimuli. (See Chapter 11 and Fig. 11.2 for a more detailed discussion of PGs.) In the kidney, PG synthesis (mainly PGE_2 and PGI_2) occurs primarily in the medulla. These PGs have a vasodilating action, thus increasing renal blood flow and promoting Na⁺ excretion. They counteract the vasoconstrictive effect of substances such as angiotensin and norepinephrine. Renal PGs may have a systemic effect in lowering BP by decreasing systemic vascular resistance. The significance of renal PGs is related to the kidneys' role in causing hypertension. In renal failure with a loss of functioning tissue, these renal vasodilator factors are also lost, which may contribute to hypertension (see Chapter 46).

Ureters

The ureters are tubes that carry urine from the renal pelvis to the bladder (Fig. 44.1). Each ureter is about 10 to 12 inches (25 to 30.5 cm) long and 0.08 to 0.3 inches (0.2 to 0.8 cm) in diameter. Arranged in a meshlike outer layer, circular and longitudinal smooth muscle fibers contract to promote the peristaltic, 1-way flow of urine through the ureters. Distention, neurologic and endocrine influences, and drugs can affect these muscle contractions.

The narrow area where each ureter joins the renal pelvis is the *ureteropelvic junction* (UPJ). Subsequently, the ureters insert into either side of the bladder base at the *ureterovesical junctions*

(UVJs). Because the ureteral lumens are narrowest at these junctions, the UPJ and UVJ are often sites of obstruction. The narrow ureteral lumens can be easily obstructed internally (e.g., urinary stones) or externally (e.g., tumors, adhesions, inflammation). Sympathetic and parasympathetic nerves, along with the vascular supply, surround the mucosal lining of the ureters. Stimulation of these nerves during passage of a stone may cause acute, severe pain, termed *renal colic.*

Because the renal pelvis holds only 3 to 5 mL of urine, kidney damage can result from a backflow of more than that amount of urine. The UVJ relies on the ureter's angle of bladder insertion and muscle fiber attachments with the bladder to prevent the backflow *(reflux)* of urine, which predisposes a person to an ascending infection. The distal ureter enters the bladder laterally at its base, courses along obliquely through the bladder wall for about 1.5 cm and intermingles with muscle fibers of the bladder base. Circular and longitudinal bladder muscle fibers adjacent to the imbedded ureter help secure it. When bladder pressure rises (e.g., during voiding or coughing), muscle fibers that the ureter shares with the bladder base contract first, promoting ureteral lumen closure. Next, the bladder contracts against its base, ensuring UVJ closure and prevention of urine reflux through the junction.

Bladder

The urinary bladder is located behind the symphysis pubis and anterior to the vagina and rectum (Fig. 44.5). Its primary functions are to serve as a reservoir for urine and to eliminate waste products from the body. Like the stomach, the bladder is a stretchable, saclike organ that contracts when it is empty.

The *trigone* is the triangular area formed by the 2 ureteral openings and bladder neck at the base of the bladder. The trigone is attached to the pelvis by many ligaments and does not change its shape during bladder filling or emptying. The bladder muscle *(detrusor)* is composed of layers of intertwined smooth muscle fibers. These fibers are capable of considerable distention during bladder filling and contraction during emptying. It is attached to the abdominal wall by an umbilical ligament, the *urachus.* Because of this attachment, as the bladder fills it rises

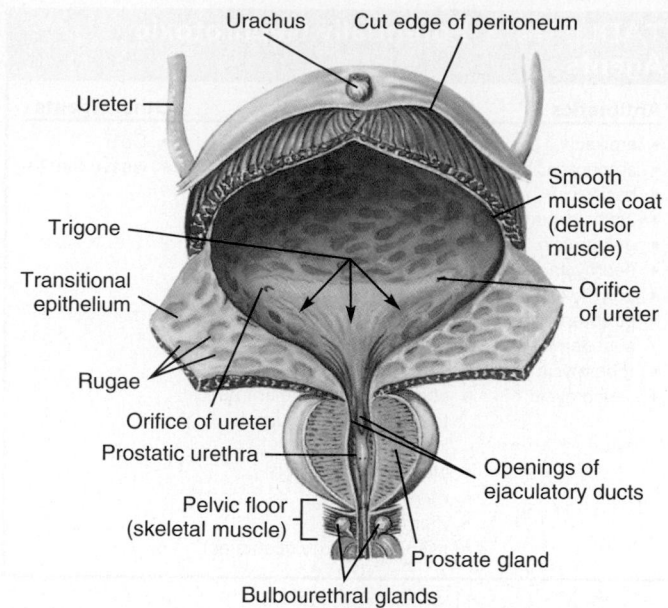

FIG. 44.5 Male urinary bladder. (Modified from Thibodeau GA, Patton KT: *Anatomy and physiology*, ed 6, St Louis, 2007, Mosby.)

toward the umbilicus. The dome and the anterior and lateral aspects of the bladder expand and contract.

Normal adult urine output is around 1500 mL/day, which varies with food and fluid intake. The volume of urine at night is less than half of that formed during the day because of hormonal influences (e.g., ADH). This diurnal pattern of urination is normal. Typically, a person will urinate 5 or 6 times during the day and occasionally at night.

On average, 200 to 250 mL of urine in the bladder cause moderate distention and the urge to urinate. When the quantity of urine reaches 400 to 600 mL, the person feels uncomfortable. Bladder capacity varies with the person, but generally ranges from 600 to 1000 mL. Evacuation of urine is termed *urination, micturition,* or *voiding.*

The bladder has the same mucosal lining as that of the renal pelvises, ureters, and bladder neck. The bladder is lined by transitional cell epithelium referred to as the *urothelium.* Unique to the urinary tract, the urothelium is resistant to absorption of urine. This means that after waste products (made by the kidneys) have left the kidneys, they cannot be reabsorbed in the urinary system. Microscopically, urothelium is only several cells deep. However, as urine enters the bladder, these cells can stretch to accommodate filling. As the bladder empties, the urothelium resumes its multicellular layer formation.

Transitional cell cancers in one section of the urinary tract can easily metastasize to other urinary tract areas given that the mucosal lining throughout the urinary tract is the same. Cancer cells may move down from upper urinary tract cancers and embed in the bladder, or large bladder tumors can invade the ureter. Cancer recurrence within the bladder is common.

Urethra

The urethra is a small tube that incorporates the smooth muscle of the bladder neck and extends to the striated muscle of the external meatus. The urethra's primary functions are to (1) control voiding and (2) serve as a conduit for urine from the bladder to the outside of the body during voiding.

The female urethra is 1 to 2 in (2.5 to 5 cm) long and lies behind the symphysis pubis but anterior to the vagina (Fig. 44.1, *C*). The male urethra, which is about 8 to 10 in (20 to 25 cm) long, starts at the bladder neck and extends the length of the penis (Fig. 44.1, *B*).

Urethrovesical Unit

Together, the bladder, urethra, and pelvic floor muscles form the *urethrovesical unit.* Voluntary control of this unit is defined as *continence.* Stimulating and inhibiting impulses are sent from the brain through the thoracolumbar (T11 to L2) and sacral (S2 to S4) areas of the spinal cord to control voiding. Bladder distention stimulates stretch receptors within the bladder wall. Impulses are transmitted to the sacral spinal cord and then to the brain, causing a desire to urinate.

If you cannot void at a given time, inhibitor impulses in the brain are stimulated and transmitted back through the thoracolumbar and sacral nerves innervating the bladder. In a coordinated fashion, the detrusor muscle accommodates to the pressure (does not contract) while the sphincter and pelvic floor muscles tighten (contract) to resist bladder pressure.

If you can void, cerebral inhibition is voluntarily suppressed. Impulses are transmitted via the spinal cord for the bladder neck, sphincter, and pelvic floor muscles to relax and for the bladder to contract. The sphincter closes, and the detrusor muscle relaxes when the bladder is empty.

Any disease or trauma that affects the function of the brain, spinal cord, or nerves that directly innervate the bladder, bladder neck, external sphincter, or pelvic floor can affect bladder function. These conditions include diabetes, multiple sclerosis, paraplegia, and tetraplegia (quadriplegia). Drugs affecting nerve transmission can affect bladder function.

Gerontologic Considerations: Effects of Aging on Urinary System

Anatomic changes in the aging kidney include a 20% to 30% decrease in size and weight between ages 30 and 90 years. By the seventh decade of life, 50% of glomeruli have lost their function.[1] Atherosclerosis accelerates the decrease of renal size with age.

Physiologic changes in the aging kidney include decreased renal blood flow, due in part to atherosclerosis, resulting in a decreased GFR. Changes in hormone levels (including ADH, aldosterone, ANP) result in decreased urinary concentrating ability and changes in the excretion of water, sodium, potassium, and acid. Despite these changes, older adults maintain homeostasis unless they encounter diseases or other physiologic stressors. After abrupt changes in blood volume, acid load, or other insults, the kidney may not be able to function effectively because much of its renal reserve has been lost.[1]

Physiologic changes occur in the aging urethra and bladder. The female urethra, bladder, vagina, and pelvic floor undergo a loss of elasticity and muscle support. Consequently, older women are more prone to bladder infections and incontinence. The prostate surrounds the proximal urethra. As men age, the prostate enlarges and may affect urinary patterns, causing hesitancy, retention, slow stream, and bladder infections.

Constipation, often experienced by older adults, can affect urination. Partial urethral obstruction may occur because of the rectum's close proximity to the urethra. Age-related changes in the urinary system and differences in assessment findings are outlined in Table 44.2.

TABLE 44.2 Gerontologic Assessment Differences

Urinary System

Gerontologic Changes	Differences in Assessment Findings
Kidney	
• ↓ Amount of renal tissue	• Less palpable
• ↓ Number of nephrons and renal blood vessels. Thickened basement membrane of Bowman's capsule and glomeruli	• ↓ Creatinine clearance, ↑ BUN level, ↑ serum creatinine
• ↓ Function of loop of Henle and tubules	• Changes in drug excretion, nocturia, loss of normal diurnal excretory pattern because of ↓ ability to concentrate urine; less concentrated urine
Ureter, Bladder, and Urethra	
• ↓ Elasticity and muscle tone	• Palpable bladder after urination because of retention
• Weakening of urinary sphincter	• Stress incontinence (especially during Valsalva maneuver), dribbling of urine after urination
• ↓ Bladder capacity and sensory receptors	• Frequency, urgency, nocturia, overflow incontinence
• Estrogen deficiency leading to thin, dry vaginal tissue	• Stress or overactive bladder, dysuria
• ↑ Prevalence of unstable bladder contractions	• Overactive bladder
• Prostatic enlargement	• Hesitancy, frequency, urgency, nocturia, straining to urinate, retention, dribbling

TABLE 44.3 Potentially Nephrotoxic Agents

Antibiotics	Other Drugs	Other Agents
• amikacin	• captopril	• Gold
• amphotericin B	• cimetidine	• Heavy metals
• bacitracin	• cisplatin	
• cephalosporins	• cocaine	
• gentamicin	• cyclosporine	
• neomycin	• ethylene glycol	
• polymyxin B	• heroin	
• streptomycin	• lithium	
• sulfonamides	• methotrexate	
• tobramycin	• nitrosoureas (e.g., carmustine)	
• vancomycin	• nonsteroidal antiinflammatory drugs (e.g., ibuprofen, indomethacin)	
	• phenacetin	
	• quinine	
	• rifampin	
	• salicylates (large quantities)	

ASSESSMENT OF URINARY SYSTEM

Subjective Data

Important Health Information

Past Health History. Ask the patient about the presence or history of kidney disease or other urologic problems. Note specific urinary problems, such as cancer, infections, benign prostatic hyperplasia (BPH), and stones. Ask about other health problems that may affect kidney function, including hypertension, diabetes, gout, connective tissue disorders (e.g., systemic lupus erythematosus), hepatitis, human immunodeficiency virus (HIV) infection, neurologic conditions (e.g., stroke, back injury), and trauma.[2]

Medications. An assessment of the patient's current and past use of medications is important. Include over-the-counter drugs, prescription drugs, and herbal therapies. Drugs affect the urinary tract in several ways. Many drugs can be nephrotoxic (Table 44.3). Certain drugs may alter the quantity and character of urine output (e.g., diuretics). Several drugs change the color of urine. Phenazopyridine (Pyridium) turns urine orange. Nitrofurantoin (Macrodantin) turns urine dark yellow to brown. Anticoagulants may cause hematuria. Many antidepressants, calcium channel blockers, antihistamines, and drugs used for neurologic and musculoskeletal disorders affect the ability of the bladder or sphincter to contract or relax normally.

Surgery or Other Treatments. Ask the patient about hospitalizations related to renal or urologic diseases and all urinary problems during past pregnancies. Inquire about the duration, severity, and patient's perception of any problem and its treatment. Document past surgeries, especially pelvic surgeries, and urinary tract instrumentation (e.g., catheterization). Ask the patient about any radiation or chemotherapy treatment for cancer.

Functional Health Patterns. Key questions to ask a patient with problems related to the renal system are listed in Table 44.4.

Health Perception–Health Management Pattern. Ask about the patient's general health. Abnormal kidney function may be suspected if the patient reports changes in weight or appetite, excess thirst, fluid retention, headache, pruritus, blurred vision, or "feeling tired all the time." An older adult may report malaise and nonlocalized abdominal discomfort as the only symptoms of a urinary tract infection (UTI). In older adults with a UTI, family members may report the patient is disoriented, has fallen, or has increased confusion.

Obtain a smoking history. Cigarette smoking is a major risk factor for bladder and kidney cancer. Smokers who also work with cancer-causing chemicals have an especially high risk for bladder cancer.

CASE STUDY

Patient Introduction

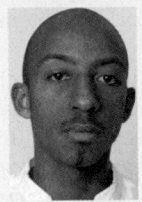

(© iStockphoto/Thinkstock.)

A.K. is a 28-yr-old black man who comes to the emergency department (ED) in acute distress with severe abdominal pain. The pain began about 6 hours ago after he finished a 10-mile run as part of his training for a marathon. He says that the pain has steadily increased and he is nauseous. His urine is a dark, smoky color.

Discussion Questions

1. What are the possible causes of A.K.'s abdominal pain, nausea, and urine color?
2. What type of assessment would be most appropriate for A.K.: comprehensive, focused, or emergency? On what basis did you make that decision?
3. What assessment questions will you ask him?

You will learn more about A.K. and his condition as you read through this assessment chapter.

(See p. 1015 for more information on A.K.)

Answers available at *http://evolve.elsevier.com/Lewis/medsurg*.

TABLE 44.4 Health History

Urinary System

Health Perception–Health Management
- How is your energy level compared with 1 yr ago?
- Do you notice any visual changes?*
- Have you ever smoked? If yes, how many packs per day?
- Tell me about the types of jobs you have had.

Nutritional-Metabolic
- How is your appetite?
- Has your weight changed over the past year?*
- Do you take vitamins, herbs, or any other supplements?*
- How much and what kinds of fluids do you drink daily?
- How many dairy products and how much meat do you eat?
- Do you drink coffee? Colas? Tea?
- Do you spice your food heavily?*

Elimination
- Are you able to sit through a 2-hr meeting or ride in a car for 2 hr without urinating?
- Do you awaken at night with the desire to urinate? If so, how many times does this occur during an average night?
- Do you ever notice blood in your urine?* If so, at what point in the urination does it occur?
- Have you noticed any change in the color or smell of your urine?*
- Do you ever pass urine when you do not intend to? When?
- Do you use special devices or supplies for urine elimination or control?*
- How often do you move your bowels?
- Do you ever have constipation or diarrhea?*
- Do you ever have problems controlling your bowels?*

Activity-Exercise
- Have you noticed any changes in your ability to perform your usual daily activities?*
- Do certain activities worsen your urinary problem?*
- Has your urinary problem caused you to alter or stop any activity or exercise?*
- Do you need help moving or getting to the bathroom?*

Sleep-Rest
- Do you awaken at night from an urge to urinate?* How does this disturb your sleep?
- Do you awaken at night from pain or other problems and urinate as a matter of routine before returning to sleep?*
- Do you have daytime sleepiness and fatigue because of nighttime urination?*

Cognitive-Perceptual
- Do you ever have pain when you urinate?* If so, where is the pain?

Self-Perception–Self-Concept
- How does your urinary problem make you feel about yourself?
- Do you perceive your body differently since you have developed a urinary problem?

Role-Relationship
- Does your urinary problem interfere with your relationships with family or friends?*
- Has your urinary problem caused a change in your job status or affected your ability to carry out job-related responsibilities?*

Sexuality-Reproductive
- Has your urinary problem caused any change in your sexual pleasure or performance?*
- Do hygiene concerns interfere with sexual activities?

Coping–Stress Tolerance
- Do you feel able to manage the problems associated with your urinary problem? If not, explain.
- What strategies are you using to cope with your urinary problem?

Values-Beliefs
- Has your present illness affected your belief system?*
- Are your treatment decisions related to your urinary problem in conflict with your value system?*

*If yes, describe.

Exposure to certain chemicals can affect the urinary system. Aromatic amines and some organic chemicals increase the risk for bladder cancer. Phenol and ethylene glycol are examples of nephrotoxic chemicals. Obtain an occupational history. Machinists, painters, hairdressers, printers, and truck drivers have an increased incidence of bladder cancer.[3]

Information about places where a patient has lived is important. Persons living in the Southeast part of the United States have the highest incidence of urinary stones. This may be caused by the higher mineral content of the soil and water.[4] A person living in Middle Eastern countries or Africa can acquire certain parasites that can cause cystitis or bladder cancer.

GENETIC RISK ALERT

- Polycystic kidney disease and congenital urinary tract abnormalities (e.g., Alport syndrome [congenital nephritis]) are genetic disorders.
- A family history of certain renal or urologic problems increases the chance of similar problems occurring in the patient.
- For any disease reported in the health history, ask if other family members also have/had the same or similar diseases.

Nutritional-Metabolic Pattern. The usual quantity and types of fluid a patient drinks are important in relation to urinary tract disease. Dehydration may contribute to UTIs, stone formation, and kidney failure. Large intake of specific foods, such as dairy products or foods high in proteins, may lead to stone formation. Asparagus may cause the urine to smell musty. Red urine caused by beet ingestion may be mistaken for bloody urine. Caffeine, alcohol, carbonated beverages, some artificial sweeteners, or spicy foods often worsen urinary inflammatory diseases. Green tea and some herbal teas cause diuresis. An unexplained weight gain may be the result of fluid retention from a kidney problem. Anorexia, nausea, and vomiting can dramatically affect fluid status and require careful monitoring.

Elimination Pattern. Questions about urine elimination patterns are the cornerstone of the health history in the patient with a lower urinary tract disorder. Begin with asking how the patient manages urine elimination. Ask about daytime (diurnal) voiding frequency and the frequency of nocturia. Pelvic organ prolapses, particularly advanced anterior vaginal prolapse, may cause suprapubic pressure, frequency, urgency, and incontinence from urinary retention. Ask about other bothersome lower urinary tract symptoms, including urgency, incontinence, or urinary retention. Table 44.5 lists some common manifestations of urinary tract disorders.

TABLE 44.5 Manifestations of Urinary System Disorders

| General Manifestations | SPECIFIC MANIFESTATIONS RELATED TO URINARY SYSTEM | | | | |
	Edema	Pain	Patterns of Urination	Urine Output	Urine Composition
• Anorexia • Blurred vision • Change in weight • Chills • Cognitive changes • Excessive thirst • Fatigue • Headaches • High BP • Nausea and vomiting	• Ankle • Ascites • Facial (periorbital) • Generalized edema • Sacral	• Dysuria • Flank or costovertebral angle • Groin • Suprapubic	• Change in stream • Dribbling • Dysuria • Frequency • Hesitancy of stream • Incontinence • Nocturia • Retention • Stress incontinence • Urgency	• Anuria • Oliguria • Polyuria	• Color (red, brown, yellowish green) • Concentrated • Dilute • Hematuria • Pyuria

Changes in the color and appearance of urine are often significant and need evaluated. If blood is visible in the urine, determine if it occurs at the beginning of, throughout, or at the end of urination. This is harder for the female patient.

Assess bowel function. Problems with fecal incontinence may signal neurologic causes for bladder problems because of shared nerve pathways. Constipation and fecal impaction can partially obstruct the urethra, causing inadequate bladder emptying, overflow incontinence, and infection.

Determine the patient's method of managing a urinary problem. A patient may already be using a catheter or collection device. Sometimes a patient must assume a specific position to urinate or perform maneuvers, such as pressing on the lower abdomen (Credé's method) or straining (Valsalva maneuver), to empty the bladder.

Activity-Exercise Pattern. Assess the patient's level of activity. A sedentary person is more likely to have stasis of urine than an active person and thus be predisposed to infection and stones. Demineralization of bones in a person with limited physical activity can cause increased urine calcium precipitation.

An active person may find that increasing activity worsens the urinary problem. The patient who has had prostate surgery or who has weakened pelvic floor muscles may leak urine when trying certain activities, such as running. Some men develop chronic inflammatory prostatitis or epididymitis after heavy lifting or long-distance driving.

Sleep-Rest Pattern. Nocturia is a common and a particularly bothersome symptom that often leads to sleep deprivation, daytime sleepiness, and fatigue. It occurs in multiple problems affecting the lower urinary tract, including urinary incontinence, urinary retention, and interstitial cystitis. Nocturia may be related to polyuria from kidney disease, poorly controlled diabetes, alcohol use, excess fluid intake, liver disease, heart failure, or obstructive sleep apnea.

When assessing nocturia, determine whether the need to urinate causes the person to arise from sleep or whether pain or other symptoms interrupt sleep. Ask if the person urinates as a matter of habit before returning to bed. Up to 1 episode of nocturia is considered normal in younger adults, and up to 2 episodes are acceptable in adults ages 65 years or older. If an older adult has more than 2 episodes during the night, assess the amount and timing of fluid intake. This information will help determine whether further investigation is needed.

Cognitive-Perceptual Pattern. Assess the level of mobility, visual acuity, and dexterity. These are important factors to evaluate in a patient with urologic problems, especially when urine retention or incontinence is a problem. Determine if the patient is alert, understands instructions, and can recall instructions when needed.

If urinary incontinence is present, ask how the patient is managing the problem. Recognize that incontinence is often distressing and embarrassing. Discuss the problem with the patient with sensitivity in a nonjudgmental manner.

A frequent symptom of renal and urologic problems is pain, including dysuria, groin pain, costovertebral pain, and suprapubic pain. Assess pain and document the location, character, and duration. The absence of pain when other urinary symptoms exist is significant. Many urinary tract cancers are painless in the early stages.

Self-Perception–Self-Concept Pattern. Problems associated with the urinary system, such as incontinence, urinary diversion procedures, and chronic fatigue (may occur with anemia), can result in loss of self-esteem and a negative body image.

Role-Relationship Pattern. Urinary problems can affect many aspects of a person's life, including the ability to work and relationships with others. These factors have important implications for future treatment and management of the patient's condition.

Urinary system problems may be serious enough to cause problems in job-related and social situations. Chronic dialysis therapy often makes regular employment or management of home and family responsibilities difficult. Concurrent poor health and negative body image can seriously affect existing roles.

Sexuality-Reproductive Pattern. Assess the effect of renal problems on the patient's sexual satisfaction. Problems related to personal hygiene and fatigue can negatively affect sexual relationships. Although urinary incontinence is not directly associated with sexual dysfunction, it often has a devastating effect on self-esteem and social and intimate relationships. Counseling both the patient and partner may be needed.

Objective Data
Physical Examination
Inspection. Assess for changes in the following:
- *Skin:* Pallor, yellow-gray cast, excoriations, changes in turgor, bruises, texture (e.g., rough, dry skin) (see Table 22.9 for assessment of dark-skinned persons)
- *Mouth:* Stomatitis, ammonia breath odor
- *Face and extremities:* Generalized edema, peripheral edema
- *Abdomen:* Abdominal contour for midline mass in lower abdomen (may indicate bladder distention and urinary retention) or unilateral mass (sometimes seen in adults, indicating kidney enlargement from large tumor or polycystic kidney)

CASE STUDY—cont'd

Subjective Data

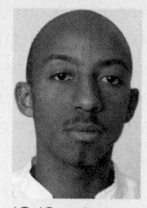

(© iStockphoto/Thinkstock.)

A focused subjective assessment of A.K. revealed the following information:

Past Medical History: History of 1 isolated incidence of gout 6 years ago. He stopped drinking alcohol with no further occurrence. Appendectomy 12 years ago.

Medications: None.

Health Perception–Health Management: A.K. states that he is usually healthy. He does not smoke or drink alcohol. He has never had this type of pain before. Describes the pain as being sharp and colicky (coming in waves). Rates the pain as 9 on a scale of 0 to 10.

Nutritional-Metabolic: A.K. is currently on a high-protein diet as he trains for the marathon. He eats a lot of chicken, beef, and seafood. He drinks milk-based protein shakes and water after exercising but admits that he does not think he drinks enough to replace fluid loss from perspiration. He drinks coffee for energy but denies eating chocolate or other sweets. He avoids sodas.

Elimination: Denies any history of problems with urination, constipation, or diarrhea. This is the first time he has ever noticed a change of color in his urine.

Activity-Exercise: Prides himself on his ability to exercise and run without difficulty.

Sleep-Rest: Does not awaken at night to urinate.

Cognitive-Perceptual: Denies pain on urination.

Self-Perception–Self-Concept: Believes he can monitor himself and maintain a healthy lifestyle.

Coping–Stress Tolerance: Worried that this pain may interfere with his marathon training.

Discussion Questions

1. Which subjective assessment findings are of most concern to you?
2. What would be your priority assessment of A.K.?
3. What should be included in the physical assessment? What would you be looking for?

You will learn more about the physical examination of the urinary system in the next section.

(See p. 1016 for more information on A.K.)

Answers available at *http://evolve.elsevier.com/Lewis/medsurg*.

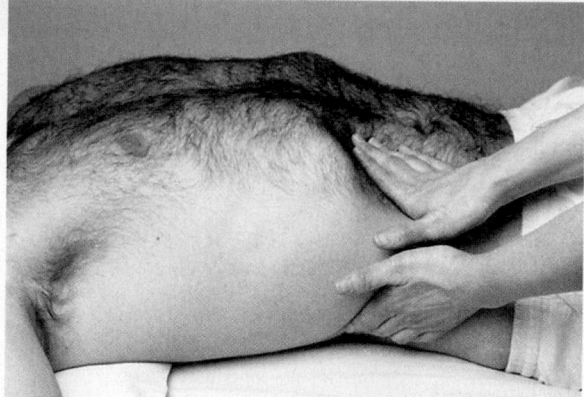

FIG. 44.6 Palpating the right kidney. (From Brundage DJ: *Renal disorders*, St Louis, 1992, Mosby.)

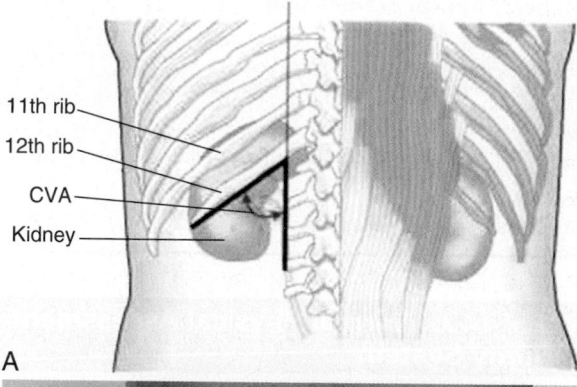

11th rib
12th rib
CVA
Kidney

A

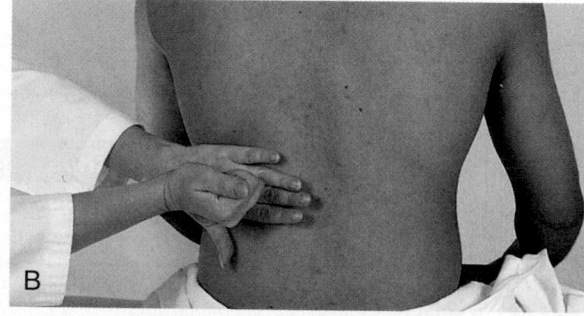

B

FIG. 44.7 **A,** Costovertebral angle. **B,** Indirect fist percussion of the costovertebral angle *(CVA)*. To assess the kidney, place one hand over the twelfth rib at the CVA on the back. Thump that hand with the ulnar edge of the other fist. (From Jarvis C: *Physical examination and health assessment*, ed 7, St Louis, 2016, Saunders.)

- *Weight:* Weight gain from edema. Weight loss and muscle wasting in kidney failure
- *General state of health:* Fatigue, lethargy, and decreased alertness

Palpation. The kidneys are posterior organs protected by the abdominal organs, ribs, and heavy back muscles. A landmark useful in locating the kidneys is the costovertebral angle (CVA) formed by the rib cage and the vertebral column. The normal-sized left kidney is rarely palpable because the spleen lies directly on top of it. Occasionally the lower pole of the right kidney is palpable.

To palpate the right kidney, place your left (anterior) hand behind and support the patient's right side between the rib cage and the iliac crest (Fig. 44.6). Elevate the right flank with the left hand. Use your right hand to palpate deeply for the right kidney. The lower pole of the right kidney may be felt as a smooth, rounded mass that descends on inspiration. If the kidney is palpable, note its size, contour, and tenderness. Kidney enlargement is suggestive of cancer or other serious renal pathologic conditions.

The urinary bladder is normally not palpable unless it is distended with urine. If the bladder is full, it may be felt as a smooth, round, firm organ and is sensitive to palpation.

Percussion. Tenderness in the flank area may be detected by fist percussion *(kidney punch)*. This technique is performed by striking the fist of one hand against the dorsal surface of the other hand, which is placed flat along the posterior CVA margin (Fig. 44.7). Normally this type of percussion should not elicit pain. If CVA tenderness and pain are present, it may indicate a kidney infection or polycystic kidney disease.[5]

A bladder does not percuss until it contains at least 150 mL of urine. If the bladder is full, dullness is heard above the symphysis pubis. A distended bladder may be percussed as high as the umbilicus.

Auscultation. Use the diaphragm of the stethoscope to auscultate bowel sounds, since the bowels can affect the urinary system.

FOCUSED ASSESSMENT
Urinary System

Use this checklist to ensure that the key assessment steps have been done.

Subjective
Ask the patient about any of the following and note responses.

Painful urination	Y	N
Changes in color of urine (blood, cloudy)	Y	N
Change in characteristics of urination (decreased, excessive)	Y	N
Problems with frequent nighttime urination (nocturia)	Y	N

Objective: Diagnostic
Check the following laboratory results for critical values.

Blood urea nitrogen	✓
Serum creatinine	✓
Urinalysis	✓
Urine culture and sensitivity	✓

Objective: Physical Examination
Inspect

Abdomen	✓
Urinary meatus for inflammation or discharge	✓

Palpate

Abdomen for bladder distention, masses, or tenderness	✓

Percuss

Costovertebral angle for tenderness	✓

TABLE 44.6 Normal Physical Assessment of Urinary System

- No costovertebral angle tenderness
- Nonpalpable kidney and bladder
- No palpable masses

Table 44.6 shows how to record the normal physical assessment findings of the urinary system. Table 44.7 describes assessment abnormalities of the urinary system. Assessment findings may vary in the older adult. Table 44.2 presents the age-related changes in the urinary system and differences in assessment findings. Use a *focused assessment* to evaluate the status of previously identified urinary system problems and to monitor for signs of new problems. A focused assessment of the urinary system is outlined in the box on this page.

CASE STUDY—cont'd
Objective Data: Physical Examination

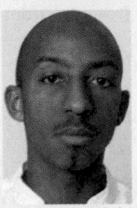

(© iStockphoto/Thinkstock.)

A focused assessment of A.K. reveals the following: A.K. is lying with his knees bent and drawn to his abdominal area. He appears restless and keeps moving from back to side to reduce his discomfort. Vital signs are as follows: BP 156/70, apical pulse 108, respiratory rate 24, temperature 37.4° C, O_2 saturation 96% on room air. Awake, alert, and oriented × 3. Lungs are clear to auscultation. Apical pulse is regular. Abdomen nondistended with + bowel sounds in all 4 quadrants. No rebound tenderness. Positive left costovertebral tenderness. Voiding small amounts of dark, smoky urine.

Discussion Questions
1. Which physical assessment findings are of most concern to you?
2. Based on the results of the subjective and physical assessment findings, what diagnostic studies do you think may be ordered for A.K.?

You will learn more about diagnostic studies related to the urinary system in the next section.

(See p. 1022 for more information on A.K.)

TABLE 44.7 Assessment Abnormalities
Urinary System

Finding	Description	Possible Etiology and Significance
Anuria	Technically no urination (24-hr urine output <100 mL)	Acute kidney injury, end-stage renal disease, bilateral ureteral obstruction
Burning on urination	Stinging pain in urethral area	Urethral irritation, UTI, urethral calculus
Dysuria	Painful or difficult urination	UTI, interstitial cystitis, urethral calculus, and wide variety of pathologic conditions
Enuresis	Involuntary nocturnal urination	Lower urinary tract disorder
Frequency	↑ Incidence of urination	Acutely inflamed bladder, retention with overflow, excess fluid intake, intake of bladder irritants, urethral calculus
Hematuria	Blood in the urine	Cancer of genitourinary tract, blood dyscrasias, kidney disease, UTI, stones in kidney or ureter, anticoagulants
Hesitancy	Delay or difficulty in initiating urination	Partial urethral obstruction, benign prostatic hyperplasia
Incontinence	Inability to voluntarily control discharge of urine	Neurogenic bladder, bladder infection, injury to external sphincter
Nocturia	Frequent urination at night	Kidney disease with impaired concentrating ability, bladder obstruction, heart failure, diabetes, post renal transplant, excess evening and nighttime fluid intake
Oliguria	↓ Amount of urine in a time period (24-hr urine output of 100–400 mL)	Severe dehydration, shock, transfusion reaction, kidney disease, end-stage renal disease
Pain	Suprapubic pain (related to bladder), urethral pain (irritation of bladder neck), flank pain, CVA tenderness	Infection, urinary retention, foreign body in urinary tract, urethritis, pyelonephritis, renal colic, stones
Pneumaturia	Passage of urine containing gas	Fistula connections between bowel and bladder, gas-forming UTI
Polyuria	Large volume of urine in a time period	Diabetes, diabetes insipidus, chronic kidney disease, diuretics, excess fluid intake, obstructive sleep apnea
Retention	Inability to urinate even though bladder contains excess amount of urine	Finding after pelvic surgery, childbirth, catheter removal, anesthesia; urethral stricture or obstruction; neurogenic bladder
Stress incontinence	Involuntary urination with ↑ pressure (sneezing or coughing)	Weakness of sphincter control, lack of estrogen, urinary retention

DIAGNOSTIC STUDIES OF URINARY SYSTEM

Many diagnostic studies are used to assess problems of the urinary system. Tables 44.8, 44.9, 44.10, and 44.11 describe the most common studies. Select studies are described in more detail here.

Many radiologic studies require the use of a bowel preparation the evening before the study to clear the lower GI tract of feces and flatus. Because the kidneys lie in a retroperitoneal location, colon contents can obstruct visualization of the urinary tract. If the bowel preparation does not adequately clear the lower GI tract, the study may be unsuccessful and need rescheduled. Common bowel preparations include enemas, magnesium citrate, and bisacodyl (Dulcolax) tablets or suppositories. Patients with kidney failure should not receive some bowel preparations, such as magnesium citrate and Fleet enema, because the kidneys cannot excrete the magnesium (see Chapter 46).

Iodine-based contrast media used in some diagnostic studies may cause contrast-induced kidney injury (CIN) and allergic reactions. Keeping the patient hydrated is important. Some patients may need IV fluids started hours before the procedure.[6] N-acetylcysteine, a renal vasodilator and antioxidant, is sometimes given to reduce the incidence of CIN. It can be given by oral or IV route.

When a patient has multiple diagnostic studies, it is important to maintain hydration.[6] The patient is at risk for dehydration when they have had nothing by mouth for consecutive days, extended time in the radiology department, and bowel preparations. Severe dehydration, especially in debilitated or older patients and patients with diabetes, may lead to acute kidney injury. Ensure that the patient is properly hydrated and given adequate nourishment between studies. Check with the HCP about insulin dosage for patients with diabetes who are NPO.

TABLE 44.8 Urinalysis

General examination of urine to establish baseline information or provide data to establish a tentative diagnosis and determine whether further studies are needed.
Before: Wash perineal area before collecting specimen.
During: Try to obtain first urinated morning specimen.
After: Ensure specimen is examined within 1 hr of urinating.

Test	Normal	Abnormal Finding	Possible Etiology and Significance
Bilirubin	None	Present	Liver disorders. May appear before jaundice is visible (see Chapter 43)
Casts	None Occasional hyaline	Present	Molds of the renal tubules that may contain protein, WBCs, RBCs, or bacteria. Noncellular casts (hyaline in appearance) occasionally found in normal urine
Color	Amber yellow	Dark, smoky color Yellow-brown to olive green Orange-red or orange-brown Cloudiness of freshly voided urine Colorless urine	Hematuria Excess bilirubin phenazopyridine (Pyridium) UTI Excess fluid intake, kidney disease, or diabetes insipidus
Culture for organisms	No organisms in bladder<10^4 organisms/mL result of normal urethral flora	Bacteria counts >10^5/mL	UTI; most common organisms are *E. coli*, enterococci, *Klebsiella*, *Proteus*, and streptococci
Glucose	None	Glycosuria	Diabetes, low renal threshold for glucose reabsorption (if blood glucose level is normal). Pituitary disorders
Ketones	None	Present	Altered carbohydrate and fat metabolism in diabetes and starvation; dehydration, vomiting, severe diarrhea
Odor	Aromatic	Ammonia-like odor Unpleasant odor	Urine allowed to stand UTI
Osmolality	50–1200 mOsm/kg (50–1200 mmol/kg)	<50 mOsm/kg >1200 mOsm/kg	Tubular dysfunction. Kidney lost ability to concentrate or dilute urine
pH	4.6–8.0 (average, 6.0)	>8.0	UTI. Urine allowed to stand at room temperature (bacteria decompose urea to ammonia)
Protein	Random protein (dipstick): 0–trace 24-hr protein (quantitative): 50–80 mg/day	Persistent proteinuria	Characteristic of acute and chronic kidney disease, especially involving glomeruli. Heart failure. In absence of disease: high-protein diet, strenuous exercise, dehydration, fever, emotional stress, contamination by vaginal secretions
RBCs	0–4/hpf	<4.0 >4/hpf	Respiratory or metabolic acidosis Stones, cystitis, cancer, glomerulonephritis, tuberculosis, kidney biopsy, UTI, trauma
Specific gravity	1.005–1.030 Maximum concentrating ability of kidney in morning urine (1.025–1.030)	Low High Fixed at about 1.010	Dilute urine, excess diuresis, diabetes insipidus Dehydration, albuminuria, glycosuria Renal inability to concentrate urine; end-stage renal disease
WBCs	0–5/hpf	>5/hpf	UTI or inflammation

hpf, High-powered field.

TABLE 44.9 Diagnostic Studies

Urine

Study	Description and Purpose	Nursing Responsibility
Composite urine collection	Measures specific components, such as electrolytes, glucose, protein, 17-ketosteroids, catecholamines, creatinine, and minerals. Composite urine specimens are collected over a period ranging from 2–24 hr.	*During:* Have patient urinate and discard this first urine specimen. Note this time as the start of the test. Save all urine from subsequent urinations in a container for designated period. At end of period, ask patient to urinate, and this urine is added to container. Remind patient to save all urine during study period. Specimens may need refrigerated or preservatives added to container used for collecting urine.
Concentration test	Evaluates renal concentration ability. Measured by specific gravity readings. *Reference interval:* 1.005–1.030.	*Before:* Have patient fast after given time in evening (in usual procedure). *During:* Collect 3 urine specimens at hourly intervals in morning.
Creatinine clearance	Creatinine is a waste product of protein breakdown (primarily body muscle mass). Clearance of creatinine by kidney approximates the GFR. Calculated as follows: $$\text{Creatinine clearance} = \frac{\text{Urine creatinine (mg/dL)} \times \text{Urine volume (mL/min)}}{\text{Serum creatinine (mg/dL)}}$$ Reference interval: *Male:* 107–139 mL/min/1.73 m^2 *Female:* 87–107 mL/min/1.73 m^2 (corrected for body surface area).	*During:* Collect 24-hr urine specimen. Discard first urination when test is started. Save urine from all subsequent urinations for 24 hr. Have patient urinate at end of 24 hr and add specimen to collection. Ensure that serum creatinine is measured during 24-hr period.
Protein determination		
• Dipstick (Albustix, Combistix)	Detects protein (primarily albumin) in urine. *Reference interval:* 0 to trace.	*During:* Dip end of stick in urine and read result by comparison with color chart on label as directed. Grading is from 0 to 4+. Interpret with caution. Positive result may not indicate significant proteinuria. Some drugs may give false-positive readings.
• Quantitative protein test	A 24-hr collection gives a more accurate indication of amount of protein in urine. Persistent proteinuria usually indicates glomerular kidney disease. *Reference interval:* 50–80 mg/day (mainly albumin).	*During:* Perform 24-hr urine collection as above.
Residual urine	Determines amount of urine left in bladder after urinating. Finding may be abnormal in problems with bladder innervation, sphincter impairment, benign prostatic hyperplasia, or urethral strictures. *Reference interval:* ≤50 mL urine (increases with age).	*During:* Immediately after patient urinates, catheterize patient or use bladder ultrasound equipment. If a large amount of residual urine is obtained, HCP may want catheter left in bladder.
Urine culture ("clean catch," "midstream")	Confirms suspected UTI and identifies causative organisms. *Normally,* bladder is sterile, but urethra contains bacteria and a few WBCs. *Reference interval:* If properly collected, stored, and handled: <10^3 organisms/mL usually indicates no infection. 10^3–10^5/mL is usually not diagnostic. Test may need repeated. >10^5/mL indicates infection.	*During:* Use sterile container for collection of urine. Touch only outside of container. *For women:* Wipe the periurethral area from front to back, dry the area thoroughly with sterile swab, separate labia with one hand. *For men:* Retract foreskin (if present), cleanse glans around urethra, replace foreskin after cleaning. After cleaning, have patient start voiding, and collect the specimen 1 to 2 seconds after voiding starts. The initial voided urine flushes out most contaminants in the urethra and perineal area. Catheterization may be needed if patient is unable to cooperate with procedure.
Urine cytologic study	Identifies abnormal cellular structures that occur with bladder cancer. Used to follow the progress of bladder cancer after treatment.	*During:* Obtain specimens by voiding, catheterization, or bladder irrigation. Do not use morning's first voided specimen because epithelial cells may change in appearance in urine held in bladder overnight. *After:* Specimen should be fresh or brought to laboratory within the hour. An alcohol-based fixative is then added to preserve the cellular structure.

Urine Studies

Urinalysis. Urinalysis is one of the first studies done to evaluate disorders of the urinary tract (Table 44.8). Results from the urinalysis may show abnormalities, suggest the need for further studies, or show progression in a previously diagnosed disorder.

Although a specimen may be collected at any time of the day for a routine urinalysis, it is best to obtain the first specimen urinated in the morning. This concentrated specimen is more likely to contain abnormal constituents if they are present in the urine. The specimen should be examined within 1 hour of urinating. Otherwise, bacteria multiply rapidly, RBCs hemolyze, *casts* (molds of renal tubules) disintegrate, and the urine becomes alkaline because of urea-splitting bacteria. If it is not possible to send the specimen to the laboratory immediately, refrigerate it. However, for the best results, coordinate specimen collection with routine laboratory hours.

Creatinine Clearance. A common test used to analyze urinary system disorders is creatinine clearance. Creatinine is a waste product made by muscle breakdown. Urinary excretion of creatinine is a measure of the amount of active muscle tissue in the

TABLE 44.10 Blood Studies

Urinary System

Test	Reference Interval	Significance
Bicarbonate	22–26 mEq/L (22–26 mmol/L).	Most patients in renal failure have metabolic acidosis and low serum HCO_3^- levels.
Blood urea nitrogen (BUN)	10–20 mg/dL (3.6–7.1 mmol/L)	Used to detect renal problems. Concentration of urea in blood is regulated by rate at which kidney excretes urea. Nonrenal factors may increase BUN (e.g., rapid cell destruction from infections, fever, GI bleeding, trauma, athletic activity, excessive muscle breakdown).
BUN/creatinine ratio	12:1–20:1	Increased ratio may be due to conditions that decrease blood flow to kidneys (e.g., heart failure, dehydration, GI bleeding) or increased dietary protein. A decreased ratio may occur with liver disease (from decreased urea formation) and malnutrition.
Calcium (total)	9.0–10.5 mg/dL (2.25–2.62 mmol/L)	Main mineral in bone and aids in muscle contraction, neurotransmission, and clotting. In kidney disease, decreased reabsorption of Ca^{2+} leads to renal osteodystrophy.
Creatinine	*Male:* 0.6–1.2 mg/dL (53–106 μmol/L) *Female:* 0.5–1.1 mg/dL (44.97 μmol/L)	More reliable than BUN as a determinant of renal function. Creatinine is a product of muscle and protein metabolism. It is released at a constant rate.
Phosphorus	3.0–4.5 mg/dL (0.97–1.45 mmol/L).	Phosphorus balance is inversely related to Ca^{2+} balance. In kidney disease, phosphorus levels are high because the kidney is the primary excretory organ.
Potassium	3.5–5.0 mEq/L (3.5–5.0 mmol/L)	Kidneys excrete majority of body's potassium. In kidney disease, K^+ determinations are critical because K^+ is one of the first electrolytes to become abnormal. High K^+ levels >6 mEq/L can lead to muscle weakness and cardiac dysrhythmias.
Sodium	136–145 mEq/L (136–145 mmol/L)	Main extracellular electrolyte determining blood volume. Values usually stay within normal range until late stages of renal failure.
Uric acid	*Male:* 4.0–8.5 mg/dL (0.24–0.51 mmol/L) *Female:* 2.7–7.3 mg/dL (0.16–0.43 mmol/L)	Used as screening test for disorders of purine metabolism. Can indicate kidney disease. Values depend on renal function, rate of purine metabolism, and dietary intake of food rich in purines.

TABLE 44.11 Diagnostic Studies

Urinary System

Study	Description and Purpose	Nursing Responsibility
Endoscopy		
Cystoscopy	Inspects interior of bladder with a tubular lighted scope (cystoscope) (Fig. 44.10). Can be used to insert ureteral catheters, remove stones, obtain biopsy specimens of bladder lesions, and treat bleeding lesions. Lithotomy position is used. Procedure may be done using local or general anesthesia, depending on patient's needs and condition. Complications include urinary retention, urinary tract hemorrhage, bladder infection, and perforation of bladder.	*Before:* Give IV fluids if general anesthesia is to be used. Ensure consent form is signed. Explain procedure to patient. Give preoperative medication. *After:* Explain that burning on urination, pink-tinged urine, and urinary frequency are expected effects. Observe for bright red bleeding, which is not normal. Help with ambulation because orthostatic hypotension may occur. Offer warm sitz baths, heat, mild analgesics to relieve discomfort.
Radiologic Procedures		
Computed tomography (CT) scan (CT urogram)	Visualizes kidneys, ureters, and bladder. Can detect tumors, abscesses, suprarenal masses (e.g., adrenal tumors), and obstructions. Done with or without contrast media. Contrast is iodine based.	*Before:* Before contrast medium used, evaluate renal function. Assess if patient is allergic to shellfish, since the contrast is iodine based. Patient may need to be NPO 4 hr prior to study. *During:* Warn patient that contrast injection may cause a feeling of being warm and flushed. Patient must lie completely still during scan. *After:* Encourage patient to drink fluids to avoid renal problems with any contrast.
Cystogram	Visualizes bladder and evaluates vesicoureteral reflux. Evaluates patients with neurogenic bladder and recurrent UTIs. Can delineate abnormalities of bladder (e.g., diverticula, stones, tumors). Contrast media is instilled into bladder via cystoscope or catheter.	*Before:* Explain procedure to patient. *During:* If done via cystoscope, follow nursing care related to cystoscopy.
Intravenous pyelogram (IVP)	Visualizes urinary tract after IV injection of contrast media. Evaluates size and shape of kidneys, ureters, and bladder. Cysts, tumors, and ureteral obstructions distort normal appearance of these structures. Patient with decreased renal function should not have IVP because contrast media can be nephrotoxic.	*Before:* Cathartic or enema given night before. Assess patient for iodine sensitivity to avoid anaphylactic reaction. *During:* Warn patient that contrast injection may cause a feeling of being warm and flushed. *After:* Force fluids to avoid renal problems with contrast.
Kidneys, ureters, bladder (KUB)	X-ray examination of abdomen and pelvis. Delineates size, shape, and position of kidneys, ureter, and bladder. Can see radiopaque stones and foreign bodies.	*Before:* No special preparation needed.

TABLE 44.11 Diagnostic Studies

Urinary System—cont'd

Study	Description and Purpose	Nursing Responsibility
Loopogram	Detects obstructions, anastomotic leaks, stones, and reflux when patient has a urinary pouch or ileal conduit. Because urinary diversions are created with bowel, there is risk for absorption of contrast media.	*Before:* Explain procedure to patient. *During:* Monitor patient for reactions to the contrast media.
Magnetic resonance angiography	Visualizes renal vasculature. Gadolinium-enhanced studies allow visualization of renal artery.	Same as renal arteriogram. Does not require femoral artery puncture
Magnetic resonance imaging (MRI)	Visualizes kidneys. Not proven useful for detecting urinary stones or calcified tumors.	*Before:* Oral and/or IV contrast injection may be used. Check for pregnancy, allergies, and renal function before test. Have patient remove all metal objects. Remove metallic foil patches. Contraindicated for persons with implanted metallic devices or other metal fragments unless noted to be MRI safe. Ask about any history of surgical insertion of staples, plates, dental bridges, or other metal appliances. Patient may need to be fasting. Assess for claustrophobia and the need for antianxiety medication. *During:* Patient must lie completely still during scan.
Nephrostogram (Antegrade pyelogram)	Evaluates upper urinary tract when patient has allergy to contrast media, decreased renal function, or abnormalities that prevent passage of a ureteral catheter. Contrast media may be injected percutaneously into renal pelvis or via a nephrostomy tube that is already in place when determining tube function or ureteral integrity after trauma or surgery.	*Before:* Explain procedure and prepare patient as for IVP. *During and after:* Watch for signs of complications (e.g., hematuria, infection, hematoma).
Renal arteriogram (angiogram)	Visualizes renal blood vessels. Can aid in diagnosing renal artery stenosis (Fig. 44.8), extra or missing renal blood vessels, and renovascular hypertension. Can aid in distinguishing between a renal cyst and renal tumor. Included in workup of a potential renal transplant donor. A catheter is inserted into the femoral artery and passed up the aorta to the level of renal arteries (Fig. 44.9). Contrast media is injected to outline renal blood supply.	*Before:* Cathartic or enema may be used the night before. Before injection of contrast material, assess for iodine sensitivity. Tell patient a transient warm feeling may be felt along the course of blood vessel when contrast media is injected. *After:* Place a pressure dressing over femoral artery injection site. Observe site for bleeding and inflammation. Have patient maintain bed rest with affected leg straight. Take peripheral pulses in the involved leg every 30–60 min to detect occlusion of blood flow (from thrombus or emboli).
Renal biopsy	Obtains renal tissue for examination to determine type of kidney disease or to follow progress of kidney disease. Usually done as a skin (percutaneous) biopsy through needle insertion into lower lobe of kidney under CT or ultrasound guidance. Absolute contraindications are bleeding disorders, single kidney, and uncontrolled hypertension. Relative contraindications include suspected renal infection, hydronephrosis, and possible vascular lesions.	*Before:* Type and crossmatch patient for blood. Ensure consent form is signed. Assess coagulation status through patient history, medication history, CBC, hematocrit, prothrombin time, and bleeding and clotting time. Patient should not be taking aspirin or warfarin. *After:* Apply pressure dressing and keep patient on affected side for 30–60 min. Bed rest for 24 hr. Vital signs every 5–10 min, first hour. Assess for flank pain, hypotension, decreasing hematocrit, fever, chills, urinary frequency, dysuria, and gross or microscopic hematuria. Inspect biopsy site for bleeding. Teach patient to avoid lifting heavy objects for 5–7 days and to not take anticoagulant drugs until allowed by HCP.

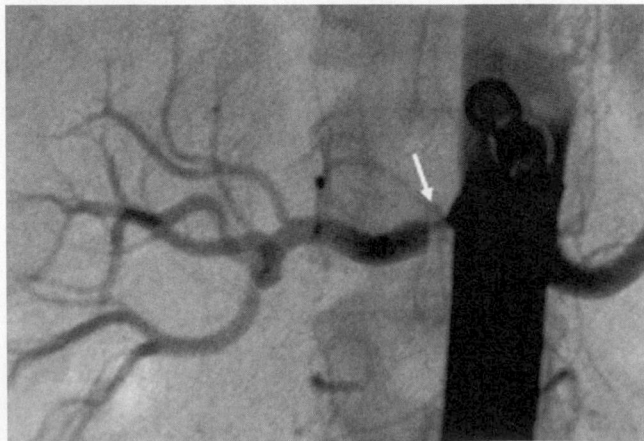

FIG. 44.8 Renal arteriogram showing stenosis of the left renal artery *(arrow)*. (From Staub D, Zeller T, Trenk D: Predicting blood pressure improvement after revascularization for renal artery stenosis, *Eur J Vasc Endovasc* 40:599, 2010.)

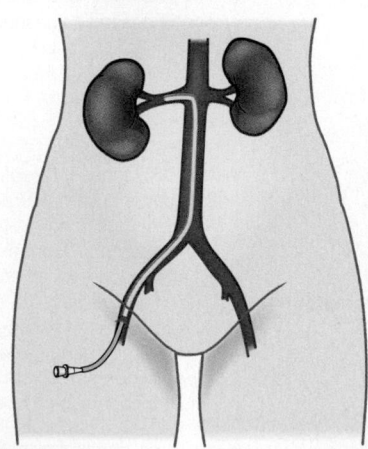

FIG. 44.9 Catheter insertion for a renal arteriogram.

TABLE 44.11 Diagnostic Studies

Urinary System—cont'd

Study	Description and Purpose	Nursing Responsibility
Renal scan	Evaluates anatomic structures, perfusion, and function of kidneys. IV radioactive isotopes are injected. Radiation detector probes are placed over kidney and scintillation counter monitors radioactive material in kidney. Radio-isotope distribution in kidney is scanned and mapped. Shows location, size, and shape of kidney and assesses blood flow, glomerular filtration, tubular function, and urinary excretion. Abscesses, cysts, and tumors may appear as cold spots because of nonfunctioning tissue. Monitors function of a transplanted kidney.	*Before:* No diet or activity restriction. Tell patient that there should not be any pain or discomfort during test.
Renal ultrasound	Detects renal or perirenal masses (tumors, cysts) and obstructions. Small external ultrasound probe is placed on patient's skin. Conductive gel is applied to skin. Noninvasive procedure involves passing sound waves into body structures and recording images as they are reflected. Computer interprets tissue density based on sound waves and displays it in picture form. Can be used safely in patients with renal failure.	*Before:* Explain procedure to patient. No bowel preparation needed. *During:* Because radiation exposure is avoided, repeated images can be obtained over a brief period.
Retrograde pyelogram	X-ray of urinary tract taken after injection of contrast material into kidneys. May be done if an IVP does not visualize the urinary tract or has decreased renal function. A cystoscope is inserted, and ureteral catheters are inserted through it into renal pelvis. Contrast media is injected through catheters.	*Before:* Prepare patient as for IVP. Tell patient that there may be pain from distention of pelvis and discomfort from cystoscope. Anesthesia may be given for procedure. *After:* Complications similar to those for cystoscopy.
Urethrogram	Similar to a cystogram. Contrast media is injected retrograde into urethra to identify strictures, diverticula, or other urethral pathologic conditions. When urethral trauma is suspected, a urethrogram is done before catheterization.	*Before:* Explain procedure to patient.
Voiding cystourethrogram (VCUG)	Voiding study of bladder opening (bladder neck) and urethra. Bladder is filled with contrast media. Fluoroscopic films are taken to visualize bladder and urethra. After urination, another film is taken to assess for residual urine. Can detect abnormalities of lower urinary tract, urethral stenosis, bladder neck obstruction, vesicoureteral reflux, and prostatic enlargement.	*Before:* Explain procedure to patient.

Urodynamic Studies

Study	Description and Purpose	Nursing Responsibility
Cystometrogram	Evaluates bladder's capacity to contract and expel urine. Involves insertion of catheter and instillation of water or saline solution into bladder. Measurements of pressure exerted against bladder wall are recorded. If abdominal pressure is measured, a second tube is inserted into rectum or vagina. This tube is attached to a small fluid-filled balloon to allow pressure recording.	*Before:* Explain procedure to patient. *During:* Ask patient about sensations of bladder filling, usually including the first desire (urge) to urinate, a strong desire to urinate, and perception of bladder fullness. *After:* Observe patient for manifestations of UTI after procedure.
Radionuclide cystography (RNC)	Detects and grades vesicoureteral reflux. Like VCUG with a small dose of radioisotope tracer instilled into the bladder via urethral catheter. More sensitive than VCUG, and radiation dose is 1/1000 that of the VCUG.	*Before:* Explain procedure to patient as in VCUG.

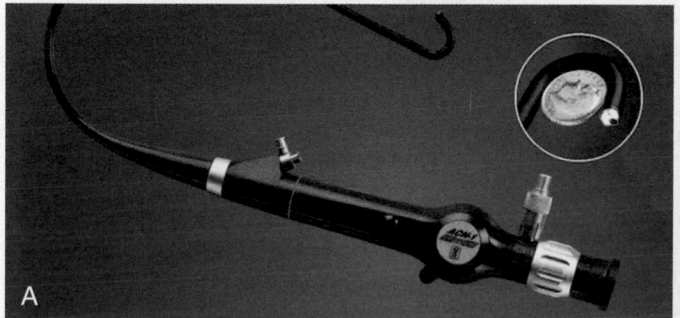
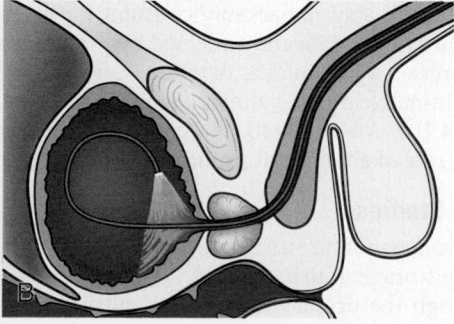

FIG. 44.10 Cystoscopic examination of the bladder in a man. A, Flexible cystonephroscope. B, Scope inserted into bladder. (*A*, Courtesy Circon Corporation, Santa Barbara, CA.)

TABLE 44.11   Diagnostic Studies

Urinary System—cont'd

Study	Description and Purpose	Nursing Responsibility
Sphincter electromyography (EMG)	Recording of electrical activity created when nervous system stimulates muscle tissue. By placing needles, percutaneous wires, or patches near the urethra, pelvic floor muscle activity can be assessed. During the cystometrogram, sphincter EMG is used to identify voluntary pelvic floor muscle contractions and response of these muscles to bladder filling, coughing, and other provocative maneuvers.	*Before:* Explain procedure to patient.
Urine flow study (uroflow)	Measures urine volume in a single voiding expelled in a period. Used to (1) assess the degree of outflow obstruction caused by such conditions as benign prostatic hyperplasia, (2) assess bladder or sphincter dysfunction effects on voiding, and (3) evaluate effects of treatment for lower urinary tract problems. Graphic displays can illustrate straining and intermittent flow patterns or other abnormal voiding disorders. *Normal maximum flow rate:* Men: 20–25 mL/sec; women: 25–30 mL/sec. Volume voided and patient's age can affect the flow rate.	*Before:* Explain procedure to patient. *During:* Ask the patient to start the test with a comfortably full bladder, urinate into a designated container, and try to empty completely. *After:* Measure residual urine volume immediately after a urinary flow study because this will help identify degree of chronic urinary retention that is often associated with abnormal flow patterns.
Videourodynamics	Combination of cystometrogram, sphincter EMG, and/or urinary flow study with anatomic imaging of the lower urinary tract, typically via fluoroscopy. Used in selected cases to identify an obstructive lesion and characterize anatomic changes in bladder and lower urinary tract	*Before:* Explain procedure to patient.
Voiding pressure flow study	Combines a urinary flow rate, cystometric pressures (intravesical, abdominal, and detrusor pressures), and sphincter EMG for detailed evaluation of micturition. It is completed by assisting the patient to a specialized toilet to urinate while the various pressure tubes and EMG apparatus remain in place.	*Before:* Explain procedure to patient.
Whitaker study	Measures the pressure differential between renal pelvis and bladder. Ureteral obstruction can be assessed. Percutaneous access to renal pelvis obtained by placing a catheter in renal pelvis. A catheter is placed in bladder. Fluid is perfused through the percutaneous tube or needle at a rate of 10 mL/min. Pressure data are then collected. Pressure measurements are combined with fluoroscopic imaging to find the level of obstruction.	*Before:* Explain procedure to patient.

body, not of body weight. Therefore people with larger muscle mass have higher values. Because almost all creatinine in the blood is normally excreted by the kidneys, creatinine clearance is the most accurate indicator of renal function. The result of a creatinine clearance test closely approximates that of the GFR. A blood specimen to measure serum creatinine should be obtained during the period of urine collection.

Creatinine levels stay remarkably constant for each person because they are not significantly affected by protein ingestion, muscular exercise, water intake, or rate of urine production. Normal creatinine clearance values range from 87 to 139 mL/min (Table 44.10). After age 40, the creatinine clearance rate decreases at a rate of about 1 mL/min/yr.

Urodynamic Studies

Urodynamic studies measure urinary tract function. Urodynamic tests study the storage of urine within the bladder and the flow of urine through the urinary tract to the outside of the body. A combination of techniques may be used for a detailed assessment of urinary function (Table 44.11).

CASE STUDY—cont'd

Objective Data: Diagnostic Studies

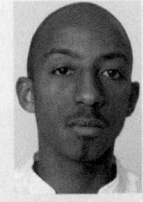

(© iStockphoto/Thinkstock.)

The HCP orders the following initial diagnostic studies for A.K.:
- CBC, basic metabolic panel (electrolytes, BUN, creatinine)
- Urinalysis, culture if indicated
- Renal ultrasound

A.K.'s CBC and metabolic panel results are within normal limits. His urinalysis shows moderate hematuria and the renal ultrasound shows several stones in the left ureter. There is no hydronephrosis at present. The HCP prescribes IV opioids for pain management and admits A.K. to a medical unit for further observation.

Discussion Questions

1. Which diagnostic study results are abnormal?
2. Which diagnostic study results are of most concern to you?

Answers available at *http://evolve.elsevier.com/Lewis/medsurg.*

BRIDGE TO NCLEX EXAMINATION

The number of the question corresponds to the same-numbered outcome at the beginning of the chapter.

1. A renal stone in the pelvis of the kidney will change kidney function by interfering with the
   a. structural support of the kidney.
   b. regulation of the concentration of urine.
   c. entry and exit of blood vessels at the kidney.
   d. collection and drainage of urine from the kidney.

2. A patient with kidney disease has oliguria and a creatinine clearance of 40 mL/min. These findings most directly reflect abnormal function of
   a. tubular secretion.
   b. glomerular filtration.
   c. capillary permeability.
   d. concentration of filtrate.

3. The nurse identifies a risk for urinary stones in a patient who relates a health history that includes
   a. hyperaldosteronism.
   b. serotonin deficiency.
   c. adrenal insufficiency.
   d. hyperparathyroidism.

4. Diminished ability to concentrate urine, associated with aging of the urinary system, is attributed to
   a. a decrease in bladder sensory receptors.
   b. a decrease in the number of functioning nephrons.
   c. decreased function of the loop of Henle and tubules.
   d. thickening of the basement membrane of Bowman's capsule.

5. During physical assessment of the urinary system, the nurse
   a. performs fist percussion to detect tenderness in the flank area.
   b. expects a dull percussion sound when 100 mL of urine is present in the bladder.
   c. percusses above the symphysis pubis to determine the level of urine in the bladder.
   d. palpates the lower pole of the right kidney as a smooth mass that descends on expiration.

6. Normal findings expected by the nurse on physical assessment of the urinary system include (*select all that apply*)
   a. nonpalpable bladder.
   b. nonpalpable left kidney.
   c. auscultation of renal artery bruit.
   d. no CVA tenderness elicited by a kidney punch.
   e. full bladder percusses as dullness above the symphysis pubis.

7. A diagnostic study that evaluates renal blood flow, glomerular filtration, tubular function, and excretion is a(n)
   a. IVP.
   b. VCUG.
   c. renal scan.
   d. loopogram.

8. On reading the urinalysis results of a dehydrated patient, the nurse would expect to find
   a. a pH of 8.4.
   b. RBCs of 4/hpf.
   c. color: yellow, cloudy.
   d. specific gravity of 1.035.

1. d, 2. b, 3. d, 4. c, 5. a, 6. a, b, d, e, 7. c, 8. d

For rationales to these answers and even more NCLEX review questions, visit *http://evolve.elsevier.com/Lewis/medsurg*.

ⓔ EVOLVE WEBSITE/RESOURCES LIST

http://evolve.elsevier.com/Lewis/medsurg
Review Questions (Online Only)
Key Points
Answer Keys for Questions
- Rationales for Bridge to NCLEX Examination Questions
- Answer Guidelines for Case Study on pp. 1012, 1015, 1016, and 1022
Conceptual Care Map Creator
Audio Glossary
Content Updates

REFERENCES

*1. Denic A, Lieske JC, Chakkera HA, et al: The substantial loss of nephrons in healthy human kidneys with aging *JASN* 28:313, 2017.
*2. Webster AC, Nagler EV, Morton RL, et al: Chronic kidney disease, *Lancet* 389:1238, 2017.
3. American Cancer Society: Bladder cancer risk factors. Retrieved from *www.cancer.org/cancer/bladder-cancer/causes-risks-prevention/risk-factors.html*.
*4. Ziemba JB, Matlaga BR: Epidemiology and economics of nephrolithiasis, *Investig Clin Urol* 58:299, 2017.
5. Jarvis C: *Physical examination and health assessment*, 7th ed, St Louis, 2016, Saunders.
*6. Fähling M, Seeliger E, Patzak A, et al: Understanding and preventing contrast-induced acute kidney injury, *Nat Rev Nephrol* 13:169, 2017.

45

Renal and Urologic Problems

Cynthia Ann Smith

*Caring about others, running the risk of feeling, and
leaving an impact on people, brings happiness.*

Harold Kushner

http://evolve.elsevier.com/Lewis/medsurg

CONCEPTUAL FOCUS

Elimination

Fluids and Electrolytes

Infection

Pain

LEARNING OUTCOMES

1. Discuss the pathophysiology, clinical manifestations, and interprofessional and nursing management of urinary tract infections, cystitis, urethritis, and pyelonephritis.
2. Distinguish the etiology, clinical manifestations, and nursing and interprofessional management of acute poststreptococcal glomerulonephritis, Goodpasture syndrome, and chronic glomerulonephritis.
3. Describe the common causes, clinical manifestations, and interprofessional and nursing management of nephrotic syndrome.
4. Compare and contrast the etiology, clinical manifestations, and interprofessional and nursing management of various types of urinary calculi.
5. Distinguish the common causes and management of renal trauma, renal vascular problems, and hereditary kidney diseases.
6. Describe the clinical manifestations and nursing and interprofessional management of kidney and bladder cancers.
7. Describe the common causes and management of urinary incontinence and urinary retention.
8. Distinguish among urethral, ureteral, suprapubic, and nephrostomy catheters regarding indications for use and nursing responsibilities.
9. Explain the nursing management of the patient undergoing nephrectomy or urinary diversion surgery.

KEY TERMS

calculus, p. 1035
cystitis, p. 1025
glomerulonephritis, p. 1032
Goodpasture syndrome, p. 1033
hydronephrosis, p. 1035
ileal conduit, p. 1055
interstitial cystitis (IC), p. 1031

lithotripsy, p. 1038
nephrolithiasis, p. 1035
nephrosclerosis, p. 1041
nephrotic syndrome, p. 1034
polycystic kidney disease (PKD), p. 1041
pyelonephritis, p. 1025
renal artery stenosis, p. 1041

stricture, p. 1040
urethritis, p. 1025
urinary incontinence (UI), p. 1045
urinary retention, p. 1050
urinary tract infection (UTI), p. 1024
urosepsis, p. 1025

A wide range of renal and urologic disorders contribute to impaired elimination. The diverse causes of these disorders are grouped by common problems, such as infectious, immunologic, obstructive, traumatic, cancerous, and neurologic mechanisms. This chapter discusses disorders of the upper urinary tract (kidneys and ureter) and lower urinary tract (bladder and urethra). Many patients are at risk fluid, electrolyte, and acid-base imbalances because of the kidneys' vital role in homeostasis. The person may have discomfort and incontinence and problems with disrupted sleep or skin integrity.

INFECTIOUS AND INFLAMMATORY DISORDERS OF URINARY SYSTEM

URINARY TRACT INFECTION

Urinary tract infections (UTIs) are infections that affect the urinary tract. They are the second most common bacterial disease and the most common bacterial infection in women.[1] *Escherichia coli* is the most common pathogen causing a UTI. It causes 70% to 95% of cases without urinary tract structural abnormalities or stones (Table 45.1). It is seen primarily in

TABLE 45.1 Common Causes of Urinary Tract Infections

- *Candida albicans*
- *Enterobacter*
- *Enterococcus*
- *Escherichia coli*
- *Klebsiella*
- *Proteus*
- *Pseudomonas*
- *Serratia*
- *Staphylococcus*
- Streptococci

TABLE 45.2 Risk Factors for Urinary Tract Infections

Anatomic Factors
- Congenital defects leading to obstruction or urinary stasis
- Fistula exposing urinary stream to skin, vagina, or fecal stream
- Obesity
- Shorter female urethra and colonization from normal vaginal flora

Factors Compromising Immune Response
- Aging
- Diabetes
- HIV infection

Factors Increasing Urinary Stasis
- Extrinsic obstruction (tumor, fibrosis compressing urinary tract)
- Intrinsic obstruction (stone, tumor of urinary tract, urethral stricture, BPH)
- Renal impairment
- Urinary retention (e.g., neurogenic bladder)

Foreign Bodies
- Catheters (indwelling, external condom catheter, ureteral stent, nephrostomy tube, intermittent catheterization)
- Urinary tract instrumentation (cystoscopy)
- Urinary tract stones

Functional Disorders
- Constipation
- Voiding dysfunction with detrusor sphincter muscle incoordination

Other Factors
- Habitual delay of urination ("nurse's bladder," "teacher's bladder")
- Pregnancy
- Menopause
- Multiple sex partners (women)
- Poor personal hygiene
- Use of spermicidal agents, contraceptive diaphragm (women), bubble baths, feminine sprays

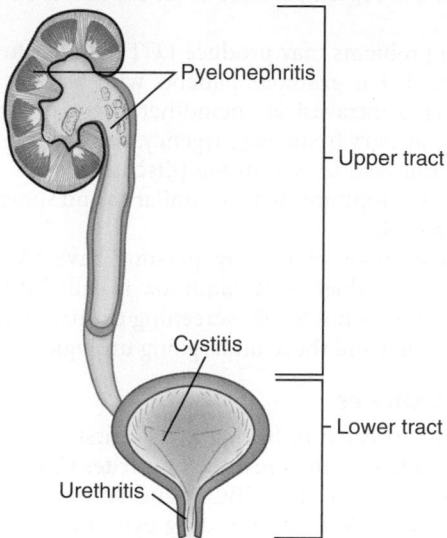

FIG 45.1 Sites of infectious processes in the upper and lower urinary tracts.

women.[2] *Candida albicans* is the second most common pathogen, causing UTIs associated with indwelling catheter use or asymptomatic colonization.

Bacterial counts of 10^5 colony-forming units per milliliter (CFU/mL) or higher typically indicate a clinically significant UTI. However, counts as low as 10^2 to 10^3 CFU/mL in a person with signs and symptoms are indicative of UTI.

Although fungal and parasitic infections may cause UTIs, this is uncommon. UTIs from these causes sometimes occur in patients who are immunosuppressed, have diabetes, have kidney problems, or received multiple courses of antibiotic therapy. These types of UTIs may occur in persons who live in or have traveled to certain developing countries.

Classification of Urinary Tract Infection

A UTI can be broadly classified as an upper or lower UTI according to its location within the urinary system (Fig. 45.1). We use specific terms to delineate the location of a UTI. For example, **pyelonephritis** implies inflammation (usually caused by infection) of the renal parenchyma and collecting system. **Cystitis** is an inflammation of the bladder, while **urethritis** is an inflammation of the urethra. **Urosepsis** is a UTI that has spread systemically. It is a life-threatening condition requiring emergency treatment.

Classifying a UTI as complicated or uncomplicated is also useful. *Uncomplicated UTIs* occur in an otherwise normal urinary tract and usually only involve the bladder. *Complicated UTIs* occur in a person with a structural or functional problem in the urinary tract. Examples include obstruction, stones, catheters, abnormal genitourinary (GU) tract, acute kidney injury (AKI), chronic kidney disease (CKD), renal transplant, diabetes,

or neurologic diseases. They can also occur when a person has developed antibiotic resistance, is immunocompromised, has pregnancy-induced changes, or has recurrent infection. The person with a complicated infection is at risk for pyelonephritis, urosepsis, and renal damage.

Etiology and Pathophysiology

The urinary tract above the urethra is normally sterile. Several mechanical and physiologic defense mechanisms aid in maintaining sterility and preventing UTIs. These defenses include normal voiding with complete emptying of the bladder, ureterovesical junction competence, and ureteral peristaltic activity that propels urine toward the bladder. Antibacterial characteristics of urine are maintained by an acidic pH (less than 6.0), high urea concentration, and abundant glycoproteins that interfere with the growth of bacteria. A change in any of these defense mechanisms increases the risk for a UTI (Table 45.2).

The organisms that usually cause UTIs originate in the perineum and are introduced via the ascending route from the urethra. Most infections are caused by gram-negative bacilli normally found in the gastrointestinal (GI) tract. However, gram-positive organisms, such as streptococci, enterococci, and *Staphylococcus saprophyticus,* can also cause UTIs.

A common factor contributing to ascending infection is urologic instrumentation (e.g., catheterization, cystoscopic

TABLE 45.3 Lower Urinary Tract Symptoms (LUTS)

Symptoms	Description
Emptying Symptoms	
Dysuria	• Painful or difficult urination
Hesitancy	• Difficulty starting urine stream
	• Delay between initiation of urination (because of urethral sphincter relaxation) and beginning of flow of urine
	• Diminished urinary stream
Intermittency	• Interruption of urinary stream while voiding
Postvoid dribbling	• Urine loss after completion of voiding
Urinary retention or incomplete emptying	• Inability to empty urine from bladder
	• Caused by atonic bladder or obstruction of urethra
	• Can be acute or chronic
Storage Symptoms	
Incontinence	• Involuntary or accidental urine loss or leakage
Nocturia	• Awakened by urge to void 2 or more times during sleep
	• May be diurnal or nocturnal depending on sleep schedule
Nocturnal enuresis	• Adults: loss of urine during sleep
Urgency	• Sudden, strong, or intense desire to void immediately
	• Often accompanied by frequency
Urinary frequency	• More than 8 times in 24-hr period
	• Often <200 mL each voiding

examinations). Instrumentation allows bacteria that are normally present at the opening of the urethra to enter the urethra or bladder. Sexual intercourse promotes "milking" of bacteria from the vagina and perineum and may cause minor urethral trauma that predisposes women to UTIs.

UTIs can result from hematogenous transmission, in which blood-borne bacteria invade the kidneys, ureters, or bladder from elsewhere in the body. For a kidney infection to occur in this manner, there must be prior injury to the urinary tract, such as obstruction of the ureter, damage caused by stones, or renal scars.

UTIs are the most common health care–associated infection (HAI). They are primarily associated with use of an indwelling catheter. *Catheter-associated urinary tract infections (CAUTIs)* are often caused by *E. coli* and, less often, *Pseudomonas* organisms. CAUTIs are often underrecognized and undertreated, leading to extended hospital stays, increased health care costs, and patient morbidity and mortality.[3]

Clinical Manifestations

Manifestations of UTIs range from painful urination in uncomplicated urethritis or cystitis to severe systemic illness associated with abdominal or back pain, fever, sepsis.

Lower urinary tract symptoms (LUTS) occur in patients who have UTIs of the upper urinary tract, as well as those confined to the lower tract. Symptoms are related to either bladder storage or bladder emptying (Table 45.3). These include dysuria, frequency (voiding more than every 2 hours), urgency, and suprapubic discomfort or pressure. The urine may contain grossly visible blood (hematuria) or sediment, giving it a cloudy appearance. Infection of the upper urinary tract (involving the renal parenchyma, pelvis, and ureters) typically causes fever,

chills, and flank pain. A UTI confined to the lower urinary tract does not usually have systemic manifestations. People with significant bacteriuria may have no symptoms or may have nonspecific symptoms, such as fatigue or anorexia.

Remember that the characteristic manifestations of a UTI are often absent in older adults. Older adults tend to have nonlocalized abdominal discomfort rather than dysuria and suprapubic pain. They may have cognitive impairment or generalized clinical deterioration. Because older adults are less likely to have a fever with a UTI, temperature is an unreliable indicator of a UTI.[4]

Multiple problems may produce LUTS similar to the symptoms of a UTI. For example, patients with bladder tumors or those receiving intravesical chemotherapy or pelvic radiation usually have urinary frequency, urgency, and dysuria. Interstitial cystitis/painful bladder syndrome (discussed on p. 1031) produces urinary symptoms that are similar to and sometimes confused with a UTI.

A small number of healthy persons have some bacteria colonizing the bladder. This condition is called *asymptomatic bacteriuria*. It does not justify screening or treatment except in pregnant women and those undergoing urologic procedures.

Diagnostic Studies

In a patient suspected of having a UTI, first obtain a dipstick urinalysis to identify the presence of nitrites (indicating bacteriuria), white blood cells (WBCs), and leukocyte esterase (an enzyme present in WBCs, indicating pyuria). Microscopic urinalysis can confirm these findings. After confirmation of bacteriuria and pyuria, a urine culture may be done. A urine culture is needed in persistent bacteriuria, recurring UTIs (more than 2 or 3 episodes per year), or complicated, CAUTI, or HAI UTIs. Urine also may be cultured when the infection is unresponsive to empiric therapy or the diagnosis is questionable.

A voided midstream technique *(clean-catch urine sample)* is preferred for obtaining a urine culture in most circumstances (see Table 44.9). When an adequate clean-catch specimen cannot be obtained, catheterization may be needed. A specimen obtained by catheterization provides more accurate results than a clean-catch specimen.

A urine culture with *sensitivity testing* can determine the bacteria's susceptibility to a variety of antibiotic drugs. The results allow the HCP to choose an antibiotic known to be capable of destroying the bacteria causing a UTI in a specific patient.

Some patients need imaging studies of the urinary tract. An ultrasound or CT scan may be done when obstruction of the urinary system is suspected or UTIs recur.

Interprofessional Care

The interprofessional care and drug therapy of UTIs are outlined in Table 45.4. Once a UTI has been diagnosed, appropriate antimicrobial therapy is started. An antibiotic may be chosen based on the HCP's best judgment *(empiric therapy)* or the results of sensitivity testing.

Uncomplicated UTIs are treated with a short-term course of antibiotics, typically for 3 days. In contrast, complicated UTIs need a longer period of treatment, lasting 7 to 14 days or more.[4,5] Many residents of long-term care facilities, especially women, have chronic asymptomatic bacteriuria. However, we usually only treat symptomatic UTIs.

First-choice drugs to treat uncomplicated or initial UTIs are trimethoprim/sulfamethoxazole (TMP/SMX), nitrofurantoin,

TABLE 45.4 Interprofessional Care

Urinary Tract Infection

Diagnostic Assessment

- History and physical examination
- Urinalysis (midstream, "clean-catch" voided specimen)
- Urine for culture and sensitivity (if indicated)
- Imaging studies of urinary tract (if indicated): CT scan , ultrasound, cystoscopy

Management

Uncomplicated UTI

- Patient teaching
- Adequate fluid intake (6 8-oz glasses/day)

Drug Therapy

- Antibiotics
  - fluconazole (in patients with fungal UTI)
  - fosfomycin (Monurol)
  - nitrofurantoin (Macrodantin, Macrobid)
  - TMP/SMX (Bactrim, Bactrim DS)
  - trimethoprim alone (in patients with sulfa allergy)
  - phenazopyridine (Pyridium)

Recurrent UTI

- Repeat urinalysis
- Urine culture and sensitivity testing
- Adequate fluid intake (6 8-oz glasses/day)
- Repeat patient teaching
- Imaging studies of urinary tract (if indicated): see above

Drug Therapy

- Antibiotic: nitrofurantoin, TMP/SMX
- Sensitivity-guided antibiotic therapy: ampicillin, amoxicillin, first-generation cephalosporin, fluoroquinolones
- 3- to 6-month trial of suppressive or prophylactic antibiotic regimen
- Postcoital antibiotic prophylaxis: cephalexin, nitrofurantoin, TMP/SMX

TABLE 45.5 Nursing Assessment

Urinary Tract Infection

Subjective Data

Important Health Information

Past health history: Previous UTI. Urinary stones, reflux, strictures, or retention. Neurogenic bladder, pregnancy, benign prostatic hyperplasia, bladder cancer, sexually transmitted infection.
Medications: Antibiotics, anticholinergics, antispasmodics
Surgery or other treatments: Recent urologic instrumentation (catheterization, cystoscopy)

Functional Health Patterns

Cognitive-perceptual: Suprapubic or low back pain, bladder spasms, dysuria, burning on urination
Elimination: Urinary frequency, urgency, hesitancy, dysuria, nocturia
Health perception–health management: Urinary hygiene practices. Lassitude, malaise
Nutritional-metabolic: Nausea, vomiting, anorexia. Chills and fever
Sexuality-reproductive: Multiple sex partners, use of spermicidal agents or contraceptive diaphragm (women)

Objective Data

General

Fever, chills, dysuria
Atypical presentation in older adults: afebrile, absence of dysuria, loss of appetite, altered mental status

Urinary

Hematuria. Cloudy, foul-smelling urine

Possible Diagnostic Findings

Leukocytosis. Urinalysis positive for bacteria, pyuria, RBCs, WBCs, and nitrites. Positive urine culture. Ultrasound, CT scan, MRI, Voiding cystourethrogram (VCUG), and cystoscopy showing urinary tract abnormalities

---

cephalexin, and fosfomycin.[5] TMP/SMX has the advantages of being inexpensive and taken twice daily. A disadvantage is *E. coli* resistance to TMP/SMX, β-lactams, and ciprofloxacin, which is an increasing problem in the United States. Nitrofurantoin can be given 3 or 4 times daily, but a twice-daily formulation is available.

Other antibiotics used in the treatment of uncomplicated UTI include ampicillin, amoxicillin, and cephalosporins. Fluoroquinolones (e.g., levofloxacin, ciprofloxacin) should be used to treat only complicated UTIs. In patients with UTIs from fungi, fluconazole (Diflucan) is the preferred therapy.

 DRUG ALERT Nitrofurantoin (Macrodantin)

- Avoid use if the patient's creatinine clearance < 30 mL/min.
- Notify HCP at once if fever, chills, cough, chest pain, dyspnea, rash, or numbness or tingling of fingers or toes develops.

A urinary analgesic, such as oral phenazopyridine, may relieve discomfort caused by severe dysuria. Phenazopyridine is an azo dye excreted in urine, where it exerts a topical analgesic effect on the urinary tract mucosa. It is taken up to 2 concurrent days. Teach patients that this drug causes the urine to turn orange or red.

Patients who have repeated UTIs may receive prophylactic or suppressive antibiotics. A low dose of TMP/SMX, nitrofurantoin, or another antibiotic taken daily may prevent recurring UTIs. A single dose may be taken after an event likely to provoke a UTI, such as sexual intercourse. Although suppressive therapy is often effective on a short-term basis, this strategy is limited

because of the risk for antibiotic resistance, which leads to breakthrough infections with increasingly virulent pathogens.

❖ NURSING MANAGEMENT: URINARY TRACT INFECTION

◆ Nursing Assessment

Subjective and objective data that should be obtained from a patient with a UTI are shown in Table 45.5.

◆ Nursing Diagnoses

Nursing diagnoses for the patient with a UTI may include:

- Impaired urinary system function
- Acute pain
- Lack of knowledge

More information on nursing diagnoses and interventions for the patient with a UTI is presented in eNursing Care Plan 45.1 (available on the website for this chapter).

◆ Planning

The overall goals are that the patient with a UTI will have (1) relief from bothersome symptoms, (2) no upper urinary tract involvement, and (3) no recurrence.

◆ Nursing Implementation

◆ **Health Promotion.** It is important to recognize people who are at risk for a UTI. These include debilitated persons, older adults, patients who are immunocompromised (e.g., cancer, diabetes), and patients treated with immunosuppressive drugs or corticosteroids. Health promotion activities can help decrease the frequency of UTIs and provide for early detection of infection. These activities include teaching preventive measures, including (1) emptying the bladder regularly and completely, (2) evacuating the bowel regularly, (3) wiping the perineal area from front to back after voiding and defecation, and (4) drinking an adequate amount of liquid each day.

To estimate the amount of fluid intake a person should have in 24 hours, take the person's weight in pounds, and divide that number in half. The result is the number of ounces of fluid a person should have per day. Thus a 150-lb person would need 75 oz/day. The person will obtain about 20% of this fluid from food, which leaves 60 oz (1775 mL) by drinking, or just over 7 8-oz glasses of fluid.

Routine and thorough perineal hygiene is important for all hospitalized patients, especially after using a bedpan, after a bowel movement, or if fecal incontinence is present. Answer call lights quickly and offer the bedpan or urinal to bedridden patients at frequent intervals. These measures can prevent incontinence and decrease the number of incontinence episodes.

Prevention of CAUTI. All patients undergoing catheterization of the urinary tract are at risk for developing CAUTI. You play a key role in preventing CAUTI. Avoiding unnecessary catheterization and early removal of indwelling catheters are the most effective means for reducing CAUTI. Always follow aseptic technique during these procedures. Wash your hands before and after contact with each patient. Wear gloves for care of urinary catheters. The American Nurses Association offers an evidence-based clinical tool for decreasing CAUTI.[6] Special measures for the care of urethral catheters are discussed later in this chapter on p. 1052.

◆ **Acute Care.** Acute care for a patient with a UTI includes ensuring adequate fluid intake unless contraindicated. Maintaining adequate fluid intake may be hard because of the patient feeling that fluid intake will make the pain and urinary frequency associated with a UTI worse. Tell patients that fluids will increase frequency of urination but will also dilute the urine, making the bladder less irritable. Fluids will help flush out bacteria before they have a chance to colonize in the bladder. Caffeine, alcohol, citrus juices, chocolate, and highly spiced foods or beverages should be avoided because they are potential bladder irritants.

Application of local heat to the suprapubic area or lower back may relieve the discomfort associated with a UTI. Have the patient apply a heating pad (turned to its lowest setting) against the back or suprapubic area. A warm shower or sitting in a tub of warm water filled above the waist can also give temporary relief.

Teach the patient about the prescribed drug therapy, including side effects. Emphasize the importance of taking the full course of antibiotics. Often patients stop antibiotic therapy once symptoms disappear. This can lead to inadequate treatment, recurrence of infection, and/or bacterial resistance to antibiotics.

Sometimes a second drug or a reduced dosage of drug is given after the first course to suppress bacterial growth in patients susceptible to recurrent UTI. Teach the patient to monitor for signs of improvement (e.g., cloudy urine becomes clear) as well as a decrease in or cessation of symptoms. Tell patients to promptly report any of the following to their HCP: (1) persistence of bothersome LUTS beyond the antibiotic treatment course, (2) onset of flank pain, or (3) fever.

TABLE 45.6 Patient & Caregiver Teaching

Urinary Tract Infection

When teaching a patient and caregiver measures to prevent a recurrence of a urinary tract infection (UTI), include:

1. Take all antibiotics as prescribed. Symptoms may improve after 1–2 days of therapy, but organisms may still be present.
2. Practice appropriate hygiene, including:
   * Carefully clean the perineal region by separating the labia in females, or in males pulling back the foreskin if present when cleansing.
   * Wipe from front to back after urinating.
   * Cleanse with warm soapy water after each bowel movement.
3. Empty the bladder before and after sexual intercourse.
4. Void regularly, about every 3–4 hours during the day.
5. Maintain adequate fluid intake.
6. Avoid vaginal douches and harsh soaps, bubble baths, powders, and sprays in the perineal area.
7. Report to the HCP symptoms or signs of recurrent UTI (e.g., fever, cloudy urine, pain on urination, urgency, frequency).

◆ **Ambulatory Care.** Home care for the patient with a UTI should emphasize the importance of adhering to the drug regimen. Your responsibility is to teach the patient and caregiver about the need for ongoing care (Table 45.6). This includes: (1) taking antimicrobial drugs as ordered, (2) maintaining adequate daily fluid intake, (3) voiding regularly (every 3 to 4 hours), (4) voiding before and after intercourse, and (5) temporarily stopping the use of a diaphragm.

If treatment is complete and the symptoms are still present, teach the patient to get follow-up care. Recurrent symptoms because of bacterial persistence or inadequate treatment typically occur within 1 to 2 weeks after completion of therapy. If the patient has followed the treatment plan, a relapse indicates the need for further evaluation.

◆ Evaluation

The expected outcomes are that the patient with a UTI will
* Have normal urinary elimination patterns
* Report relief of bothersome urinary tract symptoms
* State knowledge of the treatment plan

ACUTE PYELONEPHRITIS

Etiology and Pathophysiology

Pyelonephritis is an inflammation of the renal parenchyma (Fig. 45.2) and collecting system, including the renal pelvis. The most common cause is bacterial infection. Fungi, protozoa, or viruses can also infect the kidney.[7]

Urosepsis is a systemic infection arising from a urologic source. Its prompt diagnosis and effective treatment are critical because it can lead to septic shock and death unless promptly treated. Septic shock is discussed in Chapter 65.

Pyelonephritis usually begins with colonization and infection of the lower urinary tract via the ascending urethral route. Bacteria normally found in the intestinal tract, including *E. coli* or *Proteus*, *Klebsiella*, or *Enterobacter* species, often cause pyelonephritis. A preexisting factor can be present, like *vesicoureteral reflux* (retrograde [backward] movement of urine from lower to upper urinary tract) or dysfunction of the lower urinary tract (e.g., obstruction from benign prostatic hyperplasia [BPH], stricture, urinary stone). For residents of

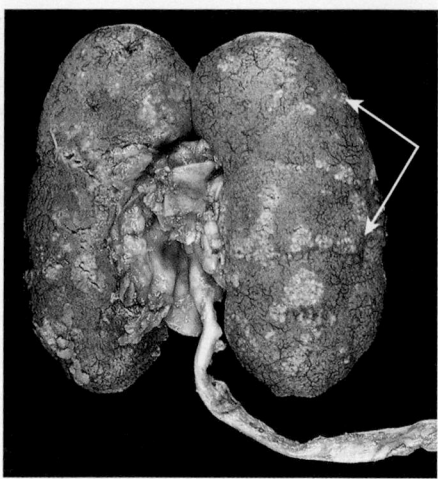

FIG 45.2 Acute pyelonephritis. Cortical surface shows grayish-white areas of inflammation and abscess formation *(arrows)*. (From Kumar V, Abbas AK, Aster JC, et al: *Robbins and Cotran pathologic basis of disease*, ed 8, Philadelphia, 2010, Saunders.)

long-term care facilities, CAUTI is a common cause of pyelonephritis and urosepsis.

Acute pyelonephritis often starts in the renal medulla and spreads to the adjacent cortex. Pregnancy-induced physiologic changes in the urinary system are one of the most important risk factors for acute pyelonephritis. Recurring episodes of pyelonephritis, especially in the presence of obstructive abnormalities, can lead to *chronic pyelonephritis* (discussed later).

Clinical Manifestations and Diagnostic Studies

The classic manifestations of acute pyelonephritis include (1) fever/chills, (2) nausea/vomiting (3) malaise, and (4) flank pain. They may include the LUTS, such as dysuria, urgency, and frequency. *Costovertebral angle tenderness* to percussion (costovertebral angle [CVA] pain) is typically present on the affected side. In some cases of pyelonephritis, renal scarring and decreased kidney function can occur, which can be potentially life-threatening.

Urinalysis results may show pyuria, bacteriuria, and varying degrees of hematuria. White blood cell (WBC) casts found in the urine may indicate involvement of the renal parenchyma. Urine cultures with sensitivities are done when pyelonephritis is suspected. Blood cultures may be done on hospitalized patients with more severe illness.

Ultrasounds may be done to identify anatomic abnormalities, hydronephrosis, renal abscesses, or an obstructing stone. CT scans are the preferred imaging studies. They can assess for signs of infection in the kidney and complications of pyelonephritis, such as impaired renal function, scarring, chronic pyelonephritis, or abscesses.

Interprofessional Care

The diagnostic tests and interprofessional care of acute pyelonephritis are outlined in Table 45.7. Patients with severe infections or complicating factors, such as nausea and vomiting with dehydration, need hospitalized.

The patient with mild symptoms may be treated as an outpatient with antibiotics for 7 to 14 days (Table 45.7). Parenteral antibiotics are often given initially in the hospital to rapidly establish high serum and urinary drug levels.[7] When initial treatment resolves acute symptoms and the patient can

---

TABLE 45.7 Interprofessional Care
Acute Pyelonephritis

Diagnostic Assessment
- History and physical examination
- Urinalysis
- Urine for culture and sensitivity
- Imaging studies: ultrasound (initially), CT scan, cystoscopy, voiding cystourethrogram (VCUG)
- CBC count with WBC differential
- Blood culture (if bacteremia is suspected)
- Percussion for flank (CVA) pain

Management
Mild Symptoms
- Outpatient management or short hospitalization
- Adequate fluid intake
- NSAIDs or antipyretic drugs
- Follow-up urine culture and imaging studies

Drug Therapy
- Empirically selected broad-spectrum antibiotics: ampicillin, fluoroquinolones (ciprofloxacin, levofloxacin), or TMP/SMX if infection expected to be susceptible
- Short course of IV antibiotics, such as aztreonam, ceftriaxone, ciprofloxacin, or levofloxacin, may be indicated
- Switch to sensitivity-guided therapy when results of urine and blood culture are available

Severe Symptoms
- Hospitalization
- Adequate fluid intake (parenteral initially; switch to oral fluids as nausea, vomiting, and dehydration subside)
- NSAIDs or antipyretic drugs to reverse fever and relieve discomfort
- Follow-up urine culture and imaging studies

Drug Therapy
- Parenteral antibiotics
  - Empirically selected broad-spectrum antibiotics: aminoglycosides without or with ampicillin, extended spectrum cephalosporins, extended-spectrum penicillin-carbapenem
  - Switch to sensitivity-guided antibiotic therapy when results of urine and blood culture are available
- Oral antibiotics when patient tolerates oral intake

---

tolerate oral fluids and drugs, the person may be discharged on a regimen of oral antibiotics for an additional 14 to 21 days. Symptoms and signs typically improve or resolve within 48 to 72 hours after starting therapy.

Relapses may be treated with a 6-week course of antibiotics. Antibiotic prophylaxis also may be used for recurrent infections. The effectiveness of therapy is based on the presence or absence of bacterial growth on urine culture.

Urosepsis is characterized by bacteriuria and bacteremia (bacteria in blood). Close observation and vital sign monitoring are essential. Prompt recognition and treatment of septic shock may prevent irreversible damage or death.

❖ NURSING MANAGEMENT: ACUTE PYELONEPHRITIS

◆ Nursing Assessment

Subjective and objective data that should be obtained from a patient with pyelonephritis are similar to those for the patient with a UTI (Table 45.5).

◆ Nursing Diagnoses

Nursing diagnoses for the patient with pyelonephritis include those for the patient with a UTI (see p. 1027).

◆ Planning

The overall goals are that the patient with pyelonephritis will have (1) normal renal function, (2) normal body temperature, (3) no complications, (4) relief of pain, and (5) no recurrence of symptoms.

◆ Nursing Implementation

Health promotion and maintenance measures are similar to those for cystitis (see p. 1031). Early treatment for cystitis can prevent ascending infections. Because patients with structural abnormalities of the urinary tract are at high risk for infection, stress the need for regular medical care.

Nursing interventions vary depending on the severity of symptoms. These include teaching the patient about the disease process with emphasis on (1) continuing medications as prescribed, (2) having a follow-up urine culture, and (3) recognizing signs of recurrence or relapse (Table 45.6). In addition to antibiotic therapy, encourage the patient to drink at least 8 glasses of fluid every day, even after the infection has been treated. Rest will increase patient comfort.

The patient who has frequent relapses or reinfections may receive long-term, low-dose antibiotics. Making certain the patient understands the reason for therapy is important to increase adherence.

◆ Evaluation

The expected outcomes for the patient with pyelonephritis are the same as for UTI (see p. 1028).

CHRONIC PYELONEPHRITIS

In *chronic pyelonephritis* the kidneys become inflamed, develop fibrosis (scarring) leading to loss of renal function, and can atrophy (shrink). Chronic pyelonephritis is usually the result of significant anatomic abnormalities, such as vesicoureteral reflux or recurring infections involving the upper urinary tract. However, it may occur in the absence of an existing infection, recent infection, or history of UTIs.

Radiologic imaging studies can confirm the diagnosis of chronic pyelonephritis and possible contributing factors. A renal biopsy can show the loss of functioning nephrons, infiltration of the parenchyma with inflammatory cells, and fibrosis.

The level of renal function in chronic pyelonephritis depends on whether 1 or both kidneys are affected, the extent of scarring, and the presence of coexisting infection. Chronic pyelonephritis can progress to end-stage renal disease (ESRD). Monitoring and treating infection and correcting any underlying contributing factors are important. Nursing and interprofessional management of the patient with CKD is discussed in Chapter 46.

URETHRITIS

Urethritis is inflammation of the urethra. Causes of urethritis include a bacterial or viral infection, *Trichomonas* or monilial infection (especially in women), chlamydial infection, and gonorrhea (especially in men).

In men, the causes of urethritis are usually sexually transmitted. Purulent discharge can indicate a gonococcal urethritis.

A clear discharge typically signifies a nongonococcal urethritis. (Sexually transmitted infections are discussed in Chapter 52.) Urethritis produces bothersome LUTS, including dysuria, urgency, and frequency, similar to those seen with cystitis.

In women, urethritis is hard to diagnose. It often produces bothersome LUTS, but urethral discharge may not be present.

Treatment of urethritis is based on identifying and treating the cause and providing symptomatic relief. Drugs used for bacterial infections include TMP/SMX, doxycycline (Vibramycin), ceftriaxone, and nitrofurantoin. Metronidazole (Flagyl) and tinidazole (Monistat) are options for treating *Trichomonas* infection. Drugs, such as nystatin, clotrimazole, or fluconazole, may be used for monilial infections. In chlamydial infections, doxycycline or azithromycin may be used. For treatment of gonococcal urethritis, the preferred first-line treatment is azithromycin 1 g orally with 250 mg intramuscular ceftriaxone. Women with negative urine cultures and no pyuria usually do not respond to antibiotics.

Warm sitz baths may temporarily relieve bothersome symptoms. Teach the patient to (1) avoid using vaginal deodorant sprays, (2) properly cleanse the perineal area after bowel movements and voiding, and (3) avoid sexual intercourse for at least 7 days. Teach patients with sexually transmitted urethritis to refer their sex partners for evaluation and testing if they had sexual contact in the 60 days before the onset of the patient's symptoms or diagnosis.

URETHRAL DIVERTICULA

Urethral diverticula are localized outpouchings of the urethra. Typically, they result from enlargement of obstructed periurethral glands. In women, who have a higher incidence than men, the diverticula protrude into the anterior vaginal wall. The rare cases reported in males usually are associated with congenital lower urinary tract anomalies or surgical trauma.

The periurethral glands are found along the entire length of the urethra, with the majority draining into the distal third of the urethra. Skene's glands are the largest of these glands. Causes of urethral diverticula include urethral trauma, vaginal delivery, urethral instrumentation, urethral dilation, and frequent infections of the periurethral glands.

Symptoms include dysuria, postvoid dribbling, frequency (voiding more often than every 2 hours), urgency, suprapubic discomfort or pressure, dyspareunia, and a feeling of incomplete bladder emptying. Urinary incontinence is often present. However, many women have no symptoms.

The urine may contain gross blood (hematuria) or sediment, which gives it a cloudy appearance. An anterior vaginal wall mass may be felt on physical examination. When palpated, the mass is often quite tender and expresses purulent discharge through the urethra.

Radiographic studies, such as ultrasound and MRI, are helpful in determining the size of the diverticulum in relation to the urethral lumen. A voiding cystourethrography (VCUG) may be done but has a lower sensitivity than that of ultrasound and MRI. A urethroscopy may be of benefit.

Surgical options include transvaginal diverticulectomy, marsupialization (creation of a permanent opening) of the diverticular sac into the vagina (*Spence procedure*), and urethroscopic surgical excision. Stress urinary incontinence, infection, bleeding, and urethral-vaginal fistula are potential complications of the surgery.

INTERSTITIAL CYSTITIS/PAINFUL BLADDER SYNDROME

Interstitial cystitis (IC) is a chronic, painful inflammatory disease of the bladder characterized by symptoms of urgency, frequency, and pain in the bladder and/or pelvis. IC is often called bladder pain syndrome or painful bladder syndrome (PBS). The term *IC/PBS* refers to cases of urinary pain that cannot be attributed to other causes, such as UTI or urinary stones. IC/PBS is more common in women, affecting about 3 to 8 million women and 1 to 4 million men each year.[8]

The cause of IC/PBS is unknown. It is likely multifactorial. Possible causes include neurogenic hypersensitivity of the lower urinary tract, changes in mast cells in the muscle and/or mucosal layers of the bladder, infection with an unusual organism (e.g., slow-growing virus), or production of a toxic substance in the urine.

Clinical Manifestations and Diagnostic Studies

The 2 primary manifestations of IC/PBS are pain and bothersome LUTS (e.g., frequency, urgency). People with severe cases may void as often as 60 times in a day, including nighttime urination. The pain is usually in the suprapubic area, but may involve the vagina, labia, or entire perineal region, including the rectum and anus. The pain varies from mild to severe. The pain can be worsened by bladder filling, postponed urination, physical exertion, pressure against the suprapubic area, certain foods, or emotional distress. Voiding temporarily relieves pain. Bothersome LUTS are similar to a UTI. The condition is often misdiagnosed as a recurring or chronic UTI or, in men, chronic prostatitis.

The patient may have periods of remission and exacerbation. Women often report pain that occurs before menstruation. Sexual intercourse or emotional stress worsen pain. Some patients have symptoms that disappear altogether after a period of weeks to months. Others have persistent symptoms over months to years.

IC/PBS is a diagnosis of exclusion. A careful history and physical examination are necessary to rule out other disorders that produce similar symptoms, such as cancer, UTI, or endometriosis. Urine cultures do not find any bacteria or other organisms in the urine. Cystoscopic examination may reveal a small bladder capacity, Hunner lesions (distinct inflammatory areas on the bladder wall), and glomerulations (superficial ulcerations with pinpoint bleeding), but these findings are not always present.

Interprofessional Care

Because the cause of IC/PBS is unknown, no single treatment consistently reverses or relieves symptoms. Various therapies have been effective, including nutritional and drug therapy. People with IC/PBS do not respond to antibiotic therapy. They rarely need surgical therapy.

Eliminating foods and beverages that are likely to irritate the bladder may provide some relief from symptoms. Typical bladder irritants include caffeine; alcohol; citrus products; carbonated drinks; chocolate; foods containing vinegar, curries, or hot peppers; and foods or beverages likely to lower urinary pH, including fruits such as cranberries. An over-the-counter (OTC) dietary supplement called *calcium glycerophosphate* (Prelief) alkalinizes the urine and may provide relief from the irritating effects of certain foods. Recipes and menus for a well-balanced diet that is specifically designed to avoid bladder-irritating foods and beverages are available at the website for the Interstitial Cystitis Association *(www.ichelp.org)*.

Because stress can worsen or cause flare-ups of IC/PBS symptoms, stress management techniques such as relaxation breathing and imagery (see Chapter 6) may be helpful. Using lubrication or changing positions may decrease pain associated with sexual intercourse.

The tricyclic antidepressants, amitriptyline (preferred) and nortriptyline, may reduce burning and urinary frequency. Pentosan (Elmiron) is the only oral agent approved for the treatment of patients with symptoms of IC. It enhances the protective effects of the glycosaminoglycan layer of the bladder and relieves pain by reducing the irritative effects of urine on the bladder wall. These drugs provide relief over time (weeks to months) but do not give the immediate relief that may be needed for an acute exacerbation of symptoms. A short course of opioid analgesics may be used for immediate relief. Antihistamine therapy, such as hydroxyzine, may be of use.

Pelvic physical therapy and bladder hypodistention therapy may be useful. Dimethyl sulfoxide (DMSO) can be directly instilled into the bladder through a small catheter. This drug desensitizes pain receptors in the bladder wall. Heparin, lidocaine, or sodium bicarbonate can be instilled into the bladder to relieve acute IC/PBS symptoms. Like pentosan, we think they enhance the protective properties of the glycosaminoglycan layer of the bladder. Intradetrusor botulism toxin and use of cyclosporine A have been found to be of some help.

While uncommon, surgery can be considered to improve severe, debilitating pain. Sacral neuromodulation or fulguration (using high-frequency energy to destroy a lesion) and resection of Hunner lesions are options. Urinary diversion, such as an ileal conduit, without or with removal of the bladder, is an option when other measures fail. Unfortunately, some patients have reported pain within the urinary diversion, which means that some factor in the urine may contribute to IC/PBS in certain cases.

❖ NURSING MANAGEMENT: INTERSTITIAL CYSTITIS/PAINFUL BLADDER SYNDROME

Assess the characteristics of the pain associated with IC/PBS. Ask the patient about specific dietary or lifestyle factors that relieve pain or make it worse. Teach the patient to keep a bladder log or voiding diary over a period of at least 3 days to determine voiding frequency and patterns of nocturia. Keeping a pain record at the same time may be useful.

A UTI may occur during IC/PBS management because of diagnostic instrumentation and frequent bladder instillations. A UTI is likely to cause an acute exacerbation of bothersome LUTS and urinary frequency, as well as dysuria (not typically associated with IC/PBS), odorous urine, and hematuria.

Review with the patient good nutrition, particularly in light of the broad dietary restrictions often necessary to control IC-related pain. Advise the patient to take a multivitamin containing no more than the recommended dietary allowance for essential vitamins and to avoid high-potency vitamins, because they may irritate the bladder. The patient should avoid clothing that creates suprapubic pressure, including pants with tight belts or restrictive waistlines. Educational materials about diet, coping with the need for frequent urination, and coping with the emotional burden of IC/PBS are available from the Interstitial

Cystitis Association *(www.ichelp.org)*. Reassurance that IC/PBS is a real condition experienced by others and that it can be treated may relieve the anxiety, anger, guilt, and frustration related to having chronic pain and voiding dysfunction in the absence of a clear-cut diagnosis and treatment strategy.

GENITOURINARY TUBERCULOSIS

Genitourinary tuberculosis (GUTB) is the second most common type of extrapulmonary tuberculosis. Between 2% and 20% of patients with pulmonary TB will develop GUTB. Onset can occur 1 to 46 years after the primary lung infection.[9,10] When the kidney is first infected with bacilli, the patient is often asymptomatic. Sometimes the patient will have fatigue and develops a low-grade fever. As the lesions ulcerate, infection descends to the bladder and other GU organs. The patient has cystitis, frequent urination, burning on voiding, and epididymitis (in men). Hematuria, pyuria, and symptoms of a UTI are the first manifestations in most patients with GUTB.

A diagnosis of GUTB is based on finding *Mycobacterium tuberculosis* bacilli in the urine. Radiographic tests include plain radiographs, CT scan, IV pyelography, and VCUG. These studies help determine the extent and severity of the disease. Tuberculin skin test results are positive in most patients, but this finding only means that the person has had previous inhalation of mycobacteria rather than active disease.

Long-term complications of GUTB depend on the duration of the disease. Scarring of the renal parenchyma, calcifications, hydronephrosis, and the development of ureteral strictures occur. The earlier treatment is started, the less likely renal failure will develop. The patient may need long-term urologic follow-up. Nursing and interprofessional management of the patient with TB is discussed in Chapter 27.

IMMUNOLOGIC DISORDERS OF KIDNEY

GLOMERULONEPHRITIS

Glomerulonephritis (inflammation of the glomeruli) affects both kidneys equally and is the third leading cause of ESRD in the United States. Although the glomerulus is the primary site of inflammation, tubular and interstitial changes as well as vascular scarring and hardening *(glomerulosclerosis)* within the kidney can occur.[11]

A variety of conditions are associated with glomerulonephritis. These range from kidney infections, drugs toxic to the kidneys, problems with the immune system, and systemic diseases (Table 45.8). Glomerulonephritis can be acute or chronic.

TABLE 45.8 Causes and Risk Factors for Glomerulonephritis (GN)

Cause or Risk Factor	Description	Cause or Risk Factor	Description
Conditions Causing Scarring of Glomeruli		**Infections**	
Diabetic nephropathy	• Primary cause of end-stage renal disease in the United States (see Chapter 46) • Microvascular changes of diffuse glomerulosclerosis involving thickening of the glomerular basement membrane	Infective endocarditis	• Bacteria can cause an infection of 1 or more of the heart valves (see Chapter 36) • People at risk include those with a heart defect, such as a damaged or artificial heart valve • Bacterial endocarditis is associated with GN, but the exact cause is not known
Focal segmental glomerulosclerosis	• Characterized by scattered scarring of glomeruli • May result from another disease or occur for unknown reasons	Poststreptococcal glomerulonephritis	• GN may develop 1–2 wk after a streptococcal throat infection or, rarely, a skin infection (impetigo) • Antibodies (Ab) to strep antigen (Ag) develop and the Ag-Ab deposit in the glomeruli, causing inflammation
Hypertension	• Nephrosclerosis is a complication of hypertension • GN can cause hypertension	Viral infections	• Viral infections can trigger GN • Common viruses include HIV, hepatitis B, and hepatitis C viruses
Immune Diseases		**Vasculitis**	
Goodpasture syndrome	• Autoimmune disorder that causes lung and kidney disease • Causes bleeding into lungs and GN	Polyarteritis	• Autoimmune disease that affects small and medium blood vessels • Can affect any organ but common in heart, kidneys, and intestines
Immunoglobulin A (IgA) nephropathy	• Results from deposits of IgA in the glomeruli • Characterized by recurrent episodes of hematuria	Wegener's granulomatosis	• Form of vasculitis affecting small and medium blood vessels • Most often affects kidneys, lungs, and upper respiratory tract
Scleroderma	• Disease of unknown cause characterized by widespread changes in connective tissue and vascular lesions in many organs (see Chapter 64) • In the kidney, vascular lesions are associated with fibrosis • Severity of renal involvement varies	**Other Causes**	
		Amyloidosis	• Caused by infiltration of tissues with amyloid (hyaline substance) • Hyaline bodies consist largely of protein • Kidney involvement is common • Proteinuria is often the first clinical manifestation
Systemic lupus erythematosus (SLE)	• Autoimmune disorder characterized by the involvement of several tissues and organs, particularly joints, skin, and kidneys (see Chapter 64) • GN often occurs in SLE and has a poor prognosis	Illegal drug use	• People who use these drugs are at increased risk for GN

GN, Glomerulonephritis.

With *acute glomerulonephritis,* symptoms come on suddenly and may be temporary or reversible. An example of this is acute poststreptococcal glomerulonephritis (discussed in the next section). *Chronic glomerulonephritis* is slowly progressive glomerulonephritis that can lead to irreversible renal failure (discussed later in this chapter).

Diagnostic studies and a comprehensive history, including any recent infection, such as a sore throat or upper respiratory tract infection, or a diagnosis of diabetes, aid in identifying the type of glomerulonephritis present.

Acute Poststreptococcal Glomerulonephritis

Acute poststreptococcal glomerulonephritis (APSGN) is a common type of acute glomerulonephritis. It is most common in children, young adults, and adults older than 60 years. APSGN develops about 1 to 2 weeks after an infection of the tonsils, pharynx, or skin (e.g., streptococcal sore throat, impetigo) by nephrotoxic strains of group A β-hemolytic streptococci.[12] The person makes antibodies to the streptococcal antigen. Although the exact mechanism is not known, tissue injury occurs as the antigen-antibody complexes are deposited in the glomeruli, complement is activated (see Chapter 11), and inflammation results.

Manifestations include generalized body edema, hypertension, oliguria, hematuria, and varying degrees of proteinuria. Fluid retention occurs because of decreased glomerular filtration. At first, edema appears in low-pressure tissues, such as those around the eyes *(periorbital edema).* Later it progresses to involve the total body, with ascites or peripheral edema in the legs. Smoky urine indicates bleeding in the upper urinary tract. The degree of proteinuria varies with the severity of the glomerulonephropathy. Hypertension primarily results from increased extracellular fluid volume. The patient may have abdominal or flank pain. Sometimes the patient may be asymptomatic, and the problem is found on routine urinalysis.

The diagnosis of APSGN is based on a complete history and physical examination. An immune response to the streptococci is often shown by assessment of antistreptolysin-O (ASO) titers. The finding of decreased complement components (especially C3 and CH50) indicates an immune-mediated response. A renal biopsy may be done to confirm the disease.

Dipstick urinalysis and urine sediment microscopy can reveal significant numbers of erythrocytes. Erythrocyte casts are highly suggestive of APSGN. Proteinuria may range from mild to severe. Blood tests include blood urea nitrogen (BUN) and serum creatinine to assess the extent of renal impairment.

❖ NURSING AND INTERPROFESSIONAL MANAGEMENT: ACUTE POSTSTREPTOCOCCAL GLOMERULONEPHRITIS

More than 95% of patients with APSGN recover completely or improve rapidly with conservative management. Accurate recognition and assessment are critical since chronic glomerulonephritis can develop if the patient is not treated appropriately.

Management focuses on symptomatic relief. Rest is recommended until the signs of glomerular inflammation (proteinuria, hematuria) and hypertension subside. Restricting sodium and fluid intake and diuretics can reduce edema. Severe hypertension is treated with antihypertensive drugs. Dietary protein intake may be restricted if there is evidence of an increase in nitrogenous wastes (e.g., increased BUN). The dietary protein restriction varies with the degree of proteinuria. Low-protein, low-sodium, fluid-restricted diets are discussed in Chapter 46.

Antibiotics should be given only if the streptococcal infection is still present. Corticosteroids and cytotoxic drugs are not of value in treating APSGN.

One of the most important ways to prevent APSGN is to encourage early diagnosis and treatment of sore throats and skin lesions. If a culture is positive for streptococci, treatment with the appropriate antibiotic therapy is essential. Encourage the patient to take the full course of antibiotics to ensure that the bacteria have been eradicated. Good personal hygiene is a key factor in preventing the spread of cutaneous streptococcal infections.

In most cases, recovery from the acute glomerulonephritis is complete. However, if progressive involvement occurs and chronic glomerulonephritis develops, ESRD can result.

Chronic Glomerulonephritis

Chronic glomerulonephritis is a syndrome of permanent and progressive renal fibrosis. It can progress to ESRD. Most types of glomerulonephritis and nephrotic syndrome can eventually lead to chronic glomerulonephritis. Some people who develop chronic glomerulonephritis have no history of kidney disease. The cause of a patient's chronic glomerulonephritis may not be found. Although not common, an inherited disorder (e.g., Alport syndrome [see p. 1043]) may be the cause.

With chronic glomerulonephritis, symptoms develop slowly over time. Patients are often unaware that progressive kidney impairment is occurring. They do not realize that they have severe kidney impairment until a diagnostic evaluation is done. Chronic glomerulonephritis is often discovered coincidentally with the finding of an abnormality on a urinalysis, high BP, or increased serum creatinine.

The syndrome is characterized by proteinuria, hematuria, and the slow development of uremia (see Chapter 46) because of decreasing renal function. Chronic glomerulonephritis progresses insidiously toward ESRD over a course of several years.

Manifestations include varying degrees of hematuria (ranging from microscopic to gross), proteinuria, and urinary excretion of various formed elements, including red blood cells (RBCs), WBCs, and casts. Increased BUN and serum creatinine levels are common. Ultrasound and CT scan are the preferred diagnostic measures. However, a renal biopsy may be done to determine the exact cause of the glomerulonephritis.

The patient's history provides vital information related to glomerulonephritis. Assess exposure to drugs (e.g., nonsteroidal anti-inflammatory drugs [NSAIDs]), microbial infections, and viral infections (e.g., hepatitis). Evaluate the patient for more generalized conditions involving immune disorders, such as systemic lupus erythematosus (SLE). The patient may not recall any history of renal problems.

Treatment depends on the cause of the chronic glomerulonephritis and includes supportive and symptomatic care. Management of CKD is discussed in Chapter 46.

Goodpasture Syndrome

Goodpasture syndrome is an autoimmune disease characterized by antibodies that attack the glomerular and alveolar basement membranes. Damage to the kidneys and lungs results when binding of the antibody causes an inflammatory reaction mediated by complement activation (see Chapter 11).

Goodpasture syndrome is a rare disease that occurs primarily in older children and adults, especially those in their 30s to 60s. The manifestations can include flu-like and pulmonary symptoms, such as cough, mild shortness of breath, hemoptysis, crackles, and pulmonary insufficiency. Renal involvement includes hematuria, weakness, pallor, and anemia. It can proceed quickly to renal failure. Pulmonary hemorrhage usually occurs and may precede glomerular abnormalities by weeks or months.

Current management includes corticosteroids, immunosuppressive drugs (e.g., cyclophosphamide, azathioprine [Imuran]), plasmapheresis (see Chapter 13), rituximab, and dialysis. Plasmapheresis removes the circulating anti–glomerular basement membrane (GBM) antibodies, and immunosuppressive therapy inhibits further antibody production. Renal transplantation can be tried after the circulating anti-GBM antibody titer decreases. Although the disease may recur in the transplanted kidney, this is not a contraindication to transplantation.

Encourage smoking cessation. The patient receives nursing care appropriate for a critically ill patient who has AKI (see Chapter 46) and respiratory distress (see Chapter 67). Death is often from hemorrhage in the lungs and respiratory failure.

Rapidly Progressive Glomerulonephritis

Rapidly progressive glomerulonephritis (RPGN) is a type of glomerular disease with glomerular crescent formations. In contrast to chronic glomerulonephritis, which develops slowly and progresses over many years, RPGN is characterized by rapid, progressive loss of renal function over days to weeks.

RPGN can occur in a variety of situations: (1) as a complication of inflammatory or infectious disease (e.g., APSGN, Goodpasture syndrome), (2) as a complication of a systemic disease (e.g., SLE), (3) or as an idiopathic disease.

Manifestations include hypertension, edema, proteinuria, hematuria, and RBC casts. Treatment is directed toward correction of fluid overload, hypertension, uremia, and inflammatory injury to the kidney. Treatment includes corticosteroids, cyclophosphamide, and plasmapheresis. Dialysis therapy and transplantation are used as maintenance therapy for the patient with RPGN who has progressed to ESRD. After kidney transplantation, RPGN may recur.

NEPHROTIC SYNDROME

Nephrotic syndrome results when the glomerulus is excessively permeable to plasma protein, causing proteinuria that leads to low plasma albumin and tissue edema.

Etiology and Clinical Manifestations

Common causes of nephrotic syndrome are listed in Table 45.9. About one third of patients with nephrotic syndrome have a systemic disease, such as diabetes or SLE.[13]

The characteristic manifestations of nephrotic syndrome include peripheral edema, massive proteinuria, hypertension, hyperlipidemia, hypoalbuminemia, and foamy urine. The increased glomerular membrane permeability found in nephrotic syndrome is responsible for the massive excretion of protein in the urine. This results in decreased total serum protein and subsequent edema formation. Ascites and *anasarca* (massive generalized edema) develop if there is severe hypoalbuminemia.

TABLE 45.9 **Causes of Nephrotic Syndrome**	
Primary Glomerular Disease • Acute glomerulonephritis • Membranous glomerulopathy • Primary nephrotic syndrome • Rapidly progressive glomerulonephritis **Extrarenal Causes** **Allergens (Minimal Change Disease)** • Bee sting • Pollen **Cancers** • Hodgkin's lymphoma • Leukemias • Solid tumors of lungs, colon, stomach, breast	**Drugs** • captopril • heroin • NSAIDs • penicillamine **Infections** • Bacterial (streptococcal, syphilis) • Protozoal (malaria) • Viral (hepatitis, HIV, mononucleosis) **Multisystem Disease** • Amyloidosis • Diabetes • SLE

The diminished plasma oncotic pressure from the decreased serum proteins stimulates hepatic lipoprotein synthesis, which results in hyperlipidemia. At first, cholesterol and low-density lipoproteins are high. Later, triglyceride levels increase. Fat bodies (fatty casts), often appear in the urine, causing foamy urine.

Immune responses are altered in nephrotic syndrome. As a result, infection is a primary cause of morbidity and mortality. Calcium and skeletal abnormalities may occur, including hypocalcemia, blunted calcium response to parathyroid hormone, hyperparathyroidism, and osteomalacia.

Hypercoagulability is a serious issue for those with nephrotic syndrome. Hypercoagulability increases the risk for arterial and venous thromboembolism, including pulmonary embolism and deep vein or renal thrombus.

❖ Interprofessional and Nursing Care

Specific treatment of nephrotic syndrome depends on the cause. The goals are to cure or control the primary disease and relieve the symptoms. Corticosteroids and cyclophosphamide may be used in the treatment of nephrotic syndrome. Prednisone has been effective to varying degrees for some causes of nephrotic syndrome (e.g., membranous glomerulonephritis, lupus nephritis). Managing diabetes is an important consideration for nephrotic syndrome related to diabetes.

Angiotensin-converting enzyme inhibitor or angiotensin receptor blocker drugs are used to try to reduce urine protein losses. Diuretics (typically loop diuretics) can improve edema.

The treatment of hyperlipidemia includes lipid-lowering agents (see Table 33.6). Anticoagulant therapy may be needed if thrombosis is present.

The patient is placed on a low-sodium (less than 2.3 g/day), moderate-protein (1 to 2 g/kg/day) diet. If urine protein losses are high (more than 10 g/day), more protein may be recommended. Patients with nephrotic syndrome are usually anorexic and have the potential to become malnourished from the excess loss of protein in the urine. Serve small, frequent meals in a pleasant setting to encourage better dietary intake.

A major nursing intervention for a patient with nephrotic syndrome focuses on the management of edema. Assess the edema by (1) weighing the patient daily, (2) accurately recording intake and output, and (3) measuring abdominal girth or extremity size. Compare this information daily to assess the effectiveness of treatment. Clean the edematous skin carefully. Avoid trauma to the skin. Monitor the effectiveness of diuretic therapy.

Because the patient with nephrotic syndrome is susceptible to infection, teach the patient to avoid exposure to persons with known infections. Support for the patient, especially in helping cope with an altered body image, is essential because of the embarrassment and shame often associated with the edematous appearance.

OBSTRUCTIVE UROPATHIES

Urinary obstruction refers to any anatomic or functional condition that blocks or impedes the flow of urine (Fig. 45.3). It may be congenital or acquired. Damaging effects from urinary tract obstruction affect the system above the level of the obstruction. The severity of these effects depends on the location, duration of obstruction, amount of pressure or dilation, and presence of urinary stasis or infection. Infection increases the risk for irreversible damage.[14]

When obstruction occurs at the level of the bladder neck or prostate, significant bladder changes can occur. Detrusor muscle fibers *hypertrophy* (increase in size) to contract harder to push urine out a narrower pathway. Over a long period, the detrusor loses its ability to compensate for this resistance, eventually leading to a large residual urine volume in the bladder.

When *bladder outlet obstruction* is present, pressure increases during bladder filling or storage and can be transmitted to the ureter. This pressure leads to *reflux* (backflow, or backward movement, of urine), *hydroureter* (ureteral dilation and distention), vesicoureteral reflux (backflow of urine from the lower to upper urinary tract), and **hydronephrosis** (dilation or enlargement of the renal pelvises and calyces) (Fig. 45.4). Chronic pyelonephritis and renal atrophy may develop. If only 1 kidney is obstructed, the other kidney may try to compensate by enlarging.

Partial obstruction may occur in the ureter or at the ureteropelvic junction (UPJ) (where the renal pelvis narrows into the ureter). If the pressure stays low or moderate, the kidney may continue to dilate with no noticeable loss of function. Urinary stasis and reflux increase the risk for pyelonephritis. If only 1 kidney is involved, and the other kidney is functioning, the patient may be asymptomatic.

If both kidneys or only 1 functioning kidney is involved (e.g., if the patient has only 1 kidney), changes in renal function (e.g., increased BUN and serum creatinine levels) occur. Progressive obstruction can lead to renal failure. Treatment requires finding and relieving the blockage. This can include insertion of a tube (e.g., urethral or ureteral), surgical correction of the primary problem, or diversion of the urinary stream above the level of blockage.

URINARY TRACT CALCULI

In their lifetime, 13% of men and 7% of women in the United States will have **nephrolithiasis,** or kidney stone disease. The term **calculus** refers to the stone, and *lithiasis* refers to stone formation.

Most patients are middle-aged adults. The risk for developing kidney stones increases with age.[15] Stone formation is more frequent in whites than in blacks, Hispanics, and Asians.

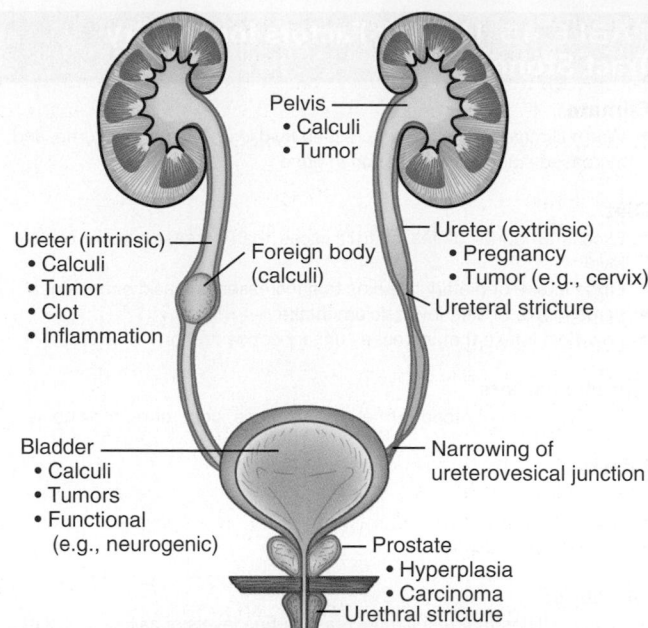

FIG 45.3 Sites and causes of upper and lower urinary tract obstruction.

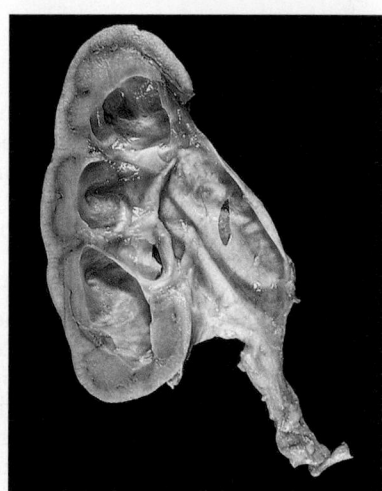

FIG 45.4 Hydronephrosis of the kidney. Note the marked dilation of the pelvis and calyces and thinning of the renal parenchyma. (From Kumar V, Abbas AK, Aster JC, et al: *Robbins and Cotran pathologic basis of disease,* ed 8, Philadelphia, 2010, Saunders.)

The incidence is higher in persons with a family history of stone formation. Stones recur in up to 50% of patients. In the United States, the incidence of stone disease is highest in the Southeast, followed by the Southwest and Midwest. Stone formation occurs more often in the summer months, supporting the possible contributing factors of a hot climate and dehydration.

GENDER DIFFERENCES
Urinary Tract Stones

Men
- Most likely to have urinary stones, except for struvite stones

Women
- More likely to have struvite stones associated with UTI

TABLE 45.10 Risk Factors for Urinary Tract Stones

Climate
- Warm climates that cause increased fluid loss, low urine volume, and increased solute concentration in urine

Diet
- Excess amounts of tea or fruit juices that increase urinary oxalate level
- Large intake of dietary proteins that increases uric acid excretion
- Large intake of salt, low calcium intake
- Low fluid intake that increases urinary concentration

Genetic Factors
- Family history of stone formation, cystinuria, gout, or renal acidosis

Lifestyle
- Immobility
- Obesity
- Sedentary occupation

Metabolic
- Abnormalities that result in increased urine levels of calcium, oxalate, uric acid, or citric acid

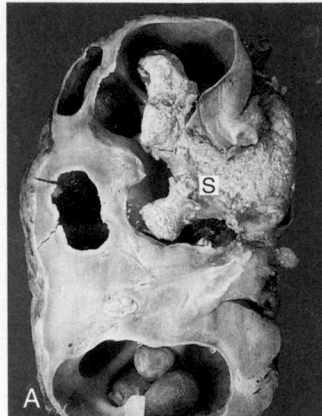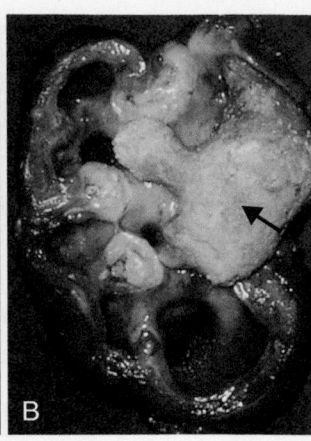

FIG 45.5 A, Renal staghorn stone. The renal pelvis is filled with a large stone that is shaped to its contours, resembling the horns of a stag *(S)*. B, Imbedded staghorn stone *(arrow)* in hydronephrotic, infected, nonfunctioning kidney. (*A,* From Stevens A, Lowe JS, Scott I: *Core pathology: Illustrated review in color,* ed 3, London, 2009, Mosby Ltd. *B,* From Bullock N, Doble A, Turner W, et al: *Urology: An illustrated colour text,* London, 2008, Churchill Livingstone.)

Etiology and Pathophysiology

Many factors are involved in the incidence and type of stone formation, including climatic, dietary, genetic, metabolic, and lifestyle influences (Table 45.10). No single theory accounts for stone formation in all cases. Crystals, when in a supersaturated concentration, can precipitate and unite to form a stone. Keeping urine dilute and free flowing reduces the risk for recurrent stone formation in many people.

We think kidney stones form when certain crystal-forming substances are not diluted by the kidney and/or there is reduced ability of the kidneys to keep the crystals from sticking together. Urinary pH, solute load, and inhibitors in the urine affect the formation of stones. The higher the pH (alkaline), the less soluble are calcium and phosphate. The lower the pH (acidic), the less soluble are uric acid and cystine. When a substance is not very soluble in fluid, it is more likely to precipitate out of solution.

Other key factors in stone formation include obstruction with associated urinary stasis and UTI with urea-splitting bacteria (e.g., *Proteus, Klebsiella, Pseudomonas,* and some species of staphylococci). These bacteria cause the urine to become alkaline and contribute to the formation of struvite stones. Infected stones, trapped in the kidney (Fig. 45.5), may assume a staghorn configuration as the stone branches to occupy a larger part of the collecting system. These stones can lead to a renal infection, hydronephrosis, and loss of kidney function.

Genetic factors may contribute to urine stone formation. Cystinuria, an autosomal recessive disorder, causes a markedly increased excretion of cystine.

🌐 PROMOTING HEALTH EQUITY
Urologic Disorders

- Urinary tract stones are more common among whites than blacks.
- Uric acid stones are more common in Jewish men.
- Bladder cancer has a higher incidence among white men than black men.
- Urinary incontinence is underreported because culturally it is seen as a social hygiene problem causing patient embarrassment.

Types of Urinary Stones

The 5 major categories of stones are (1) calcium oxalate, (2) calcium phosphate, (3) cystine, (4) struvite (magnesium ammonium phosphate), and (5) uric acid (Table 45.11). Calcium stones can exist as calcium oxalate, calcium phosphate, or a mixture of both. Although calcium stones are the most common, stone composition may be mixed. Stones can be found in various locations in the urinary tract (Figs. 45.3 and 45.5).

Clinical Manifestations

The first symptom of a kidney stone is usually severe pain that begins suddenly. Typically, a person feels a sharp, severe pain in the flank area, back, or lower abdomen. People describe the pain as the most excruciating that a person can endure. We call this pain *renal colic*. It results from the stretching, dilation, and spasm of the ureter in response to the obstructing stone. Nausea and vomiting may occur due to the severe pain.

Urinary stones cause manifestations when they obstruct urinary flow. Common sites of obstruction are at the UPJ and ureterovesical junction (UVJ). The type of pain is determined by the location of the stone. If the obstruction is in a calyx or at the UPJ, the patient may have dull costovertebral flank pain or renal colic. Pain resulting from the passage of a stone down the ureter is intense and colicky. If the stone is nonobstructing, pain may be absent.

Patients with renal colic have a hard time being still. They go from walking to sitting to lying down, and then they repeat the process. Some people refer to this as the "kidney stone dance."

The patient may be in mild shock with cool, moist skin. As a stone nears the UVJ, pain moves around toward the abdomen and down toward the lower quadrant. Men may have testicular pain, while women may have labial pain. Both men and women can have groin pain. The patient may have manifestations of a UTI with dysuria, fever, and chills.

Diagnostic Studies

Stones are easily diagnosed with either a noncontrast helical (spiral) CT scan or ultrasound. A complete urinalysis helps confirm the diagnosis of a urinary stone by assessing for hematuria

TABLE 45.11 Types of Urinary Tract Stones

Characteristics	Predisposing Factors	Treatment
Calcium Oxalate		
Small, can easily get trapped in ureter. More frequent in men than in women. *Incidence:* 35%–40%	Idiopathic hypercalciuria, hyperoxaluria, independent of urinary pH, family history	Increase hydration. Reduce dietary oxalate, animal protein, and sodium (see Table 45.12). Encourage increased intake of calcium, fruits, and vegetables. Give thiazide diuretics. Give potassium citrate to maintain alkaline urine. Avoid vitamin C and calcium supplements.
Calcium Phosphate		
Mixed stones (typically), with struvite or oxalate stones. *Incidence:* 8%–10%	Alkaline urine, primary hyperparathyroidism	Increase hydration. Treat underlying causes and other stones. Reduce dietary sodium and animal protein intake. Increase dietary calcium intake. Avoid vitamin C supplements.
Cystine		
Genetic autosomal recessive defect. Defective absorption of cystine in GI tract and kidney, excess concentrations causing stone formation. *Incidence:* 1%–2%	Acidic urine	Increase hydration. Give α-penicillamine, captopril or tiopronin to prevent cystine crystallization. Give potassium citrate to keep urine alkaline.
Struvite (Magnesium Ammonium Phosphate)		
3–4 times more common in women. Always associated with urinary tract infections. Large staghorn type (usually) (Fig. 45.5). *Incidence:* 10%–15%	Urinary tract infections (usually *Proteus*)	Give antimicrobial agents, acetohydroxamic acid. May need surgery to remove stone. Take measures to acidify urine.
Uric Acid		
Predominant in men, high incidence in Jewish men. *Incidence:* 5%–8%	Gout, acidic urine, inherited condition	Reduce urinary concentration of uric acid. Alkalinize urine with potassium citrate. Give allopurinol. Reduce dietary purines (see Table 45.12).

and crystalluria. Measuring urine pH is useful in the diagnosis of struvite stones (tendency to alkaline or high pH) and uric acid or cystine stones (tendency to acidic or low pH).

Retrieval and analysis of the stone(s) is important in the diagnosis of the underlying problem contributing to stone formation. The patient's serum calcium, phosphorus, sodium, potassium, bicarbonate, uric acid, BUN, and creatinine levels are measured. Patients who have recurrent stone formation should have a 24-hour urinary measurement of calcium, phosphorus, magnesium, sodium, oxalate, citrate, cysteine, sulfate, potassium, uric acid, and total urine volume.

Interprofessional Care

Evaluation and management of a patient with renal stones consist of 2 concurrent approaches. The first approach is directed toward managing the acute attack by treating the pain, infection, and/or obstruction. Give opioids to relieve renal colic pain. NSAIDs can be considered if there is no contraindication based upon the renal function. Most stones are 4 mm or less in size and pass spontaneously. However, it may take weeks for a stone to pass.

α-Adrenergic blockers, such as tamsulosin (Flomax) or terazosin, which relax the smooth muscle in the ureter, can help stone passage. These drugs also relax the muscle tissue in the prostate in men with BPH.

The second approach is directed toward evaluating the cause of the stone formation and preventing further stone development. Obtain information from the patient, including a family history of stone formation; geographic residence; nutritional assessment, including fluid intake and the intake of vitamins A, C, and D; activity pattern (active or sedentary); history of prolonged illness with immobilization or dehydration; and any history of disease or surgery involving the GI or genitourinary tract. Include any prior episodes of stone formation, prescribed and OTC medications, and use of dietary supplements.

Therapy for active stone formers requires a comprehensive management approach, with the primary emphasis on teaching. Adequate hydration, dietary sodium restrictions, dietary changes, and drugs are used to minimize urinary stone formation (Table 45.11). Depending on the specific problem underlying the stone formation, various drugs are prescribed. These drugs prevent stone formation in several ways. These include altering urine pH, preventing excessive urinary excretion of a substance, or correcting a primary disease (e.g., hyperparathyroidism).

Treatment of struvite stones requires control of infection. This may be difficult if the stone is still in place. In addition to antibiotics, acetohydroxamic acid may be used to treat kidney infections that result in the continual formation of struvite stones. Acetohydroxamic acid inhibits the chemical action caused by the persistent bacteria and can slow struvite stone formation. Stones may have to be removed surgically if the infection cannot be controlled.[16]

Endourology, lithotripsy, or open surgical stone removal may be used in the following situations: (1) stones too large for spontaneous passage (usually greater than 7 mm); (2) stones associated with bacteriuria or symptomatic infection; (3) stones causing impaired renal function; (4) stones causing persistent pain, nausea, or paralytic ileus; (5) inability of patient to be treated medically; and (6) patient with only 1 kidney.[16]

Endourologic Procedures. If the stone is in the bladder, a cystoscopy is done to remove small stones. For large stones (Fig. 45.6), a *cystolitholapaxy* is done. In this procedure, large stones are

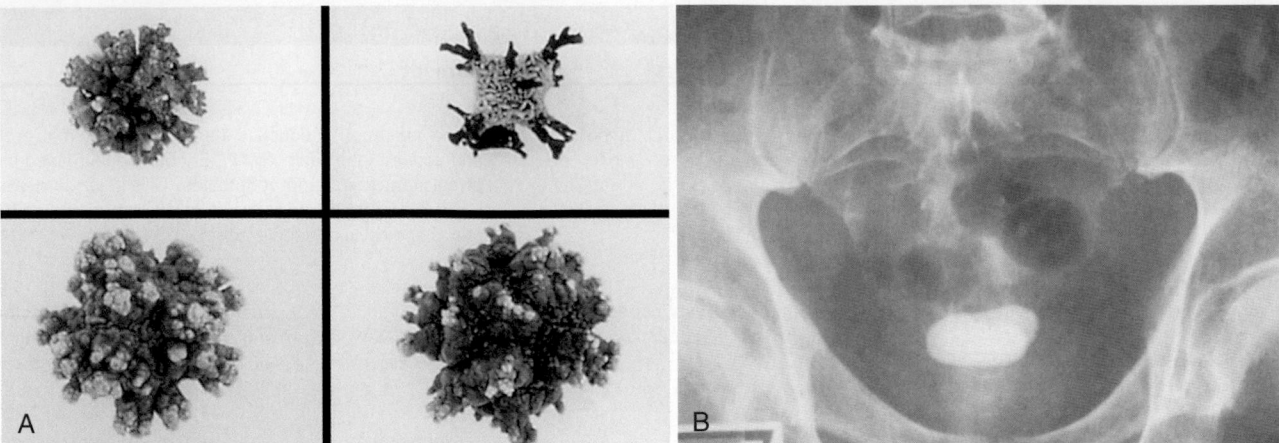

FIG 45.6 A, Calcium oxalate stones. B, Plain abdominal x-ray showing large bladder stone. (From Bullock N, Doble A, Turner W, et al: *Urology: An illustrated colour text,* London, 2008, Churchill Livingstone.)

broken up with an instrument called a *lithotrite* (stone crusher), using mechanical crushing or laser energy. The bladder is then irrigated, and the crushed stones washed out. A *cystoscopic lithotripsy* uses ultrasonic waves to break up stones. Complications associated with these procedures include hemorrhage, retained stone fragments, and infection.

Flexible *ureteroscopes* can be used to remove stones from the renal pelvis and upper urinary tract. Ultrasonic, laser, or electrohydraulic lithotripsy may be used in conjunction with ureteroscopy to break up the stone.

In *percutaneous nephrolithotomy,* a nephroscope is inserted into the kidney pelvis through a track (using a sheath) in the skin. The track is created in the patient's back. The kidney stones can be fragmented using ultrasound, electrohydraulic, or laser lithotripsy. The stone fragments are removed, and the pelvis is irrigated. A percutaneous nephrostomy tube can be left in place to make sure that the ureter is not obstructed. Complications include bleeding, injury to adjacent structures, and infection.

Lithotripsy. Lithotripsy is a procedure used to eliminate stones from the urinary tract. Lithotripsy techniques include (1) laser lithotripsy, (2) extracorporeal shock-wave lithotripsy (ESWL), (3) percutaneous ultrasonic lithotripsy, and (4) electrohydraulic lithotripsy. *Laser lithotripsy* is used to shatter ureteral and large bladder stones (bladder stones are described earlier). To access ureteral stones, a ureteroscope is used to get close to the stone. A small fiber is inserted up the scope so that the tip (which emits the laser energy) can come in contact with the stone. A holmium laser in direct contact with the stone is commonly used. The intense energy breaks the stone into small pieces, which can be extracted or flushed out. Because of the type of laser energy, no other tissue is affected. This minimally invasive treatment usually requires general anesthesia.

In *extracorporeal shock-wave lithotripsy (ESWL),* a noninvasive procedure, the patient is anesthetized (spinal or general) to ensure they maintain the same position during the procedure. The HCP uses fluoroscopy or ultrasound to focus the lithotripter over the affected kidney. Then, a high-voltage spark generator produces high-energy acoustic shock waves that shatter the stone without damaging the surrounding tissues. The small pieces of stone are then excreted in the urine. A complication of ESWL is steinstrasse, in which the ureter is blocked by those smaller pieces.

In *percutaneous ultrasonic lithotripsy* an ultrasonic probe is placed in the renal pelvis via a percutaneous nephroscope inserted through a small flank incision. The HCP positions the probe against the stone. The probe produces ultrasonic waves, which break the stone into sand-like particles. The patient receives general or spinal anesthesia.

In *electrohydraulic lithotripsy* the probe is positioned directly on a stone, but it breaks the stone into small fragments that are removed by forceps or suction. A continuous saline irrigation flushes out the stone particles, and all the outflow drainage is strained so that the particles can be analyzed. Stones can also be removed by basket extraction.

Complications of lithotripsy are rare but include hemorrhage, infection, and obstruction. Hematuria is common after lithotripsy procedures. The first few times that the patient voids, the urine is bright red. As the bleeding subsides, the urine becomes dark red or a smoky color. Antibiotics are usually given after the procedure to reduce the risk for infection.

Afterward, the patient usually has moderate to severe colicky pain. A self-retaining ureteral stent is often placed after the procedure to help the passage of sand (shattered stone) and prevent sand buildup within the ureter, which may lead to obstruction. The stent is typically removed within 2 weeks after lithotripsy. If a stone is large or positioned in the mid or distal ureter, other treatment, such as surgery, may be needed. Encourage fluids to help dilute the urine and reduce the pain from passing stone fragments.

Surgical Therapy. A small group of patients need open surgical procedures. The primary indications for surgery include pain, infection, and obstruction. The type of open surgery done depends on the location of the stone. A *nephrolithotomy* is an incision into the kidney to remove a stone. A *pyelolithotomy* is an incision into the renal pelvis for stone removal. If the stone is in the ureter, a *ureterolithotomy* is done. A *cystotomy* may be indicated for bladder stones. For open surgery on the kidney or ureter, a flank incision directly below the diaphragm and across the side is usually preferred. The most common complications after surgical procedures for stone removal are related to hemorrhage.

Nutritional Therapy. To manage an obstructing stone, the patient should drink adequate fluids to avoid dehydration. Forcing excess fluids is not advised because it does not promote spontaneous passage of stones in the urine. Forcing fluids may increase the pain or precipitate the development of renal colic.

EVIDENCE-BASED PRACTICE
Preventing Recurrent Kidney Stones

You are caring for K.D. a 41-yr-old man who is being discharged home after successful kidney stone retrieval. This was his first kidney stone and he says it was "very painful." He asks you, "Can anything be done to prevent another stone?" You see on the chart that the stone was composed of calcium oxalate and that he has gout.

Making Clinical Decisions

Best Available Evidence. Increased fluid intake (about 3 L/day) to produce 2.5 L/day of urine decreases the risk for recurrent calcium stones in patients with a prior stone. Dietary calcium intake should be 1000 to 1200 mg/day. Addition of drugs (e.g., thiazide diuretics, potassium citrate, allopurinol) for persons with recurrent calcium stones can further reduce risk. Nutritional counseling (e.g., registered dietician) for these patients is recommended.

Clinician Expertise. You know risk factors for kidney stone formation include low fluid intake and having conditions such as gout, obesity, diabetes, and/or primary hyperparathyroidism. You understand preventive measures may decrease the chance of recurrent kidney stones after the first incidence.

Patient Preferences and Values. K.D. states it may be hard to increase his fluid intake and he wants to know if a drug is available instead.

Implications for Nursing Practice

1. Why is it important for K.D. to understand the link between increased fluid intake and stone recurrence?
2. How would you help him identify ways to increase his fluid intake?
3. How would you respond to K.D.'s request for a drug to prevent recurrence?

Reference for Evidence

Dion M, Ankawi G, Chew B, et al.: CUA guideline on the evaluation and management of the kidney stone patient—2016 Update, *Can Urol Assoc J* 10:E347, 2016.

After an episode of urolithiasis, encourage a high fluid intake (around 3 L/day) to produce a urine output of at least 2.5 L/day. High urine output prevents supersaturation of minerals (i.e., dilutes the concentration of urine) and promotes excretion of minerals within the urine, thus preventing stone formation. Increasing fluid intake is particularly important for patients at risk for dehydration, including those who (1) are active in sports, (2) live in a dry climate, (3) perform physical exercise, (4) have a family history of stone formation, or (5) work outside or in an occupation that requires a great deal of physical activity. Water is the preferred fluid. Limit consumption of colas, coffee, and tea because high intake of these beverages tends to increase the risk for recurring urinary stones.

A low-sodium diet is recommended, since high-sodium intake increases calcium excretion in the urine. Foods high in calcium, oxalate, and purines are shown in Table 45.12.

❖ NURSING MANAGEMENT: URINARY TRACT CALCULI

◆ Nursing Assessment

Subjective and objective data that should be obtained from a patient with urinary tract stones are outlined in Table 45.13.

◆ Nursing Diagnoses

Nursing diagnoses for the patient with urinary tract stones include:

- Impaired urinary system function
- Acute pain
- Lack of knowledge

TABLE 45.12 Nutritional Therapy
Urinary Tract Stones

Depending on the type of stone, modifying the diet can be helpful in preventing reoccurrence.

Calcium

High: Milk, cheese, ice cream, yogurt, sauces containing milk; all beans (except green beans), lentils; fish with fine bones (e.g., sardines, kippers, herring, salmon); dried fruits, nuts; Ovaltine, chocolate, cocoa

Oxalate

High: Dark roughage, spinach, rhubarb, asparagus, cabbage, tomatoes, beets, nuts, celery, parsley, runner beans; chocolate, cocoa, instant coffee, Ovaltine, tea; Worcestershire sauce

Purine

High: Sardines, herring, mussels, liver, kidney, goose, venison, meat soups, sweetbreads
Moderate: Chicken, salmon, crab, veal, mutton, bacon, pork, beef, ham

TABLE 45.13 Nursing Assessment
Urinary Tract Stones

Subjective Data
Important Health Information

Past health history: Recent or chronic UTI. Immobilization. Previous urinary tract stones, obstruction, or kidney disease with urinary stasis. Gout, BPH, hyperparathyroidism, chronic diarrhea
Medications: Prior use of medication for prevention of stones or treatment of UTI, allopurinol, analgesics, loop diuretics, thiazide diuretics
Surgery or other treatments: External urinary diversion, long-term indwelling urinary catheter

Functional Health Patterns

Health perception–health management: Family history of urinary tract stones, sedentary lifestyle
Nutritional-metabolic: Nausea, vomiting. Dietary intake of purines, calcium ingestion, salt excess, oxalates, phosphates and use of OTC supplements. Low fluid intake. Chills
Elimination: Decreased urine output, urinary urgency, frequency, feeling of bladder fullness
Cognitive-perceptual: Acute, severe, colicky pain in flank, back, abdomen, groin, or genitalia. Burning on urination, dysuria. Anxiety

Objective Data
General

Guarding, back pain, fever, dehydration

Integumentary

Warm, flushed skin or pallor with cool, moist skin (mild shock)

Gastrointestinal

Abdominal distention, absence of bowel sounds

Urinary

Oliguria, hematuria, tenderness on palpation of renal areas, passage of stone or stones

Possible Diagnostic Findings

↑ BUN and serum creatinine levels. Urinalysis showing RBCs, WBCs, pyuria, crystals, casts, minerals, bacteria. ↑ Uric acid, calcium, phosphorus, oxalate, or cystine values on 24-hr urine sample. Stones or anatomic changes on KUB x-ray, CT scan or renal/bladder US. Direct visualization of obstruction on cystoureteroscopy

More information on nursing diagnoses and interventions for the patient with urinary tract stones is presented in eNursing Care Plan 45.2 (on the website for this chapter).

◆ Planning

The overall goals are that the patient with urinary tract stones will have (1) relief of pain, (2) no urinary tract obstruction, and (3) knowledge of ways to prevent recurrence of stones.

◆ Nursing Implementation

Most people who have had urinary stones can lower their risk for recurrence by changing their lifestyle and dietary habits. Adequate fluid intake is important to produce a urine output of around 2.5 L/day. Consult with the HCP about specific recommendations for fluid intake in a given person. The moderately active, ambulatory person should drink about 3 L/day. Fluid intake must be higher in the active person who works outdoors or who regularly engages in athletic activities.

Preventive measures for a person who is on bed rest or is immobile for a prolonged time include maintaining an adequate fluid intake, turning the patient every few hours, and helping the patient sit or stand, if possible, to maximize urinary flow.

Other preventive measures focus on reducing metabolic or secondary risk factors. For example, dietary restriction of purines may be helpful for the patient at risk for developing uric acid stones. Teach the patient the dosage, scheduling, and potential side effects of drugs used to reduce the risk for stone formation (Table 45.11). Some patients may be taught to self-monitor urinary pH or urine output.

Pain management and patient comfort are primary nursing responsibilities when managing a patient who has an obstructing stone and renal colic. To ensure that any spontaneously passed stones are retrieved, strain all urine voided by the patient using a gauze or a urine strainer. Encourage ambulation to promote movement of the stone from the upper to the lower urinary tract. To ensure safety, tell the patient who has acute renal colic to ask for help when ambulating, particularly if opioid analgesics are being given.

◆ Evaluation

The expected outcomes are that the patient with urinary tract stones will
- Maintain free flow of urine with minimal hematuria
- Report satisfactory pain relief
- State understanding of disease process and ways to prevent recurrence

STRICTURES

A ureteral or urethral stricture is a narrowing of the lumen of the ureter or urethra.

Ureteral Strictures

Ureteral strictures can affect the entire length of the ureter, from the UPJ to UVJ. While these can be congenital, they are usually from adhesions or scar formation after surgery or radiation. They may be due to extrinsic factors, such as large tumors in the peritoneal cavity. Depending on its severity, ureteral obstruction can threaten the function of the kidney.

Manifestations include mild to moderate colic, flank pain and CVA tenderness. This pain may be moderate to severe in intensity, especially if the patient drinks a large volume of fluids, such as alcohol, over a brief period. Infection is unusual unless a stone or foreign object, such as a stent or nephrostomy tube, is present.

The discomfort and obstruction of a ureteral stricture may be temporarily bypassed by placing a stent using endoscopy or by diverting urinary flow via a nephrostomy tube inserted into the renal pelvis of the affected kidney. Definitive correction requires dilation with a balloon or catheter. If the stricture is severe or recurs after initial balloon or catheter dilation, it is surgically incised using an endoscopic procedure *(endoureterotomy)*. In select patients, an open surgical approach may be needed to excise the stenotic area and reanastomose the ureter to the contralateral ureter *(ureteroureterostomy)* or to the renal pelvis. Alternatively, distal ureteral strictures may be treated by a *ureteroneocystostomy* (reimplantation of the ureter into the bladder wall).

Urethral Strictures

A *urethral stricture* is the result of fibrosis or inflammation of the urethral lumen. Causes of urethral strictures include trauma, urethritis (particularly after gonococcal infection), surgical intervention or repeated catheterizations (iatrogenic), or a congenital defect of the urethra. Once the process of inflammation and fibrosis begins, the lumen of the urethra narrows and its compliance (ability to close or open in response to bladder filling or voiding) is compromised. Meatal stenosis, a narrowing of the urethral opening, is common.

Manifestations associated with a urethral stricture include a diminished force of the urinary stream, straining to void, sprayed stream, postvoid dribbling, or a split urine stream. The patient may report feelings of incomplete bladder emptying with urinary frequency and nocturia. Moderate to severe obstruction of the bladder outlet may lead to acute urinary retention. The patient may have a history of urethritis, difficulty with insertion of a urinary catheter, or trauma involving the penis or the perineum. However, many patients are unable to recall any such events, thus leading to a diagnosis of an idiopathic stricture. A history of UTI is common, particularly if the stricture involves the distal urethra. Retrograde urethrography (RUG), ultrasound urethrography, cystourethrogram, and VCUG are used to identify stricture length, location, and caliber.

Initial management focuses on dilation. A metal instrument (urethral sound) may be placed, or a series of progressively larger stents (filiforms and followers) can be placed into the urethra to expand its lumen in a stepwise fashion. Although this process is initially successful, stenosis often recurs. Recurrences may be managed by teaching the patient to repeatedly dilate the urethra by self-catheterization using a soft (coudé-tip, red rubber) catheter every few days. Alternatively, an endoscopic or open surgical procedure *(urethroplasty)* may be a more definitive therapy for an obstructive urethral stricture. Shorter strictures may be treated by resecting the fibrotic area followed by reanastomosis of the urethra. Longer strictures may require the use of a skin flap as a substitute urethral segment.

RENAL TRAUMA

Renal trauma can be blunt or penetrating. *Blunt trauma* is the most common cause. Injury to the kidney should be considered in sports injuries, motor vehicle accidents, and falls.

Renal trauma is especially likely when the patient injures the abdomen, flank, or back. Around 10% of patients with abdominal trauma also have renal trauma. *Penetrating injuries* may result from violent encounters (e.g., gunshot, stabbing incidents).

The severity of renal trauma depends on the extent of the injury. Obtain a history of trauma to the area of the kidneys. Gross or microscopic hematuria may be present. Diagnostic studies include urinalysis, ultrasound, CT, or MRI evaluation. Renal arteriography also may be done. Both the injured kidney and the uninvolved kidney should be evaluated. Treatments range from bed rest, fluids, and analgesia to exploratory surgery and repair or nephrectomy.[17]

Nursing interventions depend on the type of trauma and the extent of any associated injuries. Interventions related to renal trauma include (1) assess the cardiovascular status and monitor for shock, especially in a penetrating injury; (2) ensure adequate fluid intake and monitor intake and output; (3) provide for pain relief and comfort measures; and (4) assess for hematuria and myoglobinuria.

RENAL VASCULAR PROBLEMS

Vascular problems involving the kidney include (1) nephrosclerosis, (2) renal artery stenosis, and (3) renal vein thrombosis.

NEPHROSCLEROSIS

Nephrosclerosis is sclerosis of the small arteries and arterioles of the kidney. The decreased blood flow results in ischemia, interstitial fibrosis, and necrosis of parts of the kidney. *Benign nephrosclerosis,* which usually occurs in adults older than 60 years of age, is caused by vascular changes from hypertension and atherosclerosis. Atherosclerotic vascular changes account for most of the loss of renal function associated with aging. The degree of nephrosclerosis is related to the severity of hypertension. In the early stages, the patient with benign nephrosclerosis may have normal renal function, with the only detectable abnormality being hypertension.

Accelerated nephrosclerosis (malignant nephrosclerosis) is associated with a significantly high BP, which can be as high as 300/150 mm/Hg, with small focal hemorrhages developing in the kidneys. It begins suddenly and is a medical emergency. It is characterized by systolic BP ≥180 and/or diastolic BP ≥120 mm/Hg with evidence of new or ongoing organ damage. Renal insufficiency progresses rapidly.

The availability and use of antihypertensive drugs have improved the prognosis for patients with benign and malignant nephrosclerosis. Treatment for benign nephrosclerosis is the same as that for essential hypertension (see Chapter 32). Malignant nephrosclerosis is treated with aggressive antihypertensive therapy. The prognosis for a patient with untreated or refractory malignant hypertension is poor. These conditions can lead to death.

RENAL ARTERY STENOSIS

Renal artery stenosis is a partial occlusion of 1 or both renal arteries and their major branches. It can be due to atherosclerotic narrowing or fibromuscular hyperplasia. Renal artery stenosis can be a cause of secondary hypertension.

When hypertension develops suddenly, renal artery stenosis should be considered, especially in patients under 30 or over 50 years of age and in those with no family history of hypertension. This contrasts with the age distribution for developing primary hypertension, which is 30 to 50 years of age.

Diagnostic tests used to assess for renal artery stenosis include a renal duplex Doppler ultrasonography, CT or MRI angiography, and renal arteriogram (the gold standard).

The goals of therapy are to control BP and restore perfusion to the kidney. Percutaneous transluminal renal angioplasty, with or without stenting, is the procedure of choice, especially in older patients who are poor surgical risks.

Surgical revascularization of the kidney is needed when decreased blood flow causes renal ischemia or when renovascular hypertension is present. Revascularization of the kidney may result in the patient's BP becoming normotensive. The surgical procedure usually involves anastomosis between the kidney and another major artery, usually the splenic artery or aorta. In certain cases of unilateral renal involvement, unilateral nephrectomy may be indicated.

RENAL VEIN THROMBOSIS

Renal vein thrombosis may occur unilaterally or bilaterally. Causes include trauma, extrinsic compression (e.g., tumor, aortic aneurysm), renal cell cancer, pregnancy, contraceptive use, and nephrotic syndrome.

The patient has flank pain, hematuria, fever, or nephrotic syndrome. Anticoagulation (e.g., heparin, warfarin [Coumadin]) is important to treat the high incidence of pulmonary emboli. Corticosteroids may be used for the patient with nephrotic syndrome. Surgical thrombectomy may be done instead of or along with anticoagulation.

HEREDITARY KIDNEY DISEASES

Hereditary kidney diseases involve developmental abnormalities of the renal parenchyma. Most inherited structural abnormalities are cystic. However, cysts may develop because of obstructive uropathies, metabolic problems, or neurologic diseases. Cysts may be evaluated to rule out tumors.

POLYCYSTIC KIDNEY DISEASE

Polycystic kidney disease (PKD) is one of the most common life-threatening genetic diseases in the world. It affects 600,000 people in the United States. PKD is the fourth leading cause of ESRD, affecting 5% of those with ESRD. A nongenetic PKD (acquired cystic kidney disease [ACKD]) is seen in those with severe kidney scarring and damage who typically require dialysis. After 5 years on dialysis, 90% of patients will have ACKD.[18]

Genetic Link

PKD has 2 hereditary forms: one manifests in childhood and one in adulthood. The childhood form of PKD is a rare autosomal recessive disorder that is often rapidly progressive (see the Genetics in Clinical Practice box). The adult form of PKD is an autosomal dominant disorder and accounts for 90% of all PKD cases (see Figs. 12.4 and 12.5). If 1 parent has the disease, there is a 50% chance that the disease will pass to the child.

🧬 GENETICS IN CLINICAL PRACTICE

Polycystic Kidney Disease (PKD)

	Adult	Child
Genetic basis	Autosomal dominant	Autosomal recessive
Incidence	1 in 400–1000	1 in 25,000
Gene location	• *PKD1* gene on chromosome 16 and *PKD2* gene on chromosome 4 • Genes code for polycystins (proteins that promote normal kidney development and function) • Mutations in genes lead to formation of thousands of cysts that disrupt the normal function of kidneys and other organs	• Polycystic kidney and hepatic disease *(PKHD1)* gene on chromosome 6 • Gene codes for fibrocystin • Mutations in gene leads to cyst formation
Genetic testing	DNA testing available	DNA testing available
Age of onset	Ages 30–40, but symptoms can start earlier	Infancy or childhood
Clinical implications	• Multisystem involvement • Systemic hypertension occurs in 60%–80% of patients • Increased risk for cerebral aneurysms • Families at risk should be screened	• Up to 30%–50% of affected newborns die shortly after birth • If infant survives the newborn period, chances of survival are good • One third need dialysis or transplantation by age 10 yr

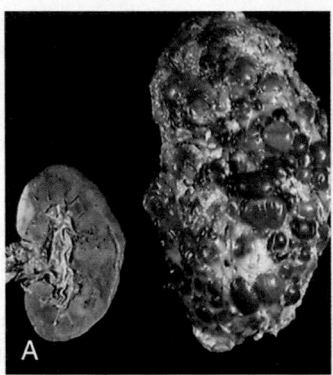 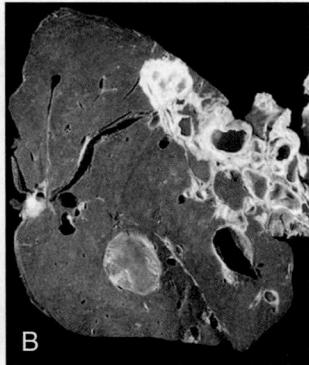

FIG 45.7 A, Comparison of polycystic kidney with normal kidney. B, Cysts in the liver. (A, From Brundage DJ: *Renal disorders*, St Louis, 1992, Mosby. B, From Kumar V, Abbas AK, Fausto N: *Robbins and Cotran pathologic basis of disease*, ed 7, Philadelphia, 2005, Saunders.)

Adult PKD involves both kidneys and occurs in both men and women. The cortex and medulla are filled with large, thin-walled cysts that are several millimeters to several centimeters in diameter (Fig. 45.7). The cysts enlarge and destroy surrounding tissue by compression. The cysts are filled with fluid and may contain blood or pus. PKD kidneys appear enlarged and look like they are filled with golf balls.

Adult PKD can be symptomless for many years. Signs and symptoms usually develop between 30 and 40 years of age.[18] Symptoms appear when the renal cysts begin to enlarge. Often the first manifestations are hypertension, hematuria (from rupture of cysts), or a feeling of pain or heaviness in the back, side, or abdomen. However, the first manifestation can be a UTI or urinary stones.

Chronic pain is the most common problem in persons with PKD. The pain can be constant and severe. Bilateral, enlarged kidneys are often palpable on physical examination. Many people have no symptoms, which can delay diagnosis.

PKD can affect the liver (liver cysts [Fig. 45.7]), heart (abnormal heart valves), blood vessels (aneurysms), and intestines (diverticulosis). The most serious complication is a cerebral aneurysm, which can rupture.

Diagnosis is based on manifestations, family history, ultrasound (best screening measure), or CT scan (provides more precise images). The disease usually progresses from loss of kidney function to ESRD by age 60 in 50% of patients.[18]

❖ Interprofessional and Nursing Care

There is no cure for PKD at present. A major aim of treatment is to prevent or treat infections of the urinary tract. Nephrectomy may be done if pain, bleeding, or infection becomes a chronic, serious problem. Dialysis and kidney transplant may be needed to treat ESRD (see Chapter 46).

When the patient begins to have progressive renal failure, the interventions depend on the remaining renal function. Nursing measures are those used for management of ESRD. They include diet modification, fluid restriction, drugs (e.g., antihypertensives), and help for the patient and family in coping with the chronic disease process and financial concerns.

The patient who has adult PKD often has children by the time the disease is diagnosed. The patient needs appropriate counseling about plans for having more children. Genetic counseling should be provided for the children. More resources can be found at the PKD Foundation website *(www.pkdcure.org)*.

❓ CHECK YOUR PRACTICE

You are doing a rotation in the dialysis unit. You have been doing vital sign checks on a 45-yr-old man who receives dialysis 3 times/wk. When you ask him why he is on dialysis, he tells you that he has polycystic kidney disease. After further discussion, he tells you that he has 1 son who is now 23 years old, but they are estranged. He does not want to tell him about his medical problems or why he is on dialysis.
• How would you respond to this patient?

MEDULLARY CYSTIC DISEASE

Medullary cystic disease is a hereditary disorder that occurs in older adults. Most cysts occur in the medulla. The kidneys are asymmetric in shape and are significantly scarred. Defects in the kidneys' concentrating ability result in polyuria. Other manifestations include hypertension, progressive renal failure, severe anemia, and metabolic acidosis. Genetic counseling may be helpful in family planning. Treatment measures are those related to ESRD (see Chapter 46). A similar disease, familial juvenile nephronophilisis, is found in young children. It can also affect the nervous system and eyes.

ALPORT SYNDROME

Alport syndrome, also known as *chronic hereditary nephritis*, is an inherited disease that primarily affects the glomeruli. The basic defect is a mutation in a gene for collagen that results in altered synthesis of the glomerular basement membrane.[19]

There are 3 genetic types of Alport syndrome: sex-linked, autosomal recessive type, and autosomal dominant type. In sex-linked, the most common type, the earliest manifestation is hematuria. These patients have progressive hearing loss and deformities of the lens of the eye. The other types of Alport syndrome cause hematuria but not deafness or lens deformities.

Males are affected earlier and more severely than females. The disease is often diagnosed in the first decade of life. Alport syndrome causes progressive kidney damage, leading to ESRD. Children with the autosomal recessive type usually develop ESRD by their teens or young adult years. People with autosomal dominant Alport syndrome usually live well into middle age before ESRD develops.

As there is no specific treatment currently available, treatment measures are supportive. Corticosteroids and cytotoxic drugs are not effective. Kidney transplantation is usually successful in people with Alport syndrome and is considered the best treatment. The disease does not recur after kidney transplantation.

URINARY TRACT TUMORS

KIDNEY CANCER

Tumors that arise from the cortex, pelvis, or calyces may be benign or cancerous. *Kidney cancer* is more common. In the United States, about 65,340 new cases of kidney cancer are diagnosed each year, and about 14,970 people die from kidney cancer.[20]

Most cases of kidney cancer are renal cell carcinomas (adenocarcinoma) (Fig. 45.8). It occurs twice as often in men as in women. The average age at diagnosis is 64 years. It is uncommon in those under 45 years old. Smoking and obesity are significant risk factors. An increased incidence is found in first-degree relatives of people who have or had renal cell cancer. Other risk factors include ACKD, hypertension, and exposure to asbestos, cadmium, and gasoline.

Clinical Manifestations and Diagnostic Studies

Early-stage kidney cancer usually has no symptoms, so many patients go undiagnosed until the disease has significantly progressed. Many kidney cancers are diagnosed as incidental findings on imaging studies used to evaluate symptoms for unrelated conditions.

Kidney tumors can cause symptoms by compressing, stretching, or invading structures near or within the kidney. The most common presenting symptoms are hematuria and flank pain. Other manifestations include weight loss, fever, hypertension, hypercalcemia, and a palpable mass in the flank or abdomen. A varicocele may be present.

About 33% of patients have metastasis at the time of diagnosis. Local extension of kidney cancer into the renal vein and vena cava is common (Fig. 45.8). The most common sites of metastases include lungs, liver, and long bones.

CT scan is often used in the diagnosis and can detect small kidney tumors. Ultrasound examinations have improved the ability to determine between a solid mass tumor and a cyst. This is significant because most masses detected on imaging are cysts. Angiography, biopsy, and MRI are used in the diagnosis of renal tumors. Radionuclide isotope scanning can detect metastases.

❖ Interprofessional and Nursing Care

Preventive measures, including quitting smoking, maintaining a healthy weight, controlling BP, and reducing exposure to toxins, can help reduce the incidence of kidney cancer. Patients in high-risk groups should be aware of their increased risk for kidney cancer. Teach them about early manifestations (e.g., hematuria, hypertension). A cure for kidney cancer may be possible when it is detected early and treated.

Interprofessional care of the patient with kidney cancer is outlined in Table 45.14. Staging of kidney cancer provides a basis for determining treatment options. The following is a simple description of staging of kidney cancer:

Stage I: The tumor can be up to 7 cm in diameter and is confined to the kidney.

Stage II: The tumor is larger than a stage I tumor and is still confined to the kidney.

Stage III: The tumor extends beyond the kidney to the surrounding tissue and may have spread to a nearby lymph node.

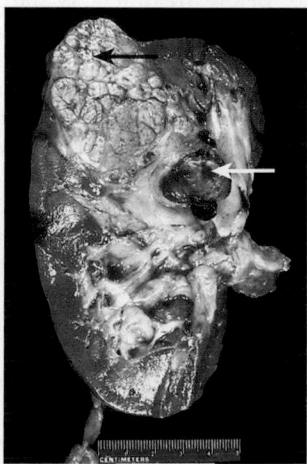

FIG 45.8 Cross section of kidney with renal cell cancer. The cancer *(black arrow)* is on the pole of the kidney. Note that the renal vein is involved and thrombosed *(white arrow)*. (From Kumar V, Abbas AK, Fausto N: *Robbins and Cotran pathologic basis of disease*, ed 7, Philadelphia, 2005, Saunders.)

⚙ TABLE 45.14 Interprofessional Care

Renal Cancer

Diagnostic Assessment	Management
• History and physical examination	• Surgical therapy
• Urinalysis	• Partial nephrectomy
• Ultrasound	• Radical nephrectomy
• Abdominal CT scan	• Ablation
• MRI	• Cryoablation
• Renal biopsy	• Radiofrequency ablation
• Renal scan	• Radiation therapy
• Angiography	• Chemotherapy
	• Immunotherapy
	• Targeted therapy

Stage IV: Cancer spreads outside the kidney to multiple lymph nodes or to distant parts of the body, such as bones, brain, liver, or lung.

The treatment of choice for some kidney cancers is a partial nephrectomy (for smaller tumors), simple total nephrectomy, or a radical nephrectomy (for larger tumors). Radical nephrectomy involves removal of the kidney, adrenal gland, surrounding fascia, part of the ureter, and draining lymph nodes. Nephrectomy can be performed by a conventional (open) approach or laparoscopically (see discussion of nephrectomy on p. 1053). Other treatment options include cryoablation (freezing technique) and radiofrequency ablation (destroying tumor by using radiofrequency heat). These procedures can be used when surgery is not an option (e.g., patient has co-morbid conditions) and for small renal tumors.

Kidney cancer is relatively resistant to most chemotherapy drugs. While kidney cancer can be resistant to radiation therapy, it may be useful in certain situations, such as metastasis to bone or lungs.

Immunotherapy, including α-interferon and interleukin-2 (IL-2), is another treatment option in metastatic disease. (The use of α-interferon and IL-2 is discussed in Chapter 15.) Another type of drug used as immunotherapy is nivolumab (Opdivo). This drug targets PD-1, a protein on T cells that normally helps keep these cells from attacking other cells in the body. By blocking PD-1, this drug boosts the immune response against cancer cells. This can shrink some tumors or slow their growth.

Targeted therapy is another treatment option for metastatic kidney cancer. Kinase inhibitors, a class of targeted therapies, block certain proteins (kinases) that play a role in tumor growth and cancer progression. Kinase inhibitors include sunitinib (Sutent), sorafenib (Nexavar), cabozantinib (Cabometyx), and axitinib (Inlyta). Bevacizumab (Avastin), sunitinib (Sutent), and pazopanib (Votrient) inhibit the formation of new blood vessel growth to the tumor. Temsirolimus (Torisel) and everolimus (Afinitor) inhibit a specific protein known as the mechanistic target of rapamycin (mTOR).[21] These drugs are discussed in Table 15.13. The mechanisms of action are shown in Fig. 15.16.

The diagnosis of kidney cancer is devastating. Often the disease may already be metastasized by the time a person is diagnosed. The nursing care of the patient with cancer is discussed in Chapter 15.

BLADDER CANCER

Bladder cancer is the most common cancer of the urinary system.[22] About 81,190 new cases of bladder cancer are diagnosed annually, and about 17,240 deaths related to bladder cancer are reported every year. Cancer of the bladder is most common in older adults; 90% of cases occur in those over the age of 55. Bladder cancer is far more common in men than in women and in whites than in blacks or Hispanics.[23]

The most frequent cancerous tumor of the urinary tract is transitional cell cancer of the bladder. Most bladder tumors are papillomatous growths within the bladder (Fig. 45.9).

About half of bladder cancers are related to cigarette smoking. Other risk factors include exposure to dyes used in the rubber and other industries. Others at risk include women treated with radiation for cervical cancer; patients who received cyclophosphamide, docetaxel, or gemcitabine; and those who have indwelling catheters for long periods.[22] People with chronic, recurrent

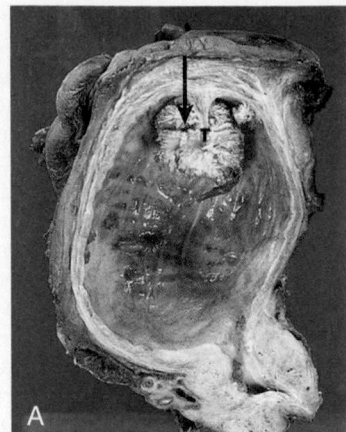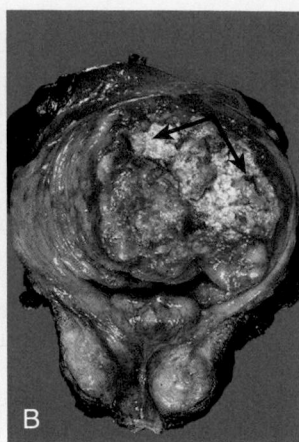

FIG 45.9 A, Papillary transitional cell cancer *(T)* seen arising from the dome of the bladder as a cauliflower-like lesion *(arrow).* B, Opened bladder showing advanced stage bladder cancer. Yellow areas are ulcerations and necrosis *(arrows).* (*A,* From Stevens A, Lowe J: *Pathology: Illustrated review in colour,* ed 2, London, 2000, Mosby. *B,* From Kumar V, Abbas AK, Fausto N: *Robbins and Cotran pathologic basis of disease,* ed 7, Philadelphia, 2005, Saunders.)

urinary tract stones, often in the bladder, and chronic lower UTIs have an increased risk for squamous cell cancer of the bladder.

Clinical Manifestations and Diagnostic Studies

Microscopic or gross, painless hematuria (chronic or intermittent) is the most common manifestation of bladder cancer. Bladder irritability with dysuria, frequency, and urgency may occur.

When cancer is suspected, obtain urine specimens to identify any cancer or atypical cells. Exfoliated cells from the bladder's epithelial surface can be detected in voided specimens. Other urine tests assess for specific factors associated with bladder cancer, such as bladder tumor antigens. Bladder cancers can be detected using CT, ultrasound, or MRI. The presence of cancer is confirmed by cystoscopy and biopsy.[24]

❖ NURSING AND INTERPROFESSIONAL MANAGEMENT: BLADDER CANCER

Most bladder cancers are diagnosed at an early stage when the cancer is treatable. Before treatment is started, bladder cancers are graded based on the cell type and staged based on the extent and invasiveness of the cancer. We use a grading system to classify the cancerous potential of tumor cells, using a scale from well differentiated (closely resembling the normal tissue) to undifferentiated (poorly differentiated) (see p. 239 in Chapter 15).

The clinical staging of bladder cancer is determined by the depth of invasion of the bladder wall and surrounding tissue. The following is a simple description of staging of bladder cancer:

Stage I: Cancer is in the inner lining of the bladder but has not invaded the bladder muscle wall.

Stage II: Cancer has invaded the bladder wall but is still confined to the bladder.

Stage III: Cancer has spread through the bladder wall to surrounding tissue. It may have spread to the prostate in men or the uterus or vagina in women.

Stage IV: Cancer has spread to the lymph nodes and other organs, such as lungs, bones, or liver.

TABLE 45.15 Interprofessional Care

Bladder Cancer

Diagnostic Assessment
- History and physical examination
- Urinalysis
- Urine cytology studies
- Cystoscopy with biopsy
- Ultrasound
- CT scan

Management
- Surgical therapy
  - Transurethral resection with fulguration
  - Laser photocoagulation
  - Open loop resection with fulguration
  - Cystectomy (segmental, partial, or radical)
- Radiation therapy
- Intravesical immunotherapy
  - Bacille Calmette-Guérin (BCG)
  - α-interferon (Intron A)
- Intravesical chemotherapy
  - doxorubicin
  - epirubicin
  - gemcitabine
  - mitomycin
  - thiotepa
  - valrubicin (Valstar)
- Systemic chemotherapy and immunotherapy

Interprofessional care of bladder cancer includes surgery, radiation, chemotherapy, and intravesical therapy (Table 45.15).

◆ Surgical Therapy

Surgical therapies include a variety of procedures. *Transurethral resection of the bladder tumor* (TURBT) is used for superficial lesions of the bladder's inner lining. The HCP uses a wire loop inserted through the cystoscope to remove the tumor and tissue, which are sent for pathologic evaluation. The base can be treated by fulguration, which burns the base of the tumor, or by use of a high-energy laser to kill the cancer cells. This procedure is also used to control bleeding in the patient who is a poor operative risk or who has advanced tumors. The primary disadvantages of this approach are reoccurrence of the bladder cancer at another site and potential for scarring and/or limited ability to hold urine with repeated TURBT procedures.[25]

A *segmental cystectomy (partial cystectomy)* is used to treat larger tumors or those that involve only 1 area of the bladder. The part of the bladder wall containing the tumor is removed along with a margin of normal tissue.

When the tumor is invasive or involves the trigone (the area where the ureters insert into the bladder) and the patient is free from metastasis beyond the pelvic area, a radical cystectomy is the treatment of choice. A *radical cystectomy* involves removal of the bladder, prostate, and seminal vesicles in men and the bladder, uterus, cervix, urethra, anterior vagina, and ovaries in women. After a radical cystectomy, a new way must be created for urine to leave the body. This surgical technique is called a *urinary diversion* (discussed later in this chapter).[25]

Postoperative instructions for any of these procedures include drinking a large volume of fluid for the first week after the procedure. Teach the patient to monitor the color and consistency of the urine. The urine is pink for the first several days after the procedure, but it should not be bright red or contain blood clots. For 7 to 10 days after tumor resection, the patient may see dark red or rust-colored flecks in the urine. These may be from the healing tumor resection site.

Give opioid analgesics and stool softeners for a brief period after the procedure. Help the patient and family cope with fears about cancer, surgery, and sexuality. Emphasize the importance of regular follow-up care. Follow-up cystoscopies are needed on a regular basis after surgery for bladder cancer.

◆ Radiation Therapy, Chemotherapy, and Immunotherapy

Radiation therapy can be used in combination with cystectomy or as the primary therapy when the cancer is inoperable or the patient refuses surgery. Chemotherapy drugs and immunotherapy can be used to treat bladder cancer.

◆ Intravesical Therapy

Chemotherapy with local instillation of immunotherapy or chemotherapy can be delivered directly into the bladder by a urethral catheter.[24] *Intravesical therapy* is usually started at weekly intervals for 6 to 12 weeks. The drug is instilled directly into the patient's bladder and retained for about 2 hours. The patient's bladder must be empty before instillation. Change the patient's position every 15 minutes during the instillation for maximum contact in all areas of the bladder. Maintenance therapy after the initial induction regimen may be beneficial.

Bacille Calmette-Guérin (BCG), a weakened strain of *Mycobacterium bovis,* is the treatment of choice for carcinoma in situ. BCG stimulates the immune system rather than acting directly on cancer cells in the bladder. When BCG fails, α-interferon, in addition to BCG, may be used. Other treatments that can be used when BCG fails include mitomycin, epirubicin, gemcitabine, valrubicin, and thiopeta (an alkylating agent).[24]

Most patients have irritative voiding symptoms and hemorrhagic cystitis after intravesical therapy. Thiotepa can significantly reduce WBC and platelet counts in some people when absorbed into the circulation from the bladder wall. BCG may cause flu-like symptoms, increased urinary frequency, hematuria, or systemic infection. Other side effects of chemotherapy (e.g., nausea, vomiting, hair loss) do not occur with intravesical chemotherapy.

Encourage patients to increase their daily fluid intake and to quit smoking. Assess the patient for secondary UTI and stress the need for routine urologic follow-up. The patient may have fears or concerns about sexual activity or bladder function that must be addressed. Because of the high rate of disease recurrence and progression in bladder cancer, follow-up studies are important.

BLADDER DYSFUNCTION

URINARY INCONTINENCE

Urinary incontinence (UI) is an involuntary leakage of urine. Although incontinence is more prevalent among older adults, it is not a natural consequence of aging. UI has traditionally been viewed as a social or hygienic problem. It has a major effect on quality of life and contributes to serious health problems, especially in older adults.

GENDER DIFFERENCES
Urinary Incontinence

Men
- A common manifestation of BPH and prostate cancer in men
- More likely to have overflow incontinence caused by urinary retention

Women
- Prevalence of UI is higher in women than men
- More likely to have stress and urge incontinence than men

Etiology and Pathophysiology

UI occurs when bladder pressure exceeds urethral closure pressure. Anything that interferes with bladder or urethral sphincter control can result in UI. Using the acronym *DRIP*, the causes can include *D*: delirium, dehydration, depression; *R*: restricted mobility, rectal impaction; *I*: infection, inflammation, impaction; and *P*: polyuria, polypharmacy. Patients may have more than 1 type of incontinence (Table 45.16). The combination of stress and urge incontinence is referred to as mixed incontinence.

Diagnostic Studies

The basic evaluation for UI includes a focused history, physical assessment, and bladder log or voiding record whenever possible. Obtain information related to the onset of UI, factors that provoke urinary leakage, and associated conditions. Pay special attention to factors known to produce transient UI, particularly when the onset of urine loss is sudden. Whenever possible, ask the patient to keep a bladder log or voiding diary documenting the timing of urinations, episodes of urinary leakage, and frequency of nocturia for a period of 1 to 7 days (minimum of 3 days if possible). This record can be kept by nursing staff if the person is in an inpatient or long-term care facility.

Begin the physical examination with an assessment of general health and functional issues associated with urination, including mobility, dexterity, and cognitive function. A pelvic examination includes careful inspection of the perineal skin for signs of erosion or rashes related to UI and existence of pelvic organ prolapse. Assess local innervation and pelvic floor muscle strength, including a digital examination of the pelvic floor muscle to determine weakness or tension.

A urinalysis can identify factors contributing to transient UI (e.g., UTI, diabetes). Measure postvoid residual (PVR) urine in the patient undergoing evaluation for UI. The PVR volume is obtained by asking the patient to void, followed by catheterization or use of a bladder ultrasound (preferably within 10 to 20 minutes).

Urodynamic testing is needed in select cases of UI. Imaging studies of the upper urinary tract (e.g., ultrasound) are done when UI is associated with UTIs or evidence of upper urinary tract involvement.

Interprofessional Care

Many cases of UI can be cured or significantly improved. Transient, reversible factors are first corrected, followed by management of the type of UI (Table 45.16). In general, less invasive treatments are tried before more invasive methods (e.g., surgery). Nevertheless, the choice of the initial treatment is patient specific, based on patient preference, the type and severity of UI, and associated anatomic defects.

Several behavioral therapies may be used to improve UI (Table 45.17). Pelvic floor muscle training (Kegel exercises) is used to manage stress, urge, or mixed UI (Table 45.18).[26] Biofeedback can help the patient identify, isolate, contract, and relax the pelvic muscles (see the Complementary & Alternative Therapies box).

COMPLEMENTARY & ALTERNATIVE THERAPIES
Biofeedback

Scientific Evidence
Biofeedback is helpful in treating a variety of medical conditions: urinary incontinence, asthma, Raynaud's disease, irritable bowel syndrome, hot flashes, headaches, hypertension, seizure disorders, and nausea and vomiting associated with chemotherapy.

Nursing Implications
- Feedback from monitoring equipment can teach patients to control certain involuntary body responses, such as urinary incontinence.
- Although biofeedback is considered safe, patients should consult a qualified professional before using biofeedback.

Drug Therapy. Drug therapy varies according to the UI type (Table 45.19). In stress UI, drugs have a limited role in the management. Bladder sphincter tone and urethral resistance can be increased with α-adrenergic agonists, but they have limited benefit. In urge and reflex UI, drugs play a key role.

Anticholinergic drugs (muscarinic receptor blockers) block the action of acetylcholine at muscarinic receptors. They relax the bladder muscle and inhibit overactive detrusor contractions (Table 45.19). Side effects include dry mouth and eyes, constipation, blurred vision, and sleepiness.

Botox (onabotulinumtoxin A) can be used to treat UI from detrusor overactivity. Botox is injected into the bladder, resulting in relaxation of the bladder, an increase in its storage capacity, and a decrease in UI.

DRUG ALERT Antimuscarinic Agents

- Overdosage can result in severe anticholinergic effects.
- These effects include GI cramping, diaphoresis, eye pain, blurred vision, and urinary urgency.

Surgical Therapy. Surgical techniques vary depending on the type of UI. Surgical correction of stress UI is aimed at making the urinary structures more receptive to intraabdominal pressure and augmenting the urethral resistance of the internal sphincter. It may involve repositioning the urethra and/or creating a backboard of support to stabilize the urethra and bladder neck and make them more receptive to changes in intraabdominal pressure. Another technique for stress UI augments the urethral resistance of the intrinsic sphincter with a sling or periurethral injectable.

Retropubic colposuspension and pubovaginal sling placement appear to be most effective. Typically, both procedures are done through low transverse incisions. Complications specific to the retropubic suspensions include postoperative voiding dysfunction, urgency, and vaginal prolapse.

Placement of a suburethral sling, using the person's own fascia, cadaveric fascia, or a synthetic material, can correct stress UI in women. Complications include vascular and bowel injury, urinary retention, mesh or sling erosion, infection, urgency, and bladder perforation. Suburethral slings have success rates

TABLE 45.16 Types of Urinary Incontinence

Description	Causes	Treatment
Functional Incontinence • Loss of urine resulting from cognitive, functional, or environmental factors	• Older adults often have problems that affect balance and mobility (e.g., severe arthritis) • Cognitive problems (e.g., dementia)	• Modifying the environment or care plan to facilitate regular, easy access to toilet and promote patient safety • Includes better lighting, ambulatory assistance equipment, clothing alterations, timed voiding, different toileting equipment
Incontinence After Trauma or Surgery • In women, vesicovaginal or urethrovaginal fistula may occur • In men, change in continence involves proximal urethral sphincter (bladder neck and prostatic urethra) and distal urethral sphincter (external striated muscle)	• Fistulas may occur during pregnancy, after delivery of baby, after hysterectomy or invasive cancer of cervix, or after radiation therapy • Incontinence is a postoperative complication of transurethral, perineal, or retropubic prostatectomy	• External condom catheter • Penile clamp • Placement of artificial implantable sphincter • Surgery to correct fistula • Urinary diversion surgery to bypass urethra and bladder
Overflow Incontinence • Occurs when pressure of urine in overfull bladder overcomes sphincter control • Leakage of small amounts of urine is frequent throughout day and night • Urination may occur frequently in small amounts • Bladder stays distended and is usually palpable	• Caused by bladder or urethral outlet obstruction (bladder neck obstruction, urethral stricture, pelvic organ prolapse) or by underactive detrusor muscle caused by myogenic or neurogenic factors (e.g., herniated disc, diabetic neuropathy) • May occur after anesthesia and surgery (e.g., hemorrhoidectomy, herniorrhaphy, cystoscopy) • Neurogenic bladder (flaccid type).	• Urinary catheterization to decompress bladder • Use Credé or Valsalva maneuver • α-Adrenergic blockers (Table 45.19) • 5α-Reductase inhibitors (Table 45.19) to decrease outlet resistance • Bethanechol (Urecholine) to enhance bladder contractions • Intermittent catheterization • Intravaginal device, such as a pessary, to support prolapse • Surgery to correct underlying problem
Reflex Incontinence • Condition occurs when no warning or stress precedes periodic involuntary urination • Urination is frequent, moderate in volume, and occurs equally during day and night	• Spinal cord lesion above S2 interferes with central nervous system inhibition • Disorder results in detrusor hyperreflexia and interferes with pathways coordinating detrusor contraction and sphincter relaxation	• Treat underlying cause • Bladder decompression to prevent ureteral reflux and hydronephrosis • Intermittent self-catheterization • Baclofen or diazepam to relax external sphincter • Prophylactic antibiotics • Surgical sphincterotomy
Stress Incontinence • Sudden increase in intraabdominal pressure causes involuntary passage of urine • Can occur during coughing, laughing, sneezing, or physical activities, such as heavy lifting, exercising • Leakage usually is in small amounts and may not be daily	• Most common in women with relaxed pelvic floor musculature (from delivery, use of instrumentation during vaginal delivery, or multiple pregnancies) • Structures of female urethra atrophy when estrogen decreases • Prostate surgery for BPH or prostate cancer	• Pelvic floor muscle exercises (e.g., Kegel exercises), weight loss if obese, cessation of smoking, topical estrogen products, external condom catheters or penile incontinence clamp in men, surgery • Urethral inserts, patches, or bladder neck support devices (e.g., incontinence pessary) to correct underlying problem

Urge Incontinence
• Often referred to as overactive bladder
• Occurs randomly when involuntary urination is preceded by urinary urgency
• Leakage is periodic but frequent and usually in large amounts
• Nocturnal frequency and incontinence are common
	• Caused by uncontrolled contraction or overactive detrusor muscle
	• Bladder escapes central inhibition and contracts reflexively
	• Conditions include:
	  • Nervous system disorders (e.g., stroke, Alzheimer's disease, brain tumor, Parkinson's disease)
	  • Bladder disorders (e.g., carcinoma in situ, radiation effects, interstitial cystitis)
	  • Interference with spinal inhibitory pathways (e.g., cancer in spinal cord, spondylosis)
	• Bladder outlet obstruction or conditions of unknown cause
		• Treat underlying cause
		• Biobehavioral interventions (bladder retraining with urge suppression, decrease in dietary irritants, bowel regularity, pelvic floor muscle exercises)
		• Anticholinergic drugs (Table 45.19)
		• Calcium channel blockers (Table 45.19)
		• mirabegron (Myrbetriq)
		• Vaginal estrogen creams
		• Containment devices (e.g., external condom catheters)
		• Absorbent products

TABLE 45.17 Interventions for Urinary Incontinence

Intervention	Description
Lifestyle Modifications	Self-management to reduce or eliminate risk factors, including: • Smoking cessation • Weight reduction • Good bowel regimen • Reduction of bladder irritants (e.g., caffeine, aspartame artificial sweetener, citrus juices) • Fluid modifications for those with urge incontinence
Scheduled Voiding Regimens	
Bladder retraining and urge-suppression strategies	Scheduled toileting with progressive voiding intervals. Includes teaching of urge-control using relaxation and distraction techniques, self-monitoring, reinforcement techniques, and other strategies, such as conscious contraction of pelvic floor muscles.
Habit retraining	Scheduled toileting with adjustments of voiding intervals (longer or shorter) based on the person's voiding pattern.
Prompted voiding	Scheduled toileting that requires prompts to void from a caregiver (typically every 3 hr). Used in conjunction with operant conditioning techniques to reward people for maintaining continence and appropriate toileting.
Timed voiding	Toileting on a fixed schedule (typically every 2–3 hr during waking hours).
Pelvic Floor Muscle Rehabilitation	
Biofeedback	See Complementary & Alternative Therapies box on p. 1046.
Electrical stimulation	Application of low-voltage electric current to sacral and pudendal afferent fibers through vaginal, anal, or surface electrodes. Used to inhibit bladder overactivity and improve awareness, contractility, and efficiency of pelvic muscle contraction.
Pelvic floor muscle (Kegel) exercises or training	Table 45.18.
Vaginal weight training	Active retention of vaginal weights (devices designed and shaped to exercise and strengthen pelvic floor muscles) at least twice a day. Typically used in combination with pelvic floor muscle exercises.
Anti-Incontinence Devices	
Incontinence clamps (penile compression devices)	Mechanical fixed compression applied to the penis to prevent any flow or leakage via the urethra. Must be released to void.
Intraurethral occlusive device (urethral plug)	Single-use device that is worn in the urethra to provide mechanical obstruction to prevent urine leakage. Removed for voiding.
Intraurethral valve pump	Replaceable urinary prosthesis for use in women who have impaired detrusor contractility (cannot contract muscles to push urine out of the bladder). Draws urine out to empty bladder and blocks urine flow when continence is desired.
Intravaginal support devices (pessaries and bladder neck support prostheses)	Devices support bladder neck, relieve minor pelvic organ prolapse, and change pressure transmission to the urethra.
Containment Devices	
Absorbent products	Variety of reusable and disposable pads and undergarment systems.
External collection devices	External catheter (condom) systems (e.g., penile sheaths) direct urine into a drainage bag. Most often used by men.

comparable to those of colposuspension or slings and are associated with shorter recovery periods. An artificial urethral sphincter can be used in men with intrinsic sphincter deficiency and severe stress UI.

A bulking agent can be injected underneath the mucosa of the urethra to correct stress UI in women or men. Bulking agents include glutaraldehyde cross-linked bovine collagen (GAX collagen), autologous fat, carbon beads, carbon hydroxyapatite, and polydimethylsiloxane injections. Although treatment with bulking agents avoids the risk associated with open surgery, reinjection is typically needed after several years.

In artificial sphincter surgery, the bladder sphincter that no longer works is replaced with an artificial one. A silicone inflatable ring is placed around the urethra (internally), and the patient inflates it to stop the flow and deflates it when the need to empty occurs. The patient must be able to work the pump that is placed internally. This procedure is usually used only as a last resort in a patient who is cognitively aware and able to use the artificial sphincter.[27]

❖ NURSING MANAGEMENT: URINARY INCONTINENCE

It is important to recognize both the physical and emotional problems associated with UI. Maintain and enhance the patient's dignity, privacy, and feelings of self-worth. This involves a 2-step approach with (1) containment devices to manage existing urinary leakage and (2) a definitive plan to reduce or resolve the factors leading to UI.

🔍 CHECK YOUR PRACTICE

You are doing BP and glucose screening at the community senior center. While you are checking the BP on a 78-yr-old woman, she starts to sob quietly. You tell her that her BP is 134/84 and gently place your hand on her arm. You ask her what is wrong. She tells you, "I have to pee all the time. I soak the bed and my husband won't sleep with me anymore. I am washing sheets and my clothes all the time. Our whole house smells like urine."

• How would you respond to her?

TABLE 45.18 Patient Teaching

Pelvic Floor Muscle (Kegel) Exercises

Include the following instructions when teaching the patient to perform Kegel exercises:

What Is the Pelvic Floor Muscle?

- Your pelvic floor muscle provides support for your bladder and rectum and, in women, the vagina and uterus.
- If it weakens or is damaged, it cannot support these organs and their position can change.
- This causes problems with the normal bladder and rectal function.
- If you have a weak pelvic floor muscle, you may want to do special exercises to make the muscle stronger, prevent unwanted urine leakage, and lessen urinary urgency.

Finding the Pelvic Floor Muscle

- Without tensing the muscles of your leg, buttocks, or abdomen, imagine that you are trying to control the passing of gas or pinching off a stool.
- Or imagine you are in an elevator full of people and you feel the urge to pass gas. What do you do?
- You tighten or pull in the ring of muscle around your rectum—your pelvic floor muscle.
- You should feel a lifting sensation in the area around the vagina or a pulling in of your rectum.

How to Do the Exercises

There are 2 different kinds of exercises—short squeezes and long squeezes.

1. To do the *short squeezes,* tighten your pelvic floor muscle quickly, squeeze hard for 2 seconds, and then relax the muscle. Also, when you have strong urinary urges, try to tighten your pelvic floor muscle quickly and hard several times in a row until the urge passes.
2. To do the *long squeezes,* tighten the muscle for 5–10 seconds before you relax.

Do both of these exercises 40–50 times each day.

When to Do These Exercises

- You can do these exercises anytime and anywhere.
- You can do these exercises in any position but sitting or lying down may be the easiest.

How Long Does It Take Before I Notice a Change?

After 4–6 weeks of doing these exercises, you should start to see less urine leakage and urinary urgency.

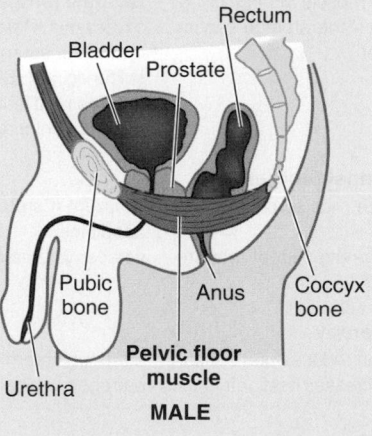

MALE

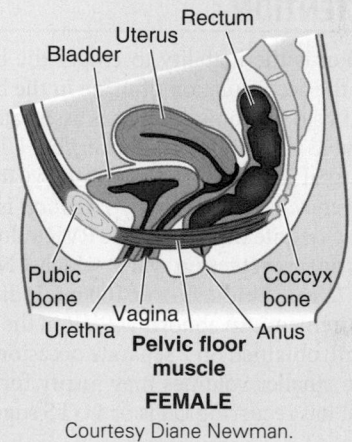

FEMALE

Courtesy Diane Newman.

Management options are reviewed in Tables 45.17 and 45.18. They include lifestyle interventions such as teaching the patient about consuming an adequate volume of fluids and reducing or eliminating bladder irritants, particularly caffeine and alcohol, from the diet. Have the patient maintain a regular, flexible schedule of urination, usually every 2 to 3 hours while awake. Advise patients to quit smoking because this habit increases the risk for stress UI. Teach patients about the relationships among constipation, UI, and urinary retention. Aggressive management of constipation is recommended. Begin with ensuring adequate fluid intake, increasing dietary fiber, lightly exercising, and judiciously using stool softeners. The management of constipation is discussed in Chapter 42.

Behavioral treatments include scheduled voiding regimens (timed voiding, habit training, prompted voiding), bladder retraining, and pelvic floor muscle training. Assess how the patient contains urine and offer alternative devices when indicated. Many women use feminine hygiene pads. Many men and women may use household products, such as rags, paper towels, or folded toilet tissue. Unfortunately, none of these products is designed to wick urine away from the skin, prevent soiling of clothing, and reduce or eliminate odor.

Provide information on products specifically designed to contain urine. For example, patients with mild to moderate UI often benefit from incontinent pads containing superabsorbent material, designed to absorb many times its weight in water. Patients with higher volume urine loss or those with both urinary and fecal incontinence may need disposable or reusable incontinence protective underwear, briefs, or pad/pant systems.

In inpatient or long-term care facilities, nursing management of UI includes maximizing toilet access. This may take the form of offering the urinal or bedpan or helping the patient to the bathroom every 2 to 3 hours or at scheduled times. Ensure that toilets are accessible to patients and provide privacy to allow effective urine elimination.

⁜⁜ NURSING MANAGEMENT
Caring for the Patient With Incontinence

All members of the interprofessional care team are responsible for decreasing the risk for incontinence and preventing complications, such as skin breakdown, in patients who have UI. The RN plays a key role in delivering interventions to prevent and manage UI.

- Assess for risk factors for incontinence or urinary retention.
- Determine type of incontinence that patient is experiencing.
- Develop plan of care to decrease incontinence.
- Teach patient ways to decrease incontinence, such as pelvic floor muscle (Kegel) exercises.
- Assist patient in choosing appropriate products to contain urine.
- Delegate to the LPN/VN:
  - Use bladder scanner to estimate the postvoid residual volume (PVR).
  - Catheterize patient and measure PVR.
  - Give medications to decrease incontinence or urinary retention.
- Oversee UAP:
  - Help incontinent patient to commode or bedpan at regular intervals.
  - Clean patient and provide skin care.
  - Notify RN about new-onset incontinence in a previously continent patient.

URINARY RETENTION

Urinary retention is the inability to empty the bladder when a person voids or the accumulation of urine in the bladder because of an inability to void. In some cases, it is associated with urinary leakage or postvoid dribbling, called *overflow UI. Acute urinary retention* is the total inability to pass urine via micturition. It is a medical emergency. *Chronic urinary retention* is an incomplete bladder emptying despite urination. The PVR volumes in patients with chronic urinary retention vary widely. Normal PVR is between 50 and 75 mL. Findings over 100 mL indicate the need to repeat the measurement. An abnormal PVR in the older patient of more than 200 mL obtained on 2 separate occasions needs further evaluation. Even smaller volumes may justify further evaluation when the patient has recurring UTIs or LUTS suggestive of UTI.

Etiology and Pathophysiology

Urinary retention is caused by 2 different dysfunctions of the urinary system: bladder outlet obstruction and deficient detrusor (bladder muscle) contraction strength. *Bladder outlet obstruction* leads to urinary retention when the blockage is so severe that the bladder can no longer evacuate its contents despite a detrusor contraction. A common cause of obstruction in men is an enlarged prostate.

Deficient detrusor contraction strength leads to urinary retention when the muscle is no longer able to contract with enough force or for enough time to completely empty the bladder. Common causes are neurologic diseases affecting sacral segments 2, 3, and 4; long-standing diabetes; overdistention; chronic alcoholism; and drugs (e.g., anticholinergic drugs).

Diagnostic Studies

The diagnostic studies for urinary retention are the same as the ones for UI (see p. 1046).

Interprofessional Care

Behavioral therapies that were described for UI may be used in the management of urinary retention. Scheduled toileting and double voiding may be effective in chronic urinary retention with moderate PVR volumes. *Double voiding* is an attempt to maximize bladder evacuation. The patient is asked to void, sit on the toilet for 3 to 4 minutes, and void again before exiting the bathroom.

For acute or chronic urinary retention, catheterization may be needed. Intermittent catheterization allows the patient to remain free of an indwelling catheter with its associated risk of CAUTI and urethral irritation. In some situations, an indwelling catheter is preferred (e.g., if the patient is unwilling or unable to perform intermittent catheterization). An indwelling catheter is also used when urethral obstruction makes intermittent catheterization uncomfortable or infeasible.

Drug Therapy. Several drugs may be given to promote bladder evacuation. For the patient with obstruction at the level of the

TABLE 45.19 Drug Therapy
Voiding Dysfunction

Class and Mechanism of Action	Drug
α-Adrenergic Agonists	
Increase urethral resistance	pseudoephedrine
α-Adrenergic Blockers	
Reduce urethral sphincter resistance to urinary outflow	alfuzosin (Uroxatral) doxazosin (Cardura) tamsulosin (Flomax) terazosin
5α-Reductase Inhibitors	
Suppress androgen resulting in epithelial atrophy and decrease in prostate size	dutasteride (Avodart) finasteride (Proscar)
β₃-Adrenergic Agonist	
Improves bladder's storage capacity by relaxing bladder muscle during filling	mirabegron (Myrbetriq)
Anticholinergics (Muscarinic Receptor Blockers)	
Reduce overactive bladder contractions in urge urinary incontinence Relax bladder muscle during filling and improves the storage capacity of bladder	darifenacin (Enablex) fesoterodine (Toviaz) flavoxate (Urispas) oxybutynin (Ditropan XL, Oxytrol Transdermal System) solifenacin (VESIcare) tolterodine (Detrol, Detrol LA) trospium chloride
Calcium Channel Blockers	
Reduce smooth muscle contraction strength May reduce burning pain of interstitial cystitis	diltiazem (Cardizem) nifedipine verapamil (Calan)
Hormone Therapy	
Local application reduces urethral irritation and increases host defenses against UTI	estrogen cream (Premarin) estrogen vaginal ring (Estring)
Tricyclic Antidepressants	
Reduce sensory urgency and burning pain of interstitial cystitis Reduce overactive bladder contractions	amitriptyline imipramine (Tofranil)

bladder neck, an α-adrenergic blocker may be prescribed. These drugs relax the smooth muscle of the bladder neck and prostatic urethra and may decrease urethral resistance. Examples of α-adrenergic blockers are listed in Table 45.19. They are indicated in patients with BPH or bladder neck or detrusor sphincter dyssynergia (muscle incoordination).

Surgical Therapy. Surgical interventions are used to manage urinary retention caused by obstruction. Transurethral or open surgical techniques are used to treat benign or cancerous prostatic enlargement, bladder neck contracture, urethral strictures, or dyssynergia of the bladder neck. Pelvic reconstruction using an abdominal or transvaginal approach can correct bladder outlet obstruction in women with severe pelvic organ prolapse.

While surgery has had a minimal role in the management of urinary retention caused by deficient detrusor contraction strength, a few new procedures may be of benefit. Sacral neuromodulation involves a stimulator device and placement of a lead wire into the S3 foramen. Placement of an intraurethral valve pump, which empties the patient's bladder on command, may be an option.

❖ NURSING MANAGEMENT: URINARY RETENTION

Acute urinary retention is a medical emergency that requires prompt recognition and bladder drainage. Insert a catheter as ordered. Use a catheter with a retention balloon in anticipation of the need for an indwelling catheter.

Teach the patient with acute urinary retention and the patient predisposed to these episodes ways to minimize risk. Teach the patient to drink small amounts throughout the day and avoid the intake of large volumes of fluid over a brief period. Tell the patient (if chilled) to warm up before trying to void. They should avoid excess alcohol intake because it leads to polyuria and a diminished awareness of the need to void until the bladder is distended.

Have the patient who is unable to void drink a cup of coffee or brewed caffeinated tea to create or maximize urinary urgency. Tell patients that sitting in a tub of warm water or taking a warm shower may help them void. If these measures do not lead to successful urination, have the patient seek immediate care.

Patients with chronic urinary retention may be managed by behavioral methods, indwelling or intermittent catheterization, surgery, or drugs. Scheduled toileting and double voiding are the primary behavioral interventions used for chronic retention. Scheduled toileting can reduce, rather than expand, bladder capacity. In this case, have the patient void every 3 to 4 hours regardless of the desire to void. This is particularly useful in the patient with chronic overdistention, diabetes, or chronic alcoholism with a large bladder capacity and diminished or delayed sensations of bladder filling and urgency.

CATHETERIZATION

INDICATIONS FOR AND COMPLICATIONS OF CATHETERIZATION

Indications for short-term urinary catheterization are listed in Table 45.20. Unacceptable reasons for catheterization include (1) routine acquisition of a urine specimen for laboratory analysis and (2) convenience of the nursing staff or the patient's family. The risk for CAUTI is too high to allow catheterization of a patient for the convenience of hospital personnel or family members.

TABLE 45.20 Indications for Urinary Catheterization

Indwelling Catheter
- Relieve urinary retention caused by lower urinary tract obstruction, paralysis, or inability to void
- Bladder decompression preoperatively and operatively for lower abdominal or pelvic surgery
- Facilitate surgical repair of urethra and surrounding structures
- Splinting of ureters or urethra to promote healing after surgery or other trauma in area
- Accurate measurement of urine output
- Contamination of stage III or IV pressure injuries with urine that has impeded healing, despite appropriate personal care for the incontinence
- Terminal illness or severe impairment, which makes positioning or clothing changes uncomfortable, or which is associated with intractable pain

Intermittent (Straight, in and out) Catheter
- Relieve urinary retention caused by lower urinary tract obstruction, paralysis, or inability to void
- Study of anatomic structures of urinary system
- Urodynamic testing
- Collect sterile urine sample in certain situations
- Instill medications into bladder
- Measure residual urine after voiding (postvoid residual [PVR]) if portable ultrasound not available

Complications that are seen with long-term use (more than 30 days) of indwelling catheters include CAUTI, bladder spasms, periurethral abscess, chronic pyelonephritis, urosepsis, urethral trauma or erosion, fistula or stricture formation, and stones. Catheterization for sterile urine specimens may be needed if the patient has a history of complicated UTI. A catheter should be the last resort to provide the patient with a dry environment to prevent skin breakdown and protect dressings or skin lesions.

Urinary catheterization is often used in the management of the hospitalized patient. However, it is not without serious complications. As previously discussed on p. 1028, CAUTIs are the most common HAI. Scrupulous aseptic technique is mandatory when a urinary catheter is inserted. After insertion, maintenance and protection of the closed drainage system are major nursing responsibilities. Do not routinely irrigate the catheter; this should be done only if ordered.

While the patient has a catheter in place, maintain catheter, manage fluid intake, provide for the patient's comfort and safety, and prevent infection. Address the psychologic implications of urinary drainage. Patient concerns can include embarrassment related to exposure of the body, an altered body image, and fear that care of the catheter will result in increased dependency.

CATHETER CONSTRUCTION

Catheter materials include Teflon-coated latex, silicone elastomer, plastic, and hydrogel-coated silicone or latex. Catheters coated with silver or antimicrobial agents may prevent CAUTIs.

Catheters vary in construction materials, tip shape (Fig. 45.10), and size of the lumen. A coudé-tip catheter is often used in men. Catheters are sized according to the French scale. Each French unit (F) equals 0.33 mm of diameter. The diameter listed is the internal diameter of the catheter. The size used varies with the patient's size and the purpose of catheterization. In women,

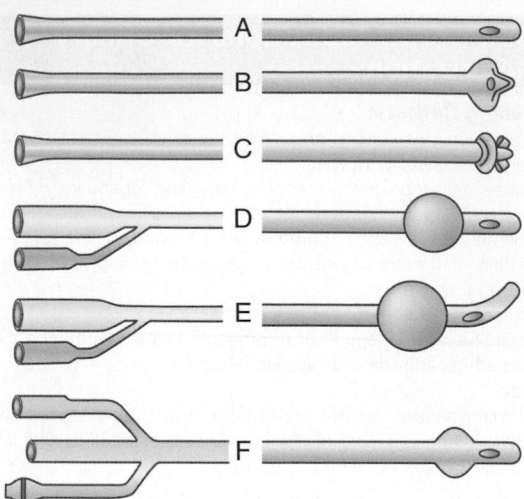

FIG 45.10 Types of urinary catheters. **A**, Simple urethral catheter. **B**, Mushroom-tip de Pezzer catheter (can be for suprapubic catheterization). **C**, Wing-tip Malecot catheter (wings hold catheter in place for temporary drainage). **D**, Indwelling urethral catheter with inflated balloon. **E**, Indwelling Tiemann catheter with coudé-tip (slightly curved tip allows for passage past obstruction). **F**, 3-way indwelling catheter (third lumen can be used for irrigation).

urethral catheter sizes 14F to 16F are the most common. In men, sizes 14F to 18F are used. Balloon sizes are either 5 or 30 mL. The primary problem resulting from too large a catheter is tissue erosion from excessive pressure on the meatus or urethra.

TYPES OF CATHETERS

Four routes are used for urinary tract catheterization: urethral, ureteral, suprapubic, and via a nephrostomy tube.

Urethral Catheterization

Urethral catheterization, the most common route of catheterization, involves the insertion of a catheter through the external meatus into the urethra, past the internal sphincter, and into the bladder.

Ureteral Catheters

The *ureteral catheter* is placed through the ureters into the renal pelvis. The catheter is inserted either (1) by being threaded up the urethra and bladder to the ureters under cystoscopic observation or (2) by surgical insertion through the abdominal wall into the ureters. The ureteral catheter is used after surgery to splint the ureters and to prevent them from being obstructed by edema. Record the urine volume from the ureteral catheter separately from that of other urinary catheters.

The patient is often kept on bed rest while a ureteral catheter is in place until the HCP orders ambulation. The self-retaining ureteral catheter is often inserted after a lithotripsy procedure or when ureteral obstruction from adjacent tumors or fibrosis threatens renal function. A double-J ureteral catheter is often used and allows the patient to ambulate. One end coils up in the kidney pelvis, while the other coils in the bladder.

Check the placement of the ureteral catheter frequently and avoid tension on the catheter. The catheter drains urine from the renal pelvis, which has a capacity of 3 to 5 mL. If the volume of urine in the renal pelvis increases, tissue damage to the pelvis will result from pressure. Do not clamp the ureteral catheter. If the HCP orders irrigation of the ureteral catheter, use strict aseptic technique. If the output is decreased, notify the HCP immediately.

◼◼ Nursing Management

Care of the Patient With a Urethral Catheter

The following measures can be used to manage patients with a urethral catheter and prevent a CAUTI.
- Determine need for catheterization, but HCP must order.
- Choose appropriate type and size of catheter.
- Insert catheter in patient with urethral trauma, pain, or obstruction.
- Develop plan of care to decrease risk for infection in patient with indwelling catheter.
- Teach catheter care to the patient, particularly one who is ambulatory.
- Use a sterile, closed drainage system in short-term catheterization.
- Do not disconnect the distal urinary catheter and proximal drainage tube except for catheter irrigation (if ordered and indicated).
- Use sterile technique whenever the collecting system is open. If frequent irrigations are necessary in short-term catheterization to maintain catheter patency, a triple-lumen catheter may be preferable, permitting continuous irrigations within a closed system.
- A routine catheter change is not needed if the patient is catheterized for less than 2 weeks. For long-term use of an indwelling catheter, replace the catheter based on patient assessment and not on a routine changing schedule.
- If ordered, aspirate small volumes of urine for culture from the catheter sampling port using a sterile syringe and needle. Prepare the puncture site with an antiseptic solution.
- With long-term use of a catheter, a leg bag may be used. If the collection bag is reused, wash it in soap and water and rinse thoroughly. When it is not reused immediately, fill it with ½ cup of vinegar and drain. Vinegar is effective against *Pseudomonas* and other organisms and eliminates odors.
- Remove the catheter as early as possible. Intermittent catheterization and external catheters are alternatives that are associated with fewer cases of bacteriuria and CAUTI.
- Ensure that UAP:
  - Maintain unobstructed downhill flow of urine.
  - Empty the collecting bag regularly and accurately record the urine output.
  - Provide perineal care (once or twice a day and when needed), cleaning the meatus-catheter junction with soap and water.
  - Do not use lotion or powder near the catheter.
  - Anchor catheter using a securement device. Anchor catheter to upper thigh in women and lower abdomen in men to prevent catheter movement and urethral tension.

Check the drainage often (at least every 1 or 2 hours). It is normal for some urine to drain around the ureteral catheter into the bladder. Accurately record the urine output from the ureteral and urethral catheters. Sometimes a ureteral catheter may be used as a stent and is not expected to drain. It is important to check with the HCP as to the type of catheter and what to expect.

Suprapubic Catheters

Suprapubic catheterization is the simplest and oldest method of urinary diversion. The 2 methods of insertion of a suprapubic catheter into the bladder are (1) through a small incision in the abdominal wall and (2) using a trocar. A suprapubic catheter is placed while the patient is under general anesthesia for another surgical procedure or at the bedside with a local anesthetic. The catheter may be sutured into place. Tape the catheter to prevent dislodgment. The care of the tube and catheter is similar to that of the urethral catheter. A pectin-base skin barrier (e.g., Stomahesive) is effective in protecting the skin around the insertion site from breakdown.

The suprapubic catheter is used in temporary situations, such as bladder, prostate, and urethral surgery. It is also used on a long-term basis in some patients.

A suprapubic catheter is prone to poor drainage because of mechanical obstruction of the catheter tip by the bladder wall, sediment, and clots. To ensure patency of the tube (1) prevent tube kinking by coiling the excess tubing and maintaining gravity drainage, (2) have the patient turn from side to side, and (3) milk the tube. If these measures are not effective, obtain an order from the HCP to irrigate the catheter using sterile technique.

If the patient has bladder spasms that are hard to control, urinary leakage may result. Oxybutynin or other oral antispasmodics or belladonna and opium (B&O) suppositories may be prescribed to decrease bladder spasms.

Nephrostomy Tubes

The *nephrostomy tube* (catheter) is inserted on a temporary basis to preserve renal function when a ureter is completely obstructed. The tube is inserted through a small flank incision directly into the pelvis of the kidney and attached to connecting tubing for closed drainage. The principle is the same as with the ureteral catheter—that is, the catheter should never be kinked, compressed, or clamped. If the patient has excessive pain in the area or if there is excess drainage around the tube, check the catheter for patency. If irrigation is ordered, use strict aseptic technique. Gently instill no more than 5 mL of sterile saline solution at one time to prevent overdistention of the kidney pelvis and renal damage. Infection and secondary stone formation are complications associated with the insertion of a nephrostomy tube.

Intermittent Catheterization

An alternative approach to a long-term indwelling catheter is *intermittent catheterization,* often referred to as "straight" catheterization or "in-and-out" catheterization. The main goal of intermittent catheterization is to prevent urinary retention, stasis, and compromised blood supply to the bladder caused by prolonged pressure.[28]

It is being used more often in conditions such as neurogenic bladder (e.g., spinal cord injuries, chronic neurologic diseases) and bladder outlet obstruction in men. This type of catheterization is used in the oliguric and anuric phases of AKI to reduce the chance of infection from an indwelling catheter. Intermittent catheterization is also used postoperatively after a surgical procedure to treat UI.

The technique consists of inserting a urethral catheter into the bladder every 3 to 5 hours. Some patients perform intermittent catheterization only once or twice a day to measure residual urine and to ensure an empty bladder.

The techniques and protocols for intermittent catheterization vary. Catheters can be sterile (single use) or clean (multiple use). Catheters can be coated (prelubricated) or uncoated. Research on intermittent catheterization shows no convincing evidence that any specific technique (sterile or clean), catheter type (coated or uncoated), method (single-use or multiple-use), person (self or other), or strategy is better than any other for all clinical settings.[28]

The design of single-use, self-lubricating, silicone-coated (closed-sterile) systems is useful for patients who have recurrent UTIs or need to catheterize while at work or during travel. Teach patients to wash and rinse the catheter and their hands with soap and water before and after catheterization. Lubricant is necessary for men and may make catheterization more comfortable for women. The patient, caregiver, or HCP may insert the catheter.

Sterile technique is used for catheterization in the hospital or long-term care facility. For home care, a clean technique that includes good hand washing with soap and water is used. Teach the patient to observe for signs of UTI so that treatment can be started early. Some patients are placed on prophylactic antibiotics. Urethral damage from intermittent catheterization in men is similar to problems seen with indwelling catheterization. Complications include urethritis, urethral sphincter damage (especially if there is a forceful catheterization against a closed sphincter), urethral stricture, and creation of a false passage.

SURGERY OF THE URINARY TRACT

RENAL AND URETERAL SURGERY

The most common indications for nephrectomy are a renal tumor, polycystic kidneys that are bleeding or severely infected, massive traumatic injury to the kidney, and the elective removal of a kidney from a donor to be transplanted. Surgery involving the ureters and kidneys is most often done to remove stones that become obstructive, correct congenital anomalies, and divert urine when necessary.

Surgical Procedure

Nephrectomy can be performed by a conventional (open) approach or laparoscopically. In the open approach, an incision of about 6 to 10 inches is made through several layers of muscle. The incision can be made in the flank or abdominal area.

Laparoscopic Nephrectomy. *Laparoscopic nephrectomy* can be done to remove a diseased kidney or obtain a kidney from a living donor for transplant into a person with ESRD. With a laparoscopic nephrectomy, there are 3 to 5 puncture sites. One incision is to view the kidney, and another to dissect it. The laparoscope has a miniature camera so that the surgeons can watch what they are doing on a video monitor. Once dissected, the kidney is maneuvered into a nylon or polyurethane impermeable sack and then safely removed from the patient. Compared with conventional nephrectomy, the laparoscopic approach is less painful, involves a shorter hospital stay, and has a much faster recovery.

Preoperative Management

The basic needs of the patient undergoing renal and ureteral surgery are similar to those of any patient who has surgery (see Chapters 17 through 19). It is important preoperatively to ensure adequate fluid intake and a normal electrolyte balance. Tell the patient that if there is a flank incision, surgery will require a hyperextended, side-lying position. This position often causes the patient to have muscle aches after surgery. If a nephrectomy is planned, it is important that the patient have 1 working kidney to maintain normal renal function.

Postoperative Management

Specific postoperative needs of a patient are related to urine output, respiratory status, and abdominal distention.

Urine Output. In the immediate postoperative period, measure and record the urine output at least every 1 or 2 hours. Measure drainage from the various catheters and record it separately. Do not clamp or irrigate the catheter or tube without a specific order. The total urine output should be at least 0.5 mL/kg/hr. It is important to assess for urine drainage on the dressing and to estimate this amount. Observe and monitor the color and consistency of urine. Urine with increased amounts of mucus, blood, or sediment may occlude the drainage tubing or catheter.

Weigh the patient daily using the same scale and have the patient wear similar clothing and dressings each time. A significant change in daily weight can indicate retention of fluids, which places the patient at cardiovascular risk for developing heart failure. Fluid retention can increase the work required of the remaining kidney to perform its functions.

Respiratory Status. A nephrectomy can be performed through a flank incision just below the diaphragm. Postoperatively, it is important to ensure adequate ventilation. The patient is often reluctant to turn, cough, and breathe deeply because of the incisional pain. Give adequate pain medication to ensure the patient's comfort and ability to perform coughing and deep-breathing exercises. Have the patient use an incentive spirometer every 2 hours while awake. Early and frequent ambulation helps maintain respiratory function.

Abdominal Distention. Abdominal distention is present to some degree in most patients who have had surgery on their kidneys or ureters. It is often due to paralytic ileus caused by

manipulation and compression of the bowel during surgery. Oral intake is restricted until bowel sounds are present (usually 24 to 48 hours after surgery). IV fluids are given until the patient can take oral fluids. Progression to a regular diet follows.

URINARY DIVERSION

Urinary diversion may be performed with or without cystectomy. Urinary diversion procedures are done when urinary flow is blocked. Common causes include bladder cancer, neurogenic bladder, congenital anomalies, strictures, trauma to the bladder, and chronic bladder inflammation. Numerous urinary diversion techniques and bladder substitutes are possible, including an incontinent urinary diversion, a continent urinary diversion catheterized by the patient, or an orthotopic neobladder bladder so that the patient voids urethrally.[29] Types of surgical procedures for urinary diversion are described in Table 45.21 and Fig. 45.11.

TABLE 45.21 **Urinary Diversion Surgery**			
Description	**Advantages**	**Disadvantages**	**Special Considerations**
Cutaneous Ureterostomy			
Ureters are excised from bladder and brought through abdominal wall, and stoma is created. Ureteral stomas may be created from both ureters, or ureters may be brought together, and one stoma created.	No need for major surgery.	External appliance necessary because of continuous urine drainage. Possibility of stricture or stenosis of small stoma.	Periodic catheterizations may be needed to dilate stomas to maintain patency.
Ileal Conduit			
Ureters are implanted into part of ileum or colon that has been resected from intestinal tract. Abdominal stoma is created.	Relatively good urine flow with few physiologic alterations.	External appliance necessary to continually collect urine.	Surgical procedure is complex. Postoperative complications may be increased. Reabsorption of urea by ileum occurs. Meticulous attention is necessary to care for stoma and collecting device.
Nephrostomy			
Catheter is inserted into pelvis of kidney. Procedure may be done to 1 or both kidneys and may be temporary or permanent. It is most often done in advanced disease as palliative procedure.	No need for major surgery.	High risk for renal infection. Predisposition to stone formation from catheter.	Nephrostomy tube may have to be changed every month. Never clamp the catheter.

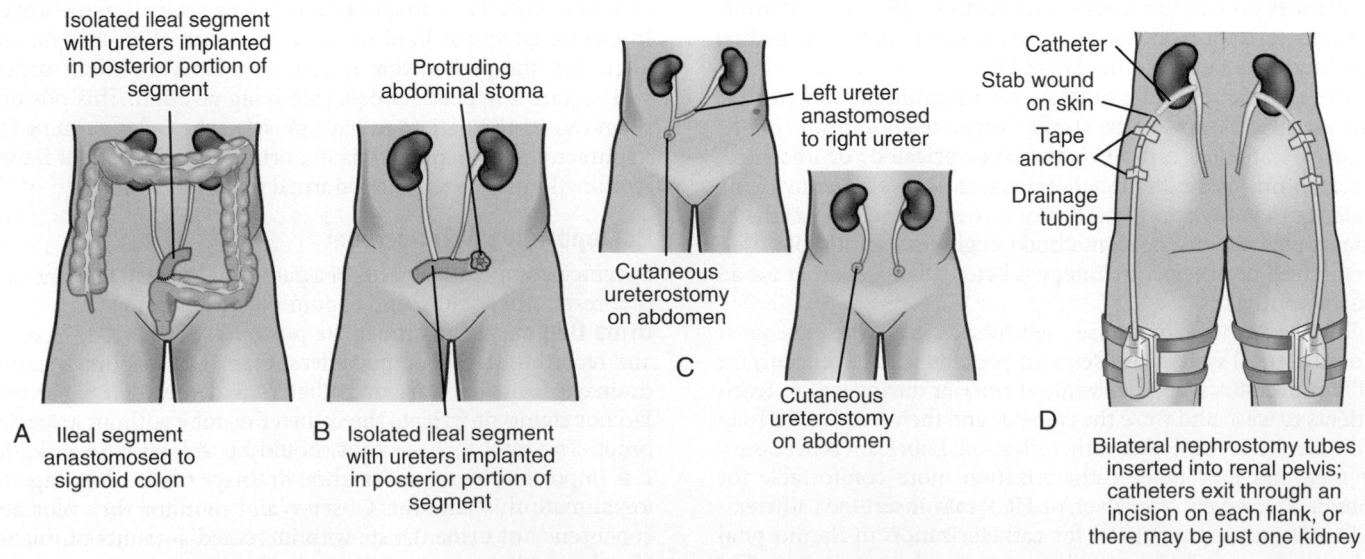

FIG 45.11 Methods of urinary diversion. A, Ureteroileosigmoidostomy. B, Ileal loop (ileal conduit). C, Ureterostomy (transcutaneous ureterostomy and bilateral cutaneous ureterostomies). D, Nephrostomy.

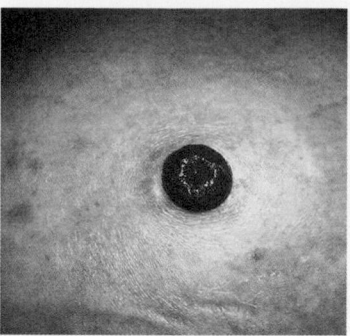

FIG 45.12 Urinary stoma. Symmetric, no skin breakdown, protrudes about 1.5 cm. Mucosa is healthy red. This configuration is flat when the patient is upright or supine. (Courtesy Lynda Brubacher, Virginia Mason Hospital, Seattle, WA.)

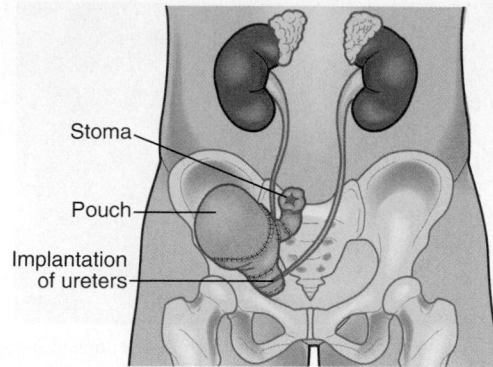

FIG 45.13 Creation of a Kock pouch with implantation of ureters into one intussuscepted part of the pouch and creation of a stoma with the other intussuscepted part.

Incontinent Urinary Diversion

Incontinent urinary diversion is diversion to the skin, requiring an appliance. The simplest form is the cutaneous ureterostomy. However, complications including scarring and strictures of the ureter, have led to the more frequent use of ileal or colonic conduits. The most common incontinent urinary diversion procedure is the **ileal conduit** (ileal loop). In this procedure a 6- to 8-in (15- to 20-cm) segment of the ileum is converted into a conduit for urinary drainage. The colon (colon conduit) can be used instead of the ileum. The ureters are anastomosed into one end of the conduit, and the other end of the bowel is brought out through the abdominal wall to form a stoma (Fig. 45.12). Although the bowel segment is still supported by the mesentery, it is completely isolated from the intestinal tract. The bowel is anastomosed and continues to function normally.

Because there is no valve and no voluntary control over the stoma, drops of urine flow from the stoma every few seconds, requiring a permanent external collecting device. The visible stoma and need for external collection devices are disadvantages of this procedure. The lifelong need to care for and deal with the stoma and collection devices may be difficult. These problems have led to the increasing use of continent diversions and neobladder bladder substitutes.

Continent Urinary Diversions

A *continent urinary diversion* is an intraabdominal urinary reservoir that can be catheterized. Continent diversions are internal pouches created similarly to the ileal conduit. Reservoirs are constructed from the ileum, ileocecal segment, or ascending colon. Large segments of bowel are altered to prevent peristaltic action. A surgically created valve and the large, low-pressure reservoir helps prevent involuntarily leakage. The patient with a continent reservoir needs to self-catheterize every 4 to 6 hours but does not need to wear external attachments. Patients may wear a small bandage on the stoma to collect any mucous drainage or excess drainage. Examples of continent diversions are the Kock (Fig. 45.13), Mainz, Indiana, and Florida pouches. The main difference among the various diversions is the segment of bowel used. For example, the Indiana pouch uses part of the ilium and right colon as a reservoir. It has become a popular form of continent urinary diversion.

Orthotopic Bladder Reconstruction

Orthotopic bladder reconstruction, or orthotopic neobladder, is the construction of a new bladder in the bladder's normal anatomic position, with discharge of urine through the urethra. The neobladder is surgically shaped from various segments of the intestines to make a low-pressure reservoir. An isolated segment of the distal ileum is often preferred. The ureters and urethra are sutured into the neobladder. Various procedures include the hemi-Kock pouch, Studer pouch, and W-shaped ileoneobladder.

Orthotopic bladder reconstruction has become a more viable option for both men and women if cancer does not involve the bladder neck or urethra. Ideal patients have normal renal and liver function, longer than 1- to 2-year life expectancy, adequate motor skills, and no history of inflammatory bowel disease or colon cancer. Obese patients and those with inflammatory bowel disease are not good candidates. The advantage of orthotopic bladder substitution is that it allows for natural micturition. Incontinence is a possible problem with this technique, and intermittent catheterization may be needed.

❖ NURSING MANAGEMENT: URINARY DIVERSION

Preoperative Management

Teaching is important for the patient awaiting cystectomy and urinary diversion surgery. Assess the patient's ability and readiness to learn before starting a teaching program. The patient's anxiety and fear may be decreased by providing more information. However, anxiety and fear may also interfere with learning. Involve the patient's caregiver and family in the teaching process.

Discuss the psychosocial aspects of living with a stoma (including clothing, changes in body image and sexuality, exercise, and odor). This may allay some fears. The patient with an orthotopic neobladder may have problems with incontinence. Discuss patients' concerns about sexual activities and let them know that counseling is available. A wound, ostomy, and continence nurse (WOCN) should be involved in the preoperative phase of the patient's care. A visit from an ostomate can be helpful. Additional interventions are discussed in eNursing Care Plan 45.3 for the patient with an ileal conduit (on the website for this chapter).

Postoperative Management

Plan nursing interventions during the postoperative period to prevent surgical complications, such as atelectasis (see Chapter 19). After pelvic surgery, there is an increased incidence of thrombophlebitis and UTI. Removal of part of the bowel increase the risk of paralytic ileus and small bowel obstruction. The patient is kept NPO, and a nasogastric tube may be needed for a few days.

Prevent injury to the stoma and maintain urine output. Tell the patient that mucus in the urine is a normal occurrence. The mucus is secreted by the mucosa of the intestine (which was

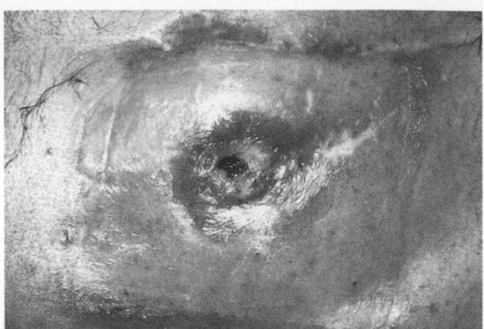

FIG 45.14 Ammonia salt encrustation from alkaline urine. (Courtesy Lynda Brubacher, Virginia Mason Hospital, Seattle, WA.)

used to create the ileal conduit) in response to the irritating effect of urine. Encourage a high fluid intake to "flush" the ileal conduit or continent diversion.

When an ileal conduit is created, provide meticulous care for the skin around the stoma. Alkaline encrustations with dermatitis may occur when alkaline urine comes in contact with exposed skin (Fig. 45.14). The urine is kept acidic to prevent alkaline encrustations. Other common peristomal skin problems include yeast infections, product allergies, and shearing-effect excoriations. Changing appliances (pouches) is described in Table 45.22. A properly fitting appliance is essential to prevent skin problems. The appliance should be about 0.1 in (0.2 cm) larger than the stoma. It is normal for the stoma to shrink within the first few weeks after surgery.

Teach the patient with a continent diversion (e.g., Indiana pouch) to catheterize at first every few hours. Over time this can be extended to every 4 to 6 hours. Irrigation of the pouch with normal saline or sterile water is often needed.

Patients with a neobladder may have postoperative urinary retention and need catheterization. It may take up to 6 months for them to regain bladder control. Patients empty their neobladders by relaxing their outlet sphincter muscles and bearing down with their abdominal muscles. Since there is no longer neurologic feedback between the reservoir and the brain, the patient should not expect a normal desire to void. To avoid bladder overdistention, patients should void at least every 2 to 4 hours, sit during voiding, and practice pelvic floor muscle relaxation to aid voiding. Follow-up x-ray studies include a "pouchogram" 3 to 4 weeks after surgery to assess for healing.

Acceptance of the surgery and changes in body image is needed to ensure the patient's best adjustment to a urinary diversion. Patient concerns include fear that the stoma will be offensive to others and will interfere with sexual, personal, professional, and recreational activities. Advise the patient that few activities will be restricted because of the urinary diversion. Meeting and sharing feelings with similar patients can help.

Discharge teaching after an ileal conduit includes teaching the patient about symptoms of obstruction or infection and care of the ostomy. The patient with an ileal conduit is fitted for a permanent appliance 7 to 10 days after surgery. It may have to be refitted later, depending on the degree of stoma healing and shrinkage.

Appliances are made of a variety of products, including natural and synthetic rubbers, plastics, and metals. Most appliances have a faceplate that adheres to the skin, a collecting pouch, and an opening to drain the pouch. The faceplate may be secured to the skin with glues, adhesives, or adherent synthetic wafers. Some appliances do not need adhesives because their design

TABLE 45.22 Patient & Caregiver Teaching

Ileal Conduit Appliances

Include the following instructions when teaching a patient or a caregiver how to change an ileal conduit appliance:

Temporary Appliance
1. Cut hole in pouch to fit over stoma (pouch 0.1 in [0.2 cm] larger than stoma).
2. Remove old pouch.
3. Clean area gently and remove old adhesive.
4. Wash area with warm water.
5. Place wick (rolled-up 4 × 4–in pad) over stoma to keep area dry during rest of procedure.
6. Dry skin around stoma.
7. Apply tincture of benzoin or other skin protectant around stoma to area where pouch will be placed.
8. Apply pouch by first smoothing its edges toward side and lower part of body.
9. Remove wick and complete application of bag.
10. If patient is usually in bed, apply bag so that it lies toward side of body.
11. If patient is ambulatory, apply bag so that it lies vertically.
12. Connect drainage tubing to pouch.
13. Keep drainage pouch on same side of bed as stoma.

Permanent Appliance*
1. Keep appliance in place for 2–14 days.
2. Change appliance when fluid intake has been restricted for several hours.
3. Sit or stand in front of mirror.
4. Moisten edge of faceplate with adhesive solvent and gently remove.
5. Clean skin with adhesive solvent.
6. Wash skin with warm water (may be done while showering).
7. Dry skin and inspect.
8. Place wick (rolled-up 4 × 4–inch pad) over stoma to keep skin free of urine.
9. Apply skin cement to faceplate and skin.
10. Place appliance over stoma.
11. Wash removed appliance with soap and lukewarm water; soak in distilled vinegar; rinse with lukewarm water and air dry.

*Many disposable appliances with self-adhesive backing are used as permanent appliances.

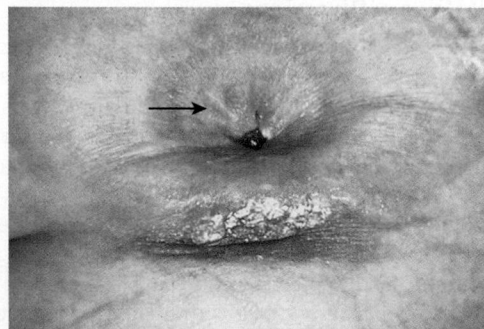

FIG 45.15 Retracted urinary stoma with pressure sore from faceplate above stoma *(arrow)*. (Courtesy Lynda Brubacher, Virginia Mason Hospital, Seattle, WA.)

relies on pressure to keep the pouch in place. If improperly fitted or applied, the faceplate may cause skin problems (Fig. 45.15). Tell the patient and caregiver about where to buy supplies, emergency telephone numbers, location of ostomy clubs, and follow-up visits with a WOCN. Follow-up with an HCP is imperative to monitor the patient's recovery, detect any complications, and assess renal function.

CASE STUDY

Painful Bladder and Frequent Urination

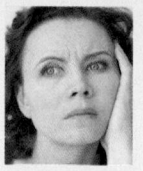

(© marilook/iStock/Thinkstock.)

Patient Profile

L.T., a 38-yr-old woman, comes to the HCP's office today for the eighth time in the past year for a history of pelvic pain with urinary frequency during the day, nocturia, and urgency to void. All previous urine cultures have been negative for bacteria. A recent evaluation by her gynecologist was negative for endometriosis.

Subjective Data

- Has a history of suprapubic and vaginal pain, urinary frequency and urgency
- Reports bladder pain that increases with bladder filling
- States this is her third attack of suprapubic pain and painful urination in 2 months
- Constant pain and discomfort has been physically and emotionally exhausting
- Is worried that she has cancer, and no one cares
- Has had 4 pregnancies with uneventful vaginal deliveries
- Normal menstrual cycles
- Her husband and she rarely have sexual intercourse because she has pain with intercourse
- Has a bowel movement every day. Denies constipation and/or diarrhea
- Recalls having many UTIs as a child

Objective Data

Physical Examination

- Lungs are clear. BP 132/86. Heart rate 86/min. Respiratory rate 18/min. Abdomen soft, tender in suprapubic region.

Diagnostic Studies

- Urinalysis obtained today: normal
- Previous urine cytology ordered to rule out cancer: normal
- Recent referral to urologist for cystoscopy which was done a few weeks ago

Interprofessional Care

- Cystoscopy results indicated glomerulations and Hunner lesions
- Urologist diagnosed interstitial cystitis
- Urologist prescribed pentosan (Elmiron), which she has not started yet
- Follow-up in 4 weeks with the urologist

Discussion Questions

1. After taking the patient's history, would you consider a UTI as a cause of her symptoms? Why or why not?
2. What additional testing and patient information would be helpful?
3. What is the significance of the cystoscopy findings?
4. What is the reason for the use of pentosan (Elmiron)?
5. *Priority Decision:* What are the priority nursing diagnoses for L.T.?
6. *Patient-Centered Care:* How can you help L.T. deal with her diagnosis and treatment plan?
7. Collaboration: Why is it important to get a dietitian involved in L.T.'s care?
8. *Evidence-Based Practice:* L.T. asks you how she can control her interstitial cystitis. How would you respond?

Answers available at *http://evolve.elsevier.com/Lewis/medsurg.*

BRIDGE TO NCLEX EXAMINATION

The number of the question corresponds to the same-numbered outcome at the beginning of the chapter.

1. The nurse teaches the female patient who has frequent UTIs that she should
   a. take tub baths with bubble bath.
   b. void before and after sexual intercourse.
   c. take prophylactic sulfonamides for the rest of her life.
   d. restrict fluid intake to prevent the need for frequent voiding.

2. One of the nurse's *most* important roles in relation to acute post-streptococcal glomerulonephritis (APSGN) is to
   a. promote early diagnosis and treatment of sore throats and skin lesions.
   b. encourage patients to obtain antibiotic therapy for upper respiratory tract infections.
   c. teach patients with APSGN that long-term prophylactic antibiotic therapy is needed to prevent recurrence.
   d. monitor patients for respiratory symptoms that indicate the disease is affecting the alveolar basement membrane.

3. The edema that occurs in nephrotic syndrome is due to
   a. increased hydrostatic pressure caused by sodium retention.
   b. decreased aldosterone secretion from adrenal insufficiency.
   c. increased fluid retention caused by decreased glomerular filtration.
   d. decreased colloidal osmotic pressure caused by loss of serum albumin.

4. A patient is admitted to the hospital with severe renal colic. The nurse's *first priority* in management of the patient is to
   a. administer opioids as prescribed.
   b. obtain supplies for straining all urine.
   c. encourage fluid intake of 3 to 4 L/day.
   d. keep the patient NPO in preparation for surgery.

5. The nurse recommends genetic counseling for the children of a patient with
   a. nephrotic syndrome.
   b. chronic pyelonephritis.
   c. malignant nephrosclerosis.
   d. adult-onset polycystic kidney disease.

6. The nurse identifies a risk factor for kidney and bladder cancer in a patient who relates a history of
   a. aspirin use.
   b. tobacco use.
   c. chronic alcohol use.
   d. use of artificial sweeteners.

7. In planning nursing interventions to increase bladder control in the patient with urinary incontinence, the nurse includes (*select all that apply*)
   a. teaching the patient to use Kegel exercises.
   b. clamping and releasing a catheter to increase bladder tone.
   c. teaching the patient biofeedback mechanisms to train pelvic floor muscles.
   d. counseling the patient concerning choice of incontinence containment device.
   e. developing a fluid modification plan, focusing on decreasing intake before bedtime.

8. A patient with a ureterolithotomy returns from surgery with a nephrostomy tube in place. Postoperative nursing care of the patient includes
   a. clamping the tube for 10 minutes every hour to decrease spasms.
   b. encouraging fluids of at least 2 to 3 L/day after nausea has subsided.
   c. notifying the provider if nephrostomy tube drainage is more than 30 mL/hr.
   d. irrigating the nephrostomy tube with 10 mL of normal saline solution as needed.

9. A patient has had a cystectomy and ileal conduit diversion. Four days after surgery, you note mucous shreds in the drainage bag. The nurse should
   a. notify the provider.
   b. notify the charge nurse.
   c. irrigate the drainage tube.
   d. document it as a normal observation.

1. b, 2. a, 3. d, 4. a, 5. d, 6. b, 7. a, c, 8. b, 9. d

For rationales to these answers and even more NCLEX review questions, visit *http://evolve.elsevier.com/Lewis/medsurg.*

ⓔ EVOLVE WEBSITE/RESOURCES LIST

http://evolve.elsevier.com/Lewis/medsurg
Review Questions (Online Only)
Key Points
Answer Keys for Questions
  • Rationales for Bridge to NCLEX Examination Questions
  • Answer Guidelines for Case Study on p. 1057
Student Case Studies
  • Patient With Bladder Cancer and Urinary Diversion
  • Patient With Glomerulonephritis and Acute Kidney Injury
Nursing Care Plans
  • eNursing Care Plan 45.1: Patient With a Urinary Tract Infection
  • eNursing Care Plan 45.2: Patient With Urinary Tract Calculi
  • eNursing Care Plan 45.3: Patient With an Ileal Conduit
Conceptual Care Map Creator
Audio Glossary
Content Updates

REFERENCES

1. National Institute of Diabetes and Digestion and Kidney Diseases: Kidney and urologic diseases statistics for the United States. Retrieved from *www.niddk.nih.gov/health-information/health-topics/urologic-disease/urinary-tract-infections-in-adults/Pages/facts.aspx.*
2. Brusch JL, Bavaro MF, Cunha BA, et al: Cystitis in females. Retrieved from *http://emedicine.medscape.com/article/233101-overview.*
3. Brusch JL, Bronze MS: Catheter-related urinary tract infection (UTI). Retrieved from *https://emedicine.medscape.com/article/2040035-overview#a1.*
4. Chu CC, Lowder J:. Diagnosis and treatment of urinary tract infections across age groups, *Am J Obstet Gynecol* 219:40, 2018.
*5. University of Rochester: Guidelines for the diagnosis and management of urinary tract infections. Retrieved from *www.rochesterpatientsafety.com/Images_Content/Site1/Files/Pages/UTI_Treatment_Guidelines.pdf.*
6. American Nurses Association: ANA CAUTI prevention tool. Retrieved from *www.nursingworld.org/practice-policy/work-environment/health-safety/infection-prevention/ana-cauti-prevention-tool/.*
*7. European Association of Urology: Urological infections guidelines. Retrieved from *http://uroweb.org/guideline/urological-infections/#3.*
8. National Institute for Diabetes and Digestive and Kidney Diseases: Interstitial cystitis/painful bladder syndrome. Retrieved from *www.niddk.nih.gov/health-information/health-topics/urologic-disease/interstitial-cystitis-painful-bladder-syndrome.*
9. Lessnau K, Kim ED, Pais VM: Tuberculosis of the genitourinary system: Overview of GUTB. Retrieved from *http://emedicine.medscape.com/article/450651-overview.*
10. Figueiredo AA, Lucon AM, Srougi M: Urogenital tuberculosis, *Microbiol Spectr.* 5, 2017.
11. National Institute of Diabetes and Digestion and Kidney Diseases: Glomerular diseases. Retrieved from *www.niddk.nih.gov/health-information/kidney-disease/glomerular-diseases.*
12. Bhimma R: Acute poststreptococcal glomerulonephritis. Retrieved from *https://emedicine.medscape.com/article/980685-overview.*
13. Cohen EP, Batuman V: Nephrotic syndrome. Retrieved from *http://emedicine.medscape.com/article/244631-overview.*
14. US National Library of Medicine: Obstructive uropathy. Retrieved from *https://medlineplus.gov/ency/article/000507.htm.*
*15. Canadian Urological Association: CUA guidelines on the evaluation and medical management of the kidney stone patient—2016 Update, *Can Urol Assoc J* 10:E347, 2016.
*16. American Urological Association/Endourology Society: Surgical management of stones: AUA/Endourology Society guidelines. Retrieved from *www.auanet.org/guidelines/surgical-management-of-stones-(aua/endourological-society-guideline-2016).*
*17. American Urological Association: Urotrauma. Retrieved from *www.auanet.org/guidelines/urotrauma-(2014-amended-2017).*
18. National Kidney Foundation: Polycystic kidney disease. Retrieved from *www.kidney.org/atoz/content/polycystic.*
19. Genetics Home Reference: Alport syndrome. Retrieved from *https://ghr.nlm.nih.gov/condition/alport-syndrome#diagnosis.*
20. American Cancer Society: Key statistics about kidney cancer 2018. Retrieved from *www.cancer.org/cancer/kidney-cancer/about/key-statistics.html.*
*21. American Urological Association: Renal mass and localized renal cancer: AUA guidelines. Retrieved from *www.auanet.org/guidelines/renal-mass-and-localized-renal-cancer-new-(2017).*
22. Farling KB: Bladder cancer: Risk factors, diagnosis, and management, *Nurse Pract* 42:26, 2017.
23. American Cancer Society: Key statistics about bladder cancer 2018. Retrieved from *www.cancer.org/cancer/bladder-cancer/about/key-statistics.html.*
*24. American Urological Association, Society of Urologic Oncology: Diagnosis and treatment of non-muscle invasive bladder cancer: AUA/SUO joint guidelines. Retrieved from *www.auanet.org/guidelines/non-muscle-invasive-bladder-cancer-(aua/suo-joint-guideline-2016).*
*25. American Urological Association, American Society of Clinical Oncology, American Society of Radiation Oncology, Society of Urologic Oncology: Treatment of non-metastatic muscle-invasive bladder cancer: AUA/ASCO/ASTRO/SUO guidelines. Retrieved from *www.auanet.org/guidelines/muscle-invasive-bladder-cancer-new-(2017).*
*26. Palmer MH, Willis-Gray MG: Overactive bladder in women, *AJN* 117:34, 2017.
*27. American Urological Association, Society of Urodynamics: Female pelvic medicine and urogenital reconstruction: Surgical treatment of female stress urinary incontinence: AUA/SUFU guidelines. Retrieved from *www.auanet.org/guidelines/stress-urinary-incontinence-(sui)-new-(aua/sufu-guideline-2017).*
*28. Southern Health National Health Services Foundation Trust: Urinary catheter care guidelines. Retrieved from www.southernhealth.nhs.uk/_resources/assets/inline/full/0/70589.pdf.
29. National Institute for Diabetes and Digestive and Kidney Diseases: Urinary diversion. Retrieved from *www.niddk.nih.gov/health-information/health-topics/urologic-disease/urinary-diversion.*

*Evidence-based information for clinical practice.

46

Acute Kidney Injury and Chronic Kidney Disease

Hazel Dennison

Too often we underestimate the power of a touch, a smile, a kind word, a listening ear, or the smallest act of caring, all of which have the potential to turn a life around.

Leo Buscaglia

http://evolve.elsevier.com/Lewis/medsurg

CONCEPTUAL FOCUS

Acid-Base Balance
Adherence

Coping
Elimination

Fluids and Electrolytes
Nutrition

LEARNING OUTCOMES

1. Outline criteria used to classify acute kidney injury using the acronym RIFLE (*R*isk, *I*njury, *F*ailure, *L*oss, *E*nd-stage renal disease).
2. Relate the clinical course of acute kidney injury.
3. Explain the interprofessional and nursing management of a patient with acute kidney injury.
4. Define chronic kidney disease and delineate its 5 stages based on the glomerular filtration rate.
5. Identify risk factors that contribute to the development of chronic kidney disease.
6. Describe the significance of cardiovascular disease in people with chronic kidney disease.
7. Explain the conservative interprofessional care and related nursing management of the patient with chronic kidney disease.
8. Distinguish among renal replacement therapy options for persons with end-stage renal disease.
9. Compare and contrast nursing interventions for patients on peritoneal dialysis and hemodialysis.
10. Discuss the role of nurses in the management of patients who receive a kidney transplant.

KEY TERMS

acute kidney injury (AKI), p. 1059
acute tubular necrosis (ATN), p. 1061
anuria, p. 1062
arteriovenous fistula (AVF), p. 1076
arteriovenous grafts (AVGs), p. 1076
automated peritoneal dialysis (APD), p. 1075
azotemia, p. 1059

chronic kidney disease (CKD), p. 1065
CKD mineral and bone disorder (CKD-MBD), p. 1068
continuous ambulatory peritoneal dialysis (CAPD), p. 1075
continuous renal replacement therapy (CRRT), p. 1079

dialysis, p. 1073
end-stage renal disease (ESRD), p. 1065
hemodialysis (HD), p. 1073
oliguria, p. 1061
peritoneal dialysis (PD), p. 1073
uremia, p. 1066

Kidney failure, also called *renal failure*, is the partial or complete impairment of kidney function. It results in an inability to excrete metabolic waste products and water. Kidney failure contributes to problems with all body systems. All patients have problems with fluid, electrolyte, and acid-base imbalance. Adhering to dietary therapies and the treatment plan can be challenging. The patient must deal with changes in lifestyle, occupation, family relationships, and self-image that can lead to withdrawal and depression. The patient grieves the loss of kidney function and independence.

Kidney failure is classified as acute or chronic (Table 46.1). Acute kidney injury (AKI) has a rapid onset. Chronic kidney disease (CKD) is gradual with a progressive decline in kidney function.

ACUTE KIDNEY INJURY

Acute kidney injury (AKI) is the term used to encompass the entire scope of the syndrome, ranging from a slight deterioration in kidney function to severe impairment. AKI is characterized by a rapid loss of kidney function. This loss is accompanied by a rise in serum creatinine and/or a reduction in urine output. AKI can develop over hours or days with progressive elevations of blood urea nitrogen (BUN), creatinine, and potassium with or without a reduction in urine output. The severity of dysfunction can range from a small increase in serum creatinine or reduction in urine output to the development of azotemia, an accumulation of nitrogenous waste products (urea nitrogen, creatinine) in the blood.

Although AKI is potentially reversible, it has a high mortality rate.[1] AKI usually affects people with other life-threatening conditions (Table 46.2).[2] AKI often follows severe, prolonged hypotension, hypovolemia, or exposure to a nephrotoxic agent. Hospitalized patients develop AKI at a high rate (1 in 5) and have a high mortality rate. When AKI develops in patients in intensive care units (ICUs), the mortality rate can be as high as 70% to 80%.[3,4]

Etiology and Pathophysiology

The causes of AKI are multiple and complex. We categorize them as prerenal, intrarenal (or intrinsic), and postrenal causes (Table 46.2 and Fig. 46.1).

Prerenal. *Prerenal* causes of AKI are factors that reduce systemic circulation, causing a reduction in renal blood flow. The decrease in blood flow leads to decreased glomerular perfusion and filtration of the kidneys.

It is important to distinguish prerenal oliguria from the oliguria of intrarenal AKI. In prerenal oliguria there is no damage to the kidney tissue (parenchyma). The oliguria is caused by a decrease in circulating blood volume (e.g., severe dehydration, heart failure [HF], decreased cardiac output). Prerenal

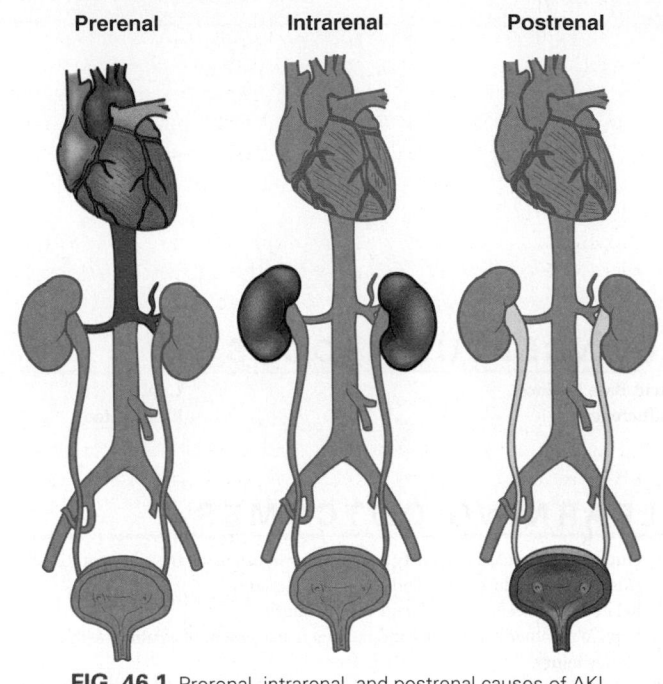

FIG. 46.1 Prerenal, intrarenal, and postrenal causes of AKI.

TABLE 46.1 Comparison of Acute Kidney Injury and Chronic Kidney Disease

	Acute Kidney Injury	Chronic Kidney Disease
Onset	Sudden	Gradual, often over many years
Most common cause	Acute tubular necrosis	Diabetic nephropathy
Diagnostic criteria	Acute reduction in urine output *AND/OR* Elevation in serum creatinine	GFR <60 mL/min/1.73 m² for >3 mo *AND/OR* Kidney damage >3 mo
Reversibility	Potentially	Progressive and irreversible
Primary cause of death	Infection	CVD

TABLE 46.2 Common Causes of Acute Kidney Injury

Prerenal	Intrarenal	Postrenal
Decreased Cardiac Output • Cardiogenic shock • Dysrhythmias • HF • MI **Decreased Peripheral Vascular Resistance** • Anaphylaxis • Neurologic injury • Septic shock **Decreased Renovascular Blood Flow** • Bilateral renal vein thrombosis • Embolism • Hepatorenal syndrome • Renal artery thrombosis **Hypovolemia** • Burns • Dehydration • Excessive diuresis • GI losses (diarrhea, vomiting) • Hemorrhage • Hypoalbuminemia	**Interstitial Nephritis** • Allergies: antibiotics (sulfonamides, rifampin), NSAIDs, ACE inhibitors • Infections: bacterial (acute pyelonephritis), viral (Epstein-Barr), fungal (candidiasis) **Nephrotoxic Injury** • Chemical exposure: ethylene glycol, lead, arsenic, carbon tetrachloride • Contrast media • Drugs: aminoglycosides (gentamicin, amikacin), amphotericin B • Hemolytic blood transfusion reaction • Severe crush injury **Other Causes** • Acute glomerulonephritis • Malignant hypertension • Prolonged prerenal ischemia • Thrombotic disorders • Toxemia of pregnancy • Systemic lupus erythematosus	• BPH • Bladder cancer • Calculi formation • Neuromuscular disorders • Prostate cancer • Spinal cord disease • Strictures • Trauma (back, pelvis, perineum)

oliguria is readily reversible with appropriate treatment.[5] With a decrease in circulating blood volume, autoregulatory mechanisms that increase angiotensin II, aldosterone, norepinephrine, and antidiuretic hormone try to preserve blood flow to essential organs. Prerenal azotemia results in a reduction in sodium excretion (less than 20 mEq/L), increased sodium and water retention, and decreased urine output.

Prerenal conditions contribute to intrarenal AKI. If decreased perfusion persists for an extended time, the kidneys lose their ability to compensate and damage to kidney parenchyma occurs (intrarenal damage).

Intrarenal. *Intrarenal* causes of AKI (Table 46.2) include conditions that cause direct damage to the kidney tissue, resulting in impaired nephron function. The damage from intrarenal causes usually results from prolonged ischemia, nephrotoxins (e.g., aminoglycoside antibiotics, contrast media), hemoglobin released from hemolyzed red blood cells (RBCs), or myoglobin released from necrotic muscle cells.

Nephrotoxins can cause obstruction of intrarenal structures by crystallizing or causing damage to the epithelial cells of the tubules. Hemoglobin and myoglobin can block the tubules and cause renal vasoconstriction. Kidney diseases, such as acute glomerulonephritis and systemic lupus erythematosus (SLE), may also cause AKI.

Acute tubular necrosis (ATN) is the most common intrarenal cause of AKI in hospitalized patients. It is primarily the result of ischemia, nephrotoxins, or sepsis. Ischemic and nephrotoxic ATN is responsible for 90% of intrarenal AKI cases.[6,7] Severe kidney ischemia causes a disruption in the basement membrane and patchy destruction of the tubular epithelium. Nephrotoxic agents cause necrosis of tubular epithelial cells, which slough off and plug the tubules. Other risks associated with developing ATN while in the hospital include major surgery, shock, blood transfusion reaction, muscle injury from trauma, and prolonged hypotension. ATN is potentially reversible if the basement membrane is not destroyed and the tubular epithelium regenerates.

Postrenal. *Postrenal* causes of AKI involve mechanical obstruction in the outflow of urine. With the flow of urine obstructed, urine refluxes into the renal pelvis, impairing kidney function. The most common postrenal causes are benign prostatic hyperplasia (BPH), prostate cancer, stones, trauma, and extrarenal tumors. Bilateral ureteral obstruction leads to *hydronephrosis* (kidney dilation), increase in hydrostatic pressure, and tubular blockage, resulting in a progressive decline in kidney function. If bilateral obstruction is relieved within 48 hours of onset, complete recovery is likely. Prolonged obstruction can lead to tubular atrophy and irreversible kidney fibrosis. Postrenal causes of AKI account for less than 10% of AKI cases.[8]

Clinical Manifestations

Prerenal and postrenal AKI that has not caused intrarenal damage usually resolves quickly with treatment. When parenchymal damage occurs due to either prerenal or postrenal causes, or when parenchymal damage occurs directly as with intrarenal causes, AKI has a prolonged course. Clinically, AKI may progress through phases: oliguric, diuretic, and recovery. When a patient does not recover from AKI, CKD may develop.

The RIFLE classification describes the stages of AKI (Table 46.3). *Risk*, the first stage of AKI, is followed by *Injury*, which is the second stage. Then AKI increases in severity to the last, or third, stage, *Failure*. The 2 outcome variables are *Loss* and *End-stage renal disease*.[9,10]

Oliguric Phase. The most common manifestations of AKI are discussed in this section.

Urinary Changes. The most common initial manifestation of AKI is oliguria, a reduction in urine output to less than 400 mL/day. Oliguria usually occurs within 1 to 7 days of the injury to the kidneys. If the cause is ischemia, oliguria often occurs within 24 hours. When nephrotoxic drugs are involved, the onset may be delayed for as long as 1 week. This phase lasts on average 10 to 14 days but can last months in some cases. The longer the oliguric phase lasts, the poorer the prognosis for complete recovery of kidney function.[1]

TABLE 46.3 RIFLE Classification for Staging Acute Kidney Injury

Stage	GFR Criteria	Urine Output Criteria	Clinical Example
Risk	Serum creatinine increased × 1.5 OR GFR decreased by 25%	Urine output <0.5 mL/kg/hr for 6 hr	• 68-yr-old black woman with type 2 diabetes, hypertension, CAD, CKD • Scheduled to undergo emergency coronary artery bypass graft • Serum creatinine is 1.8 mg/dL (increased), weight 60 kg • Calculated GFR is 35 mL/min/1.73 m² • Has stage 3b CKD
Injury	Serum creatinine increased × 2 OR GFR decreased by 50%	Urine output <0.5 mL/kg/hr for 12 hr	• During surgery, she is hypotensive for a sustained period • Diagnosed with acute tubular necrosis • After surgery: serum creatinine is 3.6 mg/dL, urine output reduced to 28 mL/hr
Failure	Serum creatinine increased × 3 OR GFR decreased by 75% OR Serum creatinine >4 mg/dL with acute rise ≥0.5 mg/dL	Urine output <0.3 mL/kg/hr for 24 hr (oliguria) OR Anuria for 12 hr	• 72 hours after surgery, develops ventilator-associated pneumonia and sepsis while in ICU • Serum creatinine rises to 5.2 mg/dL, urine output drops to 10 mL/hr • BP remains low despite dopamine therapy
Loss	Persistent acute kidney failure. Complete loss of kidney function >4 wk	—	• Starts on continuous venovenous hemodialysis • After 3 wk of therapy she has a cardiopulmonary arrest and does not survive
End-stage renal disease	• Complete loss of kidney function >3 mo	—	—

Nonoliguric AKI has a urine output greater than 400 mL/day. About 50% of patients will be nonoliguric, making the initial diagnosis more difficult.[7]

While changes in urine output generally do not correspond to changes in glomerular filtration rate (GFR), they can be helpful in distinguishing the cause of AKI. For example, anuria (no urine output) is usually seen with urinary tract obstruction. Oliguria is often seen with prerenal causes. Nonoliguric AKI occurs with acute interstitial nephritis and ATN.[8]

A urinalysis may show casts, RBCs, and white blood cells (WBCs). Casts form from mucoprotein impressions of the necrotic renal tubular epithelial cells, which slough into the tubules. The specific gravity may be fixed at around 1.010, with urine osmolality at about 300 mOsm/kg (300 mmol/kg). This is the same specific gravity and osmolality of plasma, thus reflecting tubular damage with a loss of concentrating ability by the kidney. Proteinuria may be present if AKI is related to glomerular membrane dysfunction.

Fluid Volume. Hypovolemia (volume depletion) has the potential to worsen all forms of AKI. Fluid replacement is often enough to treat many forms of AKI, especially prerenal causes. When urine output decreases, fluid retention occurs. The severity of the manifestations depends on the extent of the fluid overload. In the case of reduced urine output (anuria and oliguria), the neck veins may become distended with a bounding pulse. Edema and hypertension may develop. Fluid overload can eventually lead to HF, pulmonary edema, and pericardial and pleural effusions.

Metabolic Acidosis. In the normal kidney, excess hydrogen ions are excreted to maintain a physiologic balance of the blood pH. Impaired kidneys cannot excrete hydrogen ions or the acid products of metabolism. Serum bicarbonate (HCO_3^-) production decreases from defective reabsorption and regeneration of HCO_3^- ions. Serum HCO_3^- is depleted through buffering of acidic hydrogen ions and metabolic end products. The patient with severe acidosis may develop Kussmaul respirations (rapid, deep respirations) to try to compensate by increasing CO_2 exhalation.

Sodium Balance. Damaged tubules cannot conserve sodium. Urinary sodium excretion may increase, resulting in normal or below-normal levels of serum sodium. Excess sodium intake is avoided because it can lead to volume expansion, hypertension, and HF. Uncontrolled hyponatremia or water excess can lead to cerebral edema.

Potassium Excess. The kidneys normally excrete 80% to 90% of the body's potassium. In AKI the serum potassium level increases because the kidney's normal ability to excrete potassium is impaired. The risk for hyperkalemia increases if AKI is caused by massive tissue trauma because the damaged cells release potassium into the extracellular fluid (ECF). Bleeding and blood transfusions may cause cellular destruction, releasing more potassium into the ECF. Metabolic acidosis worsens hyperkalemia as hydrogen ions enter the cells, and potassium is driven out of the cells into the ECF.

While patients with hyperkalemia are often asymptomatic, some may have weakness with severe hyperkalemia. Because cardiac muscle is intolerant of acute increases in potassium, emergency treatment of hyperkalemia is needed.

Acute or rapid development of hyperkalemia may result in signs that are apparent on electrocardiogram (ECG). These changes include peaked T waves, widening of the QRS complex, and ST segment depression. Progressive changes in the ECG related to increasing potassium levels are shown in Fig. 16.14.

Hematologic Disorders. Several hematologic disorders occur in patients with AKI. Hospital-acquired AKI often occurs in patients who have multiorgan failure. Leukocytosis is often present. The most common cause of death in AKI is infection. The most common sites of infection are the urinary and respiratory systems.

Waste Product Accumulation. The kidneys are the primary excretory organs for urea (an end product of protein metabolism) and creatinine (an end product of endogenous muscle metabolism). BUN and serum creatinine levels are increased in kidney disease. An increased BUN level also can be caused by dehydration; corticosteroids; or catabolism resulting from infections, fever, severe injury, or GI bleeding. The best serum indicator of AKI is creatinine because it is not affected by other factors.

Neurologic Disorders. Neurologic changes can occur as the nitrogenous waste products accumulate in the brain and other nervous tissue. The manifestations can be as mild as fatigue and difficulty concentrating and escalate to seizures, stupor, and coma.

Diuretic Phase. During the diuretic phase of AKI, daily urine output is usually around 1 to 3 L but may reach 5 L or more. The nephrons are still not fully functional even as urine output increases. The high urine volume is caused by osmotic diuresis from the high urea concentration in the glomerular filtrate and the inability of the tubules to concentrate the urine. In this phase, the kidneys have recovered their ability to excrete wastes but not to concentrate the urine. Hypovolemia and hypotension can occur from massive fluid losses.

Patients who develop an oliguric phase will have greater diuresis as kidney function returns. Large losses of fluid and electrolytes require patient monitoring for hyponatremia, hypokalemia, and dehydration. The diuretic phase may last 1 to 3 weeks. Near the end of this phase, the patient's acid-base, electrolyte, and waste product (BUN, creatinine) values stabilize.

Recovery Phase. The recovery phase begins when the GFR increases, allowing the BUN and serum creatinine levels to decrease. Major improvements occur in the first 1 to 2 weeks of this phase. Kidney function may take up to 12 months to stabilize. The patient's overall health, severity of kidney injury, and number and type of complications influence the outcome of AKI. Some patients do not recover and progress to end-stage renal disease (ESRD). The older adult is less likely to have a complete recovery of kidney function. Patients who recover may achieve clinically normal kidney function but remain in an early stage of CKD.

Diagnostic Studies

A thorough history is essential for diagnosing the cause of AKI. Consider prerenal causes when there is a history of dehydration, hypotension, or blood loss. Suspect intrarenal causes if the patient has been exposed to potentially nephrotoxic drugs or contrast media used in a radiologic study. A history of changes in the urinary stream, stones, BPH, or bladder or prostate cancer suggests postrenal causes.

Although changes in urine output and serum creatinine occur relatively late in the course of AKI, they are known diagnostic indicators. An increase in serum creatinine may not be evident until there is a loss of more than 50% of kidney function. The rate of increase in serum creatinine is important as a diagnostic indicator in determining the severity of injury.

Urinalysis is an important diagnostic test. Urine sediment containing abundant cells, casts, or proteins suggests intrarenal disorders. The urine osmolality, sodium content, and specific gravity help in distinguishing the causes of AKI. Urine sediment may be normal in both prerenal and postrenal AKI. In intrarenal problems, hematuria, pyuria, and crystals may be seen. Other testing may be needed (Table 46.4). A kidney ultrasound is often the first test done. It provides imaging without exposure to potentially nephrotoxic contrast agents. It is useful for evaluating for kidney disease and obstruction of the urinary collection system. A renal scan can assess abnormalities in kidney blood flow, tubular function, and the collecting system. A CT scan can identify lesions, masses, obstructions, and vascular anomalies. A renal biopsy is the best method for confirming intrarenal causes of AKI.

Having an MRI or magnetic resonance angiography (MRA) study with the contrast media gadolinium is not advised in patients with kidney failure. Giving gadolinium can be potentially fatal.

In patients with normal kidney function, contrast media poses minimal risk. In patients with kidney disease, *contrast-induced nephropathy* (CIN) can occur when contrast media for diagnostic studies causes nephrotoxic injury. In patients with diabetes receiving metformin, the drug should be held for 48 hours prior to and after the use of contrast media to decrease the risk for lactic acidosis. The best way to avoid CIN is to avoid exposure to contrast media by using other diagnostic tests, such as ultrasound. If contrast media must be given to a high-risk patient, the patient needs to have optimal hydration and the lowest possible dose of the contrast agent. Nursing interventions to ensure adequate fluid intake and hydration can decrease the risks associated with contrast media. Other treatment options to prevent CIN are controversial, such as giving HCO_3^- or sodium chloride solutions or prophylactic *N*-acetylcysteine.

Interprofessional Care

Because AKI is potentially reversible, the primary goals of treatment are to eliminate the cause, manage the signs and symptoms, and prevent complications while the kidneys recover (Table 46.4). The first step is to determine if there is adequate intravascular volume and cardiac output to ensure adequate perfusion of the kidneys. Diuretic therapy may be given and usually includes loop diuretics (e.g., furosemide [Lasix], bumetanide [Bumex]) or an osmotic diuretic (e.g., mannitol). If AKI is already established, forcing fluids and diuretics will not be effective and may be harmful. Closely monitor fluid intake during the oliguric phase of AKI.

The general rule for calculating the fluid restriction is to add all losses for the previous 24 hours (e.g., urine, diarrhea, emesis, blood) plus 600 mL for insensible losses (e.g., respiration, diaphoresis). For example, if a patient excreted 300 mL of urine on Tuesday with no other losses, the fluid allocation on Wednesday would be 900 mL.

Hyperkalemia is one of the most serious complications in AKI because it can cause life-threatening dysrhythmias. Therapies used to treat high potassium levels are listed in Table 46.5. Both insulin and sodium bicarbonate are temporary measures for treating hyperkalemia by promoting a transient shift of potassium into the cells. Potassium will eventually diffuse back

---

TABLE 46.4 Interprofessional Care

Acute Kidney Injury

Diagnostic Assessment

- History and physical examination
- Identify precipitating cause
- Serum creatinine and BUN levels
- Serum electrolytes
- Urinalysis
- Renal ultrasound
- Renal scan
- CT scan

Management

- Treat precipitating cause
- Fluid restriction (600 mL plus previous 24-hr fluid loss)
- Nutritional therapy
  - Adequate protein intake (0.6–2 g/kg/day) depending on degree of catabolism
  - Enteral nutrition
  - Parenteral nutrition
  - Dietary restrictions (potassium, phosphate, sodium)
- Measures to lower potassium (if high) (Table 46.5)
- Calcium supplements or phosphate-binding agents
- Dialysis (if necessary)
- Continuous RRT (if necessary)

TABLE 46.5 Therapies for High Potassium Levels

Calcium Gluconate IV

- Generally used in advanced cardiac toxicity (evidence of hyperkalemic ECG changes)
- Raises the threshold for excitation, resulting in dysrhythmias

Dietary Restriction

- Potassium intake is limited to 40 mEq/day
- Primarily used to prevent recurrent elevation, not for acute elevation

Hemodialysis

- Most effective therapy to remove potassium
- Works within a short time

Patiromer (Veltassa)

- Oral suspension that binds potassium in GI tract
- Used to treat patients with CKD
- Do not use as an emergency drug for life-threatening hyperkalemia
- Has a delayed onset of action
- Do not give to a patient with a paralytic ileus as bowel necrosis can occur

Regular Insulin IV

- Potassium moves into cells when insulin is given
- IV glucose given concurrently to prevent hypoglycemia
- When effects of insulin decrease, potassium shifts back out of cells

Sodium Bicarbonate

- Can correct acidosis and cause a shift of potassium into cells

Sodium Polystyrene Sulfonate (Kayexalate)

- Given by mouth or retention enema
- When resin is in the bowel, potassium is exchanged for sodium
- Produces osmotic diarrhea, allowing for evacuation of potassium-rich stool
- Removes 1 mEq of potassium per 1 g of drug
- Do not give to a patient with a paralytic ileus as bowel necrosis can occur

into the bloodstream. Calcium gluconate raises the threshold at which dysrhythmias occur, temporarily stabilizing the myocardium. Only sodium polystyrene sulfonate (Kayexalate), patiromer (Veltassa), and dialysis remove potassium from the body.

Conservative therapy may be all that is necessary until kidney function improves. If conservative therapy is not effective in treating AKI, then *renal replacement therapy* (RRT) is used. Controversy exists about the timing of RRT in AKI.[11] The most common indications for RRT in AKI are (1) volume overload, resulting in compromised cardiac and/or pulmonary status; (2) high serum potassium level; (3) metabolic acidosis (serum HCO_3^- level less than 15 mEq/L [15 mmol/L]); (4) BUN level greater than 120 mg/dL (43 mmol/L); (5) significant change in mental status; and (6) pericarditis, pericardial effusion, or cardiac tamponade. Although laboratory values provide rough parameters, the best guideline is the clinical status of the patient.

Of the several RRT therapy options available, there is no consensus about the best approach.[10] Even though peritoneal dialysis (PD) is a viable option for RRT, it is not often used. Intermittent hemodialysis (HD) and continuous renal replacement therapy (CRRT) have both been used effectively.

CRRT is provided continuously over 24 hours through cannulation of a vein or catheter placement. CRRT has much slower blood flow rates compared with intermittent HD. HD is the method of choice when changes are needed emergently. It is technically more complicated because it requires specialized staff and equipment and vascular access. The patient needs anticoagulation therapy to prevent blood clotting when the blood makes contact with the extracorporeal dialysis circuit. Rapid fluid shifts during HD may cause hypotension. (RRT and CRRT are discussed later in this chapter on pp. 1076–1080.)

Nutritional Therapy. The goal of nutritional management in AKI is to provide adequate calories to prevent catabolism despite restrictions that prevent electrolyte and fluid problems and azotemia. Nutritional intake must maintain adequate caloric intake (providing 30 to 35 kcal/kg and 0.8 to 1.0 g of protein per kilogram of desired body weight) to prevent the breakdown of body protein.

Adequate energy should primarily be from carbohydrate and fat sources to prevent ketosis from endogenous fat breakdown and gluconeogenesis from muscle protein breakdown. Essential amino acids may be supplemented. Potassium and sodium are regulated per plasma levels. Sodium is restricted as needed to prevent edema, hypertension, and HF. Dietary fat intake is increased so that the patient receives at least 30% to 40% of total calories from fat. Fat emulsion IV infusions given as a nutritional supplement provide a good source of nonprotein calories. If a patient cannot maintain adequate oral intake, enteral nutrition is the preferred route for nutritional support (see Chapter 39). When the gastrointestinal (GI) tract is not functional, parenteral nutrition (PN) is necessary to provide adequate nutrition. The patient treated with PN may need daily HD or CRRT to remove the excess fluid. Concentrated PN formulas are available to minimize fluid volume.

❖ NURSING MANAGEMENT: ACUTE KIDNEY INJURY

◆ Nursing Assessment

A number of assessments are essential for developing an interprofessional plan of care.[12] Daily weights, strict intake and output, and vital signs are key. Daily monitoring of a patient's urine output has prognostic implications and is crucial for determining therapy and daily fluid volume replacement. Examine the urine for color, specific gravity, glucose, protein, blood, and sediment. Assess the patient's general appearance, including skin color, edema, neck vein distention, and bruises. If a patient is receiving dialysis, observe the access site for inflammation and exudate. Evaluate the patient's mental status and level of consciousness. Assess the oral mucosa for dryness and inflammation. Auscultate the lungs for crackles and wheezes or decreased breath sounds. Monitor the heart for an S_3 gallop, murmurs, or a pericardial friction rub. Assess ECG readings for dysrhythmias. Review all laboratory values and diagnostic test results.

◆ Nursing Diagnoses
Nursing diagnoses for the patient with AKI include:
- Electrolyte imbalance
- Fluid imbalance
- Risk for infection
- Anxiety

◆ Planning
The overall goals are that the patient with AKI will (1) completely recover without any loss of kidney function, (2) maintain normal fluid and electrolyte balance, (3) have decreased anxiety, and (4) adhere to and understand the need for careful follow-up care.

◆ Nursing Implementation
◆ Health Promotion.
Prevention and early recognition of AKI are the most important aspects of care. Prevention is directed primarily toward identifying and monitoring high-risk populations, controlling exposure to nephrotoxic drugs and industrial chemicals, and preventing prolonged episodes of hypotension and hypovolemia. In the hospital, factors that increase the risk for developing AKI are preexisting CKD, older age, massive trauma, major surgical procedures, extensive burns, HF, sepsis, and obstetric complications.

Carefully monitor the patient's weight, intake and output, and fluid and electrolyte balance. Assess and record extrarenal losses of fluid from vomiting, diarrhea, hemorrhage, and increased insensible losses. Prompt replacement of significant fluid losses helps prevent ischemic tubular damage associated with trauma, burns, and extensive surgery. Intake and output records and the patient's weight are valuable indicators of fluid volume status. Aggressive diuretic therapy for the patient with fluid overload from any cause can lead to a reduction in renal blood flow.

Monitor kidney function in persons who are taking drugs that are potentially nephrotoxic (see Table 44.3). Nephrotoxic drugs should be used sparingly in the high-risk patient. When these drugs must be used, they should be given in the smallest effective doses for the shortest possible periods. Caution the patient about abuse of over-the-counter (OTC) analgesics (especially nonsteroidal antiinflammatory drugs [NSAIDs]), as these may worsen kidney function in the patient with mild CKD.

Angiotensin-converting enzyme (ACE) inhibitors can decrease perfusion pressure and cause hyperkalemia. If other measures, such as diet modification and diuretics, cannot control the hyperkalemia, ACE inhibitors may have to be reduced or stopped. However, ACE inhibitors are often used to prevent proteinuria and progression of kidney disease, especially in patients with diabetes.[13]

◆ Acute Care.
The patient with AKI is critically ill and may have co-morbid diseases or conditions (e.g., diabetes, cardiovascular

disease [CVD]) in addition to kidney injury. Focus on the patient holistically since they will have many physical and emotional needs. Usually the changes caused by AKI arise suddenly. The patient needs help in understanding that kidney disease may affect the entire body's functions.

You have a key role in managing fluid and electrolyte balance during the oliguric and diuretic phases. Observe and record accurate intake and output. Take daily weights with the same scale at the same time each day to detect excessive gains or losses of body fluid (1 kg is equivalent to 1000 mL of fluid). Assess for signs and symptoms of hypervolemia (in the oliguric phase) or hypovolemia (in the diuretic phase), potassium and sodium problems, and other electrolyte imbalances that may occur in AKI (see Chapter 16).

Because infection is the leading cause of death in AKI, meticulous aseptic technique is critical. Protect the patient from those with infectious diseases. Be alert for local manifestations of infection (e.g., swelling, redness, pain) as well as systemic manifestations (e.g., fever, malaise, leukocytosis).

If a patient with renal failure has an infection, it is important to recognize that the temperature may not always be high. Patients with AKI have a blunted febrile response to an infection (e.g., pneumonia). If antibiotics are used to treat an infection, the type, frequency, and dosage must be carefully considered because the kidneys are the primary route of excretion for many antibiotics. Dosages may be decreased depending on the patient's level of kidney function if the drug is eliminated by the kidneys. Nephrotoxic drugs (see Table 44.3) should be used judiciously.

Perform skin care and take measures to prevent pressure injuries as mobility may be impaired. Mouth care is important to prevent stomatitis, which develops when ammonia (made by bacterial breakdown of urea) in saliva irritates the mucous membranes.

INFORMATICS IN PRACTICE
Computer Monitoring of Antibiotic Safety

- Many patients receiving antibiotic therapy are at risk for kidney failure.
- Set the computer to alert you about elevated creatinine levels and, if possible, send you a text message.
- By notifying the HCP early, medications can be stopped or doses decreased and the patient's kidney function preserved.

◆ **Ambulatory Care.** Recovery from AKI is highly variable and depends on whether other body systems fail, the patient's general condition and age, the length of the oliguric phase, and the severity of nephron damage. Protein and potassium intake are dictated by kidney function. Regular evaluation of kidney function is necessary. Teach the patient the signs and symptoms of recurrent kidney disease. Emphasize measures to prevent the recurrence of AKI.

The long-term convalescence of 3 to 12 months may cause psychosocial and financial hardships for the patient, caregiver, and family. Make appropriate referrals for counseling. If the kidneys do not recover, the patient will need to transition to life on chronic dialysis or possible transplantation.

◆ **Evaluation**

The expected outcomes are that the patient with AKI will
- Regain and maintain normal fluid and electrolyte balance
- Adhere to the treatment regimen
- Have no complications
- Have a complete recovery

 Gerontologic Considerations: Acute Kidney Injury

The GFR declines with age. In older adults, impaired function of other organ systems from CVD or diabetes can increase the risk for developing AKI. The aging kidney is less able to compensate for changes in fluid volume, solute load, and cardiac output.

Although the causes of AKI in older adults are similar to younger adults, they are at an increased risk for AKI. Dehydration is a predisposing factor and tends to occur more often in older adults. Dehydration can occur from polypharmacy (diuretics, laxatives, drugs that suppress appetite or consciousness), acute febrile illnesses, and immobility.

Other common causes of AKI in the older adult include hypotension, diuretic therapy, aminoglycoside therapy, obstructive disorders (e.g., BPH), surgery, infection, and contrast media. Mortality rates are similar for older and younger patients. Patients over 65 years of age are less likely to recover from AKI. Despite this, age is not a barrier to offering RRT.[11]

CHRONIC KIDNEY DISEASE

Chronic kidney disease (CKD) involves progressive, irreversible loss of kidney function. More than 26 million American adults, or 1 out of every 9, have CKD. CKD is much more common than AKI (Table 46.1). We partially attribute the increasing prevalence of CKD to increased risk factors, including an aging population, increased rates of obesity, and increased incidence of diabetes and hypertension.

Because the kidneys are highly adaptive, kidney disease is often not recognized until there has been considerable loss of nephrons. Patients with CKD are often asymptomatic, resulting in CKD being underdiagnosed and untreated. It is thought that about 70% of people with CKD are unaware that they have the disease.[14]

CKD has many different causes. The leading ones are diabetes (about 50%) and hypertension (about 25%) (Table 46.6). Less common causes include glomerulonephritis, cystic diseases, and urologic diseases.[15] Kidney diseases are discussed in Chapter 45.

Kidney Disease Improving Global Outcomes (KDIGO) Clinical Practice Guidelines defines CKD as either the presence of kidney damage or a decreased GFR less than 60 mL/min/1.73 m^2 for longer than 3 months. The stages of CKD are shown in Table 46.7. The last stage of kidney disease, end-stage renal disease (ESRD), occurs when the GFR is less than 15 mL/min.

TABLE 46.6 **Risk Factors for Chronic Kidney Disease**	
Risk Factors	**Prevention and Management**
Age >60 yr	Prevent insult or injury to kidneys
Cardiovascular disease	Institute aggressive risk factor reduction
Diabetes	Achieve optimal glycemic control
Ethnic minority (e.g., black, Native American)	Teach about ↑ risk and assist with appropriate screening (BP measurement, urinalysis)
Exposure to nephrotoxic drugs	Limit exposure and give sodium bicarbonate as treatment
Family history of CKD	Teach about ↑ risk and assist with appropriate screening
Hypertension	Maintain BP in normal range with ACE inhibitors or ARBs

TABLE 46.7 Stages of Chronic Kidney Disease

Description	GFR (mL/min/1.73 m²)	Clinical Action Plan
Stage 1 Kidney damage with normal or ↑ GFR	≥90	Diagnosis and treatment CVD risk reduction Slow progression
Stage 2 Kidney damage with mild ↓ GFR	60–89	Estimation of progression
Stage 3a Moderate ↓ GFR	45–59	Evaluation and treatment of complications
Stage 3b Moderate ↓ GFR	30–44	More aggressive treatment of complications
Stage 4 Severe ↓ GFR	15–29	Preparation for renal replacement therapy (dialysis, kidney transplant)
Stage 5 Kidney failure	<15 (or dialysis)	Renal replacement therapy (if uremia present and patient desires treatment)

Source: Alseiari M, Meyer KB, Wong JB: Evidence underlying KDIGO (Kidney Disease: Improving Global Outcomes) guideline recommendations: A systematic review, *Am J Kidney Dis* 67:417, 2016.

At this point, RRT (dialysis or transplantation) is required to maintain life.

Over half a million Americans are receiving treatment (dialysis, transplant) for ESRD. Despite all the technologic advances in life-sustaining treatment with dialysis, patients with ESRD have a high mortality rate. As the stage of kidney disease progresses, the mortality rate increases. Mortality rates are as high as 19% to 24% for patients with ESRD on dialysis.[14,16]

The prognosis and course of CKD are highly variable depending on the cause, patient's condition and age, and adequacy of health care follow-up. Some people live normal, active lives with kidney disease, while others may rapidly progress to ESRD (stage 5).

Since 1972, the United States has covered most of the costs of providing dialysis through Medicare benefits. Under Title XVIII of the Social Security Act, ESRD was recognized as a disability. Medicare pays for 80% of eligible charges. The state, private insurance, or patient covers the rest.[16]

Clinical Manifestations

As kidney function deteriorates, all body systems become affected. The manifestations result from retained urea, creatinine, phenols, hormones, electrolytes, and water. **Uremia** is a syndrome in which kidney function declines to the point that symptoms may develop in multiple body systems (Fig. 46.2). It often occurs when the GFR is 15 mL/min or less. The manifestations of uremia vary among patients depending on the cause of the kidney disease, co-morbid conditions, age, and degree of adherence to the prescribed medical regimen. Many patients

are tolerant of the changes caused by declining kidney function because they occur gradually.

Urinary System. In the early stages of CKD, patients usually do not report any change in urine output. Since diabetes is the primary cause of CKD, polyuria may be present, but not necessarily from kidney disease. As CKD progresses, patients have increasing difficulty with fluid retention and need diuretic therapy. After a period on dialysis, patients may develop anuria.

Metabolic Disturbances

Waste Product Accumulation. As the GFR decreases, the BUN and serum creatinine levels increase. The BUN increase is not only from kidney disease but also protein intake, fever, corticosteroids, and catabolism. For this reason, serum creatinine clearance determinations (calculated GFR) are considered more accurate indicators of kidney function than BUN or creatinine (Table 46.8). Significant increases in BUN contribute to nausea, vomiting, lethargy, fatigue, impaired thought processes, and headaches.

Altered Carbohydrate Metabolism. Impaired glucose metabolism, resulting from cellular insensitivity to the normal action of insulin, causes defective carbohydrate metabolism. Mild to moderate hyperglycemia and hyperinsulinemia may occur.

Insulin and glucose metabolism may improve (but not to normal values) after starting dialysis. Patients with diabetes who needed insulin before starting dialysis may need less insulin therapy when they start dialysis and their kidney disease progresses. Patients with diabetes who develop uremia may need less insulin than before the onset of CKD. Insulin, which depends on the kidneys for excretion, stays in the circulation longer. Insulin dosing must be individualized, and glucose levels monitored carefully.

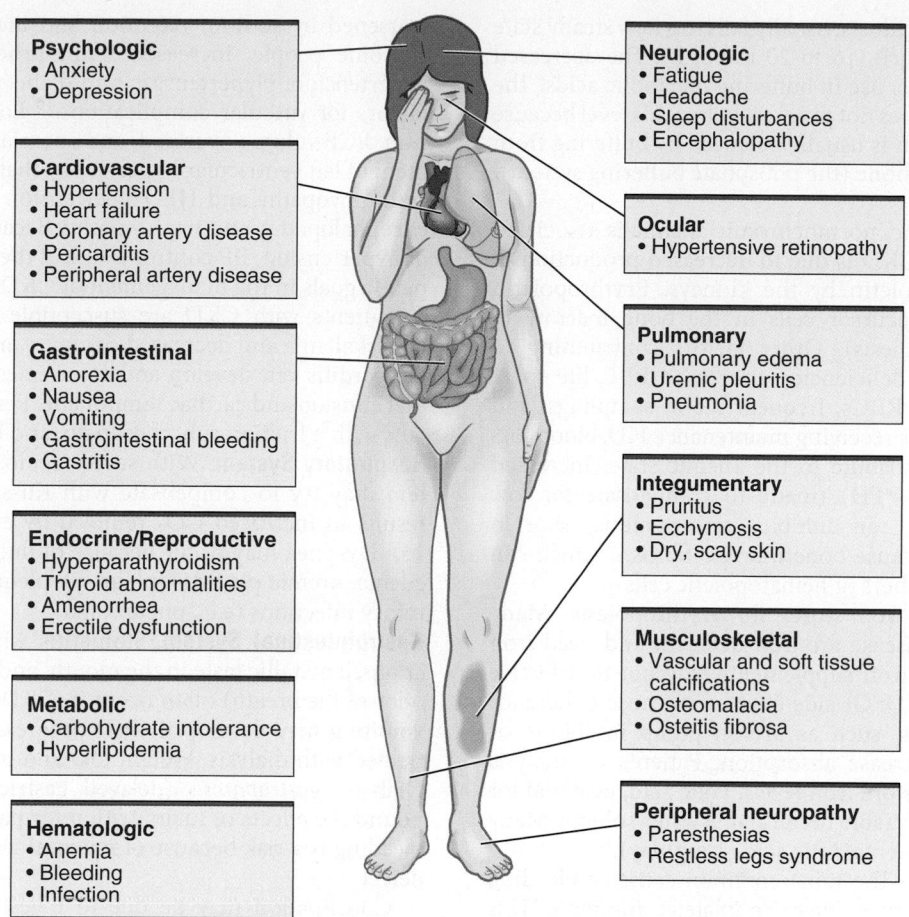

Psychologic
- Anxiety
- Depression

Cardiovascular
- Hypertension
- Heart failure
- Coronary artery disease
- Pericarditis
- Peripheral artery disease

Gastrointestinal
- Anorexia
- Nausea
- Vomiting
- Gastrointestinal bleeding
- Gastritis

Endocrine/Reproductive
- Hyperparathyroidism
- Thyroid abnormalities
- Amenorrhea
- Erectile dysfunction

Metabolic
- Carbohydrate intolerance
- Hyperlipidemia

Hematologic
- Anemia
- Bleeding
- Infection

Neurologic
- Fatigue
- Headache
- Sleep disturbances
- Encephalopathy

Ocular
- Hypertensive retinopathy

Pulmonary
- Pulmonary edema
- Uremic pleuritis
- Pneumonia

Integumentary
- Pruritus
- Ecchymosis
- Dry, scaly skin

Musculoskeletal
- Vascular and soft tissue calcifications
- Osteomalacia
- Osteitis fibrosa

Peripheral neuropathy
- Paresthesias
- Restless legs syndrome

FIG. 46.2 Possible manifestations of CKD.

TABLE 46.8 Indicators of Kidney Function

This example shows why serum creatinine alone is a poor indicator of kidney function. Calculation of GFR is considered the best index to estimate kidney function as shown by the following example.

Estimation of GFR	TYPE OF PATIENT	
	76-Yr-Old Black Woman (Weight 56 kg)	28-Yr-Old Black Man (Weight 74 kg)
Serum creatinine	1.4 mg/dL	1.4 mg/dL
GFR, estimated by the Cockcroft-Gault formula*	30.2 mL/min	82.2 mL/min
GFR, estimated by MDRD equation†	47 mL/min/1.73 m²	64 mL/min/1.73 m²

*Cockcroft-Gault GFR = (140 – Age) × (Weight in kilograms) × (0.85 if female)/(72 × Cr).
†GFR as estimated by MDRD equation calculator can be accessed at www.mdrd.com.
Cr, Creatinine; *GFR,* glomerular filtration rate; *MDRD,* modification of diet in renal disease.

Elevated Triglycerides. Hyperinsulinemia stimulates hepatic production of triglycerides. Many patients with uremia develop dyslipidemia, with increased very-low-density lipoproteins (VLDLs), increased low-density lipoproteins (LDLs), and decreased high-density lipoproteins (HDLs). The altered lipid metabolism is related to decreased levels of the enzyme lipoprotein lipase, which is important in the breakdown of lipoproteins. Most patients with CKD die from CVD.[17]

Electrolyte and Acid-Base Imbalances

Potassium. Hyperkalemia is a serious electrolyte disorder associated with CKD. Fatal dysrhythmias can occur when the serum potassium level reaches 7 to 8 mEq/L (7 to 8 mmol/L). Hyperkalemia results from the decreased excretion of potassium by the kidneys, the breakdown of cellular protein, bleeding, and metabolic acidosis. Potassium may come from foods, dietary supplements, drugs, and IV infusions.

Sodium. Sodium may be high, normal, or low in kidney disease. Because of impaired sodium excretion, sodium is retained with water. If large quantities of water are retained, dilutional hyponatremia occurs. Sodium retention can contribute to edema, hypertension, and HF. Sodium intake is patient specific but is generally restricted to 2 g/day.

Calcium and Phosphate. Calcium and phosphate changes are discussed in the section on the musculoskeletal system on pp. 1068–1069.

Magnesium. Magnesium is primarily excreted by the kidneys. Hypermagnesemia is generally not a problem unless the patient is ingesting magnesium (e.g., Milk of Magnesia, magnesium citrate, antacids containing magnesium). Manifestations can include absent reflexes, decreased mental status, dysrhythmias, hypotension, and respiratory failure.

Metabolic Acidosis. Metabolic acidosis results from the kidneys' impaired ability to excrete excess acid and from defective reabsorption and regeneration of HCO_3^-. The average adult makes 80 to 90 mEq of acid per day. This acid is normally buffered by HCO_3^-. In kidney disease, plasma HCO_3^-, which is an indirect measure of acidosis, usually falls to a new steady state at around 16 to 20 mEq/L (16 to 20 mmol/L). The decreased plasma HCO_3^- reflects its use in buffering metabolic acids. The HCO_3^- level generally does not progress below this level because hydrogen ion production is usually balanced by buffering from demineralization of the bone (the phosphate buffering system).

Hematologic System

Anemia. A normocytic, normochromic anemia is associated with CKD. Anemia in CKD is due to decreased production of the hormone erythropoietin by the kidneys. Erythropoietin normally stimulates precursor cells in the bone marrow to make RBCs (erythropoiesis). Other factors contributing to anemia are nutritional deficiencies, decreased RBC life span, increased hemolysis of RBCs, frequent blood samplings, and GI bleeding. For patients receiving maintenance HD, blood loss in the dialyzer can contribute to the anemic state. Increased parathyroid hormone (PTH) (made to compensate for low serum calcium levels) can inhibit erythropoiesis, shorten survival of RBCs, and cause bone marrow fibrosis, which can result in decreased numbers of hematopoietic cells.

We need sufficient iron stores for erythropoiesis. Many patients with kidney disease are iron deficient and need iron supplementation. Oral iron supplements may not be effective for the person with CKD. GI side effects can cause adherence difficulties. Medications, such as proton pump inhibitors or phosphate binders, decrease absorption. Patients on dialysis may need IV iron to restore iron levels. Folic acid, essential for RBC maturation, is dialyzable because it is water soluble. Many patients receive supplemental folic acid (1 mg/day).[18]

Bleeding Tendencies. The most common cause of bleeding in uremia is a qualitative defect in platelet function. This dysfunction is caused by impaired platelet aggregation and impaired release of platelet factor III. Changes in the coagulation system occur due to increased concentrations of both factor VIII and fibrinogen. The altered platelet function, hemorrhagic tendencies, and GI bleeding susceptibility can usually be corrected with regular HD or PD.

Infection. Patients with advanced CKD have an increased susceptibility to infection. This is due to changes in WBC function and altered immune response and function. Both cellular and humoral immune responses are suppressed. Other factors contributing to the increased risk for infection include hyperglycemia and external trauma (e.g., catheters, needle insertions into vascular access sites).

Cardiovascular System

The most common cause of death in patients with CKD is CVD. Leading causes of death are myocardial infarction (MI), ischemic heart disease, peripheral arterial disease, HF, cardiomyopathy, and stroke.[17] CVD and CKD are so closely linked that if patients develop cardiac events (e.g., MI, HF), kidney function is evaluated. Traditional CVD risk factors, such as hypertension and increased lipids, are common in CKD patients.

CVD may be related to vascular calcification and arterial stiffness. Calcium deposits in the vascular medial layer are associated with stiffening of the blood vessels. The mechanisms involved are multifactorial. They include (1) vascular smooth muscle cells changing into chondrocytes or osteoblast-like cells, (2) high total body amount of calcium and phosphate resulting from abnormal bone metabolism, (3) impaired renal excretion, and (4) drug therapies to treat the bone disease (e.g., calcium-phosphate binders).[19]

Hypertension, which is prevalent in patients with CKD, is both a cause and a consequence of CKD. Hypertension is worsened by sodium retention and increased ECF volume.[20] In some people, increased renin production contributes to hypertension. Hypertension and diabetes are contributing risk factors for vascular complications.[19] Long-standing hypertension, ECF volume overload, and anemia contribute to development of left ventricular hypertrophy that may eventually lead to cardiomyopathy and HF. Hypertension can cause retinopathy, encephalopathy, and nephropathy. Because of the many effects of hypertension, BP control is one of the most important therapeutic goals in the management of CKD.[20]

Patients with CKD are susceptible to dysrhythmias from hyperkalemia and decreased coronary artery perfusion. Uremic pericarditis can develop and sometimes progresses to pericardial effusion and cardiac tamponade. Pericarditis typically presents with a friction rub, chest pain, and low-grade fever.

Respiratory System

With severe acidosis, the respiratory system may try to compensate with Kussmaul breathing, which results in increased CO_2 removal by exhalation (see Chapter 16). Dyspnea may occur because of fluid overload, pulmonary edema, uremic pleuritis (pleurisy), pleural effusions, and respiratory infections (e.g., pneumonia).

Gastrointestinal System

Stomatitis with exudates and ulcerations, a metallic taste in the mouth, and *uremic fetor* (a urinous odor of the breath) often occur in CKD. Anorexia, nausea, and vomiting may develop if CKD progresses to ESRD and is not treated with dialysis. Weight loss and malnutrition may occur. Diabetic *gastroparesis* (delayed gastric emptying) can compound the effects of malnutrition for patients with diabetes. GI bleeding is a risk because of mucosal irritation and the platelet defect.

Constipation may be due to ingesting iron salts or calcium-containing phosphate binders. Limitations on fluid intake and physical inactivity can increase the risk for constipation.

Neurologic System

Neurologic changes are expected as kidney disease progresses. They are the result of increased nitrogenous waste products, electrolyte imbalances, metabolic acidosis, and atrophy and demyelination of nerve fibers.

The central nervous system (CNS) becomes depressed, resulting in lethargy, apathy, decreased ability to concentrate, fatigue, irritability, and altered mental ability. Seizures and coma may result from a rapidly increasing BUN and hypertensive encephalopathy.

Peripheral neuropathy initially manifests as a slowing of nerve conduction to the extremities. The patient may describe paresthesias in the feet and legs as a burning sensation. Eventually, motor involvement may lead to bilateral foot drop, muscular weakness and atrophy, and loss of deep tendon reflexes. Muscle twitching, jerking, *asterixis* (hand-flapping tremor), and nocturnal leg cramps may occur. In patients with diabetic neuropathy, uremic neuropathy can compound symptoms.[21] Those with advanced stage 5 CKD may develop restless legs syndrome (see Chapter 58).

Dialysis should improve general CNS manifestations and may slow or halt the progression of neuropathies. Motor neuropathy may not be reversible. The treatment for neurologic problems is dialysis or transplantation. Altered mental status, a late manifestation of CKD stage 5, rarely occurs unless the patient has chosen not to have RRT.

Musculoskeletal System

CKD mineral and bone disorder (CKD-MBD) develops as a systemic disorder of mineral and bone metabolism caused by progressive deterioration in kidney function (Fig. 46.3). Activated vitamin D is necessary to

PATHOPHYSIOLOGY MAP

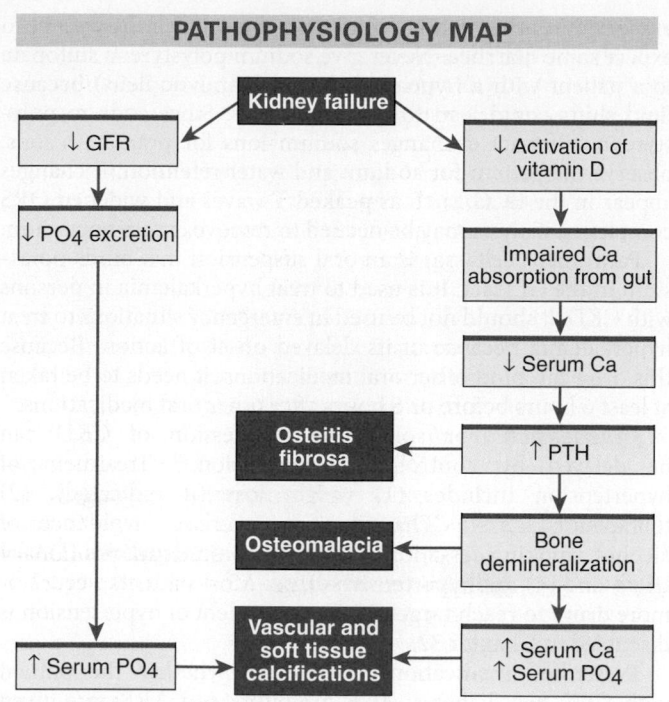

FIG. 46.3 Mechanisms of CKD-MBD. *GFR,* Glomerular filtration rate; *PTH,* parathyroid hormone.

optimize absorption of calcium from the GI tract. As kidney function deteriorates, less vitamin D is converted to its active form, resulting in decreased serum levels. Low levels of active vitamin D result in decreased serum calcium levels.[19]

Serum calcium levels are regulated primarily by PTH. When hypocalcemia occurs, the parathyroid gland secretes PTH, which stimulates bone demineralization, releasing calcium from the bones. Phosphate is also released, leading to high serum phosphate levels. Hyperphosphatemia results from decreased phosphate excretion by the kidneys. It decreases serum calcium levels and further reduces the kidneys' ability to activate vitamin D.

Low serum calcium, increased phosphate, and decreased vitamin D contribute to the stimulation of the parathyroid gland and excretion of PTH. PTH acts on the bone to increase remodeling and increase serum calcium levels. The accelerated rate of bone remodeling causes a weakened bone matrix and places the patient at a higher risk for fractures.

Normally plasma calcium is found ionized or free (physiologically active form) or bound to protein. Low ionized calcium levels can lead to tetany (see Chapter 16). However, in CKD, it is unusual for hypocalcemia to be symptomatic. In the acidotic state associated with CKD, more calcium is in the ionized form than is bound to protein.

CKD-MBD is a common complication of CKD and results in skeletal complications, vascular and soft tissue (extraskeletal) complications. Skeletal complications include (1) *osteomalacia* (results from demineralization from slow bone turnover and defective mineralization of newly formed bone) and (2) *osteitis fibrosa* (decalcification of the bone and replacement of bone tissue with fibrous tissue).

Soft tissue complications result from vascular calcifications. Vascular calcifications are a significant contributing factor to CVD. Irritation from calcium deposits in the eye can cause "uremic red eye." Intracardiac calcifications can disrupt the conduction system and cause cardiac arrest.

Integumentary System. A small number of patients develop refractory pruritus that can have a devastating impact on their well-being and quality of life. Pruritus has multiple causes, including dry skin, calcium-phosphate deposition in the skin, and sensory neuropathy. It is more common in patients receiving dialysis than in the earlier stages of CKD. The itching may be so intense that it can lead to bleeding or infection from scratching. Uremic frost is an extremely rare condition in which urea crystallizes on the skin. This is usually seen only when BUN levels are extremely high (e.g., over 200 mg/dL).

Reproductive System. Both men and women can have infertility and a decreased libido. Women usually have low levels of estrogen, progesterone, and luteinizing hormone, causing anovulation and menstrual changes (usually amenorrhea). Menses and ovulation may return after starting dialysis. Men have loss of testicular consistency, decreased testosterone levels, and low sperm counts.

Sexual dysfunction may be caused by anemia, which causes fatigue and decreased libido. Peripheral neuropathy can cause impotence in men and anorgasmia in women. Other factors that may cause changes in sexual function are psychologic problems (e.g., anxiety, depression), physical stress, and medication side effects. Sexual function may improve with maintenance dialysis and become normal with successful transplantation.

Patients who become pregnant while receiving dialysis have been able to carry a fetus to term, but there is significant risk to the mother and infant. Pregnancy in patients with a kidney transplant is more common, but there is still considerable risk to both the mother and fetus.

Psychologic Changes. Personality and behavioral changes, emotional lability, withdrawal, and depression often occur in patients with CKD. Fatigue and lethargy contribute to the feeling of illness. The changes in body image caused by edema, integumentary changes, and access devices (e.g., fistulas, catheters) may lead to anxiety and depression. Decreased ability to concentrate and slowed mental activity can give the appearance of dullness and disinterest in the environment. The patient must deal with significant changes in lifestyle, occupation, family responsibilities, and financial status. Long-term survival depends on medications, dietary restrictions, dialysis, and possibly transplantation. The patient grieves the loss of kidney function and independence.

Diagnostic Studies

Persistent proteinuria is usually the first sign of kidney damage. Screening for CKD involves a dipstick evaluation of protein in the urine or evaluation for albuminuria, which is not detected with routine urinalysis. The urine of patients with diabetes must be examined for albuminuria if no protein is present on routine urinalysis. A person with persistent proteinuria (1+ protein on standard dipstick testing 2 or more times over a 3-month period) should have further assessment of risk factors and a diagnostic workup with blood and urine tests to evaluate for CKD.

A urinalysis can detect RBCs, WBCs, protein, casts, and glucose. A renal ultrasound is usually done to detect any obstructions and determine the size of the kidneys. Other diagnostic studies (Table 46.9) help establish the diagnosis and cause of CKD. A kidney biopsy may be necessary to provide a definitive diagnosis.

Serum creatinine alone poorly reflects kidney function. GFR is the preferred measure to determine kidney function. Several

TABLE 46.9 Interprofessional Care

Chronic Kidney Disease

Diagnostic Assessment
- History and physical examination
- Identification of reversible kidney disease
- Renal ultrasound, renal scan, CT scan
- Renal biopsy
- BUN, serum creatinine, and creatinine clearance levels
- Serum electrolytes
- Lipid profile
- Urinalysis
- Protein-to-creatinine ratio in first morning voided specimen
- Hematocrit and hemoglobin levels

Management
- Correction of extracellular fluid volume overload or deficit
- RRT (dialysis, kidney transplant)
- Nutritional therapy (Tables 46.10 and 16.6)
- Measures to lower potassium (Table 46.5)

Drug Therapy
- Calcium supplementation, phosphate binders, or both
- Antihypertensive therapy
- ACE inhibitors or ARBs
- Erythropoietin therapy
- Lipid-lowering drugs
- Adjustment of drug dosages to degree of renal function

GFR calculators are available. The equations used most often to estimate GFR are the Cockcroft-Gault formula and Modification of Diet in Renal Disease (MDRD) Study equation (Table 46.8). MDRD is the preferred method.[22]

Interprofessional Care

The overall goals of CKD therapy are to preserve existing kidney function, reduce the risks for CVD, prevent complications, and provide for the patient's comfort. Early recognition, diagnosis, and treatment can prevent the progression of kidney disease. It is important that patients with CKD receive appropriate referral to a nephrologist early in the course of the disease. Every effort is made to detect and treat potentially reversible causes of kidney failure (e.g., HF, dehydration, infections, nephrotoxins, urinary tract obstruction, glomerulonephritis, renal artery stenosis).

Patients with CKD have a high incidence of CVD. More patients die from CVD than live to need dialysis. When a patient has CKD, therapy is aimed at treating CVD in addition to slowing the progression of kidney disease (Table 46.9).

A focus on stages 1 through 4 (Table 46.7) before the need for dialysis (stage 5) includes the control of hypertension, hyperparathyroidism, CKD-MBD, anemia, and dyslipidemia. The next section focuses primarily on the drug and nutritional aspects of care.

Drug Therapy

Hyperkalemia. Multiple strategies are used to manage hyperkalemia (Table 46.5). These include restricting high-potassium foods and drugs. Acute hyperkalemia may need treatment with IV glucose and insulin or IV 10% calcium gluconate.

Sodium polystyrene sulfonate, a cation-exchange resin, is often given to lower potassium levels in stage 4 CKD. Sodium polystyrene sulfonate has an osmotic laxative action and ensures evacuation of the potassium from the bowel. Tell the patient to expect some diarrhea. Never give sodium polystyrene sulfonate to a patient with a hypoactive bowel (paralytic ileus) because fluid shifts could lead to bowel necrosis. Since sodium polystyrene sulfonate exchanges sodium ions for potassium ions, observe the patient for sodium and water retention. If changes appear in the ECG, such as peaked T waves and widened QRS complexes, dialysis may be needed to remove excess potassium.

Patiromer (Veltassa) is an oral suspension that binds potassium in the GI tract. It is used to treat hyperkalemia in persons with CKD. It should not be used in emergency situations to treat hyperkalemia because of its delayed onset of action. Because this drug can bind other oral medications, it needs to be taken at least 6 hours before or 6 hours after other oral medications.

Hypertension. For some, the progression of CKD can be delayed by controlling hypertension.[20] Treatment of hypertension includes (1) weight loss (if indicated), (2) therapeutic lifestyle changes (e.g., exercise, avoidance of alcohol, smoking cessation), (3) diet recommendations (DASH Diet), and (4) antihypertensive drugs. Most patients need 2 or more drugs to reach target BP. The treatment of hypertension is discussed in Chapter 32.

Prescribed medications depend on whether the patient with CKD has diabetes. ACE inhibitors and ARBs are given to patients with diabetes and those with nondiabetic proteinuria. They decrease proteinuria and may delay the progression of CKD. They must be used with caution as they can further decrease the GFR and increase serum potassium levels.

Measure the BP with the patient in the supine, sitting, and standing positions to monitor the effect of antihypertensive drugs. Teach the patient and caregiver how to monitor the BP at home and what readings require immediate intervention.

CKD-MBD. It is hard to determine what type of bone disease a patient may have by just looking at the serum levels of calcium, phosphorus, PTH, and alkaline phosphatase. The gold standard for diagnosis is a bone biopsy.

Interventions for CKD-MBD include limiting dietary phosphorus, giving phosphate binders, supplementing vitamin D, and controlling hyperparathyroidism.[19] Phosphate intake is not usually restricted until the patient needs RRT. At that time, phosphate is usually limited to about 1 g/day, but dietary control alone is usually inadequate.

Phosphate binders include calcium-based binders, calcium acetate, and calcium carbonate. They bind phosphate in the bowel and then excrete it in the stool. Giving calcium may increase the calcium load and place the patient at increased risk for vascular calcifications. So, when calcium levels are increased or there is evidence of existing vascular or soft tissue calcifications, non–calcium-based phosphate binders may be used. These include lanthanum carbonate (Fosrenol); sevelamer carbonate (Renvela;, and iron-based, calcium-free phosphate binders, such as sucroferric oxyhydroxide (Velphoro) and ferric citrate (Auryxia).

To be most effective, give phosphate binders with each meal. Constipation is a frequent side effect of phosphate binders. Stool softeners may be needed.

Because bone disease (osteomalacia) is associated with excess aluminum, aluminum preparations should be used with caution in patients with kidney disease. Do not use magnesium-containing antacids (e.g., Maalox, Mylanta) because magnesium depends on the kidneys for excretion.

Hypocalcemia is a problem in the later stages of CKD due to the inability of the GI tract to absorb calcium in the absence of active vitamin D. If hypocalcemia persists even if the serum phosphate levels are normal, supplemental calcium and vitamin D should be given. Assess vitamin D levels to determine the need for supplementation. If the levels are low (serum values less than 30 ng/mL), vitamin D is given in the form of cholecalciferol.

Treatment of secondary hyperparathyroidism in ESRD patients requires the activated form of vitamin D because the kidneys cannot activate vitamin D. Active vitamin D is available as oral or IV calcitriol (Rocaltrol), IV paricalcitol (Zemplar), or oral or IV doxercalciferol (Hectorol). Their use can reduce the high PTH levels. Cinacalcet (Sensipar), a calcimimetic agent, is used to control secondary hyperparathyroidism. Calcimimetics mimic calcium and increase the sensitivity of the calcium receptors in the parathyroid glands. As a result, the parathyroid glands detect calcium at lower serum levels and decrease PTH secretion.

If parathyroid disease becomes severe, a subtotal or total parathyroidectomy may be done to decrease the synthesis and secretion of PTH. In most cases, a total parathyroidectomy is done and parathyroid tissue transplanted into the forearm. The transplanted cells make PTH as needed. If PTH production becomes excessive, some cells can be removed from the forearm.

Hypercalcemia may occur with calcium and vitamin D supplementation. If hypercalcemia occurs, vitamin D may be withheld, and calcium-based phosphate binders replaced with non–calcium-based phosphate binders.

Anemia. Anemia in CKD is caused by a decreased production of erythropoietin by the kidneys. Exogenous erythropoietin (EPO) is used to treat anemia. It is available as epoetin alfa (Epogen, Procrit), which can be given IV or subcutaneously, usually 2 or 3 times per week. Darbepoetin alfa (Aranesp) is longer acting and can be given weekly or biweekly.

Hemoglobin and hematocrit levels may take 2 to 3 weeks to increase. Higher hemoglobin levels (more than 12 g/dL) and higher doses of EPO are associated with a higher rate of thromboembolic events and increased risk for death from serious CV events (MI, HF, stroke). The recommendation is to use the lowest possible dose of EPO to treat anemia.

Treatment of CKD-related anemia is patient specific with the goal being to reduce the need for blood transfusions. There is no target hemoglobin or widely accepted EPO dosing strategy. Teach people who are prescribed EPO about the risks and benefits and allow them to decide about their treatment plan.

EPO can increase BP and is contraindicated in uncontrolled hypertension. The underlying mechanism is related to the hemodynamic changes (e.g., increased whole blood viscosity) that occurs as the anemia is corrected.

EPO therapy may lead to iron deficiency from the increased demand for iron to support erythropoiesis. Iron supplementation is recommended if the plasma ferritin concentrations fall below 100 ng/mL. Most CKD patients receive iron supplementation.

Although iron can be given by mouth or IV, the enteral route is limited due to GI side effects, which decrease patient adherence. Oral iron should not be taken at the same time as phosphate binders because calcium binds the iron, preventing its absorption. Tell the patient that iron may make the stool dark in color. Most patients receiving HD are prescribed IV iron sucrose (Venofer) or sodium ferric gluconate complex (Ferrlecit). Supplemental folic acid (1 mg/day) is usually given because it is needed for RBC formation and is removed by dialysis.

Blood transfusions are avoided unless the patient has an acute blood loss or has symptomatic anemia (i.e., dyspnea, excess fatigue, tachycardia, palpitations, chest pain). Transfusions increase the development of antibodies, thus making it harder to find a compatible donor for kidney transplantation. Multiple blood transfusions may lead to iron overload because each unit of blood has about 250 mg of iron.

Dyslipidemia. Dyslipidemia, a risk factor for CVD, is a common problem in CKD. Statins (HMG-CoA reductase inhibitors), such as atorvastatin (Lipitor), are used to lower LDL cholesterol levels (see Table 33.6). Statins should be used in patients with CKD, especially those with diabetes, not yet on dialysis.[23]

Fibrates (fibric acid derivatives), such as gemfibrozil (Lopid), are used to lower triglyceride levels (see Table 33.6) and can increase HDLs. Specific drugs used in these classes depend on the individual patient response and HCP recommendation.

Complications of Drug Therapy. The kidneys partially or totally excrete many drugs. CKD causes decreased elimination that leads to an accumulation of drugs and the potential for drug toxicity. Drug doses and frequency of administration are adjusted based on the severity of the kidney disease. Increased sensitivity may result as drug levels increase in the blood and tissues. Drugs of particular concern include digoxin, diabetic agents (metformin, glyburide), antibiotics (e.g., vancomycin, gentamicin), and opioid drugs.

Nutritional Therapy

Protein Restriction. The current diet for the person with CKD is designed to maintain good nutrition (Table 46.10). Calorie-protein malnutrition is a potential and serious problem that results from altered metabolism, anemia, proteinuria, anorexia, and nausea. Other factors leading to malnutrition include depression and complex diets that restrict protein, phosphorus, potassium, and sodium. Frequent monitoring of laboratory parameters, especially serum albumin, prealbumin, and ferritin, and anthropometric measurements are necessary to evaluate nutritional status. All patients with CKD should be referred to a dietitian for nutritional teaching.

For the patient undergoing dialysis, protein is not routinely restricted. For CKD stages 1 through 4, many HCPs encourage a diet with normal protein intake. Teach patients to avoid high-protein diets and supplements because they may overburden the diseased kidneys.[24]

Dietary protein guidelines for PD differ from those for HD because of protein loss through the peritoneal membrane. During PD, protein intake must be high enough to compensate for the losses so that the nitrogen balance is maintained. The recommended protein intake is at least 1.2 g/kg of ideal body weight (IBW) per day. This can be increased depending on the patient's needs.

For patients with malnutrition or inadequate caloric or protein intake, commercially prepared products that are high in protein but low in sodium and potassium are available (e.g., Nepro, Amin-Aid). As an alternative, liquid or powder breakfast drinks may be bought at the grocery store.

Fluid Restriction. Water and any other fluids are not routinely restricted in patients with CKD stages 1 to 5 who are not receiving HD. To reduce fluid retention, diuretics are often used. Patients on HD have a more restricted fluid intake than patients receiving PD. For those receiving HD, as their urine output decreases, fluids are restricted. Recommended fluid intake depends on the daily urine output. Generally, 600 mL (from insensible loss) plus an amount equal to the previous day's urine output is allowed for a patient receiving HD.

TABLE 46.10 Nutritional Therapy

Chronic Kidney Disease

	Pre-ESRD	Hemodialysis	Peritoneal Dialysis
Calcium	About 1000–1500 mg/day	Patient specific	Patient specific
Calories	30–35 kcal/kg/day	30–35 kcal/kg/day	25–35 kcal/kg/day (includes calories from dialysate glucose absorption)
Fluid allowance	As desired or depends on urine output	Urine output plus 600–1000 mL	Unrestricted if weight and BP controlled and residual renal function
Iron	Supplement recommended if receiving erythropoietin	Supplement recommended if receiving erythropoietin	Supplement recommended if receiving erythropoietin
Phosphate	Patient specific or 1.0–1.8 g/day	Patient specific or about 0.6–1.2 g/day	Patient specific or about 0.6–1.2 g/day
Potassium	Based on laboratory values	Patient specific or about 2–4 g/day	Usually not restricted
Protein	Patient specific or 0.6–1.0 g/kg/day (low protein)	1.2 g/kg/day	1.2–1.3 g/kg/day
Sodium	Patient specific or 1–3 g/day	Patient specific or 2–3 g/day	Patient specific or 2–4 g/day

Foods that are liquid at room temperature (e.g., gelatin, ice) are counted as fluid intake. Space fluid allotment throughout the day so that the patient does not become thirsty. Teach patients to limit fluid intake so that weight gains are no more than 1 to 3 kg between dialyses *(interdialytic weight gain).*

Sodium and Potassium Restriction. Teach patients with CKD to restrict sodium. Sodium-restricted diets may vary from 2 to 4 g/day. Teach the patient to avoid high-sodium foods, such as cured meats, pickled foods, canned soups and stews, frankfurters, cold cuts, soy sauce, and salad dressings (see Table 34.8). Potassium restriction depends on the kidneys' ability to excrete potassium. Salt substitutes should be avoided in potassium-restricted diets because they contain potassium chloride.

Dietary restrictions for potassium range from about 2000 to 3000 mg (39 mg = 1 mEq). Teach patients receiving HD which foods are high in potassium and to avoid them (see Table 16.6). Patients using PD do not usually need potassium restrictions. They may need oral potassium supplementation because of the loss of potassium with dialysis exchanges.

Phosphate Restriction. As kidney function deteriorates, phosphate elimination by the kidneys is decreased and the patient begins to develop hyperphosphatemia. By the time a patient reaches ESRD, phosphate is limited to around 1 g/day. Foods that are high in phosphate include meat and dairy products (e.g., milk, ice cream, cheese, yogurt, pudding). Many foods that are high in phosphate are also high in protein. Since patients on dialysis are encouraged to eat a diet containing protein, phosphate binders are essential to control the phosphate level.

❖ NURSING MANAGEMENT: CHRONIC KIDNEY DISEASE

◆ Nursing Assessment

Obtain a complete history of any existing kidney disease or family history of kidney disease. Some kidney disorders, including Alport syndrome and polycystic kidney disease, have a genetic component. Other disorders that can lead to CKD are diabetes, hypertension, and SLE.

Because many drugs are potentially nephrotoxic, ask the patient about both current and past use of prescription and OTC drugs and herbal preparations. Decongestants and antihistamines that contain pseudoephedrine and phenylephrine cause vasoconstriction and lead to an increase in BP. Magnesium and

aluminum from antacids can accumulate in the body because they cannot be excreted. Some antacids have high levels of salt, contributing to hypertension.

NSAIDs (aspirin, ibuprofen, naproxen) can contribute to the development of AKI and progression of CKD, especially when taken in higher doses than recommended. If taken as prescribed, these analgesics are usually considered safe.

Assess the patient's dietary habits and discuss any problems with intake. Measure the patient's height and weight and evaluate any recent weight changes.

The chronicity of kidney disease and the long-term treatment affect virtually every area of a person's life, including family relationships, social and work activities, self-image, and emotional state. Assess the patient's support systems. The choice of treatment modality may be related to support systems available.

◆ Nursing Diagnoses

Nursing diagnoses for patients with CKD include:
- Fluid imbalance
- Electrolyte imbalance
- Impaired nutritional status
- Difficulty coping

More information on nursing diagnoses and interventions for the patient with CKD is presented in eNursing Care Plan 46.1, available on the website for this chapter.

◆ Planning

The overall goals are that a patient with CKD will (1) show knowledge of and ability to adhere to the therapeutic plan, (2) take part in decision making for the plan of care and future treatment modality, (3) have effective coping strategies, and (4) continue with activities of daily living within physiologic limitations.

◆ Nursing Implementation

◆ Health Promotion. Identify those at risk for CKD. At-risk persons include those diagnosed with diabetes or hypertension and people with a history (or a family history) of kidney disease or repeated urinary tract infections (UTIs). They should have regular checkups that include a routine urinalysis and calculation of the estimated GFR.

People with diabetes need to have their urine checked for albuminuria if routine urinalysis is negative for protein. Teach patients with diabetes to report any changes in urine appearance

TABLE 46.11 Patient & Caregiver Teaching

Chronic Kidney Disease

Include the following information in the teaching plan for the patient and caregiver:

1. Dietary (sodium, potassium, phosphate) and fluid restrictions.
2. Common problems patient will encounter in modifying diet and fluid intake.
3. Signs and symptoms of electrolyte imbalance, especially high potassium.
4. Alternative ways of reducing thirst, such as sucking on ice cubes, lemon, or hard candy.
5. Reasons for prescribed drugs and common side effects. *Examples:*
   - Phosphate binders (including calcium supplements used as phosphate barriers) should be taken with meals.
   - Take calcium supplements prescribed to treat hypocalcemia on an empty stomach, but not at the same time as iron supplements.
   - Iron supplements should be taken between meals.
6. The importance of reporting any of the following: weight gain >4 lb (2 kg), increasing BP, shortness of breath, edema, increasing fatigue or weakness, or confusion or lethargy
7. Need for support and encouragement. Share concerns about lifestyle changes, living with a chronic illness, and decisions about type of dialysis or transplantation.

(color, odor), frequency, or volume to the HCP. If a patient needs a potentially nephrotoxic drug, it is important to monitor kidney function with serum creatinine, BUN, and GFR. Those at risk must take measures to prevent or delay the progression of CKD. Most important are measures to reduce the risk or progression of CVD. These include glycemic control for patients with diabetes (see Chapter 48), BP control (see Chapter 32), and lifestyle modifications, including smoking cessation.

 PROMOTING POPULATION HEALTH

Prevention and Detection of Chronic Kidney Disease

- Early detection and treatment are the primary methods for reducing CKD.
- Ensure proper diagnosis and treatment of diabetes as it is the leading cause of CKD.
- Monitor BP to detect elevations so that treatment can be started early.
- Treat hypertension appropriately and aggressively as it is the second leading cause of CKD.

◆ **Acute Care.** Most of the care of the patient with CKD occurs on an outpatient basis. In-hospital care is needed for management of complications and for kidney transplantation (if applicable).

◆ **Ambulatory Care.** Encourage patients to take part in their care. Teach the patient and caregiver about the diet, drugs, and follow-up medical care (Table 46.11). The patient needs to understand the drugs and common side effects. Because patients with CKD take many medications, a pillbox organizer or a list of the drugs and the times of administration may be helpful. Tell the patient to avoid OTC medications, such as NSAIDs and aluminum- and magnesium-based laxatives and antacids. Teach the patient to take daily BP readings and watch for signs and symptoms of fluid overload, hyperkalemia, and other electrolyte imbalances.

The dietitian should meet with the patient and caregiver on a regular basis for diet planning. A diet history and consideration of cultural variations help with diet planning and adherence. The rate of progression of CKD is dependent on the type of kidney disease and presence of other co-morbid conditions.

The patient can complete an evaluation for a kidney transplant prior to the need to start dialysis. Patients may receive a transplant before ever having to start dialysis. Even though transplantation offers the best therapeutic management for many ESRD patients, the critical shortage of donor organs limits this option for many patients.

Most patients need either PD or HD. Most patients use HD. Explain to the patient and caregiver what is involved in PD or HD and home HD modalities, transplantation, and palliative care. Offer information about all treatment options so that the patient can be involved in the decision-making process, giving a sense of control over life-altering decisions. Tell the patient that even while on dialysis, transplant is still an option. Let the patient know that if a transplanted organ fails, the patient can return to dialysis.

It is important to respect the patient's choice to not receive treatment. Patients themselves often start the conversation about palliative care. Focus the discussion on moving from the curative approach to promotion of comfort care and consideration of hospice care. Listen to the patient and caregiver, allowing them to do most of the talking and pay special attention to their hopes and fears. (Palliative and end-of-life care is discussed in Chapter 9.)

◆ **Evaluation**

The expected outcomes are that the patient with CKD will maintain

- Fluid and electrolyte levels within normal ranges
- An acceptable weight with no more than a 10% weight loss

DIALYSIS

Dialysis is the movement of fluid and molecules across a semipermeable membrane from one compartment to another. Clinically, dialysis is a technique in which substances move from the blood through a semipermeable membrane and into a dialysis solution *(dialysate)*. It corrects fluid and electrolyte imbalances and removes waste products in kidney failure. It also can be used to treat drug overdoses.

The 2 methods of dialysis available are **peritoneal dialysis (PD)** and **hemodialysis (HD)** (Table 46.12). In PD the peritoneal membrane acts as the semipermeable membrane. In HD an artificial membrane (usually made of cellulose-based or synthetic materials) is used as the semipermeable membrane and is in contact with the patient's blood.

Dialysis is begun when the patient's uremia can no longer be adequately treated with conservative medical management. Generally, this is when the GFR is less than 15 mL/min/1.73 m². This criterion can vary widely in different clinical situations. The nephrologist determines when to start dialysis based on the patient's clinical status. Certain uremic complications, including encephalopathy, neuropathies, uncontrolled hyperkalemia, pericarditis, and accelerated hypertension, indicate a need for immediate dialysis.

Most patients with ESRD are treated with dialysis because (1) there is a lack of donated organs, (2) some patients are physically or mentally unsuitable for transplantation, or (3) some

TABLE 46.12 Comparison of Peritoneal Dialysis and Hemodialysis

Advantages	Disadvantages
Peritoneal Dialysis (PD)	
• Immediate initiation in almost any hospital	• Bacterial or chemical peritonitis
• Less complicated than hemodialysis	• Protein loss into dialysate
	• Exit site and tunnel infections
• Portable system with CAPD	• Self-image problems with catheter placement
• Fewer dietary restrictions	• Hyperglycemia
• Rather short training time	• Surgery for catheter placement
• Usable in patient with vascular access problems	• Contraindicated in patient with multiple abdominal surgeries, trauma, unrepaired hernia
• Less cardiovascular stress	
• Home dialysis possible	• Requires completion of education program
• Preferable for patient with diabetes	• Catheter can migrate
	• Best instituted with willing partner
Hemodialysis (HD)	
• Rapid fluid removal	• Vascular access problems
• Rapid removal of urea and creatinine	• Dietary and fluid restrictions
	• Heparinization may be necessary
• Effective potassium removal	
• Less protein loss	• Extensive equipment necessary
• Lowering of serum triglycerides	• Hypotension during dialysis
• Home dialysis possible	• Added blood loss that contributes to anemia
• Temporary access can be placed at bedside	• Specially trained personnel necessary
	• Surgery for permanent access placement
	• Self-image problems with permanent access

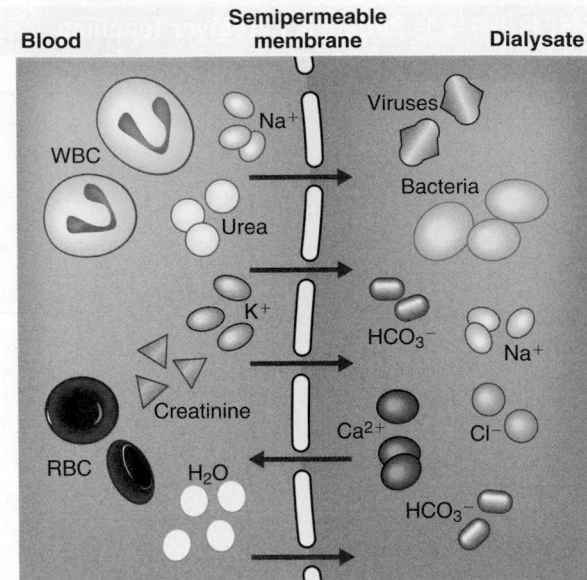

FIG. 46.4 Osmosis and diffusion across a semipermeable membrane.

the dialysate (osmotic gradient) with the addition of glucose. In HD, the gradient is created by increasing pressure in the blood compartment (positive pressure) or decreasing pressure in the dialysate compartment (negative pressure). ECF moves into the dialysate because of the pressure gradient. The excess fluid is removed by creating a pressure differential between the blood and the dialysate solution with a combination of positive pressure in the blood compartment and negative pressure in the dialysate compartment.

PERITONEAL DIALYSIS

Although PD was first used in 1923, it did not come into widespread use for chronic treatment until the 1970s with the development of soft, pliable peritoneal solution bags and the introduction of the concept of continuous PD. In the United States, about 12% of patients receiving dialysis treatments are on PD.

Catheter Placement

Peritoneal access is obtained by inserting a catheter through the anterior abdominal wall (Fig. 46.5). The catheter is about 24 in (60 cm) long and has 1 or 2 Dacron cuffs. The cuffs act as anchors and prevent the migration of microorganisms into the peritoneum. Within a few weeks, fibrous tissue grows into the Dacron cuff, holding the catheter in place and preventing bacterial penetration into the peritoneal cavity. The tip of the catheter rests in the peritoneal cavity. It has many perforations spaced along the distal end of the tubing, allowing fluid movement through the catheter.

The technique for catheter placement varies. It is usually placed surgically so that the catheter can be seen directly, minimizing potential complications. Patient preparation for catheter insertion includes emptying the bladder and bowel, weighing the patient, and obtaining a signed consent form. After placement, PD may be started at once with low-volume exchanges or delayed for 2 weeks pending healing and sealing of the exit site. Once the catheter incision site is healed, the patient may shower and then pat the catheter and exit site dry.[25] Daily catheter

patients do not want transplants. An increasing number of people, including older adults and those with complex medical problems, are receiving maintenance dialysis. A patient's age is not a factor in determining candidacy for dialysis.

General Principles of Dialysis

Solutes and water move across the semipermeable membrane from the blood to the dialysate or from the dialysate to the blood per concentration gradients. The principles of diffusion, osmosis, and ultrafiltration are involved in dialysis (Fig. 46.4). *Diffusion* is the movement of solutes from an area of greater concentration to an area of lesser concentration. In kidney failure, urea, creatinine, uric acid, and electrolytes (potassium, phosphate) move from the blood to the dialysate with the net effect of lowering their concentration in the blood. RBCs, WBCs, and plasma proteins are too large to diffuse through the pores of the membrane. Small-molecular-weight substances can pass from the dialysate into a patient's blood, so the purity of the water used for dialysis is monitored and controlled.

Osmosis is the movement of fluid from an area of lesser concentration to an area of greater concentration of solutes. Glucose is added to the dialysate and creates an osmotic gradient across the membrane, pulling excess fluid from the blood.

Ultrafiltration (water and fluid removal) results when there is an osmotic gradient or pressure gradient across the membrane. In PD, excess fluid is removed by increasing the osmolality of

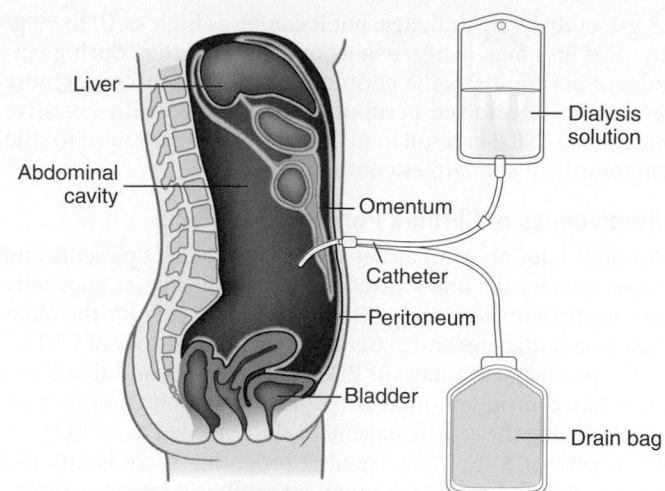

FIG. 46.5 Peritoneal dialysis showing peritoneal catheter inserted into peritoneal cavity.

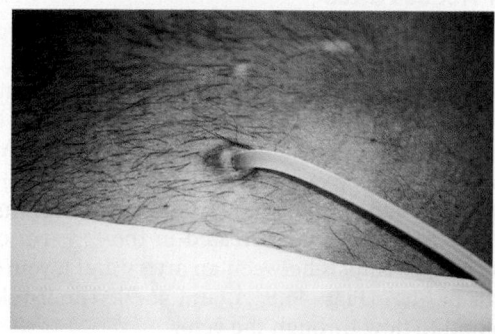

FIG. 46.6 Peritoneal catheter exit site. (Courtesy Mary Jo Holechek, Baltimore, MD.)

care varies. Some patients just wash with soap and water and go without a dressing (Fig. 46.6). Others need daily dressing changes. Showering is preferred to bathing.

In PD it is critical to maintain aseptic technique to avoid peritonitis. Several tubing connections and devices are commercially available to help maintain an aseptic system. Teach all patients to examine their catheter site for signs of infection.

Dialysis Solutions and Cycles

PD is done by putting dialysis solution into the peritoneal space. The 3 phases of the PD cycle are inflow (fill), dwell (equilibration), and drain. Together, the 3 phases are an *exchange.* For manual PD, a period of about 30 to 50 minutes is needed to complete an exchange. During *inflow,* a prescribed amount of solution, usually 2 L, is infused through an established catheter over about 10 minutes. The flow rate may be decreased if the patient has pain. After the solution has been infused, the inflow clamp is closed.

The next part of the cycle is the *dwell* phase, or equilibration, during which diffusion and osmosis occur between the patient's blood and peritoneal cavity. The duration of the dwell time is usually between 4 and 6 hours. *Drain* time takes 15 to 30 minutes. It may be facilitated by gently massaging the abdomen or changing position. The cycle starts again with the infusion of another 2 L of solution.

PD solutions vary. The choice of the exchange volume is primarily determined by the size of the peritoneal cavity. An

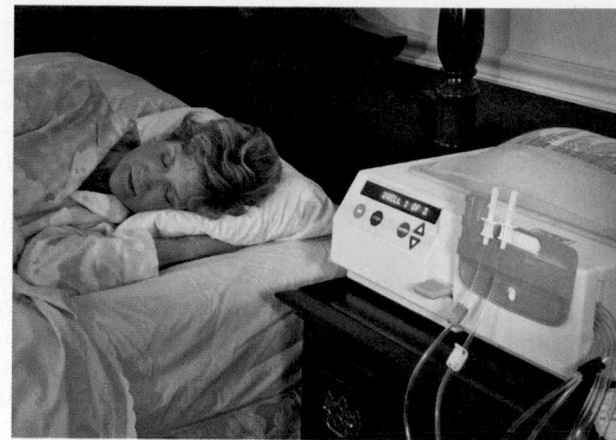

FIG. 46.7 Automated PD that can be used while the patient is sleeping.

average-size person typically uses a 2-L exchange. A larger person may need a 3-L exchange volume. Smaller exchange volumes are used for patients with a smaller body, pulmonary compromise (the added pressure of the large volume may cause respiratory problems), or inguinal hernias.

Ultrafiltration (fluid removal) during PD depends on osmotic forces. Dextrose is the most commonly used osmotic agent in PD solutions. It is relatively safe and inexpensive. It is associated with high rates of peritoneal glucose absorption, leading to problems with hypertriglyceridemia, hyperglycemia, and long-term peritoneal membrane dysfunction.

Alternatives to dextrose PD solution include icodextrin and amino acid solutions. Icodextrin is a commercially available iso-osmolar preparation. It induces ultrafiltration by its oncotic effect. Amino acid PD solutions are available and used mainly for patients who need nutritional supplementation.

Peritoneal Dialysis Systems

Automated Peritoneal Dialysis. Automated peritoneal dialysis (APD) is the most popular form of PD because it allows patients to do dialysis while they sleep. An automated device called a *cycler* delivers the dialysate for APD (Fig. 46.7). The size of a cycler is similar to a DVD player. The automated cycler times and controls the fill, dwell, and drain phases. The machine cycles 4 or more exchanges per night with 1 to 2 hours per exchange. Alarms and monitors are built into the system to make it safe for the patient to sleep while dialyzing. The patient disconnects from the machine in the morning and usually leaves fluid in the abdomen during the day.

It is hard to achieve the required solute and fluid clearance solely with nighttime APD. One or 2 daytime manual exchanges may be prescribed to ensure adequate dialysis.

Continuous Ambulatory Peritoneal Dialysis. Continuous ambulatory peritoneal dialysis (CAPD) is done every few hours during the day. The patient may perform an exchange of 2 L of peritoneal dialysate 4 times daily, with dwell times averaging 4 hours. A common schedule includes exchanges at 7 AM, 12 noon, 5 PM, and 10 PM.

In CAPD, the person instills 2 to 3 L of dialysate from a plastic bag into the peritoneal cavity through a disposable administration line. The bag and line are then disconnected. After the equilibration period, the line is reconnected to the catheter, the dialysate (effluent) is drained from the peritoneal cavity, and a new 2- to 3-L bag of dialysate solution is infused.

Complications of Peritoneal Dialysis

Exit Site Infection. Infection of the peritoneal catheter exit site is most often caused by *Staphylococcus aureus* or *Staphylococcus epidermidis* (from skin flora). Manifestations include redness at the site, tenderness, and drainage. Superficial exit site infections caused by these organisms generally resolve with antibiotic therapy. If not treated immediately, subcutaneous tunnel infections may progress and may cause peritonitis, necessitating catheter removal.

Peritonitis. Peritonitis results from contact contamination or an exit site or tunnel infection. Most often it occurs because of improper technique when connections for exchanges are contaminated. Peritonitis is usually caused by *S. aureus* or *S. epidermidis*. It rarely results from bacteria in the intestine crossing into the peritoneal cavity.

The main manifestations are abdominal pain, rebound tenderness, and cloudy peritoneal effluent with a WBC count greater than 100 cells/μL (more than 50% neutrophils) or bacteria in the peritoneal effluent shown by Gram stain or culture. GI manifestations may include diarrhea, vomiting, abdominal distention, and hyperactive bowel sounds. Fever may or may not be present. To determine if the peritoneal effluent is cloudy, drain the effluent and place the drained bag on reading material, such as a newspaper. If you cannot read the print through the effluent, it is cloudy.

Cultures, Gram stain, and a WBC differential of the peritoneal effluent are used to confirm the diagnosis of peritonitis. Antibiotics can be given orally, IV, or intraperitoneally. In most cases, the patient is treated on an outpatient basis.

The formation of adhesions in the peritoneum can result from repeated infections and interferes with the peritoneal membrane's ability to act as a dialyzing surface. Repeated infections may require the removal of the peritoneal catheter and a temporary or permanent change of modality to HD.

Hernias. Increased intraabdominal pressure from the dialysate volume can cause hernias to develop in predisposed persons, such as multiparous women and older men. After hernia repair, PD often can be resumed after several days using small dialysate volumes and keeping the patient supine.

Lower Back Problems. Increased intraabdominal pressure can cause or worsen lower back pain. The lumbosacral curvature is increased by intraperitoneal infusion of dialysate. Orthopedic binders and a regular exercise program for strengthening the back muscles are helpful for some patients.

Bleeding. After peritoneal catheter placement, it is common for the PD effluent drained after the first few exchanges to be pink or slightly bloody from trauma associated with catheter insertion. Bloody effluent over several days or the new appearance of blood in the effluent can indicate active intraperitoneal bleeding. If this occurs, check the BP and hematocrit. Blood may be present in the effluent of women who are menstruating or ovulating. This requires no intervention.

Pulmonary Complications. Atelectasis, pneumonia, and bronchitis may occur from repeated upward displacement of the diaphragm, resulting in decreased lung expansion. Longer dwell times increase the risk for pulmonary problems. Frequent repositioning and deep-breathing exercises can help. When the patient is lying in bed, elevate the head of the bed to prevent these problems.

Protein Loss. The peritoneal membrane is permeable to plasma proteins, amino acids, and polypeptides. These substances are lost in the dialysate fluid. The amount of loss is usually about 0.5 g/L of dialysate drainage, but it can be as high as 10 to 20 g/day. This loss may increase to as much as 40 g/day during episodes of peritonitis as the peritoneal membrane becomes more permeable. Unresolved peritonitis is associated with excessive protein loss that can result in malnutrition. PD may need to stop temporarily or sometimes permanently.

Effectiveness of Chronic Peritoneal Dialysis

Mortality rates are similar between in-center HD patients and PD patients for the first few years. After about 2 years, mortality rates for patients receiving PD increase, especially for the older person with diabetes and patients with a prior history of CVD.[25]

The primary advantage of PD is its simplicity and that it is a home-based program, increasing patient participation in their care. Learning the self-management skills needed to do PD usually involves a 3- to 7-day training program. There is no need for special water systems. Equipment setup is relatively simple.

HEMODIALYSIS

Vascular Access Sites

HD requires a very rapid blood flow and access to a large blood vessel. Obtaining vascular access is one of the hardest problems associated with HD. Enough time is needed for evaluation and consideration of the best arteriovenous (AV) access for HD. The types of vascular access include AV fistulas (AVFs), AV grafts (AVGs), and temporary vascular access.[26]

Arteriovenous Fistulas and Grafts. A subcutaneous arteriovenous fistula (AVF) is usually created in the forearm or upper arm with an anastomosis between an artery and a vein (usually cephalic or basilic) (Figs. 46.8, *A*, and 46.9). The fistula allows arterial blood to flow through the vein.

The vein becomes "arterialized," increasing in size and developing thicker walls. The arterial blood flow is essential to provide the rapid blood flow needed for HD. As the fistula matures, it is more amenable to repeated venipunctures. Maturation may take 6 weeks to months. AVF should be placed at least 3 months before starting HD. A fistula is the preferred access for HD.[26]

Normally, a *thrill* (buzzing sensation) can be felt by palpating the fistula, and a *bruit* (rushing sound) can be heard with a stethoscope. The thrill and bruit are created by arterial blood moving at a high velocity through the vein.

⍰ CHECK YOUR PRACTICE

You are rotating to the inpatient dialysis unit today. It is your first time working with HD patients. You are helping a hemodialysis tech "hook-up" a 56-yr-old man to HD. He has been on HD for 5 years due to polycystic kidney disease. You take his vital signs, palpate his AV fistula, and then use your stethoscope to auscultate the AV fistula. You are concerned because you feel a super-strong pulse and hear a very loud "whoosh" sound. The patient turns to you and just smirks, "I bet you have never had a thrill like that."

- You are very flustered and not sure how to respond. What should you say to him?

AVFs are harder to create in patients with a history of severe peripheral vascular disease (e.g., people with diabetes), those with prolonged IV drug use, and obese women. These persons may need a synthetic graft.

Arteriovenous grafts (AVGs) are made of synthetic materials (polytetrafluoroethylene [PTFE, Teflon]) and form a "bridge" between the arterial and venous blood supplies. Grafts are

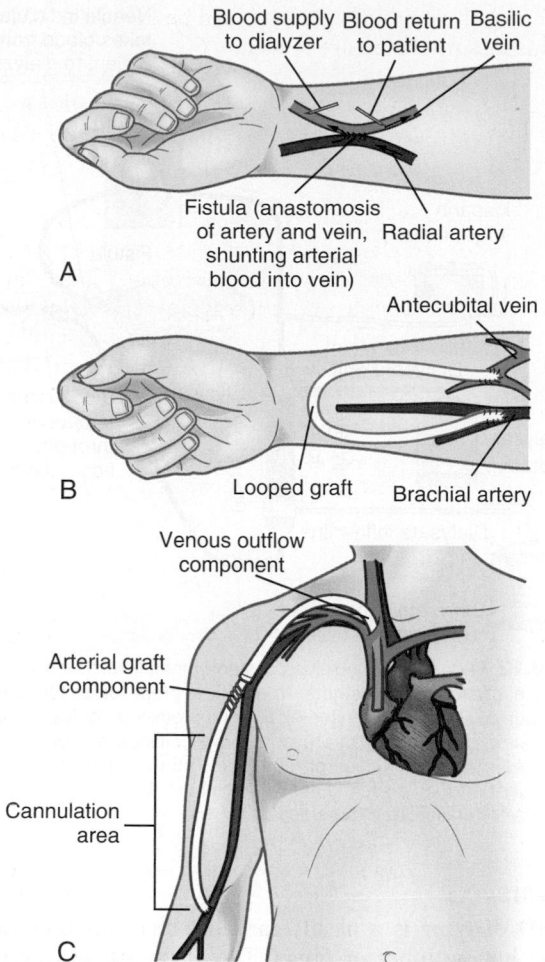

FIG. 46.8 Vascular access for hemodialysis. A, AVF. B, AVG. C, HeRO Graft.

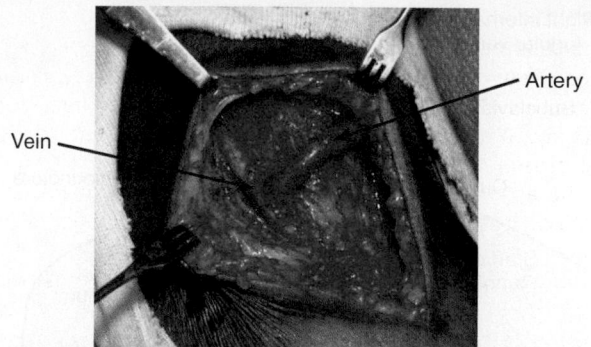

FIG. 46.9 AVF created by anastomosing an artery and a vein. (Courtesy Dr. Stephen Van Voorst, MD.)

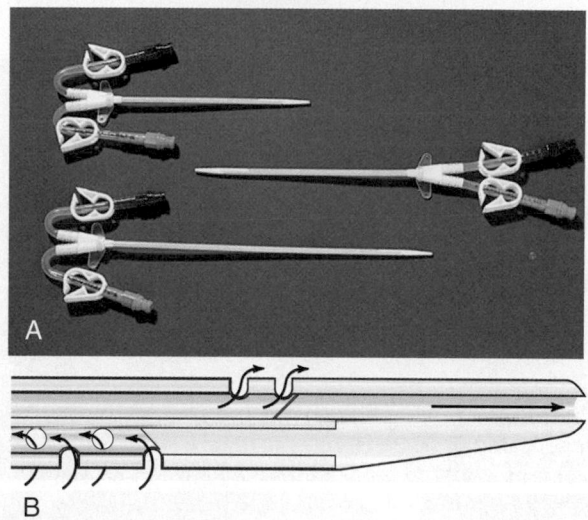

FIG. 46.10 Temporary double-lumen vascular access catheter for acute hemodialysis. A, Soft, flexible double-lumen tube is attached to a Y hub. B, The distance between the arterial intake lumen and the venous return lumen typically provides recirculation rates of 5% or less. (A, Courtesy Quinton Instrument Co., Seattle, WA.)

placed under the skin and are surgically anastomosed between an artery (usually brachial) and a vein (usually antecubital) (Fig. 46.8, *B*). An interval of 2 to 4 weeks is usually needed to allow the graft to heal, but it may be used earlier. Because grafts are made of artificial materials, they are more likely than AVFs to become infected and tend to form clots. When AVG infections occur, they may need surgical removal, since it is hard to completely resolve the infection from the synthetic material.

A common problem in patients on HD is central venous stenosis (CVS) or occlusion. CVS is serious and has a greater impact than peripheral venous stenosis because the central veins are the final pathway for blood flow to the heart. As CVS progresses, vascular access for HD is often lost.

HeRO (Hemodialysis Reliable Outflow) *Graft* is a special bridge access used in patients when other access options are exhausted. It consists of 2 pieces: a reinforced tube to bypass blockages in veins and a dialysis graft anastomosed to an artery to be accessed for HD (Fig. 46.8, *C*). The HeRO Graft is placed under the skin, like both a fistula and standard graft. The HeRO Graft bypasses the venous system and provides blood flow directly from a target artery to the heart. It may be harder to auscultate the bruit or feel the thrill in this type of access because of the absence of a venous anastomosis.

Surgical creation of AV access for HD has several risks. These include distal ischemia *(steal syndrome)* and pain because too

much arterial blood is being shunted or "stolen" from the distal extremity. Manifestations of steal syndrome are pain distal to the access site, numbness or tingling of fingers that may worsen during dialysis, and poor capillary refill. Aneurysms can develop in the AV access and can rupture if left untreated.

> **! SAFETY ALERT** AV Fistulas and Grafts
> • Never perform BP measurements, IV line insertion, or venipuncture in an extremity with AV access.
> • These special precautions are taken to prevent infection and clotting of the vascular access.
> • When a patient is hospitalized, place signs in patient's room and label the arm with a band that says, "No BP, blood draws, or IV in this arm."

Temporary Vascular Access. When immediate vascular access is needed, catheterization of the internal jugular or femoral vein is done. A flexible catheter inserted at the bedside into 1 of these large veins gives access to the circulation without surgery (Fig. 46.10). The catheters usually have a double external lumen with an internal septum separating the 2 internal segments. One lumen is used for blood removal and the other for blood return (Fig. 46.11, *A* and *B*). Temporary catheters have high rates of infection, dislodgment, and malfunction. A patient should not be discharged from the hospital with a temporary catheter in place.

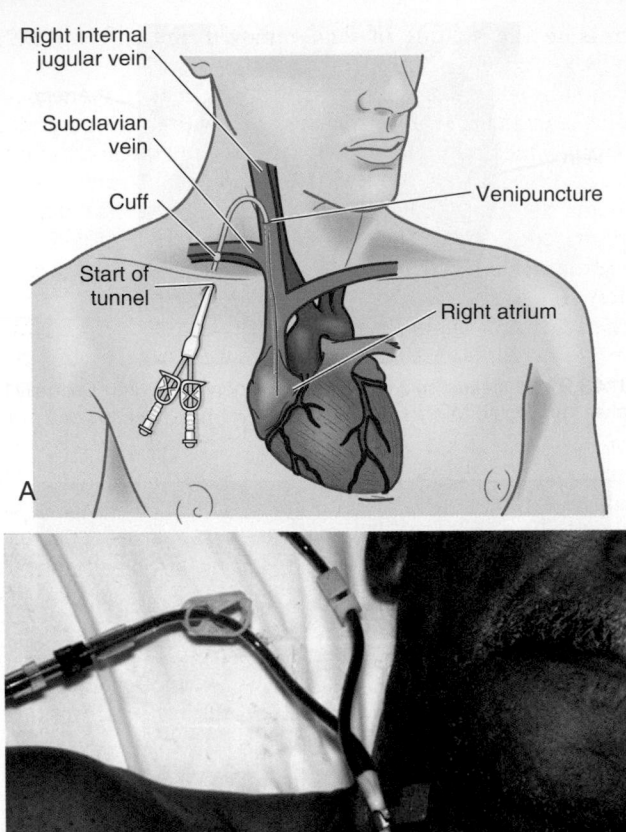

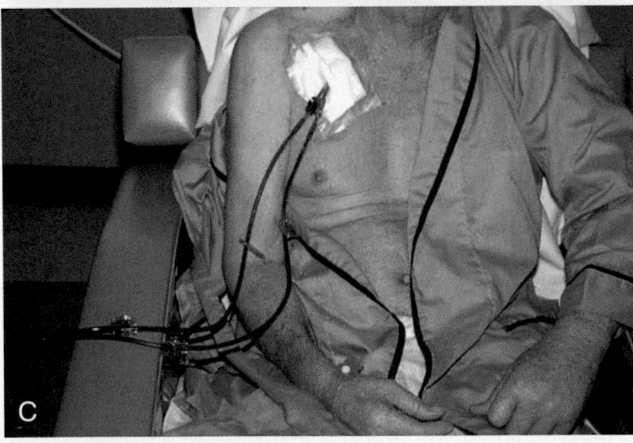

FIG. 46.11 A, Right internal jugular placement for a tunneled, cuffed semipermanent catheter. B, Temporary hemodialysis catheter in place. C, Long-term cuffed hemodialysis catheter. (B and C, Courtesy Dr. Stephen Van Voorst, MD.)

Long-term cuffed HD catheters are often used for temporary vascular access. These catheters give temporary access while the patient is waiting for fistula placement or as long-term access when other forms of access have failed. They exit on the upper chest wall and are tunneled subcutaneously to the internal or external jugular vein (Fig. 46.11, C). The catheter tip rests in the right atrium. It has 1 or 2 subcutaneous Dacron cuffs that prevent infection from tracking along the catheter and anchor the catheter, eliminating the need for sutures.

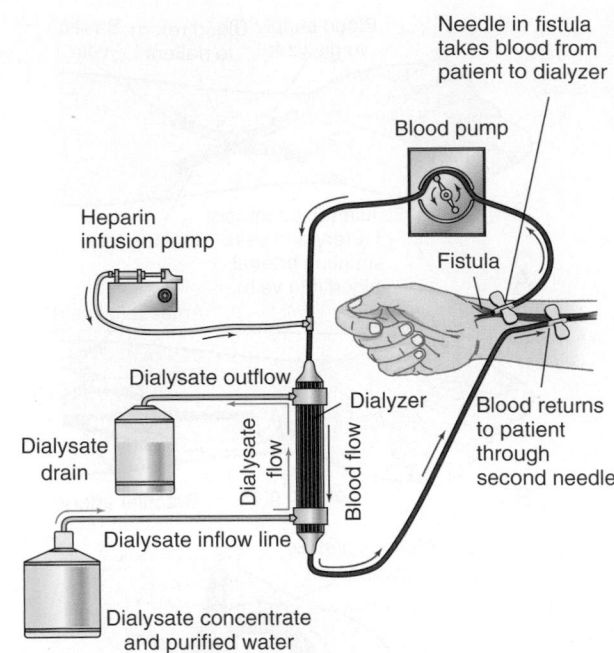

FIG. 46.12 Parts of a hemodialysis system. Blood is removed via a needle inserted in a fistula or via catheter lumen. It is propelled to the dialyzer by a blood pump. Heparin is infused either as a predialysis bolus or through a heparin pump continuously to prevent clotting. Dialysate is pumped in and flows in the opposite direction of the blood. The dialyzed blood is returned to the patient through a second needle or catheter lumen. Old dialysate and ultrafiltrate are drained and discarded.

Dialyzers

The HD dialyzer is a plastic cartridge that has thousands of parallel hollow tubes or fibers. The fibers are semipermeable membranes made of cellulose-based or other synthetic materials. The blood is pumped into the top of the cartridge and dispersed into all the fibers. Dialysis fluid (*dialysate*) is pumped into the bottom of the cartridge and bathes the outside of the fibers. Ultrafiltration, diffusion, and osmosis occur across the pores of this semipermeable membrane. When the dialyzed blood reaches the end of the thousands of semipermeable fibers, it converges into a single tube that returns it to the patient. Dialyzers differ in surface area, membrane composition and thickness, clearance of waste products, and removal of fluid.

Procedure for Hemodialysis

The needles used for HD are large bore, usually 14 to 16 gauge. They are inserted into the fistula or graft to obtain vascular access. One needle is placed to pull blood from the circulation to the HD machine, and the other needle is used to return the dialyzed blood to the patient. The needles are attached via tubing to dialysis lines. If a patient has a catheter, the 2 blood lines are attached to the 2 catheter lumens. The needle closer to the fistula (red catheter lumen) pulls blood from the patient to the dialyzer using a blood pump. Blood is returned from the dialyzer to the patient through the second needle (blue catheter lumen).[27]

When blood comes in contact with a foreign material, such as the dialyzer, it tends to clot. Heparin is added to the blood to prevent clotting.

In addition to the dialyzer, a dialysate delivery and monitoring system is used (Fig. 46.12). This system pumps the dialysate through the dialyzer, countercurrent to the blood flow. To end

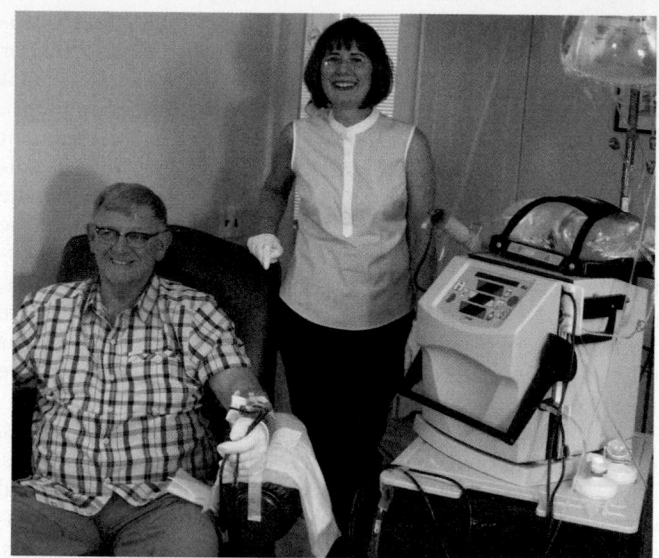

FIG. 46.13 Home hemodialysis is growing in popularity, and machines are more compact. (From NxStage Medical, Inc, Lawrence, MA.)

the treatment, a saline solution is used to return the blood in the extracorporeal circuit back to the patient through the vascular access. The needles are removed from the patient, and firm pressure is applied to the venipuncture sites until the bleeding stops.

Before beginning treatment, assess fluid status (weight, BP, peripheral edema, lung and heart sounds), condition of vascular access, and temperature. The difference between the last postdialysis weight and the present predialysis weight determines the ultrafiltration or the amount of weight (from fluid) to be removed. While the patient is on dialysis, take vital signs at least every 30 to 60 minutes because rapid BP changes may occur.

Settings and Schedules for Hemodialysis. Most HD patients are treated in a community-based center and dialyze for 3 to 4 hours 3 days per week. Most people sleep, read, talk, or watch television during HD.

Other schedule options for HD are short daily HD and long nocturnal HD. The patient receiving long nocturnal HD has the advantage of sleeping while dialyzing. Each nocturnal treatment lasts 6 to 8 hours, and the patient dialyzes up to 6 times per week.

In addition to in-center HD, home HD is available (Fig. 46.13). The use of home HD often depends on a patient's family support. One of the main advantages of home HD is that it allows greater freedom in choosing dialysis times. In short daily HD, the patient dialyzes for 2½ to 3 hours per session 5 to 6 days per week. Short daily HD is usually done at home.

Patients who choose daily dialysis or nocturnal dialysis may have fewer uremic symptoms, tend to need fewer medications, and have fewer dialysis-related side effects (e.g., hypotension, cramps). In addition, they have more autonomy. Although daily home HD offers the potential of significant health benefits, only about 2% of HD patients dialyze at home.

Complications of Hemodialysis

Hypotension. Hypotension that occurs during HD primarily results from rapid removal of vascular volume (hypovolemia), decreased cardiac output, and decreased systemic vascular resistance. The drop in BP may cause light-headedness, nausea, vomiting, seizures, vision changes, and chest pain from cardiac ischemia. The usual treatment for hypotension includes

decreasing the volume of fluid removed and infusing 0.9% saline solution.

Muscle Cramps. We do not completely understand the cause of muscle cramps in HD. Factors associated with developing muscle cramps include hypotension, hypovolemia, high ultrafiltration rate, and low-sodium dialysis solution. Treatment includes reducing the ultrafiltration rate and giving fluids (saline, glucose, mannitol). Hypertonic saline is not recommended since the sodium load can be problematic. Hypertonic glucose is preferred.

Loss of Blood. Blood loss may result from blood not being completely rinsed from the dialyzer, accidental separation of blood tubing, dialysis membrane rupture, or bleeding after removing the needles at the end of HD. If a patient has received too much heparin or has clotting problems, postdialysis bleeding can occur. It is essential to rinse back all blood, avoid excess anticoagulation, and hold firm but nonocclusive pressure on access sites until the risk for bleeding has passed.

Hepatitis. Hepatitis B used to have an unusually high prevalence in dialysis patients, but the incidence today is low. Lower transfusion requirements, screening, and recommendations for vaccinations have lowered the incidence. Outbreaks of hepatitis B still occur, likely from breaks in infection control practices. To prevent transmission, all patients and personnel in dialysis units receive hepatitis B vaccine.

Currently, hepatitis C virus (HCV) causes most cases of hepatitis in dialysis patients. (Hepatitis is discussed in more detail in Chapter 43.) About 10% of patients undergoing dialysis in the United States are positive for anti-HCV, which indicates a previous infection. Infection control precautions are mandated in caring for the patient with hepatitis C to protect the patient and staff (see Chapter 14). Currently no vaccine is available for hepatitis C.

Effectiveness of Hemodialysis

HD is still an imperfect therapy for management of ESRD. It cannot fully replace the normal biologic functions of the kidneys. It can ease many of the symptoms of CKD and, if started early, can prevent certain complications. It does not alter the accelerated rate of CVD and the related high mortality rate.

The yearly death rate of patients receiving maintenance HD is around 19% to 24%. CVD (stroke, MI) causes most deaths. Infectious complications are the second leading cause of death.[27]

Adaptation to maintenance HD varies considerably. At first, many patients feel positive about the dialysis because it makes them feel better and keeps them alive, but there is often great ambivalence about whether it is worthwhile. Dependence on a machine is a reality. In response to their illness, dialysis patients may be nonadherent or depressed and show suicidal tendencies. The primary nursing goals are to (1) help the patient to maintain a healthy self-image and (2) return the patient to the highest level of function possible, including returning to work.

CONTINUOUS RENAL REPLACEMENT THERAPY

Continuous renal replacement therapy (CRRT) is a method for treating AKI. It provides a means by which uremic toxins and fluids are removed while acid-base status and electrolytes are adjusted slowly and continuously in a hemodynamically unstable patient. The principle of CRRT is to dialyze patients in a more physiologic way (over 24 hours), just like the kidneys. CRRT is contraindicated if a patient has life-threatening manifestations of uremia (hyperkalemia, pericarditis) that need rapid treatment. CRRT can be used in conjunction with HD.

Several types of CRRT are available (Table 46.13). CRRT often uses the venovenous approaches of continuous venovenous hemofiltration (CVVH), continuous venovenous hemodialysis (CVVHD), and continuous venovenous hemodiafiltration (CVVHDF).

Vascular access for CRRT is achieved by using a double-lumen catheter (as used in HD [Fig. 46.10]) placed in the jugular or femoral vein. A blood pump propels the blood through the circuit. A highly permeable, hollow-fiber hemofilter removes plasma water and nonprotein solutes, which are collectively termed *ultrafiltrate*. The ultrafiltration rate (UFR) may range from 0 to 500 mL/hr. Under the influence of hydrostatic pressure and osmotic pressure, water and nonprotein solutes pass out of the filter into the extracapillary space and drain through the ultrafiltrate port into a collection device (drainage bag) (Fig. 46.14). The remaining fluid continues through the filter and returns to the patient via the return port of the double-lumen catheter.

TABLE 46.13 Continuous Renal Replacement Therapies

Therapy	Abbreviation	Purpose
Continuous venovenous hemofiltration	CVVH	Removes fluid and solutes Requires replacement fluid
Slow continuous ultrafiltration	SCUF	Simplified version of CVVH Removes fluid No fluid replacement required
Continuous venovenous hemodialysis	CVVHD	Removes fluids and solutes Requires dialysate and replacement fluid
Continuous venovenous hemodiafiltration	CVVHDF	Removes fluids and solutes Requires dialysate and replacement fluid

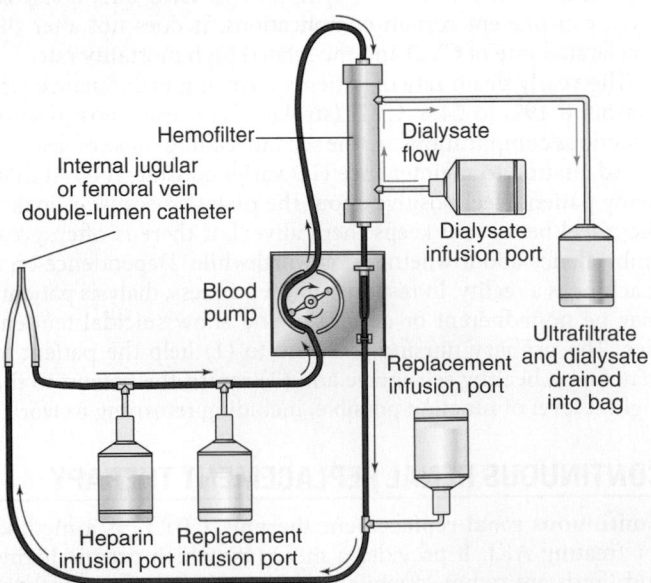

FIG. 46.14 Basic schematic of continuous venovenous therapies. A blood pump is required to pump blood through the circuit. Replacement ports are used for instilling replacement fluids and can be given prefilter or postfilter. Dialysate port is used for infusing dialysis solution. Regardless of modality, ultrafiltrate is drained via the ultrafiltration drain port.

As ultrafiltrate drains out of the hemofilter, fluid and electrolyte replacements can be infused through a port found before or after the filter as the blood returns to the patient. Replacement fluid is designed to replace volume and solutes, such as sodium, chloride, HCO_3^-, and glucose. The infusion rate of replacement fluid is determined by the degree of fluid and electrolyte imbalance. Replacement fluid infused into the infusion port before the hemofilter allows for greater clearance of urea and can decrease filter clotting. An infusion port after the filter dilutes intravascular fluid and decreases the concentration of unwanted solutes, such as BUN, creatinine, and potassium. Anticoagulants are given to prevent blood clotting. They may be infused as a bolus at the initiation of CRRT or through an infusion port before the hemofilter.

The type of CRRT can be customized to the patient's needs. Some types involve the introduction of replacement fluids. CVVHD and CVVHDF use dialysate. Dialysis fluid is attached to the distal end of the hemofilter, and the fluid is pumped countercurrent to the blood flow (Fig. 46.14). As in hemodialysis, diffusion of solutes and ultrafiltration via hydrostatic pressure and osmosis occur. This is an ideal treatment for a patient who needs both fluid and solute control but cannot tolerate the rapid fluid shifts associated with HD.

Several features of CRRT differ from HD:
- The blood pump in CRRT runs at a slower (150 mL/min average) rate. This may improve hemodynamic stability.
- Continuous rather than intermittent. Fluid volume can be removed over days (24 hours to more than 2 weeks) versus hours (3 to 4 hours).
- Solute removal can occur by *convection* (no dialysate required) in addition to osmosis and diffusion.
- Causes less hemodynamic instability (e.g., hypotension)
- Does not need constant monitoring by a specialized HD nurse but does require a trained ICU nurse
- Does not require complicated HD equipment

CRRT can be continued as long as 30 to 40 days. The hemofilter should be changed every 24 to 48 hours because of loss of filtration efficiency or potential for clotting. The ultrafiltrate should be clear yellow. Specimens may be obtained for serum chemistries. If the ultrafiltrate becomes bloody or blood tinged, suspect a rupture in the filter membrane. Stop treatment to prevent blood loss.

Specific nursing interventions include obtaining weights and monitoring and documenting laboratory values daily to ensure adequate fluid and electrolyte balance. Assess hourly intake and output, vital signs, and hemodynamic status. Although reductions in central venous pressure and pulmonary artery pressure are expected, there should be little change in mean arterial pressure or cardiac output. Assess and maintain the patency of the CRRT system. Care for the patient's vascular access site to prevent infection. Once the patient's AKI is resolved or there is a decision to withdraw treatment, CRRT is stopped and the needle(s) removed.

WEARABLE ARTIFICIAL KIDNEY

The wearable artificial kidney (WAK) has recently been developed and is approved for use to improve the quality of life of an ESRD patient. The WAK is a miniaturized dialysis machine that can be worn on the body. The carrier resembles a tool belt. The device connects to a patient via a catheter. Like conventional dialysis machines, it is designed to filter the blood of

ESRD patients. Unlike current portable or stationary dialysis machines, it can run continuously on batteries. The present version weighs about 10 lb, but future modifications could make it lighter and more streamlined.[28]

KIDNEY TRANSPLANTATION

Major advances have been made in kidney transplantation since the first live donor kidney transplant was done in 1954 between identical twins. These advances include organ procurement and preservation, surgical techniques, tissue typing and matching, immunosuppressant therapy, and prevention and treatment of graft rejection. A general discussion of organ transplantation is in Chapter 13.

Even though kidney transplantation is the best treatment option available to patients with ESRD, fewer than 4% ever receive a transplant. This is due to the large disparity between the supply and demand for kidneys. Every year thousands are waiting for kidney transplants (more than 100,000 are currently on the list), yet only about 17,000 transplants take place every year. Most die while waiting. Transplants from a deceased (cadaveric) donor usually require a prolonged waiting period, with differences in waiting time depending on age, gender, and race. Average wait times in the United States for a deceased kidney usually range from 2 to 5 years.[29-31]

Kidney transplantation is very successful, with 1-year graft survival rates over 90% for deceased donor transplants and 95% for live donor transplants.[30] An advantage of kidney transplantation when compared with dialysis is that it reverses many of the pathophysiologic changes associated with renal disease. It eliminates the dependence on dialysis and the accompanying dietary and lifestyle restrictions. Transplantation is less expensive than dialysis after the first year.

Recipient Selection

Appropriate recipient selection is important for a successful outcome. Candidacy is determined by a variety of medical and psychosocial factors that vary among transplant centers. Some transplant programs exclude patients who are morbidly obese or who continue to smoke despite smoking cessation interventions. A careful evaluation is done to identify and minimize potential complications after transplantation. Certain patients, particularly those with CVD and diabetes, are considered high risk. They must be carefully evaluated and then monitored closely after transplantation.

For a small number of patients who are approaching ESRD, a *preemptive transplant* (before dialysis is required) is possible if they have a living donor. This approach is best for patients with diabetes, who have a much higher mortality rate on dialysis than nondiabetics.

Contraindications to transplantation include advanced cancer, refractory or untreated heart disease, chronic respiratory failure, extensive vascular disease, chronic infection, and unresolved psychosocial disorders (e.g., nonadherence to medical regimens, alcohol use, drug use). Being HIV-positive or having hepatitis B or C infection is not a contraindication to transplantation.

Surgical procedures may be done before transplantation based on the results of the recipient evaluation. Coronary artery bypass or coronary angioplasty may be needed for advanced coronary artery disease. Cholecystectomy may be necessary for patients with a history of gallstones, biliary obstruction, or

cholecystitis. On rare occasions, bilateral nephrectomies are done for patients with refractory hypertension, recurrent UTIs, or grossly enlarged kidneys from polycystic kidney disease. In general, the recipient's own kidneys are not removed before receiving a kidney transplant.

Histocompatibility Studies

Histocompatibility studies, including human leukocyte antigen (HLA) testing and crossmatching, are discussed in Chapter 13 on p. 205.

Donor Sources

Kidneys for transplantation are obtained from compatible blood-type deceased donors, blood relatives, emotionally related (close and distant) living donors (e.g., spouses, distant cousins,), and altruistic living donors who are known (friends) or unknown to the recipient. Living donation accounts for around 27% of all kidney transplants in the United States. Most transplant centers regard them as the preferred donation modality.[31]

Live Donors. Live donors undergo an extensive evaluation to ensure that they are in good health and have no history of disease that would place them at risk for developing kidney disease or operative complications. Crossmatches are done at the time of the evaluation and about a week before the transplant to ensure that no antibodies to the donor are present or that the antibody titer is below the allowed level. Advantages of a live donor kidney include (1) better patient and graft survival rates regardless of histocompatibility match, (2) immediate organ availability, (3) immediate function due to minimal *cold time* (kidney out of body and not getting blood supply), and (4) the opportunity to have the recipient in the best possible medical condition because the surgery is elective.

The potential donor sees a nephrologist for a complete history and physical examination and laboratory and diagnostic studies. Laboratory studies include a 24-hour urine study for creatinine clearance and total protein, complete blood count, and chemistry and electrolyte profiles. Hepatitis B and C, HIV, and cytomegalovirus (CMV) testing is done to assess for transmitted diseases. An ECG and chest x-ray are done. A renal ultrasound and renal arteriogram or 3-dimensional CT scan is done to ensure that the blood vessels supplying each kidney are adequate and that no anomalies exist and to determine which kidney will be used in the transplant.

A transplant psychologist or social worker determines if the person is emotionally stable and able to deal with the issues related to organ donation. All donors must be informed about the risks and benefits of donation, the potential short- and long-term complications, and what to expect during the hospitalization and recovery phases. Kidney donation is considered safe without any long-term health consequences. Although the recipient's insurance covers the costs of the evaluation and surgery, no compensation is available for lost wages during the posthospitalization recovery period. This period can last 6 weeks or longer.

When there is ABO incompatibility between a donor and recipient, paired donor exchange is a viable alternative. *Paired organ donation,* in which one donor/recipient pair who are incompatible or poorly matched with each other find another donor/recipient pair with whom they can exchange kidneys. Thus a spouse (person A) who wants to donate a kidney to his wife (person B) but is incompatible is paired with another donor/recipient pair involving a son with ESRD (person C) and his mother (person D). In this example, person A would donate his kidney to person C, and person D would donate her kidney to person B. Paired organ donation is the practice of matching biologically incompatible donor/recipient pairs to permit transplantation of both candidates with a well-matched organ.

Another option for ABO incompatibility or a positive crossmatch between the donor and recipient is to use plasmapheresis to remove antibodies from the recipient. This allows transplant candidates to receive kidneys from live donors with blood types that we have traditionally considered incompatible. After the transplant, the patient undergoes more plasmapheresis treatments.

Deceased Donors. Deceased (cadaver) kidney donors are relatively healthy persons who have an irreversible brain injury and are declared brain dead. The most common causes of injury are cerebral trauma from motor vehicle accidents or gunshot wounds, intracerebral or subarachnoid hemorrhage, and anoxic brain damage caused by cardiac arrest. The brain-dead donor must have effective CV function and be supported on a ventilator to preserve the organs.

Even if the donor carried a signed donor card, permission from the donor's legal next of kin is still requested after brain death has been declared. That is why it is important for you to talk with your family about your wishes before losing the capacity to convey your desires.

In deceased kidney donation, the kidneys are removed and preserved. They can be preserved for up to 72 hours. Most transplant surgeons prefer to transplant kidneys before the cold time (time outside of the body when being transported from the deceased donor to the recipient) reaches 24 hours. Prolonged cold time increases the chance that the kidney will not function immediately, and ATN may develop.

The United Network for Organ Sharing (UNOS) distributes deceased donor kidneys using an objective computerized point system. A new kidney allocation system (KAS) started in early 2015 after several years of refinement. All donor kidneys receive a kidney donor profile index (KDPI). The KDPI includes 10 donor factors that evaluate the risk for a kidney transplant failure. The KDPI can help predict how long a kidney may function. Each kidney transplant candidate gets an individual Estimated Post-Transplant Survival (EPTS) score. This score ranges from 0 to 100 percent. The score is related to how long a candidate will need a functioning kidney transplant when compared with other candidates. For example, a person with an EPTS score of 20% is likely to need a kidney longer than 80% of other candidates. The EPTS score is based on age, length of time on dialysis, previous transplants, and having diabetes.[32]

When a donor becomes available, the donor's key information is compared with the data of all patients awaiting transplantation locally and nationwide. When a kidney arrives at the recipient's transplant center, a final crossmatch is done. It must be negative for the deceased donor transplantation to proceed.

The only exception is if a patient needs an emergency transplant or if a donor and recipient match on all 6 HLA antigens (zero antigen mismatch). The patient meeting either of these criteria goes to the top of the list. Emergency transplants receive priority because the patient is facing imminent death if not transplanted. If a zero antigen mismatch patient is found nationally, since statistically these grafts have better survival rates, one of the donor kidneys must be sent to that recipient's transplant center regardless of location.

Surgical Procedure

Live Donor. A transplant surgeon performs the live donor nephrectomy. The donor's surgery begins 1 to 2 hours before the recipient's surgery. The recipient is surgically prepared for the kidney transplant in a nearby operating room.

Laparoscopic donor nephrectomy is the most common technique for removing a kidney in a living donor. (Laparoscopic nephrectomy is discussed in Chapter 45.) After the kidney is removed, it is flushed with a chilled, sterile electrolyte solution and prepared for immediate transplant into the recipient. The use of a laparoscopic donor nephrectomy procedure is minimally invasive, with fewer risks and shorter recovery time than an open procedure. The laparoscopic approach significantly decreases hospital stay, pain, operative blood loss, debilitation, and length of time off work. For these reasons, the number of people willing to donate a kidney has increased significantly.

For an *open (conventional) nephrectomy,* the donor is placed in the lateral decubitus position on the operating table so that the flank is exposed laterally. An incision is made at the level of the eleventh rib. The rib may have to be removed to give adequate visualization of the kidney.

Kidney Transplant Recipient. The transplanted kidney is usually placed extraperitoneally in the iliac fossa. The right iliac fossa is preferred to facilitate anastomoses of the blood vessels and ureter and minimize the occurrence of paralytic ileus. A urinary catheter is placed into the bladder, and an antibiotic solution is instilled to distend the bladder and decrease the risk for

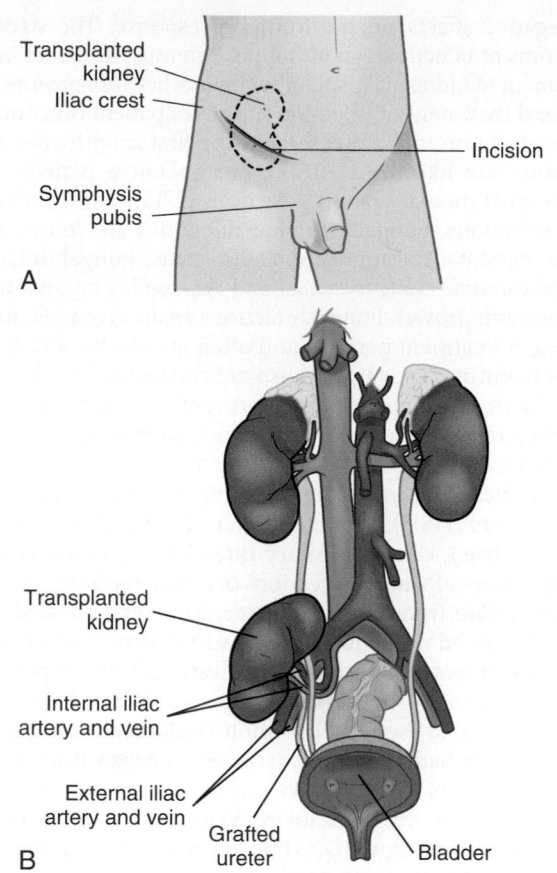

FIG. 46.15 A, Surgical incision for a renal transplant. B, Surgical placement of transplanted kidney.

infection. A crescent-shaped incision is made extending from the iliac crest to the symphysis pubis (Fig. 46.15).

Rapid revascularization is critical to prevent ischemic injury to the kidney. The donor artery is anastomosed to the recipient's internal iliac (hypogastric) or external iliac artery. The donor vein is anastomosed to the recipient's external iliac vein. When the anastomoses are complete, the clamps are released, and blood flow to the kidney is reestablished. The kidney should become firm and pink. Urine may begin to flow from the ureter at once. The donor ureter is then tunneled through the bladder submucosa before entering the bladder cavity and being sutured in place. This approach is called *ureteroneocystostomy*. This allows the bladder wall to compress the ureter as it contracts for micturition, thereby preventing reflux of urine up the ureter into the transplanted kidney. Transplant surgery takes about 3 to 4 hours.

❖ NURSING MANAGEMENT: KIDNEY TRANSPLANT RECIPIENT

◆ Preoperative Care

Nursing care of the patient in the preoperative phase includes emotional and physical preparation for surgery. Because the patient and caregiver may have been waiting years for the kidney transplant, a review of the operative procedure and what can be expected in the immediate postoperative recovery period is necessary. Stress that there is a chance the kidney may not function at once, and dialysis may be needed for days to weeks. Review the need for immunosuppressive drugs and measures to prevent infection.

To ensure the patient is in the best physical condition for surgery, an ECG, chest x-ray, and laboratory studies are done. Dialysis may be needed before surgery for fluid overload or hyperkalemia. Because dialysis may be needed after transplantation, the patency of the vascular access must be maintained. Label the vascular access extremity "dialysis access, no procedures" to prevent use of that extremity for BP measurement, blood drawing, or IV infusions. A patient on PD must empty the peritoneal cavity of all dialysate solution before going to surgery and have the PD catheter capped.

◆ Postoperative Care

◆ Live Donor.
Postoperative care for the donor is similar to that after open (conventional) or laparoscopic nephrectomy (see Chapter 45). Closely monitor renal function to assess for impairment and the hematocrit to assess for bleeding. Donors usually have more pain than the recipient. Donors who had an open surgical approach may have more pain than those after a laparoscopic approach.

Donors who had an open approach are usually discharged from the hospital in 4 or 5 days and return to work in 6 to 8 weeks. With a laparoscopic approach, donors are discharged from the hospital in 2 to 4 days and return to work in 4 to 6 weeks. The surgeon sees the donor 1 to 2 weeks after discharge.

Nurses caring for the living donor must acknowledge the precious gift that this person has given. The donor has taken physical, emotional, and financial risks to help the recipient. It is vital that the donor is not forgotten after surgery. The donor will need support if the donated organ does not work at once or for some reason fails.

◆ Kidney Transplant Recipient.
The priority during the postoperative period is maintaining fluid and electrolyte balance. Kidney transplant recipients require close monitoring and spend the first 12 to 24 hours in the ICU. Large volumes of urine may be made soon after the blood supply to the transplanted kidney is reestablished. This diuresis is due to the (1) new kidney's ability to filter BUN, which acts as an osmotic diuretic; (2) abundance of fluids given during the surgery; and (3) initial renal tubular dysfunction, which inhibits the kidney from concentrating urine normally. Urine output during this phase may be as high as 1 L/hr and gradually decreases as the BUN and serum creatinine levels return toward normal. Urine output is replaced with fluids milliliter for milliliter hourly for the first 12 to 24 hours.

Central venous pressure readings are essential for monitoring fluid status. Dehydration must be avoided to prevent renal hypoperfusion and renal tubular damage. Electrolyte monitoring to assess for hyponatremia and hypokalemia often associated with rapid diuresis is critical. Treatment with potassium supplements or infusion of 0.9% normal saline may be needed. IV sodium bicarbonate may be given if the patient develops metabolic acidosis from a delay in the return of kidney function.

ATN in the transplanted kidney can occur because of prolonged cold times causing ischemic damage or the use of marginal cadaveric donors (those who are medically suboptimal). While the patient is in ATN, dialysis is needed to maintain fluid and electrolyte balance. Some patients have high-output ATN with the ability to excrete fluid but not metabolic wastes or electrolytes. Other patients have oliguric or anuric ATN. These patients are at risk for fluid overload in the immediate postoperative period and must be assessed closely for the need for dialysis. ATN can last from days to weeks, with gradually improving kidney function. Most patients with ATN are discharged from the hospital on dialysis. This is extremely discouraging for the patient, who needs reassurance that renal function usually improves. Dialysis is discontinued when urine output increases and serum creatinine and BUN begin to normalize.

A sudden decrease in urine output in the early postoperative period is a cause for concern. It may be due to dehydration, rejection, a urine leak, or obstruction. A common cause of early obstruction is a blood clot in the urinary catheter. Catheter patency must be maintained since the catheter stays in the bladder for 3 to 5 days to allow the ureter-bladder anastomosis to heal. If you suspect blood clots, gentle catheter irrigation (if ordered) can reestablish patency.

With a hospital length of stay averaging 4 to 5 days, identify and address discharge planning and teaching needs early. Patient teaching ensures a smooth transition from the hospital to home. Include how to recognize signs of rejection, infection, and any complications of surgery. Frequent blood tests and clinic visits help to detect rejection early.

Immunosuppressive Therapy

The goal of immunosuppression is to adequately suppress the immune response to prevent rejection of the transplanted kidney while maintaining sufficient immunity to prevent overwhelming infection. Immunosuppressive therapy is discussed in Chapter 13.

Complications of Transplantation

Complications of PD, HD, and kidney transplantation are compared in Table 46.14.

Rejection. Rejection is one of the major problems after kidney transplantation. Rejection can be hyperacute, acute, or chronic. The types of rejection are discussed in Chapter 13 on p. 206. Patients with chronic rejection may be placed on the transplant list to be retransplanted before dialysis is required.

Infection. Infection is a significant cause of morbidity and mortality after transplantation.[32] The transplant recipient is at risk for infection because of suppression of the body's normal defense mechanisms by surgery, immunosuppressive drugs, and the effects of ESRD. Underlying systemic illness, such as diabetes or SLE, malnutrition, and older age, can further compound

the negative effects on the immune response. The signs and symptoms of infection can be subtle. You must be astute in your assessment of kidney transplant recipients because prompt diagnosis and treatment of infection improves patient outcomes.

The common infections seen in the first month after transplantation are like those of any postoperative patient. These include pneumonia, wound infections, UTIs, and IV line and drain infections. Fungal and viral infections are common due to the patient's immunosuppressed state. Fungal infections include *Candida, Cryptococcus,* and *Aspergillus* organisms and *Pneumocystis jiroveci.* Fungal infections are hard to treat, require prolonged treatment periods, and often involve the administration of nephrotoxic drugs. Transplant recipients usually receive prophylactic antifungal drugs to prevent these infections, such as clotrimazole, fluconazole (Diflucan), and trimethoprim/sulfamethoxazole (Bactrim).

Viral infections, including CMV, Epstein-Barr virus, herpes simplex virus (HSV), varicella-zoster virus, and polyomavirus (e.g., BK virus), can be primary infections or reactivations of existing disease. Primary infections occur as new infections after transplantation from an exogenous source such as the donated organ or a blood transfusion. Reactivation occurs when a virus exists in a patient and becomes reactivated after transplantation because of immunosuppression.

CMV is one of the most common viral infections. If a recipient has never had CMV and receives an organ from a donor with a history of CMV, antiviral prophylaxis will be needed (e.g., ganciclovir, valganciclovir [Valcyte]). To prevent HSV infections, oral acyclovir (Zovirax) is given for several months after the transplant.

Cardiovascular Disease. CVD is the leading cause of death after renal transplantation.[32] Transplant recipients have an increased incidence of atherosclerotic vascular disease. Hypertension, dyslipidemia, diabetes, smoking, rejection, infections, and increased homocysteine levels (many of which existed prior to the transplant) can all contribute to CVD. Immunosuppressants can worsen hypertension and dyslipidemia.

Teach the patient to control risk factors, such as high cholesterol, triglycerides, and blood glucose and weight gain. Adherence to the prescribed antihypertensive regimen is essential to prevent CV events and damage to the new kidney.

Cancers. The overall incidence of cancer in kidney transplant recipients is greater than in the general population, primarily because of immunosuppressive therapy. Not only do immunosuppressants suppress the immune system to prevent rejection, they also suppress the ability to fight infection and the production of abnormal cells, including cancer cells.

The most common types of cancer after transplant are (1) skin cancers—basal and squamous cell cancers and melanoma—and (2) *posttransplant lymphoproliferative disorder (PTLD).* Most PTLDs are of B-cell origin, associated with Epstein-Barr virus (EBV), and cause aggressive lymphomas (Hodgkin's and non-Hodgkin's lymphoma). Most cases of PTLD occur within the first year of transplant.

Patients are also at risk for cancers of the colorectum, breast, cervix, liver, stomach, oropharynx, anus, vulva, and penis. Regular screening for cancer is an important part of the transplant recipient's preventive care. Teach the patient to avoid sun exposure by using protective clothing and sunscreens to minimize the incidence of skin cancers.

Recurrence of Original Kidney Disease. Recurrence of the original disease that destroyed the native kidneys occurs in

TABLE 46.14 Complications of Dialysis and Transplantation

Peritoneal Dialysis (PD)	Hemodialysis (HD)	Transplantation
• Abdominal pain	• CVD	• Cancers
• Carbohydrate abnormalities	• Disequilibrium syndrome	• Corticosteroid-related complications
• Catheter outflow	• Exsanguination	• CVD
• CVD	• Hepatitis	• Recurrence of kidney disease
• Encapsulating sclerosing peritonitis	• Hypotension	• Susceptibility to infection
• Exit site infection	• Infection, including sepsis	• Transplant rejection
• Hernias	• Muscle cramp	• Hyperacute
• Lipid abnormalities		• Acute
• Lower back pain		• Chronic
• Peritonitis		
• Protein loss		
• Pulmonary problems		
• Atelectasis		
• Pneumonia		
• Bronchitis		

some kidney transplant recipients. It is most common with certain types of glomerulonephritis, immunoglobulin A (IgA) nephropathy, diabetic nephropathy, and focal segmental sclerosis. Disease recurrence can result in the loss of a functioning kidney transplant. Patients must be advised before transplantation if they have a disease known to recur.

Corticosteroid-Related Complications. Aseptic necrosis of the hips, knees, and other joints can result from chronic corticosteroid therapy and renal osteodystrophy. Other significant problems related to corticosteroids include peptic ulcer disease, diabetes, cataracts, dyslipidemia, infections, and cancers. The use of tacrolimus and other immunosuppressants has allowed corticosteroid doses to be much lower than they were in the past.

Many transplant programs have started corticosteroid-free drug regimens because of the problems of long-term corticosteroid use. Other centers withdraw patients from corticosteroids after transplantation. For patients who stay on corticosteroids, vigilant monitoring for side effects and prompt treatment is essential. Corticosteroid therapy as immunosuppression is discussed in Chapter 13 on p. 207.

Gerontologic Considerations: Chronic Kidney Disease

The incidence of CKD in the United States is increasing most rapidly in older adults. The most common diseases leading to renal disease in older adults are hypertension and diabetes.[33]

The care of older patients is particularly challenging, not only because of the normal physiologic changes of aging but also because of the disabilities, chronic diseases, and co-morbid conditions that occur with aging. Physiologic changes include decreased cardiopulmonary function, bone loss, immunodeficiency, altered protein synthesis, impaired cognition, and altered drug metabolism. Malnutrition is common in these patients for a variety of reasons, including lack of mobility, social isolation, physical disability, and impaired cognitive function.

When conservative therapy for CKD is no longer effective, the older patient needs to consider the best treatment modality based on physical and emotional health, personal preferences, and availability of support. Quality-of-life measures show no justification for excluding the older adult from dialysis programs. Rationing dialysis based on age alone is not a reasonable decision for health care professionals to make. Older adults have successfully used dialysis, especially PD. Many choose treatment with in-center HD due to a lack of help in the home and reluctance to manage the technology of home HD or PD. Establishing vascular access for HD may be difficult because of atherosclerotic changes.

Although transplantation is an option, older adults must be carefully screened to ensure that the benefits of transplantation outweigh the risks.[34] Although a living donor is preferable, this may not be an option for many older patients.

The most common cause of death in older ESRD patients is CVD (MI, stroke), followed by withdrawal from dialysis. If a competent patient decides to withdraw from dialysis, it is essential to support the patient and family. Ethical issues (see the Ethical/Legal Dilemmas box) to consider in this situation include patient competency, benefit versus burden of treatment, and futility of treatment. Withdrawal from treatment is not a failure if the patient is well informed and comfortable with the decision.

ETHICAL/LEGAL DILEMMAS
Withdrawing Treatment

Situation

L.R., a 70-yr-old patient with diabetes and ESRD, has been on dialysis for 10 years. He tells you that he wants to stop his dialysis. His quality of life has diminished during the past 2 years since his wife died. He is not a transplant candidate.

Ethical/Legal Points for Consideration

- Informed consent includes the legal right to refuse treatment. However, the right to refuse may be more difficult if (1) it is contrary to the wishes of family and friends, (2) the treatment still appears to have effectiveness, and (3) the treatment has been in place for some time.
- Quality-of-life decisions often outweigh the benefit against the burden of treatment. When a treatment becomes too burdensome, the patient, if competent, may request to withdraw the treatment.
- It must be determined whether some other treatable problem, such as depression, may be clouding the patient's judgment.
- Although there is no ethical or legal difference between withdrawing treatment and withholding treatment, withdrawing treatment feels different because it requires an action.
- Some health care professionals become conflicted when asked to withdraw treatment, since they may think they are contributing to the patient's premature death.
- If a decision is made to withdraw treatment, the interprofessional care team, patient, and family should develop a follow-up plan that includes palliative care and hospice support.

Discussion Questions

1. How should you respond to L.R.'s request?
2. What is the American Nurses Association's position on withdrawing or withholding treatment that no longer benefits the patient or causes suffering?

CASE STUDY
Chronic Kidney Disease

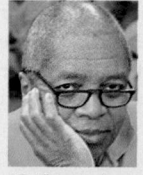
(© iStockphoto/ Thinkstock.)

Patient Profile

M.B. is a 56-yr-old black college professor. He is seen by his primary care provider for a routine physical examination. He has not seen an HCP in a little over a year. He reports generalized malaise, frequent urination, and "increasing thirst." His medical history is significant for borderline hypertension and dyslipidemia. He smokes 1 pack of cigarettes per day. His efforts to quit have been unsuccessful.

Subjective Data

- Family history: father died of an MI at age 62, brother had coronary artery bypass graft (CABG) at age 50, mother died from complications of diabetes
- Becomes "winded" when walking from his car to his office at the university
- Wakes up at night to urinate and has more frequent urination
- Increasing thirst

Continued

Chronic Kidney Disease—cont'd

Objective Data

Laboratory Data

- Calculated creatinine clearance using the MDRD equation: 42 mL/min/1.73 m²
- Serum creatinine 2.5 mg/dL
- BUN 35 mg/dL
- Serum glucose 264 mg/dL
- Hgb 13 g/dL
- Serum cholesterol 236 mg/dL

Physical Examination

- Weight 220 lb, height 5 ft, 11 in
- BP 168/104 mm Hg

Discussion Questions

1. What do you think caused M.B.'s kidney disease?
2. What stage of chronic kidney disease does he have?
3. Identify the abnormal diagnostic study results and why each would occur.
4. *Priority Decision:* Based on the assessment data provided, what are the priority nursing diagnoses? Are there any collaborative problems?
5. What are the most important treatment measures that the interprofessional team can provide for M.B.?
6. *Patient-Centered Care:* What are the nursing interventions that would help promote M.B.'s self-management of his disease process?
7. *Collaboration:* How can the interprofessional team work together with M.B. to decide on the best form of renal replacement therapy?
8. *Evidence-Based Practice:* M.B. tells you that he has not been taking his BP medications regularly. When he asks you how important they are, what will you tell him?

Answers available at *http://evolve.elsevier.com/Lewis/medsurg.*

BRIDGE TO NCLEX EXAMINATION

The number of the question corresponds to the same-numbered outcome at the beginning of the chapter.

1. RIFLE defines the first 3 stages of AKI based on changes in
   a. blood pressure and urine osmolality.
   b. fractional excretion of urinary sodium.
   c. estimation of GFR with the MDRD equation.
   d. serum creatinine or urine output from baseline.

2. During the oliguric phase of AKI, the nurse monitors the patient for *(select all that apply)*
   a. hypotension.
   b. ECG changes.
   c. hypernatremia.
   d. pulmonary edema.
   e. urine with high specific gravity.

3. If a patient is in the diuretic phase of AKI, the nurse must monitor for which serum electrolyte imbalances?
   a. Hyperkalemia and hyponatremia
   b. Hyperkalemia and hypernatremia
   c. Hypokalemia and hyponatremia
   d. Hypokalemia and hypernatremia

4. A patient is admitted to the hospital with chronic kidney disease. The nurse understands that this condition is characterized by
   a. progressive irreversible destruction of the kidneys.
   b. a rapid decrease in urine output with an elevated BUN.
   c. an increasing creatinine clearance with a decrease in urine output.
   d. prostration, somnolence, and confusion with coma and imminent death.

5. Nurses can screen patients at risk for developing chronic kidney disease. Those considered to be at increased risk include *(select all that apply)*
   a. older black patients.
   b. patients more than 60 years old.
   c. those with a history of pancreatitis.
   d. those with a history of hypertension.
   e. those with a history of type 2 diabetes.

6. Patients with chronic kidney disease have an increased incidence of cardiovascular disease related to *(select all that apply)*
   a. hypertension.
   b. vascular calcifications.
   c. a genetic predisposition.
   d. hyperinsulinemia causing dyslipidemia.
   e. increased high-density lipoprotein levels.

7. Nutritional support and management are essential across the entire continuum of chronic kidney disease. Which statements are true related to nutritional therapy? *(select all that apply)*
   a. Sodium and salt may be restricted in someone with advanced CKD.
   b. Fluid is not usually restricted for patients receiving peritoneal dialysis.
   c. Decreased fluid intake and a low-potassium diet are part of the diet for a patient receiving hemodialysis.
   d. Decreased fluid intake and a low-potassium diet are part of the diet for a patient receiving peritoneal dialysis.
   e. Decreased fluid intake and a diet in protein-rich foods are part of a diet for a patient receiving hemodialysis.

8. An ESRD patient receiving hemodialysis is considering asking a relative to donate a kidney for transplantation. In helping the patient decide about treatment, the nurse informs the patient that
   a. successful transplantation usually provides better quality of life than that offered by dialysis.
   b. if rejection of the transplanted kidney occurs, no further treatment for the renal failure is available.
   c. hemodialysis replaces the normal functions of the kidneys, and patients do not have to live with the continual fear of rejection.
   d. the immunosuppressive therapy after transplantation makes the person ineligible to receive other treatments if the kidney fails.

9. To assess the patency of a newly placed arteriovenous graft for dialysis, the nurse should *(select all that apply)*
   a. monitor the BP in the affected arm.
   b. irrigate the graft daily with low-dose heparin.
   c. palpate the area of the graft to feel a normal thrill.
   d. listen with a stethoscope over the graft to detect a bruit.
   e. assess the pulses and neurovascular status distal to the graft.

10. A kidney transplant recipient has had fever, chills, and dysuria over the past 2 days. What is the *first* action that the nurse should take?
    a. Assess temperature and initiate workup to rule out infection.
    b. Reassure the patient that this is common after transplantation.
    c. Provide warm covers to the patient and give 1 gram oral acetaminophen.
    d. Notify the nephrologist that the patient has manifestations of acute rejection.

1. d, 2. b, 3. c, 4. a, 5. a, b, d, 6. a, b, d, e, 7. a, b, d, 8. c, 9. c, d, e, 10. a

For rationales to these answers and even more NCLEX review questions, visit *http://evolve.elsevier.com/Lewis/medsurg*.

ⓔ EVOLVE WEBSITE

http://evolve.elsevier.com/Lewis/medsurg
Review Questions (Online Only)
Key Points
Answer Keys for Questions
- Rationales for Bridge to NCLEX Examination Questions
- Answer Guidelines for Case Study on p. 1085
- Answer Guidelines for Managing Care of Multiple Patients Case Study (Section 10) on p. 1088

Student Case Studies
- Patient With Glomerulonephritis and Acute Kidney Injury
- Patient With Kidney Transplant

Nursing Care Plan
- eNursing Care Plan 46.1: Patient With Chronic Kidney Disease

Conceptual Care Map Creator
Audio Glossary
Content Updates

REFERENCES

*1. Moriama N, Saito S, Ishihara S, et al: Early development of acute kidney injury is an independent predictor of in-hospital mortality in patients with acute myocardial infarction, *J Cardiol* 69:1, 2017.

2. Thornburg B: Acute kidney injury, *Nursing* 46:24, 2016.

3. Bevc S, Ekart R, Hois R: The assessment of acute kidney injury in critically ill patients, *Eur J Int Med* 45:54, 2017.

*4. Omotoso BA, Abdel-Rahman EM, Xin W, et al: Dialysis requirement, long-term major adverse cardiovascular events (MACE) and all-cause mortality in hospital acquired acute kidney injury (AKI): A propensity-matched cohort study, *J Nephrol* 29:847, 2016.

*5. Nash DM, Przech S, Wald R, et al: Systematic review and meta-analysis of renal replacement therapy modalities for acute kidney injury in the intensive care unit, *J Crit Care* 41:138, 2017.

*6. Abdel-Basset E, Walid A, Maha A, et al: Early versus delayed initiation of continuous renal replacement therapy in critically ill patients with acute kidney injury, *Egy J Hosp Med* 69:2219, 2017.

*7. Perez-Fernandez X, Sabater-Riera J, Sileanu F, et al: Renal: Clinical variables associated with poor outcome from sepsis-associated acute kidney injury and the relationship with timing of initiation of renal replacement therapy, *J Crit Care* 40:154, 2017.

*8. Greer R, Yang L, Crews D, et al: Hospital discharge communications during care transitions for patients with acute kidney injury: A cross-sectional study, *BMC Health Serv Res* 16:449, 2016.

*9. Zarbock A, Gerb J, Van Aken H, et al: Early versus late initiation of renal replacement therapy in critically ill patients with acute kidney injury, *JAMA* 148:558, 2016.

*10. Izawa J, Uchino S, Takinami M: A detailed evaluation of the new acute kidney injury criteria by KDIGO in critically ill patients, *J Anesthesiol* 30:215, 2016.

11. Loiselle M: Decisional needs assessment to help patients with advanced chronic kidney disease make better dialysis choices, *Nephrol Nurs J* 43:463, 2016.

*12. Alseiari M, Meyer KB, Wong JB: Evidence underlying KDIGO guideline recommendations: A systematic review, *Am J Kidney Dis*, 67:417, 2016.

*13. Flack JM, Calhoun D, Schifrin EL: The new ACC/AHA hypertension guidelines for the prevention, detection, evaluation, and management of high blood pressure in adults, *Am J Hypertension* 31:133, 2018.

*14. Galbraith L, Jacobs C, Hemmelgarn B, et al: Chronic disease management interventions for people with chronic kidney disease in primary care: a systematic review and meta-analysis, *Neph Dialysis Transpl* 33:112, 2017.

15. National Institute of Diabetes and Digestive and Kidney Diseases: US Renal Data System: 2017 annual data report: Epidemiology of kidney disease in the US. Retrieved from *www.usrds.org/adr.aspx*.

16. US Department of Health and Human Services: ESRD: General information. Retrieved from *www.cms.gov/Medicare/End-Stage-Renal-Disease/ESRDGeneralInformation/index.html*.

*17. Ettehad D, Emdin CA, Kiran A, et al: Blood pressure lowering for prevention of cardiovascular disease and death: A systematic review and meta-analysis, *Lancet* 387:10022, 2016.

18. Coyne D, Goldsmith D, Macdougall L: New options for the anemia of chronic kidney disease, *Kidney Int* 7:157, 2017.

*19. Ketteler M, Block GA, Evenepoel P: Executive summary of the 2017 KDIGO CKD-MBD guideline update: What's changed and why it matters, *Kidney Int* 92:26, 2017.

*20. Malhotra R, Nguyen H, Benevente, et al: Association between more intensive versus less intensive blood pressure lowering and risk of mortality in chronic kidney disease stages 3-5: A systematic review and meta-analysis, *JAMA Int Med* 177:1498, 2017.

*21. Natale P, Ruospo M, Saglimbene VM, et al: Interventions for improving sleep quality with chronic kidney disease. *Cochrane Database Syst Rev*, CD012625, 2017.

22. Saran R, Robinson B, Abbott KC, et al: US Renal Data System 2016 annual data report: Epidemiology of kidney disease in the United States, *Am J Kidney Dis* 69:S688, 2017.

23. National Kidney Foundation: NKF Kidney Disease Outcomes Quality Initiative. Retrieved from *www.kidney.org/professionals/guidelines/guidelines_commentaries*.

*24. Perez-Torres A, Garcia EG, Garcia-Llana H, et al: Improvement in nutritional status in patients with chronic kidney disease by a nutritional program with no impact on renal function and determined by male sex. *J Renal Nutrition* 27:303, 2017.

25. National Kidney and Urologic Diseases Information Clearinghouse: Treatment methods for kidney disease: Peritoneal dialysis. Retrieved from *http://kidney.niddk.nih.gov/health-information/kidney-failure/peritoneal-dialysis*.

26. Debus ES, Grundmann RT: *Evidence-based therapy in vascular surgery*, New York, 2017, Springer.

27. National Kidney and Urologic Diseases Information Clearinghouse: Treatment methods for kidney disease: hemodialysis. Retrieved from *http://kidney.niddk.nih.gov/health-information/kidney-disease/kidney-failure/hemodialysis*.

28. Lee CJ, Rossi PJ: Portable and wearable dialysis devices for the treatment of patients with ESRD. In: Shalhub S, Dua A, Shin S, eds: *Hemodialysis access: Fundamentals and advanced management*, Basel, Switzerland, 2017, Springer.

29. Hart A, Smith JM, Skeans MA, et al: OPTN/SRTR 2016 annual data report: Kidney, *Amer J Transplant* 18:18, 2018.

*30. Neuberger JM, Bechstein WO, Kuypers DR, et al: Practical recommendations for long term management of modifiable risk factors in kidney and liver transplant recipients: A guidance report and clinical checklist on managing modifiable risk in transplantation, *Transplantation* 101:S1, 2017.

*31. Mathur AK, Chang YH, Steidley DE, et al: Patterns of care and outcomes in cardiovascular disease after kidney transplantation in the United States, *Transplant Direct* 3:e26, 2017.

32. Organ procurement and transplant network kidney allocation system. Retrieved from *https://optn.transplant.hrsa.gov/learn/professional-education/kidney-allocation-system/*.

*33. Wongrakpanich S, Susantitaphong P, Isaranuwatchai S, et al: Dialysis therapy and conservative management of advanced chronic kidney disease in the elderly: A systematic review, *Nephron* 137:178, 2017.

34. O'Hare AM, Song MK, Moss AH: Research priorities for palliative care for older adults with advanced kidney disease, *J Palliative Med* 20:453, 2017.

*Evidence-based information for clinical practice.

CASE STUDY

Managing Care of Multiple Patients

You are working on the medical-surgical unit and have been assigned to care for the following 4 patients. You are also assigned to receive the next new admission to the clinical unit. You have 1 UAP on your team to help you.

Patients

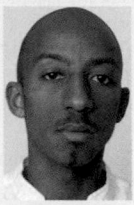

A.K., a 28-yr-old black man, was admitted for observation after a renal ultrasound found several stones in the left ureter. A.K. came to the ED with sharp, colicky left flank pain for which the HCP prescribed IV opioids. His last pain medication was given 2 hours ago. His current pain level is 4 on a scale of 1 to 10. He is voiding dark, smoky-colored urine. His vital signs are within normal limits. He has positive costovertebral tenderness.

(© iStockphoto/Thinkstock.)

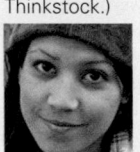

S.U., a 29-yr-old Hispanic woman with type 1 diabetes, was admitted with acute pyelonephritis following a recent UTI. She has bilateral flank pain and has abdominal tenderness to palpation. Her temperature is 101.5°F (38.6°C). Her urinalysis shows pyuria and hematuria. The WBC is high at 14,800/μL. Blood culture results are pending. IV antibiotics have been started. Most recent blood glucose is 215 mg/dL.

(© iStockphoto/Thinkstock.)

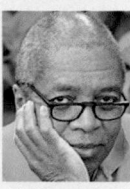

M.B., a 56-yr-old black college professor, was admitted with uncontrolled hypertension. He was recently diagnosed with CKD. He smokes at least 1 pack of cigarettes per day and is having some nicotine withdrawal symptoms. His BP on admission was 224/102 mm Hg. He is receiving IV metoprolol (Lopressor) 5 mg q4hr prn for SBP >180 mm Hg. His most recent BP 3 hr ago was 174/86 mm Hg. Laboratory results show a BUN of 66 mg/dL and serum creatinine of 3.2 mg/dL.

(© iStockphoto/Thinkstock.)

D.M., an 82-yr-old woman, was admitted to the ED with severe dehydration, heart failure, and acute kidney injury. Her daughter found her unconscious and lying on the floor. She is confused. Her serum potassium is 6.3 mEq/L. Her urine output for the past 8 hours was 90 mL.

(© iStockphoto/Thinkstock.)

Discussion Questions

1. **Priority Decision:** After receiving report, which patient should you see first? Second? Provide a rationale for your decision.
2. **Collaboration:** Which tasks could you delegate to the UAP (select all that apply)?
   a. Obtain vital signs on M.B.
   b. Strain A.K.'s voided urine.
   c. Report D.M.'s potassium level to the HCP.
   d. Measure D.M.'s urine output and report the results to the RN.
   e. Assess S.U. for manifestations of sepsis and diabetic ketoacidosis.

3. **Priority Decision:** As you are assessing D.M., the UAP tells you that M.B.'s BP is 190/96. He is asymptomatic. Additionally, the charge nurse tells you that you will be receiving a patient with heart failure from the ED within the next 20 minutes. Which action would be *most* appropriate?
   a. Ask the charge nurse to assign the new admission to someone else.
   b. Have the UAP admit the new patient while you administer M.B.'s IV metoprolol.
   c. Call the ED and have them hold the new admission until after you have assessed all your patients.
   d. Ask the charge nurse to give M.B.'s IV metoprolol while you complete your assessment of D.M. and S.U.

Case Study Progression

As you complete your assessment of D.M., you note her apical pulse is irregular. She has 1+ pitting edema in her lower extremities. Her BP is 160/90 mm Hg, heart rate 108 beats/min, and respiratory rate 28/min. Auscultation of her lungs reveals crackles in the bases and O₂ saturation is 92% on room air. You notify her HCP.

4. Which interventions would you expect the HCP to order for D.M.? *(select all that apply)*
   a. Administer IV Kayexalate.
   b. Obtain arterial blood gas levels.
   c. Administer 40 mg of furosemide IV push.
   d. Prepare her for hemodialysis and notify her family.
   e. Obtain a 12-lead ECG and start continuous ECG monitoring.
5. **Priority Decision:** Which concern has the *highest* priority when planning care for A.K.?
   a. Acute pain
   b. Infection risk
   c. Risk for injury
   d. Difficulty coping
6. **Priority Decision:** You begin S.U.'s scheduled infusion of IV ceftriaxone. Which parameters are the *most* important to monitor while she is receiving this drug?
   a. PT and INR
   b. BUN and creatinine
   c. CBC with differential
   d. Liver function studies
7. Which statement would be *most* appropriate when teaching S.U. about her kidney infection?
   a. "The damage to your kidneys will likely require dialysis."
   b. "You will need to be in the hospital for a 2-week course of IV antibiotics."
   c. "It is very important that you maintain adequate hydration to flush your kidneys."
   d. "You will not need further antibiotics once you are discharged from the hospital."
8. **Collaboration:** As the UAP prepares the room for the patient being admitted from the ED, you overhear her telling a co-worker that she does all your work for you. What is your *best* initial action?
   a. Report the incident to the charge nurse for follow-up.
   b. Ask the UAP to discuss her concerns with you in private.
   c. Tell the UAP how much you appreciate and value her input on your team.
   d. Immediately clarify the situation by telling the UAP all the tasks you are completing.

Answers available at *http://evolve.elsevier.com/Lewis/medsurg.*

Assessment: Endocrine System

Julia A. Hitch

> *Our compassion and acts of selflessness take us to the deeper truths.*
>
> ***Amma***

http://evolve.elsevier.com/Lewis/medsurg

CONCEPTUAL FOCUS

Homeostasis
Hormonal Regulation

Reproduction
Stress

LEARNING OUTCOMES

1. Describe the common characteristics and functions of hormones.
2. Identify the locations of the endocrine glands.
3. Describe the functions of hormones secreted by the pituitary, thyroid, parathyroid, and adrenal glands and the pancreas.
4. Describe the locations and roles of hormone receptors.
5. Obtain significant subjective and objective assessment data related to the endocrine system from a patient.
6. Perform a physical assessment of the endocrine system using the appropriate techniques.
7. Link age-related changes in the endocrine system to differences in assessment findings.
8. Distinguish normal from common abnormal findings of a physical assessment of the endocrine system.
9. Describe the purpose, significance of results, and nursing responsibilities related to diagnostic studies of the endocrine system.

KEY TERMS

aldosterone, p. 1095
antidiuretic hormone (ADH), p. 1093
catecholamines, p. 1094
circadian rhythm, p. 1090
corticosteroid, p. 1095

cortisol, p. 1095
hormones, p. 1089
insulin, p. 1095
negative feedback, p. 1090
positive feedback, p. 1090

thyroxine (T_4), p. 1094
triiodothyronine (T_3), p. 1094
tropic hormones, p. 1093

STRUCTURES AND FUNCTIONS OF ENDOCRINE SYSTEM

Glands

Endocrine glands include the hypothalamus, pituitary, thyroid, parathyroids, adrenals, pancreas, ovaries, testes, and pineal gland (Fig. 47.1). These glands make and release special chemical messengers called *hormones*. The endocrine system has 5 general functions: (1) a role in reproductive and central nervous system (CNS) development in the fetus, (2) stimulating growth and development during childhood and adolescence, (3) sexual reproduction, (4) maintaining homeostasis, and (5) responding to emergency demands.[1]

Hormones

Hormones are chemical substances made by endocrine glands that control and regulate the activity of certain target cells or organs. Many are made in one part of the body and control and regulate the activity of certain cells or organs in another part of the body. The thyroid gland makes the hormone thyroxine, which affects many body tissues when released directly into the circulation. Other hormones act locally on cells where they are released and never enter the bloodstream. We call this local effect *paracrine action*. The action of sex steroids on the ovary is an example of paracrine action.

Most hormones have common characteristics, including (1) secretion in small amounts at variable but predictable rates,

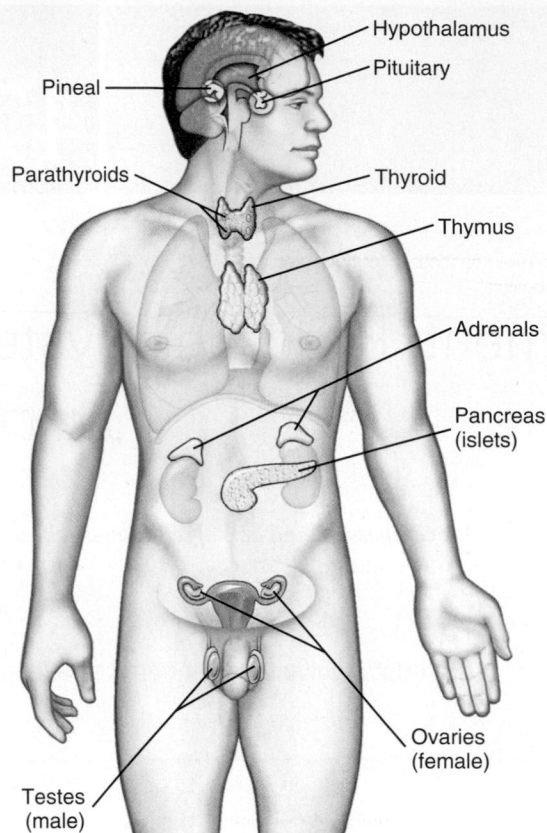

FIG. 47.1 Location of the major endocrine glands. The parathyroid glands lie on the posterior surface of the thyroid gland. (Modified from Patton KT, Thibodeau GA: *Anatomy and physiology*, ed 8, St Louis, 2013, Mosby.)

(2) regulation by feedback systems, and (3) ability to bind to specific target cell receptors. Table 47.1 reviews the major hormones, the glands or tissues that make the hormones, their target organs or tissues, and their functions.

There is a strong connection between the endocrine system and nervous system. *Catecholamines* (e.g., epinephrine), secreted by the adrenal gland, travel through the bloodstream and affect multiple organ systems. These same substances, when secreted by nerve cells in the brain and peripheral nervous system, act as neurotransmitters, sending important impulses across nerve synapses.[1]

Organs can act as endocrine glands by secreting hormones. For example, the kidneys secrete erythropoietin, a substance that stimulates red blood cell production. The heart secretes atrial natriuretic peptide (ANP). The gastrointestinal (GI) tract secretes many peptide hormones (e.g., gastrin), that aid in digestion. These hormones are discussed in their respective assessment chapters.

Hormone Receptors. Hormones exert their effects by recognizing their target tissues and attaching to receptor sites in a "lock-and-key" type of mechanism. This means a hormone will act only on cells that have a receptor specific for that hormone (Fig. 47.2).

Lipid-Soluble and Water-Soluble Hormones. We classify hormones by their chemical structure as either lipid soluble or water soluble. The differences in solubility become important in understanding how the hormone interacts with the target cell (Fig. 47.3). Lipid-soluble hormones (steroids, thyroid) are bound to plasma proteins as they travel to target cells. They

cross the cell membrane by simple diffusion. Water-soluble hormones (insulin, growth hormone, prolactin) circulate freely in the blood and act directly on target tissues.

Regulation of Hormonal Secretion. Specific mechanisms control endocrine activity by either stimulating or inhibiting hormone synthesis and secretion. These include positive and negative feedback, nervous system control, and physiologic rhythms.

Simple Feedback. Negative feedback relies on the blood level of a hormone or other chemical compound regulated by the hormone (e.g., glucose). It is the most common type of endocrine feedback system. It results in the gland increasing or decreasing the release of a hormone. Negative feedback functions like a thermostat. Cold air in a room activates the thermostat to release heat. Warm air signals the thermostat to turn off the heater. An example of negative feedback is calcium and parathyroid hormone (PTH) regulation. Low blood levels of calcium stimulate the parathyroid gland to release PTH. PTH acts on the bone, intestine, and kidneys to increase blood calcium levels. The increased blood calcium level then inhibits further PTH release (Fig. 47.4).

With positive feedback, increasing hormone levels cause another gland to release a hormone that then stimulates further release of the first hormone. Something must stop the release of the first hormone (e.g., follicle death) or its release will continue. The ovarian hormone estradiol works by this type of feedback. Increased levels of estradiol made by the follicle during the menstrual cycle result in the production and release of follicle-stimulating hormone (FSH) by the anterior pituitary. FSH causes further increases in estradiol until the death of the follicle. This results in a drop of FSH serum levels.

Nervous System Control. Nervous system activity directly affects some endocrine glands. Pain, fear, sexual excitement, and other stressors can stimulate the nervous system to control hormone secretion. For example, when the CNS senses or perceives stress, the sympathetic nervous system (SNS) secretes catecholamines (e.g., epinephrine), which maximize heart and lung function and vision to deal with the stress more effectively. Chronic exposure to some stressors can cause persistent increases in heart rate and BP and changes in the endocrine system. This puts patients at risk for chronic disease, such as hypertension and heart disease. Stress-related effects are discussed in Chapter 6.

Rhythms. A common physiologic rhythm is the circadian rhythm. It is a 24-hour rhythm that is driven by sleep-wake or dark-light 24-hour (diurnal) cycles. Hormone levels and the responsiveness of target tissues fluctuate predictably during these cycles. Cortisol, made by the adrenal cortex, rises early in the day, declines toward evening, and rises again toward the end of sleep to peak by morning (Fig. 47.5). Growth hormone, thyroid-stimulating hormone, and prolactin levels peak during sleep. Reproductive cycles are often longer than 24 hours *(ultradian)*. An example is the menstrual cycle. These rhythms are important to consider when interpreting laboratory results for hormone levels.

Hypothalamus

Although many refer to the pituitary gland as the "master gland" of the endocrine system, most of its functions rely on its interrelationship with the hypothalamus, which lies next to the pituitary gland. The hypothalamus releases substances that either stimulate or inhibit the production and release of

TABLE 47.1 Endocrine Glands and Hormones

Hormones	Target Tissue	Functions
Anterior Pituitary (Adenohypophysis)		
Adrenocorticotropic hormone (ACTH)	Adrenal cortex	Fosters growth of adrenal cortex Stimulates corticosteroid secretion
Gonadotropic hormones • Follicle-stimulating hormone (FSH) • Luteinizing hormone (LH)	Reproductive organs	Stimulate sex hormone secretion, reproductive organ growth, reproductive processes
Growth hormone (GH), or somatotropin	All body cells	Promotes protein anabolism (growth, tissue repair) and lipid mobilization and catabolism
Melanocyte-stimulating hormone (MSH)	Melanocytes in skin	↑ Melanin production in melanocytes to make skin darker
Prolactin	Ovary and mammary glands in women	Stimulates milk production in lactating women. ↑ Response of follicles to LH and FSH
	Testes in men	Stimulates testicular function in men
Thyroid-stimulating hormone (TSH), or thyrotropin	Thyroid gland	Stimulates synthesis and release of thyroid hormones, growth and function of thyroid gland
Posterior Pituitary (Neurohypophysis)		
Antidiuretic hormone (ADH)	Renal tubules, vascular smooth muscle	Promotes reabsorption of water from the renal tubules, vasoconstriction
Oxytocin	Uterus, mammary glands	Stimulates milk secretion, uterine contractility
Thyroid		
Calcitonin	Bone tissue	Regulates calcium and phosphorus serum levels. ↓ Serum Ca^{2+} levels
Thyroxine (T_4)	All body tissues	Precursor to T_3
Triiodothyronine (T_3)	All body tissues	Regulates metabolic rate of all cells and processes of cell growth and tissue differentiation
Parathyroids		
Parathyroid hormone (PTH) or parathormone	Bone, intestine, kidneys	Regulates calcium and phosphorus serum levels. Promotes bone demineralization and ↑ intestinal absorption of Ca^{2+}. ↑ Serum Ca^{2+} levels
Adrenal Medulla		
Epinephrine (adrenaline)	Catecholamine	↑ In response to stress. Enhances and prolongs effects of sympathetic nervous system
Norepinephrine (noradrenaline)	Catecholamine	↑ In response to stress. Enhances and prolongs effects of sympathetic nervous system
Adrenal Cortex		
Androgens (e.g., dehydroepiandrosterone [DHEA], androsterone) and estradiol	Reproductive organs	Promote growth spurt in adolescence, secondary sex characteristics, and libido in both sexes
Corticosteroids (e.g., cortisol, hydrocortisone)	All body tissues	Promote metabolism. ↑ In response to stress. Antiinflammatory
Mineralocorticoids (e.g., aldosterone)	Kidney	Regulate sodium and potassium balance and thus water balance
Pancreas (Islets of Langerhans)		
Amylin (from β cells)	Liver, stomach	↓ Gastric motility, glucagon secretion, and endogenous glucose release from liver. ↑ Satiety
Glucagon (from α cells)	General	Stimulates glycogenolysis and gluconeogenesis
Insulin (from β cells)	General	Promotes glucose transport from the blood into the cell
Pancreatic polypeptide	General	Influences regulation of pancreatic exocrine function and metabolism of absorbed nutrients
Somatostatin	Pancreas	Inhibits insulin and glucagon secretion
Gonads		
Women: Ovaries		
Estrogen	Reproductive system, breasts	Stimulates development of secondary sex characteristics, preparation of uterus for fertilization and fetal development. Stimulates bone growth
Progesterone	Reproductive system	Maintains lining of uterus needed for successful pregnancy
Men: Testes		
Testosterone	Reproductive system	Stimulates development of secondary sex characteristics, spermatogenesis

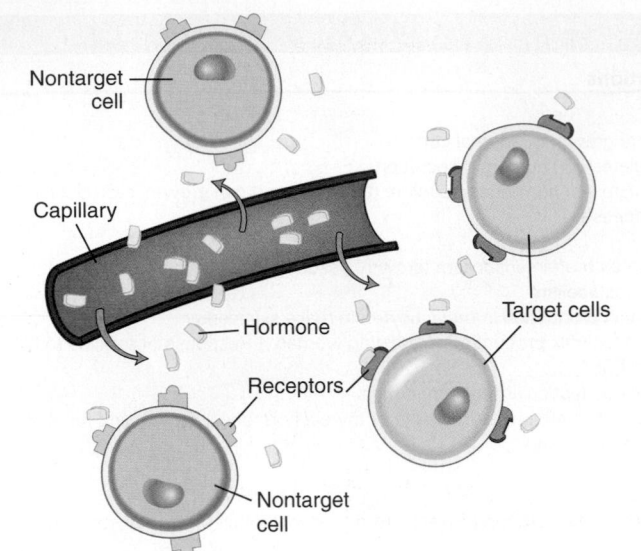

FIG. 47.2 The target cell concept. Hormones act only on cells that have receptors specific to that hormone, since the shape of the receptor determines which hormone can react with it. This is an example of the lock-and-key model of biochemical reactions.

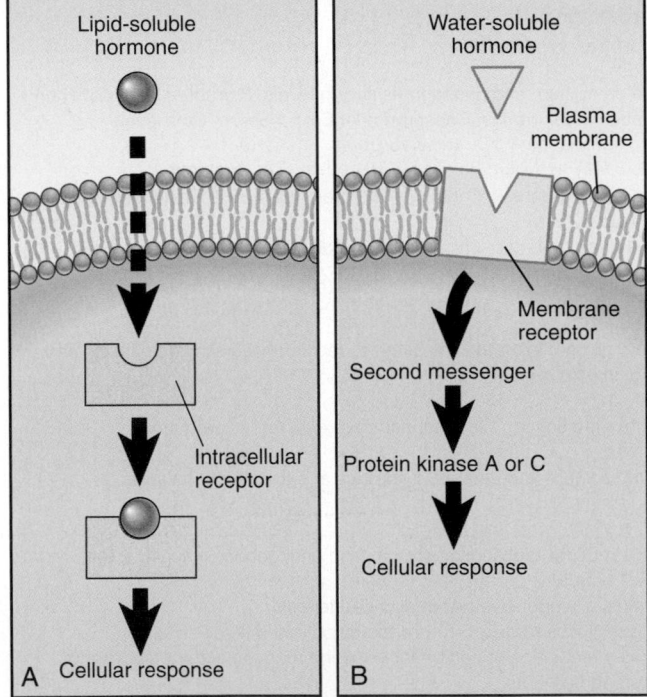

FIG. 47.3 A, Lipid-soluble hormones (e.g., steroid hormones) penetrate the cell membrane and interact with intracellular receptors. B, Water-soluble hormones (e.g., protein hormones) bind to receptors in the cell membrane. The hormone-receptor interaction stimulates various cell responses. (Modified from McCance KL, Huether SE: *Pathophysiology: The biologic basis for disease in adults and children*, ed 6, St Louis, 2010, Mosby.)

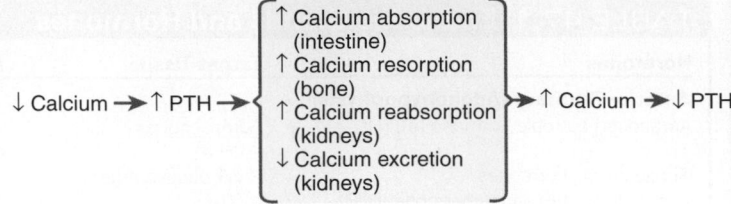

FIG. 47.4 Feedback mechanism between PTH and calcium.

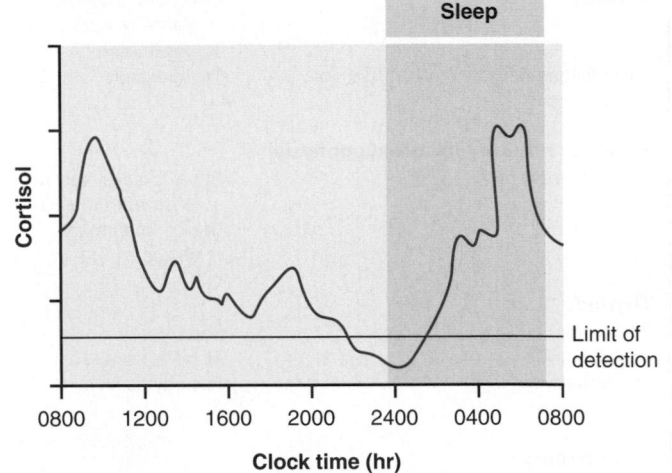

FIG. 47.5 Circadian rhythm of cortisol secretion.

TABLE 47.2 **Hormones of the Hypothalamus**

The following hormones from the hypothalamus target the anterior pituitary:

Releasing Hormones
- Corticotropin-releasing hormone (CRH)
- Thyrotropin-releasing hormone (TRH)
- Growth hormone–releasing hormone (GHRH)
- Gonadotropin-releasing hormone (GnRH)
- Prolactin-releasing factor (PRF)

Inhibiting Hormones
- Somatostatin (inhibits growth hormone release)
- Prolactin-inhibiting factor (PIF)

hormones from the pituitary gland (Table 47.2). Examples of these hormones include corticotropin-releasing hormone and thyrotropin-releasing hormone. Somatostatin inhibits growth hormone release.

Neurons in the hypothalamus receive input from the CNS, including the brainstem, limbic system, and cerebral cortex. These neurons create a circuit that helps coordinate the endocrine system and autonomic nervous system (ANS). The hypothalamus also coordinates the expression of complex behavioral responses, such as anger, fear, and pleasure.

Pituitary

The pituitary gland *(hypophysis)* is in the sella turcica under the hypothalamus at the base of the brain above the sphenoid bone (Fig. 47.1). The infundibular *(hypophyseal)* stalk connects the pituitary and hypothalamus. This stalk relays information between the hypothalamus and pituitary, creating a strong neuroendocrine connection. The pituitary consists of 2 major parts, the anterior lobe *(adenohypophysis)* and posterior lobe *(neurohypophysis)*. A smaller intermediate lobe makes melanocyte-stimulating hormone (MSH).

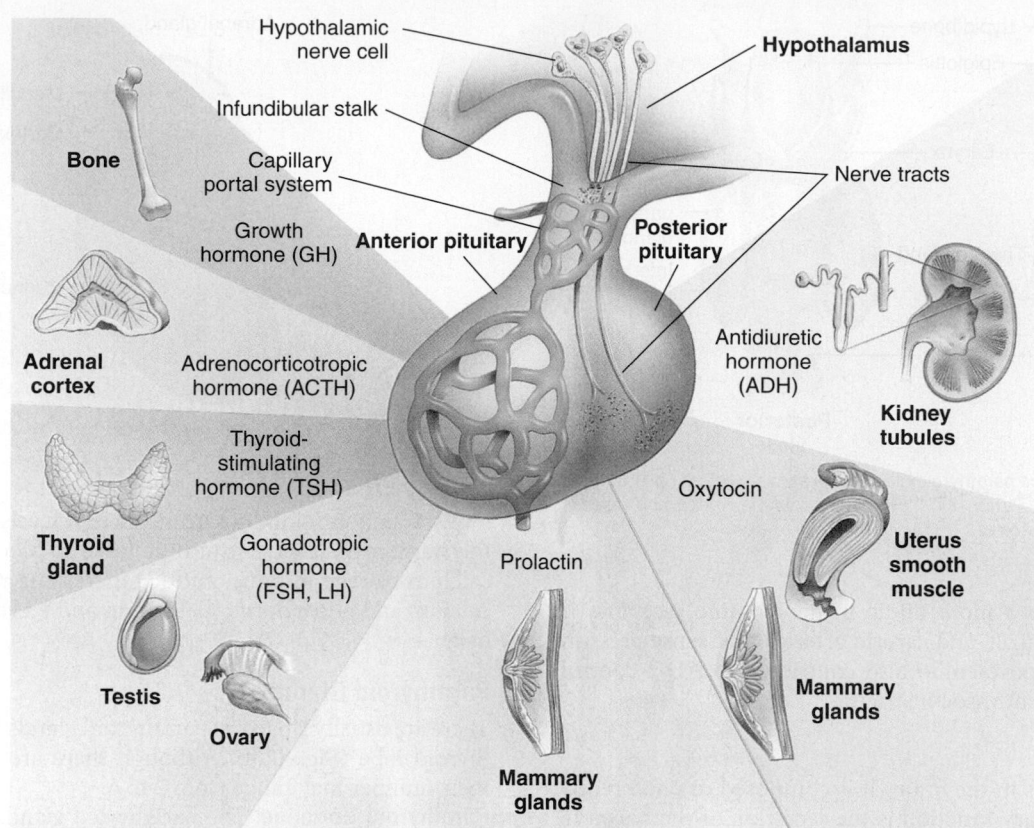

FIG. 47.6 Relationship between the hypothalamus, pituitary, and target organs. The hypothalamus communicates with the anterior pituitary via a capillary system and with the posterior pituitary via nerve tracts. The anterior and posterior pituitary hormones are shown with their target tissues. (Modified from Patton KT, Thibodeau GA: *Anatomy and physiology,* ed 8, St Louis, 2013, Mosby.)

Anterior Pituitary. The anterior lobe of the pituitary accounts for 80% of the gland by weight. The hypothalamus regulates the anterior lobe through releasing and inhibiting hormones. These hypothalamic hormones reach the anterior pituitary through a network of capillaries known as the *hypothalamus-hypophyseal portal system.* These releasing and inhibiting hormones in turn affect the secretion of 6 hormones from the anterior pituitary (Fig. 47.6).

We refer to several hormones secreted by the anterior pituitary as tropic hormones. Tropic hormones control the secretion of hormones by other glands. Thyroid-stimulating hormone (TSH) stimulates the thyroid gland to secrete thyroid hormones. Adrenocorticotropic hormone (ACTH) stimulates the adrenal cortex to secrete corticosteroids. FSH stimulates secretion of estrogen and the development of ova in women and sperm in men. Luteinizing hormone (LH) stimulates ovulation in women and secretion of sex hormones in both men and women.

Growth hormone (GH) affects the growth and development of all body tissues. It has many biologic actions, including a role in protein, fat, and carbohydrate metabolism. *Prolactin,* or lactogenic hormone, stimulates the breast development needed for lactation after childbirth.

Posterior Pituitary. The posterior pituitary is composed of nerve tissue and is essentially an extension of the hypothalamus. Communication between the hypothalamus and posterior pituitary occurs through nerve tracts. The hormones secreted by the posterior pituitary, antidiuretic hormone (ADH) and oxytocin, are made in the hypothalamus. These hormones travel down the

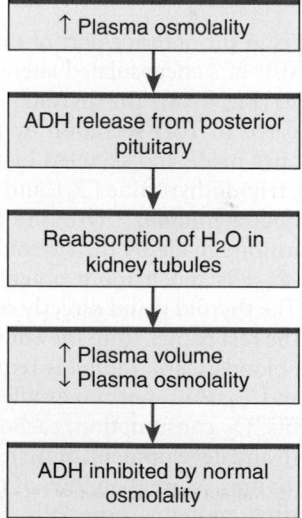

FIG. 47.7 Relationship of plasma osmolality to ADH release and action.

nerve tracts from the hypothalamus to the posterior pituitary and are stored there until stimuli trigger their release (Fig. 47.6).

The major physiologic role of ADH (also called *arginine vasopressin*) is to regulate fluid volume. It causes the renal tubules to reabsorb water, making the urine more concentrated. A rise in plasma osmolality or hypovolemia causes specialized neurons in the hypothalamus, known as *osmoreceptors,* to stimulate ADH release from the posterior pituitary (Fig. 47.7). When ADH release is inhibited, renal tubules do not reabsorb

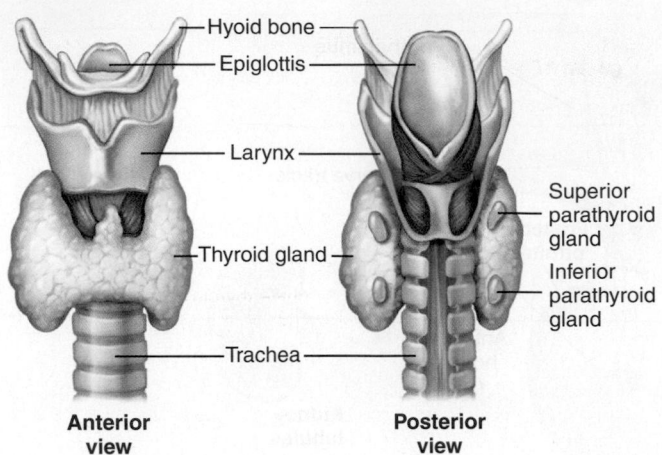

FIG. 47.8 Thyroid and parathyroid glands. Note the surrounding structures. (From Thibodeau GA, Patton KT: *The human body in health and disease,* ed 4, St Louis, 2005, Mosby.)

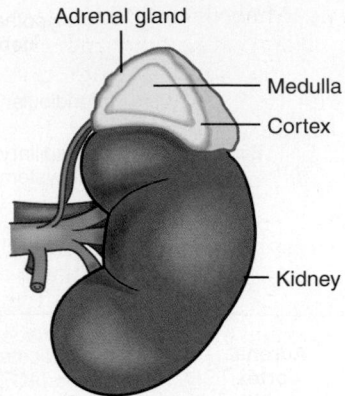

FIG. 47.9 The adrenal gland is composed of the adrenal cortex and the adrenal medulla.

water, resulting in a more dilute urine. Volume receptors in large veins, heart atria, and carotid arteries that sense pressure changes (from hypovolemia) also contribute to ADH control. ADH is also a potent vasoconstrictor.

Pineal Gland

The pineal gland is in the brain. It is composed of photoreceptive cells. Its primary function is the secretion of the hormone *melatonin.* Melatonin secretion increases in response to exposure to the dark and decreases in response to light exposure. The gland helps to regulate circadian rhythms and the reproductive system at the onset of puberty.

Thyroid Gland

The thyroid gland is in the anterior part of the neck in front of the trachea. It consists of 2 encapsulated lateral lobes connected by a narrow isthmus (Fig. 47.8). The thyroid gland is highly vascular. Its size is related to TSH secretion by the anterior pituitary. The 3 hormones made and secreted by the thyroid gland are thyroxine (T_4), triiodothyronine (T_3), and calcitonin.

Thyroxine and Triiodothyronine. Thyroxine (T_4) accounts for 90% of thyroid hormone made by the thyroid gland. However, triiodothyronine (T_3) is much more potent and has greater metabolic effects. The thyroid gland directly secretes about 20% of circulating T_3. The rest comes from the conversion of T_4 after its release into the bloodstream. Iodine is required for the synthesis of both T_3 and T_4. Both hormones affect metabolic rate, caloric requirements, O_2 consumption, carbohydrate and lipid metabolism, growth and development, brain function, and other nervous system activities. More than 99% of thyroid hormones are bound to plasma proteins, especially thyroxine-binding globulin made by the liver. Only the unbound "free" hormones are biologically active.

TSH from the anterior pituitary gland stimulates thyroid hormone production and release. When circulating levels of thyroid hormone are low, the hypothalamus releases thyrotropin-releasing hormone (TRH). TRH causes the anterior pituitary to release TSH. High circulating thyroid hormone levels inhibit the secretion of both TRH from the hypothalamus and TSH from the anterior pituitary gland.

Calcitonin. *Calcitonin* is made by C cells (parafollicular cells) of the thyroid gland in response to high circulating calcium

levels. Calcitonin lowers serum calcium levels by (1) inhibiting the transfer of calcium from the bone to blood, (2) increasing calcium storage in bone, and (3) increasing renal excretion of calcium and phosphorus. Calcitonin and PTH regulate calcium balance.

Parathyroid Glands

There are usually 2 pairs of parathyroid glands lying behind each thyroid lobe (Fig. 47.8). Although there are usually 4 glands, their number may range from 2 to 6.

Parathyroid Hormone. The parathyroid glands secrete parathyroid hormone (PTH), also called *parathormone.* Its major role is to regulate serum calcium levels. PTH increases serum calcium levels by acting on bone, the kidneys, and indirectly on the GI tract. PTH stimulates the transfer of calcium from the bone into the blood. In the kidney, PTH promotes calcium reabsorption (moving calcium from the renal tubules back into the bloodstream) and phosphate excretion. PTH stimulates the renal conversion of vitamin D to its most active form (1,25-dihydroxyvitamin D_3). This form of vitamin D promotes calcium and phosphorus absorption in the GI tract. PTH secretion is regulated by a negative feedback system. When serum calcium or magnesium levels are low, PTH secretion increases. When serum calcium or active vitamin D levels are high, PTH secretion falls.

Adrenal Glands

The adrenal glands are small, paired, highly vascular glands located on the upper part of each kidney. Each gland consists of 2 parts: medulla and cortex (Fig. 47.9). Each part has distinct functions and act independently from the other.

Adrenal Medulla. The adrenal medulla is the inner part of the adrenal gland. It consists of sympathetic postganglionic neurons. The medulla secretes the catecholamines *epinephrine* (adrenaline), *norepinephrine* (noradrenaline), and *dopamine.* We consider catecholamines neurotransmitters when they are secreted by neurons and hormones when they are secreted by the adrenal medulla. They are an essential part of the SNS's "fight or flight" response.

Adrenal Cortex. The adrenal cortex is the outer part of the adrenal gland. It secretes several steroid hormones, including *glucocorticoids, mineralocorticoids,* and *androgens.* Cholesterol is the precursor for steroid hormone synthesis. Glucocorticoids (e.g., cortisol) are named for their effects on glucose metabolism. They inhibit the inflammatory response and are considered antiinflammatory. Mineralocorticoids (e.g., aldosterone) are essential for maintaining fluid and electrolyte balance. The term **corticosteroid** refers to both glucocorticoids and mineralocorticoids.

Cortisol. Cortisol, the most abundant and potent glucocorticoid, is necessary to maintain life and protect the body from stress. It is secreted in a diurnal pattern (Fig. 47.5). A negative feedback mechanism controls cortisol secretion. The release of corticotropin-releasing hormone (CRH) from the hypothalamus stimulates the secretion of ACTH by the anterior pituitary.

A major function of cortisol is regulating blood glucose concentration by stimulating hepatic glucose formation (*gluconeogenesis*). Cortisol inhibits peripheral glucose use in the fasting state, inhibits protein synthesis, and stimulates the mobilization of glycerol and free fatty acids. It helps maintain vascular integrity and fluid volume through its action on mineralocorticoid receptors. Cortisol decreases the inflammatory response by stabilizing the membranes of cellular lysosomes and preventing increased capillary permeability. Stress, burns, infection, fever, acute anxiety, and hypoglycemia increase cortisol levels.

Aldosterone. Aldosterone is a potent mineralocorticoid that maintains extracellular fluid volume. It acts on the renal tubule to promote renal reabsorption of sodium and excretion of potassium and hydrogen ions. Hyponatremia, hyperkalemia, and angiotensin II stimulate aldosterone synthesis and secretion. ANP and hypokalemia inhibit aldosterone synthesis and release.

Adrenal Androgens. The adrenal cortex secretes small amounts of androgens. They are converted to sex steroids in peripheral tissues: testosterone in men and estrogen in women. The most common adrenal androgens are dehydroepiandrosterone (DHEA) and androstenedione. Because they are precursors to other sex steroids, their actions are like those of testosterone and estrogen. In postmenopausal women, the major source of estrogen is the peripheral conversion of adrenal androgens to estrogen.

Pancreas

The pancreas is a long, tapered, lobular, soft gland located behind the stomach and anterior to the first and second lumbar vertebrae. The pancreas has both exocrine and endocrine functions. The hormone-secreting part of the pancreas is the *islets of Langerhans*. The islets account for less than 2% of the gland. They consist of 4 types of hormone-secreting cells: α, β, delta, and F cells. The α cells make and secrete the hormone glucagon. The β cells make and secrete insulin and amylin. Delta cells make and secrete somatostatin. F (or PP) cells secrete pancreatic polypeptide.

Glucagon. Pancreatic α cells release *glucagon* in response to low blood glucose levels, protein ingestion, and exercise. Glucagon increases blood glucose, providing fuel for energy by stimulating glycogenolysis (breakdown of glycogen into glucose), gluconeogenesis (formation of glucose from noncarbohydrate molecules), and ketogenesis. Glucagon and insulin function in a reciprocal manner to maintain normal blood glucose levels.

Insulin. Insulin is the main regulator of metabolism and storage of ingested carbohydrates, fats, and proteins. Insulin facilitates glucose transport into cells, transport of amino acids across muscle membranes, and the synthesis of amino acids into protein in the peripheral tissues. However, the brain, nerves, lens of the eye, hepatocytes, erythrocytes, and cells in the intestinal mucosa and kidney tubules are not dependent on insulin for glucose uptake. After a meal, insulin is responsible for how we use and store nutrients (*anabolism*). An increased blood glucose

TABLE 47.3 Gerontologic Assessment Differences

Endocrine System

Changes	Clinical Significance
Thyroid	
Atrophy of thyroid gland	↑ Incidence of hypothyroidism with aging
↓ secretion of T_3, T_4, TSH	Most older adults maintain adequate thyroid function
↑ Nodules	Thyroid hormone replacement dose lower in older adults
Parathyroid	
↑ Secretion of PTH	↑ Calcium resorption from bone
↑ Basal level of PTH	Hypercalcemia, hypercalciuria (may reflect defective renal mechanism)
Adrenal Cortex	
Adrenal cortex becomes more fibrotic and slightly smaller	↓ Metabolic clearance rate for glucocorticoids
↓ Metabolism of cortisol	
↓ Plasma levels of adrenal androgens and aldosterone	
Adrenal Medulla	
↑ Secretion and basal level of norepinephrine	↓ Responsiveness to β-adrenergic agonists and receptor blockers
↓ β-Adrenergic receptor response to norepinephrine	May partly explain ↑ incidence of hypertension with aging
Pancreas	
↑ Fibrosis and fatty deposits in pancreas	May partly contribute to ↑ incidence of diabetes with advanced aging
↑ Glucose intolerance with ↓ sensitivity to insulin	
Gonads	
Women: ↓ Estrogen secretion	Have menopausal symptoms
	↑ Risk for arteriosclerosis and osteoporosis
Men: ↓ Testosterone secretion	Men may or may not have symptoms

level is the major stimulus for insulin synthesis and secretion. Low blood glucose levels, glucagon, somatostatin, hypokalemia, and catecholamines usually inhibit insulin secretion.

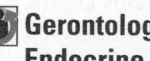 Gerontologic Considerations: Effects of Aging on Endocrine System

Normal aging has many effects on the endocrine system (Table 47.3). These include (1) decreased hormone production and secretion, (2) altered hormone metabolism and biologic activity, (3) decreased responsiveness of target tissues to hormones, and (4) changes in circadian rhythms.

Assessing the effects of aging on the endocrine system may be difficult because the subtle changes of aging may mimic manifestations of endocrine disorders. Endocrine problems may manifest differently in an older adult than in a younger person. Older adults may have multiple co-morbidities and take medications that change the body's usual response to endocrine function. Symptoms of endocrine problems, such as fatigue, constipation, or mental impairment, may be attributed to aging, resulting in delayed treatment.

ASSESSMENT OF ENDOCRINE SYSTEM

Endocrine problems generally result from too much or too little of a specific hormone. The onset of symptoms is often gradual. Subtle or vague symptoms are often attributed to other physiologic or psychologic causes. Patients may present with fluid and electrolyte imbalances, altered tissue perfusion, inadequate coping mechanisms, changes in heart rhythm, or changes in skin integrity that can be interpreted as many other conditions. Alternatively, patients may present with acute symptoms that are life threatening and demand immediate intervention.

CASE STUDY

Patient Introduction

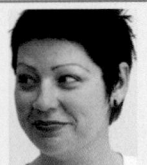

L.M. is a 35-yr-old Hispanic woman who comes to the clinic saying she is "just not feeling well." Her husband, H.M., is with her. L.M. states that she has gained a lot of weight despite trying to watch her diet and just seems to be getting more and more tired. H.M. voices concerns about the changes in his wife's energy level.

(© iStockphoto/ Thinkstock.)

Discussion Questions

1. What are the possible causes of L.M.'s weight gain, fatigue, and irritability?
2. What would be your priority assessment of L.M.?
3. What questions would you ask L.M.?

You will learn more about L.M. and her condition as you read through this assessment chapter.

(See p. 1098 for more information on L.M.)

Answers available at *http://evolve.elsevier.com/Lewis/medsurg.*

Subjective Data

Information obtained from the patient can provide important clues as to the functioning of the endocrine system. You will need to obtain a thorough history from the patient and/or a caregiver if the patient's mental acuity is compromised.

Important Health Information

Past Health History. Patients with endocrine disorders often present with nonspecific complaints. The chief complaint may relate to not just one but a group of symptoms. The most common presenting problems include fatigue, weakness, menstrual irregularities, and weight changes. It is important to determine if the onset of symptoms has been gradual or sudden and what the patient has done about them.

Because some of the more general signs of problems are the easiest to overlook, you must evaluate any reported or observed changes in weight, appetite, skin, libido, mental acuity, emotional stability, or energy levels.

Medications. Ask about the use of all medications (both prescription and over-the-counter), herbs, and dietary supplements. Ask about the reason for taking the drug, the dosage, and the length of time the drug has been taken. In particular, ask about the use of hormone replacements. Knowing that the patient is currently taking hormone replacements, such as insulin, thyroid hormone, or corticosteroids (e.g., prednisone), should alert you to potential adverse drug events. For example, corticosteroids may increase blood glucose levels and cause bone loss with long-term use. Thyroid preparations may cause tachycardia or dysrhythmias. Drug-to-drug interactions and adverse effects of nonhormonal medications can contribute to endocrine problems.

Surgery or Other Treatments. Ask about past medical, surgical, and obstetric history, including number of pregnancies and live births. Assess growth patterns and stages of physical and emotional development. For example, knowing about radiation therapy to the head and neck is important when you suspect thyroid or pituitary problems.

Functional Health Patterns. Key questions to ask the patient with an endocrine problem are outlined in Table 47.4.

Health Perception–Health Management Pattern. Heredity plays a key role in the development of endocrine problems. Ask about first-degree relatives with diabetes, thyroid disease, or endocrine gland cancers, since these conditions have a familial tendency. A genetic assessment of family members may be needed.

GENETIC RISK ALERT

Pituitary

- Nephrogenic diabetes insipidus can be inherited as a sex-linked or autosomal disorder.

Thyroid

- Genetics has a role in many cases of hypothyroid and hyperthyroid disorders.
- Hashimoto's thyroiditis, the most common cause of hypothyroidism, and Graves' disease, a cause of hyperthyroidism, are autoimmune disorders. Both likely result from a combination of genetic and environmental factors.[2]

Multiple Endocrine Neoplasia

- Multiple endocrine neoplasia (MEN) involves tumors in 2 or more different endocrine glands.
- There are several types of MEN. Mutations of *MEN1, RET,* and *CDKN1B* genes determine the type.
- The features of MEN are relatively consistent within a family.
- A common tumor associated with MEN type 2 is medullary thyroid cancer.[2]

Diabetes

- Genetics has a strong role in the development of type 1 and type 2 diabetes.

Nutritional-Metabolic Pattern. Changes in appetite and weight can indicate an endocrine problem. Ask about a history of weight distribution and changes. Weight loss with increased appetite may occur with hyperthyroidism or diabetes. Weight gain may occur with hypothyroidism or hypocortisolism. Obese persons are more likely to develop type 2 diabetes.

Ask if there have been problems with nausea, vomiting, or diarrhea. An enlarged thyroid gland can cause difficulty swallowing or a change in neck size. Increased SNS activity, including nervousness, palpitations, sweating, and tremors, may occur with thyroid problems or a rare tumor of the adrenal medulla (*pheochromocytoma*). Heat or cold intolerance occur with hyperthyroidism or hypothyroidism, respectively.

Ask about changes in the patient's skin, especially on the face, neck, hands, or body creases. Changes in skin texture and skin that seems thicker or drier may suggest an endocrine problem. A patient with hypothyroidism or excess GH may have skin that feels coarse or leathery. Ask if the patient has noticed any change in the distribution of hair anywhere on the body.

TABLE 47.4 Health History

Endocrine System

Health Perception–Health Management	**Cognitive-Perceptual**
• What is your usual day like? • Have you noticed any changes in your ability to perform your usual activities compared with last year? 5 years ago?*	• How is your memory? Have you noticed any changes?* • Have you had any blurring or double vision?* • When was your last eye examination?

Nutritional-Metabolic

- What are your weight and height?
- How much do you want to weigh?
- Have there been any changes in your appetite or weight?*
- Have you noticed any changes in the distribution of the hair anywhere on your body? *
- Have you noticed any changes in the color of your skin, especially on your face, neck, hands, or body creases? *
- Has the texture of your skin changed? For example, does it seem thicker and drier than it used to?*
- Have you noticed any difficulty swallowing, throat pain, or hoarseness? Is the top button on your shirt or blouse hard to button?*
- Do you feel more nervous than you used to? Do you notice your heart pounding or that you sweat when you do not think you should be sweating?
- Do you have difficulty holding things because of shakiness of your hands?*
- Do you feel that most rooms are too hot or too cold? Do you often have to put on a sweater, or feel as though you need to open windows when others in the room seem comfortable?*
- Do you have, or have you had any wounds that were slow to heal?*

Elimination

- Do you have to get up at night to urinate? If so, how many times? Do you keep water by your bed at night?
- Have you ever had a kidney stone?*
- Describe your usual bowel pattern. Have you noted any bowel changes?*
- Do you use anything, such as laxatives, to help you move your bowels?*

Activity-Exercise

- What is your usual activity pattern during a typical day?
- Do you have a planned exercise program? If yes, what is it and have you had to make any changes in this routine lately? If so, why, and what kinds of changes?
- Do you have fatigue with or without activity?*
- Have you had any trouble with breathing?*

Sleep-Rest

- How many hours do you sleep at night? Do you feel rested on awakening?
- Are you ever awakened by sweating during the night?*
- Do you have nightmares?*

Self-Perception–Self-Concept

- Have you noticed any changes in your physical appearance or size?*
- Are you concerned about your weight?*
- Do you feel you are able to do what you think you can do? If not, why not?
- Does your health problem affect how you feel about yourself?*

Role-Relationship

- Do you have a support system or partner? Are you married? Do you have any children? Do you think you are able to take care of your family and home? If not, why not?
- Where do you work? What kind of work do you do? Are you able to do what is expected of you and what you expect of yourself?
- Are you retired? What type of work did you do before you retired? How do you spend your time now that you have retired?

Sexuality-Reproductive

Women

- When did you start to menstruate? Was this earlier or later than other women in your family?
- When was your last menstrual period? Do you have scant, heavy, or irregular menstrual flows?
- How many children have you had? How much did they weigh at birth? Were you told you had diabetes during any pregnancy?*
- Are you menopausal? If so, for how long?
- Are you trying to get pregnant but cannot?*
- Are you postmenopausal? If so, do you have any bleeding from your uterus?

Men

- Have you noticed any changes in your ability to get and maintain an erection?*
- Are you trying to have children but cannot?*

Coping–Stress Tolerance

- What kind of stressors do you have?
- How do you deal with stress or problems?
- What is your support system? To whom do you turn when you have a problem?

Value-Belief

- Do you think medicine should still be taken even though you feel okay?
- Do any of your prescribed therapies cause any conflict in your value-belief system?*

*If yes, describe.

Elimination Pattern. Because maintaining fluid balance is a major role of the endocrine system, questions related to fluid intake and elimination patterns may uncover endocrine problems. For example, increased thirst and urination can indicate diabetes (pancreas disorder) or diabetes insipidus (pituitary disorder). Ask about the frequency and consistency of bowel movements. Diarrhea can occur with hyperthyroidism or thyroid cancer. Constipation occurs with hypothyroidism, hypoparathyroidism, and hypopituitarism.

Activity-Exercise Pattern. Determine if there are any acute or gradual changes in energy level or persistent fatigue. A patient with chronic fatigue secondary to hypothyroidism, hypocortisolism, or diabetes may report changes in activity level.

Sleep-Rest Pattern. Ask the patient how many hours they typically sleep, and if they feel rested on awakening. Sleep problems can result from nocturia, nightmares, anxiety, depression, or insomnia that occur with diabetes or thyroid problems.

Cognitive-Perceptual Pattern. Memory deficits may occur with hypothyroidism and changes in sodium levels. Inappropriate secretion of antidiuretic hormone (SIADH) or pituitary tumors can cause hyponatremia. These issues can occur gradually. Gathering information from patient and family about memory, cognitive abilities, and balance can increase the chances of an earlier diagnosis.

Self-Perception–Self-Concept Pattern. Many endocrine disorders may affect a patient's self-esteem because of associated changes in physical appearance. For example, weight gain associated with hypothyroidism or exophthalmos and goiter associated with hyperthyroidism can cause problems related to body image.

Role-Relationship Pattern. Questions related to roles and relationships can highlight depression, chronic fatigue, and sleep problems. With chronic fatigue, depression, and anxiety, patients and their families will have stressed relationships. Questions related to home life and the patients' ability to fulfill their role in the family will aid in identifying problems.

Sexuality-Reproductive Pattern. The endocrine system regulates GH, prolactin, LH, FSH, testosterone, and estrogen. Therefore, menstrual problems, hirsutism, infertility, decreased libido, and growth disorders can be a result of endocrine disorders. Some women develop hypothyroidism during or after menopause. Other patients begin to develop type 2 diabetes during middle age when sex hormones are changing. Document the presence of abnormal secondary sex characteristics, such as facial hair *(hirsutism)* in women. Obtain a detailed history of menstruation and pregnancy. Menstrual problems can occur with disorders of the ovaries and pituitary, thyroid, and adrenal glands. A history of large-birth-weight babies or gestational diabetes increases the risk for developing type 2 diabetes later in life. Male sexual problems may include impotence, infertility, or the lack of development of secondary sexual characteristics. Retrograde ejaculation can occur in diabetes.

Coping–Stress Tolerance Pattern. Because stress worsens some endocrine conditions, ask patients about their stress level and usual coping patterns. Patients with adrenal insufficiency have difficulty dealing with stress. These patients are at risk for developing hypotension and fluid and electrolyte imbalance.

Value-Belief Pattern. Determining a patient's ability to make lifestyle changes is an important nursing function. Identify the patient's value-belief patterns so that you can help to determine appropriate treatment plans. This is especially important in a condition such as diabetes, which may require major lifestyle changes. Other disorders, such as hypothyroidism or hypocortisolism, may be managed with medications but need lifelong monitoring.

Objective Data

Except the thyroid and testes, most endocrine glands are inaccessible to direct examination. Assessment can be accomplished using objective data from the physical examination and diagnostic tests. It is essential to understand the actions of hormones in order to assess the function of a gland by monitoring the target tissue.

Physical Examination. Use the following general examination when evaluating endocrine function.[3] Specific clinical findings for the various endocrine problems are discussed in Chapters 48 and 49. Endocrine disorders may cause changes in mental and emotional status. Throughout the examination, assess the patient's orientation, alertness, memory, cognitive abilities, affect, personality, and appropriateness of their behavior.

Take a full set of vital signs at the beginning of the examination. Variations in temperature, heart rate, and BP can occur

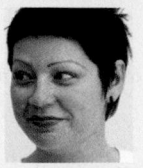
with a variety of endocrine-related problems. Obtain height and weight. Calculate body mass index (BMI) to assess nutritional status.

Integument. Assess the color and texture of the skin, hair, and nails. Note the overall skin color as well as pigmentation and bruising. Decreased skin pigmentation can occur in hypopituitarism, hypothyroidism, and hypoparathyroidism. Hyperpigmentation, or "bronzing" of the skin, especially on

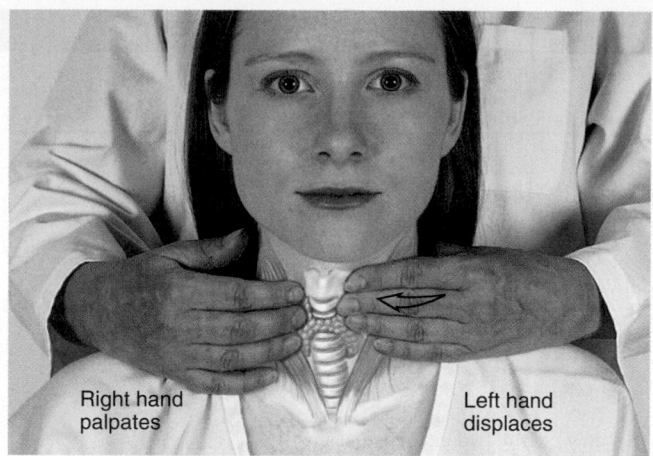

FIG. 47.10 Posterior palpation of the thyroid gland. (From Jarvis C: *Physical examination and health assessment*, ed 6, St Louis, 2012, Saunders.)

Right hand palpates

Left hand displaces

knuckles, elbows, knees, genitalia, and palmar creases, is a classic finding in a form of adrenal insufficiency known as *Addison's disease*. Palpate the skin for texture and moisture. Examine hair distribution on the head, face, trunk, and extremities. Assess the hair's appearance and texture. Hair loss, excess hair growth, or dull, brittle hair may suggest endocrine problems. Assess for delayed wound healing.

Head. Inspect the size and contour of the head. Facial features should be symmetric. Hyperreflexia and facial muscle contraction upon percussion of the facial nerve *(Chvostek's sign)* may occur in hypoparathyroidism. Inspect the eyes for position, symmetry, and shape. Large and protruding eyes (exophthalmos) are associated with hyperthyroidism. Assess visual acuity using a Snellen eye chart. Visual field loss may occur with a pituitary tumor. In the mouth, inspect the buccal mucosa, condition of teeth, and tongue size. Note hair distribution on the scalp and face. Hearing loss is common in acromegaly from excess GH.[4]

Neck. The thyroid gland is not usually visible during inspection. A feature that distinguishes the thyroid from other masses in the neck is its upward movement on swallowing. Inspect the neck while the patient swallows a sip of water. The neck should appear symmetric without lumps or bulging.

Palpate the thyroid for its size, shape, symmetry, and tenderness and for any nodules. *Goiter*, an enlarged thyroid gland, can occur with hyperthyroidism or hypothyroidism. Be careful not to press too hard or massage an enlarged thyroid gland. This can cause a sudden release of thyroid hormone into an already overloaded system. An experienced clinician should perform palpation in patients with a known diagnosis of hyperthyroidism.

Perform palpation using a posterior or anterior approach. For *anterior palpation*, stand in front of the patient, with the patient's neck flexed. Place your thumb horizontally with the upper edge along the lower border of the cricoid cartilage. Then move your thumb over the isthmus as the patient swallows water. Place your fingers laterally to the anterior border of the sternocleidomastoid muscle and palpate each lateral lobe before and while the patient swallows water.

For *posterior palpation*, stand behind the patient (Fig. 47.10). With the thumbs of both hands resting on the nape of the patient's neck, use your index and middle fingers of both hands to feel for the thyroid isthmus and for the anterior surfaces of the lateral lobes. To relax the neck muscles, ask the patient to flex the neck slightly forward and to the right. Displace the thyroid

cartilage to the right with your left hand and fingers. Palpate with your right hand after placing the thumb deep and behind the sternocleidomastoid muscle with the index and middle fingers in front of it. Ask the patient to swallow water and feel for the thyroid to move up. In a normal person, the thyroid is often not palpable. If palpable, it usually feels smooth with a firm consistency. It is not tender with gentle pressure.[5] If nodules, enlargement, asymmetry, or hardness (abnormal findings) are present, refer the patient for further evaluation. Auscultate the lateral lobes of an enlarged thyroid gland with the stethoscope bell to hear a *bruit*, a soft swishing sound that can occur with a goiter or hyperthyroidism.

Thorax. Inspect the thorax for shape and characteristics of the skin. Note the presence of breast gynecomastia in men. Auscultate lung sounds and heart sounds. Note any adventitious lung sounds (wheezing, decreased sounds) or extra heart sounds. Signs of fluid overload or heart failure may be present in patients with SIADH or hypothyroidism.

Abdomen. Inspect the contour of the abdomen and note the symmetry and color. Cushing syndrome (hypercortisolism) causes the skin to be fragile, resulting in purple-blue striae across the abdomen. Note general obesity or truncal obesity. Auscultate bowel sounds.

Extremities. Assess the size, shape, symmetry, and general proportion of hands and feet. Patients with acromegaly from pituitary tumors may have large hands and feet. Inspect the skin for changes in pigmentation, lesions, and edema. Assess muscle strength and deep tendon reflexes. In the upper extremities, assess for tremors by placing a piece of paper on the outstretched fingers, palm down. Muscular spasms of the hand elicited on application of an occlusive BP cuff for 3 minutes *(Trousseau's sign)* may occur in hypoparathyroidism.

Genitalia. Inspect the genital hair distribution pattern, since it may be changed with hormone problems.

Assessment abnormalities related to the endocrine system are outlined in Table 47.5. A focused assessment of the endocrine system is shown on p. 1101.

CASE STUDY—cont'd

Objective Data: Physical Examination

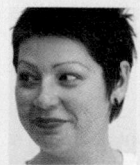

(© iStockphoto/Thinkstock.)

A focused assessment of L.M. reveals the following:
L.M. is sitting on the edge of the examination table. She appears somewhat anxious. Her BP is 190/80, heart rate 84, respiratory rate 20, temp 98.6° F (37° C). Her weight is 160 lb, and she is 5 ft, 4 in tall. L.M.'s face is reddened and puffy. She appears to have a lump on the back of her neck and shoulders. There is some acne on her face, along with some hair growth on her upper lip and chin area. Her abdomen is protruding, but her arms and legs are thin. She has +1 edema in her ankles bilaterally. There are several bruises on her upper and lower extremities, as well as purple stretch marks on her abdomen.

Discussion Questions
1. Which physical assessment findings are of most concern to you?
2. Based upon the subjective and objective assessment data presented so far, what are 3 priority nursing diagnoses?
3. What diagnostic studies would you expect to be ordered?

You will learn more about diagnostic studies related to the endocrine system in the next section.
(See p. 1106 for more information on L.M.)

Answers available at *http://evolve.elsevier.com/Lewis/medsurg*.

TABLE 47.5 Assessment Abnormalities

Endocrine System

Finding	Description	Possible Etiology and Significance
Cardiovascular		
Chest pain	Angina caused by increased metabolic demands, effusions	Hyperthyroidism, hypothyroidism
Dysrhythmias	Tachycardia, atrial fibrillation	Hypothyroidism, hyperthyroidism, hypoparathyroidism, hyperparathyroidism, pheochromocytoma
Fluid overload or signs of heart failure	Crackles in the lungs, peripheral edema, shortness of breath	SIADH, hypothyroidism, myxedema
Hypertension	High BP caused by ↑ metabolic demands and catecholamines	Hyperthyroidism, pheochromocytoma, Cushing syndrome
Gastrointestinal		
Constipation	Passage of infrequent hard stools	Hypothyroidism, hyperparathyroidism
Head and Neck		
Exophthalmos	Eyeball protrusion from orbits	Occurs in hyperthyroidism because of fluid accumulation in eye and retroorbital tissue
Goiter	Generalized enlargement of thyroid gland	Hyperthyroidism, hypothyroidism, iodine deficiency
Moon face	Periorbital edema and facial fullness	Cushing syndrome because of ↑ cortisol secretion
Myxedema	Puffiness, periorbital edema, masklike affect	Hydrophilic mucopolysaccharides infiltrating dermis in patients with hypothyroidism
Thyroid nodule(s)	Localized enlargement of thyroid gland	May be benign or malignant
Visual changes	↓ Visual acuity and/or ↓ peripheral vision	Pituitary gland enlargement or tumor leading to pressure on optic nerve
Integument		
Bruises easily	Multiple bruises over various parts of body	Cushing syndrome
Changes in hair distribution	Hair loss	Hypothyroidism, hyperthyroidism, ↓ pituitary secretion
	↓ Axillary and pubic hair	Cortisol deficiency
	Hirsutism (excess facial hair on women)	Cushing syndrome, prolactinoma (a pituitary tumor)
Changes in skin texture	Thick, cold, dry skin	Hypothyroidism
	Thick, leathery, oily skin	GH excess (acromegaly)
	Warm, smooth, moist skin	Hyperthyroidism
Depigmentation (vitiligo)	Patchy areas of light skin	May be a marker of autoimmune endocrine disorders
Edema	Generalized edema	Mucopolysaccharide accumulation in tissue in hypothyroidism
Hyperpigmentation	Darkening of the skin, especially in skinfolds and creases	Increased secretion of MSH from Addison's disease, acanthosis nigricans
Skin ulceration	Areas of ulcerated skin, most often found on legs and feet	Peripheral neuropathy and peripheral vascular disease, which are contributory factors in the development of diabetic foot ulcers
Striae	Purplish red marks below the skin surface. Usually seen on abdomen, breasts, and buttocks	Cushing syndrome
Musculoskeletal		
Changes in muscular strength or muscle mass	Generalized weakness and/or fatigue	Common with many endocrine problems, including pituitary, thyroid, parathyroid, and adrenal problems
		Diabetes, diabetes insipidus
	↓ Muscle mass	Specifically seen in GH deficiency and Cushing syndrome from protein wasting
Enlargement of bones and cartilage	Coarsening of facial features. ↑ In size of hands and feet over a period of several years	Gradual enlargement and thickening of bony tissue occurring with GH excess in adults as seen in acromegaly secondary to pituitary dysfunction
Neurologic		
↑ Deep tendon reflexes	Hyperreflexia	Hyperthyroidism, hypoparathyroidism
Lethargy	State of mental sluggishness or somnolence	Hypothyroidism
Seizure	Sudden involuntary contraction of muscles	Consequence of a pituitary tumor
		Hypervolemia and hyponatremia with SIADH
		Complications of diabetes, severe hypothyroidism
Tetany	Intermittent involuntary muscle spasms usually involving the extremities	Severe hypocalcemia that can occur with hypoparathyroidism
Nutrition		
Changes in weight	Weight loss	Hyperthyroidism caused by ↑ in metabolism, type 1 diabetes, diabetic ketoacidosis
	Weight gain	Hypothyroidism, Cushing syndrome, type 2 diabetes

TABLE 47.5   Assessment Abnormalities

Endocrine System—cont'd

Finding	Description	Possible Etiology and Significance
Glucose levels altered	↑ Serum glucose	Diabetes, Cushing syndrome, GH excess
Reproductive		
Changes in reproductive function	Menstrual irregularities, ↓ libido, ↓ fertility, impotence	Pituitary hypofunction, GH excess, thyroid problems, adrenocortical problems
Other		
↓ Urine output	↓ Water reabsorption from kidney tubules	SIADH
Polydipsia	Excessive thirst	Extreme water losses in diabetes (with severe hyperglycemia), diabetes insipidus, dehydration
Polyuria	Excess urine output	Diabetes (from hyperglycemia) or diabetes insipidus (associated with ↓ ADH)
Thermoregulation	Cold insensitivity Heat intolerance	Hypothyroidism caused by a slowing of metabolic processes Hyperthyroidism caused by excessive metabolism

FOCUSED ASSESSMENT

Endocrine System

Use this checklist to ensure the key assessment steps have been done.

Subjective

Ask the patient about any of the following and note responses.

Excessive or increased thirst	Y	N
Excess or decreased urination	Y	N
Excessive hunger	Y	N
Heat or cold intolerance	Y	N
Excessive sweating	Y	N
Recent weight gain or loss	Y	N

Objective: Diagnostic

Check the following laboratory results for critical values.

Potassium	✓
Glucose	✓
Sodium	✓
Glycosylated hemoglobin (A1C)	✓
Thyroid studies: TSH, T_3, T_4	✓
Serum osmolality	✓

Objective: Physical Examination

Inspect/Measure

Body temperature	✓
Height and weight	✓
Alertness and emotional state	✓
Skin for changes in color and texture	✓
Hair for changes in color, texture, and distribution	✓

Auscultate

Heart rate, BP	✓

Palpate

Extremities for edema	✓
Skin for texture and temperature	✓
Neck for thyroid size, shape	✓

DIAGNOSTIC STUDIES OF ENDOCRINE SYSTEM

Diagnostic studies of the endocrine system are shown in Tables 47.6 and 47.7. Pertinent findings from the history and physical examination guide the selection of diagnostic studies. Imaging studies can identify pituitary tumors, thyroid nodules, or adrenal tumors. Laboratory studies may include direct measurement of the hormone level or an indirect measure of gland function by evaluating blood or urine components affected by the hormone, such as glucose or electrolytes. We can also measure the releasing or stimulating hormone. For example, we can evaluate thyroid function by measuring TSH.

We can assess hormones with constant basal levels, such as T_4, with a single measurement. Note the time of the sample collection on the laboratory slip. Information about night shift work is important for hormones with circadian or sleep-related secretion (e.g., cortisol). Evaluating other hormones may require multiple blood samplings, such as in suppression tests (e.g., dexamethasone) and stimulation tests (e.g., glucose tolerance). In these situations, it is often necessary to obtain IV access to give the testing medication and fluids and draw multiple blood samples.

Pituitary gland problems can manifest in a wide variety of ways because of the number of hormones produced. Many diagnostic studies evaluate these hormones either directly or indirectly.

Several tests are available to evaluate thyroid function. The most sensitive and accurate laboratory test is the measurement of TSH. Thus it is often the first diagnostic test done to evaluate thyroid function.[6] Follow-up tests ordered when the TSH level is abnormal include total T_4, free T_4, and total T_3. Free T_4 is the unbound thyroxine and more accurately reflects thyroid function than total T_4.

The only hormone secreted by the parathyroid glands is PTH. Because PTH regulates serum calcium and phosphate levels, these levels reflect abnormalities in PTH secretion. For this reason, diagnostic tests for the parathyroid gland typically include PTH, serum calcium, and serum phosphate levels.

Tests associated with the adrenal cortex function focus on measuring blood plasma and urine levels of the 3 types of hormones secreted: glucocorticoids, mineralocorticoids, and androgens. Urine studies often require a 24-hour urine collection to eliminate the impact of short-term fluctuations in plasma hormone levels.

The tests used to evaluate glucose metabolism are important in the diagnosis and management of diabetes. See Chapter 48 for information about diagnostic studies for diabetes.

TABLE 47.6 Serology and Urine Studies

Endocrine System

Study	Reference Interval	Purpose and Description	Nursing Responsibility
Adrenal Studies			
Blood Studies			
Adrenal steroid precursors • Androstenediones (AD) • Dehydroepiandrosterone DHEA) • Dehydroepiandrosterone sulfate (DHEA S) • 11-Deoxycortisol	AD • *Female:* 0.05–2.05 ng/mL • *Male:* 0.04–1.06 ng/mL DHEA • *Female:* 0.14–7.88 ng/mL • *Male:* 0.11–6.73 ng/mL DHEA S • *Female:* 7–488 mcg/dL • *Male:* 7–371 mcg/dL 11-Deoxycortisol • *Adults:* 10–79 ng/dL	Assesses for congenital adrenal hyperplasia, sex hormones abnormalities, adrenal or gonadal tumors.	*Before:* Tanner stage I–V of physical development needed for accurate assessment. Determine date of last menstrual period (LMP) for females. Test should be done 1 wk before or after menstrual cycle. *After:* Note date of LMP on laboratory slip.
Adrenocorticotropic hormone (ACTH, corticotropin)	• *Female:* 6–58 pg/mL • *Male:* 7–69 pg/mL	Measures amount of ACTH made by the anterior pituitary gland. Levels determine if there is an overproduction or underproduction of cortisol, and whether cause is an adrenal gland or pituitary gland abnormality.	*Before:* Patient should be NPO after midnight. Do morning blood draw between 6 and 8 AM. *During:* Use prechilled blood tube and place on ice.
ACTH stimulation test with cosyntropin (Cortisol stimulation test)	*Rapid test:* Cortisol levels increase more than 7 mcg/dL higher than baseline *24-Hour test:* Cortisol levels >40 mcg/dL *3-Day test:* Cortisol levels greater than 40 mcg/dL	Used to evaluate cause of adrenal insufficiency. If cortisol levels increase after cosyntropin injection, the cause of adrenal insufficiency is the pituitary gland. If there is no or little rise in cortisol levels, the cause of adrenal insufficiency is the adrenal gland.	*Before:* Obtain baseline cortisol level at beginning of cosyntropin infusion. *During:* Inject bolus of IV cosyntropin with a plastic syringe. Draw cortisol samples 30 and 60 min after bolus. Monitor site and rate of IV infusion. Ensure sample collection at appropriate times.
Aldosterone	*Supine:* 3–10 ng/dL (0.08–0.30 nmol/L) *Upright:* • *Female:* 5–30 ng/dL (0.14–0.08 nmol/L) • *Male:* 6–22 ng/dL (0.17–0.61 nmol/L)	Used to identify hyperaldosteronism. Helps distinguish primary aldosteronism from adrenal disease versus secondary aldosteronism from extraadrenal disease.	*Before:* Usually morning blood sample is preferred. Tell patient that the required position (supine/sitting/standing) must be maintained for 2 hr before specimen is drawn.
Cortisol (hydrocortisone, serum cortisol)	• *8 AM:* 5–23 mcg/dL (138–635 nmol/L) • *4 PM:* 3–13 mcg/dL (83–359 nmol/L)	Measures serum cortisol level to evaluate adrenal activity. Cortisol levels are normally highest in the morning, slowly drop during the day, and are lowest around midnight.	*Before:* Sample should be drawn in morning. Note if patient works night shift. Mark time of blood draw on laboratory slip. Stress and excessive physical activity produce elevated results.
Dexamethasone suppression (DST, prolonged/rapid DST, cortisol suppression test, ACTH suppression test)	Prolonged method: • *Low dose:* >50% reduction of plasma cortisol and 17-hydroxycorticosteroid (17-OCHS) • *High dose:* >50% reduction of plasma cortisol and 17-OCHS Rapid (overnight) method: • Plasma cortisol levels suppressed to <2 mcg/dL	Helps to identify and determine cause of adrenal hyperactivity (e.g., Cushing syndrome).	*Before:* Patient should fast for 8–10 hr prior. Do not test acutely ill patients or those under stress. Stress-stimulated ACTH may override suppression. Screen patient for drugs, such as estrogen and corticosteroids, that may give false-positive results. *Overnight method:* Dexamethasone 1 mg (low dose) or 4 mg (high dose) is given at 11 PM to suppress secretion of corticotropin-releasing hormone. Plasma cortisol sample is drawn at 8 AM.
Metanephrine, plasma free (fractionated metanephrines)	*Normetanephrine:* <0.5 nmol/L or 18–111 pg/mL by HPLC *Metanephrine:* <0.9 nmol/L or 12–60 pg/mL by HPLC	Used to identify pheochromocytoma of the adrenal or extraadrenal glands.	*Before:* Ask about recent history of vigorous exercise, high stress levels, or starvation (may artificially ↑ levels). Assess for drugs (e.g., caffeine, alcohol, levodopa, nitroglycerin, acetaminophen, and those containing epinephrine or norepinephrine) that can alter results.
Urine Studies			
Cortisol (hydrocortisone, urine cortisol, free cortisol)	24-Hour specimen: <100 mcg/24 hr (<276 nmol/day)	Measures urine cortisol level to evaluate adrenal activity.	*Before:* Explain 24-hr urine collection and need to avoid stressful situations and excessive physical exercise. Assess for drug use (e.g., reserpine, diuretics, phenothiazines, insulin, amphetamines) that may alter results.

TABLE 47.6 Serology and Urine Studies—cont'd

Endocrine System

Study	Reference Interval	Purpose and Description	Nursing Responsibility
17-Hydroxycorticosteroids (17-OCHS)	24-Hour specimen: *Adults:* • *Male:* 3–10 mg/24 hr (8.3–27.6 µmol/day) • *Female:* 2–8 mg/24 hr (5.2–22.1 µmol/day)	Measures 17-OCHS, a cortisol metabolite, to evaluate adrenocortical function. Older adults may have slightly lower values.	*Before*: Explain 24-hr urine collection and need to avoid stressful situations and excessive physical exercise. Assess for drug use (e.g., erythromycin, spironolactone) that may alter results.
17-Ketosteroids (17-KS)	24-Hour specimen: • *Male:* 6–20 mg/24 hr (20–70 µmol/day) • *Female:* 6–17 mg/24 hr (20–60 µmol/day)	Evaluates adrenocortical and gonadal functions by measuring urinary androgen metabolites. Older adults may have slightly lower values.	*Before:* Explain 24-hr urine collection.
Vanillylmandelic acid (VMA)	24-Hour specimen: <6.8 mg/24 hr (<35 µmol/24 hr)	Measures the excretion of catecholamine metabolite. Used to identify catecholamine-producing tumors, such as pheochromocytoma.	*Before*: Explain 24-hr urine collection. Must follow VMA-restricted diet 2–3 days before and during the urine collection. *During*: Keep 24-hr urine collection at pH <3.0 with HCl acid as preservative. Keep on ice.

Pancreatic Studies
Blood Studies

Study	Reference Interval	Purpose and Description	Nursing Responsibility
C-Peptide (connecting peptide insulin, insulin C-peptide, proinsulin C-peptide)	*Fasting:* 0.78–1.89 ng/mL (0.26–0.62 nmol/L) *1 hour after glucose load:* 5–12 ng/mL	Measures amount of C-peptide, which is released with insulin. Distinguishes between type 1 (low levels) and type 2 diabetes (normal or high levels).	*Before:* Patient should fast 8–12 hr prior. Water intake is allowed.
Glucagon	50–100 pg/mL (50–100 ng/L)	Assesses for glucagonoma (α islet cell tumor). Evaluates pancreatic function, especially in people with diabetes who have low blood glucose (hypoglycemia).	*Before:* Patient should fast 8–12 hr prior. Water intake is allowed.
Glucose (blood sugar, fasting blood glucose [FBG])	*Fasting* (defined as no caloric intake for at least 8 hr): 74–106 mg/dL (4.1–5.9 mmol/L) *Casual* (defined as any time of day): ≤200 mg/dL (<11.1 mmol/L)	Aids in the diagnosis of diabetes.	*Before:* Patient should fast 8-12 hr prior. Water intake is allowed. Assess for the many drugs that may influence results.
Glucose, postprandial (2-hour postprandial glucose [2-hr PPG])	*0–50 yr:* <140 mg/dL (<7.8 mmol/L) *50–60 yr:* <150 md/dL *60 yr and older:* <160 mg/dL	Aids in the diagnosis of diabetes.	*Before:* Patient should fast 8–12 hr, then eat a meal of at least 75 g of carbohydrate. Patient must fast after eating this meal until blood is drawn. No exercise during test.
Glucose tolerance test (GTT, oral glucose tolerance [OGTT])	*Nonpregnancy:* *Fasting:* <110 mg/dL (<6.1 mmol/L *1 hr:* <180 mg/dL (<11.1 mmol/L) *2 hr:* <140 mg/dL (<7.8 mmol/L)	Assesses glucose levels in people with symptoms of (hypoglycemia). Aids in the diagnosis of diabetes.	*Before:* Patient should fast 8–12 hr prior. Many drugs may influence results, including caffeine and smoking. Ensure that patient's diet 3 days before test includes 150–300 g of carbohydrate with intake of at least 1500 cal/day.
Glycosylated hemoglobin (GHb, GHB, glycohemoglobin, hemoglobin A1C [Hb A1C], diabetic control index, glycated protein)	*Nondiabetic adult/child:* 4%–5.6% *Prediabetes:* 5.7%–6.4% *Good diabetic control:* <7%[7]	Measures the average blood glucose for the past 90 days. Used to diagnose and screen diabetes treatment plans.	*Before:* Tell patient that fasting is not necessary and that blood sample will be drawn.
Insulin assay	6–26 µU/mL (43–186 pmol/L)	Assesses insulin levels in people with symptoms of hypoglycemia. Assesses for insulinomas and carbohydrate and lipid absorption abnormalities.	*Before:* Patient should fast 8–12 hr prior. Water intake is allowed.

Urine Studies

Study	Reference Interval	Purpose and Description	Nursing Responsibility
Glucose (urine sugar)	*Random specimen:* negative *24-hour specimen:* 50–300 mg/day (0.3–1.7 mmol/day)	Measures amount of glucose in the urine. Assesses diabetes management.	*Before:* Use freshly voided urine. Many drugs alter glucose readings. Follow directions exactly to avoid errors.
Ketones	None or negative	Measures amount of ketones in the urine. Assesses for diabetic ketoacidosis, a life-threatening condition seen most often in people with type 1 diabetes.	*Before:* Use freshly voided urine specimen. Test is often done with glucose test. Follow directions exactly. Certain drugs can produce false-positive or false-negative results.

Continued

TABLE 47.6 Serology and Urine Studies—cont'd

Endocrine System

Study	Reference Interval	Purpose and Description	Nursing Responsibility
Parathyroid Studies			
Blood Studies			
Calcium (total)	9.0–10.5 mg/dL (2.25–2.62 mmol/L)	Assesses the function of the parathyroid gland and calcium absorption.	*Before:* Patient must fast 8–12 hr prior. Assess for drug use (e.g., albuterol, heparin, diuretics) that may alter results. *After:* Keep sample on ice.
Calcium (ionized)	4.5–5.6 mg/dL (1.05–1.3 mmol/L)	Free form of total calcium. Unchanged by inconsistent serum albumin levels that occur in certain populations, such as critically ill patients.	As above.
Parathyroid hormone (PTH, parathormone)	*Intact (whole):* 10–65 pg/mL (10–65 ng/L) *N terminal:* 8–24 pg/mL *C terminal:* 50–330 pg/mL	Used to determine the cause of changes in calcium levels caused by parathyroid or nonparathyroid problems. Monitored in patients with chronic kidney disease, especially those on dialysis.	*Before:* Patient should fast 8–12 hr prior. Obtain sample in the morning. *During:* Obtain serum calcium level at same time. *After:* Mark time of blood draw on laboratory slip.
Phosphate (PO4), phosphorus (P)	3.0–4.5 mg/dL (0.97–1.45 mmol/L)	Measures amount of inorganic phosphate in the blood. Assesses for disorders related to calcium and phosphorus disorders.	*Before:* Patient must fast 8–12 hr prior. If possible, hold IV fluids containing glucose for 8 hr prior.
Pituitary Studies			
Blood Studies			
Antidiuretic hormone (ADH, vasopressin, Arginine vasopressin [AVP])	1–5 pg/mL	Assesses for diabetes insipidus (DI) or SIADH.	*Before:* Patient must fast 8–12 hr prior.
Gonadotropins • **Follicle-stimulating hormone (FSH) assay** • **Luteinizing hormone (LH assay, Lutropin)**	*FSH (Adult)* • *Male:* 1.42–15.4 IU/L • *Female:* *Follicular phase:* 1.37–9.9 IU/L *Ovulatory phase:* 6.17–17.2 IU/L *Luteal phase:* 1.09–9.2 IU/L *Postmenopause:* 19.3–100.6 IU/L *LH (Adult)* • *Male:* 1.24–7.8 IU/L • *Female:* *Follicular phase:* 1.68–15 IU/L *Ovulatory phase:* 21.9–56.6 IU/L *Luteal phase:* 0.61–16.3 IU/L *Postmenopause:* 14.2–52.3 IU/L	Assesses for pituitary, puberty or infertility conditions and menopause.	*Before:* Tell patient that fasting is not necessary and that blood sample will be drawn. *During:* Note on the laboratory slip time of LMP or whether woman is menopausal.
Growth hormone (GH, human growth hormone [HGH], somatotropin hormone [SH])	• *Men:* <5 ng/mL • *Women:* <10 ng/mL	Evaluates GH secretion and pituitary gland function.	*Before:* Patient must fast 8–12 hours prior. Emotional and physical stress may alter results. Indicate patient fasting status and recent activity level on the laboratory slip.
GH stimulation (GH provocation, insulin tolerance test [ITT], arginine test)	GH levels >10 mg/mL	Aids in identifying GH deficiency and conditions caused from decreased pituitary hormone production.	*Before:* Patient must fast 10-12 hours prior. Water is allowed on morning of test. Establish IV access for medication administration and blood sampling. *During:* Continually assess for hypoglycemia and hypotension. Keep 50% dextrose and 5% dextrose IV solution at the bedside in case severe hypoglycemia occurs.
Insulin-like growth factor (IGF-1, somatomedin C, insulin-like growth factor binding proteins [IGF BP])	42–110 ng/mL	Evaluates GH and pituitary gland function. Provides a more accurate reflection of mean plasma concentration of GH because it is not subject to circadian rhythm and fluctuations.	*Before:* Patient must fast 8–12 hr prior.

TABLE 47.6 Serology and Urine Studies—cont'd

Endocrine System

Study	Reference Interval	Purpose and Description	Nursing Responsibility
Urine Studies			
Water deprivation (ADH stimulation)	*Neurogenic DI:* >9% rise in urine osmolality *Nephrogenic DI:* <9% rise in urine osmolality *Psychogenic polydipsia:* <9% rise in urine osmolality	Distinguishes among neurogenic, nephrogenic, or psychogenic DI.	*Before*: Obtain baseline weight and urine and plasma osmolality. Should be done only if serum sodium is normal and urine osmolality is <300 mOsm/kg. *During*: Patient may need to fast. Severe dehydration may occur. Assess urine hourly for volume and specific gravity. Send hourly urine samples to laboratory for osmolality determination. Send blood samples for sodium and osmolality every 2 hr. Stop test and rehydrate if patient's weight drops >2 kg at any time. *After*: Rehydrate with oral fluids. Check orthostatic BP and pulse to ensure adequate fluid volume.
Thyroid Studies			
Blood Studies			
Antithyroglobulin antibody (thyroid autoantibody, thyroid antithyroglobulin antibody, thyroglobulin antibody, thyroid peroxidase antibody [TPO])	<116 IU/mL	Measures thyroid antibody levels. Aids in diagnosing autoimmune thyroid disease and separates it from other forms of thyroiditis. One or more antibody tests may be ordered depending on symptoms.	*Before*: Explain blood draw procedure to the patient.
Thyroglobulin (Tg, thyrogen-stimulated thyroglobulin)	• *Male:* 0.5–53 ng/mL • *Female:* 0.5–43.0 ng/mL	Identifies functioning thyroid tissue and thyroid cancer cells. Used primarily as a tumor marker for patients being treated for thyroid cancer.	As above.
Thyroid-stimulating hormone (TSH, thyrotropin)	2–10 µU/mL	Most sensitive diagnostic test for evaluating thyroid function. Helps in distinguishing primary (thyroid), secondary (pituitary), and tertiary (hypothalamus) hypothyroidism.	As above.
Thyroxine-binding globulin (TBG, thyroid-binding globulin)	*10–19 yr:* • *Male:* 1.4–2.6 mg/dL • *Female:* 1.4–3.0 mg/dL *20 yr:* 1.7–3.6 mg/dL *Oral contraceptives:* 1.5–5.5 mg/dL	Measures TBG, the main thyroid hormone protein carrier. Used to assess thyroid function when T_4 and T_3 levels are abnormal.	As above.
Thyroxine, total and Free (T_4, thyroxine screen, FT_4)	*Free T_4:* 0.8–2.8 ng/dL (10–36 pmol/L) *Total T_4:* • *Male:* 4–12 mcg/dL (51–154 nmol/L) • *Female:* 5–12 mcg/dL (64–154 nmol/L) • *>60 yr:* 5–11 mcg/dL (64–142 nmol/L)	Used to evaluate thyroid function and monitor thyroid replacement or suppressive therapy. Free T_4 levels not affected by protein levels like total T_4 is, so it is thought to be more precise marker of thyroid function.	As above.
Triiodothyronine (total T_3 radioimmunoassay [T_3 by RIA], free T_3)	*16–20 yr:* 80–210 ng/dL *20–50 yr:* 70–205 ng/dL (1.2–3.4 nmol/L) *>50 yr:* 40–180 ng/dL (0.6–2.8 nmol/L)	Evaluates thyroid function. Free T_3 measures the active component of total T_3. Used to diagnose hyperthyroidism if TSH is abnormal and T_4 levels are normal. May be used to monitor drug therapy.	As above.
T_3 uptake (thyroid hormone–binding ratio [THBR], T_3 resin uptake)	24%–39%	Use in conjunction with T_4 to assess thyroid function. Indirectly measures binding capacity of thyroid-binding globulin	As above.

TABLE 47.7 Radiologic Studies

Endocrine System

Study	Description and Purpose	Nursing Responsibility
Adrenal arteriography (angiography; adrenal)	Assesses for arterial obstructive conditions and/or tumors of the adrenal glands.	*Before*: Assess for allergies, especially to contrast dye. Have patient fast 6–12 hr prior. Give sedative and other drugs, as ordered. *During*: Patient will feel flushed when dye is injected. *After:* Check pressure dressing site after procedure. Monitor BP, pulse, and circulation distal to injection site. Place compression device over site. Maintain IV and/or oral fluid intake.
Computed tomography (CT)	*Abdominal:* Used to detect adrenal hyperplasia and tumors or pancreatic abnormalities, such as pancreatitis, tumors, or cysts. *Brain:* Used to detect a pituitary tumor and its size. *Neck:* Can locate thyroid nodules and assess for thyroid cancer.	*Before*: Before contrast medium used, evaluate renal function. Assess if patient is allergic to shellfish since the contrast is iodine based. Patient may need to be NPO 4 hr prior to study. If the patient is taking metformin, hold it the day of the test to prevent hypoglycemia or acidosis. *During:* Warn patient that contrast injection may cause a feeling of being warm and flushed. Patient must lie completely still during scan. *After:* Encourage patient to drink fluids to avoid renal problems with any contrast.
Magnetic resonance cholangiopancrea-tography (MRCP)	Assesses for the source of pancreatitis and can detect pancreatobiliary tumors.	*Before*: Patient may need to be fasting. Oral and/or IV contrast injection may be used. Check for pregnancy, allergies, and renal function. *During*: Patient must lie completely still during scan.
Magnetic resonance imaging (MRI)	*Abdominal:* Can distinguish benign tumors from adrenal cancers. *Brain:* Study of choice for radiologic evaluation of the pituitary gland and hypothalamus. Used to identify tumors in these glands.	*Before:* Oral and/or IV contrast injection may be used. Check for pregnancy, allergies, and renal function before test. Have patient remove all metal objects. Ask about any history of surgical insertion of staples, plates, dental bridges, or other metal appliances. Remove metallic foil patches. Patient may need to be fasting. Assess for claustrophobia and the need for antianxiety medication. *During:* Patient must lie completely still during scan.
Parathyroid scan (parathyroid scintigraphy)	Used to find the parathyroid glands. Radioactive isotopes are taken up by cells in parathyroid glands. Obtains image of the glands and any abnormally active areas.	*Before:* Check for iodine allergy. Some foods and medications are restricted a few weeks before the scan.
Radioactive iodine (RAIU) uptake	Direct measure of thyroid activity and evaluates function of thyroid nodules. For 2–4 hours: 3%–19%. *For 24 hr:* 11%–30%	*Before:* Radioactive iodine given orally or IV. Check for allergies. *During:* Uptake by the thyroid gland is measured with a scanner at several time intervals, such as 2–4 hr and at 24 hr. *After:* Encourage patient to increase fluid intake as radionuclide takes 6–24 hr to be eliminated from body.
Thyroid scan	Used to evaluate nodules of thyroid. Benign nodules appear as warm spots because they take up radionuclide. Cancer tumors appear as cold spots because they tend not to take up radionuclide.	*Before:* Radioactive isotopes are given orally or IV. Check for allergies. *After*: Encourage patient to increase fluid intake as radionuclide takes 6–24 hr to be eliminated from body.
Thyroid ultrasound	Evaluates thyroid nodules to determine size and characteristics (cystic or solid tumors). Used to observe management and surveillance of nodules and unaffected portions of the gland.	*Before:* Explain that gel and a transducer will be used over the neck. The test lasts 15 min. No fasting or sedation required.

CASE STUDY—cont'd

Objective Data: Diagnostic Studies

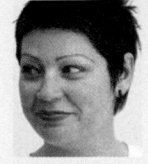
(© iStockphoto/ Thinkstock.)

The HCP orders the following initial diagnostic studies to be drawn in the morning after an 8-hr fast:

- CBC, basic metabolic panel (electrolytes, BUN, creatinine)
- Fasting blood glucose (FBG)
- TSH, free T₄
- Plasma cortisol levels
- Plasma ACTH levels

CBC results reveal a WBC of 12,200/μL and a decreased lymphocyte count at 800 cells/μL. The rest of the CBC is within normal limits (WNL). The FBG is 130 mg/dL. The plasma cortisol and ACTH levels are high. Thyroid studies are WNL.

Discussion Questions

1. Which diagnostic study results are of most concern to you?
2. Do you expect the HCP to order any other diagnostic studies for L.M.?
3. What are the interprofessional team's priorities for L.M. at this time?

Answers available at *http://evolve.elsevier.com/Lewis/medsurg*.

BRIDGE TO NCLEX EXAMINATION

The number of the question corresponds to the same-numbered outcome at the beginning of the chapter.

1. A characteristic common to all hormones is that they
   a. circulate in the blood bound to plasma proteins.
   b. influence cellular activity of specific target tissues.
   c. accelerate the metabolic processes of all body cells.
   d. enter a cell and change the cell's metabolism or gene expression.

2. A patient is receiving radiation therapy for cancer of the kidney. The nurse monitors the patient for signs and symptoms of damage to the
   a. pancreas.
   b. thyroid gland.
   c. adrenal glands.
   d. posterior pituitary gland.

3. A patient has a serum sodium level of 152 mEq/L (152 mmol/L). The normal hormonal response to this situation is
   a. release of ADH.
   b. release of ACTH.
   c. secretion of aldosterone.
   d. secretion of corticotropin-releasing hormone.

4. All cells in the body are believed to have intracellular receptors for
   a. insulin.
   b. glucagon.
   c. growth hormone.
   d. thyroid hormone.

5. When obtaining subjective data from a patient during assessment of the endocrine system, the nurse asks specifically about
   a. energy level.
   b. intake of vitamin C.
   c. employment history.
   d. frequency of sexual intercourse.

6. An appropriate technique to use during physical assessment of the thyroid gland is
   a. asking the patient to hyperextend the neck during palpation.
   b. percussing the neck for dullness to define the size of the thyroid.
   c. having the patient swallow water during inspection and palpation of the gland.
   d. using deep palpation to determine the extent of a visibly enlarged thyroid gland.

7. Endocrine disorders often go unrecognized in the older adult because
   a. symptoms are often attributed to aging.
   b. older adults rarely have identifiable symptoms.
   c. endocrine disorders are relatively rare in the older adult.
   d. older adults usually have subclinical endocrine disorders that minimize symptoms.

8. Abnormal findings during an endocrine assessment include *(select all that apply)*
   a. excess facial hair on a woman.
   b. blood pressure of 100/70 mm Hg.
   c. soft, formed stool every other day.
   d. 3-lb weight gain over last 6 months.
   e. hyperpigmented coloration in lower legs.

9. A patient has a total serum calcium level of 3 mg/dL (1.5 mEq/L). If this finding reflects hypoparathyroidism, the nurse would expect further diagnostic testing to reveal
   a. decreased serum PTH.
   b. increased serum ACTH.
   c. increased serum glucose.
   d. decreased serum cortisol levels.

1. b, 2. c, 3. a, 4. d, 5. a, 6. c, 7. a, 8. a, e, 9. a

For rationales to these answers and even more NCLEX review questions, visit *http://evolve.elsevier.com/Lewis/medsurg*.

EVOLVE WEBSITE/RESOURCES LIST

http://evolve.elsevier.com/Lewis/medsurg
Review Questions (Online Only)
Key Points
Answer Keys for Questions
- Rationales for Bridge to NCLEX Examination Questions
- Answer Guidelines for the Case Study on pp. 1096, 1098, 1099, and 1106

Conceptual Care Map Creator
Audio Glossary
Supporting Media
- Animations
  - Overview of the Endocrine System
  - Thyroid and Parathyroid Glands
  - Thyroid Secretion

Supporting Media
Content Updates

REFERENCES

1. Huether SE, McCance K: *Understanding pathophysiology*, ed 6, St Louis, 2017, Elsevier.
2. Stratakis CA: *Genetics of endocrine disorders*, St Louis, 2017, Elsevier.
3. Jarvis C: *Physical examination and health assessment*, ed 7, St Louis, 2016, Saunders.
*4. Vilar L, Vilar CF, Lyra R, et al: Acromegaly: Clinical features at diagnosis, *Pituitary* 20:22, 2017.
5. Parsa AA, Gharib H: *Thyroid nodules*, New York, 2018, Humana.
6. Pagana K, Pagana T, Pagana TN: *Mosby's manual of diagnostic and laboratory tests*, ed 13, St Louis, 2017, Mosby.
*7. American Diabetes Association: Standards of medical care in diabetes—2018, *Diabetes Care* 41:S13, 2018.

*Evidence-based information for clinical practice.

48

Diabetes Mellitus

Jane K. Dickinson

Wherever a man turns he can find someone who needs him.

Albert Schweitzer

http://evolve.elsevier.com/Lewis/medsurg

CONCEPTUAL FOCUS

Glucose Regulation
Infection
Nutrition

Self-Management
Sensory Perception

LEARNING OUTCOMES

1. Describe the pathophysiology and clinical manifestations of diabetes mellitus.
2. Distinguish between type 1 and type 2 diabetes mellitus.
3. Describe the interprofessional care of a patient with diabetes.
4. Describe the role of nutrition and exercise in managing diabetes mellitus.
5. Discuss the nursing management of a patient with newly diagnosed diabetes mellitus.
6. Describe the nursing management of a patient with diabetes mellitus in the ambulatory and home care settings.
7. Relate the pathophysiology of acute and chronic complications of diabetes mellitus to the clinical manifestations.
8. Explain the interprofessional care and nursing management of a patient with acute and chronic complications of diabetes mellitus.

KEY TERMS

basal-bolus plan, p. 1113
dawn phenomenon, p. 1118
diabetes mellitus (DM), p. 1108
diabetes-related ketoacidosis (DKA), p. 1130
diabetes-related nephropathy, p. 1137

diabetes-related neuropathy, p. 1137
diabetes-related retinopathy, p. 1136
hyperosmolar hyperglycemia syndrome (HHS), p. 1133
impaired fasting glucose (IFG), p. 1111

impaired glucose tolerance (IGT), p. 1111
insulin resistance, p. 1111
prediabetes, p. 1111
self-monitoring of blood glucose (SMBG), p. 1123
Somogyi effect, p. 1117

This chapter discusses the pathophysiology, manifestations, complications, and management of diabetes. The long-term complications associated with diabetes can make it a devastating disease. Diabetes is the leading cause of adult blindness, end-stage renal disease, and nontraumatic lower limb amputations. It is a major contributing factor to heart disease and stroke. Managing diabetes requires daily decisions about food intake, blood glucose monitoring, medication, and exercise. You play a vital role in promoting the patient's self-management of diabetes through providing comprehensive patient and caregiver education.

DIABETES MELLITUS

Diabetes mellitus (DM), most often referred to as diabetes, is a chronic multisystem disease characterized by hyperglycemia from abnormal insulin production, impaired insulin use, or both. Diabetes is a serious health problem throughout the world. Its prevalence is rapidly increasing. Currently in the United States, an estimated 29.1 million people, or 9.3% of the population, have diabetes. 86 million more people have prediabetes.[1]

About 8.1 million people with diabetes have not been diagnosed and are unaware that they have the disease. Diabetes is the seventh leading cause of death in the United States.[2] Adults with diabetes have heart disease death rates and risk for strokes that are 2 to 4 times higher than adults without diabetes. In addition, more than half of adults with diabetes have hypertension and high cholesterol levels.[2]

Etiology and Pathophysiology

Current theories link the causes of diabetes, singly or in combination, to genetic, autoimmune, and environmental factors (e.g., virus, obesity). Regardless of its cause, diabetes is primarily a disorder of glucose metabolism related to absent or insufficient insulin supply and/or poor use of the available insulin.

The American Diabetes Association (ADA) recognizes 4 different classes of diabetes. The 2 most common are type 1 and type 2 diabetes (Table 48.1). The 2 other classes are gestational diabetes and other specific types of diabetes with various causes.
Normal Glucose and Insulin Metabolism. Insulin is a hormone made by the β cells in the islets of Langerhans of the pancreas. Under normal conditions, insulin is continuously released into

TABLE 48.1 **Comparison of Type 1 and Type 2 Diabetes**

Factor	Type 1 Diabetes	Type 2 Diabetes
Age at onset	More common in young people but can occur at any age	More common in adults but can occur at any age
		Incidence increasing in children
Type of onset	Signs and symptoms usually abrupt, but disease process may be present for several years	Gradual, may go undiagnosed for years
Prevalence	Accounts for 5%–10% of all types of diabetes	Accounts for 90%–95% of all types of diabetes
Endogenous insulin	Absent	Initially increased in response to insulin resistance. Secretion decreases over time
Environmental factors	Virus, toxins	Obesity, lack of exercise
Islet cell antibodies	Often present at onset	Absent
Primary defect	Absent or minimal insulin production	Insulin resistance, decreased insulin production over time, and changes in adipokines production
Symptoms	Polydipsia, polyuria, polyphagia, fatigue, weight loss without trying	Often none. Fatigue, recurrent infections. May also have polyuria, polydipsia, and polyphagia
Ketosis	Present at onset or during insulin deficiency	Not present except during infection or stress
Insulin therapy	Required for all	Required for some. Disease is progressive and insulin treatment may need to be added to treatment plan
Nutrition status	Thin, normal, or obese	Often overweight or obese. May be normal
Nutrition therapy	Essential	Essential
Vascular and neurologic complications	Frequent	Frequent

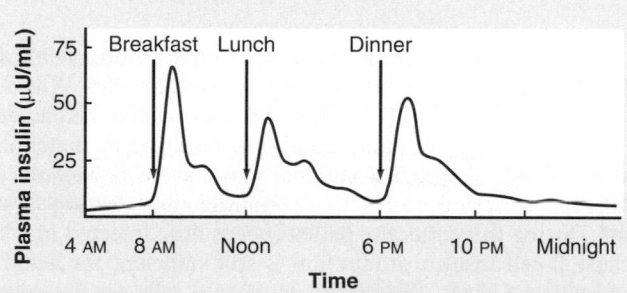

FIG. 48.1 Normal endogenous insulin secretion. After meals, insulin concentrations rise rapidly in blood and peak at about 1 hour. Then insulin concentrations promptly decline toward preprandial values as carbohydrate absorption from the GI tract declines. After carbohydrate absorption from the GI tract is complete and during the night, insulin concentrations are low and fairly constant, with a slight increase at dawn.

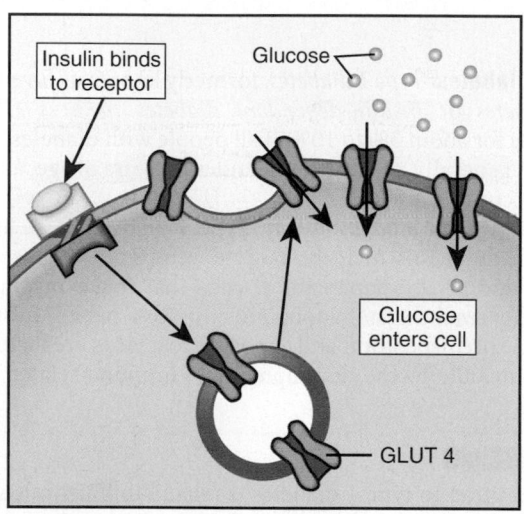

FIG. 48.2 Normal glucose metabolism. Insulin binds to receptors along the cell walls of muscle, adipose, and liver cells. Glucose transport proteins (GLUT 4s) then attach to the cell wall and allow glucose to enter the cell, where it is either stored or used to make energy.

the bloodstream in small amounts, with increased release when food is ingested (Fig. 48.1). Insulin lowers blood glucose and facilitates a stable, normal glucose range of about 74 to 106 mg/dL (4.1 to 5.9 mmol/L). The amount of insulin secreted daily by an adult is about 40 to 50 U, or 0.6 U/kg of body weight.

Insulin promotes glucose transport from the bloodstream across the cell membrane to the cytoplasm of the cell (Fig. 48.2). Cells break down glucose to make energy. Liver and muscle cells store excess glucose as glycogen. The rise in plasma insulin after a meal inhibits gluconeogenesis, enhances fat deposition of adipose tissue, and increases protein synthesis. For this reason, insulin is an *anabolic,* or storage, hormone. The fall in insulin level during normal overnight fasting promotes the release of stored glucose from the liver, protein from muscle, and fat from adipose tissue.

Skeletal muscle and adipose tissue have specific receptors for insulin and are considered insulin-dependent tissues. Insulin is required to "unlock" these receptor sites, allowing the transport of glucose into the cells to be used for energy. Other tissues (e.g., brain, liver, blood cells) do not directly depend on insulin for glucose transport but require an adequate glucose supply for normal function. Although liver cells are not considered

insulin-dependent tissue, insulin receptor sites on the liver facilitate uptake of glucose and its conversion to glycogen.

Other hormones (glucagon, epinephrine, growth hormone [GH], cortisol) work against the effects of insulin. They are *counterregulatory hormones.* These hormones increase blood glucose levels by (1) stimulating glucose production and release by the liver and (2) decreasing the movement of glucose into the cells. The counterregulatory hormones and insulin work together to maintain blood glucose levels within the normal range by regulating the release of glucose for energy during food intake and periods of fasting.

Insulin is synthesized from its precursor, proinsulin. Enzymes split proinsulin to form insulin and C-peptide, and the 2 substances are released in equal amounts. Therefore measuring C-peptide in serum and urine is a useful clinical indicator of pancreatic β-cell function and insulin levels.

GENETICS IN CLINICAL PRACTICE

Type 1 and Type 2 Diabetes and Maturity-Onset Diabetes of the Young (MODY)

Type 1 Diabetes	Type 2 Diabetes	MODY
Genetic Basis • Increased susceptibility (40%–50%) when a person has specific human leukocyte antigens (HLA-DR3, HLA-DR4) • Polygenic (>40 genes influence susceptibility)	• Polygenic (>25 genes influence susceptibility)	• Autosomal dominant • Monogenic (single gene) • Caused by mutations in any of 6 MODY genes (types 1–6) • Gene mutations lead to β-cell dysfunction
Risk to Offspring • Risk to offspring of mothers with diabetes is 1%–4% • Risk to offspring of fathers with diabetes is 5%–6% • When 1 identical twin has type 1 diabetes, the other gets the disease about 30%–40% of the time	• Risk to offspring is 8%–14% • When 1 identical twin has type 2 diabetes, the other gets it about 60%–75% of the time	• If 1 parent has MODY, a child has a 50% chance of developing disease • If 1 parent has MODY, a child has a 50% chance of being a carrier
Clinical Implications • Result of complex interaction of genetic, autoimmune, and environmental factors	• Result of complex genetic interactions and other metabolic factors • Metabolic factors are modified by environmental factors, such as body weight and exercise.	• Accounts for 1%–5% of people with diabetes • Young age of onset (often before age 25) • Not associated with obesity or hypertension • Treatment depends on the genetic mutation that caused MODY

Type 1 Diabetes. *Type 1 diabetes,* formerly known as *juvenile-onset diabetes* or *insulin-dependent diabetes mellitus (IDDM),* accounts for about 5% to 10% of all people with diabetes. Type 1 diabetes generally affects people under 40 years of age, although it can occur at any age.[3]

Etiology and Pathophysiology. Type 1 diabetes is an autoimmune disorder in which the body develops antibodies against insulin and/or the pancreatic β cells that make insulin. This eventually results in not enough insulin for a person to survive. A genetic predisposition and exposure to a virus are factors that may contribute to the development of immune-related type 1 diabetes.

Genetic Link

Predisposition to type 1 diabetes is related to human leukocyte antigens (HLAs) (see Chapter 13). In theory, when a person with certain HLA types is exposed to a viral infection, the β cells of the pancreas are destroyed, either directly or through an autoimmune process. The HLA types associated with an increased risk for type 1 diabetes include HLA-DR3 and HLA-DR4.

Idiopathic diabetes is a form of type 1 diabetes that is strongly inherited and not related to autoimmunity. It only occurs in a small number of people with type 1 diabetes, most often of Hispanic, African, or Asian ancestry.[3] *Latent autoimmune diabetes in adults* (LADA), a slowly progressing autoimmune form of type 1 diabetes. It occurs in adults and is often mistaken for type 2 diabetes.

Onset of Disease. In type 1 diabetes, the islet cell autoantibodies responsible for β-cell destruction are present for months to years before the onset of symptoms. Manifestations develop when the person's pancreas can no longer make enough insulin to maintain normal glucose. Once this occurs, the onset of symptoms is usually rapid. Patients often are initially seen with impending or actual ketoacidosis. The patient usually has a history of recent and sudden weight loss and the classic symptoms of *polydipsia* (excessive thirst), *polyuria* (frequent urination), and *polyphagia* (excessive hunger).

The person with type 1 diabetes requires insulin from an outside source *(exogenous insulin)* to sustain life. Without insulin, the patient will develop diabetes-related ketoacidosis (DKA), a life-threatening condition resulting in metabolic acidosis. Newly diagnosed patients may have a remission, or "honeymoon period," for 3 to 12 months after starting treatment. During this time, the patient needs little injected insulin because β-cell insulin production is still sufficient for healthy blood glucose levels. Eventually, as more β cells are destroyed and blood glucose levels increase, the honeymoon period ends and the patient will require insulin on a permanent basis.

Type 2 Diabetes. *Type 2 diabetes,* formerly known as *adult-onset diabetes* or *non–insulin-dependent diabetes mellitus (NIDDM),* accounts for about 90% to 95% of people with diabetes.[2] Many risk factors contribute to the development of type 2 diabetes. These include being overweight or obese, being older, and having a family history of type 2 diabetes. Although the disease is seen less often in children, the incidence is increasing due to the increasing prevalence of childhood obesity. Type 2 diabetes is more prevalent in some ethnic populations. Blacks, Asian Americans, Hispanics, Native Hawaiians or other Pacific Islanders, and Native Americans have a higher rate of type 2 diabetes than whites.[2]

PROMOTING HEALTH EQUITY
Diabetes

- Native Americans and Alaska Natives have highest prevalence for both men (14.9%) and women (15.3%).
- Pima Indians in Arizona have the highest rate of diabetes in the world (50% of adults).
- Native American and Alaska Native women are twice as likely to die from diabetes as white women.
- Rates are higher among blacks (12.7%) and Hispanics (12.1%) than among whites (7.4%) and Asians (8.0%).
- Blacks are twice as likely as whites to die from diabetes.

Etiology and Pathophysiology. Type 2 diabetes is characterized by a combination of inadequate insulin secretion and insulin resistance. The pancreas usually makes some *endogenous* (self-made) insulin. However, the body either does not make enough insulin or does not use it effectively, or both. The presence of endogenous insulin is a major distinction between type 1 and type 2 diabetes. In type 1 diabetes, there is an absence of endogenous insulin.

Genetic Link

Although we do not fully understand the genetics of type 2 diabetes, it is likely multiple genes are involved. We have found genetic mutations that lead to insulin resistance and a higher risk for obesity in many people with type 2 diabetes. Persons with a first-degree relative with the disease are 10 times more likely to develop type 2 diabetes.

Metabolic abnormalities have a role in the development of type 2 diabetes (Fig. 48.3). The first factor is insulin resistance, a condition in which body tissues do not respond to the action of insulin because insulin receptors are unresponsive, are insufficient in number, or both. Most insulin receptors are located on skeletal muscle, fat, and liver cells. When insulin is not properly used, the entry of glucose into the cell is impeded, resulting in hyperglycemia. In the early stages of insulin resistance, the pancreas responds to high blood glucose by producing greater amounts of insulin (if β cell function is normal). This

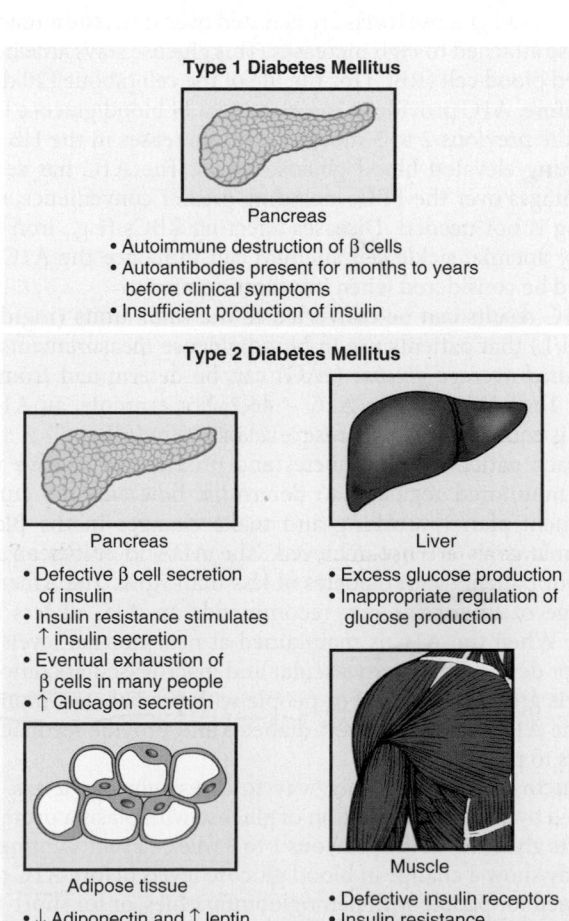

FIG. 48.3 Altered mechanisms in type 1 and type 2 diabetes.

creates a temporary state of hyperinsulinemia that coexists with hyperglycemia.

A second factor in the development of type 2 diabetes is a marked decrease in the ability of the pancreas to make insulin, as the β cells become fatigued from the compensatory overproduction of insulin or when β-cell mass is lost. The underlying basis for the failure of β cells to adapt is unknown. It may be linked to the adverse effects of chronic hyperglycemia or high circulating free fatty acids. In addition, the α cells of the pancreas increase production of glucagon.

This leads to a third factor, which is inappropriate glucose production by the liver. Instead of properly regulating the release of glucose in response to blood levels, the liver does so in a haphazard way that does not correspond to the body's needs at the time.

A fourth factor is altered production of hormones and cytokines by adipose tissue *(adipokines)*. Adipokines secreted by adipose tissue appear to play a role in glucose and fat metabolism and are likely to contribute to the development of type 2 diabetes.[4] We think adipokines cause chronic inflammation, a factor involved in insulin resistance, type 2 diabetes, and cardiovascular disease (CVD). The 2 main adipokines thought to affect insulin sensitivity are adiponectin and leptin. Finally, the brain, kidneys, and gut have roles in the development of type 2 diabetes. We are continuously learning more about metabolic factors in the development of type 2 diabetes.[4]

People with *metabolic syndrome* have an increased risk for developing type 2 diabetes. Metabolic syndrome has 5 components: increased glucose levels, abdominal obesity, high BP, high levels of triglycerides, and decreased levels of high-density lipoproteins (HDLs) (see Table 40.12). A person with 3 of the 5 components is considered to have metabolic syndrome.[5] Overweight persons with metabolic syndrome can reduce their risk for diabetes through a program of weight loss and regular physical activity. See Chapter 40 for more about metabolic syndrome.

Onset of Disease. The disease onset in type 2 diabetes is usually gradual. The person may go for many years with undetected hyperglycemia and few, if any, symptoms. Many people are diagnosed on routine laboratory testing or when they undergo treatment for other conditions, and elevated glucose or glycosylated hemoglobin (A1C) levels are found. The signs and symptoms of hyperglycemia develop when about 50% to 80% of β cells are no longer secreting insulin. At the time of diagnosis, the average person has had type 2 diabetes for 6½ years.

Prediabetes. Persons diagnosed with prediabetes are at increased risk for developing type 2 diabetes. Prediabetes is defined as impaired glucose tolerance (IGT), impaired fasting glucose (IFG), or both. It is an intermediate stage between normal glucose homeostasis and diabetes, in which the blood glucose levels are elevated but not high enough to meet the diagnostic criteria for diabetes.[6] A diagnosis of IGT is made if the 2-hour oral glucose tolerance test (OGTT) values are 140 to 199 mg/dL (7.8 to 11.0 mmol/L). IFG is diagnosed when fasting blood glucose levels are 100 to 125 mg/dL (5.56 to 6.9 mmol/L).

Persons with prediabetes usually do not have symptoms. However, long-term damage to the body, especially the heart and blood vessels, may already be occurring. It is important for patients to undergo screening and to understand risk factors for diabetes. People with prediabetes can take action to prevent or delay the development of type 2 diabetes. Encourage those with prediabetes to have their blood glucose and A1C checked regularly and monitor for symptoms of diabetes, such as fatigue, frequent infections, or slow-healing wounds. Maintaining a healthy weight, exercising regularly, and making healthy food choices reduce the risk for developing overt type 2 diabetes in people with prediabetes.

Gestational Diabetes. *Gestational diabetes* develops during pregnancy and occurs in about 2% to 10% of pregnancies in the United States.[7] Women with gestational diabetes have a higher risk for cesarean delivery, and their babies have increased risk for perinatal death, birth injury, and neonatal complications. Women who are at high risk for gestational diabetes are screened at the first prenatal visit. Those at high risk include women who are obese, are of advanced maternal age, or have a family history of diabetes. Women with an average risk for gestational diabetes are screened using an OGTT at 24 to 28 weeks of gestation. Most women with gestational diabetes have normal glucose levels within 6 weeks postpartum. Women with a history of gestational diabetes have up to a 63% chance of developing type 2 diabetes within 16 years.[7] Gestational diabetes and managing the pregnant patient with diabetes are specialized areas not covered in detail in this chapter. Consult an obstetric text for more information.

Other Specific Types of Diabetes. Diabetes occurs in some people because of another medical condition or treatment of a medical condition that causes abnormal blood glucose levels. Conditions that may cause diabetes can result from injury to, interference with, or destruction of the β-cell function in the pancreas. These include Cushing syndrome, hyperthyroidism, recurrent pancreatitis, cystic fibrosis, hemochromatosis, and parenteral nutrition. Common drugs that can induce diabetes include corticosteroids (prednisone), thiazides, phenytoin (Dilantin), and atypical antipsychotics (e.g., clozapine [Clozaril]). Diabetes caused by medical conditions or drugs can resolve when the underlying condition is treated or the drug is discontinued.

Clinical Manifestations

Type 1 Diabetes. Because the onset of type 1 diabetes is rapid, the first manifestations are usually acute. The classic symptoms are *polyuria, polydipsia,* and *polyphagia.* The osmotic effect of excess glucose in the bloodstream causes polydipsia and polyuria. Polyphagia is a result of cellular malnourishment when insulin deficiency prevents cells from using glucose for energy. Weight loss may occur because the body cannot get glucose and instead breaks down fat and protein to try to make energy. Weakness and fatigue may result because body cells lack needed energy from glucose. Ketoacidosis, a complication most common in those with untreated type 1 diabetes, is associated with additional manifestations. It is discussed later in this chapter.

Type 2 Diabetes. The manifestations of type 2 diabetes are often nonspecific. It is possible a person with type 2 diabetes will have classic symptoms associated with type 1 diabetes, including polyuria, polydipsia, and polyphagia. Some of the more common manifestations associated with type 2 diabetes are fatigue, recurrent infections, recurrent vaginal yeast or candida infections, prolonged wound healing, and vision problems.

Diagnostic Studies

The diagnosis of diabetes is made using 1 of the following 4 methods:

1. A1C of 6.5% or higher
2. Fasting plasma glucose (FPG) level of 126 mg/dL (7.0 mmol/L) or greater. *Fasting* is defined as no caloric intake for at least 8 hours

3. A 2-hour plasma glucose level of 200 mg/dL (11.1 mmol/L) or greater during an OGTT, using a glucose load of 75 g
4. In a patient with classic symptoms of hyperglycemia (polyuria, polydipsia, unexplained weight loss) or hyperglycemic crisis, a random plasma glucose level of 200 mg/dL (11.1 mmol/L) or greater

If a patient is seen with a hyperglycemic crisis or clear symptoms of hyperglycemia (polyuria, polydipsia, polyphagia) with a random plasma glucose level of 200 mg/dL or greater, repeat testing is not needed. Otherwise, criteria 1 through 3 require confirmation by repeat testing to rule out laboratory error. It is preferable for the repeat test to be the same test used initially. For example, if a random elevated blood glucose is used for the initial measurement, that same measure should be used to confirm a diagnosis.

The accuracy of laboratory results depends on adequate patient preparation and attention to the many factors that may influence the results. For example, factors that can falsely elevate values include recent severe restrictions of dietary carbohydrate, acute illness, drugs (e.g., contraceptives, corticosteroids), and restricted activity, such as bed rest. A patient with impaired gastrointestinal (GI) absorption or who has recently taken acetaminophen may have false-negative results.

A1C measures the amount of glycosylated hemoglobin (Hgb) as a percentage of total Hgb. For example, A1C of 6.5% means that 6.5% of the total Hgb has glucose attached to it. The amount of glycosylated Hgb depends on the blood glucose level. When blood glucose levels are elevated over time, the amount of glucose attached to Hgb increases. This glucose stays attached to the red blood cell (RBC) for the life of the cell (about 120 days). Therefore, A1C provides a measurement of blood glucose levels over the previous 2 to 3 months, with increases in the Hb A1C reflecting elevated blood glucose levels. The A1C has several advantages over the FPG, including greater convenience, since fasting is not needed. Diseases affecting RBCs (e.g., iron deficiency anemia, sickle cell anemia) can influence the A1C and should be considered when interpreting results.

A1C results can be converted to the same units (mg/dL or mmol/L) that patients use in blood glucose measurements. An *estimated average glucose* (eAG) can be determined from the A1C. The eAG = $28.7 \times$ A1C $- 46.7$. For example, an A1C of 8.0% is equivalent to a glucose level of 183 mg/dL.

Teach patients with diabetes and prediabetes to have their A1C monitored regularly to determine how well the current treatment plan is working and make changes in the plan if glycemic goals are not achieved. The ADA identifies an A1C goal for patients with diabetes of less than 7.0%. The American College of Endocrinology recommends an A1C of less than 6.5%. When the A1C is maintained at near-normal levels, the risk for developing microvascular and macrovascular complications is greatly reduced. For people with prediabetes, monitoring the A1C can detect overt diabetes and provide feedback on efforts to prevent diabetes.

Fructosamine is another way to assess glucose levels. It is formed by a chemical reaction of glucose with plasma protein. It reflects glycemia in the previous 1 to 3 weeks. Fructosamine levels may show a change in blood glucose levels before A1C does. It is used for people with hemoglobinopathies, or for short-term measurement of glucose levels, for instance, after a change in medication or during pregnancy.

Islet cell autoantibody testing is primarily done to help distinguish between autoimmune type 1 diabetes and diabetes from other causes. Autoantibodies can develop to 1 or several autoantigens, including GAD65, IA-2, or insulin.

Interprofessional Care

The goals of diabetes management are to reduce symptoms, promote well-being, prevent acute complications related to hyperglycemia and hypoglycemia, and prevent or delay the onset and progression of long-term complications. These goals are most likely to be met when the patient maintains blood glucose levels as near to normal as possible. Patient teaching, which enables the patient to become the most active participant in their own care, is essential to achieve glycemic goals. Nutrition therapy, drug therapy, exercise, and self-monitoring of blood glucose are the tools used in managing diabetes (Table 48.2).

The 3 major types of glucose-lowering agents (GLAs) used in the treatment of diabetes are insulin, oral agents (OAs), and noninsulin injectable agents. All persons with type 1 diabetes require insulin. For some people with type 2 diabetes, a healthy eating plan, regular physical activity, and maintaining a healthy body weight are enough to attain optimal blood glucose levels. Eventually, most people will need medication management because type 2 diabetes is a progressive disease.

Drug Therapy: Insulin

Exogenous (injected) insulin is needed when a patient has inadequate insulin to meet specific metabolic needs. People with type 1 diabetes require exogenous insulin to survive. They often use multiple daily injections of insulin (often 4 or more) or continuous insulin infusion via an insulin pump to adequately manage blood glucose levels. People with type 2 diabetes may need exogenous insulin during periods of severe stress, such as

TABLE 48.2 Interprofessional Care

Diabetes

Diagnostic Assessment
- History and physical examination
- Blood tests, including fasting blood glucose, postprandial blood glucose, A1C, fructosamine, lipid profile, BUN and serum creatinine, electrolytes, islet cell autoantibodies
- Urine for complete urinalysis, albuminuria, and acetone (if indicated)
- BP
- ECG (if indicated)
- Funduscopic examination (dilated eye examination)
- Dental examination
- Neurologic examination, including monofilament test for sensation to lower extremities
- Ankle-brachial index (ABI) (if indicated) (see Table 37.3)
- Foot (podiatric) examination
- Monitoring of weight

Management
- Patient and caregiver teaching and follow-up programs
- Nutrition therapy (Table 48.8)
- Exercise therapy (Tables 48.9 and 48.10)
- Self-monitoring of blood glucose (SMBG) (Table 48.11)

Drug Therapy
- Insulin (Fig. 48.3 and Tables 48.3 and 48.4)
- OAs and noninsulin injectable agents (Table 48.7)
- Enteric-coated aspirin (81–162 mg/day)
- ACE inhibitors (see Table 32.6)
- Angiotensin II receptor blockers (ARBs) (see Table 32.6)
- Antihyperlipidemic drugs (see Table 33.6)

illness or surgery. Since type 2 diabetes is a progressive disease, over time, the combination of nutrition therapy, exercise, OAs, and noninsulin injectable agents may no longer adequately manage blood glucose levels. At that point, exogenous insulin is added as part of the management plan. People with type 2 diabetes may also need up to 4 injections per day to adequately maintain their blood glucose levels. Insulin pumps also can be used for patients with type 2 diabetes.

Types of Insulin. Today, people use only genetically engineered human insulin made in laboratories. The insulin is derived from common bacteria (e.g., *Escherichia coli*) or yeast cells using recombinant deoxyribonucleic acid (DNA) technology. In the past, insulin was extracted from beef and pork pancreases. These forms of insulin are no longer available.

Insulins differ by their onset, peak action, and duration (Fig. 48.4). They are categorized as rapid-acting, short-acting, intermediate-acting, and long-acting insulin (Table 48.3).

Insulin Plans. Examples of insulin plans are shown in Table 48.4. The insulin approach that most closely mimics endogenous insulin production is the basal-bolus plan (often called *intensive or physiologic insulin therapy*). It consists of multiple daily insulin injections (or an insulin pump) together with frequent self-monitoring of blood glucose (or a continuous glucose monitoring system). Injections include rapid- or short-acting (bolus) insulin before meals and intermediate- or long-acting (basal) background insulin once or twice a day. The goal is to achieve a glucose level as close to normal as possible, as much of the time as possible. This is referred to as "time in range."

Other, less intense plans can promote healthy blood glucose levels for some people. Ideally, the patient and the HCP will work together to choose a plan. Selection criteria are based on the desired and feasible blood glucose levels and the patient's lifestyle, food choices, and activity patterns. If a less intense plan is not giving the person optimal results, the HCP may encourage a more intense approach.

Mealtime Insulin (Bolus). To manage postprandial blood glucose levels, the timing of rapid- and short-acting insulin in relation to meals is crucial. Rapid-acting synthetic insulin analogs, which include aspart (NovoLog), glulisine (Apidra), and lispro (Humalog), have an onset of action of about 15 minutes. They should be injected within 15 minutes of mealtime. The rapid-acting analogs most closely mimic natural insulin secretion in response to a meal.

Short-acting regular insulin has an onset of action of 30 to 60 minutes. It is injected 30 to 45 minutes before a meal to ensure that the insulin is working at the same time as meal absorption. Because timing an injection 30 to 45 minutes before a meal is hard for some people to do with their lifestyles, the flexibility that rapid-acting insulins offer is preferred by those taking insulin with their meals.[8] Short-acting insulin is more likely to cause hypoglycemia because of a longer duration of action.

Long- or Intermediate-Acting (Basal) Background Insulin. In addition to mealtime insulin, people with type 1 diabetes use a long- or intermediate-acting basal (background) insulin to maintain blood glucose levels in between meals and overnight. Without 24-hour background insulin, people with type 1 diabetes are more prone to developing DKA. Many people with type 2 diabetes who use OAs will need basal insulin to adequately manage blood glucose levels.

The long-acting insulins include degludec (Tresiba), detemir (Levemir), and glargine (Lantus, Toujeo, Basaglar). This type of insulin is released steadily and continuously. For most people,

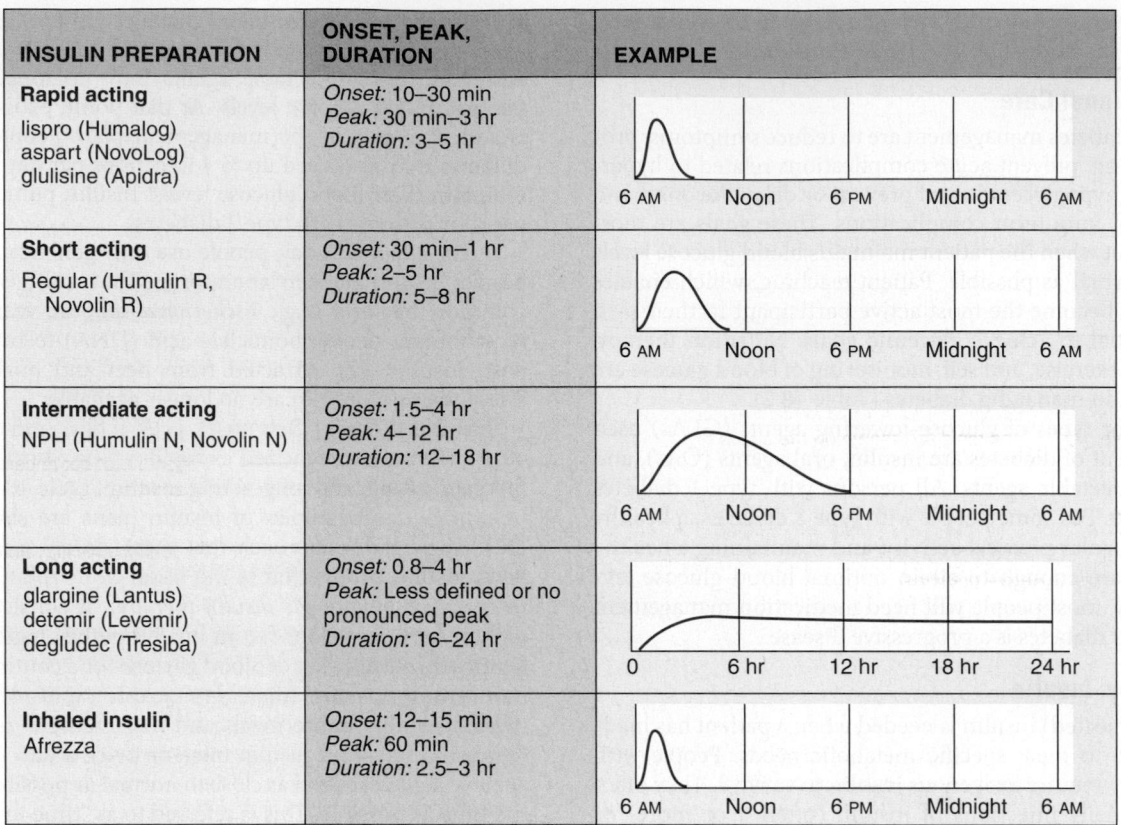

INSULIN PREPARATION	ONSET, PEAK, DURATION	EXAMPLE
Rapid acting lispro (Humalog) aspart (NovoLog) glulisine (Apidra)	*Onset:* 10–30 min *Peak:* 30 min–3 hr *Duration:* 3–5 hr	
Short acting Regular (Humulin R, Novolin R)	*Onset:* 30 min–1 hr *Peak:* 2–5 hr *Duration:* 5–8 hr	
Intermediate acting NPH (Humulin N, Novolin N)	*Onset:* 1.5–4 hr *Peak:* 4–12 hr *Duration:* 12–18 hr	
Long acting glargine (Lantus) detemir (Levemir) degludec (Tresiba)	*Onset:* 0.8–4 hr *Peak:* Less defined or no pronounced peak *Duration:* 16–24 hr	
Inhaled insulin Afrezza	*Onset:* 12–15 min *Peak:* 60 min *Duration:* 2.5–3 hr	

FIG. 48.4 Commercially available insulin preparations showing onset, peak, and duration of action. Individual patient responses to each type of insulin are different and affected by many different factors.

TABLE 48.3 Drug Therapy

Types of Insulin

Classification	Examples
Rapid-acting insulin	aspart (NovoLog) glulisine (Apidra) lispro (Humalog)
Short-acting insulin	regular (Humulin R, Novolin R)
Intermediate-acting insulin	NPH (Humulin N, Novolin N)
Long-acting insulin	degludec (Tresiba) detemir (Levemir) glargine (Basaglar, Lantus, Toujeo) insulin glargine (Basaglar)
Combination therapy (premixed)	aspart protamine/aspart 70/30* (NovoLog Mix 70/30) degludec/aspart 70/30 (Ryzodeg) lispro protamine/lispro 75/25* (Humalog Mix 75/25) lispro protamine/lispro 50/50* (Humalog Mix 50/50) NPH/regular 70/30* (Humulin 70/30, Novolin 70/30) NPH/regular 50/50* (Humulin 50/50)
More concentrated insulin	Humulin R U-500 Toujeo U-300 (insulin glargine)
Inhaled insulin	Afrezza

*These numbers refer to percentages of each type of insulin.

it does not have a peak of action. The action time for long-acting insulin varies (Fig. 48.4). Although they can be given once daily, detemir is often given twice daily. Because they lack peak action time, the risk for hypoglycemia from this type of insulin is greatly reduced. Glargine and detemir must not be diluted or

mixed with any other insulin or solution in the same syringe. If OAs and long-acting insulin are not adequate to achieve glycemic goals, mealtime insulin may be added.

Intermediate-acting insulin (NPH) can be used as a basal insulin. It has a duration of 12 to 18 hours. The disadvantage of NPH is that it has a peak ranging from 4 to 12 hours, which can result in hypoglycemia. NPH can be mixed with short- and rapid-acting insulins. It should never be given IV.

CHECK YOUR PRACTICE

You are preparing your patient's order for NPH insulin. When you look at the vial, you notice that it is cloudy. You are thinking that you should throw away the vial because has become contaminated.
- Before you take this action, what should you do?

All insulins are clear solutions except NPH, lispro protamine, and aspart protamine. They are cloudy because they contain a protein called protamine, which makes them work longer. These insulins must be gently agitated before administration.

Combination Insulin Therapy. For those who want to use only 1 or 2 injections per day, a short- or rapid-acting insulin is mixed with intermediate-acting insulin in the same syringe. This allows the patient to have both mealtime and basal coverage without having to give 2 separate injections. Although this may be more appealing to the patient, most patients achieve optimal blood glucose levels with basal-bolus therapy. Patients may mix the 2 types of insulin themselves or use a commercially premixed formula or pen (Table 48.3). Premixed formulas offer

TABLE 48.4 Drug Therapy

Insulin Regimens

Regimen	Type of Insulin and Frequency	Action Profile	Comments
Once a day Single dose	Intermediate (NPH) *At bedtime*	7 AM Noon 6 PM Midnight 7 AM	1 injection should provide nighttime coverage.
	OR Long-acting (degludec [Tresiba], detemir [Levemir], glargine [Lantus]) *In AM or at bedtime*	7 AM Noon 6 PM Midnight 7 AM	1 injection may last up to 24 hr with fewer defined peaks and less chance for hypoglycemia. Does not cover postprandial blood glucose levels.
Twice a day Split-mixed dose	NPH and regular or rapid (both regular and rapid are shown on the diagram) *Before breakfast and at dinner*	7 AM Noon 6 PM Midnight 7 AM	2 injections provide coverage for 24 hr. Patient must eat at certain times to avoid hypoglycemia.
Three times a day Combination of mixed and single dose	NPH and regular or rapid (both regular and rapid are shown on the diagram) *Before breakfast* + Regular or rapid *Before dinner* + NPH *At bedtime*	7 AM Noon 7 PM 9 PM Midnight 7 AM	3 injections provide coverage for 24 hr, especially during early AM hours. Decreased potential for 2–3 AM hypoglycemia
Basal-bolus Multiple dose	Regular or rapid (both regular and rapid are shown on the diagram) *Before breakfast, lunch, and dinner* + Long-acting (degludec, detemir, or glargine) *Once or twice a day* *OR* Regular or rapid (both regular and rapid are shown on the diagram) *Before breakfast, lunch, and dinner* + NPH *Twice a day*	7 AM Noon 6 PM Midnight 7 AM 7 AM Noon 6 PM Midnight 7 AM	More flexibility is allowed at mealtimes and for amount of food intake. Good postprandial coverage. Preprandial blood glucose checks and following an individualized plan is necessary. Patients with type 1 diabetes require basal insulin to cover 24 hr. Most physiologic approach, except for pump

———— Rapid-acting (lispro, aspart, glulisine) insulin.

———— Short-acting (regular) insulin.

- - - - - - - Intermediate-acting (NPH) or long-acting (glargine, detemir, degludec) insulin.

convenience to patients, who do not have to draw up and mix insulin from 2 different vials. This is especially helpful to those who lack the visual, manual, or cognitive skills to mix insulin themselves. However, the convenience of these formulas limits the potential for optimal blood glucose levels because there is less opportunity for flexible dosing based on need.

Storage of Insulin. As a protein, insulin has special storage considerations. Extreme temperatures alter the insulin molecule and can make it less effective. Insulin vials and pens in use may be left at room temperature for up to 4 weeks unless the room temperature is higher than 86° F (30° C) or below freezing (less than 32° F [0° C]). Teach patients to avoid prolonged exposure to direct sunlight. A patient who is traveling in hot climates may store insulin in a thermos or cooler to keep it cool (not frozen). Store unopened insulin vials and pens in the refrigerator.

Patients who are traveling or caregivers of patients who are sight impaired or who lack the manual dexterity to fill their own syringes may prefill insulin syringes. Prefilled syringes with 2 different insulins are stable for up to 1 week when stored in the refrigerator. Syringes with only 1 type of insulin are stable up to 30 days.

Teach patients to store syringes in a vertical position with the needle pointed up to avoid clumping of suspended insulin in the needle. Before injection, gently roll prefilled syringes between the palms 10 to 20 times to warm the insulin and resuspend the particles. Some insulin combinations cannot be prefilled and stored because the mixture can alter the onset, action, and/or peak times of either insulin. Consult a reference as needed when mixing and prefilling different types of insulin.

Administration of Insulin. Routine doses of insulin are given by subcutaneous injection. Regular insulin can be given IV when immediate onset of action is desired. Insulin is not taken orally because it is inactivated by gastric fluids. Teach patients to avoid injecting insulin IM because rapid and unpredictable absorption could result in hypoglycemia.

Insulin Injection. The steps in giving a subcutaneous insulin injection are outlined in Table 48.5. Teach this technique to new insulin users and review it periodically with long-term users.

TABLE 48.5 Patient & Caregiver Teaching

Preparing an Insulin Injection

Include the following instructions when teaching the patient and caregiver about insulin therapy:

1. Wash hands thoroughly.
2. Always inspect insulin bottle before using it. Make sure that it is the proper type and concentration, expiration date has not passed, and top of bottle is in perfect condition. Insulin solutions (except for NPH, lispro protamine, aspart protamine) should look clear and colorless. Discard if it appears discolored or if you see particles in the solution.
3. For intermediate-acting insulins (which are normally cloudy), gently roll the insulin bottle between the palms of hands to mix the insulin. Clear insulins do not need to be agitated.
4. Choose proper injection site (Fig. 48.5).
5. Ensure that the site is clean and dry.
6. Push the needle straight into the skin (90-degree angle). If you are very thin, muscular, or using an 8- or 12-mm needle, you may need to pinch the skin and/or use a 45-degree angle.
7. Push the plunger all the way down, leave needle in place for 5 sec to ensure that all insulin has been injected, and then remove needle.
8. Destroy and dispose of single-use syringe safely.

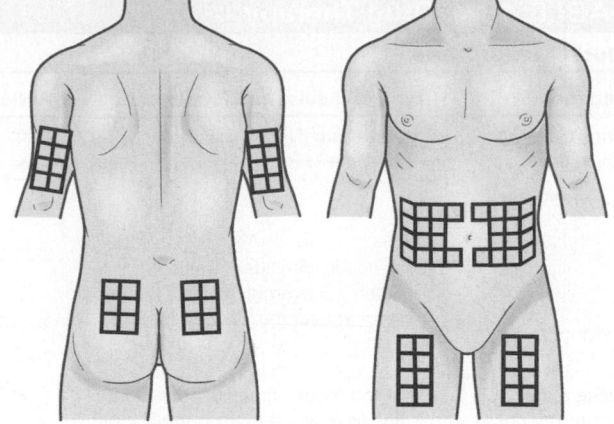

FIG. 48.5 Injection sites for insulin.

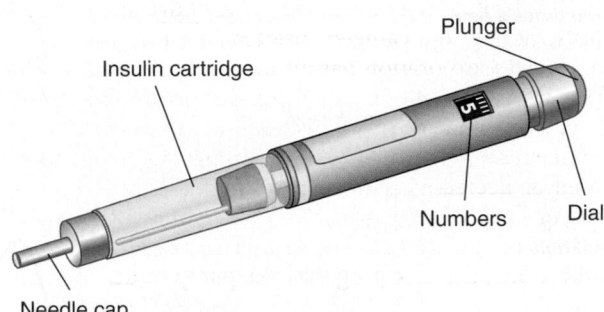

FIG. 48.6 Parts of insulin pen.

Never assume that because the patient already uses insulin, they know and practice the correct insulin injection technique. The patient may not have understood prior instructions, or changes in eyesight may result in inaccurate preparation.[9] The patient may not see air bubbles in the syringe or may improperly read the scale on the syringe. The patient receiving mixed insulins in the same syringe needs to learn the proper technique for combining them if commercially prepared premixed insulins are not used.

The speed with which peak serum concentrations are reached varies with the injection site. The fastest subcutaneous absorption is from the abdomen, followed by the arm, thigh, and buttock. Although the abdomen is often the preferred injection site, other sites work well (Fig. 48.5). Caution the patient about injecting into a site that is to be exercised. For example, injecting into the thigh and then going jogging could increase body heat and circulation. This could increase the rate of insulin absorption and speed the onset of action, resulting in hypoglycemia.

Teach patients to rotate the injection within and between sites. This allows for better insulin absorption. It may be helpful to think of the abdomen as a checkerboard, with each ½-in square representing an injection site. Injections are rotated systematically across the board, with each injection site at least ½ to 1 inch away from the previous injection site. It can be helpful to inject fast-acting insulin into faster-absorbing sites and slow-acting insulin into slower absorbing sites.

Most commercial insulin is available as U100. This means that 1 mL contains 100 U of insulin. U100 insulin must be used with a U100-marked syringe. Disposable plastic insulin syringes are available in a variety of sizes, including 1.0, 0.5, and 0.3 mL. The 0.5-mL size may be used for doses of 50 U or less. The 0.3-mL syringe can be used for doses of 30 U or less. The 0.5- and 0.3-mL syringes are in 1-unit increments. This provides more accurate delivery when the dose is an odd number. The 1.0-mL syringe is necessary for patients who inject more than 50 U of insulin. The 1.0-mL syringe is in 2-unit increments. When patients change from a 0.3- or a 0.5-mL to a 1.0-mL syringe, tell them of the dose increment difference.

Insulin syringe needles come in 3 lengths: 6 mm (½ in), 8 mm (⅝₆ in), and 12.7 mm (½ in).[10] Needle gauges vary among syringes. The needle gauges available are 28, 29, 30, and 31. The higher the gauge number, the smaller the diameter, thus resulting in a more comfortable injection. Only the person using the syringe should recap the needle; never recap a needle used for a patient. To prepare the site, routine hygiene, such as washing with soap and rinsing with water, is adequate. This applies primarily to patient self-injection technique. When injection occurs in a health care agency, policy usually mandates site preparation with alcohol to prevent health care–associated infection (HAI).

Insulin injections are typically given at a 90-degree angle. For extremely thin or muscular patients in the hospital, perform injections at a 45-degree angle. At home, patients inject at a 90-degree angle using the shortest needle desired. Pinching up of the skin to avoid IM injection is no longer done because of the use of short needles.

An insulin pen is a compact portable device loaded with an insulin cartridge that serves the same function as a needle and syringe (Fig. 48.6). Pen needles are available in lengths of 4 mm (⁵⁄₃₂ in), 5 mm (³⁄₁₆ in), 8 mm (⁵⁄₁₆ in), and 12.7 mm (½ in) and in 3 gauges: 29, 31, and 32. Insulin pens offer convenience and flexibility. They are portable and compact, are more discreet than using a vial and syringe, and provide consistent and accurate dosing. For patients with poor vision, the pen is a better option, since they can hear the clicks of the pen as the dose is selected. Insulin pens come packaged with printed instructions, including pictures of the steps to take when using the pen. These instructions are helpful when teaching new users and reviewing technique with current users of a pen.

Insulin Pump. An *insulin pump* delivers a continuous subcutaneous insulin infusion through a small device worn on the belt,

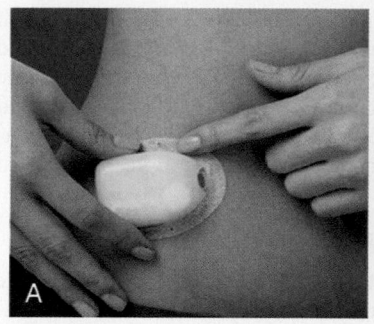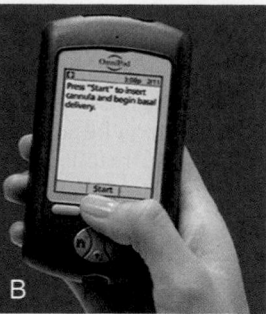

FIG. 48.7 A, OmniPod Insulin Management System. The Pod holds and delivers insulin. B, The Personal Diabetes Manager (PDM) wirelessly programs insulin delivery via the Pod. The PDM has a built-in glucose meter. (Courtesy of Insulet Corporation.)

in a pocket, or under clothing. Insulin pumps use rapid-acting insulin. It is loaded into a reservoir or cartridge and connected via plastic tubing to a catheter inserted into the subcutaneous tissue. Insulet Corporation has an insulin pump that is a tubing-free system (Fig. 48.7). All insulin pumps are programmed to deliver a continuous infusion of rapid-acting insulin 24 hours a day, known as the *basal rate*. Basal insulin can be temporarily increased or decreased based on carbohydrate intake, activity changes, or illness. Pump users need different basal rates at different times of the day.

At mealtime, the user programs the pump to deliver a bolus infusion of insulin appropriate to the amount of carbohydrate ingested and an additional amount, if needed, to bring down or "correct" high preprandial blood glucose. The infusion set is changed every 2 to 3 days and placed in a new site to avoid infection and promote good insulin absorption. Insulin pump users check their blood glucose level at least 4 times per day and/or use a continuous glucose monitoring system. Monitoring 8 times or more per day is common.

A major advantage of the insulin pump is the potential for keeping blood glucose levels in a tighter range with a goal of eliminating both high and low glucose. With careful programming and constant monitoring, this is possible because insulin delivery is similar to the normal physiologic pattern. Pumps offer users more flexibility with meal and activity patterns. Potential challenges of insulin pump therapy include infection at the insertion site, an increased risk for DKA if the insulin infusion is disrupted, the cost of the pump and supplies, and being attached to a device.[11]

Problems With Insulin Therapy. Problems associated with insulin therapy include hypoglycemia, allergic reactions, lipodystrophy, hypertrophy, and the Somogyi effect. Hypoglycemia is discussed in detail later in this chapter. Guidelines for assessing patients treated with insulin and other GLAs are outlined in Table 48.6.

Allergic Reactions. Local inflammatory reactions to insulin may occur, such as itching, erythema, and burning around the injection site. Local reactions may be self-limiting within 1 to 3 months or may improve with a low dose of antihistamine. A true insulin allergy, which is rare, is manifested by a systemic response with urticaria and possibly anaphylactic shock. Preservative in the insulin and the latex or rubber stoppers on the vials have been implicated in allergic reactions.

Lipodystrophy and Hypertrophy. Lipodystrophy (loss of subcutaneous fatty tissue) may occur if the same injection sites are used frequently. The use of human insulin has significantly reduced

TABLE 48.6 **Assessing the Patient Treated With Glucose-Lowering Agents**	
Category	**Assessment**
For Patient With Newly Diagnosed Diabetes or for Reevaluation of Medication Plan	
Affective	• What emotions and attitudes are patient and caregiver displaying concerning diagnosis of diabetes and insulin or OA treatment?
Cognitive	• Is patient or caregiver able to understand why insulin or OAs are being used as part of diabetes management?
	• Is patient or caregiver able to understand concepts of asepsis, combining insulins, and side effects of medications?
	• Is patient able to remember to take >1 dose/day?
	• Does patient take medications at right times in relation to meals?
Psychomotor	• Is patient or caregiver physically able to prepare and give accurate doses of the drugs?
For Patient Follow-up	
Effectiveness of therapy	• Is patient having symptoms of hyperglycemia?
	• Does blood glucose record show blood glucose levels in or out of the target range?
	• Is A1C in a healthy range and consistent with glucose records?
Self-management behaviors	• If patient is having hyperglycemia or hypoglycemia, how are those episodes managed?
	• Has patient determined reason for hyperglycemia or hypoglycemia?
	• How much insulin or OA is patient taking and at what time of day? Is patient adjusting insulin dose? Under what circumstances and by how much?
	• Has the exercise pattern changed?
	• Is patient making healthy food choices? Are meals taken at times corresponding to peak insulin action?
Side effects of therapy	• Is atrophy or hypertrophy present at injection sites?
	• Has patient had hypoglycemia? If so, how often? What time of day? What were the symptoms of hypoglycemia?
	• Are there reports of nightmares, night sweats, or early morning headaches?
	• Has patient had a skin rash or GI upset since taking OAs?
	• Has patient gained or lost weight?

the risk for lipodystrophy. *Atrophy*, which is uncommon, is the wasting of subcutaneous tissue and presents as indentations in injection sites. *Hypertrophy* happens more often and is a thickening of the subcutaneous tissue. It eventually regresses if the patient does not use the site for at least 6 months. Injecting into a hypertrophied site may result in erratic insulin absorption.

Somogyi Effect and Dawn Phenomenon. Hyperglycemia in the morning may be due to the Somogyi effect. A high dose of insulin causes a decline in blood glucose levels during the night. As a result, counterregulatory hormones (e.g., glucagon, epinephrine, GH, cortisol) are released. They stimulate lipolysis, gluconeogenesis, and glycogenolysis, which in turn cause rebound hyperglycemia. The danger of this effect is that when blood glucose levels are measured in the morning, hyperglycemia is apparent and the patient (or the HCP) may increase the insulin dose.

If a patient has morning hyperglycemia, checking blood glucose levels between 2:00 and 4:00 AM for hypoglycemia will help determine if the cause is the Somogyi effect. The patient may report headaches on awakening and recall having night sweats or nightmares.

The dawn phenomenon is also characterized by hyperglycemia that is present on awakening. Two counterregulatory hormones (GH and cortisol), which are excreted in increased amounts in the early morning hours, may be the cause of this phenomenon. The dawn phenomenon affects many people with diabetes and tends to be most severe when GH is at its peak in adolescence and young adulthood.

Careful assessment is needed to diagnose the Somogyi effect or dawn phenomenon because the treatment for each differs. The treatment for Somogyi effect is a bedtime snack, reducing the dose of insulin, or both. The treatment for dawn phenomenon is an increase in insulin or an adjustment in administration time. Your assessment must include insulin dose, injection sites, and variability in the time of meals or insulin administration. Ask the patient to measure and document bedtime, nighttime (between 2:00 and 4:00 AM), and morning fasting blood glucose levels on several occasions. If the predawn levels are less than 60 mg/dL (3.3 mmol/L) and signs and symptoms of hypoglycemia are present, the insulin dosage should be reduced. If the 2:00 to 4:00 AM blood glucose is high, the insulin dosage should be increased. Counsel the patient on appropriate bedtime snacks.

Inhaled Insulin. Afrezza is a rapid-acting inhaled insulin. It is given at the beginning of each meal or within 20 minutes after starting a meal. Afrezza must be used in combination with long-acting insulin in patients with type 1 diabetes. It should not be used to treat diabetic ketoacidosis. Patients with chronic lung disease, such as asthma or COPD, or who smoke, should not use Afrezza because bronchospasm can occur. Other common adverse reactions are hypoglycemia, cough, and throat pain or irritation.

Drug Therapy: Oral and Noninsulin Injectable Agents

OAs and noninsulin injectable agents work to improve the mechanisms by which the body makes and uses insulin and glucose. These drugs primarily work on 3 defects of type 2 diabetes: (1) insulin resistance, (2) decreased insulin production, and (3) increased hepatic glucose production (Fig. 48.8). These drugs may be used in combination with agents from other classes or with insulin to achieve blood glucose goals. OAs and noninsulin injectable agents are listed in Table 48.7.

Biguanides. The most widely used OA is metformin. It is the only drug in the biguanide class available in the United States. Metformin is the most effective first-line treatment for type 2 diabetes.[8] Forms of metformin include Glucophage (immediate release), Glucophage XR (extended release), Fortamet (extended release), and Riomet (liquid). The primary action of metformin is to reduce glucose production by the liver. It enhances insulin sensitivity at the tissue level and improves glucose transport into the cells. It also has beneficial effects on plasma lipids.

Because it may cause moderate weight loss, metformin may be useful for people with type 2 diabetes and prediabetes who

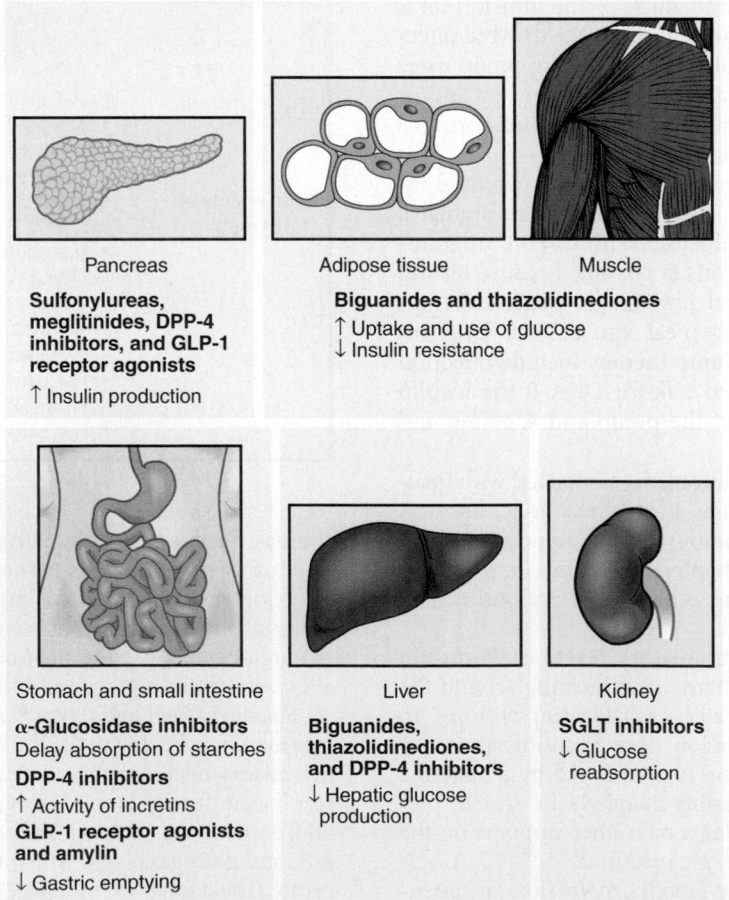

Pancreas

Sulfonylureas, meglitinides, DPP-4 inhibitors, and GLP-1 receptor agonists

↑ Insulin production

Adipose tissue

Biguanides and thiazolidinediones

↑ Uptake and use of glucose
↓ Insulin resistance

Muscle

Stomach and small intestine

α-Glucosidase inhibitors
Delay absorption of starches

DPP-4 inhibitors
↑ Activity of incretins

GLP-1 receptor agonists and amylin
↓ Gastric emptying

Liver

Biguanides, thiazolidinediones, and DPP-4 inhibitors
↓ Hepatic glucose production

Kidney

SGLT inhibitors
↓ Glucose reabsorption

FIG. 48.8 Sites and mechanisms of action of type 2 diabetes drugs. *DDP-4,* Dipeptidyl peptidase; *GLP-1,* glucagon-like peptide-1; *SGLT,* sodium-glucose co-transporter.

TABLE 48.7 **Drug Therapy**

Oral Agents and Noninsulin Injectable Agents

Type	Mechanism of Action	Side Effects
Oral Agents		
α-Glucosidase Inhibitors		
acarbose (Precose)	Delays absorption of complex carbohydrates (starches) from GI tract	Gas, abdominal pain, diarrhea
miglitol (Glyset)		
Biguanides		
metformin (Fortamet Glucophage, Glucophage XR, Glumetza, Riomet)	↓ Rate of hepatic glucose production. ↑ Insulin sensitivity. Improves glucose uptake by tissues, especially muscles *Ⱦ kidney, liver, or HF*	Diarrhea, lactic acidosis. Must be held 1–2 days before IV contrast media given and for 48 hr after *take w/ food*
Dipeptidyl Peptidase-4 (DPP-4) Inhibitors		
alogliptin (Nesina)	Enhances activity of incretins. Stimulates release of insulin from pancreatic β-cells. ↓ Hepatic glucose production	Pancreatitis, allergic reactions
linagliptin (Tradjenta)		
saxagliptin (Onglyza)		
sitagliptin (Januvia)		
Dopamine Receptor Agonists		
bromocriptine (Cycloset)	Activates dopamine receptors in central nervous system. Unknown how it improves glucose levels	Orthostatic hypotension
Meglitinides		
nateglinide (Starlix)	Stimulates a rapid and short-lived release of insulin from the pancreas	Weight gain, hypoglycemia
repaglinide (Prandin)		
Sodium-Glucose Co-Transporter 2 (SGLT2) Inhibitors		
canagliflozin (Invokana)	↓ Renal glucose reabsorption and ↑ urinary glucose excretion	↑ Risk for genital infections and UTIs. Hypoglycemia
dapagliflozin (Farxiga)		
empagliflozin (Jardiance)		
ertugliflozin (Steglatro)		
Sulfonylureas		
glimepiride (Amaryl)	Stimulates release of insulin from pancreatic islets. ↓ Glycogenolysis and gluconeogenesis. Enhances cellular sensitivity to insulin	Weight gain, hypoglycemia
glipizide (Glucotrol, Glucotrol XL)		
glyburide (DiaBeta, Glynase)		
Thiazolidinediones		
pioglitazone (Actos)	↑ Glucose uptake in muscle. ↓ Endogenous glucose production *good for insulin resistance*	Weight gain, edema
rosiglitazone (Avandia)		*pioglitazone:* May ↑ risk for bladder cancer and worsen HF.
		rosiglitazone: May ↑ risk for cardiovascular events (e.g., MI, stroke)
Combination Oral Therapy		
Actoplus Met, Actoplus Met XR	Same as for metformin and pioglitazone	See side effects for individual drugs
Duetact	Same as for pioglitazone and glimepiride	
Glucovance	Same as for metformin and glyburide	
Glyxambi	Same as for empagliflozin and linagliptin	
Janumet, Janumet XR	Same as for metformin and sitagliptin	
Jentadueto	Same as for linagliptin and metformin	
Kazano	Same as for alogliptin and metformin	
Kombiglyze	Same as for saxagliptin and metformin	
Oseni	Same as for alogliptin and pioglitazone	
PrandiMet	Same as for metformin and repaglinide	
Segluromet	Same as for metformin and ertugliflozin	
Steglujan	Same as for sitagliptin and ertugliflozin	
Synjardy	Same as metformin and empagliflozin	
Xigduo	Same as for dapagliflozin and metformin	
Noninsulin Injectable Agents		
Amylin Analogs		
pramlintide (Symlin)	Slows gastric emptying, decreases glucagon secretion and endogenous glucose output from liver. ↑ Satiety	Hypoglycemia, nausea, vomiting, ↓ appetite, headache
Glucagon-Like Peptide-1 (GLP-1) Receptor Agonists		
albiglutide (Tanzeum)	Stimulates release of insulin, ↓ glucagon secretion, and slow gastric emptying. ↑ Satiety	Nausea, vomiting, hypoglycemia, diarrhea, headache
dulaglutide (Trulicity)		
exenatide (Byetta)		
exenatide extended-release (Bydureon)		
liraglutide (Victoza)		
lixisenatide (Adlyxin)		
semaglutide (Ozempic)		

are overweight or obese. It is also used to prevent type 2 diabetes in those with prediabetes who are younger than age 60 and have risk factors, such as hypertension or a history of gestational diabetes.

Patients who are undergoing surgery or radiologic procedures that involve the use of a contrast medium need to temporarily discontinue metformin before surgery or the procedure. This reduces the risk of contrast-induced kidney injury (CIN) (see Chapter 44). They should not resume the metformin until 48 hours afterward, once their serum creatinine has been checked and is normal.

💊 DRUG ALERT Metformin

- Do not use in patients with kidney disease, liver disease, or heart failure. Lactic acidosis is a rare complication of metformin accumulation.
- IV contrast media that contain iodine pose a risk for CIN, which could worsen metformin-induced lactic acidosis.
- To reduce risk for CIN, discontinue metformin 2 days before the procedure.
- May be resumed 48 hours after the procedure, assuming kidney function is normal.
- Do not use in people who drink excess amounts of alcohol.
- Take with food to minimize GI side effects.

Sulfonylureas. Sulfonylureas include glimepiride (Amaryl), glipizide (Glucotrol, Glucotrol XL), and glyburide (DiaBeta, Glynase). The primary action of sulfonylureas is to increase insulin production by the pancreas. Therefore hypoglycemia is the major side effect.

Meglitinides. Like sulfonylureas, nateglinide (Starlix) and repaglinide (Prandin) increase insulin production by the pancreas. However, because they are more rapidly absorbed and eliminated than sulfonylureas, they are less likely to cause hypoglycemia. When taken just before meals, pancreatic insulin production increases during and after the meal, mimicking the normal response to eating. Teach patients to take meglitinides any time from 30 minutes before each meal right up to the time of the meal. These drugs should not be taken if a meal is skipped.

α-Glucosidase Inhibitors. These drugs, also known as "starch blockers," work by slowing down carbohydrate absorption in the small intestine. Acarbose (Precose) and miglitol (Glyset) are the available drugs in this class. Taken with the first bite of each main meal, they are most effective in lowering postprandial blood glucose. Their effectiveness is measured by checking 2-hour postprandial glucose levels.

Thiazolidinediones. Thiazolidinediones, sometimes called "insulin sensitizers," include pioglitazone (Actos) and rosiglitazone (Avandia). They are most effective for people who have insulin resistance. These agents improve insulin sensitivity, transport, and use at target tissues. Because they do not increase insulin production, they do not cause hypoglycemia when used alone. However, these drugs are rarely used today because of their adverse effects. Rosiglitazone is associated with adverse cardiovascular events (e.g., myocardial infarction [MI]) and can be obtained only through restricted access programs. Pioglitazone can worsen heart failure (HF) and is associated with an increased risk for bladder cancer.

Dipeptidyl Peptidase-4 (DPP-4) Inhibitors. Normally, the intestines release incretin hormones throughout the day. When glucose levels are normal or elevated, incretins increase insulin synthesis and release from the pancreas and decrease hepatic glucose production. Levels increase in response to a meal. The 2 main incretin hormones are gastric inhibitory peptide [GIP]

and glucagon-like peptide-1 [GLP-1]). They are quickly inactivated by the enzyme dipeptidyl peptidase-4 (DPP-4).

DPP-4 inhibitors (also known as *gliptins*) come in pill form. They include alogliptin (Nesina), linagliptin (Tradjenta), saxagliptin (Onglyza), and sitagliptin (Januvia). DPP-4 inhibitors block the action of DPP-4, which inactivates incretin hormones. The result is an increase in insulin release, decrease in glucagon secretion, and decrease in hepatic glucose production. Since the DPP-4 inhibitors are glucose dependent, they lower the potential for hypoglycemia. The main benefit of these drugs over other medications with similar effects is the absence of weight gain as a side effect.

Sodium-Glucose Co-Transporter 2 (SGLT2) Inhibitors. Normally, sodium glucose transporters reabsorb glucose from the kidneys back into the blood stream. Sodium-glucose co-transporter 2 (SGLT2) inhibitors work by blocking the reabsorption of glucose by the kidney, increasing urinary glucose excretion. Drugs in this class include canagliflozin (Invokana), dapagliflozin (Farxiga), and empagliflozin (Jardiance).

Dopamine Receptor Agonist. Bromocriptine (Cycloset) is a dopamine receptor agonist that improves glucose levels. The mechanism of action is unknown. We think patients with type 2 diabetes have low levels of dopamine activity in the morning. These low dopamine levels may interfere with the body's ability to control blood glucose. Bromocriptine increases dopamine receptor activity. It can be used alone or as an add-on to another type 2 diabetes treatment.

Combination Oral Therapy. Many combination drugs are currently available (Table 48.7). These drugs combine 2 different classes of medications to treat diabetes. One advantage of combination therapy is that the patient takes fewer pills, thus improving medication taking.

Glucagon-Like Peptide-1 Receptor Agonists. Albiglutide (Tanzeum), dulaglutide (Trulicity), exenatide (Byetta), exenatide extended-release (Bydureon), liraglutide (Victoza), and lixisenatide (Adlyxin) simulate GLP-1 (an incretin hormone), which is decreased in people with type 2 diabetes. These drugs increase insulin synthesis and release from the pancreas, inhibit glucagon secretion, slow gastric emptying, and reduce food intake by increasing satiety.

These drugs may be used as monotherapy or adjunct therapy for patients with type 2 diabetes who have not achieved optimal glucose levels on OAs. These drugs are given using a subcutaneous injection in a prefilled pen. Byetta is given twice daily. Liraglutide is given once daily. Albiglutide, dulaglutide, and Bydureon are given once every 7 days. The delayed gastric emptying that occurs with these drugs may affect the absorption of oral medications. Advise patients to take fast-acting oral medications at least 1 hour before injecting a GLP-1 agonist drug.

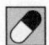 DRUG ALERT Exenatide (Byetta)

- Acute pancreatitis and kidney problems have been associated with its use.

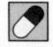 DRUG ALERT Liraglutide (Victoza) and Dulaglutide (Trulicity)

- Do not use in patients with a personal or family history of medullary thyroid cancer.
- Acute pancreatitis has been associated with its use.

Amylin Analogs. Pramlintide (Symlin) is the only available amylin analog. Amylin, a hormone secreted by the β cells of the pancreas in response to food intake, slows gastric emptying, reduces glucagon secretion, and increases satiety. Pramlintide is used in addition to mealtime insulin in patients with type 1 or type 2 diabetes who have elevated blood glucose levels on insulin therapy. It is only used concurrently with insulin and is not a replacement for insulin. Pramlintide is given before meals subcutaneously into the thigh or abdomen. It cannot be injected into the arm because absorption from this site is too variable. The drug cannot be mixed in the same syringe with insulin.

The concurrent use of pramlintide and insulin increases the risk for severe hypoglycemia during the 3 hours after injection, especially in patients with type 1 diabetes. Teach patients to eat a meal with at least 250 calories and keep a form of fast-acting glucose on hand in case hypoglycemia develops. When pramlintide is used, the bolus dose of insulin should be reduced.

 DRUG ALERT Pramlintide (Symlin)

- Can cause severe hypoglycemia when used with insulin.

Other Drugs Affecting Blood Glucose Levels. Both the patient and the HCP must be aware of drug interactions that can potentiate hypoglycemia and hyperglycemia effects. For example, β-adrenergic blockers can mask symptoms of hypoglycemia and prolong the hypoglycemic effects of insulin. Thiazide and loop diuretics can worsen hyperglycemia by inducing potassium loss, although low-dose thiazide therapy is usually considered safe.

Nutrition Therapy

Individualized nutrition therapy, consisting of counseling, education, and ongoing monitoring, is a cornerstone of care for people with diabetes and prediabetes.[12] Changing eating habits can be challenging for many people. Achieving nutrition goals requires a coordinated team effort that considers the person's behavioral, cognitive, socioeconomic, cultural, and religious backgrounds and preferences. Because of these complexities, it is recommended that a dietitian with expertise in diabetes management work with the person who has diabetes. The dietitian starts with a nutrition assessment and develops an individualized food plan. Other team members may include nurses, certified diabetes educators (CDEs), clinical nurse specialists, social workers, and other HCPs.

Guidelines from the ADA state that, within the context of an overall healthy eating plan, a person with diabetes can eat the same foods as a person who does not have diabetes. This means that the same principles of healthy nutrition that apply to the general population also apply to the person with diabetes. Table 48.8 describes nutrition guidelines for patients with diabetes. According to the ADA, the overall goal of nutrition therapy is to help people with diabetes make healthy food choices that will lead to achieving and/or maintaining safe and healthy blood glucose levels. Additional specific goals include:

- Maintain blood glucose levels as close to normal as safely possible to prevent or reduce the risk for complications of diabetes.
- Achieve lipid profiles and BP levels that reduce the risk for CVD.
- Prevent or slow the rate of development of chronic complications of diabetes by modifying nutrient intake and lifestyle.
- Address individual nutrition needs while considering personal and cultural preferences and respecting the person's willingness or ability to change eating and dietary habits.
- Maintain the pleasure of eating by encouraging a variety of healthy food choices.

TABLE 48.8 Nutrition Therapy

Diabetes

Component	Recommendations
Total carbohydrate	• Include carbohydrate from fruits, vegetables, grains, legumes, and low-fat milk • Monitor by carbohydrate counting, exchange lists, or use of appropriate proportions • Fiber intake at 25–30 g/day • Nonnutritive sweeteners are safe when consumed within FDA daily intake levels
Protein	• Individualize goals • High-protein diets are not recommended for weight loss
Fat	• Individualize goals • Minimize *trans* fat • Dietary cholesterol <200 mg/day • ≥2 servings of fish per week to provide polyunsaturated fatty acids
Alcohol	• Limit to moderate amount (maximum 1 drink per day for women, 2 drinks per day for men) • Consume alcohol with food to reduce risk for nocturnal hypoglycemia in those using insulin or drugs that promote insulin secretion • Moderate alcohol consumption has no acute effect on glucose and insulin concentrations • Carbohydrates taken with the alcohol (mixed drink) may raise blood glucose

Source: American Diabetes Association: Lifestyle management: Standards of medical care in diabetes, *Diabetes Care* 41:S38, 2018.

Type 1 Diabetes. People with type 1 diabetes base their meal planning on usual food intake and preferences balanced with insulin and exercise patterns. The patient coordinates insulin dosing with eating habits and activity pattern in mind. Day-to-day consistency in timing and amount of food eaten makes it much easier to manage blood glucose levels, especially for those using conventional, fixed insulin regimens. Patients using rapid-acting insulin can adjust the dose before each meal based on the current blood glucose level and the carbohydrate content of the meal. Intensified insulin therapy, such as multiple daily injections or the use of an insulin pump, allows considerable flexibility in food selection and can be adjusted for changes from usual eating and exercise habits. This does not diminish or replace the need for healthy food choices and a well-balanced diet.

Type 2 Diabetes. Nutrition therapy in type 2 diabetes emphasizes achieving glucose, lipid, and BP goals. Modest weight loss has been associated with improved insulin sensitivity. Therefore weight loss is recommended for all persons with diabetes who are overweight or obese.[13]

There is no one proven strategy or method. A nutritionally adequate meal plan with appropriate serving sizes, a reduction of saturated and *trans* fats, and low carbohydrates can decrease calorie consumption. Spacing meals is another strategy that spreads nutrient intake throughout the day. A weight loss of 5% to 7% of body weight often improves blood glucose levels, even if desirable body weight is not achieved. Weight loss is best achieved by a moderate decrease in calories and an increase in caloric expenditure. Regularly exercising and adopting new behaviors and attitudes can promote long-term lifestyle changes. Monitoring blood glucose levels, A1C, lipids, and BP gives feedback on how well the goals of nutrition therapy are being met.

Food Composition. A healthy balance of nutrients is essential to maintain blood glucose levels and overall health. Energy from food intake can be balanced with the patient's energy output. Teach patients to plan their individual meal plan with their lifestyle and health goals in mind. The following are general recommendations for nutrient balance.

Carbohydrate. Carbohydrates include sugars, starches, and fiber. They are an important source of energy, fiber, vitamins, and minerals and needed by all people, including those with diabetes. Foods containing carbohydrate from whole grains, fruits, vegetables, and low-fat dairy are part of a healthy meal plan. The ADA recommends individualizing carbohydrate intake as there is no ideal amount for all people with diabetes.

All persons benefit from including dietary fiber as part of a healthy meal plan. The current recommendation for the general population is 25 to 30 g/day.[13]

Nutritive and nonnutritive sweeteners may be included in a healthy meal plan in moderation. Nonnutritive sweeteners include the sugar substitutes saccharine, aspartame, sucralose, stevia, neotame, and acesulfame-K.

Fat. Dietary fat provides energy, transports fat-soluble vitamins, and provides essential fatty acids. The ADA recommends individualizing saturated fat intake. Less than 200 mg/day of cholesterol and limited *trans* fats are recommended as part of a healthy meal plan. Decreasing fat and cholesterol intake helps reduce the risk for CVD. Healthy fats are those that come from plants, such as olives, nuts, and avocados.

Protein. The amount of daily protein in the diet for people with diabetes and normal renal function is the same as for the general population. The ADA recommends individualizing protein intake. Teach patients to choose lean protein whenever possible.

Alcohol. Alcohol inhibits gluconeogenesis (breakdown of glycogen to glucose) by the liver. This can cause severe hypoglycemia in patients on insulin or OAs that increase insulin secretion. Create a trusting environment in which patients feel comfortable being honest about their alcohol use because its use can make blood glucose harder to manage.

Moderate alcohol consumption can be safely incorporated into the meal plan if the person is monitoring blood glucose levels and not at risk for other alcohol-related problems. Moderate consumption is defined as 1 drink per day for women and 2 drinks per day for men. A patient can reduce the risk for alcohol-induced hypoglycemia by eating carbohydrates when drinking alcohol. On the other hand, mixed drinks often contain sweetened mixers and can increase blood glucose levels. To decrease the carbohydrate content, recommend using sugar-free mixes and drinking dry, light wines.

Patient Teaching Related to Nutrition Therapy. Most often, the dietitian initially teaches the principles of nutrition management. Whenever possible, work with dietitians as part of an interprofessional diabetes care team. Some patients who have limited insurance coverage or live in remote areas do not have access to a dietitian. In these cases, you may need to assume responsibility for teaching basic nutrition principles to patients with diabetes.

Carbohydrate counting is a meal planning technique used to keep track of the amount of carbohydrate eaten with each meal and per day. Teach patients to keep carbohydrate intake within a healthy range. The amount of total carbohydrate per day depends on blood glucose levels, age, weight, activity level, patient preference, and prescribed medications. A serving size of carbohydrate is 15 g. A typical adult usually starts with 45 to 60 g

of carbohydrate per meal. For some patients, insulin doses are tailored to the amount of carbohydrate foods that a patient will consume at the meal, with a set number of units of insulin given per gram of carbohydrate (e.g., 1 U/15 g carbohydrate, 2 U/25 g carbohydrate). Teach the patient about the foods that contain carbohydrate, how to read food labels, and appropriate serving sizes.

Diabetes exchange lists are another method for meal planning. Instead of counting carbohydrate, the person is given a meal plan with specific numbers of helpings from a list of exchanges for each meal and snack. The exchanges are starches, fruits, milk, meats, vegetables, fats, and free foods. The patient chooses foods from the various exchanges based on the prescribed meal plan. This method may be easier for some patients than carbohydrate counting. It also encourages a well-balanced meal plan. Another advantage is that this approach helps the patient limit portion sizes and overall food intake, an important part of weight management.

MyPlate was developed by the U.S. Department of Agriculture (USDA) to represent national nutrition guidelines for people with or without diabetes. This simple method helps the patient see the amount of vegetables, starch, and meat that fills a 9-in plate. The recommendation is that each meal has half of the plate filled with nonstarchy vegetables, one fourth filled with a starch, and one fourth filled with a protein (*www.diabetes.org/food-and-fitness/food/planning-meals/create-your-plate*). An 8-oz glass of nonfat milk and a small piece of fresh fruit complete the meal.[12]

Whenever possible, include family members and caregivers in nutrition education and counseling, especially the person who cooks for the household. However, the responsibility for maintaining a healthy eating plan still belongs to the person with diabetes. Reliance on another person to make health decisions interferes with the patient's ability to develop self-care skills, which are essential in managing diabetes. Foster independence, even in patients with visual or cognitive impairment. It is important to discuss traditional foods with the patient. Individualize food choices considering the patient's preferences and culturally appropriate foods.

Exercise

Regular, consistent exercise is an essential part of diabetes and prediabetes management.[14] The ADA recommends that people with diabetes engage in at least 150 min/wk (30 minutes, 5 days/week) of a moderate-intensity aerobic physical activity (Table 48.9). The ADA encourages people with type 2 diabetes to perform resistance training 3 times a week unless contraindicated.[15]

TABLE 48.9 **Activities That Affect Caloric Expenditure**		
Light Activity (100–200 kcal/hr)	**Moderate Activity (200–350 kcal/hr)**	**Vigorous Activity (400–900 kcal/hr)**
• Fishing • Light housework • Secretarial work • Teaching • Walking casually	• Active housework • Bicycling (light) • Bowling • Dancing • Gardening • Golf • Roller skating • Walking briskly	• Aerobic exercise • Bicycling (vigorous) • Hard labor • Ice skating • Outdoor sports • Running • Soccer • Tennis • Wood chopping

Exercise decreases insulin resistance and can have a direct effect on lowering blood glucose levels. It contributes to weight loss, which further decreases insulin resistance. The therapeutic benefits of regular physical activity may result in a decreased need for diabetes medications to reach target blood glucose goals in people with type 2 diabetes. Regular exercise may also help reduce triglyceride and low-density lipoprotein (LDL) cholesterol levels, increase HDL, reduce BP, and improve circulation.

Encourage patients to be active every day and to seek medical clearance before starting a new or more intensive exercise program. Patients start slowly with gradual progression toward the desired goal. Patients who use insulin, sulfonylureas, or meglitinides are at increased risk for hypoglycemia when they increase physical activity, especially if they exercise at the time of peak drug action or eat too little to maintain adequate blood glucose levels. This can also occur if a normally sedentary patient with diabetes has an unusually active day.

The glucose-lowering effects of exercise can last up to 48 hours after the activity, so it is possible for hypoglycemia to occur long after the activity. Patients who use drugs that can cause hypoglycemia should exercise about 1 hour after a meal or have a 10- to 15-g carbohydrate snack and check their blood glucose before exercising. It is preferable not to increase caloric intake for exercise. If needed, they can eat small carbohydrate snacks every 30 minutes during exercise to prevent hypoglycemia. Patients using drugs that place them at risk for hypoglycemia should always carry a fast-acting source of carbohydrate, such as glucose tablets or hard candies, when exercising. If they have frequent lows from exercise, the medication dose may need to be lowered. Table 48.10 describes exercise guidelines for patients with diabetes.

TABLE 48.10 Patient & Caregiver Teaching
Exercise for Patients With Diabetes

Include the following information in the exercise teaching plan for the patient and caregiver:
1. Exercise does not have to be vigorous to be effective. The blood glucose-reducing effects of exercise can be reached with activity such as brisk walking.
2. Choose exercises that are enjoyable to foster regularity.
3. Use properly fitting footwear to avoid rubbing or injury.
4. The exercise session includes a warm-up period and a cool-down period. Start the exercise program gradually and increase slowly.
5. Exercise is best done after meals, when the blood glucose level is rising.
6. Exercise plans are patient specific and monitored by the HCP.
7. Monitor blood glucose levels before, during, and after exercise to determine the effect exercise has on blood glucose levels at specific times of the day.
8. Before exercise, if blood glucose ≤100 mg/dL, eat a 15-g carbohydrate snack. After 15 to 30 min, recheck blood glucose levels. Delay exercise if <100 mg/dL.
9. Before exercise, if blood glucose ≥250 mg/dL in a person with type 1 diabetes and ketones are present, delay vigorous activity until ketones are gone. Drink fluids.
10. Exercise-induced hypoglycemia may occur several hours after the completion of exercise.
11. Planned or spontaneous exercise can still occur when taking a glucose-lowering medication.
12. It is important to compensate for extensive planned and spontaneous activity by monitoring blood glucose levels and making adjustments in the insulin dose (if taken) and food intake.

The body can perceive strenuous activity as a stress, causing a release of counterregulatory hormones and a temporary elevation of blood glucose. In a person with type 1 diabetes who has hyperglycemia and ketones, exercise can worsen these conditions. Teach these patients to delay activity if the blood glucose level is over 250 mg/dL and ketones are present in the urine. If hyperglycemia is present without ketosis, it is not necessary to postpone exercise.[12]

Monitoring Blood Glucose

Self-monitoring of blood glucose (SMBG) is a critical part of diabetes management. By providing a current blood glucose reading, SMBG lets the patient make decisions about food intake, activity patterns, and medication dosages. It produces accurate records of daily glucose fluctuations and trends and alerts the patient to acute episodes of hyperglycemia and hypoglycemia. SMBG provides patients with a tool for achieving and maintaining specific glycemic goals. It is recommended for all patients who use insulin to manage their diabetes. Other patients with diabetes use SMBG to help achieve and maintain glycemic goals and monitor for acute fluctuations in blood glucose related to drugs, food, and exercise.

The frequency of SMBG depends on several factors. These include the patient's glycemic goals, type of diabetes, medication regimen, patient's ability to check blood glucose independently, access to supplies and equipment, and patient's willingness and ability to do so. The recommendation for patients who use multiple insulin injections or insulin pumps is to monitor their blood glucose 4 to 8 times each day. Patients using less frequent insulin injections, noninsulin therapy, or nutrition management will monitor as often as needed to achieve their glycemic goals.[9]

Patients who perform SMBG use portable blood glucose monitors. A wide variety of blood glucose monitors are available (Fig. 48.9). Disposable lancets are used to get a small drop of capillary blood (usually from a finger stick) that is placed in a reagent strip. After a specified time, the monitor displays a digital reading of the capillary blood glucose value. The technology of SMBG is rapidly changing. Newer, more convenient systems are introduced on an ongoing basis.

Some systems allow the user to collect blood from alternative sites, such as the forearm or palm. Alternative site use is not recommended with rapidly changing blood glucose readings, during pregnancy, or when symptoms of low blood glucose are present. The data from some glucose monitors can be uploaded

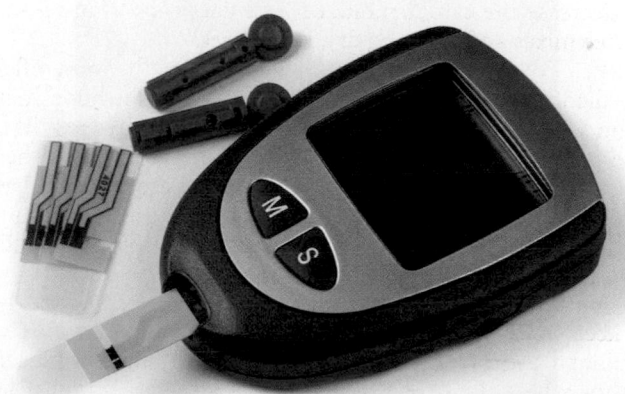

FIG. 48.9 Blood glucose monitors are used to measure blood glucose levels. (© iStock.com/kolesnikovserg.)

to a computer and reviewed by HCPs, allowing for more frequent and efficient adjustment of the plan of care if needed.

Continuous glucose monitoring (CGM) systems are another route for monitoring glucose. More people with type 1 diabetes are using CGMs. These systems are slowly being used by people with type 2 diabetes as well. Insurance coverage and cost are the most common limiting factors. Some insulin pumps have CGM integrated as part of the system. Flash glucose monitoring is another option. It allows users to wave a reader over a subcutaneous sensor and get glucose readings at any time (Fig. 48.10).

Using a sensor inserted subcutaneously, the systems display glucose values that are updated every 1 to 5 minutes. CGM assesses interstitial glucose, which lags behind blood glucose by 5 to 10 minutes.[16] The patient inserts the sensor using an automatic insertion device. Data are sent from the sensor to a transmitter, which displays the glucose value on either an insulin pump or a pager-like receiver. The CGM can be used with or without an insulin pump. Newer CGMs can "share" data with a smart phone.

CGMs help the patient and HCP identify trends and patterns in glucose levels. The goal is to increase "time in range" (70 to 180 mg/dL) and have fewer highs and lows. They are useful for managing insulin therapy or when continuous blood glucose readings are clinically important. The patient is alerted to episodes of hypoglycemia and hyperglycemia, thus allowing corrective action to be quickly taken. Some systems need finger-stick measurements using a blood glucose monitor to calibrate the sensor and to make treatment decisions. In 2016 the FDA approved making insulin dosing decisions based on a CGM reading, without first checking a finger-stick blood glucose value.

Blood glucose meters available today are reliable when used consistently and correctly. It is not necessary to compare meter readings to laboratory readings. If the A1C result does not correspond to the blood glucose readings on the home meter, it is

a good idea to troubleshoot any problems with the meter, strips, or hand washing technique.

Because errors in monitoring technique can cause errors in management strategies, comprehensive patient teaching is essential. Initial instruction should be followed with regular reassessment. Review the instructions that come with each product. If a product has a control solution, teach patients to use and interpret control solutions. Control solution should be used when first using a blood glucose meter or when there is a reason to believe that the readings are not correct. Table 48.11 lists the steps to include when teaching the patient how to perform SMBG.

People with type 1 diabetes often check their blood glucose before meals. This is because many patients use insulin pumps or multiple daily injections and base the insulin dose on the carbohydrates in a meal or make adjustments if the preprandial value is above or below target. Checking blood glucose 2 hours after the first bite of food helps a person determine if the bolus insulin dose was adequate for that meal.

Teach patients to monitor blood glucose whenever hypoglycemia is suspected and then take immediate action. During times of illness, check blood glucose levels at 4-hour intervals to determine the effects of the illness on glucose levels. Teach the patient to monitor blood glucose before and after exercise to determine the effects of exercise on blood glucose levels. This is especially important in the patient with type 1 diabetes.

A patient who is visually impaired, cognitively impaired, or limited in manual dexterity needs careful evaluation of the degree to which SMBG can be done independently. Nurses preparing patients for discharge from the hospital and nurses working in home health and outpatient settings may need to identify caregivers who can assume this responsibility. Adaptive devices are available to help patients with certain limitations. These include talking meters and other equipment for the visually impaired.

Bariatric Surgery

Bariatric surgery may be an option for patients with type 2 diabetes, especially if the diabetes or associated co-morbidities are hard to manage with lifestyle and drug therapy. Patients with

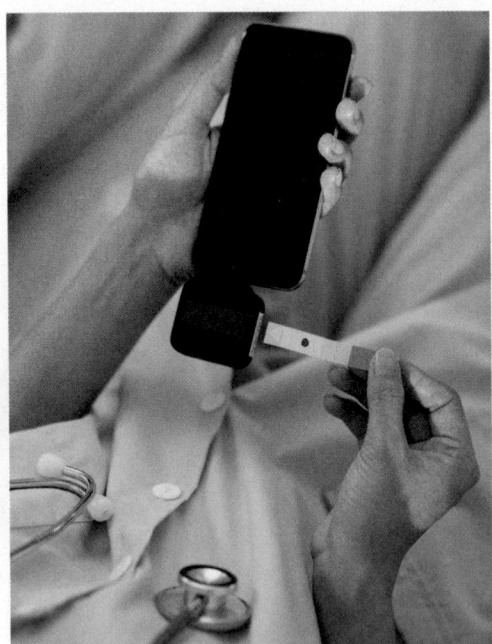

FIG. 48.10 Glucometers that connect to a smartphone allow the patient to measure blood glucose, log the measurements in an app, and share the results with health care providers. (© DragonImages/iStock.com.)

TABLE 48.11 **Patient & Caregiver Teaching**
Self-Monitoring of Blood Glucose (SMBG)

Include the following instructions when teaching the patient and caregiver about SMBG:

1. Wash and dry hands completely. It is not necessary to clean the site with alcohol, and it may interfere with test results.
2. If it is hard to get an adequate drop of blood for testing, warm the hands in warm water or let the arms hang dependently for a few minutes before making the finger puncture.
3. A lancing device is usually used. Place the lancet in the device, following the instructions that come with it. If the puncture is made on the finger, use the side of the finger pad rather than near the center. Fewer nerve endings are along the side of the finger pad. If using an alternative site (e.g., forearm), special equipment may be needed. Refer to manufacturer's instructions for alternative site use, except during hypoglycemia episodes.
4. Set lancing device to make a puncture just deep enough to get a sufficiently large drop of blood. Unnecessarily deep punctures may cause pain and bruising. Current meters need very small amounts of blood.
5. Follow instructions on monitor for checking the blood glucose level.
6. Record results. Compare with personal blood glucose goals.

type 2 diabetes who have undergone bariatric surgery need lifelong lifestyle support and monitoring. Bariatric surgery is discussed in Chapter 40.

Pancreas Transplantation

Pancreas transplantation is an option for select patients with type 1 diabetes. Usually it is done for patients who have end-stage renal disease (ESRD) and have had or plan to have a kidney transplant. Kidney and pancreas transplants are often done together, or a pancreas may be transplanted after a kidney transplant. If renal failure is not present, the ADA recommends that pancreas transplantation be considered only for patients who exhibit these 3 criteria: (1) a history of frequent, acute, and severe metabolic complications (e.g., hypoglycemia, hyperglycemia, ketoacidosis) requiring medical attention; (2) clinical and emotional problems with the use of exogenous insulin therapy that are so severe as to be incapacitating; and (3) consistent failure of insulin-based management to prevent acute complications.

Successful pancreas transplantation can improve quality of life, primarily by eliminating the need for exogenous insulin and frequent blood glucose measurements. Transplantation can eliminate acute complications experienced by patients with type 1 diabetes (e.g., hypoglycemia, hyperglycemia). However, transplantation is only partially successful in reversing the long-term renal and neurologic complications of diabetes. The patient will need lifelong immunosuppression to prevent rejection of the organ. Complications can result from immunosuppressive therapy. Immunosuppressive therapy is discussed in Chapter 13.

Pancreatic islet cell transplantation is another potential treatment measure. During this procedure, the islets are harvested from the pancreas of a deceased organ donor. Most recipients need the use of 2 or more pancreases. The islets are infused via a catheter through the upper abdomen into the portal vein of the liver. With only the islets transplanted, pain and recovery time are less than with whole pancreas transplants. Currently, this procedure is experimental in the United States. Research is continuing to investigate the best ways to implant the islet cells and prevent their rejection.

Culturally Competent Care: Diabetes

Because culture can have a strong influence on dietary preferences and meal preparation practices, culturally competent care has special relevance for the patient with diabetes. For example, certain ethnic and cultural groups, such as Hispanics, Native Americans, blacks, and Asians and Pacific Islanders have a high incidence of diabetes. The increased prevalence can be attributed to genetic predisposition, environmental factors, and dietary choices.

Explore the influences of culture on food choices and meal planning with the patient as part of the health history. When teaching about nutrition, consider the patient's cultural food preferences. Nutrition resources specifically designed for members of different cultural groups are available from the ADA.

❖ NURSING MANAGEMENT: DIABETES

◆ Nursing Assessment

Table 48.12 provides initial subjective and objective data to gather from a person with diabetes. After the initial assessment, perform periodic patient assessments on a regular basis.

TABLE 48.12 Nursing Assessment

Diabetes

Subjective Data

Important Health Information

Past health history: Mumps, rubella, coxsackievirus, or other viral infections. Recent trauma, infection, or stress. Pregnancy, gave birth to infant >9 lb. Chronic pancreatitis, Cushing syndrome, acromegaly, family history of type 1 or type 2 diabetes

Medications: Use of insulin or OAs, corticosteroids, diuretics, phenytoin (Dilantin)

Surgery or other treatments: Any recent surgery

Functional Health Patterns

Health perception–health management: Positive family history, malaise

Nutrition-metabolic: Obesity, weight loss (type 1), weight gain (type 2). Thirst, hunger, nausea and vomiting. Poor healing (especially involving the feet), eating habits

Elimination: Constipation or diarrhea, frequent urination, frequent bladder infections, nocturia, urinary incontinence

Activity-exercise: Muscle weakness, fatigue

Cognitive-perceptual: Abdominal pain, headache, blurred vision, numbness or tingling of extremities, pruritus

Sexuality-reproductive: ED, frequent vaginal infections, vaginal dryness or pain, ↓ libido

Adaptation: Depression, irritability, apathy

Value-belief: Health beliefs, commitment to lifestyle changes involving food, medication, and activity patterns

Objective Data

Eyes

Soft, sunken eyeballs.* History of vitreal hemorrhages, cataracts

Integumentary

Dry, warm, inelastic skin. Pigmented lesions (on legs), ulcers (especially on feet), loss of hair on toes, acanthosis nigricans

Respiratory

Rapid, deep respirations (Kussmaul respirations)*

Cardiovascular

Hypotension.* Weak, rapid pulse*

Gastrointestinal

Dry mouth, vomiting.* Fruity breath*

Neurologic

Altered reflexes, restlessness, confusion, stupor, coma*

Musculoskeletal

Muscle wasting*

Possible Findings

Serum electrolyte abnormalities. Fasting blood glucose level ≥126 mg/dL. OGTT >200 mg/dL, random glucose ≥200 mg/dL. Leukocytosis. ↑ BUN, creatinine, triglycerides, cholesterol, LDL, VLDL. ↓ HDL. A1C >6.0% (A1C >7.0% in those with diagnosed diabetes), glycosuria, ketonuria, albuminuria. Acidosis

*Indicates manifestations of diabetes-related ketoacidosis (DKA).

◆ Nursing Diagnoses

Nursing diagnoses related to diabetes may include:
- Lack of knowledge
- Hyperglycemia
- Hypoglycemia

- Risk for injury
- Impaired peripheral neurovascular function

Additional information on nursing diagnoses and interventions for the patient with diabetes is presented in eNursing Care Plan 48.1 available on the website.

◆ Planning

The overall goals are for the patient with diabetes to (1) engage in self-care behaviors to actively manage diabetes, (2) have few or no hyperglycemia or hypoglycemia emergencies, (3) maintain blood glucose levels at normal or near-normal levels, (4) reduce the risk for chronic complications from diabetes, and (5) adjust lifestyle to accommodate the diabetes plan with minimum stress. The goal is for the patient with diabetes to safely and effectively fit diabetes into life, rather than living life around diabetes.

◆ Nursing Implementation

◆ Health Promotion. Your role in health promotion is to identify, monitor, and teach the patient at risk for diabetes. Obesity is the main risk factor for type 2 diabetes. The ADA recommends routine screening for type 2 diabetes for all adults who are overweight or obese (BMI 25 kg/m² or greater) or have 1 or more risk factors. For people who do not have risk factors for diabetes, begin screening at age 45. Table 48.13 provides criteria to screen for prediabetes and diabetes. If results are normal, repeat screening at 3-year intervals.[3]

Many other factors put a person at an increased risk for diabetes. These include age, ethnicity (being Native American, Hispanic, black, Asian, Pacific Islander), having a baby that weighed more than 9 lb at birth, history of gestational diabetes, and a family history of diabetes. A diabetes risk test is available at *www.diabetes.org/risk-test.jsp*. The diabetes risk test

---

TABLE 48.13 **Screening for Diabetes in Asymptomatic, Undiagnosed Persons**

Who to Screen

1. Consider screening all adults who are overweight (BMI >25 kg/m²) and have additional risk factors:
   - First-degree relative with diabetes
   - Physically inactive
   - Members of a high-risk ethnic population (e.g., black, Hispanic, Native American, Asian American,* Pacific Islander)
   - Women who delivered a baby weighing >9 lb or were diagnosed with gestational diabetes
   - Hypertensive (≥140/90 mm Hg) or on therapy for hypertension
   - HDL cholesterol level ≤35 mg/dL (0.90 mmol/L) and/or a triglyceride level ≥250 mg/dL (2.82 mmol/L)
   - Women with polycystic ovary syndrome
   - A1C ≥5.7%, IGT, or IFG on previous screening
   - Other conditions associated with insulin resistance (e.g., acanthosis nigricans)
2. In the absence of the above criteria, screening for diabetes should begin at age 45 yr.
3. If results are normal, repeat screening at least every 3 years, with more frequent screening depending on initial results and risk status.

What Measurements Are Used

To screen for diabetes or to assess risk of future diabetes, A1C, FPG, or 2-hour OGTT is appropriate.

Source: American Diabetes Association: Standards of medical care in diabetes, *Diabetes Care* 41:S15, 2018.
*Consider screening Asian Americans with a BMI of 23 kg/m² or higher.

---

determines if the person is at risk for prediabetes or diabetes based on the number of risk factors present.

Primary prevention is a cost-effective approach. Current recommendations for primary prevention include lifestyle modifications for at-risk people. A modest weight loss of 5% to 7% of body weight and 150 minutes of physical activity a week lowered the risk for developing type 2 diabetes by 34% to 58%.[17]

♥ PROMOTING POPULATION HEALTH
Preventing Diabetes

- Increase level of exercise by aiming for 150 minutes of moderate activity each week.
- Maintain a healthy weight through a nutritionally balanced diet.
- If overweight, lose weight and take part in a regular exercise program.
- Follow a diet low in fat, total calories, and processed foods and high in whole grains, fruits, and vegetables.
- If overweight and over age 45, get screened for diabetes yearly.
- Avoid cigarette smoking or tobacco products.
- Limit consumption of alcohol to moderate levels.
- Follow the prescribed treatment plan for hypertension.

◆ **Acute Care.** Acute situations involving the patient with diabetes include hypoglycemia, DKA, and hyperosmolar hyperglycemic syndrome (HHS). Nursing management for these situations is discussed in more detail later in this chapter. Other areas of acute care relate to management during acute illness and surgery.

Acute Illness and Surgery. Both emotional and physical stress can increase the blood glucose level and result in hyperglycemia. Because stress is unavoidable, certain situations may require more intense treatment, such as extra insulin and more frequent blood glucose monitoring, to maintain glycemic goals and avoid hyperglycemia.

Acute illness, injury, and surgery may evoke a counterregulatory hormone response, resulting in hyperglycemia. Even common illnesses, such as a viral upper respiratory tract infection or the flu, can cause this response. Encourage patients with diabetes to check blood glucose at least every 4 hours during times of illness. Teach acutely ill patients with type 1 diabetes and a blood glucose greater than 240 mg/dL (13.3 mmol/L) to check urine for ketones every 3 to 4 hours.

Teach patients to contact the HCP when glucose levels are over 300 mg/dL twice in a row or urine ketone levels are moderate to high. A patient with type 1 diabetes may need an increase in insulin to prevent DKA. Elevated blood glucose levels can lead to poor healing and infection. Insulin therapy may be needed for a patient with type 2 diabetes to prevent or treat hyperglycemia symptoms and avoid an acute hyperglycemia emergency. In critically ill patients, insulin therapy may be started if the blood glucose is persistently greater than 180 mg/dL. These patients have a higher targeted blood glucose goal, which is usually 140 to 180 mg/dL. Food intake is important during times of stress and illness, when the body needs extra energy. If patients can eat normally, they can continue with their regular meal plan while increasing the intake of noncaloric fluids, such as water, sugar-free gelatin, and other decaffeinated beverages, and continue taking OAs, noninsulin injectable agents, and insulin as prescribed. When illness causes patients to eat less than normal, they can continue to take OAs, noninsulin injectable agents, and/or insulin as prescribed while supplementing food intake with carbohydrate-containing fluids. Examples include low-sodium soups, juices, and regular, sugar-sweetened decaffeinated soft drinks. It is important to tell the patient to contact an HCP if they are unable to keep down food or fluid.

During the intraoperative period, adjustments in the diabetes plan can be made to ensure safe and healthy blood glucose levels. The patient is given IV fluids and insulin (if needed) just before, during, and after surgery when there is no oral intake. Explain to the patient with type 2 diabetes who has been on OAs that this is a temporary measure, not a sign of worsening diabetes.

When caring for an unconscious surgical patient receiving insulin, be alert for signs of hypoglycemia, such as sweating, tachycardia, and tremors. Frequent monitoring of blood glucose can prevent episodes of severe hypoglycemia.

◆ **Ambulatory Care.** Successful diabetes management involves ongoing interaction among the patient, caregiver, and interprofessional team. It is important that a CDE be involved in the care of the patient and family. Because diabetes is a complex chronic condition, a great deal of patient contact takes place in outpatient and home settings. The major goal of patient care in these settings is to enable the patient (with the help of a caregiver as needed) to reach an optimal level of independence in self-care activities. Unfortunately, many patients face challenges in reaching these goals. Diabetes increases the risk for other chronic conditions that can affect self-care activities. These include visual impairment, lower extremity problems that affect mobility, and other functional limitations related to a stroke.

An important nursing function is to assess the ability of patients and caregivers in performing activities such as SMBG and insulin injection. Assistive devices for self-administration of insulin include syringe magnifiers, vial stabilizers, and dosing aids for the visually impaired. In some cases, referrals are made to help the patient achieve the self-care goal. These may include an occupational therapist, a social worker, a home care nurse, a home health aide, or a dietitian.

A diagnosis of diabetes affects the patient in many profound ways. Self-management of the disease is demanding. Patients with diabetes continually face lifestyle choices that affect the foods they eat, their activities, and demands on their time and energy. The requirements of scheduled meals, SMBG, medication, and insulin management may interfere with the patient's other responsibilities. Any change in the daily routine can be hard. In addition, they face the challenge of preventing or dealing with the devastating complications of diabetes.

Careful assessment of what it means to the patient to have diabetes is a good starting point for teaching. The goals of teaching are mutually determined by the patient and you, based on individual needs and therapeutic requirements. Identify the patient's support system, and include them in planning, teaching, and counseling. When family members and other persons close to the patient are included, they can support the patient's self-care behaviors. They can also provide care if self-care is not possible. Encourage the family and caregivers to provide emotional support and encouragement as the patient deals with the reality of living with a chronic disease.

Insulin Therapy. Nursing responsibilities for the patient receiving insulin include proper administration, assessment of the patient's response to insulin therapy, and teaching the patient about administration, storage, and side effects of insulin (Table 48.5). Table 48.6 lists guidelines for assessing a patient using GLAs, including insulin and OAs.

EVIDENCE-BASED PRACTICE
Interactive Self-Management and Diabetes

A.Y. is a 62-yr-old woman with a history of poorly controlled type 2 diabetes. She knows the importance of keeping blood glucose levels close to normal to prevent long-term complications. A.Y. tells you she wants to be more involved in her care. You see she is motivated and wants to learn how to better manage her diabetes.

Making Clinical Decisions

Best Available Evidence. The delivery of education and skills related to diabetes self-management includes a variety of formats. These include the use of electronic messages transmitted by phone or the Web and behavioral change techniques, such as goal-setting, problem-solving, and action planning. Evidence supports multiple benefits from using interactive self-management interventions. These include improved glycemic control as measured by A1C levels, increased knowledge and self-efficacy, and reduced diabetes-related distress.

Clinician Expertise. You know interactive self-management strategies are effective in helping patients improve glycemic control. You are aware that several options, such as text messaging and Web-based programs, can be useful for delivering information to and from patients with diabetes who manage their own care.

Patient Preferences and Values. A.Y. shows a strong interest in taking more control of her diabetes and wishes to receive information on physical activity, blood glucose monitoring, and diet.

Implications for Nursing Practice

1. What options for interactive self-management of her diabetes will you offer A.Y.?
2. As you empower A.Y. to initially manage her care, why is it important for you to assess A.Y.'s knowledge and skills?
3. What parameters will you use to assess if she is able to manage her own care?

Reference for Evidence

Cheng L, Sit JWH, Choi K-C, et al: Effectiveness of interactive self-management interventions in individuals with poorly controlled type 2 diabetes: a meta-analysis of randomized controlled trials, *Worldviews Evid Based Nurs* 14:65, 2017.

Assessment of the patient who is a new user of insulin includes evaluating their ability to safely manage this therapy. This includes the ability to understand the interaction of insulin, food, and activity and to recognize and treat the symptoms of hypoglycemia appropriately. If the patient does not have the cognitive skills to do these things, identify and teach another responsible person. The patient or caregiver must have the cognitive and manual skills needed to prepare and inject insulin. Otherwise, additional resources will be needed to assist the patient. For patients with cognitive, physical, and other barriers, consider referral to a CDE. A CDE has the specialized knowledge and skills to promote self-care behaviors for these patients.

Many patients are fearful when they first begin using insulin. Some find it hard to self-inject because they are afraid of needles or the pain associated with an injection. Others may think that they do not need insulin or that they will be hypoglycemic after an injection. Explore the patient's underlying fears before beginning the teaching. Assessing the patient's beliefs and concerns about starting insulin will guide the teaching, counseling, and plan of care. Having open discussion with patients, providing educational materials and programs, and working with a CDE are all beneficial for patients starting insulin.

Follow-up assessment of the patient who has been using insulin therapy includes inspecting injection sites for signs of lipodystrophy and other reactions, reviewing insulin preparation and injection technique, taking a history of the occurrence of hypoglycemia, and assessing how the patient managed hypoglycemia. A review of the patient's recorded blood glucose readings is vital in assessing how the patient is doing and making any needed adjustments.

Oral and Noninsulin Injectable Agents. Your responsibilities for the patient taking OAs and noninsulin injectable agents are similar to those for the patient taking insulin. Proper administration, assessment of the patient's use of and response to these drugs, and teaching the patient and family are all essential nursing actions.

Your assessment is valuable in determining the most appropriate drug for a patient. Factors such as the patient's mental status, eating habits, home environment, learning ability, resources, attitude toward diabetes, and medication history all play a significant role in determining the most appropriate drug. For example, frail older adults who live alone are at high risk for severe hypoglycemia because low blood glucose is often undetected or untreated. This is especially true if the patient has cognitive impairment. In these cases, an OA that does not cause hypoglycemia, or a shorter-acting OA, would be most appropriate.

Patient teaching is essential. Some patients may assume that their diabetes is not a serious condition if they are only taking a pill to treat it. Teach the patient that OAs will help manage blood glucose and help prevent serious long- and short-term complications of diabetes. Discuss how OAs and noninsulin injectable agents are used in addition to food choices and activity as therapy for diabetes and the importance of following their meal and activity plans. Teach patients not to take extra pills if they have overeaten. If the patient uses sulfonylureas and metformin, teach the patient about the prevention, recognition, and management of hypoglycemia.

Personal Hygiene. The potential for infection requires diligent skin and dental hygiene practices. Because of the susceptibility to periodontal disease, encourage daily brushing and flossing and regular dental visits. When having dental work done, have the patient tell the dentist they have diabetes.

Routine care includes regular bathing, with an emphasis on foot care. Advise patients to inspect their feet daily, avoid going barefoot, and wear shoes that are supportive and comfortable. If cuts, scrapes, or burns occur, treat them promptly and monitor them carefully. Wash the area and apply a nonabrasive or nonirritating antiseptic ointment. Cover the area with a dry, sterile pad. Teach patients to notify the HCP at once if the injury does not begin to heal within 24 hours or if signs of infection develop.

Medical Identification and Travel. Teach the patient to always carry medical identification indicating that they have diabetes. Police, paramedics, and many private citizens are aware of the need to look for this identification when working with sick or unconscious persons. An identification card (Fig. 48.11) can supply valuable information, such as the name of the HCP; the type of diabetes; and the type and dosage of insulin, noninsulin injectable agents, or OAs.

Travel for a patient with diabetes requires planning. Being sedentary for long periods may raise the person's glucose level. Encourage the patient to get up and walk at least every 2 hours to lower the risk for deep vein thrombosis and prevent elevation

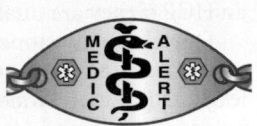

I have DIABETES

If unconscious or behaving abnormally, I may be having a reaction associated with diabetes or its treatment.

If I can swallow, give me a sweet drink, orange juice, LifeSavers, or low-fat milk.

If I do not recover promptly, call a physician or send me to the hospital.

If I am unconscious or cannot swallow, do not attempt to give me anything by mouth, but call 911 or send me to the hospital immediately.

FIG. 48.11 Medical alerts. A patient with diabetes should carry a card and wear a bracelet or necklace that indicates diabetes. If the patient with diabetes is unconscious, these measures will ensure prompt and appropriate attention.

NURSING MANAGEMENT
Caring for the Patient With Diabetes

You will need to collaborate with many health care team members to deliver, delegate, and coordinate care based on the patient's status.

- Assess for risk factors for prediabetes and type 1 and type 2 diabetes.
- Teach the patient and caregiver about diabetes management, including SMBG, insulin, noninsulin injectables, OAs, nutrition, physical activity, and managing hypoglycemia.
- Develop a plan to avoid hypoglycemia or hyperglycemia in a patient with DM who is acutely ill or having surgery.
- Assess for acute complications and implement appropriate actions for hypoglycemia, DKA, and HHS.
- In patients having acute complications, perform or directly supervise actions, including IV fluid and insulin administration.
- Assess for chronic complications, including CVD, retinopathy, nephropathy, neuropathy, and foot complications.
- Teach the patient and caregiver about prevention and management of chronic complications related to diabetes.
- Oversee LPN/VNs, and in some states and settings UAP, administer insulin, noninsulin injectable agents, and OAs to stable patients.

Collaborate With Other Team Members
Dietitian

- Obtain a diet history from the patient.
- Work with patient and caregiver to create an individualized meal plan.
- Provide instructions for meal plan as needed.

Physical Therapist

- Assess patient's current level of fitness.
- Develop an exercise plan with the patient.

Occupational Therapist

- Teach with patient with vision impairment how to use devices to draw up and measure insulin.
- Provide teaching on how to use a talking blood glucose monitor or use any blood glucose monitor one handed.
- Develop protective techniques for activities that involve exposure to heat, cold, and sharp objects.

Social Worker

- Aid the patient in finding resources to meet medical and financial needs.
- Help with coping with diabetes, including managing problems within the family or workplace.

of glucose levels. Teach the patient to have a full set of diabetes care supplies in the carry-on luggage when traveling by plane, train, or bus. This includes blood glucose monitoring equipment, insulin, noninsulin injectable agents, OAs, and syringes or insulin pens and pen needles.

Best practices for traveling with diabetes supplies and equipment change frequently. Encourage patients to check TSA guidelines before traveling at *www.diabetes.org/living-with-diabetes/know-your-rights/discrimination/public-accommodations/air-travel-and-diabetes/*. Notify screeners if an insulin pump is used so that they can inspect it while it is on the body, rather than removing it.

For patients who use insulin or OAs that can cause hypoglycemia, keep snack items and a quick-acting carbohydrate source for treating hypoglycemia in the carry-on luggage. Keep extra insulin available in case a bottle breaks or is lost. For longer trips, carry a full day's supply of food in case of canceled flights, delayed meals, or closed restaurants. If the patient is planning a trip out of the country, it is wise to have a letter from the HCP explaining that the patient has diabetes and requires all the materials, especially syringes, for ongoing health care.

When travel involves time changes, such as traveling coast to coast or across the International Date Line, the patient can contact the HCP to plan an appropriate insulin schedule. During travel, most patients find it helpful to keep watches set to the time of the city of origin until they reach their destination. The key to travel when taking insulin is to know the type of insulin being taken, its onset of action, the anticipated peak time, and mealtimes.

Patient and Caregiver Teaching. The goals of diabetes self-management education are to match the level of self-management to the patient's individual ability so that they can become the most active participant possible. Patients who actively manage their diabetes care have better outcomes than those who do not. For this reason, an educational approach that facilitates informed decision making by the patient is advocated. We call this the *empowerment approach* to education.

The empowerment approach includes eliminating messages that are judgmental and negative and replacing them with empowering, person-centered, and strengths-based language. An example includes referring to a patient as a person with diabetes versus calling them a diabetic. This places the emphasis on the person versus the disease. Other examples of words that may be perceived as negative or judgmental include compliant, uncontrolled, and poorly controlled."[18] Research has shown that people with diabetes feel the impact of negative language and would trust their HCPs more if they used empowering language and made them feel like a partner in their care.

🌿 COMPLEMENTARY & ALTERNATIVE THERAPIES

Herbs and Supplements That May Affect Blood Glucose

Scientific Evidence

Herbs and supplements that may lower blood glucose include aloe, ginger, cinnamon, St. John's wort, garlic, and ginseng. However, many studies have been small and not well designed. Further research is needed.

Nursing Implications

- Teach patients to use herbs and supplements with caution since they may affect blood glucose.
- Encourage patients with diabetes to talk with their HCP before using herbs or nutritional supplements.
- Teach patients who use herbs to regularly monitor their blood glucose levels.

Source: Gupta RC, Chang D, Nammi S, et al: Interactions between antidiabetic drugs and herbs: an overview of mechanisms of action and clinical implications, *Diabetol Metab Syndr* 9:59, 2017.

INFORMATICS IN PRACTICE
Patient Teaching Using Smart Phone Apps

- Teaching is a critical part of nursing care for patients with diabetes. Put some fun into patient teaching by using smart phone applications.
- Apps offer convenient, quick access to up-to-date information.
- Introduce patients to a variety of smart phone apps for healthy living and managing diabetes.
- Sample apps include Glooko, Health2Sync, Glucosio, MyNetDiaryPRO, Diabetes Tracker, mySugr, and BeatO.

Source: Based on a list provided by Healthline. Retrieved from *www.healthline.com/health/diabetes/top-iphone-android-apps*.

Unfortunately, patients can encounter a variety of physical, psychologic, and emotional barriers when it comes to effectively managing their diabetes. These barriers may include feelings of inadequacy about one's own abilities, unwillingness to make behavioral changes, ineffective coping strategies, and cognitive deficits. If the patient is not able to manage the disease, a family member may be able to assume part of this role. If the patient or caregiver cannot make decisions related to diabetes management, consider a referral to a CDE, social worker, or other resources within the community. These resources can help the patient and family in outlining a feasible treatment program that meets their capabilities.

An assessment of the patient's knowledge of diabetes and lifestyle preferences is useful in planning a teaching program. Tables 48.14 and 48.15 present guidelines to use for patient and caregiver teaching. Assess the patient's knowledge base frequently so that gaps in knowledge or incorrect or inaccurate ideas can be corrected.

The ADA offers resources for patients in the form of pamphlets, booklets, books, and a monthly magazine called *Diabetes Forecast*. Affiliates of the ADA are found in all states. Most can be reached by dialing 1-800-DIABETES (800-342-2383). The ADA publishes materials and sponsors conferences for health care professionals concerned with diabetes education, research, and management of patients. The ADA website *(www.diabetes.org)* has extensive information for the public and health care professionals. The ADA also recognizes education programs that meet the national standards of diabetes education and can provide a list of these programs. Most drug companies manufacturing diabetes-related products have free educational materials for patients and HCPs. It is critical that you stay current in your diabetes knowledge so that you can effectively teach and support patients with diabetes.

◆ Evaluation

The expected outcomes are that the patient with diabetes will
- State key elements of the treatment plan
- Describe self-care measures that may prevent or slow progression of chronic complications
- Maintain a balance of nutrition, activity, and insulin availability that results in stable, safe, and healthy blood glucose levels
- Have no injury from decreased sensation in the feet
- Implement measures to increase peripheral circulation

ACUTE COMPLICATIONS OF DIABETES

The acute complications of diabetes arise from events associated with hyperglycemia and hypoglycemia. Hyperglycemia (high blood glucose) occurs when there is not enough insulin working. Hypoglycemia (low blood glucose) occurs when there is too much insulin working. Many signs and symptoms of

TABLE 48.14 Patient & Caregiver Teaching
Management of Diabetes

Include the following instructions when teaching the patient and caregiver how to manage diabetes:

Component	What to Teach
Disease process	• Introduce the pancreas and the islets of Langerhans. • Describe how insulin is made and what affects its production. • Discuss the relationship of insulin and glucose. • Explain the difference between type 1 and type 2 diabetes.
Physical activity	• Discuss the effect of regular exercise on managing blood glucose and improving cardiovascular function and general health.
Menu planning	• Stress the importance of a well-balanced diet as part of a diabetes management plan. • Explain the impact of carbohydrates on blood glucose levels.
Medication	• Ensure that the patient understands the proper use of prescribed medication (e.g., insulin [Table 48.5], OAs, noninsulin injectables). • Account for a patient's physical or other limitations or inabilities for self-medication. If necessary, involve the family or caregiver in proper use of medication. • Discuss all side effects and safety issues about medication.
Monitoring blood glucose	• Teach correct blood glucose monitoring. • Include when to check blood glucose levels, how to record them, and how to adjust insulin levels, if necessary.
Risk reduction	• Ensure that the patient understands and appropriately responds to the signs and symptoms of hypoglycemia and hyperglycemia (Table 48.16). • Stress the importance of proper foot care (Table 48.21), regular eye examinations, and consistent glucose monitoring. • Teach the patient about the effect that stress can have on blood glucose.
Psychosocial	• Help the patient identify resources that are available to help with the adjustment and answer questions about living with a chronic condition such as diabetes.

TABLE 48.15 Patient & Caregiver Teaching
Instructions for Patients With Diabetes

Include the following essential instructions for diabetes management for the patient and caregiver:

Blood Glucose
- Monitor your blood glucose at home and record results in a log.
- Take your insulin, OA, and/or noninsulin injectable agent as prescribed.
- Take insulin consistently, especially when you are sick.
- Keep an adequate supply of insulin on hand at all times.
- Obtain A1C blood test every 3–6 mo as an indicator of your long-term blood glucose levels.
- Be aware of symptoms of hypoglycemia and hyperglycemia.
- Always carry a form of rapid-acting glucose so that you can treat hypoglycemia quickly.
- Teach family members how and when to use glucagon if patient becomes unresponsive because of hypoglycemia.

Exercise
- Learn how exercise and food affect your blood glucose levels.
- Remember that exercise will usually lower your blood glucose level.
- Begin an exercise program after approval from HCP.

Food
- Work with a dietitian to create a patient specific meal plan.
- Make healthy food choices and eat regular meals at regular times.
- Choose foods low in saturated and *trans* fat. Know your cholesterol level.
- Limit the amount of alcohol you drink.
- Be aware that excess amounts of alcohol may lead to unpredictable low blood glucose events.
- Avoid fad diets.
- Limit regular soda and fruit juice.

Other Guidelines
- Obtain an annual eye examination by an ophthalmologist.
- Obtain annual urine monitoring for protein.
- Examine your feet at home.
- Wear comfortable, well-fitting shoes to help prevent foot injury. Break in new shoes gradually.
- Always carry identification that says you have diabetes.
- Have other medical problems treated, especially high BP and high cholesterol.
- Have a yearly influenza vaccination.
- Quit or never start smoking cigarettes or using nicotine products.
- Avoid applying heat or cold directly to your feet.
- Avoid going barefoot.
- Keep skin moisturized by applying cream to surfaces of feet, but not between toes.

hyperglycemia and hypoglycemia overlap. It is important for the HCP to distinguish between them because hypoglycemia worsens rapidly and is a serious threat if action is not immediately taken. Table 48.16 compares the manifestations, causes, management, and prevention of hyperglycemia and hypoglycemia.

DIABETIC KETOACIDOSIS

Etiology and Pathophysiology

Diabetes-related ketoacidosis (DKA) is caused by a profound deficiency of insulin. It is characterized by hyperglycemia, ketosis, acidosis, and dehydration. It is most likely to occur in people with type 1 diabetes. DKA may be seen in people with type 2 diabetes in conditions of severe illness or stress in which the pancreas cannot meet the extra demand for insulin. Precipitating factors include illness; infection; inadequate insulin dosage; undiagnosed type 1 diabetes; lack of education, understanding, or resources; and neglect.

When the circulating supply of insulin is insufficient, glucose cannot be properly used for energy. The body compensates by breaking down fat stores as a secondary source of fuel (Fig. 48.12). Ketones are acidic by-products of fat metabolism that can cause serious problems when they become excessive in the blood. Ketosis alters the pH balance, causing metabolic acidosis to develop. Ketonuria is a process that occurs when ketone bodies are excreted in the urine. During this process, electrolytes that are cations are also excreted with the anionic ketones to try to maintain electrical neutrality.

Insulin deficiency impairs protein synthesis and causes excessive protein degradation. This results in nitrogen losses from the tissues. Insulin deficiency stimulates the production of glucose from amino acids (from proteins) in the liver and leads to further hyperglycemia. Because of the insulin deficiency, the

TABLE 48.16 Comparison of Hyperglycemia and Hypoglycemia

Hyperglycemia	Hypoglycemia
Manifestations	
• Elevated blood glucose	• Blood glucose <70 mg/dL (3.9 mmol/L)
• Increase in urination	• Cold, clammy skin
• Increase in appetite followed by lack of appetite	• Numbness of fingers, toes, mouth
• Weakness, fatigue	• Tachycardia
• Blurred vision	• Emotional changes
• Headache	• Headache
• Glycosuria	• Nervousness, tremors
• Nausea and vomiting	• Faintness, dizziness
• Abdominal cramps	• Unsteady gait, slurred speech
• Progression to DKA or HHS	• Hunger
• Mood swings	• Changes in vision
	• Seizures, coma
Causes	
• Illness, infection	• Alcohol intake without food
• Corticosteroids	• Too little food—delayed, omitted, inadequate intake
• Too much food	• Too much diabetes medication
• Too little or no diabetes medication	• Too much exercise without adequate food intake
• Inactivity	• Diabetes medication or food taken at wrong time
• Emotional, physical stress	• Loss of weight without change in medication
• Poor absorption of insulin	• Use of β-adrenergic blockers interfering with recognition of symptoms
Clinical Course	
• More gradual onset	• More rapid onset
• Definition of elevated glucose varies by person, based on personal glucose targets	• Pattern of manifestations changes over time
Treatment	
• Get medical care	• Follow the Rule of 15 (see pp. 1134–1135).
• Continue diabetes medication as prescribed	• See Table 48.19 for emergency treatment of hypoglycemia.
• Check blood glucose frequently and check urine for ketones; record results	
• Drink fluids at least on an hourly basis	
• Contact HCP about ketonuria	
Preventive Measures	
• Take prescribed dose of medication at proper time	• Take prescribed dose of medication at proper time
• Accurately give insulin, noninsulin injectables, OA	• Accurately give insulin, noninsulin injectables, OA
• Make healthy food choices	• Coordinate eating with medications
• Follow sick-day rules when ill	• Eat adequate food intake needed for calories for exercise
• Check blood glucose routinely	• Be able to recognize symptoms and treat them immediately
• Wear or carry diabetes identification	• Carry simple carbohydrates
	• Teach family and caregiver about symptoms and treatment
	• Check blood glucose routinely
	• Wear or carry diabetes identification

PATHOPHYSIOLOGY MAP

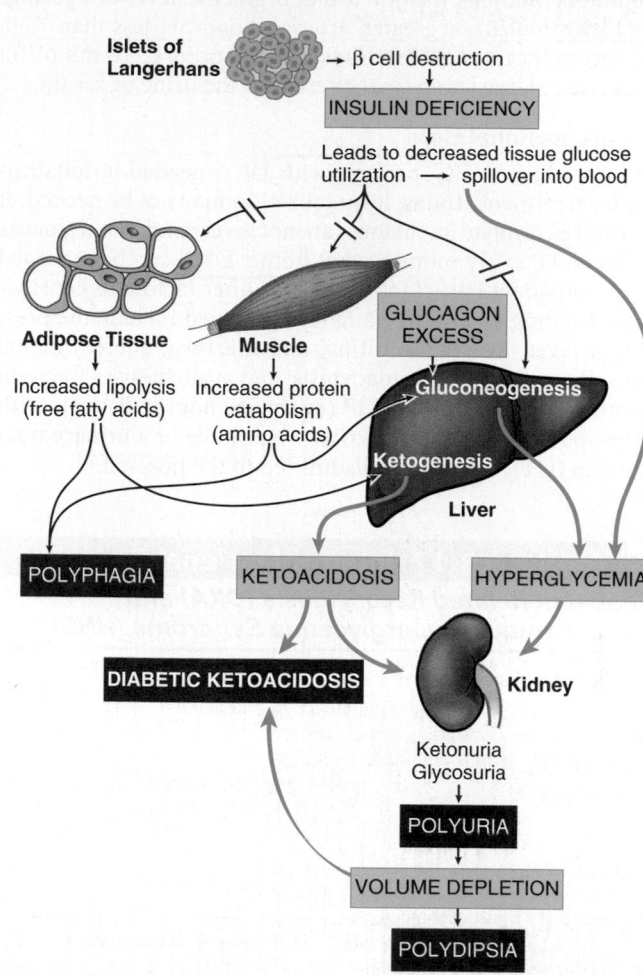

FIG. 48.12 Metabolic events leading to diabetic ketoacidosis. (Modified from Kumar V, Abbas AK, Aster JC, et al: *Robbins and Cotran pathologic basis of disease,* ed 8, Philadelphia, 2010, Saunders.)

additional glucose cannot be used and the blood glucose level rises further, adding to the osmotic diuresis.

If not treated, the patient will develop severe depletion of sodium, potassium, chloride, magnesium, and phosphate. Vomiting caused by the acidosis results in more fluid and electrolyte losses. Eventually, hypovolemia, followed by shock, will ensue. Renal failure, which may eventually occur from hypovolemic shock, causes the retention of ketones and glucose, and the acidosis progresses. Untreated, the patient becomes comatose from dehydration, electrolyte imbalance, and acidosis. If the condition is not treated, death is inevitable.

Clinical Manifestations

Dehydration occurs in DKA with manifestations of dry mucous membranes, tachycardia, and orthostatic hypotension. Early symptoms may include lethargy and weakness. As the patient becomes severely dehydrated, the skin becomes dry and loose, and the eyes become soft and sunken. Abdominal pain may be present and accompanied by anorexia, nausea, and vomiting. Acetone is noted on the breath as a sweet, fruity odor.

Kussmaul respirations (rapid, deep breathing associated with dyspnea) are the body's attempt to reverse metabolic acidosis through the exhalation of excess CO_2. (See Chapter 16 for a discussion of respiratory compensation of metabolic acidosis.) Laboratory findings include a blood glucose level of 250 mg/dL (13.9 mmol/L) or greater, arterial blood pH less than 7.30, and serum bicarbonate level less than 16 mEq/L (16 mmol/L). Moderate to large ketones are present in the urine or serum.

Interprofessional Care

Before we had SMBG, patients with DKA needed hospitalization for treatment. Today, hospitalization may not be needed. If fluid and electrolyte imbalances are not severe and blood glucose levels can be safely monitored at home, DKA can be managed on an outpatient basis (Table 48.17). Other factors to consider when deciding where the patient is managed include the presence of fever, nausea, vomiting, and diarrhea; altered mental status; the cause of the ketoacidosis; and availability of frequent communication with the HCP (every few hours). Patients with DKA who have an illness such as pneumonia or a urinary tract infection (UTI) usually need admitted to the hospital.

DKA is a serious condition that proceeds rapidly and must be treated promptly. Refer to Table 48.18 for the emergency management of a patient with DKA. Because fluid imbalance is potentially life threatening, the first goal of therapy is to establish IV access and begin fluid and electrolyte replacement. Typically, the initial fluid therapy involves an IV infusion of 0.45% or 0.9% NaCl at a rate to raise BP and restore urine output to 30 to 60 mL/hr. When blood glucose levels approach 250 mg/dL (13.9 mmol/L), 5% to 10% dextrose is added to prevent hypoglycemia and a sudden drop in glucose that can be associated with cerebral edema. Overzealous rehydration, especially with hypotonic IV solutions, can cause cerebral edema.

The aim of fluid and electrolyte therapy is to replace extracellular and intracellular water and to correct deficits of sodium, chloride, bicarbonate, potassium, phosphate, and magnesium. Monitor patients with renal or cardiac compromise for fluid overload. Obtain a serum potassium level before starting insulin. If the patient is hypokalemic, giving insulin will further decrease potassium levels, making early potassium replacement essential. Although initial serum potassium may be normal or high, levels can rapidly decrease once therapy starts as insulin drives potassium into the cells, leading to life-threatening hypokalemia.

IV insulin therapy is given to correct hyperglycemia and hyperketonemia. It is important to prevent rapid drops in serum glucose to avoid cerebral edema. A blood glucose reduction of 36 to 54 mg/dL/hr (2 to 3 mmol/L/hr) will avoid complications. Insulin allows water and potassium to enter the cell along with glucose and can lead to a depletion of vascular volume and hypokalemia, so monitor the patient's fluid balance and potassium levels.

 TABLE 48.17 Interprofessional Care

Diabetes-Related Ketoacidosis (DKA) and Hyperosmolar Hyperglycemia Syndrome (HHS)

Diagnostic Assessment
- History and physical examination
- Blood studies, including blood glucose, CBC, pH, ketones, electrolytes, BUN, arterial or venous blood gases
- Urinalysis, including specific gravity, glucose, acetone

Management
- Administration of IV fluids
- IV administration of short-acting insulin
- Electrolyte replacement
- Assessment of mental status
- Recording of intake and output
- Central venous pressure monitoring (if indicated)
- Assessment of blood glucose levels
- Assessment of blood and urine for ketones
- ECG monitoring
- Assessment of cardiovascular and respiratory status

 CHECK YOUR PRACTICE

A 22-yr-old female patient admitted with DKA has a blood glucose level of 554 mg/dL. You are trying to regulate her IV rate. You know that giving IV fluids too rapidly and quickly lowering of serum glucose can lead to cerebral edema. You also know that incorrect fluid replacement, especially with hypotonic fluids, can cause a sudden fall in serum sodium that can cause cerebral edema.
- What are the best clinical indicators of successful treatment of DKA?
- What is your role as a nurse in caring for this patient?

✚ **TABLE 48.18 Emergency Management**

Diabetes-Related Ketoacidosis

Etiology	Assessment Findings	Interventions
• Undiagnosed diabetes • Inadequate treatment of existing diabetes • Insulin not taken as prescribed • Illness, infection • Change in eating, insulin, or exercise plan • Malfunction of insulin pump/nondelivery of insulin	• Abdominal pain • Breath odor of ketones (fruity) • Dry mouth • Eyes appearing sunken • Fever • Flushed, dry skin • Glucosuria and ketonuria • Increasing restlessness, confusion, lethargy • Labored breathing (Kussmaul respirations) • Nausea and vomiting • Rapid, weak pulse • Serum glucose >250 mg/dL (13.9 mmol/L) • Thirst • Urinary frequency	**Initial** • Ensure patent airway. • Give O₂ via nasal cannula or nonrebreather mask. • Establish IV access with large-bore catheter. • Begin fluid resuscitation with 0.9% NaCl solution 1 L/hr until BP stabilized and urine output 30-60 mL/hr. • Begin continuous regular insulin drip 0.1 U/kg/hr. • Identify history of diabetes, time of last food, and time and amount of last insulin injection. **Ongoing Monitoring** • Monitor vital signs, level of consciousness, ECG, O₂ saturation, and urine output. • Assess breath sounds for fluid overload. • Monitor serum glucose and serum potassium. • Give potassium to correct hypokalemia. • Give sodium bicarbonate if severe acidosis (pH <7.0). • Add dextrose to IV fluid for blood glucose <250 mg/dL.

HYPEROSMOLAR HYPERGLYCEMIA SYNDROME ~infection~

Hyperosmolar hyperglycemia syndrome (HHS) is a life-threatening syndrome that can occur in the patient with diabetes who is able to make enough insulin to prevent DKA, but not enough to prevent severe hyperglycemia, osmotic diuresis, and extracellular fluid depletion (Fig. 48.13). HHS is less common than DKA (Table 48.17). It often occurs in patients over 60 years of age with type 2 diabetes.

Common causes of HHS are UTIs, pneumonia, sepsis, any acute illness, and newly diagnosed type 2 diabetes. HHS is often related to impaired thirst sensation and/or a functional inability to replace fluids. There is usually a history of inadequate fluid intake, increasing mental depression or cognitive impairment, and polyuria.

PATHOPHYSIOLOGY MAP

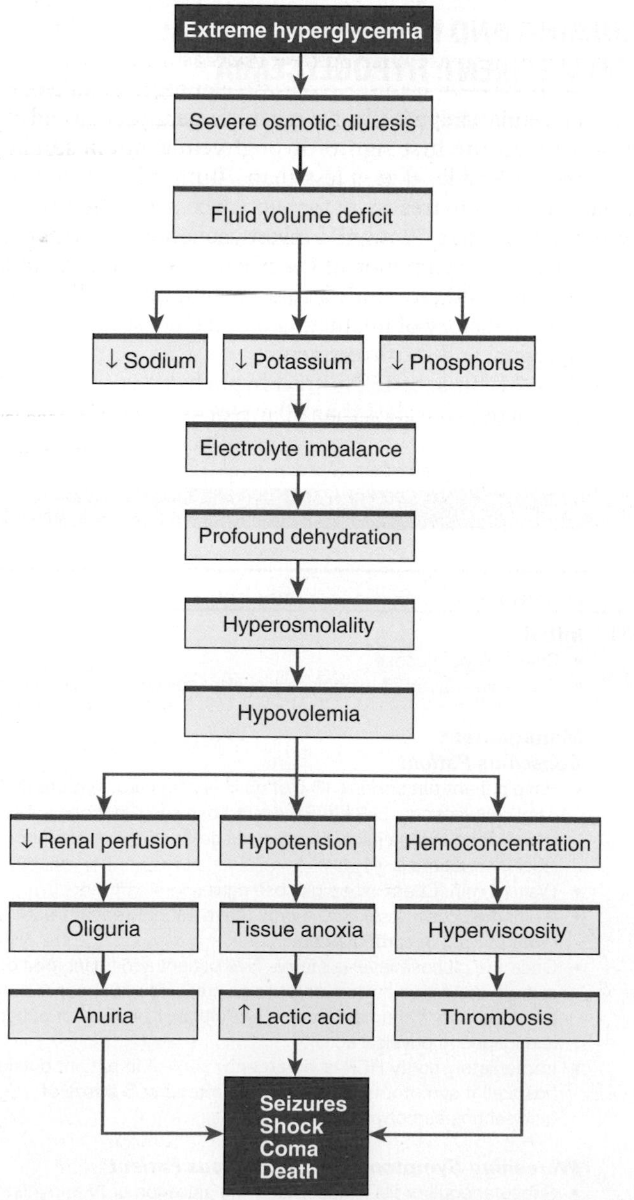

Extreme hyperglycemia
↓
Severe osmotic diuresis
↓
Fluid volume deficit
↓
↓ Sodium | ↓ Potassium | ↓ Phosphorus
↓
Electrolyte imbalance
↓
Profound dehydration
↓
Hyperosmolality
↓
Hypovolemia
↓
↓ Renal perfusion | Hypotension | Hemoconcentration
↓
Oliguria | Tissue anoxia | Hyperviscosity
↓
Anuria | ↑ Lactic acid | Thrombosis
↓
Seizures
Shock
Coma
Death

FIG. 48.13 Pathophysiology of hyperosmolar hyperglycemic syndrome. (Modified from Urden LD, Stacy KM, Lough ME: *Critical care nursing: Diagnosis and management,* ed 6, St Louis, 2010, Mosby.)

The main difference between HHS and DKA is that the patient with HHS usually has enough circulating insulin so that ketoacidosis does not occur. Because HHS has fewer symptoms in the earlier stages, blood glucose levels can climb quite high before the problem is recognized. The higher blood glucose levels increase serum osmolality and cause more severe neurologic manifestations, such as somnolence, coma, seizures, hemiparesis, and aphasia. Since these manifestations resemble a stroke, immediate determination of the glucose level is critical for correct diagnosis and treatment.

Laboratory values in HHS include a blood glucose level greater than 600 mg/dL (33.33 mmol/L) and a marked increase in serum osmolality. Ketone bodies are absent or minimal in both blood and urine.

Interprofessional Care

HHS is a medical emergency. It has a high mortality rate. The management of HHS is similar to DKA. It includes immediate IV administration of insulin and either 0.9% or 0.45% NaCl. HHS usually requires large volumes of fluid replacement. This should be done slowly and carefully. Patients with HHS are often older and may have cardiac or renal compromise, requiring hemodynamic monitoring to avoid fluid overload during fluid replacement. When blood glucose levels fall to about 250 mg/dL (13.9 mmol/L), IV fluids containing dextrose are given to prevent hypoglycemia.

Electrolytes are monitored and replaced as needed. Hypokalemia is not as significant in HHS as it is in DKA, although fluid losses may result in milder potassium deficits that require replacement. Assess vital signs, intake and output, laboratory values, and cardiac monitoring to check the efficacy of fluid and electrolyte replacement. This includes monitoring serum osmolality and frequently assessing cardiac, renal, and mental status. Once the patient is stabilized, begin attempts to detect and correct the underlying cause.

❖ NURSING MANAGEMENT: DIABETES-RELATED KETOACIDOSIS AND HYPEROSMOLAR HYPERGLYCEMIA SYNDROME

Closely monitor the hospitalized patient with appropriate blood and urine tests. You are responsible for monitoring blood glucose and urine for output and ketones and using laboratory data to determine appropriate patient care.

Monitor the administration of (1) IV fluids to correct dehydration, (2) insulin therapy to reduce blood glucose and serum ketone levels, and (3) electrolytes given to correct electrolyte imbalance. Assess renal status and cardiopulmonary status related to hydration and electrolyte levels. Monitor the level of consciousness.

Assess for signs of potassium imbalance resulting from low levels of insulin and osmotic diuresis (see Chapter 16). When insulin treatment is started, serum potassium levels may decrease rapidly as potassium moves into the cells once insulin is available. This movement of potassium into and out of extracellular fluid influences cardiac functioning. Cardiac monitoring is useful in detecting characteristic changes of potassium excess or deficit that are observable on ECG tracings (see Fig. 16.14). Assess vital signs often to identify fever, hypovolemic shock, tachycardia, and Kussmaul respirations.

HYPOGLYCEMIA

Hypoglycemia, or low blood glucose, occurs when there is too much insulin in proportion to available glucose in the blood.

This causes the blood glucose level to drop to less than 70 mg/dL (3.9 mmol/L). When glucose drops below 70 mg/dL, counterregulatory hormones are released and the autonomic nervous system is activated. Suppression of insulin secretion and production of glucagon and epinephrine provide a defense against hypoglycemia. Epinephrine release causes manifestations that include shakiness, palpitations, nervousness, diaphoresis, anxiety, hunger, and pallor. Because the brain needs a constant supply of glucose in sufficient quantities to function properly, hypoglycemia can affect mental functioning. These "neuroglycopenia" manifestations are difficulty speaking, visual changes, stupor, confusion, and coma. Manifestations of hypoglycemia can mimic alcohol intoxication. Untreated hypoglycemia can progress to loss of consciousness, seizures, coma, and death.

Hypoglycemia unawareness is a condition in which a person does not have the warning signs and symptoms of hypoglycemia until the glucose level reaches a critical point. Then the person may become incoherent and combative or lose consciousness. This is often a result of diabetes-related autonomic neuropathy that interferes with the secretion of counterregulatory hormones that cause these symptoms. Patients at risk for hypoglycemia unawareness include those who have had repeated episodes of hypoglycemia, older adults, and patients who use β-adrenergic blockers. Using intensive treatment to lower blood glucose levels in patients who have or are at risk for hypoglycemia unawareness may not be an appropriate goal. These patients usually keep blood glucose levels somewhat higher than those who can detect and manage the onset of hypoglycemia.

Causes of hypoglycemia are often related to a mismatch in the timing of food intake and the peak action of insulin or OAs that increase endogenous insulin secretion. The balance between blood glucose and insulin can be disrupted by giving too much insulin or medication, ingesting too little food, delaying the time of eating, and performing unusual or unexpected exercise. Hypoglycemia can occur at any time, but most often occurs when the OA or insulin is at its peak of action or when the patient's daily routine is disrupted without adequate adjustments in diet, drugs, and activity. Although hypoglycemia is most common with insulin therapy, it can occur with noninsulin injectable agents and OAs and may persist for an extended time because of the longer duration of action of these drugs.

Symptoms of hypoglycemia may occur when a very high blood glucose level falls too rapidly (e.g., a blood glucose level of 300 mg/dL [16.7 mmol/L] falling quickly to 150 mg/dL [10 mmol/L]). Although the blood glucose level is above normal by definition and measurement, the sudden metabolic shift can cause hypoglycemia symptoms. Aggressively managing blood glucose levels, lowering high blood glucose levels for the first time, or lowering blood glucose with insulin after a long period of hyperglycemia can cause this situation.

❖ NURSING AND INTERPROFESSIONAL MANAGEMENT: HYPOGLYCEMIA

Hypoglycemia can usually be quickly reversed with effective treatment. At the first sign of hypoglycemia, check the blood glucose, if possible. If it is less than 70 mg/dL (3.9 mmol/L), immediately begin treatment for hypoglycemia. If the blood glucose is greater than 70 mg/dL, investigate other possible causes of the signs and symptoms. If the patient has manifestations of hypoglycemia and monitoring equipment is not available or the patient has a history of fluctuating blood glucose levels, assume hypoglycemia, and start treatment.

Follow the "Rule of 15" to treat hypoglycemia (Table 48.19). A blood glucose value less than 70 mg/dL is treated by ingesting

---

✚ TABLE 48.19 Emergency Management

Hypoglycemia

Etiology	Assessment Findings	Interventions
• Too little food—delayed, omitted, inadequate intake • Too much diabetes medication • Too much exercise without adequate food intake • Diabetes medication or food taken at wrong time • Alcohol use without food intake	• Blood glucose <70 mg/dL (3.9 mmol/L) • Cold, clammy skin • Numbness of fingers, toes, mouth • Tachycardia • Emotional changes • Headache • Nervousness, tremors • Faintness, dizziness • Unsteady gait, slurred speech • Hunger • Changes in vision • Seizures, coma	**Initial** • Check blood glucose. • Determine cause of hypoglycemia (after correction of condition). **Management** ***Conscious Patient*** • Have patient eat or drink 15 g of quick-acting carbohydrate (4–6 oz of regular soda, 5–8 LifeSavers, 1 Tbsp syrup or honey, 4 tsp jelly, 4–6 oz orange juice, commercial dextrose products [per label instructions]). • Wait 15 min. Check blood glucose again. • If blood glucose is still <70 mg/dL, have patient repeat treatment of 15 g of carbohydrate. • Once the glucose level is stable, give patient additional food of carbohydrate plus protein or fat (e.g., crackers with peanut butter or cheese) if the next meal is more than 1 hr away or patient is engaged in physical activity. • Immediately notify HCP or emergency service (if patient outside hospital) if symptoms do not subside after 2 or 3 doses of quick-acting carbohydrate. ***Worsening Symptoms or Unconscious Patient*** • Subcutaneous or IM injection of 1 mg glucagon or IV administration of 20–50 mL of 50% glucose. • Turn the patient on the side to prevent aspiration.

15 g of a simple (fast-acting) carbohydrate, such as 4 to 6 oz of fruit juice or a regular soft drink. Commercial products, such as gels or tablets containing specific amounts of glucose, are convenient for carrying in a purse or pocket to be used in such situations. Recheck the blood glucose 15 minutes later. If the value is still less than 70 mg/dL, ingest 15 g more of carbohydrate and recheck the blood glucose in 15 minutes. If no significant improvement occurs after 2 or 3 doses of 15 g of simple carbohydrate, contact the HCP. After an acute episode of hypoglycemia, the patient may need a snack with carbohydrate and protein if the next meal is more than an hour away or if they are being active.

Avoid treatment with carbohydrates that contain fat, such as candy bars, cookies, whole milk, and ice cream. The fat in those foods will slow the absorption of the glucose and delay the response to treatment. Do not overtreat with large quantities of quick-acting carbohydrates because a rapid fluctuation to hyperglycemia can occur.

In an acute care setting, patients with hypoglycemia may be given 20 to 50 mL of 50% dextrose IV. If the patient is not alert enough to swallow and no IV access is available, another option is to give 1 mg of glucagon by IM or subcutaneous injection. An IM injection in a site such as the deltoid muscle will result in a quicker response. Glucagon stimulates a strong hepatic response to convert glycogen to glucose and makes glucose rapidly available. Nausea is a common reaction after glucagon injection. To prevent aspiration if vomiting occurs, turn the patient on the side until they are alert. Patients with minimal glycogen stores will not respond to glucagon. This includes patients with alcohol-related hepatic disease, starvation, and adrenal insufficiency.

Teach family members and others likely to be present if severe hypoglycemia occurs when and how to inject glucagon.

Once the acute hypoglycemia is reversed, explore with the patient the reasons why the situation developed. This assessment may indicate the need for further patient teaching to avoid future episodes of hypoglycemia.

CHRONIC COMPLICATIONS ASSOCIATED WITH DIABETES

ANGIOPATHY

Chronic complications associated with diabetes are primarily those of end-organ disease from damage to blood vessels (*angiopathy*) from chronic hyperglycemia (Fig. 48.14). Angiopathy is a leading cause of diabetes-related deaths, with about 68% of deaths caused by CVD and 16% caused by strokes for those ages 65 or older.[19] These chronic blood vessel dysfunctions are divided into 2 categories: macrovascular complications and microvascular complications.

Several theories exist as to how and why chronic hyperglycemia damages cells and tissues. Possible causes include (1) the accumulation of damaging by-products of glucose metabolism, such as sorbitol, which is associated with damage to nerve cells; (2) the formation of abnormal glucose molecules in the basement membrane of small blood vessels, such as those that circulate to the eyes and kidneys; and (3) a derangement in RBC function that leads to a decrease in oxygenation to the tissues.

The Diabetes Control and Complications Trial (DCCT), a landmark study in diabetes management, showed the risk for

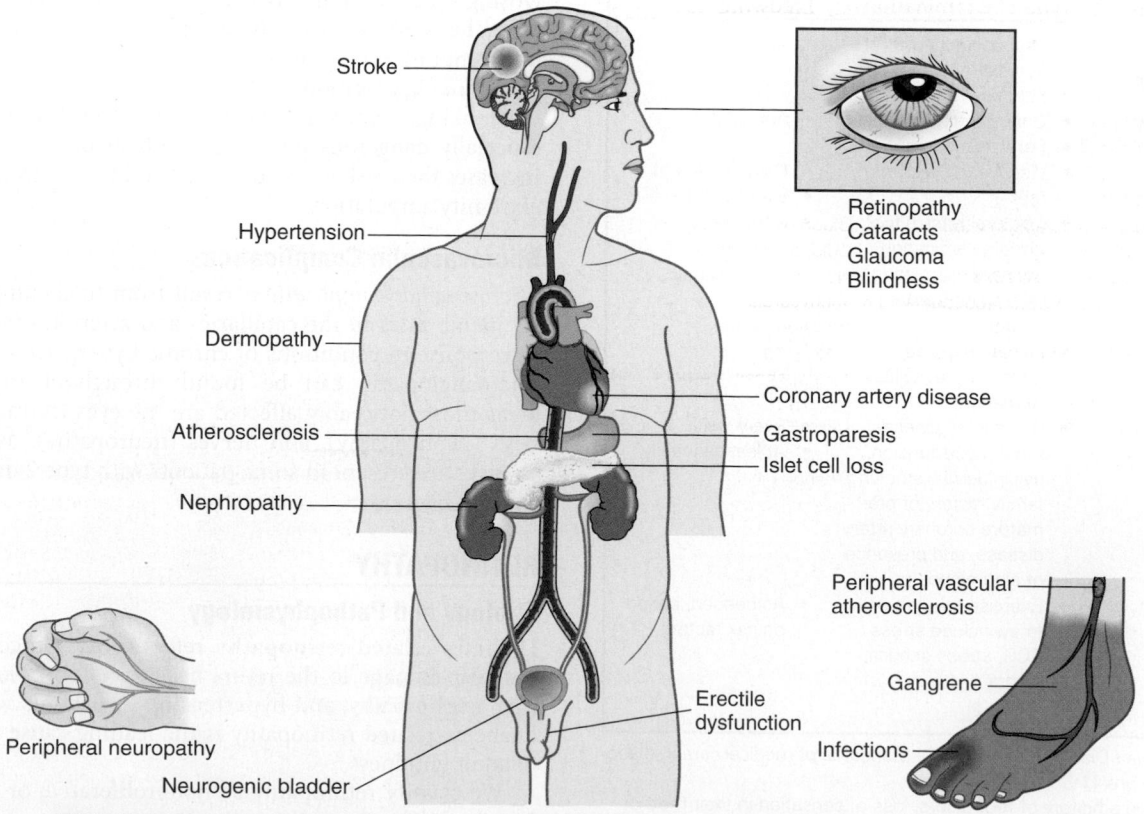

FIG. 48.14 Long-term complications of diabetes. (From Kumar V, Abbas AK, Aster JC, et al: *Robbins and Cotran pathologic basis of disease*, ed 8, Philadelphia, 2010, Saunders.)

microvascular complications could be significantly reduced in patients with type 1 diabetes by keeping blood glucose levels as near to normal as possible for as much of the time as possible *(tight or intensive therapy)*.[20] Those who maintained tight glucose levels reduced their risk for developing retinopathy and nephropathy, common microvascular complications. Based on these findings, the ADA issued recommendations for diabetes management that included treatment goals to maintain blood glucose levels as near to normal as possible. Specific targets for individual patients must consider the risk for severe or undetected hypoglycemia as a side effect of intensive management.

The United Kingdom Prospective Diabetes Study (UKPDS) showed that intensive treatment of type 2 diabetes significantly lowered the risk for developing diabetes-related eye, kidney, and neurologic problems. The findings included a 25% reduction of microvascular disease and a 16% reduction in the risk for MI in those who maintained long-term blood glucose levels.[21]

Because of the devastating effects of long-term complications, patients with diabetes need scheduled and ongoing monitoring for the detection and prevention of chronic complications. The ADA recommendations for ongoing evaluation are shown in Table 48.20. It is essential that patients understand the importance of regular follow-up visits.

Macrovascular Complications

Macrovascular complications are diseases of the large and medium-size blood vessels that occur with greater frequency and with an earlier onset in people with diabetes. Macrovascular

TABLE 48.20 Monitoring for Long-Term Complications Related to Diabetes

Complication	Type of Examination	Frequency
Retinopathy	• Funduscopic: dilated eye examination • Fundus photography	• Annually
Nephropathy	• Urine for albuminuria • Serum creatinine	• Annually
Neuropathy (foot and lower extremities)	• Visual examination of foot • Comprehensive foot: • Visual examination • Sensory examination with monofilament and tuning fork • Palpation (pulses, temperature, callus formation)	• Daily by patient • Every visit to HCP • Annually*
Cardiovascular disease	• Risk factor assessment: hypertension, dyslipidemia, smoking, family history of premature coronary artery disease, and presence of albuminuria or • Exercise stress testing (may include stress ECG, stress echocardiogram, stress nuclear imaging)	• Every visit • At least annually • As needed, based on risk factors

Source: American Diabetes Association: Standards of medical care in diabetes, *Diabetes Care* 41:S86, 2018.
*If patients have a history of foot ulcers, loss of sensation in their feet, or other foot abnormalities, the recommendation is to have a foot examination at every visit.

diseases include cerebrovascular, cardiovascular, and peripheral vascular disease. Women with diabetes have a 4 to 6 times increased risk for CVD. Men with diabetes have a 2 to 3 times increased risk for CVD compared with those without diabetes.[2]

Patients with diabetes can decrease several risk factors associated with macrovascular complications, such as obesity, smoking, hypertension, high fat intake, and sedentary lifestyle. The ADA recognizes that diabetes alone is a CVD risk factor. The ADA recommends yearly screening for CVD risk factors in people with diabetes.[22]

Insulin resistance is important in the development of CVD and implicated in the pathogenesis of essential hypertension and dyslipidemia. We do not completely understand the role of insulin resistance in the pathogenesis of CVD. It seems to combine with dyslipidemia in contributing to greater risk for CVD in patients with diabetes.

Optimizing BP control in patients with diabetes is significant in preventing CVD and renal disease. Treating hypertension in those with diabetes results in a decrease in macrovascular and microvascular complications. Hypertension in people with diabetes causes an increase in mortality greater than for those with hypertension without diabetes. The ADA recommends BP screening at every visit for people with diabetes. They recommend lifestyle counseling for BP greater than 130/80 mm Hg and treatment to achieve a target BP of less than 140/90 mm Hg for most patients with diabetes.[22] Hypertension is discussed in Chapter 32, and coronary artery disease is discussed in Chapter 33.)

Patients with diabetes have an increase in lipid abnormalities that contribute to their increased risk for CVD. The ADA recommends screening all adults for dyslipidemia at the time diabetes is diagnosed and starting statin therapy as needed. Dosing is based on the presence of age and other CVD risk factors. The ADA advocates treating hyperlipidemia with lifestyle interventions, including nutrition therapy, exercise, weight loss, and smoking cessation.

Smoking, which is detrimental to health in general, is especially dangerous for people with diabetes. It significantly increases their risk for blood vessel and CVD, stroke, and lower extremity amputation.

Microvascular Complications

Microvascular complications result from thickening of the vessel membranes in the capillaries and arterioles (small vessels) in response to conditions of chronic hyperglycemia. Although microangiopathy can be found throughout the body, the areas most noticeably affected are the eyes (retinopathy), kidneys (nephropathy), and nerves (neuropathy). Microvascular changes are present in some patients with type 2 diabetes at the time of diagnosis.

RETINOPATHY

Etiology and Pathophysiology

Diabetes-related retinopathy refers to the process of microvascular damage to the retina because of chronic hyperglycemia, nephropathy, and hypertension in patients with diabetes. Diabetes-related retinopathy is the leading cause of new cases of adult blindness.[2]

We classify retinopathy as nonproliferative or proliferative. In *nonproliferative retinopathy,* the most common form, partial occlusion of the small blood vessels in the retina causes microaneurysms to develop in the capillary walls. The walls of these microaneurysms are so weak that capillary fluid leaks out, causing retinal edema and eventually hard exudates or intra-retinal hemorrhages. This may cause mild to severe vision loss, depending on which parts of the retina are affected. If the center of the retina (macula) is affected, vision loss can be severe.

Proliferative retinopathy, the most severe form, involves the retina and vitreous. When retinal capillaries become occluded, the body compensates by forming new blood vessels to supply the retina with blood, a pathologic process known as *neovascularization.* These new vessels are extremely fragile and hemorrhage easily, producing vitreous contraction. Eventually light is prevented from reaching the retina as the vessels break and bleed into the vitreous cavity. The patient sees black or red spots or lines. If these new blood vessels pull the retina while the vitreous contracts, causing a tear, partial or complete retinal detachment will occur. If the macula is involved, vision is lost. Without treatment, more than half of patients with proliferative diabetic retinopathy will be blind.

Persons with diabetes are prone to other visual problems. Glaucoma occurs because of the occlusion of the outflow channels from neovascularization. This type of glaucoma is hard to treat and often results in blindness. Cataracts develop at an earlier age and progress more rapidly in people with diabetes.

Interprofessional Care

The earliest and most treatable stages of diabetes-related retinopathy often cause no changes in the vision. Therefore teach patients with type 2 diabetes to have a dilated eye examination by an ophthalmologist or a specially trained optometrist at the time of diagnosis and annually thereafter for early detection and treatment. Those with type 1 diabetes need to have a dilated eye examination within 5 years after the onset of diabetes and then annually.

The best approach to managing diabetes-related eye disease is to prevent it by maintaining healthy blood glucose levels and managing hypertension. Laser photocoagulation therapy can reduce the risk for vision loss in patients with proliferative retinopathy or macular edema and, sometimes, nonproliferative retinopathy. Laser photocoagulation destroys the ischemic areas of the retina that make growth factors that encourage neovascularization. A patient who develops vitreous hemorrhage and retinal detachment of the macula may need to undergo vitrectomy. *Vitrectomy* is the aspiration of blood, membrane, and fibers from the inside of the eye through a small incision just behind the cornea. (Photocoagulation and vitrectomy are discussed in Chapter 20.)

A fluocinolone acetonide intravitreal implant (Iluvien) is used to treat retinopathy. It is an injectable microinsert that provides sustained treatment through continuous delivery of corticosteroid fluocinolone acetonide for 36 months. Iluvien is injected in the back of the patient's eye with an applicator that uses a 25-gauge needle, which allows for a self-sealing wound.

Vascular endothelial growth factor (VEGF) plays a key role in the development of diabetes-related retinopathy. We are currently studying drugs injected into the eye that block the action of VEGF and reduce inflammation for their effectiveness in treating retinopathy.[23]

NEPHROPATHY

Diabetes-related nephropathy is a microvascular complication associated with damage to the small blood vessels that supply the glomeruli of the kidney. It is the leading cause of ESRD in the United States and seen in 20% to 40% of people with diabetes. Risk factors include hypertension, genetic predisposition, smoking, and chronic hyperglycemia. Keeping blood glucose levels in a healthy range is critical in the prevention and delay of diabetes-related nephropathy.[21]

Patients are screened for nephropathy annually with a random spot urine collection to assess for albuminuria and measure the albumin-to-creatinine ratio. Serum creatinine is measured to give an estimate of the glomerular filtration rate and the degree of kidney function.

Patients with diabetes who have albuminuria receive either ACE inhibitor drugs (e.g., lisinopril [Prinivil, Zestril]) or angiotensin II receptor blockers (e.g., losartan [Cozaar]). Both classifications of these drugs are used to treat hypertension and delay the progression of nephropathy in patients with diabetes. Hypertension significantly accelerates the progression of nephropathy. Therefore aggressive BP management is indicated for all patients with diabetes. See Chapter 32 for a discussion of hypertension and Chapter 46 for a discussion of renal failure.

NEUROPATHY

Diabetes-related neuropathy is nerve damage that occurs because of the metabolic imbalances associated with diabetes. About 60% to 70% of patients with diabetes have some degree of neuropathy.[2] The most common type affecting persons with diabetes is sensory neuropathy. This can lead to the loss of protective sensation in the lower extremities. Coupled with other factors, it significantly increases the risk for complications that result in a lower limb amputation. More than 60% of nontraumatic amputations in the United States occur in people with diabetes.[2] Screening for neuropathy begins at the time of diagnosis in patients with type 2 diabetes and 5 years after diagnosis in patients with type 1 diabetes.[3]

Etiology and Pathophysiology

We do not completely understand the pathophysiologic processes of diabetes-related neuropathy. Theories include metabolic, vascular, and autoimmune factors. The prevailing theory is that persistent hyperglycemia leads to an accumulation of sorbitol and fructose in the nerves that causes damage. How they cause damage is unknown. The result is reduced nerve conduction and demyelination. Ischemic damage by chronic hyperglycemia in blood vessels that supply the peripheral nerves is implicated in the development of diabetes-related neuropathy. Neuropathy can precede, accompany, or follow the diagnosis of diabetes.

Classification

The 2 major categories of diabetes-related neuropathy are *sensory neuropathy,* which affects the peripheral nervous system, and *autonomic neuropathy.* Each type has several forms.

Sensory Neuropathy. The most common form of sensory neuropathy is distal symmetric polyneuropathy, which affects the hands and/or feet bilaterally. This is sometimes called *stocking-glove neuropathy.* Characteristics include loss of sensation, abnormal sensations, pain, and paresthesias. The pain, which patients describe as burning, cramping, crushing, or tearing, is usually worse at night and may occur only at that time. The paresthesias may be associated with tingling, burning, and itching sensations. The patient may report a feeling of walking on pillows or numb feet. The skin can become so sensitive (hyperesthesia) that the patient cannot tolerate even light pressure from bed sheets. Complete or partial loss of sensitivity to touch and temperature is common. Foot injury and ulcerations can occur without the patient ever having pain (Fig. 48.15). Neuropathy can cause atrophy of the small muscles of the hands and feet, causing deformity and limiting fine movement.

Managing blood glucose is the only treatment for diabetes-related neuropathy. It is effective in many, but not all, cases. Drug therapy may be used to treat neuropathic symptoms, especially pain. At the start of therapy, symptoms usually increase, followed by relief of pain in 2 to 3 weeks.

Drugs commonly used include topical creams (e.g., capsaicin [Zostrix]), tricyclic antidepressants (e.g., amitriptyline), selective serotonin and norepinephrine reuptake inhibitors (e.g., duloxetine [Cymbalta]), and antiseizure drugs (e.g., gabapentin [Neurontin], pregabalin [Lyrica]). Capsaicin is a moderately effective topical cream made from chili peppers. It depletes the accumulation of pain-mediating chemicals in the peripheral sensory neurons. The cream is applied 3 or 4 times a day.

Tricyclic antidepressants are moderately effective in treating diabetes-related neuropathy. They work by inhibiting the reuptake of norepinephrine and serotonin, which are neurotransmitters thought to play a role in the transmission of pain through the spinal cord. We think duloxetine relieves pain by increasing the levels of serotonin and norepinephrine, which improves the body's ability to regulate pain. Antiseizure drugs decrease the release of neurotransmitters that transmit pain.[24]

Autonomic Neuropathy. Autonomic neuropathy can affect nearly all body systems and lead to hypoglycemia unawareness, bowel incontinence and diarrhea, and urinary retention. *Gastroparesis* (delayed gastric emptying) is a complication of autonomic neuropathy that can cause anorexia, nausea, vomiting, gastroesophageal reflux, and persistent feelings of fullness. Gastroparesis can trigger hypoglycemia by delaying food absorption. Cardiovascular abnormalities associated with autonomic neuropathy are postural hypotension, resting tachycardia, and painless MI. Assess patients with diabetes for postural hypotension to determine if they are at risk for falls. Teach the patient with postural hypotension to change from a lying or sitting position slowly.

Diabetes can affect sexual function in men and women. Erectile dysfunction (ED) in men with diabetes is well recognized and common, often being the first manifestation of autonomic neuropathy. ED is associated with other factors, including

vascular disease, elevated blood glucose levels, endocrine disorders, psychogenic factors, and medications. Decreased libido is a problem for some women with diabetes. Candida and nonspecific vaginitis are common. ED or sexual dysfunction requires sensitive therapeutic counseling for both the patient and the patient's partner. See Chapter 55 for more about ED.

A neurogenic bladder may develop as the sensation in the inner bladder wall decreases, causing urinary retention. A patient with retention has infrequent voiding, difficulty voiding, and a weak stream of urine. Emptying the bladder every 3 hours in a sitting position helps prevent stasis and infection. Tightening the abdominal muscles during voiding and using the Credé maneuver (mild massage downward over the lower abdomen and bladder) may help with complete bladder emptying. Cholinergic agonist drugs, such as bethanechol (Urecholine), may be used. The patient may need to learn self-catheterization (see Chapter 45).

COMPLICATIONS OF FEET AND LOWER EXTREMITIES

People with diabetes are at high risk for foot ulcerations and lower extremity amputations. The development of diabetes-related foot complications can be the result of a combination of microvascular and macrovascular diseases that place the patient at risk for injury and serious infection (Fig. 48.16). Sensory neuropathy and peripheral artery disease (PAD) are risk factors for foot complications. In addition, clotting abnormalities, impaired immune function, and autonomic neuropathy have a role. Smoking has a negative effect on the health of lower extremity blood vessels and increases the risk for amputation.

Sensory neuropathy is a major risk factor for lower extremity amputation in the person with diabetes. *Loss of protective sensation* (LOPS) often prevents the patient from being aware that a foot injury has occurred. Improper footwear and injury from stepping on foreign objects while barefoot are common causes of undetected foot injury in the person with LOPS. Because the primary risk factor for lower extremity amputation is LOPS, annual screening using a *monofilament* is important.[25] This is done by applying a thin, flexible filament to several spots on the plantar surface of the foot and asking the patient to report if it

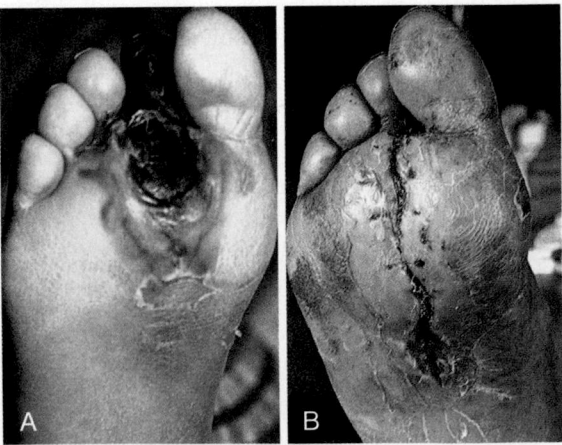

FIG. 48.16 The necrotic toe developed as a complication of diabetes. A, Before amputation. B, After amputation. (From Chew SL, Leslie D: *Clinical endocrinology and diabetes: An illustrated colour text,* Edinburgh, 2006, Churchill Livingstone.)

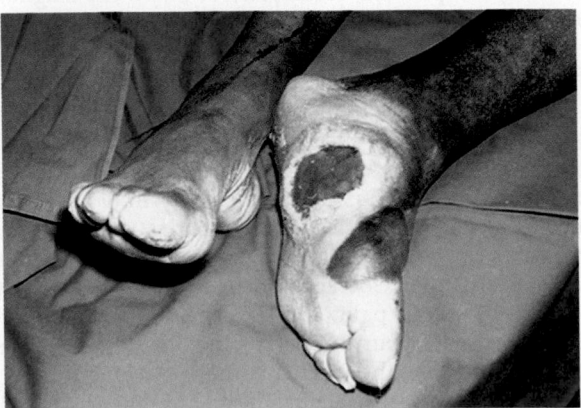

FIG. 48.15 Neuropathy: Neurotrophic ulceration.

is felt. Insensitivity to a monofilament greatly increases the risk for foot ulcers that can lead to amputation.

PAD increases the risk for amputation by causing a reduction in blood flow to the lower extremities. With decreased blood flow, oxygen, white blood cells (WBCs), and vital nutrients are not available to the tissues. Wounds take longer to heal, and the risk for infection increases. Signs of PAD include intermittent claudication, pain at rest, cold feet, loss of hair, delayed capillary filling, and dependent rubor (redness of the skin that occurs when the extremity is in a dependent position). PAD is diagnosed by history, ankle-brachial index (ABI), and angiography. Management includes reduction of risk factors, especially smoking, cholesterol intake, and hypertension. Bypass or graft surgery is indicated in some patients. PAD is discussed in Chapter 37.

If the patient has LOPS or PAD, aggressive measures must be taken to teach the patient how to prevent foot ulcers. These measures include choosing proper footwear, including protective shoes. Teach the patient to carefully avoid injury to the foot, practice diligent skin and nail care, inspect the foot thoroughly each day, and treat small problems promptly. Guidelines for patient teaching are listed in Table 48.21.

Proper care of a foot ulcer is critical for wound healing. Several forms of treatment can be used. Casting can redistribute the weight on the plantar surface of the foot. Wound care for the ulcer can include debridement, dressings, advanced wound healing products (becaplermin [Regranex]), vacuum-assisted closure, ultrasound, hyperbaric O_2, and skin grafting.

TABLE 48.21 Patient & Caregiver Teaching*
Foot Care

Include the following instructions when teaching the patient and caregiver about foot care:

1. Wash feet daily with a mild soap and warm water. First test water temperature with elbow.
2. Pat feet dry gently, especially between toes.
3. Examine feet daily for cuts, blisters, swelling, and red, tender areas. Do not depend on feeling sores. If eyesight is poor, have others inspect feet.
4. Use lanolin on feet to prevent skin from drying and cracking. Do not apply between toes.
5. Use mild foot powder on sweaty feet.
6. Do not use commercial remedies to remove calluses or corns.
7. Cleanse cuts with warm water and mild soap, covering with clean dressing. Do not use iodine, rubbing alcohol, or strong adhesives.
8. Report skin infections or nonhealing sores to HCP at once.
9. Cut toenails evenly with rounded contour of toes. Do not cut down corners. The best time to trim nails is after a shower or bath.
10. Separate overlapping toes with cotton or lamb's wool.
11. Avoid open-toe, open-heel, and high-heel shoes. Leather shoes are preferred to plastic ones. Wear slippers with soles. Do not go barefoot. Inspect feet, socks and shoes for foreign objects before putting on.
12. Wear clean, absorbent (cotton or wool) socks or stockings that have not been mended. Colored socks must be colorfast.
13. Do not wear clothing that leaves impressions, hindering circulation.
14. Do not use hot water bottles or heating pads to warm feet. Wear socks for warmth.
15. Guard against frostbite.
16. Exercise feet daily either by walking or by flexing and extending feet in suspended position. Avoid prolonged sitting, standing, and crossing of legs.

*This teaching guide is also appropriate for patients with peripheral vascular problems.

Neuropathic arthropathy, or *Charcot's foot*, results in ankle and foot changes that lead to joint dysfunction and footdrop. These changes occur gradually and promote an abnormal distribution of weight over the foot. This increases the chances of developing a foot ulcer as new pressure points appear. Foot deformity should be recognized early, and proper footwear fitted before ulceration occurs.

SKIN COMPLICATIONS

Up to two thirds of persons with diabetes develop skin problems. Diabetes-related dermopathy, the most common skin lesion, is characterized by reddish brown, round or oval patches. They initially are scaly, then they flatten out and become indented. The lesions appear most often on the shins but can occur on the front of the thighs, forearm, side of the foot, scalp, and trunk.

Acanthosis nigricans is a manifestation of insulin resistance. It can appear as a velvety light brown to black skin thickening, mainly on flexures, axillae, and the neck. *Necrobiosis lipoidica diabeticorum* usually appears as red-yellow lesions, with atrophic skin that becomes shiny and transparent, revealing tiny blood vessels under the surface (Fig. 48.17). This condition is uncommon. It occurs more often in young women. It may appear before other signs and symptoms of diabetes. Because the thin skin is prone to injury, special care must be taken to protect affected areas from injury and ulceration.

INFECTION

A person with diabetes is more susceptible to infections because of a defect in the mobilization of WBCs and an impaired phagocytosis by neutrophils and monocytes. Recurring or persistent infections, such as *Candida albicans*, boils, and furuncles in the undiagnosed patient often lead the HCP to suspect diabetes. Loss of sensation (neuropathy) may delay the detection of an infection.

Persistent glycosuria may predispose patients to bladder infections, especially patients with a neurogenic bladder. Decreased circulation resulting from angiopathy can prevent or delay the immune response. Antibiotic therapy has prevented

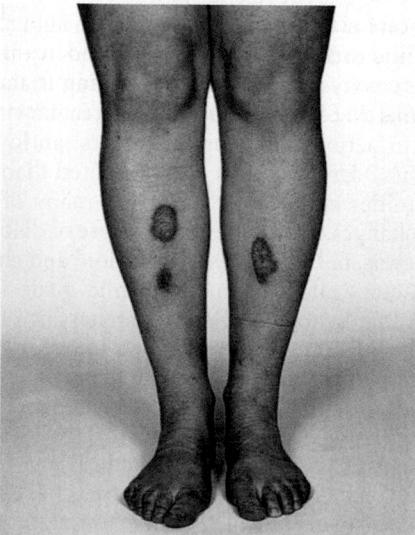

FIG. 48.17 Necrobiosis lipoidica diabeticorum. (From Chew SL, Leslie D: *Clinical endocrinology and diabetes: An illustrated colour text,* Edinburgh, 2006, Churchill Livingstone.)

infection from being a major cause of death in patients with diabetes. The treatment of infections must be prompt and vigorous. Teach patients to prevent infection by practicing good hand hygiene, avoiding exposure to persons who have a communicable illness, and getting an annual influenza vaccine and pneumococcal vaccine. (Guidelines for pneumococcal vaccine are shown in Table 27.5.)

PSYCHOLOGIC CONSIDERATIONS

Patients with diabetes have high rates of depression, anxiety, and eating disorders. Depression contributes to diminished diabetes self-care, feelings of helplessness related to chronic illness, and poor outcomes.[9] Diabetes distress is different from depression and encompasses the stress, fear, and burden of living with and managing a demanding chronic disease. Assess patients for manifestations of depression and/or diabetes distress.

Disordered eating behaviors (DEBs) can occur in people with both type 1 and type 2 diabetes. DEBs include anorexia, bulimia, binge eating, excessive restriction of calories, and intense exercise. The greatest incidence of eating disorders is seen in females. Adolescent girls with diabetes are more than twice as likely to develop DEB than those who do not have diabetes.[26] Patients may intentionally decrease their dose of insulin or omit the dose. This is called "diabulimia." It leads to weight loss, hyperglycemia, and glycosuria because the food ingested cannot be used for energy without adequate insulin. Insulin omission and DEBs can have serious consequences, including retinopathy, neuropathy, lipid abnormalities, DKA, and death.[26]

Open communication is critical to identify these behaviors early. Refer patients with eating disorders to a mental health professional with expertise in eating disorders and an understanding of diabetes management.

Gerontologic Considerations: Diabetes

Diabetes is present in more than 25% of persons over 65 years of age. This age-group is the fastest-growing segment of the population developing diabetes.[2] Older people with diabetes have higher rates of premature death, functional disability, and coexisting illnesses, such as hypertension and stroke, than those without diabetes. The prevalence of diabetes increases with age. A major reason for this is that the process of aging is associated with a reduction in β-cell function, decreased insulin sensitivity, and altered carbohydrate metabolism. Aging is also associated with conditions that are more likely to be treated with drugs that impair insulin action (e.g., corticosteroids, antihypertensives, phenothiazines). Undiagnosed and untreated diabetes is more common in older adults, partly because many of the normal physiologic changes of aging resemble those of diabetes, such as low energy levels, falls, dizziness, confusion, and chronic UTIs.

Several factors affect setting glycemic goals for an older adult. One is that hypoglycemia unawareness is more common in older adults, making them more likely to have adverse consequences from blood glucose–lowering therapy. They may have delayed psychomotor function that could interfere with the ability to treat hypoglycemia. Other factors include the patient's desire for treatment and coexisting medical problems, such as cognitive impairment. Compounding the challenge, diabetes increases the rate of decline of cognitive function. Although it is generally agreed that treatment is indicated to prevent complications, intensive diabetes management may be hard and dangerous to achieve, especially in older adults.

Meal planning and exercise are recommended therapy for older adults with diabetes. Consider functional limitations that may interfere with physical activity and the ability to prepare meals. Because of the physiologic changes that occur with aging, the therapeutic outcome for the older adult who receives OAs may be altered. Assess renal function and creatinine clearance in those over 80 years of age taking metformin. Monitor those taking sulfonylurea drugs (e.g., glipizide) for hypoglycemia and renal and liver dysfunction. Insulin therapy may be started if OAs are not effective. However, older adults are more likely to have limitations in the manual dexterity and visual acuity necessary for accurate insulin administration. Insulin pens may be a safer alternative.

Patient education issues include those related to altered vision, mobility, cognitive status, and functional ability. Plan patient teaching based on individual needs, using a slower pace with simple printed or audio materials in patients with cognitive and functional limitations. Include the family or caregivers in the teaching. Consider the patient's financial and social situation and the effect of multiple drugs, eating habits, and quality-of-life issues.

CASE STUDY

Diabetes-Related Ketoacidosis

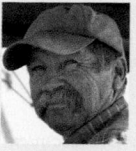
(© katrinaelena/ iStock/ Thinkstock.)

Patient Profile

N.B., a 48-yr-old farmer, was admitted to the emergency department after he was found unconscious by his wife in their barn. They live 40 miles from the nearest health care facility. He has a medical history of type 1 diabetes, hypertension, and diabetic neuropathy.

Subjective Data (Provided by Wife)

- Diagnosed with type 1 diabetes 15 years ago
- Takes 40 U/day of insulin via insulin pump: 5 U of lispro insulin bolus with breakfast, 5 U bolus with lunch, and 10 U bolus with dinner plus 20 U of basal insulin
- Has history of gastroenteritis for 1 wk with vomiting and anorexia
- Stopped taking meal time boluses 2 days ago when he was unable to eat
- Has not changed his infusion set in 5 days

Objective Data

Physical Examination

- Respirations deep with rate 36 breaths/min
- Fruity acetone smell on breath
- Skin flushed and dry
- Heart rate 118 beats/min; BP 98/60 mm Hg

Diagnostic Studies

- Blood glucose level 730 mg/dL (40.5 mmol/L)
- Blood pH 7.26

Discussion Questions

1. Briefly explain the pathophysiology behind N.B.'s diabetes-related ketoacidosis (DKA).
2. What factors precipitated his developing DKA?
3. What clinical manifestations of DKA does this patient exhibit?
4. What distinguishes this case history from one of hyperosmolar hyperglycemia syndrome (HHS) or hypoglycemia?
5. **Priority Decision:** Based on the assessment data presented, what are the priority nursing diagnoses? Are there any collaborative problems?
6. **Priority Decision:** What is the priority nursing intervention for N.B.?
7. **Priority Decision:** What is the priority teaching for this patient and his family?
8. **Evidence-Based Practice:** N.B.'s wife asks you if she should have given her husband insulin when he got sick. How would you respond?
9. **Collaboration:** How can the interprofessional team be most effective in caring for N.B?
10. **Quality Improvement:** What outcomes would indicate that the interprofessional team was effective in caring for N.B.?
11. Develop a conceptual care map for N.B.

Answers and a corresponding concept map are available at *http://evolve.elsevier.com/Lewis/medsurg*.

■ BRIDGE TO NCLEX EXAMINATION

The number of the question corresponds to the same-numbered outcome at the beginning of the chapter.

1. Polydipsia and polyuria related to diabetes are primarily due to
   a. the release of ketones from cells during fat metabolism.
   b. fluid shifts resulting from the osmotic effect of hyperglycemia.
   c. damage to the kidneys from exposure to high levels of glucose.
   d. changes in RBCs resulting from attachment of excess glucose to hemoglobin.

2. Which statement would be correct for a patient with type 2 diabetes who was admitted to the hospital with pneumonia?
   a. The patient must receive insulin therapy to prevent ketoacidosis.
   b. The patient has islet cell antibodies that have destroyed the pancreas's ability to make insulin.
   c. The patient has minimal or absent endogenous insulin secretion and requires daily insulin injections.
   d. The patient may have enough endogenous insulin to prevent ketosis but is at risk for hyperosmolar hyperglycemia syndrome.

3. Analyze the following diagnostic findings for your patient with type 2 diabetes. Which result will need further assessment?
   a. A1C 9%
   b. BP 126/80 mm Hg
   c. FBG 130 mg/dL (7.2 mmol/L)
   d. LDL cholesterol 100 mg/dL (2.6 mmol/L)

4. Which statement by the patient with type 2 diabetes is accurate?
   a. "I will limit my alcohol intake to 1 drink each day."
   b. "I am not allowed to eat any sweets because of my diabetes."
   c. "I cannot exercise because I take a blood glucose-lowering medication."
   d. "The amount of fat in my diet is not important. Only carbohydrates raise my blood sugar."

5. You are caring for a patient with newly diagnosed type 1 diabetes. What information is *essential* to include in your patient teaching before discharge from the hospital? *(select all that apply)*
   a. Insulin administration
   b. Elimination of sugar from diet
   c. Need to reduce physical activity
   d. Use of a portable blood glucose monitor
   e. Hypoglycemia prevention, symptoms, and treatment

6. What is the *priority* action for the nurse to take if the patient with type 2 diabetes reports blurred vision and irritability?
   a. Call the provider.
   b. Give insulin as ordered.
   c. Assess for other neurologic symptoms.
   d. Check the patient's blood glucose level.

7. A patient with diabetes has a serum glucose level of 824 mg/dL (45.7 mmol/L) and is unresponsive. After assessing the patient, the nurse suspects diabetes-related ketoacidosis rather than hyperosmolar hyperglycemia syndrome based on the finding of
   a. polyuria.
   b. severe dehydration.
   c. rapid, deep respirations.
   d. decreased serum potassium.

8. Which are appropriate therapies for patients with diabetes? *(select all that apply)*
   a. Use of statins to reduce CVD risk
   b. Use of diuretics to treat nephropathy
   c. Use of ACE inhibitors to treat nephropathy
   d. Use of serotonin agonists to decrease appetite
   e. Use of laser photocoagulation to treat retinopathy

1. b, 2. d, 3. a, 4. a, 5. a, 6. d, e, 7. c, 8. a, c, e

For rationales to these answers and even more NCLEX review questions, visit *http://evolve.elsevier.com/Lewis/medsurg.*

ⓔ EVOLVE WEBSITE/RESOURCES LIST

http://evolve.elsevier.com/Lewis/medsurg
Review Questions (Online Only)
Key Points
Answer Keys for Questions
• Rationales for Bridge to NCLEX Examination Questions
• Answer Guidelines for Case Study on p. 1141
Student Case Studies
• Patient With Type 1 Diabetes Mellitus and Diabetes-Related Ketoacidosis
• Patient With Type 2 Diabetes Mellitus and Hyperosmolar Hyperglycemia Syndrome
Nursing Care Plans
• eNursing Care Plan 48.1: Patient With Diabetes Mellitus
Conceptual Care Map Creator
• Conceptual Care Map for Case Study on p. 1141
Audio Glossary
Supporting Media
• Animation
• Insulin Function
Content Updates

REFERENCES

1. American Diabetes Association: Statistics about diabetes. Retrieved from *www.diabetes.org/diabetes-basics/statistics.*
2. Centers for Disease Control and Prevention: 2017 National diabetes statistics report. Retrieved from *www.cdc.gov/diabetes/pdfs/data/statistics/national-diabetes-statistics-report.pdf.*
*3. American Diabetes Association: Diagnosis and classification of diabetes mellitus, *Diab Care* 41:S13, 2018.
4. Bouzid T, Hamel FG, Lim JY: Role of adipokines in controlling insulin signaling pathways in type-2 diabetes and obesity, *Int J Diabetes Res* 5:75, 2016.
5. Ben-Shmuel S, Rostoker R, Scheinman EJ, et al: Metabolic syndrome, type 2 diabetes, and cancer: Epidemiology and potential mechanisms, *Handb Exp Pharmacol* 233:355, 2016.
6. Kawada T: Risk factors for developing prediabetes, *J Diabetes Res Clin Metab* 135:232, 2018.
7. Centers for Disease Control and Prevention: Gestational diabetes. Retrieved from *www.cdc.gov/diabetes/basics/gestational.html.*
*8. Chamberlain JJ, Herman WH, Leal S, et al. Pharmacologic therapy for type 2 diabetes: Synopsis of the 2017 ADA standards of medical care in diabetes, *Ann Intern Med* 166:572, 2017.

9. American Association of Diabetes Educators: *The art and science of self-management education desk reference,* ed 4, Chicago, 2017, The Association.
10. BD Diabetes: Syringe and needle sizes. Retrieved from *www.bd.com/en-us/offerings/capabilities/diabetes-care/insulin-syringes.*
11. Joslin Diabetes Center: The advantages and disadvantages of an insulin pump. Retrieved from *www.joslin.org/info/the_advantages_and_disadvantages_of_an_insulin_pump.html.*
*12. American Diabetes Association: Lifestyle management: Standards of medical care in diabetes, *Diabetes Care* 41:S38, 2018.
13. American Diabetes Association: Food and fitness: Create your plate. Retrieved from *www.diabetes.org/food-and-fitness/food.*
*14. US Department of Health and Human Services: Physical Activity Guidelines Advisory Committee report. Retrieved from *www.cdc.gov/nccdphp/sgr/contents.htm.*
*15. American Diabetes Association: Fitness. Retrieved from *www.diabetes.org/food-and-fitness/fitness.*
16. Wood A, O'Neal D, Furler J, et al: Continuous glucose monitoring: A review of the evidence, opportunities for future use and ongoing challenges, *Internal Med J* 48:499, 2018.
17. American Diabetes Association: Prevention or delay of type 2 diabetes, *Diab Care* 40:S44, 2017.
*18. Dickinson JK, Guzman SJ, Maryniuk MD, et al: The use of language in diabetes care and education, *Diab Care* 40:1790, 2017.
19. Boucher J, Hurrell D: Cardiovascular disease and diabetes, *Diab Spect* 21:154, 2008. (Classic)
*20. Diabetes Control and Complications Trial Research Group: The effect of intensive treatment of diabetes on the development and progression of long-term complications in insulin-dependent diabetes mellitus, *N Engl J Med* 329:977, 1993. (Classic)
*21. UK Prospective Diabetes Study (UKPDS) Group: Intensive blood-glucose control with sulphonylureas or insulin compared with conventional treatment and risk of complications in patients with type 2 diabetes, *Lancet* 352:837, 1998. (Classic)
22. American Diabetes Association: Cardiovascular disease and risk management: Standards of medical care in diabetes, *Diab Care* 41:S86, 2018.
23. Bahrami B, Hong T, Gilles MC, et al: Anti-VEGF therapy for diabetic eye diseases, *Asia Pac J Ophthalmol* 6:535, 2017.
*24. Waldfogel JM, Nesbit SA, Dy SM, et al: Pharmacotherapy for diabetic peripheral neuropathy: A systematic review, *Neurology* 88:1958, 2017.
*25. American Diabetes Association: Microvascular complications and foot care: Standards of medical care in diabetes, *Diab Care* 41:S105, 2018.
26. Doyle EA, Quinn SM, Ambrosino JM, et al: Disordered eating behaviors in emerging adults with type 1 diabetes: A common problem for both men and women, *J Pediatr Health Care* 31:327, 2017.

*Evidence-based information for clinical practice.

49

Endocrine Problems

Ann Crawford

The best way to cheer yourself up is to try to cheer somebody else up.

Mark Twain

ⓔ http://evolve.elsevier.com/Lewis/medsurg

CONCEPTUAL FOCUS

Coping
Fluids and Electrolytes
Hormonal Regulation

Nutrition
Perfusion
Reproduction

Thermoregulation
Tissue Integrity

LEARNING OUTCOMES

1. Explain the pathophysiology, clinical manifestations, and interprofessional and nursing management of the patient with an imbalance of hormones made by the anterior pituitary gland.
2. Describe the pathophysiology, clinical manifestations, and interprofessional and nursing management of the patient with an imbalance of hormones made by the posterior pituitary gland.
3. Explain the pathophysiology, clinical manifestations, and interprofessional and nursing management of the patient with thyroid dysfunction.
4. Describe the pathophysiology, clinical manifestations, and interprofessional and nursing management of the patient with parathyroid dysfunction.

5. Identify the pathophysiology, clinical manifestations, and interprofessional and nursing management of the patient with an imbalance of hormones made by the adrenal cortex.
6. Describe the pathophysiology, clinical manifestations, and interprofessional and nursing management of the patient with an excess of hormones made by the adrenal medulla.
7. List the side effects of corticosteroid therapy.

KEY TERMS

acromegaly, p. 1144
Addison's disease, p. 1165
Cushing syndrome, p. 1161
diabetes insipidus (DI), p. 1148
exophthalmos, p. 1150
goiter, p. 1149
Graves' disease, p. 1150

hyperaldosteronism, p. 1167
hyperparathyroidism, p. 1159
hyperthyroidism, p. 1150
hyperparathyroidism, p. 1161
hypoparathyroidism, p. 1161
hypopituitarism, p. 1145
hypothyroidism, p. 1156
myxedema, p. 1156

pheochromocytoma, p. 1168
syndrome of inappropriate antidiuretic hormone (SIADH), p. 1147
thyroid cancer, p. 1158
thyroiditis, p. 1149
thyrotoxicosis, p. 1150

The endocrine system is made up of several organs and glands that are involved in the synthesis and secretion of hormones that affect every body system. Because hormones have a wide range of action, problems with their regulation are associated with homeostatic changes that can affect many aspects of a person's life. The severity varies widely. There may be adverse effects on perfusion, metabolism, and nutrition. Regulating fluid and electrolyte balance, skin integrity, and temperature may be difficult. The patient may have problems with growth and fertility and reproductive processes since these are hormone dependent. There may be a wide range of psychologic responses, including anxiety and depression.

DISORDERS OF ANTERIOR PITUITARY GLAND

The pituitary gland is considered the master gland of the endocrine system. The anterior pituitary gland secretes growth hormone (GH), prolactin, and tropic hormones, adrenocorticotropic hormone (ACTH), thyroid-stimulating hormone (TSH), follicle-stimulating hormone (FSH), and luteinizing hormone (LH). These hormones affect growth, sexual maturation, reproduction, metabolism, stress response, and fluid balance. As a result, pituitary gland disorders manifest in a variety of ways.

Tumors of the pituitary gland account for 5% to 20% of primary intracranial tumors.[1] The most common, a pituitary adenoma, is a slow-growing, benign tumor. It often occurs in adults between 40 and 60 years of age. Hypersecretory pituitary adenomas secrete an excess of a specific hormone causing manifestations related to the action of that hormone. The most common are prolactinomas and GH- and ACTH-secreting adenomas.[1]

ACROMEGALY

Acromegaly is a rare condition characterized by an overproduction of GH. Around 4 of every 1 million adults in the United States are diagnosed annually.[2] It affects both genders equally. The mean age at the time of diagnosis is 40 to 45 years old.

Etiology and Pathophysiology

Acromegaly most often occurs because of a benign GH-secreting pituitary adenoma. The excess GH results in an overgrowth of soft tissues and bones in the hands, feet, and face. Because the problem develops after epiphyseal closure, the bones of the arms and legs do not grow longer.

Clinical Manifestations

The changes resulting from excess GH in adults can occur slowly, over many years, and may go unnoticed by the person, family, and friends. Thickening and enlargement of the bony and soft tissues on the face, feet, and head occur (Fig. 49.1). Patients may have proximal muscle weakness and joint pain that can range from mild to crippling. Carpal tunnel syndrome and peripheral neuropathy may be present.

Tongue enlargement results in dental and speech problems. The voice deepens because of hypertrophy of the vocal cords. Sleep apnea may occur because of upper airway narrowing and obstruction from increased amounts of pharyngeal soft tissues. The skin becomes thick, leathery, and oily with acne outbreaks.

Vision changes may occur from pressure on the optic nerve from a pituitary adenoma. Headaches are common. Since GH antagonizes the action of insulin, glucose intolerance and manifestations of diabetes may occur, including *polydipsia* (increased thirst) and *polyuria* (increased urination).

The life expectancy of those with acromegaly is reduced by 5 to 10 years. They are prone to cardiovascular disease (CVD), diabetes, and colorectal cancer.[3] Even if patients are cured or the disease is well controlled, manifestations such as joint pain and deformities often remain.

Diagnostic Studies

In addition to the history and physical examination, a diagnosis requires evaluating plasma insulin-like growth factor-1

(IGF-1) levels and GH response to an oral glucose tolerance test (OGTT). IGF-1 mediates the peripheral actions of GH. As GH levels rise, so do IGF-1 levels. Since GH is released in a pulsatile fashion, several samples are needed to obtain an accurate assessment. Serum IGF-1 levels are more constant, giving a more reliable diagnostic measure of acromegaly. During an OGTT, GH concentration normally falls because glucose inhibits GH secretion. In acromegaly, GH levels do not fall and in some cases GH levels rise.

MRI or high-resolution CT scan with contrast media can detect pituitary adenomas. A complete eye examination, including visual fields, is done because a tumor may cause pressure on the optic chiasm or optic nerves.

❖ Interprofessional and Nursing Care

The patient's prognosis depends on the age at onset, age when treatment started, and tumor size. The overall goal is to return the patient's GH levels to normal. Treatment consists of surgery, radiation therapy, drug therapy, or a combination of these therapies. Treatment can stop bone growth and reverse tissue hypertrophy. However, sleep apnea, diabetes, and cardiac problems may persist.

Surgery (hypophysectomy) is the treatment of choice. It offers the best chance for a cure and optimal symptom management, especially for smaller pituitary tumors.[4] Surgery results in an immediate reduction in GH levels. IGF-1 levels fall within a few weeks. Patients with larger tumors or those with GH levels greater than 45 ng/mL may need adjuvant radiation or drug therapy. Surgery and radiation therapy for pituitary tumors are discussed later in this chapter on p. 1145.

Drug therapy is an option for patients whose surgery did not result in a cure and/or in combination with radiation therapy. The main drug used is octreotide (Sandostatin), a somatostatin analog. It reduces GH levels to normal in many patients. Octreotide is given by subcutaneous injection 3 times a week. Long-acting somatostatin analogs, octreotide (Sandostatin LAR), pasireotide (Signifor), and lanreotide SR (Somatuline Depot), are available as IM injections given every 4 weeks. GH levels are measured every 2 weeks to guide drug dosing and then every 6 months until the desired response is achieved.

Dopamine agonists (e.g., bromocriptine, cabergoline) may be given alone or with somatostatin analogs if complete remission has not been achieved after surgery. These drugs reduce the secretion of GH from the tumor.

GH antagonists (e.g., pegvisomant [Somavert]) reduce the effect of GH in the body by blocking liver production of IGF-1. Most patients taking this drug achieve normal IGF-1 levels with symptom improvement.[3]

Serial photographs showing improvement in appearance may be helpful to the patient's recovery. Psychosocial effects of acromegaly include body image problems, sexual problems, and depression. Fatigue and sleep problems may persist after surgery. Patients will need strategies for dealing with these symptoms. Referral to a support group may be helpful.

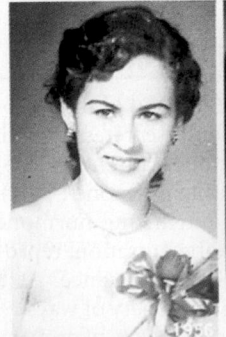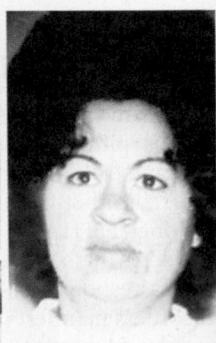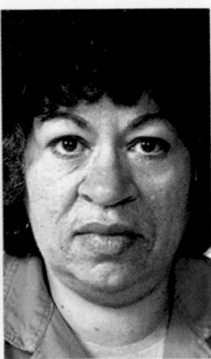

FIG. 49.1 Progressive development of facial changes associated with acromegaly. (Courtesy Linda Haas, Seattle, WA.)

EXCESSES OF OTHER TROPIC HORMONES

Excess secretion of prolactin or the tropic hormones (e.g., ACTH, TSH) by the anterior pituitary gland will cause other endocrine glands to overproduce certain hormones. An excess of these hormones (discussed later in the chapter) can cause significant problems in metabolism and general health.

A prolactin-secreting adenoma is known as a *prolactinoma*. They account for about 40% of pituitary tumors.[5] Women with prolactinomas may have galactorrhea, anovulation, infertility, infrequent or absent menses, decreased libido, and hirsutism. In men, impotence, decreased sperm density, and libido may result. Compression of the optic chiasm can cause vision changes and signs of increased intracranial pressure, including headache, nausea, and vomiting.

Because prolactinomas do not typically progress in size, drug therapy is usually the first-line treatment. The dopamine agonists cabergoline and bromocriptine are given to block the release of prolactin. Surgery may be an option, depending on the extent and size of the tumor. Radiation therapy can reduce the risk for tumor recurrence for patients with large tumors.

HYPOFUNCTION OF PITUITARY GLAND

Hypopituitarism is a rare disorder that involves a decrease in 1 or more of the pituitary hormones. A deficiency of only 1 pituitary hormone is called *selective hypopituitarism*. Total failure of the pituitary gland results in deficiency of all pituitary hormones—a condition referred to as *panhypopituitarism*. The most common hormone deficiencies associated with hypopituitarism involve GH and gonadotropins (e.g., LH, FSH).

Etiology and Pathophysiology

The usual cause of pituitary hypofunction is a pituitary tumor. Autoimmune disorders, infections, pituitary infarction (Sheehan syndrome), or destruction of the pituitary gland (from trauma, radiation, or surgical procedures) can also cause hypopituitarism. Blacks have a higher incidence of pituitary tumors than other ethnic groups.[6]

Anterior pituitary hormone deficiencies can lead to end-organ failure. TSH and ACTH deficiencies are life threatening. ACTH deficiency can lead to acute adrenal insufficiency and hypovolemic shock from sodium and water depletion. Acute adrenal insufficiency is discussed later in this chapter on pp. 1165–1166.

Clinical Manifestations and Diagnostic Studies

The manifestations vary with the type and degree of dysfunction. Early manifestations associated with a space-occupying lesion include headaches, vision changes (decreased visual acuity or decreased peripheral vision), loss of smell, nausea and vomiting, and seizures. Manifestations associated with hyposecretion of the target glands vary widely (Table 49.1).

In addition to a history and physical examination, diagnostic studies such as MRI and CT can identify a pituitary tumor. Laboratory tests generally involve the direct measurement of pituitary hormones (e.g., TSH) or an indirect determination of the target organ hormones (e.g., triiodothyronine [T_3], thyroxine [T_4]). (See Chapter 47 for more information about diagnostic studies.)

❖ Interprofessional and Nursing Care

The treatment for hypopituitarism often consists of surgery or radiation therapy followed by lifelong hormone therapy. Surgery and radiation therapy for pituitary tumors are discussed in the

TABLE 49.1 Manifestations of Hypopituitarism

Hormone Deficiency	Manifestations
Adrenocorticotropic hormone (ACTH)	Involves cortisol deficiency: weakness, fatigue, headache, dry and pale skin, ↓ axillary and pubic hair, ↓ resistance to infection, fasting hypoglycemia
Follicle-stimulating hormone (FSH) and luteinizing hormone (LH)	*Women:* Menstrual irregularities, loss of libido, changes in secondary sex characteristics (e.g., ↓ breast size) *Men:* Testicular atrophy, ↓ spermatogenesis, loss of libido, impotence, ↓ facial hair and muscle mass
Growth hormone (GH)	Subtle, nonspecific findings: truncal obesity, osteoporosis, ↓ muscle mass and strength, weakness, fatigue, depression, or flat affect
Thyroid-stimulating hormone (TSH)	Mild form of primary hypothyroidism: fatigue, cold intolerance, constipation, lethargy, weight gain

next section. Appropriate hormone therapy is used (e.g., GH, corticosteroids, thyroid hormone). Hormone therapies for thyroid hormone and corticosteroids are discussed later in this chapter on p. 1156 and p. 1167.

Somatropin (Genotropin, Humatrope, Omnitrope), recombinant human GH, is used for long-term hormone therapy in adults with GH deficiency. These patients respond well to GH replacement. They have increased energy, increased lean body mass, a feeling of well being, and improved body image. Mild to moderate side effects of GH include fluid retention with swelling in the feet and hands, myalgia, joint pain, and headache. GH is given daily as a subcutaneous injection (preferably in the evening). The dosing is variable and adjusted based on symptoms, IGF-1 levels, and the presence of adverse effects.

Although gonadal deficiency is not life threatening, hormone therapy will improve sexual function and general well-being. It is contraindicated in those with certain medical conditions, such as phlebitis, pulmonary embolism, breast cancer in women, and prostate cancer in men. Estrogen and progesterone replacement therapy may be given to hypogonadal women to treat hot flashes, vaginal dryness, and decreased libido. (Hormone therapy for women is discussed in Chapter 53.) Testosterone is used to treat men with gonadotropin deficiency. The benefits achieved with testosterone therapy include a return of male secondary sex characteristics; improved libido; and increased muscle mass, bone mass, and bone density. (Hormone therapy for men is discussed in Chapter 54.)

PITUITARY SURGERY

A *hypophysectomy* is the surgical removal of the pituitary gland. It is the treatment of choice for tumors in the pituitary area, especially smaller pituitary adenomas. Most surgeries are done by an endoscopic *transsphenoidal* approach (Fig. 49.2). When the entire pituitary gland is removed, there is permanent loss of all pituitary hormones. The patient will need lifelong replacement therapy of thyroid hormone, sex hormones, and glucocorticoids.

Radiation therapy can reduce the size of a tumor before surgery. It is also used when surgery does not produce a cure or

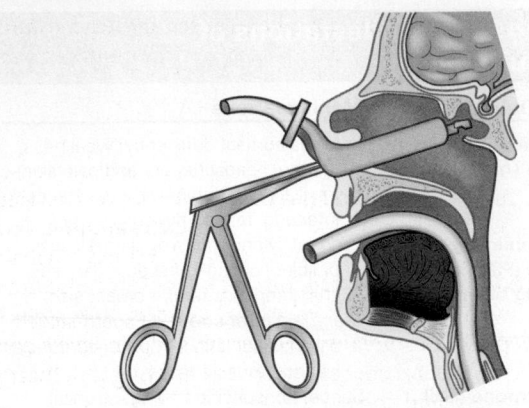

FIG. 49.2 Surgery on the pituitary gland is most often done by a trans-sphenoidal approach. An incision is made in the inner aspect of the upper lip and gingiva. The sella turcica is entered through the floor of the nose and sphenoid sinuses.

when patients are poor candidates for surgery. Its full effects may not be noted for months to years. Radiation therapy may lead to hypopituitarism, which then requires lifelong hormone replacement therapy. Stereotactic radiosurgery (gamma knife surgery, proton beam, linear accelerator) is an option for small, surgically inaccessible pituitary tumors or in place of conventional radiation.

❖ NURSING MANAGEMENT: PITUITARY SURGERY

After surgery, assess the patient for the formation of a hematoma compressing the optic nerve or optic chiasma. Monitor peripheral vision, visual acuity, extraocular movements, and pupillary response. Report changes at once because prompt intervention may prevent visual deterioration from becoming permanent (Table 49.2).

Cerebrospinal fluid (CSF) leaks and epistaxis are other common complications after surgery.[7] The HCP may place a petroleum jelly–coated ribbon of gauze or a balloon-tipped catheter (like an indwelling urinary catheter) in the sphenoid sinus. It is usually removed after 24 hours. It can be left in for 2 to 3 days if there is concern for bleeding or CSF leak. It is important that the patient does not blow the nose for at least 48 hours after surgery and avoids vigorous coughing, sneezing, and straining at stool.

Monitor the "moustache" dressing regularly for any drainage. Check any clear drainage with a urine dipstick for glucose and protein. If present, notify the HCP of a possible CSF leak. A sample can be sent to the laboratory. A glucose level greater than 30 mg/dL (1.67 mmol/L) indicates CSF leakage from an open connection with the brain. If this happens, the patient is at increased risk for meningitis.

A persistent and severe generalized or supraorbital headache may indicate CSF leakage into the sinuses. A CSF leak usually resolves within 72 hours when treated with head elevation and bed rest. If the leak persists, daily spinal taps may be done to reduce pressure to below-normal levels.

Other measures include elevating the head of the patient's bed at all times to a 30-degree angle. This avoids pressure on the sella turcica and decreases headaches. Monitor the pupillary response, speech patterns, and extremity strength to detect neurologic complications. Gentle mouth care every 4 hours is essential to keep the surgical area clean and free of debris. Have the patient avoid tooth brushing for at least 10 days to protect the suture line.

TABLE 49.2 Nursing Management

Care of the Patient After Pituitary Surgery

- Monitor vital signs. Assess peripheral pulses and watch for orthostatic hypotension.
- Monitor neurologic/cognitive status (e.g., level of consciousness, orientation, speech) hourly for the first 24 hr and then every 4 hr.
- Assess extremity strength and reflexes.
- Monitor field of vision, visual acuity, extraocular movements, and pupillary response. Notify HCP of any changes.
- Assess dressing for type and amount of drainage. Notify HCP for excessive bleeding or CSF drainage.
- Maintain strict intake and output and monitor fluid balance. Assess for DI or SIADH.
- Keep head of bed elevated at least 30 degrees at all times.
- Encourage deep breathing exercises and incentive spirometer use.
- Monitor for pain and give analgesic medications as prescribed.
- Encourage high-fiber diet to decrease potential for constipation.
- Perform oral care every 4 hr.
- Teach the patient to:
  - Avoid vigorous coughing, sneezing, and blowing the nose
  - Avoid bending over at the waist or straining at stool (Valsalva maneuver) due to potential increased intracranial pressure
  - Avoid use of toothbrushes until incision heals
  - Follow replacement hormone therapy plan

Fluid and electrolyte problems can occur from the development of diabetes insipidus (DI).[8] Transient DI may occur because of the loss of antidiuretic hormone (ADH), which is stored in the posterior lobe of the pituitary gland, or cerebral edema related to manipulation of the pituitary during surgery. DI may be permanent after surgery. To assess for DI, closely monitor urine output and measure specific gravity. Report a urine output of more than 200 mL/hr for more than 3 consecutive hours or a specific gravity level of <1.005. Patients with DI will have a high serum sodium and extreme thirst. DI is treated by giving desmopressin acetate (DDAVP). Fluid replacement may be needed to avoid hypovolemia related to high urine output. Syndrome of inappropriate antidiuretic hormone secretion (SIADH) can occur after any intracranial surgery. SIADH typically occurs later than DI, usually around the fourth postoperative day. It may occur due to manipulation of the pituitary and other structures causing release of ADH. The fluid retention caused by circulating ADH leads to dilutional hyponatremia. Sodium levels of less than 125 mEq/L will manifest as headache, vomiting, and decreased level of consciousness. The manifestations and treatment of DI and SIADH are discussed in the next section.

ADH, cortisol, and thyroid hormone replacement are needed after a hypophysectomy. Teach the patient about the need for lifelong therapy. Surgery may result in permanent loss or deficiencies in FSH and LH. This can lead to decreased fertility. Assist the patient in working through the grieving process associated with these losses.

DISORDERS OF POSTERIOR PITUITARY GLAND

The hormones secreted by the posterior pituitary are ADH and oxytocin. ADH, also referred to as *arginine vasopressin* (AVP) or vasopressin, has a key role in the regulation of water balance and serum osmolarity (see Chapter 47). The primary problems associated with ADH secretion are a result of either overproduction or underproduction of ADH.

SYNDROME OF INAPPROPRIATE ANTIDIURETIC HORMONE   Hypertonic diuretics

Etiology and Pathophysiology   Holds water

Syndrome of inappropriate antidiuretic hormone (SIADH) results from an overproduction of ADH or the release of ADH despite normal or low plasma osmolarity (Fig. 49.3). ADH increases the permeability of the renal distal tubule and collecting duct, which leads to the reabsorption of water into the circulation. Extracellular fluid volume expands, plasma osmolality declines, glomerular filtration rate increases, and sodium levels decline (dilutional hyponatremia).[8] Thus features of the disorder are fluid retention, serum hypoosmolality, dilutional hyponatremia, hypochloremia, and concentrated urine in the presence of normal or increased intravascular volume.

SIADH occurs more often in older adults. The most common cause is cancer, especially small cell lung cancer (Table 49.3).

PATHOPHYSIOLOGY MAP

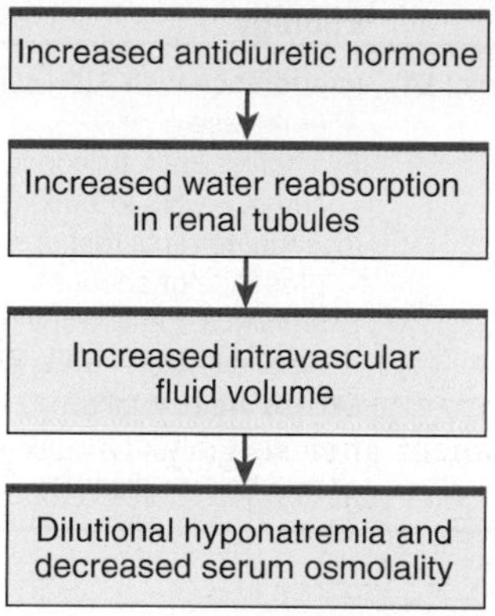

Increased antidiuretic hormone

↓

Increased water reabsorption in renal tubules

↓

Increased intravascular fluid volume

↓

Dilutional hyponatremia and decreased serum osmolality

FIG. 49.3 Pathophysiology of SIADH. (Modified from Urden LD, Stacy KM, Lough ME: *Critical care nursing: Diagnosis and management*, ed 6, St Louis, 2010, Mosby.)

TABLE 49.3 Causes of SIADH

Cancer
- Colorectal cancer
- Lymphoid cancers (Hodgkin's lymphoma, non-Hodgkin's lymphoma, lymphocytic leukemia)
- Pancreatic cancer
- Prostate cancer
- Small cell lung cancer
- Thymus cancer

CNS Disorders
- Brain tumors
- Cerebral atrophy
- Guillain-Barré syndrome
- Head injury (skull fracture, subdural hematoma, subarachnoid hemorrhage)
- Infection (encephalitis, meningitis)
- Stroke
- Systemic lupus erythematosus

Drug Therapy
- carbamazepine (Tegretol)
- Chemotherapy agents (vincristine, vinblastine, cyclophosphamide)
- chlorpropamide
- General anesthesia agents
- Opioids
- oxytocin
- Thiazide diuretics
- Selective serotonin reuptake inhibitor (SSRI) antidepressants
- Tricyclic antidepressants

Miscellaneous Conditions
- Adrenal insufficiency
- Chronic obstructive pulmonary disease
- HIV*
- Hypothyroidism
- Lung infection (pneumonia, tuberculosis, lung abscess)
- Positive pressure mechanical ventilation

SIADH tends to be self-limiting when caused by head trauma or drugs. It can be chronic when associated with tumors or metabolic diseases.

Clinical Manifestations and Diagnostic Studies

The patient with SIADH has low urine output and increased body weight. At first, the patient has thirst, dyspnea on exertion, and fatigue. Mild hyponatremia causes muscle cramping, irritability, and headache. As the serum sodium level falls (usually below 120 mEq/L [120 mmol/L]), manifestations become more severe and include vomiting, abdominal cramps, and muscle twitching. As plasma osmolality and serum sodium levels continue to decline, cerebral edema may occur, leading to lethargy, confusion, seizures, and coma.

The diagnosis is made by simultaneous measurements of urine and serum osmolality. Dilutional hyponatremia is indicated by a serum sodium less than 135 mEq/L, serum osmolality less than 280 mOsm/kg (280 mmol/kg), and urine specific gravity greater than 1.030. A serum osmolality much lower than the urine osmolality shows the body is inappropriately excreting concentrated urine in the presence of dilute serum.

❖ Interprofessional and Nursing Care

When assessing patients at risk and those who have confirmed SIADH, be alert for low urine output with a high specific gravity, a sudden weight gain without edema, or a decreased serum sodium level. Monitor intake and output, vital signs, and heart and lung sounds. Obtain daily weights. Observe for signs of hyponatremia, including seizures, headache, vomiting, and decreased neurologic function.

Once SIADH is diagnosed, treatment is directed at the underlying cause. Medications that stimulate ADH release should be avoided or discontinued (Table 49.3). If symptoms are mild and serum sodium is greater than 125 mEq/L (125 mmol/L), the only treatment may be a fluid restriction of 800 to 1000 mL/day. This restriction should result in weight reduction and a gradual rise in serum sodium concentration and osmolality. An improvement in symptoms should accompany normalization of serum sodium and osmolality. Provide the patient with frequent oral care and distractions to decrease discomfort related to thirst from the fluid restriction.

A loop diuretic, such as furosemide (Lasix), may be used to promote diuresis. The serum sodium must be at least 125 mEq/L (125 mmol/L) because it may promote further sodium loss. Because furosemide increases potassium, calcium, and magnesium losses, supplements may be needed. Demeclocycline also may be given. This drug blocks the effect of ADH on the renal tubules, resulting in more dilute urine.

Initiate seizure and fall precautions if the patient has an altered sensorium or is having seizures. Position the head of the bed flat or elevated no more than 10 degrees. This enhances venous return to the heart and increases left atrial filling pressure, thus reducing the release of ADH. Frequent turning, positioning, and range-of-motion exercises are important to maintain skin integrity and joint mobility.

In cases of severe hyponatremia (less than 120 mEq/L), especially in the presence of neurologic manifestations, such as seizures, small amounts of IV hypertonic saline solution (3% sodium chloride) may be slowly given. It is important to correct hyponatremia slowly. The level should not increase by more than 8 to 12 mEq/L in the first 24 hours. Quickly increasing levels can cause osmotic demyelination syndrome with permanent damage to nerve cells in the brain.[8] A fluid restriction of 500 mL/day may be needed for those with severe hyponatremia.

Vasopressor receptor antagonists (drugs that block the activity of ADH) are used to treat euvolemic hyponatremia in hospitalized patients. Two drugs are FDA-approved: conivaptan (Vaprisol) and tolvaptan (Samsca). Conivaptan is given IV; tolvaptan is given orally. Neither should be given to patients with liver disease because they worsen liver function.

Help the patient with chronic SIADH in self-managing the treatment plan. In chronic SIADH, a fluid restriction of 800 to 1000 mL/day is recommended. Ice chips or sugarless chewing gum help decrease thirst. Have the patient obtain a daily weight to monitor changes in fluid balance. Have the patient supplement the diet with sodium and potassium, especially if taking loop diuretics. Teach the patient the symptoms of fluid and electrolyte imbalances, particularly those involving sodium and potassium (see Chapter 16).

DIABETES INSIPIDUS _vasopressin_

Etiology and Pathophysiology

Diabetes insipidus (DI) is caused by a deficiency of production or secretion of ADH or a decreased renal response to ADH. The decrease in ADH results in fluid and electrolyte imbalances caused by increased urine output and increased plasma osmolality (Fig. 49.4). Depending on the cause, DI may be transient or a chronic, lifelong condition. There are several types of DI (Table 49.4). Central DI is the most common form.

Clinical Manifestations

Key features of DI are polydipsia and polyuria. The patient excretes large quantities of urine (2 to 20 L/day) with a very low specific gravity (less than 1.005) and urine osmolality of less than 100 mOsm/kg (100 mmol/kg). Serum osmolality is increased (usually greater than 295 mOsm/kg [295 mmol/kg]) because of hypernatremia (serum sodium greater than 145 mg/dL) caused by pure water loss in the kidneys. Most patients compensate for fluid loss by drinking large amounts of water so that serum osmolality stays normal or is moderately increased. The patient may be tired from nocturia and have generalized weakness. Uncorrected hypernatremia can cause brain shrinkage and intracranial bleeding.[8]

The onset of central DI is usually acute and accompanied by excess fluid loss. After intracranial surgery, central DI has a triphasic pattern: (1) an acute phase with an abrupt onset of polyuria, (2) an interphase in which urine volume normalizes, and (3) a third phase in which central DI may become permanent. The third phase occurs 10 to 14 days after surgery. Central DI from head trauma is often self-limiting and improves with treatment of the underlying problem. Although the manifestations of nephrogenic DI are like those of central DI, the onset and amount of fluid loss are less dramatic.

Severe dehydration can result if oral fluid intake cannot keep up with urinary losses. The patient will have hypotension, tachycardia, and hypovolemic shock. Increasing serum osmolality and hypernatremia can cause central nervous system (CNS) manifestations, ranging from irritability and mental dullness to coma.

Diagnostic Studies

Patients with DI excrete dilute urine at a rate greater than 200 mL/hr with a specific gravity of less than 1.005. Central DI is

PATHOPHYSIOLOGY MAP

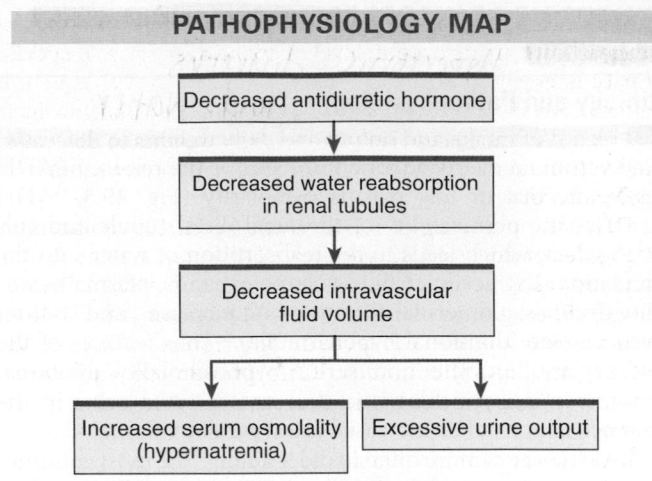

FIG. 49.4 Pathophysiology of diabetes insipidus.

TABLE 49.4 Types of Diabetes Insipidus

Type	Etiology
Central (neurogenic) DI	Interference with ADH synthesis, transport, or release _Examples:_ Brain tumor, head injury, brain surgery, CNS infections
Nephrogenic DI	Inadequate renal response to ADH despite presence of adequate ADH _Examples:_ Drug therapy (especially lithium), renal damage, hereditary renal disease
Primary DI	Excess water intake _Examples:_ Structural lesion in thirst center, psychologic disorder

diagnosed by a water deprivation test. Before the test, body weight, and urine osmolality, volume, and specific gravity are measured. The patient is deprived of water for 8 to 12 hours and then given desmopressin acetate (DDAVP) subcutaneously or nasally. Patients with central DI have a dramatic increase in urine osmolality (from 100 to 600 mOsm/kg) and a significant decrease in urine volume. The patient with nephrogenic DI will not be able to increase urine osmolality to greater than 300 mOsm/kg.

Another test to distinguish central DI from nephrogenic DI is to measure the level of ADH after an analog of ADH (e.g., desmopressin) is given. If the cause is central DI, the kidneys will respond to the hormone by concentrating urine. If the kidneys do not respond in this way, the cause is nephrogenic.

❖ Interprofessional and Nursing Care

Management of the patient with DI includes early detection, maintaining adequate hydration, and patient teaching for long-term management. A therapeutic goal is maintaining fluid and electrolyte balance.

For central DI, fluid and hormone therapy are the cornerstone of treatment. Fluids are replaced orally or IV, depending on the patient's condition and ability to drink copious amounts of fluids. In acute DI, IV hypotonic saline or dextrose 5% in water (D_5W) is given and titrated to replace urine output. If IV glucose solutions are used, monitor serum glucose levels because hyperglycemia and glycosuria can lead to osmotic diuresis, which increases the fluid volume deficit. Monitoring BP, heart rate, urine output, level of consciousness, and specific gravity is essential and may be done hourly in the acutely ill patient. Assess for signs of acute dehydration. Maintain an accurate record of intake and output and daily weights to determine fluid volume status. Adjustments in fluid replacement should be made accordingly.

DDAVP, an analog of ADH, is the hormone replacement of choice for central DI. Another ADH replacement drug is aqueous vasopressin. DDAVP can be given orally, IV, subcutaneously, or as a nasal spray. Assess the response to DDAVP by monitoring pulse, BP, level of consciousness, intake and output, and specific gravity. Chlorpropamide and carbamazepine (Tegretol) can help decrease thirst associated with central DI.

Because the kidney is unable to respond to ADH in nephrogenic DI, hormone therapy has little effect. Instead, the treatment includes a low-sodium diet and thiazide diuretics (e.g., hydrochlorothiazide, chlorothiazide [Diuril]), which may reduce flow to the ADH-sensitive distal nephrons. Limiting sodium intake to no more than 3 g/day often helps decrease urine output. If a low-sodium diet and thiazide drugs are not effective, indomethacin (Indocin) may be prescribed. Indomethacin, a nonsteroidal antiinflammatory drug (NSAID), helps increase renal responsiveness to ADH.

DISORDERS OF THYROID GLAND

Problems with thyroid function are among the most common endocrine disorders. The thyroid hormones, thyroxine (T_4) and triiodothyronine (T_3), regulate energy metabolism and growth and development. Disorders of the thyroid gland include goiter, benign and malignant nodules, inflammatory conditions leading to hyperthyroidism, and hypothyroidism (Fig. 49.5).

GOITER

A goiter is an enlarged thyroid gland. In a person with a goiter, the thyroid cells are stimulated to grow. This may result in an overactive thyroid (hyperthyroidism) or an underactive thyroid (hypothyroidism). The most common cause of goiter worldwide is a lack of iodine in the diet.[9] In the United States, where most people use iodized salt, goiter is more often due to the overproduction or underproduction of thyroid hormones or to nodules that develop in the gland itself. *Goitrogens* (foods or drugs that contain thyroid-inhibiting substances) can cause a goiter (Table 49.5).

A nontoxic goiter is a diffuse enlargement of the thyroid gland that does not result from cancer or an inflammatory process. Normal levels of thyroid hormone are associated with this type of goiter. *Nodular goiters* are thyroid hormone–secreting nodules that function independent of TSH stimulation. There may be multiple nodules (multinodular goiter) or a single nodule (solitary autonomous nodule). The nodules are usually benign follicular adenomas. If these nodules are associated

with hyperthyroidism, they are called *toxic nodular goiters.* This type of goiter is often found in patients with Graves' disease (Fig. 49.6). Toxic nodular goiters occur equally in men and women. Although they can appear at any age, they most often occur in people over 40 years of age.

TSH and T_4 levels are measured to determine whether a goiter is associated with normal thyroid function, hyperthyroidism, or hypothyroidism. Thyroid antibodies (e.g., thyroid peroxidase [TPO] antibody) show the presence of *thyroiditis* (inflammation of the thyroid). Treatment with thyroid hormone may prevent further thyroid enlargement. Surgery can remove large goiters. Goiter as a manifestation of thyroid disorders is discussed in the next sections.

THYROIDITIS

Thyroiditis, an inflammation of the thyroid gland, encompasses several clinical disorders.[10] It is a frequent cause of goiter. *Subacute granulomatous thyroiditis* is thought to be caused by a viral infection. *Acute thyroiditis* is due to bacterial or fungal infection. Subacute and acute forms of thyroiditis have an abrupt onset. The patient reports pain localized in the thyroid or radiating to the throat, ears, or jaw. Systemic manifestations include fever, chills, sweats, and fatigue.

TABLE 49.5 **Goitrogens**	
Thyroid Inhibitors	**Select Foods**
• iodine in large doses	• Broccoli
• methimazole (Tapazole)	• Brussels sprouts
• propylthiouracil (PTU)	• Cabbage
	• Cauliflower
Other Drugs	• Kale
• amiodarone	• Mustard
• lithium	• Peanuts
• *p*-aminosalicylic acid	• Strawberries
• Salicylates	• Turnips
• Sulfonamides	

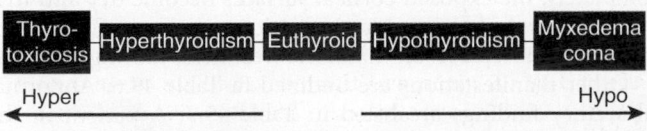

Thyro-toxicosis	Hyperthyroidism	Euthyroid	Hypothyroidism	Myxedema coma

Hyper ←————————————————————————→ Hypo

FIG. 49.5 Continuum of thyroid dysfunction.

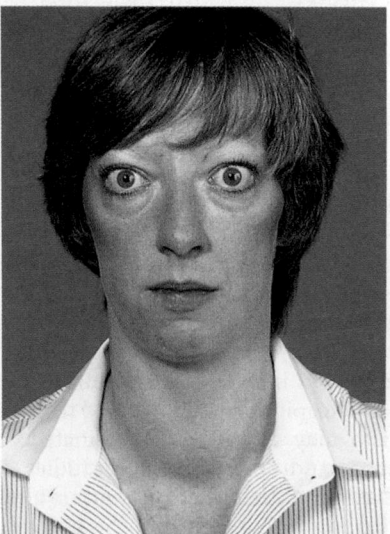

FIG. 49.6 Exophthalmos and goiter of Graves' disease. (From Forbes CD, Jackson WF: *Colour atlas and text of clinical medicine,* ed 3, London, 2003, Mosby.)

Hashimoto's thyroiditis (chronic autoimmune thyroiditis) is caused by the destruction of thyroid tissue by antibodies.[11] It is the most common cause of hypothyroid goiters in the United States. Risk factors include female gender, a positive family history, older age, and white ethnicity. The goiter, which is the hallmark of Hashimoto's thyroiditis, may develop gradually or rapidly. If it enlarges rapidly, it may compress structures in the neck (e.g., trachea, laryngeal nerves), changing the voice and affecting breathing. As thyroid tissue is destroyed by antibodies, there may be a transient phase of hyperthyroidism due to leaking thyroid hormone from the damaged tissues.

Silent, painless thyroiditis, which may be early Hashimoto's thyroiditis, can occur in postpartum women. This condition is usually seen in the first 6 months after delivery. It may be due to an autoimmune reaction to fetal cells in the mother's thyroid gland.

T_4 and T_3 levels are initially increased in subacute, acute, and silent thyroiditis but become decreased with time. Suppressed radioactive iodine uptake (RAIU) is seen in subacute and silent thyroiditis. In Hashimoto's thyroiditis, T_4 and T_3 levels are usually low and the TSH level is high. Antithyroid antibodies are present in Hashimoto's thyroiditis.

Recovery from acute or subacute thyroiditis may be complete in weeks or months without any treatment. If the thyroiditis is bacterial in origin, treatment may include specific antibiotics or surgical drainage. In the subacute and acute forms, NSAIDs (aspirin, naproxen [Aleve]) are used to relieve symptoms. With more severe pain, corticosteroids (e.g., prednisone up to 40 mg/day) can relieve discomfort. Propranolol (Inderal) or atenolol (Tenormin) may relieve cardiovascular symptoms related to a hyperthyroid condition. The patient who is hypothyroid needs thyroid hormone therapy.

Nursing care of the patient with thyroiditis includes patient teaching about the disease process and course of treatment. Teach the patient not to stop medications abruptly. Tell the patient to remain under close health care supervision so that progress can be monitored. Teach the patient to report to the HCP any change in symptoms, such as difficulty breathing or swallowing, swelling to face and extremities, or rapid weight gain or loss. Teach those receiving thyroid hormone about the expected side effects of these drugs and ways to manage them (see p. 1158).

The patient with Hashimoto's thyroiditis is at risk for other autoimmune diseases, such as Addison's disease, pernicious anemia, or Graves' disease. Teach the patient the signs and symptoms of these disorders, particularly Addison's disease.

HYPERTHYROIDISM

Hyperthyroidism is hyperactivity of the thyroid gland with sustained increase in synthesis and release of thyroid hormones. It occurs in women more than men, with the highest frequency in persons 20 to 40 years old. The most common form is Graves' disease. Other causes include toxic nodular goiter, thyroiditis, excess iodine intake, pituitary tumors, and thyroid cancer. Since hyperthyroidism may be caused by iodinated contrast media used in CT scans and other radiologic studies, monitor those who are at risk closely after iodinated contrast media exposure.[11]

The term thyrotoxicosis refers to the physiologic effects or clinical syndrome of hypermetabolism resulting from excess circulating levels of T_4, T_3, or both.[12] Hyperthyroidism and thyrotoxicosis usually occur together. Subclinical hyperthyroidism

occurs when the patient has a serum TSH level below 0.4 mU/L but normal T_4 and T_3 levels. Overt hyperthyroidism is defined by low or undetectable TSH and increased T_4 and T_3 levels. The patient may or may not have symptoms of hyperthyroidism.

Etiology and Pathophysiology

Graves' Disease. Graves' disease is an autoimmune disease of unknown cause characterized by diffuse thyroid enlargement and excess thyroid hormone secretion. It accounts for 75% of the cases of hyperthyroidism. Causative factors, such as a lack of iodine, smoking, infection, and stressful life events, may interact with genetic factors to cause Graves' disease.

In Graves' disease, the patient develops antibodies to the TSH receptor. These antibodies attach to the receptors and stimulate the thyroid gland to release T_3, T_4, or both. The excess release of thyroid hormones leads to the manifestations associated with thyrotoxicosis. The disease is characterized by remissions and exacerbations, with or without treatment. It may progress to destruction of the thyroid tissue, causing hypothyroidism. Graves' disease is associated with the presence of other autoimmune disorders, including rheumatoid arthritis, pernicious anemia, systemic lupus erythematosus, Addison's disease, celiac disease, and vitiligo.

Clinical Manifestations

The manifestations are related to the effect of excess circulating thyroid hormone. It directly increases metabolism and tissue sensitivity to sympathetic nervous system stimulation.

Palpation of the thyroid gland may reveal a goiter. When the thyroid gland is excessively large, a goiter may be seen on inspection. Auscultating the thyroid gland may reveal bruits, a reflection of increased blood supply. Another common finding is *ophthalmopathy,* a term used to describe abnormal eye appearance or function. A classic finding in Graves' disease is exophthalmos, a protrusion of the eyeballs from the orbits that is usually bilateral (Fig. 49.6). Exophthalmos results from increased fat deposits and fluid (edema) in the orbital tissues and ocular muscles. The increased pressure forces the eyeballs outward. The upper lids are usually retracted and elevated, with the sclera visible above the iris. When the eyelids do not close completely, the exposed corneal surfaces become dry and irritated. Corneal ulcers and loss of vision can occur. Changes in the ocular muscles result in muscle weakness, causing diplopia.

Other manifestations are outlined in Table 49.6. Abnormal laboratory findings are listed in Table 49.7. A patient in the early stages of hyperthyroidism may only have weight loss and

TABLE 49.6 Manifestations of Thyroid Dysfunction

Hyperfunction	Hypofunction	Hyperfunction	Hypofunction
Cardiovascular System		**Reproductive System**	
• Systolic hypertension	• ↑ Capillary fragility	• Menstrual irregularities	• Prolonged menstrual periods or
• ↑ Rate and force of cardiac contractions	• ↓ Rate and force of contractions	• Amenorrhea	amenorrhea
• Bounding, rapid pulse	• Varied changes in BP	• ↓ Libido	• ↓ Libido
• ↑ Cardiac output	• Cardiac hypertrophy	• ↓ Fertility	• Infertility
• Systolic murmurs	• Distant heart sounds	• Impotence and gynecomastia in men	
• Dysrhythmias	• Anemia		
• Palpitations	• Heart failure	**Respiratory**	
• Angina	• Angina	• Dyspnea on mild exertion	• Dyspnea
		• ↑ Respiratory rate	• ↓ Breathing capacity
Gastrointestinal System			
• ↑ Appetite, thirst	• ↓ Appetite	**Skin**	
• Weight loss	• Weight gain	• Warm, smooth, moist skin	• Dry, thick, inelastic, cold skin
• ↑ Peristalsis	• Nausea and vomiting	• Thin, brittle nails detached from nail bed (onycholysis)	• Thick, brittle nails
• Diarrhea, frequent defecation	• Constipation	• Hair loss (may be patchy)	• Dry, sparse, coarse hair
• ↑ Bowel sounds	• Distended abdomen	• Clubbing of fingers (thyroid acropachy) (Fig. 49.7)	• Poor turgor of mucosa
• Splenomegaly	• Enlarged, scaly tongue		• Generalized interstitial edema
• Hepatomegaly	• Celiac disease	• Palmar erythema	• Puffy face
		• Fine, silky hair	• ↓ Sweating
Musculoskeletal System		• Premature graying (in men)	• Pallor
• Fatigue	• Fatigue	• Diaphoresis	
• Weakness	• Weakness	• Vitiligo	
• Proximal muscle wasting	• Muscular aches and pains	• Pretibial myxedema (infiltrative dermopathy)	
• Dependent edema	• Slow movements		
• Osteoporosis	• Arthralgia	**Other**	
		• Goiter (Fig. 49.6)	• Goiter
Nervous System		• Intolerance to heat	• Intolerance to cold
• Hyperactive deep-tendon reflexes	• Prolonged relaxation of deep tendon reflexes	• Elevated basal temperature	• ↑ Risk for infection
• Depression	• Anxiety, depression	• Lid lag, stare	• ↑ Sensitivity to opioids, barbiturates, anesthesia
• Lack of ability to concentrate	• Slowed mental processes	• Eyelid retraction	
• Rapid speech	• Slow, slurred speech	• Exophthalmos	• ↓ Hearing
• Insomnia	• Sleepiness		
• Difficulty focusing eyes	• Apathy		
• Nervousness	• Lethargy		
• Fine tremor of fingers and tongue	• Forgetfulness		
	• Hoarseness		
• Lability of mood, delirium	• Stupor, coma		
• Restlessness	• Paresthesias		
• Personality changes of irritability, agitation			
• Stupor, coma			

TABLE 49.7 Laboratory Results for Hyperthyroid and Hypothyroid Patients

Test	Hyperthyroid	HYPOTHYROID	
		Primary	Secondary
Thyroid-stimulating hormone (TSH)	↓	↑	↓
T₄ (thyroxine)	↑	↓	↓
Total cholesterol	N	↑	↑
Low-density lipoproteins (LDLs)	↓	↑	↑
Triglycerides	N	↑	↑
Creatine kinase (CK)	N	↑	↑
Basal metabolic rate (BMR)	↑	↓	↓
Thyroid peroxidase (TPO) antibody	N	+ (in autoimmune hypothyroidism)	N

N, Normal; +, positive.

increased nervousness. *Acropachy* (clubbing of the digits) may occur with advanced disease (Fig. 49.7). Manifestations (e.g., palpitations, tremors, weight loss) in older adults do not differ significantly from those of younger adults (Table 49.8). In older patients who are confused and agitated, dementia may be suspected and delay the diagnosis.

Complications

Acute thyrotoxicosis (also called *thyrotoxic crisis* or *thyroid storm*) is an acute, severe, and rare condition that occurs when excess amounts of thyroid hormones are released into the circulation. Although considered a life-threatening emergency, death is rare when treatment is started early. Acute thyroiditis is thought to result from stressors (e.g., infection, trauma, surgery) in a patient with preexisting hyperthyroidism. Patients having a thyroidectomy are at risk because manipulation of the hyperactive thyroid gland results in an increase in hormones released.

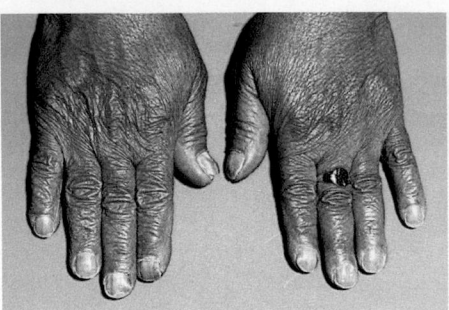

FIG. 49.7 Thyroid acropachy. Digital clubbing and swelling of fingers. (From Chew SL, Leslie D: *Clinical endocrinology and diabetes: An illustrated colour text*, Edinburgh, 2006, Churchill Livingstone.)

TABLE 49.8 Comparison of Hyperthyroidism in Younger and Older Adults

	Younger Adult	Older Adult
Common causes	Graves' disease in >90% of cases	Graves' disease or toxic nodular goiter
Common symptoms	Nervousness, irritability, weight loss, heat intolerance, warm moist skin	Anorexia, weight loss, apathy, lassitude, depression, confusion
Goiter	Present in >90% of cases	Present in about 50% of cases
Ophthalmopathy	Exophthalmos (Fig. 49.6) present in 20%–40% of cases	Exophthalmos less common
Cardiac features	Tachycardia and palpitations common, but without heart failure	Angina, dysrhythmia (especially atrial fibrillation with rapid ventricular response), heart failure may occur

In acute thyrotoxicosis, all the symptoms of hyperthyroidism are prominent and severe. Manifestations include severe tachycardia, heart failure, shock, hyperthermia (up to 106°F [41.1°C]), agitation, delirium, seizures, abdominal pain, vomiting, diarrhea, and coma.

Diagnostic Studies

The primary laboratory findings used to confirm the diagnosis of hyperthyroidism are low or undetectable TSH levels (<0.4 mU/L) and increased free thyroxine (free T_4) levels. Total T_3 and T_4 levels also may be assessed, but they are not as definitive. Total T_3 and T_4 determine both free and bound (to protein) hormone levels. The free hormone is the only biologically active form of these hormones.

The RAIU test can distinguish Graves' disease from other forms of thyroiditis. The patient with Graves' disease shows a diffuse, homogeneous uptake of 35% to 95%, while the patient with thyroiditis shows an uptake of less than 2%. The person with a nodular goiter has an uptake in the high normal range.

Interprofessional Care

The goal of management is to block the adverse effects of excess thyroid hormone, suppress oversecretion of thyroid hormone, and prevent complications. There are several treatment options, including antithyroid medications, radioactive iodine therapy,

TABLE 49.9 Interprofessional Care
Hyperthyroidism

Diagnostic Assessment
- History and physical examination
- Ophthalmologic examination
- ECG
- Laboratory tests
  - TSH levels, serum free T_4
  - Thyroid antibodies (e.g., thyroid peroxidase [TPO] antibody)
  - Total serum T_3 and T_4
- Radioactive iodine uptake (RAIU)

Management
Drug Therapy
- Antithyroid drugs
  - methimazole (Tapazole)
  - propylthiouracil
- iodine (SSKI)

Radiation Therapy
- Radioactive iodine

Surgical Therapy
- Subtotal thyroidectomy

Nutritional Therapy
- High-calorie, high-protein diet
- Frequent meals

and surgical intervention (Table 49.9). Supportive therapy is directed at managing respiratory distress, reducing fever, replacing fluid, and eliminating or managing the initiating stressor(s).

The choice of treatment is influenced by the patient's age and preferences, coexistence of other diseases, and pregnancy status.

Drug Therapy. Drugs used to treat hyperthyroidism include antithyroid drugs, iodine, and β-adrenergic blockers. These drugs are useful in treating thyrotoxic states but are not curative. Radiation therapy or surgery may be needed.

Antithyroid Drugs. The first-line antithyroid drugs are propylthiouracil and methimazole (Tapazole).[12] These drugs inhibit thyroid hormone synthesis. Reasons for use include Graves' disease in the young patient, hyperthyroidism during pregnancy, and the need to achieve a euthyroid state before surgery or radiation therapy. Propylthiouracil is generally used for patients who are in the first trimester of pregnancy, had an adverse reaction to methimazole, or need a rapid reduction in symptoms. It is the first-line therapy in thyrotoxicosis since it blocks the peripheral conversion of T_4 to T_3. An advantage of propylthiouracil is that it achieves the therapeutic goal of being euthyroid more quickly. However, it must be taken 3 times per day. Methimazole is given in a single daily dose.

Improvement usually begins 1 to 2 weeks after the start of drug therapy. Results are usually seen within 4 to 8 weeks. Therapy is usually continued for 6 to 15 months to allow for spontaneous remission, which occurs in 20% to 40% of patients. Emphasize to the patient the importance of adhering to the drug plan. Abruptly stopping drug therapy can result in a return of hyperthyroidism.

Iodine. Iodine is available as saturated solution of potassium iodide (SSKI) and Lugol's solution. Iodine is used with other antithyroid drugs to prepare the patient for thyroidectomy or for treatment of thyrotoxicosis. Rapidly giving large doses of iodine inhibits synthesis of T_3 and T_4 and blocks the release of these hormones into circulation. It also decreases the vascularity of the thyroid gland, making surgery safer and easier. The maximal effect is usually seen within 1 to 2 weeks. Because of a reduction in the therapeutic effect, long-term iodine therapy is not effective in controlling hyperthyroidism.

Iodine is mixed with water or juice and given after meals. Sipping it through a straw decreases the chance of it staining the teeth. Assess the patient for signs of iodine toxicity, such as swelling of the buccal mucosa and other mucous membranes, excess salivation, nausea and vomiting, and skin reactions. If toxicity occurs, stop administering iodine and notify the HCP.

β-Adrenergic Blockers. β-Adrenergic blockers are used for symptomatic relief of thyrotoxicosis. These drugs block the effects of sympathetic nervous stimulation, thereby decreasing tachycardia, nervousness, irritability, and tremors. Propranolol is usually given with antithyroid agents. Atenolol is the preferred β-adrenergic blocker for use in the hyperthyroid patient with asthma or heart disease.

Radioactive Iodine Therapy. Radioactive iodine (RAI) therapy is the treatment of choice for most nonpregnant adults. RAI damages or destroys thyroid tissue, thus limiting thyroid hormone secretion. RAI has a delayed response. The maximum effect may not be seen for up to 3 months. For this reason, the patient is usually treated with antithyroid drugs and propranolol before and for 3 months after starting RAI until the effects of radiation become apparent. Although RAI is usually effective, 80% of patients have posttreatment hypothyroidism, resulting in the need for lifelong thyroid hormone therapy. Teach the patient the symptoms of hypothyroidism and to seek medical help if these symptoms occur.

RAI therapy is usually given on an outpatient basis. A pregnancy test is done before starting therapy for all women who have menstrual cycles. Tell the patient that radiation thyroiditis and parotitis are possible and may cause dryness and irritation of the mouth and throat. Relief may be obtained with frequent sips of water, ice chips, or a salt and soda gargle 3 or 4 times per day. This gargle is made by dissolving 1 tsp of salt and 1 tsp of baking soda in 2 cups of warm water. The discomfort should subside in 3 to 4 days. A mixture of antacid (Mylanta or Maalox), diphenhydramine, and viscous lidocaine can be used to swish and spit, increasing patient comfort when eating.

To limit radiation exposure to others, teach the patient receiving RAI home precautions, including (1) using private toilet facilities, if possible, and flushing 2 or 3 times after each use; (2) separately laundering towels, bed linens, and clothes daily at home; (3) not preparing food for others that requires prolonged handling with bare hands; and (4) avoiding being close to pregnant women and children for 7 days after therapy.

Surgical Therapy. A thyroidectomy is done for those who have (1) a large goiter causing tracheal compression, (2) a lack of response to antithyroid therapy, or (3) thyroid cancer (Fig. 49.8). Surgery may be done when a person is not a candidate for RAI. One advantage that thyroidectomy has over RAI is a more

rapid reduction in T$_3$ and T$_4$ levels. A *subtotal thyroidectomy* is the preferred surgical procedure. It involves removing a significant portion (90%) of the thyroid gland.

Some patients may undergo minimally invasive endoscopic or robotic thyroidectomy. Endoscopic thyroidectomy is appropriate for patients with small nodules (less than 3 cm) and no evidence of cancer. Robotic surgery is best for those who are not overweight and have small nodules on only one side of the gland. Advantages of endoscopic and robotic procedures over open thyroidectomy include less scarring, less pain, and a faster return to normal activity.

Nutritional Therapy. With the increased metabolic rate in hyperthyroid patients, there is a high potential for the patient to have nutrition problems. A high-calorie diet (4000 to 5000 cal/day) may be needed to satisfy hunger, prevent tissue breakdown, and decrease weight loss. This can be achieved with 6 full meals a day and snacks high in protein, carbohydrates, minerals, and vitamins. The protein content should be 1 to 2 g/kg of ideal body weight. Increase carbohydrate intake to compensate for increased metabolism. Carbohydrates provide energy and decrease the use of body-stored protein. Teach the patient to avoid highly seasoned and high-fiber foods because they can further stimulate the already hyperactive GI tract. Have the patient avoid caffeine-containing liquids, such as coffee, tea, and cola, to decrease the restlessness and sleep problems. Refer the patient to a dietitian for help in meeting individual nutritional needs.

❖ NURSING MANAGEMENT: HYPERTHYROIDISM

◆ Nursing Assessment

Subjective and objective data you should obtain from a person with hyperthyroidism are outlined in Table 49.10.

◆ Nursing Diagnoses

Nursing diagnoses for the patient with hyperthyroidism include:
- Activity intolerance
- Impaired nutritional status

Additional information on nursing diagnoses and interventions is presented in eNursing Care Plan 49.1 for the patient with hyperthyroidism (available on the website for this chapter).

◆ Planning

The overall goals are that the patient with hyperthyroidism will (1) have relief of symptoms, (2) have no serious complications related to the disease or treatment, (3) maintain nutritional balance, and (4) cooperate with the therapeutic plan.

◆ Nursing Implementation

◆ **Acute Care.** Patients with hyperthyroidism are usually treated in an outpatient setting. However, those who develop acute thyrotoxicosis or undergo thyroidectomy need hospitalization and acute care.

Acute Thyrotoxicosis. Acute thyrotoxicosis requires aggressive treatment, often in an intensive care unit (ICU). Give medications (previously discussed) that block thyroid hormone production and the sympathetic nervous system. Provide supportive therapy, including monitoring for dysrhythmias and decompensation, ensuring adequate oxygenation, and giving IV fluids to replace fluid and electrolyte losses. This is especially important in the patient who has fluid losses from vomiting and diarrhea (Table 49.11).

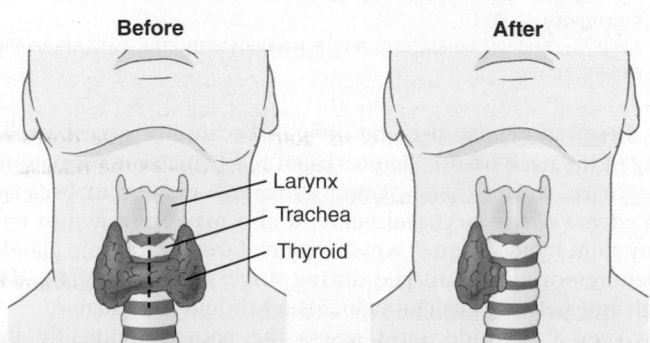

Before **After**

Larynx
Trachea
Thyroid

FIG. 49.8 Subtotal thyroidectomy. Part of the thyroid gland is removed.

TABLE 49.10 Nursing Assessment

Hyperthyroidism

Subjective Data

Important Health Information

Past health history: Preexisting goiter. Recent infection or trauma, immigration from iodine-deficient area, autoimmune disease

Medications: Thyroid hormones, herbal therapies that may contain thyroid hormone

Functional Health Patterns

Health perception–health management: Positive family history of thyroid or autoimmune disorders

Nutritional-metabolic: Iodine intake, weight loss, ↑ appetite, thirst, nausea, vomiting

Elimination: Diarrhea, polyuria, sweating

Activity-exercise: Dyspnea on exertion, palpitations, muscle weakness, fatigue

Sleep-rest: Insomnia

Cognitive-perceptual: Chest pain, nervousness, heat intolerance, pruritus

Sexuality-reproductive: ↓ Libido, impotence, gynecomastia (in men), amenorrhea (in women)

Coping–stress tolerance: Emotional lability, irritability, restlessness, personality changes, delirium

Objective Data

General Observation

Agitation, rapid speech and body movements, anxiety, restlessness, hyperthermia, enlarged or nodular thyroid gland

Eyes

Exophthalmos, eyelid retraction, infrequent blinking

Skin

Warm, diaphoretic, velvety skin. Thin, loose nails. Fine, silky hair and hair loss. Palmar erythema, clubbing, white pigmentation of skin (vitiligo), diffuse edema of legs and feet

Respiratory

Tachypnea, dyspnea on exertion

Cardiovascular

Tachycardia, bounding pulse, systolic murmurs, dysrhythmias, hypertension, bruit over the thyroid gland

Gastrointestinal

↑ Bowel sounds. Increased appetite, diarrhea, weight loss, liver and/or spleen enlargement

Neurologic

Hyperreflexia; diplopia. Fine tremors of hands, tongue, eyelids

Musculoskeletal

Muscle wasting

Reproductive

Menstrual irregularities, infertility, impotence, gynecomastia in men

Possible Diagnostic Findings

↑ T_3, ↑ T_4, ↑ T_3 resin uptake, ↓ or undetectable TSH. Chest x-ray showing enlarged heart. ECG findings of tachycardia, atrial fibrillation

Ensuring adequate rest may be a challenge because of the patient's irritability and restlessness. Provide a calm, quiet room because increased metabolism and sensitivity of the sympathetic nervous system causes sleep problems. Other interventions may include (1) placing the patient in a cool room away from very ill patients and noisy, high-traffic areas; (2) using light bed coverings and changing the linen often if the patient is diaphoretic; and (3) encouraging and assisting with exercise involving large muscle groups (tremors can interfere with small-muscle coordination) to allow the release of nervous tension and restlessness. It is important to establish a supportive, trusting relationship to promote coping by a patient who is irritable, restless, and anxious.

If exophthalmos is present, there is a potential for corneal injury related to irritation and dryness. The patient may have orbital pain. To relieve eye discomfort and prevent corneal ulceration, apply artificial tears to soothe and moisten conjunctival membranes. Restricting salt may help reduce periorbital edema. Elevate the patient's head to promote fluid drainage from the periorbital area. The patient should sit upright as much as possible.

Dark glasses reduce glare and prevent irritation from smoke, air currents, dust, and dirt. If the eyelids cannot be closed, lightly tape them shut for sleep. To maintain flexibility, teach the patient to exercise the intraocular muscles several times a day by turning the eyes in the complete range of motion. Good grooming can help reduce the loss of self-esteem from an altered body image. If the exophthalmos is severe, treatment options include corticosteroids, radiation of retroorbital tissues, orbital decompression, or corrective lid or muscle surgery.

Thyroid Surgery. When a subtotal thyroidectomy is the treatment of choice, the patient must be adequately prepared to avoid complications. Before surgery, antithyroid drugs, iodine, and β-adrenergic blockers may be given to achieve a euthyroid state. Iodine also decreases the vascularization of the thyroid gland, reducing the risk for hemorrhage.

Before surgery, teach the patient about routine postoperative care and comfort and safety measures. Show the patient how to support the head manually while turning in bed, since this minimizes stress on the suture line after surgery. The patient should practice neck range-of-motion exercises. Tell the patient that talking is likely to be difficult for a short time after surgery. Review the importance of performing leg exercises.

Postoperative Care. Postoperative complications include hypothyroidism, damage to or inadvertent removal of parathyroid glands, causing hypoparathyroidism and hypocalcemia, hemorrhage, injury to the recurrent or superior laryngeal nerve, thyrotoxicosis, and infection.[13] Recurrent laryngeal nerve damage leads to vocal cord paralysis. If both cords are paralyzed, spastic airway obstruction will occur, requiring an immediate tracheostomy.

> ⚠ **SAFETY ALERT** Airway Obstruction
> - Although not common, airway obstruction after thyroid surgery is an emergency.
> - Keep O_2, suction equipment, and a tracheostomy tray available in the patient's room.

Respiration may become difficult because of excess swelling of the neck tissues, hemorrhage, and hematoma formation. *Laryngeal stridor* (harsh, vibratory sound) may occur because of edema of the laryngeal nerve. It also may be related to tetany from hypocalcemia, which occurs if the parathyroid glands were removed or damaged during surgery. To treat tetany, IV calcium salts (e.g., calcium gluconate) should be available. After a thyroidectomy, assess the patient frequently for signs of hemorrhage or tracheal compression (Table 49.12).

✚ TABLE 49.11 Emergency Management

Acute Thyrotoxicosis

Etiology	Assessment Findings	Interventions

• Infection, surgery, trauma in a patient with hyperthyroidism
• Thyroidectomy
	• Abdominal pain
	• Agitation
	• Delirium
	• Diarrhea
	• Heart failure
	• Hyperthermia (up to 106° F [41.1° C])
	• Seizures
	• Severe tachycardia
	• Shock
	• Vomiting
		• Begin fluid replacement with isotonic saline infusions containing dextrose.
		• Monitor airway, breathing, and circulation.
		• Monitor vital signs at least every 30 min.
		• Apply continuous O₂ saturation and ECG monitoring.
		• Monitor serial serum electrolytes, serum glucose, ABGs, and serum calcium levels.
		• Monitor urine output hourly.
		• Apply ice packs and cooling blankets to reduce fever. Acetaminophen as needed.
		• Provide pulmonary hygiene.
		• Assess for manifestations of heart failure or pulmonary edema (e.g., extra heart sounds, adventitious lung sounds).
		• Decrease O₂ demands by decreasing anxiety and pain.
		• Restrict visitors, if needed.
		• Give prescribed drugs and monitor effects:
		  • β-Adrenergic blockers
		  • Antithyroid agents
		  • Iodine compounds
		  • Glucocorticoids

TABLE 49.12 Nursing Management

Care of the Patient After Thyroid Surgery

- Assess vital signs every 15 min until stable and then every 30 min for the first 24 hr after surgery.
- Monitor airway and respiratory status (patency, rate, rhythm, depth, and effort).
- Assess the patient every 2 hr for 24 hr for signs of hemorrhage or tracheal compression (e.g., irregular breathing, neck swelling, frequent swallowing, choking, blood on the dressings, and sensations of fullness at the incision site).
- Assist the patient with coughing and deep breathing.
- Apply supplemental O₂ with humidification as ordered.
- Have suction equipment and a tracheostomy kit available for immediate use.
- Assess the ability to speak aloud, noting voice quality, tone, and any problems speaking. Notify the HCP of any permanent hoarseness or loss of vocal volume.
- Monitor calcium levels and assess for signs of tetany and hypocalcemia (e.g., tingling in toes, fingers, around the mouth; muscular twitching; apprehension) and any difficulty in speaking and hoarseness. Check Trousseau's sign and Chvostek's sign (see Fig. 16.15).
- Keep calcium salts (calcium gluconate, calcium chloride) available for immediate IV use.
- Assess condition of operative site and dressing. Monitor the area under the patient's neck and shoulders for drainage.
- Place the patient in a semi-Fowler's position. Support the head and neck with pillows. Avoid neck flexion to prevent tension on the suture line.
- Provide comfort measures and give analgesic medications as prescribed.

The patient should expect some hoarseness for 3 or 4 days after surgery because of edema. Keep the patient in a semi-Fowler's position and support the patient's head with pillows. Avoid any tension on the suture lines. Monitor vital signs and assess for any signs of hypocalcemia from hypoparathyroidism. If recovery is uneventful, the patient ambulates within hours after surgery. Fluids are allowed as soon as tolerated. A soft diet starts the day after surgery.

The appearance of the incision may be distressing to the patient. Reassure the patient that the scar will fade in color and eventually look like a normal neck wrinkle. A scarf, jewelry, a high collar, or other covering can effectively camouflage the scar.

◆ **Ambulatory Care.** Teach the patient and caregiver that thyroid hormone balance will be monitored periodically. Most patients have a period of relative hypothyroidism soon after surgery because of the substantial reduction in the size of the thyroid. However, the remaining tissue usually hypertrophies over time and recovers the ability to make hormones. Giving thyroid hormone is avoided because the exogenous hormone inhibits pituitary production of TSH and delays or prevents the restoration of normal gland function and tissue regeneration.

To prevent weight gain, caloric intake must be greatly reduced below the amount that was required before surgery. Adequate iodine is needed to promote thyroid function, but excesses can inhibit the thyroid gland. Seafood once or twice a week or normal use of iodized salt should provide enough iodine intake. Encourage regular exercise to stimulate the thyroid gland. Teach the patient to avoid high environmental temperatures because they inhibit thyroid regeneration.

Regular follow-up care is needed. The patient should see the HCP biweekly for a month and then at least semiannually to assess thyroid function. Tell the patient who had a complete thyroidectomy about the need for lifelong thyroid hormone replacement. Teach the patient the signs and symptoms of thyroid failure and to seek medical care promptly if these develop.

◆ **Evaluation**

The expected outcomes are that the patient with hyperthyroidism will
- Have relief of symptoms
- Have no serious complications related to the disease or treatment
- Cooperate with the therapeutic plan
- Maintain nutritional balance

HYPOTHYROIDISM

Hypothyroidism is a deficiency of thyroid hormone that causes a general slowing of the metabolic rate. About 4% of the U.S. population has mild hypothyroidism, with about 0.3% having more severe disease. Hypothyroidism is more common in women than men. Subclinical hypothyroidism occurs when the TSH is greater than 4.5 mU/L, but the T_4 levels are normal. Up to 10% of women older than 60 years have subclinical hypothyroidism.[14] Patients with overt hypothyroidism have increased TSH and decreased T_4 levels. Critically ill patients may present with nonthyroidal illness syndrome (NTIS).[15] Those with NTIS have low T_3, T_4, and TSH levels.

Etiology and Pathophysiology

We classify hypothyroidism as primary or secondary. *Primary hypothyroidism* is caused by destruction of thyroid tissue or defective hormone synthesis. *Secondary hypothyroidism* is caused by pituitary disease with decreased TSH secretion or hypothalamic dysfunction with decreased thyrotropin-releasing hormone (TRH) secretion. Hypothyroidism can be brief and related to thyroiditis or stopping thyroid hormone therapy.

Iodine deficiency is the most common cause of hypothyroidism worldwide. In the United States, the most common cause of primary hypothyroidism is atrophy of the thyroid gland. This atrophy is the result of Hashimoto's thyroiditis or Graves' disease. These autoimmune diseases destroy the thyroid gland. Hypothyroidism can develop after treatment for hyperthyroidism, specifically thyroidectomy or RAI therapy. Drugs, such as amiodarone, which contains iodine, and lithium, which blocks hormone production, can cause hypothyroidism.

Hypothyroidism that develops in infancy *(cretinism)* results from thyroid hormone deficiencies during fetal or early neonatal life. All infants in the United States are screened for decreased thyroid function at birth.

Clinical Manifestations

The systemic effects of hypothyroidism are characterized by a slowing of body processes (Table 49.6). Manifestations vary depending on the severity and the duration of thyroid deficiency and the patient's age at the onset of the deficiency. Symptoms may develop over months to years, unless hypothyroidism occurs after a thyroidectomy, after thyroid ablation, or during treatment with antithyroid drugs.

The patient is often tired and lethargic. There may be personality and mental changes, including impaired memory, slowed speech, decreased initiative, and somnolence. Many appear depressed. Weight gain is a result of a decreased metabolic rate.

Hypothyroidism may cause significant cardiovascular problems, especially in a person with a history of CVD. It is associated with decreased cardiac contractility and decreased cardiac output. The patient may have low exercise tolerance and shortness of breath on exertion. High serum cholesterol and triglyceride levels and the accumulation of mucopolysaccharides in the intima of small blood vessels can result in coronary atherosclerosis. Anemia is common.

Patients with severe, long-standing hypothyroidism may have myxedema. Myxedema results from the accumulation of hydrophilic mucopolysaccharides in the dermis and other tissues (Fig. 49.9). It alters the physical appearance of the skin and subcutaneous tissues with puffiness, facial and periorbital

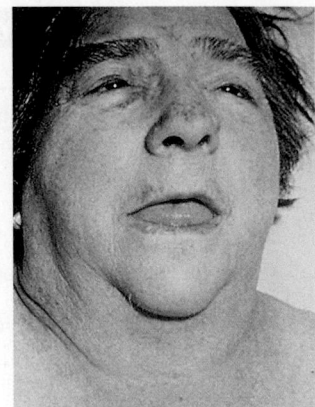

FIG. 49.9 Common features of myxedema. Dull, puffy skin; coarse, sparse hair; periorbital edema; and prominent tongue. (Courtesy Paul W. Ladenson, MD, The Johns Hopkins University and Hospital, Baltimore, MD. From Seidel HM, Ball JW, Dains JE, et al, editors: *Mosby's guide to physical examination*, ed 6, St Louis, 2006, Mosby.)

edema, and a masklike affect. Patients may have an altered self-image related to their disabilities and altered appearance.

In the older adult, we may attribute the typical manifestations of hypothyroidism (fatigue, cold and dry skin, hoarseness, hair loss, constipation, cold intolerance) to normal aging. For this reason, the patient's symptoms may not raise suspicion of an underlying condition. Older adults who have confusion, lethargy, and depression should be evaluated for thyroid disease.

Complications

The mental sluggishness, drowsiness, and lethargy of hypothyroidism may progress gradually or suddenly to a notable impairment of consciousness or coma. This situation, termed *myxedema coma*, is a medical emergency. Myxedema coma can be precipitated by infection, drugs (especially opioids, tranquilizers, and barbiturates), exposure to cold, and trauma. It is characterized by subnormal temperature, hypotension, and hypoventilation. Cardiovascular collapse can result from hypoventilation, hyponatremia, hypoglycemia, and lactic acidosis. For the patient to survive myxedema coma, vital functions must be supported and IV thyroid hormone replacement given.

Diagnostic Studies

The most reliable laboratory tests for thyroid function are TSH and free T_4. These values, correlated with symptoms obtained from the history and physical examination, confirm the diagnosis of hypothyroidism. Serum TSH levels help determine the cause of hypothyroidism. Serum TSH is high when the defect is in the thyroid and low when it is in the pituitary or the hypothalamus. The presence of thyroid antibodies suggests an autoimmune origin. Other abnormal laboratory findings are high cholesterol and triglycerides, anemia, and increased creatine kinase (Table 49.7).

Interprofessional Care

The treatment goal for a patient with hypothyroidism is to restore a euthyroid state as safely and rapidly as possible with hormone therapy (Table 49.13). A low-calorie diet can promote weight loss or prevent weight gain.

Levothyroxine (Synthroid) is the drug of choice to treat hypothyroidism. In the young and otherwise healthy patient, the maintenance replacement dosage is adjusted according to

TABLE 49.13 Interprofessional Care

Hypothyroidism

Diagnostic Assessment	Management
• History and physical examination • Serum TSH and free T_4 • Total serum T_3 and T_4 • Thyroid peroxidase (TPO) antibodies	• Thyroid hormone replacement (e.g., levothyroxine) • Monitor thyroid hormone levels and adjust dosage (if needed) • Nutritional therapy to promote weight loss • Patient and caregiver teaching (Table 49.14)

the patient's response and laboratory findings. When beginning thyroid hormone therapy, the first dosages are low to avoid increases in resting heart rate and BP. In the patient with compromised cardiac status, careful monitoring is needed when starting and adjusting the dosage because the usual dose may increase myocardial O_2 demand. This may cause angina and dysrhythmias.

 DRUG ALERT Levothyroxine (Synthroid)
• Carefully monitor patients with CVD who take this drug.
• Monitor heart rate and report pulse greater than 100 beats/min or an irregular heartbeat.
• Promptly report chest pain, weight loss, nervousness, tremors, and/or insomnia.

In a patient without side effects, the dose is increased at 4- to 6-week intervals as needed based on the TSH levels. It may take up to 8 weeks before the full effect of hormone therapy is seen. Levothyroxine has a peak of action of 1 to 3 weeks. It is important that the patient regularly take replacement medication. Lifelong thyroid therapy is usually required.

Liotrix is a synthetic mix of levothyroxine (T_4) and liothyronine (T_3) in a 4:1 combination. Liotrix has a faster onset of action with a peak of 2 to 3 days. It can be used in acutely ill patients with hypothyroidism.

❖ NURSING MANAGEMENT: HYPOTHYROIDISM

◆ Nursing Assessment

Careful assessment may reveal early and subtle changes in a patient suspected of having hypothyroidism. Note any history of hyperthyroidism and treatment with antithyroid medications, RAI, or surgery. Ask the patient about using iodine-containing medications (Table 49.5). Note any changes in appetite, weight, activity level, speech, memory, and skin (e.g., increased dryness or thickening). Assess for cold intolerance, constipation, and signs of depression. Further assessment should focus on heart rate, tenderness over the thyroid gland, and edema in the extremities and face.

◆ Nursing Diagnoses

Nursing diagnoses for the patient with hypothyroidism may include:
• Activity intolerance
• Constipation
• Impaired nutritional status

Additional information on nursing diagnoses and interventions is presented in the eNursing Care Plan 49.2 for the patient with hypothyroidism (available on the website for this chapter).

◆ Planning

The overall goals are that the patient with hypothyroidism will (1) have relief of symptoms, (2) maintain a euthyroid state, (3) maintain a positive self-image, and (4) adhere with lifelong thyroid therapy.

◆ Nursing Implementation

◆ Health Promotion.
Routine screening of thyroid function is not recommended in nonpregnant, asymptomatic adults. Risk factors include being female, white ethnicity, advancing age or having type 1 diabetes, Down syndrome, family history of thyroid disease, goiter, previous hyperthyroidism, and external beam radiation in the head and neck area.[16] High-risk populations should be screened for subclinical thyroid disease.

◆ Acute Care.
Most people with hypothyroidism are treated on an outpatient basis. The person who develops myxedema coma needs acute nursing care, often in the ICU. Mechanical respiratory support and cardiac monitoring are often needed.

Give thyroid hormone therapy and all other medications IV because severe gastric hypomotility may prevent the absorption of oral agents. Monitor the core temperature for hypothermia that often occurs in myxedema and myxedema coma. Use gentle soap and moisturize often to prevent skin breakdown. Frequent position changes and a low-pressure mattress help maintain skin integrity.

Monitor the patient's progress by assessing vital signs, body weight, fluid intake and output, and edema. Cardiac assessment is especially important because the cardiovascular response to hormone therapy determines the medication regimen. Note energy level and mental alertness, which should improve within 2 to 14 days and continue a steady progression to normal levels. Neurologic status and TSH levels are used to determine continuing treatment.

◆ Ambulatory Care.
Patient teaching about medication management and identification of complications is essential (Table 49.14). At first the hypothyroid patient may have a hard time processing complex instructions. It is important to give written instructions, repeat the information often, and assess the patient's comprehension level.

Stress the need for lifelong drug therapy and avoiding abruptly stopping drugs. Caution patients against doubling up on doses for any reason. Some patients notice weight loss and are tempted to increase dosing to achieve a desired weight. Teach the patient the expected and unexpected side effects, including the signs and symptoms of hypothyroidism and hyperthyroidism (Table 49.6). The manifestations of overdose are the same as hyperthyroidism. Tell the patient to contact the HCP at once if symptoms, such as orthopnea, dyspnea, rapid pulse, palpitations, chest pain, nervousness, or insomnia, are present.

The patient with diabetes should test blood glucose levels at least daily because the return to the euthyroid state often increases insulin requirements. Thyroid drugs increase the effects of anticoagulants and decrease the effect of digitalis compounds. Teach the patient the toxic signs and symptoms of these medications and the need to remain under close medical observation until stable. Medication interactions are an important reason for patients to consult the HCP before switching brands of thyroid replacement medication. Switching brands may change bioavailability of the drug and physiologic response.

TABLE 49.14 Patient & Caregiver Teaching

Hypothyroidism

Include the following instructions when teaching the patient and caregiver about management of hypothyroidism:

1. Discuss the importance of thyroid hormone therapy:
   - Need for lifelong therapy
   - Taking thyroid hormone in the morning before food
   - Need for regular follow-up care and monitoring of thyroid hormone levels
2. Caution the patient not to switch brands of the hormone since the bioavailability of thyroid hormones may differ.
3. Emphasize the need for a comfortable, warm environment because of cold intolerance.
4. Teach ways to prevent skin breakdown. Use soap sparingly and apply lotion to skin.
5. Caution the patient, especially if an older adult, to avoid sedatives. If they must be used, suggest that the lowest dose be used. Caregiver should closely monitor mental status, level of consciousness, and respirations.
6. Discuss ways to minimize constipation, including:
   - Gradual increase in activity and exercise
   - Increased fiber in diet
   - Use of stool softeners
   - Regular bowel elimination time
   - Tell patient to avoid using enemas. They cause vagal stimulation, which can be hazardous if heart disease is present.

With treatment, striking transformations occur in both appearance and mental function. Most adults return to a normal state. Cardiovascular conditions and psychosis may persist despite corrections of the hormonal imbalance. Relapses occur if treatment is interrupted.

◆ Evaluation

The expected outcomes are that the patient with hypothyroidism will

- Have relief from symptoms
- Maintain a euthyroid state with normal thyroid hormone and TSH levels
- Avoid complications of therapy
- Adhere to lifelong therapy

THYROID NODULES AND CANCER

A *thyroid nodule* (growth in the thyroid gland) may be benign or malignant (thyroid cancer). More than 95% of all thyroid gland nodules are benign. Prevalence of thyroid nodule development increases with age. Benign nodules are usually not dangerous, but they can cause tracheal compression if they become too large.

Thyroid cancer is the most common type of cancer of the endocrine system. An estimated 62,450 new cases of thyroid cancer are diagnosed annually. The incidence of thyroid cancer has increased significantly in the past 25 years. It is the most rapidly increasing cancer in the United States. Thyroid cancer affects more women, and the incidence is higher in whites and Asian Americans.[17] Adults at risk include those who had head and neck radiation therapy during childhood, were exposed to radioactive fallout, or have a personal or family history of goiter.

Types of Thyroid Cancer

The 4 main types of thyroid cancer are papillary, follicular, medullary, and anaplastic. *Papillary* thyroid cancer is the most common type, accounting for about 70% to 80% of all thyroid cancers. Papillary cancer tends to grow slowly. It initially spreads to lymph nodes in the neck.

Follicular thyroid cancer makes up about 15% of all thyroid cancers. It tends to occur in older patients. Follicular cancer first metastasizes into the cervical lymph nodes and then spreads to the neck, lungs, and bones.

Medullary thyroid cancer, accounts for up to 10% of all thyroid cancers. It is more likely to occur in families and be associated with other endocrine problems. It is diagnosed by genetic testing for a proto-oncogene called *RET*. Medullary thyroid cancer is a type of multiple endocrine neoplasia. It is often poorly differentiated and associated with early metastasis.

Anaplastic thyroid cancer occurs in less than 2% of patients with thyroid cancer. It is the most advanced and aggressive thyroid cancer. The patient is least likely to respond to treatment and has a poor prognosis.

Clinical Manifestations and Diagnostic Studies

The primary manifestation of thyroid cancer is a painless, palpable nodule or nodules in an enlarged thyroid gland. Most nodules are found during routine palpation of the neck. The presence of firm, palpable, cervical masses suggests lymph node metastasis. Some patients may have difficulty swallowing or breathing because of tumor growth invading the trachea or esophagus. Hemoptysis and airway obstruction may occur if the trachea is involved. Patients with thyroid cancer generally are euthyroid.

Nodular enlargement of the thyroid gland or palpation of a mass requires further evaluation. Ultrasound is often the first test used. Follow-up testing may involve CT, MRI, positron emission tomography (PET), and ultrasound-guided fine-needle aspiration (FNA). An FNA is done when a tissue sample for pathologic examination is needed. A thyroid scan may be done. The scan shows whether nodules on the thyroid are "hot" or "cold." "Hot" tumors take up radioactive iodine. They are almost always benign. If the nodule does not take up the radioactive iodine, it appears as "cold" and has a higher risk for being cancer.

Increases in serum calcitonin are associated with medullary thyroid cancer. In papillary and follicular cancers, serum thyroglobulin is high. In families with a history of medullary thyroid cancer, family members are encouraged to have genetic testing and thyroid screening on a regular basis.

❖ Interprofessional and Nursing Care

Surgical removal of the tumor is the main treatment for thyroid cancer. Surgical procedures range from unilateral total lobectomy to near-total thyroidectomy with bilateral lobectomy. Lymph nodes in the neck may be removed to determine if the cancer has spread. RAI may be given to some patients to destroy any remaining cancer cells after surgery. RAI therapy improves survival rates in patients with papillary and follicular thyroid cancer. External beam radiation may be given as palliative treatment for patients with metastatic thyroid cancer.

Many thyroid cancers are TSH dependent. Thyroid hormone therapy in high doses is often prescribed to inhibit pituitary secretion of TSH. Chemotherapy, including doxorubicin, may be used for advanced disease. Vandetanib (Caprelsa), lenvatinib (Lenvima), sorafenib tosylate (Nexavar), and cabozantinib (Cometriq) are targeted therapies used for metastatic thyroid cancer. These drugs inhibit tyrosine kinases, enzymes that are involved in the growth of cancer cells.

Nursing care for the patient with thyroid cancer is similar to that of a patient undergoing thyroidectomy (see p. 1154). Because of the surgical site location and the potential for hypocalcemia, the patient needs frequent postoperative assessment. Assess the patient for airway obstruction, bleeding, and tetany since the parathyroid gland may have been disturbed or removed during surgery.

MULTIPLE ENDOCRINE NEOPLASIA

Multiple endocrine neoplasia (MEN) is an inherited condition characterized by hormone-secreting tumors.[18] It is caused by the mutation of 1 of 2 genes, *MEN1* or *RET*, that normally control cell growth. Tumors may develop in childhood or later in life.

The 2 major types of MEN are type 1 and type 2. Both types are often inherited as autosomal dominant disorders. Persons with type 1 often have parathyroid gland hyperactivity (hyperparathyroidism). Other signs may include hyperactivity of the pituitary gland (prolactinoma) and pancreas (gastrinoma). In most cases, the tumors are initially benign. Some tumors later become malignant. Persons with type 2 neoplasia often have medullary thyroid carcinoma. They may develop pheochromocytoma (tumor of the adrenal glands). Pheochromocytoma is discussed later in this chapter on p. 1168.

Treatment includes conservative management (watchful waiting), drugs to block the effects of excess hormone, and surgical removal of the gland and/or tumor. It is important for patients to have regular screening visits with the HCP so that new tumors may be detected early and existing tumors carefully monitored.

DISORDERS OF PARATHYROID GLANDS

HYPERPARATHYROIDISM

Etiology and Pathophysiology

Hyperparathyroidism is a condition involving an increased secretion of parathyroid hormone (PTH). PTH helps regulate serum calcium and phosphate levels by stimulating bone resorption of calcium, renal tubular reabsorption of calcium, and activation of vitamin D. Thus oversecretion of PTH is associated with increased serum calcium levels.

Hyperparathyroidism is classified as primary, secondary, or tertiary. *Primary hyperparathyroidism* is due to an increased secretion of PTH leading to disorders of calcium, phosphate, and bone metabolism. The most common cause is a benign tumor (adenoma) in the parathyroid gland. Patients who have previously undergone head and neck radiation have an increased risk for developing a parathyroid adenoma. Long-term lithium therapy is also associated with primary hyperparathyroidism. Primary hyperparathyroidism affects 25 of 100,000 persons per year.[19] The peak incidence is in the 40s and 50s. It affects twice as many women as men.[19]

Secondary hyperparathyroidism is a compensatory response to conditions that induce or cause hypocalcemia, the main stimulus of PTH secretion. These include vitamin D deficiencies, malabsorption, chronic kidney disease, and hyperphosphatemia.

Tertiary hyperparathyroidism occurs when there is hyperplasia of the parathyroid glands and a loss of negative feedback (see Chapter 47) from circulating calcium levels. Thus there is

autonomous secretion of PTH even with normal calcium levels. This condition is seen in patients who have had a kidney transplant after a long period of dialysis treatment for chronic kidney disease (see Chapter 46).

Excess levels of PTH usually lead to hypercalcemia and hypophosphatemia. Multiple body systems are affected (Table 49.15). Decreased bone density can occur because of the effect of PTH on osteoclastic (bone resorption) and osteoblastic (bone formation) activity. The kidneys cannot reabsorb the excess calcium. This leads to increased urinary calcium levels (hypercalciuria). This urinary calcium, along with a large amount of urinary phosphate, can lead to stone formation.

Clinical Manifestations and Complications

Manifestations range from an asymptomatic person (diagnosed through testing for unrelated problems) to a patient with overt symptoms.[19] The manifestations are associated with hypercalcemia (Table 49.15). Loss of appetite, constipation, fatigue, emotional disorders, shortened attention span, and muscle weakness, particularly in the proximal muscles of the lower extremities, often occur. Complications include osteoporosis, renal failure, kidney stones, pancreatitis, cardiac changes, and long bone, rib, and vertebral fractures.

Diagnostic Studies

PTH levels are increased in patients with hyperparathyroidism. Serum calcium levels usually exceed 10 mg/dL (2.50 mmol/L). Because of its inverse relation with calcium, the serum phosphorus level is usually less than 3 mg/dL (0.1 mmol/L). Hypercalcemia in asymptomatic cases is often identified through a routine chemistry panel.

Increases in other laboratory tests include urine calcium, serum chloride, uric acid, creatinine, amylase (if pancreatitis is present), and alkaline phosphatase (in the presence of bone disease). Bone density measurements may be used to detect bone loss. Conversely, those with bone loss on a screening dual-energy x-ray absorptiometry (DEXA) scan should be tested for hypercalcemia. MRI, CT, and/or ultrasound can detect an adenoma.

Interprofessional Care

The goal of treatment is to relieve symptoms and prevent complications caused by excess PTH. The choice of therapy depends on the urgency of the situation, degree of hypercalcemia, and underlying cause of the disorder.

Surgical Therapy. The most effective treatment of primary and secondary hyperparathyroidism is surgical intervention. Surgery involves partial or complete removal of the parathyroid glands. The most common procedure involves endoscopy and is done on an outpatient basis. Criteria for surgery include increased serum calcium levels (more than 1 mg/dL above the upper limit of normal), hypercalciuria (greater than 400 mg/day), markedly reduced bone mineral density, overt symptoms (e.g., neuromuscular effects, kidney stones), or age under 50 years. Parathyroidectomy leads to a rapid reduction of high calcium levels.

Patients who have multiple parathyroid glands removed may undergo autotransplantation of normal parathyroid tissue in the forearm or near the sternocleidomastoid muscle. This allows PTH secretion to continue with normalization of calcium levels. If autotransplantation is not possible or if it fails, the patient will need to take calcium supplements for life.

TABLE 49.15 Manifestations of Parathyroid Dysfunction

Hyperfunction	Hypofunction	Hyperfunction	Hypofunction
Cardiovascular System		**Neurologic System**	
• Hypertension	• Hypotension	• Lethargy, weakness, fatigue	• Weakness, fatigue
• Angina	• Edema	• Psychosis, depression	• Depression
• Dysrhythmias	• Dysrhythmias	• Depressed reflexes	• Hyperreflexia, muscle cramps
• Shortened ST segment	• Elongation of ST segment	• Personality changes	• Personality changes
• Shortened QT interval	• Prolonged QT interval	• Irritability	• Irritability
• ↑ Digitalis effect	• ↓ Cardiac output	• Memory impairment	• Memory impairment
		• Delirium, confusion, coma	• Disorientation, confusion (in older adult)
Gastrointestinal System		• Headache	
• Vague abdominal pain	• Abdominal cramps	• Poor coordination	• Headache, ↑ intracranial pressure
• Anorexia	• Fecal incontinence (in older adult)	• Gait abnormalities	• Tetany, seizures
• Nausea and vomiting	• Malabsorption	• Psychomotor retardation	• Positive Chvostek's and Trousseau's sign
• Constipation		• Paresthesias	• Tremor
• Pancreatitis			• Paresthesias of lips, hands, feet
• Peptic ulcer disease			
• Cholelithiasis		**Renal/Urinary System**	
• Weight loss		• Hypercalciuria	• Urinary frequency
		• Kidney stones	• Urinary incontinence
Laboratory Findings		• Urinary tract infections	
• ↑ Calcium	• ↓ Calcium	• Polyuria	
• ↓ Phosphorus	• ↑ Phosphorus		
		Skin	
Musculoskeletal System		• Skin necrosis	• Dry, scaly skin
• Weakness, fatigue	• Weakness, fatigue	• Moist skin	• Hair loss on scalp and body
• Skeletal pain	• Painful muscle cramps		• Brittle nails, transverse ridging
• Backache	• Skeletal x-ray changes, osteosclerosis		• Lack of tooth enamel
• Pain on weight bearing	• Soft tissue calcification		
• Osteoporosis	• Difficulty walking	**Visual System**	
• Pathologic fractures of long bones		• Impaired vision	• Eye changes, including lenticular opacities, cataracts, papilledema
• Compression fractures of spine; kyphosis		• Corneal calcification	
• ↓ muscle tone, muscle atrophy			

Nonsurgical Therapy. A conservative approach is often used in patients who are asymptomatic or have mild symptoms of hyperparathyroidism. Ongoing care includes regular examination with measurements of serum PTH, calcium, phosphorus, alkaline phosphatase, creatinine and blood urea nitrogen (BUN) (to assess renal function), and urinary calcium excretion. Annual x-rays and DEXA scans assess for metabolic bone loss. Continued ambulation and avoiding immobility are important. Dietary measures include high fluid and moderate calcium intake.

Severe hypercalcemia is managed with IV sodium chloride solution and loop diuretics, such as furosemide, to increase the urinary excretion of calcium. Several drugs help to lower calcium levels, but they do not treat the underlying problem. Bisphosphonates (e.g., alendronate [Fosamax]) inhibit osteoclastic bone resorption, normalizing serum calcium levels and improving bone mineral density. IV bisphosphonates (e.g., pamidronate [Aredia]) can rapidly lower serum calcium in patients with dangerously high levels. Phosphates are given if the patient has normal renal function and low serum phosphate levels.

Calcimimetic agents (e.g., cinacalcet [Sensipar]) increase the sensitivity of the calcium receptor on the parathyroid gland, resulting in decreased PTH secretion and calcium blood levels. They are useful in treating secondary hyperparathyroidism in those with chronic kidney disease on dialysis or in patients with parathyroid cancer.

❖ NURSING MANAGEMENT: HYPERPARATHYROIDISM

Nursing care for the patient after a parathyroidectomy is similar to that for a patient after thyroidectomy. The major complications are associated with hemorrhage and fluid and electrolyte problems. *Tetany,* a condition of neuromuscular hyperexcitability associated with sudden decrease in calcium levels, is another concern. It is usually apparent early in the postoperative period but may develop over several days. Mild tetany, characterized by unpleasant tingling of the hands and around the mouth, may be present but should decrease over time. If tetany becomes more severe (e.g., muscular spasms, laryngospasms), IV calcium may be given. IV calcium gluconate should be readily available for patients after parathyroidectomy in case acute tetany occurs.

Monitor intake and output to evaluate the patient's fluid status. Assess calcium, potassium, phosphate, and magnesium levels frequently, as well as Chvostek's and Trousseau's signs (see Fig. 16.15). Encourage mobility to promote bone calcification.

If surgery is not done, treatment to relieve symptoms and prevent complications is started. Help the patient to adapt the meal plan to their lifestyle. A referral to a dietitian may be useful. Because immobility can worsen bone loss, emphasize the importance of an exercise program. Encourage the patient to keep the regular follow-up appointments. Teach the patient the symptoms of hypocalcemia and hypercalcemia and to report them if they occur. Hypocalcemia and hypercalcemia are discussed in Chapter 16.

HYPOPARATHYROIDISM

Hypoparathyroidism is an uncommon condition associated with inadequate circulating PTH. It is characterized by hypocalcemia due to a lack of PTH to maintain serum calcium levels. PTH resistance at the cellular level may also occur *(pseudohypoparathyroidism)*. This is caused by a genetic defect resulting in hypocalcemia despite normal or high PTH levels. It is often associated with hypothyroidism and hypogonadism.

The most common cause is iatrogenic. This may include accidental removal of the parathyroid glands or damage to the vascular supply of the glands during neck surgery (e.g., thyroidectomy). Idiopathic hypoparathyroidism resulting from the absence, fatty replacement, or atrophy of the glands is a rare disease. It usually occurs early in life and may be associated with other endocrine disorders. Affected patients may have antiparathyroid antibodies. Severe hypomagnesemia (e.g., malnutrition, chronic alcoholism, renal failure) can suppress PTH secretion. Other causes of parathyroid deficiency include tumors and heavy metal poisoning.

The features of acute hypoparathyroidism are due to hypocalcemia (Table 49.15). Sudden decreases in calcium concentration cause tetany, characterized by tingling of the lips and stiffness in the extremities. Painful tonic spasms of smooth and skeletal muscles can cause dysphagia and laryngospasms, which compromise breathing. Lethargy, anxiety, and personality changes may occur. Abnormal laboratory findings include decreased serum calcium and PTH levels and increased serum phosphate levels.

❖ Interprofessional and Nursing Care

Treatment goals are to treat acute complications, such as tetany, maintain normal serum calcium levels, and prevent long-term complications. Emergency treatment of tetany after surgery requires IV calcium administration.

Give IV calcium slowly. Use ECG monitoring when giving calcium because high serum calcium levels can cause hypotension, serious dysrhythmias, or cardiac arrest. The patient who takes digoxin is particularly vulnerable. It is important to assess IV patency before administration. Calcium chloride can cause venous irritation and inflammation. Extravasation may cause cellulitis, necrosis, and tissue sloughing.

Rebreathing may partially relieve acute neuromuscular symptoms associated with hypocalcemia, including muscle cramps and mild tetany. Have the patient breathe in and out of a paper bag or breathing mask. This reduces CO_2 excretion from the lungs, increases carbonic acid levels in the blood, and lowers the pH. A lower pH (acidic environment) enhances calcium ionization, which causes more total body calcium to be available in the active form.

Teach the patient how to manage long-term drug and nutritional therapy. PTH replacement is not recommended because of the expense and need for parenteral administration. Most patients receive oral calcium supplements, magnesium supplements, and vitamin D.

Vitamin D is used to enhance intestinal calcium absorption. Vitamin D (e.g., 1,25-dihydroxycholecalciferol, calcitriol [Rocaltrol]) increases calcium levels rapidly and is quickly metabolized. Rapid metabolism is desired because vitamin D is a fat-soluble vitamin and toxicity can cause irreversible renal impairment.

A high-calcium meal plan includes foods, such as dark green vegetables, soybeans, and tofu. Tell the patient to avoid foods containing oxalic acid (e.g., spinach, rhubarb) because they inhibit calcium absorption. Teach the patient about the need for follow-up care, including monitoring of calcium levels 3 or 4 times a year.

DISORDERS OF ADRENAL CORTEX

Adrenal cortex steroid hormones have 3 main classifications: glucocorticoids, mineralocorticoids, and androgens. Glucocorticoids regulate metabolism, increase blood glucose levels, and are critical in the physiologic stress response. The primary glucocorticoid is cortisol. Mineralocorticoids regulate sodium and potassium balance. The primary mineralocorticoid is aldosterone. Androgens contribute to growth and development in both genders and to sexual development in men. The term *corticosteroid* refers to any of these 3 types of hormones made by the adrenal cortex.

CUSHING SYNDROME

Etiology and Pathophysiology

Cushing syndrome is a clinical condition that results from chronic exposure to excess corticosteroids, particularly glucocorticoids.[20] Several conditions can cause Cushing syndrome. The most common cause is iatrogenic administration of exogenous corticosteroids (e.g., prednisone). About 85% of the cases of endogenous Cushing syndrome are due to an ACTH-secreting pituitary adenoma (Cushing disease). Less common causes include adrenal tumors and ectopic ACTH production by tumors (usually of the lung or pancreas) outside of the hypothalamic-pituitary-adrenal axis. Cushing disease and primary adrenal tumors are more common in women in the 20- to 40-year-old age-group. Ectopic ACTH production is more common in men.

Clinical Manifestations

Manifestations occur in most body systems and are related to excess levels of corticosteroids (Table 49.16). Although signs of glucocorticoid excess usually predominate, symptoms of mineralocorticoid and androgen excess can occur.

Corticosteroid excess causes pronounced changes in physical appearance (Fig. 49.10). Weight gain is the most common feature. It results from the accumulation of adipose tissue in the trunk (centripetal obesity), face ("moon face"), and cervical areas ("buffalo hump") (Fig. 49.11). Hyperglycemia occurs because of glucose intolerance associated with cortisol-induced insulin resistance and increased gluconeogenesis by the liver. Muscle wasting causes weakness, especially in the extremities. A loss of bone matrix leads to osteoporosis and back pain. The

TABLE 49.16 Manifestations of Adrenocortical Dysfunction

System	Cushing Syndrome	Addison's Disease
Glucocorticoids		
General appearance	Truncal obesity, thin extremities, rounding of face (moon face), fat deposits on back of neck and shoulders (buffalo hump) (Fig. 49.11)	Weight loss, emaciation
Cardiovascular	Hypervolemia, hypertension, edema of lower extremities	Hypotension, tendency to develop refractory shock, vasodilation
Gastrointestinal	↑ Secretion of pepsin and HCl acid, risk for peptic ulcer disease, anorexia	Anorexia, nausea and vomiting, cramping abdominal pain, diarrhea
Immune	Inhibition of immune response, suppression of allergic response	Tendency for coexisting autoimmune diseases
Metabolic	Hyperglycemia, negative nitrogen balance, dyslipidemia	Hyponatremia, insulin sensitivity, fever
Musculoskeletal	Muscle wasting in extremities, fatigue, osteoporosis, awkward gait, back pain, weakness, compression fractures	Fatigue
Psychologic	Euphoria, irritability, depression, insomnia, anxiety	Depression, exhaustion or irritability, confusion, delusions
Renal/urinary	Glycosuria, hypercalciuria, risk for kidney stones	
Skin	Thin, fragile skin, purplish red striae (Fig. 49.12). Petechial hemorrhages, bruises. Florid cheeks (plethora), acne, poor wound healing	Bronzed or smoky hyperpigmentation of face, neck, hands (especially creases) (Fig. 49.13), buccal membranes, nipples, genitalia, and scars (if pituitary function normal). Vitiligo, alopecia
Mineralocorticoids		
Cardiovascular	Hypertension, hypervolemia	Hypovolemia, tendency toward shock, decreased cardiac output
Fluid and electrolytes	Marked sodium and water retention, edema, marked hypokalemia, alkalosis	Sodium loss, ↓ volume of extracellular fluid, hyperkalemia, salt craving
Androgens		
Musculoskeletal	Muscle wasting and weakness	↓ Muscle size and tone
Reproductive	*Women:* Menstrual irregularities and enlargement of clitoris	*Women:* ↓ Libido in women
	Men: Gynecomastia and testicular atrophy	*Men:* No effect in men
Skin	Hirsutism, acne, hyperpigmentation	↓ Axillary and pubic hair (in women)

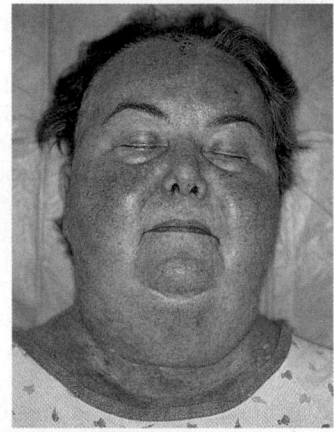

FIG. 49.10 Cushing syndrome. Facies include a rounded face ("moon face") with thin, reddened skin. Hirsutism may be present. (From Seidel HM, Ball JW, Dains JE, et al: *Mosby's guide to physical examination*, ed 6, St Louis, 2006, Mosby.)

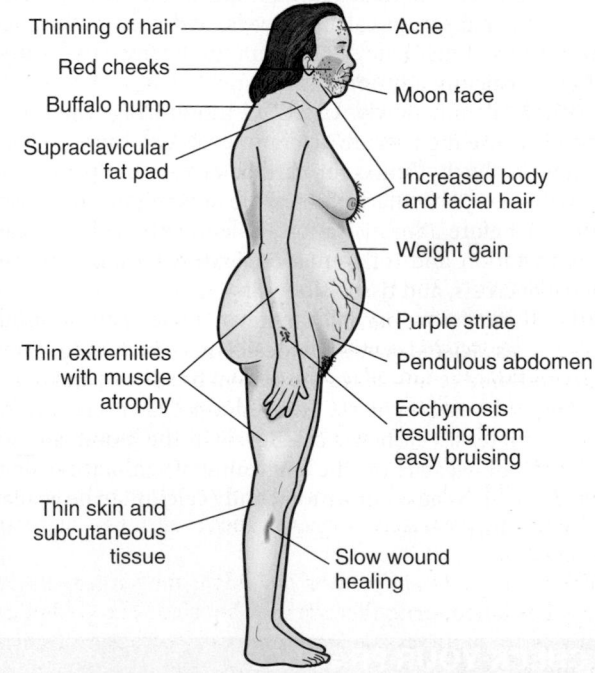

FIG. 49.11 Common characteristics of Cushing syndrome.

loss of collagen makes the skin weaker, thinner, and more easily bruised. Purplish red striae (usually depressed below the skin surface) appear on the abdomen, breast, or buttocks (Fig. 49.12). Catabolic processes lead to a delay in wound healing.

Mineralocorticoid excess may cause hypokalemia from potassium excretion and hypertension from fluid retention. Adrenal androgen excess may cause severe acne, the development of male characteristics in women, and feminization in men. Menstrual disorders and hirsutism in women and gynecomastia and impotence in men are seen more often in adrenal cancers.

Diagnostic Studies

Diagnosing Cushing syndrome begins with confirming increased plasma cortisol levels. We use 3 tests: (1) midnight or late-night salivary cortisol, (2) low-dose dexamethasone suppression test, and (3) 24-hour urine cortisol.[21] Urine cortisol

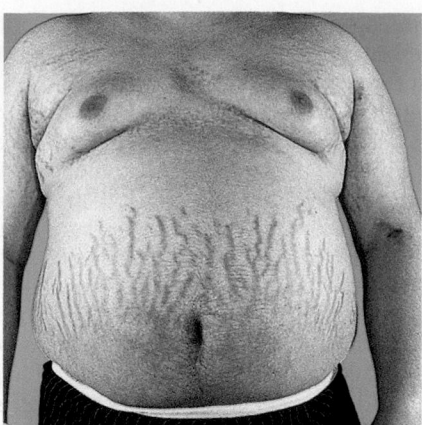

FIG. 49.12 Cushing syndrome. Truncal obesity; broad, purple striae; and easy bruising (left antecubital fossa). (From Chew SL, Leslie D: *Clinical endocrinology and diabetes: An illustrated colour text,* Edinburgh, 2006, Churchill Livingstone.)

TABLE 49.17 Interprofessional Care

Cushing Syndrome

Diagnostic Assessment
- History and physical examination
- Dexamethasone suppression test
- 24-Hr urine for free cortisol and 17-ketosteroids
- Plasma and salivary cortisol levels
- Plasma ACTH levels
- Complete blood count (CBC) with WBC differential
- Blood chemistries for sodium, potassium, glucose
- CT scan, MRI

Management
Pituitary Adenoma
- Transsphenoidal resection
- Radiation therapy

Adrenocortical Adenoma, Cancer, or Hyperplasia
- Adrenalectomy (open or laparoscopic)
- Drug therapy (e.g., ketoconazole, mitotane, mifepristone [Korlym])

Ectopic ACTH-Secreting Tumor
- Treatment of the tumor (surgical removal or radiation)

Exogenous Corticosteroid Therapy
- Discontinue or change the dose of exogenous corticosteroids

levels higher than 100 mcg/24 hr indicate Cushing syndrome. Urine levels of 17-ketosteroids may be high. A CT scan or MRI of the pituitary and adrenal glands can detect a tumor.

Plasma ACTH levels may be low, normal, or high, depending on the underlying cause of Cushing syndrome. High or normal ACTH levels indicate Cushing disease, while low or undetectable levels indicate an adrenal or medication cause. Other findings associated with, but not diagnostic of, Cushing syndrome include leukocytosis, lymphopenia, eosinopenia, hyperglycemia, glycosuria, hypercalciuria, and osteoporosis. Hypokalemia and alkalosis are seen in ectopic ACTH syndrome and adrenal cancer.

Interprofessional Care

The primary goal of treatment is to normalize hormone secretion. The specific treatment depends on the underlying cause (Table 49.17). If the underlying cause is a pituitary adenoma, the standard treatment is surgical removal of the pituitary tumor using the transsphenoidal approach.[21] (This was discussed earlier in this chapter on p. 1145.) Radiation therapy is an option for patients who are not good surgical candidates.

An adrenalectomy is done if Cushing syndrome is caused by adrenal tumors or hyperplasia. Sometimes, bilateral adrenalectomy is needed. A laparoscopic approach is used unless a malignant adrenal tumor is suspected. An open surgical adrenalectomy is usually done for adrenal cancer.

Patients with ectopic ACTH-secreting tumors are best managed by removing the tumor (usually lung or pancreas). This is usually possible when the tumor is benign. If a cancerous tumor has already metastasized, surgical removal may not be possible or successful.

When the patient is a poor candidate for surgery or prior surgery has failed, drug therapy may be tried. The goal of drug therapy is to suppress the synthesis and secretion of cortisol from the adrenal gland (*medical adrenalectomy*). Drugs used include ketoconazole and mitotane. These are used cautiously because they are often toxic at the dosages needed to reduce cortisol secretion. Hydrocortisone or prednisone may be needed to avoid adrenal insufficiency. Mifepristone (Korlym) may be used to control hyperglycemia in patients with endogenous Cushing syndrome who have type 2 diabetes.

If Cushing syndrome developed because of prolonged use of corticosteroids (e.g., prednisone), the following alternatives may be tried: (1) gradually discontinuing corticosteroid therapy, (2) reducing the corticosteroid dose, and (3) converting to alternate-day dosing. Gradual tapering of the corticosteroids is necessary to avoid potentially life-threatening adrenal insufficiency. In alternate-day dosing, twice the daily dosage of a shorter-acting corticosteroid is given every other morning to minimize hypothalamic-pituitary-adrenal suppression, growth suppression, and altered appearance. This plan is not used when the corticosteroids are given as hormone therapy.

❖ NURSING MANAGEMENT: CUSHING SYNDROME

◆ Nursing Assessment

Subjective and objective data that should be obtained from a patient with Cushing syndrome are outlined in Table 49.18.

◆ Nursing Diagnoses

Nursing diagnoses for the patient with Cushing syndrome may include:
- Risk for infection
- Impaired nutritional status
- Disturbed body image
- Impaired tissue integrity

Additional information on nursing diagnoses and interventions is presented in eNursing Care Plan 49.3 for the patient with Cushing syndrome (available on the website for this chapter).

◆ Planning

The overall goals are that the patient with Cushing syndrome will (1) have relief of symptoms, (2) avoid serious complications, (3) maintain a positive self-image, and (4) actively take part in the therapeutic plan.

TABLE 49.18 Nursing Assessment

Cushing Syndrome

Subjective Data

Important Health Information

Past health history: Pituitary tumor (Cushing disease). Adrenal, pancreatic, or pulmonary cancer. GI bleeding, frequent infections
Medications: Corticosteroids

Functional Health Patterns

Health perception–health management: Malaise
Nutritional-metabolic: Weight gain, anorexia. Prolonged wound healing, easy bruising
Elimination: Polyuria
Activity-exercise: Weakness, fatigue
Sleep: Insomnia, poor sleep quality
Cognitive-perceptual: Headache. Back, joint, bone, and rib pain. Poor concentration and memory
Self-perception–self-concept: Negative feelings about changes in personal appearance
Sexuality-reproductive: Amenorrhea, impotence, ↓ libido
Coping–stress tolerance: Anxiety, mood changes, emotional lability, psychosis

Objective Data

General

Truncal obesity, supraclavicular fat pads, buffalo hump, moon face

Skin

Hirsutism of body and face, thinning of head hair. Thin, friable skin. Acne, petechiae, purpura, hyperpigmentation. Purplish red striae on breasts, buttocks, and abdomen. Edema of lower extremities

Cardiovascular

Hypertension

Musculoskeletal

Muscle wasting, thin extremities, awkward gait

Reproductive

Gynecomastia, testicular atrophy (in men), enlarged clitoris (in women)

Possible Diagnostic Findings

Hypokalemia, hyperglycemia, dyslipidemia, polycythemia, lymphocytopenia, eosinopenia. ↑ Plasma cortisol, ↑ salivary cortisol. High, low, or normal ACTH levels. Abnormal dexamethasone suppression test. ↑ Urine free cortisol, 17-ketosteroids. Glycosuria, hypercalciuria. Osteoporosis on x-ray

◆ **Nursing Implementation**

◆ **Health Promotion.** Health promotion focuses on identifying patients at risk for Cushing syndrome. Patients receiving long-term, exogenous corticosteroids are at risk. Teaching related to using medications and monitoring side effects is an important preventive measure.

◆ **Acute Care.** The patient with Cushing syndrome is seriously ill. Because the therapy has many side effects, assessment focuses on signs and symptoms of hormone and drug toxicity and complicating conditions (e.g., CVD, diabetes, infection). Monitor vital signs, daily weight, and glucose. Assess for infection. Because signs and symptoms of inflammation (e.g., fever, redness) may be minimal or absent, assess for pain, loss of function, and purulent drainage. Monitor for signs and symptoms of thromboembolic events, such as pulmonary emboli (e.g., sudden chest pain, dyspnea, tachypnea).

Another important focus of nursing care is emotional support. Changes in appearance, such as truncal obesity, multiple bruises, hirsutism in women, and gynecomastia in men, can be distressing. The patient may feel unattractive, repulsive, or unwanted. You can help by being sensitive to the patient's feelings and offering respect and unconditional acceptance. Reassure the patient that the physical changes and much of the emotional lability will resolve when hormone levels return to normal.

If treatment involves surgical removal of a pituitary adenoma, an adrenal tumor, or one or both adrenal glands, nursing care will include preoperative and postoperative care.

Preoperative Care. Before surgery, the patient should be brought to optimal physical condition. Hypertension and hyperglycemia must be controlled. Hypokalemia must be corrected with diet and potassium supplements. A high-protein diet helps correct the protein depletion. Preoperative teaching depends on the type of surgical approach planned (hypophysectomy or adrenalectomy). Include information about the expected care after surgery.

Postoperative Care. Surgery on the adrenal glands poses great risks. Because the adrenal glands are vascular, the risk for hemorrhage is increased. After both laparoscopic and open adrenalectomy, the patient may have a nasogastric tube, a urinary catheter, IV therapy, and central venous pressure monitoring. Initiate VTE prophylaxis.

Manipulating glandular tissue during surgery may release large amounts of hormones into the circulation. This can produce marked fluctuations in the metabolic processes affected by these hormones. After surgery, BP, fluid balance, and electrolyte levels may be unstable due to these hormone fluctuations.

High doses of corticosteroids (e.g., hydrocortisone [Solu-Cortef]) are given IV during surgery and for several days afterward to ensure adequate responses to the stress of the procedure. If large amounts of endogenous hormone were released into the systemic circulation during surgery, the patient is likely to develop hypertension, increasing the risk for hemorrhage. High corticosteroid levels cause problems with glycemic control, increase risk for infection, and delay wound healing.

The critical period for circulatory instability is 24 to 48 hours after surgery. During this time, you must constantly be alert for signs of corticosteroid imbalance. Report any rapid or significant changes in BP, respirations, or heart rate. Monitor fluid intake and output carefully and assess for potential imbalances. IV corticosteroids are given, and the dosage and flow rate are adjusted to the patient's manifestations and fluid and electrolyte balance. Oral doses are given as tolerated. After IV corticosteroids are withdrawn, keep the IV line open for quick administration of corticosteroids or vasopressors. Obtain morning urine samples at the same time each morning for cortisol measurement to evaluate the surgery's effectiveness.

If corticosteroid dosage is tapered too rapidly after surgery, acute adrenal insufficiency may develop. Vomiting, increased weakness, dehydration, and hypotension are signs of hypocortisolism. The patient may have painful joints, pruritus, or peeling skin and may have severe emotional problems. Report these signs and symptoms so that drug doses can be adjusted as needed.

The patient is usually kept on bed rest until the BP stabilizes. Be alert for subtle signs of infection because the usual inflammatory responses are suppressed. To prevent infection, provide meticulous care when changing the dressing and during any other procedures that involve access to body cavities, circulation, or areas under the skin.

◆ **Ambulatory Care.** Discharge instructions are based on the patient's lack of endogenous corticosteroids and resulting inability to react physiologically to stressors. Consider a home health nurse referral, especially for older adults, because of the need for ongoing evaluation and teaching. Teach the patient to always wear a Medic Alert bracelet and carry medical identification and instructions in a wallet or purse. Teach the patient to avoid exposure to extreme temperatures, infections, and emotional situations. Stress may cause acute adrenal insufficiency because the remaining adrenal tissue cannot meet an increased hormonal demand. Teach patients to adjust their corticosteroid replacement therapy by their stress levels. Consult with the patient's HCP to determine the parameters for dosage changes if this plan is feasible. If the patient cannot adjust their own medication, or if weakness, fainting, fever, or nausea and vomiting occur, the patient should contact the HCP for a possible adjustment in corticosteroid dosage. Many patients require lifetime replacement therapy. However, patients should be prepared for it to take several months to adjust the hormone dose satisfactorily.

◆ Evaluation

The expected outcomes are that the patient with Cushing syndrome will

- Have no signs or symptoms of infection
- Maintain weight appropriate for height
- State acceptance of appearance and treatment plan
- Show healing of skin and maintaining intact skin

ADRENOCORTICAL INSUFFICIENCY

Etiology and Pathophysiology

Adrenocortical insufficiency (hypofunction of the adrenal cortex) may be from a primary cause (Addison's disease) or a secondary cause (lack of pituitary ACTH secretion). In Addison's disease, all 3 classes of adrenal corticosteroids (glucocorticoids, mineralocorticoids, and androgens) are reduced. In secondary adrenocortical insufficiency, corticosteroids and androgens are deficient but mineralocorticoids rarely are. ACTH deficiency may be caused by pituitary disease or suppression of the hypothalamic-pituitary axis because of the use of exogenous corticosteroids.

Up to 80% of Addison's disease cases in the United States are caused by an autoimmune response.[22] Autoimmune adrenalitis causes the adrenal cortex to be destroyed by antibodies. This results in loss of glucocorticoid, mineralocorticoid, and adrenal androgen hormones. Addison's disease can be present along with other endocrine conditions. This is known as *autoimmune polyglandular syndrome.* It is most common in white females. Those with autoimmune adrenalitis often have other autoimmune disorders, such as type 1 diabetes, autoimmune thyroid disease, pernicious anemia, and celiac disease.[23]

Although tuberculosis causes Addison's disease worldwide, it is now an uncommon cause in the United States. Other causes include amyloidosis, fungal infections (e.g., histoplasmosis), acquired immunodeficiency syndrome (AIDS), and metastatic cancer. Iatrogenic Addison's disease may be due to adrenal hemorrhage, often related to anticoagulant therapy, chemotherapy, ketoconazole therapy for AIDS, or bilateral adrenalectomy. Adrenal insufficiency most often occurs in adults younger than 60 years of age and affects both genders equally.

Clinical Manifestations

Because manifestations do not tend to become evident until 90% of the adrenal cortex is destroyed, the disease is often advanced before it is diagnosed. The manifestations have a slow (insidious) onset and include anorexia, nausea, progressive weakness, fatigue, and weight loss. Increased ACTH causes the striking feature of a bronze-colored skin hyperpigmentation. It is seen mainly in sun-exposed areas of the body; at pressure points; over joints; and in the creases, especially palmar creases (Fig. 49.13). The changes in the skin are likely due to increased secretion of β-lipotropin (which contains melanocyte-stimulating hormone [MSH]). MSH is increased because of decreased negative feedback and subsequent low corticosteroid levels. Other manifestations include abdominal pain, diarrhea, headache, orthostatic hypotension, salt craving, and joint pain. Irritability and depression may occur in primary adrenal hypofunction.

Patients with secondary adrenocortical hypofunction may have many signs and symptoms similar to those of patients with Addison's disease. However, they usually do not have hyperpigmented skin because ACTH levels are low.

Complications

Patients with adrenocortical insufficiency are at risk for acute adrenal insufficiency *(Addisonian crisis).* It is a life-threatening emergency caused by insufficient adrenocortical hormones or a sudden sharp decrease in these hormones. Addisonian crisis is triggered by (1) stress (e.g., from infection, surgery, psychologic distress), (2) the sudden withdrawal of corticosteroid hormone therapy, (3) adrenal surgery, or (4) sudden pituitary gland destruction.

During acute adrenal insufficiency, the patient has severe manifestations of glucocorticoid and mineralocorticoid deficiencies. These include hypotension, tachycardia, dehydration, hyponatremia, hyperkalemia, hypoglycemia, fever, weakness, and confusion. Hypotension may lead to shock. Circulatory collapse associated with adrenal insufficiency is often unresponsive to the usual treatment (vasopressors and fluid replacement). GI manifestations include severe vomiting, diarrhea, and pain in the abdomen. Pain may occur in the lower back and legs.

Diagnostic Studies

The ACTH stimulation test is a common test to diagnose adrenal insufficiency. Baseline cortisol and ACTH levels are measured, and the patient is given an IV injection of synthetic ACTH (cosyntropin). Cortisol and ACTH levels are rechecked after 30 and 60 minutes. The normal response is a rise in blood cortisol levels. People with Addison's disease have little or no

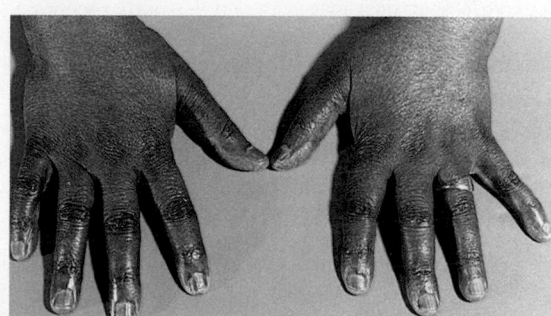

FIG. 49.13 Hyperpigmentation typically seen in Addison's disease. (From Chew SL, Leslie D: *Clinical endocrinology and diabetes: An illustrated colour text,* Edinburgh, 2006, Churchill Livingstone.)

increase in cortisol levels. Those with primary adrenal insufficiency have a high ACTH level.[22]

When the response to the ACTH test is abnormal, a corticotropin-releasing hormone (CRH) stimulation test may be done. The patient is given an IV injection of synthetic CRH, and blood is taken after 30 and 60 minutes. Those with Addison's disease have high ACTH levels but no cortisol. People with secondary adrenal insufficiency from pituitary or hypothalamus problems do not make ACTH or have a delayed response.[23]

Other abnormal laboratory findings may include hyperkalemia, hypochloremia, hyponatremia, hypoglycemia, anemia, and increased BUN levels.[23] An ECG may show low voltage and peaked T waves caused by hyperkalemia. CT scans and MRI can identify other causes, including tumors, fungal infections, tuberculosis, or adrenal calcification.

❖ Interprofessional and Nursing Care

Treatment focuses on managing the underlying cause when possible. The mainstay is often lifelong hormone therapy with glucocorticoids and mineralocorticoids (Table 49.19). Overall, patients who take their medications consistently can expect a normal life expectancy. Hydrocortisone, the most common form of hormone therapy, has both glucocorticoid and mineralocorticoid properties. Mineralocorticoids are replaced with fludrocortisone. Women need androgen replacement with dehydroepiandrosterone (DHEA) as their only source of androgen production is the adrenal glands.[23] Increased salt is added to the diet.

As a nurse, you have a key role in the long-term management of Addison's disease. The serious nature of the disease and the need for lifelong hormone therapy necessitate a comprehensive teaching plan. Table 49.20 outlines the major areas to include in a teaching plan.

Glucocorticoids are usually given in divided doses, two thirds in the morning and one third in the afternoon. Mineralocorticoids are given once daily, preferably in the morning. This schedule reflects normal circadian rhythm in endogenous hormone secretion and decreases the side effects associated with corticosteroid therapy. Teach patients using mineralocorticoid therapy (fludrocortisone) how to take their BP, increase salt intake, and report any significant changes to the HCP.

The patient with Addison's disease needs an increased dosage of corticosteroids in stressful situations to prevent Addisonian crisis. Examples of situations requiring corticosteroid adjustment are fever, influenza, tooth extraction, and rigorous physical activity, such as playing sports on a hot day or distance running. Provide written and verbal instructions on when to change the dose. Review stress management techniques. If vomiting or diarrhea occurs, as may happen with gastroenteritis, the patient should notify the HCP at once. Electrolyte replacement and parenteral administration of cortisol may be needed.

Teach patients the signs and symptoms of corticosteroid deficiency and excess (Cushing syndrome) and to report these signs to the HCP so that the drug dose can be adjusted. It is critical that the patient wear an identification bracelet (Medic Alert) and carry a wallet card saying the patient has Addison's disease so that appropriate therapy can be started in case of an emergency. The patient should always carry an emergency kit with 100 mg of IM hydrocortisone and syringes. Teach the patient and caregiver how to give an IM injection.

When the patient with Addison's disease is hospitalized, nursing management focuses on monitoring the patient while correcting fluid and electrolyte balance. Assess vital signs and neurologic status. Monitor for signs of fluid volume deficit and electrolyte imbalance. Obtain a daily weight and keep an accurate intake and output record. Take a complete medication history to determine drugs that can potentially interact with corticosteroids. These drugs include oral hypoglycemics, cardiac glycosides, oral contraceptives, anticoagulants, and NSAIDs.

Note changes in BP, weight gain, weakness, or other manifestations of Cushing syndrome. Guard the patient against exposure to infection and help with daily hygiene. Protect the patient from noise, light, and environmental temperature extremes. The patient cannot cope with these stresses because of the inability to make corticosteroids.

TABLE 49.19 Interprofessional Care
Addison's Disease

Diagnostic Assessment
- History and physical examination
- ACTH stimulation test
- Serum cortisol and ACTH
- Urine cortisol and aldosterone
- CRH suppression test
- Serum electrolytes
- CT scan, MRI

Management
- Daily glucocorticoid (e.g., prednisone, hydrocortisone) replacement (two thirds on awakening in morning, one third in late afternoon)
- Daily mineralocorticoid (fludrocortisone) in morning
- ↑ Salt in the diet
- Androgen replacement with dehydroepiandrosterone (DHEA) for women
- Salt additives for excess heat or humidity
- ↑ Doses of glucocorticoid for stress situations (e.g., surgery, hospitalization)

TABLE 49.20 Patient & Caregiver Teaching
Addison's Disease

Include the following information in the teaching plan for the patient with Addison's disease and the caregiver:

1. Names, dosages, and actions of drugs
2. Symptoms of overdosage and underdosage
3. Conditions requiring increased dosage (e.g., trauma, infection, surgery, emotional crisis)
4. Course of action to take related to changes in medication
   - Increased dose of corticosteroid
   - Self-administration of large dose of corticosteroid IM
   - Consultation with HCP
5. Preventing infection and need for prompt and vigorous treatment of existing infections
6. Need for lifelong replacement therapy
7. Need for lifelong medical supervision
8. Need to carry medical identification
9. Fall prevention
10. Adverse effects of corticosteroid therapy and prevention techniques
11. Special instruction for patients with diabetes and management of blood glucose when taking corticosteroids

Addisonian crisis is a life-threatening emergency requiring aggressive management. Treatment is directed toward shock management and high-dose hydrocortisone replacement. Large volumes of 0.9% saline solution and 5% dextrose are given to reverse hypotension and electrolyte imbalances until BP returns to normal.

CORTICOSTEROID THERAPY

Corticosteroids are effective in treating many diseases and disorders (Table 49.21). However, the long-term administration of corticosteroids at therapeutic doses often leads to serious complications and side effects (Table 49.22). For this reason, corticosteroid therapy is not recommended for minor chronic conditions. Therapy should be reserved for diseases that have a risk for death or permanent loss of function and for conditions in which short-term therapy is likely to produce remission or recovery. The potential benefits of treatment must always be weighed against the risks.

TABLE 49.21 Drug Therapy
Diseases/Disorders Treated With Corticosteroids

Hormone Therapy	Gastrointestinal Diseases
• Adrenal insufficiency	• Inflammatory bowel disease
• Congenital adrenal hyperplasia	• Celiac disease

Therapeutic Effect

Allergic Reactions	*Liver Diseases*
• Anaphylaxis	• Alcoholic hepatitis
• Bee stings	• Autoimmune hepatitis
• Contact dermatitis	
• Drug reactions	*Neurologic Diseases*
• Serum sickness	• Cerebral edema and increased
• Urticaria	intracranial pressure
	• Head trauma

Connective Tissue Diseases	*Pulmonary Diseases*
• Mixed connective tissue	• Aspiration pneumonia
disorders	• Asthma
• Polymyositis	• Chronic obstructive pulmo-
• Polyarteritis nodosa	nary disease
• Rheumatoid arthritis	
• Systemic lupus erythematosus	*Other Diseases or Disorders*
	• Skin diseases
Endocrine Diseases	• Cancer, leukemia, lymphoma
• Hypercalcemia	• Immunosuppression
• Hashimoto's thyroiditis	• Inflammation
• Thyrotoxicosis	• Nephrotic syndrome

TABLE 49.22 Drug Therapy
Effects and Side Effects of Corticosteroids

- Delayed wound healing with ↑ risk for wound dehiscence
- Fat from extremities redistributed to trunk and face
- Glucose intolerance
- Hypertension with ↑ risk for heart failure
- Hypocalcemia related to anti–vitamin D effect
- Hypokalemia
- ↑ Risk for infection
- Infection develops more rapidly and spreads more widely
- Mood and behavior changes
- Pathologic fractures, especially compression fractures of the vertebrae (osteoporosis)
- Peptic ulcer disease
- Pituitary ACTH synthesis suppressed
- Skeletal muscle atrophy and weakness
- Suppressed inflammatory response

 CHECK YOUR PRACTICE

You are working in the outpatient clinic. Your 39-yr-old female patient has Cushing syndrome from high doses of prednisone use for her severe systemic lupus erythematosus. At her office visit today, she tells you, "I looked in the mirror this morning and did not recognize the fat, ugly woman looking back at me."

- How would you respond to her?

A beneficial effect of corticosteroids in one situation may be a harmful one in another. For example, decreasing inflammation in arthritis is an important therapeutic effect, but increasing the risk for infection is a harmful effect. Suppressing inflammation and the immune response may help save lives in persons with anaphylaxis and in those receiving an organ transplant, but it can reactivate latent tuberculosis and increase the risk for infection and cancer. The vasopressive effect of corticosteroids is critical in allowing a person to function in stressful situations but can cause hypertension when used for drug therapy.

DRUG ALERT Corticosteroids
- Teach the patient not to abruptly stop these drugs.
- Monitor the patient for signs of infection.
- Have patients with diabetes closely monitor blood glucose.

Patients receive corticosteroid therapy for many reasons. Detailed instruction is needed to ensure patient adherence. When corticosteroids are used as nonreplacement therapy, they are taken once daily or once every other day. They should be taken early in the morning with food to decrease gastric irritation. Because exogenous corticosteroid use may suppress endogenous ACTH and therefore endogenous cortisol (suppression is time and dose dependent), emphasize the danger of abruptly stopping corticosteroid therapy to patients and caregivers. Corticosteroids taken for longer than 1 week will suppress adrenal production, and oral corticosteroids must be tapered. Ensure that increased doses of corticosteroids are prescribed in acute care or home care settings in situations of physical or emotional stress.

Corticosteroid-induced osteoporosis is an important concern for patients who receive corticosteroid treatment for prolonged periods (longer than 3 months).[24] Therapies to reduce bone resorption include increased calcium intake, vitamin D supplementation, bisphosphonates (e.g., alendronate), and a low-impact exercise program. Further instruction and interventions to minimize the side effects and complications of corticosteroid therapy are outlined in Table 49.23.

HYPERALDOSTERONISM

Hyperaldosteronism (Conn's syndrome) is characterized by excess aldosterone secretion. The main effects of aldosterone are (1) sodium retention and (2) potassium and hydrogen ion excretion. Thus the hallmark of this disease is hypertension with hypokalemic alkalosis. *Primary hyperaldosteronism* (PA) is most often caused by a small solitary adrenocortical adenoma. Sometimes, multiple lesions are involved and are associated with bilateral adrenal hyperplasia.

TABLE 49.23 Patient & Caregiver Teaching

Corticosteroid Therapy

Include the following instructions when teaching the patient and caregiver to manage corticosteroid therapy:

1. Follow a diet high in protein, calcium (at least 1500 mg/day), and potassium and low in fat and concentrated simple carbohydrates, such as sugar, syrups, and candy.
2. Ensure adequate rest and sleep, such as daily naps and avoiding caffeine late in the day.
3. Take part in an exercise program to help maintain bone integrity.
4. Recognize edema and ways to restrict sodium intake to <2000 mg/day if edema occurs.
5. Monitor glucose levels and recognize symptoms of hyperglycemia (e.g., polydipsia, polyuria, blurred vision). Report hyperglycemic symptoms or capillary glucose levels >120 mg/dL (10 mmol/L).
6. Notify HCP if heartburn after meals or epigastric pain that is not relieved by antacids occurs.
7. See an eye specialist yearly to assess for cataracts.
8. Use safety measures, such as getting up slowly from bed or a chair and good lighting, to avoid accidental injury.
9. Maintain appropriate hygiene practices.
10. Avoid contact with persons with colds or other contagious illnesses to prevent infection.
11. Inform all HCPs about long-term corticosteroid use.
12. Recognize need for ↑ doses of corticosteroids in times of physical and emotional stress.
13. Never abruptly stop the corticosteroids because this could lead to Addisonian crisis and death.

PA affects women more than men and usually occurs between 30 and 50 years of age. A genetic link has been found in some patients.[25] PA causes up to 2% of all cases of hypertension. *Secondary hyperaldosteronism* occurs in response to a nonadrenal cause of increased aldosterone levels, such as renal artery stenosis, renin-secreting tumors, and chronic kidney disease.

Increased aldosterone levels are associated with sodium retention and potassium excretion. Sodium retention leads to hypernatremia, hypertension, and headache. Edema does not usually occur because the rate of sodium excretion increases, preventing more severe sodium retention. Potassium wasting leads to hypokalemia, which causes generalized muscle weakness, fatigue, dysrhythmias, glucose intolerance, and metabolic alkalosis that may lead to tetany.

Hyperaldosteronism should be suspected in hypertensive patients with hypokalemia who are not being treated with diuretics. PA is associated with increased plasma aldosterone levels, increased sodium levels, decreased serum potassium levels, and decreased plasma renin activity. A CT scan or MRI can detect an adenoma.[25] If a tumor is not found, plasma 18-hydroxycorticosterone is measured after overnight bed rest. A level greater than 50 ng/dL indicates an adenoma.

❖ Interprofessional and Nursing Care

The preferred treatment for PA is surgical removal of the adenoma (adrenalectomy). A laparoscopic approach is most often used. Before surgery, patients should be treated with potassium-sparing diuretics (e.g., spironolactone, eplerenone [Inspra]) and antihypertensive agents to normalize serum potassium levels and BP. Spironolactone and eplerenone block the binding of aldosterone to the mineralocorticoid receptor in the terminal distal tubules and collecting ducts of the kidney, thus increasing

sodium and water excretion and potassium retention. Oral potassium supplements and sodium restrictions may be needed. However, potassium supplementation and a potassium-sparing diuretic should not be started simultaneously because of the risk for hyperkalemia. Teach patients taking eplerenone to avoid grapefruit juice as it may increase potential for hyperkalemia.

Patients with bilateral adrenal hyperplasia are treated with a potassium-sparing diuretic. Calcium channel blockers may be used to control BP. Dexamethasone may be used to decrease adrenal hyperplasia.

Nursing care includes careful assessment of fluid and electrolyte balance (especially potassium) and cardiovascular status. Monitor BP frequently before and after surgery because unilateral adrenalectomy is successful in controlling hypertension in only 80% of patients with an adenoma. Tell patients receiving spironolactone about the possible side effects of gynecomastia, impotence, and menstrual disorders, as well as the signs and symptoms of hypokalemia and hyperkalemia. Teach patients how to monitor their own BP and the need for frequent monitoring. Stress the need for continued health supervision.

DISORDERS OF ADRENAL MEDULLA

PHEOCHROMOCYTOMA

Pheochromocytoma is a rare condition caused by a tumor in the adrenal medulla. It affects the chromaffin cells, resulting in an excess production of catecholamines (epinephrine, norepinephrine). The most dangerous immediate effect of the disease is severe hypertension. If left untreated, it may lead to encephalopathy, diabetes, cardiomyopathy, multiple organ failure, and death. It most often occurs in young to middle-aged adults. Pheochromocytoma may be inherited in persons with MEN.[26]

The most striking findings are severe, episodic hypertension accompanied by severe, pounding headache; tachycardia with palpitations; profuse sweating; and unexplained abdominal or chest pain. Attacks can be induced by direct trauma, mechanical pressure to the tumor, stress (e.g., surgery, exercise, defecation, sexual intercourse, alcohol consumption, smoking), or many drugs, including antihypertensives, opioids, radiologic contrast media, and tricyclic antidepressants. Attacks can last from a few minutes to several hours.

The simplest and most reliable diagnostic test is measurement of urinary fractionated metanephrines (catecholamine metabolites) and fractionated catecholamines and creatinine, usually done as a 24-hour urine collection. Values are increased in at least 95% of persons with pheochromocytoma. Serum catecholamines may be increased during an "attack." CT scans and MRI can detect tumors. Do not palpate the abdomen of a patient with suspected pheochromocytoma. It may cause the sudden release of catecholamines and severe hypertension.

❖ Interprofessional and Nursing Care

The main treatment is surgical removal of the tumor. Treatment with α- and β-adrenergic receptor blockers is required before surgery to control BP and prevent an intraoperative hypertensive crisis. Therapy begins with an α-adrenergic receptor blocker (e.g., doxazosin, prazosin, phenoxybenzamine) 10 to 14 days before surgery to reduce BP.[26] After adequate α-adrenergic blockade, β-adrenergic receptor blockers (e.g., propranolol) are used to decrease tachycardia and dysrhythmias. If β-blockers are started too early, unopposed α-adrenergic stimulation can precipitate a hypertensive crisis. Therapy can cause orthostatic hypotension. Teach the patient to make postural changes cautiously.

Surgery is usually done using a laparoscopic approach. Removing the adrenal tumor often cures the hypertension, but hypertension persists in about 10% to 30% of patients. If surgery is not an option, metyrosine (Demser) can decrease catecholamine production by the tumor.

Case finding is an important nursing role. Although pheochromocytoma is associated with several symptoms, the diagnosis is often missed. Any patient with hypertension accompanied by symptoms of sympathoadrenal stimulation should be referred to an HCP for definitive diagnosis. Assess the patient for the classic triad of symptoms of pheochromocytoma: severe pounding headache, tachycardia, and profuse sweating. Monitor the BP often if the patient is having an "attack."

Make the patient as comfortable as possible. Monitor blood glucose levels to assess for diabetes. Patients need rest, nourishing food, and emotional support during this period. Surgical care is similar to that for any patient undergoing adrenalectomy. Note that BP fluctuations from catecholamine excesses tend to be severe and must be carefully monitored. Emphasize the importance of follow-up and routine BP monitoring because hypertension may persist even when the tumor is removed.

CASE STUDY

Graves' Disease

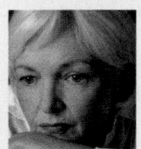

(© Hemera Technologies/ AbleStock.com/ Thinkstock.)

Patient Profile

R.D., a 52-yr-old white woman, was admitted to the hospital with a high fever. Unable to find a source of infection, the HCP does an endocrine workup. R.D. is diagnosed with Graves' disease.

Subjective Data

- Reports recent job loss because she is no longer able to tolerate work-related stress
- Reports symptoms including fatigue, unintentional weight loss, insomnia, palpitations, vision problems, and heat intolerance

Objective Data

Physical Examination

- Fever of 104° F (40° C)
- BP of 150/80 mm Hg, pulse of 116 beats/min, and respiratory rate of 26 breaths/min
- Hot, moist skin
- Fine tremors of the hands
- 4+ deep tendon reflexes and muscle strength of 1 to 2 out of 5

Interprofessional Care

- Subtotal thyroidectomy planned for 2 months later
- Started on methimazole (Tapazole) and propranolol (Inderal LA)

Discussion Questions

1. Explain the cause of R.D.'s symptoms.
2. What diagnostic studies were probably ordered? What would the results have been to establish the diagnosis of Graves' disease?
3. Why was surgery delayed?
4. **Collaboration:** What is the interprofessional team's top priority at this time for R.D.?
5. **Quality Care:** What is the expected outcome associated with drug therapy?
6. **Priority Decision:** What are her priority teaching needs at this time?
7. **Patient-Centered Care:** What teaching will you provide after surgery so that R.D. can successfully self-manage her care?
8. **Priority Decision:** Based on the assessment data presented, what are the priority nursing diagnoses pertinent to this patient while hospitalized? Are there any collaborative problems?
9. **Evidence-Based Practice:** Why is R.D. counseled to give up her long-standing cigarette smoking habit?

Answers available at *http://evolve.elsevier.com/Lewis/medsurg.*

BRIDGE TO NCLEX EXAMINATION

The number of the question corresponds to the same-numbered outcome at the beginning of the chapter.

1. After a hypophysectomy for acromegaly, immediate postoperative nursing care should focus on
   a. frequent monitoring of serum and urine osmolarity.
   b. parenteral administration of a GH-receptor antagonist.
   c. keeping the patient in a recumbent position at all times.
   d. patient teaching about the need for lifelong hormone therapy.

2. A patient with a head injury develops SIADH. Manifestations the nurse would expect to find include
   a. hypernatremia and edema.
   b. muscle spasticity and hypertension.
   c. low urine output and hyponatremia.
   d. weight gain and decreased glomerular filtration rate.

3. The health care provider prescribes levothyroxine for a patient with hypothyroidism. After teaching about this drug, the nurse determines that further instruction is needed when the patient says
   a. "I can expect the medication dose may need to be adjusted."
   b. "I only need to take this drug until my symptoms are improved."
   c. "I can expect to return to normal function with the use of this drug."
   d. "I will report any chest pain or difficulty breathing to the doctor right away."

4. After thyroid surgery, the nurse suspects damage or removal of the parathyroid glands when the patient develops
   a. muscle weakness and weight loss.
   b. hyperthermia and severe tachycardia.
   c. hypertension and difficulty swallowing.
   d. laryngospasms and tingling in the hands and feet.

5. Important nursing intervention(s) when caring for a patient with Cushing syndrome include (*select all that apply*)
   a. restricting protein intake.
   b. monitoring blood glucose levels.
   c. observing for signs of hypotension.
   d. administering medication in equal doses.
   e. protecting patient from exposure to infection.

6. An important preoperative nursing intervention before an adrenalectomy for hyperaldosteronism is to
   a. monitor blood glucose levels.
   b. restrict fluid and sodium intake.
   c. administer potassium-sparing diuretics.
   d. advise the patient to make postural changes slowly.

7. To control the side effects of corticosteroid therapy, the nurse teaches the patient who is taking corticosteroids to
   a. increase calcium intake to 1500 mg/day.
   b. perform glucose monitoring for hypoglycemia.
   c. obtain immunizations due to high risk for infections.
   d. avoid abrupt position changes because of orthostatic hypotension.

1. a, 2. c, 3. b, 4. d, 5. b, e, 6. c, 7. a

For rationales to these answers and even more NCLEX review questions, visit *http://evolve.elsevier.com/Lewis/medsurg*.

EVOLVE WEBSITE/RESOURCES LIST

REFERENCES

1. American Cancer Society: About pituitary tumors. Retrieved from *www.cancer.org/cancer/pituitary-tumors/about/what-is-pituitary-tumor.html*.
2. National Institute of Diabetes and Digestive, and Kidney Diseases: Acromegaly. Retrieved from *www.niddk.nih.gov/health-information/health-topics/endocrine/acromegaly/Pages/fact-sheet.aspx*.
3. Pituitary Network Association: About acromegaly. Retrieved from *http://acromegaly.org/en/about/about-acromegaly*.
*4. Buchfelder M, Schlaffer SM: The surgical treatment of acromegaly, *Pituitary* 20:1, 2017.
*5. Auriemma RS, Grasso LS, Pivonello R, et al: The safety of treatments for prolactinomas, *Opin Drug Saf* 15:4, 2016.
*6. Molitch ME: Diagnosis and treatment of pituitary adenomas: A review, *JAMA* 317:5, 2017.
*7. Prete A, Corsello SM, Salvatori R. Current best practice in the management of patients after pituitary surgery, *Ther Adv Endocrinol Metab* 8:3, 2017.
8. Braun MM, Mahowald M, Electrolytes: Sodium disorders, *FP Essent* 459:11, 2017.
9. Vanderpump MP: Epidemiology of iodine deficiency, *Minerva Med* 108:2, 2017.
10. Dunn D, Turner C: Hypothyroidism in women, *Nurs Womens Health* 20:1, 2016.
*11. Salman F, Oktaei H, Solomon S, et al: Recurrent Graves' hyperthyroidism after prolonged radioiodine-induced hypothyroidism, *Ther Adv Endocrinol Metab* 8:7, 2017.
12. Ross DS, Burch HB, Cooper DS, et al: 2016 American Thyroid Association guidelines for diagnosis and management of hyperthyroidism and other causes of thyrotoxicosis, *Thyroid* 26:10, 2016.
*13. Caulley L, Johnson-Obaseki S, Luo L, et al: Risk factors for postoperative complications in total thyroidectomy: A retrospective, risk-adjusted analysis from the National Surgical Quality Improvement Program, *Medicine* 96:5, 2017.
14. Chaker L, Bianco AC, Jonklaas J, et al: Hypothyroidism, *Lancet* 390:10101, 2017.
*15. Kumar E, McCurdy MT, Koch CA, et al: Impairment of thyroid function in critically ill patients in the intensive care units, *Am J Med Sci* 355:3, 2018.
*16. Hennessey JV, Garber JR, Woeber KA, et al: American Association of Clinical Endocrinologists and American College of Endocrinology position statement on thyroid dysfunction, *Endocr Pract* 22:84, 2016.
17. Bibbins-Domingo K, Grossman DC, Curry SJ, et al: Screening for thyroid cancer: US Preventive Services Task Force recommendation statement, *JAMA* 317:18, 2017.
18. National Institutes of Health: Multiple endocrine neoplasia. Retrieved from *https://ghr.nlm.nih.gov/condition/multiple-endocrine-neoplasia*.
19. Markowitz ME, Underland L, Gensure R: Parathyroid disorders, *Pediatr Rev* 37:12, 2016.
*20. Sharma ST: An individualized approach to the evaluation of Cushing syndrome, *Endocr Pract* 23:6, 2017.
*21. Lonser RR, Nieman L, Oldfield EH: Cushing's disease: Pathobiology, diagnosis, and management, *J Neurosurg* 126:404, 2017.
22. Munir S, Waseem M: Addison disease, *StatPearls*, 2018. Retrieved from *www.statpearls.com/as/endocrine%20and%20metabolic/17183/*.
23. National Institute of Diabetes and Digestive and Kidney Diseases: Addison's disease. Retrieved from *www.niddk.nih.gov/health-information/health-topics/endocrine/adrenal-insufficiency-addisons-disease/Pages/fact-sheet.aspx*.
24. Arthritis Foundation: Treating corticosteroid-induced bone loss. Retrieved from *www.arthritis.org/living-with-arthritis/treatments/medication/drug-types/corticosteroids/osteoporosis-bone-loss.php*.
25. Gyamlani G, Headley CM, Naseer A, et al: Primary aldosteronism: Diagnosis and management, *Am J Med Sci* 352:4, 2016.
26. Azadeh N, Ramakrishna H, Bhatia NL, et al: Therapeutic goals in patients with pheochromocytoma: A guide to perioperative management, *Ir J Med Sci* 185:1, 2016.

*Evidence-based information for clinical practice.

50

Assessment: Reproductive System

Kim K. Choma

Be a rainbow in someone else's cloud.

Maya Angelou

http://evolve.elsevier.com/Lewis/medsurg

CONCEPTUAL FOCUS

Hormonal Regulation   Sexuality
Reproduction

LEARNING OUTCOMES

1. Describe the structures and functions of the male and female reproductive systems.
2. Outline the functions of the major hormones essential for the functioning of the male and female reproductive systems.
3. Explain the physiologic changes during the stages of sexual response for both a man and a woman.
4. Link the age-related changes of the male and female reproductive systems to the differences in assessment findings.

5. Obtain significant subjective and objective data related to the male and female reproductive systems and information about sexual function from a patient.
6. Perform a physical assessment of the male and female reproductive systems using the appropriate techniques.
7. Distinguish normal from common abnormal findings of a physical assessment of the male and female reproductive systems.
8. Describe the purpose, significance of results, and nursing responsibilities related to diagnostic studies of the male and female reproductive systems.

KEY TERMS

amenorrhea, p. 1177   gonads, p. 1171   spermatogenesis, p. 1171
ductus deferens, p. 1172   menarche, p. 1176   testosterone, p. 1176
dyspareunia, p. 1181   menopause, p. 1177   uterus, p. 1173
epididymis, p. 1172   menstrual cycle, p. 1176   vulva, p. 1174
estrogen, p. 1175   progesterone, p. 1175

STRUCTURES AND FUNCTIONS OF MALE AND FEMALE REPRODUCTIVE SYSTEMS

The reproductive systems of males and females consist of primary (or essential) organs and secondary (or accessory) organs. The primary reproductive organs are referred to as gonads. The female gonads are the ovaries. The male gonads are the testes. The main purpose of the gonads is secretion of hormones and production of gametes (ova and sperm, sex cells that unite during fertilization to form a new cell called a *zygote*). Secondary (or accessory) organs begin their maturity at puberty under the influence of sex hormones. They are responsible for (1) transporting and nourishing the ova (eggs) and sperm and (2) preserving and protecting the fertilized ova.

Male Reproductive System

The 3 main roles of the male reproductive system are (1) sperm production and transportation, (2) deposition of sperm in the female reproductive tract, and (3) hormone secretion. The

primary male reproductive organs are the testes. Secondary reproductive organs include ducts (epididymis, ductus deferens, ejaculatory duct, urethra), sex glands (prostate gland, Cowper's glands, seminal vesicles), and the external genitalia (scrotum, penis) (Fig. 50.1).

Testes. The paired testes are ovoid, smooth, firm organs. They measure 1.4 to 2.2 in (3.5 to 5.6 cm) long and 0.8 to 1.2 in (2 to 3 cm) wide. They lie within the scrotum. It is a loose protective sac composed of a thin outer layer of skin over a tough connective tissue layer. Within the testes, coiled structures called the semi-niferous tubules form *spermatozoa* (immature sperm). The process of sperm production is called spermatogenesis. Interstitial cells lie between the seminiferous tubules. These cells make the male sex hormone testosterone.

Ducts. Sperm formed in the seminiferous tubules move through a series of ducts. These ducts transport sperm from the testes to the outside of the body. As sperm exit the testes, they enter and pass through the epididymis, ductus deferens, ejaculatory duct, and urethra.

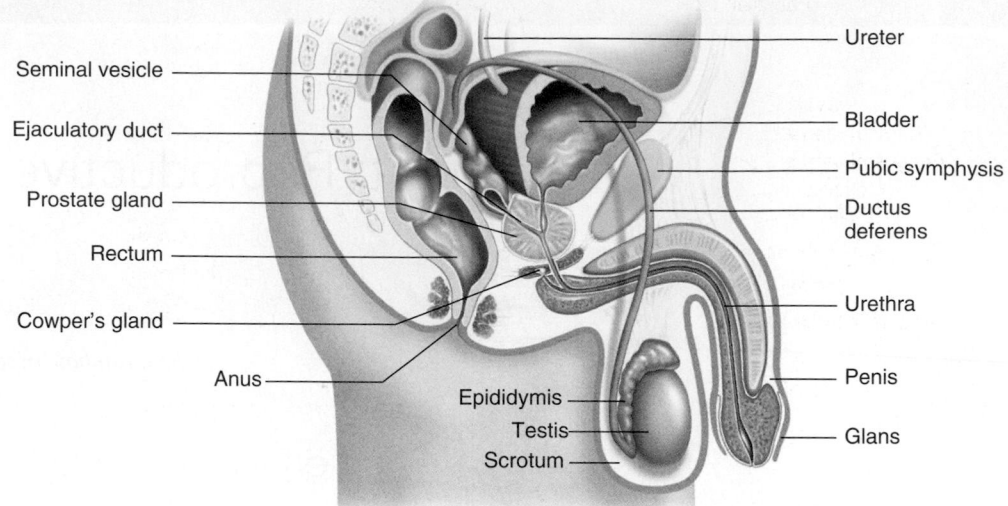

FIG 50.1 Male reproductive tract. (Modified from Patton KT, Thibodeau GA: *Anatomy and physiology*, ed 8, St Louis, 2013, Mosby.)

The **epididymis** is a comma-shaped structure found on the posterosuperior aspect of each testis within the scrotum (Figs. 50.1 and 50.2). It is a long, tightly coiled structure that measures, uncoiled, about 20 ft in length.[1] The epididymis transports sperm as they mature. Sperm exit the epididymis through a long, thick tube called the **ductus deferens**.

The ductus deferens (also called the *vas deferens*) is continuous with the epididymis within the scrotal sac. It travels upward through the scrotum and continues through the inguinal ring into the abdominal cavity. The spermatic cord is composed of a connective tissue sheath that encloses the ductus deferens, arteries, veins, nerves, and lymph vessels as it ascends through the inguinal canal (Fig. 50.2). In the abdominal cavity, the ductus deferens travels up, over, and behind the bladder. Behind the bladder the ductus deferens joins the seminal vesicle to form the ejaculatory duct (Fig. 50.1).

The ejaculatory duct passes downward through the prostate gland, connecting with the urethra. The urethra extends from the bladder, through the prostate, and ends in a slit-like opening (the meatus) on the ventral side of the *glans,* the tip of the penis. During the process of ejaculation, sperm travel through the urethra and out of the penis.

Glands. The seminal vesicles, prostate gland, and Cowper's (bulbourethral) glands are the accessory glands. These glands make and secrete seminal fluid *(semen),* which surrounds the sperm and forms the *ejaculate.* The ejaculate fluid serves as a medium for the transport of sperm and creates an alkaline, nutritious environment that promotes sperm motility and survival.

The seminal vesicles lie behind the bladder, between the bladder and rectum. The ducts of the seminal vesicles fuse with the ductus deferens to form the ejaculatory ducts that enter the prostate gland. The prostate gland lies beneath the bladder. Its posterior surface is in contact with the rectal wall. The prostate normally measures 0.8 in (2 cm) wide and 1.2 in (3 cm) long. It is divided into right and left lateral lobes and an anteroposterior median lobe. Cowper's glands lie on each side of the urethra and slightly posterior to it, just below the prostate. The ducts of these glands enter directly into the urethra.

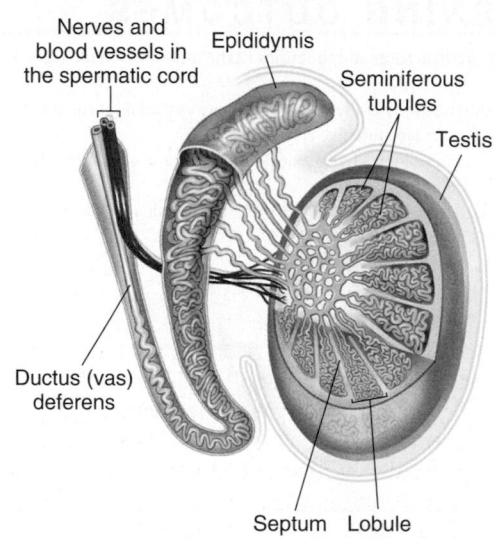

FIG 50.2 Seminiferous tubules, testis, epididymis, and ductus (vas) deferens in the male. (Modified from Patton KT, Thibodeau GA: *Anatomy and physiology*, ed 8, St Louis, 2013, Mosby.)

External Genitalia. The male external genitalia consist of the penis and scrotum. The penis consists of a shaft and tip, which is called the *glans.* The glans is covered by a fold of skin, the prepuce (or foreskin), that forms at the junction of the glans and shaft of the penis. In circumcised males the prepuce has been removed. The shaft consists of erectile tissue composed of the corpus cavernosum, corpus spongiosum (fibrous sheath that encases the erectile tissue), and urethra. The skin covering the penis is thin, loose, and hairless.

Female Reproductive System

The 3 main roles of the female reproductive system are (1) ova production, (2) hormone secretion, and (3) protect and facilitate the development of the fetus in a pregnant female. Like the male, the female has primary and secondary reproductive organs. The primary reproductive organs in the female are the

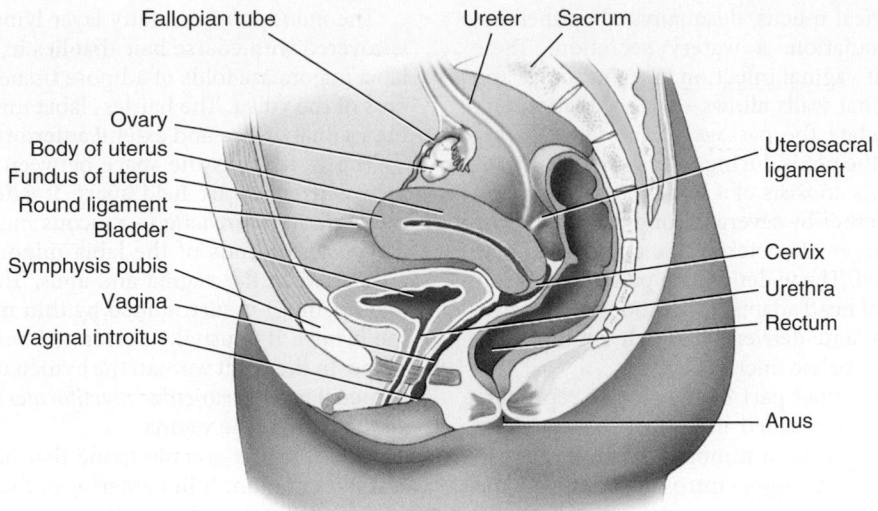

FIG 50.3 Female reproductive tract. (Modified from McKenry L, Tessier E, Hogan M: *Mosby's pharmacology in nursing*, St Louis, 2006, Mosby.)

paired ovaries. Secondary reproductive organs include the ducts (fallopian tubes), uterus, vagina, sex glands (Bartholin's glands, breasts), and external genitalia (vulva).

Pelvic Organs

Ovaries. The ovaries are found on either side of the uterus, just behind and below the fallopian tubes (Fig. 50.3). The almond-shaped ovaries are firm and solid, around 0.6 in (1.5 cm) wide and 1.2 in (3 cm) long. Their functions include ovulation and secretion of the 2 major reproductive hormones: estrogen and progesterone.

The outer zone of the ovary has follicles with germ cells, or *oocytes.* Each follicle contains a primordial (immature) oocyte surrounded by granulosa and theca cells. These 2 layers protect and nourish the oocyte until the follicle reaches maturity and ovulation occurs. However, not all follicles reach maturity. In a process termed *atresia,* most of the immature follicles become smaller and are reabsorbed by the body. Thus the number of follicles declines from 1 million at birth to about 400,000 at *menarche* (first menstruation). This is the female's lifetime supply of sex cells. In contrast, males make spermatocytes throughout their reproductive life cycle. As a woman ages, both the number and quality of the oocytes decline. Fewer than 500 oocytes are actually released by ovulation during the reproductive years of the normal healthy woman.[2]

Fallopian Tubes. The fallopian tubes transport the ovum toward the uterus, facilitating fertilization or implantation. The tubes are uterine appendages that end by curling around the ovary. The distal ends of the fallopian tubes consist of fingerlike projections called *fimbriae.* They sweep the ovum from the ruptured ovarian follicle (ovulation) into the fallopian tube. The tubes, which average 4.8 in (12 cm) in length, extend from the fimbriae to the superior lateral borders of the uterus.

Normally, each month during a woman's reproductive years, 1 ovarian follicle reaches maturity. That ovum is ovulated, or expelled, from the ovary through the stimulus of the gonadotropic hormones: follicle-stimulating hormone (FSH) and luteinizing hormone (LH). The ovum then travels through a fallopian tube, where fertilization by sperm may occur (if sperm are present). Fertilization usually takes place within the outer one third of the fallopian tubes. An ovum can be fertilized up to 72 hours after its release.

Uterus. The uterus is a pear-shaped, hollow, muscular organ found between the bladder and rectum (Fig. 50.3). In the mature *nulliparous* (never pregnant) woman, the uterus is about 2.4 to 3.2 in (6 to 8 cm) long and 1.6 in (4 cm) wide. The uterine walls consist of an outer serosal layer, the *perimetrium;* a middle muscular layer, the *myometrium;* and an inner mucosal layer, the *endometrium.*

The uterus consists of the fundus, body (or corpus), and cervix (Fig. 50.3). The body makes up about 80% of the uterus. It connects with the cervix at the isthmus, or neck. The cervix is the lower part of the uterus. It projects into the anterior wall of the vaginal canal. It makes up about 15% to 20% of the uterus in the nulliparous female. The cervix consists of the *ectocervix,* the outer part that protrudes into the vagina, and the *endocervix,* the canal in the opening of the cervix. The opening of the cervix is the *cervical os* (Fig. 50.4).

The ectocervix is covered with squamous epithelial cells. This gives it a smooth, pinkish appearance. The endocervix is lined with columnar epithelial cells, which give it a rough, reddened appearance. The junction at which the 2 types of epithelial cells (squamous and columnar) meet is the *squamocolumnar junction* (Fig. 50.4). Cells sampled from the squamocolumnar junction are examined as part of a Papanicolaou (Pap) test, which is a critical part of cervical cancer screening.

The cervical canal is 0.8 to 1.6 in (2 to 4 cm) long. It is relatively tightly closed. However, menses can be expelled and sperm can enter the uterus through the cervical os. The entrance of sperm into the uterus is facilitated by mucus made by the cervix under the influence of estrogen. Under normal conditions, the cervical mucus becomes watery, stretchy, and more abundant at ovulation. The postovulatory cervical mucus, under the influence of progesterone, is thick and inhibits sperm passage. The cervix can stretch to allow passage of a fetus during the birth process. The columnar epithelium, under hormonal influence, provides elasticity during labor.

Vagina. The vagina is a tubular structure 3 to 4 in (7.6 to 10 cm) long. The anterior vaginal wall lies along the urethra and bladder. The posterior vaginal wall is next to the rectum. It is lined with squamous epithelium. In reproductive-age women, the vagina has multiple transverse folds called *rugae.* Vaginal secretions consist of cervical mucus, desquamated epithelium, and, during sexual stimulation, a watery secretion. These fluids help protect against vaginal infection. The muscular and erectile tissue of the vaginal walls allows enough dilation and contraction to accommodate the passage of the fetus during labor and penetration of the penis during intercourse.

Pelvis. The female pelvis consists of 4 bones (2 pelvic bones, sacrum, coccyx) held together by several strong ligaments. The pelvis in females has a larger diameter and is circular. A male pelvis is more heart shaped. The wider female pelvis plays a key role in childbirth. The fetal head adapts its position to the pelvic dimensions during labor and delivery through rotation and flexion to pass through the pelvic inlet.[1]

External Genitalia. The external part of the female reproductive system (Fig. 50.5) is often called the vulva. It consists of the mons pubis, labia majora, labia minora, vestibule, clitoris, urethral meatus, Skene's glands, vaginal introitus (opening), and Bartholin's glands.

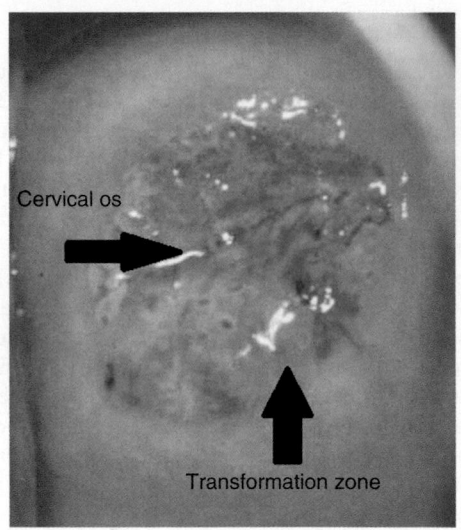

FIG 50.4 Cervical os and squamocolumnar junction (transformation zone). (Courtesy Candy Tedschi, NP, Great Neck, NY.)

The *mons pubis* is a fatty layer lying over the pubic bone. It is covered with coarse hair that lies in a triangular pattern. The labia majora are folds of adipose tissue that form the outer borders of the vulva. The hairless labia minora form the borders of the vaginal orifice and extend anteriorly to enclose the clitoris.

The *vestibule* is the space between the labia minora that is seen when they are held apart. It extends from the clitoris to the *posterior fourchette* (a mucous membrane band that forms the posterior ends of the labia minora). The perineum is the area between the vagina and anus. The vaginal introitus (vaginal opening) is surrounded by thin membranous tissue called the *hymen*. It is usually perforated and has many variations in shape. In the adult woman the hymen usually appears as folds or hymenal tags *(carunculae myrtiformes)*. It separates the external genitalia from the vagina.

The *clitoris* is erectile tissue that becomes engorged during sexual excitation. It lies anterior to the urethral meatus and the vaginal orifice and is usually covered by the prepuce. Clitoral stimulation is an important part of sexual activity for many women.

Ducts of the Skene's glands lie alongside the urinary meatus and correspond to the prostate gland in males. We think they help lubricate the urinary meatus. The Bartholin's glands are found at the posterior and lateral aspects of the vaginal orifice. They secrete a thin, mucoid material we think contributes slightly to lubrication during sexual intercourse. These glands are not usually palpable unless sebaceous-like cysts form or they are swollen from an infection, such as a sexually transmitted infection (STI). Bartholin's glands correspond to Cowper's glands in males.

Breasts. The breasts are a secondary sex characteristic that develops during puberty in response to estrogen and progesterone. Cyclic hormonal changes lead to regular changes in breast tissue to prepare it for lactation when fertilization and pregnancy occur.

The breasts extend from the second to the sixth ribs. The extension of breast tissue into the upper-outer quadrant into the axilla is an area referred to as the *tail of Spence* (Fig. 50.6). The fully mature breast is dome shaped and has a pigmented center called the *areola*. The areolar region contains Montgomery's

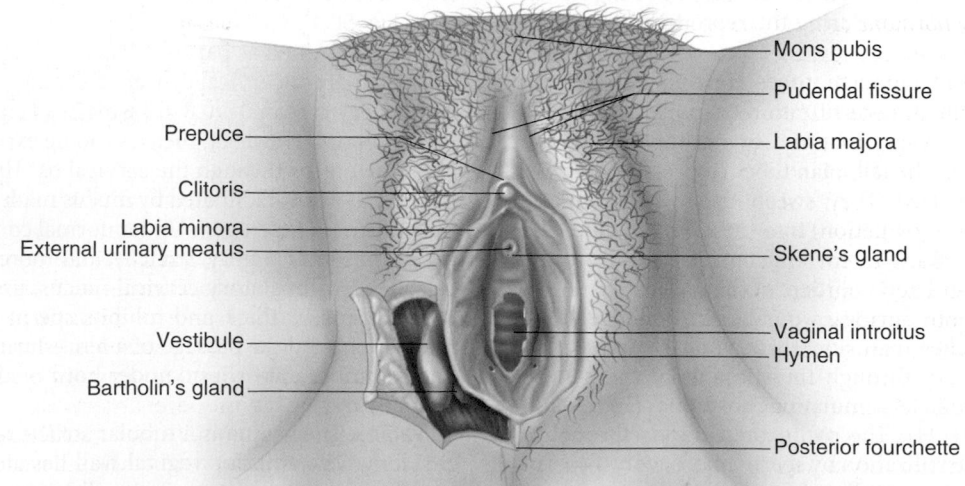

FIG 50.5 External female genitalia. (Modified from Patton KT, Thibodeau GA: *Anatomy and physiology,* ed 8, St Louis, 2013, Mosby.)

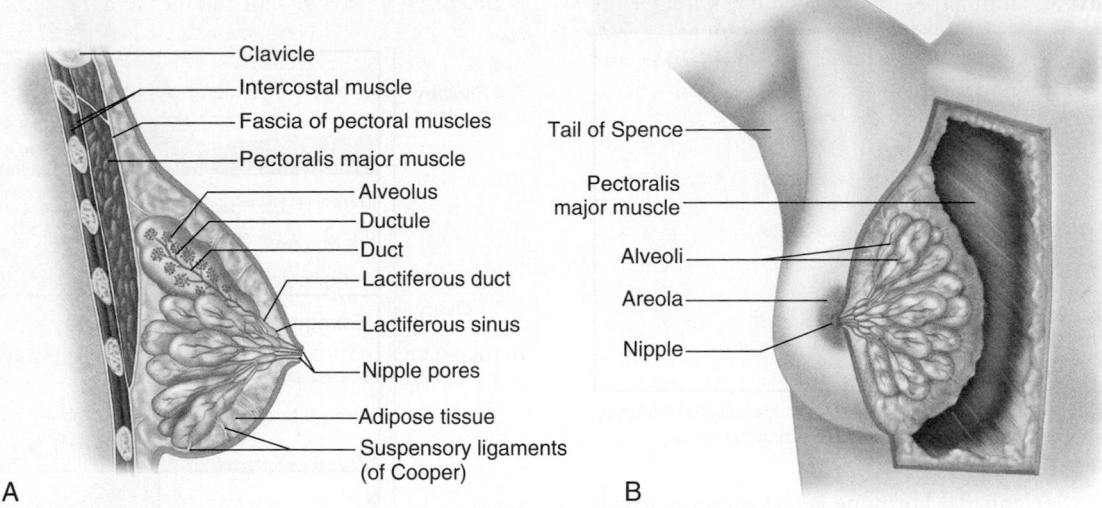

FIG 50.6 The lactating female breast. **A,** Glandular structures are anchored to the overlying skin and the pectoralis muscle by suspensory ligaments of Cooper. Each lobule of glandular tissue is drained by a lactiferous duct that eventually opens through the nipple. **B,** Anterior view of a lactating breast. In nonlactating breasts, glandular tissue is less evident, with adipose tissue making up most of the breast. (Modified from Patton KT, Thibodeau GA: *Anatomy and physiology*, ed 8, St Louis, 2013, Mosby.)

tubercles, which are similar to sebaceous glands. They help lubricate the nipple. During lactation, the alveoli secrete milk. The milk then flows into a ductal system and is transported to the lactiferous sinuses. The nipple has 15 to 20 tiny openings through which the milk flows during breastfeeding. The fibrous and fatty tissue that supports and separates the channels of the mammary duct system is primarily responsible for the varying sizes and shapes of the breasts.

Neuroendocrine Regulation of Reproductive System

The hypothalamus, pituitary gland, and gonads secrete several hormones (Fig. 50.7). (Endocrine hormones are discussed in Chapter 47.) These hormones regulate the processes of ovulation, sperm formation, and fertilization and the formation and function of the secondary sex characteristics. The hypothalamus secretes gonadotropin-releasing hormone (GnRH), which stimulates the anterior pituitary gland to secrete its hormones, including FSH and LH. LH in males is sometimes called *interstitial cell–stimulating hormone (ICSH)*. The gonadal hormones are estrogen, progesterone, and testosterone.

In women, FSH production stimulates the growth and maturity of the ovarian follicles necessary for ovulation. The mature follicle makes estrogen, which in turn suppresses the release of FSH. Another hormone, inhibin, is also secreted by the ovarian follicle. It inhibits both GnRH and FSH secretion. In men, FSH stimulates the seminiferous tubules to make sperm.

LH contributes to the ovulatory process. It causes follicles to complete maturation and undergo ovulation. It affects the development of a ruptured follicle (area where ovum exited during ovulation), which turns into a corpus luteum, which secretes progesterone. **Progesterone** plays a major role in the menstrual cycle, specifically in the secretory phase. It maintains the rich vascular state of the uterus (secretory phase) in preparation for fertilization and implantation. Adequate progesterone is necessary to maintain an implanted ovum. Like estrogen, progesterone is involved in the bodily changes associated with pregnancy. In men, LH triggers testosterone production by the

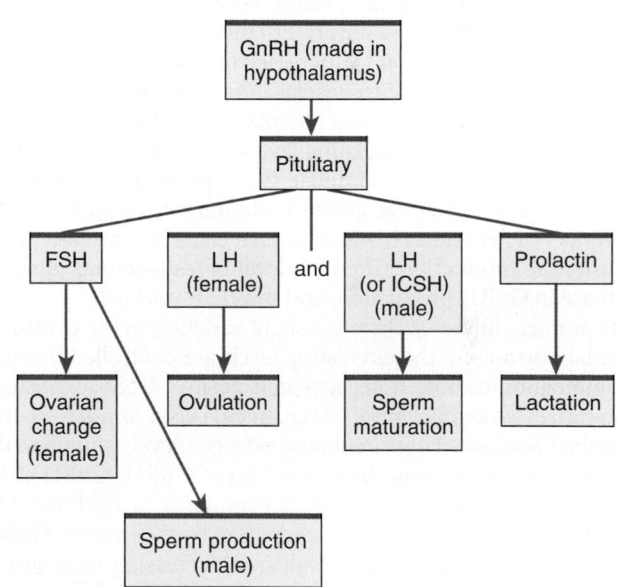

FIG 50.7 Hypothalamic-pituitary-gonadal axis. Only the major pituitary hormone actions are depicted. *FSH,* Follicle-stimulating hormone; *GnRH,* gonadotropin-releasing hormone; *ICSH,* interstitial cell–stimulating hormone; *LH,* luteinizing hormone.

interstitial cells of the testes and thus is essential for the full maturation of sperm.

In women, prolactin stimulates the development and growth of the mammary glands. During lactation, it initiates and maintains milk production. In men, prolactin has no known function.

In women the gonadal hormones, estrogen and progesterone, are made by the ovaries. Small amounts of an estrogen precursor are also made in the adrenal cortices. **Estrogen** is essential to the development and maintenance of the secondary sex characteristics, proliferative phase of the menstrual cycle immediately after menstruation, and uterine changes essential to pregnancy. In men, most estrogen is made in the adrenal cortices. We do not understand the role and importance of estrogen in men.

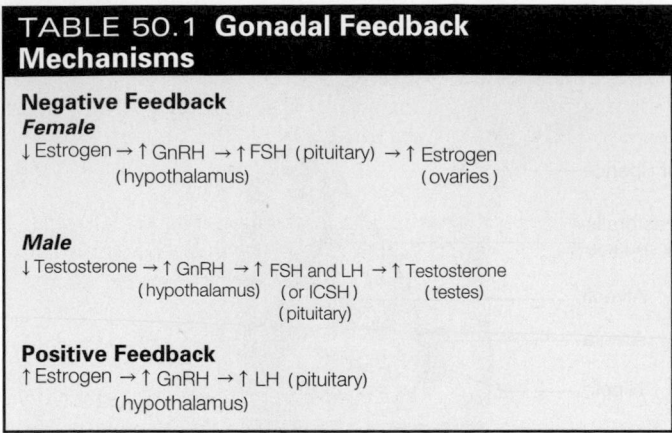

TABLE 50.1 Gonadal Feedback Mechanisms

Negative Feedback

Female

↓ Estrogen → ↑ GnRH → ↑ FSH (pituitary) → ↑ Estrogen
        (hypothalamus)   (ovaries)

Male

↓ Testosterone → ↑ GnRH → ↑ FSH and LH → ↑ Testosterone
           (hypothalamus)   (or ICSH)   (testes)
                             (pituitary)

Positive Feedback

↑ Estrogen → ↑ GnRH → ↑ LH (pituitary)
         (hypothalamus)

FSH, Follicle-stimulating hormone; *GnRH,* gonadotropin-releasing hormone; *ICSH,* interstitial cell–stimulating hormone; *LH,* luteinizing hormone.

In men, the major gonadal hormone is testosterone, which is made by the testes. Testosterone is responsible for the development and maintenance of secondary sex characteristics and adequate spermatogenesis. In women, the adrenal glands and ovaries make small amounts of androgens.

The circulating levels of gonadal hormones are controlled primarily by a *negative feedback process.* Receptors within the hypothalamus and pituitary are sensitive to the circulating blood levels of the hormones (Table 50.1). Increased hormone levels stimulate a hypothalamic response to decrease the high circulating levels. Likewise, low circulating levels provoke a hypothalamic response that increases the low circulating levels. For example, low circulating testosterone levels stimulate the hypothalamus to secrete GnRH. This triggers the anterior pituitary to secrete greater amounts of FSH and LH, which in turn cause an increase in the testosterone production. The high level of testosterone signals a decrease in GnRH production, and thus FSH and LH.

In women, however, there is a slight variation in the control of gonadal hormones. The circulating levels are controlled through a combination of both a negative and positive feedback system. A *negative feedback control* mechanism exists similar to that described for men. Low circulating estrogen levels stimulate the hypothalamus to increase its production of GnRH. GnRH stimulates the pituitary to secrete greater amounts of FSH and LH, resulting in increased estrogen production by the ovaries. Higher levels of circulating estrogen result in a decreasing secretion of GnRH and thus a decrease in the secretion of FSH by the pituitary.

Women also have a *positive feedback control* mechanism. Here, with increased levels of circulating estrogen, more GnRH is made, resulting in an increased level of LH from the pituitary. Likewise, low estrogen levels result in a lower level of LH.

Menarche

Menarche is the first episode of menstrual bleeding, indicating that a girl has reached puberty. Menarche usually occurs at around 12 to 13 years of age but can occur as early as 10 years of age in some girls. Menstrual cycles are often irregular for the first 1 to 2 years after menarche because of *anovulatory cycles* (cycles without ovulation).

Menstrual Cycle

The major functions of the ovaries are ovulation and the secretion of hormones. These functions are accomplished during the normal menstrual cycle, a monthly process mediated by the

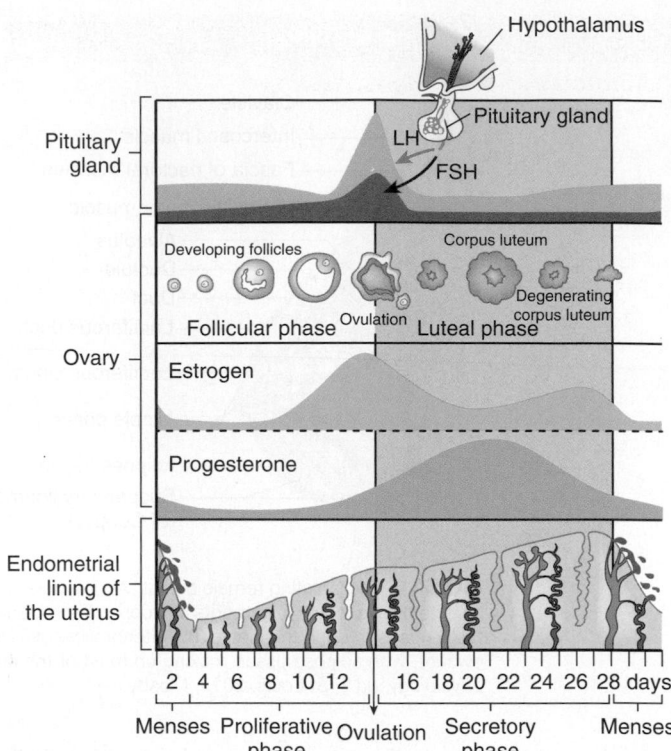

FIG 50.8 Events of the menstrual cycle. The *lines* depict the changes in blood hormone levels, the development of the follicles, and the changes in the endometrium during the cycle. (Modified from Patton KT, Thibodeau GA: *Anatomy and physiology,* ed 8, St Louis, 2013, Mosby.)

hormonal activity of the hypothalamus, pituitary gland, and ovaries. Menstruation occurs during each month in which an ovum is not fertilized (Fig. 50.8). The length of the menstrual cycle ranges from 21 to 35 days, with an average of 28 days. Most women have regular cycles. Irregular cycles may occur and can be due to a variety of factors, including hormonal fluctuations, medications, or conditions, such as uterine fibroids. Table 50.2 describes characteristics of the menstrual cycle and related teaching.

The menstrual cycle is divided into 3 phases. They are labeled in relation to uterine and ovarian changes: (1) the *proliferative,* or *follicular, phase;* (2) the *secretory,* or *luteal, phase;* and (3) the *menstrual,* or *ischemic, phase.* The menstrual cycle begins on the first day of menstruation, which usually lasts 4 to 6 days. The first day of the menstrual cycle is charted as the last menstrual period (LMP). During menstruation, estrogen and progesterone levels are low, but FSH levels begin to increase. During the follicular phase, a single follicle matures fully under FSH stimulation. The mechanism that ensures that usually only 1 follicle reaches maturity is not known. The mature follicle stimulates estrogen production, causing a negative feedback with resulting decreased FSH secretion.

Although the first stage of follicular maturation is stimulated by FSH, complete maturation and ovulation occur only in the presence of LH. When estrogen levels peak on about the 12th day of the cycle, there is a surge of LH, which triggers ovulation 1 or 2 days later. After ovulation, LH promotes the development of the corpus luteum, a temporary functional cyst that forms with the ruptured follicle.

The fully developed corpus luteum continues to secrete estrogen and initiates progesterone secretion. If fertilization occurs,

TABLE 50.2 Patient Teaching

Characteristics of Menstruation

Include the following information when teaching the patient about menstruation:

Characteristic	Teaching
Menarche • Occurs between ages 10 and 16 yr • Average age at onset is 12–13 yr	• See HCP about possible endocrine or developmental abnormality when delayed.
Interval • Usually is 21–35 days • Regular cycles as short as 17 days or as long as 45 days are considered normal if pattern is consistent for the person	• Keep track of periods via an app or calendar to identify menstrual cycle pattern • Expect some irregularity in perimenopausal period • Be aware that drugs (e.g., opioids, contraceptives) and stressful life events can result in missed periods
Duration • Menstrual flow generally lasts 2–8 days	• Realize that pattern is fairly constant but that wide variations do exist
Amount • Menstrual flow varies from 20–80 mL per menses. Average is 30 mL • Amount varies among women and in same woman at different times • It is usually heaviest first 2 days	• Count pads or tampons used per day • The average tampon or pad (when completely saturated) absorbs 20–30 mL • Very heavy flow is indicated by complete soaking of 2 pads in 1–2 hr • Flow increases and then gradually decreases in perimenopausal period • IUD or drugs, such as anticoagulants and thiazides, can cause heavy menses • Women with uterine fibroids may have increased or heavy menses
Composition • Menstrual discharge is mixture of endometrium, blood, mucus, and vaginal cells • Dark red, less viscous than blood, and usually does not clot	• Clots indicate heavy flow or vaginal pooling

estrogen and progesterone continue to be secreted because of the continued activity of the corpus luteum from stimulation by human chorionic gonadotropin (hCG). If fertilization does not take place, menstruation occurs because of a decrease in estrogen production and progesterone withdrawal.

During the *follicular phase,* the endometrial lining of the uterus undergoes change. As more estrogen is made, the endometrial lining goes through proliferative changes, including an increase in the length of blood vessels and glandular tissue.

With ovulation and the resulting increased levels of progesterone, the *luteal* (or *secretory*) *phase* begins. If the corpus luteum regresses (when fertilization does not occur) and estrogen and progesterone levels fall, the endometrial lining can no longer be supported. As a result, the blood vessels contract, and tissue begins to slough (fall away). This sloughing results in the menses and the start of the menstrual phase.

Menopause

Menopause is the physiologic cessation of menses associated with declining ovarian function. It is usually considered complete after 1 year of amenorrhea (absence of menstruation). Menopause is discussed in Chapter 53.

Phases of Sexual Response

The sexual response is a complex interplay of psychologic and physiologic phenomena. It is influenced by several variables (e.g., stress, illness). The changes that occur during sexual excitement are similar for men and women. Masters and Johnson described the sexual response in terms of the excitement, plateau, orgasmic, and resolution phases.[3]

Male Sexual Response. The penis and urethra are essential to the transport of sperm into the vagina and cervix during intercourse. This transport is facilitated by penile erection in response to sexual stimulation during the *excitement phase.* Erection results from the filling of the large venous sinuses within the erectile tissue of the penis. In the flaccid state the sinuses hold only a small amount of blood. During an erection, they are congested with blood. Because the penis is richly endowed with sympathetic, parasympathetic, and pudendal nerve endings, it is readily stimulated to erection. The loose skin of the penis becomes taut from venous congestion. This tautness allows for easy insertion into the vagina.

As the man reaches the *plateau phase,* the erection is maintained. The penis increases in diameter from a slight increase in vasocongestion. Testicle size also increases. Sometimes the glans penis becomes reddish purple.

The contractions of the penile and urethral musculature during the *orgasmic phase* propel the sperm outward through the meatus. In this process, termed *ejaculation,* sperm are released into the ductus deferens. Sperm advance through the urethra, where fluids from the prostate and seminal vesicles are added to the ejaculate. The sperm continue their path through the urethra, receiving a small amount of fluid from the Cowper's glands. They are finally ejaculated through the urinary meatus. *Orgasm* is characterized by the rapid release of vasocongestion and muscular tension through rhythmic contractions. This occurs primarily in the penis, prostate gland, and seminal vesicles. After ejaculation, a man enters the *resolution phase.* The penis undergoes involution, gradually returning to its unstimulated, flaccid state.

Female Sexual Response. The changes that occur in a woman during sexual excitation are similar to those in a man. In response to stimulation, the clitoris becomes congested and vaginal lubrication increases from secretions from the cervix, Bartholin's glands, and vaginal walls. This initial response is the excitation phase.

As excitement is maintained in the plateau phase, the vagina expands, and the uterus is elevated. In the orgasmic phase, contractions occur in the uterus from the fundus to the lower uterine segment. There is a slight relaxation of the cervical os, which helps the entrance of the sperm, and rhythmic contractions of the vagina. Muscular tension is rapidly released through rhythmic contractions in the clitoris, vagina, and uterus. A resolution

TABLE 50.3 Gerontologic Assessment Differences

Reproductive Systems

Structure	Changes	Assessment Findings Abnormalities
Male		
Breasts	Enlargement	Gynecomastia (abnormal enlargement)
Penis	↓ Subcutaneous fat	Easily retractable foreskin (if uncircumcised) ↓ Size Fewer sustained erections
Prostate	Benign hyperplasia	Enlargement, urinary obstruction, incontinence
Testes	↓ Testosterone production	↓ Size, firmness
Female		
Breasts	↓ Subcutaneous fat, increased fibrous tissue, ↓ skin turgor	Less resilient, looser, more pendulous tissue ↓ Size Duct around nipple may feel like stringy strand
Ovaries	↓ Ovarian function	Nonpalpable ovaries are normal postmenopause
Urethra	↓ Muscle tone, mucosal thinning	Possible urinary tract infections, painful urination (dysuria), urgency, frequency, incontinence
Uterus	↓ Thickness of myometrium	Uterine prolapse
Vagina	Tissue atrophy, ↓ muscle tone, alkaline pH	Mucosa becomes pale, dry, smooth and thins Vagina narrows and shortens
Vulva	↓ Skin turgor	Atrophy ↓ Amount of pubic hair ↓ Size of clitoris and labia

phase follows, in which these organs return to their preexcitation state. However, women do not have to go through the resolution (refractory) recovery state before they can be orgasmic again. They can be multiorgasmic without resolution between orgasms.

 Gerontologic Considerations: Effects of Aging on Reproductive Systems

With advancing age, changes occur in the male and female reproductive systems (Table 50.3). In women, many of these changes are related to decreased estrogen production associated with menopause.[4] Decreased estrogen and other sex steroids in postmenopausal women is associated with breast and genital atrophy, reduced bone mass, and increased rate of atherosclerosis. Vaginal dryness may occur, which can lead to urogenital atrophy and changes in the composition of the vaginal *microbiome* (the aggregate of microorganisms and their genetic material in a particular environment).[5]

Testosterone levels decline in men as they age. Manifestations of this decline are more gradual in men and can be physical, psychologic, or sexual. Changes include an increase in prostate size and a decrease in testosterone level, sperm production, muscle tone of the scrotum, and size and firmness of the testicles. Erectile dysfunction (ED) and sexual dysfunction occur in some men because of these changes.

Effects of Aging on Sexual Function

Men	Women
• ↑ Stimulation necessary for erection • ↓ Force of ejaculation • ↓ Ability to attain or sustain erection • ↓ Size and rigidity of the penis at full erection • ↓ Libido and interest in sex	• ↓ Vaginal lubrication • ↓ Sensitivity with labia shrinking and more clitoris exposed • Difficulty in maintaining arousal • Difficulty in achieving orgasm after stimulation • ↓ Libido and interest in sex

Many factors affect sexuality in later life. Gradual changes occur in the sexual responses of men and women. The cumulative effects of these changes, as well as the negative social attitude toward sexuality in older adults, can affect the sexual practices of older adults. Illness, disability, medicines, and surgeries can affect a person's ability to take part in sexual activities.

Nurses play a vital role in providing accurate and unbiased information about sexuality and age. Emphasize the normalcy of sexual activity in older adults and refer them to resources that address such issues.

ASSESSMENT OF MALE AND FEMALE REPRODUCTIVE SYSTEMS

Subjective Data

Important Health Information. In addition to general health information, elicit information specifically related to the reproductive system. Reproduction and sexual issues are often considered extremely personal and private. The extent and depth of the interview about a patient's sexuality and reproductive health depend primarily on your expertise and on the patient's needs and willingness to discuss the topic. Assess your comfort with your own sexuality because any discomfort in questioning becomes obvious to the patient.

A professional demeanor is important when taking a reproductive or sexual history. Develop trust with the patient to elicit such information. Conduct interviews in an environment that provides reassurance, confidentiality, and a nonjudgmental attitude. Be sensitive, use gender-neutral terms when asking about

Patient Introduction

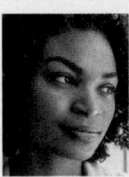

A.K. is a 21-yr-old black woman who is being evaluated for pelvic pain and irregular menstrual bleeding for the past several months. She takes oral contraceptive pills orally once daily and naproxen (Aleve) as needed for pain.

(© Benjamin A. Peterson/Mother Image/mother image/Fuse/Thinkstock.)

Discussion Questions

1. What are the possible causes for A.K.'s irregular menstrual bleeding?
2. What assessment questions would you ask A.K.?
3. How would you individualize the assessment based on her age, ethnic/cultural background, and condition?

You will learn more about A.K. and her condition as you read through this assessment chapter.
(See p. 1182 for more information on A.K.)

Answers available at *http://evolve.elsevier.com/Lewis/medsurg.*

partners, and maintain an awareness of a patient's culture and beliefs. Begin with the least sensitive information (e.g., menstrual history) before asking questions about more sensitive issues, such as sexual practices or STIs.

Past Health History. The health history should include information about major illnesses, hospitalizations, immunizations, and surgeries. Ask about any infections involving the reproductive system, including STIs. Take a complete obstetric and gynecologic history from the female patient.

Mumps and rubella affect reproductive function. The occurrence of mumps in young men is associated with an increased risk for sterility. Bilateral testicular atrophy may occur from mumps-related orchitis. Ask male patients if they have had mumps, have been immunized with the mumps vaccine, or have any signs of sterility.

Rubella is of primary concern to women of childbearing age. Having rubella during the first 3 months of pregnancy increases the risk for congenital anomalies. So, encourage immunization for all women of childbearing age who have not been immunized for rubella or have not already had the disease. Antibody titers can determine rubella immunity. Women should not be immunized if they are already pregnant.[6] Advise women to avoid becoming pregnant for 1 month after vaccination, or ideally, when their immunity has been confirmed by antibody titers.

Ask the patient about current health status and any acute or chronic health problems. Chronic illnesses, such as cardiovascular disease, respiratory problems, anemia, cancer, and kidney and urinary tract problems, may affect the reproductive system and sexual functioning.

Ask questions relating to possible endocrine disorders, particularly diabetes, hypothyroidism, and hyperthyroidism. These disorders directly interfere with women's menstrual cycles and with sexual performance. Men with diabetes may have ED and retrograde ejaculation. In women with uncontrolled diabetes, pregnancy may pose significant health risks to both the woman and unborn fetus.

Determine if the patient has a history of a stroke. In men, strokes may cause physiologic or psychologic ED. Men who have had a myocardial infarction (MI) may have ED because of fear that sexual activity could precipitate another MI. Post MI medication, such as β-blockers, may affect a man's ability to achieve an erection.[7] Although most patients have concerns about sexual activity after an MI, many are not comfortable expressing these fears to the nurse. Be sensitive to this concern.

Document the patient's allergies, especially if the patient is allergic to latex or drugs, including sulfonamides, macrolides, cephalosporins, tetracyclines, or penicillin. These drugs are often used to treat reproductive and genitourinary (GU) problems, such as STIs and urinary tract infections (UTIs). Silicone and latex are often used in diaphragms and condoms. An allergy to these substances precludes their use as contraceptive methods.

Medications. Document all prescription and over-the-counter drugs that the patient is taking, including the reason for use, dosage, and length of time that the drug has been taken. Ask the patient about the use of herbal products and dietary and nutritional supplements.

Particularly relevant is the use of diuretics (sometimes prescribed for premenstrual edema) and psychotropic agents (which may interfere with sexual performance). Antihypertensives, such as amlodipine (Norvasc), lisinopril (Prinivil), propranolol

(Inderal), and clonidine (Catapres), may cause ED. Use of drugs such as alcohol, marijuana, barbiturates, amphetamines, or cocaine can affect the reproductive system.

In women, document the use of hormonal contraceptives and hormone therapy (HT). The long-term use of combined HT (specifically a combination of oral conjugated equine estrogen and a progestin, *medroxyprogesterone acetate*) is associated with an increased risk for stroke, breast cancer, deep vein thrombosis, and gallbladder disease. These risks are higher in women who also use tobacco products.[8] For postmenopausal women who may have symptoms, such as hot flashes, newer data that suggest that HT does not increase the risk for mortality. Women will need counseling based on their degree of symptoms and associated morbidities to help balance their quality of life with menopausal symptoms.[9]

A history of cholecystitis and hepatitis is important because these conditions may be contraindications for the use of oral contraceptives. Oral contraceptives often aggravate cholecystitis. Chronic liver inflammation generally precludes the use of estrogen products because they are metabolized by the liver. Chronic obstructive pulmonary disease may be a contraindication to oral contraceptive use because progesterone thickens respiratory secretions.

Surgery or Other Treatments. Note any surgical procedures. Common surgical procedures involving the female reproductive system are listed in Table 53.14. Record any therapeutic or spontaneous abortions and type of intervention (e.g., medical versus surgical abortion).

Functional Health Patterns. The key questions to ask a patient with a reproductive problem are outlined in Table 50.4.

Health Perception–Health Management Pattern. The primary focus of this pattern is the patient's perception of his or her own health and measures that the patient takes to maintain health. Ask about self-examination practices and screenings. Mammography and periodic cervical Pap tests are integral to a woman's health. Men are at risk for testicular and prostate cancer. However, controversy exists about the benefits of routine screening for these cancers.[10] All patients should discuss the benefits and risks of screening with their HCP.

⚕ GENETIC RISK ALERT

- Breast, ovarian, uterine, and prostate cancer have known genetic risk factors.
- Having a first-degree relative with any of these cancers significantly increases the risk for cancer for the patient.
- The risk increases if several family members have had these cancers over succeeding generations.
- Persons with a known hereditary predisposition to breast or ovarian cancer can use this information to make informed decisions about how to minimize their risks.

An accurate family history is avital. Ask about a history of cancer, especially cancer of the reproductive organs. Determine if the patient has a familial tendency for diabetes, hypothyroidism, hyperthyroidism, hypertension, stroke, angina, MI, endocrine disorders, or anemia.

Assessment of the reproductive system is incomplete without knowledge of the patient's lifestyle choices. Determine whether a patient has smoked or is currently smoking, the amount (if any) of alcohol consumption, or if the patient uses illicit drugs. Risks associated with smoking include ectopic pregnancy, miscarriage, an increased risk for perinatal mortality and morbidity,

TABLE 50.4 Health History

Reproductive System

Health Perception–Health Management
- How would you describe your overall health?
- Describe the health of your family members. Any history of breast, uterine, ovarian, or prostate cancer?*

Women
- Do you perform breast self-examination? Any concerns?
- What was the date of your last Pap test and the results?*
- Any prior abnormalities with your Pap tests?
- What was the date of your last mammogram and the results?*
- Any prior abnormalities with your mammograms?

Men
- Do you perform testicular self-examination? Any concerns?

Nutritional-Metabolic
- Describe what you usually eat and drink.
- Have you had any changes in weight?*
- How do you feel about your current weight?
- Do you take any nutritional supplements, such as calcium or vitamins?*
- Do you have any dietary restrictions?*

Elimination
- Do you have problems with urination (e.g., pain, burning, dribbling, incontinence, frequency)?*
- Have you had bladder infections? If so, when? How often?
- Do you have problems with bowel movements?*
- Do you have any constipation, loose stools, or blood with stools?*
- Do you use laxatives?*

Activity-Exercise
- What activities do you typically do each day?
- Do you have enough energy for your desired activities?

Sleep-Rest
- How many hours do you typically sleep each night?
- Do you feel rested after sleep?
- Do you have any problems associated with sleeping?*

Cognitive-Perceptual
- Do you have pain? If yes, where?
- Do you have pain during sexual activity or intercourse?*

Self-Perception–Self-Concept
- How would you describe yourself?
- Have there been any recent changes that have made you feel differently about yourself?*
- Are you having any problems that are affecting your sexuality?*

Role-Relationship
- Describe your living arrangements. With whom do you live?
- Do you have a significant other? If yes, is this relationship satisfying?
- Are you having any role-related problems in your family?* At work?*
- What are the relationships among your family members?

Sexuality-Reproductive
- Are you sexually active? If so, how many partners do you have?
- What kind of sex do you engage in (e.g., oral, vaginal, anal)?
- How do you protect yourself against sexually transmitted infections and unwanted pregnancy?
- Are you satisfied with your present means of sexual expression? If not, explain.
- Have you had any recent changes in your sexual practices?*

Women
- How old were you when you had your first menstrual period? (Menarche)
- What was the first day of your last menstrual period?
- Describe your period. How many days does it last? How often does it come (e.g., every 28 days)?
- Do you have pain with your period? Do you pass clots?
- Do you feel your flow is heavy or excessive?
- How old were you when you went through menopause?
- Have you had any postmenopausal bleeding or spotting?*
- Pregnancy history: How many times have you been pregnant? How many living children do you have? Have you ever had any miscarriages or abortions? Did they need medical intervention?

Men
- Do you have any problem obtaining or sustaining an erection?
- Do you have any problems with ejaculation?

Coping–Stress Tolerance
- Have there been any major changes in your life within the past couple of years?*
- What is stressful in your life right now?
- How do you handle health problems when they occur?
- Do you feel safe in your home? Work? Has anyone ever tried to hurt or harm you?

Value-Belief
- What beliefs do you have about your health and illnesses?
- Do you use home remedies?*
- Is religion an important part of your life?*
- Do you think that any of your personal beliefs or values may be compromised because of your treatment?*

*If yes, describe.

placental abnormalities, preterm delivery, and congenital facial defects of the fetus.[11] Smoking increases the risk for morbidity and mortality in women who use oral contraceptives. Smoking in women is also associated with early menopause.[5] Decreased sperm counts and ED are seen in male smokers. Smoking is a known cofactor for persistence of *human papillomavirus* (HPV) infection for oral and anogenital cancers among men and women.[12]

Nutritional-Metabolic Pattern. Anemia is a common problem in women in their reproductive years, particularly during pregnancy and the postpartum period. Evaluate the adequacy of the diet with this condition in mind. Iron-deficiency anemia is the most common cause of anemia in menstruating females.

Take a thorough nutritional and psychologic history to assess for the presence of an eating disorder. Anorexia nervosa can cause amenorrhea and other problems, such as osteoporosis, that are related to menopause. Obesity can be related to polycystic ovarian syndrome and may be a precursor to type 2 diabetes.

From early adolescence, teach women about adequate calcium and vitamin D intake to prevent osteoporosis. Estimate the patient's daily calcium intake to determine whether supplementation is needed. Evaluate folic acid intake for women in their reproductive years because a deficiency can result in spina bifida and other fetal neural tube defects.[13]

Elimination Pattern. Many gynecologic problems can result in GU problems. Urinary incontinence is common in older women. Factors associated with female incontinence include relaxation of the pelvic musculature caused by multiple births, advancing age, fibroid tumors, diabetes, obesity, and weight gain. Condom, diaphragm, and spermicide use is associated with an increased risk for UTIs. Vaginal infections, such as bacterial vaginosis (BV), facilitate the growth of *Escherichia coli*, which causes most UTIs.[14] Men may have urethritis, an inflammation of the urethra, which may be caused by an STI. Urethritis can cause painful urination. Benign prostatic hyperplasia (BPH) is common in older men. It can cause urinary retention or difficulty in starting the urinary stream.

Activity-Exercise Pattern. Record the amount, type, and intensity of activity and exercise. Lack of weight-bearing exercise is an important factor in the development of osteoporosis, especially in postmenopausal women. Adolescent females who engage in excessive leanness sports may have *female athlete triad*. It is characterized by secondary amenorrhea, low energy availability, and osteoporosis.[15] Anemia can result in fatigue and activity intolerance and interfere with satisfactory performance of activities of daily living.

Sleep-Rest Pattern. Sleep patterns for women may be affected during the postpartum period and while raising young children. Hot flashes and sweating during perimenopause can cause serious sleep interruption when the woman awakens in a drenching sweat. The need to change her nightgown and bedding further disrupts her sleep. Insomnia is common among perimenopausal women. Daytime fatigue can result from sleep problems. In men, frequent urination at night associated with prostate enlargement or hormone therapy for prostate cancer can disturb sleep.

Cognitive-Perceptual Pattern. Pelvic pain is associated with various gynecologic disorders, such as pelvic inflammatory disease, ovarian cysts, and *endometriosis*. Dyspareunia (painful intercourse) can be problematic for women in the postmenopausal period. The pain associated with intercourse can create a reluctance to take part in sexual activity and strain relationships with sexual partners. Refer women with dyspareunia to their HCP.

Self-Perception–Self-Concept Pattern. Changes that occur with aging, such as pendulous breasts and vaginal dryness in women and decreased penis size in men, may lead to emotional distress. The subtle changes associated with sexuality and advancing age may affect self-concept.

Role-Relationship Pattern. Obtain information about the family structure and occupation. Ask about recent changes in work-related relationships or family conflict. Assess the patient's role in the family as a starting point to determine family dynamics. Roles and relationships are affected by changes within the family. The addition of a new baby may change family dynamics.

Sexuality-Reproductive Pattern. For women, obtain a menstrual and a chronologic obstetric history. The menstrual history includes the first day of the LMP, description of menstrual flow, age of menarche, and, if applicable, age at menopause. Menstrual history data are used in the detection of pregnancy, infertility, and many gynecologic problems. Have the patient describe any changes in her usual menstrual pattern

TABLE 50.5 Sexual History Format

The Five Ps of Taking a Sexual History*

The 5 Ps	Questions
1. Partners	Are you currently sexually active? (yes or no) • Do you have sex with men, women, or both? • In the past 2 months, with how many partners have you had sex? • In the past 12 months, with how many partners have you had sex?
2. Practices	To understand your risk for STIs, I need to understand the kind of sex you have had recently. • Genital (penis in the vagina) • Anal (penis in the anus) • Oral (mouth on penis, vagina, or anus)
3. Protection from STIs	Do you and your partner(s) use any protection against STIs? • What kind? • How often?
4. Past history of STIs	Have you ever been diagnosed with an STI? • What type? • When? • How were you treated?
5. Prevention of pregnancy	Are you or your partner trying to get pregnant? • If not, what are you doing to prevent pregnancy?

Adapted from *www.cdc.gov/std/treatment/sexualhistory.pdf.*
*Modify this guide as needed to be culturally appropriate based on culture or gender dynamics.

to determine whether the change is transient and unimportant or connected with a more serious gynecologic problem. Terminology that describes abnormal uterine bleeding patterns is discussed in Chapter 53.

Identify changes in menstrual patterns associated with the use of oral contraceptives, intrauterine devices (IUDs), birth control patches, vaginal rings, progestin-only implants, or medroxyprogesterone injections. Oral contraceptives usually decrease the amount and duration of flow. Some IUDs can increase menstrual flow. Some IUDs are used for both contraception and as a nonsurgical treatment for heavy menstrual bleeding.

The obstetric history includes the number of pregnancies, full-term births, preterm births, stillbirths, living children, and abortions (including spontaneous [miscarriage], ectopic, or induced). Document the course of each pregnancy, including the duration of each pregnancy, date of delivery, problems that may have occurred with each pregnancy, and any medical or surgical interventions that were needed.

Table 50.5 outlines *The 5 Ps of Sexual Health* approach for taking a sexual history. Never make an assumption about a patient's sexual orientation. Ask both men and women about their general satisfaction with their sexuality. Ask the patient about sexual beliefs and practices and whether they achieve orgasm. Explore any unexplained change in sexual practices or performance. Reproductive problems can cause physiologic or psychologic problems that can lead to painful intercourse, ED, sexual dysfunction, or infertility.

Coping–Stress Tolerance Pattern. The stress related to situations such as pregnancy or menopause increases dependence on support systems. Determine whom the support people are in the patient's life. The diagnosis of an STI can cause stress for the patient and partner. Explore ways to manage this stress with patients by encouraging them to share their fears and concerns.

Value-Belief Pattern. Sexual and reproductive functioning is closely related to cultural, religious, moral, and ethical values. Be aware of your own beliefs in these areas. Recognize and sensitively react to the patient's personal beliefs associated with reproductive and sexuality issues.

CASE STUDY—cont'd

Subjective Data

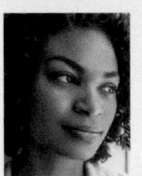

(© Benjamin A. Peterson/Mother Image/mother image/Fuse/Thinkstock.)

A focused assessment of A.K. revealed the following information:

Health Perception–Health Management: In good health. Pap smear 2 months ago was normal. Has not had any surgeries

Nutritional-Metabolic: 5 ft 4 in, 140 lb (BMI 24 kg/m²)

Elimination: Denies any changes with urination or bowel movements

Activity-Exercise: Exercises at gym 3 times a week

Cognitive-Perceptual: Denies dyspareunia

Self-Perception–Self Concept: Attends college and hopes to graduate this semester

Role-Relationship: Single, lives with 3 other young women in off-campus housing

Sexuality-Reproductive: Menarche at age 14. Last menstrual period 2 weeks ago. Menses is usually every 28 days, lasting 2 days, but has noted irregular bleeding with increased pelvic pain over past few months. Sexually active with men—3 lifetime partners. In a mutually monogamous relationship of 2 years duration. Practices vaginal and oral sex

Coping–Stress Tolerance: Denies stressors

Value-Belief: Raised Baptist, but does not attend services at school

Discussion Questions

1. Which subjective assessment findings are of most concern to you?
2. What should be included in the physical assessment?

You will learn more about physical examination of the reproductive system in the next section.
(See p. 1183 for more information on A.K.)

Answers available at *http://evolve.elsevier.com/Lewis/medsurg.*

Objective Data

Physical Examination: Male. The examination of the male external genitalia by the nurse includes inspection and palpation of the pubis, penis, and scrotum. The patient may be lying or standing. The standing position is preferred. Sit in front of the standing patient. Use gloves during examination of the male genitalia.

If breast cancer is suspected or there is a strong family history of breast cancer in a male patient, a clinical breast examination is conducted in the same pattern for a male patient as a female breast examination (see Fig. 51.1).

Pubis. Assess for hair distribution and presence of body lice. Normally, the hair is in a diamond-shaped pattern and coarser than scalp hair. The absence of hair is not a normal finding unless the man is shaving or waxing the pubic hair. Carefully assess the skin for irritation and inflammation.

Penis and Scrotum. Inspect the penis for any lesions, bleeding, or swelling. Note the location of the urethral meatus and the presence of a foreskin. If present, retract the foreskin and note any redness, discharge, irritation, lesions, or swelling from the meatus. Replace the foreskin over the glans after observation.

Inspect the scrotum by lifting each testis to inspect all sides of the scrotal sac. Palpate the testes for tenderness or masses. The left testis usually hangs lower than the right. An undescended testis *(cryptorchidism)* is a major risk factor for testicular cancer and a potential cause of male infertility.

Anus. Note if the buttocks have any lesions, swelling, or inflammation. Spread the buttocks apart with both hands to expose the anus. Inspect the anal sphincter and perineal regions for fissures, lesions, masses, and hemorrhoids. The anus should be free from inflammation or skin changes.

Physical Examination: Female. With a chaperone present, physical examination of women often begins with inspection and palpation of the breasts and axillae then proceeds to the abdomen and genitalia. Examining the abdomen provides an opportunity to detect pain or any masses that may involve the GU system. Abdominal examination is discussed in Chapter 38.

Breasts. To perform a breast examination, first examine the breasts by visual inspection. With the patient seated, inspect the breasts for symmetry, size, shape, skin color, vascular patterns, dimpling, and unusual lesions. Ask the patient to put the arms at the sides, arms overhead, lean forward, and press hands on hips. Observe for any abnormalities during these maneuvers. Palpate the axillae and clavicular areas for enlarged lymph nodes.

After the patient assumes the supine position, place a pillow under the back on the side to be examined. Ask the patient to put the arm above and behind the head. This flattens breast tissue and make palpation easier. Then palpate the breast in a systematic fashion, preferably using a vertical line (see Fig. 51.1). Use the distal finger pads of the index, middle, and ring fingers for palpation. Include the axillary tail of Spence in the examination. This area of the breast lies adjacent to the upper outer quadrant. It is where most breast cancer develops. Palpate the area around the areolae for masses. Document the color, consistency, and odor of any discharge. For patients at average risk who have no breast symptoms, the benefit of routine clinical breast examinations to detect early breast cancer is unclear. Teach patients to be familiar with how their breasts feel and report any significant changes or concerns to an HCP.[16]

External Genitalia. The examination of a woman's genitalia by the nurse includes inspection and palpation of the mons pubis, vulva, and anus. Use gloves for the examination. Assess for hair distribution, presence of body lice, lesions, redness, edema, or discharge. Many women remove hair from the genital region via shaving, waxing, or laser hair removal and may develop folliculitis (infection of the hair follicle). Separate the labia to fully inspect the clitoris, urethral meatus, and vaginal orifice. Spread the buttocks apart to inspect the anus for fissures, lesions, and hemorrhoids.

Internal Pelvic Examination. HCPs with advanced or specialized training usually do this part of the examination. During the speculum examination, the HCP inspects the walls of the vagina and cervix for inflammation, discharge, polyps, and suspicious growths. A Pap test and specimens for nucleic acid amplification tests (NAATs) for STI sampling and microscopic examination may be obtained. After the speculum examination, a bimanual examination may be done to assess the size, shape, and consistency of the uterus and ovaries. The ovaries and tubes are not normally palpable.

Table 50.6 gives an example of a recording format for the physical assessment findings for the male and female

TABLE 50.6 Normal Physical Assessment of Reproductive System

Male	Female
Breasts	
Nipples soft. No lumps, nodules, swelling, or enlarged tissue noted.	Symmetric without dimpling. Nipples soft. No drainage, retraction, or lesions noted. No masses or tenderness. No lymphadenopathy.
External Genitalia	
Diamond-shaped hair distribution. No penile lesions or discharge noted. Scrotum symmetric, no masses, descended testes. No inguinal hernia.	Triangular hair distribution. Genitalia dark pink, no lesions, redness, swelling, or inflammation in perineal region. No vaginal discharge noted. No tenderness with palpation of Skene's ducts and Bartholin's glands.
Anus	
No hemorrhoids, fissures, or lesions noted.	No hemorrhoids, fissures, or lesions noted.

CASE STUDY—cont'd
Objective Data: Physical Examination

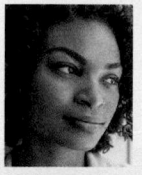

(© Benjamin A. Peterson/Mother Image/mother image/Fuse/Thinkstock.)

Focused assessment of A.K. reveals the following: BP is 118/76 mm Hg; her pulse is 70 beats/min and regular. Skin warm and dry without lesions. No cyanosis of lips, mucous membranes, or nail beds. Thyroid is not enlarged. Heart examination is normal. Abdomen soft and nontender. External genitalia examination is normal. Bimanual examination by the HCP is negative for cervical motion tenderness, uterine anomalies. She has pain on left side with palpation of a soft mass consistent with an ovarian cyst.

Discussion Questions

1. Based on the subjective and objective assessment findings, what diagnostic tests would you anticipate being ordered for A.K.?

You will learn more about diagnostic studies related to the reproductive system in the next section.

(See p. 1183 for more information on A.K.)

Answers available at *http://evolve.elsevier.com/Lewis/medsurg.*

reproductive systems. Tables 50.7 through 50.9 summarize assessment abnormalities of the breasts, female reproductive system, and male reproductive system, respectively.

A *focused assessment* is used to evaluate the status of previously identified reproductive problems and to monitor for signs of new problems. A focused assessment of the reproductive system is presented in the box on this page.

DIAGNOSTIC STUDIES OF REPRODUCTIVE SYSTEMS

The most common diagnostic studies used to assess the reproductive systems are described in Tables 50.10 through 50.14. Diagnostic studies of the endocrine system may also be done in a person with a reproductive system problem (see Tables 47.6 and 47.7).

FOCUSED ASSESSMENT
Reproductive System

Use this checklist to ensure the key assessment steps have been done.

Subjective

Ask the patient about any of the following and note responses.

Vaginal or vulvar: discharge, lesions, itching, unusual bleeding, odor	Y	N
Penile pain, lesions, discharge	Y	N
Medications: oral contraceptives, antihypertensives, psychotropics, hormones	Y	N
Clinical examinations of reproductive systems (breast, pelvis, testicular, prostate) and results	Y	N
Pain: abdomen, pelvis, or genitalia	Y	N

Objective: Diagnostic

Check the following for results and critical values.

Serum/urine hCG	✓
Serum PSA	✓
CBC	✓
Hormone studies (testosterone, progesterone, estrogen, FSH, LH, TSH)	✓
NAAT STI results (e.g., *Chlamydia*, gonorrhea, *Trichomonas*)	✓
In office testing (e.g., wet mounts, pH assessment)	✓
Mammography and/or ultrasound of breasts	✓
Ultrasound: abdominal, pelvic, transvaginal, prostate	✓

Objective: Physical Examination
Inspect

External genitalia for redness, swelling, discharge, lesions	✓
Breasts for swelling, dimpling, retraction, drainage, redness, skin changes, masses,	✓

Palpate

Breast tissue for masses or tenderness	✓
External genitalia: tenderness, pain	✓

hCG, Human chorionic gonadotropin; *PSA,* prostate-specific antigen.

CASE STUDY—cont'd
Objective Data: Diagnostic Studies

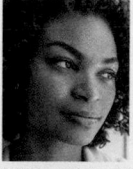

(© Benjamin A. Peterson/Mother Image/mother image/Fuse/Thinkstock.)

The following laboratory and diagnostic tests are ordered for A.K.:

Urine pregnancy test, urinalysis, pelvic and transvaginal ultrasound, complete blood count (CBC), thyroid stimulating hormone (TSH), gonorrhea and chlamydia NAAT testing. Her results are:

Urine pregnancy test: Negative

Urinalysis: Normal

CBC: hemoglobin, 13.2 g/dL, hematocrit, 36%

TSH: 2.3 IU/L

Gonorrhea and chlamydia tests: Negative

The pelvic and transvaginal ultrasound revealed a 4-cm ovarian cyst.

Discussion Questions

1. Which diagnostic and laboratory test results are of concern to you?
2. What patient teaching can you provide A.K. based on her diagnostic test results?

Answers available at *http://evolve.elsevier.com/Lewis/medsurg.*

TABLE 50.7 Assessment Abnormalities

Breast

Finding	Description	Possible Etiology and Significance
Dimpling	Unilateral, recent onset, no pain	Cancer
Nipple inversion or retraction	Recent onset, redness, pain, unilateral	Abscess, inflammation, cancer
	Recent onset (usually within past year), unilateral presentation, lack of tenderness	Cancer
Nipple scaling or irritation	Unilateral or bilateral presentation, crusting, possible ulceration	Paget's disease, eczema, infection
Nipple secretions		
• Galactorrhea (female)	Milky, no relationship to lactation, unilateral or bilateral, intermittent or consistent presentation	Drug therapy, especially phenothiazines, tricyclic antidepressants, methyldopa. Hypofunction or hyperfunction of thyroid or adrenal glands. Hypothalamus or pituitary tumor. Excess estrogen. Prolonged suckling or breast foreplay
• Galactorrhea (male)	Milky, bilateral presentation	Chorioepithelioma of testes, pituitary tumor
• Multicolored or dark green discharge	Thick, sticky, and often bilateral	Ductal ectasia (dilation of mammary ducts)
• Purulent	Gray-green or yellow color. Frequent unilateral presentation. Association with pain, redness, induration, nipple inversion	Puerperal (after birth) mastitis (inflammatory condition of breast) or abscess
	Same as above but usually without nipple inversion	Infected sebaceous cyst
• Serosanguineous or bloody drainage	Unilateral presentation	Papillomatosis (widespread development of nipple-like growths), intraductal papilloma, cancer (male and female)
• Serous discharge	Clear appearance, unilateral or bilateral, intermittent or consistent presentation	Intraductal papilloma
Nodules, lumps, or masses	Multiple, bilateral, well-delineated, soft or firm, mobile cysts. Pain. Premenstrual occurrence	Fibrocystic changes
	Rubbery consistency, fluid-filled interior, pain	Ductal ectasia
	Soft, mobile, well-delineated cyst, absence of pain	Lipoma, fibroadenoma
	Redness, tenderness, induration	Infected sebaceous cysts, abscesses
	Usually singular, hard, irregularly shaped, poorly delineated, non-mobile	Cancer

TABLE 50.8 Assessment Abnormalities

Female Reproductive System

Finding and Description	Possible Etiology and Significance
Vulvar Discharge	
Thin gray or white, copious flow, malodorous or fishy, vulvar irritation	Bacterial vaginosis infection
White, thick, curdy, frequent itching and inflammation, lack of odor or yeast-like smell	Candidiasis (*Candida* or yeast infection), vaginitis
Mucopurulent discharge; bloody discharge	*Chlamydia trachomatis* or *Neisseria gonorrhoeae* infection, menstruation, trauma, cancer
Frothy green or yellow color; malodorous	*Trichomonas vaginalis*
Vulvar Redness	
Bright or beefy red color, itching	*Candida albicans*, allergy, chemical vaginitis
Reddened base, painful vesicles or ulcerations	Genital herpes
Macules or papules, itching	Chancroid, contact dermatitis, scabies, pediculosis
Vulvar Growths	
Soft, fleshy growth, nontender	Condyloma acuminatum (genital warts)
Flat and warty appearance, nontender	Condyloma latum
Same as either of above, possible pain	Cancer
Reddened base, vesicles, and small erosions; pain	Lymphogranuloma venereum, genital herpes, chancroid
Indurated, firm ulcers, no pain	Chancre (syphilis), granuloma inguinale
Abdominal Pain, Tenderness, or Pelvic Masses	
Intermittent or consistent tenderness in right or left lower quadrant	Salpingitis (infection of fallopian tube), ectopic pregnancy, ruptured ovarian cyst, PID, tubal or ovarian abscess
Periumbilical location, consistent occurrence	Cystitis, endometritis (inflammation of endometrium), ectopic pregnancy
Abdominal or pelvic pain, especially with menses, which radiates to back, rectum or vagina.	Endometriosis (a disorder in which the endometrial lining grows on pelvic organs or outside the pelvis in rare cases)
Pelvic masses	Fibroids, ovarian cysts (typically benign); Cancer or metastases (requires additional testing and treatment)

PID, Pelvic inflammatory disease.

TABLE 50.9 Assessment Abnormalities

Male Reproductive System

Finding and Description	Possible Etiology and Significance
Penile Growths or Masses	
Indurated, smooth, disk-like appearance. Absence of pain. Singular presentation	Chancre (syphilis)
Papular to irregularly shaped ulceration with pus, lack of induration	Chancroid
Ulceration with induration and nodularity	Cancer
Flat, wartlike nodule	Condyloma latum
Raised, fleshy, moist, elongated projections with single or multiple projections	Condyloma acuminatum (genital warts)
Localized swelling with retracted, tight foreskin	Paraphimosis (inability to replace foreskin to its normal position after retraction), trauma
Vesicles, Erosions, or Ulcers	
Painful, reddened base. Vesicular or small erosions	Genital herpes, balanitis (inflammation of glans penis), chancroid
Painless, singular, small erosion with eventual lymphadenopathy	Lymphogranuloma venereum, cancer
Scrotal Masses	
Localized swelling with tenderness, unilateral or bilateral presentation	Epididymitis (inflammation of epididymis), testicular torsion, orchitis (mumps)
Swelling, tenderness	Incarcerated hernia
Swelling without pain. Unilateral or bilateral presentation. Translucent, cordlike or wormlike appearance	Hydrocele (accumulation of fluid in outer covering of testes), spermatocele (firm, sperm-containing cyst of epididymis), varicocele (dilation of veins that drain testes), hematocele (accumulation of blood within scrotum)
Firm, nodular testes or epididymis. Frequent unilateral presentation	Tuberculosis, cancer
Penile Discharge	
Clear to purulent color, minimal to copious flow	Urethritis or gonorrhea, *Chlamydia trachomatis* infection, trauma
Penile or Scrotal Redness	
Macules and papules	Scabies, pediculosis
Inguinal Masses	
Bulging unilateral presentation during straining	Inguinal hernia
1- to 3-cm nodules	Lymphadenopathy

TABLE 50.10 Serology Studies

Male and Female Reproductive Systems

Study	Reference Interval	Description and Purpose
Anti-müllerian hormone (AMH)	*Female:* 13–45 yr: 0.9–9.5 ng/mL >45 yr: <1.0 ng/mL	Measures ovarian function. Level reflects size of the remaining egg supply ("ovarian reserve"). May be done when a woman has manifestations of polycystic ovarian syndrome (PCOS). Used to monitor AMH-producing ovarian tumor. Females with high AMH levels have a better response to ovarian stimulation during fertility treatments.
Estradiol	*Female:* Follicular phase: 20–350 pg/mL (73–1285 pmol/L) Luteal phase: 30–450 pg/mL (110–1652 pmol/L) Postmenopause: ≤20 pg/mL (≤73 pmol/L) *Male:* 10–50 pg/mL (37–184 pmol/L)	Measures ovarian function. Useful in assessing estrogen-secreting tumors and states of precocious female puberty. May be used to confirm perimenopausal status. Increased levels in men may indicate testicular tumor.
Follicle-stimulating hormone (FSH)	In 24-hr urine samples: *Female:* Follicular phase: 2–15 U/24 hr Midcycle: 8–60 U/24 hr Luteal phase: 2–10 U/24 hr Postmenopause: 35–100 U/24 hr *Male:* 3–11 U/24 hr In blood: *Female:* Follicular phase: 1.37–9.9 mU/mL Ovulatory phase: 6.17–17.2 mU/mL Luteal phase: 1.09–9.2 mU/mL Postmenopause: 19.3–100.6 mU/mL *Male:* 1.42–15.4 mU/mL	Assesses gonadal function. Abnormal levels may indicate pituitary tumors or dysfunction. Increased in menopause. May be used to confirm menopausal status.

Continued

TABLE 50.10 Serology Studies

Male and Female Reproductive Systems—cont'd

Study	Reference Interval	Description and Purpose
Human chorionic gonadotropin (hCG)	Qualitative: Negative Quantitative: <5 mIU/mL (<5 IU/L) (males and non-pregnant females)	Detects pregnancy. Detects hydatidiform mole and chorioepithelioma (in men and women). Done with urine or blood.
Luteinizing hormone (LH)	*Female:* Premenopause: 5–25 IU/L, with higher peaks at ovulation Postmenopause: 14–52.3 IU/L *Male:* 1.8–8.6 IU/L	Associated with ovulation in women and testosterone production in men. Used in women in the workup of infertility and menstrual irregularities.
Progesterone	*Female:* Follicular phase: 15–70 ng/dL (0.5–2.2 nmol/L) Luteal phase: 200–2500 ng/dL (6.4–79.5 nmol/L) Postmenopause: <40 ng/dL (1.28 nmol/L) *Male:* 13–97 ng/dL (0.4–3.1 nmol/L)	Used to assess infertility, monitors success of drugs for infertility or the effect of progesterone treatment, determines whether ovulation is occurring. Diagnoses problems with adrenal glands and some types of cancer.
Prolactin	*Female:* 3.8–23.2 ng/mL (3.8–23.2 mg/L) *Male:* 3.0–14.7 ng/mL (3.0–14.7 mg/L)	Detects pituitary dysfunction that can cause amenorrhea, decreased libido, and impotence.
Prostate-specific antigen (PSA)	*Male:* <4 ng/mL (<4 mcg/L)	Detects prostate cancer. Used to monitor response to therapy.
Testosterone	In 24-hr urine samples: *Female:* 2–12 mcg/24 hr (6.9–41.6 nmol/24 hr) *Male:* 40–135 mcg/24 hr (139–469 nmol/24 hr) In blood: *Female:*15–70 ng/dL (0.52–2.43 nmol/L) *Male:* 280–1100 ng/dL (10.4–38.17 nmol/L)	Detects tumors and developmental anomalies of the testicles. Used to assess male infertility.

TABLE 50.11 Radiologic Studies

Male and Female Reproductive System

Study	Description and Purpose
CT scan of pelvis	Detects tumors in the pelvis.
Mammography	X-ray image used to assess breast tissue. Detects benign and malignant masses. Mammography screening guidelines are discussed in Chapter 51.
MRI	Radio waves and magnetic field are used to assess soft tissue. Useful after an abnormal mammogram or in women with dense breast tissue. Breast MRI may be with mammography to detect breast cancer in women at high risk for breast cancer. Used to diagnose abnormalities in female and male reproductive systems.
Ultrasound (US) (breast, pelvic, testicular, transvaginal [TV], rectal [TRUS])	Measures and records high-frequency sound waves as they pass through tissues of variable density. Breast US: Used to detect fluid-filled masses and for follow-up screening after mammography in women with dense breast tissue. Pelvic and TV US: In women, used to detect pelvic masses, such as ectopic pregnancy, ovarian cysts, fibroids, and cancer. Testicular US: Detects testicular masses and testicular torsion. TRUS: Used to diagnose prostate tumors.

TABLE 50.12 Interventional Studies

Study	Description and Purpose	Nursing Responsibility
Colposcopy	Direct visualization of cervix with binocular microscope. Allows magnification of cervix and study of cellular abnormalities. Used as follow-up for abnormal Pap test and for examination of women exposed to DES in utero. Cervical biopsy(ies) may be taken. Assesses for vaginal or vulvar dysplasia.	*Before:* Teach patient about the procedure. Tell patient this test is similar to a speculum examination. *After:* If a biopsy was done, tell patient she may have some vaginal bleeding and to avoid sexual intercourse until healed.
Conization	Cone-shaped sample of squamocolumnar tissue of cervix is removed for direct study.	*Before:* Teach patient about the procedure. Requires use of surgical facilities and anesthesia. *After:* Tell patient to avoid sexual intercourse and tampons for 3–4 wk. May have some discharge or spotting for 1 wk. 3-wk follow-up necessary.
Dilation and curettage (D&C)	Operative procedure that dilates cervix and allows curetting of endometrial lining. Used in assessment of abnormal bleeding and cytologic evaluation of lining.	*Before:* Teach patient about procedure and sedation. *After:* Assess degree of bleeding with frequent pad check during first 24 hr.

TABLE 50.12 Interventional Studies—cont'd

Study	Description and Purpose	Nursing Responsibility
Hysterosalpingo-gram (HSG)	Involves instillation of contrast media through cervix into uterine cavity and through fallopian tubes. X-ray images taken to detect abnormalities of uterus and its adnexa (ovaries and tubes) as contrast progresses through them. Most useful in diagnostic assessment of fertility (e.g., to detect adhesions near ovary, abnormal uterine shape, blockage of tubal pathways).	*Before:* Teach patient about procedure and that it may be uncomfortable. Contrast medium is used. *After:* Tell patient she may have slight vaginal bleeding and cramping. Monitor for foul-smelling vaginal discharge, severe pain, fever, or chills.
Hysteroscopy	Allows visualization of uterine lining through insertion of scope through cervix. Used to diagnose and treat abnormal bleeding, such as polyps and fibroids. Biopsy may be done during procedure. May be part of infertility assessment.	*Before:* Should be NPO for at least 6 hr prior. May be done in the HCP's office or an outpatient setting. *After:* Tell patient that mild cramping and slight bloody discharge is normal.
Laparoscopy	Allows visualization of pelvic structures via fiberoptic scopes inserted through small abdominal incisions. Instillation of CO_2 into the abdominal cavity improves visualization. Used in diagnostic assessment of uterus, tubes, and ovaries (Fig. 50.9). Often used for tubal sterilization or part of infertility assessment.	*Before:* Prepare patient for vaginal operation with preoperative teaching and sedation. *After:* Tell patient referred shoulder pain is likely from residual gas in the abdomen. A heating pad may help. A slight discharge or spotting for 2–5 days is normal.
Loop electrosurgical excision procedure (LEEP)	Excision of cervical tissue via an electrosurgical instrument. Diagnoses and treats cervical dysplasia. Minimal amount of tissue removed and preserves childbearing ability.	*Before:* Teach about procedure. May be done in the HCP's office. Patient may feel slight tingling or abdominal cramping during procedure. *After:* Tell patient that discharge, bleeding, and cramping may occur for 1–3 days.
Ultrasound-guided biopsy	Use of ultrasound guidance while performing a biopsy. Ultrasound used to direct the biopsy needle into the region of interest and obtain a sample of tissue. Can diagnose infection, inflammation, or mass.	*Before:* Teach about procedure. Usually done as an outpatient. *After:* Tell patient to monitor for signs and symptoms of infection at biopsy site.

DES, Diethylstilbestrol.

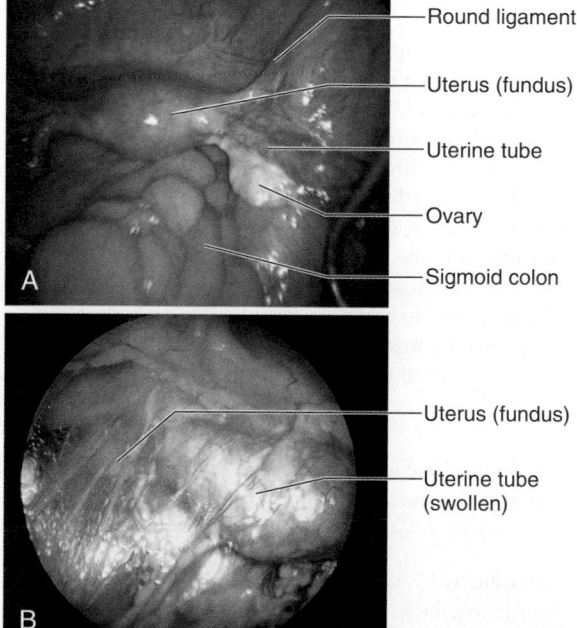

Round ligament
Uterus (fundus)
Uterine tube
Ovary
Sigmoid colon

A

Uterus (fundus)
Uterine tube (swollen)

B

FIG 50.9 Laparoscopic views of the female pelvis. A, Normal image. B, Pelvic inflammatory disease. (Note reddish inflammatory membrane covering and fixing the ovary and uterus to the surrounding structures.) (*A,* From Abrahams P, Marks S, Hutching R: *McMinn's color atlas of human anatomy,* ed 5, Philadelphia, 2003, Saunders. *B,* From Symonds EM, MacPherson MB: *Color atlas of obstetrics and gynecology,* London, 1994, Mosby Wolfe.)

TABLE 50.13 Cytology and Microbiologic Studies

Study	Description and Purpose
Cultures	Specimens from urine to assess for gonorrhea, chlamydia or UTIs. Rectal and throat cultures may be taken depending on data from sexual history.
Gram stain	Used for rapid detection of gonorrhea. Presence of gram-negative intracellular diplococci generally needs treatment. Not highly accurate for women. A valid alternative for chlamydia testing.
Nucleic acid amplification test (NAAT)	Nonculture test used to identify small amounts of DNA or RNA in test samples. Sensitivity similar to culture tests. Uses ligase or polymerase chain reaction that amplifies the signal of the nucleic acids in the test sample so that they are easier to identify. CDC preferred method to test for gonorrhea, chlamydia, and trichomoniasis. Can be done on a wide variety of samples, including vaginal, endocervical, urethral, urine, rectal, and pharyngeal.
Papanicolaou (Pap) test	Microscopic study of exfoliated cervical cells to detect abnormal cells. *Conventional cytology* entails fixing cells directly to a slide at the time of collection and sending the slide to the laboratory for interpretation. In *liquid-based cytology* the specimen is sent to the laboratory in a liquid solution that preserves it and is processed for microscopic evaluation at the laboratory. Testing for HPV may be done on specimen obtained for liquid-based Pap test (see Chapter 53).
Wet mounts	Direct microscopic examination of vaginal discharge specimen is done immediately after collection. Determines presence or absence and number of *Trichomonas* organisms, bacteria, white and red blood cells, and candidal buds or hyphae.

TABLE 50.14 Fertility Studies

Study	Description and Purpose
Basal body temperature assessment	Indirectly indicates whether ovulation has occurred. Temperature rises at ovulation and stays high during secretory phase of normal menstrual cycle.
Semen analysis	Assesses semen for volume (2–5 mL), viscosity, sperm count (>20 million/mL), sperm motility (60% motile), and percent of abnormal sperm (60% with normal structure).
Serum anti-müllerian hormone, estradiol, FSH, progesterone	Same as serology studies. See Table 50.10.
Urinary LH	Over-the-counter "ovulation predictor kits." Identifies midcycle LH surge that precedes ovulation by 1 to 2 days.

■ BRIDGE TO NCLEX EXAMINATION

The number of the question corresponds to the same-numbered outcome at the beginning of the chapter.

1. A normal male reproductive function that may be altered in a patient who undergoes an orchiectomy (removal of testes) is the production of
   a. PSA.
   b. GnRH.
   c. testosterone.
   d. seminal fluid.

2. Luteinizing hormone (LH) secretion by the anterior pituitary (*select all that apply*)
   a. results in ovulation.
   b. causes follicles to complete maturation.
   c. affects development of ruptured follicles.
   d. directly inhibits both GnRH and FSH secretion.
   e. stimulates testosterone production by interstitial cells of testes.

3. Female orgasm is characterized by
   a. resolution.
   b. increased breast size.
   c. relaxation of cervical os.
   d. vasoconstriction and dystonia.

4. An age-related finding during the assessment of the older woman's reproductive system is
   a. vaginal atrophy.
   b. increased libido.
   c. nipple enlargement.
   d. increased vulvar skin turgor.

5. Significant information about a person's health history related to the reproductive system should include (*select all that apply*)
   a. tobacco use.
   b. intellectual status.
   c. number of sexual partners.
   d. previous history of shingles.
   e. previous sexually transmitted infections.

6. Nucleic acid amplification tests (NAATs) used in the diagnosis of STIs can be obtained from (*select all that apply*)
   a. urine.
   b. vagina.
   c. urethra.
   d. rectum.
   e. endocervix.

7. An abnormal finding noted during physical assessment of the male reproductive system is
   a. descended testes.
   b. symmetric scrotum.
   c. slight clear urethral discharge.
   d. the glans covered with prepuce.

8. The nurse is caring for a patient scheduled for hysteroscopy. The nurse explains to the woman that
   a. the procedure treats cervical dysplasia.
   b. bleeding and discharge are rare after the procedure.
   c. the procedure involves curettage of the endometrial lining.
   d. the procedure allows visualization of the lining of the uterus.

1. c, 2. a, b, c, e; 3. c, 4. a, 5. a, c, e; 6. a, b, c, d, e; 7. c, 8. d

For rationales to these answers and even more NCLEX review questions, visit *http://evolve.elsevier.com/Lewis/medsurg*.

ⓔ EVOLVE WEBSITE/RESOURCES LIST

http://evolve.elsevier.com/Lewis/medsurg
Review Questions (Online Only)
Key Points
Answer Keys for Questions
 • Rationales for Bridge to NCLEX Examination Questions
Answer Guidelines for the Case Study on pp. 1178, 1182, and 1183
Conceptual Care Map Creator
Audio Glossary
Supporting Media
 • Animations
 • Ovulation

 • Reproductive System Overview
 • Spermatogenesis
Content Updates

REFERENCES

1. Patton KT, Thibodeau GA: *Structure and function of the body*, ed 15, St Louis, 2016, Elsevier.
2. Strauss J. Barbieri R: *Yen and Jaffe's reproductive endocrinology: Physiology, pathophysiology, and clinical management*, ed 8, Philadelphia, 2018, Elsevier.
3. Masters WH, Johnson E: *Human sexual response*, Boston, 1966, Little Brown. (Classic)
4. Knudtson J, McLaughlin JE: Effects of aging on the female reproductive system. Retrieved from *www.merckmanuals.com/home/women-s-health-issues/biology-of-the-female-reproductive-system/effects-of-aging-on-the-female-reproductive-system*.

*5. Cobin RH, Goodman NF: American Association of Clinical Endocrinologists and American College of Endocrinology position statement on menopause—2017 update, *Endoc Pract* 23:869, 2017.

*6. Centers for Disease Control and Prevention: Pregnancy and rubella. Retrieved from *www.cdc.gov/rubella/pregnancy.html*.

7. Male reproductive endocrinology: Effects of aging. Retrieved from *https://medlineplus.gov/ency/article/004017.htm*.

8. The American College of Obstetricians and Gynecologists: The menopause years. Retrieved from *www.acog.org/Patients/FAQs/The-Menopause-Years*.

*9. Manson JE, Aragaki AK, Rossouw JE, et al: Menopausal hormone therapy and long-term all-cause and cause-specific mortality: The Women's Health Initiative randomized trials, *JAMA* 318:927, 2017.

*10. American Cancer Society: Can prostate cancer be found early? Retrieved from *www.cancer.org/cancer/prostatecancer/detailedguide/prostate-cancer-detection*.

*11. Centers for Disease Control and Prevention: Health effects of cigarette smoking. Retrieved from *www.cdc.gov/tobacco/data_statistics/fact_sheets/health_effects/effects_cig_smoking/*.

12. deSanjose S, Brotons, M, Pavon MA: The natural history of human papillomavirus infection, *Best Pract Res Clin Obstet Gynaecol* 47:2, 2018.

*13. Centers for Disease Control and Prevention: Folic acid recommendations. Retrieved from *www.cdc.gov/ncbddd/folicacid/recommendations.html*.

14. Tonolini M: *Imaging and intervention in urinary tract infections and urosepsis*, New York, 2018, Springer.

15. American College of Obstetrics and Gynecology: Opinion on the female athletic triad. Retrieved from *https://www.acog.org/Resources-And-Publications/Committee-Opinions/Committee-on-Adolescent-Health-Care/Female-Athlete-Triad*.

16. American Cancer Society: American Cancer Society recommendations for the early detection of breast cancer. Retrieved from *www.cancer.org/cancer/breast-cancer/screening-tests-and-early-detection/american-cancer-society-recommendations-for-the-early-detection-of-breast-cancer.html*.

*Evidence-based information for clinical practice.

51

Breast Disorders

Deena Dell

Caring for others is an expression of what it means to be fully human.

Hillary Clinton

ⓔ http://evolve.elsevier.com/Lewis/medsurg

CONCEPTUAL FOCUS

Coping	Infection	Sexuality
Cellular Regulation	Pain	

LEARNING OUTCOMES

1. State screening guidelines for the early detection of breast cancer.
2. Explain the types, causes, clinical manifestations, and interprofessional and nursing management of common benign breast disorders.
3. State the risk factors for breast cancer.
4. Describe the pathophysiology and clinical manifestations of breast cancer.
5. Describe the interprofessional and nursing management of breast cancer.
6. Specify the physical and psychologic aspects of nursing management for the patient undergoing breast cancer surgery.
7. Explain the indications for, types and complications of, and nursing management after reconstructive breast surgery.

KEY TERMS

ductal ectasia, p. 1194
fibroadenoma, p. 1193
fibrocystic changes, p. 1192
galactorrhea, p. 1193

gynecomastia, p. 1194
intraductal papilloma, p. 1193
lumpectomy, p. 1199
lymphedema, p. 1199

mammoplasty, p. 1207
mastalgia, p. 1191
mastitis, p. 1192
Paget's disease, p. 1196

Breast disorders are a significant health concern for women. Whether the actual diagnosis is a benign condition or a cancer, the initial discovery of a lump or change in the breast often triggers intense feelings of anxiety and fear. The potential loss of a breast, or part of a breast, may be devastating for many women because of the significant psychologic, social, sexual, and body image implications associated with it.

The most common breast disorders in women are fibrocystic changes, fibroadenoma, intraductal papilloma, ductal ectasia, and breast cancer. In a woman's lifetime, there is a 1 in 8 (12%) chance that she will be diagnosed with breast cancer.[1] Although rare, breast cancer does occur in men. Being aware of personal risk, including genetic factors, and taking part in recommended screening are important health promotion activities.

ASSESSMENT OF BREAST DISORDERS

Breast Cancer Screening Guidelines

Screening guidelines for the early detection of breast cancer vary depending on a woman's age and risk. For women at average risk for breast cancer, these are the American Cancer Society (ACS) recommended guidelines[2]:

- Women should undergo regular screening mammography starting at age 45 years.
- Women should be offered the chance to begin screening between the ages of 40 and 44.
- Women aged 45 to 54 years should be screened annually.
- Women 55 years and older should transition to biennial screening or be able to continue screening annually.
- Women should continue screening if their overall health is good, and they have a life expectancy of 10 years or longer.
- The ACS does not recommend depending on clinical breast examination (CBE) for breast cancer screening among average-risk women at any age.

Women at increased risk for breast cancer (family history, genetic link, prior breast cancer, history of thoracic radiation therapy, or certain atypical findings on a prior breast biopsy) should talk with their HCP about the benefits and limitations of starting screening earlier with 3D mammography and breast magnetic resonance imaging (MRI) and having more frequent clinical breast encounters. A clinical encounter includes an assessment of risk factors, instruction in ways to reduce the risk factors, and a CBE.[3]

Consistent breast self-examination (BSE) may be a useful way to increase self-awareness of how one's breast normally look and feel. However, research has shown that BSE has no effect on reducing deaths from breast cancer. However, you still need to teach women the importance of knowing how their breasts look and feel and to report breast changes (e.g., nipple discharge, a lump) to their HCP.[3]

If a woman wants to learn about BSE, include information related to potential benefits, limitations, and harm (chance of a false-positive test result). Allow time for questions about the procedure and a return demonstration. For women who choose to perform BSE, teach the method described at *www.breastcancer.org/symptoms/testing/types/self_exam/bse_steps*.

Diagnostic Studies

Radiologic Studies. We use several techniques to screen for breast disorders or to help diagnose a suspicious physical finding. *Mammography* is a method used to visualize the breast's internal structure using x-rays (Fig. 51.1). This generally well-tolerated procedure can detect suspicious lumps that cannot be felt. Mammography has significantly improved the early and accurate detection of breast cancer. Improved imaging technology has reduced the radiation dose from mammography.

A comparison of current and prior mammograms may show early tissue changes. Because some tumors metastasize late, early detection by mammography allows for earlier treatment and the prevention of metastasis. In younger women, mammography is less sensitive because of the greater density of breast tissue, resulting in more false-negative results.

With digital mammography x-ray images are digitally coded and stored in a computer (Fig. 51.1). Digital mammograms are more accurate than traditional film mammography in younger women with dense breasts. The availability and associated costs of digital mammography are issues related to this technology.

3D mammography, or tomosynthesis mammography, produces a 3D image of the breast. It gives a clearer view of

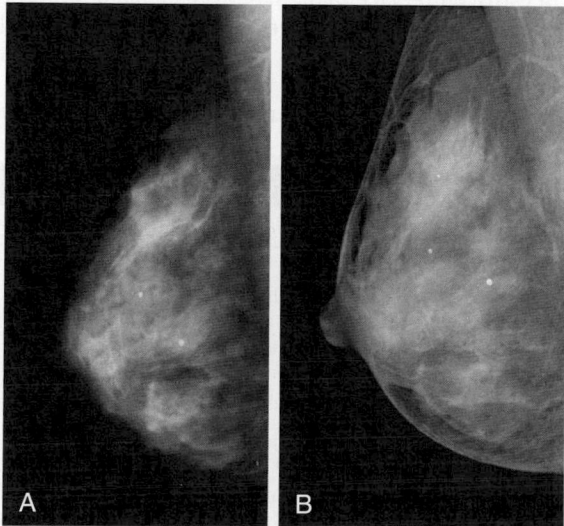

FIG. 51.1 Screening mammogram showing dense breast tissue and benign, scattered microcalcifications of a 57-year-old. **A,** Using conventional x-rays. **B,** Using digital x-rays. (From Adam A, Dixon AK, Grainger RG, et al: *Grainger and Allison's diagnostic radiology*, ed 5, St Louis, 2008, Churchill Livingstone.)

overlapping breast tissue structures. It can increase the numbers of cancers detected and decrease the number of false-positive results (a result stating a cancer is present when it is not).[3]

Calcifications are the most easily recognized mammogram abnormality (Fig. 51.1). These deposits of calcium crystals form in the breast for many reasons, such as inflammation, trauma, and/or aging. Although most calcifications are benign, they may be associated with breast cancer.

About 10% to 15% of all breast cancers cannot be seen on mammography. They may be detected by palpation or other breast imaging studies, such as ultrasound and MRI. If the clinical findings are suspicious and the mammogram is normal, an ultrasound or MRI may be done. Based on these findings, a biopsy may be done.

Ultrasound is used in conjunction with mammography to discern a solid mass from a cystic mass, to evaluate a mass in a pregnant or lactating woman, and to locate and biopsy a suspicious lesion. MRI is recommended as a screening tool in addition to mammography for women who are at high risk for breast cancer (e.g., first-degree relative with a *BRCA* mutation).[3]

Biopsies. A definitive diagnosis of a suspicious area is made by analyzing biopsied tissue. Biopsy techniques include *fine-needle aspiration* (FNA), core (core needle), vacuum-assisted, and excisional biopsies.

FNA biopsy is done by inserting a needle into a lesion to sample fluid from a breast cyst, remove cells from intercellular spaces, or sample cells from a solid mass. Before the procedure, the breast area is first locally anesthetized. Then the needle is placed into the breast, and fluid and cells are aspirated into a syringe. Usually 3 or 4 passes are made. If the results are negative with a suspicious lesion, another biopsy may be necessary.

A *core (core needle) biopsy* involves removing small samples of breast tissue using a hollow "core" needle. For palpable lesions, this is done by fixing the lesion with one hand and performing a needle biopsy with the other. In the case of nonpalpable lesions, *stereotactic mammography*, ultrasound, or MRI image guidance is used. Stereotactic mammography uses computers to pinpoint the exact location of a breast mass based on mammograms. With ultrasound, the HCP watches the needle on the ultrasound monitor to help guide it to the area of concern. Because a core biopsy removes more tissue than an FNA, it is more accurate.

Vacuum-assisted biopsy is a version of core biopsy that uses a vacuum technique to help collect the tissue sample. In core biopsy, several separate needle insertions are used to obtain multiple samples. During vacuum-assisted biopsy, the needle is inserted only once into the breast, and the needle can be rotated, which allows for multiple samples through a single needle insertion.

Minimally invasive breast biopsies have become the standard of care for diagnosing abnormalities found either on imaging studies or through CBE. However, in some cases an *excisional biopsy* is recommended. An excisional biopsy is done in an operating room.

BENIGN BREAST DISORDERS

MASTALGIA

Mastalgia, or breast pain, is the most common breast-related symptom reported in women. The most common form is *cyclic mastalgia*, which coincides with the menstrual cycle.[4] Women describe it as diffuse bilateral breast tenderness or heaviness. Breast pain may last 2 or 3 days or most of the month and is related to hormonal sensitivity. The symptoms often decrease with menopause.

Noncyclic mastalgia has no relationship to the menstrual cycle and can continue into menopause. It may be constant or intermittent throughout the month and last for several years. Symptoms include a burning, aching, or soreness in the breast. It usually affects only 1 breast. The pain may be from trauma, fat necrosis, ductal ectasia, costochondritis, or arthritic pain in the chest or neck radiating to the breast.

For patients with breast pain, mammography and targeted ultrasound are often done to exclude cancer and provide information on the cause of the pain. Evidence supporting treatments for benign breast pain have yielded conflicting results. Some relief for cyclic pain may occur by reducing intake of caffeine and dietary fat; taking vitamin E or gamma-linolenic acid (evening primrose oil); and continually wearing a supportive bra. Compresses, ice, analgesics, and antiinflammatory drugs may help. Tamoxifen may provide relief with few side effects. Danazol is an FDA approved treatment. The androgenic side effects (acne, edema, hirsutism) make this therapy unacceptable for many women. Finally, you need to reassure women that mastalgia is not a usual sign of breast cancer.[4]

BREAST INFECTIONS

Mastitis

Mastitis is an inflammatory condition of the breast that occurs most often in lactating women (Table 51.1). *Lactational mastitis* presents as a localized area that is erythematous, painful, and tender to palpation. Fever is often present. The infection develops when organisms (usually staphylococci) gain access to the breast through a cracked nipple. In its early stages, mastitis can be cured with antibiotics. Breastfeeding should continue unless an abscess is forming, or there is purulent drainage. The mother may wish to use a nipple shield or to hand-express milk from the involved breast until the pain subsides. The woman should see her HCP promptly to begin a course of antibiotic therapy. Any breast that stays red, tender, and not responsive to antibiotics requires follow-up care and evaluation for inflammatory breast cancer.[4,5]

Mastitis sometimes develops in women who are not lactating. This is called *periductal mastitis*. It is seen most often in regular smokers aged late 20s to early 30s. Treatment is the same as for lactating mastitis.

Lactational Breast Abscess

If lactational mastitis persists after several days of antibiotic therapy, a lactational breast abscess may be present. In this condition, the skin may become red and edematous over the involved breast, often with a corresponding palpable mass, and the patient may have a fever. Antibiotics alone are insufficient treatment for a breast abscess. Ultrasound-guided drainage of the abscess or surgical incision and drainage are needed. The drainage is cultured, sensitivities are obtained, and therapy with the appropriate antibiotic is begun. Breastfeeding can continue in most cases with ongoing treatment of the abscess.

FIBROCYSTIC CHANGES

Fibrocystic changes in the breast are benign conditions characterized by changes in breast tissue (Fig. 51.2).[6,7] Fibrocystic changes are the most common breast disorder, occurring in more than 50% of women in North America. They occur most often in women between 30 and 50 years of age but may begin under 21 years of age in as many as 10% of women. Fibrocystic changes most often occur in women with premenstrual abnormalities, nulliparous women, women with a history of spontaneous abortion, nonusers of oral contraceptives, and women with early menarche and late menopause.

The use of the term *fibrocystic disease* is incorrect because the cluster of problems represent benign disorders. Fibrocystic changes include the development of excess fibrous tissue, hyperplasia of the epithelial lining of the mammary ducts, proliferation of mammary ducts, and cyst formation. We think these changes are due to a heightened responsiveness of breast tissue to circulating estrogen and progesterone. They may cause pain from chronic inflammation, edema, nerve irritation, and fibrosis. Pain and nodularity often increase over time. They tend to subside after menopause unless the woman is taking high doses of estrogen replacement. Symptoms related to fibrocystic changes often worsen in the premenstrual phase and subside after menstruation.

TABLE 51.1 Common Benign Breast Disorders

Disorder	Risk Factors	Clinical Manifestations
Lactational mastitis	Occurs in up to 10% of postpartum lactating mothers (both primipara and multipara), usually within first 3 mo after birth	• Warm to touch, indurated, painful, often unilateral • Most often caused by *Staphylococcus aureus*
Fibrocystic changes	Most common between ages 30 and 50	• Not usually discrete masses—nodularity instead • Usually accompanied by cyclic pain and tenderness • Mass(es) often cyclic in occurrence (movable, soft)
Cysts	Most common over age 35. Incidence decreases after menopause. Develop in over half of women in North America	• Palpable fluid-filled mass (movable, soft) • Multiple cysts can occur and recur • Rarely associated with breast cancer
Fibroadenoma	Often occurs in teens and those in their 20s	• Palpable mass (firm, movable), usually 1–3 cm in size • Rarely associated with breast cancer
Fat necrosis	Many women report a history of trauma to breast	• Usually a hard, tender, mobile, indurated mass with irregular borders
Ductal ectasia	Most common in women over 60 yr old. Considered a normal part of aging. May be due to duct obstruction or mastitis	• Nipple fixation, usually accompanied by nipple discharge of thick gray material • Often associated with breast pain

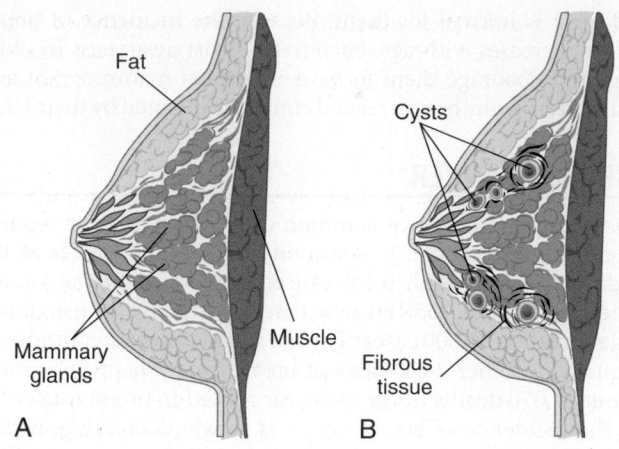

FIG. 51.2 A, Normal breast tissue. B, Fibrocystic breast tissue.

Manifestations of fibrocystic breast changes include 1 or more palpable lumps that are often round, well delineated, and freely movable within the breast (Table 51.1). Discomfort ranging from tenderness to pain may occur. The lump usually increases in size and sometimes tenderness before menstruation. Cysts may enlarge or shrink rapidly. Nipple discharge associated with fibrocystic breasts is often green or dark brown, not bloody.

Alone, fibrocystic changes are not associated with increased breast cancer risk. Masses or nodules can appear in both breasts. They often occur in the upper, outer quadrants and usually occur bilaterally.

Mammography may be helpful in distinguishing fibrocystic changes from breast cancer. However, in some women, the breast tissue is so dense that it is hard to obtain a mammogram. In these situations, ultrasound may be more useful in differentiating a fluid-filled cyst from a solid mass.

❖ **Interprofessional and Nursing Care**

With the discovery of a discrete mass in the breast by a woman or her HCP, aspiration or biopsy may be indicated. If the nodularity is recurrent, a wait of 7 to 10 days may be planned in order to note any changes that may be related to the menstrual cycle. With large or frequent cysts, an excisional biopsy may be preferred over repeated aspiration. An excisional biopsy may be done if (1) no fluid is found on aspiration, (2) the fluid is hemorrhagic, or (3) a residual mass remains after fluid aspiration. The biopsy is usually done in an outpatient surgery unit.

Severe fibrocystic changes may make palpation of the breast more difficult. Teach the woman with cystic changes to maintain regular follow-up care with her HCP and encourage breast self-awareness and to report any changes found so they can be evaluated.

Treatment for a fibrocystic condition is similar to that described earlier for mastalgia. Teach the woman with fibrocystic breasts that she may expect a recurrence of the cysts in 1 or both breasts until menopause, and that the cysts may enlarge or become painful just before menstruation. Reassure her that the cysts do not "turn into" cancer. Tell her that any new lump that does not respond in a cyclic manner over 1 to 2 weeks should be examined by her HCP.

FIBROADENOMA

Fibroadenoma is the most common cause of discrete benign breast lumps in young women. It generally occurs in women in their teens and twenties and is found more often in blacks than whites.

The possible cause of fibroadenoma may be increased estrogen sensitivity in a localized area of the breast. Fibroadenomas are usually small (but can be large [2 to 3 cm]), painless, round, well delineated, and very mobile. They are usually solid, firm, and rubbery in consistency. There is no accompanying retraction or nipple discharge. The fibroadenoma may appear as a single unilateral mass, although multiple bilateral fibroadenomas may occur. Growth is slow and often ceases when the size reaches 2 to 3 cm. Menstruation does not affect size. However, pregnancy can stimulate dramatic growth.

Fibroadenomas are easily detected by physical examination and may be visible on mammography and ultrasound. However, definitive diagnosis requires FNA, core, or excisional biopsy and tissue examination to exclude a cancer. Treatment can include observation with regular monitoring if cancer is not present, there are no symptoms, and the mass stays less than 3 cm. A fibroadenoma that increases in size and/or is symptomatic should be removed by surgical resection or, in some cases, cryotherapy. All new lesions should be evaluated by breast ultrasound and possible biopsy.[3]

NIPPLE DISCHARGE

Nipple discharge may occur spontaneously or because of nipple manipulation. A milky secretion is due to inappropriate lactation, or **galactorrhea**. It may be a result of certain medicines or endocrine or neurologic disorders. Nipple discharge may be idiopathic (no known cause).

Secretions can be serous, bloody, or brown to green. A cytology slide may be made of the secretion to determine the specific cause and recommended treatment. Disorders associated with nipple discharge include benign breast conditions, such as fibrocystic changes, intraductal papilloma, or ductal ectasia. In most cases, nipple discharge is not related to cancer.

ATYPICAL HYPERPLASIA

Atypical hyperplasia is usually found after a biopsy is done to evaluate a suspicious area found on a mammogram or during a CBE. It can be in either the ducts (atypical ductal hyperplasia) or in the lobules (atypical lobular hyperplasia). Both are associated with an increased risk for developing breast cancer. To follow up on a diagnosis of atypical hyperplasia, an excisional biopsy or lumpectomy may be done to remove all the affected tissue.[6]

INTRADUCTAL PAPILLOMA

An **intraductal papilloma** is a benign, soft or hard growth found in the mammary ducts. It is usually unilateral. Typically, the nipple has a bloody discharge that can be intermittent or spontaneous. Most intraductal papillomas are beneath the areola and may be difficult to palpate. They usually occur in women 30 to 50 years of age. A single duct or several ducts may be involved. Papillomas are associated with a slightly increased risk for developing breast cancer. So, a core biopsy should be done. If any abnormal cells are found, surgical excision of the papilloma and the involved duct or duct system is done.[8]

DUCTAL ECTASIA

Ductal ectasia (duct dilation) is a benign breast disease of perimenopausal and postmenopausal women involving the ducts in the subareolar area. It usually involves several bilateral ducts. Nipple discharge is the primary symptom. Ductal ectasia is initially painless but may progress to burning, itching, pain around the nipple, and swelling in the areolar area. Inflammatory signs are often present, and the nipple may retract. The discharge may become bloody in more advanced disease. It is not associated with cancer. If an abscess develops, warm compresses and antibiotics are usually effective treatments. Therapy consists of close follow-up examinations or surgical excision of the involved ducts.

MALE GYNECOMASTIA

Gynecomastia is a transient, noninflammatory enlargement of 1 or both breasts. It is the most common breast problem in men. The condition is usually temporary and benign. Gynecomastia itself is not a risk factor for breast cancer. The most common cause of gynecomastia is a change in the normal ratio of active androgen to estrogen in plasma or within the breast itself.[6]

Gynecomastia can occur in puberty. During puberty, there is often a transient relative imbalance between estrogen and testosterone, leading to gynecomastia. This condition usually resolves by age 20 years when adult androgen-to-estrogen ratios are reached. The treatment of pubertal gynecomastia is reassurance of the parent and teenager about the benign nature of the condition.

Gynecomastia can be a manifestation of other problems. It may accompany diseases such as testicular tumors, adrenal cancer, pituitary adenomas, hyperthyroidism, and liver disease. It can be a side effect of drug therapy, particularly with estrogen and androgen, digitalis, isoniazid, ranitidine, and spironolactone. Marijuana use can also cause gynecomastia.

Senescent Gynecomastia

Senescent gynecomastia occurs in many older men. The likely cause is high plasma estrogen levels with the increased conversion of androgens to estrogens in peripheral circulation. Although initially unilateral, the tender, firm, centrally located enlargement may become bilateral. A discrete, circumscribed mass with gynecomastia must be biopsied to determine if it is the rare breast cancer in males. Senescent hyperplasia needs no treatment. It usually regresses within 6 to 12 months.

Gerontologic Considerations: Age-Related Breast Changes

The loss of subcutaneous fat and structural support and the atrophy of mammary glands often result in pendulous breasts in the postmenopausal woman. Encourage older women to wear a well-fitting bra. Adequate support can improve physical appearance and reduce pain in the back, shoulders, and neck. It can also prevent *intertrigo*, dermatitis caused by friction between opposing surfaces of skin. Sagging breasts can be surgically lifted (mastopexy).

The decrease in glandular tissue makes a breast mass easier to palpate. This decreased density likely results from age-related decreases in estrogen. Rib margins may be palpable in a thin woman and can be confused with a mass. That is why it is so important that women become familiar with their own breasts

and what is normal for them. Because the incidence of breast cancer increases with age, encourage breast awareness in older women. Encourage them to have an annual mammogram and CBE and have any breast-related concern evaluated by their HCP.

BREAST CANCER

Breast cancer is the most common cancer in American women except for skin cancer. It is second only to lung cancer as the leading cause of death from cancer in women. In the United States, more than 255,180 new cases of invasive breast cancer and more than 60,000 cases of in situ breast cancer are diagnosed annually. Another 2470 cases of breast cancer happen in men. About 41,070 deaths occur each year related to breast cancer.[1]

The incidence of breast cancer is slowly decreasing, with a slight drop in the number of deaths related to breast cancer. This decline may be the result of the decreased use of hormone therapy after menopause as well as earlier detection and advances in treatment. Breast cancer survivors are the largest group of any cancer survivors.[1]

Etiology and Risk Factors

Although we do not completely understand the cause, several risk factors are related to breast cancer (Table 51.2). Risk factors

TABLE 51.2 Risk Factors for Breast Cancer

Risk Factor	Comments
Age ≥50 yr	Majority found in postmenopausal women
	After age 60, ↑ in incidence
Alcohol use	Drinking ≥1 alcoholic beverage per day may have an ↑ risk
Benign breast disease with atypical epithelial hyperplasia, lobular carcinoma in situ	Atypical changes in breast biopsy ↑ risk
Early menarche (before age 12), late menopause (after age 55)	A long menstrual history ↑ risk
Exposure to ionizing radiation	Radiation damages DNA (e.g., prior treatment for Hodgkin's lymphoma)
Family history	Breast cancer in a first-degree relative, particularly when premenopausal or bilateral
Female	Women account for 99% of breast cancer cases
First full-term pregnancy after age 30, nulliparity, no breastfeeding	Prolonged exposure to unopposed estrogen ↑ risk
Genetic factors (*BRCA1, BRCA2, P53, PTEN, PALB2, ATM, CHEK2, NBM*)	Gene mutations play a role in up to 10% of breast cancer cases
Hormone use	Use of estrogen and/or progesterone as hormone therapy, especially in postmenopausal women
Long-term heavy smoking	May ↑ risk, especially in women who begin smoking before first pregnancy
Personal history of breast, colon, endometrial, or ovarian cancer	Personal history significantly ↑ risk for breast cancer, risk for cancer in other breast, and recurrence
Physical inactivity	Risk ↑s most after menopause
Weight gain and obesity after menopause	Fat cells store estrogen, which ↑ the risk for developing breast cancer

appear to be cumulative and interacting. So, the presence of multiple risk factors may greatly increase the overall risk, especially for people with a positive family history.

Risk Factors for Women. The risk factors most associated with breast cancer include female gender and advancing age. Women are at far greater risk than men, with 99% of breast cancers occurring in women. Increasing age also increases the risk for developing breast cancer. The incidence of breast cancer in women under 25 years of age is very low. Risk increases gradually until age 60. After age 60, the incidence increases dramatically.

Hormonal regulation of the breast is related to breast cancer development, but the mechanisms are poorly understood. The hormones estrogen and progesterone may act as tumor promoters to stimulate breast cancer growth if cancer changes in the cells have already occurred. The Women's Health Initiative study showed that combined hormone therapy (estrogen plus progesterone) (1) increases the risk for breast cancer after as little as 2 years use and (2) increased the risk for having a larger, more advanced breast cancer at diagnosis. Using estrogen therapy alone for longer than 15 years (for women with a prior hysterectomy) increases a woman's long-term risk for breast cancer in some studies.[9] A link also exists between oral contraceptive use and increased risk for breast cancer. This risk decreases when use stops and is gone after 10 years.

Modifiable risk factors include excess weight gain during adulthood, sedentary lifestyle, smoking, dietary fat intake, obesity, and alcohol use. Environmental factors, such as radiation exposure, may play a role.

Genetic Link

Family history of breast cancer is an important risk factor, especially if the involved family member also had ovarian cancer, was premenopausal, had bilateral breast cancer, or is a first-degree relative (i.e., mother, father, sister, brother, daughter). Having any first-degree relative with breast cancer doubles a woman's risk for breast cancer, especially if the relative was diagnosed at a young age.[10,11] A breast cancer risk assessment tool for HCPs is available *(www.cancer.gov/bcrisktool)*. Genetic counseling must be considered for a person at high risk for breast cancer.

Up to 10% of all breast cancers are hereditary. This means that specific genetic abnormalities that contribute to breast cancer development have been inherited. Most inherited cases of breast cancer are associated with mutations in 2 genes: *BRCA1* and *BRCA2*. *BRCA* stands for *BR*east *CA*ncer. Everyone has *BRCA* genes. The *BRCA1* gene, found on chromosome 17, is a tumor suppressor gene that inhibits tumor development when functioning normally. Women who have *BRCA1* mutations have a 41% to 90% lifetime chance of developing breast cancer along with an increased risk for developing cancer in the other breast. The *BRCA2* gene, found on chromosome 11, is another tumor suppressor gene. Women with a mutation of this gene have a similar risk for breast cancer.[10,11]

In addition to *BRCA* gene mutations, we have identified many other abnormal genes that increase a person's risk for developing breast cancer. These include the tumor suppressor genes *p53* and *PTEN* (which inhibit tumor development when functioning normally), *ATM and NBM* (which help to repair damaged deoxyribonucleic acid [DNA]), *CHEK2* (which stops tumor growth), *PALB2* (which partners with *BRCA* to suppress tumor growth), and *CDH1* (which makes a protein to bind cells together).[12]

Most people who develop breast cancer do not have an abnormal breast cancer gene or a family history of breast cancer.

GENETICS IN CLINICAL PRACTICE

Breast Cancer

Genetic Basis
- Mutations occur in *BRCA1* and/or *BRCA2* genes.
- Normally, these genes are tumor suppressor genes involved in DNA repair.
- Transmission is autosomal dominant.
- Other genes (e.g., *ATM, CHEK-2, p53, PTEN, PALB2, NBM, NF1, STR11, CHD1*) may increase the risk for breast cancer.

Incidence
- Up to 10% of breast cancers are related to *BRCA1* and *BRCA2* gene mutations.
- As many as 1 in 300 to 800 women in the United States have *BRCA1* and *BRCA2* gene mutations.[11]
- Women with *BRCA1* and *BRCA2* gene mutations have a 41% to 90% lifetime risk for developing breast cancer.
- Mutations in *BRCA* genes may cause as many as 90% of all inherited breast cancers.
- *BRCA1* and *BRCA2* gene mutations are associated with early-onset breast cancer that is more likely to involve both breasts.
- Men with mutations in *BRCA1* and *BRCA2* have an increased risk for breast cancer and prostate cancer.
- Family history of both breast and ovarian cancer increases the risk for having a *BRCA* mutation.

Genetic Testing
- DNA testing is available for *BRCA1* and *BRCA2* gene mutations.
- Genetic tests can analyze an entire panel of genes in specific breast cancer patient populations.

Clinical Implications
- Most breast cancers (about 90%) are not inherited. They are associated with genetic changes that occur after a person is born (somatic mutations). There is no risk for passing on the mutated gene to children.
- Bilateral oophorectomy and/or bilateral mastectomy reduces the risk for breast cancer and ovarian cancer in women with *BRCA1* and *BRCA2* mutations.
- Women with *BRCA* mutations have a higher risk for developing ovarian, colon, pancreatic, and uterine cancers.[11]
- Genetic counseling and testing for *BRCA* mutations should be offered to patients whose personal or family history puts them at high risk for a genetic predisposition to breast cancer.

Ongoing research continues to look at the role of genes in the development of breast cancer.

Risk Factors for Men. Predisposing risk factors for breast cancer in men include hyperestrogenism, a family history of breast cancer, and radiation exposure. A thorough examination of the male breast should be a routine part of a physical examination. Men in *BRCA*-positive families should consider genetic testing. Teach men who test positive for a *BRCA* gene mutation to be aware of how their breasts look and feel and to report any changes to their HCP. They should have a CBE every year starting at age of 35. Screening mammography is not recommended as there is no evidence showing this to be of benefit. These men should begin prostate screening at age 35 as they have an increased risk for developing prostate cancer.[11]

Prophylactic Oophorectomy and Mastectomy. In women with *BRCA1* or *BRCA2* mutations, prophylactic bilateral oophorectomy can decrease the risk for breast and ovarian cancers. Removing the ovaries lowers the risk for breast cancer because the ovaries are the main source of estrogen in a premenopausal woman. Removing the ovaries does not reduce the risk for breast cancer in postmenopausal women because the ovaries are not the main producers of estrogen in these women. Women with *BRCA* mutations also have a higher risk for developing breast cancer in the unaffected (contralateral) breast. So, they may, as might any woman who has a high risk for developing breast cancer choose, in consultation with her HCP and genetic counselor, to undergo prophylactic bilateral mastectomy.

Pathophysiology

The main components of the breast are lobules (milk-producing glands) and ducts (milk passages that connect the lobules and the nipple). In general, breast cancer arises from the epithelial lining of the ducts *(ductal carcinoma)* or from the epithelium of the lobules *(lobular carcinoma)*. Breast cancers may be in situ (within the duct) or invasive (invading through the wall of the duct).

Metastatic breast cancer is breast cancer that has spread to other organs. The most common sites are the bone, liver, lung, and brain. Cancer growth rates can range from slow to rapid. Factors that affect cancer prognosis are tumor size, axillary node involvement (the more nodes involved, the worse the prognosis), tumor differentiation, estrogen and progesterone receptor status, and *human epidermal growth factor receptor 2* (HER-2) status. HER-2 is a protein that helps regulate cell growth.[13]

Types of Breast Cancer

Breast cancer is not just one disease, but a group of diseases characterized by different pathologic findings and clinical behaviors. Breast cancer can be classified as (1) ductal or lobular or other or (2) noninvasive or invasive (Table 51.3). We can also classify it based on hormonal status and genetic subtypes.

Noninvasive Breast Cancer. An estimated 20% of breast cancers are noninvasive. These intraductal cancers include *ductal carcinoma in situ* (DCIS) and pure Paget's disease.[13]

DCIS tends to be unilateral and may progress to invasive breast cancer if left untreated. Treatment options include breast-conserving treatment (lumpectomy) with or without radiation therapy, total mastectomy with or without sentinel lymph node biopsy, and/or hormone therapy (e.g., tamoxifen) to prevent recurrences.[14]

In the past, *lobular carcinoma in situ* (LCIS) was considered a noninvasive breast cancer. However, it has now been reclassified as a benign condition that is a risk factor for developing breast cancer.[13] No surgical or radiation treatment is indicated for LCIS. Hormone therapy may be used as a preventive measure to reduce breast cancer risk for some patients.

Invasive Ductal Carcinoma. *Invasive (infiltrating) ductal carcinoma* is the most common type of breast cancer. It accounts for about 80% of all invasive breast cancers. It starts in the milk ducts, then breaks through the walls of the duct, invading the surrounding tissue. From there it may metastasize to other parts of the body. Subtypes of invasive ductal carcinoma include

TABLE 51.3 Classification of Breast Cancer

Based on Tissue Type
- Ductal carcinoma (affects milk ducts)
  - Medullary
  - Tubular
  - Colloid (mucinous)
- Lobular carcinoma (affects milk-producing glands)
- Other
  - Inflammatory
  - Paget's disease
  - Phyllodes tumor

Based on Invasiveness
Noninvasive (In situ)
- Ductal carcinoma in situ (DCIS)
- Pure Paget's disease

Invasive (Spreading to Other Locations)
- Invasive ductal carcinoma
- Invasive lobular carcinoma

Based on Hormone Receptor and Genetic Status
Estrogen and Progesterone Receptor Status
- Estrogen receptor positive
- Estrogen receptor negative
- Progesterone receptor positive
- Progesterone receptor negative

HER-2 Genetic Status
- HER-2 positive
- HER-2 negative

medullary carcinoma, tubular carcinoma, colloid (mucinous) carcinoma, papillary carcinoma, and metaplastic carcinoma.

Invasive Lobular Carcinoma. *Invasive (infiltrating) lobular carcinoma* begins in the lobules (milk-producing glands) of the breast. It accounts for about 10% to 15% of invasive breast cancers. The cancer cells can break out of the lobule and metastasize to other areas of the body. Invasive lobular carcinoma usually presents as a subtle thickening in the upper outer quadrant of the breast. It is often not detected by mammography.

Other Types of Breast Cancer

Inflammatory Breast Cancer. *Inflammatory breast cancer* is an aggressive and fast-growing breast cancer with a high risk for metastasis. It accounts for about 1% to 3% of all breast cancers. In the early stages, it is often mistaken for mastitis. However, the inflammatory changes do not improve with antibiotics, because cancer cells block the lymph channels in the skin of the breast. Because of skin involvement, the breast looks red, feels warm, and has a thickened appearance that is often described as looking like an orange peel *(peau d'orange)*. Sometimes, the breast develops ridges and small bumps that look like hives. A breast mass may not be present. Changes may not show up on mammograms, making diagnosis difficult. Inflammatory breast cancer is associated with a worse prognosis as compared to invasive ductal and lobular breast cancers.[14]

Paget's Disease. Paget's disease is a rare breast cancer that starts in the breast ducts and spreads to the nipple and areola. It causes about 1% of all breast cancers. It is different from Paget's disease of the bone, which is discussed in Chapter 63. Most women with Paget's disease have underlying ductal carcinoma. Only in rare cases is the cancer confined to the nipple and not associated with some invasive cancer (in situ).

Itching, burning, bloody nipple discharge with superficial skin erosion and ulceration may be present. A pathologic examination of the lesion confirms the diagnosis. Nipple changes are often diagnosed as an infection or dermatitis, which can lead to treatment delays.

The treatment of Paget's disease is surgical removal of the involved tissue by either central lumpectomy or mastectomy with or without sentinel node biopsy. Radiation therapy may be used after surgery. The prognosis is good when the cancer is confined to the nipple.[14]

Phyllodes Tumor. A phyllodes tumor is a very rare tumor that develops in the connective tissue (stroma) of the breast. The tumors tend to grow quickly, within a period of weeks or months, to a size of 2 to 3 cm or sometimes larger. Although most are benign, some are cancerous. Treatment is usually excision with a wide margin. Axillary surgery is not necessary.[14]

Triple-Negative Breast Cancer. A patient whose breast cancer tests negative for all 3 receptors (estrogen, progesterone, HER-2) has *triple-negative breast cancer*. Receptor testing is discussed on p. 1198. The incidence of triple-negative breast cancer is higher in blacks, Hispanics, premenopausal women, and those with a *BRCA1* mutation. These patients tend to have more aggressive tumors with a poorer prognosis. These cancers do not respond to hormone therapy or therapy for HER-2. Chemotherapy appears to be the more successful for treating triple-negative breast cancer.

Clinical Manifestations

Breast cancer is usually detected as a lump or thickening in the breast or mammography abnormality. It occurs most often in the upper, outer quadrant of the breast, which is the location of most of the glandular tissue (Fig. 51.3). Breast cancers vary in their growth rate. If palpable, breast cancer is characteristically hard and may be irregularly shaped, poorly delineated, nonmobile, and nontender.

A small number of breast cancers cause nipple discharge. The discharge is usually unilateral and may be clear or bloody. Nipple retraction may occur. Peau d'orange may occur due to plugging of the dermal lymphatics. In large cancers, infiltration, induration, and dimpling pulling in) of the overlying skin may occur.

Complications

The main complication of breast cancer is recurrence (Table 51.4). Recurrence may be *local* or *regional* (skin or soft tissue

near the mastectomy site, axillary or internal mammary lymph nodes) or distant. Widely disseminated or metastatic disease involves the growth of cancerous breast cells in parts of the body distant from the breast (most often involving the bone, lung, brain, liver). Metastases primarily occur through the lymphatics, usually those of the axilla (Fig. 51.4). However, metastatic disease can occur anywhere.

Diagnostic Studies

In addition to radiologic and biopsy studies used to diagnose breast cancer (see earlier discussion in this chapter on p. 1191), other tests are used to predict the risk for local or systemic recurrence. These tests include axillary lymph node analysis, tumor size, estrogen and progesterone receptor status, cell-proliferative indices (number of cells that are dividing), and genomic assays.

Axillary Lymph Node Analysis. Axillary lymph node involvement is an important prognostic factor in breast cancer. *Axillary lymph nodes* are often examined to see if cancer has spread to the axilla on the same side of the breast as the cancer (Fig. 51.4). The more nodes involved, the greater the risk for recurrence.

A *sentinel lymph node biopsy* (SLNB) helps to identify the lymph node(s) that drain first from the tumor site. Those nodes are called *sentinel node(s)* (SLN). In SLNB, a radioisotope and/or blue dye, which will travel the same route as the cancer, is injected into the affected breast. Then, in surgery, the

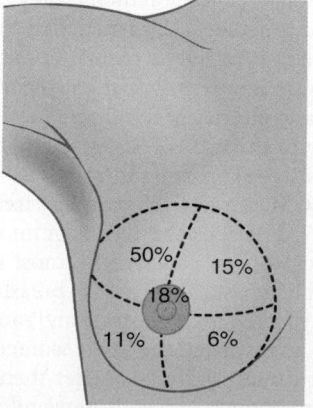

FIG. 51.3 Distribution of where breast cancer occurs.

TABLE 51.4 Sites of Breast Cancer Recurrence and Metastasis

Site	Manifestations
Local Recurrence	
Skin, chest wall	Firm, discrete nodules. Sometimes pruritic, usually painless, often in or near a scar
Regional Recurrence	
Lymph nodes	Enlarged nodes in axilla or supraclavicular area, usually nontender
Distant Metastasis	
Bone marrow	Anemia, infection, ↑ bleeding, bruising, petechiae. Weakness, fatigue, mild confusion, light-headedness, dyspnea
Brain	Headache described as "different," unilateral sensory loss, focal muscular weakness, hemiparesis, incoordination (ataxia), nausea and vomiting unrelated to medication, cognitive changes
Liver	Abdominal distention. Right lower quadrant abdominal pain sometimes radiating to scapular area. Nausea and vomiting, anorexia, weight loss. Weakness and fatigue. Hepatomegaly, ascites, jaundice. Peripheral edema. High liver enzymes
Lung (including lung nodules and pleural effusions)	Shortness of breath, tachypnea, nonproductive cough
Skeletal	Localized pain of gradually increasing intensity, percussion tenderness at involved sites, pathologic fracture caused by involvement of bone cortex
Spinal cord	Progressive back pain, localized and radiating. Change in bladder or bowel function. Loss of sensation in lower extremities

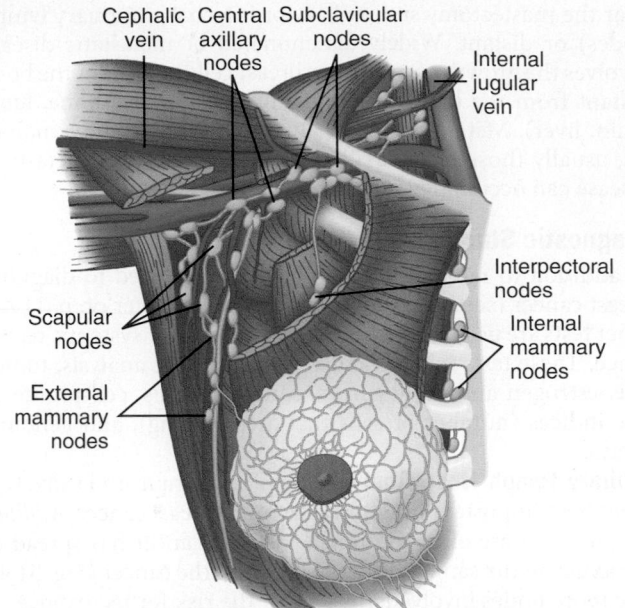

FIG. 51.4 Lymph nodes and drainage in the axilla. The sentinel lymph node is usually found in the external mammary nodes. A complete axillary dissection would remove all nodes. (From Donegan WL, Spratt JS: *Cancer of the breast*, ed 3, Philadelphia, 1988, Saunders.)

HCP determines if the radioisotope (using radioactive detector) or dye (visually see blue nodes) is found in any SLNs. A local incision is made in the axilla, and the HCP dissects the blue-stained and/or radioactive SLNs. Generally, with SLNB, 1 to 4 axillary lymph nodes are removed. The nodes are sent for pathologic analysis. If the SLNs are negative, no further axillary surgery is needed.

If the SLNs are positive, a complete *axillary lymph node dissection* (ALND) may be done. In an ALND, the HCP will typically remove 12 to 20 lymph nodes. SLNB is less invasive than ALND and is associated with lower morbidity rates compared with ALND.

Tumor Size. *Tumor size* is a prognostic variable. In general, the larger the tumor, the poorer the prognosis. The wide variety of biologic types of breast cancer explains the variability of disease behavior. In general, the more well differentiated (like the original cell type) the tumor, the less aggressive it is. The cells of poorly differentiated (unlike the original cell type) tumors appear morphologically disorganized, and they are more aggressive.

Estrogen and Progesterone Receptor Status. *Estrogen receptor (ER) and progesterone receptor (PR) status* is another diagnostic test useful for decisions about both treatment and prognosis. Receptor-positive tumors (1) often show histologic evidence of being well differentiated, (2) have a lower chance for recurrence, (3) often have a *diploid* (more normal) DNA content and low proliferative indices, and (4) are often hormone dependent and responsive to hormone therapy. Receptor-negative tumors (1) are often poorly differentiated histologically, (2) often recur, (3) have a high incidence of *aneuploidy* (abnormally high or low DNA content) and higher proliferative indices, and (4) are usually unresponsive to hormone therapy. Ploidy status (number of chromosomes in a cell) correlates with tumor aggressiveness. Diploid tumors have a much lower risk for recurrence than aneuploid tumors.

Cell-Proliferative Indices. *Cell-proliferative indices* indirectly measure the rate of tumor cell proliferation. The number of tumor cells in the synthesis (S) phase of the cell cycle (see Chapter 15, Fig. 15.1) is another important prognostic indicator. Although cell-proliferative indices are not routinely done as part of the breast cancer pathology evaluation, patients with cells that have high S-phase fractions have a higher risk for recurrence and earlier cancer death.

Genomic Assay. An important *genomic assay* is to determine HER-2, which is a prognostic indicator. Overexpression of HER-2 is associated with unusually aggressive tumor growth, a greater risk for recurrence, and a poorer prognosis. HER-2 is overexpressed in 10% to 20% of patients with breast cancer. The presence of HER-2 helps in the selection and sequence of drug therapy and predicts the patient's response to treatment.

A *genomic* test uses a sample of the breast cancer tissue to analyze the activity of a group of genes that can affect how a cancer is likely to behave and respond to treatment. Knowing whether certain genes are present or absent, or overly active or not active enough, can provide information about the risk for recurrence and the expected benefit of chemotherapy or hormone therapy. The 21-gene recurrence (OncotypeDX) test is the most often used genomic test.[15] Other genomic tests are MammaPrint, PAM50 (Prosigna), EndoPredict, and the Breast Cancer Index.

Interprofessional Care

A wide range of treatment options is available to the patient and HCPs making critical decisions about how to treat breast cancer (Table 51.5). The treatment plan is often determined by prognostic factors, the clinical stage, and biology of the cancer.

Staging of Breast Cancer. The most widely accepted staging method for breast cancer is the TNM system. This system uses traditional anatomic factors of tumor size (T), nodal involvement (N), and presence of metastasis (M) to determine the stage of disease (Table 51.6). The stages range from 0 to IV, with stage 0 being in situ cancer with no lymph node involvement and no metastasis. Stage IV indicates metastatic spread, regardless of tumor size or lymph node involvement. This system is used worldwide to communicate the size of a breast cancer and the extent to which it has spread. It provides an accurate prediction of the outcome of a group of patients.

The latest cancer staging guidelines add biologic factors in making the final determination of stage. These enable more accurate determination of prognosis and appropriate systemic therapy. These factors include tumor grade, hormone receptor expression, HER-2 overexpression and/or amplification, and genomic panels.[13]

For example, some larger tumors will now be considered stage I instead of stage II based on their biology. For patients with hormone receptor–positive, HER2-negative, lymph node–negative tumors, and a low-risk gene recurrence score, regardless of T size, place into the same prognostic category as T1a-T1b N0 M0. Patients with triple-negative tumors have survival equal to that of patients with disease 1 TNM stage higher who have ER, PR, or HER2-positive expressing tumors.

Surgical Therapy. Surgery is the primary treatment for breast cancer. Table 51.7 describes the most common surgical procedures used to treat breast cancer. The most common surgical options for operable breast cancer are (1) breast conservation surgery (lumpectomy [segmental mastectomy]) and (2) mastectomy with or without reconstruction. Most women diagnosed with early-stage breast cancer (tumors smaller than 5 cm) are candidates for either treatment choice. The overall survival rate with lumpectomy and radiation is the same as that with mastectomy.[14]

TABLE 51.5 Interprofessional Care

Breast Cancer

Diagnostic Assessment
Prediagnosis
- Health history, including risk factors
- Physical examination, including breast and lymph nodes
- Mammography
- Ultrasound (if indicated)
- Breast MRI (if indicated)
- Biopsy

Postdiagnosis
- Lymph node analysis
- Estrogen and progesterone receptor status
- Cell-proliferative indices
- HER-2 marker
- Genetic assays (e.g., MammaPrint, Oncotype DX)

Staging
- Complete blood count
- Liver function tests
- Chest x-ray (if indicated)
- CT scan of chest, abdomen, pelvis (if indicated)
- PET/CT, MRI, bone scans (if indicated)

Management
Surgical Therapy
- Breast-conserving surgery (lumpectomy) with SLNB and/or axillary lymph node dissection
- Simple (total) mastectomy with SLNB and/or axillary lymph node dissection
- Modified radical mastectomy
- Reconstructive surgery

Radiation Therapy
- External radiation
- Brachytherapy
- Palliative radiation therapy

Drug Therapy (Table 51.8)
- Chemotherapy
- Hormone therapy
- Immunotherapy
- Targeted therapy

TABLE 51.6 Staging of Breast Cancer

Stage	Tumor Size	Lymph Node Involvement	Metastasis
0	TIS (tumor in situ)	No	No
I			
A	<2 cm	No	No
B	<2 cm	<2 mm	No
II			
A	No evidence of tumor ranging to 5 cm	No, or 1–3 axillary nodes and/or internal mammary nodes	No
B	Ranging from ≤2 to >5 cm	No, or 1–3 axillary nodes and/or internal mammary nodes	No
III			
A	Ranging ≤2 to >5 cm	Yes, 1–9 axillary nodes and/or internal mammary nodes	No
B	Any size with extension to chest wall or skin	No, or 1–9 axillary nodes and/or internal mammary nodes	No
C	Any size	Yes, ≥10 axillary nodes, internal mammary nodes, or infraclavicular nodes	No
IV	Any size	Any type of nodal involvement	Yes

Adapted from Guiliano AE, Connolly JL, Edge SB, et al: Breast cancer: Major changes in the American Joint Committee on Cancer 8th edition cancer staging manual, *Cancer J Clin* 67:290, 2017.

It is important to note that breast reconstruction is an option for any woman undergoing surgical treatment for breast cancer. For women undergoing mastectomy, breast reconstruction can be done at the time of the mastectomy or delayed for months or even years. Women may opt to not have reconstruction and choose to use a breast prosthesis instead.

Breast-Conserving Surgery. Breast-conserving surgery, also called lumpectomy, involves removing the entire tumor along with a margin of normal surrounding tissue (Fig. 51.5, *A*). In some cases, it may take 2 or 3 more surgeries to remove all the cancer from the margins. After surgery, radiation therapy is usually delivered to the entire breast, ending with a boost to the tumor bed. If the risk for recurrence is high, chemotherapy may be given before radiation therapy.

Not everyone is a candidate for breast conservation surgery. Contraindications include breast size too small in relation to the tumor size to yield an acceptable cosmetic result, multifocal masses and calcifications, multicentric masses (in more than 1 quadrant), diffuse calcifications in more than 1 quadrant, or prior radiation therapy. Because of the time commitment (i.e., 3 to 7 weeks of daily radiation therapy treatments) and travel distances to access radiation therapy treatment centers, some patients may choose mastectomy over breast conservation surgery.

Axillary Lymph Node Analysis. SLNB is the preferred standard for axillary lymph node analysis and staging. It was described on p. 1197. However, if the SLN cannot be identified, or if the node is positive for cancer, ALND may have to be done.

Lymphedema. Lymphedema, an accumulation of lymph in soft tissue, can occur because of the lymph node sampling procedure or radiation therapy (Fig. 51.6). When the axillary nodes cannot return lymph fluid to the central circulation, the fluid accumulates in the arm, hand, or breast, causing obstructive pressure on the veins and venous return. The patient may have heaviness, impaired motor function in the arm, and numbness and paresthesia of the fingers. Cellulitis and progressive fibrosis of the skin can result from untreated lymphedema. (See further discussion on lymphedema later in this chapter on p. 1206.)

Mastectomy. A *total* or *simple mastectomy* removes the entire breast. A *modified radical mastectomy* includes removal of the breast and axillary lymph nodes. It preserves the pectoralis major muscle (Fig. 51.5, *B*). For women desiring breast reconstruction, a skin-sparing mastectomy provides the best cosmetic result and does not increase the chance of the cancer recurring. In a *nipple-sparing mastectomy,* the nipple and/or areola are left in place and the breast tissue under them is removed. Women who have a small, low-grade cancer near the outer part of the

TABLE 51.7 Surgical Procedures for Breast Cancer

Procedure	Side Effects	Complications	Patient Issues
Breast-Conserving Surgery (Lumpectomy) With Radiation Therapy			
Excision of tumor with no tumor at margins, sentinel lymph node biopsy (SLNB) and/or axillary lymph node dissection (ALND) Radiation therapy	• Breast soreness • Breast edema • Skin reactions • Arm swelling • Sensory changes in breast and arm	*Short-term:* moist desquamation,* hematoma, seroma, infection *Long-term:* fibrosis,* lymph-edema,† myositis, pneumoni-tis,* rib fractures*	• Prolonged treatment* • Impaired arm mobility† • Change in texture and sensitivity of breast
Mastectomy **Simple Mastectomy**	• Chest wall tightness, scar	*Short-term:* skin flap necrosis, seroma, hematoma, infection	• Loss of breast
Removal of breast, preservation of pectoralis muscle, SLNB may be done at same time **Modified Radical Mastectomy** Removal of breast with ALND, pectoralis muscle is spared	• Phantom breast sensations • Lymphedema • Sensory changes • Impaired range of motion	*Long-term:* sensory loss, muscle weakness, lymphedema	• Incision • Body image • Need for prosthesis • Impaired arm mobility
Breast Implants and Tissue Expansion			
Expander used to slowly stretch tissue. Saline gradually injected into reservoir over weeks to months Insertion of implant under muscu-lofascial layer of chest wall	• Discomfort • Chest wall tightness	*Short-term:* skin flap necrosis, wound separation, seroma, hematoma, infection *Long-term:* capsular contractions, displacement of implant	• Body image • Prolonged HCP visits to expand implants • Potential added surgeries for nipple construction, symmetry
Breast Reconstruction Tissue Flap Procedures‡			
Transverse Rectus Abdominis Musculocutaneous (TRAM) Flap			
Musculocutaneous flap (muscle, skin, fat, blood supply) is trans-posed from abdomen to the mastectomy site May be done concurrently with mastectomy	• Pain related to 2 surgical sites and extensive surgery	*Short-term:* delayed wound healing, infection, skin flap necrosis, abdominal hernia, hematoma	• Longer postoperative recovery
Deep Inferior Epigastric Artery Perforator (DIEP) Flap			
Free flap that transfers skin and fat from the abdomen to the chest. Differs from TRAM flap because no muscle is moved	• Requires more time in surgery than pedicle TRAM flap • Pain related to 2 surgical sites	Needs to be closely monitored first 24–48 hours after surgery. If flap fails, patient needs surgery	• Patients may have less pain and restriction of movement than with a pedicle TRAM flap.

*Specific to radiation therapy.
†If ALND (less likely with SLNB).
‡This list is not inclusive as other breast reconstruction options are available to patients.

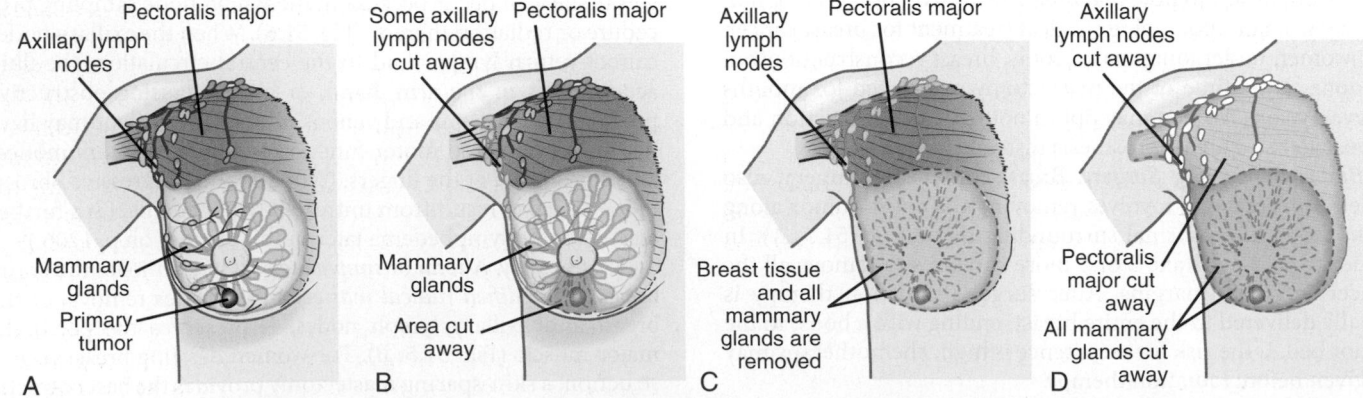

FIG. 51.5 Breast cancer surgery. A, Preoperative. B, Lumpectomy. C, Simple mastectomy. D, Modified radical mastectomy.

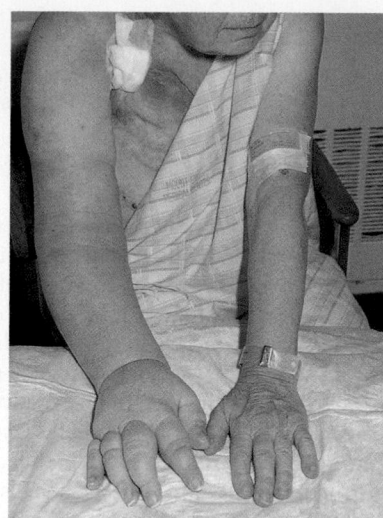

FIG. 51.6 Lymphedema. Accumulation of fluid in the tissue after excision of lymph nodes. (From Swartz MH: *Textbook of physical diagnosis: History and examination,* ed 6, Philadelphia, 2010, Saunders.)

breast, with no signs of cancer in the skin or near the nipple, may be able to have nipple-sparing surgery.[14]

For women who have a mastectomy, breast reconstruction can be done with the mastectomy or it can be delayed. Some women choose not to have reconstruction. There are 2 main types of breast reconstruction procedures: implant reconstruction or tissue flap procedures (Table 51.7). Breast reconstructive surgery is discussed on pp. 1207–1209.

Post–Breast Therapy Pain Syndrome. *Post–breast therapy pain syndrome* (PBTPS) occurs in some people who have had procedures for breast cancer. Most often it is caused by injury to nerves during surgery. However, it also can be due to chemotherapy and radiation therapy. The most common theory is that PBTPS results from injury to intercostobrachial nerves. These are sensory nerves that exit the chest wall muscles and provide sensation to the shoulder and upper arm.

Because of its multiple causes, PBTPS symptoms can range from mild to debilitating.[16] Common symptoms include chest and upper arm pain, tingling down the arm, continuous aching and burning, numbness, shooting or pricking pain, and unbearable itching that persists beyond the normal 3-month healing time. Edema may be present.

Treatment includes nonsteroidal antiinflammatory drugs (NSAIDs), low-dose antidepressants, topical anesthetics (e.g., EMLA [lidocaine and prilocaine]), and antiseizure drugs (e.g., gabapentin). Other treatments include biofeedback, physical therapy to prevent "frozen shoulder" syndrome from inadequate movement, guided imagery, and psychologic counseling with a therapist trained in the management of chronic pain syndromes.

Phantom Breast Pain. *Phantom breast pain* is feeling pain in the breast after the breast was removed via mastectomy. It occurs

❓ CHECK YOUR PRACTICE

You are working in the breast clinic and doing a postoperative assessment on a 56-yr-old woman who had a right radical mastectomy 6 weeks ago. She is reporting sharp, prickly feelings in her right arm. She tells you, "I also feel pain in the breast that was removed. Am I going crazy? That breast is not even attached to my body anymore!"
• How would you respond and what follow-up would you provide?

for the same reasons phantom limb sensation occurs after limb amputations. The brain continues to send signals to nerves in the breast area that were cut during surgery, even though the breast is no longer physically there.

Radiation Therapy. Radiation therapy is one *adjuvant (additional)* therapy that can be used after surgery. It is used for breast cancer to (1) prevent local breast cancer recurrences after breast-conserving surgery; (2) prevent local and lymph node recurrences after mastectomy; or (3) relieve pain caused by local, regional, or distant spread of cancer.

External Radiation Therapy. When radiation therapy is a primary treatment, it is usually done after surgery for the breast cancer. The decision to use radiation therapy after mastectomy is based on the chance that local, residual cancer cells are present. Radiation of the axilla and/or supraclavicular nodes may be done when lymph nodes are involved to decrease the risk for axillary recurrence. Radiating a localized area does not prevent distant metastasis.

In traditional whole breast, and in some cases regional lymph node, radiation treatment, the area is radiated 5 days per week over the course of about 5 to 7 weeks. An external beam of radiation delivers daily fractions to a total dose of 46 to 50 Gy (4500 to 5000 cGy). Patients who have had breast-conserving surgery may receive a "boost" dose of radiation to the area where the original tumor was located. It is given by external beam and adds 4 to 8 more treatments to the total number given.[14]

Newer and preferred regimens use a type of accelerated external beam radiation called hypofractionation. This type of radiation has a shortened schedule, daily for 3 to 4 weeks, with a total dose of 40 to 42.5 Gy.[14]

Fatigue, skin changes, and breast edema may be temporary side effects of external radiation therapy. Nursing management of the patient receiving radiation therapy is discussed in Chapter 15.

Brachytherapy. *Brachytherapy* (internal radiation) is used for partial-breast radiation. It is an alternative to traditional external radiation treatment for some patients with early-stage breast cancer.[14] This method has the same chance for local recurrence as whole breast radiation. However, some studies show the cosmetic results are not as good.

Brachytherapy is minimally invasive. The radiation is delivered directly into the cavity left after a tumor is surgically removed by a lumpectomy. Because the radiation is concentrated and focused on the area with the highest risk for tumor recurrence, it only requires 5 treatments. Therapy is delivered using a multicatheter method or balloon-catheter system.

In the *multicatheter method* (e.g., SAVI) many very small catheters are placed in the breast at the site of the tumor. The SAVI is inserted through a small incision, and the catheter bundle expands uniformly. The ends of the catheters stick out through little holes in the skin. Small radioactive seeds are placed in the catheters. The seeds are left in place just long enough to deliver the radiation dose (e.g., 5 to 10 minutes) then removed. The radiation does not remain in the body between treatments or after the last treatment is over.

In the *balloon-catheter system,* a balloon is placed where the tumor was located. The balloon is filled with fluid, to keep it in place, then radioactive seeds are inserted (Fig. 51.7). Radiation is emitted by a tiny radioactive seed attached by a wire to an afterloader, a computer-controlled machine. The seed travels through the MammoSite applicator into the inflated balloon. As with the multicatheter system, the radiation does not remain in

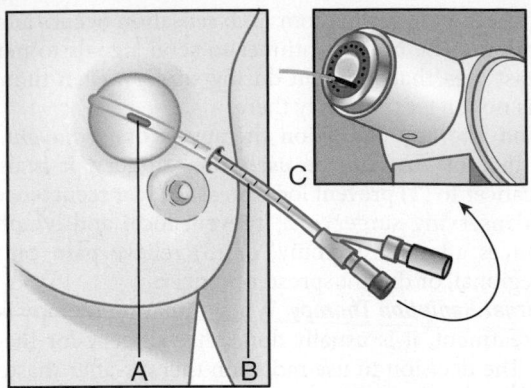

FIG. 51.7 High-dose brachytherapy for breast cancer. The MammoSite system involves the insertion of a single small balloon catheter *(B)* at the time of the lumpectomy or shortly thereafter into the tumor resection cavity (the space that is left after the HCP removes the tumor). A tiny radioactive seed *(A)* is inserted into the balloon, connected to a machine called an *after-loader (C)*, and delivers the radiation therapy.

the body between treatments or after the last treatment is over. Once the last session is done, the balloon is deflated, and the system is removed.

Palliative Radiation Therapy. In addition to reducing the primary tumor mass with a resultant decrease in pain, radiation therapy can be used to treat symptomatic metastatic lesions in such sites as bone, soft tissue organs, brain, and chest. Radiation therapy often relieves pain and is successful in controlling recurrent or metastatic disease.

Drug Therapy. Drug therapy includes chemotherapy, hormone therapy, immunotherapy, and targeted therapy. When drug therapy is given before surgery, we call it *neoadjuvant therapy*. Neoadjuvant therapy is often used to shrink the size of the tumor enough to make surgical removal possible or to allow for breast-conserving surgery in women who would have been recommended to have a mastectomy. It also allows time for genetic testing to occur (if appropriate) so a patient can make a more informed decision about what type of surgery to have. Drug therapy after surgery is called *adjuvant therapy*. Drug therapy can decrease the rate of recurrence and increase the length of survival. Because of the risk for recurrent disease, nearly all patients with evidence of node involvement, particularly those who are hormone receptor negative, will have some type of drug therapy. Some patients, particularly those with a more aggressive tumor, are known to be at higher risk for recurrent or metastatic disease. Drug therapy may be used for these patients even when there is no evidence of node involvement. Weighing the risks and benefits of drug therapy is a complex process.[14]

Chemotherapy. Chemotherapy is the use of cytotoxic drugs to destroy cancer cells. A combination of drugs is usually superior to the use of a single drug. Combination treatment is best because the drugs have different mechanisms of action and work at different parts of the cell cycle. When used in the neoadjuvant and adjuvant setting, chemotherapy is usually given for 3 to 6 months. However, when a patient has metastasis, chemotherapy may be given for the rest of the patient's life.

Common combination-therapy protocols in the adjuvant and neoadjuvant setting are (1) CMF: cyclophosphamide, methotrexate, and fluorouracil; (2) AC: doxorubicin and cyclophosphamide, with or without the addition of a taxane, such as paclitaxel (Taxol) or docetaxel (Taxotere); or (3) CEF or CAF: cyclophosphamide, epirubicin (Ellence) or doxorubicin, and fluorouracil.

 DRUG ALERT Doxorubicin

- Monitor for signs of cardiotoxicity and heart failure (e.g., shortness of breath, pedal edema, decreased activity tolerance, dysrhythmias, ECG changes).
- Tell the patient not to have immunizations without the HCP's approval.

Teach patients to avoid contact with those who recently received live virus vaccine and those with infections. Because chemotherapy affects healthy cells, many side effects accompany chemotherapy. The incidence and severity of common side effects are related to specific drug combination, drug schedule, and dosage. The most common side effects involve rapidly dividing cells in the gastrointestinal tract (nausea, anorexia, weight loss), bone marrow (anemia), and hair follicles (hair loss).

Cognitive changes during and after treatment can occur. This phenomenon is called *"chemobrain."* These changes include difficulties in concentration, memory, focus, and attention. Cognitive changes in cancer are discussed in Chapter 15 on p. 251.

EVIDENCE-BASED PRACTICE

Treatment for Breast Cancer

C.P. is a 56-yr-old woman who was diagnosed with stage IIIA breast cancer. Her treatment plan is to receive neoadjuvant chemotherapy and then have surgery and radiation. C.P. tells you that she is anxious and will have surgery and radiation but does not want chemotherapy because she is afraid of the side effects.

Making Clinical Decisions

Best Available Evidence. The use of chemotherapy before surgery reduces the size and extent of the tumor, thus making the surgery more likely to succeed. It reduces the chance a more extensive treatment will be needed.

Clinician Expertise. Neoadjuvant chemotherapy is usually recommended for stage IIIA breast cancer. The common side effects (e.g., nausea, vomiting, fatigue) can be managed with appropriate treatment.

Patient Preferences and Values. C.P. does not want chemotherapy and prefers to take her chances. If the cancer comes back, she will have chemotherapy.

Implications for Nursing Practice

1. Why is it important to discuss with C.P. the reason chemotherapy is recommended?
2. What information would you share with her about treatment side effects and how they can be managed?
3. You note her spouse appears attentive and supportive. How will you involve him in C.P.'s care?

Reference for Evidence

National Comprehensive Cancer Network: NCCN guidelines for patients: Invasive breast cancer, 2018. Retrieved from *www.nccn. org/patients/guidelines/breast-invasive/index.html.*

Hormone Therapy. Estrogen can promote the growth of breast cancer cells if the cells are ER positive. Hormone therapy can block the effect and source of estrogen, promoting tumor regression.

ER and PR status assays can identify women whose breast cancers are likely to respond to hormone therapy. These assays predict whether hormone therapy is a treatment option. Chances of tumor regression are significantly greater in women whose tumors have estrogen and progesterone receptors. The 21-gene recurrence score (OncotypeDX) is an excellent prognostic assay to identify which women with hormone-positive breast cancer can be treated with hormone therapy alone and do not need chemotherapy.

TABLE 51.8 Drug Therapy
Breast Cancer

Drug Class	Mechanism of Action	Indications
Hormone Therapy		
Aromatase Inhibitors		
anastrozole (Arimidex) exemestane (Aromasin) letrozole (Femara)	Prevents production of estrogen by inhibiting aromatase	ER-positive breast cancer in postmenopausal women only
Estrogen Receptor Blockers		
fulvestrant (Faslodex)	Blocks estrogen receptors (ERs)	ER-positive breast cancer in postmenopausal women only
tamoxifen	Blocks ERs	ER-positive breast cancer in premenopausal and postmenopausal women Used as a preventive measure in high-risk pre-menopausal and postmenopausal women
toremifene (Fareston)	Blocks ERs	ER-positive breast cancer in postmenopausal women only
Estrogen Receptor Modulator		
raloxifene (Evista)	In breast, blocks the effect of estrogen. In bone, promotes effect of estrogen and prevents bone loss	Postmenopausal women
Immunotherapy and Targeted Therapy		
ado-trastuzumab emtansine (Kadcyla)	Trastuzumab connected to a chemotherapy drug called DM1	HER-2-positive breast cancer
everolimus (Afinitor)	Binds to mechanistic target of rapamycin (mTOR), thereby suppressing T cell activation and proliferation	ER-positive, HER-2-negative breast cancer in postmenopausal women
lapatinib (Tykerb)	Inhibits HER-2 tyrosine kinase and EGFR tyrosine kinase	HER-2-positive breast cancer
abemaciclib (Verzenio) palbociclib (Ibrance) ribociclib (Kisqali)	Kinase inhibitors	ER-positive, HER-2-negative breast cancer in postmenopausal women
neratinib (Nerlynx) pertuzumab (Perjeta) trastuzumab (Herceptin) trastuzumab-pkrb (Herzuma) trastuzumab-qyyp (Trazimera)	Blocks HER-2 receptor	HER-2-positive breast cancer

Hormone therapy can (1) block ERs or (2) suppress estrogen synthesis by inhibiting aromatase, an enzyme needed for estrogen synthesis (Table 51.8). Premenopausal women with ER-positive breast cancers may benefit from the removal or suppression of their ovaries. Ovarian ablation can be done surgically or by using luteinizing hormone–releasing hormone (LHRH) analogs, such as goserelin (Zoladex) or leuprolide (Lupron).

Estrogen Receptor Blockers. ER blockers include tamoxifen, toremifene (Fareston), and fulvestrant (Faslodex). Tamoxifen has been the hormone therapy of choice in ER-positive women with all stages of breast cancer over the past 30 years. It also may be used in high-risk women to prevent breast cancer. Common side effects include hot flashes, mood swings, vaginal discharge and dryness, and other effects associated with decreased estrogen. It also increases the risk for blood clots, cataracts, stroke, and endometrial cancer in postmenopausal women.

 DRUG ALERT Tamoxifen

- Irregular vaginal bleeding or spotting may occur.
- Decreased visual acuity, corneal opacity, and retinopathy can occur in women receiving high doses (240–320 mg/day for >17 mo). These problems may be irreversible.
- Teach the patient to immediately report decreased visual acuity.
- Monitor for signs of deep vein thrombosis, pulmonary embolism, and stroke, including shortness of breath, leg cramps, and weakness.

Aromatase inhibitors. Aromatase inhibitor drugs interfere with the anastrozole enzyme aromatase, which is needed for the synthesis of estrogen. These drugs include anastrozole, letrozole (Femara), and exemestane (Aromasin). They are used in the treatment of breast cancer in postmenopausal women. Aromatase inhibitors do not block the production of estrogen by the ovaries. Thus they are of little benefit and may be harmful in premenopausal women.

Aromatase inhibitors have different side effects than tamoxifen. They rarely cause blood clots and do not cause endometrial cancer. Because they block the production of estrogen in postmenopausal women, osteoporosis and bone fractures may occur. These drugs have been associated with night sweats, nausea, arthralgias, and myalgias.

Estrogen receptor modulator and others. Raloxifene (Evista) is a selective ER modulator that has both estrogen-agonistic effects on bone and estrogen-antagonistic effects on breast tissue. (Raloxifene is discussed in the section on osteoporosis in Chapter 63.) Less common drugs that may be used to suppress hormone-dependent breast tumors include megestrol acetate, diethylstilbestrol, and fluoxymesterone.

Immunotherapy and Targeted Therapy. As more is known about the genetic changes in breast cancer, we have developed drugs that specifically target cells that have altered gene expression. One of these genetic changes is the overexpression of HER-2.

Tumors that overexpress the HER-2 protein tend to be more aggressive and are more likely to recur.

Trastuzumab (Herceptin) is a monoclonal antibody to HER-2. After the antibody attaches to the antigen, blocks signals that tell the cancer cells to proliferate. It can be used alone or in combination with chemotherapy agents. The most common side effects are flu-like symptoms (fever, chills, myalgia), nausea and vomiting, diarrhea, and infusion reactions. Another possible, but more serious side effect, is heart damage. Trastuzumab-qyyp (Trazimera) and trastuzumab-pkrb (Herzuma) are newly approved biosimiliars of trastuzamab.

 DRUG ALERT Trastuzumab (Herceptin)

- Use with caution in women with preexisting heart disease.
- Monitor for signs of ventricular dysfunction and heart failure.

Other drugs that target HER-2 include pertuzumab (Perjeta) and ado-trastuzumab emtansine (Kadcyla). Kadcyla is trastuzumab connected to a chemotherapy drug called DM1. Lapatinib (Tykerb) works inside the cell by blocking the function of the HER-2 protein. Nerotinib (Nerlynx) is an option for extended adjuvant therapy for some high-risk women. Using 2 of these agents together for neoadjuvant therapy can increase the number of tumors that become undetectable and can improve survival when used for adjuvant therapy. Other drugs that target HER-2 include pertuzumab (Perjeta), trastuzumab-qyyp (Trazimera), trastuzumab-pkrb (Herzuma), and ado-trastuzumab emtansine (Kadcyla). Kadcyla is trastuzumab connected to a chemotherapy drug called DM1. Lapatinib (Tykerb) works inside the cell by blocking the function of the HER-2 protein. Using 2 of these agents together for neoadjuvant therapy can increase the number of tumors that become undetectable.

Drugs in other classes that are used to treat breast cancer include everolimus (Afinitor) and the CDK 4 and 6 inhibitors palbociclib (Ibrance), ribociclib (Kisquali), and abemaciclib (Verzenio). Everolimus works by blocking mTOR, a protein that normally promotes cell growth and division. CDK 4 and 6 inhibitors prevent cells from dividing, thus slowing cancer growth. (The use of immunotherapy and targeted therapy is discussed in Chapter 15.)

 Culturally Competent Care: Breast Cancer

Differences exist in the incidence, mortality rates, and care issues among diverse racial and ethnic groups related to breast cancer (see Promoting Health Equity box on this page). In addition,

---

PROMOTING HEALTH EQUITY

Breast Cancer

- White and black women have the highest incidence of breast cancer.
- Black women have lower survival rates from breast cancer than white women, even when diagnosed at an early stage.
- Hispanic and black women are more likely to be diagnosed at a later stage of breast cancer than white women.
- Triple-negative breast cancer has a higher incidence in black and Hispanic women.
- Mortality rates are lower among Hispanic and Asian/Pacific Islander women than among white and black women.
- Breast cancer is the most common diagnosed cancer among Hispanic women.
- Indian/Alaskan native women have the lowest rate of breast cancer screening of any ethnic group.

---

cultural differences may involve gender roles, health beliefs, religion, family structure, socioeconomic factors (e.g., poverty) and lack of health insurance. Lack of education may influence disparities related to access to health care and having recommended surveillance examinations.[17,18]

Cultural values strongly influence how a person responds to and copes with breast cancer and treatment. Diverse cultural norms influence health beliefs and behaviors. Breast cancer screening, diagnosis, and treatment are affected by the cultural values and meanings (body image, sexuality, modesty, motherhood) associated with the breasts. Women may delay screening or treatment for varying reasons, including an acceptance of disease as inevitable fate or "God's will," a mistrust of Western medicine, lack of health care benefits, fear, or the stigma of a cancer diagnosis.

❖ NURSING MANAGEMENT: BREAST CANCER

◆ Nursing Assessment

You must consider many factors when assessing a patient with a breast problem. The history of the breast disorder helps establish a diagnosis. Investigate the presence of nipple discharge, pain, rate of growth of the lump, breast asymmetry, and correlation with the menstrual cycle.

Carefully record the size and location of the lump or lumps. Assess the physical characteristics of the lesion, including consistency, mobility, and shape. If nipple discharge is present, note the color and consistency and whether it occurs from 1 or both breasts.

Subjective and objective data to obtain from a person suspected of having or diagnosed with breast cancer are outlined in Table 51.9.

◆ Nursing Diagnoses

Nursing diagnoses related to the care of a patient diagnosed with breast cancer vary. After diagnosis and before a treatment plan has been selected, the following nursing diagnoses would apply:
- Difficulty coping
- Lack of knowledge
- Disturbed body image

If surgery is planned, the nursing diagnoses and interventions may include those in eNursing Care Plan 51.1 (available on the website for this chapter).

◆ Planning

The overall goals are that the patient with breast cancer will (1) actively take part in the decision-making process related to treatment, (2) adhere to the therapeutic plan, (3) communicate about and manage the side effects of adjuvant therapy, (4) access and benefit from the support provided by significant others and HCPs, and (5) adhere to recommended follow-up and surveillance after treatment.

◆ Nursing Implementation

◆ **Health Promotion.** Review the risk factors in Table 51.2. People can reduce their risk factors by maintaining a healthy weight, exercising regularly, limiting alcohol, eating nutritious food, and never smoking (or quitting if currently smoking).

Encourage people to adhere to the breast cancer screening guidelines shown on pp. 1190–1191. A person at high risk needs to develop a personalized plan with the HCP. Early detection

TABLE 51.9 Nursing Assessment

Breast Cancer

Subjective Data

Important Health Information

Past health history: Benign breast disease with atypical changes. Previous unilateral breast cancer. Menstrual history (early menarche with late menopause), pregnancy history (nulliparity or first full-term pregnancy after age 30). Endometrial, ovarian, or colon cancer. Hyperestrogenism and testicular atrophy (in men)

Medicines: Hormones, especially as postmenopausal hormone therapy and in oral contraceptives. Infertility treatments

Surgery or other treatments: Exposure to therapeutic radiation (e.g., Hodgkin's lymphoma or thyroid radiation)

Functional Health Patterns

Health perception–health management: Family history of breast cancer (young age at diagnosis). History of abnormal mammogram or atypical prior biopsy. Palpable change found on BSE. Known *BRCA* mutation carrier, first-degree relative of *BRCA* carrier (but untested)

Nutritional-metabolic: Obesity; unexplained severe weight loss (may indicate metastasis)

Activity-exercise: Level of usual activity

Cognitive-perceptual: Changes in cognition, headache, bone pain (may indicate metastasis)

Sexuality-reproductive: Unilateral nipple discharge (clear, milky, bloody). Change in breast contour, size, or symmetry

Coping–stress tolerance: Psychologic stress

Self-perception–self-concept: Anxiety about threat to self-esteem

Objective Data

General

Axillary and supraclavicular lymphadenopathy

Integumentary

Hard, irregular, nonmobile breast lump most often in upper, outer sector, possibly fixated to fascia or chest wall. Thickening of breast. Nipple inversion or retraction, erosion. Edema ("peau d'orange"), erythema, induration, infiltration, or dimpling (in later stages). Firm, discrete nodules at mastectomy site (may indicate local recurrence). Peripheral edema (may indicate metastasis)

Respiratory

Pleural effusions (may indicate metastasis)

Gastrointestinal

Hepatomegaly, jaundice, ascites (may indicate liver metastasis)

Possible Diagnostic Findings

Finding of mass or change in tissue on breast examination. Abnormal mammogram, ultrasound, or breast MRI. Positive results of FNA or surgical biopsy; similar results with a needle biopsy

---

can decrease the morbidity and mortality associated with breast cancer.

Along with these lifestyle choices, there are other risk-reduction options for people at high risk. Genetic testing for *BRCA* and other gene mutations is available. People with a strong family history of breast cancer should talk with their HCP about the possibility of genetic testing. There is no reason for routine screening for genetic abnormalities in women without evidence of a strong family history of breast cancer.

In women with an abnormal *BRCA1* or *BRCA2* gene, prophylactic oophorectomy may reduce their risk for developing breast cancer and ovarian cancer. In deciding whether and

when to undergo this surgical procedure, women should receive counseling about the risks and benefits of prophylactic oophorectomy, including fertility issues.

Prophylactic surgery decisions require a great deal of thought, patience, and discussion with the HCP, genetic counselor, and family. Patients need to consider these options and make decisions with which they feel comfortable. Removing both breasts and ovaries at a young age does not eliminate the risk for breast cancer. A small risk exists that cancer can develop in the areas where the breasts used to be. Close follow-up is necessary even after prophylactic surgery.

◆ **Acute Care.** The times of waiting for the initial biopsy results and waiting for the HCP to make treatment recommendations are difficult for patients and their families. Even after the HCP has discussed treatment options, the patient often relies on you to clarify and expand on these options. During this stressful time, the patient may not be coping effectively. Appropriate nursing interventions are to explore the patient's usual decision-making processes, help to evaluate the advantages and disadvantages of the options, provide information relevant to the decision, clarify unresolved issues with the HCP, and support the patient and family once the decision is made.

Provide the patient with enough information to ensure informed consent. Some patients seek extensive, detailed information to maintain a sense of control. Others avoid information to decrease anxiety and fear. Be sensitive to the person's need for and preferred type of information. These include (1) instructions on pain control and what to expect after surgery (e.g., dressing and drain care, turning, coughing, deep breathing), (2) a review of mobility restrictions and postoperative exercises, and (3) an explanation of the recovery period.

The woman who has breast-conserving surgery usually has an uncomplicated postoperative course with variable pain intensity. Pain depends primarily on the extent of the lymph node sampling procedure. If an ALND has been done or if the patient had a mastectomy, drains are generally left in place and patients are discharged home with them. Teach the patient and family, with a return demonstration, how to manage the drains at home.

Most patients are discharged from the hospital 24 to 48 hours after a mastectomy, depending on if reconstructive surgery was done. Restoring arm function on the affected side after breast cancer surgery is a key nursing goal. Arm and shoulder exercises, which are started gradually, may begin prior to discharge (Fig. 51.8). These exercises are designed to prevent contractures and muscle shortening, maintain muscle tone, and improve lymph and blood circulation. The difficulty and pain encountered in performing what used to be simple tasks may cause frustration and depression. The goal of all exercise is a gradual return to full range of motion.

Discomfort can be minimized by giving analgesics regularly when the patient is in pain and about 30 minutes before starting exercises. When the patient can shower, the warm water on the involved shoulder often relaxes the muscle and reduces joint stiffness.

Explain the specific follow-up plan to the patient and emphasize the importance of ongoing monitoring and self-care. After surgery, teach the patient to report symptoms, such as fever, inflammation at the surgical site, erythema, and unusual swelling. Other changes to report are new back pain, weakness, shortness of breath, and change in mental status, including confusion.

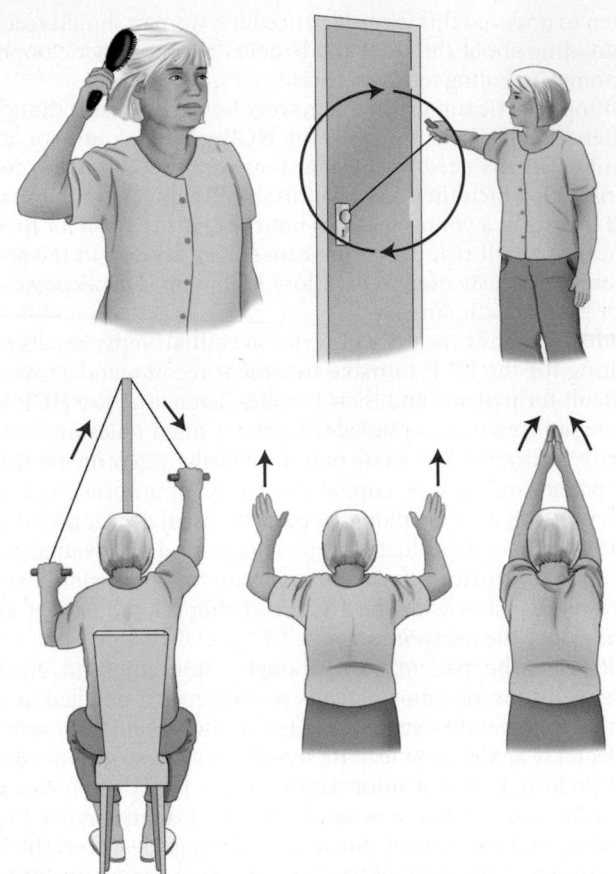

FIG. 51.8 Postoperative exercises for the patient with a mastectomy or lumpectomy with axillary lymph node sampling and/or dissection.

For women who have had a mastectomy without breast reconstruction, a variety of products are available. Your role is to present the choices and resources. Options include garments such as camisoles with soft breast prosthetic inserts or a fitted prosthesis with bra. Should the woman choose a breast prosthesis, a certified fitter can help her choose a comfortable, more permanent weighted prosthesis and bra. This is generally done 4 to 8 weeks after surgery.

Lymphedema. Upper extremity lymphedema can occur at any point after treatment for breast cancer. Teach the patient ways to prevent and reduce lymphedema. These include no BP readings, venipunctures, or injections on the affected arm, if possible. The affected arm should not be dependent for long periods. Caution should be used to prevent infection, burns, or compromised circulation on the affected side. Encourage exercise and maintaining a normal weight.

If trauma to the arm occurs, the area should be washed thoroughly with soap and water and observed. A topical antibiotic ointment and a bandage or other sterile dressing may be applied.

When lymphedema is acute (Fig. 51.6), complete decongestive therapy will be recommended. This therapy is performed by specially trained professionals. It consists of a massage-like technique to mobilize the subcutaneous accumulation of fluid. This may be followed by use of compression bandaging and an intermittent pneumatic compression sleeve. The sleeve applies mechanical massage to the arm and helps move lymph drainage up toward the heart. Elevating the arm so that it is level with the heart and performing isometric exercises reduce the fluid in the arm. To maintain maximum volume reduction, the patient may need to wear a fitted compression sleeve during waking hours and preventively during air travel.

Psychosocial Support. Throughout history, the female breast has been a symbol of beauty, femininity, sexuality, and motherhood. The potential loss of a breast, or part of a breast, may be devastating for many women because of the significant psychologic, social, sexual, and body image implications associated with it. For men diagnosed with breast cancer, isolation and embarrassment related to the diagnosis can occur. You must be aware of resources for men (*www.malebreastcancer.org*).

As hard as it is to predict which patients will develop physical effects of treatment, it can be even more difficult to foresee the psychosocial effects of treatment. In some cases, psychosocial concerns may increase the physical effects of cancer, such as pain, fatigue, sleep problems, fear of recurrence, and cognitive changes.

Screening all cancer patients for psychosocial distress is a Commission on Cancer accreditation requirement.[19] From the time of diagnosis through treatment, survivorship, or metastatic disease, the patient may have signs of distress or tension (e.g., tachycardia, increased muscle tension, sleep problems, restlessness, changes in appetite or mood). Assess the patient's body language and affect during periods of high stress and indecision so that you can begin appropriate interventions, including referral to a mental health provider.

Remain sensitive to the complex psychologic impact that a diagnosis of cancer and breast surgery can have on patients and their families. With an accepting attitude and the offer of resources, you can help the patient cope with feelings of fear, anger, anxiety, and depression. You can help to:

- Provide a safe environment for the expression of feelings.
- Identify sources of support and strength, such as the partner, family, and spiritual or religious practices.
- Encourage the patient to identify and learn personal coping strengths.
- Promote communication among the patient, family, and friends.
- Answer questions about the disease, treatment options, and reproductive, fertility, or lactation issues (if appropriate).
- Make resources available for mental health counseling.
- Offer information about local and national community resources.

Referring patients to support resources, such as *www.Breastcancer.org*, the Cancer Support Community, or local breast cancer organizations, is valuable. The ACS and National Cancer Institute can provide excellent materials to help you in meeting the special needs of patients with breast cancer. In addition to in-person and online support programs, multiple free smart phone applications are available through national cancer organizations that provide reliable and current information for the patient and his or her family.

How the loss of part or all of the breast and cancer affect the patient's sexual identity, body image, and relationships can vary. Many HCPs do not adequately address sexual concerns. If you are comfortable, begin a discussion of sexuality by inviting questions about relationships or intimacy concerns. Often the patient's partner and/or family members need help dealing with their emotional reactions to the diagnosis and surgery before they can provide effective support for the patient. There are no physical reasons why a mastectomy would prevent sexual satisfaction. A woman taking hormone therapy may have a decreased sexual

🌿 COMPLEMENTARY & ALTERNATIVE THERAPIES

Supportive Care

Many women use complementary and integrative therapies as supportive care during cancer treatment to improve quality of life and manage treatment-related side effects.

Scientific Evidence
- There is strong evidence that practicing meditation and relaxation decreases anxiety and depression and improves quality of life.
- Stress management, yoga, massage, music therapy, and meditation decrease stress, fatigue, anxiety, and depression and improve quality of life.

Nursing Implications
- Women use a variety of integrative therapies during breast cancer treatment.
- Meditation, yoga, relaxation, stress management, massage, music therapy, and energy conservation may be especially helpful in managing symptoms and improving quality of life during treatment.

Reference for Evidence
Greenlee H, DuPont-Reyes MJ, Balneaves L, et al.: Clinical practice guidelines on the evidence-based use of integrative therapies during and after breast cancer treatment, *CA Cancer J Clin* 67:1954, 2017.

---

drive or vaginal dryness. She may need to use lubrication to prevent discomfort during intercourse. If difficulty in adjustment or other problems develop, single or couples counseling may be useful to deal with the emotional side of a diagnosis of cancer.

Depression and anxiety may occur with the continued stress and uncertainty of a cancer diagnosis. A patient's self-esteem and identity may be threatened. The support of family and friends and taking part in a cancer support group and/or counseling are important aspects of care that may improve the patient's quality of life.

Survivorship. Almost 3 million breast cancer survivors are alive in the United States, making this population the largest group of cancer survivors. We expect this number to grow due to an aging population and improved methods for early detection and treatment. After treatment for breast cancer, the patient will have ongoing survivorship care.[19,20]

A history and physical examination is recommended 1 to 4 times per year as clinically appropriate for 5 years, then annually thereafter. In addition, teach breast cancer survivors to perform monthly BSE and chest wall self-examination and report any changes to their HCP. Local recurrence of breast cancer is usually at the surgical site. Breast cancer survivors should have an annual mammogram. Other breast imaging studies, such as a breast ultrasound or breast MRI, should be done only as an adjunct to mammography and not for annual routine surveillance. Cancer survivorship is discussed in Chapter 15 on p. 264.

◆ Evaluation

Expected outcomes are that the patient after breast cancer surgery will
- Identify activities that can reduce postoperative edema and improve mobility
- Show effective use of coping strategies
- Discuss feelings about and the meaning of changes in physical appearance
- Identify community and online resources, personal counseling resources, and support groups

👤 Gerontologic Considerations: Breast Cancer

A major risk for breast cancer is increasing age. More than half of all breast cancers occur in women who are age 65 or older.[1] Older women are less likely to have mammograms. Screening and treatment decisions for breast cancer should be based on a woman's general health status rather than biologic age, since health status has a greater influence on tolerance to treatment and long-term prognosis. In addition to medical co-morbidities and life expectancy, treatment decisions for the older woman with breast cancer should be based on an assessment of nutritional and functional status; vision; gait, and balance; and the presence of delirium, dementia, or depression.

Breast cancer treatment is similar for older and younger patients, including the use of surgery, radiation therapy, and drug therapy. For healthy older women, breast cancer survival rates are similar to those of younger women when matched by cancer stage.

MAMMOPLASTY

Mammoplasty is the surgical change in the size or shape of the breast. It may be done electively for cosmetic purposes to either enlarge or reduce the size of the breasts. It also may be done to reconstruct the breast after a mastectomy.

A professional, nonjudgmental attitude and clear information about surgical breast options are most useful for women engaged in decision making about mammoplasty. The desire to change the appearance of the breasts has special significance for each woman as she attempts to change or recreate her body image. Be aware of the cultural value that the woman places on the breast. Help the patient set realistic expectations about what mammoplasty can achieve and possible complications (e.g., hematoma formation, hemorrhage, infection). If an implant is involved, capsular contracture and loss of the implant are possible.

Breast Reconstruction

Breast reconstructive surgery is a type of surgery for women who have had all or part of a breast removed. It is done to achieve symmetry and to restore or preserve body image. It may be done simultaneously with a mastectomy or some time afterward. The timing of reconstructive surgery is personalized based on the patient's physical and psychologic needs.[21]

Indications. The main indication for breast reconstruction is to improve a woman's self-image, regain a sense of normalcy, and assist in coping with the loss of the breast. It restores the contour of the breast without the use of an external prosthesis. Reconstruction techniques cannot restore lactation, nipple sensation, or erectility. Although the breast will not fully resemble its premastectomy appearance, the reconstructed appearance usually is an improvement over the mastectomy scar (Fig. 51.9).

Types of Reconstruction

Breast Implants and Tissue Expansion. Implants have a silicone shell filled with either silicone gel or saline.[22] Some newer types use a cohesive gel, which is a thicker silicone gel. Implant surgery can be done in 1 or 2 stages.

In the 1-stage procedure, the implant is placed at the same time as the mastectomy. The implant is usually placed under the pectoralis muscle.

In the 2-stage procedure, a tissue expander is inserted after the mastectomy. The expander stretches the skin and muscle at the mastectomy site before inserting permanent implants (Fig. 51.10). It is placed in a pocket under the pectoralis muscle,

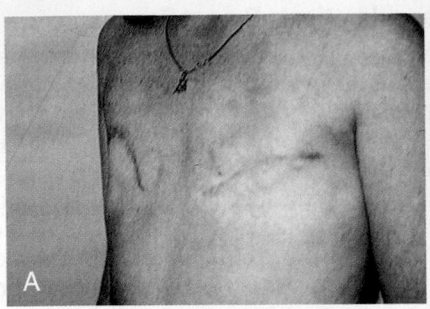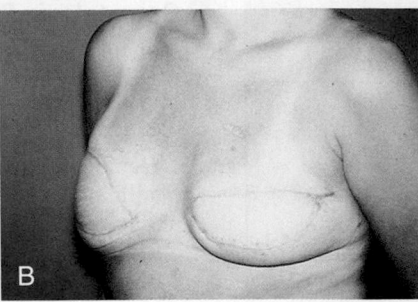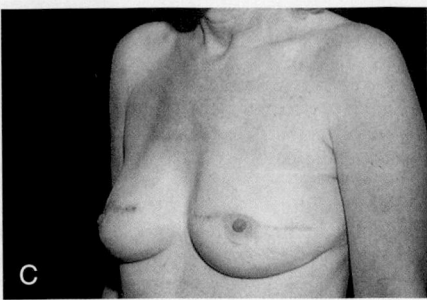

FIG. 51.9 A, Appearance of chest after bilateral mastectomy. B, Breast reconstruction before nipple-areolar reconstruction. C, Breast reconstruction after nipple-areolar reconstruction. (Courtesy Brian Davies, MD. From Fortunato N, McCullough S, eds: *Plastic and reconstructive surgery*, St Louis, 1998, Mosby.)

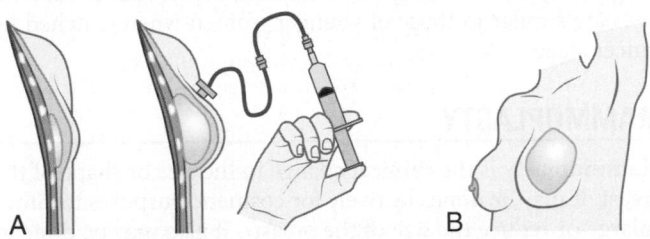

FIG. 51.10 A, Tissue expander with gradual expansion. B, Tissue expander in place after mastectomy.

which protects the implant and provides soft tissue coverage. The expander is minimally inflated, then gradually filled by weekly injections of sterile saline solution. This procedure stretches the skin and muscle and can be painful. A small magnet embedded in most expanders helps locate the port where the fluid is injected. A woman should not have an MRI with a magnet in place.

The expander can be (1) surgically removed and a permanent implant is inserted or (2) remain in place to become the implant, thus eliminating the need for a second surgical procedure. Tissue expansion does not work well in those with extensive scar tissue from surgery or radiation therapy.

The body's natural response to the presence of a foreign substance is the formation of a fibrous capsule around the implant. If excessive capsular formation occurs because of infection, hematoma, trauma, or reaction to a foreign body, a contracture can develop, resulting in deformity. Although HCPs differ in their approaches to the prevention of contracture formation, gentle manual massage around the implant is routine. Other adverse outcomes include wrinkling, scarring, asymmetry, pain, and infection at the incision site. There is a small chance of anaplastic large cell lymphoma occurring. This has mostly been associated with textured implants.[19]

Tissue Flap Procedures. Another type of breast reconstruction uses autologous (person's own) tissue to recreate a breast mound. In autologous reconstruction, tissue from the abdomen, back, thighs, or buttocks is used to create a reconstructed breast. The most common types of tissue flap procedures are *transverse rectus abdominis musculocutaneous (TRAM) flap, deep inferior epigastric artery perforator (DIEP) flap*, and *latissimus dorsi flap*.

The TRAM flap is a common flap surgery. The rectus abdominis muscles are paired flat muscles running from the rib cage down to the pubic bone. Arteries running inside the muscles provide branches at many levels, and these branches supply the fat and skin across a large expanse of the abdomen.

There are 2 different types of TRAM flaps: pedicle and free. In a pedicle flap, the tissue stays attached to the rectus muscle and is tunneled under the skin to the patient's chest (Fig. 51.11). In a free flap, the tissue is completely separated from the muscle and its blood supply and moved to the new place on the patient's chest. The tissue is molded and fashioned to form a breast. The abdominal incision is closed, giving the patient a result that is similar to having an abdominoplasty ("tummy tuck"). The procedure can last 6 to 8 hours with recovery taking 6 to 8 weeks. Some patients have report pain and fatigue for up to 3 months. Complications include bleeding, seroma, hernia, infection, and low back pain.

Perforator flaps are a type of free flap (a perforator artery connects a superficial artery with a deep one) that do not use muscle tissue. A *DIEP flap* is the type done most often. With the DIEP flap, only the skin and fat are taken from the same lower abdominal area as the TRAM flap. Patients may have less pain and restriction of movement with this procedure. The *superficial inferior epigastric artery perforator (SIEAP)* is another option using the abdominal area.

The *latissimus dorsi flap* is a pedicle flap. In this type of flap, a block of skin and muscle from the patient's back replaces tissue removed during mastectomy. A small implant may be needed under the flap to gain reasonable breast shape and size. A disadvantage of this technique is a scar on the back.

Less often, flaps are taken from the buttocks, hips, or thighs. The transverse upper gracilis flap, or inner thigh flap, is one type of free flap. Tissue, including the gracilis muscle, is taken from the bottom fold of the buttock extending into the inner thigh. The inferior or superior gluteal artery perforators are used for flaps taken from the buttocks.

Nipple-Areolar Reconstruction. Many patients undergoing breast reconstruction also have nipple-areolar reconstruction. Nipple reconstruction gives the reconstructed breast a much more natural appearance (Fig. 51.9, *C*). Nipple-areolar reconstruction is usually done a few months after breast reconstruction. Tissue to construct a nipple may be taken from the opposite breast or from a small flap of tissue on the reconstructed breast mound. Most often, the areola is tattooed with a permanent pigmented dye. Improved techniques now allow skilled tattoo artists to create a complete 3D nipple-areola complex. Polyurethane removable nipples are also available.

Breast Augmentation

In *augmentation mammoplasty* (procedure to enlarge the breasts), an implant is placed in a surgically created pocket between the capsule of the breast and pectoral fascia, or

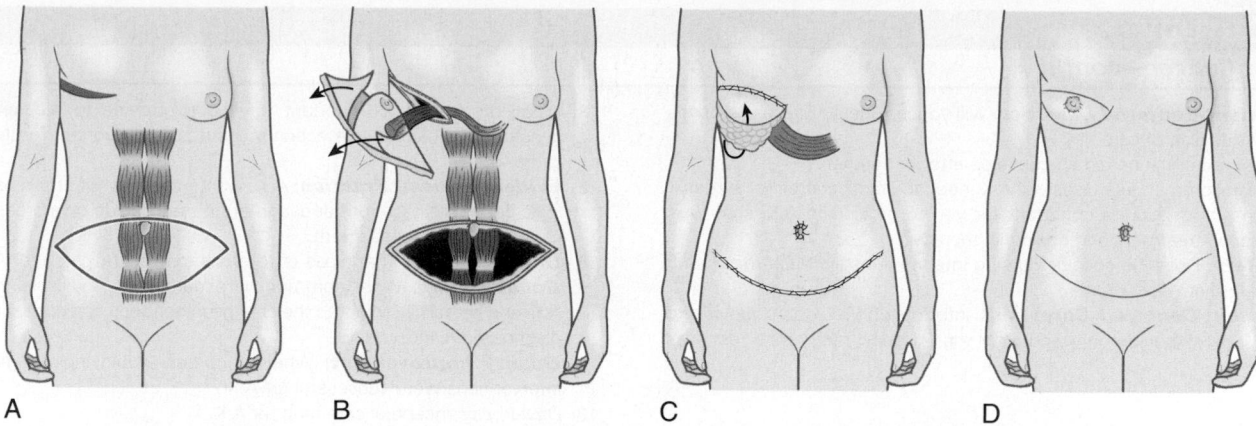

FIG. 51.11 Transverse rectus abdominis musculocutaneous (TRAM) flap. **A**, TRAM flap is planned. **B**, The abdominal tissue, while attached to the rectus muscle, nerve, and blood supply, is tunneled through the abdomen to the chest. **C**, The flap is trimmed to shape the breast. The lower abdominal incision is closed. **D**, Nipple and areola are reconstructed after the breast is healed.

ideally under the pectoralis muscle. (Implants are discussed on p. 1207.)

Breast Reduction

For some women, large breasts can be a source of physical and psychologic discomfort. They can interfere with normal daily activities, such as walking, using a computer, and driving a car. The weight of large breasts can lead to back, shoulder, and neck problems, including degenerative nerve changes. Overly large breasts can interfere with self-esteem, self-image, and comfort in wearing some clothing. Reducing breast size can have positive effects on the patient's psychologic and physical health.

Reduction mammoplasty is done by resecting wedges of tissue from the upper and lower quadrants of the breast. The excess skin is removed, and the areola and nipple are relocated on the breast. Lactation usually can be accomplished if massive amounts of tissue are not removed and the nipples are left connected during surgery.

❖ NURSING MANAGEMENT: BREAST AUGMENTATION AND REDUCTION

Breast augmentation and breast reduction may be done in the outpatient surgical area or involve overnight hospitalization. General anesthesia is used. Drains are generally placed in the surgical site to prevent hematoma formation and then removed when drainage is under 20 to 30 mL/day. Examine drainage for color and odor to detect infection or hemorrhage. Monitor the temperature. Change dressings as needed using sterile technique.

After surgery, assure the woman that the breast's appearance will improve when healing is complete. Depending on HCP preference, the patient may be told to wear a bra that provides good support continuously for 2 or 3 days after breast reduction or augmentation. Depending on the extent of the surgery, most women resume normal activities within 2 to 3 weeks. Strenuous exercise must often be avoided for several weeks.

CASE STUDY

Breast Cancer

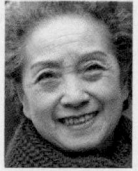

(© XiXinXing/
iStock/
Thinkstock.)

Patient Profile

A.K., a 68-yr-old married Asian American woman, has been diagnosed with a 1.3-cm estrogen- and progesterone-positive, HER-2–negative breast cancer. She is scheduled in the morning for a lumpectomy and sentinel lymph node biopsy (SLNB) with possible axillary node dissection.

Interprofessional Care

Preoperative

• When she is seen in the clinic 1 week before surgery, she is crying uncontrollably and says, "My husband does not want to look at me anymore. He is afraid of what I am going to look like with a flat chest."

• She says, "I cannot sleep, and I just pace the floor at night."

• "My mother died of breast cancer when she was 60, and my sister got it when she was 40."

• Expresses concern that her 2 daughters (34 and 32) and their daughters are going to get "this horrible disease."

Operative Procedure

• Lumpectomy and SLNB are done
• Tumor was removed with clear margins
• No cancer cells in her sentinel lymph nodes
• 4 lymph nodes are removed
• Tissue specimen sent for a 21-gene recurrence score genomic test

Postoperative

• Does not want to leave hospital and refuses to get out of bed
• Swelling and restricted range of motion in right arm
• Pain not controlled well with pain medication

Follow-Up Findings and Treatment

• 21-Gene recurrence score is 11, low risk
• Scheduled for external radiation and a consult with medical oncologist to discuss hormone therapy

Discussion Questions

1. What in A.K.'s breast cancer experience with her family members may influence her coping response?

Continued

CASE STUDY

Breast Cancer—cont'd

2. **Patient-Centered Care:** How will you include cultural preferences in A.K.'s plan of care?
3. What complication did she develop after her surgery?
4. Which common exercises will A.K. need to practice after her surgery?
5. What information is important for you to provide to A.K. about her radiation treatment and hormonal therapy?
6. **Safety:** Describe specific nursing interventions aimed at minimizing risk for harm for A.K.
7. **Patient-Centered Care:** What information would you provide to A.K. about her surgery and why the 21-gene recurrence test was done?

8. What information is important for you to provide to A.K. and her daughters? What early detection measures are important for them to know?
9. **Evidence-Based Practice:** A.K. wants to know what the psychologic benefit may be for her daughters if they decide on a breast cancer genetic risk assessment.
10. **Collaboration:** What types of referrals may be indicated for A.K.?
11. **Collaboration:** What community resources are available to help A.K. and her family adjust to the change in her body and cope with the diagnosis of cancer?
12. **Quality Improvement:** What outcomes would indicate nursing interventions were successful for A.K.?
13. Develop a conceptual care map for A.K.

Answers and a corresponding conceptual care map available at *http://evolve.elsevier.com/Lewis/medsurg.*

BRIDGE TO NCLEX EXAMINATION

The number of the question corresponds to the same-numbered outcome at the beginning of the chapter.

1. You are a community health nurse planning a program on breast cancer screening guidelines for women in the neighborhood. Which recommendations you would include? *(select all that apply)*
   a. Women over age 55 may have biennial screening.
   b. Screening should end when the women reaches age 65.
   c. Women aged 45 to 54 years should be screened annually.
   d. Regular screening mammography should start at age 45 years.
   e. Clinical breast examinations can be used if the woman has average risk.

2. You are caring for a young woman who has painful fibrocystic breast changes. Management of this patient would include
   a. scheduling a biopsy to rule out the presence of breast cancer.
   b. teaching that symptoms will subside if she stops using oral contraceptives.
   c. preparing her for surgical removal of the lumps, since they will become larger and more painful.
   d. explaining that restricting coffee and chocolate and supplementing with vitamin E may relieve some discomfort.

3. When discussing risk factors for breast cancer with a group of women, you emphasize that the greatest known risk factor for breast cancer is
   a. being a woman over age 60.
   b. experiencing menstruation for 30 years or more.
   c. using hormone therapy for 5 years for menopausal symptoms.
   d. having a paternal grandmother with postmenopausal breast cancer.

4. A patient with breast cancer has a lumpectomy with sentinel lymph node biopsy that is positive for cancer. You explain that, of the other tests done to determine the risk for cancer recurrence or spread, the results that support the more favorable prognosis are *(select all that apply)*
   a. well-differentiated tumor.
   b. estrogen receptor–positive tumor.
   c. overexpression of HER-2 cell marker.
   d. involvement of two to four axillary nodes.
   e. aneuploidy status from cell proliferation studies.

5. You are caring for a patient with breast cancer following a simple mastectomy. Postoperatively, to restore arm function on the affected side, you would
   a. apply heating pads or blankets to increase circulation.
   b. place daily ice packs to minimize the risk for lymphedema.
   c. teach passive exercises with the affected arm in a dependent position.
   d. emphasize regular exercises for the affected shoulder to increase range of motion.

6. Preoperatively, to meet the psychologic needs of a woman scheduled for a simple mastectomy, you would
   a. discuss the limitations of breast reconstruction.
   b. include her significant other in all conversations.
   c. promote an environment for expression of feelings.
   d. explain the importance of regular follow-up screening.

7. To prevent capsular formation after breast reconstruction with implants, teach the patient to
   a. gently massage the area around the implant.
   b. bind the breasts tightly with elastic bandages.
   c. avoid strenuous exercise until the implant has healed.
   d. exercise the arm on the affected side to promote drainage.

1. a, c, 2. d, 3. a, 4. a, b, 5. d, 6. c, 7. a

For the rationale for these answers and even more NCLEX review questions, visit *http://evolve.elsevier.com/Lewis/medsurg.*

ⓔ EVOLVE WEBSITE/RESOURCES LIST

http://evolve.elsevier.com/Lewis/medsurg
Review Questions (Online Only)
Key Points
Answer Keys for Questions
- Rationales for Bridge to NCLEX Examination Questions
- Answer Guidelines for Case Study on p. 1209

Student Case Study
- Patient With Breast Cancer

Nursing Care Plan
- eNursing Care Plan 51.1: Patient After Breast Surgery

Conceptual Care Map Creator
- Conceptual Care Map for Case Study on p. 1209

Audio Glossary
Content Updates

REFERENCES

1. American Cancer Society: Cancer facts and figures 2017. Retrieved from *www.cancer.org/content/dam/cancer-org/research/cancer-facts-and-statistics/annual-cancer-facts-and-figures/2017/cancer-facts-and-figures-2017.pdf*.

*2. American Cancer Society: ACS recommendations for early detection of breast cancer. Retrieved from *www.cancer.org/cancer/breast-cancer/screening-tests-and-early-detection/american-cancer-society-recommendations-for-the-early-detection-of-breast-cancer.html*.

*3. National Comprehensive Cancer Network: NCCN guidelines, version1, 017: Breast cancer screening and diagnosis. Retrieved from *www.nccn.org/professionals/physician_gls/pdf/breast-screening.pdf*.

4. Liu J, Jacobs L: The management of benign breast disease. In: Cameron J, Cameron A: *Current surgical therapy,* ed 12, Atlanta, 2017, Elsevier.

5. Nordqviist C. Mastitis: Treatment, causes, and symptoms. Retrieved from *www.medicalnewstoday.com/articles/163876.php*.

6. Bland KI, Copeland EM, Klimberg VS, et al: *The breast comprehensive management of benign and malignant diseases,* ed 5, Philadelphia, 2018, Elsevier.

7. Smith R: Fibrocystic breast changes. In: *Netter's obstetrics and gynecology,* ed 3, Philadelphia, 2018, Elsevier.

*8. American College of Obstetricians and Gynecologists: Practice bulletin: Diagnosis and management of benign breast disorders, *Obstet & Gynecol* 127:e141, 2016.

9. American Cancer Society: Breast cancer: Risk factors and prevention. Retrieved from *www.cancer.org/cancer/breast-cancer/risk-and-prevention.html*.

10. National Cancer Institute: *Genetics and breast and gynecologic cancers PDQ®—Health professional version.* Retrieved from *www.cancer.gov/types/breast/hp/breast-ovarian-genetics-pdq*.

11. National Comprehensive Cancer Network: *NCCN guidelines, version 2, 2017: Genetic/familial high-risk assessment: Breast and ovarian.* Retrieved from *www.nccn.org/professionals/physician_gls/pdf/genetics_screening.pdf*.

12. Breastcancer.org: Gene testing. Retrieved from *www.breastcancer.org/symptoms/testing/genetic*.

13. Guiliano AE, Connelly JL, Edge SB, et al: Breast cancer—Major changes in the American Joint Committee on Cancer 8th edition cancer staging manual, *Cancer J Clin* 67:290, 2017.

*14. National Comprehensive Cancer Network: *NCCN guidelines, version 2, 2017: Breast cancer.* Retrieved from *www.nccn.org/professionals/physician_gls/pdf/breast.pdf*.

15. About OncotypeDX breast DCIS score. Retrieved from *www.oncotypeiq.com/en-US/breast-cancer/patients-and-caregivers/stage-0-dcis/about-the-test*.

16. Post-breast therapy pain syndrome. Retrieved from *www.cancersupportivecare.com/neuropathicpain.php*.

17. Who gets triple negative breast cancer? Retrieved from *www.breastcancer.org/symptoms/diagnosis/trip_neg/who_gets*.

*18. Koç H, O'Donnell O, Van Ourti T: What explains education disparities in screening mammography in the United States? A comparison with the Netherlands, *Int J Environ Res Public Health* 15:1961, 2018.

19. American College of Surgeons Commission on Cancer: Cancer program standards 2016 edition: Ensuring survivor-centered care. Retrieved from *www.facs.org/~/media/files/quality%20programs/cancer/coc/2016%20coc%20standards%20manual_interactive%20pdf.ashx*.

20. Runowicz CD, Leach CR, Henry LH. et al: ACS/American Society of Clinical Oncology breast cancer survivorship care guideline, *J Clin Oncol* 34:611, 2016.

21. American Cancer Society: Breast reconstructive surgery. Retrieved from *www.cancer.org/cancer/breast-cancer/reconstruction-surgery.html*.

22. Food and Drug Administration: Breast implants. Retrieved from *www.fda.gov/MedicalDevices/ProductsandMedicalProcedures/ImplantsandProsthetics/BreastImplants/default.htm*.

*Evidence-based information for clinical practice.

52

Sexually Transmitted Infections

Daniel P. Worrall

The meaning of life is to find your gift. The purpose of life is to give it away.

Pablo Picasso

ⓔ http://evolve.elsevier.com/Lewis/medsurg

CONCEPTUAL FOCUS

Infection

Pain

Reproduction

Sexuality

LEARNING OUTCOMES

1. Identify factors contributing to sexually transmitted infections (STIs) in the United States.
2. Describe the etiology, clinical manifestations, complications, and diagnostic studies for chlamydia, gonorrhea, trichomoniasis, genital herpes, genital warts, and syphilis.
3. Compare and contrast primary genital herpes with recurrent genital herpes.

4. Explain the interprofessional care and treatment of chlamydia, gonorrhea, trichomoniasis, genital herpes, genital warts, and syphilis.
5. Discuss the nursing assessment for patients who have an STI.
6. Describe the nursing management of patients with STIs.
7. Summarize the nursing role in the prevention and control of STIs.

KEY TERMS

chlamydial infections, p. 1213
genital herpes, p. 1217
genital warts, p. 1218

gonorrhea, p. 1215
sexually transmitted infections (STIs), p. 1212

syphilis, p. 1220
trichomoniasis, p. 1216

Sexually transmitted infections (STIs) are infectious diseases that are spread through sexual contact with the penis, vagina, anus, mouth, or sexual fluids of an infected person. Many do not view STIs as a serious health threat because they are easily treated. However, the complications are serious and can include infertility and cancer. Having an STI can affect persons' well-being, their relationships, and their sexual lives. Patient education, counseling, and referral are essential nursing roles for promoting health and optimal sexual well-being.

Mucosal tissues in the genitals (urethra in men, vagina in women), rectum, and mouth are especially susceptible to the bacteria and viruses that cause STIs. A list of common STIs is shown in Table 52.1. Some STIs, such as genital human papillomavirus (HPV), can spread from direct skin-to-skin contact with an infected person. Other STIs, such as human immunodeficiency virus (HIV), may be contracted via blood or blood products or be transmitted from mother to baby during pregnancy or labor and delivery. Some STIs can spread through *autoinoculation* (spread of infection by touching or scratching an infected area and transferring it to another part of the body). STIs cannot typically be transmitted from casual contact or inanimate objects.

FACTORS AFFECTING INCIDENCE OF STIs

STIs are quite common. There are nearly 20 million new STIs diagnosed in the United States each year, resulting in an estimated 16 billion in health care costs.[1] More than 110 million Americans are infected with an STI at any given time. Having 1 STI increases the risk for getting another. A person can have more than 1 STI at the same time.

All STIs have an *incubation period*. It is the time from initial infection to the time when symptoms first appear or screening tests for the infection are positive. This can lead to the transmission of disease from an asymptomatic (but infected) person to another person, even before any symptoms or signs begin.

In the United States, all cases of gonorrhea, chlamydia, and syphilis must be reported to public health authorities for surveillance purposes for federally funded control programs and partner notification. Surveillance and partner notification are a major part of the effort to prevent and control the spread of STIs. Nurses and other HCPs play a vital role, as they are mandated to report these STIs to public health authorities. Despite this requirement, only a small number of infections are reported. This is especially important when considering that the

TABLE 52.1 Causes of Sexually Transmitted Infections (STIs)

STI	Cause
Bacterial Infections	
Chlamydial	*Chlamydia trachomatis*
Gonorrhea	*Neisseria gonorrhoeae*
Syphilis	*Treponema pallidum*
Viral Infections	
Genital herpes	Herpes simplex virus (HSV 1 or 2)
Genital warts (*condylomata acuminata*)	Human papillomavirus (HPV)
Human immunodeficiency virus infection (HIV)	Human immunodeficiency virus (HIV) (see Chapter 14)
Hepatitis B and C	Hepatitis B and C viruses (see Chapter 43)
Molluscum	Molluscum contagiosum
Parasitic/Protozoan Infection	
Trichomoniasis	*Trichomonas vaginalis*

TABLE 52.2 Risk Factors for STIs

High-Risk Behaviors
- Alcohol or drug use (inhibits judgment)
- Having new or multiple sexual partners
- Having more than 1 sexual partner
- Having sexual partners who have/have had multiple partners
- Inconsistent or incorrect use of condoms or other barrier methods
- Sharing needles used to inject drugs

High-Risk Medical History
- Having 1 STI is a risk factor for getting another
- Not being vaccinated for STIs or other infections that may be transmitted through some forms sexual activity (HPV, hepatitis A and B)
- Receiving multiple courses of nonoccupational postexposure prophylaxis for HIV infection

High-Risk Populations
- Adolescents and young adults (age <25)
- Ethnicity (e.g., black, American Indian/Alaskan Native, Native Hawaiian/Other Pacific Islander, Hispanic)[1]
- Men who have sex with men
- Persons in correctional facilities
- Transgender persons
- Victims of sexual assault
- Women

more than 2 million cases of gonorrhea, chlamydia, and syphilis reported in the United States annually do not represent the actual number of infections.

Many factors contribute to the high rate of STIs.[2,3] Earlier reproductive maturity and increased longevity make for a longer sexual life span. Other factors include (1) greater sexual freedom, (2) inconsistent or incorrect use of barrier methods (e.g., condoms) during sexual activity, and (3) the media's increasing emphasis on sexuality without mentioning safer sex. Substance use can further contribute to unsafe sexual practices by impairing judgment. Risk factors for STIs are outlined in Table 52.2.

STIs affect certain groups of people disproportionately. This includes youth under age 25 and those who are socially and economically disadvantaged.

Trends in methods of contraceptive use also affect the rate of STIs. The male condom is the best form of protection (other than abstinence) against STIs. Although condom use has increased in the United States, condoms are not often used in the general population. Most women use hormonal (e.g., oral contraceptive pills, patch, injectables) or long-acting reversible contraceptives (e.g., intrauterine devices, implantable devices).[4] These do not provide barrier protection against STIs.[5]

This chapter covers the most common forms of STIs. HIV infection is covered in Chapter 14. Anyone who contracts an STI may also be at risk for HIV infection. HIV preexposure prophylaxis (PrEP) or nonoccupational postexposure prophylaxis (nPEP) may be appropriate for these persons.[6] See Chapter 14 for more about PrEP and nPEP.

STIs CHARACTERIZED BY DISCHARGE, CERVICITIS, OR URETHRITIS

CHLAMYDIAL INFECTIONS

Chlamydia is the most common reportable STI in the United States. Nearly 1.6 million cases are reported annually, and incidence is on the rise. As many infections are asymptomatic, the actual number of infections is significantly higher.[1]

Etiology and Pathophysiology

Chlamydial infections are caused by *Chlamydia trachomatis*, a gram-negative bacterium and intracellular pathogen. *Chlamydia* is transmitted through exposure to sexual fluids during vaginal, anal, or oral sex. Ejaculation does not have to occur for it to be transmitted. The incubation period for chlamydia is 1 to 3 weeks. Infection with *Chlamydia* does not provide protection from reinfection. This means that people who were treated for chlamydial infection can always be reinfected.

The most common site for infection in men is the urethra. Infections in the male urethra are called *urethritis*. The most

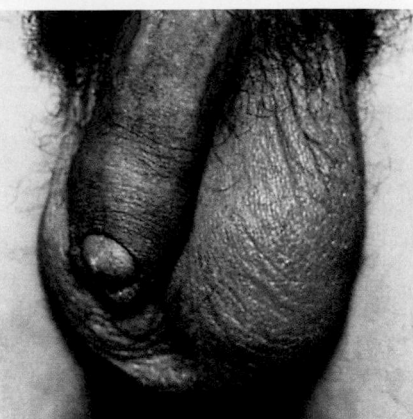

FIG. 52.1 Chlamydial epididymitis. Red, swollen scrotum. (From Morse S, Moreland A, Holmes K: *Atlas of sexually transmitted diseases and AIDS*, London, 1996, Mosby-Wolfe.)

 TABLE 52.3 Interprofessional Care
Chlamydial Infections

Diagnostic Assessment
- History and physical examination
- Nucleic acid amplification test (NAAT)
- Testing for other STIs (gonorrhea, HIV, syphilis)

Management
- Azithromycin (Zithromax) or doxycycline (Vibramycin)
- Alternative regimen: erythromycin, ofloxacin, or levofloxacin (Levaquin)
- Teach to abstain from sexual contact for 7 days after completing treatment
- Treat all sexual partners, who must also wait 7 days before resuming sexual contact

common site for infection for women is the cervix. Infections in the female cervix are called *cervicitis*. Both men and women can get chlamydia of the rectum from receptive anal sex or the oropharynx from giving oral sex. Because the vagina acts as a natural reservoir for infectious secretions, STI transmission is often more efficient from men to women than it is from women to men.

There are many serotypes of the *C. trachomatis* bacteria. A subset of these strains can cause another STI, lymphogranuloma venereum (LGV). More common serotypes are often the cause of nongonococcal urethritis (NGU).

Clinical Manifestations

Patients with chlamydia often have no symptoms. However, if symptoms develop in men, they may have pain with urination or a urethral discharge. Rarely, men can have pain or swelling of the testicles caused by infection of the epididymis (Fig. 52.1). Symptoms of cervicitis include mucopurulent discharge (mucus with pus), bleeding, dysuria, and pain with intercourse. Symptoms of rectal chlamydia include anorectal pain, discharge, bleeding, pruritus, tenesmus, mucus-coated stools, or painful bowel movements.

Complications

Complications often develop from poorly managed, inaccurately diagnosed, or undiagnosed chlamydia. Chlamydia is often not diagnosed until complications occur. While men rarely have long-term complications from infection, epididymitis can result in male infertility. More often, chlamydia can affect a woman's reproductive tract, resulting in *pelvic inflammatory disease* (PID).[7] PID can damage fallopian tubes and increases a woman's risk for an ectopic pregnancy (pregnancy outside of uterus), infertility, and chronic pelvic pain. The risk for developing PID increases with repeated infection The more episodes of PID, the more likely a woman will experience infertility. Both men and women can develop a rare reactive arthritis, an autoimmune response to infection with *C. trachomatis*.

Diagnostic Studies

Diagnosis of any STI requires an accurate sexual history, a physical examination, and laboratory tests specific to each infection. The preferred method for diagnosing chlamydia is through a nucleic acid amplification test (NAAT) (Table 52.3). NAAT is used to identify small amounts of DNA or RNA in test samples. NAAT can be done on endocervical or vaginal swabs from women, urethral swabs from men, and urine from both men and women. NAATs are the recommended test for rectal and oropharyngeal screening and diagnosis.[8]

Interprofessional Care

Because of the high prevalence of asymptomatic infections, regular screening for chlamydia in high-risk populations is recommended (Table 52.2). Anyone diagnosed and treated for chlamydia needs to return for testing 3 months after treatment to be sure that they have not been reinfected or to detect treatment failure.

Drug Therapy. The preferred treatment is a single dose of azithromycin (Zithromax) or doxycycline (Vibramycin) twice a day for 7 days (Table 52.3). All sexual contacts within 60 days should be evaluated and treated to prevent reinfection and further transmission. Teach patients to abstain from sexual contact for 7 days after treatment or until all partners have been treated and have also abstained from sexual contact for 7 days. Review the ways to reduce risk for acquiring a repeat or new STI in the future. Tell patients to return if symptoms persist or recur.

> **DRUG ALERT** Doxycycline (Vibramycin)
> - Patients should avoid prolonged or excessive exposure to sunlight.
> - Take doses on an empty stomach either 1 hour before eating or 2 hours after eating.
> - Avoid taking with antacids, iron products, or dairy products.
> - Pregnant women should not take doxycycline.

Unfortunately, there is a high rate of recurrence for chlamydia. This often occurs when the sexual partners of infected people are not treated. This "ping-pong" effect (treatment, reexposure, then reinfection) can end only when both partners are treated appropriately. Because of this issue, the CDC recommends *expedited partner therapy* (EPT).[8,9] EPT means HCPs can give drugs or prescriptions to patients with STIs to give to partners without their examining the partner. The legality of EPT varies from state to state, but few states prohibit EPT. EPT is not routinely recommended for men who have sex with men (MSM) because of a higher risk for coexisting infections in partners of MSM, especially undiagnosed syphilis or HIV. It is not recommended for female partners who are symptomatic because of the risk for PID.

GONOCOCCAL INFECTIONS

Gonorrhea is the second most common reportable STI in the United States. The incidence is on the rise. There are an estimated 820,000 cases each year, though only 468,000 cases are reported.[1]

Etiology and Pathophysiology

Gonorrhea is caused by *Neisseria gonorrhoeae,* a gram-negative, diplococcus bacterium. Gonorrhea can be transmitted by exposure to sexual fluids during vaginal, anal, or oral sex. Ejaculation does not have to occur for it to be transmitted. The incubation period ranges from 1 to 14 days. As in chlamydia, prior infection does not provide protection from reinfection. The most common site for infection for men is the urethra and for women, the cervix. Both men and women can get gonorrhea of the rectum from anal sex or of the oropharynx from oral sex.

Clinical Manifestations

The initial site of infection in men is usually the urethra. Most men will be symptomatic within a few days. The most common symptoms of gonococcal urethritis are dysuria, purulent urethral discharge (Fig. 52.2), or epididymitis. Most women who contract gonorrhea are asymptomatic or have minor symptoms that they often overlook. For women, common symptoms are increased vaginal discharge, dysuria, frequency of urination, or bleeding after sex. Often, redness and swelling can occur at the cervix or urethra along with a purulent exudate (Fig. 52.3).

Both men and women can contract rectal gonorrhea during anal intercourse or oropharyngeal gonorrhea during oral sex. Symptoms of rectal infection include mucopurulent rectal discharge or bleeding, anorectal pain, pruritus, tenesmus, mucus-coated stools, or painful bowel movements. Most patients with gonorrhea in the throat have few symptoms. Some may have a sore throat within days of performing oral sex.

Complications

Because men are often symptomatic and seek treatment early in the course of gonorrhea, they are less likely to develop serious complications than women. The complication in men is epididymitis, which can result in infertility.

Because many women are asymptomatic and seldom seek treatment, serious complications are more common and usually the reason for seeking medical care. Untreated gonorrhea can cause an infection in the Bartholin's glands or Skene's glands or result in PID. PID increases risk for ectopic pregnancy, infertility, and chronic pelvic pain.

Although rare, both men and women can develop disseminated gonococcal infection (DGI). DGI is associated with skin lesions, fever, arthralgia, arthritis, and/or endocarditis (Fig. 52.4).

Neonates can develop gonococcal conjunctivitis *(ophthalmia neonatorum)* from exposure to an infected mother during

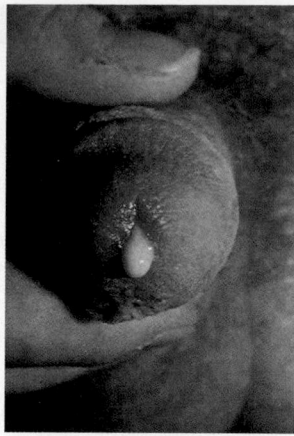

FIG. 52.2 Profuse, purulent drainage in a patient with gonorrhea. (From Marx J, Walls R, Hockberger R: *Rosen's emergency medicine: Concepts and clinical practice,* ed 7, St Louis, 2010, Mosby.)

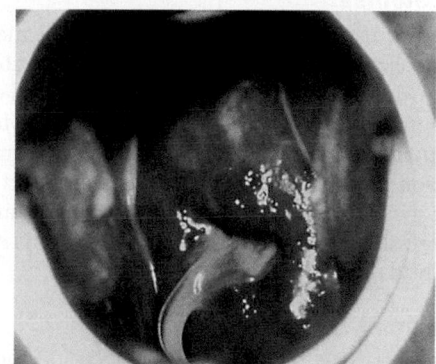

FIG. 52.3 Endocervical gonorrhea. Cervical redness and edema with discharge. (From Morse S, Moreland A, Holmes K: *Atlas of sexually transmitted diseases and AIDS,* London, 1996, Mosby-Wolfe.)

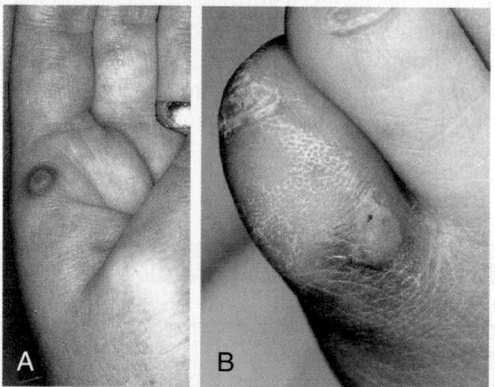

FIG. 52.4 Skin lesions with disseminated gonococcal infection. **A,** On the hand. **B,** On the fifth toe. (*A,* From Cohen J, Powderly WG: *Infectious diseases,* ed 2, St Louis, 2004, Mosby. *B,* From Mandell GL, Bennett JE, Dolin R: *Mandell, Douglas, and Bennett's principles and practice of infectious diseases,* ed 7, Philadelphia, 2010, Churchill Livingstone.)

delivery that can result in permanent blindness. Almost all states have laws or health department regulations requiring the use of prophylactic eye treatment of all newborns to prevent such infections. Because of both improved prenatal screening for gonorrhea and prophylactic treatment regimens, *ophthalmia neonatorum* caused by gonorrhea is rare.

Diagnostic Studies

For men, a presumptive diagnosis of gonorrhea is made if there is a history of sexual contact with a new or infected partner followed within a few days by urethral discharge. For women, making a diagnosis based on symptoms is difficult. Most women are asymptomatic or have symptoms that may be confused with other conditions, such as chlamydial or urinary tract infection.

A culture may be used to diagnose infection. Gram stains of urethral secretions can be used, but the sensitivity is not as good as other methods.

Interprofessional Care

Drug Therapy. Because of a short incubation period and high rates of infectivity, treatment is often given without waiting for positive test results. The first-line treatment is dual therapy with IM ceftriaxone with oral azithromycin (Zithromax) as a single dose (Table 52.4). Over the years, *N. gonorrhoeae* has developed resistance to many classes of antibiotics, including fluoroquinolones (e.g., ciprofloxacin [Cipro], levofloxacin) and tetracyclines (e.g., doxycycline [Vibramycin]).[10] Given the increasing rate of drug resistance, all patients with gonorrhea must receive treatment with at least 2 antibiotics. Patients treated with a preferred regimen but who have a positive test 7 days after treatment need antibiotic sensitivity testing.

TABLE 52.4 Interprofessional Care
Gonococcal Infections

Diagnostic Assessment

- History and physical examination
- Gram-stained smears of urethral or endocervical exudate
- Culture for *Neisseria gonorrhoeae*
- Nucleic acid amplification test (NAAT) to detect *N. gonorrhoeae*
- Testing for other STIs (syphilis, HIV, chlamydial infection)

Management

- Uncomplicated gonorrhea: ceftriaxone IM with azithromycin (Zithromax)
- Treatment of sexual contacts
- Teach to abstain from sexual contact for 7 days after treatment
- Treat all sexual partners, who must also wait 7 days before resuming sexual contact
- Reexamination if symptoms persist or recur after treatment

As with chlamydia, all sexual contacts within 60 days should be evaluated and treated to prevent reinfection and further transmission. Teach patients to abstain from sexual contact for 7 days after treatment, or until all partners have been treated and have also abstained from sexual contact for 7 days. Review the ways to reduce risk for acquiring a repeat or new STI in the future.

TRICHOMONIASIS

Trichomoniasis ("trich") is an STI caused by the protozoan parasite *Trichomonas vaginalis*. It is another common STI in the United States, affecting an estimated 3.7 million people.[1] This infection is often overlooked compared to other STIs. However, better testing methods have improved detection. It is much more common among women than men, especially among women with HIV.

Etiology and Pathophysiology

Trichomonas can be transmitted by exposure to sexual fluids during vaginal, anal, or oral sex, even if ejaculation does not occur. The incubation period is usually 1 week to 1 month but can be much longer. Prior infection does not provide protection from reinfection.

The most common site for infection in men is the urethra and in women is the cervix. It is uncommon for *Trichomonas* to infect the rectum. It is not known to infect the oropharynx. Routine screening should be considered for women in high-risk populations, including HIV-positive women and women seeking care for vaginal discharge.[8]

Clinical Manifestations

Most people do not have symptoms. Men may report burning with urination, ejaculation, or urethral discharge. Women may report painful urination, vaginal itching, painful intercourse, bleeding after sex, or a yellow-green discharge with a foul odor. The cervix can have a "strawberry" appearance.

Complications

The main complications of untreated infection are related to the inflammation and irritation that it causes in the genital tract. This inflammation makes an infected person more likely to contract or transmit another STI, particularly HIV. While gonorrhea and chlamydia are responsible for most PID, trichomoniasis is associated with PID in women with HIV.

Diagnostic Studies

The preferred method of diagnosing trichomoniasis is by NAAT testing of vaginal or endocervical secretions or urine. Other methods include culture, point-of-care testing, or direct visualization of trichomonads under the microscope. Identification of motile trichomonads in the vaginal secretions confirms infection. Tests can be done on liquid-based cervical Pap samples. In men, NAAT testing is recommended.[8]

Interprofessional Care

Drug Therapy. Patients and their partners should be treated with either metronidazole (Flagyl) or tinidazole (Tindamax). Teach patients to abstain from sexual contact for 7 days after treatment or until all sexual partners have completed a full course of treatment and abstained from sexual contact for 7 days. Tell patients to return if symptoms persist or recur. Any sexual partner within the preceding 60 days should be treated. Teach patients to use condoms or other barrier methods with every sexual contact. Because of a high rate of recurrence, repeat testing 3 months after treatment is recommended.

STIs CHARACTERIZED BY GENITAL LESIONS OR ULCERS

GENITAL HERPES INFECTIONS

Genital herpes is a common, lifelong, incurable infection. There are 2 strains of herpes: herpes simplex virus type 1 (HSV-1) and herpes simplex virus type 2 (HSV-2). Although both forms of HSV may cause anogenital infection, HSV-1 is usually associated with oral lesions. HSV-2 is more common in the genitals or anus.[8] However, an increasing proportion of anogenital herpes infections are caused by HSV-1. It is possible, but rare, to have HSV-2 infection of the mouth. Having 1 type does not protect against getting the other.

Around 50 million people in the United States have HSV-2. Most new infections are transmitted by someone who is unaware they are infected. The prevalence of new genital HSV-2 infections is twice as high among women compared to men. Hispanic and black persons are more likely to be infected.[1]

Etiology and Pathophysiology

The virus enters through the mucous membranes or breaks in the skin during contact with an infected person. The virus reproduces inside the cell and spreads to the surrounding cells. Then the virus enters the peripheral or autonomic nerve endings and ascends to the sensory or autonomic nerve ganglion near the infection site, where it often becomes dormant. Viral reactivation (recurrence or "outbreak") occurs when the virus descends to that initial site of infection, either the mucous membranes or skin.

When a person is infected with HSV-1 or HSV-2, the virus persists within the person for life. Transmission of either strain of HSV to others occurs easiest through direct contact with skin or mucous membranes when an infected person is symptomatic. However, both can be transmitted without any apparent symptoms, called *asymptomatic viral shedding*. It is impossible to predict when asymptomatic shedding will occur or for how long. HSV-2 is more likely to shed than HSV-1.

HSV-1 was primarily associated with orolabial disease, known as "cold sores" or "fever blisters" (Fig. 52.5) and HSV-2 with anogenital disease. However, there has been a shift in understanding that either HSV-1 or HSV-2 can cause genital, anal, or orolabial infections. In most cases, HSV-1 infections are more common "above the waist," involving the gingivae, dermis, upper respiratory tract, and, rarely the central nervous system (CNS). HSV-2 almost always infects sites "below the waist," the genital tract, perineum, or anus. It is important to understand that there is no absolute, single site for either virus.

Clinical Manifestations

Primary Episode. A *primary (initial) episode* of genital herpes has an incubation of 2 to 12 days. Most people do not have any recognizable symptoms of primary HSV genital infection. If symptoms do occur, they follow a series of stages. During the *prodromal stage*, the period before lesions appear, the patient may have burning, itching, or tingling at the site of inoculation. In the *vesicular stage*, few to multiple small, often painful

vesicles (blisters) may appear on the buttock, inner thigh, penis, scrotum, vulva, perineum, perianal region, vagina, or cervix. The vesicles have large quantities of infectious viral particles. Next, in the *ulcerative stage,* the lesions rupture and form shallow, moist ulcerations. In the *final stage,* spontaneous crusting and epithelialization of the erosions occur (Fig. 52.6).

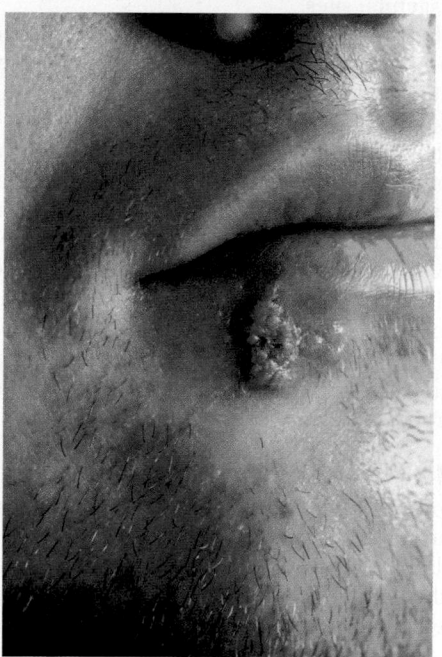

FIG. 52.5 Herpes simplex virus (HSV). (© iStock.com/zeleno.)

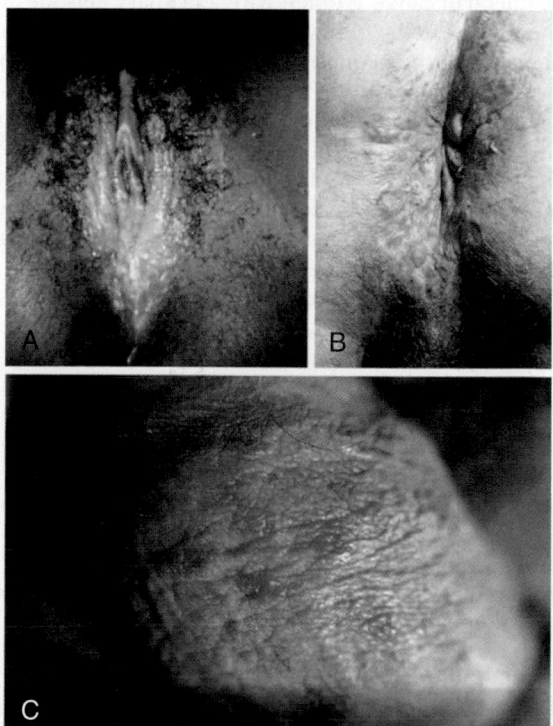

FIG. 52.6 Unruptured vesicles of herpes simplex virus type 2 (HSV-2). A, Vulvar area. B, Perianal area. C, Penile herpes simplex, ulcerative stage. (*A* and *C,* From Centers for Disease Control and Prevention. Courtesy Susan Lindsley. *B,* From Morse S, Moreland A, Holmes K: *Atlas of sexually transmitted diseases and AIDS,* London, 1996, Mosby-Wolfe.)

Regional (inguinal node) lymphadenopathy and systemic flu-like symptoms, including fever, headache, malaise, and myalgia may occur with the primary episode. Urination may be painful from the urine touching active lesions. The whole process from prodrome to healing varies and can take up to 3 weeks. Autoinoculation can occur if active lesions are touched or scratched, causing additional and potentially recurrent infection at extragenital sites.

Recurrent Episodes. *Recurrent genital herpes* occurs in many people during the year after the primary episode. The symptoms of recurrent episodes are less severe, and the lesions usually heal more quickly. HSV-1 genital infections recur less often than HSV-2 genital infections. Over time, both decrease in frequency.

Common triggers of recurrence include stress, fatigue, sunburn, general illness, immunosuppression, and menses. Many patients can predict a recurrence by noticing the prodromal symptoms of tingling, burning, and itching at the site where the lesions will recur. The greatest risk for transmitting infection exists when active lesions are present. However, it is possible to transmit the virus when no visible lesions or symptoms are present. Most HSV transmission occurs during these asymptomatic periods.

Complications

Both HSV-1 and HSV-2 can cause rare but serious complications, including blindness, encephalitis, and aseptic meningitis. Autoinoculation can result in the development of extragenital lesions in the buttocks, groin, thighs, fingers, and eyes. Genital ulcers increase the risk for contracting HIV. HSV lesions can be more severe and more persistent in HIV-infected patients.

Pregnant women with HSV can transmit the virus to the baby, especially if the virus is shed while the infant passes though the birth canal. Women with a primary episode of HSV near the time of delivery have the highest risk for transmitting genital herpes to the neonate. The virus can infect the neonate's skin, eyes, mouth, or the CNS or become widespread and cause significant morbidity and mortality. An active genital lesion at the time of delivery is an indication for cesarean delivery.[8]

One of the most profound consequences for people with genital herpes is the overall impact it can have on their psychologic well-being, their relationships, and their sexual lives. You can help teach patients to understand how to talk to sexual partners about HSV. Refer patients who need counseling. Teach patients with herpes that it is a common, manageable, non–life-threatening condition and help them to understand their treatment options.

Diagnostic Studies

Diagnosis is often based on the patient's reported symptoms, then confirmed by visual examination. Culture from open skin eruptions can be used to diagnose HSV and distinguish between HSV-1 and HSV-2. Highly accurate blood tests for antibodies are available for HSV-1 and HSV-2, but do not show the location of the infection. These antibodies usually appear by 12 weeks after exposure.

Interprofessional Care

Drug Therapy. Although not a cure, antiviral drugs can shorten the duration of HSV viral shedding, shorten the healing time of eruptions, and reduce the frequency of outbreaks by up to 80%.[8] Treatment of HSV should start before diagnostic results are available because early treatment reduces the duration of the ulcers and risk for transmission (Table 52.5).

TABLE 52.5 **Interprofessional Care**
Genital Herpes

Diagnostic Assessment
- History and physical examination
- Antibody assay for HSV type
- Viral isolation by tissue culture

Management
- Identify triggering factors
- Abstain from sexual contact while lesions are present and until fully healed
- Symptomatic care
- Confidential counseling and testing for HIV

Primary (Initial) Infection
- Acyclovir (Zovirax), valacyclovir (Valtrex) or famciclovir (Famvir)

Recurrent Episodic Infection
- Acyclovir, valacyclovir, or famciclovir for shorter duration

Suppressive Therapy
- Acyclovir, valacyclovir, or famciclovir daily at a lower dose

Severe Infection
- IV acyclovir until clinical improvement, followed by oral antiviral therapy

Three antiviral agents are available for the treatment of HSV: acyclovir (Zovirax), famciclovir (Famvir), and valacyclovir (Valtrex). These drugs inhibit herpetic viral replication. They are prescribed for both primary and recurrent infections. Taken daily at a lower dose, they can be used as suppressive therapy to decrease frequent anogenital recurrences. Teach patients with active outbreaks to maintain good hygiene, wear loose-fitting cotton undergarments, and avoid sexual contact until the outbreak has completely healed to reduce transmission to others.

The main goal is to keep eruptions clean and dry. Techniques to reduce pain with urination include pouring water onto the perineal area while voiding to dilute the urine or voiding in the shower. Pain may need a local anesthetic, such as lidocaine gel, or analgesics, such as ibuprofen, acetaminophen, acetaminophen with codeine, or aspirin. Ice packs to the affected area can give some relief.

IV acyclovir is reserved for severe or life-threatening infections in which hospitalization is needed for the treatment of ocular or widespread infections, CNS infections (e.g., meningitis), or pneumonitis.

GENITAL WARTS

Genital warts *(condylomata acuminata)* are caused by the HPV. There are around 100 types of papillomavirus, of which at least 40 strains are sexually transmitted.[8] "Low-risk" strains of the virus can cause warts on the skin. "High-risk" strains can lead to cancers of the genital tract, anus, or oropharynx in some patients. HPV types 6 and 11 cause about 90% of genital and anal wart cases. About 355,000 people are diagnosed each year. Most sexually active men and women will be infected with some type of HPV at some point in their lives. In most states, HPV is not a reportable infection. (Cervical HPV infection is discussed in Chapter 53.)

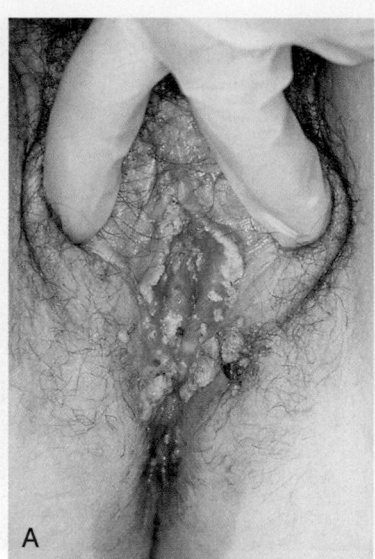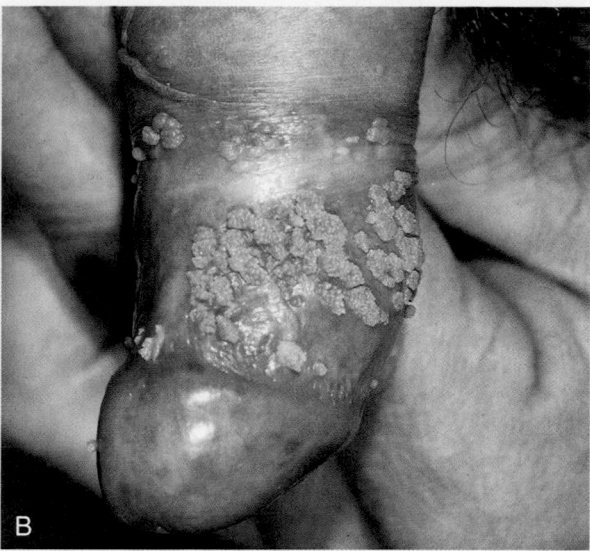

FIG. 52.7 Genital warts. **A,** Vulvar warts. **B,** Multiple warts on the penis. (From Habif TP: *Clinical dermatology,* ed 6, St Louis, 2015, Mosby.)

Etiology and Pathophysiology

HPV is transmitted by skin-to-skin contact, most often during vaginal, anal, or oral sex. It can be transmitted during nonpenetrating sexual activity. The basal epithelial cells infected with HPV undergo transformation and proliferation to form a warty growth (Fig. 52.7). The incubation period can range from weeks to months to years. Infection with 1 type of HPV does not prevent infection with another type.

In most people, HPV is considered transient (virus is "cleared" or resolves spontaneously after 1 to 2 years). However, it can persist even when the warts themselves are not visible after treatment. It is unclear whether removing visible warts helps a person to clear the virus, cures the virus, or reduces a person's ability to transmit the virus.[8]

Clinical Manifestations

Most people with HPV do not know that they are infected because they are asymptomatic. Genital or anal warts are discrete single or multiple papillary growths that are white to gray, are pink-flesh colored, or can be hyperpigmented depending on the skin type. They may grow and coalesce to form large, cauliflower-like masses. Most patients have 1 to 10 genital warts.

In men, warts occur on the penis and scrotum, inside or around the anus, or in the urethra. In women, warts occur on the inner thighs, vulva, vagina, or cervix, in the perianal area, including in the internal anal canal (Fig. 52.7). There are usually no other signs or symptoms. Itching may occur with anogenital warts. Bleeding on defecation may occur with anal warts.

Diagnostic Studies

Most early lesions caused by HPV are undetectable by visual examination. A diagnosis of genital warts can be made based on the characteristic appearance of the lesions (Fig. 52.7). Warts may be confused with *condylomata lata* of secondary syphilis, cancer, or benign growths. Testing should be done to rule out

other conditions. At present, the only definitive diagnostic procedure is biopsy of any questionable growth. Testing for cervical HPV is discussed in Chapter 53.

Complications

Although genital and anal warts can grow, spread, or be transmitted to others, they have few long-term complications and are not associated with the development of cancer. Infection with "high-risk" strains of HPV (types 16 and 18) can lead to cancers of the cervix, vagina, vulva, penis, anus, and oropharynx. For some people, HPV lesions can cause psychosocial burden due to the cosmetic appearance of lesions or the need for long courses of HPV-related treatment. During pregnancy, warts tend to grow rapidly and increase in size.

Interprofessional Care

HPV Vaccines. It may be possible to eradicate some cancerous HPV types over the next few decades, especially if both girls and boys are vaccinated. Currently 3 vaccines are available to protect against HPV. A quadrivalent vaccine (Gardasil) protects against types 6, 11, 16, and 18. The bivalent vaccine Cervarix offers protection against HPV types 16 and 18. A 9-valent vaccine (Gardasil 9) protects against HPV types 6, 11, 16, 18 and 5 other HPV types. These vaccines are given in 2 or 3 IM doses over a 6-month period and have few side effects. The CDC recommends that all children, male and female, be vaccinated at age 11 to 12, but vaccination can be started as early as age 9.[11] The bivalent and quadrivalent vaccines are approved for persons up to age 26. The 9-valent vaccine is approved for girls 9 to 26 and boys 9 to 15.

These vaccines do not treat active HPV infection. Ideally, persons should receive the vaccine before the start of sexual activity. Those who are infected with HPV can still get protection against HPV types not already contracted. HPV vaccines offer protection against strains causing 90% of genital warts and 70% (Gardasil) to 90% (Gardasil-9) of cervical cancers. They may offer protection from anal and certain types of throat cancer.

HPV Vaccine and Young Males

T.N. is a 19-yr-old man who is being seen in the health care center for signs and symptoms of a urinary tract infection. After reviewing his health history, you learn he has not received the HPV vaccine. When asked, he shares with you that he is sexually active and that he does not need to get the vaccine because his girlfriend already has.

Making Clinical Decisions

Best Available Evidence. Males ages 15 to 26 can be vaccinated with 9-valent/9vHPV (Gardasil 9) to reduce the incidence of HPV infections and HPV-related cancers (e.g., anal, oropharyngeal, cervical, penile). HPV infections are caused by HPV types 6, 11, 16, 18, 31, 33, 45, 52, or 58. The HPV vaccine also protects against the 2 HPV types (6 and 11) that cause 90% of anogenital warts. Vaccination rates for HPV lag behind most all other vaccinations for young people.

Clinician Expertise. You know younger men may be unaware of the recommendations for the HPV vaccine. The vaccine was originally approved to prevent cervical, vulvar, and vaginal cancer in females ages 9 through 26. Since there is no routine screening for HPV-related cancers except cervical cancer, a vaccine that prevents most of these cancers is critical. You know that T.N. will need a 3-dose series (0, 1 to 2, 6 months) to complete his immunization.

Patient Preferences and Values. T.N. states he never has unprotected sex and does not like injections.

Implications for Nursing Practice

1. Why is it important to discuss the risks and benefits of the vaccine to T.N.?
2. How would you respond to T.N., who has heard that if you are already sexually active the vaccine will not be effective?
3. How can you address T.N.'s concerns about his dislike of injections?

Reference for Evidence

Centers for Disease Control and Prevention: Human Papillomavirus Vaccination and Cancer Prevention. Retrieved from *www.cdc.gov/vaccines/vpd/hpv/index.html*.

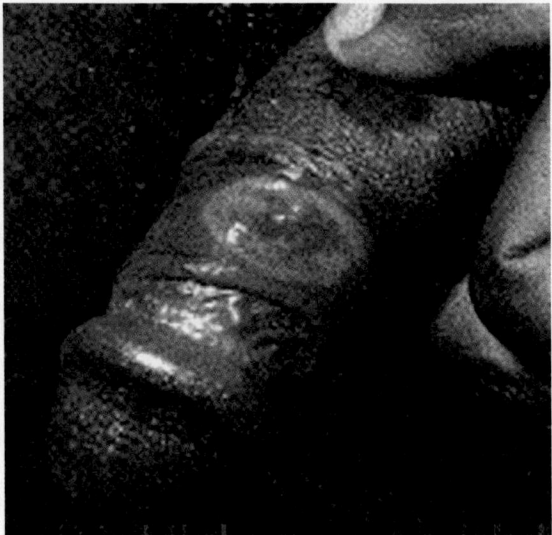

FIG. 52.8 Primary syphilis chancre. (From Morse S, Holmes K, Ballard R: *Atlas of sexually transmitted diseases and AIDS*, ed 4, London, 2010, Saunders.)

Therapy should be modified if a patient has not improved or cannot tolerate the side effects of certain treatments.

If the warts do not resolve with topical therapies, treatments such as cryotherapy with liquid nitrogen, electrocautery, laser therapy, local α-interferon injections, or surgical excision may be needed. Teach patients that because treatment does not destroy the virus (merely the infected tissue), recurrence and reinfection are possible. Long-term follow-up is advised.

SYPHILIS

Syphilis is a sexually transmitted bacterial infection that can cause serious long-term complications if not identified and treated appropriately. Over 88,000 cases of syphilis are reported annually in the United States, with a sharp increase seen in recent years. The population most affected by syphilis is MSM, with the highest rates among black MSM between 25 and 29 years old.[1]

Etiology and Pathophysiology

Syphilis is caused by *Treponema pallidum,* a bacterial spirochete. It is transmitted by direct contact with a syphilitic ulcer called a *chancre.* A chancre can occur externally on the genitals, anus, or lips or internally in the vagina, rectum, or mouth or tongue (Fig. 52.8) or through the mucosal membranes of an infected person. Transmission can occur during vaginal, anal, or oral sex. The incubation period can range from 10 to 90 days (average 21 days). Having the infection does not provide protection from reinfection, even after successful treatment. An infected pregnant woman can transmit syphilis to her fetus during her pregnancy. There is a high risk for stillbirth or having babies who develop complications after birth, including seizures and death.

Clinical Manifestations

Syphilis is called "*The Great Imitator*" because it can present with a variety of signs and symptoms that mimic other diseases.

Drug Therapy. Treatment of genital or anal warts is hampered by the high proportion of asymptomatic and undiagnosed infections and lack of curative treatment. The primary goal of treatment is the removal of symptomatic warts.

In-office treatment consists of chemical or ablative (removal with laser or electrocautery) methods. A common treatment is the use of trichloroacetic acid (TCA) or bichloroacetic acid (BCA) applied directly to the wart surface. Petroleum jelly applied with a cotton swab to the surrounding normal skin can minimize irritation. A sharp, stinging pain is often felt with initial acid contact, but this quickly subsides.

Patient-applied treatments are also available. Podofilox liquid and gel are available by prescription (Condylox, Condylox Gel). The patient applies the solution or gel for 3 successive days. Treatment can be repeated for up to 4 weeks or until resolution of the lesions. Imiquimod cream (Aldara, Zyclara) is an immune response modifier that is applied at bedtime, either 3 times per week (Aldara) or nightly for up to 16 weeks (Zyclara). Sinecatechin ointment (Veregen) is made from the extract of green tea leaves and has antioxidant properties. It is applied 3 times daily for up to 16 weeks.

Treatment of warts may or may not decrease infectivity as the HPV causing these may still be present. Anogenital warts are hard to treat and often need more than 1 treatment or modality.

TABLE 52.6 Stages of Syphilis

Primary
- *Infectivity:* Highly infectious
- Duration of stage: 3–6 wk
- Single or multiple chancres (painless indurated lesions) of penis, vulva, lips, mouth, vagina, and rectum (Fig. 52.8). Occurs 10–90 days after inoculation
- Regional lymphadenopathy (microorganisms drain into the lymph nodes)
- Exudate and blood from chancre are highly infectious

Secondary
- *Infectivity:* Highly infectious
- *Duration of stage:* Occurs a few weeks after primary chancre heals, lasts 1–2 yr
- Flu-like symptoms: malaise, fever, sore throat, headaches, fatigue, arthralgia, generalized adenopathy
- Mucous patches in mouth (Fig. 52.9), tongue, or cervix
- Symmetric, nonpruritic rash bilaterally that appears on trunk, palms, and/or soles (Fig. 52.10)
- *Condylomata lata* (moist, weeping papules) in the anogenital area
- Weight loss, alopecia

Latent
- *Infectivity:* Early (<1 yr)—infectious; late (≥1 yr)—noninfectious
- *Duration of stage:* Throughout life or progression to late stage
- Absence of signs or symptoms
- Diagnosis based on positive specific treponemal antibody test together with normal CSF and absence of clinical manifestations

Late
- *Infectivity:* Noninfectious
- *Duration of stage:* Chronic (without treatment), occurs 1–20 years after initial infection
- Gummas (chronic, destructive lesions affecting any organ of body, especially skin, bone, liver, mucous membranes) (Fig. 52.11)
- *Cardiovascular:* Aneurysms, heart valve insufficiency, heart failure, aortitis
- *Neurosyphilis:* Can occur at any stage of syphilis
- *General paresis:* Personality changes from minor to psychotic, tremors, physical and mental deterioration
- *Tabes dorsalis* (ataxia, areflexia, paresthesias, lightning pains, damaged joints)

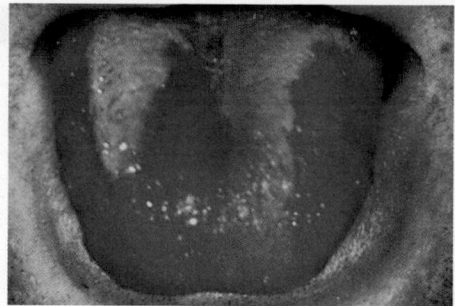

FIG. 52.9 Secondary syphilis. Mucous patch in the mouth. (From Mandell GL, Bennett JE, Dolin R: *Mandell, Douglas, and Bennett's principles and practice of infectious diseases,* ed 7, Philadelphia, 2010, Churchill Livingstone.)

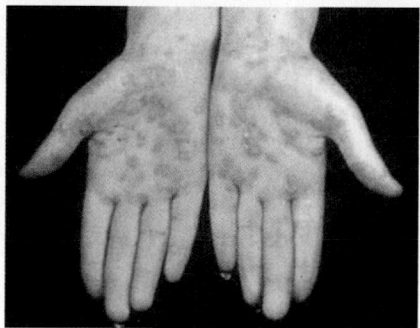

FIG. 52.10 Secondary syphilis. Palmar rash. (From Centers for Disease Control and Prevention Public Health Image Library. Courtesy Robert Sumpter.)

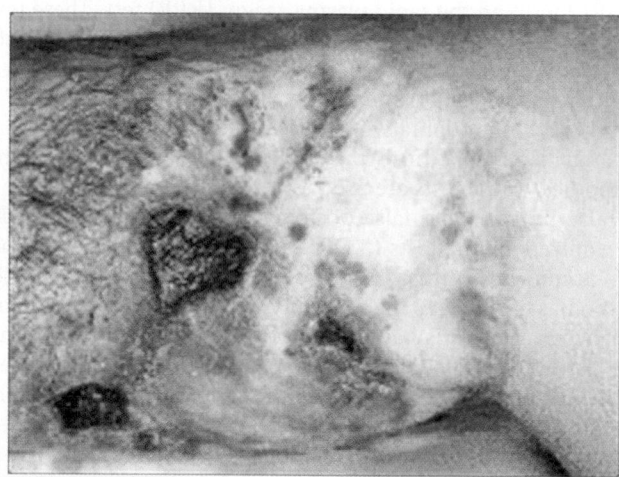

FIG. 52.11 Destructive skin gummas associated with tertiary syphilis. (From Gawkrodger D, Ardern-Jones M: *Dermatology,* ed 6, St Louis, 2016, Mosby.)

Compared with other STIs, syphilis is harder to recognize, which can delay treatment. If it is not diagnosed and treated, specific clinical stages occur with the progression of the disease (Table 52.6).

The primary stage is the development of a chancre at the site of transmission. This can appear days to months following infection. In most patients, it occurs by 3 weeks. Chancres can be found on the genitals but often go unnoticed when inside the mouth, vagina, or anus. As the chancre begins to heal or shortly after, patients will progress to the secondary stage of infection if untreated. This stage is usually characterized by a maculopapular rash. It may be coupled with other systemic symptoms. The classic rash appears on the palms of the hands or soles of the feet, but often involves the trunk or extremities. Without treatment, the rash will resolve, but the patient still has syphilis and will remain infectious for some time.

Tertiary, or late syphilis, is the final stage. Patients will not have obvious symptoms. During this stage, the organism is silently causing organ damage over many years. The formation of gummas can lead to serious complications.

Complications

Gummas may cause irreparable damage to skin, bone, or liver. In cardiovascular syphilis, the resulting aneurysm may press on structures such as the intercostal nerves, causing pain. The risk for rupture exists as the aneurysm increases in size. Scarring of the aortic valve can cause aortic valve insufficiency and heart failure.

Neurosyphilis occurs when *T. pallidum* invades the CNS. It can occur at any stage of syphilis. Visual impairment, *tabes dorsalis* (progressive locomotor ataxia), and dementia are rare, extreme manifestations.

TABLE 52.7 Interprofessional Care
Syphilis

Diagnostic Assessment
- History and physical examination
- Dark-field microscopy
- Nontreponemal and/or treponemal serologic testing
- Testing for other STIs (HIV, gonorrhea, chlamydial infection)

Management
- Antibiotic therapy:
  - Penicillin G benzathine (Bicillin LA)
  - Doxycycline or tetracycline (if penicillin contraindicated)
- Confidential counseling and testing for HIV infection
- Surveillance
- Repeat of nontreponemal tests at 6 and 12 mo
- Examination of cerebrospinal fluid at 1 yr if treatment involves alternative antibiotics or treatment failure has occurred.

Chancres on or inside the genitalia or anus enhance HIV transmission. Patients with HIV and syphilis appear to be at greatest risk for clinically significant CNS involvement and may need more intensive treatment than other patients with syphilis.

Diagnostic Studies

Syphilis is most often diagnosed by a blood test. We classify tests for syphilis as those done for screening and those done to confirm a positive screening test. Nontreponemal tests used for screening detect antibodies that are not specific for syphilis. These tests include the Venereal Disease Research Laboratory (VDRL) test and the rapid plasma reagin (RPR) test. These tests usually become positive 10 to 14 days after the appearance of a chancre. We call the fluorescent treponemal antibody absorption (FTA-Abs) test, *T. pallidum* particle agglutination (TP-PA) test, and syphilis qualitative enzyme-linked immunoassay (EIA) *treponemal tests* because they specifically detect treponemal antibodies. These tests are used to confirm a diagnosis.[8]

False-negative and false-positive test results can occur with the nontreponemal tests (VDRL, RPR). A false-negative result may occur with primary syphilis if the test is done before the person has had time to make antibodies. A false-positive finding may occur if patients have various other diseases or inflammatory conditions. Positive nontreponemal test results are always confirmed by treponemal tests. In the cerebrospinal fluid (CSF), changes such as an increased WBC count, increased total protein, and a positive treponemal antibody test are diagnostic of neurosyphilis.

If treatment with antibiotics is started early in the course of the disease based on the history and the symptoms, the serologic testing may not show syphilis. If the patient tests positive with screening serology (RPR), it will take time for this to normalize after treatment. This test is often used to ensure cure in patients. Once a person tests positive for syphilis via syphilis-specific testing (TP-PA, EIA), these findings may stay positive for an indefinite period despite successful treatment.

Interprofessional Care

Because of the serious complications associated with untreated syphilis, screening programs for high-risk groups are important for reducing morbidity and mortality. The evaluation of all patients with syphilis should include HIV testing. The CDC recommends annual syphilis testing for HIV patients (Table 52.7).[8]

Drug Therapy. Management is aimed at starting treatment early. Penicillin G benzathine (Bicillin L-A) is the recommended treatment for all stages (Table 52.7). When penicillin is contraindicated, doxycycline or tetracycline may be used. Aqueous procaine penicillin G is the treatment of choice for neurosyphilis. Treatment cannot reverse damage that is already present in the later stages of the disease. All sexual contacts from the preceding 90 days should be treated. Reexamination and follow-up testing are recommended every 6 months for up to 2 years to ensure cure. Repeat HIV testing should be done on all HIV-negative patients diagnosed with primary or secondary syphilis given the higher risk for HIV transmission during these stages.

❖ NURSING MANAGEMENT: STIs
◆ Nursing Assessment

Subjective and objective data that should be obtained from a person with an STI are outlined in Table 52.8. You must be aware of patients' gender identity and current anatomy. Screen patients based on risk history and sexual behaviors. Assess the patient's risk for contracting an STI. Questions to ask include number of partners (in the last month, year?), types of partners ("Do you have sex with men, women, or both?"), type of birth control used (if applicable), use of condoms or other barrier methods, history of an STI, use of drugs and alcohol, exchange of sex for drugs or money, and risk for violence and personal safety.[12] Plan teaching based on the responses to these questions.

Interpersonal skills necessary for this interview include respect, compassion, and a nonjudgmental attitude. Tailor your counseling to the patient. Start by asking patients how they define themselves, including their gender identity and sexual preferences. Do not assume someone is heterosexual, MSM, or women who have sex with women (WSW) based on appearance. Do not assume MSM engage in the same sexual practices. Finally, do not assume that older people are not at risk. Sex and sexuality are dynamic across the life cycle, and sexually active older adults can be at risk for STIs.[13]

🅀 CHECK YOUR PRACTICE

You are working on the medicine unit caring for a 68-yr-old man admitted for IV penicillin for neurosyphilis. The nurse that you are working with says, "I can't believe a man that old could get syphilis."
- How would you respond?
- What should you discuss with your colleague?

◆ Nursing Diagnoses

Nursing diagnoses for the patient with an STI include:
- Impaired sexual functioning
- Risk for infection
- Lack of knowledge

◆ Planning

The overall goals are that the patient with an STI will (1) understand the mode of transmission of STIs and the risks associated with STIs, (2) complete treatment and return for appropriate follow-up, (3) notify or assist in notifying sexual contacts about their need for testing and treatment, (4) abstain from sexual contact until infection is resolved, and (5) demonstrate knowledge of safer sex practices.

TABLE 52.8 Nursing Assessment

STIs

Subjective Data

Important Health Information

Sexual health history: Sexual activity, history of STIs, multiple sexual partners, unsafe sexual practices

Medications: Allergy to antibiotics

Functional Health Patterns

Health perception–health management: Unsafe sexual practices, drug and/or alcohol use

Nutritional-metabolic: Nausea, vomiting, anorexia. Pharyngitis, oral lesions, chills. Alopecia

Elimination: Dysuria, urinary frequency, urethral discharge, pain with bowel movements

Cognitive-perceptual: Arthralgia, headache, painful, burning lesions, itching or irritation at infected site

Sexuality-reproductive: Dyspareunia, vaginal or penile discharge, bleeding with sex, genital or perianal lesions

Objective Data

General

Fever, lymphadenopathy (generalized or inguinal)

Integumentary

Syphilis: Primary: Painless, indurated genital, oral, or perianal lesions

Secondary: Bilateral, symmetric rash on palms, soles, or entire body. Mucous patches on mouth or tongue; alopecia

Genital herpes: Painful genital or anal vesicular lesions

Genital warts: Single or multiple gray or white genital or anal warts

Gastrointestinal

Rectal discharge, rectal lesions

Urinary

Urethral discharge, erythema

Reproductive

Cervical mucopurulent discharge, cervical erythema, cervical bleeding; penile purulent discharge, epididymitis, proctitis, genital lesions

Possible Diagnostic Findings

Chlamydia: Positive culture or NAAT cervical, urethral, anal, oropharyngeal, or urine samples

Gonorrhea: Positive cultures or NAAT from cervical, urethral, anal, oropharyngeal, or urine samples

Genital herpes: Positive HSV-1 or HSV-2 serum antibody test. Positive culture from active lesion indicating HSV-1 or HSV-2

Syphilis: Positive findings on VDRL and RPR, spirochetes on dark-field microscopy

Trichomoniasis: Positive increased pH and positive motile protozoa on wet preparation of discharge. Positive FDA–approved rapid test or liquid-based Pap positive for trichomoniasis

TABLE 52.9 Understanding Risk for STIs in Special Populations

When dealing with the following populations at risk for STIs, it is important to consider cultural, behavioral, and other risk factors that may place them at increased risk for STIs or not receiving appropriate screening.

Women Who Have Sex With Women (WSW)

- WSW should not be presumed to be at low or no risk for STIs based on sexual orientation.
- WSW are at risk for acquiring bacterial, viral, and protozoal infections from current and prior partners, both male and female.
- Practices involving digital-vaginal or digital-anal contact, particularly with shared penetrative sex items, present a means for transmission of infected cervicovaginal secretions.
- Female-to-female transmission of chlamydia, trichomoniasis, HIV, HPV, HSV, and syphilis have been reported.
- Report of same-sex behavior in women should not deter HCPs from screening for all STIs.

Men Who Have Sex With Men (MSM)

- MSM are at higher risk for HIV, syphilis, hepatitis C, and other viral and bacterial STIs compared to the general population.
- HIV-uninfected MSM who are diagnosed with an STI should be counseled about the options for HIV prevention, including preexposure prophylaxis (PrEP) and nonoccupational postexposure prophylaxis (nPEP).
- Rates of syphilis, gonorrhea, and chlamydia are increasing in MSM, particularly in HIV-infected MSM.
- Assess risk for STIs among MSM patients and be comfortable asking questions about sexual identity and practices, including insertive and receptive anal sex.

Transgender Persons

- *Transgender man* is a term used to describe a person born anatomically female but who identifies as male. *Transgender woman* is a term used to describe a person born anatomically male but who identifies as female.
- Rates of certain STIs, including HIV, are higher among transgender women, compared to the general population.
- Not all transgender persons have had genital reassignment surgery and may still have the genitals they were assigned at birth. Therefore screen these persons for STIs based on both risk history and current anatomy. For example, a transgender man may still have a vagina and cervix.

Source: Centers for Disease Control: Sexually transmitted disease treatment guidelines. Retrieved from *www.cdc.gov/std/tg2015/specialpops.htm.*

in which both partners have been tested for STIs can reduce the risk. Addressing issues related to drug and alcohol use is important for promoting healthy sexual behavior.

Be prepared to teach special populations, including MSM, WSW, and transgender persons, about their risks (Table 52.9). Encourage routine testing in people who are at higher risk, so STIs can be identified early. This will help decrease the potential for complications and reduce transmission to others. A teaching guide for the patient with an STI is shown in Table 52.10.

Measures to Prevent Infection. Encourage patients to take notice of a sexual partner's genitalia before sex, paying attention to any discharge, sores, blisters, lesions, or rashes. Help patients to be aware of specific signs and symptoms of infection. This can help them to make good decisions about whether to continue sexual activity with safer-sex modifications or to choose not to have sexual contact at all. Remind patients that most STIs may have no symptoms but can still be transmitted. Emphasize with patients that when they have sex, they are exposed to the infections of everyone with whom their partner has ever had sex.

◆ **Nursing Implementation**

◆ **Health Promotion.** Many approaches to stopping the spread of STIs have had varying degrees of success. Be prepared to discuss "safer" sex practices and harm reduction with all patients, not only those who are perceived to be at risk. These practices include abstinence, monogamy, avoiding high-risk sexual behaviors, and correctly using condoms and other barriers with every sexual act. Sexual abstinence is the only certain method of avoiding all STIs, but few people consider this option. Limiting sexual contacts to an established, monogamous relationship

---

TABLE 52.10 Patient Teaching

STIs

When teaching the patient with STIs:

1. Explain precautions to take, such as
   - Using condoms and other barrier methods with every sexual encounter
   - Being monogamous, defining what monogamy means with your partner
   - Asking potential partners about their sexual history
   - Asking potential partners if they have been tested for STIs
   - Avoiding sex with partners who have visible oral, inguinal, genital, perineal, or anal lesions or those who use IV drugs
   - Voiding and washing genitalia and surrounding area after sex to flush out/wash away organisms to reduce potential for transmitting infection
2. Explain the importance of taking all antibiotics or antiviral agents as prescribed. Symptoms will improve after 1–2 days of treatment, but organisms may still be present.
3. Teach patients diagnosed with gonorrhea, chlamydia, syphilis, or trichomoniasis that all sexual partners need to be treated to prevent transmission and reinfection.
4. Teach patients to abstain from sexual contact during and for 7 days after treatment and to use condoms or other barrier methods when sexual activity is resumed to prevent spread of infection and reinfection.
5. Explain the importance of follow-up examination and retesting at least once after treatment (if appropriate) to confirm complete cure and prevent relapse.
6. Allow patients and partners to voice their concerns and clarify areas that need explanation.
7. Teach patients about the signs and symptoms of complications and need to report problems to their HCP to ensure proper follow-up and early treatment of reinfection.
8. Tell patients of the infectious nature of these infections to avoid a false sense of security, which may result in careless sexual practices or poor personal hygiene.
9. Tell patients about health department requirements for anonymously reporting certain STIs.

Proper use of a condom is a highly effective mechanical barrier to several infections that may be transmitted by or to a penis. Partners should openly discuss any objections to condom use, such as interference with spontaneity and the presence of a barrier. Information about the mechanics of sexual arousal and incorporating a condom into sex can help in overcoming the resistance to its use. Refusing sexual activity with any partner who will not use a condom is a safe and legitimate option.

The *female condom,* a lubricated polyurethane sheath designed for vaginal use, is another option for some women. Teach patients to avoid the spermicide nonoxynol 9 (N-9), which can be used alone to prevent pregnancy or as a condom

lubricant. Nonoxynol 9 is one of the least effective methods of birth control when used alone. It can be irritating to the vagina and rectum, increasing the risk for acquiring an STI.

Screening Programs. Screening programs are an effective means of identifying, treating, preventing, and controlling the spread of STIs. At present, there are CDC-recommended screening programs for certain populations, including young people, MSM, pregnant women, and anyone at increased risk for exposure to an STI (e.g., new partners, nonmonogamous relationships, not using condoms).[8]

Case Finding. Interviewing and case finding are other methods used to control the spread of STIs. These activities are directed toward finding and examining all sexual contacts of patients with reportable STIs so that effective treatment can be started. Public health professionals, often nurses, are aware of the social implications of STIs and the need for discretion in finding partners. Sexual contacts are not told about the origin of the information naming them as a contact or the timing of exposure to ensure patient privacy mandates.

Partner notification and treatment impose a heavy burden on public health departments. As a result, the notification often becomes the responsibility of the infected partner. The infected partner may choose not to tell sexual partners, and the partners may choose not to seek treatment. Unfortunately, this perpetuates the disease.

Educational and Research Programs. Actively encourage your community to provide better education about STIs for its citizens. High-risk populations (e.g., young people under age 25, MSM) should be a prime target for such educational programs. STI rates are rising in older adults.[13] Older adults are less likely to use condoms and often have a hard time starting discussions of sexual health issues.

Knowledge and understanding can decrease the incidence of STIs. Encourage the HPV vaccine that protects against genital warts and cervical cancer for boys and girls before the start of sexual activity. Accurate and current information may help reduce parental fears related to the vaccine. Consider stressing the prevention of cancer as a reason for the vaccine, which may be more productive and less controversial, thus making the parent and adolescent more receptive.

Acute Care

Psychologic Support. The diagnosis of an STI may be met with a variety of emotions, such as embarrassment, shame, guilt, anger, or even a desire for vengeance. Encourage the patient to voice feelings. Couples in marital or committed relationships have an added problem when an STI is diagnosed if they must face the implication of sexual activity outside the relationship. The STI raises other concerns about their relationship and may serve as an incentive for further problem solving. A referral for professional counseling to explore the impact of the STI on their relationship may be indicated.

A patient who has genital herpes is faced with the fact that future outbreaks will occur and that no cure is available. This can be frustrating and disruptive to the patient's physical, emotional, social, and sexual life. Help the patient identify and avoid any factors that may precipitate outbreaks, such as stress, local trauma, or sun exposure. Tell the patient that the frequency and severity of recurrences will decrease over time. It is important to stress that herpes is manageable and does not pose a risk to their overall health.

Genital or anal warts involve a prolonged course of treatment. Clearing the virus takes time and is not always possible. Patients

---

🔲 **PROMOTING POPULATION HEALTH**

Preventing Sexually Transmitted Infections

- Follow "safer" sex practices every time you have sexual contact and be responsible for your own protection.
- Have sexual activity only in an established, monogamous relationship.
- Obtain vaccinations to help prevent some types of HPV.
- Know your sex partners. Be comfortable saying "no" to sexual activity.
- Limit alcohol use to moderate levels.
- If you are at risk, obtain testing regularly and encourage partners to do the same.

can become frustrated and distressed due to frequent office visits, associated costs, potential for unpleasant side effects because of treatment, and effects of the infection on future health and sexual relationships. Support and a willingness to listen to the patient's concerns are needed. Local or online support groups are available for almost all STIs. Help patients to connect with support groups.

Follow-up. If you work in public health facilities, clinics, or other outpatient settings, you are more likely to care for a patient with an STI than if you work in a hospital setting. Whatever the setting, as a nurse, you are in a position to explain and interpret treatment measures, such as the purpose and possible side effects of prescribed drugs and the need for follow-up care (Table 52.10).

Single-dose treatment for gonorrhea, chlamydia, and syphilis helps prevent the problems associated with nonadherence with drug therapy. Give special instructions to the patient receiving multiple-dose therapy to complete the prescribed treatment. Teach the patient about problems resulting from nonadherence. All patients should return to the treatment center for a repeat culture from the infected sites or for serologic testing at designated times to determine the effectiveness of the treatment.

ETHICAL/LEGAL DILEMMAS
Confidentiality and HIPAA

Situation

P.H. is a 22-yr-old woman who recently tested positive for chlamydia. You tell her to tell her sexual partners of the infection. She refuses to tell her boyfriend because he will know that she has had sex with another partner. You later learn that the nursing student who was in the clinic for the day is a friend of her boyfriend and told him that he should have STI testing.

Ethical/Legal Points for Consideration

- Each state has requirements for reporting communicable diseases and other health-related data. Inform the patient of the reporting requirements for communicable diseases.
- Nurses and other HCPs have both a legal and an ethical obligation to maintain confidentiality of patient information. The Health Insurance Portability and Accountability Act (HIPAA) ensures the privacy of personal health information.
- The duty to maintain confidentiality is not absolute and may be limited, as needed, to protect the patient or other parties, or by law or regulation, such as mandated reporting for safety or public health reasons.
- Your main obligation is to the patient seeking care. Patient teaching is one way to establish a partnership with this woman. Share information about the effects of the disease, the consequences of reinfection, and the effect of the disease on others who may not know that they are infected. Then encourage the patient to tell her partners of the diagnosis and discuss the option of expedited partner therapy (EPT) where applicable.

Discussion Questions

- What are your state's requirements for reportable conditions?
- In your opinion, what is the best way to balance the needs of an individual patient with those of the public?
- What are the risks to agencies for the breach of confidentiality and HIPAA?

Reference

Code of Ethics for Nurses. Retrieved from *www.nursingworld.org/practice-policy/nursing-excellence/ethics/code-of-ethics-for-nurses/*.

Explaining to the patient that cures are not always obtained on the first treatment can reinforce the need for a follow-up visit. Advise the patient to inform sexual partners of the need for testing and treatment as a contact, regardless of whether they are free of symptoms or experiencing symptoms.

Hygiene Measures. Emphasize to the patient with an STI the importance of certain hygiene measures, such as frequent hand washing. Tell the patient not to scratch infection sites to avoid autoinoculation of STIs that can be spread to other parts of the body. Washing with soap and water and voiding after sex may have some benefit in decreasing the exposure to STIs but does not give adequate protection against transmission. Teach patients not to douche after sex. It can push bacteria higher into the reproductive tract or undermine local immune responses.

Sexual Activity. Sexual abstinence is needed during the communicable phase of any STI. Long-term precautions must be taken with those STIs that are chronic or recurrent. Emphasize that even single-dose treatments can take up to 1 week to clear the infection. Thus the patient is infectious during this period and should avoid all sexual contact. Emphasize the importance of using condoms or other barrier methods to help prevent the spread of infection and reinfection after treatment. Remind patients that complications can follow if sexual activity occurs before treatment completion. Patients need to discuss re-treatment or continued treatment with an HCP. During treatment, the patient can choose to relate to a partner in an intimate way that avoids penetrative, oral-genital contact, or skin-to-skin contact.

◆ **Ambulatory Care.** Because many STIs are cured with a single dose or short course of antibiotic therapy, many patients are casual about the outcome of these infections. The consequences of this attitude can include delays in treatment, nonadherence with instructions, and the development of complications, treatment failure, or reinfection. Complications are serious and costly and can include future infertility.

Surgery and prolonged therapy are needed for many patients with infection-related complications. Major surgical procedures, such as resection of an aneurysm or aortic valve replacement, may be needed to treat cardiovascular problems caused by syphilis. Pelvic surgery and procedures to correct fertility problems from an STI may be needed. If not successful, patients may need assisted reproductive technologies to achieve future pregnancy. Because young people ages 15 to 24 represent about 50% of new STIs annually, it is important to know that almost every state and the District of Columbia have laws that allow minors to consent to STI services without parental involvement (the minimum age varies by state).[8]

◆ **Evaluation**

Expected outcomes for the patient with an STI are that the patient will

- Understand the course, modes of transmission, and treatment options for the STI
- Relate the potential long-term complications of untreated infection
- Adhere with drug regimens and the follow-up protocol
- Understand the importance of partner notification and treatment
- Have no reinfection and understand STI risk-reducing behaviors and practices going forward

CASE STUDY
Gonococcal and Chlamydial Infection

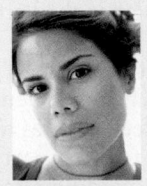

(© Eyecandy Images/ Thinkstock.)

Patient Profile

C.R. is a 24-yr-old Hispanic woman seen in the outpatient clinic reporting increased yellow vaginal discharge and bleeding after sex for the past 2 weeks. She is sexually active with a new partner. She was treated in the past for chlamydial infection at age 20.

Subjective Data

- She and her partner use condoms "sometimes"
- Last menstrual period was 3 weeks ago
- Noticed her partner had some unusual discharge before they had sex
- Appears anxious and teary

Objective Data

- Cervix: erythematous
- Mucopurulent cervical discharge
- Urine pregnancy test is negative
- NAAT of the cervix is positive for *N. gonorrhoeae* and *C. trachomatis*

Interprofessional Care

- ceftriaxone 250 mg IM × 1 dose
- azithromycin 1 g PO × 1 dose

Discussion Questions

1. What were C.R.'s risk factors for acquiring gonorrhea and chlamydial infection?
2. What complications could occur if C.R.'s infections are not treated?
3. *Priority Decision:* What is the priority of care for C.R.?
4. *Priority Decision:* Based on the assessment data presented, what are the priority nursing diagnoses?
5. *Patient-Centered Care:* What instructions should C.R. receive to ensure successful treatment? To prevent reinfection? To prevent further transmission of the infection?
6. *Patient-Centered Care:* What impact is her diagnosis likely to have on C.R.'s self-image? On her relationship with her sexual partner?
7. *Safety:* C.R. tells you she is worried about how her partner will react when she discloses this information. What safety precautions should be considered?
8. *Evidence-Based Practice:* C.R. mentions she is using the spermicide nonoxynol-9 (N-9) to protect herself against STIs. Would you advise her to continue to use it?

Answers available at *http://evolve.elsevier.com/Lewis/medsurg.*

▮ BRIDGE TO NCLEX EXAMINATION

The number of the question corresponds to the same-numbered outcome at the beginning of the chapter.

1. Which populations have a higher risk for acquiring sexually transmitted infections (STIs)? *(select all that apply)*
   a. Transgender persons
   b. Young adults (age < 25)
   c. Men who have sex with men
   d. Men in long-term care facilities
   e. Women in correctional facilities

2. The nurse is obtaining a subjective data assessment from a woman reported as a sexual contact of a man with chlamydial infection. The nurse understands that symptoms of chlamydial infection in women
   a. are often absent.
   b. are similar to those of genital herpes.
   c. include a macular palmar rash in the later stages.
   d. may involve chancres inside the vagina that are not visible.

3. A primary HSV infection differs from recurrent HSV episodes in that *(select all that apply)*
   a. only primary infections are sexually transmitted.
   b. symptoms are less severe during recurrent episodes.
   c. transmission of the virus to a fetus is less likely during primary infection.
   d. systemic manifestations, such as fever and myalgia, are more common in primary infection.
   e. lesions from recurrent HSV are more likely to transmit the virus than lesions from primary HSV.

4. Explain to the patient with gonorrhea that treatment will include both ceftriaxone and azithromycin because
   a. azithromycin helps prevent recurrent infections.
   b. some patients do not respond to oral drugs alone.
   c. coverage with more than one antibiotic will prevent reinfection.
   d. the increasing rates of drug resistance requires using at least 2 drugs.

5. In assessing patients for STIs, the nurse needs to know that many STIs can be asymptomatic. Which STIs can be asymptomatic? *(select all that apply)*
   a. Syphilis
   b. Gonorrhea
   c. Genital warts
   d. Genital herpes
   e. Chlamydial infection

6. To prevent the infection and transmission of STIs, the nurse's teaching plan would include an explanation of
   a. the appropriate use of oral contraceptives.
   b. the need for annual Pap tests for women with HPV.
   c. sexual positions that can be used to avoid infection.
   d. sexual practices that are considered high-risk behaviors.

7. Provide emotional support to a patient with an STI by
   a. offering information on how safer sexual practices can prevent STIs.
   b. showing concern when listening to the patient who expresses negative feelings.
   c. reassuring the patient that the disease is highly curable with appropriate treatment.
   d. helping the patient who received an STI from their sexual partner in forgiving the partner.

1. a, b, c, e, 2. a, 3. b, d, 4. d, 5. a, b, c, d, e, 6. d, 7. b.

For rationales to these answers and even more NCLEX review questions, visit *http://evolve.elsevier.com/Lewis/medsurg.*

ⓔ EVOLVE WEBSITE/RESOURCES LIST

http://evolve.elsevier.com/Lewis/medsurg
Review Questions (Online Only)
Key Points
Answer Keys for Questions
- Rationales for Bridge to NCLEX Examination Questions
- Answer Guidelines for Case Study on p. 1226

Conceptual Care Map Creator
Audio Glossary
Content Updates

REFERENCES

1. Centers for Disease Control and Prevention: Sexually transmitted disease surveillance. Retrieved from *www.cdc.gov/std/stats/*.
2. Shannon CL, Klausner JD: The growing epidemic of sexually transmitted infections in adolescents: A neglected population, *Curr Opin Pediatr* 30:137, 2018.
3. Poteat TC, Malik M, Beyrer C: Epidemiology of HIV, sexually transmitted infections, viral hepatitis, and tuberculosis among incarcerated transgender people: A case of limited data, *Epidemiol Rev* 40:27, 2018.
4. Copen CE: Condom use during sexual intercourse among women and men aged 15-44 in the United States: 2011-2015 national survey of family growth, *Natl Health Stat Rep* 105:1, 2017.
*5. Centers for Disease Control and Prevention: US Public Health Service: Preexposure prophylaxis for the prevention of HIV infection in the United States—2017 Update. Retrieved from *www.cdc.gov/hiv/pdf/risk/prep/cdc-hiv-prep-guidelines-2017.pdf*.
*6. Centers for Disease Control and Prevention: *Updated guidelines for antiretroviral postexposure prophylaxis after sexual, injection drug use, or other nonoccupational exposure to HIV—United States*. Retrieved from *https://stacks.cdc.gov/view/cdc/38856*.
7. Centers for Disease Control and Prevention: *Pelvic inflammatory disease (PID)—CDC fact sheet*. Retrieved from *www.cdc.gov/std/pid/stdfact-pid-detailed.htm*.
*8. Centers for Disease Control and Prevention: *Sexually transmitted diseases treatment guidelines*. Retrieved from *www.cdc.gov/std/tg2015/default.htm*.
9. Centers for Disease Control and Prevention: *Expedited partner therapy*. Retrieved from *www.cdc.gov/std/ept/*.
10. Weston EJ, Wi T, Papp J: Strengthening global surveillance for antimicrobial drug-resistant *Neisseria gonorrhoeae* through the enhanced gonococcal antimicrobial surveillance program, *Emerg Infect Dis* 23:S47, 2017.
*11. Meites E, Kempe A, Markowitz LE: Use of a 2-dose schedule for human papillomavirus vaccination—Updated recommendations of the Advisory Committee on Immunization Practices, *MMWR* 65:1405, 2016.
12. Centers for Disease Control and Prevention: A guide to taking a sexual history. Retrieved from *www.cdc.gov/std/treatment/sexualhistory.pdf*.
13. Syme ML, Cohn TJ, Barnack-Tavlaris J: A comparison of actual and perceived sexual risk among older adults, *J Sex Res* 54:149, 2017.

*Evidence-based information for clinical practice.

53

Female Reproductive Problems

Kim K. Choma

Never believe that a few caring people can't change the world.

Margaret Mead

(e) http://evolve.elsevier.com/Lewis/medsurg

CONCEPTUAL FOCUS

Cellular Regulation	Inflammation	Reproduction
Hormonal Regulation	Pain	Sexuality
Infection		

LEARNING OUTCOMES

1. Summarize the etiologies of infertility and the strategies for diagnosis and treatment of the infertile woman.
2. Describe the etiology, clinical manifestations, and interprofessional and nursing management of menstrual problems and abnormal uterine bleeding.
3. Identify the risk factors, clinical manifestations, and nursing and interprofessional management of ectopic pregnancy.
4. Describe the changes related to menopause and interprofessional and nursing management of the patient with menopausal symptoms.
5. Describe the assessment and interprofessional and nursing management of women with pelvic inflammatory disease and endometriosis.
6. Explain the clinical manifestations, diagnostic studies, interprofessional care, including surgical therapy for cervical, endometrial, ovarian, and vulvar cancers.
7. Discuss the nursing management of the patient requiring surgery of the female reproductive system.
8. Distinguish among the common problems that occur with cystoceles, rectoceles, and fistulas and the related interprofessional and nursing management.
9. Summarize the clinical manifestations of sexual assault and the nursing and interprofessional management of the patient who has been sexually assaulted.

KEY TERMS

abnormal uterine bleeding (AUB), p. 1232
abortion, p. 1229
amenorrhea, p. 1232
cystocele, p. 1248
dysmenorrhea, p. 1231
ectopic pregnancy, p. 1233

endometriosis, p. 1238
hysterectomy, p. 1240
infertility, p. 1228
leiomyomas, p. 1240
menopause, p. 1234
pelvic inflammatory disease (PID), p. 1237

perimenopause, p. 1234
premenstrual syndrome (PMS), p. 1230
sexual assault, p. 1249
uterine prolapse, p. 1247

This chapter discusses several disorders, many of which are related to hormonal regulation, infection, inflammation, and cancer. Problems of the female reproductive and genital system can profoundly affect sexuality and reproduction. The consequences of these problems vary widely. Besides the obvious manifestations, a diagnosis of ovarian cancer often triggers intense feelings of anxiety and fear. An infertile couple can struggle with grief and the stress of infertility treatments. Pain and sexual dysfunction from prolapse or endometriosis can cause psychologic, social, and body image problems. We close with discussing sexual assault and the multiple physical and psychologic effects of intimate violence.

INFERTILITY

Infertility is the inability of a couple to conceive after at least 1 year of regular unprotected intercourse. Around 12% to 18%

of women are not pregnant after 12 months of trying to conceive.[1] *Fecundability,* the probability of achieving a pregnancy in 1 menstrual cycle, is a more accurate label because it recognizes varying degrees of infertility. Impaired fecundity refers to women who have difficulty getting pregnant or carrying a pregnancy to term.

Etiology and Pathophysiology

Infertility may be caused by male, female, or combined factors. Of couples with infertility, 25% have male factors that affect their chances of conceiving. Conditions that cause male infertility are discussed in Chapter 54. Sometimes the cause of infertility may not be found.

Female infertility may be due to problems with ovulation, the fallopian tubes, or conditions that affect the uterus or cervix. In women the risk for infertility begins around age 30. By the time a woman reaches the age of 40, the chances of

TABLE 53.1 Interprofessional Care

Infertility

Diagnostic Assessment

- History and physical examination of both partners, including psychosocial functioning
- Review of menstrual and gynecologic history
- Assessment of possible sexually transmitted infections
- Hormone levels
  - Serum hormone levels (e.g., FSH, LH, prolactin)
  - Urinary LH
- Pap test with HPV test as indicated by age
- Ovulatory study
- Tubal patency study
  - Hysterosalpingogram
- Semen analysis
- Pelvic ultrasound
- Genetic screening

Management

- Hormone therapy
- Drug therapy (Table 53.2)
- Intrauterine insemination
- Assisted reproductive technologies (ARTs)

TABLE 53.2 Drug Therapy

Infertility

Drug	Mechanism of Action
Follicle-Stimulating Hormone Agonists	
follitropin (Gonal-f) urofollitropin (Bravelle)	Stimulates follicle growth and maturation by mimicking the body's natural FSH.
GnRH Agonists	
leuprolide (Lupron) nafarelin (Synarel)	Suppresses release of LH and FSH with continuous use. May be used in the treatment of endometriosis.
GnRH Antagonists	
cetrorelix (Cetrotide) ganirelix	Prevents premature LH surges and premature ovulation in women undergoing ovarian stimulation.
Human Chorionic Gonadotropin (hCG)	
Novarel Pregnyl Profasi	Induces ovulation by stimulating release of eggs from follicles.
Menotropins (Human Menopausal Gonadotropin)	
Humegon Pergonal Repronex	Product made of FSH and LH to promote the development and maturation of follicles in ovaries.
Selective Estrogen Receptor Modulator	
clomiphene (Clomid)	Stimulates hypothalamus to ↑ production of GnRH, which ↑ release of LH and FSH. End result is stimulation of ovulation.

conceiving are 10% or less. For both genders, chronic diseases, genital infections, and exposure to environmental toxins can affect fertility.[2]

Diagnostic Studies

Formal evaluation of the infertile couple is usually done after 1 year of regular unprotected intercourse. Earlier evaluation may occur in women over age 35 or based on medical or physical findings. Couples who are being evaluated usually have a detailed history and physical examination. Based on the findings, diagnostic testing may be ordered (Table 53.1).

A comprehensive evaluation of the female reproductive system includes cervical, uterine, endometrial, tubal, peritoneal, and ovarian factors that could be the source of infertility. A semen sample is done to determine if the cause is related to the male partner.

❖ Interprofessional and Nursing Care

Infertility management depends on the cause. If the cause is due to ovarian function, supplemental hormone therapy may be used. Table 53.2 reviews drugs commonly used for women with infertility. Couples should be involved in fertility treatment decisions. The choices involve 4 major aspects: effectiveness (e.g., live birth rate), burdens of treatments (office visits, frequent injections), safety, (e.g., risk for multiple gestation), and costs.[3]

Assisted reproductive technology (ART) can be used to help women who are having difficulty becoming pregnant. ART includes fertility drugs for ovulation induction, artificial insemination, and surrogacy. Types of ART include (1) in vitro fertilization (IVF), (2) gamete intrafallopian transfer (GIFT), (3) zygote intrafallopian transfer (ZIFT), (4) donor gametes, (5) freezing of ova, and (6) intracytoplasmic sperm injection (ICSI), a type of IVF that is often used for couples with male factor infertility. Some types of ART, such as IVF, are expensive and can be emotionally stressful. Assisting couples with infertility is critical. You can provide teaching about the physiology of reproduction and an overview of infertility evaluation and treatments.

TABLE 53.3 Types of Spontaneous Abortion

Type	Description
Complete abortion	All products of conception (POC) are expelled
Incomplete abortion	Parts of POC are retained
Inevitable abortion	Cervix is open and pregnancy loss cannot be prevented
Infected (septic) abortion	Endometrium (uterine lining) and POC become infected
Missed abortion	Fetus has died but has not been expelled
Threatened abortion	Unexplained bleeding with or without pain. Suggests pregnancy loss may occur

EARLY PREGNANCY LOSS

Early pregnancy loss is a term used to describe the loss of a pregnancy before 20 weeks of gestation.[4] **Abortion** is another term we use to describe the loss of pregnancy. Abortions are classified as *spontaneous* (those occurring naturally [e.g., miscarriage]) or *induced* (those occurring from medical intervention). *Miscarriage* is the common term for the unintended loss of a pregnancy.

Spontaneous Abortion

Spontaneous abortion is the natural loss of pregnancy before 20 weeks of gestation (Table 53.3). Nearly 20% of pregnancies result in miscarriage. The loss can be devastating for both the

TABLE 53.4 Methods for Inducing Abortions

Method	Length of Pregnancy	Description
Dilation and evacuation (D&E)	10–16 wk	Cervix is dilated, and contents of uterus are removed by vacuum cannula and use of other instruments as needed.
Medical vacuum aspiration	Usually up to 2 wk after first missed period	Catheter is inserted through cervix into uterus, and suction is applied. Contents of uterus are aspirated.
Mifepristone (Mifeprex) with misoprostol (Cytotec)	Up to 49–63 days*	Mifepristone is given orally, followed by misoprostol orally 48 hr later.
Suction aspiration (curettage)	Up to 12 wk	Cervix is dilated, uterine aspirator is introduced, and suction is applied, removing contents of uterus.

*FDA recommends 49 days. The American Congress of Obstetricians and Gynecologists guidelines state it is safe to use up to 63 days.

mother and her partner. Fetal chromosomal abnormalities cause many miscarriages before 8 weeks of gestation. Testing for chromosomal anomalies is now available for products of conception (POC) from a miscarriage. Other causes of miscarriage include endocrine abnormalities, maternal infection, uterine abnormalities (e.g., uterine fibroids, endometriosis), immunologic factors, and environmental factors.

Treatment to prevent miscarriage is limited. Although bed rest and avoiding vaginal intercourse are often recommended, there is no evidence that these measures improve the outcome. Women are told to report any bleeding to the HCP.

If the pregnancy is not viable, 2 options are considered: expectant management or medical management. *Expectant management* refers to monitoring the patient to see if the POC are expelled naturally without complications. *Medical management* may be needed if the POC do not pass completely or bleeding becomes excessive. This may involve a *dilation and curettage (D&C)* or the use of medications (e.g., misoprostol [Cytotec]) to expel the remaining contents from the uterus. The D&C involves surgically dilating the cervix and scraping the endometrium of the uterus to empty the contents of the uterus.

Women who have moderate-to-heavy bleeding and the passage of clots during pregnancy may need emergency care at a hospital. Vital signs and blood loss are monitored along with an assessment of psychologic well-being. Any heavy bleeding, severe pain, or fever that occurs after medical management should be reported to the HCP. Ovulation can occur as soon as 2 weeks after early pregnancy loss. Normal menses should return within 4 to 6 weeks.

Provide grief support as the couple deals with the psychologic distress of their loss. Encourage them to share their feelings. Referral to a pregnancy loss support group may be helpful.

Induced Abortion

Induced abortion is an elective termination of a pregnancy.[5] There are several ways to induce an abortion (Table 53.4). Deciding which method to use depends on the length of the pregnancy and the woman's condition.

Once the woman makes the decision to have an abortion, she and her partner need support and acceptance. Prepare the patient for what to expect both emotionally and physically. Grief and sadness are normal emotions after an abortion. Nursing care for a woman who terminates her pregnancy includes assessment of a woman's need for counseling and support, providing for privacy, maintaining her physical comfort, and monitoring her vital signs.

After the abortion, teach the patient the signs and symptoms of complications. These includes abnormal vaginal bleeding, severe abdominal cramping, fever, and foul-smelling drainage. Stress to the patient that as soon as 1 week after having an abortion she can become pregnant again. Normal menstruation returns in 4 to 6 weeks.

Teach patients to refrain from intercourse and putting anything into the vagina for 1 week after the abortion. The exception is for women who use NuvaRing birth control. Oral contraception can be started the day of the abortion or 1 to 2 weeks after the procedure, depending on the patient's needs and desires.

PROBLEMS RELATED TO MENSTRUATION

The normal menstrual cycle is discussed in Chapter 50. The menstrual cycle may be irregular the first few years after menarche and in the years preceding menopause. Although most women have a predictable menstrual cycle, considerable normal variation exists among women in cycle length and in duration, amount, and character of the menstrual flow (see Table 50.2). During the perimenopausal period (the years prior to menopause) as ovarian function begins to decrease, women may note a change in their menstrual patterns.

PREMENSTRUAL SYNDROME

Premenstrual syndrome (PMS) refers to a group of symptoms that occur during a woman's menstrual cycle. Many women have symptoms of PMS. They may be severe enough to affect interpersonal relationships, work responsibilities, academic performance, and social activities.

PMS includes a variety of physical, psychologic, and somatic symptoms. As many as 150 symptoms are associated with PMS. (PMDD) is the term used to describe PMS associated with a severe mood disorder.

Etiology and Pathophysiology

We do not completely understand the cause of PMS. PMS is likely due to a combination of biologic and psychosocial factors. Genetics, hormone and neurotransmitter (e.g., serotonin) imbalances, and nutrition problems are all thought to be causes of PMS.

Clinical Manifestations

PMS is extremely variable in its manifestations, frequency, and severity. Symptoms may also vary from one cycle to another. Common symptoms include breast discomfort, peripheral edema, abdominal bloating, sensation of weight gain, episodes of binge eating, headaches, anxiety, depression, irritability and moodiness, back pain, insomnia, menstrual cramps, fatigue, and generalized muscle pain.

Diagnostic Studies and Interprofessional Care

A focused health history and physical examination are done to identify any underlying conditions which may account for symptoms. These include thyroid problems, uterine fibroids, anemia, nutritional and vitamin deficiencies, autoimmune disorders, endometriosis, and depression.

To accurately diagnose PMS or PMDD, 4 factors are critical: (1) consistency of the syndrome complex, (2) occurrence of the symptoms in the luteal phase and resolution after the beginning of menses, (3) documented ovulatory cycles, and (4) symptoms that disrupt the woman's life.

A holistic approach to managing PMS symptoms for women includes stress management, dietary changes, exercise, teaching, and cognitive behavioral therapy. Mindfulness activities can help women deal with the discomforts of PMS.[6]

Drug Therapy. Selective serotonin reuptake inhibitors (SSRIs) (e.g., sertraline [Zoloft], fluoxetine [Prozac]) have provided relief to women who have anxiety, irritability, and mood changes associated with PMS. Many women choose to take oral contraceptives (OCPs) and/or nonsteroidal antiinflammatory drugs (NSAIDs) to reduce cramping, blood flow, and back pain. Vitamin B$_6$, calcium, and magnesium have been recommended for mood changes associated with PMS.

> ### ❓ CHECK YOUR PRACTICE
>
> You are working in the gynecology outpatient clinic. Your patient is a 28-yr-old woman who reporting symptoms of PMS. She tells you, "My PMS has gotten so bad lately that I spend the entire day in bed due to pain. I am very anxious and overwhelmed. I can't function like this anymore."
> - How would you respond?
> - What are things she can do to relieve symptoms?

❖ NURSING MANAGEMENT: PREMENSTRUAL SYNDROME

Nursing care for the patient with PMS includes teaching her about the symptoms associated with PMS and how to manage them (Table 53.5). Acknowledging that she has PMS can be therapeutic and empowering. Teaching the woman's partner about the nature of PMS helps the partner better understand PMS and its effects. Provide the patient with support and reassure her that PMS is not an emotional disorder, but one that has a physiologic basis and can be managed.

👥 TABLE 53.5 Interprofessional Care

Premenstrual Syndrome (PMS)

Diagnostic Assessment
- History and physical examination
- Symptom diary

Management
- Stress management
- Nutritional therapy
- Aerobic exercise

Drug Therapy
- Diuretics
- Combined OCPs
- Prostaglandin inhibitors (e.g., ibuprofen)
- SSRIs (e.g., sertraline [Zoloft])

DYSMENORRHEA

Dysmenorrhea is painful menses with abdominal cramping. The 2 types of dysmenorrhea are *primary* (no pathologic condition exists) and *secondary* (pelvic disease is the underlying cause). Dysmenorrhea is one of the most common gynecologic problems.

Etiology and Pathophysiology

Primary dysmenorrhea begins in the first few years after menarche, typically with the onset of regular menstrual cycles. It is usually related to increased levels of prostaglandin, a hormone that is found in the endometrium. Endometrial stimulation by estrogen and progesterone results in a dramatic increase in prostaglandin production. Prostaglandin stimulates the uterus to contract. Uterine contractions and constriction of small endometrial blood vessels result in tissue ischemia and increased sensitization of the pain receptors. This results in painful menstrual cramps. As menstruation continues, prostaglandin levels decrease each day and menstrual cramping lessens.

Secondary dysmenorrhea usually occurs after adolescence, most commonly at 30 to 40 years of age and worsens as a woman ages. Common pelvic conditions that cause secondary dysmenorrhea include endometriosis, chronic pelvic inflammatory disease (PID), and uterine fibroids. Because secondary dysmenorrhea can be caused by many conditions, the manifestations and severity vary. However, painful menses is the main manifestation.

Clinical Manifestations

Manifestations include menstrual pain that is most severe during the first few days of menses. Painful menstruation rarely lasts more than 2 days. Typical symptoms include lower, colicky abdominal pain that often radiates to the lower back and upper thighs. Nausea, diarrhea, fatigue, and headache may occur.

Secondary dysmenorrhea usually occurs after the woman has little to no pain during the menstrual cycle. The pain, which may be unilateral, is often more constant and continues longer than in primary dysmenorrhea. Depending on the cause, symptoms such as *dyspareunia* (painful intercourse), painful defecation, or irregular bleeding may occur at times other than menstruation.

Diagnostic Studies

Evaluation begins with a complete health history and pelvic examination. A probable diagnosis of primary dysmenorrhea is given if the history reveals an onset shortly after menarche with symptoms that are associated only with menses. The pelvic examination is otherwise normal. If the HCP finds an underlying cause of dysmenorrhea, the diagnosis is secondary dysmenorrhea.

❖ Interprofessional and Nursing Care

Treatment for primary dysmenorrhea includes pharmacologic and nonpharmacologic therapy. NSAIDs (e.g., naproxen [Naprosyn]) inhibit prostaglandins. OCPs may be used to decrease estrogen and progesterone. This results in lower prostaglandin levels, decreased monthly endometrial lining proliferation, and decreased menstrual flow.

Nonpharmacologic interventions include applying heat to the lower abdomen or back and physical exercise. Regular exercise helps to reduce prostaglandin production. Acupuncture and transcutaneous nerve stimulation may be used for women who have inadequate relief from drugs or who prefer not to take drugs.

Treatment of secondary dysmenorrhea depends on the etiology. Some patients are helped by the approaches used for primary dysmenorrhea. However, if a gynecologic problem is the main cause of secondary dysmenorrhea, then treating that underlying problem is the priority. For example, women with endometriosis who have secondary dysmenorrhea may benefit from OCPs.

Nursing interventions include teaching women with dysmenorrhea about the cause, symptoms, and treatment. This will provide women with a basis for coping with the problem and increase feelings of self-control. Teach women that during acute pain, relief may be obtained by applying heat to the abdomen or back and taking NSAIDs. Suggest noninvasive pain-relieving practices, such as relaxation breathing and guided imagery, yoga, and meditation. Other measures to reduce discomfort include regular exercise and good nutrition.

ABNORMAL UTERINE BLEEDING

Abnormal uterine bleeding (AUB) is any change in a woman's menstrual flow, including volume, duration, or cycle pattern. AUB can be classified based on the cause of bleeding (Fig. 53.1). *Heavy menstrual bleeding* (HMB) (instead of the term *menorrhagia*) describes excessive bleeding. *Intermenstrual bleeding* (instead of the term *metrorrhagia*) refers to bleeding between regular menstrual cycles.

Chronic AUB is classified as uterine bleeding that is abnormal in volume, timing, or regularity and has been present for most of the past 6 months. *Acute AUB* is an episode of heavy bleeding that requires immediate treatment.

In reproductive-age women, causes of AUB include uterine fibroids, polyps, ovulatory dysfunction, endometrial problems, or cancer. Other causes include bleeding disorders (e.g., thrombocytopenia), leukemia, medications, eating disorders, or liver failure.[7] For postmenopausal women, endometrial cancer must be considered whenever bleeding or spotting occurs after menstrual bleeding has ceased for 1 year or longer.

Anovulation is the most common reason for missing menses. Ovulation is often erratic for several years after menarche and before menopause. Bleeding in between periods (spotting) is common for women who start taking OCPs. If spotting continues beyond the first few months on OCPs, a different pill formulation may be prescribed. Spotting with long-acting progestin therapies (e.g., intrauterine devices [IUDs], Nexplanon implant, progestin-only pills [levonorgestrel, norethindrone], progesterone injections [medroxyprogesterone acetate]) is common and not usually associated with any serious complications.

Amenorrhea is the absence or abnormal interruption of menstruation (Table 53.6). *Primary amenorrhea* refers to the failure of menstrual cycles to begin by 16 years of age. *Secondary amenorrhea* occurs when menstrual cycles stop for 3 to 6 months in menstruating women. Primary amenorrhea is often associated with chromosomal or congenital abnormalities and the female athletic triad. Causes of secondary amenorrhea include primary ovarian insufficiency, polycystic ovary syndrome (PCOS), hypothalamic disorders, and hyperprolactinemia.

Diagnostic Studies and Interprofessional Care

Once it is determined that a patient has AUB, the HCP will determine if the AUB is related to a structural cause or nonstructural cause. A comprehensive history and physical examination are done to find the cause of AUB (Table 53.7). Laboratory evaluation and diagnostic procedures are based on findings from the history and physical examination. Treatment depends on the cause of the problem, degree of threat to the patient's health, her quality of life, and whether children are desired in the future.

Combined OCPs may be prescribed for a woman with amenorrhea to ensure regular shedding of the endometrium. Tranexamic acid (Lysteda) may be used during the menstrual cycle to treat heavy menstrual bleeding. This drug stabilizes a protein that helps blood to clot. The use of tranexamic acid is contraindicated in women who use combined OCPs.

Estradiol valerate/dienogest (Natazia) is the only combined OCP approved for treatment of heavy menstrual bleeding. It may be given to women who want an OCP to prevent pregnancy. Other options for treatment of heavy menstrual bleeding include NSAIDs and the Mirena IUD (progestin IUD).

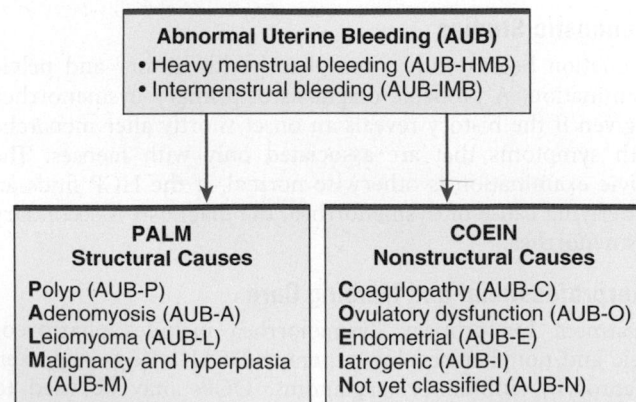

FIG. 53.1 PALM-COIEN classification system for abnormal uterine bleeding. (Used with permission. Munro MG, Critchley HO, Broder MS, et al: FIGO classification system [PALM–OEIN] for causes of AUB in nongravid women of reproductive age, *Int J Gynecol Obstet* 11:3, 2011.)

TABLE 53.6 **Causes of Amenorrhea**	
Genetic	**Medications**
• Congenital absence or doubling of reproductive organ(s)	• Antidepressants
• Turner's syndrome	• Antihypertensives
	• Antipsychotics
Hormonal Imbalance	• Chemotherapy
• Polycystic ovary syndrome (PCOS)	• Hormone therapy (oral or injectable contraceptives, intrauterine devices)
• Pituitary tumors	
• Thyroid dysfunction	**Natural Amenorrhea**
	• Breastfeeding
Lifestyle	• Menopause
• Acute and chronic illness	• Pregnancy
• Excess exercise	
• Low body weight	**Structural Problems**
• Stress	• Damage or scarring to reproductive organs from infection, trauma, radiation

TABLE 53.7 Interprofessional Care
Abnormal Uterine Bleeding

Diagnostic Assessment
- History, including surgical history and medication history
- Age of menarche/menopause
- Bleeding patterns and perceived severity of bleeding (clots, soaking through clothing)
- Evaluation for obesity/hirsutism (suggestive of polycystic ovary syndrome)
- Pelvic examination
- Pregnancy test
- Complete blood count (CBC)
- Thyroid-stimulating hormone (TSH)
- STI screening
- Screening for bleeding disorders (if indicated)
- Imaging studies and tissue sampling
  - Transvaginal/pelvic ultrasound
  - Saline infusion sonohysterography
  - Endometrial biopsy
  - Hysteroscopy

Management
Based on the cause, may include:
- OCPs
- Hormonal therapy
- NSAIDS
- Mirena IUD

❖ NURSING MANAGEMENT: ABNORMAL UTERINE BLEEDING

Teach women about the characteristics of the menstrual cycle to help them identify variations (see Table 50.2). This knowledge can decrease apprehension and dispel misconceptions about the menstrual cycle. Encourage the patient to report excessive bleeding, passing of clots, and unusually long duration of menstrual cycles.

Teach women to avoid the prolonged use of superabsorbent tampons that can increase the risk for toxic shock syndrome (TSS). TSS is an acute life-threatening condition caused by a toxin from *Staphylococcus aureus*. TSS causes high fever, vomiting, diarrhea, weakness, myalgia, and a sunburn-like rash.

ECTOPIC PREGNANCY

An **ectopic pregnancy** is the implantation of the fertilized ovum anywhere outside the uterus. Almost all ectopic pregnancies occur within the fallopian tube. Around 3% of all pregnancies are ectopic (Fig. 53.2). Ectopic pregnancy is a life-threatening condition. Early detection can lead to successful management and reduce morbidity and mortality.

Etiology and Pathophysiology

Ectopic pregnancy can be caused by blockage of the fallopian tube(s) or reduction of tubal peristalsis that impedes or delays the fertilized ovum from passing to the uterus. After the fertilized egg implants itself in the fallopian tube, the growth of the gestational sac expands the tubal wall. Eventually the fallopian tube ruptures, leading to acute peritonitis. This occurs 6 to 8 weeks after the last normal menstrual period. Often the woman presents due to bleeding and/or pelvic pain or pressure.

Risk factors or causes for ectopic pregnancy include a history of PID, prior ectopic pregnancy, current progestin-releasing

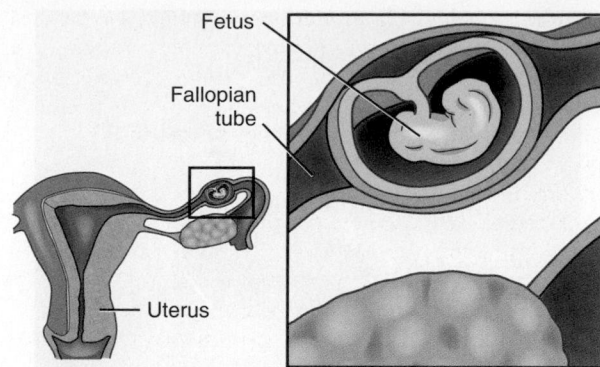

FIG. 53.2 Ectopic pregnancy occurring in the fallopian tube.

IUD, and prior pelvic or tubal surgery. Procedures used in infertility treatment (e.g., IVF, embryo transfer, ovulation induction) increase the risk.

Clinical Manifestations

The classic manifestations are abdominal or pelvic pain, missed menses, and/or irregular vaginal bleeding. Others include morning sickness, breast tenderness, gastrointestinal (GI) symptoms, malaise, and syncope. Often, the symptoms of pregnancy (e.g., nausea) decrease as the hormones level off, offering a clue early on that something is not right.

Pelvic and/or abdominal pain is almost always present. It is caused by distention of the fallopian tube. The character of the pain varies among women. It can be colicky or vague, unilateral or bilateral.

Symptom severity does not necessarily correlate with the extent of vaginal bleeding. Vaginal bleeding that may accompany ectopic pregnancy is usually described as spotting. However, bleeding may be heavier and can be confused with menses. If tubal rupture occurs, there is risk for hemorrhage and hypovolemic shock. This situation is an emergency.

Diagnostic Studies

Diagnosing an ectopic pregnancy can be challenging because of the manifestations. If the HCP suspects an ectopic pregnancy, a pelvic examination, vaginal ultrasound, and serum pregnancy test (quantitative human chorionic gonadotropin [β-hCG]) are done. Serum β-hCG levels can be measured every few days until ultrasound testing can confirm or rule out ectopic pregnancy. This is usually about 5 to 6 weeks after conception.

❓ CHECK YOUR PRACTICE

You are working in the ED. Your patient is a 29-yr-old woman who presented with acute abdominal pain. She has had in vitro fertilization. Her pain is 7 (on 0 to 10 pain scale). The HCP suspects an ectopic pregnancy. She is crying, "I am going to lose this baby, and we have been trying so hard to have one."
- As her nurse, what are your priorities?
- How would you respond to her?

❖ Interprofessional and Nursing Care

There are 2 ways to treat ectopic pregnancies: drug therapy or surgery.[8] Drug therapy is used (1) when an ectopic pregnancy is confirmed on ultrasound, (2) the woman is hemodynamically

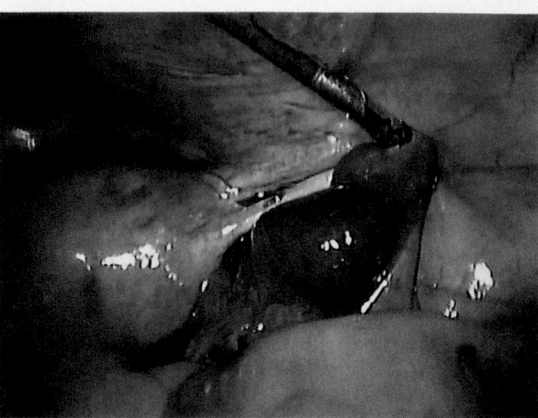

FIG. 53.3 Laparoscopic treatment of ectopic pregnancy in the right fallopian tube. (From Katz V: *Comprehensive gynecology*, ed 5, St Louis, 2007, Mosby.)

TABLE 53.8 Manifestations of Perimenopause and Postmenopause

Perimenopause	Postmenopause
• Irregular menstrual cycles	• Atrophy of genitourinary tissue (e.g., vulvar, vaginal epithelium) with decreased support
• Mood changes	
• Occasional vasomotor symptoms (e.g., hot flashes)	• Breast tenderness
• Sleep problems	• Cessation of menses
• Vaginal dryness	• Osteopenia, osteoporosis
	• Vasomotor instability (e.g., hot flashes, night sweats)
	• Stress and urge incontinence

TABLE 53.9 Manifestations of Estrogen Deficiency

Cardiovascular	Psychologic
• ↓ High-density lipoproteins (HDLs)	• Emotional lability
• ↑ Increased low-density lipoproteins (LDLs)	• Change in sleep pattern
	• ↓ REM sleep
Genitourinary	**Vasomotor**
• Atrophic vaginitis	• Hot flashes
• Dyspareunia from poor lubrication	• Night sweats
• Incontinence	**Other**
Musculoskeletal	• ↓ Collagen content of skin
• ↑ Fracture rate, especially vertebral bodies but also humerus, distal radius, and upper femur	• Breast tissue changes

stable, (3) the woman is compliant with follow-up, and (4) the pregnancy is small and the fallopian tube has not ruptured.

Methotrexate therapy is the drug therapy of choice. Methotrexate stops the growth of rapidly dividing cells, such as embryonic, fetal, and early placenta cells, by inhibiting DNA synthesis and disrupting cell multiplication. Methotrexate can be given as a single shot or as several injections. The most common side effect is cramping abdominal pain. It usually occurs during the first 2 to 3 days of treatment. Other side effects may include vaginal bleeding, nausea, vomiting, indigestion, or dizziness.

Serum β-hCG levels are measured on posttreatment days 4 and 7. A 15% reduction in β-hCG is expected. Weekly β-hCG tests are done until negative. If at any time serum β-hCG levels plateau or increase, methotrexate may be repeated. If an ectopic pregnancy continues after 2 or 3 doses of methotrexate, surgical treatment is needed to remove the ectopic pregnancy.

If surgery is needed, a conservative approach that limits damage to the reproductive system is the goal. If the pregnancy is small, the pregnancy is removed laparoscopically (Fig. 53.3). If the tube ruptures, emergent surgery is done to stabilize the patient.

Nursing care includes closely monitoring vital signs and observing for signs of shock. Provide patient teaching to prepare her for the diagnostic procedures and drug therapy. Explain the side effects of methotrexate and tell her to avoid NSAIDs. Follow-up with weekly β-hCG tests is required. If the patient needs laparoscopic surgery, provide patient teaching and emotional support.

PERIMENOPAUSE AND POSTMENOPAUSE

Perimenopause is a normal life transition for women that begins with the first signs of change in menstrual cycles and ends after cessation of menses. Menstrual changes can include shorter or longer cycles, less frequent cycles, lighter cycles, or heavier cycles.

Menopause is a normal physiologic cessation of menses associated with declining ovarian function that ends in cessation of the menstrual cycle and ovulation. *Natural menopause* is diagnosed retrospectively after 12 months of no periods. The average age for a woman is 52 years. The age can vary from 40 to 58 years.

Induced menopause occurs after surgical intervention to remove the ovaries or from side effects of chemotherapy, radiation therapy, or other drugs. *Postmenopause* is a term that refers to the time in a woman's life after menopause.

Clinical Manifestations

Manifestations of perimenopause and menopause are outlined in Table 53.8. Perimenopause is a time of erratic hormonal fluctuation and irregular menstrual cycles. With the decrease in function of the ovaries, estrogen levels drop, and hot flashes and other symptoms begin. The signs and symptoms of decreased estrogen are listed in Table 53.9.

The loss of estrogen plays a significant role in age-related changes. Changes most critical to a woman's well-being are the increased risks for coronary artery disease (CAD) and osteoporosis (from bone density loss). Other changes include a redistribution of fat, a tendency to gain weight more easily, muscle and joint pain, loss of skin elasticity, changes in hair amount and distribution, and atrophy of external genitalia and breast tissue.

Vasomotor instability (hot flashes) and irregular menses are the main manifestations associated with menopause. A hot flash is a sudden sensation of intense heat along with perspiration and flushing. Atrophy of the vulva and vagina may occur due to decreased estrogen levels. Decreased estrogen also causes thinning of the vaginal mucosa and the disappearance of rugae. This results in a decrease in vaginal secretions and causes the secretions to become more alkaline. Because of these changes, the vagina is easily traumatized. The woman can have dyspareunia and be more susceptible to infection.

Vaginal atrophy can lead to unnecessary and premature cessation of sexual activity. This can be corrected with water-soluble lubricants or, if needed, hormonal creams (vaginal estrogen) or oral hormone replacement therapy. About half of midlife women have vaginal atrophy, but few seek care.

The woman can have atrophic changes in the lower urinary tract and the vulva, which can result in a regression of the labia minora and majora. Bladder capacity decreases. The bladder and urethral tissue lose tone. These changes can cause symptoms that mimic a bladder infection (e.g., dysuria, urgency, frequency) when no infection is present. Decreasing blood serum estrogen levels can cause an array of physical and cognitive changes during menopause that include depression, irritability, insomnia, and memory loss.

Interprofessional Care

The diagnosis of menopause should be made only after careful consideration of other possible causes for a woman's symptoms. Testing of follicle-stimulating hormone (FSH) levels in the perimenopause period is not recommended because hormone levels change throughout the menstrual cycle. However, once a woman has no periods for at least a year, FSH testing can confirm a diagnosis of menopause. FSH levels are increased in menopause. When a woman's FSH blood level is consistently elevated to 30 mIU/mL or higher, and she has not had a menstrual period for a year, it is generally accepted that she has reached menopause.

Drug Therapy. Hormone replacement therapy (HRT) using estrogen, with or without progesterone, is prescribed for some women. Women may choose to use HRT for short-term symptom management and treatment for several years (4 to 5 years) of menopausal symptoms. The risks (e.g., increased risk for breast and endometrial cancer, risk for blood clots) and benefits (e.g., minimizes bone loss, hot flashes, vaginal atrophic changes) must be carefully considered.[9]

Nonhormonal Therapy. Because of the risks associated with HRT, some women choose to use nonhormonal and nonpharmacologic interventions to manage their symptoms. For significant menopausal symptoms, nonhormonal pharmacologic agents may be used. For example, the SSRI antidepressants paroxetine (Paxil), fluoxetine, and venlafaxine (Effexor XR) are effective alternatives to HRT to reduce hot flashes.

Clonidine (Catapres), an antihypertensive drug, and gabapentin (Neurontin), an antiseizure drug, also have been shown to manage vasomotor symptoms during menopause. Selective estrogen receptor modulators (SERMs), such as raloxifene (Evista), are also used to manage menopausal symptoms. SERMs have positive benefits of estrogen, including preventing bone loss, without the negative effects (e.g., endometrial hyperplasia).

Some women seek herbal therapies to ease the symptoms they experience during menopause. While you will see a number of supplements marketed for menopause, there is no research showing that the use of any herb as a treatment for menopause symptoms is effective.

Nutritional Therapy. Good nutrition can decrease the risk for cardiovascular disease (CVD) and osteoporosis and help with vasomotor symptoms. A decrease in metabolic rate and careless eating habits can cause the weight gain and fatigue often attributed to menopause. An adequate intake of calcium and vitamin D helps maintain healthy bones and counteracts loss of bone density.

COMPLEMENTARY & ALTERNATIVE THERAPIES
Herbs and Supplements for Menopause

Herb	Scientific Evidence	Nursing Implications
Black cohosh	Mixed evidence for use in the treatment of menopausal symptoms	• Generally well tolerated in recommended doses for up to 6 mo. • Should not be used by women with a liver disorder.
Soy	Mixed evidence for treatment of menopausal symptoms	• Women with a history of breast, ovarian, or uterine cancer or endometriosis should consult with their HCP before using soy or soy products. • Soy may interact with warfarin. Patients taking warfarin should consult with their HCP before using soy or soy products.

Source: *www.nlm.nih.gov/medlineplus/herbalmedicine.html#summary.*

Postmenopausal women not taking supplemental HRT should have a daily calcium intake of at least 1500 mg. Women taking estrogen replacement need at least 1000 mg/day. Calcium supplements are best absorbed when taken with meals, but not taken as a single dose. The woman should divide the calcium she needs into 2 doses per day so that it is absorbed properly. Either dietary calcium or calcium supplements may be used (see Table 63.14).

❖ NURSING MANAGEMENT: PERIMENOPAUSE AND POSTMENOPAUSE

Menopause is a time of great transition for a woman both physically and psychologically. Many women have symptoms for years during the perimenopausal period while others transition without any difficulty. Menopause may be occurring simultaneously with role changes in the woman's personal and professional life. The combination of menopause and these changes can cause great emotional distress or a renewed sense of self and well-being.

Women in their perimenopausal and menopausal years need a lot of emotional support. Provide reassurance that symptoms can be treated and managed with either hormonal or nonhormonal therapies. It is important to teach them about strategies to prevent or reduce the risk for CVD and osteoporosis.

INFECTIONS OF LOWER GENITAL TRACT

Etiology and Pathophysiology

The female genital tract is susceptible to different types of infections, especially when the pH of the genital tract is altered. In most women, the vaginal pH is typically below 4.5, which helps prevent certain bacterial infections from occurring. The pH level of the vagina is maintained through a combination of sufficient levels of estrogen and *Lactobacillus*, a naturally occurring bacteria that colonizes the vagina.

Infection and inflammation of the vagina, cervix, and vulva often occur when estrogen levels decrease or medication use (e.g., contraceptives, antibiotics, corticosteroids) affects the microbiome of the vagina, leading to changes in the pH balance of the genital tract. For example, *Candida albicans* may be present in small numbers in the vagina. Women who take an

TABLE 53.10 Infections of the Lower Genital Tract

Infection and Etiology	Manifestations	Treatment Considerations
Bacterial Vaginosis *Corynebacterium vaginale* *Gardnerella vaginalis*	Watery discharge with fish-like odor. May or may not have other symptoms	Drug therapy based on cause: • clindamycin (Clindesse)—vaginal • metronidazole (Flagyl)—oral or intravaginal • tinidazole (Tindamax)—oral • *Lactobacillus acidophilus* taken orally by diet (e.g., yogurt, fermented soy products) or supplements can ↓ unwanted vaginal bacteria
Cervicitis *Chlamydia trachomatis* *Neisseria gonorrhoeae* (most often)	Sexually transmitted. Mucopurulent discharge with postcoital spotting from cervical inflammation	Drug therapy based on cause, common agents include azithromycin (Zithromax) and ceftriaxone. Treat patient and partner. May be reportable according to state laws.
Severe Recurrent Vaginitis (more than 4 episodes per year) *Candida albicans* (most often) or non-*albicans* strains	Depend on cause	Drug therapy based on cause. All women who are unresponsive to first-line treatment should be offered HIV testing. Common in women with uncontrolled diabetes or HIV infection.
Trichomonas Vaginitis *Trichomonas vaginalis* (protozoa)	Sexually transmitted. Itching, frothy greenish or gray discharge. Hemorrhagic spots on cervix or vaginal walls	Antifungal agents • metronidazole (Flagyl) • tinidazole (Tindamax) Treat patient and partner
Vulvovaginal Candidiasis *Candida albicans* (fungus)	Itching, thick white curd-like discharge	Antifungal agents • clotrimazole (Gyne-Lotrimin, Mycelex) • fluconazole (Diflucan) • miconazole (Monistat) • terconazole (Terazol)

antibiotic for another type of infection may have an overgrowth of *C. albicans*. This leads to a condition called *vulvovaginal candidiasis* (often called a "yeast infection").

Organisms gain entrance to the lower genital tract through contaminated hands, clothing, douching, and intercourse. Women should not douche. Douching changes the natural acidity and microbiome of the vagina, causing an overgrowth of bacteria. Most lower genital tract infections are related to sexual intercourse. Intercourse can transmit organisms, injure tissue, and change the acid-base balance of the vagina.

Table 53.10 presents the causes, manifestations, and interprofessional care of common infections of the female lower genital tract.

Clinical Manifestations

The manifestations of lower genital tract infections depend on the type of infection. Abnormal vaginal discharge and a reddened vulva are common. Women with vulvovaginal candidiasis have a curd-like discharge with intense itching and pain with urination. Women with bacterial vaginosis often have vaginal discharge that has a fishy odor. With cervicitis, there may be spotting (bleeding) after intercourse.

Common vulvar lesions include herpes infection and genital warts. Initial or primary herpes infections may be extremely painful. Herpes infections begin as a small vesicle followed by a superficial red, painful, ulcer. Genital warts, caused by the

human papillomavirus (HPV), vary in appearance. Irregularly shaped "cauliflower" lesions are common. Genital warts are painless unless traumatized. (Herpes infection and genital warts are discussed in Chapter 52.)

Postmenopausal women may develop vulvar changes, such as *lichen sclerosis*. This chronic inflammatory skin condition is associated with intense itching in the genital skin area (e.g., labia minora, clitoris). Although the vulvar changes are white with a "tissue paper" appearance initially, scratching causes changes in the appearance. The cause is unknown.

Interprofessional Care

Evaluation of genital problems includes a history, physical examination, and appropriate laboratory and diagnostic studies. Because many problems relate to sexual activity, a sexual history is essential. The nature of the problem determines the extent of the evaluation. When ulcerative lesions are present, the HCP will usually obtain a culture for herpes and a blood test for syphilis. Genital warts are usually identified by their clinical appearance. Vulvar skin conditions may be examined by colposcopy and biopsy of the skin lesion.

Problems involving vaginal discharge are evaluated by examining the discharge under a microscope or by obtaining specimens for testing. To assess for cervicitis, specimens are obtained for chlamydial, gonorrhea, and trichomonal infections. (Sexually transmitted infections [STIs] are discussed in Chapter 52.)

Drug therapy is based on the diagnosis (Table 53.10). Antibiotics taken as directed will cure bacterial infections. Teach patients how to properly take their medications and get follow-up care. Partners should be treated so that reinfection does not occur.

Women with vaginal conditions or cervical infection should abstain from intercourse for at least 1 week. Sexual partners must be evaluated and treated if the patient is diagnosed with trichomoniasis, chlamydial infection, gonorrhea, syphilis, or HIV.

Treatment of vulvar skin conditions is symptomatic because no cures are available. Treatment involves controlling the "itch-scratch cycle." High-potency topical corticosteroid ointments (e.g., clobetasol), help relieve itching. Stopping the itch-scratch cycle prevents further damage to the skin.

❖ NURSING MANAGEMENT: INFECTIONS OF LOWER GENITAL TRACT

Teach women about common infections of the genital tract and how to reduce their risks for infection. Recognize symptoms that indicate a problem, and help women seek care promptly. Discussing problems that concern the patient's genitalia or sexual intercourse is often hard. Use a nonjudgmental attitude to make women feel more comfortable while empowering them to ask questions.

When a woman is diagnosed with a genital infection, ensure that she fully understands the treatment. If a woman is using a vaginal medication for the first time, show her the applicator and how to fill it. Teach where and how the applicator should be inserted using visual aids or models. Vaginal creams should be inserted before going to bed so the medication will remain in the vagina for a long period.

PELVIC INFLAMMATORY DISEASE (PID)

Pelvic inflammatory disease (PID) is an infectious condition of the pelvic cavity. It may involve the fallopian tubes (salpingitis), ovaries (oophoritis), and pelvic peritoneum (peritonitis). A tubo-ovarian abscess may form (Fig. 53.4).

Etiology and Pathophysiology

PID is often the result of an untreated cervical infection. The organism infecting the cervix can spread into the uterus, fallopian tubes, ovaries, and peritoneal cavity. *C. trachomatis* and *N. gonorrhoeae* are the most common causative organisms of PID.[10] Other organisms include anaerobes, mycoplasma, streptococci, and enteric gram-negative rods. It is important to remember that not all cases of PID are the result of an STI. Organisms can gain entrance during sexual intercourse or after pregnancy termination, pelvic surgery, or childbirth.

Women at increased risk for chlamydia infection (e.g., younger than 24 years of age, have multiple sex partners, have a new sex partner) should be routinely tested. The infection can be asymptomatic and unknowingly transmitted during intercourse.

Clinical Manifestations

Lower abdominal pain is a common. The pain typically starts gradually and then becomes constant. The intensity may vary from mild to severe. Movement, such as walking, can increase the pain. The pain is often associated with intercourse. Spotting after intercourse and purulent cervical or vaginal discharge may occur. Fever and chills may be present.

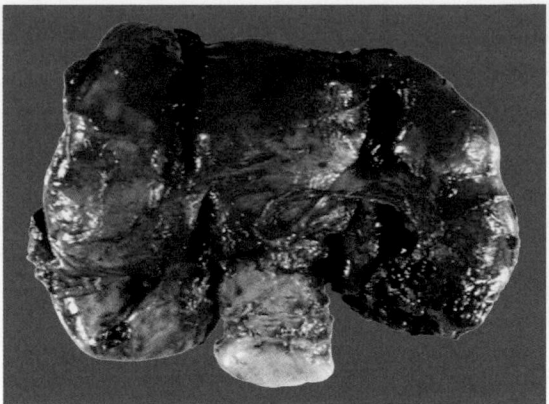

FIG. 53.4 Pelvic inflammatory disease. Acute infection of the fallopian tubes and the ovaries. The tubes and the ovaries have become an inflamed mass attached to the uterus. A tubo-ovarian abscess is present. (From Kumar V, Abbas AK, Aster JC, Fausto N: *Robbins and Cotran pathologic basis of disease*, ed 8, Philadelphia, 2010, Saunders.)

Women with less acute symptoms often notice increased cramping pain with menses, irregular bleeding, and some pain with intercourse. Women who have mild symptoms may go untreated either because they did not seek care or the HCP misdiagnoses their symptoms.

Complications

Complications of PID include septic shock, perihepatitis, tubo-ovarian abscess, peritonitis, and embolism. PID can cause adhesions and strictures in the fallopian tubes, which may lead to ectopic pregnancy. After 1 episode of PID, the risk for having an ectopic pregnancy increases nearly 10 times. Further damage can obstruct the fallopian tubes and cause infertility.

Interprofessional Care

A pelvic examination aids in the diagnosis of PID. Women with PID have lower abdominal tenderness, adnexal tenderness, and positive cervical motion tenderness.

Diagnostic testing includes examination for *N. gonorrhoeae* and *C. trachomatis* and a pregnancy test to rule out an ectopic pregnancy. When the patient's pain or obesity compromises the pelvic examination, a vaginal ultrasound may be done.

PID is usually treated on an outpatient basis. The patient is given a combination of antibiotics to provide broad coverage against the causative organisms. With effective antibiotic therapy, the pain should subside. The patient should abstain from intercourse for 3 weeks. Her partner(s) must be examined and treated. An important part of care is physical rest and oral fluids. Reevaluation in 48 to 72 hours, even if symptoms are improving, is an essential part of outpatient care.

If outpatient treatment is unsuccessful, a tubo-ovarian abscess is present, or the patient is acutely ill or in severe pain, admission to a hospital is needed. IV antibiotics are given in the hospital. Corticosteroids may be added to the antibiotic regimen to reduce inflammation, allowing for faster recovery and optimizing the chances for fertility. Application of heat to the lower abdomen or sitz baths may improve circulation and decrease pain. Bed rest in the semi-Fowler's position promotes drainage of the pelvic cavity by gravity and may prevent the development of abscesses high in the abdomen. Analgesics to relieve pain and IV fluids to prevent dehydration are used.

TABLE 53.11 Nursing Assessment

Pelvic Inflammatory Disease (PID)

Subjective Data

Important Health Information

Past health history: Use of IUD. Previous PID, gonorrhea, or chlamydial infection. Multiple sexual partners. Exposure to partner with urethritis. Infertility

Medications: Use of and allergy to any antibiotics

Surgery or other treatments: Recent abortion or pelvic surgery

Functional Health Patterns

Health perception–health management: Malaise

Nutritional-metabolic: Nausea, vomiting; chills, fever

Elimination: Urinary frequency, urgency

Cognitive-perceptual: Lower abdominal and pelvic pain, low back pain, onset of pain just after a menstrual cycle. Dysmenorrhea, dyspareunia, dysuria, vulvar pruritus

Sexuality-reproductive: Abnormal vaginal bleeding and menstrual irregularity. Vaginal discharge

Objective Data

Reproductive

Mucopurulent cervicitis, vulvar maceration, vaginal discharge (heavy and purulent to thin and mucoid), tenderness on motion of cervix and uterus. Presence of inflammatory masses on palpation

Possible Diagnostic Findings

Leukocytosis, ↑ erythrocyte sedimentation rate, positive culture of secretions or endocervical fluid, pelvic inflammation and positive endometrial biopsy on laparoscopic examination, abscess or inflammation on ultrasonography

Surgery is needed for abscesses that do not resolve with IV antibiotics. The abscess may be drained by laparoscopy or laparotomy. In extreme cases of infection or severe chronic pelvic pain, a hysterectomy may be done. When surgery is done, the capacity for childbearing is preserved whenever possible.

❖ NURSING MANAGEMENT: PELVIC INFLAMMATORY DISEASE

Subjective and objective data that should be obtained from the woman with PID are outlined in Table 53.11. Prevention, early recognition, and prompt treatment of vaginal and cervical infections can help prevent PID and its serious complications. Give accurate information about factors that place a woman at increased risk for PID. Urge women to seek medical attention for any unusual vaginal discharge or possible infection of their reproductive organs. Tell patients that not all vaginal discharge indicates infection, but early diagnosis and treatment of an infection, if present, can prevent serious complications. Teach patients methods to decrease the risk for getting STIs and to recognize the signs of infection in their partner(s).

The patient may feel guilty about having PID, especially if it is associated with an STI. She may be concerned about the complications associated with PID, such as infertility, and the increased incidence of ectopic pregnancy. Discuss with the patient her feelings and concerns to help her cope with them more effectively.

For hospitalized patients, you have a key role in implementing drug therapy, monitoring the patient's health status, and providing symptom relief and patient teaching. Record vital signs and the character, amount, color, and odor of the vaginal discharge. Assess the degree of abdominal pain to determine the effectiveness of drug therapy.

CHRONIC PELVIC PAIN

Chronic pelvic pain refers to pain in the pelvic region (below the umbilicus and between the hips) that lasts 6 months or longer. The cause of chronic pelvic pain is often hard to find. Many different conditions can cause pelvic pain. Gynecologic etiologies include PID, endometriosis, ovarian cysts, uterine fibroids, pelvic adhesions, and ectopic pregnancies. Abdominal causes include irritable bowel syndrome, interstitial cystitis, and colitis. Psychologic factors (e.g., depression, chronic stress, history of sexual or physical abuse) may increase the risk for developing chronic pelvic pain. Emotional distress makes pain worse. Living with chronic pain contributes to emotional distress.

Chronic pelvic pain has many different manifestations. These include severe and steady pain, intermittent pain, dull and achy pain, pelvic pressure or heaviness, and sharp pain or cramping. Pain may occur during intercourse or while having a bowel movement.

Determining the cause of chronic pelvic pain often involves a process of elimination. In addition to a detailed history and physical examination (including a pelvic examination), the patient may be asked to keep a journal of the onset of symptoms and any precipitating factors.

Diagnostic tests may include specimens from the cervix or vagina (used to detect STIs), ultrasound, CT scan, or MRI to detect abnormal structures or growths. Laparoscopy may be used to see the pelvic organs. This procedure is especially useful in detecting endometriosis and chronic PID.

If the cause of chronic pelvic pain is found, treatment focuses on that cause. If no cause can be found, treatment involves managing the pain. Over-the-counter pain drugs (e.g., aspirin, ibuprofen, acetaminophen) may give some relief. Sometimes stronger pain drugs may be needed. OCPs or other hormonal drugs may help relieve cyclic pelvic pain related to menstrual cycles. If an infection is the source of the problem, antibiotics are used.

Tricyclic antidepressants (e.g., amitriptyline, nortriptyline [Pamelor]) have pain-relieving and antidepressant effects. These drugs may help improve chronic pelvic pain even in women who do not have depression. Counseling can help the woman live with chronic pain.

Laparoscopic surgery may be used to remove pelvic adhesions or endometrial tissue. As a last resort, a hysterectomy may be done.

ENDOMETRIOSIS

Endometriosis is a condition in which endometrial tissue accumulates outside the endometrium of the uterus. Endometriosis is a common gynecologic problem.

The most frequent sites for endometrial tissue growth are in or near the ovaries, uterosacral ligaments, and uterovesical peritoneum (Fig. 53.5). The tissue responds to the hormones of the ovarian cycle and undergoes a "mini-menstrual cycle" similar to the uterine endometrium. Although it is not a life-threatening condition, endometriosis can cause considerable pain. It can significantly affect a woman's quality of life and ability to conceive. It also increases the risk for ovarian cancer.

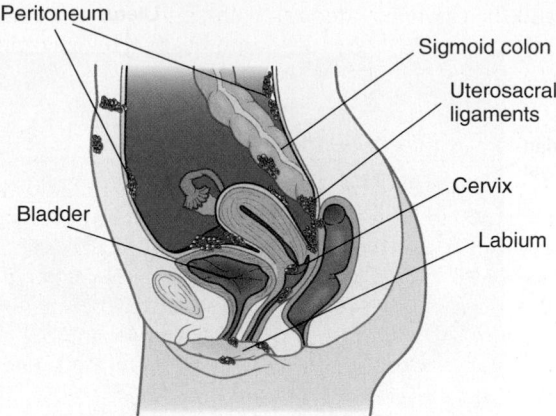

FIG. 53.5 Common sites of endometriosis.

Etiology and Pathophysiology

We have several theories as to the cause of endometriosis. One theory is that the disorder is due to retrograde (backward) flow of endometrial tissue. Instead of flowing out the cervix, the endometrial tissue flows through the fallopian tubes, depositing endometrial tissue into the pelvis.

Other theories suggest that endometrial tissue spreads to the pelvic area through the lymph system or bloodstream. Or, there is an increased sensitivity and production of prostaglandins, which are released prior to onset of menses. Other proposed causes include a genetic predisposition and altered immune function.

Clinical Manifestations

Patients with endometriosis have a wide range of manifestations. The severity of symptoms does not always correlate with the degree of disease found. The most common ones are secondary dysmenorrhea, infertility, pelvic pain, dyspareunia, and AUB. Less common ones include backache, painful bowel movements, and dysuria. With menopause, the ovaries no longer make estrogen and the symptoms may disappear.

❖ Interprofessional and Nursing Care

Endometriosis may be suspected based on a woman's history of the characteristic symptoms and the HCP's palpation of firm nodular lumps in the adnexa on bimanual examination. Laparoscopy with a biopsy is needed for a definitive diagnosis. MRI is now being used more often prior to surgery to determine if gynecologic symptoms the woman is having are from endometriosis.

Treatment is influenced by the patient's age, desire for pregnancy, symptom severity, and extent and location of the disease. When endometriosis is the probable cause of infertility, therapy proceeds more rapidly. When symptoms are not disruptive, a "watch and wait" approach is used (Table 53.12). Teach the patient about comfort measures that may be helpful. Reassure the woman that endometriosis is not life threatening and treatment options exist. Women who have severe disabling pain, sexual difficulties from dyspareunia, and infertility may need psychologic support.

Drug Therapy. Drug therapy does not cure endometriosis but can reduce symptoms. The most common drugs used to control symptoms and cause regression of endometrial tissue are

---

TABLE 53.12 Interprofessional Care
Endometriosis

Diagnostic Assessment
- History and physical examination
- Pelvic examination
- Laparoscopy
- Pelvic ultrasound
- MRI

Management
Conservative Therapy
- Watch and wait

Drug Therapy
- Danazol (use is limited by the occurrence of androgenic side effects)
- GnRH agonists (e.g., leuprolide [Lupron])
- NSAIDs
- OCPs

Surgical Therapy
- Laparotomy to remove implanted tissue and adhesions
- TAH-BSO after childbearing

---

combined OCPs. Their continuous use causes regression of endometrial tissue. NSAIDs, such as ibuprofen, naproxen (Naprosyn), and diclofenac (Voltaren) can relieve pain.

Another class of drugs used is gonadotropin-releasing hormone (GnRH) agonists (e.g., leuprolide [Lupron], nafarelin [Synarel]). These drugs result in amenorrhea. Side effects are usually the same as those of menopause (hot flashes, vaginal dryness, emotional lability). Loss of bone density can occur in women who stay on the therapy longer than 6 months. "Add-back" therapy with norethindrone acetate (Aygestin) can ease side effects.

 DRUG ALERT Leuprolide (Lupron)

- Assess patient for pregnancy before starting therapy.
- Monitor patient for dysrhythmias, palpitations.
- Teach patient to use nonhormonal contraceptive measures during therapy.

Surgical Therapy. The only cure for endometriosis is surgical removal of all endometrial tissue.[11] It involves removal or destruction of endometrial tissue and excision of adhesions by laparoscopic laser surgery or laparotomy. Definitive surgery involves removal of the uterus, fallopian tubes, ovaries, and as many endometrial implants as possible. GnRH agonist therapy can be given for 4 to 6 months to reduce the size of the lesions before surgery.

For women wishing to get pregnant, conservative surgical therapy can remove implants blocking the fallopian tube. Adhesions are removed from the tubes, ovaries, and pelvic structures. Efforts are made to conserve all tissues necessary to maintain fertility.

Patients should be actively involved in making the decision about preserving part or all their ovaries, if surgically possible. Explore the patient's feelings about maintaining her ovarian function. The HCP should assess the woman's risk for ovarian cancer and provide this information for her consideration.

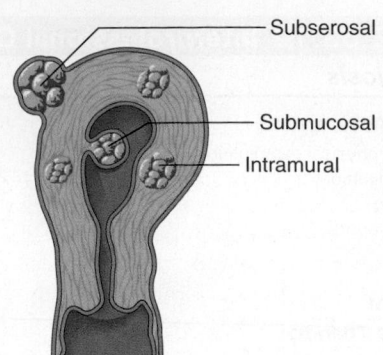

FIG. 53.6 Leiomyomas. Uterine section showing whorl-like appearance and locations of leiomyomas. (From McCance KL, Huether SE: *Pathophysiology: The biologic basis for disease in adults and children,* ed 6, St Louis, 2010, Mosby.)

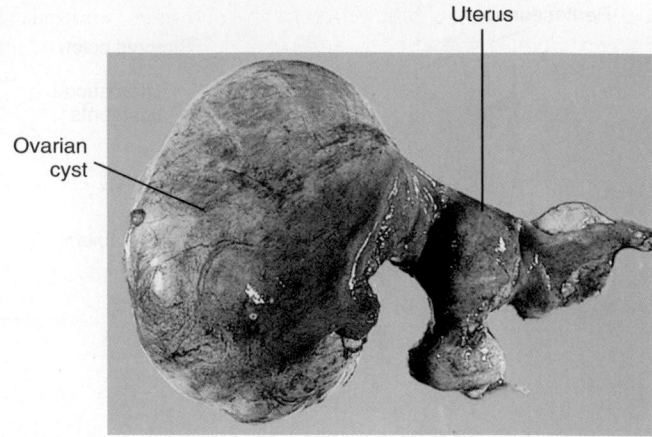

FIG. 53.7 Large ovarian cyst. (From Symonds EM, McPherson MBA: *Colour atlas of obstetrics and gynecology,* London, 1994, Mosby.)

BENIGN TUMORS OF THE FEMALE REPRODUCTIVE SYSTEM

LEIOMYOMAS

Etiology and Pathophysiology

Leiomyomas (usually called uterine fibroids) are benign smooth-muscle tumors (noncancerous) that occur during the childbearing years. Fibroids do not increase a woman's risk for endometrial cancer. They may be present inside the uterus within the endometrium, within the muscle of the uterus (myometrium), or outside on the surface of the uterus (subserosal). The size, shape, location, and number of fibroids vary among women. Some fibroids grow in spurts, while others slowly grow during the reproductive years (Fig. 53.6). They can occur at any age but often occur in women ages 30 to 40 years.

The cause of fibroids is unknown. Their growth appears to depend on estrogen and progesterone because they grow during the reproductive years and undergo atrophy after menopause. Fibroids have more estrogen and progesterone receptors than normal uterine tissue. So, they are more sensitive and grow in response to the release of these hormones.

Genetics may play a role. Identical twins and women with mothers and sisters with leiomyomas have an increased risk. Black women have increased incidence. They present with larger uterine fibroids and ones at an early age compared to other women. Other risk factors include early age of menarche, alcohol use, and a diet high in red meat and low in green vegetables.

Clinical Manifestations

Most women who have fibroids do not report any symptoms. Those who do may have abdominal and pelvic pain (i.e., dull, heaving, and/or achy pain and with pelvic pressure), painful sexual intercourse, pressure or dysuria, or frequent urination. If the fibroids are large, women may report constipation and difficulty passing stool. AUB can present as increased duration, more frequent, or increased menstrual bleeding. The pain associated with a fibroid seems to be caused from uterine blood vessel compression as the fibroid grows or from the fibroid pressing on surrounding organs.

❖ Interprofessional and Nursing Care

Diagnosis is based on the characteristic pelvic examination findings of an enlarged uterus distorted by nodular masses. Ultrasound can confirm the diagnosis. In some cases, small fibroids are found during a hysteroscopy, laparoscopy, or hysterosalpingogram when a woman is having a comprehensive workup for other gynecologic conditions, especially infertility.

The treatment depends on the manifestations, patient's age, her desire to conceive, and the location and size of the fibroid. If the symptoms are minimal, the HCP may choose to follow the patient closely for a period of time. Treatment may be needed if a woman is seeking conception, is having AUB, has pelvic pain and pressure, has anemia, or has difficulty with urination and defecation.

The most common and least invasive treatment for fibroids is the use of OCPs to maintain and slow growth and manage AUB. If surgical intervention is needed, options include a myomectomy (surgical removal of the uterine fibroid only) or a hysterectomy (surgical removal of the uterus with or without the ovaries and fallopian tubes). Myomectomies are typically done when the fibroids are small and few in number and the woman would like to preserve her uterus. Hysterectomies are done when there are multiple fibroids s, if they are large, or if their location is affecting bowel and/or bladder function.

Uterine artery embolization (UAE) is increasingly being used as an alternative treatment to treat fibroids. UAE is the process by which embolic material (small plastic or gelatin beads) is injected into the uterine artery. This process blocks blood flow to the uterus and shrinks the fibroid. Because UAE's effects on future fertility are unknown, the procedure is offered to women who no longer want children.

OVARIAN CYSTS

Ovarian cysts are usually soft and surrounded by a thin capsule. Follicular and corpus luteum cysts are common ovarian cysts (Fig. 53.7). Multiple small ovarian follicles may occur with PCOS. They are not cancerous.

Ovarian cysts are often asymptomatic until they are large enough to cause pressure in the pelvis. Depending on the tumor's size and location, constipation, menstrual irregularities, urinary frequency, a full feeling in the abdomen, anorexia, an increase in abdominal girth, and peripheral edema may occur.

Pelvic pain may be present if the tumor is growing rapidly. Severe pain results when the cyst twists on its pedicle (ovarian torsion). In some cases, an ovarian cyst can rupture. A ruptured ovarian cyst is not only extremely painful, but it can lead to serious complications, such as hemorrhage and infection, especially if large.

Pelvic examination may reveal a mass or an enlarged ovary. A pelvic ultrasound can help determine a diagnosis. In premenopausal women, ovarian cysts often resolve on their own. If the mass is cystic (does not appear cancerous) and smaller than 5 cm, the patient is asked to return for reexamination in 4 to 6 weeks. This is called "watchful waiting."

In postmenopausal women, watchful waiting may be an option depending on the results of the ultrasound. If the mass is cystic and greater than 5 cm or is solid, laparoscopic surgery or laparotomy is done. Immediate surgery is needed if ovarian torsion occurs, causing the ovary to rotate and cutting off circulation. Surgical techniques are used to save as much of the ovary as possible (if indicated).

Polycystic Ovary Syndrome

Polycystic ovary syndrome (PCOS) is a disorder that includes ovulatory dysfunction, polycystic ovaries, and hyperandrogenism.[12] It most often occurs in women under 30 years old and is a cause of infertility.

The cause of PCOS is unknown. We think it is due to the ovaries producing estrogen and excess testosterone but not progesterone. Because of this hormonal imbalance, ovulation fails, and multiple fluid-filled cysts develop from mature ovarian follicles (Fig. 53.8).

Classic manifestations of PCOS include irregular menstrual periods, amenorrhea, hirsutism, and obesity (80% of women). Of these, obesity is associated with severe symptoms, such as excess androgens, amenorrhea, and infertility. Many women start with normal menstrual periods, which become irregular after 1 to 2 years, and then the periods become infrequent. Untreated PCOS can lead to CVD and abnormal insulin resistance with type 2 diabetes.

Successful management includes early diagnosis and treatment to improve quality of life and decrease the risk for complications. Pelvic ultrasound reveals enlarged ovaries with multiple small cysts. Treatment is based on symptoms. OCPs are useful in regulating menstrual cycles. Hirsutism may be treated with spironolactone. Hyperandrogenism can be treated with flutamide and a GnRH agonist, such as leuprolide. Metformin reduces

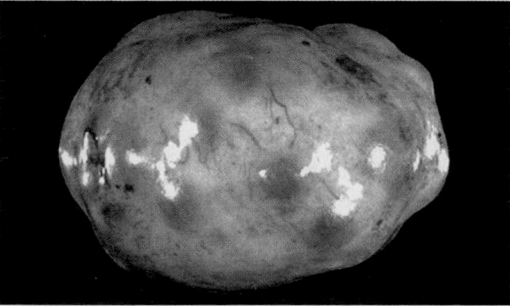

FIG. 53.8 Polycystic ovary syndrome. Multiple fluid-filled cysts in the ovary. (From Kumar V, Abbas A, Fausto N: *Robbins and Cotran pathologic basis of disease,* ed 7, Philadelphia, 2005, Saunders.)

hyperinsulinemia, improves hyperandrogenism, and can restore ovulation. For women wishing to become pregnant, fertility drugs (e.g., clomiphene [Clomid]) may induce ovulation.

Nursing management includes teaching about the importance of weight management and exercise to decrease insulin resistance. Obesity worsens problems related to PCOS. Monitor lipid profile and fasting glucose levels. Hirsutism is cosmetically distressing for many women. Support the patient as she explores measures to remove unwanted hair (e.g., depilating agents, electrolysis). Stress the importance of regular follow-up care to monitor the effectiveness of therapy and to detect any complications.

CERVICAL POLYPS

Cervical polyps are benign pedunculated (stalked) lesions that generally arise from the endocervical mucosa. Polyps are a characteristic bright cherry red and are soft and fragile. They are usually small, measuring less than 3 cm in length. They may be single or multiple. Their cause is unknown. Symptoms are usually not present, but intermenstrual bleeding after straining for a bowel movement and coitus can occur. Polyps are prone to infection.

Polyps may be seen protruding through the cervical os during a speculum examination. When the polyp is small, it can be excised in an outpatient procedure. If the point of attachment cannot be found and is not accessible to cautery, a polypectomy is done in an operating room. All tissue removed is biopsied as polyps, on rare occasion, are malignant.

CANCERS OF THE FEMALE REPRODUCTIVE SYSTEM

CERVICAL CANCER

Around 13,240 women in the United States are diagnosed with cervical cancer each year and 4100 women will die. While Hispanic women are the most likely to be diagnosed with cervical cancer, black women have the highest mortality rate from cervical cancer.[13]

Cervical cancer was once a common cause of cancer death. However, with early detection (Pap test, HPV testing), the mortality rate from cervical cancer has significantly declined.

⊕ PROMOTING HEALTH EQUITY

Cancers of the Female Reproductive System

Ovarian Cancer
- The mortality rate for black women is higher than any other ethnic group.

Endometrial Cancer
- The mortality rate for black women is higher than any other ethnic group.

Cervical Cancer
- The incidence rate is highest among Hispanic women
- Mortality rates are twice as high among black women.

Etiology and Pathophysiology

Risk factors for cervical cancer include (1) infection with high-risk strains of HPV 16 and 18, (2) immunosuppression, (3) using OCPs for a long period of time, (4) being exposed to the drug diethylstilbestrol (DES), (5) giving birth to many children, and (6) smoking.

The cervix is the lower third of the uterus that projects into the vagina. It is made up of glandular cells that line the uterine cavity and endocervical canal. Squamous epithelium lines the vagina and outer part of the cervix. These 2 cell types meet and undergo a normal physiologic process known as *squamous metaplasia*. This is the transformation of columnar epithelium into squamous epithelium, which results in an area called the *transformation zone*. This process begins at puberty and continues throughout a women's reproductive life cycle. The transformation zone moves in and out the endocervical canal, depending upon hormonal status and other factors. While the entire anogenital tract can be infected by HPV, the transformation zone is an area that is particularly susceptible to HPV-associated carcinogenesis.

Clinical Manifestations

Early cervical cancer often has no symptoms. An unusual discharge, AUB, or postcoital bleeding eventually occurs. The discharge is usually thin and watery but becomes dark and foul smelling as the disease advances. Vaginal bleeding first presents as spotting. As the tumor enlarges, bleeding becomes heavier and more frequent (Fig. 53.9). Pain is a late symptom. It is followed by weight loss, anemia, and cachexia.

Diagnostic Studies

The 2 tests used for cervical cancer screening are the Papanicolaou (Pap) test and the HPV test. The Pap test helps find changes in cervical cells that may indicate precancerous changes. Cells are obtained from the cervix during a speculum examination. HPV testing can identify high-risk HPV types 16 and 18, of which 80% are associated with cervical cancer, more than any other high-risk HPV types. The use of the HPV test is age-dependent and Pap result–dependent. To do an HPV test, cervical scrapings are tested for viral DNA or RNA.

All women should begin cervical cancer screening at age 21. Women ages 21 to 29 years should get a Pap test every 3 years. Women between the ages of 30 and 65 should have a Pap test and HPV test every 5 years. This is the preferred approach, but the woman may choose to get a Pap test without an HPV test every 3 years.[14] If both tests are negative, the risk for cervical

cancer is very low, and women can wait 5 years before another screening. HPV tests may be used to provide more information when a Pap test has unclear results. Women found to have an abnormal Pap test typically need a *colposcopy* (an examination of the cervical tissue under magnification). Typically, a cervical biopsy(s) is taken and sent for further analysis by a pathologist. Other tests for gonorrhea, chlamydia, and trichomonas can be run off the Pap test.

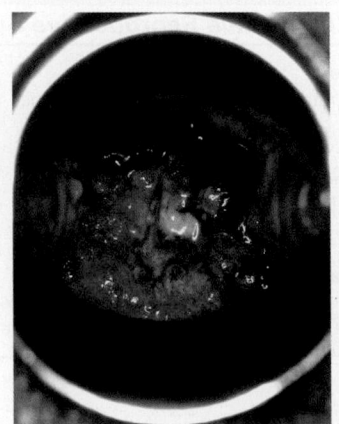

FIG. 53.9 Cervical cancer. View through a speculum inserted into the vagina. (From Drake RL, Vogl W, Mitchell AWM: *Gray's anatomy for students,* ed 2, Edinburgh, 2010, Churchill Livingstone.)

Interprofessional Care

Vaccination against HPV provides for primary prevention of cervical cancer. Teach both parents and patients about the need to complete the HPV vaccination series prior to first sexual contact. The CDC recommends that all children, males and females, be vaccinated at age 11 to 12, when the immune system has a better uptake of the vaccine. Vaccines can be given as early as age 9.

Currently 3 vaccines are available to protect against HPV. Gardasil, protects against types 6, 11, 16, and 18. Gardasil 9 protects against HPV types 6, 11, 16, 18, and 5 other HPV types. Cervarix offers protection against HPV types 16 and 18. These vaccines are given in 2 or 3 IM doses (depending upon the patient's age) over a 6-month period. They have few side effects. More specific information about HPV vaccines is discussed in Chapter 52 on p. 1219.

Women diagnosed with cervical cancer are typically referred to a gynecologic oncologist for treatment recommendations.[15] Treatment options can include surgery or a combination of chemotherapy and radiation. For patients with advanced disease, bevacizumab (Avastin), a targeted therapy drug, may be used in addition to cisplatin-based chemotherapy. Bevacizumab is an angiogenesis inhibitor. It works by interfering with the blood vessels that supply nutrients to cancer cells. (Chemotherapy, radiation therapy, and targeted therapy are discussed in Chapter 15.)

ENDOMETRIAL CANCER

Endometrial cancer is the most common gynecologic cancer. About 63,000 women are diagnosed each year with endometrial cancer, and 11,300 will die.[16] If endometrial cancer is diagnosed in the early stage, it has a low mortality rate, with survival rates over 88%. The average age of a woman diagnosed with endometrial cancer is 60. It is rare in women under the age of 45.

Etiology and Pathophysiology

The major risk factor for endometrial cancer is exposure to estrogen, especially unopposed estrogen. Obesity is a risk factor because adipose cells store estrogen, thus increasing the amount of circulating estrogen. Other risk factors include increasing age, never being pregnant, early menarche, late menopause, smoking, diabetes, and a personal or family history of hereditary nonpolyposis colorectal cancer (HNPCC) (see the Genetics in Clinical Practice box for HNPCC in Chapter 42 on p. 949). Pregnancy, use of OCPs and IUDs, and physical exercise are associated with reduced risk.

Endometrial cancer arises from the lining of the endometrium within the uterus. Most tumors are adenocarcinomas. If endometrial cancer is not diagnosed in early stages, it can invade the myometrium (muscle of the uterus) and the regional lymph nodes. If metastasis occurs, common sites include the lung, liver, bone, and brain. Prognosis depends on tumor size, cell type, degree of invasion into the myometrium, and any metastasis.[17]

Clinical Manifestations

Early manifestations include AUB, especially in postmenopausal women. Later symptoms can include dysuria, dyspareunia, unintentional weight loss, and pelvic pain.

Interprofessional Care

No routine screening test is available for endometrial cancer. Most cases are diagnosed at an early stage because of postmenopausal bleeding. An endometrial biopsy is the main diagnostic test for identifying endometrial cancer. This procedure is typically done in the office.

The National Comprehensive Cancer Network (NCCN) recommends surveillance and risk reduction for women with Lynch syndrome, a hereditary cancer associated with endometrial cancer. Hysterectomy and bilateral salpingo-oophorectomy should be offered to women who have completed childbearing and carry *MLH1, MLH2, or MLH6* mutations. For carriers of *MLH1 or MLH2*, annual endometrial biopsy is advised.

Treatment of endometrial cancer in the early stage is a total hysterectomy and bilateral salpingo-oophorectomy with lymph

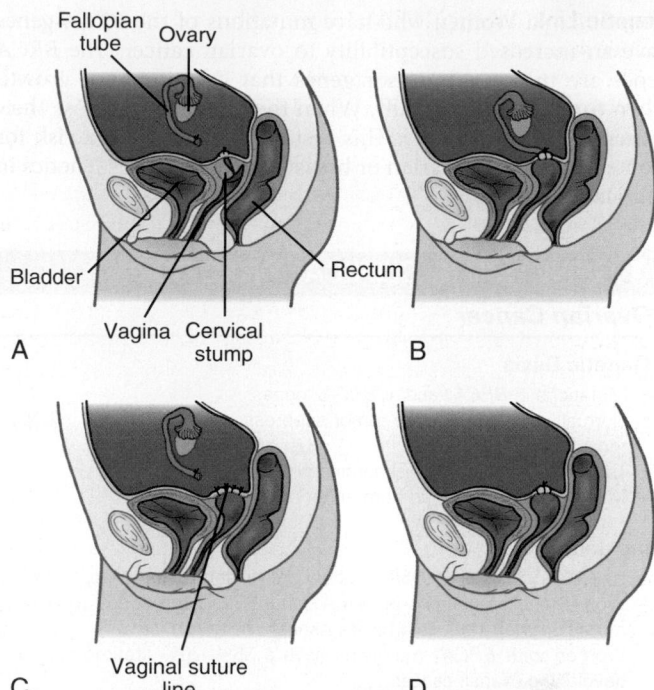

FIG. 53.10 Hysterectomies. **A,** Cross section of subtotal hysterectomy. The cervical stump, fallopian tubes, and ovaries remain. **B,** Cross section of total hysterectomy. The fallopian tubes and ovaries remain. **C,** Cross section of vaginal hysterectomy. The fallopian tubes and ovaries remain. **D,** Total hysterectomy, salpingectomy, and oophorectomy. The uterus, fallopian tubes, and ovaries are completely removed.

node biopsies. These may be done by less invasive types of surgery, including robotics and laparoscopy. (Various types of hysterectomies are shown in Fig. 53.10.) External radiation either to the pelvis or abdomen or internal radiation (brachytherapy) intravaginally follows surgery if there is local or distant metastasis.

The woman with advanced or recurrent disease may receive chemotherapy and hormonal therapy. The 5-year survival rate for stage 1 cancer is 90%, with reductions seen as the grade of the cancer increases.

OVARIAN CANCER

Ovarian cancer is the deadliest gynecologic cancer in the United States. Around 22,240 women will receive an ovarian cancer diagnosis in 2018, and about 14,070 women die. It is the fifth leading cause of cancer deaths in women in the United States. Half of women diagnosed are age 63 and older. Overall the 5- and 10-year survival rates are 45% and 35%, respectively. Most women with ovarian cancer are diagnosed when the disease is advanced, for which the 5-year survival rate is 27%.

Etiology and Pathophysiology

The cause of ovarian cancer is not known. The major risk factor is family history (1 or more first-degree relatives). A family history of breast or colon cancer is also a risk factor. Other risk factors include a personal history of breast or colon cancer and HNPCC (see the Genetics in Clinical Practice box on HNPCC in Chapter 42 on p. 949).

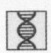 **Genetic Link.** Women who have mutations of the *BRCA* genes have an increased susceptibility to ovarian cancer. The *BRCA* genes are tumor suppressor genes that inhibit tumor growth when functioning normally. When they mutate, they lose their tumor suppressor ability. This results in an increased risk for women to develop ovarian or breast cancer (see the Genetics in Clinical Practice box).

GENETICS IN CLINICAL PRACTICE

Ovarian Cancer

Genetic Basis
- Mutations in *BRCA1* and/or *BRCA2* genes
- Normally these genes are tumor suppressor genes involved in DNA repair
- Transmission is autosomal dominant
- Mutations passed down from either mother or father

Incidence
- 5%–10% of cases of ovarian cancer are related to hereditary factors.
- Women with mutations in *BRCA1* and *BRCA2* are about 10 times more common in those who are Ashkenazi Jewish.
- Women with *BRCA1* mutations have a 35%–70% lifetime risk for developing ovarian cancer.
- Women with *BRCA2* mutations have a 10%–30% lifetime risk for developing ovarian cancer.
- Family history of both breast and ovarian cancer increases the risk for having a BRCA mutation.
- *BRCA* mutations occur in 10%–20% of patients with ovarian cancer who have no family history of breast or ovarian cancer.[18]

Genetic Testing
- DNA testing is available for *BRCA1* and *BRCA2* genetic mutations.

Clinical Implications
- Bilateral salpingectomy-oophorectomy reduces the risk for ovarian cancer in women with *BRCA1* and *BRCA2* mutations.
- Genetic counseling and testing for *BRCA* mutations should be offered to women whose personal or family history puts them at high risk for ovarian cancer.
- Women with *BRCA* mutations have a higher risk for developing breast, colon, pancreatic, and uterine cancers.

Women who have never been pregnant (nulliparity) are at higher risk. Other risk factors include increasing age, high-fat diet, increased number of ovulatory cycles (usually associated with early menarche and late menopause), HRT, and possibly the use of infertility drugs.

Breastfeeding, multiple pregnancies, OCP use (more than 5 years), and early age at first birth reduce the risk for ovarian cancer. These factors may have a protective effect because they reduce the number of ovulatory cycles and thus reduce the exposure to estrogen.

There are 3 major types of ovarian cancer. About 90% of ovarian cancers are epithelial cancers that arise from malignant transformation of the surface epithelial cells. Germ cell tumors account for another 3%, and sex cord stromal, 2%. Histologic grading is important to determine the prognosis of the disease. Tumor cells are graded according to the level of differentiation, ranging from well differentiated (grade I) to poorly differentiated (grade III) to undifferentiated (grade IV). Grade IV cells have a poorer prognosis than the other grades.

Intraperitoneal dissemination is a common characteristic of ovarian cancer. It metastasizes to the uterus, bladder, bowel, and

TABLE 53.13 Interprofessional Care

Ovarian Cancer

Diagnostic Assessment
- History and physical examination
- Pelvic examination
- Abdominal and transvaginal ultrasound
- CA-125 level
- Laparotomy for diagnostic staging

Management
- Surgery
  - TAH-BSO with pelvic lymph node biopsies
  - Debulking for advanced disease
- Chemotherapy
  - Adjuvant and palliative
- Radiation therapy
  - Adjuvant and palliative

omentum. In advanced disease, it can spread to the stomach, colon, liver, and other parts of the body.

Clinical Manifestations

Early ovarian cancer usually has no obvious symptoms. Most manifestations are vague and nonspecific. These include pelvic or abdominal pain, bloating, urinary urgency or frequency, and difficulty eating or feeling full quickly. Late-stage disease typically presents with abdominal enlargement with ascites (fluid in the abdominal cavity), unexplained weight loss or gain, and menstrual changes.

Diagnostic Studies

No accurate screening test exists for early detection of ovarian cancer. For women at high risk for ovarian cancer, screening using a combination of the tumor marker CA-125, ultrasound, and yearly pelvic examination is recommended. However, this approach is not proven to be effective in reducing ovarian cancer mortality.[18] The CA-125 test is positive in 80% of women with epithelial ovarian cancer. CA-125 is also used to monitor the course of the disease and response to treatment. The problem is that CA-125 levels can be high with other cancers (e.g., pancreatic cancer) or with benign gynecologic conditions, including fibroids and endometriosis.

Since postmenopausal women should not have palpable ovaries, a mass of any size found during a bimanual pelvic examination is considered suspicious. An abdominal or a transvaginal ultrasound can be done to detect ovarian masses (Table 53.13). An exploratory laparotomy may be used to establish the diagnosis and stage the disease.

Interprofessional Care

Options for women at high risk based on family and health history include prophylactic removal of the ovaries and fallopian tubes and the use of OCPs. While salpingo-oophorectomy significantly reduces the risk for ovarian cancer, it does not completely eliminate the risk for cancer in the peritoneum.

The initial treatment for all stages of ovarian cancer is a total abdominal hysterectomy and bilateral salpingo-oophorectomy (TAH-BSO) with removal of the omentum and as much of the tumor as possible (i.e., tumor debulking). Depending on the grade and stage of cancer, treatment options include intraperitoneal and systemic chemotherapy, intraperitoneal instillation of radioisotopes, and external abdominal and pelvic radiation therapy. Combination chemotherapy and radiation therapy should be considered before a single-modality treatment.

The chemotherapy agents most commonly used are taxanes (paclitaxel or docetaxel) and platinum agents (carboplatin or cisplatin). (See Table 15.7 for more about these drugs.)

Targeted therapy used to treat advanced ovarian cancer includes bevacizumab (Avastin) (discussed on p. 1243), rucaparib (Rubraca), and olaparib (Lynparza). Rucaparib and olaparib are poly ADP-ribose polymerase (PARP) inhibitors. They block enzymes involved in repairing damaged DNA. They are used for women with ovarian cancer that is associated with defective *BRCA* genes.

VAGINAL CANCER

Vaginal cancers are rare, with about 5170 new cases reported annually. They usually occur in women between ages 50 and 70. Vaginal tumors can be secondary sites or metastases of other gynecologic cancers, such as cervical or endometrial cancer. About 70% of vaginal cancers are squamous cell carcinomas, which begin in the squamous epithelium. Intrauterine exposure to diethylstilbestrol (DES) places a woman at risk for clear cell adenocarcinoma of the vagina.

Treatment depends on the type of cells involved, stage of the disease, and the size and location of the tumor.[19] Squamous cell carcinomas can be treated with both surgery and radiation. The process of transitioning from precancer to cancer can take many years. The term for the precancerous condition of squamous cells is *vaginal intraepithelial neoplasia* (VAIN.) There are 3 types of VAIN: VAIN 1, VAIN 2, and VAIN 3. VAIN 3 progresses closest to a true cancer.

VULVAR CANCER

Vulvar cancer is rare. There are about 6020 new cases reported each year, with an estimated 1150 deaths for 2017. Preinvasive lesions are referred to as *vulvar intraepithelial neoplasia (VIN)*, which precedes invasive vulvar cancer. The 3 types of VIN are VIN 1, VIN 2, and VIN 3. The invasive form occurs mainly in women over 60 years of age, with the highest incidence being in women in their 70s.

Patients with vulvar cancer may have symptoms of vulvar itching or burning, pain, bleeding, or discharge. Women who are immunosuppressed and/or have diabetes, hypertension, or chronic vulvar dystrophies have the highest risk for developing vulvar cancer. HPV DNA have been identified in some, but not all, vulvar cancers.

Diagnosis is based on physical examination, colposcopy, and biopsy results of the suspicious lesion. VIN can be treated topically with imiquimod cream (Aldara) or laser surgery. Surgery is the most common treatment for vulvar cancer. The goal is to remove all the cancer without any loss of the woman's sexual function.

If a woman has extensive lesions, a vulvectomy is recommended. Various types of vulvectomies are described in Table 53.14. As adjuvant measures, the patient may have chemotherapy or radiation therapy after surgery.

❖ NURSING AND INTERPROFESSIONAL MANAGEMENT: CANCERS OF FEMALE REPRODUCTIVE SYSTEM

◆ Nursing Assessment

Women with cancer of the reproductive system may have a variety of manifestations. These include leukorrhea, AUB,

TABLE 53.14 Surgical Procedures Involving the Female Reproductive System

Type of Surgery	Description
daVinci	Minimally invasive surgery using robotics for major gynecologic procedures.
Dilation and Curettage (D&C)	Dilation of cervix and scraping of endometrium.
Endometrial Ablation	An outpatient procedure using hot or cold energy to destroy the endometrial lining of the uterus in cases of AUB.
Hysterectomy	
Abdominal supracervical hysterectomy	Removal of uterus only with cervix remaining intact.
Radical hysterectomy	Panhysterectomy, partial vaginectomy, and dissection of lymph nodes in pelvis.
Total abdominal hysterectomy (TAH)	Uterus and cervix removed using a pfannenstiel incision (bikini cut).
Total abdominal hysterectomy and bilateral salpingo-oophorectomy (TAH-BSO)	Uterus, cervix, fallopian tubes, and ovaries removed using a pfannenstiel or a vertical incision.
Vaginal hysterectomy	Uterus and cervix removed through a cut in the top of vagina.
Laparoscopic hysterectomy	Laparoscope (video camera and small surgical instruments).
• Laparoscopic-assisted vaginal hysterectomy (LAVH)	Incision made at top of vagina. Uterus and cervix removed through the vagina. Laparoscope inserted into abdomen to assist in the procedure.
• Laparoscopic supracervical hysterectomy	Uterus removed using only laparoscopic instruments. Cervix is left intact.
Hysteroscopy	Video done with D&C to check for abnormal uterine lining, AUB, polyps.
Myomectomy	Removal of fibroid from the uterus, leaving the uterus in place.
Pelvic Exenteration	Radical hysterectomy, total vaginectomy, removal of bladder with diversion of urinary system and resection of colon and rectum with colostomy.
Vaginectomy	Removal of vagina.
Vulvectomy	Removal of part or all the vulva.
• Skinning vulvectomy	Removal of top layer of vulvar skin where the cancer is found. Skin grafts from other parts of the body may be needed to cover the area.
• Simple vulvectomy	Entire vulva is removed.
• Radical vulvectomy	Entire vulva, including clitoris, labia majora and minora, and nearby tissue, is removed. Nearby lymph nodes may be removed.

vaginal discharge, abdominal pain and pressure, bowel and bladder dysfunction, and vulvar itching and burning. Assessment for these signs and symptoms is an important nursing responsibility.

◆ Nursing Diagnoses

Nursing diagnoses for the female patient with cancer of the reproductive system include:

- Anxiety
- Acute pain
- Disturbed body image
- Impaired sexual functioning

◆ Planning

The overall goals are that the patient with cancer of the female reproductive system will (1) actively take part in treatment decisions, (2) achieve satisfactory pain and symptom management, (3) recognize and report problems promptly, (4) maintain preferred lifestyle as long as possible, and (5) continue to practice cancer detection strategies.

◆ Nursing Implementation

◆ **Health Promotion.** Through your contact with women in a variety of settings, teach women the importance of routine screening for cancers of the reproductive system. Cancer can be prevented when screening reveals precancerous conditions. Routine screening increases the chance that a cancer will be found in an early stage.

Teach women about risk factors for cancers of the reproductive system. Limiting sexual activity during adolescence, using condoms, having fewer sexual partners, and not smoking reduce the risk for cervical cancer. When high-risk behaviors are identified, help women in changing their lifestyles to decrease risk.

◆ **Acute Intervention Related to Surgery.** Types of surgery of the female reproductive tract are described in Table 53.14 and Fig. 53.10. All patients have a degree of anxiety when expecting surgery. The prospect of major gynecologic surgery increases these concerns. Some women may focus on the effect the surgery will have on their appearance and sexual functions. Discuss the woman's feelings and concerns about her surgery. Assess each patient individually. Be willing to listen since this can provide considerable psychologic support.

Preoperatively, prepare the patient physically for surgery with the standard perineal or abdominal preparation. A vaginal douche and enema may be given (based on the HCP's preference). The bladder should be emptied before the patient goes to the operating room. An indwelling catheter is often inserted.

Hysterectomy. After a hysterectomy, abdominal distention may develop from the sudden release of pressure on the intestines when a large tumor is removed or from paralytic ileus due to anesthesia and pressure on the bowel. Food and fluids may be restricted if the patient is nauseated. Ambulation will help relieve flatus.

Initiate venous thromboembolism (VTE) prophylaxis. Apply intermittent pneumatic compression devices and administer anticoagulant therapy. Frequent position changes, avoiding high-Fowler's position, and avoiding pressure under the knees minimize stasis and pooling of blood. Pay special attention to patients with varicosities. Encourage leg exercises to promote circulation.

Discharge teaching includes what to expect after surgery (e.g., she will not menstruate). Review specific activity restrictions. Intercourse should be avoided until the wound is healed (about 4 to 6 weeks). However, intercourse is not contraindicated once healing is complete. If a vaginal hysterectomy was done, tell the patient that she may have a temporary loss of vaginal sensation. Reassure her that the sensation will return in several months.

Physical restrictions are needed for a short time. Heavy lifting should be avoided for 2 months. Teach her to avoid activities that may increase pelvic congestion, such as dancing and walking swiftly, for several months. However, activities such as swimming may be both physically and mentally helpful. Assure her that once healing is complete, all previous activity can be resumed.

Salpingectomy and Oophorectomy. Care of the woman who had removal of a fallopian tube (salpingectomy) or an ovary (oophorectomy) is like that for any patient having abdominal surgery. However, if a large ovarian cyst is removed, she may have abdominal distention caused by the sudden release of pressure in the intestines. An abdominal binder may provide relief until the distention subsides.

When both ovaries are removed (bilateral oophorectomy), surgical menopause results. The symptoms are similar to those of regular menopause but may be more severe because of the sudden withdrawal of hormones.

Vulvectomy. It is important to know the extent of the vulvectomy and the significant effect it is likely to have on the patient's life. Because the surgery causes mutilation of the perineal area and the healing process is slow, the patient is likely to become discouraged. Provide opportunities for the patient to express her feelings and concerns about the operation.

Pay special attention to bowel and bladder care. A low-residue diet and stool softeners prevent straining and wound contamination. An indwelling catheter is used to provide urinary drainage. Be careful not to dislodge the catheter because extensive edema makes its reinsertion difficult. Heavy, taut sutures are often used to close the wounds, resulting in severe discomfort. In other instances, the wound may heal by granulation. Give analgesics to control pain. Carefully position the patient using strategically placed pillows to provide comfort. Initiate VTE prophylaxis.

Discharge teaching includes specific instructions in self-care. Teach her to report any unusual odor, fresh bleeding, breakdown of incision, or perineal pain. Home care nursing can help the patient during her adjustment period.

Sexual function is often retained. Whether clitoral sensation is retained may be critical to some women, particularly if it was the source of orgasmic satisfaction. Discussing alternative methods of achieving sexual satisfaction may be needed.

Pelvic Exenteration. When other forms of therapy do not control the spread of cancer and no metastases have been found outside of the pelvis, pelvic exenteration may be done. This radical surgery usually involves removal of the uterus, ovaries, fallopian tubes, vagina, bladder, urethra, and pelvic lymph nodes (Fig. 53.11). In some situations, the descending colon, rectum, and anal canal also are removed. Women who have this procedure are selected based on their likelihood of surviving the surgery and their ability to adjust to and accept the resulting limitations.

Postoperative care is similar to that of a patient who has had a radical hysterectomy, an abdominal perineal resection, and an ileostomy or a colostomy. The physical, emotional, and social adjustments to life by the woman and her family are great. There are urinary or fecal diversions in the abdominal wall, a reconstructed vagina, possible lymphedema, and the onset of menopausal symptoms.

Assess the patient's physical and emotional adjustment to the changes in body image from the surgery and her ability to carry out any treatment measures. The patient's rehabilitative process should keep pace with her acceptance of the situation. You need to provide understanding and support during a long recovery period. Gently encourage the patient to regain her independence. She needs to share her feelings about her altered body structure. Include her caregiver and family in the plan of care. Careful follow-up monitoring is needed so that early recurrence of the cancer can be identified and treated.

◆ **Acute Intervention With Radiation Therapy.** Teach the patient who is to receive external radiation to urinate immediately before the treatment to minimize radiation exposure to the bladder. Review the side effects of radiation, including enteritis and cystitis. Discuss measures that can be used to reduce their impact.

Nursing management of the patient receiving internal radiation therapy requires special considerations. Do not stay in the immediate area any longer than is necessary to give proper care and attention. (Radiation therapy is discussed in Chapter 15.)

◆ **Evaluation**

The expected outcomes are that the patient with cancer of the female reproductive system will
- Actively take part in treatment decisions
- Achieve satisfactory pain and symptom management
- Recognize and report problems promptly
- Maintain preferred lifestyle as long as possible
- Continue to practice cancer detection strategies

PELVIC ORGAN PROLAPSE

Pelvic organ prolapse (POP) involves the descent of 1 or more aspects of the uterus and vagina, allowing nearby organs, such as the bladder and rectum, to herniate into the vaginal space.[20] Although vaginal birth increases the risk for POP, it can occur in women who never went through childbirth. Obesity, chronic coughing, and straining during bowel movements can increase the risk for POP. The decreased estrogen that normally accompanies perimenopause decreases connective tissue support and increases the risk.

UTERINE PROLAPSE

Uterine prolapse is the downward displacement of the uterus into the vaginal canal(Fig. 53.12). Prolapse is rated by degrees. In first-degree prolapse, the cervix rests in the lower part of the vagina. Second-degree prolapse means the cervix is at the

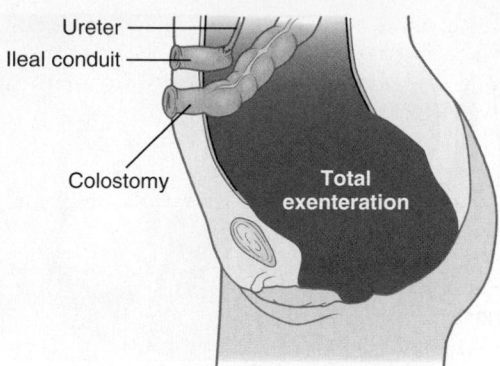

FIG. 53.11 Total exenteration is removal of all pelvic organs with creation of an ileal conduit and a colostomy.

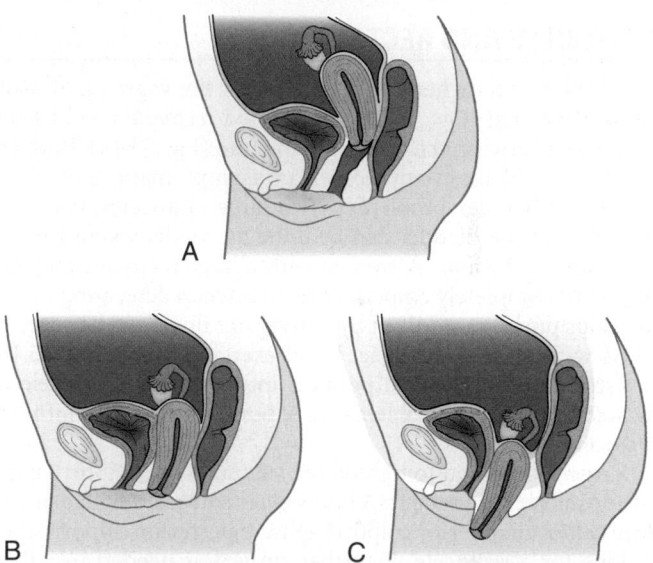

FIG. 53.12 Uterine prolapse. **A,** First-degree prolapse. **B,** Second-degree prolapse. **C,** Third-degree prolapse.

vaginal opening. Third-degree prolapse means the uterus protrudes through the introitus.

Symptoms vary with the degree of prolapse. The patient may describe a feeling of "something coming down." She may have dyspareunia, a dragging or heavy feeling in the pelvis, and a backache. Stress incontinence is a common and troubling problem. When third-degree uterine prolapse occurs, the protruding cervix and vaginal walls are subjected to constant irritation, and tissue changes may occur.

Therapy depends on the degree of prolapse and how much the woman's daily activities have been affected.[20] Pelvic muscle strengthening exercises (Kegel exercises) may be effective for some women (see Table 45.18). If not, a pessary may be used. A *pessary* is a device that is placed in the vagina to help support the uterus. A wide variety of shapes exist, including rings, arches, and balls. Most are made of plastic or wire coated with plastic. When a woman first receives a pessary, she needs instructions on how to clean it. Pessaries that are left in place for long periods are associated with erosion, fistulas, and vaginal cancer.

If more conservative measures are not successful, surgery is indicated. Surgery generally involves a vaginal hysterectomy with anterior and posterior repair of the vagina and the underlying fascia.

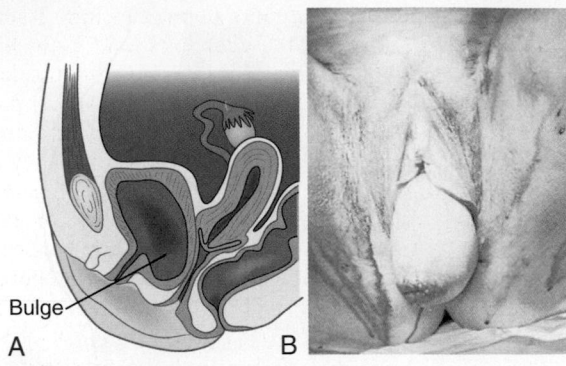

FIG. 53.13 A, Cystocele. B, Bladder has prolapsed into the vagina, causing a uterine prolapse.

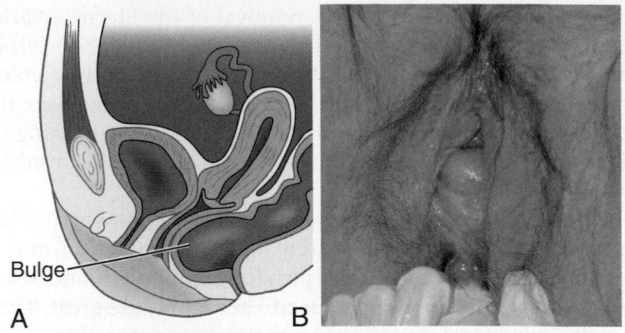

FIG. 53.14 A, Rectocele. B, Rectum has prolapsed into the vagina. (*B*, From Townsend CM: *Sabiston textbook of surgery*, ed 18, St Louis, 2009, Mosby.)

CYSTOCELE AND RECTOCELE

Cystocele occurs when support between the vagina and bladder is weakened (Fig. 53.13). Similarly, a *rectocele* results from weakening between the vagina and rectum (Fig. 53.14). Both are common problems. Many women are asymptomatic. Some have bowel and bladder problems. With large cystoceles, complete emptying of the bladder can be difficult, predisposing women to bladder infections. A woman with a large rectocele may not be able to completely empty her rectum when defecating unless she helps push the stool out by putting her fingers in her vagina.

As with uterine prolapse, Kegel exercises (see Table 45.18) can strengthen weakened perineal muscles if the cystocele or rectocele is not too problematic. A pessary may be helpful for cystoceles.

Surgery designed to tighten the vaginal wall (colporrhaphy) is the preferred treatment. A cystocele is corrected with a procedure called an anterior colporrhaphy. A posterior colporrhaphy is done for a rectocele. If further surgery is needed to relieve stress incontinence, procedures to support the urethra and restore the proper angle between the urethra and the posterior bladder wall are done.

❖ NURSING AND INTERPROFESSIONAL MANAGEMENT: PELVIC ORGAN PROLAPSE

Help women avoid or decrease problems with pelvic support by teaching them how to do Kegel exercises.[21] Women of all ages may benefit from these exercises. Teach the patient to pull in or contract her muscles as if she were trying to stop the flow of urine, control the passing of gas, or pinch off a stool (see Table 45.18).

With vaginal surgery, the preoperative preparation usually includes a cleansing douche the morning of surgery. A cleansing enema is usually given before a rectocele repair. A perineal shave may be done.

After surgery, the goals of care are to prevent wound infection and pressure on the vaginal suture line. Perineal care must be done at least twice a day and after each urination or defecation. Apply an ice pack locally to help relieve perineal discomfort and swelling. A disposable glove filled with ice and covered with a cloth works well to create an ice pack. Later, sitz baths may be used.

After an anterior colporrhaphy, an indwelling catheter is usually left in the bladder for 4 days to allow the local edema to subside. The catheter keeps the bladder empty, preventing strain on the sutures. Twice-daily catheter care with an

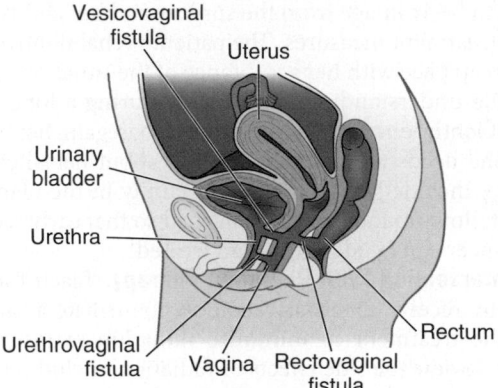

FIG. 53.15 Common fistulas involving the vagina.

antiseptic is generally done. To prevent constipation after a posterior colporrhaphy, a high-fiber diet and stool softener may be used.

Review discharge instructions before the patient leaves the hospital. These include the (1) use of mild laxative as needed; (2) restrictions on heavy lifting and prolonged standing, walking, or sitting; and (3) avoiding intercourse until the HCP gives permission. There may be a temporary loss of vaginal sensation, which can last for several months.

FISTULA

A *fistula* is an abnormal opening between internal organs or between an organ and the exterior of the body (Fig. 53.15). Gynecologic procedures cause most urinary tract fistulas. Other causes include injury during childbirth and disease processes such as cancer. Fistulas may develop between the vagina and bladder, urethra, ureter, or rectum. When *vesicovaginal* fistulas (between the bladder and vagina) develop, some urine leaks into the vagina. With *rectovaginal* fistulas (between the rectum and vagina), flatus and feces escape into the vagina. In both instances, excoriation and irritation of the vaginal and vulvar tissues occur and may lead to severe infections. In addition to wetness, offensive odors may develop, causing embarrassment and severely limiting socialization.

❖ Interprofessional and Nursing Care

Because small fistulas may heal spontaneously within a matter of months, treatment may not be needed. If the fistula does not heal, surgical repair is needed. Inflammation and tissue edema must be eliminated before surgery, which may involve a wait of many months. The fistulectomy may result in the patient having an ileal conduit or temporary colostomy. (See Chapter 45 for care of a patient with an ileal conduit and Chapter 42 for care of a patient with a colostomy.)

Perineal hygiene is of great importance before and after surgery. Cleanse the perineum every 4 hours. Warm sitz baths should be taken 3 times daily if possible. After surgery, emphasize ways to avoid stress on the repaired areas and prevent infection. Make sure the indwelling catheter, usually in place for 7 to 10 days, is draining at all times. Encourage the patient to maintain an adequate fluid intake to provide for internal catheter irrigation. Use minimal pressure and strict asepsis if catheter irrigation is needed. Change perineal pads often. The first stool after bowel surgery may be purposely delayed to prevent wound contamination. Later, give stool softeners or mild laxatives (as ordered).

Surgical repair of fistulas is not always effective, even in the best conditions. Therefore supportive nursing care for the patient and her significant others is especially important. Encouragement and reassurance are needed to help the patient cope with her problems.

SEXUAL ASSAULT

Sexual assault is the forcible perpetration of a sexual act on a person without their consent. It is a crime of violence and aggression. It can include any of the following actions: sodomy (anal or oral copulation with a person of the same or opposite sex); forced vaginal intercourse; assault with a foreign object; unwanted kissing, touching, or fondling; and serial battery and rape. The Federal Bureau of Investigation's (FBI's) definition of *rape* includes female or male victims who have experienced sexual assault that includes oral or anal penetration.

Sexual assault may be committed by a stranger or by an intimate partner. *Intimate partner violence (IPV)* is a major health problem in the United States.[22] Sexual assault that is perpetrated by a family member is termed *incest*. *Statutory rape* is consensual sexual intercourse with someone younger than a specific age. This age usually varies state to state. Most states use the criteria of a person younger than 16 years of age. Most states consider that an adolescent who is 16 years of age or older can consent to consensual sexual intercourse.

The involvement of children 14 years of age or younger in sexual activity, either consensual or forced, is termed *child sexual abuse*. Child sexual abuse is defined as the employment, persuasion, inducement, enticement, or even coercion of a person younger than 14 years of age in any sexually explicit conduct or simulation of sexual conduct. It includes behaviors that are forced onto the child for the purpose of producing video material, as well as rape, molestation, prostitution, or other forms of exploitation involving any sexual behavior.

Every 98 seconds, an American is sexually assaulted. Annually, 1.3 million rape or rape-related assaults occur to women. 18% of women report that they had been victims of an attempted or completed rape during their lifetime. Most (80%) reported that they were assaulted before the age of 25. Survivors have an array of physical and psychologic health consequences, such as suicidal thoughts and depression, after sexual violence.[23]

Clinical Manifestations

Physical. Some female victims of assault have more injuries than others. Factors that influence the severity of injury include the woman's age, if the perpetrator used a weapon, and if the victim knew the perpetrator. Physical injuries may include fractures, subdural hematomas, cerebral concussions, and intraabdominal injuries. Sexual injuries may include bruising and lacerations of the perineum, hymen, vulva, vagina, cervix, and anus. Sexual assault places women at risk for STIs and pregnancy.

Psychologic. Immediately after the assault, women may show signs of shock, numbness, denial, or withdrawal. Some women may seem unnaturally calm, while others may cry or express anger. Feelings of humiliation, degradation, embarrassment, anger, self-blame, and fear of another assault are often expressed.

These symptoms usually decrease after 2 weeks, and victims may appear to have adjusted. Yet any time from 2 to 3 weeks to months or years after the assault, symptoms may return and become more severe.

Rape trauma syndrome is a classification of posttraumatic stress disorder. Flashbacks, intrusive recall, sleep problems, GI symptoms, and numbing of feelings are common initial symptoms. Women feel embarrassment, self-blame, and powerlessness. Later symptoms include mood swings, irritability, and anger. Feelings of despair, shame, and hopelessness may be internalized and lead to depression, and the risk for suicide may increase.

Interprofessional Care

The highest priority for the victim of assault is her emotional and physical safety. Table 53.15 outlines the emergency management of the patient who has been sexually assaulted. Most emergency departments (EDs) have identified personnel who have received special training to work with women who have been assaulted. The sexual assault nurse examiner (SANE) is a registered nurse who is certified to provide care to victims of sexual assault, while ensuring evidence is safeguarded. Special procedures are followed in taking the history and conducting the examination to preserve all evidence in case of future prosecution. When the victim of an assault is in the ED or clinic, a specific chain of events occurs to collect legal evidence if the woman chooses to pursue legal action (Tables 53.15 and 53.16).

The SANE takes a comprehensive gynecologic and sexual history and an account of the assault (who, what, when, and where) and does a general physical and pelvic examination. Laboratory tests are done to identify sperm in the vagina and to screen for STIs or pregnancy. The patient receives preventive treatment for pregnancy and STIs and treatment for injuries sustained in the assault.

Follow-up physical and psychologic care is recommended. Women should return weekly for the first month after the assault. This includes the time period when a woman's psychologic reactions may be the most severe.

❖ NURSING MANAGEMENT: SEXUAL ASSAULT

Nursing care for a sexual assault victim is complex. Provide emotional and nonjudgmental support. Obtain referrals as needed for follow-up care. Part of the role of the SANE is to discuss the risk for pregnancy and STIs and offer the patient an emergency contraception pill and antibiotics (Table 53.17). A social worker or nurse case manager referral should be made by the primary nurse in the ED. They can assist the patient in securing financial compensation to help them pay for emergency services as a result of the assault, counseling services, and any missed work.

✚ TABLE 53.15 Emergency Management

Sexual Assault

Etiology	Assessment Findings	Interventions
• Assault involving genitalia (male or female) without consent • Sexual molestation • Sodomy	• Anger • Crying • ↓ Level of consciousness • Emotional or physical manifestations of shock • Extragenital injuries • Hyperventilation • Hysteria • Pain in genital or extragenital area • Silence • Vaginal, oral, and rectal injuries	**Initial** • Treat shock and other urgent medical problems (e.g., head injury, hemorrhage, wounds, fractures). • Assess emotional state. • Contact support person (i.e., social worker, rape advocate, sexual assault nurse examiner). • Do *not* clean the patient until all evidence is collected. Make sure the patient does not wash, douche, urinate, brush teeth, or gargle. • Place sheet on floor. Then have patient stand on sheet to remove clothing. Place sheet with clothing in paper bag. • Obtain forensic evidence per local protocol (e.g., body hair, nail scrapings, tissue, dried semen, vaginal washing, blood samples). • Maintain chain of evidence for all legal specimens. Clearly label evidence and keep in locked cabinet until given to law enforcement agency. • Obtain baseline HIV, syphilis, and other STI screening. • Determine method of contraception, date of last menstrual period, and date of last tetanus immunization. • Consider tetanus prophylaxis if lacerations contain soil or dirt. • Vaccinate against hepatitis B if not already done. **Ongoing Monitoring** • Monitor vital signs and emotional status. • Provide clothing as needed. • Counsel patient about confidential HIV and STI testing.

TABLE 53.16 Evaluation of Alleged Sexual Assault

1. Medicolegal
• Valid written consent for examination, photographs, laboratory tests, release of information, and laboratory samples
• Appropriate "chain of evidence" documentation

2. History
• History of assault (who, what, when, where)
• Penetration, ejaculation, extragenital acts
• Activities since assault (e.g., changed clothes, bathed, douched)
• Inquire about safety
• Menstrual and contraceptive history
• Medical history
• Emotional status
• Current symptoms

3. General Physical Examination
• Vital signs and general appearance
• Extragenital trauma: mouth, breasts, neck
• Cuts, bruises, scratches (photographs taken)

4. Pelvic Examination
• Vulvar trauma, redness. Hymen, anal, and rectal status
• Matted hairs or free hairs
• Vaginal examination with unlubricated speculum for discharge, blood, lacerations
• Uterine size
• Adnexa, especially hematomas

5. Laboratory Samples
• Vaginal vault content sampling
• Vaginal smears: microscope evaluation for trichomonads and semen
• Oral or rectal swabs and smears (if indicated)
• Blood samples: pregnancy test; serologic testing for syphilis, HIV, and hepatitis B infection
• Freeze serum sample for later testing
• Cultures: cervix and other areas (if indicated) for gonorrhea and chlamydia infection
• Fingernail scrapings
• Pubic hair scrapings
• Clipping of matted pubic hairs

6. Treatment
• Care of injuries and emotional trauma
• Prophylaxis for STIs, tetanus, and hepatitis B (see appropriate chapters)
• If appropriate, consider levonorgestrel (Plan-B One-Step) emergency contraceptive pill up to 72 hr after assault; follow-up for pregnancy test in 2–3 wk
• Testing for HIV, syphilis, and hepatitis B may be done at 6–8 wk
• Protection of legal rights
• Recommendation of continued follow-up and services of rape crisis center

TABLE 53.17 Patient Teaching

Sexual Assault Prevention

Include the following instructions when teaching measures to prevent sexual assault:

1. Be proactive and take a self-defense class.
2. Be aware of date-rape drugs (e.g., GHB, Rohypnol, ketamine). Never leave your beverage unattended when socializing.
3. Place and maintain lights at all entrances to your home.
4. Keep your doors locked and do not open them to a stranger. Ask for identification if a service person comes to the door.
5. Do not advertise that you live alone. List only your initials with your last name in the telephone directory or on the mailbox. Never reveal to a caller that you are home alone.
6. Avoid walking alone in deserted areas. Walk to the parking lot with a friend. Be sure you see each other leave.
7. Have your keys ready as you approach your car or home.
8. Keep all doors locked and the windows up when driving.
9. Never get on an elevator with a suspicious person. Pretend you have forgotten something and get off.
10. Say what you mean in social situations. Be sure your voice and body language reflect your response.
11. Be cautious with online correspondence.
12. Carry a loud whistle and use it when you think you are in danger.
13. Yell "Fire!" if you are attacked and run toward a lighted area

CASE STUDY

Uterine Fibroids and Endometrial Cancer

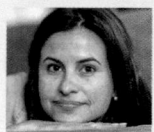

(© Juanmonino/ iStock.com.)

Patient Profile

B.C. is a 49-yr-old Latina woman who has lower pelvic discomfort and anemia. She has hypertension and hypothyroidism. B.C. is the mother of 2 teenage children. She has had abnormal uterine bleeding for 5 months. Large multiple uterine fibroids were diagnosed on ultrasound. She comes to the hospital for an abdominal hysterectomy.

Subjective Data

- Was initially reluctant about surgery
- Concerned about her dyspareunia and her husband's reaction to the surgery
- States she has pelvic discomfort and vaginal spotting

Objective Data (Preoperative)

- BP 140/92 mm Hg, pulse 82 beats/min, respirations 14 breaths/min
- Height 5ft, 6 in; weight 145 lb.

Operative

- During surgery, abnormal-looking endometrial tissue was sent for pathologic analysis. The results were positive for endometrial cancer.
- Had total hysterectomy and bilateral salpingo-oophorectomy with lymph node biopsies. 5 large fibroids were found in the uterus.

Postoperative Status

- Returned to room with indwelling urinary catheter in place
- Abdominal incision
- Intermittent pneumatic compression devices on lower extremities
- Patient-controlled analgesia (PCA) pump for pain management

Discussion Questions

1. Can the manifestations of uterine fibroids be distinguished from endometrial cancer?
2. **Patient-Centered Care:** Preoperatively, B.C. asks you about the effect of the surgery on her sexuality. How would you respond, and what type of patient teaching would you do?
3. **Patient-Centered Care:** When she is told about the diagnosis of endometrial cancer, she is shocked. She cannot believe that it was not discovered before surgery. How would you respond to her?
4. **Priority Decision:** What are priorities of care for B.C.?
5. **Safety:** When assessing B.C. after you got her out of bed, you note that her abdominal dressing is saturated with blood and she says she feels weak and dizzy. What would you do?
6. What other complications (including reasons for their development) can occur after an abdominal hysterectomy?
7. **Priority Decision:** Based on the assessment data presented, what are the priority nursing diagnoses? Are there any collaborative problems?
8. Her 17-yr-old daughter asks you if she is at risk for endometrial cancer. How would you respond?

Answers available at *http://evolve.elsevier.com/Lewis/medsurg.*

■ BRIDGE TO NCLEX EXAMINATION

The number of the question corresponds to the same-numbered outcome at the beginning of the chapter.

1. In telling a patient with infertility what she and her partner can expect, the nurse explains that
   a. ovulatory studies can help determine tube patency.
   b. a hysterosalpingogram is a common diagnostic study.
   c. for most couples, the cause of infertility is usually not found.
   d. semen analysis is performed only if testosterone levels are low.

2. An appropriate question to ask the patient with painful menstruation to distinguish primary from secondary dysmenorrhea is
   a. "Does your pain become worse with activity or overexertion?"
   b. "Have you had a recent personal crisis or change in your lifestyle?"
   c. "Is your pain relieved by nonsteroidal antiinflammatory medications?"
   d. "When in your menstrual history did the pain with your period begin?"

3. The nurse should advise the woman recovering from surgical treatment of an ectopic pregnancy that
   a. she has an increased risk for salpingitis.
   b. maintaining bed rest for 12 hours will assist in healing.
   c. having an ectopic pregnancy increases her risk for another.
   d. intrauterine devices and infertility treatments must be avoided.

4. To prevent or decrease age-related changes that occur after menopause in a patient who chooses not to take hormone therapy, the *most* important self-care measure to teach is
   a. maintaining usual sexual activity.
   b. increasing the intake of dairy products.
   c. performing regular aerobic, weight-bearing exercise.
   d. taking vitamin E and B-complex vitamin supplements.

5. In caring for a patient with endometriosis, the nurse teaches the patient that interventions used to treat or cure this condition may include (*select all that apply*)
   a. radiation.
   b. antibiotic therapy.
   c. oral contraceptive pills.
   d. surgical removal of tissue.
   e. total abdominal hysterectomy and salpingo-oophorectomy.

6. Nursing care for the patient with endometrial cancer who had a total abdominal hysterectomy and salpingectomy and oophorectomy includes
   a. maintaining absolute bed rest.
   b. keeping the patient in high-Fowler's position.
   c. need for supplemental estrogen after removal of ovaries.
   d. encouraging movement and walking as much as tolerated.

7. Postoperative care for the patient who had an abdominal hysterectomy includes (*select all that apply*)
   a. monitoring urine output.
   b. changing position frequently.
   c. restricting all food for 24 hours.
   d. observing perineal pad for bleeding.
   e. encouraging leg exercises to promote circulation.

8. Postoperative nursing care for the woman with a gynecologic fistula includes (*select all that apply*)
   a. bed rest.
   b. bladder training.
   c. warm sitz baths.
   d. perineal hygiene.
   e. use of daily enemas.

9. The *first* nursing intervention for the patient who has been sexually assaulted is to
   a. treat urgent medical problems.
   b. contact support person for the patient.
   c. provide supplies for the patient to cleanse self.
   d. document bruises and lacerations of the perineum and the cervix.

1. b, 2. d, 3. c, 4. c, 5. c, d, e, 6. d, 7. a, b, e, 8. c, d, 9. a

For rationales to these answers and even more NCLEX review questions, visit *http://evolve.elsevier.com/Lewis/medsurg*.

ⓔ EVOLVE WEBSITE/RESOURCES LIST

REFERENCES

1. National Institutes of Health: How common is infertility? Retrieved from *www.nichd.nih.gov/health/topics/infertility/conditioninfo/common*.
2. Centers for Disease Control and Prevention: What is infertility? Retrieved from *www.cdc.gov/reproductivehealth/infertility/index.htm*.
3. Barbieri RL: Female infertility. In: Strauss JF, Barbieri RL, eds: *Yen and Jaffe's reproductive endocrinology, physiology, pathophysiology, and clinical management,* ed 8, Philadelphia, 2019, Elsevier.
4. American Congress of Obstetricians and Gynecologists: Early pregnancy loss. Retrieved from *www.acog.org/~/media/For%20Patients/faq090.pdf*.
5. American Congress of Obstetricians and Gynecologists: Induced abortion. Retrieved from *www.acog.org/-/media/For-Patients/faq043.pdf?dmc=1&ts=20150208T1033249676*.

*6. Lustyk M, Gerrish W, Douglas H, et al: Relationships among premenstrual symptom reports, menstrual attitudes, and mindfulness. Retrieved from *www.uptodate.com/contents/treatments-for-female-infertility?-search=treatrnents-for-female-infertility&source=search_result&selected Title=3~132&usage_type=default&display_rank=3.*

7. American Congress of Obstetricians and Gynecologists: Abnormal uterine bleeding. Retrieved from *www.acog.org/Patients/FAQs/Abnormal-Uterine-Bleeding#abnormal.*

8. Tulundi T: Ectopic pregnancy: Choosing a treatment and methotrexate therapy. Retrieved from *www.uptodate.com/contents/ectopic-pregnancy-choosing-a-treatment-and-methotrexate-therapy?source=search_result&search=ectopic+pregnancy&selectedTitle=2~150.*

*9. Shifren JL, Gass LS: The North American Menopause Society recommendations for clinical care of midlife women. Retrieved from *www.menopause.org/publications/clinical-care-recommendations.*

10. Centers for Disease Control and Prevention: *Pelvic inflammatory disease.* Retrieved from *www.cdc.gov/std/pid/stdfact-pid-detailed.htm.*

11. Rosin M, Abrao MS: Endometriosis: From diagnosis to surgical management. In: Gomes-da-Silveira G, da Silveira G, Pessini S, eds: *Minimally invasive gynecology,* New York, 2018, Springer.

*12. Polycystic ovary syndrome guidelines. Retrieved from *https://emedicine.medscape.com/article/256806-guidelines.*

13. American Cancer Society: Cancer facts and figures 2018. Retrieved from *www.cancer.org/research/cancer-facts-statistics/all-cancer-facts-figures/cancer-facts-figures-2018.html.*

*14. American Cancer Society: The American Cancer Society guidelines for the prevention and early detection of cervical cancer. Retrieved from *www.cancer.org/cancer/cervical-cancer/prevention-and-early-detection/cervical-cancer-screening-guidelines.html.*

15. National Cancer Institute: Cervical cancer treatment. Retrieved from *www.cancer.gov/types/cervical/patient/cervical-treatment-pdq#link/_117.*

16. American Cancer Society: Key statistics for endometrial cancer. Retrieved from *www.cancer.org/cancer/endometrial-cancer/about/key-statistics.html.*

17. National Cancer Institute: Endometrial cancer treatment (PDQ)—Health professional version. Retrieved from *www.cancer.gov/types/uterine/hp/endometrial-treatment-pdq.*

18. American Cancer Society: Special section: Ovarian cancer. Retrieved from *www.cancer.org/content/dam/cancer-org/research/cancer-facts-and-statistics/annual-cancer-facts-and-figures/2018/cancer-facts-and-figures-special-section-ovarian-cancer-2018.pdf.*

19. National Cancer Institute: *Vaginal cancer treatment (PDQ)—Health professional version.* Retrieved from *www.cancer.gov/types/vaginal/hp/vaginal-treatment-pdq.*

20. American College of Obstetrics and Gynecology: Practice bulletin #176: Pelvic organ prolapse. Retrieved from *www.acog.org/Clinical%20 Guidance%20and%20Publications/Practice%20Bulletins/Committee%20 on%20Practice%20Bulletins%20Gynecology/Pelvic%20Organ%20 Prolapse.aspx.*

21. American College of Obstetrics and Gynecology: Pelvic support problems. Retrieved from *www.acog.org/Patients/FAQs/Pelvic-Support-Problems.*

22. Centers for Disease Control and Prevention: Intimate partner violence. Retrieved from *www.cdc.gov/violenceprevention/intimatepartnerviolence.*

23. Rape, Abuse, and Incest National Network: Victims of sexual violence: Statistics. Retrieved from *www.rainn.org/statistics/victims-sexual-violence.*

*Evidence-based information for clinical practice

54

Male Reproductive Problems

Anthony Lutz

I would like my life to be a statement of love and compassion—and where it isn't, that's where my work lies.

Ram Dass

http://evolve.elsevier.com/Lewis/medsurg

CONCEPTUAL FOCUS

Cellular Regulation	Pain	Sexuality
Infection	Reproduction	

LEARNING OUTCOMES

1. Describe the pathophysiology, clinical manifestations, and interprofessional and nursing management of benign prostatic hyperplasia.
2. Describe the pathophysiology, clinical manifestations, and interprofessional care of prostate cancer.
3. Explain the nursing management of prostate cancer.
4. Specify the pathophysiology, clinical manifestations, and interprofessional and nursing management of prostatitis and problems of the penis and scrotum.

5. Explain the clinical manifestations and interprofessional care of testicular cancer.
6. Describe the pathophysiology, clinical manifestations, and interprofessional and nursing management of problems related to male sexual function.
7. Discuss the psychologic and emotional implications related to male reproductive problems.

KEY TERMS

benign prostatic hyperplasia (BPH), p. 1254
epididymitis, p. 1271
erectile dysfunction (ED), p. 1273
orchitis, p. 1271
paraphimosis, p. 1270

phimosis, p. 1270
prostate cancer, p. 1262
prostatitis, p. 1269
radical prostatectomy, p. 1265
testicular cancer, p. 1272

testicular torsion, p. 1272
transurethral resection of the prostate (TURP), p. 1260
vasectomy, p. 1273

This chapter discusses problems of the male reproductive system. These involve a variety of structures, including the prostate, penis, urethra, ejaculatory duct, scrotum, testes, epididymis, ductus (vas) deferens, and rectum (Fig. 54.1). Many of these problems can profoundly affect sexuality and reproduction. Sexual dysfunction from prostate problems or erectile dysfunction (ED) can cause psychologic and body image problems. The patient may have anxiety because of a perceived loss of his sex role, self-esteem, or quality of sexual interaction with his partner. Patient education and counseling are essential nursing roles for promoting health and optimal sexual well-being.

PROBLEMS OF THE PROSTATE GLAND

BENIGN PROSTATIC HYPERPLASIA

Benign prostatic hyperplasia (BPH) is a condition in which the prostate gland increases in size, disrupting the outflow of urine from the bladder through the urethra. Half of men will have some signs of BPH by the age of 50. That number increases to more than 70% for men 60 to 69 years old.[1] Symptoms of BPH can include bothersome lower urinary tract symptoms (LUTS), such as difficulty starting a urine stream, a decreased/weaker flow of urine, or urinary frequency. BPH with LUTS does not cause or lead to an increased risk for prostate cancer.[2]

Etiology and Pathophysiology

There are several potential factors that may play a role in the development and progression of BPH. We think that hormonal changes associated with aging are a contributing factor. Dihydroxytestosterone (DHT), one of several sex hormones, stimulates prostate cell growth. Excess amounts of DHT can cause overgrowth of prostate tissue. As men age, they have a decrease in testosterone but continue to make and accumulate high levels of DHT, resulting in prostate enlargement.

Another possible cause of BPH is an increased proportion of estrogen (as compared to testosterone). Throughout their lives, men make both testosterone and small amounts of estrogen. As men age, the amount of active testosterone in the blood decreases, leaving a higher proportion of estrogen. A higher

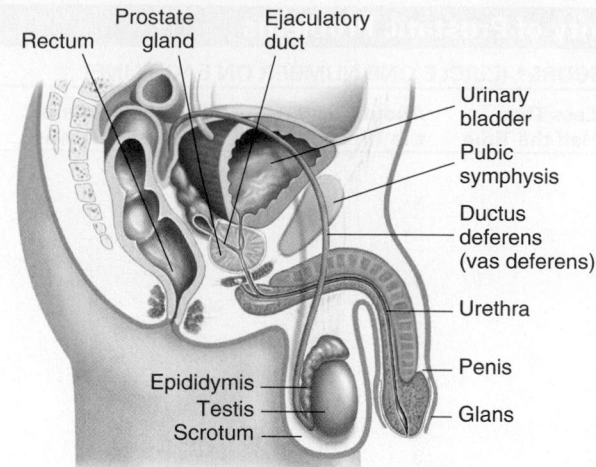

FIG. 54.1 Areas of the male reproductive system in which problems are likely to develop.

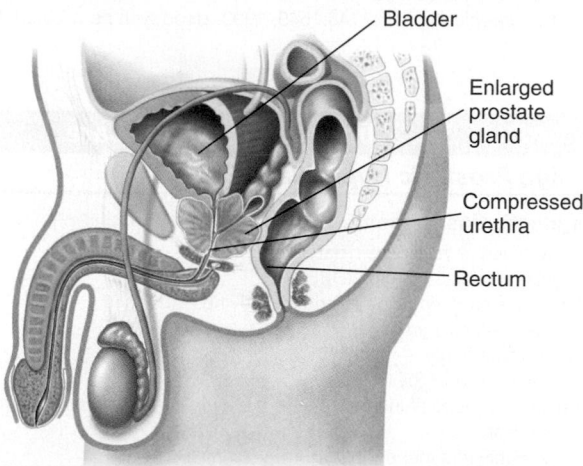

FIG. 54.2 BPH. The enlarged prostate compresses the urethra.

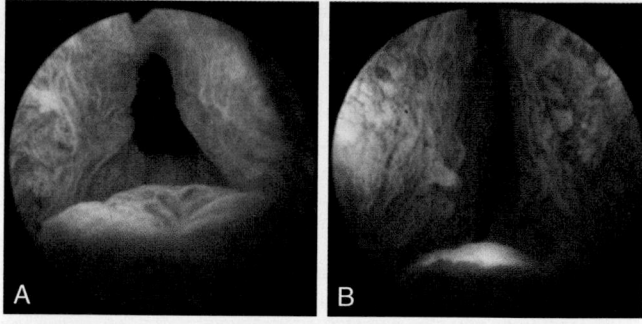

FIG. 54.3 Views of the prostate by cystoscopy. **A,** Normal appearance. **B,** Moderate BPH with urethral obstruction. (From Townsend CM, Beauchamp RD, Evers BM, et al: *Sabiston textbook of surgery,* ed 19, Philadelphia, 2012, Saunders.)

Clinical Manifestations

Manifestations occur gradually and may not be noticed until prostate enlargement has been present for some time. Early symptoms may not cause many problems because the bladder can compensate for a small amount of resistance to urine flow. As the severity of urethral obstruction increases, symptoms gradually worsen.

Symptoms can be divided into 2 groups: irritative and obstructive. *Irritative symptoms* include nocturia, urinary frequency, urgency, dysuria, bladder pain, and incontinence. These symptoms are related to inflammation or infection. Nocturia is often the first symptom that the patient notices. *Obstructive symptoms,* caused by prostate enlargement, include a decrease in the caliber and force of the urinary stream, difficulty in starting a stream, intermittency (stopping and starting stream several times while voiding), and dribbling at the end of urination. These symptoms are due to the increased effort of the bladder as it tries to empty through the decreased diameter of the urethra. As a group, both irritative and obstructive symptoms are considered LUTS.

The American Urological Association (AUA) symptom index for BPH (Table 54.1) is a widely used tool to assess voiding symptoms from obstruction.[4] Although this tool is not diagnostic, it helps determine the extent of symptoms and guide treatment. Higher scores on this tool mean greater symptom severity.

Complications

Complications of BPH are relatively rare. Some men may have acute urinary retention. This complication is manifested by the sudden and painful inability to urinate. Treatment involves the insertion of a catheter to drain the bladder. Surgery may be indicated in severe situations.

Urinary tract infection (UTI) can be a complication of BPH. Since the bladder is unable to empty completely, bacteria can grow in the residual urine that remains in the bladder and cause infection. In more severe cases, infection can progress into the kidney and cause pyelonephritis. In severe cases, infection can spread into the bloodstream and sepsis can develop. Bladder calculi (stones) may develop because of the alkalinization of the residual urine. So, the finding of bladder stones often indicates obstruction related to BPH. The risk for kidney stones is not significantly increased in this population.

Other complications include renal failure caused by *hydronephrosis* (distention of the renal pelvis and calyces by urine that cannot flow through the ureter to the bladder) and bladder damage if treatment for acute urinary retention is delayed.

amount of estrogen within the prostate gland increases the activity of substances (including DHT) that promote prostate cell growth.

BPH usually develops in the inner part of the prostate, called the transition zone. (Prostate cancer is most likely to develop in the outer part, called the peripheral zone). As the transition zone of the prostate enlarges, it gradually compresses the urethra, leading to partial or complete obstruction (Fig. 54.2). This compression of the urethra leads to the development of clinical manifestations. There is no direct relationship between overall prostate size and the severity of manifestations or degree of obstruction.[3] The location of the enlargement is most significant in the development of obstructive symptoms (Fig. 54.3). For example, it is possible for mild prostate enlargement to cause severe obstructive symptoms or for extreme prostate enlargement to cause few obstructive symptoms.

Risk factors for BPH include aging, obesity (especially increased waist circumference), lack of physical activity, a high amount of dietary animal protein, alcohol use, ED, smoking, and diabetes. A family history of BPH in a first-degree relative also may be a risk factor.

TABLE 54.1 AUA Symptom Index to Determine Severity of Prostatic Problems

Questions	AUA SYMPTOM SCORE* (CIRCLE ONE NUMBER ON EACH LINE)					
	Not At All	Less Than 1 Time in 5	Less Than Half the Time	About Half the Time	More Than Half the Time	Almost Always
Over the Past Month						
1. How often do you have the sensation that your bladder is not completely empty after you finish urinating?	0	1	2	3	4	5
2. How often do you have to urinate again, less than 2 hr after you finish urinating?	0	1	2	3	4	5
3. How often do you stop and start again several times when you urinate?	0	1	2	3	4	5
4. How often do you find it difficult to postpone urination?	0	1	2	3	4	5
5. How often do you have a weak urinary stream?	0	1	2	3	4	5
6. How often do you have to push or strain to begin urination?	0	1	2	3	4	5
7. How many times do you usually get up to urinate from the time you go to bed at night until the time you get up in the morning?	0 (None)	1 (1 time)	2 (2 times)	3 (3 times)	4 (4 times)	5 (5 times or more)
Sum of circled numbers (AUA Symptom Score): _____*						

Source: Barry MJ, Fowler FJ, O'Leary MP, et al: The AUA symptom index for benign prostatic hyperplasia, *J Urol* 148:1549, 1992. Used with permission.
*Score is interpreted as follows: 0–7, mild; 8–19, moderate; 20–35, severe.
AUA, American Urological Association.

Diagnostic Studies

A detailed history and physical examination are both important in the diagnosis. Diagnostic studies are outlined in Table 54.2. A digital rectal examination (DRE) is done to estimate the prostate size, symmetry, and consistency. In BPH, the prostate is symmetrically enlarged, firm, and smooth.

Other diagnostic testing may include a urinalysis and urine culture and sensitivities to look for bacteria, nitrites, leukocyte esterase, white blood cells (WBCs), or microscopic hematuria (RBCs), which could indicate infection or inflammation.

A prostate-specific antigen (PSA) blood test may be done to screen for prostate cancer. PSA levels may be slightly increased in patients with BPH, as PSA is released into the bloodstream by both benign and malignant prostate cells. Serum creatinine levels can assess for renal insufficiency. If creatinine levels are high, a renal ultrasound may be done to evaluate for hydronephrosis. Because symptoms of BPH are similar to those of a neurogenic bladder, a neurologic examination may be done.

In patients with an abnormal DRE and high PSA, a transrectal ultrasound (TRUS) is typically ordered. This examination allows for accurate assessment of prostate size and can help to distinguish BPH from prostate cancer. Biopsies can be taken during the ultrasound procedure. A pelvic MRI with attention to the prostate is an alternative imaging test that can be done in the setting of abnormal DRE and high PSA. If abnormal areas are seen on MRI, these areas can be specially targeted on a TRUS prostate biopsy using new software and equipment (called an MRI-fusion targeted biopsy). Currently insurance coverage of pelvic MRI can sometimes be an issue. However, recent studies have shown risk assessment with MRI prior to biopsy and MRI-targeted biopsy is superior to standard TRUS biopsy in men at risk for prostate cancer.[5]

Uroflowmetry, a study that measures the volume of urine expelled from the bladder, is helpful to determine the extent of urethral blockage and the type of treatment needed. Postvoid

TABLE 54.2 Interprofessional Care
Benign Prostatic Hyperplasia

Diagnostic Assessment
- History and physical examination
- Digital rectal examination (DRE)
- Urinalysis and urine culture and sensitivities
- Prostate-specific antigen (PSA)
- Serum creatinine
- Postvoid residual (by ultrasound)
- Renal ultrasound (if increased serum creatinine/to evaluate for hydronephrosis)
- Transrectal ultrasound (TRUS)
- Uroflowmetry
- Cystoscopy
- Urodynamic/pressure flow studies

Management
Active Surveillance
- Annual PSA and DRE
- Repeat IPSS score and postvoid residual if any symptoms change

Drug Therapy
- 5α-Reductase inhibitors (e.g., dutasteride [Avodart], finasteride [Proscar])
- α-Adrenergic receptor blockers (e.g., alfuzosin, doxazosin, tamsulosin [Flomax])
- Combination 5α-reductase inhibitor and α-adrenergic receptor blocker (e.g., dutasteride plus tamsulosin [Jalyn])
- Erectogenic drugs (e.g., tadalafil [Cialis])

Minimally Invasive Therapy
- Laser enucleation of the prostate (HoLEP or ThuLEP)
- Photoselective vaporization of the prostate (PVP)
- Prostatic urethral lift (PUL)
- Transurethral microwave thermotherapy (TUMT)
- Transurethral needle ablation (TUNA)
- Water vapor thermal therapy

Invasive (Surgery) Therapy
- Transurethral incision of the prostate (TUIP)
- Transurethral resection of the prostate (TURP)
- Simple prostatectomy (open, laparoscopic, or robotic-assisted)

residual urine volume is can determine the degree of urine flow obstruction. Cystoscopy, a procedure allowing internal visualization of the urethra and bladder, is done if the diagnosis is unclear or to see the degree of prostatic enlargement. If the diagnostic picture is unclear, urodynamic/pressure flow studies can be done to help evaluate bladder function and assess for obstruction.

Interprofessional Care

The goals of interprofessional care are to (1) restore bladder drainage, (2) relieve the patient's symptoms, and (3) prevent or treat the complications of BPH. Treatment is generally based on the degree to which the symptoms bother the patient or the presence of complications, rather than the size of the prostate. Alternatives to surgical intervention for some patients include surveillance, drug therapy, and minimally invasive procedures.

The most conservative treatment that is recommended for some patients with BPH is referred to as *active surveillance,* or watchful waiting. When the patient has mild symptoms (AUA symptom scores of 0 to 7), a wait-and-see approach is taken. Teaching patients to make lifestyle changes can help relieve early or mild symptoms. Making dietary changes (decreasing intake of bladder irritants, like caffeine, alcohol, carbonated drinks, artificial sweeteners, and spicy or acidic foods), avoiding certain drugs (e.g., decongestants, anticholinergics), and restricting evening fluid intake may improve symptoms.

In addition, a timed voiding schedule (also referred to as "bladder re-training") may reduce symptoms, eliminating the need for further intervention. If the patient begins to have signs or symptoms that indicate an increase in obstruction, further treatment is needed.

Drug Therapy. The 2 main classes of drugs that are used to treat BPH include 5α-reductase inhibitors and α-adrenergic receptor blockers. Combination therapy using both types of drugs may be more effective in reducing symptoms than using 1 drug alone. A medication in the erectogenic class of drugs also can be used to help treat BPH.

5α-Reductase Inhibitors. 5α-Reductase inhibitors work by reducing the size of the prostate gland. They block the 5α-reductase type 1 and 2 isoenzymes, which are necessary for the conversion of testosterone to DHT (main intraprostatic androgen). Prostate size is directly related to the amount of DHT. By blocking DHT, overly enlarged prostates can decrease in size. This class of medication is more effective for men with larger prostates who have bothersome symptoms.

Finasteride (Proscar) inhibits only the type 2 isoenzyme. It is an appropriate treatment option for men who have a moderate to severe symptom score on the AUA symptom index (Table 54.1). Although most men who are treated with the drug have symptom improvement, it can take up to 6 months to be effective. It must be taken on a regular basis to have an effect. Because it blocks the enzyme needed for conversion of testosterone to DHT, a common side effect is decreased libido.

Serum PSA levels may appear decreased by almost 50% when taking finasteride. Therefore, to "correct" for the apparent decrease caused by the finasteride, the HCP should double the PSA value for a patient who has been on a 5α-reductase inhibitor for at least 6 months. This allows for an accurate comparison to premedication levels, in order to track trends more accurately in the PSA.

Dutasteride (Avodart) has the same effect on prostatic tissue as finasteride. It is a dual inhibitor of 5α-reductase types 1 and 2 isoenzymes. The combination of a 5α-reductase inhibitor (dutasteride) and an α-adrenergic receptor blocker (tamsulosin) is available in a single oral medication (Jalyn).

These drugs may lower the risk for some prostate cancers. However, using them to prevent prostate cancer is not been recommended and research is currently ongoing. Patients who develop a high PSA level while taking these drugs should be referred to their HCP. Encourage the patient to discuss the need for prostate cancer screening with the HCP.

DRUG ALERT Finasteride (Proscar)

- Women who may be or are pregnant should not handle tablets due to potential risk to male fetus (anomaly).

α-Adrenergic Receptor Blockers. α-Adrenergic receptor blockers are another drug treatment option for BPH. These drugs selectively block α$_1$-adrenergic receptors, which are abundant in the prostate, and are increased in hyperplastic prostate tissue. They offer symptom relief by relaxing the smooth muscle of the prostate that surrounds the urethra, thus facilitating urinary flow through the urethra. These medications do not decrease the overall size of the prostate.

α-adrenergic blockers used include alfuzosin (Uroxatral), doxazosin (Cardura), prazosin (Minipress), tamsulosin (Flomax), and silodosin (Rapaflo). Symptom improvement can often be seen within days to weeks of starting α-adrenergic blockers. Because they relax the smooth muscle of the prostatic urethra, one of the most common side effects is retrograde ejaculation.

Erectogenic Drugs. Tadalafil (Cialis) can be used in men who have symptoms of BPH alone or in combination with ED. It is effective in reducing symptoms for both conditions.

Herbal Therapy. Some patients take plant extracts, such as saw palmetto (*Serenoa repens*). However, research shows that saw palmetto has no benefit over a placebo.[6] Advise patients to discuss herbal therapies with their HCP.

Minimally Invasive Therapy. Minimally invasive therapies are becoming more common as an alternative to watchful waiting and invasive treatment (Table 54.3). They generally do not involve hospitalization or catheterization. They are associated with few adverse events. Many minimally invasive therapies have outcomes comparable to invasive techniques.

Photoselective Vaporization of the Prostate. Photoselective vaporization of the prostate (PVP) uses a high-power green laser light to vaporize prostate tissue. The use of laser therapy through visual or ultrasound guidance is an effective alternative to transurethral resection of the prostate (TURP) in treating BPH.[7] The laser beam is delivered transurethrally through a fiber instrument inserted into the meatus and through the urethra. It can cut, coagulate, and vaporize prostatic tissue. Improvements in urine flow and symptoms are almost immediate after the procedure. PVP works well for larger prostate glands, but irritative voiding symptoms may persist for several weeks.

Laser Enucleation of the Prostate. Laser enucleation involves delivering a laser beam transurethrally through a fiber instrument. It is used for rapid coagulation and vaporization of prostatic tissue, with better coagulative properties in the tissue compared with TURP. There are 2 types of lasers in this class: holmium laser enucleation of the prostate (HoLEP) and thulium

TABLE 54.3 Treatment for Benign Prostatic Hyperplasia

Description	Advantages	Disadvantages
Minimally Invasive		
Laser Enucleation of the Prostate Laser beams used to rapidly vaporize and coagulate prostate tissue. Laser does not penetrate deep tissue. 2 types of lasers in this class: holmium laser enucleation of the prostate (HoLEP), thulium laser enucleation of the prostate (ThuLEP).	• Outpatient procedure • Better coagulative properties in tissue compared with TURP • Comparable results to TURP and PVP • Minimal bleeding • Fast recovery time	• Catheter needed after for 24–48 hr • Irritative voiding symptoms, urinary incontinence • Hematuria • Retrograde ejaculation • May be more difficult to perform compared with PVP
Photoselective Vaporization of the Prostate (PVP) Procedure uses a laser beam to cut or destroy part of the prostate. May be more effective for small to moderate-sized prostates.	• Short procedure • Comparable results to TURP • Minimal bleeding • Fast recovery time • Rapid symptom improvement • Very effective	• Catheter needed up to 7 days after due to edema and urinary retention • Delayed sloughing of tissue • Takes several weeks to reach optimal effect • Retrograde ejaculation
Prostatic Urethral Lift (PUL) Permanent transprostatic implants/tension sutures placed transurethrally via cystoscope. Mechanically open the prostatic urethra by compressing the prostate tissue/parenchyma.	• Outpatient procedure • Erectile dysfunction, urinary incontinence, and retrograde ejaculation are minimal • No change in PSA since no prostate tissue ablated	• Lack of long-term durability/results • Treatment response rates slightly lower when compared with TURP • If unsuccessful, may need repeat PUL or TURP in the future
Transurethral Microwave Thermotherapy (TUMT) Use of microwave radiating heat to produce coagulative necrosis of the prostate.	• Outpatient procedure • Erectile dysfunction, urinary incontinence, and retrograde ejaculation are rare • Mild effects: bladder spasm, hematuria, dysuria	• Potential for damage to surrounding tissue • Urinary catheter needed after for 2–7 days • Not appropriate for men with rectal problems
Transurethral Needle Ablation (TUNA) Low-wave radiofrequency used to heat the prostate, causing necrosis.	• Outpatient procedure • Erectile dysfunction, urinary incontinence, and retrograde ejaculation are rare • Precise delivery of heat to desired area • Very little pain • Early return to activities	• Urinary retention common • Irritative voiding symptoms • Hematuria for up to a week • May need a catheter for a short time after
Transurethral Vaporization of Prostate (TUVP) Electrosurgical modification of the standard TURP. Vaporization and desiccation are used together to destroy prostatic tissue. Can use a variety of energy delivery mediums (e.g., button, rollerball, or vaportrode).	• Minimal risks • Minimal bleeding and sloughing	• Retrograde ejaculation • Intermittent hematuria
Water Vapor Thermal Therapy Heated water vapor/steam used to destroy obstructive prostate tissue. Delivered transurethrally via handheld device with a retractable needle that releases the water vapor in 9-second doses.	• Outpatient procedure • Can be done in an outpatient office setting • Erectile dysfunction, urinary incontinence, and retrograde ejaculation are rare • Precise delivery of steam to desired area • Very little pain	• Relatively new, so lack of long-term durability/results • Irritative voiding symptoms and UTI • Hematuria
Invasive (Surgery)		
Transurethral Incision of Prostate (TUIP) Involves transurethral incisions into prostatic tissue to relieve obstruction. Effective for men with small to moderate prostates.	• Outpatient procedure • Minimal complications • Low occurrence of erectile dysfunction or retrograde ejaculation • Outcomes similar to TURP	• Urinary catheter needed after procedure

TABLE 54.3 Treatment for Benign Prostatic Hyperplasia—cont'd

Description	Advantages	Disadvantages
Transurethral Resection of Prostate (TURP)		
Use of excision and cauterization to remove prostate tissue via cystoscope. Standard for treatment of BPH.	• Erectile dysfunction unlikely	• Bleeding, clot retention • Retrograde ejaculation • Catheter needed after
Simple Prostatectomy (open, laparoscopic, or robotic-assisted)		
Surgery of choice for men with large prostates (often >100 g), bladder damage, or other complicating factors. If open, involves an external incision with 2 possible approaches (either retropubic or perineal; see Fig. 54.6). If laparoscopic and/or robotic-assisted, involves several small abdominal incisions and 1 slightly larger incision near the umbilicus.	• Complete visualization of the prostate and surrounding tissue	• Erectile dysfunction • Bleeding • Pain • Risk for infection

laser enucleation of the prostate (ThuLEP). Neither penetrate deep tissue, which decreases side effects.

Prostatic Urethral Lift. Prostatic urethral lift (PUL) involves permanent transprostatic implants or tension sutures delivered transurethrally via cystoscope. They mechanically open the prostatic urethra by compressing the prostate tissue. This alters prostate anatomy without ablation of any tissue. This is a relatively new minimally invasive treatment for BPH. So far, it has been studied only in prostates less than 80 g in size and in prostates without an obstructive median lobe. This means there is a current lack of long-term data on the durability of this treatment over time and the rates of needing either repeat treatment or progression to TURP in the future.

Transurethral Microwave Thermotherapy. Transurethral microwave thermotherapy (TUMT) is an outpatient procedure that involves the delivery of microwaves directly to the prostate through a transurethral probe. The microwaves increase the temperature of the prostate tissue to about 113° F (45° C). The heat causes death of tissue, relieving the obstruction. A rectal temperature probe is used during the procedure to ensure that the temperature in the rectum is kept below 110° F (43.5° C) to prevent rectal tissue damage. The procedure takes about 90 minutes.

Urinary retention is a common complication. Patients who have a TUMT are generally sent home with an indwelling catheter for 2 to 7 days to maintain urinary flow and facilitate the passing of small clots or necrotic tissue. Antibiotics, pain medication, and bladder antispasmodic medications are used to treat and prevent postprocedure problems. Anticoagulant therapy should be stopped 10 days before treatment.

Transurethral Needle Ablation. Transurethral needle ablation (TUNA) is another procedure that increases the temperature of prostate tissue, thus causing localized necrosis. TUNA differs from TUMT in that low-wave radiofrequency is used to heat the prostate. Only prostate tissue in direct contact with the needle is affected, which allows for more precise removal of the target tissue. Most patients undergoing TUNA have an improvement in symptoms. It is done in an outpatient unit or HCP's office using local anesthesia and IV or oral sedation. The TUNA procedure lasts about 30 minutes.

Transurethral Vaporization of the Prostate. Transurethral vaporization of the prostate (TUVP) is an electrosurgical

> **? CHECK YOUR PRACTICE**
>
> You are caring for a patient who is scheduled for a transurethral needle ablation for BPH. He appears anxious. He tells you, "I'm afraid of the pain after the procedure. They told me I might have to have a tube in my bladder. I don't know how I'll manage at home."
> • What type of information and teaching would you provide him?

modification of the standard TURP, where vaporization and desiccation are used together to destroy obstructive prostatic tissue. There are a variety of energy delivery mediums that can be used to deliver the energy (e.g., button, rollerball, vaportrode). This is why it is referred to as a "button TURP." The results, side effects, and long-term outcomes are equivalent to TURP. Because TUVP uses a bipolar energy delivery surface, an energy current is not passed through the patient's body to a grounding pad. This allows for saline to be used during the procedure for irrigation, which dramatically decreases the risk for TUR syndrome (discussed on p. 1260.).

Water Vapor Thermal Therapy. Water vapor thermal therapy is another relatively new minimally invasive treatment for BPH. It uses heated water vapor/steam to destroy obstructive prostate tissue. The steam is delivered transurethrally directly into the prostate by a hand-held device with a retractable needle. It releases the heated water vapor in 9-second doses. It is potentially a good option for a patient who is looking to minimize the risk for postprocedure ED. This treatment has been studied only on prostates less than 80 g in size thus far. It lacks long-term durability data.

Invasive (Surgery) Therapy. Invasive treatment of symptomatic BPH involves surgery. The choice of the treatment approach depends on the size and location of the prostatic enlargement and patient factors, such as age and surgical risk. Invasive treatments are described in Table 54.3.

Invasive therapy is indicated when a decrease in urine flow causes discomfort, persistent residual urine, acute urinary retention because of obstruction with no reversible precipitating cause, or hydronephrosis. Intermittent catheterization or insertion of an indwelling catheter can temporarily reduce symptoms and bypass the obstruction. However, avoid long-term catheter use because of the increased risk for infection.

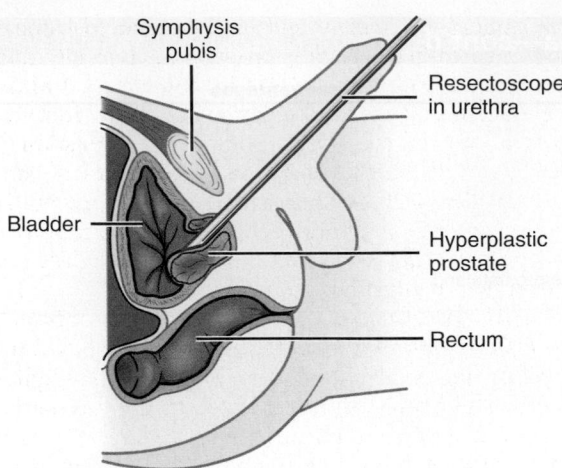

FIG. 54.4 Transurethral resection of the prostate.

Transurethral Incision of the Prostate. Transurethral incision of the prostate (TUIP) is a surgical procedure done under local anesthesia for men with moderate to severe symptoms. Several small incisions are made into the prostate gland to expand the urethra, which relieves pressure on the urethra and improves urine flow. TUIP is an option for patients with a small or moderately enlarged prostate gland.

Transurethral Resection of the Prostate. Transurethral resection of the prostate (TURP) is a surgical procedure involving the removal of prostate tissue using a resectoscope inserted through the urethra. TURP has long been considered the gold standard for surgical treatment of obstructing BPH. Most patients have marked improvements in symptoms and urinary flow rates. While in the past many TURP procedures required a longer hospital stay, many TURP procedures now are done on an outpatient basis.

In TURP no external surgical incision is made. A resectoscope is inserted through the urethra to excise and cauterize obstructing prostatic tissue (Fig. 54.4). A large 3-way indwelling catheter with a 30-mL balloon is inserted into the bladder after the procedure to provide hemostasis and to facilitate urinary drainage. If there is a large amount of hematuria with clots after surgery, then the bladder can be irrigated, either continuously or intermittently, for the first 24 hours to prevent obstruction from blood clots.

TURP was classically done with a monopolar resectoscope/loop. It sends a current through the patient during the resection to a grounding pad, so iso-osmolar fluid is used for irrigation. TURP has a relatively low risk, but caregivers must be vigilant for signs or symptoms of transurethral resection syndrome (TUR or TURP syndrome). This condition is manifested by nausea, vomiting, confusion, bradycardia, and hypertension. TUR syndrome is the result of hyponatremia due to longer operative times and prolonged intraoperative bladder irrigation with the iso-osmolar fluid. However, it is now common practice for a TURP to be done with a bipolar resectoscope/loop. This allows for saline to be used for irrigation and dramatically decreases the risk for TUR syndrome.

Other complications include bleeding and clot retention. Because bleeding is a common complication, patients taking aspirin, warfarin (Coumadin), or other anticoagulants must

stop taking medications several days before surgery. BPH medications are stopped after the procedure.

❖ NURSING MANAGEMENT: BENIGN PROSTATIC HYPERPLASIA

Because you will be most directly involved in care of patients with BPH having invasive therapies, the focus of nursing management in this section is on preoperative and postoperative care.

◆ Nursing Assessment

Subjective and objective data that should be obtained from a patient with BPH are outlined in Table 54.4.

Nursing Diagnoses

Nursing diagnoses for the patient with BPH before surgery may include:

- Acute pain
- Risk for infection
- Impaired urinary system function

Nursing diagnoses and interventions for the patient with BPH who has invasive therapy (surgery) are presented in eNursing Care Plan 54.1 (available on the website for this chapter).

◆ Planning

The overall preoperative goals for the patient having invasive procedures are to have (1) restoration of urinary drainage; (2)

TABLE 54.4 Nursing Assessment
Benign Prostatic Hyperplasia

Subjective Data
Important Health Information
Medications: Testosterone supplementation
Surgery or other treatments: Previous treatment for BPH

Functional Health Patterns
Health perception–health management: Knowledge of the condition
Nutritional-metabolic: Voluntary fluid restriction
Elimination: Urinary urgency, diminution in caliber and force of urinary stream. Hesitancy in starting voiding. Postvoid dribbling, urinary retention, urinary incontinence
Sleep-rest: Nocturia
Cognitive-perceptual: Dysuria, sensation of incomplete voiding, bladder discomfort
Sexuality-reproductive: Anxiety about sexual dysfunction

Objective Data
General
Older adult male

Urinary
Distended bladder on palpation. Smooth, firm, elastic enlargement of prostate on rectal examination

Possible Diagnostic Findings
Enlarged prostate on ultrasonography, bladder neck obstruction on cystoscopy, residual urine with postvoiding ultrasound or catheterization. WBCs, bacteria, or microscopic hematuria with bladder infection. ↑ Serum creatinine levels with renal involvement

resolution of any UTI; and (3) understanding of the upcoming procedure, implications for sexual function, and urinary control. The overall postoperative goals are to have (1) no complications, (2) restoration of urinary control, (3) complete bladder emptying, and (4) satisfying sexual expression.

◆ Nursing Implementation

◆ **Health Promotion.** The cause of BPH is largely attributed to the aging process. Health promotion focuses on early detection and treatment. The AUA currently recommends that men age 55 to 69 have the greatest potential benefit from PSA screening. The recommended screening interval is every 2 years.[8] When symptoms of BPH are present, further diagnostic screening may be needed (Table 54.2).

Some men find that consuming alcohol, caffeine, or other bladder irritants tends to increase prostatic voiding symptoms because the diuretic effect increases bladder distention and overactivity. Compounds found in common cough and cold remedies, such as pseudoephedrine (e.g., Sudafed) and phenylephrine (e.g., Allerest PE, Coricidin D), often worsen the symptoms of BPH. These drugs are α-adrenergic agonists that cause smooth muscle contraction. If this occurs, the patient should avoid these drugs.

Teach patients with obstructive symptoms to urinate every 2 to 3 hours and when they first feel the urge. This will minimize urinary stasis and acute urinary retention. Teach patients to maintain a normal level of fluid so that they do not become dehydrated. The patient may think that if he restricts his fluid intake, symptoms will be less severe, but this only increases the chances of an infection while concentrating his urine.

◆ **Acute Care.** The following discussion focuses on preoperative and postoperative care for the patient undergoing a TURP.

◆ *Preoperative Care.* Antibiotics are usually given before any invasive genitourinary (GU) procedure. Any infection of the urinary tract must be treated before surgery. Restoring urinary drainage and encouraging a high fluid intake (2 to 3 L/day unless contraindicated) are helpful in managing the infection. Prostatic obstruction may result in acute retention or inability to void. Urinary drainage must be restored before surgery.

A urethral catheter, such as a coudé (curved-tip) catheter, may be needed to restore bladder drainage. In many health care settings, 2% lidocaine gel is inserted into the urethra before catheter placement. The lidocaine gel acts as a lubricant, provides local anesthesia, and helps open the urethral lumen. If a sizable obstruction of the urethra exists, the HCP may insert a filiform catheter with enough rigidity to pass the obstruction. Aseptic technique is important to avoid introducing bacteria into the bladder. (Urinary catheters are discussed in Chapter 45.)

Patients may be concerned about the impact of the impending surgery on sexual function. Provide an opportunity for the patient and his partner to express their concerns. Tell the patient that his ejaculate volume may be decreased or absent after the procedure. Most types of prostatic surgery result in some degree of *retrograde ejaculation*. This is a condition in which some semen travels back into the bladder during orgasm instead of traveling out of the penis. This may decrease orgasmic sensations felt during ejaculation. Retrograde ejaculation is not harmful. The semen is voided during the next urination.

Postoperative Care. The main complications after surgery are hemorrhage, bladder spasms, urinary incontinence, and infection. Adjust the plan of care to the type of surgery, reasons for surgery, and patient's response to surgery.

After surgery, the patient will have a standard catheter or a triple-lumen catheter. Bladder irrigation is typically done to remove clotted blood from the bladder and ensure drainage of urine. The bladder is irrigated either manually on an intermittent basis or more often, as continuous bladder irrigation (CBI) with sterile normal saline solution or another prescribed solution. If the bladder is manually irrigated, instill 50 mL of irrigating solution and then withdraw with a syringe to remove clots that may be in the bladder and catheter. Painful bladder spasms often occur with manual irrigation.

With CBI, irrigating solution is continuously infused and drained from the bladder. The rate of infusion is based on the color of drainage. Ideally the urine drainage should be light pink without clots. Continuously monitor the inflow and outflow of the irrigant. If outflow is less than inflow, assess the catheter patency for kinks or clots. If the outflow is blocked and patency cannot be reestablished by manual irrigation, stop the CBI, and notify the HCP.

▓▓ NURSING MANAGEMENT
Patient Receiving Bladder Irrigation

- Assess for bleeding and clots.
- Assess catheter patency by measuring intake and output and presence of bladder spasms.
- Manually irrigate catheter if bladder spasms or decreased outflow occurs.
- Give antispasmodics and analgesics as needed.
- Monitor catheter drainage for increased blood or clots.
- Discontinue CBI and notify HCP if obstruction occurs.
- Teach patient Kegel exercises after catheter removal.
- Provide care instructions for patient discharged with indwelling catheter.

Use careful aseptic technique when irrigating the bladder because bacteria can be easily introduced into the urinary tract. Secure the catheter to the leg with tape or a catheter strap to prevent urethral irritation and minimize the risk for bladder infection. The catheter should be connected to a closed-drainage system. Do not disconnect unless it is being removed, changed, or irrigated.

Blood clots are expected after prostate surgery for the first 24 to 36 hours. However, large amounts of bright red blood in the urine can indicate hemorrhage. Hemorrhage may occur from displacement of the catheter, dislodgment of a large clot, or increases in abdominal pressure.

Release or displacement of the catheter dislodges the balloon that provides counterpressure on the operative site. Traction on the catheter may be applied to provide counterpressure (tamponade) on the bleeding site in the prostate, thereby decreasing bleeding. Such traction can result in local necrosis if pressure is applied for too long. Pressure should be relieved on a scheduled basis by qualified personnel.

Activities that increase abdominal pressure should be avoided in the recovery period. These include sitting or walking for prolonged periods and straining to have a bowel movement (Valsalva maneuver).

Bladder spasms are a distressing complication for the patient after transurethral procedures. They occur because of irritation of the bladder mucosa from the insertion of the resectoscope, presence of a catheter, or clots leading to obstruction of the catheter. If bladder spasms develop, check the catheter for clots. If present, remove the clots by irrigation so that urine can flow freely. Tell the patient not to urinate around the catheter because this increases the chance of spasm. Belladonna and opium suppositories or other antispasmodics (e.g., oxybutynin [Ditropan XL]), along with relaxation techniques, are used to relieve the pain and decrease spasm.

The catheter is often removed 2 to 4 days after surgery. The patient should have a voiding trial after catheter removal. If he cannot urinate, he will have a catheter reinserted for a day or so or be taught to perform clean intermittent self-catheterization (see Chapter 45).

Sphincter tone may be poor right after catheter removal, resulting in urinary incontinence or dribbling. This is a common but distressing situation for the patient. Sphincter tone can be strengthened by having the patient practice Kegel exercises (pelvic floor muscle technique) 10 to 20 times per hour while awake. (Kegel exercises are discussed in Table 45.18.) Encourage the patient to practice starting and stopping the stream several times during urination. This helps the patient to target the correct pelvic floor muscles when doing Kegel exercises.

It can take several weeks to achieve urinary continence. In some instances, control of urine may never be fully regained. Continence can improve for up to 12 months. If continence has not been achieved by that time, the patient may be referred to a continence clinic. A variety of methods, including biofeedback, have been used to achieve positive results.

Teach the patient how to use a penile clamp, a condom catheter, or incontinence pads or briefs to avoid embarrassment from dribbling. In severe cases, an occlusive cuff that serves as an artificial sphincter can be surgically implanted to restore continence. Help the patient find ways to manage the problem that allow him to continue socializing and interacting with others. (Urinary incontinence is discussed in Chapter 45.)

Observe the patient for signs of infection. If an external wound is present (e.g., from an open, laparoscopic, or robotic-assisted prostatectomy), assess the area for redness, heat, swelling, and purulent drainage. Special care must be taken if a perineal incision is present because of the proximity of the anus. Avoid rectal procedures, such as rectal temperatures and enemas. The insertion of well-lubricated belladonna and opium suppositories is acceptable.

Dietary intervention and stool softeners are important to prevent the patient from straining while having bowel movements. Straining increases the intraabdominal pressure, which can lead to bleeding at the operative site. A diet high in fiber promotes the passage of stool.

◆ **Ambulatory Care.** Discharge planning and home care issues are important aspects of care after prostate surgery. Patient teaching includes (1) caring for an indwelling catheter (if one is in place), (2) managing urinary incontinence, (3) maintaining adequate oral fluid intake, (4) observing for signs and symptoms of urinary tract and wound infection, (5) preventing constipation, (6) avoiding heavy lifting (more than 10 lb [4.5 kg]), and (7) refraining from driving or intercourse after surgery as directed by the HCP.

The patient may have a change in sexual function after surgery. Recovery depends on the type of surgery done and the interval of time between when symptoms first appeared and the date of surgery. For example, it may take up to 1 to 2 years for complete sexual function to return after nerve-sparing prostatectomy. Many men have retrograde ejaculation because of trauma to the internal urethral sphincter. ED may occur if the nerves are cut or damaged during surgery. The patient may have

anxiety over the change because of a perceived loss of his sex role, self-esteem, or quality of sexual interaction with his partner. Discuss these changes with the patient and his partner and allow them to ask questions and express their concerns. Sexual counseling and treatment options may be needed if ED becomes a chronic issue. (ED is discussed later in this chapter).

The bladder may take up to 2 months to return to its normal capacity. Teach the patient to drink at least 2 to 3 L of fluid per day and urinate every 2 to 3 hours to flush the urinary tract. Teach the patient to avoid or limit the amounts of bladder irritants, such as caffeine products, citrus juices, and alcohol. Because the patient may have incontinence or dribbling, he may incorrectly believe that decreasing fluid intake will relieve this problem.

Urethral strictures may result from instrumentation or catheterization. Treatment may include teaching the patient intermittent clean self-catheterization or having a urethral dilation.

Tell the patient to discuss the need for a yearly DRE with his HCP if he has had any procedure other than complete removal of the prostate. Hyperplasia or cancer can occur in the remaining prostatic tissue.

◆ **Evaluation**

The expected outcomes are that the patient with BPH who has surgery will
- Report acceptable pain control
- Report improved urinary function with no pain or incontinence

PROSTATE CANCER

Prostate cancer is a tumor of the prostate gland. Prostate cancer is the most common cancer among men, excluding skin cancer. It is the second leading cause of cancer death in men, exceeded only by lung cancer. The American Cancer Society estimates that in 2018 there will be 164,690 men diagnosed with prostate cancer, and 29,430 men will die from prostate cancer. A man has a 1 in 9 risk for developing prostate cancer in his lifetime. More than 2.9 million men in the United States are survivors of prostate cancer.[9]

Etiology and Pathophysiology

Prostate cancer is a slow-growing, androgen-dependent cancer. It can spread by 3 routes: by direct extension, through the lymph system, or through the bloodstream. Spread by direct extension involves the seminal vesicles, urethral mucosa, bladder wall, and external sphincter. The cancer later spreads through the lymphatic system to the regional lymph nodes. The bloodstream is the mode of spread to the axial skeleton (e.g., pelvic bones, head of the femur, lower lumbar spine), liver, and lungs.

Age, ethnicity, and family history are known risk factors for prostate cancer. The incidence of prostate cancer rises markedly after age 50. The median age at diagnosis is 66 years old. However, many cases occur in younger men, who sometimes have a more aggressive type of cancer.

Dietary factors and obesity may be related to prostate cancer. A diet high in red and processed meat and high-fat dairy products along with a low intake of vegetables and fruits may increase the risk for prostate cancer. Environment may play a role. There is an increased prevalence of prostate cancer in farmers and commercial pesticide applicators, possibly due to chemicals found in pesticides. It is not clear if smoking is a risk factor for prostate cancer.

🧬 Genetic Link

Currently no known single gene causes prostate cancer. Some genes or gene mutations are more common in men with prostate cancer. From a genetics viewpoint, prostate cancer can be classified into 3 categories.

Most prostate cancers (about 75%) are considered *sporadic,* which means that damage to the genes occurs by chance after a person is born. Prostate cancer that runs in a family, called *familial prostate cancer,* is less common (about 20%). It occurs because of a combination of genes and environment or lifestyle factors. Familial prostate cancer is when 2 or more first-degree relatives (father, brother, son) are diagnosed with prostate cancer.

Hereditary (inherited) prostate cancer is rare (5% to 10%) and occurs when gene mutations are passed down in a family from 1 generation to the next. In hereditary prostate cancer, a family has any of the following characteristics: (1) 3 or more first-degree relatives with prostate cancer, (2) prostate cancer in 3 generations on the same side of the family, and (3) 2 or more close relatives (father, brother, son, grandfather, uncle, nephew) on the same side of the family diagnosed with prostate cancer before age 55.

Having a family history does not mean that a man will develop prostate cancer. It means that he has an increased risk. Men with a family history of prostate cancer should talk with their HCP about their concerns. It is important for the HCP to obtain a detailed family history. Depending on the findings, a referral to a genetic counselor may be appropriate.

Hereditary breast and ovarian cancer (HBOC) syndrome is associated with mutations in the *BRCA1* and/or *BRCA2* genes (BRCA stands for *BR*east *CA*ncer). Women with HBOC have an increased risk for breast and ovarian cancer. Men with HBOC have an increased risk for breast cancer and prostate cancer. Mutations in *BRCA1* and *BRCA2* cause only a small number of familial prostate cancers. Genetic testing may be appropriate for families with prostate cancer that have HBOC.

Clinical Manifestations and Complications

Prostate cancer typically has no symptoms in the early stages. Eventually, the patient may have LUTS similar to those of BPH. Pain in the lumbosacral area that radiates down to the hips or the legs, when combined with urinary symptoms, may indicate metastasis.

The tumor can spread to pelvic lymph nodes, bones, bladder, lungs, and liver. Once the tumor has spread to distant sites, the major problem becomes pain management. As the cancer

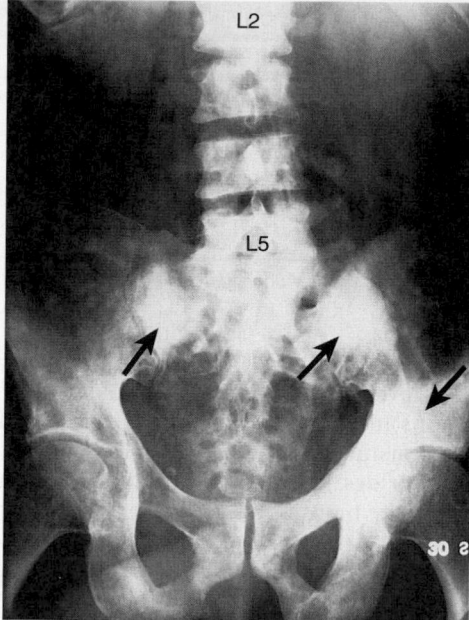

FIG. 54.5 Metastasis of prostate cancer to the pelvis and lumbar spine, indicated by *arrows.* (From Mettler F: *Essentials of radiology,* ed 2, Philadelphia, 2004, Saunders.)

spreads to the bones (common site of metastasis), pain can become severe, especially in the back and legs because of spinal cord compression and bone destruction (Fig. 54.5).

Diagnostic Studies

Most men in the United States with prostate cancer are diagnosed by PSA screening. As prostate cancer screening has become more widespread, smaller cancers are being found in older men. In most cases, slow-growing cancers probably do not need to be treated. Many men live and die *with* prostate cancer, but most will not die *from* it.

Men have a chance to make an informed decision with their HCP about whether to be screened for prostate cancer. Men should be told about the potential risks (e.g., subsequent evaluation and treatment that may not be needed) and benefits (early detection of prostate cancer) of PSA screening before being tested. After this discussion, men who want to be screened may have an annual PSA test and DRE. On DRE, an abnormal prostate may feel hard, nodular, and asymmetric.

The AUA thinks that men age 55 to 69 have the greatest potential benefit from PSA screening and recommend screening every 2 years.[8] Men at higher risk (black men, men with a first-degree relative with prostate cancer) will have an individualized screening schedule.

The American Cancer Society recommends that men should have a discussion with their HCP about screening for prostate cancer. Men should not be screened unless they have received this information. The discussion about screening should take place at:
- Age 50 for men who are at average risk for prostate cancer and are expected to live at least 10 more years.
- Age 45 for men at high risk for developing prostate cancer. This includes blacks and men who have a first-degree relative (father, brother, or son) diagnosed with prostate cancer at an early age (younger than age 65).
- Age 40 for men at even higher risk (those with more than 1 first-degree relative who had prostate cancer at an early age).

TABLE 54.5	**Staging of Prostate Cancer**				
Stage	**Tumor Size**	**Lymph Node Involvement**	**Metastasis**	**PSA Level**	**Gleason Score**
I	Not felt on DRE. Not seen by visual imaging.	No	No	<10	≤6
II	Felt on DRE. Seen by imaging. Tumor confined to prostate.	No	No	10–20	6–7
III	Cancer outside prostate. Possible spread to seminal vesicles.	No	No	Any level	Any score
IV	Any size.	Any nodal involvement.	Yes	Any level	Any score

Adapted from American Cancer Society: How is prostate cancer staged? Retrieved from *www.cancer.org/Cancer/ProstateCancer/DetailedGuide/prostate-cancer-staging*.

High PSA levels do not always indicate prostate cancer. Mild elevations in PSA may occur with aging, BPH, recent ejaculation, constipation, acute or chronic prostatitis, or after long bike rides. Cystoscopy, indwelling urethral catheters, and prostate biopsies may cause transient increases in PSA levels.

Neither PSA nor DRE is a definitive diagnostic test for prostate cancer. If PSA levels are continually high or if the DRE is abnormal, a biopsy of the prostate tissue is usually done. Biopsy of prostate tissue is necessary to confirm the diagnosis of prostate cancer. The biopsy is typically done using a transrectal approach. In a transrectal ultrasound (TRUS) procedure, an ultrasound probe allows the HCP to see abnormalities in the prostate. When a suspicious area is found, biopsy needles are inserted through the wall of the rectum into the prostate to obtain tissue samples. A pathologic examination of the specimen is done to assess for malignant changes. For patients at a high risk for infection with a transrectal biopsy, or with a history of prior postbiopsy sepsis, a transperineal approach is another option if it is available at the agency. There can be a lower risk for infection with the transperineal approach as the biopsy needles do not pierce the rectal wall. It is typically done in the operating room.

Another approach for biopsies is to use an MRI/ultrasound fusion biopsy. In this approach, pelvic MRI 3-dimensional images are fused with real-time, transrectal ultrasound images. This new technique is more accurate than the traditional approach. Typically, men who are candidates for this procedure have a history of a previous negative ultrasound-guided biopsy and increasing PSA. This approach may also be used for men who are on active surveillance. However, as discussed earlier in this chapter, recent studies show risk assessment with MRI prior to biopsy and MRI-targeted biopsy to be superior to standard TRUS biopsy in men at risk for prostate cancer who have never had a prostate biopsy before.[5]

PSA is used to monitor the success of treatment. When treatment has been successful, with either prostatectomy or hormone therapy, PSA levels should fall to undetectable levels. With successful radiation therapy, the PSA level should decrease to a very low number (the nadir) and remain stable near that number. The regular measurement of PSA levels after treatment is important to evaluate the effectiveness of treatment and possible recurrence of prostate cancer.[10]

With advanced prostate cancer, serum alkaline phosphatase can be increased because of bone metastases. Other tests used to determine the location and extent of the spread of the cancer may include a nuclear medicine whole body bone scan, a CT scan of the abdomen and pelvis, and an MRI of the pelvis with special attention to the prostate.

Interprofessional Care

Chemoprevention of prostate cancer is an active area of research. As discussed earlier in this chapter, finasteride and dutasteride, used to treat BPH, may reduce the chance for getting prostate cancer. Men who are concerned about prostate cancer should discuss with their HCP the potential risks and benefits of taking finasteride or dutasteride.

Early recognition and treatment are important to control tumor growth, prevent metastasis, and preserve quality of life. Most patients (93%) with prostate cancer are diagnosed when the cancer is at a local or regional stage.[9,11] The 5-year survival rate with a diagnosis at this stage is almost 100%.

The most common classification system for determining the extent of prostate cancer is the tumor, node, and metastasis (TNM) system (Table 54.5). The tumor is graded based on tumor histology using 2 different grading systems: the Gleason scale and the Grade Group.[12] The Gleason scale grades the tumor from 1 to 5 based on the degree of glandular differentiation. Grade 1 represents the most well-differentiated or lowest grade (most like the original cells), and grade 5 represents the most poorly differentiated (unlike the original cells) or highest grade. The 2 most commonly occurring patterns of cells are graded, and the 2 scores are added together to create a Gleason score. Gleason score ranges from 6 to 10. Currently the lowest risk Gleason score is Gleason 6 (3+3).

The Grade Group system grades the cells based on their differentiation. The Grade Group assigns the tumor a number on a scale from 1 to 5. Grade Group 1 is the lowest risk and Grade Group 5 the highest risk. Currently, the Gleason score and the Grade Group system are used together. A low-risk, well-differentiated prostate cancer specimen may be graded a Grade Group 1, Gleason 6 (3+3) prostate cancer. The trend is moving toward Grade Group scoring only.

The PSA level at diagnosis and the patient's Gleason score and Grade Group are used with the TNM system to determine the stage of the tumor, which is vital to determine treatment options.

The interprofessional care of the patient with prostate cancer depends on the stage of the cancer and the patient's overall health (Table 54.6). None of these diagnostic options can predict the progression of prostate cancer. At all stages, there is more than one treatment option depending on the stage, Gleason score, and PSA. The decision of which treatment course to pursue should be made jointly by patients, their partners, and the interprofessional care team.[10,11]

Active Surveillance. Low-grade prostate cancer is relatively slow growing. Therefore a conservative approach to management of prostate cancer is active surveillance, or "watchful waiting." This strategy is appropriate when the patient has (1)

TABLE 54.6 Interprofessional Care

Prostate Cancer

Diagnostic Assessment
- History and physical examination
- Digital rectal examination (DRE)
- Prostate-specific antigen (PSA)
- Transrectal ultrasound (TRUS) or pelvic MRI
- Prostate biopsy
- CT abdomen and pelvis with contrast (to assess for metastatic disease)

Management

Active Surveillance
- Closely monitor PSA and DRE (annually, at minimum)
- Repeat/surveillance prostate biopsies
- Repeat imaging
- Consider genomic testing on biopsy tissue, if appropriate

Surgery
- Radical prostatectomy
- Cryotherapy
- Orchiectomy (for metastatic disease)

Radiation Therapy
- External beam for primary, adjuvant, and recurrent disease
- Brachytherapy

Drug Therapy
- Androgen deprivation therapy (Table 54.7)
- Chemotherapy for metastatic disease

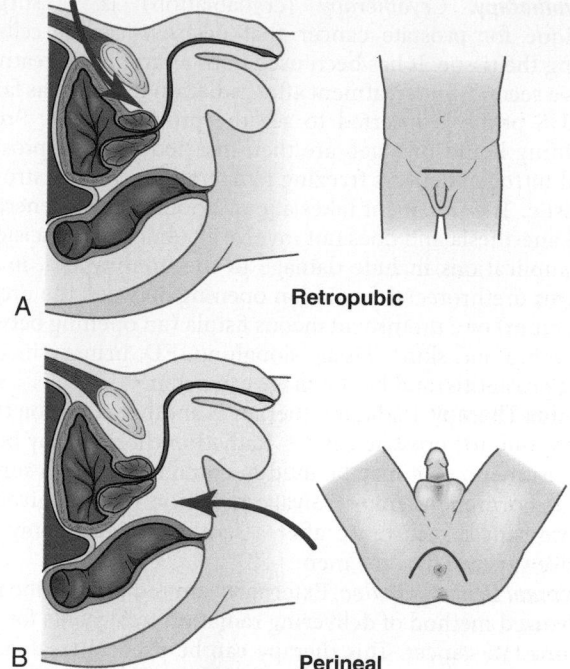

FIG. 54.6 Common approaches used to perform a prostatectomy. A, Retropubic approach involves a midline abdominal incision. B, Perineal approach involves an incision between the scrotum and the anus.

a life expectancy of less than 10 years (low risk for dying of the disease); (2) a low-grade, low-stage tumor; and (3) serious coexisting medical conditions. With active surveillance, patients are typically followed with frequent PSA measurements and DRE to monitor the progress of the disease. Significant changes in the PSA level, the DRE, or the development of symptoms, warrant a reevaluation of treatment options.

Surgical Therapy

Radical Prostatectomy. With radical prostatectomy, the entire prostate gland, seminal vesicles, and part of the bladder neck (ampulla) are removed. The entire prostate is removed because the cancer tends to be in many different places within the gland. A pelvic lymph node dissection is typically done at the same time as prostatectomy to pathologically assess for nodal metastases in the local pelvic area. Typically, a higher number of lymph nodes are removed and dissected if the prostate cancer is higher grade/higher risk on biopsy. Surgery is usually not an option for advanced-stage disease except to relieve symptoms associated with obstruction.

Traditional surgical approaches for an open radical prostatectomy include retropubic and perineal approaches (Fig. 54.6). With the *retropubic* approach, a low midline abdominal incision is made to access the prostate gland and the pelvic lymph nodes can be dissected. With the *perineal* resection, an incision is made between the scrotum and anus.

A *robotic-assisted* (e.g., da Vinci system) prostatectomy is a type of surgery in which the HCP sits at a computer console while controlling high-resolution cameras and microsurgical instruments. Robotics is being used more often since it allows for increased precision, visualization, and dexterity by the HCP when removing the prostate gland. It results in less bleeding, less pain, and a faster recovery compared with other approaches.[13]

After surgery, the patient has a large indwelling catheter with a 20-mL or 30-mL balloon placed in the bladder via the urethra. A drain is left in the surgical site to aid in removing drainage from the area. This drain is typically removed after a few days. Because the perineal approach has a higher risk for infection (because of the location of the incision related to the anus), careful dressing changes and perineal care after each bowel movement are important for comfort and to prevent infection. Depending on the type of surgery, the length of hospital stay ranges from 1 to 3 days.

Two major adverse outcomes after a radical prostatectomy are ED and urinary incontinence. The incidence of ED depends on the patient's age, preoperative sexual function, whether nerve-sparing surgery was done, and the HCP's expertise. Sexual function after surgery tends to return gradually over at least 24 months or more. Phosphodiesterase type 5 (PDE5) inhibitor medications may help improve sexual function.

Problems with urinary control may occur for the first few months after surgery because the bladder must be reattached to the urethra after the prostate is removed. Over time, the bladder adjusts, and most men regain urinary continence. Kegel exercises strengthen the pelvic floor muscles and the urinary sphincter and may help improve continence. (Kegel exercises are discussed in Table 45.18.) Other complications associated with surgery include hemorrhage, seroma, lymphocele, urinary retention, infection, wound dehiscence, and VTE.[14]

Nerve-Sparing Procedure. Near the prostate gland are neurovascular bundles that maintain erectile functioning. The preservation of these bundles during a prostatectomy is possible while still removing all the cancer. Nerve-sparing prostatectomy is not indicated for patients with cancer outside of the prostate gland. Although the risk for ED is reduced with this procedure, there is no guarantee that potency will be maintained.

Cryotherapy. *Cryotherapy* (cryoablation) is a surgical technique for prostate cancer that destroys cancer cells by freezing the tissue. It has been used both as an initial treatment and as a second-line treatment after radiation therapy has failed. A TRUS probe is inserted to see the prostate gland. Probes containing liquid nitrogen are then inserted into the prostate. Liquid nitrogen delivers freezing temperatures, thus destroying the tissue. The treatment takes about 2 hours under general or spinal anesthesia and does not involve an abdominal incision.

Complications include damage to the urethra and, in rare cases, an urethrorectal fistula (an opening between the urethra and rectum) or a urethrocutaneous fistula (an opening between the urethra and skin). Tissue sloughing, ED, urinary incontinence, prostatitis, and hemorrhage can occur.

Radiation Therapy. Radiation therapy is another common treatment option for prostate cancer. Radiation therapy may be the only treatment, or it may be used in combination with surgery or with hormone therapy. Salvage radiation therapy given for prostate cancer recurrence after a radical prostatectomy may improve survival in some men.

External Beam Radiation. External beam radiation is the most widely used method of delivering radiation treatments for men with prostate cancer. This therapy can be used to treat cancer confined to the prostate and/or surrounding tissue. Patients are usually treated on an outpatient basis 5 days a week for 4 to 8 weeks. Each treatment lasts less than 1 hour.

Side effects from radiation can be acute (occurring during treatment or within 90 days that follow) or delayed (occurring months or years after treatment). The most common side effects involve changes to the skin (dryness, redness, irritation, pain), gastrointestinal tract (diarrhea, abdominal cramping, bleeding, radiation proctitis), urinary tract (dysuria, hematuria, frequency, hesitancy, urgency, nocturia, radiation cystitis), and sexual function.[15] Fatigue may occur. There is a rare risk for secondary cancers after radiation to the pelvic area (e.g., bladder cancer, rectal cancer). In patients with localized prostate cancer, cure rates with external beam radiation are comparable to those with radical prostatectomy.

Brachytherapy. *Brachytherapy* involves placing radioactive seed implants into the prostate gland. This delivers high doses of radiation directly to the tissue while sparing the surrounding tissue (rectum and bladder). The radioactive seeds are placed in the prostate gland with a needle through a grid template guided by TRUS (Fig. 54.7) to ensure accurate placement of the seeds.

Because brachytherapy is a one-time outpatient procedure, many patients find this more convenient than external beam radiation treatment. Brachytherapy is best suited for patients with early-stage disease. The most common side effect is the development of urinary irritative or obstructive problems. Some men may have ED. The AUA Symptom Index (Table 54.1) can be used to measure urinary function for patients undergoing brachytherapy and can be incorporated into nursing management. For those with more advanced tumors, brachytherapy may be offered in combination with external beam radiation treatment.[16] (Brachytherapy is discussed in Chapter 15.)

Drug Therapy. The forms of drug therapy available for the treatment of advanced or metastatic prostate cancer are androgen deprivation (hormone) therapy, chemotherapy, or a combination of both.

Androgen Deprivation Therapy. Prostate cancer growth is largely dependent on the presence of androgens. *Androgen deprivation therapy* (ADT) reduces the levels of circulating androgens to reduce the tumor growth.[17] Androgen deprivation

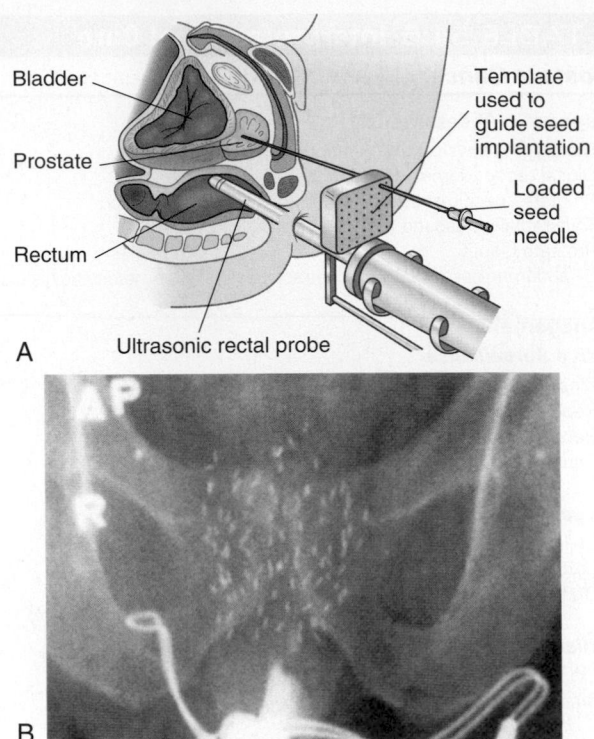

FIG. 54.7 A, Prostate brachytherapy. Implantation of radioactive seeds with a needle guided by ultrasound and a template grid. **B,** Radioactive seeds. (*B*, From Abeloff MD, Armitage JO, Niederhuber JE, et al, eds: *Abeloff's clinical oncology,* ed 4, 2008, Churchill Livingstone.)

can be produced by inhibiting androgen production or blocking androgen receptors (Table 54.7).

One of the biggest challenges with ADT is that almost all tumors treated become resistant to this therapy (*hormone refractory*) within a few years. A high PSA level is often the first sign that this therapy is no longer effective. Patients taking ADT have an increased risk for cardiovascular side effects, including high serum cholesterol and triglyceride levels and coronary artery disease.

Osteoporosis and fractures may occur in those receiving ADT. Drugs recommended to reduce bone mineral loss include zoledronic acid (Reclast) and raloxifene (Evista). Zoledronic acid is a bisphosphonate therapy given IV. A rare complication of therapy is osteonecrosis of the jaw. Denosumab (Prolia, Xgeva), a drug that slows the breakdown of bone, may be used to increase bone mass in men with nonmetastatic prostate cancer.

Androgen synthesis inhibitors. The hypothalamus produces luteinizing hormone–releasing hormone (LHRH), which stimulates the anterior pituitary to produce luteinizing hormone (LH) and follicle-stimulating hormone (FSH). LH stimulates the testicular Leydig cells to make testosterone. *LHRH agonists* super stimulate the pituitary, downregulating the LHRH receptors and leading to a refractory condition in which the anterior pituitary is unresponsive to LHRH. These drugs cause an initial, transient increase in LH and FSH; testosterone abruptly rises resulting in a *flare.* Symptoms may worsen during this time. However, with continued administration, LH and testosterone levels decrease.

LHRH agonists include goserelin (Zoladex), leuprolide (Lupron Depot, Eligard), and triptorelin (Trelstar) (Table 54.7). These drugs essentially produce a chemical castration similar to the effects of an orchiectomy. They are given by subcutaneous or IM injections on a regular basis. Viadur is an implant that is placed subcutaneously and delivers leuprolide continuously for 1 year.

TABLE 54.7 Drug Therapy

Androgen Deprivation Therapy for Prostate Cancer

Therapy	Mechanism of Action	Side Effects
Androgen Receptor Blockers bicalutamide (Casodex) enzalutamide (Xtandi) flutamide nilutamide (Nilandron)	• Block action of testosterone by competing with receptor sites	• Loss of libido, erectile dysfunction, and hot flashes • Breast pain and gynecomastia
Androgen Synthesis Inhibitors ***CYP17 Enzyme Inhibitor*** abiraterone (Zytiga)	• Inhibits CYP17, an enzyme needed to produce testosterone • Inhibits testosterone synthesis from testes, adrenal glands, and prostate cancer cells	• Joint swelling, fluid retention • Muscle discomfort • Hot flashes • Diarrhea
LHRH Agonists goserelin (Zoladex) leuprolide (Eligard , Lupron Depot) triptorelin (Trelstar)	• ↓ Secretion of LH and FSH • ↓ Testosterone production	• Hot flashes, gynecomastia, ↓ libido, erectile dysfunction • Depression and mood changes
LHRH Antagonist degarelix (Firmagon)	• Blocks LH receptors • Immediate testosterone suppression	• Pain, redness, and swelling at injection site • High liver enzymes

Degarelix (Firmagon) is an *LHRH antagonist* that lowers testosterone levels to castration levels. Unlike the LHRH agonists, degarelix does not cause a testosterone flare because it acts directly to block LH and FSH receptors. It is given as a subcutaneous injection. Results are seen in 3 days.

Abiraterone (Zytiga) works by inhibiting an enzyme, CYP17, which is needed to produce testosterone. This drug is given orally to men with castration-resistant prostate cancer, usually in combination with prednisone. It improves overall survival by 4 to 5 months.

Androgen receptor blockers. Androgen receptor blockers are another classification of antiandrogen drugs that compete with circulating androgens at the receptor sites. Flutamide, nilutamide (Nilandron), bicalutamide, and enzalutamide (Xtandi) are androgen receptor blockers. They are taken daily as an oral medication and can be used in combination with an LHRH agonist (e.g., goserelin, leuprolide). Combining an androgen receptor blocker with an LHRH agonist results in combined androgen blockade.

Chemotherapy. The use of chemotherapy is limited to treatment for those with hormone-refractory prostate cancer (HRPC) in late-stage disease. In HRPC the cancer is progressing despite treatment. This occurs in patients who have taken an antiandrogen for a certain period. The goal of chemotherapy is mainly palliative.

Some commonly used chemotherapy drugs for prostate cancer include cabazitaxel (Jevtana), cyclophosphamide, docetaxel (Taxotere), estramustine (Emcyt), mitoxantrone, paclitaxel (Abraxane), and vinblastine.

Men with advanced prostate cancer who have HRPC may receive a vaccine (sipuleucel-T [Provenge]). We do not know exactly how, but the vaccine stimulates the patient's system against the cancer. Use prolongs survival by about 4 months but does not reduce tumor burden. It is individually prepared for each man by a process that combines his own WBCs with granulocyte-macrophage colony-stimulating factor (GM-CSF), which then attacks the prostate tumor cells.

Radiotherapy. Radium-223 dichloride (Xofigo) can be used in the treatment of patients with castration-resistant prostate cancer, symptomatic bone metastases, and no known visceral metastatic disease. It is an alpha particle–emitting radiotherapy drug that mimics calcium and forms complexes with hydroxyapatite at areas of increased bone turnover, such as bone metastases.

Orchiectomy. A bilateral orchiectomy is the surgical removal of the testes. It may be done alone or after prostatectomy. It is the gold standard for androgen deprivation. There are no side effects to be managed. It is very low cost when compared with other options. For advanced stages of prostate cancer, an orchiectomy is an option for cancer control, with rapid relief of bone pain associated with advanced tumors.

Orchiectomy may shrink the prostate, thus relieving urinary obstruction in the later stages of disease when surgery is not an option. After an orchiectomy, weight gain and loss of muscle mass can change a man's physical appearance. These physical changes can affect self-esteem, leading to grief and depression. Because this procedure is permanent, many men prefer drug therapy over an orchiectomy.

 ## Culturally Competent Care: Prostate Cancer

Nurses need to be aware of ethnic and cultural considerations when providing information about the risk for prostate cancer and screening recommendations. Consider not only the ethnic differences in the incidence of prostate cancer but also differences in health promotion practices.

Black men have the highest mortality rates from prostate cancer, in part because their prostate cancer often is more advanced at the time of diagnosis. Despite the availability of screening measures (PSA and DRE), black men and those in lower socioeconomic groups may not access these services. This is only partially related to knowledge levels about prostate cancer. In comparison to white men, black men with prostate cancer report more problems with financial access to transportation and health care costs. They describe using more religious coping strategies. White men are perceived as receiving more favorable treatment from their HCPs than black men.[18]

Although exposure to electronic and print media is successful in informing some men about prostate cancer, the effectiveness differs significantly based on demographic variables, such as ethnicity, age, education level, and socioeconomic level. Ideally, all men should be aware of the risks associated with prostate cancer and the screening methods available. Consider the best method to communicate this information to men of all cultures and ethnicities to promote understanding and participation in prostate cancer screening for men in at-risk groups.

❖ NURSING MANAGEMENT: PROSTATE CANCER

◆ Nursing Assessment

Subjective and objective data that should be obtained from a patient with prostate cancer are outlined in Table 54.8.

◆ Nursing Diagnoses

Nursing diagnoses for the patient with prostate cancer depend on the stage of the cancer. General ones may include:

- Lack of knowledge
- Acute pain
- Urinary retention and impaired urinary system function
- Impaired sexual functioning
- Anxiety

◆ Planning

The overall goals are that the patient with prostate cancer will (1) be an active participant in the treatment plan, (2) have acceptable pain control, (3) follow the therapeutic plan, (4) understand the effect of the therapeutic plan on sexual function, and (5) find an acceptable way to manage the impact on bladder and bowel function.

◆ Nursing Implementation

◆ **Health Promotion.** One of the most important roles in relation to prostate cancer is to encourage patients, in consultation with their HCPs, to have annual prostate screening (PSA and DRE). The age at which to begin screening was discussed earlier on p. 1263. Because of their increased risk for prostate cancer, black men and other men at high risk, such as those with a family history of prostate cancer, should discuss the need for annual PSA and DRE beginning at age 45.[9]

◆ **Acute Care.** Care of the patient having a radical prostatectomy is similar to surgical procedures for BPH. Nursing interventions for the patient who has radiation therapy and chemotherapy are discussed in Chapter 15. Another consideration is the patient's psychologic response to a diagnosis of cancer. Provide sensitive, caring support for the patient and his family to help them cope with the diagnosis. Prostate cancer support groups are available for men and their families to encourage them to be active, informed participants in their own care.

◆ **Ambulatory Care.** Teach catheter care if the patient is discharged with an indwelling catheter in place. Teach the patient to clean the urethral meatus with soap and water once a day; maintain a high fluid intake; keep the collecting bag lower than the bladder at all times; and keep the catheter securely anchored to the inner thigh or abdomen. Tell them to report any signs of bladder infection, such as bladder spasms, fever, or hematuria.

If urinary incontinence is a problem, encourage the patient to practice pelvic floor muscle exercises (Kegel exercises) at every urination and throughout the day. Continuous practice during the 4- to 6-week healing process improves the success

---

TABLE 54.8 Nursing Assessment
Prostate Cancer

Subjective Data
Important Health Information
Medications: Testosterone supplements. Use of any medications affecting urinary tract such as morphine, anticholinergics, monoamine oxidase inhibitors, and tricyclic antidepressants

Functional Health Patterns
Health perception–health management: Positive family history. ↑ Fatigue and malaise
Nutritional-metabolic: High-fat diet. Anorexia, weight loss (may indicate metastasis)
Elimination: Hesitancy or straining to start stream, urinary urgency, frequency, retention with dribbling, weak stream, hematuria
Sleep-rest: Nocturia
Cognitive-perceptual: Dysuria. Low back pain radiating to legs or pelvis, bone pain (may indicate metastasis). Pain level
Self-perception–self-concept: Anxiety about self-concept

Objective Data
General
Older adult male. Pelvic lymphadenopathy (late sign)

Urinary
Distended bladder on palpation. Unilaterally hard, enlarged, fixed prostate on rectal examination

Musculoskeletal
Pathologic fractures (metastasis)

Possible Diagnostic Findings
Serum PSA. Serum alkaline phosphatase. Nodular and irregular prostate on ultrasonography, positive biopsy results. Anemia

---

rate. Products used for incontinence specifically designed for men are available through home care product catalogs and retail stores. (Urinary incontinence is discussed in Chapter 45).

Palliative and end-of-life care are often appropriate and beneficial to the patient with advanced disease and his family (see Chapter 9). Common problems with advanced prostate cancer include fatigue, bladder outlet obstruction and ureteral obstruction (caused by compression of the urethra and/or ureters from tumor mass or lymph node metastasis), severe bone pain and fractures (from bone metastasis), spinal cord compression (from spinal metastasis), and leg edema (from lymphedema, VTE). Nursing interventions must focus on all these problems.

Pain management is one of the most important aspects of your care for these patients. Pain control involves ongoing pain assessment, giving prescribed medications (both opioid and nonopioid agents), and nonpharmacologic methods of pain relief (e.g., relaxation breathing). (Pain management is further discussed in Chapter 8).

◆ Evaluation

The outcomes are that the patient with prostate cancer will

- Be an active participant in the treatment plan
- Have acceptable pain control
- Follow the therapeutic plan
- Understand the effect of the treatment on sexual function
- Find an acceptable way to manage the impact on bladder or bowel function

PROSTATITIS

Etiology and Pathophysiology

Prostatitis is a broad term that describes a group of inflammatory and noninflammatory conditions affecting the prostate gland. Prostatitis is one of the most common urologic disorders. It is thought that 10% to 15% of all men in the United States will have prostatitis in their lifetime.[19] Almost 2 million men are treated for prostatitis every year.

The 4 categories of prostatitis syndromes are (1) acute bacterial prostatitis, (2) chronic bacterial prostatitis, (3) chronic prostatitis/chronic pelvic pain syndrome, and (4) asymptomatic inflammatory prostatitis. The most common type is nonbacterial.

Both acute and chronic bacterial prostatitis generally result from organisms reaching the prostate gland by ascending from the urethra, descending from the bladder, or invading via the bloodstream or the lymphatic channels. Common causative organisms are *Escherichia coli* (most common), *Klebsiella, Pseudomonas, Enterobacter, Proteus, Chlamydia trachomatis, Neisseria gonorrhoeae,* and group D streptococci.

Chronic bacterial prostatitis differs from acute prostatitis in that it involves recurrent episodes of infection. It is the most common reason for recurrent UTIs in adult men.

Chronic prostatitis/chronic pelvic pain syndrome describes a syndrome of prostate and urinary pain in the absence of an obvious infectious process. The cause of this syndrome is not known. It may occur after a viral illness, or it may be associated with sexually transmitted infections (STIs), especially in younger adults. A culture reveals no causative organisms, but leukocytes may be found in prostatic secretions.

Asymptomatic inflammatory prostatitis is usually diagnosed in those who have no symptoms but are found to have an inflammatory process in the prostate. These patients are usually diagnosed during the evaluation of other GU tract problems. Leukocytes are present in the seminal fluid from the prostate. The cause of this process is unclear.

Clinical Manifestations and Complications

Common manifestations of acute prostatitis include fever, chills, back pain, and perineal pain. In addition, acute urinary symptoms such as dysuria, urinary frequency, urgency, and cloudy urine may occur. The patient may progress to acute urinary retention caused by prostatic swelling if he remains untreated. With DRE, the prostate is extremely swollen, extremely tender, and boggy.

Complications of prostatitis are epididymitis and cystitis. Sexual function may be affected as manifested by postejaculation pain, libido problems, and ED. Prostatic abscess is a potential, but rare, complication.

In chronic bacterial prostatitis and chronic prostatitis/chronic pelvic pain syndrome, manifestations are similar but generally milder than those of acute bacterial prostatitis. These include irritative voiding symptoms (frequency, urgency, dysuria), backache, perineal and pelvic pain, and ejaculatory pain. Obstructive symptoms are rare unless there is coexisting BPH. With DRE, the prostate feels enlarged and soft or boggy and can be slightly tender with palpation. Chronic prostatitis can predispose the patient to recurrent UTIs.

The clinical features of prostatitis can mimic those of a UTI. However, it is important to remember that acute cystitis is not common in men.

Diagnostic Studies

Because patients with prostatitis have urinary symptoms, a urinalysis (UA) and urine culture and sensitivities are needed. Often WBCs and bacteria are present. The patient with a fever needs blood cultures and a complete blood count (CBC) to check the WBC count. The PSA test may be done to rule out prostate cancer. However, PSA levels are often increased with prostatic inflammation or infection. Thus, when inflammation or infection is present, the PSA may not be considered diagnostic.

Microscopic evaluation and culture of expressed prostate secretion can potentially be useful in the diagnosis of prostatitis. Expressed prostate secretion is obtained using a premassage and postmassage test. The patient is asked to void into a specimen cup just before and just after a vigorous prostate massage. Prostatic massage (for expressed prostate secretion) is becoming less common in clinical practice unless all other diagnostic options are exhausted. It should not be done if acute bacterial prostatitis is suspected, since compression is extremely painful and can increase the risk for bacterial spread. TRUS is not useful in the diagnosis of prostatitis. However, TRUS or MRI may be done to rule out an abscess in the prostate.

❖ Interprofessional and Nursing Care

Antibiotics commonly used for acute and chronic bacterial prostatitis include fluoroquinolones (e.g., ciprofloxacin [Cipro], levofloxacin, ofloxacin), clindamycin, cephalexin (Keflex), trimethoprim/sulfamethoxazole (Bactrim), doxycycline (Vibramycin), or tetracycline. Antibiotics are usually given orally for up to 4 weeks for acute bacterial prostatitis. However, if the patient has high fever or other signs of impending sepsis, he will be hospitalized and given IV antibiotics.

Men with chronic bacterial prostatitis may be given oral antibiotic therapy for 8 to 12 weeks. Antibiotics may be given for a lifetime if the patient is immunocompromised. A short course of oral antibiotics is usually prescribed for those with chronic prostatitis/chronic pelvic pain syndrome in case of bacterial infection. However, antibiotic therapy is often ineffective for patients whose prostatitis is not due to bacteria.

Patients with acute and chronic bacterial prostatitis tend to have a great amount of discomfort. The pain resolves as the infection is treated. However, they may have residual discomfort for several weeks after a course of antibiotics, as it takes time for the prostate to return to normal. Pain management for patients with chronic prostatitis/chronic pelvic pain syndrome is more difficult because the pain persists for weeks to months. No single approach provides relief for everyone. Antiinflammatory agents (e.g., ibuprofen, naproxen) may be used for pain control in prostatitis, but these drugs provide only moderate pain relief.

Warm sitz baths may help to relieve pain. Relaxation of muscle tissue in the prostate using α-adrenergic blockers (e.g., tamsulosin, alfuzosin) are effective in reducing discomfort for some men.

Acute urinary retention can develop in acute prostatitis, requiring insertion of a urinary catheter. However, passage of a catheter through an inflamed urethra is contraindicated in acute prostatitis. The placement of a suprapubic catheter may then be indicated. Repetitive prostatic massage may be recommended as adjunct therapy for prostatitis for men. This potentially relieves congestion within the prostate by squeezing out excess prostatic secretions, providing pain relief. Like massage, measures to stimulate ejaculation (masturbation and inter-course) may help to drain the prostate and provide some relief.

Because the prostate can serve as a source of bacteria, fluid intake should be kept at a high level. Encourage the patient to drink plenty of fluids. Men with acute bacterial prostatitis have increased fluid needs from fever and infection. Management of fever is an important nursing intervention.

PROBLEMS OF THE PENIS

Health problems of the penis are rare if STIs are excluded (see Chapter 52). Problems of the penis may be classified as congenital, problems of the prepuce, problems with the erectile mechanism, and cancer.

CONGENITAL PROBLEMS

Hypospadias is a urologic problem in which the urethral meatus is on the ventral surface of the penis. This can be anywhere from the corona to the perineum. Causes include hormonal influences in utero, environmental factors, and genetic factors. Surgical repair of hypospadias, especially those that are close to the scrotum or perineum, is usually done while the boy is young. Surgery may be done if it is associated with *chordee* (a painful downward curvature of the penis during erection) or if it prevents intercourse or normal urination. Surgery may be considered for cosmetic reasons or emotional well-being in older boys and adult men.

PROBLEMS OF PREPUCE

Problems of the prepuce (foreskin) are not as common in the United States as in most other countries because circumcision (surgical removal of the foreskin of the penis) is a routine procedure for many male infants. However, these conditions do occur and can be very painful and potentially an emergency. It is important to be familiar with these problems so appropriate treatment and pain relief can be promptly provided.

Phimosis is a tightness or constriction of the foreskin around the head of the penis, making retraction difficult (Fig. 54.8, *A*). It is caused by chronic inflammation of the foreskin. It is usually associated with poor hygiene techniques that allow bacterial and yeast organisms to become trapped under the foreskin. Topical corticosteroid cream, with or without an antifungal, applied 2 or 3 times daily to the exterior and interior of the tip of the foreskin may be effective in the initial treatment of inflammation. Definitive treatment is either circumcision or a dorsal slit surgical procedure.

Paraphimosis is tightness of the foreskin resulting in the inability to pull it forward from a retracted position, thus preventing normal return over the glans. It is a urologic emergency. A tightly retracted phimotic ring can compromise arterial flow to the glans. An ulcer can develop if the foreskin stays contracted (Fig. 54.8, *B*). Paraphimosis can occur when the foreskin is pulled back during bathing, use of urinary catheters, or intercourse and is not placed back in the forward position. Replacement of the foreskin after careful cleaning helps prevent this condition. The goal of treatment is to return the foreskin to its natural position over the glans penis through manual reduction. One strategy involves pushing the glans back through the prepuce by applying constant thumb pressure while the index fingers pull the prepuce over the glans. Ice and/or hand

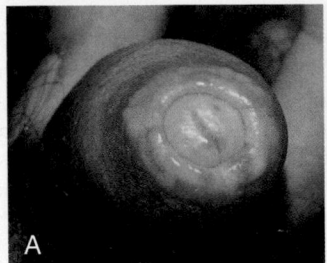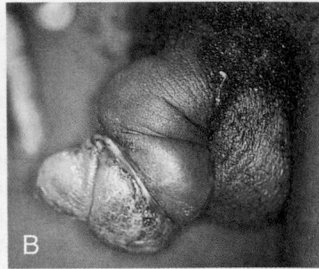

FIG. 54.8 A, Phimosis: inability to retract the foreskin due to secondary lesions on the prepuce (foreskin). **B,** Paraphimosis: ulcer with edema from foreskin remaining contracted over the prepuce (foreskin).

compression on the foreskin, glans, and penis may be applied before to reduce edema. Treatment may include antibiotics or warm soaks. Definitive treatment is either circumcision or a dorsal slit.

PROBLEMS OF ERECTILE MECHANISM

Priapism is a painful erection lasting longer than 4 hours. It is caused by complex vascular and neurologic factors that result in an obstruction of venous outflow in the penis. Conditions that may be associated with priapism include sickle cell disease, diabetes, trauma to the spinal cord, degenerative lesions of the spine, and drugs (e.g., cocaine, trazodone). Vasoactive drugs (e.g., alprostadil) injected into the corpora cavernosa for ED can cause priapism. Complications include penile tissue necrosis caused by lack of blood flow or hydronephrosis from bladder distention. Without immediate medical treatment, the risk for permanent ED is high.

Treatment varies depending on the cause. Patients with sickle cell disease may need a blood exchange transfusion. Other patients may be treated with sedatives, an injection of a smooth muscle relaxant directly into the penis, or aspiration and irrigation of the corpora cavernosa with a large-bore needle.

Peyronie's disease is caused by plaque formation in the corpora cavernosa of the penis that results in inelasticity during erection. The palpable, nontender, hard plaque formation may occur spontaneously or result from trauma to the penile shaft. The plaque prevents adequate blood flow into the spongy tissue, which results in a curvature during erection. The condition is not dangerous but can result in painful erections, ED, or embarrassment. Patients may improve slightly over time, stabilize, or need surgery. Collagenase clostridium histolyticum (Xiaflex) and intralesional verapamil (ILV) are medication options. Each is given as a series of injections into the plaque. The goal of therapy is to reduce the curvature and allow men to avoid surgery.

CANCER OF PENIS

Cancer of the penis is rare in the United States. More than 95% are squamous cell carcinoma. It occurs more often in men who have human papillomavirus (HPV) infection and phimosis or uncircumcised men.[20] The tumor may appear as a superficial ulceration or a pimple-like nodule. Pain is rare. This contributes to a delay in seeking treatment. The nontender warty lesion may be mistaken for a genital wart. Treatment in the early stages is laser removal of the growth. A radical resection of the penis may be done if the cancer has spread. Surgery, radiation, or chemotherapy are options, depending on the extent of the disease, lymph node involvement, or metastasis.

PROBLEMS OF SCROTUM AND TESTES

It is important for the patient to see his HCP if he feels any scrotal lumps or painful areas in his scrotum or testes. He would not be able to tell normal variations from cancer when performing self-examination. An incidental finding of a "scrotal lump" results in high anxiety for the patient.

INFLAMMATORY AND INFECTIOUS PROBLEMS

Skin Problems

The skin of the scrotum is susceptible to several common skin diseases. The most common are fungal infections, dermatitis (neurodermatitis, contact dermatitis, seborrheic dermatitis), and parasitic infections (scabies, lice). These conditions involve discomfort for the patient but are associated with few severe complications (see Chapter 23).

Epididymitis

Epididymitis is an acute, painful inflammatory process of the epididymis (Fig. 54.9). It is often due to an infectious process, trauma, or urinary reflux down the ductus (vas) deferens. It is usually unilateral. Swelling may progress to the point that the epididymis and testis are indistinguishable. In men younger than 35 years of age, the most common cause is gonorrhea or chlamydial infection. In men over 35, the most common cause is *E. coli* infection. BPH and prostatitis are common contributors in older men.

The use of antibiotics is important for both partners if the transmission is through sexual contact. Encourage patients to refrain from sexual intercourse until treatment is complete. They should use a condom if they do engage in intercourse. Conservative treatment consists of elevating the scrotum, ice packs, and analgesics. Ambulation places the scrotum in a dependent position and increases pain. Acute tenderness subsides within 1 week, although some discomfort and swelling may last for weeks or months.

Orchitis

Orchitis refers to an acute inflammation of the testis. In orchitis, the testis is painful, tender, and swollen. It generally occurs after an episode of bacterial or viral infection, such as mumps, pneumonia, tuberculosis, or syphilis. It can be a side effect of epididymitis, trauma, infectious mononucleosis, influenza, catheterization, or complicated UTI. Mumps orchitis is a condition contributing to infertility that can be avoided by childhood vaccination against mumps. Treatment is similar to that for epididymitis.

CONGENITAL PROBLEMS

Cryptorchidism (undescended testes) is failure of the testes to descend into the scrotal sac before birth. It is the most common congenital testicular condition and is more common on the right. It may occur bilaterally or unilaterally and may be a contributing factor to male infertility if corrective surgery is not done by 2 years of age. The incidence of testicular cancer is higher if the condition is not corrected before puberty. Surgery is done to locate and suture the testis or testes to the scrotum.

ACQUIRED PROBLEMS

Hydrocele

A *hydrocele* is a nontender, fluid-filled mass that results from interference with lymphatic drainage of the scrotum and swelling

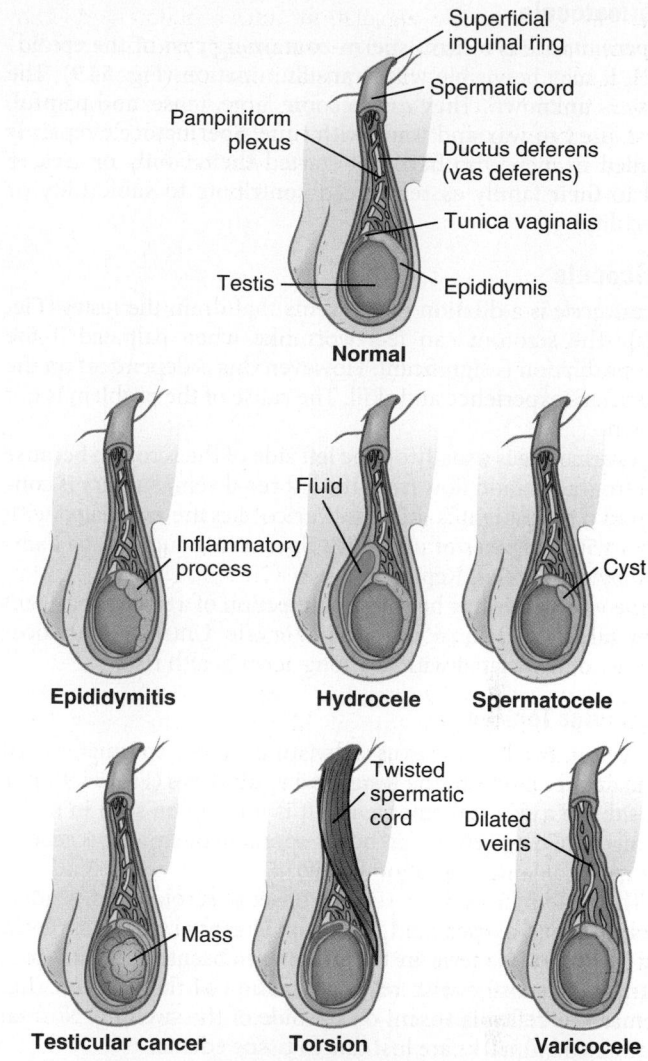

FIG. 54.9 Scrotal masses.

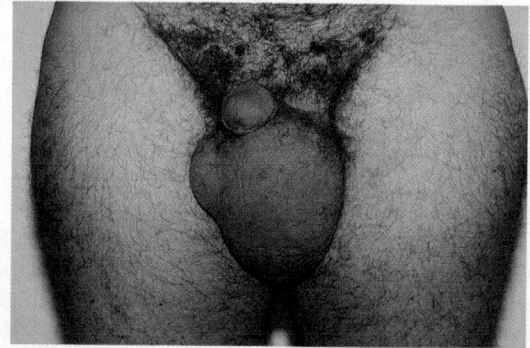

FIG. 54.10 Hydrocele. (From Swartz MH: *Textbook of physical diagnosis,* ed 6, Philadelphia, 2010, Saunders.)

of the tunica vaginalis that surrounds the testis (Fig. 54.10; also Fig. 54.9). Diagnosis is aided by shining a flashlight through the scrotum (transillumination). No treatment is needed unless the swelling becomes large and uncomfortable, then surgical repair of the hydrocele is needed. Hydrocele repair is avoided in men who have not started their family or seek to add to their family as repair can contribute to subfertility or infertility.

Spermatocele

A *spermatocele* is a firm, sperm-containing cyst of the epididymis. It may be visible with transillumination (Fig. 54.9). The cause is unknown. They can become large, tense, and painful. Their size can wax and wane with time. Spermatocele repair is avoided in men who have not started their family or seek to add to their family as repair can contribute to subfertility or infertility.

Varicocele

A *varicocele* is a dilation of the veins that drain the testes (Fig. 54.9). The scrotum can feel wormlike when palpated if the venous dilation is significant. However, this is dependent on the examiner's experience and skill. The cause of the problem is not known.

A varicocele is usually on the left side of the scrotum because of retrograde blood flow from the left renal vein. Surgery is considered if the patient is infertile. Varicoceles are associated with 40% to 50% of cases of infertility. Sperm is thought to be damaged by varicoceles. Repair of the varicocele may be through injection of a sclerosing agent or by surgical ligation of the spermatic vein. Untreated varicoceles are not associated with any long-term health risk.

Testicular Torsion

Testicular torsion involves a twisting of the spermatic cord that supplies blood to the testes and epididymis (Fig. 54.9). It is considered a surgical emergency. It is most often seen in males younger than age 20. It can occur spontaneously, or because of trauma or an anatomic abnormality.

The patient has severe, sudden onset of scrotal pain, tenderness, swelling, nausea, and vomiting. Urinary symptoms, fever, and WBCs or bacteria in the urine are absent. The pain does not usually subside with rest or elevation of the scrotum. The cremasteric reflex is absent on the side of the swelling. Normal anatomic landmarks are lost due to tissue edema.

A scrotal/testicular Doppler ultrasound is typically done to assess blood flow within the testicle. Decreased or absent blood flow confirms the diagnosis. Torsion is an emergency! If the blood supply to the affected testicle is not restored within 4 to 6 hours, ischemia to the testis will occur, leading to necrosis. Unless the torsion resolves spontaneously, surgery to untwist the cord and restore the blood supply must be done emergently.

TESTICULAR CANCER

Etiology and Pathophysiology

Testicular cancer is overall relatively rare. It accounts for less than 1% of all cancers found in males. However, it is the most common type of cancer in young men between 15 and 44 years of age. In the United States, about 8430 new cases occur annually. The median age at diagnosis is 33 years old.[21]

Testicular tumors are more common in males who have had undescended testes (cryptorchidism) or a family history of testicular cancer or anomalies. Other predisposing factors include orchitis, human immunodeficiency virus (HIV) infection, maternal exposure to exogenous estrogen, and testicular cancer in the other testis.

Most testicular cancers develop from 2 types of embryonic germ cells: seminomas and nonseminomas. Seminoma germ cell cancers are the most common but are the least aggressive. Nonseminoma testicular germ cell tumors are rare but very aggressive. Non–germ cell tumors arise from other testicular tissue. These include Leydig cell and Sertoli cell tumors. They account for less than 10% of testicular cancers.

Clinical Manifestations

Testicular cancer may have a slow or rapid onset depending on the type of tumor (Fig. 54.9). The patient may notice a painless lump in his scrotum, scrotal swelling, and a feeling of heaviness. The scrotal mass usually is nontender and firm. Some patients report a dull ache or heavy sensation in the lower abdomen, perianal area, or scrotum. Acute pain is the first symptom in about 10% of patients. Manifestations associated with advanced disease are varied and include lower back or chest pain, cough, and dyspnea.

Diagnostic Studies

Palpation of the scrotal contents is the first step in diagnosing testicular cancer. A cancerous mass is firm and does not transilluminate. Ultrasound of the testes is done if testicular cancer is suspected (e.g., palpable mass) or when persistent or painful testicular swelling is present. If testicular cancer is suspected, serum tumor markers should be checked to determine the serum levels of α-fetoprotein (AFP), lactate dehydrogenase (LDH), and human chorionic gonadotropin (hCG). (The tumor markers AFP and hCG are discussed in Chapter 15.)

If ultrasound is suspicious for testicular cancer, a radical inguinal orchiectomy should be done. A chest x-ray, CBC, basic metabolic panel, and liver function tests may be done before. Anemia may be present. Liver function levels may be increased in metastatic disease. If cancer is confirmed by pathology, then a CT scan of the abdomen and pelvis (and possibly the chest) can be done to further stage and assess for metastases.

❖ Interprofessional and Nursing Care

Testicular cancer is one of the most curable types of cancer. Interprofessional care generally involves a radical inguinal orchiectomy (surgical removal of the affected testis, spermatic cord, and regional lymph nodes). Some patients with early-stage disease do not need further treatment after an orchiectomy. Retroperitoneal lymph node dissection and removal also may be done in early-stage disease. These nodes are the primary route for metastasis.

Postorchiectomy treatment may involve radiation therapy, or chemotherapy, depending on the stage of the cancer. Radiation therapy is mainly used for patients with a seminoma, which is very sensitive to radiation. Radiation does not work well for nonseminomas.

Testicular germ cell tumors are more sensitive to systemic chemotherapy than any other adult solid tumor. Chemotherapy protocols use a combination of agents, including bleomycin, cisplatin, etoposide, and ifosfamide (Ifex). Retroperitoneal lymph node dissection may be done after chemotherapy as adjunct therapy in patients with advanced testicular cancer.

❓ CHECK YOUR PRACTICE

You are working on the urologic oncology unit caring for a 24-yr-old man who recently had an orchiectomy for testicular cancer. He appears quiet and nonengaged when you assess him. He says, "I'm never going to have a normal sex life."

- How would you respond? What kind of support or information would you provide?

The prognosis for patients with testicular cancer in recent years has greatly improved. 95% obtain complete remission if the disease is detected in the early stages. Because of treatment successes, many men with testicular cancer are long-term survivors.

However, some drugs used to treat testicular cancer can cause serious long-term side effects. These include pulmonary toxicity, kidney damage, nerve damage (which can cause numbness and tingling), and hearing loss (from nerve damage). Secondary cancers can occur due to chemotherapy (see Chapter 15).

All patients with testicular cancer require surveillance and regular physical examinations, chest x-rays, CT scans, and assessment of serum tumor markers (hCG, AFP, LDH). The goal is to detect relapse when the tumor burden is minimal.

Pretreatment subfertility or impaired fertility is identified at diagnosis. In treatment of testicular cancer, chemotherapy with cisplatin and/or pelvic radiation often damages the testicular germ cells. However, spermatogenesis can return in some patients. Because of the high risk for infertility, the cryopreservation of sperm in a sperm bank before treatment begins should be sensitively discussed and recommended for the man with testicular cancer.[22] Ejaculatory dysfunction may result from retroperitoneal lymph node dissection. These issues may be hard to discuss with the newly diagnosed patient. Men may think that the disease is a threat to their masculinity and self-worth.

SEXUAL FUNCTION

VASECTOMY

Vasectomy is the bilateral surgical ligation or resection of the ductus deferens performed for the purpose of sterilization (Fig. 54.11). The procedure takes only 15 to 30 minutes. It is usually done with the patient under local anesthesia on an outpatient basis. Although vasectomy is considered a permanent form of sterilization, successful vasectomy reversals (*vasovasotomy, vasoepididymostomy*) are common.

After vasectomy, the patient should not notice any difference in the look or feel of the ejaculate because its major components are seminal and prostatic fluid. The patient must use a different form of contraception until semen examination reveals no sperm. Sperm cells continue to be made by the testes but are stored in the epididymis and reabsorbed by the body rather than being passed through the ductus deferens. Vasectomy does not affect the hormone production, ability to ejaculate, or physiologic mechanisms related to erection or orgasm. Psychologic adjustment may be a problem after surgery. It may be hard for the patient to separate vasectomy from castration at a subconscious level. Some men may develop psychogenic ED or may feel the need to become more sexually active than they were in the past to prove their masculinity.

ERECTILE DYSFUNCTION

Erectile dysfunction (ED) is the inability to attain or maintain an erection that allows satisfactory sexual activity. Although sexual function is a topic that many persons are uncomfortable discussing, health care professionals must be able and willing to address ED.

ED is a condition that is significant because of its prevalence. More than 10 million men in the United States are thought to have ED. It can occur at any age, although the incidence

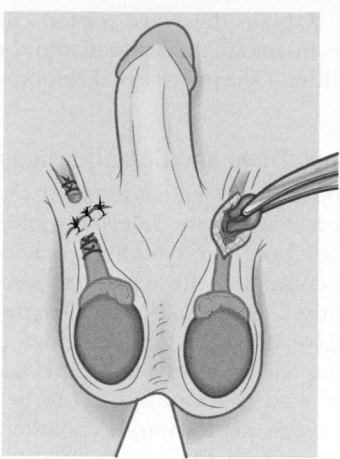

FIG. 54.11 Vasectomy procedure. The ductus deferens is ligated or resected for the purpose of sterilization.

TABLE 54.9 **Common Risk Factors for Erectile Dysfunction**	
Drug Induced	**Neurologic**
• Alcohol	• Cerebrovascular disease
• Antiandrogens	• Parkinson's disease
• Antihypertensives	• Trauma to the spinal cord
• Antilipidemic agents	• Tumors or transection of spinal cord
• Major tranquilizers (diazepam [Valium], alprazolam [Xanax])	
• Marijuana, cocaine	**Psychologic**
• Nicotine	• Anxiety
• Tricyclic antidepressants (e.g., amitriptyline [Elavil])	• Depression
	• Stress
Endocrine	**Vascular**
• Diabetes	• Atherosclerosis
• Hypogonadism	• Hypertension
• Obesity	• Peripheral vascular disease
Genitourinary	**Other**
• Radical prostatectomy	• Aging
• Renal failure	

increases with age. In fact, it is estimated that about 50% of all men between ages 40 and 70 have at least some degree of ED. ED is increasing in all sexually active males. In younger men, the increase is attributed to substance use (e.g., recreational drugs, alcohol), stress, and anxiety. Middle-aged men are more likely to have ED due to chronic medical conditions (e.g., diabetes, hypertension) or treatment for these conditions (e.g., antihypertensive drugs) that may cause ED.

Etiology and Pathophysiology

ED can be due to many factors (Table 54.9). Common causes include diabetes, vascular disease, side effects from medications, result of surgery (e.g., prostatectomy), trauma, chronic illness, stress, difficulty in a relationship, or depression. Since ED results from reduced blood flow to the penis, there is a potential association with cardiovascular disease because the risk factors for both disorders are the same.

Normal physiologic age-related changes are associated with changes in erectile function and may be an underlying cause of ED for some men. Table 50.3 lists age-related changes in sexual function. Explain these age-related changes (if necessary) to reassure an anxious older man about normal changes in his sexual abilities. (The male sexual response is discussed in Chapter 50.)

Clinical Manifestations and Complications

The typical symptom of ED is a patient's self-report of problems associated with erectile activity, describing an inability to attain or maintain an erection. The symptoms may occur only occasionally, may be continual with a gradual onset, or may occur with a sudden onset. A gradual onset of symptoms is usually associated with physiologic factors. A sudden or rapid onset of symptoms may be related to psychologic issues. It is common for younger men who seek care for ED to be diagnosed with diabetes, hypertension, depression, or cholesterol abnormalities during their evaluation for ED.[23]

A man's inability to perform sexually can cause great distress in his interpersonal relationships and may interfere with his concept of himself as a man. It can affect the relationship between the man and his partner. Problems with ED can lead to personal issues, including anger, anxiety, and depression.

Diagnostic Studies

The first step in the diagnosis and management of ED begins with a thorough sexual, health, and psychosocial history.[24] Self-administered assessment and treatment-related questionnaires may be useful as primary screening tools. For example, the International Index of Erectile Function (IIEF) identifies a man's response to 5 key areas of male sexual function: erectile function, orgasmic function, sexual desire, intercourse satisfaction, and overall satisfaction.

Second, a physical examination should focus on secondary sexual characteristics. Note if secondary sexual characteristics reflect the person's chronologic age (Tanner stage). A DRE should be done to assess prostate size, consistency, and presence of nodules. Assessment of BP with palpation and auscultation of the femoral arteries and peripheral pulses should be included.

Further examination or diagnostic testing is typically based on findings from the history and physical examination. A serum glucose, hemoglobin A1C (Hb A1C), and lipid profile are recommended to rule out diabetes. Hormonal levels for testosterone, prolactin, LH, and thyroid hormones may help identify endocrine-related problems. PSA level and a CBC may help to identify other diseases.

Other diagnostic tests may be done to diagnose ED. Nocturnal penile tumescence and rigidity testing is a noninvasive method that involves the continuous measurement of penile circumference and axial rigidity during sleep. These are used to distinguish between physiologic or psychogenic causes of ED. Vascular studies, including penile arteriography, penile blood flow study, and duplex Doppler ultrasound studies, are used to assess penile blood inflow and outflow. These tests help to identify vascular problems interfering with erection.

❖ Interprofessional and Nursing Care

The goal of ED therapy is for the patient and his partner to achieve a satisfactory sexual relationship. The treatment for ED can be based on the underlying cause. Generally, men are moved directly into treatment without a costly workup. A variety of treatment options are available (Table 54.10). Advise

TABLE 54.10 Interprofessional Care

Erectile Dysfunction

Diagnostic Assessment	Drug Therapy
• History and physical examination	• avanafil (Stendra)
• Sexual history	• sildenafil (Viagra)
• Serum glucose and lipid profile	• tadalafil (Cialis)
• Testosterone, prolactin, and thyroid hormone levels	• vardenafil (Levitra, Staxyn)
• Nocturnal penile tumescence and rigidity testing	**Devices and Implants**
• Vascular studies	• Intraurethral medication pellet
	• Intracavernosal self-injection
Management	• Penile implants
• Modify reversible causes	• Vacuum erection device (VED)
• Sexual counseling	

patients that no option will restore ejaculation or tactile sensations if they were absent before treatment.

It is important to determine if ED is reversible before treatment is started. For example, if ED appears to be a side effect of prescribed drugs, other treatments can be explored. With an established diagnosis of testicular failure (hypogonadism), androgen replacement therapy may be part of the prescribed treatment.

For men who have ED that is psychologic in nature, counseling for the patient (with or without his partner) is recommended. This counseling should be carried out by a qualified sex therapist.

The man with ED needs a great deal of emotional support for both himself and his partner. Men often do not feel comfortable discussing their problems because of their perceptions of society's expectations of a man's sexual abilities. Reassure the patient that confidentiality will be maintained. Many men delay seeking medical care and may expect immediate solutions to their problems. The interprofessional care team should provide a support system and accurate information.

Erectogenic Drugs. Avanafil (Stendra), sildenafil (Viagra), tadalafil (Cialis), and vardenafil (Levitra, Staxyn) are erectogenic drugs. These drugs are PDE5 inhibitors. They cause smooth muscle relaxation and increased blood flow into the corpus cavernosum, promoting penile erection. They are taken orally before sexual activity. These drugs have been found to be generally safe and effective for the treatment of most types of ED but are ineffective in the absence of arousal.

Side effects include headaches, leg/back pain, dyspepsia, flushing, and nasal congestion. Rare side effects are blurred or blue-green visual problems, sudden hearing loss, and an erection lasting more than 4 hours (priapism). Teach the patient to seek immediate medical attention if any of these reactions occur. Because these drugs may potentiate the hypotensive effect of nitrates, they are contraindicated for those taking nitrates (e.g., nitroglycerin).

Be aware that increasing numbers of men are seeking other ways to obtain ED medications. This include compounding pharmacies and online pharmacies. This may be due to both the cost of ED medications and the lack of insurance coverage for them.

 DRUG ALERT Phosphodiesterase Type 5 (PDE5) Inhibitors

• Should not be used with nitrates (nitroglycerin) in any form.
• Can potentiate hypotensive effects of nitrates.

Vacuum Erection Devices. Vacuum erection devices (VEDs) are suction devices that are applied to a flaccid penis then produce an erection by pulling blood up into the corporeal bodies. A penile ring or constrictive band is placed around the base of the penis to retain venous blood, preventing the erection from subsiding.

Intraurethral Devices and Intracavernosal Injections. Intraurethral devices include the use of vasoactive drugs applied as a topical gel or a medication pellet inserted into the urethra using a medicated urethral system for erection (MUSE) device. Intracavernosal self-injections may be performed, with medication injected directly into the corpus cavernosum.

Alprostadil (Caverject, Edex) is a vasoactive drug that enhances blood flow into the penile arteries. It can be given either by injection or as a transurethral pellet (suppository). When given as a suppository, the drug is placed into the opening at the tip of the penis. When injected, a needle and syringe is used to inject the drug directly into the corpus cavernosum. Trimix (a combination product) includes alprostadil, papaverine, and phentolamine.

Penile Implants. Implantation requires surgery but can sometimes be done in an outpatient setting. The devices are implanted into the corporeal bodies to provide an erection firm enough for penetration. The inflatable implant consists of cylinders in the penis, a small pump in the scrotum, and a reservoir in the lower abdomen. The main complications associated with penile prostheses are infection, erosions, and, rarely, mechanical failure.

Sexual Counseling. Sexual counseling can be recommended at any point during treatment for ED. It may be most valuable in cases with a component of psychogenic ED. Counseling should address psychologic or interpersonal factors that may enhance sexual expression, as well as other factors that are of concern. Counseling can be effective for the patient. It can include his partner, especially if he is involved in a long-term relationship.

HYPOGONADISM

Hypogonadism is a gradual decline in androgen secretion that occurs in most men as they age. The primary male androgen that is reduced is testosterone (Fig. 54.12). This has also been called *late onset-hypogonadism* or *hypogonadism of old age*. It can begin as early as age 40. It is unclear what causes a decline in testosterone. Obesity is a contributing factor.

Manifestations associated with low testosterone include decreased libido, fatigue, ED, depression and mood swings, and sleep problems. Since many of these manifestations can be associated with aging, some patients may not mention this to their HCP, or the HCP may not recognize these manifestations as signs of low testosterone. Long-term effects of low testosterone include loss of muscle mass and strength, which may contribute to an increased risk for falls and fractures.

Hypogonadism is diagnosed with a blood test and a physical examination. Normal serum testosterone levels can range from 300 to 1100 ng/dL, but often the normal ranges vary between laboratories. Replacement testosterone therapy is considered once total serum testosterone levels drop below 300 ng/dL on 2 separate early morning measurements/occasions, and the patient has manifestations of low testosterone.[25] Therapy may be started earlier depending on severity of symptoms. Testosterone replacement therapy (TRT) should not be started until the patient, in consultation with his HCP, considers the risks and benefits of therapy. Potential risks of TRT include lowered levels of high-density lipoprotein (HDL) cholesterol, increased hematocrit, and worsening sleep apnea, although these are rare. Since TRT may

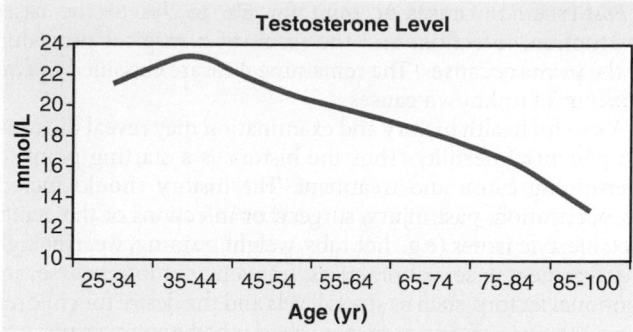

FIG. 54.12 Changes in testosterone plasma level in men as they age.

cause increased growth of prostate tissue, TRT is contraindicated in patients with unmanaged BPH or prostate cancer. Before treatment is started, a DRE and PSA test should be done. Once TRT begins, the HCP should closely monitor the patient.

Replacement therapy is available in different forms, including injection, transdermal, topical, buccal, or intranasal preparations. Oral TRT is not approved for use in the United States. IM injections, such as testosterone cypionate (Depo-Testosterone) and testosterone enanthate (Delatestryl), are available in varying doses. These drugs create a cyclic rise and fall in serum testosterone levels. The highest levels occur 2 to 3 days after the injection. Testosterone levels slowly decrease until the next injection. One side effect of this form of TRT is that men may report mood swings with the hormone fluctuations.

Transdermal preparations, including patches and gels (e.g., Androderm, Testim), are often prescribed. They are applied to the skin at product-specific sites, including the back, arm, and abdomen. Skin irritation is a common side effect. Testosterone may also be given as a buccal tablet (Striant) or intranasally (Natesto).

Emphasize to the patient the importance of hand washing with soap and water after applying testosterone preparations to the skin. Covering the area with clothing until the preparation has dried is recommended.

Women of childbearing age and children should avoid direct contact with testosterone products. Testosterone may cause early signs of puberty in young children and changes (virilization) in the external genitalia of a female fetus.

INFERTILITY

Infertility in a couple is defined as the inability to conceive after 1 year of frequent unprotected intercourse. Infertility is a disorder of a couple, not of one person. For this reason, both partners must be involved in determining the cause of infertility. Infertility is caused by factors involving the man in a significant number of cases. Some estimate 25% of cases are male-related.[26]

Problems of the hypothalamic-pituitary system, testicular disorders, and problems of the ejaculatory system can cause male infertility. The physical causes of infertility can be divided into 3 categories: pretesticular, testicular, and posttesticular. The *pretesticular* or endocrine causes occur in only about 3% of the cases. They can generally be treated with medication or surgery.

Testicular problems make up 50% of the cases. The most common cause of male infertility is a varicocele. Other factors that influence the testes include infection (e.g., mumps virus, STIs, bacterial infections), congenital anomalies, drugs, radiation, substance use (alcohol, nicotine, drugs), and environmental hazards.

Posttesticular causes account for 5% to 7% of the cases. Obstruction, infection, and the result of a surgical procedure are the primary causes. The remaining 40% are classified as *idiopathic,* or of unknown causes.

A careful health history and examination may reveal the cause of a patient's infertility. Thus the history is a starting point for determining cause and treatment. The history should include age; occupation; past injury, surgery, or infections of the genital tract; lifestyle issues (e.g., hot tubs, weight training, wearing tight undergarments); sexual practices; frequency of intercourse; and emotional factors, such as stress levels and the desire for children. Record the use of drugs, such as chemotherapeutic agents, anabolic steroids or testosterone, sulfasalazine (Azulfidine), cimetidine (Tagamet HB), and recreational drugs, since these drugs can reduce the sperm count. A physical examination may identify a varicocele, Peyronie's disease, or other physical findings.

The first test in the male infertility evaluation is a semen analysis to determine sperm concentration, motility, and morphology. Hormone studies are helpful in determining the cause, including plasma testosterone and serum LH and FSH measurements. Be tactful in dealing with the male patient undergoing infertility studies. Many cultures equate fertility and masculinity. Both male and female partners should undergo evaluation simultaneously to avoid potential treatment delays for the couple.

Treatment options for the man include drugs, conservative lifestyle changes (e.g., avoiding scrotal heat, substance use, high stress), in vitro fertilization techniques, and corrective surgery. Infertility can seriously strain a relationship. The couple may need counseling and discussion of alternatives if conception is not achieved. (Female infertility is discussed in Chapter 53.)

CASE STUDY

Benign Prostatic Hyperplasia With Acute Urinary Retention

Patient Profile

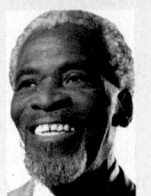

(© IPGGutenber-gUKLtd/iStock/Thinkstock.)

B.G., a 60-yr-old married black man with hypertension, COPD, and coronary artery disease, comes to the ED because of an inability to void for the past 13 hours and pain in the lower abdomen.

Subjective Data

- Reports the urge to void
- Is restless, anxious, and agitated

Objective Data

- Has prostate enlargement on digital rectal examination
- Has hematuria, bacteria, and WBCs in urine
- Has a tender and palpable bladder above the umbilicus
- PSA test: 8 ng/mL

Interprofessional Care

- Indwelling catheter inserted by a urology resident
- Admitted to the hospital for observation

Discussion Questions

1. What risk factors for prostate problems are present in B.G.?
2. Explain the cause of the manifestations that B.G. exhibited.
3. What are possible reasons for B.G.'s high PSA level?
4. Discuss the drug and surgical options available to B.G.
5. ***Patient-Centered Care:*** B.G. asks you about the effect of the various surgical options on his ability to have sex. How would you respond and what type of teaching would you provide?
6. ***Priority Decision:*** Based on the assessment data, what are the priority nursing diagnoses?
7. ***Priority Decision:*** What is the priority nursing intervention for B.G.?
8. ***Patient-Centered Care:*** On further assessment, you note that B.G. is concerned he may have incontinence if he has surgery on his prostate. How would you help him resolve this concern related to treatment options, and how would you teach him about these options?
9. ***Evidence-Based Practice:*** What information would you offer to B.G. when he asks if he should start taking saw palmetto to prevent future UTIs?

Answers available at *http://evolve.elsevier.com/Lewis/medsurg.*

▌ BRIDGE TO NCLEX EXAMINATION

The number of the question corresponds to the same-numbered outcome at the beginning of the chapter.

1. Postoperatively, a patient who has had a laser prostatectomy has continuous bladder irrigation with a 3-way urinary catheter with a 30-mL balloon. When he reports bladder spasms with the catheter in place, the nurse should
   a. deflate the balloon to 10 mL to decrease bulk in the bladder.
   b. deflate the balloon and then reinflate to ensure that the catheter is patent.
   c. explain that this feeling is normal and that he should not try to urinate around the catheter.
   d. stop the irrigation, assess the patient's vital signs, and notify the HCP of possible obstruction.

2. Which factors would place a patient at a higher risk for prostate cancer *(select all that apply)*?
   a. Older than 65 years
   b. Asian or Native American
   c. Long-term use of an indwelling urethral catheter
   d. Father diagnosed and treated for early-stage prostate cancer
   e. Previous history of undescended testicle and testicular cancer

3. A patient scheduled for a radical prostatectomy for prostate cancer expresses the fear that he will have erectile dysfunction. In responding to this patient, the nurse should keep in mind that
   a. PD5 inhibitors are not recommended in prostatectomy patients.
   b. erectile dysfunction can occur even with a nerve-sparing procedure.
   c. the most common complication of this surgery is bowel incontinence.
   d. the provider will place a penile implant during surgery to treat any dysfunction.

4. The nurse explains to the patient with chronic bacterial prostatitis who is undergoing antibiotic therapy that *(select all that apply)*
   a. all patients require hospitalization.
   b. pain will lessen once treatment has ended.
   c. the course of treatment is generally 1 to 2 weeks.
   d. long-term therapy may be needed in immunocompromised patient.
   e. if the condition is not treated appropriately, he is at risk for prostate cancer.

5. In assessing a patient for testicular cancer, the nurse understands that the manifestations of this disease often include
   a. urinary frequency.
   b. painless mass in the scrotal area.
   c. erectile dysfunction with retrograde ejaculation.
   d. rapid onset of dysuria with scrotal swelling and fever.
6. The nurse should explain to the patient who has erectile dysfunction (ED) that *(select all that apply)*
   a. the most common cause is benign prostatic hypertrophy.
   b. ED may be due to medications or conditions such as diabetes.
   c. only men who are 65 years or older benefit from PDE5 inhibitors.
   d. there are medications and devices that can be used to help with erections.
   e. this condition is primarily due to anxiety and best treated with psychotherapy.

7. To decrease the patient's discomfort related to discussing his reproductive organs, the nurse should
   a. relate his sexual concerns to his sexual partner.
   b. arrange to have male nurses care for the patient.
   c. give him written material and ask if he has questions.
   d. maintain a nonjudgmental attitude toward his sexual practices.

1. c, 2, a, 3, b, 4, b, 5, b, 6, b, d, 7, d

For rationales to these answers and even more NCLEX review questions, visit *http://evolve.elsevier.com/Lewis/medsurg*.

ⓔ EVOLVE WEBSITE/RESOURCES LIST

http://evolve.elsevier.com/Lewis/medsurg
Review Questions (Online Only)
Key Points
Answer Keys for Questions
• Rationales for Bridge to NCLEX Examination Questions
• Answer Guidelines for Case Study on p. 1276
• Answer Guidelines for Managing Care of Multiple Patients Case Study (Section 11) on p. 1278
Student Case Study
• Patient With Benign Prostatic Hyperplasia
Nursing Care Plan
• eNursing Care Plan 54.1: Patient Having Prostate Surgery
Conceptual Care Map Creator
Audio Glossary
Supporting Media
• Animations
   • Prostatectomy
   • Vasectomy
Content Updates

REFERENCES

1. Briolat G: Benign prostatic hyperplasia. In: Lajiness M, Quallich S, eds. *The Nurse Practitioner in Urology*, Basel, Switzerland, 2016, Springer International Publishing.
*2. Al-Khalil S, Boothe D, Durdin T, et al: Interactions between benign prostatic hyperplasia (BPH) and prostate cancer in large prostates. A retrospective data review, *Int Urol Nephrol* 48:91, 2016.
*3. American Urological Association: AUA guideline: Surgical management of lower urinary tract symptoms attributed to benign prostatic hyperplasia. Retrieved from *www.auanet.org/guidelines/surgical-management-of-lower-urinary-tract-symptoms-attributed-to-benign-prostatic-hyperplasia-(2018)*.
4. Barry M, Fowler F, O'Leary M, et al: The AUA symptom index for benign prostatic hyperplasia, *J Urol* 148:1549, 1992. (Classic)
*5. Kasivisvanathan V, Rannikko A, Borghi M, et al: MRI-targeted or standard biopsy for prostate-cancer diagnosis, *N Engl J Med* 378:1767, 2018.
*6. Nabavizadeh R, Zangi M, Kim M, et al: Herbal supplements for prostate enlargement. Current state of the evidence, *Urology* 112:145, 2018.
*7. Calves J, Thoulouzan M, Perroui-Verbe MA, et al: Long-term patient reported clinical outcomes and reoperation rate after photovaporization with the CPS-180W greenlight laser, *Eur Urol Focus* 17:S2405, 2017.
*8. American Urological Association: AUA guideline: Early detection of prostate cancer. Retrieved from *www.auanet.org/guidelines/prostate-cancer-early-detection-guideline*.

9. American Cancer Society: What are the key statistics about prostate cancer? Retrieved from *www.cancer.org/cancer/prostatecancer/detailedguide/prostate-cancer-key-statistics*.
*10. Loblaw A, Souter LH, Canil C, et al: Follow-up care for survivors of prostate cancer—Clinical management: A program in evidence-based care systematic review and clinical practice guidelines, *Clin Oncol (R Coll Radiol)* 29:711, 2017.
11. National Cancer Institute: Treatment choices for men with early-stage prostate cancer. Retrieved from *www.cancer.gov/types/prostate/patient/prostate-treatment-pdq*.
*12. Montironi R, Cimadamore A, Cheng L, et al: Prostate cancer grading in 2018: Limitations, implementations, cribriform morphology, and biological markers, *Int J Biol Markers* 33:331, 2018.
*13. Coughlin GD, Yaxley JW, Chambers SK, et al: Robot-assisted laparoscopic prostatectomy versus open radical prostatectomy: 24-Month outcomes from a randomized controlled study, *Lancet Oncol* 19:1051, 2018.
*14. Barocas DA, Alvarez J, Resnick MJ, et al: Association between radiation therapy, surgery, or observation for localized prostate cancer and patient-reported outcomes after 3 years, *JAMA* 317:1126, 2017.
15. Oncolink: Possible side effects of radiation treatment for prostate cancer. Retrieved from *www.oncolink.org/cancers/prostate/treatments/possible-side-effects-of-radiation-treatment-for-prostate-cancer*.
*16. Strouthos I, Chatzikonstantinou G, Zamboglou N, et al: Combined high dose rate brachytherapy and external beam radiotherapy for clinically localized prostate cancer, *Radiother Oncol* 128:301, 2018.
17. Gamat M, McNeel DG: Androgen deprivation and immunotherapy for the treatment of prostate cancer, *Endocr Relat Cancer* 12:T297, 2017.
*18. Pollack C, Armstrong K, Mitra N, et al: A multidimensional view of racial differences in access to prostate cancer care, *Cancer* 123:4449, 2017.
19. National Institute of Diabetes and Digestive and Kidney Disorders Information Clearinghouse: Prostatitis. Retrieved from *www.niddk.nih.gov/health-information/urologic-diseases/prostate-problems/prostatitis-inflammation-prostate*.
*20. Araujo LA, De Paula AA, de Paula HD, et al: Human papillomavirus genotype distribution in penile carcinoma: Association with clinic pathological factors, *PloSOne* 6:e0199557, 2018.
21. Woldu SL, Bargrodia A: Update on epidemiologic considerations and treatment trends in testicular cancer, *Curr Opin Urol* 28:440, 2018.
22. McBride A, Lipshultz LI: Male fertility preservation, *Curr Urol Rep* 19:40, 2018.
*23. Nguyen HMT, Gabrielson AT, Hellstrom WJG: Erectile dysfunction in young men—A review of the prevalence and risk factors, *Sex Med Rev* 5:508, 2017.
*24. Burnett AL, Nehra A, Breau RH, et al: Erectile dysfunction: AUA guideline, *J Urol* 200:633, 2018.
*25. American Urological Association: AUA guideline: Evaluation and management of testosterone deficiency. Retrieved from *www.auanet.org/guidelines/evaluation-and-management-of-testosterone-deficiency*.
26. Lotti F, Maggi M: Sexual dysfunction and male infertility, *Nat Rev Urol* 15:287, 2018.

*Evidence-based information for clinical practice

CASE STUDY

Managing Care of Multiple Patients

You are working on the medical-surgical unit and have been assigned to care for the following 6 patients. You have 1 LPN and 1 UAP on your team to help you.

Patients

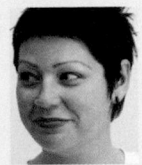

L.M. is a 35-yr-old Hispanic woman who went to the clinic 3 days ago saying she was just "not feeling well." She was admitted to the hospital for treatment of hypertension caused by newly diagnosed Cushing syndrome. She has been depressed and crying because of her physical appearance. Her last BP was 164/94 mm Hg.

(© iStockphoto/
Thinkstock.)

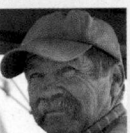

N.B. is a 48-yr-old man admitted to the ICU 2 days ago in diabetic ketoacidosis. He was transferred to the clinical unit yesterday evening. His fasting blood glucose level this morning is 296 mg/dL.

(© iStockphoto/
Thinkstock.)

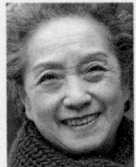

A.K. is a 68-yr-old Asian American woman recently diagnosed with adenocarcinoma of her right breast. She had a lumpectomy and axillary node dissection yesterday. She has a Jackson-Pratt drain in her right chest. Her last pain medication was given 1 hour ago, at which time she rated her pain as a 7 on a scale of 0–10.

(© XiXinXing/
iStock/
Thinkstock.)

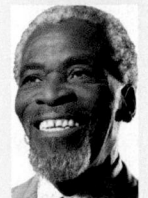

B.G. is a 60-yr-old black man who was admitted to the hospital because of an inability to void for 13 hours and pain in the lower abdomen. He has a urinary tract infection and prostatic enlargement. The urology resident inserted an indwelling catheter. B.G. is scheduled to undergo a TURP this morning.

(© IPGGutenber-
gUKLtd/iStock/
Thinkstock.)

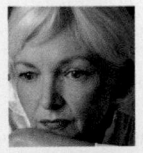

R.D. is a 52-yr-old white woman who was diagnosed with Graves' disease 2 mo ago. She was treated with antithyroid medication for 2 mo and underwent a subtotal thyroidectomy yesterday. In report it was noted that her voice has become slightly "hoarse" in the last hour.

(© Jupiterimages/
Photos.com/
Thinkstock.)

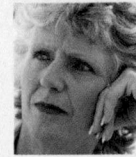

B.C. is a 49-yr-old Latina woman who had a total abdominal hysterectomy and bilateral salpingo-oo-phorectomy 1 day ago. She has a urinary catheter in place. Her vital signs are stable. She is not reporting any pain.

(© Juanmonino/
iStock.com.)

Discussion Questions

1. *Priority Decision:* After receiving report, which patient should you see first? Second? Provide a rationale.
2. *Collaboration:* Which tasks could you delegate to UAP? *(select all that apply)*
   a. Assist B.C. to ambulate in the hallway.
   b. Teach B.G. what to expect postoperatively.
   c. Take R.D.'s vital signs and report the results to you.
   d. Assess A.K.'s mastectomy incision for manifestations of infection.
   e. Listen to L.M. talk about her feelings while helping her with AM care.
3. *Priority Decision and Collaboration:* While you are assessing R.D., the LPN informs you that A.K.'s chest dressing is totally saturated with bloody drainage. Which *initial* action would be most appropriate?
   a. Ask the LPN to call the laboratory for a stat Hgb and Hct on A.K.
   b. Tell the LPN to reinforce the dressing with sterile 4× 4–gauze pads.
   c. Have the LPN stay with R.D. while you assess the patency of A.K.'s Jackson-Pratt drain.
   d. Ask the LPN to stay with A.K. and have the UAP monitor R.D. while you call A.K.'s HCP.

Case Study Progression

A.K.'s Jackson-Pratt drain was not functioning properly. You get it working and change the chest dressing. The incision is well approximated without signs of infection. When you leave the room, the Jackson-Pratt has a small amount of serosanguineous drainage in it. As you enter R.D.'s room, you notice she is having a carpal spasm on the same arm on which the LPN is taking her BP. You recognize this as a manifestation of hypocalcemia and notify the health care provider.

4. Which assessment findings would be *most* important to include in a discussion with the health care provider about R.D.? *(select all that apply)*
   a. Patient is anxious
   b. Hoarseness of voice
   c. Most recent Hgb and Hct
   d. Carpal spasm upon inflation of BP cuff
   e. Blood pressure of 138/76 and heart rate of 78
5. *Priority Decision:* Which intervention would be of *highest* priority in caring for L.M.?
   a. Assess her for fall risk.
   b. Assess her for signs and symptoms of hypoglycemia.
   c. Teach her the need for a high-carbohydrate, low-protein diet.
   d. Reassure her that her physical appearance will improve with treatment.
6. B.G. asks you what to expect when he returns from surgery. You explain that he will have a(n)
   a. dressing in his groin as well as a urinary catheter.
   b. 3-way urinary catheter connected to an irrigation system.
   c. patient-controlled analgesia (PCA) pump for pain control.
   d. abdominal and a perineal drain that will be recharged q4hr.
7. *Priority Decision and Management Decision:* The LPN is assigned to give medications to N.B., including his sliding scale Novolog insulin with breakfast. The UAP, who is also a senior nursing student, tells you that the LPN gave N.B.'s insulin at least 30 minutes after the patient ate his breakfast. What is your *best* initial action?
   a. Report the incident to the charge nurse for follow-up.
   b. Talk to the LPN about the importance of timely medication administration.
   c. Ask the LPN what time the insulin was given and when the patient ate breakfast.
   d. Ask the UAP to first discuss the concern with the LPN to follow proper channels of communication.

Answers available at *http://evolve.elsevier.com/Lewis/medsurg.*

55

Assessment: Nervous System

Tara Shaw

Act as if what you do makes a difference. It does.

William James

ⓔ http://evolve.elsevier.com/Lewis/medsurg

CONCEPTUAL FOCUS

Cognition

Functional Ability

Intracranial Regulation

Sensory Perception

LEARNING OUTCOMES

1. Distinguish between the functions of neurons and glial cells.
2. Explain the anatomic location and functions of the cerebrum, brainstem, cerebellum, spinal cord, peripheral nerves, and cerebrospinal fluid.
3. Identify the major arteries supplying the brain.
4. Describe the functions of the 12 cranial nerves.
5. Compare the functions of the 2 divisions of the autonomic nervous system.
6. Link the age-related changes in the neurologic system to the differences in assessment findings.

7. Obtain significant subjective and objective data related to the nervous system from a patient.
8. Perform a physical assessment of the nervous system using the appropriate techniques.
9. Distinguish normal from abnormal findings of a physical assessment of the nervous system.
10. Describe the purpose, significance of results, and nursing responsibilities related to diagnostic studies of the nervous system.

KEY TERMS

autonomic nervous system (ANS), p. 1284
blood-brain barrier, p. 1285
central nervous system (CNS), p. 1279
cerebrospinal fluid (CSF), p. 1283
cranial nerves (CNs), p. 1284

dermatome, p. 1284
glial cells, p. 1280
lower motor neurons (LMNs), p. 1281
meninges, p. 1286
neurons, p. 1279

neurotransmitters, p. 1280
peripheral nervous system (PNS), p. 1279
reflex, p. 1281
synapse, p. 1280
upper motor neurons (UMNs), p. 1281

The nervous system is one of the most complex systems. It controls all the body's activities. Having a general understanding of the nervous system is critical to your being able to analyze and interpret clinical findings. This chapter reviews the structures and functions, assessment, and diagnostic studies of the nervous system.

STRUCTURES AND FUNCTIONS OF NERVOUS SYSTEM

The nervous system is responsible for the control and integration of the body's many activities. It is divided into the central nervous system and peripheral nervous system. The **central nervous system (CNS)** consists of the brain, spinal cord, and cranial nerves I and II. The **peripheral nervous system (PNS)** consists of cranial nerves III to XII, spinal nerves, and peripheral components of the autonomic nervous system (ANS).

Cells of Nervous System

The nervous system is made up of 2 types of cells: neurons and supportive glial cells.

Neurons. **Neurons** are the primary functional unit of the nervous system. Although neurons come in many shapes and sizes, they share 3 characteristics: (1) *excitability,* or the ability to generate a nerve impulse; (2) *conductivity,* or the ability to transmit an impulse; and (3) *influence,* or the ability to influence other neurons, muscle cells, or glandular cells.

A typical neuron consists of a cell body, multiple dendrites, and an axon (Fig. 55.1). The *cell body* contains the nucleus and cytoplasm. It is the metabolic center of the neuron. *Dendrites*

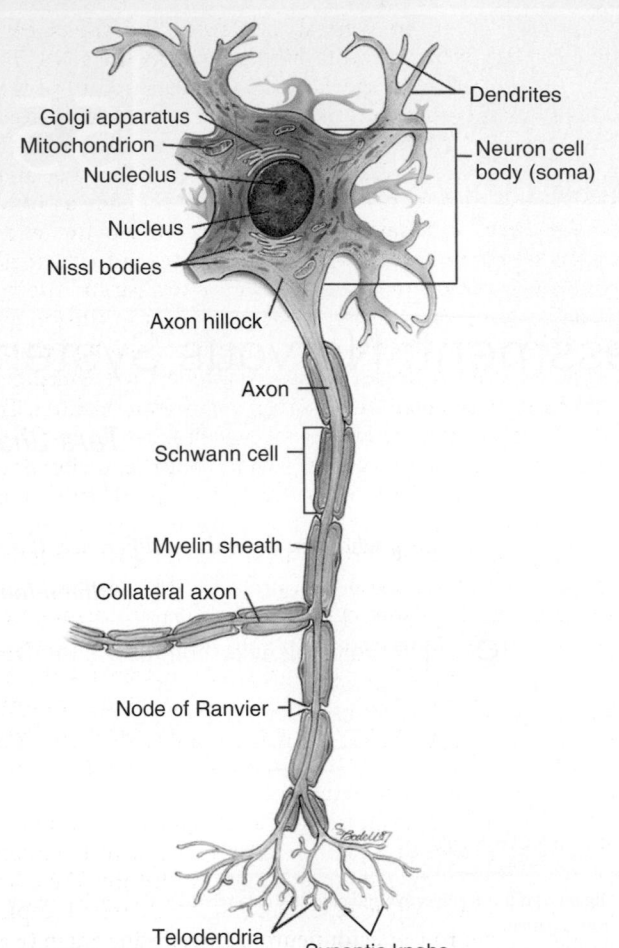

FIG. 55.1 Structural features of neurons: dendrites, cell body, and axons. (Modified from Thibodeau GA, Patton KT: *Anatomy and physiology*, ed 8, St Louis, 2013, Mosby.)

are short processes extending from the cell body. They receive impulses or signals from other neurons and conduct them toward the cell body. The *axon* projects varying distances from the cell body. The axon carries nerve impulses to other neurons or to end organs, such as smooth and striated muscles and glands.

Many axons in the CNS and PNS are covered by a *myelin sheath*, a white, lipid protein substance that acts as an insulator for the conduction of impulses. Axons may be myelinated or unmyelinated, as in the case of smaller fibers.

Glial Cells. Glial cells (glia or neuroglia) provide support, nourishment, and protection to neurons. Glial cells make up about half of the brain and spinal cord mass. Glial cells are divided into microglia and macroglia. *Microglia,* specialized macrophages capable of phagocytosis, protect the neurons. These cells are mobile within the brain and multiply when the brain is damaged.

Macroglial cells include astrocytes, oligodendrocytes, and ependymal cells. *Astrocytes* are found mainly in gray matter. They provide structural support to neurons. Their delicate processes form the *blood-brain barrier* with the endothelium of the blood vessels. They also play a role in *synaptic transmission* (conduction of impulses between neurons). When the brain is injured, astrocytes act as phagocytes for cleaning up neuronal debris. They help restore the neurochemical milieu and provide support for repair. Proliferation of astrocytes contributes to the formation of scar tissue (*gliosis*) in the CNS.

Oligodendrocytes are specialized cells that produce the myelin sheath of nerve fibers in the CNS. They are found mainly in the white matter of the CNS. *Ependymal cells* line the brain ventricles and aid in the secretion of cerebrospinal fluid (CSF).

Neuroglia are mitotic and can replicate. In general, when neurons are destroyed, the tissue is replaced by the proliferation of neuroglial cells. Most primary CNS tumors involve glial cells. Primary cancers involving neurons are rare.

Nerve Regeneration

If the axon of the nerve cell is damaged, the cell tries to repair itself. Damaged nerve cells try to grow back to their original destinations by sprouting many branches from the damaged ends of their axons. Axons in the CNS are generally less successful than peripheral axons in regeneration.[1]

Schwann cells myelinate the nerve fibers in the PNS. Injured nerve fibers in the PNS can regenerate by growing within the protective myelin sheath of the Schwann cells if the cell body is intact and the environment is optimal.[2] The final result of nerve regeneration depends on the number of axon sprouts that join with the appropriate Schwann cell columns and reinnervate appropriate end organs.

Neurons have long been thought to be nonmitotic. That is, after being damaged, neurons could not be replaced. Recent research shows a subset of glial cells (astrocytes) proliferate after certain injuries in the CNS, and neurogenesis may occur from stem cells.[3] These findings support the expectation that the patient will have a certain amount of recovery after injury involving the neurons.

Nerve Impulse

The purpose of a neuron is to initiate, receive, and process messages about events both within and outside the body. The initiation of a neuronal message (*nerve impulse*) involves the generation of an action potential. A series of action potentials travel along the axon. When the impulse reaches the end of the nerve fiber, a chemical interaction involving neurotransmitters transmits the impulse across the junction (*synapse*) between nerve cells by. This chemical interaction generates another set of action potentials in the next neuron. These events are repeated until the nerve impulse reaches its destination.

Because of its insulating capacity, myelination of nerve axons speeds the conduction of an action potential. Many peripheral nerve axons have *nodes of Ranvier* (gaps in the myelin sheath) that allow an action potential to travel much faster by jumping from node to node. We call this *saltatory* (hopping) *conduction*. In an unmyelinated fiber, conduction is slower. The wave of depolarization travels the entire length of the axon, with each part of the membrane becoming depolarized in turn.

Synapse. A synapse is the structural and functional junction between 2 neurons. It is where the nerve impulse is transmitted from 1 neuron to another. The nerve impulse also can be transmitted from neurons to glands or muscles. The essential structures of synaptic transmission are a presynaptic terminal, synaptic cleft, and receptor site on the postsynaptic cell (Fig. 55.2).

Neurotransmitters. Neurotransmitters are chemicals that affect the transmission of impulses across the synaptic cleft. *Excitatory neurotransmitters* (e.g., epinephrine, norepinephrine, glutamate) activate postsynaptic receptors that increase the chance that an action potential will be generated. *Inhibitory neurotransmitters* (e.g., serotonin, γ-aminobutyric acid [GABA],

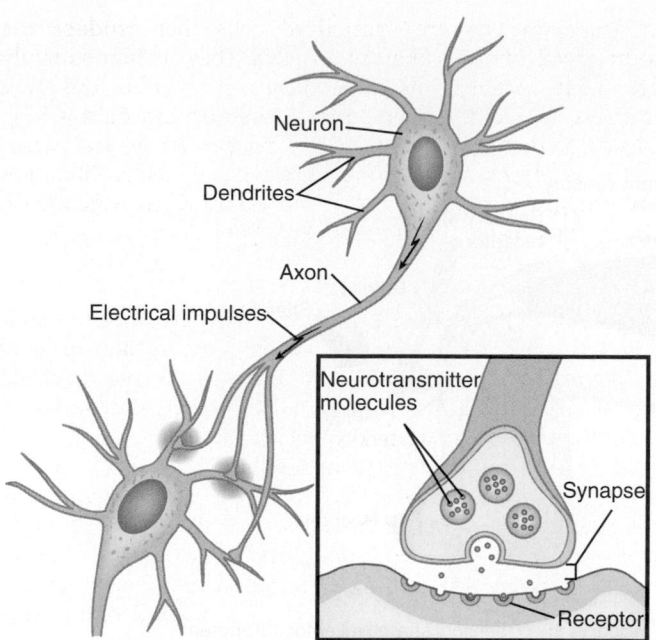

FIG. 55.2 Impulse generation between neurons. Synapse shown with neurotransmitters and receptors.

dopamine) activate postsynaptic receptors to decrease the chance that an action potential will be generated. For example, endorphins block pain transmission while substance P makes nerves more sensitive to pain.

In general, the net effect (excitatory or inhibitory) depends on the number of presynaptic neurons releasing neurotransmitters on the postsynaptic cell. A presynaptic cell that releases an excitatory neurotransmitter does not always cause the postsynaptic cell to depolarize enough to generate an action potential.

When many presynaptic cells release excitatory neurotransmitters on a single neuron, the sum of their input is enough to generate an action potential. Neurotransmitters continue to combine with the receptor sites at the postsynaptic membrane until they are inactivated by enzymes, are taken up by the presynaptic endings, or diffuse away from the synaptic region. Drugs and toxins can affect neurotransmitters by changing their function or blocking their attachment to receptor sites on the postsynaptic membrane. We can use cerebral microdialysis to measure neurotransmitter levels in the cerebral cortex (see Chapter 56).

Central Nervous System

The components of the CNS include the cerebrum (cerebral hemispheres), brainstem, cerebellum, and spinal cord.

Spinal Cord. The *spinal cord* is continuous with the brainstem and exits from the cranial cavity through the foramen magnum. A cross section of the spinal cord reveals gray matter that is centrally located in an H shape and surrounded by white matter. The gray matter contains the cell bodies of voluntary motor neurons, preganglionic autonomic motor neurons, and association neurons (interneurons). The white matter contains the axons of the ascending sensory and descending motor fibers. The myelin surrounding these fibers gives them their white appearance. The spinal pathways or tracts are named for the point of origin and the point of destination (e.g., spinocerebellar tract [ascending], corticospinal tract [descending]).

Ascending Tracts. In general, the ascending tracts carry specific sensory information to higher levels of the CNS. This information comes from special sensory receptors in the skin, muscles and joints, viscera, and blood vessels and enters the spinal cord by way of the dorsal roots of the spinal nerves. The ascending tracts are organized by sensory modality and anatomy. The fasciculus gracilis and the fasciculus cuneatus (often called the *dorsal* or *posterior columns*) carry information about touch, deep pressure, vibration, position sense, and kinesthesia (appreciation of movement, weight, and body parts). The *spinocerebellar tracts* carry information about muscle tension and body position to the cerebellum for coordination of movement. The *spinothalamic tracts* carry pain and temperature sensations.

Other ascending tracts may also carry sensory modalities. The signs and symptoms of various neurologic diseases suggest there are additional pathways for touch, position sense, and vibration.

Descending Tracts. Descending tracts carry impulses that are responsible for muscle movement. Among the most important descending tracts are the corticobulbar and corticospinal tracts, collectively termed the *pyramidal tract.* These tracts carry voluntary impulses from the cerebral cortex to the cranial and peripheral nerves. Another group of descending motor tracts carries impulses from the extrapyramidal system (all motor systems except the pyramidal) concerned with voluntary movement. It includes pathways originating in the brainstem, basal ganglia, and cerebellum. The motor output exits the spinal cord by way of the ventral roots of the spinal nerves.

Reflex Arc. A reflex is an involuntary response to stimuli. In the spinal cord, reflex arcs play an important role in maintaining muscle tone, which is essential for body posture. The components of a monosynaptic reflex arc (Fig. 55.3) are a receptor organ, afferent neuron, effector neuron, and effector organ (e.g., skeletal muscle). The afferent neuron synapses with the efferent neurons in the gray matter of the spinal cord. More complex reflex arcs have other neurons (interneurons) in addition to the afferent neuron influencing the effector neuron.

Lower and Upper Motor Neurons. Upper motor neurons (UMNs) originate in the cerebral cortex and project downward. The corticobulbar tract ends in the brainstem, and the corticospinal tract descends into the spinal cord. These neurons influence skeletal muscle movement. UMN lesions generally cause weakness or paralysis, disuse atrophy, hyperreflexia, and increased muscle tone (spasticity).

Lower motor neurons (LMNs) are the final common pathway through which descending motor tracts influence skeletal muscle. The cell bodies of LMNs, which send axons to innervate the skeletal muscles of the arms, trunk, and legs, are found in the anterior horn of the corresponding segments of the spinal cord (e.g., cervical segments contain LMNs for the arms). LMNs for skeletal muscles of the eyes, face, mouth, and throat are found in the corresponding segments of the brainstem. These cell bodies and their axons make up the somatic motor components of the cranial nerves. LMN lesions generally cause weakness or paralysis, denervation atrophy, hyporeflexia or areflexia, and decreased muscle tone (flaccidity).

Brain. The *brain* has 3 major intracranial components: cerebrum, brainstem, and cerebellum.

Cerebrum. The *cerebrum* is composed of the right and left cerebral hemispheres. It is divided into 4 lobes: frontal, temporal, parietal, and occipital (Fig. 55.4). The functions of the cerebrum are multiple and complex (Table 55.1). The *frontal lobe* controls higher cognitive function, memory retention,

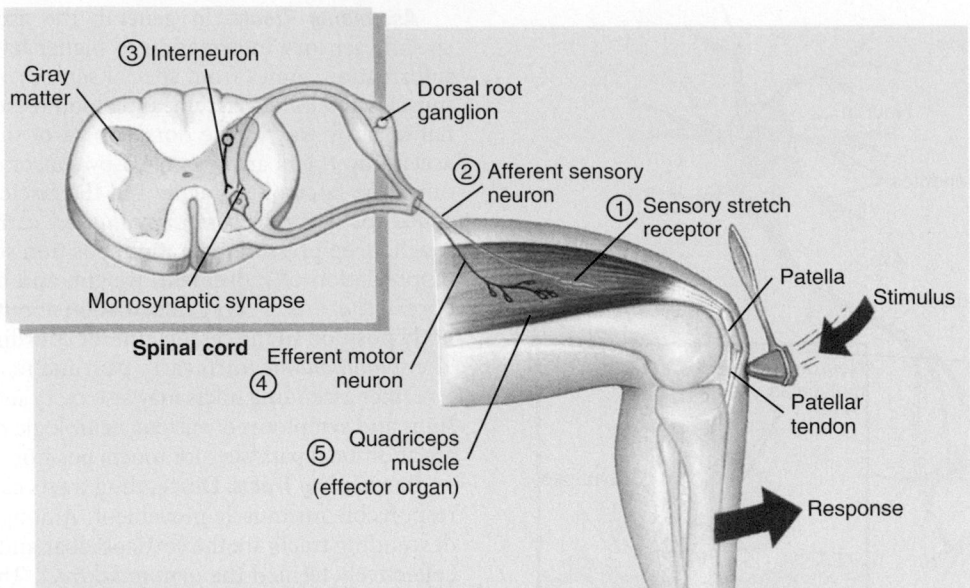

FIG. 55.3 Basic diagram of the patellar "knee jerk" reflex arc, including the (1) sensory stretch receptor, (2) afferent sensory neuron, (3) interneuron, (4) efferent motor neuron, and (5) quadriceps muscle (effector organ). (Modified from Thibodeau GA, Patton KT: *Anatomy and physiology*, ed 6, St Louis, 2007, Mosby.)

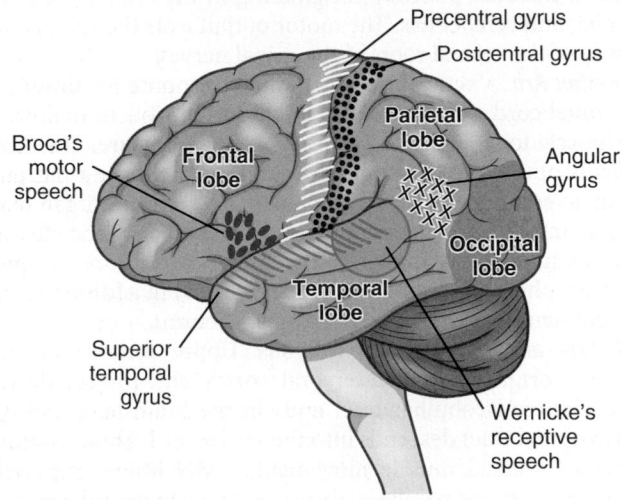

FIG. 55.4 Left hemisphere of cerebrum, lateral surface, showing major lobes and areas of the brain.

voluntary eye movements, voluntary motor movement, and motor functions involved in speech production *(Broca's area)*. The *temporal lobe* integrates somatic, visual, and auditory data and contains *Wernicke's receptive speech area*. (Language and potential functional deficits are described with strokes in Chapter 57 [see Table 57.4].)

The *parietal lobe* interprets spatial information and contains the sensory cortex. Processing of sight takes place in the *occipital lobe*.

The division of the cerebrum into lobes is useful to delineate portions of the neocortex (gray matter), which makes up the outer layer of the cerebral hemispheres. Neurons in specific parts of the neocortex are essential for various highly complex and sophisticated functions, such as language, memory, and appreciation of visual-spatial relationships.

The basal ganglia, thalamus, hypothalamus, and limbic system are also in the cerebrum. The *basal ganglia* are a group of structures found centrally in the cerebrum and midbrain. Most of them are on both sides of the thalamus. The function of the basal ganglia includes the initiation, execution, and completion of voluntary movements, learning, emotional response, and automatic movements associated with skeletal muscle activity (e.g., swallowing saliva, blinking, swinging the arms while walking).

The *thalamus* lies directly above the brainstem (Fig. 55.5). It is the major relay center for sensory input from the body, face, retina, and cochlear and taste receptors. Motor relay nuclei in the thalamus connect the cerebellum and basal ganglia to the frontal cortex.

The *hypothalamus* is just below the thalamus and slightly in front of the midbrain. It exerts a direct influence on release of hormones from the anterior pituitary gland. It has a rich capillary connection to the pituitary gland to aid in the transport of hormones. These hormones include thyroid-stimulating hormone, growth hormone, luteinizing hormone, and prolactin-releasing hormone, which play a role in regulating reproductive function. In contrast, the supraoptic and paraventricular neurons travel directly through the pituitary stalk to the posterior pituitary, where they release vasopressin and oxytocin. The hypothalamus contains the satiety center that regulates appetite. With input from the limbic system, it also regulates body temperature, water balance (through influence on vasopressin secretion), circadian rhythm, and expression of emotion. The *limbic system* is found near the inner surfaces of the cerebral hemispheres. It is concerned with emotion, aggression, feeding behavior, and sexual response.

Brainstem. The *brainstem* includes the midbrain, pons, and medulla (Fig. 55.5). Ascending and descending fibers to and from the cerebrum and cerebellum pass through the brainstem. The nuclei of cranial nerves III through XII are in the brainstem. The vital centers concerned with respiratory, vasomotor, and heart function are in the medulla.

Also in the brainstem is the *reticular formation,* a diffusely arranged group of neurons and their axons that extends from the

TABLE 55.1 Function of Cerebrum

Part	Location	Function
Cortical Areas		
Motor		
Primary	Precentral gyrus	Motor control and movement on opposite side of body
Supplemental	Anterior to precentral gyrus	Facilitates proximal muscle activity, including activity for stance and gait, and spontaneous movement and coordination
Sensory		
Association areas	Parietal lobe	Integrates somatic and sensory input
	Posterior temporal lobe	Integrates visual and auditory input for language comprehension
	Anterior temporal lobe	Integrates past experiences
	Anterior frontal lobe	Controls higher order processes (e.g., judgment, reasoning)
Auditory	Superior temporal gyrus	Registers auditory input
Somatic	Postcentral gyrus	Sensory response from opposite side of body
Visual	Occipital lobe	Registers visual images
Language		
Comprehension	Wernicke's area in dominant posterior temporal lobe	Integrates auditory language (understanding of spoken words)
Expression	Broca's area in dominant frontal lobe	Regulates motor speech
Basal Ganglia	Near lateral ventricles of both cerebral hemispheres	Controls and refines learned and automatic movements
Thalamus	Below and slightly posterior to basal ganglia	Relays sensory and motor input to and from cerebrum
Hypothalamus	Below and anterior to thalamus	Regulates endocrine and autonomic functions
Limbic System	Lateral to hypothalamus	Influences emotional behavior and basic drives, such as feeding and sexual behavior

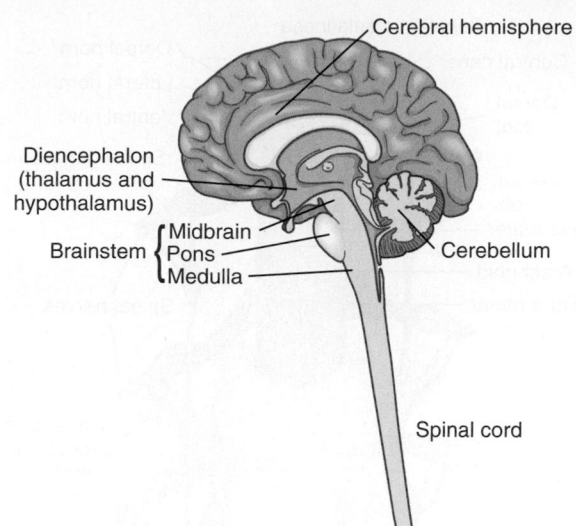

FIG. 55.5 Major divisions of the CNS.

Ventricles and Cerebrospinal Fluid. The ventricles are 4 interconnected fluid-filled cavities. The lower part of the fourth ventricle becomes the central canal in the lower part of the brainstem. The spinal canal extends centrally through the full length of the spinal cord.

Cerebrospinal fluid (CSF) is made largely in the choroid plexuses of the brain within the ventricles. It circulates within the subarachnoid space that surrounds the brain, brainstem, and spinal cord, cushioning the brain and spinal cord. CSF flows from the cranial cavity to the spinal cavity, carrying nutrients through both passive diffusion and active transport. We make CSF at an average rate of about 500 mL/day. The ventricles and central canal are filled with an average of 150 mL at any given time. Changes in the rate of CSF production or absorption can occur, leading to a change in the volume within the ventricles and central canal. Excessive buildup of CSF results in a condition known as *hydrocephalus*.

CSF circulates throughout the ventricles and seeps into the subarachnoid space surrounding the brain and spinal cord. It is absorbed primarily through the *arachnoid villi* (tiny projections into the subarachnoid space) into the intradural venous sinuses and eventually into the venous system.

The analysis of CSF composition provides useful diagnostic information related to certain nervous system diseases. We often measure CSF pressure in patients with actual or suspected intracranial injury. Increased intracranial pressure, indicated by increased CSF pressure, can force downward (central) herniation of the brain and brainstem. The signs marking this event are part of the herniation syndrome (see Chapter 56).

Peripheral Nervous System

The PNS includes all the neuronal structures that lie outside the CNS. It consists of the spinal and cranial nerves, their associated ganglia (groupings of cell bodies), and portions of the ANS.

Spinal Nerves. The spinal cord can be seen as a series of spinal segments, each on top of another with no visible boundaries. In addition to the cell bodies, each segment has a pair of dorsal (afferent) sensory nerve fibers or roots and ventral (efferent) motor fibers or roots. They innervate a specific region of the body. This combined motor-sensory nerve is called a *spinal nerve* (Fig. 55.6). The cell bodies of the voluntary motor system

medulla to the thalamus and hypothalamus. The functions of the reticular formation include relaying sensory information, influencing excitatory and inhibitory control of spinal motor neurons, and controlling vasomotor and respiratory activity. The *reticular activating system* (RAS) is a complex system that requires communication among the brainstem, reticular formation, and cerebral cortex. The RAS regulates arousal and sleep-wake transitions. The brainstem also contains the centers for sneezing, coughing, hiccupping, vomiting, sucking, and swallowing.

Cerebellum. The *cerebellum* is in the posterior cranial fossa below the occipital lobe. It coordinates voluntary movement and maintains trunk stability and equilibrium. The cerebellum receives information from the cerebral cortex, muscles, joints, and inner ear. It influences motor activity through axonal connections to the thalamus, motor cortex, and brainstem nuclei and their descending pathways.

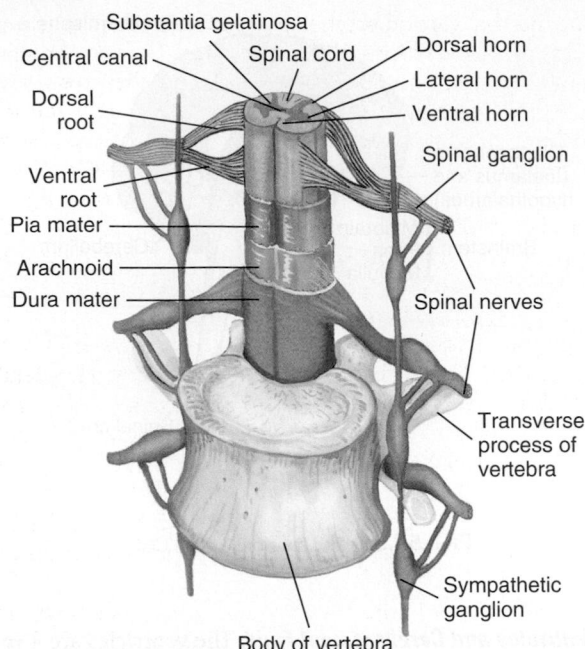

FIG. 55.6 Cross section of spinal cord showing attachments of spinal nerves and coverings of the spinal cord.

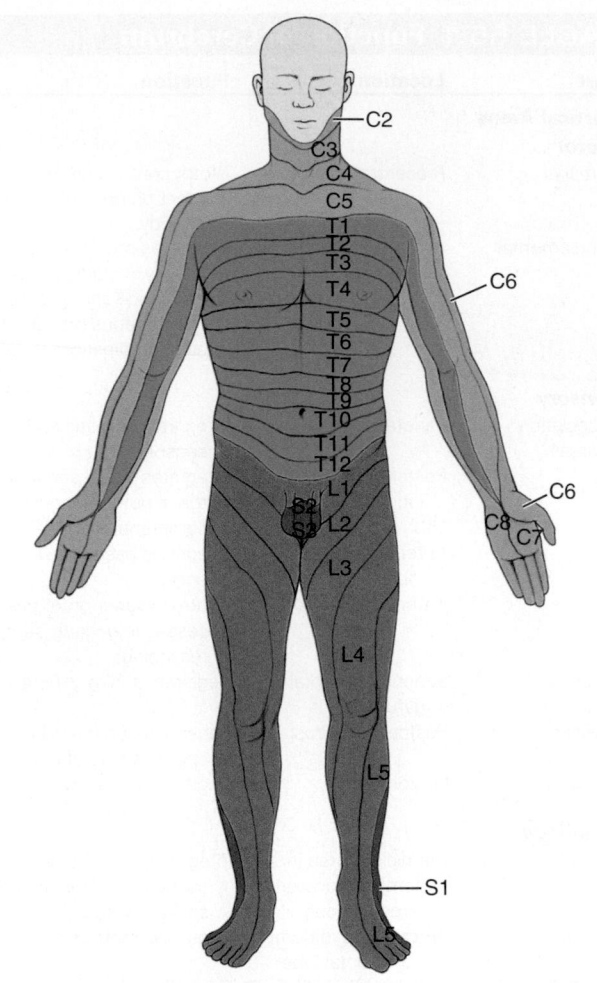

FIG. 55.7 Dermatomes of the body. (From Herlihy B: *The human body in health and illness,* ed 4, St Louis, 2011, Saunders.)

are in the anterior horn of the spinal cord gray matter. The cell bodies of the autonomic (involuntary) motor system are in the anterolateral part of the spinal cord gray matter. The cell bodies of sensory fibers are in the dorsal root ganglia just outside the spinal cord. On exiting the spinal column, each spinal nerve divides into ventral and dorsal rami, a collection of motor and sensory fibers that eventually goes to peripheral structures (e.g., skin, muscles, viscera).

A **dermatome** is the area of skin innervated by the sensory fibers of a single dorsal root of a spinal nerve (Fig. 55.7). The dermatomes give a general picture of somatic sensory innervation by spinal segments. A *myotome* is a muscle group innervated by the primary motor neurons of a single ventral root. The dermatomes and myotomes of a given spinal segment overlap with those of adjacent segments because of the development of ascending and descending collateral branches of nerve fibers.

Cranial Nerves. The **cranial nerves (CNs)** are the 12 paired nerves composed of cell bodies with fibers that exit from the cranial cavity. Unlike the spinal nerves, which always have both afferent sensory and efferent motor fibers, some CNs are only sensory, some only motor, and some both.

Table 55.4 (later in this chapter) outlines the motor and sensory components of the CNs. Fig. 55.8 shows the position of the CNs in relation to the brain and spinal cord. Just as the cell bodies of the spinal nerves are found in specific segments of the spinal cord, cell bodies (nuclei) of the CNs found in specific segments of the brainstem. Exceptions are the nuclei of the olfactory and optic nerves. The primary cell bodies of the olfactory nerve are in the nasal epithelium. The cell bodies of the optic nerve are in the retina.

Autonomic Nervous System. The **autonomic nervous system (ANS)** is divided into the sympathetic and parasympathetic systems. The ANS governs involuntary functions of heart muscle, smooth muscle, and glands through both efferent and afferent pathways. The 2 systems function together to maintain a relatively balanced internal environment. The preganglionic cell

bodies of the *sympathetic nervous system* (SNS) are found in spinal segments T1 through L2. The major neurotransmitter released by the postganglionic fibers of the SNS is norepinephrine. The neurotransmitter released by the preganglionic fibers is acetylcholine.

The preganglionic cell bodies of the *parasympathetic nervous system* (PSNS) are found in the brainstem and sacral spinal segments (S2 through S4). Acetylcholine is the neurotransmitter released at both preganglionic and postganglionic nerve endings.

SNS stimulation activates the mechanisms required for the "fight-or-flight" response that occurs throughout the body (Fig. 55.9). In contrast, the PSNS is geared to act in localized and discrete regions. It conserves and restores the body's energy stores. The ANS provides dual and often reciprocal innervation to many structures. For example, the SNS increases the rate and force of heart contraction and the PSNS decreases the rate and force.

Cerebral Circulation

Knowing the distribution of the brain's major arteries is essential for understanding and evaluating the signs and symptoms of cerebrovascular disease and trauma. The brain's blood supply arises from the internal carotid arteries (anterior circulation) and the vertebral arteries (posterior circulation). They are shown in Fig. 55.10.

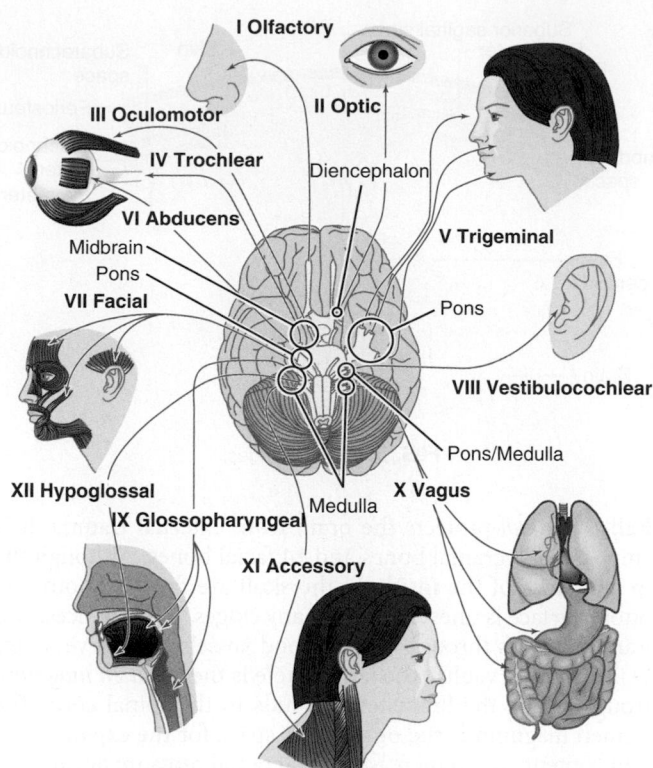

FIG. 55.8 The cranial nerves are numbered by the order in which they leave the brain. (Redrawn from McCance KL, Huether SE: Pathophysiology: *The biologic basis for disease in adults and children*, ed 6, St Louis, 2010, Mosby.)

The internal carotid arteries provide blood flow to the anterior and middle portions of the cerebrum. The vertebral arteries join to form the basilar artery, which branches to supply the middle and lower parts of the temporal lobes, occipital lobes, cerebellum, brainstem, and part of the diencephalon. The main branch of the basilar artery is the posterior cerebral artery. The *circle of Willis* is formed by communicating arteries that join the basilar and internal carotid arteries (Fig. 55.11). The circle of Willis plays a key role in cerebral blood flow. Interestingly, only 40% of us have a well-formed, complete circle of Willis. Everyone else has a degree of variation.[4]

Superior to the circle of Willis, 3 pairs of arteries supply blood to the left and right hemispheres. The anterior cerebral artery feeds the medial and anterior portions of the frontal lobes. The middle cerebral artery feeds the outer portions of the frontal, parietal, and superior temporal lobes. The posterior cerebral artery feeds the medial portions of the occipital and inferior temporal lobes. Venous blood drains from the brain through the dural sinuses, which form channels that drain into the 2 jugular veins.

Blood-Brain Barrier. The **blood-brain barrier** is a physiologic barrier between blood capillaries and brain tissue. This barrier protects the brain from harmful agents, while allowing nutrients and gases to enter. The structure of brain capillaries differs from that of other capillaries, so substances that normally pass into most tissues are prevented from entering brain tissue. Lipid-soluble compounds enter the brain easily. Water-soluble and ionized drugs enter the brain and the spinal cord slowly. Thus the blood-brain barrier affects the penetration of drugs. Only certain drugs can enter the CNS from the bloodstream.

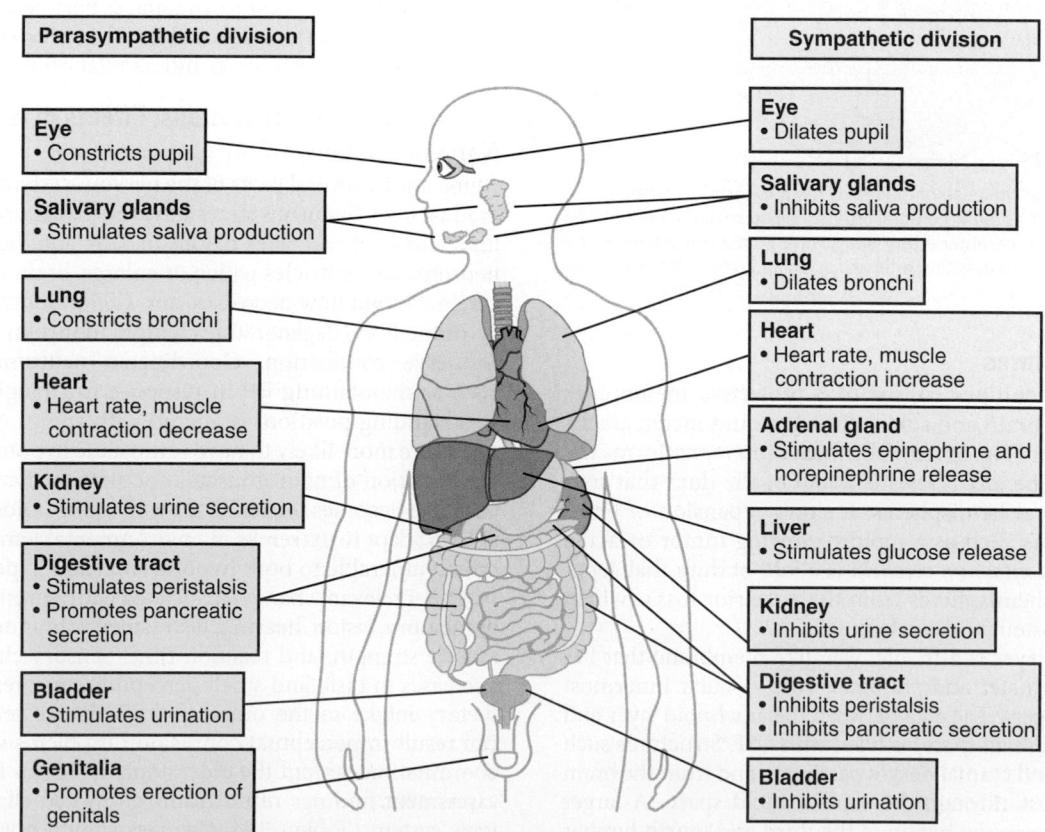

FIG. 55.9 Effects of the sympathetic and parasympathetic systems.

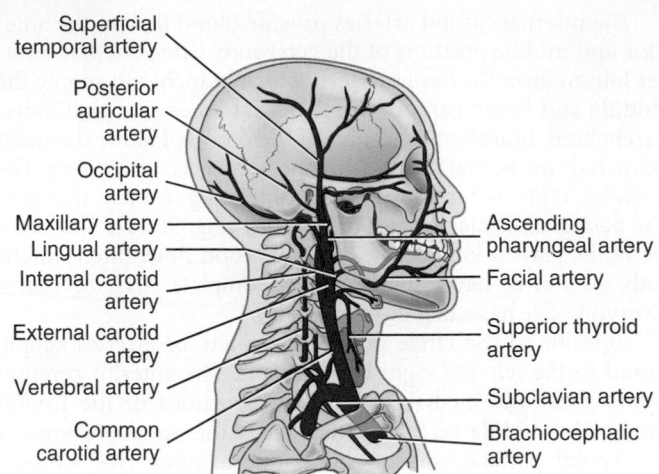

FIG. 55.10 Arteries of the head and neck. Brachiocephalic artery, right common carotid artery, right subclavian artery, and their branches. The major arteries to the head are the common carotid and vertebral arteries. (Modified from Thibodeau GA, Patton KT: *Anatomy and physiology*, ed 8, St Louis, 2013, Mosby.)

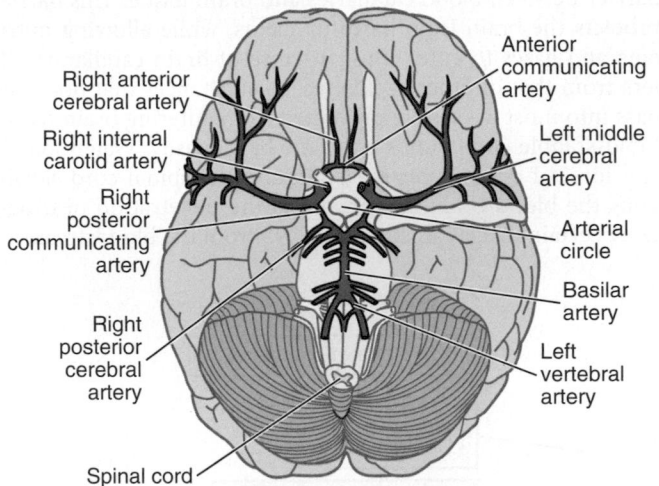

FIG. 55.11 Arteries at the base of the brain. The arteries that compose the circle of Willis are the 2 anterior cerebral arteries joined to each other by the anterior communicating cerebral artery and to the posterior cerebral arteries by the posterior communicating arteries. (Modified from Thibodeau GA, Patton KT: *Anatomy and physiology*, ed 8, St Louis, 2013, Mosby.)

Protective Structures

Meninges. The meninges consist of 3 protective membranes that surround the brain and spinal cord: the dura mater, arachnoid, and pia mater (Fig. 55.12). The thick *dura mater* forms the outermost layer. The *falx cerebri* is a fold of the dura that separates the 2 cerebral hemispheres. It slows expansion of brain tissue in conditions such as a rapidly growing tumor or acute hemorrhage. The *tentorium cerebelli* is a fold of dura that separates the cerebral hemispheres from the posterior fossa (which contains the brainstem and cerebellum).

The *arachnoid* layer is a fragile, web-like membrane that lies between the dura mater and *pia mater* (the vascular innermost layer of the meninges). The area between the arachnoid layer and pia mater *(subarachnoid space)* is filled with CSF. Structures such as arteries, veins, and cranial nerves passing to and from the brain and skull must pass through the subarachnoid space. A larger subarachnoid space in the region of the third and fourth lumbar vertebrae is the area used to obtain CSF during a lumbar puncture.

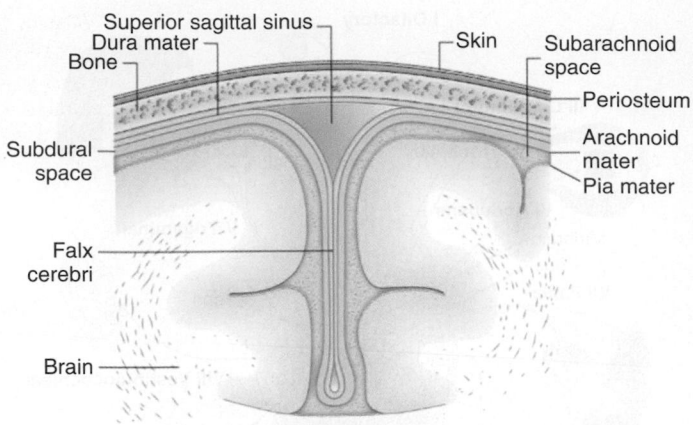

FIG. 55.12 Meninges.

Skull. The *skull* protects the brain from external trauma. It is composed of 8 cranial bones and 14 facial bones. Although the top and sides of the inside of the skull are fairly smooth, the bottom surface is uneven. It has many ridges, prominences, and foramina (holes through which blood vessels and nerves enter the intracranial vault). The largest hole is the *foramen magnum*, through which the brainstem extends to the spinal cord. The foramen magnum is the only major space for the expansion of brain contents when increased intracranial pressure occurs.

Vertebral Column. The *vertebral column* protects the spinal cord, supports the head, and provides flexibility. The vertebral column is made up of 33 individual vertebrae: 7 cervical, 12 thoracic, 5 lumbar, 5 sacral (fused into 1), and 4 coccygeal (fused into 1). Each vertebra has a central opening through which the spinal cord passes. A series of ligaments holds the vertebrae together. Intervertebral discs occupy the spaces between vertebrae, allowing movement of the column. Fig. 55.13 shows the natural curvature of the spinal column and its relation to the trunk.

Gerontologic Considerations: Effects of Aging on Nervous System

Aging affects several parts of the nervous system. In the CNS, the gradual loss of neurons in certain areas of the brainstem, cerebellum, and cerebral cortex begins in early adulthood. With loss of neurons, the ventricles widen or enlarge, brain weight decreases, cerebral blood flow decreases, and CSF production declines.

In the PNS, degenerative changes in myelin cause a decrease in nerve conduction. Coordinated neuromuscular activity, such as maintaining BP in response to changing from a lying to a standing position, is altered with aging. As a result, older adults are more likely to have orthostatic hypotension. Similarly, coordination of neuromuscular activity to maintain body temperature becomes less efficient with aging. Older adults are less able to adapt to extremes in environmental temperature and are more vulnerable to both hypothermia and hyperthermia.

Other relevant changes associated with aging include decreases in memory, vision, hearing, taste, smell, vibration, position sense, muscle strength, and reaction time. Sensory changes, including decreases in taste and smell perception, may result in decreased dietary intake in the older adult. Reduced hearing and vision can result in perceptual confusion.[5] Problems with balance and coordination can put the older adult at risk for falls.[6] Changes in assessment findings result from age-related changes in the nervous system (Table 55.2). Changes should not be attributed to aging without considering other underlying causes.

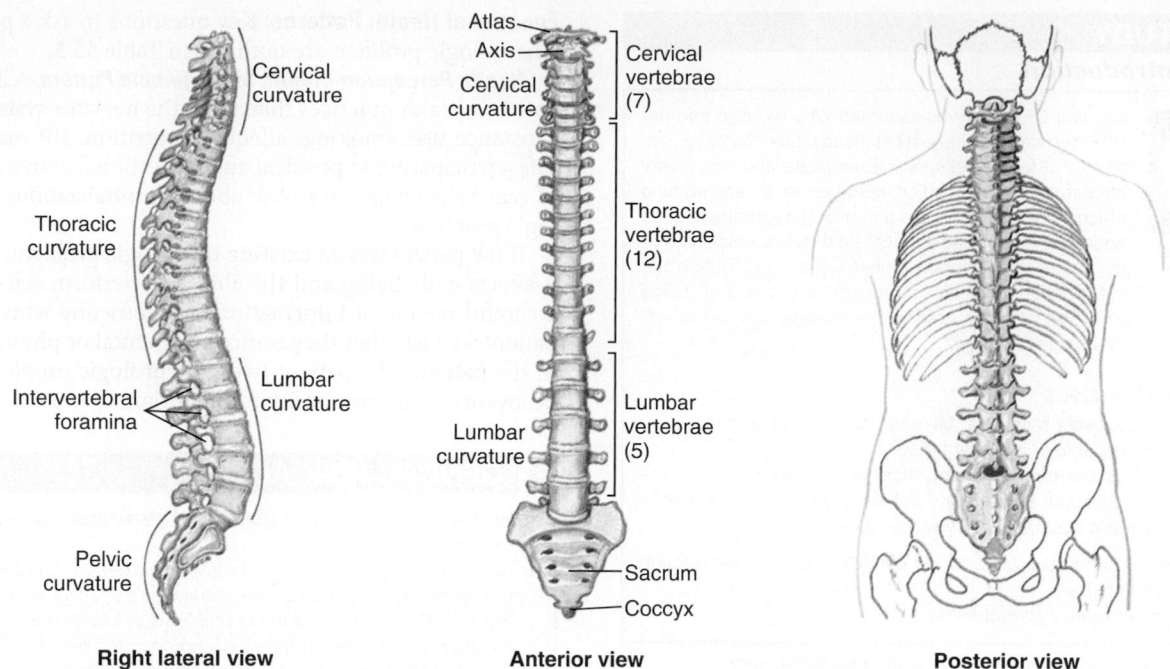

FIG. 55.13 The vertebral column (3 views). (Modified from Thibodeau GA, Patton KT: *Anatomy and physiology*, ed 8, St Louis, 2013, Mosby.)

TABLE 55.2 Gerontologic Assessment Differences

Nervous System

Component	Changes	Differences in Assessment Findings
Central Nervous System		
Brain	↓ Cerebral blood flow and metabolism Cerebral tissue atrophy and ↑ size of ventricles ↓ Efficiency of temperature-regulating mechanism ↓ Neurotransmitters, loss of neurons ↓ O$_2$ supply	• Altered balance, vertigo, syncope, ↑ postural hypotension • Changes in gait and ambulation • Changes in mental functioning • ↓ Kinesthetic sense • Impaired ability to adapt to environmental temperature • ↓ Proprioception, ↓ sensory input • Slowed conduction of nerve impulses, with slowed response time
Peripheral Nervous System		
Cranial and spinal nerves	Cell degeneration, death of neurons Loss of myelin and ↓ conduction time	• ↓ Reaction time in specific nerves • ↓ Speed and intensity of neuronal reflexes
Functional Divisions		
Motor **Sensory***	↓ Muscle bulk Atrophy of taste buds Degeneration and loss of fibers in olfactory bulb Degenerative changes in nerve cells in inner ear, cerebellum, and proprioceptive pathways ↓ Electrical activity ↓ Sensory receptors	• ↓ Strength and agility • ↓ Sense of touch, pain, and temperature • Slowing of or change in sensory reception • Signs of malnutrition, weight loss • ↓ Sense of smell • Poor ability to maintain balance, widened gait
Reflexes	↓ Deep tendon reflexes ↓ Sensory conduction velocity	• Below-average reflex score • Sluggish reflexes, slowed reaction time
Reticular Formation		
Reticular activating system	Modification of hypothalamic function ↓ Stage IV sleep	• Changes in sleep patterns
Autonomic Nervous System		
Sympathetic nervous system and parasympathetic nervous system	Morphologic features of ganglia Slowed autonomic nervous system responses	• Orthostatic hypotension, systolic hypertension

*Specific changes related to the eye are listed in Table 20.1. Specific changes related to the ear are listed in Table 21.1.

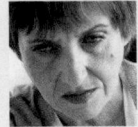
ASSESSMENT OF NERVOUS SYSTEM

Subjective Data
Important Health Information

Past Health History. When performing a neurologic examination, first determine if an emergency exists. For example, does the patient have decreasing level of consciousness? The neurologic assessment is done when an abnormality is identified during screening or can be expected based on patient history. Is the patient a reliable historian and able to give detailed information? If not, interview someone with first-hand knowledge of the patient's history and current problem. Avoid suggesting symptoms or asking leading questions.

Second, the mode of onset and course of the illness are especially important aspects of the history. Often these facts alone can reveal the nature of a neurologic disease process. Obtain all pertinent data in the history of the present illness, especially data related to the characteristics and progression of the symptoms. In some cases, the history may include birth injury (e.g., cerebral palsy from hypoxia) and/or other neurologic insults, such as a traumatic brain injury, stroke, or degenerative disease.

Growth and developmental history can be important in determining if nervous system dysfunction was present at an early age. Specifically, ask about major developmental tasks, such as walking and talking.

Medications. Obtain a careful medication history, especially the use of sedatives, opioids, tranquilizers, and mood-elevating drugs. Many other drugs can cause neurologic side effects. Ask the patient to describe the medication regimen to determine adherence to prescribed therapies.

Surgery or Other Treatments. Ask about any surgery involving any part of the nervous system, such as head, spine, or sensory organs. If a patient had surgery, determine the date, cause, procedure, recovery, and current status. Note any history of eye surgery to determine the relevance of abnormal pupil assessment.

Functional Health Patterns. Key questions to ask a patient with a neurologic problem are outlined in Table 55.3.

Health Perception–Health Management Pattern. Ask about the patient's health practices that affect the nervous system, such as substance use, smoking, adequate nutrition, BP management, safe participation in physical and recreational activities, and use of seat belts or helmets. Ask about hospitalizations for neurologic problems.

If the patient has an existing neurologic problem, assess how it affects daily living and the ability to perform self-care. After a careful review of information, ask someone who knows the patient well whether they notice any mental or physical changes in the patient. The patient with a neurologic problem may not be aware of it or may be a poor historian.

Nutritional-Metabolic Pattern. Neurologic problems can result in poor nutrition. Problems related to chewing, swallowing, facial nerve paralysis, and muscle coordination could make it difficult for the patient to ingest adequate nutrients. Certain vitamins, such as thiamine (B_1), niacin, and pyridoxine (B_6), are essential for the health of the CNS. Deficiencies in any of these can result in nonspecific problems, such as depression, apathy, neuritis, weakness, mental confusion, and irritability. Cobalamin (vitamin B_{12}) deficiency can occur in older adults, who may have problems with vitamin absorption from supplements as well as natural food sources, such as meat, fish, and poultry. Untreated, cobalamin deficiency can cause mental function decline. In the patient with brain injury, early nutritional support can markedly improve outcomes.[7]

Elimination Pattern. Bowel and bladder problems often are associated with neurologic problems, such as stroke, head injury, spinal cord injury, MS, and dementia. To plan appropriate interventions, determine if the bowel or bladder problem was present before or after the current neurologic event. Urinary retention and incontinence of urine and feces are the most common elimination problems associated with a neurologic problem or its treatment. For example, nerve root compression (as occurs in cauda equina conditions) leads to a sudden onset of incontinence. Record key details, such as number of episodes, accompanying sensations or lack of sensations, and measures to control the problem.

Activity-Exercise Pattern. Many neurologic disorders can cause problems in the patient's mobility, strength, and coordination. These problems can affect the patient's usual activity and exercise patterns and can increase the risk for falls.[6] Assess the person's activities of daily living because neurologic diseases can affect the ability to perform motor tasks, which increases the risk for injury.

Sleep-Rest Pattern. Sleep pattern changes can be both a cause and a response to neurologic problems. Pain and reduced ability to change position because of muscle weakness and paralysis

TABLE 55.3 Health History

Nervous System

Health Perception–Health Management
- What are your usual daily activities?
- Do you use alcohol, tobacco, or recreational drugs?*
- What safety practices do you follow in a car? On a motorcycle? On a bicycle?
- Do you have hypertension? If so, how is it managed?
- Have you ever been hospitalized for a neurologic problem?*
- Do you take any medication to manage neurologic problems? If so, what?

Nutritional-Metabolic
- Are you able to feed yourself?
- Do you have any problems getting adequate nutrition because of chewing or swallowing difficulties, facial nerve paralysis, or poor muscle coordination?*
- Give a 24-hr dietary recall.

Elimination
- Do you have incontinence of your bowels or bladder?*
- Do you ever have problems with urinary hesitancy, urgency, retention?*
- Do you postpone your bowel movements?*

Activity-Exercise
- Describe any problems you have with usual activities and exercise because of a neurologic problem.
- Do you have weakness or lack of coordination?*
- Are you able to perform your personal hygiene needs alone?*

Sleep-Rest
- Describe your sleep pattern.
- When you have trouble sleeping, what do you do?

Cognitive-Perceptual
- Have you noticed any changes in your memory?*
- Do you have dizziness, heat or cold sensitivity, numbness, or tingling?*
- Do you have chronic pain?*
- Do you have any problem with verbal or written communication?*
- Have you noticed any changes in vision or hearing?*

Self-Perception–Self-Concept
- How do you feel about yourself, about who you are?
- Describe your general emotional pattern.

Role-Relationship
- Have you had changes in roles such as spouse, parent, or breadwinner?*

Sexuality-Reproductive
- Are you dissatisfied with your sexual function?*
- Are problems related to your sexual function causing tension in an important relationship?*
- Do you feel the need for professional counseling related to your sexual function?*

Coping–Stress Tolerance
- Describe your usual coping pattern.
- Do you think your present coping pattern is adequate to meet the stressors of your life?*
- What needs are unmet by your current support system?

Value-Belief
- Describe any culturally specific beliefs and attitudes that may influence your care.

*If yes, describe.

could interfere with sleep quality. Hallucinations resulting from dementia or drugs can interrupt sleep. Carefully assess and record the patient's sleep pattern and bedtime routines.

Cognitive-Perceptual Pattern. Because the nervous system controls cognition and sensory integration, many neurologic problems affect these functions. Consider culture, age, and education when assessing communication because they play a role in our interaction with others. Assess memory, language, calculation ability, problem-solving ability, insight, and judgment. Ask the patient hypothetical questions such as, "What is a reasonable price for a cup of coffee?" or "What would you do if you saw a car crash outside your house?" Consider if the patient's plans and goals match the physical and mental capabilities. Note the presence of factors affecting intellectual capacity, such as cognitive impairment, hallucinations, delusions, and dementia.

Assess a person's ability to use and understand language. Appropriateness of responses is a useful indicator of cognitive and perceptual ability. Determine the patient's understanding and ability to carry out needed treatments. Neurologic-related cognitive changes can interfere with the patient's understanding of the disease and adherence to related treatment.

Pain is common with many neurologic problems and is often the reason a patient seeks care. Carefully assess the patient's pain. (Pain and pain assessment are discussed in Chapter 8.)

Self-Perception–Self-Concept Pattern. Neurologic diseases can drastically change a patient's control over life and create dependency on others for meeting daily needs. The patient's physical appearance and emotional control can be affected. Sensitively ask about the patient's evaluation of self-worth, perception of abilities, body image, and general emotional pattern.

Role-Relationship Pattern. Physical impairments, such as weakness and paralysis, can alter or limit participation in usual roles and activities. Cognitive changes can permanently alter a person's ability to maintain previous roles. These changes can dramatically affect the patient and caregiver. Ask the patient if a role change has occurred (e.g., spouse or breadwinner) because of neurologic problems and determine how long it has lasted. Caregivers should take part in decision making when neurologic deficits prevent the patient from decisions that will affect the role.

Sexuality-Reproductive Pattern. Assess the person's ability to take part in sexual activity. Many neurologic disorders can affect sexual response. Cerebral lesions may inhibit the desire phase or the reflex responses of the excitement phase. The hypothalamus stimulates the pituitary gland to release hormones that influence sexual desire. Brainstem and spinal cord lesions may partially or completely interrupt the desire or ability to have intercourse. Neuropathies and spinal cord lesions may prevent reflex activities of the sexual response or affect sensation and decrease desire. Despite neurologically related changes in sexual function, many persons can achieve satisfying expression of intimacy and affection.

Coping–Stress Tolerance Pattern. The physical sequelae of a neurologic problem can strain a patient's coping ability. Often the problem is chronic, and the patient must learn new coping skills. Assess if the patient's coping skills are adequate to deal with the stress of this problem. Also assess the patient's support system.

Value-Belief Pattern. Many neurologic problems have serious, long-term, life-changing effects. Determine what these effects are because they can strain the patient's belief system. Assess if any religious or cultural beliefs could affect the treatment plan.

CASE STUDY—cont'd

Subjective Data

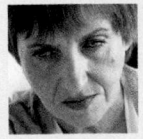

(© TatyanaGl/ iStock/ Thinkstock.)

After her admission to the hospital, a subjective assessment of J.K. revealed the following information:
Past Medical History: No history of seizures, migraine, or other headache prior to the current headaches and seizure.
Medications: lisinopril 10 mg PO daily.
Health Perception–Health Management: Never smoked. Occasional social alcohol use. Reports good health other than mild hypertension.
Nutritional-Metabolic: J.K. is 5 ft, 5 in tall; weight 145 lb.
Activity-Exercise: Moderate activity. No formal exercise or participation in sports.
Cognitive-Perceptual: Says her headaches led her to get her eyes tested. Has had only minor decrease in visual acuity.
Coping–Stress Tolerance: Is depressed and fearful. She is worried that something serious is wrong. Denies dizziness, change in hearing, or memory deficits.

Discussion Questions

1. Which subjective assessment findings are of most concern to you?
2. Based on these subjective assessment findings, what should be included in the physical assessment?

You will learn more about the physical examination of the neurologic system in the next section.
(See p. 1293 for more information on J.K.)

Answers available at http://evolve.elsevier.com/Lewis/medsurg.

Objective Data

Physical Examination. The standard neurologic examination helps determine the presence, location, and nature of nervous system disease (Fig. 55.14). The examination assesses 6 categories of function: mental status, cranial nerve function, motor function, sensory function, cerebellar function, and reflexes.[8] Develop a consistent pattern of completing the neurologic examination to remember to include each element for every patient examination.

Mental Status. Assessment of mental status (cerebral function) gives a general impression of how the patient is functioning. It involves determining complex and high-level cerebral functions governed by many areas of the cerebral cortex. Complete most of the mental status examination during your interaction with the patient. For example, assess language and memory when asking the patient for details of the illness and significant past events. Consider the patient's age, cultural background, and level of education when evaluating mental status.

The components of the mental status examination include:

- *General appearance and behavior:* This includes level of consciousness (awake, asleep, comatose), motor activity, body posture, dress and hygiene, facial expression, and speech pattern. This assessment begins when you first see the patient. A patient who has deficits in self-care as shown by poor grooming is more likely to have other cognitive deficits.

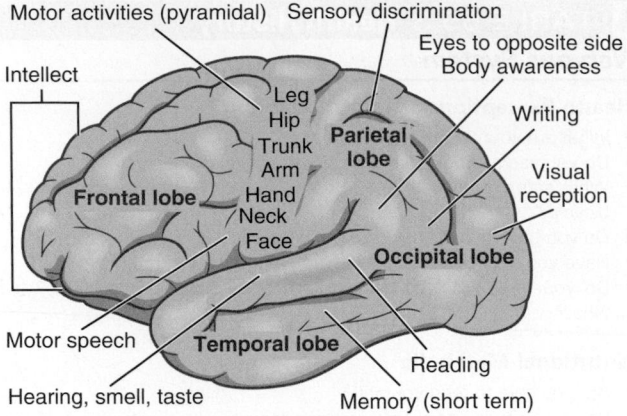

FIG. 55.14 Each area of the brain controls a particular activity.

- *Cognition:* Note orientation to time, place, person, and situation, as well as memory, general knowledge, insight, judgment, problem solving, and calculation. Common questions are "Who were the last 3 presidents?" "What do people use to cut paper?" "Can you count backward from 100 by 7s?"[8] Often a structured mental status questionnaire is used to evaluate these functions and provide baseline data for evaluating changes over time. Common tools include the Mini-Mental State Examination (MMSE) (see Table 59.10) and Montreal Cognitive Assessment (MoCA).[9] Delirium is an acute and transient disorder of cognition that can be seen at any time during a patient's illness. As discussed in Chapter 59, delirium is often an early indicator of various illnesses (see Table 59.16). The Confusion Assessment Method tool is used to assess for delirium (see Table 59.18).
- *Mood and affect:* Note any agitation, anger, depression, or euphoria, and the appropriateness of these states. Use suitable questions to reveal the patient's feelings.

Cranial Nerves. Testing each CN is an essential part of the neurologic examination (Table 55.4).

Olfactory nerve. Chronic rhinitis, sinusitis, and heavy smoking may decrease the sense of smell. Problems with the ability to smell may be associated with a tumor involving the olfactory bulb or the result of a basilar skull fracture that has damaged the olfactory fibers as they pass through the delicate cribriform plate of the skull. *Anosmia* (loss of sense of smell) is an early sign in Parkinson's disease and Alzheimer's disease.[10]

Optic nerve. Visual field defects may arise from lesions of the optic nerve, optic chiasm, or tracts that extend through the temporal, parietal, or occipital lobes. Visual field changes resulting from brain lesions include *hemianopsia* (half of the visual field is affected), *quadrantanopia* (one fourth of the visual field is affected), *bitemporal hemianopsia* (bilateral peripheral vision is affected), or monocular vision. It may be hard to test acuity if the patient does not read English or is aphasic.

Oculomotor, trochlear, and abducens nerves. Because the oculomotor (CN III), trochlear (CN IV), and abducens (CN VI) nerves help move the eye, they are tested together (Table 55.4). With weakness or paralysis of an eye muscle, the eyes do not move together, and the patient has a *disconjugate gaze.* Note the presence and direction of *nystagmus* (fine, rapid jerking movements of the eyes), even though this condition most often indicates vestibulocerebellar problems.

TABLE 55.4 Cranial Nerves

Function and Assessment

Nerve	Function	Assessment
I Olfactory	*Sensory:* from olfactory (smell)	Ask patient to close 1 nostril at a time and identify easily recognized odors (e.g., coffee). Any asymmetry in sense of smell is important.
II Optic	*Sensory:* from retina of eyes (vision)	Examine each eye independently. *Visual fields:* Position yourself opposite the patient. Ask him or her to look directly at the bridge of your nose and indicate when an object (finger, pencil tip) presented from the periphery of each of the visual fields is seen (Fig. 55.15). *Visual acuity:* Ask patient to read a Snellen chart. Record the number on the lowest line the patient can read with 50% accuracy. The patient who wears glasses should wear them during testing unless they are used only for close reading. If a Snellen chart is not available, ask the patient to read newsprint for gross assessment of acuity. Record the distance from patient to newsprint needed for accurate reading.
III Oculomotor	*Motor:* to 4 eye movement muscles and levator palpebrae muscle *Parasympathetic:* smooth muscle in eyeball	Ask the person to hold the head steady and to follow the movement of your finger, pen, or penlight only with the eyes. Hold the target back about 12 inches so that the person can focus on it comfortably. Move the target to each of the 6 positions (right and up, right, right and down, left and up, left, left and down), hold it momentarily, and then move back to center. Progress clockwise. A normal response is parallel tracking of the object with both eyes. Check for pupillary constriction and *accommodation* (pupils constricting with near vision). To test pupillary constriction, shine a light into the pupil of 1 eye; look for ipsilateral constriction of the same pupil and contralateral (consensual) constriction of the opposite eye. Note the size and shape of the pupils. The optic nerve must be intact for this reflex to occur.
IV Trochlear	*Motor:* to 1 eye movement muscle, the superior oblique muscle	See testing for CN III. Because the oculomotor (CN III), trochlear (CN IV), and abducens (CN VI) nerves help move the eye, they are tested together.
V Trigeminal		
• Ophthalmic branch	*Sensory:* from forehead, eye, superior nasal cavity	*Sensory:* Have patient close eyes and identify light touch (cotton wisp) and pinprick in each of the 3 divisions (ophthalmic, maxillary, and mandibular) of nerve on both sides of face.
• Maxillary branch	*Sensory:* from inferior nasal cavity, face, upper teeth, mucosa of superior mouth	*Motor:* Ask patient to clench teeth and then palpate masseter muscles just above the mandibular angle. Muscles should feel equally strong on both sides.
• Mandibular branch	*Sensory:* from surfaces of jaw, lower teeth, mucosa of lower mouth, and anterior tongue *Motor:* to muscles of mastication	*Corneal (blink) reflex:* Evaluates CN V and CN VII simultaneously. Sensory component (corneal sensation) is innervated by the ophthalmic division of CN V. The motor component (eye blink) is innervated by the facial nerve (CN VII). Have patient look up and away. Then from the other side, lightly touch the cornea with cotton wisp. Look for normal blink reaction of both eyes. Repeat on other side.
VI Abducens	*Motor:* to the lateral rectus muscle of the eye (1 eye movement)	See testing for CN III. Because CN III, CN IV, and CN VI nerves help move the eye, they are tested together.
VII Facial	*Motor:* to facial muscles of expression and cheek muscle *Sensory:* taste from anterior two thirds of tongue	Ask patient to raise eyebrows, close eyes tightly, purse lips, draw back the corners of mouth in an exaggerated smile, and frown. Note any asymmetry in the facial movements because this can indicate damage to nerve.
VIII Vestibulocochlear		
• Vestibular branch	*Sensory:* from equilibrium sensory organ (vestibular apparatus)	Not routinely tested unless the patient has dizziness, vertigo, unsteadiness, or auditory dysfunction.
• Cochlear branch	*Sensory:* from auditory sensory organ (cochlea), hearing	Have patient close eyes and indicate when they hear the rustling of your fingertips. For more precise assessment of hearing, perform the Weber and Rinne tests or use an audiometer (see Table 21.6).
IX Glossopharyngeal	*Sensory:* from pharynx and posterior tongue, including taste *Motor:* to superior pharyngeal muscles	The glossopharyngeal and vagus nerves (CN IX and CN X) are tested together because both innervate the pharynx. To test the gag reflex, touch the sides of the posterior pharynx or soft palate with a tongue blade. If the reflex is weak or absent, the patient is in danger of aspirating food or secretions. Another test for the awake, cooperative patient is to ask the patient to say "ah," and note the bilateral symmetry of elevation of the soft palate. If a patient has an endotracheal tube, the cough reflex (elicited when the suction catheter contacts the *carina* of the respiratory tree) is a method of assessing the vagus nerve.
X Vagus	*Sensory:* from much of viscera of thorax and abdomen *Motor:* to larynx and middle and inferior pharyngeal muscles *Parasympathetic:* to heart, lungs, most of digestive system	See testing for CN IX. The glossopharyngeal and vagus nerves (CN IX and CN X) are tested together because both innervate the pharynx.
XI Accessory	*Motor:* to sternocleidomastoid and trapezius muscles	Ask patient to shrug the shoulders and to turn head to either side against resistance. Sternocleidomastoid and trapezius muscles should contract smoothly. Note symmetry, atrophy, or fasciculation of muscle.
XII Hypoglossal	*Motor:* to muscles of tongue	Ask to protrude tongue, which should protrude in midline. Next ask the patient to move the tongue up and down and side to side. Finally, the patient should be able to push the tongue to either side against the resistance of a tongue blade. Note any asymmetry, atrophy, or fasciculation.

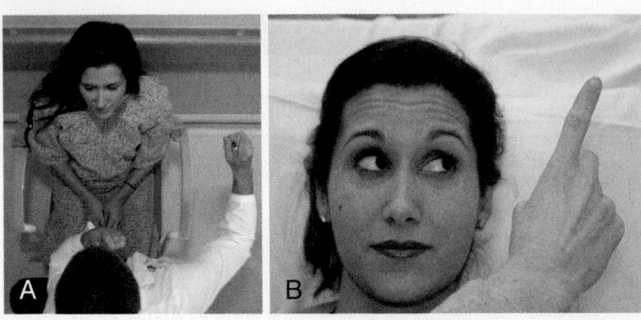

FIG. 55.15 A, Nurse checking visual fields. B, Nurse checking extraocular movement (EOM). (Courtesy DaiWai Olson, RN, PhD, CCRN, Dallas, TX.)

Because the oculomotor nerve exits at the top of the brainstem at the tentorial notch, it can be compressed easily by expanding mass lesions. When this occurs, sympathetic input to the pupil is unopposed; the pupil changes shape and becomes dilated. The lack of pupillary constriction is an early sign of central herniation (see Chapter 56).

Two abbreviations we often used to record the reaction of the pupils are *PERRL* (*P*upils are *E*qual [in size], *R*ound, and *R*eactive to *L*ight) and *PERRLA* (*P*upils are *E*qual, *R*ound, and *R*eactive to *L*ight and *A*ccommodation). The *PERRL* abbreviation is appropriate when accommodation cannot be assessed, as in an unconscious patient. Convergence and accommodation are tested by having the patient focus on the examiner's finger as it moves toward the patient's nose.

Another function of the oculomotor nerve is to keep the eyelid open. Damage to the nerve can cause *ptosis* (drooping eyelid), pupillary abnormalities, and eye muscle weakness.

Motor System. The motor system examination includes assessment of strength, tone, coordination, and symmetry of the major muscle groups. Test muscle strength by asking the patient to push and pull against the resistance of your arm as it opposes flexion and extension of the patient's muscle. Ask the patient to offer resistance at the shoulders, elbows, wrists, hips, knees, and ankles. Mild weakness of the arm is demonstrated by downward drifting of the arm or pronation of the palm (*pronator drift*). The pronator drift test is especially sensitive when the patient has a potential for vasospasm or increasing edema in 1 hemisphere of the cerebrum. Ask the patient to close the eyes and hold the arms out with palms facing up (like they are holding a large pizza). The patient should hold this position for 30 seconds. Downward drift with palm pronation indicates a problem in the opposite motor cortex. Note any weakness or asymmetry of strength between the same muscle groups of the right and left sides.

Test muscle tone by passively moving the limbs through their range of motion. You should identify a slight resistance to these movements. Abnormal tone is described as *hypotonia* (flaccidity) or *hypertonia* (spasticity). Note any involuntary movements, such as tics, tremor, *myoclonus* (spasm of muscles), *athetosis* (slow, writhing, involuntary movements of extremities), *chorea* (involuntary, purposeless, rapid motions), and *dystonia* (impairment of muscle tone).

Test cerebellar function by assessing balance and coordination. A good screening test for both balance and muscle strength is to observe the patient's stature (posture while standing) and gait. Note the pace and rhythm of the gait. Observe for normal symmetric and oppositional arm swing. The patient's ability to ambulate helps to determine the level of nursing care needed and the risk for falling.

The finger-to-nose test (having the patient alternately touch the nose, then touch the examiner's finger) and the heel-to-shin test (having the patient stroke the heel of 1 foot up and down the shin of the opposite leg) assess coordination and cerebellar function. Reposition your finger while the patient is touching the nose so that the patient must adjust to a new distance each time your finger is touched. These movements should be performed smoothly and accurately. Other tests include asking the patient to pronate and supinate both hands rapidly and to do a shallow knee bend, first on 1 leg and then on the other. Note dysarthria or slurred speech because it is a sign of incoordination of the speech muscles.

Sensory System. In the somatic sensory examination, several modalities are tested. Each modality is carried by a specific ascending pathway in the spinal cord before it reaches the sensory cortex. As a rule, perform the examination with the patient's eyes closed and avoid providing the patient with clues. Ask "How does this feel?" rather than "Is this sharp?" In the routine neurologic examination, sensory testing of the anterior torso, posterior torso, and all extremities is sufficient. However, if a problem is identified in sensory function, the boundaries of that dysfunction should be carefully delineated along the dermatome.

Touch, pain, and temperature. Light touch is usually tested first using a cotton wisp or light pinprick. Gently touch each extremity and ask the patient to indicate when they feel the stimulus. Test pain by alternately touching the skin with the sharp and dull end of a pin. Tell the patient to respond "sharp" or "dull." Evaluate each limb separately.

Extinction is assessed by simultaneously touching both sides of the body symmetrically. Normally, the simultaneous stimuli are both perceived (sensed). An abnormal response occurs when the patient perceives the stimulus on only 1 side. The other stimulus is *extinguished*.

Test the sensation of temperature by applying tubes of warm and cold water to the skin and asking the patient to identify the stimuli with the eyes closed. If pain sensation is intact, you do not have to assess temperature sensation because the same ascending pathways carry both sensations.

Vibration sense. Assess vibration sense by applying a vibrating tuning fork to the fingernails and bony prominences of the hands, legs, and feet. Ask the patient if the vibration or "buzz" is felt. Then ask the patient to indicate when the vibration ceases.

Position sense. Assess position sense (*proprioception*) by placing your thumb and forefinger on either side of the patient's forefinger or great toe and gently moving his or her digit up or down. Ask the patient to close the eyes and state the direction in which the digit is moved.

Another test of proprioception is the Romberg test. Ask the patient to stand with feet together and then close his or her eyes. If the patient can maintain balance with the eyes open but sways or falls with the eyes closed (i.e., a positive Romberg test), vestibulocochlear dysfunction or disease in the posterior columns of the spinal cord may be present. Be aware of patient safety during this test.

Cortical sensory functions. Several tests evaluate cortical integration of sensory perceptions (which occurs in the parietal lobes). Explain these tests to the patient before performing

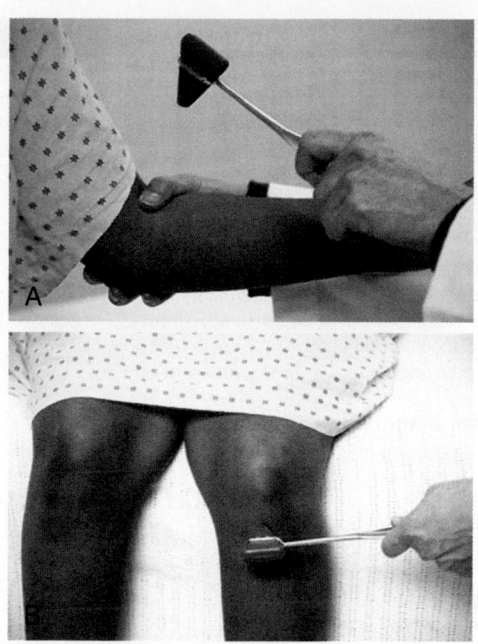

FIG. 55.16 The examiner strikes a swift blow over a stretched tendon to elicit a stretch reflex. **A,** Biceps reflex. **B,** Patellar reflex.

them, while his or her eyes are still open. Assess *two-point discrimination* by placing the 2 points of a calibrated compass on the tips of the fingers and toes. The minimum recognizable separation is 4 to 5 mm in the fingertips and a greater degree of separation elsewhere. This test is important in diagnosing diseases of the sensory cortex and PNS.

Test *graphesthesia* (ability to feel writing on skin) by having the patient identify numbers traced on the palm of the hands. Test *stereognosis* (ability to perceive the form and nature of objects) by having the patient close the eyes and identify the size and shape of easily recognized objects (e.g., coins, keys, safety pin) placed in the hands.

Reflexes. Tendons have receptors that are sensitive to stretch. A reflex contraction of the skeletal muscle occurs when the tendon is stretched. In general, we test the biceps, triceps, brachioradialis, patellar, and Achilles tendon reflexes. Initiate a simple muscle stretch reflex by briskly tapping the tendon of a stretched muscle, usually with a reflex hammer (Fig. 55.16). Measure the response (muscle contraction of the corresponding muscle) on a 0 to 5 scale as follows: 0 = absent reflex; 1 = weak response, seen only with reinforcement; 2 = normal response; 3 = brisk response; 4 = hyperreflexia with nonsustained clonus; and 5 = hyperreflexia with sustained clonus. *Clonus,* an abnormal response, is a continued rhythmic contraction of the muscle with continuous application of the stimulus.

Elicit the *biceps reflex,* with the patient's arm partially flexed and palm up, by placing your thumb over the biceps tendon in the antecubital space and striking the thumb with a hammer. The normal response is flexion of the arm at the elbow or contraction of the biceps muscle that you can feel with your thumb.

Elicit the *triceps reflex* by striking the triceps tendon above the elbow while the patient's arm is flexed. The normal response is extension of the arm or visible contraction of the triceps.

Elicit the *brachioradialis reflex* by striking the radius 3 to 5 cm above the wrist while the patient's arm is relaxed. The normal response is flexion and supination at the elbow or visible contraction of the brachioradialis muscle.

Elicit the *patellar reflex* by striking the patellar tendon just below the patella. The patient can be sitting or lying as long as the leg being tested hangs freely. The normal response is extension of the leg with contraction of the quadriceps.

Gently dorsiflex the patient's foot at the ankle. Elicit the *Achilles tendon reflex* by striking the Achilles tendon while the patient's leg is flexed at the knee. The normal response is plantar flexion at the ankle.

A *focused assessment* is used to evaluate the status of previously identified neurologic problems and to monitor for signs of new problems. A focused assessment of the neurologic system is shown in the box on p. 1294.

Table 55.5 is an example of a normal neurologic physical assessment. Abnormal assessment findings of the neurologic system are shown in Table 55.6.

CASE STUDY—cont'd
Objective Data: Physical Examination

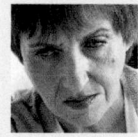

A physical assessment of J.K. reveals the following:
- BP 145/80, HR 78, RR 20, T 37° C
- Alert, oriented, and appropriate, but anxious
- Strength 5/5 on all extremities
- Visual field deficits in upper left quadrant of visual field

(© TatyanaGl/ iStock/ Thinkstock.)

Discussion Questions

1. Which physical assessment findings are of most concern to you?
2. Based on the results of the subjective and physical assessment, what diagnostic studies do you think may be ordered for J.K.?

You will learn more about diagnostic studies related to the neurologic system in the next section.

(See p. 1298 for more information on J.K.)

Answers available at *http://evolve.elsevier.com/Lewis/medsurg.*

DIAGNOSTIC STUDIES OF NERVOUS SYSTEM

Many diagnostic studies are available to assess the nervous system (Tables 55.7, 55.8, 55.9, and 55.10). CSF analysis provides information about a variety of CNS diseases. Normal CSF is clear, colorless, odorless, and free of red blood cells. It contains little protein. Normal CSF values are listed in Table 55.7. CSF may be obtained through lumbar puncture (LP) or, on occasion, ventriculostomy.

During LP, the HCP aspirates CSF through a needle inserted into the L3-4 or L4-5 interspace. A manometer attached to the needle is used to obtain CSF pressure. CSF is withdrawn in a series of tubes and sent for analysis. LP is contraindicated in the presence of increased intracranial pressure because of the risk for downward herniation from CSF removal or if there is infection at the intended puncture site. Nursing care of the patient undergoing LP is outlined in Table 55.8.

Biopsies of nerve, muscle, brain, and arterial tissues are useful in diagnosing several disorders (e.g., tumors, infectious disease, degenerative diseases, temporal artery for arteritis). A brain biopsy is usually done using a stereotactic procedure.

TABLE 55.5 Normal Physical Assessment of Nervous System*

Parameter	Findings
Mental status	• Alert and oriented, orderly thought processes. • Appropriate mood and affect.
Cranial nerves†	• Smell intact to soap or coffee. • Visual fields full to confrontation. • Intact extraocular movements. • No nystagmus. Pupils equal, round, reactive to light and accommodation. • Intact facial sensation to light touch and pinprick. • Facial movements full. • Hearing intact bilaterally. • Intact gag and swallow reflexes. Symmetric smile. Midline protrusion of tongue. • Full strength with head turning and shoulder shrugging.
Motor system	• Normal gait and station. Normal tandem walk. Negative Romberg test. • Normal and symmetric muscle bulk, tone, and strength. • Smooth performance of finger-nose, heel-shin movements.
Sensory system	• Intact sensation to light touch, position sense, pinprick, heat, and cold.
Reflexes‡	• Biceps, triceps, brachioradialis, patellar, and Achilles tendon reflexes 2/5 bilaterally. • Toes pointed down with plantar stimulation.

*If some part of the neurologic examination was not done, this should be indicated (e.g., "Smell not tested").
†May be recorded as "CN I to XII intact."
‡May also be recorded as drawing of stick figure showing reflex strength at appropriate sites.

FOCUSED ASSESSMENT
Nervous System

Use this checklist to make sure the key assessment steps have been done.

Subjective
Ask the patient about any of the following and note responses.

Blackouts/loss of memory	Y	N
Weakness, numbness, tingling in arms or legs	Y	N
Headaches, especially new onset	Y	N
Loss of balance/coordination	Y	N
Orientation to person, place, time, and situation	Y	N

Objective: Diagnostic
Check the following diagnostic results for critical values.

Lumbar puncture	✓
CT or MRI of brain	✓
EEG	✓

Objective: Physical Examination
Inspect/Observe

General level of consciousness/orientation	✓
Oropharynx for gag reflex and soft palate movement	✓
Peripheral sensation of light touch and pinprick (face, hands, feet)	✓
Smell with coffee or soap	✓
Eyes for extraocular movements, PERRLA, peripheral vision, nystagmus	✓
Gait for smoothness and coordination	✓

Palpate

Strength of neck, shoulders, arms, and legs for fullness and symmetry	✓

Percuss

Reflexes	✓

TABLE 55.6 Assessment Abnormalities

Nervous System

Finding	Description	Possible Etiology and Significance
Cranial Nerves		
Dysphagia	Difficulty in swallowing	Lesions involving motor pathways of CN IX and CN X (including lower brainstem)
Ophthalmoplegia	Paralysis of eye muscles	Lesions in brainstem
Eyes		
Anisocoria	Inequality of pupil size	Oculomotor nerve injury Sympathetic pathway injury
Diplopia	Double vision	Lesions affecting nerves of extraocular muscles, cerebellar damage
Homonymous hemianopsia	Loss of vision in one side of visual field	Lesions in the contralateral occipital lobe
Papilledema	"Choked disc," swelling of optic nerve head	Increased intracranial pressure
Mental Status		
Altered consciousness	Stuporous, mute, ↓ response to verbal cues or pain	Intracranial lesions, metabolic disorder, psychiatric disorders
Anosognosia	Inability to recognize bodily defect or disease	Lesions in right parietal cortex
Motor System		
Apraxia	Inability to perform learned movements despite having desire and physical ability to perform them	Cerebral cortex lesion
Ataxia	Lack of coordination of movement	Lesions of sensory or motor pathways, cerebellum Antiseizure drugs, sedatives, hypnotic drug toxicity (including alcohol)

TABLE 55.6 **Assessment Abnormalities**

Nervous System—cont'd

Finding	Description	Possible Etiology and Significance
Dyskinesia	Impairment of voluntary movement, resulting in fragmentary or incomplete movements	Disorders of basal ganglia, idiosyncratic reaction to psychotropic drugs
Hemiplegia	Paralysis on 1 side	Stroke and other lesions involving contralateral motor cortex
Nystagmus	Jerking or bobbing of eyes as they track moving object	Lesions in cerebellum, brainstem, vestibular system
		Antiseizure drugs, sedatives, hypnotic toxicity (including alcohol)
Reflexes		
Deep tendon reflexes	↓ or absent motor response	Lower motor neuron lesions
Extensor plantar response	Toes pointing up with plantar stimulation	Suprasegmental or upper motor neuron lesion
Sensory System		
Analgesia	Loss of pain sensation	Lesion in spinothalamic tract or thalamus. Analgesic drugs
Anesthesia	Absence of sensation	Lesions in spinal cord, thalamus, sensory cortex, or peripheral sensory nerve. Anesthesia drugs
Astereognosis	Inability to recognize form of object by touch	Lesions in parietal cortex
Paresthesia	Abnormal sensation, such as numbness or tingling	Lesions in the posterior column or sensory cortex
Speech		
Aphasia, dysphasia	Loss of or impaired language faculty (comprehension, expression, or both)	Left cerebral cortex lesion
Dysarthria	Lack of coordination in articulating speech	Cerebellar or cranial nerve lesion
		Antiseizure drugs, sedatives, hypnotic drug toxicity (including alcohol)
Spinal Cord		
Bladder dysfunction		
• Atonic (autonomous)	Absence of muscle tone and contractility, enlargement of capacity, no sensation of discomfort, overflow with large residual, inability to voluntarily empty	Early stage of spinal cord injury
• Hypertonic	↑ Muscle tone, ↓ capacity, reflex emptying, dribbling, incontinence	Lesions in pyramidal tracts (efferent pathways)
• Hypotonic	More ability than atonic bladder but less than normal	Interruption of afferent pathways from bladder
Paraplegia	Paralysis of lower extremities	Spinal cord transection or mass lesion (thoracolumbar region)
Tetraplegia (quadriplegia)	Paralysis of all extremities	Spinal cord transection or mass lesion (cervical region)

TABLE 55.7 **Cerebrospinal Fluid Analysis**

Parameter	Normal Value
Specific gravity	1.007
pH	7.35
Appearance	Clear, colorless
Red blood cells (RBCs)	None
White blood cells (WBCs)	0–5 cells/μL (0–5 × 10^6 cells/L)
Protein	
• Lumbar	15–45 mg/dL (0.15–0.45 g/L)
• Cisternal	15–25 mg/dL (0.15–0.25 g/L)
• Ventricular	5–15 mg/dL (0.05–0.15 g/L)
Glucose	40–70 mg/dL (2.2–3.9 mmol/L)
Microorganisms	None
Pressure	60–150 mm H_2O

TABLE 55.8 Nursing Management

Care of the Patient Undergoing Lumbar Puncture

Preprocedure	Postprocedure
• Obtain vital signs and a baseline neurologic assessment. Notify HCP of signs of increased intracranial pressure.	• Monitor neurologic signs and vital signs. Monitor for headache intensity and drainage from the puncture site.
• Assess coagulation studies to reduce the risk for epidural hematoma.	• Apply pressure and a pressure dressing to the puncture site.
• Teach patient and caregiver about procedure. Tell the patient they may feel temporary, sharp pain or tingling radiating down the leg as a sterile needle is passed between 2 lumbar vertebrae.	• Keep the patient in a reclining position for 1 hour or up to several hours to decrease the risk for spinal headache. The patient may to turn from side to side as long as the head is not raised.
• Give sedative and analgesia, as ordered.	• Ensure proper labeling of CSF specimens and send to laboratory.
• Have patient void.	• Teach the patient to report numbness, tingling, and movement of the extremities; pain at the injection site; and the inability to void.
• Place patient in a side-lying position.	• Encourage fluids with a straw to replace the CSF that was removed.
	• Give ordered analgesia, as needed.

TABLE 55.9 Radiologic Studies

Nervous System

Study	Description and Purpose	Nursing Responsibility
Cerebral angiography	Serial x-ray visualization of intracranial and extracranial blood vessels done to detect vascular lesions (aneurysms, hematomas, arteriovenous malformations) and brain tumors (Fig. 55.17). Catheter is inserted into the femoral (sometimes brachial) artery and passed through the aortic arch into the base of a carotid or a vertebral artery for injection of contrast medium. Timed-sequence radiographic images are obtained as contrast flows through arteries, smaller vessels, and veins.	*Before:* Assess patient for stroke risk because thrombi may be dislodged during procedure. May need to be NPO. *During:* Warn patient that contrast injection may cause a feeling of being warm and flushed. Patient must lie completely still during scan. *After:* Monitor neurologic signs and VS every 15–30 min for first 2 hr, every hour for next 6 hr, then every 2 hr for 24 hr. Maintain bed rest for 6 hr (1 hr if a closure device is used). Assess for bleeding. Report any neurologic status changes.
CT scan	Provides a rapid means of obtaining radiographic images of the brain (Fig. 55.18, *A*). Computer-assisted x-ray of multiple cross sections of body parts to detect problems such as hemorrhage, tumor, cyst, edema, infarction, brain atrophy, and other abnormalities. Contrast medium may be used to enhance visualization of brain structures.	*Before:* Evaluate renal function before contrast medium used. Assess if patient is allergic to shellfish since the contrast is iodine based. Patient may need to be NPO 4 hr prior. If the patient is taking metformin, hold it the day of the test to prevent hypoglycemia or acidosis. *During:* Warn patient that contrast injection may cause a feeling of being warm and flushed. Patient must lie completely still during scan. *After:* Encourage patient to drink fluids to avoid renal problems with any contrast.
• CT angiography (CTA)	Noninvasive imaging of vascular system (e.g., aneurysms). Evaluates blood volume, flow, and mean transit time as a measure of perfusion. Has fewer complications than cerebral angiography and is less expensive.	Similar to CT (see above).
MRI	Imaging of brain, spinal cord, and spinal canal by means of magnetic energy (Fig. 55.18, *B*). Used to detect strokes, MS, tumors, trauma, herniation, and seizures. Provides greater detail than CT and improved resolution (detail) of intracranial structures. Takes a longer time to complete and may not be appropriate in life-threatening emergencies. Contrast medium may be used to enhance visualization. The contrast agent *gadolinium* has a lower incidence of allergy than iodine used in CT.	*Before:* Oral and/or IV contrast injection may be used. Check for pregnancy, allergies, and renal function. Have patient remove all metal objects. Ask about any history of surgical insertion of staples, plates, dental bridges, or other metal appliances. Remove metallic foil patches. Patient may need to be fasting. Assess for claustrophobia and the need for antianxiety medication. *During:* Patient must lie completely still.
• Magnetic resonance angiography (MRA)	Uses differential signal characteristics of flowing blood to evaluate extracranial and intracranial blood vessels. Provides both anatomic and hemodynamic information. Can be used in conjunction with contrast medium.	Similar to MRI (see above).
• Functional MRI (fMRI)	MRI technique that provides time-related (temporal) images that can evaluate how the brain responds to various stimuli. Makes it possible to detect the brain areas that are involved in a task, process, or an emotion.	Similar to MRI (see above).

TABLE 55.9 Radiologic Studies

Nervous System—cont'd

Study	Description and Purpose	Nursing Responsibility
• MR spectroscopy (MRS)	Noninvasive test for measuring biochemical changes in the brain, especially the presence of tumors. Compares the chemical composition of normal brain tissue with abnormal tumor tissue. Can detect tissue changes in stroke and epilepsy.	Similar to MRI (see above).
Myelogram	X-ray of spinal cord and vertebral column after injection of contrast medium into subarachnoid space. Used to detect spinal lesions (e.g., herniated or ruptured disc, spinal tumor).	*Before:* Give sedative as ordered. Have patient empty bladder. Tell patient that test is done with patient on tilting table that is moved during test. *After:* Patient should lie flat for 1–2 hours to prevent spinal headache. Encourage fluids. Monitor neurologic signs and VS. Headache, nausea, and vomiting may occur.
Positron emission tomography (PET)	Measures metabolic activity of brain to assess cell death or damage. Uses radioactive material that shows up as a bright spot on the image (see Fig. 15.7). Used for patients with stroke, Alzheimer's disease, seizure disorders, Parkinson's disease, and tumors.	*Before:* Explain procedure to patient. Tell patient not to take sedatives or tranquilizers. Have patient empty bladder. Insert 2 IV lines. *During:* Patient may be asked to perform different activities during test.
Single-photon emission computed tomography (SPECT)	Method of scanning similar to PET but uses more stable substances and different detectors. Radiolabeled compounds are injected, and their photon emissions can be detected. Resulting images are accumulation of labeled compound. Assesses blood flow and O_2 and glucose metabolism in the brain. Used to diagnose strokes, brain tumors, and seizure disorders.	Similar to PET (see above).
Skull and spine x-rays	Simple x-ray of skull and spinal column. Done to detect fractures, bone erosion, calcifications, abnormal vascularity.	*Before:* Remove any radiopaque objects that can interfere with results. Explain procedure to patient. *During:* Avoid excessive exposure of patient and self.
Ultrasound		
Carotid artery duplex scan	Noninvasive study that evaluates the degree of stenosis of carotid and vertebral arteries. Combines ultrasound and Doppler technology. Probe is placed over the carotid artery and slowly moved along the course of common carotid artery. Frequency of reflected ultrasound signal corresponds to blood velocity. Increased blood flow velocity can indicate stenosis of a vessel.	*Before:* Explain procedure to patient.
Transcranial Doppler	Same technology as carotid duplex but evaluates blood flow velocities of intracranial blood vessels. Probe is placed on skin at various "windows" in the skull (areas in the skull that have only a thin bony covering) to record velocities of the blood vessels.	*Before:* Explain procedure to patient.

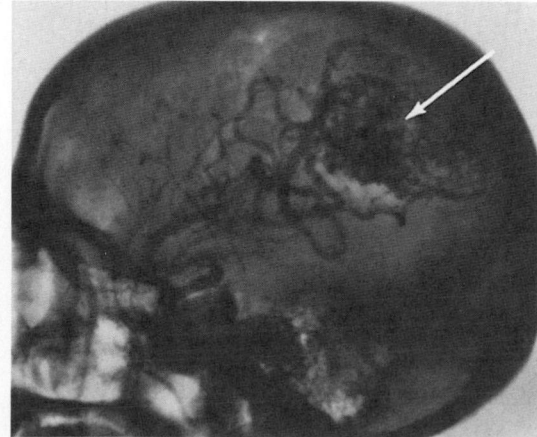

FIG. 55.17 Cerebral angiogram illustrating an arteriovenous malformation *(arrow)*. (From Chipps E, Clanin N, Campbell V: *Neurologic disorders,* St Louis, 1992, Mosby.)

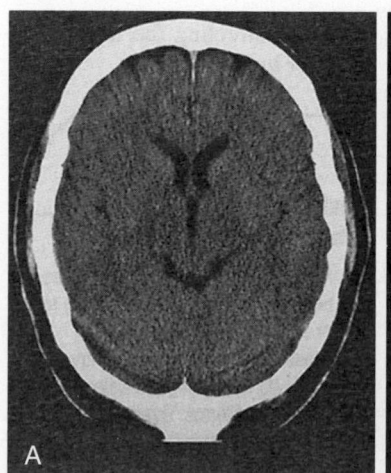
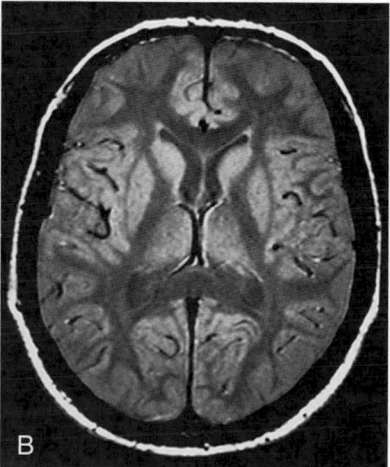

FIG. 55.18 Normal images of the brain. A, CT scan. B, MRI. (From Fuller G, Manford M: *Neurology: An illustrated colour text,* ed 3, New York, 2010, Churchill Livingstone.)

TABLE 55.10 Electrographic Studies

Nervous System

Electroencephalography (EEG)	Electrical activity of brain is recorded using scalp electrodes. Evaluates seizure disorders, cerebral disease, CNS effects of systemic diseases, brain injury, brain death. Specific tests may be done to evaluate brain's electrical response to lights and loud noises.	*Before:* Tell patient procedure is noninvasive and without danger of electric shock. Determine if any medications (e.g., tranquilizers, antiseizure drugs) should be withheld. *After:* Resume medications and have patient wash electrode paste out of hair.
Electromyography (EMG)	Recording of electrical activity associated with innervation of skeletal muscle. Needle electrodes are inserted into the muscle to record specific motor units. Normal muscle at rest shows no electrical activity. Electrical activity occurs only when the muscle contracts. Activity may be altered in diseases of muscle (e.g., myopathic conditions) or in disorders of muscle innervation (e.g., segmental or LMN lesions, peripheral neuropathic conditions).	*Before:* Explain procedure. Tell patient that pain and discomfort are associated with insertion of needles. HCPs may restrict stimulants (e.g., caffeine) 2–3 hr prior. *After:* Assess needle sites for hematoma or inflammation. Give as-needed analgesics.
Electroneurography (nerve conduction studies)	Measures nerve conduction velocity of peripheral nerves. Involves applying a brief electrical stimulus to a distal portion of a sensory nerve and recording the resulting wave of depolarization at a point proximal to the stimulation. The time between the stimulus onset and the first wave of depolarization at the recording electrode is measured. Damaged nerves have slower conduction velocities.	*Before:* Explain procedure to patient. For example, a stimulus can be applied to the forefinger and a recording electrode placed over the median nerve at the wrist will detect the speed of the conduction.
Evoked potentials	Electrical activity associated with nerve conduction along sensory pathways is recorded by electrodes placed on skin and scalp. A stimulus generates the impulse. Increases in the normal time from stimulus onset to a given peak (latency) indicate slowed nerve conduction or nerve damage. Used to diagnose disease (e.g., MS), locate nerve damage, and monitor function during surgery. Can diagnose disorders of the visual or auditory systems because it shows if a sensory impulse is reaching the right part of brain.	*Before:* Explain procedure to patient. Have patient shampoo hair before test.
Magnetoencephalography (MEG)	Uses a biomagnetometer to detect magnetic fields generated by neural activity. Can accurately pinpoint the part of the brain involved in a stroke, seizure, or other disorder or injury. Measures extracranial magnetic fields and scalp electric field (EEG).	*Before:* Explain procedure to patient. MEG, a passive sensor, does not make physical contact with patient.

CNS, Central nervous system; *LMN,* lower motor neuron.

CASE STUDY—cont'd

Objective Data: Diagnostic Studies

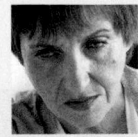

MRI/MRA results show a temporal-parietal glioblastoma that has extended into margins of the occipital lobes.

Discussion Questions

1. Are these the diagnostic studies that you expected to be ordered?
2. Why are these diagnostic study results of concern to you?

(© TatyanaGl/ iStock/ Thinkstock.)

This case study is continued in Chapter 57 on p. 1350.

Answers available at *http://evolve.elsevier.com/Lewis/medsurg.*

▉ BRIDGE TO NCLEX EXAMINATION

The number of the question corresponds to the same-numbered outcome at the beginning of the chapter.

1. In a patient with a disease that affects the myelin sheath of nerves, such as multiple sclerosis, the glial cells affected are the
   a. microglia.
   b. astrocytes.
   c. ependymal cells.
   d. oligodendrocytes.

2. Drugs or diseases that impair the function of the extrapyramidal system may cause loss of
   a. sensations of pain and temperature.
   b. regulation of the autonomic nervous system.
   c. integration of somatic and special sensory inputs.
   d. automatic movements associated with skeletal muscle activity.

3. During the admitting neurologic examination, the nurse determines the patient has speech difficulties with weakness of the right arm and lower face. The nurse would expect a CT scan to show pathology in the distribution of the
   a. basilar artery.
   b. left middle cerebral artery.
   c. right anterior cerebral artery.
   d. left posterior communicating artery.

4. A patient is seen in the emergency department after diving into the pool and hitting the bottom with a blow to the face that hyperextended the neck and scraped the skin off the nose. The patient describes "having double vision" when looking down. During the neurologic examination, the nurse finds the patient is unable to abduct either eye. The nurse recognizes this finding is related to
   a. a basal skull fracture.
   b. an injury to CN VI on both sides.
   c. a stiff neck from the hyperextension injury.
   d. facial swelling from the scrape on the bottom of the pool.

5. Stimulation of the parasympathetic nervous system results in *(select all that apply)*
   a. constriction of the bronchi.
   b. dilation of skin blood vessels.
   c. increased secretion of insulin.
   d. increased blood glucose levels.
   e. relaxation of the urinary sphincters.

6. The nurse is assessing the muscle strength of an older adult. The nurse knows the findings cannot be compared with those of a younger adult because
   a. nutritional status is better in young adults.
   b. muscle tone and strength decrease in older adults.
   c. muscle strength should be the same for all adults.
   d. most young adults exercise more than older adults.

7. A patient is admitted with a headache, fever, and general malaise. The HCP has asked that the patient be prepared for a lumbar puncture. What is a *priority* nursing action to avoid complications?
   a. Evaluate laboratory results for changes in the white cell count.
   b. Give acetaminophen for the headache and fever before the procedure.
   c. Notify the provider if signs of increased intracranial pressure are present.
   d. Administer antibiotics before the procedure to treat the potential meningitis.

8. During neurologic testing, the patient can perceive pain elicited by pinprick. Based on this finding, the nurse may omit testing for
   a. position sense.
   b. patellar reflexes.
   c. temperature perception.
   d. heel-to-shin movements.

9. A patient's eyes jerk while the patient looks to the left. The nurse will record this finding as
   a. nystagmus.
   b. CN VI palsy.
   c. ophthalmic dyskinesia.
   d. oculocephalic response.

10. The nurse is caring for a patient with peripheral neuropathy who is scheduled for EMG studies tomorrow morning. The nurse should
    a. ensure the patient has an empty bladder.
    b. instruct the patient about the risk for electric shock.
    c. ensure the patient has no metallic jewelry or metal fragments.
    d. teach the patient that pain may be experienced during the study.

1. d, 2. d, 3. b, 4. b, 5. a, b, c, e, 6. b, 7. c, 8. c, 9. a, 10. d

For rationales to these answers and even more NCLEX review questions, visit *http://evolve.elsevier.com/Lewis/medsurg*.

ⓔ EVOLVE WEBSITE/RESOURCES LIST

http://evolve.elsevier.com/Lewis/medsurg
Review Questions (Online Only)
Key Points
Answer Keys for Questions
- Rationales for Bridge to NCLEX Examination Questions
- Answer Guidelines for Case Study on pp. 1288, 1290, 1293, and 1298
Conceptual Care Map Creator
Audio Glossary
Supporting Media
- Animations
- Cervical Nerves
- Overview of Nervous System
- Parts of the Brain
- Synaptic Transmission
- The Synapse
- Vertebral Column and Spinal Nerves
- Content Updates

REFERENCES

*1. Curcio M, Bradke F: Axon regeneration in the central nervous system: Facing the challenges from the inside, *Annu Rev Cell Dev B* 8:46, 2018.

*2. Boerboom A, Dion V, Chariot A, et al: Molecular mechanisms involved in Schwann cell plasticity, *Front Mol Neurosci* 10:38, 2017.

3. Falk S, Götz M: Glial control of neurogenesis, *Curr Opin Neurobiol* 47:188, 2017.

*4. Mukherjee D, Jani ND, Narvid J, et al: The role of circle of Willis anatomy variations in cardio-embolic stroke: A patient-specific simulation-based study, *Ann Biomed Eng* 46:1128, 2018.

5. NIH MedlinePlus: Aging changes in the senses. Retrieved from *www.nlm.nih.gov/medlineplus/ency/article/004013.htm*.

6. Cuevas-Trisan R: Balance problems and fall risks in the elderly, *Phys Med Rehab Clin N Amer* 28:727, 2017.

*7. Blaser AR, Starkopf J, Alhazzani W, et al: Early enteral nutrition in critically ill patients: ESICM clinical practice guidelines, *Intens Care Med* 43:380, 2017.

8. Daroff RB, Jankovic J, Mazziotta JC, et al: *Bradley's neurology in clinical practice*, ed 7, St Louis, 2016, Elsevier.

9. Finney GR, Minagar A, Heilman KM: Assessment of mental status, *Neurol Clin* 34:1, 2016.

*10. Marin C, Vilas D, Langdon C, et al: Olfactory dysfunction in neurodegenerative diseases, *Curr Allergy Asthm R* 18:42, 2018.

*Evidence-based information for clinical practice.

56

Acute Intracranial Problems

Kristen Keller

If you want others to be happy, practice compassion.
If you want to be happy, practice compassion.

Dalai Lama XIV

http://evolve.elsevier.com/Lewis/medsurg

CONCEPTUAL FOCUS

Cognition	Intracranial Regulation	Safety
Functional Ability	Mobility	Sensory Perception

LEARNING OUTCOMES

1. Explain the physiologic mechanisms that maintain normal intracranial pressure.
2. Describe the common etiologies, clinical manifestations, and interprofessional care of the patient with increased intracranial pressure.
3. Describe the nursing management of the patient with increased intracranial pressure.
4. Distinguish types of head injury by mechanism of injury and clinical manifestations.
5. Describe the interprofessional and nursing management of the patient with a head injury.
6. Compare the types, clinical manifestations, and interprofessional care of patients with brain tumors.
7. Discuss the nursing management of the patient with a brain tumor.
8. Describe the nursing management of the patient undergoing cranial surgery.
9. Distinguish among the primary causes and interprofessional and nursing management of brain abscess, meningitis, and encephalitis.

KEY TERMS

brain abscess, p. 1326
cerebral edema, p. 1302
coma, p. 1303
concussion, p. 1312
contusion, p. 1313
diffuse axonal injury (DAI), p. 1313

encephalitis, p. 1327
epidural hematoma, p. 1313
Glasgow Coma Scale (GCS), p. 1308
head injury, p. 1311
intracerebral hematoma, p. 1314
intracranial pressure (ICP), p. 1300

meningitis, p. 1324
nuchal rigidity, p. 1324
subdural hematoma, p. 1313
unconsciousness, p. 1303

The body has various mechanisms by which it regulates the intracranial space to promote optimal brain function. Acute intracranial problems can disrupt these processes, leading to increased intracranial pressure (ICP), reduced blood flow to the brain, and brain tissue damage. This chapter discusses the mechanisms that maintain normal ICP and problems that lead to increased ICP. Head injury, brain tumors, and cerebral infections and inflammatory disorders are common problems that disrupt intracranial regulation.

INTRACRANIAL REGULATION

Understanding the dynamics associated with ICP is important in caring for patients with different neurologic problems. The skull is an enclosed space with 3 essential volume components: brain tissue, blood, and cerebrospinal fluid (CSF) (Fig. 56.1). The intracellular and extracellular fluids of brain tissue make up about 78% of this volume. Blood in the arterial, venous, and capillary network makes up 12% of the volume. The remaining 10% is the volume of the CSF.

Primary versus secondary injury is an important concept in understanding ICP. *Primary injury* occurs at the initial time of an injury (e.g., impact of car accident, blunt-force trauma). It results in displacement, bruising, or damage to any of the components (brain tissue, blood, CSF).

Secondary injury is the resulting hypoxia, ischemia, hypotension, edema, or increased ICP that follows the primary injury. Secondary injury, which can occur several hours to days after the initial injury, is a concern when managing brain injury. Nursing management of the patient with an acute intracranial problem must include management of secondary injury and increased ICP.

Normal Intracranial Pressure

Intracranial pressure (ICP) is the hydrostatic force measured in the brain CSF compartment. Under normal conditions in which intracranial volume stays relatively constant, the balance

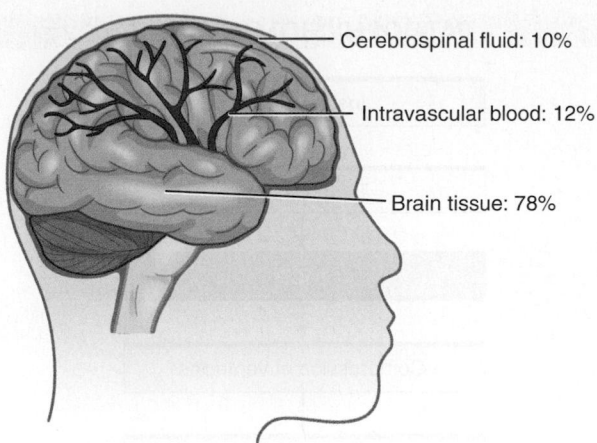

Cerebrospinal fluid: 10%

Intravascular blood: 12%

Brain tissue: 78%

FIG. 56.1 Components of the brain.

TABLE 56.1 **Calculation of Cerebral Perfusion Pressure**
CPP = MAP − ICP
MAP = DBP + 1/3 (SBP − DBP)
OR
MAP = $\dfrac{SBP + 2\,(DBP)}{3}$
Example: Systemic BP = 122/84 mm Hg MAP = 97 mm Hg ICP = 12 mm Hg CPP = 85 mm Hg

CPP, Cerebral perfusion pressure; *DBP,* diastolic blood pressure; *MAP,* mean arterial pressure; *SBP,* systolic blood pressure.

among the 3 components (brain tissue, blood, CSF) maintains ICP. Factors that influence ICP under normal circumstances are changes in (1) arterial pressure; (2) venous pressure; (3) intraabdominal and intrathoracic pressure; (4) posture; (5) temperature; and (6) blood gases, particularly CO_2 levels. The degree to which these factors increase or decrease the ICP depends on the brain's ability to adapt to changes.

The Monro-Kellie doctrine states that the 3 components must stay at a relatively constant volume within the closed skull structure. If the volume of any 1 of the 3 components increases within the cranial vault and the volume from another component is displaced, the total intracranial volume will not change.[1] This hypothesis is applicable only in situations in which the skull is closed. The hypothesis is not valid in persons with displaced skull fractures or craniectomy (removal of part of the skull).

We can measure ICP in the ventricles, subarachnoid space, subdural space, epidural space, or brain tissue using a pressure transducer.[2] Normal ICP ranges from 5 to 15 mm Hg. A sustained pressure greater than 20 mm Hg is considered abnormal and must be treated.

Normal Compensatory Adaptations

In applying the Monro-Kellie doctrine, the body can adapt to volume changes within the skull in 3 different ways to maintain a normal ICP. The first compensatory mechanisms can include changes in the CSF volume. CSF volume can be changed by altering CSF absorption or production and by displacing CSF into the spinal subarachnoid space. Second, changes in intracranial blood volume can occur through the collapse of cerebral veins and dural sinuses, regional cerebral vasoconstriction or dilation, and changes in venous outflow. Third, brain tissue volume compensates through distention of the dura or compression of brain tissue.

Initially an increase in volume produces no increase in ICP because of these compensatory mechanisms. However, there is limited ability to compensate for changes in volume. As the volume increase continues, ICP rises and decompensation occurs, resulting in compression and ischemia.

Cerebral Blood Flow

Cerebral blood flow (CBF) is the amount of blood in milliliters passing through 100 g of brain tissue in 1 minute. The global CBF is about 50 mL/min/100 g of brain tissue. Maintaining blood flow to the brain is critical because the brain requires a constant supply of O_2 and glucose. The brain uses 20% of the body's O_2 and 25% of its glucose.[3]

Autoregulation of Cerebral Blood Flow. The brain regulates its own blood flow in response to its metabolic needs despite wide fluctuations in systemic arterial pressure. *Cerebral autoregulation* is the automatic adjustment in the diameter of the cerebral blood vessels by the brain to maintain a constant blood flow during changes in arterial BP. The purpose of autoregulation is to ensure a consistent CBF to provide for the metabolic needs of brain tissue and maintain cerebral perfusion pressure within normal limits.

The lower limit of systemic arterial pressure at which autoregulation is effective in a normotensive person is a mean arterial pressure (MAP) of 70 mm Hg. Below this, CBF decreases, and symptoms of cerebral ischemia, such as syncope and blurred vision, occur. The upper limit of systemic arterial pressure at which autoregulation is effective is a MAP of 150 mm Hg. When this pressure is exceeded, the vessels are maximally constricted, and further vasoconstrictor response is lost.

The *cerebral perfusion pressure* (CPP) is the pressure needed to ensure blood flow to the brain. CPP is equal to the MAP minus the ICP (CPP = MAP − ICP) (see the example in Table 56.1). Normal CPP is 60 to 100 mm Hg. As the CPP decreases, autoregulation fails and CBF decreases. A CPP of less than 50 mm Hg is associated with ischemia and neuronal death. A CPP of less than 30 mm Hg results in ischemia and is incompatible with life.

Though CPP is clinically useful, it does not consider the effect of cerebrovascular resistance. Cerebrovascular resistance, generated by the arterioles within the cranium, links CPP and blood flow as follows:

$$CPP = Flow \times Resistance$$

When cerebrovascular resistance is high, blood flow to brain tissue is impaired. Transcranial Doppler is a noninvasive technique used in intensive care units (ICUs) to monitor changes in cerebrovascular resistance.

Normally, autoregulation maintains an adequate CBF and CPP by adjusting the diameter of cerebral blood vessels and metabolic factors that affect ICP. It is critical to maintain MAP when ICP is increased.

Remember that CPP may not reflect perfusion pressure in all parts of the brain. There may be local areas of swelling and compression limiting regional perfusion pressure. Thus a higher

CPP may be needed for these patients to prevent localized tissue damage. For example, a patient with an acute stroke may need a higher BP, increasing MAP and CPP, to increase perfusion to the brain and prevent further tissue damage.

Factors Affecting Cerebral Blood Flow. CO_2, O_2, and hydrogen ion concentration affect cerebral blood vessel tone. An increase in the partial pressure of CO_2 in arterial blood ($PaCO_2$) relaxes smooth muscle, dilates cerebral vessels, decreases cerebrovascular resistance, and increases CBF. A decrease in $PaCO_2$ constricts cerebral vessels, increases cerebrovascular resistance, and decreases CBF.

Cerebral O_2 tension of less than 50 mm Hg results in cerebrovascular dilation. This dilation decreases cerebrovascular resistance, increases CBF, and increases O_2 tension. However, if O_2 tension is not increased, anaerobic metabolism begins, resulting in an accumulation of lactic acid. As lactic acid increases and hydrogen ions accumulate, the environment becomes more acidic. Within this acidic environment, further vasodilation occurs in a continued attempt to increase blood flow. The combination of a severely low partial pressure of O_2 in arterial blood (PaO_2) and increased hydrogen ion concentration (acidosis), which are both potent cerebral vasodilators, may produce a state in which autoregulation is lost and compensatory mechanisms do not meet tissue metabolic demands.

CBF can be affected by cardiac or respiratory arrest, systemic hemorrhage, and other pathophysiologic states (e.g., diabetic coma, encephalopathies, infections, toxicities). Regional CBF can be affected by trauma, tumors, cerebral hemorrhage, or stroke. When regional or global autoregulation is lost, CBF is no longer maintained at a constant level but is directly influenced by changes in systemic BP, hypoxia, or catecholamines.

INCREASED INTRACRANIAL PRESSURE

Any patient who becomes unconscious acutely, regardless of the cause, should be suspected of having increased ICP.

Mechanisms of Increased Intracranial Pressure

Increased ICP is a potentially life-threatening situation that results from an increase in any or all the 3 components (brain tissue, blood, CSF) within the skull. Increased ICP is clinically significant because it decreases CPP, increases risks for brain ischemia and infarction, and is associated with a poor prognosis.[4] Common causes of increased ICP include a mass (e.g., hematoma, contusion, abscess, tumor) and cerebral edema (from brain tumors, hydrocephalus, head injury, brain inflammation).

These cerebral insults, which may result in hypercapnia, cerebral acidosis, impaired autoregulation, and systemic hypertension, increase the formation and spread of cerebral edema. This edema distorts brain tissue, further increasing the ICP, and leads to even more tissue hypoxia and acidosis. Fig. 56.2 shows the progression of increased ICP.

It is critical to maintain CBF to preserve tissue and thus minimize secondary injury. Sustained increases in ICP result in brainstem compression and herniation of the brain. *Herniation* occurs as the brain tissue is forcibly shifted from the compartment of greater pressure to a compartment of lesser pressure.

Displacement and herniation of brain tissue can cause a potentially reversible process to become irreversible. Ischemia and edema are further increased, compounding the preexisting problem. Compression of the brainstem and cranial nerves may

PATHOPHYSIOLOGY MAP

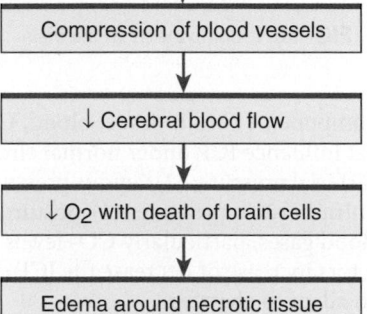
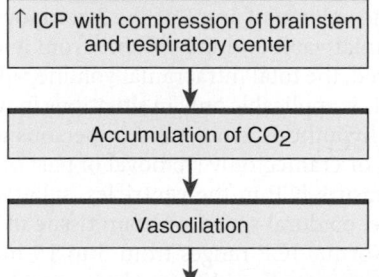

Insult to brain

↓

Tissue edema

↓

↑ ICP

↓

Compression of ventricles

↓

Compression of blood vessels

↓

↓ Cerebral blood flow

↓

↓ O_2 with death of brain cells

↓

Edema around necrotic tissue

↓

↑ ICP with compression of brainstem and respiratory center

↓

Accumulation of CO_2

↓

Vasodilation

↓

↑ ICP resulting from ↑ blood volume

↓

Death

FIG. 56.2 Progression of increased ICP.

be fatal. Fig. 56.3 shows types of herniation. Herniation forces the cerebellum and brainstem downward through the foramen magnum. If compression of the brainstem is unrelieved, respiratory arrest will occur due to compression of the respiratory control center in the medulla. In this situation, intense pressure is placed on the brainstem. If herniation continues, brainstem death is imminent.

Cerebral Edema

There are a variety of causes of cerebral edema (increased accumulation of fluid in the extravascular spaces of brain tissue) (Table 56.2). Regardless of the cause, cerebral edema results in an increase in tissue volume that can increase ICP. The extent and severity of the original insult are factors that determine the degree of cerebral edema.

There are 3 types of cerebral edema: vasogenic, cytotoxic, and interstitial. The same patient may have more than 1 type.

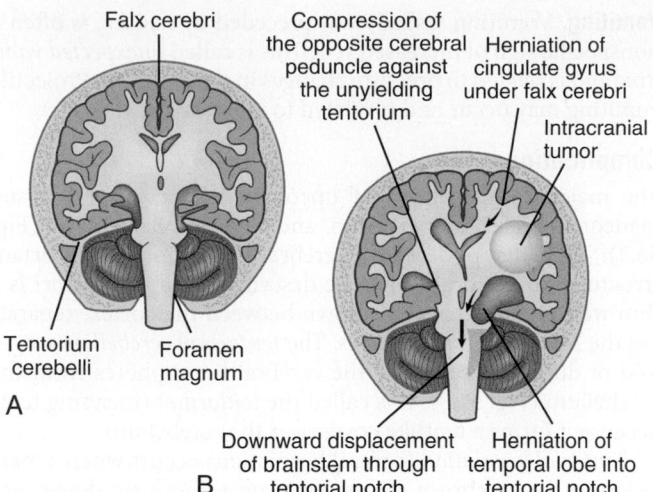

FIG. 56.3 Herniation. A, Normal relationship of intracranial structures. B, Shift of intracranial structures. (Modified from McCance KL, Huether SE: *Pathophysiology: The biologic basis for disease in adults and children*, ed 6, St Louis, 2010, Mosby.)

TABLE 56.2 Causes of Cerebral Edema

Cerebral Infections	Toxic or Metabolic Encephalopathic Conditions
• Encephalitis • Meningitis	• Hepatic encephalopathy • Lead or arsenic intoxication • Uremia
Head Injuries and Brain Surgery	
• Contusion • Hemorrhage • Posttraumatic brain swelling	**Vascular Insult** • Anoxic and ischemic episodes • Cerebral infarction (thrombotic or embolic) • Venous sinus thrombosis
Mass Lesions	
• Brain abscess • Brain tumor (primary, metastatic) • Hematoma (intracerebral, subdural, epidural) • Hemorrhage (intracerebral, cerebellar, brainstem)	

Vasogenic Cerebral Edema. *Vasogenic cerebral edema,* the most common type of cerebral edema, occurs mainly in the white matter. It is characterized by leakage of large molecules from the capillaries into the surrounding extracellular space. This results in an osmotic gradient that favors the flow of fluid from the intravascular to extravascular space. A variety of problems, such as brain tumors, abscesses, and ingested toxins, may increase in the permeability of the blood-brain barrier and produce an increase in the extracellular fluid volume. The speed and extent of the spread of the edema are influenced by the systemic BP, site of the brain injury, and extent of the blood-brain barrier defect.

This edema may produce a continuum of symptoms, ranging from headache to a decrease in consciousness, including coma (profound state of unconsciousness) and focal neurologic deficits.

It is important to recognize that although a headache may seem to be a benign symptom, in cases of cerebral edema it can quickly progress to coma and death. So, you must be vigilant in your assessment.

Cytotoxic Cerebral Edema. *Cytotoxic cerebral edema* results from disruption of the integrity of the cell membranes. It develops from destructive lesions or trauma to brain tissue, resulting in cerebral hypoxia or anoxia and syndrome of inappropriate antidiuretic hormone (SIADH) secretion. In this type of edema, the blood-brain barrier stays intact. Cerebral edema occurs from fluid and protein shifts from the extracellular space directly into the cells, with subsequent swelling and loss of cellular function.

Interstitial Cerebral Edema. *Interstitial cerebral edema* is usually a result of hydrocephalus. *Hydrocephalus* is a buildup of fluid in the brain. It is manifested by ventricular enlargement. It can be due to excess CSF production, obstruction of flow, or an inability to reabsorb the CSF. Hydrocephalus treatment usually consists of a ventriculostomy or ventriculoperitoneal shunt. Management of hydrocephalus is discussed later in this chapter on p. 1319.

Clinical Manifestations

The manifestations of increased ICP can take many forms, depending on the cause, location, and rate of increases in ICP.

Change in Level of Consciousness. The *level of consciousness* (LOC) is the most sensitive and reliable indicator of the patient's neurologic status. Changes in LOC are a result of impaired CBF, which causes O_2 deprivation to the cells of the cerebral cortex and reticular activating system (RAS). The RAS is found in the brainstem, with neural connections to many parts of the nervous system. An intact RAS can maintain a state of wakefulness even in the absence of a functioning cerebral cortex. Interruptions of impulses from the RAS or changes in functioning of the cerebral hemispheres can cause unconsciousness, an abnormal state of complete or partial unawareness of self or environment.

The patient's state of consciousness is defined by the patient's clinical responses and pattern of brain activity (recorded by an electroencephalogram [EEG]). A change in consciousness may be dramatic (as in coma) or subtle (e.g., flattening of affect, change in orientation, decrease in level of attention). In the deepest state of unconsciousness (e.g., coma), the patient does not respond to painful stimuli. Corneal and pupillary reflexes are absent. The patient cannot swallow or cough and is incontinent of urine and feces. The EEG pattern shows suppressed or absent neuronal activity.

Changes in Vital Signs. Increasing pressure on the thalamus, hypothalamus, pons, and medulla causes changes in vital signs.

Manifestations such as *Cushing's triad* (systolic hypertension with a widening pulse pressure, bradycardia with a full and bounding pulse, irregular respirations) may be present but often do not appear until ICP has been increased for some time or is suddenly and markedly increased (e.g., head trauma). Always recognize Cushing's triad as a medical emergency as it is a sign of brainstem compression and impending death. A change in body temperature may occur because increased ICP affects the hypothalamus.

🔓 CHECK YOUR PRACTICE

You are monitoring the vital signs of an 82-yr-old woman who was admitted for a head injury after she fell while walking on the sidewalk. She hit her head on a fire hydrant. She was confused on admission, but vital signs were stable at BP 150/86, pulse 84, respirations 14/min. 2 hours after admission, her vital signs are now BP 166/74, pulse 54, respirations 10 to 16/min.
• What is your interpretation of her vital signs?

Ocular Signs. Compression of cranial nerve (CN) III, the oculomotor nerve, results in dilation of the pupil on the same side (*ipsilateral*) as the mass lesion, sluggish or no response to light, inability to move the eye upward and adduct, and ptosis of the eyelid. These signs can be the result of the brain shifting from midline, compressing the trunk of CN III, and paralyzing the muscles controlling pupillary size and shape. In this situation, a fixed, unilateral, dilated pupil is considered a neurologic emergency that indicates brain herniation.

Other cranial nerves may be affected, including the optic (CN II), trochlear (CN IV), and abducens (CN VI) nerves. Signs of problems with these cranial nerves include blurred vision, diplopia, and changes in extraocular eye movements. *Central herniation* may initially manifest as sluggish but equal pupil response. *Uncal herniation* may cause a dilated unilateral pupil. *Papilledema* (an edematous optic disc seen on retinal examination) is a nonspecific sign associated with persistent increases in ICP.

Decrease in Motor Function. As the ICP continues to rise, the patient has changes in motor ability. A *contralateral* (opposite side of the mass lesion) hemiparesis or hemiplegia may develop, depending on the location of the source of the increased ICP. If painful stimuli are used to elicit a motor response, the patient may localize to the stimuli or withdraw from it.

Noxious stimuli may elicit *decorticate* (flexor) or *decerebrate* (extensor) posturing (Fig. 56.4). Decorticate posture consists of internal rotation and adduction of the arms with flexion of the elbows, wrists, and fingers. It is a result of interruption of voluntary motor tracts in the cerebral cortex. Extension of the legs may be seen. A decerebrate posture may indicate more serious damage. It results from disruption of motor fibers in the midbrain and brainstem. In this position, the arms are stiffly extended, adducted, and hyperpronated. There is hyperextension of the legs with plantar flexion of the feet.

Headache. Although the brain itself is insensitive to pain, compression of other intracranial structures, such as arteries, veins, and cranial nerves, can cause a headache. A nocturnal headache and/or a headache in the morning is cause for concern and may indicate a tumor or other space-occupying lesion that is causing increased ICP. Straining, agitation, or movement may worsen the pain.

Vomiting. Vomiting, usually not preceded by nausea, is often a nonspecific sign of increased ICP. This is called *unexpected vomiting* and is related to pressure changes in the cranium. Projectile vomiting may occur and is related to increased ICP.

Complications

The major complications of uncontrolled increased ICP are inadequate cerebral perfusion and cerebral herniation (Fig. 56.3). To better understand cerebral herniation, 2 important structures in the brain must be described. The *falx cerebri* is a thin wall of dura that folds down between the cortex, separating the 2 cerebral hemispheres. The *tentorium cerebelli* is a rigid fold of dura that separates the cerebral hemispheres from the cerebellum (Fig. 56.3). It is called the *tentorium* (meaning tent) because it forms a tentlike cover over the cerebellum.

Tentorial herniation (central herniation) occurs when a mass lesion in the cerebrum forces the brain to herniate downward through the opening created by the brainstem. *Uncal herniation* occurs when there is lateral and downward herniation. *Cingulate herniation* occurs when there is lateral displacement of brain tissue beneath the falx cerebri.

Diagnostic Studies

Diagnostic studies can be used to identify the cause of increased ICP (Table 56.3). CT and MRI are used to discern the many conditions that can cause increased ICP and assess the effect of treatment.

TABLE 56.3 Interprofessional Care
Increased Intracranial Pressure

Diagnostic Assessment
- History and physical examination
- Vital signs, neurologic assessments, ICP measurements
- Skull, chest, and spinal x-ray studies
- CT scan, MRI, cerebral angiography, EEG, PET
- Transcranial Doppler studies
- Infrascanner
- ECG
- Evoked potential studies
- Lumbar puncture (should not be done if there is a risk for herniation)
- Laboratory studies, including CBC, coagulation profile, electrolytes, serum creatinine, ABGs, ammonia level, drug and toxicology screen, CSF analysis (for protein, WBC, and glucose)

Management
- Elevation of head of bed to 30 degrees with head in a neutral position
- Intubation and mechanical ventilation
- ICP monitoring
- Cerebral oxygenation monitoring ($PbtO_2$, $SjvO_2$)
- Maintain PaO_2 ≥100 mm Hg
- Maintain fluid balance and assess osmolality
- Maintain systolic arterial pressure between 100 and 160 mm Hg
- Maintain CPP >60 mm Hg
- Reduction of cerebral metabolism (e.g., high-dose barbiturates)

Drug Therapy
- Osmotic diuretic (mannitol)
- Hypertonic saline
- Antiseizure drugs (e.g., phenytoin [Dilantin])
- Corticosteroids (dexamethasone) for brain tumors, bacterial meningitis
- Histamine (H_2)-receptor antagonist (e.g., cimetidine) or proton pump inhibitor (e.g., pantoprazole to prevent GI ulcers and bleeding

---

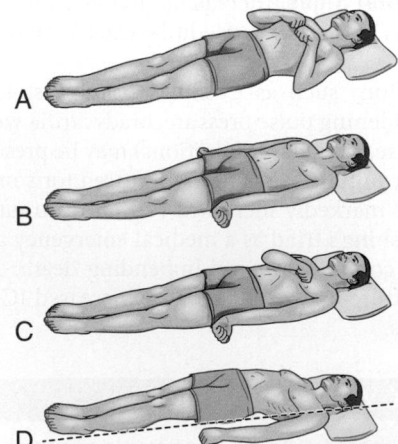

FIG. 56.4 Decorticate and decerebrate posturing. **A,** Decorticate response. Flexion of arms, wrists, and fingers with adduction in upper extremities. Extension, internal rotation, and plantar flexion in lower extremities. **B,** Decerebrate response. All 4 extremities in rigid extension, with hyperpronation of forearms and plantar flexion of feet. **C,** Decorticate response on right side of body and decerebrate response on left side of body. **D,** Opisthotonic posturing.

Other tests include EEG, cerebral angiography, ICP measurement, brain tissue oxygenation measurement via the LICOX catheter (described later), positron emission tomography (PET), transcranial Doppler studies, and evoked potential studies. In general, a lumbar puncture (LP) is not done when increased ICP is suspected. The reason for this is that cerebral herniation could occur from the sudden release of the pressure in the skull from the area above the LP.

In some agencies, a hand-held near-infrared scanner (Infrascanner) is used to detect life-threatening intracranial bleeding. The scanner directs a wavelength of light that can penetrate tissue and bone. Blood from intracranial hematomas absorbs the light differently from other areas of the brain.

Monitoring ICP and Cerebral Oxygenation

Indications for Intracranial Pressure Monitoring. ICP monitoring is used to guide clinical care when the patient is at risk for or has elevations in ICP.[4] It may be used in patients with a variety of neurologic problems, including hemorrhage, stroke, tumor, infection, or traumatic brain injury (TBI). ICP should be monitored in patients admitted with a *Glasgow Coma Scale* (GCS) score of 8 or less and an abnormal CT scan or MRI. These results indicate that the patient may have bleeding, contusion, edema, or other problems. The GCS is discussed later on p. 1308.

Methods of Measuring ICP. Patients with conditions known to elevate ICP, except those with irreversible problems or advanced neurologic disease, usually undergo ICP monitoring in an ICU. Multiple methods and devices are available to monitor ICP in various sites (Fig. 56.5).

The gold standard for monitoring ICP is the *ventriculostomy*, in which a specialized catheter is inserted into the lateral ventricle and coupled to an external transducer (Figs. 56.6 and 56.7). This technique directly measures the pressure within the ventricles, facilitates removal and/or sampling of CSF, and allows for intraventricular drug administration. In this system the transducer is external. It is important to ensure that the transducer is level with the foramen of Monro (interventricular foramen). The system must also be at the ideal height (Fig. 56.8, *A*). A reference point for this foramen is the tragus of the ear. Every time the patient is repositioned, assess the system to ensure it is level.

The *fiberoptic catheter*, an alternative technology, uses a sensor transducer found within the catheter tip. The sensor tip is placed within the ventricle or the brain tissue and gives a direct measurement of brain pressure.

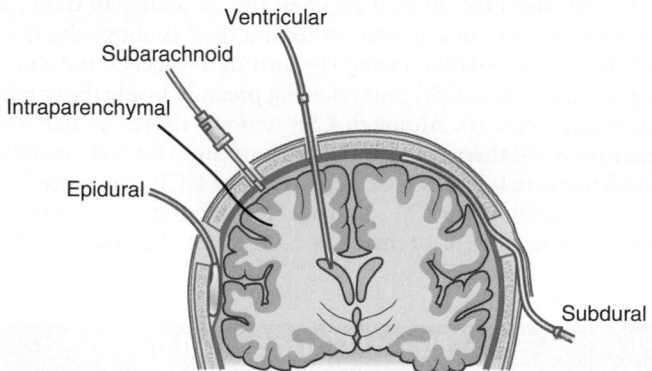

FIG. 56.5 Coronal section of brain showing potential sites for placement of ICP monitoring devices.

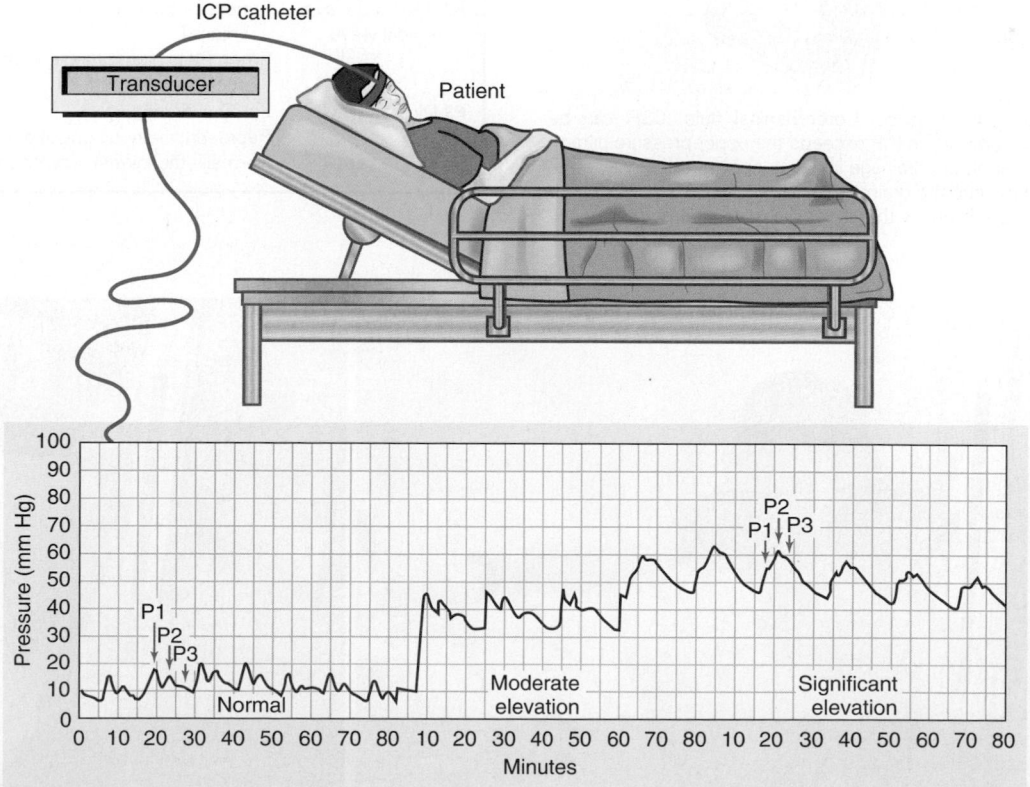

FIG. 56.6 ICP monitoring can be used to continuously measure ICP. The ICP tracing shows normal, elevated, and plateau waves. At high ICP, the P2 peak is higher than the P1 peak, and the peaks become less distinct and plateau. (Modified from Copstead-Kirkhorn LC, Banasik JL: *Pathophysiology*, ed 5, St Louis, 2013, Mosby.)

The *air pouch/pneumatic technology,* another system for monitoring ICP, has an air-filled pouch at the tip of the catheter that maintains a constant volume. The pressure changes within the cranium are transmitted through the changes exerted on this pouch to the monitor.

ICP is represented on the monitor as a mean pressure in millimeters of mercury (mm Hg). If a CSF drainage device is in place, the drain must be closed for at least 6 minutes to ensure an accurate reading. Record the waveform strip along with other pressure monitoring waveforms. The normal ICP waveform has 3 phases (Fig. 56.6 and Table 56.4). It is important to monitor the ICP waveform and the mean CPP. When ICP is normal, P1, P2, and P3 resemble a staircase. As ICP increases, P2 rises above P1. This indicates poor ventricular compliance (Fig. 56.6). Consider the rate at which changes occur and the patient's clinical condition. Neurologic deterioration may not occur until ICP elevation is pronounced and sustained. Immediately report to the HCP any ICP elevation, either as a mean increase in pressure or as an abnormal waveform configuration.

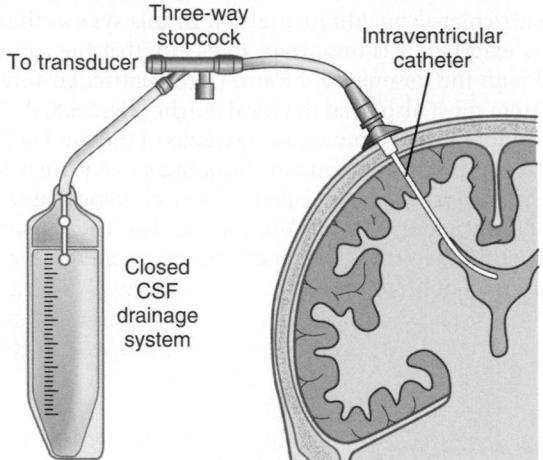

FIG. 56.7 Ventriculostomy in place. Cerebrospinal fluid (CSF) can be drained via a ventriculostomy when ICP exceeds the upper pressure parameter set by the HCP. Intermittent drainage involves opening the 3-way stopcock to allow CSF to flow into the drainage bag for brief periods (30 to 120 seconds) until the pressure is below the upper pressure parameters.

Inaccurate ICP readings can be caused by CSF leaks around the monitoring device, obstruction of the intraventricular catheter (from tissue or blood clot), a difference between the height of the catheter and the transducer, kinks in the tubing, and incorrect height of the drainage system relative to the patient's reference point. Bubbles or air in the tubing can dampen the waveform.

Infection is a serious complication with ICP monitoring. Factors that contribute to infection include ICP monitoring more than 5 days, use of a ventriculostomy, a CSF leak, and a concurrent systemic infection. Routinely assess the insertion site, use aseptic technique, and monitor the CSF for a change in drainage color or clarity.

Cerebrospinal Fluid Drainage. With the ventricular catheter, it is possible to control ICP by removing CSF (Fig. 56.7). The HCP typically orders a specific level at which to start drainage (e.g., if ICP is greater than 20 mm Hg) and the frequency of drainage (intermittent or continuous). When the ICP is above the indicated level, the system is opened by turning a stopcock and allowing the drainage of CSF, thus relieving pressure inside the cranial vault (Fig. 56.8, *B*). Although CSF removal decreases ICP and improves CPP, there are no universal guidelines for CSF removal. Guidelines are typically based on agency or HCP preference.[5]

The 2 options for CSF drainage are intermittent or continuous. If intermittent drainage is used, open the system at the

TABLE 56.4 Normal Intracranial Pressure Waveforms*

Waveform	Meaning
P1 Percussion wave	Represents arterial pulsations. Normally the highest of the 3 waveforms.
P2 Rebound wave or tidal wave	Reflects intracranial compliance or relative brain volume. When P2 is higher than P1, intracranial compliance is compromised.
P3 Dicrotic wave	Follows dicrotic notch. Represents venous pulsations. Normally the lowest waveform.

*See Fig. 56.6.

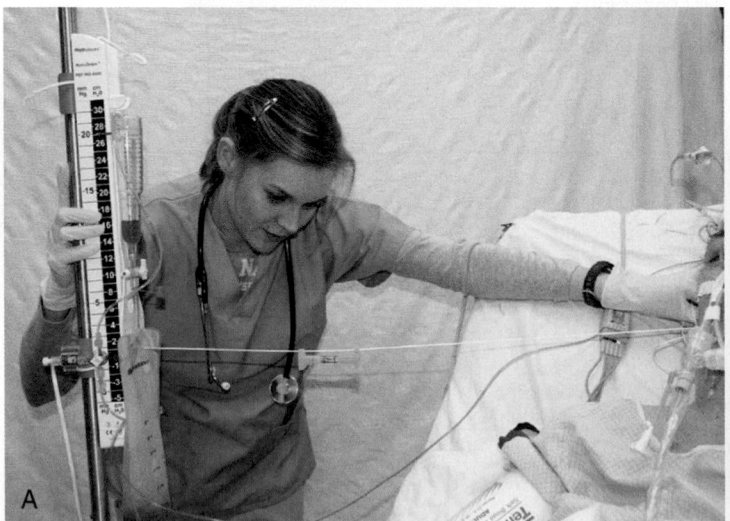
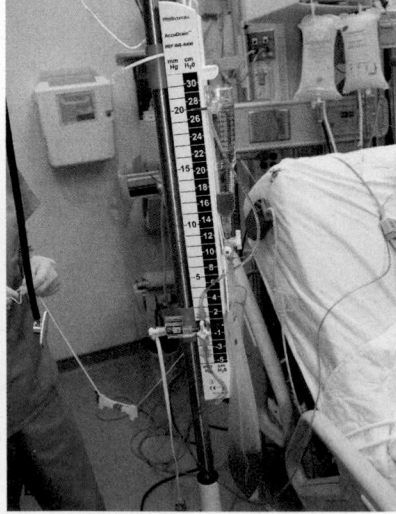

FIG. 56.8 A, Leveling a ventriculostomy. B, Cerebrospinal fluid is drained into a drainage system. (Courtesy Meg Zomorodi, RN, PhD, CNL, Raleigh, NC.)

indicated ICP and allow CSF to drain for 2 to 3 minutes. Then close the stopcock to return the ventriculostomy to a closed system. If continuous ICP drainage is ordered, carefully monitor the volume of CSF drained. Keep in mind that normal CSF production is about 20 to 30 mL/hr. There is a total CSF volume of about 150 mL within the ventricles and subarachnoid space. Post a sign above the patient's bed to notify anyone before turning, moving, or suctioning the patient to prevent the removal of too much CSF, which can result in other complications.

Complications include ventricular collapse, infection, and herniation or subdural hematoma formation from rapid decompression. Strict aseptic technique during dressing changes or sampling of CSF is crucial to prevent infection. The system must stay intact to ensure that the ICP readings are accurate because treatment is based on the pressures.

Cerebral Oxygenation Monitoring. Technology is available to measure cerebral oxygenation and assess perfusion. Three intracranial devices used in ICU settings are the LICOX catheter, Neurovent catheter, and jugular venous bulb catheter.

The LICOX and Neurovent catheters are placed in healthy white matter of the brain (Fig. 56.9). These catheters measure brain oxygenation and temperature. These systems provide continuous monitoring of the pressure of O_2 in brain tissue ($PbtO_2$). The normal range for $PbtO_2$ is 20 to 40 mm Hg. A low $PbtO_2$ level indicates ischemia.[2] These catheters can also measure brain temperature. A cooler brain temperature (96.8° F [36° C]) may produce better outcomes.

Jugular venous bulb oximetry, which measures global O_2 extraction, is used in some agencies. The jugular venous bulb catheter is placed in the internal jugular vein and positioned so that the catheter tip is in the jugular bulb. An x-ray verifies placement. This catheter provides a measurement of jugular venous O_2 saturation ($SjvO_2$), which indicates total venous brain tissue extraction of O_2. This is a measure of cerebral O_2 supply and demand. The normal $SjvO_2$ range is 60% to 75%. Values less than 50% indicate impaired cerebral oxygenation.[2]

In addition to measuring ICP and brain oxygenation, many HCPs are now looking at multimodality monitoring in TBI and intracranial hypertension. This technology includes brain microdialysis (measurement of small molecules), continuous EEG, and blood flow monitoring.

Interprofessional Care

The goals of interprofessional care (Table 56.3) are to (1) identify and treat the underlying cause of increased ICP and (2) support brain function. The earlier the condition is recognized and treated, the better the patient outcome. A careful history is important in the search for the underlying cause. The underlying cause of increased ICP is usually an increase in blood (hemorrhage), brain tissue (tumor or edema), or CSF (hydrocephalus) in the brain.

For any patient with increased ICP, it is important to maintain adequate oxygenation to support brain function and prevent secondary injury. An endotracheal tube or tracheostomy may be needed to maintain adequate ventilation. Arterial blood gas (ABG) analysis guides the O_2 therapy. The goal is to maintain the PaO_2 at 100 mm Hg or greater and to keep $PaCO_2$ in normal range at 35 to 45 mm Hg. The patient may need to be on a mechanical ventilator to ensure adequate oxygenation.

If increased ICP is caused by a mass lesion (e.g., tumor, hematoma), surgical removal of the mass is the best treatment. See the sections on brain tumors and cranial surgery later in this chapter. In aggressive situations, a craniectomy (removal of part of skull) may be done to reduce ICP and prevent herniation.

Drug Therapy. Drug therapy plays an important part in the management of increased ICP. Mannitol (Osmitrol) (25%) is an osmotic diuretic given IV. Mannitol decreases ICP in 2 ways: plasma expansion and osmotic effect. The immediate plasma-expanding effect reduces the hematocrit and blood viscosity. This increases CBF and cerebral O_2 delivery. A vascular osmotic gradient is created by mannitol. Thus fluid moves from the tissues into the blood vessels, reducing the ICP because of the decrease in the total brain fluid content. Monitor fluid and electrolyte status when osmotic diuretics are used. Mannitol may be contraindicated if renal disease is present and serum osmolality increased.

Hypertonic saline solution is another option. It produces massive movement of water out of edematous swollen brain cells and into blood vessels. This movement can reduce swelling and improve cerebral blood flow. Care during an infusion includes frequent monitoring of BP and serum sodium levels because intravascular fluid volume excess can occur. Hypertonic saline infusion is just as effective as mannitol when treating increased

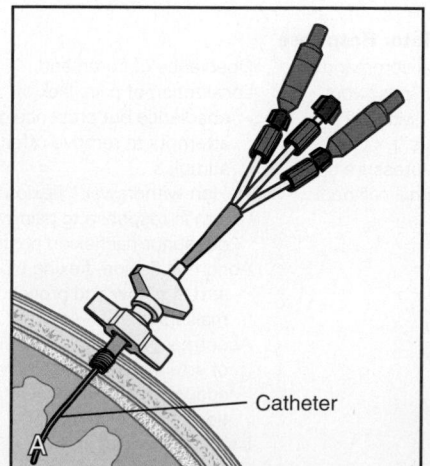
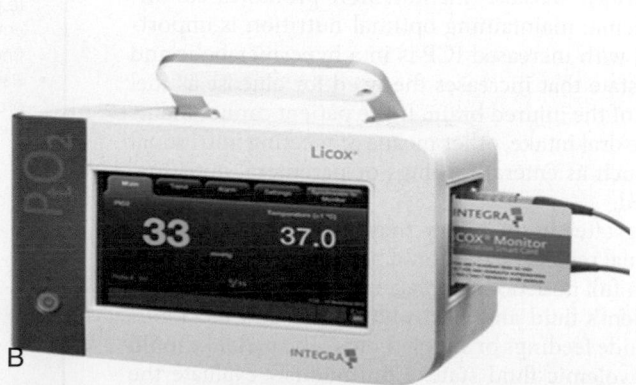

FIG. 56.9 A, The LICOX brain tissue O_2 system involves insertion of a catheter. B, The system measures O_2 in the brain ($PbtO_2$), brain tissue temperature, and ICP. (B, Courtesy of Integra LifeSciences Corporation, Plainsboro, NJ.)

ICP. They are often used concurrently when caring for a patient with a severe brain injury.[6]

Corticosteroids (e.g., dexamethasone) are used to treat vasogenic edema around tumors and abscesses. These drugs are not recommended for TBI. Corticosteroids stabilize the cell membrane and inhibit the synthesis of prostaglandins (see Fig. 11.2), preventing the formation of proinflammatory mediators. Corticosteroids also improve neuronal function by improving CBF and restoring autoregulation.

Complications associated with the use of corticosteroids include hyperglycemia, increased incidence of infections, and gastrointestinal (GI) bleeding. Regularly monitor fluid intake and sodium levels. Perform blood glucose monitoring at least every 6 hours. Patients receiving corticosteroids should receive antacid, histamine (H_2)-receptor blockers (e.g., cimetidine, ranitidine), or proton pump inhibitors (e.g., pantoprazole) to prevent GI ulcers and bleeding.

IV 0.9% sodium chloride is the preferred solution for giving secondary medications. If 5% dextrose in water or 0.45% sodium chloride is used, serum osmolarity decreases and an increase in cerebral edema may occur.

Metabolic demands, such as fever (greater than 100.4° F [38° C]), agitation or shivering, pain, and seizures, can increase ICP. Implement measures to reduce these metabolic demands to lower the ICP in the at-risk patient. Monitor patients for seizure activity. They may need prophylactic antiseizure medication. Maintain the temperature at 96.8° to 98.6° F (36° to 37° C) by using antipyretics (e.g., acetaminophen), cool baths, cooling blankets, ice packs, or intravascular cooling devices as needed. Avoid letting the patient shiver or shake, since this increases the metabolic workload on the brain. If this occurs, the patient may need sedatives or a different cooling method.

Drug therapy for reducing cerebral metabolism may be an effective way to control ICP. Reducing the metabolic rate decreases the CBF and therefore the ICP. High doses of barbiturates (e.g., pentobarbital, thiopental) are used in patients with increased ICP refractory to other treatments. Barbiturates decrease cerebral metabolism, causing a decrease in ICP and a reduction in cerebral edema. With this treatment, monitor the patient's ICP, blood flow, and EEG. Barbiturate dosing is typically based on analysis of the bedside EEG tracing and the ICP. The HCP orders the barbiturate infusion at a rate that achieves a desired level of brain wave suppression to control ICP. *Total burst suppression*, recognized by the absence of spikes showing brain activity on the EEG monitor, shows that maximal therapeutic effect has been achieved.

Nutritional Therapy. Because malnutrition promotes continued cerebral edema, maintaining optimal nutrition is important. The patient with increased ICP is in a hypermetabolic and hypercatabolic state that increases the need for glucose as fuel for metabolism of the injured brain. If the patient cannot maintain an adequate oral intake, other means of meeting nutritional requirements, such as enteral feedings or parenteral nutrition, should be started.

Early feeding after brain injury may improve patient outcome.[5] Nutritional replacement should begin within 3 days after injury and reach full nutritional replacement within 7 days after injury. The patient's fluid and electrolyte status and metabolic needs should guide feedings or supplements. The patient should be kept in a euvolemic fluid state. Continuously evaluate the patient based on clinical factors such as urine output, insensible fluid loss, serum and urine osmolality, and serum electrolytes.

❖ NURSING MANAGEMENT: INCREASED INTRACRANIAL PRESSURE

◆ Nursing Assessment

Subjective data about the patient with increased ICP can be obtained from the patient, caregiver, or family member who is familiar with the patient. Describe the LOC by noting the specific behaviors seen. Assess the LOC using the GCS. Assess body functions, especially circulation and respiration.

◆ **Glasgow Coma Scale.** The Glasgow Coma Scale (GCS) is a quick, practical, and standard system for assessing the LOC. The 3 areas assessed in the GCS are the patient's ability to (1) open the eyes when a verbal or painful stimulus is applied, (2) speak, and (3) obey commands. Specific assessments evaluate the patient's response to varying degrees of stimulus. Three indicators of response are evaluated: (1) opening of the eyes, (2) best verbal response, and (3) best motor response (Table 56.5).

TABLE 56.5 Glasgow Coma Scale

Appropriate Stimulus	Response	Score
Eyes Open		
• Approach to bedside	Spontaneous response.	4
• Verbal command	Opening of eyes to name or command.	3
• Pain	Lack of opening of eyes to previous stimuli but opening to pain.	2
	Lack of opening of eyes to any stimulus.	1
	Untestable.*	U
Best Verbal Response		
• Verbal questioning with maximum arousal	Appropriate orientation, conversant. Correct identification of self, place, year, and month.	5
	Confusion. Conversant, but disorientation in 1 or more spheres.	4
	Inappropriate or disorganized use of words (e.g., cursing), lack of sustained conversation.	3
	Incomprehensible words, sounds (e.g., moaning).	2
	Lack of sound, even with painful stimuli.	1
	Untestable.*	U
Best Motor Response		
• Verbal command (e.g., "raise your arm, hold up 2 fingers")	Obedience of command.	6
	Localization of pain, lack of obedience but presence of attempts to remove offending stimulus.	5
• Pain (pressure on proximal nail bed)	Flexion withdrawal,* flexion of arm in response to pain without abnormal flexion posture.	4
	Abnormal flexion, flexing of arm at elbow and pronation, making a fist.	3
	Abnormal extension, extension of arm at elbow usually with adduction and internal rotation of arm at shoulder.	2
	Lack of response.	1
	Untestable.*	U

*Added to the original scale by some centers.

Specific behaviors observed as responses to the testing stimulus are given a numeric value. Your responsibility is to elicit the best response on each of the scales: the higher the scores, the higher the level of brain functioning. The subscale scores are particularly important if a patient is untestable in an area. For example, severe periorbital edema may make eye opening impossible.

The total GCS score is the sum of the numeric values assigned to each of the 3 areas. The highest GCS score is 15 for a fully alert person, and the lowest possible score is 3. A GCS score of 8 or less generally indicates coma, and mechanical ventilation should be considered. Plot the results of the GCS scores on a graph, which can be used to determine whether the patient is stable, improving, or deteriorating.

The GCS offers several advantages in the assessment of the unconscious patient. It allows different health care professionals to arrive at the same conclusion about the patient's status. It can be used to determine between different or changing states.

Although the GCS is the gold standard assessment tool for LOC, other scales, such as the *Full Outline of Unresponsiveness (FOUR) scale,* are also used.[7] In cases of stroke or hemorrhage associated with increased ICP, use the NIH Stroke Scale (see Table 57.10). Other key neurologic assessments include cranial nerve assessment and motor and sensory testing. Cranial nerve assessment is outlined in Table 55.4.

◆ **Neurologic Assessment.** Compare the pupils with one another for size, shape, movement, and reactivity (Fig. 56.10). If the oculomotor nerve (CN III) is compressed, the pupil on the affected side *(ipsilateral)* becomes larger until it fully dilates. If ICP continues to increase, both pupils dilate.

Test pupillary reaction with a penlight. The normal reaction is brisk constriction when the light is shone directly into the eye. Note a consensual response (slight constriction in the opposite pupil) at the same time. A sluggish reaction can indicate early pressure on CN III. A fixed pupil unresponsive to light stimulus usually indicates increased ICP. However, note that there are other causes of a fixed pupil, including direct injury to CN III, previous eye surgery, atropine administration, and use of mydriatic eye drops.

In some agencies, HCPs are using a hand-held device *(pupillometer)* to measure the pupil reactivity and size. The device removes any subjectivity from the pupil evaluation.

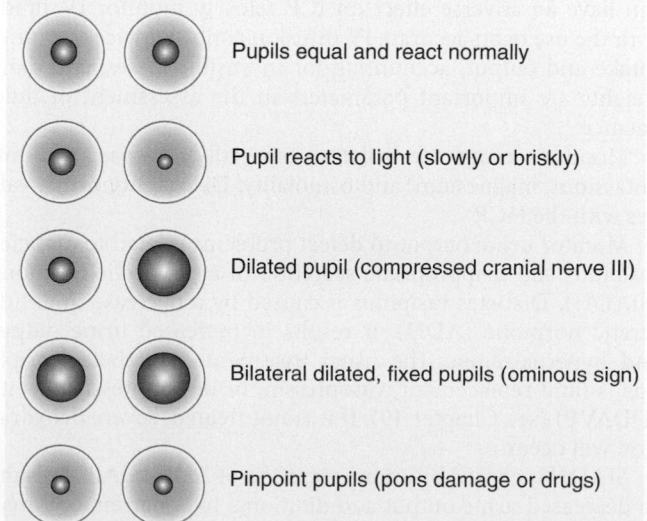

Pupils equal and react normally

Pupil reacts to light (slowly or briskly)

Dilated pupil (compressed cranial nerve III)

Bilateral dilated, fixed pupils (ominous sign)

Pinpoint pupils (pons damage or drugs)

FIG. 56.10 Pupillary check for size and response.

Assess eye movements controlled by CN III, CN IV, and CN VI in the patient who is awake and able to follow commands. They can be used to assess brainstem function. Testing the corneal reflex gives information about the functioning of CN V and CN VII. If this reflex is absent, start routine eye care to prevent corneal abrasion (see Chapter 20).

Eye movements of the uncooperative or unconscious patient can be elicited by reflex with the use of head movements (oculocephalic) and caloric stimulation (oculovestibular). To test the oculocephalic reflex (doll's eye reflex), turn the patient's head briskly to the left or right while holding the eyelids open. A normal response is movement of the eyes across the midline in the direction opposite that of the turning. Next, quickly flex and then extend the neck. Eye movement should be opposite to the direction of head movement—up when the neck is flexed and down when it is extended. Abnormal responses can help locate an intracranial lesion. This test should not be done if a cervical spine problem is suspected.

To test the oculovestibular reflex (cold caloric), the patient is positioned with the head of bed elevated. A syringe of ice-cold water is instilled into the external auditory ear canal. The patient's eyes are assessed for a total of 1 minute. The absence of eye movement or response indicates severe neurologic demise. This test requires patent external auditory ear canals and tympanic membranes.

Test motor strength by asking the awake and cooperative patient to squeeze your hands to compare strength in the hands. The pronator drift test is an excellent measure of strength in the upper extremities. The patient raises the arms in front of the body with the palms facing upward and eyes closed. If there is any weakness in the upper extremity, the palmar surface turns downward and the arm drifts down. This would indicate a problem in the opposite motor cortex. Asking the patient to raise the foot from the bed or to bend the knees up in bed is a good assessment of lower extremity strength. Test all 4 extremities for strength and for any asymmetry in strength or movement.

Assess the motor response of the unconscious or uncooperative patient by observation of spontaneous movement. If no spontaneous movement is possible, apply a pain stimulus to the patient and note the response. Resistance to movement during passive range-of-motion exercises is another measure of strength. Do not include hand squeezing as part of the assessment of motor movement in the unconscious or uncooperative patient, since this is a reflex action and can misrepresent the patient's status.

Record vital signs, including BP, pulse, respiratory rate, and temperature. Be aware of Cushing's triad, which indicates severely increased ICP. Besides recording respiratory rate, note the respiratory pattern. Specific respiratory patterns are associated with severely increased ICP (Fig. 56.11).

◆ **Nursing Diagnoses**

Nursing diagnoses for the patient with increased ICP include:
- Decreased intracranial adaptive capacity
- Ineffective tissue perfusion
- Risk for injury

Additional information on nursing diagnoses and interventions for patients with increased ICP is presented in eNursing Care Plan 56.1 (available on the website for this chapter).

◆ **Planning**

The overall goals for the patient with increased ICP are to (1) maintain a patent airway; (2) have ICP within normal limits; (3) have normal fluid, electrolyte, and nutritional balance; and (4) prevent complications from immobility and decreased LOC.

Pattern	Location of Lesion	Description
1. Cheyne-Stokes 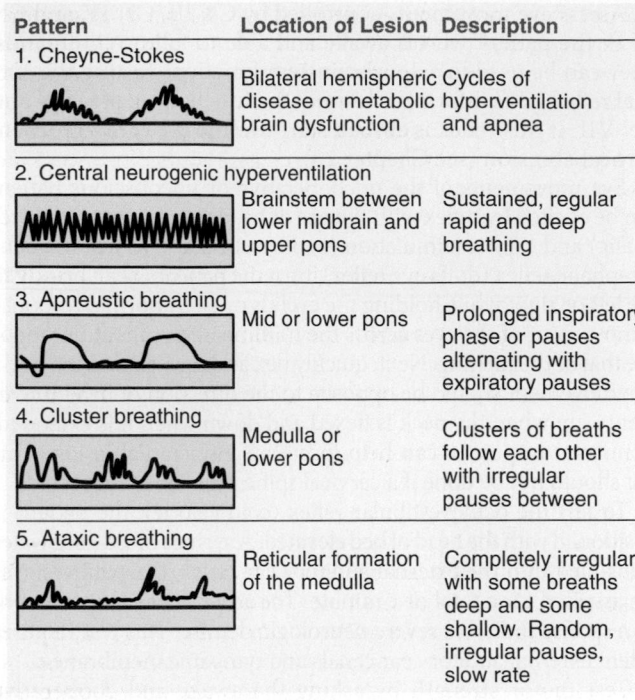	Bilateral hemispheric disease or metabolic brain dysfunction	Cycles of hyperventilation and apnea
2. Central neurogenic hyperventilation	Brainstem between lower midbrain and upper pons	Sustained, regular rapid and deep breathing
3. Apneustic breathing	Mid or lower pons	Prolonged inspiratory phase or pauses alternating with expiratory pauses
4. Cluster breathing	Medulla or lower pons	Clusters of breaths follow each other with irregular pauses between
5. Ataxic breathing	Reticular formation of the medulla	Completely irregular with some breaths deep and some shallow. Random, irregular pauses, slow rate

FIG. 56.11 Common abnormal respiratory patterns associated with coma.

◆ Nursing Implementation

◆ Acute Care

Respiratory Function. Maintaining a patent airway is critical in the patient with increased ICP and is a major nursing responsibility. As the LOC decreases, the patient is at an increased risk for airway obstruction from the tongue dropping back and occluding the airway or from accumulation of secretions.

> **⚠ SAFETY ALERT Altered Breathing**
> • Be alert to altered breathing patterns in a patient with increased ICP.
> • Snoring sounds indicate obstruction and require immediate intervention.

Remove accumulated secretions by suctioning as needed. An oral airway facilitates breathing and provides an easier suctioning route in the comatose patient. In general, any patient with a GCS of 8 or less or an altered LOC who is unable to maintain a patent airway or effective ventilation needs intubation and mechanical ventilation.

Frequently monitor and evaluate the ABG values. Take measures to maintain the levels within prescribed or acceptable parameters. The appropriate ventilatory support can be ordered based on the PaO_2 and $PaCO_2$ values.

Prevent hypoxia and hypercapnia to minimize secondary injury. Suctioning and coughing cause transient decreases in the PaO_2 and increases in the ICP. Keep suctioning to a minimum and less than 10 seconds in duration. Give 100% O_2 before and after to prevent decreases in the PaO_2. To avoid cumulative increases in the ICP with suctioning, limit suctioning to 2 passes per suction procedure, if possible. Patients with increased ICP are at risk for lower CPP during suctioning.

Try to prevent abdominal distention, since it can interfere with respiratory function. Inserting a nasogastric (NG) tube to aspirate the stomach contents can prevent distention, vomiting, and aspiration. However, in patients with facial and skull fractures, an NG tube is contraindicated due to risk for inadvertent intracranial placement. Oral insertion of a gastric tube is preferred.

Sedation. Pain, anxiety, and fear related to the primary injury, therapeutic procedures, or noxious stimuli can increase ICP and BP, thus complicating the patient's management and recovery. The appropriate choice or combination of sedatives, paralytics, and analgesics for symptom management is a challenge. Giving these agents may alter the neurologic state, thus masking true neurologic changes. It may be necessary to temporarily stop drug therapy to appropriately assess neurologic status. The choice, dose, and combination of agents may vary depending on the patient's history, neurologic state, and overall clinical presentation.

Opioids, such as morphine sulfate and fentanyl, are rapid-onset analgesics with minimal effect on CBF or O_2 metabolism. The IV sedative propofol (Diprivan) is used to manage anxiety and agitation in the ICU because of its rapid onset and short half-life. An accurate neurologic assessment can be done soon after stopping an infusion of propofol.

Dexmedetomidine (Precedex), an α_2-adrenergic agonist, is used for continuous IV sedation of intubated and mechanically ventilated patients in the ICU setting for up to 24 hours. When using continuous IV sedatives, be aware of the side effects of these drugs, especially hypotension, since this can lower CPP.

Nondepolarizing neuromuscular blocking agents (e.g., vecuronium, cisatracurium besylate [Nimbex]) are useful for achieving complete ventilatory control in the treatment of refractory intracranial hypertension. Because these agents paralyze muscles without blocking pain or noxious stimuli, they are used in combination with sedatives, analgesics, or benzodiazepines.

Benzodiazepines, although useful for sedation, are usually avoided in the managing the patient with increased ICP because of the hypotensive effect and long half-life. They are usually given as an adjunct to neuromuscular blocking agents.

The patient should be in a quiet, calm environment with minimal noise and interruptions. Observe the patient for signs of agitation, irritation, or frustration. Teach the caregiver and family about decreasing stimulation. Coordinate with team members to minimize procedures that may cause agitation.

Fluid and Electrolyte Balance. Fluid and electrolyte problems can have an adverse effect on ICP. Closely monitor IV fluids with the use of an accurate IV infusion control device or pump. Intake and output, accounting for insensible losses, and daily weights are important parameters in the assessment of fluid balance.

Monitor serum electrolytes, especially glucose, sodium, potassium, magnesium, and osmolality. Discuss abnormal values with the HCP.

Monitor urine output to detect problems related to diabetes insipidus and inappropriate secretion of antidiuretic hormone (SIADH). Diabetes insipidus is caused by a decrease in antidiuretic hormone (ADH). It results in increased urine output and hypernatremia. The usual treatment of diabetes insipidus is fluid replacement, vasopressin, or desmopressin acetate (DDAVP) (see Chapter 49). If it is not treated, severe dehydration will occur.

SIADH is caused by excess secretion of ADH. SIADH results in decreased urine output and dilutional hyponatremia. It may result in cerebral edema, changes in LOC, seizures, and coma. (Treatment of SIADH is described in Chapter 49.)

Monitoring ICP. ICP monitoring is used in combination with other physiologic parameters to guide the care of the patient and assess the patient's response to treatment. Suctioning, hypoxemia, and arousal from sleep are factors that can increase ICP. Be alert to these factors and try to minimize them. Increased intrathoracic pressure can increase ICP by impeding the venous return. So, coughing, straining, sneezing, and the Valsalva maneuver should be avoided.

Body Position. Proper head positioning is important. Maintain the patient with increased ICP in the head-up position. Keep the head in a midline position, avoiding extreme neck flexion. Flexion can cause venous obstruction and contribute to increased ICP. Adjust the body position to decrease the ICP and improve the CPP. Elevating the head of the bed promotes drainage from the head and decreases the vascular congestion that can produce cerebral edema. However, raising the head of the bed above 30 degrees may decrease the CPP by lowering systemic BP. Carefully evaluate the effects of elevating the head of the bed on both ICP and CPP. Position the bed so that it lowers the ICP while optimizing the CPP and other indices of cerebral oxygenation.

Take care to turn the patient with slow, gentle movements. Rapid changes in position may increase ICP. Prevent discomfort when turning and positioning the patient because pain or agitation increases pressure. Avoid extreme hip flexion to decrease the risk for raising the intraabdominal pressure, which increases ICP. Decorticate or decerebrate posturing is a reflex response in some patients with increased ICP. Turning, skin care, and even passive range of motion can elicit these posturing reflexes.

Provide the physical care to minimize complications of immobility, such as atelectasis and contractures. Turn the patient at least every 2 hours.

Protection From Injury. The patient with increased ICP and decreased LOC needs protection from self-injury. Confusion, agitation, and the possibility of seizures increase the risk for injury. Use restraints judiciously in the agitated patient. If restraints are necessary to keep the patient from removing tubes or falling out of bed, they should be secure enough to be effective. Observe the skin area under the restraints regularly for irritation. Agitation may increase with the use of restraints, which indicates the need for other measures to protect the patient from injury. Light sedation with sedative agents may be needed. Having a family member stay with the patient may have a calming effect.

For the patient with seizures or the patient at risk for such activity, institute seizure precautions. These include padded side rails, an Ambu bag at the bedside, readily available suction, accurate and timely administration of antiseizure drugs, and close observation. Antiseizure prophylaxis against early seizures (within the first 7 to 10 days) is recommended in severe brain injury. This practice is controversial for mild to moderate brain injury.[8]

The patient can benefit from a quiet, nonstimulating environment. Always use a calm, reassuring approach. Touch and talk to the patient, even one who is in a coma.

Psychologic Considerations. In addition to carefully planned physical care, be aware of the psychologic well-being of patients and their families. Anxiety over the diagnosis and the prognosis can be distressing to the patient, caregiver and family, and nursing staff. Your competent and assured manner in performing care is reassuring to everyone involved. Short, simple explanations are appropriate and allow the patient and caregiver to acquire the amount of information they desire. There is a need for support, information, and teaching of both patients and families. Assess the family members' desires to help with providing care for the patient and allow for their participation as appropriate. Encourage interprofessional management (e.g., social work, chaplain) involving the patient and family in decision-making as much as possible.

◆ **Evaluation**

The expected outcomes are that the patient with increased ICP will

- Maintain ICP and cerebral perfusion within normal parameters
- Have no serious increases in ICP during or after care activities
- Have no complications of immobility

HEAD INJURY

Head injury includes any injury or trauma to the scalp, skull, or brain. A serious form of head injury is *traumatic brain injury* (TBI). Statistics about the occurrence of head injury are incomplete because many victims die at the injury scene or the condition is considered minor and health care services are not sought. An estimated 2.8 million persons are treated each year in U. S. emergency departments (EDs) for TBI. Of those, 57,000 die and 282,000 are hospitalized. Of those hospitalized, 20% will die.[9] At least 5.3 million Americans (2% of the U.S. population) currently live with disabilities resulting from TBI.

The most common causes of head injury are falls and motor vehicle accidents. Other causes of head injury include firearms, assaults, sports-related trauma, recreational injuries, and war-related injuries.[9] Men are twice as likely to sustain a TBI as women.

Head trauma has a high potential for a poor outcome. Deaths from head trauma occur at 3 points after injury: immediately after the injury, within 2 hours after injury, and about 3 weeks after injury.[10] Most deaths occur immediately after the injury, either from the direct head trauma or from massive hemorrhage and shock. Deaths occurring within a few hours of the trauma are caused by progressive worsening of the brain injury or internal bleeding.[11]

Deaths occurring 3 weeks or more after the injury result from multisystem failure. Expert nursing care in the weeks after the injury is crucial in decreasing the mortality risk and in optimizing patient outcomes.[12]

Types of Head Injuries

Scalp Lacerations. *Scalp lacerations* are an easily recognized type of external head trauma. Because the scalp contains many blood vessels with poor constrictive abilities, most scalp lacerations are associated with profuse bleeding. Even relatively small wounds can bleed significantly. The major complications associated with scalp laceration are blood loss and infection.

Skull Fractures. *Skull fractures* often occur with head trauma. Skull fractures are described in several ways: (1) linear or depressed; (2) simple, comminuted, or compound; and (3) closed or open (Table 56.6). Fractures may be closed or open, depending on the presence of a scalp laceration or extension of the fracture into the air sinuses or dura. The type and severity of a skull fracture depend on the velocity, momentum, direction, and shape (blunt or sharp) of the injuring agent and site of impact.

TABLE 56.6 Types of Skull Fractures

Type	Description	Cause
Comminuted	Multiple linear fractures with fragmentation of bone into many pieces	Direct, high-momentum impact
Compound	Depressed skull fracture and scalp laceration with communicating pathway to intracranial cavity	Severe head injury
Depressed	Inward indentation of skull	Powerful blow
Linear	Break in continuity of bone without change of relationship of parts	Low-velocity injuries
Simple	Linear or depressed skull fracture without fragmentation or communicating lacerations	Low to moderate impact

TABLE 56.7 Manifestations of Skull Fractures

Fracture Location	Manifestations
Basilar	CSF or brain otorrhea, bulging of tympanic membrane caused by blood or CSF, Battle's sign, tinnitus or hearing difficulty, rhinorrhea, facial paralysis, conjugate deviation of gaze, vertigo
Frontal	Exposure of brain to contaminants through frontal air sinus, possible association with air in forehead tissue, CSF rhinorrhea, pneumocranium (air between cranium and dura mater)
Orbital	Periorbital bruising (raccoon eyes), optic nerve injury
Parietal	Deafness, CSF or brain otorrhea, bulging of tympanic membrane caused by blood or CSF, facial paralysis, loss of taste, Battle's sign
Posterior fossa	Occipital bruising resulting in cortical blindness, visual field defects, rare appearance of ataxia or other cerebellar signs
Temporal	Boggy temporal muscle because of extravasation of blood, oval-shaped bruise behind ear in mastoid region (Battle's sign), CSF otorrhea, middle meningeal artery disruption, epidural hematoma

The location of the fracture determines the manifestations (Table 56.7). For example, a basilar skull fracture is a specialized type of linear fracture involving the base of the skull. Manifestations can evolve over the course of several hours and vary with the location and severity of fracture. These may include cranial nerve deficits, Battle's sign (postauricular bruising), and periorbital bruising (raccoon eyes) (Fig. 56.12). This fracture is often associated with a tear in the dura and subsequent leakage of CSF.

Rhinorrhea (CSF leakage from the nose) or *otorrhea* (CSF leakage from the ear) generally confirms that a fracture has traversed the dura (Fig. 56.12). Rhinorrhea may also manifest as postnasal sinus drainage. Rhinorrhea may be overlooked unless the patient is specifically assessed for this finding. The risk for meningitis is high with a CSF leak. Antibiotics should be given as a preventive measure.

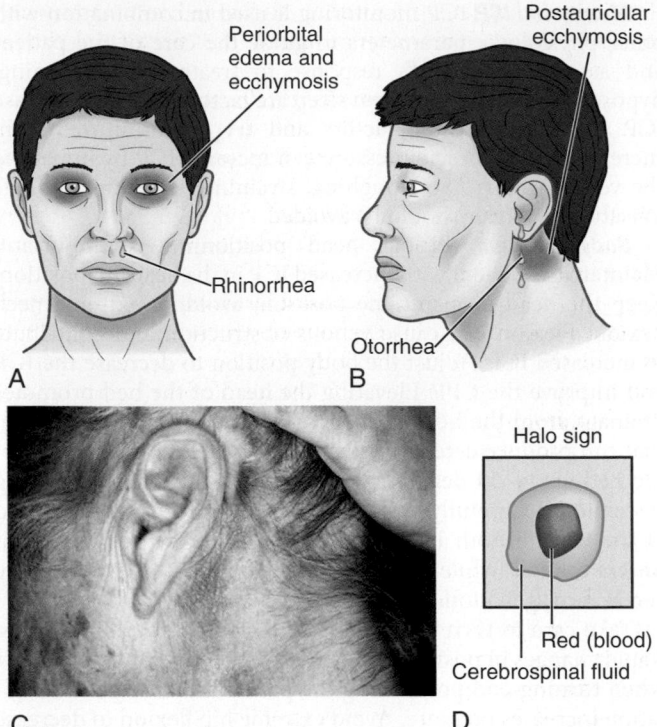

FIG. 56.12 A, Raccoon eyes and rhinorrhea. B, Battle's sign (postauricular bruising) with otorrhea. C, Battle's sign. D, Halo or ring sign (see text). (C, From Bingham BJG, Hawke M, Kwok P: *Clinical atlas of otolaryngology*, St Louis, 1992, Mosby.)

Two methods of testing can be used to determine whether the fluid leaking from the nose or ear is CSF. The first method is to test the leaking fluid with a Dextrostix or Tes-Tape strip to determine whether glucose is present. CSF gives a positive reading for glucose. If blood is present in the fluid, testing for glucose is unreliable because blood also contains glucose. In this event, look for the *halo* or *ring* sign (Fig. 56.12, *D*). Allow the leaking fluid to drip onto a white gauze pad (4 × 4) or towel, and then observe the drainage. Within a few minutes, the blood coalesces into the center, and a yellowish ring encircles the blood if CSF is present. Note the color, appearance, and amount of leaking fluid because both tests can give false-positive results.

The major complications of skull fractures are intracranial infections, hematoma, and meningeal and brain tissue damage. When a basilar skull fracture is suspected, an orogastric tube should be inserted rather than a NG tube.

Head Trauma. Brain injuries are categorized as diffuse (generalized) or focal (localized). In a *diffuse* injury (e.g., concussion, diffuse axonal injury), damage to the brain is not localized to one area. In a *focal injury* (e.g., contusion, hematoma), damage is localized to a specific area of the brain. Brain injury can be classified as *minor* (GCS 13 to 15), *moderate* (GCS 9 to 12), or *severe* (GCS 3 to 8).

Diffuse Injury. Concussion, a sudden transient mechanical head injury with disruption of neural activity and a change in the LOC, is considered a minor diffuse head injury. The patient may or may not lose total consciousness with this injury.

Typical signs include a brief disruption in LOC, amnesia about the event (retrograde amnesia), and headache. The manifestations are generally of short duration. If the patient has not lost consciousness, or if the loss of consciousness lasts less than

5 minutes, the patient is usually discharged with instructions to notify the HCP if symptoms persist or if behavioral changes are noted.

Postconcussion syndrome may develop in some patients, usually from 2 weeks to 2 months after the injury. Manifestations include persistent headache, lethargy, personality and behavioral changes, shortened attention span, decreased short-term memory, and changes in intellectual ability. This syndrome can significantly affect the patient's abilities to perform activities of daily living.

Concussion is generally considered benign and usually resolves spontaneously. For some, the signs and symptoms may be the beginning of a more serious, progressive problem, especially in a patient with a history of prior concussion or head injury. At the time of discharge, it is important to give the patient and caregiver instructions for observation and accurate reporting of symptoms or changes in neurologic status.

Diffuse axonal injury. Diffuse axonal injury (DAI) is widespread axonal damage occurring after a mild, moderate, or severe TBI. The damage occurs primarily around axons in the subcortical white matter of the cerebral hemispheres, basal ganglia, thalamus, and brainstem.[13] Initially, we thought DAI occurred because the tensile forces of trauma sheared axons, resulting in axonal disconnection. There is increasing evidence that axonal damage is not preceded by an immediate tearing of the axon from the traumatic impact. Instead, the trauma changes the function of the axon, resulting in axon swelling and disconnection. This process takes 12 to 24 hours to develop and may persist longer.

The clinical signs of DAI vary. They may include a decreased LOC, increased ICP, decortication or decerebration, and global cerebral edema. About 90% of patients with DAI stay in a persistent vegetative state.[13] Patients with DAI who survive the initial event are rapidly triaged to an ICU. There, they will be vigilantly watched for signs of increased ICP and treated accordingly.

Focal Injury. Focal injury can be minor to severe and localized to an area of injury. Focal injury consists of lacerations, contusions, hematomas, and cranial nerve injuries.

Lacerations involve actual tearing of the brain tissue. They often occur in association with depressed and open fractures and penetrating injuries. Tissue damage is severe, and surgical repair of the laceration is impossible because of the nature of brain tissue. Medical management consists of antibiotics (until meningitis is ruled out) and preventing secondary injury related to increased ICP. If bleeding is deep into the brain tissue, focal and generalized signs develop.

With major head trauma, many delayed responses can occur. These include hemorrhage, hematoma formation, seizures, and cerebral edema. Intracerebral hemorrhage is generally associated with cerebral laceration. This hemorrhage manifests as a space-occupying lesion accompanied by unconsciousness, hemiplegia on the contralateral side, and a dilated pupil on the ipsilateral side. As the hematoma expands, signs of increased ICP become more severe. Subarachnoid hemorrhage and intraventricular hemorrhage can occur from head trauma.

A contusion is bruising of the brain tissue within a focal area. It is usually associated with a closed head injury and often occurs at a fracture site. A contusion may have areas of hemorrhage, infarction, necrosis, and edema.

With contusion, the phenomenon of *coup-contrecoup injury* is often noted (Fig. 56.13). Injuries can range from minor to severe. Damage from coup-contrecoup injury occurs when the

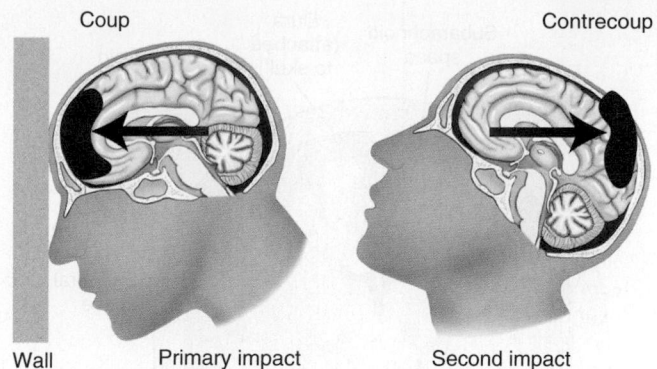

FIG. 56.13 Coup-contrecoup injury. After the head strikes the wall, a coup injury occurs as the brain strikes the skull (primary impact). The contrecoup injury (the second impact) occurs when the brain strikes the skull surface opposite the site of the original impact.

brain moves inside the skull due to high-energy or high-impact injury mechanisms. Contusions or lacerations occur both at the site of the direct impact of the brain on the skull *(coup)* and at a second area of damage on the opposite side away from injury *(contrecoup)*, leading to multiple contused areas. *Contrecoup* injuries tend to be more severe. The overall prognosis depends on the amount of bleeding around the contusion site.

Contusions may continue to bleed or rebleed and appear to "blossom" on subsequent CT scans of the brain. Bleeding worsens the neurologic outcome. Neurologic assessment may show focal and generalized manifestation, depending on the contusion's size and location. Seizures can occur because of a brain contusion, particularly when the injury involves the frontal or temporal lobes. Anticoagulant use and coagulopathy are associated with increased hemorrhage, more severe head injury, and an increased mortality rate.[14] This is especially important with older adults who are taking anticoagulants. If they fall, their contusion is likely to be more severe due to anticoagulant use. Assess for risk for falls in all patients taking anticoagulants.

Complications

Epidural Hematoma. An epidural hematoma results from bleeding between the dura and inner surface of the skull (Figs. 56.14 and 56.15). An epidural hematoma is a neurologic emergency. It is usually associated with a linear fracture crossing a major artery in the dura, causing a tear. It can have a venous or an arterial origin. Venous epidural hematomas are associated with a tear of the dural venous sinus and develop slowly. With arterial hematomas, the middle meningeal artery lying under the temporal bone is often torn. Hemorrhage occurs into the epidural space, which lies between the dura and inner surface of the skull (Fig. 56.14). Because this is an arterial hemorrhage, the hematoma develops rapidly.

Classic signs of an epidural hematoma include an initial period of unconsciousness at the scene, with a brief lucid interval followed by a decrease in LOC. Other manifestations may be a headache, nausea and vomiting, or focal findings. Rapid surgical intervention to evacuate the hematoma and prevent cerebral herniation, along with medical management for increasing ICP, dramatically improves outcomes.

Subdural Hematoma. A subdural hematoma occurs from bleeding between the dura mater and arachnoid layer of the meninges (Fig. 56.14). A subdural hematoma usually results from injury to the brain tissue and its blood vessels. The veins

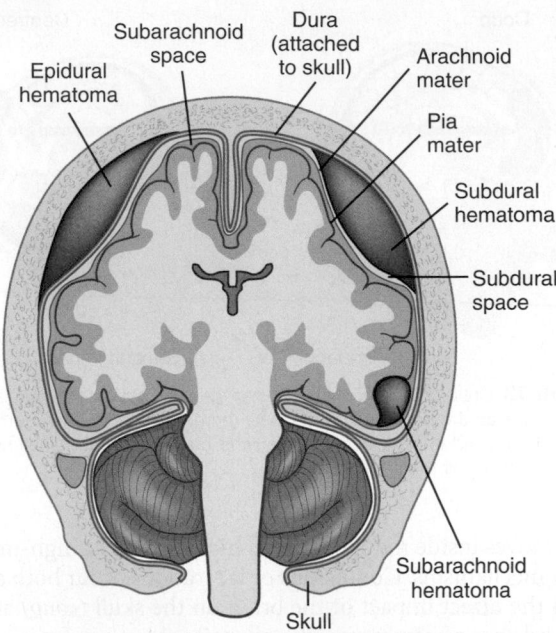

FIG. 56.14 Locations of epidural, subdural, and subarachnoid hematomas. (From Copstead-Kirkhorn LC, Banasik JL: *Pathophysiology*, ed 4, St Louis, 2010, Mosby.)

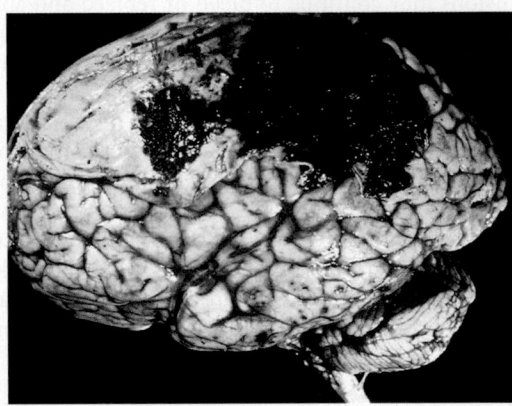

FIG. 56.15 Epidural hematoma covering a portion of the dura. Multiple small contusions are seen in the temporal lobe. (From Kumar V, Abbas AK, Aster JC, et al: *Robbins and Cotran pathologic basis of disease*, ed 8, Philadelphia, 2010, Saunders.)

that drain from the surface of the brain into the sagittal sinus are the source of most subdural hematomas. Because it is usually venous in origin, a subdural hematoma may be slower to develop. However, an arterial hemorrhage can cause a subdural hematoma, in which case it develops more rapidly.

Subdural hematomas may be acute, subacute, or chronic (Table 56.8). An *acute subdural hematoma* manifests within 24 to 48 hours of the injury.[15] The signs and symptoms are similar to those associated with brain tissue compression in increased ICP. They include decreasing LOC and headache. The size of the hematoma determines the patient's presentation and prognosis. The patient's appearance may range from drowsy and confused to unconscious. The ipsilateral pupil dilates and becomes fixed if ICP is significantly increased. Blunt-force injuries that produce acute subdural hematomas may cause significant underlying brain injury, resulting in cerebral edema. The resulting increase in ICP from the cerebral edema can increased morbidity and mortality despite surgery to evacuate the hematoma.

TABLE 56.8 Types of Subdural Hematomas

Occurrence After Injury	Progression of Symptoms	Treatment
Acute		
24–48 hr after severe trauma	Immediate deterioration	Craniotomy, evacuation, and decompression
Subacute		
48 hr–2 wk after severe trauma	Decline in mental status as hematoma develops. Progression dependent on size and location of hematoma	Evacuation and decompression
Chronic		
Weeks or months, usually >20 days after injury. Often injury seemed trivial or was forgotten by patient	Nonspecific, nonlocalizing progression. Progressive change in level of consciousness	Evacuation and decompression, membranectomy

A *subacute subdural hematoma* usually occurs within 2 to 14 days of the injury. After the initial bleeding, this hematoma may appear to enlarge over time as the breakdown products of the blood draw fluid into the subdural space.

A *chronic subdural hematoma* develops over weeks or months after a seemingly minor head injury.[15] They are more common in older adults because of a potentially larger subdural space from brain atrophy. With atrophy, the brain stays attached to the supportive structures and tension is increased. This makes it subject to tearing. Because the subdural space is larger, the presenting problem is focal symptoms (specific to a certain area of the brain) rather than signs of increased ICP.[15] Patients with a history of alcohol use are prone to subdural hematomas because of an increased incidence of falls.

Diagnosis of a subdural hematoma in the older adult may be delayed because symptoms mimic other health problems in this age-group, such as somnolence, confusion, lethargy, and memory loss. The manifestations of a subdural hematoma are often attributed to vascular disease (stroke, transient ischemic attack [TIA]) or dementia.

❓ CHECK YOUR PRACTICE

You are doing BP screenings in the senior center when you meet a 76-yr-old man and his wife. As you perform their BP screening, the wife tells you that her husband has been getting severe headaches, is dizzy, and sometimes has difficulty talking. Based on your advice, they go to an urgent care center, where a CT scan is done. The results show he has a chronic subdural hematoma. When you find out the diagnosis, you are puzzled because you thought he was having a stroke and cannot understand how he got a subdural hematoma.

• If you had been the nurse, what would you have done differently when screening this man?

Intracerebral Hematoma. Intracerebral hematoma occurs from bleeding within the brain tissue. It occurs in about 16% of head injuries. It usually happens in the frontal and temporal lobes, possibly from rupture of intracerebral vessels at the

✚ TABLE 56.9 Emergency Management

Head Injury

Etiology	Assessment Findings	Interventions
Blunt • Assault • Fall • Motor vehicle collision • Sports injury **Penetrating** • Arrow • Gunshot • Knife	**Surface Findings** • Bruises or contusions on face, Battle's sign (bruising behind ears) • Fracture or depressions in skull • Raccoon eyes (dependent bruising around eyes) • Scalp lacerations **Central Nervous System** • Asymmetric facial movements • Combativeness • Confusion • CSF leaking from ears or nose • Decerebrate or decorticate posturing • Decreased level of consciousness • Depressed or hyperactive reflexes • Dilated or unequal pupils, photophobia • Flaccidity • Garbled speech, abusive speech • GCS score <12 • Incontinence • Involuntary movements • Seizures **Respiratory** • Central neurogenic hyperventilation • Cheyne-Stokes respirations • Decreased O_2 saturation • Pulmonary edema	**Initial** • If unresponsive, assess circulation, airway, and breathing. • If responsive, monitor airway, breathing, and circulation. • Assume neck injury with head injury. • Stabilize cervical spine. • Apply O_2 via nonrebreather mask. • Establish IV access with 2 large-bore catheters to infuse normal saline or lactated Ringer's solution. • Intubate if GCS score <8. • Control external bleeding with sterile pressure dressing. • Remove patient's clothing. **Ongoing Monitoring** • Maintain normothermia using blankets, warm IV fluids, as needed. • Monitor vital signs, level of consciousness, O_2 saturation, cardiac rhythm, GCS score, pupil size and reactivity. • Expect intubation if gag reflex is impaired or absent. • Assess for rhinorrhea, otorrhea, scalp wounds. • Give fluids cautiously to prevent fluid overload and increasing ICP.

time of injury. The size and location of the hematoma are key in determining the patient's outcome.

Diagnostic Studies and Interprofessional Care. In general, the diagnostic studies are similar to those used for a patient with increased ICP (Table 56.3). CT scan is the best diagnostic test to evaluate for head trauma. It allows for rapid diagnosis and intervention in the acute care setting. MRI, PET, and evoked potential studies may be used to diagnose head injuries. An MRI scan is more sensitive than the CT scan in detecting small lesions. Transcranial Doppler studies allow for the measurement of cerebral blood flow (CBF) velocity. A cervical spine x-ray series, CT scan, or MRI of the spine may be done since cervical spine trauma often occurs at the same time as a head injury.

Emergency management of the patient with a head injury is outlined in Table 56.9. The principal treatment of head injuries is prompt diagnosis and surgery (if needed), In addition, we institute measures to prevent secondary injury by treating cerebral edema and managing increased ICP. For the patient with concussion and contusion, observation and management of increased ICP are the main management strategies.

The treatment of skull fractures is usually conservative. For depressed fractures and fractures with loose fragments, a craniotomy is done to elevate the depressed bone and remove the free fragments. If large amounts of bone are destroyed, the bone may be removed (craniectomy) and a cranioplasty will be needed later (see pp. 1321–1322).

In cases of large acute subdural and epidural hematomas or those associated with significant neurologic impairment, the blood must be removed through surgical evacuation. A craniotomy is generally done to see and allow control of the bleeding vessels. Burr-hole openings may be used in an extreme emergency

for a more rapid decompression, followed by a craniotomy. A drain may be placed after surgery for several days to prevent blood from reaccumulating. In cases in which extreme swelling is expected (e.g., DAI, hemorrhage), a craniectomy may be done. This involves removing a piece of skull to reduce the pressure inside the cranial vault. It reduces the risk for herniation.

❖ NURSING MANAGEMENT: HEAD INJURY

◆ **Nursing Assessment.** A patient with a head injury always has the potential to develop increased ICP, which is associated with higher mortality rates and poorer functional outcomes. Objective data are obtained by applying the GCS (Table 56.5), assessing and monitoring the neurologic status, and determining whether a CSF leak has occurred. Nursing assessment related to increased ICP is discussed on pp. 1308–1309. Nursing assessment of the patient with a head injury is outlined in Table 56.10.

◆ **Nursing Diagnoses**

Nursing diagnoses for the patient who has sustained a head injury may include:

• Decreased intracranial adaptive capacity
• Ineffective tissue perfusion
• Hyperthermia
• Risk for injury
• Anxiety

◆ **Planning**

The overall goals are that the patient with an acute head injury will (1) maintain adequate cerebral oxygenation and perfusion;

TABLE 56.10 Nursing Assessment

Head Injury

Subjective Data

Important Health Information

Past health history: Mechanism of injury: motor vehicle collision, sports injury, industrial incident, assault, falls
Medications: Anticoagulant drugs

Functional Health Patterns

Health perception–health management: Alcohol or recreational drugs. Risk-taking behaviors
Cognitive-perceptual: Headache, mood or behavioral change, mentation changes, aphasia, dysphasia, impaired judgment
Coping–stress tolerance: Fear, denial, anger, aggression, depression

Objective Data

General

Altered mental status

Integumentary

Lacerations, contusions, abrasions, hematoma, Battle's sign, periorbital edema and bruising, otorrhea, exposed brain matter

Respiratory

Rhinorrhea, impaired gag reflex, inability to maintain a patent airway. Impending herniation: altered/irregular respiratory rate and pattern

Cardiovascular

Impending herniation: Cushing's triad (systolic hypertension with widening pulse pressure, bradycardia with full and bounding pulse, irregular respirations)

Gastrointestinal

Vomiting, projectile vomiting, bowel incontinence

Urinary

Bladder incontinence

Reproductive

Uninhibited sexual expression

Neurologic

Altered level of consciousness, seizure activity, pupil dysfunction, cranial nerve deficit(s)

Musculoskeletal

Motor deficit/impairment, weakness, palmar drift, paralysis, spasticity, decorticate or decerebrate posturing, muscular rigidity or increased tone, flaccidity, ataxia

Possible Diagnostic Findings

Location and type of hematoma, edema, skull fracture, and/or foreign body on CT scan and/or MRI; abnormal EEG; positive toxicology screen or alcohol level, ↓ or ↑ blood glucose level; ↑ ICP

ETHICAL/LEGAL DILEMMAS

Brain Death

Situation

The emergency nurse receives a call from emergency response system (ERS) personnel, who are in route with R.G., a young man involved in a motorcycle crash. He was not wearing a helmet and has a large open skull fracture. Transport from the accident scene was delayed by 45 min because of a severe thunderstorm and traffic congestion. R.G. has fixed, dilated pupils and is in cardiac arrest. Estimated arrival at the hospital is still another 45 min because of the severe weather. EMS personnel request permission to stop resuscitation efforts.

Ethical/Legal Points for Consideration

- Criteria for brain death include coma or unresponsiveness, absence of brainstem reflexes, and apnea (see Chapter 9).
- The definition of death has changed with the advent of new technology, monitoring devices, and interventions.
- In a situation in which the professional responsible for determining a state of death is in remote contact with the patient, but the monitoring devices available provide virtual contact with the patient, a remote diagnosis of death may be legally acceptable.
- Brain death criteria do not address patients in a permanent vegetative state since the brainstem activity in these patients is adequate to maintain heart and lung function.
- CPR is not appropriate when survival is not expected or the patient is expected to survive without the ability to communicate. Quantitative futility implies that survival is not expected after CPR under given circumstances. In the absence of mitigating factors, prolonged resuscitative efforts are unlikely to be successful and can be stopped if there is no return of spontaneous circulation at any time during 30 minutes of cumulative advanced life support.
- It is ethical for ED personnel to stop treatment started by ERS personnel in the prehospital setting if there is valid, after-the-fact evidence that these interventions are now inappropriate.

Discussion Questions

- What are your feelings about cessation of brain function vs. cessation of heart and lung function as the criteria for death of a patient?
- What are your state's laws or practices about stopping CPR efforts by ERS personnel in the field?

♥ PROMOTING POPULATION HEALTH

Reducing the Risk for Head Injuries

- Always wear car seat belts in motor vehicles.
- Do not drive after using drugs or alcohol.
- Do not text and drive or drive distracted.
- Wear helmets while bicycling, skating, skateboarding, skiing, and playing contact sports.
- Athletes should follow safe playing techniques and the rules of the game.
- Assess home safety and implement any corrective measures needed.
- Older adults should continue to exercise regularly to improve strength and balance.
- Follow workplace safety precautions, including wearing helmets and protective gear.

(2) stay afebrile; (3) be free of discomfort; (4) be free from infection; (5) have adequate nutrition; and (6) attain maximal cognitive, motor, and sensory function.

❖ Nursing Implementation

◆ **Health Promotion.** One of the best ways to prevent head injuries is to prevent car and motorcycle accidents. Be active in campaigns that promote driving safety. Speak to driver education classes about the dangers of distracted driving and driving after drinking alcohol or using drugs. Helmets for motorcycle riders is the most effective measure for increasing survival after crashes.

◆ **Acute Care.** Management at the injury scene can have a significant impact on the outcome of a head injury. Emergency management of head injury is outlined in Table 56.9. The general goal of nursing management of the patient with head injury is to

TABLE 56.11 Patient & Caregiver Teaching

Head Injury

Include the following instructions when teaching the patient and caregiver about care during the first 2 or 3 days after a head injury:

1. Notify your HCP immediately if you have signs and symptoms that may indicate complications. These include:
   - Increased drowsiness (e.g., difficulty arousing, confusion)
   - Nausea or vomiting
   - Worsening headache or stiff neck
   - Seizures
   - Vision difficulties (e.g., blurring) or sensitivity to light (photophobia)
   - Behavioral changes (e.g., irritability, anger)
   - Motor problems (e.g., clumsiness, difficulty walking, slurred speech, weakness in arms or legs)
   - Sensory problems (e.g., numbness)
   - A heart rate <60 beats/min
2. Have someone stay with you.
3. Abstain from alcohol.
4. Check with your HCP before taking drugs that may increase drowsiness, including muscle relaxants, tranquilizers, and opioid analgesia.
5. Avoid driving, using heavy machinery, playing contact sports, and taking hot baths.

maintain cerebral oxygenation and perfusion and prevent secondary cerebral ischemia.

Surveillance or monitoring for changes in neurologic status is critically important because the patient's condition may deteriorate rapidly, requiring emergency surgery. Appropriate nursing interventions are started if surgery is anticipated. Because of the close association between hemodynamic status and cerebral perfusion, be aware of any coexisting injuries or conditions.

Explain the need for frequent neurologic assessments to both the patient and caregiver. Behavioral manifestations associated with head injury can result in a frightened, disoriented patient who is combative and resists help. Your approach should be calm and gentle. A family member may be available to stay with the patient and thus decrease anxiety and fear. An important need of the caregiver and family members in the acute injury phase is information about the patient's diagnosis, treatment plan, and reason for the interventions. Other teaching points are described in Table 56.11.

Perform neurologic assessments at intervals based on the patient's condition. The GCS is useful in assessing the LOC (Table 56.5). Report any signs of a deteriorating neurologic state, no matter how subtle, such as a decreasing LOC or decreasing motor strength, to the HCP. Monitor the patient's condition closely.

The major focus of nursing care for the patient with a brain injury relates to increased ICP (see eNursing Care Plan 56.1). However, some problems need specific nursing intervention.

Eye problems may include loss of the corneal reflex, periorbital bruising and edema, and diplopia. Loss of the corneal reflex may require lubricating eye drops or taping the eyes shut to prevent abrasion. Periorbital bruising and edema decrease with time. Cold and, later, warm compresses provide comfort and hasten the process. Wearing an eye patch can relieve diplopia. Consider a consult with an ophthalmologist.

Fever may occur from injury to or inflammation of the hypothalamus. Fever can cause increased CBF, cerebral blood volume, and ICP. Increased metabolism from fever increases metabolic waste, which in turn causes further cerebral vasodilation. Avoid fever with a goal of a temperature of 96.8° to 98.6° F (36° to 37° C) as the standard of care. Use interventions to

reduce temperature as previously discussed (see p. 1308) in conjunction with sedation to prevent shivering.

If CSF rhinorrhea or otorrhea occurs, inform the HCP at once. The head of the bed may be raised to decrease the CSF pressure so that a tear can seal. A loose collection pad may be placed under the nose or over the ear. Do not place a dressing in the nasal or ear cavities. Document the amount of drainage each shift. Teach the patient not to sneeze or blow the nose. Do not use NG tubes. Do not perform nasotracheal suctioning on these patients because of the high risk for meningitis.

Nursing measures specific to the care of the immobilized patient, such as those related to bladder and bowel function, skin care, and infection, are needed. Nausea and vomiting may be a problem and can be alleviated by antiemetic drugs. Headache can usually be controlled with acetaminophen or small doses of codeine.

If the patient's condition deteriorates, intracranial surgery may be needed (see the section on cranial surgery on pp. 1321–1323). A burr-hole opening or craniotomy may be done, depending on the underlying injury that is causing the problems. The emergency nature of the surgery may hasten the usual preoperative preparation. Consult with the HCP to determine specific preoperative nursing measures.

The patient is often unconscious before surgery, making it necessary for a family member to sign the consent form for surgery. This is a difficult and frightening time for the patient's caregiver and family and requires sensitive nursing management. The suddenness of the situation makes it especially hard for the family to cope. Use a team approach, including social workers, to help the patient and family throughout the hospitalization and recovery time.

◆ **Ambulatory Care.** Once the condition has stabilized, the patient is usually transferred for acute rehabilitation management. There may be chronic problems related to motor and sensory deficits, communication, memory, and intellectual functioning. Conditions that may need nursing and interprofessional management include nutrition problems, bowel and bladder problems, spasticity, dysphagia, and hydrocephalus. Many of the principles for managing the patient with a stroke are appropriate for these patients (see Chapter 57).

Seizure disorders may occur in patients with nonpenetrating head injury. Seizures may develop during the first week after the head injury or not until years later. Antiseizure drugs may be used prophylactically to manage posttraumatic seizure activity, but this practice is controversial.

The mental and emotional sequelae are often the most incapacitating problems. One of the consequences of TBI is that the person may not realize that a brain injury has occurred. Many patients with head injuries who were comatose for more than 6 hours undergo some personality change. They may have loss of concentration and memory and defective memory processing. Personal drive may decrease. Apathy may increase. Euphoria and mood swings, along with a seeming lack of awareness of the seriousness of the injury, may occur. The patient's behavior may indicate a loss of social restraint, judgment, tact, and emotional control.

Progressive recovery may continue for years. Specific nursing management in the posttraumatic phase depends on specific residual deficits. Being able to return to work and maintaining employment is one of the challenges during the recovery period.[16] The patient's outward physical appearance does not necessarily reflect what has happened in the brain. It is not a

TABLE 56.12 Types of Brain Tumors

Type	Tissue of Origin	Characteristics
Acoustic neuroma (schwannoma)	Cells that form myelin sheath around nerves. Often affects cranial nerve VIII	Many grow on both sides of the brain. Usually benign or low-grade.
Gliomas		
• Astrocytoma	Supportive tissue, glial cells, and astrocytes	Can range from low-grade to moderate-grade.
• Ependymoma	Ependymal epithelium	Range from benign to highly malignant. Most are benign and encapsulated.
• Glioblastoma	Primitive stem cell (glioblast)	Highly malignant and invasive. Among the most devastating of primary brain tumors.
• Medulloblastoma	Primitive neuroectodermal cell	Highly malignant and invasive. Metastatic to spinal cord and remote areas of brain.
• Oligodendroglioma	Oligodendrocytes	Benign (encapsulation and calcification).
Hemangioblastoma	Blood vessels of brain	Rare and benign. Surgery is curative.
Meningioma	Meninges	Can be benign or malignant. Most are benign.
Metastatic tumors	Lungs and breast (most common)	Malignant.
Pituitary adenoma	Pituitary gland	Usually benign.
Primary central nervous system lymphoma	Lymphocytes	Increased incidence in transplant recipients and acquired immunodeficiency syndrome (AIDS) patients.

good indicator of how well the patient will ultimately function in the home or work environment.

Give the family special consideration. They need to understand what is happening. Provide guidance and referrals for financial aid, child care, and other personal needs. Help the family in involving the patient in family activities whenever possible. Help the patient and family remain hopeful. The family often has unrealistic expectations of the patient as the coma begins to recede. The family expects full return to pretrauma status. In reality, the patient usually has a reduced awareness and ability to interpret environmental stimuli. Prepare the family for the patient's emergence from coma and explain that the process of awakening often takes several weeks. In addition, arrange for social work and chaplain consultations for the family.

When it is the time for discharge planning, the patient, caregiver, and family may benefit from specific instructions to avoid family-patient friction. Special "no" policies that may be suggested by the HCP, neuropsychologist, and nurse include no drinking of alcoholic beverages, no driving, no use of firearms, no working with hazardous implements and machinery, and no unsupervised smoking. Family members, particularly spouses, go through role transition as the role changes from that of spouse to that of caregiver.

◆ Evaluation

The expected outcomes are that the patient with a head injury will
- Maintain normal CPP
- Achieve maximal cognitive, motor, and sensory function
- Have no infection or fever

BRAIN TUMORS

There are an estimated 23,400 people diagnosed each year with brain tumors in the United States. The brain is also a frequent site for metastasis from other sites.[17] Males have a slightly higher incidence of brain tumors than females. Brain tumors most often occur in middle-aged persons, but they may be seen at any age.

🌐 PROMOTING HEALTH EQUITY
Brain Tumors

- Whites have a higher incidence of malignant brain tumors than blacks.
- White males have the highest incidence of malignant brain tumors.
- Blacks have the highest incidence of benign brain tumors (e.g., meningiomas).

Types

Brain tumors can occur in any part of the brain or spinal cord. Tumors of the brain may be *primary*, arising from tissues within the brain, or *secondary*, resulting from a metastasis of cancer from elsewhere in the body.[18]

Metastatic brain tumors are the most common brain tumor. The cancers that most often metastasize to the brain are lung and breast.

Primary brain tumors are generally classified according to the tissue from which they arise (Table 56.12). Meningiomas are the most common primary brain tumor. Other common brain tumors are gliomas (e.g., astrocytoma, glioblastoma [most common form of glioma]).

More than half of brain tumors are malignant. They infiltrate the brain tissue and are not amenable to complete surgical removal. Other tumors may be histologically benign but are located such that complete removal is not possible.

Brain tumors rarely metastasize outside the central nervous system (CNS) because they are contained by structural (meninges) and physiologic (blood-brain) barriers. Table 56.12 compares the most common brain tumors. A glioblastoma and meningioma are shown in Fig. 56.16.

Clinical Manifestations and Complications

The manifestations of brain tumors depend mainly on their location and size (Table 56.13). A wide range of manifestations are possible. Headache is common. Tumor-related headaches tend to be worse at night and may awaken the patient. The headaches are usually dull and constant but sometimes throbbing. Seizures are common in gliomas and brain metastases. Brain tumors can cause nausea and vomiting from increased ICP.

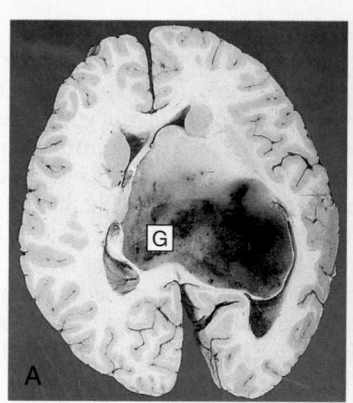
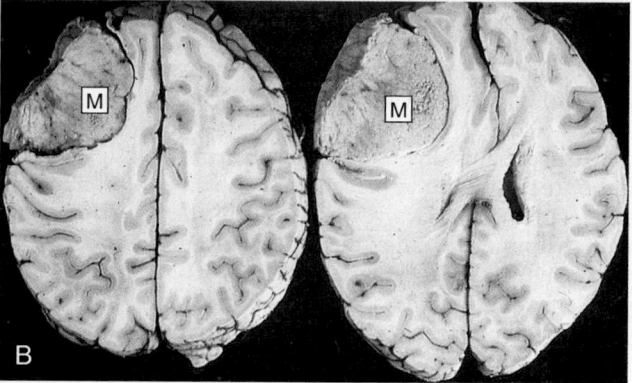

FIG. 56.16 A, A large glioblastoma *(G)* arises from one cerebral hemisphere and has grown to fill the ventricular system. B, Meningioma. These 2 different sections from different levels in the same brain show a meningioma *(M)* compressing the frontal lobe and distorting underlying brain. (From Stevens A, Lowe J: *Pathology: Illustrated review in colour,* ed 2, London, 2000, Mosby.)

TABLE 56.13 Manifestations of Brain Tumors

Tumor Location	Manifestations
Brainstem tumors	Headache on awakening, drowsiness, vomiting, ataxic gait, facial muscle weakness, hearing loss, dysphagia, dysarthria, "crossed eyes" or other visual changes, hemiparesis
Cerebellopontine tumors	Tinnitus and vertigo, deafness
Cerebral hemisphere	
• Frontal lobe (unilateral)	Unilateral hemiplegia, seizures, memory deficit, personality and judgment changes, visual changes
• Frontal lobe (bilateral)	Symptoms associated with unilateral frontal lobe tumors. Ataxic gait
• Parietal lobe	Speech problems (if tumor is in the dominant hemisphere), inability to write, spatial disorders, unilateral neglect
• Occipital lobe	Vision changes and seizures
• Temporal lobe	Few symptoms. Seizures, dysphagia, hallucinations, auras
Fourth ventricle and cerebellar tumors	Headache, nausea, and papilledema (occur from ↑ ICP). Ataxic gait and changes in coordination
Meningeal tumors	Symptoms associated with compression of the brain and depend on tumor location
Metastatic tumors	Headache, nausea, or vomiting (occur from ↑ ICP). Other symptoms depend on tumor location
Subcortical	Hemiplegia; other symptoms may depend on area of infiltration
Thalamus and sellar tumors	Headache, nausea, vision changes, papilledema, and nystagmus (occur from ↑ ICP). Diabetes insipidus may occur

Cognitive dysfunction, including memory problems and mood or personality changes, is common, especially in patients with brain metastases. Muscle weakness, sensory losses, aphasia, and visual-spatial dysfunction may occur.

If the tumor mass obstructs the ventricles or occludes the outlet, ventricular enlargement (hydrocephalus) can occur. As the brain tumor expands, it may produce manifestations of increased ICP, cerebral edema, or obstruction of the CSF pathways. Unless treated, all brain tumors eventually cause death from increasing tumor volume leading to increased ICP.

Diagnostic Studies

An extensive history and a comprehensive neurologic examination is done in the workup of a patient with a suspected brain tumor. The history and physical examination may provide data with respect to location. New onset of seizures or adult-onset migraines may indicate a brain tumor and should be investigated. Diagnostic studies are similar to those used for a patient with increased ICP (Table 56.3).

The sensitivity of techniques such as MRI and PET scans allows for detection of small tumors and may provide more reliable diagnostic information than a CT scan. CT with contrast and MRI are used to identify the lesion's location. Other tests include magnetic resonance spectroscopy, functional MRI (fMRI), and single-photon emission computed tomography (SPECT). An EEG can rule out seizures but is of less importance. An LP is seldom diagnostic and carries with it the risk for cerebral herniation. Cerebral angiography can determine blood flow to the tumor and further localize the tumor. Other studies are done to rule out a primary lesion elsewhere in the body. Endocrine studies are helpful when a pituitary adenoma is suspected (see Chapter 49).

The correct diagnosis of a brain tumor can be made by obtaining tissue for histologic study. In most patients, tissue is obtained at the time of surgery. Computer-guided stereotactic biopsy is also an option. A smear or frozen section can be done in the operating room for a preliminary interpretation of the histologic type. With this information, the HCP can make a better decision about the extent of surgery.

Interprofessional Care

Treatment goals are aimed at (1) identifying the tumor type and location, (2) removing or decreasing tumor mass, and (3) preventing or managing increased ICP.

Surgical Therapy. Surgical removal is the preferred treatment for brain tumors. Stereotactic surgical techniques are used with greater frequency to perform a biopsy and remove small brain tumors. The outcome of surgery depends on the tumor's type, size, and location. Meningiomas and oligodendrogliomas can usually be completely removed. The more invasive gliomas and medulloblastomas may only be partially removed. Computer-guided stereotactic biopsy, ultrasound, fMRI, and cortical mapping can localize brain tumors during surgery.

Complete surgical removal of brain tumors is not always possible because the tumor is not always accessible or may involve vital parts of the brain. Surgery can reduce tumor mass, which decreases ICP, provides relief of symptoms, and extends survival time.

Ventricular Shunts. Hydrocephalus due to a tumor obstructing the CSF flow can be treated with the placement of a ventricular shunt. A catheter with 1-way valves is placed in the lateral ventricle and then tunneled under the skin to drain CSF into the peritoneal cavity. Rapid decompression of ICP can cause total body collapse and weakness. Headache may be prevented by gradually introducing the patient to the upright position.

Manifestations of shunt malfunction, which are related to increased ICP, include decreasing LOC, restlessness, headache, blurred vision, or vomiting. This may require shunt revision or replacement. Infection may occur, as exhibited by high fever, persistent headache, and stiff neck. Antibiotics are used to treat the infection. In some situations, the shunt must be replaced. CSF drainage is managed with an extraventricular drainage system while the infection is treated.

Radiation Therapy and Stereotactic Radiosurgery. Radiation therapy may be used as a follow-up measure after surgery. Radiation seeds can be implanted into the brain. Cerebral edema and rapidly increasing ICP may be a complication of radiation therapy. These problems can usually be managed with high doses of corticosteroids (e.g., dexamethasone, methylprednisolone). Radiation therapy is discussed in Chapter 15.

Stereotactic radiosurgery is a method of delivering a highly concentrated dose of radiation to a precise location within the brain. Stereotactic radiosurgery may be used when conventional surgery has failed or is not an option because of the tumor location. (Radiosurgery is discussed on p. 1322.)

Chemotherapy and Targeted Therapy. The effectiveness of chemotherapy has been limited by the difficulty with getting drugs across the blood-brain barrier, tumor cell heterogeneity, and tumor cell drug resistance. Chemotherapy drugs called *nitrosoureas* (e.g., carmustine, lomustine) are used to treat brain tumors. Normally the blood-brain barrier prohibits the entry of most drugs into the brain. Cancer tumors can cause a breakdown of the blood-brain barrier in the area of the tumor, thus allowing chemotherapy agents to be used to treat the cancer. Chemotherapy-laden biodegradable wafers (e.g., Gliadel wafer [polifeprosan with carmustine implant]) implanted at the time of surgery can deliver chemotherapy directly to the tumor site. Other drugs being used include methotrexate and procarbazine (Matulane). One way used to deliver chemotherapy drugs directly to the CNS is intrathecal administration via an Ommaya reservoir.

Temozolomide (Temodar) is an oral chemotherapy agent that can cross the blood-brain barrier. In contrast with many chemotherapy drugs, which require metabolic activation to exert their effects, temozolomide can convert spontaneously to a reactive agent that directly interferes with tumor growth. It does not interact with other common drugs taken by patients with brain tumors, such as antiseizure drugs, corticosteroids, and antiemetics.

DRUG ALERT Temozolomide (Temodar)

- Causes myelosuppression. Before using, the absolute neutrophil count should be ≥1500/µL and platelet count should be ≥100,000/µL.
- To reduce nausea and vomiting, take on empty stomach or at bedtime.

Bevacizumab (Avastin) is used to treat patients with glioblastoma that continues to progress after standard therapy. Bevacizumab is a targeted therapy that inhibits the action of vascular endothelial growth factor, which helps form new blood vessels. These vessels can feed a tumor, helping it to grow, and provide a pathway for cancer cells to circulate in the body. Targeted therapy is discussed in Chapter 15 and Table 15.13.

Other Therapies. A medical device system, the Optune System, is used to treat glioblastoma that recurs or progresses after receiving chemotherapy and radiation therapy. With this system, electrodes are placed on the surface of the patient's scalp to deliver low-intensity, changing electrical fields called *tumor treatment fields* (TTFs) to the tumor site.

❖ NURSING MANAGEMENT: BRAIN TUMORS

◆ Nursing Assessment

Interview data are as important as the actual physical assessment. Ask about the medical history, intellectual abilities and educational level, and history of nervous system infections and trauma. Structure the initial assessment to provide baseline data of the patient's neurologic status. Use this information to design a realistic, patient specific care plan.

Assess the patient's LOC, motor abilities, sensory perception, integrated function (including bowel and bladder function), and balance and proprioception. Determine the presence of seizures, syncope, nausea and vomiting, and headaches or other pain. Assess the coping abilities of the patient, caregiver, and family. Watching a patient perform activities of daily living and listening to the patient's conversation can be part of the neurologic assessment. Having the patient or caregiver explain the problem can be helpful to determine the patient's limitations and obtain information about the patient's insight into the problems. Record all initial data to provide a baseline for comparison to determine whether the patient's condition is improving or deteriorating.

◆ Nursing Diagnoses

Nursing diagnoses for the patient with a brain tumor may include:

- Ineffective tissue perfusion
- Acute pain
- Anxiety
- Risk for injury

◆ Planning

The overall goals are that the patient with a brain tumor will (1) maintain normal ICP, (2) maximize neurologic functioning, (3) achieve control of pain and discomfort, and (4) be aware of the long-term implications with respect to prognosis and cognitive and physical functioning.

◆ Nursing Implementation

A tumor of the frontal lobe can cause behavioral and personality changes. Loss of emotional control, confusion, disorientation, memory loss, impulsivity, and depression may be signs of a frontal lobe lesion. The patient often does not perceive these changes. They can be disturbing and frightening to the caregiver and family. These changes can also cause a distancing to occur between the family and patient. Help the caregiver and family understand what is happening to the patient and support the family.

The confused patient with behavioral instability can be a challenge. Protecting the patient from self-harm is an important part of nursing care. Essential interventions include close supervision of activity, use of side rails, judicious use of restraints, appropriate sedatives, padding of the rails and the area around the bed, and a calm, reassuring approach.

Perceptual problems associated with frontal and parietal lobe tumors contribute to a patient's disorientation and confusion. Minimize environmental stimuli, create a routine, and use reality orientation for the confused patient. Tumors in the temporal lobe can cause hallucinations, which may be confused with dementia or delirium.

Seizures, which often occur with brain tumors, are managed with antiseizure drugs. Use seizure precautions for the patient's protection. Some behavioral changes seen in the patient are a result of seizure disorders and can improve with adequate seizure control. Patients at risk for seizures may be unable to drive, so be aware of the extra resources needed and collaborate with the social worker and family. Seizure disorders are discussed in Chapter 58.

Motor and sensory dysfunctions interfere with activities of daily living. Encourage the patient to provide as much self-care as physically possible. Self-image often depends on the patient's ability to take part in care within the limitations of the physical deficits.

Language deficits may be present. Motor (expressive) or sensory (receptive) dysphasia may occur. The problem with communication can be frustrating for the patient and may interfere with your ability to meet the patient's needs. Try to establish a communication system that both the patient and staff can use.

Nutritional intake may be decreased because of the patient's inability to eat, loss of appetite, or loss of desire to eat. Assess nutritional status and ensure adequate nutritional intake. Encourage the patient to eat. Some patients may need enteral or parenteral nutrition (see Chapter 39).

Provide help and support during the adjustment phase and in long-range planning. Social work and home health nurses may be needed to aid the caregiver with discharge planning and to help the family adjust to role changes and psychosocial and socioeconomic factors. Issues related to palliative and end-of-life care must be discussed with both the patient and family (see Chapter 9).

◆ Evaluation

The expected outcomes are that the patient with a brain tumor will

- Achieve control of pain, vomiting, and other discomforts
- Maintain ICP within normal limits
- Have maximal neurologic function given the location and extent of the tumor
- Maintain optimal nutritional status
- Accept the long-term consequences of the tumor and its treatment

CRANIAL SURGERY

Indications for cranial surgery are related to brain tumors, CNS infection (e.g., abscess), vascular abnormalities, craniocerebral trauma, seizure disorder, or intractable pain (Table 56.14).

Types

Various types of cranial surgical procedures are outlined in Table 56.15.

TABLE 56.14 Indications for Cranial Surgery

Indication	Cause	Surgical Procedure
Aneurysm repair	Dilation of weak area in arterial wall (usually near anterior portion of circle of Willis)	Dissection and clipping or coiling of aneurysm
Arteriovenous (AV) malformation	Congenital tangle of arteries and veins (often in middle cerebral artery)	Excision of malformation
Brain abscess	Bacteria that caused intracranial infection	Excision or drainage of abscess
Brain tumors	Benign or malignant cell growth	Excision or partial resection of tumor
Hydrocephalus	Overproduction of cerebrospinal fluid, obstruction to flow, defective reabsorption	Placement of ventriculoperitoneal or (rarely) ventriculoatrial shunt
Intracranial bleeding	Rupture of cerebral vessels because of trauma or stroke	Surgical evacuation through burr holes or craniotomy
Skull fractures	Trauma to skull	Debridement of fragments and necrotic tissue, elevation and realignment of bone fragments

TABLE 56.15 Types of Cranial Surgery

Type	Description
Burr hole	Opening into the cranium with a drill. Used to remove localized fluid and blood beneath the dura.
Craniectomy	Excision into the cranium to cut away bone flap.
Cranioplasty	Repair of cranial defect resulting from trauma, malformation, or previous surgical procedure. Artificial material used to replace damaged or lost bone.
Craniotomy	Opening into cranium with removal of bone flap and opening the dura to remove a lesion, repair a damaged area, drain blood, or relieve ↑ ICP.
Shunt procedures	Alternative pathway to redirect cerebrospinal fluid from one area to another using a tube or implanted device. Examples include ventricular shunt and Ommaya reservoir.
Stereotactic procedure	Precise localization of a specific area of the brain using a frame or frameless system based on 3-dimensional coordinates. Used for biopsy, radiosurgery, or dissection.

Craniotomy. Depending on the location of the pathologic condition, a *craniotomy* may be frontal, parietal, occipital, temporal, suboccipital, or a combination of any of these. The HCP drills a set of burr holes and uses a saw to connect the holes to remove the bone flap (Fig. 56.17). Sometimes operating microscopes are used to magnify the site. After surgery, the bone flap is secured with small plates or wired shut. Sometimes drains are placed to remove fluid and blood. Patients are usually cared for in an ICU until stable.

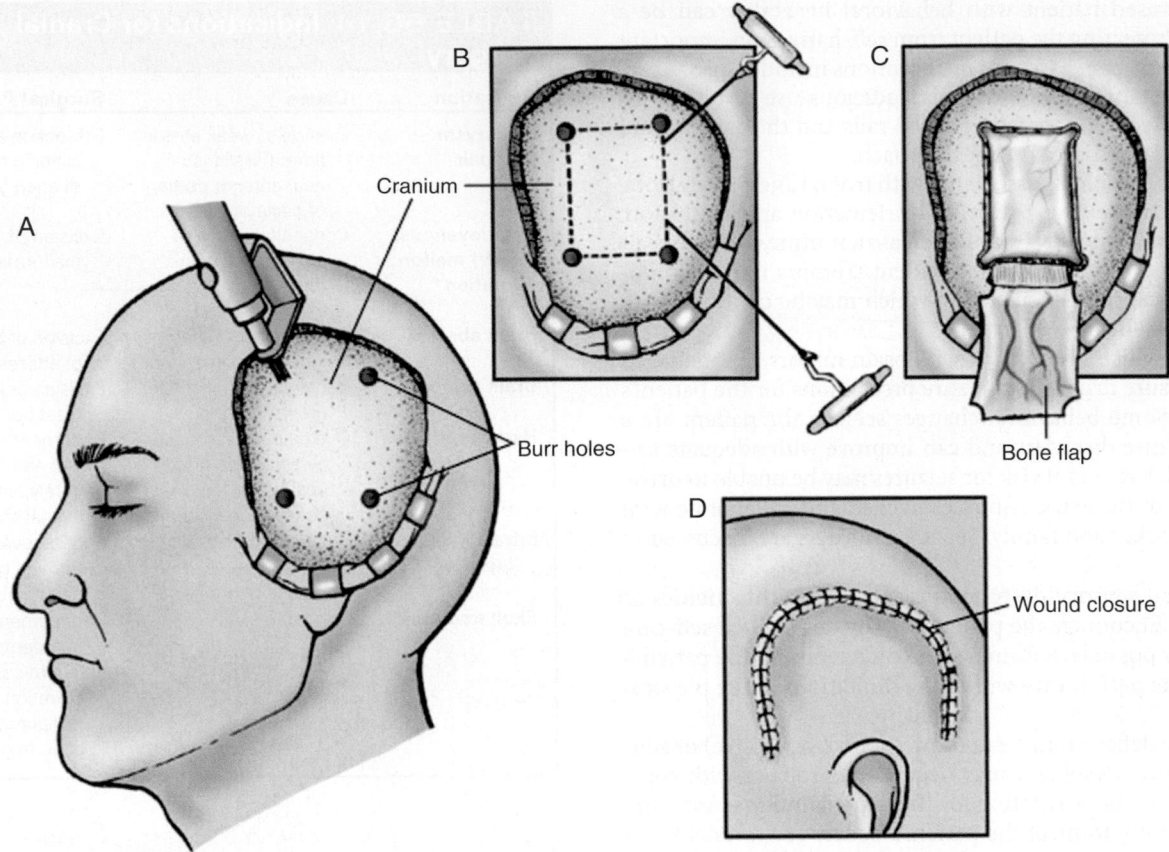

FIG. 56.17 Craniotomy. **A**, Burr holes are drill into skull. **B**, Skull is cut between burr holes with a surgical saw. **C**, Bone flap is turned back to expose cranial contents. **D**, Bone flap is replaced and wound closed. (From Monahan F, Sands J, Neighbors M, et al: *Phipps' medical-surgical nursing: Health and illness perspectives,* ed 9, St Louis, 2007, Mosby.)

Stereotactic Radiosurgery. Stereotactic procedures use a precision apparatus (often computer guided) to help the HCP precisely target an area of the brain. Stereotactic biopsy can be done to obtain tissue samples for histologic examination. CT scanning and MRI are used to image the targeted tissue. With the patient under general or local anesthesia, the HCP drills a burr hole or creates a bone flap for an entry site and then introduces a probe and biopsy needle. Stereotactic procedures are used for removal of small brain tumors and abscesses, drainage of hematomas, ablative procedures for extrapyramidal diseases (e.g., Parkinson's disease), and repair of arteriovenous malformations. A major advantage of the stereotactic approach is a reduction in damage to surrounding tissue.

Stereotactic radiosurgery is not a form of surgery in the traditional sense. Instead, radiosurgery uses precisely focused radiation to destroy tumor cells and other abnormal growths in the brain. Computers create 3-dimensional images of the brain. These images are used to guide the focused radiation while the patient's head is held still in a stereotactic frame (Fig. 56.18). Radiosurgical techniques can use ionizing radiation generated by a linear accelerator, gamma knife, or CyberKnife. In these procedures, a high dose of cobalt radiation is delivered to precisely targeted tumor tissue. The dose of radiation is delivered in a single treatment lasting a few hours or in multiple sessions. Side effects include fatigue, headache, and nausea.

In combination with stereotactic procedures to identify and localize tumor sites, surgical lasers can be used to destroy tumors. Lasers work by creating thermal energy, which destroys

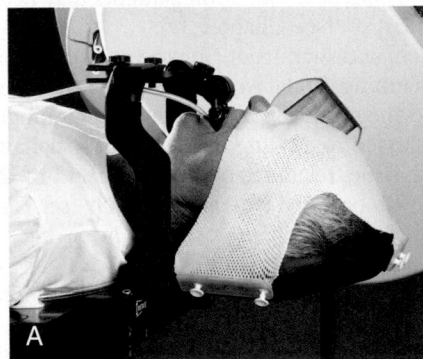

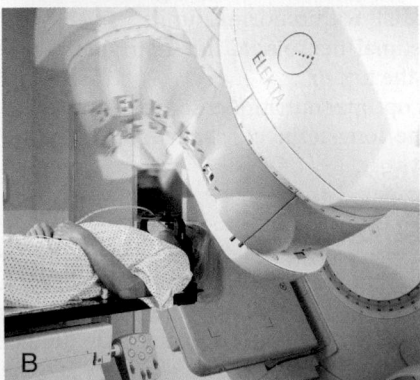

FIG. 56.18 A, Patient in a stereotactic frame. **B**, Elekta's Fraxion head frame helps ensure accuracy and precision in stereotactic radiation therapy (SRT) of cancer targets in the brain and cranium. (Courtesy Elekta, Stockholm, Sweden.)

the tissue on which it is focused. Laser therapy provides the benefit of reducing damage to surrounding tissue.

❖ NURSING MANAGEMENT: CRANIAL SURGERY

◆ Nursing Implementation

◆ **Acute Care.** The general preoperative and postoperative nursing care for the patient undergoing cranial surgery is similar regardless of the cause. It is similar to that for the patient with increased ICP. The patient (if conscious and coherent), caregiver, and family will be concerned about the potential physical and emotional problems that can result from surgery. The uncertainty about the prognosis and outcome requires compassionate nursing care in the preoperative period.

Preoperative teaching is important in allaying the fears of the patient, caregiver, and family and in preparing them for the postoperative period. Provide general information about the type of operation that will be done and what can be expected right after the operation. Explain that some hair may be shaved to allow for better exposure and to prevent contamination. The hair is usually removed in the operating room after induction of anesthesia. Tell them that the patient will be in an ICU or special care unit after surgery.

The main goal of care after cranial surgery is preventing increased ICP. Nursing management of the patient with increased ICP was outlined on pp. 1308–1311. Frequent assessment of the patient's neurologic status is essential during the first 48 hours. Closely monitor fluid and electrolyte levels and serum osmolality to detect changes in sodium regulation, the onset of diabetes insipidus, or severe hypovolemia.

Monitor the patient for pain and nausea. Nausea and vomiting are common after surgery and are usually treated with antiemetics. The use of promethazine is discouraged because it can increase somnolence and alter the accuracy of a neurologic assessment.

Although the brain itself does not have pain receptors, patients often report headache caused by edema or pain at the incision site. Control pain with short-acting opioids and monitor neurologic status.

The surgical dressing is usually in place for a few days. With an incision over the skull in the anterior or middle fossa, the patient will return from the operating room with the head elevated at an angle of 30 to 45 degrees. The head of the bed should stay elevated at least 30 degrees unless the surgical approach is in the posterior fossa or a burr hole has been made. In these cases, the patient is generally kept flat or at a slight elevation (10 to 15 degrees) during the postoperative phase.

Turning and positioning the patient will depend on the site of the operation. If a bone flap has been removed (craniectomy), do not position the patient on the operative side. Place a sign at the head of the bed, alerting everyone of the craniectomy site and position of the surgical site. Observe the dressing for color, odor, and amount of drainage. Notify the HCP immediately of any excess bleeding or clear drainage. Checking drains for placement and assessing the area around the dressing are important. Scalp care should include meticulous care of the incision to prevent wound infection. Cleanse the area and treat it following agency protocol or the HCP's orders. Once the dressing is removed, use an antiseptic soap for washing the scalp. The psychologic impact of hair removal can be lessened by using a wig, turban, scarves, or cap. For the patient who is receiving radiation, teach the patient to use a sunblock and head covering if any sun exposure is expected.

◆ **Ambulatory Care.** The rehabilitative potential for a patient after cranial surgery depends on the reason for the surgery,

postoperative course, and patient's general state of health. Base your nursing interventions on a realistic appraisal of these factors. Specific rehabilitation potential cannot be determined until cerebral edema and increased ICP subside postoperatively. An overall goal is to foster independence for as long as possible and to the highest degree possible.

Take care to maintain as much function as possible through measures such as careful positioning, meticulous skin and mouth care, regular range-of-motion exercises, bowel and bladder care, and adequate nutrition. Address the needs and problems of each patient individually because many variables affect the plan.

Collaborate with other specialists. The physical therapist may provide an exercise plan to regain functional deficits. A speech therapist will help the patient regain communication skills. The patient's mental and physical deterioration, including seizures, personality disorganization, apathy, and wasting, is difficult for both family and health care professionals. Cognitive and emotional residual deficits are often harder to accept than are motor and sensory losses. Social workers can help the patient and family adapt to changes in their home life, work, and financial circumstances.

ETHICAL/LEGAL DILEMMAS
Withholding Treatment

Situation
C.J., a 26-yr-old patient in a permanent vegetative state, is diagnosed with her 15th bladder infection. As her home care nurse, you must determine whether to seek antibiotics for this infection. The family members have expressed a concern that no heroic measures be used to extend the life of their daughter and sister. However, they have been unwilling to stop providing enteral nutrition through a gastrostomy tube. Should antibiotics be withheld?

Ethical/Legal Points for Consideration
- Patients in a persistent vegetative state do not recover.
- The main legal issue here is who has the legal right to refuse or consent to treatment for this incapacitated patient. You need to know if a guardian has been appointed by the court or if her parents retain a form of guardianship to make health care decisions for her.
- You need to know when the vegetative state began; that is, did the patient ever have the right to consent having reached the age of majority as a competent adult or did the vegetative state begin while she was a minor? If the patient did become a competent adult before the vegetative state, did she ever express any preference for quality-of-life and end-of-life decision making?
- The courts have widespread legal precedents for accepting the decision of the patient's guardian or parents or the patient's clearly expressed preferences for quality-of-life decision making.
- Life-sustaining treatment is any treatment that serves to prolong life without reversing the underlying medical condition. Life-sustaining treatment may include, but is not limited to, mechanical ventilation, renal dialysis, chemotherapy, antibiotics, and artificial nutrition and hydration.
- There is no ethical distinction between withdrawing and withholding life-sustaining treatment. If there is not adequate evidence of the incompetent patient's preferences and values, the decision should be based on the best interests of the patient (i.e., what outcome will most likely promote the patient's well-being).

Discussion Questions
1. How would you approach C.J.'s family?
2. What are your feelings about providing nutrition, hydration, and treatments that will prolong life in a patient for whom there is no hope of recovery?
3. What options are available to the family for the care of their daughter once a decision is made about withholding antibiotics?

INFLAMMATORY CONDITIONS OF THE BRAIN

Brain abscesses, meningitis, and encephalitis are the most common inflammatory conditions of the brain and spinal cord (Table 56.16). Inflammation can be caused by bacteria, viruses, fungi, and chemicals (e.g., contrast media used in diagnostic tests, blood in the subarachnoid space). CNS infections may occur via the bloodstream, by extension from a primary site, or along cranial and spinal nerves.

The mortality rate for inflammatory conditions of the brain is about 10% to 15% in the general population, with higher rates in older and immunosuppressed patients. Some who recover have long-term neurologic deficits, including hearing loss.[19]

BACTERIAL MENINGITIS

Meningitis is an acute inflammation of the meningeal tissues surrounding the brain and spinal cord. Meningitis usually occurs in fall, winter, or early spring. It is often related to a viral respiratory disease. Older adults and persons who are debilitated are affected more often than the general population. College students living in dormitories and people living in institutions (e.g., prisoners) have a high risk for contracting meningitis. Untreated bacterial meningitis has a mortality rate of 50% to 100%.[20]

Etiology and Pathophysiology

Streptococcus pneumoniae and *Neisseria meningitidis* are the leading causes of bacterial meningitis. *N. meningitides* has at least 13 different subtypes (serogroups) with 5 of them (A, B, C, Y, W) causing most cases. *Haemophilus influenzae* was once the most common cause of bacterial meningitis. However, the use of *H. influenzae* vaccine has resulted in a significant decrease in meningitis from this organism.

The organisms usually gain entry to the CNS through the upper respiratory tract or bloodstream. However, they may enter by direct extension from penetrating wounds of the skull or through fractured sinuses in basilar skull fractures.

The inflammatory response to the infection tends to increase CSF production with a moderate increase in ICP. In bacterial meningitis the purulent secretions quickly spread to other areas of the brain through the CSF and cover the cranial nerves and other intracranial structures. If this process extends into the brain parenchyma or if concurrent encephalitis is present, cerebral edema and increased ICP become more of a problem. Closely observe all patients for manifestations of increased ICP. ICP can increase from swelling around the dura and increased CSF volume.

Clinical Manifestations

Fever, severe headache, nausea, vomiting, and nuchal rigidity (neck stiffness) are key signs of meningitis. Photophobia, a decreased LOC, and signs of increased ICP may be present. Coma is associated with a poor prognosis. It occurs in 5% to 10% of patients with bacterial meningitis. Seizures occur in one third of all cases. The headache becomes progressively worse and may be accompanied by vomiting and irritability.

If the infecting organism is a meningococcus, a skin rash is common. Petechiae may be seen on the trunk, lower extremities, and mucous membranes. A *tumbler test* can be done by pressing the base of a drinking glass against the rash. The rash does not blanch or fade under pressure.

Complications

The most common acute complication of bacterial meningitis is increased ICP. Most patients have increased ICP. It is the major cause of an altered mental status.

Another complication is residual neurologic dysfunction. It often involves many cranial nerves. Cranial nerve irritation can have serious sequelae. The optic nerve (CN II) is compressed by increased ICP. Papilledema is often present, and blindness may occur. When CN III, CN IV, and CN VI are irritated, ocular movements are affected. Ptosis, unequal pupils, and diplopia are common. Irritation of CN V results in sensory losses and loss of the corneal reflex. Irritation of CN VII results in facial paresis.

TABLE 56.16 Comparison of Cerebral Inflammatory Conditions

	Meningitis	Encephalitis	Brain Abscess
Cause	Bacteria (*Streptococcus pneumoniae, Neisseria meningitidis*, group B streptococci, viruses, fungi)	Bacteria, fungi, parasites, herpes simplex virus (HSV), other viruses (e.g., West Nile virus)	Streptococci, staphylococci through bloodstream
Cerebrospinal Fluid (Reference Interval)			
• Pressure (<20 mm H_2O)	Increased *Bacterial:* 200–500 *Viral:* ≤250	Normal to slight increase	Increased
• WBC count (0–5 cells/μL)	*Bacterial:* >1000/μL (mainly neutrophils) *Viral:* 25–500/μL (mainly lymphocytes)	500/μL, neutrophils (early), lymphocytes (later)	25–300/μL (neutrophils)
• Protein (15–45 mg/dL [0.15–0.45 g/L])	*Bacterial:* >500 mg/dL *Viral:* 50–500 mg/dL	Slight increase	Normal
• Glucose (50–77 mg/dL [2.2–3.9 mmol/L])	*Bacterial:* Decreased 5–40 *Viral:* Normal or low >40	Normal	Low or absent
• Appearance	*Bacterial:* Turbid, cloudy *Viral:* Clear or cloudy	Clear	Clear
Diagnostic Studies	CT scan, Gram stain, smear, culture, PCR	CT scan, EEG, MRI, PET, PCR, IgM antibodies to virus in serum or CSF	CT scan
Treatment	Antibiotics, dexamethasone, supportive care, prevention of ↑ ICP	Supportive care, prevention of ↑ ICP, acyclovir (Zovirax) for HSV	Antibiotics, incision and drainage Supportive care

*PCR is used to detect viral RNA or DNA.
IgM, immunoglobulin M; *PCR*, polymerase chain reaction.

Irritation of CN VIII causes tinnitus, vertigo, and deafness. The dysfunction usually disappears within a few weeks. However, hearing loss may be permanent.

Hemiparesis, dysphasia, and hemianopsia may occur. These signs usually resolve over time. If they do not, suspect a cerebral abscess, subdural empyema, subdural effusion, or persistent meningitis. Acute cerebral edema may cause seizures, CN III palsy, bradycardia, hypertensive coma, and death.

Headaches may occur for months after the diagnosis of meningitis until the irritation and inflammation have completely resolved. It is important to implement pain management for chronic headaches.

A noncommunicating hydrocephalus may occur if the exudate causes adhesions that prevent the normal flow of CSF from the ventricles. CSF reabsorption by the arachnoid villi may be obstructed by the exudate. In this situation, surgical implantation of a shunt is the only treatment.

Waterhouse-Friderichsen syndrome is a complication of meningococcal meningitis. The syndrome is manifested by petechiae, disseminated intravascular coagulation (DIC), adrenal hemorrhage, and circulatory collapse. DIC and shock, which are some of the most serious complications of meningitis, are associated with meningococcemia. DIC is discussed in detail in Chapter 30.

Diagnostic Studies

When a patient has manifestations suggestive of bacterial meningitis, a blood culture and CT scan should be done. Diagnosis is usually verified by doing an LP with analysis of the CSF (Table 56.16). An LP should be done only after the CT scan has ruled out an obstruction in the foramen magnum to prevent a fluid shift resulting in herniation.

Specimens of the CSF, sputum, and nasopharyngeal secretions are taken for culture before the start of antibiotic therapy to identify the causative organism. A Gram stain is done to detect bacteria. The predominant white blood cell type in the CSF with bacterial meningitis is neutrophils.

X-rays of the skull may show infected sinuses. CT scans and MRI may be normal in uncomplicated meningitis. In other cases, CT scans may reveal evidence of increased ICP or hydrocephalus.

Interprofessional Care

Bacterial meningitis is a medical emergency. Rapid diagnosis based on history and physical examination is crucial because the patient is usually in a critical state when health care is sought. When meningitis is suspected, antibiotic therapy is begun after the collection of specimens for cultures, even before the diagnosis is confirmed (Table 56.17).

Ampicillin, penicillin, vancomycin, cefuroxime (Ceftin), cefotaxime, ceftriaxone, ceftizoxime, and ceftazidime are the main drugs given to treat bacterial meningitis. Dexamethasone may be given before or with the first dose of antibiotics. Collaborate with the HCP to manage the headache, fever, and nuchal rigidity often associated with meningitis.

❖ NURSING MANAGEMENT: BACTERIAL MENINGITIS

◆ Nursing Assessment

Initial assessment should include vital signs, neurologic assessment, fluid intake and output, and evaluation of the lungs and skin.

◆ Nursing Diagnoses

Nursing diagnoses for the patient with bacterial meningitis may include:

- Decreased intracranial adaptive capacity
- Ineffective tissue perfusion
- Hyperthermia
- Acute pain

Additional information on nursing diagnoses and interventions for the patient with bacterial meningitis is presented in eNursing Care Plan 56.2 (available on the website for this chapter).

◆ Planning

The overall goals for the patient with bacterial meningitis are to (1) return to maximal neurologic functioning, (2) resolve the infection, and (3) control pain and discomfort.

◆ Nursing Implementation

◆ Health Promotion.
Prevention of respiratory tract infections through vaccination programs for pneumococcal pneumonia and influenza is important. Meningococcal vaccines are available that protect against the serogroups of meningococcal disease that are most often seen in the United States. They will not prevent all cases. Two types of meningococcal vaccines are available in the United States:

- Meningococcal conjugate vaccines (MCV4) (Menactra, Menveo)
- Serogroup B meningococcal vaccines (Bexsero, Trumenba)

Early and vigorous treatment of respiratory tract and ear infections is important. Persons who have close contact with anyone who has bacterial meningitis should receive prophylactic antibiotics.

◆ Acute Care.
The patient with bacterial meningitis is usually acutely ill. The fever is high, and head pain is severe. Irritation of the cerebral cortex may result in seizures. The changes in mental

---

TABLE 56.17 Interprofessional Care
Bacterial Meningitis

Diagnostic Assessment

- History and physical examination
- Analysis of CSF (for protein, WBC, and glucose), Gram stain, and culture
- CBC, coagulation profile, electrolyte levels, glucose, platelet count
- Blood culture
- CT scan, MRI, PET scan
- Skull x-ray studies

Management

- Rest
- IV fluid
- Hypothermia

Drug Therapy

- IV antibiotics
  - ampicillin, penicillin
  - cephalosporin (e.g., cefotaxime, ceftriaxone)
- codeine for headache
- dexamethasone
- acetaminophen or aspirin for temperature >100.4° F (38° C)
- phenytoin IV
- mannitol (Osmitrol) IV for diuresis

status and LOC depend on the degree of increased ICP. Assess and record vital signs, neurologic status, fluid intake and output, skin, and lung fields at regular intervals based on the patient's condition.

Head and neck pain with movement requires attention. Codeine provides some pain relief without undue sedation for most patients. Assist the patient to a position of comfort, often curled up with the head slightly extended. The head of the bed should be slightly elevated. A darkened room and a cool cloth over the eyes relieve the discomfort of photophobia.

For the patient with delirium, low lighting may decrease hallucinations. All patients have some degree of mental distortion and hypersensitivity. They may be frightened and misinterpret the environment. Make every attempt to minimize environmental stimuli and prevent injury. A familiar person at the bedside may have a calming effect. Be efficient with care while conveying an attitude of caring and unhurried gentleness. The use of touch and a soothing voice to give simple explanations of activities is helpful. If seizures occur, make appropriate observations and take protective measures. Give antiseizure drugs, such as phenytoin (Dilantin) or levetiracetam (Keppra), as ordered. Manage problems associated with increased ICP (see the section on increased ICP on pp. 1308–1311).

Fever is vigorously treated because it increases cerebral edema and the risk for seizures. In addition, neurologic damage may result from an extremely fever over a prolonged time. Acetaminophen or aspirin may be used to reduce fever. If the fever is resistant to aspirin or acetaminophen, more vigorous means are needed (e.g., cooling blanket). Take care not to reduce the temperature too rapidly because shivering may result, causing a rebound effect and increasing the temperature and ICP. Wrap the extremities in soft towels or a blanket covered with a sheet to reduce shivering. If a cooling blanket is not available or desirable, tepid sponge baths with water may be effective in lowering the temperature. Protect the skin from excessive drying and injury and prevent breaks in the skin.

Because high fever increases the metabolic rate and thus insensible fluid loss, assess the patient for dehydration and adequacy of fluid intake. Diaphoresis further increases fluid losses and should be noted on the output record. Calculate replacement fluids as 800 mL/day for respiratory losses and 100 mL for each degree of temperature above 100.4° F (38° C). Supplemental feeding (e.g., enteral nutrition) to maintain adequate nutritional intake may be needed. Follow the designated antibiotic schedule to maintain therapeutic blood levels.

Meningitis generally requires respiratory isolation until the cultures are negative. Meningococcal meningitis is highly contagious, while other causes of meningitis may pose minimal to no infection risk with patient contact. However, standard precautions are essential to protect the patient and nurse.

◆ **Ambulatory Care.** After the acute period has passed, the patient needs several weeks of recovery before resuming normal activities. In this period, stress the importance of adequate nutrition, with an emphasis on a high-protein, high-calorie diet in small, frequent feedings.

Muscle rigidity may persist in the neck and backs of the legs. Progressive range-of-motion exercises and warm baths are useful. Have the patient gradually increase activity as tolerated but encourage adequate rest and sleep.

Residual effects can result in sequelae such as dementia, seizures, deafness, hemiplegia, and hydrocephalus. Assess vision, hearing, cognitive skills, and motor and sensory abilities after

recovery, with appropriate referrals as indicated. Throughout the acute and recovery periods, be aware of the anxiety and stress felt by the caregiver and other family members.

◆ **Evaluation**

The expected outcomes are that the patient with bacterial meningitis will

* Have appropriate cognitive function
* Be oriented to person, place, and time
* Maintain body temperature within normal range
* Report satisfaction with pain control

VIRAL MENINGITIS

The most common causes of viral meningitis are enteroviruses, arboviruses, human immunodeficiency virus, and herpes simplex virus (HSV). Enteroviruses most often spread through direct contact with respiratory secretions. Viral meningitis usually presents as a headache, fever, photophobia, and stiff neck.[19] The fever may be moderate or high.

The Xpert EV test can rapidly diagnose viral meningitis. A sample of CSF is used to determine if enterovirus is present, and results are available within hours of symptom onset.[20]

The CSF can be clear or cloudy, and the typical finding is lymphocytosis. Organisms are not seen on Gram stain or acid-fast smears. Polymerase chain reaction (PCR) used to detect viral-specific deoxyribonucleic acid (DNA) or ribonucleic acid (RNA) is a sensitive method for diagnosing CNS viral infections.

Antibiotics should be given after the LP while awaiting the results of the CSF analysis. Antibiotics are the best defense for bacterial meningitis. We can easily discontinue them if the meningitis is found to be viral.

Viral meningitis is managed symptomatically because the disease is self-limiting. Full recovery is expected. Rare sequelae include persistent headaches, mild mental impairment, and incoordination.

BRAIN ABSCESS

Brain abscess is an accumulation of pus within the brain tissue from a local or systemic infection. Direct extension from an ear, tooth, mastoid, or sinus infection is the main cause. Other causes for brain abscess formation include spread from a distant site (e.g., pulmonary infection, bacterial endocarditis), skull fracture, and prior brain trauma or surgery. Streptococci and *Staphylococcus aureus* are the most common infective organisms.

Manifestations are similar to those of meningitis and encephalitis and include headache, fever, and nausea and vomiting. Signs of increased ICP may include drowsiness, confusion, and seizures. Focal symptoms may reflect the local area of the abscess. For example, visual field defects or psychomotor seizures are common with a temporal lobe abscess. Visual impairment and hallucinations may accompany an occipital abscess. CT and MRI are used to diagnose a brain abscess.

Antimicrobial therapy is the primary treatment for brain abscess. Other manifestations are treated symptomatically. If drug therapy is not effective, the abscess may have to be drained or removed if it is encapsulated.

Nursing measures are similar to those for management of meningitis or increased ICP. If surgical drainage or removal is the treatment of choice, nursing care is similar to that of a patient having cranial surgery.

ENCEPHALITIS

Encephalitis, an acute inflammation of the brain, is a serious and sometimes fatal disease. Several thousand cases occur in the United States each year. It is usually caused by a virus. Many different viruses can cause encephalitis. Some are associated with certain seasons of the year or endemic to certain geographic areas.

Ticks and mosquitoes transmit epidemic encephalitis. Examples of encephalitis include eastern equine, La Crosse, St. Louis, West Nile, and western equine.[21] Nonepidemic encephalitis may occur as a complication of measles, chickenpox, or mumps. HSV encephalitis is the most common cause of acute nonepidemic viral encephalitis. Cytomegalovirus encephalitis occurs in patients with acquired immunodeficiency syndrome (AIDS).

Clinical Manifestations and Diagnostic Studies

Encephalitis can be acute or subacute. The onset is typically nonspecific, with fever, headache, nausea, and vomiting. Signs of encephalitis appear on day 2 or 3 and may vary from minimal changes in mental status to coma. Virtually any CNS abnormality can occur, including hemiparesis, tremors, seizures, cranial nerve palsies, personality changes, memory impairment, amnesia, and dysphasia.

Early diagnosis and treatment of viral encephalitis are essential for favorable outcomes. Diagnostic findings are shown in Table 56.16. Brain imaging techniques include CT, MRI, and PET. PCR tests allow for early detection of HSV and West Nile encephalitis. West Nile virus should be strongly considered in adults over 50 years old who develop encephalitis or meningitis in summer or early fall. The best diagnostic test for West Nile virus is a blood test that detects viral RNA. This test is also used to screen donated blood, organs, cells, and tissues.

❖ Interprofessional and Nursing Care

Prevention of encephalitis focuses on mosquito control. Measures include cleaning rain gutters, removing old tires, draining bird baths, and removing water where mosquitoes can breed. Insect repellent should be used during mosquito season.

Interprofessional and nursing management of encephalitis, including West Nile virus infection, is symptomatic and supportive. In the initial stages of encephalitis, many patients need intensive care.

Acyclovir (Zovirax) is used to treat encephalitis caused by HSV infection. Its use reduces mortality rates, although neurologic complications may still occur. For maximal benefit, treatment should start before the onset of coma. Treat seizure disorders with antiseizure drugs. Prophylactic treatment with antiseizure drugs may be used in severe cases of encephalitis. Treatment of cytomegalovirus encephalitis in AIDS patients is discussed in Chapter 14.

CASE STUDY

Traumatic Brain Injury

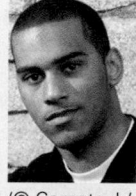

(© Comstock/Thinkstock.)

Patient Profile

C.G. is a 24-yr-old black man who has just returned from a 15-month army deployment to Afghanistan. He comes to the outpatient clinic with a report of chronic headaches (pain rating of 8 [0- to 10-point scale]) and trouble sleeping. His wife has noticed some personality changes since his return from deployment and is concerned that he has posttraumatic stress disorder (PTSD).

Subjective Data

* Reports that he has been depressed lately but attributes it to headache and difficulty returning home
* Headache is worse in the morning or when he lies down
* Uses tobacco and drinks coffee throughout the day
* Has trouble sleeping
* Reports "incidents" of heavy combat and blasts with a loss of consciousness. Cannot remember how many times
* Unable to obtain a more through history as he becomes quite agitated

Objective Data

* During your assessment, you note that C.G. is looking around the room and jumps when the phone rings next door
* Loss of short-term memory (remembers 1 of 3 items)
* Heart rate ranges from 100 to 130 beats/min
* ECG strip is shown below:

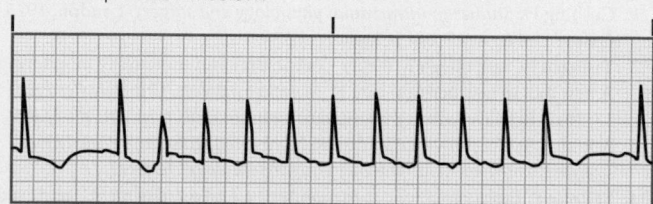

* Systolic BP ranges from 120 to 160 mm Hg
* Right pupil, 3 mm sluggishly reactive; left pupil, 3 mm briskly reactive

Diagnostic Studies

* CT of the head: negative for skull fracture, hematoma, or hemorrhage. Cerebral edema present, with cingulate herniation on the right side
* MRI of the head: Mild diffuse axonal injury

Discussion Questions

1. What could be the cause of C.G.'s hypertension, tachycardia, and ECG rhythm?
2. In addition to PTSD, what do his manifestations suggest?
3. **Priority Decision:** Based on the assessment data presented, what are the priority nursing diagnoses? Are there any collaborative problems?
4. **Priority Decision:** What are the priority nursing interventions that should be implemented?
5. **Collaboration:** How can the interprofessional team work together to meet his needs?
6. **Safety:** Are there any safety concerns for this patient or his wife?
7. **Evidence-Based Practice:** What interventions and support can help his wife?

Answers available at *http://evolve.elsevier.com/Lewis/medsurg.*

BRIDGE TO NCLEX EXAMINATION

The number of the question corresponds to the same-numbered outcome at the beginning of the chapter.

1. Vasogenic cerebral edema increases intracranial pressure by
   a. shifting fluid in the gray matter.
   b. altering the endothelial lining of cerebral capillaries.
   c. leaking molecules from the intracellular fluid to the capillaries.
   d. altering the osmotic gradient flow into the intravascular component.

2. A patient with intracranial pressure monitoring has a pressure of 12 mm Hg. The nurse understands that this pressure reflects
   a. a severe decrease in cerebral perfusion pressure.
   b. an alteration in the production of cerebrospinal fluid.
   c. the loss of autoregulatory control of intracranial pressure.
   d. a normal balance among brain tissue, blood, and cerebrospinal fluid.

3. A nurse plans care for the patient with increased intracranial pressure with the knowledge that the *best* way to position the patient is to
   a. keep the head of the bed flat.
   b. elevate the head of the bed to 30 degrees.
   c. maintain patient on the left side with the head supported on a pillow.
   d. use a continuous-rotation bed to continuously change patient position.

4. The nurse is alerted to a possible acute subdural hematoma in the patient who
   a. has a linear skull fracture crossing a major artery.
   b. has focal symptoms of brain damage with no recollection of a head injury.
   c. develops decreased level of consciousness and a headache within 48 hours of a head injury.
   d. has an immediate loss of consciousness with a brief lucid interval followed by decreasing level of consciousness.

5. During admission of a patient with a severe head injury to the emergency department, the nurse places the *highest* priority on assessment for
   a. patency of airway.
   b. presence of a neck injury.
   c. neurologic status with the Glasgow Coma Scale.
   d. cerebrospinal fluid leakage from the ears or nose.

6. A patient is suspected of having a brain tumor. The signs and symptoms include memory deficits, visual changes, weakness of right upper and lower extremities, and personality changes. The nurse determines that the tumor is *most* likely located in the
   a. frontal lobe.
   b. parietal lobe.
   c. occipital lobe.
   d. temporal lobe.

7. Nursing management of a patient with a brain tumor includes *(select all that apply)*
   a. discussing with the patient methods to control inappropriate behavior.
   b. using diversion techniques to keep the patient stimulated and motivated.
   c. assisting and supporting the family in understanding any changes in behavior.
   d. limiting self-care activities until the patient has regained maximum physical functioning.
   e. planning for seizure precautions and teaching the patient and the caregiver about antiseizure drugs.

8. The nurse on the clinical unit is assigned to four patients. Which patient should she assess *first*?
   a. Patient with a skull fracture whose nose is bleeding
   b. An older patient with a stroke who is confused and whose daughter is present
   c. Patient with meningitis who is suddenly agitated and reporting a headache of 10 on a 0- to 10 scale
   d. Patient 2 days postoperative after a craniotomy for a brain tumor who has had continued vomiting

9. A nursing measure that can reduce the potential for seizures and increased intracranial pressure in the patient with bacterial meningitis is
   a. administering codeine for relief of head and neck pain.
   b. controlling fever with prescribed drugs and cooling techniques.
   c. maintaining strict bed rest with the head of the bed slightly elevated.
   d. keeping the room dark and quiet to minimize environmental stimulation.

1. b, 2. d, 3. b, 4. c, 5. a, 6. a, 7. c, e, 8. c, 9. b

For rationales to these answers and even more NCLEX review questions, visit *http://evolve.elsevier.com/Lewis/medsurg*.

ⓔ EVOLVE WEBSITE/RESOURCES LIST

http://evolve.elsevier.com/Lewis/medsurg
Review Questions (Online Only)
Key Points
Answer Keys for Questions
- Rationales for Bridge to NCLEX Examination Questions
- Answer Guidelines for Case Study on p. 1327
Student Case Studies
- Patient With Head Injury
- Patient With Meningitis
Nursing Care Plans
- eNursing Care Plan 56.1: Patient With Increased Intracranial Pressure
- eNursing Care Plan 56.2: Patient With Meningitis
Conceptual Care Map Creator

Audio Glossary
Supporting Media
- Animation
  - Parts of the Brain Controlling Body Function
Content Updates

REFERENCES

1. Cushing H: *Studies in intracranial physiology and surgery,* London, 1925, Oxford University Press. (Classic)
*2. Tasneem N, Samaniego E, Pieper C, et al: Brain multimodality monitoring: A new tool in neurocritical care of comatose patients, *Crit Care Res Pract* 17, 2017. Retrieved from *www.hindawi.com/journals/ccrp/2017/6097265/*.
3. Seidman R: Cerebrovascular disease. Retrieved from *https://medicine.stonybrookmedicine.edu/pathology/neuropathology/chapter2*.
*4. LeRoux P: Intracranial pressure monitoring and management. Retrieved from *www.hindawi.com/journals/ccrp/2017/6097265/*.

*5. Brain Trauma Foundation: Guidelines for the management of severe traumatic brain injury. Retrieved from *https://braintrauma.org/uploads/03/12/Guidelines_for_Management_of_Severe_TBI_4th_Edition.pdf.*

*6. Peters NA, Farrell LB, Smith JP: Hyperosmolar therapy for the treatment of cerebral edema, *US Pharm* 43:HS8, 2018.

*7. Nair SS, Surendran A, Prabhakar RB, et al: Comparison between FOUR score and GCS in assessing patients with traumatic head injury: A tertiary centre study, *Int Surg J* 4:656, 2017.

*8. Surgical Critical Care: Seizure prophylaxis in patients with traumatic brain injury. Retrieved from *www.surgicalcriticalcare.net/Guidelines/Seizure%20prophylaxis%20in%20TBI%202017.pdf.*

9. Taylor CA, Bell JM, Breiding MJ, et al: Traumatic brain injury–related emergency department visits, hospitalizations, and deaths—United States, 2007 and 2013, *MMWR* 66:1, 2017.

*10. Sobrino J, Shafi S: Timing and causes of death after injuries, *Proc Bayl Univ Med Cent* 26:2, 2013. (Classic)

11. American Association of Neurological Surgeons: Traumatic brain injury. Retrieved from *www.aans.org/Patients/Neurosurgical-Conditions-and-Treatments/Traumatic-Brain-Injury.*

*12. Varghese R, Chakrabarty J, Menon G: Nursing management of adults with severe traumatic brain injury: A narrative review, *Indian J Crit Care Med* 21:10, 2017.

13. Wasserman J, Koenigsberg RA: Diffuse axonal injury. Retrieved from *https://emedicine.medscape.com/article/339912-overview.*

*14. Narun S, Brors O, Stokland O, et al: Mortality among head trauma patients taking preinjury antithrombotic agents: A retrospective cohort analysis from a level 1 trauma centre, *BMC Emerg Med* 16:29, 2016.

15. Subdural hematoma. Retrieved from *https://emedicine.medscape.com/article/1137207-overview.*

*16. Rumrill P, Hendriks DJ, Elias E, et al: Cognition and return to work after mild/moderate traumatic brain injury: A systematic review, *Work* 58:1, 2017.

17. National Cancer Institute. Brain tumor. Retrieved from *www.cancer.gov/cancertopics/types/brain.*

18. National Brain Tumor Society: Understanding brain tumors. Retrieved from *http://braintumor.org/brain-tumor-information/understanding-brain-tumors/.*

19. National Institute of Neurological Disorders and Stroke: Meningitis and encephalitis fact sheet. Retrieved from *www.ninds.nih.gov/Disorders/Patient-Caregiver-Education/Fact-Sheets/Meningitis-and-Encephalitis-Fact-Sheet.*

20. World Health Organization: Meningococcal meningitis. Retrieved from *www.who.int/mediacentre/factsheets/fs141/en/.*

21. National Institute of Neurologic Disorders and Stroke: Meningitis and encephalitis. Retrieved from *www.ninds.nih.gov/Disorders/Patient-Caregiver-Education/Fact-Sheets/Meningitis-and-Encephalitis-Fact-Sheet.*

*Evidence-based information for clinical practice.

57

Stroke

Michelle Bussard

One person caring about another represents life's greatest value.

John Rohn

http://evolve.elsevier.com/Lewis/medsurg

CONCEPTUAL FOCUS

Family Dynamics   Intracranial Regulation   Safety

Functional Ability   Mobility   Sensory Perception

LEARNING OUTCOMES

1. Describe the incidence of and risk factors for stroke.
2. Explain mechanisms that affect cerebral blood flow.
3. Compare and contrast the etiology and pathophysiology of ischemic and hemorrhagic strokes.
4. Correlate the clinical manifestations of stroke with the underlying pathophysiology.
5. Identify diagnostic studies done for patients with strokes.
6. Distinguish among the interprofessional care, drug therapy, and surgical therapy for patients with ischemic strokes and hemorrhagic strokes.
7. Describe the acute nursing management of a patient with a stroke.
8. Describe the rehabilitative nursing management of a patient with a stroke.
9. Explain the psychosocial impact of a stroke on the patient, caregiver, and family.

KEY TERMS

aneurysm, p. 1335

aphasia, p. 1336

cerebrovascular accident (CVA), p. 1330

dysarthria, p. 1336

dysphasia, p. 1336

embolic stroke, p. 1333

hemorrhagic strokes, p. 1334

intracerebral hemorrhage, p. 1334

ischemic stroke, p. 1333

stroke, p. 1330

subarachnoid hemorrhage (SAH), p. 1335

thrombotic stroke, p. 1333

transient ischemic attack (TIA), p. 1332

Stroke occurs when there is (1) *ischemia* (inadequate blood flow) to a part of the brain or (2) *hemorrhage* (bleeding) into the brain that results in death of brain cells. In a stroke, functions such as movement, sensation, thinking, talking, or emotions that were controlled by the affected area of the brain are lost or impaired. The severity of the loss of function varies according to the location and extent of the brain damage.

The terms *brain attack* and cerebrovascular accident (CVA) are also used to describe stroke. The term *brain attack* communicates the urgency of recognizing the warning signs of a stroke and treating it as a medical emergency, as we would do with a heart attack (Table 57.1). After the onset of a stroke, immediate medical attention is crucial to decrease disability and the risk for death.

Stroke is a major public health concern. An estimated 7 million people over the age of 20 in the United States have had a stroke.[1] With an aging population, we can expect a further increase in the incidence of strokes. However, stroke can occur at any age. About 34% of strokes occur in people younger than 65 years old.[2]

Stroke is currently the fifth most common cause of death in the United States. More than 137,000 deaths occur each year from stroke.[3] While deaths due to stroke have declined, stroke is the leading cause of serious long-term disability. About 800,000 people have a stroke each year, and 15% to 30% have a permanent disability.[4]

Common long-term disabilities include *hemiparesis* (partial paralysis on one side), inability to walk, complete or partial dependence for activities of daily living (ADLs), *aphasia* (dysfunction in communication), and depression. In addition to the physical, cognitive, and emotional impact of the stroke on the survivor, the stroke affects the lives of the stroke victim's caregiver and family. A stroke is a lifelong change for both the stroke survivor and family. Be mindful of this impact when caring for patients who survive stroke.

PATHOPHYSIOLOGY OF STROKE

Anatomy of Cerebral Circulation

Blood is supplied to the brain by 2 major pairs of arteries: internal carotid arteries (anterior circulation) and vertebral arteries (posterior circulation). The carotid arteries branch to supply most of the (1) frontal, parietal, and temporal lobes; (2) basal

TABLE 57.1 Patient & Caregiver Teaching

FAST for Warning Signs of Stroke

FAST is an easy way to remember the signs of stroke. Include the following information in the teaching plan for a patient at risk for stroke and the patient's caregiver:

F	Face drooping	Does one side of the face droop or is it numb? Ask the person to smile. Is the smile uneven?
A	Arm weakness	Is one arm weak or numb? Ask the person to raise both arms. Does one arm drift downward?
S	Speech difficulties	Is speech slurred? Is the person unable to speak or hard to understand? Ask the person to repeat a simple sentence like "The sky is blue." Is the sentence repeated correctly?
T	Time	Time is CRITICAL! If someone shows any of these signs (even if they go away), call 911 and get the person to the hospital. Note the time when the signs first appeared.

In addition, report the sudden onset of the following:
- Confusion
- Numbness or weakness, especially in 1 side of the body
- Severe headache with no known cause
- Trouble seeing in one or both eyes
- Trouble walking, dizziness, loss of balance or coordination

Source: American Stroke Association: FAST. Retrieved from *www.strokeassociation.org/STROKEORG/WarningSigns/Stroke-Warning-Signs-and-Symptoms_UCM_308528_SubHomePage.jsp.*

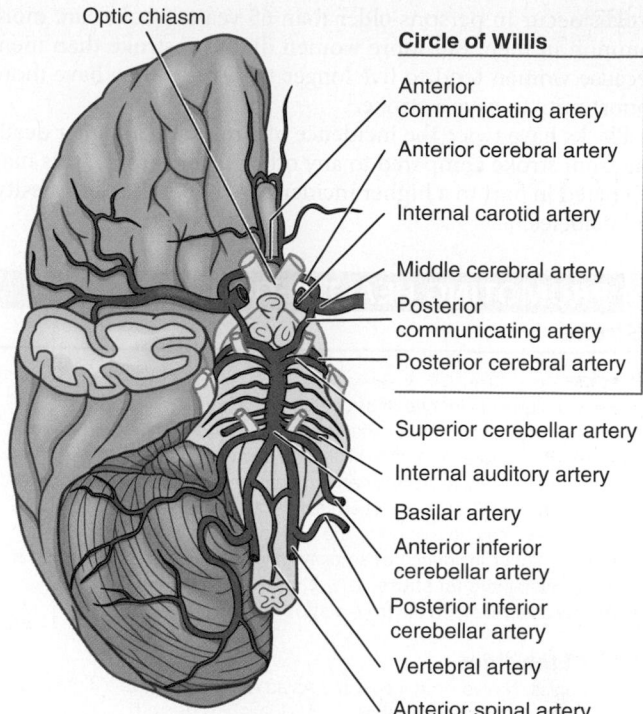

FIG. 57.1 Cerebral arteries and the circle of Willis. The top of the temporal lobe has been removed to show the course of the middle cerebral artery.

ganglia; and (3) part of the diencephalon (thalamus and hypothalamus). The major branches of the carotid arteries are the middle cerebral and anterior cerebral arteries. The vertebral arteries join to form the basilar artery, which branches to supply the middle and lower parts of the temporal lobes, occipital lobes, cerebellum, brainstem, and part of the diencephalon. The main branch of the basilar artery is the posterior cerebral artery. The anterior and posterior cerebral circulation is connected at the *circle of Willis* by the anterior and posterior communicating arteries (Fig. 57.1). Fig. 55.11 shows the arteries at the base of the brain. Genetic variations in this area are common, and all connecting vessels may not be present.

Regulation of Cerebral Blood Flow

The brain needs a continuous supply of blood to provide the O_2 and glucose that neurons need to function. Blood flow must be maintained at 750 to 1000 mL/min (55 mL/100 g of brain tissue), or 20% of the cardiac output, for optimal brain functioning. If blood flow to the brain is totally interrupted (e.g., cardiac arrest), neurologic metabolism is altered in 30 seconds, metabolism stops in 2 minutes, and cell death occurs in 5 minutes.

The brain is normally protected from changes in mean systemic arterial BP over a range from 50 to 150 mm Hg by a mechanism known as *cerebral autoregulation*. This involves changes in the diameter of cerebral blood vessels in response to changes in pressure so that the blood flow to the brain stays constant. When cerebral ischemia occurs, autoregulation may be impaired, making the brain dependent on systemic BP. CO_2 is a potent cerebral vasodilator. Changes in arterial CO_2 levels have a dramatic effect on cerebral blood flow (CBF). Increased CO_2 levels increase CBF. Decreased CO_2 levels decrease CBF. Very low arterial oxygen (O_2) levels (partial pressure of arterial

O_2 less than 50 mm Hg) or increases in hydrogen ion concentration also increase CBF.

Factors that affect blood flow to the brain include systemic BP, cardiac output, and blood viscosity. During normal activity, O_2 requirements vary considerably. Changes in cardiac output, vasomotor tone, and distribution of blood flow normally maintain adequate blood flow to the brain. Cardiac output must be reduced by one third before CBF is reduced. Changes in blood viscosity affect CBF, with decreased viscosity increasing blood flow.

Collateral circulation may develop over time to compensate for a decrease in CBF. An area of the brain can potentially receive blood supply from another blood vessel even if blood supply from the original vessel has been cut off (e.g., because of thrombosis). In other words, the vessels in the brain make an "alternative route" for blood flow to reach damaged areas, thus preventing a stroke.

Intracranial pressure (ICP) influences CBF. Increased ICP causes brain compression and reduced CBF. One of your major goals when caring for a stroke patient is to reduce secondary injury related to increased ICP (see Chapter 56).

RISK FACTORS FOR STROKE

The most effective way to decrease the burden of stroke is prevention and teaching, especially about risk factors. We divide risk factors into nonmodifiable and modifiable. Stroke risk increases with multiple risk factors. Thus, the primary prevention of stroke focuses on reducing modifiable risk factors, which can dramatically reduce the morbidity and mortality of stroke.[5]

Nonmodifiable Risk Factors

Nonmodifiable risk factors include age, gender, ethnicity or race, and family history or heredity. Stroke risk increases with age, doubling each decade after 55 years of age. Two thirds of all strokes occur in persons older than 65 years. Strokes are more common in men, but more women die from stroke than men. Because women tend to live longer than men, they have more opportunity to have a stroke.[2]

Blacks have twice the incidence of stroke and a higher death rate from stroke compared to any other ethnic group. This may be related in part to a higher incidence of hypertension, obesity, and diabetes.[2]

Genetic risk factors are important in the development of all vascular diseases, including stroke. A person with a family history of stroke has an increased risk for having a stroke. We think that genes encoding products involved in lipid metabolism, thrombosis, and inflammation are genetic factors for stroke. People who have at least 2 first-degree relatives with a history of subarachnoid hemorrhage (SAH) or aneurysm should be screened to rule out anomalies in their cerebral vasculature.[6]

Modifiable Risk Factors

Modifiable risk factors are those that can potentially be altered through lifestyle changes and medical treatment, thus reducing the risk for stroke. They include hypertension, heart disease, diabetes, smoking, obesity, sleep apnea, metabolic syndrome, lack of physical exercise, poor diet, and drug and alcohol use. We think modifiable risk factors cause 90% of strokes.[6]

Hypertension is the single most important modifiable risk factor. It is often undetected and inadequately treated. Increases in systolic BP (SBP) and diastolic BP (DBP) independently increase stroke risk. The proper treatment of hypertension reduces stroke risk up to 50%. New recommendations by the American Heart Association (AHA) include home BP monitoring with a goal of SBP less than 140 mm Hg.[4]

Heart disease, including atrial fibrillation, myocardial infarction (MI), cardiomyopathy, cardiac valve abnormalities, and congenital heart defects, such as patent foramen ovale, is a risk factor for stroke. Atrial fibrillation is responsible for about 25% of all strokes.[7] People with atrial fibrillation are 5 times more likely to have a stroke than people with a regular heart rhythm.[8] The incidence of atrial fibrillation increases with age. Oral anticoagulants (e.g., warfarin, dabigatran) and adherence to their therapy play a vital role in stroke prevention.[4,9]

Diabetes is a significant risk factor for stroke. Stroke risk in people with diabetes is 5 times higher than in the general population.[7]

Smoking nearly doubles the risk for ischemic stroke. Smokers are 4 times as likely to have a hemorrhagic stroke than nonsmokers.[5] The risk associated with smoking decreases substantially over time after the smoker quits. After 5 to 10 years of no tobacco use, former smokers have the same risk for stroke as nonsmokers.

The effect of alcohol on stroke risk appears to depend on the amount consumed. Women who drink more than 1 alcoholic drink per day and men who drink more than 2 alcoholic drinks per day are at higher risk for hypertension, which increases their chance of stroke. Illicit drug use, especially cocaine use, increases stroke risk.[6]

A waist circumference to hip circumference ratio equal to or above the mid-value for the population increases the risk for ischemic stroke 3-fold. In addition, obesity is associated with hypertension, high blood glucose, and increased blood lipid levels, all of which increase stroke risk.[6] An association of physical inactivity and increased stroke risk is present in both men and women. Benefits of physical activity can occur with even light to moderate regular activity. The American Stroke Association recommends 40 minutes of exercise 3 to 4 days per week to reduce risk for stroke.[9] Nutrition teaching is important, since a diet high in fat and low in fruits and vegetables may increase stroke risk.

The early forms of birth control pills that had high levels of progestin and estrogen increased a woman's chance of having a stroke, especially if the woman smoked heavily. Newer, low-dose oral contraceptives have lower risks for stroke except in those who have hypertension and smoke. The AHA recommends smoking cessation and alternatives to estrogen oral contraceptives for those women to reduce the incidence of stroke.[4]

Women who have migraines with aura have an increased risk for stroke. Other conditions that may increase the stroke risk include inflammatory conditions (e.g., rheumatoid arthritis), sickle cell disease, and blood clotting disorders, such as factor V Leiden mutation.[5]

Transient Ischemic Attack

Another risk factor associated with stroke is a history of a transient ischemic attack (TIA). A TIA is a transient episode of neurologic dysfunction caused by focal brain, spinal cord, or retinal ischemia, but without acute infarction of the brain. Symptoms typically last less than 1 hour.

It is important to teach the patient to seek treatment for any stroke symptoms, since there is no way to predict if a TIA will resolve or if it will progress to a stroke. In general, one third of those who had a TIA do not have another, one third have more TIAs, and one third progress to stroke.[10]

TIAs may be due to microemboli that temporarily block the blood flow. TIAs are a warning sign of progressive cerebrovascular disease. The signs and symptoms of a TIA depend on the blood vessel that is involved and the area of the brain that is ischemic. If the carotid system is involved, patients may have a temporary loss of vision in 1 eye (*amaurosis fugax*), transient hemiparesis, numbness or loss of sensation, or a sudden inability to speak. Signs of a TIA involving the vertebrobasilar system may include tinnitus, vertigo, darkened or blurred vision, diplopia, ptosis, dysarthria, dysphagia, ataxia, and unilateral or bilateral numbness or weakness.

CHECK YOUR PRACTICE

You are talking with your uncle at your family reunion. He knows that you are a nurse and seems very eager to talk with you. He tells you that earlier this morning he was having problems talking, got dizzy, and then "blanked" out for a while. He found himself just lying on the floor in his room.

- He says, "I think it is just all the excitement of the reunion, but what do you think?"

A TIA is treated as a medical emergency since it can lead to an ischemic stroke. Teach people at risk for TIAs to seek medical attention at once with any stroke-like symptom and to identify the time of onset of symptoms. The ABCD[2] score is a tool used to predict stroke risk for a person after a TIA (Table 57.2).[11]

TYPES OF STROKE

Unlike a TIA, in which ischemia occurs without infarction, a stroke results in infarction (cell death). Strokes are classified as ischemic or hemorrhagic based on the cause and underlying pathophysiologic findings (Fig. 57.2 and Table 57.3).

Ischemic Stroke

An ischemic stroke results from inadequate blood flow to the brain from partial or complete occlusion of an artery.[12] Ischemic strokes are classified as thrombotic or embolic strokes.

Thrombotic Stroke. A thrombotic stroke occurs from injury to a blood vessel wall and formation of a blood clot (Fig. 57.2, A). The lumen of the blood vessel becomes narrowed, and, if it becomes occluded, infarction occurs. Thrombosis develops readily where atherosclerotic plaques have already narrowed blood vessels. Thrombotic stroke is the most common cause of stroke. It accounts for about 60% of strokes.[2] They are more common in older adults, especially those with high cholesterol, atherosclerosis, or diabetes. Most thrombotic strokes are associated with hypertension or diabetes, both of which accelerate atherosclerosis. Many times, a TIA precedes thrombotic strokes.[7]

The extent of the stroke depends on rapidity of onset, size of the damaged area, and presence of collateral circulation. Most patients with ischemic stroke do not have a decreased level of consciousness (LOC) in the first 24 hours, unless it is due to a brainstem stroke or other condition, such as seizure, increased ICP, or hemorrhage. Manifestations of ischemic stroke may progress in the first 72 hours as infarction and cerebral edema increase.

Embolic Stroke. Embolic stroke occurs when an embolus lodges in and occludes a cerebral artery, resulting in infarction and edema of the area supplied by the involved vessel (Fig. 57.2, B). Embolism is the second most common cause of stroke.[2] Most emboli originate in the endocardial (inside) layer of the heart, when a plaque breaks off from the endocardium and enters the circulation. The embolus travels upward to the cerebral circulation and lodges where a vessel narrows or bifurcates (splits). Heart conditions, including atrial fibrillation, MI, infective endocarditis, rheumatic heart disease, valvular heart prostheses, patent foramen ovale, and atrial septal defects, account for most embolic ischemic strokes.[2] Less common causes of emboli include air and fat from long bone (e.g., femur) fractures.

TABLE 57.2 ABCD[2] Score

The ABCD[2] score is a risk assessment tool. It is designed to predict the risk for stroke 2 days after a transient ischemic attack (TIA). Calculate the score by adding up points for 5 factors.

Risk Factor	Points
Age ≥60 yr	1
Systolic BP ≥140 mm Hg *OR* diastolic BP ≥90 mm Hg	1
Clinical features of TIA (choose 1)	
Unilateral weakness with or without speech impairment *OR*	2
Speech impairment without unilateral weakness	1
Duration	
TIA duration ≥60 min *OR*	2
TIA duration 10–59 min	1
Diabetes	1
Total ABCD[2] Score	0–7

ABCD[2] score	2-Day Stroke Risk (%)	Care Needed
0–3	1.0	Hospitalization not needed unless there is another indication (e.g., new atrial fibrillation)
4–5	4.1	Hospitalization in most situations
6–7	8.1	Hospitalization

Permission obtained from National Stroke Association. Retrieved from *www.stroke.org.*

The patient with an embolic stroke often has severe manifestations that occur suddenly. Embolic strokes can affect any age-group. Rheumatic heart disease is a cause of embolic stroke in young to middle-aged adults. An embolus arising from an atherosclerotic plaque is more common in older adults.

Warning signs are less common with embolic than with thrombotic stroke. The embolic stroke often occurs rapidly, giving little time to accommodate to an obstructed blood vessel with the development of collateral circulation. The patient is usually conscious, although they may have a headache. The effects of the emboli are initially characterized by severe neurologic deficits, which can be temporary if the clot breaks up and allows blood to flow. Smaller emboli then continue to obstruct

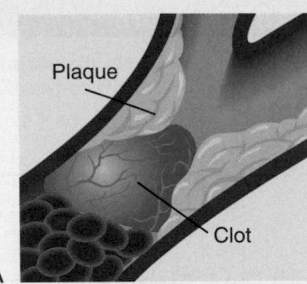

A Thrombotic stroke. The process of clot formation (thrombosis) results in a narrowing of the lumen, which blocks the passage of the blood through the artery.

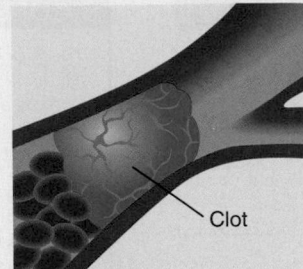

B Embolic stroke. An embolus is a blood clot or other debris circulating in the blood. When it reaches an artery in the brain that is too narrow to pass through, it lodges there and blocks the flow of blood.

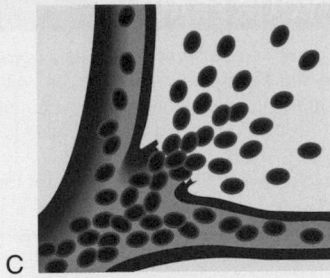

C Hemorrhagic stroke. A burst blood vessel may allow blood to seep into and damage brain tissues until clotting shuts off the leak.

FIG. 57.2 Major types of stroke.

TABLE 57.3 Types of Stroke

Gender and Age	Warning and Onset	Prognosis
Ischemic		
Incidence: Accounts for 87% of strokes		
Embolic		
Men more than women	*Warning:* TIA (uncommon) *Onset:* Sudden onset, most likely to occur during activity	Single event, signs and symptoms develop quickly, usually some improvement, recurrence common without aggressive treatment of underlying disease.
Thrombotic		
Men more than women Oldest median age	*Warning:* TIA (30%–50% of cases) *Onset:* Often during or after sleep	Stepwise progression, signs and symptoms develop slowly, usually some improvement, recurrence in 20%–25% of survivors.
Hemorrhagic		
Incidence: Accounts for 13% of strokes		
Intracerebral		
Slightly higher in women	*Warning:* Headache (25% of cases) *Onset:* Activity (often)	Progression over 24 hr. Poor prognosis, fatality more likely with presence of coma.
Subarachnoid		
Slightly higher in women Youngest median age	*Warning:* Headache (common) *Onset:* Activity (often), sudden onset, most often related to head trauma	Usually single sudden event, fatality more likely with presence of coma.

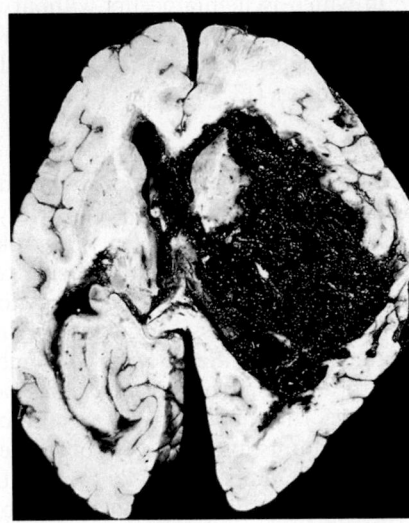

FIG. 57.3 Massive hypertensive hemorrhage rupturing into a lateral ventricle of the brain. (From Kumar V, Abbas AK, Aster JC, et al: *Robbins and Cotran pathologic basis of disease*, ed 8, Philadelphia, 2010, Saunders.)

Hemorrhagic Stroke

Hemorrhagic strokes result from bleeding into the brain tissue itself (intracerebral or intraparenchymal hemorrhage) or into the subarachnoid space or ventricles (SAH or intraventricular hemorrhage).

Intracerebral Hemorrhage. Intracerebral hemorrhage is bleeding within the brain caused by a rupture of a vessel (usually in the basal ganglia) (Fig. 57.2, C). The prognosis of patients with intracerebral hemorrhage is poor. The 30-day mortality rate is 40% to 80%. Half of the deaths occur within the first 48 hours.[2]

Hypertension is the most common cause of intracerebral hemorrhage (Fig. 57.3). Other causes include vascular malformations, coagulation disorders, anticoagulant and thrombolytic drugs, trauma, brain tumors, and ruptured aneurysms. Hemorrhage often occurs during periods of activity. Most often there is a sudden onset of symptoms, with progression over minutes to hours because of ongoing bleeding.

Manifestations include neurologic deficits, headache, nausea, vomiting, decreased LOC, and hypertension. The extent of the symptoms varies depending on the amount, location, and

smaller vessels, which in turn involve smaller portions of the brain with fewer deficits noted.

The prognosis is related to the amount of brain tissue deprived of its blood supply. Recurrence of embolic stroke is common unless the underlying cause is aggressively treated.

duration of the bleeding. A blood clot within the closed skull can result in a mass that causes pressure on brain tissue, displaces brain tissue, and decreases CBF, leading to ischemia and infarction.

Most intracerebral hemorrhages occur in the cerebral lobes, cerebellum, pons, thalamus, subcortical white matter, internal capsule, or a part of the basal ganglia called the putamen. At first, patients have a severe headache with nausea and vomiting. Manifestations of putaminal and internal capsule bleeding include weakness of one side (including the face, arm, and leg), slurred speech, and deviation of the eyes. Progression of symptoms related to a severe hemorrhage includes hemiplegia, fixed and dilated pupils, abnormal body posturing, and coma. Thalamic hemorrhage results in hemiplegia with more sensory than motor loss. Bleeding into the subthalamic areas of the brain leads to problems with vision and eye movement. Cerebellar hemorrhages are characterized by severe headache, vomiting, loss of ability to walk, dysphagia, dysarthria, and eye movement changes.

Hemorrhage in the pons is the most serious because basic life functions (e.g., respiration) are rapidly affected. Hemorrhage in the pons can be characterized by hemiplegia leading to complete paralysis, coma, abnormal body posturing, fixed pupils, hyperthermia, and death.

Subarachnoid Hemorrhage. Subarachnoid hemorrhage (SAH) occurs when there is intracranial bleeding into the cerebrospinal fluid (CSF)–filled space between the arachnoid and pia mater membranes on the surface of the brain. SAH is often caused by rupture of a cerebral aneurysm (congenital or acquired weakness and ballooning of vessels). Aneurysms may be saccular or berry aneurysms, ranging from a few millimeters to 20 to 30 mm in size, or fusiform atherosclerotic aneurysms. Most aneurysms are in the circle of Willis. Other causes of SAH include trauma and illicit drug (cocaine) use. The incidence of SAH increases with age and is higher in women than men.

The patient may have warning signs and symptoms if the ballooning artery applies pressure to brain tissue. Minor warning symptoms may result from leaking of an aneurysm before major rupture. In general, cerebral aneurysms are viewed as a "silent killer," since people do not have warning signs or symptoms of an aneurysm until rupture has occurred.

CHECK YOUR PRACTICE

You are watching your husband's "for fun" soccer game. He leaves the game and is kneeling on the ground. When you try to assess what is going on he says, "I've got a terrible headache. It just started." Knowing that he sometimes gets headaches when he is stressed, you ask him if he is feeling stressed. He almost screams back at you, "NO! This is the worst headache of my life!"

• What should you do?

Loss of consciousness may or may not occur. The patient's LOC may range from alert to comatose, depending on the severity of the bleed. Other manifestations include focal neurologic deficits (including cranial nerve deficits), nausea, vomiting, seizures, and stiff neck.

Complications of aneurysmal SAH include rebleeding before surgery or other therapy is started and cerebral vasospasm (narrowing of the blood vessels), which can result in cerebral infarction. Cerebral vasospasm is likely due to an interaction between the metabolites of blood and the vascular smooth muscle. This occurs when the subarachnoid blood clots break

---

TABLE 57.4 Stroke Manifestations Related to Artery Involvement

Artery	Manifestations
Anterior cerebral	Motor and/or sensory deficit (contralateral), sucking or rooting reflex, rigidity, gait problems, loss of proprioception and fine touch
Middle cerebral	*Dominant side:* Aphasia, motor and sensory deficit, hemianopsia
	Nondominant side: Neglect, motor and sensory deficit, hemianopsia
Posterior cerebral	Hemianopsia, visual hallucination, spontaneous pain, motor deficit
Vertebral	Cranial nerve deficits, diplopia, dizziness, nausea, vomiting, dysarthria, dysphagia, and/or coma

---

down or dissolve, releasing metabolites that can cause endothelial damage and vasoconstriction. The release of endothelin (a potent vasoconstrictor) may play a key role in the induction of cerebral vasospasm after SAH. Patients with SAH who are at risk for vasospasm are often kept in the intensive care unit (up to 14 days) until the threat of vasospasm is reduced. Peak time for vasospasm is 6 to 10 days after the initial bleed.

Despite improvements in surgical techniques and management, many patients with SAH die. Some die almost immediately when a rupture occurs. Others die from subsequent bleeding. Survivors may be left with significant morbidity, including cognitive problems.

CLINICAL MANIFESTATIONS OF STROKE

Neurologic manifestations do not significantly differ between ischemic and hemorrhagic stroke. The reason for this is that destruction of neural tissue is the basis for neurologic dysfunction caused by both types of stroke. The manifestations are related to the location of the stroke. Specific manifestations related to the type of stroke were discussed in the previous section. The general manifestations of ischemic and hemorrhagic stroke are discussed together here.

A stroke can affect many body functions, including motor activity, bladder and bowel elimination, intellectual function, spatial-perceptual changes, personality, affect, sensation, swallowing, and communication. The functions affected are directly related to the artery involved and area of the brain that it supplies (Table 57.4). Manifestations related to right- and left-brain damage differ somewhat. These are shown in Fig. 57.4.

Motor Function

Motor deficits are the most obvious effect of stroke. Motor deficits include impairment of (1) mobility, (2) respiratory function, (3) swallowing and speech, (4) gag reflex, and (5) self-care abilities. Symptoms are caused by the destruction of motor neurons in the pyramidal pathway (nerve fibers from the brain that pass through the spinal cord to the motor cells). The characteristic motor deficits include loss of skilled voluntary movement (*akinesia*), impaired integration of movements, changes in muscle tone, and altered reflexes. The initial *hyporeflexia* (depressed reflexes) progresses to *hyperreflexia* (hyperactive reflexes) for most patients.

Motor deficits after a stroke follow certain specific patterns. Because the pyramidal pathway crosses at the level of the

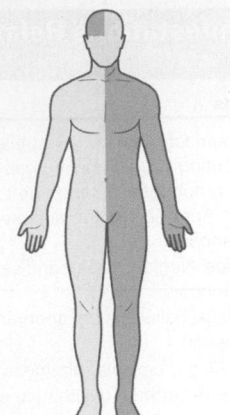
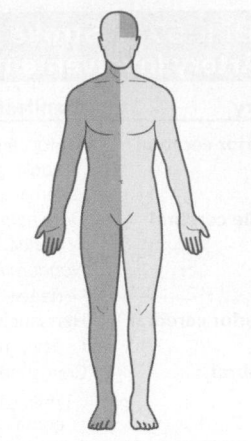

Right-brain damage (stroke on right side of the brain)	**Left-brain damage** (stroke on left side of the brain)
• Paralyzed left side: hemiplegia	• Paralyzed right side: hemiplegia
• Left-sided neglect	• Impaired speech/language aphasias
• Spatial-perceptual deficits	• Impaired right/left discrimination
• Tends to deny or minimize problems	• Slow performance, cautious
• Rapid performance, short attention span	• Aware of deficits: depression, anxiety
• Impulsive, safety problems	• Impaired comprehension related to language, math
• Impaired judgment	
• Impaired time concepts	

FIG. 57.4 Manifestations of right-brain and left-brain stroke.

medulla, a lesion on one side of the brain affects motor function on the opposite side of the body (contralateral). The arms and legs of the affected side may be weakened or paralyzed to different degrees depending on which part of and to what extent the cerebral circulation was compromised. A stroke affecting the middle cerebral artery leads to a greater weakness in the upper extremity than the lower extremity. The affected shoulder tends to rotate internally, and the hip rotates externally. The affected foot is plantar flexed and inverted. An initial period of flaccidity may last from days to several weeks and is related to nerve damage. Spasticity of the muscles, which follows the flaccid stage, is related to interruption of upper motor neuron influence.

Communication

The left hemisphere is dominant for language skills in right-handed persons and in most left-handed persons.[12] Language disorders involve expression and comprehension of written and spoken words. The patient may have aphasia. Types of aphasia include *receptive aphasia* (loss of comprehension), *expressive aphasia* (inability to produce language), or *global aphasia* (total inability to communicate). Aphasia occurs when a stroke damages the dominant hemisphere of the brain.

Dysphasia refers to impaired ability to communicate. However, in most settings the terms *aphasia* and *dysphasia* are used interchangeably. Aphasia is the more common term used. Patterns of aphasia may differ since the stroke affects different portions of the brain. Aphasia may be classified as *nonfluent* (minimal speech activity with slow speech that requires obvious effort) or *fluent* (speech is present but has little meaningful communication) (Table 57.5). Most types of aphasia are mixed, with impairment in both expression and understanding. A massive stroke may result in global aphasia.

TABLE 57.5 Types of Aphasia

Type	Characteristics
Broca's	• Type of nonfluent aphasia • Damage to frontal lobe of brain • Often speak in short phrases that make sense but take great effort • Often omit small words (e.g., is, and, the) • May say, "Walk dog," meaning, "I will take the dog for a walk," or "Book 2 table," for "There are 2 books on the table" • Typically understands others' speech • Often aware of their difficulties and can become easily frustrated
Global	• Type of nonfluent aphasia • Results from damage to extensive portions of language areas of brain • Have severe communication difficulties • May be extremely limited in ability to speak or understand language
Wernicke's	• Type of fluent aphasia • Damage occurs in left temporal lobe, although it can result from damage to right lobe • May speak in long sentences that have no meaning, add unnecessary words, and even create made-up words • May say, "You know that smoodle pinkered and that I want to get him round and take care of him like you want before" • Usually have great difficulty understanding speech • Often unaware of their mistakes • Often difficult to follow what person is trying to say
Other	• Results from damage to different language areas in brain • Some may have difficulty repeating words and sentences, even though they can speak and understand the meaning of the word or sentence • May have difficulty naming objects, even though they know what the object is and what its use is

Many stroke patients have dysarthria, a problem with the muscular control of speech. Impairment may involve pronunciation, articulation, and phonation. Dysarthria does not affect the meaning of communication or the comprehension of language, but it does affect the mechanics of speech. Some patients have a combination of aphasia and dysarthria.

Affect

Patients who had a stroke may have a hard time controlling their emotions. Emotional responses may be exaggerated or unpredictable. Depression and feelings associated with changes in body image and loss of function can make this worse.[13] Mobility and communication problems increase frustration.

❓ CHECK YOUR PRACTICE

You are working in the outpatient stroke clinic, counseling the family of one of your favorite patients. He is a well-respected 65-yr-old business man who has returned home after a stroke. His family tells you that during meals he becomes frustrated and begins to cry because of the difficulty getting food into his mouth and chewing. His family cannot understand why a previously very competent man is so emotional.

• How should you counsel the family? What teaching is needed?

Intellectual Function

A stroke may impair both memory and judgment. These impairments can occur with strokes affecting either side of the brain. A left-brain stroke is more likely to result in memory problems related to language. Patients with a left-brain stroke often are cautious in making judgments.

The patient with a right-brain stroke tends to be impulsive and to move quickly. An example is that they try to rise quickly from a wheelchair without locking the wheels or raising the footrests. On the other hand, people with a left-brain stroke would move slowly and cautiously from the wheelchair. Patients with either type of stroke may find it hard to make generalizations, interfering with their ability to learn.

Spatial-Perceptual Problems

Those who had a stroke on the right side of the brain are more likely to have problems with spatial-perceptual orientation. However, this can also occur in people with left-brain stroke.

Spatial-perceptual problems may be divided into 4 categories.
- The first results from damage of the parietal lobe. It causes the patient to have an incorrect perception of self and illness. In this situation, patients may deny their illnesses or not recognize their own body parts.
- The second category occurs when the patient neglects all input from the affected side (erroneous perception of self in space). This may be worsened by *homonymous hemianopsia,* in which blindness occurs in the same half of the visual fields of both eyes. The patient also has difficulty with spatial orientation, such as judging distances.
- The third spatial-perceptual deficit is *agnosia,* the inability to recognize an object by sight, touch, or hearing.
- The fourth deficit is *apraxia,* the inability to carry out learned sequential movements on command. Patients may or may not be aware of their spatial-perceptual problems. You need to assess for this potential problem as it will affect rehabilitation and recovery.

Elimination

Most problems with urinary and bowel elimination are temporary. When a stroke affects one hemisphere of the brain, the prognosis for normal bladder function is excellent. At least partial sensation for bladder filling remains, and voluntary urination is present. At first the patient may have frequency, urgency, and incontinence. Although motor control of the bowel is usually not a problem, patients are often constipated. Constipation is associated with immobility, weak abdominal muscles, dehydration, and decreased response to the defecation reflex. Elimination problems may also be related to inability to state the need to eliminate and difficulty managing clothing (resulting in incontinence). Scheduled toileting and clothes that are easily removed encourage independence.

DIAGNOSTIC STUDIES FOR STROKE

When manifestations of a stroke occur, diagnostic studies (Table 57.6 and 57.7) are done to (1) confirm that it is a stroke and not another type of brain lesion and (2) identify the likely cause of the stroke. Diagnostic study results also guide decisions about therapy. A key assessment is to determine the time of the onset of symptoms. This is important for all types of stroke, especially ischemic strokes since the time can affect treatment decisions.

TABLE 57.6 Diagnostic Studies

Stroke

Diagnosis of Stroke (Including Extent of Involvement)
- CT scan
- CT angiography (CTA)
- CT/MRI perfusion and diffusion imaging
- MRI
- Magnetic resonance angiography (MRA)

Cerebral Blood Flow
- Carotid angiography
- Carotid duplex scanning
- Cerebral angiography
- Digital subtraction angiography
- Transcranial Doppler ultrasonography

Cardiac Assessment
- Cardiac markers (troponin, creatine kinase-MB)
- Chest x-ray
- Echocardiography (transthoracic, transesophageal)
- ECG

Additional Studies
- Coagulation studies: prothrombin time, activated partial thromboplastin time
- CBC (including platelets)
- Electrolyte panel with blood glucose
- Lipid profile
- Renal and hepatic studies

Once the person suspected of TIA or stroke arrives in the emergency department, it is important for the patient to rapidly undergo either a noncontrast head CT or MRI. These important diagnostic tests can rapidly distinguish between ischemic and hemorrhagic stroke. They help determine the size and location of the stroke and treatment options. MRI is more effective in identifying ischemic stroke than CT scans. However, a CT scan is a rapid diagnostic tool to rule out hemorrhage. Serial scans may be used to assess the effectiveness of treatment and to evaluate recovery.

CT angiography (CTA) provides visualization of cerebral blood vessels. It can be done after or at the same time as the noncontrast CT scan. CTA can give an estimate of perfusion and detect filling defects in the cerebral arteries. Magnetic resonance angiography (MRA) can detect vascular lesions and blockages, similar to CTA. CT/MRI perfusion and diffusion imaging may be done.

If the suspected cause of the stroke includes emboli from the heart, diagnostic cardiac tests should be done. Cardiac imaging is recommended because many strokes are caused by blood clots from the heart. Blood tests can help identify conditions contributing to stroke and to guide treatment (Table 57.6).

Angiography can identify cervical and cerebrovascular occlusion, atherosclerotic plaques, and malformation of vessels. Cerebral angiography can definitively identify the source of SAH. Risks of angiography include dislodging an embolus, causing vasospasm, inducing further hemorrhage, and provoking an allergic reaction to contrast media.

Intraarterial digital subtraction angiography (DSA) involves the injection of a contrast agent to visualize blood vessels in the neck and the large vessels of the circle of Willis. It reduces the dose of contrast material, uses smaller catheters, and shortens

TABLE 57.7 Interprofessional Care

Acute Stroke

Diagnostic Assessment
- History and physical examination
- Diagnostic studies (Table 57.6)

Management

Drug Therapy
- Platelet inhibitors (e.g., aspirin)
- Anticoagulation therapy for patients with atrial fibrillation

Surgical Therapy
- Carotid endarterectomy
- Stenting of carotid artery
- Transluminal angioplasty
- Surgical interventions for aneurysms at risk for bleeding

Acute Care
- Maintenance of airway
- Fluid therapy
- Treatment of cerebral edema
- Prevention of secondary injury

Ischemic Stroke
- Tissue plasminogen activator (tPA) IV or intraarterial
- Endovascular therapy

Hemorrhagic Stroke
- Surgical decompression if indicated
- Clipping or coiling of aneurysm

Role of Interprofessional Team Members

Speech Therapy
- Assess swallowing reflex
- Evaluate patient for communication defects (e.g., aphasia)

Occupational Therapy
- Evaluate ability to perform self-care
- Teach to perform activities of daily living and adapting tasks

Physical Therapy
- Recommend functional position
- Assess function and together with patient, plan a rehabilitation program

the length of the procedure compared with conventional angiography. It is considered safer than cerebral angiography because there is less vascular manipulation.

Transcranial doppler (TCD) ultrasonography is a noninvasive study that measures the velocity of blood flow in the major cerebral arteries. TCD is effective in detecting microemboli and vasospasm. It is ideal for the patient suspected of having an SAH. Carotid duplex scanning is used to detect the cause of the stroke and stratify patients for either medical management or carotid intervention if they have carotid stenosis.

An LP can determine if red blood cells are present in the CSF if we suspect a SAH but the CT does not show hemorrhage. An LP is avoided if the patient is suspected of having an obstruction in the foramen magnum or other signs of increased ICP because of the danger of herniation of the brain downward. This could lead to pressure on cardiac and respiratory centers in the brainstem and potentially death.

The LICOX system may be used as a diagnostic tool to evaluate the progression of stroke. LICOX measures brain

oxygenation and temperature (see discussion in Chapter 56 on p. 1307 and Fig. 56.9). Secondary brain injury adds significantly to mortality risk and poor functional outcome after a stroke.

INTERPROFESSIONAL CARE FOR STROKE

Preventive Therapy

Primary prevention is a priority for decreasing morbidity and mortality risk from stroke. The goals of stroke prevention include health promotion for a healthy lifestyle and management of modifiable risk factors to prevent a stroke. Health promotion focuses on (1) healthy diet, (2) weight control, (3) regular exercise, (4) no smoking, (5) limiting alcohol consumption, (6) BP management, and (7) routine health assessments. Patients with known risk factors (e.g., diabetes, hypertension, obesity, high serum lipids, cardiac dysfunction) need close management.

 PROMOTING POPULATION HEALTH

Stroke Prevention

- Reduce salt and sodium intake.
- Maintain a normal body weight.
- Follow a diet low in saturated fat and high in fruits and vegetables.
- Limit alcohol use to moderate levels.
- Maintain an SBP less than 140 mm Hg.
- Exercise 40 minutes 3 to 4 days per week.
- Avoid cigarette smoking and tobacco products.
- Maintain a normal blood glucose level and control diabetes.
- Follow the prescribed treatment plan for diagnosed cardiac problems.

Preventive Drug Therapy. Measures to prevent the development of a thrombus or an embolus are used in patients with TIAs, since they are at high risk for stroke. Antiplatelet drugs are usually the chosen treatment to prevent stroke in patients who had a TIA. Aspirin, at a dose of 81 mg/day, is the most often used antiplatelet agent. Other agents include ticlopidine, clopidogrel (Plavix), dipyridamole (Persantine), and combined dipyridamole and aspirin (Aggrenox).

 DRUG ALERT Ticlopidine and Clopidogrel (Plavix)

- Inform all HCPs and dentists that the medication is being taken before scheduling surgery or major dental procedures.
- They may have to be discontinued 10 to 14 days before surgery if antiplatelet effect is not desired.

For patients with atrial fibrillation, oral anticoagulation can include warfarin (Coumadin) and the direct factor Xa inhibitors: rivaroxaban (Xarelto), dabigatran (Pradaxa), and apixaban (Eliquis). The primary advantage of direct factor Xa inhibitors compared to warfarin is that they do not need close monitoring or dosage adjustments. Statins (e.g., simvastatin, lovastatin) are effective in stroke prevention for those with high cholesterol levels who had a TIA.[10]

Left Atrial Appendage Occlusion. The left atrial appendage (LAA) is a pouch that extends off the left atrium. We think the LAA is the source of many stroke-causing emboli in patients with atrial fibrillation. Removing or occluding the LAA decreases the incidence of strokes. LAA occlusion is a treatment strategy to prevent blood clot formation in patients with atrial fibrillation. It is an alternative for patients who cannot use oral anticoagulants, such as warfarin. After LAA occlusion, patients may be able to stop taking anticoagulants.[9]

A special stapler can be used to remove the LAA. Or, the HCP can place sutures that manually occlude the LAA. There are also special LAA occlusion devices (e.g., AtriClip, Watchman).[9] These devices are positioned around the LAA and then closed, like a clamp that is used to shut off the blood supply. This prevents blood from flowing into and out of the LAA.

Patent Foramen Ovale. Patients with a patent foramen ovale are at increased risk for an ischemic stroke. In this condition, there is a hole between the left and right atriums. Blood clots can pass through this opening and go to the brain, leading to ischemia. An occlusion device implanted in this opening can prevent clot dislodgment (e.g. Amplatzer PFO).[14]

Surgical/Endovascular Therapy for TIA and Stroke Prevention. Surgical interventions for the patient with TIAs due to carotid disease include carotid endarterectomy, transluminal angioplasty, and stenting. In a *carotid endarterectomy* (CEA), the atheromatous lesion is removed from the carotid artery to improve blood flow.

Transluminal angioplasty is the insertion of a balloon to open a stenosed artery in the brain and improve blood flow. The balloon is threaded up to the carotid artery through a catheter inserted in the femoral artery.

Stenting involves intravascular placement of a stent to try to maintain patency of the artery (Fig. 57.5). The stent can be inserted during an angioplasty. Once in place, the system can be used with a tiny filter that opens like an umbrella. The filter catches and removes the debris that is stirred up during the stenting procedure before it floats to the brain, where it can trigger a stroke. Stenting is a less invasive strategy for revascularization in patients unable to withstand the CEA because of coexisting medical conditions.

Postoperative nursing care includes neurovascular assessment and BP management. Assess for complications, including stent occlusion and retroperitoneal hemorrhage. Minimize the risk for bleeding at the insertion site by keeping the patient's leg straight for the prescribed time.

Acute Care for Ischemic Stroke

During initial evaluation, the single most important point in the patient's history is the time of onset of symptoms. Interprofessional goals during the acute phase are preserving life, preventing further brain damage, and reducing disability (Table 57.7).

Table 57.8 outlines the emergency management of the patient with a stroke. In the unresponsive person, acute care begins with assessing circulation, airway, and breathing. Patients may have difficulty keeping an open and clear airway because of a decreased level of consciousness or decreased or absent gag and swallowing reflexes. Maintaining adequate oxygenation is important. O_2 administration, artificial airway insertion, intubation, and mechanical ventilation may be needed. Baseline neurologic assessment is carried out, and patients are monitored closely for signs of increasing neurologic deficit. Many patients may worsen in the first 24 to 48 hours.

For emergency care, patients should be transported to the closest certified stroke center. If one is not available, they should be sent to the closest facility offering emergency stroke care.[15] The AHA recommends that acute care facilities have stroke teams in place. The stroke team generally consists of a registered nurse, neurologist, radiologist, and radiologic technician.

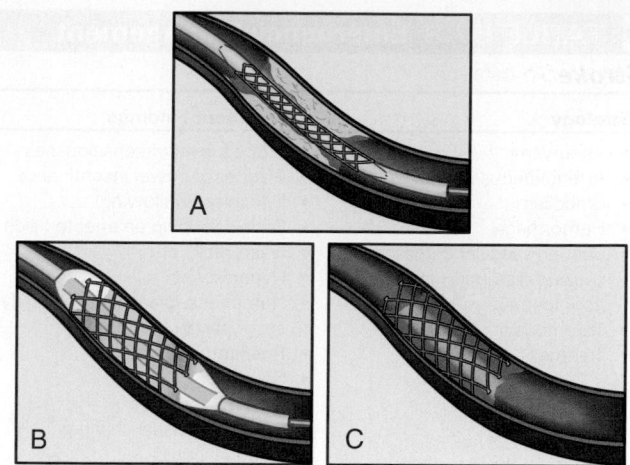

FIG. 57.5 Brain stent used to treat blockages in cerebral blood flow. **A,** A balloon catheter is used to implant the stent into an artery of the brain. **B,** The balloon catheter is moved to the blocked area of the artery and then inflated. The stent expands due to inflation of the balloon. **C,** The balloon is deflated and withdrawn, leaving the stent permanently in place holding the artery open and improving the flow of blood.

Elevated BP is common immediately after a stroke. It may be a protective response to maintain cerebral perfusion. However, it can be detrimental. In patients with an ischemic stroke who do not receive fibrinolytic therapy (discussed later), the use of drugs to lower BP is recommended only if BP is markedly increased (SBP greater than 220 mm Hg or DBP greater than 120 mm Hg). In a patient who is going to have fibrinolytic therapy, the BP must be less than 185/110 mm Hg and then maintained at or below 180/105 mm Hg for at least 24 hours after fibrinolytic therapy. In an acute stroke, IV antihypertensives, such as labetalol and nicardipine (Cardene), are preferred. Although low BP right after a stroke is uncommon, we correct hypotension and hypovolemia if present.

Fluid and electrolyte balance must be controlled carefully. The goal is to keep the patient adequately hydrated to promote perfusion and decrease further brain injury. Overhydration may compromise perfusion by increasing ICP and cerebral edema. Adequate fluid intake during acute care via oral, IV, or tube feedings is a priority. Monitor urine output to make sure the patient does not become dehydrated.

If secretion of antidiuretic hormone (ADH) increases in response to the stroke, urine output decreases and fluid is retained. Low serum sodium (hyponatremia) may occur. IV solutions with glucose and water are avoided because they are hypotonic and may further increase cerebral edema and ICP. Glycemic control should be maintained to avoid extreme hypoglycemia or hyperglycemia. In general, decisions about fluid and electrolyte replacement therapy are based on the extent of intracranial edema, manifestations of increased ICP, central venous pressure levels, electrolyte levels, and intake and output.

Increased ICP is more likely to occur with hemorrhagic strokes but can occur with ischemic strokes. Increased ICP from cerebral edema usually peaks in 72 hours and may cause brain herniation. Management of increased ICP includes practices that improve venous drainage. These include elevating the head of the bed, keeping head and neck in alignment, and avoiding hip flexion. Other measures for reducing ICP include managing fever (goal temperature of 96.8° to 98.6° F [36° to 37° C]), drug therapy to prevent seizures, pain management, and preventing

✚ TABLE 57.8 Emergency Management

Stroke

Etiology	Assessment Findings	Interventions
• Aneurysm • Arteriovenous malformation • Embolism • Hemorrhage • Sudden vascular compromise causing disruption of blood flow to brain • Thrombosis • Trauma	• Altered level of consciousness • Bladder or bowel incontinence • Difficulty swallowing • Facial drooping on affected side • Heart rate ↑ or ↓ • Hypertension • Numbness, weakness, or paralysis of part of body • Respiratory distress • Seizures • Severe headache • Speech or visual changes • Unequal pupils • Vertigo	**Initial** • If unresponsive, assess circulation, airway, and breathing. • If responsive, monitor airway, breathing, and circulation. • Call stroke code or stroke team. • Remove dentures. • Perform pulse oximetry. • Maintain adequate oxygenation (SaO_2 >95%) with supplemental O_2, if needed. • Establish IV access with normal saline. • Maintain BP according to guidelines. • Remove clothing. • Obtain CT scan or MRI. • Perform baseline laboratory tests (including blood glucose) immediately and treat if hypoglycemic. • Position head in midline. • Elevate head of bed 30 degrees if no symptoms of shock or injury. • Institute seizure precautions. • Anticipate thrombolytic therapy for ischemic stroke. • Keep patient NPO until swallow reflex evaluated. **Ongoing Monitoring** • Monitor vital signs and neurologic status, including level of consciousness (NIH Stroke Scale), motor and sensory function, pupil size and reactivity, SaO_2, and cardiac rhythm. • Reassure patient and family.

NIH, National Institutes of Health; *SaO₂,* arterial O_2 saturation.

constipation. CSF drainage may be used in some patients to reduce ICP. The specific management of increased ICP is discussed in Chapter 56.

Drug Therapy for Ischemic Stroke. Fibrinolytic therapy should not be delayed. Recombinant tissue plasminogen activator (tPA) is used to produce localized fibrinolysis by binding to the fibrin in the thrombi. The fibrinolytic action of tPA occurs as the plasminogen is converted to plasmin, whose enzymatic action then digests fibrin and fibrinogen, thus breaking down the clot. Other fibrinolytic agents cannot be substituted for tPA. (Fibrinolytic [thrombolytic] therapy is discussed in Chapter 33.)

tPA is given IV to reestablish blood flow through a blocked artery to prevent cell death in patients with the acute onset of ischemic stroke. tPA must be given within 3 to 4½ hours of the onset of signs of ischemic stroke.[16] Patients are screened carefully before tPA can be given. Screening includes a noncontrast CT scan or MRI to rule out hemorrhagic stroke; blood tests for coagulation disorders; screening for recent history of gastrointestinal (GI) bleeding, stroke, or head trauma within the past 3 months; major surgery within 14 days; or recent active internal bleeding within 22 days.[16]

During tPA infusion, closely monitor the patient's vital signs and neurologic status to assess for improvement or for potential deterioration related to intracerebral hemorrhage. Control of BP (SBP less than 185 mm Hg) is critical during treatment and for 24 hours following.

Intraarterial infusion of tPA may be used for patients with an ischemic stroke when mechanical thrombectomy is not an option. To be effective, intraarterial tPA must be given within 6 hours of the onset of stroke symptoms. In the intraarterial tPA procedure, the neurovascular specialist inserts a thin, flexible catheter into an artery (usually the femoral artery) and guides

the catheter (using angiogram) to the area of the clot. The tPA is given through the catheter and immediately targets the clot. Less tPA is needed when it is delivered directly to the clot, which can reduce the chance for intracranial hemorrhage.

The use of anticoagulants (e.g., heparin) in the emergency phase after an ischemic stroke is not recommended because of the risk for intracranial hemorrhage. Aspirin at a dose of 325 mg may be started within 24 to 48 hours after the onset of an ischemic stroke. Complications of higher dose aspirin include GI bleeding. Aspirin should be given cautiously if the patient has a history of peptic ulcer disease.

After the patient has stabilized and to prevent further clot formation, patients with strokes caused by thrombi and emboli may be treated with anticoagulants and platelet inhibitors (see discussion on stroke prevention on p. 1338.). For patients with atrial fibrillation, oral anticoagulants include warfarin and the direct factor Xa inhibitors: rivaroxaban (Xarelto), dabigatran (Pradaxa), and apixaban (Eliquis). Platelet inhibitors include aspirin, ticlopidine, clopidogrel, and dipyridamole. The use of statins is effective for the patient after an ischemic stroke.[9]

Endovascular Therapy for Ischemic Stroke. Stent retrievers are a way of opening blocked arteries in the brain by using a removable stent system.[17] During the procedure, a catheter is used to guide the small stent from the femoral artery in the groin area to the affected artery in the brain. The stent is guided (using neuroimaging) into the part of the artery where a blood clot has formed. The stent expands the interior walls of the artery and allows blood to get to the patient's brain immediately to prevent as much brain damage as possible. The clot seeps into the mesh of the stent. Then, after a few minutes the stent and clot are removed together. Stent retrievers are becoming the most effective way of managing ischemic stroke.[17]

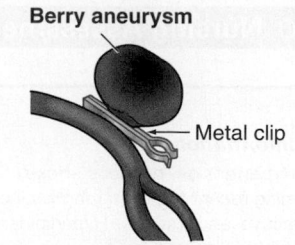

FIG. 57.6 Clipping of aneurysms.

The ENROUTE device accesses the carotid arteries through the neck, rather than the groin. It allows the surgeon to maintain blood flow to the brain while performing carotid angioplasty and stenting.[18]

Acute Care for Hemorrhagic Stroke

Drug Therapy for Hemorrhagic Stroke. Anticoagulants and platelet inhibitors are contraindicated in patients with hemorrhagic strokes. The main drug therapy for patients with hemorrhagic stroke is the management of hypertension. Oral and IV agents may be used to maintain BP within a normal to high-normal range (SBP less than 160 mm Hg). Seizure prophylaxis in the acute period after intracerebral and subarachnoid hemorrhages is situation specific and decided among the interprofessional care team.[19]

Surgical Therapy for Hemorrhagic Stroke. Surgical interventions for hemorrhagic stroke include immediate evacuation of aneurysm-induced hematomas or cerebellar hematomas larger than 3 cm. Those who have an arteriovenous malformation (AVM) may have a hemorrhagic stroke if the AVM ruptures. The treatment of AVM is surgical resection and/or radiosurgery (i.e., gamma knife). Interventional neuroradiology to embolize the blood vessels that supply the AVM may be done prior.

With SAH, bleeding from a damaged vessel causes blood to accumulate between the brain and skull. The leaked blood can irritate, damage, or destroy the surrounding brain cells. When blood enters the subarachnoid space, it mixes with the CSF. This can block CSF circulation, thus causing increased pressure on the brain. The open spaces in the brain (ventricles) may enlarge, resulting in hydrocephalus. This further increases ICP (due to the large accumulation of blood) and can result in further brain injury. Inserting a ventriculostomy for CSF drainage can dramatically improve these situations by reducing the ICP.[20] Goals for managing ICP are the same for patients with SAH as they are for patients dealing with acute stroke. The management of ICP is discussed in Chapter 56.

SAH is usually caused by a ruptured aneurysm. Patients may have multiple aneurysms. Treatment of an aneurysm involves clipping or coiling the aneurysm to prevent rebleeding (Figs. 57.6 and 57.7). In *clipping* the aneurysm, the neurosurgeon places a metallic clip on the neck of the aneurysm to block blood flow and prevent rupture. The clip stays in place for life.

In the procedure known as *coiling*, a hydrogel-coated platinum coil is inserted into the lumen of the aneurysm via interventional neuroradiology (Fig. 57.7). Guglielmi detachable coils (GDCs) give immediate protection against hemorrhage by reducing the blood pulsations within the aneurysm. Eventually, a thrombus forms within the aneurysm. Then the aneurysm becomes sealed off from the parent vessel by the formation of an endothelialized layer of connective tissue.

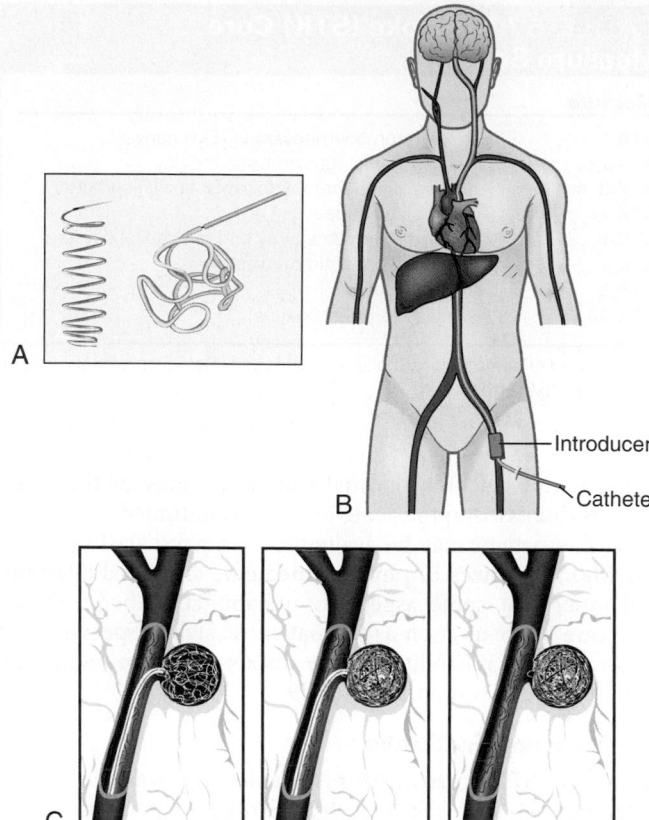

FIG. 57.7 Guglielmi detachable coil (GDC). **A,** A coil is used to occlude an aneurysm. Coils are made of soft, springlike platinum. The softness of the platinum allows the coil to assume the shape of irregularly shaped aneurysms while posing little threat of rupture of the aneurysm. **B,** A catheter is inserted through an introducer (small tube) in an artery in the leg. The catheter is threaded up to the cerebral blood vessels. **C,** Platinum coils attached to a thin wire are inserted into the catheter and then placed in the aneurysm until the aneurysm is filled with coils. Packing the aneurysm with coils prevents the blood from circulating through the aneurysm, reducing the risk for rupture.

After aneurysmal occlusion via clipping or coiling, hyperdynamic therapy (hemodilution-induced hypertension using vasoconstricting agents, such as phenylephrine or dopamine, and hypervolemia) may be started to increase the mean arterial pressure and cerebral perfusion. Volume expansion is achieved with crystalloid or colloid solutions.

Patients with SAH may receive the calcium channel blocker nimodipine to treat cerebral vasospasms and minimize cerebral damage. It may be given either before or after aneurysm clipping or coiling. Nimodipine restricts the influx of calcium ions into cells by reducing the number of open calcium channels. Although nimodipine is a calcium channel blocker, we do not know its exact mechanism of action in reducing vasospasm.

DRUG ALERT Nimodipine

- Assess BP and apical pulses before administration.
- If pulse is ≤60 beats/min or SBP is <90 mm Hg, hold the medication and contact the provider.

Rehabilitation Care

After the stroke patient has stabilized for 12 to 24 hours, interprofessional care shifts from preserving life to lessening

TABLE 57.9 Stroke (STK) Core Measure Set

Measure	Topic
STK-1	Venous thromboembolism (VTE) prophylaxis
STK-2	Discharged on antithrombotic therapy
STK-3	Anticoagulation therapy for atrial fibrillation/flutter
STK-4	Thrombolytic therapy
STK-5	Antithrombotic therapy by end of hospital day 2
STK-6	Discharged on statin medication
STK-8	Stroke education
STK-10	Assessed for rehabilitation

Source: The Joint Commission. Stroke core measures. Retrieved from *www.joint-commission.org/stroke*.

disability and reaching optimal function. Many of the interventions discussed in the acute phase are continued during this phase. The patient may be evaluated by a physiatrist (a physician who specializes in physical medicine and rehabilitation). Remember that some aspects of rehabilitation begin in the acute care phase as soon as the patient is stable. Specific measures related to rehabilitation are discussed in the section on Ambulatory Care on pp. 1347–1349.

Core Measures for Stroke

The stroke (STK) core measures (Table 57.9) were developed in partnership with the American Stroke Association (ASA) for use by primary stroke centers. These measures are used by hospitals for accreditation and certification. The measures align with guidelines supported by the AHA Get With The Guidelines (GWTG) stroke patient management tool and the CDC's Paul Coverdell National Acute Stroke Registry (PCNASR).

❖ NURSING MANAGEMENT: STROKE

◆ Nursing Assessment

Subjective and objective data that you should obtain from a person who has had a stroke are detailed in Table 57.10. Primary assessment focuses on cardiac and respiratory status and neurologic assessment. If the patient is stable, the nursing history is obtained as follows: (1) description of the current illness with attention to initial symptoms, especially symptom onset and duration, nature (intermittent or continuous), and changes; (2) history of having had similar symptoms previously; (3) current medications; (4) history of risk factors and other illnesses, such as hypertension; and (5) family history of stroke, aneurysm, or cardiovascular diseases. Obtain this information through interviewing the patient and caregivers.

Secondary assessment includes a comprehensive neurologic examination. The primary assessment tool to evaluate and document neurologic status in acute stroke patients is the NIHSS, which measures stroke severity (Table 57.11).[21] The NIHSS is a predictor of both short- and long-term outcomes of stroke patients. It also serves as a data collection tool for planning patient care and exchanging information among HCPs. Other assessment data includes (1) LOC; (2) cognition; (3) motor abilities; (4) cranial nerve function; (5) sensation; (6) proprioception; (7) cerebellar function; and (8) deep tendon reflexes. Clear documentation of initial and ongoing neurologic examinations is essential to note changes in the patient's status.

TABLE 57.10 Nursing Assessment

Stroke

Subjective Data

Important Health Information

Past health history: Hypertension, previous stroke, TIA, aneurysm, cardiac disease (including recent MI, dysrhythmias, heart failure, valvular heart disease, infective endocarditis. Hyperlipidemia, polycythemia, blood clotting disorders, diabetes, gout

Family history: Neurologic disorders, aneurysms, stroke, TIA, diabetes, hypertension, coronary artery disease

Medications: Oral contraceptives; use of and adherence with antihypertensive and anticoagulant therapy; illicit substance use

Functional Health Patterns

Health perception–health management: Alcohol use, smoking, drug use

Nutritional-metabolic: Anorexia, nausea, vomiting. Dysphagia, altered sense of taste and smell

Elimination: Change in bowel and bladder patterns

Activity-exercise: Loss of movement and sensation. Syncope, weakness on one side, generalized weakness, easy fatigability

Cognitive-perceptual: Numbness, tingling of one side of the body, loss of memory. Change in speech, language, problem-solving ability. Pain, headache (possibly sudden and severe) (hemorrhage). Visual changes. Denial of illness

Objective Data

General

Emotional lability, lethargy, apathy or combativeness, fever

Respiratory

Loss of cough reflex, labored or irregular respirations, tachypnea, wheezes (aspiration), airway occlusion (tongue), apnea, coughing when eating or delayed coughing

Cardiovascular

Hypertension, tachycardia, carotid bruit

Gastrointestinal

Loss of gag reflex, bowel incontinence, decreased or absent bowel sounds, constipation

Urinary

Frequency, urgency, incontinence

Neurologic

Contralateral motor and sensory deficits, including weakness, paresis, paralysis, anesthesia. Unequal pupils, hand grasps. Akinesia, aphasia (expressive, receptive, global), dysarthria (slurred speech), agnosia, apraxia, visual deficits, perceptual or spatial problems, altered level of consciousness (drowsiness to deep coma) and Babinski's sign, ↓ followed by ↑ deep tendon reflexes, flaccidity followed by spasticity, amnesia, ataxia, personality change, nuchal rigidity, seizures

Possible Diagnostic Findings

Positive CT, CTA, MRI, MRA, or other neuroimaging scans showing size, location, and type of lesion. Positive Doppler ultrasonography and angiography showing stenosis

◆ Nursing Diagnoses

Nursing diagnoses for the person with a stroke may include:
- Decreased intracranial adaptive capacity
- Impaired communication
- Difficulty coping
- Risk for aspiration
- Impaired physical mobility
- Risk for injury

TABLE 57.11 National Institutes of Health Stroke Scale (NIHSS)

Description

The NIH Stroke Scale (NIHSS) is a 15-item neurologic examination used to evaluate the effect of an acute stroke. Total scores on the NIHSS range from 0 to 42, with higher values reflecting more severity.

Procedure for Use

A trained observer rates the patient's ability to answer questions and perform activities. Ratings for each item are scored, and there is an allowance for untestable (UN) items. If an item is left untested, a detailed explanation must be clearly written on the form. Training can be completed free at *www.nihstrokescale.org*.

Item	Scale Definition
Level of consciousness	0 = Alert 1 = Not alert, but arousable by minor stimulation 2 = Not alert, requires repeated stimulation to get attention 3 = Responds only with reflex motor or autonomic effects or totally unresponsive, flaccid, areflexic
Level of consciousness questions	0 = Answers both questions correctly 1 = Answers 1 question correctly 2 = Answers neither question correctly
Level of consciousness commands	0 = Performs both tasks correctly 1 = Performs 1 task correctly 2 = Performs neither task correctly
Best gaze	0 = Normal 1 = Partial gaze palsy 2 = Forced deviation, or total gaze paresis
Visual	0 = No visual loss 1 = Partial hemianopsia 2 = Complete hemianopsia 3 = Bilateral hemianopsia or blind
Facial palsy	0 = Normal symmetric movement 1 = Minor paralysis 2 = Partial paralysis 3 = Complete paralysis of 1 or both sides
Motor and drift (for each extremity)	0 = No drift 1 = Drift 2 = Some effort against gravity 3 = No effort against gravity, limb falls 4 = No movement UN = Amputation
Limb ataxia	0 = Absent 1 = Present in 1 limb 2 = Present in 2 limbs
Sensory	0 = Normal 1 = Mild to moderate sensory loss 2 = Severe to total sensory loss
Best language	0 = No aphasia, normal 1 = Mild to moderate aphasia 2 = Severe aphasia 3 = Mute, no usable speech or auditory comprehension
Dysarthria	0 = Normal 1 = Mild to moderate 2 = Severe UN = Intubated or other physical barrier
Extinction or inattention	0 = No abnormality 1 = Inattention or extinction to bilateral stimulation 2 = Does not recognize own hand
Distal motor function	0 = Normal (no flexion after 5 sec) 1 = At least some extension but not fully extended 2 = No voluntary extension after 5 sec

Source: National Institutes of Health: NIH stroke scale. Retrieved from *www.stroke.nih.gov/resources/scale.htm.*

Additional information on nursing diagnoses and interventions are presented in eNursing Care Plan 57.1 (available on the website for this chapter).

◆ Planning

Establish the goals of nursing care together with the patient, caregiver, and family. Typical goals are that the patient will (1) maintain a stable or improved level of consciousness, (2) attain maximum physical functioning, (3) attain maximum self-care abilities and skills, (4) maintain stable body functions (e.g., bladder control), (5) maximize communication abilities, (6) maintain adequate nutrition, (7) avoid complications of stroke, and (8) maintain effective personal and family coping.

◆ Nursing Implementation

◆ Health Promotion.

You have a key role in promoting a healthy lifestyle. Teaching should focus on stroke prevention, especially for persons with known risk factors. Most strokes are caused by modifiable risk factors. Nursing measures to reduce risk factors for stroke are similar to those for coronary artery disease (see Chapter 33) and were discussed earlier in this chapter on p. 1338.

Uncontrolled or undiagnosed hypertension is the primary cause of stroke. Therefore you need to be involved in BP screening and ensuring that patients adhere to using their antihypertensive drugs and home BP monitoring. If a person has diabetes, it is important that it is well controlled. If a person has atrial fibrillation, an anticoagulant (see p. 1338) or aspirin may reduce the risk for stroke. Because smoking is a major risk factor for stroke, you need to be actively involved in helping patients to stop smoking (see Chapter 10, Tables 10.4 to 10.6).

Another important aspect of health promotion is teaching patients and families about early symptoms associated with stroke or TIA. Table 57.1 presents information on when to seek health care for these symptoms.

◆ Acute Care

Respiratory System. During the acute phase after a stroke, management of the respiratory system is a nursing priority. Stroke patients are vulnerable to respiratory problems. Advancing age and immobility increase the risk for atelectasis and pneumonia.

Nursing interventions to support adequate respiratory function are tailored to meet the patient's specific needs (Table 57.12). Some stroke patients, especially those with brainstem or hemorrhagic stroke, may need endotracheal intubation and mechanical ventilation. An oropharyngeal airway in a comatose patient may prevent the tongue from falling back and obstructing the airway and provide access for suctioning. Alternatively, a nasopharyngeal airway may be used to provide airway protection and access. When an artificial airway is needed for a prolonged time, a tracheostomy may be done.

Nursing interventions include frequently assessing airway patency and function, providing oxygenation, suctioning, promoting patient mobility, positioning the patient to prevent aspiration, and encouraging deep breathing. In patients who are on mechanical ventilation, oral care at least every 2 hours reduces the occurrence of ventilator-assisted pneumonia.

Risk for aspiration pneumonia is high because of impaired consciousness or dysphagia. Dysphagia after stroke is common. Airway obstruction can occur because of problems with chewing and swallowing, food pocketing (food remaining in the buccal cavity of the mouth), and the tongue falling back. Enteral nutrition (EN) places the patient at risk for aspiration

TABLE 57.12 Nursing Management

Caring for the Patient With an Acute Stroke

- Assess manifestations of stroke and determine when the they started.
- Screen patient for contraindications for tissue plasminogen activator (tPA) therapy.
- Infuse tPA for patients with ischemic stroke who meet the criteria for tPA administration.
- Assess respiratory status and start needed actions, such as O_2, oropharyngeal or nasopharyngeal airways, suctioning.
- Position patient to prevent aspiration and atelectasis.
- Assess neurologic status, including intracranial pressure (ICP), if needed.
- Monitor cardiovascular status, including hemodynamic monitoring, if needed.
- Calculate intake and output, noting imbalances.
- Regulate IV infusions and adjust fluid intake to patient needs.
- Assess patient's ability to swallow in conjunction with the speech therapist.
- Give scheduled anticoagulant and antiplatelet drugs.
- Implement measures to prevent VTE and skin breakdown.
- Delegate to UAP:
  - Obtain vital signs and report these to RN.
  - Measure and record urine output.
  - Help with proper positioning and turning patient at least every 2 hr.
  - Perform passive and active ROM exercises.

pneumonia. Screen all patients for their ability to swallow. Keep them NPO until dysphagia is ruled out.

Patients who have an unclipped or uncoiled aneurysm may have rebleeding and further increased ICP with coughing or suctioning, so nursing management is aimed at reducing these interventions while maintaining a proper airway.

Neurologic System. Perform ongoing neurologic assessments, including the NIHSS, mental status, pupillary response, and extremity movement and strength. Closely monitor vital signs. A decreasing level of consciousness may indicate increasing ICP. Monitor ICP and cerebral perfusion pressure if the patient is in a critical care environment. Record your nursing assessment promptly to communicate the patient's neurologic status to the stroke team.

Cardiovascular System. Nursing goals for the cardiovascular system are aimed at maintaining homeostasis. Many patients with stroke have decreased cardiac reserves from cardiac disease. Fluid retention, overhydration, dehydration, or BP changes may further compromise cardiac efficiency. Central venous pressure, pulmonary artery pressure, or hemodynamic monitoring may be used to monitor fluid balance and cardiac function in the critical care unit.

Nursing interventions include (1) monitoring vital signs frequently; (2) monitoring cardiac rhythms; (3) calculating intake and output, noting imbalances; (4) regulating IV infusions; (5) adjusting fluid intake to individual patient needs; (6) monitoring lung sounds for crackles and wheezes, indicating pulmonary congestion; and (7) monitoring heart sounds for murmurs. Bedside monitors or telemetry may record cardiac rhythms.

Hypertension sometimes occurs after a stroke as the body tries to increase CBF. It is important to monitor for orthostatic hypotension before ambulating the patient for the first time. Neurologic changes can occur with a sudden decrease in BP.

The patient is at risk for venous thromboembolism (VTE), especially in the weak or paralyzed lower extremity. VTE is related to immobility, loss of venous tone, and decreased muscle

pumping activity in the leg. The most effective prevention is to keep the patient moving. Teach the patient active range-of-motion (ROM) exercises if the patient has voluntary movement in the affected extremity. For the patient with hemiplegia, perform passive ROM exercises several times a day. Other measures to prevent VTE include positioning to minimize the effects of dependent edema and using intermittent pneumatic compression devices. VTE prophylaxis may include low-molecular-weight heparin (e.g., enoxaparin [Lovenox]).[22] The nursing assessment includes measuring the calf and thigh daily, observing for swelling of the lower extremities, noting unusual warmth of the leg, and asking the patient about pain in the calf.

Musculoskeletal System. The nursing goal for the musculoskeletal system is to maintain optimal function by preventing joint contractures and muscular atrophy. In the acute phase, ROM exercises and positioning are important nursing interventions. Passive ROM exercise is begun on the first day of hospitalization. Muscle atrophy from lack of innervation and activity can develop after stroke, so exercise is an important intervention for rehabilitation and recovery.

The paralyzed or weak side needs special attention when the patient is positioned. Position each joint higher than the joint proximal to it to prevent dependent edema. Specific deformities on the weak or paralyzed side that may be present in patients with stroke include internal rotation of the shoulder; flexion contractures of the hand, wrist, and elbow; external rotation of the hip; and plantar flexion of the foot. Subluxation of the shoulder on the affected side is common. Careful positioning and moving of the affected arm may prevent development of a painful shoulder condition. Immobilization of the affected upper extremity may precipitate a painful shoulder-hand syndrome.

Nursing interventions to optimize musculoskeletal function include (1) trochanter roll at the hip to prevent external rotation; (2) hand cones (not rolled washcloths) to prevent hand contractures; (3) arm supports with slings and lap boards to prevent shoulder displacement; (4) avoidance of pulling the patient by the arm to avoid shoulder displacement; (5) posterior leg splints, footboards, or high-top tennis shoes to prevent footdrop; and (6) hand splints to reduce spasticity.

Using a footboard for the patient with spasticity is controversial. Rather than preventing plantar flexion (footdrop), the sensory stimulation of a footboard against the bottom of the foot increases plantar flexion. Likewise, experts disagree on whether hand splints decrease spasticity. The decision about using footboards or hand splints is made on an individual patient basis.

Integumentary System. The skin of the patient with stroke is susceptible to breakdown related to loss of sensation, decreased circulation, and immobility. Advanced age, poor nutrition, dehydration, edema, and incontinence compound the risk.

Measures to prevent skin breakdown includes (1) pressure relief by position changes, special mattresses, or wheelchair cushions; (2) good skin hygiene; (3) emollients applied to dry skin; and (4) early mobility. An example of a position change schedule is side-back-side, with a maximum duration of 2 hours for any position. Position the patient on the weak or paralyzed side for only 30 minutes. Controlling pressure is the main factor in both preventing and treating skin breakdown. Use pillows under lower extremities to reduce pressure on the heels. See more information on preventing pressure injuries in Chapter 11.

Gastrointestinal System. The most common bowel problem for the stroke patient is constipation. Fluid and fiber intake goals are determined with the stroke team based on the patient's nutritional and fluid status. Patients may be prophylactically placed on stool softeners and/or fiber (psyllium [Metamucil]). Laxatives, suppositories, or additional stool softeners may be ordered if the patient does not respond to increased fluid and fiber. Enemas are used only if suppositories and digital stimulation are ineffective because they cause vagal stimulation and increase ICP. Physical activity promotes bowel function. If a patient has liquid stools, check for stool impaction.

Bowel retraining may be needed and continued into the rehabilitation phase. A bowel management program consists of placing the patient on the bedpan or bedside commode or taking the patient to the bathroom at a regular time daily to reestablish bowel regularity. A good time for a bowel movement is 30 minutes after breakfast because eating stimulates the gastrocolic reflex and peristalsis. The timing may have to be adjusted as individual bowel habits may vary.

Urinary System. In the acute stage of stroke, the primary urinary problem is poor bladder control, resulting in incontinence. Take steps to promote normal bladder function and avoid the use of indwelling catheters. If an indwelling catheter is used initially, remove it as soon as the patient is medically and neurologically stable. Long-term use of an indwelling catheter is associated with urinary tract infections and delayed bladder retraining.

Avoid bladder overdistention. An intermittent catheterization program may be used for patients with urinary retention to lower the incidence of urinary infections. An alternative to intermittent catheterizations for a male patient is an external catheter. External catheters do not address problems with urine retention.

Often the patient has functional incontinence, which is associated with communication, mobility, and dressing problems. A bladder retraining program consists of (1) adequate fluid intake, with most of it given between 7:00 AM and 7:00 PM; (2) scheduled toileting every 2 hours using bedpan, commode, or bathroom while encouraging the usual position for urinating (standing for men and sitting for women); (3) observing for signs of restlessness, which may indicate the need for urination; and (4) assessing for bladder distention by palpation. Encourage patients to wear pants without drawstrings, buttons, or zippers. These can be hard to manage if motor or sensory deficits exist.

Assessing postvoid residual volume is often done using bladder ultrasound. The ultrasound measures how much urine is in the bladder after voiding. If urine stays in the bladder, incomplete emptying is a problem and may cause urinary tract infections. A coordinated program by the entire nursing staff is needed to achieve urinary continence.

Nutrition. The patient's nutritional needs require quick assessment and treatment. The patient may initially receive IV infusions to maintain fluid and electrolyte balance and to give drugs. Patients with severe impairment may need EN or parenteral nutrition. Patients should have their nutritional needs addressed in the first 24 hours of admission to the hospital because nutrition is important for recovery and healing.[23]

Many patients have dysphagia after a stroke. Keep patients NPO until a speech therapist performs a swallowing evaluation. This should be done in the first 24 hours after the stroke.[23] You or another member of the interprofessional team may perform the screen if a speech therapist cannot perform the formal evaluation.

! SAFETY ALERT Oral Feeding After Stroke
- Dysphagia is common after stroke.
- Keep the patient on NPO status until a speech therapist does a swallowing evaluation.

Before starting feeding, assess the gag reflex by gently stimulating the back of the throat with a tongue blade. If the gag reflex is present, the patient will gag spontaneously. If it is absent, defer the feeding and begin exercises to stimulate swallowing. The speech therapist or occupational therapist is usually responsible for designing this program. However, you may be involved in helping to develop the program in some clinical settings.

To assess swallowing ability, elevate the head of the bed to an upright position (unless contraindicated). Give the patient a small amount of crushed ice or ice water to swallow. If the gag reflex is present and the patient can swallow safely, you may proceed with feeding.

The speech therapist may recommend various dietary items. Foods should be easy to swallow and provide enough texture, temperature (warm or cold), and flavor to stimulate a swallow reflex. Crushed ice can be used as a stimulant. Pureed foods are not usually the best choice because they are often bland or too smooth. Thin liquids are often hard to swallow and may promote coughing. We can thicken thin liquids with a commercially available thickening agent (e.g., Thick-It). Avoid milk products because they tend to increase the viscosity of mucus and increase salivation.

Mouth care before feeding helps stimulate sensory awareness and salivation and can help swallowing. Keep the patient in the high-Fowler's position, preferably in a chair, for the feeding and 30 minutes afterward. While feeding, keep the head flexed forward. Place food in the unaffected side of the mouth. Teach the patient to swallow and then swallow again. Follow feedings with good oral hygiene because food may collect in the affected side of the mouth.

During the acute and rehabilitation phase of the stroke, a dietitian can help determine the appropriate daily caloric intake based on the patient's size, weight, and activity level. If the patient is unable to take in an adequate oral diet and dysphagia persists, a percutaneous endoscopic gastrostomy (PEG) tube may be used for nutritional support. EN is described in Chapter 39.

The inability to feed one's self can be frustrating and may result in malnutrition and dehydration. Interventions to promote self-feeding include using the unaffected upper extremity to eat; employing assistive devices, such as rocker knives, plate guards, and nonslip pads for dishes (Fig. 57.8); and removing unnecessary items from the tray or table, which can reduce spills. Provide a calm environment (e.g., turn off the television) to decrease sensory overload and distraction. The effectiveness of the dietary program is evaluated in terms of maintenance of weight, adequate hydration, and patient satisfaction. Introduce these interventions in the acute care setting so that maximum rehabilitation can occur once the patient is discharged.

Communication. During the acute stage of stroke, your role in meeting the patient's psychologic needs is primarily supportive. Speech, comprehension, and language deficits are the most difficult problems for the patient and caregiver. Assess the patient for both the ability to speak and the ability to understand. The patient's response to simple questions can guide you in structuring explanations and instructions. If the patient cannot understand words, use gestures to support verbal cues. Collaborate with the speech therapist to assess and formulate a plan of care to enhance communication.

Nursing interventions that support communication include (1) communicating often and meaningfully; (2) allowing time for the patient to comprehend and answer; (3) using simple,

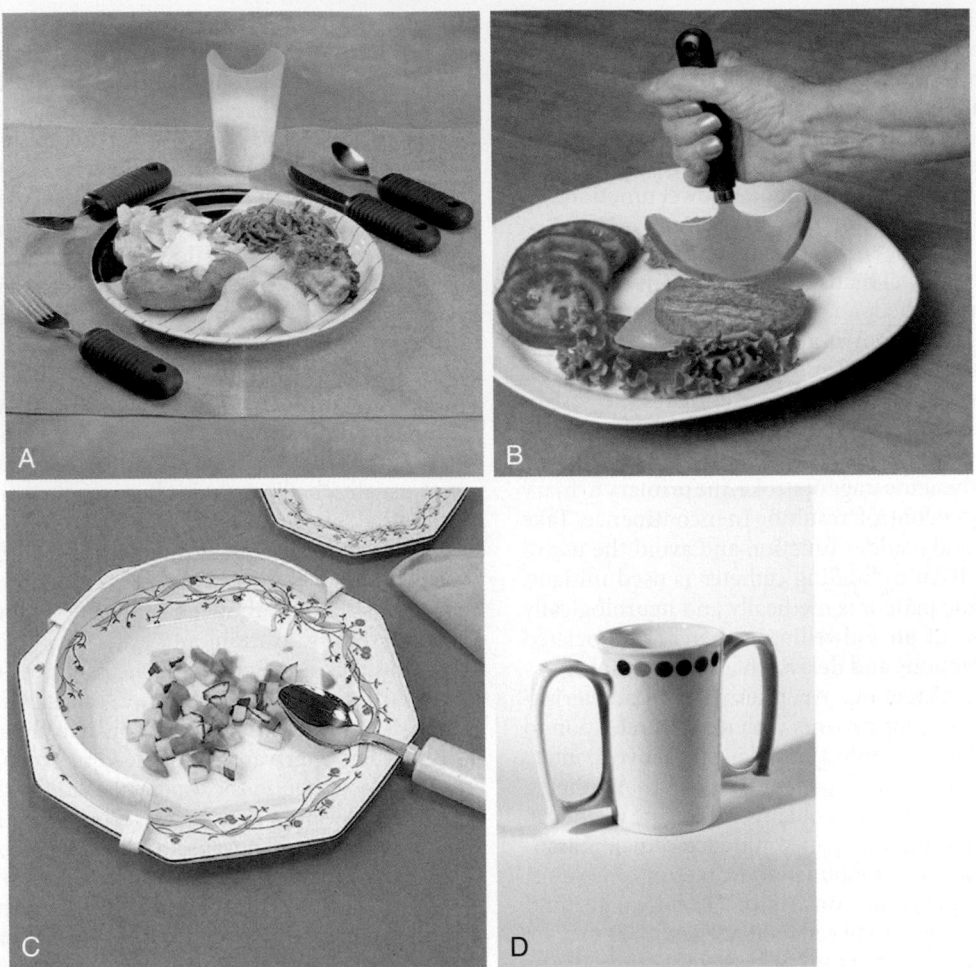

FIG. 57.8 Assistive devices for eating. **A,** The rounded plate helps keep food on the plate. Special grips and weighted handles are helpful for some persons. The cup shape allows drinking without having to tilt the head. **B,** Knives with rounded blades are rocked back and forth to cut food. The person does not need a fork in one hand and a knife in the other. **C,** Plate guards help keep food on the plate. **D,** Cup with special handles promotes independence. (Products *A, B,* and *C* courtesy of Performance Health, Warrenville, IL. *D,* Courtesy of Granny Jo Products, Lakeland, FL.)

short sentences; (4) using visual cues; (5) structuring conversation so that it permits simple answers by the patient; and (6) praising the patient honestly for improvements with speech.

An alert patient is usually anxious because of lack of understanding about what has happened and because of problems with communication or the inability to communicate. Verbal stimuli can easily overwhelm the patient with aphasia. Give the patient extra time to understand and respond to communication. Guidelines for communicating with a patient who has aphasia are outlined in Table 57.13. A picture board may be helpful for communicating with the stroke patient. The speech therapist often does further evaluation and treatment of language and communication deficits once the patient has stabilized. It is important to teach the caregiver and family these communication strategies.

Sensory-Perceptual Problems. Patients who had a stroke often have perceptual deficits. Patients with a stroke on the right side of the brain usually have difficulty judging position, distance, and rate of movement. These patients are often impulsive and impatient and tend to deny problems related to strokes. They may fail to correlate spatial-perceptual problems with the inability to perform activities, such as guiding a wheelchair through the doorway. They best understand directions given verbally. Break

down the task into simple steps for ease of understanding. The patient with a right-brain stroke and left hemiplegia is at higher risk for injury because of mobility problems. Environmental control (e.g., removing clutter, using good lighting) aids in concentration and safer mobility. Provide nonslip socks at all times. One-sided neglect is common for people with right-brain stroke. You may need to help or remind the patient to dress the weak or paralyzed side or shave the forgotten side of the face.

Patients with a left-brain stroke (right hemiplegia) often are slower in organizing and performing tasks. They tend to have impaired spatial discrimination. These patients usually admit to deficits and have a fearful, anxious response to a stroke. Their behaviors are slow and cautious. Nonverbal cues and instructions are helpful for patients who had a left-brain stroke.

Homonymous hemianopsia (blindness in the same half of each visual field) is common after a stroke. Persistent disregard of objects in part of the visual field should alert you to this possibility. At first, help the patient to compensate by arranging the environment within the patient's perceptual field, such as arranging the food tray so that all foods are on the right side or the left side to accommodate for field of vision (Fig. 57.9). Later, the patient learns to compensate for the visual defect by consciously attending to or by scanning the neglected side. Weak

TABLE 57.13 Communicating With a Patient With Aphasia

The following are guidelines for communicating with a patient with aphasia:

1. Decrease environmental stimuli that may be distracting and disrupting to communication efforts.
2. Treat the patient as an adult.
3. Speak with normal volume and tone.
4. Present a single thought or idea at a time.
5. Keep questions simple or ask questions that can be answered with "yes" or "no."
6. Let the person speak. Do not interrupt. Allow time for the person to complete thoughts.
7. Make use of gestures as an alternative form of communication. Encourage this by saying, "Show me . . . ." or "Point to what you want."
8. Do not pretend to understand the person if you do not. Calmly say you do not understand. Encourage the use of nonverbal communication or ask the person to write out what they want.
9. Give the patient time to process information and generate a response before repeating a question or statement.
10. Allow body contact (e.g., clasp of a hand, touching) as much as possible. Realize that touching may be the only way the patient can express feelings.
11. Organize the patient's day by preparing and following a schedule (the more familiar the routine, the easier it will be).
12. Do not push communication if the person is tired or upset. Aphasia worsens with fatigue and anxiety.
13. Teach communication techniques to caregiver and family members.

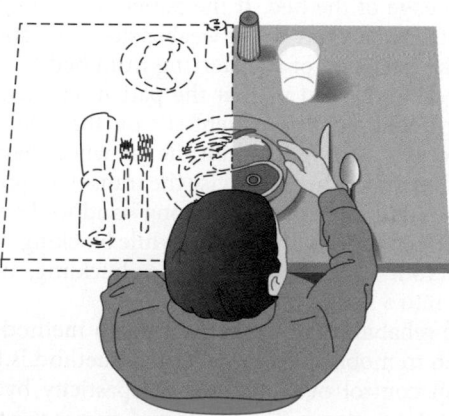

FIG. 57.9 Spatial and perceptual deficits in stroke. Perception of a patient with homonymous hemianopsia shows that food on the left side is not seen and thus is ignored. (Modified from Hoeman SP: *Rehabilitation nursing*, ed 2, St Louis, 1995, Mosby.)

or paralyzed extremities are carefully checked for adequacy of dressing, hygiene, and trauma.

In the clinical situation, it is often hard to distinguish between a visual field cut and a neglect syndrome. Both problems may occur with strokes affecting either the right or the left side of the brain. A person may be unfortunate enough to have both homonymous hemianopsia and a neglect syndrome, which increases the inattention to the weak or paralyzed side. A neglect syndrome results in decreased safety awareness and places the patient at high risk for injury. Immediately after the stroke, anticipate safety hazards and provide protection from injury. Safety measures include closely observing the patient, elevating side rails, lowering the height of the bed, and using video monitors. Avoid using restraints and soft vests because this may agitate the patient.

Other visual problems may include *diplopia* (double vision), loss of the corneal reflex, and *ptosis* (drooping eyelid), especially if the stroke is in the vertebrobasilar distribution. Diplopia is often treated with an eye patch. If the corneal reflex is absent, the patient is at risk for corneal abrasion and should be observed closely and protected against eye injuries. Prevent corneal abrasions with artificial tears or gel to keep the eyes moist and an eye shield (especially at night). We usually do not treat ptosis unless it inhibits vision.

Coping. A stroke is usually a sudden, extremely stressful event for the patient, caregiver, family, and significant others. Stroke is often a family disease, affecting the family emotionally, socially, and financially and changing roles and responsibilities within the family. The stroke patient and family may perceive the stroke as a threat to life and their accustomed lifestyle. Reactions to this threat vary considerably but may involve fear, apprehension, denial of the severity of stroke, depression, anger, and sorrow. During the acute phase of caring for the stroke patient and caregiver, nursing interventions designed to promote coping involve providing information and emotional support.

Explanations to the patient about what has happened and diagnostic and therapeutic procedures should be clear and understandable. Reinforce as needed. Decision making and upholding the patient's wishes during this challenging time are of upmost importance. Advance directives should be honored. Update the family daily and hold family meetings about feeding tube placement or tracheostomy.

Give the caregiver and family a careful, detailed explanation of what has happened to the patient. However, if the family is extremely anxious and upset during the acute phase, explanations may have to be repeated later. Because family members usually have not had time to prepare for the illness, they may need help in arranging care for family members or pets and for transportation and finances. A social services referral is often helpful.

It is challenging to keep the patient with aphasia adequately informed. Use demeanor and touch to convey support. When communicating with a patient who has a communication deficit, speak in a normal volume and tone, keep questions simple, and present one thought or idea at a time. To decrease frustration, always let the patient speak without interruption and make use of gestures. Use writing and communication boards.

◆ Ambulatory Care

Care Transitions. The patient is usually discharged from the acute care setting to home, an intermediate- or long-term care facility, or a rehabilitation facility. Ideally, discharge planning with the patient and caregiver starts early in the hospitalization and promotes a smooth transition between care settings. The stroke team provides guidance for the appropriate care needed after discharge. Factors that are considered include the patient's medical needs and independence in performing ADLs, caregiver's capacity to provide care, and community setting.[24] If the patient needs a short- or long-term health care facility, the team can make appropriate referrals that allow time to select and arrange for care.

If the patient is returning home, the team can make referrals for needed equipment and services in preparation for discharge. You can prepare the patient and caregiver for discharge through teaching and evaluating the transition plan for any barriers. Follow-up care is carefully planned to allow continuing nursing care; physical, occupational, and speech therapy; and medical care. Identify community resources to provide recreational activities, group support, spiritual assistance, respite care, adult day care, and home assistance based on the patient's needs.

Rehabilitation. *Rehabilitation* is the process of maximizing the patient's capabilities and resources to promote optimal functioning related to physical, mental, and social well-being. The goals of rehabilitation are to prevent deformity and maintain and improve function. Ongoing rehabilitation is essential to maximize the patient's abilities. Most patients recover in the first 6 months after a stroke, with maximum benefit 1 year after a stroke.[1]

Rehabilitation requires a team approach so that the patient and caregiver can benefit from the combined, expert care of an interprofessional team. The team must communicate and coordinate care to achieve the patient's goals. As a nurse, you can facilitate this process and are often the key to successful rehabilitation efforts. The rehabilitation team is composed of many members. These include nurses, physicians, psychiatrist, physical therapist, occupational therapist, speech therapist, registered dietitian, respiratory therapist, vocational therapist, recreational therapist, social worker, psychologist, pharmacist, and chaplain.

Physical therapy focuses on mobility, progressive ambulation, transfer techniques, and equipment needed for mobility. Occupational therapy emphasizes retraining for skills of daily living, including eating, dressing, hygiene, and cooking. Occupational therapists are skilled in cognitive and perceptual evaluation and training. Speech therapy focuses on speech, communication, cognition, and eating abilities.

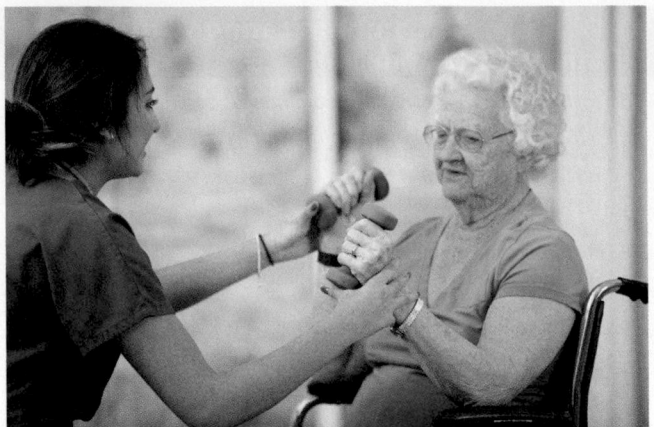

FIG. 57.10 A patient who had a stroke works with a physical therapist to improve arm strength. (© Thinkstock 78783452.)

INFORMATICS IN PRACTICE

Video Games for Stroke Recovery

- Patients dealing with the effects of a stroke often find it hard to perform activities of daily living.
- Playing active video games, such as Nintendo Wii or Xbox Kinect, brings some fun into stroke recovery and may get patients to spend more time in therapy.
- Gaming helps patients regain lost strength, improve motor skills, and improve problem solving and short- and long-term memory.
- Patients can play with their families, including children, making gaming a way to involve others in rehabilitation.

The rehabilitation nurse assesses the patient, caregiver, and family with attention to the (1) patient's rehabilitation potential, (2) physical status of all body systems, (3) complications caused by the stroke or other chronic conditions, (4) patient's cognitive status, (5) family resources and support, and (6) expectations of the patient and caregiver related to the rehabilitation program. Many interventions started in the acute phase of care continue throughout rehabilitation.

Musculoskeletal Function. The initial assessment consists of determining the stage of recovery of muscle function. If the muscles are still flaccid several weeks after the stroke, the prognosis for regaining function is poor, and care focuses on preventing further loss.

Most patients begin to show signs of spasticity with exaggerated reflexes within 48 hours after the stroke. Spasticity at this phase denotes progress toward recovery. As improvement continues, small voluntary movements of the hip or shoulder may be accompanied by involuntary movements in the rest of the extremity *(synergy)*. The last stage of recovery occurs when the patient has voluntary control of isolated muscle groups.

Interventions for the musculoskeletal system advance in a manner of progressive activity. Balance training is the first step. It begins with the patient sitting up in bed or dangling the legs over the edge of the bed. Assess tolerance by noting dizziness or syncope caused by vasomotor instability. Loss of postural stability is common after stroke. When the nondominant hemisphere is involved, walking apraxia and loss of postural control are usually apparent. The patient may be unable to sit upright and tends to fall sideways. Provide proper support with pillows or cushions.

Assess whether patients autocorrect their posture when sitting on the edge of the bed. If the patient can straighten their posture instead of leaning to the weaker side, the patient may be ready for the next step of transferring from bed to chair. Place the chair beside the bed so that the patient can lead with the stronger arm and leg. The patient sits on the side of the bed, stands, places the strong hand on the far wheelchair arm, and sits down. You may either supervise the transfer or provide minimal aid by guiding the patient's strong hand to the wheelchair arm, standing in front of the patient while blocking the patient's knees with your knees to prevent knee buckling, and guiding the patient into a sitting position.

In some rehabilitation units, the Bobath method is used as an approach to mobility. The goal of this method is to help the patient gain control over patterns of spasticity by inhibiting abnormal reflex patterns. Therapists and nurses use the Bobath approach to encourage normal muscle tone, normal movement, and bilateral function of the body. An example is to have the patient transfer into the wheelchair using the weak or paralyzed side and the stronger side to facilitate more bilateral functioning.

Another approach to stroke rehabilitation is *constraint-induced movement therapy* (CIMT). CIMT encourages the patient to use the weakened extremity by restricting movement of the normal extremity. This approach can be challenging for patients. It is used only under the supervision of physical or occupational therapy. Movement training, skill acquisition, stretching, and exercise are other therapies offered for rehabilitation of the stroke patient.[25]

Supportive or assistive equipment, such as canes, walkers, and leg braces, may be needed on a short- or long-term basis for mobility. The physical therapist usually selects the proper supportive device(s) to meet individual needs and instructs the patient about use. Incorporate physical therapy activities into the patient's daily routine for added practice and repetition of rehabilitation efforts (Fig. 57.10).

EVIDENCE-BASED PRACTICE
Virtual Reality Training and Stroke

You are a nurse working in an outpatient rehabilitation setting with C.W., a 62-yr-old woman who had a stroke 2 months ago. She has left-sided weakness especially in her lower extremity that affects her balance and mobility. She tells you she misses not being able to fully engage with friends with whom she regularly walked with each morning until her stroke.

Making Clinical Decisions

Best Available Evidence. Impaired gait is highly linked with balance disorders in patients with stroke. Reduced balance is a major obstacle to achieving independence in activities of daily living after stroke. A loss of balance often results in falls and even serious injuries. Virtual reality (VR) training on gait and balance ability showed significant benefits on gait speed, Berg Balance Scale scores, and Timed "Up & Go" scores when compared to traditional physical therapy. VR training can improve mobility and daily functioning in patients undergoing rehabilitation for stroke.

Clinician Expertise. You know that a walking program can be an important part of stroke rehabilitation. Improvements in mobility reach their maximum potential in the first year after a stroke. You note the benefit of VR training for practicing daily activities that may currently be unsafe, such as walking, showering, and dressing.

Patient Preferences and Values. C.W. states that she is willing to "try something new" as part of her treatment.

Implications for Nursing Practice

1. What parameters will you use to assess C.W.'s progress with the VR training?
2. Why is it important for you to determine with C.W. if VR training translates into the actual performance of her previous activities?
3. As you coordinate her rehabilitation care, how will you promote communication among interprofessional team members?

References for Evidence

de Rooij IJM, van de Port IGL, Meijer J-WG: Effect of virtual reality training on balance and gait ability in patients with stroke: Systematic review and meta-analysis, *Phys Ther* 96:1905, 2016.

Li Z, Han XG, Sheng J, et al: Virtual reality for improving balance in patients after stroke: A systematic review and meta-analysis, *Clin Rehabil* 30:432, 2016.

Stroke Survivorship and Coping. Patients who had a stroke often have emotional responses that are not appropriate or typical for the situation. They may appear apathetic, depressed, fearful, anxious, weepy, frustrated, and angry. Some patients, especially those with a stroke on the left side of the brain (right hemiplegia), have exaggerated mood swings. The patient may be unable to control emotions and may suddenly burst into tears or laughter. This behavior is out of context and often is unrelated to the patient's underlying emotional state. Nursing interventions for atypical emotional response are to (1) distract the patient who suddenly becomes emotional, (2) explain to the patient and family that emotional outbursts may occur after a stroke, (3) maintain a calm environment, and (4) avoid shaming or scolding the patient during emotional outbursts.

The patient with a stroke may have many losses, including sensory, intellectual, communicative, functional, role behavior, emotional, social, and vocational losses. The patient, caregiver, and family often go through the process of grief and mourning associated with the losses. Some patients develop long-term depression with symptoms, including anxiety, weight loss, fatigue, poor appetite, and sleep problems. The time and energy needed to perform previously simple tasks can result in anger and frustration.

The patient, caregiver, and family need help coping with the losses associated with stroke. Provide assistance by (1) supporting communication between the patient and family; (2) discussing lifestyle changes resulting from stroke deficits; (3) discussing changing roles and responsibilities within the family; (4) being an active listener to allow the expression of fear, frustration, and anxiety; (5) including the family and patient in short- and long-term goal planning and patient care; (6) supporting family conferences, and (7) identifying support groups and referrals as needed.

Maladjusted dependence with inadequate coping occurs when the patient does not maintain optimal functioning for self-care, family responsibilities, decision making, or socialization. This situation can cause resentment from both the patient and family with a negative cycle of interpersonal dependency and control. Caregivers and family members must cope with 3 aspects of the patient's behavior: (1) recognition of behavioral changes resulting from neurologic deficits that are not changeable, (2) responses to multiple losses by both the patient and family, and (3) behaviors that may have been reinforced during the early stages of stroke as continued dependency.

The patient, caregiver, and family may express guilt over not living healthy lifestyles or not seeking professional help sooner. Family therapy is a helpful adjunct to rehabilitation. Open communication, information about the total effects of stroke, teaching about stroke treatment, and therapy are helpful. Stroke support groups in rehabilitation facilities and the community are helpful in terms of mutual sharing, education, coping skills, and understanding.

Sexual Function. A patient who had a stroke may be concerned about the loss of sexual function. Many patients are comfortable talking about their anxieties and fears about sexual function if you are comfortable and open to the topic. You can start a discussion about the topic with the patient and spouse or significant other. Common concerns include impotence and the chance of another stroke occurring during sex. Nursing interventions include teaching about (1) optional positioning of partners, (2) timing for peak energy periods, and (3) patient and partner counseling.

Community Integration. Traditionally, successful community integration after stroke is hard for the patient because of persistent problems with cognition, coping, physical deficits, and emotional changes that interfere with functioning. Older adults who had a stroke often have more severe deficits and multiple health problems. Failure to continue the rehabilitation regimen at home may result in deterioration and further complications.

Community resources can be an asset to patients and their families. The National Stroke Association provides information, resources, referral services, and quarterly newsletters on stroke. The American Stroke Association, a division of the AHA, has information about stroke, hypertension, diet, exercise, and assistive devices. This association sponsors self-help groups in many areas. Easter Seals supplies wheelchairs and other assistive devices for stroke patients. Local groups can offer more daily help with meals and transportation.

Gerontologic Considerations: Stroke

Stroke is a significant cause of death and disability. The majority (66%) of strokes that require hospitalization occur in adults over age 65.[4] Stroke can result in a profound disruption in the life of an older adult. The magnitude of disability and changes in total function can leave patients wondering if they can ever return to their "old self." Loss of independence may be a major concern. The ability to perform ADLs may require many adaptive changes because of physical, emotional, perceptual, and cognitive deficits. Home management may be challenging if the patient's caregiver is also older or has health problems. There may be limited family members, including adult children, living nearby to provide help.

The rehabilitative phase and helping the older patient deal with the residual deficits of stroke, as well as aging, can be a challenging nursing experience. Patients may become fearful and depressed because they think they may have another stroke or die. The fear can become immobilizing and interfere with effective rehabilitation.

Changes may occur in the patient-spouse relationship. The dependency resulting from a stroke may threaten the relationship. The spouse may have chronic medical problems that can affect their ability to care for the stroke survivor. The patient may not want anyone other than the spouse to provide care, thus putting a significant burden on the spouse.

You can help the patient and caregiver in the transition through acute hospitalization, rehabilitation, long-term care, and home care. The needs of the patient, caregiver, and family require ongoing nursing assessment and adaptation of interventions in response to changing needs to optimize quality of life for them all.

CASE STUDY

Stroke

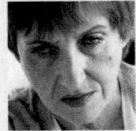

Patient Profile

J.K. is a 57-yr-old white woman who was referred to the neurosurgery service for management of a temporal-parietal glioblastoma (see the Case Study in Chapter 55 on p. 1298). She was diagnosed after presenting with

(© iStockphoto/ Thinkstock.)

persistent headaches, a seizure in her HCP's office, and left-side upper visual field loss and neglect. Her MRI/MRA showed a temporal-parietal glioblastoma that extends into the occipital lobes. She was scheduled for surgery to debulk the tumor. J.K. lives alone and holds a management position. She was concerned about her ability to return to work after her surgery.

J.K. returned from surgery to the neurosurgery unit drowsy but following commands. Her pupils were equal and responded to light. During the night J.K. developed left-sided weakness of both arm and leg. She is now having difficulty with answering questions.

Subjective Data

- Left arm and leg are weak and feel numb
- She is trying to answer questions but looks confused and cannot follow commands

Objective Data

- BP 150/90 mm Hg
- Right gaze preference
- Left homonymous hemianopsia
- Left arm weakness (3/5) greater than leg weakness (4/5)

- Decreased sensation on both left arm and leg
- Has speech but not clear. Difficulty with word finding and following commands
- CT scan shows a hemorrhagic stroke into the site of the tumor bed, and temporal-parietal and anterior occipital areas extending into the thalamus

Discussion Questions

1. How did J.K.'s diagnosis (glioblastoma) put her at risk for a stroke?
2. **Priority Decision:** What potential complications is J.K. at highest risk for developing?
3. **Priority Decision:** Based on the assessment data provided, what are the priority nursing diagnoses? Are there any collaborative problems?
4. **Priority Decision:** What are the priority nursing interventions for J.K.?
5. **Collaboration:** What nursing interventions for J.K. can the RN delegate to UAP?
6. What strategies can you implement to improve communication for J.K.?
7. **Collaboration:** How would you involve other interprofessional team members in J.K.'s care?
8. **Safety:** How can you ensure safety for J.K. in light of her homonymous hemianopsia and left-sided neglect?
9. **Patient-Centered Care:** How can you address J.K.'s concerns about her finances and self-care?
10. Develop a conceptual care map for J. K.

Answers available at *http://evolve.elsevier.com/Lewis/medsurg.*

BRIDGE TO NCLEX EXAMINATION

The number of the question corresponds to the same-numbered outcome at the beginning of the chapter.

1. Which patient has the highest risk for a having a stroke?
   a. An obese 45-yr-old Native American.
   b. A 65-yr-old black man with hypertension.
   c. A 35-yr-old Asian American woman who smokes.
   d. A 32-yr-old white woman taking oral contraceptives.
2. The factor related to cerebral blood flow that *most* often determines the extent of cerebral damage from a stroke is the
   a. O_2 content of the blood.
   b. amount of cardiac output.
   c. level of CO_2 in the blood.
   d. degree of collateral circulation.
3. Information provided by the patient that would help distinguish a hemorrhagic stroke from a thrombotic stroke includes
   a. sensory changes.
   b. a history of hypertension.
   c. presence of motor weakness.
   d. sudden onset of severe headache.
4. A patient is having word finding difficulty and weakness in his right arm. What area of the brain is *most* likely involved?
   a. brainstem.
   b. vertebral artery.
   c. left middle cerebral artery.
   d. right middle cerebral artery.

5. The nurse explains to the patient with a stroke who is scheduled for angiography that this test is used to determine the
   a. presence of increased ICP.
   b. site and size of the infarction.
   c. patency of the cerebral blood vessels.
   d. presence of blood in the cerebrospinal fluid.

6. A patient having TIAs is scheduled for a carotid endarterectomy. The nurse explains that this procedure is done to
   a. decrease cerebral edema.
   b. reduce the brain damage that occurs during a stroke in evolution.
   c. prevent a stroke by removing atherosclerotic plaques blocking cerebral blood flow.
   d. provide a circulatory bypass around thrombotic plaques obstructing cranial circulation.

7. For a patient who is suspected of having a stroke, the *most* important piece of information that the nurse can obtain is
   a. time of the patient's last meal.
   b. time at which stroke symptoms first appeared.
   c. patient's hypertension history and management.
   d. family history of stroke and other cardiovascular diseases.

8. Bladder training in a male patient who has urinary incontinence after a stroke includes
   a. limiting fluid intake.
   b. helping the patient to stand to void.
   c. keeping a urinal in place at all times.
   d. catheterizing the patient every 4 hours.

9. Common psychosocial problems a patient may have post stroke include *(select all that apply)*
   a. depression.
   b. disassociation.
   c. sleep problems.
   d. intellectualization
   e. denial of severity of stroke.

1. b, 2. d, 3. d, 4. c, 5. c, 6. c, 7. b, 8. b, 9. a, c, e

For rationales to these answers and even more NCLEX review questions, visit *http://evolve.elsevier.com/Lewis/medsurg.*

ⓔ EVOLVE WEBSITE/RESOURCES LIST

http://evolve.elsevier.com/Lewis/medsurg
Review Questions (Online Only)
Key Points
Answer Keys for Questions
- Rationales for Bridge to NCLEX Examination Questions
- Answer Guidelines for Case Study on p. 1350
Student Case Studies
- Patient With Hypertension and Stroke
- Patient With Stroke
eNursing Care Plans
- eNursing Care Plan 57.1: Patient With Stroke
Conceptual Care Map Creator
- Conceptual Care Map for Case Study on p. 1350
Audio Glossary
Content Updates

REFERENCES

1. National Stroke Association: *Stroke survivors.* Retrieved from *www.stroke.org/we-can-help/survivors.*
2. Center for Disease Control and Prevention: *Stroke facts.* Retrieved from *www.cdc.gov/stroke/facts.htm.*
3. American Heart Association: Stroke falls to no. 5 killer in US. Retrieved from *www.heart.org/en/news/2018/05/01/stroke-falls-to-no-5-killer-in-us.*
4. Vega C: Updated guidelines available for primary prevention of stroke. Retrieved from *www.medscape.org/viewarticle/834329.*
*5. Boehme AK, Esenwa C, Elkind MS: Stroke risk factors, genetics, and prevention, *Cir Res* 120:472, 2017.
*6. O'Donnell MJ, Chin SL, Rangarajan, et al: Global and regional effects of potentially modifiable risk factors associated with acute stroke in 32 countries: A case-control study, *Lancet* 388:761, 2016.
*7. Meschia J, Bushnel C, Boden-Albala B, et al: Guidelines for the primary prevention of stroke: A statement for healthcare professionals from the AHA/American Stroke Association, *Stroke* 45:12, 2014. (Classic).
8. National Institute of Neurological Disorders and Stroke: Brain basics: Preventing stroke. Retrieved from *www.ninds.nih.gov/Disorders/Patient-Caregiver-Education/Preventing-Stroke.*
9. Watchman: Left atrial appendage closure implant. Retrieved from *www.watchman.com/atrial-fibrillation-stroke/atrial-fibrillation-afib.html.*
10. American Heart Association/American Stroke Association: Transient ischemic attacks. Retrieved from *www.strokeassociation.org/STROKE-ORG/AboutStroke/TypesofStroke/TIA/TIA-Transient-Ischemic-Attack_UCM_310942_Article.jsp.*
11. National Stroke Association: ABCD[2] score. Retrieved from *www.stroke.org/tia-abcd2-tool/.*
12. American Heart Association/American Stroke Association: Ischemic strokes. Retrieved from *www.strokeassociation.org/STROKEORG/AboutStroke/TypesofStroke/IschemicClots/Ischemic-Strokes-Clots_UCM_310939_Article.jsp.*
*13. Eriksen S, Gay C, Lerdal A: Acute phase factors associated with the course of depression during the first 18 months after first ever stroke, *Disabil Rehabil* 38:30, 2016.
14. Amplatzer PFO Occluder. Retrieved from *www.pfoamplatzer.com.*
*15. Gross H, Grose N. Emergency neurological life support: Acute ischemic stroke, *Neurocrit Care* 27:102, 2017.
16. Anderson JA: Acute ischemic stroke: The golden hour, *Nursing2017 CritCare* 11:36, 2016.
*17. Hentschel KA, Daou B, Chalouhi N, et al: Comparison of non–stent retriever and stent retriever mechanical thrombectomy devices for the endovascular treatment of acute ischemic stroke, *JNS* 126:1123, 2017.
18. Malas MB, Leal J, Kashyap V, et al: Technical aspects of transcarotid artery revascularization using the ENROUTE transcarotid neuroprotection and stent system, *J Vasc Surg* 31:916, 2017.
*19. Al-Mufti F, Dancour E, Amuluru K, et al: Neurocritical care of emergent large-vessel occlusion: The era of a new standard of care, *J Intensive Care Med* 19:373, 2016.
20. Watson J: Subarachnoid hemorrhage surgery. Retrieved from *https://emedicine.medscape.com/article/247090-overview.*
21. American Stroke Association: NIH Stroke Scale International. Retrieved from *www.nihstrokescale.org.*
*22. Goshgarian C, Gorelick PB: DVT prevention in stroke, *Curr Neurol Neurosci* 17:81, 2017.
*23. Fedder WN: Review of evidenced-based nursing protocols for dysphagia assessment, *Stroke* 48:e99, 2017.
*24. Camicia M, Lutz BJ: Nursing's role in successful transitions across settings, *Stroke* 47:e246, 2016.
*25. Han P, Zhang W, Kang L, et al: Clinical evidence of exercise benefits for stroke. In: Xiao J, ed: *Exercise for cardiovascular disease prevention and treatment,* Singapore, 2017, Springer.

*Evidence-based information for clinical practice.

58

Chronic Neurologic Problems

Madona D. Plueger and Dottie Roberts

Compassion is a verb.

Thich Nhat Hanh

🄴 http://evolve.elsevier.com/Lewis/medsurg

CONCEPTUAL FOCUS

Cognition	Inflammation	Safety
Coping	Intracranial Regulation	
Functional Ability	Mobility	

LEARNING OUTCOMES

1. Compare and contrast the etiology, clinical manifestations, and interprofessional and nursing management of tension-type, migraine, and cluster headaches.
2. Distinguish the etiology, clinical manifestations, diagnostic studies, and interprofessional and nursing management of seizure disorder, multiple sclerosis, Parkinson's disease, and myasthenia gravis.
3. Describe the clinical manifestations and nursing and interprofessional management of restless legs syndrome, amyotrophic lateral sclerosis, and Huntington's disease.
4. Explain the potential impact of chronic neurologic disease on physical and psychologic well-being.
5. Outline the major goals of treatment for the patient with a chronic, progressive neurologic disease.

KEY TERMS

This chapter discusses headaches, chronic neurologic disorders, and degenerative neurologic disorders. Chronic neurologic disorders include seizure disorder and restless legs syndrome (RLS). *Degenerative nerve diseases* lead to nerve damage that worsens as the diseases progress. Most of these neurologic problems have no cure. Treatment aims to reduce symptoms and help the patient maintain optimal function. Many have a genetic basis.

Degenerative nerve diseases include multiple sclerosis, Parkinson's disease, myasthenia gravis, amyotrophic lateral sclerosis, and Huntington's disease. They affect many activities, including balance, movement, speech, and respiratory and heart function. Patients with these diseases have similar concerns and problems. They must deal not only with their disease but also with the impact of the disease on their quality of life. Many patients have concerns about safety, mobility, self-care, and coping. Patients and their caregivers often need psychosocial support, especially as the disease progresses and disability gets worse.

HEADACHES

Headache is the most common type of pain that people have. Most people have functional headaches, such as migraine or tension-type headaches. Others have organic headaches caused by intracranial or extracranial disease. Headaches tend to occur more often in women than in men.

Pain-sensitive structures in the head include venous sinuses, dura, and cranial blood vessels. In addition, there are 3 divisions of the trigeminal nerve (cranial nerve [CN] V), facial nerve (CN VII), glossopharyngeal nerve (CN IX), vagus nerve (CN X), and the first 3 cervical nerves. Because these nerves have both motor and sensory functions, increased pain intensity and symptoms can occur when a person moves.

Headaches are classified as primary or secondary headache. *Primary headache* includes tension-type, migraine, and cluster headaches. Primary headaches are not caused by a disease or another medical condition. The type of primary headache is determined using the International Headache Society

(IHS) guidelines based on characteristics of the headache (Table 58.1).[1] *Secondary headaches* are caused by another condition or disorder, such as sinus infection, neck injury, and brain tumor.

A patient may have more than 1 type of headache. The history and neurologic examination are diagnostic keys to determine the type of headache. The examination of a person with a headache is often normal. Unexplained abnormal findings require further diagnostic studies to identify the underlying cause.

TENSION-TYPE HEADACHE

Tension-type headache (TTH), also called *stress headache,* is the most common type of headache. This type of headache is characterized by its bilateral location and pressing or tightening quality. TTH is usually of mild or moderate intensity. It can last from minutes to days. TTHs are divided by frequency into episodic or chronic.[1] Chronic TTH can become a serious problem that leads to decreased quality of life and severe disability.

Etiology and Pathophysiology

We do not know the cause TTH. It may have a neurobiologic basis similar to migraine headaches. For some, episodic headaches evolve into chronic headaches. Increased frequency, though, does not necessarily increase headache intensity. Headaches may occur intermittently for weeks, months, or even years.

Clinical Manifestations

Patients often have a bilateral frontal-occipital headache described as a constant, dull pressure or a bandlike headache associated with neck pain. There may be increased tone in the cervical and neck muscles. The headache may involve sensitivity to light (*photophobia*) or sound (*phonophobia*) but not nausea or vomiting. There are no *premonitory symptoms* (warning symptoms of impending headache). Physical activity does not worsen symptoms.

Many patients have a combination of migraine headache and TTH, with features of both occurring together. Patients with migraine headaches may have TTH between migraine attacks. Fig. 58.1 shows the location of pain for common headache syndromes.

Diagnostic Studies

Careful history taking may be the most useful tool for diagnosing TTH (Table 58.2). If TTH is present during physical examination, increased resistance to passive movement of the head and tenderness of the head and neck may be seen. Electromyography (EMG) may show sustained contraction of neck, scalp, or facial muscles. However, the patient may not have increased muscle tension with an EMG, even when it is done during a headache. Imaging is ordered when symptoms raise concern about a possible pathologic cause.

MIGRAINE HEADACHE

Migraine headache is a recurring headache characterized by unilateral throbbing pain. Migraines are most common between the ages of 25 and 55. 12% of the population has migraines.[2] Many people who have migraines have a family history of migraines. Other risk factors include age, female gender, obesity, low level of education, depression, and stressful life events. Overuse of medications for acute migraine or ineffective acute treatment can contribute to chronic migraine headache.[3]

The IHS subdivides migraines into categories. *Migraine without aura* (formerly called *common migraine*) is the most common type. *Migraine with aura* (formerly called *classic migraine*) occurs in 25% to 30% of migraine headache episodes.[4]

GENDER DIFFERENCES
Headaches

Men
- Cluster headaches are 3 times more common than in women.
- Have more exercise-induced headaches than women.

Women
- Migraine headaches are 3 times more common than in men.
- Have more tension headaches than men.

Etiology and Pathophysiology

Although there are many theories about the cause of migraine headaches, we do not know the exact cause. Current theory suggests a complex series of neurovascular events starts the headache. People who have migraines have a state of neuron hyperexcitability in the cerebral cortex, especially in the occipital cortex. Genetics appear to play a role. Risk for migraine headache increases 50% to 75% if even 1 parent has a history of migraine.[5]

Migraine is associated with seizure disorder, ischemic stroke, asthma, depression, anxiety, myocardial infarction, Raynaud's syndrome, and irritable bowel syndrome. In many cases, migraine headaches have no known precipitating events. For some patients, specific factors may trigger a headache. *Triggers* for migraine headaches include bright lights, sound, hormone fluctuations, certain smells, poor sleep, or high stress.[6] Common food triggers include chocolate, cheese, oranges, tomatoes, onions, monosodium glutamate, aspartame, and alcohol (especially red wine).

Clinical Manifestations

Premonitory symptoms and an aura may precede the headache phase by several hours or days. Premonitory symptoms occur before the onset of aura or headache. They may include sensory experiences (e.g., photophobia, phonophobia); mood, sleep, or cognitive changes (e.g., poor concentration, irritability, fatigue); and homeostatic changes (e.g., thirst and cravings, change in bowel habits).[7] An aura is a complex of neurologic symptoms that occur before a headache for some patients. Visual symptoms, such as bright lights, scotomas (patchy blindness), visual distortions, or zigzag lines, are the most common type of aura.[1] They occur in over 90% of patients in at least some attacks. Sensory (voices or sounds that do not exist, strange smells) and/or motor phenomena (e.g., weakness, paralysis, feeling that limbs are moving) may be part of an aura.

A migraine headache may last 4 to 72 hours. Patients often describe the headache as a steady, throbbing pain that is synchronous with the pulse. Although the headache is usually unilateral, it may switch to the opposite side in another episode. During the headache, patients may try to avoid noise, light, odors, people, and problems.

TABLE 58.1 Interprofessional Care

Headaches

Tension-Type Headaches	Migraine Headache	Cluster Headache
Location		
Bilateral, bandlike pressure at base of skull	Unilateral in 60%, may switch sides; often anterior location	Unilateral, radiating up or down from 1 eye
Quality		
Constant, squeezing tightness	Throbbing, synchronous with pulse	Severe, bone crushing
Frequency		
Cycles for many years	Periodic, cycles of several months and years	May have months or years between attacks Attacks occur in clusters over a period of 2–12 wk
Duration		
30 min–7 days	4–72 hr	5 min–3 hr
Time and Mode of Onset		
Not related to time	May be preceded by premonitory symptoms or aura Onset after awakening Improves with sleep	Nocturnal, often awakens person from sleep
Associated Symptoms		
Palpable neck and shoulder muscle tension Stiff neck Tenderness	Irritability, sweating Nausea, vomiting Photophobia Phonophobia Premonitory symptoms: sensory, motor, or psychic phenomena	Facial flushing or pallor Unilateral lacrimation, ptosis, rhinitis
Treatment: Abortive and Symptomatic Drugs		
Nonopioid analgesics: aspirin, acetaminophen, NSAIDS Analgesic combinations • butalbital/acetaminophen/caffeine • butalbital/aspirin/caffeine (Fiorinal) • dichloralphenazone/acetaminophen/isometheptene Muscle relaxants	Nonopioid analgesics: aspirin, NSAIDs Serotonin receptor agonists • almotriptan (Axert) • eletriptan (Relpax) • frovatriptan (Frova) • naratriptan (Amerge) • rizatriptan (Maxalt) • sumatriptan (Imitrex) • zolmitriptan (Zomig) Combination • sumatriptan/naproxen (Treximet) α-Adrenergic blockers • ergotamine tartrate (Ergomar) • dihydroergotamine nasal spray (Migranal) Analgesic combinations • acetaminophen/caffeine/aspirin Corticosteroids • dexamethasone	α-Adrenergic blockers • ergotamine tartrate Serotonin receptor agonists • almotriptan • eletriptan • frovatriptan • naratriptan • rizatriptan • sumatriptan • zolmitriptan O_2 100% inhalation via mask
Treatment: Preventive		
Tricyclic antidepressants • amitriptyline • nortriptyline (Pamelor) • doxepin Selective serotonin reuptake inhibitors • fluoxetine (Prozac) • paroxetine (Paxil) β-Adrenergic blocker: • propranolol (Inderal) Antiseizure drugs • topiramate (Topamax) • divalproex (Depakote) Other drugs • mirtazapine (Remeron) Biofeedback Psychotherapy Muscle relaxation training	β-Adrenergic blocker • propranolol (Inderal) Antidepressants • amitriptyline (Elavil) • imipramine (Tofranil) Antiseizure drugs • divalproex • gabapentin • topiramate • valproic acid (Depakene) Botulinum toxin A Calcium channel blocker • nifedipine (Procardia) • verapamil Biofeedback Relaxation therapy Cognitive-behavioral therapy	α-Adrenergic blockers • ergotamine tartrate Corticosteroid • prednisone Calcium channel blocker • verapamil Lithium Biofeedback

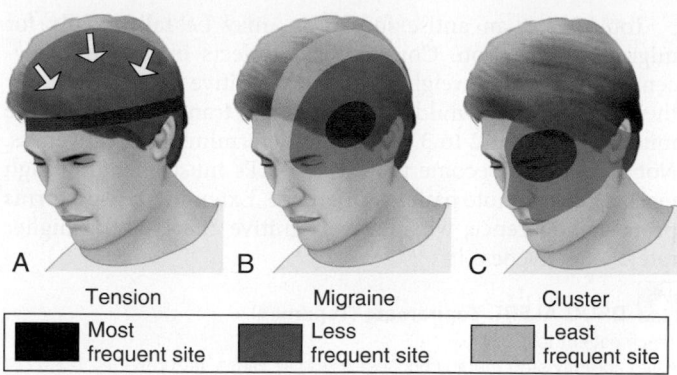

FIG. 58.1 Location of pain for common headache syndromes. A, Tension headache is often described as feeling of a weight in or on the head or a band squeezing the head. B, Migraine headache is usually unilateral, in the temple on 1 side of the head. The pain can be bilateral. C, Cluster headache pain is focused in and around 1 eye.

TABLE 58.2 Diagnostic Studies

Headaches

History and Physical Examination
- Neurologic examination (often negative)
- Inspection for local infection
- Palpation of head for tenderness, bony swellings
- Auscultation for bruits over major arteries, especially neck

Routine Laboratory Studies
- CBC (may show anemia, infection)
- Electrolytes (may show dehydration, other illnesses)
- Urinalysis (may show infection, other medical diagnoses [e.g., diabetes])
- Other diagnostic studies to assess evidence of disease, deformity, or infection: angiography, EMG, EEG, MRA, MRI, LP

Diagnostic Studies

The diagnosis of migraine headache is usually based on the patient history. Neurologic and other diagnostic examinations are often normal (Table 58.2).

No specific laboratory or radiologic test can diagnose migraine headache. Neuroimaging techniques (e.g., head CT scan with or without contrast, MRI) are not part of the routine evaluation of headache unless the neurologic examination is abnormal. If atypical features are present, further testing is done to rule out a secondary headache.

CLUSTER HEADACHE

Cluster headache is the most severe form of primary headache. It is classified as a trigeminal autonomic cephalalgia (TAC). This reflects its effect on the trigeminal nerve (CN V) and associated autonomic symptoms (e.g., runny or stuffy nose).[8] Repeated headaches occur in clusters, generally at the same time of day or night. Age at onset is typically 20 to 50 years, but they can start at any age. They affect men more than women. They occur more often in persons who smoke.[9] Less than 1% of people in the United States have cluster headache.

Etiology and Pathophysiology

Neither the cause nor how cluster headache occurs is fully known. The patterns of cluster headache suggest dysfunction of the hypothalamus. Many attacks occur at night, waking the person 1 to 2 hours after falling asleep. This may mean there is a circadian rhythm problem. Alcohol is a dietary trigger. Pain often starts within an hour of a drink. Strong odors (e.g., gasoline, paint fumes) can trigger cluster headache.[10]

Clinical Manifestations

Patients with cluster headache have severe, intense pain lasting from a few minutes to 3 hours. In contrast to the pulsing pain of migraine headache, the pain of cluster headache is sharp and stabbing. The pain is usually around the eye, radiating to the temple, forehead, cheek, nose, or gums. Other manifestations may include swelling around the eye, lacrimation (tearing), facial flushing or pallor, nasal congestion, and miosis (pupil constriction). Most patients have at least 3 of these symptoms. During the headache, the patient may be agitated and restless, unable to sit still or relax.

Cluster headaches can occur every other day and as often as 8 times a day. A cluster typically lasts 2 weeks to 3 months, and then the patient goes into remission for months to years. Typically, 2 cluster periods a year may be separated by months without symptoms. Because cluster periods often occur seasonally, headaches may be mistaken for symptoms of allergies. A small number of patients (10% to 15%) have chronic headaches without remission.[1]

Diagnostic Studies

The diagnosis of cluster headache is based on the patient history according to IHS criteria.[1] Asking patients to keep a headache diary can be useful. CT scan, MRI, or magnetic resonance angiography (MRA) may rule out an aneurysm, tumor, or infection. A lumbar puncture (LP) may rule out other disorders that may cause similar symptoms.

OTHER TYPES OF HEADACHES

Other types of headaches can occur. A headache may be the first symptom of a more serious illness. Headache can accompany subarachnoid hemorrhage; brain tumors; intracranial masses; vascular abnormalities; trigeminal neuralgia (tic douloureux); diseases of the eyes, nose, and teeth; and systemic illness (e.g., infection, carbon monoxide poisoning, altitude sickness, polycythemia vera). Because of the varied causes of headache, thorough clinical evaluation is important. It should include assessment of personality, life adjustment, environment, and living situation, as well as a comprehensive evaluation of neurologic and physical condition.

INFORMATICS IN PRACTICE
Social Media Use for Patients With Migraine Headaches

- Many people with migraine headaches think others do not understand their pain and its impact on their quality of life.
- Encourage patients to take part in a social media outlet where people who have migraines share their experiences.
- Patients can describe their physical and emotional pain on social media. It can help them cope better and improve their quality of life.

INTERPROFESSIONAL CARE FOR HEADACHES

If no systemic disease is the cause, the type of headache guides therapy. Table 58.2 outlines the general assessment of a patient with headaches to rule out any intracranial or extracranial disease. Table 58.1 shows therapies for preventing and managing different types of headaches.

Cognitive-behavioral therapy and relaxation therapy used alone or in conjunction with drug therapy may help some patients (see Chapter 6). Biofeedback involves the use of physiologic monitoring equipment that gives the patient information about muscle tension and peripheral blood flow (e.g., skin temperature of the fingers). The patient is trained to relax the muscles and raise the finger temperature. Reinforcement occurs when the patient makes these changes. Acupuncture, acupressure, and hypnosis are options for some patients.

Drug Therapy

Tension-Type Headache. Drug therapy for TTH usually involves aspirin, acetaminophen (Tylenol), or nonsteroidal antiinflammatory drugs (NSAIDs) used alone or in combination with caffeine, a sedative, or a muscle relaxant. Treatment is often disappointing. These analgesics may be only partly effective, even with use of the maximum dose. Stronger analgesics provide no additional benefit. For some, analgesics can make the headache worse.[11]

Many of these drugs have serious side effects. Caution the patient about the long-term use of aspirin or aspirin-containing drugs because they can cause gastrointestinal (GI) bleeding and coagulation abnormalities in some patients. Drugs containing acetaminophen can cause kidney damage with chronic use and liver damage when taken in large doses or when combined with alcohol. To decrease the recurrence of TTH, many patients take an antidepressant. Common drugs include tricyclic agents (e.g., amitriptyline, nortriptyline); mirtazapine (Remeron), a nonadrenergic serotonergic antidepressant; and venlafaxine (Effexor XR). Antiseizure drugs, such as topiramate (Topamax) or divalproex (Depakote), also may be used.

Migraine Headache. The aim of drug treatment of an acute migraine is stopping or decreasing the symptoms. Many people with mild or moderate migraine headache can get relief with NSAIDs, aspirin, or caffeine-containing analgesics. For moderate to severe headaches, triptans are the first line of therapy.

Triptans (e.g., sumatriptan [Imitrex]) affect selected serotonin receptors. They reduce neurogenic inflammation of cerebral blood vessels and cause vasoconstriction (Table 58.1). Some patients respond better to a certain triptan than to others. Triptans are most effective when taken at the start of a migraine headache or during the aura. Sumatriptan is available in several dosage forms and delivery systems (oral, subcutaneous, nasal spray, transdermal). It is also the only ultrafast-acting triptan. A combination of oral sumatriptan and naproxen sodium (Treximet) is more effective for symptom relief than either medication alone. Because triptans cause vasoconstriction, they may not be appropriate for people with heart disease (e.g., hypertension, high cholesterol) or history of stroke. When triptans are contraindicated or ineffective, other drugs can be used (Table 58.1).

 DRUG ALERT Sumatriptan (Imitrex)
- Should not be given to patients with a history of:
  - Ischemic cardiac, cerebrovascular, or peripheral vascular problems.
  - Uncontrolled hypertension (may increase BP).
- Excess dosage may cause tremor and decrease respirations.

Preventive treatment is important in managing migraine headache. The decision to start preventive treatment is made based on frequency, severity, and disability related to headaches. Several different classes of medications are used.

Topiramate, an antiseizure drug, may be taken daily for migraine prevention. Common side effects include hypoglycemia, paresthesia, weight loss, and cognitive changes. Usually these side effects are mild to moderate and transient. Topiramate must be taken for 2 to 3 months to determine its effectiveness. Not all patients become pain free. HCPs must offer thorough teaching to promote patient adherence. Extended-release forms promote adherence, with fewer cognitive effects and a higher rate of effectiveness.[12]

 DRUG ALERT Topiramate (Topamax)
Teach patient to:
- Not abruptly stop therapy because this may cause seizures.
- Avoid tasks that require alertness (e.g., driving, operating heavy machinery) until response to the drug is known.
- Take adequate fluids to decrease risk for developing renal stones.
- Tell the HCP if you are pregnant or want to become pregnant.

β-Blockers have been effective in migraine prevention. Commonly prescribed agents include metoprolol (Lopressor) and propranolol (Inderal). Propranolol is similar to amitriptyline in its efficacy. Atenolol (Tenormin) and nadolol (Corgard) are other options for migraine prevention.

Botulinum toxin A (Botox) may be an effective prophylactic treatment for adults who have chronic migraines at least 15 days each month or migraines that do not respond to other medications. Botox is given by multiple injections around the head and neck into the pain fibers involved in headaches. Maximum benefit may not be seen for up to 6 months. During this time, the patient should continue their regular medications. Injections are usually given every 3 months. The most common reactions are neck pain and headache. A slight risk exists for the toxin to migrate from the injection site to other areas of the face and neck, causing swallowing and breathing difficulties. Teach the patient to seek immediate medical attention if this occurs.

Cluster Headache. Triptans are the standard of treatment for occasional cluster headache. Nasal administration or subcutaneous injection is appropriate. However, as discussed earlier, they are contraindicated for patients with vascular risk factors due to their vasoconstrictive effects.

High-flow 100% O_2 by non-rebreather mask is well-tolerated, safe, and effective as an alternative treatment. O_2 delivered at a rate of 6 to 8 L/min for 10 minutes may relieve headache by causing vasoconstriction and increasing synthesis of serotonin in the central nervous system (CNS). Treatment can be repeated after a 5-minute rest. A drawback to this treatment is that the patient must have continuous access to the O_2 supply.

Those with chronic cluster headache often need preventive treatment. High-dose verapamil is the first-choice drug. It is typically given at double or more the dose used for other disorders.[8] Because of its effects on cardiac conduction, verapamil should be started only after careful consideration of the risks. Careful monitoring is needed during treatment. An electrocardiogram (ECG) should be done with every dose increase and every 6 months during treatment for patient safety. Other drug options may include lithium, ergotamine, antiseizure drugs (e.g., topiramate), and melatonin. Options for patients with refractory cluster headaches include invasive nerve blocks, deep brain stimulation, and ablative neurosurgical procedures (e.g., percutaneous radiofrequency).

Other Headaches. Patients with frequent headaches may overuse analgesics or other medications used for headache treatment. *Medication overuse headache* (MOH) is the term used to describe a new type of headache or marked worsening of a preexisting headache condition. Drugs known to cause this problem are acetaminophen, aspirin, NSAIDs (e.g., ibuprofen), triptans, ergotamine, and opioids.[1] Headache often occurs daily and is present on wakening. Patients may have nausea, restlessness, weakness, lack of energy, decreased memory, difficulty concentrating, depression, and irritability. Treatment involves abrupt withdrawal of the offending drug (except for opioids, which must be tapered) and using alternative drugs, such as amitriptyline.

Some people have chronic headaches that are difficult to treat. IV medication administration with novel therapies, such as ketamine and lidocaine, and neurostimulation are emerging as options.

❖ NURSING MANAGEMENT: HEADACHES

◆ Nursing Assessment

Table 58.3 outlines subjective and objective data to obtain from a patient with headaches. The history is key and focused on specific details of the headaches. These include location and type of pain, onset, frequency, duration, relation to events (emotional, psychologic, physical), and time of day of the occurrence. Ask about illnesses, surgery, trauma, allergies, family history, and response to medication. A thorough history may suggest headache is due to other drug therapies or a condition other than headache. For example, estrogen withdrawal headache is possible during the drug-free interval of an oral contraceptive.

Ask the patient to keep a diary of headaches with specific details. This record can help identify the type of headache and precipitating events. If there is a history of migraine, TTH, or cluster headache, ask the patient if the character, intensity, or location of the headache has changed. The answer may be an important clue about the cause of the headache.

◆ Nursing Diagnoses

Nursing diagnoses for the patient with headaches may include:
- Acute pain
- Lack of knowledge

Additional information on nursing diagnoses and interventions is presented in eNursing Care Plan 58.1 for the patient with headaches (available on the website for this chapter).

◆ Planning

The overall goals are that the patient with headaches will (1) have reduced or no pain, (2) understand triggering events and treatments, (3) use positive coping strategies to deal with pain, and (4) have increased quality of life and decreased disability.

◆ Nursing Implementation

An inability to cope with daily stresses can cause headaches. Thus effective treatment may involve helping the patient examine the daily routine, recognize stressful situations, and develop effective coping strategies. Help the patient identify precipitating factors and develop ways to avoid or minimize them. Encourage daily exercise, relaxation periods, and socialization as ways to decrease headaches. Suggest relaxation, medication, yoga, and other ways to address headache pain.

TABLE 58.3 Nursing Assessment

Headaches

Subjective Data

Important Health Information

Past health history: Seizures, cancer, recent fall or other trauma, cranial infection, stroke. Asthma or allergies. Relationship of headache to overwork, stress, menstruation, exercise, food, sexual activity, travel, bright lights, or noxious environmental stimuli

Medications: Hydralazine, bromides, nitroglycerin, ergotamine (withdrawal), NSAIDs (in high daily doses), estrogen preparations, oral contraceptives, OTC medications

Surgical interventions or other treatments: Craniotomy, sinus surgery, facial surgery

Functional Health Pattern

Health perception–health management: Positive family history. Malaise

Nutritional-metabolic: Ingestion of alcohol, caffeine, cheese, chocolate, monosodium glutamate, aspartame, lunch meats (nitrites in cured meats), sausage, hot dogs, onions, avocados. History of anorexia, nausea, vomiting (migraine premonitory symptom); unilateral lacrimation (cluster)

Activity-exercise: Vertigo, fatigue, weakness, paralysis, fainting

Sleep-rest: Insomnia

Cognitive-perceptual
- *Tension type:* Bilateral, bandlike, dull and persistent, base-of-skull headache, neck tenderness
- *Migraine:* Aura. Unilateral, severe, throbbing headache (possible switching of side). Visual changes, photophobia, phonophobia, dizziness, tingling or burning sensations
- *Cluster:* Unilateral and severe, nocturnal headache. Nasal stuffiness

Self-perception–self-concept: Depression

Coping–stress tolerance: Stress, anxiety, irritability, withdrawal

Objective Data

General

Anxiety, apprehension

Integumentary

Migraine: Generalized edema (premonitory symptom) pallor, diaphoresis

Cluster: Forehead diaphoresis, pallor, unilateral facial flushing with cheek edema, conjunctivitis

Neurologic

Horner's syndrome, restlessness (cluster), hemiparesis (migraine)

Musculoskeletal

Resistance of head and neck movement, nuchal rigidity (meningeal, tension type), palpable neck and shoulder muscle tension (tension type)

Possible Diagnostic Findings

Evidence of disease, deformity, or infection on brain imaging (CT, MRI, MRA), cerebral angiogram, LP, EEG, EMG

Teach the patient about drugs prescribed for preventive and symptomatic treatment of headache. The patient should be able to describe the purpose, action, dosage, and side effects of the drugs. To prevent accidental overdose, urge the patient to make a written note of each dose of drug or headache remedy. In addition to using analgesics and analgesic combinations to relieve headache, encourage the patient with migraines to seek a quiet, dimly lit environment. Massage and moist hot packs to the neck and head can help a patient with TTH.

Provide dietary counseling for the patient with headaches triggered by food. Encourage the patient to eliminate foods that

TABLE 58.4 Patient & Caregiver Teaching

Headaches

Include the following instructions when teaching the patient with a headache and the patient's caregiver:

1. Keep a diary or calendar of headaches and possible precipitating events.
2. Avoid possible triggers for a headache:
   - Foods containing amines (cheese, chocolate), nitrites (meats, such as hot dogs), vinegar, onions, monosodium glutamate
   - Fermented or marinated foods
   - Caffeine
   - Oranges
   - Tomatoes
   - Aspartame
   - Nicotine
   - Ice cream
   - Alcohol (especially red wine)
   - Emotional stress
   - Fatigue
   - Drugs, such as ergot-containing preparations (ergotamine tartrate) and monoamine oxidase inhibitors (e.g., rasagiline [Azilect])
3. Learn the purpose, action, dosage, and side effects of drugs taken.
4. Self-administer sumatriptan subcutaneously, if prescribed.
5. Use stress management techniques (see Chapter 6).
6. Take part in regular exercise.
7. Contact HCP if any of the following occur:
   - Symptoms become more severe, last longer than usual, or are resistant to medication
   - Nausea and vomiting (if severe or not typical), change in vision, or fever occurs with the headache
   - Problems occur with any drugs

may provoke headaches. Active challenge and provocative testing (designed specifically to provoke symptoms) with suspect foods may help determine specific causative agents. However, teach the patient that food triggers may change over time.

Teach patients to avoid smoking and exposure to triggers, such as strong perfumes and gasoline fumes. Cluster headaches may occur at high altitudes with low O_2 levels during air travel. Ergotamine, taken before the plane takes off, may decrease this risk. See Table 58.4 for a teaching guide for the patient with a headache.

◆ Evaluation

Expected outcomes are that the patient with headaches will
- Report satisfaction with pain management
- Use drug and nondrug measures appropriately to manage pain

CHRONIC NEUROLOGIC DISORDERS

SEIZURE DISORDER

Seizure disorder, also known as *epilepsy,* is a group of neurologic diseases marked by recurring seizures. It is the fourth most common neurologic disorder. Only migraine, stroke, and Alzheimer's disease occur more often. About 3.4 million Americans have seizure disorder. 1 in 26 people will develop seizure disorder during their lifetime.[13]

Seizure is a transient, uncontrolled electrical discharge of neurons in the brain that interrupts normal function. Seizures may accompany a variety of disorders, or they may occur without any apparent cause. Seizures from systemic and metabolic

problems are not considered seizure disorder if they stop when the underlying problem is corrected. Metabolic problems that may cause seizures include acidosis, electrolyte imbalances, hypoglycemia, hypoxia, alcohol and barbiturate withdrawal, dehydration, and water intoxication. Extracranial disorders that may cause seizures include systemic lupus erythematosus; diabetes; hypertension; sepsis; and heart, lung, liver, or kidney diseases.

Etiology and Pathophysiology

Seizure disorder has many possible causes. The most common ones vary by age. Common causes during the first 6 months of life are severe birth injury, congenital defects involving the CNS, infection, and inborn errors of metabolism. In those 2 to 20 years of age, the main causes are birth injury, infection, head trauma, and genetic factors. In young adults 20 to 30 years of age, seizure disorder usually occurs from structural lesions, such as trauma, brain tumors, or vascular disease. After 50 years of age, the main causes are stroke and metastatic brain tumors. However, one third of all cases are idiopathic. This means they cannot be attributed to a specific cause. These cases are known as *idiopathic generalized epilepsy (IGE).*

Seizure disorder is characterized by a group of abnormal neurons that seem to fire without a clear cause. Any stimulus that causes the neuron's cell membrane to depolarize can cause this firing. It spreads by physiologic pathways to involve near or distant areas of the brain. Localization of the *seizure focus* (the place where the seizure originates) is critical to the success of any possible surgical treatment.

Besides neuron alterations, changes in the function of astrocytes may play several key roles in recurring seizures. Activation of astrocytes by hyperactive neurons is one of the crucial factors that causes nearby neurons to generate an epileptic discharge. We continue to learn about abnormal neural antibodies that can cause seizures. *N*-methyl-D-aspartate (NMDA) receptor antibodies are present in the cerebrospinal fluid (CSF) in 80% of patients. The emerging concept of autoimmune seizure disorder may lead to better outcomes for those resistant to drug therapy.[14]

Genetic Link

Genetic abnormalities may be an important factor contributing to IGE. The role of genetics in seizure disorder is complex because it is hard to separate genetic from environmental or acquired influences. In some types, families carry a predisposition to seizure disorder through a naturally low threshold to stimuli, such as trauma, disease, and high fever. Other types of IGE are related to changes in specific genes that control the flow of ions in and out of cells, regulate neuron signaling, or are involved with protein and carbohydrate metabolism.

Sometimes seizure disorder is related to a specific genetic disorder that affects various parts of the body and causes seizures. Many cause brain abnormalities or metabolic disorders (e.g., phenylketonuria [PKU]) and have seizures as a major feature. Other seizures are known to have a genetic basis, but we have not found the gene that causes them.[15]

Clinical Manifestations

Specific manifestations of seizure are determined by the site of the electrical disturbance. The preferred way of classifying seizures is based on the clinical and electroencephalographic (EEG) manifestations. This system divides seizures into 3 major

TABLE 58.5 Classification of Seizures

Generalized Onset Seizure	Focal-Onset Seizure
(Involves both hemispheres of brain)	(Limited to 1 hemisphere of brain)
• Motor seizure	• Aware (no impairment of awareness/consciousness)
• Tonic	• Impaired awareness (impairment of awareness/consciousness)
• Clonic	
• Tonic-clonic	• Motor onset
• Myoclonic	• Automatisms
• Myoclonic-tonic-clonic	• Atonic
• Myoclonic-atonic	• Clonic
• Atonic	• Epileptic spasms
• Epileptic spasms	• Hyperkinetic
• Nonmotor (Absence) seizure	• Myoclonic
• Typical	• Tonic
• Atypical	• Nonmotor onset
• Myoclonic	• Autonomic
• Eyelid myoclonia	• Behavior arrest
	• Cognitive
	• Emotional
	• Sensory
	Unknown Onset Seizure
	(Due to inadequate information or inability to assign to other categories above)

Adapted from Fisher RS, Cross JH, D'Souza C, et al: Instruction manual for the ILAE 2017 operational classification of seizure types, *Epilepsia* 58:4, 2017.

classes: *generalized onset, focal onset,* and *unknown onset* (Table 58.5).[16] They are further described under each classification as *motor* or *nonmotor.* Descriptors address what occurs during the seizure.

Depending on the type, a seizure may occur in four phases: (1) *prodromal phase,* with sensations or behavior changes that precede a seizure by hours or days; (2) *aural phase,* with a sensory warning that is similar each time a seizure occurs and is considered part of the seizure; (3) *ictal phase,* from first symptoms to the end of seizure activity; and (4) *postictal phase,* the recovery period after the seizure.

Generalized-Onset Seizures. Generalized-onset seizures start over wide areas of both sides of the brain. They are characterized by bilateral, synchronous epileptic discharges from the onset of the seizure. In most cases, the patient has impaired awareness for a few seconds to several minutes.

Tonic-Clonic Seizure. Tonic-clonic seizure (formerly called grand mal) is the most common generalized-onset motor seizure. During a tonic-clonic seizure, the patient loses consciousness and falls to the ground, if upright. The body stiffens (tonic phase) for 10 to 20 seconds and the extremities jerk (clonic phase) for another 30 to 40 seconds. Cyanosis, excessive salivation, tongue or cheek biting, and incontinence may occur during the seizure.

In the postictal phase, the patient usually has muscle soreness, feels tired, and may sleep for several hours. Some patients may not feel normal for several hours or days after a seizure. The patient has no memory of the seizure.

Other Generalized-Onset Motor Seizures. Other types of generalized-onset motor seizures include tonic and clonic. A tonic seizure involves a sudden onset of increased tone in the extensor muscles, contributing to sudden stiff movements.

Tonic seizures most often occur in sleep and affect both sides of the body. Patients will fall if they are standing when the seizure occurs. Tonic seizures usually last less than 20 seconds. The patient usually stays aware. Clonic seizures begin with loss of awareness and sudden loss of muscle tone, followed by rhythmic limb jerking that may or may not be symmetric. Clonic seizures are rare.

A generalized *atonic seizure* (or *drop attack*) involves either a tonic episode or a paroxysmal loss of muscle tone. It begins suddenly with the person falling to the ground. Seizures typically last less than 15 seconds. The person usually stays conscious and can resume normal activity immediately. Patients with atonic seizure are at great risk for head injury. They often have to wear protective helmets.

Generalized-Onset Nonmotor (Absence) Seizures. Absence seizure usually occurs only in children and rarely beyond adolescence. This type of seizure may stop altogether as the child matures, or it may evolve into another type of seizure. A *typical absence seizure* is marked by a brief staring spell that resembles daydreaming. It often goes unnoticed because it lasts less than 10 seconds. Usually the patient is unresponsive when spoken to during the seizure.[16] The EEG has a classic spike-wave pattern with 3 per second.

In *atypical absence seizure,* the staring spell is accompanied by other signs and symptoms, such as eye blinking or jerking movements of the lips. This type of seizure often lasts more than 10 seconds (as much as 30 seconds), with a gradual beginning and end. If the patient has existing cognitive impairment, it may be hard to tell seizure activity from usual behavior. Atypical absence seizures usually continue into adulthood. An EEG shows atypical spike-and-wave patterns, with fewer than 3 per second.

Other generalized-onset nonmotor seizures include myoclonic and eyelid myoclonia. The *myoclonic absence seizure* is characterized by rhythmic arm abduction (3 movements per second) leading to progressive arm elevation. It usually lasts 10 to 60 seconds. *Eyelid myoclonia* refers to jerking of the eyelids (at least 3 per second), often with upward eye deviation. It usually lasts less than 10 seconds.[16]

Focal-Onset Seizures. Focal-onset seizures (formerly called *partial* or *partial focal seizures*) are the other major class of seizures (Table 58.5). Focal seizures begin in 1 hemisphere of the brain in a specific region of the cortex, as shown by the EEG. They cause sensory, motor, cognitive, or emotional manifestations based on the function of the involved area of the brain. For example, if the discharging focus is in the medial aspect of the postcentral gyrus, the patient may have paresthesia in the leg on the side opposite the focus. This can help distinguish the type of seizure event.

Focal-onset seizures may be described by level of awareness (*aware* or *impaired awareness*). However, this is optional and applied only when awareness is known. *Focal awareness seizures* were called simple partial seizures. Patients are conscious and alert but have unusual feelings or sensations that can take many forms. They may have sudden and unexplainable feelings of joy, anger, sadness, or nausea. They may hear, smell, taste, see, or feel things that are not real.

In a *focal impaired awareness seizure* (previously called complex partial seizures), patients have a loss of consciousness or a change in their awareness, producing a dreamlike state. Their eyes are open. They make movements that may seem purposeful, but they cannot interact with observers. During a seizure, some people may do things that can be dangerous or embarrassing, such as walking into traffic or removing their clothes. They may continue an activity started before the seizure, such as counting coins or choosing items from a grocery shelf. After the seizure they do not remember the activity performed during the seizure. Seizures usually last 1 to 2 minutes. Patients may be tired or confused after the seizure and may not return to normal activity for hours.

The degree of awareness can be unspecified, and a seizure classified as *motor* or *nonmotor*. Motor activities include atonic (loss of tone), tonic (sustained stiffening), clonic (rhythmic jerking), myoclonic (irregular, brief jerking), or epileptic spasms (flexion or extension of arms with flexion of trunk). Some people show strange behavior, such as lip smacking or other repetitive, purposeless actions *(automatisms)*. With a focal nonmotor seizure, the patient can have emotional manifestations, such as fear or joy, strange feelings, or symptoms such as a racing heart, goose bumps, or waves of heat or cold.

Psychogenic Nonepileptic Seizures (PNES). Because of the close resemblance, psychogenic seizures may be misdiagnosed as seizure disorder. Proper diagnosis usually requires video-EEG monitoring to identify associated events. If the diagnosis of seizure disorder is excluded, history of emotional or physical abuse or a specific traumatic event often emerges. Some patients may have both psychogenic seizures and seizure disorder. Care provided by a specialist is essential. Once the diagnosis is made, the treatment of choice is psychological intervention.[17]

Complications

Physical. Status epilepticus (SE) is a state of continuous seizure activity or a condition in which seizures recur in rapid succession without return to consciousness between seizures. SE is defined as any seizure lasting longer than 5 minutes. The longer a seizure lasts, the less likely it is to stop without drug therapy.

SE is a neurologic emergency that can occur with any type of seizure. The highest incidence occurs in children and older adults. During repeated seizures, the brain uses more energy than can be supplied. As neurons become exhausted and cease to function, permanent brain damage may result. *Convulsive status epilepticus* (CSE) is the most common form. It occurs with prolonged or repeated tonic-clonic seizures. The goal of therapy is to rapidly end clinical and electrical seizure activity. Without effective, timely treatment, CSE can lead to fatal respiratory insufficiency, hypoxemia, dysrhythmias, hyperthermia, and systemic acidosis. The prognosis for CSE is related to its duration and the patient's age.[18]

The term *nonconvulsive status epilepticus* is used to described long or repeated focal impaired awareness seizures. Symptoms may be subtle, making it hard to tell recovery from seizure symptoms. No consistent time frame dictates when this state is considered an emergency. It depends on the length and frequency of seizure activity.

Refractory status epilepticus (RSE) is continuous seizure activity despite administration of first- and second-line therapy. RSE carries a high risk for mortality and neurologic damage. This highlights the need for careful, rapid escalation of treatment for CSE to avoid progression. *Super refractory SE* is a refractory condition that continues or recurs 24 hours or more after starting anesthetic treatment. It also includes cases in which seizure activity returns after withdrawal of anesthetic drugs or persists after 7 days of continuous general anesthesia. About 15% of patients who enter the hospital with SE become super-refractory.[19]

Subclinical seizures are a form of SE in which a sedated patient seizes but there are no external signs because of sedative use. For example, a patient under sedation for ventilatory support in the intensive care unit (ICU) could have a seizure without physical movements and we miss the seizure occurrence.

People with seizure disorder have a higher mortality rate than the general population. Severe injury, and even death, can result from trauma suffered during a seizure. Patients who lose consciousness during a seizure are at greatest risk. Other deaths are due to accidents during seizures, suicide, treatment-related death, death from an underlying disease, or sudden unexpected death in epilepsy (SUDEP).

SUDEP affects about 1 in 150 persons with uncontrolled seizures each year.[20] It is almost always associated with tonic-clonic seizures. Occurrence is higher in males, in persons taking multiple antiseizure drugs, and patients with poorly managed seizure activity. The exact cause is not known. It could be related to respiratory dysfunction, dysrhythmias, or cerebral depression. Specific teaching about medication adherence and disease awareness is critical for at-risk people.

Psychosocial. Perhaps the most common complication of seizure disorder is the effect on a patient's lifestyle. Patients may have ineffective coping methods because of psychosocial problems related to having seizure disorder. An increased incidence of depression occurs in people who have seizures that are difficult to control. Many antiseizure drugs have side effects that overlap with depressive symptoms.

Although attitudes have improved in recent years, a diagnosis of seizure disorder still carries a social stigma. Patients may be victims of discrimination in employment and educational opportunities. Transportation may be difficult if state law does not allow the person to drive. Screen patients often for depression. Encourage them to pursue available treatment options.

Diagnostic Studies

A diagnosis of seizure disorder may have many socioeconomic, physical, and psychologic consequences for the patient. Accurate diagnosis is crucial. The most useful diagnostic tool is an accurate, comprehensive description of seizures and the patient's health history (Table 58.6). Information from caregivers can be helpful.

The EEG is useful, but only if it shows abnormalities. Abnormal findings help determine the type of seizure and

TABLE 58.6 Interprofessional Care

Seizure Disorder

Diagnostic Assessment	Diagnostic Studies
History and Physical Examination	• CBC, urinalysis, electrolytes, creatinine, fasting blood glucose
• Birth and developmental history	• LP for CSF analysis
• Significant illnesses and injuries	• CT, MRI, MRA, MRS, PET scan
• Family history	• EEG
• Febrile seizures	
• Comprehensive neurologic assessment	**Management**
	• Antiseizure drugs (Table 58.8)
Seizure History	• Surgery
• Precipitating factors	• Vagal nerve stimulation
• Antecedent events	• Psychosocial counseling
• Seizure description (including onset, duration, frequency, postictal state)	• Physical therapy

pinpoint the seizure focus. Ideally, an EEG should be done within 24 hours of a suspected seizure. However, only a small number of patients with seizure disorder have abnormal EEG findings the first time the test is done. Repeated EEGs or continuous EEG monitoring may be needed to detect abnormalities. An EEG is not a definitive test because some patients without seizure disorder have abnormal patterns on their EEGs. Many patients with seizure disorder have normal EEG results between seizures. If abnormal discharges do not occur during the 30 to 40 minutes of sampling during EEG, the test may not show an abnormality. Magnetoencephalography (MEG) may be done with the EEG. This test has greater sensitivity in detecting small magnetic fields of neuron activity.

A complete blood count (CBC), serum chemistries, studies of liver and kidney function, and urinalysis should be done to rule out metabolic disorders. A CT scan or MRI should be done in any new-onset seizure to rule out a structural lesion. Cerebral angiography, single-photon emission computed tomography (SPECT), magnetic resonance spectroscopy (MRS), MRA, and positron emission tomography (PET) may be done in certain situations. If an MRI shows a spot or lesion but EEG results differ, MEG can determine if the brain waves are coming from the lesion. MEG can be helpful in a patient with prior brain surgery as EEG results may be affected by changes in the scalp and brain.

The International League Against Epilepsy has developed specific diagnostic criteria for each type of seizure, including conditions that resolve over time *(www.ilae.org)*. If a patient is diagnosed with seizure disorder, the seizure type must be correctly identified to determine the appropriate treatment.

Interprofessional Care

Most seizures do not require emergency medical care because they are self-limiting and rarely cause bodily injury. However, if SE or significant bodily harm occurs, or if the event is a first-time seizure, medical care should be sought immediately. Table 58.6 outlines the diagnostic studies and interprofessional care of seizure disorder. Table 58.7 summarizes emergency care of the patient with a tonic-clonic seizure, the seizure most likely to need emergency medical care.

Drug Therapy. The main treatment for seizure disorder is antiseizure drugs (Table 58.8). Because a cure is not possible, the goal of therapy is to prevent seizures with minimal drug side effects. Drugs generally stabilize nerve cell membranes and prevent spread of the epileptic discharge. Therapy should begin with a single drug based on the patient's age and weight and type, frequency, and cause of seizure. Dosage should be increased until seizures are under control or toxic side effects occur. Antiseizure drugs successfully control seizures for about 70% of patients.

✚ TABLE 58.7 Emergency Management

Tonic-Clonic Seizures

Etiology	Assessment Findings	Interventions
Drug-Related Processes • Ingestion, inhalation • Overdose • Withdrawal of alcohol, opioids, antiseizure drugs **Head Trauma** • Cerebral contusion • Epidural hematoma • Intracranial hematoma • Subdural hematoma • Traumatic birth injury • Idiopathic **Infectious Processes** • Encephalitis • Meningitis • Sepsis **Intracranial Events** • Brain tumor • Hypertensive crisis • Increased ICP due to clogged shunt • Stroke • Subarachnoid hemorrhage **Medical Disorders** • Heart, liver, lung, or kidney disease • Systemic lupus erythematosus **Metabolic Imbalances** • Fluid and electrolyte imbalance • Hypoglycemia **Other** • Cardiac arrest • High fever • Psychiatric disorders	**Aural Phase** • Bowel and bladder incontinence • Diaphoresis • Loss of consciousness • Pallor, flushing, or cyanosis • Peculiar sensations that precede seizure • Tachycardia • Warm skin **Tonic Phase** • Continuous muscle contractions **Hypertonic Phase** • Extreme muscular rigidity lasting 5–15 sec **Clonic Phase** • Rigidity and relaxation alternating in rapid succession **Postictal Phase** • Altered level of consciousness, lethargy • Confusion and headache • Repeated tonic-clonic seizures for several min	**Initial** • Ensure patent airway. • Protect patient from injury during seizure. *Do not restrain.* Pad side rails. • Remove or loosen tight clothing. • Establish IV access. • Stay with patient until seizure has passed. • Anticipate giving phenobarbital, phenytoin (Dilantin), benzodiazepines (e.g., diazepam [Valium], midazolam [Versed], lorazepam [Ativan]) to try to stop seizures. • Suction as needed. • Assist ventilations if patient does not breathe spontaneously after seizure. • Anticipate need for intubation if gag reflex absent. **Ongoing Monitoring** • Monitor vital signs, level of consciousness, O₂ saturation, Glasgow Coma Scale results, pupil size and reactivity. • Reassure and orient patient after seizure. • Never force an airway between patient's clenched teeth. • Give IV dextrose for hypoglycemia.

If seizure control is not achieved with a single drug, dosage or timing of administration may be changed or a second drug may be added. About one third of patients need a combination regimen for enough control. Patients should discuss new treatments with their HCPs to provide the best control with the least amount of medication.

The therapeutic range for each drug is the serum level above which most patients have toxic side effects and below which most continue to have seizures. Therapeutic drug ranges are only guides for therapy. If the patient's seizures are well controlled with a subtherapeutic level, the drug dosage does not have to be increased. Likewise, if a drug level is above the therapeutic range and the patient has good seizure control without toxic side effects, the drug dosage does not have to be decreased. Serum drug levels are monitored if seizures continue to occur, frequency increases, or drug adherence is questioned. Because they have a large therapeutic range, many newer drugs do not require drug-level monitoring.

The main drugs to treat tonic-clonic and focal-onset seizures are phenytoin (Dilantin), carbamazepine (Tegretol), phenobarbital, and divalproex. The drugs used most often to treat generalized-onset nonmotor and myoclonic seizures include ethosuximide (Zarontin), divalproex, and clonazepam (Klonopin). Table 58.8 lists other drugs used for seizure treatment. Some drugs are effective for multiple seizure types. Pregabalin (Lyrica) is used as an additional treatment for focal aware or impaired awareness seizures not successfully controlled with 1 medication.

 DRUG ALERT Carbamazepine (Tegretol)
- Do not take with grapefruit juice.
- Teach patient to report visual changes (e.g., blurry or double vision).
- Abrupt withdrawal after long-term use may cause seizures.

Treatment of SE requires a rapid-acting IV antiseizure drug. The drugs most often used are lorazepam (Ativan) and diazepam (Valium). Because these are short-acting drugs, their administration is followed with long-acting drugs, such as phenytoin or phenobarbital.

Because many antiseizure drugs (e.g., phenytoin, phenobarbital, ethosuximide, lamotrigine, topiramate) have a long half-life, they can be given once or twice a day. This simplifies the drug plan and increases the patient's adherence because the drug does not have to be taken at work or school. Unnecessary combination therapy is avoided whenever possible. Medications

TABLE 58.8 Drug Therapy
Seizure Disorder

- brivaracetam (Briviact)
- carbamazepine (Tegretol)
- clonazepam (Klonopin)
- daclizumab (Zinbryta)
- diazepam (Diastat)
- divalproex (Depakote)
- eslicarbazepine (Aptiom)
- ethosuximide (Zarontin)
- ezogabine (Potiga)
- felbamate (Felbatol)
- gabapentin (Neurontin)
- lacosamide (Vimpat)
- lamotrigine (Lamictal)
- levetiracetam (Keppra)
- lorazepam (Ativan)
- oxcarbazepine (Trileptal)
- perampanel (Fycompa)
- phenytoin (Dilantin)
- pregabalin (Lyrica)
- primidone (Mysoline)
- tiagabine (Gabitril)
- topiramate (Topamax)
- valproic acid (Depakene)
- vigabatrin (Sabril)
- zonisamide (Zonegran)

should be reviewed routinely and the least effective medication discontinued by tapering.

 DRUG ALERT Antiseizure Drugs
- Abrupt withdrawal after long-term use may cause seizures.
- If weaning is to occur, the patient must be seizure free for a prolonged period (e.g., 2 to 5 yr) and have a normal neurologic examination and EEG.

Side effects of antiseizure drugs involve the CNS. They include diplopia, drowsiness, ataxia, and mental slowness. Neurologic assessment for dose-related toxicity involves testing the eyes for nystagmus and evaluating hand and gait coordination, cognitive functioning, and general alertness.

As a nurse, you need to be knowledgeable about drug side effects, so you can teach patients and start proper treatment. For example, common side effects of phenytoin are gingival hyperplasia (excess growth of gingival tissue) and hirsutism, especially in young adults. Good dental hygiene, including regular tooth brushing and flossing, can decrease gingival hyperplasia. If gingival hyperplasia is extensive, the hyperplastic tissue may be surgically removed (gingivectomy) and phenytoin replaced with another antiseizure drug.

Medication nonadherence can be a problem in people with seizure disorder, often due to undesirable side effects. Take measures to increase adherence to the prescribed drug plan. If HCPs are aware of nonadherence, they can work with the patient to find an acceptable drug plan. For example, using pregabalin as an adjunct medication in some cases may allow a decreased dose of the primary antiseizure drug and thus decrease side effects.

 ### Gerontologic Considerations: Drug Therapy for Seizure Disorder

Many older adults have a first single seizure, then do not have another seizure. To be considered for antiseizure drug therapy, older adults should have recurrent seizures, an obvious structural predisposition for seizures, or onset of seizure disorder presenting as SE. Older adults are more responsive to antiseizure drugs than younger adults, but they also are more likely to have side effects at lower serum drug concentrations.

Age-related changes in liver enzymes decrease the liver's ability to metabolize drugs. Because the liver metabolizes phenytoin, it should not be used in older patients with liver problems. The potential effects on cognitive function make phenobarbital, carbamazepine, and primidone less desirable for older adults. Carbamazepine, phenytoin, phenobarbital, or primidone can increase the risk for osteomalacia, osteopenia, and osteoporosis. Several newer antiseizure drugs offer greater treatment benefit to older adults. Compared with older drugs, gabapentin, lamotrigine, oxcarbazepine (Trileptal), and levetiracetam may be safer, have fewer effects on cognitive function, and have fewer interactions with other drugs.

Surgical Therapy. Despite availability of newer drugs with fewer side effects, no solution has been found for *medically refractory epilepsy* (not responsive to drug therapy). About 30% of patients do not respond to antiseizure drugs. For people with a defined site of seizure origin (epileptogenic zone), research shows the benefit of surgical resection of that focal area over continued use of different antiseizure drugs. About 80% are seizure free 5 years after surgery, with 72% still seizure free at 10 years.

Not all patients benefit from surgery. An extensive preoperative evaluation is important, including continuous EEG monitoring and other tests to ensure precise localization of the focal point. Surgical candidates must meet 3 requirements: (1) a confirmed diagnosis of seizure disorder, (2) an adequate trial with drug therapy without satisfactory results, and (3) a defined electroclinical syndrome (type of seizure disorder).

Other Therapies. *Vagal nerve stimulation* (VNS), a form of neuromodulation, is used as an adjunct to drugs when an accessible focal point cannot be identified for surgical removal. The exact mechanism of action is unknown. It may increase blood flow to specific brain areas. It could raise levels of neurotransmitters important to seizure control and change EEG patterns during a seizure. In VNS, a surgically implanted electrode in the neck is programmed to deliver electrical impulses to the vagus nerve, usually on the left side. The patient activates the electrode with a magnet when they sense a seizure is imminent. Newer devices respond to an increasing heart rate, which is often associated with seizures. Adverse effects include coughing, hoarseness, dyspnea, and tingling in the neck. Battery life is 5 to 10 years, and surgical replacement is needed. Benefits of VNS can be seen within 24 months after implantation. Contraindications include a history of dysrhythmias or sleep apnea.

Responsive neurostimulation (Neuropace RNS System) is similar to a cardiac pacemaker. It continually monitors the EEG to detect abnormalities, then responds to seizure activity by delivering electrical stimulation to a precise location. The device is placed under the skin, outside the skull, with connections to electrodes over the area of seizure focus. The HCP uses a programmable wand to download information about seizure activity. This is used to assess treatment efficacy and guide care. This modality is an option for persons who are not surgical candidates or have multiple areas of seizure focus.

A *ketogenic diet* is a special high-fat, low-carbohydrate diet that helps control seizures in some people. A person on this diet produces ketones that pass into the brain, where they replace glucose as an energy source. Meals are carefully planned to restrict the amount of protein and carbohydrate in the diet. Patients on this diet who use anticoagulants need close monitoring for bleeding. Although HCPs are more likely to recommend the diet for children than adults, the diet can work equally well in both age-groups. Most people must continue their use of antiseizure medication but may take smaller doses or fewer medications. Seizures may worsen if the diet is stopped abruptly. Long-term effects of the diet are not clear.

Biofeedback to control seizures is aimed at teaching the patient to maintain a certain brain wave frequency that is refractory to seizure activity. Further trials are needed to assess the effectiveness of biofeedback for seizure control.

❖ NURSING MANAGEMENT: SEIZURE DISORDER

◆ Nursing Assessment

Subjective and objective data to obtain from a patient with seizure disorder are outlined in Table 58.9. Obtain data related to a specific seizure episode from a witness.

TABLE 58.9 Nursing Assessment
Seizure Disorder

Subjective Data

Important Health Information

Past health history: Seizures, birth defects or injuries, anoxic episodes. CNS trauma, tumors, or infections. Stroke, metabolic disorders, alcohol use, exposure to metals and carbon monoxide, hepatic or renal failure, fever, pregnancy, systemic lupus erythematosus

Medications: Adherence to antiseizure medication plan. Barbiturate or alcohol withdrawal. Use and overdose of cocaine, amphetamines, lidocaine, theophylline, penicillin, lithium, phenothiazines, tricyclic antidepressants, benzodiazepines

Functional Health Patterns

Health perception–health management: Positive family history
Cognitive-perceptual: Headaches, aura, mood or behavioral changes before seizure. Mentation changes. Abdominal pain, muscle pain (postictal)
Self-perception–self-concept: Anxiety, depression. Loss of self-esteem, social isolation
Sexuality-reproductive: Decreased sexual drive, erectile dysfunction. Increased sexual drive (postictal)

Objective Data

General

Precipitating factors, including severe metabolic acidosis or alkalosis, hyperkalemia, hypoglycemia, dehydration, or water intoxication

Integumentary

Bitten tongue, soft tissue damage, cyanosis, diaphoresis (postictal)

Respiratory

Abnormal respiratory rate, rhythm, or depth. Apnea (ictal). Absent or abnormal breath sounds, possible airway occlusion

Cardiovascular

Hypertension, tachycardia or bradycardia (ictal)

Gastrointestinal

Bowel incontinence, excessive salivation

Urinary

Incontinence

Neurologic

Generalized Onset

Tonic-clonic: Loss of consciousness, muscle tightening, then jerking. Dilated pupils. Hyperventilation, then apnea. Postictal somnolence
Absence: Altered consciousness (5–30 sec), minor facial motor activity

Focal Onset

Aware: Aura. Focal sensory, motor, cognitive, or emotional phenomena (focal motor)
Impaired awareness: Altered consciousness with inappropriate behaviors, automatisms, amnesia of event

Musculoskeletal

Weakness, paralysis, ataxia (postictal)

Possible Diagnostic Findings

Positive toxicology screen or blood alcohol level. Altered serum electrolytes, acidosis or alkalosis, very low blood glucose, ↑ blood urea nitrogen or serum creatinine, abnormal liver function tests, ammonia; abnormal CT scan or MRI of head, abnormal findings from LP. Abnormal discharges on EEG

◆ Nursing Diagnoses

Nursing diagnoses for the patient with seizure disorder may include:

- Impaired breathing
- Difficulty coping
- Risk for fall-related injury

Additional information on nursing diagnoses and interventions for the patient with seizure disorder is presented in eNursing Care Plan 58.2 (available on the website for this chapter).

◆ Planning

The overall goals are that the patient with seizure disorder will (1) be free from injury during a seizure, (2) have optimal mental and physical functioning while taking antiseizure drugs, and (3) have satisfactory psychosocial functioning.

◆ Nursing Implementation

◆ **Health Promotion.** Following general safety measures (e.g., wearing helmets in situations involving risk for head injury) can prevent some seizure disorders. Improved perinatal care has reduced fetal trauma and hypoxia and thus brain damage leading to seizure disorder.

The patient with seizure disorder should practice good general health habits (e.g., maintain proper diet, get adequate rest, exercise). Help the patient identify events or situations that cause seizures and provide suggestions for avoiding them or handling them better. Teach the patient to avoid excess alcohol use, fatigue, and loss of sleep. Help the patient handle stress constructively.

◆ **Acute Care.** Nursing care for a hospitalized patient with seizure disorder or a patient who has had seizures due to other factors involves observation and treatment of the seizure, patient and caregiver teaching, and psychosocial intervention.

> **? CHECK YOUR PRACTICE**
>
> You are making your morning rounds and go to check your 22-yr-old female patient, who was admitted the night before with increased seizure activity. When you go to her room, her roommate is yelling, "Help, help!" You find the patient is on the floor jerking and stiffening and not responding to you.
> - What should you do?

When a seizure occurs, carefully observe and record details of the event because the diagnosis and subsequent treatment often rest on the seizure description. What events preceded the seizure? When did the seizure occur? How long did each phase (aural [if any], ictal, postictal) last? What occurred during each phase?

All subjective data (usually the only type of data in the aural phase) and objective data are important. Note the exact onset of the seizure (which body part was affected first and how); the course and nature of the seizure activity (loss of consciousness, tongue biting, automatisms, stiffening, jerking, total lack of muscle tone); body parts involved and their sequence of involvement; and autonomic signs, such as dilated pupils, excessive salivation, altered breathing, cyanosis, flushing, diaphoresis, or incontinence. Assessment of the postictal period should include a detailed description of the level of consciousness, vital signs, pupil size and position of the eyes, memory loss, muscle soreness, speech disorders (aphasia, dysarthria), weakness or paralysis, sleep period, and the duration of each sign or symptom.

> **! SAFETY ALERT** Seizure
>
> During a seizure, you should:
> - Maintain a patent airway for the patient.
> - Protect the patient's head, turn the patient to the side, loosen constrictive clothing, ease patient to the floor (if seated).
> - Do not restrain the patient.
> - Do not place any objects in the patient's mouth

After the seizure, the patient may need repositioning (to open and maintain the airway), suctioning, and O_2. A seizure can be frightening for the patient and others who witnessed it. Assess their level of understanding and provide information about how and why the event occurred. This is an excellent chance for you to dismiss many common misconceptions about seizures.

> ### ■ NURSING MANAGEMENT
> #### *Caring for the Patient With Seizure Disorder*
>
> **Role of the RN**
> - Teach patient about factors that increase risk for seizures.
> - Teach patient about prescribed antiseizure medications, including drug plan, side effects, and monitoring of drug levels.
> - Assess and record details of seizure events, including events preceding the seizure; length of each phase of the seizure; course and nature of seizure activity; and level of consciousness, vital signs, and activity during the postictal period.
> - Assess airway patency, and position patient to maintain airway during and after seizures.
> - Give IV antiseizure medications to the patient with SE.
> - Give oral antiseizure medications as scheduled.
> - Make appropriate referrals to community agencies to help the patient with the financial impact of seizure disorder, work training, employment, and living arrangements.
> - Teach caregivers about management of seizures and SE.
> - In the ambulatory and home care setting, evaluate patient self-management of medications and lifestyle.
> - Oversee UAP:
>   - Place suction equipment, bag-valve-mask, and O_2 at the patient's bedside.
>   - Remove potentially harmful objects from the bedside and pad side rails.
>   - Immediately report any seizure activity to the RN.
>   - Obtain vital signs during the postictal period.
>
> **Collaborate With Other Team Members**
> ***Respiratory Therapist***
> - Assess airway patency and suction as needed.
> - Assist ventilations if patient does not breathe spontaneously after seizure.
> - Assist with intubation if gag reflex absent.
>
> ***Occupational Therapist***
> - Help patient with increasing self-care measures, including eating and dressing.
>
> ***Social Worker***
> - Help patient identify and obtain needed resources.
> - Offer counseling to develop positive coping skills.

◆ **Ambulatory Care.** Prevention of recurring seizures is the major goal of treatment. Help the patient understand that for treatment to be effective, drugs must be taken regularly and consistently. Review details of the drug plan and what to do if a dose is missed. Usually the dose is made up if the omission is remembered within 24 hours. Caution the patient not to adjust drug dosages without HCP guidance because this can increase seizure frequency and cause SE. Encourage the patient to report any medication side effects and keep regular appointments with the HCP.

TABLE 58.10   Patient & Caregiver Teaching

Seizure Disorder

Include the following information in the teaching plan for the patient with seizure disorder:

1. Take antiseizure medications as prescribed. Report all drug side effects to the HCP.
2. When needed, blood is drawn to ensure therapeutic drug levels. Schedule regular visits with the HCP to discuss treatment options.
3. Use nondrug techniques, such as relaxation therapy, to try to reduce the number of seizures.
4. Be aware of community and online resources for education and help with tracking and explaining seizure activity.
5. Wear a medical alert bracelet or necklace and carry an identification card.
6. Avoid excess alcohol use, fatigue, and loss of sleep.
7. Eat regular meals and snacks in between if feeling shaky, faint, or hungry.
8. Be knowledgeable as a woman of childbearing age about antiseizure medications and contraceptive use.

Caregivers should receive the following information:

Focal-Onset Seizures

1. Stay calm. Guide patient to safety to prevent injury but do not restrain.
2. Observe for asymmetry of activity and focus on specific actions, such as lip smacking and abnormal movements.
3. Assess patient's level of consciousness and ability to converse and respond appropriately.
4. Note the time the seizure started and stopped. Take note of the time of return to baseline.
5. Provide respect and explanation of occurrence.

Generalized-Onset Tonic-Clonic Seizures

1. When seizure occurs outside the hospital setting, activate ERS if (1) the duration is greater than 5 minutes; (2) events recur without the patient recovering to baseline; (3) the patient is unable to establish a normal breathing pattern, is injured or pregnant; or (4) you do not know if this is a first-time seizure event.
2. Maintain patient safety. Lower the patient to the floor or bed, remove glasses if worn, and loosen restrictive clothing.
3. Do not place anything in the patient's mouth. Patient's teeth/dentures may be damaged, and caregiver may be bitten.
4. Position patient on side (if possible) to improve the patient's ability to release oral secretions.
5. Note the time the seizure started and stopped. Take note of the time of return to baseline.
6. Assess for any injury and lingering motor weakness.

You have a vital role in teaching the patient and caregiver. Review the guidelines for teaching shown in Table 58.10. Teach caregivers the emergency management of tonic-clonic seizures (Table 58.7). Remind them it is not necessary to call an ambulance or send a person to the hospital after a single seizure unless the seizure is prolonged, another seizure immediately follows, extensive injury has occurred, or it is unknown if this was a first-time seizure.

Patients with seizure disorder may have concerns or fears related to recurrent seizures, incontinence, or loss of self-control. Support patients through teaching and by helping them use effective coping mechanisms.

Perhaps the greatest challenge for a patient with seizure disorder is adjusting to the limitations imposed by the illness. Discrimination in employment is a serious problem facing the person with seizure disorder. For issues relating to job discrimination, refer patients to the state department of vocational rehabilitation or the U.S. Equal Employment Opportunity Commission (EEOC).

Help the patient find appropriate resources. If you think associating with others who have seizure disorder would be beneficial, refer the patient to the local chapter of the Epilepsy Foundation (EF). This volunteer agency offers varied services to patients with a seizure disorder *(www.epilepsy.com)*. Refer the patient who is an eligible veteran to a Department of Veterans Affairs medical center that provides comprehensive care. If intensive psychologic counseling is needed, refer the patient to a community mental health center.

Social workers and welfare agencies can help with financial implications and living arrangements. State agencies specializing in vocational rehabilitation services can provide vocational assessment, counseling, and funding for training. They can help with job placement for patients whose seizures are not well controlled. They offer financial assistance for transportation and medical costs related to vocational rehabilitation or job maintenance.

Driving laws for patients who have had a seizure vary from state to state. For example, some states require a 3-month seizure-free period before issuing or reissuing a driver's license. Others require up to 1 year. The EF provides current information on driving laws for each state.

Tell the patient that medical alert bracelets, necklaces, and identification cards are available through the EF, local pharmacies, or companies specializing in identification devices (e.g., Medic Alert). Using medical identification is optional. Some patients have found them beneficial, but others do not want to be identified as having seizure disorder.

Encourage the patient to learn more about seizures through self-education. The EF provides informational pamphlets, has an extensive website, and may offer support groups. Many agencies that offer services to patients with seizure disorder offer teaching aids and support.

◆ Evaluation

Expected outcomes are that the patient with seizure disorder will

- Have a breathing pattern adequate to meet O_2 needs
- Have no seizure-related injury
- Express acceptance of seizure disorder by adhering to treatment plan

RESTLESS LEGS SYNDROME

Etiology and Pathophysiology

Restless legs syndrome (RLS) *(Willis-Ekbom disease)* is a relatively common sleep and movement disorder with unpleasant sensory (paresthesia) and motor abnormalities of 1 or both legs. About 8% of the U.S. population has RLS.[21] A small number have severe symptoms that affect their quality of life and require medication for treatment. RLS is more common in older adults and in women.

There are 2 distinct types of RLS: primary (idiopathic) and secondary. Most people have primary RLS. Secondary RLS can occur with metabolic problems associated with iron deficiency, renal disease and hemodialysis, and neuropathy. Sleep deprivation, sleep apnea, pregnancy (especially third trimester), and use of certain medications (e.g., antiemetics, antidepressants that increase serotonin), can cause or worsen symptoms.

We do not know the exact pathophysiology of primary RLS. We think it is related to a dysfunction in the brain's basal ganglia circuits that use the neurotransmitter dopamine (DA), which controls movements. In RLS, this dysfunction causes the urge to move the legs. RLS has a genetic link. Those with primary RLS often report a positive family history, with symptoms that start before age 40.[21]

Clinical Manifestations

The severity of RLS sensory symptoms ranges from infrequent minor discomfort (numbness, tingling, "pins and needles" sensation) to severe pain. Sensory symptoms often appear first. Some patients compare the sensations to bugs creeping or crawling on the legs. The leg pain is localized within the calf muscles. Patients can have pain in the upper extremities and trunk. The discomfort occurs when the patient is inactive. It is most common in the evening or at night.

Pain at night can disrupt sleep. Physical activity, such as walking, stretching, rocking, or kicking, often relieves the pain. In the most severe cases, patients sleep only a few hours at night. This causes daytime fatigue and disrupts the daily routine. Motor problems associated with RLS include voluntary restlessness and stereotyped, periodic, involuntary movements. The involuntary movements usually occur during sleep. Fatigue further worsens symptoms. RLS worsens over time. Symptoms become more frequent and last longer.

Diagnostic Studies

RLS is diagnosed largely based on the patient's history or the report of the bed partner about nighttime activities. Diagnosis of RLS can be made when the patient meets all 5 specific criteria: (1) overwhelming urge to move the legs, often accompanied by uncomfortable or unpleasant sensations in the legs; (2) urge to move the legs worsens during rest or inactivity; (3) urge to move the legs is partially or totally relieved by movement, as long as the activity continues; (4) urge to move the legs becomes worse in the evening or night; and (5) these features are not due to another medical or behavioral condition.[21]

The patient may have polysomnography studies during sleep to distinguish RLS from other clinical conditions that can disturb sleep (e.g., sleep apnea). While periodic leg movements in sleep can support the diagnosis of RLS, they are not exclusive to RLS. Blood tests, such as a CBC, serum ferritin, and renal function tests (e.g., serum creatinine), may help exclude secondary causes of RLS. A patient with diabetes may have paresthesia caused by peripheral neuropathy related to diabetes or RLS.

❖ Interprofessional and Nursing Care

The goal of interprofessional management is to reduce patient discomfort and distress and improve sleep quality. When RLS is due to renal failure or iron deficiency, treating these conditions may decrease symptoms. Lifestyle changes may help persons with mild to moderate RLS. For example, decreasing the use of alcohol or tobacco, maintaining regular sleep habits, exercising, and massaging and stretching the legs may be helpful. The patient should avoid antihistamine-containing medications (e.g., diphenhydramine).

If nondrug measures fail, drug therapy is an option. No single medication effectively manages RLS for all patients. The main drugs used to treat RLS aim to increase the amount of DA in the brain. They include DA precursors (e.g., carbidopa/levodopa) and DA agonists (e.g., ropinirole [Requip], pramipexole [Mirapex], rotigotine [Neupro]). The antiseizure drug gabapentin enacarbil (Horizant) may decrease the sensory sensations and nerve pain. The patient with iron-deficiency anemia may need to start iron supplementation.

Other drugs may relieve some symptoms of RLS. Very low doses of opioids (e.g., oxycodone) may help patients with severe symptoms who do not respond to other drug therapies. The main side effect of opioids is constipation, so patients may need to take a stool softener or laxative. Clonidine (Catapres) and propranolol (Inderal) are effective in some patients. Benzodiazepines (e.g., lorazepam [Ativan]) may help patients obtain more restful sleep. However, they are last-line treatments due to their side effects.[21]

Using a Relaxis device may help some patients. It produces vibration, providing counter stimulation that competes with and decreases RLS sensations. The patient places the legs on the Relaxis pad. It provides 30 minutes of uninterrupted vibration after being activated, then it slowly winds down over another 5 minutes to complete a 35-minute therapy cycle. If needed, it may be restarted one more time. The patient chooses the vibration intensity based on symptoms.

▌DEGENERATIVE NEUROLOGIC DISORDERS

MULTIPLE SCLEROSIS

Multiple sclerosis (MS) is a chronic, progressive, degenerative disorder of the CNS characterized by disseminated demyelination of nerve fibers of the brain and spinal cord. MS can affect people of any age. The onset of MS is usually between 20 and 50 years of age, with symptoms first appearing at an average of 30 to 35 years of age. People diagnosed at 50 years of age or older generally have more progressive disease. MS affects women 2 to 3 times more often than men. Around 400,000 people in the United States have MS, with 10,000 new cases diagnosed annually.[22]

MS is more prevalent in temperate climates (between 45 and 65 degrees of latitude), such as those found in the northern United States, Canada, and Europe. People who are born in a high-risk area and move to a low-risk area before age 15 assume the risk of their new home. We suspect exposure to some environmental agent before puberty may cause a person to develop MS later in life. MS is less common in Hispanics, Asians, and people of African descent. It rarely occurs in some ethnic groups, including Alaskan Natives and Aborigines.

Etiology and Pathophysiology

While we do not know the cause of MS, it is unlikely due to a single cause. We think MS develops in a genetically susceptible person after an environmental exposure, such as an infection. The inherited susceptibility to MS likely involves multiple genes. Having a first-degree relative with MS increases a person's risk for developing the disease. We have found common genetic factors in families with more than 1 affected member.[23]

Possible precipitating factors include infection, smoking, physical injury, emotional stress, excessive fatigue, pregnancy, and a poor state of health. The role of factors such as exposure to pathogens is controversial. We have investigated more than a dozen viruses and bacteria but have not proven any cause MS.

MS is marked by 3 processes: chronic inflammation, demyelination, and gliosis in the CNS. The primary condition is an autoimmune process driven by activated T cells. An unknown trigger in a genetically susceptible person may start this process.

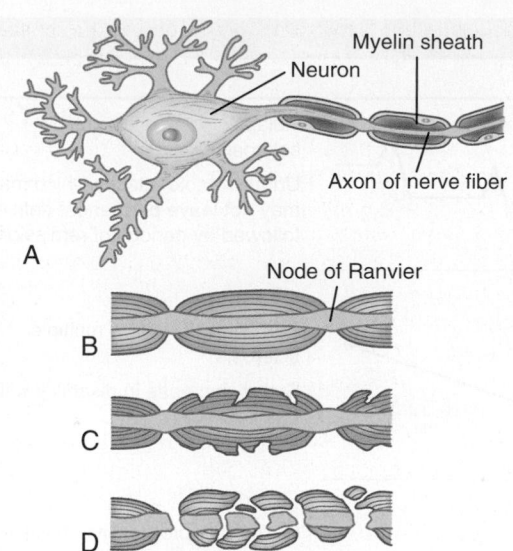

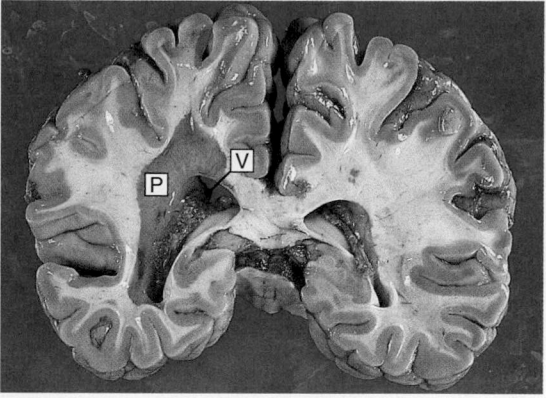

FIG. 58.3 Chronic multiple sclerosis. Demyelination plaque *(P)* at gray-white junction and adjacent partially remyelinated shadow plaque *(V)*. (From Stevens A, Lowe J: *Pathology: Illustrated review in colour*, ed 2, London, 2000, Mosby.)

FIG. 58.2 Pathogenesis of multiple sclerosis. **A,** Normal nerve cell with myelin sheath. **B,** Normal axon. **C,** Myelin breakdown. **D,** Myelin totally disrupted; axon not functioning.

The activated T cells in the systemic circulation go to the CNS and disrupt the blood-brain barrier. This may be the first event in the development of MS. Subsequent antigen-antibody reaction within the CNS activates the inflammatory response and leads to axon demyelination.

Attacks on the myelin sheaths of the neurons in the brain and spinal cord first cause damage to the myelin sheath (Fig. 58.2, *A to C*). The nerve fiber is not affected. Transmission of nerve impulses still occurs, but it is slowed. The patient may have a noticeable impairment of function (e.g., weakness). However, myelin can still regenerate. When it does, symptoms disappear. At that point, the patient has a remission.

As inflammation continues, nearby oligodendrocytes are affected. Myelin loses the ability to regenerate. Eventually damage occurs to the underlying axon. Nerve impulse transmission is disrupted, and nerve function is lost permanently (Fig. 58.2, *D*). As inflammation subsides, glial scar tissue replaces damaged tissue. This leads to the formation of hard, rigid plaques (Fig. 58.3). These plaques are found throughout the white matter of the CNS.

The average life expectancy after the onset of symptoms is more than 25 years. Death usually occurs due to infectious complications of immobility (e.g., pneumonia) or because of an unrelated disease.

Clinical Manifestations

The onset of MS is often slow and gradual. Vague symptoms occur periodically over months or years. Because they do not prompt the patient to seek medical attention, MS may not be diagnosed until long after the first symptom. For some patients, MS is marked by rapid, progressive deterioration. Others have remissions and exacerbations. With repeated exacerbations, the overall trend is progressive deterioration in neurologic function.

Because changes from MS have a spotty distribution in the CNS, symptoms vary with each patient based on the areas of the CNS involved. Some patients have severe, long-lasting symptoms early in the course of the disease. Others have only occasional, mild symptoms for several years after onset. A classification scheme of MS, with 4 primary patterns, has been developed based on the clinical course (Table 58.11).

The first symptom of MS may be blurred or double vision, red-green color distortion, or even blindness in 1 eye (Fig. 58.4). Many patients describe extremity muscle weakness and problems with coordination and balance. Those symptoms may affect walking or standing. MS can cause partial or complete paralysis in the worst cases. Most have numbness and tingling. *Lhermitte's sign* is a temporary sensory symptom described as an electric shock going down the spine or into the limbs with neck flexion. Some patients report pain, especially in the low thoracic and abdominal regions. Other frequent problems include speech impairments, hearing loss, tremors, and dizziness. Possible cerebellar signs include nystagmus, ataxia, dysarthria, and dysphagia. Many patients have severe, even disabling fatigue. This is worsened by heat, humidity, deconditioning, and medication side effects.

A rigid plaque is in areas of the CNS that control elimination can bowel and bladder function. Bowel problems usually involve constipation. Urinary problems vary. A common problem in patients with MS is a *spastic* (uninhibited) bladder. The bladder has a small capacity for urine, and its contractions are unchecked. The result is urinary urgency and frequency, often with dribbling or incontinence.

A *flaccid* (hypotonic) bladder occurs with a lesion in the reflex arc controlling bladder function. The patient generally has urinary retention because there is no sensation or desire to void, no pressure, and no pain. Urgency and frequency may be present. A combination of spastic and flaccid bladder can occur. Urinary problems can be diagnosed with urodynamic studies.

Sexual problems occur in many people with MS. Physiologic erectile dysfunction may result from spinal cord involvement in men. Women may have decreased desire for sexual activity (libido), difficulty with orgasm, painful intercourse, and decreased vaginal lubrication. Decreased sensation can prevent a normal sexual response in men and women. The emotional effects of chronic illness and the loss of self-esteem contribute to loss of sexual response. Some women with MS have remission or an improvement in their symptoms during pregnancy. Hormonal changes associated with pregnancy appear to affect the immune system.

About half of people with MS have problems with cognitive function. Most involve problems with short-term memory, attention, information processing, planning, visual perception, and word finding. General intellect stays unchanged and

TABLE 58.11   Patterns of Multiple Sclerosis

Category	Characteristics		
Relapsing-remitting	• Clearly defined attacks of worsening neurologic function *(relapses)* with partial or complete recovery *(remission)*. • 85% of people first diagnosed with this type of MS.		**Relapsing-remitting multiple sclerosis** Unpredictable attacks which may or may not leave permanent deficits followed by periods of remission
Primary-Progressive	• Steadily worsening neurologic function from the beginning with minor improvements but no distinct relapses or remissions. • 10% of people first diagnosed with this type of MS.		**Primary progressive multiple sclerosis** Steady increase in disability without attacks.
Secondary-progressive	• A relapsing-remitting initial course, followed by progression with or without occasional relapses, minor remissions, and plateaus. • New treatments may slow progression. • Most people initially diagnosed with relapsing-remitting MS eventually transition to this type.		**Secondary progressive multiple sclerosis** Initial relapsing-remitting multiple sclerosis that suddenly begins to have decline without periods of remission.
Progressive-relapsing	• Progressive disease from onset, with clear acute relapses, with or without full recovery. Periods between relapses are characterized by continuing progression. • 5% of people with MS.		**Progressive-relapsing multiple sclerosis** Steady decline since onset with super-imposed attacks.

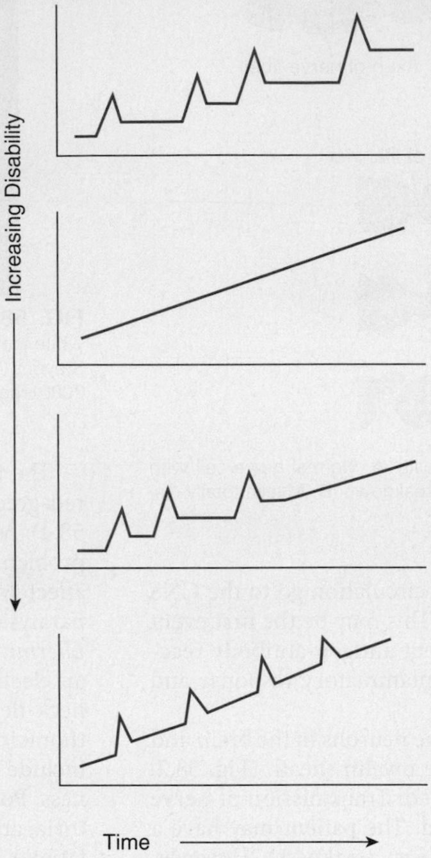

(Vertical axis: Increasing Disability; horizontal axis: Time)

intact. This includes long-term memory, conversational skills, and reading comprehension. Symptoms can be mild and thus easily overlooked. However, about 5% to 10% of patients with MS have such severe cognitive changes that they significantly impair the person's ability to perform activities of daily living (ADLs). Most of the time, cognitive difficulties occur later in the course of the disease. However, they can occur early and sometimes are present at the onset of MS.

People with MS may have emotional changes, such as anger, depression, or euphoria. Physical and emotional trauma, fatigue, and infection may worsen or trigger signs and symptoms.

Diagnostic Studies

Because there is no definitive diagnostic test for MS, the history, manifestations, and results of certain diagnostic tests are important (Table 58.12). Imaging in MS is vital. An MRI of the brain and spinal cord may show plaques, inflammation, atrophy, and tissue breakdown and destruction. CSF analysis may show an increase in immunoglobulin G and the presence of oligoclonal banding.[24] Evoked potential responses are often delayed because of decreased nerve conduction from the eye and ear to the brain.

To be diagnosed with MS, the patient must have (1) evidence of at least 2 inflammatory demyelinating lesions in at least 2 different locations within the CNS, (2) damage or an attack occurring at different times (usually 1 month or more apart), and (3) all other possible diagnoses ruled out. If evidence exists for only 1 lesion, or only 1 clinical attack has occurred, the HCP will monitor the patient for another attack or for an attack at a different site in the CNS.

Interprofessional Care

Drug Therapy. Because no cure currently exists for MS, interprofessional care is aimed at treating the disease process and providing symptomatic relief (Table 58.12). No cases of MS are alike, so we tailor therapy to the disease pattern and symptoms of each patient (Table 58.13). Disease-modifying therapy has been found to be more effective when started early in the course of MS. Delays in treatment are linked to poor outcomes.

Treatment of MS begins with use of immunomodulator drugs to modify disease progression and prevent relapses. These drugs include (1) interferon β-1a (Rebif, Plegridy, Avonex), (2) interferon β-1b (Betaseron, Extavia), and (3) glatiramer acetate (Copaxone, Glatopa).

 DRUG ALERT β-Interferon

- Rotate injection sites with each dose.
- Assess for depression and suicidal ideation.
- Teach patient to wear sunscreen and protective clothing when exposed to sun.
- Tell the patient that flu-like symptoms are common after starting therapy.

Teriflunomide (Aubagio) is an immunomodulatory agent with antiinflammatory properties. The exact mechanism of

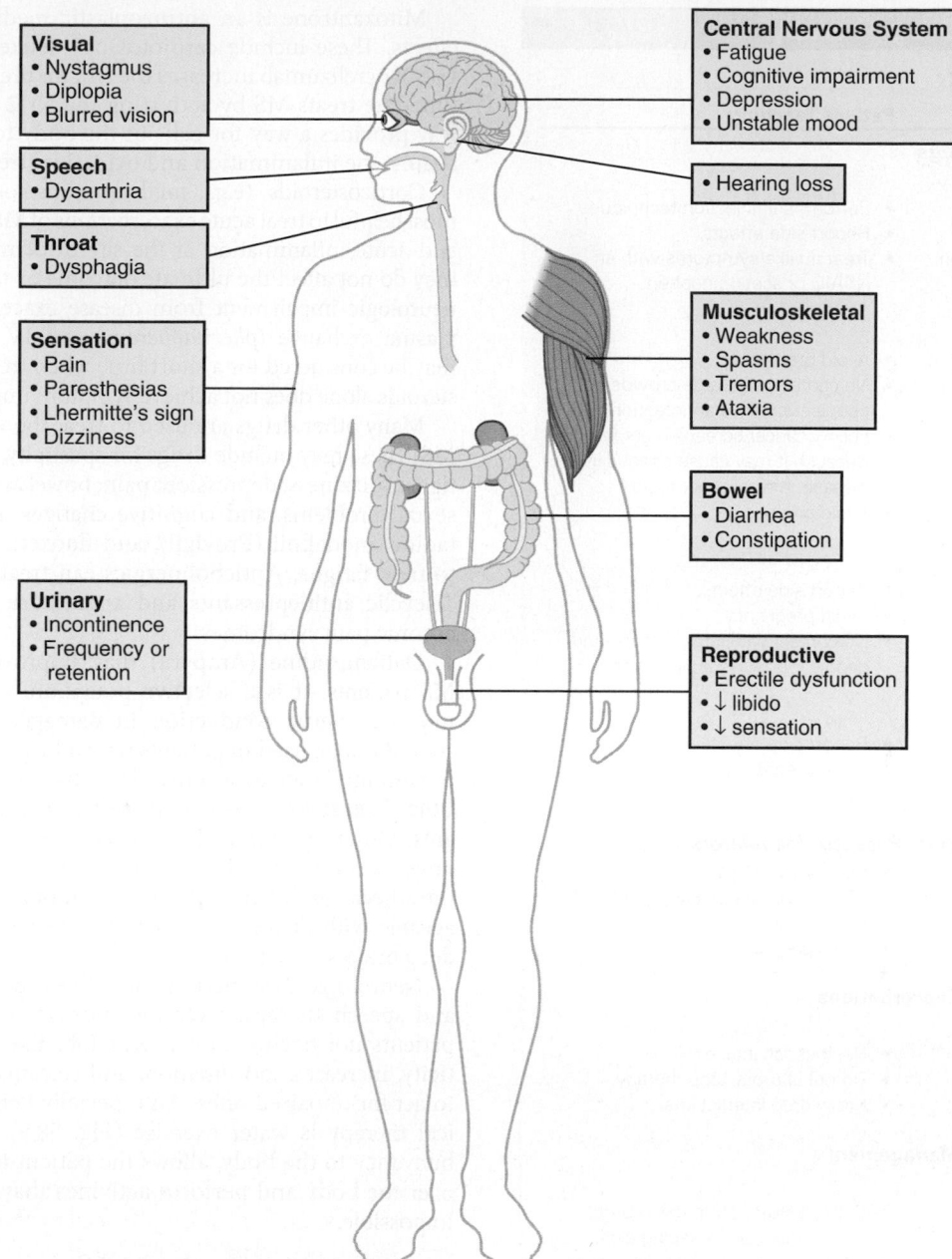

Visual
• Nystagmus
• Diplopia
• Blurred vision

Speech
• Dysarthria

Throat
• Dysphagia

Sensation
• Pain
• Paresthesias
• Lhermitte's sign
• Dizziness

Urinary
• Incontinence
• Frequency or retention

Central Nervous System
• Fatigue
• Cognitive impairment
• Depression
• Unstable mood

• Hearing loss

Musculoskeletal
• Weakness
• Spasms
• Tremors
• Ataxia

Bowel
• Diarrhea
• Constipation

Reproductive
• Erectile dysfunction
• ↓ libido
• ↓ sensation

FIG. 58.4 Manifestations of multiple sclerosis.

TABLE 58.12 Interprofessional Care

Multiple Sclerosis

Diagnostic Assessment	Management
• History and physical examination	• Drug therapy (Table 58.13)
• CSF analysis	• Surgical therapy
• CT scan	• Thalamotomy (unmanageable tremor)
• MRI, MRS (magnetic resonance spectroscopy)	• Neurectomy, rhizotomy, cordotomy (unmanageable spasticity)
• Evoked potential testing	• Physical therapy
• Somatosensory evoked potential (SSEP)	• Occupational therapy
• Auditory evoked potential (AEP)	
• Visual evoked potential (VEP)	

action is unknown. It may reduce the number of activated lymphocytes in the CNS. Fingolimod (Gilenya) and siponimod (Mayzent) reduce MS disease activity by preventing lymphocytes from reaching the CNS and causing damage. These drugs are used to treat relapsing forms of MS.

For more active and aggressive forms of MS, natalizumab (Tysabri), alemtuzumab (Lemtrada), mitoxantrone, ocrelizumab (Ocrevus), and dimethyl fumarate (Tecfidera) may be used. Natalizumab is given when patients have had an inadequate response to other drugs. An adverse effect of natalizumab is the increased risk for a potentially fatal viral infection of the brain (progressive multifocal leukoencephalopathy). Because of its safety profile, alemtuzumab is reserved for patients who have an inadequate response to 2 or more drugs used for the treatment of MS.

TABLE 58.13 Drug Therapy

Multiple Sclerosis

Drug	Patient Teaching
Disease-Modifying Drugs	
Immunomodulators	
β-1a interferon (Rebif, Plegridy, Avonex)	• Perform self-injection techniques.
β-1b interferon (Betaseron, Extavia)	• Report side effects.
	• Treat flu-like symptoms with an NSAID or acetaminophen.
glatiramer acetate (Copaxone)	
mavenclad (Cladribine)	• Avoid pregnancy.
teriflunomide (Aubagio)	• No contact with large crowds and people who have an infection.
	• Follow cancer screening guidelines.
	• Because it may cause serious liver disease, monitor liver tests.
	• Avoid pregnancy.
Immunosuppressants	
dimethyl fumarate (Tecfidera)	• Report side effects.
mitoxantrone	• Avoid pregnancy.
	• No contact with large crowds and people who have an infection.
Monoclonal Antibody	
alemtuzumab (Lemtrada)	• Report side effects.
daclizumab (Zinbryta)	• Avoid pregnancy.
natalizumab (Tysabri)	
Sphingosine 1-Phosphate Receptor Modulators	
fingolimod (Gilenya)	• Report side effects.
siponimod (Mayzent)	• Monitor blood pressure and heart rate regularly.
	• Avoid pregnancy.
Drugs for Managing Exacerbations	
Corticosteroids	
ACTH	• Restrict salt intake.
methylprednisolone	• Do not abruptly stop therapy.
prednisone	• Know drug interactions.
Drugs for Symptom Management	
Anticholinergics	
oxybutynin (Ditropan XL)	• Consult HCP before using other drugs, especially sleeping aids, antihistamines (possibly leading to potentiated effect).
propantheline	
Cholinergics	
bethanechol (Urecholine)	• Consult with HCP before using other drugs, including OTC drugs.
neostigmine	
Muscle Relaxants	
baclofen (Lioresal)	• Avoid driving and similar activities because of sedative effects.
dantrolene (Dantrium)	
diazepam (Valium)	• Do not abruptly stop therapy.
tizanidine (Zanaflex)	• Do not use with tranquilizers and alcohol.
Nerve Conduction Enhancer	
dalfampridine (Ampyra)	• Be aware that it may cause seizures, especially at higher doses.
	• Take the tablet whole. Do not take more than 2 in 24 hr.

Mitoxantrone is an antineoplastic medication with serious effects. These include cardiotoxicity, leukemia, and infertility. Use of ocrelizumab increases the risk for breast cancer. Dimethyl fumarate treats MS by activating the Nrf2 pathway. This pathway provides a way for cells in the body to defend themselves against the inflammation and oxidative stress caused by MS.

Corticosteroids (e.g., methylprednisolone, prednisone) are most helpful to treat acute exacerbations of MS. They reduce edema and acute inflammation at the site of demyelination. However, they do not affect the ultimate outcome or the degree of residual neurologic impairment from disease exacerbation. Therapeutic plasma exchange *(plasmapheresis)* and IV immunoglobulin G may be considered for a short time when treatment with corticosteroids alone does not achieve symptom improvement.

Many other drugs are used to treat the various symptoms of MS. These may include drugs for spasticity, fatigue, tremor, vertigo or dizziness, depression, pain, bowel and bladder problems, sexual problems, and cognitive changes. For example, amantadine, modafinil (Provigil), and fluoxetine (Prozac) are used to treat fatigue. Anticholinergics can treat bladder symptoms. Tricyclic antidepressants and antiseizure drugs are used for chronic pain syndromes.

Dalfampridine (Ampyra) may improve walking speed in MS patients. It is a selective potassium channel blocker that improves nerve conduction in damaged nerve segments. It should not be used in patients with a history of seizure disorder or with moderate to severe kidney disease.

Other Therapies. Spasticity is treated mainly with muscle relaxants. Other options include surgery (e.g., neurectomy, rhizotomy, cordotomy), dorsal-column electrical stimulation, or intrathecal baclofen (Lioresal). Tremors that become unmanageable with drugs are sometimes treated by thalamotomy or deep brain stimulation.

Neurologic dysfunction sometimes improves with physical and speech therapy. Exercise improves daily functioning for patients not having an exacerbation. Exercise decreases spasticity, increases coordination, and retrains unaffected muscles to act for impaired ones. An especially beneficial type of physical therapy is water exercise (Fig. 58.5). Water, which gives buoyancy to the body, allows the patient to have more control over the body and perform activities that would otherwise be impossible.

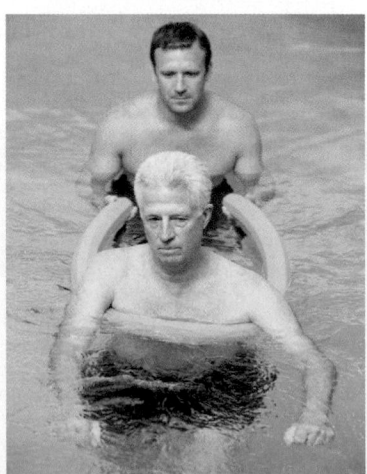

FIG. 58.5 Water therapy provides exercise and recreation for the patient with a chronic neurologic disease. (© Photos.com/AbleStock.com/Thinkstock.)

❖ NURSING MANAGEMENT: MULTIPLE SCLEROSIS

◆ Nursing Assessment

Subjective and objective data that should be obtained from a patient with MS are outlined in Table 58.14.

◆ Nursing Diagnoses

Nursing diagnoses for the patient with MS may include:

- Impaired physical mobility
- Difficulty coping
- Urinary retention

Additional information on nursing diagnoses and interventions for the patient with MS is presented in the eNursing Care Plan 58.3 (available on the website for this chapter).

◆ Planning

The overall goals are that the patient with MS will (1) maximize neuromuscular function, (2) maintain independence in ADLs for as long as possible, (3) manage fatigue, (4) optimize psychosocial well-being, (5) adjust to the illness, and (6) reduce factors that precipitate exacerbations.

TABLE 58.14 Nursing Assessment

Multiple Sclerosis

Subjective Data

Important Health Information

Past health history: Recent or past viral infections or vaccinations, other recent infections, residence in cold or temperate climates, recent physical or emotional stress, pregnancy, exposure to extremes of heat and cold

Medications: Adherence to regimen of corticosteroids, immunomodulators, immunosuppressants, cholinergics, anticholinergics, antispasmodics

Functional Health Patterns

Health perception–health management: Positive family history; malaise
Nutritional-metabolic: Weight loss; difficulty in chewing, dysphagia
Elimination: Urinary frequency, urgency, dribbling or incontinence, retention; constipation
Activity-exercise: Generalized muscle weakness, muscle fatigue; tingling and numbness; ataxia (clumsiness)
Cognitive-perceptual: Eye, back, leg, joint pain; painful muscle spasms; vertigo; blurred or lost vision; diplopia; tinnitus
Sexuality-reproductive: Impotence, decreased libido
Coping–stress tolerance: Anger, depression, euphoria, social isolation

Objective Data

General

Apathy, inattentiveness

Integumentary

Pressure ulcers

Neurologic

Nystagmus, ataxia, tremor, spasticity, hyperreflexia, decreased hearing

Musculoskeletal

Muscle weakness, paresis, paralysis, spasms, foot dragging, dysarthria

Possible Diagnostic Findings

↓ T suppressor cells, demyelinating lesions on MRI or MRS scans, ↑ IgG or oligoclonal banding in CSF, delayed evoked potential responses

IgG, Immunoglobulin G; *MRS,* magnetic resonance spectroscopy.

◆ Nursing Implementation

The patient with MS should be aware of triggers that may cause worsening of the disease. These include infection (especially upper respiratory and urinary tract infections [UTIs]), trauma, immunization, childbirth, stress, and change in climate. Each person responds differently to triggers. Help the patient identify triggers and develop ways to avoid them or decrease their effects.

During the diagnostic phase, reassure the patient that certain diagnostic studies must be done to rule out other neurologic disorders, even if a tentative diagnosis of MS has been made. Help the patient to deal with anxiety caused by a diagnosis of a disabling illness. The patient with recently diagnosed MS may need help with the grieving process.

During an acute exacerbation, the patient may be immobile and confined to bed. The focus of nursing interventions at this phase is to prevent complications of immobility. These include respiratory and UTIs and pressure injuries.

Focus patient teaching on general resistance to illness. This includes avoiding fatigue, extremes of heat and cold, and exposure to infection. Encourage early treatment of infection when it occurs. Teach the patient to seek a good balance of exercise and rest; minimize caffeine intake; and eat nutritious, well-balanced meals. The patient should know the treatment plan, drug side effects, how to identify and manage side effects, and drug interactions with over-the-counter (OTC) drugs. The patient should consult the HCP before taking any OTC drugs.

Bladder control is a major problem for many patients with MS. Anticholinergics may help some patients to decrease spasticity. You may need to teach others self-catheterization. Constipation is common. A diet high in fiber may help relieve constipation.

The patient with MS and caregivers need to make many emotional adjustments because of disease unpredictability, the need for lifestyle changes, and the challenge of avoiding or decreasing precipitating factors. The uncertainty of disease progression, along with fatigue and decreased mobility, can cause anxiety and depression. The National Multiple Sclerosis Society and its local chapters offer a variety of services to meet the needs of patients with MS.

◆ Evaluation

The expected outcomes are that the patient with MS will

- Maintain or improve muscle strength and mobility
- Use assistive devices appropriately for ambulation and mobility
- Maintain urinary continence
- Make decisions about health and lifestyle modifications to manage MS

PARKINSON'S DISEASE

Parkinson's disease (PD) is a chronic, progressive neurodegenerative disorder characterized by slowness in the initiation and execution of movement (*bradykinesia*), increased muscle tone (*rigidity*), tremor at rest, and gait changes. It is the most common form of *parkinsonism* (a syndrome characterized by similar symptoms).

Up to 1 million Americans will be living with PD by 2020. 60,000 persons are diagnosed each year. Incidence of PD increases with age, though 4% of people with PD are diagnosed before age 50 years. Men are 1.5 times more likely to have PD than women.[25]

Etiology and Pathophysiology

The exact cause of PD is unknown. Although we do not consider PD a hereditary condition, genetic risk factors should be evaluated for their interplay with environmental factors. Exposure to well water, pesticides, herbicides, industrial chemicals, and wood pulp mills may increase risk for PD. Rural residence is considered a risk factor.[25]

Many forms of secondary *(atypical)* parkinsonism exist other than PD. Symptoms of parkinsonism have occurred after exposure to a variety of chemicals, including carbon monoxide and manganese (among copper miners). Drug-induced parkinsonism can follow therapy with metoclopramide (Reglan), reserpine, methyldopa, lithium, haloperidol (Haldol), and chlorpromazine. It can be seen after the use of illicit drugs, including amphetamine and methamphetamine. After stopping these drugs, symptoms of parkinsonism generally disappear. One notable exception is irreversible parkinsonism that follows exposure to the product of meperidine analog synthesis (MTPT). Other causes include hydrocephalus, other neurodegenerative disorders, hypoparathyroidism, infections, stroke, tumor, and trauma.

Many changes found in the brains of people with PD may play a part in development of the disease, including a lack of DA. The pathologic process of PD involves degeneration of the DA-producing neurons in the substantia nigra of the midbrain (Figs. 58.6 to 58.8). This in turn disrupts the normal balance between DA and acetylcholine (ACh) in the basal ganglia. The neurotransmitter DA is essential for normal functioning of the extrapyramidal motor system, including control of posture, support, and voluntary motion. Manifestations of PD do not occur until 80% of neurons in the substantia nigra are lost.

Unusual clumps of protein called *Lewy bodies* are found in the brains of patients with PD. It is not known what causes Lewy bodies to form. Their presence indicates abnormal brain functioning. Lewy body dementia is discussed in Chapter 59.

🧬 Genetic Link

We do not fully understand how genetic changes cause PD or influence the risk for developing PD. Around 15% of patients with PD have a family history of PD. Many autosomal dominant and recessive genes are linked to familial PD. Autosomal dominant PD is rare, affecting only 1% to 2% of people with PD. Examples include the *SNCA* and *LRRK2* genes.[25] Mutations in the *LRRK2* gene also appear to have a role in noninherited (sporadic) cases of PD. Recessive genes include parkin *(PARK2, PARK7),* and *PINK1.* Mutations in these genes are often associated with a younger age of disease onset. They also have more manifestations compared to those typically seen with age-related PD. *PINK1* mutations are related to a rare, early-onset form of PD.

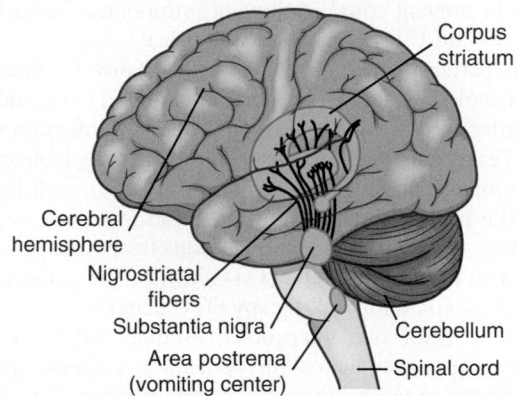

FIG. 58.6 Nigrostriatal disorders produce parkinsonism. Left-sided view of the human brain showing the substantia nigra and the corpus striatum *(shaded area)* lying deep within the cerebral hemisphere. Nerve fibers extend upward from the substantia nigra, divide into many branches, and carry dopamine to all regions of the corpus striatum.

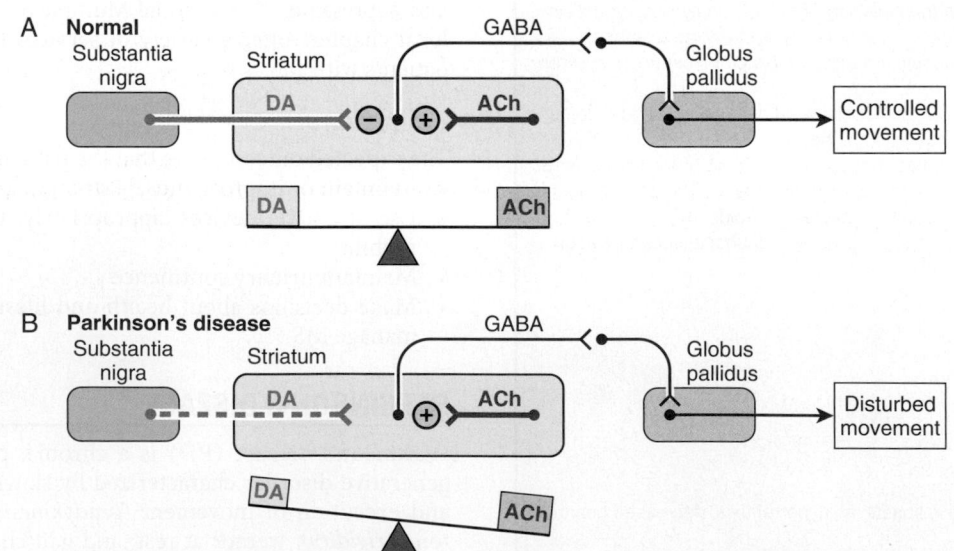

FIG. 58.7 A deficit in dopamine *(DA)* exists in Parkinson's disease. This deficit creates an imbalance between DA and the excitatory neurotransmitter acetylcholine. **A,** In a healthy person, DA released from neurons in the substantia nigra inhibits the firing of neurons in the striatum that release γ-aminobutyric acid *(GABA).* Conversely, neurons in the striatum, which release acetylcholine *(ACh),* excite the GABAergic neurons. Under normal conditions, inhibitory actions of DA are balanced by excitatory actions of ACh, and controlled movement results. **B,** In Parkinson's disease, neurons in the substantia nigra that supply DA to the striatum degenerate. When a deficit of DA occurs, excitatory effects of ACh go unopposed and disturbed movements (tremor, rigidity) result. (From Lehne RA: *Pharmacology for nursing care,* ed 8, St Louis, 2013, Saunders.)

Clinical Manifestations

The onset of PD is gradual, with an ongoing progression. Only 1 side of the body may be involved at first. Classic manifestations can be remembered by the mnemonic *TRAP* (**t**remor, **r**igidity, **a**kinesia, **p**ostural instability). Early in the disease, only a mild tremor, a slight limp, or a decreased arm swing may be seen. Later, the patient may have a shuffling gait and appear unable to stop. The patient's arms are flexed, and postural reflexes seem to be lost. The patient may have speech problems *(hypokinetic dysarthria)* that can affect communication and quality of life.

Tremor. *Tremor* is often the first sign. It may be minimal at first, so the patient is the only one who notices it. This tremor can affect handwriting, causing it to trail off, especially toward the ends of words. Parkinsonian tremor is more prominent at rest. It is worsened by emotional stress or increased concentration. The hand tremor is described as "pill rolling" because the thumb and forefinger appear to move in a rotary fashion as if rolling a pill, coin, or other small object. Tremor can involve the diaphragm, tongue, lips, and jaw. It rarely causes shaking of the head.

Unfortunately, in many people a benign *essential tremor* is mistakenly diagnosed as PD. Essential tremor occurs during voluntary movement, has a more rapid frequency than parkinsonian tremor, and is often familial.

Rigidity. *Rigidity* is the increased resistance to passive motion when the limbs are moved through their range of motion (ROM). Parkinsonian rigidity is typified by a jerky quality *(cogwheel rigidity),* as if there were occasional catches in the passive movement of a joint. Sustained muscle contraction causes the rigidity and results in muscle soreness; feeling tired and achy; or pain in the head, upper body, spine, or legs. Slow movement is another result of rigidity because the alternating contraction and relaxation in opposing muscle groups (e.g., biceps and triceps) is inhibited.

Akinesia. *Akinesia* is the absence or loss of control of voluntary muscle movements. In PD, *bradykinesia* (slowness of movement) is especially evident in the loss of automatic movements. This occurs because of the physical and chemical change of the basal ganglia and other structures in the extrapyramidal portion of the CNS. In the unaffected patient, automatic movements are involuntary and occur subconsciously. They include blinking of the eyelids, swinging of the arms while walking, swallowing saliva, using facial and hand movements for self-expression, and making minor movements to adjust posture.

The patient with PD does not perform these movements and lacks natural activity. This accounts for the stooped posture, masked face (deadpan expression), drooling of saliva, and shuffling gait *(festination)* that are typical of a person with PD. The posture is that of a slowed "old man" image, with the head and trunk bent forward and the legs constantly flexed (Fig. 58.9).

Postural Instability. *Postural instability* is common. Patients may describe being unable to stop themselves from going forward *(propulsion)* or backward *(retropulsion)*. Assessment of postural instability includes the "pull test." The examiner stands behind the patient and gives a tug backward on the shoulder, causing the patient to lose their balance and fall backward.

Many nonmotor symptoms are common. They include depression, anxiety, apathy, fatigue, pain, urinary retention, constipation, erectile dysfunction, and memory changes. Sleep problems are common. They include difficulty staying asleep at night, restless sleep, nightmares, and drowsiness or sudden sleep onset during the day. Rapid eye movement (REM) sleep behavior disorder is a preparkinsonian state that occurs in about one third of patients with PD. It is characterized by violent dreams and potentially dangerous motor activity during REM sleep. It may cause harm to the patient or bed partner.[26]

Complications

As PD progresses, complications increase. These include motor symptoms (e.g., dyskinesias [spontaneous, involuntary movements], weakness, neurologic problems (e.g., dementia), and neuropsychiatric problems (e.g., depression, hallucinations, psychosis). As PD progresses, dementia often results and is associated with increased mortality.

As swallowing becomes more difficult (dysphagia), malnutrition or aspiration may result. Increasing weakness may lead to pneumonia, UTIs, and skin breakdown. Orthostatic hypotension is common. Along with loss of postural reflexes, it can cause falls or other injury. The patient's increased fall risk means caregivers must be aware of environmental conditions that may contribute to falls.

Diagnostic Studies

Because no specific diagnostic test exists for PD, diagnosis is based on the patient's history and clinical features. Clinical diagnosis requires the presence of TRAP and asymmetric onset. Confirmation of PD is a positive response to antiparkinsonian drugs (levodopa or DA agonist). MRI and CT have a limited role in diagnosis of PD because they do not show a specific pathologic finding. However, they can rule out a stroke or brain tumor.

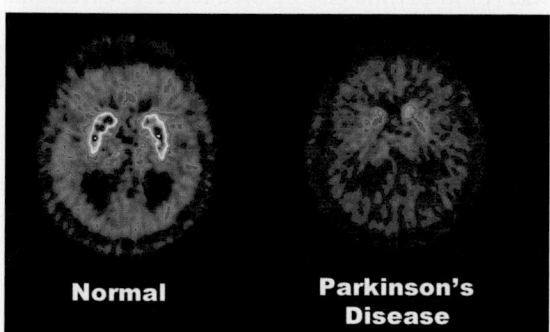

FIG. 58.8 In Parkinson's disease, PET scan showing reduced fluorodopa uptake in the basal ganglia *(right)* compared with a normal control *(left)*. (From Aminoff MJ, Daroff RB: *Encyclopedia of the neurological sciences,* Waltham, MA, 2003, Academic Press.)

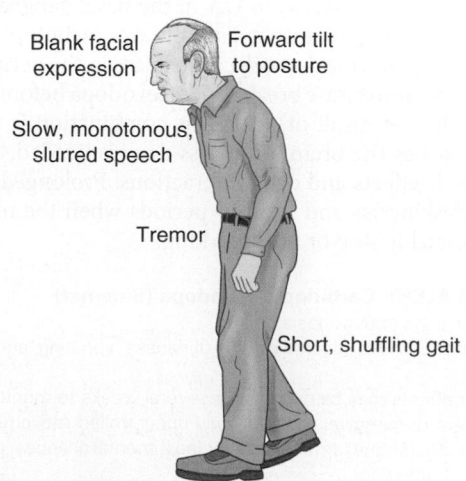

FIG. 58.9 Characteristic appearance of a patient with Parkinson's disease.

EVIDENCE-BASED PRACTICE

Exercise and Parkinson's Disease

You are a nurse working with T.K, a 77-yr-old man who has had Parkinson's disease (PD) for 5 years. You note he has a moderate tremor, shuffling gait, and decreased arm flexion. He asks you what types of physical activity he can do to improve his mobility and balance.

Making Clinical Decisions

Best Available Evidence. Patients with mild to moderately severe PD have improvements in gait performance and health-related quality of life after taking part in exercise programs. Facility-based programs produce greater effects on improving balance and mobility over the short and long term. Exercise training to improve balance and gait ability may prevent falls in people with PD.

Clinician Expertise. You know it is important to promote and encourage patients with PD to take part in physical exercise to help improve or maintain functional mobility and prevent falls. You are aware that we should design exercise programs around physical activities the person enjoys.

Patient Preferences and Values. T.K. says that in years past, he enjoyed dancing with his wife and currently likes to walk in his neighborhood.

Implications for Nursing Practice

1. What information will you provide to T.K. about muscle atrophy and joint contractures and the importance of physical activity?
2. How will you help T.K. and his wife in exploring community resources and programs related to physical activities that support his interests?

References for Evidence

Lee JH, Choi M, Yoo Y: A meta-analysis of nonpharmacological interventions for people with Parkinson's disease, *Clin Nurs Res* 26:608, 2017.

Shen X, Wong-Yu IS, Mak MK: Effects of exercise on falls, balance, and gait ability in Parkinson's disease: A meta-analysis, *Neurorehabil Neural Repair* 30:512, 2016.

Interprofessional Care

Because PD has no cure, interprofessional care focuses on symptom management (Table 58.15).

Drug Therapy. Drug therapy for PD is aimed at correcting the imbalance of neurotransmitters within the CNS. Antiparkinsonian drugs either enhance the release or supply of DA (dopaminergic) or block the effects of the overactive cholinergic neurons in the striatum (anticholinergic) (Fig. 58.7). Levodopa with carbidopa (Sinemet) is the primary treatment for symptomatic patients. Levodopa is a chemical precursor of DA and can cross the blood-brain barrier. It is converted to DA in the basal ganglia. Sinemet is the preferred drug because it also contains carbidopa, an agent that inhibits the enzyme dopa-decarboxylase in the peripheral tissues. Dopa-decarboxylase breaks down levodopa before it reaches the brain. The net result of using this combination is that more levodopa reaches the brain. Thus less drug is needed. Levodopa has many side effects and drug interactions. Prolonged use often results in dyskinesias and "off/on" periods when the medication will unpredictably stop or start working.

 DRUG ALERT Carbidopa/Levodopa (Sinemet)

- Monitor for signs of dyskinesia.
- Monitor for short-term adverse effects of nausea, vomiting, and light-headedness.
- Stress that effects may be delayed for several weeks to months.
- Teach patient or caregiver to report any uncontrolled movement of face, eyelids, mouth, tongue, arms, hands, or legs; mental changes; palpitations; and difficulty urinating.
- Do not give levodopa with food because protein reduces absorption.

Many patients receive Sinemet early in the disease course for the management of motor symptoms. However, some HCPs think that, after a few years of therapy, the effectiveness of Sinemet wears off. Therefore they prefer to start therapy with a DA receptor agonist, a drug that directly stimulates DA receptors. Ropinirole (Requip) and pramipexole (Mirapex) may be used alone or in combination with Sinemet. Many of these medications are available in extended-release forms that improve patients' ability to adhere to treatment plans. Rotigotine (Neupro), another DA receptor agonist, is available as a transdermal patch applied once daily. It is an adjunctive therapy for patients taking Sinemet.

 DRUG ALERT Pramipexole (Mirapex)

- Take the drug with food to decrease nausea.
- Notify the HCP immediately if uncontrollable urges, confusion, muscle rigidity, excess urination, shortness of breath, or vision changes occur.

The antiviral agent amantadine is a weak antagonist of NMDA-type glutamate receptors. It increases DA release and blocks DA reuptake. It may be useful as a single therapy for early PD. It can be used later with levodopa. As a single treatment, amantadine often becomes less effective after a few months.[27] Withdrawal of amantadine even after extended therapy can worsen dyskinesia.

Anticholinergic drugs, such as trihexyphenidyl and benztropine (Cogentin), decrease the activity of ACh, providing balance between cholinergic and dopaminergic actions.[27] Antihistamines (e.g., diphenhydramine) with anticholinergic properties may be used to manage tremors.

Selegiline (Eldepryl), rasagiline (Azilect), and safinamide (Xadago) are monoamine oxidase type B (MAO-B) inhibitors that may be used in combination with Sinemet.[27] By inhibiting MAO-B, the enzyme that degrades DA, these agents increase the levels of DA and prolong the half-life of levodopa. Rasagiline can be used alone as therapy in early PD. However, MAO-B inhibitors are less effective at treating motor symptoms than DA receptor agonists.

Entacapone (Comtan) and tolcapone (Tasmar) block the enzyme catechol *O*-methyltransferase (COMT), which breaks down levodopa in the peripheral circulation. Thus, they prolong the effect of Sinemet and are used only as adjuncts. They are often used when the patient's response to levodopa is wearing off at the end of the dosing interval. Tolcapone is rarely prescribed because it is associated with fatal hepatotoxicity.[27]

Rivastigmine (Exelon) or donepezil (Aricept) is used to treat dementia. Amitriptyline may be used to treat depression.

🧑‍🤝‍🧑 TABLE 58.15 Interprofessional Care

Parkinson's Disease

Diagnostic Assessment	Management
• History and physical examination	• Antiparkinsonian drugs (Table 58.16)
• TRAP (tremor, rigidity, akinesia, postural instability)	• Surgical therapy
• Positive response to antiparkinsonian drugs	• Deep brain stimulation
• MRI	• Ablation surgery
• Rule out side effects of phenothiazines, reserpine, benzodiazepines, haloperidol	• Physical therapy
	• Occupational therapy
	• Dietitian consult for nutritional therapy

Table 58.16 outlines the drugs commonly used in PD. The use of only 1 drug is preferred because fewer side effects occur and the drug dosage is easier to adjust than when several drugs are used. However, as PD progresses, combination therapy is often needed. Excessive amounts of dopaminergic drugs can worsen rather than relieve symptoms (*paradoxical intoxication*).

Within 3 to 5 years of standard PD treatments, many patients have episodes of hypomobility (e.g., inability to rise from chair, speak, or walk; also called *off episodes*). Off episodes can occur toward the end of a dosing interval with standard medications (so-called *end-of-dose wearing off*) or at unpredictable times (spontaneous "on/off"). A combination of carbidopa, levodopa, and entacapone (Stalevo) is available for patients with end-of-dose wearing off. It can be prescribed to make dosing easier, with 1 pill substituting for 3. Stalevo is typically prescribed for patients with advanced PD with intense motor fluctuations. The injectable DA receptor agonist apomorphine (Apokyn) can improve movement in hypomobility episodes. Apomorphine must be taken with an antiemetic drug because it causes severe nausea and vomiting when taken alone. It cannot be taken with antiemetics in the serotonin (5-HT3) receptor antagonist class (e.g., ondansetron [Zofran]). This combination can lead to very low BP and loss of consciousness.

TABLE 58.16 Drug Therapy

Parkinson's Disease

Drug	Mechanism of Action
Dopaminergics	
Dopamine Precursors	
levodopa (L-dopa) levodopa/carbidopa (Sinemet)	Converted to dopamine in basal ganglia
Dopamine Receptor Agonists	
pramipexole (Mirapex) ropinirole (Requip, Requip XL) rotigotine (Neupro [transdermal patch])	Stimulate dopamine receptors
Dopamine Agonists	
amantadine	Blocks NMDA-type glutamate receptors, increases dopamine release, and blocks dopamine reuptake
apomorphine (Apokyn)	Stimulates postsynaptic dopamine receptors
Anticholinergics	
benztropine (Cogentin) trihexyphenidyl	Block cholinergic receptors, thus helping to balance cholinergic and dopaminergic activity
Antihistamine	
diphenhydramine	Has anticholinergic effect
Monoamine Oxidase Inhibitors	
rasagiline (Azilect) safinamide (Xadago) selegiline (Eldepryl)	Block breakdown of dopamine
Catechol O-Methyltransferase (COMT) Inhibitors	
entacapone (Comtan) tolcapone (Tasmar)	Block COMT and slow the breakdown of levodopa, thus prolonging the action of levodopa

Surgical Therapy. Surgical procedures to relieve symptoms of PD are usually used in patients who are not responsive to drug therapy or who have developed severe motor complications. Surgical procedures fall into 3 categories: deep brain stimulation (DBS), ablation (destruction), and transplantation. The most common surgical treatment is DBS. This involves placing an electrode in the thalamus, globus pallidus, or subthalamic nucleus and connecting it to a generator placed in the upper chest (similar to a pacemaker) (Fig. 58.10). The device is programmed to deliver a specific current to the targeted brain location. DBS is preferred to ablation procedures because it is reversible and programmable. It can be safely done bilaterally. DBS reduces the increased neuronal activity produced by DA depletion. It can improve motor function and reduce dyskinesia and medication use. DBS is most effective when patients are carefully selected and screened.[27]

Ablation surgery involves finding, targeting, and destroying an area of the brain affected by PD. The goal is to destroy tissue that produces abnormal chemical or electrical impulses leading to tremors or other symptoms. Typical targets of ablation are the thalamus (*thalamotomy*) and globus pallidus (*pallidotomy*).[27] Newer treatments, such as the gamma knife and focused ultrasound, are noninvasive options.

Transplantation of fetal neural tissue into the basal ganglia was designed to provide DA-producing cells in the brains of patients with PD. Research of this therapy was largely abandoned after mixed results over several decades. In the last few years, better transplant techniques have renewed interest in this as a potential option.

Nutritional Therapy. Diet is of major importance to patients with PD because malnutrition and constipation can result from poor nutrition. Patients who have dysphagia and bradykinesia need appetizing foods that are easy to chew and swallow. The diet should contain adequate fiber and fruit to reduce constipation.

Eating 6 small meals a day may be less tiring than eating 3 large meals a day. Plan ample time for eating to avoid frustration. Cut food into bite-sized pieces. Protein ingestion and vitamin B_6 can impair the absorption of levodopa. Limiting protein intake to the evening meal can decrease this problem. They may need to consult with the HCP about including vitamin B_6 in a multivitamin and fortified cereals.

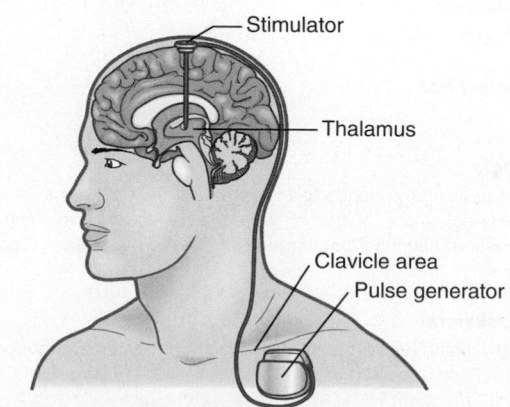

FIG. 58.10 Deep brain stimulation (DBS) can be used to treat tremors and uncontrolled movements of Parkinson's disease. Electrodes are surgically placed in the brain and connected to a neurostimulator (pacemaker device) in the chest.

❖ NURSING MANAGEMENT: PARKINSON'S DISEASE

◆ Nursing Assessment

Subjective and objective data that should be obtained from a patient with PD are outlined in Table 58.17.

◆ Nursing Diagnoses

Nursing diagnoses for the patient with PD may include:

- Impaired physical mobility
- Impaired nutritional status
- Risk for fall-related injury
- Impaired sleep pattern

Additional information on nursing diagnoses and interventions for the patient with PD is presented in eNursing Care Plan 58.4 (available on the website for this chapter).

TABLE 58.17 Nursing Assessment

Parkinson's Disease

Subjective Data
Important Health Information
Past health history: CNS trauma, cerebrovascular disorders, exposure to metals and carbon monoxide, encephalitis or other infections
Medications: Major tranquilizers, especially haloperidol (Haldol), and phenothiazines, reserpine, methyldopa, amphetamines

Functional Health Patterns
Health perception–health management: Fatigue
Nutritional-metabolic: Excessive salivation, dysphagia, weight loss
Elimination: Constipation, incontinence, excessive sweating
Activity-exercise: Difficulty in initiating movements, frequent falls, loss of dexterity, micrographia (handwriting deterioration)
Sleep-rest: Insomnia, nightmares, daytime sleepiness
Cognitive-perceptual: Diffuse pain in head, shoulders, neck, back, legs, and hips. Muscle soreness and cramping
Self-perception–self-concept: Depression, mood swings, hallucinations

Objective Data
General
Blank (masked) facial expression, slow and monotonous speech, infrequent blinking

Integumentary
Seborrhea, dandruff; ankle edema

Cardiovascular
Postural hypotension

Gastrointestinal
Drooling

Neurologic
Tremor at rest, first in hands (pill rolling), later in legs, arms, face, and tongue. Aggravation of tremor with anxiety, absence in sleep. Poor coordination, cognitive impairment and dementia, impaired postural reflexes

Musculoskeletal
Cogwheel rigidity, dysarthria, bradykinesia, contractures, stooped posture, shuffling gait

Possible Diagnostic Findings
No specific tests. Diagnosis based on history and physical findings and ruling out of other diseases

◆ Planning

The overall goals are that the patient with PD will (1) maximize neurologic function, (2) maintain independence in ADLs for as long as possible, and (3) optimize psychosocial well-being.

◆ Nursing Implementation

Because PD is a chronic degenerative disorder with no acute exacerbations, teaching and nursing care are directed toward maintaining good health, encouraging independence, and avoiding complications, such as contractures and falls. Problems due to bradykinesia can be addressed by relatively simple measures.

❓ CHECK YOUR PRACTICE

You are working in a rehabilitation facility with a new patient, a 78-yr-old man with Parkinson's disease. He was at your facility briefly 6 months ago with a fractured hip after falling in his yard. The family has asked to talk with you about their fear of taking him for a walk in the hallways because he is so unstable.

- What advice would you give to the family?

Promoting physical exercise and a well-balanced diet are major nursing concerns. Exercise can limit the effects of decreased mobility, such as muscle atrophy, contractures, and constipation. The American Parkinson Disease Association (*www.apdaparkinson.org*) publishes booklets and fact sheets with helpful exercises that can be used by caregivers and health care professionals.

A physical therapist can design a personal exercise program to strengthen and stretch specific muscles. Overall muscle tone and specific exercises to strengthen the muscles involved with speaking and swallowing should be included. Although exercise will not stop disease progress, it will enhance the patient's functional ability. An occupational therapist can help the patient with ways to increase self-care measures, including eating and dressing.

⚠ SAFETY ALERT Preventing Falls
For patients who are at risk for falling and tend to "freeze" while walking, have them do the following:
- Consciously think about stepping over an imaginary object on the floor.
- Rock from side to side before stepping forward.
- Walk to a beat, such as with music.
- Try to swing both arms from front to back.
- Take 1 step backward and 2 steps forward.

Work closely with the patient's caregivers to find creative ways to promote independence and self-care. The patient can get out of a chair better by using an upright chair with arms and placing the back legs of the chair on small (2-inch) blocks. Encourage environmental changes to improve safety. These include removing rugs and excess furniture to avoid stumbling, using an elevated toilet seat to help the patient get on and off the toilet, and elevating the legs of an ottoman to decrease dependent ankle edema. Clothing can be simplified by using slip-on shoes and Velcro hook-and-loop fasteners or zippers on clothing, instead of buttons.

Effective management of sleep problems can greatly improve the quality of life for patients with PD. Some patients find the use of satin nightwear or satin sheets helpful. Information on teaching about sleep hygiene practices is discussed in Chapter 7.

In the early stages of PD, many patients have depression and anxiety. Patients need to adjust their lifestyle, including work and home responsibilities. As PD progresses, the impact on the patient's psychologic well-being increases. Assist the patient by listening, providing teaching, gently correcting distorted thoughts, and encouraging social interactions. Psychologic therapy and counseling can be helpful. Ensure that patients with PD receive prescribed medications on time to avoid on-off effects.

In the early stage of PD, the patient may have subtle changes in cognitive function that can progress to dementia. This causes increased caregiver burden and may lead to long-term care placement. Information on care of the patient with dementia is provided in Chapter 59.

Family members (e.g., spouse, children) care for most patients with PD. Their burden increases as the disease progresses. This often occurs while the caregiver's physical and mental health also decline. Help them find appropriate resources.

◆ Evaluation

The expected outcomes are that the patient with PD will
- Maintain optimal muscle function
- Use assistive devices appropriately for ambulation and mobility
- Maintain nutritional intake adequate for metabolic needs
- Have unimpaired swallowing of fluids and/or solids
- Use methods of communication that allow interaction with others

MYASTHENIA GRAVIS

Myasthenia gravis (MG) is an autoimmune disease of the neuromuscular junction marked by fluctuating weakness of certain skeletal muscle groups. This weakness increases with muscle use. MG can occur in anyone. An estimated 60,000 people have MG in the United States. In women, the MG starts before age 40 years. Men usually develop MG after age 60.[28]

Etiology and Pathophysiology

MG is caused by an autoimmune process in which antibodies attack ACh receptors. This results in fewer ACh receptor (AChR) sites at the neuromuscular junction. This prevents ACh molecules from attaching to receptors and stimulating muscle contraction. Anti-AChR antibodies are found in the serum of 90% of patients with generalized MG. In the 10% of patients who lack autoantibodies to AChR, muscular weakness may be related to autoantibodies to muscle-specific tyrosine kinase or to other unknown antigens.[29] Thymic hyperplasia and tumors are common in patients with MG, suggesting autoantibody production occurs in the thymus.[28]

Clinical Manifestations and Complications

The key feature is fluctuating weakness of skeletal muscles. MG usually affects multiple muscle groups. This includes muscles used to move the eyes and eyelids, chew, swallow, speak, and breathe. Muscles are generally strongest in the morning and become exhausted with continued activity. Muscle weakness is prominent by the end of the day. A period of rest usually restores strength.

In more than half of patients, the first muscles involved are the ocular muscles, causing ptosis (drooping of the eyelids) in 1 or both eyes and double vision (Fig. 58.11).[29] MG does not progress beyond the ocular muscles in about 20% of patients. When facial muscles are affected, facial mobility and expression can be impaired. Patients may have difficulty chewing and swallowing food. Speech is affected, and the voice often fades after a long conversation. The muscles of the trunk and limbs are sometimes affected. Of these, the proximal muscles of the neck, shoulder, and hip are more often affected than the distal muscles. No other neural problems accompany MG. No sensory loss occurs, reflexes are normal, and muscle atrophy is rare.

The course of MG is highly variable. Some patients may have short-term remissions, and others may stabilize. Others may have severe, progressive involvement. Fatigue, pregnancy, illness, trauma, temperature extremes, stress, and hypokalemia can exacerbate MG. Certain drugs, including β-adrenergic blockers, quinidine, phenytoin (Dilantin), certain anesthetics, and aminoglycoside antibiotics, can worsen MG.[29]

Myasthenic crisis is an acute worsening of muscle weakness triggered by respiratory infection, surgery, emotional distress, pregnancy, exposure to certain drugs, or beginning treatment with corticosteroids. The major complications of MG result from muscle weakness in areas that affect swallowing and breathing. This results in aspiration, respiratory insufficiency, and respiratory tract infection.

Diagnostic Studies

The diagnosis of MG can be made based on history and physical examination. Other tests may be used for confirmation. EMG may show a decreased response to repeated stimulation of the hand muscles that shows muscle fatigue. Single-fiber EMG is sensitive in confirming MG. Use of drugs and serologic testing for specific antibodies is useful.

The response to a Tensilon test can indicate MG. A patient with MG has rapid improvement in muscle strength after IV injection of edrophonium chloride (Tensilon). Edrophonium is an anticholinesterase agent. It blocks the enzyme acetylcholinesterase, the enzyme that breaks down ACh. This test also helps diagnose a cholinergic crisis (from an overdose of anticholinesterase drug), which occurs due to excessive cholinesterase inhibition. In a cholinergic crisis, edrophonium may increase muscle weakness. Atropine, a cholinergic antagonist, should be readily available to counteract the effects of edrophonium when it is used diagnostically. In patients with a confirmed diagnosis of MG, a chest CT scan may be done to evaluate the thymus.

Interprofessional Care

Drug Therapy. Drug therapy for MG includes anticholinesterase drugs, alternate-day corticosteroids, and immunosuppressants

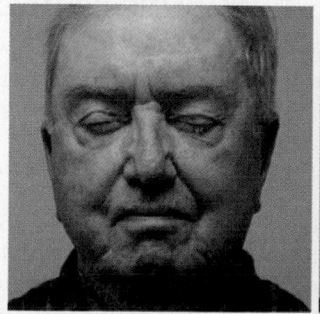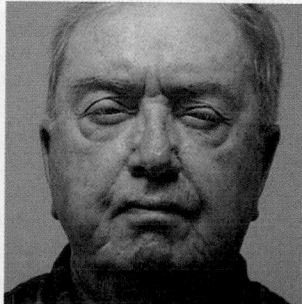

FIG. 58.11 "Peek" sign in myasthenia gravis. During sustained forced eyelid closure, he is unable to bury his eyelashes *(left)* and, after 30 sec, he is unable to keep the lids fully closed *(right)*. (From Sanders DB, Massey JM: Clinical features of myasthenia gravis. In AG Engel, ed: *Neuromuscular junction disorders: Handbook of clinical neurology,* New York, 2008, Elsevier.)

TABLE 58.18 Interprofessional Care

Myasthenia Gravis

Diagnostic Assessment	Management

• History and physical examination
• Fatigability with prolonged upward gaze (2–3 min)
• Muscle weakness
• EMG
• Tensilon test
• Acetylcholine receptor antibodies
• Chest x-ray
	• Drug therapy
	  • Anticholinesterase agents
	  • Corticosteroids
	  • Immunosuppressive agents
	• Surgery (thymectomy)
	• Plasmapheresis
	• IV immunoglobulin G

TABLE 58.19 Comparison of Myasthenic and Cholinergic Crises

Myasthenic Crisis	Cholinergic Crisis
Causes	
Exacerbation of myasthenia after precipitating factors, failure to take drug as prescribed, or drug dose too low	Overdose of anticholinesterase drugs resulting in ↑ acetylcholine at the receptor sites, remission (spontaneous or after thymectomy)
Differential Diagnosis	
Improved strength after IV administration of anticholinesterase drugs	Weakness within 1 hr after ingestion of anticholinesterase drugs
↑ Weakness of skeletal muscles manifesting as ptosis, bulbar signs (e.g., difficulty swallowing, difficulty articulating words), or dyspnea	↑ Weakness of skeletal muscles manifesting as ptosis, bulbar signs, dyspnea Effects on smooth muscle include pupillary miosis, salivation, diarrhea, nausea or vomiting, abdominal cramps, ↑ bronchial secretions, sweating, or lacrimation

(Table 58.18). Anticholinesterase drugs enhance transmission at the neuromuscular junction. Inhibiting acetylcholinesterase with an anticholinesterase inhibitor prolongs the action of ACh and improves impulse transmission at the neuromuscular junction. Pyridostigmine (Mestinon) is the most successful drug of this group in the long-term treatment of MG.

Tailoring the dose to avoid a myasthenic or cholinergic crisis often presents a clinical challenge. Corticosteroids (specifically prednisone) are used to suppress the immune response. Other drugs used for immunosuppression include azathioprine (Imuran), mycophenolate (CellCept), and cyclosporine (Sandimmune). Up to 80% of patients who receive corticosteroids have complete cessation of symptoms or marked improvement. Some patients become weaker for a brief time before regaining strength. These benefits must be weighed with concerns about chronic use of these medications.

Surgical Therapy. Because the thymus gland in the patient with MG appears to enhance the production of AChR antibodies, removing the thymus gland causes improvement in most patients. Thymectomy is indicated for almost all patients with thymoma, patients with generalized MG between puberty and about age 65 years, and patients with purely ocular MG.

Other Therapies. Plasmapheresis and IV immunoglobulin G can yield short-term improvement in symptoms. They are indicated for patients in myasthenic crisis or in preparation for surgery when corticosteroids must be avoided. Plasmapheresis directly removes circulating AChR antibodies, leading to a decrease in symptoms. (Plasmapheresis is discussed in Chapter 13.) It is not certain how IV immunoglobulin works. It is probably related to a decrease in antibody production.

❖ NURSING MANAGEMENT: MYASTHENIA GRAVIS

◆ Nursing Assessment

Assess the severity of MG by asking the patient about fatigue, what body parts are affected, and how severely they are affected. Some patients become so fatigued they are no longer able to work or even walk. Assess the patient's coping abilities and understanding of MG.

Obtain a thorough medication history. Many drugs are contraindicated or must be used with caution in patients with MG. Classes of drugs that should be carefully evaluated before use include β-adrenergic blockers, quinidine, phenytoin (Dilantin), certain anesthetics, and aminoglycoside antibiotics.[29]

Objective data should include respiratory rate and depth, O_2 saturation, arterial blood gas analyses, and pulmonary function tests. Assess for any evidence of respiratory distress in patients with acute myasthenic crisis. Assess muscle strength of all face and limb muscles, swallowing, speech (volume and clarity), and cough and gag reflexes.

◆ Nursing Diagnoses

Nursing diagnoses for the patient with MG may include:
- Impaired airway clearance
- Activity intolerance
- Risk for aspiration
- Disturbed body image

◆ Planning

The overall goals are that the patient with MG will (1) have a return of normal muscle strength, (2) manage fatigue, (3) avoid complications, and (4) maintain a quality of life appropriate to the disease course.

◆ Nursing Implementation

The patient with MG who is admitted to the hospital usually has a respiratory tract infection or is in acute myasthenic crisis. Nursing care is aimed at maintaining adequate ventilation, continuing drug therapy, and watching for side effects of therapy. Be able to distinguish cholinergic from myasthenic crisis (Table 58.19) because the causes and treatment of these conditions differ greatly. Features of a cholinergic crisis include involuntary muscle contraction, sweating, excessive salivation, and constricted pupils.

As with other chronic illnesses, focus care on the neurologic deficits and their impact on daily living. Teach the patient about a balanced diet that can easily be chewed and swallowed. Semisolid foods may be easier to eat than solids or liquids. Scheduling doses of drugs to reach peak action at mealtime may make eating easier. Arrange diversional activities that need little physical effort and match the patient's interests. Help the patient plan ADLs to avoid fatigue. Focus teaching on adherence to the treatment plan, complications, potential adverse reactions to specific drugs, complications of therapy (crisis conditions), and what to do about them. Explore community resources, such as the Myasthenia Gravis Foundation of America and MG support groups.

◆ **Evaluation**

The expected outcomes are that the patient with MG will

- Maintain optimal muscle function
- Be free from side effects of drugs
- Have no complications (myasthenic or cholinergic crises) from MG
- Maintain a quality of life appropriate to the disease course

AMYOTROPHIC LATERAL SCLEROSIS

Amyotrophic lateral sclerosis (ALS) is a rare progressive neuromuscular disorder marked by loss of motor neurons. ALS usually leads to death 2 to 5 years after diagnosis, but a few patients may survive for more than 10 years. This disease became known as *Lou Gehrig's disease* after the famous baseball player was stricken with it in 1939. Perhaps the best-known patient with ALS is British theoretical physicist Stephen Hawking. He was diagnosed at age 21 years and lived with ALS for over 50 years, dying at age 76. The typical onset is between age 55 and 75 years. ALS is most common in whites, men, and veterans of the Gulf War. About 20,000 Americans have ALS.[30]

In ALS, motor neurons in the brainstem and spinal cord gradually degenerate for unknown reasons. Dead motor neurons cannot produce or transport signals to muscles. Consequently, electrical and chemical messages originating in the brain do not reach the muscles to activate them.

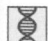 **Genetic Link**

About 5% to 10% of ALS cases are genetic. Mutations in more than a dozen genes have been found to cause familial ALS (FALS). One gene is "chromosome 9 open reading frame 72," or *C9ORF72*. People with FALS from a *C9ORF72* mutation often develop ALS earlier. This same gene also causes frontotemporal dementia (FTD). A few people have both ALS and dementia (ALS-FTD). Other times FALS results from mutations in the gene that gives instructions to make the enzyme copper-zinc superoxide dismutase 1 (*SOD1*).[31]

Progressive muscle weakness and atrophy are the classic sign of ALS. Early symptoms of weakness vary. For some, symptoms initially affect the arms or legs ("limb-onset" ALS). The person may have trouble with tasks requiring fine motor skills (e.g., writing, typing) or notice they are tripping, dropping things, or stumbling more often. Those who first have problems with slurred speech or swallowing have "bulbar onset" ALS.

Muscle wasting and involuntary contractions result from the denervation of the muscles and lack of stimulation and use. Other symptoms include pain, sleep disorders, spasticity and hyperreflexia, drooling, emotional lability, constipation, and esophageal reflux. ALS does not affect a patient's intelligence but affected people may have depression and problems with decision making and memory. Death often results from compromised respiratory function due to muscle weakness and paralysis.

No cure exists for ALS. Treatment options are limited. Riluzole (Rilutek) slows the progression of ALS. This drug reduces damage to motor neurons by decreasing the release of glutamate (an excitatory neurotransmitter) in the brain. Edaravone (Radicava), approved by FDA in May 2017, is the first new drug treatment for ALS in 20 years. This drug is given IV daily for 14 days, followed by a 14-day drug-free period. Subsequent dosing is over 10 to 14 days, again followed by a 14-day drug-free period. Edaravone is a free radical scavenger that we think relieves effects of oxidative stress, a likely factor in progression of ALS.[32]

The illness trajectory for ALS is devastating because the patient is cognitively intact while wasting away. Guide the patient in the use of moderate-intensity, endurance-type exercises for the trunk and limbs because this may help to reduce ALS spasticity. Nursing interventions include (1) facilitating communication, (2) reducing aspiration risk, (3) early identification of respiratory insufficiency, (4) decreasing pain from muscle weakness, (5) decreasing risk for fall-related injury, and (6) providing diversional activities, such as reading and companionship.

Support the patient and caregivers emotionally. This includes grieving related to the loss of motor function and impending death. Discuss advance directives and artificial methods of ventilation with the patient and caregiver.

HUNTINGTON'S DISEASE

Huntington's disease (HD) is a progressive, degenerative brain disorder. It is a genetically transmitted, autosomal dominant disorder. The offspring of a person with HD have a 50% risk for inheriting it. The onset of HD is usually between ages 30 and 50 years. Diagnosis is often made after the affected person has had children. About 25,000 to 30,000 Americans are symptomatic and 150,000 or more are at risk for HD.[33] It affects men and women equally across races.

The diagnostic process begins with a review of the family history and clinical symptoms. Genetic testing confirms the disease in a person with symptoms. People who are asymptomatic but who have a positive family history of HD must decide if they want genetic testing. If the test is positive, the person will develop HD. However, when the disease will develop cannot be determined.

Like PD, the pathologic process of HD involves the basal ganglia and extrapyramidal motor system. However, instead of a deficiency of DA, HD involves a deficiency of the neurotransmitters ACh and γ-aminobutyric acid (GABA). The net effect is an excess of DA, which leads to symptoms that are the opposite of those of parkinsonism.

Manifestations include movement disorder and cognitive and psychiatric problems. The movement disorder is marked by abnormal and excessive involuntary movements *(chorea)*. These are writhing, twisting movements of the face, limbs, and body. The movements get worse as the disease progresses. Because facial movements involving speech, chewing, and swallowing are affected, aspiration and malnutrition are likely. The gait deteriorates, and ambulation eventually becomes impossible. Eventually all psychomotor processes, including the ability to eat and talk, are impaired.

Psychiatric symptoms are often present in the early stage of HD, even before the onset of motor symptoms. Depression is common. Other psychiatric symptoms include anxiety,

GENETICS IN CLINICAL PRACTICE

Huntington's Disease (HD)

Genetic Basis
- Autosomal dominant disorder.
- Caused by mutation in *HTT* gene found on chromosome 4.
- A single copy of altered gene (heterozygous) is enough to cause HD.
- Offspring of a person with HD have a 50% chance of inheriting the disease-causing allele.

Incidence
- Occurs in 3 to 7 in 100,000 people of European ancestry.
- Less common in other populations, including people of Japanese, Chinese, and African descent.

Genetic Testing
- DNA testing is available.
- DNA testing can be done on fetal cells obtained by amniocentesis or chorionic villus sampling.
- Preimplantation genetic diagnosis can be done on embryos before implantation and pregnancy.
- No test is available to predict when symptoms will develop.

Clinical Implications
- Consider genetic counseling if there is a family history of HD.
- Because HD is an autosomal dominant disorder, those at risk have a strong motivation to seek genetic testing.
- A positive result is not considered a diagnosis because it may be obtained decades before symptoms begin.
- A negative test means the person does not carry the mutated gene and will not develop HD.

agitation, impulsivity, apathy, social withdrawal, and obsessiveness. Cognitive deterioration is more variable. It involves perception, memory, attention, and learning.

Death usually occurs 10 to 30 years after the onset of symptoms.[33] The most common cause of death is pneumonia, followed by suicide. Other causes of death include injuries related to falls and other complications.

Because HD has no cure, treatment is palliative. Drugs are available to control movements and behavioral problems. Tetrabenazine (Xenazine) is used to treat chorea. It decreases the amount of DA available at synapses in the brain and thus reducing the involuntary movements of chorea. If chorea is accompanied by other symptoms, tetrabenazine may not be the treatment of choice. For example, tetrabenazine can worsen depression. Deutetrabenazine (Austedo) is related to tetrabenazine. It is also approved for the treatment of chorea. Research suggests this drug is better tolerated than tetrabenazine.[34] Other medications for the movement disorder include neuroleptics (e.g., haloperidol, risperidone), benzodiazepines, and DA-depleting agents, such as reserpine.

Cognitive disorders are treated as needed with nondrug therapies (e.g., counseling, memory books). Psychiatric disorders can be treated with selective serotonin reuptake inhibitors, such as sertraline (Zoloft) and paroxetine (Paxil). Antipsychotic medication, such as haloperidol or risperidone, may be needed.

HD presents a great challenge to health care professionals. The goal of nursing management is to provide the most comfortable environment possible for the patient and caregiver by maintaining physical safety, treating physical symptoms, and providing emotional and psychologic support.

Because of the chorea, caloric requirements are high. The patient may need as many as 4000 to 5000 cal/day to maintain body weight. As HD progresses, meeting caloric needs becomes a greater challenge when the patient has difficulty swallowing and holding the head still. Depression and mental deterioration can compromise nutritional intake. Enteral or parenteral nutrition may be needed as the disease progresses.

End-of-life issues need to be discussed with the patient and caregiver. These include care in the home or long-term care facility, artificial methods of feeding, advance directives and cardiopulmonary resuscitation (CPR), use of antibiotics to treat infections, and guardianship. Address these topics throughout the course of the disease as the patient and caregiver adapt to increasing disability.

CASE STUDY

Seizure Disorder With Headache

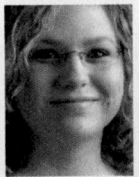

(© Purestock/ Thinkstock.)

Patient Profile

C.S. is a 24-yr-old woman who was diagnosed with seizure disorder at age 15. At that time, she had a generalized-onset tonic-clonic seizure and was given a prescription for valproate (Depakote). She had a second witnessed seizure 4 months later but has since been seizure free. C.S. now reports headaches and says she is afraid her seizures are going to return. She is single, lives alone, and describes her job as stressful.

Subjective Data
- Describes headache pain on the left side of her forehead as throbbing
- Has vomited with headache
- Describes changes in vision, including flashing lights
- Headache occurs nearly every month on a regular cycle

Objective Data
- Alert and oriented to person
- Neurologic examination negative
- Serum valproate levels within normal limits
- EEG normal
- CT of head normal

Discussion Questions

1. What is seizure disorder?
2. What is the pathophysiology of seizure disorder?
3. What is the significance of the laboratory and diagnostic findings?
4. Is the headache related to seizure activity?
5. **Safety:** To ensure C.S.'s safety, what nursing interventions are needed?
6. **Patient-Centered Care:** What teaching will you include in the plan of care for C.S. about the course of the disease?
7. **Priority Decision:** Based on the assessment data, what are the priority nursing diagnoses?
8. **Evidence-Based Practice:** Based on current treatment guidelines, what medication may be effective in managing both C.S.'s seizure disorder and her migraine headaches?
9. Develop a conceptual care map for C.S.

Answers available at *http://evolve.elsevier.com/Lewis/medsurg.*

BRIDGE TO NCLEX EXAMINATION

The number of the question corresponds to the same-numbered outcome at the beginning of the chapter.

1. A 50-yr-old man reports recurring headaches. He describes them as sharp, stabbing, and around his left eye. He says his left eye seems to swell and get teary when these headaches occur. Based on this history, you suspect he has
   a. cluster headaches.
   b. tension headaches.
   c. migraine headaches.
   d. medication overuse headaches.

2. A 65-yr-old woman was just diagnosed with Parkinson's disease. The priority nursing intervention is
   a. searching the Internet for educational videos.
   b. helping the caregiver explore respite care options.
   c. promoting physical exercise and a well-balanced diet.
   d. teaching about the benefits and risks of ablation surgery.

3. The nurse finds an 87-yr-old patient is continually rubbing, flexing, and kicking her legs throughout the day. The night shift reports this same behavior escalates at night, preventing her from obtaining sleep. The next step the nurse should take is to
   a. ask the provider for a daytime sedative for the patient.
   b. request soft restraints to prevent her from falling out of her bed.
   c. ask the provider for a nighttime sleep medication for the patient.
   d. perform an assessment, suspecting a disorder such as restless legs syndrome.

4. Possible social effects of a chronic neurologic disease include (select all that apply)
   a. divorce.
   b. job loss.
   c. depression.
   d. role changes.
   e. loss of self-esteem.

5. The nurse is reinforcing teaching with a patient newly diagnosed with amyotrophic lateral sclerosis (ALS). Which statement would be appropriate to include in the teaching?
   a. "Even though the symptoms you have are severe, most people recover with treatment."
   b. "ALS results from excess chemicals in the brain, so symptoms can be controlled with medication."
   c. "You need to consider advance directives now, because you will lose cognitive function as the disease progresses."
   d. "This is a progressing disease that eventually results in permanent paralysis, though you will not lose any cognitive function."

1. a, 2, c, 3, d, 4, a, b, c, d, e, 5, d

For rationales to these answers and even more NCLEX review questions, visit *http://evolve.elsevier.com/Lewis/medsurg*.

EVOLVE WEBSITE/RESOURCES LIST

http://evolve.elsevier.com/Lewis/medsurg
Review Questions (Online Only)
Key Points
Answer Keys for Questions
- Rationales for Bridge to NCLEX Examination Questions
- Answer Guidelines for Case Study on p. 1380
Student Case Studies
- Patient With Parkinson's Disease and Hip Fracture
- Patient With Seizures
Nursing Care Plans
- eNursing Care Plan 58.1: Patient With Headaches
- eNursing Care Plan 58.2: Patient With Seizure Disorder
- eNursing Care Plan 58.3: Patient With Multiple Sclerosis
- eNursing Care Plan 58.4: Patient With Parkinson's Disease
Conceptual Care Map Creator
- Conceptual Care Map for Case Study on p. 1380
Audio Glossary
Content Updates

REFERENCES

1. Headache Classification Committee of the International Headache Society: *The international classification of headache disorders*. Retrieved from *www.ichd-3.org/*.
2. Migraine Research Foundation: Migraines. Retrieved from *http://migraineresearchfoundation.org/about-migraine/migraine-facts/*.
3. May A, Schulte LH: Chronic migraine: Risk factors, mechanisms, and treatment, *Nat Rev Neurol* 12:8, 2016.
4. American Migraine Foundation: Understanding migraine with aura. Retrieved from *https://americanmigrainefoundation.org/understanding-migraine/understanding-migraine-aura/*.
5. American Migraine Foundation: The genetics of migraine. Retrieved from *https://americanmigrainefoundation.org/understanding-migraine/the-genetics-of-migraine/*.
6. American Migraine Foundation: Living with migraine. Retrieved from *https://americanmigrainefoundation.org/living-with-migraine/*.
7. Karsan N, Prabhakar P, Goadsby PJ: Premonitory symptoms of migraine in children and adolescents, *Curr Pain Headache Rep* 21:7, 2017.
8. American Migraine Foundation: Cluster headache. Retrieved from *https://americanmigrainefoundation.org/understanding-migraine/cluster-headache/*.
9. National Institute of Neurological Disorders and Stroke: Headache: Hope through research. Retrieved from *www.ninds.nih.gov/Disorders/Patient-Caregiver-Education/Hope-Through-Research/Headache-Hope-Through-Research*.
10. The Migraine Trust: Cluster headache. Retrieved from *www.migrainetrust.org/about-migraine/types-of-migraine/other-headache-disorders/cluster-headache/*.
11. Warren E: Neurological symptoms in primary care: Part 3: Headache, *Pract Nurs* 47:3, 2017.
12. Silberstein SD: Topiramate in migraine prevention: A 2016 perspective, *Headache* 57:1, 2017.
13. Centers for Disease Control and Prevention: Epilepsy fast facts. Retrieved from *www.cdc.gov/epilepsy/about/fast-facts.htm*.
14. Gaspard N: Autoimmune epilepsy, *CONTINUUM* 22:1, 2016.
15. Epilepsy Foundation: Genetic testing. Retrieved from *www.epilepsy.com/learn/diagnosis/genetic-testing*.
16. Fisher RS, Cross JH, D'Souza C, et al: Instruction manual for the ILAE 2017 operational classification of seizure types, *Epilepsia* 58:4, 2017.
*17. Hingray C, El-Hage W, Duncan R, et al: Access to diagnostic and therapeutic facilities for psychogenic nonepileptic seizures: An international survey by the ILAE PNES Task Force, *Epilepsia* 59:1, 2018.
18. Epilepsy Foundation: Status epilepticus. Retrieved from *www.epilepsy.com/information/professionals/about-epilepsy-seizures/classifying-seizures/status-epilepticus*.

*19. Glauser T, Shinnar S, Gloss D, et al: Evidence-based guideline: Treatment of convulsive status epilepticus in children and adults: Report of the Guideline Committee of the American Epilepsy Society, *Epilepsy Curr* 16:1, 2016.

*20. Harden C, Tomson T, Gloss D, et al: Practice guideline summary: Sudden unexpected death in epilepsy incidence rates and risk factors, *Neurol* 88:17, 2017.

21. National Institute of Neurological Disorders and Stroke: Restless legs syndrome fact sheet. Retrieved from *www.ninds.nih.gov/Disorders/Patient-Caregiver-Education/Fact-Sheets/Restless-Legs-Syndrome-Fact-Sheet*.

22. Multiplesclerosis.net: MS statistics. Retrieved from *http://multiplesclerosis.net/what-is-ms/statistics*.

23. National Multiple Sclerosis Society: What causes MS? Retrieved from *www.nationalmssociety.org/What-is-MS/What-Causes-MS*.

*24. Thompson AJ, Banwell BL, Barkhof F, et al: Diagnosis of multiple sclerosis: 2017 Revisions of the McDonald criteria, *Lancet* 391:1622, 2018.

25. Parkinson's Foundation: Statistics. Retrieved from *http://parkinson.org/Understanding-Parkinsons/Causes-and-Statistics/Statistics*.

*26. Jennum P, Christensen JA, Zoetmulder M: Neurophysiological basis of rapid eye movement sleep behavior disorder: Informing future drug development, *Nat Sci Sleep* 15:107, 2018.

27. Gonzalez-Usigli HA: Parkinson disease. Retrieved from *www.merckmanuals.com/professional/neurologic-disorders/movement-and-cerebellar-disorders/parkinson-disease#section_15*.

28. National Institute of Neurological Disorders and Stroke: Myasthenia gravis fact sheet. Retrieved from *www.ninds.nih.gov/Disorders/Patient-Caregiver-Education/Fact-Sheets/Myasthenia-Gravis-Fact-Sheet#4*.

29. Mayo Clinic: Myasthenia gravis. Retrieved from *www.mayoclinic.org/diseases-conditions/myasthenia-gravis/symptoms-causes/syc-20352036*.

30. ALS Association: ALS. Retrieved from *www.alsa.org/*.

31. National Institute of Neurological Disorders and Stroke: Amyotrophic lateral sclerosis fact sheet. Retrieved from *www.ninds.nih.gov/disorders/amyotrophiclateralsclerosis/detail_ALS.htm*.

32. Almeida MJ: Edaravone (Radicava) for amyotrophic lateral sclerosis. Retrieved from *https://alsnewstoday.com/edaravone-radicava-for-als/*.

33. Mayo Clinic: Huntington's disease. Retrieved from *www.mayoclinic.org/diseases-conditions/huntingtons-disease/symptoms-causes/syc-20356117*.

34. Heo YA, Scott LJ. Deutetrabenazine: A review in chorea associated with Huntington's disease, *Drugs* 77:1857, 2017.

*Evidence-based information for clinical practice.

59

Dementia and Delirium

Janice Smolowitz

You treat a disease you win, you lose. You treat a person,
I guarantee you'll win, no matter what the outcome.

Patch Adams

ⓔ http://evolve.elsevier.com/Lewis/medsurg

CONCEPTUAL FOCUS

Cognition	Functional Ability	Stress
Family Dynamics	Safety	

LEARNING OUTCOMES

1. Define *dementia* and *delirium*.
2. Classify the different etiologies of dementia.
3. Explain the pathophysiology for different types of dementia
4. Discuss the clinical manifestations of mild cognitive impairment.
5. Describe the clinical manifestations, diagnostic studies, and nursing and interprofessional care for a patient with dementia.
6. Discuss the clinical manifestations, diagnostic studies, and nursing and interprofessional care for a patient with Alzheimer's disease.
7. Explain the etiology, pathophysiology, clinical manifestations, diagnostic studies, and nursing and interprofessional care for a patient with delirium.

KEY TERMS

Alzheimer's disease (AD), p. 1386
delirium, p. 1398
dementia, p. 1383
dementia with Lewy bodies (DLB), Table 59.3, p. 1385

frontotemporal lobar degeneration (FTLD), Table 59.3, p. 1385
mild cognitive impairment (MCI), p. 1389
mixed dementia, p. 1384
neurofibrillary tangles, p. 1387

retrogenesis, p. 1388
sundowning, p. 1395

This chapter discusses the cognitive disorders of dementia and delirium, with a focus on the nursing management of patients with Alzheimer's disease (AD). Cognitive impairment refers to any deficit in intellectual functioning, including problems with memory, orientation, attention, and concentration. The consequences of cognitive impairment can be devastating for the person and caregivers. Ultimately, dementia adversely affects functional ability and the person's ability to work, fulfill responsibilities, and perform activities of daily living (ADLs). There is a high risk for many problems, including injury, impaired nutrition, and social isolation.

Persons with dementia and delirium may have symptoms of depression. Depression and dementia are often mistaken for each another, especially among older adults. Manifestations of depression, especially among older adults, may include sadness, difficulty concentrating, fatigue, apathy, feelings of despair, and inactivity. When depression is severe, poor concentration and attention may result, causing memory and functional impairment. When dementia and depression occur together there can be marked intellectual deterioration. Table 59.1 compares key features of dementia, delirium, and depression. Your ability to interview the patient and family members about presenting symptoms and signs can aide in early diagnosis and treatment.

DEMENTIA

Dementia is a disorder characterized by a decline from previous level of function in 1 or more cognitive domains: complex attention, executive function, language, learning and memory, perceptual-motor, and social cognition.[1] The cognitive decline interferes with ability to function and perform daily activities. This decline does not occur with onset of an acute state of confusion, such as delirium, or the onset of another major mental disorder, such as depression.

As the average life span increases, the number of patients diagnosed with dementia is increasing. AD is the most common form of dementia. It accounts for 60% to 80% of all cases of dementia (Fig. 59.1). In 2018, 5.7 million Americans over age 65 were living with AD. We expect this number to reach 14 million by 2050.[2]

TABLE 59.1 Comparison of Dementia, Delirium, and Depression

Feature	Dementia	Delirium	Depression
Onset	Usually insidious	Abrupt, although initially can be subtle	Often coincides with life changes. Often abrupt
Progression	Slow	Abrupt. Can fluctuate from day to day	Variable, rapid to slow but may be uneven
Duration	Years (average of 8 yr but can be much longer)	Hours to days to weeks. Can be prolonged in some	Can be several months to years, especially if not treated
Thinking	Difficulty with abstract thinking, impaired judgment, words difficult to find	Disorganized, distorted. Slow or accelerated incoherent speech	Intact but with apathy, fatigue. May be indecisive. Feels sense of hopelessness. May not want to live
Perception	Misperceptions often present. Delusions and hallucinations	Distorted. Delusions and hallucinations	May deny or be unaware of depression. May have feelings of guilt
Psychomotor behavior	May pace or be hyperactive. As disease progresses, may not be able to perform tasks or movements when asked	Variable. Can be hyperactive or hypoactive, or mixed	Often withdrawn and hypoactive
Sleep-wake cycle	Sleeps during day. Frequent awakenings at night. Fragmented sleep	Disturbed sleep. Reversed sleep-wake cycle	Disturbed, often with early morning awakening

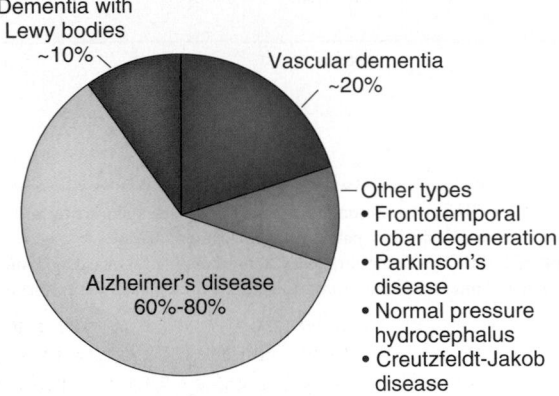

FIG. 59.1 Causes of dementia.

Dementia with Lewy bodies ~10%

Vascular dementia ~20%

Alzheimer's disease 60%-80%

Other types
- Frontotemporal lobar degeneration
- Parkinson's disease
- Normal pressure hydrocephalus
- Creutzfeldt-Jakob disease

Etiology and Pathophysiology

Dementia is caused by treatable and untreatable conditions. Table 59.2 describes the types of dementia and their underlying causes. Treatable causes may initially be reversible. However, with prolonged exposure or disease, irreversible changes may occur.

The most common causes of dementia are neurodegenerative conditions that cannot be reversed (Table 59.3). Most of these are due to AD. Other causes include dementia with Lewy bodies (DLB), frontotemporal dementia (FTD), and Parkinson's disease with dementia (PDD). Vascular, or multiinfarct dementia (VaD), is a loss of cognitive function caused by cardiovascular disease (CVD). The prevalence of VaD is higher among blacks and those with hypertension and diabetes. VaD may be caused by a single infarct (stroke) or multiple strokes.

Mixed dementia occurs when 2 or more types of dementia are present at the same time. It is characterized by the hallmark abnormalities of AD and another type of dementia. Usually the other type of dementia is VaD, but it can be other types.

Normal pressure hydrocephalus is a rare disorder characterized by an obstruction in the flow of cerebrospinal fluid (CSF). This causes a buildup of CSF in the brain. Manifestations include dementia, urinary incontinence, and difficulty walking. Meningitis, encephalitis, or head injury may cause the condition. If diagnosed early, it is treatable by surgery in which a shunt is inserted to divert the fluid away from the brain.

TABLE 59.2 Causes of Dementia

Type of Dementia	Cause
Neurodegenerative disorders	• AD • Amyotrophic lateral sclerosis (ALS) • Dementia with Lewy bodies (DLB) • Down syndrome • Frontotemporal lobar degeneration (FTLD) • Huntington's disease • Parkinson's disease
Vascular diseases	• Chronic subdural hematoma* • Subarachnoid hemorrhage* • Vascular (multiinfarct) dementia
Immunologic diseases or infections	• Multiple sclerosis • Systemic exertion intolerance disease • Infections (e.g., Creutzfeldt-Jakob disease) • Acquired immunodeficiency syndrome (AIDS) • Meningitis* • Encephalitis* • Neurosyphilis* • Systemic lupus erythematosus*
Medications†	• Anticholinergics • Antiparkinsonian drugs • Cardiac drugs: digoxin, methyldopa • Cocaine • Heroin • Hypnotics • Opioids • phenytoin (Dilantin) • Tranquilizers
Metabolic or nutritional diseases	• Alcohol use disorder • Cobalamin (vitamin B_{12}) deficiency* • Folate deficiency* • Hyperthyroidism* • Hypothyroidism* • Thiamine (vitamin B_1) deficiency*
Systemic diseases	• Dialysis dementia* • Hepatic encephalopathy* • Uremic encephalopathy* • Wilson's disease
Trauma	• Head injury*
Tumors	• Brain tumors (primary)* • Metastatic tumors*
Ventricular disorders	• Hydrocephalus*

*Potentially reversible.
†These are examples of drugs that may cause cognitive impairment that is potentially reversible.

TABLE 59.3 Neurodegenerative Causes of Dementia

Neurodegenerative Disorder	Characteristics	Management
Dementia With Lewy Bodies (DLB) • Characterized by presence of Lewy bodies (abnormal deposits of protein α-synuclein) in brainstem and cortex • Has features of both AD and Parkinson's disease. • Imperative that a correct diagnosis is made	• Diagnosis is based on manifestations • Typically have manifestations of parkinsonism (extrapyramidal signs [bradykinesia, rigidity, postural instability, but not always a tremor]), hallucinations, short-term memory loss, unpredictable cognitive shifts, and sleep problems • Pneumonia is a common complication	• Drugs may include levodopa/carbidopa and acetylcholinesterase inhibitors • Manage dementia and problems related to dysphagia and immobility • Swallowing problems can lead to impaired nutrition • At risk for falls from impaired mobility and balance
Down Syndrome • Genetic disorder caused by presence of all or part of a third copy of chromosome 21	• Typically associated with physical growth delays, characteristic facial features, and mild to moderate intellectual disability	• Much higher risk for developing dementia • Estimated 80% will develop dementia
Frontotemporal Lobar Degeneration (FTLD) • Associated with atrophy of frontal and temporal lobes of brain • In Pick's disease, a type of FTLD, brain may have abnormal microscopic deposits called *Pick bodies* • Often misdiagnosed as a psychiatric problem because of strange behaviors	• Changes in behavior, sleep, and eventually memory • Progresses relentlessly and may lead to language impairment, erratic behavior, and dementia • Tends to occur at a younger age than does AD, typically about age 60	• No specific treatment • Antidepressants and antipsychotics to treat behavioral manifestations
Parkinson's Disease, Huntington's Disease, and Amyotrophic Lateral Sclerosis • Chronic, progressive, and incurable diseases	• Associated with development of dementia in the later stages of disease	• See Chapter 58

Clinical Manifestations

The onset of manifestations varies depending on the cause. Manifestations associated with neurologic degeneration usually occur gradually and progress over time. Symptoms of VaD may appear abruptly or progress in a stepwise pattern. While the cause of dementia cannot be determined based only on the history of symptom progression, patterns can guide your thinking about the different causes. An acute change that occurs over days to weeks or subacute change that occurs over weeks to months may indicate an infectious or metabolic cause of dementia, such as encephalitis, meningitis, hypothyroidism, or drug-related dementia. Other manifestations of dementia are discussed in the section on clinical manifestations of AD on p. 1387.

Diagnostic Studies

The diagnosis of dementia is focused on determining the cause (e.g., reversible versus irreversible factors). An important first step is a thorough medical, neurologic, and psychologic history. During the history, special attention is given to reviewing the cognitive and behavioral changes that have occurred. Family members and significant others can give important information. Elicit information about (1) problems with judgment; (2) reduced interest in hobbies/activities; (3) repeating questions, stories, or statements; (4) trouble learning how to use a tool or appliance; (5) forgetting the correct month or year; (6) problems handling financial affairs; (7) difficulty remembering appointments; and (8) consistent problems with thinking and/or memory.

Obtain a complete medication history, including the use of prescribed and over-the-counter medications, herbal supplements, and recreational substances. Ask about drugs that can impair cognition, such as analgesics, anticholinergics, psychotropics, and sedative-hypnotics.

A thorough physical assessment is done to rule out other potential medical conditions. For example, slow movement, rigidity, asymmetric tremor of an extremity, and shuffling gait are suggestive of Parkinsonism. Dementia, urinary incontinence, and ataxic gait suggest normal pressure hydrocephalus. The neurologic assessment includes a mental status examination or screening test. Agreement among findings from the assessment, screening tests, and history can help confirm the presence of dementia.

Based on history and physical assessment findings, diagnostic studies are ordered to confirm the most likely cause and exclude other possible conditions. The American Academy of Neurology (AAN) recommends routine screening tests, including an electrolyte panel, liver function tests, serum vitamin B_{12} level, complete blood count, and thyroid function tests.[3] Specialized laboratory tests, such as red blood cell folate in a patient with alcoholism or ionized serum calcium in a patient with multiple myeloma, are ordered based on history. Neuroimaging with a head CT or MRI scan is important for patients with acute onset of cognitive impairment, rapid neurologic deterioration, or findings that suggest a subdural hematoma, thrombotic stroke, or cerebral hemorrhage.

❖ Interprofessional and Nursing Care

Management of patients with dementia is similar to the management of patients with AD, which is described later in this chapter. Preventive measures for VaD include treatment of risk factors, such as hypertension, diabetes, smoking, hypercholesterolemia, and dysrhythmias. Stroke is discussed in Chapter 57. Drugs that are used for patients with AD are also useful for patients with VaD. Drug therapy is discussed on p. 1392 later in this chapter.

ALZHEIMER'S DISEASE

Alzheimer's disease (AD) is a chronic, progressive, neurodegenerative brain disease. It is thought that 11% of people age 65 and older, and nearly one third of those over age 85, have AD. Only a small number of people younger than 60 years of age develop AD. When AD develops in someone younger than 60 years, it is referred to as *early-onset AD*. AD that occurs in people over 60 years old is called *late-onset AD*.

Ultimately the disease is fatal. Death typically occurs 4 to 8 years after diagnosis, although some patients have lived for 20 years. AD is the sixth leading cause of death in the United States.[2] It is the only cause of death among the top 10 in the United States that cannot be prevented or cured, nor its progression slowed.

The burden of caring for a patient with AD is well documented. 25% of AD caregivers are caring for both someone with the disease and a child or grandchild. 60% of family caregivers describe high or very high emotional stress.[2] More than 1 in 6 family caregivers report they had to stop working due to caregiving responsibilities. 74% of caregivers described becoming "somewhat concerned" to "very concerned" about maintaining their own health since becoming caregivers.

GENDER DIFFERENCES
Alzheimer's Disease and Dementia

Men
- Men have a higher incidence of VaD than women.

Women
- Nearly two thirds of people with AD are women.
- Women are more likely to develop AD than men, mainly because they live longer.
- About twice as many women as men die each year from AD.

🌐 PROMOTING HEALTH EQUITY
Alzheimer's Disease

- Older blacks are about twice as likely to have AD as older whites.
- Older Hispanics are about 1½ times as likely to have AD as older whites.
- Variations in health, lifestyle, and socioeconomic risk factors across ethnic groups account for most of the differences in risk.
- Increased rates of CVD and diabetes may be related to the increased prevalence of AD in blacks and Hispanics.
- Lower levels of education and other socioeconomic characteristics may increase risk.[2]

Source: Alzheimer's Association: 2018 Alzheimer's disease facts and figures, *Alzheimers Dement* 14:367, 2018.

Etiology

The exact cause of AD is unknown. It is likely a combination of multiple factors.

Aging. The greatest risk factor for AD is age. Most people with AD are diagnosed at age 65 or older. While age is the greatest risk factor, AD is not a normal part of aging and age alone does not cause the disease.[2]

Family History. Family history of AD is an important risk factor.[1] Persons with a first-degree relative (parent or sibling) with dementia are more likely to develop the disease. Those who have more than 1 first-degree relative with dementia are at even higher risk for developing AD.

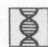 Genetic Link

Persons with a clear pattern of inheritance within a family have familial AD (FAD). FAD is associated with onset before age 60 and a more rapid disease course. Cases are referred to as sporadic when there is no familial connection. The pathogenesis of FAD and sporadic AD is similar.

The first gene associated with late-onset and sporadic forms of AD was the epsilon (E)-4 allele of the apolipoprotein E *(ApoE)* gene on chromosome 19. *ApoE* contains the instructions to make a protein that helps to carry cholesterol and other types of fat in the bloodstream. *ApoE* may have a role in clearing amyloid plaques. Mutations in this gene result in more amyloid deposits.

ApoE comes in several different alleles or forms. Three alleles occur most often. People inherit 1 allele (e.g., *ApoE-2, ApoE-3, ApoE-4*), from each parent. The presence of *ApoE-4*, which is a risk-factor gene, increases the risk for developing late-onset AD. *ApoE* testing is controversial. Not all people with *ApoE-4* develop AD. Among patients with dementia who meet the clinical criteria for AD, finding *ApoE-4* increases the reliability of diagnosis.

In patients with early-onset AD, 3 genes have been identified as important: presenilin-1 *(PSEN1)*, presenilin-2 *(PSEN2)*, and amyloid precursor protein *(APP)* (see the Genetics in Clinical Practice box). When these genes mutate, they cause brain cells to overproduce β-amyloid.[2] *PSEN1* mutations cause AD before age 60 and often before age 50. *PSEN2* causes early-onset FAD.

Cardiovascular Factors. Brain health is closely linked to the health of the heart and blood vessels. Brain functioning depends on a good blood supply and nutrients delivered to it by that blood supply.

Many factors increase the risk for CVD. These include diabetes, hypertension, obesity, hypercholesterolemia, and smoking. Diabetes dramatically increases the risk for developing AD and other types of dementia. Diabetes can contribute to dementia in several ways. Chronic high levels of insulin and glucose may be directly toxic to brain cells. Insulin resistance, which causes high blood glucose and can lead to type 2 diabetes, may interfere with the body's ability to break down amyloid, a protein that forms brain plaques in AD. High blood glucose and high cholesterol have a role in atherosclerosis, which contributes to VaD.[4]

Diabetes may contribute to poor memory and decreased mental function in other ways. The disease causes microangiopathy, which damages small blood vessels throughout the body. Ongoing damage to blood vessels in the brain may be one reason why people with diabetes are at a higher risk for cognitive problems as they age.[5] People with diabetes may lose brain volume, especially gray matter, as the disease progresses.

Head Trauma. Head trauma is a risk factor for dementia. Professional football players and military veterans who had traumatic brain injury or posttraumatic stress disorder have an increased risk for AD and other types of dementia.[6]

Pathophysiology

Characteristic findings of AD related to changes in the brain's structure and function include (1) amyloid plaques, (2) neurofibrillary tangles, (3) loss of connections between neurons, and (4) neuron death.[7] Fig. 59.2 shows the pathologic changes in AD.

As part of aging, people develop some plaques in their brain tissue. In AD, more plaques appear in certain parts of

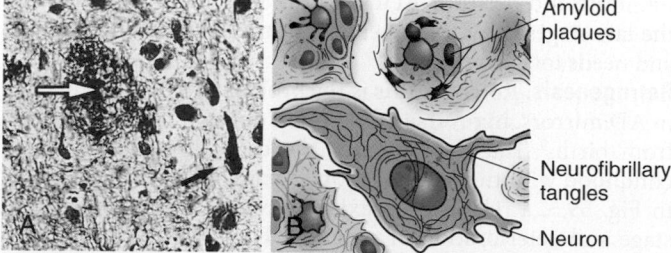

FIG. 59.2 Pathologic changes in AD. **A,** Plaque with central amyloid core *(white arrow)* next to a neurofibrillary tangle *(red arrow)* on the histologic specimen from a brain autopsy. **B,** Schematic representation of amyloid plaque and neurofibrillary tangle.

the brain. These plaques consist of clusters of insoluble deposits of a protein called β-amyloid, other proteins, remnants of neurons, non-nerve cells such as microglia (cells that surround and digest damaged cells or foreign substances), and other cells, such as astrocytes.

β-Amyloid is cleaved from amyloid precursor protein (APP), which is associated with the cell membrane (Fig. 59.3). The normal function of APP is unknown. Genetic factors may play a critical role in how the brain processes the β-amyloid protein. Overproduction of β-amyloid is an important risk factor for AD. Abnormally high levels of β-amyloid cause cell damage either directly or by eliciting an inflammatory response and ultimately neuron death.

In AD, plaques develop first in areas of the brain used for memory and cognitive function, including the hippocampus (a structure that is important in forming and storing short-term memories). Eventually AD attacks the cerebral cortex, especially the areas responsible for language and reasoning.

Neurofibrillary tangles are abnormal collections of twisted protein threads inside nerve cells. The main component of these structures is a protein called tau. Tau proteins in the central nervous system (CNS) are involved in providing support for intracellular structure through their support of microtubules. Tau proteins hold the microtubules together like railroad ties. In AD tau protein is altered. As a result, the microtubules twist together in a helical fashion (Fig. 59.3). This ultimately forms the neurofibrillary tangles found in the neurons of people with AD.

Plaques and neurofibrillary tangles are not unique to patients with AD or dementia. They are also found in the brains of people without cognitive impairment. However, they are more abundant in the brains of those with AD.

The other feature of AD is the loss of connections between neurons and neuron death. These processes result in structural damage. Affected parts of the brain begin to shrink in a process called brain atrophy. By the final stage of AD, brain tissue has shrunk significantly (Fig. 59.4).

Clinical Manifestations

Research suggests AD causes pathologic changes in the brain at least 15 years before the manifestations of AD appear.[8] The Alzheimer's Association has developed a list of 10 warning signs that are common manifestations of AD (Table 59.4).

Symptoms do not always directly relate to abnormal changes in the brain caused by AD. The stages of AD can be categorized as mild, moderate, and severe (Table 59.5). The rate of progression from mild to severe is highly variable and ranges from 3 to 20 years.

The initial manifestations are usually related to changes in cognitive functioning. The person may have memory loss, mild disorientation, or trouble with words and numbers. Often a family member reports the patient's declining memory to the HCP.

Normal age-related memory decline is characterized by mild changes that do not interfere with ADLs (Table 59.6). In AD the memory loss initially relates to recent events, with remote memories still intact. With time and progression of AD, memory loss includes both recent and remote memory and affects the ability to perform self-care.

As AD progresses, personal hygiene deteriorates, as does the ability to concentrate and maintain attention. Ongoing loss of neurons in AD can cause the person to act in unpredictable ways. Behavioral manifestations, such as agitation or aggression, result from changes that take place within the brain. These behaviors are neither intentional nor controllable by the person with the disease. Some people develop delusions and hallucinations.

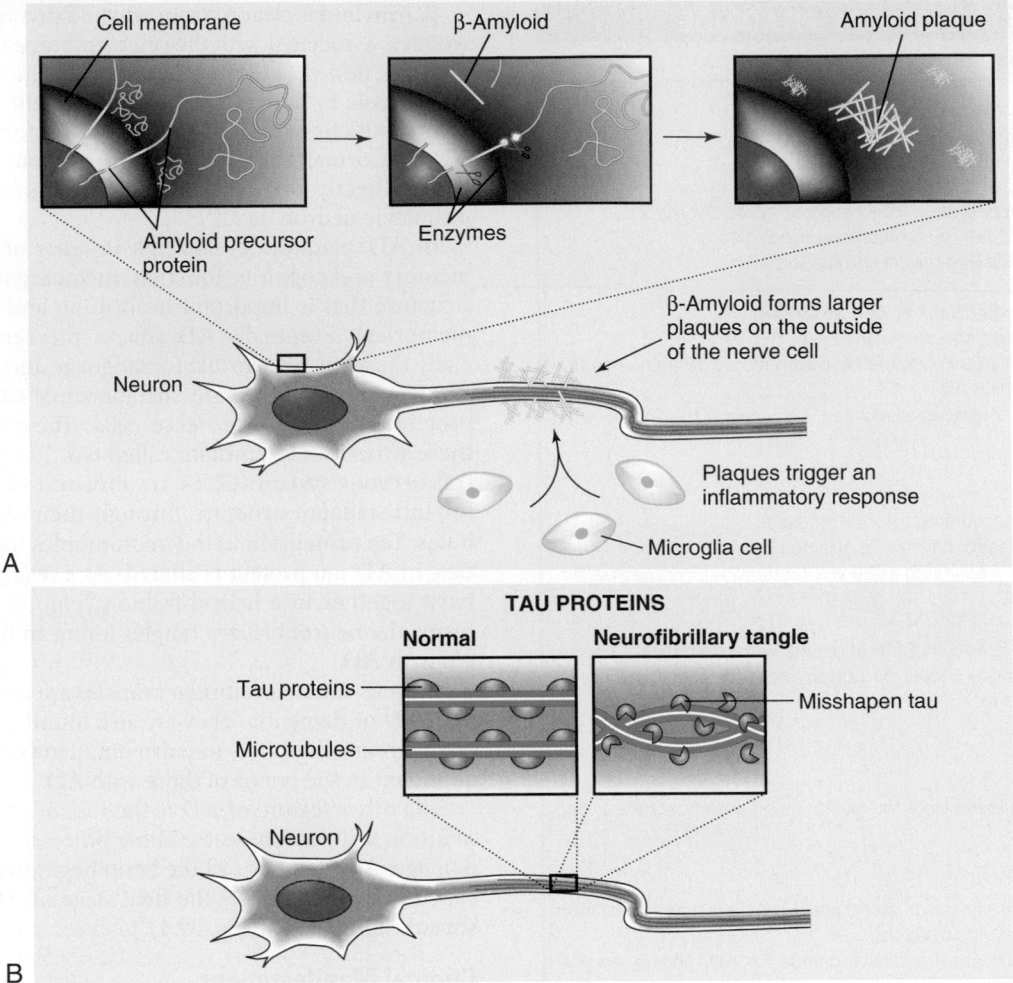

FIG. 59.3 Current theories about the development of AD. **A,** Abnormal amounts of β-amyloid are cleaved from the amyloid precursor protein *(APP)* and released into the circulation. The β-amyloid fragments come together in clumps to form plaques that attach to the neuron. Microglia react to the plaque, and an inflammatory response results. **B,** Tau proteins provide structural support for the neuron microtubules. Chemical changes in the neuron cause structural changes in tau proteins. This results in twisting and tangling (neurofibrillary tangles).

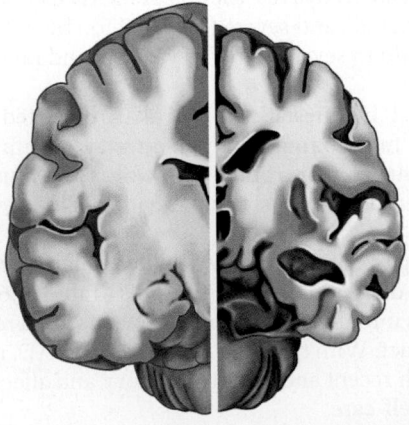

FIG. 59.4 Effects of AD on the brain. This figure compares a normal brain *(left)* with a brain affected by AD *(right)*.

With progression of AD, more cognitive impairments occur. These include dysphasia (difficulty comprehending language and oral communication), apraxia (inability to manipulate objects or perform purposeful acts), visual agnosia (inability to recognize objects by sight), and dysgraphia (difficulty communicating by writing). Eventually long-term memories cannot be recalled, and the person may not recognize family members and friends. Later in the disease, the ability to communicate and perform ADLs is lost. Some tend to wander. In the late stages of AD, the person is unresponsive, incontinent, and needs total care.

Retrogenesis. Retrogenesis is the process in which the decline in AD mirrors, in reverse order, brain development that occurs from birth.[9] Thus it compares the developmental stages of childhood with the deterioration of patients with AD. As seen in Fig. 59.5, a relationship exists between the developmental stage and deterioration of function. For example, it is appropriate for a patient with AD in the moderate stage to feel good about putting together puzzles that belong to his 3-yr-old grandson. In fact, they may play well together on the same task or project.

Diagnostic Criteria for Alzheimer's Disease

The National Institute on Aging and the Alzheimer's Association have criteria and guidelines for diagnosing AD.[10] Guidelines address the use of imaging and biomarkers that may help determine whether changes are due to AD.

TABLE 59.4 Patient & Caregiver Teaching

Early Warning Signs of Alzheimer's Disease

Include the following information in the teaching plan for the patient with Alzheimer's disease:

1. Memory loss that affects job skills
   - Frequent forgetfulness or unexplainable confusion at home or in the workplace may signal that something is wrong.
   - This type of memory loss goes beyond forgetting an assignment, colleague's name, deadline, or phone number.
2. Problems with abstract thinking
   - For the patient with AD, this goes beyond challenges, such as balancing a checkbook.
   - The patient with AD may not be able to recognize numbers or do basic calculations.
3. Difficulty doing familiar tasks
   - It is normal for most people to become distracted and to forget something (e.g., leave something on the stove too long).
   - People with AD may cook a meal, then forget not only to serve it but also that they made it.
4. Poor or decreased judgment
   - Many people from time to time may choose not to dress appropriately for the weather (e.g., not bringing a coat or sweater on a cold evening).
   - The patient with AD may dress inappropriately in more noticeable ways, such as wearing a bathrobe to the store or a sweater on a hot day.
5. Problems with language
   - Most people have trouble finding the "right" word from time to time.
   - People with AD may forget simple words or substitute inappropriate words, making their speech difficult to understand.
6. Misplacing things
   - For many people, temporarily misplacing keys, purses, or wallets is a normal, albeit frustrating, event.
   - The patient with AD may put items in inappropriate places (e.g., eating utensils in clothing drawers) but have no memory of how they got there.
7. Changes in mood
   - Most people have mood changes.
   - The patient with AD tends to have more rapid mood swings for no apparent reason.
8. Changes in personality
   - As most people age, they may have some change in personality (e.g., become less tolerant).
   - The patient with AD can change dramatically, either suddenly or over time. For example, someone who is easygoing may become angry, suspicious, or fearful.
9. Loss of initiative
   - The patient with AD may become and remain uninterested and uninvolved in many or all of his or her usual pursuits.

Adapted from Alzheimer's Association: *Early warning signs*, Chicago, The Association. Retrieved from *www.alz.org/alzheimers_disease_know_ the_10_signs.asp.*

AD is considered on a spectrum (Table 59.7). The stages are preclinical AD, mild cognitive impairment, and dementia due to AD.[10] Dementia marks the terminal stage of the disease.

Preclinical Stage. A long lag exists between pathologic changes in the brain and manifestations of AD. The future goal would be to modify the disease process of AD before it becomes symptomatic. Once plaques and tangles have formed in sufficient quantity, it may be too late to intervene to prevent the disease or its progression. Although current attempts at modifying the disease process have not been successful, research is ongoing.

Mild Cognitive Impairment. Mild cognitive impairment (MCI) is the second stage in the AD spectrum. It is a state of cognitive function in which persons have problems with memory, language, or other essential cognitive functions. The problems are severe enough to be noticed by the person having them and by others and can be found on screening tests. Family members may see changes in the person's abilities (Table 59.6). To the casual observer, the person with MCI may seem normal. Because the problems do not interfere with daily activities, the patient does not meet the criteria for being diagnosed with dementia.

We classify MCI based on the cognitive skills affected. MCI that primarily affects memory is called amnestic MCI. With amnestic MCI, a person may forget important information that they would have recalled easily, such as appointments. The person is often aware of the change in memory.

MCI that affects other cognitive skills is nonamnestic MCI. Skills that may be affected include the ability to make sound decisions or complete a complex task.[11]

Between 15% and 20% of people 65 years and older have MCI. They are at high risk for developing AD. Some people with MCI show no progression and do not go on to develop AD. An estimated 15% of people with MCI will eventually develop AD.[2]

No drugs have been approved for the treatment of MCI. There is little evidence that drugs used in AD, such as cholinesterase inhibitors, affect progression to dementia or improve cognitive test scores in people with MCI.[11]

The primary treatment of MCI consists of ongoing monitoring. Monitoring the patient with MCI for changes in memory and thinking skills that indicate a worsening of symptoms or a progression to AD or other dementia is critical (Table 59.4).

Diagnostic Studies

No definitive diagnostic test exists for AD. The diagnosis is primarily a diagnosis of exclusion. In patients with cognitive impairment, there is increased emphasis on early and careful evaluation. As discussed earlier, many conditions can cause

TABLE 59.5 Stages of Alzheimer's Disease

Mild	Moderate	Severe
• Forgetfulness beyond what is seen in a normal patient	• Memory loss and confusion become more obvious	• Severe impairment of all cognitive functions
• Short-term memory impairment, especially for new learning	• Has more trouble organizing, planning, and following directions	• Little memory, unable to process new information
• Loss of initiative and interests	• May need help getting dressed	• Unable to perform self-care activities
• May forget recent events or the names of people or things	• May start having episodes of incontinence	• Often needs help with daily needs
• Impatient	• Trouble recognizing family members and friends	• May not be able to talk
• May no longer be able to solve simple math problems	• Agitation, restlessness	• Cannot understand words
• Slowly loses the ability to plan and organize	• May lack judgment and begin to wander, gets lost	• May have problems eating, swallowing
	• May have trouble sleeping	• May not be able to walk or sit up without help
	• Delusions, hallucinations, paranoia	• Immobility
	• Behavioral problems	• Incontinence

TABLE 59.6 Comparison of Normal Forgetfulness and Memory Loss

Normal Forgetfulness	Memory Loss in Mild Cognitive Impairment	Memory Loss in Alzheimer's Disease
• Sometimes misplaces keys, eyeglasses, or other items	• Often misplaces items	• Forgets what an item is used for or puts it in an inappropriate place
• Momentarily forgets an acquaintance's name	• Often forgets people's names and is slow to recall them	• May not remember knowing a person
• Sometimes has to search for a word	• Has increasing difficulty finding desired words	• Begins to lose language skills and may withdraw from social interaction
• Sometimes forgets to run an errand	• Begins to forget important events and appointments	• Loses sense of time, does not know what day it is
• May forget an event from the distant past	• May forget recent events or newly learned information	• Seriously impaired recent memory and problems learning and remembering new information
• When driving, may momentarily forget where to turn, but quickly orients self	• Becomes temporarily lost more often, may have trouble understanding and following a map	• Becomes easily disoriented or lost in familiar places, sometimes for hours
• Jokes about memory loss	• Worries about memory loss, family and friends notice lapses	• May have little or no awareness of cognitive problems

Adapted from Rabins P: Memory. In *The Johns Hopkins white papers,* Baltimore, 2007, Johns Hopkins University.

Stage	Alzheimer's Disease	Reisberg Stage*	Developmental Age	Diversion/Distraction Activities
Mild	No difficulty at all	1		
	Some memory trouble begins to affect job/home. Forgets familiar names.	2		
	Much difficulty maintaining job performance. Withdrawal from difficult situations.	3	12+ yr	Can function with understanding. Enjoy things previously enjoyed—watch TV, play and listen to music, play games.
	Can no longer hold a job, plan and prepare meals, handle personal finances, etc. Driving becomes difficult, although can drive to familiar places.	4	8–12 yr	Can still enjoy simple games, watch TV and videos. Enjoys family photos and memories.
Moderate	Can no longer select proper clothing for occasion or season. Needs help to remain safe in home. Forgets to bathe.	5	5–7 yr	Needs age-appropriate toys and games.
	Requires assistance with dressing.	6a	4–5 yr	Enjoy many of the same activities as preschoolers.
	Requires assistance with bathing.	6b	4–5 yr	
	Can no longer use toilet without assistance.	6c	4 yr	
	Urinary incontinence	6d	3–4.5 yr	
	Fecal incontinence	6e	2–3 yr	
Severe	Speech now limited to about words per day.	7a	15 mo	Enjoys infant toys, mobiles, dangling ribbons.
	Speech now limited to 1 word per day.	7b	1 yr	
	Can no longer walk without assistance.	7c	1 yr	
	Can no longer sit up without assistance.	7d	6–10 mo	
	Can no longer smile.	7e	2–4 mo	
	Can no longer hold up head.	7f	1–3 mo	

FIG. 59.5 Retrogenesis (back to birth) in AD. (*Based on Functional Assessment Staging. From Reisberg B: Functional assessment staging [FAST], *Psychopharmacol Bull* 24:653, 1988.)

TABLE 59.7 Diagnostic Criteria for Alzheimer's Disease

	Stage and Description	Recommendations for Biomarkers
Preclinical Alzheimer's disease (AD)	• Brain changes, including amyloid buildup and other early neuron changes, may already be in process • At this point, significant symptoms are not yet evident • In some people, amyloid buildup can be detected with PET scans and cerebrospinal fluid (CSF) analysis	• Use of imaging and biomarker tests at this stage are recommended only for research • Biomarkers are still being developed and standardized, and are not used by clinicians in general practice
Mild cognitive impairment (MCI) due to AD	• MCI stage is marked by symptoms of memory problems, enough to be noticed and measured, but not compromising a patient's independence • May or may not progress to AD	• Used primarily by researchers • May be used in specialized clinical settings to supplement standard tests to help determine possible causes of MCI • May help confirm that the patient's impairment is related to AD
Dementia due to Alzheimer's disease	• Characterized by memory, thinking, and behavioral symptoms that impair a patient's ability to function in daily life • Dementia marks the terminal stage of AD • Encompasses all stages shown in Table 59.5	• Can increase the level of certainty about a diagnosis of AD • May be used to distinguish AD from other dementias

Source: National Institute on Aging: Diagnostic criteria for Alzheimer's disease. Retrieved from *www.nia.nih.gov/health/alzheimers-disease-diagnostic-guidelines*.

manifestations of dementia, some of which are treatable or reversible (Table 59.2).

When all other possible conditions that can cause cognitive impairment have been excluded, a clinical diagnosis of AD can be made. A comprehensive evaluation includes a complete health history, physical examination, neurologic and mental status assessments, and laboratory tests (Table 59.8). A definitive diagnosis of AD requires an examination of brain tissue at autopsy and findings of neurofibrillary tangles and plaques.

Neuroimaging techniques allow for detection of changes early in the disease and monitoring of treatment response. In AD, multiple brain structures atrophy and the volume of the brain correlates with neurodegeneration. Brain imaging tests, such as CT or MRI, may show brain atrophy in the later stages of the disease. This finding occurs in other diseases and can be seen in people without cognitive impairment. PET scanning can help distinguish AD from other forms of dementia (Fig. 59.6). PET determines brain metabolism using glucose tracers. PET can also detect amyloid.

Guidelines identify 2 biomarker categories: (1) biomarkers showing the level of β-amyloid accumulation in the brain and (2) biomarkers showing that nerve cells in the brain are injured or actually degenerating. Biomarkers include (1) CSF neurochemical markers: β-amyloid and tau proteins, and (2) imaging biomarkers: volumetric MRI and PET. The level of tau in the CSF is an indication of neurodegeneration. Plasma levels of tau or β-amyloid are not of any value in diagnosing AD.

Some imaging biomarkers are used in specialized clinical settings. CSF biomarkers are mainly used for research. Biomarkers may be used in some cases to increase the level of certainty about a diagnosis of AD and to distinguish AD from other dementias. However, we need to do more research with biomarkers before they can be routinely used in practice.

Neuropsychologic testing is important for diagnostic purposes and to establish a baseline for evaluating changes over time. They are repeated at regular intervals during the course of care to assess changes in the patient's cognitive status. Common tools include the Mini-Cog (Table 59.9), Mini-Mental State Examination (MMSE) (Table 59.10), and Montreal Cognitive Assessment (MoCA). Brief screenings, such as the Mini-Cog, are useful for ongoing screening, especially when time is limited. The clock drawing test can be used as part of the Mini-Cog or by itself to assess cognitive

TABLE 59.8 Interprofessional Care

Alzheimer's Disease

Diagnostic Assessment
• History and physical assessment, including psychologic evaluation
• Neuropsychologic testing, including Mini-Cog (Table 59.9), Mini-Mental State Examination (Table 59.10)
• Brain imaging tests: CT, MRI, MRS, PET
• CBC
• ECG
• Serum glucose, creatinine, blood urea nitrogen
• Serum levels of vitamins B_1, B_6, B_{12}
• Thyroid function tests
• Liver function tests
• Screening for depression

Management
• Drug therapy for cognitive problems (Table 59.11)
• Behavioral modification
• Moderate exercise
• Assistance with functional independence
• Assistance and support for caregiver

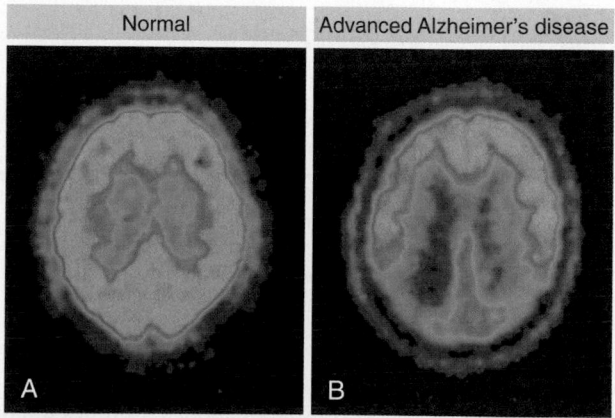

FIG. 59.6 PET scan assist in diagnosing AD. Radioactive fluorine is applied to glucose (fluorodeoxyglucose), and the yellow areas show metabolically active cells. **A,** A normal brain. **B,** Advanced AD is recognized by hypometabolism in many areas of the brain. (From Roberts GS: *Neuropsychiatric disorders,* London, 1993, Mosby-Wolfe.)

TABLE 59.9 The Mini-Cog

The Mini-Cog is used as a brief assessment tool for cognitive impairment. It can be quickly administered and can guide the need for further evaluation.

Administration

- Tell the patient to listen carefully to and remember 3 unrelated words and then to repeat the words. *Example:* apple, table, penny. (This initial step is not scored.) The same 3 words may be repeated to the patient up to 3 tries to register all 3 words.
- Tell the patient to draw the face of a clock, either on a blank sheet of paper or on a sheet with the clock circle already drawn on the page. After the patient puts the numbers on the clock face, ask them to draw the hands of the clock to read a specific time (11:10). The test is considered normal if all numbers are present in the correct sequence and position and the hands readably display the requested time.
- Ask the patient to repeat the 3 previously stated words.

Scoring (out of total of 5 points)

Give 1 point for each recalled word after the clock drawing test.
- Patients recalling none of the 3 words are classified as cognitively impaired (score = 0).
- Patients recalling all 3 words are classified as not cognitively impaired (score = 3).
- Patients with intermediate word recall of 1 or 2 words are classified on the clock drawing test:
  The clock drawing test is scored 2 if normal and 0 if abnormal.

Interpretation of results

0–2: Positive screen for dementia

3–5: Negative screen for dementia

Source: Borson S, Scanlan J, Brush M, et al: The Mini-Cog: A cognitive "vital signs" measure for dementia screening in multi-lingual elderly, *Intern J Geriatr Psychiatry* 15:1021, 2000.

TABLE 59.10 Mini-Mental State Examination (MMSE)

Sample Items

Orientation to Time

"What is the date?"

Registration

"Listen carefully, I am going to say 3 words. You say them back after I stop. Ready? Here they are . . . HOUSE (pause), CAR (pause), LAKE (pause). Now repeat those words back to me." (Repeat up to 5 times but score only the first trial.)

Naming

"What is this?" (Point to a pencil or pen.)

Reading

"Please read this and do what it says." (Show examinee the words CLOSE YOUR EYES on the stimulus form.)

Reproduced by special permission of the Publisher, Psychological Assessment Resource, Inc., 16204 North Florida Avenue, Lutz, FL. 33549, from the Mini-Mental State Examination, by Marshal Folstein and Susan Folstein, Copyright 1975, 1998, 2001 by Mini-Mental, LLC, Inc. Published 2001 by Psychological Assessment Resources, Inc. Further reproduction is prohibited without permission from PAR, Inc. The MMSE can be purchased from PAR, Inc., by calling 813-968-3003.

function (Fig. 59.7). The MMSE takes about 7 minutes to complete. It gives information about orientation, recall, attention, calculation, language manipulation, and constructional praxis. The MoCA takes about 10 minutes to do. It assesses memory, language, attention, visuospatial, and executive functions.

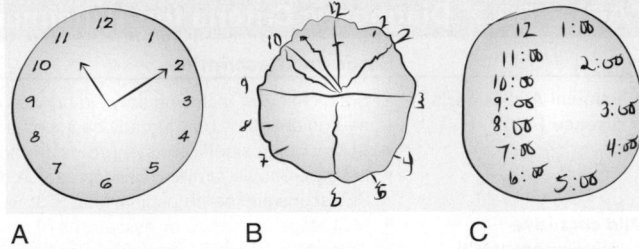

FIG. 59.7 Clock drawing is a simple test that can be used as an assessment technique in dementia. The patient is asked to draw a clock, put in all the numbers, and set the hands at 11:10. **A,** A clock drawn by a patient with no dementia. **B** and **C** Clocks drawn by people with AD. (Modified from Stern TA: *Massachusetts General Hospital comprehensive clinical psychiatry,* Philadelphia, 2008, Mosby.)

TABLE 59.11 Drug Therapy

Alzheimer's Disease

Problem	Drugs
Decreased memory and cognition	Cholinesterase inhibitors • donepezil (Aricept) • galantamine (Razadyne) • rivastigmine (Exelon) N-methyl-D-aspartate (NMDA) receptor antagonist • memantine (Namenda)
Depression	Selective serotonin reuptake inhibitors (SSRIs) • citalopram (Celexa) • fluoxetine (Prozac) • sertraline (Zoloft) • fluvoxamine (Luvox) Atypical antidepressants • mirtazapine (Remeron) • trazodone
Behavioral problems (e.g., agitation, physical aggression, disinhibition)	Antipsychotics* • aripiprazole (Abilify) • haloperidol (Haldol) • olanzapine (Zyprexa) • quetiapine (Seroquel) • risperidone (Risperdal) Benzodiazepines • clonazepam (Klonopin) • lorazepam (Ativan)
Sleep problems	• zolpidem (Ambien)

*The use of these drugs in older patients with dementia is associated with an increased risk for death.

Interprofessional Care

At this time there is no cure for AD. Treatment does not stop the deterioration of brain cells. Interprofessional care of patients with AD is aimed at controlling undesirable behavioral manifestations and providing support for family caregivers.

Drug Therapy. Although medication for AD is available (Table 59.11), these drugs do not cure or reverse the progression of the disease. They help many people for a period of time by leading to a modest decrease in the rate of decline of cognitive function. There is no effect on overall disease progression.[2]

Cholinesterase inhibitors block cholinesterase, the enzyme responsible for the breakdown of acetylcholine in the synaptic cleft (Fig. 59.8). Cholinesterase inhibitors include donepezil (Aricept), rivastigmine (Exelon), and galantamine (Razadyne). Rivastigmine is available as a patch.

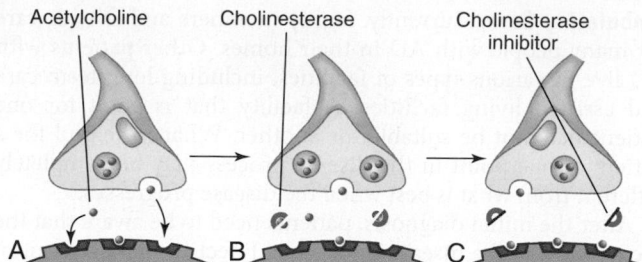

FIG. 59.8 Mechanism of action of cholinesterase inhibitors. **A**, Acetylcholine is released from the nerve synapses and carries a message across the synapse. **B**, Cholinesterase breaks down acetylcholine. **C**, Cholinesterase inhibitors block cholinesterase, thus giving acetylcholine more time to transmit the message.

Memantine (Namenda) protects the brain's nerve cells against excess amounts of glutamate, which is released in large amounts by cells damaged by AD. The attachment of glutamate to *N*-methyl-D-aspartate (NMDA) receptors permits calcium to flow freely into the cell, which in turn may lead to cell degeneration. Memantine may prevent this destructive sequence by blocking the action of glutamate.

Treating the depression that is often associated with AD may improve cognitive ability. Depression is often treated with selective serotonin reuptake inhibitors, including fluoxetine (Prozac), sertraline (Zoloft), fluvoxamine (Luvox), and citalopram (Celexa). The antidepressant trazodone may help with problems related to sleep.

Antipsychotic drugs approved for treating psychotic conditions have been used for the management of agitation and aggressive behavior, which occurs in some patients with AD. These drugs have been shown to increase the risk for death and cognitive decline in patients with AD. They should be used only in patients with AD when agitation and psychosis symptoms are severe, are dangerous, and/or cause significant distress to the patient.[12]

❖ NURSING MANAGEMENT: ALZHEIMER'S DISEASE

◆ Nursing Assessment

Subjective and objective data that should be obtained from a patient with AD are outlined in Table 59.12. Useful questions for the patient and caregiver are, "When did you first notice the memory loss?" and "How has the memory loss progressed since then?"

◆ Nursing Diagnoses

Nursing diagnoses for AD may include:
- Confusion
- Risk for injury
- Altered perception

Additional information on nursing diagnoses and interventions for the patient with AD is presented in eNursing Care Plan 59.1 (available on the website for this chapter).

◆ Planning

The overall goals are for the patient with AD to (1) maintain functional ability for as long as possible, (2) be in a safe environment with a minimum of injuries, (3) have personal care needs met, and (4) have dignity maintained. The overall goals for the caregiver of a patient with AD are to (1) reduce caregiver stress, (2) maintain personal, emotional, and physical health, and (3) cope with the long-term effects of caregiving.

TABLE 59.12 Nursing Assessment
Alzheimer's Disease

Subjective Data

Important Health Information

Past health history: Repeated head trauma, stroke, CNS infection, family history of dementia

Medications: Use of any drug to decrease symptoms (e.g., tranquilizers, hypnotics, antidepressants, antipsychotics)

Functional Health Patterns

Health perception–health management: Positive family history. Emotional lability

Nutritional-metabolic: Anorexia, malnutrition, weight loss

Elimination: Incontinence

Activity-exercise: Poor personal hygiene, gait instability, weakness, inability to perform activities of daily living

Sleep-rest: Frequent nighttime awakening, daytime napping

Cognitive-perceptual: Forgetfulness, inability to cope with complex situations, difficulty with problem solving (early signs), depression, withdrawal, suicidal ideation (early)

Objective Data

General

Disheveled appearance, agitation

Neurologic

Mild: Loss of recent memory, disorientation to date and time, flat affect, lack of spontaneity. Impaired abstraction, cognition, and judgment

Moderate: Agitation, impaired ability to recognize close family and friends, loss of remote memory, confusion, apraxia, agnosia, alexia (inability to understand written language); aphasia, inability to do simple tasks

Severe: Inability to do self-care, incontinence, immobility, limb rigidity, flexor posturing

Possible Diagnostic Findings

Diagnosis by exclusion, cerebral cortical atrophy on CT scan, poor scores on mental status tests, hippocampal atrophy on MRI scan, abnormal changes on PET

◆ Nursing Implementation

◆ Health Promotion.
Can AD be prevented? Although there is no known definitive way to prevent AD, there are several things that we can do to keep our brain healthy and modify the risk for developing dementia (Table 59.13).

Early recognition and treatment of AD are important. You have a responsibility to inform patients and their families about the early signs of AD (Table 59.4). In the early stages of AD, patients are often aware that their memory is faulty and do things to mask the problem.

◆ Acute Care.
The diagnosis of AD is traumatic for both the patient and family. It is not unusual for the patient to have depression, denial, worry, fear, and feelings of loss and dread.[13] You are in an important position to assess for depression. Antidepressant drugs and counseling may be needed. Family caregivers may be in denial and may not seek medical attention early in the disease. You can assess family caregiver's ability to accept and cope with the diagnosis.

Although there is no treatment that reverses AD, ongoing monitoring of both the patient and caregiver is important. Patients with AD move through the stages at variable rates. HCPs collaborate with caregivers and patients to manage manifestations, which change over time.

TABLE 59.13 Patient & Caregiver Teaching

Decreasing Risk for Cognitive Decline

The following are tips to reduce the risk for cognitive decline and dementia:

1. Avoid harmful substances

   Excessive drinking and drug use can damage brain cells. Stop smoking because it increases the risk for cognitive decline.

2. Challenge your mind

   Read often, do crossword puzzles. Keep mentally active. Learn new skills. Go back to school. This strengthens the brain connections and promotes new ones.

3. Exercise regularly

   Even low to moderate level activity, such as walking or gardening 3 to 5 times per week, can make you feel better. Daily physical activity, even in older adults, can decrease the risk for cognitive decline.

4. Stay socially active

   Pursue social activities that have meaning to you. Family, friends, church, and a sense of community may all contribute to better brain health.

5. Avoid trauma to the brain

   Because traumatic brain injury may be a risk factor for developing AD, promote safety in physical activities and driving. Use the car seat belt. Wear a helmet when playing contact sports or riding a bike. Fall proof your home.

6. Take care of mental health

   Recognize and treat depression early. Depression may cause or worsen memory loss and other cognitive impairment.

7. Treat diabetes.

   Better blood glucose control can help to prevent the cognitive decline associated with diabetes.

8. Take care of your heart

   Risk factors for cardiovascular disease and stroke (hypertension, obesity) negatively affect your cognitive health. Heart health is linked to brain health.

9. Get enough sleep

   Not getting enough sleep may result in problems with memory and thinking.

10. Get the right fuel

    A healthy and balanced diet low in fats and high in vegetables and fruits helps to reduce the risk for cognitive decline.

Adapted from Alzheimer's Association: 10 Ways to love your brain. Retrieved from *www.alz.org/help-support/brain_health/10_ways_to_love_ your_brain;* and Baumgart M, Snyder HM, Carrillo MC, et al: Summary of evidence on modifiable risk factors for cognitive decline and dementia: A population-based perspective, *Alzheimers Dement* 11:718, 2015.

The nursing care needed by the patient with AD changes as the disease progresses, which emphasizes the need for regular assessment and support. The severity of the problems and amount of nursing care needed increase over time. The specific manifestations of the disease depend on the area of the brain involved. Nursing care focuses on decreasing manifestations, preventing harm, and supporting the patient and caregiver throughout the disease process.

Patients with AD may have other acute and chronic illnesses that require hospitalization or surgical interventions. Hospitalization can be traumatic for the patient with AD and the caregiver. Hospitalization can precipitate a worsening of dementia or development of delirium among patients with AD. Caregivers and health care professionals need to help patients who have difficulty explaining their symptoms or recalling their health and medical histories. In the acute care setting, patients with AD need to be observed more closely because of concerns for their safety. They should be frequently reassured and oriented to place and time. Anxiety or disruptive behavior may be reduced with using consistent nursing staff.

◆ **Ambulatory Care.** Currently, family members and friends care for many people with AD in their homes. Other patients with AD live in various types of facilities, including long-term care and assisted living facilities. A facility that is good for one patient may not be suitable for another. What is helpful for a patient at one point in the disease process may be completely different from what is best when the disease progresses.

After the initial diagnosis, patients need to be aware that the progression of the disease is variable. Effective management of the disease may slow symptom progression and decrease the burden on the patient, caregiver, and family. Decisions related to care should be made with the patient, family members, and interprofessional care team early in the disease. You have a role in advising the patient and caregiver to initiate health care decisions, including advance directives, while the patient has the capacity to do so. This can ease the burden for the caregiver as the disease progresses.

In the early stages of AD, memory aids, such as calendars, may be beneficial. Patients often become depressed during this phase. Depression may be related to the diagnosis of an incurable disorder and the impact of the disease on ADLs, including driving, socializing, and taking part in recreational activities. Nurses teach caregivers to perform tasks needed to maximize quality of life and safety of the patient with AD.

Adult day care is one of the options available to the patient with AD. Although programs vary in size, structure, physical environment, and staff experience, the common goals of all day care programs are to provide respite for the family and a protective environment. During the early and moderate stages of AD, the patient can still benefit from stimulating activities that encourage independence and decision making in a protective environment. The patient returns home tired, content, less frustrated, and ready to be with the family. The respite from the demands of care allows the caregiver to be more responsive to the patient's needs.

As the disease progresses, the demands on the caregiver eventually exceed the resources, and the patient with AD may need to be placed in a long-term care facility. Special dementia units are becoming increasingly common. The dementia unit is designed with an emphasis on safety. Many facilities have designated areas that allow the patient to walk freely within the unit, while the unit is secured so that the patient cannot wander outside.

As the disease progresses to the late stage, the patient is severely impaired, having difficulty with basic functions, including walking and talking. Total care is needed for this patient. Specific problems relate to the care of the patient with AD in all phases of the disease. These problems are described next.

Behavioral Problems. Behavioral problems occur in about 90% of patients with AD. These problems include repetitiveness or asking the same question repeatedly, delusions, hallucinations, agitation, aggression, altered sleeping patterns, wandering, hoarding, and resisting care. Many times, these behaviors are unpredictable and may challenge caregivers. Caregivers must be aware that these behaviors are not intentional and are often difficult to control. Behavioral problems are often the reason that patients are placed in institutional care settings.[14]

These behaviors are often the patient's way of responding to pain, frustration, temperature extremes, or anxiety. When these behaviors become problematic, you must plan interventions carefully. Assess the patient's physical status. Check for changes in vital signs, urinary and bowel patterns, and pain that could account for behavioral problems. Assess the environment to identify factors that may trigger behavior disruptions. Extremes in temperature or excessive noise may lead to behavior changes. When environmental conditions are agitating the patient, either move the patient or remove the stimulus.

When a patient resists or pulls tubes or dressings, cover these items with stretch tube gauze or remove them from the visual field. Reassure the patient that you are present to keep him or her safe. Do not ask challenging "why" questions. The patient with AD cannot think logically. If the patient cannot state distress, validate their mood. Rephrase the patient's statement to validate its meaning. Closely observe the patient's emotional state.

Nursing strategies that address difficult behavior include redirection, distraction, and reassurance. When a patient is restless or agitated, redirecting involves changing the patient's focus by having them perform activities, such as sweeping, raking, or dusting. Providing snacks, taking a car ride, sitting on a porch swing or rocker, listening to favorite music, watching videotapes, looking at family photographs, or walking may distract an agitated patient. Reassure patients by telling them that they will be protected from danger, harm, or embarrassment. Repetitive activities, including songs, poems, music, massage, aromas, or a favorite object can be soothing.

Do not threaten to restrain an agitated patient. Ask a calming family member to stay with the patient. Monitor the patient frequently and record all interventions. As verbal skills decline, you and the caregiver must rely more on the patient's body language to communicate care needs. The use of positive nursing actions can reduce the use of chemical (drug therapy) restraints.

Disruptive behaviors have been treated with antipsychotic drugs (Table 59.11). However, as discussed on p. 1393, these have adverse side effects. All other measures of treating behavioral issues should be exhausted before drug treatment is started.

? CHECK YOUR PRACTICE

You are working in a secure Alzheimer's unit. While making rounds at 4 PM you see Dan, one of the UAPs, screaming at an 84-yr-old male resident. When you approach Dan and the resident, you ask what is going on. Dan responds, "Every day about this time he gets so agitated and starts yelling at me, so I yell back."
• How would you handle the situation? What teaching does Dan need?

A specific type of agitation, termed *sundowning*, is when the patient becomes more confused and agitated in the late afternoon or evening. Behaviors related to sundowning include agitation, aggressiveness, wandering, resistance to redirection, and increased verbal activity, such as yelling. The cause of sundowning is unclear. It may be due to a disruption of circadian rhythms. Other causes include pain, hunger, unfamiliar environment and noise, medications, reduced lighting, and fragmented sleep.[15]

Managing sundowning can be challenging for you, the patient, and the family. When a patient has sundowning, remain calm and avoid confrontation. Assess the situation for possible causes of the agitation. Nursing interventions that may be helpful include (1) creating a quiet, calm environment; (2) maximizing exposure to daylight by opening blinds and turning on lights during the day; (3) evaluating medications to determine if any could cause sleep problems; (4) limiting naps and caffeine; and (5) consulting with the HCP about drug therapy.

▓▓ NURSING MANAGEMENT
Caring for the Patient With Alzheimer's Disease

The RN is responsible for ongoing assessment of the patient's level of function and for developing the plan of care. Since most patients with AD are cared for at home or in long-term care settings, many routine nursing activities are performed by licensed practical/vocational nurses (LPN/VNs), unlicensed assistive personnel (UAP), or family caregivers.

• Assess patients' memory and level of function.
• Teach patients and caregivers about using memory enhancement aids, such as calendars or notes.
• Monitor for physiologic problems, such as pain, swallowing difficulties, urinary tract infection, pneumonia, skin breakdown, and constipation.
• Assess nutritional and fluid intake and develop a plan to ensure adequate intake.
• Evaluate safety risk factors.
• Determine possible precipitating factors for behavioral changes and develop strategies to address difficult behavior.
• Assess family caregivers' stress level and coping strategies.
• Make referrals for community services, such as adult day care and respite care.
• Delegate to LPN/VN:
  • Monitor for behavioral changes that may indicate physiologic problems.
  • Check the environment for potential safety hazards.
  • Give enteral feedings to patients who are unable to swallow, if ordered.
  • Give ordered medications.
• Oversee UAP:
  • Help patients to use the toilet, commode, or bedpan at frequent intervals.
  • Provide personal hygiene, skin care, and oral care.
  • Help patients with eating.
  • Aid patients with daily activities.
  • Use bed alarms and surveillance to decrease risk for falls.

Collaborate With Other Team Members
Dietitian
• Assess nutrition status and provide prescribed nutritional support.
• Offer practical suggestions to enhance dietary intake.
Occupational Therapist
• Suggest ways to help patients retain self-care ability as long as possible.
Social Worker
• Help caregivers identify and obtain needed resources.
• Provide support and counseling to caregivers.

Safety. The patient with AD is at risk for problems related to personal safety. Potential hazards include falling, ingesting dangerous substances, wandering, injuring others and self with sharp objects, being burned, and being unable to respond to crisis situations. These concerns require careful attention in the home environment to minimize risk. Supervision is needed. As the patient's cognitive function declines over time, they may have problems navigating physical spaces and interpreting environmental cues. Help the caregiver assess the home environment for safety risks.

! SAFETY ALERT Preventing Falls
Teach the caregiver to take the following steps:
• Have stairwells well lit.
• Make sure the patient can grasp the handrails.
• Tack down carpet edges.
• Remove throw rugs and extension cords.
• Use nonskid mats in tub or shower.
• Install handrails in the bath and by the commode.

Wandering is a major concern for caregivers. Wandering may be related to loss of memory or to side effects of medications. It may be an expression of a physical or emotional need, restlessness, curiosity, or stimuli that trigger memories of earlier routines. As with other behaviors, observe for factors or events that may precipitate wandering. For example, the patient may be sensitive to stress and tension in the environment. In such cases, wandering may reflect an attempt to leave.

When someone with AD is discovered missing, every second counts. To assist caregivers with finding them, the Alzheimer's Association and the MedicAlert Foundation have created an alliance called MedicAlert + Alzheimer's Association Safe Return.[16] This program includes identification products (e.g., bracelet, necklace, wallet cards), a national photo and information database, a 24-hour toll-free emergency crisis line, local chapter support, and wandering behavior education and training for caregivers and families.

Tracking devices (e.g., global positioning system [GPS]) can be used to find people who wander. These devices can be placed in shoes, sewn into pockets, worn as a bracelet or pendant, or clipped to a belt.

Pain Management. Because of difficulties with oral and written language, patients with AD may have a hard time expressing physical problems, including pain. You need to rely on other clues, such as the patient's behavior. Pain can result in changes in behavior, including increased vocalization, agitation, withdrawal, and changes in function. Pain should be recognized and treated promptly and the patient's response monitored.

Eating and Swallowing Difficulties. Undernutrition is a problem in the moderate and severe stages of AD. Loss of interest in food and decreased ability to self-feed (*feeding apraxia*), as well as co-morbid conditions, can result in significant nutritional problems. In long-term care facilities, inadequate aid with feeding may add to the problem.

Use pureed foods, thickened liquids, and nutritional supplements when chewing and swallowing become problematic for the patient. The patient may need reminders to chew their food and to swallow. A quiet and unhurried environment without distractions (e.g., television) at mealtimes can be helpful. Low lighting, music, and simulated nature sounds may improve eating behaviors. Easy-grip eating utensils and finger foods may allow the patient to self-feed. Liquids should be offered frequently.

When oral feeding is not possible, explore alternative routes. Nasogastric (NG) feeding may be used for short periods. However, for the long term, the NG tube is uncomfortable and may add to the patient's agitation. A percutaneous endoscopic gastrostomy (PEG) tube is another option (see Fig. 39.7). PEG tubes can be problematic since patients with AD are vulnerable to aspiration of feeding formula and tube dislodgment. The potential positive outcomes to be gained from nutritional therapies are considered in light of overall outcome goals and potential adverse effects of the specific therapy. Nutritional support therapies are described in Chapter 39.

Oral Care. In the late stages of AD, the patient is unable to perform oral self-care. With decreased tooth brushing and flossing, dental problems are likely to occur. Because of swallowing difficulties, patients may retain food in the mouth, adding to the potential for tooth decay. Dental caries and tooth abscess can cause discomfort or pain and increase agitation. Inspect the mouth regularly and provide mouth care to those patients unable to perform self-care.

Infection Prevention. Urinary tract infection and pneumonia are the most common infections in patients with AD. Such infections are the cause of death in many patients with AD. Because of feeding and swallowing problems, the patient is at risk for aspiration pneumonia. Immobility can predispose the patient to pneumonia.

Reduced fluid intake, prostate enlargement in men, poor hygiene, and urinary drainage devices can predispose patients to bladder infection. Any manifestations of infection, such as a change in behavior, fever, cough, or pain on urination, require prompt evaluation and treatment.

Skin Care. It is important to monitor the patient's skin over time. Note and treat rashes, areas of redness, and skin breakdown. In the late stages, incontinence along with immobility and undernutrition can place the patient at risk for skin breakdown. Keep the skin clean and dry. Change the patient's position regularly to avoid areas of pressure over bony prominences.

Elimination Problems. During the moderate and severe stages of AD, urinary and fecal incontinence lead to increased need for nursing care. When possible, behavioral retraining of bladder and bowel function by scheduled toileting may help decrease episodes of incontinence.

Another common elimination problem is constipation. Causes may relate to immobility, reduced fiber intake, and decreased fluid intake. Increased dietary fiber, fiber supplements, and stool softeners are the first lines of management. The combination of aging, other health problems, and swallowing difficulties may increase the risk for complications associated with the use of mineral oil, stimulants, osmotic agents, and enemas. Management of constipation is discussed in Chapter 42.

Caregiver Support. More than 16 million Americans provide unpaid care for people with AD or other dementias.[2] Most of these are family members providing care in the home (Fig. 59.9). AD disrupts all aspects of patient and family life. Caregivers for people with AD describe it as very stressful. They often have adverse consequences relating to their own emotional and physical health.

The chronic and often severe stress associated with dementia caregiving increases the risk for the development of dementia in spouse caregivers.[17] One mechanism proposed is that the detrimental effects of the chronic stress of caregiving can affect the hippocampus, a region of the brain responsible for memory.

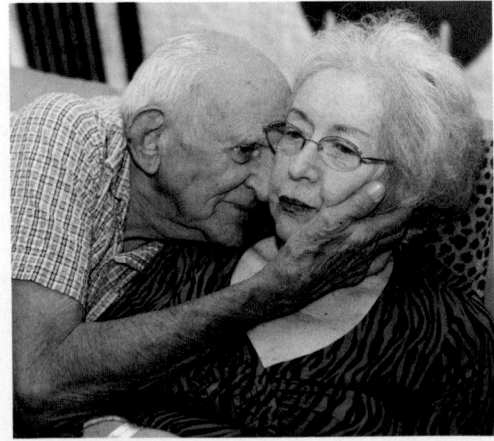

FIG. 59.9 Caregivers of patients with dementia face an incredible challenge that often causes deterioration in their own physical and emotional health. (© iStock/Thinkstock.)

As the disease progresses, the relationship between the caregiver and patient with AD changes. Family roles may be altered or reversed. A child may care for a parent. Decisions must be made, including when to tell the patient about the diagnosis, have the patient stop driving or doing activities that may have become dangerous, ask for assistance, and place the patient in adult day care or a long-term care facility. With early-onset AD, the patient is affected during their most productive years in terms of career and family. The consequences can be devastating to the patient and family.

Sexual relations for couples are seriously affected by AD. As the disease progresses, sexual interest may decline for both the patient and partner. Several reasons account for this, including fatigue, memory impairment, and episodes of incontinence. Some patients become sexually driven and uninhibited as the disease progresses.

Work with the caregiver to assess stressors and identify coping strategies to reduce the burden of caregiving. For example, ask which behaviors are most disruptive to family life at a given time. This is likely to change as the disease progresses. Determining what is most disruptive or distressful to the caregiver can help establish priorities.

Patient safety is a high priority. It is important to assess what the caregiver's expectations are about the patient's behavior.

Are the expectations reasonable given the progression of the disease? A family and caregiver teaching guide based on the disease stages is provided in Table 59.14. Other tips for caregivers are listed in Table 59.15. A nursing care plan for the family caregiver (eNursing Care Plan 59.2) is available on the website for this chapter.

Support groups for caregivers and family members (Fig. 59.10) can provide an atmosphere of understanding and give current information about the disease itself and related topics, such as safety, legal, ethical, and financial issues. The Alzheimer's Association has many educational and support systems available to help family caregivers (www.alz.org).

TABLE 59.14 Patient & Caregiver Teaching

Alzheimer's Disease

Include the following instructions when teaching families and caregivers the management of the patient with Alzheimer's disease:

Mild Stage

- Many treatable (and potentially reversible) conditions can mimic dementia (Table 59.2). Try to establish a diagnosis.
- Get the patient to stop driving. Confusion and poor judgment can impair driving skills and potentially put others at risk.
- Encourage activities such as visiting with friends and family, listening to music, enjoying hobbies, and exercising.
- Provide cues in the home, establish a routine, and determine a specific location where essential items (e.g., glasses) must be kept.
- Do not correct misstatements or faulty memory.
- Register with MedicAlert + Alzheimer's Association Safe Return, a program established by the MedicAlert Foundation and the Alzheimer's Association to locate those who wander from their homes.
- Make plans in terms of advance directives, care options, financial concerns, and personal preference for care.

Moderate Stage

- Install door locks for patient safety.
- Provide protective wear for urinary and fecal incontinence.
- Ensure that the home has good lighting, install handrails in stairways and bathroom, and remove area rugs.
- Label drawers and faucets (hot and cold) to ensure safety.
- Develop ways, such as distraction and diversion, to cope with behavioral problems. Identify and reduce potential triggers (e.g., reduce stress, extremes in temperature) for disruptive behavior.
- Provide memory triggers, such as pictures of family and friends.

Severe Stage

- Follow a regular schedule for toileting to reduce incontinence.
- Provide care to meet needs, including oral care and skin care.
- Monitor diet and fluid intake to ensure their adequacy.
- Continue communication through talking and touching.
- Consider placement in a long-term care facility when providing total care becomes too difficult.

TABLE 59.15 Nursing Management

Assisting Patients With Dementia

Do

- Treat the adult with respect and dignity, even when behavior is childlike.
- Use gentle touch and direct eye contact.
- Remain patient, flexible, calm, and understanding.
- Expect challenging behaviors, since the patient's ability to think logically is affected.
- Give directions using gestures or pictures.
- Simplify tasks. Focus on one thing at a time.
- Avoid questions or topics that require extensive thought, memory, or words.
- Be flexible. If one approach does not work, try another.
- Use distraction, changing the subject, redirecting to another activity.
- Provide reassurance. Praise sincerely for success.

Do Not

- Criticize, correct, or argue.
- Rush or hurry the patient.
- Force participation in activities or events.
- Talk about the patient as if they are not there.
- Blame the patient with AD. Instead, blame the disease.
- Take challenging behaviors patiently. These behaviors are due to the disease.
- Use condescending terms, such as "honey" or "sweetie."
- Use threatening gestures.
- Overreact to the patient with AD.
- Try to explain "why" or rationalize.

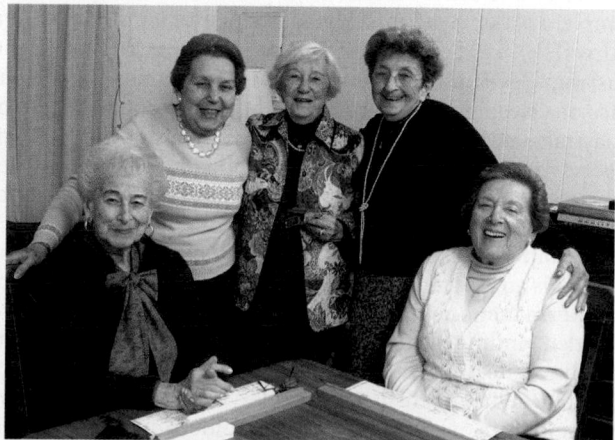

FIG. 59.10 Support groups are an effective way to help caregivers cope. (© iStockphoto/Thinkstock.)

◆ **Evaluation**

Expected outcomes are that the patient with AD will:
- Function at the highest level of cognitive ability
- Perform basic personal care ADLs, by self or with assistance, as needed
- Have no injury
- Stay in a restricted area during ambulation and activity

DELIRIUM

Delirium is a state of confusion that develops over days to hours.[1] The patient has decreased ability to direct, focus, sustain, and shift attention and awareness. Deficits in memory, orientation, language, visuospatial ability, or perception may be present. The patient may be hypoactive or hyperactive. Emotional problems include fear, depression, euphoria, or perplexity. Sleep may be disturbed.

These symptoms represent a change from the patient's baseline and tend to fluctuate throughout the day. They do not occur in the context of a severely reduced level of arousal, such as coma, and cannot be explained by another preexisting, evolving, or established neurocognitive disorder.

Etiology and Pathophysiology

We do not know the exact cause of delirium. A main contributing factor is impairment of cerebral oxidative metabolism, in which the brain gets less oxygen and has problems using it. Multiple neurotransmitter abnormalities may be involved. Cholinergic deficiency, excess release of dopamine, and both increased and decreased serotonin activity may contribute to delirium. Proinflammatory cytokines, including interleukin-1 (IL-1), IL-2, IL-6, tumor necrosis factor-α (TNF-α), cytokines, and interferon, appear to play a role.

Delirium is rarely caused by a single factor. It most often occurs among hospitalized older adults. Up to 60% of older adults hospitalized for medical conditions have delirium at some time during their hospitalization.[18] Stress, surgery, and sleep deprivation have been linked to delirium. Delirium is the most common surgical complication among older adults. The incidence is 15% to 25% after major elective surgery and 50% after high-risk procedures, such as hip fracture repair and heart surgery.[19] Pain and depression contribute to delirium, especially among older adults.[19]

Delirium is often the result of the interaction of the patient's underlying condition with a precipitating event. Delirium can occur after a relatively minor insult in a vulnerable patient. For example, a patient with underlying health problems, such as heart failure (HF), cancer, cognitive impairment, or sensory limitations, may develop delirium in response to a minor change, such as use of a sleeping medication. In other less vulnerable patients, it may take a combination of factors, such as anesthesia, major surgery, mechanical ventilation, infection, and prolonged sleep deprivation, to precipitate delirium. Delirium can be a symptom of a serious medical illness, such as bacterial meningitis.

Dementia is the leading risk factor for delirium. Furthermore, delirium is a risk factor for developing dementia. Delirium may cause permanent neuronal damage and lead to dementia.[20]

Understanding factors that can lead to delirium can help determine effective interventions. Common factors that can precipitate delirium are listed in Tables 59.16 and 59.17. Many of these factors are more common among older adults. Older adults have limited compensatory mechanisms to deal with physiologic insults, such as hypoxia, hypoglycemia, and dehydration. They

TABLE 59.16 Factors That Precipitate Delirium

Demographic Characteristics • Age 65 year or older • Male gender	**Functional Status** • Functional dependence • History of falls • Immobility
Cognitive Status • Cognitive impairment • Dementia • Depression • History of delirium	**Medical Conditions** • Acute infection, sepsis, fever • Chronic kidney or liver disease • Electrolyte imbalances • Fracture or trauma • History of stroke • Neurologic disease • Severe acute illness • Terminal illness
Decreased Oral Intake • Dehydration • Malnutrition	
Drugs • Alcohol or drug use or withdrawal • Aminoglycosides • Anticholinergics • Opioids • Sedative-hypnotics • Treatment with multiple drugs	**Sensory** • Sensory deprivation • Sensory overload • Visual or hearing impairment
	Surgery • Cardiac surgery • Noncardiac surgery • Orthopedic surgery • Prolonged cardiopulmonary bypass
Environmental • Admission to ICU • Emotional stress • Pain (especially untreated) • Sleep deprivation • Use of physical restraints	

TABLE 59.17 Mnemonic for Causes of Delirium

Dementia, dehydration
Electrolyte imbalances, emotional stress
Lung, liver, heart, kidney, brain
Infection, intensive care unit
Rx drugs
Injury, immobility
Untreated pain, unfamiliar environment
Metabolic disorders

are more susceptible to drug-induced delirium, in part because of their increased use of multiple drugs. Many drugs, including sedative-hypnotics, opioids (especially meperidine [Demerol]), benzodiazepines, and anticholinergics, can cause or contribute to delirium, especially in older or vulnerable patients.[21]

Clinical Manifestations

Patients with delirium can have a variety of manifestations, ranging from hypoactivity and lethargy to hyperactivity, agitation, and hallucinations. Patients can have mixed delirium, with both hypoactive and hyperactive symptoms. Delirium can develop over the course of hours to days. It usually develops over a 2- to 3-day period. The early manifestations often include inability to concentrate, disorganized thinking, irritability, insomnia, loss of appetite, restlessness, and confusion. Later manifestations may include agitation, misperception, misinterpretation, and hallucinations.

Delirium can last from 1 to 7 days. However, delirium may persist for months or years. Some patients do not completely recover.

TABLE 59.18 Confusion Assessment Method (CAM)

Delirium is diagnosed with the presence of features 1 and 2, and either 3 or 4.

Feature 1
Acute Onset and Fluctuating Course
Data usually obtained from a family member or nurse.
Shown by positive responses to the following questions:

- Is there evidence of an acute change in mental status from the patient's baseline?
- Did the (abnormal) behavior fluctuate during the day (i.e., tend to come and go, or increase and decrease in severity)?

Feature 2
Inattention
Shown by positive response to the following question:

- Did the patient have problem focusing attention (e.g., being easily distractible, or having problem keeping track of what was being said)?

Feature 3
Disorganized Thinking
Shown by a positive response to the following question:

- Was the patient's thinking disorganized or incoherent, such as rambling or irrelevant conversation, unclear or illogical flow of ideas, or unpredictable switching from subject to subject?

Feature 4
Altered Level of Consciousness
Shown by any answer other than "alert" to the following question:

- Overall, how would you rate this patient's level of consciousness (alert [normal], vigilant [hyper alert], lethargic [drowsy, easily aroused], stupor [difficult to arouse], or coma [unarousable])?

Adapted from Inouye S, van Dyck C, Alessi C, et al: Clarifying confusion: The Confusion Assessment Method, *Ann Intern Med* 113:941, 1990.

Manifestations of delirium are sometimes confused with those of dementia. A key distinction between them is that the patient who has sudden cognitive impairment, disorientation, or clouded sensorium is more likely to have delirium rather than dementia. A comparison of delirium and dementia is shown in Table 59.1.

Diagnostic Studies

Diagnosing delirium is complicated because many critically ill patients cannot communicate their needs. A careful medical and psychologic history and physical assessment are the first steps in diagnosing delirium and its underlying cause. This includes careful attention to medications, both prescription and OTC. The Confusion Assessment Method (CAM) is a reliable tool for assessing delirium (Table 59.18). The version of the CAM may vary depending on the clinical setting. It is important to distinguish whether the delirium is part of underlying dementia.

Once delirium has been diagnosed, explore potential causes. Carefully review the patient's health history and medication record. Laboratory tests include complete blood count, serum electrolytes, blood urea nitrogen, and creatinine levels; ECG; urinalysis; liver and thyroid function tests; and oxygen saturation level. Drug and alcohol levels may be obtained. If unexplained fever or nuchal rigidity is present and meningitis or encephalitis is suspected, a lumbar puncture may be done. CSF is examined for glucose, protein, and bacteria. If the patient's history includes head injury, appropriate x-rays or scans may be ordered. In general, brain imaging studies, such as CT and MRI, are used only when head injury is known or suspected.

ETHICAL/LEGAL DILEMMAS
Board of Nursing Disciplinary Action

Situation
The state board of nursing has received multiple complaints about J.R., an RN who works in a long-term care facility. J.R. has signed off on 3 controlled substances count sheets that have been determined to be inaccurate. During an investigation it was discovered that several members of the nursing staff knew about J.R.'s reported behavior, but they did not report their observations to the unit administrator because the administrator is J.R.'s aunt. After the investigation, the board of nursing subpoenas J.R. to a meeting to discuss charges in preparation for a disciplinary hearing.

Ethical/Legal Points for Consideration
Regulation of professional nursing practice is the right of each of the 50 states. Most have regulatory agencies charged with writing regulations and rules to implement the state nurse practice act. The regulations approved by these agencies carry the weight of law. Failure to behave accordingly places a nurse at risk for disciplinary action.

The RN who is charged with unprofessional behavior has been charged with an offense and is entitled to the same legal rights as any other person, including a fair and timely hearing, opportunity to confront the accusers, right to be represented by an attorney, and right to prepare a defense.

Possible disciplinary actions include temporary suspension of the nursing license, revocation of the nursing license, mandatory rehabilitation for substance use, and mandated supervision and evaluation of practice. Sometimes the disciplinary action includes fines and requires reeducation. The state board of nursing may report the action to the state attorney general if evidence suggests that a crime has been committed. The RN who is found guilty of unprofessional practice must report this action on all future applications for nursing positions.

All RNs should be familiar with their state's nurse practice act and regulations, and the composition and actions of the state board of nursing. Nurses should pay attention to the regulation that lists examples of actionable behavior and disciplinary actions sanctioned by the state.

RNs have a legal and ethical obligation to report suspected illegal behavior to their administrators and to continue reporting until the situation is resolved. By failing to report, the RN may be charged as an accessory to the act or aiding and abetting the behavior. This RN may be charged with unprofessional behavior and risks losing his or her nursing license. Shifting the obligation to someone else to report or failure to continue reporting each incident does not satisfy this duty.

Discussion Questions
1. How would you handle a situation in which retaliation for reporting unprofessional behavior may occur?
2. What would you do if the nurse suspected of illegal behavior is related to someone in the administrative hierarchy?

❖ NURSING AND INTERPROFESSIONAL MANAGEMENT: DELIRIUM

Treatment is important as many cases of delirium are potentially reversible. In caring for the patient with delirium, you are responsible for prevention, early recognition, and treatment. Prevention of delirium involves recognition of patients at high risk, including those with neurologic disorders, such as dementia, stroke, CNS infection, and Parkinson's disease.[22] Other risk factors include sensory impairment, older age, surgery, hospitalization in an intensive care unit (ICU), and untreated pain. Risk factors are listed in Table 59.16.

Care of the patient with delirium focuses on eliminating precipitating factors. If it is drug induced, medications are discontinued. Keep in mind that delirium can accompany drug and alcohol withdrawal. Depending on the history, drug screening may be done. Fluid and electrolyte imbalances and nutritional deficiencies (e.g., thiamine) are corrected if appropriate. If the problem is related to an overstimulating or understimulating environment, then changes should be made. If delirium is from infection, appropriate antibiotic therapy is started. Similarly, if delirium is due to chronic illness, such as chronic kidney disease or HF, treatment focuses on these conditions.

Care of the patient with delirium includes protecting the patient from harm. Give priority to creating a calm and safe environment. This may include encouraging family members to stay at the bedside, providing familiar objects and family photos, transferring the patient to a private room or one closer to the nurses' station, and planning for consistent nursing staff if possible. Use reorientation and behavioral interventions in patients with delirium. Provide the patient with reassurance and reorienting information as to place, time, and procedures. Clocks, calendars, and lists of scheduled activities are helpful. Reduce environmental stimuli, including noise and light levels.

Personal contact through touch and verbal communication can be an important reorienting strategy. If the patient uses eyeglasses or a hearing aid, they should be readily available because sensory deprivation can precipitate delirium. Avoid the use of restraints. Other interventions, including relaxation techniques, music therapy, and massage, may be appropriate for some patients with delirium.

Comprehensive interventions to prevent delirium should be implemented by the health care team.[23] The team may address issues related to polypharmacy, pain, nutritional status, and potential for incontinence. The patient with delirium is at risk for the adverse consequences of immobility, including skin breakdown. Give attention to increasing physical activity or providing range-of-motion exercises, when appropriate, and maintaining skin integrity.

Focus on supporting the family and caregivers during episodes of delirium. Family members need to understand factors that may have precipitated the delirium, as well as the potential outcomes. Patient education materials are available at *www. ICUdelirium.org.*

◆ Drug Therapy

Drug therapy is reserved for patients with severe agitation, especially when it interferes with needed medical treatments. Agitation can put the patient at risk for falls and injury. Medication therapy is used cautiously because many of the drugs used to manage agitation have psychoactive properties.

Drugs should be used only when nonpharmacologic interventions have failed.

Dexmedetomidine (Precedex), an α-adrenergic receptor agonist, has been used in ICU settings for sedation. The use of low-dose antipsychotics (e.g., haloperidol, risperidone [Risperdal], olanzapine [Zyprexa], quetiapine [Seroquel]), though common practice, is controversial.[24] Research suggests their use does not change the duration of delirium or the length of hospitalization.[24]

Haloperidol can be given IV, IM, or orally and will produce sedation. Other side effects include hypotension; extrapyramidal side effects, including *tardive* dyskinesia (involuntary muscle movements of face, trunk, and arms) and *athetosis* (involuntary writhing movements of the limbs); muscle tone changes; and anticholinergic effects. Carefully monitor older patients receiving antipsychotic agents.

Short-acting benzodiazepines (e.g., lorazepam [Ativan]) can be used to treat delirium associated with sedative and alcohol withdrawal or in conjunction with antipsychotics to reduce extrapyramidal side effects. However, these drugs may worsen delirium caused by other factors and must be used cautiously.

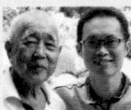

BRIDGE TO NCLEX EXAMINATION

The number of the question corresponds to the same-numbered outcome at the beginning of the chapter.

1. Dementia is defined as a
   a. syndrome that results only in memory loss.
   b. disease associated with abrupt changes in behavior.
   c. disease that is always due to reduced blood flow to the brain.
   d. syndrome characterized by cognitive dysfunction and loss of memory.

2. Vascular dementia is associated with
   a. transient ischemic attacks.
   b. bacterial or viral infection of neuronal tissue.
   c. cognitive changes secondary to cerebral ischemia.
   d. abrupt changes in cognitive function that are irreversible.

3. Dementia with Lewy bodies (DLB) is characterized by
   a. remissions and exacerbations over many years.
   b. memory impairment, muscle jerks, and blindness.
   c. parkinsonian symptoms, including muscle rigidity.
   d. increased intracranial pressure from decreased CSF drainage.

4. Which statement(s) accurately describe(s) mild cognitive impairment? *(select all that apply)*
   a. Cannot be detected by screening tests
   b. The person may appear normal to the casual observer
   c. Family members may see changes in the patient's abilities
   d. Problems that the person is experiencing interfere with daily activities
   e. The person is usually aware that there is a problem with his or her memory

5. The clinical diagnosis of dementia is based on
   a. CT or MRS.
   b. brain biopsy.
   c. electroencephalogram.
   d. patient history and cognitive assessment.

6. A *priority* goal of treatment for the patient with Alzheimer's disease is to
   a. maintain patient safety.
   b. maintain or increase body weight.
   c. return to a higher level of self-care.
   d. enhance functional ability over time.

7. Which patient is *most* at risk for developing delirium?
   a. A 50-yr-old woman with cholecystitis
   b. A 19-yr-old man with a fractured femur
   c. A 42-yr-old woman having an elective total hysterectomy
   d. A 78-yr-old man admitted to the medical unit with complications of heart failure

1. d, 2. c, 3. c, 4. b, c, e, 5. d, 6. a, 7. d

For rationales to these answers and even more NCLEX review questions, visit *http://evolve.elsevier.com/Lewis/medsurg.*

EVOLVE WEBSITE/RESOURCES LIST

http://evolve.elsevier.com/Lewis/medsurg
Review Questions (Online Only)
Key Points
Answer Keys for Questions
- Rationales for Bridge to NCLEX Examination Questions
- Answer Guidelines for Case Study on p. 1400
Student Case Study
- Patient With Alzheimer's Disease
eNursing Care Plans
- eNursing Care Plan 59.1: Patient With Alzheimer's Disease
- eNursing Care Plan 59.2: Family Caregivers
Conceptual Care Map Creator
Audio Glossary
Content Updates

REFERENCES

1. American Psychiatric Association: *Diagnostic and statistical manual of mental disorders,* ed 5, Arlington, VA, 2013, American Psychiatric Association. (Classic)
2. Alzheimer's Association: 2018 *Alzheimer's Association facts and figures report.* Retrieved from *www.alz.org/alzheimers-dementia/facts-figures.*
3. American Academy of Neurology: Detection, diagnosis, and management of dementia. Retrieved from *http://tools.aan.com/professionals/practice/pdfs/dementia_guideline.pdf.*
*4. Yang T, Sun Y, Lu Z, et al: The impact of cerebrovascular aging on vascular cognitive impairment and dementia, *Ageing Res Rev* 34:15, 2017.
5. Munshi MN: Cognitive dysfunction in older adults with diabetes: What a clinician needs to know, *Diabetes Care* 40:461, 2017.

*6. Mendez MF: What is the relationship of traumatic brain injury to dementia? *J Alzheimers Dis* 57:667, 2017.
7. Heuther S, McCance KL: *Understanding pathophysiology,* ed 6, St Louis, 2017, Elsevier.
8. Aisen PS, Cummings J, Jack CR, et al: On the path to 2025: Understanding the Alzheimer's disease continuum, *Alzheimers Res Ther* 1:60, 2017.
*9. Ahmed S, Kaur A, Venigalla H, et al: The retrogenesis model in Alzheimer's disease: Evidence and practical applications, *Curr Psych Rev* 13:35, 2017.
*10. McKhann GM, Knopman DS, Chertkow H, et al: The diagnosis of dementia due to Alzheimer's disease: Recommendations from the National Institute on Aging and the Alzheimer's Association workgroup, *Alzheimers Dement* 7:263, 2011. (Classic)
11. Alzheimer's Association: Mild cognitive impairment. Retrieved from *www.alz.org/alzheimers-dementia/what-is-dementia/related_conditions/mild-cognitive-impairment.*
*12. Reus VI, Fochtmann LJ, Eyler AE, et al: The American Psychiatric Association practice guideline on the use of antipsychotics to treat agitation or psychosis in patients with dementia, *Amer J Psych* 173:543, 2016.
*13. Kristiansen PJ, Normann HK, Norberg A, et al: How do people in the early stage of Alzheimer's disease see their future? *Dementia* 16:145, 2017.
*14. Connors MH, Ames D, Woodward M, et al: Psychosis and clinical outcomes in Alzheimer disease: A longitudinal study, *Amer J Geriat Psychiat* 26:304, 2018.
*15. Canevelli M, Valletta M, Trebbastoni A, et al: Sundowning in dementia: Clinical relevance, pathophysiological determinants, and therapeutic approaches, *Front Med (Lausanne)* 27:73, 2016.
16. Alzheimer's Association: MedicAlert + Alzheimer's Association Safe Return. Retrieved from *https://alz.org/help-support/caregiving/safety/medicalert-safe-return.*
*17. Dassel KB, Carr DC, Vitaliano P: Does caring for a spouse with dementia accelerate cognitive decline? Findings from the Health and Retirement Study, *Gerontologist* 57:319, 2017.

18. Oh ES, Fong TG, Hshieh TT, et al: Delirium in older persons: Advances in diagnosis and treatment, *JAMA* 318:1161, 2017.

19. Marcantonio ER: Delirium in hospitalized older adults, *NEJM* 377:1456, 2017.

*20. Oldham MA, Flanagan NM, Khan A, et al: Responding to ten common delirium misconceptions with best evidence: An educational review for clinicians, *J Neuropsychiatry Clin Neurosci* 30:51, 2017.

*21. American Geriatrics Society Expert Panel on Postoperative Delirium in Older Adults: Postoperative delirium in older adults: Best practice statement from the American Geriatrics Society, *J Am Coll Surg* 220:136, 2015. (Classic)

22. Delirium prevention and safety: Starting with the ABCDEF's. Retrieved from *www.icudelirium.org/medicalprofessionals.html*.

23. Flaherty JH, Yue J, Rudolph JL: Dissecting delirium: Phenotypes, consequences, screening, diagnosis, prevention, treatment, and program implementation, *Clin Ger Med* 33:393, 2017.

*24. Neufeld KJ, Yue J, Robinson TN et al: Antipsychotic medication for prevention and treatment of delirium in hospitalized adults: A systematic review and meta-analysis, *J Am Geriatric Soc* 64:705, 2016.

*Evidence-based information for clinical practice.

60

Spinal Cord and Peripheral Nerve Problems

Cindy Sullivan

It only takes a split second to smile and forget, yet to someone that needed it, it can last a lifetime.

Steve Maraboli

http://evolve.elsevier.com/Lewis/medsurg

CONCEPTUAL FOCUS

Family Dynamics	Mobility	Sensory Perception
Functional Ability	Pain	

LEARNING OUTCOMES

1. Outline the classification of spinal cord injuries and associated clinical manifestations.
2. Describe the clinical manifestations and interprofessional and nursing management of neurogenic and spinal shock.
3. Relate the clinical manifestations of spinal cord injury to the level of disruption and rehabilitation potential.
4. Describe the nursing management of the patient with a spinal cord injury.
5. Explain the types, clinical manifestations, and interprofessional and nursing management of spinal cord tumors.

6. Explain the etiology, clinical manifestations, and interprofessional and nursing management of trigeminal neuralgia and Bell's palsy.
7. Describe the etiology, clinical manifestations, and interprofessional and nursing management of Guillain-Barré syndrome/acute inflammatory demyelinating polyneuropathy.
8. Explain the etiology, clinical manifestations, and interprofessional and nursing management of chronic inflammatory demyelinating polyneuropathy.

KEY TERMS

acute inflammatory demyelinating polyneuropathy (AIDP), p. 1424
autonomic dysreflexia, p. 1414
Bell's palsy, p. 1423
botulism, p. 1426
chronic inflammatory demyelinating polyneuropathy (CIDP), p. 1425

Guillain-Barré syndrome (GBS), p. 1424
neurogenic bladder, p. 1407
neurogenic bowel, p. 1407
neurogenic (vasogenic) shock, p. 1404
paraplegia, p. 1405
spinal cord injury (SCI), p. 1403
spinal shock, p. 1404

tetanus, p. 1425
tetraplegia, p. 1405
trigeminal neuralgia (TN), p. 1421

This chapter discusses spinal cord and peripheral nerve problems, including spinal cord injuries, spinal cord tumors, cranial nerve disorders, and polyneuropathies. A focus of this chapter is the nursing management of the problems encountered by the patient with spinal cord injury (SCI). The potential for disruption of individual growth and development, altered family dynamics, economic loss from unemployment, and the high cost of rehabilitation and long-term health care make SCI a major problem. While many people with SCI can care for themselves independently, those with the highest level of injury need around-the-clock care at home or in a long-term care facility. The nurse's role in providing holistic care can have a significant impact on the patient's general health and well-being.

SPINAL CORD PROBLEMS

SPINAL CORD INJURY

Spinal cord injury (SCI) is caused by trauma or damage to the spinal cord. It can result in temporary or permanent alteration in the function of the spinal cord. About 17,000 Americans have SCIs each year. Some 282,000 persons in the United States are living with SCI. The average life expectancy for persons with SCI is less than those without SCI and has not improved since the 1980s. Mortality rates are high in the first year after injury with a 30% rehospitalization rate.[1]

Etiology and Pathophysiology

SCI is usually a result of trauma. The 4 most common causes are motor vehicle collisions (38%), falls (30.5%), violence (13.5%), and sports injuries (9%).[1]

Types of Injury. Neurologic damage caused by SCI occurs in 2 phases: *primary injury* (initial physical disruption of the spinal cord) and *secondary injury* (from processes, such as ischemia, hypoxia, hemorrhage, edema).

Primary Injury. Primary injury results from direct physical trauma to the spinal cord due to blunt or penetrating trauma. Trauma can cause spinal cord compression by bone displacement, interruption of blood supply, or distraction from pulling. Penetrating trauma, such as gunshot and stab wounds, can cause tearing and transection.

Secondary Injury. Secondary injury refers to the ongoing, progressive damage that occurs after the primary injury. Secondary injury causes further permanent damage. It begins a few minutes after injury and lasts for months. Fig. 60.1 shows the cascade of events causing secondary injury. These events result in edema, ischemia, and inflammation. They result in cell death, disruption of the blood-brain barrier, and demyelination. This can extend the level of deficit and worsen long-term outcome.

Seconds after the insult, mechanical disruption leads to small hemorrhages in the white and gray matter, damage to the axons, and cell membrane destruction.[2,3] Over the next minutes to hours, neuron destruction occurs. Blood-spinal barrier disruption allows for an influx of inflammatory cytokines. This further increases spinal cord edema and promotes ongoing inflammation.[4] Edema due to the inflammatory response is especially harmful because of limited space for tissue expansion. Thus compression of the spinal cord occurs. Edema extends above and below the injury, increasing ischemic damage. Within 24 hours, permanent damage may occur from edema.

The resulting hypoxia reduces O_2 levels below the metabolic needs of the spinal cord. Lactate metabolites and an increase in vasoactive substances, including norepinephrine, serotonin, and dopamine, occur. High levels of these substances cause vasospasms and hypoxia with subsequent necrosis. Unfortunately, the spinal cord has minimal ability to adapt to vasospasm.

Apoptosis (programmed cell death) continues for weeks. It contributes to postinjury demyelination. The inflammatory response at the site of the initial injury focuses on clearing up the initial cellular debris without damaging normal tissue. This results in a central non-neural core of connective tissue that we refer to as a glial scar (Fig. 60.2). The glial scar creates a physical barrier. It restricts the cells in the spinal cord from migration and regeneration. This leads to irreversible nerve damage and permanent neurologic deficit.

Spinal and Neurogenic Shock. Spinal shock may occur shortly after acute SCI. It is characterized by loss of deep tendon and sphincter reflexes, loss of sensation, and flaccid paralysis below the level of injury. This syndrome lasts days to weeks. It often masks postinjury neurologic function.[3]

In contrast to spinal shock, neurogenic (vasogenic) shock can occur in cervical or high thoracic injury (T6 or higher). It occurs from unopposed parasympathetic response due to loss of sympathetic nervous system (SNS) innervation. It causes peripheral vasodilation, venous pooling, and decreased cardiac output. Manifestations include significant hypotension (< 90 mmHg), bradycardia, and temperature dysregulation. Neurogenic shock can continue for 1 to 3 weeks.[5] Hypotension can result in poor perfusion and oxygenation to the spinal cord and worsen spinal cord ischemia.[6]

Classification of Spinal Cord Injury. SCI is classified by the (1) mechanism of injury, (2) level of injury, and (3) degree of injury.

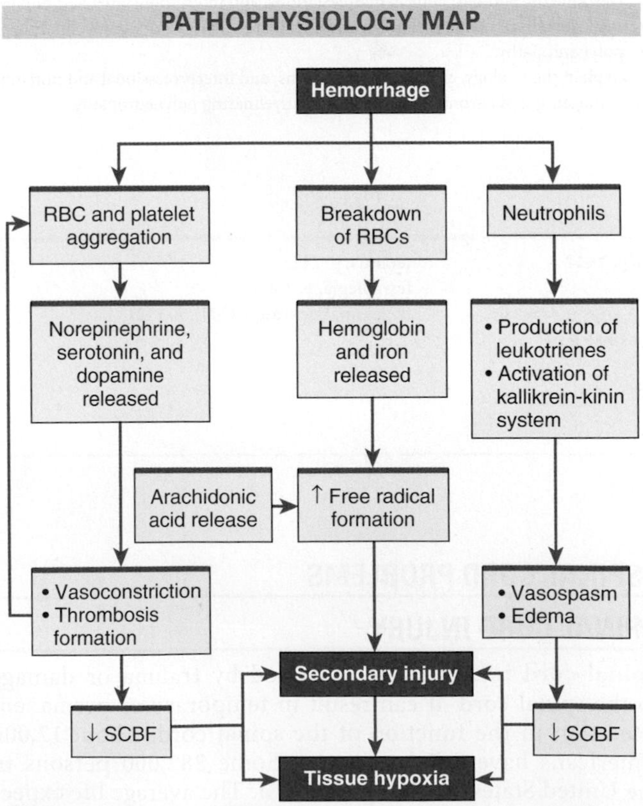

PATHOPHYSIOLOGY MAP

Hemorrhage

- RBC and platelet aggregation
- Breakdown of RBCs
- Neutrophils

- Norepinephrine, serotonin, and dopamine released
- Hemoglobin and iron released
- • Production of leukotrienes • Activation of kallikrein-kinin system

- Arachidonic acid release
- ↑ Free radical formation

- • Vasoconstriction • Thrombosis formation
- • Vasospasm • Edema

- ↓ SCBF
- Secondary injury
- ↓ SCBF

- Tissue hypoxia

FIG. 60.1 Cascade of metabolic and cellular events that leads to spinal cord ischemia and hypoxia of secondary injury. *RBCs,* Red blood cells; *SCBF,* spinal cord blood flow. (Modified from Marciano FF, Greene KA, Apostolides PJ, et al: Pharmacologic management of spinal cord injury: Review of the literature, *BNI Q* 11:11, 1995. In KL McCance, SE Huether, editors: *Pathophysiology: The biologic basis for disease in adults and children,* ed 5, St Louis, 2006, Mosby.)

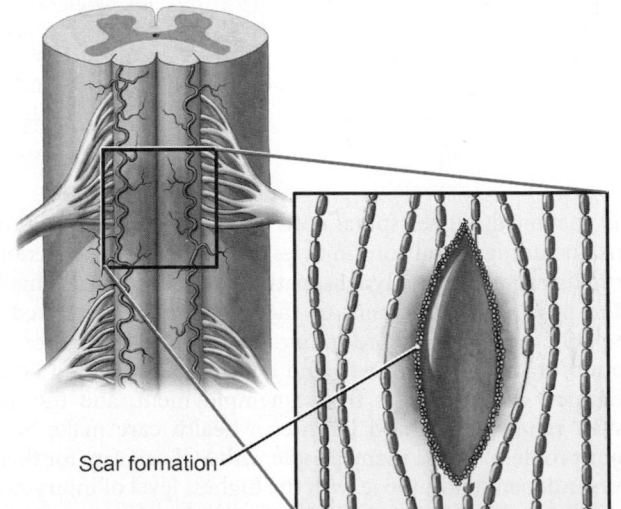

Scar formation

FIG. 60.2 1 to 2 days following the injury, astrocytes proliferate and surround the edges of the fibrotic scar to confine inflammation to the area of injury. This process may take 7 to 10 days. It protects neighboring neural tissue from further damage. (Used with permission from Barrow Neurological Institute, Phoenix, AZ.)

Mechanisms of Injury. The major mechanisms of injury include flexion, flexion-rotation, hyperextension, vertical compression, extension-rotation, and lateral flexion (Fig. 60.3). Flexion-rotation injury is the most unstable because ligaments that stabilize the spine are torn. This injury most often contributes to severe neurologic deficits.

Level of Injury. *Skeletal level* of injury is the vertebral level with the most damage to vertebra and related ligaments. *Neurologic level* is the lowest segment of the spinal cord with normal sensory and motor function on both sides of the body. The level of injury may be cervical, thoracic, lumbar, or sacral. Cervical and lumbar injuries are most common because those areas of the spine are associated with the greatest flexibility and movement.

Injury from C1 to T1 can cause paralysis of all 4 extremities, resulting in tetraplegia (formerly called *quadriplegia*). The degree of impairment in the arms after cervical injury depends on the level of injury. The lower the level, the more function is retained in the arms.

Paraplegia (paralysis and loss of sensation in the legs) can occur in SCI below the level of T2.[2] Fig. 60.4 shows affected structures and functions at different levels of cord injury.

Degree of Injury. The degree of spinal cord involvement may be complete or incomplete (partial). *Complete cord involvement* results in total loss of sensory and motor function below the level of injury. *Incomplete cord involvement* results in a mixed loss of voluntary motor activity and sensation and leaves some tracts intact. The degree of sensory and motor loss depends on the level of injury and reflects specific damaged nerve tracts.

Five major syndromes are associated with incomplete injuries: central cord syndrome, anterior cord syndrome, Brown-Séquard syndrome, cauda equina syndrome, and conus medullaris syndrome (Table 60.1).

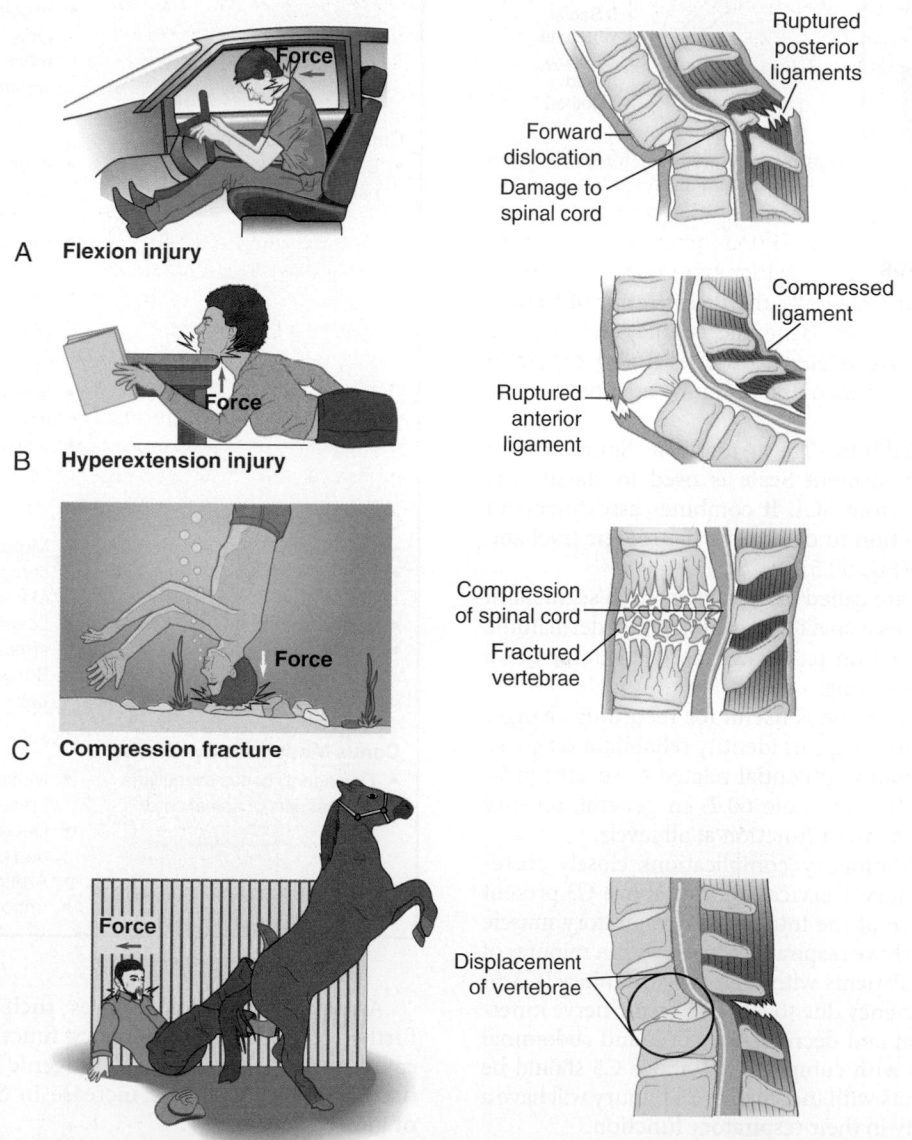

A Flexion injury

B Hyperextension injury

C Compression fracture

D Flexion-rotation injury

FIG. 60.3 Examples of mechanisms of spinal cord injury. **A,** Flexion injury of the cervical spine ruptures the posterior ligaments. **B,** Hyperextension injury of the cervical spine ruptures the anterior ligaments. **C,** Compression fractures crush the vertebrae and force bony fragments into the spinal canal. **D,** Flexion-rotation injury of the cervical spine often results in tearing of ligamentous structures that normally stabilize the spine. (*A, B,* and *C,* From Copstead-Kirkhorn LC, Banasik JL: *Pathophysiology,* ed 5, St Louis, 2014, Mosby.)

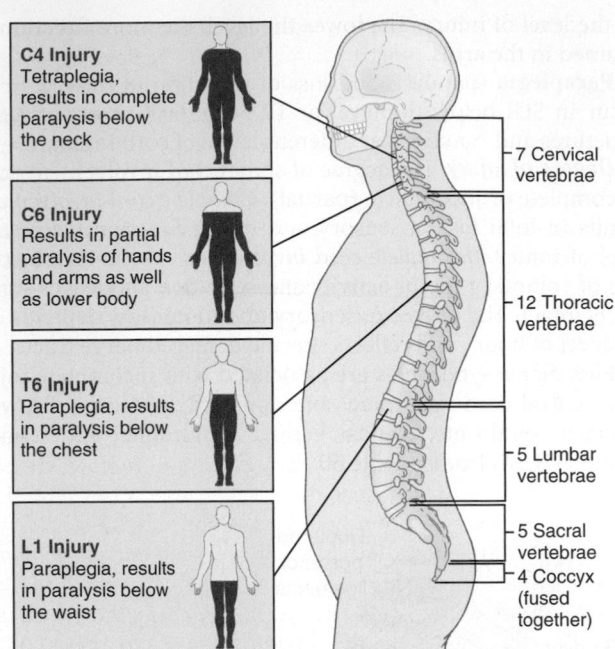

FIG. 60.4 Symptoms, degree of paralysis, and potential for rehabilitation depend on level of spinal injury.

C4 Injury
Tetraplegia, results in complete paralysis below the neck

C6 Injury
Results in partial paralysis of hands and arms as well as lower body

T6 Injury
Paraplegia, results in paralysis below the chest

L1 Injury
Paraplegia, results in paralysis below the waist

7 Cervical vertebrae

12 Thoracic vertebrae

5 Lumbar vertebrae

5 Sacral vertebrae

4 Coccyx (fused together)

Clinical Manifestations

Manifestations of SCI are generally the direct result of trauma that causes cord compression, ischemia, edema, and possible cord transection. They are related to the level and degree of injury. The patient with an incomplete injury may have a mix of manifestations.

Motor and Sensory Effects. The American Spinal Injury Association (ASIA) Impairment Scale is used to classify the severity of impairment from SCI. It combines assessments of motor and sensory function to determine neurologic level and completeness of injury (Fig. 60.5).[7]

The sensory regions are called *dermatomes*. Each segment of the spinal cord innervates a specific area of skin. A dermatome map is shown in Fig. 55.7 on p. 1284. Each dermatome has a recommended point for testing.

The ASIA Impairment Scale is useful for recording changes in neurologic status. It also helps us identify rehabilitation goals. Movement and rehabilitation potential related to specific locations of SCI are described in Table 60.2. In general, sensory function closely matches motor function at all levels.

Respiratory System. Respiratory complications closely correspond to the level of injury. Cervical injuries above C3 present special problems because of the total loss of respiratory muscle function. These patients have respiratory arrest within minutes of injury if not intubated. Patients with high cervical injury (C3-5) have respiratory insufficiency due to loss of phrenic nerve innervation to the diaphragm and decreases in chest and abdominal wall strength.[8] Patients with complete SCI above C5 should be intubated at once. Patients with incomplete SCI injury will have a high degree of variability in their respiratory function.

Cervical and thoracic injuries cause paralysis of abdominal muscles and often the intercostal muscles. The patient cannot cough effectively enough to remove secretions, increasing the risk for aspiration, atelectasis, and pneumonia. Hypoventilation and impairment of the intercostal muscles lead to a decrease in vital capacity and tidal volume.

TABLE 60.1 **Incomplete Spinal Cord Injury Syndromes**	
Description	**Manifestations**
Anterior Cord Syndrome	
• Damage to anterior spinal artery • Results in compromised blood flow to anterior spinal cord • Typically results from acute compression of anterior part of the spinal cord • Common with flexion injury	• Motor paralysis and loss of pain and temperature sensation below level of injury • Since posterior cord tracts are not injured, sensations of touch, position, vibration, and motion remain intact
Brown-Séquard Syndrome	
• Damage to half of the spinal cord • Typically results from penetrating injury to spinal cord	• *Contralateral* (opposite side of injury): Loss of pain and temperature sensation below level of injury • *Ipsilateral* (same side as injury): Loss of motor function, light touch, pressure, position, and vibratory sense
Cauda Equina Syndrome	
• Damage to cauda equina (lumbar and sacral nerve roots)	• Asymmetric distal weakness, patchy sensation in lower extremities • May cause flaccid paralysis of lower extremities • Complete loss of sensation between legs and over buttocks, inner thighs, and backs of legs (*saddle area*) • Areflexic (flaccid) bladder and bowel • Severe, radicular, asymmetric pain
Central Cord Syndrome	
• Damage to central spinal cord • Occurs most often in cervical cord region • More common in older adults • Caused by hyperextension injury in people with degenerative disease	• Motor weakness and altered sensation present in upper extremities • Lower extremities not usually affected • Burning pain in upper extremities
Conus Medullaris Syndrome	
• Damage to conus medullaris (lowest part of spinal cord)	• Motor function in legs may be preserved, weak, or flaccid • Decrease in or loss of sensation in perianal area • Areflexic bowel and bladder • Impotence

Associated traumatic injuries, such as lung contusions, can further compromise pulmonary function. Fluid overload can cause pulmonary edema. Neurogenic pulmonary edema may occur due to a dramatic increase in SNS activity at the time of injury.

Maintaining an arterial saturation above 92% reduces hypoxemia, which can lead to bradycardia and worsen secondary injury. Patients are assessed for manifestations of respiratory distress, including dyspnea, decreased vital capacity, and pCO_2 > 20mm Hg above baseline, which would indicate the need for intubation.

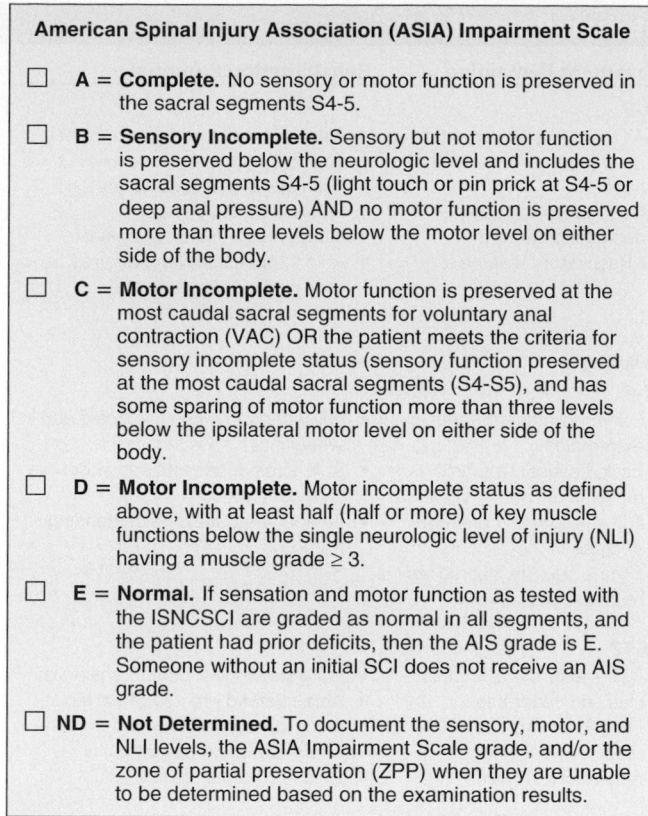

American Spinal Injury Association (ASIA) Impairment Scale

☐ **A = Complete.** No sensory or motor function is preserved in the sacral segments S4-5.

☐ **B = Sensory Incomplete.** Sensory but not motor function is preserved below the neurologic level and includes the sacral segments S4-5 (light touch or pin prick at S4-5 or deep anal pressure) AND no motor function is preserved more than three levels below the motor level on either side of the body.

☐ **C = Motor Incomplete.** Motor function is preserved at the most caudal sacral segments for voluntary anal contraction (VAC) OR the patient meets the criteria for sensory incomplete status (sensory function preserved at the most caudal sacral segments (S4-S5), and has some sparing of motor function more than three levels below the ipsilateral motor level on either side of the body.

☐ **D = Motor Incomplete.** Motor incomplete status as defined above, with at least half (half or more) of key muscle functions below the single neurologic level of injury (NLI) having a muscle grade ≥ 3.

☐ **E = Normal.** If sensation and motor function as tested with the ISNCSCI are graded as normal in all segments, and the patient had prior deficits, then the AIS grade is E. Someone without an initial SCI does not receive an AIS grade.

☐ **ND = Not Determined.** To document the sensory, motor, and NLI levels, the ASIA Impairment Scale grade, and/or the zone of partial preservation (ZPP) when they are unable to be determined based on the examination results.

FIG. 60.5 The ASIA Impairment Scale. (From American Spinal Injury Association.)

Cardiovascular System. Any cord injury above T6 leads to dysfunction of the SNS. The result may be bradycardia, peripheral vasodilation, and hypotension (neurogenic shock). Peripheral vasodilation causes relative hypovolemia because of the increase in the capacity of the dilated veins. It reduces venous return of blood to the heart. Cardiac output then decreases, leading to hypotension. Other injuries can cause hemorrhagic shock and further reduce BP. It is important to identify all causes of hypotension in the person with SCI. Those on β-blockers, young healthy patients, and older adults may not be tachycardic with hemorrhage.[8]

Urinary System. Urinary dysfunction occurs in most patients after SCI. **Neurogenic bladder** describes any type of bladder dysfunction related to abnormal or absent bladder innervation. After SCI, the ability for the bladder muscles and the micturition center in the brain to transmit information is impaired. Both the detrusor muscle (bladder wall) and sphincter muscle (a valve around the top of the urethra) may be overactive due to the lack of brain control. This may cause high bladder pressures and urinary retention. Incontinence results from reflex emptying and failure to store urine.

Depending on the injury, a neurogenic bladder may (1) have no reflex detrusor contractions (*flaccid, hypotonic*), which can result in bladder stretching from overdistention; (2) have hyperactive reflex detrusor contractions (*spastic*), seen in SCI above T12, leading to incontinence; or (3) lack coordination between detrusor contraction and urethral relaxation (*dyssynergia*), resulting in reflux of urine into the kidneys. Reflux into the kidneys can lead to stone formation, hydronephrosis, pyelonephritis, and renal failure.[9]

Gastrointestinal System. Decreased gastrointestinal (GI) motor activity contributes to gastric distention and the development of paralytic ileus. Gastric emptying may be delayed, especially in patients with higher level SCI. Excessive release of hydrochloric acid (HCl) in the stomach may cause stress ulcers. Dysphagia may be present in patients who need mechanical ventilation, tracheostomy, and anterior spine surgery.

Intraabdominal bleeding may be hard to diagnose because the person with SCI may not have pain or tenderness. Continued hypotension and decreases in hemoglobin and hematocrit may be the only signs of bleeding. Expanding abdominal girth may be seen.

Loss of voluntary control of the bowel after SCI results in **neurogenic bowel**. SCI above the level of the conus medullaris results in a *hyperreflexic* bowel with increased rectal and sigmoid compliance. Combined with increased anal sphincter tone and the inability to sense a full rectum, this causes stool retention and constipation.[10] SCI at or below the conus medullaris causes the bowel to be *areflexic*. Peristalsis is impaired and stool movement is slow. The defecation reflex may be damaged and anal sphincter tone relaxed. This leads to constipation, increased risk for incontinence, and possible impaction, ileus, or megacolon. Hemorrhoids can occur over time.

Integumentary System. The risk for skin breakdown over bony prominences in areas of decreased or absent sensation is a major consequence of immobility related to SCI. Pressure injuries can occur quickly and lead to infection and sepsis.

Thermoregulation. *Poikilothermia* is the inability to maintain a constant core temperature, with the patient assuming the temperature of the environment. It occurs in SCI because interruption of the SNS prevents peripheral temperature sensations from reaching the hypothalamus. There is a decreased ability to sweat or shiver below the level of injury, which affects the ability to regulate body temperature. The degree of poikilothermia depends on the level of injury. Cervical injuries are associated with a greater loss of ability to regulate temperature than are thoracic or lumbar injuries.

Metabolic Needs. The person with SCI has increased nutritional needs due to increased metabolism and more protein breakdown. Lean body mass decreases and muscles atrophy, leading to weight loss. In the acute injury phase, stress on the body from hemodynamic instability and medical interventions, such as surgery, can worsen stress. Nutritional support should start early. Enteral nutrition (EN) or parenteral nutrition (PN) can supply the person's caloric, protein, and micronutrient requirements needs.[11] Adequate nutrition helps prevent skin breakdown, reduce infection, and decrease the rate of muscle atrophy.

Peripheral Vascular Problems. Venous thromboembolism (VTE) is a common problem after SCI due to hypercoagulability, venous stasis, and venous endothelial injury.[12] Immobilization promotes venous stasis and thrombi of the lower extremities. Detecting a deep venous thrombosis (DVT) may be hard in a person with SCI because usual signs and symptoms, such as pain and tenderness, are not present.

Pain. Pain after SCI differs in type and severity. The patient's physical functioning and emotions influence pain. The pain can be nociceptive or neuropathic.

Nociceptive pain in SCI can result from musculoskeletal, visceral, and/or other types of injury (e.g., skin ulceration, headache). Patients often describe musculoskeletal pain as dull or aching. It starts or worsens with movement. Visceral pain is in

TABLE 60.2   Level of Spinal Cord Injury and Rehabilitation Potential

Movement Remaining	Rehabilitation Potential	Movement Remaining	Rehabilitation Potential
Tetraplegia		*C7-8*	
C1-3		• All triceps to elbow extension, finger extensors and flexors	• Able to transfer self to wheelchair
• Often fatal	• Able to drive electric wheelchair equipped with portable ventilator by using chin control or mouth stick, headrest to stabilize head	• Good grasp with some decreased strength	• Roll over and sit up in bed
• Movement in neck and above, loss of innervation to diaphragm, absence of independent respiratory function	• Computer use with mouth stick, head wand, or noise control	• ↓ Respiratory reserve	• Push self on most surfaces
	• Attendant care 24 hr/day, able to instruct others		• Perform most self-care
			• Independent use of wheelchair
			• Able to drive car with powered hand controls (in some patients)
			• Attendant care 0–6 hr/day
C4		**Paraplegia**	
• Sensation and movement in neck and above	• Same as C1-3	*T1-6*	
• May be able to breathe without ventilator		• Full innervation of upper extremities	• Full independence in self-care and in wheelchair
		• Back, essential intrinsic muscles of hand	• Able to drive car with hand controls (in most patients)
C5		• Full strength and dexterity of grasp	• Independent standing in standing frame
• Full neck, partial shoulder, back, biceps	• Able to drive electric wheelchair with mobile hand supports	• ↓ Trunk stability, decreased respiratory reserve	
• Gross elbow, inability to roll over or use hands	• Indoor mobility in manual wheelchair		
• ↓ Respiratory reserve	• Able to feed self with setup and adaptive equipment	*T6-12*	
	• Attendant care 10 hr/day	• Full, stable thoracic muscles and upper back	• Full independent use of wheelchair
		• Functional intercostal muscles, resulting in ↑ respiratory reserve	• Able to stand erect with full leg brace, ambulate on crutches with swing (although gait difficult)
C6			• Unable to climb stairs
• Shoulder and upper back abduction and rotation at shoulder	• Able to help with transfer and perform some self-care	*L1-2*	
• Full biceps to elbow flexion, wrist extension, weak grasp of thumb	• Feed self with hand devices	• Varying control of legs and pelvis	• Good sitting balance
• ↓ Respiratory reserve	• Push wheelchair on smooth, flat surface	• Instability of lower back	• Full use of wheelchair
	• Drive adapted van from wheelchair		• Ambulation with long leg braces
	• Independent computer use with adaptive equipment	*L3-4*	
	• Attendant care 6 hr/day	• Quadriceps and hip flexors	• Completely independent ambulation with short leg braces and canes
		• Absence of hamstring function, flail ankles	• Unable to stand for long periods

the thorax, abdomen, and/or pelvis. It may be dull, tender, or cramping.

Neuropathic pain in SCI occurs from damage to the spinal cord or nerve roots. The pain can be at or below the level of injury. Patients often describe the pain as hot, burning, tingling, pins and needles, cold, and/or shooting. They may be extremely sensitive to stimuli. Even light touch can cause significant pain. (Pain is discussed in Chapter 8.)

Diagnostic Studies

CT scan is the preferred imaging study to diagnose the location and degree of injury and the degree of spinal canal compromise. Cervical x-rays are done when CT scan is not readily available. However, it is hard to see C7 and T1 on a cervical x-ray, decreasing the ability to fully evaluate a cervical spine injury.

MRI is used to assess soft tissue injury, neurologic changes, unexplained neurologic deficits, or worsening neurologic condition. MRI results guide clinical decisions about surgery.[2] Perform a comprehensive neurologic examination with assessment of the head, chest, and abdomen for other injuries or trauma. Patients with cervical injuries who have altered mental status may need a CT angiogram to rule out vertebral artery damage. Table 37.9 presents the diagnostic studies used to determine the site or location and extent of a VTE.

Interprofessional Care

Prehospital. Goals immediately after injury include maintaining a patent *airway*, adequate ventilation/*breathing*, and adequate *circulating* blood volume (ABCs) and preventing extension of spinal cord damage (secondary injury). Table 60.3 outlines emergency management of the patient with SCI. Spinal motion should be restricted with a combination of a rigid cervical collar and a supportive backboard with straps. Patients should be kept supine and may be logrolled for transfers. Uncooperative patients may need chemical sedation or physical restraints to protect them from further injury.[13] Reverse Trendelenburg position may be used if necessary. Spinal immobilization in patients with penetrating trauma should be tried as long as it does not affect resuscitation efforts.[13]

Intubation to secure the airway is done as soon as possible for patients with respiratory distress. Using end-tidal CO_2 monitoring can help determine the need for rapid sequence intubation (RSI). Patients with stable airways in the field may need intubation at the medical facility. Systemic and neurogenic shock are treated with IV fluids and vasopressors to maintain systolic BP (SBP) greater than 90 mm Hg. After cervical injury, all body systems must be maintained until the full extent of the damage can be evaluated. After stabilization at the injury scene, the person should be transferred to the nearest medical facility.

➕ TABLE 60.3 Emergency Management

Spinal Cord Injury

Etiology	Assessment Findings	Interventions
Blunt Trauma • Compression, flexion, extension, or rotation injuries to spinal column • Diving • Falls • Motor vehicle crash • Pedestrian accidents • Sports injuries **Penetrating Trauma** • Gunshot wounds • Stab wounds • Stretched, torn, crushed, or lacerated spinal cord	• Respiratory distress/difficulty breathing • Neurogenic shock: hypotension, bradycardia, cool or warm dry skin • Spinal shock • Muscle weakness, paralysis, or flaccidity • Changes in sensation: temperature, light touch, deep pressure, proprioception • Numbness, paresthesia • Pain, tenderness, deformities, or muscle spasms adjacent to vertebral column • Cuts; bruises; open wounds on head, face, neck, or back • Bowel and bladder incontinence • Urinary retention • Priapism • Decreased rectal sphincter tone	**Initial** • Ensure patent airway and adequate breathing. • Maintain SaO_2 >90%: • Apply O_2 via nasal cannula, nonrebreather mask, or endotracheal tube. • Maintain SBP >90 mm Hg. • Establish IV access with 2 large-bore catheters to infuse normal saline or lactated Ringer's solution. • Immobilize and stabilize cervical spine. • Assess for other injuries. • Control external bleeding. • Obtain appropriate imaging. **Ongoing Monitoring** • Monitor vital signs, level of consciousness, motor and sensory function, O_2 saturation, cardiac rhythm, urine output. • Anticipate need for intubation if in respiratory distress or gag reflex absent. • Maintain normal temperature.

The preferred facility is one that specializes in acute SCI care. A thorough assessment determines the degree of deficit and the level and degree of injury.

Acute Care. Interprofessional care during the acute phase for a patient with a cervical injury is described in Table 60.4. Compared to cervical injury, patients with SCI of the thoracic and lumbar vertebrae need less intense support. At this level of injury, respiratory compromise is not as severe, and bradycardia is usually not a problem. Other problems are treated symptomatically.

Obtain a history, with emphasis on how the incident occurred. Assess the extent of injury perceived by the patient or by the emergency response system (ERS) personnel right after the event. Initial assessment occurs in the emergency department (ED). It includes managing the person's ABCs and vital signs to ensure a secure airway and maintain oxygenation saturation (SaO_2) greater than 92% and mean arterial pressure (MAP) greater than 85 mm Hg. Avoid SBP less than 90 mm Hg. Appropriate medical interventions and diagnostics are implemented to ensure the patient is hemodynamically stable.

Perform a complete neurologic assessment using the ASIA tool (Fig. 60.5). Muscle groups are tested with and against gravity, alone and against resistance, on both sides of the body. Record strength, symmetry, and spontaneous movement. Complete a sensory examination, including touch and pain, as tested by pinprick. Start at the toes and work upward toward the head. Assess rectal tone and note the presence of *priapism*. Voluntary anal contractions indicate incomplete SCI. If time and conditions permit, assess position sense and vibration.

Mechanisms of injury that cause spinal cord trauma, especially involving the cervical cord, may result in brain injury and/or vertebral artery injury. Assess for a history of unconsciousness, signs of concussion, and increased intracranial pressure (see Chapter 56). Carefully assess for musculoskeletal injuries and trauma to internal organs. Because the patient may have altered or no muscle, bone, or visceral sensations below the level of injury, the only clue to internal trauma with hemorrhage may be a rapidly decreasing BP and increasing pulse. Check urine for hematuria, which indicates internal injuries.

Move the patient in alignment as a unit *(logroll)* during transfers and when repositioning to prevent further injury. Monitor respiratory, cardiac, urinary, and GI functions. The patient may go directly to surgery after the initial evaluation or to the intensive care unit (ICU) for monitoring and management.

Nonoperative Stabilization. Nonoperative treatments involve stabilization of the injured spinal segment and decompression, either through traction or realignment. Stabilization eliminates damaging motion at the injury site. It is meant to prevent secondary spinal cord damage caused by narrowing of the spinal canal, or continued contusion or compression of the spinal cord at the level of the injury. Early realignment of an unstable fracture-dislocation injury by closed reduction through craniocervical traction is effective and safe.

Surgical Therapy. Surgical treatment after acute SCI is used to manage instability and decompress the spinal cord. It may reduce secondary injury and improve the patient's outcome. Early surgery (within 24 hours after the injury) is recommended for persons with central cord syndrome and for adults with an acute SCI at any level.[2] The type of surgery depends on the severity and level of the injury, mechanism of injury, and location and degree of compression.

Surgery to stabilize the spine can be done from the back of the spine *(posterior approach)* or from the front of the spine *(anterior approach)*. In some cases, both approaches may be needed. Fixation involves attaching metal screws, plates, or other devices to the bones of the spine to help keep them aligned. This procedure is usually done when 2 or more vertebrae are injured. Small pieces of bone may be attached to the injured bones to help them fuse into 1 solid piece. The bone used is obtained from the patient's spinal bone harvested during surgery, from another bone in the patient's body, or from donor bone. (Specific surgical and nursing interventions for these techniques are discussed in Chapter 63 on pp. 1488–1489.)

Drug Therapy. Current evidence for the use of methylprednisolone is mixed. Guidelines for managing spinal cord injuries issued by both the American Association of Neurological Surgeons and Congress of Neurological Surgeons do not recommend its use for treating acute SCI.[14] The FDS no longer approves its use either. However, recommendations in the AOSPine 2017 Guidelines suggest a 24-hour infusion of high-dose methylprednisolone within 8 hours of acute SCI.[2] So, some HCPs may consider this option.

VTE prophylaxis with low-molecular-weight heparin (LMWH) (e.g., enoxaparin [Lovenox]) or fixed, low-dose heparin should start within 72 hours after injury, unless contraindicated. Contraindications include internal or external bleeding and recent surgery. For those with abnormal kidney function, heparin is best as LMWH is mainly excreted via the kidneys.

Vasopressor agents (e.g., phenylephrine, norepinephrine) are used in the acute phase of injury as adjuvants to treatment. They maintain the MAP to improve perfusion to the spinal cord. Use of vasopressors has significant risk for complications. These include ventricular tachycardia, troponin elevation, metabolic acidosis, and atrial fibrillation. Dopamine has more complications than phenylephrine in SCI. Considerations for vasopressor selection include level of injury, patient age, and comorbidities (e.g., heart problems).

TABLE 60.4 Interprofessional Care

Cervical Cord Injury

Diagnostic Assessment
- History and physical examination, including complete neurologic examination
- ABGs
- Electrolytes, serum glucose, coagulation profile, hemoglobin and hematocrit
- Urinalysis
- CT scan, MRI, EMG (measure evoked potentials)
- Anteroposterior, lateral, and odontoid spinal x-rays
- Serial bedside pulmonary function tests (PFTs)

Management
Acute Care
- Immobilization and stabilization of vertebral column
- ABCs (airway, breathing, circulation)
- O$_2$ by high-humidity mask (PaO$_2$ >60 mm Hg)
- Intubation (if indicated by ABGs and PFTs)
- Maintain heart rate (e.g., atropine) and BP (e.g., dopamine) (SBP >90 mm Hg, MAP >85)
- Administer IV fluids
- Insert NG tube and attach to suction.
- Assessment and management of nutrition
- Maintain normal body temperature
- Indwelling urinary catheter
- Pain management
- VTE prophylaxis
- Pressure injury prevention
- Stress ulcer prophylaxis
- Bowel and bladder care and training
- Mobilization once spine stabilized
- Physical, occupational, speech therapy and physiatrist consults

Rehabilitation and Home Care
- Physical therapy (ROM, mobility, strength, equipment)
- Occupational therapy (splints, ADLs training)
- Speech therapy (swallow and cognition)
- Pain management
- Spasticity management
- Bowel and bladder training
- Autonomic dysreflexia prevention
- Pressure injury prevention
- Recreational therapy
- Patient and caregiver teaching

❖ NURSING MANAGEMENT: SPINAL CORD INJURY

◆ Nursing Assessment

Subjective and objective data you should obtain from a patient with recent SCI are outlined in Table 60.5.

TABLE 60.5 Nursing Assessment

Spinal Cord Injury

Subjective Data
Important Health Information
Past health history: Motor vehicle crash, sports injury, industrial incident, gunshot or stabbing injury, falls

Functional Health Patterns
Health perception–health management: Use of alcohol or recreational drugs. Risk-taking behaviors
Activity-exercise: Loss of strength, movement, and sensation below level of injury. Dyspnea, inability to breathe adequately ("air hunger")
Cognitive-perceptual: Tenderness, pain at or above level of injury. Numbness, tingling, burning, twitching of extremities
Coping–stress tolerance: Fear, denial, anger, depression

Objective Data
General
Poikilothermia (unable to regulate body heat)

Integumentary
Warm, dry skin below level of injury (neurogenic shock)

Respiratory
Injury at C1-3: Apnea, inability to cough
Injury at C4: Poor cough, diaphragmatic breathing, hypoventilation
Injury at C5-T6: ↓ Respiratory reserve

Cardiovascular
Injury above T6: Bradycardia, hypotension, postural hypotension, absence of vasomotor tone

Gastrointestinal
↓ Or absent bowel sounds (paralytic ileus in injuries above T5), abdominal distention, constipation, fecal incontinence, fecal impaction

Urinary
Retention (for injuries at T1-L2), flaccid bladder (acute stages), spasticity with reflex bladder emptying (later stages)

Reproductive
Priapism, altered sexual function

Neurologic
Complete: Areflexic, flaccid paralysis and anesthesia below level of injury resulting in tetraplegia (injuries above C8) or paraplegia (injuries below C8), hyperactive deep tendon reflexes and bilaterally positive Babinski test (after resolution of spinal shock)
Incomplete: Mixed loss of voluntary motor activity and sensation

Musculoskeletal
Muscle atony (in flaccid state), contractures (in spastic state)

Pain
Neuropathic, musculoskeletal, and/or visceral

Possible Diagnostic Findings
Location of level and type of bony involvement on spinal x-ray. Injury, edema, compression on CT scan and MRI; positive finding on myelogram

Nursing Diagnoses

Nursing diagnoses for the patient with SCI depend on the severity of the injury and level of dysfunction. Nursing diagnoses for a patient with SCI may include:

- Impaired breathing
- Impaired nutritional status
- Ineffective tissue perfusion
- Impaired tissue integrity
- Impaired urinary system function
- Constipation
- Difficulty coping

Additional information on nursing diagnoses and interventions for the patient with complete cervical SCI is presented in eNursing Care Plan 60.1 (available on the website for this chapter).

Planning

Overall goals are that the patient with an SCI will (1) maintain an optimal level of neurologic functioning; (2) have minimal or no complications of immobility; (3) learn new skills, gain new knowledge, and acquire new behaviors to be able to care for self or direct others to do so; and (4) return home at an optimal level of functioning.

Nursing Implementation

Health Promotion. Nursing interventions for the prevention of SCI include identifying high-risk persons and providing teaching. Support measures to combat distracted and impaired driving. Teach people to use child safety seats and helmets for motorcyclists and bicyclists. Promote programs for older adults (e.g., STEADI) aimed at preventing accidental death and injury.[15]

Emphasize the importance of health promotion and screening behaviors after SCI. Health-promoting behaviors after SCI can have significant impact on the general health and well-being of the person with SCI. Nursing interventions include (1) teaching and counseling; (2) referring to programs such as smoking cessation classes, recreation programs, and alcohol treatment programs; and (3) performing routine physical examinations for non-neurologic problems. Promotion and screening programs must be accessible to and accommodate people with SCI. Nurses should advocate for wheelchair-accessible examination rooms, adjustable-height examination tables, and appointment scheduling that allows extra time if needed.

Acute Care. High cervical cord injury caused by flexion-rotation is the most complex SCI. It is the focus of this section. Interventions for this type of injury can be modified for patients with less severe injuries.

Immobilization. To restrict spinal motion, maintain the neck in a neutral position. For cervical injuries, closed reduction with skeletal traction is used for early realignment *(reduction)* of the injury. Crutchfield (Fig. 60.6) or Gardner-Wells tongs or halo (halo ring) can provide this type of traction. A rope extends from the center of the device over a pulley to weights attached at the end. Traction must be maintained at all times. Possible displacement of the skull pins is a disadvantage of tongs. If pin displacement occurs, hold the patient's head in a neutral position and get help. Immobilize the head while the HCP reinserts the tongs.

> **! SAFETY ALERT Cervical Spine Injuries**
> - Always keep the patient's body in correct alignment.
> - Turn the patient as a unit (e.g., logrolling) to prevent movement of the spine.

No specific guidelines address the maximum weight for traction. The HCP may start with 10 lb and add 5 lb for each level to the injury. The goal is spinal reduction. Awake patients are monitored with x-ray and neurologic and pain assessment. Comatose patients need serial x-rays to evaluate the effects of traction. The need for surgery is determined after the spine is reduced. After cervical fusion or other stabilization surgery, the patient may have a hard cervical collar or sternal-occipital-mandibular immobilizer brace (Fig. 60.7).

Some patients with spinal fractures with or without acute SCI may not be able to have surgery but still need immobilization for their cervical fracture. In these patients, the halo frame can be attached to a special vest (Halo vest) (Fig. 60.8). This allows the patient to move and ambulate while cervical bones fuse. Surgery is used instead of the halo if the patient has ligament instability from the injury; has severe cervical deformity; or is morbidly obese, older, cachectic, or noncompliant.

Infection at the tong or pin insertion sites is a potential problem. Preventive care is based on agency protocol. A common protocol involves cleansing sites twice a day with chlorhexidine. Antibiotic ointment is then applied to act as a mechanical barrier to the entrance of bacteria. Patient and caregiver teaching for a patient with a halo vest is outlined in Table 60.6.

Patients with stable thoracic or lumbar spine injuries may be immobilized with a custom thoracolumbar sacral orthosis (TLSO or body jacket) to limit spinal flexion, extension, and rotation. A Jewett brace may be used instead to restrict forward flexion. Unstable injuries may require surgical decompression and fusion in addition to the TLSO or lumbosacral orthotic (LSO).

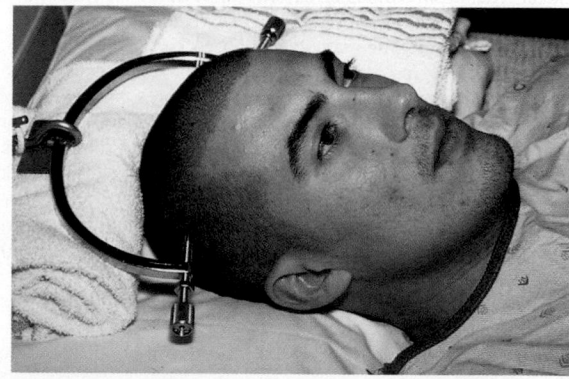

FIG. 60.6 Cervical traction is attached to tongs inserted in the skull. (Courtesy Michael S. Clement, MD, Mesa, AZ.)

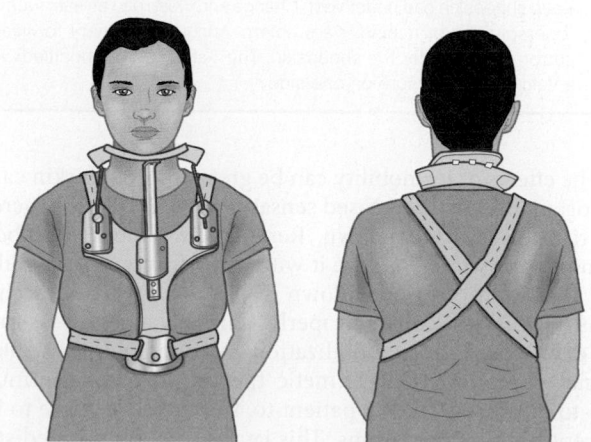

FIG. 60.7 Sternal-occipital-mandibular immobilizer brace.

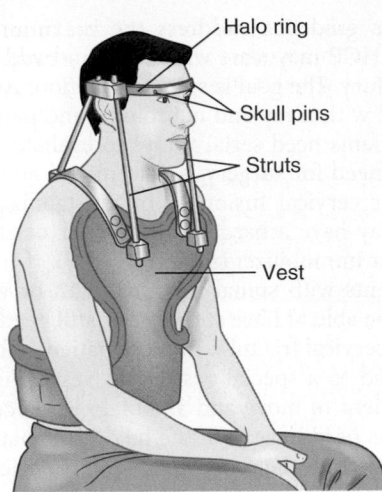

FIG. 60.8 Halo vest. The halo traction brace immobilizes the cervical spine, which allows the patient to ambulate and take part in self-care. (Modified from Urden LD, Stacy KM, Lough ME: *Priorities in critical care nursing,* ed 6, St Louis, 2012, Mosby.)

TABLE 60.6   Patient & Caregiver Teaching

Halo Vest Care

Include the following instructions when teaching the patient and caregiver management of a halo vest:

1. Inspect the pins on the halo traction ring. Report to HCP if pins are loose or signs of infection are present, including redness, tenderness, swelling, or drainage at insertion sites.
2. Clean around pin sites carefully with chlorhexidine, water, or half-strength peroxide on a cotton swab as directed.
3. Apply antibiotic ointment as prescribed.
4. For skin care, have patient lie down with the head resting on a pillow to reduce pressure on the brace. Loosen 1 side of the vest. Gently wash the skin under the vest with soap and water, rinse area, and then dry it thoroughly. At the same time, check the skin for pressure points, redness, swelling, bruising, or chafing. Close the open side and repeat the procedure on the other side.
5. If the vest becomes wet or damp, carefully dry it with a blow dryer.
6. Encourage patient to use assistive device (e.g., cane, walker) to improve balance; encourage use of flat shoes.
7. Teach patient to turn the entire body, not just the head and neck, when trying to look sideways.
8. In case of an emergency, always keep a set of wrenches close to the halo vest.
9. Mark the vest strap to maintain consistent buckling and fit.
10. Avoid grabbing bars or vest to help the patient.
11. Keep sheepskin pad under vest. Change and wash pad at least weekly.
12. If perspiration or itching is a problem, encourage patient to wear a cotton T-shirt under the sheepskin. The T-shirt can be modified with a Velcro seam closure on one side.

The effects of immobility can be great. Thorough skin care is important because decreased sensation and circulation increase the risk for skin breakdown. Remove the patient's backboard as soon as possible. Replace it with other forms of immobilization to prevent skin breakdown in the coccygeal and occipital areas. Fit cervical collars properly. Carefully assess areas under any device used for immobilization. We often place patients on special beds (Fig. 60.9). Kinetic therapy involves continuous side-to-side rotation of a patient to 40 degrees or more to help prevent lung complications. This lateral rotation also redistributes pressure, helping prevent pressure injuries.

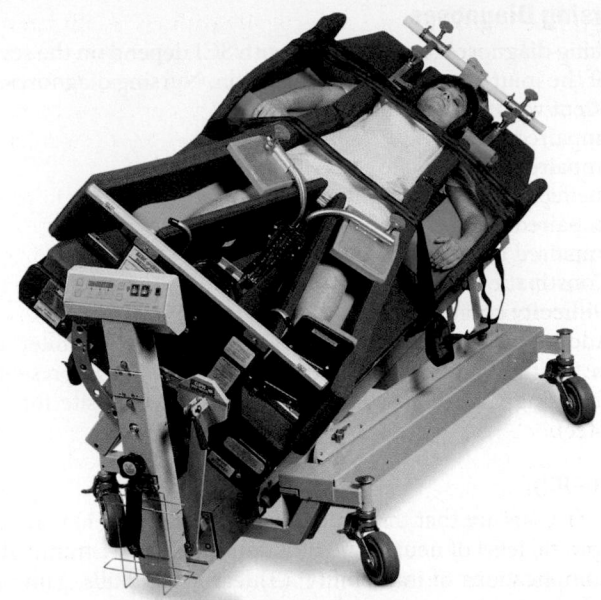

FIG. 60.9 The RotoRest Therapy System helps prevent and treat lung complications for immobile patients, including those with unstable cervical, thoracic, and lumbar fractures. Kinetic therapy, the continual side-to-side bilateral rotation of the patient, redistributes pulmonary blood flow and mobilizes secretions to improve ventilation and perfusion matching. The therapy system helps to prevent pressure injuries. (Courtesy Arjo Huntleigh, Addison, IL.)

Respiratory Dysfunction. Respiratory complications are the leading acute and chronic causes of morbidity and mortality in SCI.[16] Respiratory dysfunction is present in up to 65% of patients with cervical SCI. During the first 48 hours after injury, spinal cord edema may increase the level of dysfunction, and respiratory distress may occur. Injury at or above C4 affects the phrenic nerve, which leads to the diaphragm, and breathing can stop.

Monitor the patient carefully for respiratory compromise and be prepared for quick action if arrest occurs. Regularly assess (1) breath sounds, (2) arterial blood gases (ABGs), (3) tidal volume, (4) vital capacity, (5) skin color, (6) breathing patterns (especially use of accessory muscles), (7) subjective comments about the ability to breathe, and (8) amount and color of sputum. A PaO_2 greater than 60 mm Hg and a $PaCO_2$ less than 45 mm Hg are acceptable values in a patient with uncomplicated tetraplegia. A patient who is unable to count to 20 aloud without taking a breath needs immediate attention.

In addition to ongoing assessment, intervene to maintain ventilation. Apply O_2 and provide appropriate ventilatory support until ABGs stabilize. If the patient is exhausted from labored breathing or ABGs show inadequate oxygenation or ventilation, endotracheal intubation or tracheostomy and mechanical ventilation is needed. Patients who have chest trauma or difficulty weaning from the ventilator may need a tracheostomy for airway management.

Clearing secretions is vital in reducing the risk for lung complications and possible respiratory failure.[16] Perform tracheal suctioning if crackles or coarse breath sounds are present. Chest physiotherapy and assisted (augmented) coughing can help. Perform assisted coughing either manually, by placing the heels of both hands just below the xiphoid process and exert firm upward pressure to the area timed with the patient's efforts to cough (see Fig. 67.6), or mechanically with an insufflation-exsufflation device. Encourage the use of incentive spirometry.

The older adult has more difficulty responding to hypoxia and hypercapnia. Thus aggressive chest physiotherapy, adequate oxygenation, and proper pain management are essential to maximize respiratory function and gas exchange.

Cardiovascular Instability. Heart rate is slowed, often to less than 60 beats/min, because of unopposed vagal response. Any increase in vagal stimulation, as occurs with turning or suctioning, can cause cardiac arrest. Loss of SNS tone in peripheral vessels results in chronic low BP with potential orthostatic hypotension. The lack of muscle tone to aid venous return can cause sluggish blood flow and predispose the patient to VTE. Dysrhythmias may occur.

Frequently assess vital signs. If bradycardia is symptomatic, give an anticholinergic drug, such as atropine. A temporary or permanent pacemaker may be inserted in some patients. Maintain SBP greater than 90 mm Hg and keep MAP between 85 and 90 mm Hg for the first 7 days after SCI. Manage hypotension with fluid replacement and a vasopressor agent, such as phenylephrine or norepinephrine.

Maintain a normal blood volume. If blood loss has occurred from other injuries, monitor hemoglobin and hematocrit and give blood according to protocol. Assess the patient for signs of hypovolemic shock from hemorrhage.

Orthostatic hypotension is likely to occur in the patient with injury at T6 and above. The patient may have light headedness, dizziness, and nausea. Assess orthostatic BP when mobilizing the patient. Some lose consciousness when moved from the bed to a chair. For symptomatic patients, use an abdominal binder and graduated compression stockings to promote venous return. Drugs used to increase intravascular volume include salt tablets and fludrocortisone. Midodrine may be given to promote blood vessel contraction and increase venous return.

Consider the effects of aging on the cardiovascular system of the older adult. The older patient is less able to manage the stress of traumatic injury because heart contractions weaken, and cardiac output is reduced. Maximum heart rate is reduced. The older adult may also have cardiovascular disease.

Use LMWH or low-dose heparin in combination with intermittent pneumatic compression devices or graduated compression stockings to promote venous return and reduce the risk for VTE. Remove stockings every 8 hours for skin care. Assess thighs and calves every shift for signs of VTE. Regularly perform range-of-motion (ROM) exercises and stretching. Continue VTE prophylaxis for 3 months after injury.

Fluid and Nutritional Management. During the first 48 to 72 hours after the injury, the GI tract may stop functioning (*paralytic ileus*). A nasogastric (NG) tube must be inserted if ileus occurs. Because the patient cannot have oral intake, monitor fluid and electrolyte status.

Nutrition should be started within the first 72 hours after injury. Specific solutions and additives are determined by individual requirements. Due to severe catabolism, a high-protein, high-calorie diet is needed for energy and tissue repair. If the patient cannot be fed through the GI system, either orally or through EN, PN should be started to reduce nitrogen losses that occur during the hypermetabolic state.

Once bowel sounds are present or flatus is passed, and the patient is not receiving mechanical ventilation, a formal swallow evaluation is done. If no risk for aspiration is identified, gradually introduce oral food and fluids. If the patient fails the

swallow evaluation or is unable to eat due to an endotracheal tube or tracheostomy, a more secure feeding tube may be placed in the stomach or jejunum (see Chapter 39).

Patients may have anorexia due to depression, boredom with agency food, or discomfort at being fed (often by a hurried person). Some patients have a normally small appetite. Sometimes refusal to eat is a way of asserting control. If the patient is not eating adequately, assess the cause.

Based on assessment findings, make a contract with the patient with mutual goal setting for the diet. This contract gives the patient increased control and often results in improved nutritional intake. General measures also may be effective. For example, provide a pleasant eating environment, allow adequate time to eat (including any self-feeding the patient can achieve), encourage the family to bring in special foods, and plan social rewards for eating.

Consult a dietitian to ensure evaluation of the appropriate laboratory markers and develop the treatment plan. Keep a calorie count and record the patient's daily weight to evaluate progress. If possible, the patient should take part in recording calorie intake. Dietary supplements may be needed to meet nutritional goals. Include increased dietary fiber to promote bowel function.

Bladder and Bowel Management. Immediately after the injury, urine retention occurs because of the loss of autonomic and reflex control of the bladder and sphincter (*neurogenic bladder*). Because there is no sensation of fullness, overdistention of the bladder can result in reflux into the kidney and cause renal failure. Bladder overdistention may even result in rupture of the bladder. Thus an indwelling catheter may be inserted soon after injury. Ensure patency of the catheter by frequent inspection and irrigation, if needed. In some agencies, an HCP's order is required for this procedure. Strict aseptic technique for catheter care is essential to prevent infection. During the period of indwelling catheterization, encourage a large fluid intake. Check the catheter to prevent kinking and ensure free flow of urine.

Catheter-acquired urinary tract infection (CAUTI) is a common problem. The best way to prevent CAUTI is regular and complete bladder drainage. Once the patient is stabilized, assess the best means of managing long-term urinary function. Clean intermittent catheterization (CIC) is the preferred method for emptying the bladder. CAUTI and CIC are discussed in Chapter 45.

CIC should be done 4 to 6 times daily to prevent bacterial overgrowth from urinary stasis. Keep urine residuals under 500 mL to prevent bladder distention. If the urine is cloudy or has a strong odor or if the patient develops symptoms of a urinary tract infection (UTI) (e.g., chills, fever, malaise), send a specimen for culture.

Consider age-related changes in renal function. The older adult is more likely to develop renal stones. Older men may have benign prostatic hyperplasia, which may interfere with urinary flow and complicate management of urinary problems. It can affect the ability to complete CIC.

Start a bowel program to combat constipation from neurogenic bowel. This involves inserting a rectal stimulant (suppository or small-volume enema) daily at a regular time, followed by gentle digital stimulation or manual evacuation until evacuation is complete. At first, the program may be done in bed with the patient in the side-lying position. However, as soon as the patient has resumed sitting, the patient should be in the upright position on a padded bedside commode chair. These programs typically take 30 to 60 minutes to complete. Measures to reduce constipation include adequate fluid intake, a diet high in fiber and vegetables, and increased activity and exercise.

Temperature Control. Monitor the environment closely to maintain an appropriate temperature. Regularly assess the patient's body temperature. Do not use excess covers or unduly expose the patient (e.g., during bathing). If an infection with high fever develops, more aggressive methods for temperature control may be needed (e.g., a cooling blanket).

Stress Ulcers. Stress ulcers can occur in the patient with SCI because of the physiologic response to severe trauma and psychologic stress. Peak incidence of stress ulcers is 6 to 14 days after injury. Test stool and gastric contents daily for blood. Monitor the hematocrit for a slow drop. Histamine (H_2)-receptor blockers (e.g., ranitidine) or proton pump inhibitors (e.g., pantoprazole, omeprazole) given prophylactically decreases the secretion of HCl acid and prevents ulcers.

Sensory Deprivation. To prevent sensory deprivation, compensate for the patient's absent sensations by stimulating the patient above the level of injury. Conversation, music, and interesting foods can be a part of the nursing care plan. If the head of the bed must stay flat, provide prism glasses to help the patient read and watch television.

Help the patient avoid withdrawing from the environment. Promote adequate rest and sleep. Assess for changes in mood. Depression is common (discussed later in chapter on p. 1418).

Pain Management. Musculoskeletal nociceptive pain can develop from injuries to bones, muscles, and ligaments. The pain is worse with movement or palpation. Antiinflammatory drugs, such as ibuprofen (Motrin), may help with pain. Opioids may be used to manage nociceptive pain.

Visceral nociceptive pain is a dull, tender, or cramping pain in the thorax, abdomen, or pelvis. It may originate in the bladder or bowel. Assess the patient's bowel and bladder function to avoid bladder distention or constipation. Other causes of nociceptive pain include UTI and renal stones. Notify the HCP if the patient has persistent pain despite treatment. Diagnostic imaging may be needed to determine the cause.

Neuropathic pain in the initial phase is usually at the level of SCI. It may occur on 1 or both sides of the body within the affected dermatome and up to 3 levels below. The patient will describe hot, burning, tingling, shooting, electric pain. Pregabalin (Lyrica) is used to reduce symptoms.

Neuropathic pain can occur months or years after SCI, become chronic, and negatively affect sleep. The patient's mood, sudden noise, constipation, and infection can affect the pain. Teach the patient and caregiver about possible pain triggers and offer relaxation therapy. Other modes of treatment may include tricyclic antidepressants, intrathecal drugs, antiseizure drugs, epidural stimulation, and destructive surgical intervention.

Skin Care. The most common long-term complication in SCI is pressure injury (PI) formation. Healthy skin requires adequate blood circulation. Constant pressure in 1 position can compress blood vessels and limit blood supply, causing cell death and PI. Little evidence addresses interventions for prevention and treatment of PI in SCI.[17] Factors associated with increased risk for PI formation include heart and renal disease, smoking, alcohol or drug use, diabetes, hypoxia, hypotension, and pneumonia, UTI, and other infections.[18]

Prevention of PI requires diligent nursing care. Perform a risk assessment for PI formation with a daily comprehensive visual and tactile examination of the skin. Areas most vulnerable to breakdown include the sacrum, ischia, trochanters, and heels. Assess surgical incisions for healing and skin integrity under collars and braces. Regularly assess nutritional status. Both weight loss and gain can contribute to skin breakdown. Teach the patient and caregiver about the causes and risk factors for PI development.[19]

A consult with the wound, ostomy, continence nurse (WOCN) can assist with prevention and management strategies (e.g., surface overlays).[19] Monitor incontinence and implement appropriate neurogenic bowel and bladder management interventions. Apply skin barrier creams.

Carefully position and reposition the patient at least every 2 hours. Gradually increase the times between turns if no redness over bony prominences is seen when turning. While the patient is supine in bed, float the heels to reduce pressure. Consider prophylactic dressings to prevent sacral and heel wounds. Move the patient carefully during turns and transfers to avoid stretching and folding of soft tissues *(shear)* or abrasion.

Many patients are placed on specialty mattresses.[17] When the patient is moved to a chair or wheelchair, use pressure-relieving cushions. Pressure relief should be scheduled every 15 to 20 minutes when the patient is in a chair and should last 30 to 60 seconds each time.

Reflexes. Once spinal cord shock is resolved, return of reflexes may complicate rehabilitation. Lacking control from the higher brain centers, reflexes are often hyperactive and have exaggerated responses. Penile erection can occur from a variety of stimuli, causing embarrassment and discomfort. Spasms ranging from mild twitches to convulsive movements below the level of injury may occur. The patient or caregiver may interpret this reflex activity as a return of function. Tactfully explain the reason for the activity. Tell the patient of the positive use of these reflexes in sexual, bowel, and bladder retraining. Antispasmodic drugs, such as baclofen (Lioresal), dantrolene (Dantrium), and tizanidine (Zanaflex), may help control spasms. Botulism toxin injections may be given to treat severe spasticity.

Autonomic Dysreflexia. The return of reflexes after the resolution of spinal shock means patients with injury at T6 or higher may develop autonomic dysreflexia. Autonomic dysreflexia (AD) is a massive, uncompensated cardiovascular reaction mediated by the SNS. It involves stimulation of sensory receptors below the level of the SCI. The intact SNS below the level of injury responds to the stimulation with a reflex arteriolar vasoconstriction that increases BP. The parasympathetic nervous system is unable to directly counteract these responses via the injured spinal cord. Baroreceptors in the carotid sinus and aorta sense the hypertension and stimulate the parasympathetic system. This causes a decrease in heart rate. Visceral and peripheral vessels do not dilate because efferent impulses cannot pass through the injured spinal cord. It most often presents in the chronic phase after SCI.[20]

The most common precipitating cause of AD is a distended bladder or rectum. However, any sensory stimulation, including contraction of the bladder or rectum, stimulation of the skin, or stimulation of pain receptors can cause AD. AD is a life-threatening condition that requires immediate resolution. Proper identification and elimination of the inciting stimulus for AD can resolve the event. If uncorrected, it can lead to status epilepticus, stroke, myocardial infarction, and even death.

Manifestations include hypertension, throbbing headache, marked diaphoresis above the level of injury, bradycardia (30 to 40 beats/min), piloerection from pilomotor spasm, flushing of the skin above the level of injury, blurred vision or spots in the visual fields, nasal congestion, anxiety, and nausea. Measure BP when a patient with SCI reports a headache. Suspect AD in adults with SBP elevation of 20 to 40 mm Hg above baseline.[20]

Immediate nursing interventions include elevating the head of the bed 45 degrees or sitting the patient upright (to lower the BP) and determining the cause (bowel impaction, urinary retention, UTI, PI, tight clothing). Notify the HCP. The most common cause is bladder irritation. Immediate catheterization to relieve bladder distention may be needed. Instill lidocaine jelly in the urethra before catheterization. If a catheter is already in place, check it for kinks or folds. If it is plugged, perform small-volume irrigation slowly and gently to open the catheter or insert a new catheter.

Stool impaction can cause AD. Apply an anesthetic ointment to avoid increasing symptoms, then perform a digital rectal examination (if trained). Remove all skin stimuli, such as constrictive clothing and tight shoes. Monitor BP often during the episode. If symptoms persist after the source has been relieved, give a rapid-onset and short-duration agent, such as nitroglycerin, nitroprusside, or hydralazine. Continue careful monitoring until vital signs stabilize.

Teach the patient and caregiver to recognize causes and symptoms of AD (Table 60.7). They must understand the life-threatening nature of AD, know how to relieve the cause, and activate the ERS, if needed.

Rehabilitation and Home Care. Rehabilitation of the person with SCI is complex. With physical and psychologic care and intensive and specialized rehabilitation, the patient with SCI can learn to function at the highest level of wellness. All patients with a new SCI should receive comprehensive inpatient rehabilitation in a rehabilitation unit or center that specializes in SCI rehabilitation.[2] Rehabilitation is an interprofessional team effort. Team members include rehabilitation nurses, HCPs, physical therapists, occupational therapists, speech therapists, vocational counselors, psychologists, therapeutic recreation specialists, prosthetists, orthotists, case managers, social workers, and dietitians.

Many of the problems that begin in the acute period become chronic and continue throughout life. Rehabilitation focuses on retraining physiologic processes as well as extensive patient and caregiver teaching about how to manage the physiologic and life changes resulting from the injury (Fig. 60.10).

Rehabilitation care is organized around the patient's goals and needs. The patient is expected to be involved in therapies and learn self-care for several hours each day. Such intensive work at a time when the patient is dealing with the sudden change in health and function can be stressful. Progress may be slow. The rehabilitation nurse has a key role in providing encouragement, specialized nursing care, and patient and caregiver teaching and in helping to coordinate efforts of the rehabilitation team.

Respiratory Rehabilitation. The patient with mechanical ventilation will need around-the-clock caregivers who are knowledgeable about respiratory hygiene and tracheostomy care. The rehabilitation nurse and respiratory therapist should teach patients and caregivers about home ventilator and tracheostomy care. The patient may need chest percussion or postural drainage to manage secretions to lower the risk for atelectasis and pneumonia. Refer to appropriate community agencies as needed.

Some patients with high cervical SCI have improved respiratory function with phrenic nerve stimulators or electronic diaphragmatic pacemakers.[21] These devices are not appropriate for all ventilator-dependent patients but are safe and effective for those with an intact phrenic nerve. Some ventilators are portable, allowing ventilator-dependent patients with tetraplegia to be mobile and less dependent.

If the patient was weaned from the ventilator during hospitalization, downsizing (gradual decrease in size) and removal of the tracheostomy will be done during rehabilitation. Teach assisted coughing, regular use of incentive spirometry, and

TABLE 60.7 Patient & Caregiver Teaching

Autonomic Dysreflexia

For a patient at risk for autonomic dysreflexia, include the following information in the teaching plan for the patient and caregiver:

1. Signs and symptoms
   - Sudden onset of acute headache.
   - Elevation in BP and/or reduction in pulse rate.
   - Flushed face and upper chest (above level of injury) and pale extremities (below level of injury).
   - Sweating above level of injury.
   - Nasal congestion.
   - Feeling of apprehension.
   - Immediate interventions.
   - Raise the person to a sitting position.
   - Remove the noxious stimulus (fecal impaction, kinked urinary catheter, tight clothing).
   - Call the HCP if above actions do not relieve the signs and symptoms.
2. Measures to decrease the incidence of autonomic dysreflexia
   - Maintain regular bowel function.
   - If manual rectal stimulation is used to promote bowel function, use a local anesthetic to prevent autonomic dysreflexia.
   - Monitor urine output.
   - Teach the patient to wear a Medic Alert bracelet indicating a history of risk for autonomic dysreflexia.

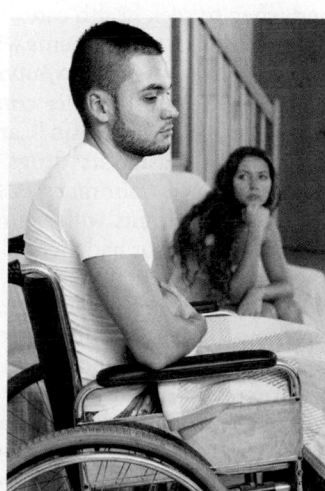

FIG. 60.10 A spinal cord injury has a major effect on a person's physical, emotional, and psychologic health.

TABLE 60.8 Types of Neurogenic Bladder

Type	Characteristics	Causes	Manifestations
Uninhibited bladder (spastic, overactive)	• No inhibitions influence time and place of voiding • Bladder empties in response to stretching of bladder wall	• Results from lesions above the pons • Observed in stroke, brain tumor, brain trauma	• Incontinence, frequency, urgency • Voiding is unpredictable and incomplete

Upper motor neuron bladder (flaccid, spastic/overactive)	• *Mixed A type* (most common):
	  • Bladder is flaccid and external sphincter is spastic, leading to urinary retention.
	• *Mixed B type:*
	  • Bladder is spastic with flaccid external sphincter leading to urinary incontinence.
		• Results from lesions between pons and sacral spinal cord
		• Seen in SCI or multiple sclerosis involving the cervicothoracic spinal cord
			• Detrusor-sphincter dyssynergia
			• Can lead to high bladder pressures and kidney damage from urinary reflux
			• Sensory function impaired

Lower motor neuron bladder (flaccid, underactive, areflexic)	• Bladder acts as if all motor functions were paralyzed • Bladder fills without emptying	• Results from lower motor neuron injury caused by trauma involving S2-4 or below • Lesions of cauda equina, pelvic nerves	• If sensory function intact, patient feels bladder distention and hesitancy • No control of micturition, resulting in urinary retention, over distention of bladder, overflow incontinence, and UTI

breathing exercises to the patient who is not ventilator dependent. They should limit exposure to persons with fever, cold, and cough. Adhering to swallowing precautions (e.g., proper positioning of head and neck) and diet recommendations can prevent aspiration.

Neurogenic Bladder. Types of neurogenic bladder are described in Table 60.8. The type of bladder dysfunction determines management options. After the patient's overall condition is stable and assessment shows return of neurologic reflexes, urodynamic testing (see Table 44.11) and a urine culture may be done. Diagnostic and interprofessional care of neurogenic bladder is described in Table 60.9.

The patient with SCI and a neurogenic bladder needs a comprehensive program to manage bladder function. The goal is to improve quality of life and safety through preserving renal function, minimizing UTI and bladder stones, and developing a plan for urinary continence. Many factors are considered when selecting a bladder management strategy. These include patient preference, upper extremity function, and caregiver availability. For the selected strategy, teach the patient and caregiver successful self-management. Teach them about the various management techniques, how to obtain supplies, care of supplies and equipment, and when to seek health care.

Various drugs can be used to treat patients with a neurogenic bladder. Anticholinergic drugs (e.g., oxybutynin, tolterodine [Detrol]) may be used to suppress bladder contraction. α-Adrenergic blockers (e.g., terazosin, doxazosin [Cardura]) can relax the urethral sphincter. Antispasmodic drugs (e.g., baclofen) may decrease spasticity of pelvic floor muscles. *Botulinum toxin* is an effective alternative in patients with neurogenic detrusor overactivity who cannot tolerate or had an inadequate response to anticholinergic drugs.[22]

Numerous drainage methods are possible. These include bladder reflex retraining (if partial voiding control remains), indwelling catheter, CIC, and external catheter (condom catheter). Evaluate long-term use of an indwelling catheter because of the associated high incidence of CAUTI, fistula formation, and diverticula. However, this is the best option for some patients. Patients with indwelling catheters need to have adequate fluid intake (at least 3 to 4 L/day). Regularly check the patency of the indwelling catheter. Frequency of routine catheter changes

 TABLE 60.9 Interprofessional Care

Neurogenic Bladder

Diagnostic Assessment

• History and physical examination, including neurologic and pelvic examinations
• Laboratory: Urinalysis, urine culture and sensitivity, blood urea nitrogen, serum creatinine, creatinine clearance
• Urodynamic testing (postvoid residual, cystometric testing, EMG, urethral pressure profile)

Management

• Patient teaching
• Voiding diary
• Bladder retraining: time voiding, manual expression, intermittent catheterization
• Fluid schedule: intake of 1800–2000 mL/day
• Indwelling urinary catheter

Drug Therapy

• Tricyclic antidepressants
• Anticholinergic drugs
• α-Adrenergic blockers
• Antispasmodics
• Botulinum toxin injection into bladder wall

Bladder and/or Urethral Surgical Therapy

• Bladder augmentation
• Sphincter resection or removal *(sphincterotomy)*
• Electrode placement for electrical stimulation
• Urinary diversion
• Urethral stents and balloon dilation
• Artificial urinary sphincter

ranges widely depending on the type of catheter used and agency policy.

CIC is recommended as the first-line option for bladder management (see Chapter 45). Nursing assessment is important in selecting the time interval between catheterizations. At first, catheterization is done every 4 hours. Measure bladder volume before catheterization using a bladder ultrasound machine. If less than 200 mL of urine is present, the time interval until

TABLE 60.10   Patient & Caregiver Teaching

Bowel Management After Spinal Cord Injury

For the patient with a spinal cord injury, include the following information about bowel management in the teaching plan for the patient and caregiver:

1. Optimal nutritional intake includes the following:
   - 3 well-balanced meals each day
   - 2 servings from the milk group
   - 2 or more servings from the meat group, including beef, pork, poultry, eggs, fish
   - 4 or more servings from the vegetable and fruit groups
   - 4 or more servings from the bread and cereal group
2. Fiber intake should be about 20–30 g/day. Increase the amount of fiber eaten gradually over 1–2 wk.
3. Consume at least 2–3 L of fluid per day unless contraindicated. Drink water or fruit juices (fluid softens hard stools). Limit caffeinated beverages, such as coffee, tea, and cola (caffeine stimulates fluid loss through urination).
4. Avoid foods that produce gas (e.g., beans) or upper GI upset (e.g., spicy foods).
5. *Timing:* Follow a regular schedule for bowel elimination. A good time is 30 min after the first meal of the day.
6. *Position:* If possible, an upright position with feet flat on the floor or on a step stool enhances bowel evacuation. Staying on the toilet, commode, or bedpan for longer than 20–30 min may cause skin breakdown. Based on stability, someone may need to stay with the patient.
7. *Activity:* Exercise is important for bowel function. In addition to improving muscle tone, it increases appetite and GI transit time. Exercise muscles, including stretching, ROM, position changing, and functional movement.
8. *Drug treatment:* Suppositories may be needed to stimulate a bowel movement. Manual stimulation of the rectum may be helpful in starting defecation. Use stool softeners as needed to regulate stool consistency. Use oral laxatives only if necessary.

---

catheterization may be extended. If more than 500 mL of urine is present, the time interval is shortened. CIC is usually done 4 to 6 times daily.

Suprapubic catheters are a safe option in select patients. Because of personal preference or the inability to catheterize due to neurologic dysfunction, 30% of patients with SCI use indwelling urethral or suprapubic catheters. The incidence of bacteriuria after catheter introduction is 5% to 10% per day.

Traditional bladder management options include *urinary diversion surgery* for the recurrent UTI patient with renal involvement or repeated stones. Surgical treatment of neurogenic bladder includes bladder neck revision (sphincterotomy), bladder augmentation (augmentation cystoplasty), perineal ureterostomy, cystotomy, vesicostomy, and anterior urethral transplantation. Placement of a sacral cord stimulator, penile prosthesis, or artificial sphincter is possible. Urinary diversion procedures are discussed in Chapter 45.

Neurogenic Bowel. Careful management of bowel evacuation is necessary in the patient with SCI because voluntary control may be lost. Usual measures for preventing constipation include high-fiber diet and adequate fluid intake (see Table 42.10). Patient and caregiver teaching is needed to promote successful independent bowel management. Guidelines related to bowel management are outlined in Table 60.10.

These measures may not be adequate to stimulate evacuation. Suppositories (e.g., bisacodyl [Dulcolax], glycerin) or small-volume enemas and digital stimulation (done 20 to 30 minutes

after suppository insertion) by the nurse or patient may be needed. In the patient with an upper motor neuron injury, digital stimulation can relax the external sphincter to promote defecation. A stool softener, such as docusate sodium (Colace), can help regulate stool consistency. Oral stimulant laxatives should be used only if absolutely necessary and not on a regular basis.

Valsalva maneuver and manual stimulation are useful in patients with lower motor neuron injuries. Because the Valsalva maneuver requires intact abdominal muscles, it is used in patients with injuries below T12. In general, a bowel movement every other day is considered adequate. However, consider pre-injury patterns. Fecal incontinence can result from too much stool softener or a fecal impaction.

Timing of defecation is important. Planning bowel evacuation for 30 to 60 minutes after the first meal of the day may enhance success by taking advantage of the gastrocolic reflex induced by eating. This reflex may also be stimulated by drinking a warm beverage right after the meal. Discuss timing of the bowel program among the interprofessional team so there are no interruptions when the patient is doing therapy (e.g., swimming pool therapy).

Record all bowel movements, including amount, time, and consistency. Consider using the International Spinal Cord Injury Bowel Function Data Set. This is a 16-item, comprehensive, standardized format for assessing bowel function in the patient with SCI.[23]

Spasticity. Spasticity can be both beneficial and undesirable. It aids with mobility, especially for the patient with incomplete SCI. Spasticity improves circulation by promoting venous return, decreasing orthostatic hypotension and the risk for VTE. Unfortunately, the patient with marked spasticity and tone may have difficulty with positioning and mobility from spasms. Spasms can cause significant pain and make activities of daily living (ADLs) difficult for the patient.

The Ashworth and Modified Ashworth Scales are used to evaluate spasticity. Treatment includes ROM exercises to prevent muscle and joint tightness and reduce the risk for contracture. Antispasmodic drugs, such as baclofen or tizanidine, may be given. Botulinum toxin injection is useful for specific muscle involvement.

Skin Care. Prevention of PI is part of the lifelong treatment plan after SCI. Nurses in rehabilitation are responsible for teaching the patient and caregiver about daily skin care. PI may not be noticed until severe damage has occurred. Include information on the importance of adequate nutrition to skin condition. Anticipatory guidance about potential risks is essential. Patient and caregiver teaching related to skin care is outlined in Table 60.11.

Pain Management. The acute pain of the initial injury may persist during the first few weeks of rehabilitation. Chronic pain can result from overuse of muscles in the shoulders and arms for movement and repositioning. Pain often disrupts sleep. Assess, evaluate, and treat pain routinely. Use analgesics and interventions, such as massage and repositioning, to help the patient during therapy. Patients may benefit from referral to a pain management specialist.

Sexuality. Sexuality is an important issue regardless of the patient's age or sex. Open discussion with the patient about sexual rehabilitation is essential. A nurse or other rehabilitation professional trained in sexual counseling should provide support for the patient and the partner. Alternative methods of obtaining sexual satisfaction, such as oral-genital sex, may be

TABLE 60.11 Patient & Caregiver Teaching

Skin Care After Spinal Cord Injury

To prevent skin breakdown in a patient with spinal cord injury, include the following instructions when teaching the patient and caregiver:

Change Position Frequently
- If in a wheelchair, lift self and shift weight every 15–30 min.
- If in bed, change position with a regular turning schedule (at least every 2 hr) that includes sides, back, and abdomen.
- Use pressure-reducing mattresses and wheelchair cushions (not egg-crate).
- Use pillows to protect bony prominences when in bed.

Monitor Skin Condition
- Inspect skin often for areas of redness, swelling, and breakdown.
- If a wound develops, follow standard wound care procedures.

Protect Skin
- Do not sit too close to fires, space heaters, or other sources of heat.
- Use sunscreen liberally when outdoors.
- Keep fingernails trimmed to avoid scratches and abrasions.
- Do not wear clothes that are too tight or too loose.
- Dress warmly in cold weather to prevent frostbite.
- Do not put hot foot in your lap without protection.

suggested. Explicit films may help, such as a film showing sexual activities of a patient with paraplegia and a nondisabled partner. Use graphics cautiously because they may focus too much on the mechanics of sex rather than on the relationship.

Knowledge of the level and completeness of injury is needed to understand the male patient's potential for orgasm, erection, and fertility, and the patient's capacity for sexual satisfaction. Men normally have 2 types of erections: psychogenic and reflex. The process of *psychogenic erection* begins in the brain with sexual thoughts. Signals from the brain are sent through the nerves of the spinal cord to the T10-L2 levels. The signals are then relayed to the penis and trigger an erection. Men with low-level incomplete injuries are more likely to have psychogenic erection than men with higher level incomplete injuries. Men with complete injuries are less likely to have psychogenic erection.[24]

A *reflex erection* occurs with direct physical contact to the penis or other erotic areas. This short lived, uncontrolled, erection is involuntary and does not require sexually stimulating thoughts. Most men with SCI can have a reflex erection with physical stimulation if the S2-S4 nerve pathways are not damaged.

Treatment for erectile dysfunction includes drugs, vacuum devices, and surgical procedures. Phosphodiesterase inhibitors (e.g., sildenafil [Viagra]) have become the first-line treatment in men with SCI between T6 and L5. Sexual stimulation is needed to get an erection after taking the medication. Penile injection of vasoactive substances (papaverine, alprostadil, or a combination) is another medical treatment. Risks include scarring, bruising, and infection. Use may lead to priapism. Vacuum suction devices use negative pressure to encourage blood flow into the penis. Erection is maintained by a constriction band placed at the base of the penis. The main surgical option is implantation of a penile prosthesis.[24] (Erectile dysfunction is discussed in Chapter 54.)

SCI affects male fertility, causing poor sperm motility and ejaculatory dysfunction. Recent advances in methods of sperm retrieval include penile vibratory stimulation and rectal probe electroejaculation. Surgical removal of sperm is a last resort for sperm retrieval. Once retrieved, sperm can be directly injected into an egg via intracytoplasmic sperm injection (ICSI). These techniques have changed the prognosis for men with SCI to father children from unlikely to a reasonable chance of successful outcomes.[24]

The effect of SCI on female sexual response is less clear. A woman of childbearing age with SCI usually stays fertile. The injury does not affect the ability to become pregnant or deliver normally through the birth canal. Menses may cease for as long as 6 months after injury. If sexual activity is resumed, protection against unplanned pregnancy is needed. Pregnancy is associated with increased risk for diabetes and UTI and higher rates of AD, PI, increased spasticity, and catheter-related issues. Labor and delivery have high rates of complications.[25]

Care should be taken not to dislodge an indwelling catheter during sexual activity. A patient with an external catheter should refrain from fluids and remove the catheter before sexual activity. Teach patients about the risk for AD. The bowel program should include evacuation the morning of sexual activity. Encourage the patient to tell the partner that incontinence is always possible. The woman may need a water-soluble lubricant to supplement decreased vaginal secretions and ease vaginal penetration. Women with some residual pelvic innervation can achieve normal orgasm. Use of the Eros device may help with orgasmic dysfunction.[25]

Grief and Depression. Depression after SCI is common and disabling. Patients with SCI may feel an overwhelming sense of loss. They may temporarily lose control over everyday activities as they depend on others for ADLs and for life-sustaining measures. Patients may feel they are useless and burdens to their families. At a life stage when independence is of great importance, they may be totally dependent on others.

Working through grief is a hard, lifelong process for which the patient needs support and encouragement. Table 60.12 outlines the grief response to SCI and appropriate nursing interventions. Your role in grief work is to support the patient and family and to allow mourning as part of the rehabilitation process. Maintaining hope is important during the grieving process and should not be interpreted as denial. With recent advances in rehabilitation, the patient is often independent physically and discharged from the rehabilitation center before completing the grief process.

The goal of recovery is related more to adjustment than to acceptance. *Adjustment* implies the ability to go on with living with certain limitations. Problem-based strategies are effective in supporting positive adjustment. When the patient accepts the current new normal, levels of coping and adjustment are improved. Nonacceptance is more predictive of psychologic distress, disengagement, denial, fantasy, and dependence on drugs and alcohol.

When the patient is depressed, be patient. Sympathy is not helpful. Treat the patient as an adult and encourage participation in care planning.[26] A primary nurse relationship is helpful. To adjust, the patient needs continual support throughout the rehabilitation process in the form of acceptance, affection, and caring. Be attentive when the patient needs to talk and sensitive to needs at various stages of the grief process.

Although depression during the grief process usually lasts days to weeks, some patients become clinically depressed and need treatment for depression. Evaluation by a psychiatric nurse or psychiatrist is recommended. Treatment may include drugs and therapy. Treatment is maximized when the patient's personal preferences are identified, and care is tailored to patient needs.

ETHICAL/LEGAL DILEMMAS
Right to Refuse Treatment

Situation

R.D., a 25-yr-old man, had a SCI to C7-8 after a motorcycle accident. He was diagnosed with anterior cord syndrome and has motor paralysis, which may prevent him from riding motorcycles again. He has become extremely depressed and no longer wishes to live. Because of his emotional state, R.D. is now refusing to eat. Can he be forced to receive EN?

Ethical/Legal Points for Consideration

- Withholding treatment in a newly injured but otherwise healthy young adult may present an ethical dilemma for some nurses. They may consider it assisted suicide and believe that it violates the ethical principles of beneficence and nonmaleficence.
- A competent adult has the right to consent to or refuse medical treatment under the right to privacy, the Fourteenth Amendment of the Constitution, and case law.[*]
- Case law has supported the concept that forced treatment is battery (unlawful use of force on somebody). A mentally competent, physically incapacitated adult can refuse EN. The health agency must follow the patient's wishes.[†]
- To be competent to take part in informed consent or refusal, an adult must be able to understand the information provided about the procedure or treatment, consider choices among available alternatives, and make a choice based on his values and preferences. Depression may not be a factor in determining competency to make informed treatment choices.
- If, after adequate evaluation and treatment for pain, depression, or other medical conditions, the patient persists in his refusal, his wishes must be respected.
- Refusal to eat or drink has never been upheld as illegal, and the alternative—forced eating and drinking—is clearly a violation of patient rights and the criminal act of battery.

Discussion Questions

1. What are your feelings about requests to withhold treatment in a young person with a newly acquired disability?
2. What resources are available to help R.D., his family, and nursing staff deal with this emotionally charged and ethically complex situation?

[*]*Cruzan v. Director, Missouri Department of Health*, 497 U.S. 261, 1990. Retrieved from *www.supreme.justia.com/cases/federal/us/497/261*.
[†]*Bouvia v. Superior Court*, 1986. Retrieved from *http://law.justia.com/cases/california/calapp3d/179/1127.html*.

TABLE 60.12 Grief Response in Spinal Cord Injury

Patient Behavior	Nursing Intervention
Shock and Denial Struggle for survival, complete dependence, excessive sleep, withdrawal, fantasies, unrealistic expectations	• Provide honest information. • Use simple diagrams to explain injury. • Encourage patient to begin road to recovery. • Establish agreement to use and improve all current abilities while not denying the possibility of future improvement.
Anger Refusal to discuss paralysis, ↓ self-esteem, manipulation, hostile and abusive language	• Coordinate care with patient and encourage self-care. • Support family members. • Use humor appropriately. • Allow patient outbursts of emotions. • Do not allow fixation on injury.
Depression Sadness, pessimism, anorexia, nightmares, insomnia, agitation, "blues," suicidal preoccupation, refusal to take part in any self-care activities	• Encourage family involvement and use of community resources. • Plan graded steps in rehabilitation to give success with minimal opportunity for frustration. • Give cheerful and willing assistance with ADLs: • Avoid sympathy. • Use firm kindness.
Adjustment and Acceptance Planning for future, actively taking part in therapy, finding personal meaning in experience and continuation of growth, returning to premorbid personality	• Remember patients have unique personalities. • Balance support systems to encourage independence. • Set goals with patient input. • Emphasize potential.

Caregivers need counseling to avoid promoting dependency in the patient through guilt or misplaced sympathy. They have intense grieving. A support group of family members and friends of patients with SCI can help them increase their participation and knowledge of the grieving process, physical problems, rehabilitation plan, and meaning of the disability.

◆ Evaluation

Expected outcomes are that the patient with SCI will

- Maintain adequate ventilation and have no signs of respiratory distress
- Maintain adequate circulation and BP
- Maintain intact skin over bony prominences
- Maintain adequate nutrition
- Establish a bowel management program based on neurologic function and personal preference
- Establish a bladder management program based on neurologic function, caregiver status, and lifestyle choices
- Have no episodes of AD

Gerontologic Considerations: Spinal Cord Injury

Because of increased work and recreational activities among older adults, more of them have SCI (Fig. 60.11). Falls are the leading cause of SCI for people age 65 and older. Older adults with traumatic injuries have more complications than younger patients, are hospitalized longer, and have higher mortality rates.

Chronic illnesses associated with aging can have a serious impact on older adults living with SCI. As patients with SCI age, both individual aging changes and length of time since injury can affect functional ability. For example, bowel and bladder dysfunction can increase with the duration and severity of SCI.

Health promotion and screening are important for the older patient with SCI. Daily skin inspections and UTI prevention measures are critical. Regular breast examinations for women and prostate cancer screening for men are recommended. Heart disease is the most common cause of morbidity and mortality among older adults with SCI. The lack of sensation, including chest pain, in persons with high-level injuries may mask acute myocardial ischemia. Altered autonomic nervous system function and decreases in physical activity can place patients at risk for heart problems, including hypertension.

Rehabilitation for the older adult with SCI may take longer because of preexisting conditions and poorer health status at the time of initial injury. An interprofessional approach to rehabilitation is essential in preventing secondary complications.

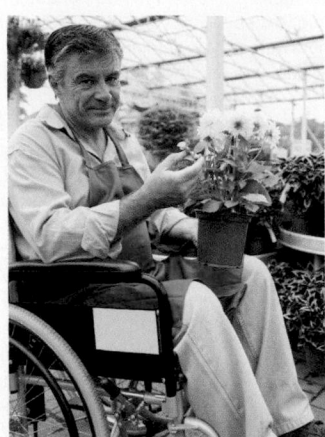

FIG. 60.11 An increasing number of older adults are living with a chronic spinal cord injury. (© WavebreakmediaLtd/WavebreakMedia/Thinkstock.)

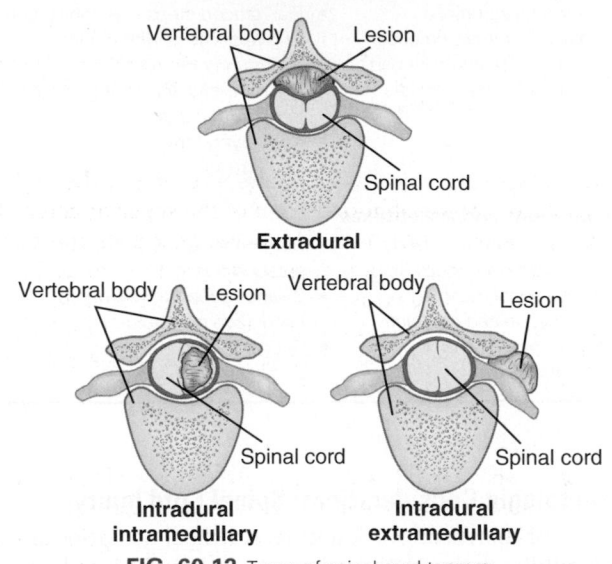

FIG. 60.12 Types of spinal cord tumors.

SPINAL CORD TUMORS

Spinal cord tumors can have a devastating impact due to spinal compression and neurologic dysfunction. Tumors are classified as *primary* (arising from some part of spinal cord, dura, nerves, or vessels) or *secondary* (from primary growths in other places in the body that have metastasized to the spinal cord).

Etiology and Pathophysiology

Spinal cord tumors are either *extradural* (outside the dura), *intradural-extramedullary* (between the spinal cord and dura), and *intramedullary* (within the substance of spinal cord itself) (Fig. 60.12 and Table 60.13).

Extradural tumors include metastatic cancer and benign schwannomas. Many patients with cancer will have metastasis to the spine. Metastatic lesions can invade intradurally and compress the spinal cord. Tumors that often metastasize to the spinal epidural space are those that spread to bone, such as prostate, breast, lung, and kidney cancer. Intradural-extramedullary lesions include meningiomas that develop in the arachnoid membrane, schwannomas and neurofibromas that extend from the nerve root, and ependymomas found at the end of the spinal cord. Intramedullary tumors arise from glial or ependymal cells found throughout the entire spinal cord. The most common lesions are astrocytes and ependymomas.[27]

Many spinal cord tumors are slow growing. Their symptoms are due to the mechanical effects of slow compression and irritation of nerve roots, displacement of the spinal cord, or gradual obstruction of the blood supply. The slowness of growth does not cause secondary injury as in traumatic SCI. Thus complete functional restoration may be possible when the tumor is removed.

Clinical Manifestations

Both sensory and motor problems may result, with the location and extent of the tumor determining the severity and extent of the problem. The most common early symptom of a spinal cord tumor is back pain or pain radiating along the compressed nerve route.[28] Location of the pain depends on the level of compression. Pain may worsen with activity, coughing, straining, and/or lying down. There may be slowly increasing clumsiness, weakness, and spasticity. Paralysis can develop. Sensory disruption occurs as coldness, numbness, and tingling

TABLE 60.13 Classification of Spinal Cord Tumors

Type	Incidence	Treatment	Prognosis
Extradural Outside spinal cord in extradural space	Metastatic lesions and benign schwannomas	Relief of cord pressure by surgical laminectomy, radiation, chemotherapy, or combination approach	*Benign:* Excellent with resection *Metastatic:* Poor, treatment usually palliative
Intradural Extramedullary Within dura mater but outside spinal cord	Mostly benign. Meningiomas, neurofibromas, schwannomas	Complete surgical removal of tumor (if possible) Partial removal followed by radiation	Usually very good if no damage to cord from compression
Intramedullary Within spinal cord	Mostly benign. Astrocytomas, ependymomas	Complete surgical removal of tumor (if possible) Partial removal followed by radiation	Usually very good if no damage to cord from compression Complete surgical resection of astrocytomas difficult

in 1 or more extremities. Neurogenic bowel and bladder are marked by incontinence, constipation, and urgency with difficulty in starting the flow, progressing to retention with overflow incontinence.

❖ Interprofessional and Nursing Care

Extradural tumors can be seen on routine spinal x-rays. Intradural extramedullary and intramedullary tumors require MRI, CT scan, or CT myelogram for detection. CSF analysis may reveal tumor cells. Patients with tumors suspicious for metastatic disease need an oncology referral and further diagnostic testing to identify the primary cancer.[27]

Spinal cord compression is an emergency. Relief of ischemia related to the compression is the goal of therapy. Corticosteroids (e.g., dexamethasone) are generally given immediately to relieve tumor-related edema.[29]

Indications for surgery depend on the type of tumor and neurologic deficit. Emergency surgery may be needed to decompress the spinal cord, obtain tissue for biopsy, and help to determine appropriate treatment.[27] Primary spinal tumors may be removed with the goal of cure. In patients with metastatic tumors, treatment is mainly palliative. The goal is to restore or preserve neurologic function, stabilize the spine, and alleviate pain. Radiation and/or chemotherapy may be used to treat the tumor.

Relieving pain and maximizing neurologic function are the ultimate goals of treatment. Assess the patient's neurologic status before and after treatment. Giving analgesia as needed is an important nursing responsibility. Depending on the amount of neurologic dysfunction, care of the patient may be similar to that of a patient recovering from SCI.

CRANIAL NERVE DISORDERS

Cranial nerve disorders are often classified as peripheral neuropathies. The 12 pairs of cranial nerves are considered the peripheral nerves of the brain. The disorders usually involve the motor and/or sensory branches of a single nerve (*mononeuropathies*). Causes of cranial nerve problems include tumors, trauma, infection, inflammatory processes, and idiopathic (unknown) causes. The 2 cranial nerve disorders discussed here are trigeminal neuralgia and Bell's palsy.

TRIGEMINAL NEURALGIA

Trigeminal neuralgia (TN) *(tic douloureux)* is characterized by sudden, usually unilateral, severe, brief, stabbing, recurrent episodes of pain in the distribution of the trigeminal nerve. It occurs in about 12 per 100,000 Americans each year. TN affects more women than men. It occurs most often in people over age 50.

We classify TN as *classic* (TN 1) or *atypical* (TN 2). Patients may have both types. The pain intensity and lifestyle disruption that accompany TN can cause marked physical and psychologic dysfunction.

Etiology and Pathophysiology

The trigeminal nerve, the fifth cranial nerve (CN V), has both motor and sensory branches. TN most often affects the sensory (afferent) branches of the second and third division (maxillary and mandibular branches) of CN V (Fig. 60.13).

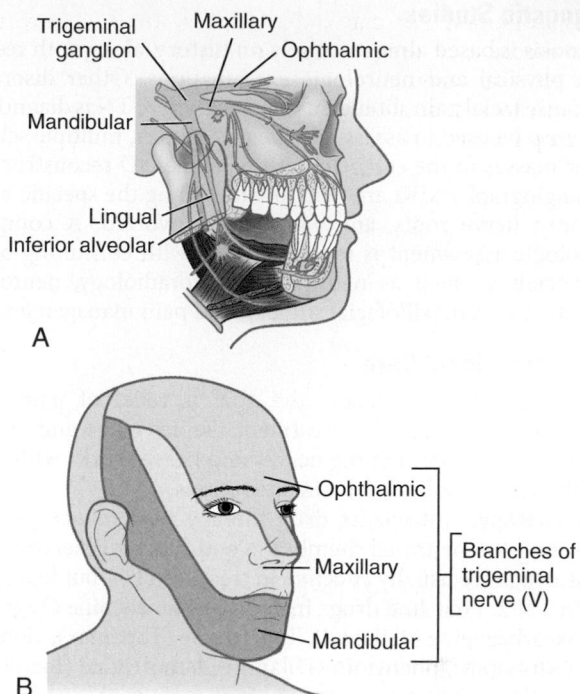

FIG. 60.13 A, Trigeminal (fifth cranial) nerve and its 3 main divisions: ophthalmic, maxillary, and mandibular nerves. B, Cutaneous innervation of the head. (Modified from Patton KT, Thibodeau GA: *Anatomy and physiology,* ed 8, St Louis, 2013, Mosby.)

Most cases result from vascular compression of the trigeminal nerve root by an abnormal loop of the superior cerebellar artery. This artery compresses the nerve as it exits the brainstem. Constant compression appears to lead to chronic injury, causing flattening and atrophy of the nerve and damage to the myelin sheath.[30] In some cases, TN may be related to underlying pathology, such as multiple sclerosis, shingles, or masses in the cerebellum or brainstem.

Clinical Manifestations

The first episode of TN is sudden with a memorable onset. In TN 1, the patient has an abrupt onset of waves of excruciating pain. It is described as a burning, knifelike, or lightning-like shock in the lips, upper or lower gums, cheek, forehead, or side of the nose.[31] Facial twitching, grimacing, and frequent blinking and tearing of the eye can occur during the acute attack (giving rise to the term *tic douloureux*). Some patients may have facial sensory loss. Attacks are usually brief, lasting only seconds to 2 or 3 minutes. Frequency ranges from 1 to over 50 times a day.[31]

Pain episodes are usually started by a triggering mechanism of light touch at a specific point *(trigger zone)* along the distribution of the nerve branches. Precipitating stimuli include chewing, brushing the teeth, feeling a hot or cold blast of air on the face, washing the face, yawning, or even talking. As a result, the patient may eat improperly, neglect hygienic practices, wear a cloth over the face, and withdraw from interaction with others. The patient may sleep excessively as a means of coping with pain.

TN 2 manifests as constant aching, burning, crushing, or stabbing pain. The pain has a lower intensity and does not subside completely.[32] The distinct attacks associated with TN 1 do not occur in TN 2.

Diagnostic Studies

Diagnosis is based almost entirely on history, along with results from physical and neurologic examinations. Other disorders that cause facial pain should be ruled out before TN is diagnosed. MRI may be used to assess for sinusitis, cancer, multiple sclerosis, or masses in the cerebellopontine angle. 3D reconstruction and angiography MRI are helpful with seeing the specific brain anatomy, nerve roots, and vasculature involved. A complete neurologic assessment is required along with consulting other subspecialties, such as neurology, neuroradiology, neurosurgery, dentistry, maxillofacial surgery, and pain management.

Interprofessional Care

Once a diagnosis is made, the goal is relief of pain with either medical or surgical treatment (Tables 60.14 and 60.15). Electrical stimulation of the nerves and nerve blocks with local anesthetics or botulinum toxin are options.

Drug Therapy. Antiseizure drug therapy may reduce pain by stabilizing the neuronal membrane and blocking nerve firing. These drugs are usually effective in treating TN 1 but less effective in TN 2. First-line drugs include carbamazepine (Tegretol) and oxcarbazepine (Trileptal). Topiramate (Topamax), clonazepam (Klonopin), phenytoin (Dilantin), lamotrigine (Lamictal), gabapentin, and valproic acid are other options.[30]

Tricyclic antidepressants, such as amitriptyline or nortriptyline, can help treat the constant burning or aching pain. Analgesics or opioids are usually not effective in controlling pain in TN 1 but may help with pain in TN 2.[30]

Surgical Therapy. If a conservative approach is ineffective or the patient is unable to tolerate adverse effects of medications, surgical therapy is available (Table 60.15). In percutaneous procedures, affected nerve fibers are damaged to eliminate pain. Although most patients are pain-free after any of the procedures, pain relief lasts longest with microvascular decompression. About half of treated patients develop recurrent pain within 12 to 15 years.[30]

◆ NURSING MANAGEMENT: TRIGEMINAL NEURALGIA

Patients usually receive outpatient treatment. Assess the attacks in detail, including triggering factors, characteristics, frequency, and pain management techniques. This information helps you to plan patient care. Evaluate the degree of pain and its effects on the patient's lifestyle, drug use, emotional state, and suicidal tendencies. Note behavior (including withdrawal).

TABLE 60.14 Interprofessional Care

Trigeminal Neuralgia

Diagnostic Assessment
- History and physical examination (including neurologic examination)
- MRI

Management
- Drug therapy
  - Antiseizure drugs (e.g., carbamazepine, oxcarbazepine [Trileptal], gabapentin [Neurontin])
  - Tricyclic antidepressants (e.g., amitriptyline)
- Local nerve block
- Surgical therapy (Table 60.15)

Monitor the patient's response to drug therapy and note any side effects. Discuss complementary pain management measures, such as acupuncture, biofeedback, and yoga. Environmental assessment is essential during an acute period to decrease triggering stimuli. The room should be kept at an even, moderate temperature and free of drafts. The patient may prefer to complete all self-care activities, fearing someone else will inadvertently cause injury.

Assess the patient's nutritional status and hygiene (especially oral). Teach the patient about the importance of nutrition, hygiene, and oral care. Convey understanding if oral neglect is apparent. A small, soft-bristled toothbrush or a warm mouthwash helps promote oral care. Hygiene activities are best done when analgesia is at its peak.

TABLE 60.15 Surgical Therapy for Trigeminal Neuralgia

Procedure	Description
Percutaneous Procedures	
Balloon compression	• Cannula is inserted through cheek and guided to a natural opening in the base of skull.
	• Soft catheter with a balloon tip is threaded through cannula.
	• Balloon is inflated and mechanical compression damages trigeminal nerve.
Glycerol rhizotomy (injection into 1 or more branches of trigeminal nerve) (Fig. 60.14)	• Thin needle inserted through puncture in cheek and guided through natural opening in base of skull.
	• Glycerol is injected into trigeminal ganglion.
	• Procedure can be repeated multiple times.
Radiofrequency thermal lesioning	• Needle is passed through cheek thorough a natural opening in base of skull.
	• Patient is awakened, then a small electric current is passed through the needle, causing tingling.
	• When the needle is positioned so the tingling occurs in the same area of pain, patient is sedated again, then radiofrequency current is used to destroy part of the nerve.
	• Can result in facial numbness (although some degree of sensation may be retained), corneal anesthesia, and trigeminal motor weakness
Surgical Procedures	
Microvascular decompression, with or without neurectomy	• Small craniotomy done behind the ear (suboccipital craniotomy).
	• Blood vessels that appear to be compressing the nerve at the root entry zone where it exits the pons are then displaced and repositioned.
	• If there is no compression, cutting of the nerve (neurectomy) may be done.
Stereotactic radiosurgery (gamma knife, cyber knife)	• Uses stereotactic localization to focus high doses of radiation to area where trigeminal nerve exits the brainstem.
	• Radiation causes slow formation of a lesion on nerve and disrupts transmission of pain signals to brain.
	• Pain relief from this procedure may take several months. (Radiosurgery is discussed in Chapter 56.)

Encourage food that is high in protein and calories and easy to chew. Food should be served lukewarm and offered frequently. If oral intake is sharply reduced and the patient's nutritional status is compromised, an NG tube can be inserted on the unaffected side for EN.

Appropriate teaching related to surgical procedures depends on the type of procedure planned (e.g., percutaneous). The patient needs to know they will be awake during local procedures in order to cooperate when corneal and ciliary reflexes and facial sensations are checked. After the procedure, compare the patient's pain with the preoperative intensity. Evaluate the corneal reflex, extraocular muscles, hearing, sensation, and facial nerve function often (see Chapter 55). If the corneal reflex is impaired, take special care to protect the eyes. This includes using artificial tears or eye shields.

After a percutaneous radiofrequency procedure, apply an ice pack to the jaw on the operative side for 3 to 5 hours. To avoid injuring the mouth, the patient should not chew on the operative side until sensation has returned. If intracranial surgery was done, general postoperative nursing care after a craniotomy is appropriate. (Nursing care related to craniotomy is discussed in Chapter 56.)

Plan for regular follow-up care. Teach the patient about any medications. Although pain may be relieved, encourage the patient to keep environmental stimuli to a moderate level and to use stress management techniques. Long-term management after surgical intervention depends on residual effects of the procedure. If anesthesia is present or the corneal reflex is altered, teach the patient to (1) chew on the unaffected side; (2) avoid hot foods or beverages, which can burn the mucous membranes; (3) check the oral cavity after meals to remove food particles; (4) practice meticulous oral hygiene and continue with semiannual dental visits; (5) protect the face against extremes of temperature; (6) use an electric razor; (7) wear a protective eye shield and avoid rubbing eyes; and (8) examine eye regularly for symptoms of infection or irritation.

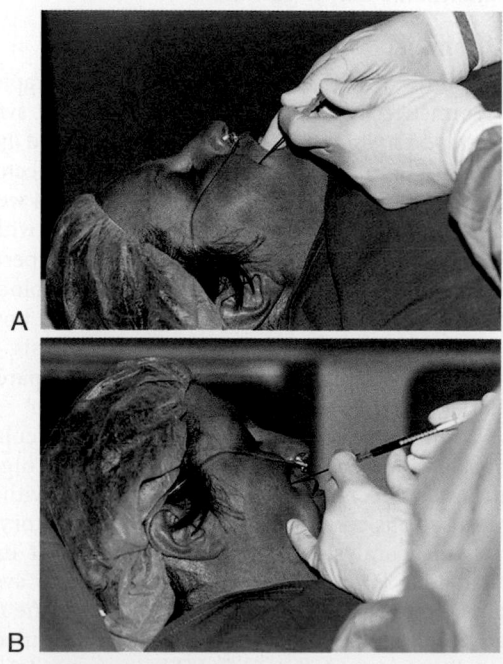

FIG. 60.14 Glycerol rhizotomy for the treatment of trigeminal neuralgia. **A**, Patient with trigeminal neuralgia having needle placed. **B**, HCP injecting glycerol. (Courtesy Joe Rothrock, Media, PA.)

BELL'S PALSY

Bell's palsy is an acute, usually temporary, facial paresis (or palsy) resulting from damage or trauma of the facial nerve (CN VII). It usually affects only 1 side of the face, but both sides can be affected.

Bell's palsy is the most common facial nerve disorder.[33] Each year about 40,000 Americans are diagnosed with Bell's palsy. It occurs equally between men and women and can affect any age-group. The peak incidence is between ages 15 and 60 years. There is a high incidence during pregnancy and in persons with upper respiratory tract conditions (e.g., flu, colds), obesity, diabetes, and hypertension.[33]

Etiology and Pathophysiology

We do not know the exact cause. Several theories exist. Some think it is a reactivation of herpes simplex virus isoform (HSV-1) and/or herpes zoster virus (HZV). The viral infection causes inflammation, leading to nerve compression and the subsequent clinical features (Fig. 60.15). Another cause may be acute demyelination similar to what happens in Guillain-Barré syndrome.

The prognosis for persons with Bell's palsy is generally very good. The extent of nerve damage determines the extent of recovery. Most begin to get better within 2 weeks after the onset and recover some or all facial function within 6 months. In some cases, there may be residual effects, including facial asymmetry or abnormal facial movements.

Clinical Manifestations

CN VII is a mixed cranial nerve with motor, sensory, and autonomic function, which accounts for the manifestations. The key feature of Bell's palsy is the acute onset of unilateral lower motor facial weakness. 50% to 60% have pain around and behind the ear and neck. Other manifestations include drooping of the eyelid and corner of the mouth, drooling, facial twitching, dryness of the eye or mouth, facial numbness, altered taste, hearing loss, and excessive tearing in 1 eye.[33] Most often these symptoms begin suddenly and reach their peak within 48 to 72 hours.

Quality of life is often decreased due to problems with eating, swallowing, speech, and taste. Patients may have psychologic withdrawal because of changes in appearance, malnutrition, dehydration, mucous membrane trauma, corneal abrasions, muscle stretching, and facial spasms and contractures.

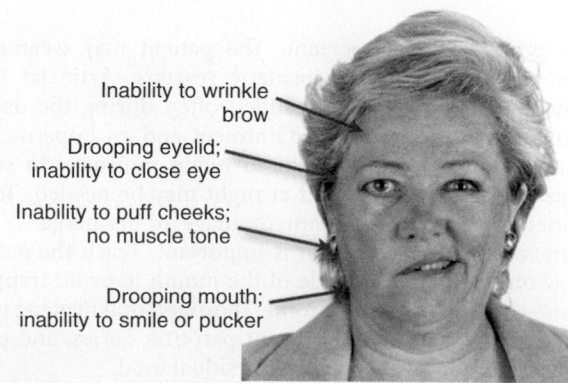

Inability to wrinkle brow

Drooping eyelid; inability to close eye

Inability to puff cheeks; no muscle tone

Drooping mouth; inability to smile or pucker

FIG. 60.15 Facial characteristics of a person with Bell's palsy. (© Jo Ann Snover/123RF Stock Photo/123rf.com.)

Diagnostic Studies

Bell's palsy is a clinical diagnosis. No definitive diagnostic test exists. The diagnosis and prognosis are indicated by clinical examination and observing the typical pattern of onset. Current guidelines do not support routine laboratory, imaging, or neurophysiologic testing at first presentation of Bell's palsy. If indicated, MRI and CT can eliminate other causes for facial paralysis. Blood tests can diagnose infections or other diseases. Electromyography (EMG) can confirm the presence of nerve damage. Patients should be referred to a neurologist or otolaryngologist as soon as possible to exclude other neurologic conditions.

Interprofessional Care

The patient with Bell's palsy is treated as an outpatient. Care focuses on relieving symptoms, preventing complications, and protecting the eye on the affected side.

Treatment is often started to try to improve the chance of a complete recovery. Oral corticosteroid therapy to reduce inflammation and swelling should be started within 72 hours of onset.[34] Some patients should receive an antiviral agent, such as acyclovir (Zovirax), in addition to the steroid therapy. Surgical decompression of the facial nerve is controversial but is considered in refractory cases.

❖ NURSING MANAGEMENT: BELL'S PALSY

Mild analgesics can relieve pain. Moist heat can reduce discomfort and aid circulation. Electrical stimulation of the nerve, facial massage, and physical therapy help maintain muscle tone and ease pain. A facial sling may be helpful to support affected muscles, improve lip alignment, and facilitate eating. The facial sling is usually made and fitted by a physical or occupational therapist. When function begins to return, active facial muscle exercises are done several times a day. Tell the patient to protect the face from cold and drafts because trigeminal *hyperesthesia* (extreme sensitivity to pain or touch) may occur.

❓ CHECK YOUR PRACTICE

You are working in the outpatient neurology clinic. Your patient is a 68-yr-old woman with Bell's palsy. Her main problem today is dry eyes. When you are doing an assessment, she tells you, "I hate the way I look. I cannot go anywhere, and I am afraid to leave the house. I am ugly and scary looking."
- How can you help her cope with her disorder?
- What can you suggest to increase moisture in the affected eye?

Eye protection is important. The patient may wear dark glasses for protective and cosmetic reasons. Artificial tears (methylcellulose) should be instilled often during the day to prevent drying of the cornea. Ointment and an impermeable eye shield can be used at night to retain moisture. In some patients, taping the lids closed at night may be needed. Teach the patient to report ocular pain, drainage, or discharge.

Maintaining good nutrition is important. Teach the patient to chew on the unaffected side of the mouth to avoid trapping food and to enjoy the taste of food. Thorough oral hygiene must be done after each meal to prevent parotitis, caries, and periodontal disease from accumulated residual food.

The change in physical appearance from Bell's palsy can be devastating. Reassure the patient that a stroke did not occur and that chances for a full recovery are good. Enlisting support from family and friends is important. Tell the patient most people recover within 3 to 6 months after onset of symptoms.

🔲 POLYNEUROPATHIES

GUILLAIN-BARRÉ SYNDROME

Guillain-Barré syndrome (GBS) is an autoimmune process that occurs a few days or weeks after a viral or bacterial infection. GBS is rare, affecting about 1 person in every 100,000.[35] It can occur at any age, but those over age 50 are at greatest risk.[36] The most common type of GBS is acute inflammatory demyelinating polyneuropathy (AIDP). Other types include acute motor axonal neuropathy (AMAN) and acute motor sensory axonal neuropathy (AMSAN). AMAN is more common in children.

Etiology and Pathophysiology

The cause of GBS is unknown. Both cellular and humoral immune responses likely play a role in AIDP. Humoral responses appear to cause AMAN.[36] Following an infection, immune responses cause injury to either the myelin sheath (AIDP) or the nerve axon itself (AMAN). There is edema and inflammation of affected nerves. The result is segmental loss of the myelin sheath with exposed nerve membranes in nerve terminals and the nodes of Ranvier. Transmission of nerve impulses is stopped or slowed. This leads to flaccid paralysis with muscle denervation and atrophy. In the recovery phase, remyelination occurs slowly. Neurologic function returns in a proximal-to-distal pattern.

Most cases of GBS follow a viral or bacterial infection of the GI or upper respiratory tract. Cytomegalovirus is the most common viral cause. *Campylobacter jejuni* gastroenteritis is the most common bacterial cause, especially for AMAN. Other related infections include Epstein-Barr virus, *Mycoplasma pneumoniae*, *Haemophilus influenza*, hepatitis (A, B, E), and Zika virus.[35] Surgery and trauma may trigger GBS.

Clinical Manifestations and Complications

The main features of GBS include acute, ascending, rapidly progressive, symmetric weakness of the limbs. The first symptoms are weakness, *paresthesia* (numbness and tingling), and *hypotonia* (reduced muscle tone) of the limbs. Reflexes in the affected limbs are weak or absent. Maximal weakness is reached in 4 weeks.

Autonomic nervous system dysfunction occurs with AIDP and AMSAN, causing orthostatic hypotension, hypertension, and abnormal vagal responses (bradycardia, heart block, asystole). Other autonomic dysfunction effects include bowel and bladder dysfunction, facial flushing, and diaphoresis. Cranial nerve involvement manifests as facial weakness and paresthesia, extraocular eye movement problems, and dysphagia.

Pain is common. It can include paresthesia, muscular aches and cramps, and hyperesthesia. It is often worse at night. Pain may contribute to decreased appetite and interfere with sleep.

The most serious complication of GBS is respiratory failure. It occurs if the paralysis progresses to nerves that innervate the thoracic area. Frequently assess the respiratory system by checking respiratory rate and depth to determine the need for immediate intervention, including intubation and mechanical ventilation. Respiratory infection or UTI may occur. Immobility from paralysis can cause paralytic ileus, muscle atrophy, VTE, PIs, orthostatic hypotension, and nutritional deficiencies.[37]

Diagnostic Studies

Diagnosis is based mainly on the patient's history and clinical signs. Clinical features required for diagnosis include progressive weakness of more than 1 limb and decreased or absent reflexes. Electrolyte levels, liver function tests, creatinine phosphokinase, and erythrocyte sedimentation rates are evaluated. Cerebrospinal fluid (CSF) analysis helps exclude other causes. In GBS the CSF has more protein than normal.[37] Results of EMG and nerve conduction studies (NCS) are used after 2 weeks to confirm the diagnosis. NCS allow the HCP to diagnose the subtype. NCS in AIDP show demyelination. This information helps with prognosis, as patients with demyelination often need mechanical ventilation and have a poorer outcome.[38]

❖ Interprofessional and Nursing Care

The management of GBS is supportive. Ventilatory support is critical during the acute phase. Patients may be in ICU for hemodynamic monitoring. Immunomodulating treatments, such as plasma exchange (PE) *(plasmapheresis)* or high-dose IV immunoglobulin (IVIG), are most effective if used within the first 2 weeks of symptom onset. They are equally effective. PE removes antibodies and other immune factors. It is used 5 times either daily or every other day in the first 2 weeks. (PE is discussed in Chapter 13.) IVIG interferes with antigen presentation. It is given over 5 days. It is readily available and is the preferred treatment in many centers.[39] After 4 weeks past disease onset, PE and IVIG therapies have little value. Corticosteroids have little effect on the prognosis or duration of the disease.

Assessment is the most important aspect of nursing care during the acute phase. During the neurologic assessment, evaluate motor and sensory function. Report changes in motor function (e.g., ascending paralysis), reflexes, cranial nerve function (gag, cornea, swallow), and level of consciousness.

Carefully assess respiratory and cardiac function. Monitor ABGs and vital capacity. Closely monitor BP and cardiac rate and rhythm during the acute phase because dysrhythmias, orthostatic hypotension, and increased or decreased BP and heart rate may occur. Vasopressor agents and volume expanders may be needed to treat the low BP. If fever develops, obtain sputum and blood cultures to identify the pathogen. Appropriate antibiotic therapy is then started.

Nutritional needs must be met despite possible problems associated with delayed gastric emptying, paralytic ileus, and potential for aspiration if the gag reflex is lost. In addition to testing for the gag reflex, note drooling and other problems with secretions that may indicate an inadequate gag reflex. EN or PN may be used to ensure adequate caloric intake.

Throughout the course of the illness, provide support and encouragement to the patient and caregivers. Early referrals should be made for physical, occupational, and speech therapy. Counseling may help the patient adjust to the sudden disabling syndrome and dependence on others.

Most patients with GBS will start to recover spontaneously at about 28 days. 80% of patients walk independently at 6 months with 60% making a full recovery in 1 year. GBS patients who have a GI infection, are older in age, have a rapid clinical onset, have a hospital length of stay longer than 11 days, have poor upper extremity motor strength, or need mechanical ventilation have a poorer prognosis.[39]

CHRONIC INFLAMMATORY DEMYELINATING POLYNEUROPATHY

Chronic inflammatory demyelinating polyneuropathy (CIDP) is a motor and sensory neuropathy. CIDP is a rare autoimmune disorder, affecting 1 to 2 persons per 100,000.[40] CIDP is more common in those in their 50s and 60s and in men more than women.[41]

Like GBS, there are different types of CIDP. CIDP differs from GBS in that symptoms gradually occur over 8 weeks and there is not an acute onset. CIDP is not self-limiting (with an end to the acute phase). Early recognition and treatment can help the patient avoid significant disability.

Etiology and Pathophysiology

We do not know the exact cause of CIDP. There is evidence to support the theory that like GBS, it has an autoimmune basis.[40] CIDP seems to be associated with infection, HIV, hepatitis C, Sjögren's syndrome, inflammatory bowel disease, melanoma, lymphoma, and diabetes.

Clinical Manifestations and Diagnostic Studies

It is important to recognize the differences between CIPD and GBS to prevent incorrect or delayed treatment. The classic presentation of patients with CIPD includes progressive symptoms lasting over 2 months, more weakness than sensory deficits, symmetric weakness in the arms and legs, impaired sensation (from distal to proximal), paresthesia and dysesthesia, and absent or decreased reflexes in all extremities. Tremors, facial weakness, and papilledema may be present. Sensory ataxia and impaired vibration and pinprick sensation occur more often in CIDP.

CIDP diagnostic tests are similar to those for GBS. CSF shows high protein levels. MRI may show changes. Key identifying features of CIDP include nerve conduction block and slowed conduction velocity, possibly due to demyelination. Nerve biopsy is done when other studies do not confirm a diagnosis.[41]

❖ Interprofessional and Nursing Care

Early recognition and diagnosis of CIDP are key to reducing permanent disability. The goal of treatment is to halt the immune response and stop nerve inflammation and demyelination. Use of IVIG, high-dose corticosteroids, or plasma exchange are all effective treatments.[41]

Patients continue therapy until maximum clinical improvement is achieved or until they reach a clinical plateau. Patients will need maintenance therapy to prevent relapse or progression. Appropriate referrals to rehabilitation should be made early in the patient's care to promote maximum recovery. Therapy may improve muscle strength, function, and mobility while minimizing muscle atrophy and joint distortion.[40]

TETANUS

Tetanus (lockjaw) is a severe infection of the nervous system affecting spinal and cranial nerves. In the United States, because of widespread immunization and careful wound care, there are only about 30 cases per year.[42] The annual worldwide incidence is between 500,000 and 1 million cases.[43]

Tetanus results from the effects of a potent neurotoxin (tetanospasmin) released by the anaerobic bacillus *Clostridium tetani*. The spores of the bacillus are present in soil, garden mold, and manure. Tetanospasmin binds to motor nerves and enters the axons. From there it can travel to the brain and spinal cord and stop the release of inhibitory neurotransmitters. The result is sustained muscle contraction. If the toxin reaches the blood or lymph system, many different muscles can be affected.[42]

C. tetani enters the body through a wound that provides an appropriate low-O_2 environment for the organisms to mature and make toxin. Examples of such wounds include IV drug use injection sites, human and animal bites, puncture wounds from stepping on a nail, gardening injuries, burns, frostbite, open fractures, and gunshot wounds. The incubation period is typically 4 to 14 days. The shorter the period, the more severe the symptoms.

The hallmark feature of generalized tetanus is muscle rigidity and spasms. Patients may have muscle soreness, cramping, or difficulty swallowing. Facial muscles are affected first with stiffness in the jaw *(trismus)*. Patients may have a sardonic smile *(risus sardonicus)* due to facial muscle contractions. As the disease progresses, the neck muscles, back, abdomen, and extremities become increasingly rigid. In severe forms, continuous tonic seizures may occur with *opisthotonos* (extreme arching of the back and retraction of the head).[42] Laryngeal and respiratory spasms cause apnea and anoxia. The slightest noise, jarring motion, or bright light can set off a painful seizure.

Tetanus prevention and immunizations, which are the most important factors influencing incidence, are outlined in Table 68.6. Adults should receive a tetanus and diphtheria toxoid booster every 10 years.[43] Teach the patient that immediate, thorough cleansing of all wounds with soap and water is important to prevent tetanus. If an open wound occurs and the patient has not been immunized within 5 years, contact the HCP so that a tetanus booster can be given.

Tetanus is a medical emergency that requires hospitalization. Patients are given immediate treatment with tetanus immune globulin (TIG). It provides temporary immunity by directly providing antitoxin.[43] Drugs to control spasms are essential.

Diazepam (Valium) or barbiturates are given to promote sedation and skeletal muscle relaxation. In severe cases, neuromuscular blocking agents (e.g., vecuronium) are given to paralyze skeletal muscles. Opioid analgesics, such as morphine or fentanyl, are used for pain management. A 10- to 14-day course of penicillin, metronidazole (drug of choice), tetracycline, or doxycycline is recommended to inhibit further growth of *C. tetani*.

Because of laryngospasm and the potential need for neuromuscular blocking drugs, the patient is placed on mechanical ventilation. Sedative agents and opioid analgesics are given to all patients who are pharmacologically paralyzed. IV fluids are needed for proper hydration due to sustained muscle contraction. Any wound should be debrided or abscess drained. Antibiotics may be given to prevent secondary infections.

BOTULISM

Botulism is a rare, but the most serious type, of food poisoning. It is caused by GI absorption of a neurotoxin made by *Clostridium botulinum*. This organism is found in the soil, and the spores are hard to destroy. It can grow in any food contaminated with the spores. Improper home canning of foods is often the cause.

We think the neurotoxin destroys or inhibits the neurotransmission of acetylcholine at the myoneural junction, resulting in disturbed muscle innervation. Neurologic manifestations can develop rapidly or evolve over several days. They include a descending paralysis with muscle incoordination and weakness, difficulty swallowing, and seizures. Respiratory muscle weakness can quickly lead to respiratory and/or cardiac arrest.

The manifestations, prevention, and treatment are described in Table 41.24. Patient and caregiving teaching related to food poisoning are outlined in Table 41.25. Nursing care during the acute illness is like that for GBS. Supportive nursing interventions include rest, activities to maintain respiratory function, adequate nutrition, and preventing loss of muscle mass.

Spinal Cord Injury

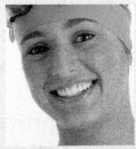

(© Comstock-Images/ Stockbyte/ Thinkstock.)

Patient Profile

Acute Phase

S.W., an 18-yr-old white woman, is admitted to the ED with the diagnosis of a cervical spinal cord injury (SCI). S.W. was swimming at a neighbor's backyard pool. She dove into the shallow end, striking her head on the bottom of the pool. Her friends noticed she did not resurface. They rescued her and brought her to the side of the pool. They maintained neck immobilization until the rescue crews arrived.

Subjective Data

- Awake and alert
- Reporting neck pain
- Anxious and asking why she cannot move her legs
- Asking to see her family

Objective Data

Physical Examination

- Weak elbow flexion (biceps) movement bilaterally
- No triceps movement bilaterally
- Gross shoulder movement present bilaterally

- No movement in bilateral lower extremities
- Decreased sensation from the shoulders down
- No bladder or bowel control
- BP 85/50 mm Hg; pulse 56 beats/min; respirations 32 breaths/min and labored

Diagnostic Studies

- CT C-spine shows C5 subluxation and compression fracture
- MRI C-spine shows severe spinal cord compression at C5-6

Interprofessional Care

- Intubated in the ED
- Started on mechanical ventilation
- Placed in tongs and traction on arrival to the ICU

Discussion Questions (Acute Phase)

1. ***Priority Decision:*** What nursing activities would be a priority on S.W.'s arrival in the ICU?
2. What physiologic problems are causing S.W. to have hypotension and bradycardia?
3. What would be the initial treatment for S.W.'s hypotension and bradycardia?

CASE STUDY—cont'd
Spinal Cord Injury

4. **Safety**: What signs and symptoms would indicate respiratory distress? What physiologic problem would cause respiratory distress in S.W.'s injury state?
5. **Collaboration**: What can the interprofessional team do to decrease S.W.'s anxiety?
6. **Priority Decision:** Based on the assessment data provided, what are the priority nursing diagnoses? What are the collaborative problems?
7. **Collaboration:** Identify activities that can be delegated to unlicensed assistive personnel (UAP).

Patient Profile
Rehabilitation Phase

S.W. is now 1-month postinjury and has been admitted to a local inpatient SCI rehabilitation agency. She has been extubated and uses a wheelchair to mobilize. She eats 3 meals a day with help and is on a strict bowel and bladder program.

Subjective Data
- Awake and alert but anxious
- Reporting a severe headache, blurred vision, and nausea

Objective Data
Physical Examination
- Flushed and diaphoretic above the level of injury
- No bowel movement for 2 days
- BP 235/106 mm Hg, pulse 32 beats/min, respirations 30 breaths/min and labored

Discussion Questions (Rehabilitation Phase)

1. **Priority Decision:** What initial priority nursing interventions would be appropriate?
2. What physiologic problem is causing S.W.'s hypertension and bradycardia?
3. Once the HCP has been notified, what other interventions would be appropriate?
4. **Quality Improvement:** What outcomes would indicate that nursing interventions were successful?
5. **Patient-Centered Care:** Patient and caregiver involvement in the rehabilitation process is vital. What teaching will you provide about bowel management?
6. **Evidence-Based Practice:** S.W. and her family are concerned about the risk for autonomic dysreflexia. What effective strategies to prevent autonomic dysreflexia would you discuss with them?

Answers available at http://evolve.elsevier.com/Lewis/medsurg.

■ BRIDGE TO NCLEX EXAMINATION

The number of the question corresponds to the same-numbered outcome at the beginning of the chapter.

1. During rehabilitation, a patient with spinal cord injury begins to ambulate with long leg braces. Which level of injury does the nurse associate with this degree of recovery?
   a. L1-2
   b. T6-7
   c. T1-2
   d. C7-8

2. A patient with a T4 spinal cord injury has neurogenic shock due to sympathetic nervous system dysfunction. What would the nurse recognize as characteristic of this condition?
   a. Tachycardia
   b. Hypotension
   c. Increased cardiac output
   d. Peripheral vasoconstriction

3. A patient with spinal cord injury has severe neurologic deficits. What is the *most* likely mechanism of injury for this patient?
   a. Compression
   b. Hyperextension
   c. Flexion-rotation
   d. Extension-rotation

4. A patient undergoing rehabilitation for a C7 spinal cord injury tells the nurse he must have the flu because he has a bad headache and nausea. The nurse's *first priority* is to
   a. call the health care provider.
   b. check the patient's temperature.
   c. measure the patient's blood pressure.
   d. elevate the head of the bed to 90 degrees.

5. The most common early symptom of a spinal cord tumor is
   a. urinary incontinence.
   b. back pain that worsens with activity.
   c. paralysis below the level of involvement.
   d. impaired sensation of pain, temperature, and light touch.

6. During assessment of the patient with trigeminal neuralgia, the nurse should (*select all that apply*)
   a. inspect all aspects of the mouth and teeth.
   b. assess the gag reflex and respiratory rate and depth.
   c. lightly palpate the affected side of the face for edema.
   d. test for temperature and sensation perception on the face.
   e. ask the patient to describe factors that initiate an episode.

7. During routine assessment of a patient with Guillain-Barré syndrome, the nurse finds the patient is short of breath. The patient's respiratory distress is caused by
   a. elevated protein levels in the CSF.
   b. immobility resulting from ascending paralysis.
   c. degeneration of motor neurons in the brainstem and spinal cord.
   d. paralysis ascending to the nerves that stimulate the thoracic area.

8. A nurse is caring for a patient newly diagnosed with chronic inflammatory demyelinating polyneuropathy (CIDP). Which statement can the nurse accurately use to teach the patient about CIDP?
   a. "Corticosteroids have little effect on this disease."
   b. "Maintenance therapy will be needed to prevent relapse."
   c. "You will go into remission in approximately eight weeks."
   d. "You should be able to walk without help within three months."

1. a, 2. b, 3. c, 4. c, 5. b, 6. a, d, e, 7. d, 8. b.

For rationales to these answers and even more NCLEX review questions, visit *http://evolve.elsevier.com/Lewis/medsurg.*

ⓔ EVOLVE WEBSITE/RESOURCES LIST

http://evolve.elsevier.com/Lewis/medsurg
Review Questions (Online Only)
Key Points
Answer Keys for Questions
- Rationales for Bridge to NCLEX Examination Questions
- Answer Guidelines for Case Study on p. 1426

Student Case Study
- Patient With Spinal Cord Injury

Nursing Care Plan
- eNursing Care Plan 60.1: Patient With a Spinal Cord Injury

Conceptual Care Map Creator
Audio Glossary
Content Updates

REFERENCES

1. The National SCI Statistical Center: Spinal cord injury (SCI) facts and figures at a glance. Retrieved from *www.nscisc.uab.edu/Public/Facts%20 2016.pdf*.

*2. Fehlings MG, Tetreault LA, Wilson JR, et al: A clinical practice guideline for the management of acute spinal cord injury: Introduction, rationale, and scope, *AOspine* 7:845, 2017.

3. Hachem LD, Ahuja CS, Fehling MG: Assessment and management of acute spinal cord injury: From point of injury to rehabilitation, *J Spinal Cord Med* 40:665, 2017.

4. Ulndreaj A, Chio JC, Ahuja CS, et al : Modulating the immune response in spinal cord injury, *Expert Re Neurother* 16:1127, 2016.

5. Ruiz IA, Squair JW, Phillips AA, et al: Incidence and natural progression of neurogenic shock after traumatic spinal cord injury, *J Neurotrauma* 35:461, 2018.

6. Dave S, Cho JJ: Shock: Neurogenic shock, Treasure Island, FL, 2018, StatPearls Publishing. Retrieved from *www.ncbi.nlm.nih.gov/books/ NBK459361/*.

7. Roberts TT, Leonard GR, Cepela DJ : Classifications in brief: ASIA Impairment Scale, *Clin Orthop Relat Res* 475:1499, 2017.

8. Stein DM, Knight WA: Emergency neurological life support: Traumatic spine injury, *Neurocrit Care* 27:S170, 2017.

*9. Neseyo U, Santiago-Lastra Y: Long-term complications of the neurogenic bladder, *Ur Clin N Am* 44:355, 2017.

10. Martinez L, Neshatican L, Khavari R: Neurogenic bowel dysfunction in patients with neurogenic bladder, *Curr Bladder Dysfunct Rep* 11:334, 2017.

*11. Felleiter P, Krebs J: Post-traumatic changes in energy expenditure and body composition in patients with acute spinal cord injury, *J Rehabil Med* 49:579, 2017.

*12. Fehlings MG, Tetreault LA, Jefferson RW, et al: A clinical practice guideline for management of patients with acute spinal cord injury: Recommendations on the type and timing of anticoagulant thromboprophylaxis, *AOspine* 7:2125, 2017.

13. Yue JK, Winkler EA, Rick JW, et al: Update on critical care for acute spinal cord injury in the setting of polytrauma, *Neurosurg Focus* 43:E19, 2017.

*14. Evanie N, Belley-Cote EP, Falla N, et al: Methylprednisolone for the treatment of patients with acute spinal cord injuries: A systematic review and meta-analysis, *J Neurotraum* 33:468, 2016.

15. STEADI: Stopping elderly accidents, deaths and injuries. Retrieved from *www.cdc.gov/steadi/index.html*.

*16. Kumar N, Pieri-Davies S, Chowdury JR, et al: Evidence-based respiratory management strategies required to preen complications and improve outcome in acute spinal cord injury patients, *Trauma* 19:23, 2017.

*17. Atkinson RA, Cullum NA: Interventions for pressure ulcers: A summary of evidence for prevention and treatment, *Spin Cord* 56:186, 2017.

*18. Brienza D, Krishnan S, Karg P, et al: Predictors of pressure ulcer incidence following traumatic spinal cord injury: A secondary analysis of a prospective longitudinal study, *Spin Cord* 56:28, 2018.

*19. Wound, Ostomy and Continence Nurses Society: Guidelines for prevention and management of pressure ulcers, *J Wound Ostomy Continence Nurs* 44:241, 2017.

*20. Eldahan KC, Rabchevsky AG: Autonomic dysreflexia after spinal cord injury: Systemic pathophysiology and methods of management, *Auton Neurosci* 209:59, 2018.

*21. Garara B, Wood A, Marcus HJ, et al: Intramuscular diaphragmatic stimulation for patient with traumatic high cervical injuries and ventilator dependent respiratory failure: A systematic review of safety and effectiveness, *Injury* 47:539, 2016.

*22. Cho YS, Kim KH: Botulinum toxin in spinal cord injury patients with neurogenic detrusor overactivity, *J Exerc Rehabil* 12:624, 2018.

23. Krogh K, Emmanuel A, Perrouin-Verbe B, et al: International Spinal Cord Bowel Function Basic Data Set (Version 2.0), *Spin Cord* 55:692, 2017.

24. Christopher & Dana Reeve Foundation Paralysis Resource Center: Sexual health for men. Retrieved from *www.christopherreeve.org/living-with-paralysis/health/sexual-health/sexual-health-for-men*.

25. Christopher & Dana Reeve Foundation Paralysis Resource Center: Sexual health for women. Retrieved from *www.christopherreeve.org/ living-with-paralysis/health/sexual-health/sexual-health-for-women*.

*26. Kornhabe R, Mclean L, Betivas V, et al: Resilience and the rehabilitation of adult spinal cord injury survivors: A qualitative systematic review, *J Adv Nurs* 74:23, 2018.

27. Kretzer RM: Intradural spinal cord tumors, *Spine* 42:22, 2017.

28. American Association of Neurological Surgeons: Spinal tumors. Retrieved from *www.aans.org/Patients/Neurosurgical-Conditions-and-Treatments/Spinal-Tumors*.

29. Kumar A, Weber MH, Gokaslan Z, et al: Metastatic spinal cord compression and steroid treatment, *Clin Spine Surg* 30:156, 2017.

30. National Institute of Health: Trigeminal neuralgia fact sheet. Retrieved from *www.ninds.nih.gov/Disorders/Patient-Caregiver-Education/Fact-Sheets/Trigeminal-Neuralgia-Fact-Sheet*.

*31. Crucca G, Finnerup NB, Jensen TS, et al: Trigeminal neuralgia: New classification of diagnostic grading for practice and research, *Am Acad Neurol* 87:220, 2016.

*32. Spina A, Mortini P, Alemanno F, et al: Trigeminal neuralgia: Toward a multimodal approach, *World Neurosurg* 103:220, 2017.

33. National Institute of Neurologic Disorders and Stroke: Bell's palsy information page. Retrieved from *www.ninds.nih.gov/Disorders/All-Disorders/ Bells-Palsy-Information-Page*.

*34. Thielker J, Geibler K, Granitzka T, et al: Acute management of Bells palsy, *Curr Otorhinolaryngol Rep* 6:161, 2018.

35. National Institute of Neurologic Disorders and Stroke: Guillain-Barré fact sheet. Retrieved from *www.ninds.nih.gov/Disorders/Patient-Caregiver-Education/Fact-Sheets/Guillain-Barr%C3%A9-Syndrome-Fact-Sheet*.

36. Centers for Disease Control and Prevention (CDC): Guillain-Barré syndrome. Retrieved from *www.cdc.gov/campylobacter/guillain-barre.html*.

37. Andary MT, Klein MJ: Guillain-Barré syndrome updated. Retrieved from *https://emedicine.medscape.com/article/315632-overview*.

38. Wilson HJ, Jacobs BC, van Doorn PA: Guillain-Barre syndrome, *Lancet* 388:717, 2016.

39. Verboon C, van Doorn PA, Jacobs BC. Treatment dilemma in Guillain-Barr syndrome, *J Neurol Neurosurg Psychiatry* 88:346, 2017.

40. National Institute of Neurologic Disorders and Stroke: Chronic inflammatory demyelinating polyneuropathy. Retrieved from *www.ninds. nih.gov/Disorders/All-Disorders/Chronic-Inflammatory-Demyelinating-Polyneuropathy-CIDP-Information-Page*.

41. Daroff RB, Jankovic J, Mazziotta JC, et al: Bradley's neurology in clinical practice, ed 7, St Louis, 2016, Elsevier.

42. Davis DP, Stoppler MC: Tetanus. Retrieved from *www.emedicinehealth. com/tetanus/article_em.htm#facts_on_tetanus*.

43. Centers for Disease Control and Prevention (CDC): Tetanus. Retrieved from *www.cdc.gov/tetanus/clinicians.html*.

*Evidence-based information for clinical practice.

61

Assessment: Musculoskeletal System

Colleen Walsh

It takes strength to be gentle and kind.

Steven Morrissey

℮ http://evolve.elsevier.com/Lewis/medsurg

CONCEPTUAL FOCUS

Functional Ability
Mobility

Safety

LEARNING OUTCOMES

1. Describe the gross and microscopic anatomy of bone.
2. Explain the classification system for joints and movements at synovial joints.
3. Describe the functions of cartilage, muscles, ligaments, tendons, fascia, and bursae.
4. Link age-related changes in the musculoskeletal system to the differences in assessment findings.
5. Obtain significant subjective and objective assessment data related to the musculoskeletal system from a patient.

6. Perform a physical assessment of the musculoskeletal system using appropriate techniques.
7. Distinguish normal from abnormal findings of a physical assessment of the musculoskeletal system.
8. Describe the purpose, significance of results, and nursing responsibilities related to diagnostic studies of the musculoskeletal system.

KEY TERMS

ankylosis, Table 61.6, p. 1439
arthrocentesis, Table 61.9, p. 1442
arthroscopy, Table 61.9, p. 1442
atrophy, Table 61.6, p. 1439
bone remodeling, p. 1430

contracture, Table 61.6, p. 1439
crepitation, Table 61.6, p. 1439
isometric contractions, p. 1432
isotonic contractions, p. 1432
kyphosis, Table 61.6, p. 1439

lordosis, Table 61.6, p. 1439
range of motion (ROM), p. 1437
scoliosis, p. 1438
x-ray, p. 1440

The musculoskeletal system is composed of voluntary muscle and 6 types of connective tissue: bone, cartilage, ligaments, tendons, fascia, and bursae. The purpose of the musculoskeletal system is to protect body organs, provide support and stability for the body, store minerals, and allow coordinated movement. This chapter reviews the structure and function of the musculoskeletal system to facilitate nursing assessment and evaluation of the assessment findings.

STRUCTURES AND FUNCTIONS OF MUSCULOSKELETAL SYSTEM

Bone

Function. The main functions of bone are support, protection of internal organs, voluntary movement, blood cell production, and mineral storage. Bones provide the supporting framework that keeps the body from collapsing. It allows the body to bear weight. Bones protect underlying vital organs and tissues. For example, the skull encloses the brain and vertebrae surround the spinal cord. The rib cage protects the lungs and heart.

Bones serve as a point of attachment for muscles and ligaments. Muscles are connected to bones by tendons. Bones act as a lever for muscles. Movement occurs because of muscle contractions applied to these levers. Ligaments provide stability to joints. Bone marrow contains hematopoietic tissue responsible for making red and white blood cells. Bones serve as a storage site for inorganic minerals, including calcium and phosphorus.

Bone is a dynamic tissue that continuously changes form and composition. It contains both organic material (collagen) and inorganic material (calcium, phosphate). The internal and external growth and remodeling of bone are ongoing processes. **Microscopic Structure.** Bone is classified according to structure as *cortical* (compact and dense) or *cancellous* (spongy). In *cortical bone*, cylindrical structural units called *osteons (Haversian systems)* fit closely together to create a dense bone structure (Fig. 61.1, *A*). Within the systems, the Haversian canals run parallel to the bone's long axis. They contain the blood vessels that travel to the bone's interior from the periosteum. Surrounding each osteon are concentric rings known as *lamellae*, which

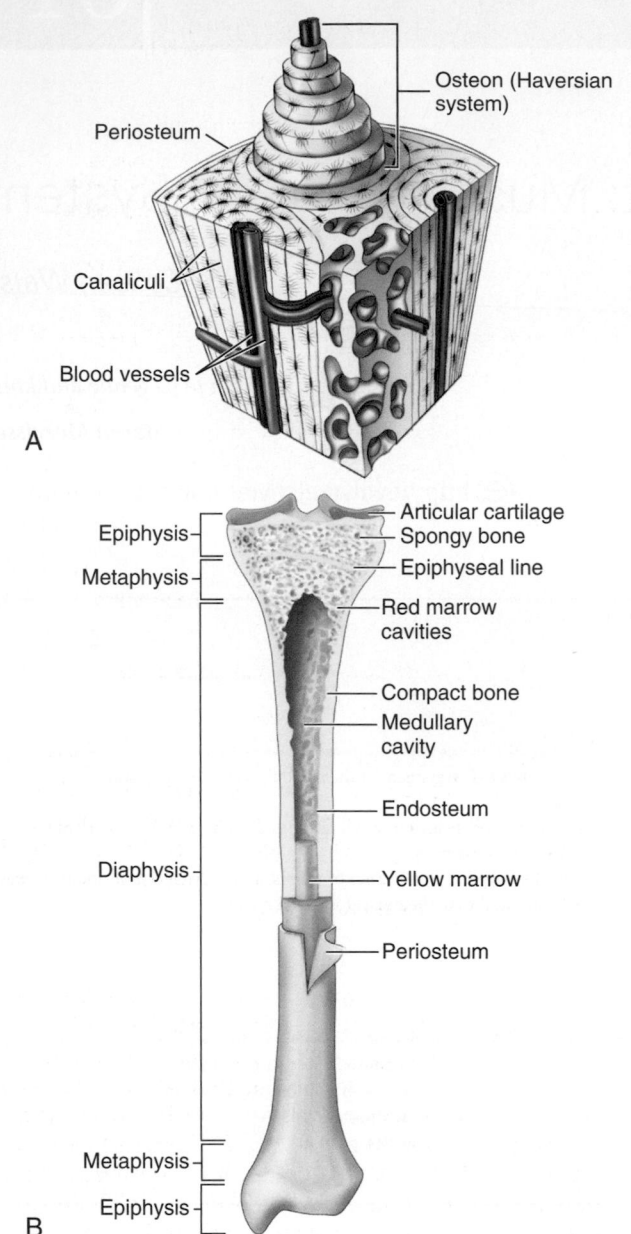

FIG. 61.1 Bone structure. **A,** Cortical bone showing numerous structural units called osteons. **B,** Anatomy of a long bone (tibia) showing cancellous and compact bone. (A, From Herlihy B, Maebius N: *The human body in health and illness,* ed 4, Philadelphia, 2011, Saunders. B, From Patton KT, Thibodeau GA: *Anatomy and physiology,* ed 8, St Louis, 2013, Mosby.)

indicate mature bone. Smaller canals *(canaliculi)* extend from the Haversian canals to the *lacunae,* where mature bone cells are embedded.

Cancellous bone has a different structure than cortical bone. The lamellae are not arranged in concentric rings. Instead, they occur along the lines of maximum stress placed on the bone. Cancellous bone is filled with red or yellow marrow. Blood reaches the bone cells by passing through spaces in the marrow.

The 3 types of bone cells are osteoblasts, osteocytes, and osteoclasts.[1] *Osteoblasts* synthesize organic bone matrix (collagen) and are the basic bone-forming cells. *Osteocytes* are mature bone cells. *Osteoclasts* take part in bone remodeling by helping in the breakdown of bone tissue. Bone remodeling is the removal of old bone by osteoclasts *(resorption)* and the deposit

of new bone by osteoblasts *(ossification).* The inner layer of bone is made mostly of osteoblasts with a few osteoclasts.

Gross Structure. The anatomic structure of bone is best represented by a typical long bone, such as the tibia (Fig. 61.1, *B*). Each long bone consists of the epiphysis, diaphysis, and metaphysis. The *epiphysis,* the widened area at each end of a long bone, is made mostly of cancellous bone. The wide epiphysis allows greater weight distribution and provides stability for the joint. The epiphysis is a primary location of muscle attachment. Articular cartilage covers the ends of the epiphysis. It provides a smooth, low-friction surface for joint movement.

The *diaphysis* is the main shaft of the long bone. It provides structural support and is composed of cortical bone. The tubular structure of the diaphysis allows it to withstand bending and twisting forces more easily.

The *metaphysis* is the flared area between the epiphysis and diaphysis. Like the epiphysis, it is composed of cancellous bone.

The *epiphyseal plate* (physis or growth plate) is the cartilaginous area between the epiphysis and metaphysis. In skeletally immature children who still have open growth plates, the epiphyseal plate actively makes chondrocytes that become mature bone. Division of the chondrocytes causes longitudinal bone growth in children. Injury to the epiphyseal plate in a growing child can cause the formation of new bone to stop at the growth plate. This leads to a shorter extremity and may contribute to significant functional problems. In the adult, the metaphysis and epiphysis become joined when chondrocyte formation at the growth plate stops and bone formation is complete.

The *periosteum* is composed of fibrous connective tissue that covers the bone. Tiny blood vessels penetrate the periosteum to bring nutrition to underlying bone. Musculotendinous fibers attach to the outer layer of the periosteum. Collagen bundles attach the inner layer of the periosteum to the bone. There is no periosteum on the articular surfaces of long bones. These bone ends are covered by articular cartilage.

The medullary *(marrow)* cavity in the center of the diaphysis contains either red or yellow bone marrow.[2] In adults, red marrow is found mainly in the *flat bones,* such as the pelvis, skull, sternum, cranium, ribs, vertebrae, and scapulae, and *cancellous* ("spongy") bone at the epiphyseal ends of long bones, such as the femur and humerus. Red bone marrow is involved in blood cell production (hematopoiesis). In the adult, the medullary cavity of long bones contains yellow bone marrow (mainly adipose tissue). Yellow marrow is involved in hematopoiesis in times of great blood cell need.

Types. The skeleton consists of 206 bones. They are classified according to shape as long, short, flat, or irregular.

Long bones have a central shaft *(diaphysis)* and 2 widened ends *(epiphyses)* (Fig. 61.1, *B*). Examples include the femur, humerus, and tibia. *Short bones* are composed of cancellous bone covered by a thin layer of compact bone. Examples include the carpals in the hand and tarsals in the foot.

Flat bones have 2 layers of compact bone separated by a layer of cancellous bone. Examples include the ribs, skull, scapula, and sternum. The spaces in the cancellous bone contain bone marrow. *Irregular bones* appear in a variety of shapes and sizes. Examples include the sacrum, mandible, and ear ossicles.

Joints

A *joint* (articulation) is a place where the ends of 2 bones are close and move in relation to each other. Joints are classified by the degree of movement that they allow (Fig. 61.2).

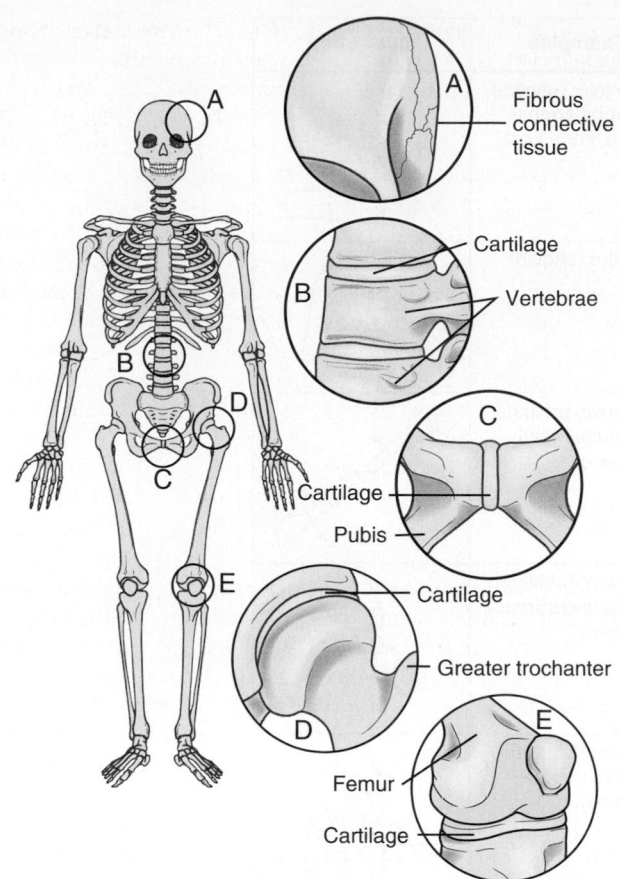

FIG. 61.2 Classification of joints. **A** to **C,** Synarthrotic (immovable) and amphiarthrotic (slightly movable) joints. **D** and **E,** Diarthrodial (*freely* movable) joints.

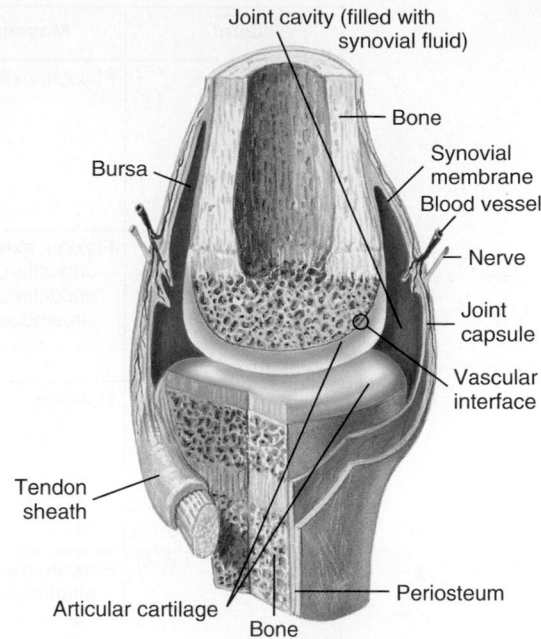

FIG. 61.3 Structure of diarthrodial (synovial) joint.

The most common joint is the freely movable *diarthrodial* (synovial) type. Each joint is enclosed in a capsule of fibrous connective tissue, which joins the 2 bones together to form a cavity (Fig. 61.3). The capsule is lined by a synovial membrane, which secretes thick synovial fluid. This fluid lubricates the joint, reduces friction, and allows opposing surfaces to slide smoothly over each other. The end of each bone is covered with articular (hyaline) cartilage. Supporting structures (e.g., ligaments, tendons) reinforce the joint capsule. They provide limits and stability to joint movement. Types of diarthrodial joints are shown in Fig. 61.4.

Cartilage

The 3 types of *cartilage* are hyaline, elastic, and fibrous. *Hyaline cartilage* is the most common. It has a moderate amount of collagen fibers. It is found in the trachea, bronchi, nose, epiphyseal plate, and articular surfaces of bones.

Elastic cartilage, which has both collagen and elastic fibers, is more flexible than hyaline cartilage. It is found in the ear, epiglottis, and larynx.

Fibrous cartilage (fibrocartilage) consists mostly of collagen fibers. It is a tough tissue that often functions as a shock absorber. Fibrous cartilage is found between the vertebral discs. It also forms a protective cushion between the bones of the pelvic girdle, knee, and shoulder.

Cartilage in synovial joints serves as a support for soft tissue and provides the articular surface for joint movement. It protects underlying tissues. Because articular cartilage is avascular, it must receive nourishment by the diffusion of material from the synovial fluid. The lack of a direct blood supply contributes to the slow metabolism of cartilage cells and explains why healing and repair of cartilage tissue occur slowly. The cartilage in the epiphyseal plate is also involved in the growth of long bones before physical maturity is reached.

Muscle

Types. The 3 types of muscle tissue are cardiac (striated, involuntary), smooth (nonstriated, involuntary), and skeletal (striated, voluntary) muscle. *Cardiac muscle* is found only in the heart. Its spontaneous contractions pump blood through the circulatory system. *Smooth muscle* is found in the walls of hollow structures, such as airways, arteries, gastrointestinal (GI) tract, urinary bladder, and uterus. Smooth muscle contraction is controlled by neuronal and hormonal influences. *Skeletal muscle,* which requires neuronal stimulation for contraction, accounts for about half of a human's body weight. It is the focus of the following discussion.

Structure. The skeletal muscle is enclosed by the *epimysium,* a continuous layer of deep fascia. The epimysium helps muscles slide over nearby structures. Connective tissue surrounding and extending into the muscle can be subdivided into fiber bundles *(fasciculi).* These bundles are covered by *perimysium* and an innermost connective tissue layer called the *endomysium* that surrounds each fiber (Fig. 61.5).

The structural unit of skeletal muscle is the muscle cell or muscle fiber. It is highly specialized for contraction. Skeletal muscle fibers are long, multinucleated cylinders that contain many mitochondria to support their high metabolic activity. Muscle fibers are composed of myofibrils, which in turn are made up of protein contractile filaments. The *sarcomere* is the contractile unit of the myofibrils. Each sarcomere consists of *myosin* (thick) filaments and *actin* (thin) filaments. The arrangement of the thin and thick filaments causes the characteristic banding of muscle seen under a microscope. Muscle contraction occurs as thick and thin filaments slide past each other, causing the sarcomeres to shorten.

Joint	Movement	Examples	Illustration
Hinge joint	Flexion, extension	Elbow joint (shown), interphalangeal joints, knee joint	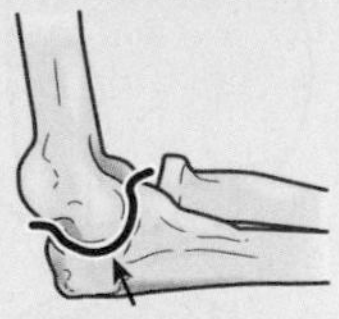
Ball and socket (spheroidal)	Flexion, extension; adduction, abduction; circumduction	Shoulder (shown), hip	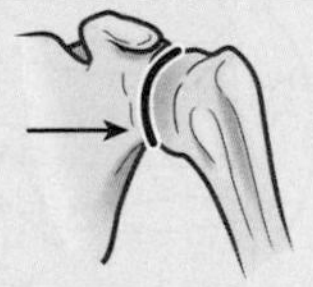
Pivot (rotary)	Rotation	Atlas-axis, proximal radioulnar joint (shown)	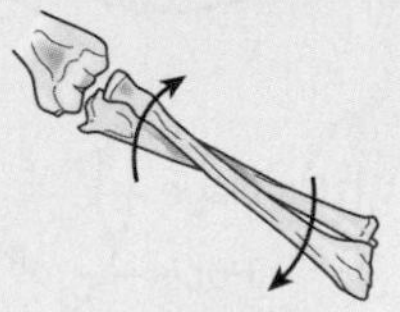
Condyloid	Flexion, extension; abduction, adduction; circumduction	Wrist joint (between radial and carpals) (shown)	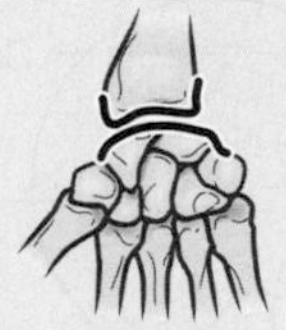
Saddle	Flexion, extension; abduction, adduction; circumduction, thumb-finger opposition	Carpometacarpal joint of thumb (shown)	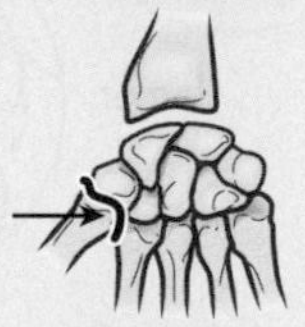
Gliding	One surface moves over another surface	Between tarsal bones, sacroiliac joint, between articular processes of vertebrae, between carpal bones (shown)	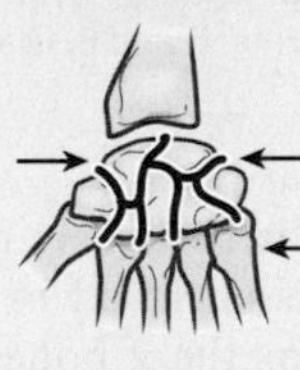

FIG. 61.4 Types of diarthrodial (synovial) joints.

Contractions. Skeletal muscle contractions allow posture maintenance, body movement, and facial expressions. Isometric contractions increase the tension within a muscle but do not produce movement. Isotonic contractions shorten a muscle to produce movement. Most contractions are a combination of tension generation *(isometric)* and shortening *(isotonic)*. Repeated isometric and/or isotonic contractions provide stress to stimulate muscle growth. Muscular *atrophy* (decrease in size) occurs with the absence of contractions that results from immobility or decreased neuronal stimulation. Increased muscular activity leads to *hypertrophy* (increase in size).

Skeletal muscle fibers are divided into 2 groups based on the type of activity they show. *Slow-twitch muscle fibers* support prolonged muscle activity, such as marathon running. Because they also support the body against gravity, they help in posture maintenance. *Fast-twitch muscle fibers* are used for rapid muscle contraction needed for activities, such as blinking the eye, jumping, or sprinting. Fast-twitch fibers tend to tire more quickly than slow-twitch fibers.

Neuromuscular Junction. Skeletal muscle fibers require a nerve impulse to contract. A nerve fiber and the skeletal muscle fibers

it stimulates are called a *motor endplate.* The junction between the axon of the nerve cell and the adjacent muscle cell is called the *myoneural* or *neuromuscular junction* (Fig. 61.6).

Presynaptic neurons release acetylcholine. It diffuses across the neuromuscular junction to bind with receptors on the motor endplate of the muscle. In response to this stimulation, the sarcoplasmic reticulum releases calcium ions into the cytoplasm. The presence of calcium triggers the contraction in the myofibrils. When calcium is low, *tetany* (involuntary contractions of skeletal muscle) can occur.

Energy Source. The direct energy source for muscle fiber contractions is adenosine triphosphate (ATP). ATP is synthesized by cellular oxidative metabolism in the numerous mitochondria found close to the myofibrils. It is rapidly depleted through conversion to adenosine diphosphate (ADP) and must be rephosphorylated. Phosphocreatine provides a rapid source for the resynthesis of ATP, but it is, in turn, converted to creatine. Glycolysis can serve as a source of ATP when the O_2 supply is inadequate for metabolic needs of the muscle tissue. In this process, 1 glucose molecule is broken down to 2 ATP molecules.

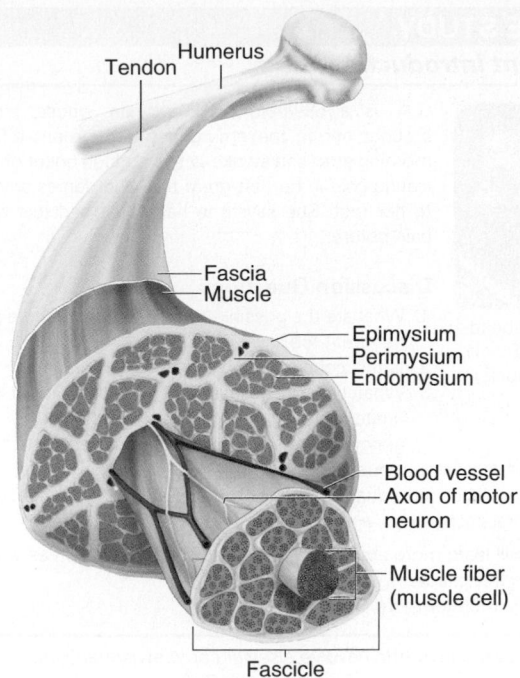

FIG. 61.5 Structure of a muscle. (From Patton KT, Thibodeau GA, Douglas M: *Essentials of anatomy and physiology*, St Louis, 2012, Mosby.)

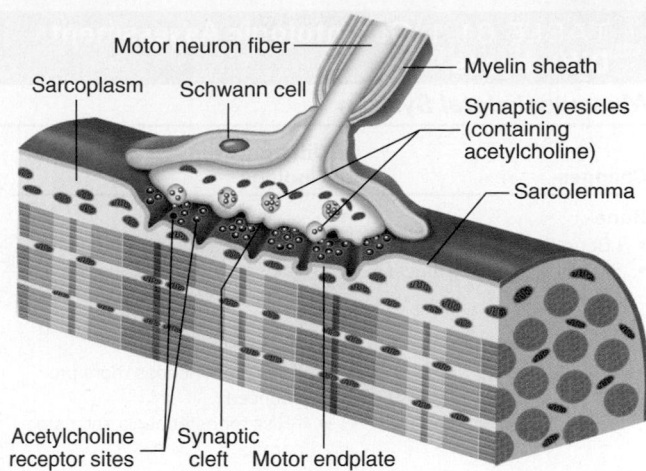

FIG. 61.6 Neuromuscular junction. (From Patton KT, Thibodeau GA: *Anatomy and physiology*, ed 8, St Louis, 2013, Mosby.)

Ligaments and Tendons

Ligaments and tendons are composed of dense, fibrous connective tissue with bundles of closely packed collagen fibers arranged in the same plane for additional strength. *Tendons* attach muscles to bones as an extension of the muscle sheath that adheres to the periosteum. *Ligaments* connect bones to bones (e.g., tibia to femur at knee joint). They have a higher elastic content than tendons.[3] Ligaments provide stability while allowing controlled movement at joints.

Ligaments and tendons have a relatively poor blood supply. This can make tissue repair a slow process after injury. For example, the stretching or tearing of ligaments that occurs with a sprain may require a long time to mend.

Fascia

Fascia refers to layers of connective tissue with intermeshed fibers that can withstand limited stretching. Superficial fascia lies right under the skin. Deep fascia is a dense, fibrous tissue that surrounds muscle bundles, nerves, and blood vessels. It also encloses individual muscles, allowing them to act independently and to glide over each other during contraction. In addition, fascia provides strength to muscle tissues.

Bursae

Bursae are small sacs of connective tissue lined with synovial membrane and containing viscous synovial fluid. They are found at bony prominences or joints to relieve pressure and decrease friction between moving parts.[4] For example, bursae are found between the (1) patella and skin (prepatellar bursae), (2) olecranon process of the elbow and skin (olecranon bursae), (3) head of the humerus and acromion process of the scapula (subacromial bursae), and (4) greater trochanter of the proximal femur and skin (trochanteric bursae). *Bursitis* is an inflammation of a bursa sac. The inflammation may be acute or chronic.

Gerontologic Considerations: Effects of Aging on Musculoskeletal System

Many functional problems experienced by the older adult are related to changes in the musculoskeletal system. Although some changes begin in early adulthood, obvious signs of musculoskeletal impairment may not appear until later adult years. Changes may affect the older adult's ability to complete self-care tasks and pursue other usual activities. Effects of musculoskeletal changes may range from mild discomfort and decreased ability to perform ADLs to severe, chronic pain and immobility.

The bone remodeling process changes in the aging adult. Increased bone resorption and decreased bone formation cause a loss of bone density. This contributes to the development of osteopenia and osteoporosis (see Chapter 63). Muscle mass and strength decrease. Almost 30% of muscle mass is lost by age 70. A loss of motor neurons can cause problems with skeletal muscle movement. Tendons and ligaments become less flexible, making movement more rigid.

Perform a musculoskeletal assessment with an emphasis on exercise practices. Obtain information on the type of exercise performed, including frequency and warm-up activities. Determine the impact of age-related changes of the musculoskeletal system on functional status. Specifically ask about changes in self-care habits and ability to be independent in the home environment. Functional limitations that are accepted by the older adult as a normal part of aging can often be addressed with appropriate preventive strategies (see Table 62.1).

The risk for falls increases in the older adult due in part to loss of strength. Aging can also bring changes in the patient's balance, making the person unsteady. *Proprioception* (awareness of self in relation to the environment) may be altered. Identify any musculoskeletal changes that increase the patient's risk for falls. Discuss fall prevention strategies.

Osteoarthritis is more likely to affect joints in the aging adult (see Chapter 64).[5] Metabolic bone diseases involve the deterioration of bone tissue (osteoporosis) and destruction of cartilage (osteoarthritis). Carefully distinguish between expected changes and the effects of disease in the aging adult. Symptoms of disease can be treated in many cases, helping the older adult to return to a higher functional level. Age-related changes in the musculoskeletal system and differences in assessment findings are outlined in Table 61.1.

TABLE 61.1 Gerontologic Assessment Differences

Musculoskeletal System

Changes	Differences in Assessment Findings
Bone	
• ↓ Bone density and strength • Slowed remodeling process	• Loss of height and deformity, such as dowager's hump (kyphosis), from vertebral compression and degeneration • Back pain, stiffness • Bony prominences more pronounced • ↑ Risk for osteopenia and osteoporosis
Joints	
• ↑ Risk for cartilage erosion that leads to direct contact between bone ends and overgrowth of bone around joint margins • Loss of water from discs between vertebrae, ↓ height of intervertebral spaces	• Joint stiffness, ↓ mobility, limited ROM, possible crepitation on movement • Pain with motion and/or weight bearing • Loss of height and shortening of trunk from disc compression. Posture change
Muscles	
• ↓ Number and diameter of muscle cells. Replacement of muscle cells by fibrous connective tissue • Loss of elasticity and deterioration of cartilage • ↓ Ability to store glycogen. ↓ Ability to release glycogen as quick energy during stress • ↓ Basal metabolic rate	• ↓ Muscle strength and mass • Abdominal protrusion • ↑ Rigidity in neck, shoulders, back, hips, and knees • ↓ Fine motor dexterity, ↓ agility • Slowed reaction times and reflexes from slowed conduction of nerve impulses along motor units • Earlier fatigue with activity

ASSESSMENT OF MUSCULOSKELETAL SYSTEM

Subjective Data

Important Health Information.

Past Health History. The most common manifestations of musculoskeletal impairment include pain, weakness, deformity, limitation of movement, stiffness, and joint crepitation (crackling sound). Ask the patient about changes in sensation or in the size of a muscle.

Questions should focus on symptoms of arthritic and connective tissue diseases (e.g., gout, psoriatic arthritis, systemic lupus erythematosus [SLE]), osteomalacia, osteomyelitis, and fungal infection of bones or joints. Ask the patient about sources of a secondary bacterial infection, such as ears, tonsils, teeth, sinuses, lungs, or genitourinary tract. These infections can enter the bones, resulting in osteomyelitis or joint destruction. Get a detailed account of the course and treatment of any of these problems.

Certain illnesses are known to affect the musculoskeletal system directly or indirectly. Ask the patient about medical problems, such as tuberculosis, poliomyelitis, diabetes, parathyroid problems, hemophilia, rickets, soft tissue infection, and neuromuscular disability.

Trauma to the musculoskeletal system is a common reason for seeking medical care. The patient who is a good historian

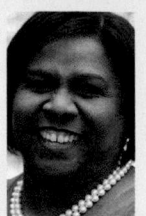
can recount minor and major injuries of the musculoskeletal system. Record information chronologically and include:

- Mechanism and circumstances of the injury (e.g., twist, crush, stretch)
- Methods and duration of treatment
- Current status related to the injury
- Need for assistive devices
- Interference with ADLs

Medications. Ask the patient about prescription and over-the-counter drugs, herbal products, and nutritional supplements. Get detailed information about each treatment, including its name, dose and frequency, length of time it was taken, reason for use, and any possible side effects. Ask about the use of skeletal muscle relaxants, opioids, nonsteroidal antiinflammatory drugs, corticosteroids, and calcium and vitamin D supplements.

Review the use of drugs that can have detrimental effects on the musculoskeletal system. Some of these and their potential side effects include antiseizure drugs (osteomalacia), phenothiazines (gait changes), corticosteroids (avascular necrosis, decreased bone and muscle mass), and potassium-depleting diuretics (muscle cramps and weakness). Ask postmenopausal women about the use of hormone therapy.

Surgery or Other Treatments. Ask about any hospitalizations related to a musculoskeletal problem. Document the reason for hospitalization; the date and duration; and the treatment, including ongoing rehabilitation. Record details of emergency treatment for musculoskeletal injuries. Get specific information about any surgical procedure, postoperative course, and complications. Ask the patient about past total knee or total hip replacement. If the patient had a period of prolonged immobilization, consider the possible development of disuse osteoporosis and muscle atrophy.

Functional Health Patterns. Past or developing musculoskeletal problems can affect the patient's overall health. The use of functional health patterns helps organize assessment data. Table 61.2 outlines specific questions to ask in relation to functional health patterns.

TABLE 61.2   Health History

Musculoskeletal System

Health Perception–Health Management Pattern
- Describe your usual daily activities.
- Do you have any problems performing these activities?* Describe what you do if you have trouble dressing, preparing meals and feeding yourself, performing basic hygiene, writing or using the phone, or maintaining your home.
- Do you have to lift heavy objects? Do your work or exercise habits require repetitive motion or joint stress? Describe any special equipment you use or wear when you work or exercise that helps protect you from injury.
- Do you take any drugs or herbal products to manage your musculoskeletal problem? If so, what are their names and what are the expected effects?

Nutritional-Metabolic Pattern
- What is your usual daily intake of food and snacks?
- Do you have problems preparing your food?
- What dietary supplements do you take? Do you take calcium or vitamin D supplements?
- What is your weight? Describe any recent weight loss or gain.

Elimination Pattern
- Does your musculoskeletal problem make it hard for you to reach the toilet in time?*
- Do you need any assistive devices or equipment to manage toileting?*
- Do you have constipation related to decreased mobility or drugs taken for your musculoskeletal problem?*

Activity-Exercise Pattern
- Do you need help in completing your usual daily activities because of a musculoskeletal problem?*
- Describe your usual exercise pattern. Do you have musculoskeletal symptoms before, during, or after exercising?*
- Are you able to move all your joints comfortably through full range of motion?
- Do you use any prosthetic or orthotic devices?*

Sleep-Rest Pattern
- Do you have any problems sleeping because of a musculoskeletal problem?*
- Do you need frequent position changes at night?*
- Do you wake up at night because of musculoskeletal pain?*
- Do you use complementary and alternative therapies to help you sleep at night?*

Cognitive-Perceptual Pattern
- Describe any musculoskeletal pain you have. How do you manage your pain? Ask about adjunctive therapies, such as heat and cold, or complementary and alternative therapies, such as acupuncture.

Self-Perception–Self-Concept Pattern
- Have changes in your musculoskeletal system (posture, walking, muscle strength) and decreased ability to do certain things affected how you feel about yourself?*
- Have these changes affected your lifestyle?*

Role-Relationship Pattern
- Do you live alone?
- Describe how family, friends, or others help you with your musculoskeletal problem.
- Describe the effect of your musculoskeletal problem on your work and your social relationships.

Sexuality-Reproductive Pattern
- Describe any sexual concerns related to your musculoskeletal problem.

Coping–Stress Tolerance Pattern
- Describe how you deal with problems such as pain, weakness, or immobility that have resulted from your musculoskeletal problem.

Value-Belief Pattern
- Describe any cultural practices or religious beliefs that may influence the treatment of your musculoskeletal problem.

*If yes, describe.

Health Perception–Health Management Pattern. Ask about the patient's health practices related to the musculoskeletal system. This includes maintaining normal body weight, avoiding excessive stress on muscles and joints, and using proper body mechanics when lifting objects. Ask the patient about tetanus, pertussis, and polio immunizations.

Safety practices can affect the patient's predisposition for certain injuries and illnesses. Ask the patient about safety practices related to the work environment, home life, recreation, and exercise. For example, if the patient is a computer programmer, ask about ergonomic adaptations in the office that decrease the risk for carpal tunnel syndrome or low back pain. Identifying problems in this area will direct your plan for patient teaching.

Get a family history of rheumatoid arthritis, SLE, ankylosing spondylitis, osteoarthritis, gout, osteoporosis, and scoliosis. A patient may have a genetic predisposition to these or other musculoskeletal disorders.

Nutritional-Metabolic Pattern. The patient's description of a typical day's diet gives clues to areas of nutritional concern that can affect the musculoskeletal system. Adequate intake of vitamins C and D, calcium, and protein is essential for a healthy musculoskeletal system. Abnormal nutritional patterns can contribute to problems such as osteomalacia and osteoporosis. Maintaining normal weight is an important nutritional goal.

⚕ GENETIC RISK ALERT

Autoimmune Diseases

- Many autoimmune diseases of the musculoskeletal system have a genetic basis involving human leukocyte antigens (HLAs).
- These diseases include ankylosing spondylitis, rheumatoid arthritis, and SLE.

Osteoporosis
- Genetic factors contribute to osteoporosis by influencing bone mineral density, and bone size, quality, and turnover.

Osteoarthritis, Gout, and Scoliosis
- A genetic predisposition is a contributing risk factor in all these diseases.

Muscular Dystrophy
- The most common types of muscular dystrophy are X-linked recessive disorders.

Obesity places added stress on weight-bearing joints, such as the knees, hips, and spine. This increases the risk for cartilage deterioration and ligament instability.

Elimination Pattern. Questions about the patient's mobility may reveal problems with ambulating to the toilet. Ask the patient if an assistive device, such as an elevated toilet seat or a grab bar, is needed to manage toileting. Decreased mobility from a musculoskeletal problem can lead to constipation. Musculoskeletal problems can contribute to bowel or bladder incontinence when ambulation is a problem.

Activity-Exercise Pattern. Many musculoskeletal problems can affect the patient's activity-exercise pattern. Get a detailed account of the type, duration, and frequency of exercise and recreational activities. Compare daily, weekend, and seasonal patterns because occasional exercise can be more of a problem than regular exercise. Ask the patient about clumsiness or limitations in movement, pain, weakness, crepitus, or any change in bones or joints that interferes with daily activities.

Extremes of activity related to occupation can affect the musculoskeletal system. For example, a desk job can negatively affect muscle flexibility and strength. Jobs that require heavy lifting or pushing can lead to damage of joints and supporting structures. Specifically ask the patient about work-related musculoskeletal injuries, including treatment and time lost from work.

Sleep-Rest Pattern. The discomfort caused by musculoskeletal problems can interfere with the patient's normal sleep pattern and lead to fatigue.[6] Ask the patient about any changes in sleep patterns. If the patient describes poor sleep related to a musculoskeletal problem, ask about the type of bedding and pillows used, bedtime routine, sleeping partner, and sleeping positions.

Cognitive-Perceptual Pattern. Fully discuss any pain reported by the patient due to a musculoskeletal problem. To give a baseline for later reassessment, ask the patient to describe the intensity of the pain on a numeric scale from 0 to 10 (0 = no pain, 10 = most severe pain imaginable). Reassessments over time help to determine the effectiveness of any treatment plan. Ask the patient about measures used to manage pain. Also ask about related problems, such as joint swelling or muscle weakness, and any adjustments that help with the problem. (Pain is discussed in Chapter 8.)

Self-Perception–Self-Concept Pattern. Many chronic musculoskeletal problems lead to deformities and a reduction in activities. This can have a serious negative impact on the patient's body image and sense of personal worth.[6] Assess the patient's feelings about these changes and any effect on interactions with family and friends.

Role-Relationship Pattern. Impaired mobility and chronic pain from musculoskeletal problems can negatively affect the patient's ability to perform in roles of spouse, parent, and/or employee. The ability to pursue and maintain meaningful social and personal relationships also can be affected by musculoskeletal problems. Carefully ask the patient about role performance and relationships.

If the patient lives alone, any musculoskeletal problem and rehabilitation may make it hard or impossible to continue to do so. Assess how much help is available from family, friends, and other caregivers. Find out if other resources are needed, such as physical therapy and home health care.

Sexuality-Reproductive Pattern. Ask women about their menstrual history. Episodes of premenopausal amenorrhea can contribute to the development of osteoporosis.[7] The pain of musculoskeletal problems can affect the patient's ability to obtain sexual satisfaction. Explore this area in a sensitive and nonjudgmental way. Help the patient feel comfortable discussing any sexual problems related to pain, movement, and positioning. More information on obtaining patient data in this area is discussed in Chapter 50.

Coping–Stress Tolerance Pattern. Mobility limitations and pain are serious potential stressors that challenge the patient's coping resources. Recognize the potential for difficulty coping in the patient and family or significant other. Additional questions will help to determine if a musculoskeletal problem is causing difficulties in coping and adjusting.

Value-Belief Pattern. Ask the patient about cultural or religious beliefs that may influence acceptance of treatment for the musculoskeletal problem. These may include recommendations for diet, exercise, medication, and lifestyle modifications.

Subjective Data

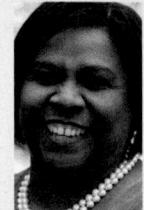

(© pixelhead-photo/iStock/Thinkstock.)

A focused subjective assessment of G.A. revealed the following information:

Past Medical History: Hypertension for 6 years. Type 2 diabetes for 11 yr, 40-pack-yr smoking history.

Medications: Metformin (Glucophage) 500 mg PO bid; glyburide (DiaBeta) 5 mg/day PO; hydrochlorothiazide 50 mg PO bid.

Health Perception–Health Management: Currently smokes 1 pack of cigarettes per day. Is trying to quit but finding it difficult. Drinks alcohol at night.

Nutritional-Metabolic: G.A. is 5 ft, 2 in tall and weighs 160 lb (BMI 29.3 kg/m²). Does not take any nutritional supplements and avoids milk and other dairy products because they make her "gassy."

Activity-Exercise: Minimally active; does not exercise. Able to perform ADLs without assistance. Denies any history of musculoskeletal problems.

Cognitive-Perceptual: Rates toe pain at 8 on a scale of 0 to 10. Describes sharp, burning pain that increases in intensity with any movement.

Coping–Stress Tolerance: Is asking for pain medicine "as strong as you can give me."

Discussion Questions

1. What subjective assessment findings are of most concern to you?
2. Is this an appropriate time to talk with G.A. about her weight?
3. Based on these subjective findings, what should be included in the physical assessment?

You will learn more about the physical assessment of the musculoskeletal system in the next section.

See p. 1438 for more information on G.A.

Answers available at *http://evolve.elsevier.com/Lewis/medsurg*.

Objective Data

Physical Examination. The basic musculoskeletal physical examination involves inspection, palpation, neurovascular assessment, and range of motion, strength, and reflex testing. Other special tests can be used to assess for specific conditions. Conduct a general overview. While obtaining a careful health history, choose areas to concentrate on during the local examination. Take specific measurements as indicated by the local examination.

Inspection. A systematic inspection is done, starting at the head and neck then moving to the upper extremities, lower extremities, and trunk. The regular use of a systematic approach is important to avoid missing important aspects of the examination. Inspect the skin for general color, scars, or other overt signs of previous injury or surgery. Certain skin lesions require further investigation because they can indicate underlying disorders. For example, butterfly rash over the cheeks and nose is characteristic of SLE.

Note the patient's general posture and body build, muscle size and symmetry, and symmetry and contour of joints. Observe for any swelling, deformity, nodules or masses, and discrepancies in limb length or muscle size. Use the patient's opposite body part for comparison when you suspect an abnormality.

If the patient can move independently, assess posture and gait by watching the patient walk, stand, and sit. Musculoskeletal and neurologic problems can result in abnormal gait patterns.

Palpation. As with inspection, palpation usually proceeds head to toe. Examine the neck, shoulders, elbows, wrists, hands, back, hips, knees, ankles, and feet. Warm your hands to prevent muscle spasm, which can interfere with identifying essential landmarks or soft tissue structures. Carefully palpate any specific areas of concern because of a subjective report or abnormal appearance on inspection.

Both superficial and deep palpation are usually done consecutively. Consider the underlying anatomy structures and landmarks you are palpating. Purposefully palpate both muscles and joints to evaluate skin temperature, local tenderness, swelling, and crepitation. Establish the relationship of adjacent structures. Evaluate the general contour, abnormal prominences, and local landmarks. Note the specific anatomic location of any abnormal findings.

Motion. When assessing the patient's joint mobility, carefully evaluate active and passive range of motion (ROM). ROM is the full movement potential of a joint. Measurements should be similar for active and passive maneuvers. *Active ROM* means the patient takes their own joints through all movements without assistance. *Passive ROM* occurs when someone else moves the patient's joints without their assistance through the full ROM. Be careful in performing passive ROM because of the risk for injury to underlying structures. If pain or resistance occurs, stop at once.

If you note deficits in active or passive ROM, assess functional ROM to determine if joint changes are affecting the ability to perform ADLs. Ask the patient if activities, such as eating, grooming, dressing, and bathing, require help or cannot be done at all.

We use a goniometer to accurately assess ROM. It measures the angle of the joint (Fig. 61.7). We do not usually measure specific degrees of ROM of all joints. If a specific musculoskeletal problem has been identified, measure ROM of the affected joint. A less exact but valuable assessment method is simply to compare the ROM of 1 extremity with that on the opposite side. Common movements that occur at the synovial joints, including *abduction, adduction, flexion,* and *extension,* are described in Table 61.3.

Muscle-Strength Testing. Grade the strength of individual muscles or groups of muscles during contraction on a 5-point scale (Table 61.4). Grade normal muscle strength with full resistance to opposition as a 5/5 bilaterally. To test resistance to opposition, have the patient apply resistance as you exert a force. For example, have the patient try to extend the elbow while you try to flex it. Compare muscle strength with the strength of the opposite extremity. Note any subtle variations in muscle strength when comparing the patient's dominant and nondominant sides. Variations in strength also exist when comparing people.

Measurement. When limb length discrepancies or subjective problems are noted, measure limb length and circumferential muscle mass. For example, when gait disorders are observed, measure leg length between the anterosuperior iliac crest and the bottom of the medial malleolus. Then compare it with the similar measurement of the opposite extremity. Measure muscle

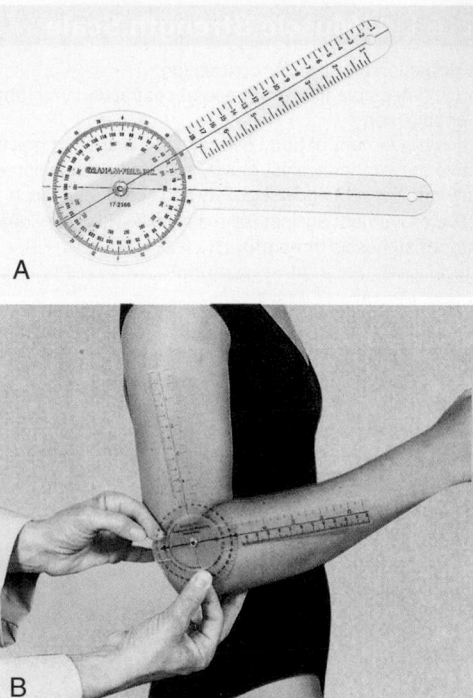

FIG. 61.7 A, Goniometer. B, Measurement of joint ROM using a goniometer. (*A,* From Wilson SF, Giddens JF: *Health assessment for nursing practice,* ed 5, St Louis, 2013, Mosby. *B,* From Barkauskas V, Baumann L, Stoltenberg-Allen K, et al: *Health and physical assessment,* ed 2, St Louis, 1998, Mosby.)

TABLE 61.3 Synovial Joint Movements

Movement	Description
Abduction	Movement of part away from midline of body
Adduction	Movement of part toward midline of body
Circumduction	Circular motion of a body part from a combination of flexion, abduction, extension, and adduction
Dorsiflexion	Flexion of the ankle and toes toward the shin
Eversion	Turning of sole outward away from midline of body
Extension	Straightening of joint that ↑ angle between 2 bones
External rotation	Movement along longitudinal axis away from midline of body
Flexion	Bending of joint from muscle contraction that causes ↓ angle between 2 bones
Hyperextension	Extension in which angle exceeds 180 degrees
Internal rotation	Movement along longitudinal axis toward midline of body
Inversion	Turning of sole inward toward midline of body
Opposition	Moving the first and fifth metacarpals anteriorly from a flattened palm ("cupping position"); makes it possible to hold objects between the thumb and fingers
Plantar flexion	Flexion of the ankle and toes toward the plantar surface of the foot ("toes pointed")
Pronation	Turning of palm downward
Supination	Turning of palm upward

mass circumferentially at the largest area of the muscle. When recording measurements, record the exact location at which the measurements were obtained (e.g., the left quadriceps muscle was measured 15 cm above the patella). This tells the next examiner of the exact area to measure and ensures consistency during reassessment.

TABLE 61.4 Muscle Strength Scale

0/5	No detection of muscular contraction
1/5	Barely detectable flicker or trace of contraction with observation or palpation
2/5	Active movement of body part with elimination of gravity
3/5	Active movement against gravity only and not against resistance
4/5	Active movement against gravity and some resistance
5/5	Active movement against full resistance without evident fatigue (normal muscle strength)

TABLE 61.5 Normal Physical Assessment of the Musculoskeletal System

- Ordinary spinal curvatures
- No muscle atrophy or asymmetry
- No joint swelling, deformity, or crepitation
- No tenderness on palpation of spine, joints, or muscles
- Full ROM of all joints without pain or laxity
- Muscle strength of 5/5

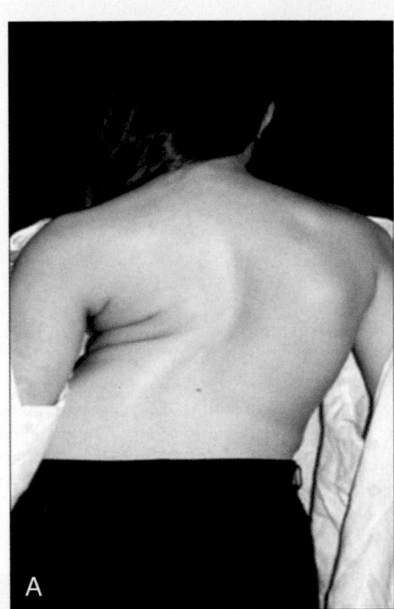 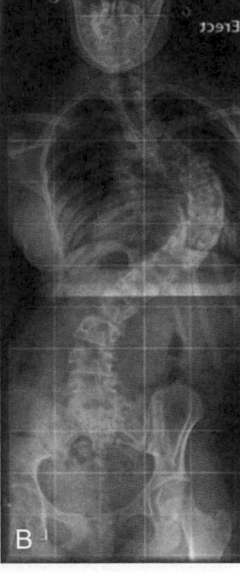

FIG. 61.8 A, Thoracic scoliosis. B, X-ray of same patient showing scoliosis greater than 90 degrees. (From Hawary R, Chukwunyerenwa C: *Update on evaluation and treatment of scoliosis, Pediatr Clin North Am* 61:1223, 2014.)

A *focused assessment* is used to evaluate previously identified musculoskeletal problems and to monitor for signs of new problems. See the Focused Assessment of the Musculoskeletal System box.

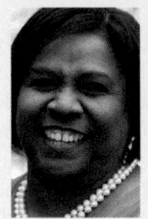
Other. Note the patient's use of an assistive device, such as a walker or cane. Assess the patient for proper fit while reviewing the safe and correct technique for using these devices. Regularly review with the patient the use of the assistive device to be sure it is still appropriate and safe. Ask the patient if the assistive device is used regularly. If not, determine possible reasons for inconsistent use.[8]

Scoliosis is a lateral S-shaped curvature of the thoracic and lumbar spine. Unequal shoulder and scapula height is usually noted when the patient is observed from the back (Fig. 61.8). Ask the patient to place the hands together above the head as if diving into a swimming pool and slowly bend forward at the waist, allowing assessment of thoracic rib prominence or paravertebral muscle prominence in the lumbar spine. Advanced scoliosis can impair lung and heart function.

The *straight-leg-raising test* is done on the supine patient with sciatica or leg pain. Passively raise the patient's leg 60 degrees or less. The test is positive if the patient reports pain along the distribution of the sciatic nerve. A positive test shows nerve root irritation from intervertebral disc prolapse and herniation, especially at level L4-5 or L5-S1.

Assessment of reflexes is discussed in Chapter 55. Table 61.5 shows an example of how to record a normal physical assessment of the musculoskeletal system. Abnormal assessment findings of the musculoskeletal system are described in Table 61.6.

FOCUSED ASSESSMENT
Musculoskeletal System

Use this checklist to be sure key assessment steps have been done.

Subjective
Ask the patient about any of the following and note responses.

Joint pain or stiffness	Y	N
Muscle weakness	Y	N
Bone pain	Y	N

Objective: Diagnostic
Check the results of the following diagnostic studies.

X-ray	✓
MRI or CT scan	✓
Bone scan	✓

Objective: Physical Examination
Inspect and Palpate

Spine and extremities (compare sides) for alignment, contour, symmetry, size, gross deformities	✓
Joints for ROM, tenderness or pain, heat, crepitus, swelling	✓
Muscles (compare sides) for size, symmetry, tone, tenderness, or pain	✓
Bones for tenderness or pain	✓

TABLE 61.6   Assessment Abnormalities

Musculoskeletal System

Finding	Description	Possible Etiology and Significance
Achilles tendonitis	Pain in ankle and posterior calf, initially when running or walking. Can progress to pain at rest.	Stress on Achilles tendon over time causing inflammation.
Ankylosis	Stiffness and fixation of a joint.	Chronic joint inflammation and destruction (e.g., rheumatoid arthritis).
Antalgic gait	Shortened stride with minimal weight bearing on the affected side, resulting in a limp.	Pain or discomfort in the lower extremity on weight bearing. Can be due to trauma or other disorders.
Ataxic gait	Staggering, uncoordinated gait often with sway.	Neurogenic disorders (e.g., spinal cord lesion).
Atrophy	↓ Size and strength of muscle leading to ↓ function and tone.	Muscle denervation, contracture, prolonged disuse from immobilization.
Boutonnière deformity	Finger abnormality, flexion of proximal interphalangeal (PIP) joint and hyperextension of the distal interphalangeal (DIP) joint of the fingers (see Fig. 64.4, *B*).	Typical deformity of rheumatoid and psoriatic arthritis caused by disruption of extensor tendons over the fingers.
Contracture	Resistance of movement of muscle or joint due to fibrosis of supporting soft tissues.	Shortening of muscle or ligaments, tightness of soft tissue, incorrect positioning of immobilized extremity.
Crepitation (crepitus)	Frequent, audible crackling sound with palpable grating that accompanies movement.	Fracture, dislocation, temporomandibular joint dysfunction, osteoarthritis.
Dislocation	Separation of 2 bones from their normal position within a joint.	Trauma, disorders of surrounding soft tissues.
Festinating gait	While walking, neck, trunk, and knees flex and the body is rigid. Delayed start with short, quick, shuffling steps. Speed may ↑ as if patient is unable to stop (festination).	Neurogenic disorders (e.g., Parkinson's disease).
Ganglion cyst	Small fluid-filled mass over a tendon sheath or joint, usually on dorsal surface of wrist or foot.	Inflammation of tissues around a joint, which can increase in size or disappear.
Kyphosis (dowager's hump)	Exaggerated thoracic curvature.	Poor posture, tuberculosis, arthritis, osteoporosis, growth disturbance of vertebral epiphyses, vertebral fractures.
Lateral epicondylitis (tennis elbow)	Dull ache along outer aspect of elbow, worsens with twisting and grasping motions.	Injury, inflammation, and/or partial tearing of tendon at its insertion on epicondyle.
Limited range of motion (ROM)	Joint does not achieve expected degrees of motion.	Injury, inflammation, contracture.
Lordosis (swayback)	Exaggerated lumbar curvature.	Other spinal deformities, muscular dystrophy, obesity, flexion contracture of hip, congenital dislocation of hip.
Muscle spasticity	↑ Muscle tone (rigidity) with sustained muscle contractions (spasms); stiffness or tightness may interfere with gait, movement, speech.	Neuromuscular disorders, such as multiple sclerosis (MS) or cerebral palsy.
Myalgia	General muscle tenderness and pain.	Chronic pain syndromes (e.g., fibromyalgia). Overuse, injury, or strain. May result from statin therapy.
Paresthesia	Numbness and tingling, often described as a "pins and needles" sensation.	Compromised sensory nerves, often due to edema in a closed space (e.g., cast, bulky dressing). Spinal stenosis.
Pes planus (flatfoot)	Abnormal flatness of the sole and arch of the foot.	Hereditary, muscle paralysis, mild cerebral palsy, early muscular dystrophy, injury to posterior tibial tendon.
Plantar fasciitis	Burning, sharp pain on heel and sole of foot. Worse in the morning with first step out of bed.	Chronic degenerative/reparative cycle resulting in inflammation.
Scoliosis	Asymmetric elevation of shoulders, scapulae, and iliac crests with lateral spine curvature (Fig. 61.8).	Idiopathic or congenital condition, neuromuscular, fracture or dislocation, osteomalacia.
Short-leg gait	A limp, unless corrective footwear used.	Leg length discrepancy ≥1 in, generally of structural origin (arthritis, fracture).
Spastic gait	Short steps with dragging of foot. Jerky, uncoordinated, cross-knee (scissor) movement.	Neurogenic (e.g., cerebral palsy, hemiplegia).
Steppage gait	↑ Hip and knee flexion to clear the foot from the floor. Foot drop is evident, foot slaps down and along walking surface.	Neurogenic disorders (e.g., peroneal nerve injury, paralyzed dorsiflexor muscles).
Subluxation	Partial dislocation of joint.	Instability of joint capsule and supporting ligaments (e.g., trauma, arthritis).
Swan neck deformity	Hyperextension of the PIP joint with flexion of the metacarpophalangeal (MCP) and DIP joints of the fingers (see Fig. 64.4, *D*).	Typical deformity of rheumatoid and psoriatic arthritis caused by contracture of muscles and tendons.
Swelling	Enlargement, often of a joint due to fluid collection. Usually leads to pain, stiffness.	Trauma or inflammation.
Tenosynovitis	Superficial swelling, pain, and tenderness along a tendon sheath.	Inflammation that often occurs with infection, injury, or overuse.
Torticollis (wryneck)	Neck is rotated and laterally bent in unusual position to one side.	Prolonged contraction of neck muscles (congenital or acquired).
Ulnar deviation (ulnar drift)	Fingers drift to ulnar side of forearm (see Fig. 64.4, *A*).	Typical deformity of rheumatoid arthritis due to tendon contracture.
Valgum deformity (knock-knees)	When knees are together and there is <1 in (2.5 cm) between the medial malleoli.	Poliomyelitis, congenital deformity, arthritis.
Varum deformity (bowlegs)	When knees are apart and the medial malleoli are together, a space of >1 in (2.5 cm) exists.	Arthritis, congenital deformity.

DIAGNOSTIC STUDIES OF MUSCULOSKELETAL SYSTEM

Many diagnostic studies are used to assess the musculoskeletal system. Tables 61.7, 61.8, and 61.9 present the most common studies. Select studies are described in more detail next.

The use of studies such as x-rays, MRI, and bone scans has greatly improved orthopedic care. The x-ray is the most common diagnostic study used to assess musculoskeletal problems and to monitor treatment effectiveness. Because bones are denser than other tissues and contain calcium, most x-rays are absorbed by the bone tissue and do not penetrate it. Dense areas show as white on the standard x-ray. X-rays provide information about bone deformity, joint congruity, bone density, and calcification in soft tissue. X-rays are useful for diagnosing fractures. They also help evaluate genetic, developmental, infectious, inflammatory, malignant, metabolic, and degenerative disorders.

Aspirated synovial fluid is assessed for volume, color, clarity, viscosity, and mucin clot formation. Normal synovial fluid is transparent and colorless or straw colored. It should be scant in amount and of low viscosity. Fluid from an infected joint may be purulent and thick or gray and thin. In gout, the fluid may be whitish yellow. Blood may be aspirated if there is hemarthrosis due to injury or a bleeding disorder.

The mucin clot test indicates the character of the protein portion of the synovial fluid. Normally a white, ropelike mucin clot is formed. In the presence of inflammation, the clot fragments easily. The fluid is examined grossly for floating fat globules, which indicate bone injury. In septic arthritis, protein content is increased, and glucose is considerably decreased. Presence of uric acid crystals suggests a diagnosis of gout. A Gram stain and culture also may be done to assess for the presence and type of infection.

TABLE 61.7 Serology Studies

Musculoskeletal System

Test	Reference Intervals	Description and Purpose
Aldolase	22–59 mU/L	Useful in monitoring muscular dystrophy, dermatomyositis.
Alkaline phosphatase	30–120 U/L (0.5–2.0 μkat/L)	Enzyme made by osteoblasts, needed for mineralization of organic bone matrix. ↑ Levels found with healing fractures, bone cancers, osteoporosis, osteomalacia, Paget's disease.
Anticyclic citrullinated peptide (anti-CCP)	Negative or <20.0 U	Assesses presence of CCP antibodies. More specific for rheumatoid arthritis than rheumatoid factor. Positive result indicates high likelihood of RA.
Anti-DNA antibody	<5 IU/mL	Detects serum antibodies that react with DNA. Most specific test for SLE.
Antinuclear antibody (ANA)	Negative at 1:40 dilution	Assesses presence of antibodies capable of destroying nucleus of tissue cells. Positive in 95% of patients with SLE. May be positive in those with scleroderma, rheumatoid arthritis, small number of normal persons.
Calcium	9.0–10.5 mg/dL (2.25–2.62 mmol/L)	Bone is primary organ for calcium storage. Calcium provides bone with rigid structure. ↓ Level found in osteomalacia, kidney disease, hypoparathyroidism. ↑ Level found in hyperparathyroidism, some bone tumors.
C-reactive protein (CRP)	<1.0 mg/dL	Used to diagnose inflammatory diseases, infections, active widespread cancer. Synthesized by liver. Present in large amounts in serum 18–24 hr after onset of tissue damage.
Creatine kinase (CK)	*Male:* 55–170 U/L *Female:* 30–135 U/L	Highest concentration found in skeletal muscle. ↑ Level in progressive muscular dystrophy, polymyositis, traumatic injuries.
Human leukocyte antigen (HLA)–B27	Negative	Antigen often present in autoimmune disorders, such as ankylosing spondylitis and rheumatoid arthritis.
Potassium	3.5–5.0 mEq/L (3.5–5.0 mmol/L)	Released into serum with cell destruction. ↑ Level with muscle trauma.
Phosphorus	3.0–4.5 mg/dL (0.97–1.45 mmol/L)	Amount present is indirectly related to calcium metabolism. ↓ Level found in osteomalacia. ↑ Level found in chronic kidney disease, healing fractures, osteolytic metastatic tumor.
Rheumatoid factor (RF)	Negative or titer <1:17	Presence of autoantibody (rheumatoid factor) in serum. Not specific for rheumatoid arthritis. Seen in other connective tissue diseases and in a small number of normal persons.

TABLE 61.8 Diagnostic Studies

Musculoskeletal System

Study	Description and Purpose	Nursing Responsibilities
Basic x-ray	Evaluates structural or functional changes of bones and joints. Can give a general impression of bone density. In anteroposterior view, x-ray beam passes from front to back, allowing 1-dimensional view. Lateral position provides 2-dimensional view.	*Before:* Remove any radiopaque objects that can interfere with results. Explain procedure to patient. *During:* Avoid excessive exposure of patient and self.
Bone scan	Involves injection of radioisotope (usually technetium [Tc]-99m) that is taken up by bone. Uniform uptake of isotope is normal. ↑ Uptake seen in osteomyelitis, primary and metastatic cancer of bone, certain fractures. ↓ Uptake seen in areas of avascular necrosis.	*Before:* Explain that radioisotope is given 2 hr before procedure. Have patient void before scan. Tell patient that no harm will result from isotopes. *During:* Patient must lie completely still during scan. *After:* Increase fluids after scan.

TABLE 61.8 Diagnostic Studies—cont'd

Musculoskeletal System

Study	Description and Purpose	Nursing Responsibilities
Computed tomography (CT) scan	X-ray beam used with a computer to provide a 3D picture. Used to identify soft tissue abnormalities, bony abnormalities, and various types of musculoskeletal trauma.	*Before:* Evaluate renal function before contrast medium used. Assess if patient is allergic to shellfish since the contrast is iodine based. Patient may need to be NPO 4 hr prior to study. If the patient is taking metformin, hold it the day of the test to prevent hypoglycemia or lactic acidosis. *During:* Warn patient that contrast injection may cause a feeling of being warm and flushed. Patient must lie completely still during scan. *After:* Encourage patient to drink fluids to avoid renal problems with any contrast.
Discogram	X-ray of cervical or lumbar intervertebral disc is done after injection of contrast media into nucleus pulposus. Permits visualization of intervertebral disc abnormalities.	*Before:* Assess patient for allergy to contrast medium. Explain procedure. *After:* May have mild back pain for 1–2 days. Use as-needed analgesics.
Dual energy x-ray absorptiometry (DEXA)	Measures bone mineral density of spine, femur, forearm, total body. Allows assessment of bone density with minimal radiation exposure. Used to diagnose metabolic bone disease (e.g., osteoporosis), monitor changes in bone density with treatment.	*Before:* Remove any radiopaque objects that can interfere with results. Explain procedure to patient.
Electromyogram (EMG)	Evaluates electrical potential associated with skeletal muscle contraction. Small-gauge needles are inserted into certain muscles. Needle probes are attached to leads that send information to EMG machine. Recordings of electrical activity of muscle are traced on audio transmitter and on oscilloscope and recording paper. Provides information related to lower motor neuron dysfunction and primary muscle disease.	*Before:* Explain procedure. Tell patient that pain and discomfort are associated with insertion of needles. Some HCPs may restrict stimulants (e.g., caffeine) 2–3 hr prior. *After:* Assess needle sites for hematoma or inflammation. Use as-needed analgesics.
MRI	Radio waves and magnetic field used to view soft tissue. Used to diagnose avascular necrosis, disc disease, tumors, osteomyelitis, ligament tears, cartilage tears. Patient placed inside scanning chamber. Gadolinium may be injected IV to enhance visualization of structures.	*Before:* Oral and/or IV contrast injection may be used. Check for pregnancy, allergies, and renal function before test. Have patient remove all metal objects. Ask about any history of surgical insertion of staples, plates, dental bridges, or other metal appliances. Remove metallic foil patches. Patient may need to be fasting. Assess for claustrophobia and the need for antianxiety medication. *During:* Patient must lie completely still during test.
Myelogram with or without CT	Involves injecting a radiographic contrast medium into sac around nerve roots. CT scan may follow to show how bone is affecting the nerve roots. Sensitive test for nerve impingement, can detect subtle lesions and injuries.	*Before:* Give sedative as ordered. Have patient empty bladder. Tell patient that test is done with patient on tilting table that is moved during test. *After:* Keep patient flat for 1–2 hr after procedure to prevent spinal headache. Encourage fluids. Monitor neurologic signs and VS. Headache, nausea, and vomiting may occur after procedure.
Somatosensory evoked potential (SSEP)	Evaluates evoked potential of muscle contractions. Electrodes are placed on skin and provide recordings of electrical activity of muscle. Used to identify subtle dysfunction of lower motor neuron and primary muscle disease. Measures nerve conduction along pathways not accessible by EMG. Transcutaneous or percutaneous electrodes applied to the skin help identify neuropathy and myopathy. Used during spinal surgery for scoliosis to detect neurologic compromise when patient is under anesthesia.	*Before:* Tell patient that procedure is like an EMG but does not involve needles. Electrodes are applied to the skin.
Thermography	Uses infrared detector to measure degree of heat radiating from skin surface. Used to evaluate cause of inflamed joint and determine patient response to antiinflammatory drug therapy.	*Before:* Tell patient that procedure is painless and noninvasive.
Quantitative ultrasound (QUS)	Evaluates bone mineral density, elasticity, and strength of bone using ultrasound rather than radiation. Used to assess heel.	*Before:* Tell patient that procedure is painless and noninvasive.

TABLE 61.9 Interventional Studies

Musculoskeletal System

Study	Description and Purpose	Nursing Responsibilities
Arthrocentesis	Incision or puncture of joint capsule to obtain samples of synovial fluid or to remove excess fluid. Local anesthesia and aseptic preparation are used before needle is inserted into joint and fluid aspirated. Used to diagnose joint inflammation, infection, meniscal tears, and subtle fractures.	*Before:* Explain procedure to patient. HCP may have patient be NPO prior. Usually done at bedside or in examination room. *After:* Send samples of synovial fluid to laboratory for examination (if indicated). Apply compression dressing and ice to decrease pain and swelling. Observe for leakage of blood or fluid on dressing. Assess the joint for any pain, fever, or swelling. Review activity restrictions.
Arthroscopy	Involves insertion of arthroscope into joint to see interior of joint cavity. Can be used for surgery (removal of loose bodies, biopsy); repair of joint structures; and diagnosis of abnormalities of meniscus, articular cartilage, ligaments, or joint capsule. Structures that can be seen through an arthroscope include knee, shoulder, elbow, wrist, jaw, hip, and ankle (Fig. 61.9).	*Before:* Explain the procedure to the patient. Can be done in outpatient setting. Local or general anesthesia may be used. HCP may have patient be NPO prior. *After:* Cover wound with sterile dressing. Apply ice to decrease pain and swelling. Observe for bleeding. Assess the joint for any pain, weakness, or swelling. Review activity restrictions.

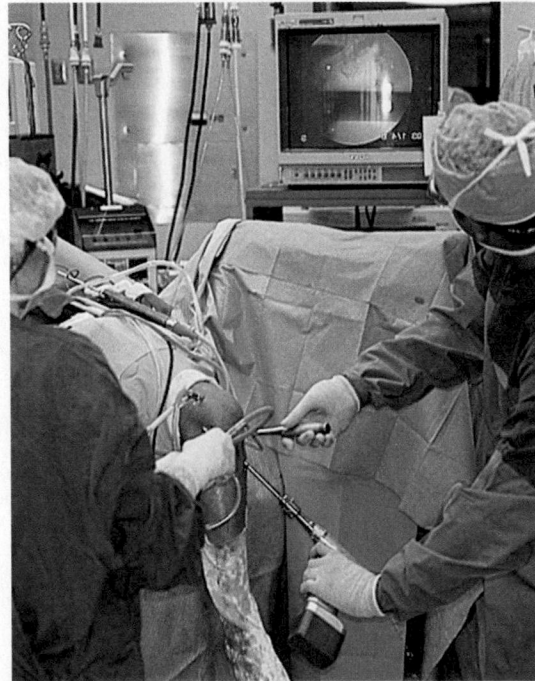

FIG. 61.9 Knee arthroscopy in progress. Notice the monitor in the background. (From Miller MD, Howard RF, Plancher KD: *Surgical atlas of sports medicine,* Philadelphia, 2003, Saunders.)

CASE STUDY—cont'd

Objective Data: Diagnostic Studies

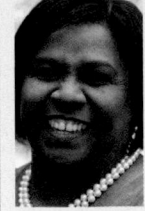

(© pixelhead-photo/iStock/ Thinkstock.)

The HCP in the ED immediately orders the following diagnostic studies:
- X-ray of left foot
- CBC, electrolytes
- Aspiration of the great toe

The x-ray of the foot shows minor soft tissue swelling but no evidence of fracture. Very mild arthritis is noted at the interphalangeal joint of the great toe. CBC and electrolytes are within normal limits.

Aspiration of the interphalangeal joint shows clear synovial fluid. Protein and glucose are within normal limits. Microscopic analysis of the synovial fluid shows urate crystals.

Discussion Questions

1. Which diagnostic results are abnormal?
2. What diagnostic study results are of most concern to you?

Answers available at *http://evolve.elsevier.com/Lewis/medsurg.*

▌ BRIDGE TO NCLEX EXAMINATION

The number of the question corresponds to the same-numbered outcome at the beginning of the chapter.

1. The bone cells that function in the formation of new bone tissue are called
   a. osteoids.
   b. osteocytes.
   c. osteoclasts.
   d. osteoblasts.
2. While performing passive range of motion for a patient, the nurse puts the elbow joint through the movements of *(select all that apply)*
   a. flexion and extension.
   b. inversion and eversion.
   c. pronation and supination.
   d. flexion, extension, abduction, and adduction.
   e. pronation, supination, rotation, and circumduction.

3. A patient with a torn ligament in the knee asks what the ligament does. The nurse's response is based on the knowledge that ligaments
   a. connect bone to bone.
   b. provide strength to muscle.
   c. lubricate joints with synovial fluid.
   d. relieve friction between moving parts.
4. The increased risk for falls in the older adult is likely due to *(select all that apply)*
   a. changes in balance.
   b. decrease in bone mass.
   c. loss of ligament elasticity.
   d. erosion of articular cartilage.
   e. decrease in muscle mass and strength.

5. The nurse is obtaining a health history of a patient with a fracture. Which condition poses the most concern related to the musculoskeletal system?
   a. Diabetes
   b. Hypertension
   c. Chronic bronchitis
   d. Nephrotic syndrome
6. When grading muscle strength, the nurse records a score of 3/5, which indicates
   a. no detection of muscular contraction.
   b. a barely detectable flicker of contraction.
   c. active movement against full resistance without fatigue.
   d. active movement against gravity but not against resistance.

7. An abnormal assessment finding of the musculoskeletal system is
   a. equal leg length bilaterally.
   b. ulnar deviation and subluxation.
   c. full range of motion in all joints.
   d. muscle strength of 5/5 in all muscles.
8. A patient is scheduled for a bone scan. The nurse explains that this diagnostic test involves
   a. incision or puncture of the joint capsule.
   b. insertion of small needles into certain muscles.
   c. administration of a radioisotope before the procedure.
   d. placement of skin electrodes to record muscle activity.

1. d, 2. a, 3. a, 4. b, 5. c, 6. d, 7. b, 8. c

For rationales to these answers and even more NCLEX review questions, visit *http://evolve.elsevier.com/Lewis/medsurg*.

ⓔ EVOLVE WEBSITE/RESOURCES LIST

REFERENCES

1. Crowther-Radulewicz CL: The musculoskeletal system. In McCance KL, Heuther SE, eds: *Pathophysiology: The biologic basis for disease in adults and children*, ed 8, St Louis, 2019, Mosby.
2. Chan BY, Gill, KG, Rebsamen SL, et al: MR imaging of pediatric bone marrow, *RadioGraphics* 36:1911, 2016.
3. Rachna C: Difference between tendons and ligaments. Retrieved from *https://biodifferences.com/difference-between-tendons-and-ligaments.html*.
4. Khodaee M: Common superficial bursitis, *Am Fam Physician* 95:224, 2017.
*5. Roberts S, Colombier P, Sowman A, et al: Ageing in the musculoskeletal system: Cellular function and dysfunction throughout life, *Acta Orthopaedica* 363:15, 2016.
*6. Hawker GA: The assessment of musculoskeletal pain, *Clinic Exp Rheumatol* 35:8, 2017.
*7. Langdahl BL: Osteoporosis in premenopausal women, *Cur Opin in Rheum* 29:410, 2017.
*8. Luz C, Bush T, Shen X: Do canes or walkers make any difference? Non-use and fall injuries, *The Gerontologist* 57:2, 2017.

*Evidence-based information for clinical practice.

62

Musculoskeletal Trauma and Orthopedic Surgery

Matthew C. Price

Never look down on anybody unless you're helping him up.

Jesse Jackson

http://evolve.elsevier.com/Lewis/medsurg

LEARNING OUTCOMES

1. Distinguish the etiology, pathophysiology, manifestations, and interprofessional and nursing management of soft tissue injuries.
2. Relate the sequence of events involved in fracture healing.
3. Compare closed reduction, cast immobilization, open reduction, and traction in terms of purpose, complications, and nursing management.
4. Assess the neurovascular condition of an injured extremity.
5. Explain common complications associated with a fracture and fracture healing.
6. Describe the interprofessional and nursing management of patients with various kinds of fractures.
7. Describe indications for and interprofessional and nursing management of the patient with an amputation.
8. Describe types of joint replacement surgery.
9. Prioritize management of the patient having joint replacement surgery.

KEY TERMS

The most common cause of musculoskeletal injury is a traumatic event resulting in fracture, dislocation, subluxation, and/or soft tissue injury. Most of these injuries are not fatal. However, the cost in terms of pain, disability, medical expense, and lost wages is enormous. Accidents are 1 of the top 3 causes of death for persons ages 1 to 64 years.[1] Nurses play a key role in teaching the public about basic principles of safety and accident prevention.

This chapter discusses musculoskeletal problems resulting from trauma and common orthopedic surgical procedures. Following trauma or surgery, the injured area is often immobilized while healing occurs. The nurse's role in preventing complications (e.g., pressure injuries, constipation, infection, venous thromboembolism [VTE]) and promoting functional ability in patients with fractures and orthopedic surgery is emphasized.

HEALTH PROMOTION

Teach people in the community to take proper safety precautions to prevent injuries while at home or work, driving, or taking part in sports. The morbidity associated with accidents can be significantly reduced if people are aware of environmental hazards, use proper safety equipment, and apply safety and traffic rules. In the work setting, teach employees and employers about use of proper safety equipment and avoiding hazardous working situations.

 PROMOTING POPULATION HEALTH

Reducing the Risk for Musculoskeletal Injuries

- Regularly wear seatbelts.
- Drive within posted speed limits.
- Avoid distracted driving (e.g., no texting, eating, talking on a cell phone).
- Do not drive under the influence of alcohol or drugs (prescribed or illicit).
- Warm up muscles before exercise.
- Use protective athletic equipment (helmets and knee, wrist, and elbow pads).
- Use proper safety equipment at work.

Encourage people, especially older adults, to take part in moderate exercise to help maintain muscle strength and balance. Ways to prevent common musculoskeletal problems in the older adult are listed in Table 62.1. To reduce risk for falls, urge them to wear nonskid, hard-soled footwear and assess their living environment for safety risks (e.g., remove throw rugs, ensure adequate lighting, maintain clear paths to the bathroom for nighttime use). Stress the importance of adequate calcium and vitamin D intake for bone health.

> ⚠️ **SAFETY ALERT Falls**
> - Falls cause many musculoskeletal injuries in the home.
> - Provide preventive teaching to high-risk persons (e.g., people with gait instability, visual or cognitive impairment).
> - Stress the importance of wearing shoes with functional, stable soles and heels.
> - Remind patients to avoid wet or slippery surfaces.
> - Encourage removal of throw rugs in the home.

TABLE 62.1 Patient & Caregiver Teaching

Prevention of Musculoskeletal Problems in Older Adults

To prevent musculoskeletal problems, include the following instructions when teaching older adults and their caregivers:
1. Use ramps in buildings and at street corners instead of steps to prevent falls.
2. Remove throw rugs from the home.
3. Treat pain and discomfort from osteoarthritis.
   - Rest in positions that decrease discomfort.
   - Use medication as prescribed for pain.
4. Use a walker or cane to help prevent falls.
5. Eat the amount and kind of foods needed to prevent weight gain. Obesity adds stress to joints, which may predispose to osteoarthritis.
6. Get regular and frequent exercise.
   - ADLs provide range-of-motion exercises. Tai Chi may be helpful.
   - Hobbies (e.g., jigsaw puzzles, needlework, model building) exercise finger joints and prevent stiffness.
   - Do daily weight-bearing exercise (e.g., walking) to improve bone health.
7. Use shoes with good support for safety and comfort.
8. Avoid sudden change in position. Rise slowly to a standing position to prevent dizziness, falls, and fractures.
9. Do not walk on uneven surfaces and wet floors.

SOFT TISSUE INJURIES

Soft tissue injuries include sprains, strains, dislocations, and subluxations. They usually result from trauma. As more people have become involved in fitness programs or sports, the incidence of soft tissue injuries has increased. Common sports-related injuries are described in Table 62.2. Sports injuries that often result in a visit to the emergency department (ED) for younger patients include sprains and strains, growth plate injuries, and repetitive motion injuries.[2]

SPRAINS AND STRAINS

Sprains and strains often result from abnormal stretching or twisting forces during vigorous activities. These injuries tend to occur around joints and in the spinal musculature.

A sprain is an injury to the ligaments surrounding a joint. Sprains are usually caused by a wrenching or twisting motion. Most occur in the ankle, wrist, and knee joints.[3] A sprain is classified according to the degree of ligament damage. A *first-degree (mild) sprain* involves tears in only a few fibers, with mild tenderness and minimal swelling. A *second-degree (moderate) sprain* results in partial disruption of the involved tissue with more swelling and tenderness. A *third-degree (severe) sprain* is a complete tear of the ligament with moderate to severe swelling.

A strain is an excessive stretching of a muscle and its fascial sheath, often involving the tendon. Most strains occur in the large muscle groups, including the lower back, calf, and hamstrings. Strains are classified as first degree (mild or slightly pulled muscle), second degree (moderate or moderately torn muscle), and third degree (severely torn or ruptured muscle). A defect in the muscle may be apparent or palpated through the skin if the muscle is torn. Because areas around joints are rich in nerve endings, the injury can be very painful.

Manifestations of sprains and strains are similar. They include pain, edema, decreased function, and bruising. Continued use of the joint, tendon, or ligament makes pain worse. Edema develops in the injured area because of the local inflammatory response.

Mild sprains and strains are usually self-limiting. Full function generally returns within 3 to 6 weeks. X-rays of the affected part may be taken to rule out a fracture. A severe sprain can

TABLE 62.2 Soft Tissue Injuries

Injury	Description	Treatment
Anterior cruciate ligament tear	Tearing of ligament by deceleration forces with pivoting or odd positions of the knee or leg.	PT with rehabilitation, knee brace. If knee instability or further injury, reconstructive surgery may be done.
Impingement syndrome	Entrapment of soft tissues and nerves under coracoacromial arch of shoulder.	NSAIDs. Rest until symptoms ↓, then begin gradual ROM and strengthening exercises.
Ligament injury	Tearing or stretching of ligament. Usually occurs from inversion, eversion, shearing, or torque applied to a joint. Characterized by sudden pain, swelling, and instability.	Rest, ice, elevation of extremity if possible, NSAIDs. Protect affected extremity by use of brace. If symptoms persist, surgical repair may be needed.
Meniscus injury	Injury to fibrocartilage discs in knee. Characterized by popping, clicking, tearing sensation, effusion, and/or swelling.	Rest, ice, elevation of extremity if possible, NSAIDs. Gradual return to regular activities. If symptoms persist, MRI to assess meniscus injury. Possible arthroscopic surgery.
Rotator cuff tear	Tear within muscle, tendons, or ligaments around shoulder.	*If minor tear:* rest, NSAIDs, and gradual mobilization with ROM and strengthening exercises. *If major tear:* surgical repair.
Shin splints	Inflammation of periosteal bone *(periostitis)* along anterior calf. Caused by improper shoes, overuse, or running on hard pavement.	Rest, ice, NSAIDs, proper shoes. Gradual ↑ in activity. If pain persists, x-ray to rule out tibial stress fracture.
Tendonitis	Inflammation of tendon due to overuse or incorrect use.	Rest, ice, NSAIDs. Gradual return to sport activity. Protective brace *(orthosis)* may be needed if symptoms recur.

cause an *avulsion fracture*, in which the ligament pulls loose a fragment of bone. The joint structure may become unstable, causing subluxation or dislocation. At the time of injury, *hemarthrosis* (bleeding into a joint space or cavity) or disruption of the synovial lining may occur. Severe strains may need surgical repair of the muscle, tendon, or surrounding fascia.

❖ NURSING MANAGEMENT: SPRAINS AND STRAINS

◆ Nursing Implementation

◆ **Health Promotion.** Warming up muscles before exercising and vigorous activity, followed by stretching, may significantly reduce the risk for sprains and strains. Strength, balance, and endurance exercises are important. Strengthening exercises that involve working against resistance build muscle strength and bone density. Balance exercises, which may overlap with some strengthening exercises, help prevent falls. Endurance exercises should start at a low level of effort and progress gradually to a moderate level.

PROMOTING POPULATION HEALTH

Health Impact of Regular Physical Activity

- Helps with weight management.
- Increases lean muscle and decreases body fat.
- Helps maintain and improve bone mass.
- Increases muscle strength, flexibility, and endurance.
- Helps prevent high BP.
- Reduces the risk for heart disease, diabetes, and colon cancer.
- Enhances sense of well-being and reduces risk for depression.

◆ **Acute Care.** If an injury occurs, immediate care focuses on (1) stopping the activity and limiting movement to the injured part, (2) applying ice packs to the injured area, (3) compressing the involved area, (4) elevating the extremity, and (5) providing analgesia as needed (Table 62.3). Most sprains and strains are treated in the outpatient setting.

RICE (Rest, Ice, Compression, Elevation) may decrease local inflammation and pain for most musculoskeletal injuries. Movement should be restricted, and the extremity rested as soon as pain is felt. Unless the injury is severe, prolonged rest is usually not needed.

There are several forms of cold therapy *(cryotherapy)* we can use. Cold causes vasoconstriction in the soft tissue and reduces the transmission and perception of nerve pain impulses. These changes also reduce muscle spasms, inflammation, and edema. Cold is most useful when applied immediately after an injury has occurred and used for 24 to 28 hours. Apply ice no more than 20 to 30 minutes at a time. Do not apply ice directly to the skin.

Compression helps decrease edema and pain. We often use an elastic compression bandage. It can be wrapped around the injured part. To prevent edema and encourage fluid return, wrap the bandage starting distally (at the point farthest from the trunk of the body) and progress proximally (toward the trunk of the body). The bandage is too tight if there is numbness or tingling below the area of compression or pain or more swelling occurs beyond the edge of the bandage. Leave the bandage in place for 30 minutes, then remove it for 15 minutes. Use of an elastic wrap may provide extra support during training, athletic, and work activities.

Elevate the injured part above heart level, even during sleep, for 24 to 48 hours to help mobilize excess fluid from the area and prevent further edema. Mild analgesics and nonsteroidal antiinflammatory drugs (NSAIDs) may be used to manage patient discomfort.

After the acute phase (usually 24 to 48 hours), apply warm, moist heat to the affected part to reduce swelling and provide comfort. Heat applications should not exceed 20 to 30 minutes, allowing a "cool-down" time between applications. Encourage the patient to use the limb if the joint is protected by a cast, brace, splint, or taping. Joint movement maintains nutrition to the cartilage. Muscle contraction improves circulation and helps

---

✚ TABLE 62.3 Emergency Management

Acute Soft Tissue Injury

Etiology	Assessment Findings	Interventions
• Crush injury • Direct blows • Falls • Motor vehicle crashes • Sports injuries	• Bruising • ↓ Movement with limited function or inability to bear weight (lower extremity) • ↓ Pulse, coolness, capillary refill >2 sec • ↓ Sensation • Edema • Muscle spasms • Pain, tenderness • Pallor • Shortening or rotation of extremity	**Initial** • Ensure airway, breathing, and circulation. • Perform neurovascular assessment of involved limb. • Elevate involved limb. • Apply compression bandage unless dislocation present. • Apply ice packs to affected area. • Immobilize affected extremity in the position found. Do *not* try to realign or reinsert protruding bones. • Anticipate x-rays of injured extremity. • Give analgesia as needed. • Give tetanus prophylaxis if there is an open fracture. • Give antibiotic prophylaxis for open fracture, large tissue defects, or mangled extremity injury. **Ongoing Monitoring** • Monitor for changes in neurovascular condition. • Implement weight-bearing restrictions as ordered for lower extremity involvement. • Anticipate compartment pressure monitoring if neurovascular assessment changes and compartment syndrome suspected.

resolve bruising and swelling. Movement also helps to prevent *contracture* (stiffening) of tendons and ligaments.

Emphasize the importance of strengthening and conditioning exercises to prevent reinjury.[4] The physical therapist may help with pain relief by using ultrasound or other interventions. The therapist may also teach the patient exercises to improve flexibility and strength.

DISLOCATION AND SUBLUXATION

Dislocation is the complete displacement or separation of the articular surfaces of the joint. Subluxation is a partial or incomplete displacement of the joint surface. Symptoms of subluxation are similar to those of a dislocation but are less severe. Multiple structures contribute to the stability of a joint. Injury to, or excessive laxity of, ligaments is a major factor in dislocations or subluxations. Weak or atrophied muscles can cause chronic joint instability. Fibrocartilage structures, such as the labrum around hip and shoulder sockets and the meniscus at the knee, play an important role in joint stability. Even small tears to these structures can result in recurrent, chronic dislocations or subluxations.

Dislocations typically result from forces on the joint that disrupt the surrounding soft tissue support structures. The joints most often dislocated in the upper extremity include the thumb, elbow, and shoulder. The shoulder most often dislocates anteriorly. Posterior shoulder dislocations are rare. They typically only happen after electrocution or seizure. In the lower extremity, the hip is vulnerable to dislocation from severe trauma, often associated with motor vehicle crashes (Fig. 62.1). The knee cap (*patella*) may dislocate because of a sharp, direct blow or after a sudden twisting inward motion while the planted foot is pointed outward.[5]

The most obvious sign of a dislocation is deformity. For example, if the hip dislocates in a posterior (or backward) direction, the affected limb may be shorter and internally rotated. Other manifestations include local pain, tenderness, loss of function of the injured part, and swelling of soft tissues near the joint. Major complications of a dislocated joint are open joint injuries, *intraarticular* fractures (within the joint), *avascular necrosis* (bone cell death from blood supply), and damage to adjacent nerves and blood vessels.

X-rays can determine the extent of displacement. The joint may be aspirated to assess for hemarthrosis or fat cells. Fat cells in the aspirate indicate a probable intraarticular fracture.

❖ Interprofessional and Nursing Care

A dislocation requires prompt attention. It is often considered an orthopedic emergency because it may be associated with significant vascular injury. The longer the joint is dislocated, the greater the risk for avascular necrosis. The femoral head of the hip joint is especially susceptible to avascular necrosis. Compartment syndrome (discussed on p. 1460) may occur after dislocation due to vascular injury and resulting ischemia. Neurovascular assessment is critical (see pp. 1455–1456).

The first goal of management of a dislocation is to realign the dislocated part of the joint to its original anatomic position. Closed reduction (no incision) may be done under local or general anesthesia or IV moderate to deep sedation. Anesthesia is often needed to relax the muscle so that the bones can be manipulated. Sometimes, open reduction (joint visualized through surgical incision) may be needed. After

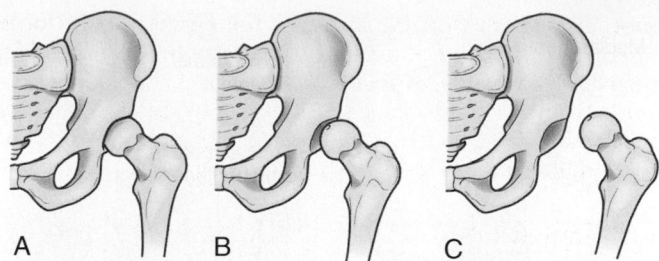

FIG. 62.1 Soft tissue injury of the hip. A, Normal. B, Subluxation (partial dislocation). C, Dislocation.

reduction, the extremity is immobilized by a brace, splint, or sling or by taping to allow torn ligaments and surrounding tissue to heal.

Nursing management is directed toward pain management and support and protection of the injured joint. After the joint has been reduced and immobilized, motion is usually restricted. A carefully monitored rehabilitation program can prevent further instability and joint dysfunction. Gentle range-of-motion (ROM) exercises may be done if the joint is stable and well supported. An exercise program slowly restores the joint to its original ROM without causing another dislocation. The patient should gradually return to normal activities.

A patient who has dislocated a joint may be at greater risk for repeated dislocations because of damage or laxity to the previously mentioned structures. Activity restrictions may be imposed on the affected joint to decrease the risk for repeated dislocations.

REPETITIVE STRAIN INJURY

Repetitive strain injury (RSI) and *cumulative trauma disorder* are terms used to describe injuries resulting from prolonged force or repetitive movements and awkward postures. RSI is also called *repetitive trauma disorder, nontraumatic musculoskeletal injury, overuse syndrome* (sports medicine), *regional musculoskeletal disorder,* and *work-related musculoskeletal disorder.* Repeated movements strain the tendons, ligaments, and muscles, causing tiny tears that become inflamed. The exact cause of these disorders is unknown. No specific diagnostic tests exist, and diagnosis is often difficult.

Persons at risk for RSI include musicians, dancers, butchers, grocery clerks, vibratory tool workers, and those who frequently use a computer mouse and keyboard. Competitive athletes and poorly trained athletes may develop RSI. Swimming, overhead throwing (e.g., baseball), weight lifting, gymnastics, tennis, skiing, and kicking sports (e.g., soccer) require repetitive motion. Overtraining compounds the effects of RSI.

Other factors related to RSI include poor posture and positioning, poor workspace ergonomics, badly designed workplace equipment (e.g., computer keyboard), and repetitive lifting of heavy objects without sufficient muscle rest. Inflammation, swelling, and pain in the muscles, tendons, and nerves of the neck, spine, shoulder, forearm, and hand may result. Symptoms of RSI include pain, weakness, numbness, or impaired motor function.

RSI can be prevented through education and *ergonomics* (the science that promotes efficiency and safety in the interaction of humans and their work environment). For example, ergonomic considerations for those who work at a desk and use a computer

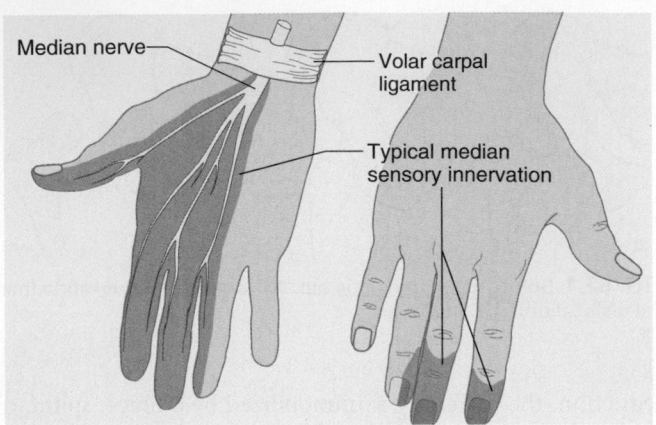

FIG. 62.2 Wrist structures involved in carpal tunnel syndrome. Median nerve distribution. *Shaded areas* show the locations of pain in carpal tunnel syndrome. (From Buttaravoli P: *Minor emergencies,* ed 3, Philadelphia, 2012, Saunders.)

Labels in figure: Median nerve · Volar carpal ligament · Typical median sensory innervation

include keeping the hips and knees flexed to 90 degrees with the feet flat, keeping the wrist straight to type, having the top of the computer monitor even with the forehead, and taking at least hourly stretch breaks.

Once RSI is diagnosed, treatment consists of (1) identifying the precipitating activity; (2) modifying equipment and/or activity; (3) pain management, including heat or cold therapy and NSAIDs; (4) rest; (5) physical therapy (PT) for strengthening and conditioning exercises; and (6) lifestyle changes.

CARPAL TUNNEL SYNDROME

Carpal tunnel syndrome (CTS) is caused by compression of the median nerve, which enters the hand at the wrist through the narrow carpal tunnel (Fig. 62.2). The carpal tunnel is formed by ligaments and bones. CTS is the most common compression neuropathy in the upper extremity. It is associated with hobbies or work that require continuous wrist movement (e.g., musicians, carpenters, computer operators).

CTS is often caused by pressure from trauma or edema (due to inflammation of a tendon [tenosynovitis]), cancer, rheumatoid arthritis (RA), or soft tissue masses, such as ganglia. Hormones may be involved because CTS often occurs during the premenstrual period, pregnancy, and menopause. Persons with diabetes, peripheral vascular disease (PVD), and RA have a higher incidence of CTS because of swelling that changes blood flow to the nerve and narrows the carpal tunnel.[6] Women are more likely than men to develop CTS, possibly because of a smaller carpal tunnel.

Manifestations of CTS are impaired sensation, pain, numbness, or weakness in the distribution of the median nerve (Fig. 62.2). Numbness and tingling may awaken the patient at night. Shaking the hands often relieves these symptoms. Clumsiness in performing fine hand movements is common.

The patient may have a positive Tinel's sign and Phalen's sign. *Tinel's sign* can be elicited by tapping over the median nerve as it passes through the carpal tunnel in the wrist. A positive response is a sensation of tingling in the distribution of the median nerve over the hand. *Phalen's sign* can be elicited by allowing the wrists to fall freely into maximum flexion and maintain the position for longer than 60 seconds. A positive response is a sensation of

tingling in the distribution of the median nerve over the hand. In late stages, atrophy of the muscles around the base of the thumb results in recurrent pain and eventual dysfunction of the hand.

❖ Interprofessional and Nursing Care

To prevent CTS, teach employees and employers to identify risk factors. Adaptive devices, such as wrist splints, may be worn to hold the wrist in a slight extension and relieve pressure on the median nerve. Special keyboard pads and computer mice that help prevent repetitive pressure on the median nerve are available for computer users. Other ergonomic changes include workstation modifications, change in body positions, and frequent breaks from work-related activities.

Care of the patient with CTS is directed toward relieving the underlying cause of the nerve compression. Early symptoms of CTS can usually be relieved by stopping the aggravating movement and by resting the hand and wrist by immobilization in a hand splint. Splints worn at night help keep the wrist in a neutral position and may reduce night pain and numbness. PT with hand and wrist exercises may lessen symptom severity. A corticosteroid injection directly into the carpal tunnel may give short-term relief. The patient may need to consider a change in occupation because of discomfort and sensory changes.

Carpal tunnel release is generally done if symptoms last more than 6 months or if there is significant impairment to conduction on electromyography (EMG). Surgery involves severing the band of tissue around the wrist to reduce pressure on the median nerve (Fig. 62.2). Surgery is done in the outpatient setting using local anesthesia. The types of carpal tunnel release surgery include open release and endoscopic surgery. In *open release surgery*, an incision is made in the wrist and then the carpal ligament is cut to enlarge the carpal tunnel. *Endoscopic carpal tunnel release* is performed through 1 or more small puncture incisions in the wrist and palm. A camera is attached to a tube, and the carpal ligament is cut. The endoscopic approach may allow a faster recovery and cause less discomfort than traditional open release surgery.

Although symptoms may be relieved right after surgery, full recovery may take months. After surgery, assess the hand's neurovascular status. Teach the patient about wound care and assessments to perform at home.

ROTATOR CUFF INJURY

The rotator cuff is made up of 4 muscles in the shoulder: the supraspinatus, infraspinatus, teres minor, and subscapularis muscles. These muscles stabilize the humeral head in the glenoid fossa while assisting with ROM of the shoulder joint and rotation of the humerus.

A tear in the rotator cuff may occur as a gradual, degenerative process due to aging, repetitive stress (especially overhead arm motions), or injury to the shoulder. In sports, repetitive overhead motions, such as in swimming, weight lifting, and swinging a racquet (tennis, racquetball), often cause injury. The rotator cuff can tear because of sudden adduction forces applied to the cuff while the arm is held in abduction. Other causes include (1) falling onto an outstretched arm and hand, (2) a blow to the upper arm, (3) heavy lifting, or (4) repetitive work motions.

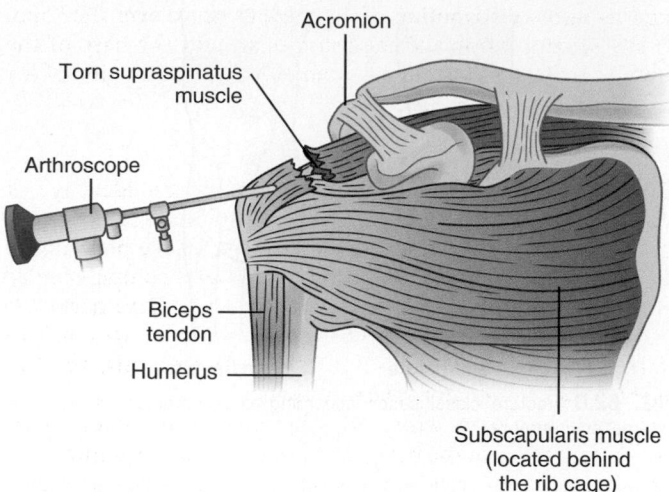

FIG. 62.3 A torn rotator cuff is repaired using arthroscopic surgery.

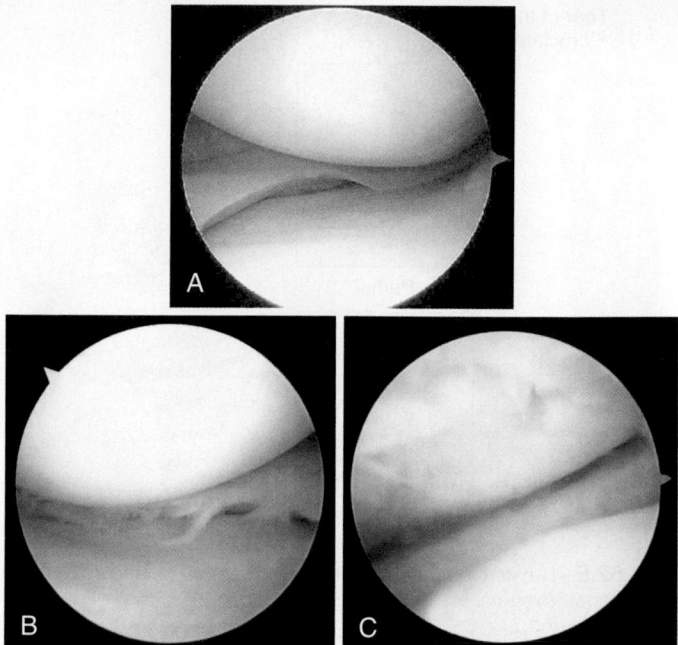

FIG. 62.4 Arthroscopic views of the meniscus. A, Normal meniscus. B, Torn meniscus. C, Surgically repaired meniscus. (A, From David Lintner, MD, Houston, TX, *www.drlintner.com.* B and C, Courtesy Peter Bonner, Placitas, NM.)

Manifestations include shoulder weakness, pain, and decreased ROM. The patient usually has severe pain when the arm is abducted between 60 and 120 degrees (the painful arc). A positive *drop arm test* is a sign of rotator cuff injury. In this test, the arm is abducted 90 degrees, and the patient is asked to slowly lower the arm to the side. If the arm falls suddenly, rotator cuff injury is suspected. An x-ray alone is not helpful in the diagnosis. A tear can usually be confirmed by MRI.

The patient with a partial tear or cuff inflammation may be treated conservatively with rest, ice and heat, NSAIDs, corticosteroid injections into the subacromial space, ultrasound, and PT. If the patient does not respond to conservative treatment or if a complete tear is present, surgical repair may be needed. Most surgical repairs are done as outpatient procedures through an arthroscope (Fig. 62.3). If the tear is extensive, part of the acromion may be surgically removed *(acromioplasty)* to relieve compression of the rotator cuff during movement. A shoulder immobilizer with an abduction pillow is typically used for 6 weeks after surgery to limit shoulder movement. However, the shoulder should not be immobilized for too long because "frozen" shoulder *(arthrofibrosis)* may occur. Pendulum exercises and other passive exercises typically begin the first postoperative day. Active PT starts after 6 weeks of immobilization. Weight restrictions for lifting are usually given. Full recovery may take 6 to 12 months.

MENISCUS INJURY

The menisci are crescent-shaped pieces of fibrocartilage in the knee. Menisci are also found in other joints, including the acromioclavicular (AC), sternoclavicular, and temporomandibular joints. Meniscus injuries are associated with ligament sprains common among athletes in sports such as basketball, football, soccer, and hockey.[7] These activities produce rotational stress when the knee is in varying degrees of flexion and the foot is planted or fixed. A blow to the knee can cause shearing of the meniscus between the femoral condyles and tibial plateau, causing a torn meniscus. Older adults and people who have jobs that require squatting or kneeling are at risk for degenerative tears.[7]

Meniscus injuries alone do not usually cause significant edema because most cartilage is avascular. However, an acutely torn meniscus may present with localized tenderness, pain, and effusion (Fig. 62.4). Pain occurs with flexion, internal rotation, and then extension of the knee *(McMurray's test).* The patient may feel that the knee is unstable and often reports that the knee "clicks," "pops," "locks," or "gives way." Quadriceps atrophy is usually present if the injury has been present for some time. Traumatic arthritis may occur from repeated meniscus injury and chronic inflammation.

MRI can confirm the diagnosis before arthroscopy. The patient's age, occupation, sport activities, degree of knee pain, and dysfunction may affect the decision whether to have surgery.

❖ Interprofessional and Nursing Care

Most meniscus injuries are treated in an outpatient setting. The acutely injured knee should be examined within 24 hours of injury. Initial care involves ice application, immobilization, and use of crutches with weight bearing as tolerated. Using a knee brace or immobilizer during the first few days after the injury protects the knee and offers some pain relief.

After acute pain has decreased, PT can help the patient regain knee flexion and muscle strength to aid in returning to full function. Teach athletes to do warm-up exercises to reduce the risk for sports-related injuries. In older adults with degenerative meniscus tears, progressive exercise therapy may improve neuromuscular function and muscle strength.[8]

Surgical repair or excision of part of the meniscus *(meniscectomy)* may be needed (Fig. 62.4). Meniscal surgery is done by arthroscopy. Pain relief may include NSAIDs or other analgesics. Rehabilitation starts soon after surgery, including quadriceps and hamstring strengthening exercises and ROM. When the patient's strength is back to its preinjury level, normal activities may be resumed.

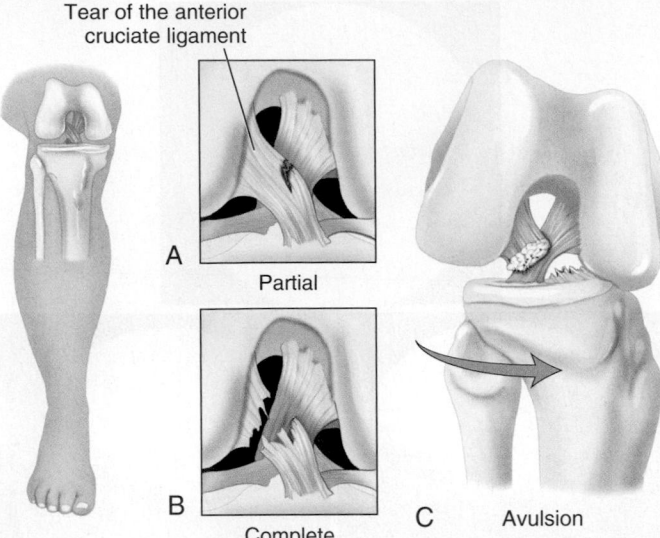

FIG. 62.5 Anterior cruciate ligament (ACL) injury. **A**, Partial tear. **B**, Complete tear. **C**, Avulsion.

ANTERIOR CRUCIATE LIGAMENT INJURY

Knee injuries account for more than 50% of all sports injuries. The most commonly injured knee ligament is the anterior cruciate ligament (ACL). ACL injuries are usually noncontact injuries that occur when the athlete pivots, lands from a jump, or stops abruptly when running. Patients often report coming down on the knee, twisting, and hearing a pop, followed by acute knee pain and swelling. The knee may feel unstable. Athletes usually cannot continue playing. Injury to the ACL can result in a partial tear, a complete tear, or an *avulsion* (tearing away) from the bones that form the knee (Fig. 62.5).

A positive *Lachman's test* suggests an ACL tear. This test is done by flexing the knee 15 to 30 degrees and pulling the tibia forward while the femur is stabilized. The test is considered positive for an ACL tear if forward motion of the tibia occurs with the feeling of a soft or indistinct endpoint. MRI is often used to diagnose an ACL tear and coexisting conditions, including a fracture, meniscus tearing, and collateral ligament injuries.

❖ Interprofessional and Nursing Care

Prevention programs can significantly reduce ACL injuries in athletes. Conservative treatment for an intact ACL injury includes rest, ice, NSAIDs, elevation, and ambulation as tolerated with crutches. If present, a tight, painful effusion may be aspirated. A knee immobilizer or hinged knee brace may provide support. PT often helps the patient maintain knee joint motion and muscle tone.

Reconstructive surgery is usually recommended for physically active patients who have sustained severe injury to the ACL and meniscus. In reconstruction, the torn ACL tissue is removed and replaced with graft tissue. ROM is encouraged soon after surgery. The knee is placed in a brace or immobilizer. Rehabilitation with PT is critical, with progressive weight bearing determined by the degree of surgical repair. A safe return to the patient's prior level of physical functioning may take 6 to 8 months.

BURSITIS

Bursae are closed sacs that are lined with synovial membrane and contain a small amount of synovial fluid. They are found at

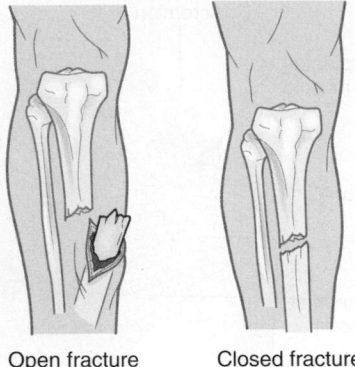

FIG. 62.6 Fracture classification according to communication with the external environment.

sites of friction, such as between tendons and bones and near the joints. **Bursitis** (inflammation of the bursa) results from repeated or excessive trauma or friction, gout, RA, or infection.

Symptoms of bursitis include warmth, pain, swelling, and limited ROM in the affected part. Common sites are the hands, elbows, shoulders, knees, and greater trochanters of the hip. Improper body mechanics, repetitive kneeling (carpet layers, coal miners, and gardeners), jogging in worn-out shoes, and prolonged sitting with crossed legs are common precipitating activities.

Try to determine and correct the cause of the bursitis. Rest is often the only treatment needed. The affected part may be immobilized in a compression dressing or splint. Ice and NSAIDs can reduce pain and inflammation.[9] Aspiration of the bursal fluid and intraarticular corticosteroid injection may be needed. If the bursal wall has become thickened and continues to interfere with normal joint function, surgical excision *(bursectomy)* may be done. Septic bursae may be treated with oral antibiotics, but usually need surgical incision and drainage.

FRACTURES

Classification

A **fracture** is a disruption or break in the continuity of bone. Although traumatic injuries cause most fractures, some fractures are due to a disease process, such as cancer or osteoporosis *(pathologic fracture)*.

We classify fractures in several ways. Fractures are described as *open* or *closed* based on communication with the external environment (Fig. 62.6). In an *open fracture*, the skin is broken and bone exposed, causing soft tissue injury. In a *closed fracture*, the skin is intact over the site.

We also describe fractures as complete or incomplete. A fracture is *complete* if the break goes completely through the bone. An *incomplete* fracture occurs partly across a bone shaft, but the bone is still intact. An incomplete fracture is often the result of bending or crushing forces applied to a bone.

Fractures are identified according to the direction of the fracture line. Types include linear, oblique, transverse, longitudinal, and spiral fractures (Fig. 62.7).

Finally, fractures can be classified as displaced or nondisplaced. In a *displaced* fracture, the 2 ends of the broken bone are separated from each other and out of their normal positions. Displaced fractures are often *comminuted* (more than 2

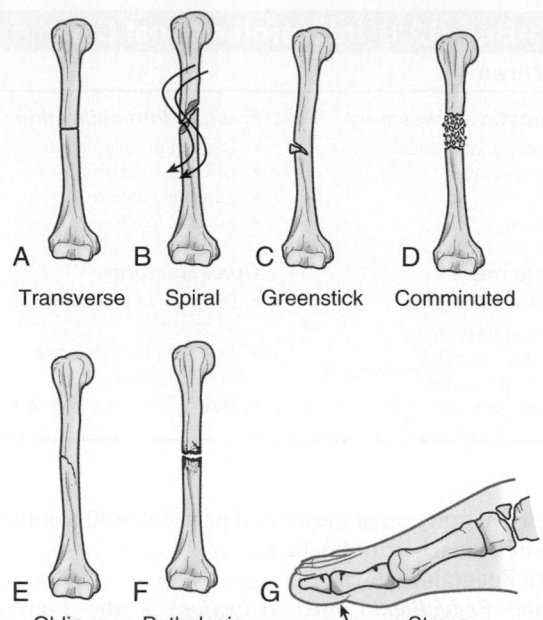

FIG. 62.7 Types of fractures. **A,** Transverse fracture: the line of the fracture extends across the bone shaft at a right angle to the longitudinal axis. **B,** Spiral fracture: the line of the fracture extends in a spiral direction along the bone shaft. **C,** Greenstick fracture: an incomplete fracture with 1 side splintered and the other side bent. **D,** Comminuted fracture: a fracture with more than 2 fragments. The smaller fragments appear to be floating. **E,** Oblique fracture: the line of the fracture extends across and down the bone. **F,** Pathologic fracture: a spontaneous fracture at the site of a diseased bone. **G,** Stress fracture: occurs in normal or abnormal bone that is subject to repeated stress, such as from jogging or running.

fragments) or *oblique* (Fig. 62.7). In a *nondisplaced* fracture, the bone fragments stay in alignment. Nondisplaced fractures are usually transverse, spiral, or greenstick (Fig. 62.7).

Manifestations

Manifestations include immediate localized pain, decreased function, and inability to bear weight or use the affected part (Table 62.4). The patient guards and protects the extremity against movement. Obvious bone deformity may be present.

Fracture Healing

Knowledge of the stages of fracture healing (Fig. 62.8) is needed to provide appropriate interventions. Bone goes through a complex multistage healing process *(union)* that occurs in 6 stages:

1. *Fracture hematoma:* When a fracture occurs, bleeding creates a hematoma that surrounds the ends of the bone fragments. The hematoma is composed of extravasated blood that changes from a liquid to a semisolid clot in the first 72 hours after injury.[10]
2. *Granulation tissue:* During this stage, active phagocytosis absorbs the products of local necrosis. The hematoma converts to granulation tissue. Granulation tissue (consisting of new blood vessels, fibroblasts, and osteoblasts) forms the basis for new bone substance *(osteoid)* during days 3 to 14 after injury.
3. *Callus formation:* As minerals (calcium, phosphorus, and magnesium) and new bone matrix are deposited in the osteoid, an unorganized network of bone is formed and woven about the fracture parts. *Callus* is primarily composed of

TABLE 62.4 Manifestations of Fracture

Manifestation	Significance
Bruising Discoloration of skin from extravasation of blood in subcutaneous tissues.	May appear immediately after injury and distal to injury. Reassure patient that process is normal, and discoloration will resolve.
Crepitation Grating or crunching of bony fragments, producing palpable or audible crunching or popping sensation.	May ↑ chance for nonunion if bone ends are allowed to move excessively. Micromovement of fragments (postfracture) helps in osteogenesis (new bone growth).
Deformity Abnormal position of extremity or part from original forces of injury and action of muscles pulling fragment into abnormal position. Seen as a loss of normal bony contours.	Classic sign of fracture. If uncorrected, it may cause problems with bony union and restoration of function of injured part.
Edema and Swelling Disruption or penetration of skin or soft tissues by bone fragments, or bleeding into surrounding tissues.	Unchecked bleeding and swelling in closed space can occlude blood vessels and damage nerves (e.g., ↑ risk for compartment syndrome).
Loss of Function Disruption of bone or joint, preventing functional use of limb or part.	Fracture must be managed properly to ensure restoration of function to limb or part.
Muscle Spasm Irritation of tissues and protective response to injury and fracture.	May displace nondisplaced fracture or prevent it from reducing spontaneously.
Pain and Tenderness Muscle spasm due to involuntary reflex action of muscle, direct tissue trauma, ↑ pressure on nerves, movement of fracture fragments.	Prompt the patient to splint muscle around fracture and reduce motion of injured area.

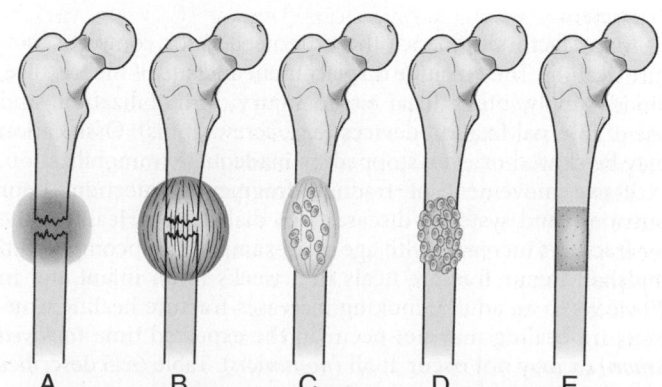

FIG. 62.8 Bone healing (schematic representation). **A,** Bleeding at fractured ends of the bone with hematoma formation. **B,** Organization of hematoma into fibrous network. **C,** Invasion of osteoblasts, lengthening of collagen strands, and deposition of calcium. **D,** Callus formation: new bone is built up as osteoclasts destroy dead bone. **E,** Remodeling is accomplished as excess callus is resorbed and trabecular bone is laid down.

TABLE 62.5 Complications of Fracture Healing

Complication	Description
Angulation	Fracture heals in abnormal position in relation to midline of structure (type of malunion).
Delayed union	Fracture healing progresses more slowly than expected. Healing eventually occurs.
Malunion	Fracture heals in expected time but in unsatisfactory position. May cause deformity or dysfunction.
Myositis ossificans	Deposition of calcium in muscle tissue at site of significant blunt muscle trauma or repeated muscle injury.
Nonunion	Fracture does not heal despite treatment. No x-ray evidence of callus formation.
Pseudoarthrosis	Type of nonunion occurring at fracture site in which a false joint is formed with abnormal movement at site.
Refracture	New fracture occurs at original fracture site.

TABLE 62.6 Interprofessional Care

Fractures

Diagnostic Assessment
- History and physical examination
- X-ray
- CT scan, MRI

Management
Fracture Reduction
- Manual traction
- Closed reduction
- Skeletal traction
- Open reduction

Fracture Immobilization
- Casting or splinting
- Skeletal traction
- External fixation
- Internal fixation

Open Fractures
- Surgical debridement and irrigation
- Tetanus and diphtheria immunization
- Prophylactic antibiotic therapy

cartilage, osteoblasts, calcium, and phosphorus. It usually appears by the end of the second week after injury. An x-ray can show evidence of callus formation.

4. *Ossification:* Ossification of the callus occurs from 3 weeks to 6 months after the fracture and continues until the fracture has healed. Callus ossification is sufficient to prevent movement at the fracture site when the bones are gently stressed. However, the fracture is still evident on x-ray. During this stage of *clinical union,* the patient may be allowed limited mobility, or the cast may be removed.

5. *Consolidation:* As callus continues to develop, the distance between bone fragments decreases and eventually closes. Ossification continues and can be equated with *radiologic union,* which occurs when an x-ray shows complete bony union. This phase can occur up to 1 year after injury.

6. *Remodeling:* Excess bone tissue is resorbed in the last stage of bone healing, and union is complete. Gradual return of the injured bone to its preinjury structural strength and shape occurs. Bone remodels in response to physical loading stress (Wolff's law). Initially, stress is provided through exercise. Weight bearing is gradually introduced. New bone is deposited in sites subjected to stress and resorbed at areas of little stress.

Many factors influence the time needed for complete fracture healing. They include displacement and site of the fracture, blood supply, other local tissue injury, immobilization, and use of internal fixation devices (e.g., screws, pins). Ossification may be slowed or even stopped by inadequate immobilization, excessive movement of fracture fragments, infection, poor nutrition, and systemic disease (e.g., diabetes).[11] Healing time for fractures increases with age. For example, an uncomplicated midshaft femur fracture heals in 3 weeks in an infant and in 20 weeks in an adult. Smoking increases fracture healing time. Fracture healing may not occur in the expected time *(delayed union)* or may not occur at all *(nonunion).* Table 62.5 describes complications of fracture healing.

Interprofessional Care

The overall goals of fracture treatment are (1) anatomic realignment of bone fragments through reduction, (2) immobilization to maintain realignment, and (3) restoration of normal or near-normal function of the injured part. Table 62.6 outlines the interprofessional care of fractures.

Fracture Reduction

Closed Reduction. Closed reduction is the nonsurgical, manual realignment of bone fragments to their anatomic position. Traction and countertraction are manually applied to the bone fragments to restore position, length, and alignment. Closed reduction is usually done while the patient is under local or general anesthesia. Traction, casting, splints, or orthoses (braces) may be used after reduction to maintain alignment and immobilize the injured part until healing occurs.

Open Reduction. Open reduction is the correction of bone alignment through a surgical incision. It usually includes internal fixation of the fracture with wires, screws, pins, plates, intramedullary rods, or nails. The type and location of the fracture, patient age, and concurrent disease influence the decision to use open reduction. The main risks of open reduction are infection, complications associated with anesthesia, and effects of preexisting medical conditions (e.g., diabetes). However, open reduction internal fixation (ORIF) facilitates early ambulation, thus decreasing the risk for complications related to prolonged immobility.

Traction. Traction is the application of a pulling force to an injured or diseased body part or extremity. Traction is used to (1) prevent or reduce pain and muscle spasm (e.g., whiplash, unrepaired hip fracture), (2) immobilize a joint or part of the body, (3) reduce a fracture or dislocation, and (4) treat a pathologic joint condition (e.g., tumor, infection). Traction is also used to (1) provide immobilization to prevent soft tissue damage, (2) promote active and passive exercise, (3) expand a joint space during arthroscopic procedures, and (4) expand a joint space before major joint reconstruction.

Traction devices apply a pulling force on a fractured extremity to attain realignment while *countertraction* pulls in the opposite direction. The most common types of traction are skin traction and skeletal traction. *Skin traction* is generally used for short-term treatment (48 to 72 hours) until skeletal traction or surgery is possible. Tape, boots, or splints are applied directly to the skin, mainly to help decrease muscle spasms in the injured extremity. Traction weights are usually 5 to 10 lb (2.3 to 4.5 kg). *Buck's traction* is a type of skin traction sometimes used for the patient with a hip, knee, or femur fracture (Fig. 62.9).[12] Pelvic or cervical skin traction may require heavier weights applied intermittently. In skin traction, regular assessment of the skin is a priority because pressure points

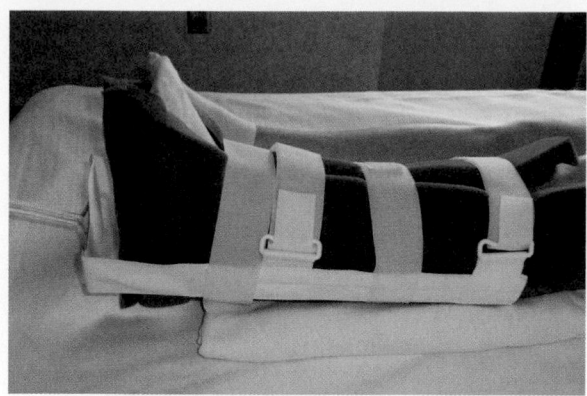

FIG. 62.9 Buck's traction is most often used for fractures of the hip and femur. (Courtesy Mary Wollan, RN, BAN, ONC, Spring Park, MN.)

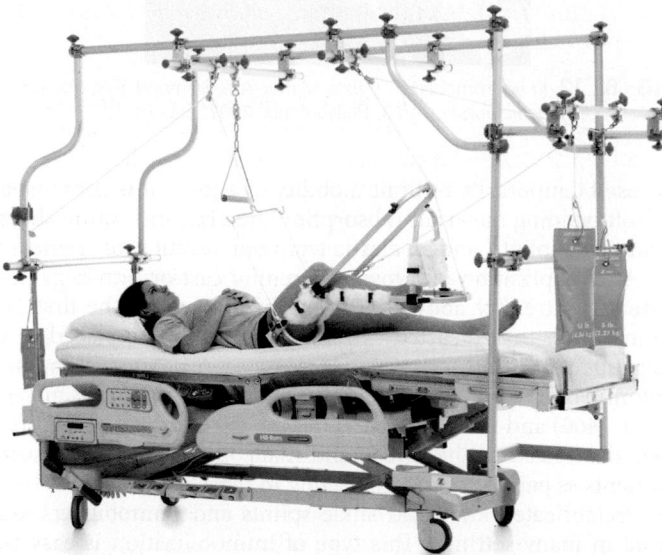

FIG. 62.10 Balanced suspension skeletal traction. Most often used for fractures of the femur, hip, and lower leg. (Courtesy Zimmer, Inc.)

and skin breakdown may develop quickly. Assess key pressure points every 2 to 4 hours.

Skeletal traction is used to align injured bones and joints or to treat joint contractures and congenital hip dysplasia. It provides a long-term pull that keeps the injured bones and joints aligned. To apply skeletal traction, the HCP inserts a pin or wire into the bone, and weights are attached to align and immobilize the injured body part. Weight for skeletal traction ranges from 5 to 45 lb (2.3 to 20.4 kg). The use of too much weight can result in delayed union or nonunion. The major complications of skeletal traction are infection at the pin insertion site and the effects of prolonged immobility.

A common type of skeletal traction is balanced suspension traction (Fig. 62.10). Fracture alignment depends on the correct positioning and alignment of the patient while the traction forces stay constant. For extremity traction to be effective, forces also must be pulling in the opposite direction *(countertraction)*. Countertraction is supplied by the patient's body weight or by weights pulling in the opposite direction. Elevating the end of the bed can help. Traction must be maintained continuously. Keep the weights off the floor and moving freely through the pulleys.

Fracture Immobilization. Fracture immobilization is achieved with casts, braces, splints, immobilizers, and external and internal fixation devices.

Casts. A *cast* is a temporary immobilization device often applied after closed reduction. It allows the patient to perform many normal ADLs while providing enough immobilization to ensure stability. A cast generally immobilizes the joints above and below a fracture. This restricts tendon and ligament movement, thus assisting with joint stabilization while the fracture heals. The 2 most common cast materials are natural (plaster of Paris) and fiberglass. We use fiberglass casts most often because they are lighter, relatively waterproof, and longer wearing than plaster of Paris.[13] They also allow early weight bearing. Plaster of Paris is now used primarily for contact casting in the treatment of diabetic foot ulcers.[14]

To apply a cast on an extremity, first cover the affected part with stockinette that is cut longer than the extremity. Then place cotton padding over the stockinette, with extra padding for bony prominences. If using plaster of Paris, immerse it in warm water and then wrap and mold it around the affected part. The number of layers of plaster bandage and the technique of application determine the strength of the cast. The plaster sets within 15 minutes, so the patient may move around without difficulty. However, it is not strong enough for weight bearing until about 36 to 72 hours after application.[13] The decision about the patient's weight bearing is made by the HCP. Casts made of fiberglass or other synthetic materials (thermolabile plastic, thermoplastic resins, polyurethane) are activated by submersion in cool or tepid water. Then they are molded to fit the torso or extremity.

Leave a fresh plaster cast uncovered to allow air circulation. Covering the cast allows heat to build up in the cast. This may cause a burn and delay drying. Avoid direct pressure on the cast during the drying period. Handle the cast gently with an open palm to avoid denting the cast. Once the cast is thoroughly dry, the rough edges may be *petaled* to minimize skin irritation. Petaling also prevents plaster of Paris debris from falling into the cast and causing irritation or pressure necrosis. Place several strips (petals) of tape over the rough areas to ensure a smooth cast edge.

Upper extremity injuries. An acute fracture or soft tissue injury of the upper extremity can be immobilized by using a (1) sugar-tong splint, (2) posterior splint, (3) short arm cast, or (4) long arm cast (Fig. 62.11). The *sugar-tong splint* is applied for acute wrist injuries or injuries that may result in significant swelling. Splints are placed over a well-padded forearm, beginning at the phalangeal joints of the hand, extending up the dorsal aspect of the forearm around the distal humerus, and then down the volar aspect of the forearm to the distal palmar crease. The splinting material is wrapped with either elastic bandage or bias stockinette. The sugar-tong posterior splint accommodates early swelling in the fractured extremity.

The *short arm cast* is often used for the treatment of stable wrist or metacarpal fractures. An aluminum finger splint can be built into the short arm cast for treatment of phalangeal injuries. The short arm cast is a circular cast extending from the distal palmar crease to the proximal forearm. This cast immobilizes the wrist and allows unrestricted elbow motion.

The *long arm cast* is often used for stable forearm or elbow fractures and unstable wrist fractures. It is similar to the short arm cast but extends to the proximal humerus, restricting motion at the wrist and elbow. Support the extremity and

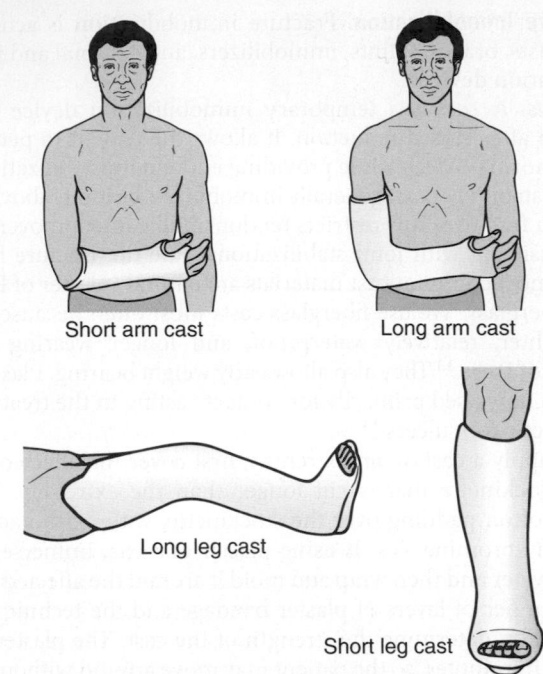

Short arm cast

Long arm cast

Long leg cast

Short leg cast

FIG. 62.11 Common types of casts.

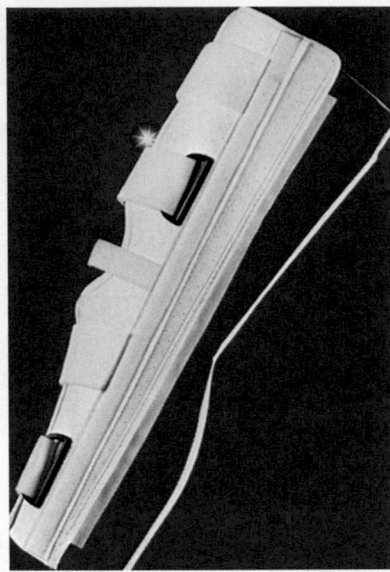

FIG. 62.12 Knee immobilizer. (From Maher AB, Salmond SW, Pellino T, editors: *Orthopedic nursing*, ed 3, Philadelphia, 2002, Saunders.)

reduce edema by elevating the extremity with a sling. However, when a hanging arm cast is used for a proximal humerus fracture, avoid elevation or use of a supportive sling. The hanging provides traction and maintains fracture alignment.

When a sling is used, ensure the axillary area is well padded to prevent skin breakdown from direct skin-to-skin contact. Apply the sling carefully to avoid putting undue pressure on the neck. Encourage movement of the fingers (unless contraindicated) to decrease edema by enhancing the pumping action of blood vessels. Teach the patient to actively move joints of the upper extremity if not immobilized to prevent stiffness and contractures.

Vertebral injuries. The *body jacket brace* is used for immobilization and support for stable spine injuries of the thoracic or lumbar spine. The brace goes around the chest and abdomen, extending from above the nipple line to the pubis. After application of the brace, assess the patient for the development of superior mesenteric artery syndrome *(cast syndrome)*. This condition occurs if the brace is too tight, compressing the superior mesenteric artery against the duodenum. The patient generally has abdominal pain, abdominal pressure, nausea, and vomiting. Assess the abdomen for decreased bowel sounds (there may be a window in the brace over the umbilicus). Treatment of cast syndrome includes gastric decompression with a nasogastric (NG) tube and suction. Assess respiratory status, bowel and bladder function, and areas of pressure over the bony prominences, especially the iliac crest. The brace may have to be adjusted or removed if any complications occur.

Lower extremity injuries. Injuries to the lower extremity can be immobilized with a long leg cast, short leg cast, cylinder cast, or prefabricated splint or immobilizer. The usual indications for a long leg cast are an unstable ankle fracture, soft tissue injuries, a fractured tibia, and knee injuries. The cast usually extends from the base of the toes to the groin and gluteal crease. The short leg cast is used for stable ankle and foot injuries. A cylinder cast is used for knee injuries or fractures. It extends from the groin to the malleoli of the ankle. A Robert Jones dressing may

be used temporarily to limit mobility of a joint. It is composed of soft padding materials (absorption dressing and cotton sheet wadding), splints, and an elastic wrap or bias-cut stockinette.

After application of a lower extremity cast or dressing, elevate the extremity above the heart on pillows for the first 24 hours. After that, a casted extremity should not be placed in a dependent position as this may increase edema. After cast application, observe for signs of compartment syndrome (discussed on p. 1460) and increased pressure, especially in the heel, anterior tibia, head of the fibula, and malleoli. Increased pressure presents as pain or a burning feeling in these areas.

Prefabricated knee and ankle splints and immobilizers are used in many settings. This type of immobilization is easy to apply and remove, which allows close observation of the affected joint for swelling and skin breakdown (Fig. 62.12). Depending on the injury, removal of the splint or immobilizer promotes ROM of the affected joint and faster return to function.

The *hip spica cast* is mainly used for femur fractures in children to immobilize the affected extremity and trunk. It extends from above the nipple line to the base of the foot (single spica) and may include the opposite extremity up to an area above the knee (spica and a half) or both extremities (double spica). Assess the patient with a hip spica cast for the same problems associated with the body jacket brace.

External Fixation. An *external fixator* is composed of metal pins and wires that are inserted into the bone and attached to external rods to stabilize the fracture while it heals (Fig. 62.13). It can be used to apply traction or to compress fracture fragments and immobilize reduced fragments when the use of a cast or traction is not appropriate. The external device holds fracture fragments in place similar to a surgically implanted internal device. External fixation is used mainly for complex fractures with extensive soft tissue damage, correction of congenital bony defects, nonunion or malunion, and limb lengthening.

External fixation is often used to try to salvage extremities that otherwise may require amputation. Because the use of an external device is a long-term process, ongoing assessment for pin loosening and infection is critical. Infection may require removal of the device. Teach the patient and caregiver about

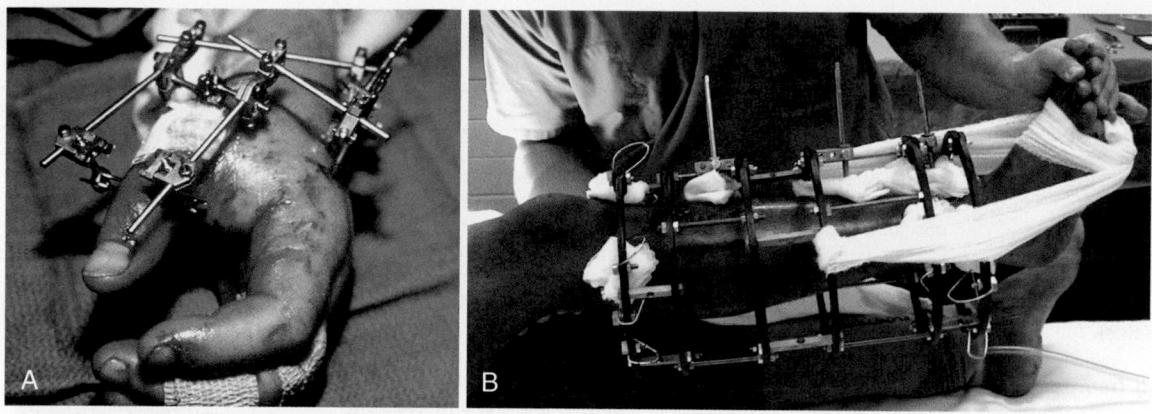

FIG. 62.13 External fixators. **A,** Stabilization of hand injury. **B,** Stabilization of a tibial fracture. (*A,* Courtesy Howmedica, Inc, Allendale, PA. *B,* From Canale ST, Beaty JH: *Campbell's operative orthopedics,* ed 12, Philadelphia, 2013, Mosby.)

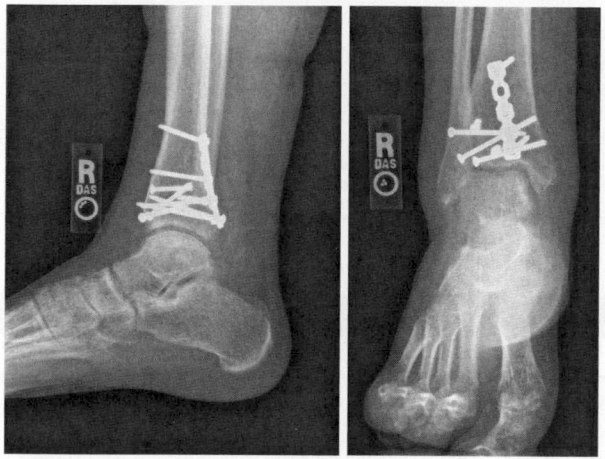

FIG. 62.14 Views of internal fixation devices to stabilize a fractured tibia and fibula. (From Jeremy Lewis, MD, Albuquerque, NM.)

meticulous pin care. Although each HCP has a protocol for pin care cleaning, chlorhexidine is often used.[15]

Internal Fixation. Internal fixation devices (pins, plates, intramedullary rods, metal and bioabsorbable screws) are surgically inserted to realign and maintain position of bony fragments (Fig. 62.14). These metal devices are biologically inert and made from stainless steel, vitallium, or titanium. Proper alignment and bone healing are evaluated regularly by x-rays.

Electrical Bone Growth Stimulation. Electrical bone growth stimulation can promote healing, especially with fracture nonunion or delayed union. The mechanism of action may include (1) increasing calcium uptake and the production of bone growth factors, (2) increasing collagen synthesis, and (3) promoting the growth of new blood vessels.[16]

There are noninvasive, semi-invasive, and invasive methods of electrical bone growth stimulation. Noninvasive stimulators use direct current or pulsed electromagnetic fields (PEMFs) to generate a weak electrical current. Electrodes are typically in a band applied over the patient's skin or cast and worn 10 to 12 hours each day, usually while the patient is sleeping. Semi-invasive or percutaneous bone growth stimulators use an external power supply and electrodes that are inserted through the skin and into the bone. Invasive stimulators require surgical implantation of a current generator in an IM or subcutaneous space. An electrode is implanted in the bone fragments.

Drug Therapy. Patients with fractures have varying degrees of pain associated with muscle spasms. Central and peripheral muscle relaxants, such as carisoprodol (Soma), cyclobenzaprine, or methocarbamol (Robaxin), may be given to manage pain associated with muscle spasms.

Give tetanus and diphtheria toxoid or tetanus immunoglobulin to the patient with an open fracture who has not been previously immunized or whose immunization is expired (see Table 68.6). Bone-penetrating antibiotics, such as a cephalosporin (e.g., cefazolin), are used prophylactically before surgery.

Nutritional Therapy. Proper nutrition is essential to ensure optimal soft tissue and bone healing. An adequate energy source is needed to promote muscle strength and tone, build endurance, and provide energy for ambulation and gait-training skills. The patient's dietary requirements must include adequate protein (e.g., 1 g/kg of body weight), vitamins (especially B, C, and D), calcium, phosphorus, and magnesium. Low serum protein and vitamin C deficiencies interfere with tissue healing. Immobility and bone healing increase calcium needs.

A fluid intake of 2000 to 3000 mL/day promotes optimal bladder and bowel function. Adequate fluid and a high-fiber diet with fruits and vegetables prevent constipation. If immobilized in bed with skeletal traction or in a body jacket brace, the patient should eat 6 small meals. This helps avoid overeating that can cause abdominal pressure and cramping.

❖ NURSING MANAGEMENT: FRACTURES

◆ Nursing Assessment

A brief history of the traumatic episode, mechanism of injury, and position in which the patient was found can be obtained from the patient or witnesses. As soon as possible, the patient should be transported to an ED, where thorough assessment can be done and treatment started (Table 62.7). Subjective and objective data that should be obtained from a person with a fracture are outlined in Table 62.8.

If a fracture is suspected, the extremity is immobilized in the position in which it is found. Unnecessary movement increases risk for damage to adjacent nerves and blood vessels. It may also convert a closed fracture to an open fracture.

◆ Neurovascular Assessment. A thorough neurovascular assessment of the affected extremity, distal to the fracture site, is a primary concern. Musculoskeletal injuries may cause changes in the neurovascular status of an injured extremity. Poor

✚ TABLE 62.7 Emergency Management

Fractured Extremity

Etiology	Assessment Findings	Interventions
Blunt Trauma • Direct blow • Fall • Forced flexion or hyper-extension • Motor vehicle crash • Pedestrian event • Twisting force **Penetrating Trauma** • Blast • Gunshot **Other** • Pathologic condition • Violent muscle contraction (seizures) • Crush injury	• Bruising • ↓ Distal pulses • Deformity or unnatural position of affected limb • Edema • Grating (crepitus) • Loss of function • Muscle spasm • Numbness, tingling • Tenderness, pain • Warmth at site • Wound over injured site, exposure of bone	**Initial** • Treat life-threatening injuries first. • If unresponsive, assess circulation, airway, and breathing. • If responsive, monitor airway, breathing, and circulation. • Control external bleeding with direct pressure or sterile pressure dressing and elevation of the extremity. • Assess neurovascular condition distal to injury before and after splinting. • Elevate injured limb if possible. • Do not try to straighten fractured or dislocated joints. • Do not manipulate protruding bone ends. • Apply ice packs to affected area. • Obtain x-rays of affected limb. • Give tetanus prophylaxis if there is a break in skin integrity. • Mark location of pulses to aid repeat assessment. • Splint fracture site, including joints above and below fracture site. **Ongoing Monitoring** • Assess vital signs, level of consciousness, O$_2$ saturation, neurovascular condition, pain. • Assess for compartment syndrome (excessive pain, pain with passive stretch of the affected extremity muscles, pallor, paresthesia, with late signs of paralysis and pulselessness). • Assess for FES (dyspnea, chest pain, temperature elevation).

TABLE 62.8 Nursing Assessment

Fracture

Subjective Data

Important Health Information

Past health history: Traumatic injury, long-term repetitive forces (stress fracture), bone or systemic diseases, prolonged immobility, osteopenia, osteoporosis

Medications: Corticosteroids (osteoporotic fractures); analgesics

Surgery or other treatments: First aid treatment of fracture, musculoskeletal surgeries

Functional Health Patterns

Health perception–health management: Calcium and vitamin D supplementation

Activity-exercise: Loss of motion or weakness of affected part, muscle spasms

Cognitive-perceptual: Sudden and severe pain in affected area; numbness, tingling, loss of sensation distal to injury; ongoing pain that increases with activity (stress fracture)

Objective Data

General

Apprehension, guarding of injured site

Integumentary

Skin lacerations, pallor and cool skin or bluish and warm skin distal to injury; bruising, edema at fracture site

Cardiovascular

Reduced or absent pulse distal to injury, ↓ skin temperature, delayed capillary refill

Neurovascular

Paresthesia, absent or ↓ sensation, hypersensation

Musculoskeletal

Restricted or lost function of affected part; local bony deformities, abnormal angulation; shortening, rotation, or crepitation of affected part; muscle weakness

Possible Diagnostic Findings

Identification and extent of fracture on x-ray, bone scan, CT scan, or MRI

---

positioning, physiologic responses to the traumatic injury, and application of a cast or constrictive dressing can cause nerve or vascular damage, usually distal to the injury. Record clinical findings before fracture treatment. This way if a problem occurs later, it will help determine if it was missed during the original examination or a result of treatment.

The neurovascular assessment consists of *peripheral vascular assessment* (color, temperature, capillary refill, peripheral pulses, edema) and *peripheral neurologic assessment* (sensation, motor function, pain). Throughout the neurovascular assessment, compare both extremities to obtain an accurate assessment.

Assess an extremity's color (pink, pale, cyanotic) and temperature (hot, warm, cool, cold) around the injury. Pallor or a cool-to-cold extremity below the injury could indicate arterial insufficiency. A warm, cyanotic extremity could indicate poor venous return. Next, assess capillary refill. A delay in returning to its original color (greater than 3 seconds) can occur with arterial insufficiency.[17]

Compare pulses on the unaffected and injured extremities to identify differences in rate or quality. This contralateral evaluation is critical. A decreased or absent pulse distal to the injury can indicate vascular dysfunction and insufficiency. Assess peripheral edema. Pitting edema may be present with severe injury.

Assess ulnar, median, and radial nerve function to evaluate sensation and motor innervation in the upper extremity. Assess motor function by asking the patient to (1) abduct the fingers (ulnar nerve), (2) oppose the thumb and small finger (median nerve), and (3) flex and extend the wrist (or the fingers, if in a cast) (radial nerve). In the lower extremity, assess the patient's ability to perform dorsiflexion (peroneal nerve) and plantar flexion (tibial nerve). Evaluate sensory function of the peroneal nerve by touching the web space between the great and second toes. Stroke the plantar surface (sole) of the foot to assess sensory function of the tibial nerve.

The patient may report *paresthesia* (abnormal sensation [e.g., numbness, tingling]) and hypersensation or hyperesthesia. Partial or full loss of sensation (paresis or paralysis) may be a late sign of neurovascular damage. Teach the patient to immediately report any changes in sensation or the ability to move the digits in the affected extremity.

◆ Nursing Diagnoses

Nursing diagnoses for the patient with a fracture may include:
- Impaired physical mobility
- Risk for infection
- Acute pain

Additional information on nursing diagnoses and interventions for the patient with a fracture is presented in cNursing Care Plan 62.1 (on the website for this chapter).

◆ Planning

The overall goals are that the patient with a fracture will (1) have healing with no associated complications, (2) have acceptable pain relief, and (3) achieve maximal rehabilitation potential.

◆ Nursing Implementation

Acute Care. Patients with fractures may be treated in an ED or an HCP's office and released to home care. They also may need hospitalization for varying amounts of time. Specific nursing measures depend on the setting and type of treatment.

Preoperative Care. If surgical intervention is needed to treat a fracture, patients must be prepared. In addition to the usual preoperative nursing care (see Chapter 17), teach the patient about the type of immobilization and assistive devices that will be used. Discuss expected activity limitations after surgery. Assure them that nursing staff will help meet their personal needs until they can resume self-care. Review pain management strategies.

Postoperative Care. In general, nursing care after surgery involves monitoring vital signs and applying general principles of postoperative nursing care (see Chapter 19). Frequent neurovascular assessment of the affected extremity is needed to detect early and subtle changes. Carefully follow any limitations related to turning, positioning, and extremity support. Minimize pain and discomfort through proper alignment and positioning. Frequently observe dressings or casts for any signs of bleeding or drainage. Report a significant increase in size of the drainage area to the HCP. If a wound drainage system is in place, regularly measure the volume of drainage and assess its character (e.g., bloody, purulent). Report increased or purulent drainage at once to the HCP. Maintain the patency of any drainage systems, using aseptic technique to avoid contamination.

Other nursing responsibilities depend on the type of immobilization used. A blood salvage and reinfusion system may be used to allow recovery and reinfusion of the patient's own blood. The blood is retrieved from a joint space or cavity; then the patient receives this blood in the form of an autotransfusion. (Autotransfusion is discussed in Chapter 30.)

Other Measures. Patients often have reduced mobility because of a fracture. Plan care to decrease risk for the many possible complications of immobility. Prevent constipation by increasing patient activity. Maintain high fluid intake (more than 2500 mL/day unless contraindicated by the patient's health status) and a diet high in bulk and roughage (fresh fruits and vegetables). If these measures are not effective in continuing the patient's normal bowel elimination pattern, give stool softeners, laxatives, or suppositories. Maintain a regular time for elimination to promote bowel regularity.

Renal stones can develop from bone demineralization due to reduced mobility. Hypercalcemia from demineralization causes a rise in urine pH and stone formation from calcium precipitation. Unless contraindicated, maintain a fluid intake of 2500 mL/day to decrease the risk for stone formation. (Renal stones are discussed in Chapter 45.)

Rapid deconditioning of the cardiopulmonary system can occur from prolonged bed rest, resulting in orthostatic hypotension and decreased lung capacity. Unless contraindicated, decrease these effects by having the patient sit on the side of the

---

NURSING MANAGEMENT

Caring for the Patient With a Cast or Traction

- Perform neurovascular assessment on the affected extremity.
- Monitor pain intensity and give prescribed analgesics.
- Determine correct body alignment to enhance traction.
- Monitor skin integrity around cast and at traction pin sites.
- Monitor cast during drying for denting or flattening.
- Teach patient and caregiver about cast care or traction and measures to prevent complications (e.g., ROM exercises).
- Assess for complications associated with immobility (e.g., constipation, VTE, kidney stones, atelectasis) and develop a plan to minimize those complications.
- Oversee unlicensed assistive personnel (UAP):
  - Position casted extremity above heart level as directed by RN.
  - Apply ice to cast as directed by RN.
  - Maintain body position and integrity of traction (if trained in this procedure).
  - Help patient with passive and active ROM exercises.
  - Notify RN about patient reports of pain, tingling, or decreased sensation in the affected extremity.

Collaborate With Physical Therapist

- Assess patient's current mobility and need for assistance.
- Teach safe ambulation with assistive device based on patient's weight-bearing restrictions.
- Establish exercise plan and teach patient to perform exercises safely.
- Coordinate PT with RN so that patient can receive timely analgesia.
- Discuss home environment with patient and identify modifications to promote safety (e.g., stair training).

Collaborate With Occupational Therapist

- Assess impact of patient's condition on ability to perform ADLs.
- Teach patient use of assistive devices (e.g., long-handled reacher, shoe donner) to promote self-care while maintaining activity restrictions.

bed, allowing the patient's lower limbs to dangle over the bedside, and having the patient perform standing transfers. When the patient is allowed to increase activity, assess for orthostatic hypotension. Assess patients for signs of VTE. VTE is discussed in Chapter 37.

Traction. When slings are used with traction, regularly inspect exposed skin areas. Pressure over a bony prominence created by wrinkled sheets or blankets may cause pressure necrosis. Persistent skin pressure may impair blood flow and cause injury to peripheral nerves and blood vessels. Assess skeletal traction or external fixation pin sites for signs of infection. Pin site care may vary. It often includes regularly cleansing with chlorhexidine, rinsing with sterile saline, and drying the area with sterile gauze.

External rotation of the affected extremity is a classic assessment finding for a patient with unrepaired hip fracture. If skin traction is ordered before surgery, apply traction without trying to reposition or realign the extremity. Movement of fracture fragments can occur during repositioning, causing increased pain and possible nerve impingement. Keep the patient in the center of the bed in a supine position to provide adequate countertraction.

Discuss specific patient activity with the HCP. If exercise is allowed, encourage patient participation in a simple exercise program based on activity restrictions. Have the patient perform frequent position changes, ROM exercises of unaffected joints, deep-breathing exercises, and isometric exercises. These activities should be done several times each day. Teach the patient to use the trapeze bar (if permitted) to raise the body off the bed for linen changes and placement of the bedpan. Encourage and help the hospitalized patient to stay connected with friends and family by telephone or through social media resources.

◆ **Ambulatory Care**

Cast Care. Most uncomplicated fractures are treated in an outpatient setting. Whatever the type of cast material, a cast can interfere with circulation and nerve function if it is applied too tightly or excess edema occurs after application. Frequent neurovascular assessment of the immobilized extremity is critical. Teach the patient to recognize and promptly report tightness of the cast and areas of pressure or discomfort. Explain the importance of elevating the extremity above heart level to promote venous return and applying ice to control or prevent edema during the initial phase. However, if compartment syndrome is suspected, do not elevate the extremity above the heart.

Patient and caregiver teaching is important to prevent complications. Table 62.9 describes patient and caregiver instructions for cast care. Teach the patient to exercise joints above and below the cast. Tell the patient not to scratch or place anything inside the cast because this may cause skin injury and infection. For itching, direct a hair dryer on a cool setting under the cast. Confirm the patient's and caregiver's understanding of these instructions before discharge. A follow-up phone call is appropriate. Home care nursing visits may be needed, especially for the patient with a body jacket brace.

The cast is typically removed in the outpatient setting. Patients often fear being cut by the oscillating blade of the cast saw. Reassure the patient that damage to the skin is unlikely. Teach the patient about possible changes in the appearance of the extremity beneath the cast (e.g., dry, wrinkled skin; atrophied muscle; foul odor). The patient may be scared to use the injured extremity after cast removal.

Ambulation. Know the overall goals of PT in relation to the patient's abilities, needs, and tolerance. The physical therapist

---

TABLE 62.9 Patient & Caregiver Teaching

Cast Care

After a cast is applied, include the following instructions when teaching the patient and the caregiver:

Do

1. Apply ice directly over fracture site for first 24 hr (avoid getting cast wet by keeping ice in plastic bag and protecting cast with cloth).
2. Check with HCP before getting fiberglass cast wet.
3. Dry cast thoroughly if inadvertently exposed to water.
   - Blot dry with towel.
   - Use hair dryer on low setting until cast is thoroughly dry.
4. Elevate extremity above heart level for first 48 hr.
5. Regularly move joints above and below cast.
6. Use hair dryer on cool setting for itching inside the cast.
7. Report signs of possible problems to HCP:
   - Increasing pain despite elevation, ice, analgesia.
   - Swelling associated with pain and discoloration of toes or fingers.
   - Pain during movement.
   - Burning or tingling under cast.
   - Sores or foul odor under cast.
8. Keep appointment to have fracture and cast checked.

Do Not

1. Get cast wet.
2. Remove any padding.
3. Insert any objects inside cast.
4. Bear weight on new cast for 48 hr (not all casts are made for weight bearing; check with HCP when unsure).
5. Cover cast with plastic for prolonged periods.

---

is responsible for mobility training and teaching about the use of assistive aids (cane, crutches, walker). Reinforce these instructions to the patient. The patient with lower extremity fractures usually starts mobility training when able to sit in bed and dangle the feet over the side. Work with the physical therapist to give analgesia before a PT session.

When the patient begins to ambulate, know the patient's weight-bearing status and the correct technique if the patient is using an assistive device. Ambulation occurs in different degrees of weight-bearing: (1) non–weight bearing (no weight on the involved extremity), (2) touch-down/toe-touch weight bearing (contact with floor for balance but no weight borne), (3) partial–weight-bearing ambulation (25% to 50% of patient's weight borne), (4) weight bearing as tolerated (based on patient's pain and tolerance), and (5) full–weight-bearing ambulation (no limitations).

Assistive Devices. Devices for ambulation range from a cane (can relieve up to 40% of the weight normally borne by a lower limb) to a walker or crutches (may allow for complete non–weight-bearing ambulation). The HCP decides which device is best, balancing the need for maximum stability and safety with the need for maneuverability in small spaces, such as bathrooms. Discuss with the patient lifestyle requirements and help select a device that allows the patient to feel most secure and independent. The technique for using assistive ambulation devices varies. The involved limb is usually advanced at the same time or immediately after advance of the device. The uninvolved limb is advanced last. Canes are held in the hand opposite the involved extremity.

Place a transfer belt (gait belt) around the patient's waist to provide stability while teaching the patient how to use an assistive device. Discourage the patient from reaching for furniture or relying on another person for support. A patient with inadequate upper limb strength or poorly fitted crutches bears weight at the axilla rather than at the hands. This can damage the neurovascular bundle that passes across the axilla. If verbal coaching does not correct the problem, teach the patient another form of ambulation (e.g., walker) until strength is adequate.

Patients who must ambulate without weight bearing need enough upper limb strength to lift their own weight at each step. Because the muscles of the shoulder girdle and upper arm may not be accustomed to this work, patients require focused training for this task. Push-ups, pull-ups using the overhead trapeze bar, and weight lifting develop the triceps and biceps muscles. Straight-leg raises and quadriceps-setting exercises strengthen the quadriceps muscles.

Psychosocial Concerns. Short-term rehabilitative goals address the transition from dependence to independence in performing simple ADLs. They are directed at preserving or increasing strength and endurance. Long-term rehabilitative goals are aimed at preventing problems associated with musculoskeletal injury (Table 62.10). During the rehabilitative phase, help the patient adjust to any problems caused by the injury (e.g., separation from family, financial impact of medical care, loss of income from inability to work, potential for disability). Assess patients for posttraumatic stress disorder. This is especially important if significant injury to others or fatalities were associated with the patient's injuries.

The caregiver may have a key role in providing long-term care. Teach the caregiver how to help with strength and endurance exercises, mobility, and promoting activities that enhance the quality of daily living. Offer support and encouragement while actively listening to the patient's and caregiver's concerns.

◆ Evaluation

The expected outcomes are that the patient with a fracture will
- Report satisfactory pain management
- Show proper care of cast or immobilizer
- Have uncomplicated bone healing

COMPLICATIONS OF FRACTURES

Most fractures heal without complications. Complications of fractures may be direct or indirect. *Direct complications* include problems with bone infection, bone union, and avascular necrosis. *Indirect complications* include compartment syndrome, VTE, fat embolism syndrome (FES), breakdown of skeletal muscle *(rhabdomyolysis)*, and hypovolemic shock. Most musculoskeletal injuries are not life threatening. Death after a fracture is usually due to damage to underlying organs and vascular structures or complications of the fracture or immobility. Open fractures, fractures with severe blood loss, and fractures that damage vital organs (e.g., lung, heart) are medical emergencies requiring immediate attention.

Infection

Open fractures and soft tissue injuries have a high rate of infection. An open fracture usually results from severe external forces. Communication of the fracture site with the outside environment can contaminate the fracture site with microorganisms or foreign bodies. Damage to the surrounding soft tissue and blood vessels impairs the ability of defense mechanisms to respond to microorganisms.[18] Dying or contaminated tissue is an ideal medium for many common pathogens, including anaerobic bacilli, such as *Clostridium tetani*. Measures to prevent infection and osteomyelitis are important.

TABLE 62.10 Problems Associated With Musculoskeletal Injuries

Problem	Description	Nursing Considerations
Atrophy	• ↓ Muscle mass occurs from disuse after prolonged immobilization. • Loss of nerve function can cause muscle atrophy.	• Isometric muscle-strengthening exercises as able with immobilization device helps reduce amount of atrophy. • Muscle atrophy interferes with and prolongs rehabilitation process.
Contracture	• Abnormal condition of joint characterized by flexion and fixation. • Caused by atrophy and shortening of muscle fibers and ligaments or by loss of normal elasticity of skin over joint.	• Can be prevented by frequent position change, correct body alignment, active-passive ROM exercises several times a day. • Intervention requires gradual progressive stretching of muscles or ligaments in region of joint.
Footdrop	• Plantar-flexed position of the foot occurs when Achilles tendon in ankle shortens because it has been allowed to assume an unsupported position. • Peroneal nerve palsy (a compression neuropathy) can cause footdrop and spinal nerve compression.	• For patient with long-term injuries, support foot in neutral position to ↓ risk for footdrop. • Once footdrop has developed, can significantly hinder ambulation and gait training. • May need splint to keep feet in neutral position. • High-top athletic shoes may help. Apply at scheduled times to keep feet in neutral position.
Muscle spasms	• Caused by involuntary muscle contraction after fracture, muscle strain, or nerve injury. • May last several weeks. • Pain associated with muscle spasms is often intense and can last from several seconds to several minutes.	• Measures to ↓ intensity of muscle spasms are similar to actions for pain management. • Do not massage muscle spasms. Massage may stimulate muscle tissue contraction that ↑ spasm and pain. • Thermotherapy, especially heat, may reduce muscle spasm.
Pain	• Common with fractures, edema, muscle spasm. • May be mild to severe and described as aching, dull, burning, throbbing, sharp, or deep.	• Causes include incorrect positioning and alignment of extremity, incorrect support of extremity, sudden movement of extremity, immobilization device that is applied too tightly or incorrectly, constrictive dressings, motion at fracture site. • Determine causes of pain so that corrective action can be taken.

Open fractures require aggressive surgical debridement. The wound is initially cleaned by saline lavage in the operating room. Gross contaminants are irrigated and mechanically removed. Contused, contaminated, and devitalized tissue (muscle, subcutaneous fat, skin, and bone fragments) is surgically excised (*debridement*). The amount of soft tissue damage determines if the wound is closed at the time of surgery or if it needs repeat debridement, closed suction drainage, and/or skin grafting. During surgery, the open wound may be irrigated with antibiotic solution. Antibiotic-impregnated beads also may be placed in the surgical site. Patients usually receive IV antibiotics for at least 3 days.[18] In conjunction with aggressive surgical management, antibiotics have greatly reduced the occurrence of infection.

Compartment Syndrome

Compartment syndrome is a condition in which swelling causes increased pressure within a limited space (muscle compartment). Because the fascia surrounding the muscle has limited ability to stretch, continued swelling can cause pressure that compromises the function of blood vessels and nerves in the compartment. Capillary perfusion is reduced below a level needed for tissue life. Compartment syndrome often involves the leg but can occur in any muscle group.

There are 38 compartments in the upper and lower extremities. Two basic causes of compartment syndrome are (1) decreased compartment size resulting from restrictive dressings, splints, casts, excessive traction, or premature closure of fascia; and (2) increased compartment contents due to bleeding, inflammation, edema, or IV infiltration.

Edema can create enough pressure to obstruct circulation and cause venous occlusion, which further increases edema. Arterial flow is eventually compromised, causing ischemia in the extremity. As ischemia continues, muscle and nerve cells are destroyed. Fibrotic tissue eventually replaces healthy tissue. Contracture, disability, and loss of function can occur. Delays in diagnosis and treatment may lead to irreversible muscle and nerve ischemia. The extremity may become functionally useless or severely impaired.

Compartment syndrome is usually associated with fractures (especially of long bones), extensive soft tissue damage, and crush injury.[19] Fractures of the distal humerus and proximal tibia are the most common fractures associated with compartment syndrome. Compartment injury can also occur after knee or leg surgery. Prolonged pressure on a muscle compartment may result when someone is trapped under a heavy object or a person's limb is trapped beneath the body because of response to drugs or alcohol.

Clinical Manifestations. Compartment syndrome may occur initially from the body's physiologic response to the injury, or it may be delayed for several days after the original insult or injury. Ischemia can occur within 4 to 8 hours after the onset of compartment syndrome.

One or more of the "6 *Ps*" are specific to compartment syndrome: (1) *pain* out of proportion to the injury that is not managed by opioid analgesics, and *pain* on passive stretch of muscle in the compartment; (2) increasing *pressure* in the compartment; (3) *paresthesia* (numbness and tingling); (4) *pallor*, coolness, and loss of normal color of the extremity; (5) *paralysis* or loss of function; and (6) *pulselessness* (decreased or absent peripheral pulses).

Interprofessional Care. Prompt diagnosis of compartment syndrome is critical.[19] Perform and document regular neurovascular assessment on all patients with fractures, especially those with injury of the extremities or soft tissue in these areas. Early recognition and effective treatment of compartment syndrome are essential to avoid permanent damage to muscles and nerves.

Carefully assess the location, quality, and intensity pain (see Chapter 8). Evaluate the patient's pain intensity on a scale of 0 to 10. Pain unrelieved by drugs and out of proportion to the level of injury is one of the *first* signs of compartment syndrome. Paresthesia is also an early sign. Notify the HCP immediately of these changes in the patient's condition. Relieving the source of pressure (e.g., cast is cut [bivalved] or dressing loosened by order of the HCP) typically decreases pain and paresthesia and can avoid compartment syndrome. Reducing traction weight may also decrease external pressures on the extremity. Pulselessness and paralysis are later signs of compartment syndrome. Do not wait until these late signs occur to contact the HCP. Amputation may be needed due to prolonged ischemia.

With suspected compartment syndrome, do not elevate the extremity above the heart. Similarly, do not apply cold compresses. They may cause vasoconstriction and worsen compartment syndrome.

Surgical decompression (e.g., fasciotomy) of the involved compartment may be needed (Fig. 62.15).[19] The fasciotomy site is left open for several days to allow adequate soft tissue decompression. Infection resulting from delayed wound closure is a potential problem after fasciotomy. In severe cases of compartment syndrome, amputation is done.

⊘ CHECK YOUR PRACTICE

Your 22-yr-old male patient had a fall while mountain climbing. He returned from surgery 8 hours ago with a long leg cast placed for open fractures of the femur and tibia. He continually reports pain that IV morphine does not seem to help.

- How will you assess his neurovascular condition?
- What signs and symptoms would suggest the development of compartment syndrome?
- What is the most likely intervention if compartment syndrome is developing?

Venous Thromboembolism

Veins of the lower extremities and pelvis are at great risk for clot (thrombus) formation after a fracture, especially a hip fracture. VTE may also occur after total hip or total knee replacement surgery. In patients with limited mobility, inactivity of muscles that normally help pump venous blood from the extremities to the heart worsens venous stasis.

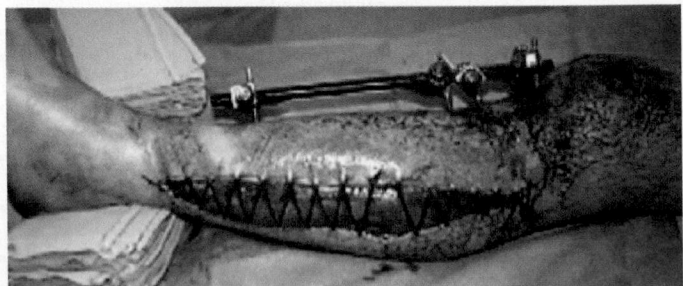

FIG. 62.15 Fasciotomy associated with compartment syndrome. Stabilization of fracture with external fixator. (From Browner BD, Jupiter JB, Levine AM, Trafton P: *Skeletal trauma: Fractures, dislocations, ligamentous injuries*, ed 4, Philadelphia, 2009, Saunders.)

Because of the high risk for VTE in the orthopedic surgical patient, prophylactic anticoagulant drugs should be given for at least 10 to 14 days.[20] The most common agents used include (1) warfarin (Coumadin), (2) low-molecular-weight heparin (LMWH) (e.g., enoxaparin [Lovenox], fondaparinux), (3) aspirin, or (4) a factor Xa inhibitor (e.g., rivaroxaban [Xarelto], apixaban).[20] Besides wearing compression gradient stockings (antiembolism hose) or using intermittent pneumatic compression devices, the patient should dorsiflex and plantar flex the ankle of an affected lower extremity against resistance and perform ROM exercises on the unaffected leg. For upper extremity injuries, have the patient flex and extend the wrist if not immobilized by a cast or splint and perform ROM exercises on the unaffected arm. VTE is discussed in Chapter 37.

> **⚠ SAFETY ALERT** Anticoagulant Therapy
> - Monitor for signs of external bleeding (e.g., nosebleeds) or internal bleeding (e.g., tea-colored urine).
> - Teach patient signs of bleeding and what to do if bleeding occurs.
> - Teach patient safe self-injection if taking an injectable anticoagulant after discharge.
> - Encourage patient to keep appointments for laboratory testing to monitor effects of warfarin (if prescribed).

Fat Embolism Syndrome

Fat embolism syndrome (FES) is characterized by fat globules entering the circulatory system from fractures. They collect in areas with abundant blood vessels, especially the lungs and brain.[21] FES contributes to mortality associated with fractures. The fractures most often associated with FES are those of the long bones, ribs, tibia, and pelvis. FES can also occur after total joint replacement, spinal fusion, liposuction, crush injuries, and bone marrow transplantation.

Two theories about FES exist. According to the mechanical theory, fat emboli originate from fat released from the marrow of injured bone. The fat enters systemic circulation, where it travels to other organs. As fat droplets become stuck in small blood vessels, local ischemia and inflammation occur. The biochemical theory suggests hormonal changes caused by trauma or sepsis stimulate systemic release of free fatty acids (e.g., chylomicrons) that form the fat emboli.

Clinical Manifestations. Early recognition of FES is crucial to prevent patient death. Most patients have symptoms within 24 to 48 hours after injury. Severe forms have occurred within hours of injury. Fat emboli in the lungs cause hemorrhagic interstitial pneumonitis with signs and symptoms of acute respiratory distress syndrome (ARDS). These include chest pain, tachypnea, cyanosis, dyspnea, apprehension, tachycardia, and hypoxemia.[21] These symptoms are caused by poor O_2 exchange. Changes in mental status due to hypoxemia are common. Petechiae on the neck, anterior chest wall, axilla, buccal membrane, and conjunctiva of the eye may help distinguish FES from other problems. They may appear due to intravascular thromboses caused by decreased oxygenation. However, petechiae occur in only 20% to 60% of cases of FES. They may fade before they are noticed.[21]

The clinical course of FES may be rapid and acute. In a short time, skin color can change from pallor to cyanosis. The patient may become comatose. No specific laboratory tests aid in the diagnosis. However, certain abnormalities may be present.

These include fat cells in blood, urine, or sputum; a decrease of PaO_2 to less than 60 mm Hg; ST segment and T-wave changes on ECG; decreased platelet count and hematocrit; and high erythrocyte sedimentation rate (ESR). A chest x-ray may show bilateral pulmonary infiltrates.

Interprofessional Care. Management of FES is supportive and related to managing symptoms. Treatment includes fluid administration to prevent hypovolemic shock, correction of acidosis, and blood transfusions. Dobutamine and nitrous oxide may be given for hemodynamic support.[21] Use of corticosteroids to prevent or treat FES is controversial.

The patient needs appropriate respiratory support. Administer O_2 to treat hypoxia. Intubation or intermittent positive pressure ventilation may be an option if satisfactory PaO_2 cannot be obtained with supplemental O_2 alone. Some patients develop pulmonary edema and/or ARDS, leading to increased mortality. Most persons survive FES with few complications.

Preventing the development of FES is important. Careful immobilization and handling of a long bone fracture are the most important factors in preventing FES. Reposition the patient as little as possible before fracture immobilization or stabilization to decrease the risk of dislodging fat droplets into the general circulation.

 CHECK YOUR PRACTICE

> You are caring for a 24-yr-old male patient who had a femur fracture in a motorcycle accident last night. He is scheduled for ORIF later today. While doing your assessment, you notice that he seems very restless. You note some axillary petechiae.
> - What complication would you suspect is occurring?
> - Why is this patient particularly at risk for this complication?
> - What is the most important intervention for a patient with this complication?

Rhabdomyolysis

Rhabdomyolysis is a syndrome caused by the breakdown of damaged skeletal muscle cells. This breakdown causes the release of myoglobin into the bloodstream. Myoglobin precipitates and causes obstruction in renal tubules. This results in acute tubular necrosis and acute kidney injury (AKI). Because of possible muscle damage, assess urine output. Common signs are dark reddish-brown urine and symptoms of AKI (see Chapter 46).

TYPES OF FRACTURES

COLLES' FRACTURE

A *Colles' fracture* is a fracture of the distal radius. The styloid process of the ulna may be involved as well. The injury usually occurs when the patient falls on an outstretched arm and hand. It is one of the most common types of fractures in adults. It most often occurs in patients over 50 years old whose bones are osteoporotic *(fragility fracture)* (Fig. 62.16). A younger person with a Colles' fracture caused by a low-energy force should be referred for an osteoporosis evaluation.

Symptoms include pain in the immediate area of injury, pronounced swelling, and dorsal displacement of the distal fragment (silver-fork deformity). This displacement appears as an

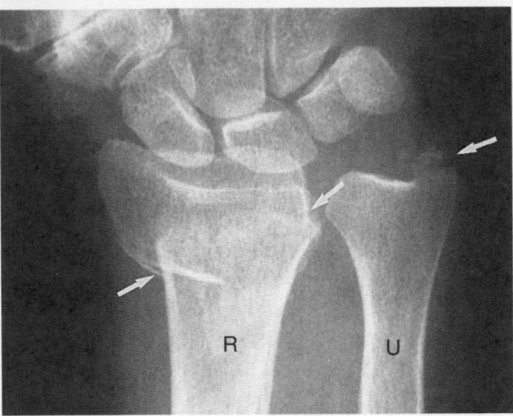

FIG. 62.16 Colles' fracture. Fracture of the distal radius (R) and ulnar (U) styloid from patient falling on the outstretched hand. (From Mettler FA: *Essentials of radiology*, ed 2, Philadelphia, 2005, Saunders.)

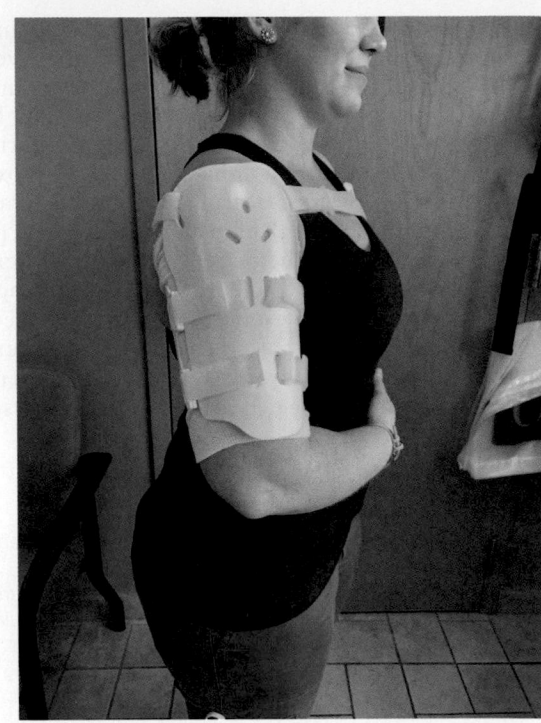

FIG. 62.17 Humeral cuff brace. (Courtesy Matthew C. Price, MS, RN, CNP, ONP-C, RNFA, Columbus, OH.)

obvious deformity of the wrist. The major complication is vascular insufficiency from edema. CTS can be a later complication.

A Colles' fracture is usually managed with closed reduction of the fracture and application of a splint or cast. If displaced, the fracture is typically managed with open reduction and internal or external fixation. Nursing management includes frequent neurovascular assessment and measures to reduce edema. Provide support and protect the extremity. Encourage active movement of the thumb and fingers to reduce edema and increase venous return. Teach the patient to perform active movements of the shoulder to prevent stiffness or contracture.

HUMERAL SHAFT FRACTURE

Fractures involving the shaft of the humerus are common among young and middle-aged adults. The most common symptoms are obvious displacement of the humeral shaft, shortened extremity, abnormal mobility, and pain. Complications associated include radial nerve injury and injury to the brachial artery due to laceration, transection, or muscle spasm.

Treatment depends on the specific fracture location and displacement. Nonoperative treatment may include a hanging arm cast, shoulder immobilizer, sling and swathe (a type of immobilizer that prevents shoulder movement), or humeral cuff brace (Fig. 62.17).

The humeral cuff brace is typically used to stabilize midshaft humerus fractures. Two pieces of molded plastic are fitted together in a clam-shell configuration and held together with Velcro straps. The humeral cuff brace is a good option for nonoperative fracture management if the patient is at increased risk for intraoperative complications.

When these devices are used, elevate the head of the bed to assist gravity in reducing the fracture. Allow the arm to hang freely when the patient is sitting or standing. Provide measures to protect the axilla and prevent skin breakdown. Carefully place absorbable composite dressing pads (e.g., ABD pads) in the axilla. Change them twice daily or as needed. Skin or skeletal traction may be used for reduction and immobilization.

During the rehabilitative phase, an exercise program to improve strength and motion of the injured extremity is extremely important. Exercises should include assisted motion of the hand and fingers. The shoulder can be exercised if the fracture is stable. This helps prevent stiffness from frozen shoulder or fibrosis of the shoulder capsule.

PELVIC FRACTURE

Pelvic fractures range from relatively minor to life threatening, depending on the mechanism of injury and associated vascular damage. Although only a small number of fractures are pelvic fractures, this type of injury is associated with a high mortality rate. Attention to more obvious injuries at the time of a traumatic event may result in oversight of pelvic injuries.

Pelvic fractures may cause serious intraabdominal injury, including laceration and hemorrhage of the urethra, bladder, or colon. They can cause acute pelvic compartment syndrome. Paralytic ileus may occur after pelvic fracture. Patients may survive the pelvic injury, only to die from sepsis, FES, or VTE.

Abdominal assessment may show local swelling, tenderness, deformity, unusual pelvic movement, and bruising. Assess the neurovascular condition of the lower extremities and determine associated injuries. Pelvic fractures are diagnosed by x-ray and CT scan.

Treatment depends on the severity of the injury. Stable, nondisplaced fractures require little intervention. Ambulation with weight bearing as tolerated is typically encouraged.[22] Complex or displaced fractures (e.g., open book fracture) need external fixation alone or combined with ORIF (e.g., screws), often done emergently. Use extreme care in handling or moving the patient, to prevent further injury. Turn the patient only when ordered by the HCP. Because a pelvic fracture can damage other organs, assess bowel and urinary elimination. Regularly perform distal neurovascular assessment. Provide back care with adequate help or while the patient is raised from the bed by independent use of a trapeze.

ETHICAL/LEGAL DILEMMAS
Entitlement to Treatment

Situation

D.C., a 35-yr-old English tourist, was in a hang-gliding accident while touring the United States. She was taken to the regional trauma center for treatment of internal injuries, blood loss, and severe pelvic fractures. She has become septic, is now in renal failure, and has ARDS. She has no health insurance. Despite a poor chance of survival, her husband and parents want all possible measures to be taken.

Ethical/Legal Points for Consideration

- Federal law requires hospitals receiving federal funds through Medicare and Medicaid to provide emergency evaluation and treatment to stabilize patients (Emergency Medical Treatment and Active Labor Act [EMTALA]). Once the patient is stabilized, they are under no obligation to continue treatment and may transfer the patient to another facility.
- Discussions with the family must occur to clarify treatment goals (e.g., recovery, survival, continued biologic existence, nonabandonment of the patient) and what they mean by wanting "everything done." There is no legal or ethical obligation to continue medical treatment when treatment goals cannot be met.
- Contact with the English consulate may result in collaboration to stabilize the patient and transport her to England.
- Neither HCPs nor hospitals are required to provide medically futile care (care that provides no benefit to the patient).
- Although her home country (England) offers universal health care, D.C. assumed the risk when engaging in a potentially dangerous activity and did not obtain international health insurance coverage for her visit to a foreign country.

Discussion Questions

1. How can the nurse facilitate discussions with the family about treatment goals for D.C.?
2. Are family members able to state D.C.'s wishes for her own care in such a situation?

HIP FRACTURE

Hip fractures are common in older adults. 95% of hip fractures result from a fall.[23] More than 320,000 patients are admitted to hospitals each year because of a hip fracture. Up to 37% of those patients die within 1 year of injury. Many older adults develop disabilities that require long-term care. By age 90, about 33% of all women and 17% of all men will have had a hip fracture. In adults over 65 years old, hip fracture occurs more often in women than in men because of osteoporosis.

Hip fracture refers to a fracture of the proximal (upper) third of the femur, which extends 5 cm below the lesser trochanter (Fig. 62.18). Fractures within the hip joint capsule are *intracapsular fractures*. Intracapsular fractures are further identified by their specific locations: (1) *capital* (fracture of the head of the femur), (2) *subcapital* (fracture just below the head of the femur), and (3) *transcervical* (fracture of the femoral neck). These fractures, which are often associated with osteoporosis and minor trauma, are called *fragility fractures*.

Extracapsular fractures occur outside the joint capsule. They are either (1) *intertrochanteric* (in a region between the greater and lesser trochanter) or (2) *subtrochanteric* (below the lesser trochanter). Most are caused by severe direct trauma or a fall.

Clinical Manifestations

Manifestations include external rotation, muscle spasm, shortening of the affected extremity, and severe pain and tenderness

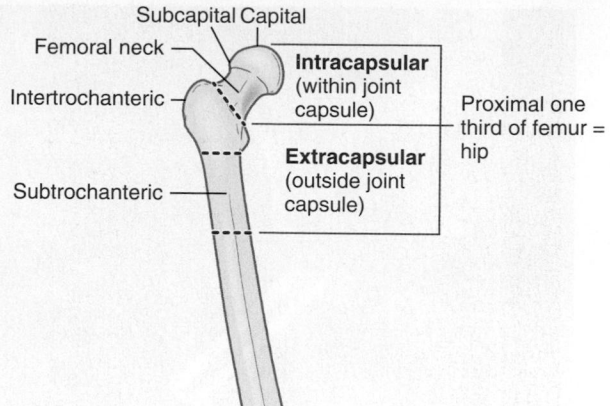

FIG. 62.18 Femur with location of various types of fracture.

around the fracture site. Displaced femoral neck fractures may disrupt blood supply to the femoral head, resulting in avascular necrosis of the femoral head.

Interprofessional Care

Immediate surgery is the standard of care. Initially the affected extremity may be immobilized with Buck's traction (Fig. 62.9) if the patient's physical condition needs stabilized before surgery can be done. Buck's traction can be used for 24 to 48 hours to relieve painful muscle spasms.

Surgical treatment allows early mobilization and decreases the risk for major complications. The type of surgery depends on the location and severity of the fracture and the person's age. Surgical options include (1) closed reduction with percutaneous pinning (CRPP) (minimally invasive surgery to stabilize the femoral neck and head with screws), (2) repair with internal fixation devices (e.g., hip compression screw, intramedullary devices), (3) replacement of the femoral head with a prosthesis (partial hip replacement or *hemiarthroplasty*, often used for fracture of the femoral neck) (Fig. 62.19), and (4) total hip replacement (involves both the femur and acetabulum) (Fig. 62.20).

❖ NURSING MANAGEMENT: HIP FRACTURE

◆ Nursing Implementation

◆ **Preoperative Care.** In addition to the usual preoperative nursing care (see Chapter 17), teaching may be done in the ED. Most patients are medically stable and thus do not have an overnight preoperative period in which to receive instructions. Most people who have hip fractures are older adults. When planning treatment of the hip fracture, consider the patient's chronic health problems (e.g., diabetes, heart and pulmonary disease). Surgery may be delayed briefly until the patient's general health is stabilized. Begin to consider discharge plans because the length of stay after surgery will be no more than a few days.

Before surgery, severe muscle spasms can increase pain. Analgesics or muscle relaxants, comfortable positioning (unless contraindicated), and properly applied traction (if used) can help to manage the spasms.

◆ **Postoperative Care.** Similar principles of patient care apply to any of the surgical procedures for hip fractures. In the initial postoperative period, assess vital signs, intake, and output. Monitor respiratory function and encourage deep breathing and coughing. Assess pain and give pain medication. Observe

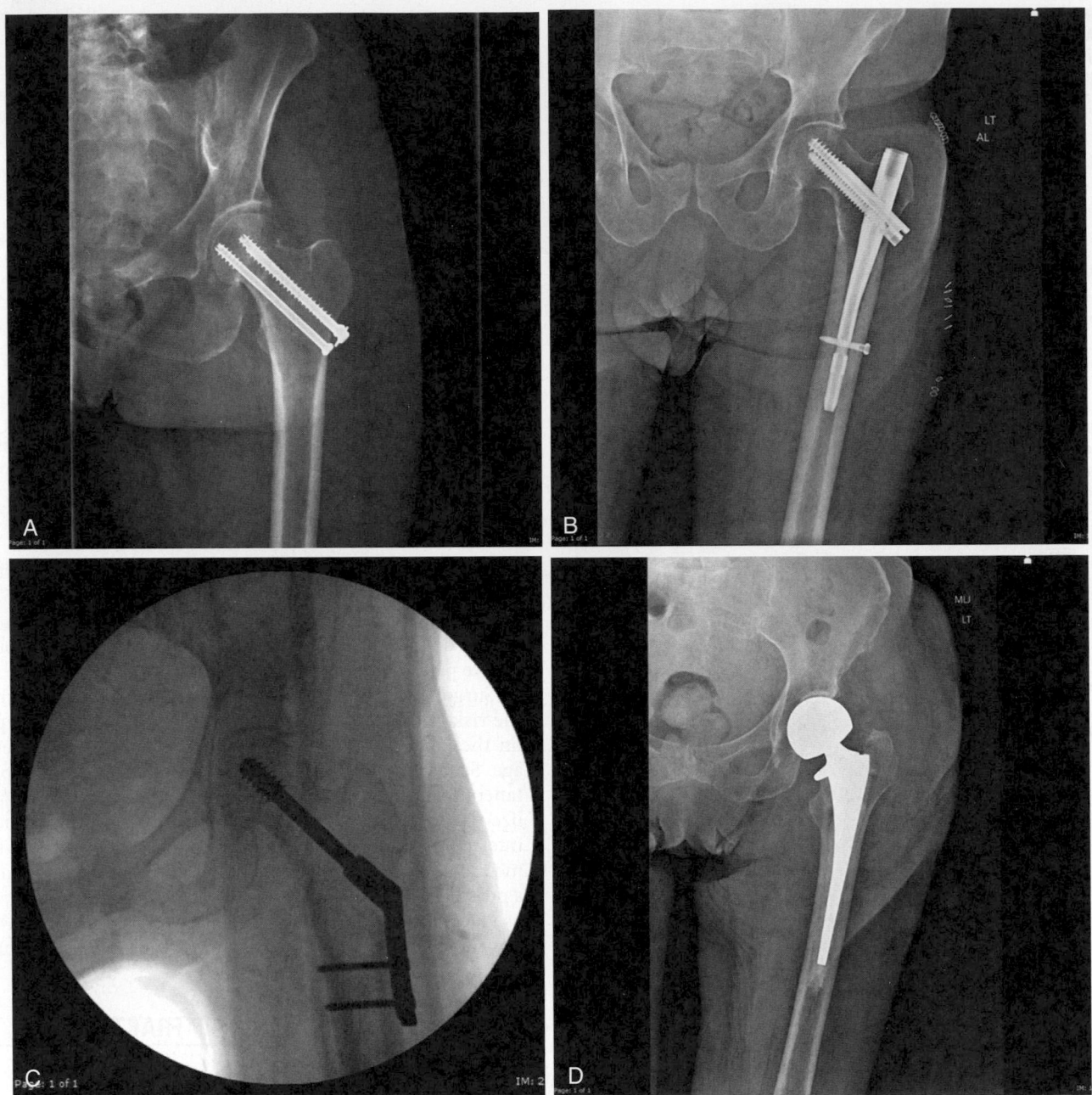

FIG. 62.19 Types of surgical repair for a hip fracture: **A**, Closed reduction with percutaneous pinning. **B**, Intramedullary nail. **C**, Sliding hip screw. **D**, Hemiarthroplasty. (Courtesy Matthew C. Price, MS, RN, CNP, ONP-C, RNFA, Columbus, OH.)

the dressing and incision for signs of bleeding. See eNursing Care Plan 62.2 for the orthopedic surgical patient (available on the website for this chapter).

Neurovascular impairment is possible. Assess the patient's extremity for (1) color, (2) temperature, (3) capillary refill, (4) distal pulses, (5) edema, (6) sensation, (7) motor function, and (8) pain. Decrease edema by elevating the leg when the patient is in bed or in a chair. Pain in the affected extremity can be reduced by maintaining limb alignment with pillows between the patient's knees when turning the patient to the nonoperative side.

Encourage the patient to use the overhead trapeze bar and the opposite side rail to help in position changes. Avoid turning the patient to the affected side unless approved by the HCP. A

physical therapist can teach the patient how to transfer out of the bed to a chair. Have the patient exercise the unaffected leg and both arms

If hemiarthroplasty or total joint replacement was done by a *posterior approach* (incision posterior to the midline of the greater trochanter down the femoral shaft), measures to prevent dislocation must be used (Table 62.11). Tell the patient and caregiver about positions and activities that increase the patient's risk for dislocation (more than 90 degrees of flexion, adduction across the midline [crossing of legs and ankles], internal rotation of hip). Many daily activities may reproduce these positions: (1) putting on shoes and socks, (2) crossing the legs or feet while seated, (3) assuming the side-lying position incorrectly, (4) standing up or sitting down while the hip is flexed more than

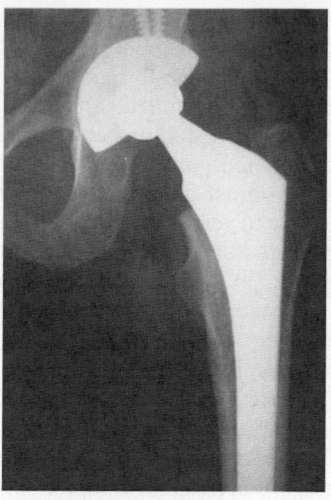

FIG. 62.20 Total hip replacement (arthroplasty) with cementless femoral prosthesis of metal alloy with plastic acetabular socket.

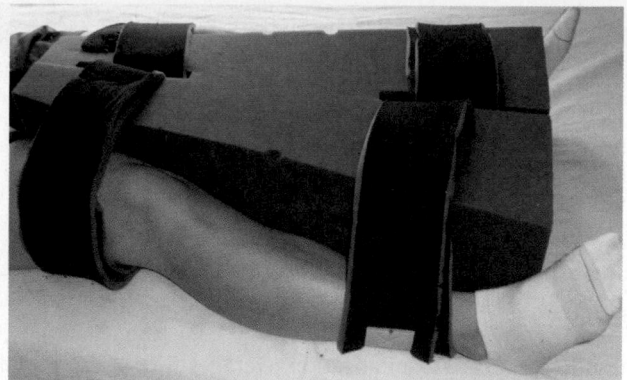

FIG. 62.21 Maintaining abduction after total hip replacement. (Courtesy Mary Wollan, RN, BAN, ONC, Spring Park, MN.)

TABLE 62.11 Patient & Caregiver Teaching

Posterior Hip Replacement

After a hip replacement by posterior surgical approach, include the following instructions when teaching a patient and caregiver:

Do
- Use an elevated toilet seat.
- Place chair inside shower or tub and remain seated while washing.
- Use pillow between legs for first 6 wk after surgery when lying on nonoperative side or when supine.
- Keep hip in neutral, straight position when sitting, walking, or lying.
- Notify HCP at once if severe pain, deformity, or loss of function occurs.
- Discuss personal risk factors for prosthetic joint infection with HCP and dentist before dental work.

Do Not
- Flex hip greater than 90 degrees (e.g., sitting in low chairs or toilet seats).
- Adduct hip (e.g., bring legs together at knees).
- Internally rotate hip (e.g., turn toward planted foot on affected side).
- Cross legs at knees or ankles.
- Put on own shoes or stockings without adaptive device (e.g., long-handled shoehorn or stocking-helper) for 4–6 wk after surgery.
- Sit on chairs without arms. The arms of chairs will help the patient rise to a standing position.

90 degrees relative to the chair, and (5) sitting on low seats, especially low toilet seats. Teach the patient to avoid these activities until the soft tissue capsule around the hip has healed enough to stabilize the prosthesis (usually at least 6 weeks).

Elevated toilet seats and chair alterations (e.g., raising the seat with a folded blanket, keeping a straight back) are needed. Avoid placing a soft pillow in the patient's seat because sitting on it can cause internal rotation. If a foam abduction wedge is ordered to prevent joint dislocation, place it between the patient's legs (Fig. 62.21). Apply the top straps above the knee to avoid putting pressure on the peroneal nerve at the lateral tibial tubercle. Some HCPs want the patient to keep the abductor wedge in place except when bathing or walking.

If hemiarthroplasty or total joint replacement was done by an *anterior approach* (incision is made in the front of the hip with patient lying on the back), the hip muscles are left intact. This approach generally provides a more stable hip in the postoperative period with a lower rate of complications. Precautions related to motion and weight bearing are few. They typically include instructions to avoid hyperextension.

Weight bearing on the involved extremity varies. Limited weight bearing is typically the only restriction for the patient who had ORIF of the hip fracture. Weight bearing after ORIF is generally restricted until x-ray examination shows adequate healing, usually 6 to 12 weeks. Tell the patient and caregiver about the weight-bearing status after surgery.

Taking a tub bath and driving a car are not allowed for 4 to 6 weeks. An occupational therapist (OT) may teach the patient to use assistive devices, such as long-handled shoehorns, sock assists, and reachers or grabbers, to avoid bending over to pick up something on the floor. The knees must be kept apart. Teach the patient to never cross the legs or twist to reach behind.

The physical therapist usually supervises exercises for the affected extremity and ambulation when the HCP allows it. The patient is usually out of bed the first postoperative day. In collaboration with the physical therapist, monitor the patient's ambulation for proper use of crutches or a walker. To be discharged home, the patient must show proper use of crutches or a walker over a functional distance (about 150 ft). The patient must be able to transfer to and from a chair and bed and to go up and down stairs.

Complications associated with femoral neck fracture include nonunion, avascular necrosis, dislocation, and osteoarthritis (OA). The affected leg may be shorter if the patient had an intertrochanteric fracture. A cane or shoe lift may be needed for safe ambulation.

Sudden severe pain, a lump in the buttock, limb shortening, and external rotation indicate prosthesis dislocation. This requires closed reduction with moderate to deep sedation or open reduction under general anesthesia to realign the femoral head in the acetabulum. If any of these signs occur (regardless of the setting), keep the patient NPO in anticipation of surgical intervention.

Help the patient and caregiver to adjust to restrictions and dependence because of the hip fracture. Anxiety and depression can easily occur, but creative nursing care and awareness of potential problems can help to prevent them. Tell the patient and caregiver about community services that can help with rehabilitation after hospital discharge.

◆ **Ambulatory Care.** Hospitalization averages 3 or 4 days. Older adults or patients who live alone may require care in a subacute rehabilitation unit, at a skilled nursing facility, or in an acute rehabilitation facility for a few weeks before returning home. If the patient has skilled nursing needs or is homebound for PT after discharge from postacute care, the HCP may order follow-up home health care.

Home care considerations include ongoing assessment of pain management, monitoring for infection, and prevention of VTE. If incision is closed with metal staples, they will be removed at the HCP's office. Teach the patient who is receiving an anticoagulant to report signs of bleeding to the HCP (see Chapter 37). Review how to administer an injectable anticoagulant (if needed). Teach the patient receiving warfarin about required laboratory testing.

Exercises to restore strength and tone in the quadriceps and muscles around the hip are essential to improve function and ROM. These include quadriceps setting (e.g., pressing the kneecap down), gluteal muscle setting (e.g., tightening the buttocks), leg raises in supine and prone positions, and abduction exercises from the supine and standing positions (e.g., swinging the leg out but never crossing midline). The patient continues these exercises for many months after discharge. Teach the exercise program to the caregiver who will be encouraging the patient at home.

A physical therapist assesses ROM, ambulation, and adherence to the exercise program. The patient gradually increases the number of exercise repetitions and may add ankle weights. Swimming and stationary cycling may tone quadriceps and improve cardiovascular fitness. Teach the patient to avoid high-impact exercises and sports, such as jogging and tennis, because they may loosen the implant. A physical therapist may perform a home assessment to identify hazards that may cause the patient to fall again.

◆ **Evaluation**

The expected outcomes are that the patient with a hip fracture will
• Report satisfactory pain management
• Have uncomplicated bone healing
• Take part in exercise therapy

Gerontologic Considerations: Hip Fracture

Factors that increase the risk for a hip fracture in older adults include (1) increased risk for falling due to an altered center of gravity and inability to correct a postural imbalance, (2) decreased fat and muscle to act as local tissue shock absorbers, and (3) reduced skeletal strength. Other factors that increase the older adult's risk for falling include (1) gait and balance problems, (2) altered vision and hearing, (3) slowed reflexes, (4) orthostatic hypotension, and (5) medication use. Homes can be made safer by (1) eliminating tripping hazards (e.g., throw rugs, uneven surfaces), (2) adding grab bars inside and outside the tub or shower, and beside the toilet, (3) adding railings on both sides of the stairs, and (4) installing better lighting.[23]

Many falls occur when getting in or out of a chair or bed. Falls to the side, the most common type seen in frail older adults, are more likely to result in a hip fracture than a forward fall. External hip protectors may help prevent hip fractures in the frail older patient.[24] Older adults may have low bone density (*osteopenia*) or osteoporosis, which increases their risk for fragility fractures.

Calcium and vitamin D supplementation are given to patients with osteopenia or osteoporosis. A bisphosphonate drug (e.g., alendronate [Fosamax]) may be prescribed to decrease bone loss or increase bone density. This reduces the chance of fracture. (Osteoporosis is discussed in Chapter 63.)

FEMORAL SHAFT FRACTURE

Because the femur can bend slightly to absorb stress, femoral shaft fracture occurs from a severe direct force. The force exerted to cause the fracture (e.g., from a motor vehicle crash or gunshot wound) often also damages the adjacent soft tissue. These injuries may be more serious than the bone injury. Young adults have a high incidence of this type of fracture.

Displacement of fracture fragments often causes increased soft tissue damage. Considerable blood loss (1 to 1.5 L) can occur. The most common types of femoral shaft fracture include transverse, spiral, comminuted, oblique, and open (Figs. 62.6 and 62.7).

A femoral shaft fracture is marked by pain, notable deformity and angulation, shortening of the extremity, and inability to move the hip or knee. Complications include FES; nerve and vascular injury; and problems associated with bone union, open fracture, and soft tissue damage.

Initial management involves patient stabilization and fracture immobilization. Traction may be used as a temporary measure before surgery or in the patient unable to have surgery. Placement of an *intramedullary rod* is the most common surgical treatment for femoral shaft fracture. The metal rod is placed into the marrow canal of the femur. The rod passes across the fracture to keep fragments in position. Plates and screws also may be used. Internal fixation is preferred because it reduces the hospital stay and complications associated with prolonged bed rest. External fixation may be used for an open fracture.

After surgery, gluteal and quadriceps isometric exercises will promote and maintain strength in the affected extremity. Encourage the patient to perform ROM and strengthening exercises for all uninvolved extremities to prepare for ambulation. The patient may be allowed to begin non–weight-bearing activities with an assistive device (e.g., walker, crutches). Full weight bearing is usually restricted until x-rays show union of fracture fragments. Teach the patient to carefully follow the HCP's instructions for weight bearing.

TIBIAL FRACTURE

Although the tibia is vulnerable to injury because it lacks a covering of anterior muscle, strong force is needed to cause a fracture. As a result, soft tissue damage, devascularization, and open fracture are common. The tibia is also a common site for stress fracture. Complications of tibial fractures include compartment syndrome, FES, delayed union or nonunion, and possible infection with an open fracture.

Recommended management for closed tibial fractures is closed reduction followed by immobilization in a long leg cast. ORIF with intramedullary rods, plate fixation, or external fixation is needed for complex fractures and those with extensive soft tissue damage. An emphasis of care is maintaining quadriceps strength.

Assess the neurovascular condition of the affected extremity at least every 2 hours during the first 48 hours. Have the patient perform active ROM exercises with the uninvolved leg and the upper extremities to build the strength needed for crutch walking. When the HCP has determined the patient is ready for gait training, review principles of crutch walking introduced by the physical therapist. The patient may be non–weight bearing for 6 to 12 weeks, depending on healing. Home nursing visits may be needed to monitor the patient's progress if the patient is homebound.

STABLE VERTEBRAL FRACTURE

In a stable fracture, the fracture fragments are unlikely to move or cause spinal cord damage. This type of injury is often confined to the vertebral body (anterior part of the spinal column) in the lumbar region. Sometimes it involves the cervical and thoracic regions. Vertebral bodies are usually protected from displacement by intact spinal ligaments. Stable fractures of the vertebral column are usually caused by motor vehicle crashes, falls, diving, or sports injuries. Patients with osteoporosis have more than 700,000 vertebral compression fractures annually, many of which are stable.

Most patients with stable fractures have only brief periods of disability. However, if spinal ligaments are significantly disrupted, dislocation of the vertebrae may occur. Instability and injury to the spinal cord may result (unstable fracture). These injuries generally require surgery. The most serious complication of vertebral fractures is fracture displacement, which can cause damage to the spinal cord (see Chapter 60). Although stable vertebral fractures are not associated with abnormal spinal cord pathology, all spinal injuries should be considered unstable and potentially serious until diagnostic tests determine the fracture to be stable.

The patient usually has pain and tenderness in the affected region of the spine. There may be a kyphotic deformity (flexion angulation of thoracic vertebrae) known as a *dowager's hump*. This deformity is readily identified during the physical examination (see Fig. 63.9). *Lordosis* (extreme inward curve of lumbar spine) and cervical spine involvement are possible. Sudden loss of function below the fracture indicates spinal cord impingement and paraplegia. Bowel and bladder dysfunction may occur if there is interruption of the autonomic nervous system nerves or injury to the spinal cord.

The overall goal in managing stable vertebral fractures is to keep the spine in good alignment until union is achieved. Many nursing interventions are aimed at assessing for spinal cord trauma (see Chapter 60). Regularly evaluate vital signs and bowel and bladder function. Monitor the motor and sensory function of peripheral nerves distal to the injured region. Promptly report any deterioration in the patient's neurovascular condition.

Treatment includes pain medication followed by early mobilization and bracing. The patient's mattress should be firm to support the spinal column, relax muscles, decrease edema, and prevent potential compression on nerve roots. Teach the patient to keep the spine straight when turning by moving the shoulders and pelvis together. The patient will need nursing help to learn the technique of logrolling. Several days after the initial injury, the HCP may apply a specially constructed orthotic device (e.g., thoracolumbar sacral orthosis [TLSO]), a jacket cast, or a removable corset if there is no evidence of neurologic deficit. The device gives extra support during healing and is used for a short period of time.

Lightweight bracing (e.g., Jewett or Bähler-Vogt brace) may be used for patients with stable vertebral compression fractures due to osteoporosis. Patients with osteoporosis also may be treated with 2 outpatient procedures: vertebroplasty or balloon kyphoplasty. *Vertebroplasty* uses radioimaging to guide the injection of bone cement into a fractured vertebral body. When hardened, the cement stabilizes the vertebra and prevents further compression. *Balloon kyphoplasty* involves first inserting a balloon into the vertebral body and then inflating it. This creates a cavity that is filled with bone cement under low pressure to restore the height of the vertebral body. Kyphoplasty is now the surgical treatment of choice for compression fractures. This is due to the decreased incidence of bone cement leakage into nearby structures (e.g., colon, lung) compared to vertebroplasty. Patients have decreased pain almost at once with these procedures. However, later compression fractures of adjacent vertebrae are a risk.

If the fracture is in the cervical spine, the patient may wear a hard cervical collar. Some cervical fractures are immobilized by use of a halo vest (see Fig. 60.8). This consists of a plastic jacket or cast fitted about the chest and attached to a halo held in place by skeletal pins inserted into the cranium. These devices immobilize the spine in the fracture area while allowing the patient to ambulate.

The patient with a stable vertebral fracture is discharged after (1) showing safe ambulation, (2) learning care of the cast or orthotic device, and (3) stating ways to address safety and security concerns related to the injury and treatment. Unstable vertebral fractures and spinal cord injuries are the subject of Chapter 60.

FACIAL FRACTURE

Any bone of the face can be fractured from trauma, such as a motor vehicle crash, an assault, or a fall. After facial injury it is critically important to establish and maintain a patent airway and provide adequate ventilation. Suctioning may be needed to remove foreign material and blood. A surgically created airway (*tracheostomy*) may be needed if a patent airway cannot be maintained.

Facial fractures and cervical spine injuries often occur together. All patients with facial injuries should be treated as if they have a cervical injury until proven otherwise by examination and CT scan or x-ray. Table 62.12 describes clinical manifestations of common facial fractures.

Related soft tissue injury often makes assessment of facial injury difficult. Perform oral and facial examinations after any life-threatening situations have been treated. Carefully assess ocular muscles and cranial nerves III, IV, and VI. X-rays help determine the extent of the injury. CT scanning helps distinguish between bone and soft tissue injury.

Suspect injury to the eye when facial injury occurs, especially if the injury is near the orbit. If an eye-globe rupture is suspected, stop and place a protective shield over the eye. Signs

TABLE 62.12 Manifestations of Facial Fractures

Fracture	Manifestation
Frontal bone	Rapid edema that may mask underlying fractures
Mandible	Tooth fractures, bleeding, limited motion of mandible
Maxilla	Segmental motion (instability) of maxilla and tooth fracture at socket
Nasal bone	Displacement of nasal bones, nosebleed (epistaxis)
Periorbital bone	Possible frontal sinus involvement, entrapment of ocular muscles
Zygomatic arch	Depression of cheek bone (zygomatic arch) and entrapment of ocular muscles

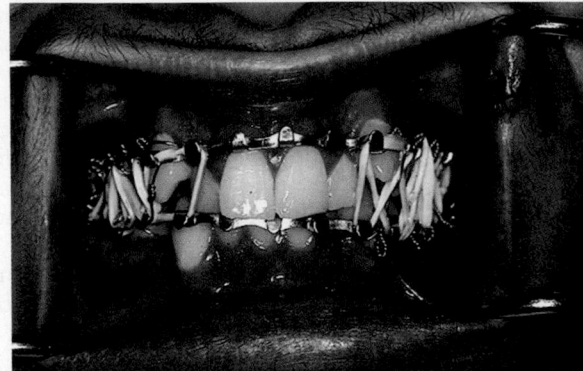

FIG. 62.22 Intermaxillary fixation. (Courtesy R.A. Weinstein, Denver, CO.)

of rupture include vitreous humor forced out of the eye. Brown tissue (iris or ciliary body) may be seen on the surface of the globe or penetrating through a laceration, with an off-center or teardrop-shaped pupil.

Specific treatment depends on the site and extent of the facial fracture and associated soft tissue injury. Immobilization or surgical stabilization may be needed. Maintain a patent airway and adequate nutrition throughout the recovery period.

Be sensitive about changes in appearance that may occur after facial fracture. Changes in appearance may be drastic. Edema and discoloration subside with time, but soft tissue injuries can cause permanent scarring.

MANDIBULAR FRACTURE

Mandibular fracture may result from trauma to the face or jaw. Maxillary fractures may also occur, but they are less common than mandibular fractures. The mandibular fracture may be simple, with no bone displacement, or may involve loss of tissue and bone. The fracture may need immediate treatment to ensure the patient's survival. Long-term treatment is sometimes needed to restore satisfactory appearance and function.

Mandibular fractures may be done therapeutically to correct an underlying alignment problem (malocclusion) that cannot be adjusted by orthodontics alone. The mandible is resected during surgery and manipulated forward or backward to correct the occlusion problem.

Surgery for a mandibular fracture includes immobilization, usually by wiring the jaws (intermaxillary fixation). Internal fixation may be done with screws and plates. In a simple fracture with no loss of teeth, the lower jaw is wired to the upper jaw. Wires are placed around the teeth, and then cross-wires or rubber bands are used to hold the lower jaw tight against the upper jaw (Fig. 62.22). Arch bars may be placed on the maxillary and mandibular arches of the teeth. Vertical wires placed between the arch bars hold the jaws together. If teeth are missing or bone is displaced, other forms of fixation may be needed (e.g., metal arch bars in the mouth or insertion of a pin in the bone). Bone grafting may be needed. Immobilization is usually needed for only 4 to 6 weeks because the fractures often heal rapidly.

❖ NURSING MANAGEMENT: MANDIBULAR FRACTURE

Teach the patient before surgery about what is involved in the surgical procedure, how the face will look afterward, and

changes caused by the surgery. Reassure the patient about the ability to breathe normally, speak, and swallow liquids. Hospitalization for respiratory monitoring is brief unless there are other injuries or problems.

Postoperative care focuses on a patent airway, oral hygiene, communication, pain management, and adequate nutrition. Two potential problems in the immediate postoperative period are airway obstruction and aspiration of vomitus. Because the patient cannot open the jaws, an airway must be maintained. Observe for signs of respiratory distress (e.g., dyspnea; changes in rate, quality, and depth of respirations). After surgery place the patient on the side with the head slightly elevated.

Tape a wire cutter or scissors (for rubber bands) to the head of the bed. Send it with the patient to all appointments and examinations away from the bedside. The wire cutter or scissors may be used to cut the wires or elastic bands in case of an emergency requiring access to the pharynx or lungs (e.g., cardiac arrest or respiratory distress). In the care plan include a picture with the appropriate wires to cut in an emergency. In some cases, cutting the wires may cause the entire facial and upper jaw structure to shift or collapse and worsen the problem. A tracheostomy or endotracheal tray should always be available.

If the patient begins to vomit or choke, try to clear the mouth and airway. Suction via the nasopharyngeal or oral route, depending on the extent of injury and type of repair. An NG tube can remove fluids and gas from the stomach to help prevent vomiting and aspiration. The NG tube can later be used as a feeding tube. Antiemetics may be given. Teach the patient to clear secretions and vomitus.

Oral hygiene is very important. Teach the patient to remove food debris by rinsing the mouth often, especially after meals and snacks. Warm normal saline solution, water, or alkaline mouthwashes may be used. A syringe and soft irrigation catheter or a Water Pik may be effective for thorough oral cleansing. Inspect the mouth several times a day to see that it is clean. Use a tongue depressor to retract the cheeks. Keep the lips, corners of the mouth, and buccal mucosa moist. Cover any sharp edges of the wires with dental wax to prevent irritation of the buccal mucosa.

Communication may be a problem, especially in the early postoperative period. Establish an effective way of communicating before surgery (e.g., use of dry erase board, pad and pencil). Usually the patient can speak well enough to be understood, especially a few days after surgery.

Intake of adequate nutrients may be a challenge because the diet must be liquid. The patient easily tires of sucking through a straw or laboriously using a spoon. Work with the dietitian and patient to plan a diet with adequate calories, protein, and fluids. Liquid protein supplements may improve the patient's nutrition. The low-bulk, high-carbohydrate diet and intake of air through the straw contribute to constipation and gas. Ambulation, prune juice, and bulk-forming laxatives may help relieve these problems.

The patient is usually discharged with the wires in place. Encourage the patient to share feelings about the changes in appearance. Discharge teaching should include oral care, diet, how to handle secretions, how and when to use wire cutters or scissors, and when to notify the HCP about concerns and problems.

AMPUTATION

An **amputation** is the removal of a body extremity by trauma or surgery. About 2 million Americans are living with limb loss.[25] About 185,000 amputations occur each year in the United States. Most amputations are done due to PVD, especially in older patients with diabetes. These patients often have peripheral neuropathy that progresses to deep ulcers and gangrene. Amputation in young people is usually due to trauma (e.g., motor vehicle crashes, farm-related injury). Battle injuries have affected over 1700 veterans since 2003, with several losing more than 1 limb.[26] Other common reasons for amputation include thermal injuries, tumors, osteomyelitis, and congenital limb disorders.

Diagnostic Studies

Diagnostic studies depend on the underlying reason for the amputation (Table 62.13). An increased white blood cell (WBC) count with abnormal differential may show infection. Vascular tests such as arteriography, Doppler studies, and venography give information about circulation in the extremity.

Interprofessional Care

If amputation is planned or elective, as for the patient with PVD, carefully assess the patient's general health. Chronic illnesses and infection must be managed before an amputation is done. Help the patient and caregiver understand the need for the amputation. Assure them that rehabilitation can help with quality of life. If the amputation is done emergently after trauma, patient management is physically and emotionally more complicated.

The goal of surgery is to preserve the greatest extremity length and function while removing all infected, pathologic, or ischemic tissue. Levels of amputation of upper and lower extremities are shown in Fig. 62.23. The type of amputation depends on the reason for the surgery. A closed amputation creates a weight-bearing *residual limb* (or stump). An anterior skin flap with dissected soft tissue padding covers the bony part of the residual limb. The skin flap is sutured posteriorly so that the suture line will not be in a weight-bearing area. Take special care to prevent accumulation of drainage, which can cause pressure and harbor bacteria that may cause infection.

Disarticulation is an amputation done through a joint. A *Syme's amputation* is a form of disarticulation at the ankle. After an open amputation *(guillotine amputation),* the surface of the residual limb is left uncovered with skin. This type of surgery is generally done to control actual or potential infection. The wound is usually closed later by a second surgical procedure or closed by skin traction surrounding the residual limb.

TABLE 62.13 Interprofessional Care
Amputation

Diagnostic Assessment	Management
• History and physical examination	**Medical**
• Physical appearance of soft tissues	• Appropriate management of underlying disease
• Skin temperature	• Stabilization of trauma victim
• Sensory function	
• Quality of peripheral pulses	**Surgical**
• Arteriography	• Residual limb management
• Venography	• Immediate or delayed prosthesis fitting
• Plethysmography (measures blood flow in the arms or legs)	
• Transcutaneous ultrasonic Doppler recordings	**Rehabilitation**
	• Coordination of prosthesis-fitting and gait-training activities
	• Coordination of muscle-strengthening and PT programs

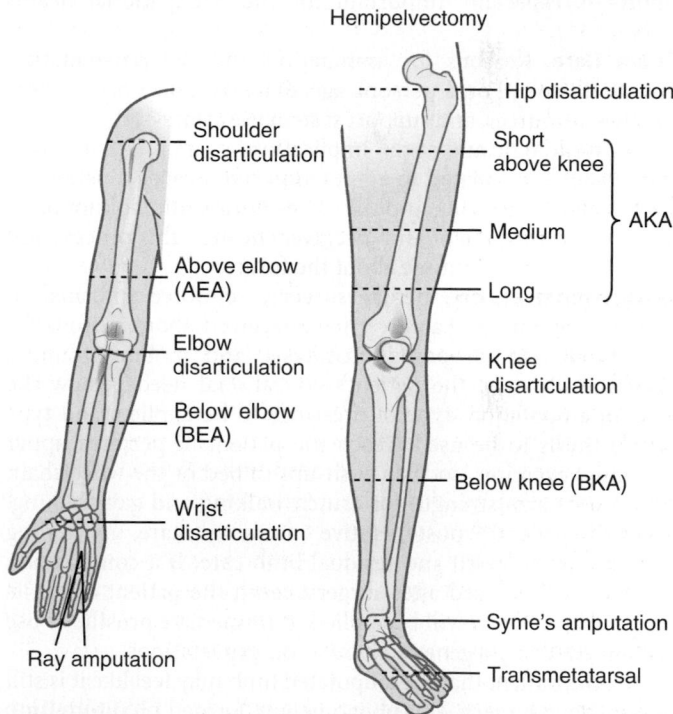

FIG. 62.23 Location and description of amputation sites of the upper and lower extremities. *AKA,* Above-the-knee amputation.

❖ NURSING MANAGEMENT: AMPUTATION

◆ Nursing Assessment

Assess for any preexisting illnesses. Because most amputations are done for vascular problems, assessment of vascular and neurologic condition is especially important (see Chapters 31 and 55).

◆ Nursing Diagnoses

Nursing diagnoses for the patient with an amputation may include:
• Disturbed body image
• Impaired tissue integrity
• Chronic pain
• Impaired physical mobility

◆ **Planning**

The overall goals are that the patient with an amputation will (1) have adequate relief from the underlying health problem, (2) have satisfactory pain management, (3) reach maximum rehabilitation potential (with the use of a prosthesis, if indicated), (4) cope with the body image changes, and (5) make satisfying lifestyle adjustments.

◆ **Nursing Implementation**

◆ **Health Promotion.** Control of illnesses, such as PVD, diabetes, chronic osteomyelitis, and pressure injuries, can eliminate or delay the need for amputation. Teach patients with these problems to carefully examine their lower extremities daily for signs of infection or skin breakdown. If the patient cannot do this, the caregiver should help. Teach the patient and caregiver to report changes in the feet or toes to the HCP. These include decreased or absent sensation, tingling, burning pain, cuts, or abrasions, and changes in skin color or temperature.

Review safety precautions for people taking part in recreational activities and potentially hazardous work. This responsibility is especially important for the occupational health nurse.

◆ **Acute Care.** Reasons for amputation and the rehabilitation potential depend on a person's age, diagnosis, occupation, personality, resources, and support system. Be aware of the tremendous psychologic and social implications of amputation. Body image problems related to amputation often cause a patient to go through a grieving process. Use therapeutic communication to help the patient and caregiver through this process and develop a realistic attitude about the future.

Preoperative Care. Before surgery, reinforce information that the patient and caregiver have received about reasons for the amputation, proposed prosthesis, and mobility-training program. To meet the patient's educational needs, know the level of amputation, type of dressings to be applied, and type of prosthesis to be used. Teach the patient to perform upper extremity exercises, such as push-ups in bed or the wheelchair, to promote arm strength for crutch walking and gait training. Discuss general postoperative nursing care, including positioning, support, and residual limb care. If a compression bandage will be used after surgery, teach the patient about its purpose and how it will be applied. If immediate prosthesis use is planned, discuss general ambulation expectations.

Tell the patient that the amputated limb may feel like it is still present after surgery. This phenomenon, termed **phantom limb sensation**, occurs in many amputees. (Nursing management of phantom limb sensation is discussed in the next section.)

Postoperative Care. General care for the patient who had an amputation depends largely on the patient's age and general state of health and the reason for the amputation. Monitor patients who had an amputation due to a traumatic injury for posttraumatic stress disorder because they may have had no time to prepare or even take part in the decision to have a limb amputated.

Prevention and detection of complications are important after surgery. Carefully monitor the patient's vital signs. Assess dressings for hemorrhage. Use sterile technique during dressing changes to reduce the risk for wound infection.

If an *immediate* postoperative prosthesis has been applied, carefully observe the surgical site. If excess bleeding occurs, notify the HCP at once. Keep a surgical tourniquet available for emergency use.

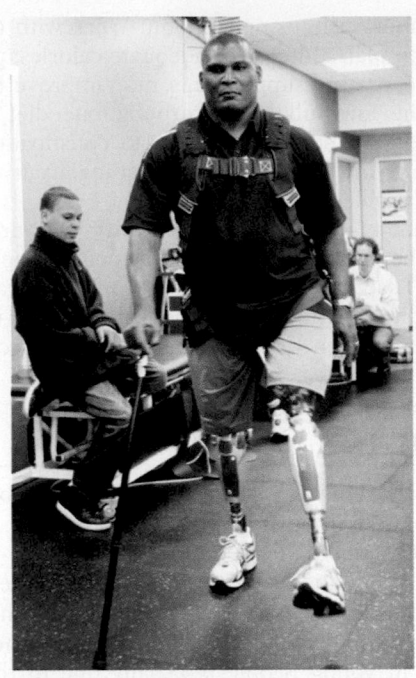

FIG. 62.24 A double amputee fitted with prostheses. (Photo courtesy US Army.)

The *delayed* prosthetic fitting may be the best choice for older adults, patients with infection, or patients who have had amputations above the knee or below the elbow (Fig. 62.24). Appropriate timing for the use of a prosthesis depends on satisfactory healing of the residual limb and the patient's general condition. A temporary prosthesis may be used for partial weight bearing after sutures are removed. If there are no problems, the patient can bear full weight on a permanent prosthesis about 3 months after amputation.

Not all patients are candidates for prostheses. The seriously ill or debilitated patient may not have the upper body strength and energy needed to use a lower extremity prosthesis. Mobility with a wheelchair may be the most realistic goal for this patient.

Patients are often extremely worried about phantom limb sensation because they still perceive pain in the missing part of the limb. As recovery and ambulation progress, phantom limb sensation and pain usually subside. However, the pain may become chronic. The patient may have shooting, burning, or crushing pain as well as feelings of coldness, heaviness, and cramping,

Unfortunately, there is no one therapy for phantom limb sensation. Mirror therapy reduces symptoms in some patients (Fig. 62.25).[27] We do not know why looking in the mirror at the remaining limb would improve symptoms. The mirror is thought to give visual information to the brain, replacing sensory feedback expected from the missing limb. Mirror therapy may also improve patient function after a stroke.

Success of the rehabilitation program depends on the patient's physical and emotional health. Chronic illness and deconditioning can complicate rehabilitation. Physical and occupational therapy must be a central part of the patient's overall plan of care.

Flexion contractures may delay rehabilitation. The most common and debilitating contracture is hip flexion. Hip adduction contracture is rare. To prevent flexion contractures, have patients avoid sitting in a chair for more than 1 hour with hips

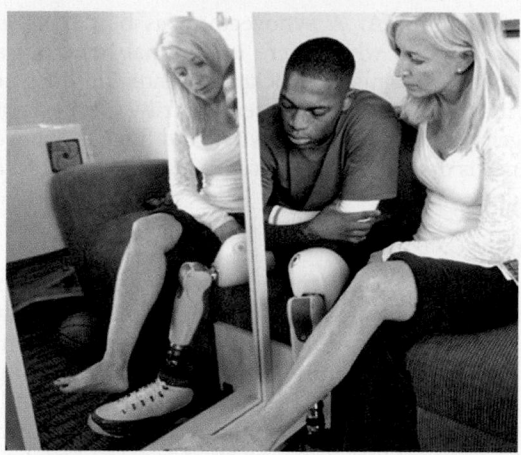

FIG. 62.25 Mirror therapy, a type of treatment that may reduce phantom limb sensation and pain. (US Navy photo courtesy Mass Communication Specialist Seaman Joseph A. Boomhower.)

Start of second bandage

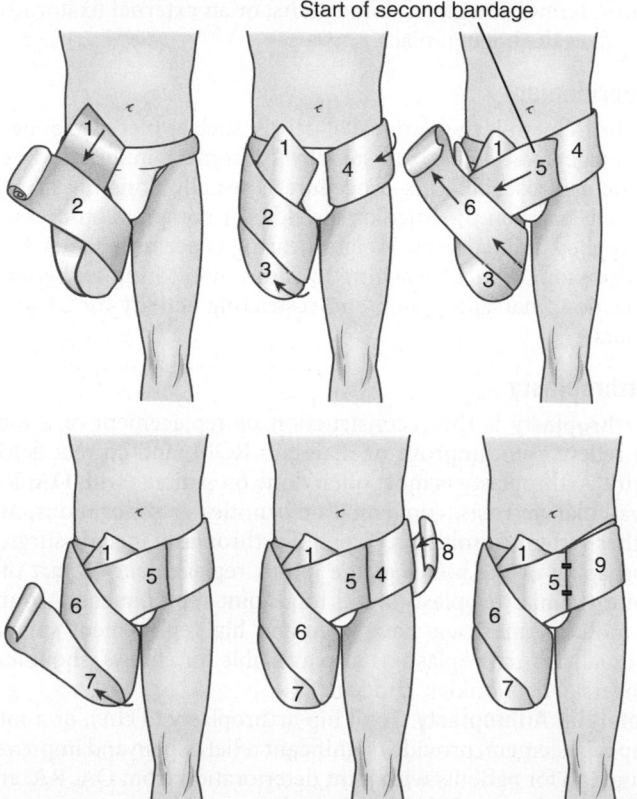

FIG. 62.26 Bandaging for the above-the-knee amputation residual limb. Figure-8 style covers progressive areas of the residual limb; 2 elastic wraps used.

flexed or having pillows under the surgical extremity. Unless contraindicated, patients should lie on their abdomen for 30 minutes 3 or 4 times each day and position the hip in extension while prone.

Proper bandaging ensures the residual limb is shaped and molded for eventual prosthesis fitting (Fig. 62.26). The HCP usually orders a compression bandage to be applied right after surgery to support soft tissues, reduce edema, hasten healing, and minimize pain. Compression also promotes residual limb

TABLE 62.14 **Patient & Caregiver Teaching**
Lower Extremity Amputation
After lower extremity amputation, include the following instructions when teaching the patient and caregiver:
1. Inspect the residual limb daily for signs of skin irritation, especially redness, abrasion, and odor. Especially evaluate areas prone to pressure.
2. Stop using the prosthesis if irritation develops. Have the area checked before resuming use of the prosthesis.
3. Wash the residual limb thoroughly each night with warm water and bacteriostatic soap. Rinse thoroughly and dry gently. Expose the residual limb to air for 20 min.
4. Do not use lotions, alcohol, powders, or oil on residual limb unless prescribed by the HCP.
5. Wear only a residual limb sock in good condition and supplied by the prosthetist.
6. Change residual limb sock daily. Launder in mild soap, squeeze, lay flat to dry.
7. Use prescribed pain management techniques.
8. Perform ROM to all joints daily. Perform general strengthening exercises (including for upper extremities) daily.
9. Do not elevate residual limb on a pillow.
10. Lay prone with hip in extension for 30 min 3 or 4 times daily.

shrinkage and maturation. This bandage may be an elastic roll applied to the residual limb or a residual limb shrinker, which is an elastic stocking that fits tightly over the residual limb.

At first, the patient always wears the compression bandage except during PT and bathing. Remove and reapply the bandage several times daily. Take care to apply it snugly but not so tight as to interfere with circulation. Wash and change shrinker bandages daily. After the residual limb is healed, bandage it only when the patient is not wearing the prosthesis. Teach the patient to avoid dangling the residual limb over the bedside to decrease edema.

As the patient's overall condition improves, the HCP and physical therapist start and supervise an exercise program. Active ROM exercises for all joints should be started as soon as possible after surgery. To prepare for mobility, the patient should increase triceps and shoulder strength for lower limb support. The patient will need to learn to balance the altered body. The lost weight of an amputated limb requires adaptation of the patient's proprioception and coordination to prevent falls and injury.

Crutch walking starts as soon as the patient is physically able. Follow orders for weight bearing carefully to avoid injury to the skin flap and delay of tissue healing. Before discharge, teach the patient and caregiver about residual limb care, ambulation, contracture prevention, recognition of complications, exercise, and follow-up care (Table 62.14).

◆ **Ambulatory Care.** When healing has occurred satisfactorily, and the residual limb is well molded, the patient is ready for prosthesis fitting. A prosthetist makes a mold of the residual limb and measures landmarks for creation of the prosthesis. The molded limb socket allows the residual limb to fit snugly into the prosthesis. The residual limb is covered with a stocking to ensure good fit and prevent skin breakdown. If the limb continues to shrink, causing a loose fit, a new socket has to be made. The patient may need to have the prosthesis adjusted to prevent rubbing and friction between the residual limb and socket. Excessive movement of a loose prosthesis can cause severe skin irritation, breakdown, and gait problems.

Artificial limbs become an integral part of the patient's changed body image. Teach the patient to clean the prosthesis socket daily with mild soap and rinse thoroughly to remove irritants. Leather and metal parts of the prosthesis should not get wet. Encourage the patient to have regular maintenance on the prosthesis. Consider the condition of the patient's shoe. A badly worn shoe alters the gait and can damage the prosthesis.

◆ **Special Considerations in Upper Limb Amputation.** Emotional implications of an upper limb amputation are often more devastating than for lower limb amputation. Despite technologic advances, we cannot replicate the movements and functional capacity of our hands with upper extremity prostheses.[28] The enforced dependency due to being 1-handed may be depressing and frustrating to the patient. Because most upper extremity amputations result from trauma, the patient likely had little time to adjust psychologically or be a part of the decision-making process.

Both immediate and delayed prosthetic fittings are possible for the below-the-elbow amputee. Prosthetic fitting is delayed for the above-the-elbow amputee. The usual functional prosthesis is the arm and hook. A cosmetic hand is available but has limited functional value. As with the lower limb prosthesis, patient motivation and perseverance are major factors contributing to a satisfactory outcome.

◆ **Evaluation**

The expected outcomes are that the patient with an amputation will

* Accept changed body image and integrate changes into lifestyle
* Have no evidence of skin breakdown
* Have reduction or absence of pain
* Become mobile within limitations imposed by amputation

Gerontologic Considerations: Amputation

If a lower limb amputation has been done on an older adult, the patient's previous ability to ambulate may affect the extent of recovery. Using a prosthesis requires significant strength and energy for ambulation. For example, walking with a below-the-knee prosthesis requires 40% more energy than walking on 2 legs. An above-the-knee prosthesis requires 60% more. Older adults whose general health is weakened by disorders such as heart or lung disease may not be able to use a prosthesis. The patient's ability to ambulate may be limited. If possible, discuss these issues with the patient and caregiver before surgery so that realistic expectations can be set.

COMMON JOINT SURGICAL PROCEDURES

Surgery plays a vital role in the treatment and rehabilitation of patients with various joint problems. The goals of surgery are to relieve chronic pain, improve joint motion, correct deformity and misalignment, and remove diseased cartilage. If the joint problem is not corrected, contraction with permanent limitation of motion may occur. Limited joint motion can be noted on physical examination. Joint-space narrowing can be seen on x-rays.

TYPES OF JOINT SURGERIES

Synovectomy

Synovectomy (removal of synovial membrane) is done to remove inflamed tissue that is causing unacceptable pain or limiting ROM in RA. A synovectomy is best done early in the disease process when there is minimal bone or cartilage destruction. Removing the thickened synovium does not cure RA but may relieve symptoms temporarily. Common sites for this surgery include the elbow, wrist, and fingers. Synovectomy in the knee is done less often because knee joint replacement is usually done.

Osteotomy

An osteotomy involves removing a wedge or slice of bone to restore alignment (joint and vertebral) and to shift weight bearing, thus relieving pain. Cervical osteotomy may be used to correct a kyphotic deformity in patients with ankylosing spondylitis. Halo vests and body jacket braces are worn until fusion occurs (3 to 4 months). Osteotomy is not effective in patients with inflammatory joint disease. However, femoral osteotomy may provide some pain relief and improve motion in select patients with hip osteoarthritis (OA). Tibial osteotomy also provides pain relief in some patients with knee instability or OA.[29]

Care of a patient who had an osteotomy is similar to that of a patient with ORIF of a fracture at a comparable site. Internal wires, screws and plates, bone grafts, or an external fixator usually fixes the bone in place.

Debridement

Debridement is the removal of debris, such as pieces of bone or cartilage (loose bodies) or osteophytes, from a joint using a fiberoptic arthroscope. This procedure is usually done on an outpatient basis on the knee or shoulder. A compression dressing is applied after surgery. Weight bearing is permitted after knee arthroscopy. Patient teaching includes monitoring for signs of infection, managing pain, and restricting activity for 24 to 48 hours.

Arthroplasty

Arthroplasty is the reconstruction or replacement of a joint to relieve pain, improve or maintain ROM, and correct deformity. Arthroplasty is most often done on patients with OA, RA, avascular necrosis, congenital deformities or dislocations, and other systemic problems. Types of arthroplasty include surgical reshaping of the bones of the joints, replacement of part of a joint (hemiarthroplasty), and total joint replacement. Around 1 million Americans have knee and hip replacement surgery annually.[30] Arthroplasty is also available for elbows, shoulders, fingers, wrists, ankles, and feet.

Total Hip Arthroplasty. Total hip arthroplasty (THA), or a total hip replacement, provides significant relief of pain and improved function for patients with joint deterioration from OA, RA, and other conditions. THA is also used to treat hip fractures.

In THA, the prosthesis (implant) replaces the ball-and-socket joint formed by the upper shaft of the femur and pelvis (Fig. 62.27). Both the ball-and-socket components can be cemented in place with polymethyl methacrylate, which bonds to the bone. They may also be inserted without cement (cementless). Cementless THA may provide longer stability by enabling ingrowth of new bone tissue into the porous surface coating of the prosthesis. Cementless devices are recommended for younger, more active patients and patients with good bone quality so that bone ingrowth into the components can be readily achieved.

The nursing care for a patient who had a THA is discussed in the section on nursing management of a patient with a hip fracture on pp. 1463–1466.

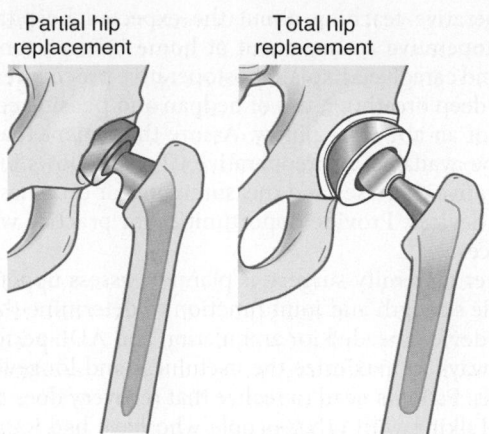

FIG 62.27 Types of hip replacements.

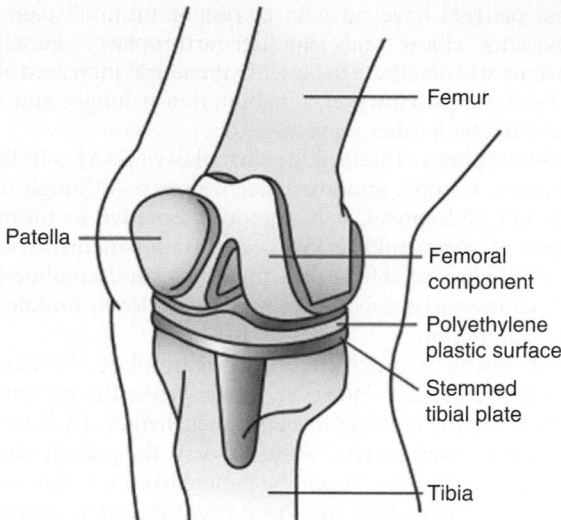

FIG. 62.28 Knee arthroplasty components. Up to 3 bone surfaces can be replaced in a total knee replacement. (Modified from Odom-Forren J: *Drain's perianesthesia nursing,* ed 7, St Louis, 2018, Elsevier.)

INFORMATICS IN PRACTICE

Web-Based Knee and Hip Replacement Community

- Most hospitals offer preoperative classes for patients undergoing joint replacement surgery, but fewer resources are available after discharge.
- Online knee and hip replacement communities offer the patient a place to share experiences and receive social support. The patient is likely to feel relieved knowing that others have similar experiences.
- Encourage patients to confirm any advice with the HCP before taking action.

Hip Resurfacing Arthroplasty. An alternative to hip replacement is hip resurfacing arthroplasty. It preserves and reshapes the femoral head (ball) rather than replacing it as in THA. The resurfaced femoral head is then capped by a metal prosthesis. Hip resurfacing may be an option for patients younger than age 60 with larger frames. A small number of patients will have a femoral neck fracture after hip resurfacing. This is not possible with THA. In addition, metal ions may be released into the bloodstream from the prosthesis. Patients may develop sensitivity or allergy to these ions.[31] Patients receiving a smaller femoral head (including many women) have a higher failure rate with a resurfaced implant when compared with patients receiving THA.

Knee Arthroplasty. Unrelieved pain and instability due to severe deterioration of the knee joint are the main reasons for total knee arthroplasty (TKA), or a total knee replacement (Fig. 62.28). Partial arthroplasty can be done on a patient with osteoarthritis limited to 1 part (compartment) of the knee.

Immediately after surgery a compression dressing may be used to immobilize the knee in extension. This dressing is removed before discharge. If the patient is unable to perform a straight-leg raise, a knee immobilizer or posterior plastic shell to maintain extension may be used during ambulation and at rest for about 4 weeks.

After surgery, emphasis is on pain management and PT. Managing pain is a primary nursing goal. Doing so decreases the patient's risk for complications and hastens the return to function.[32] Adequate analgesia should be ordered at discharge to allow the patient to continue with the exercise program. Effective pain management is key to achieving positive rehabilitation outcomes.

PT begins early with isometric quadriceps setting. Therapy progresses to straight-leg raises and gentle ROM to increase muscle strength and obtain 90-degree knee flexion. Active flexion exercises or passive flexion exercises with a continuous passive motion (CPM) machine may promote joint mobility. Ambulation starts early and typically progresses to full weight bearing before discharge. An active home exercise program involves progressive ROM with muscle strengthening and flexibility exercises. After TKA, many older patients with advanced OA show significant improvement in mobility, motor function tests, and ability to complete daily tasks.

Finger Joint Arthroplasty. A silicone rubber arthroplastic device is used to restore function in the fingers of the patient with RA. Ulnar deviation often causes severe functional limitations of the hand. The goal of hand surgery is primarily to restore function related to grasp, pinch, stability, and strength rather than to correct cosmetic deformity. Before surgery, the patient is taught hand exercises, including flexion, extension, abduction, and adduction of the fingers.

After surgery, a bulk dressing is placed and the hand is kept elevated. Perform regular neurovascular assessment and monitor for signs of infection. Success of the surgery depends largely on the postoperative treatment plan, which is usually implemented by an OT. After the dressing is removed, a guided splinting program is started. The patient is discharged with splints to use while sleeping and hand exercises to do at least 3 or 4 times a day for 10 to 12 weeks. Teach the patient to avoid lifting heavy objects.

Elbow and Shoulder Arthroplasty. Total replacement of elbow and shoulder joints is not as common as other forms of arthroplasty. Shoulder replacements are done in patients with severe pain because of RA, OA, avascular necrosis, or trauma. A specialized type of shoulder replacement, called a reverse total shoulder arthroplasty, may be done for pain and dysfunction caused by massive, irreparable, rotator cuff tears. Shoulder replacement is usually considered if the patient has adequate surrounding muscle strength and bone density. If joint replacement is needed for both elbow and shoulder, the elbow is usually done first because a severely painful elbow interferes with the shoulder rehabilitation program.

Most patients have no pain at rest or minimal pain with activity after elbow and shoulder arthroplasty. Functional improvements contribute to better hygiene and increased ability to perform ADLs. However, rehabilitation is longer and more difficult than with other joint surgeries.

Ankle Arthroplasty. Total ankle arthroplasty (TAA) is indicated for RA, OA, trauma, and avascular necrosis. Although use of TAA is not widespread, it is a good alternative to fusion for treatment of severe ankle arthritis in certain patients. Available devices include several fixed-bearing devices and a mobile-bearing cementless prosthesis. This device more closely imitates natural ankle function.

Ankle fusion is often done over arthroplasty because the result is more durable. However, fusion leaves the patient with a stiff foot and the inability to change heel height. TAA achieves a more normal gait pattern. After surgery, the patient may not bear weight for 6 weeks. Teach the patient to elevate the extremity to reduce edema, take steps to prevent infection, and maintain immobilization as directed by the HCP.

Arthrodesis

Arthrodesis is the surgical fusion of a joint. This procedure is done only if articular surfaces are too severely damaged or infected to allow joint replacement or if reconstructive surgery fails. Arthrodesis relieves pain and provides a stable but immobile joint. The fusion is usually done by removing the articular hyaline cartilage and adding bone grafts across the joint surface. The affected joint must be immobilized until bone healing has occurred. Common areas fused are wrist, ankle, cervical spine, lumbar spine, and metatarsophalangeal (MTP) joint of the great toe.

Complications of Joint Surgery

Infection is a serious complication of joint surgery, especially joint replacement surgery. The most common causative organisms are gram-positive aerobic streptococci and staphylococci. Infection may lead to pain and loosening of the prosthesis, generally requiring further surgery. Efforts to reduce infection include the use of specially designed self-contained operating suites, operating rooms with laminar airflow, and prophylactic antibiotic administration.

VTE is another potentially serious complication after joint surgeries, especially those involving the lower extremities. Provide prophylactic measures, such as anticoagulant drugs, use of intermittent pneumatic compression devices, and early ambulation. Assess patients for signs of VTE. VTE is discussed in Chapter 37.

NURSING AND INTERPROFESSIONAL MANAGEMENT: JOINT SURGERY

Preoperative Management

The primary goal of preoperative assessment is to identify risk factors for postoperative complications so we can implement measures to promote optimal outcomes. A careful history includes (1) medical diagnoses and complications, such as diabetes and VTE; (2) pain tolerance and management preferences; (3) current functional level and expectations after surgery; (4) current social support; and (5) home care needs after discharge. The patient should be free from infection and acute joint inflammation.

Preoperative teaching about the expected hospital course and postoperative management at home is important for the patient and caregiver. Explain postoperative procedures, such as turning, deep breathing, use of bedpan and bedside commode, and use of an abductor pillow. Assure the patient that analgesia will be available. A preoperative PT visit allows practice of postoperative exercises and measurement for crutches or other assistive devices. Provide opportunities for practice with assistive devices.

If lower extremity surgery is planned, assess upper extremity muscle strength and joint function to determine the type of assistive devices needed for ambulation and ADL performance. Discuss ways to maximize the usefulness and longevity of the prosthesis. Patients need to realize that recovery does not occur rapidly. Talking with other people who have had joint arthroplasty may help the patient better understand the reality of rehabilitation.

Discharge planning begins immediately. Discuss the duration of the hospital stay and the expected postoperative events so that the patient and caregiver can prepare. Discuss the safety and accessibility of the home environment (e.g., throw rugs, cords). Are the bathroom and bedroom on the first floor? Are door frames wide enough to accommodate a walker? Assess the patient's social support. Is a friend or family member available to help the patient at home? Will the patient need homemaker or meal services? The older patient may need to be discharged to a subacute or extended care facility for a few weeks to regain independent living skills.

Postoperative Management

Regularly perform neurovascular assessment postoperatively. Give ordered anticoagulant medication, analgesia, and parenteral antibiotics. Pain management strategies may include epidural or intrathecal analgesia, femoral nerve block, patient-controlled IV analgesia, and oral opioids or NSAIDs. Assess patient comfort often during the postoperative period. Monitor for postoperative complications. Nursing interventions for the patient having orthopedic surgery are presented in eNursing Care Plan 62.2 (available on the website for this chapter).

Assess ROM at regular intervals to facilitate the goal of improved functional performance. In general, the affected joint is exercised and ambulation is encouraged as early as possible to prevent complications of immobility. Specific protocols vary according to the patient, type of prosthesis, and HCP preference. Depending on the surgical approach, an abduction pillow may be used after THA.

The hospital stay after arthroplasty is about 3 days depending on the patient's course and need for PT. Some patients are discharged in 1 to 2 days. Some knee replacement surgeries are done at ambulatory surgical centers. Teach the patient to report complications, including infection (e.g., fever, increased pain, drainage) and dislocation of the prosthesis (e.g., pain, loss of function, shortening or malalignment of an extremity).

PT and ambulation enhance mobility, build muscle strength, and reduce the risk for VTE. Prophylactic anticoagulant drugs should be given for at least 10 to 14 days.[20] Some patients need therapy for up to 35 days. If the patient is taking warfarin, therapy starts on the day of surgery and the INR and prothrombin times are measured daily. Therapy with LMWH (e.g., enoxaparin), apixaban, or rivaroxaban usually starts the morning after surgery.[33]

CASE STUDY

Periprosthetic Hip Fracture and Revision Arthroplasty

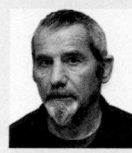

Patient Profile

M.C. is a 64-yr-old white man who has had both hips replaced (left 6 years ago, right 2 years ago). He has a history of hypothyroidism. He was admitted to the ED after tripping over a short retaining wall in his backyard while gardening. He landed on his right side.

(© aronaze/ iStock.com.)

Subjective Data

- Acute, severe pain in right hip, unable to bear weight on right leg
- Takes cholecalciferol (vitamin D₃) 1000 IU every day without calcium supplement. States calcium upsets his stomach
- Reports loss of about 30 lb in the last year through diet and exercise. Exercises 3 times a week
- Lives in multilevel house with his wife. Bedrooms are on the second level
- Has smoked ½ pack of cigarettes a day for the past 30 years
- Describes himself as "a very light social drinker"

Objective Data

- 5 ft, 9 in tall, 175 lb

Diagnostic Studies

- X-rays show periprosthetic right proximal femur fracture at the greater trochanter with loss of fixation in the femoral part of the THA
- Normal CBC, chest x-ray
- Serum calcium 8.1 mg/dL

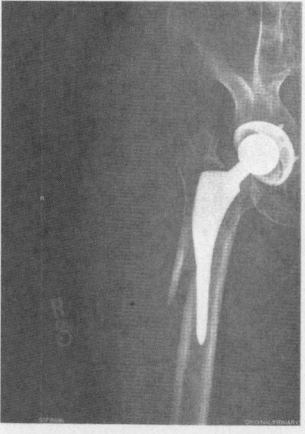

Interprofessional Care

- Revision of femoral part of his right total hip replacement with open reduction of the femoral fracture and fixation with 3 wires
- IV hydromorphone (Dilaudid) 1 mg IV every 3 hr as needed
- Cefazolin 1 gram IV every 8 hr for 24 hr
- Enoxaparin (Lovenox) 40 mg subcutaneous daily for 4 wk
- Calcium citrate 600 mg plus 800 IU vitamin D orally daily
- Levothyroxine (Synthroid) 125 mcg orally daily
- PT for transfers, gait, and stair training
- Occupational therapy for ADLs training
- Discharge planning based on mobility limitations and need for continued PT and OT

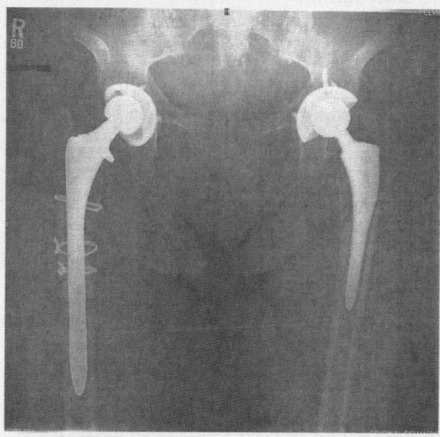

Discussion Questions

1. ***Patient-Centered Care:*** How do M.C.'s previous total joint surgeries affect his recovery after this surgery?
2. ***Priority Decision:*** As you plan care for M.C., what are the perioperative priority nursing interventions?
3. What are the most likely postoperative complications M.C. could develop?
4. In considering M.C.'s patient profile, what issues can you identify that may affect his bone healing?
5. ***Priority Decision:*** What are the priority assessments that should be done prior to discharge?
6. ***Collaboration:*** What is the interprofessional team's top priority at this time for M.C.?
7. ***Quality Improvement:*** What outcomes would indicate interprofessional care was effective?
8. ***Safety:*** What safety precautions should be considered for M.C.?
9. ***Evidence-Based Practice:*** Why is satisfactory pain management an important postoperative nursing goal for M.C.?

Answers available at *http://evolve.elsevier.com/Lewis/medsurg.*

BRIDGE TO NCLEX EXAMINATION

The number of the question corresponds to the same-numbered outcome at the beginning of the chapter.

1. The nurse suspects an ankle sprain when a patient at the urgent care center describes
   a. being hit by another soccer player during a game.
   b. having ankle pain after sprinting around the track.
   c. dropping a 10-lb weight on his lower leg at the health club.
   d. twisting his ankle while running bases during a baseball game.

2. A patient with a humeral fracture is returning for a 4-week checkup. The nurse explains that initial evidence of healing on x-ray is indicated by
   a. formation of callus.
   b. complete bony union.
   c. hematoma at the fracture site.
   d. presence of granulation tissue.

3. A patient with a comminuted fracture of the tibia is to have an open reduction with internal fixation (ORIF) of the fracture. The nurse explains that ORIF is indicated when
   a. the patient is unable to tolerate prolonged immobilization.
   b. the patient cannot tolerate the surgery for a closed reduction.
   c. other nonsurgical methods cannot achieve adequate alignment.
   d. a temporary cast would be too unstable to provide normal mobility.

4. The nurse suspects a neurovascular problem based on assessment of
   a. exaggerated strength with movement.
   b. increased redness and heat below the injury.
   c. decreased sensation distal to the fracture site.
   d. purulent drainage at the site of an open fracture.

5. A patient with a stable, closed humeral fracture has a temporary splint with bulky padding applied with an elastic bandage. The nurse notifies the provider of possible early compartment syndrome when the patient has
   a. increasing edema of the limb.
   b. muscle spasms of the lower arm.
   c. bounding pulse at the fracture site.
   d. pain when passively extending the fingers.

6. A patient with a pelvic fracture should be monitored for
   a. changes in urine output.
   b. petechiae on the abdomen.
   c. a palpable lump in the buttock.
   d. sudden increase in blood pressure.

7. The nurse teaches the patient with an above-the-knee amputation that the residual limb should not be routinely elevated because this position promotes
   a. hip flexion contracture.
   b. clot formation at the incision.
   c. skin irritation and breakdown.
   d. increased risk for wound dehiscence.

8. A patient with osteoarthritis is scheduled for total hip arthroplasty. The nurse explains the purpose of this procedure is to (select all that apply)
   a. fuse the joint.
   b. replace the joint.
   c. prevent further damage.
   d. improve or maintain ROM.
   e. decrease the amount of destruction in the joint.

9. A patient is scheduled for total ankle replacement. The nurse should tell the patient that after surgery he should avoid
   a. lifting heavy objects.
   b. sleeping on the back.
   c. abduction exercises of the affected ankle.
   d. bearing weight on the affected leg for 6 weeks.

1. d, 2. a, 3. c, 4. c, 5. d, 6. a, 7. a, 8. b, d, 9. d

For rationales to these answers and even more NCLEX review questions, visit *http://evolve.elsevier.com/Lewis/medsurg*.

EVOLVE WEBSITE/RESOURCES LIST

http://evolve.elsevier.com/Lewis/medsurg
Review Questions (Online Only)
Key Points
Answer Keys for Questions
- Rationales for Bridge to NCLEX Examination Questions
- Answer Guidelines for Case Study on p. 1475
Student Case Studies
- Patient With Musculoskeletal Trauma
- Patient With Parkinson's Disease and Hip Fracture
Nursing Care Plans
- eNursing Care Plan 62.1: Patient With a Fracture
- eNursing Care Plan 62.2: Patient Having Orthopedic Surgery
Concept Map Creator
Audio Glossary
Supporting Media
- Animations
  - ORIF Ankle
  - Total Knee Replacement
Content Updates

REFERENCES

1. Centers for Disease Control and Prevention (CDC): Leading causes of death, 2016. Retrieved from *www.cdc.gov/injury/wisqars/facts.html*.
2. National Institute of Arthritis and Musculoskeletal and Skin Diseases: Preventing sports injuries in youth: A guide for parents. Retrieved from *www.niams.nih.gov/Health_Info/Sports_Injuries/child_sports_injuries.asp*.
3. American Academy of Orthopaedic Surgeons (AAOS): Sprains, strains, and other soft-tissue injuries. Retrieved from *www.orthoinfo.org/topic.cfm?topic=A00111*.
*4. Silva PV, Kamper SJ, Costa LD: Exercise-based intervention for prevention of sports injuries (PEDro synthesis), *Br J Sports Med* 52:408, 2018.
5. American Academy of Orthopaedic Surgeons (AAOS): Common knee injuries. Retrieved from *http://orthoinfo.aaos.org/topic.cfm?topic=A00325*.
6. Mayo Clinic: Carpal tunnel syndrome. Retrieved from *www.mayoclinic.org/diseases-conditions/carpal-tunnel-syndrome/basics/definition/con-20030332*.
7. Mayo Clinic: Rotator cuff injury: Diagnosis and treatment. Retrieved from *www.mayoclinic.org/diseases-conditions/rotator-cuff-injury/symptoms-causes/syc-20350225*.
8. Mayo Clinic: Torn meniscus: Diagnosis and treatment. Retrieved from *www.mayoclinic.org/diseases-conditions/torn-meniscus/symptoms-causes/syc-20354818*.

9. Mayo Clinic: Bursitis. Retrieved from *www.mayoclinic.org/diseases-conditions/bursitis/basics/definition/con-20015102.*

10. Schell H, Duda GN, Peters A, et al: The hematoma and its role in bone healing, *J Exp Orthop* 4:5, 2017.

11. Pountos I, Giannoudis PV: Fracture healing: Back to basics and latest advances. In *Fracture reduction and fixation techniques,* New York, 2018, Springer.

*12. Matullo KS, Gangavalli A, Nwachuku C: Review of lower extremity traction in current orthopedic trauma, *JAAOS* 24:600, 2016.

13. Szostakowski B, Smitham P, Khan WS: Plaster of Paris: Short history of casting and injured limb immobilization, *Open Orthop J* 11:291, 2017.

14. American Orthopedic Foot and Ankle Society: Foot ulcers and the total contact cast. Retrieved from *www.aofas.org/footcaremd/conditions/diabetic-foot/Pages/Foot-Ulcers-and-the-Total-Contact-Cast.aspx.*

*15. Kazmers NH, Fragomen AT, Rozbruch SR: Prevention of pin site infection in external fixation: A review of the literature, *Strategies Trauma Limb Reconstr* 11:75, 2016.

*16. Gichuru M, Philips M, Yardley D, et al: A network meta-analysis evaluating different bone stimulation technologies on fracture healing outcomes, *Ann Orthop Trauma Rehab* 1:117, 2017.

17. Curtis K, Ramsden C: *Emergency and trauma care for nurses and nurse practitioners,* ed 2, St Louis, 2016, Elsevier.

*18. Zalavras CG: Prevention of infection in open fractures, *Infect Dis Clin* 31:339, 2017.

19. American Academy of Orthopaedic Surgeons (AAOS): Compartment syndrome. Retrieved from *https://orthoinfo.aaos.org/en/diseases--conditions/compartment-syndrome/.*

*20. Lieberman JR, Heckmann N: VTE in total hip arthroplasty and total knee arthroplasty patients: From guidelines to practice, *JAAOS* 25:789, 2017.

21. Fukumoto LE, Fukumoto KD: Fat embolism syndrome, *Nurs Clin* 53:335, 2018.

22. Baumgartner RE, Billow DG, Olson SA: Pelvic ring injury. In *Orthopedic traumatology,* New York, 2018, Springer.

23. Centers for Disease Control and Prevention (CDC): Hip fractures among older adults. Retrieved from *www.cdc.gov/HomeandRecreationalSafety/Falls/adulthipfx.html.*

*24. Santesso N, Carrasco-Labra A, Brignardello-Petersen R: Hip protectors for preventing hip fracture in older people. Retrieved from *www.cochrane.org/CD001255/MUSKINJ_hip-protectors-for-preventing-hip-fractures-in-older-people.*

25. Amputee Coalition: Limb loss statistics. Retrieved from *www.amputee-coalition.org/limb-loss-resource-center/resources-by-topic/limb-loss-statistics/limb-loss-statistics.*

26. Armstrong AJ, Hawley CE, Darter B, et al: Operation Enduring Freedom and Operation Iraqi Freedom veterans with amputation: An exploration of resilience, employment, and individual characteristics, *JVR* 48:167, 2018.

*27. Ambron E, Miller A, Kuchenbecker KJ, et al: Immersive low-cost virtual reality treatment for phantom limb pain: Evidence from two cases, *Front Neurol* 9:67, 2018.

28. Pierrie SN, Gaston RG, Loeffler BJ: Current concepts in upper-extremity amputation, *J Hand Surg* 43:657, 2018.

*29. Saltzman BM, Rao A, Erickson BJ, et al: A systematic review of 21 tibial tubercle osteotomy studies and more than 1000 knees: Indications, clinical outcomes, complications, and reoperations, *Pathology* 6:10, 2017.

30. American Joint Replacement Registry: Fourth AJRR annual report on hip and knee arthroplasty data. Retrieved from: *www.ajrr.net/images/annual_reports/AJRR-2017-Annual-Report---Final.pdf.*

31. American Academy of Orthopaedic Surgeons (AAOS): Hip resurfacing. Retrieved from *http://orthoinfo.aaos.org/topic.cfm?topic=A00586.*

*32. McDonald LT, Corbiere NC, DeLisle JA, et al: Pain management after total joint arthroplasty, *AORN J* 103:605, 2016.

33. Lieberman JR: Deep vein thrombosis prophylaxis: State of the art, *J Arthroplasty* 33:3107, 2018.

*Evidence-based information for clinical practice.

63

Musculoskeletal Problems

Diane Ryzner

Courage is very important. Like a muscle, it is strengthened by use.

Ruth Gordon

http://evolve.elsevier.com/Lewis/medsurg

CONCEPTUAL FOCUS

Functional Ability　　　　　　　　**Pain**
Mobility　　　　　　　　　　　　　**Safety**

LEARNING OUTCOMES

1. Describe the pathophysiology, clinical manifestations, and interprofessional and nursing management of osteomyelitis.
2. Distinguish among the types, pathophysiology, clinical manifestations, and interprofessional management of bone cancer.
3. Distinguish between the causes and characteristics of acute and chronic low back pain.
4. Explain the conservative and surgical treatment of intervertebral disc damage.
5. Describe the postoperative nursing management of a patient who has undergone vertebral disc surgery.
6. Discuss the etiology and nursing management of common foot disorders.
7. Describe the etiology, pathophysiology, clinical manifestations, and nursing and interprofessional management of osteomalacia, osteoporosis, and Paget's disease.

KEY TERMS

degenerative disc disease (DDD), p. 1486
hallux valgus, p. 1490
herniated disc, p. 1486
low back pain, p. 1484
muscular dystrophy (MD), p. 1483

osteochondroma, p. 1482
osteomalacia, p. 1491
osteomyelitis, p. 1478
osteopenia, p. 1493
osteoporosis, p. 1492

osteosarcoma, p. 1482
Paget's disease, p. 1495
sarcoma, p. 1482

We were made to move! This chapter reviews a variety of acute and chronic musculoskeletal problems unrelated to trauma that affect the musculoskeletal system. These include osteomyelitis, bone cancer, foot disorders, back pain, and metabolic bone diseases. These problems can lead to changes in mobility that affect almost every system in the body. They are a common source of pain and physical limitations that restrict the ability to fully take part in activities of daily living (ADLs), leading to disability. The nurse plays a key role in assessing pain and functional ability and initiating interventions to prevent injury and maintain mobility.

OSTEOMYELITIS

Etiology and Pathophysiology

Osteomyelitis is a severe infection of the bone, bone marrow, and surrounding soft tissue. Although *Staphylococcus aureus* is the most common cause of infection, a variety of pathogens can cause osteomyelitis (Table 63.1).[1]

Infecting microorganisms can invade by indirect or direct entry. *Indirect entry* (hematogenous) is usually associated with infection with 1 microorganism. Indirect injury accounts for only 20% of all cases. It most often affects children younger than 17 years. Risk factors in adults are older age, debilitation, hemodialysis, sickle cell disease, and IV drug use. The vertebrae are the most common site of infection in adults.[2]

Direct entry osteomyelitis most often affects adults. It can occur when an open wound (e.g., penetrating wounds, fractures, surgery) allows microorganisms to enter the body. Osteomyelitis also may be related to a foreign body, such as an implant or an orthopedic prosthetic device (e.g., plate, total joint prosthesis). It may occur in the feet of patients with diabetes or vascular disease–related ulcers or in the hips or sacrum near a pressure injury. More than 1 microorganism is usually involved.[1]

After entering the blood, microorganisms grow and pressure increases because of the nonexpanding nature of most bone. This increasing pressure eventually leads to ischemia and vascular compromise of the periosteum. The infection spreads

TABLE 63.1 Organisms Causing Osteomyelitis

Organism	Predisposing Problem
Staphylococcus aureus	Pressure injury, penetrating wound, open fracture, orthopedic surgery, disorders with vascular insufficiency (e.g., diabetes, atherosclerosis)
Staphylococcus epidermidis	Indwelling prosthetic devices (e.g., joint replacements, fracture fixation devices)
Streptococcus viridans	Abscessed tooth, gingival disease
Escherichia coli	Urinary tract infection
Mycobacterium tuberculosis	Tuberculosis
Neisseria gonorrhoeae	Gonorrhea
Pseudomonas	Puncture wounds, IV drug use
Salmonella	Sickle cell disease
Fungi, mycobacteria	Immunocompromised host

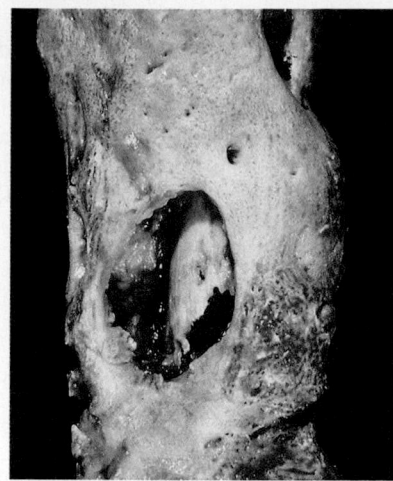

FIG. 63.2 Resection of femur due to osteomyelitis. (From Thibodeau GA, Patton KT: *The human body in health and disease*, ed 5, St Louis, 2010, Mosby.)

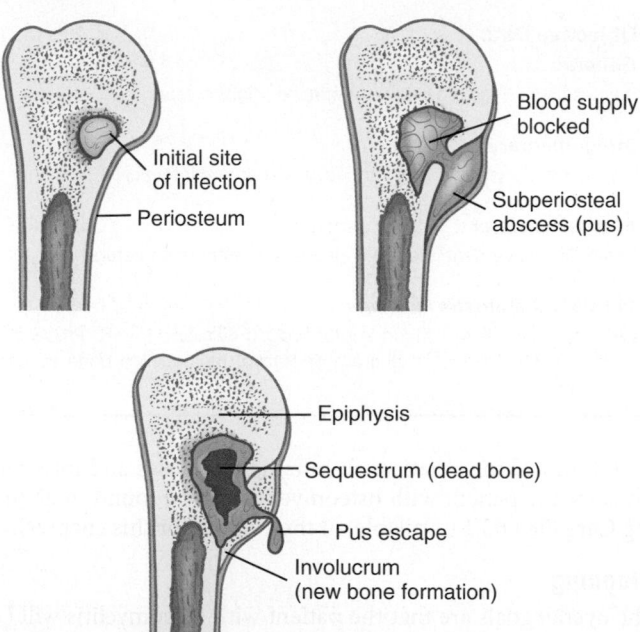

FIG. 63.1 Development of osteomyelitis infection with involucrum and sequestrum.

through the bone cortex and marrow cavity, obstructing blood flow and causing and necrosis.

Bone death occurs due to ischemia. The area of dead bone eventually separates from the surrounding living bone, forming *sequestra*. The part of the periosteum that continues to have a blood supply forms new bone called *involucrum* (Fig. 63.1). Antibiotics or white blood cells (WBCs) have difficulty reaching the sequestrum through the blood. Thus sequestrum may become a reservoir for microorganisms that spread to other sites, including the lungs and brain. If the sequestrum does not resolve or is not debrided surgically, a sinus tract may develop. Chronic, purulent cutaneous drainage from the tract results.

Clinical Manifestations and Complications

Acute osteomyelitis refers to the initial infection or an infection of less than 1 month in duration. Local manifestations of acute osteomyelitis include constant bone pain that worsens with activity and is unrelieved by rest; swelling, tenderness,

and warmth at the infection site; and restricted movement of the affected part. Systemic manifestations include fever, night sweats, chills, restlessness, nausea, and malaise. Later signs include drainage from cutaneous sinus tracts or the fracture site.

Chronic osteomyelitis refers to a bone infection that lasts longer than 1 month or an infection that did not respond to initial antibiotic treatment. Chronic osteomyelitis may be a continuous, persistent problem (a result of inadequate acute treatment) or a process of exacerbations and remissions (Fig. 63.2). Systemic manifestations are lessened. Local signs of infection become more common, including constant bone pain and swelling and warmth at the infection site. Over time, granulation tissue turns to scar tissue. The avascular scar tissue is an ideal site for continued microorganism growth because it cannot be penetrated by antibiotics.

Long-term, and mostly rare, complications of osteomyelitis include septicemia, septic arthritis, pathologic fractures, and amyloidosis.

Diagnostic Studies

Bone or soft tissue biopsy is the definitive way to identify the causative agent. The patient's blood and wound cultures are often positive. Increased WBC count and erythrocyte sedimentation rate (ESR) may occur. High C-reactive protein (CRP) may occur with acute infection. Signs of osteomyelitis usually do not appear on x-rays until 2 to 4 weeks after the initial clinical symptoms. By this time, the disease will have progressed. Compared to x-rays, CT scan may be more helpful in assessing the extent of infection. In the acute phase, MRI may be more sensitive than CT in detecting bone marrow edema, which is an early sign of osteomyelitis. Radionuclide bone scans (technetium-99m) also show abnormalities earlier than x-rays. A WBC scan (indium-111–labeled cells) may help pinpoint the area of infection.[2]

Interprofessional Care

Aggressive, prolonged IV antibiotic therapy is the treatment of choice for acute osteomyelitis if bone ischemia has not yet occurred. Cultures or a bone biopsy should be done, if possible, before starting drug therapy. Any related soft tissue abscess or ulceration often needs surgical debridement or drainage.

IV antibiotic therapy starts in the hospital and then continues at home for 4 to 6 weeks. A few persons need therapy for 3 to 6 months. Patients may be discharged to home care or a skilled nursing facility so the antibiotics can be given through a central venous access device (CVAD). (CVADs are discussed in Chapter 16.) A variety of antibiotics are used, depending on the culture results and likelihood of resistance. These include oxacillin, nafcillin, clindamycin, vancomycin, ceftriaxone, cefazolin, ceftazidime, gentamicin, and linezolid.

🗊 DRUG ALERT   Gentamicin

- Assess patient for dehydration before starting therapy.
- Ensure renal function testing is done before starting therapy, especially in older patients.
- Monitor peak and trough blood levels to achieve therapeutic effect and minimize renal and inner ear toxicity.
- Teach patient to notify HCP if any vision, hearing, or urinary problems develop.

Treatment of chronic osteomyelitis includes (1) surgical removal of the poorly perfused tissue and dead bone and (2) extended use of antibiotics. In adults with chronic osteomyelitis, oral therapy with a fluoroquinolone (e.g., ciprofloxacin [Cipro]) for 6 to 8 weeks may be prescribed instead of IV antibiotics. Oral antibiotics also may be given for 4 to 8 weeks after acute IV therapy is done to ensure the infection is resolved. The patient's response to drug therapy is monitored through bone scans and ESR testing.

Acrylic bead chains containing antibiotics may be implanted to help combat the infection. After debridement of the dead, infected tissue, a suction irrigation system may be inserted, and the wound closed. Intermittent or constant irrigation of the area with antibiotics may be used. Another option for wound management is negative-pressure wound therapy (discussed in Chapter 11). Casts or braces may be applied to protect the limb or the surgical site.

Hyperbaric O_2 may be given as an adjunct therapy in refractory cases of chronic osteomyelitis. It stimulates new blood growth and healing in the infected tissue (see p. 167 in Chapter 11).

If an orthopedic prosthetic device is the source of chronic infection, it must be removed. Muscle flaps or skin grafts provide wound coverage over the dead space (cavity) in the bone. Bone grafts may help to restore blood flow. However, flaps or grafts should never be placed in the presence of active or suspected infection.

Amputation of the extremity may be needed if bone destruction is extensive. Amputation should improve quality of life and may save the patient's life if systemic complications are developing.

❖ NURSING MANAGEMENT: OSTEOMYELITIS

◆ Nursing Assessment

Subjective and objective data that should be obtained from a person with osteomyelitis are outlined in Table 63.2.

◆ Nursing Diagnoses

Nursing diagnoses for the patient with osteomyelitis may include:

- Acute pain
- Impaired physical mobility
- Lack of knowledge

TABLE 63.2   Nursing Assessment

Osteomyelitis

Subjective Data

Important Health Information

Past health history: Bone trauma, open fracture, open or puncture wounds, other infections (e.g., streptococcal sore throat, bacterial pneumonia, sinusitis, skin or tooth infection, chronic urinary tract infection)

Medications: Analgesics or antibiotics

Surgery or other treatments: Bone surgery

Functional Health Patterns

Health perception–health management: IV drug and alcohol use. Malaise

Nutritional-metabolic: Anorexia, weight loss. Chills

Activity-exercise: Weakness, paralysis, muscle spasms around affected area

Cognitive-perceptual: Local tenderness over affected area, increased pain with movement of affected area

Coping–stress tolerance: Irritability, withdrawal, dependency, anger

Objective Data

General

Restlessness. High, spiking temperature. Night sweats

Integumentary

Diaphoresis. Erythema, warmth, edema at site of infection

Musculoskeletal

Restricted movement; wound drainage. Spontaneous fracture

Possible Diagnostic Findings

Leukocytosis, positive blood and/or wound cultures, ↑ ESR. Presence of sequestrum and involucrum on x-rays, radionuclide bone scans, CT, and MRI

Additional information on nursing diagnoses and interventions for the patient with osteomyelitis can be found in eNursing Care Plan 63.1 (available on the website for this chapter).

◆ Planning

The overall goals are that the patient with osteomyelitis will (1) have satisfactory pain and fever management, (2) not have any complications associated with osteomyelitis, (3) adhere to the treatment plan, and (4) maintain a positive outlook on the outcome of the disease.

◆ Nursing Implementation

◆ **Health Promotion.** Control of other current infections (e.g., urinary or respiratory tract, pressure injuries) is important in preventing osteomyelitis. Persons at risk for osteomyelitis are those who are immunocompromised or have diabetes, orthopedic prosthetic implants, or vascular insufficiency. Teach the at-risk patient about the local and systemic signs of osteomyelitis. Encourage the patient to contact the HCP about bone pain, fever, swelling, and restricted limb movement so that treatment can be started. Teach caregivers about their role in monitoring the patient's health.

◆ **Acute Care.** Some immobilization of the affected limb (e.g., splint, traction) is usually needed to decrease pain and reduce risk for further injury. Carefully handle the limb and avoid undue manipulation. This may increase pain and cause a pathologic fracture. Assess the patient's pain. Muscle spasms may cause minor to severe pain. Nonsteroidal antiinflammatory

NURSING MANAGEMENT
Caring for the Patient With Osteomyelitis

- Give IV antibiotics as ordered.
- Assess wound for signs of worsening infection.
- Teach patient and caregiver about antibiotic side effects and length of treatment, signs and symptoms of worsening infection, and use of hyperbaric O_2 if ordered.
- Assess for muscle spasms and give muscle relaxant as ordered. Assess patient response.
- Assess pain intensity and give analgesics as ordered. Assess patient response.
- Handle affected limb carefully to decrease pain and additional injury.
- Assess neurovascular condition of affected limb and immediately inform HCP of significant changes.
- Oversee UAP:
  - Handle affected limb carefully based on RN instruction.
  - Help patient with passive ROM of adjacent joints and active ROM exercises of unaffected limb.
  - Notify RN about patient reports of pain, tingling, or decreased sensation in the affected extremity.

Collaborate With Physical Therapist

- Assess patient's current mobility and need for aid.
- Teach safe ambulation with assistive device based on patient's weight-bearing restrictions.
- Establish exercise plan and teach patient to perform exercises safely.
- Coordinate PT so that patient can receive timely analgesia.
- Discuss home environment with patient and identify modifications to promote recovery (e.g., stair training, bed placement on first level).

Collaborate With Occupational Therapist

- Assess impact of patient's condition on ability to perform ADLs.
- Teach patient use of assistive devices (e.g., long-handled reacher, shoe donner) to promote self-care while maintaining activity restrictions.

drugs (NSAIDs), opioid analgesics, and muscle relaxants may be given. Encourage nondrug approaches to pain management (e.g., guided imagery, relaxation breathing) (see Chapter 6).

Dressings are used to absorb drainage from wounds and debride dead tissue from the wound bed. These include dry, sterile dressings; dressings saturated in saline or antibiotic solution; wet-to-dry dressings; and dressings applied with negative-pressure wound therapy. Sterile technique is essential when changing the dressing. Handle soiled dressings carefully to prevent transfer of bacteria to other areas of the wound. Discard dressings appropriately to prevent spread of infection to other patients.

The patient is often placed on bed rest in the early stages of acute infection. Good body alignment and frequent position changes promote comfort and prevent complications related to immobility. Flexion contracture of the affected lower extremity is common as the patient often positions the leg in a flexed position to promote comfort. Footdrop can develop quickly due to Achilles tendon contracture if the foot is not supported in a neutral position by a splint or boot. A tight splint or dressing may compress and injure the peroneal nerve.

Teach the patient the possible adverse and toxic reactions associated with prolonged high-dose antibiotic therapy. These reactions include hearing deficit, impaired renal function, and neurotoxicity (e.g., limb weakness or numbness, cognitive changes, vision changes, headache, behavioral problems). Reactions associated with cephalosporins (e.g., cefazolin) include hives, severe or watery diarrhea, blood in stools, and throat or mouth sores.

Tendonitis or tendon rupture (especially the Achilles tendon) can occur with use of fluoroquinolones (e.g., ciprofloxacin). Monitor peak and trough blood levels of most antibiotics to avoid adverse effects. Lengthy antibiotic therapy can cause an overgrowth of *Candida albicans* and *Clostridium difficile* in the genitourinary (GU) and gastrointestinal (GI) tracts, especially in immunosuppressed and older adult patients. Teach the patient to report any changes in the oral cavity (e.g., whitish yellow, curdlike lesions) or the GU tract (e.g., perianal itching, discharge).

 CHECK YOUR PRACTICE

Your patient on the orthopedic unit is a 22-yr-old man who was in a serious all-terrain vehicle accident in a remote area 4 days ago. He is now slowly recovering from his head injury and surgical repair of an open fracture of the femur. Yesterday, he was diagnosed with acute osteomyelitis. He is very angry and at times disoriented. When you try to assess his leg, he yells at you, "It hurts. Leave it alone!"
- What are your priorities of care?
- What signs and symptoms would suggest the patient's condition is worsening?

The patient and caregivers may be anxious and discouraged because of the serious nature of osteomyelitis, the uncertainty of the outcome, and the long, costly treatment. Continued psychologic and emotional support is an integral part of nursing management.

◆ **Ambulatory Care.** IV antibiotics can be given to the patient in a skilled nursing facility or home setting. If at home, teach the patient and caregiver how to manage the CVAD. Review how to administer the antibiotic and reinforce the need for follow-up laboratory testing. Stress the importance of continuing to take the full course of antibiotics prescribed, even after symptoms have improved.

Dressing changes are often needed if the patient has an open wound. The patient and caregiver may need supplies and instruction for completing the dressing change. If the osteomyelitis becomes chronic, the patient needs continued physical and psychologic support.

◆ **Evaluation**

The expected outcomes are that the patient with osteomyelitis will
- Have satisfactory pain management
- Adhere to the recommended treatment plan
- Show a consistent increase in mobility and range of motion

BONE TUMORS

Primary bone tumors, both benign and malignant, are rare in adults. They account for only about 3% of all tumors. Metastatic bone cancer, in which cancer has spread from another site, is a more common problem.

BENIGN BONE TUMORS

Benign bone tumors are more common than primary malignant tumors. The main types of benign bone tumors are osteochondroma, osteoclastoma, and enchondroma (Table 63.3). They are often removed surgically.

Osteochondroma

Osteochondroma is the most common primary benign bone tumor. It is characterized by an overgrowth of cartilage and bone near the end of the bone at the growth plate. They most often occur in the pelvis, scapula, or long bones of the leg.

Manifestations include a painless, hard, immobile mass; shorter-than-normal height for age; soreness of muscles close to the tumor; one leg or arm longer than the other; and pressure or irritation with exercise. Some may be asymptomatic. Diagnosis is confirmed using x-ray, CT scan, and MRI.

No treatment is needed for asymptomatic osteochondroma. Patients should have regular screening examinations to detect progression to cancer as soon as possible. If the tumor is causing pain or neurologic manifestations because of compression, surgical removal is usually done.

MALIGNANT BONE TUMORS

A sarcoma is a malignant tumor that develops in bone, muscle, fat, nerve, or cartilage. The most common types of sarcomas are osteosarcoma, chondrosarcoma, and Ewing's sarcoma (Table 63.3). In 2018, 3450 new cases of bone and joint cancer are expected in the United States, with an estimated 1590 deaths.[3] Primary malignant tumors occur most often during childhood and young adulthood. They cause bone destruction and have rapid metastasis.

Osteosarcoma

Osteosarcoma is an extremely aggressive primary bone cancer that rapidly spreads to distant sites. It usually occurs in the pelvis or metaphyseal region of the long bones of extremities, especially in the distal femur, proximal tibia, and proximal humerus (Fig. 63.3, *A*). Osteosarcoma is the most common bone cancer affecting children and young adults. It can occur in older adults, but not as often. It is most often associated with Paget's disease (discussed on p. 1495) and prior radiation.

The gradual onset of pain and swelling in the affected bone are the most common manifestations. The pain may be worse at night and increase with activity. A minor injury does not cause the cancer but may bring it to medical attention. Metastasis is present in 10% to 20% of people at the time of diagnosis.

Diagnosis is confirmed from tissue biopsy, increased serum alkaline phosphatase and calcium, x-ray, CT or PET scans, and MRI.

Preoperative chemotherapy may be used to decrease tumor size before surgery. Limb salvage procedures are usually considered if a clear (no cancer present) 6- to 7-cm margin surrounds the lesion. Limb salvage is usually not possible if the patient has major nerve or blood vessel involvement, pathologic fracture, infection, or extensive muscle involvement.

The use of adjunct chemotherapy after amputation or limb salvage has increased the 5-year survival rate to 70% in people without metastasis. Chemotherapy includes combinations of methotrexate, doxorubicin, cisplatin, ifosfamide, cyclophosphamide, and etoposide.[4]

Metastatic Bone Cancer

The most common type of malignant bone tumor occurs because of spread *(metastasis)* from a primary tumor at another site. Common primary sites include breast, colon, prostate, lungs, kidney, and thyroid.[5] Metastatic cancer cells travel from the primary tumor to the bone via the lymph and blood supply.

TABLE 63.3	Types of Primary Bone Tumors
Types	**Description**
Benign	
Enchondroma	• Intramedullary cartilage tumor usually found in cavity of a single hand or foot bone
	• Rarely transforms to cancer
	• If tumor becomes painful, surgical resection is done
	• Peak incidence in people ages 10–20 yr
Osteochondroma	• Most common benign bone tumor
	• Often found in pelvis, scapula, or metaphyseal part of long bones
	• Occurs most often in people ages 10–25 yr
	• May transform to cancer (chondrosarcoma)
Osteoclastoma (giant cell tumor)	• Arises in cancellous ends of arm and leg bones
	• About 10% are locally aggressive and may spread to lungs
	• High rate of local recurrence after surgery and chemotherapy
Malignant	
Chondrosarcoma	• Most often occurs in cartilage in arm, leg, and pelvic bones of adults ages 50–70 yr
	• Can arise from benign bone tumors (osteochondromas)
	• Wide surgical resection is typically done as tumor rarely responds to radiation and chemotherapy
	• Survival rate depends on stage, size, and grade of tumor (Fig. 63.3, *B*)
Ewing's sarcoma	• Develops in medullary cavity of pelvis and long bones, especially femur, humerus, and tibia
	• Usually occurs in children and teenagers
	• Use of wide surgical resection, radiation, and chemotherapy has improved 5-yr survival rate to 60%
Osteosarcoma	• Most common primary bone cancer
	• Occurs mostly in males ages 10–25
	• Most often in pelvis or bones of arms, legs (Fig. 63.3, *A*)

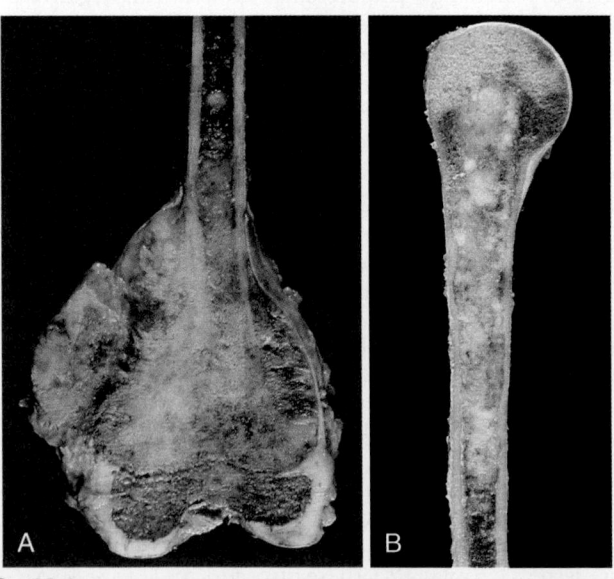

FIG. 63.3 A, Osteosarcoma. B, Chondrosarcoma. (From Damjanov I, Linder J: *Anderson's pathology*, ed 10, St Louis, 1996, Mosby.)

Metastatic bone lesions often occur in the spine, ribs, or pelvis.[5] Pathologic fractures at the site of metastasis are common because the bone is weakened. High serum calcium occurs as damaged bones release calcium.

Once a primary lesion has been found, radionuclide bone scans are often done to detect metastatic lesions before they are visible on x-ray. Metastatic bone lesions may occur at any time (even years later) after diagnosis and treatment of the primary tumor. Bone metastasis should be suspected in any patient who has local bone pain and a history of cancer. Surgical stabilization of the bone may be indicated for fracture or to prevent fracture in a high-risk patient. Prognosis depends on the primary type of cancer and any other sites of metastasis. Possible palliative treatment consists of radiation and pain management (see Chapter 15).

❖ NURSING MANAGEMENT: BONE CANCER

Nursing care of the patient with bone cancer does not differ significantly from the care provided to the patient with cancer of any other body system (see Chapter 15). Monitor the tumor site for swelling, changes in circulation, and decreased movement, sensation, or joint function.

Use special care to prevent pathologic fractures and reduce the complications associated with them. Prevent fractures by careful handling and support of the affected extremity and log-rolling the patient on bed rest. Note weakness caused by anemia and decreased mobility.

Treatment for hypercalcemia may be started if bone decalcification occurs. The patient may be unwilling to exercise or take part in activities because of weakness from the disease and treatment, fear of falling and fracturing a bone, and fear of pain. Provide regular rest periods between activities.

Assess the patient for the location and severity of pain. The pain associated with bone cancer can be severe. It is often caused by the tumor pressing against nerves and other organs near the bone. New onset or changes in pain severity may indicate pathologic fracture. Ensure adequate pain medication is provided. Sometimes radiation therapy is used as a palliative therapy to shrink the tumor and decrease pain.

Assist the patient and caregiver in accepting the prognosis associated with bone cancer. Give special attention to problems of pain and disability, side effects of chemotherapy, and postoperative care (e.g., after spinal cord decompression or amputation). As with all types of cancer, stress the importance of follow-up examinations.

MUSCULAR DYSTROPHY

Muscular dystrophy (MD) is a group of genetic diseases characterized by progressive symmetric wasting of skeletal muscles without evidence of neurologic involvement. A gradual loss of strength with increasing disability and deformity occurs with all forms of MD. The types of MD differ in the groups of muscles affected, age of onset, rate of progression, and mode of genetic inheritance (Table 63.4). Duchenne MD is the most common type.

Genetic Link

Duchenne and Becker MD are X-linked recessive disorders usually seen only in males. (X-linked recessive disorders are discussed in Chapter 12.) These disorders are caused by a mutation of the dystrophin *(DMD)* gene. Dystrophin is a protein that

TABLE 63.4 Select Types of Muscular Dystrophy

Type	Genetic Basis	Manifestations
Becker	• X-linked • Mutation of dystrophin gene	• Very similar but less severe than Duchenne MD • Onset ages 5–15 • Slower course of pelvic and shoulder muscle wasting than Duchenne • Cardiomyopathy • Respiratory failure • May survive into 50s
Duchenne	• X-linked • Mutation of dystrophin gene	• Most common form of MD • Primarily affects boys • Onset before age 5 • Progressive weakness of pelvic and shoulder muscles • Unable to walk by age 12 • Cardiomyopathy • Respiratory failure in 20s • Mental impairment
Facioscapulohumeral	• Autosomal dominant • Deletion of chromosome 4q35	• Onset before age 20 • Slowly progressive weakness of face, shoulder muscles, and upper arms and lower legs • Can affect vision and hearing
Limb-girdle	• Autosomal recessive or autosomal dominant • Mutation in any of at least 15 genes affecting proteins needed for muscle function	• Group of disorders affecting voluntary muscles, especially those of hips and shoulders • Onset ranges from early childhood to early adulthood or later • Slow progressive weakness of hip and shoulder muscles

helps keep skeletal muscle fibers intact. Abnormal dystrophin can cause defects in the muscle fiber and muscle fiber degeneration. Genetic testing can detect a mutation in the *DMD* gene and confirm a diagnosis.[6]

Other diagnostic studies for MD include muscle serum enzymes (especially creatine kinase), electromyogram (EMG) testing, and muscle fiber biopsy. Classic findings on muscle biopsy include fat and connective tissue deposits, muscle fiber degeneration and necrosis, and a deficiency of dystrophin. An ECG may show abnormalities that suggest cardiomyopathy.

No definitive therapy is available to stop progressive muscle wasting of MD. Corticosteroid therapy is part of the standard of care. It may slow disease progression for up to 2 years.[7] In 2017 the FDA approved 2 new medications to treat MD. Deflazacort (Emflaza) is the first corticosteroid approved to treat Duchene MD. Eteplirsen (Exondys 51) is the first disease-modifying drug to treat Duchene MD patients who have a certain dystrophin gene mutation.[8] Other clinical trials underway involve gene therapy and stem cell transplantation.

The main treatment goals are to preserve mobility and independence through exercise, physical therapy, and use of assistive devices. Progressive muscle weakening around the trunk can cause spinal collapse. The patient may be fitted early with an orthotic jacket to give stability and prevent further deformity or injury.[9]

Life expectancy is increasing due to advances in cardiac and respiratory care. Cardiomyopathy often occurs and causes heart failure. Dysrhythmias are a frequent cause of death.[6] Gradual decreases in respiratory function often lead to the use of continuous positive airway pressure (CPAP). Eventually tracheostomy and mechanical ventilation are needed to support respiratory function.

Encourage communication between the patient and family to cope with the emotional and physical demands of MD. Teach the patient and caregiver range-of-motion (ROM) exercises, principles of good nutrition, and signs of disease progression. Genetic testing and counseling may be recommended for persons with a family history of MD.

🧬 GENETICS IN CLINICAL PRACTICE

Duchenne and Becker Muscular Dystrophy (MD)

Genetic Basis
- Caused by various mutations in the dystrophin *(DMD)* gene
- Gene provides instructions for making dystrophin, a protein that helps keep muscle fibers intact
- Dystrophin is found mainly in skeletal and cardiac muscle
- Inherited in an X-linked recessive pattern
- Females in affected families have a 50% chance of inheriting and passing the defective gene to their children

Incidence
- Between 400 and 600 boys are born with MD each year in the United States.
- Together these disorders affect 1 in 3500 to 5000 newborn males worldwide.

Genetic Testing
- DNA testing for mutations in dystrophin gene is available.
- Genetic testing and counseling should be considered for those with a family history of MD.

Clinical Implications
- Because there are many types of MD with different genetic bases, knowing the type of MD is important to determine treatment and possible genetic counseling recommendations.

Focus care on keeping the patient active as long as possible. Prolonged bed rest should be avoided because immobility can cause more muscle wasting. As the disease progresses, teach the patient to limit sedentary periods to prevent skin breakdown and respiratory complications. Ongoing medical and nursing care is needed throughout the patient's life.

The *Muscular Dystrophy Association (www.mda.org)* is an important resource with information about support services for the patient and caregivers. The website gives updates about the latest clinical trials and treatment advances.

⚠️ SAFETY ALERT Muscular Dystrophy
- Support respiratory function as needed.
- Fit patient with an orthotic jacket or brace to prevent deformity or injury.

LOW BACK PAIN

Low back pain is most often due to a musculoskeletal problem. It may be localized or diffuse. In *localized pain,* patients feel soreness or discomfort when a specific area of the lower back is palpated or pressed. *Diffuse pain* occurs over a larger area and comes from deep tissue.

Low back pain may be radicular or referred. *Radicular pain* is caused by irritation of a nerve root. Radicular pain is not isolated to a single location. Instead, it radiates or moves along a nerve distribution. Sciatica is an example of radicular pain. *Referred pain* is felt in the lower back, but the source of the pain is another location (e.g., kidneys, lower abdomen).

Low back pain affects about 80% of adults in the United States at least once during their lives. Backache is second only to headache as the most common pain problem. It is the leading cause of job-related disability and a major contributor to missed work days.[10]

Low back pain is common because the lumbar region (1) bears most of the weight of the body, (2) is the most flexible region of the spinal column, (3) has nerve roots that are at risk for injury or disease, and (4) has a naturally poor biomechanical structure. Risk factors include lack of muscle tone, excess body weight, stress, poor posture, smoking, pregnancy, prior compression fracture of the spine, spinal problems since birth, and a family history of back pain. Jobs that require repetitive heavy lifting, vibration (such as a jackhammer operator), and extended periods of sitting are associated with low back pain.

The causes of low back pain of musculoskeletal origin include (1) acute lumbosacral strain, (2) instability of the lumbosacral bony mechanism, (3) osteoarthritis of the lumbosacral vertebrae, (4) degenerative disc disease, and (5) herniation of an intervertebral disc.

Health care personnel who perform direct patient care activities are at high risk for developing low back pain.[11] Lifting and moving patients, excessive bending or leaning forward, and frequent twisting can result in low back pain that causes lost time and productivity and disability. Nurses should follow the agency's safe patient handling standards to avoid injury.[12]

ACUTE LOW BACK PAIN

Acute low back pain lasts 4 weeks or less. Most acute low back pain is caused by trauma or an activity that produces undue stress (often hyperflexion) on the lower back. Examples of trauma or activities that cause acute back pain are heavy lifting; overuse of back muscles during yard work; a sports injury; or a sudden jolt, as in a motor vehicle crash.

Often symptoms do not appear at the time of injury. They develop later (usually within 24 hours) because of a gradual increase in pressure on the nerve from an intervertebral disc and/or associated edema. Symptoms may range from muscle ache to shooting or stabbing pain, limited flexibility or ROM, or an inability to stand upright.

Few definitive diagnostic abnormalities are present with nerve irritation and muscle strain. One test is the straight-leg-raising test (see Chapter 61, p. 1438). MRI and CT scans are not done unless trauma or systemic disease (e.g., cancer, spinal infection) is suspected. MRI findings may be limited in the acute phase of an injury due to increased edema near the injury.

❖ NURSING AND INTERPROFESSIONAL MANAGEMENT: ACUTE LOW BACK PAIN

◆ Nursing Assessment

Subjective and objective data that should be obtained from the patient with low back pain are outlined in Table 63.5.

TABLE 63.5 Nursing Assessment

Low Back Pain

Subjective Data

Important Health Information

Past health history: Acute or chronic lumbosacral strain/trauma, osteoarthritis, degenerative disc disease, obesity

Medications: Opioid analgesics and NSAIDs, muscle relaxants, corticosteroids, over-the-counter remedies (e.g., topical ointments, patches)

Surgery or other treatments: Back surgery, epidural corticosteroid injections

Functional Health Patterns

Health perception–health management: Smoking, lack of exercise
Nutritional-metabolic: Obesity
Activity-exercise: Poor posture, muscle spasms, activity intolerance
Elimination: Constipation
Sleep-rest: Interrupted sleep
Cognitive-perceptual: Pain in back, buttocks, or leg associated with walking, turning, straining, coughing, leg raising. Numbness or tingling of legs, feet, toes
Role-relationship: Occupations requiring heavy lifting, vibrations, or extended driving. Change in role within family structure due to inability to work and provide income

Objective Data

General

Guarded movement

Neurologic

Depressed or absent Achilles tendon reflex or patellar tendon reflex. Positive straight-leg-raising test, positive crossover straight-leg-raising test, positive Trendelenburg test

Musculoskeletal

Tense, tight paravertebral muscles on palpation, ↓ range of motion in spine

Possible Diagnostic Findings

Localization of site of lesion or disorder on myelogram, CT scan, or MRI. Determination of nerve root impingement on EMG

TABLE 63.6 Patient & Caregiver Teaching

Low Back Problems

Include the following instructions when teaching the patient and caregiver how to manage low back problems:

Do

- Maintain healthy body weight.
- Maintain a neutral pelvic position if standing. Place 1 foot on a low stool if standing for long periods.
- Choose a seat with good lower back support, armrests, and a swivel base. Place a pillow at the lumbar spine to maintain normal curvature. Keep knees and hips level.
- Sleep in a side-lying position with knees and hips bent, and a pillow between the knees for support.
- Sleep on back with a lift under knees and legs or on back with 10-in–high pillow under knees to flex hips and knees.
- Use proper body mechanics when lifting heavy objects. Bend at the knees, not at the waist, and stand up slowly while holding object close to your body.
- Take part in regular strength and flexibility training and low-impact aerobic exercise.
- Use local heat and cold application to relieve muscle tension.

Do Not

- Lean forward without bending knees.
- Lift anything above level of elbows.
- Stand unmoving for prolonged time.
- Sleep on abdomen or on back or side with legs out straight.
- Exercise without consulting HCP if having severe pain.
- Exceed prescribed amount and type of exercises without consulting HCP.
- Smoke or use tobacco products.

◆ **Nursing Implementation**

◆ **Health Promotion.** Serve as a role model by always using proper body mechanics. This includes increasing the patient's bed height, bending at the knees, asking for help in lifting and moving patients, and using lifting devices.

Assess the patient's use of body mechanics and offer advice when the person does activities that could produce back strain. Some HCPs refer patients with back pain to a program called "Back School." This formal program is usually taught by an HCP, nurse, or physical therapist. It is designed to teach the patient how to minimize back pain and avoid repeat episodes of pain. Tips for prevention of back injury are listed in Table 63.6. Referral to a physical therapist or personal trainer to address posture and core and abdomen strength may be appropriate. Recommend flat shoes or shoes with low heels and shock-absorbing shoe inserts for women.

Advise patients to maintain a healthy body weight. Excess body weight places more stress on the lower back. It weakens abdominal muscles that support the lower back. Sleeping position is important in preventing low back pain. Teach patients to avoid sleeping in a prone position because it causes excessive lumbar lordosis, placing stress on the lower back. Sleeping in

a supine or side-lying position with knees and hips flexed prevents pressure on support muscles, ligaments, and lumbosacral joints. Recommend use of a firm mattress.

Teach patients the importance of smoking cessation. Tobacco use impairs circulation to the intervertebral discs and contributes to low back pain.

◆ **Acute Care.** If acute muscle spasms and accompanying pain are not severe and unbearable, the patient is treated as an outpatient with NSAIDs and muscle relaxants (e.g., cyclobenzaprine). Massage and back manipulation, acupuncture, and the application of cold and hot compresses may help some patients. Severe pain may require a brief course of corticosteroids or opioid analgesics.

Some people may need a brief period (1 to 2 days) of rest at home but should avoid prolonged bed rest. Most patients do better if they continue their regular activities. Patients should refrain from activities that increase the pain, including lifting, bending, twisting, and prolonged sitting. Symptoms of acute low back pain usually improve within 2 weeks and often resolve without treatment.

Teach the patient about the cause of the pain and ways to prevent further episodes. Muscle stretching and strengthening exercises may be part of the management plan. Although the physical therapist often teaches the exercises, reinforce the type and frequency of prescribed exercise and the reason for the program.

Other nursing interventions for the patient with low back pain are detailed in eNursing Care Plan 63.2 (available on the website for this chapter).

Ambulatory Care. The goal of management is to make an episode of acute low back pain an isolated incident. If the lumbosacral area is unstable, repeated episodes are likely. Obesity, poor posture, poor muscle support, older age, or trauma may weaken the lumbosacral spine, so it is unable to meet the demands placed on it without strain. Exercise is aimed at strengthening the supporting muscles.

Persistent use of poor body mechanics may result in repeated episodes of low back pain. If the strain is work related, occupational counseling may be needed. Low back pain can cause frustration, pain, and disability. Provide emotional support and understanding care of the patient.

CHRONIC LOW BACK PAIN

Chronic low back pain lasts more than 3 months or involves a repeated incapacitating episode. It is often progressive, and the cause can be hard to determine. Causes include (1) degenerative conditions, such as arthritis or disc disease; (2) osteoporosis or other metabolic bone diseases; (3) weakness from the scar tissue of prior injury; (4) chronic strain on lower back muscles from obesity, pregnancy, or stressful postures on the job; and (5) congenital spine problems.

Spinal Stenosis

Spinal stenosis is a narrowing of the spinal canal, which holds the spinal cord. Stenosis in the lumbar spine is a common cause of chronic low back pain. Spinal stenosis can be acquired or inherited. A common acquired cause is osteoarthritis. Arthritic changes (bone spurs, calcification of spinal ligaments, disc degeneration) narrow the space around the spinal canal and nerve roots, eventually leading to compression. Inflammation caused by the compression results in pain, weakness, and numbness.

Other acquired conditions that may cause spinal stenosis include rheumatoid arthritis, spinal tumors, Paget's disease, and traumatic damage to the vertebral column. Inherited conditions that lead to spinal stenosis include congenital spinal stenosis and scoliosis.

The pain associated with lumbar spinal stenosis often starts in the lower back and then radiates to the buttock and leg. It is worse with walking or prolonged standing. Numbness, tingling, weakness, and heaviness in the legs and buttocks may be present. History of decreased pain when the patient bends forward or sits is often a sign of spinal stenosis. In most cases, stenosis slowly progresses.

❖ Interprofessional and Nursing Care

The management and treatment of chronic low back pain are similar to those for acute low back pain. Manage the patient's pain and stiffness with mild analgesics, such as NSAIDs, for daily comfort. Antidepressants (e.g., duloxetine [Cymbalta]) may help with pain management and sleep problems. The antiseizure drug gabapentin (Neurontin) may improve walking and relieve leg symptoms.

Weight reduction, rest periods, local heat or cold application, physical therapy, and exercise and activity throughout the day help keep the muscles and joints mobilized. Cold, damp weather worsens the back pain. Pain can be decreased with rest and local heat application. Complementary and alternative therapies, such as biofeedback, acupuncture, and yoga, may help reduce the pain. "Back School" (discussed on p. 1485) can significantly reduce pain and improve body posture.

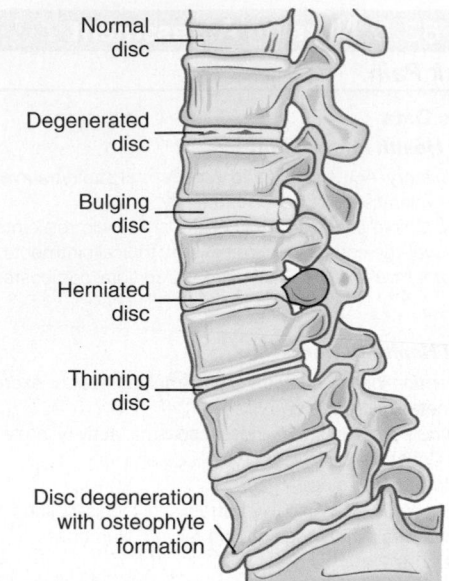

FIG. 63.4 Common causes of degenerative disc damage.

Minimally invasive treatments, such as epidural corticosteroid injections and implanted devices that deliver pain medication, are options for those with chronic low back pain that does not respond to the usual therapeutic options. Surgical intervention may be indicated in patients with severe chronic low back pain who receive no benefit from conservative care and/or have continued neurologic deficits. (Surgery for low back pain is discussed on p. 1488.)

INTERVERTEBRAL DISC DISEASE

Intervertebral discs separate the vertebrae and help absorb shock for the spine. *Intervertebral disc disease* involves the deterioration, herniation, or other dysfunction of the intervertebral discs. Disc disorders can affect the cervical, thoracic, and lumbar spine.

Etiology and Pathophysiology

Degenerative disc disease (DDD) results from loss of fluid in the intervertebral discs with aging. The discs lose their elasticity, flexibility, and shock-absorbing abilities. Unless it is accompanied by pain, DDD is a normal process.[13] The discs become thinner as the *nucleus pulposus* (gelatinous center of the disc) starts to dry out and shrink. This change limits the disc's ability to distribute pressure between vertebrae. The pressure is then transferred to the *annulus fibrosus* (strong outside part of the disc), causing progressive destruction. When the disc is damaged, the nucleus pulposus may seep through a torn or stretched annulus. This is called a herniated disc *(slipped disc),* a condition in which a spinal disc bulges outward between the vertebrae (Fig. 63.4).

A herniated disc can result from degeneration with age or repeated stress and trauma to the spine. The most common sites of herniation are the lumbosacral discs, specifically L4-5 and L5-S1. Disc herniation may also occur at C5-6 and C6-7. It may be the result of spinal stenosis, in which narrowing of the spinal canal forces the intervertebral disc to bulge.

The spinal nerves emerge from the spinal column through an opening *(intervertebral foramen)* between adjacent vertebrae.

TABLE 63.7 Manifestations of Lumbar Disc Herniation*

Intervertebral Level	Pain	Affected Reflex	Motor Function	Sensation
L3-4	Back to buttocks to posterior thigh to inner calf	Patellar	Quadriceps, anterior tibialis	Inner aspect of lower leg, anterior part of thigh
L4-5	Back to buttocks to dorsum of foot and big toe	None	Anterior tibialis, extensor hallucis longus, gluteus medius	Dorsum of foot and big toe
L5-S1	Back to buttocks to sole of foot and heel	Achilles	Gastrocnemius, hamstring, gluteus maximus	Heel and lateral foot

*A disc herniation can involve pressure on more than 1 nerve root.

Herniated discs can press against these nerves ("pinched nerve") causing *radiculopathy* (radiating pain, numbness, tingling, decreased strength and/or range of motion).

Osteoarthritis (OA) of the spine is associated with DDD and the stresses placed on the vertebrae. As the poorly lubricated joints rub against each other, the protective cartilage is damaged and painful bone spurs occur as one of the changes found in OA.

Clinical Manifestations

In *lumbar disc disease,* the most common manifestation is low back pain. Radicular pain that radiates down the buttock and below the knee, along the distribution of the sciatic nerve, generally indicates disc herniation. Specific manifestations of lumbar disc herniation are outlined in Table 63.7. A positive straight-leg-raising test may indicate nerve root irritation (see Chapter 61, p. 1438). Back or leg pain may be reproduced by raising the leg.

Low back pain from other causes may not be accompanied by leg pain. Reflexes may be depressed or absent, depending on the spinal nerve root involved. Numbness and tingling *(paresthesia)* or muscle weakness in the legs, feet, or toes may occur.

Multiple lumbar nerve root compressions *(cauda equina syndrome)* from a herniated disc, tumor, or an epidural abscess may be marked by (1) severe low back pain, (2) progressive weakness, (3) increased pain, and (4) bowel and bladder incontinence or retention. Saddle anesthesia (loss of or altered sensation of the perineum, buttocks, inner thighs and back of the legs [saddle area]) may be present. Symptoms of cauda equina syndrome may develop suddenly or evolve slowly over time. They may vary in intensity. Cauda equina is a medical emergency that requires surgical decompression to reduce pressure on the nerves and prevent permanent paralysis.[14]

In *cervical disc disease,* pain radiates into the arms and hands, following the pattern of the involved nerve. Like lumbar disc disease, reflexes may or may not be present. The handgrip is often weak. Because manifestations of cervical disc disease may include shoulder pain and dysfunction, the HCP must rule out shoulder disorders as part of the diagnosis.

Diagnostic Studies

X-rays are done to detect any structural defects. A myelogram, MRI, or CT scan is helpful in localizing the damaged site. An epidural venogram or diskogram may be needed if other diagnostic studies are inconclusive. An EMG of the extremities can be done to determine the severity of nerve irritation or to rule out other conditions, such as peripheral neuropathy.

TABLE 63.8 Interprofessional Care

Intervertebral Disc Disease

Diagnostic Assessment
- History and physical examination
- X-ray
- CT scan
- MRI
- Myelogram
- Diskogram
- EMG

Management
Conservative Therapy
- Restricted activity for several days, limited total bed rest
- Local ice or heat
- Physical therapy
- Analgesics (e.g., tramadol [Ultram])
- NSAIDs
- Muscle relaxants (e.g., cyclobenzaprine)
- Antiseizure drugs (e.g., gabapentin)
- Antidepressants (e.g., pregabalin)
- Epidural corticosteroid injections

Surgical Therapy
- Intradiscal electrothermoplasty (IDET)
- Radiofrequency discal nucleoplasty
- Interspinous process decompression system (X-Stop)
- Laminectomy with or without spinal fusion
- Discectomy
- Percutaneous laser discectomy
- Artificial disc replacement (e.g., Charité disc)
- Spinal fusion with instrumentation (e.g., plates, screws) or without instrumentation

Interprofessional Care

The patient with suspected disc damage is usually managed with conservative therapy (Table 63.8). This includes limitation of extremes of spinal movement (e.g., brace, corset, belt), local heat or ice, ultrasound and massage, traction, and transcutaneous electrical nerve stimulation (TENS). Drug therapy to manage pain includes NSAIDs, short-term oral corticosteroids, opioid analgesics, muscle relaxants, antiseizure drugs, and antidepressants.[15] Epidural corticosteroid injections may reduce inflammation and relieve acute pain. However, pain tends to recur if the underlying cause remains.

When symptoms subside, the patient should begin back-strengthening exercises twice a day and continue for life. Teach the patient the principles of good body mechanics. Discourage extremes of flexion and torsion. With a conservative treatment plan, most patients heal after 6 months.

Surgical Therapy. If conservative treatment is unsuccessful, radiculopathy becomes worse, or loss of bowel or bladder control occurs, surgery may be considered. Surgery for a damaged disc is generally done if the patient is in constant pain and/or has a persistent neurologic deficit.

Intradiscal electrothermoplasty (IDET) is a minimally invasive outpatient procedure for treatment of back and sciatic pain. A needle is inserted into the affected disc with x-ray guidance. A wire is then threaded through the needle and into the disc. As the wire is heated, small nerve fibers that have invaded the degenerating disc are destroyed. The heat also partially melts the annulus fibrosus. This causes the body to generate new reinforcing proteins in the fibers of the annulus.

Another outpatient technique is *radiofrequency discal nucleoplasty* (coablation nucleoplasty). A needle is inserted into the disc similar to IDET. Instead of a heated wire, a special radiofrequency probe is used. The probe generates energy that breaks the molecular bonds of the gel in the nucleus pulposus. Up to 20% of the nucleus is removed. This decompresses the disc and reduces pressure on the disc and surrounding nerve roots. Subsequent pain relief varies.

A third procedure involves use of an *interspinous process decompression system* (X-Stop). This titanium device fits onto a mount that is placed on vertebrae in the lower back. The X-Stop is used in patients with pain due to lumbar spinal stenosis. The device works by lifting vertebrae off the pinched nerve.

Laminectomy is a common, traditional surgical procedure for lumbar disc disease. It involves surgical excision of part of the vertebra (referred to as the *lamina*) to access and remove the protruding disc.[13] Laminectomy is often done as an outpatient procedure. However, a hospital stay of 1 to 3 days is not uncommon.

Discectomy also can be done to decompress the nerve root. Microsurgical discectomy is a version of the standard procedure. The HCP uses a microscope to better see the disc and disc space, which helps in removal of the damaged portion. This helps maintain bony stability of the spine.

Percutaneous discectomy is a safe and effective outpatient surgical procedure. A tube is passed through the retroperitoneal soft tissues to the disc with the aid of fluoroscopy. A laser is then used on the damaged part of the disc. Minimal blood loss occurs because of access through small stab wounds. The procedure decreases rehabilitation time.

The goals of artificial disc replacement surgery are to restore movement and eliminate pain. The *Charité disc* is used in patients with lumbar disc damage associated with DDD. This artificial disc has a high-density core sandwiched between 2 cobalt-chromium endplates (Fig. 63.5). After removing the damaged disc, the device is surgically placed in the spine (usually through a small incision below the umbilicus). The disc restores movement at the level of the implant. The *ProDisc-L* is another type of artificial lumbar disc used to treat DDD.[16]

Options for treatment of DDD of the cervical spine include the Prestige cervical disc, Mobi-C disc, and Secure-C artificial cervical disc.

A *spinal fusion* may be needed if the spine is unstable. The spine is stabilized by creating *ankylosis* (fusion) of adjacent vertebrae with a bone graft from the patient's fibula or iliac crest (*autograft*) or from donated cadaver bone (*allograft*). Metal fixation with rods, plates, or screws may be placed to give more stability and decrease vertebral motion. A posterior lumbar fusion may be done to give extra support for bone grafting or a prosthetic device.

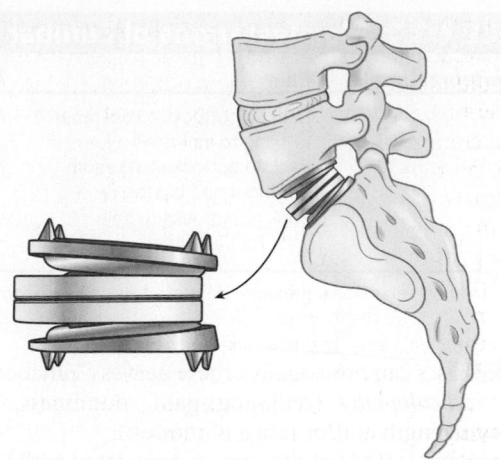

FIG. 63.5 The Charité artificial disc, used to replace a damaged intervertebral disc in degenerative disc disease of the lumbar spine. A movable high-density plastic core is placed between 2 cobalt-chromium alloy endplates. The disc's design helps realign the spine and preserve movement.

Bone morphogenetic protein (BMP), a genetically engineered protein, may be used to stimulate bone growth of the graft in spinal fusions.[17] A dissolvable sponge soaked with BMP is implanted into the spine. BMP on the sponge stimulates the body's cells to become active and produce bone, promoting fusion. The body absorbs the sponge, leaving living bone behind.

❖ NURSING MANAGEMENT: VERTEBRAL DISC SURGERY

After vertebral disc surgery, a key focus of nursing interventions is maintaining proper alignment of the spine until it has healed. Depending on the type and extent of surgery and the HCP's preference, the patient may be able to dangle the legs at the side of the bed, stand, or even ambulate the day of surgery.

After lumbar fusion, place pillows under the patient's thighs when supine and between the legs when in the side-lying position to provide comfort and ensure alignment. The patient often fears turning or any movement that may increase pain by stressing the surgical area. Have the patient logroll when changing position in bed. Reassure the patient that proper technique is being used to maintain body alignment. Remove the bed trapeze, if present, since use is contraindicated for spinal surgery patients. Enough staff should be available to move the patient without undue pain or strain for the patient or staff.

After surgery, most patients need opioids, such as morphine IV, for 24 to 48 hours. Patient-controlled analgesia (PCA) allows maintenance of optimal analgesic levels and is the preferred method of continuous pain management. Once the patient receives oral fluids, oral drugs, such as acetaminophen with codeine, hydrocodone, or oxycodone (Percocet), may be used. Diazepam (Valium) may be prescribed for muscle relaxation. Assess and document pain intensity and pain management effectiveness.

Because the spinal canal may be entered during surgery, cerebrospinal fluid (CSF) leakage is possible. Immediately report leakage of CSF on the dressing or if the patient reports a severe headache. CSF appears as clear or slightly yellow drainage on the dressing. It has a high glucose concentration and is positive for glucose when tested with a dipstick. Note the amount, color, and characteristics of drainage.

Frequently assess the patient's peripheral neurologic condition. Movement of the arms and legs and assessment of sensation should at least equal the preoperative status. Repeat these assessments every 2 to 4 hours during the first 48 hours after surgery and compare with the preoperative assessment. Paresthesia may not be relieved right after surgery. Report any new muscle weakness or paresthesia at once to the HCP and record this finding in the patient's medical record. Assess extremity circulation using skin temperature, capillary refill, and pulses.

Paralytic ileus and interference with bowel function may occur for several days. Opioids can slow bowel elimination. Assess if the patient is passing gas, has bowel sounds in all quadrants, and has a flat, soft abdomen. Stool softeners (e.g., docusate [Colace]) and laxatives may prevent and relieve constipation.

Emptying the bladder may be hard due to activity restrictions, opioids, or anesthesia. Encourage men to dangle the legs over the side of the bed or stand to urinate if allowed by the HCP. Urge patients to use a bedside commode or ambulate to the bathroom when allowed to promote bladder emptying. Intermittent catheterization or an indwelling urinary catheter may be needed by patients who have problems urinating.

Loss of sphincter tone or bladder tone may indicate nerve damage. Monitor for incontinence or problems with bowel or bladder elimination. Immediately report problems to the HCP.

In addition to nursing care appropriate for a patient who had a laminectomy, other nursing activities are needed if the patient has also had a spinal fusion. Because a bone graft is usually involved, the healing time is prolonged compared with a laminectomy. Activity limitations may be needed for an extended time. A rigid orthosis (thoracolumbar sacral orthosis [TLSO] or chairback brace) is often used during this period. Some HCPs want patients to learn to apply and remove the brace by logrolling in bed. Others allow their patients to apply the brace in a sitting or standing position. Verify the preferred method before starting this activity.

With cervical spine surgery, be alert for signs of spinal cord edema, such as respiratory distress and a worsening neurologic condition of the upper extremities. After surgery, the patient's neck may be immobilized in a soft or hard cervical collar.

In addition to the primary surgical site, regularly assess the bone graft donor site. The posterior iliac crest is the most often used donor site, although the fibula may be used. The donor site usually causes greater pain than the spinal fusion area. The donor site is bandaged with a pressure dressing to prevent excessive bleeding. If the donor site is the fibula, frequent neurovascular assessment of the extremity is a key nursing intervention.

After spinal fusion, the patient may have some immobility of the spine at the fusion site. Teach the patient to use proper body mechanics and avoid sitting or standing for prolonged periods. Encourage activities that include walking, lying down, and shifting weight from one foot to the other when standing. Teach the patient about any lifting restrictions. Encourage the patient to think through an activity before starting any potentially injurious task, such as bending or stooping. Any twisting movement of the spine is contraindicated. Teach the patient to use the thighs and knees, rather than the back, to absorb the shock of activity and movement. A firm mattress or bed board is essential.

NECK PAIN

Neck pain occurs almost as often as low back pain, affecting 10% to 20% of adults at any point in time.[18] Neck pain may result from many different conditions, including benign (e.g., poor posture) and serious (e.g., herniated cervical disc) (Table 63.9).

TABLE 63.9 Causes of Neck Pain

- Degenerative disc disease, including herniation
- Meningitis
- Osteomyelitis
- Osteoporosis
- Poor posture
- Rheumatoid arthritis
- Spondylosis
- Strain or sprain
- Trauma (e.g., fractures, subluxation)
- Tumor

TABLE 63.10 Patient & Caregiver Teaching

Neck Exercises

When teaching the patient exercises for neck pain, include the following instructions for the patient and caregiver:

- Bend your head backward until you are looking up at the ceiling. Repeat slowly 5 times. Stop if dizziness occurs.
- Bring your head forward so that your chin touches your chest and your face is looking down at the floor. Repeat slowly 5 times.
- With your head facing forward, bend your ear down toward one shoulder. Alternate this movement with your other ear. Repeat slowly 5 times on each side.
- Turn your head slowly around to one side as far as it will go. Repeat toward the other side. Repeat exercise 5 times on each side.

Cervical neck sprains and strains occur from hyperflexion and hyperextension injuries. Patients have stiffness and neck pain with possible radicular pain into the arm and hand. Pain may radiate to the head, anterior chest, thoracic spine region, and shoulders. Weakness or paresthesia of the arm and hand suggests cervical nerve root compression from stenosis, DDD, or herniation.

The cause of neck pain is diagnosed by history, physical examination, x-ray, MRI, CT scan, and myelogram. An EMG of the upper extremities may diagnose cervical radiculopathy.

Conservative treatment for neck pain in patients without an underlying disorder includes head support using a soft cervical collar, gentle traction, heat and ice applications, massage, rest until symptoms subside, ultrasound, and NSAIDs. Therapeutic neck exercises and acupuncture also may be used for pain relief.[19] Most neck pain resolves without surgical intervention.

Preventing neck pain that occurs with everyday activities, such as prolonged sitting at a computer or television, sleeping in nonaligned spinal positions, or making jarring movements during exercise, is important. Encourage patients to practice good posture and maintain neck flexibility (Table 63.10).

FOOT DISORDERS

The foot is the platform that supports the weight of the body and absorbs shock when the person ambulates. It is a complicated structure composed of bony structures, muscles, tendons, and ligaments. The foot can be affected by (1) congenital conditions; (2) structural weakness; (3) traumatic and stress injuries; and (4) systemic conditions, such as diabetes and rheumatoid arthritis. Table 63.11 outlines common foot disorders.

Footwear is used to (1) provide support, foot stability, protection, shock absorption, and a foundation for orthotics; (2) increase friction with the walking surface; and (3) treat foot abnormalities. Poorly fitting shoes cause or worsen a great deal of the pain, deformity, and disability from foot disorders.[20] Shoes may cause crowding and angulation of the toes and inhibit normal movement of foot muscles.

TABLE 63.11 Common Foot Disorders

Disorder	Description	Treatment
Forefoot		
Hallux rigidus	Painful stiffness of first MTP joint caused by osteoarthritis or local trauma.	• Conservative treatment includes intraarticular corticosteroids and passive manual stretching of first MTP joint. • Shoe with a stiff sole decreases pain in the joint during walking. • Surgical treatment is joint fusion or arthroplasty with silicone rubber implant.
Hallux valgus (bunion)	Painful deformity of great toe with lateral angulation of great toe toward second toe, bony enlargement of medial side of first metatarsal head, swelling of bursa and formation of callus over bony enlargement (Fig. 63.6).	• Conservative treatment includes wearing shoes with wide forefoot or "bunion pocket" and use of bunion pads to relieve pressure on bursal sac. • Surgical treatment involves removal of bursal sac and bony enlargement and correction of lateral angulation of great toe. • May include temporary or permanent internal fixation.
Hammer and claw toes	Hammer toe is a deformity of PIP joint on 2nd to 5th toes causing toe to be permanently bent, resembling a hammer. Mallet toe is a similar condition affecting the DIP joint. Claw toe is a similar deformity with dorsiflexion of the proximal phalanx on the MTP joint combined with flexion of both PIP and DIP joints. Symptoms include burning on bottom of foot and pain and difficulty walking when wearing shoes.	• Conservative treatment includes passive manual stretching of PIP joint and use of metatarsal arch support. • Surgical correction consists of resection of base of middle phalanx and head of proximal phalanx, bringing raw bone ends together. • Kirschner wire maintains straight position.
Morton's neuroma (Morton's toe or plantar neuroma)	Neuroma in web space between third and fourth metatarsal heads, causing sharp, sudden attacks of pain and burning sensations.	• Surgical excision is the usual treatment.
Midfoot		
Pes cavus	Elevation of longitudinal arch of foot resulting from contracture of plantar fascia or bony deformity of arch.	• Surgical correction is needed if condition interferes with ambulation.
Pes planus (flatfoot)	Loss of metatarsal arch causing pain in foot or leg.	• Symptoms are relieved by use of resilient longitudinal arch supports. • Surgical treatment consists of triple arthrodesis or fusion of subtalar joint.
Hindfoot		
Calcaneus stress fracture	Heel pain after moderate walking. Common causes are overtraining, running on hard surfaces, or osteoporosis.	• Rest, ice, shoe heel pad, and NSAIDs. • See HCP to assess for osteoporosis.
Heel pain	Heel pain with weight bearing. Common causes are plantar bursitis, plantar fasciitis, or bone spur.	• Corticosteroids are injected locally into inflamed bursa, and sponge-rubber heel cup is used. • Surgical excision of bursa or spur is done. • Stretching exercises, ice, shoe heel cup, shock-wave therapy, NSAIDs, and corticosteroids are used for plantar fasciitis.
Other Problems		
Callus	Localized thickening of skin. Covers wide area and usually found on weight-bearing part of foot.	• Softened with warm water or preparations containing salicylic acid and trimmed with razor blade or scalpel. • Pressure on bony prominences caused by shoes is relieved.
Corn	Localized thickening of skin caused by continual pressure over bony prominences, especially metatarsal head, often causing localized pain.	• Same as with callus.
Plantar wart	Painful papillomatous growth caused by virus that may occur on any part of skin on sole of foot. Warts tend to cluster on pressure points.	• Remedies containing salicylic acid (e.g., Compound W), excision with electrocoagulation, or surgical removal. • Laser treatments. • May disappear without treatment.
Soft corn	Painful lesion caused by bony prominence of a toe pressing against adjacent toe. Usual location is web space between toes. Softness caused by secretions keeping web space relatively moist.	• Pain is relieved by placing cotton or spacers between toes to separate them. • Surgical treatment is excision of projecting bone spur (if present).

DIP, Distal interphalangeal; *MTP,* metatarsophalangeal; *PIP,* proximal interphalangeal.

❖ NURSING MANAGEMENT: FOOT DISORDERS

◆ Nursing Implementation

◆ **Health Promotion.** Well-made and properly fitted shoes are essential for healthy, pain-free feet. Women's footwear is often influenced by current styles instead of comfort and support. Stress the importance of having a shoe that conforms to the foot rather than to fashion trends. The shoe must be long enough and wide enough to avoid crowding the toes and forcing the great toe into a position of hallux valgus (Fig. 63.6). At the metatarsal head, the shoe should be wide enough to allow foot muscles to move freely and toes to bend. The shank (narrow part of sole under the instep) of the shoe should be rigid enough to give good support. The height of the heel should be realistic in relation to the shoe's purpose. Ideally, the heel of the shoe should not rise more than 1 inch higher than the forefoot

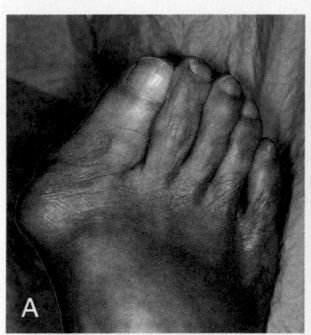 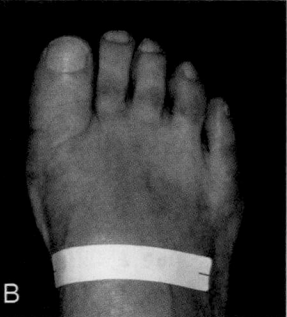

FIG. 63.6 **A,** Severe hallux valgus with bursa formation. **B,** Postoperative correction. (From Canale ST, Beaty JH: *Campbell's operative orthopaedics,* ed 12, Philadelphia, 2013, Mosby.)

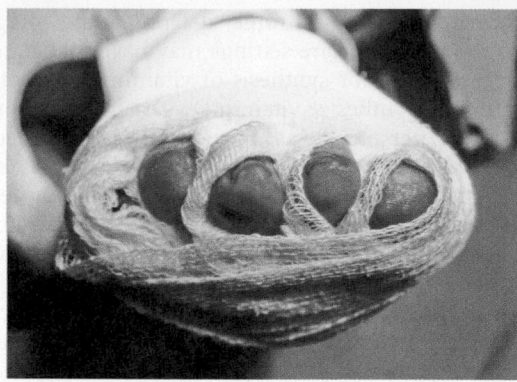

FIG. 63.7 Postoperative supportive dressing for treatment of moderate forefoot deformity. Dressing must be conforming and binding enough to hold toe in exact position. (From Canale ST, Beaty JH: *Campbell's operative orthopaedics,* ed 12, Philadelphia, 2013, Mosby.)

support. Wearing higher heeled shoes with a narrow toe box will cause hammertoes and corns over time.

Prolonged use of improper footwear can also cause a *Morton's neuroma.* They cause compression of an intermetatarsal plantar nerve, resulting in paresthesia and burning. At first, patients with Morton's neuroma may describe feeling as if a sock is rolled up under their toes. Neuromas usually occur between the third and fourth toes.

◆ **Acute Care.** Many foot problems require referral to a podiatrist. Depending on the problem, conservative therapies are tried first (Table 63.11). These include NSAIDs, ice, physical therapy, footwear changes, stretching, warm soaks, orthotics, ultrasound, and corticosteroid injections. If these methods do not help, surgery may be needed.

? CHECK YOUR PRACTICE

A 53-yr-old woman is scheduled for surgical correction of a bunion after a diagnosis of hallux valgus. You are doing her preoperative assessment. She asks you, "Do you think I caused this problem? I love shoes and have a whole closet full of fancy ones. Now I have to wear this ugly bunion shoe. I am not sure I can handle taking care of myself after surgery."
• How will you respond to the patient?
• What teaching will you provide about her postoperative care?

Depending on the type of surgery, pins or wires may extend through the toes, or a protective splint may be placed over the end of the foot. After surgery, the foot is usually immobilized by a bulky dressing (Fig. 63.7), short leg cast, slipper (plaster) cast, or a platform shoe that fits over the dressing and has a rigid sole (also known as a *bunion shoe*).

Elevate the foot with the heel off the bed to reduce discomfort and prevent edema. Assess neurovascular condition frequently during the immediate postoperative period. Inserted devices may interfere with assessment for movement. Be aware that evaluating sensation may be hard because the patient may be unable to distinguish surgical pain from pain caused by nerve pressure or circulatory impairment.

The type and extent of surgery determine the orders for ambulation. Crutches, a walker, or a cane may be needed. The patient may have pain or a throbbing sensation when lowering the affected leg. Reinforce instructions from the physical therapist. Teach the patient the importance of walking with an erect posture with proper weight distribution. Report gait problems or continued pain to the HCP. Encourage frequent rest periods with the foot elevated.

◆ **Ambulatory Care.** Teach the patient to perform daily hygienic foot care and wear clean stockings. Stockings should be long enough to avoid wrinkling and causing pressure areas. Trimming toenails straight across helps prevent ingrown toenails and reduces the risk for infection. Provide detailed instruction to patients with impaired circulation or diabetes to prevent serious complications from blisters, pressure areas, and infection. (See Table 48.21 for guidelines on foot care.)

Gerontologic Considerations: Foot Problems

The older adult is prone to foot problems because of poor circulation, atherosclerosis, and decreased sensation in the lower extremities. This is especially true for those with diabetes. A patient may develop an open wound but not feel it because of altered sensation from peripheral vascular disease or diabetic neuropathy. Teach older adults to inspect their feet daily and report any open wounds or breaks in the skin to their HCP.[21]

Untreated wounds may become infected, lead to osteomyelitis, and need surgical debridement. If the infection becomes widespread, lower limb amputation may be needed. Teach the caregiver of the older adult who needs help with hygiene practices the importance of carefully assessing the feet at regular intervals.

METABOLIC BONE DISEASES

Normal bone metabolism is affected by hormones, nutrition, and genetics. When dysfunction occurs in any of these factors, generalized reduction in bone mass and strength may result. Metabolic bone diseases include osteomalacia, osteoporosis, and Paget's disease.

OSTEOMALACIA

Osteomalacia is caused by a vitamin D deficiency that causes bone to lose calcium and become soft. The disease is uncommon in the United States. It is the same disorder as rickets in children, except the epiphyseal growth plates are closed in adults. Vitamin D is required for the absorption of calcium from the intestine. Insufficient vitamin D intake can interfere with normal bone mineralization. With little or no calcification, bones become soft.

Causes include limited sun exposure (ultraviolet rays needed for vitamin D synthesis), GI malabsorption (post weight loss surgery, celiac disease), chronic diarrhea, and pregnancy. Residents of long-term care settings may have inadequate sun exposure and thus poor synthesis of vitamin D. Persons with dark skin do not synthesize vitamin D as easily as persons with fair skin. Obese persons are at higher risk because of decreased physical activity. Chronic liver, kidneys, and small intestine disease may contribute to vitamin D deficiency. Long-term use of antiseizure drugs (e.g., phenytoin) and phosphate-binding antacids (e.g., Maalox) may decrease calcium and vitamin D absorption.[22]

Common manifestations are bone pain and muscle weakness. The pain is often worse at night and affects the lower back, pelvis, hips, legs, and ribs.[23] Muscle weakness and progressive deformity of weight-bearing bones (e.g., spine, extremities) can lead to problems walking and a waddling gait. Fractures are common and indicate delayed bone healing.

Laboratory findings include decreased serum calcium or phosphorus, decreased serum 25-hydroxyvitamin D, and increased serum alkaline phosphatase. X-rays may show effects of generalized bone demineralization, especially loss of calcium in the bones of the pelvis and associated bone deformity. *Looser's transformation zones* (ribbons of decalcification in bone found on x-ray) are diagnostic of osteomalacia. However, significant osteomalacia may exist without x-ray changes.

Interprofessional care is directed toward correcting the vitamin D deficiency. The patient often has a dramatic response when vitamin D_3 (cholecalciferol) and vitamin D_2 (ergocalciferol) supplements are used. Calcium or phosphorus supplements may be prescribed. Encourage dietary intake of eggs, meat, and oily fish (e.g., salmon, tuna). Milk and breakfast cereals fortified with calcium and vitamin D should be part of the diet. Exposure to sunlight and weight-bearing exercise are valuable as well. Assess patients who had weight loss surgery to treat obesity for osteomalacia. Any vitamin D deficiencies should be corrected.[24]

OSTEOPOROSIS

Osteoporosis is a chronic, progressive metabolic bone disease marked by low bone mass and deterioration of bone tissue, leading to increased bone fragility (Fig. 63.8). More than 54 million persons in the United States have decreased bone density or osteoporosis.[25] Osteoporosis is known as the "silent thief" because it slowly robs the skeleton of its banked resources. Bones eventually become so fragile that they cannot withstand normal mechanical stress.

Osteoporosis is more common in women. This is for several reasons: (1) women tend to have lower calcium intake than men throughout their lives (men between 15 and 50 years of age consume twice as much calcium as women); (2) women have less bone mass because of their generally smaller frames; (3) bone resorption begins at an earlier age in women and becomes more rapid at menopause; (4) pregnancy and breastfeeding deplete a woman's skeletal reserve unless calcium intake is adequate; and (5) longevity increases the risk for osteoporosis.

Current guidelines recommend an initial bone density test in all women over age 65 years. If results are normal and the person is at low risk for osteoporosis, another test is not needed for 15 years. Women who are younger than 65 and at high risk (e.g., low body weight, smoker, prior fractures) should have a bone density test earlier. Testing should also start earlier and be done more often if a person is at high risk for fractures. Currently there is not enough evidence that shows any benefit for screening men.[26]

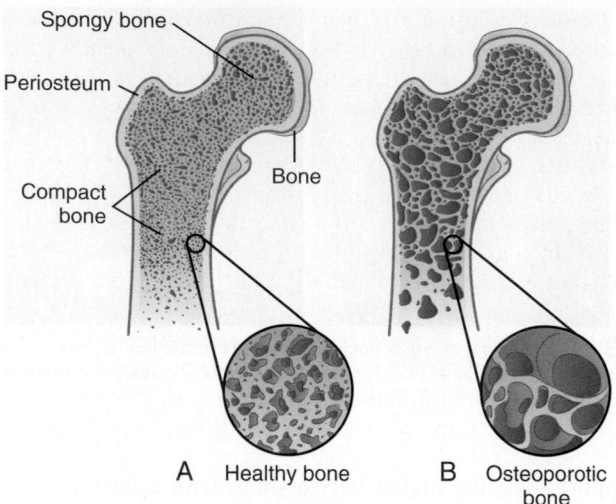

FIG. 63.8 A, Normal bone. B, Osteoporotic bone.

TABLE 63.12 **Risk Factors for Osteoporosis**
• Advancing age (>65 yr)
• Female gender
• Low body weight
• White or Asian ethnicity
• Cigarette smoking
• Sedentary lifestyle
• Estrogen deficiency in women (surgical or age-related menopause)
• Family history of osteoporosis
• Diet low in calcium or vitamin D deficiency
• Excess use of alcohol (>2 drinks/day)
• Low testosterone in men
• Long-term use of corticosteroids, thyroid replacement, heparin, long-acting sedatives, or antiseizure drugs

⊕ PROMOTING HEALTH EQUITY
Osteoporosis

- White and Asian American women have the highest incidence of osteoporosis.
- Black women begin menopause with more bone mass and have the lowest rate of bone loss after menopause.
- Risk for fracture is highest in white women.

Etiology and Pathophysiology

Risk factors for osteoporosis are listed in Table 63.12. Decreased risk is associated with regular weight-bearing exercise and adequate intake of fluoride, calcium, and vitamin D. Low testosterone is a major risk factor in men.

Peak bone mass (maximum bone tissue) is typically achieved before age 20. It is largely determined by 4 factors: heredity, nutrition, exercise, and hormone function. Heredity may be responsible for up to 70% of a person's peak bone mass. Genetic factors also influence bone size, quality, and turnover. Bone loss from midlife (ages 35 to 40 years) onward is inevitable, but the rate of loss varies. At menopause, women have rapid bone loss when the decline in estrogen production is the greatest. The rate of loss then slows and eventually matches the rate of bone lost by men ages 65 to 70 years.

Bone is continuously being deposited by osteoblasts and resorbed by osteoclasts, a process called *remodeling*. Rates of bone deposition and resorption are normally equal, so total bone mass stays constant.[27] In osteoporosis, bone resorption exceeds bone deposition.

Diseases associated with osteoporosis include inflammatory bowel disease, intestinal malabsorption, kidney disease, rheumatoid arthritis, hyperthyroidism, alcohol use disorder, cirrhosis, hypogonadism, and diabetes. Many drugs can interfere with bone metabolism, including corticosteroids, antiseizure drugs (e.g., divalproex sodium [Depakote], phenytoin), aluminum-containing antacids, heparin, some chemotherapy drugs, and excess thyroid hormones. When one of these drugs is prescribed, teach the patient about this possible side effect. Long-term corticosteroid use is a major contributor to osteoporosis.

GENDER DIFFERENCES

Osteoporosis

Men	Women
• Men are underdiagnosed and undertreated for osteoporosis compared with women. • 1 in 4 men over age 50 will have an osteoporosis-related fracture in his lifetime.	• Osteoporosis is 8 times more common in women than in men. • 1 in 2 women over age 50 years will have an osteoporosis-related fracture in her lifetime.

Clinical Manifestations

Osteoporosis occurs most often in bones of the spine, hips, and wrists. Typical early manifestations are back pain and spontaneous fractures. The loss of bone mass causes the bone to become mechanically weaker and prone to spontaneous fractures or fractures from minimal trauma. A person who has a vertebral fracture due to osteoporosis has an increased risk for having a second vertebral fracture within 1 year. Over time, vertebral fractures and wedging cause gradual loss of height and a humped thoracic spine (*kyphosis,* or "dowager's hump") (Fig. 63.9).

Diagnostic Studies

Osteoporosis often goes unnoticed because it cannot be detected by conventional x-ray until 25% to 40% of calcium in the bone is lost. Serum calcium, phosphorus, and alkaline phosphatase levels usually are normal. Alkaline phosphatase may be increased after a fracture.

Bone mineral density (BMD) measurements are typically expressed as grams of mineral per unit volume. BMD is determined by peak bone mass and amount of bone loss. (Procedures for BMD measurement are described in Table 61.8.) BMD may be measured by quantitative ultrasound (QUS) and dual-energy x-ray absorptiometry (DEXA). QUS uses sound waves to measure bone density in the heel, kneecap, or shin. DEXA (considered the gold standard of BMD studies by the World Health Organization) measures bone density in the spine, hips, and forearm.[28] These represent the most common sites of fragility fractures from osteoporosis. DEXA studies are useful to evaluate changes in bone density over time and assess effectiveness of osteoporosis treatment.

The BMD test results are compared to the ideal or peak bone mineral density of a healthy 30-yr-old adult and reported as T-scores. A T-score of 0 means the BMD is equal to the norm for a healthy young adult. Differences between the BMD and that of the healthy young adult norm are measured in units called *standard deviations (SDs)*. The more standard deviations below 0 (indicated as negative numbers), the lower the BMD and the higher the risk for fracture.

A T-score between +1 and –1 is normal. A T-score between –1 and –2.5 indicates osteopenia (bone loss that is more than normal, but not yet at the level for a diagnosis of osteoporosis). A T-score of –2.5 or lower indicates osteoporosis. The greater the negative number, the more severe the osteoporosis.[28]

Sometimes the HCP uses a Z-score instead of a T-score. In this case a person is compared with someone their own age, gender, and/or ethnic group instead of a healthy 30-yr-old person. Among older adults, Z-scores can be misleading because decreased bone density is common. If the Z-score is –2 or lower, it may suggest that something other than aging is causing abnormal bone loss.

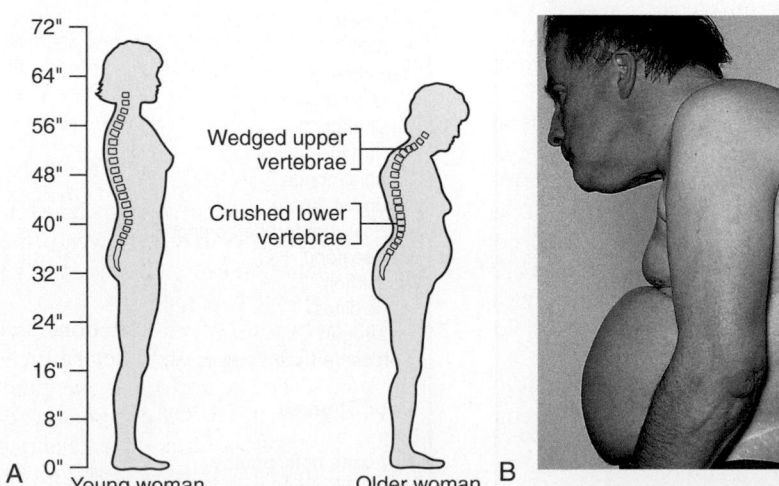

FIG. 63.9 The effects of osteoporosis. A, Comparison of young woman with an older woman. B, Severe fixed kyphosis producing a question-mark appearance. (*A,* From Phillips N: *Berry & Kohn's operating room technique,* ed 12, St Louis, 2013, Mosby. *B,* Courtesy Mir MA. In Kanski JJ: *Clinical diagnosis in ophthalmology,* St Louis, 2006, Mosby.)

❖ NURSING AND INTERPROFESSIONAL MANAGEMENT: OSTEOPOROSIS

Interprofessional care focuses on proper nutrition, calcium and vitamin D supplementation, exercise, prevention of falls and fractures, and drugs (Table 63.13). The National Osteoporosis Foundation recommends treatment for osteoporosis for postmenopausal women with (1) a T-score of less than −2.5, (2) a T-score between −1 and −2.5 with additional risk factors (Table 63.12), or (3) prior history of a hip or vertebral fracture.

A patient's risk for fracture from osteoporosis also can be calculated with the Fracture Risk Assessment (FRAX) tool. The FRAX considers BMD and other clinical factors when assessing fracture risk.[29]

The recommended calcium intake is 1000 mg/day for women ages 19 to 50 years and men ages 19 to 70 years and 1200 mg/day in women age 51 years or older and men 71 years or older. Foods high in calcium include milk, yogurt, turnip greens, cottage cheese, ice cream, sardines, and spinach (Table 63.14). If dietary intake of calcium is inadequate, supplemental calcium may be given.

It is difficult for us to absorb calcium in single doses greater than 500 mg. Teach the patient the importance of taking calcium supplements as divided doses to increase absorption. The amount of elemental calcium varies in calcium preparations. Calcium carbonate has 40% elemental calcium. It should be taken with meals because stomach acid is needed to dissolve and absorb this supplement. Calcium citrate has about 20% elemental calcium but is less dependent on stomach acid for absorption. It is better absorbed by patients taking a proton pump inhibitor (e.g., esomeprazole [Nexium]) or histamine receptor blocker (e.g., cimetidine) for acid reflux. Calcium lactate and calcium gluconate are not recommended because they have small amounts of elemental calcium.

Vitamin D is important in calcium absorption and function and may have a role in bone formation. Most people get enough vitamin D from their diet or naturally through synthesis in the skin from exposure to sunlight. Being in the sun for 20 minutes a day is generally enough. However, supplemental vitamin D (800 IU) is recommended for postmenopausal women, older men, persons who are homebound or in long-term care settings, and those in northern climates due to decreased sun exposure.

Regular physical activity is important to build and maintain bone mass. Exercise increases muscle strength, coordination, and balance. The best exercises are weight-bearing exercises that force a person to work against gravity. These include walking, hiking, weight training, stair climbing, tennis, and dancing. Walking is preferred to high-impact aerobics or running. Both may put too much stress on the bones and cause stress fractures. Encourage patients to walk 30 minutes 3 times a week. Teach patients to quit smoking and decrease alcohol use to minimize negative effects on bone mass.

Encourage patients with osteoporosis to remain ambulatory to prevent further loss of bone density due to immobility. Treatment may also involve the use of a gait aid to walk safely and protect areas of potential pathologic fractures. For example, a TLSO may be used to maintain the spine in proper alignment after fracture or treatment of a vertebral fracture. (Fractures are discussed in Chapter 62.)

Vertebroplasty and *kyphoplasty* are minimally invasive procedures used to treat osteoporotic vertebral fractures (see Chapter 62).[30] In vertebroplasty, bone cement is injected into

---

🔬 TABLE 63.13   Interprofessional Care
Osteoporosis

Diagnostic Assessment
- History and physical examination
- Serum calcium, phosphorus, alkaline phosphatase, vitamin D
- Bone mineral densitometry
- Dual-energy x-ray absorptiometry (DEXA)

Management
- Adequate dietary calcium (Table 63.14)
- Calcium supplements
- Sun exposure or vitamin D supplements
- Exercise program

Drug Therapy
- Bisphosphonates (recommended)
  - alendronate (Fosamax, Binosto)
  - risedronate (Actonel)
  - zoledronic acid (Reclast)
- Monoclonal antibodies
  - denosumab (Prolia)
  - romosozumab (Evenity)
- Bisphosphonates (other available agents)
  - etidronate (Didronel)
  - ibandronate (Boniva)
  - pamidronate (Aredia)
- Recombinant parathyroid hormone (e.g., teriparatide [Forteo], abaloparatide [Tymlos])

Minimally Invasive Procedures
- Vertebroplasty
- Kyphoplasty

🍐 TABLE 63.14   Nutritional Therapy
Sources of Calcium

Food	Calcium (mg)
Good Sources	
1 cup milk	
• Whole	279
• Skim	299
1 oz cheese	
• Mozzarella	222
• Cheddar	214
• Cottage	138
1 cup almonds	304
1 cup ice cream	168
6 oz calcium-fortified orange juice	261
3 oz seafood	
• Salmon	181
• Sardines	325
8 oz yogurt	313–384
Soft serve frozen yogurt	206
Poor Sources	
Egg	28
3 oz beef, pork, poultry	10
Apple, banana	10
1 med carrot	14
1 med potato	14
¼ head lettuce	27

the collapsed vertebra to stabilize the spine and improve the patient's pain. This procedure does not restore vertebral height or correct deformity. In kyphoplasty, a small balloon is inserted into the collapsed vertebra and inflated to restore vertebral body height before injection of bone cement. Kyphoplasty is the preferred surgical treatment for vertebral compression fractures.

◆ Drug Therapy

The recommended drug therapies for the prevention and treatment of osteoporosis are the bisphosphonates alendronate, risedronate, and zoledronic acid, or denosumab. Bisphosphonates inhibit osteoclast-mediated bone resorption and slow the cycle of bone remodeling. Although a modest increase in BMD is typical, bone remodeling may be suppressed to the extent that normal bone formation is impaired and fracture risk increases. Treatment should continue for 5 years (Table 63.13).[31]

Common side effects are anorexia, weight loss, and gastritis. Teach the patient to take the medication correctly to improve its absorption (see Drug Alert). These precautions also decrease GI side effects (especially esophageal irritation). A rare, but serious, side effect of bisphosphonates is *osteonecrosis* (bone death) of the jaw. Its cause is unknown. Those with dental disease, cancer, Paget's disease, or renal disease are most at risk for this complication. Patients should see a dentist before beginning treatment and then annually to ensure good oral health.

 DRUG ALERT Bisphosphonates

Teach patient to:
- Take with full glass of water.
- Take 30 min before food or other medications.
- Remain upright for at least 30 min after taking.

Alendronate (Fosamax) is available as a daily or weekly oral tablet. The immediate-release form of risedronate (Actonel) is given daily, weekly, or monthly, based on the dose. Zoledronic acid (Reclast) is given as a once-yearly or every-other-year IV infusion. Renal function tests and serum calcium must be assessed before administration. Other bisphosphonates are shown in Table 63.13.

Denosumab (Prolia) may be given to postmenopausal women with osteoporosis who are at high risk for fractures. It is a monoclonal antibody that binds to a protein (RANKL) involved in the formation and function of osteoclasts. Denosumab is given as a subcutaneous injection every 6 months.

Other agents used include the new monoclonal antibody romosozumab (Evenity). It inhibits the action of sclerostin, a regulatory factor in bone metabolism. This increases bone formation and, to a lesser extent, decreases bone resorption. It is given by subcutaneous injection every month for a total of 12 doses.

Raloxifene (Evista)is a selective estrogen receptor modulator (SERM). This drug mimics the effect of estrogen on bone by reducing bone resorption without stimulating the tissues of the breast or uterus. Raloxifene reduces the risk for vertebral, but not hip, fractures. Side effects, including leg cramps, hot flashes, and increased risk for blood clots, limit use.[31]

Teriparatide (Forteo) is a recombinant form of human parathyroid hormone (PTH) that increases the action of osteoblasts. This drug is used to treat osteoporosis in men and postmenopausal women at high risk for fractures, including risk related to long-term corticosteroid use.[31] Side effects include leg cramps

and dizziness. Teriparatide is the first drug approved to stimulate new bone formation in osteoporosis. Most drugs only prevent further bone loss. It is self-administered daily by subcutaneous injection from a preloaded pen.

Women no longer routinely use estrogen replacement therapy or estrogen with progesterone after menopause to prevent osteoporosis because of the increased risk for heart disease and breast and uterine cancer. A woman who takes short-term estrogen therapy to treat menopausal symptoms, such as hot flashes, may receive some protection against bone loss and hip and vertebrae fractures.[32] We think estrogen inhibits osteoclast activity, leading to decreased bone resorption.

Medical management of patients receiving corticosteroids includes prescribing the lowest effective dose for the shortest possible time. Ensure an adequate intake of calcium and vitamin D, including supplements, when osteoporosis drugs are prescribed. If osteopenia is present on bone densitometry in people who are taking corticosteroids, treatment with bisphosphonates may be considered.

PAGET'S DISEASE

Paget's disease *(osteitis deformans)* is a chronic skeletal bone disorder in which excessive bone resorption is followed by replacement of normal marrow by vascular, fibrous connective tissue. The new bone is larger, disorganized, and weaker. Areas commonly affected include the pelvis, long bones, spine, ribs, sternum, and skull. Up to 5% of adults in the United States are affected by Paget's disease.[33] Men are affected twice as often as women. Paget's disease is uncommon in people under age 40.

We do not know exactly what causes Paget's disease. The cause may be viral or genetic. Up to 40% of all patients with the disease have at least 1 relative with the disorder.

In milder forms of Paget's disease, patients do not have any symptoms. The disease may be found incidentally through x-ray or serum chemistry findings of high alkaline phosphatase.[34] Bone pain may develop gradually and progress to severe intractable pain. Other early manifestations include fatigue and progressive development of a waddling gait. Patients report becoming shorter or their heads are becoming larger. Headaches, dementia, vision deficits, and loss of hearing can result from an enlarged, thickened skull. Increased bone volume in the spine can cause spinal cord or nerve root compression.

Pathologic fracture is the most common complication and may be the first sign of Paget's disease. Other complications include osteosarcoma, fibrosarcoma, and osteoclastoma (giant cell) tumors.

Serum alkaline phosphatase is markedly increased in advanced disease, showing high bone turnover.[34] X-rays may show curvature of an affected bone. The bone cortex becomes thicker and irregular, especially in weight-bearing bones and the cranium. Bone scans using a radiolabeled bisphosphonate show increased uptake in the affected skeletal areas.

Interprofessional care is usually limited to symptomatic and supportive care, with correction of secondary deformities by surgical intervention or braces. Bisphosphonate drugs (Table 63.13) are used to slow bone resorption. Zoledronic acid may be given specifically to build bone. Calcium and vitamin D can decrease hypocalcemia, a common side effect of drug therapy. Monitor drug effectiveness by regular assessment of serum alkaline phosphatase.

Calcitonin is an option for patients who cannot tolerate bis-phosphonates. Human calcitonin inhibits osteoclastic activity, prevents bone resorption, relieves acute symptoms, and lowers serum alkaline phosphatase. This drug is available as a subcutaneous injection. Salmon calcitonin is 1 form. It has a longer half-life and greater milligram potency than human calcitonin. Response to calcitonin therapy is not permanent and often ends when therapy stops.

Pain is usually managed with NSAIDs. Orthopedic surgery for fractures, hip and knee replacement, and knee realignment may be needed.

A firm mattress can provide back support and relieve pain. The patient may need to wear a corset or light brace to relieve back pain and give support when upright. Teach the patient to correctly apply the device and regularly examine the skin for friction damage. Discourage lifting and twisting. Good body mechanics are essential. Physical therapy may increase muscle strength. A well-balanced diet is important in management of metabolic bone disorders. Vitamin D, calcium, and protein are especially important to ensure available components for bone formation. To decrease risk for falls and related fractures, teach the patient to use an assistive device and make environmental changes (e.g., do not use throw rugs).

 SAFETY ALERT   Paget's Disease

To reduce the risk for patient harm from falls:
- Assess environmental fall risk factors (poor lighting, clutter, pets in the home).
- Identify personal risk factors for falls, including drugs and uncorrected vision.
- Take action to address any identified risks.

Gerontologic Considerations: Metabolic Bone Diseases

Osteoporosis and Paget's disease are common in older adults. Teach patients proper nutrition to decrease risk for further bone loss. Keep the patient as active as possible to slow demineralization of bone from disuse or extended immobilization.

Because metabolic bone disorders increase the risk for pathologic fractures, use extreme caution when turning or moving the patient. Hip fractures, in particular, may decrease quality of life and lead to admission to a long-term care facility. A supervised exercise program is essential to osteoporosis treatment. Encourage ambulation if the patient's condition permits.

CASE STUDY
Metastatic Bone Tumor/Pathologic Fracture

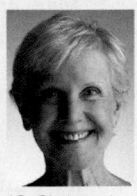

(© Christopher-Robbins/Photodisc/Thinkstock.)

Patient Profile

L.R. is a 60-yr-old white woman with a history of hypertension, hypothyroidism, and osteoporosis. Four years ago, she was diagnosed with stage 3a breast cancer and treated with surgery, radiation therapy, and chemotherapy. Today she was admitted to the emergency department after falling down 2 stairs.

Subjective Data

- Denies hitting her head or loss of consciousness
- States she was able to bear weight on her lower extremities but has significant left thigh pain after the fall
- Describes recent insidious onset of generalized weakness and fatigue
- Denies alcohol or tobacco use
- Takes levothyroxine (Synthroid) and atenolol (Tenormin) every morning. Takes risedronate (Actonel) once a month

Objective Data

- Left lower extremity slightly shorter and externally rotated compared to right lower extremity
- Moderate edema with associated ecchymosis on left thigh
- Thigh soft, compressible to palpation
- Reports pain with internal/external rotation of left lower extremity
- 2+ dorsalis pedis and posterior tibialis pulses bilaterally
- Gross motor/sensation intact in affected extremity

Diagnostic Studies

- X-ray shows oblique mid-shaft left femur fracture with lytic lesion in the femoral neck
- Normal CBC and blood chemistry results, slightly increased liver function tests
- CT scans of the chest, abdomen, and pelvis show multiple bony metastases throughout the pelvis, as well as lesions of the liver and spleen, widespread abdominal cancer, compression fractures with lesions of T11 vertebral body, and bilateral rib fractures with associated lesions.

- Whole body bone scan consistent with findings from x-ray and CT
- CT-guided biopsy of femur fracture site showed poorly differentiated cells consistent with breast cancer

Interprofessional Care

- Diagnosed with stage IV breast cancer
- Intramedullary nail for femur fracture
- Pain management
- Postoperative chemotherapy and hormone therapy
- High-protein, high-calcium, nutrient-rich diet
- Depression assessment and management
- Ambulation evaluation with gait aids as needed

Discussion Questions

1. Why did a relatively low-energy injury cause L.R.'s fracture?
2. **Patient-Centered Care:** What factors could result in inadequate caloric intake after surgery? How could you help L.R. increase her intake of protein and calcium?
3. What factors increase L.R.'s risk for delayed union or nonunion of the fracture?
4. **Priority Decision:** What are the priority teaching needs for L.R.?
5. **Collaboration:** Which persons on the interprofessional team should be responsible for L.R.'s home care instructions? Who should be responsible for ambulation and home safety teaching and assessments? Who should help L.R. with transfers and ambulation during her hospital stay?
6. **Priority Decision:** Based on the assessment data, what are the priority nursing diagnoses?
7. **Quality Improvement:** What outcomes would indicate that interprofessional care was effective?
8. **Safety:** What safety precautions should be considered for this patient?
9. **Evidence-Based Practice:** L.R asks why it is important for her to have daily injections of enoxaparin after surgery. How do you respond?

Answers available at *http://evolve.elsevier.com/Lewis/medsurg.*

■ BRIDGE TO NCLEX EXAMINATION

The number of the question corresponds to the same-numbered outcome at the beginning of the chapter.

1. A patient with osteomyelitis undergoes surgical debridement with implantation of antibiotic beads. When the patient asks why the beads are used, the nurse answers *(select all that apply)*
   a. "Oral or IV antibiotics are not effective in most cases of bone infection."
   b. "The beads are an adjunct to debridement and antibiotics for deep infections."
   c. "The beads are used to deliver antibiotics directly to the site of the infection."
   d. "This is the safest method to deliver long-term antibiotic therapy for bone infection."
   e. "Ischemia and bone death related to osteomyelitis are impenetrable to IV antibiotics."

2. A patient with osteosarcoma of the humerus shows understanding of his treatment options when he states
   a. "I accept that I have to lose my arm with surgery."
   b. "The chemotherapy before surgery will shrink the tumor."
   c. "This tumor is related to the melanoma I had 3 years ago."
   d. "I'm glad they can take out the cancer with such a small scar."

3. Which persons are at high risk for chronic low back pain? *(select all that apply)*
   a. A 63-yr-old man who is a long-distance truck driver
   b. A 30-yr-old nurse who works on an orthopedic unit and smokes
   c. A 55-yr-old construction worker who is 6 ft, 2 in and weighs 250 lb
   d. A 44-yr-old female chef with prior compression fracture of the spine
   e. A 28-yr-old female yoga instructor who is 5 ft, 6 in and weighs 130 lb

4. A patient with suspected disc herniation has acute pain and muscle spasms. The nurse's responsibility is to
   a. encourage total bed rest for several days.
   b. teach principles of back strengthening exercises.
   c. stress the importance of straight-leg raises to decrease pain.
   d. promote use of cold and hot compresses and pain medication.

5. In caring for a patient after a spinal fusion, the nurse would report which finding to the health care provider?
   a. The patient has a single episode of emesis.
   b. The patient is unable to move the lower extremities.
   c. The patient is nauseated and has not voided in 4 hours.
   d. The patient reports of pain at the bone graft donor site.

6. A patient who has had surgical correction of bilateral hallux valgus is being discharged from the same-day surgery unit. The nurse will teach the patient to
   a. rest frequently with the feet elevated.
   b. wear shoes continually except when bathing.
   c. soak the feet in warm water several times a day.
   d. expect the feet to be numb for the next few days.

7. What is most important to include in the teaching plan for a patient with osteopenia?
   a. Lose weight.
   b. Stop smoking.
   c. Eat a high-protein diet.
   d. Start swimming for exercise.

1. b, c, 2. b, 3. a, b, c, d, 4. d, 5. b, 6. a, 7. b

For rationales to these answers and even more NCLEX review questions, visit *http://evolve.elsevier.com/Lewis/medsurg*.

ⓔ EVOLVE WEBSITE/RESOURCES LIST

http://evolve.elsevier.com/Lewis/medsurg
Review Questions (Online Only)
Key Points
Answer Keys for Questions
  • Rationales for Bridge to NCLEX Examination Questions
  • Answer Guidelines for Case Study on p. 1496
Student Case Study
  • Patient With Osteoporosis
Nursing Care Plans
  • eNursing Care Plan 63.1: Patient With Osteomyelitis
  • eNursing Care Plan 63.2: Patient With Low Back Pain
Conceptual Care Map Creator
Audio Glossary
Supporting Media
  • Animations
    • Diskectomy
    • Kyphoplasty
Content Updates

REFERENCES

1. Kavanagh N, Ryan EJ, Widaa A, et al: Staphylococcal osteomyelitis. Disease progression, treatment challenges, and future directions, *Clinical Microbiology Reviews* 31:e84, 2018.
2. Schmitt S: Osteomyelitis. Retrieved from *www.merckmanuals.com/professional/musculoskeletal-and-connective-tissue-disorders/infections-of-joints-and-bones/osteomyelitis#*.
*3. Siegel RL, Miller KD, Jemal, A: Cancer statistics, *CA Cancer J Clin* 68:1, 2018.
4. American Cancer Society: Osteosarcoma. Retrieved from *www.cancer.org/cancer/osteosarcoma.html*.
5. Itano JK: *Core curriculum for oncology nursing*, ed 5, St Louis, 2016, Elsevier.
6. Muscular Dystrophy Association: Duchenne muscular dystrophy. Retrieved from *www.mda.org/disease/duchenne-muscular-dystrophy*.
*7. Matthews E, Brassington R, Kuntzer T, et al: Corticosteroids for the treatment of Duchenne muscular dystrophy, *The Cochrane Library* May 5(5):CD003725, 2016.
8. Sarepta Therapeutics: Exondys 51. Retrieved from *www.exondys51hcp.com/*.
9. Centers for Disease Control and Prevention: Duchene muscular dystrophy care considerations. Retrieved from *www.cdc.gov/features/muscular-dystrophy-care*.
10. National Institute of Neurological Disorders and Stroke: Low back pain fact sheet. Retrieved from *www.ninds.nih.gov/disorders/backpain/detail_backpain.htm*.
*11. Nourollahi M, Afshari D, Dianat I: Awkward trunk postures and their relationship with low back pain in hospital nurses, *Work* 59:317, 2018.
*12. Andrews VD, Southard EP: Safe patient handling: Keeping health care workers safe, *Med-Surg Matters* 26:4, 2017.
13. Cleveland Clinic: Degenerative back conditions. Retrieved from *https://my.clevelandclinic.org/health/diseases/16912-degenerative-back-conditions*.
14. American Academy of Orthopedic Surgeons: Cauda equina syndrome. Retrieved from *https://orthoinfo.aaos.org/en/diseases--conditions/cauda-equina-syndrome/*.
15. Mayo Clinic: Herniated disc. Retrieved from *www.mayoclinic.org/diseases-condtions/herniated-disc/diagnosis/treatment/drc-20354101*.
16. An HS, Juarez KK: Artificial disc replacement. Retrieved from *www.spineuniverse.com/treatments/surgery/artificial-disc-replacement*.

*17. Lee DD, Kim YM: A comparison of radiographic and clinical outcomes of anterior lumbar interbody fusion performed with either a cellular bone allograft containing multipotent adult progenitor cells or recombinant human bone morphogenetic protein-2, *J Orthop Surg Res* 12:126, 2017.

*18. Blanpied PR, Gross AR, Elliott JM, et al: Neck pain: Clinical practice guidelines linked to the international classification of functioning, disability and health from the orthopedic section of the American Physical Therapy Association, *J Orthop Sports Phys Ther* 47:A1, 2017.

*19. Gross AR, Paquin JP, Dupont G, et al: Exercises for mechanical neck disorders: A Cochrane review update, *Man Ther* 24:25, 2016.

*20. Buldt AK, Menz HB: Incorrectly fitted footwear, foot pain and foot disorders: A systematic search and narrative review of the literature, *JFAR* 11:43, 2018.

*21. Guidelines abstracted from the American Geriatrics Society Guidelines for improving the care of older adults with diabetes mellitus: 2013 Update, *JAGS* 61:2020, 2013. (Classic)

22. Bartl R, Bartl C: Drug-induced osteomalacia. In *Bone disorders,* New York, 2017, Springer.

23. Mayo Clinic: Osteomalacia. Retrieved from *www.mayoclinic.org/diseases-conditions/osteomalacia/symptoms-causes/syc-20355514?p=1.*

*24. Liu C, Wu D, Zhang JF, et al: Changes in bone metabolism in morbidly obese patients after bariatric surgery: A meta-analysis, *Obes Surg* 26:91, 2016.

25. National Osteoporosis Foundation: What is osteoporosis and what causes it? Retrieved from *www.nof.org/patients/what-is-osteoporosis/.*

*26. US Preventive Services Task Force: Osteoporosis to prevent fractures: Screening. Retrieved from *www.uspreventiveservicestaskforce.org/Page/Document/UpdateSummaryFinal/osteoporosis-screening1.*

27. Cleveland Clinic: Osteoporosis. Retrieved from *https://my.clevelandclinic.org/health/diseases/4443-osteoporosis.*

28. World Health Organization: WHO criteria for diagnosis of osteoporosis. Retrieved from *www.4bonehealth.org/education/world-health-organization-criteria-diagnosis-osteoporosis/.*

29. McCloskey EV, Harvey NC, Johansson H, et al: FRAX updates 2016, *Curr Opin Rheumatol* 28:433, 2016.

30. McCarthy J, Davis A: Diagnosis and management of vertebral compression fractures, *Am Fam Physician* 94:44, 2016.

*31. Qaseem A, Forciea MA, McLean RM, et al: Treatment of low bone density or osteoporosis to prevent fractures in men and women: A clinical practice guideline update from the American College of Physicians, *Ann Intern Med* 166:818, 2017.

*32. Schmidt P: The 2017 hormone therapy position statement of the North American Menopause Society, *Menopause* 24:728, 2017.

33. NIH Osteoporosis and Related Bone Diseases National Resource Center: What is Paget's disease of bone? Retrieved from *www.bones.nih.gov/health-info/bone/pagets/pagets-disease-ff#who.*

*34. Appelman-Dijkstra NM, Papapoulos SE: Paget's disease of bone. *Best Pract Res Clin Endocrinol Metab* 32:657, 2018.

*Evidence-based information for clinical practice.

64

Arthritis and Connective Tissue Diseases

Dottie Roberts

> *No one is useless in the world who lightens the burdens of another.*
>
> **Charles Dickens**

http://evolve.elsevier.com/Lewis/medsurg

CONCEPTUAL FOCUS

Fatigue	Mobility	Stress
Functional Ability	Pain	
Inflammation	Self-Management	

LEARNING OUTCOMES

1. Outline the sequence of events leading to joint destruction in osteoarthritis and rheumatoid arthritis.
2. Detail the clinical manifestations and interprofessional and nursing management of osteoarthritis and rheumatoid arthritis.
3. Describe the pathophysiology, clinical manifestations, and interprofessional care of gout, Lyme disease, and septic arthritis.
4. Discuss the pathophysiology, clinical manifestations, and interprofessional and nursing management of ankylosing spondylitis, psoriatic arthritis, and reactive arthritis.
5. Describe the pathophysiology, clinical manifestations, and interprofessional and nursing management of systemic lupus erythematosus, scleroderma, polymyositis, dermatomyositis, and Sjögren's syndrome.
6. Explain the drug therapy and related nursing management associated with arthritis and connective tissue diseases.
7. Relate possible etiologies, clinical manifestations, and interprofessional and nursing management of fibromyalgia and systemic exertion tolerance disease.

KEY TERMS

ankylosing spondylitis (AS), p. 1517
arthritis, p. 1499
CREST syndrome, p. 1523
dermatomyositis (DM), p. 1525
fibromyalgia, p. 1527
gout, p. 1513
Lyme disease, p. 1515

myofascial pain syndrome, p. 1527
osteoarthritis (OA), p. 1499
polymyositis (PM), p. 1525
psoriatic arthritis (PsA), p. 1518
Raynaud's phenomenon, p. 1523
rheumatoid arthritis (RA), p. 1505
septic arthritis, p. 1516

scleroderma, p. 1523
Sjögren's syndrome, p. 1526
spondyloarthropathies, p. 1517
systemic exertion intolerance disease (SEID), p. 1528
systemic lupus erythematosus (SLE), p. 1519

This chapter discusses *rheumatic diseases,* which primarily affect body joints, tendons, ligaments, muscles, and bones. These diseases are often marked by inflammation, pain, and loss of function in 1 or more of the body's connecting or supporting structures. The patient may be challenged by problems of limited function and fatigue, loss of self-esteem, altered body image, and fear of disability. More than 100 kinds of rheumatic diseases have been identified.[1] Over 54 million people in the United States have rheumatic conditions.[2]

ARTHRITIS

Arthritis involves inflammation of a joint or joints. Most forms of arthritis affect women more often than men in every age-group.[2] Osteoarthritis is the most common chronic condition of the joints.[3] Other forms include rheumatoid arthritis (RA), fibromyalgia, systemic lupus erythematosus (SLE), and gout.

OSTEOARTHRITIS

Osteoarthritis (OA) is a slowly progressive noninflammatory disorder of the diarthrodial *(synovial)* joints. Currently OA affects 30 million Americans. This number is expected to greatly increase as the population ages.[2]

Etiology and Pathophysiology

OA involves the gradual loss of articular cartilage with formation of bony outgrowths (spurs or osteophytes) at the joint margins.[3] OA is not a normal part of the aging process, but aging is one risk factor for disease development. Cartilage destruction

TABLE 64.1 Causes of Osteoarthritis

Cause	Effects on Joint Cartilage
Drugs	Drugs, such as indomethacin, colchicine, and corticosteroids, can stimulate collagen-digesting enzymes in joint synovium.
Hematologic or endocrine disorders	Chronic hemarthrosis (e.g., from hemophilia) contributes to cartilage deterioration.
Inflammation	Release of enzymes in response to local inflammation can affect cartilage health.
Joint instability	Damage to supporting structures causes instability, placing uneven stress on joint cartilage.
Mechanical stress	Repetitive physical activities (e.g., sports) cause cartilage deterioration.
Neurologic disorders	Pain and loss of reflexes from neurologic disorders, such as diabetic neuropathy and Charcot joint, cause abnormal movements that contribute to cartilage deterioration.
Skeletal deformities	Congenital or acquired conditions (e.g., dislocated hip) contribute to cartilage deterioration.
Trauma	Dislocations or fractures may lead to avascular necrosis or uneven stress on cartilage.

likely begins between ages 20 and 30. Most adults are affected by age 40. Few patients have symptoms until after age 50 or 60. More than half of those over age 65 have x-ray evidence of OA in at least 1 joint.[2]

OA may be caused by a known event or condition that directly damages cartilage or causes joint instability (Table 64.1). However, we cannot identify a single cause for many persons with OA. In these situations, various genetic traits may contribute to the development of cartilage defects. People with hand OA are more likely to develop knee OA.[2]

Decreased estrogen at menopause may contribute to the increased incidence of OA in aging women. Obesity is a modifiable risk factor that contributes to hip and knee OA. It increases mechanical stress on the joints. Regular moderate exercise, which helps with weight management, decreases the risk for disease development and progression. Anterior cruciate ligament injury from quick stops and pivoting, as in football and soccer, are linked to an increased risk for knee OA.[3] Work that requires frequent kneeling and stooping also increase the risk for knee OA.

GENDER DIFFERENCES
Osteoarthritis (OA)

Men
- Except for traumatic arthritis, men do not have OA as often as women until age 70 or 80 years.
- Hip OA is more common in men.

Women
- OA affects women more often.
- Hand OA (interphalangeal joints and thumb base) is more common in women.
- Knee OA is more common in women, especially after menopause. It is likely to be more severe.

The development of OA is complex. Genetic, metabolic, and local factors interact to cause cartilage deterioration from damage at the level of the chondrocytes (Fig. 64.1). The normally smooth, white, translucent articular cartilage becomes dull, yellow, and granular as the disease progresses. Affected cartilage steadily becomes softer and less elastic. It is less able to resist wear with heavy use.

The body's attempts at cartilage repair cannot keep up with the destruction of OA. As the collagen structure in the cartilage changes, articular surfaces become cracked and worn. While central cartilage becomes thinner, cartilage at the joint edges becomes thicker and osteophytes form. Joint surfaces become uneven, affecting the distribution of stress across the joint and causing reduced motion.

Although inflammation is not typical of OA, secondary synovitis may occur when phagocytes try to rid the joint of small pieces of cartilage torn from the joint surface. These changes cause the early pain and stiffness of OA. Pain in later disease occurs when articular cartilage is lost, and bony joint surfaces rub each other.

Clinical Manifestations

Joints. Manifestations range from mild discomfort to significant disability. Joint pain is the main symptom and the typical reason the patient seeks medical attention. Pain generally gets worse with joint use. In early stages of OA, joint pain is relieved by rest. However, the patient with advanced disease may have pain at rest or have trouble sleeping due to increased joint pain. Pain may worsen as the barometric pressure falls before the onset of severe weather.

As OA progresses, increasing pain can contribute greatly to disability and loss of function. The pain of OA may be referred to the groin, buttock, or outside of the thigh or knee. Sitting down becomes hard, as does rising from a chair when the hips are lower than the knees. As OA develops in the intervertebral (*apophyseal*) joints of the spine, local pain and stiffness are common.

Unlike pain, which typically worsens with activity, joint stiffness occurs after periods of rest or an unchanged position. Early morning stiffness is common. It generally resolves within 30 minutes. This distinguishes OA from inflammatory joint disorders, such as RA. Overactivity can cause a mild joint swelling that temporarily increases stiffness. *Crepitation,* a grating sensation caused by loose cartilage particles in the joint cavity, can cause stiffness. Crepitation is common in patients with knee OA.

OA usually affects joints on 1 side of the body (*asymmetrically*) rather than in pairs. For example, the left knee may be affected and the right knee unchanged. The distal interphalangeal (DIP) and proximal interphalangeal (PIP) joints of the fingers, and the metacarpophalangeal (MCP) joint of the thumb are often affected. Weight-bearing joints (hips, knees), the metatarsophalangeal (MTP) joint of the foot, and the cervical and lower lumbar vertebrae are often involved (Fig. 64.2).

Deformity. Deformity or instability associated with OA is specific to the involved joint. For example, *Heberden's nodes* occur on the DIP joints due to osteophyte formation and loss of joint space (Fig. 64.1, *D*). They can appear as early as age 40 and tend to be seen in family members. *Bouchard's nodes* on the PIP joints indicate similar disease involvement. Heberden's and Bouchard's nodes are often red, swollen, and tender. Although they usually do not cause significant loss of function, the visible deformity may bother the patient.

Knee OA often leads to obvious joint deformity due to cartilage loss in 1 joint compartment. For example, the patient

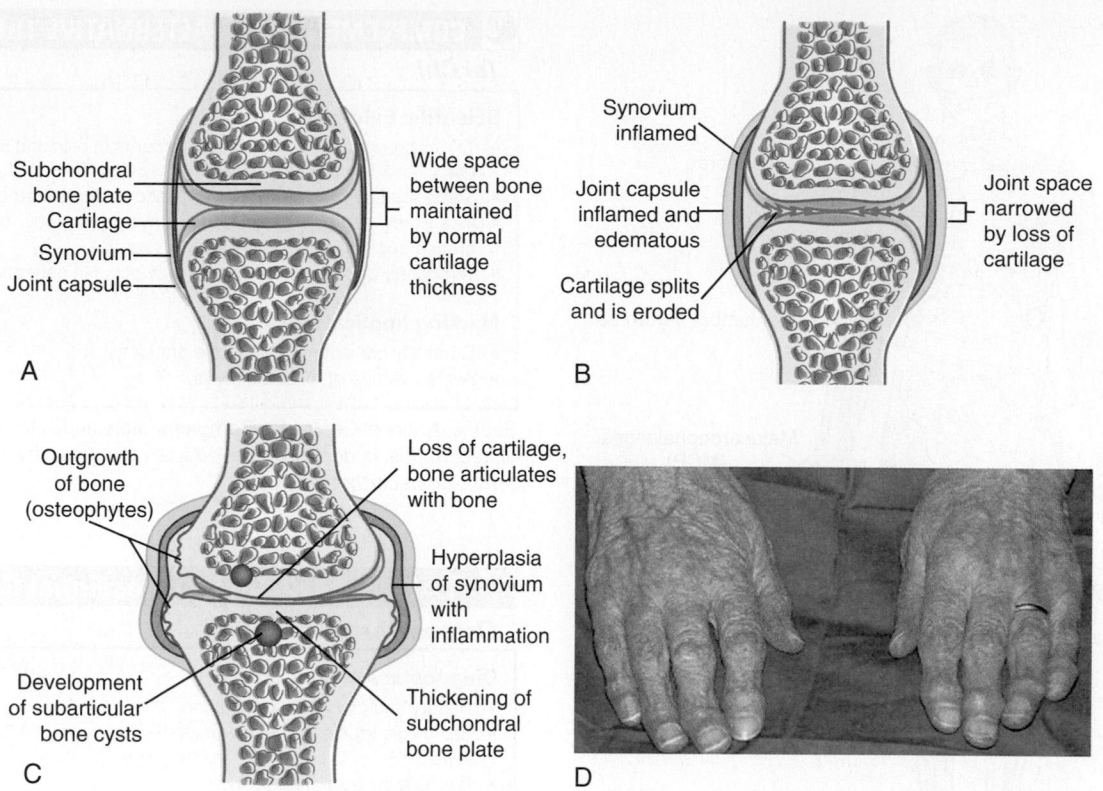

FIG. 64.1 Pathologic changes in osteoarthritis. **A,** Normal synovial joint. **B,** Early change in osteoarthritis is destruction of articular cartilage and narrowing of the joint space. There is inflammation and thickening of the joint capsule and synovium. **C,** With time, thickening of subarticular bone occurs, caused by constant friction of the 2 bone surfaces. Osteophytes form around the periphery of the joint by irregular overgrowths of bone. **D,** In osteoarthritis of the hands, osteophytes on the distal interphalangeal joints of the fingers, termed *Heberden's nodes,* appear as small nodules. (*D,* From Forbes CD, Jackson WF: *Color atlas and text of clinical medicine,* ed 3, London, 2003, Mosby.)

becomes bowlegged *(varus deformity)* in response to medial joint arthritis. Lateral joint arthritis causes a knock-kneed appearance *(valgus deformity).* In advanced hip OA, 1 leg may become shorter as the joint space narrows.

Systemic. Fatigue, fever, and organ involvement are not present in OA. This is an important distinction between OA and inflammatory joint disorders, such as rheumatoid arthritis.

Diagnostic Studies

A bone scan, CT scan, or MRI may be used to diagnose OA. These tests can detect early joint changes. X-rays help confirm disease and stage joint damage. As OA progresses, x-rays often show joint space narrowing and increasingly dense bone. Osteophytes may be visible. However, these changes do not always reflect the degree of pain the patient has. Despite strong x-ray evidence of disease, the patient may be relatively free of symptoms. Another patient may have severe pain with only slight x-ray changes.

No laboratory tests or biomarkers can be used to diagnose OA. The erythrocyte sedimentation rate (ESR) is normal except for slight increases during acute inflammation. Other routine blood tests (e.g., CBC, renal and liver function tests) are useful only in screening for related conditions or for establishing baseline values before starting treatment. Synovial fluid analysis helps distinguish OA from other types of inflammatory arthritis. In OA, the fluid is clear yellow with little or no sign of inflammation.

Interprofessional Care

OA has no cure. Interprofessional care focuses on managing pain and inflammation, preventing disability, and maintaining and improving joint function (Table 64.2). Nondrug interventions are the basis of OA management. They should be maintained throughout the patient's treatment. Drug therapy supplements nondrug treatments.

Rest and Joint Protection. Teach the patient with OA to balance rest and activity. Encourage rest of the affected joint during periods of acute inflammation. Keep joints in a functional position with splints or braces if needed. Avoid immobilization for more than 1 week because of the risk for joint stiffness with inactivity. Review how to modify usual activities to decrease stress on affected joints. Teach the patient with knee OA to avoid standing, kneeling, or squatting for long periods. Using an assistive device, such as a cane, walker, or crutches, can decrease joint stress.

Heat and Cold Applications. Apply heat and cold to help reduce pain and stiffness. Ice is not used as often as heat in OA treatment. Ice can be helpful if the patient has acute inflammation. Heat therapy is especially useful for stiffness. Treatments include hot packs, whirlpool baths, ultrasound, and paraffin wax baths.

Nutritional Therapy and Exercise. If the patient is overweight, a weight-reduction program is a critical part of the treatment plan. Help the patient evaluate the current diet to make needed changes. (Chapter 40 discusses ways to help the patient attain and maintain a healthy body weight.) Since mobilizing the joint

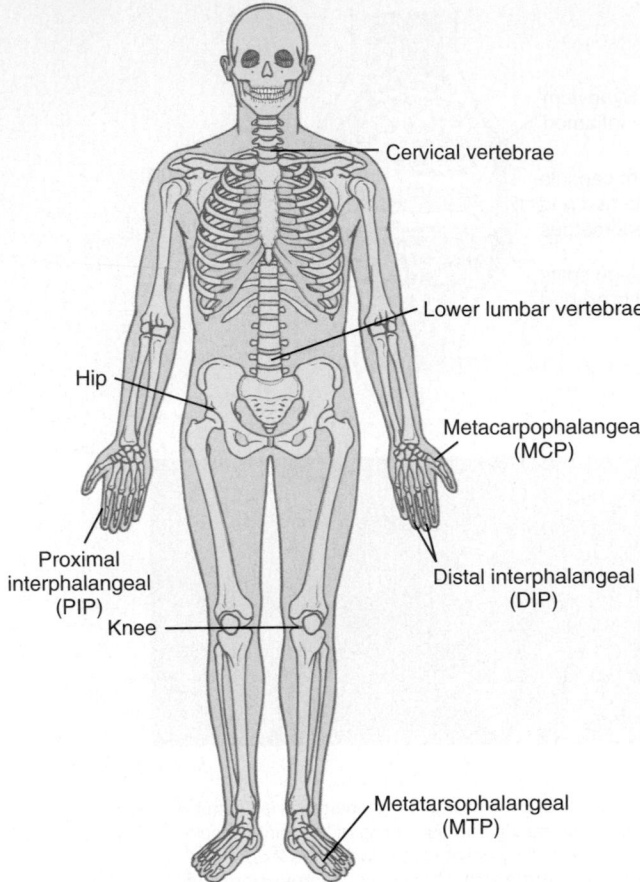

Cervical vertebrae

Lower lumbar vertebrae

Hip

Metacarpophalangeal (MCP)

Proximal interphalangeal (PIP)

Distal interphalangeal (DIP)

Knee

Metatarsophalangeal (MTP)

FIG. 64.2 Joints most often involved in osteoarthritis.

preserves articular cartilage health, exercise is an important part of OA management. Aerobic conditioning, range-of-motion (ROM) exercises, and programs to strengthen muscles around the affected joint help many patients.

Complementary and Alternative Therapies. Complementary and alternative therapies for OA symptom management are popular with patients who have not found relief through traditional medical care. Teach the patient to carefully research any alternative therapies and avoid replacing conventional OA treatments with unproven complementary approaches. Acupuncture, massage, and Tai Chi may reduce arthritis pain and improve joint mobility.

Some nutritional supplements may have antiinflammatory effects (e.g., fish oil, ginger, SAM-e). However, results of studies on glucosamine and chondroitin are mixed. The American College of Rheumatology (ACR) and American Academy of Orthopaedic Surgeons (AAOS) does not recommend their use.[4] Teach patients to discuss any supplement use with their HCP to identify possible interactions with prescribed medications.

Drug Therapy. Drug therapy is based on the severity of the patient's symptoms (Table 64.3). The patient with mild to moderate joint pain may get relief from acetaminophen (Tylenol).

A topical agent, such as capsaicin cream, may be helpful, alone or with acetaminophen. It blocks pain by locally interfering with substance P. It is responsible for the transmission of pain impulses. A concentrated product is available by prescription. Creams of 0.025% to 0.075% capsaicin are available over the counter (OTC). OTC products that contain camphor, eucalyptus oil, and menthol (e.g., Bengay, Arthricare) may provide

---

Tai Chi

Scientific Evidence
- Tai Chi brought short-term improvements in pain and stiffness in knee OA.
- Some studies found improved balance or decreased depression.
- In a study comparing Tai Chi to physical therapy, patients in both groups had improved pain for a full year.
- Temporary increase of knee pain may occur in patients with knee OA.

Nursing Implications
- Generally considered to be safe practices.
- Avoid overuse of affected joints.

Source: National Center for Complementary and Alternative Medicine: Osteoarthritis: in depth. Retrieved from *www.nccih.nih.gov/health/arthritis/osteoarthritis#hed3.*

👥 **TABLE 64.2 Interprofessional Care**

Osteoarthritis

Diagnostic Assessment
- History and physical examination
- Radiologic studies of involved joints (e.g., x-ray, CT scan, MRI, bone scan)
- Possible synovial fluid analysis

Management
- Nutritional and weight management counseling
- Rest and joint protection, use of assistive devices
- Therapeutic exercise
- Heat and cold applications
- Complementary and alternative therapies
  - Herbs and nutritional supplements (e.g., fish oil, ginger, SAM-e)
  - Movement therapies (e.g., yoga, Tai Chi)
  - Acupuncture
  - Massage
- Transcutaneous electrical nerve stimulation (TENS)
- Reconstructive joint surgery

Drug Therapy (Table 64.3)
- acetaminophen
- NSAIDs
- Intraarticular corticosteroids

temporary pain relief. Topical salicylates (e.g., Aspercreme) may be an option for patients who cannot take aspirin-containing medication. Several applications may be needed daily because topical agents have short-acting effects.

If a patient does not get adequate pain management with acetaminophen, has moderate to severe OA pain, or has signs of joint inflammation, a nonsteroidal antiinflammatory drug (NSAID) may be more effective. NSAID therapy typically is started in low-dose OTC strengths (e.g., ibuprofen 200 mg up to 4 times daily). The dose may be increased if needed. If the patient is at risk for or develops gastrointestinal (GI) side effects with an NSAID, adding a protective agent, such as misoprostol (Cytotec), may be needed. Arthrotec, a combination of misoprostol and the NSAID diclofenac, is available. Diclofenac gel may be applied to the affected joint. Teach the patient who is taking an oral NSAID to avoid use of a topical NSAID because of increased risk for adverse effects.

TABLE 64.3 Drug Therapy

Osteoarthritis

Drug	Mechanism of Action	Nursing Considerations
Corticosteroids		
Intraarticular Injections		
methylprednisolone acetate (Depo-Medrol) triamcinolone (Aristospan)	Antiinflammatory Analgesic Act by inhibiting synthesis and/or release of inflammatory mediators	Use strict aseptic technique for corticosteroid injection. Tell patient that joint may temporarily feel worse right after injection. Teach patient to avoid overusing affected joint right after injection. Tell patient improvement lasts weeks to months after injection.
Systemic		
dexamethasone hydrocortisone (Solu-Cortef) methylprednisolone (Solu-Medrol) prednisone triamcinolone	Antiinflammatory Analgesic Act by inhibiting synthesis and/or release of inflammatory mediators	Use only in life-threatening exacerbation or when symptoms persist after treatment with less potent antiinflammatory drugs. Give for limited time only, tapering dose slowly. Be aware that worsening of symptoms occurs with abrupt withdrawal of drug. Monitor BP, weight, CBC, and serum potassium. Limit sodium intake. Report signs of infection.
Nonsteroidal Antiinflammatory Drugs (NSAIDs)		
celecoxib (Celebrex) diclofenac ibuprofen (Advil) indomethacin ketoprofen meclofenamate meloxicam (Mobic) nabumetone naproxen (Aleve) oxaprozin (Daypro) piroxicam (Feldene) sulindac tolmetin	Antiinflammatory Analgesic Fever reducer (antipyretic) Act by inhibiting prostaglandin synthesis	Give drug with food, milk, or antacids (as prescribed). Report signs of bleeding (e.g., tarry stools, bruising, petechiae, nosebleeds), edema, skin rashes, persistent headaches, visual problems. Monitor BP for elevations related to fluid retention. Must be used regularly for maximal effect.
Salicylate		
aspirin, salicylate (salsalate)	Antiinflammatory Analgesic Fever reducer (antipyretic) Act by inhibiting prostaglandin synthesis	Give with food, milk, antacids (as prescribed), or full glass of water. May use enteric-coated aspirin. Report signs of bleeding (e.g., tarry stools, bruising, petechiae, nosebleeds).
Topical Analgesics		
capsaicin cream	Depletes substance P from nerve endings, interrupting pain signals to the brain	Must be used at regular intervals for maximal effect. Aloe vera cream may decrease burning sensation. Teach patient not to use cream with external heat source (heating pad) because of risk for burns. Available in OTC and prescriptive strengths.
diclofenac sodium (Voltaren gel)	Antiinflammatory Analgesic	Teach patient to avoid sun and ultraviolet (UV) light exposure. Should not be used in combination with oral NSAIDs or aspirin due to risk for increased side effects.

All NSAIDs inhibit the production of cyclooxygenase-1 (COX-1) and cyclooxygenase-2 (COX-2). These enzymes convert arachidonic acid into prostaglandins (see Fig. 8.5). Inhibiting COX-1 causes many of the untoward effects of NSAIDs, including the risk for bleeding and GI irritation.[5] Patients taking an anticoagulant (e.g., warfarin [Coumadin]) and an NSAID are at high risk for bleeding. Long-term NSAID treatment may affect cartilage metabolism, especially in older patients who may have poor cartilage integrity. As an alternative to traditional NSAIDs, the COX-2 inhibitor celecoxib (Celebrex) may be considered in selected patients.

When given in equivalent doses, all NSAIDs are comparably effective but vary widely in cost. Individual responses to NSAIDs also vary. Some patients still prefer aspirin, but it is no longer a common treatment. It should be used cautiously with NSAIDs because both inhibit platelet function and prolong bleeding time. Intraarticular injections of corticosteroids may be needed for those with local inflammation and swelling. Four or more injections without relief suggest the need for more intervention. Systemic corticosteroids are not used as they may actually hasten the disease process.

Injection of hyaluronic acid (viscosupplementation) has been a common treatment for knee OA. However, its effectiveness is not clear. Neither the ACR nor the AAOS recommends against using hyaluronates.[6] Research on the long-term effects continues.

Drugs thought to slow the progression of OA or support joint healing are known as disease-modifying osteoarthritis drugs (DMOADs). To date, no drugs have been approved to modify OA progression despite many clinical trials. Strontium ranelate, an approved treatment for osteoporosis, is being researched for effects on OA. Because it reduces levels of a cartilage turnover marker, it may be helpful in OA treatment.[5]

Surgical Therapy. Symptoms of disease are often managed conservatively for many years. However, the patient's loss of joint function, unmanaged pain, and decreased independence in self-care may lead to consideration of surgery. Patients with knee OA used to undergo arthroscopy to remove loose bodies from the joint. However, it does not have any benefit over physical therapy and medical treatment.[7] Reconstructive surgical procedures (e.g., hip and knee replacements) are discussed in Chapter 62.

❖ NURSING MANAGEMENT: OSTEOARTHRITIS

◆ Nursing Assessment

Carefully assess and document the type, location, severity, frequency, and duration of the patient's joint pain and stiffness. Determine what makes the pain better or worse. Ask the patient how these symptoms affect the ability to perform activities of daily living (ADLs). Review the patient's pain management practices. Ask about success of each treatment. Assess tenderness, swelling, limitation of movement, and crepitation of affected joints. Compare an involved joint with the opposite joint if it is not affected.

◆ Nursing Diagnoses

Nursing diagnoses for the patient with OA may include:
- Acute and chronic pain
- Impaired physical mobility
- Difficulty coping

◆ Planning

Overall goals are that the patient with OA will (1) maintain or improve joint function through a balance of rest and activity, (2) use joint protection measures (Table 64.4) to improve activity tolerance, (3) achieve independence in self-care and maintain optimal role function, and (4) use drug and nondrug strategies to manage pain satisfactorily.

◆ Nursing Implementation

◆ **Health Promotion.** Prevention of OA is possible in some cases. Focus community education on altering modifiable risk factors. For example, encourage the patient to lose weight and reduce occupational or recreational hazards. For athletic instruction and physical fitness programs, include safety measures that protect and reduce trauma to the joints. Prompt treatment of traumatic joint injuries decreases the risk for OA.

 PROMOTING POPULATION HEALTH

Preventing Osteoarthritis

- Avoid cigarette smoking.
- Promptly treat any joint injury.
- Maintain healthy weight and eat a balanced diet.
- Use safety measures to protect and decrease risk for joint injury.
- Exercise regularly, including strength and endurance training.

Acute Care. The patient with OA usually is treated as an outpatient. The interprofessional team involved may include an internal medicine physician or family HCP, a rheumatologist, a nurse, an occupational therapist, and a physical therapist. Health assessment questionnaires can pinpoint areas of decreased function. They are completed at regular intervals to

---

TABLE 64.4 Patient & Caregiver Teaching

Joint Protection and Energy Conservation

Include the following instructions when teaching patients with arthritis to protect joints and conserve energy:
- Maintain healthy weight.
- Use assistive devices, if needed.
- Avoid forceful repetitive joint movements.
- Avoid awkward positions that stress joints.
- Use good posture and body mechanics.
- Seek help with needed tasks that may cause pain.
- Organize routine tasks and pace yourself to decrease fatigue and joint pain.
- Modify home and work environment to perform tasks in less stressful ways.

---

document disease and treatment progression. Treatment goals can be based on data from the questionnaires and physical examination, with specific interventions for identified problems. The patient is usually hospitalized only if having joint surgery (see Chapter 62).

Drugs are given for the treatment of pain and inflammation. Nondrug strategies to decrease pain and disability may include massage, use of heat (thermal packs) or cold (ice packs), meditation, and yoga.[8] Splints may be prescribed to rest and stabilize painful or inflamed joints.

Once an acute flare has subsided, a physical therapist can give valuable assistance in planning an exercise program. The therapist may recommend Tai Chi as a low-impact form of exercise. Tai Chi can be done by patients of all ages and may be done in a wheelchair. Stress the importance of warming up before any exercise to decrease risk for injury.

Patient and caregiver teaching related to OA is an important nursing responsibility. Provide information about the nature and treatment of the disease, pain management, body mechanics, correct use of assistive devices (e.g., cane, walker), principles of joint protection and energy conservation (Table 64.4), nutritional choices, weight and stress management, and an exercise program.

Assure the patient that OA is a localized disease and severe deforming arthritis is not the usual course. The patient may gain support and understanding of the disease process through community resources, such as the Arthritis Foundation's self-help course *(www.arthritis.org)*.

🔲 CHECK YOUR PRACTICE

A 54-yr-old woman has OA of the left knee. She received an intraarticular corticosteroid injection in the left knee and a prescription for diclofenac 50 mg twice daily. She receives a prescription for physical therapy.
- What information will you provide about diclofenac to ensure the patient's safe, effective use?
- What type of exercises will be appropriate for this patient?
- The patient asks about complementary therapies for osteoarthritis. What will you tell her?

Ambulatory Care. Adjust home management goals to meet the patient's needs. Include the caregiver, family members, and significant others in goal setting and teaching. Discuss home and work environment modification for patient safety, accessibility, and self-care. Measures include removing throw rugs, placing rails at the stairs and bathtub, using night-lights, and wearing well-fitting supportive shoes. Assistive devices, such as canes, walkers, elevated toilet seats, and grab bars, reduce the load on an affected joint and promote safety. Urge the patient to continue all prescribed therapies at home and be open to new approaches to symptom management.

Sexual counseling may help the patient and significant other to enjoy physical closeness by introducing the idea of alternative positions and timing for sexual activity. Discussion also increases awareness of each partner's needs. Encourage the patient to take analgesics or a warm bath to decrease joint stiffness before sexual activity.

◆ Evaluation

The expected outcomes are that the patient with OA will
- Have adequate rest and activity
- Achieve acceptable pain management
- Maintain joint flexibility and muscle strength through joint protection and therapeutic exercise

RHEUMATOID ARTHRITIS

Rheumatoid arthritis (RA) is a chronic, systemic autoimmune disease characterized by inflammation of connective tissue in the diarthrodial (synovial) joints. RA is typically marked by periods of remission and exacerbation. RA often has extraarticular manifestations. RA has long been considered one of the most disabling forms of arthritis. Symptoms and outcomes can vary greatly. Without adequate treatment, patients may need mobility aids or joint reconstruction. They may have loss of independence and self-care ability.

RA occurs globally, affecting all ethnic groups. It can occur at any time of life. However, incidence increases with age, peaking between ages 30 and 50 years. RA affects around 1.5 million adult Americans. Almost 3 times as many women have the disease as men.[9]

Etiology and Pathophysiology

We do not know the exact cause of RA. It likely results from a combination of genetics and environmental triggers. An autoimmune cause is currently the most widely accepted theory. This theory suggests changes of RA begin when a genetically susceptible person has an initial immune response to an antigen. Although a bacterium or virus could be the possible antigen, no infection or organism has been found to date.

⊕ PROMOTING HEALTH EQUITY

Arthritis and Connective Tissue Disorders

- Arthritis is most common in whites and blacks.
- Hispanics and blacks have the highest incidence of arthritis-related activity limitations.
- Some Native Americans (e.g., Pima, Chippewa, Yakima) have a higher incidence of RA than other ethnic groups in North America.
- Ankylosing spondylitis is most common in whites and certain Native American groups.
- SLE is more common and more severe among black, Hispanic, Asian American, and Native American women than white women.
- Black and Hispanic women are at greater risk than white women for developing scleroderma.

The antigen, which is probably not the same in all patients, triggers formation of an abnormal immunoglobulin G (IgG). RA is marked by autoantibodies to this abnormal IgG. The autoantibodies are known as *rheumatoid factor (RF)*. They combine with IgG to form immune complexes that initially deposit on synovial membranes or superficial articular cartilage in the joints. Immune complex formation leads to the activation of complement and an inflammatory response. (Complement activation is discussed in Chapter 11. Immune complex formation is discussed in Chapter 13.)

Neutrophils are attracted to the site of inflammation, where they release proteolytic enzymes that damage articular cartilage and cause the synovial lining to thicken (Fig. 64.3). Other inflammatory cells include T helper (CD4) cells, which stimulate cell-mediated immune responses. Activated CD4 cells cause monocytes, macrophages, and synovial fibroblasts to secrete the proinflammatory cytokines interleukin-1 (IL-1), IL-6, and tumor necrosis factor (TNF). These cytokines drive the inflammatory response in RA.

Some patients report a precipitating stressful event, such as infection, work stress, physical exertion, childbirth, surgery, or emotional upset. However, research has been unable to directly correlate such events with RA onset.

⬢ Genetic Link

Genetic predisposition is important in the development of RA. The strongest evidence for a genetic influence is the role of human leukocyte antigens (HLA), especially the HLA-DR4 and HLA-DR1 antigens. (HLA is discussed in Chapter 13.) Smoking increases the risk for RA for persons who are genetically predisposed to the disease. It may interfere with treatment for diagnosed persons.[10]

Clinical Manifestations

Joints. The onset of RA is typically subtle. Nonspecific manifestations, such as fatigue, anorexia, weight loss, and generalized stiffness, may precede the onset of joint symptoms. Stiffness becomes more localized in the following weeks to months.

Specific joint involvement is marked by pain, stiffness, limited motion, and signs of inflammation (e.g., heat, swelling, tenderness). Joint symptoms occur symmetrically and often affect the small joints of the hands (PIP and MCP) and feet (MTP). Larger peripheral joints such as wrists, elbows, shoulders, knees, hips, ankles, and jaw may be involved. The cervical spine may be affected, but the axial skeleton (spine and bones connected to it) is generally spared. Table 64.5 compares RA and OA.

The patient typically has joint stiffness after periods of inactivity. Morning stiffness may last from 60 minutes to several hours or more, depending on disease activity. MCP and PIP joints are typically swollen. In early disease, the fingers may become spindle shaped from synovial hypertrophy and thickening of the joint capsule. Joints are tender, painful, and warm to the touch. Joint pain increases with motion. It varies in intensity. It may not be related to the degree of inflammation. Tenosynovitis often affects the extensor and flexor tendons around the wrists. This causes symptoms of carpal tunnel syndrome and makes it hard for the patient to grasp objects.

As the disease progresses, inflammation and fibrosis of the joint capsule and supporting structures may cause deformity and disability. Muscle atrophy and tendon destruction cause 1 joint surface to slip past the other (subluxation). Metatarsal head dislocation and subluxation in the feet may cause pain and walking disability (Fig. 64.3, *D*). Ulnar drift ("zig-zag deformity"), swan neck, and boutonnière deformities are common in the hands (Fig. 64.4).

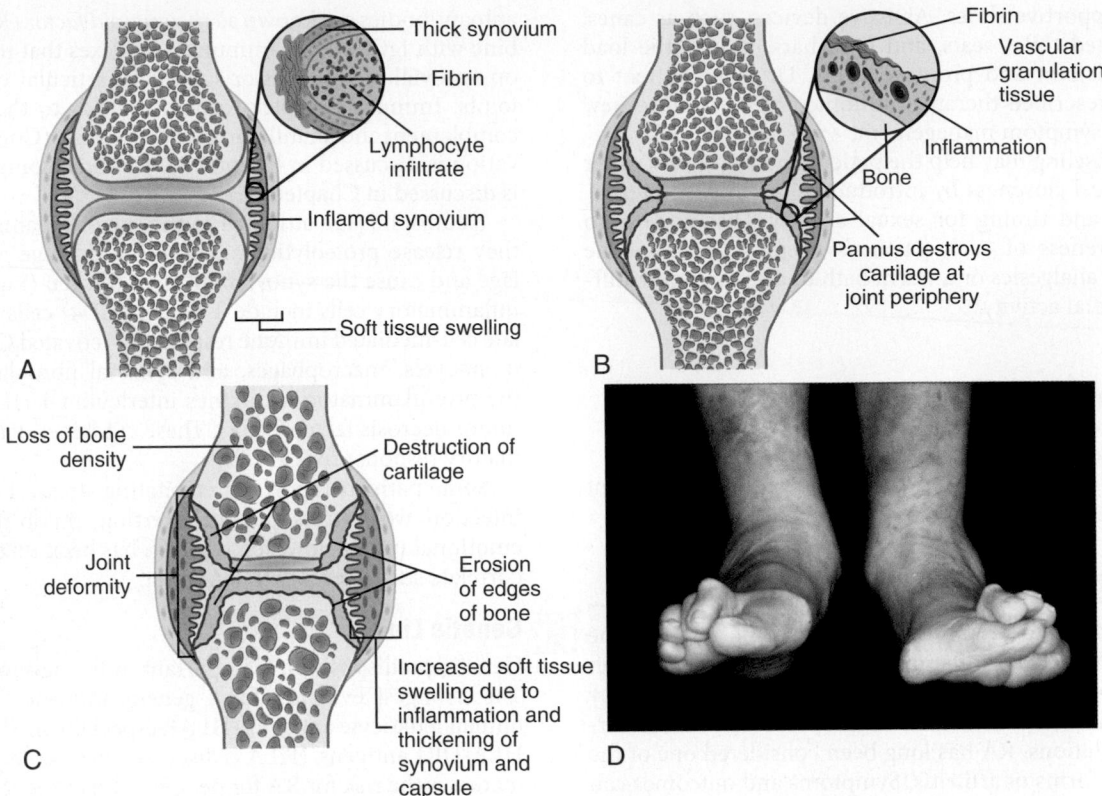

FIG. 64.3 RA. **A,** Early pathologic change is rheumatoid synovitis. Synovium becomes inflamed. Lymphocytes and plasma cells increase greatly. **B,** Over time, articular cartilage destruction occurs, and vascular granulation tissue grows across the cartilage surface (pannus) from the edges of the joint. Joint surface shows loss of cartilage beneath the extending pannus, most marked at joint margins. **C,** Inflammatory pannus causes focal destruction of bone. Osteolytic destruction of bone occurs at joint edges, causing erosions seen on x-rays. This phase is associated with joint deformity. **D,** Multiple deformities of the foot from rheumatoid arthritis. (*D,* From Canale ST, Beaty JH: *Campbell's operative orthopaedics,* ed 12, Philadelphia, 2013, Mosby.)

TABLE 64.5 Comparison of Rheumatoid Arthritis and Osteoarthritis

Parameter	Rheumatoid Arthritis	Osteoarthritis
Age at onset	Young to middle age.	Usually older than 40 years.
Gender	Female-to-male ratio is 2:1 or 3:1. Less marked sex difference after age 60.	Females 2:1 after age 60; except for traumatic arthritis, men less affected until age 70 or 80.
Weight	Lost or maintained weight.	Often overweight or obese.
Disease	Systemic disease with exacerbations and remissions.	Localized disease with variable, progressive course.
Affected joints	Small joints typically affected first (PIPs, MCPs, MTPs), wrists, elbows, shoulders, knees. Usually bilateral, symmetric joint involvement.	Weight-bearing joints of knees and hips, small joints (MCPs, DIPs, PIPs), cervical and lumbar spine. Often asymmetric.
Pain characteristics	Stiffness lasts 1 hr to all day and may ↓ with use. Pain is variable, may disrupt sleep.	Stiffness occurs on arising but usually subsides after 30 min. Pain gradually worsens with joint use and disease progression, relieved with joint rest but may disrupt sleep.
Effusions	Common.	Uncommon.
Nodules	Present, especially on extensor surfaces.	Heberden's (DIPs) and Bouchard's (PIPs) nodes.
Synovial fluid	WBC count 5000–60,000/µL with mostly neutrophils; ↓ viscosity.	WBC count <2000/µL (mild leukocytosis); normal viscosity.
X-rays	Joint space narrowing and erosion with bony overgrowths, subluxation with advanced disease. Osteoporosis related to decreased activity, corticosteroid use.	Joint space narrowing, osteophytes, subchondral cysts, sclerosis.
Laboratory findings	Rheumatoid factor positive in 70%–90% of patients; negative titers in early disease for about 25% of patients. ↑ In ANA titer likely. Positive anti-CCP in 60%–80% of patients ↑ ESR, CRP indicative of active inflammation.	Rheumatoid factor negative. ANA negative. Anti-CCP negative. Transient elevation in ESR related to synovitis.

ANA, Antinuclear antibodies; *anti-CCP,* anti-citrullinated peptide; *DIPs,* distal interphalangeal; *MCPs,* metacarpophalangeals; *MTPs,* metatarsophalangeals; *PIPs,* proximal interphalangeals.

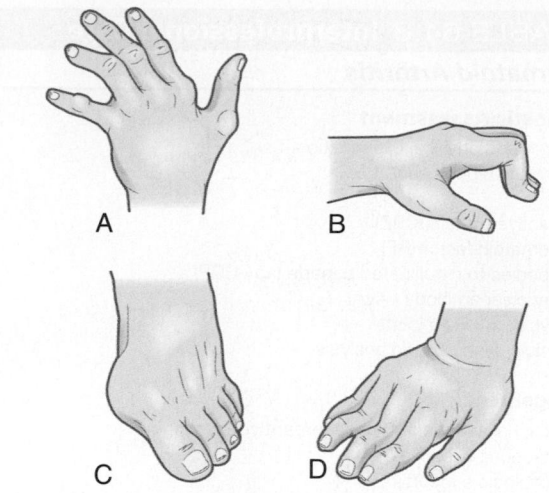

FIG. 64.4 Typical deformities of RA. **A,** Ulnar drift. **B,** Boutonnière deformity. **C,** Hallux valgus. **D,** Swan neck deformity.

Extraarticular Manifestations. RA can affect nearly every body system (Fig. 64.5). Extraarticular manifestations are more likely to occur in the person with high levels of biomarkers, such as RF.

Rheumatoid nodules develop in about half the patients with RA.[11] Rheumatoid nodules appear under the skin as firm, nontender masses. They are often found on bony areas exposed to pressure, such as the fingers and elbows. Nodules at the base of the spine and back of the head are common in older adults. Treatment is usually not needed. However, these nodules can break down, like pressure injuries. Cataracts and vision loss can result from scleral nodules. Nodular myositis and muscle fiber degeneration can cause pain like that of vascular insufficiency. In later disease, nodules in the heart and lungs can cause pleurisy, pleural effusion, pericarditis, pericardial effusion, and cardiomyopathy.

Sjögren's syndrome can occur by itself or with other arthritic disorders, such as RA and SLE. The inflammation of RA can damage the tear-producing (lacrimal) glands, making the eyes feel dry and gritty.[11] Affected patients may have photosensitivity. (Sjögren's syndrome is discussed later in this chapter on p. 1526.)

Felty syndrome is rare but can occur in those with long-standing RA. It is characterized by an enlarged spleen and low white blood cell (WBC) count. Patients with Felty syndrome are at increased risk for infection and lymphoma.

Flexion contractures and hand deformities cause decreased grasp strength and affect the patient's ability to perform self-care tasks. Depression may occur. However, it is unclear if the patient becomes depressed from struggling with chronic pain and disability or if depression is part of the autoimmune disease process. Levels of C-reactive protein (CRP), a marker of inflammation, are higher in patients with depression compared to those with no symptoms of depression.[12]

Diagnostic Studies

Accurate diagnosis is critical to prompt initiation of treatment to decrease the risk for disability. A diagnosis is often made based on history and physical findings. Criteria for diagnosis of RA in a newly presenting patient are described in Table 64.6. Laboratory tests are used to confirm diagnosis and monitor disease progression (Tables 64.7 and 64.8).

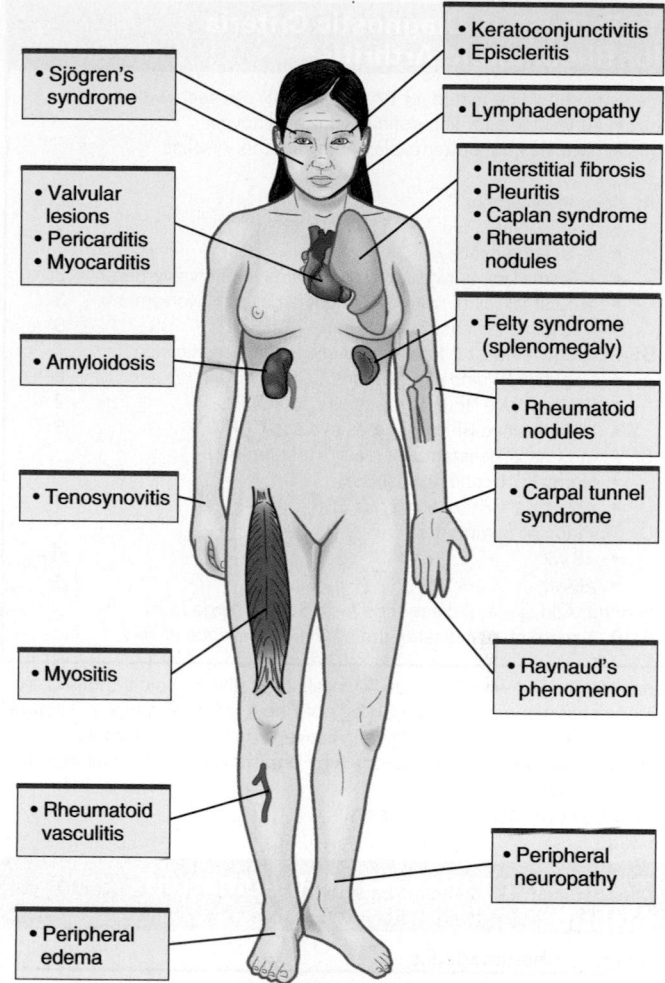

FIG. 64.5 Extraarticular manifestations of RA.

Positive RF occurs in 80% of adults with RA. Titers rise during active disease. ESR and CRP are increased as general indicators of active inflammation. Testing for the antibodies to citrullinated peptide (anti-CCP) is more specific than RF for RA. Anti-CCP is present in 60% to 80% of patients with RA. It can be found in patients' blood 5 to 10 years before they have symptoms of RA. If the patient's symptoms are consistent with RA, the presence of anti-CCP and RF makes a strong case for early, accurate diagnosis. An increase in antinuclear antibody (ANA) titers is an indicator of autoimmune reaction.

Synovial fluid analysis in early disease often shows slightly cloudy, straw-colored fluid with many fibrin flecks. The enzyme MMP-3 is increased in the synovial fluid. It may be a marker of progressive joint damage. The WBC count of synovial fluid is increased. Tissue biopsy can confirm inflammatory changes in the synovial membrane.

X-rays alone are not diagnostic of RA. They may show only soft tissue swelling and possible bone demineralization in early disease. A narrowed joint space, articular cartilage destruction, erosion, subluxation, and deformity are seen in later disease. Poor alignment and fusion may be seen in advanced disease. Baseline x-rays may be used to monitor disease progression and treatment effectiveness. Bone scans are more useful in detecting early joint changes and confirming diagnosis so that RA treatment can be started.

TABLE 64.6 Diagnostic Criteria for Rheumatoid Arthritis*

Patients should be tested for RA who initially are seen with:
- At least 1 joint with definite clinical synovitis
- Synovitis not better explained by another disease

	Score
A. Joint Involvement	
• 1 large joint	0
• 2–10 large joints	1
• 1–3 small joints (with or without large joint involvement)	2
• 4–10 small joints (with or without large joint involvement)	3
• >10 joints (at least 1 small joint)	5
B. Serology (at least 1 test result needed for classification)	
• Negative RF *and* negative anti-CCP	0
• Low-positive RF *or* low-positive anti-CCP	2
• High-positive RF *or* high-positive anti-CCP	3
C. Acute Phase Reactants (at least 1 test needed)	
• Normal CRP *and* normal ESR	0
• Abnormal CRP *or* abnormal ESR	1
D. Duration of Symptoms	
• <6 wk	0
• ≥6 wk	1

Scoring: Add score of categories A–D. Scores range from 0–10. A score of ≥6 indicates the definitive presence of RA.

From Aletaha D, Neogi T, Silman AJ, et al: 2010 Rheumatoid arthritis classification criteria: An American College of Rheumatology/European League Against Rheumatism Collaborative Initiative, *Arthr Rheum* 62:2569, 2010. Retrieved from *www.rheumatology.org/Portals/0/Files/2010_revised_criteria_classification_ra.pdf.*

*Used for newly diagnosed patients.

TABLE 64.7 Stages of Rheumatoid Arthritis

Stage	Characteristics

I	• Synovitis marked by:
	  • Synovial membrane swelling with excess blood
	  • Membrane containing small areas of lymphocyte infiltration
	  • High WBC counts in synovial fluid (5000–60,000/μL)
	  • X-ray results: soft tissue swelling, possible osteoporosis; no evidence of joint destruction

II	• ↑ Joint inflammation, spreading across cartilage into joint cavity • Signs of gradual destruction in joint cartilage • Narrowing joint space from loss of cartilage
III	• Formation of synovial pannus • Joint cartilage becomes eroded, bone exposed • X-ray results: extensive cartilage loss, erosion at joint margins, possible deformity
IV	• End-stage: inflammatory process subsides • Loss of joint function • Formation of subcutaneous nodules

Source: Rheumatoid Arthritis.net: A health union community: Understanding RA stages and progressions. Retrieved from *http://rheumatoidarthritis.net/what-is-ra/stages-and-progression.*

Interprofessional Care

An individualized treatment plan considers disease activity, joint function, age, sex, family and social roles, and response to previous treatment (Table 64.8). Treatment advances have improved the prognosis for patients with newly diagnosed RA. The progression of joint damage can be slowed or stopped with aggressive, early treatment.[13] A caring, long-term relationship with an interprofessional health care team can promote the patient's self-esteem and positive coping.

TABLE 64.8 Interprofessional Care

Rheumatoid Arthritis

Diagnostic Assessment
- History and physical examination
- Complete blood count (CBC)
- ESR
- C-reactive protein (CRP)
- Rheumatoid factor (RF)
- Antibodies to citrullinated peptide (anti-CCP)
- Antinuclear antibody (ANA)
- X-rays of involved joints
- Possible synovial fluid analysis

Management
- Nutritional and weight management counseling
- Therapeutic exercise
- Psychologic support
- Rest and joint protection, use of assistive devices
- Heat and cold applications
- Complementary and alternative therapies
  - Herbal products and nutritional supplements
  - Acupuncture
- Reconstructive surgery

Drug Therapy
- Disease-modifying antirheumatic drugs (DMARDs) (Table 64.9)
- Biologic response modifiers (BRMs) (Table 64.9)
- NSAIDs (Table 64.3)
- Intraarticular or systemic corticosteroids (Table 64.3)

Drug Therapy

Disease-Modifying Antirheumatic Drugs. Drugs are the cornerstone of RA treatment (Table 64.9). Because irreversible joint changes can occur as early as the first year of RA, HCPs aggressively prescribe disease-modifying antirheumatic drugs (DMARDs). These drugs may slow disease progression and decrease risk for joint erosion and deformity. The choice of drug is based on disease activity, the patient's functional level, and lifestyle considerations, such as the wish to become pregnant.

Methotrexate is preferred for early treatment of patients diagnosed with RA.[13] It has a lower risk for toxicity than other drugs. Rare but serious side effects include bone marrow suppression and hepatotoxicity. Methotrexate therapy requires frequent laboratory monitoring, including CBC and blood chemistry. The patient begins to see therapeutic effects within 4 to 6 weeks. However, not everyone gets adequate relief from methotrexate alone. It can be given with other DMARDs or biologic response modifiers.

Sulfasalazine (Azulfidine) and the antimalarial drug hydroxychloroquine (Plaquenil) may be effective DMARDs for mild to moderate disease. They are rapidly absorbed, relatively safe, and well-tolerated. Teach the patient taking sulfasalazine to drink adequate fluids to avoid crystal formation in the urine. Urge the patient to wear sunscreen with sun exposure. For those taking hydroxychloroquine, a baseline eye examination with follow-up every 6 to 12 months is needed because of the risk for vision loss.

The synthetic DMARD leflunomide (Arava) blocks immune cell overproduction. Its efficacy and side effects are similar to those of methotrexate and sulfasalazine. Because the drug is teratogenic, pregnancy in women of childbearing age must be excluded before therapy is started. Using 2 kinds of birth control is recommended during treatment.

Tofacitinib (Xeljanz), a JAK (Janus kinase) inhibitor, is used to treat moderate to severe active RA. The drug interferes with JAK enzymes that contribute to joint inflammation in RA. Live vaccinations should not be given to the patient receiving tofacitinib.

Biologic Response Modifiers. Biologic response modifiers (BRMs) (also called *biologics* or *immunotherapy*) are used to slow disease progression in RA. BRMs are classified based on their mechanism of action (Table 64.9). They can be used to treat patients with moderate to severe RA who have not responded to DMARDs. They can be used alone or in combination therapy with a DMARD, such as methotrexate.[13]

TNF inhibitors include etanercept (Enbrel), infliximab (Remicade), adalimumab (Humira), certolizumab (Cimzia), and golimumab (Simponi). Etanercept is a biologically engineered copy of the TNF cell receptor. It binds to TNF in circulation before TNF can bind to the cell surface receptor. Thus it inhibits the inflammatory response. This drug is given as a subcutaneous injection.

Infliximab and adalimumab are monoclonal antibodies that bind to TNF, preventing it from binding to TNF receptors on cells. Infliximab is given IV in combination with methotrexate. Adalimumab is given subcutaneously.

Certolizumab and golimumab are TNF inhibitors that improve symptoms in patients with moderate to severe RA. Both drugs are given in combination with methotrexate.

 DRUG ALERT Tumor Necrosis Factor Inhibitors

- Perform tuberculin test and chest x-ray before starting therapy.
- Monitor for signs of infection. Stop the drug temporarily and notify HCP if acute infection develops.
- Teach patients to avoid live vaccination while taking drug.
- Report bruising, bleeding, or persistent fever and other signs of infection.

Anakinra (Kineret) is an IL-1 receptor antagonist (IL-1Ra) created from new combinations of genetic material. It blocks the biologic activity of IL-1 by competitively inhibiting its ability to bind to the IL-1 receptor. Anakinra is given as a subcutaneous injection. It is used to reduce pain and swelling of moderate to severe RA. It can be used in combination with DMARDs but not with other TNF inhibitors. Using these agents together can lead to serious infection and neutropenia.

Tocilizumab (Actemra) and sarilumab (Kevzara) block the action of IL-6, a cytokine that contributes to inflammation. They are used to treat patients with moderate to severe RA who have not responded to or cannot tolerate other drugs for the disease.

Abatacept (Orencia) blocks T-cell activation. It is recommended for patients who have inadequate response to DMARDs or TNF inhibitors. It is given IV. Like anakinra, it should not be used with TNF inhibitors.

Rituximab (Rituxan) is a monoclonal antibody that targets B cells. It may be used in combination with methotrexate for patients with moderate to severe RA not responding to TNF inhibitors. It is given IV.

Other Drug Therapy. Other DMARDS include immunosuppressants (azathioprine), penicillamine (Cuprimine), and gold preparations. These medications are used less often because they are weak treatments compared to other DMARDs and biologics.

Corticosteroid therapy can be used to manage symptoms during disease flares. Intraarticular injections may temporarily reduce acute pain and inflammation. Low-dose oral corticosteroids may be used for a limited time to decrease disease activity until the effects of DMARDs or biologics are seen. However, they are inadequate as a sole therapy because they do not affect disease progression. Their long-term use should not be a mainstay of RA treatment. Complications include osteoporosis and avascular necrosis.

Various NSAIDs and salicylates are used to treat arthritis pain and inflammation. Aspirin may be used in dosages of 3 to 4 g/day in 3 to 4 doses. Blood salicylate levels should be monitored in a patient taking more than 3600 mg daily. NSAIDs have antiinflammatory and analgesic effects. Some relief may be seen within days of starting treatment with NSAIDs. Full effect may take 2 to 3 weeks. NSAIDs may be used when the patient cannot tolerate aspirin. The patient may be able to better follow the treatment plan if using an antiinflammatory drug that can be taken only once or twice a day (Table 64.3). Celecoxib (Celebrex), the only available COX-2 inhibitor, is effective in RA as well as OA. All nonaspirin NSAIDs can increase the risk for blood clots, heart attack, and stroke.

Nutritional Therapy. Although no special diet is needed for RA, balanced nutrition is important. Fatigue, pain, and depression may cause a loss of appetite. Limited endurance and mobility may make it hard to shop for and prepare food. Weight loss may result. The occupational therapist can help the patient modify the home environment and use assistive devices for easier food preparation.

Corticosteroid therapy and decreased mobility due to pain may cause unwanted weight gain. Corticosteroids increase the appetite, leading to higher caloric intake. A sensible weight loss program with balanced nutrition and exercise reduces stress on affected joints. The patient taking corticosteroids may become distressed as signs and symptoms of Cushing syndrome (e.g., moon face, redistribution of fatty tissue to the trunk) change the physical appearance. Encourage the patient not to change the dose or stop therapy abruptly. Weight will return to normal several months after treatment ends. Remind the patient to continue to eat a balanced diet.

Surgical Therapy. Surgery may be needed to relieve severe pain and improve the function of severely deformed joints. Removal of the joint lining (*synovectomy*) is one type of surgery. Total joint replacement (*arthroplasty*) can be done for many different joints in the body. Joint surgery is discussed in Chapter 62.

❖ NURSING MANAGEMENT: RHEUMATOID ARTHRITIS

◆ Nursing Assessment

Subjective and objective data to obtain from the patient with RA are outlined in Table 64.10. Begin with a careful physical assessment (e.g., joint pain, swelling, ROM, general health status). Assess psychosocial needs (e.g., family support, sexual satisfaction, emotional stress, financial constraints, vocational and career limitations). Assess for environmental concerns (e.g., transportation, home or work modifications). After identifying the patient's problems, carefully plan a program for rehabilitation and education with the interprofessional care team.

◆ Nursing Diagnoses

Nursing diagnoses for the patient with RA may include:
- Impaired physical mobility
- Chronic pain
- Disturbed body image

Additional information on nursing diagnoses and interventions for the patient with RA is provided in eNursing Care Plan 64.1 (available on the website for this chapter).

TABLE 64.9 Drug Therapy

Rheumatoid Arthritis

Drug	Mechanism of Action	Nursing Considerations
Disease-Modifying Antirheumatic Drugs (DMARDs)		
Antimalarial		
hydroxychloroquine (Plaquenil)	Exact mechanism unknown but may suppress formation of antigens	Monitor CBC and liver function. Tell patient therapeutic response may not occur for up to 6 mo. Teach patient to report visual changes, muscular weakness, and ↓ hearing or tinnitus.
Gold Compounds		
Oral: auranofin (Ridaura) *Parenteral:* gold sodium thiomalate, myochrysine, aurothioglucose	Alter immune responses, suppressing synovitis of active RA	Rule out pregnancy before beginning treatment. Monitor CBC, urinalysis, and liver and renal function. Tell patient therapeutic response may not occur for 3–6 mo. Teach patient to report pruritus, rash, sore mouth, indigestion, or metallic taste.
Immunosuppressants		
azathioprine (Imuran) cyclophosphamide	Inhibit DNA, RNA, protein synthesis	Assess for ↓ pain, swelling, stiffness, and ↑ joint mobility. Teach patient to report unusual bleeding or bruising. Tell patient therapeutic response may take up to 12 wk. Teach women of childbearing age to avoid pregnancy. Encourage ↑ fluid intake to ↓ risk for hemorrhagic cystitis.
mycophenolate mofetil (CellCept)	Inhibits DNA synthesis	Monitor blood count and liver function tests every 2–4 wk for first 3 mo of treatment, thereafter every 1–3 mo. Teach patient about ↑ infection risk. Tell patients not to take antacids at same time because they may interfere with drug absorption.
JAK (Janus Kinase) Inhibitor		
tofacitinib (Xeljanz)	Inhibits action of JAK enzymes, signaling pathways inside the cell with a key role in inflammation of RA	Tell patient of ↑ infection risk, including opportunistic infections. Monitor patient for any sign or symptom of infection for early treatment.
Miscellaneous		
leflunomide (Arava)	Antiinflammatory Immunomodulatory agent that inhibits proliferation of lymphocytes	Monitor liver function. Assess for ↓ pain, swelling, stiffness, and ↑ joint mobility. Teach women of childbearing age to avoid pregnancy.
methotrexate (Trexall)	Antimetabolite Inhibits DNA, RNA, protein synthesis	Monitor CBC and liver and renal function. Teach patient to report signs of anemia (fatigue, weakness). Keep patient well hydrated. Due to teratogenic effects, have female patient use effective contraception during and 3 mo after treatment.
penicillamine (Cuprimine, Depen)	Antiinflammatory Exact mechanism unknown but may suppress cell-mediated immune response	Monitor WBC count, platelets, urinalysis. Tell patient to take medication 1 hr before or 2 hr after meals, and at least 1 hr away from any other drug, food, or milk.
sulfasalazine (Azulfidine)	Sulfonamide Antiinflammatory Blocks prostaglandin synthesis	Tell patient drug may cause orange-yellow discoloration of urine or skin. Space doses evenly around the clock, taking drug after food with 8 oz water. Treatment may be continued even after symptoms are relieved. Monitor CBC.
Biologic Response Modifiers (Biologics, Immunotherapy)		
B-Cell Depleting Agent		
rituximab (Rituxan)	Monoclonal antibody that binds to CD20, an antigen on B cells, destroying B cells and suppressing immune response	Monitor for infection and bleeding. Tell patient to not receive live virus vaccines with treatment. Monitor for low BP if taking BP medication. Teach patient fatigue is common.
Interleukin-1 Receptor Antagonist		
anakinra (Kineret)	Blocks the action of interleukin-1, ↓ inflammatory response	Assess for ↓ pain, swelling, stiffness, and ↑ joint mobility. Injection site reaction generally occurs in first month of treatment and decreases with continued therapy. Assess renal function. Monitor for infection. Tell patient to not take drug with TNF inhibitors.
Interleukin-6 Receptor Antagonist		
sarilumab (Kevzara) tocilizumab (Actemra)	Blocks action of interleukin-6, thus ↓ inflammatory response	Given to patients with RA for whom other therapies have failed. Monitor BP and for infection. Tell patient of GI effects (e.g., perforation). Monitor liver enzyme and serum low-density lipoprotein (LDL).
T-Cell Activation Inhibitor		
abatacept (Orencia)	Inhibits T-cell activation, thus suppressing immune response	Not recommended for concomitant use with TNF inhibitors. Assess for ↓ pain, swelling, stiffness, and ↑ joint mobility.

TABLE 64.9 Drug Therapy—cont'd
Rheumatoid Arthritis

Drug	Mechanism of Action	Nursing Considerations
Tumor Necrosis Factor (TNF) Inhibitors		
adalimumab (Humira) certolizumab (Cimzia) etanercept (Enbrel) golimumab (Simponi) infliximab (Remicade)	Bind to TNF, blocking its interaction with cell surface receptors. Decrease inflammatory and immune responses	Assess for ↓ pain, swelling, stiffness, and ↑ joint mobility. Tell patient of ↑ risk for tuberculosis. Teach patient to have yearly PPD. Monitor for infection, bleeding, and emergence of cancers. Injection site reaction generally occurs in first month of treatment and ↓ with continued therapy. Teach patient to not receive live virus vaccines during treatment.
Other Agents **Antibiotics**		
doxycycline (Vibramycin)	↓ Action of enzymes on cartilage degradation	Possible treatment alternative for mild disease.
minocycline (Minocin)	Antirheumatic effect possibly related to immunomodulatory/antiinflammatory properties	

TABLE 64.10 Nursing Assessment
Rheumatoid Arthritis

Subjective Data

Important Health Information

Past health history: Recent infections. Precipitating factors, such as emotional upset, infections, overwork, childbirth, surgery. Pattern of remissions and exacerbations

Medications: Aspirin, NSAIDs, corticosteroids, DMARDs, BRMs

Surgery or other treatments: Any joint surgery

Functional Health Patterns

Health perception–health management: Positive family history for RA or other autoimmune disorders. Malaise, ability to take part in treatment plan. Impact of disease on functional ability

Nutritional-metabolic: Anorexia, weight loss, dry mucous membranes of mouth and pharynx

Activity-exercise: Stiffness and joint swelling, muscle weakness, difficulty walking, fatigue

Cognitive-perceptual: Paresthesia of hands and feet, loss of sensation; symmetric joint pain and aching that ↑ with motion or stress on joint, may interfere with rest

Objective Data

General

Lymphadenopathy, fever

Integumentary

Scleritis, uveitis, Sjögren's syndrome. Subcutaneous rheumatoid nodules on forearms, elbows. Skin ulcers. Shiny, taut skin over involved joints. Peripheral edema

Cardiovascular

Symmetric pallor and cyanosis of fingers (Raynaud's phenomenon). Distant heart sounds, murmurs, dysrhythmias

Respiratory

Bronchiectasis, pleural effusion, tuberculosis, interstitial lung disease

Gastrointestinal

Splenomegaly (Felty syndrome)

Musculoskeletal

Symmetric joint involvement with swelling, erythema, heat, tenderness. Deformities (with later disease). Enlargement of PIP and MCP joints. Limitation of joint movement, muscle contractures, muscle atrophy

Possible Diagnostic Findings

Positive RF, ANA, Anti-CCP. ↑ ESR; anemia. ↑ WBCs in synovial fluid. On x-ray evidence of joint space narrowing, bony erosion, deformity, possible osteoporosis

ANA, Antinuclear antibody; *anti-CCP,* antibodies to citrullinated peptide; *BRMs,* biologic response modifiers; *DMARDs,* disease-modifying antirheumatic drugs; *MCP,* metacarpophalangeal; *PIP,* proximal interphalangeal; *RF,* rheumatoid factor.

◆ Planning

The overall goals are that the patient with RA will (1) have acceptable pain management, (2) have minimal loss of function of affected joints, (3) take part in planning and implementing the treatment plan, (4) maintain a positive self-image, and (5) perform self-care to the maximum amount possible.

◆ Nursing Implementation

◆ **Health Promotion.** Prevention of RA is not possible. Early treatment can help prevent further joint damage. Community education programs should focus on symptom recognition to promote early diagnosis and treatment. The Arthritis Foundation offers many publications, classes, and support activities to help persons with RA.

◆ **Acute Care.** The patient newly diagnosed with RA is usually treated on an outpatient basis. Hospitalization may be needed for the patient who has systemic complications or needs surgery for decreased functional ability. Work closely with the HCP, physical and occupational therapists, and social worker to help the patient regain function and adjust to chronic illness.

◼ NURSING MANAGEMENT
Caring for the Patient With Rheumatoid Arthritis

- Give drug therapy as ordered.
- Teach patient and caregiver about drug therapy, including increased risk for infection with disease-modifying agents.
- Assess disease impact on quality of life and joint function.
- Assess pain intensity and give analgesics as ordered. Assess patient response.
- Develop program for rehabilitation and education with the interprofessional team.
- Teach patient about need for balance of rest and activity, with use of joint protective strategies.
- Oversee UAP
  - Aid patient with passive ROM of affected joints.
  - Help patient with self-care needs.

Collaborate With Interprofessional Team Members
Physical Therapist
- Assess patient's current mobility and need for assistance (e.g., walker).
- Develop exercise plan and teach patient to perform exercises safely.
- Coordinate PT with RN so that patient can receive timely analgesia.
- Recommend and apply thermal therapies.

Occupational Therapist
- Assess impact of patient's condition on ability to perform ADLs.
- Teach patient in use of assistive devices (e.g., long-handled reacher, long-handled shoe horn) to improve self-care ability without increasing stress on joints.
- Identify modifications to improve role performance (e.g., kitchen modifications for meal preparation).

Social Worker
- Assist with obtaining durable medical equipment (e.g., walker).
- Assess psychosocial and financial impact of disease. Arrange vocational retraining if needed.

Ambulatory Care. Care of the patient with RA includes a broad program of drug therapy, balance of rest and activity with joint protection, use of heat and cold applications, exercise, and patient and caregiver teaching. Nondrug management may include the use of therapeutic heat and cold, rest, relaxation techniques, joint protection (Tables 64.4 and 64.11), biofeedback, transcutaneous electrical nerve stimulation (see Chapter 8), and hypnosis. Allow the patient and caregiver to choose therapies that promote optimal comfort and fit their lifestyle.

Rest. Alternating scheduled rest periods with activity throughout the day helps relieve fatigue and pain. The amount of rest needed varies based on disease severity and the patient's limitations. The patient should rest before becoming exhausted. Total bed rest is rarely necessary. It should be avoided to prevent stiffness and other effects of immobility. A patient with mild disease may need daytime rest plus 8 to 10 hours of sleep at night.

Help the patient find ways to change daily activities to avoid overexertion and fatigue, which can worsen disease activity. For example, the patient may be able to prepare meals more easily while sitting on a high stool in front of the sink.

Teach the patient to maintain good body alignment during rest through use of a firm mattress or bed board. Encourage positions of extension. Teach the patient to avoid positions of flexion. To decrease the risk for joint contracture, never place pillows under the knees. Use a small, flat pillow under the head and shoulders if needed.

TABLE 64.11 **Patient & Caregiver Teaching**
Protection of Small Joints

Include the following instructions when teaching the patient with arthritis how to protect small joints:

1. Maintain joint in neutral position to minimize deformity.
   - Press water from a sponge instead of wringing.
2. Use strongest joint available for any task.
   - When rising from chair, push with palms rather than fingers.
   - Carry laundry basket in both arms rather than with fingers.
3. Distribute weight over many joints instead of stressing a few.
   - Slide objects instead of lifting them.
   - Hold packages close to body for support.
4. Change positions often.
   - Do not hold book or grip steering wheel for long periods without resting.
   - Avoid grasping pencil or cutting vegetables with knife for extended periods.
5. Avoid repetitive movements.
   - Do not knit or sew for long periods.
   - Rest between rooms when vacuuming.
   - Use faucets and doorknobs that are pushed rather than turned.
6. Modify chores to avoid stress on joints.
   - Avoid heavy lifting.
   - Sit on stool instead of standing during meal preparation.

Joint Protection. Protecting joints from stress is important. Help the patient find ways to alter routine tasks to put less stress on joints (Table 64.11). Energy conservation requires careful planning. The emphasis is on work simplification. Work for short periods with scheduled rest breaks to avoid fatigue (pacing). Organize activities to avoid going up and down stairs repeatedly. Use carts to carry supplies. Store frequently used materials in a convenient, easy-to-reach area. Use joint-protective devices (e.g., electric can opener) whenever possible. Teach patients to delegate tasks to other family members.

An occupational therapist helps the patient maintain upper extremity function and encourages use of splints or other assistive devices for joint protection. Lightweight splints may be prescribed to rest an inflamed joint and prevent deformity from muscle spasms and contractures. Remove the splints regularly to assess skin and perform ROM exercises. After assessment and supportive care, reapply splints as prescribed.

Occupational therapy may increase patient independence with assistive devices that simplify tasks (e.g., built-up utensils, buttonhooks, modified drawer handles, lightweight plastic dishes, raised toilet seats). Encourage the patient to make dressing easier by wearing shoes with Velcro fasteners and clothing with buttons or a zipper in the front instead of the back. Use a cane or a walker for support and decreased pain when walking.

Cold and Heat Therapy and Exercise. Cold and heat applications can help relieve stiffness, pain, and muscle spasm. Heat and cold can be used several times a day as needed. Ice is especially helpful during periods of increased disease activity. Cold application should not exceed 10 to 15 minutes at a time. Plastic bags of small frozen vegetables (peas or kernel corn) can easily mold around the shoulder, wrists, or knees to be an effective home treatment. The patient can use ice cubes or small paper cups of frozen water to massage areas on either side of a painful joint. Moist heat offers better relief for chronic stiffness. However, heat application should not exceed 20 minutes at a time.

Heating pads, moist hot packs, paraffin baths, and warm baths or showers can relieve stiffness to allow the patient to take part in therapeutic exercise. Alert the patient to the risk for a burn and the need to avoid using a heat-producing cream (e.g., capsaicin) with an external heat device. Sitting or standing in a warm shower, sitting in a tub with warm towels around the shoulders, or simply soaking the hands in a basin of warm water may relieve joint stiffness and allow the patient to perform ADLs more comfortably.

Individualized exercise is an important part of the treatment plan. A physical therapist may develop a therapeutic exercise program to improve flexibility and strength of affected joints and increase the patient's endurance. Encourage program participation and reinforce correct performance of the exercises. Progressive joint immobility and muscle weakness can occur if the patient does not move the joints. Overaggressive exercise can cause increased pain, inflammation, and joint damage. Emphasize that taking part in a recreational exercise program (e.g., walking, swimming) or doing usual daily activities does not take the place of therapeutic exercise to maintain adequate joint motion.

Gentle ROM exercises are usually done daily to keep joints functional. The patient should practice exercises with supervision. Exercising in warm water (78° to 86° F [25° to 30° C]) allows easier joint movement because of the buoyancy and warmth of the water. Although movement seems easier, water provides 2-way resistance that makes muscles work harder than they would on land. During acute inflammation, limit exercise to 1 or 2 repetitions.

Patient and Caregiver Teaching. Care of the patient with RA begins with a thorough program of education and drug therapy. Teach the patient and caregiver about the disease process and home management strategies. Inflammation may be managed through administration of NSAIDs, DMARDs, and BRMs. Careful timing of drug administration is critical to maintain a therapeutic drug level and reduce early morning stiffness. Discuss the action and side effects of each prescribed drug and any needed laboratory monitoring. Many patients with RA take several different drugs, so make the drug regimen as understandable as possible. Encourage patients to develop a way to remember to take their medications (e.g., pill containers).

Psychologic Support. For effective self-management and adherence to an individualized home treatment program, help the patient understand the nature and course of RA and the goals of therapy. Consider the patient's value system and perception of the disease.

Discuss changes in sexuality. Chronic pain or loss of function may make the patient vulnerable to claims of false advertising about unproven or even dangerous remedies. Help the patient recognize fears and concerns faced by all people who live with chronic illness.

Evaluate the family support system. Financial planning may be needed. Consider community resources, such as a home care nurse, homemaker services, and vocational rehabilitation. Self-help groups are helpful for some patients.

Living with chronic pain may lead to depression. To decrease depressive symptoms, suggest activities such as listening to music, reading, exercising, and counseling. Hypnosis and biofeedback may be useful.

Gerontologic Considerations: Arthritis

The prevalence of arthritis in older adults is high. The disease is accompanied by problems unique to this age-group. Areas of concern for older adults include:

- The high incidence of OA in older adults may keep the HCP from considering other types of arthritis.
- Age alone causes changes that make interpretation of laboratory values, such as RF and ESR, more difficult. Drugs taken for co-morbid conditions can affect laboratory values.
- Musculoskeletal pain syndromes and weakness may have no physical cause. Instead, they may be related to depression and physical inactivity.
- Diseases such as SLE, which often occur in younger adults, can develop in a milder form in older adults.

Physical and metabolic changes of aging may increase the older patient's sensitivity to both therapeutic and toxic effects of some drugs. The older adult who takes NSAIDs has an increased risk for side effects, especially GI bleeding and renal toxicity. Using NSAIDs with a shorter half-life may need more frequent dosing and have fewer side effects in the older patient with altered drug metabolism.

Polypharmacy in the older adult is a concern. Use of drugs in RA treatment may increase the chance of unexpected drug interactions. The drug regimen should be as simple as possible to increase adherence (e.g., limited number of drugs with decreased frequency of administration). This is especially important for those who lack regular assistance.

Osteopenia from corticosteroid use can worsen the problem of decreased bone density from aging and inactivity. The risk for pathologic fractures is increased, especially vertebral compression fractures. Myopathy related to corticosteroid use can be minimized by an age-appropriate exercise program. An adequate support system for the older adult is critical to the ability to follow a treatment plan.

GOUT

Gout is a type of arthritis characterized by elevation of uric acid *(hyperuricemia)* and the deposit of uric acid crystals in 1 or more joints. Sodium urate crystals may be found in articular, periarticular, and subcutaneous tissues. Unlike other forms of arthritis, gout is marked by painful flares lasting days to weeks followed by long periods without symptoms. More than 8 million Americans have gout. Blacks have a higher incidence compared to whites.[14]

GENDER DIFFERENCES

Gout

Men
- Occurs 3 times more often in men than in women until age 60.
- Usually develops in men ages 30 to 50.

Women
- Rarely develop gout before menopause.

Etiology and Pathophysiology

Uric acid is the major end product of purine catabolism. It is primarily excreted by the kidneys. Gout occurs when either the kidneys cannot excrete enough uric acid or there is too much being made for the kidneys to handle effectively.

We classify hyperuricemia as primary or secondary. *Primary hyperuricemia* is genetic. A hereditary error of purine metabolism leads to the overproduction or retention of uric acid. *Secondary hyperuricemia* may be caused by conditions that

TABLE 64.12 Causes of Hyperuricemia

- Acidosis or ketosis
- Alcohol use, especially beer and red wine
- Cancer
- Chemotherapy drugs
- Diabetes
- Drug-induced renal impairment
- Hyperlipidemia
- Hypertension
- Lead exposure
- Metabolic syndrome
- Myeloproliferative disorders
- Obesity
- Renal insufficiency
- Sickle cell anemia
- Starvation
- Use of certain common drugs (aspirin, ACE inhibitors, β-blockers, loop or thiazide diuretics, niacin)

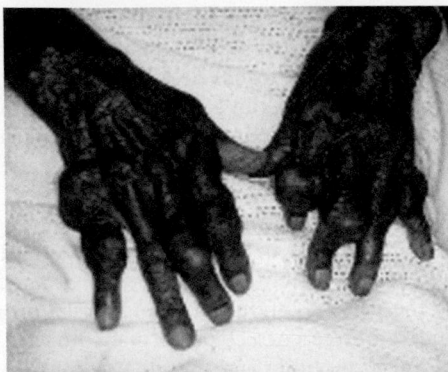

FIG. 64.6 Tophi associated with chronic gout. Painless nodules are filled with uric acid crystals. (Courtesy John Cook, MD. From Goldstein BG, Goldstein AE: *Practical dermatology*, ed 2, St Louis, 1997, Mosby.)

increase uric acid production or decrease uric acid excretion or drugs that inhibit uric acid excretion (e.g., loop diuretics, β-blockers). Organ transplant recipients receiving immunosuppressive agents are at risk for hyperuricemia (Table 64.12).

Gout is likely caused by the interaction of several factors. The most important is metabolic syndrome (obesity, insulin resistance, hypertension, hyperlipidemia). Increased intake of foods containing purines (e.g., red and organ meat, shellfish, fructose drinks) can trigger gout. High uric acid may result from prolonged fasting or excessive alcohol use because they increase the production of keto acids, which inhibit uric acid excretion.

Not everyone with high uric acid levels develops gout. Two processes are essential for a person to develop gout: crystallization and inflammation. As urate levels increase and saturate the synovial fluid or soft tissues, the excess urate coalesces into crystals. These trigger inflammation. Monocytes and macrophages try to remove the crystals through phagocytosis. This causes the release of inflammatory mediators into the surrounding area, causing more inflammation and tissue damage.[15]

Clinical Manifestations and Complications

Gout may occur acutely in 1 or more joints (usually less than 4). Inflammation of the great toe *(podagra)* is the most common initial problem. Other affected joints may include wrists, knees, ankles, and the midfoot. Olecranon bursae may be involved. Affected joints may appear dusky or cyanotic and are extremely tender. Acute gout arthritis is usually triggered by events such as trauma, surgery, alcohol use, or systemic infection. Symptom onset typically occurs at night with sudden swelling and severe pain peaking within several hours. The painful area is highly sensitive to light touch. Low-grade fever is common.

An attack usually ends in 2 to 10 days with or without treatment. The affected joint returns to normal, and patients have no symptoms between attacks.

Chronic gout is characterized by multiple joint involvement and visible deposits of sodium urate crystals called tophi. Tophi are hard white nodules. They are typically seen in subcutaneous tissue, synovial membranes, tendons, and soft tissues (Fig. 64.6). Tophi generally occur many years after the onset of disease.

The severity of gout arthritis varies. The clinical course may involve infrequent mild attacks or multiple severe episodes (up to 12 per year) marked by slowly progressive disability. In general, tophi appear earlier, and the patient has more frequent,

severe episodes of gout if serum uric acid is high. Chronic inflammation may cause joint deformity, and cartilage destruction may lead to secondary OA. Large urate crystal deposits may pierce overlying skin, producing draining sinuses that often become infected.

Excessive uric acid excretion may lead to stone formation in the kidneys or urinary tract. Pyelonephritis related to sodium urate deposits and obstruction contributes to kidney disease.

Diagnostic Studies

In gout, serum uric acid is usually increased above 6 mg/dL. However, hyperuricemia is not specifically diagnostic of gout because serum values may be normal during an acute gout attack.[15] Increased uric acid may be related to various drugs or an asymptomatic abnormality in the general population A 24-hour urine uric acid can determine if the disease is caused by decreased renal excretion or overproduction of uric acid.

The gold standard for diagnosis of gout is synovial fluid aspiration. Affected fluid contains needle-like monosodium urate crystals. This procedure is done in only a small number of patients because diagnosis can typically be made on clinical symptoms alone. However, it is the only reliable way to tell gout from septic arthritis or *pseudogout* (calcium phosphate crystal formation). Aspiration may decrease pain by relieving pressure in a swollen joint capsule.

X-rays appear normal in the early stages of gout. In chronic disease, tophi may appear as eroded areas in the bone.

❖ INTERPROFESSIONAL AND NURSING MANAGEMENT: GOUT

Goals for the care of the patient with gout (Table 64.13) include ending an acute attack with an antiinflammatory agent, such as colchicine. Hyperuricemia and gout are chronic problems that can be controlled with effective patient education and careful adherence to a treatment program. Drug therapy is the primary way to treat acute and chronic gout.

◆ Drug Therapy

Acute gout is treated with oral colchicine (Colcrys, Mitigare) and NSAIDs. Because colchicine has antiinflammatory effects but is not an analgesic, an NSAID is added for pain management. Colchicine generally produces dramatic pain relief when given within 12 hours of an attack. This helps in diagnosis because good response to this drug is further evidence of gout.

TABLE 64.13 Interprofessional Care

Gout

Diagnostic Assessment
- History and physical examination
- Family history of gout
- Sodium urate crystals in synovial fluid
- Increased serum uric acid
- Increased uric acid in 24-hr urine
- X-ray of affected joints

Management
- Joint immobilization
- Local application of heat and cold
- Joint aspiration and intraarticular corticosteroids
- Avoid food and fluids with high purine content (e.g., anchovies, liver, wine, beer)

Drug Therapy
- colchicine
- NSAIDs (e.g., naproxen [Naprosyn])
- Xanthine oxidase inhibitors: allopurinol (Zyloprim), febuxostat (Uloric)
- Uricosurics: probenecid, lesinurad (Zurampic)
- pegloticase (Krystexxa)
- Corticosteroids (e.g., prednisone)
- Intraarticular corticosteroids (methylprednisolone)
- Adrenocorticotropic hormone (ACTH)

Corticosteroids (orally or by intraarticular injection) can be helpful in treating an acute attack. Systemic corticosteroids may be used only if routine therapies are contraindicated or ineffective. Adrenocorticotropic hormone (ACTH) may be used for acute treatment of patients for whom NSAIDs, colchicine, or steroids may be problematic.

Future attacks of gout are prevented in part by a maintenance dose of a xanthine oxidase inhibitor. These drugs decrease the production of uric acid. Allopurinol is the most commonly used drug and the first choice for therapy. It is used for patients with uric acid kidney stones or renal impairment. Serious adverse effects limit the use of febuxostat (Uloric).

 DRUG ALERT Febuxostat

- May cause heart-related death and liver failure.
- Encourage patient with cardiovascular disease to take low-dose aspirin therapy.
- Monitor liver function tests before starting therapy and during treatment.
- Teach patient to notify HCP if symptoms of liver or heart problems occur.

The ACR recommends therapy with probenecid if allopurinol or febuxostat are contraindicated or the patient has intolerance to either.[15] Probenecid is a uricosuric, increasing uric acid excretion in the urine. Aspirin inactivates its effect, resulting in urate retention, and must be avoided during treatment. Acetaminophen can be used safely if analgesia is needed. Lesinurad (Zurampic), a new uricosuric agent, can be taken with a xanthine oxidase inhibitor for those with persistent, increased uric acid levels. Duzallo, a fixed-dose combination of lesinurad and allopurinol, is taken once daily.

Uricosurics can cause renal impairment. They are ineffective when creatinine clearance is reduced, as can occur in patients over age 60 years or with renal impairment. They should be taken in the morning with food and water. Teach patients to stay well hydrated and to drink about 2 L of liquid a day when taking the drug.

Patients who cannot take or do not respond to drugs that lower serum uric acid may be given pegloticase (Krystexxa). This drug is an enzyme that metabolizes uric acid into a harmless chemical excreted in the urine. It is given IV, usually for at least 6 months. Life-threatening anaphylactic and infusion reactions can occur.

The angiotensin II receptor antagonist losartan (Cozaar) may be effective for treating older patients with gout and hypertension. Losartan promotes urate excretion and may normalize serum urate. Combination therapy with losartan and allopurinol may be used.

Serum uric acid must be checked regularly to monitor treatment effectiveness. Explain the importance of drug therapy and the need for regular assessment of serum uric acid. Dietary restrictions that limit alcohol and foods high in purine help minimize uric acid production (see Table 45.12). Adequate urine volume with normal renal function (2 to 3 L/day) must be maintained to prevent precipitation of uric acid in the renal tubules. Teach obese patients in a carefully planned weight-reduction program (see Chapter 40). Teach the patient about other factors that may cause an attack, including fasting, drug use (e.g., diuretics), and major medical events (e.g., surgery, heart attack).

Nursing interventions for the patient with acute gout include supportive care of the inflamed joints. Avoid causing pain by careless handling of an inflamed joint. Bed rest may be appropriate to immobilize affected joints as needed. Use a cradle or footboard to protect a painful lower extremity from the weight of bed linens. Assess motion limitations and degree of pain.

❓ CHECK YOUR PRACTICE

A patient is admitted to the medical unit with acute gout. The right great toe is swollen, red, and painful. He is prescribed colchicine.
- What nursing interventions will you use to protect the foot and decrease pain?
- What will you discuss with the patient about possible dietary changes to decrease risk for future attacks?

LYME DISEASE

Lyme disease is an infection caused by the spirochete *Borrelia burgdorferi*. It is transmitted by the bite of an infected deer tick. It was first identified in 1975 in Lyme, Connecticut, after an unusual occurrence of arthritis in children. It is the most common vector-borne disease in the United States, with 7.9 cases per 100,000 persons.[16] The tick typically feeds on mice, dogs, cats, cows, horses, deer, and humans. Person-to-person transmission does not occur.

The summer months are the peak season for human infection. Most U.S. cases occur in 3 areas: along the northeastern states from Maryland to northern Massachusetts, in the midwestern states of Wisconsin and Minnesota, and along the northwestern coast of California and Oregon.[16] Reinfection is common.

Symptoms mimic those of other diseases, such as multiple sclerosis, mononucleosis, and meningitis. The most characteristic clinical symptom of early localized disease is *erythema migrans* (EM). This "bull's-eye rash" occurs in about 80% of infected persons. It appears at the site of the tick bite within 1 month after exposure (Fig. 64.7). It may occur anywhere else on the body as the disease progresses. The EM lesion begins as

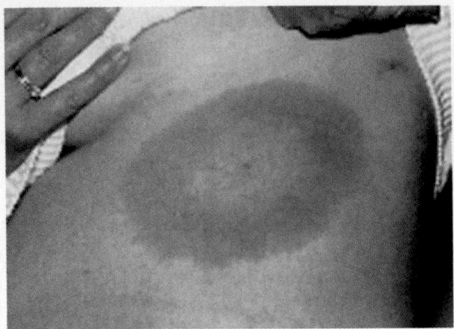

FIG. 64.7 Erythema migrans. Typical skin lesion of Lyme disease occurs at the site of tick bite. (From Marx J, Hockberger R, Walls R: *Rosen's emergency medicine,* ed 7, Philadelphia, 2009, Mosby.)

a central red macule or papule that slowly expands to include a red outer ring of up to 12 in, resembling a bull's eye. It may be warm to the touch but is not itchy or painful. The rash often occurs with acute flu-like symptoms: (1) low-grade fever, (2) headache, (3) neck stiffness, (4) fatigue, (5) loss of appetite, and (6) migratory joint and muscle pain. Flu-like symptoms generally resolve over weeks or months, even if untreated.

If not treated, the spirochete can spread within several weeks or months to the heart, joints, heart, and central nervous system (CNS). Arthritis is the second most common manifestation of Lyme disease. About 60% of persons with untreated infection develop chronic arthritic pain and swelling in the large joints, mainly the knee. Cardiac symptoms, such as heart block and pericarditis, may require hospitalization.[16] Bell's palsy is the most common neurologic effect. Other problems include short-term memory loss, cognitive impairment, shooting pains, and numbness and tingling in the feet.

Diagnosis is often based on the manifestations, especially EM, and a history of exposure in an at-risk area. The CDC recommends a 2-step laboratory testing process to confirm the diagnosis.[17] The first step is the enzyme immunoassay (EIA). It will be positive for most people with Lyme disease. If the EIA is positive or inconclusive, then a Western blot test is done. Results are diagnostic of Lyme disease only if both tests are positive. The CDC does not recommend the Western blot test alone. False-positive results lead to incorrect diagnosis and treatment. In those with neurologic involvement, cerebrospinal fluid should be examined.

Active lesions are treated with oral antibiotics. Doxycycline (Vibramycin), cefuroxime, and amoxicillin are often effective in treating early-stage infection and preventing later stages of the disease. Short-term therapy of 10 to 21 days of doxycycline is preferred. It treats both Lyme disease and human granulocytic anaplasmosis, which can be transmitted as a co-infection with a single tick bite. While other antibiotics can be used for those who cannot tolerate any of these drugs, they all are less effective. Patients with certain neurologic or cardiac complications may need IV therapy with ceftriaxone or penicillin.

A small number of persons treated with antibiotics may have lingering fatigue or joint and muscle pain. Antibiotic treatment should be extended as needed because the risks of untreated Lyme disease outweigh those of long-term antibiotic therapy.[18]

Reducing exposure to ticks is the best way to prevent Lyme disease. Patient and caregiver teaching for people living in endemic areas is outlined in Table 64.14. No vaccine is available for Lyme disease.

TABLE 64.14 Patient & Caregiver Teaching

Prevention and Early Treatment of Lyme Disease

Include the following instructions when teaching patients how to prevent Lyme disease:
- Do not walk through tall grasses and low brush or sit on logs.
- Mow grass. Remove brush around paths, buildings, and campsites to create tick-safe zones.
- Move woodpiles and bird feeders away from your house. Discourage deer (main source of food for adult ticks) from being in the area.
- Wear long pants or nylon tights of tightly woven, light-colored fabric so that you can easily see ticks.
- Tuck pants into boots or long socks, wear long-sleeved shirts tucked into pants, and wear closed toed shoes when hiking.
- Check often for ticks crawling from pant legs to open skin.
- Thoroughly inspect and wash clothes. Placing clothing in dryer on high heat kills ticks.
- Spray insect repellent containing DEET sparingly on skin or clothing. Apply permethrin to clothing and camping gear; protects for several hours.
- Have pets wear tick collars and inspect them often. Do not allow pets on furniture or beds.

Include the following instructions when teaching patients and caregivers living in endemic areas:
- Remove attached ticks with fine-tipped tweezers (not fingers). Grasp tick's mouth parts as close to skin as possible and pull straight out with steady, even pressure. Do not twist or jerk. Avoid folk solutions, such as painting the tick with nail polish or petroleum jelly (see Fig. 68.5).
- Save the tick in a bottle of alcohol (if you need it later for identification). Never crush a tick with your fingers.
- Wash bitten area with soap and water, iodine scrub, or rubbing alcohol. Apply antiseptic. Wash hands.
- See an HCP if flu-like symptoms or a bull's-eye rash appears within 2–30 days after removal of tick.

Adapted from Centers for Disease Control and Prevention: Prevent Lyme disease. Retrieved from *www.cdc.gov/features/lymedisease;* and Centers for Disease Control and Prevention: Tick removal and testing. Retrieved from *www.cdc.gov/lyme/removal/index.html.*
DEET, N,N-diethyl-m-toluamide.

SEPTIC ARTHRITIS

Septic arthritis (infectious or bacterial arthritis) is caused by microorganisms invading the joint cavity. Bacteria can travel through the bloodstream from another site of active infection, resulting in seeding of the joint. Organisms also can be introduced directly through trauma or surgical incision.

Any infectious agent can cause septic arthritis (bacteria, viruses, mycobacteria, fungi), especially in the immunocompromised patient. *Staphylococcus aureus* is the most common causative organism. Factors that increase the risk for infection include (1) diseases with decreased host resistance (e.g., RA, SLE), (2) treatment with corticosteroids or immunosuppressive drugs, and (3) debilitating chronic illness (e.g., diabetes).

Large joints, such as the knee and hip, are most often affected. Inflammation of the joint cavity causes severe pain, redness, and swelling. Septic arthritis of the hip can cause avascular necrosis. Because infection has often spread from a primary site elsewhere in the body, fever or shaking chills often accompany joint problems. Diagnosis may be made by joint aspiration *(arthrocentesis)* and synovial fluid culture. WBC count may be low early in the infectious process, especially in those who are immunosuppressed, so diagnosis is not possible solely based on WBC count. Blood cultures for aerobic and anaerobic organisms should be obtained.

Emergent aspiration or surgical drainage is a cornerstone of successful treatment. Irreversible joint damage can occur without rapid, appropriate treatment of septic arthritis. In some cases, damage can occur despite treatment. Broad-spectrum antibiotics are typically started before culture results have been received. Once the organism is identified, more specific treatment can be determined. IV antibiotics are typically transitioned to oral antibiotics, with total treatment of 4 to 6 weeks.

Assess and monitor joint inflammation, pain, and fever. To manage pain, use resting splints or traction to immobilize affected joints. Local hot compresses can decrease pain. Start gentle ROM exercises as soon as tolerated to prevent muscle atrophy and joint contractures. Explain the need for antibiotics and the importance of their continued use until the infection is resolved. Support the patient who needs joint drainage. Use strict aseptic technique when assisting with joint aspiration.

SPONDYLOARTHROPATHIES

The spondyloarthropathies are a group of multisystem inflammatory disorders that affect the spine, peripheral joints, and periarticular structures. These disorders include ankylosing spondylitis, psoriatic arthritis, and reactive arthritis. They are all negative for RF so we call them *seronegative arthropathies*.

Inheritance of human leukocyte antigen (HLA) B27 is strongly associated with these diseases. Both genetic and environmental factors play a role in their development. (HLAs and their relationship to autoimmune diseases are discussed in Chapter 13.)

The spondyloarthropathies share clinical and laboratory characteristics that may make it hard to distinguish among them in early disease. These include absence of antibodies in the serum, peripheral joint involvement (mainly of the lower extremities), low back pain *(sacroiliitis)*, pain and redness of the eyes *(uveitis)*, intestinal inflammation, and psoriasis.[19]

ANKYLOSING SPONDYLITIS

Ankylosing spondylitis (AS) is a chronic inflammatory disease that primarily affects the axial skeleton, including the sacroiliac joints, intervertebral disc spaces, and costovertebral articulations. Onset of AS is usually in the third decade of life, but onset in adolescence is fairly common. Men are 3 times more likely to develop AS. The disease may go undetected in women because of a milder course.

Etiology and Pathophysiology

We do not know the exact cause of AS. HLA-B27 antigen is found in about 90% of whites with AS, but only 8% of whites without the disease.[20] This suggests genes play a key role in AS. Along with whites, Asians and Hispanics are more likely to have AS than other ethnic groups. Inflammation in the joints and adjacent tissue causes the formation of granulation tissue *(pannus)* and dense fibrous scars that can cause joint fusion. Inflammation can affect the eyes, lungs, heart, kidneys, and peripheral nervous system.

Clinical Manifestations and Complications

AS is characterized by symmetric sacroiliitis and progressive inflammatory arthritis of the axial skeleton. Symptoms of inflammatory spine pain are the first clues to AS. The patient often has low back pain, stiffness, and limitation of motion that

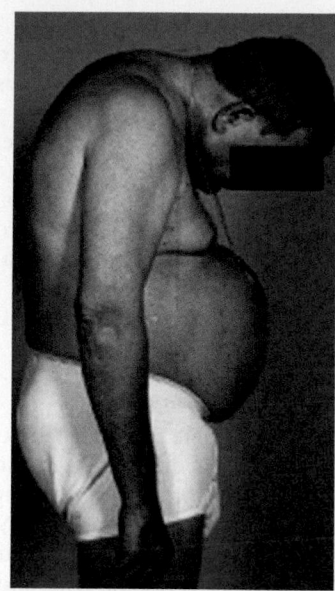

FIG. 64.8 Advanced ankylosing spondylitis. Kyphotic posture causes many patients to have a bulging abdomen due to pulmonary restriction. (From Kim DH, Henn J, Vaccaro AR, Dickman C: *Surgical anatomy and techniques to the spine*, Philadelphia, 2006, Saunders.)

GENETICS IN CLINICAL PRACTICE

Ankylosing Spondylitis

Genetic Basis
- Inheritance of HLA-B27 increases susceptibility to developing AS.
- We do not know how HLA-B27 increases the risk for AS.

Incidence
- HLA-B27 antigen is found in about 90% of whites with AS.
- Inheriting HLA-B27 does not mean a person will develop AS.
- 80% of those who inherit HLA-B27 from a parent do not develop the disease.

Genetic Testing
- Testing for HLA-B27 antigen is available.

Clinical Implications
- Diagnosis of AS usually occurs in the third decade of life.
- Multiple genetic and environmental factors play a role in pathogenesis of disease.

is worse during the night and in the morning but improves with mild activity. In women, early symptoms may include pain and stiffness in the neck rather than the lower back. Uveitis is the most common nonskeletal symptom. It can appear as an initial presentation of the disease years before arthritic symptoms develop. Patients with AS may have distressing chest pain and sternal/costal cartilage tenderness.

Severe postural abnormalities and deformity can cause significant disability (Fig. 64.8). Impaired spinal ROM and fusion, along with vision problems, raise concerns about safe ambulation. Aortic insufficiency and pulmonary fibrosis are common complications. Cauda equina syndrome (compression of the nerves at the end of the spinal cord) can occur. This contributes to lower extremity weakness and bladder dysfunction. The patient is at risk for spinal fracture from associated osteoporosis.

Diagnostic Studies

X-rays are the most important radiographic technique for the diagnosis and follow up of AS. However, x-rays are limited in detecting early sacroiliitis or subtle changes in posterior vertebrae. MRI is useful in assessing early cartilage abnormalities. CT scan is appropriate in specific situations (e.g., cases with subtle x-ray changes). Changes on later spinal films include the appearance of "bamboo spine," the result of calcifications *(syndesmophytes)* that bridge from one vertebra to another. An increased ESR and mild anemia may be seen. When the suspicion for AS is high, the presence of the HLA-B27 antigen improves the likelihood of the diagnosis.

❖ Interprofessional and Nursing Care

Prevention of AS is not possible. Families with other diagnosed HLA-B27–positive rheumatic diseases (e.g., psoriatic arthritis, juvenile spondyloarthritis) should be alert to signs of low back pain for early identification and treatment of AS.

Care of the patient with AS is aimed at maintaining maximal skeletal mobility while decreasing pain and inflammation. Heat applications can help relieve local symptoms. NSAIDs and salicylates are often prescribed. DMARDs, such as sulfasalazine or methotrexate, have little effect on spinal disease but help with peripheral joint disease. Local corticosteroid injections may be helpful in relieving symptoms.

TNF, which promotes inflammation, is increased in the blood and certain tissues of patients with AS. Etanercept, a BRM, binds TNF and inhibits its action. Etanercept reduces active inflammation and improves spinal mobility. Other anti-TNF inhibitors (infliximab, adalimumab, golimumab) may be effective.

Once pain and stiffness are managed, exercise is essential. Good posture is important to minimize spinal deformity. The exercise plan should include back, neck, and chest stretches. Hydrotherapy (e.g., sauna, steam bath) can decrease pain and facilitate spinal extension. Surgery may be needed for severe deformity and mobility impairment. Spinal osteotomy and total joint replacement are the most common procedures (see Chapter 62).

A key nursing responsibility is to teach the patient with AS about the disease and principles of therapy. The home management program should include regular exercise and attention to posture, local moist heat applications, and informed use of drugs.

Assess chest expansion (using breathing exercises) as part of baseline ROM assessment. Encourage smoking cessation to decrease the risk for lung complications in persons with reduced chest expansion. Ongoing PT includes gentle, graded stretching and strengthening exercises. These preserve ROM and improve thoracolumbar flexion and extension.

Discourage excessive physical exertion during periods of increased disease activity. Proper positioning at rest is essential. Encourage the patient to use a firm mattress. They should sleep on the back with a flat pillow, avoiding positions that encourage flexion deformity. Emphasize the need to avoid spinal flexion (e.g., leaning over a desk); heavy lifting; and prolonged walking, standing, or sitting. Encourage sports that involve natural stretching, such as swimming and racquet games. Family counseling and vocational rehabilitation are important.

PSORIATIC ARTHRITIS

Psoriatic arthritis (PsA) is a progressive inflammatory disease that affects about 30% of people with psoriasis.[21] *Psoriasis* is a common, benign, inflammatory skin disorder characterized by red, irritated, and scaly patches. Both PsA and psoriasis appear to have a genetic link with HLA antigens in many patients. Although the exact cause of PsA is unknown, we suspect a combination of immune, genetic, and environmental factors.

PsA can occur in different forms. *Distal arthritis* mainly involves the ends of the fingers and toes, with pitting and color changes in the fingernails and toenails. *Asymmetric arthritis* involves different joints on each side of the body. *Symmetric psoriatic arthritis* resembles RA. It affects joints on both sides of the body at the same time. It accounts for about 50% of cases. *Psoriatic spondylitis* is marked by pain and stiffness in the spine and neck. *Arthritis mutilans* affects only 5% of people with PsA. It is the most severe form of the disease, causing complete destruction of small joints.[21]

On x-ray, the cartilage loss and erosion are similar to RA. Advanced cases often show widened joint spaces. A "pencil in cup" deformity is common in the DIP joints due to thinning, weakened bone. In this deformity, the narrowed ends of the metacarpals or phalanges insert into the expanded end of the other bone sharing the joint. Increased ESR, mild anemia, and increased serum uric acid can be seen in some patients. Thus the diagnosis of gout must be excluded.

Treatment includes splinting, joint protection, and PT. NSAIDs given early in the course of the disease may help with inflammation. Drug therapy includes the DMARDs, such as methotrexate, which is effective for both articular and cutaneous manifestations. Sulfasalazine, cyclosporine, and BRMs (e.g., etanercept, golimumab, adalimumab, infliximab) may be used. Apremilast (Otezla), an inhibitor of the enzyme phosphodiesterase-4, can treat adults with active PsA.

REACTIVE ARTHRITIS

Reactive arthritis (Reiter's syndrome) occurs more often in young men. It is associated with a symptom complex that includes urethritis, conjunctivitis, and mucocutaneous lesions. Although we do not know the exact cause, it appears to be a reaction triggered in the body after exposure to specific genitourinary or GI tract infections. *Chlamydia trachomatis* spreads by sexual contact. Reactive arthritis is associated with GI infections from *Shigella, Salmonella, Campylobacter,* or *Yersinia* species and other pathogens.[22]

Those who are positive for HLA-B27 are at increased risk for developing reactive arthritis after sexual contact or exposure to certain GI pathogens. This finding supports the suggestion of genetic predisposition.

Urethritis develops within 1 to 2 weeks after sexual contact or GI infection. In women, symptoms include cervicitis. Low-grade fever, conjunctivitis, and arthritis may occur over the next several weeks. This type of arthritis tends to be asymmetric. It often involves the toes and the large joints of the lower extremities. Lower back pain may occur with severe disease. Lesions involving the skin and mucous membranes often occur as small, painless, superficial ulcerations on the tongue, oral mucosa, and glans penis. Soft tissue manifestations include Achilles tendinitis or plantar fasciitis. Few laboratory abnormalities occur, although the ESR may be increased.

Most patients recover within a few months of initial symptoms. Because reactive arthritis is often associated with *C. trachomatis* infection, treatment with doxycycline is widely recommended for patients and their sexual partners. Antibiotics have no effect on arthritis or other symptoms. Topical ophthalmic corticosteroids may be prescribed for treatment of uveitis. Conjunctivitis and lesions generally do not need treatment. NSAIDs and DMARDs may be used if joint symptoms do not resolve. PT may be helpful during recovery.

Most patients have complete remission with return of full joint function. Some patients may develop chronic arthritis, but the condition is often mild. X-ray changes in chronic reactive arthritis closely resemble those of AS. Treatment is based on symptoms.

SYSTEMIC LUPUS ERYTHEMATOSUS

Systemic lupus erythematosus (SLE) is a multisystem inflammatory autoimmune disease. It is a complex disorder of multifactorial origin resulting from interactions among genetic, hormonal, environmental, and immunologic factors. SLE typically affects the skin, joints, and serous membranes (pleura, pericardium). Renal, hematologic, and neurologic systems are also affected. SLE is marked by a chronic unpredictable course with alternating periods of remission and exacerbation.

About 1.5 million people in the United States have SLE. Blacks, Asian Americans, Hispanics, and Native Americans are more likely than whites to develop the disease. While SLE can affect anyone, 90% of those with SLE are women ages 15 to 45 years.[23]

Etiology and Pathophysiology

The cause of the abnormal immune response in SLE is unknown. Based on the high prevalence of SLE among family members, we suspect a genetic influence. Multiple genes from the HLA complex, including *HLA-DR2* and *HLA-DR3*, are associated with SLE.

Hormones are known to play a role in SLE. Onset or worsening of disease symptoms may occur after the start of menses, with the use of oral contraceptives, and during and after pregnancy. The disease tends to become worse in the immediate postpartum period.

Environmental factors are thought to contribute to SLE. These include sun or ultraviolet light exposure, stress, and exposure to some chemicals and toxins. Infectious agents, such as viruses, may stimulate immune hyperactivity. More than 45 drugs currently in use may trigger SLE. Most cases have been related to procainamide, hydralazine, and quinidine. Drug-induced SLE should not be confused with medication side effects, which typically occur within a few hours or days of short-term drug use. SLE generally occurs months to years after continuous therapy with a causative drug.[24]

In SLE, varied autoantibodies are made against nucleic acids (e.g., single- and double-stranded DNA), erythrocytes, coagulation proteins, lymphocytes, platelets, and many other self-proteins. Autoimmune reactions (antinuclear antibodies [ANA]) are typically directed against elements of the cell nucleus, especially DNA.

Circulating immune complexes with antibodies against DNA are deposited in the basement membranes of capillaries in the kidneys, heart, skin, brain, and joints. These complexes trigger inflammation that causes tissue destruction. Overaggressive autoimmune responses are related to activation of B and T cells. Specific disease effects depend on the involved cell types or organs. SLE is a type III hypersensitivity response (see Chapter 13).

Clinical Manifestations and Complications

Severity of SLE is extremely variable. It ranges from a relatively mild disorder to a rapidly progressive disease affecting many body systems (Fig. 64.9). No characteristic pattern occurs in the progression of SLE. The circulating immune complexes can affect any organ. The most commonly involved tissues are the skin and muscle, lining of the lungs, heart, nervous tissue, and kidneys. General complaints, such as fever, weight loss, joint pain, and excessive fatigue, may precede worsened disease activity.

Dermatologic Problems. Vascular skin lesions can appear anywhere. They are most likely to develop on sun-exposed areas. Severe skin reactions can occur in people who are sensitive to sunlight (*photosensitivity*). The classic butterfly rash over the cheeks and bridge of the nose occurs in about half of patients at some time during the disease (Fig. 64.10). SLE-specific skin disease can occur in people who do not have full-blown SLE, but the presence of skin disease increases the risk for developing SLE later in life. Some patients have *chronic cutaneous lupus* (CCLE) with discoid (round, coin-shaped) lesions. About 10% of patients have *subacute cutaneous lupus* (SCLE). Lesions in SCLE usually do not scar or itch and are not thick and scaly.[25]

Oral or nasopharyngeal ulcers occur in one third of patients with SLE. Alopecia is common, with or without related scalp lesions. The hair may grow back during remission, but hair loss may be permanent over lesions. The scalp becomes dry, scaly, and atrophied.

Musculoskeletal Problems. Arthritis occurs in many patients with SLE. Pain in multiple joints (*polyarthralgia*) with morning stiffness is often the first complaint. It may precede the onset of multisystem disease by many years. Diffuse swelling occurs with joint and muscle pain and some stiffness. SLE-related arthritis is generally nonerosive but may cause deformities (e.g., swan neck deformity of the fingers [Fig. 64.4, *D*], ulnar deviation, subluxation with joint laxity). Patients have increased risk for bone loss and fracture.

Cardiopulmonary Problems. Tachypnea and cough suggest the presence of lung disease. Pleurisy is possible. Cardiac involvement may include dysrhythmias due to fibrosis of the sinoatrial and atrioventricular nodes. This shows advanced disease and is the leading cause of death among patients with SLE. Inflammation can lead to pericarditis, myocarditis, and endocarditis. Hypertension and hypercholesterolemia from steroid use need aggressive treatment and careful monitoring. People with SLE are at risk for secondary *antiphospholipid syndrome*. This coagulation disorder causes clots in the arteries and veins. It increases the risk for stroke, gangrene, and heart attack.

Renal Problems. About 40% of persons with SLE develop kidney problems that need medical evaluation and treatment. Renal involvement is usually present within the first 5 years after diagnosis.[26] Manifestations vary from mild proteinuria to rapidly progressive glomerulonephritis. Scarring and permanent damage can lead to end-stage renal disease (ESRD).

The main goal is to slow the progression of nephropathy and preserve renal function by managing the underlying disease. The need for a renal biopsy is controversial, but findings can help guide treatment. Effective treatments include corticosteroids,

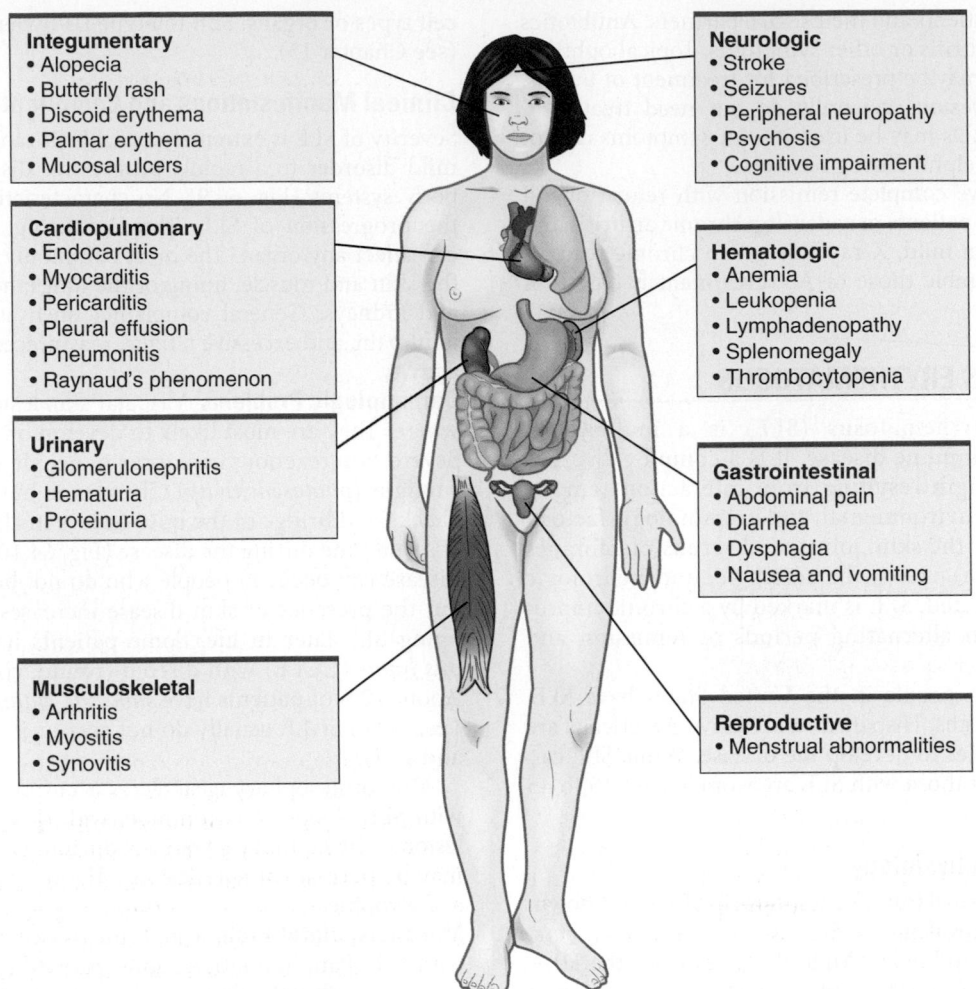

Integumentary
- Alopecia
- Butterfly rash
- Discoid erythema
- Palmar erythema
- Mucosal ulcers

Cardiopulmonary
- Endocarditis
- Myocarditis
- Pericarditis
- Pleural effusion
- Pneumonitis
- Raynaud's phenomenon

Urinary
- Glomerulonephritis
- Hematuria
- Proteinuria

Musculoskeletal
- Arthritis
- Myositis
- Synovitis

Neurologic
- Stroke
- Seizures
- Peripheral neuropathy
- Psychosis
- Cognitive impairment

Hematologic
- Anemia
- Leukopenia
- Lymphadenopathy
- Splenomegaly
- Thrombocytopenia

Gastrointestinal
- Abdominal pain
- Diarrhea
- Dysphagia
- Nausea and vomiting

Reproductive
- Menstrual abnormalities

FIG. 64.9 Multisystem involvement in SLE.

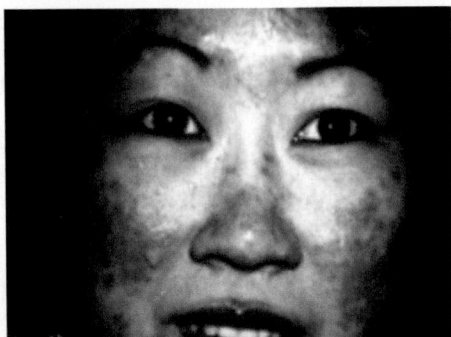

FIG. 64.10 Butterfly rash of SLE. (From Firestein GS, Budd RC, Gabriel SE, McInnes IB: *Kelley's textbook of rheumatology,* ed 9, Philadelphia, 2012, Saunders.)

cytotoxic agents (cyclophosphamide), and immunosuppressive agents (azathioprine, cyclosporine, mycophenolate mofetil [CellCept]). Oral prednisone or pulsed IV methylprednisolone may be used, especially in the initial treatment period when cytotoxic agents have not yet taken effect.

Nervous System Problems. Neuropsychiatric manifestations are common in SLE. About 15% of patients with SLE have generalized-onset or focal-onset seizures. Seizures are generally controlled by corticosteroids or antiseizure drugs. Peripheral neuropathy can occur, leading to sensory and motor deficits.

Cognitive problems may result from the deposit of immune complexes within the brain. There may be disordered thinking, disorientation, and memory deficits. Various psychiatric problems may occur, including depression, mood disorders, anxiety, and psychosis. However, they may be related to the stress of having a major illness or to associated drug therapies. Sometimes SLE may cause a stroke or aseptic meningitis. Headaches are common and can become severe during a disease flare.

Hematologic Problems. Blood problems are common due to formation of antibodies against blood cells. Anemia, leukopenia, thrombocytopenia, and coagulation disorders (excess bleeding or clotting) are often present.[27] Many patients benefit from high-intensity treatment with warfarin.

Infection. Patients with SLE appear to have increased susceptibility to infection. Risk may be due to impaired ability to eliminate invading bacteria, deficient antibody production, and immunosuppressive effects of many antiinflammatory drugs. Pneumonia is the most common infection. Fever may indicate an underlying infection rather than SLE activity alone. Vaccinations are generally safe for patients with SLE. Patients receiving corticosteroids or cytotoxic drugs must avoid live virus vaccines.

Diagnostic Studies

Diagnosis of SLE is based on distinct criteria (Table 64.15). No specific test is diagnostic for SLE, but a variety of abnormalities

TABLE 64.15 Diagnostic Criteria for Systemic Lupus Erythematosus

A person is classified as having SLE if 4 or more of the criteria are present, serially or simultaneously, during any interval of observation:

- Antinuclear antibody: abnormal titer
- Discoid rash: raised patches with scaling follicular plugging; scarring in older lesions
- Hematologic disorder: hemolytic anemia, leukopenia, lymphopenia, or thrombocytopenia
- Immunologic disorder: anti-DNA antibody or antibody to Sm (Smith) nuclear antigen or positive antiphospholipid antibodies
- Malar rash: fixed erythema, flat or raised (butterfly rash)
- Oral ulcers: usually painless
- Nonerosive arthritis: 2 or more peripheral joints with tenderness, swelling, effusion
- Pleuritis or pericarditis
- Neurologic disorder: seizures or psychosis (in the absence of causative drugs or known metabolic disorders)
- Photosensitivity: skin rash as unusual reaction to light
- Renal disorder: persistent proteinuria or cellular casts in urine

Source: American College of Rheumatology: 1997 Update of the 1982 American College of Rheumatology revised criteria for classification of systemic lupus erythematosus. Retrieved from *www.rheumatology.org/ Portals/0/Files/1997%20Update%20of%201982%20Revised.pdf.*

TABLE 64.16 Interprofessional Care
Systemic Lupus Erythematosus

Diagnostic Assessment

- History and physical examination
- Antibodies (e.g., ANA, anti-DNA, anti-Sm, antiphospholipid)
- CBC count
- Serum complement
- Urinalysis
- X-ray of affected joints
- Chest x-ray
- ECG to determine cardiac involvement

Management
Drug Therapy

- NSAIDs for mild disease
- Steroid-sparing drugs (e.g., methotrexate)
- Antimalarials (e.g., hydroxychloroquine [Plaquenil])
- Corticosteroids for flares and severe disease
- Immunosuppressive drugs (e.g., cyclophosphamide, mycophenolate mofetil [CellCept])

---

may be present in the blood. SLE is marked by the presence of ANA in 97% of persons with the disease.[28]

Anti-DNA antibodies are found in half the persons with SLE. Anti-Smith (Sm) antibodies are found in 30% to 40% of persons with SLE and are almost always considered diagnostic. Nearly 30% of people with SLE will have antiphospholipid antibodies. Antibodies to histone are most often seen in people with drug-induced SLE. Increased ESR and CRP indicate inflammation but are not diagnostic of SLE. They may be used to monitor disease activity and treatment effectiveness.[28]

Interprofessional Care

A major challenge in the treatment of SLE is managing active disease while preventing complications of treatment. Age, race, sex, socioeconomic status, co-morbid conditions, and disease severity influence survival. Prognosis can be improved with early diagnosis, ongoing assessment and prompt recognition of serious organ involvement, and effective treatment plans.

Drug Therapy. NSAIDs continue to be an important intervention, especially for patients with mild joint pain. Monitor the patient on long-term NSAID therapy for GI and renal effects.

Antimalarial agents, such as hydroxychloroquine and chloroquine, are often used to treat fatigue and skin and joint problems. They repress the immune system but do not cause immunosuppression. These drugs may reduce occurrence of flares. Patients taking hydroxychloroquine should have eye examinations by an ophthalmologist every 6 to 12 months. Retinopathy can develop with high doses of these drugs. It generally reverses when they are stopped. If the patient cannot tolerate an antimalarial agent, an antileprosy drug, such as dapsone, may be used.

Use of corticosteroids should be limited to the lowest dose for the shortest possible time. For example, steroids can be used for a few weeks until a slower acting medication becomes effective. Taper the patient's dose of steroid slowly rather than stopping the medication abruptly. High doses of corticosteroids may be especially appropriate for the patient with severe cutaneous SLE.

Immunosuppressive drugs, such as azathioprine and cyclophosphamide, may be used to suppress the immune system and reduce end-organ damage. Monitor closely to decrease the risk for drug toxicity and side effects. Because blood clots can be a life-threatening complication of SLE, anticoagulants, such as warfarin, may be prescribed. Belimumab (Benlysta) is a B-lymphocyte stimulator that inhibits the inflammation of SLE.

Topical immunomodulators can be used instead of corticosteroids to treat serious skin conditions. Tacrolimus (Protopic, Prograf) and pimecrolimus (Elidel) suppress immune activity in the skin, affecting the butterfly rash and discoid lesions.

Disease management is appropriately monitored by serial anti-DNA titers and serum complement (Table 64.16). Simpler, less costly tests, such as ESR or CRP, may be helpful.

❖ NURSING MANAGEMENT: SYSTEMIC LUPUS ERYTHEMATOSUS

◆ Nursing Assessment

Subjective and objective data to obtain from the patient with SLE are outlined in Table 64.17. In particular, assess the effect of pain and fatigue on ability to perform ADLs.

◆ Nursing Diagnoses

Nursing diagnoses for the patient with SLE may include:

- Fatigue
- Impaired tissue integrity
- Difficulty coping

Additional information on nursing diagnoses and interventions for the patient with SLE is presented in eNursing Care Plan 64.2 (available on the website for this chapter).

◆ Planning

Overall goals are that the patient with SLE will (1) have acceptable pain management, (2) show awareness of and avoid activities that worsen the disease, and (3) maintain optimal role function and positive self-image.

◆ Nursing Implementation

The unpredictable nature of SLE presents many challenges for the patient and caregiver. Physical, psychologic, and sociocultural

TABLE 64.17 Nursing Assessment

Systemic Lupus Erythematosus

Subjective Data

Important Health Information

Past health history: Exposure to ultraviolet light, drugs, chemicals, viral infections. Physical or psychologic stress. States of ↑ estrogen activity, including early onset of menses, pregnancy, and postpartum period. Pattern of remissions and flares

Medications: Oral contraceptives, procainamide, hydralazine, isoniazid, antiseizure drugs, antibiotics, corticosteroids, NSAIDs

Functional Health Patterns

Health perception–health management: Family history of autoimmune disorders, frequent infections, malaise, impact of disease on functional ability

Nutritional-metabolic: Weight loss, oral and nasal ulcers, nausea and vomiting, dry mouth *(xerostomia),* dysphagia, photosensitivity with rash, frequent infections

Elimination: ↓ Urine output, diarrhea or constipation

Activity-exercise: Morning stiffness, joint swelling and deformity, shortness of breath *(dyspnea),* excessive fatigue

Sleep-rest: Insomnia

Cognitive-perceptual: Vision problems, vertigo, headache, arthralgia, chest pain (pericardial, pleuritic), abdominal pain. Painful, throbbing, cold fingers with numbness and tingling

Sexuality-reproductive: Amenorrhea, irregular menstrual periods

Coping–stress tolerance: Depression, withdrawal

Objective Data

General

Fever, lymphadenopathy, periorbital edema

Integumentary

Alopecia. Dry, scaly scalp. Keratoconjunctivitis, butterfly rash, palmar or discoid erythema, hives (urticaria), erythema at fingernails or toenails, purpura, or petechiae. Leg ulcers

Respiratory

Pleural friction rub, ↓ breath sounds

Cardiovascular

Vasculitis, pericardial friction rub, hypertension, edema, dysrhythmias, murmurs. Bilateral, symmetric pallor and cyanosis of fingers (Raynaud's phenomenon)

Gastrointestinal

Oral and pharyngeal ulcers; splenomegaly

Neurologic

Facial weakness, peripheral neuropathies, papilledema, dysarthria, confusion, hallucination, disorientation, psychosis, seizures, aphasia, hemiparesis

Musculoskeletal

Myopathy, myositis, arthritis

Urinary

Proteinuria

Possible Diagnostic Findings

Presence of anti-DNA, anti-Sm, and antinuclear antibodies. Anemia, leukopenia, thrombocytopenia. ↑ ESR, ↑ serum creatinine. Microscopic hematuria, cellular casts in urine. Pericarditis or pleural effusion on chest x-ray

---

problems linked to long-term management require varied approaches and skills from the interprofessional team.

During a disease flare, the patient may quickly become very ill. Assess fever pattern, joint inflammation, limitation of motion, location and degree of discomfort, and fatigue. Monitor the patient's weight and fluid intake and output. This is especially important if corticosteroids are prescribed because of related fluid retention and possible renal failure. Collect 24-hour urine samples for protein and creatinine clearance as ordered. Observe for signs of bleeding due to drug therapy (e.g., pallor, skin bruising, petechiae, tarry stools).

Carefully assess neurologic function. Observe for vision problems, headaches, personality changes, seizures, and memory loss. Psychosis may result from CNS disease or be an effect of corticosteroid therapy. Nerve irritation of the extremities *(peripheral neuropathy)* may cause numbness, tingling, and weakness of the hands and feet.

Explain the nature of the disease, treatments, and all diagnostic procedures. When teaching patients about their prescribed drugs, include indications for use, proper administration, and side effects. Help patients understand that abruptly stopping a medication may worsen disease activity. Provide emotional support for the patient and caregiver, especially during a disease flare.

Emphasize the importance of patient involvement for successful home management. Help the patient understand that even strong adherence to the treatment plan is no guarantee against flares in this unpredictable disease. Several factors may increase disease activity, such as fatigue, sun exposure,

TABLE 64.18 Patient & Caregiver Teaching

Systemic Lupus Erythematosus

Include the following information in the teaching plan for a patient with SLE and the caregiver:

- Disease process
- Names of drugs, actions, side effects, dosage, administration
- Pain management strategies
- Energy conservation and pacing techniques
- Therapeutic exercise, heat therapy for arthralgia
- Relaxation therapy
- Avoid physical and emotional stress
- Avoid exposure to those with infection
- Avoid drying soaps, powders, household chemicals
- Use sunscreen protection (at least SPF 15) and protective clothing, with minimal sun exposure from 11:00 AM to 3:00 PM
- Regular medical and laboratory follow-up
- Marital and pregnancy counseling as needed
- Community resources and health care agencies

SPF, Sun protection factor.

emotional stress, infection, drugs, and surgery. Help the patient and caregiver eliminate or reduce exposure to such factors (Table 64.18).

SLE and Pregnancy. Because SLE is most common in women of childbearing age, treatment during pregnancy must be considered. The HCP and obstetrician should discuss with the woman her desire to become pregnant. Infertility may have resulted from renal involvement and use of high-dose corticosteroids and immunosuppressive drugs. The patient should understand spontaneous abortion, stillbirth, and intrauterine growth restriction are common problems. They occur because immune complexes are deposited in the placenta and inflammation occurs in placental blood vessels.

Renal, cardiovascular, lung, and central nervous systems may be affected during pregnancy. Women who already show serious effects in these systems should be counseled against pregnancy. For the best outcome, pregnancy should be planned when disease activity is minimal. Flares are common during the postpartum period. Therapeutic abortion offers the same risk for postdelivery exacerbation as carrying the fetus to term.

Psychosocial Issues. The patient with SLE may face many psychosocial issues. Disease onset and symptoms may be vague, and SLE may be undiagnosed for a long time. Supportive therapies may be as important as medical treatment in helping the patient cope with the disease. Tell the patient and caregiver that SLE has a good prognosis for most people.

Stress the importance of planning both recreational and work activities. The young adult may find sun restrictions and physical limitations hard to follow. Help the patient develop and achieve reasonable goals for improving or maintaining mobility, energy, and self-esteem.

Families worry about hereditary aspects and want to know if their children will have SLE. Many couples need pregnancy and sexual counseling. Those making decisions about marriage and careers worry how SLE will interfere with their plans. Teach employers, teachers, and co-workers as needed about the impact of SLE.

◆ Evaluation

The expected outcomes are that the patient with SLE will
- Use energy-conservation techniques
- Adapt lifestyle to current energy
- Maintain skin integrity with use of topical treatments
- Prevent disease flare with use of sunscreens and limited sun exposure

SCLERODERMA

Scleroderma *(systemic sclerosis)* is a disorder of connective tissue characterized by fibrotic, degenerative, and, sometimes, inflammatory changes in the skin, blood vessels, synovium, skeletal muscle, and internal organs.

Scleroderma occurs in all ethnic groups. It is more common in blacks, Native Americans, and persons of Japanese descent. Although symptoms may begin at any age, the usual age at onset is between 30 and 50 years. Scleroderma is relatively rare. Only about 300,000 Americans have the disease. Incidence in women is 4 times more common than in men.[3]

Two types of disease exist: *localized scleroderma,* which is the more common form, and *systemic scleroderma.* Skin changes of localized disease are usually limited to a few places on the skin or muscle without involvement of the trunk or internal organs. The prognosis of patients with limited disease is better than for those with systemic disease. Skin and connective tissue changes progress rapidly during the first months of systemic scleroderma, which is associated with internal organ involvement.[29]

Etiology and Pathophysiology

The exact cause of scleroderma is unknown. We think immunologic and vascular abnormalities play a role in the development of systemic disease. Risk factors include environmental or occupational exposure to coal, plastics, and silica dust.

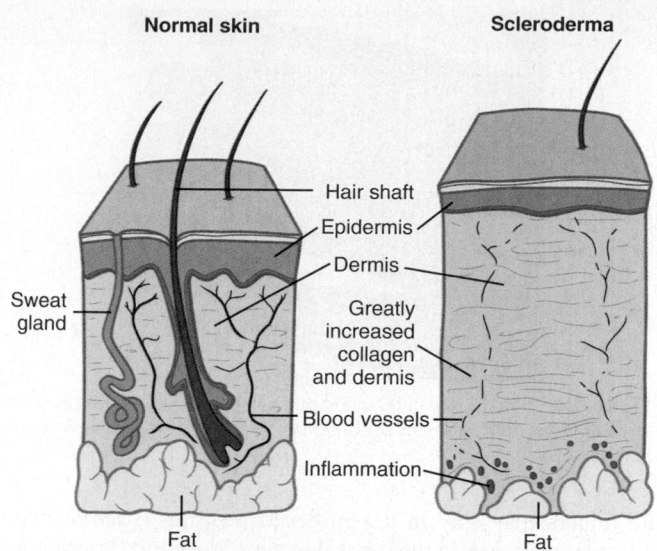

FIG. 64.11 Skin changes in scleroderma.

In scleroderma, the body makes too much collagen (protein that gives normal skin its strength and elasticity) (Fig. 64.11). This leads to progressive tissue fibrosis and occlusion of blood vessels. Collagen overproduction also disrupts normal function of internal organs, such as the lungs, kidney, heart, and GI tract.

Vascular problems, which mainly involve the small arteries and arterioles, are almost always present. These changes are some of the earliest changes in scleroderma.

Clinical Manifestations

Manifestations of scleroderma range from benign limited skin disease to diffuse skin thickening with rapidly progressive and widespread organ involvement. Localized disease is often marked by the **CREST syndrome**:

Calcinosis: painful deposits of calcium in skin of fingers, forearms, pressure points

Raynaud's phenomenon: intermittent vasospasm of fingertips in response to cold or stress

Esophageal dysfunction: difficulty swallowing due to internal scarring

Sclerodactyly: tightening of skin on fingers and toes

Telangiectasia: red spots on hands, forearms, palms, face, and lips from capillary dilation

Raynaud's Phenomenon. **Raynaud's phenomenon** (sudden vasospasm of the digits) is the most common first complaint in localized scleroderma. Patients have decreased blood flow to the fingers and toes when exposed to cold *(blanching or white phase)*. This is followed by cyanosis as hemoglobin releases O_2 to the tissues *(blue phase)*, then erythema during rewarming *(red phase)*. Numbness and tingling often occur. Raynaud's phenomenon may precede the onset of systemic disease by months, years, or even decades. Raynaud's phenomenon is described in detail in Chapter 37.

Skin and Joint Changes. Symmetric painless swelling or thickening of the skin of the fingers and hands may progress to diffuse scleroderma of the trunk. In localized disease, skin thickening generally does not extend above the elbow or knee, although the face may be affected. In diffuse disease, the skin loses elasticity and becomes taut and shiny. This causes the typical expressionless face with tightly pursed lips. Skin changes in the face may contribute to reduced ROM in the temporomandibular joint.

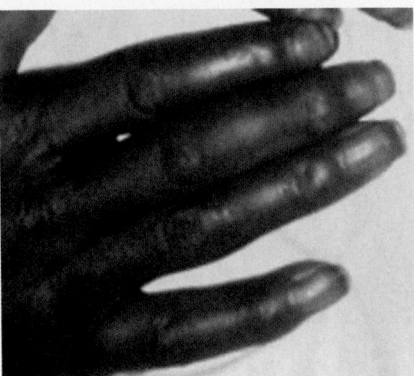

FIG. 64.12 Sclerodactyly in the hand of a patient with scleroderma. (From Zitelli BJ, Davis HW: *Atlas of pediatric physical diagnosis*, ed 4, St Louis, 2002, Mosby.)

The fingers may stay in a semiflexed position *(sclerodactyly)*, with tightened skin to the wrist (Fig. 64.12). Reduced peripheral joint function may be an early symptom of arthritis.

Internal Organ Involvement. About 20% of people with systemic scleroderma and a few with localized disease develop secondary Sjögren's syndrome, a condition associated with dry eyes and dry mouth. Dysphagia, gum disease, and dental decay can result. Frequent reflux of gastric acid can occur due to esophageal fibrosis. If swallowing becomes difficult, the patient is likely to decrease food intake and lose weight. GI effects include constipation from colonic hypomotility and diarrhea due to malabsorption from bacterial overgrowth.

Lung problems include pleural thickening, pulmonary fibrosis, and abnormal pulmonary function. The patient develops a cough and dyspnea. Pulmonary arterial hypertension and interstitial lung disease may occur. Lung disease is the main cause of death in scleroderma.

Heart disease includes pericarditis, pericardial effusion, and dysrhythmias. Heart failure from myocardial fibrosis occurs most often in patients with systemic disease.

Renal disease was a major cause of death in systemic scleroderma. Because malignant hypertension associated with rapidly progressive, irreversible renal insufficiency can occur, early recognition of renal involvement and initiation of therapy are critical. Recent improvements in dialysis, bilateral nephrectomy in patients with uncontrollable hypertension, and kidney transplant have offered hope to patients with renal failure. Use of angiotensin-converting enzyme (ACE) inhibitors (e.g., lisinopril [Prinivil]) has had a marked effect on the ability to treat renal disease.

Diagnostic Studies

Laboratory results in scleroderma are relatively normal. Blood studies may show mild hemolytic anemia from RBC damage in diseased small vessels. Anticentromere antibodies related to CREST syndrome are found in about 45% to 50% of people with localized scleroderma. They are rare in people with systemic disease. Antibodies to topoisomerase-1 are present in about 30% of people with diffuse disease.[30] Presence of either antibody is highly specific for diagnosis. If renal involvement is present, urinalysis may show proteinuria, microscopic hematuria, and casts. Serum creatinine may be increased. X-ray evidence of subcutaneous calcification, distal esophageal hypomotility, or bibasilar pulmonary fibrosis is diagnostic of scleroderma. Pulmonary function studies show decreased vital capacity and lung compliance.

TABLE 64.19 Interprofessional Care

Scleroderma

Diagnostic Assessment
- History and physical examination
- Antibodies to topoisomerase-1
- Anticentromere antibody
- Nail bed capillary microscopy
- Chest x-ray
- Skin or organ biopsy
- Urinalysis (proteinuria, hematuria, casts)
- Pulmonary function tests
- ECG

Management
- Physical therapy
- Occupational therapy

Drug Therapy
- Vasoactive agents: reserpine, bosentan, epoprostenol
- Calcium channel blockers: diltiazem, nifedipine
- ACE inhibitors: lisinopril (Prinivil)
- Immunosuppressive drugs: cyclophosphamide, mycophenolate mofetil (CellCept)

Interprofessional Care

There is no specific treatment (Table 64.19). Supportive care is directed toward preventing or treating secondary complications of involved organs. PT helps to maintain joint mobility and preserve muscle strength. Occupational therapy assists the patient in maintaining functional abilities.

Drug Therapy. Vasoactive agents are often prescribed in early disease. Calcium channel blockers (nifedipine [Procardia], diltiazem [Cardizem]) and the angiotensin II blocker losartan are common treatments for Raynaud's phenomenon. Reserpine, an α-adrenergic blocking agent, increases blood flow to the fingers. Bosentan (Tracleer), an endothelin-receptor antagonist, and the vasodilator epoprostenol (Flolan) may improve blood flow to the lung.[31]

NSAIDs and topical agents may give some relief from joint pain. Capsaicin cream may be useful, not only as a local analgesic but also as a vasodilator. Other therapies prescribed to treat specific systemic problems include (1) tetracycline for diarrhea caused by bacterial overgrowth, (2) histamine (H_2) receptor blockers (e.g., cimetidine) and proton pump inhibitors (e.g., omeprazole) for esophageal symptoms, and (3) antihypertensive agent (e.g., captopril, propranolol, methyldopa) for hypertension with renal involvement. Immunosuppressive drugs (e.g., cyclophosphamide, mycophenolate mofetil) are used in severe cases.

❖ NURSING MANAGEMENT: SCLERODERMA

Nursing interventions often begin during hospitalization for diagnosis. Assess vital signs, weight, intake and output, respiratory and bowel function, and joint ROM regularly to plan appropriate care. Emotional stress and cold ambient temperatures may aggravate Raynaud's phenomenon. Teach patients with scleroderma to avoid finger-stick blood testing because of compromised circulation and poor healing.

Teaching is an important nursing intervention throughout the disease. Obvious changes in the face and hands often lead to poor self-image and loss of mobility and function. Teach the patient to regularly take part in therapeutic exercises at home to prevent skin retraction and promote vascularization. Mouth excursion (yawning with an open mouth) is a good exercise to help with temporomandibular joint function. Isometric exercises are best if the patient has arthropathy because no joint movement occurs. Encourage the use of moist heat applications or paraffin baths to promote skin flexibility in the hands and feet. Teach the patient to use assistive devices as needed and organize activities to preserve strength and reduce disability.

Teach the patient to protect the hands and feet from cold exposure. Protect against burns or cuts that may heal slowly. Encourage the patient to avoid smoking because of its vasoconstricting effect. Report signs of infection promptly. Use alcohol-free lotions to improve skin dryness and cracking. They must be rubbed in for a long time to be absorbed through the thick skin.

Remind the patient to reduce dysphagia by eating small, frequent meals, chewing carefully and slowly, and drinking fluids. A consultation with a dietitian is helpful. Decrease risk for heartburn by using antacids 45 to 60 minutes after each meal and sitting upright for at least 2 hours after eating. Using extra pillows or raising the head of the bed on blocks may reduce gastroesophageal reflux during the night.

Job alterations are often needed due to problems with climbing stairs, using a computer, writing, and being exposed to cold. The patient may be socially withdrawn as skin tightening changes the appearance of the face and hands. Dining out may become socially embarrassing because of the patient's small mouth, swallowing difficulty, and reflux. Some persons with scleroderma wear gloves to protect fingertip ulcers and provide extra warmth. Emphasize daily oral hygiene to avoid increased tooth and gum problems. The patient needs a dentist who is familiar with scleroderma and able to adapt care to a small mouth.

Psychologic support, biofeedback training, and relaxation can reduce stress and improve sleeping habits. Sexual problems from body changes, pain, muscular weakness, limited mobility, decreased self-esteem, erectile dysfunction, and decreased vaginal secretions may require sensitive counseling.

CHECK YOUR PRACTICE

A 34-yr-old woman hospitalized for aspiration pneumonia has a 5-year history of scleroderma.
- How could scleroderma have contributed to the aspiration pneumonia?
- What strategies will you suggest to decrease the risk for pneumonia recurrence?
- What other self-care strategies will you reinforce with this patient?

POLYMYOSITIS AND DERMATOMYOSITIS

Polymyositis (PM) is diffuse, idiopathic, inflammatory myopathy of striated muscle. It causes bilateral weakness, usually most severe in the proximal or limb girdle muscles. When muscle changes associated with PM are accompanied by distinctive skin changes, the disorder is called dermatomyositis (DM).

These relatively rare disorders can be similar in signs, symptoms, and treatment, but they are 2 distinct diseases. They typically affect adults age 20 years and older. They rarely occur in

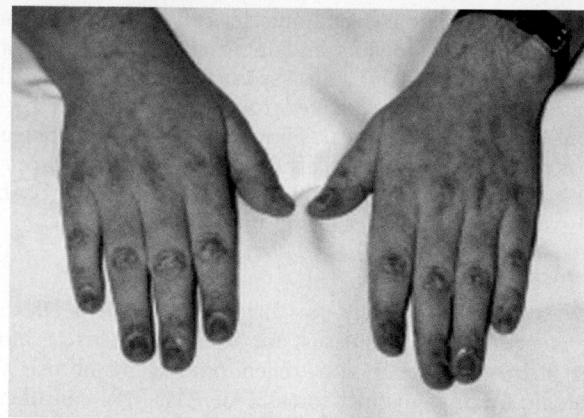

FIG. 64.13 Dermatomyositis skin changes indicating Gottron's papules. (From Firestein GS, Budd RC, Gabriel SE, McInnes IB: *Kelley's textbook of rheumatology*, ed 9, Philadelphia, 2012, Saunders.)

people under age 18 years. PM and DM occur twice as often in women as in men. Patients with PM generally have more severe disease than those with DM.

Etiology and Pathophysiology

The exact cause of PM and DM is unknown. Evidence suggests an autoimmune origin with T cell–mediated destruction of unidentified muscle antigens. Environmental factors are likely, including viral and bacterial infection, certain drugs, supplements, vaccines, medical implants, and occupational exposure.

Clinical Manifestations and Complications

Muscular. The patient with PM and DM has weight loss and increasing fatigue, with gradually developing muscle weakness that causes difficulty in performing ADLs. The most commonly affected muscles are in the shoulders, legs, arms, and pelvic girdle. The patient may have difficulty rising from a chair or bathtub, climbing stairs, combing hair, or reaching into a high cupboard. Repetitive movements are more likely to cause trouble than a single strength exercise. The patient may be unable to raise the head from a pillow as neck muscles weaken. Muscle discomfort or tenderness is uncommon. Muscle examination shows an inability to move against resistance or even gravity. Weak pharyngeal muscles may cause dysphagia and dysphonia (nasal or hoarse voice).

Dermal. Rashes are typical with DM. They usually prompt earlier recognition of DM than PM, which has no rashes. Skin changes of DM include a classic red or purple symmetric rash (*heliotrope*) with edema around the eyelids. The typical skin rash is not often found with other disorders. A scaly, smooth, or raised rash may be seen on the knuckles and sides of the hands (*Gottron's papules*) (Fig. 64.13). Reddened, smooth, or scaly patches appear with the same symmetric distribution but sparing the interphalangeal spaces (*Gottron's sign*). The rash can be confused with psoriasis or seborrheic dermatitis. A red, scaling rash (*poikiloderma*) may develop as a late finding on the back, buttocks, and a V-shaped area of the anterior neck and chest.

Hyperemia and telangiectasia are often present at the nail beds. Calcium nodules (*calcinosis cutis*) can develop throughout the skin and are especially common in long-standing DM.

Other Manifestations. Joint redness, pain, and inflammation often occur. They contribute to limited joint ROM in PM and DM. Contractures and muscle atrophy may occur with advanced disease. Weakened pharyngeal muscles can lead to poor cough effort, difficulty swallowing, and increased risk for aspiration pneumonia. Interstitial lung disease is a common complication. All patients should be evaluated routinely with a chest x-ray and pulmonary function tests. People with DM have increased risk for cancer and should receive age- and gender-appropriate screenings. PM and DM may be associated with other connective tissue disorders (e.g., scleroderma).

Diagnostic Studies

Biopsy is the gold standard for diagnosis of PM or DM after other neuromuscular diseases are excluded. Muscle biopsy shows necrosis, degeneration, regeneration, and fibrosis with pathologic findings distinct for DM or PM. MRI can identify areas of inflammation and guide the biopsy site selection.[32] Laboratory tests are helpful, but not diagnostic of either disease. Increased muscle enzymes (e.g., creatine kinase, myoglobin) reflect muscle damage but will decrease to normal or near normal with treatment. An EMG suggestive of PM shows bizarre high-frequency discharges and spontaneous fibrillation, with positive spikes at rest. Increased ESR or CRP occurs with active disease.

❖ Interprofessional and Nursing Care

PM and DM are treated initially with high-dose oral corticosteroids, with the dose tapered based on patient response. Most patients respond well to treatment. Long-term corticosteroid therapy may be needed because relapses are common when the drug is withdrawn.

Immunosuppressive drugs (methotrexate, azathioprine, tacrolimus, cyclophosphamide) may be used in combination with steroids or as a second-line therapy if the patient does not respond to steroids. IV immunoglobulin (IVIG) may be given with corticosteroids or immunosuppressants, but it is not a first-line treatment.

 DRUG ALERT IV Immunoglobulin (IVIG)

- Give by slow infusion to decrease risk for thromboembolic complications.
- Hydrate patient well during infusion to decrease risk for renal failure.
- Treat transient adverse effects, such as headache.

Injection of synthetic ACTH (repository corticotropin injection [Acthar]) helps with muscle spasms. The exact mechanism of action is unknown. Limited data are available on its effectiveness.[32]

PT can be helpful and is tailored to disease activity. Use massage and passive movement during active disease. Delay more aggressive exercises until disease activity is minimal based on low serum muscle enzymes.

Teach the patient about the disease, prescribed therapies, diagnostic tests, and the need for regular medical care. Help the patient understand that the benefits of therapy are often delayed. For example, weakness may increase during the first few weeks of corticosteroid therapy. Encourage the use of assistive devices to decrease risk for falls. To prevent aspiration, encourage the patient to rest before meals, maintain an upright position when eating, and choose easily swallowed foods.

Help the patient to organize activities and use pacing techniques to conserve energy. Encourage daily ROM exercises to prevent contractures. When inflammation is decreased, start muscle-strengthening (repetitive) exercises. Home care and bed rest may be needed during acute PM, when the patient may not be able to complete ADLs because of profound muscle weakness.

MIXED CONNECTIVE TISSUE DISEASE

Patients having a combination of clinical features of several rheumatic diseases are described as having *mixed connective tissue disease*. The term describes a disorder with features primarily of SLE, scleroderma, and PM. This disease occurs most often in women in their 20s and 30s.

About 25% of persons with a connective tissue disease develop another related disease over the course of several years, which is known as *overlap syndrome*.[33]

SJÖGREN'S SYNDROME

Sjögren's syndrome is a relatively common autoimmune disease that targets the moisture-producing exocrine glands. This leads to *xerostomia* (dry mouth) and *keratoconjunctivitis sicca* (dry eyes).[34] The nose, throat, airways, and skin can become dry. The disease may affect other glands, including those in the stomach, pancreas, and intestines (extraglandular involvement). The disease is usually diagnosed in people over age 40 but can be found in all age-groups. Women are 10 times more likely than men to have Sjögren's syndrome.

In primary Sjögren's syndrome, problems occur with lacrimal and salivary glands. However, up to 40% of patients have extended disease affecting the lungs, liver, kidneys, and skin. This occurrence increases the risk for non-Hodgkin's lymphoma.[34]

Sjögren's syndrome appears to be caused by genetic and environmental factors. A particular gene predisposes whites to the disease. Other genes are linked to the disease in people of Japanese, Chinese, and African-American ethnicity. The trigger may be a viral or bacterial infection that adversely stimulates the immune system. In Sjögren's syndrome, lymphocytes attack and damage the lacrimal and salivary glands.

Decreased tearing causes dry eyes, which leads to a gritty sensation in the eyes, burning, blurred vision, and photosensitivity. Dry mouth causes buccal membrane fissures, changes in taste, dysphagia, and increased mouth infection or dental decay. Dry skin and rashes, joint and muscle pain, and thyroid problems may be present. Other exocrine glands can be affected. For example, vaginal dryness may lead to painful intercourse (*dyspareunia*).

Autoimmune thyroid disorders, including Graves' disease and Hashimoto's thyroiditis, are common with Sjögren's syndrome. Histologic study shows lymphocyte infiltration of salivary and lacrimal glands. The disease may become more generalized and involve the lymph nodes, bone marrow, and visceral organs (pseudolymphoma).

Ophthalmologic examination (Schirmer's test for tear production), measures of salivary gland function, and lower lip biopsy of minor salivary glands aid in diagnosis. Treatment is symptomatic, including (1) instillation of preservative-free artificial tears or ophthalmic antiinflammatory drops (e.g., cyclosporine [Restasis]) as needed for adequate hydration and lubrication, (2) surgical punctal occlusion, and (3) increased fluids with meals. Dental hygiene is important.

Pilocarpine (Salagen) and cevimeline (Evoxac) can ease the dry mouth. Increased humidity at home may reduce respiratory tract infections. Vaginal lubrication with a water-soluble product, such as K-Y Jelly, may increase comfort during intercourse.

> ⚠️ **SAFETY ALERT** Sjögren's Syndrome
> To help with chewing and swallowing:
> • Moisten food with mayonnaise, sauces, gravy, or yogurt.
> • Thin foods with skim milk or broth.
> • Use a food processor or blender to finely chop or liquefy foods.
> • Try soft, creamy foods (e.g., mashed potatoes, macaroni and cheese).
> • Drink high-calorie cold liquids (e.g., breakfast drinks).
> • Avoid salty, acidic, or spicy foods.

MYOFASCIAL PAIN SYNDROME

Myofascial pain syndrome is a chronic form of muscle pain and tenderness, typically in the chest, neck, shoulders, hips, and lower back. Referred pain from these muscle groups can travel to the buttocks, hands, and head, causing severe headaches. Temporomandibular joint pain may originate in myofascial pain. Regions of pain are often within the connective tissue *(fascia)* that covers skeletal muscles. Trigger or tender points are thought to activate a characteristic pattern of pain that worsens with activity or stress.

Myofascial pain syndrome occurs more often in middle-aged adults and in women. Patients report deep, aching pain with a sensation of burning, stinging, and stiffness.

A typical PT treatment is the "spray and stretch" method. The painful area is iced or sprayed with a coolant, such as ethyl chloride and then stretched. Positive results have been seen with topical patches and injection of the trigger points with a local anesthetic (e.g., 1% lidocaine). Massage, dry needling, and ultrasound therapy have helped some patients.[35]

FIBROMYALGIA

Fibromyalgia is a chronic central pain syndrome marked by widespread, nonarticular musculoskeletal pain and fatigue with multiple tender points. Fibromyalgia is a common musculoskeletal disorder and a major cause of disability. It affects more than 3.7 million Americans. Most are women ages 40 to 75 years.[36] Fibromyalgia and systemic exertion intolerance disease (SEID) (formerly called chronic fatigue syndrome) share many common features (Table 64.20).

Etiology and Pathophysiology

Fibromyalgia involves abnormal central processing of nociceptive pain input. The increased pain is due to abnormal sensory processing in the CNS. Multiple physiologic abnormalities have been found. They include (1) increased levels of substance P in the spinal fluid, (2) low blood flow to the thalamus, (3) dysfunction of the hypothalamic-pituitary-adrenal (HPA) axis, (4) low serotonin and tryptophan, and (5) abnormal cytokine function. Serotonin and substance P play a role in mood regulation, sleep, and pain perception. Changes in the HPA axis can negatively affect a person's physical and mental health. An increased incidence of depression and decreased response to stress occur. Genetic factors contribute to the development of fibromyalgia, as a familial tendency exists. Recent illness or trauma may be a trigger in susceptible people.

TABLE 64.20 Common Features of Fibromyalgia and Systemic Exertion Intolerance Disease (SEID)

Occurrence
Previously healthy, young and middle-aged women

Etiology (Theories)
Infectious trigger, dysfunction in HPA axis, CNS problem

Clinical Manifestations
Generalized musculoskeletal pain, malaise and fatigue, cognitive problems, headaches, sleep problems, depression, anxiety, fever

Disease Course
Variable intensity of symptoms, fluctuates over time

Diagnosis
No definitive laboratory tests or joint and muscle examinations
Mainly a diagnosis of exclusion

Management
Symptomatic treatment may include antidepressant drugs, such as amitriptyline and fluoxetine (Prozac).
Nondrug measures include heat, massage, regular stretching, biofeedback, stress management, and relaxation training

HPA, Hypothalamic-pituitary-adrenal.

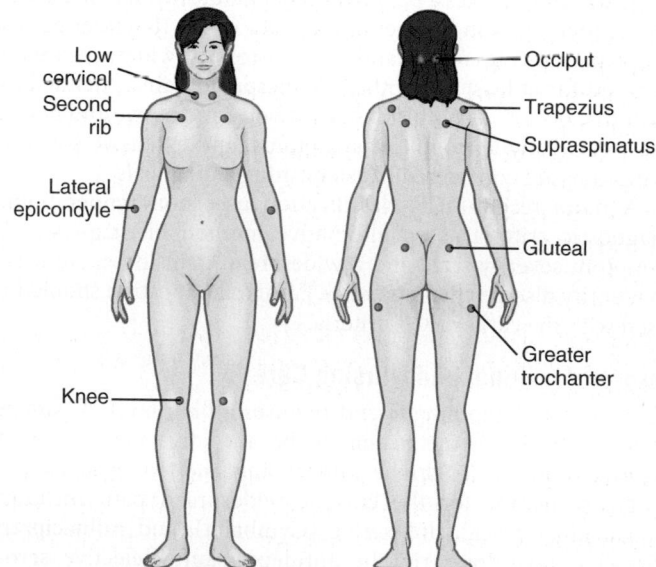

FIG. 64.14 Tender points in fibromyalgia.

Clinical Manifestations and Complications

The patient reports widespread burning pain that fluctuates through the course of a day. The patient often cannot determine if pain occurs in the muscles, joints, or soft tissues. Head or facial pain often results from stiff or painful neck and shoulder muscles. The pain can accompany temporomandibular joint dysfunction, which affects about one third of patients with fibromyalgia.

Physical examination typically shows point tenderness at 11 or more of 18 identified sites (Fig. 64.14). Patients with fibromyalgia are sensitive to painful stimuli throughout the body, not just at the identified tender sites. They may have pain in response to a stimulus that does not typically cause pain *(allodynia)*. Point tenderness can vary from day to day. Sometimes, the patient may respond to fewer than 11 tender points. At other times, palpation of all sites may cause pain.

Cognitive effects range from difficulty concentrating to memory lapses and a feeling of being overwhelmed when dealing with multiple tasks. Many report migraine headaches. Depression and anxiety often occur and may require drug therapy. Stiffness, nonrefreshing sleep, fatigue, and numbness or tingling in the hands or feet often accompany fibromyalgia. Restless legs syndrome is typical. Some describe an irresistible urge to move the legs when at rest or lying down.

Irritable bowel syndrome with constipation and/or diarrhea, abdominal pain, and bloating is common. Patients may have difficulty swallowing, perhaps because of problems in esophageal smooth muscle function. Increased frequency of urination and urinary urgency, in the absence of a bladder infection, may occur. Women with fibromyalgia may have more difficult menstruation, with disease symptoms worse during this time.

Diagnostic Studies

A definitive diagnosis of fibromyalgia is often hard to establish. Lack of knowledge about the disease and its manifestations among HCPs may cause delays in diagnosis and treatment.

Laboratory results in most cases help rule out other suspected disorders. Muscle biopsy may show a nonspecific moth-eaten appearance or fiber atrophy.

The ACR classifies a person as having fibromyalgia if 2 criteria are met: (1) pain is experienced in 11 of the 18 tender points on palpation (Fig. 64.14) and (2) a history of widespread pain is noted for at least 3 months.[37] Widespread pain is defined as pain that occurs on both sides of the body and above and below the waist. Fatigue, cognitive symptoms, and extensive somatic symptoms are considered in establishing a diagnosis.

A more recent ACR classification uses non–tender point diagnostic criteria as an alternative method of diagnosis. A symptom severity scale and a widespread pain index are used to identify disease characteristics.[38] This classification should be used with the earlier ACR criteria.

❖ Interprofessional and Nursing Care

Treatment is symptomatic and requires a high level of patient motivation. Teach the patient to be an active participant in treatment. Rest can help the pain, aching, and tenderness.

Drug therapy for the chronic widespread pain includes pregabalin (Lyrica), duloxetine (Cymbalta), and milnacipran (Savella). Low-dose tricyclic antidepressants, selective serotonin reuptake inhibitors (SSRIs), or benzodiazepines (e.g., diazepam) may be prescribed. SSRI antidepressants (e.g., sertraline [Zoloft], paroxetine [Paxil]) tend to be reserved for patients who also have depression. SSRIs may have to be prescribed at higher doses than when used to treat depression. Antidepressants and muscle relaxants (e.g., baclofen) have sedative effects that can improve nighttime rest for the patient with fibromyalgia.

Long-acting opioids are not recommended unless other therapies are not successful. In some patients, pain may be managed with OTC analgesics, such as acetaminophen, ibuprofen, or naproxen (Aleve). Nonopioids, such as tramadol (Ultram), may be used. Zolpidem (Ambien) or trazodone is sometimes given for short-term intervention in patients with severe sleep problems.

Because of the chronic nature of fibromyalgia, the patient needs consistent support from interprofessional team members. Massage is often combined with ultrasound or use of alternating heat and cold packs to soothe tense, sore muscles and increase blood circulation. Gentle stretching to relieve muscle tension and spasm can be done by a physical therapist or practiced by the patient at home. Yoga and Tai Chi are often helpful. Low-impact aerobic exercise, such as walking, can help prevent muscle atrophy.

Patients may consider limiting intake of sugar, caffeine, and alcohol because they may be muscle irritants. Vitamin and mineral supplements may help combat stress, correct deficiencies, and support the immune system. However, unproven miracle diets or supplements should be carefully investigated by the patient and discussed with the HCP before using them. Teach the patient that some foods and supplements can cause serious or even dangerous side effects when mixed with certain drugs.

Pain and the related symptoms of fibromyalgia can cause significant stress. Patients with fibromyalgia may not cope well with stress. Effective relaxation strategies include biofeedback, imagery, meditation, and cognitive-behavioral therapy. Patients need initial training for these interventions, but they can continue to practice in their own homes. (Stress management is discussed in Chapter 6.) Psychologic counseling (individual or group) and a support group may be helpful.

SYSTEMIC EXERTION INTOLERANCE DISEASE (SEID)

Systemic exertion intolerance disease (SEID), formerly called *chronic fatigue syndrome,* is a serious, complex, multisystem disease in which exertion of any sort (physical, emotional, cognitive) is impaired and accompanied by profound fatigue.[39] SEID is a poorly understood condition that can have a devastating impact on the lives of patients and their families.

SEID affects at least 1 million people in the United States. The condition is 3 to 4 times more common in women than men. SEID occurs in all ethnic and socioeconomic groups, but the illness is more common in minorities and socioeconomically disadvantaged groups. The true prevalence of SEID is unknown because many people with the disease have not been diagnosed.[39]

Etiology and Pathophysiology

Despite efforts to determine the cause and pathology of SEID, we do not know the cause. Many theories exist about the cause of SEID. Neuroendocrine abnormalities have been implicated involving a hypofunction of the HPA axis and hypothalamic-pituitary-gonadal (HPG) axis, which together regulate the stress response and reproductive hormone levels. Several microorganisms have been investigated as causative agents, including herpes viruses (e.g., Epstein-Barr virus [EBV], cytomegalovirus [CMV]), retroviruses, enteroviruses, *Candida albicans,* and mycoplasma. Because many patients have cognitive deficits (e.g., decreased memory, attention, concentration), changes in the CNS have been suggested as the cause of SEID.

Clinical Manifestations

Diagnosis of SEID requires that the patient have the following 3 symptoms

1. Impaired function with profound fatigue lasting at least 6 months

2. Malaise after exertion: total exhaustion after even minor physical or mental exertion that the patient sometimes describes as a "crash"
3. Unrefreshing sleep

At least 1 of the following manifestations is also required:

1. Cognitive impairment ("brain fog," confusion)
2. *Orthostatic intolerance* (lightheadedness, dizziness, imbalance, fainting)

Severe fatigue is the most common symptom and the problem that causes the patient to seek health care.

SEID is often hard to distinguish from fibromyalgia because many clinical features are similar (Table 64.20). In about half the cases, SEID develops slowly, or the patient may have periodic episodes that gradually become chronic. SEID can arise suddenly in a previously active, healthy person. An unremarkable flu-like illness or other acute stress is often identified as a trigger. Associated symptoms may vary in intensity over time.

The patient may become angry and frustrated with HCPs who cannot diagnose a problem. The disorder may have a major impact on work and family responsibilities. Some people may need help with ADLs.

Diagnostic Studies

Physical examination and diagnostic studies can be used to rule out other possible causes of the patient's symptoms. No laboratory test can diagnose SEID or measure its severity. SEID is a diagnosis of exclusion.

❖ Interprofessional and Nursing Care

Because no definitive treatment exists for SEID, supportive management is essential. Tell the patient what we know about the disease.

NSAIDs can be used to treat headaches, muscle and joint aches, and fever. Because many patients with SEID have allergies and sinusitis, antihistamines and decongestants can be used to treat allergic symptoms. Tricyclic antidepressants (e.g., doxepin, amitriptyline) and SSRIs (e.g., fluoxetine, paroxetine) can improve mood and sleep. Clonazepam (Klonopin) can be used to treat sleep problems and panic disorders. Use of low-dose hydrocortisone to decrease fatigue and disability is being studied.

Teach the patient to avoid total rest because it can create a self-image of the patient as an invalid. On the other hand, strenuous exertion can worsen the exhaustion. Urge the patient to plan a carefully graduated exercise program. Encourage a well-balanced diet, including fiber and fresh dark-colored fruits and vegetables for antioxidant action. Behavioral therapy may be used to promote a positive outlook and improve overall disability and fatigue.

One major problem facing many patients is loss of livelihood and economic security. When the illness strikes, they cannot work or must decrease the amount of work. Loss of a job often leads to loss of medical insurance. Obtaining disability benefits can be frustrating because of the difficulty of establishing a definitive diagnosis of SEID. Patients with SEID may have severe psychosocial losses, including social pressure and isolation from being labelled as lazy or crazy.

SEID does not appear to progress. Although most patients recover or at least gradually improve, some do not show substantial improvement. Recovery is more common in persons with a sudden onset of SEID.

CASE STUDY

Rheumatoid Arthritis

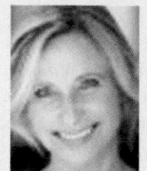

Patient Profile

K.R., a 42-yr-old married white woman, comes to the rheumatology clinic with tenderness and pain in the small joints of her hands.

Subjective Data

- Reports tenderness, joint pain, and stiffness in her hands for the last 3 mo
- Having fatigue, anorexia, and morning stiffness
- Mother diagnosed with ankylosing spondylitis 8 yr ago
- Expresses doubt about her ability to manage the disease

(© iStockphoto/Thinkstock.)

Objective Data

Physical Examination

- Swelling, warmth, and tenderness of third and fourth metacarpophalangeal joints of both hands
- Mild pain with neck motion
- Tenosynovitis

Diagnostic Studies

- Positive ESR, RF, and anti-CCP
- Mild bone demineralization present bilaterally in hand x-rays

Interprofessional Care

- Diagnosed with RA
- Started on methotrexate 7.5 mg PO once per week, etanercept (Enbrel) 50 mg subcutaneously once per week, prednisone 10 mg/day

Discussion Questions

1. How will you explain the pathophysiology of RA to K.R.?
2. K.R. asks you if genetic factors are related to a diagnosis of RA. How will you respond?
3. *Safety:* What are some home and work modifications you can suggest to K.R. to reduce her symptoms?
4. *Patient-Centered Care:* What suggestions can you make to K.R. about coping with fatigue?
5. *Collaboration:* What referrals may be needed for K.R.?
6. *Priority Decision:* Based on the assessment data presented, what are the priority nursing diagnoses?
7. *Quality Improvement*: What outcomes would indicate interprofessional care was effective?
8. *Evidence-Based Practice:* Why is an exercise program important in the treatment plan for K.R.?
9. Develop a conceptual care map for K.R.

Answers and a corresponding conceptual care map are available at *http://evolve.elsevier.com/Lewis/medsurg.*

BRIDGE TO NCLEX EXAMINATION

The number of the question corresponds to the same-numbered outcome at the beginning of the chapter.

1. In assessing the joints of a patient with osteoarthritis, the nurse understands that Bouchard's nodes
   a. are often red, swollen, and tender.
   b. indicate osteophyte formation at the PIP joints.
   c. are the result of pannus formation at the DIP joints.
   d. occur from deterioration of cartilage by proteolytic enzymes.

2. A patient with rheumatoid arthritis has articular involvement. The nurse recognizes these characteristic changes include (select all that apply)
   a. bamboo-shaped fingers.
   b. metatarsal head dislocation in feet.
   c. noninflammatory pain in large joints.
   d. asymmetric involvement of small joints.
   e. morning stiffness lasting 60 minutes or more.

3. When administering medications to the patient with chronic gout, the nurse recognizes which drug is used as a treatment for this disease?
   a. Colchicine
   b. Allopurinol
   c. Sulfasalazine
   d. Cyclosporine

4. The nurse should teach the patient with ankylosing spondylitis the importance of
   a. avoiding extremes in environmental temperatures
   b. regularly exercising and maintaining proper posture.
   c. maintaining patient's usual physical activity during flares.
   d. applying hot and cool compresses for relief of local symptoms.

5. In teaching a patient with systemic lupus erythematosus about the disorder, the nurse knows the pathophysiology includes
   a. circulating immune complexes formed from IgG autoantibodies reacting with IgG.
   b. an autoimmune T-cell reaction that results in destruction of the deep dermal skin layer.
   c. immunologic dysfunction leading to chronic inflammation in the cartilage and muscles.
   d. the production of a variety of autoantibodies directed against components of the cell nucleus.

6. In teaching a patient with Sjögren's syndrome about drug therapy for this disorder, the nurse includes instruction about the use of which drug?
   a. Pregabalin (Lyrica)
   b. Etanercept (Enbrel)
   c. Cyclosporine (Restasis)
   d. Cyclobenzaprine (Flexeril)

7. Teach the patient with fibromyalgia the importance of limiting intake of which foods? (select all that apply)
   a. Sugar
   b. Alcohol
   c. Caffeine
   d. Red meat
   e. Root vegetables

ɔ ʻq ʻɐ ʻ∠ ʻɔ ʻ9 ʻp ʻ5 ʻq ʻ4 ʻq ʻ3 ʻǝ ʻq ʻ2 ʻq ʻ1

For rationales to these answers and even more NCLEX review questions, visit *http://evolve.elsevier.com/Lewis/medsurg*.

ⓔ EVOLVE WEBSITE/RESOURCES LIST

http://evolve.elsevier.com/Lewis/medsurg
Review Questions (Online Only)
Key Points
Answer Keys for Questions
- Rationales for Bridge to NCLEX Examination Questions
- Answer Guidelines for Case Study on p. 1529
- Answer Guidelines for Managing Care of Multiple Patients Case Study (Section 12) on p. 1532
Students Case Studies
- Patient With Obesity and Osteoarthritis
- Patient With Rheumatoid Arthritis
- Patient With Systemic Lupus Erythematosus
Nursing Care Plans
- eNursing Care Plan 64.1: Patient With Rheumatoid Arthritis
- eNursing Care Plan 64.2: Patient With Systemic Lupus Erythematosus
Conceptual Care Map Creator
- Conceptual Care Map for Case Study on p. 1529
Audio Glossary
Content Updates

REFERENCES

1. Arthritis Foundation: Understanding arthritis. Retrieved from *www.arthritis.org/about-arthritis/understanding-arthritis/*.
2. Centers for Disease Control and Prevention: Arthritis. Retrieved from *www.cdc.gov/arthritis/*.
3. Arthritis Foundation: Osteoarthritis. Retrieved from *www.arthritis.org/about-arthritis/types/osteoarthritis/*.
4. National Center for Complementary and Integrative Health: Osteoarthritis: In depth. Retrieved from *https://nccih.nih.gov/health/arthritis/osteoarthritis#hed3*.
*5. Karsdal MA, Michaelis M, Ladel C, et al: Disease-modifying treatments for osteoarthritis (DMOADs) of the knee and hip: Lessons learned from failures and opportunities for the future, *Osteoarthritis Cartilage* 24:2013, 2016.
*6. American Academy of Orthopaedic Surgeons: Treatment of osteoarthritis of the knee: Evidence-based guidelines, ed 2. Retrieved from *www.aaos.org/research/guidelines/TreatmentofOsteoarthritisoftheKneeGuideline.pdf*.
7. Goodman B: Arthroscopic knee surgery little help for arthritis. Retrieved from *www.arthritis.org/living-with-arthritis/treatments/joint-surgery/types/knee/arthroscopic-knee-surgery.php*.
8. Arthritis Foundation: Other natural therapies for osteoarthritis. Retrieved from *www.arthritis.org/living-with-arthritis/treatments/natural/other-therapies/*.
9. Arthritis Foundation: What is rheumatoid arthritis? Retrieved from *www.arthritis.org/about-arthritis/types/rheumatoid-arthritis/what-is-rheumatoid-arthritis.php*.
10. Harrison P: Rheumatoid arthritis: Smoking exacerbates disease activity. Retrieved from *www.medscape.com/viewarticle/821446*.
11. Arthritis Foundation: More than just joints: How rheumatoid arthritis affects the rest of your body. Retrieved from *www.arthritis.org/about-arthritis/types/rheumatoid-arthritis/articles/rhemuatoid-arthritis-affects-body.php*.
12. Arthritis Foundation: The arthritis-depression connection. Retrieved from *www.arthritis.org/living-with-arthritis/comorbidities/depression-and-arthritis/depression-rheumatoid-arthritis.php*.
*13. Agency for Healthcare Research and Quality: Drug therapy for early rheumatoid arthritis: A systematic review update. Retrieved from *https://effectivehealthcare.ahrq.gov/topics/rheumatoid-arthritis-medicine-update/final-report-update-2018*.

*14. Kumar B, Lenert P: Gout and African Americans: Reducing disparities, *Cleve Clin J Med* 83:665, 2016.

15. Harding M: An update on gout for primary care providers, *Nurse Pract* 17:14, 2016.

*16. Armstrong AD, Hubbard MC: *Essentials of musculoskeletal care*, ed 5, Chicago, 2016, American Academy of Orthopaedic Surgeons.

17. Centers for Disease Control and Prevention: Two-step laboratory testing process. Retrieved from *www.cdc.gov/lyme/diagnosistesting/labtest/twostep/index.html*.

18. International Lyme and Associated Diseases Society: Lyme disease basics for providers. Retrieved from *www.ilads.org/research-literature/lyme-disease-basics-for-providers/*.

19. Arthritis Foundation: Spondyloarthritis: What is spondyloarthritis? Retrieved from *www.arthritis.org/about-arthritis/types/spondyloarthritis*.

20. Arthritis Foundation: What is ankylosing spondylitis? Retrieved from *www.arthritis.org/about-arthritis/types/ankylosing-spondylitis/what-is-ankylosing-spondylitis.php*.

21. Arthritis Foundation: What is psoriatic arthritis? Retrieved from *www.arthritis.org/about-arthritis/types/psoriatic-arthritis/what-is-psoriatic-arthritis.php*.

22. Arthritis Foundation: What is reactive arthritis? Retrieved from *www.arthritis.org/about-arthritis/types/reactive-arthritis/what-is-reactive-arthritis.php*.

23. Arthritis Foundation: What is lupus? Retrieved from *www.arthritis.org/about-arthritis/types/lupus/what-is-lupus.php*.

24. Lupus Foundation of America: Medications that can cause drug-induced lupus. Retrieved from *https://resources.lupus.org/entry/causes-of-drug-induced-lupus*.

25. The Johns Hopkins Lupus Center: Lupus-specific skin disease and skin problems. Retrieved from *www.hopkinslupus.org/lupus-info/lupus-affects-body/skin-lupus/*.

26. Lupus Foundation of America: Lupus kidney disease: Did you know? Retrieved from *https://resources.lupus.org/entry/lupus-kidney-disease*.

27. Feltz M, Wickam MB: Systemic lupus erythematosus, *Clin Rev* 26:38, 2016.

28. Lupus Foundation of America: Lab tests for lupus? Retrieved from *https://resources.lupus.org/entry/lab-tests*.

29. Scleroderma Foundation: *What is scleroderma?* Retrieved from *www.scleroderma.org/site/PageNavigator/patients_whatis.html#.W4nYpLgnZPY*.

30. Jimenez SA: Scleroderma. Retrieved from *https://emedicine.medscape.com/article/331864.overview*.

31. The Johns Hopkins Scleroderma Center: Scleroderma treatment options. Retrieved from *www.hopkinsscleroderma.org/patients/scleroderma-treatment-options/*.

32. National Organization for Rare Disorders: Polymyositis. Retrieved from *https://rarediseases.org/rare-diseases/polymyositis/*.

33. Cleveland Clinic: Mixed connective tissue disease. Retrieved from *https://my.clevelandclinic.org/health/diseases/15039-mixed-connective-tissue-disease*.

*34. Papageorgiou A, Ziogas DZ, Mavragani CP, et al: Predicting the outcome of Sjögren's syndrome-associated non-Hodgkin's lymphoma patients, *PLosONE* 10:e0116189, 2015.

35. Mayo Clinic: Myofascial pain syndrome. Retrieved from *www.mayoclinic.org/diseases-conditions/myofascial-pain-syndrome/diagnosis-treatment/drc-20375450*.

36. Arthritis Foundation: What is fibromyalgia? Retrieved from *www.arthritis.org/about-arthritis/types/fibromyalgia/what-is-fibromyalgia.php*.

37. Wolfe F, Smythe HA, Yunus MB, et al: The American College of Rheumatology 1990 criteria for the classification of fibromyalgia, *Arthr Rheum* 33:160, 1990. (Classic)

38. Wolfe F, Clauw DJ, Fitzcharles MA, et al: 2016 Revisions to the 2010/2011 fibromyalgia diagnostic criteria, *Semin Arthritis Rheum* 46:319, 2016.

39. Institute of Medicine of the National Academies: Beyond myalgic encephalomyelitis/chronic fatigue syndrome: Redefining an illness. Retrieved from *www.nationalacademies.org/hmd/~/media/Files/Report%20Files/2015/MECFS/MECFScliniciansguide.pdf*.

*Evidence-based information for clinical practice.

CASE STUDY

Managing Care of Multiple Patients

You are working on the medical-surgical unit and have been assigned to care for the following 5 patients. You have 1 LPN/VN and 1 UAP on your team to help you.

Patients

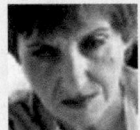

© iStockphoto/ Thinkstock.

J.K. is a 57-yr-old white woman who had debulking surgery for a temporal-parietal glioblastoma. Her MRI/MRA showed a temporal-parietal glioblastoma that extended into the occipital lobes. 4 days ago, she had a hemorrhagic stroke into the site of the tumor bed extending into the thalamus. She now has left homonymous hemianopsia and left-sided weakness.

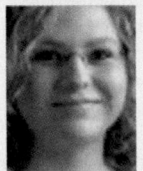

© Purestock/ Thinkstock.

J.P. is a 24-yr-old woman who fell and hit her head during a tonic-clonic seizure. Her boyfriend found her lying unconscious on the floor of her apartment. She had an emergency evacuation of a subdural hematoma and was initially in the ICU. She was transferred to the medical-surgical unit yesterday and is scheduled for a rehabilitation evaluation. She is oriented to person only and is somewhat restless. A safety sitter is at the bedside at all times.

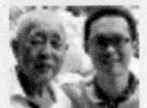

© iStockphoto/ Thinkstock.

M.Y., an 78-yr-old Asian American man, had an ORIF 2 days ago for a fractured left hip. He has a 3-yr history of Alzheimer's disease and is confused to place and time. He has been pleasant and cooperative. He has a personal alarm and bed alarm on for safety. His hip dressing is dry and intact and the drainage in the Hemovac drain is minimal.

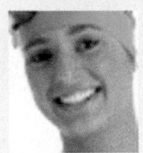

© iStockphoto/ Thinkstock.

S.W., an 18-yr-old woman, sustained a C5 cervical spinal cord injury when she dove into the shallow end of a pool and struck her head on the bottom. She was initially placed in cervical traction, intubated, and mechanically ventilated. She has since undergone surgical stabilization and the traction was removed. After spending 1 week in an inpatient SCI rehabilitation facility, she was transferred to the medical-surgical unit this morning with severe headache, blurred vision, and nausea.

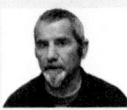

© aronaze/ iStock.com.

M.C. is a 64-yr-old white man who had a right femoral fracture of the greater trochanter after falling while gardening. He previously had both hips replaced. He had surgery 4 days ago to repair the femoral component of his right total hip replacement. Discharge home is planned today.

Discussion Questions

1. **Priority Decision:** After receiving report, which patient should you see first? Provide a rationale.
2. **Collaboration:** Which tasks could you delegate to UAP? *(select all that apply)*
   a. Explain discharge instructions to M.C.
   b. Change the dressing on M.Y.'s left hip.
   c. Obtain vital signs on M.C. before discharge.
   d. Sit with J.P. while the safety sitter takes a break.
   e. Assess J.K.'s ability to swallow before feeding her breakfast.

3. **Priority and Collaboration:** When you enter the room to assess S.W., you find her diaphoretic with a flushed face and pale extremities. Her BP is 200/102 mm Hg. Which 2 initial actions would be *most* appropriate?
   a. Ask the UAP to obtain a stat bladder scan.
   b. Have the LPN administer her oral antihypertensive meds stat.
   c. Elevate the head of the bed while assessing for any noxious stimuli.
   d. Ask the LPN to stay with S.W. while you stat page S.W.'s provider.
   e. Insert rectal suppository after applying lidocaine to the area around the rectum.

Case Study Progression

S.W.'s bladder scan showed 700 mL of urine. After you have the LPN catheterize her using a local anesthetic gel, her symptoms subside. You take this time to further teach S.W. about the manifestations of autonomic dysreflexia and the need to report any symptom as soon as it appears. You discuss bladder training strategies and how to avoid bladder distention. S.W. is grateful for the information and your caring attitude. Just as you are finishing, the UAP tells you that M.Y. has pulled out his Hemovac drain.

4. What should be your *initial* intervention for M.Y.?
   a. Reinsert the Hemovac drain.
   b. Assess the incision site for a hematoma.
   c. Notify M.Y.'s provider that the drain was removed.
   d. Apply pressure to the incisional site where the drain had been placed.
5. Which intervention would be *most* appropriate in caring for J.K.?
   a. Place her left arm in a sling for support.
   b. Arrange the food tray so that all foods are on the right side.
   c. Position her left leg so that the ankle is lower than the knee.
   d. Call the provider to get an order of warfarin to prevent VTE.
6. When teaching J.P.'s boyfriend about what to expect during recovery from a head injury, which statement is *most* accurate?
   a. "You can tell by how great she looks physically that she will ultimately function well at the home."
   b. "One good thing that will come out of this injury is that her seizures should occur less frequently."
   c. "Most patients are transferred out of the hospital for acute rehabilitation management to prepare them for going home."
   d. "She can expect a full recovery without any chronic problems, but it may take a few months to achieve that goal."
7. **Priority Decision:** You receive the morning laboratory data. Which finding should you report to the provider immediately?
   a. J.K. has a platelet level of 170,000 μ/L.
   b. M.C.'s INR after his first dose of warfarin is 1.4.
   c. M.Y.'s WBC has increased from 7000 yesterday to 10,800.
   d. S.W. who is receiving enteral nutrition, has a glucose level of 142 mg/dL.
8. **Management Decision:** As you enter M.C.'s room to discuss his discharge plans, you find him all packed up and ready to go. He tells you the UAP already told him what he needed to do. What is your *best* initial action?
   a. Ask M.C. if he has any further questions.
   b. Call the UAP to M.C.'s room to find out what she told him.
   c. Review discharge instructions with M.C. to ascertain correct understanding.
   d. Give M.C. a telephone number to call in case he has any concerns when he gets home.

Answers and rationales available at *http://evolve.elsevier.com/Lewis/medsurg.*

Critical Care

Megan Ann Brissie

Those who are happiest are those who do the most for others.

Booker T. Washington

ⓔ http://evolve.elsevier.com/Lewis/medsurg

CONCEPTUAL FOCUS

Cognition	Perfusion	Sleep
Gas Exchange	Sensory Perception	Technology and Informatics
Nutrition		

LEARNING OUTCOMES

1. Discuss the various certification opportunities for critical care registered nurses.
2. Select appropriate nursing interventions to manage common problems and needs of critically ill patients.
3. Develop strategies to manage issues related to caregivers of critically ill patients.
4. Apply the principles of hemodynamic monitoring to the nursing and interprofessional management of patients receiving monitoring.
5. Discern the purpose of, indications for, and function of circulatory assist devices and related nursing and interprofessional management.
6. Distinguish the indications for and modes of mechanical ventilation.
7. Select appropriate nursing interventions related to the care of an intubated patient.
8. Relate the principles of mechanical ventilation to the nursing and interprofessional management of patients receiving this intervention.

KEY TERMS

arterial pressure–based cardiac output (APCO), p. 1541

assist-control ventilation (ACV), p. 1554

circulatory assist devices (CADs), p. 1545

continuous positive airway pressure (CPAP), p. 1547

endotracheal (ET) intubation, p. 1548

hemodynamic monitoring, p. 1537

high-frequency oscillatory ventilation (HFOV), p. 1557

intraaortic balloon pump (IABP), p. 1545

mechanical ventilation, p. 1553

negative pressure ventilation, p. 1553

positive end-expiratory pressure (PEEP), p. 1556

positive pressure ventilation (PPV), p. 1553

pressure support ventilation (PSV), p. 1556

synchronized intermittent mandatory ventilation (SIMV), p. 1556

ventricular assist device (VAD), p. 1547

volume ventilation, p. 1553

weaning, p. 1561

This chapter focuses on the role of the critical care registered nurse (RN) in the management of critically ill patients in an intensive care setting. The chapter reviews concepts related to cardiovascular and respiratory dynamics that support perfusion and gas exchange. We emphasize the interprofessional care and nursing management of ill patients requiring advanced care modalities. These include hemodynamic monitoring, circulatory assist devices (CADs), artificial airways, and mechanical ventilation.

CRITICAL CARE NURSING

The American Association of Critical-Care Nurses (AACN) defines *critical care nursing* as a specialty that manages human responses to life-threatening problems.[1] Critical care RNs care for patients with acute and unstable physiologic problems and their caregivers. This involves assessing life-threatening conditions, starting appropriate interventions, evaluating the outcomes of interventions, and providing teaching and emotional support to caregivers.

Critical Care Units

Critical care units (CCUs) or *intensive care units* (ICUs) are designed to meet the special needs of acutely and critically ill patients. In many hospitals, the concept of ICU care has expanded from delivering care in a standard unit to bringing care to patients wherever they may be. For example, the *electronic* or *teleICU* helps the bedside ICU team by monitoring the patient from a remote location (Fig. 65.1).

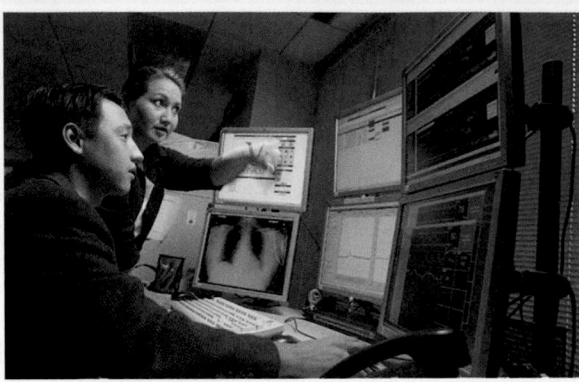

FIG. 65.1 eICU team members monitor patients from a remote site. (From Amelung PJ, Doerfler, ME: VISICU and the e ICU Program. In Le Roux PD, Levine J, Kofke WA: *Monitoring in neurocritical care,* St Louis, 2013, Elsevier.)

Similarly, *rapid response teams* (RRTs) deliver advanced care by an interprofessional team. The team is usually composed of a critical care RN, critical care physician or an advanced practice registered nurse (APRN), and a respiratory therapist (RT). RRTs bring rapid and immediate care to unstable patients in noncritical care settings. Patients often show early and subtle signs of deterioration (e.g., mild confusion, tachypnea, vital sign changes) 6 to 8 hours before cardiac or respiratory arrest. RRT intervention has made significant advances in reducing mortality rates in these patients.[2]

The technology available in the ICU is extensive and always evolving. It is possible to continuously monitor a patient's electrocardiogram (ECG), BP, O_2 saturation, cardiac output (CO), intracranial pressure (ICP), and temperature. Advanced monitoring devices can measure cardiac index (CI), stroke volume (SV), stroke volume variation (SVV), ejection fraction (EF), end-tidal carbon dioxide (EtCO$_2$), and O_2 consumption. Patients may receive ongoing support from mechanical ventilators, intraaortic balloon pumps (IABPs), CADs, or dialysis machines.

Progressive care units (PCUs), also called *intermediate care* or *step-down units,* are a transition between the ICU and the general unit. Generally, PCU patients are at risk for serious complications, but their risk is lower than that of ICU patients. Examples of patients in PCUs include those scheduled for interventional heart procedures (e.g., stent placement), awaiting heart transplant, receiving stable doses of vasoactive IV drugs (e.g., diltiazem [Cardizem]), being weaned from prolonged mechanical ventilation, or who recently had tracheostomy placement. Monitoring capabilities in PCUs may include continuous ECG, arterial BP, O_2 saturation, and EtCO$_2$.

Critical Care Registered Nurse

A critical care RN has in-depth knowledge of anatomy, physiology, pathophysiology, and pharmacology; advanced assessment skills; and the ability to use advanced technology. As a critical care RN, you perform frequent assessments to monitor trends in the patient's physiologic parameters (e.g., BP, ECG, O_2 saturation). This allows you to rapidly recognize and manage complications while aiding healing and recovery. You provide psychologic support to the patient and/or caregiver. To be effective, you must be able to communicate and collaborate with all interprofessional team members.

As a critical care RN, you will face ethical dilemmas related to the care of your patients. Moral distress over perceived issues

of delivering futile or nonbeneficial care can lead to emotional exhaustion or burnout. Consequently, it is important that all members of the interprofessional care team coexist in a healthy work environment.

Specialization in critical care nursing requires a preceptored clinical orientation, often over several months. The AACN Certification Corporation offers (1) critical care certification (CCRN) in direct care adult, pediatric, and neonatal critical care nursing; (2) progressive care certification (PCCN); (3) critical care certification knowledge (CCRN-K) or progressive care certification knowledge (PCCN-K) for those who do not provide direct care but influence care delivery in their role; and (4) teleICU certification (CCRN-E). Other certifications are available in cardiac medicine (CMC) and cardiac surgery (CSC). Certification requires RN licensure, practice experience in the related area, and successful completion of a written test. It validates basic knowledge of critical or progressive care nursing.

APRNs in critical care function in a variety of roles: patient and staff educators, consultants, administrators, researchers, or expert practitioners.[3] The APRN who is a clinical nurse specialist (CNS) typically provides advanced nursing care to meet the needs of adult-gerontology, pediatric, or neonatal patient populations. Certification for the CNS in acute and critical care is available through the AACN.

Another APRN role is the adult-gerontology acute care nurse practitioner (AG-ACNP). This APRN provides comprehensive care to select critically ill patients and their caregivers. The AG-ACNP conducts comprehensive assessments, orders and interprets diagnostic tests, manages health problems, prescribes treatments, and coordinates care among interprofessional care teams and during transitions in care settings. Certification as an AG-ACNP is available through the AACN. Prescriptive authority and licensure regulations for APRNs vary by state.

Critical Care Patient

A critically ill patient is one whose need for care is acute in nature, requiring intense and vigilant nursing care. A patient is generally admitted to the ICU for 1 of 3 reasons. First, the patient may be physiologically unstable, requiring advanced clinical judgments by you or another HCP. Second, the patient may be at risk for serious complications and need frequent assessments and often invasive interventions. Third, the patient may need intensive and complicated nursing support related to the use of IV medications (e.g., sedation, drugs requiring titration [e.g., vasopressors], or thrombolytics) and advanced technology (e.g., hemodynamic monitoring, mechanical ventilation, continuous renal replacement therapy [CRRT], ICP monitoring). The incidence of death is higher in ICU patients than in non-ICU patients. In general, nonsurvivors are older, have co-morbidities (e.g., liver disease, obesity), and have longer ICU stays.

ICU patients may be clustered by disease condition (e.g., cardiology, burns, neurology) or age-group (e.g., neonatal, pediatrics, adult). Those with medical emergencies (e.g., sepsis, diabetic ketoacidosis, drug overdoses) are treated in a medical ICU. Sometimes we cluster patients by acuity (e.g., critical and unstable versus chronic but technology dependent and stable). Patients commonly treated in the ICU include those with respiratory failure, myocardial infarction (MI), or acute neurologic impairment or those requiring care after major surgery (e.g., heart or brain surgery, organ transplantation). Fig. 65.2 shows a typical ICU bed with monitors.

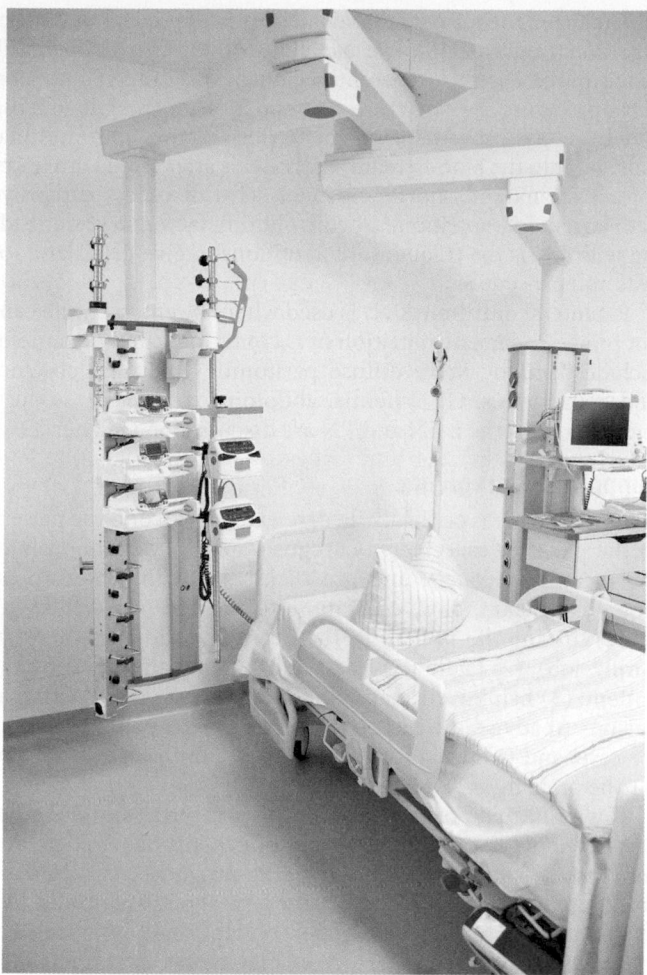

FIG. 65.2 Typical ICU bed with monitors. (© danutela/iStock.com.)

The patient who we do not expect to recover from an illness is usually not admitted to an ICU. For example, the ICU is not typically used to care for the patient in a persistent, vegetative state or to prolong the natural process of death. ICUs will manage patients who have brain death or who meet criteria for donation after cardiac death to optimize the opportunity for organ donation. Sometimes patients may be managed in the ICU to allow for end-of-life decisions or transitions of care to occur in a private, dignified setting. So, it is important that critical care RNs are skilled in palliative and end-of-life care (see Chapter 9).

Common Problems of Critical Care Patients. The patient in the ICU is at risk for many complications and special problems. Critically ill patients are often intubated and mechanically ventilated, immobile, and at high risk for skin problems (see Chapter 23) and venous thromboembolism (VTE) (see Chapter 37). The use of multiple, invasive devices predisposes the patient to health care–associated infections (HAIs). Sepsis and multiple organ dysfunction syndrome (MODS) may follow (see Chapter 66). Other special problems relate to anxiety, pain, impaired communication, sensory-perceptual problems, sleep, and nutrition.

Anxiety. Anxiety is a common problem for ICU patients. The main sources of anxiety include the perceived or expected threat to health or life, loss of control of body functions, and a foreign environment. Many patients and caregivers feel uncomfortable in the ICU with its complex equipment, high noise and

light levels, and intense pace of activity. Pain, impaired communication, sleeplessness, immobilization, and loss of control all enhance anxiety.

To help reduce anxiety, have patients and caregivers express concerns, ask questions, and state their needs. Include them in all conversations and explain the purpose of equipment and procedures. Structure the patient's environment in a way that decreases anxiety. For example, encourage caregivers to bring in photographs and personal items. Antianxiety drugs (e.g., lorazepam [Ativan]) and relaxation techniques (e.g., music therapy) may reduce the stress response that anxiety can trigger.

Pain. The control of pain in the ICU patient is very important. Unrelieved pain is common among ICU patients and can lead to poor outcomes.[4] Inadequate pain control is linked with agitation, fear, and anxiety and adds to the stress response. ICU patients at high risk for pain include those who (1) have medical conditions that include ischemic, infectious, or inflammatory processes; (2) are immobilized; (3) have invasive monitoring devices, including endotracheal tubes (ETs); and (4) undergo procedures.

For many critically ill patients (e.g., those intubated), continuous IV sedation (e.g., propofol [Diprivan]) and an analgesic agent (e.g., fentanyl) are used for sedation and pain control. However, patients getting deep sedation are often unresponsive. This prevents you and other HCPs from fully assessing the patient's neurologic status. To address this issue, all patients who can safely tolerate an interruption in sedation usually receive a daily, scheduled interruption of sedation, or "sedation holiday." These allow you to awaken the patient to conduct a neurologic examination.[5] Pain management is discussed in Chapter 8.

Impaired Communication. Inability to communicate is distressing for patients who cannot speak because of sedative and paralyzing drugs, an ET, or the inability to communicate from a neurologic impairment. As part of every procedure, explain what will happen or is happening to the patient. When the patient cannot speak, explore other methods of communication, such as picture boards, notepads, magic slates, or computers. When speaking with the patient, look directly at the patient and use hand gestures when appropriate. For those who do not speak English, you must use an approved interpreter or interpreter phone service when providing care or instructions (see Chapter 2).

Nonverbal communication is important. High levels of procedure-related touch and lower levels of comfort-related touch often characterize the ICU environment. Patients have different levels of tolerance for being touched, usually related to culture and personal history. If appropriate, use comforting touch with ongoing evaluation of the patient's response. Encourage the caregiver to talk to the patient, even if the patient is intubated, is sedated, or appears comatose. Hearing is often the last sense to decrease. Even if the patient cannot respond, they may still be able to hear.

Sleep. Nearly all ICU patients have sleep problems. Patients may have difficulty falling asleep or have disrupted sleep because of noise, anxiety, pain, frequent monitoring, treatments, or care needs. Sleep problems can cause delirium and delayed recovery.

Arrange the environment to promote the patient's sleep-wake cycle. Measures include scheduling rest periods, bundling care, limiting noise and visitors, getting physiologic measurements without disturbing the patient, opening curtains during the daytime and dimming lights at nighttime, providing eye masks/ear plugs to encourage sleep, and providing comfort measures (e.g., massage).[6] If needed, use benzodiazepines (e.g., temazepam), benzodiazepine-like drugs (e.g., zolpidem [Ambien]), or natural hormones (e.g., melatonin), especially for an older adult, to aid and maintain sleep. Promoting sleep is discussed in Chapter 7.

Sensory-Perceptual Problems. Acute and reversible sensory-perceptual changes are common in ICU patients. We used to call the combination of changes in mentation (e.g., delusions, short attention span, loss of recent memory), psychomotor behavior (e.g., restlessness, lethargy), and sleep-wake cycle (e.g., daytime sleepiness, nighttime agitation) *ICU psychosis.* The patient with these changes is not psychotic but has *delirium.* Delirium is an acute change in mental status. The prevalence of delirium in ICU patients is as high as 87%.[7] It is associated with longer hospital stays and higher mortality rates.

Major risk factors for delirium include increased age, pre-existing dementia, hypertension, alcohol use, and severe illness on admission. Environmental factors that can contribute to delirium include sleep deprivation, anxiety, sensory overload, and immobilization. Physical conditions such as hemodynamic instability, hypoxemia, electrolyte imbalances, and severe infections can lead to delirium. Last, certain drugs (e.g., sedatives [benzodiazepines], analgesics [opioids], vasopressors) are linked with delirium. Chapter 59 discusses delirium.

Monitor all ICU patients for delirium using a valid tool and initiate prevention strategies. Assessment tools for adult ICU patients include the Confusion Assessment Method for the ICU (CAM-ICU) (see Table 59.18) and the Intensive Care Delirium Screening Checklist (ICDSC). It is critical to address physiologic factors (e.g., correction of oxygenation, perfusion, electrolyte problems). Clocks and calendars can help orient the patient. Reorient patients who are confused during assessments to provide comfort and direction. The presence of a caregiver may help. Removing lines no longer needed and early mobility are effective.[8] If the patient has hyperactivity, insomnia, or delusions, treatment with sedative drugs with anxiolytic effects (e.g., dexmedetomidine [Precedex]) can be used.

Sensory overload can result in patient distress and anxiety. Environmental noise levels are high in the ICU. Help the patient understand we cannot prevent noise. Conversation is an especially stressful noise, especially when the discussion concerns the patient and is held in the presence of, but without participation from, the patient. Reduce this source of stress by finding suitable places for patient-related discussions. Whenever possible, include the patient and caregiver in the discussion.

You can limit noise levels by muting phones, setting alarms based on the patient's condition, and reducing unnecessary alarms. For example, silence the BP alarm when handling invasive lines and then reset the alarm when done. Similarly, silence ventilator alarms when suctioning. Last, limit overhead paging and all unnecessary noise in patient care areas.

Nutrition. Patients often arrive at ICUs with conditions that result in either hypermetabolic states (e.g., burns, sepsis) or catabolic states (e.g., acute kidney injury). Other times, patients are in severely malnourished states (e.g., chronic heart, lung, or liver disease). In general, inadequate nutrition increases mortality and morbidity rates. Determining whom to feed, what to feed, when to feed, and how to feed (e.g., route of administration) is crucial when caring for critically ill patients.[9] Collaborate with the HCP and dietitian to decide how best to meet the nutritional needs of the ICU patient.

The main goal of nutritional support is to prevent or correct nutritional deficiencies. We usually do this through the early provision of enteral or parenteral nutrition. Enteral nutrition (EN) preserves the structure and function of the gut mucosa and stops the movement of gut bacteria across the intestinal wall and into the bloodstream. Early EN is associated with fewer complications and shorter hospital stays. It is less expensive than parenteral nutrition.[9] A contributing factor to underfeeding with EN is the frequent interruptions to give drugs and for tests and procedures.

Parenteral nutrition (PN) is used when the enteral route cannot provide adequate nutrition or is contraindicated.[9] Examples include paralytic ileus, diffuse peritonitis, intestinal obstruction, pancreatitis, GI ischemia, abdominal trauma or surgery, and severe diarrhea. EN and PN are discussed in Chapter 39.

Supporting Caregivers

When someone is critically ill, care extends beyond the patient to the patient's caregivers. Caregivers play a valuable role in the patient's recovery and are members of the interprofessional care team. They contribute to the patient's well-being by (1) linking the patient to the outside world (e.g., news of family, job); (2) facilitating decision making and advising the patient; (3) helping with activities of daily living; (4) acting as liaisons to advise the health care team of the patient's wishes for care; and (5) providing safe, caring, familiar relationships for the patient.

Having a friend or relative in the ICU is physically and emotionally difficult, often to the point of exhaustion. Anxiety and concerns about the patient's condition, prognosis, and pain are common. Caregivers may have concern about financial issues related to hospital stay. They often disrupt their daily routines to support the patient. Caregivers may be far from their own home, friends, and relatives. Consulting with the case manager or social worker is helpful in these instances.

Caregivers of the critically ill are in crisis, and family-centered care is essential. Caregivers need your guidance and support. You must be skilled in crisis intervention to provide effective family-centered care. Conduct a family assessment and intervene as needed. Strategies include active listening, reduction of anxiety, and support for those who become upset or angry. Recognize the caregivers' feelings, listen to them openly and without being judgmental, and acknowledge their decisions. Consult other team members (e.g., chaplains, psychologists, patient representatives) as needed to help caregivers cope.

The major needs of caregivers of critically ill patients include information, communication, and access.[10] Lack of information is a major source of anxiety. Assess their understanding of the patient's status, treatment plan, and prognosis and provide information as appropriate. Identify a spokesperson to help coordinate information exchange between the interprofessional care team and caregivers.

Holding routine interprofessional conferences with caregivers improves satisfaction with communication and trust in clinicians and reduces conflict between clinicians and family members.[10] Have them meet the interprofessional care team. Include them in rounds and patient care conferences. It helps caregivers accept and cope with problems when they see that the team is caring and competent, decisions are deliberate, and their input is valued. If the patient has an advance directive, the caregiver needs to see that the patient's wishes are followed. If the patient has a durable power of attorney for health care, this person must be involved in the patient's plan of care.

Caregivers need access to the patient. The AACN strongly recommends less restrictive and more individualized visiting policies. Achieve this goal by assessing the patient's and caregiver's needs and preferences and incorporating these into the patient's plan of care.

ETHICAL/LEGAL DILEMMAS
Visitation and Caregiver Presence in the Adult ICU

Situation

B.W., a new RN, is undergoing orientation in the surgical ICU. He asks his preceptor why the patients' families are allowed on the unit throughout the day and even the night. B.W. states that, in his last position, visiting hours in the ICU were 10 AM to 12 PM and 4 PM to 6 PM. He adds that families make him nervous when they watch what he is doing and ask him many questions. B.W. says that he plans to tell the visitors to leave the patient's room when he is giving care.

Ethical/Legal Points for Consideration

- We used to think that visitation caused the patient stress, interfered with care, was mentally exhausting to patients and caregivers, and contributed to increased infection rates. Evidence does not support any of these beliefs.[1,2]
- Evidence suggests several positive benefits of flexible visitation for the patient: decreased anxiety, confusion, and agitation; fewer cardiovascular complications; shorter ICU length of stay; and reports that patients feel more secure and satisfied with care.[1]
- Similar evidence exists for the benefits of flexible visitation for caregivers: increased satisfaction, decreased anxiety, better communication, and increased opportunities for patient and caregiver teaching as caregivers are more involved in care.[1]
- Some conditions may require restricting visitation: a documented legal reason; visitor behavior presents a risk to the patient, staff, or others; visitor behavior disrupts the functioning of the unit; visitor has a contagious illness or has been exposed to a contagious disease that could endanger the patient's health; or the patient requests fewer or no visitors.

Discussion Questions

1. How should the preceptor respond to B.W.'s statement of his intentions?
2. Does B.W. have an ethical or legal obligation to allow visitation regardless of his personal concerns? Defend your position.

References

1. Davidson JE, Aslakson RA, Long AC, et al.: Guidelines for family-centered care in the neonatal, pediatric, and adult ICU, *CCM* 45:103, 2017.
2. Clark AP, Guzzetta CE: A paradigm shift for patient/family-centered care in intensive care units: Bring in the family, *Crit Care Nurse* 37(96), 2017.

The first time that caregivers visit, it is important for you to prepare them for the experience. Briefly describe the patient's appearance and physical environment (e.g., equipment, noise). Join caregivers as they enter the room. Observe the responses of the patient and caregivers. Invite the caregivers to take part in the patient's care if they want. Be prepared that people may respond differently to seeing their loved one in the ICU for the first time.

In some ICUs, visitation includes animal-assisted therapy or pet visitation, most often therapy dogs. The positive benefits (e.g., decreases in BP and anxiety) far outweigh the risks (e.g., transmission of infection from animal to patient). Pet therapy should be a part of the ICUs visitation policy.

Caregivers should also have the option to be present at the bedside when patients are undergoing invasive procedures (e.g., central line insertion) or cardiopulmonary resuscitation (CPR). Even when the outcomes are not favorable, being present helps caregivers to (1) overcome doubts about the patient's condition, (2) reduce their anxiety and fear, (3) meet their need to be together with and to support their loved one, and (4) begin the grief process if death occurs. Be a part of initiatives to develop policies and procedures that offer the option of caregiver presence during invasive procedures and CPR.[11]

Culturally Competent Care: Critical Care Patients

Providing culturally competent care to critically ill patients and caregivers can be challenging. Often, meeting the patient's physiologic needs is a priority and overshadows the influence of the patient's culture on the illness experience. It is important to consider the cultural aspects of the meaning of sickness and health, pain, dying and death, and grief when caring for critically ill patients and their caregivers (see Chapter 2).

Cultural perspectives on dying and death are complex. Some view a discussion about advance directives as a legal way to withhold, withdraw, or deny care. Customs surrounding dying and death vary. Caregiver requests may range from asking you to leave a window open so that the spirit of the deceased can leave to giving the final bath for the deceased. Ask caregivers about their cultural traditions when caring for the dying patient.

Several variables influence the expressions of grief that follow the loss of a loved one. These include the relationship between the grieving person and the deceased, whether the loss is sudden or expected, the support systems available to the grieving person, past experiences with loss, and the person's religious and cultural beliefs. Proceed cautiously when approaching patients facing death and their caregivers. Asking patients, "What do you want to know?" and "Who do you want with you when discussing options?" are good starting points. Chapter 9 provides detailed information about end-of-life care.

HEMODYNAMIC MONITORING

Hemodynamic monitoring is the measurement of pressure, flow, and oxygenation within the cardiovascular system. The purpose of hemodynamic monitoring is to assess heart function, fluid balance, and the effects of fluids and drugs on CO. Both invasive (internally placed devices) and noninvasive (externally placed devices) obtain hemodynamic parameters (values). These include systemic and pulmonary arterial pressures, central venous pressure (CVP), pulmonary artery wedge pressure (PAWP) (also known as pulmonary artery occlusive pressure [PAOP]), CO/CI, SV/SV index (SVI), SVV, O_2 saturation of the hemoglobin of arterial blood (SaO_2), and mixed venous O_2 saturation (SvO_2).

From these measurements, you can calculate several values. These include the resistance of the systemic and pulmonary arterial vasculature and O_2 content, delivery, and consumption. When you combine these data, you get a picture of the patient's hemodynamic status and the effect of therapy over time (trends). Take all measurements with attention to accuracy. Inaccurate data can result in unnecessary or inappropriate treatment.

Hemodynamic Terminology

Cardiac Output and Cardiac Index. *Cardiac output* (CO) is the volume of blood in liters pumped by the heart in 1 minute. *Cardiac index* (CI) is the measurement of CO adjusted for body surface area (BSA). It is a more precise measurement of the efficiency of the heart's pumping action. Although minor beat-to-beat variations may occur, the left and right ventricles pump the same volume. The volume ejected with each heartbeat is the SV. Like CI, *stroke volume index* (SVI) is the measurement of SV adjusted for BSA.

CO and the forces opposing blood flow determine BP. *Systemic vascular resistance* (SVR) (opposition encountered by the left ventricle) or *pulmonary vascular resistance* (PVR) (opposition encountered by the right ventricle) is the resistance to blood flow by the vessels. Preload, afterload, and contractility determine SV, and thus CO (see Chapter 31). It is essential that you understand these concepts and the physiologic effects of manipulating each of these variables. Table 65.1 presents the formulas and values for common hemodynamic parameters.

Preload. *Preload* is the volume within the ventricle at the end of diastole. Unfortunately, chamber volume measurements are hard to obtain. Instead, we use various pressures to estimate the volume. Left ventricular preload is called *left ventricular end-diastolic pressure*. PAWP, a measurement of pulmonary capillary pressure, reflects left ventricular end-diastolic pressure under normal conditions (i.e., when there is no mitral valve dysfunction, intracardiac defect, or dysrhythmia). CVP is measured in the right atrium or in the vena cava close to the heart. It is the right ventricular preload or right ventricular end-diastolic pressure when there is no tricuspid valve dysfunction, intracardiac defect, or dysrhythmia.

Frank-Starling's law explains the effects of preload. It says that the more a myocardial fiber is stretched during filling, the more it shortens during systole and the greater the force of the contraction. As preload increases, force generated in the subsequent contraction increases and SV and CO increase. The greater the preload, the greater the myocardial stretch and the greater the myocardial O_2 requirement. Thus increases in CO from increased preload require increased delivery of O_2 to the myocardium. The clinical measurement made is not a direct measurement of the muscle length. The measurement is of the pressure at the time of the peak stretch (end diastole) (Table 65.1). This pressure indirectly indicates the amount of stretch and the volume. It is also important because it indicates pressure in the blood vessels of the lungs or in the blood returning to the heart. Diuresis and vasodilation decrease preload. Fluid administration increases preload.

Afterload. *Afterload* refers to the forces opposing ventricular ejection. These forces include systemic arterial pressure, the resistance offered by the aortic valve, and the mass and density of the blood. SVR and arterial pressure are indices of left ventricular afterload, though clinically they do not include all the components of afterload. Similarly, PVR and pulmonary arterial pressure are indices of right ventricular afterload. Increased afterload often results in a decreased CO and increased O_2 demand. CO can be improved and myocardial O_2 needs reduced by decreasing afterload (i.e., decreasing forces opposing contraction). For example, vasodilator drug therapy (e.g., milrinone) can reduce afterload.

Vascular Resistance. SVR is the resistance of the systemic vascular bed. PVR is the resistance of the pulmonary vascular bed. Both these measures reflect afterload as described earlier and can be adjusted for body size (Table 65.1).

Contractility. *Contractility* describes the strength of contraction. Contractility increases when preload is unchanged and the heart contracts more forcefully. Epinephrine, norepinephrine, isoproterenol (Isuprel), dopamine, dobutamine, digitalis-like drugs, calcium, and milrinone increase or improve contractility. We call these drugs *positive inotropes*. Increased contractility results in increased SV and increased myocardial O_2 requirements. *Negative inotropes* reduce contractility. These include certain drugs (e.g., calcium channel blockers, β-adrenergic blockers) and clinical conditions (e.g., acidosis).

There are no direct clinical measures of cardiac contractility. Measuring the patient's preload (PAWP) and CO and graphing the results indirectly indicate contractility. If preload, heart rate (HR), and afterload remain constant and CO changes, contractility is changed. Contractility is reduced in the failing heart.

Principles of Invasive Pressure Monitoring

Invasive lines are used in the ICU to measure systemic and pulmonary BPs. Fig. 65.3 shows the parts of a typical invasive arterial BP monitoring system. The catheter, pressure tubing, flush system, and transducer are disposable.

Pressure monitoring equipment is referenced and zero balanced to the environment, and dynamic response characteristics are optimized for accuracy.[12] *Referencing* means placing the transducer so that the zero-reference point is at the level of the atria of the heart. The stopcock nearest the transducer is used for the zero reference. To place this level with the atria, use an external landmark, the phlebostatic axis. To find the *phlebostatic axis*, draw 2 imaginary lines with the patient supine (Fig. 65.4, *A*). Draw a horizontal line down from the axilla, midway between the anterior and posterior chest walls. Draw a vertical line laterally through the fourth intercostal space along the chest wall. The phlebostatic axis is the intersection of the 2 imaginary lines. Mark this location on the patient's chest with a permanent marker. Position the port of the stopcock nearest the transducer level at the phlebostatic axis. Tape the transducer to the patient's chest at the phlebostatic axis or ideally mount it on a bedside pole (Fig. 65.4, *B*).

Zeroing confirms that when pressure within the system is zero, the monitor reads 0. To do this, open the reference stopcock to room air (off to the patient) and observe the monitor for a reading of 0. This allows the monitor to use

TABLE 65.1 Resting Hemodynamic Parameters

Indicators	Normal Range
Preload	
Pulmonary artery diastolic pressure (PADP)	4–12 mm Hg
Pulmonary artery wedge pressure (PAWP) or left atrial pressure (LAP)	6–12 mm Hg
Right atrial pressure (RAP) or central venous pressure (CVP)	2–8 mm Hg
Right ventricular end - diastolic volume (RVEDV) = $\dfrac{\text{Stroke volume (SV)}}{\text{Right ventricular ejection fraction (RVEF)}}$	100–160 mL
Afterload	
MAP = $\dfrac{\text{Systolic blood pressure} + 2\ (\text{Diastolic blood pressure})}{3}$*	70–105 mm Hg
PAMP = $\dfrac{\text{Pulmonary artery styolic pressure (PASP)} + 2\text{PADP}}{3}$*	10–20 mm Hg
Pulmonary vascular resistance (PVR) = $\dfrac{(\text{Pulmonary artery pressure [PAMP]} - \text{PAWP}) \times 80}{\text{Cardiac output (CO)}}$	<250 dynes/sec/cm^{-5}
Pulmonary vascular resistance index (PVRI) = $\dfrac{[\text{PAMP} - \text{PAWP}] \times 80}{\text{Cardiac index (CI)}}$	160–380 dynes/sec/cm^{-5}/m^2
Systemic vascular resistance (SVR) = $\dfrac{(\text{Mean arterial pressure [MAP]} - \text{CVP}) \times 80}{\text{CO}}$	800–1200 dynes/sec/cm^{-5}
Systemic vascular resistance index (SVRI) = $\dfrac{(\text{MAP} - \text{CVP}) \times 80}{\text{CI}}$	1970–2390 dynes/sec/cm^{-5}/m^2
Other	
CI = $\dfrac{\text{CO}}{\text{Body surface area (BSA)}}$	2.2–4 L/min/m^2
CO = SV × HR	4–8 L/min
Heart rate	60–100 beats/min
RVEF = $\dfrac{\text{SV}}{\text{RVEDV} \times 100}$	40%–60%
Stroke volume = $\dfrac{\text{CO}}{\text{Heart rate}}$	60–150 mL/beat
Stroke volume index (SVI) = $\dfrac{\text{CI}}{\text{Heart rate}}$	30–65 mL/beat/m^2
Stroke volume variation (SVV) = $\dfrac{\text{SV}_{max} - \text{SV}_{min}}{\text{SV}_{mean}}$	<13%
Oxygenation	
Arterial hemoglobin O$_2$ saturation	95%–100%
Mixed venous hemoglobin O$_2$ saturation	60%–80%
Venous hemoglobin O$_2$ saturation	70%

*This formula is an approximation because it does not take into consideration the heart rate. The monitor looks at the area under the pressure curve, as well as the heart rate, to calculate MAP and PAMP.

the atmospheric pressure as a reference for 0. Zero the transducer during the initial setup, immediately after insertion of the arterial line, when the transducer has been disconnected from the pressure cable or the pressure cable has been disconnected from the monitor and when the accuracy of the measurements is questioned. Always follow the manufacturer's guidelines.

Optimizing dynamic response characteristics involves checking that the equipment reproduces, without distortion, a signal that changes rapidly. Perform a *dynamic response test (square wave test)* every 8 to 12 hours, when the system is opened to air, or when you question the accuracy of the measurements. It involves activating the fast flush and checking that the equipment reproduces a distortion-free signal (Fig. 65.5).

⚠ SAFETY ALERT Positioning the Zero Reference Stopcock
- Mark the location of the phlebostatic axis on the patient's chest with a permanent marker.
- Recheck the leveling of the zero-reference stopcock to the phlebostatic axis with any change in the patient's position.
- Transducers placed higher than the phlebostatic axis will produce falsely low BP readings.
- Transducers placed lower than the phlebostatic axis will produce falsely high BP readings.

Types of Invasive Pressure Monitoring
Arterial BP. Continuous arterial BP monitoring is indicated for patients in many situations, including acute hypotension and hypertension, respiratory failure, shock, neurologic injury,

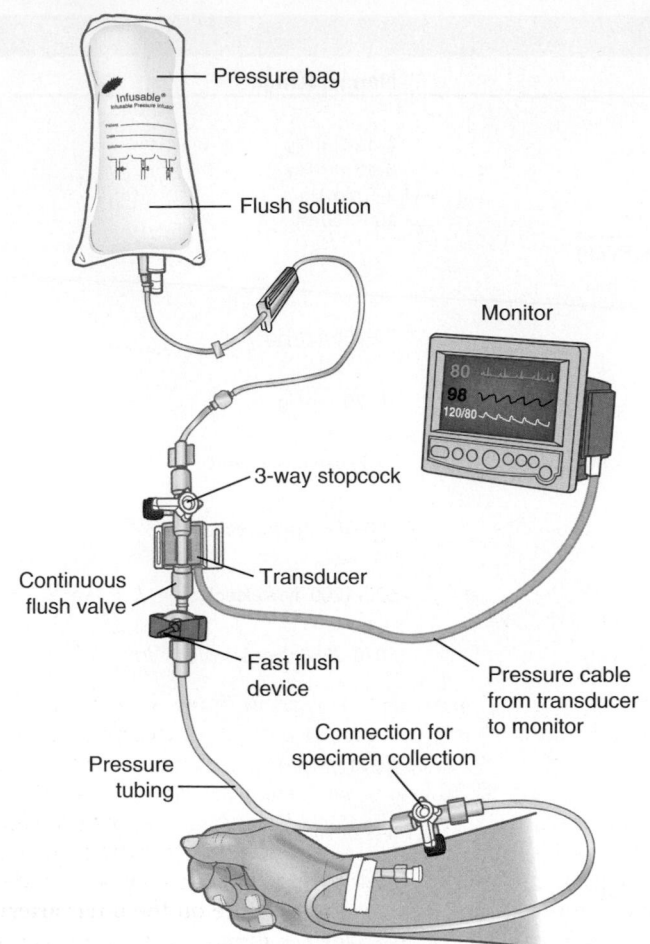

FIG. 65.3 Parts of a pressure monitoring system. The cannula, shown entering the radial artery, is connected via pressure (nondistensible) tubing to the transducer. The transducer converts the pressure wave into an electronic signal. The transducer is wired to the electronic monitoring system, which amplifies, conditions, displays, and records the signal. Stopcocks are inserted into the line for specimen withdrawal and for referencing and zero-balancing procedures. A flush system, consisting of a pressurized bag of IV fluid, tubing, and a flush device, is connected to the system. The flush system provides continuous slow (about 3 mL/hr) flushing and a mechanism for fast flushing of lines.

coronary interventional procedures, continuous infusion of vasoactive drugs (e.g., norepinephrine), and frequent arterial blood gas (ABG) sampling.[12] A nontapered Teflon catheter is typically used to cannulate an artery (e.g., radial, femoral) using a percutaneous approach. After insertion, the HCP usually sutures the catheter in place. You should immobilize the insertion site to prevent dislodging or kinking the catheter line.

Measurements. Use the arterial line to obtain systolic, diastolic, and mean arterial pressure (MAP) (Fig. 65.6). Table 65.2 outlines the steps in obtaining BP measurements with an invasive line. Obtain measurements from both digital and printed analog outputs. Readings from a printed pressure tracing at the end of expiration (to limit the effect of the respiratory cycle on arterial BP) are most accurate. When possible, position the patient supine for initial readings. Values with the head of the bed elevated up to 45 degrees are generally equal to measurements with the patient supine unless the patient's BP is extremely sensitive to orthostatic changes. It is important to keep the zero-reference stopcock level with the phlebostatic axis to ensure accurate continuous measurements.

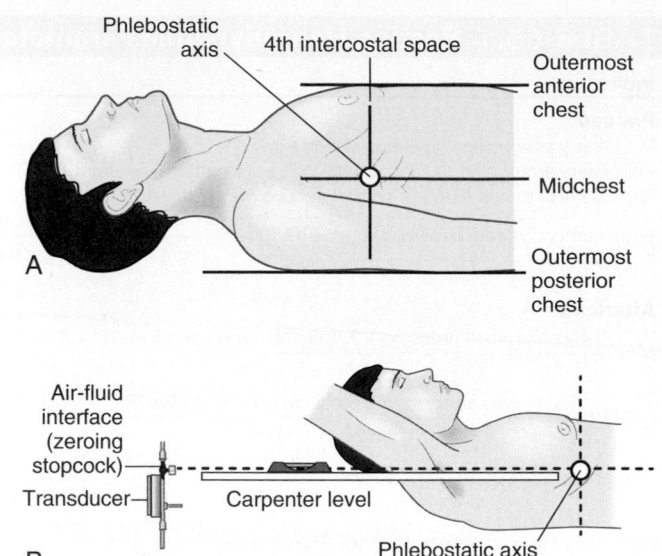

FIG. 65.4 Identification of the phlebostatic axis. **A,** Phlebostatic axis is an external landmark used to identify the level of the atria in the supine patient. It is defined as the intersection of 2 imaginary lines: 1 drawn horizontally from the axilla, midway between the anterior and posterior chest walls, and the other drawn vertically through the 4th intercostal space along the lateral chest wall. **B,** Air-fluid interface (zeroing the stopcock) is level with the phlebostatic axis using a carpenter's or laser level.

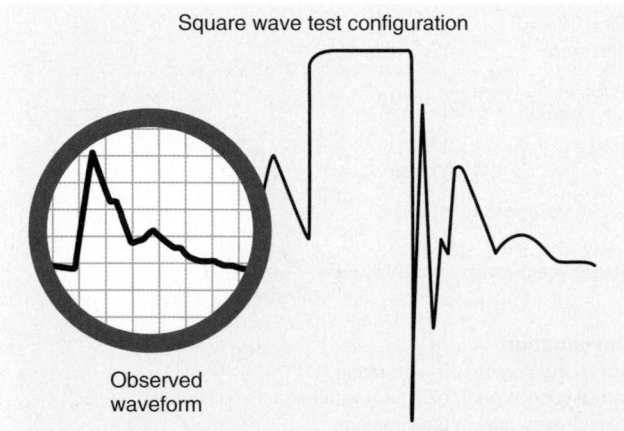

When the fast flush of the continuous flush system is activated and quickly released, a sharp upstroke terminates in a flat line at the maximal indicator on the monitor and hard copy. This is then followed by an immediate rapid downstroke extending below baseline with just 1 or 2 oscillations within 0.12 second (minimal ringing) and a quick return to a baseline. The patient's pressure waveform is also clearly defined with all components of the waveform, such as the dicrotic notch on an arterial waveform, clearly visible.

FIG. 65.5 Optimally damped system. Dynamic response test (square wave test) using the fast flush system: normal response. No adjustment in the monitoring system is needed. (From Darovic GO, Vanriper S, Vanriper J: Fluid-filled monitoring systems. In Darovic GO: *Hemodynamic monitoring,* ed 2, Philadelphia, 1995, Saunders.)

The high- and low-pressure alarms are set based on the patient's status. Various patient conditions will change the pressure tracings. In heart failure (HF), the systolic upstroke may be slower. In volume depletion, systolic pressure varies with mechanical ventilation, decreasing during inspiration. Observe simultaneous ECG and pressure tracings with dysrhythmias.

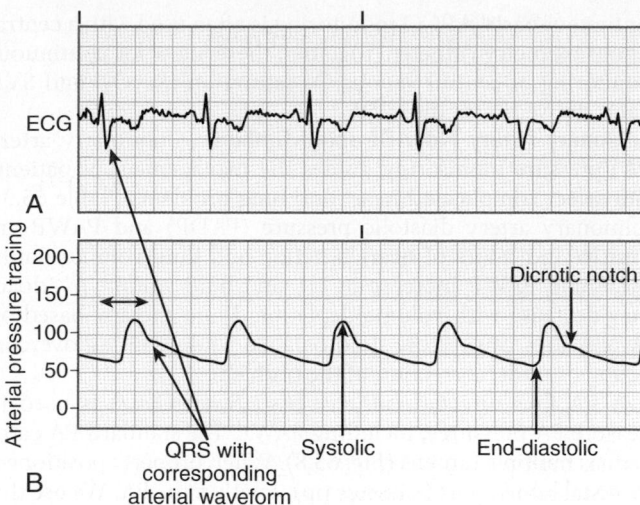

FIG. 65.6 A, Simultaneously recorded ECG tracing. **B,** Systemic arterial pressure tracing. Systolic pressure is the peak pressure. The *dicrotic notch* indicates aortic valve closure. Diastolic pressure is the lowest value before contraction. Mean pressure is the average pressure over time calculated by the monitoring equipment. (Modified from Urden LD, Stacy KM, Lough ME: *Critical care nursing: Diagnosis and management,* ed 6, St Louis, 2010, Mosby.)

TABLE 65.2 **Invasive Arterial Blood Pressure Measurement**
1. Explain the procedure to the patient.
2. Position the patient supine and flat or (if appropriate) with the head of the bed less than 45 degrees or prone.
3. Confirm that the zero reference (port of the stopcock nearest the transducer) is at the level of the phlebostatic axis (Fig. 65.4). If the reference stopcock is not taped to the patient's chest, use a leveling device to position the stopcock on a bedside pole at the point level with the phlebostatic axis.
4. Observe the monitor tracing and assess the quality of the tracing. Perform a dynamic response test (Fig. 65.5).
5. Obtain an analog printout (if available) and measure the systolic and diastolic pressures at end expiration (Fig. 65.6). If no printout is available, freeze the tracing on the oscilloscope screen and use the cursor to measure the pressures at end expiration.
6. Record the pressure measurements promptly, including (if available) the printout marked to identify the points read.

Dysrhythmias that significantly decrease arterial BP are more urgent than those that cause only a slight decrease in systolic amplitude.

Complications. Arterial lines carry the risk for hemorrhage, infection, thrombus formation, neurovascular impairment, and loss of limb. Hemorrhage is most likely to occur if the catheter dislodges or the line disconnects. To avoid this complication, use Luer-Lok connections, always check the arterial waveform, and activate alarms. If the pressure in the line falls (e.g., when the line is disconnected), the low-pressure alarm sounds immediately, allowing you to promptly correct the problem.

To limit the risk for catheter-related infection, inspect the insertion site for local signs of inflammation. Monitor the patient for signs of systemic infection. Change the pressure tubing, flush bag, and transducer every 96 hours or according to agency policy. If you suspect infection, notify the HCP, remove the catheter, and replace the equipment.

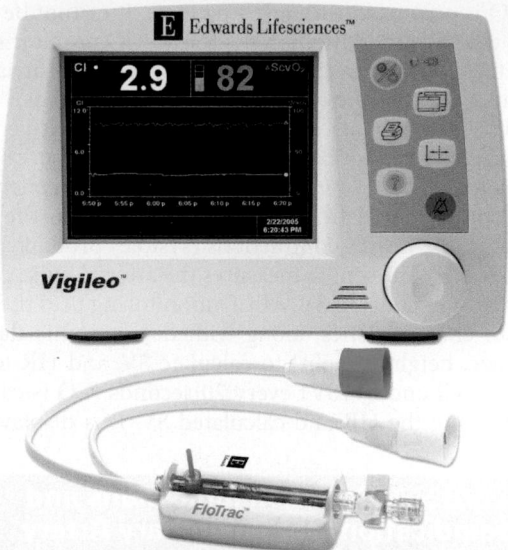

FIG. 65.7 FloTrac sensor and Vigileo monitor. (Courtesy Edwards Lifesciences, Irvine, CA.)

Circulatory impairment can result from formation of a thrombus around the catheter, release of an embolus, spasm, or occlusion of the circulation by the catheter. Before inserting a line into the radial artery, perform an *Allen test* to confirm that ulnar circulation to the hand is adequate. Apply pressure to the radial and ulnar arteries simultaneously. If the patient is able, ask the patient to open and close the hand repeatedly. The hand should blanch. Release the pressure on the ulnar artery while maintaining pressure on the radial artery. If pinkness does not return within 6 seconds, the ulnar artery is not adequate. You should not use the radial artery on that limb for line insertion.

Once the catheter is inserted, assess the neurovascular status distal to the arterial insertion site hourly. The limb with compromised arterial flow will be cool and pale, with capillary refill time longer than 3 seconds. The patient may have symptoms of neurovascular impairment (e.g., paresthesia, pain, paralysis). If present, it can result in the loss of a limb. This, this is an emergency and must be reported to the HCP at once.

To maintain line patency and limit thrombus formation, assess the flush system every 1 to 4 hours to determine that the (1) pressure bag is inflated to 300 mm Hg, (2) flush bag contains fluid, and (3) system is delivering a continuous slow (1 to 3 mL/hr) flush. Follow agency policy for adding heparin to the flush solution.[13]

Arterial Pressure–Based Cardiac Output. Arterial pressure–based cardiac output (APCO) measurement is a minimally invasive technique to determine *continuous CO* (CCO)/*continuous CI* (CCI). This technology uses a specialized sensor that attaches to a standard arterial pressure line and a monitor (Fig. 65.7).

APCO can assess a patient's ability to respond to fluids by increasing SV (*preload responsiveness*) (Table 65.1). This is determined by using SVV or by measuring the percent increase in SV after a fluid bolus.[14] SVV is the variation of the arterial pulsation caused by the heart-lung interaction. It is a sensitive indicator of preload responsiveness in certain patients. SVV helps predict whether a patient would benefit from an IV fluid challenge that may help optimize hemodynamic status.

APCO is only used with adult patients. It cannot be used in patients who are on IABP therapy. The APCO monitor may not be able to filter certain dysrhythmias, specifically atrial fibrillation, thus limiting the use of SVV in these patients.[14] SVV is used only with patients on controlled mechanical ventilation with a fixed respiratory rate and a tidal volume (V_T).

Measurements. *Arterial pressure* is the force generated by the ejection of blood from the left ventricle into the arterial circulation. The heart's contractions (systole) produce pulsatile pressure waves. The sensor measures the arterial pulse pressure, which is proportional to SV. APCO monitoring uses the arterial waveform characteristics, along with demographic data (e.g., gender, age, height, weight) to calculate SV, and HR to calculate CCO/CCI and SV/SVI every 20 seconds. CO is calculated by multiplying the HR and calculated SV. It is displayed on a continuous basis. APCO monitoring is often used with a central venous oximetry catheter. Together, these allow for continuous monitoring of central venous O_2 saturation ($ScvO_2$) and SVR that is derived from the CVP.

Pulmonary Artery Flow-Directed Catheter. Pulmonary artery (PA) pressure monitoring guides the management of patients with select complicated heart and lung problems (Table 65.3). Pulmonary artery diastolic pressure (PADP) and PAWP are sensitive indicators of heart function and fluid volume status. PADP and PAWP increase in HF and fluid volume overload. They decrease with volume depletion. Fluid therapy based on PA pressures can restore fluid balance while limiting overcorrection or undercorrection of the problem.

A PA flow-directed catheter (e.g., Swan-Ganz) is used to measure PA pressures, including PAWP. The standard PA catheter has multiple lumens (Fig. 65.8). When properly positioned, the distal lumen port (catheter tip) is within the PA. We use this port to monitor PA pressures and sample mixed venous blood (e.g., to monitor O_2 saturation).

A balloon connected to an external valve surrounds the distal lumen port. Balloon inflation has 2 purposes: (1) to allow blood to "float" the catheter forward and (2) to allow PAWP measurement. There are 1 or 2 proximal lumens, with exit ports in the right atrium or right atrium and right ventricle (if 2). The right atrium port is used for CVP measurement, injecting fluid for CO measurement, and withdrawing blood specimens. The second proximal port (if available) is for infusing fluids and drugs or for blood sampling. A temperature sensor is near the distal tip. It monitors core temperature and is used for the thermodilution method of measuring CO.[13]

An advanced technology PA catheter can continuously monitor the patient's SvO_2. CCO and right ventricular ejection fraction (RVEF) can be measured using advanced thermodilution technology. RVEF gives information about RV function and helps to assess right heart contractility. RV end-diastolic volume is assessed by dividing SV by RVEF (Table 65.1). This is a key indicator of preload.

TABLE 65.3 **Common Indications and Contraindications for Pulmonary Artery Catheterization**
Indications
• Assessment of response to therapy in patients with pulmonary hypertension and mixed types of shock
• Cardiogenic shock
• Differential diagnosis of pulmonary hypertension
• MI with complications (e.g., HF, cardiogenic shock)
• Potentially reversible systolic HF (e.g., fulminant myocarditis)
• Severe chronic HF requiring inotropic, vasopressor, and vasodilator therapy
• Transplantation workup
Contraindications
• Coagulopathy (may be overlooked in emergency situations)
• Endocardial pacemaker
• Endocarditis
• Mechanical tricuspid or pulmonic valve
• Right heart mass (e.g., thrombus, tumor)

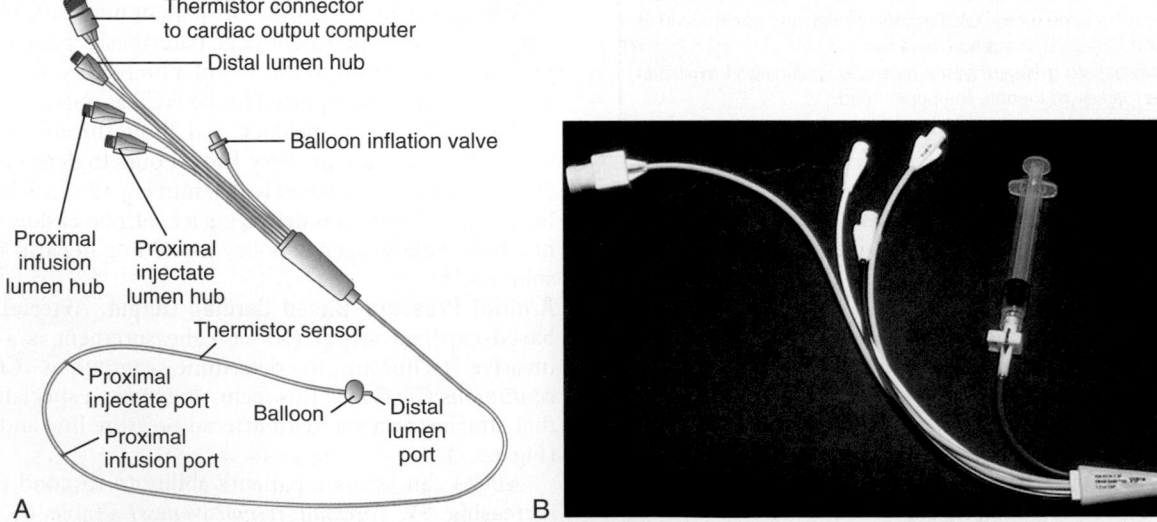

FIG. 65.8 Pulmonary artery (PA) catheter. **A,** Illustrated catheter has 5 lumens. When properly positioned, the distal lumen exit port is in the PA and the proximal lumen ports are in the right atrium and right ventricle. The distal and 1 of the proximal ports are used to measure PA and CVP, respectively. A balloon surrounds the catheter near the distal end. The balloon inflation valve is used to inflate the balloon with air to allow reading of the PAWP. A thermistor near the distal tip senses PA temperature and measures thermodilution cardiac output when solution cooler than body temperature is injected into a proximal port. **B,** Photo of an actual catheter. (*B,* Courtesy Edwards Critical Care Division, Baxter Healthcare Corporation, Santa Ana, CA.)

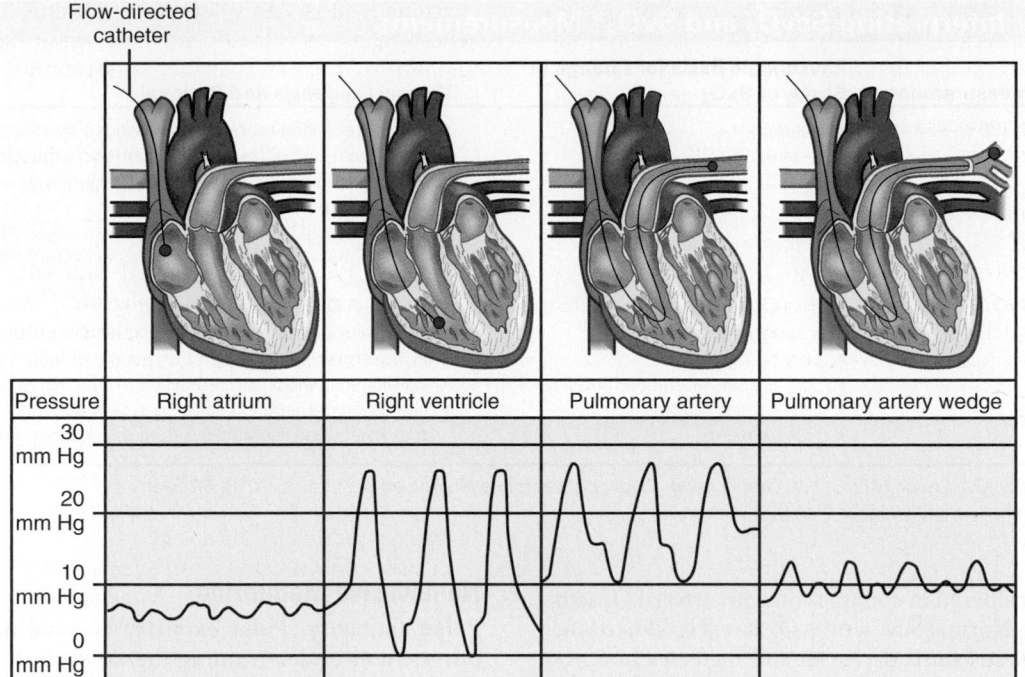

FIG. 65.9 Position of the pulmonary artery flow-directed catheter during progressive stages of insertion with corresponding pressure waveforms. (Modified from Urden LD, Stacy KM, Lough ME: *Critical care nursing: Diagnosis and management,* ed 6, St Louis, 2010, Mosby.)

The use of PA pressure monitoring has decreased dramatically. This is due, in part, to risks associated with this invasive technology (e.g., dysrhythmias, infection) and the development of less invasive techniques (e.g., APCO monitoring, bedside echocardiography).

The HCP often inserts a PA catheter at the bedside. Preparation includes arranging the monitor, cables, and infusion and pressurized flush solutions. The system is leveled and zero-referenced to the phlebostatic axis. Note the patient's electrolyte, acid-base, oxygenation, and coagulation status. Imbalances such as hypokalemia, hypomagnesemia, hypoxemia, or acidosis can make the heart more irritable. This can increase the risk for ventricular dysrhythmia during catheter insertion. Coagulopathy increases the risk for hemorrhage.

During insertion, a key nursing role is to observe the characteristic waveforms on the monitor as the HCP moves the catheter through the heart to the PA (Fig. 65.9). Monitor the ECG continuously because of the risk for dysrhythmias, especially when the catheter reaches the right ventricle. After insertion and before using the PA catheter, obtain a chest x-ray to confirm catheter placement. Note and record the measurement at the exit point. Apply an occlusive sterile dressing and change it according to agency policy.

Central Venous or Right Atrial Pressure Measurement. CVP is a measurement of right ventricular preload and reflects fluid volume status. We most often measure it with a central venous catheter placed in the internal jugular or subclavian vein. It can be measured with a PA catheter using the proximal lumen in the right atrium. CVP waveforms (Fig. 65.10) are similar to PAWP waveforms. CVP is measured as a mean pressure at the end of expiration.[13] A high CVP indicates right ventricular failure or volume overload. A low CVP indicates hypovolemia.

Venous Oxygen Saturation Monitoring. In critically ill patients, measuring the O_2 saturation of hemoglobin in venous blood

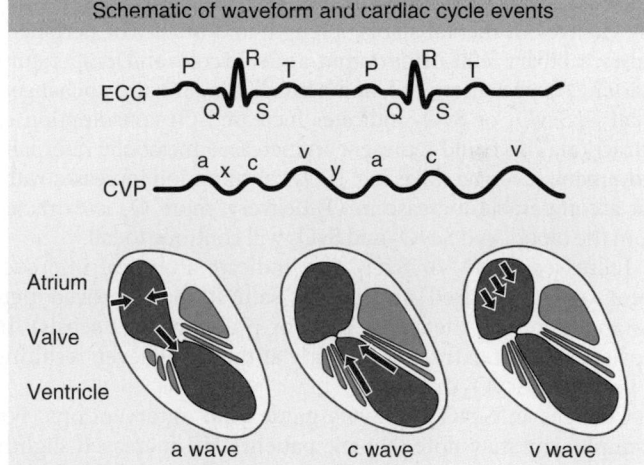

FIG. 65.10 Cardiac events that produce the CVP waveform with *a, c,* and *v* waves. The *a* wave represents atrial contraction. The *x* descent represents atrial relaxation. The *c* wave represents the bulging of the closed tricuspid valve into the right atrium during ventricular systole. The *v* wave represents atrial filling. The *y* descent represents opening of the tricuspid valve and filling of the ventricle. (Modified from Urden LD, Stacy KM, Lough ME: *Critical care nursing: Diagnosis and management,* ed 6, St Louis, 2010, Mosby.)

helps to determine the adequacy of tissue oxygenation. The O_2 saturation of venous blood from the CVP catheter is called *central venous O_2 saturation* ($ScvO_2$). Similarly, the O_2 saturation of blood from the PA catheter is the *mixed venous O_2 saturation* (SvO_2). $ScvO_2$ and SvO_2 reflect the balance among oxygenation of the arterial blood, tissue perfusion, and tissue O_2 consumption.[13] This gives a global indicator of the balance between O_2 delivery and O_2 consumption. $ScvO_2$ and SvO_2 are useful in assessing hemodynamic status and response to treatments or

TABLE 65.4 Interpreting ScvO₂ and SvO₂* Measurements

ScvO₂ and SvO₂ Measurement	Physiologic Basis for Change in ScvO₂ or SvO₂	Clinical Diagnosis and Rationale
High ScvO₂ or SvO₂ (80%–95%)	↑ O_2 supply ↓ O_2 demand	• Patient receiving more O_2 than needed by clinical condition • Anesthesia, which causes sedation and ↓ muscle movement • Hypothermia, which ↓ metabolic demand (e.g., with cardiopulmonary bypass) • Sepsis caused by ↓ ability of tissues to use O_2 at the cellular level • False high positive because pulmonary artery catheter is wedged in a pulmonary capillary (SvO₂ only)
Normal ScvO₂ or SvO₂ (60%–80%) Low ScvO₂ or SvO₂ (<60%)	Normal O_2 supply and metabolic demand ↓ O_2 supply caused by • Low hemoglobin • Low arterial saturation (SaO₂) • Low cardiac output • ↑ O_2 demand	• Balanced O_2 supply and demand • Anemia or bleeding with compromised cardiopulmonary system • Hypoxemia resulting from ↓ O_2 supply or lung disease • Cardiogenic shock caused by left ventricular pump failure • Metabolic demand exceeds O_2 supply in conditions that ↑ muscle movement and metabolic rate (e.g., seizures, fever)

Source: Urden LD, Stacy KM, Lough ME: *Critical care nursing: Diagnosis and management,* ed 8, St Louis, 2018, Elsevier.
*ScvO₂ values are generally slightly higher than SvO₂ values.

activities when considered in conjunction with arterial O_2 saturation (Table 65.4). Normal ScvO₂ or SvO₂ at rest is 60% to 80%.

Carefully review sustained decreases and increases in ScvO₂ or SvO₂. Decreased ScvO₂ or SvO₂ may indicate decreased arterial oxygenation, low CO, low hemoglobin level, or increased O_2 consumption or extraction. If the ScvO₂ or SvO₂ falls below 60%, determine which of these factors has changed. Observe for changes in arterial oxygenation (e.g., monitor pulse oximetry, ABGs) and indirectly assess CO and tissue perfusion. This is done by noting any changes in mental status, strength and quality of peripheral pulses, capillary refill, urine output, and skin color and temperature. If arterial oxygenation, CO, and hemoglobin level are unchanged, a fall in ScvO₂ or SvO₂ indicates increased O_2 consumption or extraction. This could represent an increased metabolic rate, pain, movement, fever, or shivering. If O_2 consumption increases without a comparable increase in O_2 delivery, more O_2 is extracted from the blood, and ScvO₂ and SvO₂ will continue to fall.[13]

Increased ScvO₂ or SvO₂ may indicate a clinical improvement (e.g., increased arterial O_2 saturation, improved perfusion, decreased metabolic rate) or problem (e.g., sepsis). In sepsis, O_2 is not extracted properly at the tissue level, resulting in increased ScvO₂ or SvO₂.

Changes in ScvO₂ or SvO₂ guide your interventions. For example, you may note that the patient's HR increased slightly during repositioning but that the ScvO₂ remained stable. In this case, you would conclude that the patient tolerated the position change. If the ScvO₂ dropped, this would be a sign to stop the activity until the ScvO₂ returned to baseline.

In many cases, as activity or metabolism increases, HR and CO increase, and ScvO₂ or SvO₂ stays constant or varies slightly. However, critically ill patients often have conditions (e.g., HF, shock) that prevent substantial increases in CO. In these cases, ScvO₂ or SvO₂ can be a useful indicator of the balance between O_2 delivery and consumption.

❓ CHECK YOUR PRACTICE

You are caring for a 38-yr-old woman admitted with sepsis due to a ruptured ectopic pregnancy. She has CVP and ScvO₂ monitoring in place. Trends in ScvO₂ have shown a slow, steady decline, with the most recent reading being 55%.
• What assessment data would you obtain to explain this change?

Noninvasive Monitoring

Pulse Oximetry. *Pulse oximetry* is a noninvasive, continuous method of determining the O_2 saturation of hemoglobin (SpO₂). Monitoring SpO₂ may reduce the frequency of ABG sampling (see Chapter 25). SpO₂ is normally 95% to 100%. Accurate SpO₂ measurements may be hard to obtain on patients who are hypothermic, are receiving IV vasopressor therapy (e.g., norepinephrine), or have hypoperfusion or vasoconstriction (e.g., shock).

A common use for pulse oximetry is to assess the effectiveness of O_2 therapy. Decreased SpO₂ indicates inadequate oxygenation of the blood in the pulmonary capillaries. You can correct this by increasing the fraction of inspired O_2 (FIO₂) and evaluating the patient's response. Similarly, use SpO₂ to monitor how the patient tolerates decreases in FIO₂ and responds to interventions. For example, if SpO₂ falls when you place the patient in a left lateral recumbent position, plan position changes that pose less risk for the patient.

Impedance Cardiography. *Impedance cardiography (ICG)* is a continuous or intermittent, noninvasive method of obtaining CO and assessing thoracic fluid status. Based on the concepts of *impedance* (the resistance to the flow of electric current [Ω]), ICG uses 4 sets of external electrodes to deliver a high-frequency, low-amplitude current that is like that used in apnea monitors. Blood is an excellent conductor of electricity (lower impedance), and pulsatile blood flow generates electrical impedance changes. ICG measures the change in impedance (dΩ) in the ascending aorta and left ventricle over time (dt). It is represented as dΩ/dt. Ωo is the measurement of the average impedance of the fluid in the thorax. We can calculate impedance-based hemodynamic parameters (CO, SV, SVR) from Ωo, dΩ/dt, MAP, CVP, and ECG.

Major uses of ICG include (1) detecting early signs and symptoms of pulmonary or cardiac problems, (2) determining cardiac or pulmonary cause of shortness of breath, (3) evaluating the cause and managing hypotension, (4) monitoring after removing a PA catheter or justifying insertion of a PA catheter, (5) evaluating drug therapy, and (6) diagnosing rejection after heart transplantation. ICG is not accurate in patients who have generalized edema or third spacing because the excess volume interferes with the signals.

❖ NURSING MANAGEMENT: HEMODYNAMIC MONITORING

Assessment of hemodynamic status requires integrating data from many sources and trending data over time. Comprehensive nursing observations give important clues about the patient's hemodynamic status.

Begin by obtaining baseline data about the patient's general appearance, level of consciousness, skin color and temperature, vital signs, peripheral pulses, capillary refill, and urine output. Does the patient appear tired, weak, exhausted? There may be too little cardiac reserve to sustain even minimum activity. Pallor, cool skin, and decreased pulses may indicate decreased CO. Changes in mental status may reflect problems with cerebral perfusion or oxygenation. Monitor urine output to determine the adequacy of perfusion to the kidneys. The patient with decreased perfusion to the GI tract may develop hypoactive or absent bowel sounds. If the patient is bleeding and developing shock, the BP may be stable at first. The patient may become increasingly pale and cool from peripheral vasoconstriction. Conversely, the patient with septic shock may be warm and pink yet have tachycardia and BP instability. Increased HRs are common in stressed, compromised, critically ill patients. However, sustained tachycardia increases myocardial O_2 demand and can result in decreased CO.

Always correlate observational data with data obtained from technology (e.g., ECG, arterial and PA pressures, $ScvO_2$, SvO_2). Single hemodynamic values are rarely helpful. You must monitor trends in these values over time and evaluate the whole clinical picture with the goals of recognizing early clues and intervening before problems escalate.

CIRCULATORY ASSIST DEVICES

Mechanical **circulatory assist devices (CADs)** are used to decrease cardiac work and improve organ perfusion in patients with HF when conventional drug therapy is no longer adequate. CADs include **intraaortic balloon pumps (IABPs)** and left or right ventricular assist devices (VADs).

The type of device used depends on the extent and nature of the heart problem. CADs provide support in 3 situations: (1) the left, right, or both ventricles require support while recovering from acute injury (e.g., postcardiotomy); (2) the patient must be stabilized before surgical repair of the heart (e.g., a ruptured septum); and (3) the heart has failed, and the patient is awaiting heart transplantation. All CADs decrease cardiac workload, increase myocardial perfusion, and augment circulation.

Intraaortic Balloon Pump

The IABP provides temporary circulatory assistance by reducing afterload (through reducing systolic pressure) and augmenting the aortic diastolic pressure. This improves coronary blood flow. Table 65.5 lists common indications for an IABP.

The IABP consists of a sausage-shaped balloon, a pump that inflates and deflates the balloon, a control panel for synchronizing the balloon inflation to the cardiac cycle, and fail-safe features. The balloon is inserted percutaneously or surgically into the femoral artery. It is moved toward the heart and placed in the descending thoracic aorta just below the left subclavian artery and above the renal arteries (Fig. 65.11). After placement, an x-ray confirms the position.

A pneumatic device fills the balloon with helium at the start of diastole (immediately after aortic valve closure) and deflates

TABLE 65.5 Common Indications and Contraindications for IABP Therapy

Indications
- Acute MI with any of the following*:
  - Ventricular aneurysm accompanied by ventricular dysrhythmias
  - Acute ventricular septal defect
  - Acute mitral valve dysfunction
  - Cardiogenic shock
  - Refractory chest pain with or without ventricular dysrhythmias
- High-risk interventional cardiology procedures
- Preoperative, intraoperative, and postoperative cardiac surgery (e.g., prophylaxis before surgery, failure to wean from cardiopulmonary bypass, left ventricular failure after cardiopulmonary bypass)
- Unstable angina unresponsive to drug therapy
- Short-term bridge to heart transplantation

Contraindications
- Abdominal aortic and thoracic aneurysms
- Generalized peripheral vascular disease (e.g., aortoiliac disease)†
- Irreversible brain damage
- Major coagulopathy (e.g., disseminated intravascular coagulation [DIC])
- Moderate to severe aortic insufficiency
- Terminal or untreatable diseases of any major organ system

*Allows time for emergent angiography and corrective heart surgery to be done.
†May inhibit placement of balloon and is considered a relative contraindication; sheathless insertion may be used.

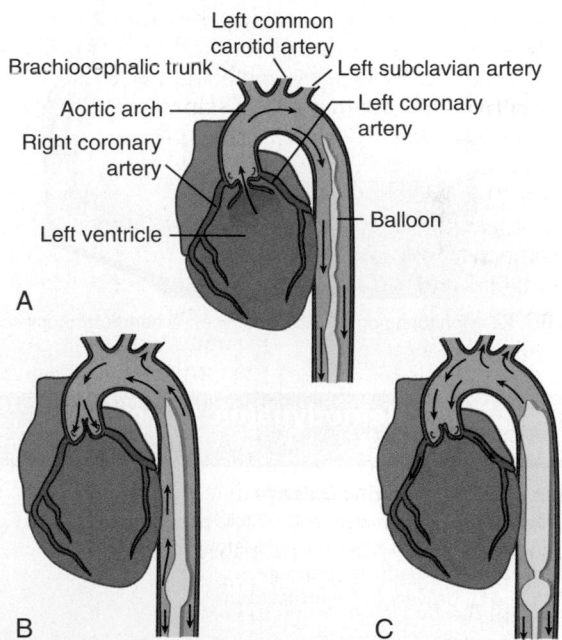

FIG. 65.11 IABP. **A,** During systole the balloon is deflated, which helps with ejection of blood into the periphery. **B,** In early diastole, the balloon begins to inflate. **C,** In late diastole, the balloon is totally inflated, which augments aortic pressure and increases the coronary perfusion pressure. This increases coronary and cerebral blood flow.

it just before the next systole. The ECG is the trigger used to start the deflation on the upstroke of the R wave (of the QRS) and inflation on the T wave. The dicrotic notch of the arterial pressure tracing is used to refine timing (Fig. 65.12).

IABP therapy is known as *counterpulsation* because the timing of balloon inflation is opposite the ventricular contraction. The IABP assist ratio is 1:1 in the acute phase of treatment, meaning that 1 IABP cycle of inflation and deflation occurs for every heartbeat.

Effects of Counterpulsation. In late diastole when the balloon is totally inflated, blood is forcibly displaced distal to the extremities and proximal to the coronary arteries and main branches of the aortic arch. Diastolic arterial pressure rises (diastolic augmentation). This increases coronary artery perfusion pressure and perfusion of vital organs. The rise in coronary artery perfusion pressure increases blood flow to the myocardium. The balloon is rapidly deflated just before systole. This creates a vacuum that causes aortic pressure to drop. When aortic resistance to left ventricular ejection is reduced (reduced afterload), the left ventricle empties more easily and completely. SV increases while myocardial O_2 consumption decreases. Table 65.6 describes the hemodynamic effects of IABP therapy.

Complications With IABP Therapy. Vascular injuries, such as aortic dissection and compromised distal circulation, are common with IABP therapy. Thrombus and embolus formation add to the risk for circulatory compromise to the extremity. The action of the IABP can destroy platelets and cause thrombocytopenia. Movement of the balloon can block the left subclavian, renal, or mesenteric arteries. This can result in a weak or absent radial pulse, decreased urine output, and reduced or absent bowel sounds. Patients receiving IABP therapy are prone to infection. Local or systemic signs of infection require catheter removal. To reduce these complications, perform cardiovascular, neurovascular, and hemodynamic assessments every 15 to 60 minutes, depending on the patient's status (Table 65.7).[13]

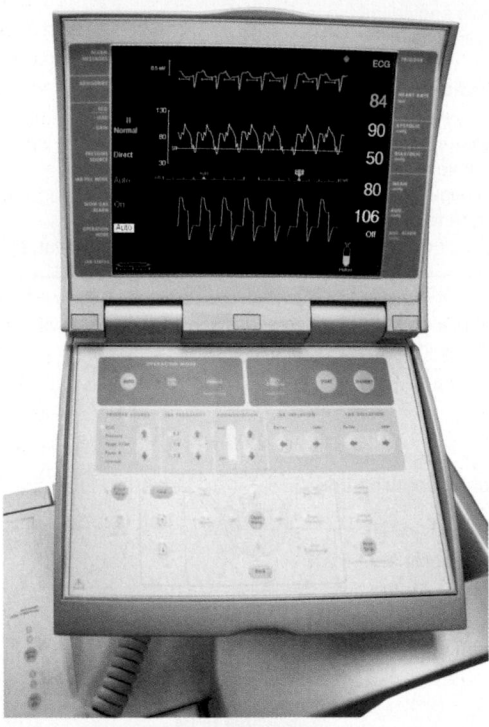

FIG 65.12 Monitoring on an IABP machine. (© beerkoff/iStock.com.)

TABLE 65.6 Hemodynamic Effects of Counterpulsation

Effects of Inflation During Diastole
- ↑ Diastolic pressure (may exceed systolic pressure)
- ↑ Pressure in the aortic root during diastole
- ↑ Coronary artery perfusion pressure
- Improved O_2 delivery to the myocardium
  - ↓ Angina
  - ↓ ECG evidence of ischemia
  - ↓ Ventricular ectopy

Effects of Deflation During Systole
- ↓ Afterload
- ↓ Peak systolic pressure
- ↓ Myocardial O_2 consumption
- ↑ Stroke volume, possibly associated with:
  - Improved mentation
  - Warm skin
  - ↑ Urine output
  - ↓ HR
- ↑ Forward flow of blood, ↓ preload
  - ↓ Pulmonary artery pressures, including PAWP
  - ↓ Crackles

TABLE 65.7 Managing Complications of IABP Therapy

Potential Complications	Nursing Interventions
Balloon leak or rupture	• Prepare for emergent removal and possible reinsertion.
Arterial trauma caused by insertion or displacement of balloon	• Assess and mark peripheral pulses before inserting balloon to use as baseline for assessing pulses after insertion. • Assess perfusion to both upper and lower extremities at least every hour. • Measure urine output at least every hour (occlusion of renal arteries causes severe ↓ in urine output). • Observe arterial waveforms for sudden changes. • Keep head of bed no higher than 45 degrees. • Do not flex cannulated leg at the hip. • Immobilize cannulated leg to prevent flexion using a draw sheet tucked under the mattress, soft ankle restraint, or knee immobilizer.
Hematologic problems due to platelet aggregation along the balloon (e.g., thrombocytopenia)	• Monitor coagulation profiles, hematocrit, and platelet count.
Hemorrhage from insertion site	• Check site for bleeding at least every hour. • Monitor vital signs for signs of hypovolemia with each check.
Infection at site	• Use strict aseptic technique for insertion and dressing changes for all lines. • Cover all insertion sites with occlusive dressings. • Give prescribed prophylactic antibiotic for entire course of therapy.
Issues related to immobilization (e.g., pressure injuries)	• Reposition patient at least q2hr, being careful to maintain proper positioning. • Use appropriate pressure-relieving devices.
VTE caused by trauma, balloon obstruction of blood flow distal to catheter	• Give prophylactic heparin therapy (if ordered). • Assess pulses, urine output, and level of consciousness at least every hour. • Check circulation, sensation, and movement in both legs at least every hour.

Mechanical complications from IABP are rare but can occur. Improper timing of balloon inflation may cause increased afterload, decreased CO, myocardial ischemia, and increased myocardial O_2 demand. If the balloon develops a leak, the pump will automatically stop. The catheter needs to be promptly removed to avoid an embolus. Signs of a leak include less effective augmentation, repeated alarms for gas loss, and blood backing up into the catheter. A malfunction of the balloon or console triggers fail-safe alarms and automatically shuts down the unit. You must be able to recognize complications immediately and report them to the HCP.

The patient with an IABP is relatively immobile, limited to side-lying or supine positions with the head of bed (HOB) elevated less than 45 degrees. The patient may be receiving mechanical ventilation and will likely have multiple invasive lines. All of this increases the risk for pressure injury and makes it hard to find comfortable positioning. The patient may have sleep problems and anxiety. Adequate sedation, pain relief, skin care, and comfort measures are essential.

As the patient improves, circulatory support provided by the IABP is gradually reduced. Weaning involves reducing the IABP assist ratio from 1:1 to 1:2 and assessing the patient's response. If the patient remains stable, the ratio is changed from 1:2 to 1:3 until the IABP catheter is removed. Pumping must continue until the line is removed even if the patient is stable. This reduces the risk for clot formation around the catheter.

Ventricular Assist Devices

A ventricular assist device (VAD) provides short- and long-term support for the failing heart and allows more mobility than the IABP. VADs are inserted into the path of flowing blood to augment or replace the action of the ventricle. Some VADs are implanted internally (e.g., peritoneum). Others are positioned externally. A typical VAD shunts blood from the left atrium or ventricle to the device and then to the aorta. Some VADs provide right or biventricular support (Fig. 65.13).

Failure to wean from cardiopulmonary bypass (CPB) after surgery is a key indicator for VAD support. VADs can support patients with HF caused by MI and patients awaiting heart transplantation. A VAD is a temporary device that can partially or totally support circulation until the heart recovers or a donor heart is found.

Appropriate patient selection for VAD therapy is critical. Indications include (1) failure to wean from CPB or postcardiotomy cardiogenic shock, (2) a bridge to recovery or heart transplantation, and (3) patients with New York Heart Association

Class IV heart disease (see Table 34.3) who have failed medical therapy. Relative contraindications for VAD therapy include (1) BSA less than manufacturer's limit (e.g., 1.2 m^2), (2) irreversible end-stage organ damage, and (3) co-morbidities that would limit life expectancy to less than 3 years.[13]

Implantable Artificial Heart

Every year, about 2200 patients receive heart transplants, yet the demand for donor hearts far exceeds the supply. Research on mechanical CADs has led to the development of a fully implantable artificial heart that can sustain the body's circulatory system. This device can provide a bridge to transplantation or replace the hearts of patients who are not eligible for a transplant and have no other treatment options. A major advantage of the artificial heart is that patients do not need immunosuppression therapy and thus avoid its inevitable, long-term effects. Risks include infection, thrombus, and stroke. Patients need lifelong anticoagulation and ongoing care from the interprofessional team.[15]

❖ NURSING AND INTERPROFESSIONAL MANAGEMENT: CIRCULATORY ASSIST DEVICES

The patient with an IABP needs highly skilled care. Perform frequent and thorough cardiovascular assessments. These include measuring hemodynamic parameters (e.g., arterial BP, CO/CI, SVR), auscultating the heart and lungs, and evaluating the ECG (e.g., rate, rhythm). Assess for adequate tissue perfusion (e.g., skin color and temperature, mental status, capillary refill, peripheral pulses, urine output, bowel sounds) at regular intervals. IABP therapy should improve these findings.

Nursing care of the patient with a VAD is like that of the patient with an IABP. Observe the patient for bleeding, cardiac tamponade, ventricular failure, infection, dysrhythmias, renal failure, hemolysis, and VTE. The patient with VAD may be mobile and need an activity plan. In some cases, patients with VADs may go home. Preparation for discharge is complex and needs in-depth teaching about the device and support equipment (e.g., battery chargers). A competent caregiver must always be present.

Ideally, patients with CADs will recover, receive an artificial heart, or undergo heart transplantation. However, many patients die, or the decision is made to no longer seek treatment and death follows. Both the patient and caregiver need emotional support. Consult other team members, such as social workers or clergy, as needed.

NONINVASIVE VENTILATION

At times, patients may need ventilator support, without the placement of an ET tube. Noninvasive ventilation (NIV) uses a mask, instead of an ET tube, to oxygenate and ventilate a patient. These masks can be full face or a nasal piece. There are 2 common modes used for NIV.

Continuous Positive Airway Pressure

Continuous positive airway pressure (CPAP) restores functional residual capacity (FRC) and is similar to positive end-expiratory pressure (PEEP). However, the pressure in CPAP is delivered continuously during spontaneous breathing, preventing the patient's airway pressure from falling to 0. For example, if CPAP is 5 cm H_2O, airway pressure during expiration is 5 cm H_2O. During inspiration, we generate 1 to 2 cm H_2O of negative pressure. This reduces airway pressure to 3 or 4 cm H_2O.

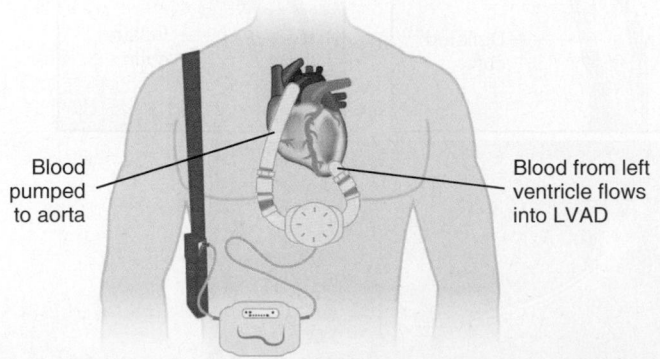

FIG. 65.13 Schematic diagram of a biventricular assist device (BVAD). (From Urden LD, Stacy KM, Lough ME: *Critical care nursing: Diagnosis and management*, ed 8, St Louis, 2018, Mosby.)

Blood pumped to aorta

Blood from left ventricle flows into LVAD

CPAP is often used to treat obstructive sleep apnea. It is a non-invasive modality, delivered through a tight-fitting face mask, nasal mask, or nasal pillows. CPAP increases *work of breathing* (WOB) because the patient must forcibly exhale against the CPAP. Therefore it must be used with caution in patients with myocardial compromise. The patient must be able to remove a mask independently due to the risk for vomiting. Those with increased secretions or the inability to control their airway are not good candidates for CPAP due to the risk for aspiration.[13]

Bilevel Positive Airway Pressure

In addition to O_2, *bilevel positive airway pressure (BiPAP)* provides 2 levels of positive pressure support: higher inspiratory positive airway pressure and lower expiratory positive airway pressure.[13] Like CPAP, the patient must be able to spontaneously breathe and cooperate with this treatment (Fig. 65.14).

BiPAP is used for COPD patients with HF and acute respiratory failure and for patients with sleep apnea. Its use after extubation can help prevent reintubation. Patients with shock, altered mental status, or increased airway secretions cannot use BiPAP because of the risk for aspiration and the inability to remove the mask.

ARTIFICIAL AIRWAYS

Patients in the ICU often need mechanical assistance to maintain airway patency. Inserting a tube into the trachea, bypassing upper airway and laryngeal structures, creates an artificial airway. The tube is placed into the trachea via the mouth or nose past the larynx (**endotracheal [ET] intubation**) or through a stoma in the neck *(tracheostomy)*. Fig. 65.15 shows the parts of an ET tube.

ET intubation is common in ICU patients requiring mechanical ventilation for short periods of time (e.g., less than 2 weeks). Other indications for intubation include (1) upper airway obstruction (e.g., burns, tumor, bleeding), (2) apnea, (3) high risk for aspiration, (4) ineffective clearance of secretions, and (5) respiratory distress. ET intubation is done quickly and safely at the bedside by an HCP or RT.

A *tracheotomy* is a surgical procedure that is done when the need for an artificial airway is expected to be prolonged. Early tracheotomy (done within 10 days) appears to have advantages over delayed tracheotomy. These include fewer ventilator dependent days, reduced length of stays, decreased pain, and improved communication.[16] Chapter 26 discusses tracheostomy tubes and related nursing management.

Endotracheal Tubes

In *oral intubation,* the ET tube is passed through the mouth and vocal cords and into the trachea with the aid of a laryngoscope or a bronchoscope. Oral ET intubation is preferred for most emergencies because the airway can be secured rapidly. A larger diameter tube is used. A larger tube reduces the WOB because of less airway resistance. It is easier to remove secretions and perform bronchoscopy, if needed. In *nasal ET intubation,* the ET is placed blindly (i.e., without seeing the larynx) through the nose, nasopharynx, and vocal cords. We rarely use nasal ET intubation. It may be done when oral intubation is not possible (e.g., unstable cervical spine injury, dental abscess, epiglottitis).

There are risks associated with oral ET intubation. It is hard to place the tube with limited head and neck mobility

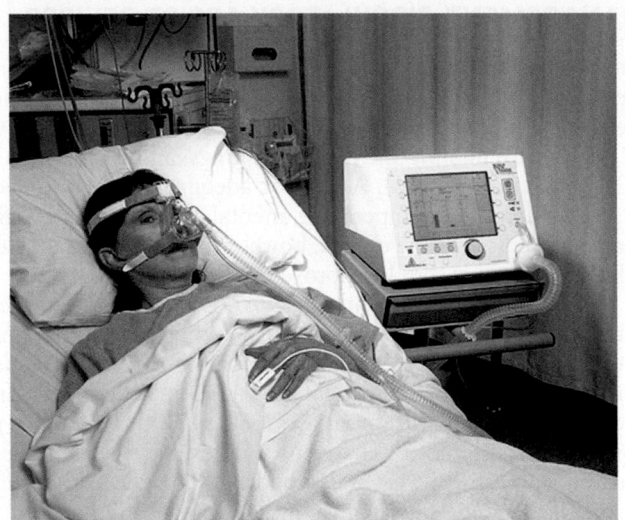

FIG. 65.14 BiPAP delivered through a face mask. (Courtesy Respironics Inc., Murrysville, PA.)

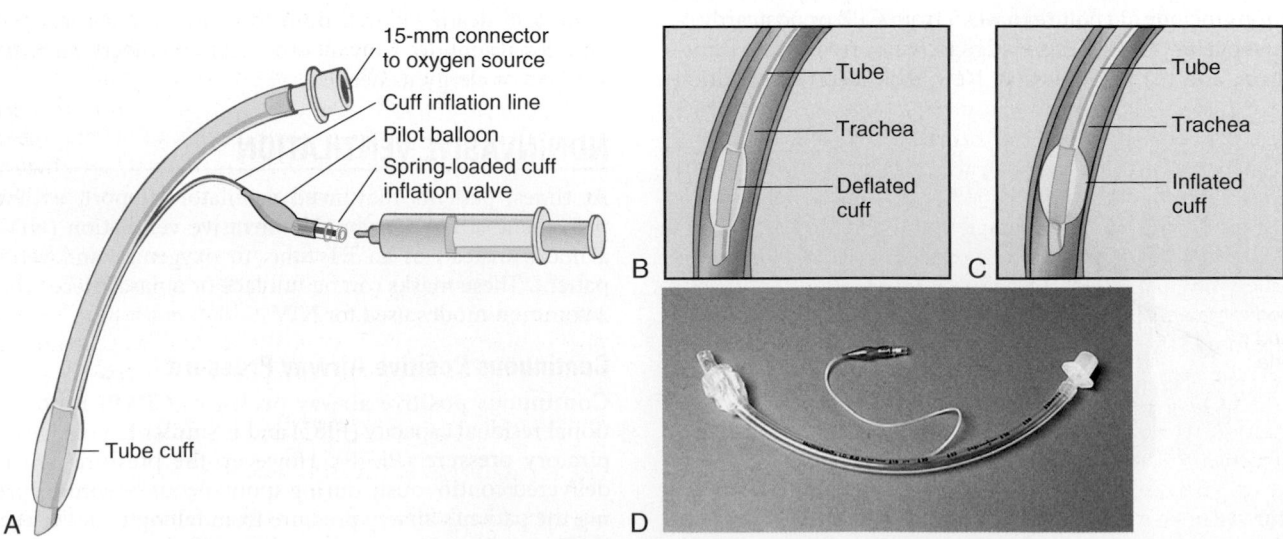

FIG. 65.15 Endotracheal tube. **A**, Parts of an endotracheal tube. **B**, Tube in place with cuff deflated. **C**, Tube in place with the cuff inflated. **D**, Photo of tube before placement. (*A,* From Beare PG, Myers JL: *Adult health nursing,* ed 3, St Louis, 1998, Mosby.)

(e.g., spinal cord injury). Teeth can be chipped or accidentally removed during the procedure. Salivation increases, and swallowing is difficult. Patients can obstruct the ET tube by biting down on the tube. Sedation, along with a bite block or oropharyngeal airway, may be used to prevent obstruction. Mouth care is a challenge because of limited space in the oral cavity.

Endotracheal Intubation Procedure

Unless ET intubation is emergent, consent for the procedure is obtained. Tell the patient and caregiver the reason for ET intubation and steps in the procedure. Explain that, while intubated, the patient will not be able to speak, but that you will provide other means of communication. Tell them that the patient's hands may have removable mitts placed or wrists may have soft restraints placed to remind them not to touch the airway.

Have a self-inflating *bag-valve-mask* (BVM) (e.g., *Ambu bag*) attached to O_2, suctioning equipment ready at the bedside, and IV access. The BVM has a reservoir that is filled with O_2 so that it delivers concentrations of 90% to 95%. The slower the bag is deflated and inflated, the higher the O_2 concentration that is delivered. Assemble and check the equipment, remove the patient's dentures or partial plates (for oral intubation), and give medications as ordered. Premedication varies depending on the patient's level of consciousness (e.g., awake, obtunded), urgency (e.g., emergent, nonemergent), and the HCP's preferences.

For oral intubation, place the patient supine with the head extended and the neck flexed ("sniffing position"). This position allows the HCP to better see the vocal cords. For nasal intubation, the nasal passages may be sprayed with a local anesthetic and vasoconstrictor (e.g., lidocaine with epinephrine) to reduce trauma and bleeding. Before intubation is started, preoxygenate the patient using the BVM and 100% O_2 for 3 to 5 minutes. Each intubation attempt is limited to less than 30 seconds. Ventilate the patient between successive attempts using the BVM and 100% O_2.

Rapid-sequence intubation (RSI) is the rapid, concurrent administration of both a sedative and a paralytic drug during emergency airway management to induce unconsciousness for intubation. It decreases the risks for aspiration and injury to the patient. RSI is not indicated in patients who are in cardiac arrest or have a known difficult airway. A sedative-hypnotic-amnesic (e.g., propofol, etomidate [Amidate]) is given to induce unconsciousness, along with a rapid-onset opioid (e.g., fentanyl) to blunt the pain of the procedure. This is followed with a drug (e.g., rocuronium) to produce skeletal muscle paralysis.[17] Monitor the patient's O_2 status during the procedure with pulse oximetry. Adhere to the agency policy about RSI medication administration.

After intubation, inflate the cuff. Confirm the placement of the ET tube while continuing to manually ventilate the patient using the BVM with 100% O_2. Use an $EtCO_2$ detector to confirm proper placement by noting the presence of exhaled CO_2 from the lungs (Fig. 65.16). Place the detector between the BVM and ET tube and look for a color change (indicating the presence of CO_2) or a number. At least 5 or 6 exhalations with a consistent CO_2 level must be present to confirm tube placement in the trachea.[13] Auscultate the lungs for bilateral breath sounds and the epigastrium for the absence of air sounds. Observe the chest for symmetric chest wall movement. SpO_2 should be stable or improved.

If the findings support proper ET tube placement, connect the ET tube to a mechanical ventilator and secure the tube per

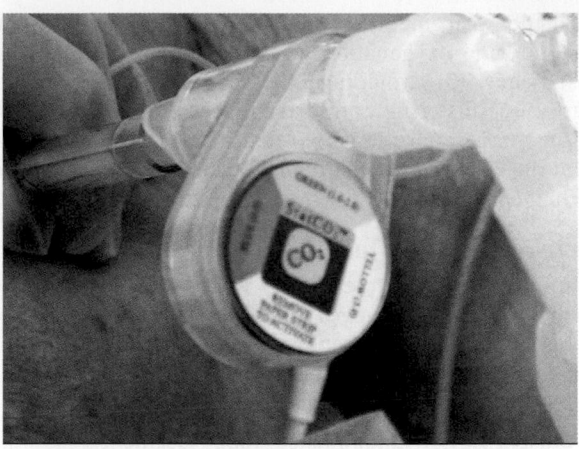

FIG. 65.16 Use an $EtCO_2$ detector to confirm proper placement of an endotracheal tube. (From Thomsen TW, Setnik GS: Orotracheal intubation, *Procedures Consult*, 2017.)

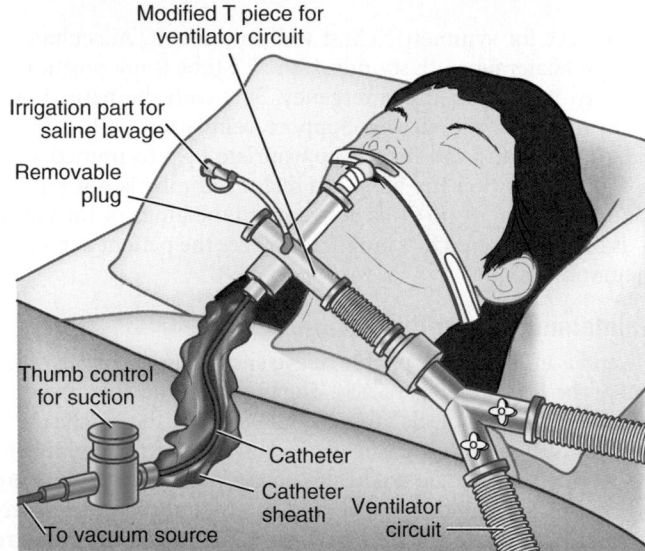

FIG. 65.17 Endotracheal tube secured to a closed tracheal suction system.

agency policy (Fig. 65.17). Suction the ET tube and pharynx. Insert a bite block, if needed, and secure it separately from the ET tube to the face. Obtain a chest x-ray to confirm tube location (2 to 6 cm above the carina in the adult). This position allows the patient to move the neck without moving the tube or causing it to enter the right mainstem bronchus. Once proper positioning is confirmed with x-ray, record and mark the position of the tube at the lip or teeth or nose.

Obtain ABGs 15 to 30 minutes after intubation to determine baseline oxygenation and ventilation status. ABG values are used to guide oxygenation and ventilation changes. Continuous pulse oximetry gives data about arterial oxygenation. $EtCO_2$ monitoring provides data related to ventilation.

❖ NURSING AND INTERPROFESSIONAL MANAGEMENT: ARTIFICIAL AIRWAY

Managing a patient with an artificial airway is often a shared responsibility between you and the RT. Agency policy dictates specific management tasks. Nursing responsibilities for the patient with an artificial airway may include: (1) maintaining correct tube placement, (2) maintaining proper cuff inflation, (3) monitoring oxygenation and ventilation, (4) maintaining tube patency, (5) providing oral care and maintaining skin integrity, (6) fostering comfort and communication, and (7) assessing for complications. See eNursing Care Plan 65.1 for the patient on a mechanical ventilator (available on the website for this chapter).

◆ Maintaining Correct Tube Placement

Continuously monitor the patient with an ET tube for proper placement. If the tube moves or is dislodged, it could end up in the pharynx or enter the esophagus or right mainstem bronchus (thus ventilating only the right lung).

> **! SAFETY ALERT Endotracheal Tube Placement**
> - Maintain proper ET tube position by recording and marking the position of the tube at the lip or teeth (usually 21 cm for women, 23 cm for men).
> - Confirm that the mark stays constant while at rest and during patient care, repositioning, and transport.

Observe for symmetric chest wall movement. Auscultate to confirm bilateral breath sounds. If the ET tube is not positioned properly, it is an airway emergency. Stay with the patient and try to maintain the airway. Support ventilation with a BVM and 100% O_2 and call for the appropriate help to immediately assess or reposition the tube. If a dislodged tube is not repositioned, minimal or no O_2 is delivered to the lungs or the entire V_T is being delivered to 1 lung. This places the patient at risk for pneumothorax.

◆ Maintaining Proper Cuff Inflation

The cuff is an inflatable, pliable sleeve encircling the lower, outer wall of the ET tube (Fig. 65.15). The high-volume, low-pressure cuff stabilizes and "seals" the ET tube within the trachea and prevents escape of ventilating gases. However, excess volume in the cuff can damage the tracheal mucosa. To prevent this, inflate the cuff with air and measure and monitor the cuff pressure. To ensure adequate tracheal perfusion, maintain cuff pressure at 20 to 25 cm H_2O.[13] Measure and record cuff pressure after intubation and on a routine basis (e.g., every 8 hours) using the *minimal occluding volume* (MOV) *technique* or *the minimal leak technique* (MLT).

To perform the MOV technique, first, in the mechanically ventilated patient, place a stethoscope over the trachea and inflate the cuff to MOV by adding air until you hear no air at peak inspiratory pressure (end of ventilator inspiration). For the spontaneously breathing intubated patient, you inflate until you hear no sound after a deep breath or after inhalation with a BVM. Second, use a manometer to verify that cuff pressure is between 20 and 25 cm H_2O and record cuff pressure in the chart. If adequate cuff pressure cannot be maintained or larger volumes of air are needed to keep the cuff inflated, there could be a leak in the cuff or tracheal dilation at the cuff site. In these situations, notify the HCP. The procedure for MLT is similar with 1 exception. You remove a small amount of air from the cuff until you hear a slight air leak at peak inflation.

◆ Monitoring Oxygenation and Ventilation

Closely monitor the patient with an ET tube for adequate oxygenation by assessing clinical findings, ABGs, SpO_2, and, if available, $ScvO_2$ or SvO_2. Assess for signs of hypoxemia, such as a change in mental status (e.g., confusion), dusky skin,

and dysrhythmias. Periodic ABGs and continuous SpO_2 provide objective data about oxygenation. Lower PaO_2 values are expected in patients with some disease states, such as chronic obstructive pulmonary disease (COPD). CVP or PA catheters with $ScvO_2$ or SvO_2 capability provide an indirect measure of the patient's tissue oxygenation status (Table 65.4).

Indicators of ventilation include clinical findings, $PaCO_2$, and continuous partial pressure of $EtCO_2$ ($PETCO_2$). Assess the patient's respirations for rate, rhythm, and use of accessory muscles. The patient who is hyperventilating will be breathing rapidly and deeply and may have circumoral and peripheral numbness and tingling. The patient who is hypoventilating will be breathing shallowly or slowly and may appear dusky. $PaCO_2$ is the best indicator of alveolar hyperventilation (e.g., decreased $PaCO_2$, increased pH indicates respiratory alkalosis) or hypoventilation (e.g., increased $PaCO_2$, decreased pH indicates respiratory acidosis).

$PETCO_2$ monitoring (*capnography*) is done by analyzing exhaled gas directly at the patient-ventilator circuit (*mainstream sampling*) or by transporting a sample of gas via a small-bore tubing to a bedside monitor (*sidestream sampling*). Continuous $PETCO_2$ monitoring can assess the patency of the airway and presence of breathing. Gradual changes in $PETCO_2$ values may accompany an increase in CO_2 production (e.g., sepsis, hypoventilation, neuromuscular blockade) or a decrease in CO_2 production (e.g., hypothermia, decreased CO, metabolic acidosis). In patients with normal ventilation-to-perfusion ratios (see Chapter 67), we can use $PETCO_2$ to estimate $PaCO_2$. $PETCO_2$ is generally 2 to 5 mm Hg lower than $PaCO_2$.[13] However, in patients with unusually large dead air space or serious mismatch between ventilation and perfusion (e.g., COPD, pulmonary embolism), $PETCO_2$ is not a reliable estimate of $PaCO_2$.

◆ Maintaining Tube Patency

Do not routinely suction a patient.[13] Regularly assess the patient to determine if suctioning is needed. Indications for suctioning include (1) visible secretions in the ET tube, (2) sudden onset of respiratory distress, (3) suspected aspiration of secretions, (4) increase in respiratory rate or frequent coughing, and (5) sudden decrease in SpO_2. Other signs that indicate the patient needs suctioning include an increase in peak airway pressure and auscultating adventitious breath sounds over the trachea or bronchi.[13]

Table 65.8 describes 2 recommended suctioning methods, the *closed-suction technique* (CST) and the *open-suction technique* (OST). The CST uses a suction catheter that is enclosed in a plastic sleeve connected directly to the patient-ventilator circuit (Fig. 65.17). With the CST, oxygenation and ventilation are maintained during suctioning, and exposure to the patient's secretions and infection is reduced for the patient's and HCP's safety. The CST should be used for patients who (1) require PEEP, (2) have high levels of FIO_2, (3) have bloody or infected pulmonary secretions, (4) require frequent suctioning, and (5) have clinical instability with the OST.[13]

Potential complications associated with suctioning include hypoxemia, bronchospasm, increased ICP, dysrhythmias, hypertension, hypotension, mucosal damage, pulmonary bleeding, pain, and infection. Closely assess the patient before, during, and after suctioning. If the patient does not tolerate suctioning (e.g., decreased SpO_2, increased or decreased BP, sustained coughing, development of dysrhythmias), stop at once. Continue to reassess the patient until hemodynamic stability is achieved,

TABLE 65.8 Suctioning Procedures for Patient on Mechanical Ventilator

General Measures for Open- and Closed-Suction Techniques

1. Gather all equipment.
2. Wash hands and don personal protective equipment and gloves.
3. Explain procedure and patient's role in assisting with secretion removal by coughing.
4. Monitor patient's cardiopulmonary status (e.g., vital signs, SpO_2, SvO_2 or $ScvO_2$, ECG, level of consciousness) before, during, and after suctioning.
5. Turn on suction and set vacuum to 100–120 mm Hg.
6. Pause ventilator alarms.

Open-Suction Technique

7. Open sterile catheter package using the inside of the package as a sterile field. NOTE: Suction catheter should be no wider than half the diameter of the ET tube (e.g., for a 7-mm ET tube, select a 10F suction catheter).
8. Fill the sterile solution container with sterile normal saline or water.
9. Don sterile gloves.
10. Pick up sterile suction catheter with dominant hand. Using nondominant hand, secure the connecting tube (to suction) to the suction catheter.
11. Check equipment for proper functioning by suctioning a small volume of sterile saline solution from the container. **(Go to step 13.)**

Closed-Suction Technique

12. Connect the suction tubing to the closed suction port.
13. Hyperoxygenate the patient for 30 seconds using 1 of the following methods:
    - Activate the suction hyperoxygenation setting on the ventilator using nondominant hand. This is the safest method to hyperoxygenate the patient and should be used when available.
    - Increase FIO_2 to 100%. NOTE: Remember to return FIO_2 to baseline level when done suctioning, if not done automatically after preset time by ventilator.
    - Disconnect the ventilator tubing from the ET tube and provide manual ventilation to the patient with 100% O_2 using a BVM device. Attach a PEEP valve to the BVM for patients on >5 cm H_2O PEEP. Give 5 or 6 breaths over 30 seconds. Having a second person deliver the manual breaths significantly increases the V_T delivered.
14. With suction off, gently and quickly insert the catheter using the dominant hand. When you meet resistance, pull back ½ in.
15. Apply continuous or intermittent suction using the nondominant thumb. Withdraw the catheter over 10 seconds or less.
16. Hyperoxygenate once more for another 30 seconds as described in step 13.
17. If secretions remain and the patient has tolerated suctioning, perform 2 or 3 suction passes as described in steps 14 and 15. NOTE: Rinse the suction catheter with sterile saline solution between suctioning passes as needed. Maintaining a closed circuit at all times is best to reduce the risk for infection.
18. Reconnect patient to ventilator (open-suction technique).
19. Rinse the catheter and connecting tubing with the sterile saline solution.
20. Suction oral pharynx. NOTE: Use a separate catheter for this step when using the closed-suction technique.
21. Discard the suction catheter and rinse the connecting tubing with the sterile saline solution (open-suction technique).
22. Reset FIO_2 (if needed) and ventilator alarms.
23. Reassess patient for signs of effective suctioning.

Adapted from Wiegand DL: *AACN procedure manual for high acuity, progressive, and critical care*, ed 7, St Louis, 2017, Elsevier.

the patient recovers, and/or the situation resolves before trying to suction again. Prevent hypoxemia by hyperoxygenating the patient before and after each suctioning pass and limiting each pass to 10 seconds or less (Table 65.8). Assess both the ECG and SpO_2 before, during, and after suctioning.

Causes of dysrhythmias during suctioning include (1) hypoxemia resulting in myocardial ischemia; (2) vagal stimulation caused by tracheal irritation; and (3) sympathetic nervous system stimulation caused by anxiety, discomfort, or pain. Dysrhythmias include tachydysrhythmias and bradydysrhythmias, premature beats, and asystole. Stop suctioning if any new dysrhythmias develop. Avoid excessive suctioning in patients with severe hypoxemia or bradycardia.

Tracheal mucosal damage may occur due to excessive suction pressures (greater than 120 mm Hg), overly vigorous catheter insertion, and the suction catheter itself. Blood streaks or tissue shreds in aspirated secretions may indicate mucosal damage. This increases the risk for infection and bleeding, especially if the patient is receiving anticoagulants. We can prevent trauma to the mucosa by following the steps described in Table 65.8.

Secretions may be thick and hard to suction because of inadequate hydration or humidification, infection, or inaccessibility of the lower airways. Maintain adequate hydration when clinically indicated (e.g., IV fluids) and provide supplemental humidification of inspired gases through the mechanical ventilator to help thin secretions. Mobilize and turn the patient (e.g., every 2 hours) to help move secretions into larger airways. If infection is the cause of thick secretions, give the patient appropriate antibiotics.

◆ Providing Oral Care and Maintaining Skin Integrity

When an oral ET tube is in place, the patient's mouth is always open. Moisten the lips, tongue, and gums with saline or water swabs to prevent mucosal drying. Proper oral care provides comfort and prevents injury to the gums and plaque formation (Table 65.9). If space is limited in the oral cavity, use smaller or pediatric-sized oral products for providing oral care.

Frequent assessment and meticulous care are needed to prevent skin breakdown on the face, lips, tongue, and nares because

TABLE 65.9 Oral Care for Patient on Mechanical Ventilator

General Measures

1. Gather all equipment.
2. Wash hands and don personal protective equipment and gloves.
3. Explain procedure to the patient and caregiver (if present).
4. Perform oral care every 2–4 hours using a suction toothbrush and toothpaste or gel for 1–2 minutes, suctioning often. Assess for plaque buildup and any potential infection.
5. Use 0.12% chlorhexidine oral rinse twice daily.
6. Apply a mouth moisturizer to oral mucosa and lips with each cleaning.
7. Suction oral cavity and pharynx when needed. Fig. 65.18 shows an endotracheal tube that can provide continuous or intermittent subglottic suctioning.
   NOTE:
   - Change all oral suction equipment and suction tubing every 24 hr.
   - Rinse nondisposable oral suction apparatus with sterile normal saline after each use and place on a dry paper towel.

Adapted from Wiegand DL *AACN procedure manual for high acuity, progressive, and critical care*, ed 7, St Louis, 2017, Elsevier.

of pressure from the ET tube or the method used to secure the ET tube to the patient's face. Ongoing assessment is shared between the RN and RT. Reposition and re-tape the ET tube (per agency policy) and as needed to prevent skin breakdown. Repositioning the ET tube may be limited to the RT. Two staff members should always perform repositioning to prevent accidental ET tube dislodgment. Monitor the patient for any signs of respiratory distress throughout the procedure.

For the nasally intubated patient, remove the old tape and clean the skin around the ET tube with saline-soaked gauze. For the orally intubated patient, remove the bite block (if present) and the old tape. Provide oral hygiene, then reposition the ET tube to the opposite side of the mouth. Replace the bite block (if appropriate) and reconfirm proper cuff inflation and tube placement. Secure the ET tube again (per agency policy).

We often use commercial ET holders. These may increase the risk for skin breakdown compared to tape.[18] If one is used, follow the manufacturer's directions for maintaining tube position, providing skin care, and preventing skin breakdown.

◆ Fostering Comfort and Communication

Intubation is a major stressor for the patient.[19] Intubated patients have stress from not being able to talk and communicate their needs. This can be frustrating for the patient, caregiver, and interprofessional care team. To communicate more effectively, use a variety of methods. (See Common Problems of Critical Care Patients earlier in this chapter on p. 1535.)

The physical discomfort associated with ET intubation and mechanical ventilation often requires sedating the patient and giving an analgesic until the ET tube is removed. Assess the drugs' effectiveness in achieving an acceptable level of patient comfort by using a valid pain scale, sedation scale (e.g., Richmond Agitation and Sedation Scale [RASS], Sedation Agitation Scale [SAS]), and/or delirium scale.[20] Consider using relaxation techniques (e.g., music therapy) to complement drug therapy.

◆ Complications of Endotracheal Intubation

Two major complications of ET intubation are unplanned extubation and aspiration. Unplanned *extubation* (i.e., removal of the ET tube from the trachea) may complicate the patient's recovery. Unplanned extubation can be due to patient removal of the ET tube or accidental removal during movement or a procedure. Usually, the unplanned extubation is obvious (i.e., the patient is holding the ET tube). Other times, the tip of the ET tube is in the hypopharynx or esophagus and the extubation is not obvious. You are responsible for preventing unplanned extubation by ensuring that the ET tube is secured and observing and supporting the ET tube during repositioning, procedures, and patient transfers. Giving adequate sedation and analgesia and using standardized weaning protocols decrease the incidence of self-extubation.[21]

The use of restraints to immobilize the patient's hands is a deterrent to self-extubation.[21] Be sure to explain to the patient and caregiver when you use short-term restraints for patient safety and discuss the use of alternatives. Reassess for the continued need of restraints (per agency policy) and limit restraint use when possible.

Should an unplanned extubation occur, stay with the patient and call for help. Interventions are aimed at maintaining the patient's airway, supporting ventilation (e.g., manually ventilating the patient with a BVM and 100% O_2), securing the

appropriate help to reintubate the patient (if needed), and providing psychologic support to the patient.

> ### ⚠ SAFETY ALERT Unplanned Extubation
>
> Observe for signs of unplanned extubation:
> - Activation of the low-pressure ventilator alarm
> - Decreased or absent breath sounds
> - Respiratory distress
> - Auditory cuff leak
>
> What to do during an unplanned extubation:
> - Stay with the patient
> - Support the patient's oxygenation as needed by applying an adjunct therapy, such as a nasal cannula or manually ventilating the patient with a BVM and 100% O_2
> - Notify the HCP and RT
> - Assess for respiratory distress and listen for stridor
> - Assess the patient's ability to cough and/or vocalize
> - Assess the patient's ability to maintain secretions
> - Assess the patient's need for reintubation
> - If the patient is unable to protect their airway or is in respiratory distress, prepare for reintubation

Aspiration is another potential hazard for the patient with an ET tube. The ET tube passes through the epiglottis, splinting it in an open position. Thus the intubated patient cannot protect the airway from aspiration. The high-volume, low-pressure ET cuff cannot totally prevent the trickle of oral or gastric secretions into the trachea.[22] Further, secretions collect above the cuff. When the cuff is deflated, those secretions can move into the lungs. Some ET tubes provide continuous suctioning of secretions above the cuff (Fig. 65.18).

Oral intubation increases salivation, yet swallowing is difficult, so suction the patient's mouth often. Use a Yankauer (tonsil-tip) suction catheter or a sterile single-use catheter. Other factors contributing to aspiration include improper cuff inflation, patient positioning, and decreased gastric mobility and bowel function if receiving EN. The patient with an ET tube is at risk for aspiration of gastric contents. Even when the cuff is properly inflated, take precautions to prevent vomiting, which can lead to aspiration.

Often, a nasogastric (NG) or an orogastric (OG) tube is inserted and connected to low, intermittent suction when a patient is first intubated. An OG tube is preferred over an NG tube to reduce the risk for sinusitis. All intubated patients who

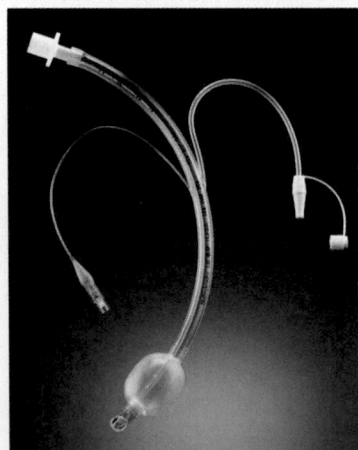

FIG. 65.18 Continuous subglottic suctioning can be provided by the Hi Lo Evac Tube. A dorsal lumen above the cuff allows for suctioning of secretions from the subglottic area. (Reprinted by permission of Nellcor Puritan Bennett Inc, Pleasanton, CA.)

are receiving EN should have the HOB elevated a minimum of 30 to 45 degrees, unless medically contraindicated.

MECHANICAL VENTILATION

Mechanical ventilation is the process by which the FIO_2 (21% [room air] or more) is moved in and out of the lungs by a mechanical ventilator. Mechanical ventilation is not curative. It is a means of supporting patients until they recover the ability to breathe independently. It can also serve as a bridge to long-term mechanical ventilation or until a decision is made to stop ventilatory support.

Indications for mechanical ventilation include (1) apnea, (2) inability to breathe or protect the airway, (3) acute respiratory failure (see Chapter 67), (4) severe hypoxia, and (5) respiratory muscle fatigue. Patients with chronic lung disease and their caregivers should be given the opportunity to discuss mechanical ventilation before end-stage respiratory failure develops. Encourage all patients, especially those with chronic illnesses, to discuss the subject of life-sustaining measures, including mechanical ventilation, with their families and HCPs. The patient's wishes about end-of-life treatment should be recorded in an advance directive.

The decision to use, withhold, or stop mechanical ventilation must be made carefully, respecting the wishes of the patient. When the interprofessional care team, patient, and/or caregiver disagree over the treatment plan that the patient desires, conferences are essential to keep the lines of communication open and discuss options. You may need to consult the agency's ethics committee for assistance.

Types of Mechanical Ventilation

The 2 major types of mechanical ventilation are negative pressure and positive pressure ventilation.

Negative Pressure Ventilation. Negative pressure ventilation involves the use of chambers that encase the chest or body and surround it with intermittent subatmospheric (or negative) pressure. The "iron lung" was the first form of negative pressure ventilation. It was developed during the polio epidemic. Intermittent negative pressure around the chest wall pulls the chest outward, reducing intrathoracic pressure. Air rushes in via the upper airway, which is outside the sealed chamber. Expiration is passive. The machine cycles off, allowing chest retraction. This type of ventilation is like normal ventilation in that decreased intrathoracic pressures produce inspiration, and expiration is passive. Negative pressure ventilation is noninvasive and does not need an artificial airway.

Several portable negative pressure ventilators are available for home use. They are mainly for patients with neuromuscular diseases, central nervous system disorders, diseases and injuries of the spinal cord, and severe COPD. They are not routinely used for acutely ill patients.

DRUG ALERT Oxygen
- O_2 is considered a drug, and overexposure can lead to O_2 toxicity.
- Mechanically ventilated patients receiving high levels of FIO_2 for prolonged periods of time (e.g., 60% FIO_2 for >24 hours) are at risk for O_2 toxicity.
- Target FIO_2 levels are to maintain SpO_2 >92% and PaO_2 between 60 and 80 mm Hg.
- Assess ABGs for evidence of excess O_2.
- Monitor patient for signs of O_2 toxicity: uncontrolled coughing, chest pain, and dyspnea.

Positive Pressure Ventilation. Positive pressure ventilation (PPV) is the main method used with acutely ill patients (Fig. 65.19). During inspiration the ventilator pushes air into the lungs under positive pressure. Unlike spontaneous ventilation, intrathoracic pressure is raised during lung inflation rather than lowered. Expiration occurs passively as in normal expiration. There are 2 categories of PPV: volume and pressure ventilation.[13]

Volume Ventilation. With volume ventilation, a predetermined V_T is delivered with each inspiration. The amount of pressure needed to deliver the breath varies based on compliance and resistance factors of the patient-ventilator system. So, the V_T is consistent from breath to breath, but airway pressures vary.

Pressure Ventilation. With *pressure ventilation*, the peak inspiratory pressure is predetermined. The V_T delivered to the patient varies based on the selected pressure and compliance and resistance factors of the patient-ventilator system. Careful attention must be given to the V_T to prevent unplanned hyperventilation or hypoventilation. For example, when the patient breathes out of synchrony with the ventilator, the pressure limit may be reached quickly, and the volume of gas delivered may be small.

Settings of Mechanical Ventilators

Mechanical ventilator settings regulate rate, V_T, O_2 concentration, and other characteristics of ventilation (Table 65.10, Fig. 65.20). Settings are based on the patient's status (e.g., ABGs, ideal body weight, current physiologic state, level of consciousness, respiratory muscle strength). Settings are evaluated and adjusted until oxygenation and ventilation targets have been reached.

It is important that you check that all ventilator alarms are always on. Alarms alert the staff to potentially dangerous situations, such as mechanical malfunction, apnea, unplanned extubation, or patient asynchrony with the ventilator (Table 65.11). On many ventilators, the alarms can be temporarily suspended or silenced for up to 2 minutes for suctioning or testing while a staff member is in the room. After that time, the alarm system automatically turns back on.

! SAFETY ALERT   Alarm Fatigue
- Alarm fatigue can develop in those who hear an excess number of alarms, resulting in sensory overload.
- This can cause a delayed response to alarms or dismissing them altogether and can lead to serious adverse events (e.g., patient death).
- One way to reduce alarm fatigue includes customizing alarm parameters based on patient specific needs.[23]

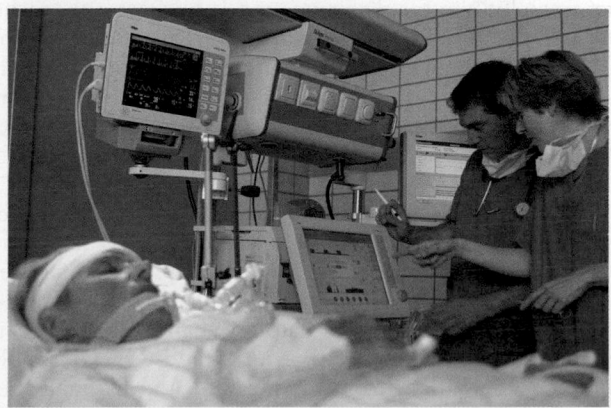

FIG. 65.19 Patient receiving mechanical ventilation. (Courtesy Draeger Medical, Houston, TX.)

TABLE 65.10 Settings of Mechanical Ventilation

Parameter	Description
Respiratory rate (f)	Number of breaths the ventilator delivers per minute. *Usual setting:* 12–20 breaths/min
Tidal volume (V_T)	Volume of gas delivered to patient during each ventilator breath. *Usual volume:* 6–8 mL/kg, 4–8 mL/kg in ARDS
O_2 concentration (FIO_2)	Fraction of inspired O_2 (FIO_2) delivered to patient. May be set between 21% (essentially room air) and 100%. *Usually adjusted* to maintain PaO_2 level >60–80 mm Hg or SpO_2 level >92%
Positive end-expiratory pressure (PEEP)	Positive pressure applied at the end of expiration of ventilator breaths. *Usual setting:* 5 cm H_2O
Pressure support	Positive pressure used to augment patient's inspiratory pressure. *Usual setting:* 5–10 cm H_2O
I/E ratio	Duration of inspiration (I) to duration of expiration (E). *Usual setting:* 1:2 to 1:1.5 unless inverse ratio ventilation is desired
Inspiratory flow rate and time	Speed with which the V_T is delivered. *Usual setting:* 40–80 L/min and time is 0.8–1.2 sec
Sensitivity	Determines the amount of effort the patient must generate to initiate a ventilator breath. It may be set for pressure triggering or flow triggering. *Usual setting:* A pressure trigger is set 0.5–1.5 cm H_2O below baseline pressure and a flow trigger is set 1–3 L/min below baseline flow
High-pressure limit	Regulates the maximal pressure the ventilator can generate to deliver the V_T. When the pressure limit is reached, the ventilator ends the breath and spills the undelivered volume into the atmosphere. *Usual setting:* 10–20 cm H_2O above peak inspiratory pressure

Adapted from Urden LD, Stacy, KM, Lough ME: *Critical care nursing: Diagnosis and management,* ed 8, St Louis, 2018, Elsevier.

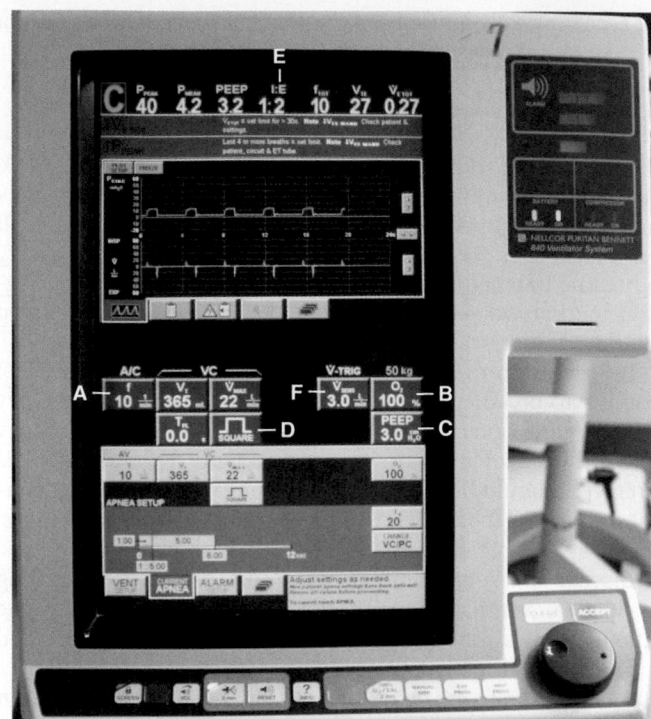

FIG. 65.20 Ventilator control panel (Puritan Bennett 840). (From Roberts JR: *Roberts and Hedges' clinical procedures in emergency medicine and acute care,* ed 7 ed, St Louis, 2019, Elsevier.)

Ventilator Alarms. Mechanical ventilators may become disconnected or malfunction. Most deaths from accidental ventilator disconnection occur while the alarm is off. Most accidental disconnections are discovered by low-pressure alarms. The most frequent site for disconnection is between the tracheal tube and the adapter. Push connections together and then twist to secure more tightly. Be certain that alarms are always set and activated. Chart that this is the case. You can pause alarms (not inactivate) during suctioning or removal from the ventilator, but you must reactivate them before leaving the patient's bedside.

Ventilator malfunction may occur. Although most agencies have emergency generators in case of a power failure and newer ventilators may have battery backup, power failure is always a possibility. Have a plan for manually ventilating all patients who depend on a ventilator. If, at any time, you decide the ventilator is malfunctioning (e.g., failure of O_2 supply), disconnect the patient from the machine and manually ventilate with a BVM and 100% O_2 until the ventilator is fixed or replaced.

Modes of Volume Ventilation

The ways by which the patient and ventilator interact to deliver effective ventilation are called *ventilator modes.* The selected ventilator mode is based on how much WOB the patient should or can perform. WOB is the inspiratory effort needed to overcome the elasticity and viscosity of the lungs along with the airway resistance. The mode is determined by the patient's ventilatory status, respiratory drive, and ABGs. Generally, ventilator modes are controlled or assisted.

With controlled ventilatory support, the ventilator does all the WOB for the patient. With assisted ventilatory support, the ventilator and patient share the WOB. Historically, volume modes, such as controlled mandatory ventilation (CMV), assist-control ventilation (ACV), and synchronized intermittent mandatory ventilation (SIMV), have been used to treat critically ill patients. Pressure modes, such as pressure support ventilation (PSV), pressure-control ventilation (PCV), and inverse ratio ventilation (PC-IRV) are becoming more common.[24] Table 65.12 describes ventilator modes.

Assist-Control Ventilation. With assist-control ventilation (ACV), the ventilator delivers a preset V_T at a preset frequency. When the patient initiates a spontaneous breath, the ventilator senses a decrease in intrathoracic pressure and then delivers the preset V_T. The patient can breathe faster than the preset rate but not slower. ACV has the advantage of allowing the patient some control over ventilation while providing some assistance. It is used in patients with a variety of conditions, including neuromuscular disorders (e.g., Guillain-Barré syndrome), pulmonary edema, and acute respiratory failure.

With ACV, the patient has the potential for hyperventilation. The spontaneously breathing patient can easily be overventilated, resulting in hyperventilation. If the volume or minimum rate is set too low and the patient is apneic or weak, the patient

TABLE 65.11 Managing Mechanical Ventilation Alarms

Alarm	Possible Causes	Interventions
High-pressure limit	• Secretions, coughing, or gagging • Patient fighting ventilator (ventilator asynchrony) • Condensate (water) in tubing • Kinked or compressed tubing (e.g., patient biting on ET tube) • ↑ Resistance (e.g., bronchospasm) • ↓ Compliance (e.g., pulmonary edema, ARDS, tension pneumothorax, atelectasis, pneumonia) • Improper alarm setting • ET tube inserted too far (e.g., right mainstem bronchus or carina)	• Clear secretions and ↑ sedation • Reassure patient • Remove water from ventilator tubing • Unkink tubing, insert bite block, or reposition patient • Give bronchodilator • Assess breath sounds, obtain chest x-ray • Adjust ET tube
Low-pressure limit	• Total or partial ventilator disconnect • Loss of airway (e.g., total or partial extubation) • ET tube or tracheotomy cuff leak (e.g., patient speaking, grunting)	• Check connections • Confirm adequate tidal volume and ET tube position with chest x-ray • Reinflate cuff
Apnea	• Respiratory arrest • Oversedation • Change in patient condition • Loss of airway (e.g., total or partial extubation)	• ↓ Sedation • ↓ Analgesia • Reverse sedation or analgesia • Confirm ET tube placement or reintubate
High V_T, minute ventilation, or respiratory rate	• Pain, anxiety • Change in patient condition (e.g., ↑ metabolic demand, fever, hypoxia, hypercapnia) • Excess condensate or secretions in tubing (i.e., false reading)	• Treat pain • Assess patient for change in condition • Obtain an ABG • Remove water or secretions from tubing
Low V_T or minute ventilation	• Change in patient's breathing efforts (e.g., rate and volume) • Patient disconnection, loose connection, or leak in circuit • ET tube or tracheotomy cuff leak (e.g., air leak) • Insufficient gas flow	• Assess patients respiratory and neurologic status. Reduce sedation. • Assess ventilator circuit for leaks • Reassess cuff to ensure cuff is adequately inflated • Check ventilator settings
Ventilator inoperative or low battery	• Machine malfunction • Unplugged, power failure, or internal battery not charged	• Ensure mechanical ventilator is plugged into right power source • Disconnect patient from mechanical ventilator and use bag-valve-mask to ventilate until machine is properly functioning

Adapted from Urden LD, Stacy KM, Lough ME: *Critical care nursing: Diagnosis and management,* ed 8, St Louis, 2018, Elsevier.

TABLE 65.12 Modes of Mechanical Ventilation

Mode of Ventilation	Ventilator Settings	Nursing Implications
Volume Modes		
Assist-control (AC) or assisted mandatory ventilation (AMV)	• Requires rate, V_T, inspiratory time, and PEEP set for the patient • The ventilator sensitivity is set, so when the patient initiates a spontaneous breath, a full-volume breath is delivered	• Hyperventilation can occur • To limit spontaneous breaths, sedation may be needed
Intermittent mandatory ventilation (IMV) and synchronized intermittent mandatory ventilation (SIMV)	• Requires rate, V_T, inspiratory time, sensitivity, and PEEP set for the patient • Between "mandatory breaths," patients spontaneously breathe at their own rates and V_T • With SIMV, the ventilator synchronizes the mandatory breaths with the patient's own inspirations	• Muscle fatigue may occur due to ↑ work of breathing
Pressure Modes		
Pressure support ventilation (PSV)	• Provides an augmented inspiration to a spontaneously breathing patient • HCP selects inspiratory pressure level, PEEP, and sensitivity • When the patient initiates a breath, a high flow of gas is delivered to the preselected pressure level, and pressure is maintained throughout inspiration • Patient determines V_T, rate, and inspiratory time	• Reduces patients work of breathing and ↑ ventilator synchrony • Monitor patient for hypercapnia
Pressure-control inverse ratio ventilation (PC-IRV)	• Combines pressure-limited ventilation with an inverse ratio of inspiration to expiration • HCP selects the pressure level, rate, inspiratory time (1:, 2:1, 3:1, 4:1), and PEEP level • With the prolonged inspiratory times, auto-PEEP may result • Auto-PEEP may be a desirable outcome of the inverse ratios	• Requires sedation and/or pharmacologic paralysis to oxygenate and ventilate patient due to discomfort • Air trapping can occur due to ↑ intra-thoracic pressure, leading to a ↓ cardiac output
Airway pressure release ventilation (APRV)	• Provides 2 levels of continuous positive airway pressure (CPAP) with timed releases • Permits spontaneous breathing throughout the respiratory cycle • HCP selects both pressure (high, low) and time (high, low). V_T is not a set variable and depends on the CPAP level, the patient's compliance and resistance, and spontaneous breathing effort	• Monitor for hypercapnia

Modified from Wiegand DL: *AACN procedure manual for high acuity, progressive, and critical care,* ed 7, St Louis, 2017, Elsevier; and Urden LD, Stacy, KM, Lough ME: *Critical care nursing: Diagnosis and management,* ed 8, St Louis, 2018, Elsevier.

can be hypoventilated. Thus these patients need vigilant assessment and monitoring of ventilatory status, including respiratory rate, ABGs, SpO_2, and $ScvO_2$ or SvO_2. It is important that the sensitivity, or amount of negative pressure needed to start a breath, is appropriate to the patient's condition. For example, if it is too hard for the patient to begin a breath, the WOB is increased and the patient may tire (i.e., the patient "rides" the ventilator) or develop ventilator dyssynchrony (i.e., the patient "fights" the ventilator).

Synchronized Intermittent Mandatory Ventilation. With synchronized intermittent mandatory ventilation (SIMV), the ventilator delivers a preset V_T at a preset frequency in synchrony with the patient's spontaneous breathing. Between ventilator-delivered breaths, the patient can breathe spontaneously through the ventilator circuit. Thus the patient receives the preset FIO_2 during the spontaneous breaths but self-regulates the rate and V_T of those breaths. SIMV is used during continuous ventilation and during weaning from the ventilator. It may be combined with PSV (described later). Potential benefits of SIMV include improved patient-ventilator synchrony, lower mean airway pressure, and prevention of muscle atrophy as the patient takes on more of the WOB.

SIMV has disadvantages. If spontaneous breathing decreases when the preset rate is low, ventilation may not be adequately supported. Only patients with regular, spontaneous breathing should use low-rate SIMV. Weaning with SIMV demands close monitoring and may take longer because the rate of breathing is gradually reduced. Patients being weaned with SIMV may have increased muscle fatigue associated with spontaneous breathing efforts.

Modes of Pressure Ventilation

Pressure Support Ventilation. With pressure support ventilation (PSV), positive pressure is applied to the airway only during inspiration and is used with the patient's spontaneous respirations. The patient must be able to initiate a breath in this modality. The level of positive airway pressure is preset so that the gas flow rate is greater than the patient's inspiratory flow rate. As the patient starts a breath, the machine senses the spontaneous effort and supplies a rapid flow of gas at the initiation of the breath and variable flow throughout the breath. With PSV, the patient determines inspiratory length, V_T, and respiratory rate. V_T depends on the pressure level and airway compliance.

PSV is used with continuous ventilation and during weaning. It also may be used with SIMV during weaning. PSV is not often used as ventilatory support during acute respiratory failure because of the risk for hypoventilation and apnea. Advantages include increased patient comfort, decreased WOB (because inspiratory efforts are augmented), decreased O_2 consumption (because inspiratory work is reduced), and increased endurance conditioning (because the patient is exercising respiratory muscles).

Pressure-Control and Pressure-Control Inverse Ratio Ventilation. *Pressure-control ventilation (PCV)* provides a pressure-limited breath delivered at a set rate. It may permit spontaneous breathing. The V_T is not set. It is determined by the pressure limit set. *Pressure-control inverse ratio ventilation (PC-IRV)* combines pressure-limited ventilation with an inverse ratio of inspiration (I) to expiration (E). Some HCPs use PC without IRV.

The *I/E ratio* is the ratio of duration of inspiration to the duration of expiration. This ratio is normally 1:2 or 1:3. With IRV, the I/E ratio begins at 1:1 and may progress to 4:1. Prolonged positive pressure is applied, increasing inspiratory time. IRV gradually expands collapsed alveoli. The short expiratory time

has a PEEP-like effect, preventing alveolar collapse. Because IRV imposes a nonphysiologic breathing pattern, the patient needs sedation and often paralysis.

PC-IRV is used for patients with acute respiratory distress syndrome (ARDS) who continue to have hypoxemia despite high levels of PEEP. Not all patients with poor oxygenation respond to PC-IRV.

Airway Pressure Release Ventilation. *Airway pressure release ventilation (APRV)* permits spontaneous breathing at any point during the respiratory cycle with a preset CPAP with short timed pressure releases. The CPAP level (pressure high, pressure low) is adjusted to keep oxygenation goals while the timed releases (time high, time low) are increased or decreased to meet ventilation goals.[25] V_T is not set. It varies depending on the CPAP level, the patient's compliance and resistance, and spontaneous breathing effort. This mode is best for patients who need high pressure levels for alveolar recruitment (open collapsed alveoli). An advantage is that it allows for spontaneous respirations. This may reduce the need for deep sedation or paralytics.

Positive End-Expiratory Pressure. Positive end-expiratory pressure (PEEP) is a ventilatory maneuver, or mechanical ventilator setting, in which positive pressure is applied to the airway during exhalation. Normally during exhalation, airway pressure drops to near 0, and exhalation occurs passively. With PEEP, exhalation is passive but pressure falls to a preset level, often 3 to 20 cm H_2O. Lung volume during expiration and between breaths is greater than normal with PEEP. This increases FRC and often improves oxygenation by restoring the lung volume that normally remains at the end of passive exhalation. The mechanisms by which PEEP increases FRC and oxygenation include increased aeration of patent alveoli, aeration of previously collapsed alveoli, and prevention of alveolar collapse throughout the respiratory cycle.

PEEP is titrated to the point that oxygenation improves without compromising hemodynamics. We call this *optimal PEEP*. Often 5 cm H_2O PEEP (referred to as *physiologic PEEP*) is used prophylactically to replace the glottic mechanism, help maintain a normal FRC, and prevent alveolar collapse. PEEP of 5 cm H_2O is used for patients with a history of alveolar collapse during weaning. PEEP improves gas exchange, vital capacity, and inspiratory force when used during weaning.

In contrast, *auto-PEEP* is not purposely set on the ventilator but is a result of inadequate exhalation time. Auto-PEEP is more PEEP over what is set by the HCP. This added PEEP may result in increased WOB, barotrauma, and hemodynamic instability. Interventions to limit auto-PEEP include sedation and analgesia, large-diameter ET tube, bronchodilators, short inspiratory times, and decreased respiratory rates. Reducing water accumulation in the ventilator circuit by frequent emptying or use of heated circuits also limits auto-PEEP. In patients with short exhalation times and early airway closure (e.g., asthma), setting PEEP above auto-PEEP can offset auto-PEEP effects by splinting the airway open during exhalation and preventing "air trapping."

FIO_2 often can be reduced when PEEP is used. PEEP is generally indicated in all patients who are mechanically ventilated. The classic indication for PEEP therapy is ARDS (see Chapter 67). PEEP is used with caution in patients with increased ICP, low CO, and hypovolemia. In these cases, the adverse effects of high PEEP may outweigh the benefits.

Other Modes. Advances in ventilator technology have led to the development of other pressure modes. However, the names and features of these other options are manufacturer specific. The superiority of these modes has not been proven. Some examples include *volume-assured pressure ventilation* and *adaptive support ventilation*.

Other Methods to Improve Oxygenation and Ventilation

Automatic Tube Compensation. *Automatic tube compensation (ATC)* is an adjunct designed to overcome WOB through an artificial airway. It is currently available on many ventilators. ATC is increased during inspiration and decreased during expiration. It is set by entering the internal diameter of the patient's airway and the desired number for compensation. ATC may be less effective in patients with excess secretions or who need longer term ventilation.

High-Frequency Oscillatory Ventilation. High-frequency oscillatory ventilation (HFOV) involves delivery of a small V_T (usually 1 to 5 mL/kg of body weight) at rapid respiratory rates (100 to 300 breaths/min). The goals are to recruit (e.g., alveolar expansion) and maintain lung volume and reduce intrapulmonary shunting. While HFOV may be a useful mode for patients with life-threatening hypoxia, it has not improved survival of patients with ARDS.[26] Patients receiving HFOV must be sedated and may need to be paralyzed to suppress spontaneous respiration.

Nitric Oxide. *Nitric oxide* (NO) is a gaseous molecule that is made intravascularly and takes part in the regulation of pulmonary vascular tone. Inhibiting NO production results in pulmonary vasoconstriction. Administering continuous inhaled NO results in pulmonary vasodilation. NO may be given through an ET tube, a tracheostomy, or a face mask. Currently, NO is used as a diagnostic screening tool for pulmonary hypertension and to improve oxygenation during mechanical ventilation in this patient population. The use of NO does not reduce mortality in patients with ARDS and may cause kidney injury.[27]

Prone Positioning. *Prone positioning* is the repositioning of a patient from a supine or lateral position to a prone (on the stomach, face down) position. This repositioning improves lung recruitment through various mechanisms. Gravity reverses the effects of fluid in the dependent parts of the lungs as the patient is moved from supine to prone. The heart rests on the sternum, away from the lungs, contributing to an overall uniformity of pleural pressures. The prone position requires increased sedation and is nurse-intensive. It is an effective supportive therapy used in critically ill patients with severe ARDS to improve oxygenation.[28]

Extracorporeal Membrane Oxygenation. *Extracorporeal membrane oxygenation* (ECMO) is an alternative form of pulmonary support for the patient with severe respiratory failure (Fig. 65.21).[13] It is used most often in the pediatric and neonatal populations but is increasingly being used in adults. ECMO is a modification of cardiac bypass. It involves partially removing

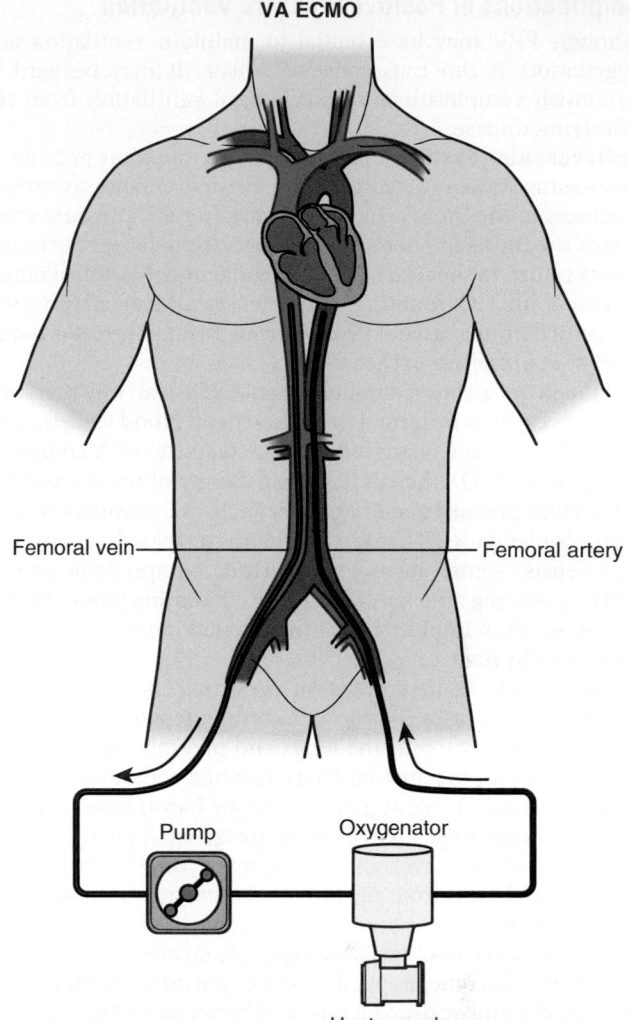

FIG. 65.21 ECMO circuit. The circuit consists of a pump, oxygenator, and heating-cooling element. Circulatory access is typically obtained through the femoral vein and artery. (From Mann DL, Zipes DP, Libby P, et al: *Braunwald's heart disease: A textbook of cardiovascular medicine,* ed 11, St Louis, 2019, Saunders.)

blood from a patient with large-bore catheters, infusing O_2, removing CO_2, and returning the blood to the patient. This intensive therapy requires systemic anticoagulation and is a time-limited intervention. A skilled team of specialists, including a perfusionist, must be continuously at the bedside.

Complications of Positive Pressure Ventilation

Although PPV may be essential to maintain ventilation and oxygenation, it can cause adverse effects. It may be hard to distinguish complications of mechanical ventilation from the underlying disease.

Cardiovascular System. PPV can affect circulation because of the transmission of increased mean airway pressure to various structures in the thorax. Increased intrathoracic pressure compresses the thoracic vessels. This compression causes decreased venous return to the heart, left ventricular end-diastolic volume (preload), and CO, resulting in hypotension. Mean airway pressure is further increased if PEEP is being titrated (greater than 5 cm H_2O) to improve oxygenation.

If the lungs are noncompliant (e.g., ARDS), airway pressures are not as easily transmitted to the heart and blood vessels. Thus effects of PPV on CO are reduced. Conversely, with compliant lungs (e.g., COPD), there is increased danger of transmission of high airway pressures and negative effects on hemodynamics.

Hypovolemia (e.g., hemorrhage) and decreased venous tone (e.g., sepsis, spinal shock) can further compromise venous return. Restoring and maintaining the circulating blood volume are important in minimizing cardiovascular complications.

Pulmonary System

Barotrauma. As lung inflation pressures increase, risk for *barotrauma* increases. Barotrauma results when the increased airway pressure distends the lungs and possibly ruptures fragile alveoli or emphysematous blebs. Patients with noncompliant lungs (e.g., COPD) are at greatest risk for barotrauma. Patients with stiff lungs (e.g., ARDS) who are given high inspiratory pressures and high levels of PEEP (greater than 5 cm H_2O) or have a lung abscess from necrotizing organisms (e.g., staphylococci) are also at risk.

Air can escape into the pleural space from alveoli or the interstitium and become trapped. Pleural pressure increases and collapses the lung, causing a pneumothorax (see Chapter 27 for more about pneumothorax.) The lungs receive air during inspiration but cannot expel it during expiration. Respiratory bronchioles are larger on inspiration than expiration. They may close on expiration, and air becomes trapped. With PPV, a simple pneumothorax can become a life-threatening tension pneumothorax. The mediastinum and contralateral lung are compressed, reducing CO. Immediate treatment of the pneumothorax is required.

Pneumomediastinum usually begins with rupture of alveoli into the lung interstitium. Progressive air movement occurs into the mediastinum and subcutaneous neck tissue, and a pneumothorax often follows. New, unexplained subcutaneous emphysema is an indication for immediate chest x-ray. Pneumomediastinum and subcutaneous emphysema may be too small to detect on x-ray or clinically before the development of a pneumothorax.

Volutrauma. The concept of *volutrauma* in PPV relates to the lung injury that occurs when a large V_T is used to ventilate noncompliant lungs. Volutrauma results in alveolar rupture and movement of fluids and proteins into the alveolar spaces. Low-volume ventilation should be used in patients with ARDS to protect the lungs.

Alveolar Hypoventilation. *Alveolar hypoventilation* can be caused by inappropriate ventilator settings, leakage of air from the ventilator tubing or around the ET tube or tracheostomy cuff, lung secretions or obstruction, and low ventilation/perfusion ratio. A low V_T or respiratory rate decreases minute ventilation. This results in hypoventilation, atelectasis, and respiratory acidosis. A leaking cuff or tubing that is not secured may cause air leakage and lower V_T. Mobilizing the patient, turning the patient at least every 2 hours, encouraging deep breathing and coughing, and suctioning (as needed) may limit lung secretions. Increasing the V_T, adding small increments of PEEP, and adding a preset number of *sighs* to the ventilator settings (i.e., a deeper than normal breath incorporated into the respiratory cycle) can help reduce the risk for atelectasis.

Alveolar Hyperventilation. Respiratory alkalosis can occur if the respiratory rate or V_T is set too high *(mechanical overventilation)* or if the patient receiving assisted ventilation is *hyperventilating*. It is easy to overventilate a patient on PPV. Especially at risk are patients with chronic alveolar hypoventilation and CO_2 retention. For example, the patient with COPD may have a chronic $PaCO_2$ elevation (acidosis) and compensatory bicarbonate retention by the kidneys. When the patient is ventilated, the patient's "normal baseline" rather than the standard normal values is the therapeutic goal. If the COPD patient is returned to a standard normal $PaCO_2$, the patient will develop alkalosis because of the retained bicarbonate. Such a patient could move from compensated respiratory acidosis to serious metabolic alkalosis.

The presence of alkalosis makes weaning from the ventilator difficult. Alkalosis, especially if the onset is abrupt, can have serious consequences, including hypokalemia, hypocalcemia, and dysrhythmias. Usually the patient with COPD who is supported on the ventilator does better with a short inspiratory and longer expiratory time.

If hyperventilation is spontaneous, it is important to determine the cause and treat it. Common causes include hypoxemia, pain, fear, anxiety, or compensation for metabolic acidosis. Patients who fight the ventilator or breathe out of synchrony may be anxious or in pain. If the patient is anxious and fearful, sitting with the patient and verbally coaching the patient to breathe with the ventilator or weaning the ventilator to a more appropriate setting may help. If these measures fail, manually ventilating the patient slowly with a BVM and 100% O_2 may slow breathing enough to bring it in synchrony with the ventilator.

Ventilator-Associated Pneumonia. The risk for HAI pneumonia is highest in patients requiring mechanical ventilation because the ET or tracheostomy tube bypasses normal upper airway defenses. Poor nutrition, immobility, and the underlying disease process (e.g., immunosuppression, organ failure) make the patient more prone to infection. *Ventilator-associated pneumonia* (VAP) is pneumonia that occurs 48 hours or more after ET intubation.[29] It occurs in as many as 27% of all intubated patients. Patients who develop VAP have significantly longer hospital stays and higher mortality rates than those who do not. Half of the patients develop early VAP (VAP that occurs within 96 hours of mechanical ventilation).

In those with early VAP, sputum cultures often grow gram-negative bacteria (e.g., *E coli, Klebsiella, Streptococcus pneumoniae, H influenzae*). Organisms associated with late VAP include antibiotic-resistant organisms, such as *Pseudomonas aeruginosa* and oxacillin-resistant *Staphylococcus aureus*. These organisms are abundant in the hospital environment and the patient's GI tract. They can spread in a number of ways, including contaminated respiratory equipment, inadequate hand washing, adverse environmental factors (e.g., poor room ventilation, high traffic flow), and decreased patient ability to cough and clear secretions. Colonization of the oropharynx tract by gram-negative organisms predisposes the patient to gram-negative pneumonia.

Clinical signs that suggest VAP include fever, high white blood cell count, purulent or odorous sputum, crackles or wheezes on auscultation, and pulmonary infiltrates noted on chest x-ray. The patient is given antibiotics after appropriate cultures are taken by tracheal suctioning or bronchoscopy and when infection is evident.

Guidelines for VAP prevention include (1) minimizing sedation, including daily spontaneous awakening trials (SATs) and daily spontaneous breathing trials (SBTs), (2) early exercise and mobilization, (3) use of ET tubes with subglottic secretion drainage ports for patients likely to be intubated greater than 48 to 72 hours, (4) HOB elevation at a minimum of 30 to 45 degrees unless medically contraindicated, (5) oral care with chlorhexidine, and (6) no routine changes of the patient's ventilator circuit tubing.[30]

Other preventive measures include strict hand washing before and after suctioning, whenever ventilator equipment is touched, and after contact with any respiratory secretions (see Nursing Management: Artificial Airway earlier in this chapter). Always wear gloves when in contact with the patient and change gloves between activities (e.g., emptying urinary catheter drainage, hanging an IV drug). Last, always drain the water that collects in the ventilator tubing away from the patient as it collects.

⚠ SAFETY ALERT VAP Prevention Strategies
- Practice good hand hygiene techniques before and after suctioning.
- Wear gloves when providing oral hygiene.
- Suction patients as needed for comfort.
- Keep the HOB elevated >30 to 45 degrees.
- Turn patient according to agency policy (e.g., side to side every 2 hours).
- Initiate early mobilization.
- Follow agency policy for limiting sedation with SAT.
- Perform daily SBT unless contraindicated.[31]

Psychosocial Needs. The patient receiving mechanical ventilation often has physical and emotional stress. In addition to the problems related to critical care patients discussed at the beginning of this chapter, the patient supported by a mechanical ventilator is unable to speak, eat, move, or breathe normally. Tubes and machines cause pain, fear, and anxiety. Usual activities, such as eating, elimination, and coughing, are extremely complicated.

The ABCDEF Bundle is an evidence-based practice of providing care that strives to attain an environment in which all patients receiving mechanical ventilation are calm, delirium free, and able to express their needs for pain control, positioning, and reassurance. The ABCDEF Bundle ensures (1) **A**ssessment, (2) **B**oth SATs and SBTs are done, (3) correct **C**hoice of analgesia and sedation, (4) **D**elirium prevention and management, (5) **E**arly mobility, and (6) **F**amily engagement.[32]

Feeling safe is an overpowering need of patients on mechanical ventilation. Work to strengthen the various factors that affect feeling safe. Encourage hope, as appropriate, and build trusting relationships with both the patient and caregiver. Involve them in decision making as much as possible.[19]

Sedation and Analgesia. Patients receiving PPV may need sedation (e.g., propofol) and/or analgesia (e.g., fentanyl) to help with optimal ventilation. Before starting sedation or analgesia in the mechanically ventilated patient who is agitated or anxious, identify the cause of distress. Common problems that can result in patient agitation or anxiety include PPV, nutritional

deficits, pain, hypoxemia, hypercapnia, drugs, and environmental stressors (e.g., sleep deprivation).

At times, the decision is made to paralyze the patient with a neuromuscular blocking agent (e.g., cisatracurium [Nimbex]) to provide more effective synchrony with the ventilator and improve oxygenation. Remember that the paralyzed patient can hear, see, and feel. It is essential to give IV sedation and analgesia concurrently when the patient is paralyzed. Sedated or paralyzed patients may be aware of their surroundings. You should always address them as if they were awake and alert.

Monitoring patients receiving these drugs is challenging. Assess the patient using train-of-four (TOF) peripheral nerve stimulation, physiologic signs of pain or anxiety (e.g., changes in HR and BP), and ventilator synchrony. The TOF assessment involves using a peripheral nerve stimulator to deliver 4 successive stimulating currents to elicit muscle twitches (Fig. 65.22).[33] The number of twitches varies with the amount of neuromuscular blockade. The usual goal is 1 or 2 twitches out of 4 currents.

Noninvasive electroencephalogram technology (e.g., bispectral index monitoring [BIS]) can be used to guide sedative and analgesic therapy.[34] Excess administration of neuromuscular blocking agents may predispose the patient to prolonged paralysis and muscle weakness even after these agents are stopped.

Neurologic System. In patients with head injury, PPV, especially with PEEP, can impair cerebral blood flow. The increased intrathoracic positive pressure impedes venous drainage from the brain. This results in jugular venous distention. The patient may have increases in ICP due to the impaired venous return and subsequent increase in cerebral volume. Elevating the HOB and keeping the patient's head in alignment may reduce the harmful effects of PPV on ICP.

Sodium and Water Imbalance. Progressive fluid retention often occurs after 48 to 72 hours of PPV, especially PPV with PEEP. Fluid retention is associated with decreased urine output and increased sodium retention. Fluid balance changes may be due to decreased CO, which causes decreased renal perfusion. This stimulates the release of renin with the subsequent production of angiotensin and aldosterone (see Chapter 44, Fig. 44.4). This results in sodium and water retention. It is possible that pressure changes within the thorax are associated with decreased release of atrial natriuretic peptide, which also causes sodium retention. Less insensible water loss occurs via the airway because ventilated

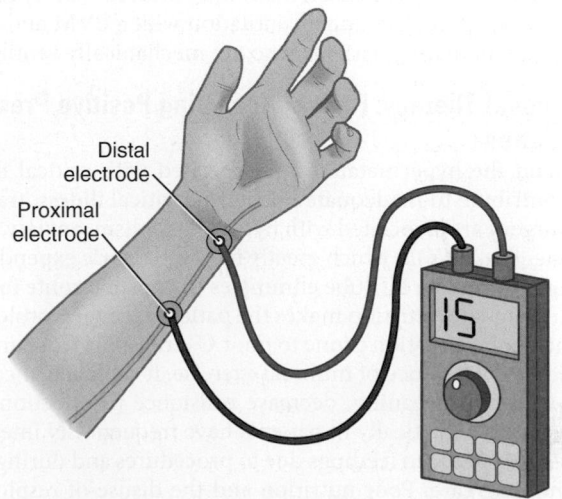

FIG. 65.22 Placement of electrodes along ulnar nerve.

delivered gases are humidified with body-temperature water. As a part of the stress response, release of antidiuretic hormone (ADH) and cortisol contributes to sodium and water retention.

Gastrointestinal System. Patients receiving PPV are stressed because of the serious illness, immobility, or discomforts associated with the ventilator. This places the patient at risk for developing stress ulcers and GI bleeding. Patients with a preexisting ulcer or those receiving corticosteroids have a higher risk. Any circulatory compromise, including reduced CO caused by PPV, may contribute to ischemia of the gastric and intestinal mucosa and increase the risk for translocation of GI bacteria.

Stress ulcer prophylaxis includes giving histamine (H_2)-receptor blockers (e.g., ranitidine), proton pump inhibitors (PPIs) (e.g., esomeprazole), or EN to decrease gastric acidity and reduce the risk for stress ulcer and hemorrhage. PPIs may increase the risk for *Clostridium difficile infection*.[35] (This is discussed in Chapter 41 on p. 898.)

Gastric and bowel dilation may occur because of gas accumulation in the GI tract from swallowed air. The irritation of an artificial airway may cause excessive air swallowing and gastric dilation. Gastric or bowel dilation may put pressure on the vena cava, decrease CO, and prohibit adequate diaphragmatic excursion during spontaneous breathing. Elevation of the diaphragm from a paralytic ileus or bowel dilation leads to compression of the lower lobes of the lungs. This may cause atelectasis and compromise respiratory function. Decompression of the stomach is done by inserting an OG or NG tube.

Immobility, sedation, circulatory impairment, decreased oral intake, use of opioid pain medicines, and stress contribute to decreased peristalsis. The patient's inability to exhale against a closed glottis may make defecation difficult. As a result, the ventilated patient is at risk for constipation. A bowel regimen should be started to help with motility.

Musculoskeletal System. Maintaining muscle strength and preventing complications associated with immobility are important. Adequate analgesia and nutrition can enhance exercise tolerance. Plan for early and progressive mobility of appropriate patients receiving PPV.[8] In collaboration with physical and occupational therapy, perform passive and active exercises to maintain muscle tone in the upper and lower extremities. Simple maneuvers, such as leg lifts, knee bends, or arm circles, are appropriate. Prevent contractures, pressure injuries, footdrop, and external rotation of the hip and legs by proper positioning and using specialized mattresses or beds. Use a portable ventilator or provide manual ventilation with a BVM and 100% O_2 when ambulating patients who are mechanically ventilated.

Nutritional Therapy: Patient Receiving Positive Pressure Ventilation

PPV and the hypermetabolism associated with critical illness can contribute to inadequate nutrition. Critical illness, trauma, and surgery are associated with hypermetabolism, anxiety, pain, and increased WOB, which greatly increase caloric expenditure. The presence of an ET tube eliminates the normal route for eating. Inadequate nutrition makes the patient receiving prolonged mechanical ventilation prone to poor O_2 transport from anemia and to poor tolerance of minimal exercise. It can delay mechanical ventilation weaning, decrease resistance to infection, and slow recovery. Critically ill patients have frequent EN interruptions. We often hold feedings due to procedures and during routine nursing care. Poor nutrition and the disuse of respiratory muscles contribute to decreased respiratory muscle strength.

Serum protein levels (e.g., albumin, prealbumin, transferrin, total protein) are usually decreased.

Patients unlikely to be able to eat independently for 3 to 5 days should have a nutritional assessment and EN started within 24 to 48 hours of admission.[9] EN is the preferred method to meet caloric needs of mechanically ventilated patients (see Chapter 39 for discussion of EN). Consult the dietitian to determine the caloric and nutrient needs of these patients.

▪▪ NURSING MANAGEMENT

Caring for the Patient Requiring Mechanical Ventilation

In the critically ill patient who requires mechanical ventilation, the RN and RT provide most of the care. Some patients who need chronic mechanical ventilation may be in long-term care settings or at home. In these settings, the RN and RT assess the patient and plan and evaluate care, but implementation of some activities may be delegated.

- Develop plan for communication with the patient who has an ET tube or tracheostomy.
- Give sedatives, analgesics, and paralytic drugs as needed.
- Teach patient and caregiver about mechanical ventilation and weaning procedures.
- Auscultate breath sounds and respiratory effort, assessing for decreased ventilation or adventitious sounds.
- Monitor ventilator settings and alarms.
- Determine need for ET tube suctioning and suction patients as needed.
- Reposition and secure ET tube (based on agency policy).
- Monitor oxygenation level and signs of respiratory fatigue during weaning procedure.
- Provide enteral nutrition.
- Oversee UAP:
  - Obtain vital signs and report to the RN.
  - Provide personal hygiene, skin care, and oral care, as directed by RN.
  - Assist with frequent position changes, including ambulation, as directed by the RN.
  - Help to perform passive or active range-of-motion (ROM) exercises.

Collaborate With Respiratory Therapist (RT)

- Auscultate breath sounds and respiratory effort, assessing for decreased ventilation or adventitious sounds.
- Monitor ventilator settings and alarms.
- Change ventilator settings as needed or ordered by HCP.
- Maintain appropriate cuff inflation on ET tube.
- Determine need for ET tube suctioning and suction patients as needed.
- Reposition and secure ET tube (based on agency policy).
- Monitor oxygenation level and signs of respiratory fatigue during weaning procedure.

Collaborate With Physical and Occupational Therapist

- Perform ROM exercises.
- Assist with early and progressive ambulation as directed by the RN.

Collaborate With Dietitian

- Assess and monitor patient's nutritional status.
- Recommend formulations for enteral and/or parenteral nutrition as needed.

Collaborate With Speech Therapist

- Perform swallowing studies.
- Assess patient's cognitive function and assist with communication.
- Provide teaching for patient with a long-term tracheostomy.

Collaborate With Social Worker

- Work with the patient and caregiver to identify care needs.
- Help the patient with transitions through the health care system.
- Teach the patient the various levels of care and seek to optimize outcomes in a cost-effective manner.

When eating with a tracheostomy tube in place, the patient should tilt the head slightly forward to assist with swallowing and to prevent aspiration. The diet may be restricted to soft foods (e.g., puddings, ice cream) and thickened liquids. Patients with a long-term tracheostomy will likely have a tube placed in the stomach (gastrostomy) or small bowel (jejunostomy) for nutritional support (see Chapter 39). Patients may be able to eat normally once the tracheostomy site heals and they meet criteria that will allow them to take oral intake. Swallowing studies and a speech therapy consultation are done to assess the patient's readiness for oral intake.

Weaning From Positive Pressure Ventilation and Extubation

Weaning is the process of reducing ventilator support and resuming spontaneous breathing. The weaning process differs for patients on short-term ventilation (up to 3 days) versus long-term ventilation (longer than 3 days). Those with short-term ventilation (e.g., after heart surgery) have a linear weaning process. Patients with prolonged PPV (e.g., patients with COPD who develop respiratory failure) often have a weaning process that consists of alternating gains and losses. Preparation

for weaning begins when PPV is started and involves a team approach (e.g., HCP, RT, RN, patient).

Weaning consists of 3 phases: the *preweaning phase*, the *weaning process*, and the *outcome phase*. The preweaning, or assessment phase, looks at the patient's ability to breathe spontaneously. Assessment depends on a combination of respiratory and non-respiratory factors (Table 65.13). Note the resolution of the primary problem that prompted patient admission. The patient's lungs should be reasonably clear on auscultation and chest x-ray. Weaning assessment parameters should include criteria to assess muscle strength (negative inspiratory force) and endurance (spontaneous V_T, vital capacity, minute ventilation, rapid shallow breathing index). There should be minimal secretions, the ability to cough and gag, and a cuff leak when the ET tube cuff is deflated.

Nonrespiratory factors include the patient's neurologic status; hemodynamics; fluid, electrolytes, and acid-base balance; nutrition; and hemoglobin. It is important to have an alert, well-rested, and well-informed patient relatively free from pain and anxiety who can cooperate with the weaning plan. This does not mean complete withdrawal from sedatives or analgesics. Instead, drugs should be titrated to achieve comfort without causing excessive drowsiness.

TABLE 65.13 Indicators for Weaning

Weaning Readiness

Patients receiving mechanical ventilation for respiratory failure should undergo a formal assessment of weaning potential if the following are satisfied*:

1. Reversal of the underlying cause of respiratory failure
2. Adequate oxygenation
   - PaO_2/FIO_2 >150–200
   - SpO_2 ≥90%
   - PEEP ≤5–7 cm H_2O
   - FIO_2 ≤40%–50%
   - pH ≥7.25

3. Hemodynamically stabile
   - Absence of myocardial ischemia
   - Absence of clinically significant hypotension (low dose or no vasopressor therapy)
4. Patient ability to initiate respirations
5. Optional criteria
   - Hemoglobin ≥7–10 g/dL
   - Core temperature ≤100.4° F (38° C) to 101.3° F (38.5° C)
   - Mental status awake and alert or easily arousable

WEANING ASSESSMENT

Measurement	Significance	Normal Values	Indices for Weaning
Spontaneous respiratory rate (RR)	Respiratory rate/frequency over 1 min.	12–20 breaths/min	<35 breaths/min
Spontaneous tidal volume (V_T)	Amount of air exchanged during normal breathing at rest. Measure of muscle endurance.	>5–7 mL/kg	≥5 mL/kg
Minute ventilation (V_E)	V_T multiplied by respiratory rate over 1 min. *For example:* 0.350 (V_T) × 28 (f) = 9.8 L/min.	>10 L/min	>10 L/min
Negative inspiratory force or pressure (NIF, NIP)	Amount of negative pressure that a patient can generate to initiate spontaneous respirations. *Measured by clinician:* After complete occlusion of inspiratory valve, a pressure manometer is attached to airway or mouth for 10–20 sec while negative inspiratory efforts are noted.	<−50 cm H_2O	<−20 cm H_2O The more negative the number, the better indication for weaning.
Positive expiratory pressure (PEP)	Measure of expiratory muscle strength and ability to cough. *Measured by clinician:* After complete occlusion of expiratory valve, a pressure manometer is attached to the airway or mouth for 10–20 sec while positive expiratory efforts are noted.	60–85 cm H_2O	≥30 cm H_2O
Rapid shallow breathing index RSBI (f/V_T)	Spontaneous respiratory rate over 1 min divided by V_T (in liters). *For example:* 30 (f)/0.400 (V_T) = 75/L	<40/L	<105/L
Spontaneous breathing trial (SBT)	If patient passes daily weaning screen, assess patient during SBT with little or no ventilator assistance. Trial should be at least 30 min to a maximum of 120 min.		Successful completion of trial is based on an integrated patient assessment.
Vital capacity (VC)	Maximum inspiration and then measurement of air during maximal forced expiration. Measure of respiratory muscle endurance or reserve or both. Requires patient cooperation.	65–75 mL/kg	≥10–15 mL/kg

Adapted from Urden LD, Stacy, KM, Lough ME: *Critical care nursing: Diagnosis and management*, ed 8, St Louis, 2018, Elsevier.
*The decision to use these criteria are personalized to the patient.

A SAT and an SBT are recommended in patients who meet a daily safety screen. A SAT should be done by stopping all sedatives and, in patients without active pain, all opioids. Sedation should be restarted at 50% of the previous dose in patients who "fail" the SAT and remain off in patients who "pass."

EVIDENCE-BASED PRACTICE

Early Mobilization and Critically Ill Patients

W.R. is a 68-yr-old man who has been in the ICU for 2 days. He is receiving mechanical ventilation, and weaning trials are planned. You have started passive exercises and dangling with W.R. You prepare to discuss early mobilization with him and his partner.

Making Clinical Decisions

Best Available Evidence. Implementing an early exercise and mobilization protocol for stable, mechanically ventilated patients is safe and well tolerated. Early mobilization improves patient outcomes (e.g., prevention of ICU-acquired weakness, maintenance of long-term function, preservation of quality of life) and reduces the length of hospital stays. Involving patients and families in decision-making around care (e.g., early mobilization) is an identified priority among this group.

Clinician Expertise. Your unit has successfully implemented AACN's **ABCDEF** bundle related to delirium, immobility, sedation/analgesia, and ventilator management in the ICU. You know that patients and their families often worry about ambulating with complex equipment attached to them.

Patient Preferences and Values. W.R. writes on the computer that he does not want to get out of bed until his "breathing tube is out." His partner tells you he is "afraid of falling."

Implications for Nursing Practice

1. What will you tell W.R. and his partner about the benefits of and protocol for early mobilization?
2. How will you involve them in the decision to take part in the program?

Reference for Evidence

McKenzie E, Potestio ML, Boyd JM, et al.: Reconciling patient and provider priorities for improving the care of critically ill patients: a consensus method and qualitative analysis of decision making, *Health Expect* 20:1367, 2017.

An SBT should last at least 30 minutes but no more than 120 minutes.[13] It may be done with low levels of PEEP, low levels of PSV, or FIO_2. Tolerance of the trial may lead to extubation. Failure to tolerate an SBT should prompt a search for reversible or complicating factors and a return to a nonfatiguing ventilator modality. The SBT should be tried daily, unless contraindicated.

All health care team members should be familiar with the weaning plan. The use of a weaning protocol decreases ventilator days.[13] The ventilator settings are not as important as the use of a daily protocol to prevent delays in weaning. The patient receiving SIMV can have the ventilator breaths gradually reduced as ventilatory status permits. PEEP or PSV can be added to SIMV. PSV is thought to provide gentle, slow respiratory muscle conditioning. It may be especially beneficial for patients who are deconditioned or have heart problems.

Weaning may be tried at any time of day. It is usually done after a period of time when the patient has been ventilated in a rest mode. The rest mode should be a stable, nonfatiguing, and comfortable form of support for the patient. It is important to allow the patient's respiratory muscles to rest between weaning trials. Once the respiratory muscles become fatigued, they may need 12 to 24 hours to recover.

The patient and caregiver need ongoing emotional support. Explain the weaning process to them to keep them informed of progress. Place the patient in a comfortable sitting or semirecumbent position. Obtain baseline vital signs and respiratory parameters. During the weaning trial, closely monitor the patient for signs and symptoms that may signal a need to end the trial (e.g., tachypnea, dyspnea, tachycardia, dysrhythmias, sustained desaturation [SpO_2 less than 90%], hypertension or hypotension, agitation, diaphoresis, anxiety, sustained V_T less than 5 mL/kg, changes in mental status). Record the patient's tolerance throughout the weaning process. Include statements about the patient's and the caregiver's feelings.

The weaning outcome phase is the period when the patient is ready for extubation or weaning is stopped because progress is not being made. The patient who is ready for extubation should receive hyperoxygenation and suctioning (e.g., oropharynx, ET tube) prior to extubation. Loosen the ET tapes or commercial holder. Have the patient take a deep breath, and at the peak of inspiration, deflate the ET tube cuff and remove the tube in one motion. After removal, encourage the patient to deep breath and cough. Suction the oropharynx as needed. Have the patient say their name to assess vocalization. Give supplemental O_2 and provide naso-oral care. Carefully monitor vital signs, respiratory status, and oxygenation immediately after extubation, within 1 hour, and per agency policy. If the patient does not tolerate extubation (e.g., decreased SpO_2 levels, tachypnea or bradypnea, tachycardia, decreased level of consciousness, decrease in PaO_2, increase in $PaCO_2$), immediate reintubation or a trial of noninvasive ventilation may be needed.

Chronic Mechanical Ventilation

Mechanical ventilators are now a part of long-term and home care. In some instances, terminally ill, ventilated patients may be discharged to hospice. The emphasis on controlling hospital costs has increased the number of patients discharged early from the acute care setting and the need to provide highly technical care, such as mechanical ventilation, in home settings. The success of home mechanical ventilation depends, in part, on careful predischarge assessment and planning for the patient and caregivers. Patients must first meet criteria to be discharged on mechanical ventilation (e.g., tracheostomy, stabile mechanical ventilator settings).

Both negative pressure and positive pressure ventilators can be used in the home. Negative pressure ventilators do not require an artificial airway and are less complicated to use. Several types of small, portable (battery-powered) positive pressure ventilators are available. They can be attached to a wheelchair or placed on a bedside table. Settings and alarms on these ventilators are simpler to use than on the standard ICU ventilators.

Home mechanical ventilation has advantages and disadvantages. Having the patient in the home eliminates the strain that the hospital setting imposes on family dynamics. Caregivers may feel helpless when they first hear about the need for long-term mechanical ventilation. However, these feelings are often balanced by the opportunity to take part in the patient's care in the home setting. At home, the patient may be able to take part in more activities of daily living around a personalized schedule. Because of the smaller size of the home ventilator, the patient may be more mobile. Another advantage is a lower risk for HAIs.

Disadvantages include problems related to equipment, reimbursement, caregiver stress and fatigue, and the patient's complex needs. Ventilated patients are usually dependent, requiring extensive nursing care, at least initially. Disposable products may not be reimbursable. Carefully assess financial resources when arranging home ventilation. Schedule a meeting with the interprofessional care team (e.g., social worker, home health care RN, RT) before starting a discharge teaching plan. Caregivers may seem enthusiastic about caring for their loved one in the home but may not understand the sacrifices they may have to make financially and in personal time and commitment. Encourage caregivers to consider respite care to periodically relieve their stress and fatigue.

OTHER CRITICAL CARE CONTENT

Table 65.14 lists critical care content discussed in other chapters of this book.

TABLE 65.14 Cross-References to Critical Care Content

Topic	Discussed in Chapter	Topic	Discussed in Chapter
Acute coronary syndrome (ACS)	33	Enteral nutrition (EN)	39
Acute heart failure	34	Head injury and ICP monitoring	56
Acute respiratory distress syndrome (ARDS)	67	Multiple organ dysfunction syndrome (MODS)	66
Acute respiratory failure	67	Myocardial infarction (MI)	33
Basic life support and CPR	Appendix A	Oxygen delivery	28
Burns	24	Pain management	8
Cardiac pacemakers	35	Parenteral nutrition (PN)	39
Cardiac surgery	33	Pulmonary edema	34
Central venous access device (CVAD)	16	Renal dialysis	46
Continuous renal replacement therapy (CRRT)	46	Shock	66
Delirium	59	Stroke	57
Dysrhythmias	35	Systemic inflammatory response syndrome (SIRS)	66
Emergencies	68	Tracheostomy	26
End-of-life (EOL) care	9	Trauma	68

CASE STUDY

Critical Care and Mechanical Ventilation

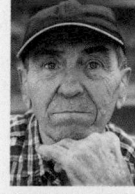
(© Thinkstock.)

Patient Profile

R.K. is a 72-yr-old white man who collapsed in his home. He was found by his daughter, and she activated the emergency response system. He was unresponsive on admission to the emergency department and is still unresponsive on arrival to the ICU. He has an oral ET tube in place and is receiving mechanical ventilation. A large-bore, peripheral IV has been placed and fluids are infusing.

Subjective Data

None. Patient has no eye opening. He is intubated and is unresponsive to painful stimuli.

Objective Data

Physical Examination

- Noninvasive BP 100/75 mm Hg; apical-radial HR 128; temperature 102° F (38.8° C); SpO$_2$ is 98%
- ECG: atrial fibrillation with a rapid ventricular response
- Purulent secretions suctioned from ET tube
- Breath sounds: coarse crackles bilaterally, decreased breath sounds on the right
- Weight: 168 lb. (76 kg)

Diagnostic Studies

- Chest x-ray shows right lower lung consolidation
- ABGs: pH 7.48; PaO$_2$ 94 mm Hg; PaCO$_2$ 30 mm Hg; HCO$_3$ 34 mEq/L
- CT scan is positive for a hemorrhagic stroke

Interprofessional Care

- Positive pressure ventilation settings: assist-control mode
- Settings: FIO$_2$ 70%, V$_T$ 700 mL, respiratory rate 16 breaths/min, PEEP 5 cm H$_2$O

- Orogastric tube. EN at 25 mL/hr, increase by 20 mL/hr every 2 hr with a goal of 80 mL/hr to start on day 2
- External condom catheter for urinary drainage and measurement
- HOB elevated at 40 degrees
- Reposition at least every 2 hr
- Azithromycin (Zithromax) 500 mg IV q24hr
- Cefotaxime 2 gram IV q6hr
- NS at 75 mL/hr

Discussion Questions

1. Identify 2 reasons for intubating and providing mechanical ventilation for R.K.
2. What does R.K.'s ABG indicate, and which ventilator setting(s) should be changed to prevent barotrauma?
3. R.K.'s BP drops to 80 mm Hg. Despite increasing doses of vasopressors and fluid challenges, his BP is still low. A central venous catheter and an arterial line are inserted. Arterial pressure–based cardiac output (APCO) monitoring is started. What would be the purpose of hemodynamic monitoring in this patient?
4. **Priority Decision:** What are 2 priority nursing considerations for a patient with invasive monitoring?
5. R.K.'s pulmonary condition deteriorates. PaO$_2$ drops to 60 mm Hg, and SpO$_2$ is 89%. PEEP is increased to 7.5 cm H$_2$O. What implications does this have for R.K. given his hemodynamic status? What other intervention could be done to improve oxygenation?
6. **Collaboration:** What patient care activities can you delegate to unlicensed assistive personnel?
7. **Evidence-Based Practice:** R.K.'s caregivers want to know why he is to receive tube feedings. What would you tell them? What is the evidence to support the use of EN?
8. **Patient-Centered Care:** After 4 days, R.K. is still unresponsive and has developed renal failure. The HCP thinks the patient will not recover from his neurologic injury and wishes to discuss goals of care with the patient's caregivers. What would be your role in this meeting?

Answers available at *http://evolve.elsevier.com/Lewis/medsurg*.

BRIDGE TO NCLEX EXAMINATION

The number of the question corresponds to the same-numbered outcome at the beginning of the chapter.

1. Certification in critical care nursing (CCRN) by the American Association of Critical-Care Nurses indicates that the nurse
   a. is an advanced practice nurse who cares for acutely and critically ill patients.
   b. may practice independently to provide symptom management for the critically ill.
   c. has earned a master's degree in the field of advanced acute and critical care nursing.
   d. has practiced in critical care and successfully completed a test of critical care knowledge.

2. What are appropriate nursing interventions for the patient with delirium in the ICU? (select all that apply)
   a. Use clocks and calendars to maintain orientation.
   b. Encourage round-the-clock presence of caregivers at the bedside.
   c. Silence all alarms, reduce overhead paging, and avoid conversations around the patient.
   d. Sedate the patient with appropriate drugs to protect the patient from harmful behaviors.
   e. Identify physiologic factors that may be contributing to the patient's confusion and irritability.

3. The critical care nurse recognizes that an ideal plan for caregiver involvement includes
   a. having a caregiver at the bedside at all times.
   b. allowing caregivers at the bedside at preset, brief intervals.
   c. a personally devised plan to involve caregivers with care and patient needs.
   d. restriction of visiting in the ICU because the environment is overwhelming to caregivers.

4. To establish hemodynamic monitoring for a patient, the nurse zeros the
   a. cardiac output monitoring system to the level of the left ventricle.
   b. pressure monitoring system to the level of the catheter tip in the patient.
   c. pressure monitoring system to the level of the atrium, or the phlebostatic axis.
   d. pressure monitoring system to the level of the atrium, or the midclavicular line.

5. The hemodynamic changes the nurse expects to find after successful initiation of intraaortic balloon pump therapy in a patient with cardiogenic shock include (select all that apply)
   a. decreased SV.
   b. decreased SVR.
   c. decreased PAWP.
   d. increased diastolic BP.
   e. decreased myocardial O_2 consumption.

6. The purpose of adding PEEP to positive pressure ventilation is to
   a. increase functional residual capacity and improve oxygenation.
   b. increase FIO_2 to try to help wean the patient and avoid O_2 toxicity.
   c. determine if the patient can be weaned and avoid pneumomediastinum.
   d. determine if the patient is in synchrony with the ventilator or needs to be paralyzed.

7. The nursing management of a patient with an artificial airway includes
   a. maintaining ET tube cuff pressure at 35 cm H_2O.
   b. routine suctioning of the tube at least every 2 hours.
   c. observing for cardiac dysrhythmias during suctioning.
   d. preventing tube dislodgment by limiting mouth care to lubrication of the lips.

8. The nurse monitors the patient with positive pressure mechanical ventilation for
   a. paralytic ileus because pressure on the abdominal contents affects bowel motility.
   b. diuresis and sodium depletion because of increased release of atrial natriuretic peptide.
   c. signs of cardiovascular insufficiency because pressure in the chest impedes venous return.
   d. respiratory acidosis in a patient with COPD because of alveolar hyperventilation and increased PaO_2 levels.

1. d, 2. a, d, e, 3. c, 4. c, 5. b, c, d, e, 6. a, 7. c, 8. c

For rationales to these answers and even more NCLEX review questions, visit http://evolve.elsevier.com/Lewis/medsurg.

---

e EVOLVE WEBSITE/RESOURCES LIST

REFERENCES

1. American Association of Critical-Care Nurses: AACN scope and standards for acute and critical care nursing. Retrieved from www.aacn.org/nursing-excellence/standards/aacn-scope-and-standards-for-acute-and-critical-care-nursing-practice.
*2. Tirkkonen J, Tamminen T, Skrifvars MB: Outcome of adult patients attended by rapid response teams: A systematic review of the literature, Resuscitation 112:43, 2017.
3. American Association of Critical-Care Nurses: Frequently asked questions about APRN Consensus Model—For nurse practitioners. Retrieved from www.aacn.org/wd/certifications/content/aprn-nurses-np-faqs.pcms?menu=certification.
4. Papathanassoglou ED, Hadjibalassi M, Miltiadous P, et al: Effects of an integrative nursing intervention on pain in critically ill patients, Amer J Crit Care 27:172, 2018.
5. Hariharan U, Garg R: Sedation and analgesia in critical care, J Anesth Crit Care Open Access 7:262, 2017.
*6. Boyko Y, Jennum P, Toft P: Sleep quality and circadian rhythm disruption in the intensive care unit: A review, Nat Sci Sleep 9:277, 2017.

*7. Kanova M, Sklienka P, Kula R, et al: Incidence and risk factors for delirium development in ICU patients. A prospective observational study, *Biomedical Paper* 161:187, 2017.

*8. Blair GJ, Mehmood T, Rudnick M, et al: Nonpharmacologic and medication minimization strategies for the prevention and treatment of ICU delirium: A narrative review, *J Intensive Care Med* 34:183, 2019.

*9. McClave SA, Taylor BE, Martindale RG, et al: Guidelines for the provision and assessment of nutrition support therapy in the adult critically ill patient, *J Parenter Enteral Nutr* 40:159, 2016.

*10. Davidson JE, Aslakson RA, Long AC, et al: Guidelines for family-centered care in the neonatal, pediatric, and adult ICU, *CCM* 45:103, 2017.

11. Clark AP, Guzzetta CE: A paradigm shift for patient/family-centered care in intensive care units: Bring in the family, *Crit Care Nurse* 37:96, 2017.

12. Edwards Lifesciences: Hemodynamic monitoring. Retrieved from *www.edwards.com/devices/hemodynamic-monitoring*.

*13. Wiegand DL: *AACN procedure manual for high acuity, progressive, and critical care*, ed 7, St Louis, 2017, Elsevier.

14. Baird MB: *Manual of critical care nursing*, ed 7, St Louis, 2016, Elsevier.

*15. Cook JL, Colvin M, Francis GS, et al: Recommendations for the use of mechanical circulatory support. Ambulatory and community patient care. A scientific statement from the AHA, *Circulation* 135:e1, 2017.

16. Herritt B, Chaudhuri D, Thavorn K, et al: Early vs. late tracheostomy in intensive care settings: Impact on ICU and hospital costs, *J Crit Care* 44:285, 2018.

17. Dean C, Chapman E: Induction of anaesthesia, *Anaesth Intensive Care*, 19:383, 2018.

*18. Hampson J, Green C, Stewart J, et al: Impact of the introduction of an endotracheal tube attachment device on the incidence and severity of oral pressure injuries in the intensive care unit: A retrospective observational study, *BMC Nursing* 17:4, 2018.

*19. Holm A, Dreyer P: Intensive care unit patients' experience of being conscious during endotracheal intubation and mechanical ventilation, *Nurs Crit Care* 22:81, 2017.

20. Au G, Johnson JR, Chlan LL: Time for a paradigm shift: Assessing for anxiety in patients receiving mechanical ventilation, *Heart & Lung* 46:135, 2017.

21. Mohammed HM, Ali AA: Nursing issues of unplanned extubation in ICU, *IJNSS* 8:17, 2018.

*22. Sousa AS, Ferrito C, Paiva JA: Intubation-associated pneumonia: An integrative review, *Intensive Crit Care Nurs* 44:45, 2018.

*23. Allan SH, Doyle PA, Sapirstein A, et al: Data-driven implementation of alarm reduction interventions in a cardiovascular surgical ICU, *Jt Comm J Qual Patient Saf* 43:62, 2017.

24. Pham T, Brochard LJ, Slutsky AS: Mechanical ventilation: State of the art, *Mayo Clin Proc* 92:1382, 2017.

25. Bein T, Wrigge H: Airway pressure release ventilation (APRV): Do good things come to those who can wait? *J Thorac Dis* 10:667, 2018.

26. Ng J, Ferguson ND: High-frequency oscillatory ventilation: Still a role? *Curr Opin Crit Care* 23:175, 2017.

*27. Karam O, Gebistorf F, Wetterslev J, et al: The effect of inhaled nitric oxide in acute respiratory distress syndrome in children and adults: A Cochrane systematic review with trial sequential analysis, *Anaesthesia* 72:106, 2017.

*28. Fan E, Del Sorbo L, Goligher E, et al: An official American Thoracic Society/European Society of Intensive Care Medicine/Society of Critical Care Medicine Clinical Practice guideline: Mechanical ventilation in adult patients with acute respiratory distress syndrome, *Amer J Resp Crit Care Med* 195:1253, 2017.

29. Centers for Disease Control and Prevention (CDC): Pneumonia (ventilator-associated [VAP] and non-ventilator-associated pneumonia [PNEU]) event. Retrieved from *www.cdc.gov/nhsn/pdfs/pscmanual/6pscvapcurrent.pdf*.

*30. American Association of Critical Care Nurses: Ventilator assisted pneumonia. Retrieved from *www.aacn.org/clinical-resources/practice-alerts/ventilator-associated-pneumonia-vap*.

31. Larrow V, Klich-Heartt EI: Prevention of ventilator-associated pneumonia in the intensive care unit: Beyond the basics, *J Neuroscience Nurs* 48:160, 2016.

*32. Marra A, Ely EW, Pandharipande PP, Patel MB: The ABCDEF bundle in critical care, *Crit Care Clin* 33:225, 2017.

33. Naguib M, Brull SJ, Johnson KB: Conceptual and technical insights into the basis of neuromuscular monitoring, *Anaesthesia* 72:16, 2017.

34. Faritous Z, Barzanji A, Azarfarin R, et al: Comparison of bispectral index monitoring with the critical-care pain observation tool in the pain assessment of intubated adult patients after cardiac surgery, *Anesthesiol Pain Med* 6:e38334, 2016.

*35. Watson T, Hickok J, Fraker S, et al: Evaluating the risk factors for hospital-onset *Clostridium difficile* infections in a large healthcare system. *Clin Infect Dis* 66:1957, 2018.

*Evidence-based information for clinical practice.

66

Shock, Sepsis, and Multiple Organ Dysfunction Syndrome

Helen Miley

*You have not lived until you have done something for
someone who can never repay you.*

John Bunyen

ⓔ http://evolve.elsevier.com/Lewis/medsurg

CONCEPTUAL FOCUS

Anxiety	**Gas Exchange**	**Perfusion**
Fluids and Electrolytes	**Immunity**	

LEARNING OUTCOMES

1. Relate the pathophysiology to the clinical manifestations of the different types of shock: cardiogenic, hypovolemic, distributive, and obstructive.
2. Compare the effects of shock, sepsis, systemic inflammatory response syndrome, and multiple organ dysfunction syndrome on the major body systems.
3. Compare the interprofessional care, drug therapy, and nursing management of patients with different types of shock.
4. Describe the interprofessional care and nursing management of a patient experiencing multiple organ dysfunction syndrome.

KEY TERMS

anaphylactic shock, p. 1569
cardiogenic shock, p. 1566
hypovolemic shock, p. 1568
multiple organ dysfunction syndrome
   (MODS), p. 1584

neurogenic shock, p. 1568
obstructive shock, p. 1571
sepsis, p. 1569
septic shock, p. 1569
shock, p. 1566

systemic inflammatory response syndrome
   (SIRS), p. 1583

Shock, systemic inflammatory response syndrome (SIRS), sepsis, and multiple organ dysfunction syndrome (MODS) are serious and interrelated problems (Fig. 66.1). **Shock** is a syndrome characterized by decreased tissue perfusion and impaired cellular metabolism. This results in an imbalance between the supply of and demand for O_2 and nutrients. The exchange of O_2 and nutrients at the cellular level is essential to life. When cells are hypoperfused, the demand for O_2 and nutrients exceeds the supply at the microcirculatory level. Ischemia can occur, leading to cell injury and death. Thus shock of any cause is life-threatening. This chapter gives an overview of the different types of shock, SIRS, sepsis, and MODS and the related management of each.

SHOCK

Classification of Shock

The 4 main categories of shock are cardiogenic, hypovolemic, distributive, and obstructive (Table 66.1). Although the cause, initial presentation, and management vary for each type, the physiologic responses of the cells to hypoperfusion are similar.

Cardiogenic Shock. Cardiogenic shock occurs when either systolic or diastolic dysfunction of the heart's pumping action results in reduced cardiac output (CO), stroke volume (SV), and BP. These changes compromise myocardial perfusion, further depress myocardial function, and decrease CO and perfusion. Causes of cardiogenic shock are shown in Table 66.1. Mortality rates for patients with cardiogenic shock are around 50%.[1] It is the leading cause of death from acute myocardial infarction (MI).[1]

The heart's inability to pump the blood forward is called *systolic dysfunction*. This inability results in a low CO (less than 4 L/min) and *cardiac index* (less than 2.5 L/min/m²). Systolic dysfunction primarily affects the left ventricle since systolic pressure is greater on the left side of the heart. The most common cause of systolic dysfunction is acute MI. When systolic dysfunction affects the right side of the heart, blood flow through the pulmonary circulation is reduced. Decreased filling of the heart results in decreased SV. Causes of diastolic dysfunction are shown in Table 66.1.

Fig. 66.2 describes the pathophysiology of cardiogenic shock. Whether the first event is myocardial ischemia, a structural

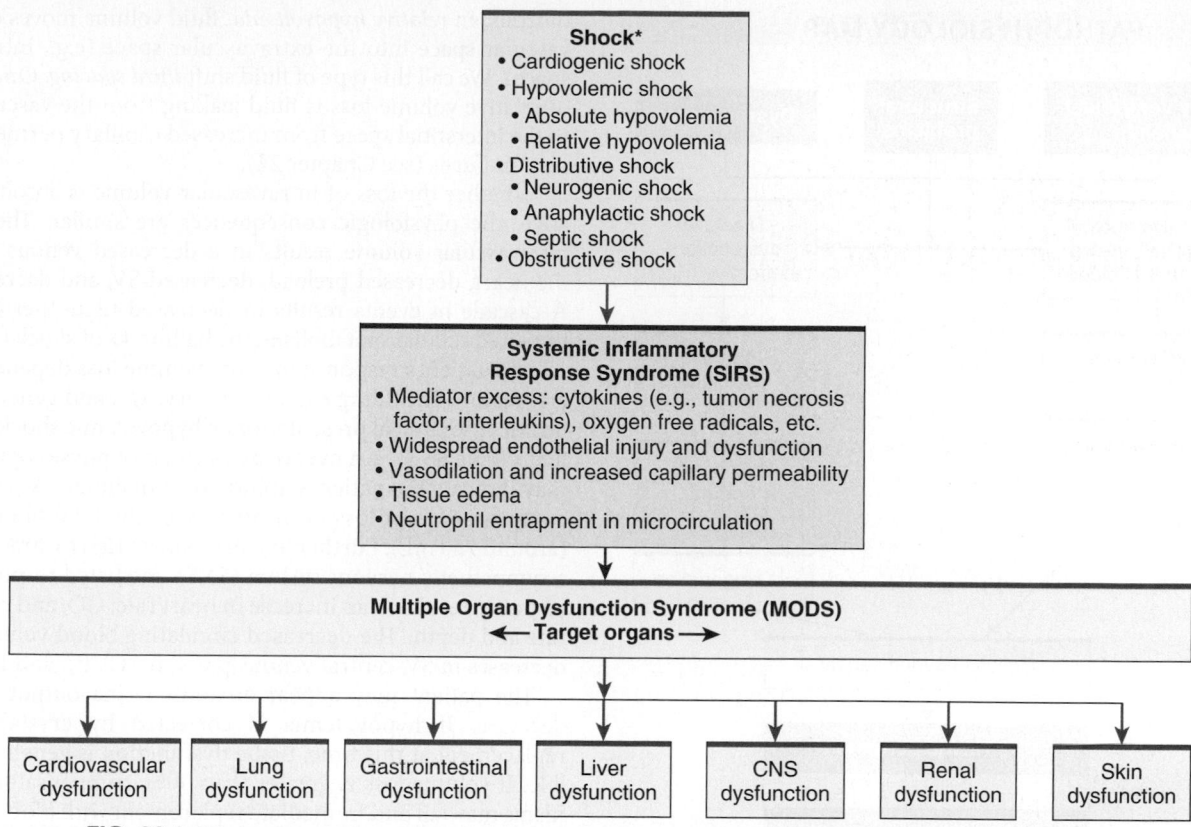

FIG. 66.1 Relationship of shock, systemic inflammatory response syndrome, and multiple organ dysfunction syndrome. (*See Table 66.1 for causes of shock states.)

TABLE 66.1 Classification of Shock States

Types and Causes	Associated Conditions	Types and Causes	Associated Conditions
Cardiogenic Shock		**Distributive Shock**	
• Diastolic dysfunction: inability of the heart to fill	Cardiac tamponade, ventricular hypertrophy, cardiomyopathy	**Anaphylactic Shock**	
• Dysrhythmias	Bradydysrhythmias, tachydysrhythmias	• Hypersensitivity (allergic) reaction to a sensitizing substance	Contrast media, blood or blood products, drugs, insect bites, anesthetic agents, food or food additives, vaccines, environmental agents, latex
• Structural factors	Valvular stenosis or regurgitation, ventricular septal rupture, tension pneumothorax		
• Systolic dysfunction: inability of the heart to pump blood forward	MI, cardiomyopathy, blunt cardiac injury, severe systemic or pulmonary hypertension, myocardial depression from metabolic problems	**Neurogenic Shock**	
		• Hemodynamic consequence of spinal cord injury and/or disease at or above T5	Severe pain, drugs, hypoglycemia, injury
Hypovolemic Shock		• Spinal anesthesia	
Absolute Hypovolemia		• Vasomotor center depression	
• External loss of whole blood	Hemorrhage from trauma, surgery, GI bleeding		
• Loss of other body fluids	Vomiting, diarrhea, excessive diuresis, diabetes insipidus, diabetes	**Septic Shock**	
		• Infection	Pneumonia, peritonitis, urinary tract, invasive procedures, indwelling lines and catheters
Relative Hypovolemia		• At-risk patients	Older adults, patients with chronic diseases (e.g., diabetes, chronic kidney disease, HF), patients receiving immunosuppressive therapy or who are malnourished or debilitated
• Fluid shifts	Burn injuries, ascites		
• Internal bleeding	Fracture of long bones, ruptured spleen, hemothorax, severe pancreatitis		
• Massive vasodilation	Sepsis		
• Pooling of blood or fluids	Bowel obstruction		
		Obstructive Shock	
		• Physical obstruction impeding the filling or outflow of blood resulting in reduced CO	Cardiac tamponade, tension pneumothorax, superior vena cava syndrome, abdominal compartment syndrome, pulmonary embolism

PATHOPHYSIOLOGY MAP

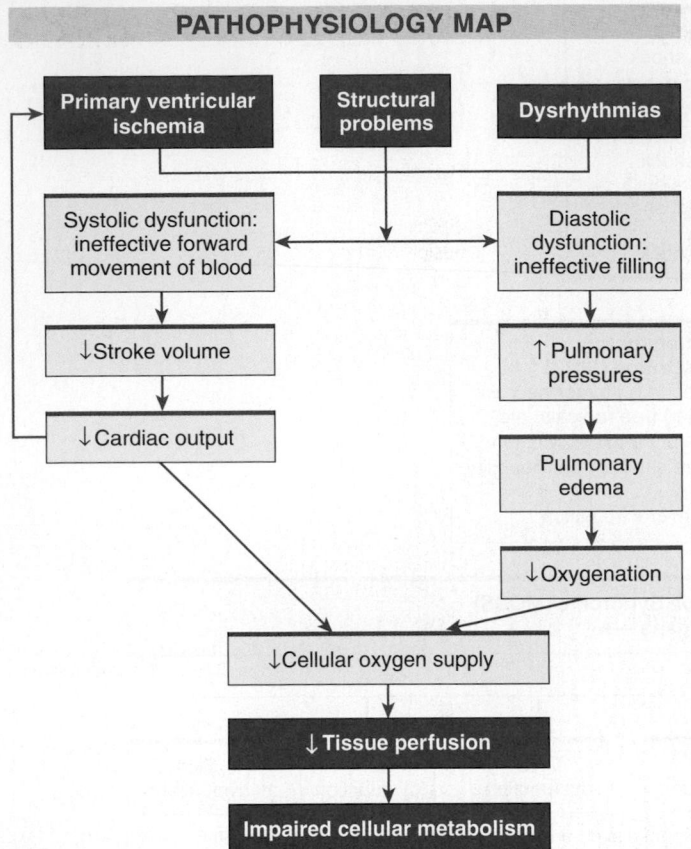

FIG. 66.2 The pathophysiology of cardiogenic shock. (Modified from Urden LD, Stacy KM, Lough ME: *Critical care nursing: Diagnosis and management,* ed 6, St Louis, 2010, Mosby.)

problem (e.g., valvular disorder, ventricular septal rupture), or dysrhythmias, the physiologic responses are similar. The patient has impaired tissue perfusion and cellular metabolism.

The early presentation of a patient with cardiogenic shock is similar to that of a patient with acute decompensated heart failure (HF) (see Chapter 34). The patient may have tachycardia and hypotension. Pulse pressure may be narrowed due to the heart's inability to pump blood forward during systole and increased volume during diastole. An increase in systemic vascular resistance (SVR) increases the workload of the heart. This increases myocardial O_2 consumption.

On assessment, the patient is tachypneic and has crackles on auscultation of breath sounds because of pulmonary congestion. The hemodynamic profile shows an increase in the pulmonary artery wedge pressure (PAWP), stroke volume variation (SVV), and pulmonary vascular resistance.

Signs of peripheral hypoperfusion (e.g., cyanosis, pallor, diaphoresis, weak peripheral pulses, cool and clammy skin, delayed capillary refill) occur. Decreased renal blood flow results in sodium and water retention and decreased urine output. Anxiety, confusion, and agitation may develop with impaired cerebral perfusion. Tables 66.2 and 66.3 describe the laboratory findings and clinical presentation of a patient with cardiogenic shock.

Hypovolemic Shock. Hypovolemic shock occurs from inadequate fluid volume in the intravascular space to support adequate perfusion (Table 66.1).[2] The volume loss may be either an absolute or a relative volume loss. *Absolute hypovolemia* results when fluid is lost through hemorrhage, gastrointestinal (GI) loss (e.g., vomiting, diarrhea), fistula drainage, diabetes insipidus, or

diuresis. In *relative hypovolemia,* fluid volume moves out of the vascular space into the extravascular space (e.g., intracavitary space). We call this type of fluid shift *third spacing.* One example of relative volume loss is fluid leaking from the vascular space to the interstitial space from increased capillary permeability, as seen in burns (see Chapter 24).

Whether the loss of intravascular volume is absolute or relative, the physiologic consequences are similar. The reduced intravascular volume results in a decreased venous return to the heart, decreased preload, decreased SV, and decreased CO. A cascade of events results in decreased tissue perfusion and impaired cellular metabolism, the hallmarks of shock (Fig. 66.3).

The patient's response to acute volume loss depends on several factors, including extent of injury, age, and general state of health. The clinical presentation of hypovolemic shock is consistent (Table 66.3). An overall assessment of physiologic reserves may indicate the patient's ability to compensate. A patient may compensate for a loss of up to 15% of the total blood volume (around 750 mL). Further loss of volume (15% to 30%) results in a sympathetic nervous system (SNS)–mediated response.[2] This response results in an increase in heart rate, CO, and respiratory rate and depth. The decreased circulating blood volume causes decreases in SV, central venous pressure (CVP), and PAWP.[3]

The patient may appear anxious. Urine output begins to decrease. If hypovolemia is corrected by crystalloid fluid replacement at this time, tissue dysfunction is generally reversible. If volume loss is greater than 30%, compensatory mechanisms may fail and immediate replacement with blood products should be started. Loss of autoregulation in the microcirculation and irreversible tissue destruction occur with loss of more than 40% of the total blood volume. Common laboratory studies and assessments that are done include serial measurements of hemoglobin and hematocrit levels, electrolytes, lactate, blood gases, mixed central venous O_2 saturation (SvO_2), and hourly urine outputs (Table 66.2).

Distributive Shock

Neurogenic Shock. Neurogenic shock is a hemodynamic phenomenon that can occur within 30 minutes of a spinal cord injury and last up to 6 weeks. Neurogenic shock related to spinal cord injuries is generally associated with a cervical or high thoracic injury. The injury results in a massive vasodilation without compensation because of the loss of SNS vasoconstrictor tone.[4] This massive vasodilation leads to a pooling of blood in the blood vessels, tissue hypoperfusion, and impaired cellular metabolism (Fig. 66.4).

In addition to spinal cord injury, spinal anesthesia can block transmission of impulses from the SNS. Depression of the vasomotor center of the medulla from drugs (e.g., opioids, benzodiazepines) can decrease the vasoconstrictor tone of the peripheral blood vessels, resulting in neurogenic shock (Table 66.1).

The classic manifestations are hypotension (from the massive vasodilation) and bradycardia (from unopposed parasympathetic stimulation).[4] The patient may not be able to regulate body temperature. Combined with massive vasodilation, the inability to regulate temperature promotes heat loss. At first, the patient's skin is warm due to the massive vasodilation. As the heat disperses, the patient is at risk for hypothermia. Later, the patient's skin may be cool or warm depending on the ambient temperature (*poikilothermia,* taking on the temperature of the environment). In either case, the skin is usually dry. Tables 66.2 and 66.3 further describe the laboratory findings and clinical presentation of a patient with neurogenic shock.

TABLE 66.2 Diagnostic Studies

Shock

Study	Finding	Significance of Finding
Arterial blood gasses	Respiratory alkalosis	Found in early shock due to hyperventilation
	Metabolic acidosis	Occurs later in shock when lactate accumulates in blood from anaerobic metabolism
Base deficit	>−6	Acid production due to hypoxia
Blood cultures	Growth of organisms	May grow organisms in patients who are in septic shock
BUN	↑	Impaired kidney function caused by hypoperfusion from severe vasoconstriction, or occurs due to cell catabolism (e.g., trauma, infection)
Creatine kinase	↑	Trauma, MI in response to cellular damage and/or hypoxia
Creatinine	↑	Impaired kidney function caused by hypoperfusion because of severe vasoconstriction
DIC screen		Acute DIC can develop within hours to days after an initial assault on the body (e.g., shock)
• Fibrin split products (FSP)	↑	
• Fibrinogen level	↓	
• Platelet count	↓	
• PTT and PT	↑	
• INR	↑	
• Thrombin time	↑	
• D-dimer	↑	
Glucose	↑	Found in early shock because of release of liver glycogen stores in response to sympathetic nervous system stimulation and cortisol. Insulin insensitivity develops
	↓	Depleted glycogen stores with liver dysfunction possible as shock progresses
Electrolytes (serum)		
• Sodium	↑	Found in early shock because of ↑ secretion of aldosterone, causing renal retention of sodium
	↓	May be iatrogenic if excess hypotonic fluid is given after fluid loss
• Potassium	↑	Results when dead cells release potassium. Occurs in acute kidney injury and acidosis
	↓	Found in early shock because of ↑ secretion of aldosterone, causing renal excretion of potassium
Lactate level	↑	Usually ↑ once significant hypoperfusion and impaired O_2 use at the cellular level have occurred. By-product of anaerobic metabolism
Liver enzymes (ALT, AST, GGT)	↑	Liver cell destruction in progressive stage of shock
Procalcitonin (PCT)	↑	Biomarker released in response to bacterial infections
RBC count, hematocrit, hemoglobin	Normal	Remains within normal limits in shock because of relative hypovolemia and pump failure and in hemorrhagic shock before fluid resuscitation
	↓	Hemorrhagic shock after fluid resuscitation when fluids other than blood are used
	↑	Nonhemorrhagic shock caused by actual hypovolemia and hemoconcentration
Troponin	↑	MI
White blood cell count	↑, ↓	Infection, septic shock

ALT, Alanine aminotransferase; *AST,* aspartate aminotransferase; *GGT,* γ-glutamyl transferase; *INR,* international normalized ratio; *PT,* prothrombin time; *PTT,* partial thromboplastin time.

Although spinal shock and neurogenic shock often occur in the same patient, they are not the same disorder. *Spinal shock* is a transient condition that is present after an acute spinal cord injury (see Chapter 60). The patient with spinal shock has an absence of all voluntary and reflex neurologic activity below the level of the injury.

Anaphylactic Shock. Anaphylactic shock is an acute, life-threatening hypersensitivity (allergic) reaction to a sensitizing substance (e.g., drug, chemical, vaccine, food, insect venom).[5] The reaction quickly causes massive vasodilation, release of vasoactive mediators, and an increase in capillary permeability. As capillary permeability increases, fluid leaks from the vascular space into the interstitial space.

Anaphylactic shock can lead to respiratory distress due to laryngeal edema or severe bronchospasm and circulatory failure from the massive vasodilation. The patient has a sudden onset of symptoms, including dizziness, chest pain, incontinence, swelling of the lips and tongue, wheezing, and stridor. Skin changes include flushing, pruritus, urticaria, and angioedema. The patient may be anxious and confused and have a sense of impending doom.

A patient can have a severe allergic reaction, possibly leading to anaphylactic shock, after contact, inhalation, ingestion, or injection with an antigen (allergen) to which the person has previously been sensitized (Table 66.1). IV administration of the antigen (allergen) is the route most likely to cause anaphylaxis. However, oral, topical, and inhalation routes can cause anaphylactic reactions. Tables 66.2 and 66.3 describe the laboratory findings and clinical presentation of a patient in anaphylactic shock. Quick and decisive action is critical to prevent an allergic reaction from progressing to anaphylactic shock. (Anaphylaxis is discussed in Chapter 13.)

Septic Shock. Sepsis is a life-threatening syndrome in response to an infection. It is characterized by a dysregulated patient response along with new organ dysfunction related to the infection (Table 66.4).[6] In as many as 30% of patients with sepsis, the causative organism is not identified. Sepsis and septic shock have a high incidence worldwide, with a mortality rate of 25% or higher.[7]

Septic shock is a subset of sepsis. It has an increased mortality risk due to profound circulatory, cellular, and metabolic abnormalities. Septic shock is characterized by persistent hypotension, despite adequate fluid resuscitation, and inadequate tissue perfusion that results in tissue hypoxia.[6,7] The main organisms that cause sepsis are gram-negative and gram-positive bacteria.

TABLE 66.3 Clinical Presentation of Types of Shock

		DISTRIBUTIVE SHOCK			
Cardiogenic Shock	**Hypovolemic Shock**	**Neurogenic Shock**	**Anaphylactic Shock**	**Septic Shock**	**Obstructive Shock**
Cardiovascular System					
Tachycardia	Tachycardia	Bradycardia	Tachycardia	Tachycardia	Tachycardia
↓ BP	↓ Preload	↓ BP	↑ CO	↓/↑ Temperature	↓ BP
↓ SV, CO	↓ CO, CVP, PAWP	↓ CO, CVP, SVR	↑ CVP, PAWP	Myocardial dysfunction	↓ Preload
↑ SVR, PAWP, CVP	↑ SVR	↓/↑ Temperature	Chest pain	Biventricular dilation	↓ CO
↓ Capillary refill	↓ Capillary refill		Third spacing of fluid	↓ Ejection fraction	↑ SVR, CVP
Respiratory System					
Tachypnea	Tachypnea →	Dysfunction related	Shortness of breath	Hyperventilation	Tachypnea →
Crackles	bradypnea (late)	to level of injury	Edema of larynx and	Crackles	bradypnea (late)
Cyanosis			epiglottis	Respiratory alkalosis →	Shortness of
			Wheezing	respiratory acidosis	breath
			Stridor	Hypoxemia	
			Rhinitis	Respiratory failure	
				ARDS	
				Pulmonary hypertension	
Renal System					
↑ Na⁺ and H₂O retention	↓ Urine output	Bladder dysfunction	Incontinence	↓ Urine output	↓ Urine output
↓ Renal blood flow					
↓ Urine output					
Skin					
Pallor	Pallor	↓ Skin perfusion	Flushing	Warm and flushed →	Pallor
Cool, clammy	Cool, clammy	Cool or warm	Pruritus	cool and mottled	Cool, clammy
		Dry	Urticaria	(late)	
			Angioedema		
Neurologic System					
↓ Cerebral perfusion:	↓ Cerebral perfusion:	Flaccid paralysis	Anxiety	Change in men-	↓ Cerebral
• Anxiety	• Anxiety	below the level	Feeling of impending	tal status (e.g.,	perfusion:
• Confusion	• Confusion	of the lesion	doom	confusion)	• Anxiety
• Agitation	• Agitation	Loss of reflex	Confusion	Agitation	• Confusion
		activity	↓ LOC	Coma (late)	• Agitation
			Metallic taste		
Gastrointestinal System					
↓ Bowel sounds	Absent bowel sounds	Bowel dysfunction	Cramping	GI bleeding	↓ To absent bowel
Nausea, vomiting			Abdominal pain	Paralytic ileus	sounds
			Nausea		
			Vomiting		
			Diarrhea		
Diagnostic Findings*					
↑ Cardiac biomarkers	↓ Hematocrit		Sudden onset	↑/↓ WBC	Specific to cause
↑ b-Type natriuretic pep-	↓ Hemoglobin		History of allergies	↓ Platelets	of obstruction
tide (BNP)	↑ Lactate		Exposure to contrast	↑ Lactate	
↑ Blood glucose	↑ Urine specific gravity		media	↑ Blood glucose	
↑ BUN	Changes in electro-			↑ Procalcitonin	
ECG (e.g., dysrhythmias)	lytes			↑ Urine specific gravity	
Echocardiogram (e.g., left				↓ Urine Na⁺	
ventricular dysfunction				Positive blood cultures	
Chest x-ray (e.g., pulmo-					
nary infiltrates)					

*Also see Table 66.2.

Parasites, fungi, and viruses can also cause sepsis and septic shock.[6] Fig. 66.5 presents the pathophysiology of septic shock.

When a microorganism enters the body, the normal immune or inflammatory responses are triggered. However, in sepsis and septic shock the body's response to the microorganism is exaggerated. Both proinflammatory and antiinflammatory responses are activated, coagulation increases, and fibrinolysis decreases.[6] Endotoxins from the microorganism cell wall stimulate the release of cytokines. These include tumor necrosis factor (TNF), interleukin-1 (IL-1), and other proinflammatory mediators that act through secondary mediators, such as platelet-activating factor, IL-6, and IL-8.[6] (See Chapter 11 for discussion of the inflammatory response.) The release of platelet-activating factor results in

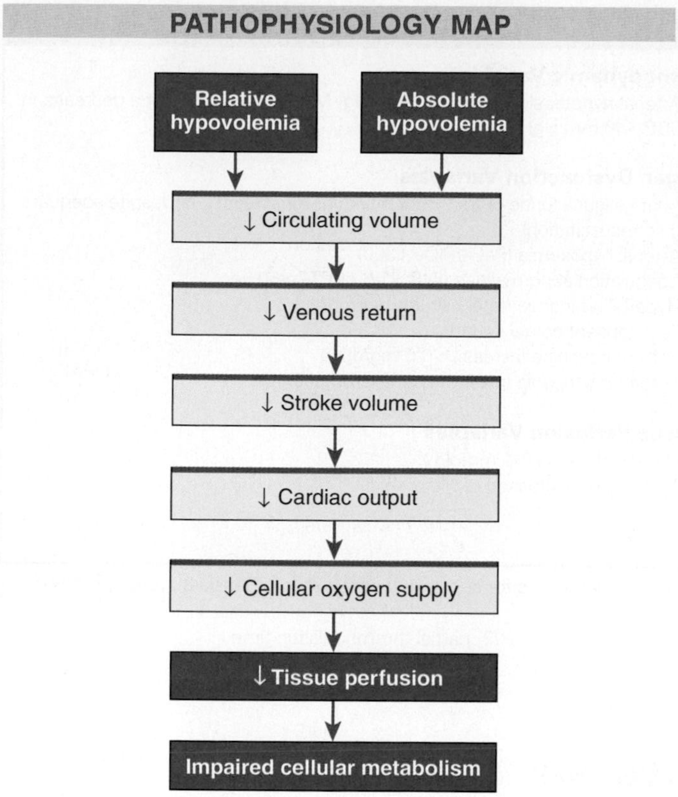

PATHOPHYSIOLOGY MAP

FIG. 66.3 The pathophysiology of hypovolemic shock. (Modified from Urden LD, Stacy KM, Lough ME: *Critical care nursing: Diagnosis and management,* ed 6, St Louis, 2010, Mosby.)

PATHOPHYSIOLOGY MAP

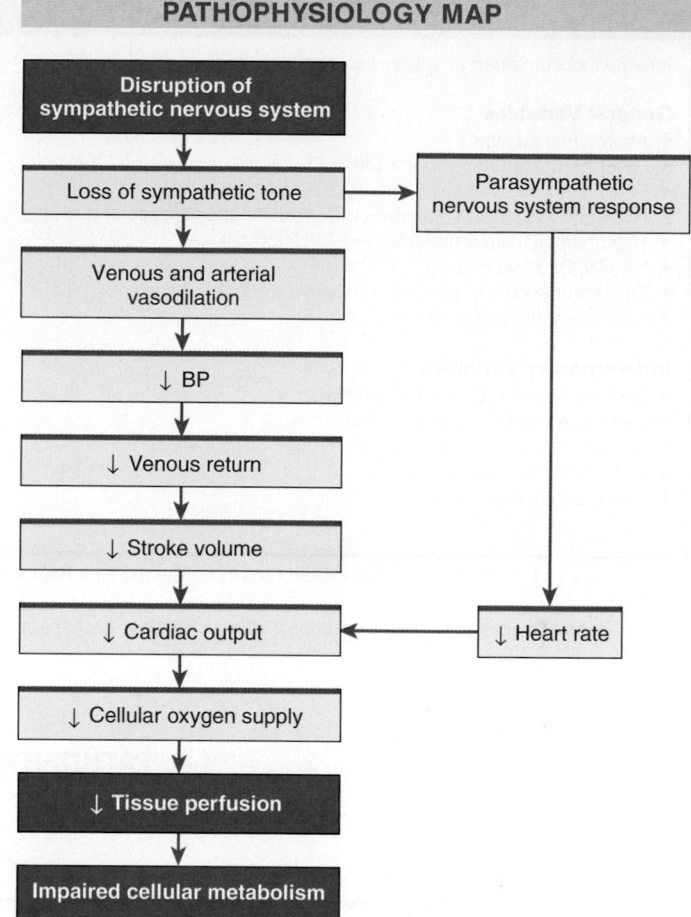

FIG. 66.4 The pathophysiology of neurogenic shock. (Modified from Urden LD, Stacy KM, Lough ME: *Critical care nursing: Diagnosis and management,* ed 6, St Louis, 2010, Mosby.)

the formation of microthrombi and obstruction of the microvasculature. The combined effects of the mediators result in damage to the endothelium, vasodilation, increased capillary permeability, and neutrophil and platelet aggregation and adhesion to the endothelium.

Septic shock has 3 major pathophysiologic effects: vasodilation, maldistribution of blood flow, and myocardial depression. Patients may be euvolemic, but because of acute vasodilation and shifting of fluids out of the intravascular space, relative hypovolemia and hypotension occur. Blood flow in the microcirculation is decreased, causing poor O_2 delivery and tissue hypoxia. We think the combination of TNF and IL-1 has a role in sepsis-induced myocardial dysfunction. The ejection fraction (EF) is decreased for the first few days after the initial insult. Because of a decreased EF, the ventricles dilate to maintain the SV. The EF typically improves, and ventricular dilation resolves over 7 to 10 days. Persistent high CO and a low SVR beyond 24 hours is an ominous finding. It is often associated with an increased development of hypotension and MODS. Coronary artery perfusion and myocardial O_2 metabolism are not primarily altered in septic shock.

Respiratory failure is common. The patient initially hyperventilates as a compensatory mechanism, causing respiratory alkalosis. Once the patient can no longer compensate, respiratory acidosis develops. Respiratory failure develops in 85% of patients with sepsis, and 40% develop acute respiratory distress syndrome (ARDS) (see Chapter 67). These patients may need to be intubated and mechanically ventilated.

Other signs of septic shock include changes in neurologic status, decreased urine output, and GI dysfunction, such as GI

bleeding and paralytic ileus. Table 66.3 gives the clinical presentation of a patient with septic shock.

Obstructive Shock. Obstructive shock develops when a physical obstruction to blood flow occurs with a decreased CO (Fig. 66.6). This can be caused by restricted diastolic filling of the right ventricle from compression (e.g., cardiac tamponade, tension pneumothorax, superior vena cava syndrome). Other causes include *abdominal compartment syndrome,* in which increased abdominal pressures compress the inferior vena cava. This decreases venous return to the heart. Pulmonary embolism and right ventricular thrombi cause an outflow obstruction as blood leaves the right ventricle through the pulmonary artery. This leads to decreased blood flow to the lungs and decreased blood return to the left atrium.

Patients have a decreased CO, increased afterload, and variable left ventricular filling pressures depending on the obstruction. Other signs include jugular venous distention and pulsus paradoxus. Rapid assessment and treatment are important to prevent further hemodynamic compromise and possible cardiac arrest (Fig. 66.6).

Stages of Shock

In addition to understanding the underlying pathogenesis of the type of shock the patient has, management is guided by knowing where the patient is on the shock "continuum." We categorize

TABLE 66.4 Diagnostic Criteria for Sepsis

Infection, documented or suspected, and some of the following:

General Variables

- Altered mental status
- Fever (temperature >100.9°F [38.3°C])
- Heart rate >90 beats/min
- Hyperglycemia (blood glucose >140 mg/dL) in the absence of diabetes
- Hypothermia (core temperature <97.0°F [36°C])
- Systolic BP ≤100 mm Hg
- Significant edema or positive fluid balance (>20 mL/kg over 24 hr)
- Tachypnea (respiratory rate ≥22/min)

Inflammatory Variables

- Leukocytosis (WBC count >12,000/μL)
- Leukopenia (WBC count <4000/μL)
- Normal WBC count with >10% immature forms (bands)
- Elevated C-reactive protein
- Elevated procalcitonin

Hemodynamic Variables

- Arterial hypotension (SBP <90 mm Hg, MAP <70 mm Hg, or a decrease in SBP >40 mm Hg)

Organ Dysfunction Variables

- Acute oliguria (urine output <0.5 mL/kg/hr for at least 2 hr despite adequate fluid resuscitation)
- Arterial hypoxemia (PaO_2/FIO_2 <300)
- Coagulation abnormalities (INR >1.5 or PTT >60 sec)
- Hyperbilirubinemia (total bilirubin >4 mg/dL)
- Ileus (absent bowel sounds)
- Serum creatinine increase >0.5 mg/dL
- Thrombocytopenia (platelet count <100,000/μL)

Tissue Perfusion Variables

- Hyperlactatemia (>1 mmol/L)
- Mottling or decreased capillary refill

Source: Singer M, Deutschman CS, Seymour CW, et al: The third international consensus definitions for sepsis and septic shock (Sepsis-3), *JAMA* 315:801, 2016.
FIO₂, Fraction of inspired O_2; *INR*, international normalized ratio; *PaO₂*, partial pressure of arterial O_2; *PTT*, partial thromboplastin time.

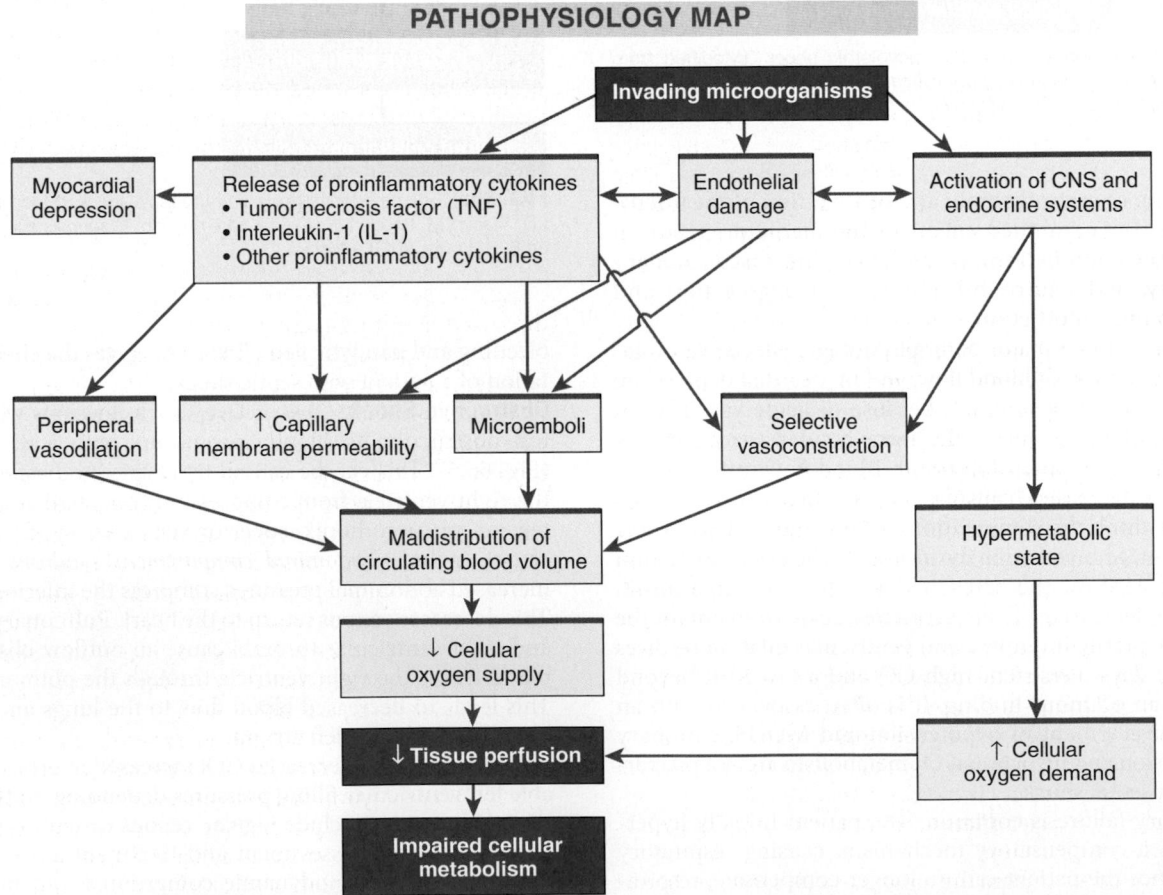

FIG. 66.5 The pathophysiology of septic shock. (Modified from Urden LD, Stacy KM, Lough ME: *Critical care nursing: Diagnosis and management,* ed 6, St Louis, 2010, Mosby.)

PATHOPHYSIOLOGY MAP

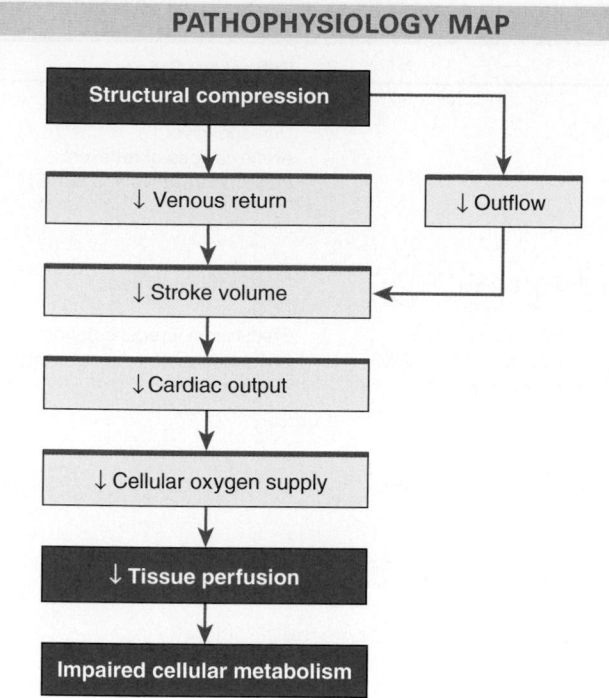

FIG. 66.6 The pathophysiology of obstructive shock.

shock into 4 overlapping stages: (1) initial stage, (2) compensatory stage, (3) progressive stage, and (4) refractory stage.[6]

Initial Stage. The continuum begins with the *initial stage* of shock that occurs at a cellular level. This stage is usually not clinically apparent. Metabolism changes at the cellular level from aerobic to anaerobic, causing lactic acid buildup. Lactic acid is a waste product that is removed by the liver. However, this process requires O_2, which is unavailable because of the decrease in tissue perfusion.

Compensatory Stage. In the *compensatory stage* the body activates neural, hormonal, and biochemical compensatory mechanisms to try to overcome the increasing consequences of anaerobic metabolism and maintain homeostasis. The patient's clinical presentation begins to reflect the body's responses to the imbalance in O_2 supply and demand (Table 66.5).

A classic sign of shock is a drop in BP. This occurs because of a decrease in CO and a narrowing of the pulse pressure. The baroreceptors in the carotid and aortic bodies immediately respond by activating the SNS. The SNS stimulates vasoconstriction and the release of the potent vasoconstrictors epinephrine and norepinephrine. Blood flow to the heart and brain is maintained. Blood flow to the nonvital organs, such as kidneys, GI tract, skin, and lungs, is diverted or shunted.

The myocardium responds to the SNS stimulation and the increase in O_2 demand by increasing the heart rate and contractility. Increased contractility increases myocardial O_2 consumption. The coronary arteries dilate to try to meet the increased O_2 demands of the myocardium.

Shunting blood away from the lungs has an important clinical effect in the patient in shock. Decreased blood flow to the lungs increases the patient's physiologic dead space. *Physiologic dead space* is the anatomic dead space (the amount of air that will not reach gas-exchanging units) and any inspired air that cannot take part in gas exchange. The clinical result of an increase in dead space ventilation is a *ventilation-perfusion mismatch*. Some

areas of the lungs that are being ventilated will not be perfused because of the decreased blood flow to the lungs. Arterial O_2 levels will decrease, and the patient will have a compensatory increase in the rate and depth of respirations (see Chapter 67).

The shunting of blood from other organ systems results in clinically important changes. The decrease in blood flow to the GI tract results in impaired motility and a slowing of peristalsis. This increases the risk for a paralytic ileus.

Decreased blood flow to the skin results in the patient feeling cool and clammy. The exception is the patient in early septic shock who may feel warm and flushed because of a hyperdynamic state. Decreased blood flow to the kidneys activates the renin-angiotensin system. Renin stimulates angiotensinogen to make angiotensin I, which is then converted to angiotensin II (see Fig. 44.4). Angiotensin II is a potent vasoconstrictor that causes both arterial and venous vasoconstriction. The net result is an increase in venous return to the heart and an increase in BP. Angiotensin II stimulates the adrenal cortex to release aldosterone. This results in sodium and water reabsorption and potassium excretion by the kidneys. The increase in sodium reabsorption raises the serum osmolality and stimulates the release of antidiuretic hormone (ADH) from the posterior pituitary gland. ADH increases water reabsorption by the kidneys, further increasing blood volume. The increase in total circulating volume results in an increase in CO and BP.

A multisystem response to decreasing tissue perfusion starts during the compensatory stage of shock. At this stage, the body can compensate for the changes in tissue perfusion. If the cause of the shock is corrected, the patient will recover with little or no residual effects. If the cause of the shock is not corrected and the body is unable to compensate, the patient enters the progressive stage of shock.

Progressive Stage. The *progressive stage* of shock begins as compensatory mechanisms fail. Changes in the patient's mental status are important findings in this stage. Patients must be moved to the intensive care unit (ICU), if not already there, for advanced monitoring and treatment.

The cardiovascular system is profoundly affected in the progressive stage of shock. CO begins to fall, resulting in a decrease in BP and coronary artery, cerebral, and peripheral perfusion. Continued decreased cellular perfusion and resulting altered capillary permeability are the distinguishing features of this stage. Altered capillary permeability allows fluid and protein to leak out of the vascular space into the surrounding interstitial space. In addition to the decrease in circulating volume, there is an increase in systemic interstitial edema. The patient may have *anasarca* (diffuse profound edema). Fluid leakage from the vascular space affects the solid organs (e.g., liver, spleen, GI tract, lungs) and peripheral tissues by further decreasing perfusion.

Sustained hypoperfusion results in weak peripheral pulses, and ischemia of the distal extremities eventually occurs. Myocardial dysfunction from decreased perfusion results in dysrhythmias, myocardial ischemia, and possibly MI. The result is a complete deterioration of the cardiovascular system.

The pulmonary system is often the first system to display signs of critical dysfunction. During the compensatory stage, blood flow to the lungs is already reduced. In response to the decreased blood flow and SNS stimulation, the pulmonary arterioles constrict, resulting in increased pulmonary artery (PA) pressure. As the pressure within the pulmonary vasculature increases, blood flow to the pulmonary capillaries decreases and ventilation-perfusion mismatch worsens.

TABLE 66.5 Manifestations of Stages of Shock*

Compensatory Stage	Progressive Stage	Refractory Stage
Neurologic System		
Oriented to person, place, time Restless, apprehensive, confused Change in level of consciousness	↓ Cerebral perfusion pressure ↓ Cerebral blood flow ↓ Responsiveness to stimuli Delirium	Unresponsive Areflexia (loss of reflexes) Pupils nonreactive and dilated
Cardiovascular System		

Sympathetic nervous system response:
• Release of epinephrine/norepinephrine
  (vasoconstriction)
• ↑ MVO_2
• ↑ Contractility
• ↑ HR
Coronary artery dilation
Narrowed pulse pressure
↓ BP
	↑ Capillary permeability → systemic interstitial edema
	↓ CO → ↓ BP and ↑ HR
	MAP <60 mm Hg (or 40 mm Hg drop in BP from baseline)
	↓ Coronary perfusion → dysrhythmias, myocardial ischemia, MI
	↓ Peripheral perfusion → ischemia of distal extremities,
	  ↓ pulses, ↓ capillary refill
		Profound hypotension
		↓ CO
		Bradycardia, irregular rhythm
		↓ BP inadequate to perfuse vital
		  organs

Respiratory System		
↓ Blood flow to the lungs: • ↑ Physiologic dead space • ↑ Ventilation-perfusion mismatch • Hyperventilation • ↑ Minute ventilation (V_E) • Tachypnea	ARDS: • ↑ Capillary permeability • Pulmonary vasoconstriction • Pulmonary interstitial edema • Alveolar edema • Diffuse infiltrates • Tachypnea • ↓ Compliance • Moist crackles	Severe refractory hypoxemia Respiratory failure
Gastrointestinal System		
↓ Blood supply ↓ GI motility Hypoactive bowel sounds ↑ Risk for paralytic ileus	Vasoconstriction and ↓ perfusion → ischemic gut (e.g., stomach, small and large intestines, gallbladder, pancreas): • Erosive ulcers • GI bleeding • Translocation of GI bacteria • Impaired absorption of nutrients	Ischemic gut
Renal System		

↓ Renal blood flow
↑ Renin resulting in release of
  angiotensin (vasoconstrictor)
↑ Aldosterone resulting in Na^+ and
  H_2O reabsorption
↑ Antidiuretic hormone resulting in
  H_2O reabsorption
	Renal tubules become ischemic → acute tubular necrosis
	↓ Urine output
	↑ BUN-to-creatinine ratio
	↑ Urine sodium
	↓ Urine osmolality and specific gravity
	↓ Urine potassium
	Metabolic acidosis
		Anuria

Hepatic System		

	Failure to metabolize drugs and waste products
	Cell death (↑ liver enzymes)
	Jaundice (↓ clearance of bilirubin)
	↑ NH_3 (ammonia) and lactate
		Metabolic changes from accu-
		  mulation of waste products
		  (e.g., NH_3, lactate, CO_2)

Hematologic System		
	DIC: • Thrombin clots in microcirculation • Consumption of platelets and clotting factors	DIC progresses
Temperature		
Normal or abnormal	Hypothermia or hyperthermia	Hypothermia
Skin		
Pale and cool Warm and flushed	Cold and clammy	Mottled, cyanotic

*The shock continuum begins with the *initial stage* of shock. This stage occurs at the cellular level and is usually not clinically apparent. Also see Table 66.2 and Table 66.3.
MVO_2, myocardial O_2 consumption.

Another key response in the lungs is the movement of fluid from the pulmonary vasculature into the interstitial space. As capillary permeability increases, the movement of fluid to the interstitial spaces results in interstitial edema, bronchoconstriction, and a decrease in functional residual capacity. With further increases in capillary permeability, fluid moves into the alveoli, causing alveolar edema and a decrease in surfactant production. The combined effects of pulmonary vasoconstriction and bronchoconstriction are impaired gas exchange, decreased compliance, and worsening ventilation-perfusion mismatch. Clinically, the patient has tachypnea, crackles, and an overall increased work of breathing.

The GI system is affected by prolonged decreased tissue perfusion. As the blood supply to the GI tract is decreased, the normally protective mucosal barrier becomes ischemic. This ischemia predisposes the patient to ulcers and GI bleeding (see Chapter 41). It increases the risk for bacterial migration from the GI tract to the blood and lungs. The decreased perfusion to the GI tract leads to a decreased ability to absorb nutrients.

The effect of prolonged hypoperfusion on the kidneys is renal tubular ischemia. The resulting acute tubular necrosis may lead to acute kidney injury (AKI). This can be worsened by nephrotoxic drugs (e.g., certain antibiotics, anesthetics, diuretics) (see Chapter 46). The patient has decreased urine output and increased blood urea nitrogen (BUN) and serum creatinine. Metabolic acidosis occurs from the kidneys' inability to excrete acids (especially lactic acid) and reabsorb bicarbonate.

The sustained hypoperfusion in the progressive stage of shock greatly affects other organs. The loss of the functional ability of the liver leads to a failure of the liver to metabolize drugs and waste products (e.g., lactate, ammonia). Jaundice results from an accumulation of bilirubin. As the liver cells die, liver enzymes increase. The liver loses its ability to function as an immune organ. Kupffer cells no longer destroy bacteria from the GI tract. Instead, they are released into the bloodstream, increasing the possibility of bacteremia.

Dysfunction of the hematologic system adds to the complexity of the clinical picture. The patient is at risk for disseminated intravascular coagulation (DIC). The consumption of the platelets and clotting factors with secondary fibrinolysis results in clinically significant bleeding from many orifices. These include the GI tract, lungs, and puncture sites (see Chapter 30). Altered laboratory values in DIC are shown in Table 66.3.

In this stage, aggressive interventions are needed to prevent the development of MODS.

Refractory Stage. In the last stage of shock, the *refractory stage,* decreased perfusion from peripheral vasoconstriction and decreased CO worsen anaerobic metabolism. The accumulation of lactic acid contributes to increased capillary permeability and dilation. Increased capillary permeability allows fluid and plasma proteins to leave the vascular space and move to the interstitial space. Blood pools in the capillary beds due to the constricted venules and dilated arterioles. The loss of intravascular volume worsens hypotension and tachycardia and decreases coronary blood flow. Decreased coronary blood flow leads to worsening myocardial depression and a further decline in CO. Cerebral blood flow cannot be maintained and cerebral ischemia results.

The patient in this stage of shock has profound hypotension and hypoxemia. The failure of the liver, lungs, and kidneys results in an accumulation of waste products, such as lactate, urea, ammonia, and CO_2. The failure of 1 organ system affects several other organ systems. Recovery is unlikely in this stage. The organs are in failure and the body's compensatory mechanisms are overwhelmed (Table 66.5).

Diagnostic Studies

There is no single diagnostic study to determine whether a patient is in shock. The diagnosis starts with a history and physical examination. Obtaining a thorough medical and surgical history and a history of recent events (e.g., surgery, chest pain, trauma) gives valuable data.

Decreased tissue perfusion in shock leads to an increased lactate with a base deficit (the amount needed to bring the pH back to normal). These laboratory changes reflect an increase in anaerobic metabolism.[8] Table 66.2 outlines laboratory findings seen in shock.

Other diagnostic studies include a 12-lead electrocardiogram (ECG), continuous ECG monitoring, chest x-ray, continuous pulse oximetry, and invasive and noninvasive hemodynamic monitoring. Chapter 65 discusses hemodynamic monitoring)

Interprofessional Care

Critical factors in the successful management of a patient in shock relate to the early recognition and treatment of the shock state. Prompt intervention in the early stages of shock may prevent the decline to the progressive or irreversible stage. Successful management of the patient in shock includes (1) identification of patients at risk for the development of shock; (2) integration of the patient's history, physical examination, and clinical findings to establish a diagnosis; (3) interventions to control or eliminate the cause of the decreased perfusion; (4) protecting target and distal organs from dysfunction; and (5) providing multisystem supportive care.

Table 66.6 provides an overview of the initial assessment findings and interventions for the emergency care of patients in shock. General management strategies begin with ensuring that the patient is responsive and has a patent airway. Once the airway is established, either naturally or with an endotracheal tube, O_2 delivery must be optimized. Supplemental O_2 and mechanical ventilation may be needed to maintain an arterial O_2 saturation of 90% or more (PaO_2 greater than 60 mm Hg) to avoid hypoxemia (see Chapter 65). The mean arterial pressure (MAP) and circulating blood volume are optimized with fluid replacement and drug therapy.

Oxygen and Ventilation. O_2 delivery depends on CO, available hemoglobin, and arterial O_2 saturation (SaO_2). Methods to optimize O_2 delivery are directed at increasing supply and decreasing demand. Supply is increased by (1) optimizing the CO with fluid replacement and/or drug therapy, (2) increasing the hemoglobin through transfusion of whole blood or packed red blood cells (RBCs), and/or (3) increasing the arterial O_2 saturation with supplemental O_2 and mechanical ventilation.

Plan care to avoid disrupting the balance of O_2 supply and demand. Space activities that increase O_2 consumption (e.g., endotracheal suctioning, position changes) appropriately for O_2 conservation. Intermittent or continuous monitoring of $ScvO_2$ by a central venous catheter or mixed venous O_2 saturation (SvO_2) may be helpful. Both reflect the dynamic balance between O_2 supply and demand. Assess these values along with related hemodynamic measures (e.g., arterial pressure–based cardiac output [APCO], O_2 consumption, hemoglobin) to evaluate the patient's response to treatments and activities (see Chapter 65).

➕ **TABLE 66.6 Emergency Management**

Shock

Etiology*	Assessment Findings	Interventions
Surgical • Aortic dissection • GI bleeding • Postoperative bleeding • Ruptured ectopic pregnancy or ovarian cyst • Ruptured organ or vessel • Vaginal bleeding **Medical** • Addisonian crisis • Dehydration • Diabetes • Diabetes insipidus • MI • Pulmonary embolus • Sepsis **Trauma** • Fractures, spinal injury • Multiorgan injury • Ruptured or lacerated vessel or organ (e.g., spleen)	• Anxiety • Chills • Confusion • Cool, clammy skin (warm skin in early onset of septic and neurogenic shock) • Cyanosis • Decreased level of consciousness • Decreased O_2 saturation • Dysrhythmias • Extreme thirst • Feeling of impending doom • Hypotension • Narrowed pulse pressure • Nausea and vomiting • Obvious hemorrhage or injury • Pallor • Rapid, weak, thready pulses • Restlessness • Tachypnea, dyspnea, or shallow, irregular respirations • Temperature dysregulation • Weakness	**Initial** • If unresponsive, assess circulation, airway, and breathing (CAB). • If responsive, monitor airway, breathing, and circulation (ABC). • Stabilize cervical spine as appropriate. • Control any external bleeding with direct pressure or pressure dressing. • Give high-flow O_2 (100%) by nonrebreather mask or bag-valve-mask. • Anticipate need for intubation and mechanical ventilation. • Establish IV access with 2 large-bore catheters (14- to 16-gauge) or an intraosseous access device; aid with central line insertion. • Begin fluid resuscitation with crystalloids (e.g., 30 mL/kg repeated until hemodynamic improvement is seen). • Draw blood for laboratory studies (e.g., blood cultures, lactate, WBC). • Assess for life-threatening injuries (e.g., cardiac tamponade, liver laceration, tension pneumothorax). • Consider vasopressor therapy if hypotension persists after fluid resuscitation. • Insert an indwelling urinary catheter and nasogastric tube. • Start antibiotic therapy after blood cultures if sepsis is suspected. • Obtain 12-lead ECG and treat dysrhythmias. **Ongoing Monitoring** • ABCs • Level of consciousness • Vital signs, including pulse oximetry; peripheral pulses, capillary refill, skin color and temperature • Respiratory status • Heart rate and rhythm • Urine output

*See Table 66.1 for other causes of shock.

Fluid Resuscitation. The cornerstone of therapy for septic, hypovolemic, and anaphylactic shock is volume expansion with administration of the appropriate fluid (Table 66.7). Fluid resuscitation should start using 1 or 2 large-bore (e.g., 14- to 16-gauge) IV catheters, an intraosseous (IO) access device, or a central venous catheter.

⚠ **SAFETY ALERT Intraosseous (IO) Access**
• Use an IO access device for emergency resuscitation when IV access cannot be obtained.
• Insertion sites include the sternum, proximal and distal tibia, and proximal and distal humerus.
• Remove IO devices within 24 hours of insertion or as soon as possible after peripheral or central IV access is obtained.
• Monitor for complications: extravasation of drugs and fluids into the soft tissue, fractures caused during insertion, and osteomyelitis.

The choice of resuscitation fluid is based on the type and volume of fluid lost and the patient's clinical status. The ideal choice of fluid is controversial. Currently, normal saline is most often used in the initial resuscitation of shock. Large-volume resuscitation with normal saline can lead to hyperchloremic metabolic acidosis. Lactated Ringer's solution can cause serum lactate levels to increase because the failing liver cannot convert lactate to bicarbonate.[9] Transfusions of RBCs may be given to treat hypovolemic shock due to bleeding. Colloids (4% to 5%) have not been shown to improve patient outcomes.[9]

Fluid responsiveness is determined by clinical assessment. This includes vital signs, cerebral and abdominal perfusion pressures, capillary refill, skin temperature, and urine output. Hemodynamic parameters, such as SVV or CO, are also used. Monitor trends in BP with an automatic BP cuff or an arterial catheter to assess the patient's response. Use an indwelling urinary catheter to monitor urine output during resuscitation.

The goal for fluid resuscitation is to restore tissue perfusion. Although BP helps determine whether the patient's CO is adequate, an assessment of end-organ perfusion (e.g., urine output, neurologic function, peripheral pulses) provides more relevant data.

⚠ **SAFETY ALERT Complications of Fluid Resuscitation**
• Warm crystalloid and colloid solutions during massive fluid resuscitation to prevent hypothermia.
• When giving large volumes of packed RBCs, remember that they do not contain clotting factors.
• Replace clotting factors based on the clinical situation and laboratory studies.

Drug Therapy. The goal of drug therapy for shock is to correct decreased tissue perfusion. Decisions on which drug to use should be based on the physiologic goal. Drugs used to improve perfusion in shock are given IV via an infusion pump and central venous line. Many of these drugs have vasoconstrictor properties that are harmful if the drug leaks into the tissues while being infused peripherally (Table 66.8).

TABLE 66.7 Fluid Therapy in Shock

Fluid Type	Mechanism of Action	Type of Shock	Nursing Implications
Crystalloids			
Isotonic			
• 0.9% NaCl, normal saline solution (NSS) • Lactated Ringer's (LR) solution	Fluid primarily stays in the intra-vascular space, ↑ intravascular volume.	Used for initial volume replacement in most types of shock.	Monitor patient closely for circulatory overload. Do not use LR in patients with liver failure. LR may be used if hyperchloremic acidosis develops from use of NSS in fluid resuscitation.
Hypertonic			
• 1.8%, 3%, 5% NaCl	Fluid stays in the intravascular space, increases serum osmolarity, shifts fluid volume from intracellular space to extracellular space to intravascular space.	May be used for initial volume expansion in hypovolemic shock.	Monitor patient closely for signs of hypernatremia (e.g., disorientation, seizures). Central line preferred for infusing saline solutions ≥3%, since these may damage veins.
Blood or Blood Products			
Packed red blood cells	Replaces blood loss, increases O_2-carrying capability.	All types.	Same precautions as any blood administration (see Chapter 30).
Fresh frozen plasma Platelets	Replaces coagulation factors. Helps control bleeding caused by thrombocytopenia.		
Colloids			
Human serum albumin (5% or 25%)	Can increase plasma colloid osmotic pressure. Rapid volume expansion.	All types except cardiogenic and neurogenic shock.	Use 5% solution in hypovolemic patients. Use 25% solution in patients with fluid and sodium restrictions. Monitor for circulatory overload. Mild side effects of chills, fever, and urticaria may develop. More expensive than crystalloids.
dextran (dextran 40)	Hyperosmotic glucose polymer.	Limited use because of side effects, including reducing platelet adhesion, diluting clotting factors.	Increases risk for bleeding. Monitor patient for allergic reactions and AKI. Has maximum volume recommendations per manufacturer.

Sympathomimetic Drugs. Many of the drugs used in the treatment of shock influence the SNS. Drugs that mimic the action of the SNS are called *sympathomimetic*. The effects of these drugs are mediated through their binding to α- or β-adrenergic receptors. The various drugs differ in their relative α- and β-adrenergic effects.[10]

Many of these drugs cause peripheral vasoconstriction and are called *vasopressor drugs* (e.g., norepinephrine, dopamine, phenylephrine). These drugs can cause severe peripheral vasoconstriction and an increase in SVR, further risking tissue perfusion. The increased SVR increases the workload of the heart and myocardial O_2 demand. It can harm a patient in cardiogenic shock by causing further myocardial damage and increasing the risk for dysrhythmias.[1] Use of vasopressor drugs is limited to patients who do not respond to fluid resuscitation. Adequate fluid resuscitation must be achieved before starting vasopressors because the vasoconstrictor effects in patients with low blood volume will cause further reduction in tissue perfusion. Typically, if the patient has persistent hypotension after adequate fluid resuscitation, a vasopressor (e.g., norepinephrine, dopamine) and/or an inotrope (e.g., dobutamine) is given.

The goal of vasopressor therapy is to achieve and maintain a MAP of greater than 65 mm Hg.[10] Continuously monitor end-organ perfusion (e.g., urine output, level of consciousness) and serum lactate levels (e.g., every 3 hours for the first 6 hours) to ensure that tissue perfusion is adequate.

Vasodilator Drugs. Patients in cardiogenic shock have decreased myocardial contractility, and vasodilators may be needed to decrease afterload. This reduces myocardial workload and O_2 requirements. Although generalized sympathetic vasoconstriction is a useful compensatory mechanism for maintaining BP, excessive constriction can reduce tissue blood flow and increase the workload of the heart. The reason for using vasodilator therapy for a patient in shock is to break the harmful cycle of widespread vasoconstriction causing a decrease in CO and BP, resulting in further sympathetic-induced vasoconstriction.

The goal of vasodilator therapy, as in vasopressor therapy, is to maintain the MAP greater than 65 mm Hg. Monitor hemodynamic parameters (e.g., CVP, CO, $ScvO_2/SvO_2$, SV, PA pressures) and assessment findings so that fluids can be increased or vasodilator therapy decreased if a serious fall in CO or BP occurs. The vasodilator agent most often used for the patient in cardiogenic shock is nitroglycerin. Vasodilation may be enhanced with nitroprusside or nitroglycerin in noncardiogenic shock.

Nutritional Therapy. Protein-calorie malnutrition is common because of hypermetabolism. Nutrition is vital to reducing mortality. Enteral nutrition (EN) should be started within the first 24 hours. However, full calorie replacement is not recommended for previously well-nourished adults early in a critical illness.[11] Start the patient on a *trophic feeding*. This is a small amount of EN (e.g., 10 mL/hr). Early EN enhances the perfusion of the

TABLE 66.8 Drug Therapy

Shock

Drug*	Mechanism of Action	Type of Shock	Nursing Implications
angiotensin II (Giapreza)	↑ BP, ↑ MAP ↑SVR	Septic and other distributive shock	Give via central line. Monitor for thromboembolic events. VTE prophylaxis is recommended.
dobutamine	↑ Myocardial contractility ↓ Ventricular filling pressures ↓ SVR, PAWP ↑ CO, SV, CVP ↑/↓ HR	Used in cardiogenic shock with severe systolic dysfunction Used in septic shock to increase O_2 delivery and raise $ScvO_2$ or SvO_2 to 70% if Hgb >7 g/dL or Hct ≥30%	Give via central line (infiltration leads to tissue sloughing). Do not give in same line with $NaHCO_3$. Monitor HR, BP (hypotension may worsen, requiring addition of a vasopressor). Stop infusion if tachydysrhythmias develop.
Dopamine	Positive inotropic effects: ↑ Myocardial contractility ↑ Automaticity ↑ Atrioventricular conduction ↑ HR, CO ↑ BP, ↑ MAP ↑ MVO_2 Can cause progressive vasoconstriction at high doses	Cardiogenic shock	Give via central line (infiltration leads to tissue sloughing). Do not give in same line with $NaHCO_3$. Monitor for tachydysrhythmias. Monitor for peripheral vasoconstriction (e.g., paresthesias, coldness in extremities) at moderate to high doses.
epinephrine (Adrenalin)	*Low doses:* β-Adrenergic agonist (cardiac stimulation, bronchodilation, peripheral vasodilation) ↑ HR, contractility, CO ↓ SVR *High doses:* α-Adrenergic agonist (peripheral vasoconstriction) ↑ SV, SVR ↑ Systolic/↓ diastolic BP, widened pulse pressure ↑ CVP, PAWP	Cardiogenic shock Anaphylactic shock Septic shock, if 2nd agent needed after norepinephrine Cardiac arrest, pulseless ventricular tachycardia, ventricular fibrillation, asystole	Monitor for HR >110 beats/min. Monitor for dyspnea, pulmonary edema. Monitor for chest pain, dysrhythmias from ↑ MVO_2. Monitor for renal failure due to ischemia.
hydrocortisone (Solu-Cortef)	↓ Inflammation, reverses ↑ capillary permeability ↑ BP, HR	Septic shock requiring vasopressor therapy (despite fluid resuscitation) to maintain adequate BP Anaphylactic shock if hypotension persists after initial therapy	Monitor for hypokalemia, hyperglycemia. Consider use as continuous infusion.
nitroglycerin	Venous dilation Dilates coronary arteries ↓ Preload, MVO_2, SVR, BP	Cardiogenic shock	Continuously monitor BP and HR, since reflex tachycardia may occur. Glass bottle recommended for infusion.
norepinephrine (Levophed)	$β_1$-Adrenergic agonist (cardiac stimulation) α-Adrenergic agonist (peripheral vasoconstriction) Renal and splanchnic vasoconstriction ↑ BP, MAP, CVP, PAWP, SVR ↑/↓ CO	Cardiogenic shock after MI Septic shock—first drug of choice for BP unresponsive to adequate fluid resuscitation	Give via central line (infiltration leads to tissue sloughing). Monitor for dysrhythmias due to ↑ MVO_2 requirements.
phenylephrine	α-Adrenergic agonist (peripheral vasoconstriction) Renal, mesenteric, splanchnic, cutaneous, and pulmonary blood vessel constriction ↑ HR, BP, SVR ↑/↓ CO	Neurogenic shock	Monitor for reflex bradycardia, headache, restlessness. Monitor for renal failure from ↓ renal blood flow. Give via central line (infiltration leads to tissue sloughing).
sodium nitroprusside	Arterial and venous vasodilation ↓ Preload, afterload ↓ CVP, PAWP ↑/↓ CO ↓ BP	Cardiogenic shock with ↑ SVR	Continuously monitor BP. Protect solution from light. Wrap infusion bottle with opaque covering. Give with D_5W only. Monitor serum cyanide levels and for signs of cyanide toxicity (e.g., metabolic acidosis, tachycardia, altered level of consciousness, seizures, coma, almond smell on breath).
vasopressin	Antidiuretic hormone Nonadrenergic vasoconstrictor ↑ MAP ↑ Urine output	Shock states (most often septic shock) refractory to other vasopressors	Given with norepinephrine and in low doses. Infusions are not titrated. Monitor hemodynamic pressures and urine output.

*Consult agency guidelines, pharmacist, pharmacology references, and drug manufacturer's materials for more information and dosing recommendations.
CVP, Central venous pressure; *MVO_2,* myocardial O_2 consumption; *PAWP,* pulmonary artery wedge pressure; *PT,* prothrombin time; *PTT,* partial thromboplastin time; *SVR,* systemic vascular resistance.

GI tract and helps maintain the integrity of the gut mucosa. Advance feedings as tolerated and as prescribed. Parenteral nutrition (PN) is used only if EN is contraindicated. Chapter 39 discusses enteral and parenteral nutrition.

Weigh the patient daily on the same scale (usually the bed scale) at the same time of day. If the patient has a significant weight loss, rule out dehydration before adding more calories. Large weight gains are common because of third spacing of fluids. Therefore daily weights serve as a better indicator of fluid status than caloric needs. Serum protein, total albumin, prealbumin, BUN, serum glucose, and serum electrolytes are all used to assess nutritional status.

Measures Specific to Type of Shock

Cardiogenic Shock. For a patient in cardiogenic shock, the overall goal is to restore heart function and the balance between O_2 supply and demand in the myocardium. Cardiac catheterization is done as soon as possible after the initial insult.[1] Specific measures to restore blood flow include angioplasty with stenting, emergency revascularization, and valve replacement (see Chapter 33). Until these interventions are done, we must support the heart to optimize SV and CO to achieve optimal perfusion (Tables 66.8 and 66.9).

Hemodynamic management of a patient in cardiogenic shock aims to reduce the workload of the heart through drug therapy and/or mechanical interventions. Drug choice is based on the clinical goal and a thorough understanding of each drug's mechanism of action. Drugs can be used to decrease the workload of the heart by dilating coronary arteries (e.g., nitrates), reducing preload (e.g., diuretics), afterload (e.g., vasodilators), and heart rate and contractility (e.g., β-adrenergic blockers).

The patient may benefit from a circulatory assist device (e.g., intraaortic balloon pump, ventricular assist device [VAD]) (see Chapter 65). The goals of this intervention are to decrease SVR and left ventricular workload so that the heart can heal.[12] A VAD may be used as a temporary measure for the patient in cardiogenic shock who is awaiting heart transplantation. Heart transplantation is an option for a small, select group of patients with cardiogenic shock.

Hypovolemic Shock. The underlying principles of managing patients with hypovolemic shock focus on stopping the loss of fluid and restoring the circulating volume. We often calculate the initial fluid resuscitation using a 3:1 rule (3 mL of isotonic crystalloid for every 1 mL of estimated blood loss). Table 66.7 describes types of fluid used for volume resuscitation, the mechanisms of action, and specific nursing implications for each fluid type.

Septic Shock. Patients in septic shock need large amounts of fluid replacement. The overall goal of fluid resuscitation is to restore the intravascular volume and organ perfusion. Initial volume resuscitation is achieved by giving 30 mL/kg of an isotonic crystalloid solution. Albumin 4% to 5% may be added when patients need substantial volumes.

A fluid challenge technique (e.g., a minimum of 30 mL/kg of crystalloids) may be used and repeated until hemodynamic improvement (e.g., increase in MAP and/or CVP, change in SVV) is seen. Table 66.9 shows predetermined end points of fluid resuscitation along with methods to reassess volume status.

One of these methods is a *passive leg raise* (PLR) challenge along with hemodynamic measures to monitor response.[13] A PLR challenge provides a transient increase in fluid volume of 150 to 500 mL by placing the patient supine and raising the legs

to 45 degrees (Fig. 66.7). Response is monitored within 1 to 2 minutes by measuring CO, CI, SV, SVV, or other parameters for improvement. If the response is positive, the patient is fluid responsive and should receive more fluids. To optimize and evaluate large-volume fluid resuscitation, hemodynamic monitoring with various noninvasive or invasive monitors is needed.

If the patient is hypotensive after initial volume resuscitation and no longer fluid responsive, vasopressors may be added. The first drug of choice is norepinephrine.[14] Vasodilation and low CO, or vasodilation alone, can cause low BP despite adequate fluid resuscitation. Vasopressin may be added for those who are refractory to initial vasopressor therapy.[14] Exogenous vasopressin can replace the stores of physiologic vasopressin that are often depleted in septic shock.

 DRUG ALERT Vasopressin
- Given along with norepinephrine.
- Infuse at low doses (e.g., 0.03 units/min) using an IV pump.
- Do not titrate infusion.
- Use cautiously in patients with coronary artery disease.

Vasopressor drugs may increase BP but can decrease SV. An inotropic agent (e.g., dobutamine) may be added to offset the decrease in SV and increase tissue perfusion (Table 66.8). IV corticosteroids may be considered for patients in septic shock who cannot maintain an adequate BP despite vasopressor therapy and fluid resuscitation.

To try to meet the increasing tissue demands coupled with a low SVR, the patient initially has a normal or high CO. If the patient is unable to achieve and maintain an adequate CO and has unmet tissue O_2 demands, CO may have to be increased using drug therapy (e.g., dopamine). $ScvO_2$ or SvO_2 monitoring is used to assess the balance between O_2 delivery and consumption, and the adequacy of the CO (see Chapter 65). If balance is maintained, the tissue demands will be met.

Broad-spectrum antibiotics are an important and early part of therapy. They should be started within the first hour of sepsis or septic shock.[15] Obtain cultures (e.g., blood, wound, urine, stool, sputum) before antibiotics are started. However, this should not delay the start of antibiotics within the first hour. Specific antibiotics may be ordered once the organism has been identified.

Glucose levels should be maintained below 180 mg/dL (10.0 mmol/L) for patients in shock.[16] Monitor glucose levels in all patients in septic shock according to agency policy. Stress ulcer prophylaxis with proton pump inhibitors (e.g., pantoprazole) and VTE prophylaxis (e.g., heparin, enoxaparin [Lovenox]) are recommended.[17]

Neurogenic Shock. The specific treatment of neurogenic shock is based on the cause. If the cause is spinal cord injury, general measures to promote spinal stability (e.g., spinal precautions, cervical stabilization with a collar) are initially used. Once the spine is stabilized, treatment of the hypotension and bradycardia is essential to prevent further spinal cord damage. Treatment involves the use of vasopressors (e.g., phenylephrine) to maintain BP and organ perfusion (Table 66.8). Bradycardia may be treated with atropine. Infuse fluids cautiously as the cause of the hypotension is not related to fluid loss. The patient with a spinal cord injury is monitored for hypothermia caused by hypothalamic dysfunction (Table 66.9).

Anaphylactic Shock. The first strategy in managing patients at risk for anaphylactic shock is prevention. A thorough history

TABLE 66.9 Interprofessional Care

Shock

Oxygenation	Circulation	Drug Therapies	Supportive Therapies
Cardiogenic Shock • Provide supplemental O_2 (e.g., nasal cannula, nonrebreather mask) • Intubation and mechanical ventilation, if needed • Monitor $ScvO_2$ or SvO_2	• Restore blood flow with angioplasty with stenting, emergent coronary revascularization • Reduce workload of heart with circulatory assist devices: IABP, VAD	• Nitrates (e.g., nitroglycerin) • Inotropes (e.g., dobutamine) • Diuretics (e.g., furosemide) • β-Adrenergic blockers (contraindicated with ↓ ejection fraction)	• Treat dysrhythmias

Hypovolemic Shock
• Provide supplemental O_2
• Monitor $ScvO_2$ or $ScvO_2$
	• Rapid fluid replacement using 2 large-bore (14–16 gauge) peripheral IV lines, an intraosseous access device, or central venous catheter
	• Restore fluid volume (e.g., blood or blood products, crystalloids)
	• End points of fluid resuscitation:
	  • CVP 15 mm Hg
	  • PAWP 10–12 mm Hg
		• No specific drug therapy	• Correct the cause (e.g., stop bleeding, GI losses)
			• Use warmed IV fluids, including blood products (if appropriate)

Septic Shock
• Provide supplemental O_2
• Intubation and mechanical ventilation, if needed
• Monitor $ScvO_2$ or SvO_2
	• Aggressive fluid resuscitation (e.g., 30 mL/kg of crystalloids repeated if hemodynamic improvement is noted)
	• End points of fluid resuscitation are based on:
	  • Focused physical examination including vital signs, cardiopulmonary assessment, capillary refill, peripheral pulses, and skin or any 2 of the following:
	    • $ScvO_2$ >70 or SvO_2 >65
	    • CVP 8–12 mm Hg
	    • Cardiovascular ultrasound
	    • Assessment of fluid responsiveness with passive leg raise or fluid challenge
		• Antibiotics as ordered
		• Vasopressors (e.g., norepinephrine)
		• Inotropes (e.g., dobutamine)
		• Anticoagulants (e.g., low-molecular-weight heparin)
			• Obtain cultures (e.g., blood, wound) before beginning antibiotics
			• Monitor temperature
			• Control blood glucose
			• Stress ulcer prophylaxis

Neurogenic Shock • Maintain patent airway • Provide supplemental O_2 • Intubation and mechanical ventilation (if needed)	• Cautious administration of fluids	• Vasopressors (e.g., phenylephrine) • Atropine (for bradycardia)	• Minimize spinal cord trauma with stabilization • Monitor temperature
Anaphylactic Shock • Maintain patent airway • Optimize oxygenation with supplemental O_2 • Intubation and mechanical ventilation, if needed	• Aggressive fluid resuscitation with colloids	• Epinephrine (IM or IV) • Antihistamines (e.g., diphenhydramine) • Histamine (H_2)-receptor blockers (e.g., ranitidine [Zantac]) • Bronchodilators: nebulized (e.g., albuterol) • Corticosteroids (if hypotension persists)	• Identify and remove offending cause • Prevent via avoidance of known allergens • Premedicate with history of prior sensitivity (e.g., contrast media)
Obstructive Shock • Maintain patent airway • Provide supplemental O_2 • Intubation and mechanical ventilation, if needed	• Restore circulation by treating cause of obstruction • Fluid resuscitation may provide temporary improvement in CO and BP	• No specific drug therapy	• Treat cause of obstruction (e.g., pericardiocentesis for cardiac tamponade, needle decompression or chest tube insertion for tension pneumothorax, embolectomy for pulmonary embolism)

CVP, central venous pressure; *PAWP*, pulmonary artery wedge pressure.

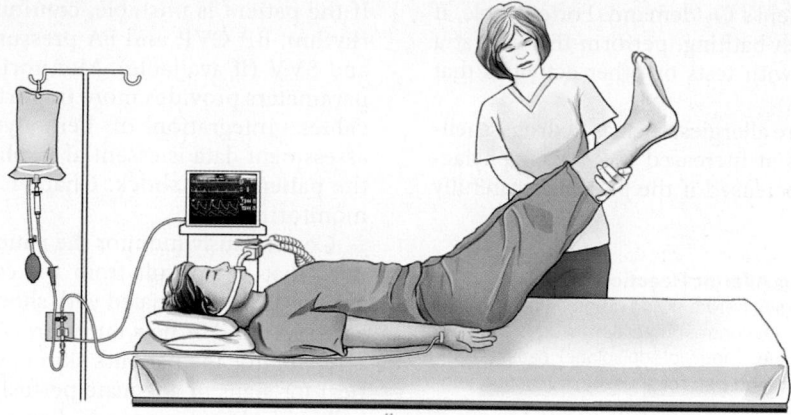

FIG. 66.7 Passive leg raise challenge in a patient with septic shock. (From Lough, M.E. *Hemodynamic monitoring: Evolving technologies and clinical practice*, Philadelphia, 2016, Elsevier.)

is key to avoiding risk factors for anaphylaxis (Table 66.1). The clinical presentation of anaphylactic shock is dramatic, and immediate intervention is required. Epinephrine is the first drug of choice to treat anaphylactic shock.[5] It causes peripheral vasoconstriction and bronchodilation and opposes the effect of histamine. Diphenhydramine and histamine receptor blockers (e.g., famotidine) are given as adjunctive therapies to block the ongoing release of histamine from the allergic reaction.

Maintaining a patent airway is important because the patient can quickly develop airway compromise from laryngeal edema or bronchoconstriction. Nebulized bronchodilators are highly effective. Aerosolized epinephrine can reduce treat laryngeal edema. Endotracheal intubation may be needed to secure and maintain a patent airway.

Hypotension results from leakage of fluid out of the intravascular space into the interstitial space because of increased vascular permeability and vasodilation. Aggressive fluid resuscitation, usually with crystalloids, is needed. IV corticosteroids may be helpful in anaphylactic shock if significant hypotension persists after 1 to 2 hours of aggressive therapy (Tables 66.8 and 66.9).

Obstructive Shock. The main strategy in treating obstructive shock is early recognition and treatment to relieve or manage the obstruction (Table 66.1). Mechanical decompression for pericardial tamponade, tension pneumothorax, and hemopneumothorax may be done by needle or tube insertion. Obstructive shock from a pulmonary embolism requires immediate anticoagulation therapy or pulmonary embolectomy. Superior vena cava syndrome, a compression or obstruction of the outflow tract of the mediastinum, may be treated by radiation, debulking, or removal of the mass or cause. A decompressive laparotomy may be done for abdominal compartment syndrome for patients with high intraabdominal pressures and hemodynamic instability.

❖ NURSING MANAGEMENT: SHOCK

◆ Nursing Assessment

Your role is vital in caring for patients who are at risk for developing shock or are in a state of shock. Focus your assessment on the ABCs: airway, breathing, and circulation. Next, assess for tissue perfusion. This includes evaluating vital signs, level of consciousness, peripheral pulses, capillary refill, skin (e.g., temperature, color, moisture), and urine output. As shock

progresses, the patient's neurologic status declines, urine output decreases, skin becomes cooler and mottled, and peripheral pulses decrease.

To understand the complexity of the patient's clinical status, integrate all the assessment data. It is essential to obtain a brief history from the patient or caregiver, including a description of the events leading to the shock state, time of onset and duration of symptoms, and health history (e.g., medications, allergies). In addition, obtain details about any care the patient received before hospitalization.

◆ Nursing Diagnoses

Nursing diagnoses for the patient in shock may include:
- Impaired cardiac output
- Ineffective tissue perfusion
- Anxiety

Additional information on nursing diagnoses and interventions for the patient with shock is presented in eNursing Care Plan 66.1 (available on the website for this chapter).

◆ Planning

The overall goals for a patient in shock include (1) evidence of adequate tissue perfusion, (2) restoration of normal or baseline BP, (3) recovery of organ function, (4) avoiding complications from prolonged states of hypoperfusion, and (5) preventing health care–associated complications of disease management and care.

◆ Nursing Implementation

◆ Health Promotion. You have a vital role in the prevention of shock, beginning with the identification of patients at risk. In general, patients who are older, are immunocompromised, or have chronic illnesses are at an increased risk. Any person who has surgery or trauma is at risk for shock resulting from hemorrhage, spinal cord injury, sepsis, and other problems (Table 66.1).

Planning is essential to help prevent shock after you identify an at-risk person. For example, a person with an acute anterior wall MI is at high risk for cardiogenic shock.[1] The main goal for this patient is to limit the infarct size. This is done by restoring coronary blood flow through percutaneous coronary intervention, thrombolytic therapy, or surgical revascularization. Rest, analgesics, and sedation can reduce the myocardial demand for O_2. Modify the ICU environment to provide care at intervals that will not increase the patient's O$_2$ demand. For example, if the patient becomes tired with bathing, perform this care at a time that does not interfere with tests or other activities that may also increase O$_2$ demand.

A person with certain severe allergies, such as to drugs, shellfish, insect bites, and latex, is at increased risk for anaphylactic shock. This risk can be decreased if the patient is carefully assessed for allergies.

> ## ⚠ SAFETY ALERT Preventing Allergic Reactions
> - Always confirm the patient's allergies before giving drugs or starting diagnostic procedures (e.g., CT scan with contrast media).
> - Premedicate (e.g., diphenhydramine, methylprednisolone) patients who need a drug to which they are at high risk for an allergic reaction (e.g., contrast media).
> - Encourage patients with allergies to obtain and wear a medical alert device and report their allergies to their HCPs.
> - Tell patients about the availability of kits that contain equipment and drugs (e.g., epinephrine [EpiPen]) for the treatment of acute allergic reactions.

Careful monitoring of fluid balance can help prevent hypovolemic shock. Ongoing monitoring of intake and output and daily weights is important. Identifying trends in the patient's condition is more meaningful than any single piece of clinical information.

Carefully monitor all patients for infection. Progression from an infection to sepsis and septic shock depends on the patient's defense mechanisms. Patients who are immunocompromised are at high risk for opportunistic infections. Strategies to decrease the risk for health care–associated infections (HAIs) include decreasing the number of invasive catheters (e.g., central lines, bladder catheters), using aseptic technique during invasive procedures, and paying strict attention to hand washing. Change equipment per agency policy. Thoroughly sanitize or discard (if disposable) equipment between patient use.

Evidence-based guidelines are available to reduce the risk for HAIs (e.g., ventilator-associated pneumonia, central line infections, catheter-associated urinary tract infections). These guidelines, called *care bundles,* outline key interventions aimed at reducing infections.[18]

◆ **Acute Care.** Your role in shock involves (1) monitoring the patient's ongoing physical and emotional status, (2) identifying trends to detect changes in the patient's condition, (3) planning and implementing nursing interventions and therapy, (4) evaluating the patient's response to therapy, (5) providing emotional support to the patient and caregiver, and (6) collaborating with other members of the interprofessional team to coordinate care.

Neurologic Status. Assess the patient's neurologic status, including orientation and level of consciousness using a valid tool, at least every 1 to 2 hours. The patient's neurologic status is the best indicator of cerebral blood flow. Be aware of the clinical manifestations of neurologic involvement (e.g., changes in behavior, restlessness, blurred vision, confusion, paresthesias). Note any subtle changes in the patient's mental status (e.g., mild agitation) and report them to the HCP.

Orient the patient to person, place, time, and events on a regular basis. Orientation to the ICU environment is especially important. Reduce noise and light levels to control sensory input. Keep a day-night cycle of activity and rest as much as possible. Sensory overload and disruption of the patient's diurnal cycle may contribute to delirium (see Chapter 59).

Cardiovascular Status. Most of the therapy for shock is based on information about the patient's cardiovascular status.

If the patient is unstable, continuously assess heart rate and rhythm, BP, CVP, and PA pressures, including CO, SVR, SV, and SVV (if available). Monitoring trends in hemodynamic parameters provides more important information than single values. Integration of hemodynamic data with physical assessment data is essential in planning strategies to manage the patient with shock. Chapter 65 discusses hemodynamic monitoring.

Continuously monitor the patient's ECG to detect dysrhythmias that may result from the cardiovascular and metabolic abnormalities associated with shock. Assess heart sounds for an S$_3$ or S$_4$ sound or new murmurs. An S$_3$ sound usually indicates HF. Monitor the patient's skin (e.g., upper and lower extremities) for signs of adequate perfusion. Changes in temperature, pallor, flushing, cyanosis, diaphoresis, and piloerection may indicate hypoperfusion.

Give the prescribed therapy to correct cardiovascular system problems. Assess the patient's response to fluid and drug administration as often as every 5 to 10 minutes. Make appropriate adjustments (e.g., drug titration) as needed. Once tissue perfusion is restored and the patient is stabilized, you can decrease the frequency of monitoring and slowly wean the patient off drugs to support BP and tissue perfusion.

> ## ❓ CHECK YOUR PRACTICE
> A 69-yr-old male patient has just been admitted to the ICU with a diagnosis of sepsis. Your assessment shows that he is confused, with weak peripheral pulses and a BP of 84/50.
> - What fluids would you expect to be ordered?
> - How much fluid would you expect to infuse to improve his BP?
> - Despite aggressive fluid resuscitation, the patient is still hypotensive. What drug would you expect to be given to improve tissue perfusion?

Respiratory Status. Frequently assess the respiratory status of the patient in shock to ensure adequate oxygenation, detect complications early, and provide data about the patient's acid-base status. At first, monitor the rate, depth, and rhythm of respirations as often as every 15 to 30 minutes. Increased rate and depth provide information about the patient's attempts to correct metabolic acidosis. Assess breath sounds every 1 to 2 hours and as needed for any changes that may indicate fluid overload or accumulation of secretions.

Use pulse oximetry to continuously monitor O$_2$ saturation. Pulse oximetry using a patient's finger may not be accurate in a shock state because of poor peripheral circulation. Instead, attach the probe to the ear, nose, or forehead (according to the manufacturer's guidelines). Arterial blood gases (ABGs) give definitive information on ventilation and oxygenation status and acid-base balance. Initial interpretation of ABGs is often your responsibility. A PaO$_2$ below 60 mm Hg (in the absence of chronic lung disease) indicates hypoxemia and the need for higher O$_2$ concentrations or for a different mode of O$_2$ administration. Low PaCO$_2$ with a low pH and low bicarbonate level may mean that the patient is trying to compensate for metabolic acidosis from increasing lactate levels.

A rising PaCO$_2$ with a persistently low pH and PaO$_2$ indicates the need for advanced pulmonary management. Many patients in shock are intubated and on mechanical ventilation. Maintaining a patent airway and monitoring for ventilator-related complications are critical. Chapter 65 discusses artificial airways and mechanical ventilation.

Renal Status. At first, measure urine output every 1 to 2 hours to assess the adequacy of renal perfusion. Inserting an indwelling urinary catheter helps measure during resuscitation. Urine output below 0.5 mL/kg/hr may indicate inadequate perfusion of the kidneys. Use trends in serum creatinine values to assess renal function. Serum creatinine is a better indicator of renal function than BUN levels, since BUN is affected by the patient's catabolic state.

Body Temperature. Monitor temperature every 4 hours if normal. In the presence of a high or subnormal temperature, obtain hourly core temperatures (e.g., urinary, esophageal, PA catheter). Use light covers and control the room temperature to keep the patient comfortably warm. If the patient's temperature rises above 101.5°F (38.6°C) and the patient becomes uncomfortable or shows cardiovascular compromise, treat the fever with antipyretic drugs (e.g., ibuprofen, acetaminophen) and remove some of the patient's covers. Consider a cooling device if fever persists despite treatment.

Gastrointestinal Status. Auscultate bowel sounds at least every 4 hours. Monitor for abdominal distention. If a nasogastric tube is present, measure drainage and check for occult blood. Check all stools for occult blood.

Skin Integrity. Hygiene is especially important for the patient in shock because impaired tissue perfusion predisposes the patient to skin breakdown and infection. Perform bathing and other nursing measures carefully because a patient in shock has problems with O_2 delivery to tissues. Use clinical judgment in determining priorities of care to limit the demands for increased O_2. Monitor trends in O_2 consumption (e.g., SpO_2, $ScvO_2/SvO_2$) during all nursing interventions to assess the patient's tolerance of activity.

The increased O_2 demand that occurs during bathing and repositioning of patients with limited O_2 reserves makes the prevention of pressure injuries challenging. Turn the patient at least every 1 to 2 hours. Maintain good body alignment. Use a pressure-relieving or pressure-reducing mattress or a specialty bed as needed. Perform passive range of motion 3 or 4 times a day to maintain joint mobility and help prevent breakdown.

Oral care is essential because mucous membranes may become dry and fragile in the volume-depleted patient. The intubated patient usually has difficulty swallowing, resulting in pooled secretions in the mouth. Apply a water-soluble lubricant to the lips to prevent drying and cracking. Brush the patient's teeth or gums with a soft toothbrush every 12 hours. Swab the lips and oral mucosa with a moisturizing solution every 2 to 4 hours.

Emotional Support and Comfort. Do not underestimate the effects of fear and anxiety when the patient and caregiver are faced with a critical, life-threatening situation (see Chapter 65). Fear, anxiety, and pain may worsen respiratory distress and increase the release of catecholamines. When implementing care, monitor the patient's mental state and level of pain using valid assessment tools. Give drugs to decrease anxiety and pain as needed. Continuous infusions of a benzodiazepine (e.g., lorazepam) and an opioid or sedative (e.g., morphine, propofol [Diprivan]) are extremely helpful in decreasing anxiety and pain.[19]

Do not overlook the patient's spiritual needs. Patients may want a visit from a chaplain, priest, rabbi, or minister. One way to provide support is to offer to call a member of the clergy rather than wait for the patient or caregiver to express a wish for spiritual counseling.

Caregivers need to be kept informed of the patient's condition. Give the patient and caregiver simple explanations of all procedures before you carry them out and information about

the plan of care. If they ask questions about progress and prognosis, give simple and honest answers.

If possible, the same nurses should continually care for the patient. This decreases anxiety, limits conflicting information, and increases trust. If the prognosis becomes grave, support the patient's caregiver when making tough decisions, such as withdrawing life support. The interprofessional care team must promote realistic expectations and outcomes. Remember, compassion is as essential as scientific and technical expertise in the total care of the patient and caregiver.

Ensure that the caregiver can spend time with the patient, provided the patient perceives this time as comforting.[20] Explain in simple terms the purpose of any tubes and equipment attached to or surrounding the patient. Tell them what they may and may not touch. If possible, place the patient's hands and arms outside the sheets to encourage therapeutic touch. Encourage caregivers to perform simple comfort measures if desired. Provide privacy as much as possible while assuring the patient and caregiver that help is readily available should it be needed. Always position the call light in reach of the patient or caregiver.

◆ **Ambulatory Care.** Rehabilitation of the patient who had a critical illness requires (1) correction of the precipitating cause, (2) prevention or early treatment of complications, and (3) teaching focused on disease management or prevention of recurrence based on the initial cause of shock. Continue to monitor the patient for complications throughout the recovery period. These may include decreased range of motion, muscle weakness, decreased physical endurance, AKI (see Chapter 46), and fibrotic lung disease (from ARDS) (see Chapter 67). Patients recovering from shock often need diverse services after discharge. These can include admission to transitional care units (e.g., for mechanical ventilation weaning), rehabilitation centers (inpatient or outpatient), or home health care agencies. Start planning for a safe transition from hospital to home as soon as the patient is admitted to the hospital.

◆ **Evaluation**

The expected outcomes are that the patient who has shock will have:

• Adequate tissue perfusion with restoration of normal or baseline BP
• Normal organ function with no complications from hypoperfusion
• Decreased fear and anxiety and increased psychologic comfort

SYSTEMIC INFLAMMATORY RESPONSE SYNDROME AND MULTIPLE ORGAN DYSFUNCTION SYNDROME

Etiology and Pathophysiology

Systemic inflammatory response syndrome (SIRS) is a systemic inflammatory response to a variety of insults, including infection (referred to as *sepsis*), ischemia, infarction, and injury.[21] Generalized inflammation in organs remote from the initial insult characterizes SIRS. Many different mechanisms can trigger SIRS. These include:

- Mechanical tissue trauma: burns, crush injuries, surgical procedures
- Abscess formation: intraabdominal, extremities
- Ischemic or necrotic tissue: pancreatitis, vascular disease, MI
- Microbial invasion: bacteria, viruses, fungi, parasites
- Endotoxin release: gram-negative and gram-positive bacteria
- Global perfusion deficits: postcardiac resuscitation, shock states
- Regional perfusion deficits: distal perfusion deficits

Multiple organ dysfunction syndrome (MODS) is the failure of 2 or more organ systems in an acutely ill patient such that homeostasis cannot be maintained without intervention.[22] MODS results from SIRS. These 2 syndromes represent the ends of a continuum. Transition from SIRS to MODS does not occur in a clear-cut manner (Fig. 66.1).

Organ and Metabolic Dysfunction. When the inflammatory response is activated, consequences include the release of mediators, direct damage to the endothelium, and hypermetabolism. Vascular permeability increases. This allows mediators and protein to leak out of the endothelium and into the interstitial space. White blood cells begin to digest the foreign debris, and the coagulation cascade is activated (see Chapter 29). Hypotension, decreased perfusion, microemboli, and redistributed or shunted blood flow eventually compromise organ perfusion.

The respiratory system is often the first system to show signs of dysfunction in SIRS and MODS.[22] Inflammatory mediators have a direct effect on the pulmonary vasculature. The endothelial damage from the release of inflammatory mediators causes increased capillary permeability. This causes movement of fluid from the pulmonary vasculature into the pulmonary interstitial spaces. The fluid then moves to the alveoli, causing alveolar edema. Type I pneumocytes (alveolar cells) are destroyed. Type II pneumocytes are damaged, and surfactant production is decreased. The alveoli collapse. This creates an increase in *shunt* (blood flow to the lungs that does not take part in gas exchange) and worsening ventilation-perfusion mismatch. The result is ARDS. Patients with ARDS need aggressive pulmonary management with mechanical ventilation. See Chapter 67 for a complete discussion of ARDS.

Cardiovascular changes include myocardial depression and massive vasodilation in response to increasing tissue demands. Vasodilation results in decreased SVR and BP. The baroreceptor reflex causes release of *inotropic* (increasing force of contraction) and *chronotropic* (increasing heart rate) factors that enhance CO. To compensate for hypotension, CO increases by an increase in heart rate and SV. Increases in capillary permeability cause a shift of albumin and fluid out of the vascular space. This further reduces venous return and thus preload. The patient becomes warm and tachycardic with a high CO and a low SVR. Other signs include decreased capillary refill, skin mottling, increased CVP and PAWP, and dysrhythmias. ScvO$_2$ or SvO$_2$ may be abnormally high because the patient is perfusing areas not consuming much O$_2$ (e.g., skin, nonworking muscle). Other areas may have blood shunted away from them. Eventually, either perfusion of vital organs becomes insufficient or the cells are unable to use O$_2$ and their function is further compromised.

Neurologic dysfunction in SIRS and MODS often presents as mental status changes. These acute changes can be an early sign of SIRS or MODS. The patient may be confused and agitated, combative, disoriented, lethargic, or comatose. These changes are due to hypoxemia, the effects of inflammatory mediators, and impaired perfusion.

AKI is common in SIRS and MODS. Hypoperfusion and the effects of the mediators can cause AKI. Decreased perfusion to the kidneys activates the SNS and the renin-angiotensin system.[22] Stimulation of the renin-angiotensin system causes systemic vasoconstriction and aldosterone-mediated sodium and water reabsorption. Another risk factor for the development of AKI is the use of nephrotoxic drugs. Many antibiotics used to treat gram-negative bacteria (e.g., aminoglycosides) can be nephrotoxic. Careful monitoring of drug levels is essential to avoid the nephrotoxic effects.

The GI tract plays a key role in the development of MODS. GI motility is often decreased in critical illness, causing abdominal distention and paralytic ileus. In the early stages of SIRS and MODS, blood is shunted away from the GI mucosa, making it highly vulnerable to ischemic injury. Decreased perfusion leads to a breakdown of this normally protective mucosal barrier. This increases the risk for ulceration, GI bleeding, and bacterial movement from the GI tract into circulation.[21]

Metabolic changes are pronounced in SIRS and MODS. Both syndromes trigger a hypermetabolic response. Glycogen stores are rapidly converted to glucose (glycogenolysis). Once glycogen is depleted, amino acids are converted to glucose (gluconeogenesis), reducing protein stores. Fatty acids are mobilized for fuel. Catecholamines and glucocorticoids are released and cause hyperglycemia and insulin resistance. The net result is a catabolic state with a loss of lean body mass (muscle).

The hypermetabolism associated with SIRS and MODS may last for several days and cause liver dysfunction. Liver dysfunction in MODS may begin long before clinical evidence of it is present. Protein synthesis is impaired. The liver cannot make albumin, one of the key proteins in maintaining plasma oncotic pressure. This changes plasma oncotic pressure, causing fluid and protein to leak from the vascular spaces to the interstitial space. At this point, giving albumin does not normalize oncotic pressure in these patients.

As the state of hypermetabolism persists, the patient cannot convert lactate to glucose and lactate accumulates (lactic acidosis). Despite increases in glycogenolysis and gluconeogenesis, eventually the liver cannot maintain an adequate glucose level and the patient becomes hypoglycemic. Hypoglycemia can also develop due to acute adrenal insufficiency.

DIC may result from dysfunction of the coagulation system. DIC causes microvascular clotting and bleeding at the same time because of the depletion of clotting factors and excessive fibrinolysis. (Chapter 30 discusses DIC.)

Electrolyte imbalances are common and result from the hormonal and metabolic changes and fluid shifts. These changes worsen mental status changes, neuromuscular dysfunction, and dysrhythmias. The release of ADH and aldosterone results in sodium and water retention. Aldosterone increases urinary potassium loss, and catecholamines cause potassium to move into the cell, resulting in hypokalemia. Hypokalemia is associated with dysrhythmias and muscle weakness. Metabolic acidosis results from impaired tissue perfusion, hypoxia, and the shift to anaerobic metabolism. This increases lactate levels. Progressive renal dysfunction also contributes to metabolic acidosis. Hypocalcemia, hypomagnesemia, and hypophosphatemia are common.

Clinical Manifestations of SIRS and MODS

The clinical manifestations of SIRS and MODS are described in Table 66.10.

❖ NURSING AND INTERPROFESSIONAL MANAGEMENT: SIRS AND MODS

The prognosis for the patient with MODS is poor, with mortality rates of 40% to 60%.[22] Mortality increases as more organ systems fail. The most common cause of death continues to be sepsis. Survival improves with early, goal-directed therapy. So, the most important goal is to prevent SIRS from progressing to MODS.

A critical part of your role is vigilant assessment and ongoing monitoring to detect early signs of deterioration or organ dysfunction. Interprofessional care for patients with SIRS and MODS focuses on (1) prevention and treatment of infection, (2) maintaining tissue oxygenation, (3) nutritional and metabolic support, and (4) appropriate support of individual failing organs. Table 66.10 outlines the management for patients with SIRS and MODS.

TABLE 66.10 Manifestations and Management of SIRS and MODS

Manifestations	Management
Respiratory System	
Development of ARDS (see Chapter 67): • Bilateral fluffy infiltrates on chest x-ray • Decreased compliance • Dyspnea (severe) • Increased minute ventilation • PaO_2/FIO_2 ratio <200 • PAWP <18 mm Hg • Pulmonary hypertension • Refractory hypoxemia • Tachypnea • Ventilation-perfusion (V/Q) mismatch	Optimize O_2 delivery and minimize O_2 consumption Mechanical ventilation (see Chapter 65) • Positive end-expiratory pressure • Lung protective modes (e.g., pressure-control inverse ratio ventilation, low tidal volumes) • Permissive hypercapnia • Positioning (e.g., continuous lateral rotation therapy, prone positioning)
Cardiovascular System	
Biventricular failure ↓ BP, MAP, SVR ↑ HR, CO, SV Massive vasodilation Myocardial depression Systolic, diastolic dysfunction	Volume management to ↑ preload Hemodynamic monitoring Arterial pressure monitoring to maintain MAP >65 mm Hg Vasopressors Intermittent or continuous $ScvO_2$ or SvO_2 monitoring Balance O_2 supply and demand Continuous ECG monitoring Circulatory assist devices VTE prophylaxis
Central Nervous System	
Acute change in neurologic status Confusion, disorientation, delirium Fever Hepatic encephalopathy Seizures	Evaluate for hepatic or metabolic encephalopathy Optimize cerebral blood flow ↓ Cerebral O_2 requirements Prevent secondary tissue ischemia Calcium channel blockers (reduce cerebral vasospasm)
Endocrine System	
Hyperglycemia → hypoglycemia	Provide continuous infusion of insulin and glucose to maintain blood glucose 140–180 mg/dL (7.77–10.0 mmol/L)

Manifestations	Management
Renal System	
Prerenal: renal hypoperfusion • BUN/creatinine ratio >20:1 • ↓ Urine Na+ <20 mEq/L • ↑ Urine osmolality • Urine specific gravity >1.020 *Intrarenal:* acute tubular necrosis • BUN/creatinine ratio <10:1–15:1 • ↑ Urine Na+ >20 mEq/L • ↓ Urine osmolality • Urine specific gravity ~1.010	Diuretics • Loop diuretics (e.g., furosemide [Lasix]) • May need to ↑ dosage due to ↓ glomerular filtration rate Continuous renal replacement therapy (see Chapter 46)
GI System	
GI bleeding Hypoperfusion → ↓ peristalsis, paralytic ileus Mucosal ischemia • ↓ Intramucosal pH • Potential translocation of gut bacteria • Potential abdominal compartment syndrome Mucosal ulceration on endoscopy	Stress ulcer prophylaxis • Antacids (e.g., Maalox) • Proton pump inhibitors (e.g., omeprazole [Prilosec]) • sucralfate (Carafate) Monitor abdominal distention, intraabdominal pressures Dietitian consult Enteral nutrition Stimulate mucosal activity Provide essential nutrients and optimal calories
Hepatic System	
Bilirubin >2 mg/dL (34 µmol/L) Hepatic encephalopathy Jaundice ↑ Liver enzymes (ALT, AST, GGT) ↓ Serum albumin, prealbumin, transferrin ↑ Serum NH_3 (ammonia)	Maintain adequate tissue perfusion Provide nutritional support (e.g., enteral nutrition) Careful use of drugs metabolized by liver
Hematologic System	
↑ Bleeding times, ↑ PT, ↑ PTT ↑ D-dimer ↑ Fibrin split products ↓ Platelet count (thrombocytopenia)	Observe for bleeding from obvious and/or occult sites Replace factors being lost (e.g., platelets) Minimize traumatic interventions (e.g., IM injections, multiple venipunctures)

ALT, Alanine aminotransferase; *AST,* aspartate aminotransferase; *GGT,* γ-glutamyl transferase; *PA,* pulmonary artery; *PAWP,* pulmonary artery wedge pressure; *PT,* prothrombin time; *PTT,* partial thromboplastin time; *ScvO₂,* O_2 saturation in venous blood; *SvO₂,* O_2 saturation in mixed venous blood; *SVR,* systemic vascular resistance.

◆ **Prevention and Treatment of Infection**

Aggressive infection control strategies are essential to decrease the risk for HAIs. Early, aggressive surgery is recommended to remove necrotic tissue (e.g., early debridement of burn tissue) that can provide a culture medium for microorganisms. Aggressive pulmonary management, including early mobilization, can reduce the risk for infection. Strict asepsis can decrease infections related to intraarterial lines, endotracheal tubes, indwelling urinary catheters, IV lines, and other invasive devices or procedures. Daily assessment of the ongoing need for invasive lines and other devices is an important strategy to prevent or limit HAIs.

Despite aggressive strategies, infection may develop. Once an infection is suspected, begin interventions to treat the cause. Send appropriate cultures and start broad-spectrum antibiotic therapy, as ordered. Adjust therapy based on the culture results, if needed.

◆ **Maintenance of Tissue Oxygenation**

Hypoxemia often occurs because patients have greater O_2 needs and decreased O_2 supply to the tissues. Interventions that decrease O_2 demand and increase O_2 delivery are essential. Sedation, mechanical ventilation, analgesia, and rest may decrease O_2 demand and should be considered. Treating fever, chills, and pain decrease O_2 demand. O_2 delivery may be optimized by using individualized tidal volumes with positive end-expiratory pressure, increasing preload (e.g., fluids) or myocardial contractility to enhance CO, or reducing afterload to increase CO.

◆ **Nutritional and Metabolic Needs**

Hypermetabolism can result in profound weight loss, cachexia, and further organ failure. Protein-calorie malnutrition is a key sign of hypermetabolism. Total energy expenditure is often increased 1.5 to 2.0 times the normal metabolic rate. Because of their short half-life, monitor plasma transferrin and prealbumin levels to assess hepatic protein synthesis.

The goal of nutritional support is to preserve organ function. Providing early and optimal nutrition decreases morbidity and mortality rates. EN is preferred. If it cannot be used, PN should be considered. (Chapter 39 discusses EN and PN.) Provide glycemic control with a goal of ≤180 mg/dL with insulin infusions in these patients.[21]

◆ **Support of Failing Organs**

Support of any failing organ is a goal of therapy. For example, the patient with ARDS requires aggressive O_2 therapy and mechanical ventilation (see Chapter 67). DIC should be treated appropriately (e.g., blood products) (see Chapter 30). Renal failure may require dialysis. Continuous renal replacement therapy is better tolerated than hemodialysis, especially in a patient with hemodynamic instability (see Chapter 46).

A final consideration may be that further interventions are futile. It is important to maintain communication between the health care team and the patient's caregiver about realistic goals and likely outcomes for the patient with MODS. Withdrawal of life support and starting end-of-life care may be the best options for the patient.

CASE STUDY

Shock

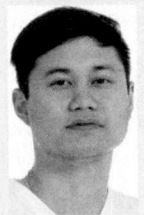
(© Thinkstock.)

Patient Profile

K.L., a 25-yr-old Korean American, was not wearing his seat belt when he was driving a motor vehicle involved in a crash. The windshield was broken, and K.L. was found 10 ft from his car. He was face down, conscious, and moaning. His wife and daughter were in the car with their seat belts on. They sustained minor injuries and were very frightened and upset. All passengers were taken to the ED. This information pertains to K.L.

Subjective Data

* States, "I can't breathe"
* Cries out when abdomen is palpated

Objective Data
Physical Examination

* *Cardiovascular:* BP 80/56 mm Hg; apical pulse 138 but no palpable radial or pedal pulses; carotid pulse 1+. ECG is below:

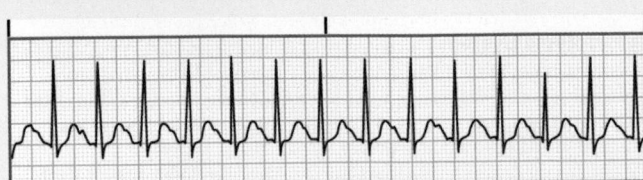

* *Respiratory:* respiratory rate 35 breaths/min; labored breathing with shallow respirations; asymmetric chest wall movement; absence of breath sounds on left side. Trachea deviated slightly to the right
* *Abdomen:* slightly distended and left upper quadrant painful on palpation
* *Musculoskeletal:* open compound fracture of the lower left leg

Diagnostic Studies

* Chest x-ray: hemothorax and 6 rib fractures on left side
* Hematocrit: 28%

Interprofessional Care (in the ED)

* Intraosseous access in right proximal tibia placed prehospital
* Left chest tube placed, draining bright red blood
* Fluid resuscitation started with crystalloids
* High-flow O_2 via nonrebreather mask

Emergency Surgical Procedures

* Splenectomy
* Repair of torn intercostal artery
* Repair of compound fracture

Discussion Questions

1. What types of shock is K.L. experiencing? What clinical manifestations did he display that support your answer?
2. What were the causes of K.L.'s shock states? What are other causes of these types of shock?
3. *Priority Decision:* What are the priority nursing responsibilities for K.L.?
4. *Priority Decision:* What ongoing nursing assessment parameters are essential for this patient?
5. What are his potential complications?
6. *Patient-Centered Care:* K.L.'s parents arrive. English is their second language. They are very anxious and asking about their son. What can you do to provide culturally competent family-centered care?
7. *Priority Decision:* Based on the assessment data presented, what are the priority nursing diagnoses?
8. *Collaboration:* Identify the tasks that could be delegated to unlicensed assistive personnel (UAP).
9. *Evidence-Based Practice:* You are orienting a new graduate RN. He asks you why crystalloids are used for fluid resuscitation. What is your response?

Answers available at *http://evolve.elsevier.com/Lewis/medsurg.*

■ BRIDGE TO NCLEX EXAMINATION

The number of the question corresponds to the same-numbered outcome at the beginning of the chapter.

1. A patient has a spinal cord injury at T4. Vital signs include falling blood pressure with bradycardia. The nurse recognizes that the patient is experiencing
   a. a relative hypervolemia.
   b. an absolute hypovolemia.
   c. neurogenic shock from low blood flow.
   d. neurogenic shock from massive vasodilation.

2. A 78-yr-old man with a history of diabetes has confusion and temperature of 104°F (40°C). There is a wound on his right heel with purulent drainage. After an infusion of 3 L of normal saline solution, his assessment findings are BP 84/40 mm Hg; heart rate 110; respiratory rate 42 and shallow; CO 8 L/min; and PAWP 4 mm Hg. This patient's symptoms are *most* likely indicative of
   a. sepsis.
   b. septic shock.
   c. multiple organ dysfunction syndrome.
   d. systemic inflammatory response syndrome.

3. Treatment modalities for the management of cardiogenic shock include (select all that apply)
   a. dobutamine to increase myocardial contractility.
   b. vasopressors to increase systemic vascular resistance.
   c. circulatory assist devices such as an intraaortic balloon pump.
   d. corticosteroids to stabilize the cell wall in the infarcted myocardium.
   e. Trendelenburg positioning to facilitate venous return and increase preload.

4. The *most* accurate assessment parameters for the nurse to use to determine adequate tissue perfusion in the patient with MODS are
   a. blood pressure, pulse, and respirations.
   b. breath sounds, blood pressure, and body temperature.
   c. pulse pressure, level of consciousness, and pupillary response.
   d. level of consciousness, urine output, and skin color and temperature.

1. d, 2. b, 3. a, c, 4. d

For rationales to these answers and even more NCLEX review questions, visit *http://evolve.elsevier.com/Lewis/medsurg*.

EVOLVE WEBSITE/RESOURCES LIST

http://evolve.elsevier.com/Lewis/medsurg
Review Questions (Online Only)
Key Points
Answer Keys to Questions
- Rationales for Bridge to NCLEX Examination Questions
- Answer Guidelines for Case Study on p. 1586
Student Case Studies
- Patient With Acute Pancreatitis and Septic Shock
- Patient With Cardiogenic Shock
- Patient With Sepsis
Nursing Care Plan
- eNursing Care Plan 66.1: Patient in Shock
Conceptual Care Map Creator
Audio Glossary
Content Updates

REFERENCES

1. Tewelde SZ, Liu SS, Winters ME: Cardiogenic shock, *Cardiol Clin* 28:53, 2018.
2. Good VS, Kirkwood PL: *Advanced critical care nursing*, ed 2, St Louis, 2017, Elsevier.
3. Hamlin S, Strauss P, Chen H, et al: Microvascular fluid resuscitation in circulatory shock, *Nurs Clin North Am* 52:291, 2017.
4. Taylor MP, Wrenn P, O'Donnell AD: Presentation of neurogenic shock within the emergency department, *Emerg Med J* 34:157, 2016.
*5. Lee SE: Management of anaphylaxis, *Otolaryngol Clin North Am* 50: 1175, 2017.
6. Kleinpell R, Schorr C, Balk R: The new sepsis definitions: Implications for critical care practitioners, *Amer J Crit Care* 25:457, 2016.
*7. Singer M, Deutschman C, Seymour C, et al: The third international consensus definitions for sepsis and septic shock (Sepsis-3), *JAMA* 315:801, 2016.
8. O'Shaughnessy J, Grzelak M, Dontsova A, et al: Early sepsis identification, *MEDSURG Nursing* 26:248, 2017.
*9. Winters ME, Sherwin R, Vilke GM, et al: What is the preferred resuscitation fluid for patients with severe sepsis and septic shock? *J Emerg Med* 53:928, 2017.
*10. Stratton L, Verlin D, Arbo J: Vasopressors and inotropes in sepsis. *Emerg Med Clin North Am* 35:75, 2017.
11. McClave SA, Taylor BE, Martindale RG, et al: Guidelines for the provision and assessment of nutrition support therapy in the adult critically ill patient: Society of Critical Care Medicine (S.C.C.M.) and American Society for Parenteral and Enteral Nutrition (A.S.P.E.N.), *J Parenter Enteral Nutr* 40:159, 2016.
12. Jakovijevi D, Lip-Burn M, Scheueler S, et al: Left ventricular assist device as a bridge to recovery for patient with advanced heart failure, *J Am Coll Cardiol* 69:1924, 2017.
*13. Pickett J, Bridges E, Kritek P, et al: Passive leg-raising and prediction of fluid responsiveness: Systematic review, *Crit Care Nurse* 37:32, 2017.
14. Timmerman RA: Managing vasoactive infusions to restore hemodynamic stability, *Nursing2019 Critical Care*, 11:35, 2016.
15. Sherwin R, Winters ME, Vilke GM, et al: Does early and appropriate antibiotic administration improve mortality in patients with severe sepsis or septic shock? *J Emerg Med* 53:588, 2017.
16. Gunst J, Van den Berghe G: Blood glucose control in the ICU. How tight? *Ann Transl Med* 5:76, 2017.
*17. Rhodes A, Evans LE, Alhazzani W, et al: Surviving sepsis campaign. International guidelines for management of sepsis and septic shock, *Intens Care Med* 43:304, 2017.
18. Institute for Healthcare Improvement: Evidence-based care bundles. Retrieved from *www.ihi.org/topics/Bundles/Pages/default.aspx*.
19. Hariharan U, Garg R: Sedation and analgesia in critical care, *J Anesth Crit Care Open Access* 7:262, 2017.
20. Davidson JE, Aslakson RA, Long AC, et al: Guidelines for family-centered care in the neonatal, pediatric, and adult ICU, *Crit Care Med* 45:103, 2017.
21. Sauaia A, Moore FA, Moore EE: Postinjury inflammation and organ dysfunction, *Crit Care Clin* 33:167, 2017.
22. Gordy S: Multiple organ failure. In Moore L, Todd S, eds: *Common problems in acute care surgery*, New York, 2017, Springer.

*Evidence-based information for clinical practice.

67

Acute Respiratory Failure and Acute Respiratory Distress Syndrome

Eugene Mondor

The closest thing to being cared for is to care for someone else.

Carson McCullers

(e) http://evolve.elsevier.com/Lewis/medsurg

CONCEPTUAL FOCUS

Acid-Base Balance
Anxiety

Gas Exchange

LEARNING OUTCOMES

1. Discuss the etiology, pathophysiology, and clinical manifestations of hypoxemic and hypercapnic acute respiratory failure.
2. Describe the nursing and interprofessional management of hypoxemic or hypercapnic respiratory failure.

3. Discuss the pathophysiology and clinical manifestations of acute respiratory distress syndrome (ARDS).
4. Describe the nursing and interprofessional management of ARDS.
5. Select measures to prevent and manage complications of acute respiratory failure and ARDS.

KEY TERMS

acute respiratory distress syndrome (ARDS), p. 1597
acute respiratory failure (ARF), p. 1588
alveolar hypoventilation, p. 1590
chronic respiratory failure, p. 1589

hypercapnic respiratory failure, p. 1588
hypoxia, p. 1591
hypoxemia, p. 1588
hypoxemic respiratory failure, p. 1588
PaO_2/FIO_2 (P/F) ratio, p. 1599

permissive hypercapnia, p 1601
refractory hypoxemia, p. 1598
shunt, p. 1590
V/Q mismatch, p. 1589
work of breathing (WOB), p. 1591

This chapter discusses acute respiratory failure (ARF) and acute respiratory distress syndrome (ARDS). Nursing and interprofessional management of patients with ARF and ARDS focus on interventions to promote adequate oxygenation, ensure effective ventilation, identify and treat the underlying causes, and prevent complications. When respiratory function is insufficient, all body systems are affected

ACUTE RESPIRATORY FAILURE

The major function of the respiratory system is gas exchange. Acute respiratory failure (ARF) occurs when oxygenation, ventilation, or both are inadequate. ARF is not a disease. It is a symptom that reflects lung function. For example, not enough O_2 is transferred to the blood or inadequate CO_2 is removed from the lungs (Fig. 67.1). ARF occurs because of disorders involving the lungs or other body systems (Table 67.1).

Conditions that interfere with adequate O_2 transfer result in hypoxemia. This causes a decrease in arterial O_2 (PaO_2) and saturation (SaO_2) to less than the normal values. Insufficient CO_2 removal results in hypercapnia. It causes an increase in arterial CO_2 ($PaCO_2$). Arterial blood gases (ABGs) are used to assess changes in pH, PaO_2, $PaCO_2$, bicarbonate, and SaO_2. We use pulse oximetry to assess arterial O_2 saturation (SpO_2).

We classify ARF as hypoxemic or hypercapnic (Fig. 67.2). Hypoxemic respiratory failure is a PaO_2 less than 60 mm Hg when the patient is receiving an inspired O_2 concentration of 60% or more.[1] In hypoxemic respiratory failure (also called *oxygenation failure*), the main problem is inadequate exchange of O_2 between the alveoli and pulmonary capillaries. The PaO_2 level shows inadequate O_2 saturation. A less than optimal PaO_2 level exists despite supplemental O_2.

Hypercapnic respiratory failure (or *ventilatory failure*) is a $PaCO_2$ greater than 50 mm Hg with acidemia (arterial pH less than 7.35).[2] The main problem is insufficient CO_2 removal. This causes the $PaCO_2$ to be higher than normal. For whatever reason, the body is unable to compensate for the increase. This allows acidemia to occur.

Patients may have both types of respiratory failure at the same time. For example, a patient with chronic obstructive

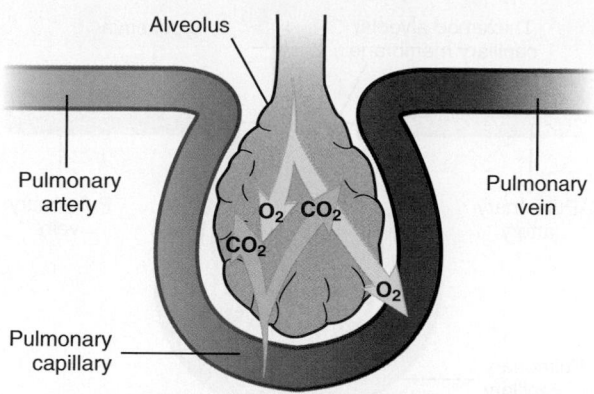

FIG. 67.1 Normal gas exchange unit in the lung.

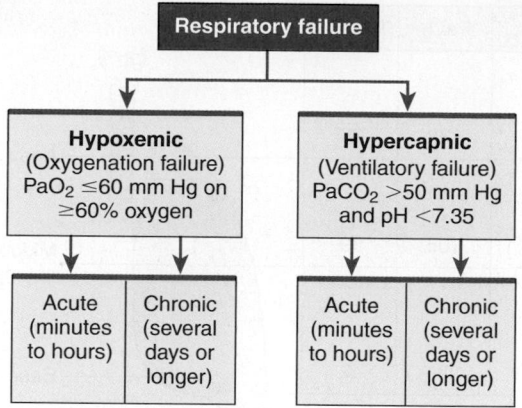

FIG. 67.2 Classification of respiratory failure.

TABLE 67.1 Common Causes of Respiratory Failure

Hypoxemic Respiratory Failure	Hypercapnic Respiratory Failure
Respiratory System • ARDS • Hepatopulmonary syndrome (e.g., low-resistance flow state, V/Q mismatch) • Massive pulmonary embolism (e.g., thrombus emboli, fat emboli) • Pneumonia • Pulmonary artery laceration and hemorrhage • Toxic inhalation (e.g., smoke inhalation)	**Respiratory System** • Asthma • COPD • Cystic fibrosis **Central Nervous System** • Brainstem injury or infarction • Sedative and opioid overdose • Spinal cord injury • Severe head injury
Cardiac System • Anatomic shunt (e.g., ventricular septal defect) • Cardiogenic pulmonary edema • Cardiogenic shock (decreasing blood flow through pulmonary vasculature) • High cardiac output states: diffusion limitation	**Chest Wall** • Kyphoscoliosis • Pain • Severe obesity • Thoracic trauma (e.g., flail chest) **Neuromuscular System** • Amyotrophic lateral sclerosis • Critical illness polyneuropathy • Guillain-Barré syndrome • Muscular dystrophy • Multiple sclerosis • Myasthenia gravis • Phrenic nerve injury • Poliomyelitis • Toxin exposure or ingestion (e.g., tree tobacco, acetylcholinesterase inhibitors, carbamate or organophosphate poisoning)

pulmonary disease (COPD) who has pneumonia could have "acute-on-chronic" respiratory failure. In other words, the patient has an underlying chronic respiratory problem. The new infection, in addition to the chronic problem, results in the "acute-on-chronic" clinical picture.

Significant changes in PaO_2 and $PaCO_2$ occur with ARF. These may develop over several minutes to a few hours to 1 or 2 days. The patient may have hemodynamic instability (e.g. tachycardia, hypotension), increased respiratory effort, and decreased level of consciousness. Urgent intervention is required. Chronic respiratory failure develops more slowly, over days to weeks. The patient is usually more stable as the

body had time to compensate for the small, but subtle, changes that have occurred.

Etiology and Pathophysiology

Hypoxemic Respiratory Failure. Four physiologic mechanisms may cause hypoxemia and hypoxemic respiratory failure: (1) mismatch between ventilation (V) and perfusion (Q), often referred to as V/Q mismatch; (2) shunt; (3) diffusion limitation; and (4) alveolar hypoventilation. The most common causes are V/Q mismatch and shunt.

Ventilation-Perfusion Mismatch. In normal lungs, the volume of blood perfusing the lungs and the amount of gas reaching the alveoli are almost identical. So, when you compare normal alveolar ventilation (4 to 6 L/min) to pulmonary blood flow (4 to 6 L/min), you have a V/Q ratio of 0.8 to 1.2.[3] In a perfect match, ventilation and perfusion would yield a V/Q ratio of 1:1, expressed as V/Q = 1. When the match is not 1:1, a V/Q mismatch occurs.

This example implies that ventilation and perfusion are perfectly matched in all areas of the lung. This situation does not normally exist. In reality, some regional mismatch occurs. For example, at the apex of the lung, V/Q ratios are greater than 1 (more ventilation than perfusion). At the base of the lung, V/Q ratios are less than 1 (less ventilation than perfusion). Because changes at the lung apex balance changes at the base, the net effect is a close overall match (Fig. 67.3).

Many diseases and conditions cause a V/Q mismatch (Fig. 67.4). The most common are those in which increased secretions are present in the airways (e.g., COPD) or alveoli (e.g., pneumonia) or bronchospasm is present (e.g., asthma). V/Q mismatch may result from pain, alveolar collapse (atelectasis), or pulmonary emboli.

Pain interferes with chest and abdominal wall movement and increases muscle tension. This often compromises ventilation. The patient is often unwilling to take big, deep breaths. As a result, short, shallow respirations contribute to the development of atelectasis. This worsens V/Q mismatch.

Pain activates the stress response, increasing baseline metabolic state. This increases O_2 consumption and CO_2 production (as a by-product of cellular and tissue metabolism). The increased O_2 demand, increased CO_2, and decreased O_2 supply increase ventilation demands. Since there is no effect on blood flow to the lungs, the result is V/Q mismatch.

Pulmonary emboli affect the perfusion part of the V/Q relationship. When a pulmonary embolus occurs, it limits blood

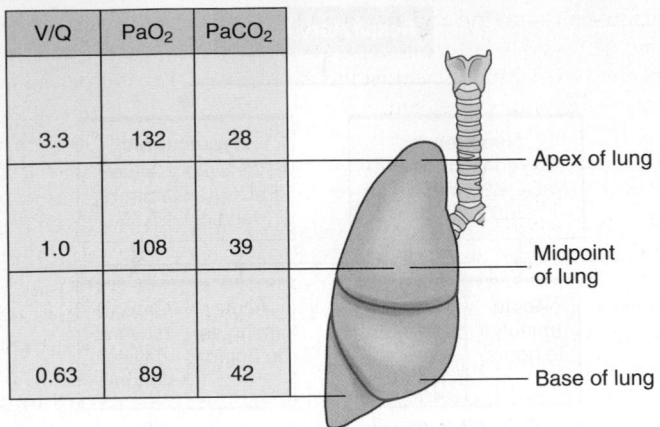

V/Q	PaO₂	PaCO₂
3.3	132	28
1.0	108	39
0.63	89	42

— Apex of lung

— Midpoint of lung

— Base of lung

FIG. 67.3 Regional V/Q differences in the normal lung. This difference causes the PaO_2 to be higher at the apex of the lung and lower at the base. Values for $PaCO_2$ are the opposite (i.e., lower at the apex and higher at the base). Blood that exits the lung is a mixture of these values.

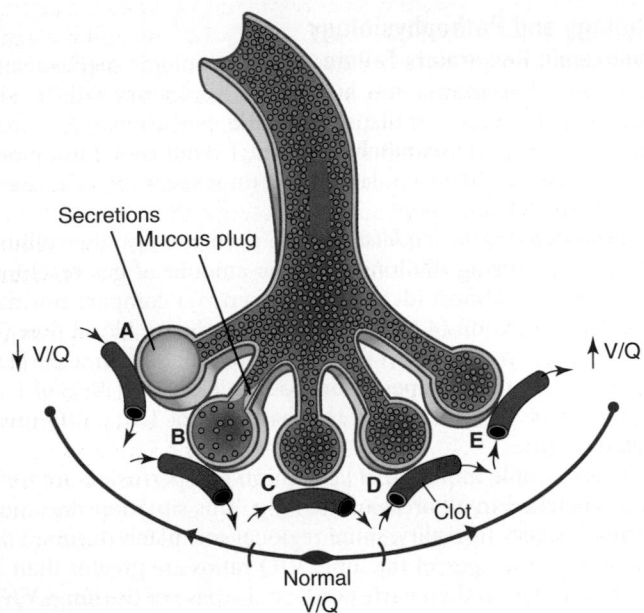

Secretions
Mucous plug
↓V/Q
A
↑V/Q
B
E
C   D
Clot
Normal
V/Q

FIG. 67.4 Range of ventilation to perfusion (V/Q) relationships. *A,* Absolute shunt, no ventilation because of fluid filling the alveoli. *B,* V/Q mismatch, ventilation partially compromised by secretions in the airway. *C,* Normal lung unit. *D,* V/Q mismatch, perfusion partially compromised by emboli obstructing blood flow. *E,* Dead space, no perfusion because of obstruction of the pulmonary capillary.

flow distal to the occlusion. Areas of normal lung ventilation remain, but there is decreased perfusion due to the vessel occlusion. This results in a V/Q mismatch. If the embolus is large, it can cause hemodynamic instability due to blockage of a large pulmonary artery.

O_2 therapy is an appropriate first step to reverse hypoxemia caused by V/Q mismatch. O_2 therapy increases the PaO_2 in the blood leaving normal gas exchange units, causing a higher-than-normal PaO_2. This blood mixes with the poorly oxygenated blood from damaged areas, raising the overall PaO_2 level in the blood leaving the lungs. The best way to treat hypoxemia caused by a V/Q mismatch is to treat the cause.

Shunt. A **shunt** occurs when blood exits the heart without having taken part in gas exchange. A shunt is an extreme V/Q mismatch. There are 2 types of shunt: anatomic and

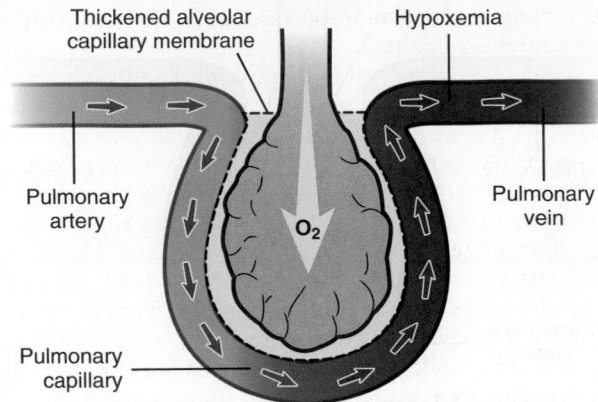

Thickened alveolar capillary membrane   Hypoxemia

Pulmonary artery

O₂

Pulmonary vein

Pulmonary capillary

FIG. 67.5 Diffusion limitation. Exchange of CO_2 and O_2 cannot occur because of the thickened alveolar-capillary membrane.

intrapulmonary. An *anatomic shunt* occurs when blood passes through an anatomic channel in the heart (e.g., a ventricular septal defect) and bypasses the lungs.[4] An *intrapulmonary shunt* occurs when blood flows through the pulmonary capillaries without taking part in gas exchange.[4] It is seen in conditions in which the alveoli fill with fluid (e.g., pneumonia) and gas exchange is severely impaired at the alveolar-capillary membrane.

O_2 therapy alone is not effective at increasing the PaO_2 if hypoxemia is due to shunt. Patients with a shunt are usually more hypoxemic than patients with V/Q mismatch. They often need mechanical ventilation with a high fraction of inspired O_2 (FIO_2) to improve gas exchange.

Diffusion Limitation. *Diffusion limitation* occurs when gas exchange across the alveolar-capillary membrane is compromised by a process that damages or destroys the alveolar membrane or affects blood flow through the pulmonary capillaries (Fig. 67.5).[5] Conditions that cause the alveolar-capillary membrane to become thicker (fibrotic) slow gas transport. These include pulmonary fibrosis, interstitial lung disease, and ARDS. The accumulation of fluid, white blood cells, or protein in the alveoli can decrease gas exchange between the alveolus and the capillary bed. A common example is pulmonary edema.

The classic sign of diffusion limitation is hypoxemia that is present during exercise but not at rest. During exercise, blood moves more quickly through the lungs. This decreases the time for diffusion of O_2 across the alveolar-capillary membrane. Diffusion limitation can occur in conditions in which CO is markedly increased (e.g., high-output heart failure [HF], severe traumatic brain injury [TBI]). As blood circulates rapidly through the pulmonary capillary bed, there is less time for gas exchange to occur.

Alveolar Hypoventilation. Alveolar hypoventilation is a decrease in ventilation that results in an increase in the $PaCO_2$. It may be caused by central nervous system (CNS) conditions, chest wall dysfunction, acute asthma, or restrictive lung diseases. Although alveolar hypoventilation is mainly a mechanism of hypercapnic respiratory failure, it contributes to hypoxemia.

Interrelationship of Mechanisms. Rarely is acute hypoxemic respiratory failure caused by a single factor. More often, it is a combination of 2 or more factors. For example, the patient with ARF from pneumonia may have a V/Q mismatch and shunt. Inflammation, edema, and exudate obstruct the airways (V/Q mismatch) and fill the alveoli with exudate (shunt). Other contributing factors include increases in O_2 demand with anxiety and unrelieved pain.

Consequences of Hypoxemia. Hypoxemia can lead to hypoxia if not corrected. Hypoxia occurs when the PaO_2 falls enough to cause signs and symptoms of inadequate oxygenation. If hypoxia or hypoxemia is severe, the cells shift from aerobic to anaerobic metabolism. Anaerobic metabolism uses more fuel, produces less energy, and is less efficient than aerobic metabolism. The waste product of anaerobic metabolism is lactic acid. Lactic acid is harder to remove from the body than CO_2, because it must be buffered with sodium bicarbonate. When the body does not have enough sodium bicarbonate to buffer the lactic acid, metabolic acidosis occurs. Left uncorrected, tissue and cell dysfunction, and ultimately cell death, occurs.

Hypercapnic Respiratory Failure. In acute hypercapnic respiratory failure, sometimes referred to as *ventilatory failure*, the lungs are often normal. In this situation, the respiratory system cannot keep CO_2 levels maintained within normal limits. This often occurs from an increase in CO_2 production or a decrease in alveolar ventilation. Hypercapnic respiratory failure can be acute or chronic. It often reflects significant problems with the respiratory system.

Many conditions can cause impaired ventilation. We group into 4 categories: (1) CNS problems, (2) neuromuscular conditions, (3) chest wall abnormalities, and (4) problems affecting the airways and/or alveoli. Acute hypercapnic respiratory failure can occur with CNS problems, neuromuscular conditions, and chest wall abnormalities in the presence of normal lungs.

Central Nervous System Problems. A number of CNS problems can suppress the drive to breathe. A common example is an overdose of a respiratory depressant drug (e.g., opioids). In a dose-related manner, CNS depressants decrease CO_2 reactivity in the brainstem. This allows arterial CO_2 levels to rise. A brainstem infarction or TBI may interfere with normal function of the respiratory center in the medulla. Patients are then at risk for acute hypercapnic respiratory failure because the medulla does not change the respiratory rate in response to a change in $PaCO_2$.

High-level spinal cord injuries can affect nerve supply to the respiratory muscles of the chest wall and diaphragm. Brain injury with a decreased level of consciousness can hinder the patient's ability to protect the airway, breathe, or manage secretions.

Neuromuscular Conditions. Various neuromuscular problems place patients at risk for respiratory failure. For example, patients with Guillain-Barré syndrome and multiple sclerosis have respiratory muscle weakness or paralysis. As a result, they cannot eliminate CO_2 and maintain normal $PaCO_2$ levels. Exposure to toxins (e.g., carbamate/organophosphate pesticides, chemical nerve agents) can interfere with the nerve supply to muscles and lung ventilation. Respiratory muscle weakness can occur from muscle wasting during a critical illness or peripheral nerve damage.

Chest Wall Abnormalities. Several conditions can prevent normal movement of the chest wall or diaphragm and limit lung expansion. In patients with flail chest, fractures prevent the rib cage from expanding normally. With kyphoscoliosis, the change in spinal configuration compresses the lungs and prevents normal expansion of the chest wall. In those with severe obesity, the weight of the chest and abdominal contents limit lung expansion.

Problems of the Airway and Alveoli. Patients with asthma, COPD, and cystic fibrosis have a high risk for hypercapnic respiratory failure because the underlying pathophysiology results in airflow obstruction and air trapping. Respiratory muscle fatigue and ventilatory failure occur from the added work of breathing needed to inspire air against increased airway resistance and air trapped within the alveoli.

Consequences of Hypercapnia. The body can tolerate increased CO_2 levels far better than low O_2 levels. This is because with slow changes in $PaCO_2$, the body may have time for compensation to occur. For example, consider the patient with COPD who has a slow increase in $PaCO_2$ after an upper respiratory tract infection. Because the change occurred over several days, there is time for the kidneys to compensate (e.g., by retaining bicarbonate). This will initially minimize the change in arterial pH. Unless the primary cause is identified and corrected, the patient's condition will likely get worse. (See Chapter 16 for a discussion of renal compensation for acid-base disorders.)

Clinical Manifestations

Respiratory failure may develop suddenly (acute, minutes or hours) or gradually (chronic, several days or weeks). A sudden decrease in PaO_2 and/or a rapid rise in $PaCO_2$ implies a serious respiratory condition, which can rapidly become a life-threatening emergency. An example is the patient with asthma who develops severe bronchospasm and a marked decrease in airflow, resulting in respiratory muscle fatigue, acidemia, and ARF.

Signs of respiratory failure are related to the extent of change in PaO_2 or $PaCO_2$, the speed of change (acute versus chronic), and the patient's ability to compensate for this change. When the patient's compensatory mechanisms fail, respiratory failure occurs. Because clinical signs vary, frequent patient assessment is a priority.

A lack of O_2 affects all body systems (Table 67.2). For example, a decreased level of consciousness may occur without enough blood, O_2, and glucose supplied to the brain. Permanent brain damage can result if hypoxia is severe and prolonged. Gastrointestinal (GI) system changes include tissue ischemia and increased intestinal wall permeability. Bacteria can migrate from the GI tract into systemic circulation. Renal function may be impaired. Sodium retention, peripheral edema, and acute kidney injury may occur.

One of the first signs of acute hypoxemic respiratory failure is a change in mental status. Mental status changes occur early because the brain is extremely sensitive to changes in O_2 (and to a lesser degree CO_2) levels and acid-base balance. Restlessness, confusion, and agitation suggest inadequate O_2 delivery to the brain. On the other hand, a morning headache and slow respiratory rate with decreased level of consciousness may indicate problems with CO_2 removal.

Tachycardia, tachypnea, slight diaphoresis, and mild hypertension are early signs of ARF.[6] These changes indicate attempts by the heart and lungs to compensate for decreased O_2 delivery and rising CO_2 levels. It is important to understand that cyanosis is an unreliable indicator of hypoxemia. It is a late sign in ARF. It often does not occur until hypoxemia is severe (PaO_2 45 mm Hg or less).[7]

The priority for the patient with ARF is immediate assessment of the patient's ability to breathe and providing any assistive measures needed. Depending on the severity of the respiratory failure and hemodynamic status, this may involve intubation and starting mechanical ventilation.

Observing the patient's position helps assess the effort associated with the work of breathing (WOB). WOB is the effort needed by the respiratory muscles to inhale air into the lungs.

TABLE 67.2 Common Manifestations of Hypoxemia and Hypercapnia

Specific	Nonspecific
Hypoxemia	
Respiratory	**Central Nervous**
Dyspnea	Agitation
Tachypnea	Confusion
Prolonged expiration	Disorientation
Nasal flaring	Restless, combative behavior
Intercostal muscle retraction	Delirium
Use of accessory muscles in respiration	↓ Level of consciousness
↓ SpO_2 (<90%)	Coma (late)
Paradoxical chest or abdominal wall movement with respiratory cycle (late)	**Cardiovascular**
	Tachycardia
Cyanosis (late)	Hypertension
	Skin cool, clammy, and diaphoretic
	Dysrhythmias (late)
	Hypotension (late)
	Other
	Fatigue
	Inability to speak in complete sentences without pausing to breathe
Hypercapnia	
Respiratory	**Central Nervous**
Dyspnea	Morning headache
Use of tripod position	Disorientation, confusion
Pursed-lip breathing	Agitation
Limited chest wall movement	Progressive somnolence
↓ Respiratory rate or rapid rate with shallow respirations	↑ ICP
	Coma (late)
↓ Tidal volume	
↓ Minute ventilation	**Cardiovascular**
	Dysrhythmias
	Hypertension
	Tachycardia
	Bounding pulse
	Neuromuscular
	Muscle weakness
	↓ Deep tendon reflexes
	Tremors, seizures (late)

Patients with mild distress may be able to lie down. In moderate distress, patients may be able to lie down but prefer to sit. With severe distress they may be unable to breathe unless sitting upright. The tripod position helps decrease the WOB in patients with moderate to severe COPD and ARF. The patients sit with the arms propped on the overbed table or on the knees. Propping the arms increases the anteroposterior diameter of the chest and changes pressure in the thorax.

The patient in ARF may have a rapid, shallow breathing pattern (hypoxemia) or a slower respiratory rate (hypercapnia). Both changes predispose the patient to insufficient O_2 delivery and CO_2 removal. Increased respiratory rates require a substantial amount of work and can lead to respiratory muscle fatigue. A change from a rapid rate to a slower rate in a patient in respiratory distress, such as that seen with acute asthma, suggests severe respiratory muscle fatigue. There is an increased chance for respiratory arrest.

The patient's ability to speak is related to the severity of dyspnea. The dyspneic patient may be able to speak only a few words at a time between breaths. For example, the patient may have "2-word" or "3-word" dyspnea. This means the patient can say only 2 or 3 words before pausing to breathe.

You may see dyspneic patients using pursed-lip breathing (see Table 28.12). This technique increases SaO_2 by slowing respirations, increasing time for expiration, and preventing small bronchioles from collapsing. You may see *retraction* (inward movement) of the intercostal spaces or supraclavicular area and use of the accessory muscles (e.g., sternocleidomastoid) during inspiration or expiration. Use of the accessory muscles often signifies a moderate degree of respiratory distress.

Paradoxical breathing occurs with severe respiratory distress. Normally, the thorax and abdomen move outward on inspiration and inward on exhalation. With paradoxical breathing, the abdomen and chest move in the opposite manner—outward during exhalation and inward during inspiration. Paradoxical breathing results from maximal use of the accessory muscles of respiration. The patient may be extremely diaphoretic from the increased WOB.

Auscultate breath sounds. Note the presence and location of any abnormal breath sounds. Fine crackles may occur with pulmonary edema. Coarse crackles heard on expiration indicate fluid in the airways. This may be a sign of pneumonia or a degree of HF. Absent or decreased breath sounds occur with atelectasis, pleural effusion, or hypoventilation. Bronchial breath sounds over the lung periphery occur with lung consolidation from pneumonia. You may hear a pleural friction rub if pneumonia involves the pleura.

Diagnostic Studies

The most common diagnostic studies used to evaluate ARF are chest x-ray and ABG analysis. A chest x-ray helps identify possible causes of respiratory failure (e.g., atelectasis, pneumonia). ABGs evaluate oxygenation (PaO_2) and ventilation ($PaCO_2$) status and acid-base (pH, bicarbonate) balance. Pulse oximetry monitors oxygenation status indirectly.

Other diagnostic studies that may be done include a complete blood cell count, serum electrolytes, urinalysis, and 12-lead ECG. Blood and sputum cultures (Gram stain, culture and sensitivity) may reveal infection. A CT scan or V/Q lung scan may be done if a pulmonary embolus is suspected. For the patient in severe ARF who needs intubation, end-tidal CO_2 (EtCO$_2$) may be used during ventilator management to assess trends in lung ventilation.[8]

❖ NURSING AND INTERPROFESSIONAL MANAGEMENT: ACUTE RESPIRATORY FAILURE

Because many different problems cause ARF, initial management and specific care varies. Factors taken into consideration include patient age, severity of onset of respiratory failure, underlying co-morbidities, and suspected or most likely cause of the respiratory failure. We then tailor management strategies to what best meets the patient's unique needs. This section discusses general assessment and interventions most commonly used for patients with ARF. In acute care settings, collaboration between nursing and the interprofessional team (e.g., ICU physicians, respiratory therapists, pharmacists) is essential.

In severe ARF, the patient will be cared for in an intensive care unit (ICU). ICU care will include central venous pressure (CVP) and arterial BP monitoring. Arterial BP will be monitored at least hourly. Central or mixed venous O_2 saturation

[ScvO$_2$ or SvO$_2$] data help determine the adequacy of tissue perfusion and the patient's response to treatment. The patient may need advanced hemodynamic monitoring to evaluate parameters such as CO and pulmonary capillary wedge pressure (PCWP). Chapter 65 discusses hemodynamic monitoring.

◆ Nursing Assessment

Table 67.3 presents subjective and objective data that you should obtain from the patient with ARF. A thorough assessment may result in early detection of respiratory insufficiency. This allows us to intervene sooner and can prevent worsening respiratory failure. Monitor patients with preexisting cardiac and/or respiratory disease closely. A slight change in their overall condition can cause significant decompensation.

It is important to observe trends in ABGs, pulse oximetry, and assessment findings. You must identify the changes that are occurring from hypoxemia or hypercarbia. Your ability to detect problems, notify the HCP, implement appropriate treatment, and evaluate response to therapy is essential.

◆ Nursing Diagnoses

Nursing diagnoses for the patient with ARF may include:
- Impaired gas exchange
- Impaired respiratory system function

Additional information on nursing diagnoses and interventions for the patient with ARF is presented in eNursing Care Plan 67.1 (available on the website for this chapter).

◆ Planning

The overall goals for the patient with ARF include (1) independently maintain a patent airway, (2) absence of dyspnea or recovery to baseline breathing patterns, (3) effectively cough and able to clear secretions, (4) normal ABG values or values within the patient's baseline, and (5) breath sounds within the patient's baseline.

◆ Nursing Implementation

◆ Prevention.
For the patient at risk for ARF, prevention and early recognition of respiratory distress are important. This is especially important for patients with neuromuscular diseases, cardiac problems, or respiratory problems (e.g., COPD). Do a thorough history and physical assessment to identify risk factors, then start appropriate interventions. Early strategies may include teaching patients about deep breathing and coughing, use of incentive spirometry, and early ambulation.

Preventing atelectasis, pneumonia, and complications of immobility, and optimizing hydration and nutrition, can decrease the risk for ARF. Those patients at high risk should be assessed more often with attention given to preventive measures.

◆ Respiratory Therapy

The goals of respiratory care include maintaining adequate oxygenation and ventilation and correcting acid-base imbalance. Interventions include O$_2$ therapy, mobilization of secretions, and positive pressure ventilation (PPV) (Table 67.4).

TABLE 67.3 Nursing Assessment

Acute Respiratory Failure

Subjective Data

Important Health Information

Past health history: Age, weight, altered level of consciousness, tobacco use (pack-years), alcohol or drug use, hospitalizations related to either acute or chronic lung disease, thoracic or spinal cord trauma, occupational exposures to lung toxins

Medications: Use of home O$_2$, inhalers (bronchodilators), home nebulization, over-the-counter drugs; immunosuppressant (e.g., corticosteroid) therapy, CNS depressants, illicit substances

Surgery or other treatments: Intubation and mechanical ventilation, recent thoracic or abdominal surgery

Functional Health Patterns

Health perception–health management: Exercise, self-care activities, immunizations (flu, pneumonia, hepatitis)

Nutritional-metabolic: Eating habits, bloating, indigestion; recent weight gain or loss, change in appetite. Use of vitamins or herbal supplements

Activity-exercise: Fatigue, dizziness, dyspnea at rest or with activity, wheezing, cough (productive or nonproductive), sputum (volume, color, viscosity), palpitations, swollen feet, change in exercise tolerance

Sleep-rest: Changes in sleep pattern, use of CPAP

Cognitive-perceptual: Headache, chest pain or tightness, chronic pain

Coping–stress tolerance: Anxiety, depression, feelings of hopelessness. Risk for drug and/or alcohol use, nicotine withdrawal

Objective Data

General

Restlessness, agitation

Integumentary

Pale, cool, clammy skin or warm, flushed skin. Peripheral and central cyanosis. Peripheral dependent edema

Respiratory

Shallow, increased respiratory rate progressing to decreased rate. Use of accessory muscles with evidence of retractions, increased diaphragmatic excursion or asymmetric chest expansion, paradoxical chest and abdominal wall movement. Tactile fremitus, crepitus, or deviated trachea on palpation. Absent, decreased, or adventitious breath sounds. Pleural friction rub. Bronchial or bronchovesicular sounds heard in other than normal location, inspiratory stridor

Cardiovascular

Tachycardia progressing to bradycardia, dysrhythmias, extra heart sounds (S$_3$, S$_4$). Bounding pulse. Hypertension progressing to hypotension. Pulsus paradoxus, jugular venous distention, pedal edema

Gastrointestinal

Abdominal distention, ascites, epigastric tenderness, hepatojugular reflex

Neurologic

Somnolence, confusion, slurred speech, restlessness, delirium, agitation, tremors, seizures, coma, asterixis, ↓ deep tendon reflexes, papilledema

Possible Diagnostic Findings

↓/↑ pH, ↑/↓ PaCO$_2$, ↑/↓ bicarbonate, ↓ PaO$_2$, ↓ SaO$_2$, abnormal hemoglobin, ↑ WBC count, changes in serum electrolytes. Abnormal findings on chest x-ray. Abnormal central venous or pulmonary artery pressures. Initially cardiac output may be ↑ due to the stress response. As hypoxemia, hypercapnia, and acidosis become more severe, cardiac output will ↓.

TABLE 67.4 Interprofessional Care

Acute Respiratory Failure

Diagnostic Assessment

- Vital signs
- History and physical examination
- Arterial blood gases (ABGs)
- Pulse oximetry
- Chest x-ray
- CBC and differential
- Serum electrolytes
- 12-Lead ECG
- Blood, sputum, and/or urine cultures (if indicated)
- Hemodynamic monitoring: CVP, SVV, PAWP (if indicated)

Management

Respiratory Therapy

- O_2 therapy
- Mobilization of secretions
  - Positioning
  - Effective coughing
  - Chest physiotherapy
  - Suctioning of the airway
  - Oral and/or IV hydration
  - Humidification (of O_2)
  - Ambulation (early mobility)
  - Positioning: head of bed elevated
- Positive pressure ventilation (PPV)
  - Noninvasive positive pressure ventilation (e.g. CPAP, BiPAP)
  - Intubation with positive pressure ventilation

Drug Therapy

- Reduce airway inflammation (e.g., corticosteroids)
- Relief of bronchospasm (e.g., albuterol)
- Reduce pulmonary congestion (e.g., furosemide [Lasix], morphine)
- Treat pulmonary infections (e.g., antibiotics)
- Reduce anxiety, pain, and restlessness (e.g., lorazepam, fentanyl, morphine)

Supportive Therapy

- Management of the underlying cause of respiratory failure
- Monitor hemodynamic status
- Optimize balance between activity and rest
- Monitor for deterioration in patient condition

CVP, Central venous pressure; *SVV,* stroke volume variation; *PAWP,* pulmonary artery wedge pressure.

◆ **Oxygen Therapy.** The primary goal of O_2 therapy is to correct hypoxemia. This requires O_2 administration. Always administer O_2 at the lowest possible FIO_2 (O_2 concentration) needed to keep SpO_2 and PaO_2 within patient-specific goals. Never withhold O_2 from a patient. It is essential to observe the patient's response to O_2 therapy. Closely monitor patients for changes in mental status, respiratory rate, and ABGs, until their PaO_2 level has reached their baseline normal value.

Several methods are available to provide O_2 to patients in ARF. Chapter 28 and Table 28.19 discuss O_2 delivery devices. The device selected depends upon the patient's overall condition, degree of respiratory failure, ability to maintain a patent airway, the amount of FIO_2 that the device can deliver, and, most importantly, the patient's ability to breathe spontaneously. Ideally, the selected O_2 delivery device must maintain PaO_2 at 60 mm Hg or higher and SaO_2 at 90% or higher.

The patient is often agitated, disoriented, and restless. A face mask, though appropriate, may cause anxiety from feelings of claustrophobia. Anxiety can cause dyspnea and increase O_2 consumption and CO_2 production. The patient may try to remove the mask. In this case, you need to explore other O_2 therapy options.

Breathing high O_2 concentrations for prolonged periods is not without potential adverse effects. Exposure to higher FIO_2 (greater than 60%) for longer than 48 hours poses a risk for O_2 *toxicity.* In this situation, oxygen free radicals from the high O_2 levels cause inflammation and cell death, by disrupting the alveolar-capillary membrane. *Absorption atelectasis* is another risk. O_2 has the ability to replace nitrogen and other gases normally present in the alveoli. Without nitrogen to help maintain size and shape of the alveolus, structural support is lost and the alveolus collapses. Other effects of prolonged exposure to high levels of O_2 include increased pulmonary capillary permeability, decreased surfactant production, surfactant inactivation, and fibrotic changes in the alveoli.[9]

Another risk of O_2 therapy is specific to patients with chronic hypercapnia (e.g., patient with COPD). Chronic hypercapnia blunts the response of chemoreceptors to high CO_2 levels as a respiratory stimulant. Initial O_2 therapy may be provided to patients with chronic hypercapnia through a low-flow device, such as a nasal cannula at 1 to 2 L/min or a Venturi mask at 24% to 28%. The patient with COPD who does not respond to O_2 therapy or other interventions may need mechanical ventilation with higher FIO_2.

◆ **Mobilization of Secretions.** Retained pulmonary secretions may cause or worsen ARF. This occurs because the movement of O_2 into the alveoli and removal of CO_2 is severely limited or blocked. Secretions can be mobilized by proper positioning, effective coughing, chest physiotherapy, suctioning, humidification, hydration, and, when possible, early ambulation.

Patient Positioning. Position the patient upright, either by elevating the head of the bed at least 30 degrees or by using a reclining chair or chair bed. This helps maximize respiratory expansion, decrease dyspnea, and mobilize secretions. A sitting position improves pulmonary function by promoting downward movement of the lungs. When lungs are upright, ventilation and perfusion are best in the lung bases. If there is a chance for aspiration, position the patient side-lying.

Patients with one-sided lung disorders may be placed in a lateral or side-lying position. This position, called *good lung down,* allows for improved V/Q matching in the affected lung. Pulmonary blood flow and ventilation are better in dependent lung areas. This position allows secretions to drain out of the affected lung so they can be removed with suctioning. For example, place a patient with right-sided pneumonia on the left side. This will maximize ventilation and perfusion in the "good" lung and aid in secretion removal from the affected lung (postural drainage). Patients with ARF often have problems with both lungs. They may need repositioning at regular intervals on both sides to optimize air movement and drainage of secretions.

Effective Coughing. When secretions are present, encourage the patient to cough. Unfortunately, not all patients will have enough strength or force to produce a cough that will clear the airway of secretions. *Augmented coughing (quad coughing)* may benefit some patients. To aid with augmented coughing, place 1 or both hands at the anterolateral base of the patient's lungs (Fig. 67.6). As you observe deep inspiration end and expiration begin, move your hands forcefully upward. This increases abdominal pressure and helps the patient cough. It increases expiratory flow and promotes secretion clearance.

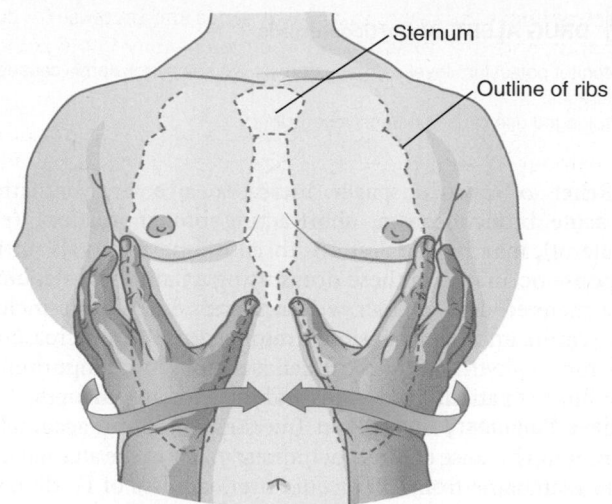

FIG. 67.6 Augmented coughing is performed by placing 1 or both hands on the anterolateral base of the lungs. After the patient takes a deep inspiration and at the beginning of expiration, move the hand(s) forcefully upward. This increases abdominal pressure and helps produce a forceful cough. (From American Association of Critical Care Nurses: *AACN advanced critical care nursing*, St Louis, 2009, Mosby.)

Huff coughing is a series of coughs performed while saying the word "huff" (see Table 28.21).[10] This technique prevents the glottis from closing during the cough. The patient takes a deep breath, holds the breath for 2 or 3 seconds, and then exhales. The huff cough is effective in clearing central airways. It may help move secretions upward. COPD patients generate higher flow rates with a huff cough than with a normal cough, and it is less tiring.

The *staged cough* also helps clear secretions. To perform a staged cough, the patient assumes a sitting position, breathes in and out 3 or 4 times through the mouth, then coughs while bending forward and pressing a pillow inward against the diaphragm.

Chest Physiotherapy. Chest physiotherapy is indicated for all patients who are producing sputum or have evidence of severe atelectasis or pulmonary infiltrates on chest x-ray. Postural drainage, percussion, and vibration to the affected lung segments help move secretions to the larger airways. Then, they can be removed by coughing or suctioning. Chest physiotherapy is discussed in Chapter 28.

Contraindications include TBI and increased intracranial pressure (ICP), unstable orthopedic injuries (e.g., spinal fractures, fractured ribs, fractured sternum), and recent hemoptysis.[11]

Suctioning. Suctioning may be needed if the patient is unable to expectorate secretions. Suctioning through an artificial airway (e.g., endotracheal tube [ET], tracheostomy) is done only as needed (see Chapters 26 and 65). Perform suctioning beyond the posterior oropharynx with caution, while monitoring the patient for complications. These include hypoxia, increased ICP, dysrhythmias, hypotension (from sudden elevation in intrathoracic pressure), hypertension and tachycardia (from noxious stimulation), and bradycardia (possible vasovagal response).

Humidification. Humidification is an adjunct in secretion management. We can thin secretions with aerosols of sterile normal saline or mucolytic drugs (e.g., acetylcysteine mixed with a bronchodilator) given by nebulizer. O_2 given by aerosol mask can thin secretions and promote their removal. Aerosol therapy may cause bronchospasm and severe coughing, causing

a decrease in PaO_2. Frequent assessment of the patient's tolerance to therapy is critical. Closely monitor the patient's respiratory status.

Hydration. Thick, viscous secretions are hard to expel. Unless contraindicated, adequate fluid intake (2 to 3 L/day) keeps secretions thin and easier to remove. The patient who is unable to take enough fluids orally needs IV hydration. Assess cardiac and renal status to determine whether the patient can tolerate the IV fluid volume and avoid HF and pulmonary edema. Regularly assess for signs of fluid overload (e.g., crackles, dyspnea, increased CVP).

◆ **Positive Pressure Ventilation.** If initial measures do not improve oxygenation and ventilation, enhanced ventilatory assistance may be needed. Noninvasive positive pressure ventilation (NIPPV) is one option for patients with acute or chronic respiratory failure. During NIPPV, a mask is placed tightly over the patient's nose or nose and mouth (Fig. 67.7). When the patient breathes spontaneously, a mechanical ventilator or table-top unit delivers PPV to the patient. With NIPPV, it is possible to provide O_2 and decrease WOB, avoiding the need for endotracheal intubation.

NIPPV is most useful in managing chronic respiratory failure in those with chest wall or neuromuscular problems. It may be used with patients with a chronic respiratory problem that is worse due to cardiac problems or infection. It is an option for patients who refuse intubation, but still want some degree of ventilatory support (e.g., patients with end-stage COPD). NIPPV is not appropriate for patients who have a decreased level of consciousness, high O_2 requirements, facial trauma, hemodynamic instability, or excessive secretions. NIPPV used after extubation can help avoid reintubation.

There are 2 forms of NIPPV used for patients with ARF. Continuous positive airway pressure (CPAP) delivers 1 level of pressure—a constant pressure—to the patient's airway during inspiration and expiration. Bilevel positive airway pressure (BiPAP) uses 2 different levels of positive pressure (one on inspiration, another on expiration) (Fig. 67.8). With both CPAP and BiPAP, the patient must be awake and alert, have stable vital signs, and be able to support spontaneous ventilation.

The most often used NIPPV for ARF is BiPAP.[12] BiPAP provides O_2 therapy and humidification, decreases WOB, and reduces respiratory muscle fatigue. It helps open collapsed airways and decrease shunt. If respiratory status worsens with NIPPV, PPV via mechanical ventilation and higher O_2 concentrations is needed. Chapter 65 discusses mechanical ventilation.

◆ **Drug Therapy**

Drug therapy depends on several factors. These include the cause of ARF, the patient's preexisting medical condition, and whether infection is present. Goals of drug therapy include to (1) reduce airway inflammation and bronchospasm, (2) relieve

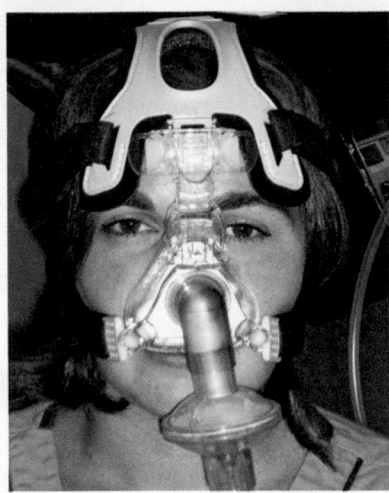

FIG. 67.7 Noninvasive bilevel positive airway pressure ventilation. A mask is placed over the nose or nose and mouth. Positive pressure from a mechanical ventilator aids the patient's breathing efforts, decreasing the work of breathing. (Courtesy Richard Arbour, RN, MSN, CCRN, CNRN, CCNS, FAAN and Anna Kirk, RN, MSN.)

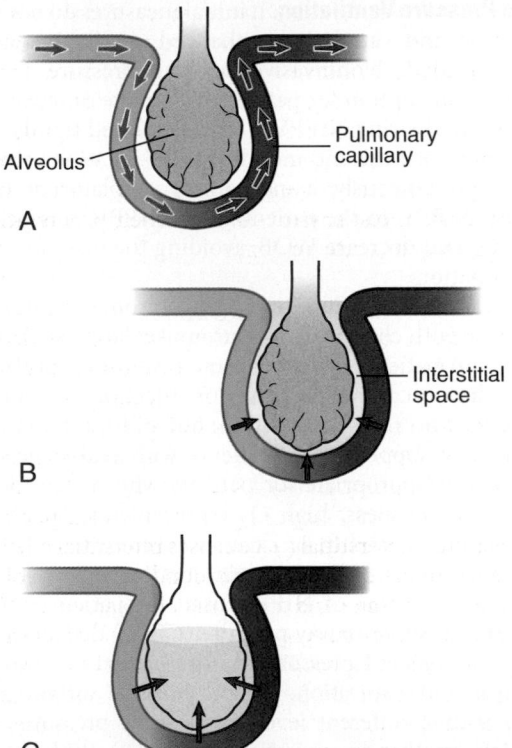

FIG. 67.8 Stages of edema formation in ARDS. **A,** Normal alveolus and pulmonary capillary. **B,** Interstitial edema occurs with increased flow of fluid into the interstitial space. **C,** Alveolar edema occurs when the fluid crosses the alveolar-capillary membrane.

pulmonary congestion; (3) treat infection; and (4) reduce anxiety, pain, and restlessness.

◆ **Reduce Airway Inflammation and Bronchospasm.** Corticosteroids (e.g., IV methylprednisolone [Solu-Medrol]) are often used in combination with other drugs, such as bronchodilators, for relief of inflammation and bronchospasm. It may take several hours to see their effects. Inhaled corticosteroids require 4 to 5 days for optimum therapeutic effects, so they will not relieve ARF.

 DRUG ALERT IV Corticosteroids

• Monitor potassium levels. Corticosteroids worsen hypokalemia caused by diuretics.
• Prolonged use causes adrenal insufficiency.

Relief of bronchospasm increases alveolar ventilation. In acute bronchospasm, short-acting bronchodilators (e.g., albuterol), may be given at 15- to 30-minute intervals until a response occurs. Give these drugs using a hand-held nebulizer or a metered-dose inhaler with a spacer. Side effects include tachycardia and hypertension. Prolonged use can increase the risk for dysrhythmias and cardiac ischemia. It is important to monitor the patient's vital signs and ECG for any changes.

◆ **Relieve Pulmonary Congestion.** Interstitial fluid can accumulate in the lungs because of direct or indirect injury to the alveolar capillary membrane from HF or fluid overload. Use of IV diuretics (e.g., furosemide [Lasix]), morphine, or nitroglycerin can decrease pulmonary congestion caused by HF. Use extreme caution when giving these drugs. Changes in heart rate and rhythm and significant decreases in BP are common. (Chapter 34 discusses HF.)

◆ **Treat Infection.** Lung infections (e.g., pneumonia, acute bronchitis) can result in excessive mucus production, fever, increased O_2 consumption, and inflamed, fluid-filled, and/or collapsed alveoli. Alveoli that are fluid filled or collapsed cannot take part in gas exchange. Consequently, pulmonary infections can either cause or worsen ARF. IV antibiotics are often given to treat infection. Chest x-rays can show the location and extent of an infection. Sputum cultures help identify the organisms causing the infection and their sensitivity to antimicrobial drugs.

◆ **Reduce Anxiety, Pain, and Restlessness.** Anxiety, pain, and restlessness may result from hypoxia. They increase O_2 consumption and CO_2 production (from an increased metabolic rate) and increase WOB. For the nonintubated patient, this may cause tachypnea and ineffective ventilation. For the intubated patient, this may cause ventilator dyssynchrony and increase the risk for unplanned extubation. We promote patient comfort in several ways.

Benzodiazepines (e.g., lorazepam, midazolam), and opioids (e.g., morphine, fentanyl) may decrease anxiety, restlessness, and pain. They are often given IV. For the nonintubated patient, they should be started at the lowest dose possible. Address treatable causes of restlessness (e.g., hypoxemia, pain, delirium). Often, restlessness and mental status changes are the first signs of hypoxemia or ventilator dyssynchrony. You should address the causes and not depend solely on the use of analgesics and sedatives.

SAFETY ALERT Managing Restlessness and Sedation

• Pain, hypoxemia, electrolyte imbalance, TBI, and drug reactions can cause restlessness.
• Assess and aggressively treat all reversible causes of restlessness.
• Monitor patients closely for CNS, cardiac, and respiratory depression when giving sedative and analgesic drugs, especially in the nonintubated patient.
• Sedative and analgesic drugs may have a prolonged effect in critically ill patients. This can delay weaning from mechanical ventilation and increase length of stay.

◆ **Medical Supportive Therapy**

Goals and interventions targeted to improving the patient's oxygenation and ventilation status are essential to improve O_2 delivery. The primary goal is to treat the underlying cause of the

ARF. Patients with V/Q mismatch, shunting, or diffusion limitation are managed differently, depending on the underlying cause. Patients are continuously monitored for their response to therapy, including changes in respiratory status, trends in ABGs, and signs of clinical improvement.

◆ Nutritional Therapy

Maintaining protein and energy stores is especially important in patients with ARF. The hypermetabolic state in critical illness increases the caloric requirements needed to maintain a stable body weight and muscle mass. Nutritional depletion causes a loss of muscle mass, including the respiratory muscles, which may delay recovery. The dietitian often determines the best method of feeding and optimal caloric and fluid requirements. Ideally, enteral or parenteral nutrition should be started within 24 to 48 hours (see Chapter 39).

◆ Evaluation

The expected outcomes are that the patient with ARF will
- Independently maintain a patent airway
- Achieve normal or baseline respiratory system function
- Maintain adequate oxygenation as shown by normal or baseline ABGs
- Have normal hemodynamic status

Gerontologic Considerations: Acute Respiratory Failure

Many factors contribute to an increased risk for respiratory failure in older adults. The reduced ventilatory capacity that accompanies aging places the older adult at risk for ARF. Physiologic changes in the lungs include alveolar dilation, larger air spaces, and loss of surface area for gas exchange. Decreased elastic recoil within the airways, decreased chest wall compliance, and decreased respiratory muscle strength occur.[13]

In older adults, the PaO_2 falls further and the $PaCO_2$ rises to a higher level before the respiratory system is stimulated to change the rate and depth of breathing. This delayed response contributes to the development of respiratory insufficiency. A history of tobacco use is a major risk factor that can accelerate age-related respiratory changes. Poor nutritional status and less physiologic reserve in the cardiopulmonary system increases the risk for further compromising respiratory function and leading to ARF.

ACUTE RESPIRATORY DISTRESS SYNDROME

Acute respiratory distress syndrome (ARDS) is a sudden and progressive form of ARF in which the alveolar-capillary membrane becomes damaged and more permeable to intravascular fluid (Fig. 67.8). Next to septic shock, ARDS is one of the most common conditions seen in the adult ICU. ARDS accounts for about 10% of all adult ICU admissions.[14] The incidence of ARDS in the United States is estimated at more than 200,000 cases each year.[14] Despite supportive therapy, the mortality rate from ARDS is around 50%.

Etiology

Table 67.5 lists conditions that predispose patients to developing ARDS. The most common cause is sepsis. ARDS may also develop because of multiple organ dysfunction syndrome (MODS). Patients with multiple risk factors are 3 or 4 times more likely to develop ARDS.

Either a direct or indirect lung injury causes ARDS. In direct lung injury, the pathogen comes into contact with the tissue of

TABLE 67.5 Predisposing Conditions to ARDS	
Direct Lung Injury	**Indirect Lung Injury**
Common Causes	
• Aspiration of gastric contents or other substances • Bacterial or viral pneumonia • Sepsis	• Sepsis (especially gram-negative infection) • Severe massive trauma • Severe TBI • Shock states (hypovolemic, cardiogenic, septic)
Less Common Causes	
• Chest trauma (blunt or penetrating) • Embolism: fat, air, amniotic fluid, thrombus • Inhalation of toxic substances • Near-drowning • O_2 toxicity • Radiation pneumonitis	• Acute pancreatitis • Cardiopulmonary bypass • Disseminated intravascular coagulation • Opioid drug overdose (e.g., heroin) • Transfusion-related acute lung injury (e.g., multiple blood transfusions) • Urosepsis

the lung. For example, aspiration of gastric contents into the lung will immediately initiate the inflammatory response. In an indirect injury, ARDS develops due to a problem somewhere else in the body. For example, necrotizing pancreatitis or bowel obstruction with perforation cause widespread inflammation and infection. As a result, septic mediators gain entrance to the bloodstream and often move toward the lungs, which provide a favorable, dark, moist environment for their proliferation. This is the beginning of acute lung injury.

Pathophysiology

The pathophysiologic changes in ARDS are divided into 3 phases: (1) injury or exudative phase, (2) reparative or proliferative phase, and (3) fibrotic or fibroproliferative phase. The pathophysiology of ARDS is shown in Fig. 67.9.

Injury or Exudative Phase. The *injury or exudative phase* usually occurs 24 to 72 hours after the initial insult (direct or indirect).[15] It generally lasts up to 7 days. Engorgement of the peribronchial and perivascular interstitial space causes interstitial edema. Fluid in the parenchyma of the lung surrounding the alveoli crosses the alveolar membrane and enters the alveolar space. V/Q mismatch and intrapulmonary shunt develop because the alveoli fill with fluid. Blood in the capillary network cannot be oxygenated.

The exact cause for the damage to the alveolar-capillary membrane is not known. Some think it is caused by stimulation of the inflammatory and immune systems. This stimulation attracts neutrophils to the pulmonary interstitium. The neutrophils release biochemical, humoral, and cellular mediators that produce changes in the lung. These changes include increased pulmonary capillary membrane permeability, destruction of collagen, formation of pulmonary microemboli, and pulmonary artery vasoconstriction.

Hypoxemia and the stimulation of juxtacapillary receptors in the stiff lung parenchyma *(J reflex)* initially cause an increase in respiratory rate and a decrease in tidal volume (V_T). This breathing pattern increases CO_2 removal, producing respiratory alkalosis. CO increases in response to hypoxemia, a compensatory effort to increase pulmonary blood flow. However, as atelectasis, pulmonary edema, and pulmonary shunt increase, compensation fails and hypoventilation, decreased CO, and decreased tissue O_2 perfusion occur.

PATHOPHYSIOLOGY MAP

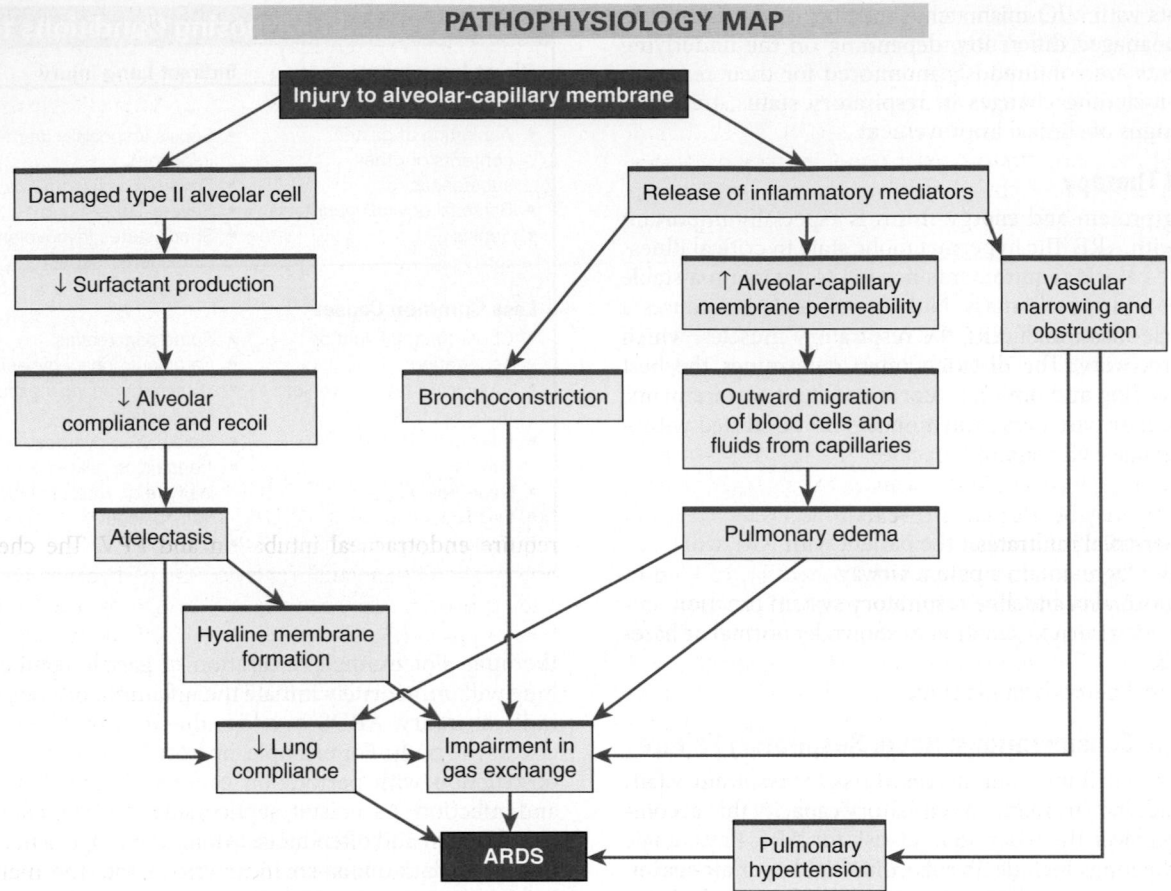

FIG. 67.9 Pathophysiology of ARDS.

The changes caused by ARDS damage both alveolar type I cells and alveolar type II cells (which make surfactant). This damage, in addition to fluid and protein accumulation, results in surfactant dysfunction. The function of *surfactant* is to maintain alveolar stability and prevent alveolar collapse. When surfactant synthesis is decreased or surfactant becomes inactivated, alveoli become unstable and collapse *(atelectasis)*. Widespread atelectasis further decreases lung compliance, compromises gas exchange, and contributes to hypoxemia.

Necrotic cells, protein, and fibrin form hyaline membranes that line the inside of each alveolus. These thick hyaline membranes contribute to the development of fibrosis and atelectasis, leading to a further decrease in gas exchange capability and reduced lung compliance.

Severe V/Q mismatch and shunting of pulmonary capillary blood result in hypoxemia unresponsive to increasing concentrations of O_2. This is the classic signs of ARDS, called **refractory hypoxemia**. In other words, despite receiving higher concentrations of O_2, the patient's condition does not improve but continues to get worse. Diffusion limitation, caused by hyaline membrane formation, contributes to and worsens hypoxemia. As the lungs become less compliant because of decreased surfactant, pulmonary edema, and atelectasis, the patient must generate higher airway pressures to inflate "stiff" lungs. Reduced lung compliance increases the patient's WOB. At this point, the patient needs mechanical ventilation.

Reparative or Proliferative Phase. The *reparative* or *proliferative phase* of ARDS begins 1 to 2 weeks after the initial lung injury.[16] During this phase, there continues to be an influx of

neutrophils, monocytes, lymphocytes, and fibroblasts as part of the inflammatory response. Increased pulmonary vascular resistance and pulmonary hypertension may occur because fibroblasts and inflammatory cells destroy the pulmonary vasculature. Lung compliance continues to decrease due to interstitial fibrosis. Hypoxemia worsens because of the thickened alveolar membrane. This causes V/Q mismatch, diffusion limitation, and shunting. Airway resistance is severely increased from fluid in the lungs and secretions in the airways. The proliferative phase is complete when the diseased lung is replaced by dense, fibrous tissue. If the reparative phase persists, widespread fibrosis results. If the reparative phase stops, the lesions will often resolve.

Fibrotic or Fibroproliferative Phase. The *fibrotic phase (chronic or late phase)* of ARDS occurs 2 to 3 weeks after the initial lung injury. Not all patients who develop ARDS enter the fibrotic stage. For those who never fully recover from ARDS, the lung is completely remodeled by collagenous and fibrous tissues. Diffuse scarring of the lungs, interstitial fibrosis, and alveolar duct fibrosis result in decreased lung compliance.[17] This reduces the surface area for gas exchange because the interstitium is fibrotic, and hypoxemia continues. Varying degrees of pulmonary hypertension may result from pulmonary vascular destruction and fibrosis.

Clinical Progression

Progression of ARDS varies among patients. Some survive the acute phase of lung injury. Pulmonary edema resolves, and complete recovery occurs within a week or so. The chance for survival is poorer in those who enter the fibrotic stage. Patients may need several weeks of long-term mechanical ventilation. It is not known why injured lungs repair and recover in some patients and in others ARDS progresses. Several factors are important in determining the course of ARDS. These include the nature of the initial injury, extent and severity of comorbidities, and pulmonary complications (e.g., pneumothorax). Genetics may account for a person's predisposition to developing ARDS.[18]

Clinical Manifestations and Diagnostic Studies

The initial presentation of ARDS is often subtle. At the time of the initial injury, and for 24 to 72 hours, the patient may not have respiratory symptoms or may have only mild dyspnea, tachypnea, cough, and restlessness. Lung auscultation may be normal or reveal fine, scattered crackles. ABGs may show mild hypoxemia and respiratory alkalosis caused by hyperventilation. The chest x-ray may be normal or reveal diffusely scattered, but minimal, interstitial infiltrates.

As ARDS progresses, symptoms worsen because of fluid in the lung parenchyma and alveoli and increased secretion accumulation in the airways. Respiratory distress becomes evident as WOB increases. Tachypnea and intercostal and suprasternal retractions may be present. Tachycardia, diaphoresis, changes in mental status, cyanosis, and pallor may occur. Lung auscultation usually reveals scattered to diffuse crackles and coarse crackles on expiration. After 72 hours, the chest x-ray often shows diffuse and extensive bilateral interstitial and alveolar infiltrates (Fig. 67.10).

As ARDS progresses, ABGs reflect changes in oxygenation and ventilation. Refractory hypoxemia is the hallmark characteristic of ARDS. Hypercapnia often signifies that respiratory muscle fatigue and hypoventilation have severely affected gas exchange, and respiratory failure is imminent.

To help evaluate the severity of hypoxemia in ARDS, we can calculate the **PaO$_2$/FIO$_2$ (P/F) ratio**. This measure reflects the ratio of the patient's PaO$_2$ to the FIO$_2$ that the patient is receiving. Under normal circumstances (e.g., PaO$_2$ 80 to 100 mm Hg; FIO$_2$ 0.21 [room air]), the P/F ratio is greater than 400 (e.g., 95/0.21 = 452). With the onset and progression of lung injury

and impairment in O$_2$ delivery through the alveolar-capillary membrane, the PaO$_2$ may remain lower than expected despite increased FIO$_2$. The P/F ratio distinguishes among mild (<300), moderate (<200), and severe (<100) ARDS (Table 67.6).

❓ CHECK YOUR PRACTICE

You are caring for a 26-yr-old woman with ARDS who experienced near-drowning 4 days ago. She is mechanically ventilated and receiving continuous IV infusions of analgesia and sedation. The ventilator settings are: full support (control mode), FIO$_2$ = 90%, PEEP = 15 cm H$_2$O, V$_T$ = 350 mL, respiratory rate 12 breaths/min (patient taking no breaths above the set rate on the ventilator), peak pressure = 35 cm H$_2$O. The patient's PaO$_2$ is 83 mm Hg.

• Calculate and interpret the PaO$_2$/FIO$_2$ (P/F) ratio.

As ARDS progresses, it is associated with profound dyspnea, hypoxemia, increased WOB, and respiratory distress, which require endotracheal intubation and PPV. The chest x-ray is often called "whiteout" (or white lung) because consolidation and infiltrates are widespread throughout the lungs, leaving few recognizable air spaces. Pleural effusions may be present. Severe hypoxemia, hypercapnia, metabolic acidosis, and organ dysfunction often accompany ARDS and provide additional challenges.

Complications

Complications may develop because of ARDS itself or its treatment (Table 67.7). Besides the lungs, the vital organs most often involved are the kidneys, liver, and heart. The main cause of death in ARDS is MODS, often accompanied by sepsis.

Abnormal Lung Function. Most patients will recover from ARDS within 6 months. Many will have normal to near normal lung function. However, not all patients regain normal lung function. Sometimes, abnormal lung function can persist for years. The severity of scarring and changes within the lungs are key factors. Mechanical ventilation, the duration of time ventilated, and use of extracorporeal life support (ECLS) may be contributing factors.[19] Patients may report extreme tiredness, chest pain, shortness of breath after minimal activity, and persistent dyspnea post-ARDS.

Ventilator-Associated Pneumonia. Risk factors for ventilator-associated pneumonia (VAP) include impaired host defenses, invasive monitoring devices, aspiration of GI contents (especially in patients receiving enteral nutrition), and

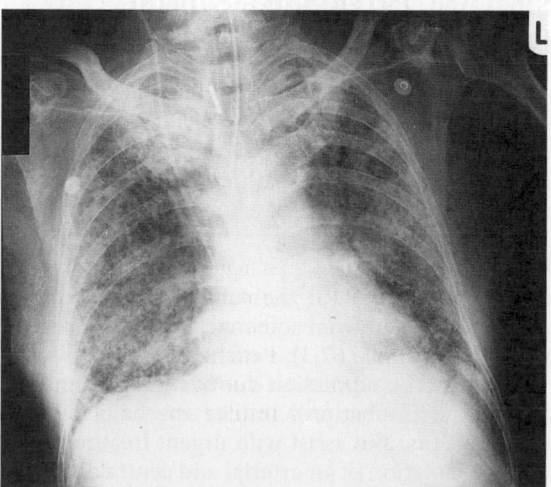

FIG. 67.10 Chest x-ray of a patient with ARDS. The x-ray shows new, bilateral, diffuse, homogeneous pulmonary infiltrates without cardiac failure, fluid overload, chest infection, or chronic lung disease. (From Cohen J, Powderly WG: *Infectious diseases*, ed 2, St Louis, 2004, Mosby.)

TABLE 67.6 Berlin Definition of ARDS

Timing
Within 1 week of a known clinical insult or new or worsening respiratory symptoms

Chest X-Ray
Bilateral opacities: not fully explained by effusions, lobar/lung collapse, or nodules

Oxygenation
Mild ARDS: PaO$_2$/FIO$_2$ ratio ≤300 with PEEP or CPAP ≥5 cm H$_2$O
Moderate ARDS: PaO$_2$/FIO$_2$ ratio ≤200 with PEEP or CPAP ≥5 cm H$_2$O
Severe ARDS: PaO$_2$/FIO$_2$ ratio <100 with PEEP or CPAP ≥5 cm H$_2$O

Modified from Pneumatikos L, Papaioannou VE: The new Berlin definition: What is, finally, the ARDS? *Pneumon* 25:365, 2012.

prolonged mechanical ventilation. Implement a ventilator bundle protocol (Table 67.8).

Common strategies to prevent VAP include elevating the head of bed 30 to 45 degrees, strict infection control measures (e.g., hand washing, sterile technique during endotracheal suctioning) and frequent oral care.

Barotrauma. *Barotrauma* occurs when fragile alveoli are overdistended with excess pressure during mechanical ventilation. The high peak airway pressures needed to ventilate the lungs predispose patients with ARDS to this complication. Barotrauma results in alveolar air escaping from ruptured alveoli. This can lead to pulmonary interstitial emphysema, pneumothorax, subcutaneous emphysema, pneumopericardium, and tension pneumothorax. Providing ventilation with a smaller V_T (e.g., 4 to 8 mL/kg) and varying amounts of PEEP minimizes the risk for barotrauma.

Stress Ulcers. Patients with ARF and ARDS are at high risk for stress ulcers because of blood being diverted from the GI to respiratory system to help meet the body's demand for O_2. Management strategies include correcting predisposing conditions, such as hypotension, shock, and acidosis. Prophylactic management includes antiulcer drugs, such as proton pump inhibitors (e.g., pantoprazole [Protonix]) and mucosal-protecting drugs (e.g., sucralfate [Carafate]). Early initiation of enteral nutrition helps prevent mucosal damage.

Venous Thromboembolism (VTE). ARDS patients are susceptible to the effects of immobility and venous stasis. They are at risk for deep vein thrombosis (DVT) and pulmonary emboli. Prophylactic management may include intermittent pneumatic compression stockings, anticoagulation (e.g. low-molecular-weight heparin), and, when possible, early ambulation.

Acute Kidney Injury. Acute kidney injury (AKI) can occur from decreased renal perfusion and subsequent decreased delivery of O_2 to the kidneys. This most often occurs in ARDS because of hypotension in septic shock. It may also result from hypoxemia or nephrotoxic drugs (e.g., vancomycin) used to treat ARDS-related infections. Management strategies for AKI include careful monitoring of intake and output, obtaining daily creatinine and urea levels, and, when needed, dialysis therapy.

Continuous renal replacement therapy (CRRT) is often used. Patients with ARDS are often hemodynamically unstable and need vasopressors and/or inotropes to maintain heart rate and BP. They cannot tolerate the large volumes of fluid that would be removed during traditional hemodialysis. CRRT is slow, gentle, and continuous. The patient can receive CRRT 24 hours a day. The overall mortality rate for ARDS patients is higher in those who need CRRT.[20]

Psychological Issues. Recovery is far from complete for the patient who survives ARDS. Survivors may have anxiety, issues with memory and attention, inability to focus, nightmares, depression, and in some instances, various degrees of posttraumatic stress disorder (PTSD). PTSD can occur in ARDS survivors up to 5 years later.[21]

❖ NURSING AND INTERPROFESSIONAL MANAGEMENT: ARDS

Management of a patient with ARF (Table 67.4) and the nursing care plan for ARF (eNursing Care Plan 67.1 [available on the website for this chapter]) apply to patients with ARDS. The next section discusses additional interprofessional care for the patient with ARDS (Table 67.9).

◆ Nursing Assessment

Because ARDS causes ARF, the subjective and objective data that you should obtain from someone with ARDS are the same as those for ARF (Table 67.3). Patient information may not be possible to obtain on admission due to the urgent need to protect the airway (intubation), initiate mechanical ventilation, monitor vital signs, and assist with urgent treatments and procedures (e.g., insertion of an arterial and central line).

◆ Planning

With appropriate therapy, overall goals include a PaO_2 of 60 mm Hg or higher and adequate lung ventilation to maintain normal pH. Specific goals for a patient with ARDS include (1)

TABLE 67.7 Complications Associated With ARDS

Cardiac
- ↓ Cardiac output
- Dysrhythmias

Central Nervous System and Psychologic
- Delirium
- PTSD

Gastrointestinal
- Hypermetabolic state, dramatically ↑ nutrition requirements
- Paralytic ileus
- Pneumoperitoneum
- Stress ulceration and hemorrhage

Hematologic
- Anemia
- Disseminated intravascular coagulation
- Thrombocytopenia
- VTE

Infection
- Catheter-related infection (e.g., central and peripheral IV catheters, urinary catheters)
- Sepsis

Renal
- AKI

Respiratory
- Pulmonary emboli
- Pulmonary fibrosis
- Ventilator associated: volutrauma, barotrauma
- VAP

TABLE 67.8 Components of a Ventilator Bundle

- Good hand washing before, during (as needed), and after delivery of patient care
- Elevate head of the bed 30 to 45 degrees
- Daily assessment of readiness for extubation (see Chapter 65)
- Stress ulcer prophylaxis (see Chapter 41)
- VTE prophylaxis (see Chapter 37)
- Daily oral care with chlorhexidine (0.12%) solution (see Table 65.9)

Source: Institute for Healthcare Improvement: How-to guide: Prevent VAP. Retrieved from *www.ihi.org/resources/Pages/Tools/HowtoGuidePreventVAP.aspx*.

TABLE 67.9 Interprofessional Care

Acute Respiratory Distress Syndrome

Diagnostic Assessment

See Table 67.6.

Management

General Care

- Identify and treat underlying cause
- Hemodynamic monitoring
- Proper patient positioning

Respiratory Therapy

- O_2 administration
- Mechanical ventilation (see Chapter 65)
- Low V_T ventilation
- Permissive hypercapnia
- PEEP
- Positioning strategies (e.g., prone)
- Extracorporeal membrane oxygenation (ECMO)

Supportive Care

- Nutrition therapy
- VTE prophylaxis
- VAP prophylaxis
- Inotropic and vasopressor drugs
  - norepinephrine (Levophed)
  - dopamine
  - dobutamine
- IV fluid administration
- Analgesia and sedation
- Neuromuscular blocking agents

PaO_2 within normal limits for age or at baseline on room air, (2) SaO_2 greater than 90%, (3) resolution of the precipitating factor(s), and (4) clear lungs on auscultation.

Implementation

Patients with moderate to severe ARDS receive care in an ICU. Even with appropriate therapy, the clinical course of ARDS is complex and unpredictable. Patients with ARDS often need several days of mechanical ventilation to allow time for the overwhelming inflammation and fluid accumulation in the lungs to begin resolving. Best practices for care of the patient with ARDS include (1) O_2 administration, (2) mechanical ventilation, (3) low V_T ventilation, (4) permissive hypercapnia, (5) PEEP, (6) prone positioning, and (7) extracorporeal membrane oxygenation (ECMO). Many of these practices are detailed in the *Acute Respiratory Distress Syndrome Clinical Network (ARDSNet) protocol.*[22]

Respiratory Therapy

Oxygen Administration. The primary goal of O_2 therapy is to correct hypoxemia. Initially, the use of a high-flow system that delivers higher O_2 concentrations to maximize O_2 delivery may be all that is needed. Continuously monitor SpO_2 to assess the effectiveness of O_2 therapy. However, for most patients diagnosed with ARDS, high-flow O_2 delivery, including BiPAP, is only a temporary measure. As respiratory failure worsens, high-flow O_2 will be not be able to keep the PaO_2 within acceptable ranges. Patients with moderate to severe ARDS and refractory hypoxemia need mechanical ventilation to keep the PaO_2 at or close to near-normal levels. However, even with mechanical ventilation, the patient may need an FIO_2 of 70%, 80%, or

higher to keep the PaO_2 at least 60 mm Hg. Most HCPs agree that in the injury and reparative phases, they may have to accept a lower than normal PaO_2 (e.g. PaO_2 55 to 80 mm Hg) and SpO_2 (88% to 95%).

Mechanical Ventilation. Mechanical ventilation is often delivered via a pressure-control type of ventilation. Pressure-control ventilation helps to keep the inspiratory and plateau pressures from becoming too high. This prevents alveolar overdistention and rupture. By reducing the amount of pressure going into the stiff, noncompliant lungs, we can help prevent further lung injury. However, no mode of mechanical ventilation is superior to the others.[23] Chapter 65 provides additional information on mechanical ventilation.

Low Tidal Volume (V_T) Ventilation. Patients with ARDS are ventilated with a low V_T of 4 to 8 mL/kg.[22] The delivery of a large V_T into stiff lungs is associated with volutrauma and barotrauma. Volutrauma causes *alveolar fractures* (damage or tears in the alveoli) and movement of fluids and protein into the alveolar spaces. Low V_T ventilation has reduced mortality and the risk for volutrauma.

Permissive Hypercapnia. As a result of delivering a lower than normal V_T to the patient with ARDS, the $PaCO_2$ level will slowly rise above normal limits. This is known as **permissive hypercapnia**. A $PaCO_2$ of up to 60 mm Hg is acceptable in the early phase of ARDS. The patient usually tolerates this rise in $PaCO_2$ if it is gradual, allowing the brain and systemic circulation to compensate. Permissive hypercapnia is not used for the patient with TBI or increased ICP.

Frequent ABG samples are needed, with careful monitoring of the pH, PaO_2, and $PaCO_2$ values. As per the ARDSNet protocol, the pH is kept between 7.30 and 7.45. CO_2 is a powerful stimulant to breathe. When permissive hypercapnia is used, the patient is usually given continuous IV analgesia and sedation.

Positive End-Expiratory Pressure (PEEP). During PPV, it is common to apply PEEP at 5 cm H_2O to compensate for loss of glottic function caused by the ET. PEEP increases functional residual capacity, or the volume of air left in the lungs at the end of a normal expiration. PEEP also helps open up ("recruit") collapsed alveoli.

We typically apply PEEP in increments of 3 to 5 cm H_2O until oxygenation is adequate, with an FIO_2 of 60% or less (if possible). PEEP may improve ventilation in respiratory units that collapse at low airway pressures, thus allowing the FIO_2 to be lowered. Patients with ARDS may need higher levels of PEEP (e.g., 10 to 20 cm H_2O). There is no identified optimal level of PEEP for patients with ARDS.

PEEP is not without complications. The added intrathoracic and intrapulmonic pressures generated by positive pressure remaining in the lungs and transmitted to surrounding structures (e.g., inferior vena cava, heart) at end expiration can compromise venous return. This in turn has the potential to decrease the amount of blood returning to both the right and left sides of the heart. Dramatic reductions in preload, CO, and BP can occur. High levels of PEEP or excess inspiratory pressures can cause barotrauma and volutrauma.

Prone Positioning. In the early phases of ARDS, fluid moves freely throughout the lung. Because of gravity, fluid pools in dependent regions of the lung. As a result, some alveoli are fluid filled (dependent areas) while others are air filled (nondependent areas). When the patient is supine, the heart and mediastinal contents place added pressure on the lungs. Consequently, the supine position predisposes all patients, including those with ARDS, to atelectasis.

Prone positioning is an option for patients with refractory hypoxemia who do not respond to other strategies to increase PaO_2. By turning the patient prone, perfusion may be better matched to ventilation. Air-filled alveoli in the anterior part of the lung become dependent. Alveoli in the posterior part of the lungs are "recruited" (given the opportunity to reexpand), improving oxygenation.

Some patients will have a big improvement in PaO_2 when prone with no change in FIO_2. The improvement in ventilation may be enough to allow a reduction in FIO_2 or PEEP. You may see hemodynamic instability (dysrhythmias, a decrease in BP) from fluid shifts when the patient is prone. There may be more need for airway suctioning as secretions are mobilized. Best practice suggests that patients be positioned prone early in the course of ARDS. They can stay in the prone position for up to 16 hours per day.[24] Placing a patient prone requires the presence of an ICU intensivist, respiratory therapist, and at least 3 to 4 nurses. Special attention must be given to securing the airway. Once prone, the patient should be positioned in a side-lying position.

◆ **Extracorporeal Membrane Oxygenation (ECMO).** Extracorporeal membrane oxygenation (ECMO) is used most often in specialized ICUs in major cities. Like hemodialysis, a large blood vessel is cannulated (most often the internal jugular, femoral artery, or femoral vein) and a catheter is inserted. The catheter is then connected to a device that allows the blood to exit the patient and pass across a gas-exchanging membrane outside the body. Within the ECMO unit, O_2 is delivered into the blood and CO_2 removed. Oxygenated blood is returned back to the patient. $ECCO_2R$ is like ECMO. It does not require as high of blood flow rates. It is only used to enhance oxygenation. Both ECMO and $ECCO_2R$ are expensive and require specially trained nurses and other personnel.

◆ **Medical Supportive Therapy**

The entire interprofessional team have important roles in the care of the patient with ARDS. All mechanically ventilated patients with ARDS in the ICU will have continuous heart rate, respiratory rate, BP, MAP, and SpO_2 monitoring. $EtCO_2$ monitoring is standard in the care of ARDS patients.[8]

Other positioning strategies for patients with ARDS include continuous lateral rotation therapy (CLRT) and kinetic therapy. CLRT provides continuous, slow, side-to-side turning of the patient by rotating the actual bed frame less than 40 degrees. The bed's lateral movement is maintained for 18 of every 24 hours to simulate postural drainage and help mobilize pulmonary secretions. The bed may contain a vibrator pack that provides chest physiotherapy. This feature assists with secretion mobilization and removal (Fig. 67.11). Kinetic therapy is like CLRT in that patients are rotated side-to-side 40 degrees or more. It is important to obtain baseline assessments of the patient's pulmonary status (e.g., respiratory rate and rhythm, breath sounds, ABGs, SpO_2) and continue to monitor the patient throughout the therapy.

Analgesia and Sedation. Analgesia and sedation, either by direct IV or continuous IV infusion, are important. Analgesia and sedation decrease the discomfort associated with the presence of an ET tube, help reduce WOB, and prevent ventilator dyssynchrony.

Patients who breathe asynchronously with mechanical ventilation may benefit from an adjustment of ventilator inspiratory flow rates or other settings. Patients who stay asynchronous with mechanical ventilation despite aggressive analgesia and sedation

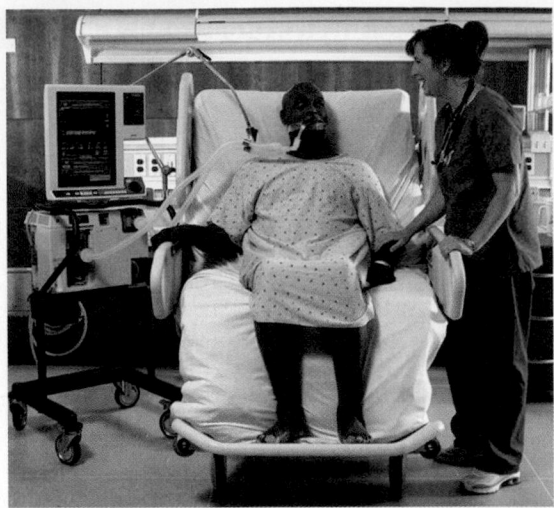

FIG. 67.11 TotalCare SpO2RT Bed System offers continuous lateral rotation therapy and percussion and vibration therapies. Patients can easily and quickly be repositioned. (© 2006 Hill-Rom Services, Inc. Reprinted with permission. All rights reserved.)

may need a neuromuscular blocking agent (NMBA). These drugs, such as vecuronium, pancuronium (Pavulon) or cisatracurium (Nimbex), relax skeletal muscles and promote synchrony with mechanical ventilation. Remember that a patient receiving neuromuscular blockade can appear to be asleep, but still be awake and in pain. For this reason, simultaneous administration of analgesia and sedation with NMBAs is essential.

> **[!] SAFETY ALERT Neuromuscular Blockade**
> - Always give concurrent analgesia and sedation to patients receiving a NMBA. This eliminates patient awareness, ensures patient comfort, and avoids the terrifying experience of being awake and in pain while paralyzed.
> - Use a NMBA for the shortest duration and at the lowest dose possible to avoid complications.

Monitoring levels of sedation in patients receiving NMBA is challenging. Levels of drug paralysis are monitored primarily by clinical assessment, including heart rate and BP, but more importantly, respiratory rate and whether the patient is taking breaths above the set rate on the ventilator.

◆ **Promoting Tissue Perfusion.** Patients with ARDS are at risk for hemodynamic compromise. Those on PPV and PEEP often have decreased CO. One cause is decreased venous return from the PEEP-induced increase in intrathoracic pressure. Impaired contractility and decreased preload can decrease CO. Changes in intrathoracic or intrapulmonary pressures from PPV can also decrease CO. Patients with an exacerbation of COPD or asthma and those receiving PPV are at risk for alveolar hyperinflation, increased right ventricular afterload, and excess intrathoracic pressures. These changes can limit blood flow from the right side of the heart, through the pulmonary vasculature, to the left side of the heart, and cause hemodynamic compromise (e.g., decreased CO). Blood return from the systemic circulation to the right side of the heart may be impaired, decreasing preload and CO.

Hemodynamic monitoring (e.g., CVP, CO, $ScvO_2$, SvO_2) is essential. This allows you to see trends, detect changes, and adjust therapy as needed. BP and mean arterial pressure (MAP) are important indicators of the adequacy of CO. Closely monitor BP and indicators of CO and tissue perfusion (SaO_2, mixed venous O_2 saturation) with the start of or changes in mechanical ventilation. A decrease in CO is treated by giving IV fluids, drugs, or both. (Chapter 66 discusses drugs used to treat decreased CO and shock.)

◆ **Maintaining Fluid Balance and Nutrition.** Maintaining fluid balance and nutrition is challenging. Increasing pulmonary capillary permeability results in fluid in the lungs and causes pulmonary edema. At the same time, the patient may be intravascularly volume depleted and at risk for hypotension and decreased CO from mechanical ventilation and PEEP.

Monitor hemodynamic parameters (e.g., CVP, stroke volume variation) and daily weights to assess the patient's fluid volume status. Monitor intake and output hourly. Keep the ARDS patient on the "dry" side. In other words, avoid aggressive resuscitation with IV fluids. ARDS patients typically have increased WOB because the alveoli, lungs, and spaces between the alveoli are partially or completely fluid filled. Since ARDS is an inflammatory process, diuretics play a minimal role.

Maintaining protein and energy stores is important. Nutritional depletion causes a loss of muscle mass, including the respiratory muscles, which may prolong mechanical ventilation and delay recovery. Ideally, enteral or parenteral nutrition should be started within 24 to 48 hours.

◆ Evaluation

The expected outcomes for the patient with ARDS are similar to those for a patient with ARF (see p. 1597). It is essential that the patient with ARDS be able to maintain and sustain adequate oxygenation and ventilation with decreasing amounts of O_2, be hemodynamically stable, and be free of complications.

CASE STUDY

Acute Respiratory Distress Syndrome

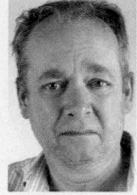

(© Thinkstock.)

Patient Profile
J.N. is a 58-yr-old white man who was admitted 36 hours ago to the surgical ICU after emergent surgery for a small-bowel obstruction, acute ischemic bowel, and perforated colon.

Past Medical History
* Mild obesity, hypertension, type 2 diabetes
* Lumbar spine surgery 5 years ago
* Chronic back pain controlled with oxycodone (Oxy-Contin) 15 mg PO 3 times daily

Operative Procedure
* Surgical procedure relieved small bowel obstruction, resected 2 feet of intestine, repaired the perforated colon, irrigated the abdominal cavity
* HR was 102 to 135, BP dropped to 70 mm Hg for 6 minutes, SpO₂ was greater than 90% for the duration of surgery
* Received 6 units of packed red blood cells and 4 L of 0.9% saline

Postoperative Status
J.N.'s pulmonary status worsened over the first 24 hours in the ICU. He required progressively higher FIO₂ via the mechanical ventilator. J.N. continued to have declining SaO₂ levels, increased WOB, and worsening hemodynamic status. He became more tachycardic. Despite direct IV analgesia and sedation, his respiratory rate increased and he was often "out-of-sync" with the ventilator. A chest x-ray showed bilateral pleural effusions and a right-sided pneumothorax, requiring chest tube placement. Immediately after chest tube placement, his SpO₂ decreased to 80% for 4 minutes. J.N. stayed dyssynchronous with the ventilator so continuous IV analgesia and sedation infusions were ordered. Neuromuscular blockade was started to decrease his WOB and achieve ventilator synchrony.

Current Status
J.N.'s oxygenation continues to worsen. He is still mechanically ventilated and is receiving 100% FIO₂ with PEEP 15 cm H₂O. Urine output has greatly decreased over the past 6 hours. He was diagnosed with AKI. His wife has brought in a copy of his advance directives. They state he does not want to be kept alive by artificial means. His wife and 2 adult children are at the bedside and voicing concerns about his status.

Objective Data
Physical Examination
* *General:* Sedated, paralyzed. Head of bed elevated 30 degrees. Skin cool, temperature 101° F (38.3° C) rectally
* *Respiratory:* ET tube in place with PPV. No accessory muscle use, retractions, or paradoxical breathing. Respiratory rate 18 breaths/min and in sync with ventilator. SpO₂ 88%, coarse crackles bilaterally throughout all lung fields. Ventilator settings: V$_T$ 350 mL, FIO₂ 100%, rate 18/min, PEEP 15 cm H₂O, peak inspiratory pressure 35 cm H₂O
* *Cardiovascular:*
* Apical-radial pulse equal, BP 96/54 mm Hg. 2+ carotid, radial, and femoral pulses; 1+ dorsalis pedis pulses. ECG is below:

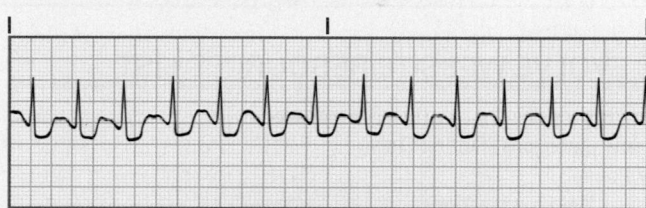

* *Gastrointestinal:* Surgical dressing dry and intact; colostomy draining a moderate amount of serosanguineous drainage
* *Urologic:* Indwelling bladder catheter draining concentrated, dark amber urine less than 30 mL/hr

Diagnostic Findings
* Current ABG: pH 7.23, PaO₂ 59 mm Hg, PaCO₂ 57 mm Hg, HCO₃ 16 mEq/L, O₂ saturation 88%.
* Hemoglobin 6.9 g/dL (69g/L), WBC 20.6/μL (20.6 × 10⁹/L)
* BUN and creatinine values are increased
* Chest x-ray: Bilateral, scattered interstitial infiltrates compatible with ARDS

Discussion Questions
1. What is the cause of ARDS for J.N? Is this a direct or indirect cause?
2. How does the pathophysiology of ARDS predispose him to refractory hypoxemia?
3. What manifestations does J.N. have that support a diagnosis of ARDS?
4. Calculate the PaO₂/FIO₂ ratio. What does this value tell you about the seriousness of his condition?
5. What other complications is J.N. at risk for developing from ARDS?
6. *Evidence-Based Practice:* You are orienting a new nurse, who asks you why you allowed J.N.'s family to stay at the bedside during your physical assessment and morning rounds with the ICU team. How would you respond?
7. *Priority Decision:* What priority interventions should be implemented to improve J.N.'s respiratory status and hypoxemia?
8. *Patient-Centered Care:* What information would you give to J.N.'s family about his status?
9. *Patient-Centered Care:* Given the guidelines in the patient's advance directive, what ethical/legal issues could you encounter?

Answers available at *http://evolve.elsevier.com/Lewis/medsurg.*

BRIDGE TO NCLEX EXAMINATION

The number of the question corresponds to the same-numbered outcome at the beginning of the chapter.

1. Which signs and symptoms distinguish hypoxemic from hypercapnic respiratory failure? *(select all that apply)*
   a. Cyanosis
   b. Tachypnea
   c. Morning headache
   d. Paradoxical breathing
   e. Use of pursed-lip breathing

2. An important consideration in selecting an O_2 delivery device for the patient with acute hypoxemic respiratory failure is to
   a. always start with noninvasive positive pressure ventilation.
   b. apply a low-flow device, such as a nasal cannula or face mask.
   c. be able to correct the PaO_2 to a normal level as quickly as possible.
   d. base the selection on the patient's condition and amount of FIO_2 needed.

3. The *most* common early clinical manifestations of ARDS that the nurse may see are
   a. dyspnea and tachypnea.
   b. cyanosis and apprehension.
   c. respiratory distress and frothy sputum.
   d. bradycardia and increased work of breathing

4. Interventions used in managing the patient with ARDS include *(select all that apply)*
   a. IV injection of surfactant.
   b. aggressive IV fluid resuscitation.
   c. giving adequate analgesia and sedation.
   d. elevating the head of bed 30 to 45 degrees when supine.
   e. monitoring hemodynamic parameters and daily weights.

5. Which intervention is *most* likely to prevent or limit volutrauma in the patient with ARDS who is mechanically ventilated?
   a. Increasing PEEP
   b. Increasing the inspiratory flow rate
   c. Use of low tidal volume ventilation
   d. Suctioning the patient via endotracheal tube hourly

1. a, b, d, 2. d, 3. a, 4. c, d, e, 5. c

For rationales to these answers and even more NCLEX review questions, visit *http://evolve.elsevier.com/Lewis/medsurg*.

ⓔ EVOLVE WEBSITE/RESOURCES LIST

http://evolve.elsevier.com/Lewis/medsurg
Review Questions (Online Only)
Key Points
Answer Keys to Questions
- Rationales for Bridge to NCLEX Examination Questions
- Answer Guidelines for Case Study on p. 1603
Student Case Studies
- Patient With Acute Respiratory Failure and Ventilatory Management
- Patient With Pulmonary Embolism and Respiratory Failure
Nursing Care Plans
- eNursing Care Plan 67.1: Patient With Acute Respiratory Failure
Conceptual Care Map Creator
Audio Glossary
Content Updates

REFERENCES

1. Kaynar AM: Respiratory failure. Retrieved from *https://emedicine.medscape.com/article/167981-overview*.
2. Baird MS: *Manual of critical care nursing: Nursing interventions and collaborative management*. 7 ed, St Louis: Elsevier; 2016.
3. Levitzky MG: *Pulmonary physiology*, 9th ed, New York: McGraw-Hill; 2018.
4. Hess DR, Kacmarek RM: *Essentials of mechanical ventilation*, ed 3, New York, 2014, McGraw-Hill.
5. Sarkar M, Nirarjan N, Banyal PK: Mechanisms of hypoxemia, *Lung India* 34:47, 2017.
6. Patel BK: Acute hypoxemic respiratory failure. Retrieved from *www.merckmanuals.com/en-ca/professional/critical-care-medicine/respiratory-failure-and-mechanical-ventilation/acute-hypoxemic-respiratory-failure-ahrf,-ards*.
7. Davis TM, Olff C: Acute respiratory failure and acute lung injury. In Good VS, Kirkwood PL: *Advanced critical care nursing*, ed 2, St Louis, 2018, Elsevier.
8. Kerslake I, Kelly F: Uses of capnography in the critical care unit, *BMJ Education* 17:178, 2017.
9. DeWit S, Stromberg H, Dallred C: *Medical-surgical nursing: Concepts and practice*, ed 3, St Louis, 2017, Elsevier.
10. Cystic Fibrosis Foundation: Coughing and huffing. Retrieved from *www.cff.org/Life-With-CF/Treatments-and-Therapies/Airway-Clearance/Coughing-and-Huffing/*.
11. Field JB: Chest physiotherapy. Retrieved from *www.merckmanuals.com/en-ca/professional/pulmonary-disorders/pulmonary-rehabilitation/chest-physiotherapy*.
12. Scala R, Pisani L: Non-invasive ventilation in acute respiratory failure: Which recipe for success? *Eur Resp Rev* 27:180029, 2018.
13. Knight J, Nigam Y: Anatomy and physiology of ageing 2: The respiratory system, *Nurs Times* 113:53, 2017.
14. Fan E, Brodie D, Slutsky AS: Acute respiratory distress syndrome: Advances in diagnosis and treatment, *JAMA* 319:698, 2018.
15. Stacy KM: Pulmonary disorders. In Urden LD, Stacy KM, Lough ME: *Critical care nursing: Diagnosis and management*, ed 8, St Louis, 2018, Elsevier.
16. European Respiratory Society: Acute respiratory distress syndrome. Retrieved from *www.erswhitebook.org/chapters/acute-respiratory-distress-syndrome/*.
17. Adigun M, McIntosh C, Onyilofor C: Treatment considerations for acute respiratory distress syndrome, *US Pharm* 41:HS6, 2016.
18. Reilly JP, Christie JD, Meyer NJ: Fifty years of research in ARDS: Genomic contributions and opportunities, *Am J Respir Crit Care Med* 196:1113, 2017.
19. Herridge MS, Moss M, Hough CL, et al: Recovery and outcomes after the acute respiratory distress syndrome (ARDS) in patients and their family caregivers, *Intensive Care Med* 42:725, 2016.
20. Tignanelli CJ, Wiktor AJ, Vatsaas CJ: Outcomes of acute kidney injury in patients with severe ARDS due to influenza A (H1N1) pdmo9 virus, *Am J Crit Care* 27:67, 2018.
21. Bienvenu OJ, Friedman LA, Colantuoni E: Psychiatric symptoms after acute respiratory distress syndrome: A 5-year longitudinal study, *Intensive Care Med* 44:38, 2018.
22. Fan E, Del Sorbo L, Goligher EC, et al: An official American Thoracic Society/European Society of Intensive Care Medicine/Society of Critical Care Medicine clinical practice guideline: Mechanical ventilation in adult patients with acute respiratory distress syndrome, *Am J Respir Crit Care Med* 195:1253, 2017.
23. Bein T, Grasso S, Moerer O, et al: The standard of care of patients with ARDS: Ventilatory settings and rescue therapies for refractory hypoxemia, *Intensive Care Med* 42:699, 2016.
24. Chiumello D, Coppola S, Froio S: Prone position in ARDS: A simple maneuver still underused, *Intensive Care Med* 44: 241, 2018.

68

Emergency and Disaster Nursing

Cathy Edson and Amy Meredith

The simple act of caring is heroic.

Edward Albert

http://evolve.elsevier.com/Lewis/medsurg

CONCEPTUAL FOCUS

Gas Exchange

Interpersonal Violence

Perfusion

Thermoregulation

LEARNING OUTCOMES

1. Apply the steps in triage, the primary survey, and the secondary survey to a patient with a medical, surgical, or traumatic emergency.
2. Relate the pathophysiology to the assessment and interprofessional care of select environmental emergencies.
3. Relate the pathophysiology to the assessment and interprofessional care of select toxicologic emergencies.

4. Select appropriate nursing interventions for victims of violence.
5. Distinguish among the responsibilities of health care providers, the community, and select federal agencies in emergency and mass casualty incident preparedness.

KEY TERMS

drowning, p. 1615
emergency, p. 1620
family presence, p. 1607
frostbite, p. 1613
heat cramps, p. 1611

heat exhaustion, p. 1611
heatstroke, p. 1612
hypothermia, p. 1613
jaw-thrust maneuver, p. 1607
mass casualty incident (MCI), p. 1620

primary survey, p. 1607
secondary survey, p. 1609
submersion injury, p. 1615
terrorism, p. 1620
triage, p. 1606

Entire books are dedicated to the nursing care of emergency patients. It is a unique specialty that requires a solid understanding of basic nursing concepts and specific approaches to patient problems. Nurses unaccustomed to the emergency department (ED) often describe the flow as "chaotic" and uncertain. Certainly, it may have this appearance. The challenge of the ED is that the nurse does not know what patient will come through the doors. The trained ED nurse must be prepared to meet this challenge. This chapter presents an overview of the triage process and care of select emergency patients. Common emergency situations discussed include heat- and cold-related emergencies, submersion injuries, bites and stings, and various types of poisonings. The chapter concludes with a discussion of terrorism, mass casualty incidents, and the methods of response.

The emergency management of various medical, surgical, and traumatic emergencies is discussed throughout this book. Tables outline the emergency management of specific problems. Table 68.1 lists these emergency management tables by title, chapter number, and page.

More than 141 million people visit EDs each year.[1] Of these, 11.2 million patients are admitted to the hospital. This number is increasing for several reasons. These include (1) the inability to see

a HCP, (2) an aging population, (3) shorter hospital stays resulting in frequent readmissions, (4) acute mental health crises, (5) ED and hospital closures, and (6) lack of or inadequate health insurance or a HCP. These factors result in overcrowding and long wait times.[2]

ED nurses care for patients of all ages with a variety of problems. However, some EDs specialize in certain patient populations or conditions, such as pediatric ED or trauma ED. The Emergency Nurses Association (ENA) is the specialty organization aimed at advancing emergency nursing practice. The ENA provides standards of care for nurses working in the ED. They offer a certification process that allows nurses to become certified emergency nurses (CENs).[3]

CARE OF EMERGENCY PATIENT

Recognizing life-threatening illness or injury is one of the most important goals of emergency nursing. Initiating interventions to reverse or prevent a crisis is often a priority before making a medical diagnosis. This process begins with your first contact with a patient. Prompt identification of patients who need immediate treatment and determining appropriate interventions are essential nurse competencies.

Triage

Triage, a French word meaning "to sort," refers to the process of rapidly determining patient acuity.[4] It is one of the most important assessment skills needed by ED nurses. Most often you will confront multiple patients who have a variety of problems. The triage process works on the premise that we must treat patients who have a threat to life before other patients.

A *triage system* identifies and categorizes patients so that the most critically ill are treated first. The ENA and American College of Emergency Physicians support the use of a 5-level triage system.[5] The *Emergency Severity Index* (ESI) is a 5-level triage system that incorporates concepts of illness severity and resource use (e.g., electrocardiogram [ECG], laboratory tests, radiology studies, IV fluids) to determine who should be treated first (Table 68.2). The ESI includes a triage algorithm that directs you to assign an ESI level to patients coming into the ED. The triage algorithm can be found in the ESI Implementation Handbook.[5]

First, assess the patient for any threats to life (ESI-1). Ask "Is the patient in imminent danger of dying?" Or, for ESI-2, is this a high-risk patient who should not wait to be seen? Next, evaluate patients who do not meet the criteria for ESI-1 or ESI-2 for the number of anticipated resources they may need. Assign patients to ESI-3, ESI-4, or ESI-5 based on this determination. Vital signs are important. Patients assigned to ESI-3 must have normal vital signs. Patients with abnormal vital signs may be reassigned to ESI-2.[5]

➕ TABLE 68.1 Emergency Management

Emergency Management Tables

Title	Chapter	Page
Abdominal Trauma	42	936
Acute Abdominal Pain	42	934
Acute GI Bleeding	41	919
Acute Soft Tissue Injury	62	1446
Acute Thyrotoxicosis	49	1155
Anaphylactic Shock	13	199
Chemical Burns	24	438
Chest Injuries	27	523
Chest Pain	33	723
Chest Trauma	27	523
Depressant Toxicity	10	149
Diabetic Ketoacidosis	48	1132
Dysrhythmias	35	760
Electrical Burns	24	437
Eye Injury	21	361
Fractured Extremity	62	1446
Head Injury	56	1315
Hyperthermia	68	1612
Hypoglycemia	48	1134
Hypothermia	68	1614
Inhalation Injury	24	437
Sexual Assault	53	1246
Shock	66	1576
Spinal Cord Injury	60	1409
Stimulant Toxicity	10	148
Stroke	57	1340
Submersion Injuries	68	1616
Thermal Burns	24	436
Tonic-Clonic Seizures	58	1361

❓ CHECK YOUR PRACTICE

You are working in the ED with your preceptor, who is a triage nurse. A 24-yr-old man arrives and states, "I think I have food poisoning. I've been vomiting all night and now I have diarrhea." The patient reports abdominal cramping that he rates as 6/10. He denies fever or chills. Vital signs: T = 97.8°F (36.6°C), HR = 94, RR = 16, BP = 121/74 mm Hg.
• Assign a triage acuity rating using the ESI.

After you complete the initial focused assessment to determine the presence of actual or potential threats to life, proceed with a more detailed assessment. A systematic approach to this assessment decreases the time needed to identify potential threats to life and limits the risk for overlooking a life-threatening condition. A primary and secondary survey is the approach used for all trauma patients. For nontrauma patients, the primary survey is followed by a focused assessment. Focused assessments are discussed in Chapter 3.

TABLE 68.2 Five-Level Emergency Severity Index (ESI)

Definition	ESI-1	ESI-2	ESI-3	ESI-4	ESI-5
Stability of vital functions (ABCs)	Unstable	Threatened	Stable	Stable	Stable
Life threat or organ threat	Obvious	Likely but not always obvious	Unlikely but possible	No	No
How soon should the HCP see the patient	Immediately	Within 10 min	Up to 1 hr	Could be delayed	Could be delayed
Expected resource intensity	High resource intensity Staff at bedside continuously Often mobilization of team response	High resource intensity Multiple, often complex diagnostic studies Frequent consultation Continuous monitoring	Medium to high resource intensity Multiple diagnostic studies (e.g., multiple laboratory studies, x-rays) or brief observation Complex procedure (e.g., IV fluids, drugs)	Low resource intensity 1 simple diagnostic study (e.g., x-ray) or simple procedure (e.g., sutures)	Low resource intensity Examination only
Examples	Cardiac arrest, intubated trauma patient, overdose with bradypnea, severe respiratory distress	Chest pain from ischemia, multiple trauma unless responsive	Abdominal pain or gynecologic disorders unless in severe distress, hip fracture in older patient	Closed extremity trauma, simple laceration, cystitis	Cold symptoms, minor burn, recheck (e.g., wound), prescription refill

Modified and reprinted with permission. © 1999, Richard C. Wuerz, MD, and David R. Eitel, MD.

Primary Survey

The primary survey (Table 68.3) focuses on airway, breathing, circulation (ABC), disability, exposure, facilitation of adjuncts and family, and other resuscitation aids. If uncontrolled external hemorrhage is noted, the usual ABC assessment format may be reprioritized to <C>ABC. The <C> stands for catastrophic hemorrhage. If present, it must be controlled first.[6] Apply direct pressure with a sterile dressing followed by a pressure dressing to any obvious bleeding sites.

The primary survey aims to identify life-threatening conditions so that appropriate interventions can be started (Table 68.4). You may identify life-threatening conditions related to ABCs at any point during the primary survey. When this occurs, start interventions immediately, before moving to the next step of the survey.

A = Alertness and Airway. Nearly all immediate trauma deaths occur because of airway obstruction. Saliva, bloody secretions, vomitus, laryngeal trauma, dentures, facial trauma, fractures, and the tongue can obstruct the airway. Patients at risk for airway compromise include those who drown or have seizures, anaphylaxis, foreign body obstruction, or cardiopulmonary arrest. If an airway is not maintained, obstruction of airflow, hypoxia, and death will result. Signs and symptoms in a patient with a compromised airway include dyspnea, inability to speak, gasping (agonal) breaths, foreign body in the airway, and trauma to the face or neck. The patient's alertness level is a crucial factor for choosing the right airway interventions. Determine level of consciousness (LOC) by assessing the patient's response to verbal and/or painful stimuli. A simple mnemonic to remember is *AVPU: A* = alert, *V* = responsive to voice, *P* = responsive to pain, and *U* = unresponsive.[6]

Airway maintenance should progress rapidly from the least to the most invasive method. Treatment includes opening the airway using the jaw-thrust maneuver (avoiding hyperextension of the neck) (Fig. 68.1), suctioning and/or removal of foreign body, inserting a nasopharyngeal or oropharyngeal airway (in unconscious patients only), and endotracheal intubation. If intubation is impossible because of airway obstruction, an emergency cricothyroidotomy or tracheotomy is done (see Chapter 26). Ventilate patients with 100% O$_2$ using a bag-valve-mask (BVM) device before intubation or cricothyroidotomy.[6]

Rapid-sequence intubation is the preferred procedure for securing an unprotected airway in the ED. It involves the use of sedatives and paralytic drugs. These drugs aid in intubation and reduce the risk for aspiration and airway trauma. (See Chapter 65 for more information on intubation.)

If the patient has a suspected spinal cord injury and is not already immobilized, the cervical spine must be stabilized at the same time as the assessment of the airway. This can be done with manual stabilization or the use of a rigid cervical collar (C collar). Keep the bed flat and continue to monitor airway patency and breathing effectiveness.

B = Breathing. Adequate airflow through the upper airway does not ensure adequate ventilation. Many problems cause breathing changes. Common ones include fractured ribs, pneumothorax, penetrating injury, allergic reactions, pulmonary emboli, and asthma attacks. Patients with these conditions may have a variety of signs and symptoms. The patient may have dyspnea, paradoxical or asymmetric chest wall movement, decreased or absent breath sounds on the affected side, visible wounds to the chest wall, cyanosis, tachycardia, and hypotension.

Every critically injured or ill patient has an increased metabolic and O$_2$ demand and should receive supplemental O$_2$. Give high-flow O$_2$ (100%) via a nonrebreather mask and monitor the patient's response. Life-threatening conditions (e.g., flail chest, tension pneumothorax) can severely and quickly compromise ventilation. Interventions may include BVM ventilation with 100% O$_2$, needle decompression, intubation, and treatment of the underlying cause.

C = Circulation. An effective circulatory system includes the heart, intact blood vessels, and adequate blood volume. Uncontrolled internal or external bleeding places a person at risk for hemorrhagic shock (see Chapter 66). Check either a femoral or carotid pulse. Peripheral pulses may be absent due to direct injury or vasoconstriction. Assess the quality and rate of the pulse if found. Assess the skin for color, temperature, and moisture. Altered mental status and delayed capillary refill (longer than 3 seconds) are common signs of shock. When evaluating capillary refill in cold environments, remember that a cold temperature delays refill.

Insert IV lines into veins in the upper extremities unless contraindicated, such as in an open fracture or an injury that affects limb circulation. Insert 2 large-bore (14- to 16-gauge) IV catheters. Start aggressive fluid resuscitation using normal saline or lactated Ringer's solution. Consider intraosseous or central venous access if unable to rapidly obtain venous access. (See Chapter 66 for more information on hypovolemic shock and fluid resuscitation.)

The HCP may order type-specific packed red blood cells if needed. In an emergency (life-threatening) situation, give blood that is not cross-matched (e.g., O negative) if immediate transfusion is needed.

D = Disability. Conduct a brief neurologic examination as part of the primary survey. The patient's LOC is a measure of the degree of disability. Use the Glasgow Coma Scale (GCS) to determine the LOC (see Table 56.5).[7] This allows for consistent communication among the interprofessional care team. Remember! The GCS is not accurate for intubated or aphasic patients. Last, assess the pupils for size, shape, equality, and reactivity.

E = Exposure and Environmental Control. Remove clothing from all trauma patients to perform a thorough physical assessment. This often requires cutting off the patient's clothing. Be careful not to cut through any area that is forensic evidence (e.g., bullet hole). Do not remove any impaled objects (e.g., knife). Removing these could result in serious bleeding and further injury. Once the patient is exposed, use warming blankets, overhead warmers, and warmed IV fluids to limit heat loss, prevent hypothermia, and maintain privacy.

Obtain a full set of vital signs, including BP, heart rate, respiratory rate, O$_2$ saturation, and temperature after the patient is exposed. If the patient has sustained or is suspected of having sustained chest trauma, or if the BP is abnormally high or low, obtain a BP in both arms.

F = Facilitate Adjuncts and Family. Research supports the benefits for patients, caregivers, and staff of allowing family presence during resuscitation and invasive procedures.[8] Patients report that caregivers provide comfort, serve as advocates for them, and help remind the care team of their "personhood." Caregivers who wish to be present during invasive procedures and resuscitation view themselves as active participants in the care process. They believe that they comfort the patient and that it is their right to be with the patient. Nurses report that family members serve as "patient helpers" and "staff

TABLE 68.3 **Emergency Assessment**

Primary Survey

Assessment	Interventions
Alertness and Airway With Cervical Spine Stabilization and/or Immobilization	
• Assess for catastrophic external bleeding. • Assess alertness (e.g., AVPU). • Assess for respiratory distress. • Determine airway patency. • Check for loose teeth or foreign bodies. • Assess for bleeding, vomitus, or edema.	• Control bleeding with direct pressure and pressure dressings. • Open airway using jaw-thrust maneuver. • Remove or suction any foreign bodies. • Insert oropharyngeal or nasopharyngeal airway, tracheostomy. • Initiate rapid sequence intubation. • Immobilize cervical spine using rigid cervical collar and cervical immobilization device.
Breathing	
• Assess ventilation. • Scan chest for signs of breathing. • Look for paradoxical movement of the chest wall during inspiration and expiration. • Note use of accessory muscles or abdominal muscles. • Observe and count respiratory rate. • Note color of nail beds, mucous membranes. • Auscultate lungs. • Assess for jugular venous distention and trachea position.	• Give supplemental O_2 via appropriate delivery system (e.g., nonrebreather mask). • Ventilate with bag-valve-mask with 100% O_2 if respirations are inadequate or absent. • Prepare to intubate if severe respiratory distress (e.g., agonal breaths) or arrest. • Have suction available. • If absent breath sounds, prepare for needle thoracostomy and chest tube insertion.
Circulation	
• Check carotid or femoral pulse. • Palpate pulse for quality and rate. • Assess skin color, temperature, moisture. • Check capillary refill.	• If absent pulse, start cardiopulmonary resuscitation and advanced life support measures. • If shock symptoms or hypotensive, start 2 large-bore (14- to 16-gauge) IVs and start infusions of normal saline or lactated Ringer's solution. • Consider intraosseous or central venous access if IV access cannot be rapidly obtained. • Give blood products if ordered.
Disability	
• Assess level of consciousness by determining response to verbal and/or painful stimuli (e.g., Glasgow Coma Scale). • Assess pupils for size, shape, equality, and reactivity.	• Periodically reassess level of consciousness, mental status, and pupil size and reactivity.
Exposure and Environmental Control	
• Assess full body for determination of additional or related injuries. • Assess environment.	• Remove clothing for adequate examination. • Stabilize any impaled objects. • Keep patient warm with blankets, warmed IV fluids, overhead lights to prevent heat loss, if appropriate. • Maintain privacy.
Facilitate Adjuncts and Family	
• Assess vital signs and pulse oximetry. • Determine caregiver's desire to be present during invasive procedures and/or cardiopulmonary resuscitation.	• Obtain bilateral blood pressures if patient has sustained or is suspected of having sustained chest trauma, or if the BP is abnormal. • Assign health team member to support caregiver(s). • Provide emotional support to patient and caregiver.
Get Resuscitation Adjuncts	
• Determine need for adjunct measures for monitoring the patient's condition.	• Obtain laboratory tests, such as type and crossmatch, CBC and metabolic panel, blood alcohol, toxicology screening, ABGs, coagulation profile, cardiac biomarkers, pregnancy. • Continuously monitor ECG. • Insert NG tube; insert orogastric tube in a patient with significant head or facial trauma. • Monitor oxygenation and ventilation (e.g., continuous pulse oximetry, capnography). • Manage pain with pharmacologic (e.g., NSAIDs, IV opioids) and nonpharmacologic (e.g., distraction, positioning, music) pain management strategies. • Provide comfort measures as appropriate (e.g., ice, position of comfort, warm blanket).

AVPU, A = alert, V = responsive to voice, P= responsive to pain, and U = unresponsive.

TABLE 68.4 Potential Life-Threatening Conditions Found During Primary Survey*

Airway
- Inhalation injury (e.g., fire victim)
- Obstruction (partial or complete) from foreign bodies, debris (e.g., vomitus), or tongue
- Penetrating wounds and/or blunt trauma to upper airway structures

Breathing
- Anaphylaxis
- Flail chest with pulmonary contusion
- Hemothorax
- Pneumothorax (e.g., open, tension)

Circulation
- Direct cardiac injury (e.g., myocardial infarction, trauma)
- Pericardial tamponade
- Shock (e.g., massive burns, hypovolemia)
- Uncontrolled external hemorrhage
- Hypothermia

Disability
- Head injury
- Stroke

* List is not all-inclusive.

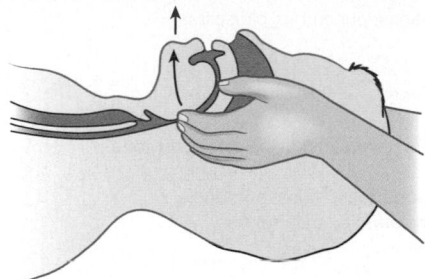

FIG. 68.1 Jaw-thrust maneuver is the recommended procedure for opening the airway of an unconscious patient with a possible neck or spinal injury. With the patient lying supine, kneel at the top of the head. Place 1 hand on each side of the patient's head, resting your elbows on the surface. Grasp the angles of the patient's lower jaw and lift the jaw forward with both hands without tilting the head.

helpers." It is essential to assign an interprofessional team member to explain the care being delivered and answer questions if a caregiver is present during resuscitation or invasive procedures.

G = Get Resuscitation Adjuncts. Start adjunct measures for monitoring the patient's condition, if not already done. Use the mnemonic "LMNOP" to remember these resuscitation aids:

L: Laboratory tests, such as type and crossmatch, complete blood count (CBC) and metabolic panel, blood alcohol, toxicology screening, arterial blood gases (ABGs), coagulation profile, cardiac biomarkers, pregnancy test, and urinalysis.

M: Monitor ECG for heart rate and rhythm.

N: Nasogastric (NG) tube to decompress and empty the stomach, reduce the risk for aspiration, and test the contents for blood. Place an orogastric tube in a patient with significant head or facial trauma since an NG tube could enter the brain.

O: Oxygenation and ventilation assessment. Continuously monitor O_2 saturation and end-tidal CO_2 (EtCO$_2$) if the patient is intubated (see Chapter 65).

P: Pain assessment and management

Most patients who come to the ED report pain.[9] Providing comfort measures is critical when caring for patients in the ED. Many EDs have pain management protocols for nurses to use to treat pain early, beginning at triage. Pain management strategies should include a combination of pharmacologic and nonpharmacologic measures. You are the advocate in ensuring comfort measures for the patient.

Secondary Survey

The secondary survey begins after addressing each step of the primary survey and starting any lifesaving interventions. The secondary survey is a brief, systematic process that aims to identify *all* injuries (Table 68.5). It is valuable for discovering unknown problems in patients with a poor or confusing history.[6]

H = History and Head-to-Toe Assessment. Obtain a history and mechanism of the injury or illness. These details provide clues to the cause and guide specific assessment and interventions. The patient may not be able to give a history. However, caregivers, friends, bystanders, and prehospital personnel can often give necessary information.

SAMPLE is a memory aid that prompts you to ask about:

S: Symptoms associated with the injury or illness

A: Allergies (e.g., drugs, food, latex, environment) and tetanus status

M: Medication history

P: Past health history (e.g., preexisting medical or psychiatric conditions, surgeries, smoking history, recent use of drugs or alcohol, last menstrual period, baseline mental status)

L: Last meal/oral intake

E: Events or environmental factors leading to the illness or injury

Details of the incident are important because the mechanism of injury and injury patterns can predict specific injuries. For example, a restrained front-seat passenger may have knee or femur fractures from hitting the dashboard and a chest injury from the airbag. Those who fell off a ladder or roof may have fractures, spinal cord injury, or head trauma.

Head, Neck, and Face. Check eyes for extraocular movements. A disconjugate gaze is a sign of neurologic damage. Battle's sign, or bruising directly behind the ears, may indicate a fracture of the base or posterior part of the skull. "Raccoon eyes," or periorbital bruising, usually occurs with a fracture of the base of the frontal part of the skull. Check the ears for blood and cerebrospinal fluid. Do not block clear drainage from the ear or nose.

Chest. Inspection and palpation of the chest will clue the nurse for heart and lung injuries. These may be life threatening and need immediate intervention.

Abdomen and Flanks. Frequent evaluation for subtle changes in the abdomen is essential. Motor vehicle crashes and assaults can cause blunt trauma. Penetrating trauma tends to injure specific organs. Stabilize, but do not remove, any impaled objects. They must be removed in a controlled environment, such as the operating room.

If the patient has blunt abdominal trauma or you suspect intraabdominal hemorrhage, perform a *focused abdominal sonography for trauma* (FAST).[6] This procedure can identify blood in the peritoneal space and assess cardiac function. It is noninvasive and done quickly at the bedside. However, a FAST cannot rule out a retroperitoneal bleed. If one is suspected, a CT scan is usually done.

Pelvis and Perineum. Inspect and gently palpate the pelvis. Do not rock the pelvis. Pain may indicate a pelvic fracture and the need for imaging. Assess for bladder distention, hematuria, dysuria, or inability to void. The HCP may perform a rectal examination to check for blood, prostate gland problems, and loss of sphincter tone (e.g., spinal cord injury).

Extremities. Assess the upper and lower extremities for point tenderness, crepitus, and deformities. If not done prehospital,

TABLE 68.5 Emergency Assessment

Secondary Survey

Assessment	Interventions
History and Head-to-Toe Assessment	
History	• Obtain details of the incident/illness, mechanism and pattern of injury, length of time since incident occurred, injuries suspected, treatment provided and patient's response, level of consciousness.
	• Use the mnemonic **SAMPLE** to determine **S**ymptoms associated with injury or illness; **A**llergies, including tetanus status; **M**edication history; **P**ast health history (e.g., preexisting medical/psychiatric conditions, last menstrual period); **L**ast meal/oral intake; and **E**vents/Environment preceding illness or injury.
Head, neck, and face	• Note general appearance, including skin color.
	• Assess face and scalp for lacerations, bone or soft tissue deformity, tenderness, bleeding, foreign bodies.
	• Inspect eyes, ears, nose, and mouth for bleeding, foreign bodies, drainage, pain, deformity, bruising, lacerations.
	• Palpate head for depressions of cranial or facial bones, contusions, hematomas, areas of softness, bony crepitus.
	• Assess neck for stiffness, pain in cervical vertebrae, tracheal deviation, distended neck veins, bleeding, edema, difficulty swallowing, bruising, subcutaneous emphysema, bony crepitus.
Chest	• Observe rate, depth, and effort of breathing, including chest wall movement and use of accessory muscles.
	• Palpate for bony crepitus and subcutaneous emphysema.
	• Auscultate breath sounds.
	• Obtain 12-lead ECG and chest x-ray.
	• Inspect for external signs of injury: petechiae, bleeding, cyanosis, bruises, abrasions, lacerations, old scars.
Abdomen and flanks	• Look for symmetry of abdominal wall and bony structures.
	• Inspect for external signs of injury: bruises, abrasions, lacerations, punctures, old scars.
	• Auscultate for bowel sounds.
	• Palpate for masses, guarding, femoral pulses.
	• Note type and location of pain, rigidity, or distention of abdomen.
Pelvis and perineum	• Gently palpate pelvis.
	• Assess genitalia for blood at the meatus, priapism, bruising, rectal bleeding, anal sphincter tone.
	• Determine ability to void.
Extremities	• Inspect for signs of external injury: deformity, bruising, abrasions, lacerations, swelling.
	• Observe skin color and palpate skin for pain, tenderness, temperature, and crepitus.
	• Evaluate movement, strength, and sensation in arms and legs.
	• Assess quality and symmetry of peripheral pulses.
Inspect posterior surfaces	• Logroll and inspect and palpate back for deformity, bleeding, lacerations, bruises. Maintain cervical spine immobilization, if appropriate.

splint injured extremities above and below the injury to decrease further soft tissue injury and pain. The HCP should realign grossly deformed, pulseless extremities before splinting. Check pulses before and after movement or splinting of an extremity. A pulseless extremity is a time-critical emergency. Immobilize and elevate injured extremities and apply ice packs. Antibiotics are given for open fractures to prevent infection.

Assess extremities for *compartment syndrome*. This occurs over several hours as pressure and swelling increase inside a muscle compartment of an extremity. This compromises the viability of the muscles, nerves, and arteries. Potential causes include crush injuries, fractures, edema, and hemorrhage.

I = Inspect Posterior Surfaces. An often overlooked part of the assessment is the back of the patient. Logroll the trauma patient while protecting the cervical spine. Up to 4 or more people with 1 person supporting the head may be needed to complete this assessment.

Acute Care and Evaluation

Once the secondary survey is complete, record all findings. Give tetanus prophylaxis based on vaccination history and the condition of any wounds (Table 68.6).[10]

Ongoing monitoring and evaluation are critical. Provide appropriate care and assess the patient's response. The evaluation of airway patency and the effectiveness of breathing is always the highest priority. Monitor respiratory rate and rhythm, O_2 saturation, and ABGs (if ordered) to evaluate the patient's respiratory status. A portable chest x-ray is done to confirm exact placement of tubes.

Closely monitor LOC; vital signs; quality of peripheral pulses; and skin temperature, color, and moisture for key information about circulation and perfusion. When indicated, insert an indwelling catheter to decompress the bladder, monitor urine output, and check for hematuria. Notify the HCP for any changes that may occur to the patient during this ongoing assessment process.

Depending on the patient's injuries or illness, the patient may be (1) transported for diagnostic tests (e.g., CT scan, angiography) or to the operating room for immediate surgery; (2) admitted; or (3) transferred to another facility. You may go with critically ill patients on transports. You are responsible for monitoring the patient during transport, notifying the HCP should the patient's condition become unstable, and starting life-support measures as needed.

Cardiac Arrest and Targeted Temperature Management

Many patients arrive at the ED in cardiac arrest. Patients with nontraumatic, out-of-hospital cardiac arrest benefit from a combination of good chest compressions and rapid defibrillation (see Appendix A), targeted temperature management (TTM), and supportive care. TTM for at least 24 hours after the return of spontaneous circulation (ROSC) decreases mortality rates and improves neurologic outcomes in many patients.[11] It is recommended for all patients who are comatose or who do not follow commands after ROSC.

TTM, also called therapeutic hypothermia, involves 3 phases: induction, maintenance, and rewarming. The induction phase begins in the ED. The goal core temperature is 89.6°

TABLE 68.6 Tetanus Vaccines and TIG for Wound Management

Vaccination History	TYPE OF WOUND	
	Clean, Minor Wounds	All Other Wound
Age 11 and Older*		
Unknown or <3 doses of tetanus toxoid-containing vaccine	Tdap and recommend catch-up vaccination	Tdap and recommend catch-up vaccination TIG
≥3 doses of tetanus toxoid-containing vaccine *and* <5yr since last dose	No indication	No indication
≥3 doses of tetanus toxoid-containing vaccine *and* 5–10yr since last dose	No indication	Tdap preferred (if not yet received) or Td
≥3 doses of tetanus toxoid–containing vaccine *and* >10yr since last dose	Tdap preferred (if not yet received)	Tdap preferred (if not yet received) or Td or Td

Source: Centers for Disease Control and Prevention: Tetanus. Retrieved from *www.cdc.gov/tetanus/clinicians.html.*

*Pregnant women: As part of standard wound management care to prevent tetanus, a tetanus toxoid–containing vaccine might be recommended for wound management in a pregnant woman if ≥5 yr have elapsed since previous Td booster. If a Td booster is indicated for a pregnant woman, Tdap should be given.

Td, Tetanus-diphtheria toxoid absorbed; *Tdap,* tetanus toxoid, reduced diphtheria toxoid, and acellular pertussis vaccine; *TIG,* tetanus immune globulin (human).

to 96.8°F (32° to 36°C). We use a variety of methods to cool patients. These include cold saline infusions and surface cooling devices (e.g., Arctic Sun).[12] Patients need intubation, mechanical ventilation, and invasive monitoring and require continuous assessment.[12] Protocols often direct the care of these patients.

Death in the Emergency Department

The loss of life in the ED is a stressful event. Many times, death is sudden and happens after an accident or unexpected illness (e.g., myocardial infarction [MI]). Sudden death is by its nature unexpected and thus shocking for family and friends.[13] It is important for you to identify and manage your feelings about sudden death so you can help them begin the grieving process (see Chapter 9).

You play a key role in providing comfort. Provide a private area for them to say goodbye, and, if appropriate, arrange for a visit from a chaplain. Assist the family by collecting the personal belongings and making mortuary arrangements. At times, you may need to contact the medical examiner or coroner. An autopsy may be done at the family's request, or if death occurred within 24 hours of ED admission, from suspected trauma or violence, or in an unusual way.

Many patients who die in the ED could potentially be candidates for *non–heart-beating donation*. We can harvest certain tissues and organs (e.g., corneas, heart valves, skin, bone, and kidneys) from patients after death. *Organ procurement organizations* aid in screening potential donors, counseling donor families, obtaining informed consent, and harvesting organs from patients who are on life support or who die in the ED.[14] Approaching caregivers about donation after an unexpected death can be distressing to both the staff and caregivers. However, for many, the act of donation may be the first positive step in the grieving process.

 Gerontologic Considerations: Emergency Care

People older than 65 account for 16% of all ED visits.[15] Regardless of a patient's age, aggressive interventions are provided for all injuries or illnesses unless the patient has a preexisting terminal illness, an extremely low chance for survival, or an advance directive indicating a different course of action.

Understanding the physiologic and psychosocial aspects of aging will improve the care delivered to older adults in the ED (see Chapter 5). Many older adults dismiss their symptoms as simply "normal for their age." It is important to fully explore any complaint by an older adult.

The older population is at high risk for injury because of the many changes that occur with aging. Falls are the leading cause of injury.[16] The most common causes of falls in older adults are generalized weakness, environmental hazards, syncope, and orthostatic hypotension. When assessing a patient who has fallen, determine whether the physical findings may have caused the fall or are due to the fall itself. For example, a patient may come to the ED with acute confusion. The confusion may be due to a stroke that caused the patient to fall. Or, the patient may have a head injury because of a fall from tripping on a rug.

ENVIRONMENTAL EMERGENCIES

Increased interest in outdoor activities, such as running, cycling, skiing, and swimming, has increased the number of environmental emergencies seen in the ED. Illness or injury may be caused by the activity, exposure to weather, or attack from various animals or humans. Specific environmental emergencies discussed in this section include heat-related emergencies, cold-related emergencies, submersion injuries, bites, stings, and envenomation.

HEAT-RELATED EMERGENCIES

Brief exposure to intense heat or prolonged exposure to less intense heat leads to heat stress. This occurs when thermoregulatory mechanisms, such as sweating, vasodilation, and increased respirations, cannot compensate for exposure to increased ambient temperatures. Ambient temperature is a product of environmental temperature and humidity. Strenuous activities in hot or humid environments, clothing that interferes with perspiration, high fevers, and preexisting illnesses predispose people to heat stress (Table 68.7). Table 68.8 presents the management of heat-related emergencies.

Heat Cramps

Heat cramps are severe cramps in large muscle groups fatigued by heavy work. Cramps are brief and intense and tend to occur during rest after exercise or heavy labor. Nausea, tachycardia, pallor, weakness, and profuse diaphoresis are often present. The condition is seen most often in healthy, acclimated athletes with inadequate fluid intake. Cramps resolve rapidly with rest and oral or parenteral replacement of sodium and water. Elevation, gentle massage, and analgesia minimize pain associated with heat cramps. Tell the patient to avoid strenuous activity for at least 12 hours. Discharge teaching should emphasize salt replacement during strenuous exercise in hot, humid environments. You can recommend the use of commercially prepared electrolyte solutions.

Heat Exhaustion

Prolonged exposure to heat over hours or days leads to **heat exhaustion**. This is a clinical syndrome characterized by fatigue, nausea, vomiting, extreme thirst, and feelings of anxiety. Hypotension, tachycardia, elevated body temperature, dilated pupils, mild confusion, ashen color, and profuse diaphoresis are present. Heat exhaustion usually occurs in people engaged in strenuous activity in hot, humid weather.

Always correlate fluid replacement to clinical and laboratory findings. Place a moist sheet over the patient to decrease core

TABLE 68.7 Risk Factors for Heat-Related Emergencies

Alcohol

Age
- Infants
- Older adults

Environmental Conditions
- High environmental temperatures
- High relative humidity

Preexisting Illness
- Cardiovascular disease
- Cystic fibrosis
- Dehydration
- Diabetes
- Obesity
- Skin disorders (e.g., large burn scars)
- Stroke or other CNS lesion

Prescription Drugs
- Anticholinergics
- Antihistamines
- Antiparkinsonian drugs
- Antispasmodics
- β-Adrenergic blockers
- Butyrophenones
- Diuretics
- Phenothiazines
- Tricyclic antidepressants

Street Drugs
- Amphetamines
- Jimson weed
- Lysergic acid diethylamide (LSD)
- Phencyclidine (PCP)
- 3,4-Methylenedioxymethamphetamine (MDMA, Ecstasy)

Adapted from Howard PK, Steinmann RA, eds: *Sheehy's emergency nursing*, ed 6, St Louis, 2010, Mosby.

temperature through evaporative heat loss. Consider hospital admission for older adults, the chronically ill, or those who do not improve within 3 to 4 hours.

Heatstroke

Heatstroke is the most serious form of heat stress and is a medical emergency. It results from failure of the hypothalamic thermoregulatory processes. Increased sweating, vasodilation, and increased respiratory rate deplete fluids and electrolytes, specifically sodium. Eventually, sweat glands stop functioning. Core temperature increases rapidly, within 10 to 15 minutes. The brain is extremely sensitive to thermal injuries. Cerebral edema and hemorrhage may occur from direct thermal injury to the brain and decreased cerebral blood flow. Death from heatstroke is directly related to the amount of time that the patient's body temperature is high.[6] Prognosis is related to age, baseline health status, and length of exposure. Older adults and those with diabetes, chronic kidney disease, heart disease, pulmonary disease, or other physiologic compromise are particularly prone.

Interprofessional Care. Treatment focuses on stabilizing the patient's ABCs, rapidly reducing the core temperature, and monitoring for dysrhythmias. Give 100% O_2 to compensate for the patient's hypermetabolic state. Ventilation with a BVM or intubation and mechanical ventilation may be needed. Place the patient on continuous ECG monitoring and pulse oximetry. Monitor laboratory findings. Correcting electrolyte imbalances and coagulation abnormalities is critical.

Place the patient in a cool environment. Promote evaporative cooling by removing clothing and spraying the patient with lukewarm water in front of a large fan.[6] Other cooling methods include conductive cooling (e.g., immersing the patient in a cool

TABLE 68.8 Emergency Management

Hyperthermia

Etiology	Assessment Findings	Interventions
Environmental - Lack of acclimatization - Physical exertion, especially during hot weather - Prolonged exposure to extreme temperatures **Trauma** - Head injury - Spinal cord injury **Metabolic** - Dehydration - Diabetes - Thyrotoxicosis **Drugs** - Amphetamines - Antihistamines - β-Adrenergic blockers - Diuretics - Phenothiazines - Tricyclic antidepressants **Other** - Alcohol - Cardiovascular disease - CNS disorders	**Heat Cramps** - Severe muscle contractions in exerted muscles - Thirst **Heat Exhaustion** - Altered mental status (e.g., anxiety) - Ashen, pale skin - Extreme thirst - Fatigue, weakness - Hypotension - Profuse sweating - Tachycardia - Temperature (99.6° to 105.8°F [37.5° to 41°C]) - Weak, thready pulse **Heatstroke** - Altered mental status (ranging from confusion to coma) - Hot, dry skin - Hypotension - Tachycardia - Tachypnea - Temperature >105.8°F (41°C) - Weakness	**Initial** - Manage and maintain ABCs. - Provide high-flow O_2 via nonrebreather mask or BVM. - Establish IV access and begin fluid replacement for significant heat injury. - Place patient in a cool environment. - For patient with heatstroke, start rapid cooling measures: remove patient's clothing, place wet sheets over patient, and place in front of fan; immerse in a cool water bath; give cool IV fluids or lavage with cool fluids. - Obtain 12-lead ECG. - Obtain blood for electrolytes and CBC. - Insert urinary catheter. **Ongoing Monitoring** - Monitor ABCs, temperature and vital signs, level of consciousness. - Monitor heart rhythm, O_2 saturation, and urine output. - Replace electrolytes as needed. - Monitor urine for development of myoglobinuria. - Monitor clotting studies for development of disseminated intravascular coagulation.

water bath); applying ice packs to the groins and axillae; and, in refractory cases, peritoneal or rectal lavage with iced fluids.

Closely monitor the patient's temperature and control shivering. Shivering increases core temperature due to the heat generated by muscle activity. This complicates cooling efforts. The HCP may order drugs to control shivering.

Heat stroke places the patient at risk for kidney injury due to *rhabdomyolysis*. It is a serious syndrome caused by the breakdown of skeletal muscle. Carefully monitor the urine for color, amount, pH, and myoglobin.

Patient and caregiver teaching focuses on how to avoid future problems. Stress the importance of proper hydration during hot weather and physical exercise. Teach patients the early signs of and interventions for heat-related stress.

COLD-RELATED EMERGENCIES

Cold injuries may be localized (e.g., frostbite) or systemic (e.g., hypothermia). Contributing factors include age, duration of exposure, environmental temperature, homelessness, preexisting conditions, drugs that suppress shivering, and alcohol intoxication. Smokers have an increased risk for cold-related injury because of the vasoconstrictive effects of nicotine.

Frostbite

Frostbite is true tissue freezing that results in the formation of ice crystals in the tissues and cells. Peripheral vasoconstriction is the first response to cold stress and results in a decrease in blood flow and vascular stasis. As cell temperature decreases, and ice crystals form in intracellular spaces, the organelles are damaged, and the cell membrane destroyed. This results in edema.

Depth of frostbite depends on ambient temperature, length of exposure, type and condition (wet or dry) of clothing, and contact with metal surfaces. Other factors that affect severity include skin color (those with dark skin are more prone to frostbite), lack of acclimatization, previous episodes, exhaustion, and poor peripheral vascular status.

Superficial frostbite involves the skin and subcutaneous tissue, usually the ears, nose, fingers, and toes. The skin appearance ranges from waxy pale yellow to blue to mottled. The skin feels crunchy and frozen. The patient may report tingling, numbness, or a burning sensation. Handle the area carefully and never squeeze, massage, or scrub the injured tissue because it is easily damaged. Swelling will occur with thawing. So, remove clothing and jewelry as they may constrict the extremity and decrease circulation.

Immerse the affected area in circulating water that is temperature controlled (98.6° to 104°F) [37° to 40°C]). Use warm soaks for the face. The patient often has a warm, stinging sensation as tissue thaws. Blisters form within a few hours (Fig. 68.2). The blisters should be debrided, and a sterile dressing applied.[17] Avoid heavy blankets and clothing because friction and weight can lead to sloughing of damaged tissue. Rewarming is extremely painful. Residual pain may last weeks or even years. Give analgesia and tetanus prophylaxis as appropriate. Evaluate the patient with superficial frostbite for systemic hypothermia.

Deep frostbite involves muscle, bone, and tendon. The skin is white, hard, and insensitive to touch. The area has the appearance of deep thermal injury with mottling gradually progressing to gangrene (Fig. 68.3). Immerse the affected extremity in a temperature-controlled, circulating water bath (98.6° to 104°F [37° to 40°C]) until flushing occurs distal to the injured area.

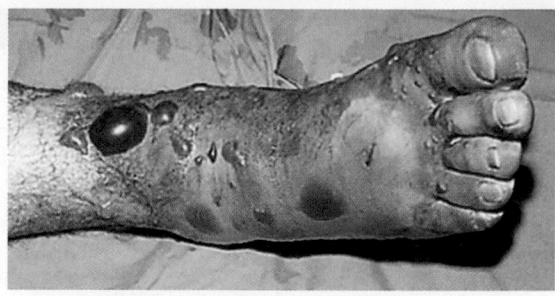

FIG. 68.2 Edema and blister formation 24 hours after frostbite injury occurring in an area covered by a tightly fitted boot. (Courtesy Cameron Bangs, MD. From Auerbach PS, Donner HJ, Weiss EA: *Field guide to wilderness medicine,* ed 2, St Louis, 2003, Mosby.)

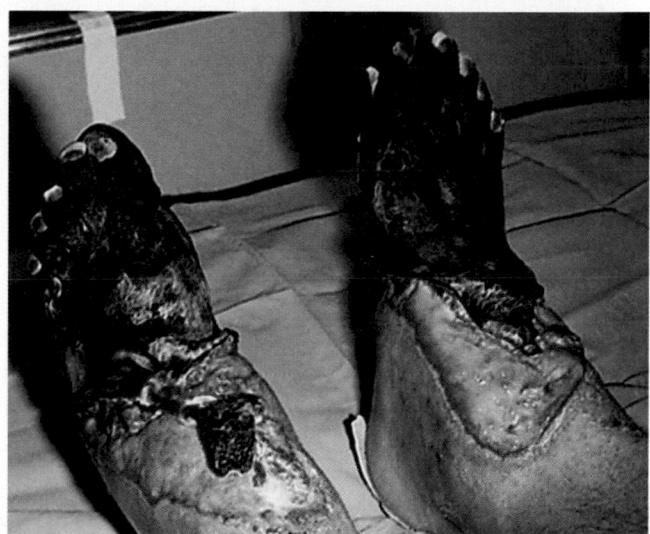

FIG. 68.3 Gangrenous necrosis 6 weeks after the frostbite injury shown in Fig. 68.2. (Courtesy Cameron Bangs, MD. From Auerbach PS, Donner HJ, Weiss EA: *Field guide to wilderness medicine,* ed 2, St Louis, 2003, Mosby.)

After rewarming, elevate the extremity to reduce edema. Significant edema may begin within 3 hours, with blistering in 6 hours to days. IV analgesia is needed in severe frostbite because of the pain associated with tissue thawing. All patients should start on nonsteroidal antiinflammatory drugs (NSAIDs) because of their dual affect as an analgesic and antiinflammatory. Give tetanus prophylaxis and evaluate the patient for systemic hypothermia.

Amputation may be needed if the injured area is untreated or treatment is unsuccessful. It may take as long as 90 days to determine the final necrotic area. The patient may be admitted to the hospital for observation with bed rest, elevation of the injured part, and prophylactic antibiotics if the wound is at risk for infection.

Hypothermia

Hypothermia is a core temperature below 95°F (35°C).[6] It occurs when heat produced by the body cannot compensate for heat lost to the environment. Most body heat is lost as radiant energy, with the greatest loss from the head, thorax, and lungs (with each breath). Wet clothing increases evaporative heat loss to 5 times greater than normal. Immersion in cold water (e.g., drowning) increases evaporative heat loss to 25 times greater than normal. Environmental exposure to freezing temperatures,

✚ TABLE 68.9 Emergency Management

Hypothermia

Etiology	Assessment Findings	Interventions

Environmental
 • Inadequate clothing for environmental temperature
 • Prolonged exposure to cold
 • Prolonged immersion or near-drowning
 	
 Metabolic
 • Hypoglycemia
 • Hypothyroidism
 	
 Health Care Associated
 • Administration of neuromuscular blocking agents
 • Blood administration
 • Cold IV fluids
 • Inadequate warming or rewarming in the ED or operating room
 	
 Other
 • Alcohol
 • Barbiturates
 • Phenothiazines
 • Shock
 • Trauma
	• Core body temperature:
	  • *Mild hypothermia:* 93° to 95°F (33.9° to 35°C)
	  • *Moderate hypothermia:* 86° to 93°F (30° to 33.9°C)
	  • *Severe hypothermia:* <86°F (30°C)
	 • Shivering, decreased or absent at core body temperatures ≤86°F (30°C)
	 • Altered mental status (ranging from confusion to coma)
	 • Areflexia (absence of reflexes)
	 • Blue, white, or frozen extremities
	 • Cyanotic, pale skin
	 • Dysrhythmias: bradycardia, atrial fibrillation, ventricular fibrillation, asystole
	 • Fixed, dilated pupils
	 • Hypotension
	 • Hypoventilation
		Initial
		 • Remove patient from cold environment.
		 • Manage and maintain ABCs.
		 • Provide high-flow O$_2$ via nonrebreather mask or BVM.
		 • Anticipate intubation for decreased or absent gag reflex.
		 • Establish IV access with 2 large-bore catheters for fluid resuscitation.
		 • Rewarm patient:
		  • *Passive:* Remove wet clothing, apply dry clothing and warm blankets, use radiant lights.
		  • *Active external:* Apply heating devices (e.g., air or fluid-filled warming blankets), use warm water immersion.
		  • *Active internal:* Provide warmed IV fluids; heated, humidified O$_2$. Peritoneal lavage with warmed fluids. Extracorporeal circulation (e.g., cardiopulmonary bypass, rapid fluid infuser, hemodialysis).
		 • Obtain 12-lead ECG.
		 • Anticipate need for defibrillation.
		 • Warm central trunk first in patients with severe hypothermia to limit rewarming shock.
		 • Assess for other injuries.
		 • Keep patient's head covered with warm, dry towels or stocking cap to limit loss of heat.
		 • Treat patient gently to avoid increased cardiac irritability.
		
		 Ongoing Monitoring
		 • Monitor ABCs, temperature, level of consciousness, vital signs
		 • Monitor O$_2$ saturation, heart rate and rhythm.
		 • Monitor electrolytes, glucose.

cold winds, and wet terrain plus physical exhaustion, inadequate clothing, and inexperience predisposes people to hypothermia. Older adults are prone to hypothermia because of decreased body fat, decreased energy reserves, decreased basal metabolic rate, decreased shivering response, chronic medical conditions, and drugs that alter body defenses. Peripheral vasoconstriction is the body's first attempt to conserve heat. As cold temperatures persist, shivering and movement are the body's only mechanisms for producing heat.

Assessment findings are variable and depend on core temperature (Table 68.9). Patients with *mild hypothermia* (93° to 95°F [33.9° to 35°C]) have shivering, lethargy, confusion, rational to irrational behavior, and minor heart rate changes. *Moderate hypothermia* (86° to 93°F [30° to 33.9°C]) causes rigidity, bradycardia, slowed respiratory rate, BP obtainable only by Doppler, metabolic and respiratory acidosis, and hypovolemia. Shivering decreases or disappears at core temperatures of 86°F (30°C).[6]

As core temperature drops, metabolic rate decreases 2 to 3 times. The cold myocardium is extremely irritable, making it vulnerable to dysrhythmias (e.g., atrial and ventricular fibrillation). Decreased renal blood flow decreases glomerular filtration rate, which impairs water reabsorption and leads to dehydration. The hematocrit increases as intravascular volume decreases. Cold blood becomes thick and acts as a thrombus, placing the patient at risk for stroke, MI, pulmonary emboli, and renal failure. Decreased blood flow leads to hypoxia, anaerobic metabolism, lactic acid accumulation, and metabolic acidosis.

Severe hypothermia (below 86°F [30°C]) makes the person appear dead and is a potentially life-threatening situation. Metabolic rate, heart rate, and respirations are so slow that they may be hard to detect. Reflexes are absent, and the pupils fixed and dilated. Profound bradycardia, ventricular fibrillation, or pulseless electrical activity may be present. Effort is made to try to warm the patient to at least 86°F (30°C) before the person is pronounced dead. The cause of death is usually refractory ventricular fibrillation.

Interprofessional Care. Treatment focuses on managing and maintaining ABCs, rewarming the patient, correcting dehydration and acidosis, and treating dysrhythmias. Mildly hypothermic patients may be rewarmed with passive and active external measures since their risk for dysrhythmia is low. Those with more severe hypothermia need active internal rewarming measures.

Carefully monitor core temperature during rewarming procedures. Rewarming places the patient at risk for *afterdrop*, a further drop in core temperature. This occurs when cold peripheral blood returns to the central circulation. Rewarming shock can produce hypotension and dysrhythmias. Thus patients with moderate to severe hypothermia should have the core warmed before the extremities. Discontinue active rewarming once the core temperature reaches 90° to 95°F (32.2° to 35°C).

Patient teaching focuses on how to avoid future cold-related problems. Essential information includes dressing in layers for cold weather, covering the head, carrying high-carbohydrate foods for extra calories, and developing a plan for survival should an injury occur when in an extreme environment.

CHECK YOUR PRACTICE

You are working in the ED when the paramedics arrive with a patient who was found lying on the sidewalk outside the downtown bus station. He is wearing only a lightweight shirt and pants. The outdoor temperature is 12°F (−11.1°C). The patient is unresponsive. Initial vital signs are as follows: rectal temperature = 89.5°F (31.9°C), HR = 38, RR = 8, BP (by Doppler) = 86 mm Hg.

- What are your priority interventions for this patient?

SUBMERSION INJURIES

Submersion injury results when a person becomes hypoxic from submersion in a liquid, usually water.[6] Around 3500 deaths from drowning occur each year in the United States. Most of the victims are children younger than 5 years of age or boys and men between ages 15 and 25.[18] The main risk factors for submersion injury include inability to swim, use of alcohol or drugs, trauma, seizures, hypothermia, stroke, and child neglect. Aggressive resuscitation efforts (e.g., airway and ventilation management), especially in the prehospital phase, improve survival of drowning victims.

Drowning is the process of experiencing respiratory impairment after submersion in water or other fluid. Submersion in cold water (below 32°F [0°C]) may slow the progression of hypoxic brain injury.

Most drowning victims do not aspirate any liquid due to laryngospasm. If liquid is aspirated, it is in small amounts. Drowning victims who do aspirate water develop pulmonary edema, which can cause acute respiratory distress syndrome (see Chapter 67).

The osmotic gradient caused by aspirated fluid leads to fluid imbalances in the body (Fig. 68.4). Hypotonic fresh water is rapidly absorbed into the circulatory system through the alveoli. Fresh water is often contaminated with chlorine, mud, or algae. This causes the breakdown of lung surfactant, fluid seepage, and pulmonary edema.

Hypertonic saltwater draws fluid from the vascular space into the alveoli, impairing alveolar ventilation and causing hypoxia. The body tries to compensate for hypoxia by shunting blood to the lungs. This results in increased pulmonary pressures and deteriorating respiratory status. More and more blood is shunted through the alveoli. Since the blood is not adequately oxygenated, and hypoxemia worsens. This can result in cerebral injury, edema, and brain death.

Interprofessional Care

Treatment focuses on correcting hypoxia and fluid imbalances, supporting basic physiologic functions, and rewarming when hypothermia is present. Initial evaluation involves assessment of airway, cervical spine, breathing, and circulation (Table 68.10). Mechanical ventilation with positive end-expiratory pressure or continuous positive airway pressure can improve gas exchange across the alveolar-capillary membrane when significant pulmonary edema is present. Ventilation and oxygenation are the main techniques for treating respiratory failure (see Chapters 65 and 67).

Deterioration in neurologic status suggests cerebral edema, worsening hypoxia, or profound acidosis. Drowning victims may have head and neck injuries that cause changes in the LOC. Complications can develop in patients who are free of symptoms immediately after the drowning episode. Consequently, observe all victims of drowning in a hospital for a minimum of 23 hours. Additional observation is needed for patients with co-morbidities.

Patient teaching focuses on water safety and how to reduce the risks for drowning. Remind patients and caregivers to lock all swimming pool gates; use life jackets on all watercrafts, including inner tubes and rafts; and learn water survival skills. Emphasize the dangers of combining alcohol and drugs with swimming and other water sports.

PATHOPHYSIOLOGY MAP

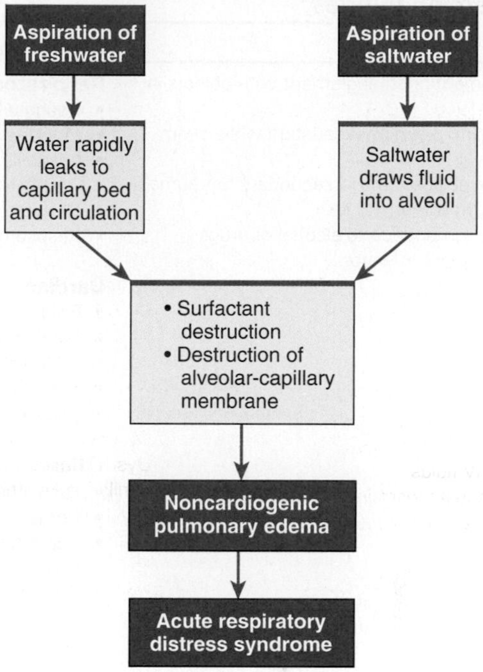

FIG. 68.4 Pathophysiology of submersion injury.

STINGS AND BITES

Animals, spiders, snakes, and insects cause injury and even death by biting or stinging. Morbidity is a result of either direct tissue damage or lethal toxins. Direct tissue damage is a product of animal size, characteristics of the animal's teeth, and strength of the jaw. Tissue is lacerated, crushed, or chewed, while teeth, fangs, stingers, spines, or tentacles release toxins that have local or systemic effects. Death associated with animal bites is due to blood loss, allergic reactions, or lethal toxins. Injuries caused by select insects, ticks, animals, and humans are described here.

Hymenopteran Stings

The *Hymenoptera* family includes bees, yellow jackets, hornets, wasps, and fire ants. Stings can cause mild discomfort or life-threatening anaphylaxis (see Chapter 66). Venom may be cytotoxic, hemolytic, allergenic, or vasoactive. Symptoms may begin immediately or be delayed up to 48 hours. Reactions are more severe with multiple stings. Most hymenopterans sting repeatedly. However, the domestic honey bee stings only once, usually leaving a barbed stinger with an attached venom sac in the skin so that venom release continues.

African honey bees (killer bees) look like domestic bees. If threatened, these bees aggressively swarm and can repeatedly sting their victims. These attacks can be fatal.

TABLE 68.10 Emergency Management

Submersion Injuries

Etiology	Assessment Findings	Interventions
• Entrapment or entanglement with objects in water • Inability to swim or exhaustion while swimming • Loss of ability to move secondary to trauma, stroke, hypothermia, MI • Poor judgment due to alcohol or drugs • Seizure while in water	**Respiratory** • Cough with pink-frothy sputum • Crackles, rhonchi • Cyanosis • Dyspnea • Respiratory distress • Respiratory arrest **Cardiac** • Bradycardia • Dysrhythmia • Hypotension • Tachycardia • Cardiac arrest **Other** • Exhaustion • Coma • Coexisting illness (e.g., MI) or injury (e.g., cervical spine injury) • Core temperature slightly elevated or below normal, depending on water temperature and length of submersion • Panic	**Initial** • Manage and maintain ABCs. • Assume cervical spine injury in all drowning victims and stabilize or immobilize cervical spine. • Provide 100% O_2 via nonrebreather mask or BVM. • Anticipate need for intubation and mechanical ventilation if airway is compromised (e.g., absent gag reflex). • Establish IV access with 2 large-bore catheters for fluid resuscitation and infuse warmed fluids, if appropriate. • Obtain 12-lead ECG. • Assess for other injuries. • Remove wet clothing and cover with warm blankets. • Obtain temperature and begin rewarming, if needed. • Obtain cervical spine and chest x-rays. • Insert gastric tube and urinary catheter. **Ongoing Monitoring** • Monitor ABCs, vital signs, level of consciousness. • Monitor O_2 saturation, heart rate and rhythm. • Monitor temperature and maintain normothermia. • Monitor for signs of acute respiratory failure.

BVM, Bag-valve-mask.

Manifestations of mild reactions include stinging, burning, swelling, and itching. More severe reactions may present with edema, headache, fever, syncope, malaise, nausea, vomiting, wheezing, bronchospasm, laryngeal edema, and hypotension. Treatment depends on the severity of the reaction. Treat mild reactions with elevation, cool compresses, antipruritic lotions, and oral antihistamines. More severe reactions require IM or IV antihistamines, subcutaneous epinephrine, and corticosteroids. Chapter 13 discusses allergic reactions and related patient teaching.

Snake Bites

There are more than 45,000 snakebites each year in the United States. *Envenomation* (poisoning by venom) occurs in only 8000 cases, with only 5 to 10 deaths each year.[19] The 2 families of venomous snakes found in the United States are Crotalidae or pit vipers (rattlesnakes, copperheads, cottonmouths) and Elapidae (coral snakes). Almost all the venomous bites are from pit vipers.

Snake venom may be hemolytic, neurotoxic, vascular toxic, or any combination of these. When bites occur, you will see fang or puncture marks. The patient often has severe pain at the site. There may be swelling, discoloration and blistering. If moderate envenomation has occurred, the patient will have paresthesias, lymphadenopathy, and nausea and vomiting. Treatment includes wound care and tetanus prophylaxis. Immobilize the affected extremity. Remove potentially constricting clothing. Most bites are minor and resolve without antivenom therapy. Patients with suspected envenomation are observed for at least 8 hours to ensure no life- or limb-threatening symptoms develop.

Manifestations of severe envenomation include profound edema, tachycardia, blurred vision, headache, chills, paresthesias, hypotension, and muscle twitching. The patient may report a metallic taste in the mouth. As symptoms progress, pulmonary edema, coagulopathy, thrombocytopenia, and hemorrhage may develop. Treatment of severe envenomation requires close patient monitoring. The ABCs are the most vital part of nursing management. Limb circumference and the advancing edema should be marked and monitored every 30 minutes. Anticipate fluid resuscitation, respiratory support, monitoring of laboratory results, and antivenom therapy. On rare occasions, the patient will need a fasciotomy.[6] The need to give antivenom is made in conjunction with a snake venom expert. Antivenom is given only if symptom progression occurs and platelet and coagulation studies are abnormal.

Snakebites from exotic snake species are primarily neurotoxic. They result in autonomic dysfunction, paralysis, and dysrhythmias. The bite should be discussed with your regional poison control center as there is specific antivenom therapy, often obtained from a zoo, for each species.

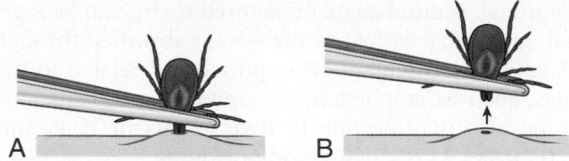

FIG. 68.5 Tick removal. **A,** Use tweezers to grasp the tick close to the skin. **B,** With a steady motion, pull the tick's body up and away from the skin. Do not be alarmed if the tick's mouthparts stay in the skin. Once the mouthparts are removed from the rest of the tick, it can no longer transmit disease.

Tick Bites

Ticks live throughout the United States. Specific types are more prevalent in certain regions. Tick-borne pathogens can be passed to humans by the bite of an infected tick. Common tick-borne illnesses include Lyme disease, Rocky Mountain spotted fever, anaplasmosis, Southern tick-associated rash illness, tick-borne relapsing fever, and tularemia.

Ticks transmit pathogens that cause disease through their feeding process. The infected tick attaches to its host and can slowly feed for up to several days. During this time, saliva from the tick can be transferred to the host. Tick saliva may harbor pathogens acquired by the tick from a prior host. The tick should be removed as soon as possible to stop the flow of saliva. Use forceps or tweezers to grasp the tick close to the point of attachment and pull upward in a steady motion (Fig. 68.5). After you remove the tick, clean the skin with soap and water. Do not use a hot match, petroleum jelly, nail polish, or other products to remove the tick. These measures may cause a tick to salivate, thus increasing the risk for infection.[20]

Lyme disease is the most common tick-borne disease in the United States. In 2016, more than 22,500 confirmed and 37,000 probable cases were reported to the CDC.[20] It is caused by the bacterium *Borrelia burgdorferi* that lives on the tick. In most cases, the tick must be attached for at least 36 hours to transmit the bacterium. Symptoms usually appear in about 7 days. The first stage begins with flu-like symptoms (e.g., headache, stiff neck, fatigue). Some patients may develop a characteristic bull's-eye rash. This is a circular area of redness 5 cm or more in diameter. Treatment at this stage includes doxycycline, cefuroxime, or amoxicillin.[20] The rash, if it develops, will disappear even if the patient is not treated.

Monoarticular arthritis, meningitis, and neuropathies occur days or weeks after the initial manifestations. Treatment at this stage involves IV ceftriaxone or penicillin. Chronic arthritis, heart disease, and peripheral nerve problems occur with the later stage of the disease. These illnesses can last several months to years after the initial skin lesion. (Chapter 64 discusses Lyme disease.)

Rocky Mountain spotted fever is caused by *Rickettsia rickettsia*. It is a bacterium that is spread to humans by the ixodid tick. The incubation period is 2 to 14 days. A pink, macular rash appears on the palms, wrists, soles, feet, and ankles within 10 days of exposure. Other symptoms include fever, chills, malaise, muscle pain, and headache. It is hard to diagnosis in the early stages. Without treatment, the disease can be fatal. Antibiotic therapy with doxycycline is the treatment of choice.

Animal and Human Bites

Every year more than 5 million animal bites are reported in the United States. Animal bites from dogs and cats are most

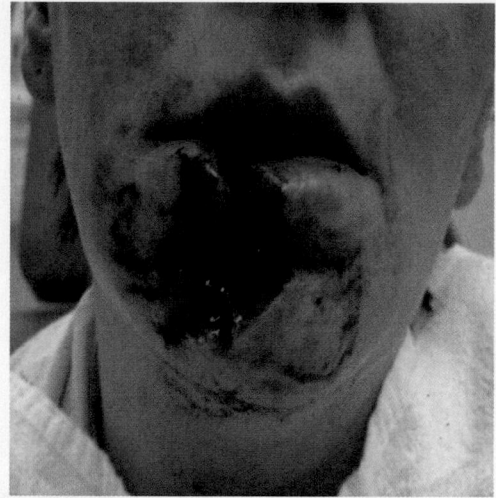

FIG. 68.6 Dog bite wound. (From Mannion C, Kanatas A, Telfer MR: One dog bite too far, *Brit J Oral Max Surg* 49:159, 2011.)

common. Wild or domestic rodents (e.g., squirrels, hamsters) follow as the third most common offenders. The few bite deaths (15 to 20) are mostly from dogs. The greatest problems associated with animal bites are infection and mechanical destruction of skin, muscle, tendons, blood vessels, and bone. The bite may cause a simple laceration or be associated with crush injury, puncture wound, or tearing of multiple layers of tissue (Fig 68.6). The severity of injury depends on animal size, victim size, and anatomic location of the bite. Children are at greatest risk.

Dog bites usually occur on the extremities. Facial bites are common in small children. Cat bites result in deep puncture wounds. They can involve tendons and joint capsules. There is a greater risk for infection than with dog bites. Septic arthritis, osteomyelitis, and tenosynovitis can occur. The most common infectious organisms from dog and cat bites are the *Pasteurella* species (e.g., *Pasteurella multocida*). Most healthy cats and dogs carry this organism in their mouths.

The human jaw has great crushing ability, causing laceration, puncture, crush injury, soft tissue tearing, and even amputation (Fig. 68.7). Hands, fingers, ears, nose, vagina, and penis are the most common sites of human bites. Often these injuries are due to violence or sexual activity. There is a high risk for infection from oral bacterial flora, most often *Staphylococcus aureus*, *Streptococcus* organisms, and hepatitis virus. Infection rates are as high as 50% when victims do not seek medical care within 24 hours of injury.

Interprofessional Care. Initial treatment for animal and human bites includes cleaning, copious irrigation, debridement, tetanus prophylaxis, and analgesics as needed. Prophylactic antibiotics are used for animal and human bites at risk for infection, such as wounds over joints, those older than 6 to 12 hours, puncture wounds, and bites of the hand or foot. People at greatest risk for infection are infants, older adults, immunosuppressed patients, patients with substance or alcohol use disorder, people living with diabetes, or those taking corticosteroids.

Leave puncture wounds open. Splint wounds over joints. Lacerations may be loosely sutured. Plastic surgery consultation may be needed for disfiguring facial wounds. The patient often receives prophylactic antibiotics. Report animal and human bites to the police as required.

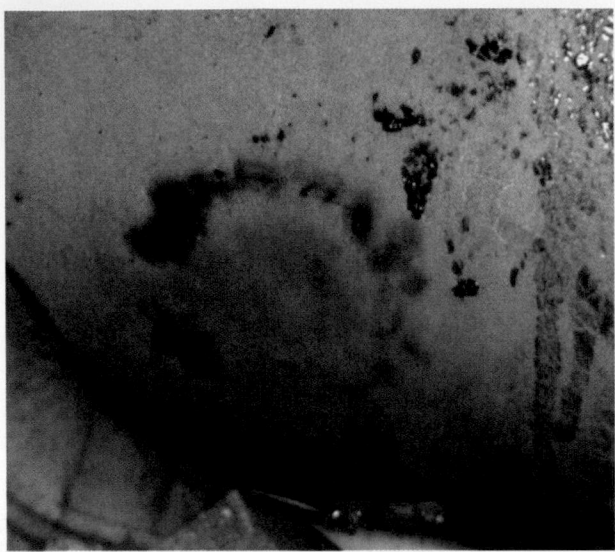

FIG. 68.7 Human bite injury. (From Stevens MR, Emam HA, Cunningham L: *Oral & maxillofacial trauma,* ed 4, St Louis, 2013, Elsevier.)

Consider *rabies postexposure prophylaxis* in the management of all animal bites. Rabies is caused by a neurotoxic virus in the saliva of an infected animal. Most rabies carriers are wild animals, like raccoons, skunks, bats, foxes, and coyotes. Rabies is usually transmitted through the saliva via a bite by the infected animal. If the saliva from the infected animal has come in contact with its claws, theoretically rabies may be transmitted through a scratch. The virus spreads through the central nervous system (CNS) via peripheral nerves. People who develop rabies may have flu-like symptoms, confusion, paresthesias, or numbness resulting in death.

Consider rabies exposure if an animal attack was not provoked, involves a wild animal, or involves a domestic animal not immunized against rabies. Always provide postexposure vaccinations when the animal is not found or a wild animal causes the bite. The series of 4 injections of rabies vaccine (human diploid cell rabies vaccine [HDCV, Imovax Rabies]) are given on days 0, 3, 7, and 14 to provide active immunity.[21] Give an initial, weight-based dose of rabies immune globulin (RIG [HyperRab S/D]) to provide passive immunity at the same time as the first dose of vaccine.

Since rabies is nearly always fatal, management efforts are directed at preventing the transmission and onset of the disease. Although death from rabies is significant worldwide, it is rare in the United States. Rabies vaccine is encouraged for persons who travel globally, since it is a serious world health concern. Notify your local health department for any suspected cases.

 DRUG ALERT Rabies Postexposure Prophylaxis
- If possible, give the calculated dose of RIG via infiltration around the wound edges.
- Give any remaining volume of RIG IM at a site distant from the vaccine site (e.g., gluteal site for bite wounds on the arm).
- Give the HDCV IM in the deltoid.

POISONINGS

A poison is any chemical that harms the body. More than 5 million cases of human poisonings occur each year in the United States. Poisonings can be accidental, occupational, recreational, or intentional. Natural or manufactured toxins can be ingested, inhaled, injected, splashed in the eye, or absorbed through the skin. Chapter 10 discusses other poisonings related to the use of drugs, such as amphetamines, opioids, and hallucinogens. Poisoning also may be due to toxic plants or contaminated foods. (Chapter 41 discusses food poisoning.)

Severity of the poisoning depends on type, concentration, and route of exposure (Table 68.11). Toxins can affect every tissue of the body, so symptoms can be seen in any body system. Specific management of toxins involves decreasing absorption, enhancing elimination, and implementing toxin-specific interventions. Consult the local poison control center (available 24 hours a day) for the most current treatment protocols for specific poisons.[22]

Decontamination takes priority over all interventions except those needed for life support. Wear *personal protective equipment (PPE)* for decontamination to prevent secondary exposure. In some cases, decontamination is done by those specially trained in hazardous material decontamination before the patient arrives at the hospital and again at the hospital, if needed.

Skin and ocular decontamination involves removing the toxins from skin and eyes using copious amounts of water or saline. Most toxins can be safely removed with water or saline. As a rule, brush dry substances from the skin and clothing before using water. Do not remove powdered lime or mustard gas with water. Lime should just be brushed off. Water mixes with mustard gas and releases chlorine gas.

Under the guidance of the Poison Control Center, binding agents, such as activated charcoal, cathartics, whole-bowel irrigation, hemodialysis, urine alkalinization, chelating agents, and antidotes, may be given to increase the elimination of poisons.[22] Focus patient teaching for toxic emergencies on how the poisoning occurred. Arrange for an evaluation and follow-up by a mental health professional for all patients who have poisoning because of a suicide attempt or substance use.

Many health care workers (e.g., nurses, housekeepers) are at risk for exposure to hazardous materials (e.g., antineoplastic drugs, cleaning agents). Always consult the Material Safety Data Sheet (required by the Occupational Health and Safety Administration [OSHA]) for specific information about hazardous agents in the workplace. OSHA should evaluate all poisoning related to a workplace hazard.

VIOLENCE

Violence is the acting out of the emotions of fear and/or anger to cause harm to someone or something. It may be the result of organic disease (e.g., temporal lobe epilepsy), psychosis (e.g., schizophrenia), or criminal behavior (e.g., assault, murder). The patient cared for in the ED may be the victim or the perpetrator of violence. Violence can take place in a variety of settings, including the home, community, and workplace.

EDs are high-risk areas for *workplace violence.*[23] Measures to protect staff include the use of on-site security personnel and police officers, metal detectors, surveillance cameras, self-defense training, and locked access doors. The ENA recommends comprehensive workplace violence prevention plans be in place in every ED.[24]

Awareness of *family and intimate partner violence* (IPV) along with the possibility of a patient being a victim or perpetrator of human trafficking is a critical part of the ED nurse's role. IPV and human trafficking are patterns of coercive behavior

TABLE 68.11 Common Poisons

Poison	Manifestations	Treatment
acetaminophen (Tylenol)	*Phase 1* (within 24 hr of ingestion): Malaise, diaphoresis, nausea and vomiting *Phase 2* (24–28 hr after ingestion): Right upper quadrant pain, ↓ urine output, ↓ nausea, increase in LFTs *Phase 3* (72–96 hr after ingestion): Nausea and vomiting, malaise, jaundice, hypoglycemia, enlarged liver, possible coagulopathies, including DIC *Phase 4* (7-8 days after ingestion): Recovery, resolution of symptoms or permanent liver damage, LFT results remain high	Activated charcoal, *N*-acetylcysteine (oral form may cause vomiting, IV form can be used)
Acids and Alkalis • *Acids:* Toilet bowl cleaners, antirust compounds • *Alkalis:* Drain cleaners, dishwashing detergents, ammonia	Excess salivation, dysphagia, epigastric pain, pneumonitis; burns of mouth, esophagus, and stomach	Immediate dilution (water, milk), corticosteroids (for alkali burns), induced vomiting is contraindicated
• Aspirin and aspirin-containing drugs	Tachypnea, tachycardia, fever, seizures, pulmonary edema, occult bleeding or hemorrhage, metabolic acidosis	Activated charcoal, gastric lavage, urine alkalinization, hemodialysis for severe acute ingestion, intubation and mechanical ventilation, supportive care
Bleaches	Irritation of lips, mouth, and eyes, superficial injury to esophagus; chemical pneumonia and pulmonary edema	Washing of exposed skin and eyes, dilution with water and milk, gastric lavage, prevention of vomiting and aspiration
Carbon monoxide	Dyspnea, headache, tachypnea, confusion, impaired judgment, cyanosis, respiratory depression	Remove from source, apply 100% O_2 via nonrebreather mask, BVM, or intubation and mechanical ventilation; consider hyperbaric O_2 therapy
Cyanide	Almond odor to breath, headache, dizziness, nausea, confusion, hypertension, bradycardia followed by hypotension and tachycardia, tachypnea followed by bradypnea and respiratory arrest	Amyl nitrate (nasally), IV sodium nitrate, IV sodium thiosulfate, supportive care
Ethylene glycol	Sweet aromatic odor to breath, nausea and vomiting, slurred speech, ataxia, lethargy, respiratory depression	Activated charcoal, gastric lavage, supportive care
Iron	Vomiting (often bloody), diarrhea (often bloody), fever, hyperglycemia, lethargy, hypotension, seizures, coma	Gastric lavage, chelation therapy (deferoxamine [Desferal])
NSAIDs	Gastroenteritis, abdominal pain, drowsiness, nystagmus, hepatic and renal damage	Activated charcoal, gastric lavage, supportive care
Tricyclic antidepressants (e.g., amitriptyline)	*In low doses:* Anticholinergic effects, agitation, hypertension, tachycardia *In high doses:* CNS depression, dysrhythmias, hypotension, respiratory depression	Multidose activated charcoal, gastric lavage, serum alkalinization with sodium bicarbonate, intubation and mechanical ventilation, supportive care; never induce vomiting
Alcohol, barbiturates, benzodiazepines, cocaine, hallucinogens, stimulants	See Chapter 10	See Chapter 10

BVM, Bag-valve-mask; *DIC,* disseminated intravascular coagulation; *LFT,* liver function test.

in relationships that involve fear, humiliation, intimidation, neglect, or intentional physical, emotional, financial, or sexual injury (see Chapter 53 for information on sexual assault). Trafficking can involve being kidnapped or even being sold by family. It may also involve coercion of runaways into a "safe" situation that results in anything but safety.

IPV is found in all cultures, socioeconomic groups, age-groups, and genders. Although men can be victims of family violence and IPV, most victims are women, children, and older adults. Each year, more than 5 million women and 3 million men are treated in EDs for *battery* (assault) by spouses, caregivers, or persons known to them. IPV is most common among women of reproductive age.[25]

In the ED, screening for family violence and IPV (e.g., Do you feel safe at home? Is anyone hurting you?) is required. Barriers to effective screening include lack of privacy, fear of offending the patient, lack of time, and discomfort with the topic. Developing and implementing policies, procedures, and staff education programs improve screening practices.

With over 100 million people worldwide affected by human trafficking, it is likely that the ED nurse will come in contact with either a victim or perpetrator of human trafficking. Interviews with former victims suggest that over 85% had come in contact with the health care system at some time during their captivity.[26] ED nurses are uniquely positioned to help identify and report a trafficking victim or perpetrator to the appropriate authorities.

Be sensitive when gathering information about suspected abuse and trafficking as it may have potential for increasing the patient's risk. Start appropriate interventions for patients who you suspect or find are victims of abuse or trafficking. This includes making referrals, notifying appropriate agencies, providing emotional support, and informing victims about their options. The ENA encourages ED nurses to become certified *sexual assault nurse examiners* (SANEs). SANEs provide expert emergency care, collect and document evidence, take part in staff and community education, and advocate for sexual assault and rape victims.[27]

AGENTS OF TERRORISM

Terrorism involves overt actions, such as the dispensing of nuclear, biologic, or chemical (NBC) agents as weapons, for the express purpose of causing harm. Prompt recognition and identification of potential health hazards are essential in the preparedness of health care professionals.

Biologic agents most often used in terrorist attacks include anthrax, smallpox, botulism, plague, tularemia, and hemorrhagic fever. Anthrax, plague, and tularemia are treated effectively with antibiotics if enough supplies are available and the organisms are not resistant.[28] Vaccines are available for most of these agents.

Chemicals used as agents of terrorism are categorized by their target organ or effect. For example, sarin is a highly toxic nerve gas that can cause death within minutes of exposure.[29] The radioactive dust and smoke can spread and cause illness if inhaled. Since radiation cannot be seen, smelled, felt, or tasted, you should start measures to limit contamination and provide for decontamination. *Ionizing radiation,* such as that from a nuclear bomb or damage to a nuclear reactor, is a serious threat to the safety of victims and the environment. Exposure to ionizing radiation may include skin contamination with radioactive material. Begin decontamination procedures immediately if external radioactive contaminants are present.

Explosive devices cause blast, crush, and/or penetrating injuries. Blast injuries result from the supersonic pressurization shock wave caused by the explosion. This shock wave primarily damages the lungs, GI tract, and middle ear. Crush injuries often result from explosions in confined spaces causing structural collapse. Some explosive devices contain materials that are projected during the explosion, leading to penetrating injuries.

PENETRATING TRAUMA

Penetrating trauma is an injury that occurs when an object pierces the skin and enters the body creating an open wound. When the object goes all the way through, creating and entry and exit wound, it is a perforating injury. The most common causes of penetrating and perforating injuries in the United States are gunshot and stab wounds. The severity of the injury largely depends on the body part involved. Patients with penetrating trauma have the best outcome when they are thoroughly evaluated and promptly treated. All victims must first have a primary assessment to maintain airway, breathing, and circulation; control bleeding; and evaluate neurologic status.

Penetrating head trauma is a traumatic brain injury (TBI) that has a high mortality rate. Most deaths from TBI are from gunshot wounds. Other causes include stab wounds, motor vehicle accidents, or occupational accidents. Those who survive penetrating head trauma often have permanent neurologic deficits.

Patients with penetrating neck trauma are at risk for injury to major blood vessels, airway, and spinal cord. Anticipate bleeding, respiratory, and neurologic problems. Chest wounds can damage the heart, lungs, esophagus, diaphragm, or trachea. Penetrating wounds to the heart are almost 80% fatal. Lung injury can cause pneumothorax or hemothorax requiring emergent decompression and chest tube insertion.

Penetrating wounds to the abdomen often result from gunshot wounds. Severity and prognosis depend on the organs injured. Mortality from abdominal wounds is about 5%. Death usually occurs later due to hemorrhage or infection.

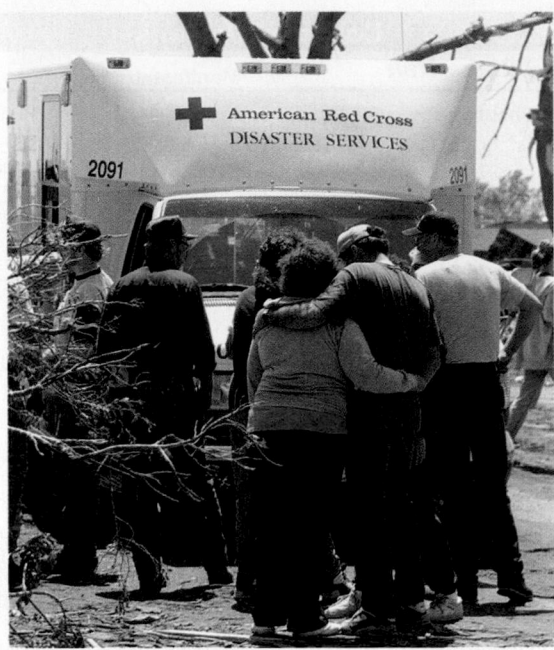

FIG. 68.8 American Red Cross. (Photo used with the permission of the American Red Cross.)

Extremity trauma is usually not life threatening but can cause permanent disability. Blood vessels may be affected, leading to hemorrhage. Angulated fractures can cause penetrating trauma. Nerves, tendons, ligaments, and muscles can be injured. Early interventions include control of bleeding and stabilization of the injured extremity.

EMERGENCY AND MASS CASUALTY INCIDENT PREPAREDNESS

The term emergency usually refers to any extraordinary event that requires a rapid and skilled response and that the community's existing resources can manage. An emergency is different from a mass casualty incident (MCI) in that an MCI is a human-made (e.g., involving NBC agents) or natural (e.g., hurricane) event or disaster that overwhelms a community's ability to respond with existing resources. MCIs usually involve large numbers of victims, physical and emotional suffering, and permanent changes within a community. MCIs always require assistance from resources outside the affected community (Fig. 68.8).

When an emergency or an MCI occurs, first responders are sent to the scene. Triage of victims of an emergency or an MCI differs from the usual ED triage. Several systems exist. Many use colored tags to designate both the seriousness of the injury and the chance for survival. One system uses green for minor injuries and yellow for urgent but not life-threatening injuries. Red means a life-threatening injury requiring immediate intervention. Blue indicates those who are expected to die, and black identifies the dead.[30]

Triage of victims of an emergency or an MCI must be done in less than 15 seconds. Victims need to be treated and stabilized and, if there is known or suspected contamination, decontaminated at the scene. After this, they are moved to hospitals. Many other victims arrive at hospitals on their own. The total number of victims a hospital can expect is estimated by doubling the number of victims who arrive in the first hour.

ETHICAL/LEGAL DILEMMAS

Good Samaritan

Situation

You are a registered nurse, employed as a charge nurse at a subacute rehabilitation facility. It is midnight, and you are driving home from work when you see a motor vehicle crash with a person at the side of the road waving and yelling for help. You stop and call 911 to report the incident. What do you do next?

Ethical/Legal Points for Consideration

- As a licensed health care professional, you are under no legal obligation to stop and give aid.
- If you do stop, you assume an obligation not to leave the scene until sufficiently trained first responders arrive and assume control.
- Many states encourage health care professionals to stop and give aid by having "Good Samaritan" laws. These laws, which vary somewhat from state to state, offer immunity from lawsuit for bystanders who offer aid in emergencies except in the case of gross negligence.
- A Good Samaritan must not be in the place of employment or under employment conditions.
- An example of gross negligence may be refusing to help someone who obviously had a serious hemorrhage in favor of a person with a minor injury because the bleeding person looked old or disheveled.
- Immunity covers only the scene of the accident and not later care under the supervision of HCPs.
- If there is a national disaster, an act of terrorism, or a major emergent need for HCPs, you may be required to go to an assigned site to offer aid. You would not be covered by the Good Samaritan Act under these circumstances.

Discussion Questions

1. What factors do you think contribute to a health care professional's decision whether to stop to provide aid?
2. What basic aid would you feel comfortable providing if you do not have an emergency or trauma background?
3. Would your professional liability (malpractice) insurance cover you if someone claimed that you acted negligently while giving aid?

In addition to the services provided by first responders, many communities have developed *community emergency response teams* (CERTs). CERTs are recognized by the Federal Emergency Management Agency (FEMA) as important partners in emergency preparedness. The CERT training helps citizens understand their personal responsibility in preparing for a natural or human-made disaster. Participants learn what to expect after a disaster and how to safely help themselves, their family, and their neighbors. Training includes lifesaving skills with emphasis on decision making and rescuer safety. CERTs are an extension of the first responder services. They can offer immediate help to victims and organize untrained volunteers to assist until professional services arrive.[31]

All HCPs have a role in emergency and MCI preparedness. Knowledge of the hospital's *emergency response plan* is essential. This includes individual roles and responsibilities of the members of the response team plus participation in emergency/MCI preparedness drills on a regular basis. Several types of drills can assess a hospital's level of emergency preparedness. These include hospital disaster drills, computer simulations, and table-top exercises. Drills allow HCPs to become familiar with the emergency response procedures.

Response to MCIs often requires the aid of a federal agency. The National Incident Management System (NIMS), American Red Cross, FEMA, and National Disaster Medical System (NDMS) are examples of federal resources.

All disasters result in psychologic stress to those involved. This stress can persist for an extended period. It is influenced, in part, by the nature of the event, the person's age, preexisting coping mechanisms, role in the event, and medical and mental health history. Many hospitals have a *critical incident stress management unit.* This unit arranges group discussions to allow participants to share their feelings about the experience. This is important for emotional recovery.

CASE STUDY

Trauma

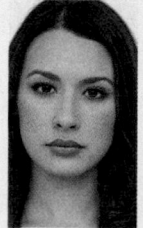

(© Thinkstock.)

Patient Profile

D.F., a 20-yr-old Hispanic female trauma victim, is brought to the ED in an ambulance. She was the driver in a motor vehicle crash and was not wearing a seat belt. Two unrestrained children in the car were pronounced dead at the scene. The paramedics said there was significant damage to the car on the driver's side.

Subjective Data

- Patient asks, "What happened? Where am I?"
- Reports of shortness of breath and leg pain

Objective Data

Physical Examination

- Vital signs: BP = 85/40 mm Hg, HR = 140 beats/min, RR = 36 breaths/min; O$_2$ saturation = 85% with 100% nonrebreather mask
- Decreased breath sounds on left side of chest
- Asymmetric chest wall movement
- Glasgow Coma Score = 14; pupils slightly unequal
- Badly deformed left lower leg with significant swelling and a pedal pulse by Doppler only
- 4-cm head laceration, bleeding controlled

Discussion Questions

1. What are D.F.'s most likely life-threatening injuries?
2. *Priority Decision:* What is the priority of care for D.F.?
3. *Priority Decision:* What interventions does this patient need immediately?
4. What other interventions should you consider?
5. *Collaboration:* What activities could you delegate to unlicensed assistive personnel (UAP)?
6. *Patient-Centered Care:* Several family members have arrived in the ED, including the mother of 1 of the children who died. The second child who died was the patient's child. How should you approach the family?
7. *Priority Decision:* Based on assessment data presented, what are the priority nursing diagnoses? Are there any collaborative problems?
8. *Evidence-Based Practice:* What are the best practice guidelines for fluid resuscitation in patients with hypovolemic shock?

Answers available at *http://evolve.elsevier.com/Lewis/medsurg.*

BRIDGE TO NCLEX EXAMINATION

The number of the question corresponds to the same-numbered outcome at the beginning of the chapter.

1. An older man arrives in triage disoriented and dyspneic. His skin is hot and dry. His wife states that he was fine earlier today. The nurse's next *priority* would be to
   a. assess his vital signs.
   b. obtain a brief medical history from his wife.
   c. start supplemental O_2 and have the provider see him.
   d. determine the kind of insurance he has before treating him.

2. A patient has a core temperature of 90°F (32.2°C). The *most* appropriate rewarming technique would be
   a. passive rewarming with warm blankets.
   b. active internal rewarming using warmed IV fluids.
   c. passive rewarming using air-filled warming blankets.
   d. active external rewarming by submersing in a warm bath.

3. What are effective interventions to decrease absorption or increase elimination of an ingested poison? *(select all that apply)*
   a. Hemodialysis
   b. Eye irrigation
   c. Hyperbaric O_2
   d. Gastric lavage
   e. Activated charcoal

4. An older woman arrives in the ED reporting severe pain in her right shoulder. The nurse notes her clothes are soiled with urine and feces. She tells the nurse that she lives with her son and that she "fell." She is tearful and asks you if she can be admitted. What possibility should the nurse consider?
   a. Dementia
   b. Possible cancer
   c. Family violence
   d. Orthostatic hypotension

5. A chemical explosion occurs at a nearby industrial site. First responders report that victims are being decontaminated at the scene and about 125 workers will need medical evaluation and care. The first action of the nurse receiving this report should be to
   a. issue a code blue alert.
   b. activate the hospital's emergency response plan.
   c. notify the Federal Emergency Management Agency (FEMA).
   d. arrange for the American Red Cross to provide aid to victims.

1. a, 2. b, 3. a, d, e, 4. c, 5. b

For rationales to these answers and even more NCLEX review questions, visit *http://evolve.elsevier.com/Lewis/medsurg*.

ⓔ EVOLVE WEBSITE/RESOURCES LIST

http://evolve.elsevier.com/Lewis/medsurg
Review Questions (Online Only)
Key Points
Answer Keys for Questions
- Rationales for Bridge to NCLEX Examination Questions
- Answer Guidelines for Case Study on p. 1621
- Answer Guidelines for Managing Care of Multiple Patients Case Study (Section 13) on p. 1623

Student Case Study
- Patient With Musculoskeletal Trauma

Conceptual Care Map Creator
Audio Glossary
Content Updates

REFERENCES

1. Centers for Disease Control and Prevention (CDC): Emergency department visits. Retrieved from *www.cdc.gov/nchs/fastats/emergency-department.htm*.
2. American College of Emergency Physicians: Only 5.5% of emergency visits are nonurgent and wait times continue to improve, CDC says. Retrieved from *http://newsroom.acep.org/2018-04-23-ACEP-Only-5-5-Percent-of-Emergency-Visits-Are-Nonurgent-and-Wait-Times-Continue-to-Improve-CDC-Says*.
3. Board of Certification for Emergency Nurses: Get certified—CEN. Retrieved from *www.bcencertifications.org/Get-Certified/CEN.aspx*.
4. Rund DA, Rausch TS: *Triage*, St Louis, 1981, Mosby. (Classic)
*5. Gilboy N, Tanabe P, Travers DA, et al: Emergency Severity Index (ESI): A triage tool for emergency department care. Retrieved from *www.ahrq.gov/professionals/systems/hospital/esi/esihandbk.pdf*.
6. Sweet V: Emergency nursing core curriculum, ed 7, St Louis, 2018, Elsevier.
*7. Nair SS, Surendran A, Prabhakar RB, et al: Comparison between FOUR score and GCS in assessing patients with traumatic head injury: A tertiary centre study, *Int Surg J* 4:656, 2017.
*8. Davidson JE, Aslakson RA, Long AC, et al: Guidelines for family-centered care in the neonatal, pediatric, and adult ICU, *CCM* 45:103, 2017.
*9. Motov SM, Nelson LS: Advanced concepts and controversies in emergency department pain management, *Anesthesiol Clin* 34:271, 2016.
10. Centers for Disease Control and Prevention (CDC): Tetanus: Prevention. Retrieved from *www.cdc.gov/tetanus/about/prevention.html*.
*11. Tisherman SA: Targeted temperature management after cardiac arrest: When, how deep, how long? *JTD* 9:4840, 2017.
*12. Madden LK, Hill M, May TL, et al: The implementation of targeted temperature management: An evidence-based guideline from the Neurocritical Care Society, *Neurocrit Care* 27:468, 2017.
*13. Mayer D: Improving the support of the suddenly bereaved, *Curr Opin Support Palliat Care* 11:1, 2017.
14. United Network for Organ Sharing: What every patient needs to know. Retrieved from *www.unos.org/wp-content/uploads/unos/WEPNTK.pdf*.
15. Centers for Disease Control and Prevention (CDC): National hospital ambulatory medical care survey: 2015 Emergency department summary tables. Retrieved from *www.cdc.gov/nchs/data/nhamcs/web_tables/2015_ed_web_tables.pdf*.
16. National Council on Aging: Fall prevention facts. Retrieved from *www.ncoa.org/news/resources-for-reporters/get-the-facts/falls-prevention-facts/*.
17. Handford C, Thomas O, Imray CH: Frostbite, *Emerg Med Clin North Am* 35:281, 2017.
18. Centers for Disease Control and Prevention (CDC): Unintentional drowning. Retrieved from *www.cdc.gov/homeandrecreationalsafety/water-safety/waterinjuries-factsheet.html*.
19. Centers for Disease Control and Prevention (CDC): Venomous snakes. Retrieved from *www.cdc.gov/niosh/topics/snakes/default.html*.
20. Centers for Disease Control and Prevention (CDC): Tick removal. Retrieved from *www.cdc.gov/ticks/removing_a_tick.html*.
21. Centers for Disease Control and Prevention (CDC): Rabies VIS. Retrieved from *www.cdc.gov/vaccines/hcp/vis/vis-statements/rabies.html*.
22. National Capital Poison Control Center: Act fast. Retrieved from *www.poison.org*.
*23. Nikathil S, Olaussen A, Gocentas RA, et al: Workplace violence in the emergency department: A systematic review and meta analysis, *EMA* 29:265, 2017.

*24. Emergency Nurses Association: Workplace violence. Retrieved from *www.ena.org/practice-resources/workplace-violence.*

25. Agency for Healthcare Research and Quality: Intimate partner violence screening. Retrieved from *www.ahrq.gov/professionals/prevention-chronic-care/healthier-pregnancy/preventive/partnerviolence.html.*

26. Gibbons P, Stoklosa H: Identification and treatment of human trafficking victims in the emergency department, *JEM* 50:715, 2016.

*27. Emergency Nurses Association: Joint position statement: Adult and adolescent sexual assault patients in the emergency setting. Retrieved from *www.ena.org/docs/default-source/resource-library/practice-resources/position-statements/joint-statements/adultandadolescentsexualassaultpatientser.pdf?sfvrsn=234258f1_6.*

28. Centers for Disease Control and Prevention (CDC): Anthrax. Retrieved from *www.cdc.gov/anthrax/medical-care/prevention.html.*

29. Agency for Toxic Substances and Disease Registry: Medical management guidelines for nerve agents: Tabun, sarin, soman, and VX. Retrieved from *www.atsdr.cdc.gov/mmg/mmg.asp?id=523&tid=93.*

30. Ryan JM, Doll D, Giannou C: Mass casualties and triage in military and civilian environment. In Velmahos G, Degiannis E, Doll D: *Penetrating trauma,* Berlin, 2017, Springer.

31. Department of Homeland Security: Community emergency response team. Retrieved from *www.ready.gov/community-emergency-response-team.*

*Evidence-based information for clinical practice.

CASE STUDY

Managing Care of Multiple Patients

You are working in a 12-bed ICU and have been assigned to care for the following 2 patients. There is 1 UAP available to help as needed.

Patients

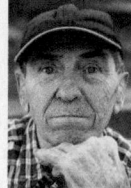

(© Thinkstock.)

R.K. is a 72-yr-old white man who was admitted with a massive stroke after collapsing at his home. He is unresponsive, even to painful stimuli. He has an oral endotracheal (ET) tube in place and is receiving mechanical ventilation (assist-control mode, FIO_2 70%, V_T 700 mL, respiratory rate 16 breaths/min, PEEP 7.5 cm H_2O). His chest x-ray shows right lower lung consolidation. A subclavian central line was placed to monitor central venous pressure (CVP) and give fluids and IV antibiotics. His cardiac rhythm on admission was atrial fibrillation with a rapid ventricular response. He is receiving IV diltiazem (Cardizem), and his ventricular response has slowed to 84 bpm. His temperature is increased despite receiving acetaminophen (Tylenol) q4hr. Enteral nutrition is running at 25 mL/hr via orogastric feeding tube. R.K. has a catheter for urinary drainage.

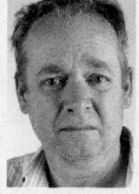

(© Thinkstock.)

J.N. is a 58-yr-old white man who was admitted 24 hours ago after emergent surgery for an acutely ischemic bowel. The surgical procedure involved extensive abdominal surgery to repair a perforated colon, irrigate the abdominal cavity, and provide hemostasis. During surgery, his systolic BP dropped to 70 mm Hg and is still in the low 90s. He is in sinus tachycardia at a rate of 128 bpm. His pulmonary status worsened over the first 24 hr in ICU. He developed a right-sided pneumothorax and a chest tube was placed at that time. His hypoxemia has rapidly progressed and is now refractory to 100% FIO_2 and 15 cm H_2O PEEP. His laboratory tests show kidney and liver failure. He has an advance directive that states he does not want to be kept alive by artificial means, but he currently is full code status. He is sedated, paralyzed, and unable to communicate. His urinary catheter is draining concentrated urine <30 mL/hr. He has a central line in place with 0.9% saline running at 125 mL/hr. His most recent ABGs are as follows: pH 7.12, PaO_2 59 mm Hg, $PaCO_2$ 62 mm Hg, HCO_3^- 17 mEq/L, and O_2 saturation 84%, and his chest x-ray shows worsening bilateral interstitial infiltrates compatible with an ARDS pattern.

Discussion Questions

1. *Priority Decision:* After receiving report, which patient should you see first? Provide rationale.
2. *Collaboration:* Which tasks could you delegate to the UAP? *(select all that apply)*
   a. Record vital signs on R.K. and J.N.
   b. Drain the water from J.N.'s ventilator tubing.
   c. Change suction tubing on R.K.'s ET tubes as needed.
   d. Titrate the diltiazem IV drip based on R.K.'s heart rate.
   e. Talk to J.N.'s family about his advance directive and current code status.
3. *Priority Decision and Collaboration:* As you are assessing J.N., the UAP informs you that R.K. just vomited all over his bed. Which *initial* action would be *most* appropriate?
   a. Ask the UAP to give R.K. a bath while you finish assessing J.N.
   b. Turn off R.K.'s enteral nutrition pump and auscultate his breath sounds.
   c. Ask the UAP to inform the HCP about J.N.'s ABG results while you assess R.K.
   d. Finish assessing R.K., then suction R.K.'s endotracheal tube to remove any emesis.

Case Study Progression

R.K.'s lungs are clear to auscultation. Evaluation of his GI status reveals minimal bowel sounds and a gastric residual of 200 mL even after his emesis. You elevate the head of his bed to 60 degrees, place the enteral nutrition on hold, and notify his HCP.

4. Which intervention would you expect the HCP to order for R.K.?
   a. Morphine sulfate 2 mg IV stat
   b. Metoclopramide (Reglan) 10 mg IV every 6 hr
   c. Restart enteral nutrition and maintain HOB elevation at 90 degrees
   d. Hold enteral nutrition for 1 hour and restart with half-strength fluid at same rate
5. J.N.'s ABG results reflect a worsening of his ARDS. You correctly identify that these results demonstrate
   a. uncompensated respiratory acidosis.
   b. uncompensated respiratory alkalosis.
   c. partially compensated respiratory acidosis.
   d. partially compensated respiratory alkalosis.
6. Calculate and interpret J.N.'s PaO_2/FIO_2 ratio.
7. What aspects of care would be the same for J.N. and R.K. since they are both receiving mechanical ventilation? *(select all that apply)*
   a. Obtaining daily arterial blood gasses.
   b. Monitoring pulse oximetry continuously.
   c. Administering an IV proton-pump inhibitor.
   d. Suctioning the endotracheal tube every 2 hours.
   e. Applying intermittent pneumatic compression stockings.
8. *Management Decision:* You walk into J.N.'s room and find his wife whispering in his ear with her hand on the ventilator tubing, appearing to be ready to disconnect him from life support. What is your *best* initial action?
   a. Ask J.N.'s wife to leave the room immediately.
   b. Report the incident to the charge nurse and security at once.
   c. Ask J.N.'s wife if you could talk to her about her husband's condition.
   d. Report the incident to J.N.'s health care provider to address J.N.'s code status.

Answers and rationales available at *http://evolve.elsevier.com/Lewis.*

Basic Life Support for Health Care Providers

Mariann M. Harding

Basic life support (BLS) for health care professionals consists of a series of actions and skills performed by the rescuer(s) based on assessment findings. The first action the rescuer performs upon finding an adult victim is assessing for responsiveness. This is done by tapping or shaking the victim's shoulder and asking, "Are you all right?" If the victim does not respond, simultaneously scan the victim's chest for signs of breathing and perform a pulse check (described later).

If the rescuer is alone, the rescuer shouts for help. If someone responds, the rescuer asks him or her to activate the *emergency response system* (ERS) (e.g., through the use of a mobile phone) and get an *automatic external defibrillator* (AED) (if available). If no one responds and the rescuer does not have a mobile phone, the rescuer should leave to activate the ERS, get an AED (if available), and return to the victim before beginning *cardiopulmonary resuscitation* (CPR) and defibrillation if necessary.[1]

CARDIOPULMONARY RESUSCITATION

Cardiac arrest is characterized by the absence of a pulse and breathing in an unconscious victim. The current approach for CPR is the chest *compressions-airway-breathing* (CAB) sequence.[1]

The first step in CPR is to perform a pulse check by palpating the carotid pulse for at least 5 but no more than 10 seconds. While maintaining a head-tilt position with 1 hand on the victim's forehead, locate the victim's trachea using 2 or 3 fingers of your other hand. Slide these fingers into the groove between the trachea and neck muscles where the carotid pulse can be felt. The technique is more easily performed on the side nearest you.

If a pulse is felt, give 1 rescue breath every 5 to 6 seconds (10 to 12 breaths/min) and recheck the pulse every 2 minutes (Fig. A.1). If no pulse is felt, start CAB.[1,2]

Chest Compressions

The proper technique for providing chest compressions is shown in Fig. A.2. Chest compression technique consists of fast and deep applications of pressure on the lower half of the sternum. The victim must be in the supine position when compressions are performed. The victim must be lying on a flat, hard surface, such as a CPR board (specially designed for use in CPR), a headboard from a unit bed, or, if necessary, the floor. Position yourself close to the side of the victim's chest. More frequently, mechanical chest compression devices are being used to provide chest compressions both prehospital and in the emergency department.

Chest compressions are combined with rescue breathing for an effective resuscitation effort of the adult victim of cardiac arrest. The compression-to-ventilation ratio for 1- or 2-rescuer CPR is 30 compressions to 2 breaths (Table A.1). However, if the patient has an advanced airway (e.g., endotracheal tube, laryngeal mask airway), do not pause between compressions for breaths and deliver 1 breath every 6 seconds (10 breaths/min).[1]

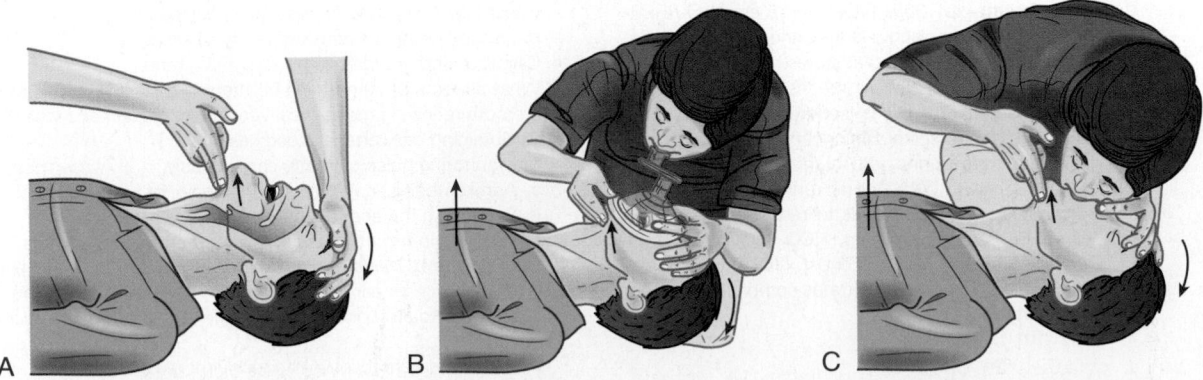

FIG. A.1 The head tilt–chin lift maneuver is used to open the victim's airway to give rescue breaths. **A,** Rescuer places 1 hand on the victim's forehead and applies firm, backward pressure with the palm to tilt the head back. The chin is lifted and brought forward with the fingers of the other hand. **B,** Mouth-to-barrier device: Rescuer places the device tightly over the victim's mouth and nose and delivers a regular breath. **C,** Mouth-to-mouth technique: Rescuer pinches the victim's nostrils, tightly seals mouth over victim's mouth, and delivers a regular breath. *NOTE:* Rescuer should observe for a rise in the victim's chest *(black arrows)*.

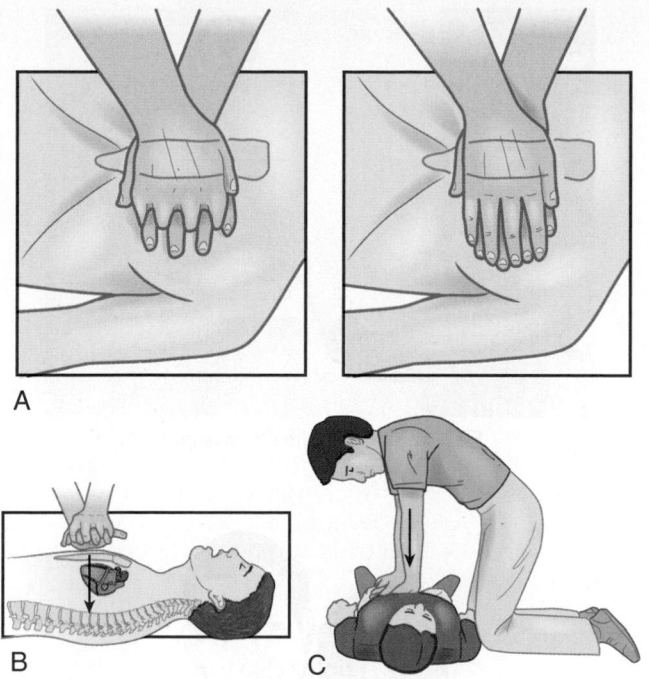

FIG. A.2 CPR. **A,** Position of the hands on the lower half of the sternum during chest compressions. **B,** When pressure is applied, the sternum is displaced posteriorly with the heel of the hand. **C,** Arms are kept straight, and the rescuer pushes deep (at least 2 in [5 cm]) and fast (a rate of 100 to 120 compressions per minute).

If a mechanical chest compression device is not used, it is preferable to have 2 persons performing CPR. One rescuer, positioned at the victim's side, performs chest compressions while the second rescuer, positioned at the victim's head, maintains an open airway and performs ventilations. To maintain the quality and rate of compressions, rescuers should change roles every 2 minutes.[2] Interruptions in CPR should be limited.

Defibrillation

When the AED or advanced cardiovascular life support (ACLS) team arrives, assess the victim's rhythm. If the victim has a shockable rhythm (e.g., ventricular tachycardia, ventricular fibrillation), deliver 1 shock and immediately resume CPR for about 2 minutes before checking the rhythm again. If the rhythm is not a shockable rhythm, immediately resume CPR and recheck the rhythm after 2 minutes. CPR should continue between rhythm checks and shocks and until the ACLS team arrives or the victim shows signs of movement.[1]

The American Heart Association includes training in the use of AEDs with BLS instruction of HCPs and laypersons. Survival from cardiac arrest is the highest when immediate CPR is provided and defibrillation occurs within 3 to 5 minutes.[2] AEDs are found in many out-of-hospital, public settings (Fig. A.3).

Airway and Breathing

If a victim has a pulse but is gasping (e.g., agonal breathing) or not breathing, establish an open airway and begin rescue breathing. Open an adult's airway by hyperextending the head (Fig. A.1). Use the *head tilt–chin lift maneuver.* This involves tilting the head back with 1 hand and lifting the chin forward with the fingers of the other hand. Use the *jaw-thrust maneuver* if you suspect a cervical spine injury (see Fig. 68.1). Try to

---

TABLE A.1 Adult 1- and 2-Rescuer Basic Life Support With Automatic External Defibrillator (AED)

Assess
- Determine unresponsiveness: tap or shake victim's shoulder; shout, "Are you all right?"
- Check for no breathing or abnormal breathing (e.g., gasping) while simultaneously performing a pulse check (5–10 sec).

Activate Emergency Response System (ERS)
- Activate ERS (e.g., call 911) and get the AED (if available) (outside of hospital).
- Call a code and ask for the AED or crash cart (in hospital).

Begin High-Quality CPR
- If victim has a pulse but is not breathing or not breathing adequately, begin rescue breathing at a rate of 1 breath every 3–5 sec, or about 12–20/min (Fig. A.1). Recheck the pulse every 2 min.*
- If there is no pulse, expose the victim's chest and immediately begin chest compressions (Fig. A.2).
- Deliver compressions at a rate of 100–120/min.
- Compress the chest at least 2 in (5 cm) but not greater than 2.4 in (6 cm).
- Allow for complete chest recoil after each compression.
- Deliver a compression-ventilation ratio of 30 compressions to 2 breaths.†
- Minimize interruptions in compressions by delivering the 2 breaths in <10 sec.

Deliver Effective Breaths
- Open airway adequately (Fig. A.1, *A*).
- Deliver breath to produce a visible chest rise (Fig. A.1, *B, C*).
- Avoid excessive ventilation.

Integrate Prompt Use of the AED
- Use AED as soon as possible.
- If rhythm is shockable, deliver 1 shock and then resume chest compressions immediately after delivery of shock.
- If the rhythm is not shockable, resume CPR and recheck rhythm every 5 cycles.

Continue CPR
- Continue CPR between rhythm checks and shocks, and until ACLS providers arrive or the victim shows signs of movement.

Source: American Heart Association: *BLS for healthcare providers: student manual,* Dallas, 2015, The Association.
ACLS, Advanced cardiovascular life support.
*If possible opioid overdose, give naloxone if available and per protocol.
†For patients with ongoing CPR and an advanced airway in place, a ventilation rate of 1 breath every 6 seconds (10 breaths per minute) with no interruption in compressions is recommended.

---

provide ventilation to the victim using a mouth-to-barrier (recommended) device (e.g., face mask or bag-valve-mask) or mouth-to-mouth resuscitation (Fig. A.1, *B, C*).[2]

For mouth-to-mouth resuscitation give ventilations with the victim's nostrils pinched. Take a regular (not deep) breath and tightly seal your lips around the victim's mouth. Give 1 breath and watch for a rise in the victim's chest. Continue rescue breaths at a rate of 10 to 12 per minute. When the victim has a tracheostomy, give ventilations through the stoma.

If the victim cannot be ventilated, proceed with CPR. When providing the next rescue breaths, look for any objects in the victim's mouth. If any objects are visible, remove them (Table A.2).

TABLE A.2 Management of the Adult Choking Victim

Conscious Adult Choking Victim

Assess Victim for Severe Airway Obstruction
  Look for any of the following signs:
- Poor or no air exchange
- Clutching the neck with the hands, making the universal choking sign
- Weak, ineffective cough or no cough at all
- High-pitched noise while inhaling or no noise at all
- Increased respiratory difficulty
- Possible cyanosis

  Ask the victim if he or she is choking. If the victim nods yes and cannot talk or has any of the symptoms noted above, severe airway obstruction is present and you must take immediate action.

Abdominal Thrusts (Heimlich Maneuver) With Standing or Sitting Victim (Fig. A.4)

1. Stand or kneel behind victim and wrap arms around the victim's waist.
2. Make fist with 1 hand.
3. Place thumb side of fist against victim's abdomen. Position fist midline, slightly above navel and well below breastbone.
4. Grasp fist with other hand and press fist into victim's abdomen with a quick, forceful upward thrust.
5. Give each new thrust with a separate, distinct movement to relieve the obstruction. *Caution:* If victim is pregnant or obese, give chest thrusts instead of abdominal thrusts. Position hands (as described) over lower portion of the breastbone and apply quick backward thrusts.
6. Repeat thrusts until object is expelled or victim becomes unresponsive.

Unconscious Adult Choking Victim

If you see a choking victim collapse and become unresponsive:
1. Activate the emergency response system.
2. Lower the victim to the ground and begin CPR, starting with compressions (do not check for a pulse).
3. Open the victim's mouth wide each time you prepare to give breaths. Look for the object. If you see the object and can easily remove it, do so with your fingers. If you do not see the object, continue with CPR using the chest compression–airway–breathing sequence (Table A.1).
4. If efforts to ventilate are unsuccessful, continue with CPR.

Source: American Heart Association: *BLS for healthcare providers: Student manual*, Dallas, 2015, The Association.

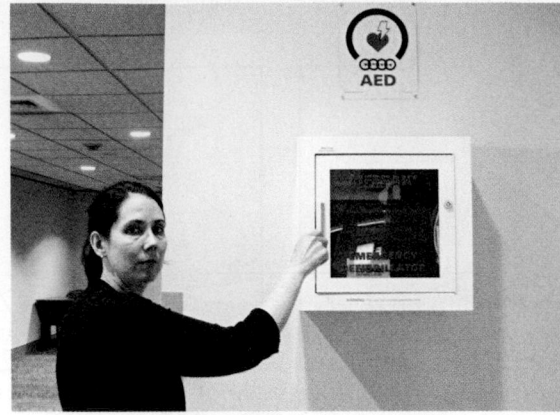

FIG. A.3 AED located in an airport.

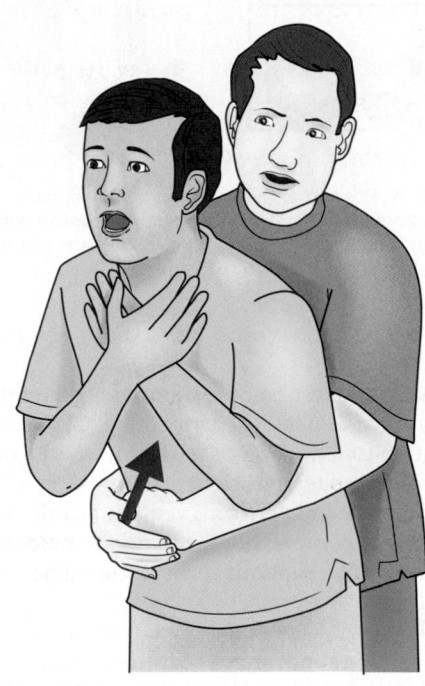

FIG. A.4 Abdominal thrusts (Heimlich maneuver) administered to a conscious (standing) choking victim.

HANDS-ONLY CPR

Hands-only CPR can be used to help adult victims who suddenly collapse from cardiac arrest outside of a health care setting. If an untrained person witnesses the event, the person should provide compression-only CPR. If you are trained and witness the event (as a bystander), you should provide conventional CPR (described previously). If you are unable to do so, provide chest compressions only (push fast and deep in the center of the chest). Both methods are effective when done in the first few minutes of an out-of-hospital cardiac arrest.[1]

REFERENCES*

1. American Heart Association: *Highlights of the 2015 American Heart Association guidelines update for CPR and ECC*, Dallas, 2015, The Association.
2. American Heart Association: *BLS for healthcare providers: Student manual*, Dallas, 2015, The Association.

*CPR guidelines are updated on an ongoing basis and are available at *https://eccguidelines.heart.org/index.php/circulation/cpr-ecc-guidelines-2*.

Nursing Diagnoses

1. Activity Intolerance: Lack of ability or energy to endure or complete daily activities.
2. Acute Confusion: Confusion occurring abruptly, over a short time interval.
3. Acute Pain: Pain occurring abruptly, over a short time interval.
4. Altered Blood Pressure: Any change in the systolic or diastolic BP.
5. Altered Perception: Change in the response to sensory stimuli, awareness of objects, or other data through the senses.
6. Anxiety: Feelings of threat, fear, apprehension, danger, or distress.
7. Chronic Pain: Pain occurring over time, long-standing.
8. Confusion: Memory impairment with disorientation in relation to person, place, or time.
9. Constipation: Decrease in the frequency of defecation accompanied by difficult or incomplete passage of stool; passage of excessively hard, dry stool.
10. Death Anxiety: Anxiety associated with the awareness of death.
11. Decreased Intracranial Adaptive Capacity: Compromised intracranial fluid volumes.
12. Diarrhea: Passage of loose, liquid, unformed stools, increased frequency of elimination accompanied by increased bowel sounds, cramping, and urgency of defecation.
13. Difficulty Coping: Inadequate personal ability to manage problems, stress, or responsibilities.
14. Disturbed Body Image: Disturbance in the mental picture of one's own body or physical appearance.
15. Electrolyte Imbalance: High or low serum electrolyte levels.
16. Fatigue: Feelings of decreased strength or endurance, weariness, mental or physical tiredness, and listlessness with lower capacity for physical or mental work.
17. Fluid Imbalance: Any change in or modification of body fluid balance.
18. Hyperglycemia: Increased serum glucose levels.
19. Hyperthermia: Increased body temperature.
20. Hypoglycemia: Decreased serum glucose levels.
21. Hypothermia: Reduced body temperature.
22. Impaired Airway Clearance: Impaired ability to keep air passage open from mouth to lung alveoli due to inability to clear secretions or obstructions from the respiratory tract.
23. Impaired Breathing: Inadequate inhalation or exhalation.
24. Impaired Cardiac Output: Any change in or modification of the pumping action of the heart.
25. Impaired Communication: Impediment or blockage to exchanging thoughts, messages, or information.
26. Impaired Gas Exchange: Impairment of the alveolar exchange of oxygen and carbon dioxide.
27. Impaired Hearing: Change in the ability to hear.
28. Impaired Nutritional Intake: Impaired ability to take in nutrients necessary for growth, normal functioning, and maintaining of life.
29. Impaired Nutritional Status: Impairment of weight and body mass in relation to intake of nutrition and specific nutrients estimated according to height, body build, and age.
30. Impaired Peripheral Neurovascular Function: Change in or modification of neurovascularization of the extremities.
31. Impaired Mobility: Diminished ability to perform independent movement.
32. Impaired Respiratory System Function: Any change in respiratory system function that influences oxygenation and breathing.
33. Impaired Sexual Functioning: Change negatively affecting a person's sexual response and the ability to participate in intercourse.
34. Impaired Sleep Pattern: Imbalance in the normal sleep/wake cycle.
35. Impaired Tissue Integrity: Damage, inflammation, or lesion to the skin or underlying structures.
36. Ineffective Tissue Perfusion: Change in the movement of blood through periphery tissues resulting in ineffective delivery of oxygen, fluids, and nutrients at the cellular level.
37. Impaired Urinary System Function: Any change in urinary system function that affects the ability to excrete waste.
38. Lack of Knowledge: Lack of information, understanding, skills, or comprehension.
39. Nausea: Sensation of feeling sick with an inclination to vomit.
40. Obesity: Condition of high body weight and body mass usually of more than 20% over ideal weight, abnormal increase in proportion of fat cells mainly in viscera and subcutaneous tissues.
41. Risk for Aspiration: Risk for inhaling gastric or external substances into the trachea or lungs.
42. Risk for Bleeding: Risk for loss of blood, externally or internally.
43. Risk for Fall-Related Injury: Risk for injury from the descent of a body from higher to lower level.
44. Risk for Infection: Risk for invasion of the body by pathogenic microorganisms that cause disease.
45. Risk for Injury: Risk for intentional or accidental physical harm or damage to tissues.

46. Sleep Deprivation: Lack of a normal sleep/wake cycle.
47. Substance Abuse: Misuse of chemically active substance for a nontherapeutic effect that may be harmful to health and cause addiction.
48. Surgical Wound: Cut of tissue made by sharp surgical instrument to create an opening into a body space or an organ.
49. Urinary Retention: Involuntary accumulation of urine in the bladder or incomplete emptying of the bladder.
50. Vomiting: Expulsion of stomach contents through the esophagus and out of mouth.

REFERENCES

International Council of Nurses: *ICNP*—*English*, Geneva, 2017, The Association.

International Council of Nurses: International Classification for Nursing Practice catalogue: CCC-ICNP equivalency table for nursing diagnoses. Retrieved from *www.icn.ch/sites/default/files/inline-files/CCC-ICNP_Equivalency_Table_for_Nursing_Diagnoses.pdf*.

International Council of Nurses: Nursing diagnoses and outcome statements. Retrieved from *www.icn.ch/sites/default/files/inline-files/icnp2017-dc.pdf*.

Laboratory Reference Intervals

The tables in this appendix list some of the most common tests, their reference intervals (formally referred to as *normal values*), and possible etiologies of abnormal results. Laboratory results may vary depending on different techniques or different laboratories. Abbreviations appearing in the tables are defined as follows:

mEq = milliequivalent
mm Hg = millimeter of mercury
mm = millimeter
mOsm = milliosmole
L = liter
dL = deciliter (10^{-1} liter)
mL = milliliter (10^{-3} liter)
μL = microliter (10^{-6} liter, 10^{-3} milliliter)
fL = femtoliter (10^{-15} liter, 10^{-12} milliliter)
g = gram

mg = milligram (10^{-3} gram)
mcg = microgram (10^{-6} gram)
ng = nanogram (10^{-9} gram)
pg = picogram (10^{-12} gram)
U = unit
μU = microunit
IU = international unit
mU = milliunit
mmol = millimole (10^{-3} mole)
μmol = micromole (10^{-6} mole)
nmol = nanomole (10^{-9} mole)
pmol = picomole (10^{-12} mole)
kPa = kilopascal
μkat = microkatal

Source: Rafai N, Horvath AR ER, Wittwer CT: *Tietz textbook of clinical chemistry and molecular diagnostics*, ed 6, St Louis, 2018, Elsevier.

TABLE C.1 Serum, Plasma, and Whole Blood Chemistries

Test	REFERENCE INTERVALS		POSSIBLE ETIOLOGY	
	Conventional Units	SI Units	High	Low
Aldolase	22–59 mU/L	22–59 mU/L	Skeletal muscle disease	Muscle-wasting disease
α_1-Antitrypsin	85–213 mg/dL	0. 85–2.13 g/L	Acute and chronic inflammation, arthritis	Early-onset emphysema, malnutrition, nephrotic syndrome
α_1-Fetoprotein	<40 ng/mL	<40 mcg/L	Cancer of testes, ovaries, and liver	
Ammonia	10–80 mcg/dL	6–47 µmol/L	Severe liver disease	
Amylase	60–120 Somogyi U/dL	30–220 U/L	Acute and chronic pancreatitis, salivary gland disease, perforated ulcers	Acute alcoholism, cirrhosis of liver, extensive destruction of pancreas
Bicarbonate	21–28 mEq/L	21–28 mmol/L	Compensated respiratory acidosis, metabolic alkalosis	Compensated respiratory alkalosis, metabolic acidosis
b-Type natriuretic peptide (BNP)	<100 pg/mL	<100 pmol/L	Heart failure	
Bilirubin			Biliary obstruction, hemolytic anemia, impaired liver function, pernicious anemia	
• Total	0.3–1.0 mg/dL	5.1–17 µmol/L		
• Indirect	0.2–0.8 mg/dL	3.4–12.0 µmol/L		
• Direct	0.1–0.3 mg/dL	1.7–5.1 µmol/L		
Blood gases*				
• Arterial pH	7.35–7.45	7.35–7.45	Alkalosis	Acidosis
• Venous pH	7.31–7.41	7.31–7.41		
• $PaCO_2$	35–45 mm Hg	4.66–5.98 kPa	Compensated metabolic alkalosis	Compensated metabolic acidosis
• $PvCO_2$	40–50 mm Hg	5.06–7.32 kPa	Respiratory acidosis	Respiratory alkalosis
• PaO_2	80–100 mm Hg	10.6–13.33 kPa	Administration of high concentration of O_2	Chronic lung disease, decreased cardiac output
• PvO_2	40–50 mm Hg	5.04–5.57 kPa		
Calcium (total)	9.0–10.5 mg/dL	2.25–2.62 mmol/L	Hyperthyroidism, hyperparathyroidism, vitamin D intoxication, multiple myeloma	Pancreatitis, hypoparathyroidism, malabsorption syndrome, renal failure, vitamin D deficiency
Calcium (ionized)	4.5–5.6 mg/dL	1.05–1.3 mmol/L	Acidosis	Alkalosis
Chloride	98–106 mEq/L	98–106 mmol/L	Metabolic acidosis, respiratory alkalosis, corticosteroid therapy, uremia	Addison's disease, vomiting, metabolic alkalosis, respiratory acidosis

Continued

TABLE C.1 Serum, Plasma, and Whole Blood Chemistries—cont'd

Test	REFERENCE INTERVALS		POSSIBLE ETIOLOGY	
	Conventional Units	SI Units	High	Low
Cholesterol	<200 mg/dL	<5.2 mmol/L	Biliary obstruction, hypothyroidism, idiopathic hypercholesterolemia, renal disease, uncontrolled diabetes	Extensive liver disease, hyperthyroidism, malnutrition, malabsorption
• High-density lipoproteins (HDLs)	*Male:* >45 mg/dL *Female:* >55 mg/dL	*Male:* >0.75 mmol/L *Female:* >0.91 mmol/L	Excessive exercise	Metabolic syndrome, liver disease
• Low-density lipoproteins (LDLs)	*Recommended:* <130 mg/dL		Chronic liver disease, familial hypercholesterolemia, nephrotic syndrome	Hyperthyroidism
• Very low-density lipoproteins (VLDLs)	7–32 mg/dL		Familial hypercholesterolemia, nephrotic syndrome	Hyperthyroidism
Cortisol	8 AM: 5–23 mcg/dL 4 PM: 3–13 mcg/dL	8 AM: 138–635 nmol/L 4 PM: 83–359 nmol/L	Cushing syndrome, hyperthyroidism	Adrenal insufficiency, panhypopituitary states
Creatine kinase (CK)	*Male:* 55–170 U/L *Female:* 30–135 U/L	*Male:* 55–170 U/L *Female:* 30–135 U/L	Musculoskeletal injury or disease, myocardial infarction, severe myocarditis, exercise, numerous IM injections	
• CK-MB	<4%–6% of total CK	<0.4–0.6	Acute myocardial infarction	
Creatinine	*Male:* 0.6–1.2 mg/dL *Female:* 0.5–1.1 mg/dL	*Male:* 53–106 µmol/L *Female:* 44–97 µmol/L	Severe renal disease	Decreased muscle mass, dehabilitation
Ferritin	*Male:* 12-300 ng/mL *Female:* 10-150 ng/mL	*Male:* 12–300 mcg/L *Female:* 10-150 mcg/L	Anemia of chronic disease, sideroblastic anemia	Iron-deficiency anemia
Folic acid (folate)	5–25 ng/mL	11–57 nmol/L	Hypothyroidism, pernicious anemia	Alcoholism, hemolytic anemia, inadequate diet, malabsorption syndrome, megaloblastic anemia
γ-Glutamyl transferase (GGT)	*Male and Female >45:* 8–38 U/L *Female <45:* 5–27 U/L	*Male and Female >45:* 8–38 U/L *Female <45:* 5–27 U/L	Liver disease, infectious myocardial infarction, pancreatitis, hyperthyroidism	Hypothyroidism
Glucose (fasting)	74–106 mg/dL	4.1–5.9 mmol/L	Acute stress, Cushing disease, diabetes, hyperthyroidism, pancreatic insufficiency	Addison's disease, hepatic disease, hypothyroidism, insulin overdosage, pancreatic tumor, pituitary hypofunction
Haptoglobin	50–220 mg/dL	0.5–2.2 g/L	Infectious and inflammatory processes, cancer	Hemolytic anemia, malnutrition, chronic liver disease
Insulin (fasting)	6–26 µU/mL	43–186 pmol/L	Acromegaly, adenoma of pancreatic islet cells, Cushing syndrome	Diabetes, hypopituitarism
Iron, total	*Male:* 80–180 mcg/dL *Female:* 60-160 mcg/dL	*Male:* 14–32 µmol/L *Female:* 11–29 µmol/L	Excess RBC destruction, hepatitis, massive blood transfusion	Anemia of chronic disease, iron-deficiency anemia, cancer
(Total) iron-binding capacity	250–460 mcg/dL	45–82 µmol/L	Iron-deficient state, polycythemia	Cirrhosis, chronic infections, pernicious anemia
Lactic acid (L-Lactate), venous	5–20 mg/dL	0.6–2.2 mmol/L	Acidosis, liver disease, sepsis, shock	
Lactic dehydrogenase (LDH)	100–190 U/L	100–190 U/L	Heart failure, hemolytic disorders, hepatitis, metastatic cancer of liver, myocardial infarction, pernicious anemia, pulmonary embolus, skeletal muscle damage	
Lactic dehydrogenase isoenzymes				
• LDH$_1$	17%–27%	0.17–0.27	Myocardial infarction, pernicious anemia	
• LDH$_2$	27%–37%	0.27–0.37	Pulmonary embolus, sickle cell crisis	
• LDH$_3$	18%–25%	0.18–0.25	Malignant lymphoma, pulmonary embolus	
• LDH$_4$	3%–8%	0.03–0.08	Systemic lupus erythematosus, pulmonary infarction	

TABLE C.1 **Serum, Plasma, and Whole Blood Chemistries—cont'd**

Test	REFERENCE INTERVALS		POSSIBLE ETIOLOGY	
	Conventional Units	SI Units	High	Low
• LDH$_5$	0%–5%	0.00–0.05	Heart failure, hepatitis, pulmonary embolus and infarction, skeletal muscle damage	
Lipase	0–160 U/L	0–160 U/L	Acute pancreatitis, hepatic disorders, perforated peptic ulcer	
Magnesium	1.3–2.1 mEq/L	0.65–1.05 mmol/L	Addison's disease, hypothyroidism, renal failure	Chronic alcoholism, severe malabsorption
Osmolality	285–295 mOsm/kg	285–295 mmol/kg	Chronic renal disease, diabetes, diabetes insipidus	Addison's disease, diuretic therapy, SIADH, hypervolemia
O$_2$ saturation (arterial) (SaO$_2$)	>95%	>0.95	Polycythemia	Anemia, cardiac decompensation, respiratory disorders
Phosphatase, alkaline	30–120 U/L	0.5–2.0 μkat/L	Biliary system obstruction, bone diseases, marked hyperparathyroidism, rickets	Excess vitamin D ingestion, hypothyroidism
Phosphorus (phosphate)	3.0–4.5 mg/dL	0.97–1.45 mmol/L	Bone cancer, hypoparathyroidism, renal disease, vitamin D intoxication, hypocalcemia	Diabetes, hyperparathyroidism, vitamin D deficiency
Potassium	3.5–5.0 mEq/L	3.5–5.0 mmol/L	Addison's disease, diabetic ketosis, massive tissue destruction, renal failure, infection, dehydration	Cushing syndrome, diarrhea (severe), diuretic therapy, gastrointestinal fistula, starvation, vomiting
Progesterone (Female)				
• Follicular phase	<50 ng/dL	0.5–2.2 nmol/L	Adrenal hyperplasia, choriocarcinoma of ovary, pregnancy, cysts of ovary	Threatened abortion, hypogonadism, amenorrhea, ovarian tumor
• Luteal phase	300-2500 ng/dL	6.4–79.5 nmol/L		
• Postmenopause	<40 ng/dL	1.28 nmol/L		
Prostate-specific antigen (PSA)	<4.0 ng/ml	<4.0 mcg/L	Prostate cancer, prostatitis, benign prostatic hypertrophy	
Proteins			Burns, cirrhosis (globulin fraction), dehydration	Liver disease, malabsorption
• Total	6.4–8.3 g/dL	64–83 g/L		
• Albumin	3.5–5.0 g/dL	35–50 g/L		
• Globulin	2.3–3.4 g/dL	23–34 g/L		
• Albumin/globulin ratio	1.5:1–2.5:1	1.5:1–2.5:1	Multiple myeloma (globulin fraction), shock, vomiting	Malnutrition, nephrotic syndrome, proteinuria, renal disease, severe burns
Sodium	136–145 mEq/L	136–145 mmol/L	Dehydration, impaired renal function, primary aldosteronism, corticosteroid therapy	Addison's disease, diabetic ketoacidosis, diuretic therapy, excessive loss from GI tract, excessive perspiration, water intoxication
Testosterone (total)	Male: 280–1080 ng/dL Female: <70 ng/dL	Male: 280–1080 ng/dL Female: <70 ng/dL	Hyperthyroidism Polycystic ovary, virilizing tumors	Hypofunction of testes, hypogonadism
T$_4$ (thyroxine), total	Male: 4–12 mcg/dL Female: 5–12 mcg/dL	Male: 59–135 nmol/L Female: 71–142 nmol/L	Hyperthyroidism, thyroiditis, hepatitis, Graves' disease, thyroid cancer	Cretinism, hypothyroidism, myxedema, Cushing syndrome, renal failure
T$_4$ (thyroxine), free	0.8–2.8 ng/dL	10–36 pmol/L		
T$_3$ uptake	24%–34%	0.24–0.34	Hyperthyroidism	Hypothyroidism
T$_3$ (triiodothyronine), total	Age 20–50: 70–205 ng/dL Age >50: 40–180 ng/dL	1.2–3.4 nmol/L 0.60–2.8 nmol/L	Hyperthyroidism	Hypothyroidism
Thyroid-stimulating hormone (TSH)	2.0–10 μU/mL	2.0–10 mU/L	Myxedema, primary hypothyroidism	Secondary hypothyroidism, hyperthyroidism
Transaminases				
• Aspartate aminotransferase (AST)	0–35 U/L	0–0.58 μkat/L	Liver disease, myocardial infarction, pulmonary infarction, acute hepatitis	Acute renal disease, diabetic ketoacidosis
• Alanine aminotransferase (ALT)	4–36 U/L	4–36 U/L	Liver disease, shock	
Transferrin	Male: 215–365 mg/dL Female: 250–380 mg/dL	Male: 2.15–3.65 g/L Female: 2.5–3.8 g/L	Iron-deficiency anemia, polycythemia vera	Cirrhosis, pernicious anemia, sickle cell disease
Transferrin saturation (%)	Male: 20%–50% Female: 15%–50%	Male: 20%–50% Female: 15%–50%	Hemolytic anemia, iron overdose	Malnutrition

Continued

TABLE C.1 Serum, Plasma, and Whole Blood Chemistries—cont'd

| Test | REFERENCE INTERVALS | | POSSIBLE ETIOLOGY | |
	Conventional Units	SI Units	High	Low
Triglycerides	*Male*: 40–160 mg/dL *Female*: 35–135 mg/dL	*Male*: 0.45–1.81 g/L *Female*: 0.40–1.52 g/L	Diabetes, hyperlipidemia, hypothy-roidism, liver disease	Malnutrition
Troponins (cardiac)			Myocardial infarction, myocardial injury	
• Troponin T (cTnT)	<0.1 ng/mL	<0.1 mcg/L		
• Troponin I (cTnI)	<0.03 ng/mL	<0.03 mcg/L		
Urea nitrogen (BUN)	10–20 mg/dL	3.6–7.1 mmol/L	Increase in protein catabolism (fever, sepsis, stress), renal disease, heart failure, myocardial infarction	Malnutrition, severe liver damage
Uric acid	*Male:* 4.0–8.5 mg/dL *Female:* 2.7–7.3 mg/dL	*Male:* 0.24–0.51 mmol/L *Female:* 0.16–0.43 mmol/L	Gout, gross tissue destruction, high-protein weight reduction diet, leukemia, renal failure	Administration of uricosuric drugs
Vitamin B$_{12}$ (cobalamin)	160–950 pg/mL	118–701 pmol/L	Chronic myeloid leukemia	Strict vegetarianism, malabsorption syndrome, pernicious anemia, total or partial gastrectomy
Vitamin C (ascorbic acid)	0.4–2.0 mg/dL	23–114 µmol/L	Excessive ingestion of vitamin C	Connective tissue disorders, hepatic disease, renal disease, rheumatic fever, vitamin C deficiency
Vitamin D	25–80 ng/dL	25–80 ng/dL	Excess dietary supplement	Liver disease, malabsorption syndromes, osteoporosis, renal disease

*Because arterial blood gases are influenced by altitude, the value for PaO$_2$ decreases as altitude increases. The lower value is normal for an altitude of 1 mile.
PaCO$_2$, Partial pressure of CO$_2$ in arterial blood; *PaO$_2$*, partial pressure of oxygen in arterial blood; *PvCO$_2$*, partial pressure of CO$_2$ in venous blood; *PvO$_2$*, partial pressure of oxygen in venous blood; *RBC*, red blood cell; *SaO$_2$*, arterial oxygen saturation.

TABLE C.2 Hematology

Test	REFERENCE INTERVALS		POSSIBLE ETIOLOGY	
	Conventional Units	SI Units	High	Low
Bleeding time	1–9 min	60–540 sec	Aspirin ingestion, ineffective platelet function, thrombocytopenia, vascular disease, von Willebrand disease	
Activated partial thromboplastin time (aPTT)	30–40 sec*	30–40 sec*	Deficiency of factors I, II, V, VIII, IX, X, XI, XII; hemophilia, heparin therapy, liver disease	Early DIC, extensive cancer
Prothrombin time (protime, PT)	11–12.5 sec*	11–12.5 sec*	Deficiency of factors I, II, V, VII, and X; liver disease; vitamin K deficiency; warfarin therapy	
Fibrinogen	200–400 mg/dL	2–4 g/L	Burns (after first 36 hr), inflammatory disease, stroke, myocardial infarction	Burns (during first 36 hr), DIC, severe liver disease, malnutrition
Fibrin split (degradation) products	<10 mcg/mL	<10 mg/L	Acute DIC, massive hemorrhage, primary fibrinolysis	
D-Dimer	<250 ng/mL	<250 mcg/L	DIC, myocardial infarction, VTE, unstable angina, cancer	
Erythrocyte count† (altitude dependent)	*Male:* 4.7–6.1 × 10⁶/μL *Female:* 4.2–5.4 × 10⁶/μL	*Male:* 4.7–6.1 × 10¹²/L *Female:* 4.2–5.4 × 10¹²/L	Dehydration, high altitudes, polycythemia vera, severe COPD	Anemia, leukemia, hemorrhage, cancer, chronic illness, kidney disease
Red blood indices				
• Mean corpuscular volume (MCV)	80–95 fL	80–95 fL	Alcoholism, liver disease, macrocytic anemia	Microcytic anemia, thalassemia
• Mean corpuscular hemoglobin (MCH)	27–31 pg	27–31 pg	Macrocytic anemia	Microcytic anemia
• Mean corpuscular hemoglobin concentration (MCHC)	32%–36%	32–36 g/dL	Spherocytosis	Iron deficiency anemia, thalassemia
Erythrocyte sedimentation rate (ESR)	<20 mm/hr (some gender variation)	<20 mm/hr (some gender variation)	*Moderate increase:* acute hepatitis, myocardial infarction; rheumatoid arthritis *Marked increase:* acute and severe bacterial infections, cancer, pelvic inflammatory disease	Malaria, severe liver disease, sickle cell anemia
Hematocrit† (altitude dependent)	*Male:* 42%–52% *Female:* 37%–47%	*Male:* 0.42–0.52 *Female:* 0.37–0.47	Dehydration, high altitudes, polycythemia, COPD	Anemia, hemorrhage, overhydration, cirrhosis, kidney disease
Hemoglobin† (altitude dependent)	*Male:* 14–18 g/dL *Female:* 12–16 g/dL	*Male:* 140–180 g/L *Female:* 120–160 g/L	COPD, high altitudes, polycythemia, dehydration, burns	Anemia, hemorrhage, kidney disease, cancer
Hemoglobin, glycosylated (A1C)	4.0%–5.6%	4.0%–5.6%	Diabetes, pre-diabetes	Sickle cell anemia, chronic renal failure, pregnancy
Platelets (thrombocytes)	150–400 × 10³/μL	150–400 × 10⁹/L	Acute infections, chronic granulocytic leukemia, chronic pancreatitis, cirrhosis, collagen disorders, polycythemia, postsplenectomy	Acute leukemia, DIC, thrombocytopenic purpura
Reticulocyte count	0.5%–2.0% of RBC	0.5%–2.0% of RBC	Hemolytic anemia, polycythemia vera	Hypoproliferative anemia, macrocytic anemia, microcytic anemia
White blood cell count†	5000–10000/mm³	5.0–10.0 × 10⁹/L	Inflammatory and infectious processes, leukemia	Aplastic anemia, side effects of chemotherapy and irradiation
WBC differential				
• Segmented neutrophils	55%–70%	0.55–0.70	Bacterial infections, collagen diseases, Hodgkin's lymphoma	Aplastic anemia, viral infections
• Band neutrophils	0–8%	0–0.08	Acute infections	
• Lymphocytes	20%–40%	0.20–0.40	Chronic infections, lymphocytic leukemia, mononucleosis, viral infections	Corticosteroid therapy, whole body irradiation
• Monocytes	2%–8%	0.02–0.08	Chronic inflammatory disorders, malaria, monocytic leukemia, acute infections, Hodgkin's lymphoma	
• Eosinophils	1%–4%	0.01–0.04	Allergic reactions, eosinophilic and chronic granulocytic leukemia, parasitic disorders, Hodgkin's lymphoma	Corticosteroid therapy
• Basophils	0.5%–1%	0.005–0.01	Hypothyroidism, ulcerative colitis, myeloproliferative diseases	Hyperthyroidism, stress

*Values depend on reagent and instrumentation used.
†Components of complete blood count (CBC).
COPD, Chronic obstructive pulmonary disease; *DIC,* disseminated intravascular coagulation.

TABLE C.3 Serology-Immunology

Test	REFERENCE INTERVALS		POSSIBLE ETIOLOGY	
	Conventional Units	SI Units	High/Positive	Low
Antinuclear antibody (ANA)	Negative at 1:40 dilution	Negative at 1:40 dilution	Chronic hepatitis, rheumatoid arthritis, scleroderma, systemic lupus erythematosus	
Anti-DNA antibody	<5 IU/mL	<5 IU/mL	Systemic lupus erythematosus	
Anti-Sm (Smith)	Negative	Negative	Systemic lupus erythematosus	
C-reactive protein (CRP)	<1.0 mg/dL	<10.0 mg/L	Acute infections, any inflammatory condition, widespread cancer	
Carcinoembryonic antigen (CEA)	*Nonsmoker:* <3 ng/mL *Smoker:* <5 ng/mL	*Nonsmoker:* <3 mcg/L *Smoker:* <5 mcg/L	Cancer of colon, liver, pancreas; cigarette smoking; inflammatory bowel disease	
Complement, total hemolytic (CH$_{50}$)	30–75 U/mL	30–75 U/mL	Cancer, ulcerative colitis	Bacterial endocarditis, glomerulonephritis, rheumatoid arthritis, systemic lupus erythematosus
Direct Coombs or direct antihuman globulin test (DAT)	Negative	Negative	Acquired hemolytic anemia, drug reactions, transfusion reactions	
Fluorescent treponemal antibody absorption (FTA-Abs)	Negative or nonreactive	Negative or nonreactive	Syphilis	
Hepatitis A antibody	Negative	Negative	Hepatitis A	
Hepatitis B surface antigen (HB$_s$Ag)	Negative	Negative	Hepatitis B	
Hepatitis C antibody	Negative	Negative	Hepatitis C	
Monospot or monotest	Negative	Negative	Infectious mononucleosis	
Rheumatoid factor (RF)	Negative or titer <1:17	Negative or titer <1:17	Rheumatoid arthritis, Sjögren's syndrome, systemic lupus erythematosus	
RPR	Negative or nonreactive	Negative or nonreactive	Leprosy, malaria, rheumatoid arthritis, systemic lupus erythematosus, syphilis,	
VDRL	Negative or nonreactive	Negative or nonreactive	Syphilis	

RPR, Rapid plasma reagin test; *VDRL,* Venereal Disease Research Laboratory test.

TABLE C.4 Urine Chemistry

Test	Specimen	REFERENCE INTERVALS		POSSIBLE ETIOLOGY	
		Units	SI Units	High	Low
Acetone	Random	Negative	Negative	Diabetes, high-fat and low-carbohy-drate diets, starvation	
Aldosterone	24 hr	2–26 mcg/day	6–72 nmol/day	*Primary aldosteronism:* adrenocortical tumors *Secondary aldosteronism:* cirrhosis, heart failure hyperkalemia, hyponatremia	ACTH deficiency, Addison's disease, corticosteroid therapy, hypokalemia
Amylase	24 hr	<5000 Somogyi U/day	6.5–48.1 U/hr	Acute pancreatitis	
Bence Jones protein	Random	<0.68 mg/dL	<0.68 mg/dL	Multiple myeloma	
Bilirubin	Random	Negative	Negative	Liver disorders	
Catecholamines	24 hr			Heart failure, pheochromocytoma, progressive muscular dystrophy	
• Epinephrine		<20 mcg/day	<109 nmol/day		
• Norepinephrine		<100 mcg/day	<590 nmol/day		
Cortisol	24 hr	<100 mcg/day	<276 nmol/day	Adrenal cancer, Cushing syndrome, hyperthyroidism, obesity, stress	Addison's disease, hypothyroidism, liver disease
Creatinine clearance	24 hr	*Male*: 107–139 mL/min *Female*: 87–107 mL/min	*Male*: 1.78–2.32 mL/sec *Female*: 1.45–1.78 mL/sec	Exercise, pregnancy	Cirrhosis, heart failure, renal disease
Estrogens	24 hr				Endocrine disturbance, ovarian dysfunction, menopause
• Female				Gonadal or adrenal tumor	
• Nonpregnant		4–60 mcg/day	4–60 mcg/day		
• Postmenopause		<20 mcg/day	<20 mcg/day		
• Male		4–25 mcg/day	4–25 mcg/day		
Glucose	Random	Negative	Negative	Diabetes, pituitary disorders	
Hemoglobin	Random	Negative	Negative	Extensive burns, glomerulonephritis, hemolytic anemia, hemolytic transfusion reaction	
5-Hydroxyindole acetic acid (5-HIAA)	24 hr	2–8 mg/day	10–40 μmol/day	Malignant carcinoid syndrome	
Ketones	Random	Negative	Negative	Diabetes, starvation, dehydration	
Metanephrine	24 hr	<1.3 mg/day	<7 μmol/day	Pheochromocytoma	
Myoglobin	Random	Negative	Negative	Crushing injuries, electric injuries, extreme physical exertion	
Osmolality	Random	50–1200 mOsm/kg	50–1200 mmol/kg	Heart failure, liver disease, shock, SIADH	Aldosteronism, diabetes insipidus, hypokalemia, pyelonephritis
pH	Random	4.6–8.0	4.6–8.0	Urinary tract infection, urine allowed to stand at room temperature	Respiratory or metabolic acidosis
Protein	Random	0–8 mg/dL	0–8 mg/dL	Acute and chronic renal disease, heart failure	
Protein (quantitative)	24 hr	50–80 mg/day	50–80 mg/day	Heart failure, inflammatory process of urinary tract, nephritis, nephrosis, strenuous exercise	
Sodium	24 hr	40–220 mEq/day	40–220 mmol/day	Acute tubular necrosis	Hyponatremia
Specific gravity	Random	1.005–1.030	1.005–1.030	Albuminuria, dehydration, glycosuria, fever	Diabetes insipidus, hypothermia, diuresis
Uric acid	24 hr	250–750 mg/day	1.48–4.43 mmol/day	Gout, leukemia	Nephritis
Urobilinogen	Random	Negative	Negative	Hemolytic disease, hepatic parenchymal cell damage, liver disease	Complete bile duct obstruction
Vanillylmandelic acid	24 hr	<6.8 mg/day	<35 μmol/day	Pheochromocytoma	

ACTH, Adrenocorticotropic hormone.

TABLE C.5 Fecal Analysis

	REFERENCE INTERVALS		POSSIBLE ETIOLOGY
Test	**Conventional Units**	**SI Units**	**High**
Fecal fat	2–6 g/24 hr	7–21 mmol/day	Common bile duct obstruction, malabsorption syndrome, pancreatic disease
Mucus	Negative	Negative	Mucous colitis, spastic constipation
Pus	Negative	Negative	Chronic bacillary dysentery, chronic ulcerative colitis, localized abscesses
Blood*	Negative	Negative	Anal fissures, gastrointestinal cancer, hemorrhoids, inflammatory bowel disease, peptic ulcer disease
Color			
• Brown			Various color depending on diet
• Clay			Biliary obstruction, presence of barium sulfate
• Tarry			More than 100 mL of blood in gastrointestinal tract
• Red			Blood in large intestine
• Black			Blood in upper gastrointestinal tract, iron medication

*Ingestion of meat may produce false-positive results. Patient may be placed on a meat-free diet for 3 days before the test.

TABLE C.6 Cerebrospinal Fluid Analysis

	REFERENCE INTERVALS		POSSIBLE ETIOLOGY	
Test	**Conventional Units**	**SI Units**	**High**	**Low**
Pressure	<20 mm H_2O	<20 mm H_2O	Hemorrhage, intracranial tumor, meningitis	Head injury, spinal tumor, subdural hematoma
Blood	Negative	Negative	Intracranial hemorrhage	
Cell count (age dependent)			CNS infection or inflammation	
• WBC	0–5 cells/µL	0–5 × 10^6 cells/L		
• RBC	Negative	Negative		
Chloride	700–750 mg/dL	118–132 mmol/L	Uremia	CNS bacterial infection
Glucose	50–75 mg/dL	2.2–3.9 mmol/L	CNS viral infection, diabetes	Bacterial infection, CNS tuberculosis
Protein				
• Lumbar	15–45 mg/dL	0.15–0.45 g/L	Guillain-Barré syndrome, poliomyelitis, trauma	
• Cisternal	15–25 mg/dL	0.15–0.25 g/L	CNS syphilis	
• Ventricular	5–15 mg/dL	0.05–0.15 g/L	Acute meningitis, brain tumor, chronic CNS infection, multiple sclerosis	

CNS, Central nervous system.

Note: Disorder names and key terms are in **boldface**. Page numbers in **boldface** indicate main discussions. Page numbers followed by *f* or *b* indicate figures or boxes/tables, respectively.

ABBREVIATIONS

ABG	arterial blood gas		DM	diabetes mellitus; diastolic murmur
ACE	angiotensin-converting enzyme		DRE	digital rectal examination
ACLS	advanced cardiac life support		DVT	deep vein thrombosis
ACS	acute coronary syndrome		ECF	extracellular fluid
ACTH	adrenocorticotropic hormone		ECG	electrocardiogram
ADH	antidiuretic hormone		ED	emergency department; erectile dysfunction
AED	automatic external defibrillator		EEG	electroencephalogram
AIDS	acquired immunodeficiency syndrome		EMG	electromyogram
AKA	above-knee amputation		EMS	emergency medical services
AKI	acute kidney injury		ENT	ear, nose, and throat
ALI	acute lung injury		ERCP	endoscopic retrograde cholangiopancreatography
ALL	acute lymphocytic leukemia		ERT	estrogen replacement therapy
ALS	amyotrophic lateral sclerosis		ESKD	end-stage kidney disease
AMI	acute myocardial infarction		ESR	erythrocyte sedimentation rate
ANA	antinuclear antibody		ET	endotracheal
ANS	autonomic nervous system		FEV	forced expiratory volume
AORN	Association of periOperative Room Nurses		FRC	functional residual capacity
APD	automated peritoneal dialysis		FUO	fever of unknown origin
aPTT	activated partial thromboplastin time		GCS	Glasgow Coma Scale
ARDS	acute respiratory distress syndrome		GERD	gastroesophageal reflux disease
ATN	acute tubular necrosis		GFR	glomerular filtration rate
BCLS	basic cardiac life support		GH	growth hormone
BKA	below-knee amputation		GI	glycemic index
BMI	body mass index		GTT	glucose tolerance test
BMR	basal metabolic rate		GU	genitourinary
BMT	bone marrow transplantation		GYN, Gyn	gynecologic
BPH	benign prostatic hyperplasia		HAI	health care–associated infection
BSE	breast self-examination		HAV	hepatitis A virus
BUN	blood urea nitrogen		Hb, Hgb	hemoglobin
CABG	coronary artery bypass graft		HBV	hepatitis B virus
CAD	coronary artery disease; circulatory assist device		Hct	hematocrit
CAPD	continuous ambulatory peritoneal dialysis		HCV	hepatitis C virus
CAVH	continuous arteriovenous hemofiltration		HD	hemodialysis, Huntington's disease
CBC	complete blood count		HDL	high-density lipoprotein
CCU	coronary care unit; critical care unit		HF	heart failure
CDC	Centers for Disease Control and Prevention		HIV	human immunodeficiency virus
CIS	carcinoma in situ		H&P	history and physical examination
CKD	chronic kidney disease		HPV	human papillomavirus
CLL	chronic lymphocytic leukemia		HSCT	hematopoietic stem cell transplantation
CML	chronic myelocytic leukemia		IABP	intraaortic balloon pump
CMP	cardiomyopathy		IBS	irritable bowel syndrome
CN	cranial nerve		ICP	intracranial pressure
CNS	central nervous system		I&D	incision and drainage
CO	cardiac output		IE	infective endocarditis
COPD	chronic obstructive pulmonary disease		IFG	impaired fasting glucose
CPAP	continuous positive airway pressure		IGT	impaired glucose tolerance
CPR	cardiopulmonary resuscitation		INR	international normalized ratio
CRRT	continuous renal replacement therapy		IOP	intraocular pressure
CRNA	certified registered nurse anesthetist		IPPB	intermittent positive-pressure breathing
CSF	cerebrospinal fluid		ITP	idiopathic thrombocytopenic purpura
CT	computed tomography		IUD	intrauterine device
CVA	cerebrovascular accident; costovertebral angle		IV	intravenous
CVAD	central venous access device		IVP	intravenous push; intravenous pyelogram
CVI	chronic venous insufficiency		JVD	jugular venous distention
CVP	central venous pressure		KS	Kaposi sarcoma
D&C	dilation and curettage		KUB	kidney, ureters, and bladder (x-ray)
DDD	degenerative disk disease		KVO	keep vein open
DI	diabetes insipidus		LAD	left anterior descending
DIC	disseminated intravascular coagulation		LDL	low-density lipoprotein
DJD	degenerative joint disease		LGV	lymphogranuloma venereum
DKA	diabetic ketoacidosis		LLQ	left lower quadrant